Effects of Disease on Clinical Laboratory Tests

FOURTH EDITION

VOLUME TWO
Listing by Disease

Donald S. Young, MD, PhD
Vice-Chair for Laboratory Medicine
Department of Pathology and Laboratory Medicine
University of Pennsylvania
Philadelphia, Pennsylvania

Richard B. Friedman, MD, FACP
Vice-President of Medical Affairs
Queens Medical Center
Honolulu, Hawaii

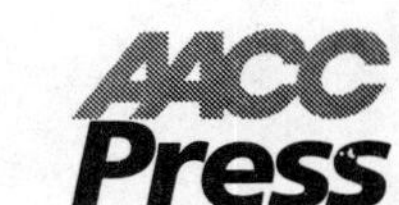

2101 L Street, NW
Suite 202
Washington, DC 20037-1558
www.aacc.org

ISBN 1-890883-45-X

Database design, book assembly, and typography by Lexi-Comp Inc., Hudson, Ohio, www.lexi.com

INTRODUCTION

This compilation is a revised and expanded version of *Effects of Disease on Clinical Laboratory Tests,* whose third edition was published in 1997. Several obsolete tests and entries of marginal value have been eliminated from this edition which contains about 12,000 new entries. The format remains the same as for the three previous editions and is compatible with that used in the other books published by the American Association for Clinical Chemistry relating to the Effects of Drugs and Preanalytical Variables on Clinical Laboratory Tests.

In this compilation of the Effects of Disease on Clinical Laboratory Tests we have attempted to bring together, in one resource, information that is scattered in many textbooks and clinical journals. This listing is neither exhaustive nor selective. The contents include information from several standard textbooks of medicine supplemented by information from recent issues of general and specialty clinical journals. However, as with any task as large as this, some important interactions must have been omitted. No attempts have been made to verify the information or to select only the most significant interactions. Where possible, information concerning the frequency and importance of the abnormality has been included. In those cases where there is reported information as to when in the course of the disease the test result changes, we have also included this information. The authors have focused their reading on topics in internal medicine, although some disorders treated by specialists are also included.

Some may criticize the non-selective nature of the file, and the fact that an abnormal increase and decrease for the same test is often listed in association with a single disease. This, in reality, reflects what has been observed clinically as tests results may sometimes be either increased or decreased during the course of a disease. Where authors differ on the direction of the abnormality, both entries have been included to highlight this discrepancy. So that the reader can make his/her own decision about which abnormality is appropriate in a particular clinical situation, we have included part of the original text together with the appropriate reference.

The information in this book should always be reviewed in conjunction with a patient's history and physical examination, and should never be applied without question to a particular patient. In attempting to determine the cause of a test abnormality in a specific patient, one should always be aware that normality is a statistical concept and therefore a certain proportion of "abnormal" results is to be expected in patients without discernible pathology. One should also remember that many patients have more than one disease, and therefore a reported test-disease relationship may really be ascribable to a co-existent disease, or to the interaction of multiple diseases. Furthermore, when tests results are described as normal or abnormal the report may not be pertinent to the actual stage of the disease in a particular patient for whom a physician is providing care.

If an abnormal test-disease relationship is not reported in the file, then either published reports show that this test is usually normal in that disease or no report of an abnormality could be found. Only in those cases where the authors of a publication have made a specific effort to study the effects of a disease on a particular test and have found the test to be normal is a normal result listed.

Structure of the File

The file is divided into five parts:

Laboratory Test Index (Alphabetical*)
Disease Keyword Index (Alphabetical)
Laboratory Test Listings (Alphabetical*)
Disease Listings by ICD-9-CM Classification
References

*Test names beginning with a **numeral** are listed first.

Laboratory Test Index

This is an alphabetized listing of all tests contained in the file. Where a test has two or more acceptable names, additional names are included with a reference to the preferred name (e.g. SGOT [see aspartate aminotransferase]). The user will find the test in the alphabetic test listing under the name most accepted in American use (e.g. aspartate aminotransferase). Some test names represent groupings of individual tests (e.g. amino acids). In these cases, entries will be included under the more general heading (e.g. amino acids) if the reference article only referred to the general grouping, and under the more specific test name if the article described the effect on a specific test (e.g., alanine). To assist the user in finding specific tests contained in a general group, but listed separately, entries in this category are listed after the term *see also* following the general heading (e.g., amino acids [*see also* alanine, asparagine, arginine, leucine, etc]).

Disease Keyword Index

This file includes an alphabetized keyword listing of all diseases in the file. Included as a keyword is any major term in all the commonly used names for that particular disease. After each entry one will find the ICD-9-CM *(The International Classification of Disease--9th revision--Clinical Modification)* code for the disease. Since the **Disease Listings by ICD-9-CM Classification** file is arranged by ICD-9-CM code, this number should be used to find entries in that file. Some of the ICD-9 codes have been modified so that all have two numbers after the decimal point, and should not be used for any purpose other than searching entries in this publication. If the user cannot find a disease in the file, he/she is encouraged to consult a current ICD-9-CM manual for more exhaustive indexing of disease names. Because the **Disease Listings by ICD-9-CM Classification** is compatible with ICD-9-CM coding, one can go directly from that index to the file. Where no ICD-9-CM code exists for a disease, a code has been created to place that disease in the relevant section of the listing or a generic 00.00 has been used.

Laboratory Test Listings

The file contains information on over 500 of the most commonly performed clinical laboratory tests listed in alphabetical order. We have attempted to prepare a comprehensive listing of diseases associated with abnormalities in results of the most commonly performed tests; however, the listing of diseases associated with the less commonly performed tests may not be as exhaustive. No attempt has been made to differentiate tests by the various techniques used to perform them. Therefore, the listing for acid phosphatase includes the techniques of Bodansky, King-Armstrong, etc as well as more modern methods. The user is encouraged to check which technique is used in his/her own laboratory and then compare this with the technique cited in the reference article before assuming that a true association exists. Yet, in the absence of drugs that interfere with a specific analytical method, an effect reported with an obsolete procedure is still likely to be pertinent.

For a particular test, the associated diseases are arranged by ICD-9-CM code. This should facilitate cross checking between diseases of common etiology or similar organ system as well as provide access to the **Disease Listings by ICD-9-CM Classification** file.

Entries for a particular test are arranged first by specimen type and then by nature of the abnormality. For each individual entry, a discussion of the course, extent, and frequency of the abnormality is included, when available, as well as a reference to the appropriate literature.

Disease Listings by ICD-9-CM Classification

How best to organize a disease file requires considerable thought. If one organized it by common disease name, then the choice of preferred name becomes crucial and associations by etiology or organ system are lost. We, therefore, decided to organize this listing by ICD-9-CM code number. This method makes the file compatible with the most commonly used classification system. The advantages of such compatibility are considerable; it not only permits use of existing comprehensive ICD-9-CM indexes, but also makes the file compatible with many existing disease and laboratory data bases.

The ICD-9-CM coding system is not perfect but, given its widespread use and the opportunity to make this listing compatible with a wealth of existing files, we elected to adopt the system for our disease categorization. It condenses several diseases into a single classification when they should be separate and separates into different categories some diseases which should be combined. Because updates of the coding system require approval of many groups, it is never totally current and therefore may not reflect the latest thinking in disease etiology. In addition, some of the most recently identified diseases are not included. Where necessary, new classification numbers have been created for diseases that are not in the existing coding system. Some categories in which two or more diseases have been lumped under a single classification number have been subdivided. Such "new" diseases and subdivided categories can usually be identified by the presence of a two-decimal place number.

For a particular disease, all tests are listed in alphabetical order. If more than one entry exists for a test it is re-sorted, first by specimen type then by direction. Each entry consists of the test name, the specimen type, the nature of the abnormality and, if available, an explanation about that abnormality. This explanation will contain any information found about the occurrence, extent, and frequency of the abnormality. After each entry, a number is included. This number can be used to look up the source of this information in the reference file.

References

References are listed in alphabetical order. Each entry consists of the name of the author, the title of the article, and the journal or text citation. Readers are encouraged to study these sources to obtain greater detail about the issues necessarily described succinctly in the text.

Interpretation of Data

This file is intended to provide assistance in the interpretation of laboratory data, in particular to assist in explaining unexpected results or changes in data. It should not be assumed that, because an entry exists in the file, it necessarily explains an abnormal test result in a given patient. Nor should it be assumed that, because no entry exists, a disease is not the cause of an abnormal laboratory result.

We have tried to include most of the relevant information in the file, although it is unlikely that we have been able to obtain all pertinent literature or facts. We would be pleased to receive any additional information that users of the file possess. Although the authors have attempted to ensure that information has been entered correctly into the file, errors may have occurred, and we would be most grateful if these could be pointed out to us. All correspondence should be sent to:

Dr. Donald S. Young
(donaldyo@mail.med.upenn.edu)
or
Dr. Richard B. Friedman
(rfriedman@queens.org)

We would like to thank David Marcus and Kenneth Hughes of Lexi-Comp, Inc. and Joanna Grimes of AACC for their assistance and encouragement in pursuing this project. We hope that with their continued support this file will be adapted for presentation in a variety of electronic media formats. Further information may be obtained from:

Joanna Grimes
Manager of Publications
American Association for Clinical Chemistry
2101 L Street, NW
Suite 202
Washington, DC 20037-1558

She may also be contacted by telephone at 202-835-8740 or 800-892-1400, extension 740.

— Donald S. Young

— Richard B. Friedman
April, 2001

1 DISEASE INDEX

A

B

C

D

E

F

G

H

J

K

L

M

N

O

P

Q

R

S

T

U

V

W

X

Y

Z

2 TEST INDEX

A

B

C

D

E

F

G

H

I

K

L

M

N

O

P

Q

R

S

T

U

V

W

X

Z

3 DISEASE LISTINGS BY ICD-9-CM CLASSIFICATION

MISCELLANEOUS

0.00 Crow-Fukase Syndrome

Soluble E-Selectin *Serum* *Increase* Mean concentrations of 95 and 68 ng/mL in 2 patients significantly higher than 30 ± 9 ng/mL in 12 healthy control individuals *3885*

0.00 Euthyroid Sick Syndrome

Thyroid Stimulating Hormone *Serum* *Increase* In 25 patients with euthyroid sick syndrome mean concentration of 1.59 ± 0.3 mU/L significantly different from reference interval of 0.3 - 4.0 mU/L *829*

Thyroxine (T4), Free *Serum* *No Effect* In 25 patients with euthyroid sick syndrome mean concentration of 17.8 ± 0.1 pmol/L not significantly different from reference interval of 7.0 - 21.8 pmol/L *829*

Tri-iodothyronine, Free (fT3) *Serum* *Decrease* In 25 patients with euthyroid sick syndrome mean concentration of 1.6 ± 0.2 pmol/L significantly less than reference interval of 3.3 - 8.2 pmol/L *829*

0.00 Hepatitis B Carrier

Alanine Aminotransferase *Serum* *No Effect* In 20 asymptomatic hepatitis B carriers mean activity of 21 ± 5 U/L not significantly different from 14 ± 8 U/L in 20 healthy volunteers *2372*

Anti-Hepatitis B Surface Antigen *Serum* *Increase* Persistence of marker beyond 24 weeks is associated with chronic carrier state *3625*

Bilirubin *Serum* *No Effect* In 20 asymptomatic hepatitis B carriers mean concentration of 0.4 ± 0.3 mg/dL not significantly different from 0.5 ± 0.3 mg/dL in 20 healthy volunteers *2372*

γ-Globulin *Serum* *No Effect* In 20 asymptomatic hepatitis B carriers mean concentration of 12 ± 2 g/L not significantly different from 11 ± 2 g/L in 20 healthy volunteers *2372*

γ-Glutamyltransferase *Serum* *No Effect* In 20 asymptomatic hepatitis B carriers mean activity of 14 ± 8 U/L not significantly different from 10 ± 3 U/L in 20 healthy volunteers *2372*

Macrophage Colony Stimulating Factor *Serum* *No Effect* In 20 asymptomatic hepatitis B carriers mean concentration of 1.98 ± 0.04 ng/mL not significantly different from 1.95 ± 0.44 ng/mL in 20 healthy volunteers *2372*

Neopterin *Urine* *No Effect* Excretion normal in healthy patients who are hepatitis B surface antigen carriers *121*

0.00 Kennedy-Alter-Sung Disease

Amyloid β-Protein *Cerebrospinal Fluid* *No Effect* In 1 patient concentration was 5.32 pmol/mL not significantly different from mean concentration of 4.00 ± 2.92 pmol/mL *3716*

Amyloid β-Protein Precursor *Cerebrospinal Fluid* *Increase* In 1 patient concentration was 3.22 integrated OD units significantly different from mean concentration of 1.35 ± 0.38 integrated OD units in 25 normal controls *3716*

α_1-Antichymotrypsin *Cerebrospinal Fluid* *No Effect* In 1 patient concentration was 3.90 µg/mL not significantly different from mean concentration of 2.27 ± 1.40 µg/mL in 25 normal controls *3716*

Cells *Cerebrospinal Fluid* *No Effect* In 1 patient concentration of 2.0 cells/µL not significantly different from normal of 3 cells/µL *3716*

Protein *Cerebrospinal Fluid* *No Effect* In 1 patient concentration of 48 mg/dL not significantly different from normal of 28 mg/dL in 25 healthy controls *3716*

0.00 Kimura's Disease

Eosinophils *Blood* *Increase* In 4 patients with Kimura's disease and eosinophilia, mean concentration of 2,620 ± 1,530 /µL compared with less than 500 /µL in 100 normal individuals *5776*

Granulocyte-Macrophage Colony Stimulating Factor *Serum* *No Effect* Not detected in the serum of either of 2 patients with condition *2744*

Interleukin-3 *Serum* *No Effect* Not detected in the serum of either of 2 patients with condition *2744*

Interleukin-5 *Serum* *No Effect* Not detected in the serum of 2 patients with Kimura's disease *2744*

Myelin Basic Protein *Serum* *Increase* In 4 patients with Kimura's disease and eosinophilia mean concentration of 488 ± 414 ng/mL compared with mean of 41 ± 19 ng/mL in 100 normal individuals *5776*

0.00 Multiple System Atrophy

Amyloid β-Protein *Cerebrospinal Fluid* *Increase* In 2 patients with multiple system atrophy concentrations were 2.55 and 8.07 pmol/mL significantly different from mean concentration of 4.00 ± 2.92 pmol/mL in one and normal in the other *3716*
Cerebrospinal Fluid *No Effect* In 2 patients with multiple system atrophy concentrations were 2.55 and 8.07 pmol/mL significantly different from mean concentration of 4.00 ± 2.92 pmol/mL in one and normal in the other *3716*

Amyloid β-Protein Precursor *Cerebrospinal Fluid* *Increase* In 2 patients with multiple system atrophy concentrations were 1.46 and 2.74 integrated OD units significantly different from mean concentration of 1.35 ± 0.38 integrated OD units in 25 normal controls in one but normal in the other *3716*
Cerebrospinal Fluid *No Effect* In 2 patients with multiple system atrophy concentrations were 1.46 and 2.74 integrated OD units significantly different from mean concentration of 1.35 ± 0.38 integrated OD units in 25 normal controls in one but normal in the other *3716*

0.00 Multiple System Atrophy *(continued)*

Angiotensin-converting Enzyme *Cerebrospinal Fluid* *No Effect* In 18 patients with untreated multiple system atrophy mean concentration of 0.80 ± 0.26 U/L not significantly different from 0.81 ± 0.18 U/L in 20 healthy controls *2758*

α_1-Antichymotrypsin *Cerebrospinal Fluid* *Increase* In 2 patients with multiple system atrophy concentrations were 4.60 and 6.85 μg/mL significantly different from mean concentration of 2.27 ± 1.40 μg/mL in 25 normal controls *3716*

Cells *Cerebrospinal Fluid* *No Effect* In 2 patients with multiple system atrophy concentrations of 0.3 and 0.0 cells/μL not significantly different from normal of 3 cells/μL *3716*

Protein *Cerebrospinal Fluid* *No Effect* In 18 patients with untreated Parkinson's mean concentration of 0.50 ± 0.31 g/L not significantly different from 0.38 ± 0.09 g/L in 20 healthy controls *2758* In 2 patients with multiple system atrophy concentrations of 31 and 31 mg/dL not significantly different from normal mean of 29 mg/dL *3716*

0.00 Noninflammatory Disease

Alkaline Phosphatase *Serum* *No Effect* In 14 patients with ankylosing spondylitis median activity of 6.1 KA U/dL not significantly different from upper limit of normal in healthy controls *430*

Alkaline Phosphatase, Bone Isoenzyme *Serum* *No Effect* In 14 patients with ankylosing spondylitis median concentration of 12.7 ng/mL not significantly different from upper limit of normal in healthy controls *430*

Viscosity *Plasma* *Decrease* In 14 patients with ankylosing spondylitis median viscosity of 1.62 ± 0.06 mPa not significantly different from 1.72 mPa in healthy controls *430* In 14 patients with noninflammatory disease median of 1.62 mPa significantly different from upper limit of normal of 1.72 mPa in healthy controls *430*

0.00 Organ Transplantation

Lymphocytes *Blood* *Decrease* In 1,042 hospitalized patients with lymphocytopenia 73 had had an organ transplant *730*

0.00 T-Lymphotropic Virus Type I Carrier

Dehydroepiandrosterone *Plasma* *No Effect* Mean concentration of 3.16 ± 1.24 ng/mL in 7 men aged 40 - 49 y not significantly different from 4.39 ± 1.69 ng/mL in 10 healthy men of the same age: comparable difference seen in women and in men of other ages *5369*

Dehydroepiandrosterone Sulfate *Plasma* *No Effect* Mean concentration of 1,311.7 ± 437.8 ng/mL in 10 men aged 40 - 49 y decreased nonsignificantly compared with 1,372.7 ± 469.6 ng/mL in 10 healthy men of the same age: comparable difference seen in women and in men of other ages *5369*

0.00 T-Lymphotropic Virus Type I (HTLV-1) Carrier

Interleukin-6 *Serum* *No Effect* In 32 adults who were T-lymphotropic virus type-1 carriers median concentration of 4.2 (range < 1.0 - 13.3) pg/mL not significantly higher than concentrations in 30 healthy adults of < 1.0 to 3.5 pg/mL with median < 1.0 pg/mL *5779*

0.00 Vitamin D Resistance

Ammonium Ions *Urine* *Increase* May lead to proximal renal tubular acidosis which is associated with hypokalemia, hyperchloremic metabolic acidosis, urine pH < 5.5, increased urinary ammonium ion excretion, a negative urine anion gap, increased urinary osmol gap, normal urinary citrate, normal urinary calcium excretion and Fanconi syndrome *4071*

Anion Gap *Urine* *Decrease* May lead to proximal renal tubular acidosis which is associated with hypokalemia, hyperchloremic metabolic acidosis, urine pH < 5.5, increased urinary ammonium ion excretion, a negative urine anion gap, increased urinary osmol gap, normal urinary citrate, normal urinary calcium excretion and Fanconi syndrome *4071*

Bicarbonate *Serum* *Decrease* May lead to proximal renal tubular acidosis which is associated with hypokalemia, hyperchloremic metabolic acidosis, urine pH < 5.5, increased urinary ammonium ion excretion, a negative urine anion gap, increased urinary osmol gap, normal urinary citrate, normal urinary calcium excretion and Fanconi syndrome *4071*

Calcium *Urine* *No Effect* May lead to proximal renal tubular acidosis which is associated with hypokalemia, hyperchloremic metabolic acidosis, urine pH < 5.5, increased urinary ammonium ion excretion, a negative urine anion gap, increased urinary osmol gap, normal urinary citrate, normal urinary calcium excretion and Fanconi syndrome *4071*

Chloride *Serum* *Increase* May lead to proximal renal tubular acidosis which is associated with hypokalemia, hyperchloremic metabolic acidosis, urine pH < 5.5, increased urinary ammonium ion excretion, a negative urine anion gap, increased urinary osmol gap, normal urinary citrate, normal urinary calcium excretion and Fanconi syndrome *4071*

Citrate *Urine* *No Effect* May lead to proximal renal tubular acidosis which is associated with hypokalemia, hyperchloremic metabolic acidosis, urine pH < 5.5, increased urinary ammonium ion excretion, a negative urine anion gap, increased urinary osmol gap, normal urinary citrate, normal urinary calcium excretion and Fanconi syndrome *4071*

Glucose *Urine* *Increase* May lead to proximal renal tubular acidosis which is associated with hypokalemia, hyperchloremic metabolic acidosis, urine pH < 5.5, increased urinary ammonium ion excretion, a negative urine anion gap, increased urinary osmol gap, normal urinary citrate, normal urinary calcium excretion and Fanconi syndrome *4071*

Osmolal Gap *Urine* *Increase* May lead to proximal renal tubular acidosis which is associated with hypokalemia, hyperchloremic metabolic acidosis, urine pH < 5.5, increased urinary ammonium ion excretion, a negative urine anion gap, increased urinary osmol gap, normal urinary citrate, normal urinary calcium excretion and Fanconi syndrome *4071*

pH *Urine* *Decrease* May lead to proximal renal tubular acidosis which is associated with hypokalemia, hyperchloremic metabolic acidosis, urine pH < 5.5, increased urinary ammonium ion excretion, a negative urine anion gap, increased urinary osmol gap, normal urinary citrate, normal urinary calcium excretion and Fanconi syndrome *4071*

Phosphate *Serum* *Decrease* May lead to proximal renal tubular acidosis which is associated with hypokalemia, hyperchloremic metabolic acidosis, urine pH < 5.5, increased urinary ammonium ion excretion, a negative urine anion gap, increased urinary osmol gap, normal urinary citrate, normal urinary calcium excretion and Fanconi syndrome *4071*

Potassium *Serum* *Decrease* May lead to proximal renal tubular acidosis which is associated with hypokalemia, hyperchloremic metabolic acidosis, urine pH < 5.5, increased urinary ammonium ion excretion, a negative urine anion gap, increased urinary osmol gap, normal urinary citrate, normal urinary calcium excretion and Fanconi syndrome *4071*

Uric Acid *Serum* *Decrease* May lead to proximal renal tubular acidosis which is associated with hypokalemia, hyperchloremic metabolic acidosis, urine pH < 5.5, increased urinary ammonium ion excretion, a negative urine anion gap, increased urinary osmol gap, normal urinary citrate, normal urinary calcium excretion and Fanconi syndrome *4071*

INFECTIOUS AND PARASITIC DISEASES

Intestinal Infectious Diseases

1.90 Cholera

Anti-Streptolysin-O Titer *Serum* *Increase* Above normal titers may occur *3953*

Bicarbonate *Feces* *Increase* Fecal carbonate concentration is higher than in plasma *367*

Chloride *Feces* *Increase* Fecal concentrations are above normal, but are consistently lower than the plasma values *367*
Serum *Increase* Due to marked loss of fluid and electrolytes *5545*

Erythrocytes *Blood* *Increase* Due to severe dehydration *2033*

Hematocrit *Blood* *Increase* Due to severe dehydration *367*

Hemoglobin *Blood* *Increase* Due to severe dehydration *2033*

Leukocytes *Blood* *Increase* Due to severe dehydration *367* Acute infections cause leukocytosis *5544*

pH *Blood* *Decrease* Metabolic acidosis *367*

Potassium *Feces* *Increase* Fecal potassium concentrations are higher than in plasma *367*
Serum *Decrease* Marked loss of fluid and electrolytes *5545* Renal wasting leads to hypokalemic state *3735*

Sodium *Feces* *Increase* Fecal concentrations are increased above normal, but are consistently lower than the plasma values *367*
Serum *Increase* Marked loss of fluid and electrolytes occurs *5545*

Specific Gravity *Serum* *Increase* Due to severe dehydration *367*

Urea Nitrogen *Serum* *Increase* Due to severe dehydration *2033*

2.00 Typhoid Fever

Adenosine Deaminase *Serum* *Increase* Found to be significantly elevated in children *4264*

Agglutination Tests *Serum* *Positive* The diagnostic value of the Widal reaction has been diminished by the widespread use of TAB vaccination. In an unimmunized patient, it does not become positive until after 7 - 10 days of illness *900*

Albumin *Urine* *Increase* Common during the febrile period *367*

Alkaline Phosphatase *Serum* *Increase* Increased due to complications *5545*

Alkaline Phosphatase Isoenzymes *Serum* *Increase* Increased incidence of the Regan (placental) isoenzyme *1497*

Aspartate Aminotransferase *Serum* *Increase* Frequently seen due to complications *5545*

Copper *Serum* *Increase* Before the onset of overt clinical illness *4062*

Creatine Kinase *Serum* *Increase* Occurs in some patients *5545*

Erythrocyte Sedimentation Rate *Blood* *No Effect* Rate typically normal *413*

γ-Globulin *Serum* *Increase* Moderate hypergammaglobulinemia, especially IgA *1792*

Hematocrit *Blood* *Decrease* Normochromic anemia is common present late in illness and during convalescence *1980* Normochromic anemia usually develops and may be aggravated by blood loss in stools *367*

Hemoglobin *Blood* *Decrease* Commonly present late in illness and during convalescence *1980* Normochromic anemia usually develops and may be aggravated by blood loss in the stools *367*

immunoglobulin A *Serum* *Increase* Moderate hypergammaglobulinemia, especially IgA *1792*

Interleukin-6 *Serum* *Increase* In 38 children aged 6 months to 14 years concentration increased in more than 50% cases and correlated with severity of illness. Mean concentration in severe category 898 ± 542 pg/mL, 263 ± 367 pg/mL in moderate category and 84 ± 116 pg/mL in mild category *435*

Iron *Serum* *Decrease* Both serum iron and zinc concentrations became significantly depressed in experimentally infected volunteers *4062*

Lactate Dehydrogenase *Serum* *Increase* Due to complications *5545*

Leukocytes *Blood* *Decrease* Counts range from 4,000 - 6,000 /µL during the first 2 weeks and 3,000 - 5,000 /µL during the 3rd and 4th week. Leukopenia is generally moderate, rarely falling below 2,500 /µL *2192* Frequent, with a decrease in neutrophilic granulocytes *1980* A low count with a relative lymphocytosis commonly seen *900*
Blood *Increase* Moderate leukocytosis to 12,000 /µL may be observed in some patients *2192*

Lymphocytes *Blood* *Increase* A low WBC count with a relative lymphocytosis is commonly seen *900*

Malate Dehydrogenase *Serum* *Increase* Slight increase *1290*

Neutrophils *Blood* *Decrease* Significant neutropenia may occur *3671*

Occult Blood *Feces* *Increase* May occur and lead to normochromic anemia later in the disease *367* Frequent during the 3rd and 4th weeks *2192*

Phospholipase A_2 Type II *Serum* *Increase* Increase in concentration observed of 1,444 µg/L compared with 2 and 4 µg/L in healthy controls *3767*

Protein *Urine* *Increase* Proteinuria is seen during febrile periods *1722*

Thyroxine Binding Globulin *Serum* *Decrease* Patients with fever had significantly lowered levels *5152*

Thyroxine (T4) *Serum* *Increase* During fever both percentage of free T4 and absolute free T4 were elevated *5152* Slightly increased in all patients *3229*

Tri-iodothyronine (T3) *Serum* *Decrease* Patients with fever had significantly lowered levels *5152* Significantly low in all patients. Fall in T3 was inversely related to the degree of fever *3229*

Tumor Necrosis Factor-α *Serum* *Increase* In 38 children aged 6 months to 14 years concentration increased in more than 50% cases and correlated with severity of illness. Mean concentration in severe category of 28 ± 18 pg/mL, 18 ± 8 pg/mL in moderate category and 18 ± 7 pg/mL in mild category *435*

Zinc *Serum* *Decrease* Both serum iron and zinc were significantly depressed in experimentally infected volunteers *4062*

3.90 Salmonellosis

Potassium *Serum* *Decrease* 40 of 248 Medicare patients with salmonellosis as first listed diagnosis hypokalemia observed *35*

Rheumatoid Factor *Serum* *Increase* Mean concentration increased in patients with salmonellosis *2472* Rheumatoid factor may be observed in certain patients *2473*

4.90 Bacillary Dysentery

Chloride *Serum* *Decrease* Fluid and electrolyte loss may be quite significant, particularly in pediatric and geriatric populations *2192*

Erythrocytes *Blood* *No Effect* Anemia is uncommon *2033*

Hemagglutination Inhibition *Serum* *Increase* Generally demonstrable *2192*

Hematocrit *Blood* *No Effect* Anemia is uncommon *2033*

Hemoglobin *Blood* *No Effect* Anemia is uncommon *2033*

Leukocytes *Blood* *Decrease* The total peripheral WBC count is not characteristic in this disease; a leukopenia, leukocytosis, or a normal count may be seen *900*
Blood *Increase* The total peripheral WBC count is not characteristic in this disease; a leukopenia, leukocytosis, or a normal count may be seen *900*
Feces *Increase* During the acute phase, examination of the stool will reveal clumps of polymorphonuclear leukocytes and RBCs, and the stool culture will be positive *1980*

Neutrophils *Blood* *Decrease* Significant neutropenia may occur *5475*
Blood *Increase* In many cases there is a significant increase in the number of immature neutrophils, so that the ratio of band to segmented neutrophils often is reversed *900*

Occult Blood *Feces* *Increase* During the acute phase, examination of the stool will reveal clumps of polymorphonuclear leukocytes and RBCs, and the stool culture will be positive *1980*

Potassium *Serum* *Decrease* Fluid and electrolyte loss may be quite significant, particularly in pediatric and geriatric populations *2192*

4.90 Bacillary Dysentery *(continued)*

Sodium *Serum* *Decrease* Fluid and electrolyte loss may be quite significant, particularly in pediatric and geriatric populations *2192*
Serum *Increase* Fluid and electrolyte loss may be quite significant, particularly in pediatric and geriatric populations *2192*

4.90 Shigellosis

Potassium *Serum* *Decrease* 2 of 22 Medicare beneficiaries hospitalized with first listed diagnosis of shigellosis had hypokalemia *35*

6.00 Amebiasis

Alanine Aminotransferase *Serum* *Increase* With liver involvement *2192*

Alkaline Phosphatase *Serum* *Increase* Becomes elevated earliest with liver abscess *900*

Aspartate Aminotransferase *Serum* *Increase* With liver involvement *2192*

Bilirubin *Serum* *No Effect* With liver involvement, jaundice is uncommon and bilirubin is usually normal *2192*

CA 195 *Serum* *Increase* False positive results occurred in 50% of patients with Amoebic liver abscess *3228*

Complement Fixation *Serum* *Increase* Usually positive during active (especially hepatic) disease. Significant positive titer is > 1:16 *5545*

Erythrocyte Sedimentation Rate *Blood* *Increase* The general rule *2192* Increased with liver abscess *5545*

γ-Glutamyltransferase *Serum* *Increase* With liver involvement *2192*

Hemagglutination Inhibition *Serum* *Increase* Test for E. histolytica has been found to be positive in over 90% of patients with proven amebic liver abscess *1980* Positive test is > 1:128 *5545* Usually positive in the presence of tissue invasion and approach 100% with extracolonic disease such as liver abscess *2039*

Hematocrit *Blood* *Decrease* Mild degree of anemia is common, either normochromic or hypochromic. Severity is related to duration of symptoms *29* Normochromic or hypochromic anemia is found in 75% of cases *2192*

Hemoglobin *Blood* *Decrease* Mild degree of anemia is common, either normochromic or hypochromic. Severity is related to duration of symptoms *29* Normochromic or hypochromic anemia is found in 75% of cases *2192*

Lactate Dehydrogenase *Serum* *Increase* Normal levels returned after complete cure in 92% of cases. Appears to be more useful than antibodies to detect cure or new infection *3227*

Leukocytes *Blood* *Increase* Increased in the majority of cases *29* A leukocytosis with a predominance of immature forms is common *900*

Neutrophils *Blood* *Increase* Moderate neutrophilia present in 75% of cases *2192*

5'-Nucleotidase *Serum* *Increase* With liver involvement *2192*

pH *Pleural Fluid* *Decrease* The pleural aspirate from an amebic empyema due to rupture of an amebic liver abscess has an acidic pH. Pleural aspirates of nonamebic etiology were noted to have an alkaline pH *4269*

Protein *Pleural Fluid* *Increase* Parasitic disease most often associated with an effusion. Exudate *126*

Specific Gravity *Pleural Fluid* *Increase* Exudate (> 1.016) *126*

6.30 Liver Abscess (Amebic)

Bilirubin *Serum* *Increase* Regardless of cause may be associated with moderate increase in concentration, to a lesser extent than with pyogenic infections *3406*

7.10 Giardiasis

Antibody Titer *Serum* *Increase* Anti-Giardia IgM and IgG by ELISA was found. Specificity and Sensitivity was 96% *1773*

Potassium *Serum* *Decrease* In 3.8% of all Medicare beneficiaries with a discharge diagnosis of giardiasis and in 23.6% of those older than 65 years hypokalemia observed *35*

Vitamin B_{12} *Serum* *Decrease* Vitamin B_{12} absorption is decreased *2035*

Tuberculosis

11.00 Tuberculosis

Antinuclear Antibodies *Pleural Fluid* *No Effect* ANA antibodies observed in 0 of 5 pleural fluid specimens *2665*

CA 19-9 *Serum* *Increase* The percentage of patients with positive serum levels was 42.3% with pulmonary disease (14.5% in asbestosis, 27.3% in bronchial asthma, 59.4% in bronchiectasis, 81.3% in idiopathic pulmonary fibrosis and 61.5% in pulmonary tuberculosis) *2026*

Calcium *Serum* *No Effect* In 40 patients with tuberculosis mean concentration of 2.30 ± 0.10 mmol/L not significantly different from 2.30 ± 0.15 mmol/L in 40 healthy controls *3319*
Urine *Increase* In 40 patients with tuberculosis mean concentration of 0.28 ± 0.10 mmol/L GFR significantly different from 0.20 ± 0.07 mmol/L GFR in 40 healthy controls *3319*

Carcinoembryonic Antigen *Pleural Fluid* *Increase* Mean concentration increased in 1 of 38 effusions in patients with tuberculosis *1649*
Serum *Increase* In 30 patients with tuberculosis 63% had concentrations less than 2.5 ng/mL, 35% had concentrations between 2.6 and 5.0 ng/mL, 2% had concentrations between 5.1 and 10.0 ng/mL and 0% had concentrations greater than 10.0 ng/mL *2010*

Cortisol *Plasma* *Decrease* Relative hypoadrenalism observed with partial destruction of the adrenal cortex *2901*

1,25-Dihydroxy Vitamin D *Serum* *Increase* In 40 patients with tuberculosis mean concentration of 68.4 ± 22.7 pmol/L not significantly different from 60.0 ± 17.7 pmol/L in 40 healthy controls *3319*

25-Hydroxy Vitamin D *Serum* *Decrease* In 40 patients with tuberculosis mean concentration of 27.9 ± 14.9 nmol/L significantly different from 50.0 ± 17.5 nmol/L in 40 healthy controls *3319*

ionized Calcium *Serum* *No Effect* In 40 patients with tuberculosis mean concentration of 1.26 ± 0.07 mmol/L not significantly different from 1.25 ± 0.06 mmol/L in 40 healthy controls *3319*

Lactate Dehydrogenase *BAL Fluid* *Increase* Mean activity in 25 patients with active pulmonary tuberculosis of 199 U/L compared with 45 U/L in control patients *1354*
Pleural Fluid *Increase* In 42 patients with tuberculous pleural effusions mean activity 535.1 ± 394.5 U/L not significantly different from 543.1 ± 468.4 U/L in 41 patients with carcinomatous effusions but significantly higher than 69.5 ± 27.0 U/L in 10 patients with transudative effusions *779*
Serum *Increase* Mean activity in 25 patients with active pulmonary tuberculosis increased in 48% *1354*

Leukocytes *Pleural Fluid* *Increase* In 42 patients with tuberculous pleural effusions mean concentration of 2,496 ± 1,524 /μL not significantly higher than 1,907 ± 1,789 /μL in 41 patients with carcinomatous effusions but significantly higher than 574 ± 648 /μL in 10 patients with transudative effusions *779*

Lymphocytes *Pleural Fluid* *Increase* In 42 patients with tuberculous pleural effusions mean concentration of 2,166 ± 1,255 /μL not significantly higher than 1,607 ± 1,432 /μL in 41 patients with carcinomatous effusions but significantly higher than 441 ± 594 /μL in 10 patients with transudative effusions *779*

Neopterin *Serum* *Increase* Increased concentration observed as in other intracellular bacterial infections *121*

Neutrophils *Pleural Fluid* *Increase* In 42 patients with tuberculous pleural effusions mean concentration of 329 ± 405 /μL not significantly higher than 302 ± 497 /μL in 41 patients with carcinomatous effusions but significantly higher than 133 ± 81 /μL in 10 patients with transudative effusions *779*

Parathyroid Hormone, Intact *Plasma* *No Effect* In 40 patients with tuberculosis mean concentration of 1.70 ± 0.71 mmol/L not significantly different from 1.95 ± 0.60 mmol/L in 40 healthy controls *3319*

Phosphate *Serum* *No Effect* In 40 patients with tuberculosis mean concentration of 1.00 ± 0.20 mmol/L not significantly different from 1.00 ± 0.10 mmol/L in 40 healthy controls *3319*

Protein *Pleural Fluid* *Increase* In 42 patients with tuberculous pleural effusions mean concentration of 41.5 ± 8.7 g/L significantly higher than 39.5 ± 7.7 g/L in 41 patients with carcinomatous effusions and 16.9 ± 3.4 g/L in 10 patients with transudative effusions *779*

Rheumatoid Factor *Serum* *Increase* Rheumatoid factor may be observed in certain patients *2473* Mean concentration increased in patients with tuberculosis *2472* Concentration may be increased as in other diseases with chronic inflammation *2952*

Soluble Interleukin-2 Receptor *Pleural Fluid* *Increase* In 42 patients with tuberculous pleural effusions mean concentration of 3.72 ± 0.09 U/mL not significantly higher than 3.36 ± 0.16 U/mL in 41 patients with carcinomatous effusions but significantly higher than 2.89 ± 0.12 U/mL in 10 patients with transudative effusions *779*
Serum *Increase* In 42 patients with tuberculous pleural effusions mean plasma concentration of 3.13 ± 0.26 U/mL not significantly higher than 2.68 ± 0.19 U/mL in 41 patients with carcinomatous effusions but significantly higher than 2.19 ± 0.09 U/mL in 10 patients with transudative effusions *779*

11.90 Pulmonary Tuberculosis

Albumin *Serum* *Decrease* Tends to be reduced to a degree proportional to the severity of the lesions *4707* *4136* In 36% of 26 patients at initial hospitalization for this disorder *1576*

Alkaline Phosphatase *Serum* *Increase* Isolated elevation suggests liver involvement in the absence of other causes *900* In 25% of 26 patients at initial hospitalization for this disorder *1576* Elevated in 50% of cases, ranging from 25 - 270 U/L, with only 10% of cases having values > 100 U/L *1025*

Amylase *Pleural Fluid* *Increase* Pleural fluid levels may be high *3482*

Angiotensin-converting Enzyme *Serum* *No Effect* No difference in levels found between control group of 108 and TB group of 100 *1846*

Anti-Streptolysin-O Titer *Serum* *Increase* Above normal titers may occur *3953*

Antibody Titer *Serum* *Increase* Used to differentiate pulmonary sarcoidosis from tuberculosis. Antituberculous antibodies were found in TB in 83%; in sarcoidosis in 22% *2786*

Antidiuretic Hormone *Plasma* *Increase* Inappropriate secretion of ADH with consequent water retention can occur *1980*

Antituberculous Glycolipid Antigen *Serum* *Increase* Mean normal concentration less than 1.7 U/mL: Sensitivity of 90% and specificity of 98% for active pulmonary tuberculosis *2600*

Arylsulfatase *Urine* *Increase* Considerable increase *1279*

Aspartate Aminotransferase *Serum* *Increase* In 35% of 26 patients at initial hospitalization for this disorder *1576*

Bicarbonate *Serum* *Increase* In 64% of 23 patients at initial hospitalization for this disorder *1576*

Calcium *Serum* *Increase* In one study of 40 patients with nonmalignant causes of hypercalcemia and low intact PTH concentration, 1 was attributable to pulmonary tuberculosis *3280*

Carcinoembryonic Antigen *Pleural Fluid* *Increase* Benign inflammatory effusions (tuberculosis, empyema, pneumonia) had mean CEA activity of 6.2 ± 3.4 ng/mL, higher than effusions caused by congestive heart failure (2.9 ± 1.5) and other noninflammatory effusions *4369*
Serum *Increase* 37% of patients had values > 2.5 ng/mL *4891*

Cells *Peritoneal Fluid* *Increase* Cell count in the peritoneal fluid varies from 2,000 - 10,000 /µL and shows a marked predominance of lymphocytes *1980*

Cholesterol *Pleural Fluid* *Increase* Rarely *869*
Serum *Decrease* In 34% of 26 patients at initial hospitalization for this disorder *1576*

Complement Fixation *Serum* *Increase* Used to differentiate pulmonary sarcoidosis from tuberculosis. Antituberculous antibodies were found in TB is 83%; in sarcoidosis 22% *2786*

Copper *Red Blood Cells* *Increase* Characteristically elevated levels *501*
Serum *Increase* Characteristically elevated in whole blood, plasma, and erythrocytes *501*

C-Reactive Protein *Serum* *Increase* Increased inconsistently *5544*

1,25-Dihydroxy Vitamin D_3 *Serum* *Increase* Observed effect *126*

Erythrocyte Sedimentation Rate *Blood* *Increase* Normal rates may be seen on occasion in patients with active tuberculosis *1980* Usually elevated *900*

Erythrocytes *Pleural Fluid* *Increase* < 100,000 /µL *4493* *1980*

γ-Globulin *Serum* *Increase* Advanced pulmonary and extrapulmonary tuberculosis *4707*

Glucose *Ascitic Fluid* *Decrease* Seen with tuberculous peritonitis *413*
Pleural Fluid *Decrease* Levels less than 3.3 mmol/L (60 mg/dL) *3142*

Granulocyte-Macrophage Colony Stimulating Factor
Serum *No Effect* In 17 patients with minimal severity pulmonary tuberculosis median concentration of 10 pg/mL, 11 pg/mL in 14 patients with moderate severity and 12 pg/mL in 9 patients with far-advanced disease not significantly different from 10 pg/mL in 9 healthy controls *1318*

Hematocrit *Blood* *Decrease* Anemia is common because of the effects of the infection on RBC production and survival and because of coexistent iron and nutritional deficiencies *900*

Hemoglobin *Blood* *Decrease* Anemia is common because of the effects of the infection on RBC production and survival and because of coexistent iron and nutritional deficiencies *900*

immunoglobulin A *Serum* *No Effect* Concentration usually normal *5544*

Immunoglobulin M *Serum* *No Effect* Concentration usually normal *5544*

Interleukin-6 *Serum* *Increase* In 17 patients with minimal severity pulmonary tuberculosis median concentration of 5 pg/mL, 5 pg/mL in 12 patients with moderate severity not significantly different, but 15 pg/mL in 9 patients with far-advanced disease significantly greater than 5 pg/mL in 11 healthy controls *1318*

Isocitrate Dehydrogenase *Serum* *No Effect* No effect on activity observed *5008*

Lactate Dehydrogenase *Pleural Fluid* *Decrease* Decreased values in primary and post-primary tuberculosis *1373*
Pleural Fluid *Increase* Moderate elevation occurred in 50% of cases, especially in active tuberculosis *1005*

Leukocytes *Blood* *Increase* Leukocytosis and rarely a leukemoid reaction may occur; however, the WBC is frequently normal. In more acute forms of the disease, the ratio of leukocytes may be increased with decreased lymphocytes *900*
Blood *No Effect* Leukocytosis and rarely a leukemoid reaction may occur; however, the WBC is frequently normal. In more acute forms of the disease, the ratio of leukocytes may be increased with decreased lymphocytes *900* Usually not elevated. Leukocytosis suggests the presence of secondary infection but may occur in acute tuberculous pneumonia *1980*

Leukotriene B_4 *Plasma* *Increase* In 13 patients with minimal severity pulmonary tuberculosis median concentration of 250 pg/mL, 500 pg/mL in 13 patients with moderate severity and 500 pg/mL in 7 patients with far-advanced disease significantly greater than 150 pg/mL in 12 healthy controls *1318*
White Blood Cells *No Effect* In patients with pulmonary tuberculosis mean concentration of 19.4 ± 4.9 pmol/10^6 cells not significantly different from 22.7 ± 9.4 pmol/10^6 cells in healthy controls *1318*

Leukotriene C_4 *White Blood Cells* *No Effect* In patients with pulmonary tuberculosis mean concentration of 8.4 ± 3.9 pmol/10^6 cells not significantly different from 7.4 ± 3.7 pmol/10^6 cells in healthy controls *1318*

Lymphocyte T-Cells *Blood* *Decrease* Normal *1588*

Lymphocytes *Ascitic Fluid* *Increase* Characteristic of chronic inflammatory disease, especially tuberculosis *4891*

11.90 Pulmonary Tuberculosis *(continued)*

Lymphocytes *(continued)*
Peritoneal Fluid *Increase* Cell count in the peritoneal fluid varies from 2,000 - 10,000 /µL and shows a marked predominance of lymphocytes *1980*
Pleural Fluid *Decrease* In patients with pulmonary tuberculosis, pulmonary malignancy or nonspecific pleuritis, the percentages and absolute numbers of B lymphocytes were significantly lower in pleural fluid than in peripheral blood *4104*
Pleural Fluid *Increase* The percentage and absolute numbers of B lymphocytes were significantly lower in pleural fluid than in peripheral blood *4104* Both the percentage and absolute numbers of lymphocytes in pleural fluid were significantly higher than in peripheral blood *4104* 43 of 46 patients had effusions with > 50% small lymphocytes *3052* A preponderance of lymphocytes is consistent with tuberculosis, carcinoma, or lymphoma *1980* Characterized by a protein content of 3 g/dL and the presence of lymphocytes *1980*

Lysozyme *Serum* *Increase* Isolated cases *2012*

Monocytes *Ascitic Fluid* *Increase* Characteristic of chronic inflammatory disease, especially tuberculosis *4891* Seen with tuberculous peritonitis *413*
Blood *Increase* Frequently elevated in active disease. Monocytosis of 8 - 15% may be seen in severe or overwhelming tuberculosis *367*
Pleural Fluid *Increase* Predominant cell type *4493*

Neopterin *Urine* *Increase* Levels were measured in 55 patients with pulmonary TB. A positive correlation between mean levels, extent and activity of disease was apparent *1586*

Neutrophils *Pleural Fluid* *Increase* Neutrophils predominate in very early stages *3052*

Oxygen Partial Pressure *Pleural Fluid* *Decrease* Empyema or tuberculous effusion *1604*

Oxygen Saturation *Blood* *Decrease* Empyema or tuberculous effusion *1604*

Parathyroid Hormone *Plasma* *Decrease* In a study of 40 patients with low intact PTH concentrations and hypercalcemia 1 was attributable to pulmonary tuberculosis *3280*

pH *Pleural Fluid* *Decrease* May occur in non-neoplastic inflammatory pleural effusion (empyema, rheumatoid disease, tuberculosis) *1604*
Pleural Fluid *No Effect* pH < 7.3 is rarely encountered in tuberculous effusions *1980*

Platelets *Blood* *Increase* In 49% of 12 patients at initial hospitalization for this disorder *1576*

Precipitins *Serum* *Increase* Found in approximately 40% of patients *5619*

Protein *Peritoneal Fluid* *Increase* Usually, but not always, over 3 g/dL *1980*
Pleural Fluid *Increase* Concentrations > 6.0 g/dL indicate tuberculosis *3052* Characterized by a protein content of 3 g/dL and the presence of lymphocytes *1980*
Serum *Decrease* Hypoproteinemia may be present. There is no specific diagnostic value to patterns of protein distribution in tuberculosis *1980*

Rheumatoid Factor *Serum* *Increase* 11% positivity *1980* The incidence of seropositivity exceeds that of a normal population *4551* 11% positivity *874* *306*

Sodium *Serum* *Decrease* Occasionally found, due to inappropriate secretion of ADH with consequent water retention *1980* Sometimes found in extensive chronic disease. Usually caused by abnormal retention of water *367* May be decreased (110 - 125 mmol/L) especially in aged or in overwhelming infection *5545*

Specific Gravity *Pleural Fluid* *Increase* Exudate (> 1.016) *126*

Tissue Polypeptide Antigen *Serum* *No Effect* In 8 patients with pulmonary tuberculosis mean concentration of 88.4 ± 43.0 U/L not significantly different from 72.7 ± 19.2 U/L in 19 healthy controls *5845*

Uric Acid *Serum* *Increase* In 48% of 26 patients at initial hospitalization for this disorder *1576*

VDRL *Serum* *Positive* False positive serologic tests may be seen *2039*

Zinc *Serum* *Decrease* Decreased levels are characteristic *501*

13.00 Tuberculous Meningitis

Adenosine Deaminase *Cerebrospinal Fluid* *Increase* In 30 cases of tuberculous mengitis activity higher than 4 U/L in all, and higher than 6 U/L in 90% cases compared with normals in whom activity was less than 4 U/L *3244* In 20 patients with tuberculous meningitis median concentration of 12.0 U/L significantly different from 1 U/L in 117 individuals without meningitis *3122*

Antidiuretic Hormone *Plasma* *Increase* Inappropriate secretion of ADH with consequent water retention *1980*

Apolipoprotein H *Cerebrospinal Fluid* *No Effect* In 15 patients with tuberculous meningitis median concentration and that in control individuals (patients with noninfectious neurological diseases) below detection limit of method *3341*

Cells *Cerebrospinal Fluid* *Increase* 25 - 500 /µL; chiefly lymphocytes *1980*

Chloride *Cerebrospinal Fluid* *Decrease* May be due mainly to the associated fall in the plasma level following vomiting, but may be associated with alteration in the plasma/CSF barrier *1290* 525 - 675 mg/dL *1980*
Serum *Decrease* Fall may be due to vomiting *1290*

Erythrocyte Sedimentation Rate *Blood* *Increase* Over 100 mm/h indicate serious disease *1098*

γ-Globulin *Serum* *Increase* Advanced pulmonary and extrapulmonary tuberculosis *4707*

Glucose *Cerebrospinal Fluid* *Decrease* Falls to < 50% of blood glucose *5545* 40 mg/dL *2039* Normal or moderately decreased *1980*

Interferon-γ *Cerebrospinal Fluid* *Increase* Proinflammatory cytokines are present in CSF of patients with tuberculous meningitis for weeks or months, not declining with treatment *5172* In 15 patients with tuberculous meningitis median concentration of 56.7 pg/mL significantly greater than in control individuals of patients with noninfectious neurological diseases (less than 5 pg/mL) *3341*

Interleukin-1 *Cerebrospinal Fluid* *Increase* Present at low concentrations in CSF of patients with tuberculous meningitis for weeks or months, but declining significantly during 4 weeks of treatment *5172*

Interleukin-6 *Cerebrospinal Fluid* *Increase* Proinflammatory cytokines are present in CSF of patients with tuberculous meningitis for weeks or months *5172*

Interleukin-8 *Cerebrospinal Fluid* *Increase* Concentration in CSF of patients with tuberculous meningitis similar to that in patients with bacterial meningitis *5172*

Interleukin-10 *Cerebrospinal Fluid* *Increase* In 15 patients with tuberculous meningitis median concentration of 46 pg/mL significantly greater than in control individuals of patients with noninfectious neurological diseases (less than 2 pg/mL) *3341*

Lactate Dehydrogenase *Cerebrospinal Fluid* *Increase* Increased in all cases in the range of 80 - 265 U/L (normal of 0 - 35 U/L), higher in those who were seriously ill and having acute onset of the disease *2664*

Leukocytes *Cerebrospinal Fluid* *Increase* Up to 1,000 /µL, the cells being 30 - 100% lymphocytes *2039* In 20 patients with tuberculous meningitis median concentration of 193 x 10^9/L significantly different from < 5 x 10^9/L in 117 individuals without meningitis *3122* Cell count usually varies between 10 - 500 /µL and consists mainly of lymphocytes, except in the early stage when neutrophils predominate *1980*

Lymphocytes *Cerebrospinal Fluid* *Increase* 30 - 100% of CSF cells are lymphocytes *2039* Count usually varies between 10 - 500 /µL and consists mainly of lymphocytes, except in the early stage when neutrophils predominate *1980*

Magnesium *Cerebrospinal Fluid* *Decrease* Low levels associated with convulsions *234*

Monocytes *Cerebrospinal Fluid* *Increase* Usually range from 50-200/µL *367*

Protein *Cerebrospinal Fluid* *Increase* In 20 patients with tuberculous meningitis median concentration of 1,220 mg/L significantly different from 220 mg/L in 117 individuals without meningitis *3122* Slightly increased in early stages but continues to increase, reaching levels > 300 mg/dL in advanced disease, and much higher levels when block of CSF occurs *2039*
Serum *Decrease* Hypoproteinemia may be present. There is no specific diagnostic value to patterns of protein distribution in tuberculosis *1980*

Rheumatoid Factor *Serum* *Increase* 11% positivity *306* *874* Positive tests may be seen in connective tissue diseases such as tuberculosis *2039*

Sodium *Serum* *Decrease* Occasionally found, due to inappropriate secretion of ADH with consequent water retention *1980* May be decreased (110 - 125 mmol/L) especially in aged or in overwhelming infection *5545*

Soluble Tumor Necrosis Factor Receptor *Cerebrospinal Fluid* *Increase* Present for prolonged periods in CSF of patients with tuberculous meningitis with increased ratio of TNF receptor to TNF-α *5172*

Soluble Tumor Necrosis Factor Receptor-p55 *Cerebrospinal Fluid* *Increase* In 15 patients with tuberculous meningitis median concentration of 2.4 ng/mL significantly greater than in control individuals of patients with noninfectious neurological diseases (less than 0.1 ng/mL) *3341*

Soluble Tumor Necrosis Factor Receptor-p75 *Cerebrospinal Fluid* *Increase* In 15 patients with tuberculous meningitis median concentration of 6.8 ng/mL significantly greater than in control individuals of patients with noninfectious neurological diseases (less than 0.5 ng/mL) *3341*

Tryptophan *Cerebrospinal Fluid* *Increase* Observed effect *5545*

Tumor Necrosis Factor-α *Cerebrospinal Fluid* *Increase* In 15 patients with tuberculous meningitis median concentration of 94.7 pg/mL significantly greater than in control individuals of patients with noninfectious neurological diseases (less than 3 pg/mL) *3341* Present at low concentrations in CSF of patients with tuberculous meningitis for weeks or months, not declining with treatment *5172*

Uric Acid *Cerebrospinal Fluid* *Increase* Markedly increased with decreased CSF:blood ratio, possibly due to cellular breakdown and nucleoprotein catabolism *5100*
Serum *Increase* Increased in both blood and CSF with a lowered blood:CSF ratio, possibly due to cellular breakdown and nucleoprotein catabolism *5100*
Urine *Increase* Increased excretion in neurological and psychiatric disorders; progressive rise in urinary level following slight rise in blood, due to disturbed purine metabolism *5100*

VDRL *Serum* *Positive* False positive serologic tests for syphilis may be seen *2039*

14.00 Peritoneal Tuberculosis

Adenosine Deaminase *Ascitic Fluid* *Increase* Mean concentration in ascitic fluid of patients with peritoneal tuberculosis of 47.9 ± 21.9 U/L compared with 9.6 ± 5 U/L in healthy controls *1463*
Serum *Increase* Both in serum and ascitic fluid of patients with peritoneal tuberculosis concentration increased. Activities above 54 U/L in serum suggest tuberculosis *433*

18.00 Miliary Tuberculosis

Adenosine Deaminase *Serum* *Increase* Value in patients with leukemia, hepatitis, miliary tuberculosis and cirrhosis were higher than in a patient with carcinoma of the liver who had the highest result in the cancer series *1784*

Alanine Aminotransferase *Serum* *Increase* In 5 cases of hepatic granuloma, ALT was 70 U/L with a range of 50 - 115 U/L *3161*

Alkaline Phosphatase *Serum* *Increase* Reported effect *2039* Constant clinical finding due to diffuse involvement of the liver with granulomas *1980* Marked elevation in all 5 cases of granuloma of liver. Maximum upper limit of normal is 85 U/L. Average elevated value 425 U/L (range 191 - 700 U/L) *3161*

Anti-Streptolysin-O Titer *Serum* *Increase* Above normal titers may occur *3953*

Arylsulfatase *Urine* *Increase* Considerable increase in urinary activity in pulmonary and renal tuberculosis *4295* Observed effect *1279*

Aspartate Aminotransferase *Serum* *Increase* In 5 cases of granuloma of liver, activities in 100% were mildly elevated, showing a mean elevation of 36 U/L over the normal maximum limit of 24 U/L *3161*

Bilirubin *Serum* *Increase* Reported effect *992* *5677* Bilirubin usually only minimally elevated *2039*

Calcium *Serum* *Increase* In one patient with miliary tuberculosis concentration of 3.25 mmol/L on admission to hospital with decline to 2.67 mmol/L after treatment for one week with antituberculosis medication *763*

Cells *Cerebrospinal Fluid* *Increase* Spinal fluid shows predominantly mononuclear pleocytosis (up to several hundred cells /μL) *2039*

Cholesterol *Pericardial Fluid* *Increase* High levels (2.6 - 5.2 mmol/L; 100 to 200 mg/dL) *566*

1,25-Dihydroxy Vitamin D_3 *Serum* *Increase* Observed effect *126*

Erythrocyte Sedimentation Rate *Blood* *Increase* Increased in disseminated or advanced tuberculosis but is not used as an index of activity *5545*

Erythrocytes *Ascitic Fluid* *Increase* > 10,000 cells/μL seen in about 5% of patients *233*
Blood *Decrease* Pancytopenia is a common feature *5677*

γ-Globulin *Serum* *Increase* Observed effect *2039*

Glucose *Cerebrospinal Fluid* *Decrease* Observed effect *2039*
Peritoneal Fluid *Decrease* Usually < 1.7 mmol/L *599*

γ-Glutamyltransferase *Serum* *Increase* In 5 patients with liver granulomas, including miliary tuberculosis and sarcoidosis, serum GGT levels were all elevated, mean activity of 303 U/L, range 116 - 740 U/L *3161*

Hematocrit *Blood* *Decrease* Observed effect *992* *5677*

Hemoglobin *Plasma* *Increase* Reported observation *5677* Reported finding *992*

Leucine Aminopeptidase *Serum* *Increase* In 12 patients with granulomatous hepatitis, all showed elevated LAP levels, varying from 380 - 1,000 U/L, with a mean of 622 U/L (normal 322 U/L) *579*

Leukocytes *Ascitic Fluid* *Increase* > 1000 /μL, usually over 70% lymphocytes *233*
Blood *Decrease* May be low or normal to markedly elevated with the leukemoid reaction *1980* Pancytopenia is a common feature *5677* Leukopenia, sometimes as low as 3,500 - 4,000 /μL, with a large number of immature forms *367* Observed in some patients *2039* Observed effect in some patients *5544*
Blood *Increase* May be low or normal to markedly elevated with the leukemoid reaction *1980* Active tuberculosis is usually accompanied by a moderate leukocytosis. Extreme leukocytosis occasionally occurs in patients seriously ill with widespread, necrotizing disease *5701* Observed effect *5677* Leukocytosis up to 20,000 /μL (leukemoid reaction) *2039*

Lymphocyte T-Cells *Blood* *Decrease* Normal *1588*

Lymphocytes *Ascitic Fluid* *Increase* Characteristic of chronic inflammatory disease, especially tuberculosis *4891*
Cerebrospinal Fluid *Increase* Predominantly mononuclear pleocytosis (up to several hundred cells/μL) *2039*

Lysozyme *Serum* *Increase* Isolated cases *2012*

Monocytes *Ascitic Fluid* *Increase* Characteristic of chronic inflammatory disease, especially tuberculosis *4891*
Blood *Increase* Frequently elevated in active disease. Monocytosis of 8 - 15% may be seen in severe or overwhelming tuberculosis *367*

Neutrophils *Blood* *Increase* Observed effect *1098* Increase was observed in two cases of tuberculosis of the liver *2803* Active tuberculosis is usually accompanied by a moderate leukocytosis. Extreme leukocytosis occasionally occurs in patients seriously ill with widespread, necrotizing disease *5701*

5'-Nucleotidase *Serum* *Increase* 2 cases were reported in which the tests were 25 and 118 U/L (normal 2 - 11 U/L) *2803* Serum 5'-nucleotidase was significantly elevated in 2 of 3 patients with liver granulomata *2803*

Platelets *Blood* *Decrease* Pancytopenia is a common feature *5677*

Protein *Ascitic Fluid* *Increase* Often > 2.5 g/dL in ascitic fluid *233*
Cerebrospinal Fluid *Increase* Observed effect *2039*
Serum *Decrease* Hypoproteinemia may be present. There is no specific diagnostic value to patterns of protein distribution in tuberculosis *1980*

Rheumatoid Factor *Serum* *Increase* The incidence of seropositivity exceeds that of a normal population *4551* 11% positivity *306* *874*

18.00 Miliary Tuberculosis *(continued)*

Sodium *Serum Decrease* Often occurs, frequently caused by inappropriate secretion of antidiuretic hormone *367*

VDRL *Serum Positive* False positive serologic tests may be seen *2039*

Vitamin A *Serum Decrease* Impaired absorption *1290*

Bacterial Diseases

20.90 Plague

Erythrocytes *Blood No Effect* Usually normal *2035*

Leukocytes *Blood Increase* Observed effect *2035* Significantly higher *1775*

21.00 Tularemia

Agglutination Tests *Serum Positive* Positive between the 1st and 3rd weeks, and a rising titer is usually demonstrable between acute and convalescent sera *1980* Agglutination reaction becomes positive in 2nd week of infection. Significant titer is 1:40; usually it becomes > 1:320 by 3rd week. Peaks at 4 - 7 weeks 1:100), then gradually decreases during next year *5545*

Albumin *Urine Increase* Mild albuminuria may occur at the height of illness *367*

C-Reactive Protein *Serum Increase* Elevated in proportion to the activity of the disease *900*

Erythrocyte Sedimentation Rate *Blood Increase* Elevated in proportion to the activity of the disease *900* During the active stages *367*

Insulin *Plasma Increase* Observed in patients with tularemia *4294* Characteristically observed with tularemia *4755*

Leukocytes *Blood Decrease* Usually normal or low *367*
Blood Increase Usually normal or slightly increased *1980*
Blood No Effect Usually normal, may be low or slightly increased *1980 367*

23.00 Brucellosis

Agglutination Tests *Serum Positive* Agglutinins appear 1 - 2 weeks after onset of infection *1980* Of 200 cases of symptomatic brucella infection, 198 had titers of 160 or > in the standard tube agglutination test *619* Becomes positive during 2nd to 3rd week of illness; 90% of patients have titers of > 1:320, and may remain positive long after infection has been cured *5545*

Alanine Aminotransferase *Serum Increase* In 5 cases of hepatic granuloma, ALT was elevated to a mean value of 70 U/L (normal = 50 U/L) and a range of 50 - 115 U/L *3161*

Alkaline Phosphatase *Serum Increase* Marked elevation in all 5 cases of granuloma of liver. Maximum upper limit of normal is 85 U/L. Average elevated value 425 U/L (range 191 to 700 U/L) *3161*

Antibody Titer *Serum Increase* Antibodies elicited early in natural infection are predominantly IgM, with lesser quantities of IgG. As the disease progresses, IgM declines, and IgG increases, reaching its height at the period of maximum resistance to reinfection *4551*

Aspartate Aminotransferase *Serum Increase* In 5 cases of granuloma of liver, 100% had mildly elevated activities, showing a mean elevation of 36 U/L over the normal maximum limit of 24 U/L *3161*

Brucella Antibody *Serum Increase* A titer of > /- 1:160 highly suggests active infection *2952*

Complement Fixation *Serum Increase* In late active disease, usually 1:16 or higher *2192*

Coombs' Test *Serum Positive* The modified Coombs' test overcomes the blocking antibody and prozone phenomenon *4551*

Erythrocyte Sedimentation Rate *Blood Increase* Occurs in < 25% of patients and usually in nonlocalized type *5545*

Hemagglutination Inhibition *Serum Increase* When a series of known positive sera were submitted to 6 recognized laboratories highly variable reports were received, ranging from negative to titers as high as 1:640 for the same serum. In view of many variables there can hardly be a titer considered to be diagnostic. In general a titer of 1:320 or higher in the presence of significant symptoms and a reasonable exposure history may be considered presumptive evidence of the disease *900*

Immunoglobulin G *Serum Increase* Antibodies elicited early in natural infection are predominantly IgM, with lesser quantities of IgG. As the disease progresses, IgM declines, and IgG increases, reaching its height at the period of maximum resistance to reinfection *4551*

Immunoglobulin M *Serum Increase* Antibodies elicited early in natural infection are predominantly IgM, with lesser quantities of IgG. As the disease progresses, IgM declines, and IgG increases, reaching its height at the period of maximum resistance to reinfection *4551*

Immunoglobulins *Serum Increase* Antibodies elicited early in natural infection are predominantly IgM, with lesser quantities of IgG. As the disease progresses, IgM declines, and IgG increases, reaching its height at the period of maximum resistance to reinfection *4551*

Leucine Aminopeptidase *Serum Increase* In 12 patients with granulomatous hepatitis, all showed elevated LAP levels, varying from 380 - 1,000 U/L, with a mean of 622 (normal = 322) *579*

Leukocytes *Blood Decrease* Leukopenia is seen in infections especially bacterial infections. Usually < 10,000 /µL with significant decreases occurring in 33% of patients *5545* May be normal or slightly elevated in the acute disease but a moderate leukopenia with a relative lymphocytosis is commonly observed *900*
Blood Increase May be normal or slightly elevated in the acute disease but a moderate leukopenia with a relative lymphocytosis is commonly observed *900*

Lymphocytes *Blood Increase* Relative lymphocytosis in some cases *1980*

Monocytes *Blood Increase* Occurs in certain bacterial infections *5544*

Neutrophils *Blood Decrease* Significant neutropenia may occur *729*

5'-Nucleotidase *Serum Increase* Significantly elevated in 2 of 3 patients with liver granulomata *2803*

Oligoclonal Banding *Cerebrospinal Fluid Increase* Oligoclonal IgG bands detected in patients with neurobrucellosis *3261*

Rheumatoid Factor *Serum Increase* Mean concentration increased in patients with brucellosis *2472* Rheumatoid factor may be observed in certain patients *2473*

VDRL *Serum Positive* False positive serologic tests are sometimes seen *2039*

30.00 Lepromatous Leprosy

Soluble CD23 *Serum Increase* In 12 patients with lepromatous leprosy median concentration of 17.4 arb U/mL significantly different from 10.1 arb U/mL in matched healthy controls *280*

30.00 Leprosy

Albumin *Serum Decrease* Markedly decreased in lepromatous leprosy and lepra reaction *4572*

Angiotensin-converting Enzyme *Serum Increase* Reported effect *4488* Observed effect *3041* Increased activities observed in patients with leprosy *2952*

Antinuclear Antibodies *Serum Increase* Found in 30% *4551*

Arginase *Lymphocytes Increase* Correlated with the degree of impairment in the protective cell mediated immune response *235*
Serum Increase Correlated with the degree of impairment in the protective cell mediated immune response *235*

Calcium *Serum Decrease* Significantly decreased in all types of leprosy except tuberculoid *4870*

Cholesterol *Serum Decrease* Slightly decreased *5545*

Complement C_3 *Serum Increase* High levels of both C_2 and C_3 have been recorded *4551*

Complement, Total *Serum Increase* Sarcoidosis, leprosy, and Wegener's granulomatosis have elevated levels *3804*

Cryoglobulins *Serum Increase* Found in 95% *4551*

Erythrocyte Sedimentation Rate *Blood Increase* ESR directly correlates with the increase in plasma fibrinogen in lepromatous leprosy *4274*

Fibrin Degradation Products *Plasma Decrease* In lepromatous leprosy *4274*

Fibrinogen *Plasma Increase* Significant increases were noted in cases with lepra reaction, particularly those manifesting necrotizing skin, kidney, and sclerodermic lesions *4274*

α_1-Globulin *Serum Decrease* Decreased in dimorphic leprosy *4572*

γ-Globulin *Serum Increase* In 50 cases of leprosy, (10 tuberculoid, 25 lepromatous leprosy, 10 lepra reaction, 5 dimorphic leprosy, all showed a rise) *4572* Often present *1980* Lepromatous leprosy *4707*

Hematocrit *Blood Decrease* Anemia, when present, is usually mild *1980*

Hemoglobin *Blood Decrease* Anemia, when present, is usually mild *1980*

Histamine *Plasma Increase* Both histamine and histaminase levels are significantly elevated, especially in cases of long duration. Patients with leprosy in reaction had highest levels, whereas tuberculoid, borderline and lepromatous cases had moderate rises *4280*

immunoglobulin A *Serum Increase* Reported effect *5327* High levels have been described but appear to be more variable than IgG *4551*

Immunoglobulin G *Serum Increase* High levels are consistently found in the sera of untreated lepromatous patients *4551*

Immunoglobulin M *Serum Increase* High levels have been described but appear to be more variable than IgG *4551* Reported effect *5327*

Interleukin-1β *Serum Increase* In 30 patients with lepromatous leprosy range 70 - 5,000 pg/mL (328 $\pm$ 184) in comparison to other groups with other forms of leprosy and normal controls (9 $\pm$ 3 pg/mL) *4004*

LE Cells *Blood Positive* Found in 8% *4551*

Leukocytes *Blood Increase* Moderate leukocytosis may occur during exacerbations *1980*

Lymphocyte T-Cells *Blood Decrease* Normal *1588*

Magnesium *Serum Decrease* Decrease was highly significant in tuberculoid, lepromatous and borderline lepromatous cases *4870*

Neopterin *Serum Increase* Increased concentration observed as in other intracellular bacterial infections *121*

Plasma Cells *Blood Increase* High levels of precipitating antimycobacterial antibodies in lepromatous leprosy are paralleled by marked plasma cell proliferation *4551*

Precipitins *Serum Increase* Found in the sera of lepromatous patients and in 50% of the patients with tuberculoid lesions that were bacillary-positive. Not found in the sera of bacillary-negative tuberculoid patients *4551*

Rheumatoid Factor *Serum Increase* Observed effect *1980* Mean concentration increased in patients with leprosy *2472* Found in 24% of patients *306* Found in 50% *4551* Rheumatoid factor may be observed in certain patients *2473* Found in 24% of patients *874* The incidence of seropositivity exceeds that of a normal population *4551*

Tumor Necrosis Factor-α *Serum Increase* In 30 patients with lepromatous leprosy mean concentration of 399 $\pm$ 189 pg/mL, in 14 with tuberculoid-tuberculoid leprosy range from 15 - 160 pg/mL. In patients exhibiting type 1 and type 2 lepra reactions concentrations of 15 to 2,100 pg/mL observed *4004*

VDRL *Serum Positive* Frequent biological false positive reactions *5252* False positive serologic test occurs in 40% of patients *5545* Found in 70% *4551*

30.10 Tuberculoid Leprosy

Soluble CD23 *Serum No Effect* In 8 patients with tuberculoid leprosy median concentration of 7.7 arb U/mL not significantly different from 10.1 arb U/mL in matched healthy controls *280*

32.00 Diphtheria

Albumin *Urine Increase* Common, particularly in severe forms of the disease *900*

Casts *Urine Increase* Frequently present *5545*

Cells *Cerebrospinal Fluid Increase* With neuritis, a pleocytosis can occur *2192*

γ-Globulin *Serum Increase* May occur *900*

Glucose *Serum Decrease* Occurs frequently *5545*

Hemagglutination Inhibition *Serum Increase* Antitoxin titer of patient's serum showed 4-fold increase between titer in acute and convalescent sera confirming diagnosis *5545*

Hematocrit *Blood Decrease* Moderate anemia persisting into convalescence is common *900*

Hemoglobin *Blood Decrease* Moderate anemia persisting into convalescence is common *900*

Leukocytes *Blood Decrease* In severe cases *900* *Blood Increase* Slight leukocytosis with neutrophilia usually is noted, although in severe cases leukopenia may occur *900* Mild to moderate leukocytosis of about 15,000 /µL with increase in immature neutrophils *1980* WBC is slightly increased (< 15,000 /µL) *5545*

Monocytes *Cerebrospinal Fluid Increase* Following paralysis *900*

Neutrophils *Blood Increase* WBC is slightly increased (< 15,000 /µL) *5545* Slight leukocytosis with neutrophilia usually is noted, although in severe cases leukopenia may occur *900*

Protein *Cerebrospinal Fluid Increase* With neuritis *2192* Prolonged elevation following paralysis *900*

Urea Nitrogen *Serum Increase* Elevation with increase in serum globulins may occur *900*

33.00 Whooping Cough

Agglutination Tests *Serum Positive* These antibodies are produced in low titer and appear only after the second week of disease *1980*

Complement Fixation *Serum Increase* These antibodies are produced in low titer and appear only after the second week of disease *1980*

Leukocytes *Blood Increase* WBC > 20,000 /µL with > 70% small lymphocytes indicates this disease *900* Leukemoid reactions (> 50,000 /µL) are frequently associated with severe complications *900* Begins late in the catarrhal stage and rises steeply *5252* Moderate to severe leukocytosis, ranging from 15,000 - 40,000 /µL with a differential of 60 - 90% lymphocytes *1980*

Lymphocytes *Blood Increase* Though the WBC count and the differential counts may be quite variable, > 20,000 /µL with more than 70% small lymphocytes indicates this disease *900* Begins late in the catarrhal stage and rises steeply *5252* Moderate to severe leukocytosis, ranging from 15,000 - 40,000 /µL with a differential of 60 - 90% lymphocytes *1980*

Neutralizing Antibodies *Serum Increase* These antibodies are produced in low titer and appear only after the 2nd week of disease *1980*

34.00 Streptococcal Pharyngitis

$CD3^+$ Lymphocytes *Blood No Effect* In 15 patients with streptococcal pharyngitis mean concentration of 3.70 $\pm$ 0.54 x 10^3cells /µL not significantly different from 3.64 $\pm$ 0.58 x 10^3 cells /µL in 15 healthy controls *3737*

$CD4^+$:$CD8^+$ Lymphocyte Ratio *Blood No Effect* In 15 patients with chronic rheumatic heart disease mean ratio of 1.13 $\pm$ 0.48 not significantly different from 1.10 $\pm$ 0.21 in 15 healthy controls *3737*

34.00 Streptococcal Pharyngitis (continued)

CD4+ Lymphocytes *Blood* *No Effect* In 15 patients with streptococcal pharyngitis mean concentration of 1.70 ± 0.30 x 10^3 cells/µL not significantly different from 1.74 ± 0.32 x 10^3 cells/µL in 15 healthy controls *3737*

CD8+ Lymphocytes *Blood* *Increase* In 15 patients with streptococcal pharyngitis mean concentration of 1.62 ± 0.14 x 10^3 cells/µL significantly different from 1.60 ± 0.14 x 10^3 cells/µL in 15 healthy controls *3737*

CD16+ Lymphocytes *Blood* *No Effect* In 15 patients with acute chronic rheumatic heart disease mean concentration of 0.80 ± 0.10 x 10^3 cells/µL not significantly different from 0.84 ± 0.166 x 10^3 cells/µL in 15 healthy controls *3737*

CD19+ Lymphocytes *Blood* *No Effect* In 15 patients with streptococcal pharyngitis mean concentration of 0.74 ± 0.24 x 10^3 cells /µL not significantly different from 1.10 ± 0.09 x 10^3 cells/µL in 15 healthy controls *3737*

CD25+ Lymphocytes *Blood* *No Effect* In 15 patients with streptococcal pharyngitis mean concentration of 0.28 ± 0.14 x 10^3 cells/µL not significantly different from 0.55 ± 0.14 x 10^3 cells/µL in 15 healthy controls *3737*

Interleukin-1α *Serum* *No Effect* In 15 patients with chronic rheumatic heart disease mean concentration of 2.1 ± 1.4 pg/mL not significantly different from 3.1 ± 1.4 pg/mL in 15 healthy controls *3737*

Interleukin-2 *Serum* *No Effect* In 15 patients with streptococcal pharyngitis mean concentration of 0.3 ± 0.05 pg/mL not significantly different from 0.3 ± 0.47 pg/mL in 15 healthy controls *3737*

Tumor Necrosis Factor-α *Serum* *No Effect* In 15 patients with streptococcal pharyngitis mean concentration of 10.9 ± 7.8 pg/mL not significantly different from 6.4 ± 4.6 pg/mL in 15 healthy controls *3737*

36.00 Meningococcal Meningitis

Albumin *Urine* *Increase* May occur *5545*

Cells *Cerebrospinal Fluid* *Increase* Cell count is elevated to thousands /µL, mostly neutrophils *367*

Erythrocytes *Urine* *Increase* May show increase *5545*

Fibrinogen *Plasma* *Increase* In 26 patients with acute meningitis without shock mean concentration of 5,200 mg/L and in 13 with meningitis with shock mean concentration of 2,400 g/L significantly higher than in healthy individuals *5401*

Glucose *Cerebrospinal Fluid* *Decrease* Usually < 35 mg/dL *2192*

Interleukin-1 Receptor Antagonist
Cerebrospinal Fluid *Increase* In 26 patients with acute meningitis without shock mean concentration of 26,500 pg/mL and in 13 with meningitis with shock mean concentration of 5.500 pg/mL significantly higher than in healthy individuals *5401*
Serum *Increase* In 26 patients with acute meningitis without shock mean concentration of 6.750 pg/mL and in 13 with meningitis with shock mean concentration of 10.600 pg/mL significantly higher than in healthy individuals *5401*

Interleukin-1 Receptor Antagonist Type II
Cerebrospinal Fluid *Increase* In 26 patients with acute meningitis without shock mean concentration of 36.3 ng/mL and in 13 with meningitis with shock mean concentration of 9.1 ng/mL significantly higher than in healthy individuals *5401*
Serum *Increase* In 26 patients with acute meningitis without shock mean concentration of 23.9 ng/mL and in 13 with meningitis with shock mean concentration of 29.6 ng/mL significantly higher than in healthy individuals *5401*

Interleukin-1β *Cerebrospinal Fluid* *Increase* In 26 patients with acute meningitis without shock mean concentration of 1,750 pg/mL and in 13 with meningitis with shock mean concentration of 490 pg/mL significantly higher than in healthy individuals *5401*
Serum *Increase* In 26 patients with acute meningitis without shock mean concentration of 55 pg/mL and in 13 with meningitis with shock mean concentration of 70 pg/mL significantly higher than in healthy individuals *5401*

Lactate *Plasma* *Increase* In 26 patients with acute meningitis without shock mean concentration of 2,123 µmol/L and in 13 with meningitis with shock mean concentration of 3,142 µmol/L significantly higher than in healthy individuals *5401*

Leukocytes *Blood* *Increase* In 26 patients with acute meningitis without shock mean concentration of 10.5 x 10^9/L and in 13 with meningitis with shock mean concentration of 11.4 x 10^9/L significantly higher than in healthy individuals *5401* Up to 40,000 /µL with 80 - 90% neutrophils almost always occurs *367*
Cerebrospinal Fluid *Increase* Markedly increased (2,500-10,000 /µL), almost all polymorphonuclear leukocytes *5545* In 26 patients with acute meningitis without shock mean concentration of 12,300 x 10^6/L and in 13 with meningitis with shock mean concentration of 434 x 10^6/L significantly higher than in healthy individuals *5401*

Neutrophils *Blood* *Increase* Leukocytosis up to 40,000 /µL with 80 - 90% neutrophils is almost always present *367*
Cerebrospinal Fluid *Increase* Cell count is elevated to thousands/µL, mostly neutrophils *367*

Platelets *Blood* *Increase* In 13 with meningitis with shock mean concentration of 701 x 10^9/L significantly higher than in healthy individuals *5401*
Blood *No Effect* In 26 patients with acute meningitis without shock mean concentration of 158 x 10^9/L not significantly different from that in healthy individuals *5401*

Protein *Cerebrospinal Fluid* *Increase* Values of 80-500 mg/dL *2192*

Thyroxine (T4) *Serum* *Increase* Slightly increased in all patients *3229*

Tri-iodothyronine (T3) *Serum* *Decrease* Significantly low in all patients. Fall in T3 is inversely related to the degree of fever *3229*

36.20 Systemic Meningococcal Disease

Tissue Factor Pathway Inhibitor *Plasma* *Increase* Concentration significantly increased in patients with disease *4807*

36.30 Adrenalitis, Meningococcal Hemorrhagic

Cortisol *Plasma* *Decrease* In critically ill patients relative hypoadrenalism observed with acute partial destruction of the adrenal cortex due to bacterial (meningococcemia), viral or fungal infections *2901*

37.00 Tetanus

Alanine Aminotransferase *Serum* *Increase* Mainly in the more severe cases *900*

Albumin *Urine* *Increase* Some patients show proteinuria *900*

Aldolase *Serum* *Increase* Very high serum levels are found in severe cases *1290*

Aspartate Aminotransferase *Serum* *Increase* Elevation occurred in 2 of 5 cases *3733* Mainly in the more severe cases *900*

Bicarbonate *Serum* *Decrease* The lowest values are found in the more severe cases *900*
Serum *Increase* Metabolic alkalosis may occur with potassium loss *1980*

Carbon Dioxide Partial Pressure *Blood* *Increase* At the onset of mild forms, blood gases may be within normal values. Later, when spasms appear and high dosages of sedatives are given, hypoxemia, acidosis plus hypercapnia and metabolic acidosis are present *900* Metabolic alkalosis may occur with potassium loss *1980*

Catecholamines *Plasma* *Increase* Found in patients with severe disease. It is believed that this increase is caused by autonomic nervous system overactivity *900*
Urine *Increase* Usually found in patients with severe disease. It is believed that this increase is caused by autonomic nervous system overactivity *900*

Cholinesterase *Serum* *Decrease* Activity may be decreased in severe cases due to inhibition by the tetanus toxin *900* Reduced levels correlate with degree of severity of disease *4177*

Creatine Kinase *Serum* *Increase* Levels were found to be elevated in 75 cases and related to the clinical severity of disease. Values higher than 2.97 mU/mL were found to be highly suggestive of disease *5382*

Erythrocyte Sedimentation Rate *Blood* *Increase* Is often increased *900*

Lactate Dehydrogenase *Serum* *Increase* Elevated above the upper limit of normal in 3 of 5 cases *3733*

Leukocytes *Blood* *Increase* Probably caused by bacterial superimposed infections in the respiratory tract or in the injured tissues responsible for the infection (focus) *900*
Urine *Increase* Some patients show degenerate leukocytes *900*

Lymphocytes *Blood* *Decrease* Lymphopenia is more usual than lymphocytosis *900*

Neutrophils *Blood* *Increase* Granulocytosis and the appearance of less mature forms of neutrophils *900*

Oxygen Partial Pressure *Blood* *Decrease* At the onset of mild forms, blood gases may be within normal values. Later when spasms appear and high dosages of sedatives are given, hypoxemia, acidosis plus hypercapnia and metabolic acidosis are present, mainly because of inadequate or improper therapeutic management *900*

pH *Blood* *Decrease* At the onset of mild forms, blood gases may be within the normal values. Later, when spasms appear and high dosages of sedatives are given, hypoxemia, acidosis plus hypercapnia and metabolic acidosis are present *900*
Blood *Increase* Metabolic alkalosis may occur with potassium loss *1980*

38.00 Septicemia

Adenosine Deaminase *Serum* *Increase* A correlation with severe infections and high assays *1784* *2737*

Alanine *Plasma* *Increase* Concentrations determined in 10 burned patients with gram-negative sepsis and 9 burned patients without sepsis revealed an increase in the gluconeogenic precursors alanine, glycine, methionine and phenylalanine in those patients with sepsis *5683*

Alanine Aminotransferase *Serum* *Increase* Elevations observed in 6 cases of extrahepatic sepsis *3748*

Albumin *Serum* *Decrease* Decreased in 6 cases of extrahepatic sepsis *3748* In 54% of 11 patients at initial hospitalization for this disorder *1576*
Urine *Increase* Transient slight increase *5545*

Alkaline Phosphatase *Serum* *Increase* Elevated in 5 of 6 cases of extrahepatic sepsis, with levels as high as 460 U/L recorded *3748* In 27% of 11 patients at initial hospitalization for this disorder *1576*
White Blood Cells *Increase* Usually increased in untreated disease *5544*

Anti-Streptolysin-O Titer *Serum* *Increase* Appear in the serum 10 - 21 days after onset of acute streptococcal infection *1980*

Apolipoprotein A-I *Serum* *Decrease* Sepsis causes the concentration to decrease *100*

Apolipoprotein B *Serum* *Decrease* Sepsis causes the concentration to decrease *100*

Aspartate Aminotransferase *Serum* *Increase* In 27% of 11 patients at initial hospitalization for this disorder *1576* Elevations observed in 6 cases of extrahepatic sepsis *3748*

Catecholamines *Plasma* *Increase* Severe stress resulting from sepsis, hypovolemia or hypercapnia causes hypersecretion *4957*
Urine *Increase* Increased due to severe stress *5544* Severe stress resulting from sepsis, hypovolemia or hypocapnia causes hypersecretion *4957*

Cholesterol *Serum* *Decrease* May fall *100* May fall, during convalescence the level rises, sometimes to above the normal range *1290* In 54% of 11 patients at initial hospitalization for this disorder *1576*

Cholinesterase *Serum* *Decrease* In conditions which may have decreased serum albumin *5544*

Complement C_1 *Serum* *No Effect* Mean concentration typically normal or slightly increased in patients with bacteremia with shock *4682*

Complement C_1q *Serum* *No Effect* Normal concentrations of C_1, C_3, and C_4 *5651* Mean concentration typically normal or slightly increased in patients with bacteremia with shock *4682*

Complement C_2 *Serum* *No Effect* Normal concentrations of C_1, C_2, and C_4 *5651* Mean concentration typically normal or slightly increased in patients with bacteremia with shock *4682*

Complement C_3 *Serum* *Decrease* In severe gram-negative infection associated with shock, depression of C_3, C_5, C_6, and C_9 may occur, with normal concentrations of C_1, C_2, and C_4. Abnormalities develop early, before shock. C_3 concentration correlates with mortality *2694* *5651* *931* *785*
Serum *No Effect* Mean concentration typically normal or slightly increased in patients with bacteremia with shock *4682*

Complement C_4 *Serum* *No Effect* In severe gram-negative infection associated with shock, depression of C_3, C_5, C_6, and C_9 may occur, with normal concentrations of C_1, C_2, and C_4. Abnormalities develop early, before shock. C_3 concentration correlates with mortality *5651* Mean concentration typically normal or slightly increased in patients with bacteremia with shock *4682*

Complement C_5 *Serum* *No Effect* Mean concentration typically normal or slightly increased in patients with bacteremia with shock *4682*

Complement CH50 *Serum* *No Effect* Mean concentration typically normal or slightly increased in patients with bacteremia with shock *4682*

Complement, Total *Serum* *Decrease* In 51 patients, 24% had decreased values *4925* In severe gram-negative infection associated with shock, depression of C_3, C_5, C_6, and C_9 may occur, with normal concentrations of C_1, C_2, and C_4. Abnormalities develop early, before shock. C_3 concentration correlates with mortality *5651*
Serum *Increase* In 51 patients, 27% had increased values *4925*

Copper *Serum* *Increase* Increased in acute and chronic infections *5544*

C-Reactive Protein *Serum* *Increase* Increased inconsistently *5544*

Creatine *Urine* *Increase* Increased breakdown of muscle *5544*

Creatinine *Serum* *Increase* In 49% of 12 patients at initial hospitalization for this disorder *1576*

Epinephrine *Plasma* *Increase* In patients with septicemic, traumatic or hemorrhagic shock, plasma epinephrine and norepinephrine concentrations were increased above the normal range *385*

Erythrocyte Casts *Urine* *Increase* Transient slight increase *5545*

Erythrocyte Sedimentation Rate *Blood* *Increase* Increased in most bacterial infections; reflects the activity of the infectious process *1980*

Factor II *Plasma* *Decrease* May be associated with defibrination resulting in platelet and coagulation factor consumption in severe gram-positive septicemia *5677*

Factor IV *Plasma* *Decrease* May be associated with defibrination resulting in platelet and coagulation factor consumption in severe gram-positive septicemia *5677*

Fibrin Degradation Products *Plasma* *Increase* Elevation is much more common in fatal cases than in survivors *4881* Raised levels are common with other evidence of enhanced fibrinolysis *2646*

Fibrinogen *Plasma* *Decrease* May be associated with defibrination resulting in platelet and coagulation factor consumption in severe gram-positive septicemia *5677*

Follistatin *Serum* *Increase* Median concentration of 15.2 μg/L in 9 patients with septicemia significantly greater than 5.4 μg/L in healthy blood donors *3474*

γ-Globulin *Serum* *Increase* Increased in 6 cases of extrahepatic sepsis *3748*

Glucose *Serum* *Increase* Fasting hyperglycemia, impaired glucose tolerance and relative hyperinsulinemia are found *4755* In 56% of 12 patients at initial hospitalization for this disorder *1576* Fasting hyperglycemia, impaired glucose tolerance and relative hyperinsulinemia are found *4294*

Glucose Tolerance *Serum* *Decrease* Fasting hyperglycemia, impaired glucose tolerance and relative hyperinsulinemia are found *4755* *4294*

38.00 Septicemia *(continued)*

Glycine *Plasma* *Increase* Concentrations determined in 10 burned patients with gram-negative sepsis and 9 burned patients without sepsis revealed an increase in the gluconeogenic precursors alanine, glycine, methionine and phenylalanine in those patients with sepsis *5683*

HDL-Cholesterol *Serum* *Decrease* Sepsis causes the concentration to decrease *100*

Hematocrit *Blood* *Decrease* Mild to moderate anemia may occur during the course of chronic infections *900*

Hemoglobin *Blood* *Decrease* Mild to moderate anemia may occur during the course of chronic infections *900*

Hyaluronic Acid *Serum* *Increase* Elevated in septicemia *395*

17-Hydroxycorticosteroids *Urine* *Increase* Increased due to severe stress *5544*

immunoglobulin A *Serum* *Increase* Perinatal infections *1290*

Immunoglobulin D *Serum* *Increase* Moderately increased *5544*

Insulin *Plasma* *Increase* Fasting hyperglycemia, impaired glucose tolerance, and relative hyperinsulinemia are found *4294* *4755*

Insulin-like Growth Factor Binding Protein-3 Protease *Serum* *Increase* Reportedly increased activity in the plasma following severe illnesses such as septicemia *2103*

Iron *Serum* *Decrease* Decreased with acute and chronic infection. Frequently develops within of onset *1290*

Iron-binding Capacity, Total *Serum* *Decrease* Acute and chronic infections. The serum iron falls proportionately more than the transferrin content *1290*

17-Ketogenic Steroids *Urine* *Increase* Increased due to severe stress *5544*

Lactate Dehydrogenase *Serum* *Increase* In 72% of 11 patients at initial hospitalization for this disorder *1576*

Leukocytes *Blood* *Decrease* Although leukocytosis generally accompanies acute bacterial infection, leukopenia may be found, and in general, the WBC is not diagnostic *900*
Blood *Increase* Moderate to marked leukocytosis with a shift to left generally occurs *1980* Although leukocytosis generally accompanies acute bacterial infection, leukopenia may be found, and in general, the WBC is not diagnostic *900* Total counts may become extremely high *5677* In 63% of 14 patients at initial hospitalization for this disorder *1576*

Lipids *Serum* *Decrease* Sepsis causes the concentration to decrease *100*

Lymphocytes *Blood* *Decrease* In 78% of 14 patients at initial hospitalization for this disorder *1576*
Blood *Increase* In convalescence from acute infection *5544*

Methionine *Plasma* *Increase* Concentrations determined in 10 burned patients with gram-negative sepsis and 9 burned patients without sepsis revealed an increase in the gluconeogenic precursors alanine, glycine, methionine and phenylalanine in those patients with sepsis *5683*

Monocytes *Blood* *Increase* In acute infection *5544*

Neopterin *Urine* *Increase* Increased in people with bacterial septicemias *4772*

Neutrophils *Blood* *Decrease* In early onset group B streptococcal disease 39 (87%) had abnormal absolute neutrophil counts, 25 with neutropenia and 14 with neutrophilia. The absolute immature neutrophil count was elevated in 19 infants (42%) *3281*
Blood *Increase* In 49% of 14 patients at initial hospitalization for this disorder *1576* Increased WBC (15,000 - 30,000 /μL) and polymorphonuclear leukocyte counts are found *5545*

Norepinephrine *Plasma* *Increase* In patients with septicemic, traumatic or hemorrhagic shock, epinephrine and norepinephrine concentrations were increased above the normal range. In nonsurvivors norepinephrine concentrations remained persistently elevated while in survivors there was a rapid decline towards the normal range *385*

5'-Nucleotidase *Serum* *Increase* 4 patients with extrahepatic infection showed elevated levels, ranging from 21 - 75 U/L (normal 3 - 17 U/L) *3748*

Phenylalanine *Plasma* *Increase* Concentrations determined in 10 burned patients with gram-negative sepsis and 9 burned patients without sepsis revealed an increase in the gluconeogenic precursors alanine, glycine, methionine and phenylalanine in those patients with sepsis *5683*

Phosphate *Serum* *Decrease* In 54 patients with gram-negative septicemias; either absolute 2 mg/dL) or relative (P/BUN = 0.04) hypophosphatemia was found in 69% of all determinations *4352* Septicemia is a less common cause of hypophosphatemia due to shift of phosphate into cells *969*

Phospholipase A *Serum* *Increase* Increased activities in association with a wide variety of nonpancreatic disorders *2615* In certain cases this was the first parameter which could have shown the beginning of a septic process *4634*

Platelets *Blood* *Decrease* May be associated with defibrination resulting in platelet and coagulation factor consumption in severe gram-positive septicemia *5677*

Properdin Factor B *Plasma* *No Effect* Mean concentration typically normal or slightly increased in patients with bacteremia with shock *4682*

Prothrombin Consumption *Blood* *Increase* May be associated with defibrination resulting in platelet and coagulation factor consumption in severe gram-positive septicemia *5677*

Prothrombin Time *Plasma* *Increase* May be associated with defibrination resulting in platelet and coagulation factor consumption in severe gram-positive septicemia *5677*

Reticulocytes *Blood* *Decrease* The absolute count is reduced *900*

Triglycerides *Serum* *Increase* Sepsis causes the concentration to increase *100*

Troponin T *Serum* *Increase* Mean concentration increased above 0.2 μg/L in 67% patients with septic infections *334*

Urea Nitrogen *Serum* *Increase* In 49% of 12 patients at initial hospitalization for this disorder *1576* A condition that may be associated with excessive protein catabolism *1025*

Uric Acid *Serum* *Increase* In 54% of 11 patients at initial hospitalization for this disorder *1576*

Xylose Tolerance Test *Urine* *Abnormal* An inverse association between amount of xylose excreted and serum γ-globulin and IgG concentrations was significant *915*

38.90 Sepsis

Adenosine Triphosphate *Red Blood Cells* *Decrease* In surgical septic patients a significant decrease was observed in the last two days before death *2804*

Adrenomedullin *Plasma* *Increase* Mean concentration in 12 patients admitted to an ICU of 107 ± 39 fmol/mL compared with 7.9 ± 8 fmol/mL in 16 healthy age-matched controls *2171* In 16 patients with severe sepsis mean concentration of 59.9 ± 11.2 fmol/mL significantly different from 5.1 ± 0.2 fmol/mL in healthy controls *5343*

Albumin *Serum* *Decrease* In 22 patients with sepsis on admission to hospital mean concentration of 26 ± 4 g/L significantly lower than in healthy adults *5364* In 6 patients with postoperative sepsis mean concentration of 28.5 g/L compared with 37.5 g/L in 20 patients in early days following uncomplicated gastrointestinal surgery *754*

Angiotensin-converting Enzyme *Serum* *Decrease* In three patients with sepsis all demonstrated low enzyme activity *2155*

α_2-Antiplasmin *Plasma* *No Effect* Median concentration in 45 patients with sepsis of 1.00 IU/mL not significantly different from median of 0.97 IU/mL in 30 healthy controls *1245*

Antithrombin III *Plasma* *Decrease* Average lowest concentration in 152 septic patients of 50 ± 17% compared with 79 ± 22% in 248 patients without sepsis *5691* Median concentration in 45 patients with sepsis of 0.71 IU/mL significantly different from median of 1.00 IU/mL in 30 healthy controls *1245*

Atrial Natriuretic Peptide *Plasma* *Increase* Mean concentration increased to 120 pg/mL from normal of 32 pg/mL in patients with sepsis and acute respiratory failure: positive correlation with mean pulmonary artery pressure and pulmonary vascular resistance but not with other variables *3520* In 18 patients with sepsis on admission to hospital mean concentration of 415.6 ± 134.8 ng/L significantly higher than 40.1 ± 14.3 ng/L in 15 matched hospital control individuals with acute illness *5458*

C_1-Esterase Inhibitor *Serum* *Increase* Significant increase observed in uncomplicated sepsis but came back to normal or was slightly decreased in septic shock *3320*

Calcitonin *Plasma* *No Effect* No significant effect of sepsis observed although procalcitonin concentration significantly increased *201*

Calcitonin Gene-related Peptide *Serum* *Increase* In 22 patients with sepsis at onset of hypotension mean concentration of 55 ± 14 pmol/L significantly higher than 16 ± 1 pmol/L in healthy adults *5364* Significant increase to mean of 14.9 ± 3.2 pg/mL compared with 2.0 ± 0.3 pg/mL in healthy control volunteers *2500*

Catalase *Red Blood Cells* *Increase* In 32 patients with sepsis mean activity of 25.3 ± 5.4 mg/g hemoglobin significantly increased compared with 16.5 ± 4.7 mg/g hemoglobin in 7 healthy controls *5576*
Serum *Increase* In 32 patients with sepsis mean activity of 40.2 ± 18.8 mg/L significantly increased compared with 4.7 ± 4.6 mg/L in 7 healthy controls *5576*

Cells *Pleural Fluid* *Increase* Concentration of 583 ± 276 /µL in 15 septic patients not significantly different from 373 ± 83 /µL in 9 nonseptic patients *3298*

Complement C_3 *Serum* *Decrease* In 6 patients with postoperative sepsis mean concentration reduced to 79% compared with 121% in early postoperative days with uncomplicated gastrointestinal surgery *754*

Complement C_3a *Serum* *Increase* Increased concentrations observed in patients with sepsis *4093* Concentration increased in multiple tissue trauma and sepsis associated with further increase *4663*

Complement C_3dg *Serum* *Increase* Highest concentrations observed in patients with sepsis *4093*

Complement, Total Hemolytic *Serum* *Decrease* When sepsis occurred in 6 patients mean concentration reduced to 69% of healthy controls compared with 90% in early postoperative days following uncomplicated gastrointestinal surgery in other patients *754*

Corticotropin *Plasma* *Increase* In 18 patients with sepsis on admission to hospital mean concentration of 130.0 ± 38.2 pmol/L significantly higher than 15.6 ± 5.8 pmol/L in 15 matched hospital control individuals with acute illness *5458*
Plasma *No Effect* Mean concentration of 8.89 ± 5.2 pg/mL 12 patients with sepsis and 7.11 ± 3.7 pg/mL in 14 patients with septic syndrome although still in normal range of 6 - 11 pg/mL *2978*

Cortisol *Plasma* *Increase* In 15 male patients highest concentrations of 1,096 pmol/L were observed in those who failed to recover from septic shock *383* During severe illness plasma cortisol concentrations tend to be higher than in other conditions, e.g. with sepsis concentrations tend to be about 50 µg/dL when patients first hospitalized decreasing to about 38 µg/dL after 8 days *2901* In 18 patients with sepsis on admission to hospital mean concentration of 1.32 ± 0.21 µmol/L significantly higher than 0.37 ± 0.08 µmol/L in 15 matched hospital control individuals with acute illness *5458*
Plasma *No Effect* Mean concentration of 24 ± 8.4 µg/dL 12 patients with sepsis and 28.5 ± 12.3 µg/dL in 14 patients with septic syndrome not significantly different from normal range of 5 - 25 µg/dL *2978*

Creatinine *Serum* *Increase* In 22 patients with sepsis on admission to hospital mean concentration of 113 ± 30 µmol/L significantly higher than in healthy adults *5364* In 16 patients with severe sepsis mean concentration of 1.48 ± 0.48 mg/dL significantly different from that in healthy controls *5343*

11-Dehydro-thromboxane B_2 *Urine* *Increase* In 224 patients with sepsis and acute failure of at least one organ system mean excretion increased by approximately 15% *409*

3,3'-Di-iodothyronine *Serum* *Increase* In 24 patients with sepsis mean concentration of 57.0 ± 36.9 pmol/L not significantly different from that in 24 healthy age and sex-matched controls in whom the mean plasma concentration was 41.6 ± 16.7 pmol/L *4138*

Di-iodotyrosine *Serum* *Increase* In patients with sepsis mean concentration of 1.38 nmol/L (range of 0.32 - 5.14 nmol/L) compared with normal range of 0.02 - 0.55 nmol/L *3443*

2,3-Dinor-6-Keto-Prostaglandin $F_{1\alpha}$ *Urine* *Increase* In 224 patients with sepsis and acute failure of at least one organ system mean excretion increased by approximately 40% *409*

Elastase-α_1-Proteinase Inhibitor *Plasma* *Increase* Median concentration in 45 patients with sepsis of 320 ng/mL significantly different from median of 80 ng/mL in 30 healthy controls *1245*

Elastase-α_1-Proteinase Inhibitor Complex *Serum* *Increase* Concentration increased in trauma and further increased in patients with sepsis *4663*

β-Endorphin *Plasma* *No Effect* Mean concentration of 21.1 ± 11.3 pg/mL 12 patients with sepsis and 23.5 ± 12 pg/mL in 14 patients with septic syndrome although still in normal range of < 30 pg/mL *2978*

Endothelial Cell Protein C Receptor *Plasma* *Increase* In 16 patients with sepsis mean concentration of 224.9 ± 74.5 ng/mL significantly different from 133.4 ± 53.4 ng/mL in 18 controls *2862*

Endothelin-1 *Plasma* *Increase* In the septic group plasma endothelin-like immunoreactivity was five-fold higher (11.3 ± 2.8 pmol/L) compared to that in volunteers (2.4 ± 0.07 pmol/L) (p less than 0.01) *5624* In 18 patients with sepsis on admission to hospital mean concentration of 26.6 ± 10.1 ng/L significantly higher than 4.2 ± 1.2 ng/L in 15 matched hospital control individuals with acute illness *5458* Significant increase to 19.9 ± 2.2 pg/mL in 11 septic patients compared with 6.1 ± 0.3 pg/mL in 14 healthy volunteers and 11.9 ± 0.7 pg/mL in 15 nonseptic postoperative cardiac surgery patients *4149* Mean endothelin-1 plasma concentrations were significantly (p less than 0.001) increased in septic patients (19.9 ± 2.2 pg/mL, mean ± standard error) compared to concentrations found in postoperative cardiac patients (11.9 ± 0.7 pg/mL) or in healthy volunteers (6.1 ± 0.3 pg/mL) *3163*

Endotoxin *Serum* *Increase* At the onset of severe infection in 52 patients with severe sepsis mean concentration of 37 ± 10 pg/mL significantly different from < 5 pg/mL in 40 healthy controls *1906* In 15 patients with sepsis and multiple organ failure mean concentration of 6.5 ± 5.1 pg/mL compared with 5.4 ± 4.0 pg/mL in 15 patients with sepsis but without multiple organ failure *1363* In 5 patients with meningococcal disease and septicemia mean concentration greater than 200 ng/L in contrast to concentration of no greater than 25 ng/L in 6 patients with meningococcemia but without sepsis *561*

Eosinophils *Blood* *Increase* In 41 trauma patients with sepsis mean concentration of 909 ± 780 /µL significantly greater than 314 ± 312 /µL in 59 patients who did not develop sepsis: difference even more marked in patients with severe sepsis *1177*

Erythropoietin *Serum* *Increase* In 16 patients with sepsis or septic shock mean concentration of 120 ± 26 mIU/mL significantly higher than 10 ± 2 mIU/mL in 10 healthy controls *2808*

Estradiol *Plasma* *Increase* In 15 male patients highest levels of 1030 pmol/L were found in those patients who failed to recover from shock *383*

Estrone *Plasma* *Increase* In 15 male patients with septic shock highest concentrations of 4330 pmol/L were found in men who did not recover from shock *383*

Fibrinogen *Plasma* *Increase* Median concentration in 45 patients with sepsis of 4.6 g/L significantly different from median of 3.0 g/L in 30 healthy controls *1245*

Fibrinopeptide A *Plasma* *Increase* In patients with multiple trauma in whom concentration increased sepsis associated with further increase *4663*

Fibronectin *Plasma* *Decrease* In newborn sepsis concentration significantly decreased *3570* In 6 patients with sepsis mean concentration of 47% compared with 70% in early days with uncomplicated gastrointestinal surgery *754* In 47 septic patients mean concentration of 162 ± 88 µg/mL compared with 285 ± 138 µg/mL in 62 nonseptic patients *5691* Significantly reduced concentrations observed in patients with septicemia *980* In both septic infants and older children concentration significantly less than in healthy children of the same age *1204*
Plasma *Increase* In 220 neonates with suspected sepsis plasma fibronectin concentration had a sensitivity of 100 %, specificity of 83%, positive predictive value of 83% and negative predictive value of 100% *1706*

Glutathione Peroxidase *Serum* *Decrease* In 3 newborns with jaundice due to sepsis mean activity of 0.346 ± 0.160 U/mL not significantly different from 0.429 ± 0.084 U/mL in 12 healthy control babies *222*

38.90 Sepsis *(continued)*

Hematocrit *Blood Decrease* In 22 patients with sepsis on admission to hospital mean value of 34.6 ± 2.3% significantly lower than in healthy adults *5364*
Blood No Effect Concentration of 29 ± 0.8% in 15 septic patients not significantly different from 29 ± 1.5% in 9 nonseptic patients *3298*

Hemoglobin *Blood Decrease* In 22 patients with sepsis on admission to hospital mean concentration of 111 ± 6 g/L significantly lower than in healthy adults *5364*

Hep 3B Erythropoietin *Plasma Increase* In 16 patients with sepsis or septic shock mean concentration of 216 ± 23 mIU/mL significantly higher than 152 ± 11 mIU/mL in 10 healthy controls *2808*

Hyaluronic Acid *Serum Increase* Concentration significantly higher in patients without septic shock when compared with controls. In those with septic shock concentration even higher *395*

Immunoglobulin E *Serum Increase* In 41 trauma patients with sepsis mean concentration significantly greater than in 59 patients who did not develop sepsis *1177*

Inhibin *Plasma No Effect* No significant correlation observed *1209*

Interferon-γ *Serum Increase* In 4 patients with sepsis syndrome mean concentration of 4.1 ± 3.1 U/mL significantly different from 0.5 ± 1.2 U/mL in 30 controls *5256*

Interleukin-1 *Serum Increase* In patients with bacterial septicemia in whom high concentrations of lipopolysaccharide were present concentration of IL-1 increased: highest concentrations were associated with fatal outcome *5502* In 37% of 97 patients with sepsis detectable amounts of IL-1 observed (median 20 pg/mL) with no significant difference between those who lived and those who died: mean concentration in Gram-negative bacteremia of 189 ± 70 pg/mL and 438 ± 189 pg/mL in Gram-positive bacteremia *714*

Interleukin-1 Receptor Antagonist *Pleural Fluid No Effect* Mean concentration of 13.1 ± 2.8 ng/mL in pleural fluid of 15 septic patients not significantly different from that in 9 nonseptic critically ill patients *3298*
Serum Increase In 11 newborns with severe infections or sepsis mean concentration of 5,635 ± 411 ng/L significantly higher than 273 ± 88 ng/L in 8 healthy newborns *1049*
Serum No Effect Mean concentration of 22.3 ± 4.2 ng/mL in 15 septic patients not significantly different concentration in serum of 9 critically ill patients without sepsis but different from 13.1 ± 2.8 ng/mL in pleural fluid of 15 septic patients *3298*

Interleukin-1α *Serum Increase* Mean concentration in 10 neonates with sepsis 6.2 ± 3.5 pg/mL significantly higher than 2.1 ± 0.4 pg/mL in healthy newborn controls and 1.25 ± 0.2 pg/mL in healthy adults *3960*
Serum No Effect No significant change observed with endotoxin infusion or in septic shock *4093*

Interleukin-1β *Serum Increase* At the onset of severe infection in 52 patients with severe sepsis mean concentration of 32.1 ± 6.3 pg/mL significantly different from < 10 pg/mL in 40 healthy controls *1906* Mean concentration in 10 neonates with sepsis of 12.7 ± 2.8 pg/mL significantly higher than 6.3 ± 1.1 pg/mL in healthy newborn controls and 5.7 ± 0.45 pg/mL in healthy adults *3960* Increased twofold after endotoxin infusion and 3 - 4 fold increased in septic shock with higher levels observed in survivors *4093* In 11 newborns with severe infections or sepsis mean concentration of 78 ± 27 ng/L significantly higher than 37 ± 7 ng/L in 28 newborns suspected as having sepsis and in controls *1049*
Serum No Effect In 40 critically ill surgical patients including 19 who developed surgical shock IL-1β not detected *1003*

Interleukin-6 *Pleural Fluid No Effect* Mean concentration of 76.0 ± 26.3 ng/L in pleural fluid of 15 septic patients not significantly different from that in 9 nonseptic critically ill patients *3298*
Serum Increase In 40 critically ill surgical patients concentration increased to 500,000 pg/mL and concentration correlated well with APACHE II score and mortality increased significantly in patients with concentrations above 1,000 pg/mL *1003* In patients with bacterial septicemia and high concentrations of lipopolysaccharide concentration increased: fatal outcome associated with highest concentrations *5502* In 18 patients with clinically defined sepsis concentration increased on first day after admission *5459* Mean concentration in 10 neonates with sepsis of 361 ± 152 pg/mL significantly higher than 11.6 ± 2.5 pg/mL in healthy newborn controls and 3.4 ± 0.2 pg/mL in healthy adults *3960* In 80% of 97 patients with sepsis detectable amounts of IL-6 observed (median concentration of 415 pg/mL) with concentration significantly higher in those who died than in those who lived: mean concentration in Gram-negative bacteremia 780 ± 234 pg/mL and 1,029 ± 178 pg/mL in Gram-positive bacteremia *714* In 15 newborns with confirmed sepsis mean concentration of about 80,000 pg/mL significantly higher than about 80 pg/mL in 22 healthy control neonates *1050* At the onset of severe infection in 52 patients with severe sepsis mean concentration of 662 ± 127 pg/mL significantly different from < 3 pg/mL in 40 healthy controls *1906* In 16 patients with sepsis or septic shock mean concentration of 12,405 ± 6,662 pg/mL significantly higher than 7 ± 1 pg/mL in 10 healthy controls *2808*
Serum No Effect Mean concentration of 18.5 ± 16.2 ng/L in 15 septic patients not significantly different from concentration in serum of 9 critically ill patients without sepsis but much less than 76.0 ± 26.3 ng/L in pleural fluid of 15 septic patients *3298*

Interleukin-8 *Pleural Fluid No Effect* Mean concentration of 1.5 ± 0.9 ng/mL in pleural fluid of 15 septic patients not significantly different from that in 9 nonspetic critically ill patients *3298*
Pulmonary Edema Fluid Increase In 11 patients with acute respiratory distress syndrome with sepsis mean concentration of 84.2 ng/mL significantly different from 6.7 ng/mL in 11 patients with hydrostatic pulmonary edema *3490*
Serum Increase In 11 patients with acute respiratory distress syndrome with sepsis mean concentration of 6.1 ± 10.9 ng/mL significantly different from 2.0 ± 3.8 ng/mL in 11 patients with hydrostatic pulmonary edema *3490* In 40 patients with sepsis mean concentration of 0.35 ± 0.35 ng/mL higher than less than 0.01 ng/mL in 20 normal volunteers *1362* Levels on admission were elevated in 42 of the 47 patients (89%) *1949*
Serum No Effect Mean concentration of 4.5 ± 2.5 ng/L in 15 septic patients not significantly different concentration in serum of 9 critically ill patients without sepsis but different from 1.5 ± 0.9 ng/L in pleural fluid of 15 septic patients *3298*

Interleukin-10 *Serum Increase* In 39 of 69 patients with Gram-negative (25) or Gram-positive (44) septicemia plasma interleukin-10 increased (range 12 - 2,740 pg/mL) compared with undetectable amounts of interleukin-10 in 29 of 33 control patients without infection and in 20 healthy volunteers *3287*

Kallistatin *Plasma Decrease* Mean concentration in 10 patients with septic syndrome of 7.7 ± 3.5 μg/mL significantly less compared with 21.2 ± 3.5 μg/mL in 30 healthy controls *781*

6-Keto-Prostaglandin $F_{1\alpha}$ *Plasma Increase* Concentration in mixed venous and arterial blood significantly increased in patients with active sepsis *5429*

Lactate *Blood Increase* In 224 patients with sepsis and acute failure of at least one organ system mean concentration of 3.0 ± 3.0 mmol/L *409*

Lactoferrin *Plasma Increase* In 23 patients with sepsis mean concentration of 1,523 ± 293 ng/mL significantly different from mean of 557 ± 181 ng/mL in 9 normal controls *2606*

Leukocytes *Blood Increase* In 22 patients with sepsis on admission to hospital mean concentration of 18.6 ± 2.2 10^9/L significantly higher than in healthy adults *5364* In 9 patients with sepsis mean concentration of 19.7 ± 9.4 x 10^3/μL *3868* Concentration of 16,886 ± 1,957 x 10^3/μL in 15 septic patients not significantly different from 12,538 ± 1,412 x 10^3/μL in 9 nonseptic patients *3298*

Lipopolysaccharides *Serum Increase* Increased concentration observed in patients with septicemia *5502* In 89% of 97 patients with sepsis detectable amounts of lipopolysaccharide observed (median 2.6 EU/mL) with no significant difference between those who lived and those who died: mean concentration of 3.6 ± 0.7 EU/mL in Gram-negative bacteremia and 1,029 ± 178 EU/mL in Gram-positive bacteremia *714*

Lymphocytes *Blood Decrease* In 1,042 hospitalized patients with lymphocytopenia 250 had bacterial or fungal sepsis *730*
Blood No Effect Concentration of 7 ± 1% in 15 septic patients not significantly different from 7 ± 1% in 9 nonseptic patients *3298*
Pleural Fluid Decrease Concentration of 22 ± 5% in 15 septic patients not significantly different from 39 ± 9% in 9 nonseptic patients *3298*

Lyso-Platelet Activating Factor *Plasma Decrease* Mean concentration in 13 male patients with clinical sepsis mean concentration of 18 ± 6 ng/mL significantly different less than concentration in 10 normal males *1838*

Macrophage Colony Stimulating Factor *Serum* *No Effect* In 50 patients with sepsis syndrome and thrombocytopenia mean concencentration of 539 ± 141 IU/mL significantly different from 208 ± 82 IU/mL in 59 healthy individuals *1551*

Methemoglobin *Blood* *Increase* In 9 patients with sepsis mean concentration of 1.0% higher than 0.6 - 0.7% in patients without infections *3868*

Myeloperoxidase *Serum* *Increase* In 23 patients with sepsis mean concentration of 169 ± 66.6 ng/mL significantly different from mean of 49.0 ± 15.1 ng/mL in 9 normal controls *2606*

Neopterin *Serum* *Increase* Very high concentrations may be observed that correlate with the severity of the sepsis *121*

Neuropeptide Y *Plasma* *Increase* In 22 patients with sepsis at onset of hypotension mean concentration of 17 ± 4 pmol/L significantly higher than 9 ± 2 pmol/L in healthy adults *5364*

Neutrophil Elastase *Plasma* *Increase* In 40 patients with sepsis mean concentration of 345.5 ± 120.1 ng/mL significantly higher than 72.3 ± 35.3 ng/mL in 20 normal volunteers *1362*

Neutrophils *Blood* *No Effect* Concentration of 85 ± 2% in 15 septic patients not significantly different from 81 ± 3% in 9 nonseptic patients *3298*
Pleural Fluid *Increase* Concentration of 67 ± 7% in 15 septic patients significantly different from 20 ± 6% in 9 nonseptic patients *3298*

Nitrate *Serum* *Increase* In patients with sepsis, systolic blood pressure below 90 mm Hg and neutrophilia mean concentration of 152 ± 51.5 µmol/L significantly different from 33.1 ± 1.6 µmol/L in healthy controls *3754*
Serum *No Effect* In patients with sepsis and neutropenia mean concentration of 43.9 ± 5 µmol/L not significantly different from 33.1 ± 1.6 µmol/L in healthy controls *3754*

Nitrate plus Nitrite *Serum* *Increase* In 4 patients with sepsis syndrome mean concentration of 44.4 ± 4.2 µmol/L significantly different from 28.5 ± 5.4 µmol/L in 30 controls *5256*

Nitrogen Balance *Patient* *Negative* Negative balance occurs with augmented protein catabolism *1959*

Phosphate *Serum* *Decrease* Hypophosphatemia occured in 60 of 134 patients with clinical risk of hypophosphatemia. Sepsis identified as risk factor *5847*

Phospholipase A_2 *Serum* *Increase* Increased concentrations reported *46* Increased catalytic activity observed in sepsis, Gram-negative infections and septic shock *3766*

Phospholipase A_2 Type I *Serum* *Increase* Concentration reported as high as 479 µg/L in sepsis compared with 2 and 4 µg/L in healthy controls *3767*

Plasminogen *Plasma* *Decrease* Median concentration in 45 patients with sepsis of 0.62 IU/mL significantly different from median of 0.98 IU/mL in 30 healthy controls *1245*

Plasminogen Activator Inhibitor-1 Antigen
Plasma *Increase* Median concentration in 45 patients with sepsis of 65 ng/mL significantly different from median of 15 ng/mL in 30 healthy controls *1245*

Plasminogen Activator Inhibitor Activity *Plasma* *Increase* Median concentration in 45 patients with sepsis of 20 IU/mL significantly different from median of 4 IU/mL in 30 healthy controls *1245*

Plasminogen:α_2-Antiplasmin Ratio *Plasma* *Decrease* Median ratio in 45 patients with sepsis of 0.6 significantly different from median of 1.0 in 30 healthy controls *1245*

Platelet Activating Factor *Serum* *No Effect* In 13 male patients with clinical sepsis mean concentration of 0.22 ± 0.04 ng/mL not significantly different from 0.25 ± 0.05 ng/mL in 10 normal males *1838*

Platelet Volume *Blood* *Increase* In 18 infants in whom coagulase-negative staphylococci sepsis developed significant increase in mean platelet volume to 9.5 ± 1.51 fL from preinfection value of 8.2 ± 0.97 fL and to 8.8 ± 1.02 fL after infection *3856*

Platelets *Blood* *Decrease* In 50 patients with sepsis syndrome and thrombocytopenia mean concencentration of 66 ± 25 x 10^9/L significantly different from that in 59 healthy individuals *1551*
Blood *Increase* Concentration of 189 ± 33 x 10^6/µL in 15 septic patients not significantly different from 168 ± 37 x 10^6/µL in 9 nonseptic patients *3298* In 18 infants in whom coagulase-negative staphylococci sepsis developed mean concentration increased from 246,000 ± 74,000 /µL preinfection to 295,000 ± 191,000 /µL during infection and 472,000 ± 192,000 /µL after infection *3856*

Prekallikrein *Plasma* *Decrease* Average lowest concentration in 64 patients with sepsis of 34 ± 17% compared with 69 ± 21% in 68 patients without sepsis *5691*

Procalcitonin *Plasma* *Increase* Significant increase observed in blood of all patients with sepsis with increase appearing at the same time as that of tumor necrosis factor-α: increase of procalcitonin from normal of less than 0.1 ng/mL to 5 - 500 ng/mL *201*

Protein *Pleural Fluid* *No Effect* Ratio of pleural fluid to serum concentration of 0.50 ± 0.02 in 15 septic patients not significantly different from 0.59 ± 0.02 in 9 nonseptic patients *3298*
Pulmonary Edema Fluid *Decrease* In 11 patients with acute respiratory distress syndrome with sepsis mean concentration of 4.2 ± 1.1 g/dL less than 4.6 ± 1.2 g/dL in 11 patients with ARDS without sepsis *3490*
Serum *No Effect* In 11 patients acute respiratory distress syndrome with sepsis mean concentration of 5.0 ± 0.8 g/dL not different from 5.0 ± 1.1 g/dL in 11 patients with ARDS without sepsis but low compared with healthy individuals *3490* Concentration of 47 ± 2 g/L in 15 septic patients not significantly different from 50 ± 5 g/L in 9 nonseptic patients *3298*

Protein C *Plasma* *Decrease* Median concentration in 45 patients with sepsis of 0.49 IU/mL significantly different from median of 1.00 IU/mL in 30 healthy controls *1245*

Protein S *Plasma* *Decrease* Median concentration in 45 patients with sepsis of 0.81 IU/mL significantly different from median of 1.00 IU/mL in 30 healthy controls *1245*

Retinol *Urine* *Increase* In 11 patients with pneumonia mean excretion of 1.10 µmol/d compared with less than 0.01 µmol/d in 8 healthy controls *5007*

Secretory Non-pancreatic Phospholipase A_2
Serum *Increase* At the onset of severe infection in 52 patients with severe sepsis mean concentration of 77.9 ± 17.2 nmol/min/mL significantly different from 3.5 ± 2 nmol/min/mL in 40 healthy controls *1906*

Selenium *Serum* *No Effect* In 3 newborns with jaundice due to sepsis mean concentration of 32.2 ± 1.6 ng/mL not significantly different from 40.3 ± 8.2 ng/mL in 12 healthy control babies *222*

Soluble E-Selectin *Serum* *Increase* In 15 patients with sepsis and multiple organ failure mean concentration of 345 ± 103 ng/mL compared with 266 ± 111 ng/mL in 15 patients with sepsis but without multiple organ failure *1363* In 23 patients with sepsis mean concentration of 231 ± 41.8 ng/mL significantly different from mean of 40.5 ± 4.5 ng/mL in 9 normal controls *2606*

Soluble Intercellular Adhesion Molecule-1 *Serum* *Increase* In 23 patients with sepsis mean concentration of 868 ± 131 ng/mL significantly different from mean of 208 ± 20.5 ng/mL in 9 normal controls *2606* In 2 patients with sepsis mean concentration of 920 ng/mL significantly higher than mean concentration of 270 ± 47 ng/mL in 10 healthy controls: no significant differences between concentrations in patients with active and inactive vasculitis *2461* In 15 patients with sepsis and multiple organ failure mean concentration of 1,103 ± 342 ng/mL compared with 863 ± 321 ng/mL in 15 patients with sepsis but without multiple organ failure *1363*

Soluble Interleukin-6 Receptor *Pleural Fluid* *No Effect* Mean concentration of 19.2 ± 3.9 ng/mL in pleural fluid of 15 septic patients not significantly different from that in 9 nonseptic critically ill patients *3298*
Serum *No Effect* Mean concentration of 86.3 ± 13.3 ng/mL in 15 septic patients not significantly different from the concentration in serum of 9 critically ill patients without sepsis but different from 19.2 ± 3.9 ng/mL in pleural fluid of 15 septic patients *3298*

Soluble Tumor Necrosis Factor Receptor-I
Pleural Fluid *No Effect* Mean concentration of 26.7 ± 1.7 ng/mL in pleural fluid of 15 septic patients not significantly different from that in 9 nonseptic critically ill patients *3298*
Serum *No Effect* Mean concentration of 13.3 ± 2.5 ng/mL in 15 septic patients not significantly different from concentration in serum of 9 critically ill patients without sepsis but different from 26.7 ± 1.7 ng/mL in pleural fluid of 15 septic patients *3298*

38.90 Sepsis *(continued)*

Soluble Tumor Necrosis Factor Receptor-II
Pleural Fluid *No Effect* Mean concentration of 38.8 ± 4.2 ng/mL in pleural fluid of 15 septic patients not significantly different from that in 9 nonseptic critically ill patients *3298*
Serum *No Effect* Mean concentration of 26.6 ± 5.9 ng/mL in 15 septic patients not significantly different concentration in serum of 9 critically ill patients without sepsis but different from 38.8 ± 4.2 ng/mL in pleural fluid of 15 septic patients *3298*

Soluble Vascular Cell Adhesion Molecule-1
Serum *Increase* In 15 patients with sepsis and multiple organ failure mean concentration of 2,655 ± 1,784 ng/mL compared with 2,045 ± 1,297 ng/mL in 15 patients with sepsis but without multiple organ failure *1363*

Substance P *Plasma* *Decrease* In 22 patients with sepsis at onset of hypotension mean concentration of 45 ± 5 pmol/L significantly lower than 117 ± 7 pmol/L in healthy adults *5364*

Superoxide Dismutase *Red Blood Cells* *Increase* In 32 patients with sepsis mean activity of 19.5 ± 4.6 kU/g hemoglobin significantly increased compared with 14.8 ± 14 kU/g hemoglobin in 7 healthy controls *5576*
Serum *Increase* In 32 patients with sepsis mean activity of 5.5 ± 5.8 kU/L significantly increased compared with 1.0 ± 2.5 kU/L in 7 healthy controls *5576*

Testosterone *Serum* *Decrease* Concentrations depressed and inversely correlated with sepsis (r = -0.33) *1209*

Thrombin/Antithrombin III Complex *Plasma* *Increase* Median concentration in 45 patients with sepsis of 7.0 µg/mL significantly different from median of 1.5 µg/mL in 30 healthy controls *1245*

Thrombomodulin *Plasma* *No Effect* In 16 patients with sepsis mean concentration of 10.6 ± 6.1 ng/mL not significantly different from 10.7 ± 11.0 ng/mL in 18 controls *2862*

Thromboxane B_2 *Plasma* *Increase* Concentration significantly increased in arterial and mixed venous plasma in patients with active sepsis *5429* At the onset of severe infection in 52 patients with severe sepsis mean concentration of 740 ± 280 pg/mL significantly different from < 40 pg/mL in 40 healthy controls *1906*

Tissue Factor Antigen *Plasma* *Increase* In 2 patients with sepsis mean concentration of 288 ± 87 pg/mL significantly greater than 126 ± 41 pg/mL in 12 healthy volunteers *5511*

Tissue Factor Pathway Inhibitor *Plasma* *Increase* High concentrations observed with fulmitant DIC complicating sepsis *2376*

Tissue Plasminogen Activator *Plasma* *Increase* Median concentration in 45 patients with sepsis of 11 ng/mL significantly different from median of 2 ng/mL in 30 healthy controls *1245*

Triglycerides *Serum* *Increase* In 41 of 239 patients with septicemia or endocarditis triglyceride concentration exceeded 2.2 mmol/L (mean 3.1 mmol/L): increased triglyceride concentration was more common in infections with gram-negative rods than with gram-positive cocci *2504*

Troponin T *Serum* *Increase* Increased concentration above 0.2 µg/L observed in 18 of 26 patients with sepsis *4959*

Tumor Necrosis Factor *Serum* *Increase* In patients with bacterial septicemia in whom high concentrations of lipopolysaccharide were present had increased concentrations of TNF: highest concentrations associated with fatal outcome *5502*

Tumor Necrosis Factor-α *Serum* *Increase* Concentration increased after endotoxin administration and in septic shock where concentration correlates with severity of illness *4093* In 54% of 97 patients with sepsis median concentration of 26 pg/mL with no difference in concentration between those who died and those who lived: mean concentration with Gram-negative bacteremia 120 ± 81 pg/mL and 83 ± 12 pg/mL in those with Gram-positive bacteremia *714* In 40 critically ill surgical patients concentration increased to some extent but not to above 100 pg/mL except in patients who developed septic shock in whom concentration was higher *1003* In 15 newborns with confirmed sepsis mean concentration of about 650 pg/mL significantly higher than about 50 pg/mL in 22 healthy control neonates *1050* Mean concentration in 10 neonates with sepsis of 292 ± 65 pg/mL significantly higher than 11.4 ± 2.4 pg/mL in healthy newborn controls and 8.8 ± 3.2 pg/mL in healthy adults *3960* Significant increase observed with the onset of sepsis *201* Mean concentration increased to 73.2 pg/mL in 24 patients with sepsis compared with 8.5 pg/mL in nonseptic patients. Maximum concentration in sepsis of 156.9 pg/mL compared with 20.2 pg/mL in controls. Mortality increased with highest serum TNF-α concentrations *1990* At the onset of severe infection in 52 patients with severe sepsis mean concentration of 107 ± 18.7 pg/mL significantly different from < 8 pg/mL in 40 healthy controls *1906* Mean concentration of 154 pg/mL observed in 24 preterm and 25 full-term newborns with sepsis significantly different from 61.5 pg/mL in 20 preterm and 20 full-term healthy control neonates *209*

Urea *Serum* *Increase* In 22 patients with septic shock on admission to hospital mean concentration of 10.4 ± 3.1 µmol/L significantly higher than in healthy adults *5364*

Vasoactive Intestinal Polypeptide *Plasma* *Increase* In patients with sepsis and meningococcal disease mean concentration above 4 pmol/L compared with concentrations of less than 2.5 pmol/L in 6 patients with meningococcemia but without sepsis *561*

von Willebrand Factor Antigen *Plasma* *Increase* In 23 patients with sepsis mean concentration of 632 ± 57.5% significantly different from mean of 115 ± 26.7% in 9 normal controls *2606*

39.00 Actinomycosis

Alanine Aminotransferase *Serum* *Increase* Liver involvement *2192*

Alkaline Phosphatase *Serum* *Increase* May be elevated in cases with osteomyelitis *900*

Erythrocyte Sedimentation Rate *Blood* *Increase* Almost always elevated *900*

γ-Glutamyltransferase *Serum* *Increase* Liver involvement *2192*

Hematocrit *Blood* *Decrease* A mild to moderate normocytic, normochromic anemia frequently accompanies this disease *900*

Hemoglobin *Blood* *Decrease* A mild to moderate normocytic, normochromic anemia frequently accompanies this disease *900*

Lactate Dehydrogenase *Serum* *Increase* Liver involvement *2192*

Leukocytes *Blood* *Increase* In uncomplicated disease the peripheral WBC usually ranges between 8,000 - 14,000 /µL. Counts over 15,000 /µL are unusual except in cases with secondary superinfection *900* May occur when destructive tissue lesions are present *1980*

Oxygen Partial Pressure *Blood* *Decrease* Pulmonary involvement *2192*

Urea Nitrogen *Serum* *Increase* Kidney involvement *2192*

40.20 Whipple's Disease

Albumin *Serum* *Decrease* In patients with severe diarrhea and malabsorption *4891* Excessive loss into GI tract and decreased production *2034* A low serum albumin will reflect possible malabsorption of protein or protein-losing enteropathy *1980*

Alkaline Phosphatase *Serum* *Decrease* An indication of vitamin D and calcium malabsorption *1980*
Serum *Increase* An indication of vitamin K malabsorption *1980*

Calcium *Serum* *Decrease* An indication of vitamin D and calcium malabsorption *1980* In patients with severe diarrhea and malabsorption *4891*

Carotene *Serum* *Decrease* Common *4891* A useful indication of fat malabsorption low levels are found in as many 80% of patients with steatorrhea *1980*

Cholesterol *Serum* *Decrease* Common *4891*

Fat *Feces* *Increase* In small intestinal disease *4891*

Folate *Serum* *Decrease* In some cases *4891*

Glucose Tolerance *Serum* *Increase* Flat peak. Poor absorption from the GI tract (normal IV GTT curve) *5544*

Hematocrit *Blood* *Decrease* Anemia is common and is usually associated with iron deficiency *4891*

Hemoglobin *Blood* *Decrease* Anemia is common and is usually associated with iron deficiency *4891*

17-Hydroxycorticosteroids *Urine* *Decrease* Reduced 24 h excretion of 17-hydroxycorticosteroids and 17-ketosteroids has been found in debilitated patients *4891*

5-Hydroxyindoleacetic Acid *Urine* *Increase* Modest increases observed in patients with Whipple's disease *2952*

Iron *Serum* *Decrease* Microcytic, hypochromic red cells and a low serum iron accompany the anemia *4891*

Iron-binding Capacity, Total *Serum* *Increase* Iron deficiency anemia is common *4891*

Iron Saturation *Serum* *Decrease* Iron deficiency anemia is common *4891*

17-Ketogenic Steroids *Urine* *Decrease* Reduced 24 h excretion of 17-hydroxycorticosteroids and 17-ketosteroids has been found in debilitated patients *4891*

17-Ketosteroids *Urine* *Decrease* Reduced 24 h excretion of 17-hydroxycorticosteroids and 17-ketosteroids has been found in debilitated patients *4891*

Leukocytes *Blood* *Increase* Mild to moderate leukocytosis may be present, especially in febrile patients *4891* Seen in the period of clinical activity *2039*

Lymphocytes *Blood* *Decrease* An absolute lymphopenia due to loss of lymphocytes into the small intestine *1980*

Magnesium *Serum* *Decrease* In patients with severe diarrhea and malabsorption *4891*

MCH *Blood* *Decrease* Anemia is common and is usually associated with iron deficiency *4891*

MCHC *Blood* *Decrease* Anemia is common and is usually associated with iron deficiency *4891*

MCV *Blood* *Decrease* Microcytic, hypochromic red cells and a low serum iron accompany the anemia *4891*
Blood *Increase* In some patients there is macrocytosis caused by folate deficiency *4891*

Occult Blood *Feces* *Increase* 30% of patients have this finding *2039*

Oligoclonal Banding *Cerebrospinal Fluid* *Increase* Oligoclonal IgG bands detected with CNS Whipple's disease *3261*

Phosphate *Serum* *Decrease* An indication of vitamin D and calcium malabsorption *1980*

Potassium *Serum* *Decrease* In patients with severe diarrhea and malabsorption *4891*

Protein *Serum* *Decrease* Enteric loss of plasma protein *4891*

Triolein ^{131}I Test *Feces* *Positive* Positive test for lipid droplets in the stool, but results are inconsistent *1980*

Xylose Tolerance Test *Urine* *Abnormal* Abnormal absorption observed *2039*

40.89 Toxic Shock

Calcitonin *Plasma* *Increase* In two patients with toxic shock syndrome inappropriately high concentrations of calcitonin observed (in one case as high as 179,000 pg/mL) *4958*

Calcium *Serum* *Decrease* Hypocalcemia frequently observed as a complication but mechanism not understood *4958*

41.84 Clostridium difficile Infection

Antithrombin *Plasma* *Decrease* In patients with clostridium difficile-associated diarrhea and colitis mean concentration of 0.70 ± 0.21 compared with 0.90 ± 0.17 in healthy controls *186*

Protein C *Plasma* *Decrease* In patients with clostridium difficile-associated diarrhea and colitis mean concentration of 0.70 ± 0.30 compared with 1.28 ± 0.23 in controls *186*

Protein S, Free *Plasma* *Decrease* In patients with clostridium difficile-associated diarrhea and colitis mean concentration of 0.27 ± 0.06 compared with 0.37 ± 0.08 in healthy controls *186*

41.90 Bacterial Infection

Alanine Aminotransferase *Peritoneal Fluid* *Increase* Mean activity of 52 U/L in fluid from 8 patients with bacterial infection significantly different from 83 U/L in fluids from 36 patients without infection *4852*
Peritoneal Fluid *No Effect* Mean activity of 74.8 U/L in fluid from 8 patients with bacterial infection not significantly different from 40.0 U/L in fluids from 32 patients without infection *4852*

Albumin *Peritoneal Fluid* *No Effect* Mean concentration of 19.3 g/L in fluid from 10 patients with bacterial infection not significantly different from 21.2 g/L in fluids from 31 patients without infection *4852*

Alkaline Phosphatase *Peritoneal Fluid* *No Effect* Mean activity of 92 U/L in fluid from 7 patients with bacterial infection not significantly different from 112 U/L in fluids from 34 patients without infection *4852*

Amylase *Peritoneal Fluid* *No Effect* Mean activity of 608 U/L in fluid from 11 patients with bacterial infection not significantly different from 304 U/L in fluids from 37 patients without infection *4852*

Amyloid A *Serum* *Increase* Median concentration in patients with bacterial infection of 15 mg/dL significantly higher than approximately 5.75 mg/dL in transplant patients in stable phase *3653*

Bilirubin *Peritoneal Fluid* *Decrease* Mean concentration of 59 µmol/L in fluid from 10 patients with bacterial infection not significantly different from 305 µmol/L in fluids from 38 patients without infection *4852*

Calcium *Peritoneal Fluid* *No Effect* Mean concentration of 3.14 mmol/L in fluid from 11 patients with bacterial infection not significantly different from 1.78 mmol/L in fluids from 57 patients without infection *4852*

Chloride *Peritoneal Fluid* *No Effect* Mean concentration of 71.7 mmol/L in fluid from 3 patients with bacterial infection not significantly different from 95.3 mmol/L in fluids from 6 patients without infection *4852*

Cholesterol *Peritoneal Fluid* *No Effect* Mean concentration of 1.77 mmol/L in fluid from 12 patients with bacterial infection not significantly different from 1.71 mmol/L in fluids from 33 patients without infection *4852*

C-Reactive Protein *Serum* *Increase* In 64 children with bacterial respiratory infection mean concentration on admission to hospital of 54 mg/L significantly different from normal *2773* In 23 patients with acute bacterial infection mean serum concentration of 155.0 ± 123.4 mg/L *5757* In 40 patients with bacterial infection mean concentration of 154 ± 122 mg/L significantly greater than normal concentration of less than 10 mg/L *4038*
Urine *Increase* In 21 patients with nonrenal bacterial infection mean concentration of 47 µg/L significantly different from < 6 µg/L in 34 renal transplant patients with normal courses *4994*

Creatine Kinase *Peritoneal Fluid* *Decrease* Mean activity of 200 U/L in fluid from 11 patients with bacterial infection significantly different from 1,043 U/L in fluids from 37 patients without infection *4852*

Creatine Kinase MB-Isoenzyme *Peritoneal Fluid* *No Effect* Mean activity of 52.1 U/L in fluid from 11 patients with bacterial infection not significantly different from 56.2 U/L in fluids from 36 patients without infection *4852*

Creatinine *Peritoneal Fluid* *Decrease* Mean concentration of 94 µmol/L in fluid from 12 patients with bacterial infection significantly different from 132 µmol/L in fluids from 37 patients without infection *4852*

γ-Glutamyltransferase *Peritoneal Fluid* *Decrease* Mean activity of 16 U/L in fluid from 8 patients with bacterial infection significantly different from 57 U/L in fluids from 32 patients without infection *4852*

Granulocyte Colony Stimulating Factor *Serum* *Increase* In 34 patients with bacterial infection mean concentration of 799 ± 1501 ng/L significantly greater than normal concentration of less than 39 ng/L *4038*

Interleukin-6 *Serum* *Increase* In 40 patients with bacterial infection mean concentration of 639 ± 907 ng/L significantly greater than normal concentration of less than 20 ng/L *4038*

Lactate *Peritoneal Fluid* *Increase* Mean concentration of 17.2 mmol/L in fluid from 11 patients with bacterial infection significantly different from 7.93 mmol/L in fluids from 36 patients without infection *4852*

41.90 Bacterial Infection *(continued)*

Lactate Dehydrogenase *Peritoneal Fluid* *Increase* Mean activity of 7,998 U/L in fluid from 8 patients with bacterial infection significantly different from 2,021 U/L in fluids from 32 patients without infection *4852*

Lactoferrin *Plasma* *Increase* In 23 patients with bacterial infection mean concentration of 215 ± 135 µg/L significantly greater than normal concentration of 40 - 215 µg/L *4038*

Leukocytes *Blood* *Increase* In 39 patients with bacterial infection mean count of 14,400 ± 6,100 /µL significantly greater than normal count of 4,000 - 9,000 /µL *4038*

α_2-Macroglobulin *Urine* *No Effect* In 21 patients with nonrenal bacterial infection mean concentration of < 180 µg/L significantly different from < 180 µg/L in 34 renal transplant patients with normal courses *4994*

Magnesium *Peritoneal Fluid* *Increase* Mean concentration of 1.39 mmol/L in fluid from 3 patients with bacterial infection significantly different from 0.69 mmol/L in fluids from 27 patients without infection *4852*

Monocytes *Blood* *No Effect* In 37 patients with bacterial infection mean count of 2,200 ± 1,500 /µL not different from normal count of 2,000 - 3,000 /µL *4038*

Myeloperoxidase *Serum* *Increase* In 40 patients with bacterial infection mean concentration of 2,075 ± 1,145 µg/L significantly greater than normal concentration of 107 - 678 µmg/L *4038*
Urine *No Effect* In 21 patients with nonrenal bacterial infection mean concentration of < 200 µg/L not significantly different from < 200 µg/L in 34 renal transplant patients with normal courses *4994*

Neopterin *Serum* *Increase* Median concentration in patients with bacterial infection of approximately 88 nmol/L significantly different from approximately 12 nmol/L in transplant patients in stable phase *3653*

Neutrophil Lipocalcin *Serum* *Increase* In 23 patients with acute bacterial infection mean serum concentration of 404.14 ± 355.02 µg/L and 145.46 ± 194.32 µg/L in plasma *5757*

Neutrophils *Blood* *Increase* In 37 patients with bacterial infection mean count of 12,400 ± 5,700 /µL significantly greater than normal count of 2,000 - 6,000 /µL *4038*

Phosphate *Peritoneal Fluid* *Increase* Mean concentration of 3.71 mmol/L in fluid from 11 patients with bacterial infection significantly different from 1.08 mmol/L in fluids from 36 patients without infection *4852*

Phospholipase A_2 Type I *Serum* *Increase* Concentration reported as high as 211 µg/L in blood-culture negative bacterial infection compared with 2 and 4 µg/L in healthy controls *3767*

Potassium *Peritoneal Fluid* *Increase* Mean concentration of 10.1 mmol/L in fluid from 11 patients with bacterial infection significantly different from 4.47 mmol/L in fluids from 56 patients without infection *4852*

Procalcitonin *Plasma* *Increase* In 10 newborn children and 9 older children with bacterial infections concentrations ranged from 6 - 53 ng/mL compared with concentrations of < 0.1 ng/mL in 21 children without infection *203*

Protein *Peritoneal Fluid* *Decrease* Mean concentration of 0.82 mmol/L in fluid from 10 patients with bacterial infection significantly different from 5.37 mmol/L in fluids from 39 patients without infection *4852*
Peritoneal Fluid *No Effect* Mean concentration of 43.2 g/L in fluid from 13 patients with bacterial infection not significantly different from 32.3 g/L in fluids from 38 patients without infection *4852*

Sodium *Peritoneal Fluid* *No Effect* Mean concentration of 127.7 mmol/L in fluid from 12 patients with bacterial infection not significantly different from 138.0 mmol/L in fluids from 56 patients without infection *4852*

Soluble CD30 *Serum* *No Effect* Concentrations of 6.9 ± 0.9 U/mL observed in 23 patients not significantly different from 8.8 ± 0.9 U/mL in 21 healthy control individuals *5561*

Triglycerides *Peritoneal Fluid* *No Effect* Mean concentration of 0.66 mmol/L in fluid from 12 patients with bacterial infection not significantly different from 0.69 mmol/L in fluids from 33 patients without infection *4852*

Urea *Peritoneal Fluid* *No Effect* Mean concentration of 9.4 mmol/L in fluid from 10 patients with bacterial infection not significantly different from 5.6 mmol/L in fluids from 38 patients without infection *4852*

Uric Acid *Peritoneal Fluid* *No Effect* Mean concentration of 279 µmol/L in fluid from 12 patients with bacterial infection not significantly different from 252 µmol/L in fluids from 33 patients without infection *4852*

42.00 Acquired Immune Deficiency Syndrome

Adenosine Deaminase *Serum* *Increase* Secondary to inflammatory response *2267* In 60 individuals with stage II disease mean activity of 41.3 ± 22.5 U/L, in 30 with stage III disease of 41.4 ± 32.8 U/L and of 61.6 ± 33.8 U/L in stage IV disease significantly higher than 13.9 ± 6.6 U/L in 30 healthy controls *3322* Secondary to inflammatory response *2267*

Alanine Aminotransferase *Serum* *Increase* Significant increase in enzyme activity related to hepatic function. About 90% of AIDS patients have antibodies to hepatitis B antigen and hepatitis B core antibody. Also significantly higher prevalence of antibodies to cytomegalovirus, herpes simplex virus, hepatitis A and EB virus *2267*

Albumin *BAL Fluid* *No Effect* No significant difference observed between concentrations in 32 healthy controls (7.69 ± 2.15 mg/dL) and in 53 patients with AIDS (7.93 ± 5.10 mg/dL) *3270*
Serum *Decrease* Observed effect *5546*
Serum *No Effect* In 44 patients with AIDS mean concentration of 38 g/L and in 40 with asymptomatic HIV infection of 43 g/L within normal range of 35 - 50 g/L although concentration in AIDS patients significantly less than in those with asymptomatic infection *4969*

Alkaline Phosphatase *Serum* *Increase* Marked increase suggests bile duct obstruction or hepatic infiltration. Marked increase observed in 17% of consecutive AIDS patients. Most common cause of increase is hepatic granulomata *268* In 44 patients with AIDS mean activity of 137 U/L slightly above upper limit of normal of 135 U/L with activity in AIDS patients significantly greater than 109 U/L in those with asymptomatic HIV infection *4969*

Amylase *Serum* *Increase* In 39 patients with AIDS 54% had hyperamylasemia (2/3 pancreatic and 1/3 salivary) and 31% pancreatitis *5716* Hyperamylasemia is common in AIDS, often of salivary origin *268*

Antibody Titer *Serum* *Increase* Using the enzyme-linked immunosorbent assay (ELISA) for HTLV-III antibodies, 82% of 88 patients with AIDS were positive, 16% borderline and 2% negative. Only 1% of 297 volunteer controls were positive, 6% borderline and 93% negative for a specificity of 98.6% and sensitivity of 97.3% *5623*

Apolipoprotein A-I *Serum* *Decrease* Observed effect *1891*

Apolipoprotein B-1000 *Serum* *Decrease* Observed effect *1891*

Apolipoproteins *Serum* *Decrease* Decreased apolipoprotein AI and B-1000 *1891*

Aspartate Aminotransferase *Serum* *Increase* Significant increase in enzyme activity related to hepatic function. About 90% of AIDS patients have antibodies to hepatitis B antigen and hepatitis B core antibody. Also significantly higher prevalence of antibodies to cytomegalovirus, herpes simplex virus, hepatitis A and EB virus *2267*

Calcium *Serum* *Decrease* In 6 patients with AIDS mean concentration of 1.22 ± 0.02 mmol/L significantly different from 1.26 ± 0.01 mmol/L in 10 normal individuals *2397*

Carnitine *Serum* *Decrease* Reduced total carnitine concentration observed in 21 of 29 AIDS patients (72%) *1076*

Carnitine, Free *Serum* *Decrease* In 21 of 29 patients with AIDS (72%) had a low concentration *1076*

β-Carotene *Serum* *Decrease* Mean concentration in 25 patients with CDC stage II disease of 0.24 ± 0.14 µmol/L and 0.21 ± 0.22 µmol/L in 18 patients with CDC stage III disease significantly different from 0.56 ± 0.29 µmol/L in 16 controls *4574*

β-Carotene:Total Lipids Ratio *Serum* *Decrease* Mean concentration in 25 patients with CDC stage II disease of 0.045 ± 0.035 and 0.038 ± 0.035 in 18 patients with CDC stage III disease significantly different from 0.082 ± 0.058 μmol/L in 16 controls *4574*

Carotenoids *Serum* *Decrease* Mean concentration in 25 patients with CDC stage II disease of 0.94 ± 0.46 μmol/L and 0.42 ± 0.37 μmol/L in 18 patients with CDC stage III disease significantly different from 1.79 ± 0.40 μmol/L in 16 controls *4574*

$CD4^+$ Lymphocytes *Blood* *Decrease* In 44 patients with AIDS mean of 140 10^6/L significantly less than 452 10^6/L in 40 patients with asymptomatic HIV infection *4969* In 37 patients with AIDS median concentration of 41 /μL significantly less than median of 923 /μL in 78 healthy controls *3816* Mean concentration of 11.0 ± 6% in 10 patients with progressing AIDS significantly different from 44.5 ± 6% in 10 healthy individuals *5843* In 33 patients with AIDS median concentration of 18 x 10^9/L compared with 670 x 10^9/L in 19 healthy controls *3826*

$CD8^+$ Lymphocytes *Blood* *Decrease* In 33 patients with AIDS median concentration of 245 x 10^9/L compared with 430 x 10^9/L in 19 healthy controls *3826*
Blood *Increase* Mean concentration of 60.1 ± 9% in 10 patients with progressing AIDS significantly different from 28.6 ± 5% in 10 healthy individuals *5843*
Blood *No Effect* In 37 patients with AIDS median concentration of 582 /μL not significantly different from median of 640 /μL in 78 healthy controls *3816*

$CD14^+$ Monocytes *Blood* *Decrease* In 17 patients with AIDS median concentration of 278 /μL significantly different from median of 425 /μL in 19 healthy controls *3816*

Cholesterol *Serum* *Decrease* Decreased in 18% of cases *1891* Hypocholesterolemia with a mean concentration of 3.9 mmol/L observed compared with 4.7 mmol/L in controls *268* Decreased 8% *1891* Mean concentration in 25 patients with CDC stage II disease of 1.74 ± 0.68 g/L and 1.75 ± 0.59 g/L in 18 patients with CDC stage III disease not significantly different from 2.12 ± 0.71 g/L in 16 controls *4574*

Complement C_3 *Serum* *No Effect* Reported effect *5546*

Complement C_4 *Serum* *No Effect* Reported effect *5546*

Creatinine *Serum* *No Effect* In 44 patients with AIDS mean concentration of 100 μmol/L and in 40 with asymptomatic HIV infection of 100 μmol/L within normal range of 50 - 120 μmol/L *4969*

1,25-Dihydroxy Vitamin D_3 *Serum* *No Effect* In 6 patients with AIDS mean concentration of 78.5 ± 17 pmol/L not significantly different from 76.5 ± 11 pmol/L in 10 normal individuals *2397*

Erythrocyte Sedimentation Rate *Blood* *Increase* Observed effect *5546*

Fibrin Degradation Products *Plasma* *Increase* In 20 patients with AIDS median concentration of 460 ng/L higher than 340 ng/L in 20 healthy controls *5266*

Fibrinogen *Plasma* *Increase* In 20 patients with AIDS median concentration of 3.68 ± 0.89 g/L higher than 2.77 ± 0.51 g/L in 20 healthy controls *5266*

Fibrinogen Degradation Products *Plasma* *Increase* In 20 patients with AIDS median concentration of 380 ng/L higher than 208 ng/L in 20 healthy controls *5266*

Follicle Stimulating Hormone *Plasma* *Decrease* Seventy-five percent of patients with low free testosterone levels had decreased LH and FSH *1190*

Glial Fibrillary Acidic Protein *Cerebrospinal Fluid* *Increase* In 2 patients with AIDS mean concentration exceeded upper limit of reference interval *119*

Glutathione Peroxidase *Red Blood Cells* *No Effect* Mean activity in 25 patients with CDC stage II disease of 42.0 ± 11.0 U/g hemoglobin and 44.2 ± 23.0 U/g hemoglobin in 18 patients with CDC stage III disease not significantly different from 42.4 ± 11.0 U/g hemoglobin in 16 controls *4574*
Serum *Decrease* Mean activity in 25 patients with CDC stage II disease of 310 ± 71 U/L and 238 ± 81 U/L in 18 patients with CDC stage III disease significantly different from 375 ± 78 U/L in 16 controls *4574*

Granulocyte-Macrophage Colony Stimulating Factor *Cerebrospinal Fluid* *Increase* In 30 HIV-infected patients classified as AIDS dementia complex (ADC), and 20 subjects with other neurological diseases (OND) a high incidence of detectable IL-6 and GM-CSF in the CSF of ADC patients was found compared with OND patients *4085*

HDL-Cholesterol *Serum* *Decrease* Decreased 37% *1891* Decreased in 37% of patients *1891*

Hemoglobin *Blood* *Decrease* In 20 patients with AIDS mean concentration of 108 g/L significantly less than 144 g/L in 20 healthy controls *5266*

Hepatitis Core Antigen *Blood* *Increase* Positive in over 90% of AIDS patients *5546*

25-Hydroxy Vitamin D_3 *Serum* *No Effect* In 6 patients with AIDS mean concentration of 61.2 ± 13.5 nmol/L not significantly different from 49.9 ± 6.5 nmol/L in 10 normal individuals *2397*

immunoglobulin A *Serum* *Increase* Elevated levels of at least one immunoglobulin was found in 78% of patients *1348* Frequently a polyclonal hypergammaglobulinemia is present, usually of IgG and IgA *5678*

Immunoglobulin G *Serum* *Increase* 27 of 29 children tested *3972* Elevated levels of at least 1 immunoglobulin found in 78% of patients *1348* Frequently a polyclonal hypergammaglobulinemia is present, usually of IgG and IgA *5678*

Interferon-γ *Serum* *Increase* In 7 children with AIDS mean concentration of 49.2 ± 110.5 pg/mL significantly higher than 0.7 ± 1.8 pg/mL in 10 healthy control children *5257*

Interleukin-1 *Cerebrospinal Fluid* *Increase* In 30 patients with AIDS dementia complex (ADC), and in 20 HIV-seronegative subjects with other neurological diseases (OND), CSF levels of IL-1α were more frequently detectable in ADC patients than in OND subjects. These cytokines were also detectable in CSF of ADC patients with minimal symptoms *4084*
Serum *No Effect* We evaluated cerebrospinal fluid (CSF) and serum concentrations of 30 patients with AIDS dementia complex (ADC), and in 20 HIV-seronegative subjects with other neurological diseases (OND). The majority of serums from both ADC and OND patients did not contain detectable levels of cytokines *4084*

Interleukin-1α *Serum* *Increase* Found in 63% of homosexual AIDS patients *5546*

Interleukin-1β *Serum* *Increase* In 7 children with AIDS mean concentration of 37.5 ± 23.6 pg/mL significantly higher than 1.5 ± 4.1 pg/mL in 10 healthy control children *5257*

Interleukin-6 *Cerebrospinal Fluid* *Increase* In 30 patients with AIDS dementia complex (ADC), and in 20 HIV-seronegative subjects with other neurological diseases (OND), CSF levels were more frequently detectable in ADC patients than in OND subjects. These cytokines were also detectable in CSF of ADC patients with minimal symptoms *4084* In 30 HIV-infected patients classified as AIDS dementia complex (ADC), and 20 subjects with other neurological diseases (OND) we have found a high incidence of detectable IL-6 and GM-CSF in the CSF of ADC patients compared with OND patients *4085*
Serum *No Effect* Cerebrospinal fluid (CSF) and serum concentrations of 30 patients with AIDS dementia complex (ADC), and in 20 HIV-seronegative subjects with other neurological diseases (OND) were studied. The majority of both ADC and OND patients did not contain detectable serum levels of cytokines *4084*

Interleukin-8 *Serum* *Increase* The means and 95% confidence intervals of IL-8 in sera of 36 HIV-infected individuals and 32 matched controls were 275 and 216 - 349 pg/mL, and 8 and 4 - 14 pg/mL, respectively, showing a 34-fold increase in IL-8 in the circulation of HIV-infected individuals *3368*

ionized Calcium *Serum* *No Effect* In 44 patients with AIDS mean concentration of 1.25 mmol/L and in 40 with asymptomatic HIV infection of 1.25 mmol/L within normal range of 1.19 - 1.31 mmol/L *4969*

Lactate Dehydrogenase *Serum* *Increase* In 27 of 33 patients with AIDS or AIDS-related complex activity significantly increased *4840* Significant increase in enzyme activity related to hepatic function. About 90% of AIDS patients have antibodies to hepatitis B antigen and hepatitis B core antibody. Also significantly higher prevalence of antibodies to cytomegalovirus, herpes simplex virus, hepatitis A and EB virus *2267*
Serum *No Effect* In 6 of 16 adults with AIDS or AIDS-related complex activity remained within normal range *4840*

42.00 Acquired Immune Deficiency Syndrome *(continued)*

LDL-Cholesterol *Serum* *Decrease* Calculated LDL-cholesterol decreased in 30% of patients *1891*

Leptin *Serum* *No Effect* In 33 patients with AIDS mean concentration of 1.16 ± 0.25 ng/mL not significantly different from < 1.60 ± 0.36 ng/mL in 22 non-infected controls *1892*

Leukocytes *Blood* *Decrease* Less than 4,500 cells/µL in 25 of 37 patients *1348*

Lipid Hydroperoxide *Serum* *Increase* Mean concentration in 25 patients with CDC stage II disease of 176 ± 58 µmol/L (significant) and 155 ± 67 µmol/L (nonsignificant) in 18 patients with CDC stage III disease different from 127 ± 14 µmol/L in 16 controls *4574*

Luteinizing Hormone *Plasma* *Decrease* Seventy-five percent of patients with low free testosterone levels had decreased LH and FSH *1190*

Lymphocyte T-Cells *Blood* *Decrease* The risk of AIDS is clearly predicted by the total number of circulating OKTA positive lymphocytes (T4) *1770*

Lymphocytes *Blood* *Decrease* Absolute lymphopenia in 1 of 29 children tested *3972* In 20 patients with AIDS mean concentration of 1,295 x 10^6/L significantly less than 2,430 x 10^6/L in 20 healthy controls *5266* Lymphopenia less than 1,500 cells/mL is often present and the absolute number of cells in the T helper/inducer subset is depressed *5678* < 1,500 cells/µL in 26 of 35 patients. 91.6% of patients had decreased concentration of T-Helper cells *1348*

β_2-Macroglobulin *Serum* *Increase* Elevated > 2.5 mg/L in 29 or 37 patients *1348* Found frequently *2821*

Macrophage Inflammatory Protein-1α *Serum* *Increase* Mean positivity of 4 in 10 patients with progressing AIDS significantly different from 0 of 10 in healthy individuals *5843*

Magnesium *Serum* *No Effect* In 6 patients with AIDS mean concentration of 0.83 ± 0.04 mmol/L not significantly different from 0.79 ± 0.02 mmol/L in 10 normal individuals *2397*

β_2-Microglobulin *Serum* *Increase* In 37 patients with AIDS median concentration of 4 mg/L significantly greater than median of 1.6 mg/L in 78 healthy controls *3816*

Monocytes *Blood* *Decrease* In 17 patients with AIDS median concentration of 299 /µL significantly different from median of 493 /µL in 19 healthy controls *3816*

N^2, N^2-Dimethylguanosine *Urine* *Increase* Mean excretion of 26.8 µmol/d in 4 patients with AIDS compared with 16.9 µmol/d in pooled normal urine *3720*

Neopterin *Cerebrospinal Fluid* *Increase* In 95 HIV-1 positive patients with neurological disease mean concentration of 6.68 ± 10.6 ng/mL and in 15 patients with non-neurological AIDS mean concentration of 1.24 ± 0.95 ng/mL was greatly increased compared with concentration in 40 HIV-negative controls (0.26 ± 0.17 ng/mL) *2092*
Serum *Increase* Extremely high concentrations may be observed in patients with AIDS with concentrations increased before symptoms observed in most patients *121* In 33 patients with AIDS median concentration of 50.3 nmol/L compared with 8.2 nmol/L in 19 healthy controls *3826*
Urine *Increase* Secondary to inflammatory response *2267* Extremely high concentrations may be observed in patients with AIDS with concentrations increased before symptoms in most patients *121*

Neutrophils *Cerebrospinal Fluid* *Increase* In 6 patients with AIDS numerous (> 10 /hpf) neutrophils present and all were associated with cytomegalovirus infection *1847*

Nitrite *Serum* *Increase* In 7 children with AIDS mean concentration of 0.5 ± 0.3 µmol/L and in 14 children seronegative for HIV-1 mean concentration of 0.48 µmol/L significantly higher than 0.2 ± 0.3 µmol/L in 10 healthy control children *5257*

Parathyroid Hormone *Plasma* *Decrease* In 6 patients with AIDS mean concentration of intact parathyroid hormone of 14 ± 2 ng/L significantly different from 23 ± 3 ng/L in 10 normal individuals *2397* In 8 of 23 patients with AIDS, PTH concentration less than 1.0 pmol/L compared with 1 in 20 patients with asymptomatic HIV infection (mean values in AIDS patients of 1.5 pmol/L and 2.6 pmol/L in asymptomatic patients) *2183*
Plasma *No Effect* In 44 patients with AIDS mean concentration of 1.5 pmol/L and in 40 with asymptomatic HIV infection of 2.6 pmol/L within normal range of 1.0 - 5.5 pmol/L although concentration in AIDS patients significantly less than in asymptomatic patients *4969*

Partial Thromboplastin Time *Plasma* *Increase* Observed effect *487* In 10 patients with AIDS all had elevated times *873*

Phosphate *Serum* *No Effect* In 44 patients with AIDS mean concentration of 1.3 mmol/L and in 40 with asymptomatic HIV infection of 1.1 mmol/L within normal range of 0.8 - 1.5 mmol/L although concentration in AIDS patients significantly higher than in asymptomatic patients *4969*

Phosphohexoseisomerase *Serum* *Increase* Significant increase in enzyme activity related to hepatic function. About 90% of AIDS patients have antibodies to hepatitis B antigen and hepatitis B core antibody. Also significantly higher prevalence of antibodies to cytomegalovirus, herpes simplex virus, hepatitis A and EB virus *2267*

Phospholipase A *Serum* *Increase* Reported effect *2200*

Plasmin-α_2-Plasmin Inhibitor Complex *Plasma* *Increase* In 20 patients with AIDS median concentration of 580 ng/mL higher than 325 ng/mL in 20 healthy controls *5266*

Plasminogen *Plasma* *Increase* In 20 patients with AIDS median concentration of 1.02 ± 0.17 U/mL higher than 0.94 ± 0.11 U/mL in 20 healthy controls *5266*

Platelets *Blood* *Decrease* Consequence of disease *5546* In 20 patients with AIDS mean concentration of 195 x 10^9/L significantly less than 235 x 10^9/L in 20 healthy controls *5266* In 7,498 patients with clinical AIDS one year incidence of platelet counts less than 50,000 /µL was 8.7% *5076*
Blood *Increase* Observed effect *5546*

Porphyrin, Total *Serum* *Increase* Of a population of 167 individuals, in patients positive for AIDS and hepatitis C median concentration of 2.31 nmol/L, 1.99 nmol/L in individuals positive for AIDS and negative for hepatitis C, 1.31 nmol/L in AIDS negative hepatitis C positive individuals and 1.14 nmol/L in AIDS and hepatitis C negative patients *3821*

Potassium *Serum* *Increase* Hyperkalemia observed in up to 21% of hospitalized patients. This may be associated with a metabolic acidosis and impaired renal function. Drug therapy, particularly trimethoprim combined with dapsone or sulfamethoxazole used to treat pneumocystis carnii pneumonia, may cause hyperkalemia *268*

Protein *BAL Fluid* *No Effect* No sgnificant difference observed between concentrations in 32 healthy controls (mean 15.59 ± 4.66 mg/dL) and in 53 patients with AIDS (17.65 ± 13.90 mg/dL) *3270*

Prothrombin Time *Plasma* *Increase* Three of seven patients studied *873*

Pseudouridine *Urine* *Increase* In 4 patients with AIDS mean excretion in 4 patients of 330 µmol/d compared with 207 µmol/d in pooled normal urine *3720*

Quinolinic Acid *Cerebrospinal Fluid* *Increase* Three fold higher concentrations than that in age matched controls (58.3 pmol/mL versus 18.4 pmol/mL) *2141* Increased two fold in patients in the early stages of the disease and averaged 3.8 times above normal in later stage patients. However in patients with either clinically overt AIDS dementia complex, aseptic meningitis, opportunistic infections, or neoplasms, CSF levels were elevated over 20 fold, generally paralleling the severity of the cognitive and motor dysfunction *2140*

RANTES *Serum* *Increase* Mean concentration of 66.0 ± 30 ng/mL in 10 patients with progressing AIDS significantly different from 17.9 ± 5 ng/mL in 10 healthy individuals *5843*

Retinol *Serum* *Decrease* Mean concentration in 25 patients with CDC stage II disease of 2.17 ± 0.69 µmol/L and 1.96 ± 0.87 µmol/L in 18 patients with CDC stage III disease significantly different from 2.77 ± 0.67 µmol/L in 16 controls *4574*

Selenium *Serum* *Decrease* Mean concentration in 25 patients with CDC stage II disease of 0.93 ± 0.19 µmol/L (not significant) and 0.59 ± 0.25 µmol/L in 18 patients with CDC stage III disease significantly different from 0.96 ± 0.17 µmol/L in 16 controls *4574*

Sodium *Serum* *Decrease* Thirty-six of one hundred and three patients (35%) had values less than 130 mEq/L. Causes included intravascular depletion and inappropriate arginine vasopressin levels for the serum osmolality *40*

Soluble CD4⁺ *Serum Increase* In 37 patients with AIDS median concentration of 25.6 U/mL significantly greater than median of 7.6 U/mL in 78 healthy controls *3816*

Soluble CD8⁺ *Serum Increase* In 37 patients with AIDS median concentration of 1,287 U/mL significantly greater than median of 555 U/mL in 78 healthy controls *3816*

Soluble CD14⁺ *Serum Increase* In 37 patients with AIDS median concentration of 5.7 ± 2.5 mg/L significantly greater than median of 2.2 ± 0.47 mg/L in 78 healthy controls *3816* Mean concentrations in patients with CDC grade C (AIDS) of about 6 µg/mL higher than mean of about 2 µg/mL in controls *3048*

Soluble CD71⁺ *Serum No Effect* In 86 patients with AIDS mean concentration of 2,534 ± 109 ng/mL not significantly different from 2,308 ± 147 ng/mL in 39 normal individuals *4302*

Soluble E-Selectin *Serum No Effect* In 33 patients with AIDS median concentration of 42.8 ng/mL compared with 47.7 ng/mL in 19 healthy controls *3826*

Soluble Intercellular Adhesion Molecule-1 *Serum Increase* In 33 patients with AIDS median concentration of 727 ng/mL compared with 243 ng/mL in 19 healthy controls *3826*

Soluble Vascular Cell Adhesion Molecule-1 *Serum Increase* In 33 patients with AIDS median concentration of 1,386 ng/mL compared with 515 ng/mL in 19 healthy controls *3826*

Testosterone, Free *Serum Decrease* Below normal in 18 of 40 (45%) patients. Seventy-five percent of patients with low levels had decreased LH and FSH *1190* Below normal in 45% of patients *1190*

Thiobarbituric Acid-reacting Substances *Serum Increase* Mean concentration in 25 patients with CDC stage II disease of 2.73 ± 0.35 µmol/L (significant) and 2.68 ± 0.40 µmol/L (non-significant) in 18 patients with CDC stage III disease different from 2.51 ± 0.30 µmol/L in 16 controls *4574*

Thymosin-α_1 *Serum Decrease* Less than 1% of normal in 70 - 80% of AIDS patients *5546*

α-Tocopherol *Serum Decrease* Mean concentration in 25 patients with CDC stage II disease of 26.8 ± 5.3 µmol/L (not significant) and 18.6 ± 5.9 µmol/L in 18 patients with CDC stage III disease significantly different from 31.1 ± 6.7 µmol/L in 16 controls *4574*

α-Tocopherol:Lipids Ratio *Serum Decrease* Mean ratio in 25 patients with CDC stage II disease of 5.07 ± 1.22 (not significant) and 3.89 ± 1.33 in 18 patients with CDC stage III disease significantly different from 5.00 ± 1.17 in 16 controls *4574*

Tranaminine *Serum Increase* Reported effect *5546*

Triglycerides *Serum Increase* Twice the levels compared to controls due to increased levels of very low density lipoprotein *1890* Hypertriglyceridemia (although quite variable) with a mean concentration of 2.3 mmol/L observed compared with 1.1 mmol/L in controls: hypertriglyceridemia appears to correlate with interferon-α concentration: increase due to increased hepatic synthesis of VLDL and decreased clearance due to decreased lipoprotein lipase activity *268* Mean concentration in 25 patients with CDC stage II disease of 1.57 ± 1.27 g/L (not significant) and 1.88 ± 0.91 g/L (significant) in 18 patients with CDC stage III disease different from 0.88 ± 0.47 g/L in 16 controls *4574*

Tumor Necrosis Factor-α *Cerebrospinal Fluid Increase* In 30 patients with AIDS dementia complex (ADC) and in 20 HIV-seronegative subjects with other neurological diseases (OND), CSF levels were more frequently detectable in ADC patients than in OND subjects. These cytokines were also detectable in CSF of ADC patients with minimal symptoms *4084*
Serum Increase In hemophilia patients infected with HIV significant increase observed in those who were HIV+ compared with those who were HIV-. HIV- and control patients had concentrations of about 2 pg/mL whereas those who were HIV+ had concentrations about 11 pg/mL *3829* In 7 children with AIDS mean concentration of 91.2 ± 45.1 pg/mL significantly higher than 2.8 ± 7.5 pg/mL in 10 healthy control children *5257* In 33 patients with AIDS median concentration of 28.4 pg/mL compared with undetecable amount in 19 healthy controls *3826*
Serum No Effect Cerebrospinal fluid (CSF) and serum concentrations of 30 patients with AIDS dementia complex (ADC), and in 20 HIV-seronegative subjects with other neurological diseases (OND) were evaluated. The majority of both ADC and OND patients did not contain detectable serum levels of cytokines *4084*

Zinc *Serum Decrease* Mean concentration in 25 patients with CDC stage II disease of 10.46 ± 2.74 µmol/L and 7.87 ± 1.4 µmol/L in 18 patients with CDC stage III disease significantly different from 12.3 ± 2.5 µmol/L in 16 controls *4574*

42.00 AIDS Related Complex

CD4⁺ Lymphocytes *Blood Decrease* In 53 patients with ARC median concentration of 182 /µL significantly less than median of 923 /µL in 78 healthy controls *3816*

CD8⁺ Lymphocytes *Blood No Effect* In 53 patients with ARC median concentration of 735 /µL significantly less than median of 640 /µL in 78 healthy controls *3816*

CD14⁺ Monocytes *Blood Increase* In 13 patients with ARC median concentration of 539 /µL significantly different from median of 425 /µL in 19 healthy controls *3816*

β_2-Microglobulin *Serum Increase* In 53 patients with ARC median concentration of 3.7 mg/L significantly greater than median of 1.6 mg/L in 78 healthy controls *3816*

Monocytes *Blood Increase* In 13 patients with ARC median concentration of 555 /µL significantly different from median of 493 /µL in 19 healthy controls *3816*

Neopterin *Serum Increase* High concentrations may be observed in patients with AIDS-related complex *121*

Soluble CD4⁺ *Serum Increase* In 53 patients with ARC median concentration of 19.3 U/mL significantly greater than median of 7.6 U/mL in 78 healthy controls *3816*

Soluble CD8⁺ *Serum Increase* In 53 patients with ARC median concentration of 1,379 U/mL significantly greater than median of 555 U/mL in 78 healthy controls *3816*

Soluble CD14⁺ *Serum Increase* In 53 patients with ARC mean concentration of 3.8 ± 1.1 mg/L significantly greater than median of 2.2 ± 0.47 mg/L in 78 healthy controls *3816*

42.00 Autoimmune Immune Deficiency Syndrome

CD4⁺ Lymphocytes *Blood Decrease* Median concentration in 8 patients with AIDS 115 x 10^6/L *3420*

CD8⁺ Lymphocytes *Blood Decrease* Median concentration in 8 patients with AIDS of 960 x 10^6/L *3420*

Cysteine *Plasma Decrease* Median concentration of 208 µmol/L in 45 men with AIDS compared with 240 µmol/L in 71 HIV-seronegative controls *2276*

Macrophage Inflammatory Protein-1α *Serum No Effect* Median concentration in 4 patients with early of AIDS 35.5 pg/mL and 39.3 pg/mL in late AIDS within the normal range of < 46.9 pg/mL *3420*

Macrophage Inflammatory Protein-1β *Serum No Effect* Median concentration in 4 patients with early AIDS of 61.6 pg/mL and 64.7 pg/mL in late AIDS within the normal range of < 46.9 pg/mL *3420*

RANTES *Serum No Effect* Median concentration in 4 patients with early AIDS of 28.4 ng/mL and 26.3 ng/mL in late AIDS within the normal range of < 46.9 ng/mL *3420*

Soluble HLA-I *Cerebrospinal Fluid Increase* Known to be present in CSF of people with varicella meningitis *216*

42.10 HIV-1 Infection

Activated T Lymphocytes *Blood Increase* In 67 HIV positive drug users mean concentration of 184.0 ± 156.4 /µL (9.9 ± 6.5%) ratio compared with 90.3 ± 61.2 /µL (3.6 ± 2.3%) in 47 HIV negative drug using controls *690*

Alanine *Plasma Decrease* In wasting syndrome associated with HIV-1 infection significantly decreased concentration observed *3675*
Plasma No Effect Mean concentration of 406 ± 76 µmol/L in 20 HIV-infected individuals not significantly different from 398 ± 92 µmol/L in 20 healthy controls *2240*

Alanine Aminotransferase *Serum Increase* In 31 of 52 patients with HIV-infection (60%) with increased pancreatic enzyme activity aminotransferase activity increased *173*

42.10 **HIV-1 Infection** *(continued)*

Albumin *Cerebrospinal Fluid* *Increase* In 4 patients with HIV infection mean concentration of 554 ± 369 mg/L not significantly higher than 179 ± 53 mg/L in 5 controls *429*
Serum *Decrease* In 54 patients with HIV-1 infection median concentration of 36.0 g/L significantly different from reference values of 40 - 45 g/L *2063*

Alkaline Phosphatase *Serum* *Decrease* In 40 patients with HIV infection mean activity of 109 U/L below upper limit of normal of 135 U/L and activity of 137 U/L in 44 AIDS patients *4969*

Alkaline Phosphatase Band-10 Isoenzyme *Serum* *Increase* In infants as young as 2 months presence of band-10 isoenzyme showed excellent correlation with presence of HIV-1 infection *3682*

β-Aminobutyric Acid *Plasma* *Decrease* In wasting syndrome associated with HIV-1 infection significantly decreased concentration observed *3675*
Plasma *Increase* In 20 HIV-infected individuals mean concentration of 17 ± 10 μmol/L nonsignificantly greater than 15 ± 10 μmol/L in 20 healthy controls *2240*

δ-Aminolevulinic Acid *Urine* *Increase* In 12 of 23 patients with HIV infection mean concentration ranged from 2.4 to 4.4 μmol/mmol creatinine significantly different from mean of 1.5 ± 0.6 μmol/mmol creatinine in normal controls *3633*

Amylase *Serum* *Increase* In 163 (149 men, 14 women) consecutive asymptomatic HIV-infected outpatients of whom only 6 were receiving dideoxyinosine, known to cause pancreatitis, 39 (24%) had increased serum amylase activity *1525* Activity increased in 10 of 47 HIV-infected children *705* 17.5% of 76 HIV-positive patients had increased activity greater than 125 U/L (mean 159 U/L) *173*

Amylase, Pancreatic Isoenzyme *Serum* *Increase* Activity increased in 6 of 47 HIV-infected children *705* In 163 (149 men, 14 women) consecutive asymptomatic HIV-infected outpatients of whom only 6 were receiving dideoxyinosine, known to cause pancreatitis, 39 (24%) had increased serum amylase activity. In 11 (28%) of these the increase was due to increased pancreatic isoamylase alone and in 6 (17%) due to increases of both pancreatic and salivary amylases *1525*

Amylase, Salivary Isoenzyme *Serum* *Increase* In 163 (149 men, 14 women) consecutive asymptomatic HIV-infected outpatients of whom only 6 were receiving dideoxyinosine, known to cause pancreatitis, 39 (24%) had increased serum amylase activity. In 17 (42%) of these the increase was due to increased pancreatic isoamylase alone and in 6 (17%) due to increases of both pancreatic and salivary amylases *1525*

Angiotensin-converting Enzyme *Serum* *Increase* Significant increases to 55.4 ± 11.4 U/L observed in patients with acquired immunodeficiency syndrome and in patients with intermediate stage of HIV infection of 57.2 ± 25.3 U/L compared with 31.9 ± 14.0 U/L in controls *3952*

Anti-Protein S Antibodies *Serum* *Positive* In a study of 35 HIV positive patients specific anti-protein S antibodies detected in 28.6% patients with a higher prevalence in symptomatic than asymptomatic patients *4943*

Anticardiolipin Antibodies *Serum* *Increase* In 35 HIV-1infected patients anticardiolipin antibodies detected in 77.1% in both symptomatic and asymptomatic individuals *4943* In 43 patients with HIV infection mean concentrations of greater than 15 GPL/mL and 15 MPL/mL were observed in 26 patients with no correlation with CD4 and platelet concentrations *1127*

Arginine *Plasma* *Decrease* In 20 HIV-infected individuals mean concentration of 58 ± 16 μmol/L not significantly less than 67 ± 27 μmol/L in 20 healthy controls *2240*

Ascorbic Acid *Serum* *No Effect* In wasting syndrome associated with HIV-1 infection no significant difference in concentration observed *3675*

Asparagine *Plasma* *Decrease* Mean concentration in 20 HIV-infected individuals mean concentration of 34 ± 10 μmol/L nonsignificantly less than 45 ± 22 μmol/L in 20 healthy controls *2240*

Aspartate Aminotransferase *Serum* *Increase* In 31 of 52 patients with HIV-infection (60%) with increased pancreatic enzyme activity aminotransferase activity increased *173*

Calcitonin *Plasma* *No Effect* In 54 patients with HIV-1 infection median concentration of 2.10 pmol/L not significantly different from reference values of < 4.5 pmol/L *2063*

Calprotectin *Cerebrospinal Fluid* *No Effect* In 15 HIV patients with CNS symptoms the 10 with HIV associated encephalopathy had concentrations within the normal range in contrast to those with opportunistic infections in whom CSF calprotectin concentration was increased *1264*

$CD4^+$:$CD8^+$ Lymphocyte Ratio *Blood* *Decrease* In 67 HIV positive drug users mean ratio of 0.55 ± 0.39 compared with 1.82 ± 0.72 in 47 HIV negative drug using controls *690*

$CD4^+$ Lymphocytes *Blood* *Decrease* In 47 HIV-1 infected men mean concentration of 359.6 ± 286.6 /μL *5840* In 10 of 20 patients with counts < 200 cells/mm^2 relative risk of progressing to AIDS 9.88%, with counts of 200 - 500 cells/mm^2 relative risk 6.37% and in 4 of 79 patients with counts > 500 cells/mm^2 no relative risk *5831* In 26 patients of CDC group A1 mean concentration of 691 ± 161 /μL, 367 ± 72 /μL in 29 of group A2, 736 ± 281 /μL in 14 of group B2 and 321 ± 94 /μL in 26 of group B2 *2185* Counts of > 200 /μL predicted the absence of AIDS in 94% HIV-infected patients *4186* In 12 asymptomatic HIV-infected patients mean concentration of 364 cells/μL compared with 62 cells/μL in 12 patients with symptomatic HIV infection and 26 cells/μ/L in 12 patients with HIV infection and diarrhea *4513* In 14 patients with HIV-1 infection pretreatment concentration of 275 x 10^6/L *1742* In 14 patients with HIV infection and wasting mean concentration of 19.8 ± 35.2 cells/μL slightly less than 59.5 ± 31.0 cells/μL in 18 patients with HIV infection and no wasting and normal range of 800 - 2000 cells/μL *912* In 67 HIV positive drug users mean concentration of 440 ± 267 /μL (24.1 ± 10.6%) compared with 1,110 ± 345 /μL (45.5 ± 7.2%) in 47 HIV negative drug using controls *690* In 250 intravenous drug users with HIV1-infection median concentration of 484.5 x 10^6/L significantly decreased compared with normal range of 500 - 1650 x 10^6/L and median proportion of 28.0% compared with normal of 33 - 60% *69* In 198 seroconverters intermediate tercile concentration of 774 - 1077 cells/μL prior to seroconversion and 563 - 830 cells/μLwith seroconversion *4787* 44 of 63 patients with HIV infection (34 asymptomatic) had concentrations less than the lower limit of normal of 485 x 10^6/L. Median count of 318 x 10^6/L *5839* B_{12} concentration reduced to below 132 pmol/L in 61 of 200 patients (30.3%) with HIV-1 virus, with significantly decreased CD4 count of 223 /μL in these patients compared with 292 /μL in those without B_{12} deficiency *3985* In 19 asymptomatic HIV-1 infected patients median concentration of 270 x 10^9/L compared with 670 x 10^9/L in 19 healthy controls *3826* Median concentration in 4 patients with non-progressing HIV-infection 1,233 x 10^6/L *3420* In 54 patients with HIV-1 infection median concentration of 66 x 10^6/L significantly different from reference values of 670 - 1000 x 10^6/L *2063* In 25 HIV-positive asymptomatic patients median concentration of 568 /μL not significantly less than median of 923 /μL in 78 healthy controls *3816*

$CD8^+$ Lymphocytes *Blood* *Decrease* Median concentration in 4 patients with non-progressing HIV-infection of 1,551 x 10^6/L *3420*
Blood *Increase* In 54 patients with HIV-1 infection median concentration of 455 x 10^6/L significantly different from reference values of 340 - 530 x 10^6/L *2063* In 25 HIV-positive asymptomatic patients median concentration of 1052 /μL not significantly greater than median of 640 /μL in 78 healthy controls *3816* In 67 HIV positive drug users mean concentration of 930 ± 578 /μL (49.5 ± 12.0%) compared with 693 ± 336 /μL (27.6 ± 7.7%) in 47 HIV negative drug using controls *690* In 19 asymptomatic HIV-1 infected patients median concentration of 750 x 10^9/L compared with 430 x 10^9/L in 19 healthy controls *3826*

$CD14^+$ Monocytes *Blood* *Increase* In 13 asymptomatic HIV-positive patients median concentration of 546 /μL significantly different from median of 425 /μL in 19 healthy controls *3816*

Cholesterol *Serum* *Decrease* Median plasma concentration in 63 patients with HIV infection (34 asymptomatic) of 168 mg/dL (4.34 mmol/L). 2 of 63 (3.2%) had concentrations less than 110 mg/dL (2.84 mmol/L) *5839* Hypocholesterolemia with a mean concentration of 3.9 mmol/L observed compared with 4.7 mmol/L in controls *268*

Complement C_3 *Cerebrospinal Fluid* *Increase* Mean concentrations in 7 patients with HIV infection of 3.2 ± 1.5 mg/L by TR-IFMA and 4.3 ± 1.8 mg/L by EID compared with mean concentrations in 30 normal individuals of 2.4 ± 0.9 mg/L by TR-IFMA and 3.6 ± 1.0 mg/L by EID *1623*

Copper *Serum* *No Effect* In wasting syndrome associated with HIV-1 infection no significant difference in concentration observed *3675*

Coproporphyrin *Urine Increase* In 5 of 23 patients with HIV infection mean concentration ranged from 21 to 380 nmol/mmol creatinine significantly different from mean of 10 ± 5 nmol/mmol creatinine in normal controls *3633*

Cortisol *Plasma No Effect* Basal concentrations are usually normal despite histological involvement of adrenals and features of adrenocortical deficiency *268* In 14 HIV infected patients with wasting mean concentration of 15.6 ± 2.3 µg/dL and 9.2 ± 1.9 µg/dL in 18 patients without wasting not different from normal range of 5 - 25 µg/dL *912*

Creatinine *Serum Increase* In 3 of 52 patients with HIV-infection (6%) with increased pancreatic enzyme activity renal failure also observed *173*
Serum No Effect In 54 patients with HIV-1 infection median concentration of 78 µmol/L not significantly different from reference values of 62 - 110 µmol/L *2063*

Cysteine *Plasma Decrease* Median concentration of 217 µmol/L in 92 asymptomatic HIV-positive men compared with 240 µmol/L in 71 HIV-seronegative controls *2276*
Plasma No Effect In 24 HIV-infected children mean concentration of 251 ± 13 µmol/L not significantly different from mean concentration of 286 ± 29 µmol/L in 24 healthy control children *4400*

Cysteine-Glycine *Plasma No Effect* In 24 HIV-infected children mean concentration of 29,95 ± 5.97 µmol/L not significantly different from mean concentration of 30.51 ± 6.23 µmol/L in 24 healthy control children *4400*

Cystine *Plasma Decrease* In 20 HIV-infected individuals mean concentration of 15 ± 13 µmol/L significantly less than 46 ± 20 µmol/L in 20 healthy controls *2240*

1,25-Dihydroxy Vitamin D_3 *Serum Decrease* In 54 patients with HIV-1 infection median concentration of 48 pmol/L significantly different from reference values of 80 - 110 pmol/L *2063*

β-Endorphin *White Blood Cells Increase* Concentration increased in HIV-positive patients *633*

Eosinophils *Blood Increase* Significant eosinophilia may be observed in patients with advanced HIV and who have CD4 counts of less than 100 cells/µL *4884*

Erythropoietin *Serum Increase* In 72 children with untreated HIV median concentration of 22 IU/L compared with 11 IU/L in 24 healthy controls *82*

Ferritin *Red Blood Cells Increase* In 86 HIV positive asymptomatic patients mean concentration of 320 µg/L packed red blood cells, in 22 asymptomatic patients but meeting CDC criteria for AIDS 773 µg/L packed red blood cells and in 60 with AIDS with complications requiring hospitalization of 453 µg/L packed red blood cells compared with normal range of 120 - 550 µg/L packed red blood cells *4355*
Serum Increase Mean concentration in 74 HIV-1 positive pregnant women during first 6 to 14 weeks of 112.8 µg/L compared with 58.8 µg/L in 148 seronegative women *4126* In patients with HIV infection concentration increased with clinical worsening of infection. In 86 asymptomatic HIV positive patients mean concentration of 112 µg/L, in 22 asymptomatic patients with CDC criteria for AIDS239 µg/L, and in 60 with an acute complication requiring hospitalization 487 µg/L *4355*

Fibrin Degradation Products *Plasma Increase* In 20 patients with HIV infection median concentration of 395 ng/L higher than 340 ng/L in 20 healthy controls *5266*

Fibrinogen *Plasma Increase* In 20 patients with HIV infection median concentration of 3.49 ± 0.68 g/L higher than 2.77 ± 0.51 g/L in 20 healthy controls *5266*

Fibrinogen Degradation Products *Plasma Increase* In 20 patients with HIV infection median concentration of 343 ng/L higher than 208 ng/L in 20 healthy controls *5266*

Folate *Red Blood Cells No Effect* In 54 patients with HIV-1 infection median concentration of 545 nmol/L not significantly different from reference values of 637 - 918 nmol/L *2063*
Serum Increase In 54 patients with HIV-1 infection median concentration of 12.5 nmol/L significantly different from reference values of 8.9 - 13.5 nmol/L *2063*

Follicle Stimulating Hormone *Plasma No Effect* Mean concentration of 5.0 ± 3.2 mIU/mL in 14 patients with HIV infection and 8.3 ± 2.0 mIU/mL in 18 HIV patients without wasting and normal range of 2 - 18 mIU/mL *912*

Ganglioside GD3 *Cerebrospinal Fluid Increase* In 22 patients with HIV-infection mean concentration of 56.7 nmol/L significantly different from 40.1 nmol/L in 44 age-matched control patients, with 7 of the 22 patients having concentrations greater than mean + 2 SD in controls *119*

Glial Fibrillary Acidic Protein *Cerebrospinal Fluid No Effect* In 20 patients with HIV-infection mean concentration of 317 ± 224 ng/L fell within normal range *119*

Globulin *Serum Increase* In 52 patients with HIV-infection with increased pancreatic enzyme activity mean concentration of 44 g/L *173*

Glutamine *Plasma No Effect* Mean concentration of glutamine and glutamic acid in 20 HIV-infected individuals of 595 ± 87 µmol/L not different from 598 ± 105 µmol/L in 20 healthy controls *2240*

Glutathione *Plasma Decrease* In 24 HIV-infected children mean concentration of 2.96 ± 0.31 µmol/L significantly less than mean concentration of 6.62 ± 0.58 µmol/L in 24 healthy control children *4400*

Glycine *Plasma Increase* In 20 HIV-infected individuals mean concentration of 117 ± 25 µmol/L nonsignificantly higher than 207 ± 49 µmol/L in 20 healthy controls *2240*

Granulocytes *Blood Decrease* B_{12} concentration reduced to below 132 pmol/L in 61 of 200 patients (30.3%) with HIV-1 virus, with significantly decreased granulocyte count of 2,530 /µL in these patients compared with 3,020 /µL in those without B_{12} deficiency *3985*

HDL-Cholesterol *Serum Decrease* Median plasma concentration in 63 patients with HIV infection (34 asymptomatic) of 35 mg/dL (0.91 mmol/L). 29 of 63 (46%) had concentrations less than 35 mg/dL (0.91 mmol/L) *5839*

Hemoglobin *Blood Decrease* In 72 children with untreated HIV median concentration of 106 g/L compared with 120 g/L in 24 healthy controls *82*
Blood No Effect In 20 patients with HIV infection mean concentration of 140 g/L not significantly less than 144 g/L in 20 healthy controls *5266*

Histidine *Plasma No Effect* Mean concentration of 74 ± 15 µmol/L in 20 HIV-infected individuals not significantly different from 71 ± 6 µmol/L in 20 healthy controls *2240*

HIV-1 p24 Antigen *Serum Increase* In 218 HIV-1 infected children mean concentration of 307 pg/mL *3544*

HIV-1 RNA *Serum Increase* In 218 HIV-1 infected children mean concentration of 105,247 copies/mL *3544* In 47 HIV-1 infected men median concentration of 4.73 log copies/mL *5840*

HIV p24 Antibody *Serum Increase* In 218 HIV-1 infected children concentrations ranged from < 1 (undetectable) to 390,625 RTU (median concentration at baseline 3.8 RTU and mean 16.6 RTU). In 35% patients at baseline concentrations were undetectable, between 1 - 4 RTU in 15%, between 5 - 124 RTU in 23% and above 125 RTU in 27% children *3544*

HIV p24 Antigen *Serum Increase* In 7 of 15 patients who were p24 antigen positive relative risk of progressing to AIDS 2.96% and in 15 of 95 patients who were p24 antigen negative no relative risk *5831*

Homocysteine *Plasma Increase* B_{12} concentration reduced to below 132 pmol/L in 61 of 200 patients (30.3%) with HIV-1 virus, with significantly increased homocysteine concentration of 9.09 µmol/L in these patients compared with 7.35 µmol/L in those without B_{12} deficiency *3985*

Homovanillic Acid *Cerebrospinal Fluid Increase* In 14 patients with HIV-1 infection median pretreatment concentration of 38 ng/mL compared with reference interval of 25 - 73 ng/mL increased by 15% after 3 - 30 months treatment *1742*
Cerebrospinal Fluid No Effect In 14 patients with HIV-1 infection median pretreatment concentration of 38 ng/mL compared with reference interval of 25 - 73 ng/mL *1742*

4-Hydroxy-3-Methoxy-Phenylglycol
Cerebrospinal Fluid No Effect In 14 patients with HIV-1 infection median pretreatment concentration of 6.4 ng/mL compared with reference interval of 6.0 - 16 ng/mL *1742*

25-Hydroxy Vitamin D_2 *Serum No Effect* In 54 patients with HIV-1 infection median concentration of 70.1 pmol/L not significantly different from reference values of 50 - 90 pmol/L *2063*

5-Hydroxyindoleacetic Acid *Cerebrospinal Fluid No Effect* In 14 patients with HIV-1 infection median pretreatment concentration of 20 ng/mL compared with reference interval of 13 - 42 ng/mL *1742*

42.10 **HIV-1 Infection** *(continued)*

5-Hydroxytryptamine *Blood* *No Effect* In 14 patients with HIV-1 infection median pretreatment concentration of 199 ng/mL compared with reference interval of 97 - 374 ng/mL *1742* In 14 patients with HIV-1 infection median pretreatment concentration of 199 ng/mL compared with reference interval of 97 - 374 ng/mL and concentration increased by 7.8% after 3 - 14 months treatment and decreased by 1.8% after 14 - 30 months treatment *1742*

IgG Index *Cerebrospinal Fluid* *Increase* In 9 of 14 patients with HIV-1 infection pretreatment concentration increased above upper limit of 0.7 *1742*

Immunoglobulin E *Serum* *Increase* Mean baseline concentration of 136.3 ng/mL in 20 asymptomatic patients and 9 with ARC not significantly different from that in healthy controls, although one patient had a concentration of 2,400 ng/mL *3389*
Serum *No Effect* Mean baseline concentration of 136.3 ng/mL in 20 asymptomatic patients and 9 with ARC not significantly different from that in healthy controls, although one patient had a concentration of 2,400 ng/mL *3389*

Immunoglobulin G *Cerebrospinal Fluid* *Increase* In 4 patients with HIV-infection mean concentration of 224 ± 190 mg/L not significantly higher than 21 ± 4.6 mg/L in 5 controls *429*

Intercellular Adhesion Molecule-1 *Serum* *Increase* In 53 HIV-positive patients with lymphadenopathy mean concentration of 473 ± 33 ng/mL, in 8 patients with ARC 538 ± 111 ng/mL and in 85 with AIDS 601 ± 32 ng/mL compared with 288 ± 16 ng/mL in 50 HIV-negative controls *4303*

Interleukin-4 *Serum* *No Effect* No significant difference observed between concentrations in 23 HIV-infected and 21 uninfected children *4288*

Interleukin-6 *Cerebrospinal Fluid* *Increase* Proinflammatory cytokines expressed in CSF of HIV-infected patients with symptoms of AIDS *5172*
Serum *Increase* Concentration significantly increased in 23 HIV infected children compared with that in 21 uninfected children *4288*
Serum *No Effect* In 10 HIV-1 infected patients without symptoms mean concentration of 7.3 ± 2.4 pg/mL not significantly different from that in 10 healthy individuals *1080* No significant difference observed between concentrations in 23 HIV-infected and 21 uninfected children *4288*

Interleukin-8 *Serum* *Increase* Mean concentration and 95% confidence interval of 275 (216 - 349) pg/mL in 36 HIV-infected individuals compared with 8 (4 - 14) pg/mL in 32 matched controls *3368* Concentration in 6 of 49 patients with stage II HIV-1, 2 of 20 stage III patients and 3 of 23 stage IV patients significantly higher than mean ± 2 SD of 2.25 ± 0.9 pg/mL in 20 healthy controls *2187*

ionized Calcium *Serum* *Decrease* In 54 patients with HIV-1 infection median concentration of 1.19 mmol/L significantly different from reference values of 1.23 - 1.27 mmol/L *2063*

Isoleucine *Plasma* *No Effect* In 20 HIV-infected individuals mean concentration of 64 ± 15 µmol/L not significantly different from 69 ± 20 µmol/L in 20 healthy controls *2240*

Isoniazid *Serum* *No Effect* In 12 asymptomatic HIV-infected patients mean maximum concentration of 6.01 µg/mL and 6.06 µg/mL in 12 patients with symptomatic HIV infection not significantly different when compared with 5.97 µg/mL in 12 healthy volunteers *4513*

LDL-Cholesterol *Serum* *Decrease* Median plasma concentration in 63 patients with HIV infection (34 asymptomatic) of 94 mg/dL (2.43 mmol/L). 35 of 63 (55.6%) had concentrations less than 100 mg/dL (2.26 mmol/L) *5839*

Leucine *Plasma* *Decrease* In wasting syndrome associated with HIV-1 infection significantly decreased concentration observed *3675*
Plasma *No Effect* In 20 HIV-infected individuals mean concentration of 123 ± 28 µmol/L not significantly different from 131 ± 31 µmol/L in 20 healthy controls *2240*

Leukocytes *Blood* *Decrease* B_{12} concentration reduced to below 132 pmol/L in 61 of 200 patients (30.3%) with HIV-1 virus, with significantly decreased WBC of 4,360 /µL in these patients compared with 5,070 /µL in those without B_{12} deficiency *3985* Counts of > 1,250 /µL predicted the absence of AIDS in 90% HIV-infected patients *4186*
Blood *No Effect* In 260 intravenous drug users with HIV1-infection median concentration of 5.0 x 10^3/L not significantly different from normal range of 4.8 - 10.8 x 10^3/L *69*

Lipase *Serum* *Increase* 18.5% of 76 HIV-positive patients had increased activity greater than 70 U/L (mean 147 U/L) *173* Activity increased in 7 of 47 HIV-infected children *705*

Luteinizing Hormone *Plasma* *Increase* Mean concentration in 18 male patients with HIV infection but without wasting of 7.28 ± 1.10 mIU/mL higher than in 14 patients with HIV infection and wasting 5.63 ± 1.35 mIU/mL and normal range of 0 - 6.5 mIU/mL *912*

Lymphocytes *Blood* *Decrease* In 20 patients with HIV infection mean concentration of 1,840 x 10^6/L less than 2,430 x 10^6/L in 20 healthy controls *5266* In 1,042 hospitalized patients with lymphocytopenia 13 had HIV infection *730*

Lysine *Plasma* *Increase* Mean concentration of 225 ± 37 µmol/L in 20 HIV-infected individuals significantly higher than 173 ± 35 µmol/L in 20 healthy controls *2240*

Macroamylase *Serum* *Increase* In 163 (149 men, 14 women) consecutive asymptomatic HIV-infected outpatients of whom only 6 were receiving dideoxyinosine, known to cause pancreatitis, 39 (24%) had increased serum amylase activity. In 5 patients (13%) the increase was due to macroamylase *1525*

Macrophage Inflammatory Protein-1α *Serum* *No Effect* Median concentration in 4 patients with early HIV-infection of 36.1 pg/mL and 35.5 pg/mL in late infection within the normal range of < 46.9 pg/mL *3420*

Macrophage Inflammatory Protein-1β *Serum* *No Effect* Median concentration in 4 patients with early HIV-infection 78.5 pg/mL and 69.8 pg/mL in late infection within the normal range of < 200 pg/mL *3420*

Magnesium *Serum* *No Effect* In 54 patients with HIV-1 infection median concentration of 0.80 mmol/L not significantly different from reference values of 0.80 - 0.90 mmol/L *2063*

MCV *Blood* *Increase* B_{12} concentration reduced to below 132 pmol/L in 61 of 200 patients (30.3%) with HIV-1 virus, with significantly increased MCV of 99.6 fL in these patients compared with 95.4 fL in those without B_{12} deficiency *3985*

Methionine *Plasma* *Decrease* In 20 HIV-infected individuals mean concentration of 19 ± 6 µmol/L significantly less than 28 ± 8 µmol/L in 20 healthy controls *2240* In wasting syndrome associated with HIV-1 infection significantly decreased concentration observed *3675*

$β_2$-Microglobulin *Serum* *Increase* In 198 seroconverters intermediate tercile concentration of 1.40 - 1.72 mg/dL prior to seroconversion and change to 1.86 - 2.42 mg/dL with seroconversion *4787* In 25 HIV-positive asymptomatic patients median concentration of 2.9 mg/L significantly greater than median of 1.6 mg/L in 78 healthy controls *3816* In 250 intravenous drug users with HIV1-infection median concentration of 4.9 mg/dL significantly increased compared with normal range of 0 - 2 mg/dL *69* In 47 HIV-1 infected men median concentration of 3.3 mg/L *5840* 45 of 63 (71.4%) of patients with HIV infection (34 asymptomatic) had concentrations greater than the upper limit of normal of 2.5 mg/L *5839* In 21 of 66 patients with concentration > 3.0 mg/L relative risk of progressing to AIDS 6.79% and in 3 of 64 patients with concentrations < 3.0 mg/L no relative risk *5831*

Monocytes *Blood* *No Effect* In 13 asymptomatic HIV-positive patients median concentration of 572 /µL not significantly different from median of 493 /µL in 19 healthy controls *3816*

Neopterin *Cerebrospinal Fluid* *Increase* In 14 patients with HIV-1 infection median pretreatment concentration of 15.2 nmol/L compared with reference interval of < 4.2 nmol/L *1742*
Serum *Increase* In 26 asymptomatic HIV-1 positive patients mean concentration of 2.81 ± 1.39 ng/mL was greatly increased compared with concentration in 31 patients with non-immune neurological diseases (1.40 ± 1.29 ng/mL) and 0.84 ± 0.25 ng/mL in 26 normal controls *2092* In 47 HIV-1 infected men median concentration of 12.7 nmol/L *5840* In 19 asymptomatic HIV-1 infected patients median concentration of 19.4 nmol/L compared with 8.2 nmol/L in 19 healthy controls *3826* Higher concentrations are associated with more rapid development of AIDS *121* In 14 patients with HIV-1 infection median pretreatment concentration of 19.0 nmol/L compared with reference interval of < 8.4 nmol/L *1742* In 198 seroconverters intermediate tercile concentration of 6.17 - 8.50 nmol/L prior to seroconversion and change to 9.04 - 12.90 nmol/L with seroconversion *4787*

Urine *Increase* 60 of 63 patients with HIV infection (34 asymptomatic) had concentrations greater than the upper limit of normal of 200 µmol/mol creatinine *5839*

Nitrite *Serum* *Increase* Mean concentration of 36.2 ± 26.2 µmol/L in 9 patients with pulmonary involvement, significantly different from 0.1 ± 0.1 µmol/L in 21 healthy volunteer controls *5258*
Serum *No Effect* Mean concentration of 0.4 ± 0.5 µmol/L in 10 asymptomatic patients, 0.2 ± 0.3 µmol/L in 12 patients with HIV-1 encephalopathy, 0.7 ± 0.3 µmol/L in 4 patients with cytomegalovirus retinitis and 0.4 ± µmol/L in 4 patients with lymphoma not significantly different from 0.1 ± 0.1 µmol/L in 21 healthy volunteer controls *5258*

Ornithine *Plasma* *Increase* Mean concentration of 121 ± 38 µmol/L in 20 HIV-infected individuals nonsignificantly higher than 94 ± 22 µmol/L in 20 healthy controls *2240*

Parathyroid Hormone *Plasma* *Decrease* In 54 patients with HIV-1 infection median concentration of 2.00 pmol/L significantly different from reference values of 1.99 - 3.67 pmol/L *2063*

Phenylalanine *Plasma* *No Effect* In 20 HIV-infected individuals mean concentration of 57 ± 14 µmol/L not significantly different from 56 ± 16 µmol/L in 20 healthy controls *2240*

Phosphate *Serum* *No Effect* In 54 patients with HIV-1 infection median concentration of 1.10 mmol/L not significantly different from reference values of 1.06 - 1.31 mmol/L *2063*

Plasmin-α_2-Plasmin Inhibitor Complex *Plasma* *Increase* In 20 patients with HIV infection median concentration of 438 ng/mL higher than 325 ng/mL in 20 healthy controls *5266*

Plasminogen *Plasma* *Increase* In 20 patients with HIV infection median concentration of 1.07 ± 0.18 U/mL higher than 0.94 ± 0.11 U/mL in 20 healthy controls *5266*

Platelets *Blood* *Decrease* In 30,214 patients with HIV infection one year incidence of platelet counts less than 50,000 /µL was 3.7% and was associated with stage of disease *5076* In 20 patients with HIV infection mean concentration of 231 x 10^9/L not significantly less than 235 x 10^9/L in 20 healthy controls *5266*
Blood *No Effect* In 260 intravenous drug users with HIV1-infection median concentration of 205.5 x 10^3/L not significantly different from normal range of 130 - 400 x 10^3/L *69*

Prealbumin *Serum* *Decrease* In 54 patients with HIV-1 infection median concentration of 0.21 g/L significantly different from reference values of 0.26 - 0.34 g/L *2063*

Prolactin *Plasma* *Increase* In 14 male patients with HIV infection and wasting mean concentration of 21.2 ± 3.8 ng/mL higher than 9.9 ± 3.4 ng/mL in 18 patients with HIV infection but no wasting and normal range of 0 - 20 ng/mL *912*

Protein *Cerebrospinal Fluid* *Increase* In 5 patients seropositive for HIV mean concentration of 0.89 ± 0.46 g/L not significantly higher than 0.21 ± 0.06 g/L in 7 controls *429*

Protein S Antigen *Plasma* *Decrease* In 35 patients with HTLV-1 infection mean concentration significantly less than in healthy controls: Effect most marked when CD4+ counts < 100 cells/µL *4943*

Protein S, Functional *Plasma* *Decrease* In 35 HIV-1 infected patients concentration significantly less than in control population: effect most marked in individuals in whom CD+ count < 100 cells/µL *4943*

Pyrazinamide *Serum* *Decrease* In 12 asymptomatic HIV-infected patients mean maximum concentration of 25.0 µg/mL and 25.0 µg/mL in 12 patients with symptomatic HIV infection markedly different when compared with 29.2 µg/mL in 12 healthy volunteers *4513*

RANTES *Serum* *No Effect* Median concentration in 4 patients with early HIV-infection 28.4 ng/mL and 35.1 ng/mL in late infection within the normal range of 24.2 - 85.9 ng/mL *3420*

Rifampin *Serum* *Decrease* In 12 asymptomatic HIV-infected patients mean maximum concentration of 5.92 µg/mL and 5.30 µg/mL in 12 patients with symptomatic HIV infection markedly different when compared with 9.29 µg/mL in 12 healthy volunteers *4513*

S-100b Protein *Cerebrospinal Fluid* *Increase* Mean concentration of 2.16 ± 3.4 ng/mL in 106 HIV-infected patients significantly different from 0.22 ± 0.08 ng/mL in 30 healthy controls *1856*

Selenium *Serum* *Decrease* In wasting syndrome associated with HIV-1 infection significantly decreased concentration observed *3675* In 11% of 70 asymptomatic HIV positive men concentration below 85 µg/L *3285* In 57 HIV-infected patients mean concentration of 58.7 ± 12.2 µg/L in 18 patients with CDC stage II and 47.6 ± 11.3 µg/L in 19 patients with stage III disease significantly different from 80.6 ± 9.6 µg/L in 48 healthy controls *3116*
Serum *Increase* 66% of 70 asymptomatic HIV positive men had normal selenium concentrations but 23% had a high concentration (greater than 120 µg/L) and 11% had a low concentration (less than 85 µg/L) *3285*

Serine *Plasma* *No Effect* Mean concentration of 117 ± 25 µmol/L in 20 HIV-infected individuals mean nonsignificantly greater than 103 ± 26 µmol/L in 20 healthy controls *2240*

Sex-Hormone Binding Globulin *Serum* *No Effect* Mean concentration of 1.59 ± 0.18 µg/dL in 14 males with HIV infection and wasting not significantly different from 1.05 ± 0.15 µg/dL in 18 HIV-infected but not wasted patients and normal range of 0.5 - 1.5 µg/dL *912*

Sodium *Serum* *Decrease* Hyponatremia observed in 31 - 58% positive patients and is associated with a high mortality *268*

Soluble CD4+ *Serum* *Increase* In 25 HIV-positive asymptomatic patients median concentration of 21.3 U/mL significantly greater than median of 7.6 U/mL in 78 healthy controls *3816*

Soluble CD8+ *Serum* *Increase* In 25 HIV-positive asymptomatic patients median concentration of 1,439 U/mL significantly greater than median of 555 U/mL in 78 healthy controls *3816*

Soluble CD14+ *Serum* *Increase* In 25 HIV-positive asymptomatic patients with lymphadenopathy mean concentration of 2.9 ± 0.8 mg/L significantly greater than median of 2.2 ± 0.47 mg/L in 78 healthy controls *3816* Mean concentrations in patients with CDC grades A and B of about 3 µg/mL higher than mean of about 2 µg/mL in controls *3048*

Soluble CD35+ *Serum* *Increase* In 18 HIV-positive asymptomatic homosexuals mean concentration of 46.4 ± 2.4 ng/mL, in 54 HIV-positive patients with lymphadenopathy mean concentration of 51.5 ± 2.0 ng/mL all significantly greater than 41.9 ± 1.9 ng/mL in 39 healthy controls, in 8 with ARC 50.3 ± 8.6 ng/mL (not significantly increased) *4302*

Soluble CD71+ *Serum* *No Effect* In 19 HIV-positive homosexuals, and 54 patients with lymphadenopathy, mean concentrations of 2,125 ± 134 ng/mL, and 2,270 ± 138 ng/mL not significantly different from 2,308 ± 147 ng/mL in 39 normal controls *4302*

Soluble E-Selectin *Serum* *Increase* In 19 asymptomatic HIV-1 infected patients median concentration of 56.1 ng/mL compared with 47.7 ng/mL in 19 healthy controls *3826*

Soluble HLA-I *Serum* *Increase* Concentration reportedly increased with viral infections including HIV-1 infection *5306*

Soluble Intercellular Adhesion Molecule-1
Cerebrospinal Fluid *Increase* In 110 HIV-1 positive patients mean concentration of 6.5 ± 6.1 ng/mL was greatly increased compared with concentration in 40 patients with non-immune neurological diseases of (1.3 ± 1.2 ng/mL). In 95 patients with HIV-1 associated neurological diseases mean concentration of 6.9 ± 6.4 ng/mL significantly higher than 3.5 ± 2.1 ng/mL in 15 patients without neurological involvement *2092*
Serum *Increase* In 136 HIV-1 positive patients mean concentration of 542.3 ± 187.9 ng/mL was greatly increased compared with concentration in HIV-negative controls and that in 26 healthy laboratory workers, mean concentration of 268.0 ± 70.9 ng/mL. This was true both for 110 symptomatic HIV-1 positive patients (565.3 ± 196.1 ng/mL) and 26 asymptomatic patients (444.7 ± 103.9 ng/mL) *2092* Range of concentrations in 108 patients with HIV-1 infections on admission to hospital of 419 - 2,399 ng/mL significantly different from 360 - 943 ng/mL in 43 controls *1625* In 19 asymptomatic HIV-1 infected patients median concentration of 537 ng/mL compared with 243 ng/mL in 19 healthy controls *3826*

Soluble Intercellular Adhesion Molecule-2 *Serum* *Increase* Range of concentrations in 132 patients with HIV-1 infections on admission to hospital of 139 - 1,955 AU significantly different from 194 - 615 AU in 52 controls *1625*

Soluble Intercellular Adhesion Molecule-3 *Serum* *Increase* Range of concentrations in 100 patients with HIV-1 infections on admission to hospital of 60 - 3,311 AU significantly different from 44 - 292 AU in 52 controls *1625*

Soluble Tumor Necrosis Factor Receptor-II
Serum *Increase* In 42 adults with HIV-infection prior to treatment for aphthous ulcers mean concentration of 3.7 ng/mL significantly greater than 2.1 ± 0.7 pg/mL in healthy controls *2393*

42.10 **HIV-1 Infection** *(continued)*

Soluble Tumor Necrosis Factor Receptor-II *(continued)*
In 23 asymptomatic patients mean concentration of 5.20 ± 1.75 ng/mL compared with mean concentration of 2.83 ± 0.70 ng/mL in 20 healthy controls with higher concentrations in patients with more advanced disease *2186* In 26 patients of CDC group A1 mean concentration of 12.6 ± 10.5 ng/mL, 5.4 ± 2.5 ng/mL in 29 of group A2, 12.4 ± 6 ng/mL in 14 of group B2 and 7.42 ± 3 ng/mL in 26 of group B2 compared with 2.83 ± 0.70 ng/mL in 20 healthy volunteer controls *2185*

Soluble Tumor Necrosis Factor Receptor-p75
Serum Decrease In 47 HIV-1 infected men median concentration of 6.7 ng/mL *5840*
Serum Increase Mean concentration in 25 patients with stage IIA HIV-1 of 5.23 ± 0.30 ng/mL and 6.05 ± 0.51 ng/mL in 24 patients with stage IIB patients significantly higher than 2.83 ± 0.15 ng/mL in 20 healthy controls *2187* 55 of 63 (87.3%) of patients with HIV infection (34 asymptomatic) had concentrations greater than the upper limit of normal of 4.8 ng/mL *5839*

Soluble Vascular Cell Adhesion Molecule-1
Serum Increase Range of concentrations in 100 patients with HIV-1 infections on admission to hospital of 447 - 2,812 ng/mL significantly different from 532 - 2,352 ng/mL in 52 controls *1625* In 19 asymptomatic HIV-1 infected patients median concentration of 903 ng/mL compared with 515 ng/mL in 19 healthy controls *3826*

Tau Protein *Cerebrospinal Fluid No Effect* Mean concentration of 57.2 ± 10.5 ng/L in 21 patients with HIV-1 infection (12 with AIDS dementia) not significantly different from that in healthy controls, 51.1 ± 7.3 ng/L *1546*

Taurine *Plasma Decrease* In wasting syndrome associated with HIV-1 infection significantly decreased concentration observed *3675*
Plasma Increase Mean concentration of 155 ± 63 µmol/L in 20 HIV-infected individuals significantly higher than 47 ± 11 µmol/L in 20 healthy controls *2240*

Testosterone *Serum Decrease* Mean concentration in 14 male patients with HIV infection and wasting of 277.4 ± 80.4 ng/dL compared with 546.3 ± 64.7 ng/dL in 18 patients with HIV infection but no wasting and normal range of 311 - 879 ng/dL *912*

Testosterone, Free *Serum Decrease* In 14 patients with HIV infection and wasting mean concentration of 44.0 ± 14.6 pg/mL less than 89.8 ± 12.1 pg/mL in 18 patients with HIV infection but no wasting and normal range of 52 - 280 pg/mL *912*

Threonine *Plasma Decrease* Mean concentration of 121 ± 34 µmol/L in 20 HIV-infected individuals not significantly different from 134 ± 41 µmol/L in 20 healthy controls *2240*

Thyroid Stimulating Hormone *Serum Increase* In 14 HIV positive patients with wasting mean concentration of 3.67 ± 0.63 mU/mL and 3.07 ± 0.54 mU/mL in 18 patients without wasting compared with normal range of 0.35 - 7.00 mU/mL *912*

Thyroxine Binding Globulin *Serum Increase* Increased concentration has been reported *268*
Serum No Effect In 14 patients with HIV infection and wasting mean concentration of 3.60 ± 0.39 mg/dL and 3.45 ± 0.33 mg/dL in 18 HIV positive patients without wasting compared with normal range of 1.8 - 4.2 mg/dL *912*

Thyroxine (T4) *Serum No Effect* In 14 HIV positive patients with wasting mean concentration of 7.3 ± 0.6 µg/dL and 7.6 ± 0.6 µg/dL in 18 HIV positive patients without wasting compared with normal range of 4 ± 12 µg/dL *912*

Thyroxine (T4), Free *Serum No Effect* Mean concentration of 0.986 ± 0.056 ng/dL in 14 patients with HIV infection and wasting and of 1.000 ± 0.048 ng/dL in 18 HIV positive patients without wasting compared with normal range of 0.71 - 1.85 ng/dL *912*

Tri-iodothyronine, Reverse (rT3) *Serum Decrease*
Reduced concentration described in association with HIV infection *268*
Serum No Effect In 14 HIV positive patients with wasting mean concentration of 21.0 ± 1.9 ng/dL and 16.7 ± 1.6 ng/dL in 18 patients with HIV infection but without wasting compared with normal range of 10 - 50 ng/dL *912*

Tri-iodothyronine (T3) *Serum No Effect* In 14 HIV positive patients with wasting mean concentration of 139.8 ± 10.0 mg/dL and 136.1 ± 10.0 mg/dL in 18 patients with HIV infection without wasting compared with normal range of 80 - 220 mg/dL *912*

Triglycerides *Serum Increase* Median plasma concentration in 63 patients with HIV infection (34 asymptomatic) of 146 mg/dL (1.65 mmol/L). 20 of 63 (31.7%) had concentrations greater than 170 mg/dL (1.92 mmol/L) the upper limit of normal *5839*

Tryptophan *Cerebrospinal Fluid Decrease* In 14 patients with HIV-1 infection median pretreatment concentration of 224 ng/mL significantly less than reference interval of 371 - 513 ng/mL *1742*
Plasma Decrease In wasting syndrome associated with HIV-1 infection significantly decreased concentration observed *3675* In 14 patients with HIV-1 infection median pretreatment blood tryptophan concentration of 6.0 µg/mL at lower limit of reference interval of 6.0 - 11 µg/mL *1742* In 20 HIV-infected individuals mean concentration of 22 ± 12 µmol/L significantly less than 46 ± 22 µmol/L in 20 healthy controls *2240*

Tumor Necrosis Factor-α *Serum Increase* In 54 patients with HIV-1 infection median concentration of 24.6 pg/mL significantly different from reference values of 0 - 10 pg/mL *2063* In 19 asymptomatic HIV-1 infected patients median concentration of 14.9 pg/mL compared with undetectable amount in 19 healthy controls *3826* In 42 adults with HIV-infection prior to treatment for aphthous ulcers mean concentration of 37.0 pg/mL significantly greater than 9.5 ± 5.7 pg/mL in healthy controls *2393* Increased concentration observed in 3 of 5 patients with HIV-associated body wasting *2909* In 23 HIV infected children concentration significantly increased compared with concentration in 21 uninfected children *4288*

Tyrosine *Plasma Decrease* In 20 HIV-infected individuals mean concentration of 50 ± 13 µmol/L nonsignificantly less than 65 ± 18 µmol/L in 20 healthy controls *2240*

Urea Nitrogen *Serum Increase* In 3 of 52 patients with HIV-infection (6%) with increased pancreatic enzyme activity renal failure also observed *173*

Uroporphyrin *Urine Increase* In 7 of 23 patients with HIV infection mean concentration ranged from 13 to 4,608 nmol/mmol creatinine significantly different from mean of 4 ± 3 nmol/mmol creatinine in normal controls *3633*

Valine *Plasma Decrease* In wasting syndrome associated with HIV-1 infection significantly decreased concentration observed *3675*
Plasma No Effect Mean concentration of 208 ± 43 µmol/L in 20 HIV-infected individuals not significantly different from 216 ± 33 µmol/L in 20 healthy controls *2240*

Vitamin A *Serum No Effect* In wasting syndrome associated with HIV-1 infection no significant difference in concentration observed *3675*

Vitamin B_{12} *Serum Decrease* Concentration reduced to below 132 pmol/L in 61 of 200 patients (30.3%) with HIV-1 virus, without any patient showing evidence of anti-intrinsic factor antibodies *3985*

Vitamin D Binding Protein *Serum No Effect* In 54 patients with HIV-1 infection median concentration of 375 mg/L not significantly different from reference values of 339 - 431 mg/L *2063*

Vitamin E *Serum No Effect* In wasting syndrome associated with HIV-1 infection no significant difference in concentration observed *3675*

Zinc *Serum Decrease* In wasting syndrome associated with HIV-1 infection significantly decreased concentration observed *3675*
Serum No Effect In 54 patients with HIV-1 infection median concentration of 12.0 µmol/L not significantly different from reference values of 12.0 - 14.0 µmol/L *2063*

Viral Diseases of the CNS

45.90 **Acute Poliomyelitis**

Aldolase *Serum No Effect* Normal activities usually observed in patients with poliomyelitis *2952*

Aspartate Aminotransferase *Cerebrospinal Fluid Increase* Always increased but does not correlate with serum level or with severity of paralysis; reaches peak in 1 week and returns to normal by 4 weeks *5545*

Serum *Increase* A mild rise was reported in all 8 cases *3733*

Bicarbonate *Serum* *Increase* Respiratory acidosis may occur *1980*

Carbon Dioxide Partial Pressure *Blood* *Increase* Respiratory acidosis may occur *1980* Neurological impairment of the respiratory drive *5863*

Cells *Cerebrospinal Fluid* *Increase* Is usually 25 - 500 /µL. At first most are polymorphonuclear leukocytes; after several days most are lymphocytes *5545* Chiefly lymphocytes *1980*

Chloride *Cerebrospinal Fluid* *Decrease* 670 - 750 mg/dL *1980*

Cerebrospinal Fluid *No Effect* Concentration unaffected *5252*

Coproporphyrin *Urine* *Increase* Possibly derived from nervous system *1290*

Creatine *Urine* *Increase* Urinary creatine may be significantly increased in patients with poliomyelitis *2952* Increased formation; myopathy *5544*

Creatine Kinase *Serum* *Increase* Mild elevation was reported in 50% of 8 cases *3733*

γ-Globulin *Cerebrospinal Fluid* *Increase* Especially IgG *413*

Glucose *Cerebrospinal Fluid* *No Effect* Disease has no effect on CSF concentration *5252* Concentration usually unaffected by disease *1980*

β-Hexosaminidase *Serum* *Increase* Increase in total concentration (hexosaminidase A and B) *3850*

Immunoglobulin G *Cerebrospinal Fluid* *Increase* Normal or decreased *413*

Lactate Dehydrogenase *Serum* *Increase* Mild elevation was recorded in all 8 cases *3733*

Leukocytes *Blood* *Increase* Occasionally a mild leukocytosis is present *1980* Blood shows early moderate increase 15,000 /µL) *5545*

Cerebrospinal Fluid *Increase* Usually 25 - 500 /µL at first. Most are polymorphonuclear leukocytes; after several days most are lymphocytes *5545*

Lymphocytes *Blood* *Decrease* The numbers of circulating lymphocytes are sharply and regularly reduced *1579*

Cerebrospinal Fluid *Increase* Cell count is usually 25 - 500 /µL at first most are polymorphonuclear leukocytes; after several days most are lymphocytes *5545*

Neutrophils *Blood* *Increase* Occasionally a mild leukocytosis is present *1980*

Cerebrospinal Fluid *Increase* Is usually 25 - 500 /µL at first most are polymorphonuclear leukocytes; after several days most are lymphocytes *5545*

Oxygen Partial Pressure *Blood* *Decrease* Neurological impairment of the respiratory drive *5863*

pH *Blood* *Decrease* Respiratory acidosis may occur *1980*

Protein *Cerebrospinal Fluid* *Increase* Often progressive increase *1980* Initial values usually fall within range of 25 - 150 mg/dL. Characteristically modest elevations are found during the first week after onset of CNS symptoms. Levels tend to decrease toward the 10th day, but may increase again in a secondary stage (100 - 400 mg/dL) in the 3rd and 4th weeks *900* May be high *5252*

46.10 Creutzfeldt-Jakob Disease

Amyloid β-Protein *Cerebrospinal Fluid* *Decrease* In 1 patient concentration was 0.81 pmol/mL significantly different from mean concentration of 4.00 ± 2.92 pmol/mL *3716*

α_1-Antichymotrypsin *Cerebrospinal Fluid* *Increase* In 1 patient concentration was 7.60 µg/mL significantly different from mean concentration of 2.27 ± 1.40 µg/mL in 25 normal controls *3716*

Cells *Cerebrospinal Fluid* *No Effect* In 1 patient concentration of 0.3 cells/µL not significantly different from normal of 3 cells/µL *3716*

Lactate *Cerebrospinal Fluid* *No Effect* Mean concentration of 1,672 ± 309 µmol/L in 2 patients with Creutzfeld-Jakob disease not significantly different from 1,850 ± 63 µmol/L in 20 controls without dementia *3823*

Protein *Cerebrospinal Fluid* *No Effect* In 1 patient concentration of 9 mg/dL not significantly different from normal of 28 mg/dL in 25 healthy controls *3716*

14-3-3 Protein *Serum* *Increase* Protein was detected in 95.4% of pathologically proved diseases but also was detected in some patients with suspected CJD *5854*

46.20 Subacute Sclerosing Panencephalitis

Oligoclonal Banding *Cerebrospinal Fluid* *Increase* Oligoclonal IgG bands detected with subacute sclerosing panencephalitis *3261*

47.00 Aseptic Meningitis

Adenosine Deaminase *Cerebrospinal Fluid* *Increase* In 62 patients with self-resolving aseptic meningitis median concentration of 2.7 U/L significantly different from 1 U/L in 117 individuals without meningitis *3122* In cases of aseptic meningitis activity greater than 4 U/L but less than 6 U/L compared with activity of less than 4 U/L in healthy controls *3244*

Amyloid A Protein *Serum* *Increase* In 21 patients mean concentration in acute phase of 1.49 ± 0.73 mg/L *3728*

Anti-Interferon-γ Autoantibodies

Cerebrospinal Fluid *Increase* Mean concentration of 0.068 ± 0.016 ng/mL in 15 patients with aseptic meningitis compared with 0.006 ± 0.005 ng/mL in 15 healthy adults *1333*

Serum *Increase* Mean concentration of 0.068 ± 0.016 ng/mL in 15 patients with aseptic meningitis compared with 0.006 ± 0.005 ng/mL in 15 healthy adults *1333*

Anti-Interleukin-4 Autoantibodies

Cerebrospinal Fluid *Increase* Mean concentration of 0.016 ± 0.0069 ng/mL in 15 patients with aseptic meningitis compared with 0.005 ± 0.004 ng/mL in 15 healthy adults *1333*

Serum *Decrease* Mean concentration of 0.05 ± 0.016 ng/mL in 15 patients with aseptic meningitis compared with 0.013 ± 0.007 ng/mL in 15 healthy adults *1333*

Anti-Interleukin-10 Autoantibodies

Cerebrospinal Fluid *Increase* Mean concentration of 0.42 ± 0.095 ng/mL in 15 patients with aseptic meningitis compared with 0.0048 ± 0.004 ng/mL in 15 healthy adults *1333*

Serum *Increase* Mean concentration of 0.13 ± 0.019 ng/mL in 15 patients with aseptic meningitis compared with 0.01 ± 0.006 ng/mL in 15 healthy adults *1333*

Anti-Tumor Necrosis Factor-α Autoantibodies

Cerebrospinal Fluid *Increase* Mean concentration of 0.69 ± 0.16 ng/mL in 15 patients with aseptic meningitis compared with 0.0046 ± 0.004 ng/mL in 15 healthy adults *1333*

Serum *Increase* Mean concentration of 0.178 ± 0.023 ng/mL in 15 patients with aseptic meningitis compared with 0.006 ± 0.005 ng/mL in 15 healthy adults *1333*

Cells *Cerebrospinal Fluid* *Increase* A pleocytosis of up to 3,000 /µL may occur. In the first day or two of illness, polymorphonuclears may predominate, but the cell differential then shifts to one predominantly of lymphocytes *2039*

C-Reactive Protein *Serum* *Increase* In 21 patients mean concentration in acute phase 0.71 ± 0.57 mg/L *3728*

Fibrin Degradation Products *Plasma* *Increase* Elevation is much more common in fatal cases than in survivors *4881*

Glucose *Cerebrospinal Fluid* *No Effect* In 20 patients with aseptic meningitis mean CSF/glucose ratio of 0 no different from 0 in 15 controls without neurological disorders *3123* Normal but may be depressed in mumps meningitis *1980*

Granulocyte-Macrophage Colony Stimulating Factor

Cerebrospinal Fluid *Increase* In 6 of 9 patients concentration above 40 pg/mL detected with range from 49 to 114 pg/mL *4804*

immunoglobulin A *Cerebrospinal Fluid* *Increase* Reported effect *1290*

Serum *Increase* IgA and IgG increased *1290*

Immunoglobulin G *Serum* *Increase* IgA and IgG increased *1290*

Immunoglobulins *Cerebrospinal Fluid* *Increase* IgA and IgG increased *1290*

Interleukin-6 *Cerebrospinal Fluid* *Increase* In 19 patients with CSF aseptic meningitis mean concentration of 1,076 ± 1,572 pg/mL significantly higher than upper limit of normal of 5

47.00 Aseptic Meningitis *(continued)*

Interleukin-6 *(continued)*
pg/mL in 21 control patients *3372* In 20 patients with aseptic meningitis mean concentration of 66 pg/mL greater than < 44 pg/mL in 15 controls without neurological disorders *3123*

Lactate Dehydrogenase *Cerebrospinal Fluid Increase* Invariably slightly elevated, with LD-1 and 2 the elevated isoenzymes *3757*

Lactate Dehydrogenase Isoenzymes
Cerebrospinal Fluid Increase Slight elevation of isoenzymes 1 and 2 invariably occurs *3757*

Leukocytes *Blood No Effect* Peripheral WBC count is generally within normal limits *1980*
Cerebrospinal Fluid Increase May increase from a few to > 1,000 /μL, mostly polymorphonuclears, in acute hemorrhagic encephalitis *367* In 20 patients with aseptic meningitis mean concentration of 130 x 10^9/L significantly greater than < 5 x 10^9/L in 15 controls without neurological disorders *3123* Count ranges from 50 - 300 /μL and rarely 2,000 /μL. Marked predominance of lymphocytes except in the earliest stage *1980* In 62 patients with self-resolving aseptic meningitis median concentration of 192 x 10^9/L significantly different from < 5 x 10^9/L in 117 individuals without meningitis *3122*

Lymphocytes *Cerebrospinal Fluid Increase* Count ranges from 50 - 300 /μL and rarely > 2,000 /μL. Marked predominance of lymphocytes except in the earliest stage *1980* After first day or two differential shifts to predominantly lymphocytes *2039* Increased in 50% of the patients *1585*

Neutrophils *Cerebrospinal Fluid Increase* May predominate in the early phase but these cells are also found in bacterial meningitis *900* In 20 patients with aseptic meningitis mean proportion of 2% greater than 0% in 15 controls without neurological disorders *3123*

Protein *Cerebrospinal Fluid Increase* In 20 patients with aseptic meningitis mean concentration of 74 mg/dL significantly greater than 16 mg/dL in 15 controls without neurological disorders *3123* Moderately elevated in acute hemorrhagic encephalitis *367* Often increased to 45 - 200 mg/dL *2039* In 62 patients with self-resolving aseptic meningitis median concentration of 440 mg/L significantly different from 220 mg/L in 117 individuals without meningitis *3122*

Tumor Necrosis Factor-α *Cerebrospinal Fluid Increase* Observed effect *3687*

47.00 Viral Meningitis

α_1-Acid Glycoprotein *Cerebrospinal Fluid Increase* In 30 patients with viral meningitis median concentration on first day of admission 8.10 mg/L *4001*
Serum Increase In 30 patients with viral meningitis median concentration on first day of admission 702 mg/L significantly different from 471 mg/L in 60 healthy controls *4001*

Adenosine Deaminase *Cerebrospinal Fluid Increase* In 29 patients with viral meningitis median concentration of 2.7 U/L significantly different from 1 U/L in 117 individuals without meningitis *3122*

Albumin *Cerebrospinal Fluid Increase* In 30 patients with viral meningitis median concentration on first day of admission 381 mg/L *4001* In 51 children with viral meningitis mean concentration of 570 mg/L *1690*

α_1-Antitrypsin *Cerebrospinal Fluid Increase* In 30 patients with viral meningitis median concentration on first day of admission of 13.9 mg/L *4001*
Serum Increase In 30 patients with viral meningitis median concentration on first day of admission of 1,760 mg/L significantly different from 1,630 mg/L in 60 healthy controls *4001*

Cells *Cerebrospinal Fluid Increase* In 51 children with viral meningitis mean concentration of 345 /mL *1690*

α_2-Ceruloplasmin *Cerebrospinal Fluid Increase* In 30 patients with viral meningitis median concentration on first day of admission of 3.51 mg/L *4001*
Serum Increase In 30 patients with viral meningitis median concentration on first day of admission of 369 mg/L significantly different from 254 mg/L in 60 healthy controls *4001*

C-Reactive Protein *Cerebrospinal Fluid Increase* In 30 patients with viral meningitis median concentration on first day of admission of 1.46 mg/L *4001*
Cerebrospinal Fluid No Effect In 9 patients with viral meningitis median concentration of 28 ng/mL (range of 0 - 147 ng/mL) compared with range of 0 - 128 ng/mL and median of 34 ng/mL in 24 control specimens *4987* Concentration not increased in comparison with controls *4988*
Serum Increase In 51 children with viral meningitis mean concentration of 13.9 mg/L *1690* In 30 patients with viral meningitis median concentration on first day of admission of 14.8 mg/L significantly different from 4.25 mg/L in 60 healthy controls *4001*

Glucose *Cerebrospinal Fluid Decrease* In 12 patients median concentration of 3.2 mmol/L (0.3 - 5.4) significantly lower than 3.6 mmol/L (1.7 - 13.3) in 84 controls *2045*
Cerebrospinal Fluid No Effect In 15 patients with viral meningitis mean CSF/serum ratio of 0 not different from 0 in 15 controls without neurological disorders *3123*

α_2-Haptoglobin *Cerebrospinal Fluid Increase* In 30 patients with viral meningitis median concentration on first day of admission 4.78 mg/L *4001*
Serum Increase In 30 patients with viral meningitis median concentration on first day of admission of 1,420 mg/L significantly different from 767 mg/L in 60 healthy controls *4001*

Interferon-γ *Cerebrospinal Fluid Increase* Detected in CSF of patients with viral meningitis at higher concentration than in bacterial meningitis *5172 5172*

Interferon-γ-inducible Protein-10
Cerebrospinal Fluid Increase Increased concentration characteristic of viral meningitis *5172*

Interferon-inducible T-cell α Chemokine
Cerebrospinal Fluid Increase Increased concentration characteristic of viral meningitis *5172*

Interleukin-1 *Cerebrospinal Fluid Increase* Detected in CSF of patients with viral meningitis but at lower concentration than in bacterial meningitis *5172*

Interleukin-6 *Cerebrospinal Fluid Increase* Detected in CSF of patients with viral meningitis at similar concentration to that in bacterial meningitis *5172* In 6 patients with proved viral meningitis concentrations ranged from 1.09 to 12.5 ng/mL compared with 0.04 to 2.65 ng/mL in controls *2054* In 12 patients median concentration of 1.18 ng/mL (0.097 - 12.5) significantly higher than 0.37 ng/mL (0.04 - 12.5) in 111 controls *2045* In 15 patients with viral meningitis mean concentration of 186 pg/mL greater than < 40 pg/mL in 15 controls without neurological disorders *3123* Concentration significantly increased in patients with acute viral meningitis *4988* In 7 patients concentrations ranged from 115 to 1,700 mg/mL (median 820 pg/mL) significantly higher than median of less than 3 pg/mL in healthy controls *4987*
Serum Increase In 51 children with viral meningitis mean concentration of 82.5 pg/mL *1690*

Interleukin-10 *Cerebrospinal Fluid Increase* Detected in CSF of patients with viral meningitis where increased concentration may persist for several days *5172*

Lactate *Cerebrospinal Fluid Increase* In 5 patients median concentration of 3.34 mmol/L (0.06 - 6.32) higher than 1.75 mmol/L (1.15 - 6.62) in 42 controls *2045*

Leukocytes *Cerebrospinal Fluid Increase* In 9 patients with viral meningitis leukocyte counts ranged from 8 to 526 /μL compared with < 5 /μL in normals. In 3 of 24 controls leukocyte count increased from 12 to 37 /μL *4987* In 29 patients with viral meningitis median concentration of 130 x 10^9/L significantly different from < 5 x 10^9/L in 117 individuals without meningitis *3122* In 15 patients with viral meningitis mean concentration of 236 x 10^9/L significantly greater than < 5 x 10^9/L in 15 controls without neurological disorders *3123* In 30 patients with viral meningitis median concentration on first day of admission of 117 /μL *4001*

α_1-Microglobulin *Cerebrospinal Fluid Increase* Of 17 patients with viral meningitis mean concentration in 10 greater than that in 15 healthy controls of 34.8 ± 16.0 μg/L *2370*

Monokine induced by Interferon-γ
Cerebrospinal Fluid Increase Increased concentration characteristic of viral meningitis *5172*

Nerve Growth Factor *Cerebrospinal Fluid Increase* Concentration increased (mean 8.5 ± 6.8 pg/mL) in 7 of 14 patients with viral meningitis or encephalitis *5091*

Neutrophils *Cerebrospinal Fluid Increase* In 15 patients with viral meningitis mean proportion of 1% greater than 0% in 15 controls without neurological disorders *3123*

Oligoclonal Banding *Cerebrospinal Fluid Increase* Oligoclonal IgG bands detected with viral meningitis (herpes, mumps, HIV, etc.) *3261*

Procalcitonin *Plasma Increase* In 51 children with viral meningitis mean concentration of 0.32 µg/L compared with a normal range of < 0.1 µg/L in the neonatal period *1690*

Protein *Cerebrospinal Fluid Increase* In 30 patients with viral meningitis median concentration on first day of admission 860 mg/L *4001* In 15 patients with viral meningitis mean concentration of 55 mg/dL greater than 16 mg/dL in 15 controls without neurological disorders *3123* In 29 patients with viral meningitis median concentration of 610 mg/L significantly different from 220 mg/L in 117 individuals without meningitis *3122* In 9 patients with viral meningitis concentration ranged from 0.3 - 3.03 g/L compared with < 0.4 g/L in healthy controls (although 3 control patients had raised concentrations from 0.46 - 1.01 g/L) *4987* In 10 patients median concentration of 0.67 g/L (0.24 - 1.22) significantly higher than 0.37 g/L (0.15 - 1.33) in 93 controls *2045*

β-Trace Protein *Cerebrospinal Fluid No Effect* In 12 patients with viral meningitis mean concentration of 17.9 ± 2.9 mg/L not significantly different from 16.6 ± 3.6 mg/L in 27 normal controls *5323*

Tumor Necrosis Factor *Cerebrospinal Fluid Increase* Small and variable increases in concentration observed in acute viral meningitis *4988* Concentration significantly increased in patients with acute infection compared with controls *4988*

Tumor Necrosis Factor-α *Cerebrospinal Fluid Increase* Detected in CSF of patients with viral meningitis but at lower concentration than in bacterial meningitis *5172* In 6 of 9 patients TNF-α detected with concentratons ranging from 16 to 231 U/mL (median 24 U/mL) compared with less than 10 U/mL in 22 of 24 control patients *4987*

Tumor Necrosis Factor-β *Cerebrospinal Fluid Increase* Detected in CSF of patients with viral meningitis where increased concentration may persist for several days *5172*

48.00 Viral Meningoencephalitis

Albumin Index *Cerebrospinal Fluid Increase* Range in 28 patients with viral meningoencephalitis of 2.4 - 27.4 significantly different from mean of 4.0 in 33 normal controls *3019*

Soluble Intercellular Adhesion Molecule-1
Cerebrospinal Fluid Increase Range in 28 patients with viral meningoencephalitis of 1.1 - 22.9 ng/mL significantly different from mean of 1.51 ng/mL in 33 normal controls *3019*
Serum No Effect Range in 28 patients with viral meningoencephalitis of 144.6 - 533.3 ng/mL not significantly different from mean of 285.1 ng/mL in 33 normal controls *3019*

49.00 Lymphocytic Choriomeningitis

Complement Fixation *Serum Increase* Develops within 2 - 4 weeks *5252 2192*

γ-Globulin *Cerebrospinal Fluid Increase* May be found in the 2nd week *5252*

Glucose *Cerebrospinal Fluid No Effect* Normal or low normal *5252*

Leukocytes *Blood Decrease* Moderate leukopenia *5252*
Blood No Effect Usually within normal limits in all types *5252*

Lymphocytes *Blood Increase* Relative lymphocytosis *5252*
Cerebrospinal Fluid Increase Cell count is between 50 - 3,500 /µL, 80 - 95% lymphocytes *5252* 100 - 3,000 /µL, occasionally up to 30,000 /µL *5545*

Neutralizing Antibodies *Serum Increase* Appear within 6 - 10 weeks and persist longer than do CF antibodies *5252 2192*

Protein *Cerebrospinal Fluid Increase* Total concentration may be high *5252*

49.80 HTLV-1 associated Myelopathy

Anti-Neutrophil Cytoplasm Antibodies *Serum No Effect* In 0 of 12 patients (0%) with HTLV-1 associated myelopathy pANCA detected *3722*

Antinuclear Antibodies *Serum Increase* In 5 of 12 patients (41.7%) with HTLV-1 associated myelopathy ANA detected *3722*

49.90 Viral Encephalitis

Amyloid β-Protein *Cerebrospinal Fluid Increase* In 1 patient with viral encephalitis concentration was 9.61 pmol/mL significantly different from mean concentration of 4.00 ± 2.92 pmol/mL *3716*

Amyloid β-Protein Precursor *Cerebrospinal Fluid Increase* In 1 patient with viral encephalitis concentration was 1.96 integrated OD units significantly different from mean concentration of 1.35 ± 0.38 integrated OD units in 25 normal controls *3716*

α_1-Antichymotrypsin *Cerebrospinal Fluid Increase* In 1 patient with viral encephalitis concentration was 5.10 µg/mL significantly different from mean concentration of 2.27 ± 1.40 µg/mL in 25 normal controls *3716*

Cells *Cerebrospinal Fluid Increase* In 1 patient with viral encephalitis concentration of 120.7 cells/µL significantly different from normal of 3 cells/µL *3716*

Oligoclonal Banding *Cerebrospinal Fluid Increase* Oligoclonal IgG bands detected with viral encephalitis (herpes, HIV, etc.) *3261*

Protein *Cerebrospinal Fluid Increase* In 1 patient with viral encephalitis concentration of 59 mg/dL significantly different from normal mean of 29 mg/dL *3716*

Soluble HLA-I *Cerebrospinal Fluid Increase* In 3 patients with viral encephalitis mean concentration of 1,328 ng/mL *216*

Soluble HLA-II *Cerebrospinal Fluid No Effect* In 3 patients with viral encephalitis, mean concentration undetectable *216*

Viral Diseases

50.00 Smallpox

Albumin *Urine Increase* With the elimination of toxic material *900*

Clotting Time *Blood Increase* Commonly found in hemorrhagic smallpox *900*

Complement Fixation *Serum Increase* Highly significant in an unvaccinated patient or when vaccination was performed years previously *900* A rising antibody titer is seen in paired sera *1980*

Hemagglutination Inhibition *Serum Increase* Only titers above 1:1000 or a great increase in titer is significant *900* A rising antibody titer is seen in paired sera *1980*

Leukocytes *Blood Decrease* Leukopenia is found in the first days of illness followed by leukocytosis with lymphocytosis and a high percentage of metamyelocytes *900* Leukopenia *2239*
Blood Increase Increased during pustular rash *5545* Leukopenia is found in the first days of illness followed by leukocytosis with lymphocytosis and a high percentage of metamyelocytes *900*

Lymphocytes *Blood Increase* Leukopenia is found in the first days of illness followed by leukocytosis with lymphocytosis and a high percentage of metamyelocytes *900*

Metamyelocytes *Blood Increase* Leukopenia is found in the first days of illness followed by leukocytosis with lymphocytosis and a high percentage of metamyelocytes *900*

Neutralizing Antibodies *Serum Increase* Only titers above 1:1,000 or a large increase in titer is significant *900* Increased titer in acute-phase and convalescent-phase sera *5545* A rising antibody titer is seen in paired sera *1980*

Neutrophils *Blood Decrease* Leukopenia frequently associated with infectious diseases *2239*

Platelets *Blood Decrease* Pronounced thrombocytopenia is commonly found in hemorrhagic smallpox *900*

52.00 Chickenpox

Albumin *Serum Decrease* May be decreased with increased β- and γ- globulins *5545*

Cells *Cerebrospinal Fluid Increase* Encephalitis *5544*

β-Globulin *Serum Increase* May be increased *5545*

γ-Globulin *Serum Increase* May be increased *5545*

Glucose *Cerebrospinal Fluid No Effect* Concentration usually unchanged *2192*

52.00 Chickenpox *(continued)*

Hemoglobin *Plasma Increase* Reported effect *4222* Observed effect *5677*

Leukocytes *Blood Decrease* Leukopenia frequently associated with infectious diseases *2239*

Lymphocytes *Blood Decrease* The numbers of circulating lymphocytes are sharply and regularly reduced *5650* *Cerebrospinal Fluid Increase* With CNS involvement the cells in the CSF number from normal to < 100 /μL and are almost exclusively lymphocytes *2192*

Neopterin *Serum Increase* Very high concentrations observed in young children with primary chicken pox *121*

Neutrophils *Blood Decrease* Leukopenia frequently associated with infectious diseases *2239*

Protein *Cerebrospinal Fluid Increase* Normal or slightly increased *2192*

53.00 Herpes Zoster Infection

Albumin *Serum Decrease* In 32% of 18 patients at initial hospitalization for this disorder *1576*

Alkaline Phosphatase *Serum Increase* In 31% of 18 patients at initial hospitalization for this disorder *1576*

Anti-Varicella Zoster Virus IgG Antibodies *Cerebrospinal Fluid Increase* In 44 patients with acute herpes zoster antibodies observed in 10 (23%) *1943*

Anti-Varicella Zoster Virus IgM Antibodies *Cerebrospinal Fluid No Effect* In 44 patients with acute herpes zoster antibodies observed in none *1943*

Antibodies to Human Leukocyte Interferon *Serum Increase* Antibodies to human leukocyte interferon occuring spontaneously without prior treatment observed in certain clinical conditions although their significance is unknown *4392*

Aspartate Aminotransferase *Serum Increase* In 36% of 18 patients at initial hospitalization for this disorder *1576*

Cells *Cerebrospinal Fluid Increase* Reported effect *1980* 40% of patients show increased cells (< 300 mononuclear cells /μL) *5545*

Cholesterol *Serum Decrease* In 21% of 18 patients at initial hospitalization for this disorder *1576*

Complement Fixation *Serum Increase* 11 of 12 children showed a rise in CF antibody during convalescence *608* A significant (4-fold or greater) anamnestic response usually occurs *2192*

Creatinine *Serum Increase* In 15% of 17 patients at initial hospitalization for this disorder *1576*

Glucose *Cerebrospinal Fluid No Effect* Concentration typically normal *1980*

Hematocrit *Blood Decrease* In 37% of 18 patients at initial hospitalization for this disorder *1576*

Hemoglobin *Blood Decrease* In 38% of 18 patients at initial hospitalization for this disorder *1576*

Homovanillic Acid *Cerebrospinal Fluid Increase* Has been reported *2456*

5-Hydroxyindoleacetic Acid *Cerebrospinal Fluid Increase* Has been reported *2456*

IgG Index *Cerebrospinal Fluid Increase* In 46 patients with acute herpes zoster increased index observed in 1 (2%), normal in all others *1943*

Lactate Dehydrogenase *Serum Increase* In 37% of 18 patients at initial hospitalization for this disorder *1576*

Leukocytes *Cerebrospinal Fluid Increase* In 46 patients with acute herpes zoster increased concentration observed in 21 (46%) *1943*

Lymphocytes *Cerebrospinal Fluid Increase* Lymphocytes pleocytosis *2192* CSF commonly shows a pleocytosis and elevation of protein, even when clinical signs of meningeal irritation or encephalomyelitis are absent *367*

Monocytes *Blood Increase* In 65% of 18 patients at initial hospitalization for this disorder *1576*

Neutralizing Antibodies *Serum Increase* A significant (4-fold or greater) anamnestic response usually occurs *2192*

Protein *Cerebrospinal Fluid Increase* In 46 patients with acute herpes zoster increased concentration observed in 12 (26%) *1943* CSF commonly shows a pleocytosis and elevation of protein, even when clinical signs of meningeal irritation or encephalomyelitis are absent *367* 20 - 110 mg/dL *1980*

Urea Nitrogen *Serum Increase* In 31% of 18 patients at initial hospitalization for this disorder *1576*

Varicella Zoster Virus DNA *Cerebrospinal Fluid No Effect* In 42 patients with acute herpes zoster VZV DNA detected in 10 (24%) *1943*

53.19 Postherpetic Neuritis

α_1-Antichymotrypsin *Serum No Effect* Mean concentration within reference interval of 47.9 ± 8.1 mg/dL in one examined patient with postherpetic neuritis *3044*

54.00 Herpes Simplex Infection

Bilirubin *Serum Increase* Observed effect *4222 5677*

Cells *Cerebrospinal Fluid Increase* Up to 500 /μL, with lymphocytes or mononuclear cells predominating *367*

Complement Fixation *Serum Increase* Increased titer of complement-fixation and neutralizing antibodies is shown in convalescent-phase compared with acute-phase sera in primary infections *5545*

Complement-fixing Antibodies *Cerebrospinal Fluid Increase* Pleural, joint, and CSF fluids contain complement-fixing antibody but in lower titer than in serum *5677* *Pleural Fluid Increase* Pleural, joint, and CSF fluids contain complement-fixing antibody but in lower titer than in serum *5677* *Serum Increase* Pleural, joint, and CSF fluids contain complement-fixing antibody but in lower titer than in serum *5677* *Synovial Fluid Increase* Pleural, joint, and CSF fluids contain complement-fixing antibody but in lower titer than in serum *5677*

Erythrocyte Sedimentation Rate *Blood Increase* 26 patients with vulval and cervical herpetic lesions showed highly significant elevations compared to normals *2690*

Erythrocytes *Cerebrospinal Fluid Increase* RBC or xanthochromia frequently found, reflecting hemorrhagic nature of the lesions *367*

Factor II *Plasma Decrease* May be associated with defibrination resulting in platelet and coagulation factor consumption *5677*

Factor IV *Plasma Decrease* May be associated with defibrination resulting in platelet and coagulation factor consumption *5677*

Fibrinogen *Plasma Decrease* May be associated with defibrination resulting in platelet and coagulation factor consumption *5677*

Herpes Simplex Virus Antibodies *Serum Increase* Increased concentrations indicate recent or past infection with herpes simplex virus *2952*

Neutralizing Antibodies *Serum Increase* Increased titer of neutralizing antibodies is shown in convalescent-phase compared with acute-phase in primary infections *5545*

Platelets *Blood Decrease* May be associated with defibrination resulting in platelet and coagulation factor consumption *5677*

Protein *Cerebrospinal Fluid Increase* Frequently elevated *367*

Prothrombin Consumption *Blood Increase* May be associated with defibrination resulting in platelet and coagulation factor consumption *5677*

Prothrombin Time *Plasma Increase* May be associated with defibrination resulting in platelet and coagulation factor consumption *5677*

54.30 Herpes Simplex Encephalitis

Amyloid β-Protein *Cerebrospinal Fluid Decrease* In 2 patients with herpes simplex encephalitis concentrations were 0.00 and 1.14 pmol/mL significantly different from mean concentration of 4.00 ± 2.92 pmol/mL *3716*

Amyloid β-Protein Precursor *Cerebrospinal Fluid Decrease* In 2 patients with herpes simplex encephalitis concentrations were 0.21 and 0.28 integrated OD units significantly different from mean concentration of 1.35 ± 0.38 integrated OD units in 25 normal controls *3716*

α_1-Antichymotrypsin *Cerebrospinal Fluid Increase* In 2 patients with herpes simplex encephalitis concentrations were 13.35 and 11.95 µg/mL significantly different from mean concentration of 2.27 ± 1.40 µg/mL in 25 normal controls *3716*

Cells *Cerebrospinal Fluid Increase* In 2 patients with herplex simplex encephalitis concentrations of 2.3 and 15.7 cells/µL significantly different from normal of 3 cells/µL in one patient and normal in the other *3716*

Cerebrospinal Fluid No Effect In 2 patients with herplex simplex encephalitis concentrations of 2.3 and 15.7 cells/µL significantly different from normal of 3 cells/µL in one patient and normal in the other *3716*

Protein *Cerebrospinal Fluid Increase* In 2 patients with herpes simplex encephalitis concentrations of 28 and 72 mg/dL significantly different from normal mean of 29 mg/dL in one and normal in the other *3716*

Cerebrospinal Fluid No Effect In 2 patients with herpes simplex encephalitis concentrations of 28 and 72 mg/dL significantly different from normal mean of 29 mg/dL in one and normal in the other *3716*

54.30 Herpes Simplex Type I Encephalitis

Albumin Index *Cerebrospinal Fluid Increase* In 3 patients with herpes simplex type I encephalitis mean CSF:serum times 10^{-1} on admission to hospital ranged from 17.7 to 35.2 *4445*

Granulocytes *Cerebrospinal Fluid Increase* In 3 patients with herpes simplex type I encephalitis mean proportions on admission to hospital ranged from 5 to 27% *4445*

IgG Index *Cerebrospinal Fluid Decrease* In 3 patients with herpes simplex type I encephalitis mean CSF:serum times 10^{-1} on admission to hospital ranged from 12.9 to 18.5 *4445*

Interleukin-8 *Cerebrospinal Fluid Increase* In 3 patients with herpes simplex type I encephalitis mean CSF concentration on admission to hospital ranged up to 4,074 pg/mL in one patient *4445*

Leukocytes *Cerebrospinal Fluid Increase* In 3 patients with herpes simplex type I encephalitis mean concentrations on admission to hospital ranged from 61 to 222 cells/µL *4445*

Lymphocytes *Cerebrospinal Fluid Increase* In 3 patients with herpes simplex type I encephalitis mean proportions on admission to hospital ranged from 33 to 86 cells/plasma cells *4445*

Macrophage Inflammatory Protein-1α
Cerebrospinal Fluid Increase In 3 patients with herpes simplex type I encephalitis mean CSF concentration on admission to hospital ranged up to 422 pg/mL in one patient *4445*

Monocyte Chemotactic Protein-1
Cerebrospinal Fluid Increase In 3 patients with herpes simplex type I encephalitis mean CSF concentration on admission to hospital ranged up to 9,450 pg/mL in one patient *4445*

Monocytes *Cerebrospinal Fluid Increase* In 3 patients with herpes simplex type I encephalitis mean proportions on admission to hospital ranged from 9 to 50% *4445*

RANTES *Cerebrospinal Fluid Increase* In 3 patients with herpes simplex type I encephalitis mean CSF concentration on admission to hospital ranged up to 10^3 pg/mL in one patient *4445*

55.00 Measles

Alanine Aminotransferase *Serum Increase* In 12 of 28 hospitalized adult patients activity was more than 5 times the upper limit of normal *5717*

Serum No Effect Activity remained within normal range for children during the entire course of the disease in 18 children *2555*

Albumin *Serum Decrease* In 11 of 14 hospitalized adult patients with measles who had hypocalcemia nadir of albumin concentration was less than or equal to 30 g/L *5717*

Aldolase *Serum Increase* Marked increase in some patients *1678* In 18 children who developed measles mean activity increased from normal (normal range of 2 - 6 U/L) to peak of 10.3 ± 0.9 U/L 2 - 3 days after onset of rash *2555*

Amylase *Serum Increase* Activity increased in 4 of 21 hospitalized adult patients with measles *5717*

Amyloid A Protein *Serum Increase* In 17 patients mean concentration in acute phase of 1.89 ± 0.31 mg/L *3728*

Aspartate Aminotransferase *Serum Increase* In 18 children mean activity increased from 35 ± 4 U/L 1 - 2 days before onset of rash to peak of 66 ± 8 U/L 2 - 3 days after rash developed *2555* In 12 of 28 hospitalized adult patients peak concentration exceeded upper limit of normal by a factor of five *5717*

Calcium *Serum Decrease* In 15 of 28 hospitalized adult patients with measles concentration fell below 2.0 mmol/L *5717*

Cells *Cerebrospinal Fluid Increase* Reported effect *5544*

Sputum Increase Wright's stain of sputum shows measles multinucleated giant cells, especially during prodrome and early rash *5545*

Complement Fixation *Serum Increase* CF antibody appeared at the same time as the rash and rose to a maximum titer of 1:512 between the 5th and 16th days after the axanthem *5252* Antibodies tend to decrease with time but may be used for diagnosing recent infection *900* Becomes positive 1 week after onset *5545*

C-Reactive Protein *Serum Increase* In 17 patients mean concentration in acute phase 0.84 ± 0.51 mg/L *3728*

Creatine Kinase *Serum Increase* Increased in 50% (n = 18) of patients. Has been reported to reside in BB or the MM fraction. May originate partly from rhabdomyolysis *2555* In 5 of 16 hospitalized patients with adult measles mean activity was more than 5 times the upper limit of normal *5717*

Creatine Kinase BB-Isoenzyme *Serum Increase* The increased activity was reported to reside in the BB fraction *5164*

Creatine Kinase MB-Isoenzyme *Serum Increase* The increased activity was reported to reside in the MB fraction *2986*

Creatinine *Serum No Effect* In 32 hospitalized adults with measles mean concentration of 68 ± 22 µmol/L not different from normal *5717*

Glucose *Cerebrospinal Fluid No Effect* In 6 hospitalized adult patients with measles mean concentration of 3.7 ± 0.4 mmol/L not significantly different from normal *5717*

Hemagglutination Inhibition *Serum Increase* Circulating antibody is present by the time the rash develops. HI antibodies and neutralizing antibodies remain indefinitely *900*

Hemoglobin *Blood No Effect* In 33 hospitalized adult patients with measles mean concentration of 145 ± 15 g/L not significantly different from normal *5717*

Plasma Increase Reported finding *4222* Observed effect *5677*

Hydroxybutyrate Dehydrogenase *Serum Increase* In 18 children with measles mean concentration rose from just above normal (upper limit 220 U/L) 1 - 2 days before onset of rash to peak of 600 U/L 2 - 3 days after onset of rash *2555*

Immunoglobulin G *Serum Increase* Maternal antibody may be differentiated from that actively produced by the infant by a steadily declining titer, since these tests primarily measure IgG *900*

Interleukin-6 *Serum Increase* Determined in 9 children with measles and in healthy children. IL-6 activity in the sera of patients was seen to increase during the acute stage *3357*

Lactate Dehydrogenase *Serum Increase* In 18 children activity increased from mean of 556 ± 34 U/L (upper limit of normal 520 U/L) 1 - 2 days before onset of rash to peak of 1,585 ± 72 U/L 2 - 3 days after rash developed *2555* In 7 of 25 hospitalized adult patients with measles activity was more than 5 times the upper limit of normal *5717*

Lactate Dehydrogenase Isoenzymes *Serum Increase* LD_1 is significantly higher than in control subjects. The increase originates from the destruction of infected lymphocytes rather than from myocardial injury *2555*

Leukocytes *Blood Decrease* Leukopenia frequently associated with infectious diseases *2239* Total WBC count is low with an absolute neutropenia *900*

55.00 Measles *(continued)*

Leukocytes *(continued)*
Blood *Increase* Slight increase at onset, then falls to 5,000 /μL with increased lymphocyte count. Increased WBC with shift to left suggests bacterial complication *5545*
Blood *No Effect* In 33 hospitalized adults with measles mean concentration of 6,800 ± 3,400 /μL not different from normal *5717*
Cerebrospinal Fluid *No Effect* In 6 hospitalized adult patients with measles mean concentration of 2,300 ± 2600 /μL not significantly different from normal *5717*

Lymphocytes *Blood* *Decrease* The numbers of circulating lymphocytes are sharply and regularly reduced *5650*

Magnesium *Serum* *No Effect* In 12 hospitalized adults with measles mean concentration of 0.74 ± 0.08 mmol/L not different from normal *5717*

Neopterin *Cerebrospinal Fluid* *Increase* Concentrations increased in CSF in children with measles encephalomyelitis *121*
Serum *Increase* Very high concentrations observed in children with peak concentration observed 1 - 3 days after onset of rash with cooncentration staying high for about 3 - 3 weeks *121*

Neutrophils *Blood* *Decrease* The total WBC count is low with an absolute neutropenia *900* Leukopenia frequently associated with infectious diseases *2239*

Phosphate *Serum* *No Effect* In 18 hospitalized adult patients with measles mean concentration of 0.84 ± 0.19 mmol/L not different from normal *5717*

Platelets *Blood* *No Effect* In 30 hospitalized adults with measles mean concentration of 173,000 ± 48,000 /μL within the reference range *5717*

Protein *Cerebrospinal Fluid* *No Effect* Mean concentration in 6 hospitalized adult patients 0.32 ± 0.05 g/L not significantly different from normal *5717*

Soluble Tumor Necrosis Factor Receptor-p60
Serum *No Effect* In 12 pediatric patients with acute measles mean concentration of 1.8 ± 0.5 ng/mL not significantly different from 1.2 ± 0.5 ng/mL in the convalescent stage and 1.5 ± 0.5 ng/mL in 30 control children *1610*

Tumor Necrosis Factor-α *Serum* *No Effect* Determined in 9 children with measles and in healthy children. Levels in patients did not increase during the acute stage *3357*

Urea *Serum* *No Effect* In 32 hospitalized adult patients with measles mean concentration of 4.0 ± 1.9 mmol/L not different from normal *5717*

VDRL *Serum* *Positive* False positive tests are sometimes seen *2039*

56.00 Rubella Infection

Cells *Cerebrospinal Fluid* *Increase* Reported effect *5544*

Complement Fixation *Serum* *Increase* Antibodies appear within 1 week after rash; therefore acute-phase serum must be collected promptly or the rise in titer may not be detected. They may last for 8 months to years *5545*

Hemagglutination Inhibition *Serum* *Increase* Change in titer from acute-phase to convalescent-phase sera is the most useful technique to demonstrate a rise in antibody titer. With rubella rash, diagnosis is established if acute sample titer is > 1:10 or if convalescent-phase serum taken 7 days after rash shows a 4-fold increase in titer *5545* Does not distinguish between IgM and IgG antibodies but absence of HI antibodies in cord blood makes diagnosis unlikely *5619*

Leukocytes *Blood* *Decrease* Leukopenia frequently associated with infectious diseases *2239* Decreased before the rash appears *5545*

Lymphocyte T-Cells *Blood* *Decrease* Normal *1588*

Lymphocytes *Blood* *Increase* Increased during the rash *5545*

Neutralizing Antibodies *Serum* *Increase* Appear within 1 - 3 days after rash and reach maximum in 2 wk. May remain positive for > 20 y *1290*

Neutrophils *Blood* *Decrease* Leukopenia frequently associated with infectious diseases *2239*

Platelets *Blood* *Decrease* Sometimes very severe in newborn infants infected with rubella *930* Decrease within 1 week of onset of rash is frequent and may be marked *5545*

60.00 Yellow Fever

Alanine Aminotransferase *Serum* *Increase* Activity was above normal in all sera tested, the degree of increase approximately proportional to the severity of disease *2477*

Albumin *Urine* *Increase* Most marked on the 3rd - 4th day of illness and declined thereafter *2477* Sudden development of intense albuminuria about day 3 - 4 g/L is characteristic, often reaching levels of 3 - 5 g/L or higher *367*

Amino Acids *Plasma* *Increase* Increased in severe cases *1290*

Anti-Mitochondrial Antibodies *Serum* *Increase* Occasionally positive in low titer *4160*

Aspartate Aminotransferase *Serum* *Increase* Activity was above normal in all sera tested, the degree of increase approximately proportional to the severity of disease *2477*

Bilirubin *Serum* *Increase* Slightly increased *5545* Has been reported *2477*

Cholesterol *Serum* *Decrease* Infections associated with liver damage *1290*

Complement Fixation *Serum* *Increase* Can be confirmed by CF antibody rises in paired sera *2477*

γ-Globulin *Serum* *Decrease* Decreased percentage during the course of the disease *3951*

Glucose *Serum* *Decrease* Deficiency in available glycogen *1290*

Leukocytes *Blood* *Decrease* Most marked by 6th day, associated with decreased lymphocytes *5545* Leukopenia frequently associated with infectious diseases *2239* In 23 cases, no consistent WBC picture was found. Leukopenia was present in a few cases, especially during the first few days of illness *2477*

Lymphocytes *Blood* *Decrease* The numbers of circulating lymphocytes are sharply and regularly reduced *5650*

Neutrophils *Blood* *Decrease* Leukopenia frequently associated with infectious diseases *2239*

Protein *Serum* *No Effect* No significant variations were found in the total protein concentrations *3951*
Urine *Increase* Occurs in severe cases *5545* Occurred in 14 of 21 cases including all 6 of the children who died *3951*

Urea Nitrogen *Serum* *Increase* Concentrations of 220 mg/dL were recorded in 3 patients, all of whom died *2477* With kidney involvement *2192*

61.00 Dengue

C-Reactive Protein *Serum* *Increase* In 49 patients with dengue mean concentration of 9.5 ± 14.4 mg/L, with the concentration in 13 significantly higher than the upper limit of normal of 10 mg/L *3769*

Phospholipase A_2 Type II *Serum* *Increase* In 49 patients with dengue mean concentration of 77.4 ± 99.9 μg/L significantly higher than the upper limit of normal of 11 μg/L *3769*

Platelets *Blood* *Decrease* In 49 patients with dengue concentrations ranged from 56 - 412 x 10^9/L, with the concentration in 13 (27%) significantly below the lower limit of normal of 150 x 10^9/L *3769*

Tumor Necrosis Factor-α *Serum* *Increase* Values as high as 50 - 400 pg/mL observed in dengue-infected children *2188*

62.10 Western Equine Encephalitis

Chloride *Cerebrospinal Fluid* *No Effect* Concentration usually unchanged *2192*

Glucose *Cerebrospinal Fluid* *No Effect* Concentration usually unchanged *2192*

Leukocytes *Blood* *Decrease* May be present early in the disease *367*
Blood *Increase* Mild leukocytosis with polymorphonuclear cells predominating is common. Leukopenia may be present early in the disease *367*

Cerebrospinal Fluid *Increase* Up to 1,000 /µL *2192*
Lymphocytes *Cerebrospinal Fluid* *Increase* Usually predominate *2192*

62.20 Eastern Equine Encephalitis

Chloride *Cerebrospinal Fluid* *No Effect* Concentration usually unchanged *2192*

Glucose *Cerebrospinal Fluid* *No Effect* Concentration usually unchanged *2192*

Leukocytes *Blood* *Decrease* Marked decrease occurs with relative lymphocytosis *5545*
Blood *Increase* May occur *900* Polymorphonuclear leukocytosis may reach 50,000 /µL *367*
Cerebrospinal Fluid *Increase* Up to 1,000 /µL *2192*

Lymphocytes *Cerebrospinal Fluid* *Increase* Usually predominate *2192*

66.00 Phlebotomus Fever

Amino Acids *Plasma* *Decrease* Basal hypoaminoacidemia. After intravenous glucose administration the total amino acid concentration rapidly decreased as much as or more than the original decline *5568*

Glucose *Serum* *Increase* Impaired glucose tolerance with relative hyperinsulinemia was observed in sandfly fever *5568*

Glucose Tolerance *Serum* *Decrease* Impaired glucose tolerance with relative hyperinsulinemia was observed in sandfly fever *5568*

Glutamine *Plasma* *Decrease* Most free serum amino acids are depressed in sandfly fever and other mild-moderate infections *305*

Insulin *Plasma* *Increase* Relative hyperinsulinemia was observed in sandfly fever *5568*

Isoleucine *Plasma* *Decrease* Most free serum amino acids are depressed in sandfly fever and other mild-moderate infections *305*

Leukocytes *Blood* *Decrease* Leukopenia frequently associated with infectious diseases *2239*

Neutrophils *Blood* *Decrease* Leukopenia frequently associated with infectious diseases *2239*

Phenylalanine *Plasma* *Increase* Increased during the viral illness in contrast with most other amino acids *5568*

Threonine *Plasma* *Decrease* Most free serum amino acids are depressed in sandfly fever and other mild-moderate infections *305*

Tyrosine *Plasma* *Decrease* Most free amino acids are depressed in sandfly fever and other mild-moderate infections *305*

Valine *Plasma* *Decrease* Most free serum amino acids are depressed in sandfly fever and other mild-moderate infections *305*

66.00 Sandfly Fever

Cortisol, Free *Urine* *Increase* 3 fold increase over basal with fever *4293*

Fatty Acids (FFA), Free *Serum* *Increase* Increased 2 fold from baseline *4293*

Glucose Tolerance *Serum* *Decrease* With fever decreased by half *4293*

Growth Hormone *Plasma* *Increase* Increased 8 fold at fasting, 18 fold at 30 minutes *4293*

Insulin *Plasma* *Increase* Increase of 2 fold at 30 minutes, 3 fold at 60 minutes *4293*

66.10 Tick-borne Fever

Complement Fixation *Serum* *Increase* Increased in sera taken during acute and convalescent phases *5545*

Hematocrit *Blood* *Decrease* Anemia develops in some patients *2192*

Hemoglobin *Blood* *Decrease* Anemia develops in some patients *2192*

Leukocytes *Blood* *Decrease* Invariably decreased. Noted by the 2nd or 3rd day of illness. Often drops to 2,000 /µL *900* Characterized by a profound leukopenia and occasional thrombocytopenia which is usually greatest during the second febrile episode *367* Initial mean count from confirmed cases of Colorado tick fever was 3,900 /µL. 67% had counts < 4,500 /µL and the mean for the leukopenic group was 2,400 /µL. No relation was found between leukopenia and age, sex, or recovery *1816*

Lymphocytes *Blood* *Increase* Relative *2192*

Neutralizing Antibodies *Serum* *Increase* Found in all patients with Colorado tick fever upon follow-up 1 month after onset. 92% showed a 4-fold rise in titer within 30 days. Peak titers were reached in the 20th week *1816* Increases are seen in sera taken during acute and convalescent phases *5545*

Neutrophils *Blood* *Decrease* There is a relative decrease in mature polymorphonuclear leukocytes with an increase in immature forms *900* Absolute neutropenia *2192*

Weil-Felix Reaction *Serum* *Positive* Agglutinins against OX-19 develop during the 2nd week *367*

70.10 Acute Hepatitis A

Alanine Aminotransferase *Serum* *Increase* In 2 patients mean activity of 1,277.0 ± 1,079 U/L significantly higher than normal range of 10 - 35 U/L *5259* In a man and a woman with hepatitis A increased ALT concentrations of 5,218 U/L and 4,526 U/L observed at the time of peak abnormalities of PSA, AST, bilirubin and reduced prothrombin time *535* Abrupt increase in activity observed within 24 to 48 h after first detected abnormality *3625*

Aspartate Aminotransferase *Serum* *Increase* Abrupt increase in activity observed within 24 to 48 h after first detected abnormality *3625* In 2 patients mean activity of 760.0 ± 565.6 U/L significantly higher than normal range of 10 - 33 U/L *5259* In a man and a woman with hepatitis A increased AST activities of 4,722 U/L and 4,316 U/L observed at the time of peak abnormalities of ALT, bilirubin and reduced prothrombin time *535*

Bilirubin *Serum* *Increase* In 2 patients mean concentration of 5.8 ± 4.8 mg/dL significantly greater than normal range of 0.1 - 1.5 mg/dL *5259* In a man and a woman with hepatitis A increased total bilirubin concentrations of 479 µmol/L and 410 µmol/L observed at the time of peak abnormalities of AST, ALT, PSA and reduced prothrombin time *535*

γ-Glutamyltransferase *Serum* *Increase* In 2 patients mean activity of 192.0 ± 43.8 U/L significantly greater than normal range of 10 - 25 U/L *5259*

Hepatitis A Virus RNA *Feces* *Increase* During the viremic phase HAV-RNA can be detected in the plasma and stools *3406*
Serum *Increase* During the viremic phase HAV-RNA can be detected in the plasma and stools *3406*

IgG Anti-HAV *Serum* *Increase* Shortly after onset of symptoms the secondary IgG antibody response begins and titers of IgG anti-HAV continue to rise for several months after recovery *3406*

IgM Anti-HAV *Serum* *Increase* Detection of antibody substantiates diagnosis: antibody first becomes detectable at the onset of clinical illness and is invariably present at onset of jaundice *3625* Onset of symptoms coincides with the development of a primary antibody, with rising titers throughout the acute phase *3406*

Neopterin *Urine* *Increase* Excretion increased in patients with hepatitis A *121*

Prostate-specific Antigen *Serum* *Increase* In a man and a woman with hepatitis A increased PSA concentrations of 28.6 ng/mL and 16.8 ng/mL observed at the time of peak abnormalities of AST, ALT, bilirubin and reduced prothrombin time *535*

Prothrombin Time *Plasma* *Decrease* In a man and a woman with hepatitis A increased prothrombin rate reduced to 60% and 64% at the time of peak abnormalities of PSA, AST, ALT and bilirubin *535*
Plasma *No Effect* In 2 patients mean time of 94.0 ± 8.4% compared with normal range of 70 - 100% *5259*

70.30 Acute Hepatitis B

Acid Ribonuclease *Serum* *Increase* Median activity in 21 patients with acute hepatitis B of 62.3 U/L significantly different from 42.0 U/L in 32 healthy controls *2566*

Adenosine Deaminase *Serum* *Increase* In 26 patients with hepatitis B infection mean concentration of 26.2 ± 11.1 U/L significantly greater than 13.9 ± 6.6 U/L in 30 healthy controls: in 38 patients with stage II AIDS and hepatitis B mean concentration of 54.2 ± 7.9 U/L *3322*

Alanine Aminotransferase *Serum* *Increase* In 32 patients mean activity of 1,442 ± 852 U/L compared with less than 30 U/L in 838 healthy controls *2374* In 10 patients with acute hepatitis mean activity of 354.80 ± 220.30 U/L significantly higher than 28.50 ± 6.55 U/L in 69 healthy blood donor controls *3591* In 20 patients with acute hepatitis B who cleared HBsAg mean activity of 1,241 ± 240 U/L and in 8 who became chronic HBsAg carriers 1,289 ± 276 U/L *841* In 8 patients mean activity of 1,955.0 ± 859.6 U/L compared with normal range of 10 - 35 U/L *5259* Median activity in 21 patients with acute hepatitis B infection 282 U/L significantly different from 22 U/L in 32 healthy controls *2566*

Albumin *Serum* *Decrease* Median concentration in 21 patients with acute hepatitis B infection of 3.3 g/dL different from 3.7 g/dL in 32 healthy controls *2566*

Alkaline Phosphatase *Serum* *Increase* Median activity in 21 patients with acute hepatitis B infection 195 U/L significantly different from 63 U/L in 32 healthy controls *2566*

Alkaline Ribonuclease *Serum* *Increase* Median activity in 21 patients with acute hepatitis B of 86.2 U/L significantly different from 67.4 U/L in 32 healthy controls *2566*

Anti-Hepatitis B Core Antibodies *Serum* *Increase* Antibody is detected approximately 2 weeks after the appearance of HBsAg *3625*

Anti-Hepatitis B Surface Antibodies *Serum* *Increase* Antibodies detected approximately some weeks after the appearance of antibodies to HBsAg *3625*

Anti-Hepatitis B Surface Antigen *Serum* *Increase* HbSAg is the first marker of hepatitis B detectable in serum preceding increases in aminotransferase activity and symptoms *3625*

Aspartate Aminotransferase *Serum* *Increase* In 8 patients with acute hepatitis B mean activity of 1,027.3 ± 535.7 U/L compared with normal range of 10 - 33 U/L *5259* In 10 patients with acute hepatitis mean activity of 782.90 ± 375.93 U/L significantly higher than 22.81 ± 7.95 U/L in 69 healthy blood donor controls *3591* In 20 patients with acute hepatitis B who cleared HBsAg mean activity of 897 ± 221 U/L and in 8 who became chronic HBsAg carriers 911 ± 260 U/L *841*

Bilirubin *Serum* *Increase* In 8 patients with acute hepatitis B mean concentration of 9.3 ± 7.1 mg/dL compared with normal range of 0.1 - 1.5 mg/dL *5259* Median concentration in 21 patients with acute hepatitis B infection 2.0 mg/dL significantly different from 0.7 mg/dL in 32 healthy controls *2566* In 20 patients with acute hepatitis B who cleared HBsAg mean concentration of 6.2 ± 2.3 mg/dL and in 8 who became chronic HBsAg carriers 6.5 ± 4.8 mg/dL *841*

CA 15-3 *Serum* *Increase* In 8 patients with acute hepatitis mean concentration of 24.7 ± 10 U/mL higher than cutoff of 22 U/mL, with 5 having concentrations greater than 22 U/mL, and 3 with concentrations above 30 U/mL and 2 with concentrations above 35 U/mL but below 40 U/mL *2076*

CD4+ Lymphocytes *Blood* *No Effect* No significant rise *3916*

CD8+ Lymphocytes *Blood* *Increase* Significantly higher as compared with normal controls *3916*

Creatinine *Serum* *No Effect* Median concentration in 21 patients with acute hepatitis B infection 0.8 mg/dL not significantly different from 0.7 mg/dL in 32 healthy controls *2566*

α-Fetoprotein *Serum* *No Effect* In 10 patients with acute hepatitis mean concentration of 3.18 ± 2.95 U/mL lower than the normal upper limit of normal of 8.5 U/mL *3591*

γ-Glutamyltransferase *Serum* *Increase* In 32 patients mean concentration of 1.7 ± 0.3 U/L compared with undetectable amounts in 838 healthy controls *2374* In 8 patients mean activity of 97.1 ± 44.9 U/L compared with normal range of 10 - 25 U/L *5259*

Hepatitis B Surface Antigen *Serum* *Increase* During the prodromal phase marked viremia develops reaching a peak before the development of symptoms with findings of HBsAg, HBeAg and HBV-DNA *3406*

Hepatitis B Virus DNA *Serum* *Increase* In 20 patients with acute hepatitis B who cleared HBsAg HBV-DNA detected in 8 (40%) and in 8 who became chronic HBsAg carriers HBV-DNA detected in all (100%) *841* At about the time of onset of symptoms the virus elicits a primary IgM antibody response to the core protein and the titer rises as the illness progresses *3406* During the prodromal phase marked viremia develops reaching a peak before the development of symptoms with findings of HBsAg, HBeAg and HBV-DNA *3406*

Hepatitis Be Antigen *Serum* *Increase* During the prodromal phase marked viremia develops reaching a peak before the development of symptoms with findings of HBsAg, HBeAg and HBV-DNA *3406*

Hepatocyte Growth Factor *Serum* *Increase* In patients with acute hepatitis mean concentration of 0.37 ng/mL compared with mean concentration in 10 normal individuals of 0.25 ± 0.06 ng/mL *3714*

Intercellular Adhesion Molecule-1 *Serum* *Increase* Mean concentration in 13 patients with acute hepatitis of approximately 3,000 μg/L significantly increased compared with mean concentration in 28 healthy blood donors of 215.5 μg/L (95% confidence limits of mean 198.1 - 232.9 μg/L) *4143*

Interferon-α *Serum* *Increase* In 20 patients with acute hepatitis B who cleared HBsAg concentrations ranged from 36 - 180 pg/mL (increased 15% patients) and in 8 who became chronic HBsAg carriers concentrations ranged from 70 - 204 pg/mL (increased in 25%) *841*

Interferon-γ *Serum* *Increase* In 20 patients with acute hepatitis B who cleared HBsAg concentrations ranged from 7 - 56 pg/mL (increased in all patients) and in 8 who became chronic HBsAg carriers concentrations ranged from 6 - 56 pg/mL (increased in 37.5%) *841*

Interleukin-1α-Autoantibody *Serum* *No Effect* In 32 patients proportion with autoantibody 15.6% compared with 12.6% in 838 healthy controls *2374*

Interleukin-6 *Serum* *Increase* In patients with acute hepatitis mean concentration of 16.6 ± 14.5 pg/mL, in those with severe acute hepatitis of 26.3 ± 19.0 pg/mL and 470.2 ± 261.4 pg/mL in patients with fulminant hepatic failure *5080*

Iron *Serum* *Increase* Increase in concentration to above 150 μg/dL observed in acute hepatitis *2952*

Neopterin *Urine* *Increase* Excretion increased in patients with hepatitis B *121*

5'-Nucleotidase *Serum* *Increase* In 5 patients mean activity of 10 U/L (range 3 - 12 U/L) compared with mean of 3.8 U/L in healthy individuals. Mean % isoforms of NTP1 32%, NTP2 14%, and NTP3 56% compared with 12%, 30%, and 58% respectively in healthy controls *3993*

Procollagen Type III Peptide *Serum* *Increase* Measured in paired serum samples from 22 patients with acute hepatitis and from 50 healthy age-matched controls. Concentrations were significantly elevated in 22 patients with acute hepatitis *4270*

Prothrombin Time *Plasma* *Increase* Prolongation of the prothrombin time usually indicates that the disease is a chronic one, such as advanced cirrhosis: if it increases in acute liver disease it usually indicates the disease is a fulminant one, for example, acute viral hepatitis, especially type B *4617* *Plasma* *No Effect* In 8 patients with acute viral hepatitis B mean time of 85.5 ± 16.1% not significantly different from normal range of 70 - 100% *5259*

Rheumatoid Factor *Serum* *Increase* Mean concentration increased in patients with acute hepatitis *2472*

Tissue Inhibitor of Metalloproteinase-1 *Serum* *Increase* In 16 patients with acute hepatitis (6 type A, 5 type B and 5 cryptogenic) mean concentration of 377.3 ± 123.2 ng/mL significantly higher than 147.8 ± 22.0 ng/mL in 53 normal individuals *3690*

Tissue Polypeptide Antigen *Serum* *Increase* In 10 patients with acute hepatitis mean concentration of 836.90 ± 642.10 U/L significantly greater than 37.73 ± 20.76 U/L in 69 healthy blood donor controls *3591*

Urea *Serum* *No Effect* Median concentration in 21 patients with acute hepatitis B infection of 34 mg/dL not significantly different from 31 mg/dL in 32 healthy controls *2566*

Urobilinogen *Urine Increase* In patients with early acute hepatitis excretion may exceed 6 mg/d compared with upper limit of normal of 4 mg/d *2952*

70.30 Hepatitis B

Interleukin-6 *Serum No Effect* In patients with chronic persistent hepatitis B and in those with primary biliary cirrhosis concentrations similar to those in controls *2532*

Neopterin *Serum Increase* In asymptomatic HBsAg carriers concentration invariably increased *997* In 37 patients mean concentration of 9.7 ± 1.3 nmol/L, with mean in 17 without cirrhosis 8.1 ± 1.4 nmol/L and 11.2 ± 2.0 nmol/L in 20 with cirrhosis different from 6.0 ± 2.2 nmol/L in healthy controls *5682* *Urine Increase* Concentration invariably increased in patients with asymptomatic HBsAg carriers *997*

Procollagen Type III Peptide *Serum Increase* All patients with chronic B virus hepatitis had raised P-III-P values in comparison with controls ($p < 0.0001$) *5183*

70.32 Chronic Hepatitis B

Alanine Aminotransferase *Serum Increase* In 20 patients with chronic hepatitis who failed to respond to interferon-alfa therapy mean baseline activity of 112 ± 18 U/L *5764* In 28 patients with chronic hepatitis B mean activity of 221 ± 10 U/L increased compared with 20 ± 2 U/L in 30 healthy controls *2269*

Albumin *Serum Decrease* In 28 patients with chronic hepatitis B mean concentration of 4.3 ± 0.1 g/dL decreased compared with 4.8 ± 0.1 g/dL in 30 healthy controls *2269* *Serum No Effect* In 20 patients with chronic hepatitis who failed to respond to interferon-alfa therapy mean baseline concentration of 3.93 ± 0.10 g/dL towards the lower limit of normal of 3.5 - 5.3 g/dL *5764*

Aspartate Aminotransferase *Serum Increase* In 20 patients with chronic hepatitis who failed to respond to interferon-alfa therapy mean baseline activity of 78 ± 15 U/L *5764* In 28 patients with chronic hepatitis B mean activity of 172 ± 8 U/L increased compared with 23 ± 1 U/L in 30 healthy controls *2269*

Bilirubin *Serum Increase* In 28 patients with chronic hepatitis B mean concentration of 2.3 ± 0.2 mg/dL increased compared with 0.6 ± 0.1 mg/dL in 30 healthy controls *2269*

CA 19-9 *Serum Increase* In 7 patients with chronic hepatitis B median concentration of 59 kU/L significantly higher than upper limit of normal of 35 kU/L, with 71% of patients having abnormal values *3218*

Carcinoembryonic Antigen *Serum No Effect* In 7 patients with chronic hepatitis B median concentration of 5 µg/L not different from upper limit of normal of 14 µg/L, and no patients had abnormal values *3218*

Cryoglobulins *Serum Increase* Cryoglobulinemia observed in 6 of 40 patients with HCV infections *3165*

Globulin *Serum Increase* In 28 patients with chronic hepatitis B mean concentration of 3.2 ± 0.2 g/dL increased compared with 2.8 ± 0.1 g/dL in 30 healthy controls *2269*

Interleukin-6 *Serum Increase* Concentration increased to mean of 38.4 ± 68.0 pg/mL in patients with chronic active hepatitis B compared with concentration in controls of 9.7 ± 6.8 pg/mL although difference not significant because of wide scatter of results *2532*

International Normalized Ratio *Plasma Increase* In 28 patients with chronic hepatitis B mean ratio of 1.5 ± 0.2 increased compared with reference range of < 1.2 *2269*

Metallopanstimulin *Serum Increase* In 11% of 18 patients with hepatitis B or C mean concentration exceeded upper limit of normal of < 10 ng/mL in healthy individuals aged 19 - 88 years *1462*

Neutrophils *Blood No Effect* In 28 patients with chronic hepatitis B mean concentration of 4.1 ± 0.4 x 10^3/µL not different when compared with 3.7 ± 0.1 x 10^3/µL in 30 healthy controls *2269*

N-terminal Peptide of Type III Procollagen *Serum Increase* Mean concentration in 19 patients with chronic hepatitis B of 0.75 ± 0.25 U/mL compared with reference interval of 0.35 - 0.65 U/mL *3669*

Procollagen Type III Peptide *Serum Increase* In 20 patients with chronic hepatitis who failed to respond to interferon-alfa therapy mean baseline concentration of 1.07 ± 0.06 U/mL greater than the upper limit of normal of < 0.8 U/mL *5764*

Prolyl 4-Hydroxylase β-subunit *Serum No Effect* Mean concentration in 19 patients with chronic hepatitis B of 60 ± 13 ng/mL compared with 38 - 74 ng/mL in 30 control individuals *3669*

Type IV Collagen 7S Domain *Serum Increase* In 20 patients with chronic hepatitis who failed to respond to interferon-alfa therapy mean baseline concentration of 6.51 ± 0.67 ng/mL greater than the upper limit of normal of < 6 ng/mL *5764*

Vitronectin *Serum Decrease* In 60 patients with chronic hepatitis B mean concentration of 150 ± 9 µg/mL significantly lower than that in 20 healthy volunteers in whom the mean concentration was 259 ± 38 µg/mL *5764*

70.51 Acute Hepatitis C

Acid Ribonuclease *Serum Increase* Median activity in 19 patients with acute hepatitis C of 53.8 U/L significantly different from 42.0 U/L in 32 healthy controls *2566*

Alanine Aminotransferase *Serum Increase* Median activity in 19 patients with acute hepatitis C infection 161 U/L significantly different from 22 U/L in 32 healthy controls *2566* Activity throughout disease usually less than 500 U/L and rarely greater than 1,000 U/L *3406* In 2 patients mean activity 663.5 ± 138.5 U/L significantly greater than normal range of 10 - 35 U/L *5259*

Albumin *Serum No Effect* Median concentration in 19 patients with acute hepatitis C infection of 3.8 g/dL not significantly different from 3.7 g/dL in 32 healthy controls *2566*

Alkaline Phosphatase *Serum Increase* Median activity in 19 patients with acute hepatitis C infection 161 U/L significantly different from 63 U/L in 32 healthy controls *2566*

Alkaline Ribonuclease *Serum Increase* Median activity in 19 patients with acute hepatitis C of 73.9 U/L significantly different from 67.4 U/L in 32 healthy controls *2566*

Aspartate Aminotransferase *Serum Increase* In 2 patients with acute hepatitis C mean activity of 138.5 ± 150.6 U/L significantly greater than normal range of 10 - 33 U/L *5259* Activity throughout disease usually less than 500 U/L and rarely greater than 1,000 U/L *3406*

Bilirubin *Serum Increase* Median concentration in 19 patients with acute hepatitis C infection 1.9 mg/dL significantly different from 0.7 mg/dL in 32 healthy controls *2566* In 2 patients mean concentration of 2.6 ± 1.2 mg/dL higher than normal range of 0.1 - 1.5 mg/dL *5259*

Complement C_4 *Serum Decrease* Consistent finding observed in patients with HCV-associated cryoglobulinemia *3100*

Creatinine *Serum No Effect* Median concentration in 19 patients with acute hepatitis C infection 0.9 mg/dL not significantly different from 0.7 mg/dL in 32 healthy controls *2566*

γ-Glutamyltransferase *Serum Increase* In 2 patients with acute hepatitis C mean activity of 72.5 ± 7.7 U/L significantly higher than normal range of 10 - 25 U/L *5259*

Interleukin-6 *Serum Increase* Measured in 72 patients with hepatitis C and hepatitis B virus infections. Significantly increased in patients with hepatitis C virus infections when compared with normal subjects and hepatitis B patients *4323*

Neopterin *Serum Increase* In 52 patients mean concentration of 12.3 ± 0.9 nmol/L, with mean in 31 without cirrhosis of 11.1 ± 1.0 nmol/L and 14.7 ± 1.7 nmol/L in 21 with cirrhosis different from 6.0 ± 2.2 nmol/L in healthy controls *5682* *Urine Increase* Excretion increased in patients with hepatitis C *121*

Prothrombin Time *Plasma No Effect* In 2 patients mean time of 85.5 ± 20.5% not different from normal range of 70 - 100% *5259*

Tumor Necrosis Factor-α *Serum Increase* Measured in 72 patients with hepatitis C and hepatitis B virus infections. Significantly increased in patients with hepatitis C virus infections when compared with normal subjects and hepatitis B patients *4323*

70.51 Acute Hepatitis C *(continued)*

Urea *Serum* *No Effect* Median concentration in 19 patients with acute hepatitis C infection of 39 mg/dL not significantly different from 31 mg/dL in 32 healthy controls *2566*

70.52 Acute Hepatitis D

Anti-Hepatitis D Antibodies *Serum* *Increase* Disease presence confirmed by detection of HDV antigen or anti-HDV antibodies *3625* Peak occurs about 4th week after infection, tailing off by 24th week *3406*

Hepatitis D Viral DNA *Serum* *Increase* Disease presence confirmed by detection of HDV antigen or anti-HDV antibodies *3625* Identifiable from 2 to 3.5 weeks following infection *3406*

IgM Anti-Hepatitis D Antibodies *Serum* *Increase* Peak occurs just before 3rd week after infection, tailing off by 6th week *3406*

70.53 Acute Hepatitis E

IgG Anti-Hepatitis E Antibodies *Serum* *Increase* Peak occurs about 90 to 100 days after infection, leveling off to a plateau by 120 days *3406*

IgM Anti-Hepatitis E Antibodies *Serum* *Increase* Peak occurs about 80 days after infection, tailing off to an undetectable amount by 170 days *3406*

70.54 Chronic Hepatitis C

Alanine Aminotransferase *Serum* *Increase* Activity throughout disease usually less than 500 U/L and rarely greater than 1,000 U/L *3406* Mean activity of 108 ± 68 U/L in 99 patients with chronic hepatitis C *1796* In 45 patients with chronic hepatitis C viral genotype 1b mean activity of 190 ± 52 U/L, in 43 with genotype 2a/2c 170 ± 35.4 U/L and in 42 with genotype 3a 165 ± 42 U/L *288* In 15 patients with chronic hepatitis C mean activity of 100 ± 49 U/L significantly greater than upper limit of normal of 55 U/L *4453* In 94 patients mean activity of 74.4 ± 47.0 U/L significantly greater than reference values of 24.0 ± 9.8 U/L *5433* Increased activity associated with increasing degree of hepatic fibrosis *3917* In 24 patients with chronic hepatitis C viral infection who were sustained responders to interferon mean activity of 98.6 ± 72.5 U/L and in 25 non-responders mean activity of 108.8 ± 52.1 U/L significantly higher than 8.2 ± 3.6 U/L in 20 healthy controls *2373* In 326 untreated patients with chronic hepatitis C mean activity of 83 ± 63 U/L significantly different from upper reference limit of 35 U/L *1901* In 22 patients with chronic hepatitis C activities ranged from 21 - 281 U/L compared with normal range of 6 - 53 U/L *2560* In 5 patients with chronic hepatitis C mean activity of 232 ± 13 U/L increased compared with 23 ± 1 U/L in 30 healthy controls *2269* Mean activity in patients with chronic hepatitis C who developed cirrhosis of 128 U/L significantly high but not different from that in those who did not, 128 U/L *4785*

Albumin *Serum* *Decrease* Reduced concentration associated with increasing degree of hepatic fibrosis *3917* In 5 patients with chronic hepatitis C mean concentration of 4.2 ± 0.2 g/dL decreased compared with 4.8 ± 0.1 g/dL in 30 healthy controls *2269* In 45 patients with chronic hepatitis C viral genotype 1b mean concentration of 39 ± 4.4 g/L, in 43 with genotype 2a/2c 41.0 ± 6.3 g/L, and in 42 with genotype 3a 40.5 ± 7.2 g/L *288*

Alkaline Phosphatase *Serum* *Increase* In 94 patients mean activity of 51.4 ± 26.6 U/L greater than reference values of 41.0 ± 15.1 U/L *5433* Increased activity associated with increasing degree of hepatic fibrosis *3917*
Serum *No Effect* In 326 untreated patients with chronic hepatitis C mean activity of 54 ± 21 U/L not significantly different from upper reference limit of 100 U/L *1901*

Amino-terminal Propeptide of Type III Procollagen
Serum *Increase* In 326 untreated patients with chronic hepatitis C mean concentration ranged from 0.75 ± 81 kU/L in the absence of histological fibrosis to 1.72 ± 0.23 kU/L with grade 4 histological fibrosis of liver, compared with reference interval of 0.41 ± 0.11 kU/L *1901*

Anti-Hepatitis C Antibodies *Serum* *Increase* Disease presence confirmed by detection of anti-HCV antibodies *3625*

Anti-Liver Cytosolic Antigen *Serum* *Increase* Occurs at high titers in some patients with active disease *1778*

Anti-LKM1 Antibodies *Serum* *No Effect* In 15 patients with chronic hepatitis C antibodies not detected in any patients prior to initiation of γ-interferon treatment *4453*

Anti-Mitochondrial Antibodies *Serum* *No Effect* In 15 patients with chronic hepatitis C antibodies not detected in any patients prior to initiation of γ-interferon treatment *4453*

Anti-Smooth Muscle Antibodies *Serum* *Increase* In 15 patients with chronic hepatitis C titers greater than 1:50 observed in 4 patients prior to initiation of γ-interferon treatment *4453*

Antinuclear Antibodies *Serum* *Increase* In 15 patients with chronic hepatitis C titers greater than 1:50 and 1:200 observed in 8 and 2 patients, respectively, prior to initiation of γ-interferon treatment *4453*

Antithyroglobulin Antibodies *Serum* *No Effect* In 15 patients with chronic hepatitis C antibodies not detected in any patients prior to initiation of γ-interferon treatment *4453*

Antithyroid Microsome Antibodies *Serum* *No Effect* In 15 patients with chronic hepatitis C antibodies not detected in any patients prior to initiation of γ-interferon treatment *4453*

Aspartate Aminotransferase *Serum* *Increase* In 5 patients with chronic hepatitis C mean activity of 181 ± 11 U/L increased compared with 23 ± 1 U/L in 30 healthy controls *2269* Increased activity associated with increasing degree of hepatic fibrosis *3917* In 326 untreated patients with chronic hepatitis C mean activity of 53 ± 36 U/L significantly different from upper reference limit of 35 U/L *1901* In 94 patients mean activity of 49.0 ± 27.4 U/L significantly greater than reference values of 22.2 ± 12.1 U/L *5433* Mean activity in patients with chronic hepatitis C who developed cirrhosis of 119 U/L significantly higher than in those who did not, 71 U/L *4785* Activity throughout disease usually less than 500 U/L and rarely greater than 1,000 U/L *3406* In 22 patients with chronic hepatitis C activities ranged from 22 - 184 U/L compared with normal range of 6 - 53 U/L *2560*

Aspartate Aminotransferase:Alanine Aminotransferase Ratio
Serum *Increase* Mean ratio in patients with chronic hepatitis C who developed cirrhosis (1.05) significantly higher than in those who did not (0.60) *4785*

Bilirubin *Serum* *Decrease* Increased concentration associated with increasing degree of hepatic fibrosis *3917*
Serum *Increase* In 5 patients with chronic hepatitis C mean concentration of 2.2 ± 0.3 mg/dL increased compared with 0.6 ± 0.1 mg/dL in 30 healthy controls *2269* In 326 untreated patients with chronic hepatitis C mean concentration of 13 ± 6 mg/L significantly different from upper reference limit of 12 mg/L *1901*

CA 19-9 *Serum* *Increase* In 19 patients with chronic hepatitis C median concentration of 79 kU/L significantly higher than upper limit of normal of 35 kU/L, with 84% of patients having abnormal values *3218*

Carcinoembryonic Antigen *Serum* *Increase* In 19 patients with chronic hepatitis C median concentration of 4 µg/L not different from upper limit of normal of 14 µg/L, but 6% of patients had abnormal values *3218*

β-Chorionic Gonadotropin *Plasma* *Increase* Mean concentration increased to about 95 ng/mL in mild cases with fibrosis to 125 ng/mL in severe cases above upper limit of normal of 78 ng/mL *5315*

Creatine Kinase *Serum* *No Effect* In 2 patients with hepatitis C-associated osteosclerosis mean activities of 40 and 89 U/L compared with upper limit of normal of 195 U/L *5659*

Creatine Kinase BB-Isoenzyme *Serum* *No Effect* In 2 patients with hepatitis C-associated osteosclerosis mean activities of < 3 and < 5 U/L (not detected %) compared with normal of 0 - 1% *5659*

Cryoglobulins *Serum* *Increase* Cryoglobulinemia observed in 69 of 127 patients with HCV infections with mean concentration of 0.33 g/L *3165*

Ferritin *Serum* *Increase* In 45 patients with chronic hepatitis C viral genotype 1b mean concentration of 170 µg/mL, in 43 with genotype 2a/2c 110 µg/mL and in 42 with genotype 3a 70 µg/mL compared with 60 µg/L in healthy controls *288*

α-Fetoprotein *Serum* *Increase* Concentrations greater than 10 ng/mL observed in 75 of 200 patients *337* Mean concentration of 11 ± 17 µg/L in 99 patients with chronic hepatitis C *1796*

Globulin *Serum* *Increase* In 5 patients with chronic hepatitis C mean concentration of 3.3 ± 0.2 g/dL increased compared with 2.8 ± 0.1 g/dL in 30 healthy controls *2269*

γ-Glutamyltransferase *Serum* *Increase* In 94 patients mean activity of 40.4 ± 42.4 U/L greater than reference values of 18.1 ± 10.2 U/L *5433* Increased activity associated with increasing degree of hepatic fibrosis *3917* In 326 untreated patients with chronic hepatitis C mean activity of 48 ± 55 U/L significantly different from upper reference limit of 40 U/L *1901* In 15 patients with chronic hepatitis C mean activity of 139 ± 116 U/L significantly greater than upper limit of normal of 80 U/L *4453*

Glutathione *Plasma* *Decrease* In 45 patients with chronic hepatitis C viral genotype 1b mean concentration of 5.5 µmol/L, in 43 with genotype 2a/2c 7 µmol/L and in 42 with genotype 3a 8 µmol/L compared with 8.5 µmol/L in healthy controls *288*

Glutathione S-Transferase *Serum* *Increase* In 94 patients mean activity of 12.0 ± 20.4 U/L greater than reference values of 3.50 ± 0.73 U/L *5433*

Hepatitis C Virus RNA *Serum* *Increase* In 22 patients with chronic hepatitis C viral RNA detected in all *2560*

Hyaluronan *Serum* *Increase* In 326 untreated patients with chronic hepatitis C mean concentration ranged from 36 ± 15 µg/L in the absence of histological fibrosis to 219 ± 89 µg/L with grade 4 histological fibrosis of liver, compared with reference interval of 27 ± 29 µg/L *1901*

Interferon-γ *Serum* *Increase* In 30 patients with chronic hepatitis C mean concentration of 0.52 ± 0.41 IU/mL compared with 0.2 ± 0.15 IU/mL in healthy donors *2450*

Interleukin-1β *Serum* *Increase* In 22 patients with chronic hepatitis C, concentrations not significantly increased in all, mean 1.1 ± 0.5 pg/mL compared with 0.73 ± 0.25 pg/mL in 20 healthy controls *2560*

Interleukin-8 *Serum* *Increase* In 22 patients with chronic hepatitis C concentrations significantly increased in all, mean 85 ± 26 pg/mL compared with 18 ± 7 pg/mL in 20 healthy controls *2560*

International Normalized Ratio *Plasma* *No Effect* In 5 patients with chronic hepatitis C mean ratio of 1.3 ± 0.3 not different when compared with reference range of < 1.2 *2269*

Lactate Dehydrogenase *Serum* *Increase* Increased activity associated with increasing degree of hepatic fibrosis *3917*

Laminin *Serum* *Increase* Mean concentration increased to about 130 ng/mL in mild cases to 185 ng/mL in severe cases, greater than upper limit of 140 ng/mL *5315*

Lipopolysaccharides *Serum* *Increase* In 16 of 89 patients (18%) with chronic hepatitis C detectable amounts of lipopolysaccharides were observed with a mean concentration of 2.72 ± 2.85 pg/mL, whereas no detectable amounts were observed in controls *2450*

Malondialdehyde *Red Blood Cells* *Increase* In 45 patients with chronic hepatitis C viral genotype 1b mean concentration of 6.5 nmol/mL, in 43 with genotype 2a/2c 6.0 nmol/mL and in 42 with genotype 3a 5.0 nmol/mL compared with 2.0 nmol/mL in healthy controls *288*

Metallopanstimulin *Serum* *Increase* In 11% of 18 patients with hepatitis B or C mean concentration exceeded upper limit of normal of < 10 ng/mL in healthy individuals aged 19 - 88 years *1462*

Neutrophils *Blood* *No Effect* In 5 patients with chronic hepatitis C mean concentration of 4.4 ± 0.5 x 10^3/µL not different when compared with 3.7 ± 0.1 x 10^3/µL in 30 healthy controls *2269*

N-terminal Peptide of Type III Procollagen *Serum* *Increase* Mean concentration in 19 patients with chronic hepatitis C of 0.86 ± 0.20 U/mL compared with reference interval of 0.35 - 0.65 U/mL *3669*

2',5'-Oligoadenylate Synthetase *Serum* *Increase* In 17 patients with chronic hepatitis C mean concentration of 79.96 ± 13.78 fmol/50 µL significantly higher than 13.78 ± 2.63 fmol/50 µL in 30 healthy age and sex matched controls *4928*

Platelets *Blood* *Decrease* Reduced concentration associated with increasing degree of hepatic fibrosis *3917*

Porphyrin, Total *Serum* *Increase* Of a population of 167 individuals, in patients positive for AIDS and hepatitis C median concentration of 2.31 nmol/L, 1.99 nmol/L in patients positive for AIDS and negative for hepatitis C, 1.31 nmol/L in AIDS negative hepatitis C positive patients and 1.14 nmol/L in AIDS and hepatitis C negative patients *3821*

Procollagen Type III Peptide *Serum* *Increase* Mean concentration increased to about 16 ng/mL in mild cases with fibrosis to 20 ng/mL in severe cases, greater than upper limit of normal of 12 ng/mL *5315*

Prolyl 4-Hydroxylase β-subunit *Serum* *No Effect* Mean concentration in 31 patients with chronic hepatitis C of 67 ± 17 ng/mL compared with 38 - 74 ng/mL in 30 control individuals *3669*

Prothrombin Time *Plasma* *Decrease* In 326 untreated patients with chronic hepatitis C mean time of 91 ± 11% different from normal *1901* Reduced time associated with increasing degree of hepatic fibrosis *3917*
Plasma *No Effect* In 45 patients with chronic hepatitis C viral genotype 1b mean time 12.0 ± 0.5 s, in 43 with genotype 2a/2c 12.0 ± 0.7 s and in 42 with genotype 3a 12.1 ± 0.6 s *288*

Rheumatoid Factor *Serum* *Increase* In 15 patients with chronic hepatitis C rheumatoid factor observed in 9 prior to initiation of γ-interferon treatment *4453*

Soluble CD14+ *Serum* *Increase* In 30 patients with chronic hepatitis C mean concentration of 4.50 ± 1.15 ng/mL compared with 2.94 ± 1.55 ng/mL in healthy donors *2450*

Soluble E-Selectin *Serum* *Increase* In 22 patients with chronic hepatitis C concentrations significantly increased in all, mean of 61.5 ± 7 ng/mL compared with 33 ± 3 ng/mL in 20 healthy controls *2560*

Soluble Intercellular Adhesion Molecule-1 *Serum* *Increase* In 22 patients with chronic hepatitis C concentrations significantly increased in all except one patient, mean 487 ± 49 ng/mL compared with 247 ± 20 ng/mL in 20 healthy controls *2560*

Soluble Tumor Necrosis Factor Receptor-p55
Serum *Increase* In 24 patients with chronic hepatitis C viral infection who were sustained responders to interferon mean concentration of 1.26 ng/mL and in 25 non-responders mean concentration of 1.32 ng/mL significantly higher than 0.85 ng/mL in 20 healthy controls *2373*

Soluble Tumor Necrosis Factor Receptor-p75
Serum *Increase* In 24 patients with chronic hepatitis C viral infection who were sustained responders to interferon mean concentration of 3.0 ng/mL and in 25 non-responders mean concentration of 3.7 ng/mL significantly higher than 1.5 ng/mL in 20 healthy controls *2373*

Soluble Vascular Cell Adhesion Molecule-1
Serum *Increase* In 22 patients with chronic hepatitis C concentrations significantly increased in all, mean of 1,527 ± 279 ng/mL compared with 672 ± 50 ng/mL in 20 healthy controls *2560*

Tissue Inhibitor of Metalloproteinase *Serum* *No Effect* Mean concentration of about 150 ng/mL in mild cases to 200 ng/mL in severe cases, less than upper limit of 250 ng/mL *5315*

Tumor Necrosis Factor-α *Serum* *Increase* In 22 patients with chronic hepatitis C concentrations significantly increased in all, mean of 32 ± 7 pg/mL compared with 12 ± 7 pg/mL in 20 healthy controls *2560*

Type IV Collagen 7S Domain *Serum* *Increase* Mean concentration increased to about 5.0 ng/mL in mild cases to 6.0 ng/mL in severe cases, greater than upper limit of 4.4 ng/mL *5315*

Type IV Collagen, Triple-helix Domain *Serum* *Increase* Mean concentration increased to about 100 ng/mL in mild cases to 170 ng/mL in severe cases, greater than upper limit of 90 ng/mL *5315*

70.59 Non A, Non B Hepatitis

Procollagen Type III Peptide *Serum* *Increase* During the acute phase the mean serum PIINP level rose significantly as compared to prehepatitis levels and to levels in a reference group not developing hepatitis *3374*

70.90 Fulminant Hepatitis

Prothrombin Time *Plasma* *Increase* Prolongation of the prothrombin time usually indicates that the disease is a chronic one, such as advanced cirrhosis: if it increases in acute liver disease it usually indicates the disease is a fulminant one *4617*

70.90 Fulminant Hepatitis *(continued)*

Tissue Plasminogen Activator *Plasma Increase* Concentration increased above 8.3 ng/mL in 86.1% of 36 patients with fulminant hepatitis *3887*

70.90 Viral Hepatitis

α_1-Acid Glycoprotein *Serum Increase* Sensitivity of 65% and a specificity of 80% with severe liver disease *1439*

Adenosine Deaminase *Serum Increase* Found to be significantly elevated in children *4264*

Alanine Aminotransferase *Serum Increase* Appears to reflect acute hepatic disease somewhat more specifically than is true of AST. Striking elevations of 220 - 1800 U/L *1025* Large increase typically observed *1576* May be elevated 2 - 4 weeks before the onset of jaundice and may reach peak levels after 1 - 2 weeks. Reflects organelle injury rather than necrosis or alteration of the permeability of the plasma membranes. Elevations as high as 2,000 - 3,000 U/L may be seen *900* Large increase in activity typically observed *5738* Markedly increased activity characteristic of disease *1980* Increases provide early indication of impending relapse, before clinically apparent *5252* In 10 active hepatitis patients mean activity of 1,205 ± 531 U/L significantly different from 14 ± 8 U/L in 20 healthy volunteers *2372* Marked elevation in nearly all patients *5008* In 22 patients with active viral hepatitis median activity of 669 U/L significantly higher than 25 U/L in their convalescent phase *1685* Significant increase observed in almost all patients *3141*

Albumin *Serum Decrease* Typical consequence of liver damage *1459* In 32% of 24 patients at initial hospitalization for this disorder *1576* Levels may be normal in the early stages of the disease process and may gradually decrease only after parenchymal damage has occurred. In severe and prolonged cases, levels bear a close relation to the clinical state and are helpful prognostically and in following results of treatment *5189*
Serum No Effect Normal in acute hepatitis; a decrease suggests chronic liver disease *1980*
Urine Increase A few RBC or mild proteinuria *900*

Aldolase *Serum Increase* Increased in 90% of patients up to 10 times normal. Activity parallels transaminase with a sharp rise before serum bilirubin rises and a return to normal 2 - 3 weeks after jaundice begins (acute icteric period) *5544* increased activity may parallel that of aminotransferases *1980* Activity increased typically with viral hepatitis *2952*

Alkaline Phosphatase *Serum Increase* Closely parallels serum bilirubin *4707* In 72% of 25 patients at initial hospitalization for this disorder *1576* Approximately 90% of patients have elevated values *1025* 40% of cases have values > 210 U/L *4707* Increased activity common *2803* Increase typically observed *5738*
White Blood Cells Increase Reported effect *5544*

Alkaline Phosphatase Isoenzymes *Serum Increase* Isoenzyme I was elevated in 12 of 12 patients. Isoenzyme IV was elevated in only 5 cases *2557*

Amino Acids *Urine Increase* Amount of urinary loss reflects degree of hepatic involvement *4707*

δ-Aminolevulinic Acid *Urine Increase* May occur *1025*

Amylase *Serum Increase* Moderate elevation found in some patients *4707* Mild pancreatitis may occur and is a contributing factor in mortality. Morphological evidence of pancreatitis found in 44% of 19 hepatitis patients at autopsy *4537*

Anti-Gliadin IgG Antibodies *Serum Increase* In 14 (13%) of the 110 patients with chronic viral hepatitis anti-gliadin IgA antibodies observed *5492*

Anti-Mitochondrial Antibodies *Serum Increase* Reported effect *4551* Transiently positive *1427* 11% of patients were positive (6% of controls) *4991* IgM smooth muscle antibody may appear as opposed to the IgG antibody found in chronic hepatitis *4160* 11% of patients were positive (6% of controls) *4176*
Serum No Effect No increase in frequency *4176*

Anti-Neutrophil Cytoplasm Antibodies *Serum Increase* In 7 of 26 patients with non-A, non-B and non-C hepatitis positive antibodies observed *2021*

Anti-Streptolysin-O Titer *Serum Increase* Above normal titers may occur *3953*

Anticardiolipin-specific IgG Antibodies *Serum No Effect* In 15 patients with acute viral hepatitis mean concentration of 5.0 ± 2.5 GPL units not significantly different from 6.3 ± 4.4 GPL units in 11 healthy controls *42*

Antinuclear Antibodies *Serum Increase* Found in 23% of patients and 2% of controls *4176*

α_1-Antitrypsin *Serum Increase* Increased *4373 4241 4763 4371 83*

Aspartate Aminotransferase *Serum Increase* Striking elevations (145 - 200 U/L) are seen in patients with acute hepatic necrosis *1025* May be elevated 2 - 4 weeks before the onset of jaundice and may reach peak levels after 1 - 2 weeks. Reflects organelle injury rather than necrosis or alteration of the permeability of the plasma membrane *900* In 22 patients with active viral hepatitis median activity of 235 U/L significantly higher than 20 U/L in their convalescent phase *1685* Increase typical of disease *2039* Marked increase typically observed *1980* In 92% of 25 patients at initial hospitalization for this disorder *1576*

Bile Acids *Serum Increase* In one study with viral hepatitis type B, bile acids and transaminase were of equal sensitivity *4891*

Bilirubin *Feces Decrease* Increased excretion typically observed but then falls at peak of disease *5544*
Feces Increase Increased excretion typically observed but then falls at peak of disease *5544*
Serum Increase Increased concentration typically observed *5738* Jaundice becomes apparent when concentration exceeds 2 mg/dL. Usually rises for 10 - 14 days to an average peak of about 10 mg/dL. But much higher levels are encountered especially when hemolysis is present. The rate of decline from the peak level is more gradual and often requires 2 - 6 weeks. The level has no prognostic significance *900* Majority of patients have increased concentration *4822* In 22 patients with active viral hepatitis median concentration of 10 mg/dL significantly higher than 1 mg/dL in their convalescent phase *1685* In 10 active hepatitis patients mean concentration of 8.2 ± 2.6 mg/dL significantly different from 0.5 ± 0.3 mg/dL in 20 healthy volunteers *2372* In 78% of 24 patients at initial hospitalization for this disorder *1576* On occasion there is severe hemolytic anemia resulting in a marked rise in the serum bilirubin, this frequently occurs in patients with glucose-6-phosphate dehydrogenase deficiency *1980*
Urine Increase Appears a few days before the onset of jaundice *900* Increased excretion usually observed *2039* Seen in anicteric hepatitis *367*

Bilirubin, Direct *Serum Increase* Direct and indirect bilirubin are equally elevated in the icteric phase *367* Typical effect observed *2039* Serum bilirubin is 50 - 75% direct in the early stage; later, indirect bilirubin is proportionately more in acute icteric period *5544* In 93% of 19 patients at initial hospitalization for this disorder *1576*

Bilirubin, Indirect *Serum Increase* In 75% of 18 patients at initial hospitalization for this disorder *1576* Serum bilirubin is 50 - 75% direct in the early stage; later, indirect bilirubin is proportionately more *5544*

Biotin *Serum Decrease* Significantly low in fulminant hepatitis compared to healthy controls *3703*

BSP Retention *Serum Increase* Useful in screening for anicteric disease and during convalescence *900* The earliest abnormality, followed by bilirubinuria, before serum bilirubin increases *5544*

CA 19-9 *Serum Increase* In one study 28% of patients with hepatitis had concentrations greater than 60 U/mL *3120*

CA 27-29 *Serum Increase* In 30% of 23 women with hepatitis concentration increased *766*

CA 72-4 *Serum Increase* In 30 patients with hepatitis or liver cirrhosis 3 (10%) had a concentration greater than cut-off of 2.5 U/mL with median concentration of 1.3 U/mL *4505*

CA 125 *Serum Increase* In one study 54% of patients with hepatitis had concentrations above cutoff value of 35 U/mL *3120* Elevated in 4% of patients *3560*

Carbon Dioxide Partial Pressure *Blood Decrease* Reduced in a high percentage of chronic as well as acute hepatitis patients *4707*

Carcinoembryonic Antigen *Serum Increase* 30% of patients had values > 2.5 ng/mL *4891* In one study 11% of patients with hepatitis had concentrations above cutoff value of

5.0 ng/mL *3120* In 30 patients with hepatitis or liver cirrhosis, 14 (47%) had a concentration greater than cut-off of 3 ng/mL with median concentration of 2.2 ng/mL *4505* In 69 patients with hepatitis 70% had concentrations less than 2.5 ng/mL, 29% had concentrations between 2.6 and 5.0 ng/mL, 1% had concentrations between 5.1 and 10.0 ng/mL and 0% had concentrations greater than 10.0 ng/mL *2010*

$CD4^+$ Lymphocytes *Blood Increase* Significantly higher as compared with normal controls *3916*

$CD8^+$ Lymphocytes *Blood Increase* Significantly higher as compared with normal controls *3916*

Chenodeoxycholic Acid *Serum Increase* Increased serum bile acids in anicteric viral hepatitis from either A or B virus. Elevated postprandial levels may persist even after transaminase and BSP retention have returned to normal *2426*

Cholesterol *Red Blood Cells Increase* 25 - 50% increase in the membrane concentration, resulting in the characteristic target cell *5699*
Serum Decrease Magnitude of depression is directly related to degree of hepatic damage. A progressive fall is a grave prognostic sign *4707* In 25% of 19 patients at initial hospitalization for this disorder *1576* Normal or mildly depressed in hepatitis; but markedly depressed in severe hepatitis *1025*

Cholesterol Esters *Serum Decrease* Striking decrease as liver involvement progresses *4707*

Cholic Acid *Serum Increase* Increased serum bile acids in anicteric viral hepatitis from either A or B virus. Elevated postprandial levels may persist even after transaminase and BSP retention have returned to normal *2426*

Cholinesterase *Serum Decrease* Tends to be more marked in patients ill with chronic liver disease, such as cirrhosis than in those ill with acute conditions, such as viral hepatitis, ascending cholangitis and acute anoxic hepatomegaly. Peaks and depressions in cholinesterase activity in acute liver disease are related to the extent of hepatic parenchymal damage *5498* Typically observed *3161* In 22 patients with active viral hepatitis median activity of 4,004 U/L significantly lower than 5,312 U/L in their convalescent phase *1685*

Cold Agglutinins *Serum Increase* Elevated titers may persist for weeks or months *4551*

Copper *Serum Increase* Significant, $p < 0.001$ *5460*

Copper Zinc Superoxide Dismutase *Serum Increase* Total activity was significantly increased in the acute phase and dropped to normal levels in the restoration phase in 29 children with cytomegalovirus hepatitis *809*

Coproporphyrin *Urine Increase* Typical observation *1290*

Creatine Kinase *Serum No Effect* No significant effect observed *1980*

Cryomacroglobulins *Serum Increase* May be observed *1774*

CYFRA 21-1 *Serum Increase* In 29 patients with hepatitis median concentration of 2.2 ng/mL significantly different from that in 50 healthy individuals with median concentration of 1.2 ng/mL and range of 0.5 - 2.4 ng/mL *3559*

Endothelin-1 *Plasma Increase* ET-1 levels (5.07 ± 2.54 pg/mL, mean ± SD), were significantly higher than those in healthy controls (2.18 ± 0.37 pg/mL) *5339*

Erythrocyte Sedimentation Rate *Blood Increase* High (mean 24.1 ± 10.7 mm/h) in cases of uncomplicated HBsAg-negative hepatitis and normal (mean < 10 mm/h) in HBsAg positive cases *3468* Nonspecific *4307*

Factor V *Plasma Decrease* Decreased factor V to below 10 - 20% of normal was useful in assessing prognosis in fulminant hepatic failure due to viral infections *5276*

Fat *Feces Increase* May be excessive amounts of fecal fat *4707*

Ferritin *Serum Increase* In one study 46% of patients with hepatitis had concentrations above cutoff value of 500 ng/mL *3120*

α-Fetoprotein *Serum Increase* Among 51 patients with fulminant hepatitis and coma, AFP was detected in 17 (85%) of 20 who survived and in only 12 (38.7%) of 31 fatal cases, ($p = 0.002$). Positivity was related to the severity of the disease and its appearance was followed by recovery. High values in severe forms are a favorable prognostic sign *2574* In some cases *2655* Levels > 30 ng/mL were found in 87% of patients with acute hepatitis and in 58% with chronic active hepatitis *75*
Serum No Effect In one study no patient with hepatitis had a concentration above cutoff value of 200 ng/mL *3120*

Folate *Serum Increase* Increased *1498* *1777*

α_1-Globulin *Serum Decrease* Concentration may be decreased in patients with acute viral hepatitis *4617* Indicates acute hepatocellular damage *5544*

α_2-Globulin *Serum Decrease* Indicates acute hepatocellular damage *5544*
Serum Increase Slight to moderate increase (related to the increase in α-lipoprotein) *1290*

β-Globulin *Serum Increase* Increased in cholangiolitis. May reach very high levels in chronic progressive disease *5189* Associated with intrahepatic biliary obstruction *1290*

γ-Globulin *Serum Increase* Frequent transiently elevated *1980* Mean total serum values were highest in acute viral hepatitis, primary hepatocellular carcinoma and cirrhosis, in that order *1459*
Serum No Effect In 10 active hepatitis patients mean concentration of 1.7 ± 0.4 g/dL not significantly different from 1.1 ± 0.3 g/dL in 20 healthy volunteers *2372*

Glucaric Acid *Urine Increase* A 3 fold increase of D-glucaric acid was found in the early stages of disease (37.13 ± 3.08 μmol/24 h vs. 9.91 ± 1.18 μmol/24 h in controls) when serum transaminases and bilirubin were very high. A lower but significantly raised level was found during recovery when the transaminases and bilirubin were greatly reduced *703*

Glucose *Serum Decrease* Concentration reduced with severe disease *4707* Can occur with various types of liver disease. Hepatic hypoglycemia is a fasting hypoglycemia and often only transiently relieved by food *1980*

Glucose Tolerance *Serum Decrease* Subnormal insulin response to oral glucose tolerance test was found in 5 of 14 patients in the icteric phase *3415*

γ-Glutamyltransferase *Saliva No Effect* Activity may be normal in normal in infectious hepatitis *2448*
Serum Increase In 77% of 14 patients at initial hospitalization for this disorder *1576* In 10 active hepatitis patients mean activity of 197 ± 93 U/L significantly different from 10 ± 3 U/L in 20 healthy volunteers *2372* The mean elevation (152 U/L) in 17 patients was 5.2 times the upper limit of normal *3161*

Glycated Protein *Serum Decrease* In acute fulminant hepatitis, the values showed a statistically significant difference between fatal (21.9 mg/dL) and surviving cases (37.4 mg/dL) *2729*

Granular Casts *Urine Increase* During the early icteric phase may reflect renal abnormalities *367*

Hematocrit *Blood Decrease* May develop late in the course of the disease *367* A mild degree of transient anemia *1980*

Hemoglobin *Blood Decrease* Mild anemia may appear late in the course of acute disease *367* A mild degree of transient anemia *1980*

Hepatitis B Surface Antigen *Serum Increase* About 80% of patients with clinical signs of viral hepatitis type B have been found to have the antigen in their blood when multiple timed sample were taken *1980* Can be present during incubation period and acute phase; occasionally may persist *5544*

β-Hexosaminidase *Serum Increase* Increase in total concentration (hexosaminidase A and B) *3850*

Hyaluronic Acid *Serum Increase* Measured concentrations in paired serum samples from 22 patients with acute hepatitis and from 50 healthy age-matched controls. Concentrations were significantly elevated in 22 patients with acute hepatitis *4270* Measured serum levels at presentation and 1 year follow-up in 37 infants who presented with hepatobiliary disease in the first 6 months of life. In patients at presentation, the hyaluronic acid concentration was raised in 6 of 11 with cryptogenic hepatitis of infancy. One year later, the 9 patients who developed progressive liver disease showed 2 - 6-fold increases in hyaluronic acid concentration while no increase was observed in the 28 with undetectable or mild disease *5283*

immunoglobulin A *Serum Increase* Mean concentration in 10 patients with acute viral hepatitis of about 400 mg/dL significantly higher than 288 ± 121 mg/dL in 18 healthy blood donors *54* Reported effect *5544*

Immunoglobulin G *Serum Increase* Slightly elevated γ-globulins, usually < 2.0 g/dL. IgG rises as illness progresses

70.90 Viral Hepatitis *(continued)*

Immunoglobulin G *(continued)*
900 Frequently transiently elevated *1980* Mean concentration in 10 patients with acute viral hepatitis of about 3,100 mg/dL significantly higher than 1,200 ± 319 mg/dL in 18 healthy blood donors *54*

Immunoglobulin M *Serum Increase* Mean concentration in 10 patients with acute viral hepatitis of about 280 mg/dL significantly higher than 80 ± 29 mg/dL in 18 healthy blood donors *54* Initial rise in IgM, followed by IgG *900* Usually increased above 400 mg/dL during acute phase *5544*

Interleukin-1α *Serum Increase* In 12 patients with acute hepatitis (A, B, and C) mean concentration of 16.0 ± 8.8 pg/mL compared with 1.1 ± 2.7 pg/mL in 18 healthy controls. Concentration decreased during recovery and became undetectable after 6 months *5259*

Interleukin-1β *Serum Increase* In 12 patients with acute viral hepatitis (A, B, and C) mean concentration of 16.0 ± 4.5 pg/mL significantly greater than 1.9 ± 5.7 pg/mL in 18 healthy controls. In all 4 patients with hepatitis B concentration decreased during recovery phase and was undetectable after 6 months *5259*

Interleukin-6 *Serum Increase* In 12 patients with acute viral hepatitis (A, B and C) mean concentration of 43.3 ± 16.0 pg/mL significantly greater than 0.5 ± 1.6 pg/mL in 18 healthy controls. In 6 patients with hepatitis B concentration decreased during recovery period and became undetectable in all patients after 6 months follow-up *5259*

Iron *Serum Increase* Increase becomes evident only after liver disease has been present for 2 - 3 weeks *369*

Iron-binding Capacity, Total *Serum Increase* May be increased with hepatitis *5544* Increases are rare other than in iron deficiency, but they may occur in viral hepatitis *1980*

Isocitrate Dehydrogenase *Serum Increase* Invariably elevated when measured within 10 days of onset of jaundice *5008* Usually elevated in the early stage (5 - 10 times normal) but returns to normal in 2 - 3 weeks *5544* 40 times normal *1025*

Isoleucine *Plasma Increase* A close relationship was found between the onset of encephalopathy and amino acid equilibrium disturbance, characterized by a fall in the molar ratio between valine, leucine and isoleucine and phenylalanine and tyrosine. All showed absolute elevations with onset of encephalopathy *1097*

Lactate Dehydrogenase *Serum Increase* 8 of 10 cases showed mild elevation *3227* Moderate elevation in most cases *5008* Slightly elevated (1 - 2 fold) values *1025* In 80% of 25 patients at initial hospitalization in this disorder *1576* Slight increase *1980*

Lactate Dehydrogenase Isoenzyme-5 *Serum Increase* Markedly elevated in 7 cases. Comprised 35.4% of the total serum LD (normal = 0 - 6%) *1756*

Lactate Dehydrogenase Isoenzymes *Serum Decrease* In 7 cases, LD_1 and LD_2 were markedly decreased (13.0% and 19.3% respectively) *1756*
Serum Increase In 7 cases, LD_4 was markedly increased (11.0%). Total LD was elevated to a mean level of 2,057 U/L *1756*

Lecithin *Red Blood Cells Increase* 25 - 50% increase in the membrane concentration, resulting in the characteristic target cell *5699*

Leucine *Plasma Increase* A close relationship was found between the onset of encephalopathy and amino acid equilibrium disturbance, characterized by a fall in the molar ratio between valine, leucine, and isoleucine, and phenylalanine and tyrosine. All showed absolute elevations with onset of encephalopathy *1097*

Leucine Aminopeptidase *Serum Increase* In 12 patients, 92% showed elevated values, ranging from 320 - 900 U/L and a mean of 592 U/L *579*

Leukocytes *Blood Decrease* Leukopenia (lymphopenia and neutropenia) is noted with onset of fever, followed by relative lymphocytosis and monocytosis *5544* There may be a slight transient drop but rarely to leukopenic levels *900* Observed in some patients *1980* *2039*

Lipase *Serum Decrease* Lack of bile salts result in the failure to activate pancreatic lipase in the intestinal lumen *4707*

Lipoprotein Lp(a) *Serum Decrease* In 22 patients with active viral hepatitis median concentration of 7 mg/dL significantly lower than 32 mg/dL in their convalescent phase *1685*

Lymphocytes *Blood Decrease* Impaired T-cell reactivity is due to a disturbed function of T-cell and not to a decrease in their number. In cases associated with significant hepatocellular damage, a reduction in the number of circulating B-cells was observed *3837*
Blood Increase Noted in some patients *900* Observed in some patients *1098* A relative lymphocytosis may result with some atypical lymphocytes *1980*

α_2-Macroglobulin *Serum Increase* Reported effect *3480*

β_2-Macroglobulin *Serum Increase* An increased serum concentration is characteristic *2586*

Macrophage Colony Stimulating Factor *Serum Increase* In 10 patients with active hepatitis mean concentration of about 5.6 ng/mL significantly different from 1.95 ± 0.44 ng/mL in 20 healthy volunteers *2372*

Magnesium *Red Blood Cells Decrease* RBC concentration was 3.18 ± 0.78 mmol/L before treatment. Normal concentration of 5.08 ± 0.25 mmol/L *508* 2 of 5 patients had abnormally low concentrations. The mean concentration for the entire group, 4.3 mmol/L packed cells, was significantly ($p < 0.001$) decreased below normal *5547*
Serum Decrease Before treatment, plasma concentration was 0.96 - 0.2 mmol/L. Normal concentration of 1.73 ± 0.13 mmol/L *508*

Malate Dehydrogenase *Serum Increase* Increase typically observed *1290*

Manganese *Serum Increase* Significant increase ($p < 0.01$) *5460* During acute phase increase up to four times that seen in normal subjects *5460* Increase becomes evident only after liver disease has been present for 2 - 3 weeks *369*

Manganese Superoxide Dismutase *Serum Increase* Total blood activity was significantly increased in the acute phase and dropped to normal levels in the restoration phase in 29 children with cytomegalovirus hepatitis *809*

Metallothionein *Serum No Effect* Since condition not associated with increased liver copper accumulation plasma concentration unaffected *3646*

β_2-Microglobulin *Serum Increase* In one study of patients with hepatitis 44% had concentrations above cutoff value of 2.0 mg/mL *3120*

Monocytes *Blood Increase* In 55% of 23 patients at initial hospitalization for this disorder *1576* Reported effect *1098*

Mucoprotein *Serum Decrease* Observed effect *1025*

Nickel *Serum Decrease* Thought to be caused by hypoalbuminemia *3428*

5'-Nucleotidase *Serum Increase* Elevations ranging from 8 - 103 U/L (normal = 2 - 11 U/L) were observed in 24 patients *2803* Increases frequently observed *367*

Ornithine Carbamoyltransferase *Serum Increase* Liver cell damage *5544*

Phenylalanine *Plasma Increase* A close relationship was found between the onset of encephalopathy and amino acid equilibrium disturbance, characterized by a fall in the molar ratio between valine leucine and isoleucine and phenylalanine and tyrosine. All showed absolute elevations with onset of encephalopathy *1097*

Phospholipids *Serum Decrease* Increased in mild but decreased in severe hepatitis *5544*
Serum Increase Increased in mild but decreased in severe hepatitis *5544*

Platelets *Blood Decrease* Patient may show anemia, leukocytosis, thrombocytopenia in fulminant hepatitis with hepatic failure *5544*

Porphyrin, Total *Urine Increase* Reported effect *5544*

Prealbumin *Serum Decrease* The mean value was 6.0 mg/dL in fatal cases, 7.4 mg/dL in survivors. The difference was not statistically significant *2729*

Procollagen Type IV Peptide *Serum Increase* The serum concentrations were 4.2 ± 0.9 ng/mL in controls, 5.1 ± 2.0 ng/mL in acute hepatitis *5765*

Prothrombin Time *Plasma Decrease* In 22 patients with active viral hepatitis median time of 90% significantly less than 100% in their convalescent phase *1685*

Plasma *Increase* May be slightly prolonged but bleeding problems are uncommon. A greatly prolonged prothrombin time heralds massive hepatic necrosis and is a sign of poor prognosis *900* Usually normal, and if prolonged, suggests severe hepatitis. If the prolongation increases, it is indicative of fulminant hepatitis *1980* Prolongation of the prothrombin time usually indicates that the disease is a chronic one, such as advanced cirrhosis: if it increases in acute liver disease it usually indicates the disease is a fulminant one, as in acute viral hepatitis *4617*

Reticulocytes *Blood* *Increase* Mild hemolytic anemia with increase in the reticulocyte count are commonly found *1980*

Rheumatoid Factor *Serum* *Increase* Observed in some patients *1980* 24% positivity *874* *306* Concentration may be increased as in other diseases with chronic inflammation *2952* Rheumatoid factor may be observed in certain patients *2473*

Soluble HLA-I *Serum* *Increase* Concentration reportedly increased with viral infections including hepatitis *5306*

Specific Gravity *Urine* *Decrease* Concentrating ability is sometimes decreased *5544*

Superoxide Dismutase *Blood* *Increase* Total activity was significantly increased in the acute phase and dropped to normal levels in the restoration phase in 29 children with cytomegalovirus hepatitis *809*

Taurine *Plasma* *Increase* Mean concentration of 2.0 mol/mL in patients with severe hepatitis significantly different from 0.12 mol/mL in healthy controls but concentration of 0.9 mol/mL in patients with mild hepatitis not significantly different from the controls *264*

Thyroxine Binding Globulin *Serum* *Increase* Not infrequently *5679* Increased level *4289* May increase TBG concentration *1965* Increased concentration observed in infectious hepatitis *206*

Thyroxine (T4) *Serum* *Increase* Increased concentration of TBG observed in infectious hepatitis which could cause increased thyroxine concentration *206* Not infrequently *5679* May increase TBG concentration *1965*

Tri-iodothyronine (T3) *Serum* *Increase* May increase TBG concentration *1965*

Triglycerides *Serum* *Increase* In 12 children a relationship was suggested between ALT and triglycerides, in which the triglycerides provide an energy substrate, thereby freeing glucose for alanine synthesis *51*

Tumor Necrosis Factor-α *Serum* *Increase* In 12 patients with acute viral hepatitis (A, B, and C) mean concentration of 41.3 ± 13.7 pg/mL significantly higher than 1.1 ± 4.7 pg/mL in 18 healthy controls. In 4 patients with hepatitis B concentration decreased during recovery. TNF-α became undetectable after a 6 months follow-up *5259*

Tyrosine *Plasma* *Increase* A close relationship was found between the onset of encephalopathy and amino acid equilibrium disturbance, characterized by a fall in the molar ratio between valine, leucine, and isoleucine, and phenylalanine and tyrosine. All showed absolute elevations with onset of encephalopathy *1097*

Uric Acid *Serum* *Increase* Mean levels were 8.0 ± 0.6 (normal concentration of 6.5 ± 0.6 mg/dL) in 16 patients. Values for the entire group were not statistically significant, but individual decreases measured upon recovery showed significant individual elevations *4295*
Urine *Increase* 24 h excretion was markedly elevated in patients (1,405 ± 149 mg/day) compared to controls (748 ± 58 mg/day) *4295*

Urobilinogen *Feces* *Decrease* Disappears at peak of disease *5544*
Urine *Increase* At peak of the disease, it disappears for days or weeks *5544* Increases during defervescent period *900*

Valine *Plasma* *Increase* A close relationship was found between the onset of encephalopathy and amino acid equilibrium disturbance, characterized by a fall in the molar ratio between valine, leucine and isoleucine, and phenylalanine and tyrosine. All showed absolute elevations with onset of encephalopathy *1097*

Vitamin A *Serum* *Decrease* In severe hepatitis *5544*

Vitamin B_{12} Binding Capacity, Unsaturated
Serum *Decrease* Decreased concentrations observed during hepatitis *2952*

VLDL-Cholesterol *Serum* *Increase* Marked elevation *126*

Zinc *Serum* *Decrease* Generally declines to values comparable to those found in other acute infections. Serum Zn exists almost entirely in a diffusible state with very little protein-bound *369*

71.00 Rabies

Albumin *Urine* *Increase* May be present *5545*

Cells *Cerebrospinal Fluid* *Increase* Usually < 1,000 /μL but counts between 1,500 - 4,000 /μL have been observed *2832*

Erythrocytes *Saliva* *Increase* May be bloody *5252*

Glucose *Serum* *Decrease* May be somewhat below normal *900*

Ketones *Serum* *Increase* Acetone may be present *900*
Urine *Increase* Acetone may be present *900*

Leukocytes *Blood* *Increase* Leukocytosis with a relative increase of neutrophils is the rule. May be moderate but high values are not unusual. The maximum count observed was 32,000 /μL *900*
Cerebrospinal Fluid *No Effect* Usually normal *900* Rreported effect *2832*

Protein *Cerebrospinal Fluid* *Increase* A slight increase *5545*
Urine *Increase* Slight *2192*

Specific Gravity *Urine* *Increase* The urine is concentrated, particularly when the body temperature is elevated and/or the kidney function is diminished *900*

72.90 Mumps

Albumin *Urine* *Increase* Proteinuria should suggest a diagnosis of mumps nephritis *900*

Amylase *Serum* *Increase* 96.2% of 224 patients showed elevations during the course of the disease. In 83.77% of patients the elevations occurred in the first week and fell progressively *675* Increased during the period of swelling and for about 10 days thereafter in 90% of patients *900*
Urine *Increase* Increased during first week *5545*

Cells *Cerebrospinal Fluid* *Increase* In meningitis and meningoencephalitis fewer than 500 /μL with only occasional cell counts exceeding 2,000 /μL. In most cases the cells are almost exclusively mononuclear from the onset: polymorphonuclear leukocytes predominate for the first few days in only a small percentage of patients. Pleocytosis may continue for as long as 5 weeks *900*

Cold Agglutinins *Serum* *Increase* Increased titer *413*

Complement Fixation *Serum* *Increase* Positive during 2nd week and remains elevated > 6 weeks; paired sera showing a 4-fold increase in titer confirm recent infection *5252* *2832* Antibodies against the S and V antigens are the most widely used serologic test. The S antibodies usually rise within the first week of illness, the V antibodies appearing 1 - 2 weeks later. A presumptive diagnosis can therefore be made when elevated S antibodies are found in the absence of V antibodies *900*

Erythrocyte Casts *Urine* *Increase* Suggests a diagnosis of mumps nephritis *900*

Erythrocyte Sedimentation Rate *Blood* *Increase* May occur with mumps arthritis and orchitis *900*

Erythrocytes *Urine* *Increase* Suggests a diagnosis of mumps nephritis *900*

Glucose *Cerebrospinal Fluid* *Decrease* Usually normal, however, recent reports have emphasized that depressed CSF concentrations (< 40 mg/dL) may be present initially and persist for several days *900*

γ-Glutamyltransferase *Saliva* *No Effect* Compared with healthy controls *2448*

Hemagglutination Inhibition *Serum* *Increase* Develops later and persists longer by several months than complement-fixation test *5545* A 4-fold difference in titer between the 1st and 3rd week is diagnostic *5252*

Leukocytes *Blood* *Decrease* May be depressed, normal or elevated, with or without a relative lymphocytosis; they are of little value in establishing a diagnosis *900*
Blood *Increase* May be depressed, normal or elevated, with or without a relative lymphocytosis; they are of little value in

72.90 Mumps *(continued)*

Leukocytes *(continued)*
establishing a diagnosis *900* Total count often reaches 15,000 - 20,000 /µL, with a high percentage of polymorphonuclear cells *367*
Blood No Effect Usually within normal limits *5252*
Cerebrospinal Fluid Increase In meningitis and meningoencephalitis, CSF usually contains fewer than 500 /µL with only occasional counts > 2,000 /µL. In most cases the cells are almost exclusively mononuclear from the onset: polymorphonuclear leukocytes predominate for the first few days in only a small percentage of patients. Pleocytosis may continue for as long as 5 weeks *900*

Lipase *Serum Increase* 11.5% of patients had slightly elevated values *675*

Lymphocytes *Blood Increase* Usually there is a slight predominance of lymphocytes but at times the reverse is true *2832*
Cerebrospinal Fluid Increase Increased T-cells and decreased B-cells in CSF were found in mumps meningitis *2544* Cell counts range from 500 to several thousand/µL, and are predominantly lymphocytes *367*

Monocytes *Blood Increase* May occur *5252*

Neutralizing Antibodies *Serum Increase* The most reliable index of the immune status of natural disease or administration of the live attenuated virus vaccine. Unfortunately their determination is impractical as a routine diagnostic procedure *900*

Neutrophils *Cerebrospinal Fluid Increase* In meningitis and meningoencephalitis fewer than 500 cells/µL with only occasional cell counts exceeding 2,000 /µL in most cases the cells are almost exclusively mononuclear from the onset: polymorphonuclear leukocytes predominate for the first few days in only a small percentage of patients. Pleocytosis may continue for as long as 5 weeks *900*

Protein *Cerebrospinal Fluid Increase* Normal or slightly elevated *900*
Urine Increase Indicates mumps nephritis *900*

73.00 Psittacosis

Alanine Aminotransferase *Serum Increase* With severe liver involvement *900*

Albumin *Urine Increase* Frequently seen *900*

Alkaline Phosphatase *Serum Increase* With severe liver involvement *900*

Angiotensin-converting Enzyme *Serum No Effect* Not elevated in active hypersensitivity pneumonitis *3400*

Aspartate Aminotransferase *Serum Increase* With severe liver involvement *900*

Cold Agglutinins *Serum No Effect* Not usually observed with disease *5545*

Complement Fixation *Serum Increase* A low titer is highly suspicious during the acute phase of the illness, and the diagnosis is confirmed by a 4-fold increase in titer *1980* Positive but not conclusive tests are presumptive in diagnosis because of false positives with other infections and cross reactions with lymphogranuloma venereum *5545*

Creatinine *Serum Increase* With severe renal involvement *900*

Erythrocyte Sedimentation Rate *Blood Increase* Usually is increased but may be normal *5545*
Blood No Effect Frequently normal *5252*

Erythrocytes *Sputum Increase* Occasionally bloody *5252*

γ-Globulin *Serum Increase* Often associated with hypergammaglobulinemia *4707*

γ-Glutamyltransferase *Serum Increase* With severe liver involvement *900*

Lactate Dehydrogenase *Serum Increase* With severe liver involvement *900*

Leukocytes *Blood Decrease* During the early stage of the illness *1980* Normal or decreased in acute phase, then increases in convalescence *5252*
Blood Increase May occur during the late or convalescent stage *1980*

Neutrophils *Blood Decrease* Rarely, profound granulocytopenia occurs *900*

Protein *Urine Increase* Common during the febrile period *5252*

Urea Nitrogen *Serum Increase* With severe renal involvement *900*

75.00 Epstein-Barr Virus Infection

Heterophile Antibody *Serum Increase* Increased concentrations indicate recent or past infection with Epstein-Barr virus *2952*

75.00 Infectious Mononucleosis

Adenosine Deaminase *Serum Increase* The highest values were found in patients with infectious mononucleosis *2737 5360*

Adenosine-N6-diethylthioether-N1-pyridinoximine 5'-phosphate *Serum No Effect* In one patient with infectious mononucleosis concentration of 168.1 nmol/dL not significantly different from concentration in healthy individuals in whom the mean concentration was 162.2 nmol/dL *5294*

Alanine Aminotransferase *Serum Increase* Elevations occur in 80 - 100% during acute illness and return to normal in 3 - 5 weeks *5677* Show abnormal results in most cases *2832* Reflected the presence and extent of hepatic damage, and the severity of subjective symptoms in 36 patients *4325*

Alkaline Phosphatase *Serum Increase* May occur; hepatic involvement is usually mild *5677* 30 (65%) had dissociation with serum bilirubin concentration. Occasionally high levels, even with normal bilirubin concentration *4822* Observed in some patients *3765* Increased in many cases, with maximum values during the 3rd week of the disease. 60 - 70% of cases are elevated ranging from 25 - 215 U/L. Only 20% of cases had values > 107 U/L *1290* Observed in some patients *1980*

Alkaline Phosphatase Isoenzymes *Serum Increase* An electrophoretically distinct isoenzyme (phosphatase N) was found in the serum of all 22 patients. Values ranged from 13 - 100% of the total activity, with 6 cases having > 80% phos-N activity *3765*

Amylase *Serum Increase* May be associated with hyperamylasemia *3024*

Anti-Mitochondrial Antibodies *Serum Increase* Reported effect *4551* IgM smooth muscle antibody may appear as opposed to the IgG antibody found in chronic hepatitis *4160* Transiently positive *2207*

Antibody Titer *Serum Increase* The presence of EB virus antibody is essential for diagnosis in heterophile-negative cases. Antibody to early antigen and EB virus-specific IgM antibody occurs in 75 - 85% of acute cases *2114*

Antinuclear Antibodies *Serum Increase* 65% of patients were positive *4068* May be present without positive LE cell test *1290*

Aspartate Aminotransferase *Serum Increase* In 80% of patients moderate (50 - 300 U/L) increases are observed. Usual values of 25 - 400 U/L *1025* In 90% of 11 patients at initial hospitalization for this disorder *1576* Elevations occur in 80 - 100% during acute illness and return to normal in 3 - 5 weeks *5677*

Bilirubin *Serum Increase* Over 1 mg/dL in 37% of patients *900* May occur; hepatic involvement is usually mild *5677*

BSP Retention *Serum Increase* May occur; hepatic involvement is usually mild *5677*

Cholesterol *Serum Decrease* In 60% of 10 patients at initial hospitalization for this disorder *1576*

Cold Agglutinins *Serum Increase* Occur frequently; they are present mostly in the IgM fraction and have anti-I specificity *1024* Elevated titers may persists for weeks or months *4551 666*

Erythrocyte Sedimentation Rate *Blood Decrease* Low readings may reflect the intracellular nature of the offending organism or liver involvement that causes decreased synthesis of fibrinogen *1980*

γ-Globulin *Serum Increase* Often associated with hypergammaglobulinemia *4707*

γ-Glutamyltransferase *Serum* *Increase* Levels correlate with serum alkaline phosphatase and 5'-nucleotidase levels *1290*

Hematocrit *Blood* *Decrease* Anemia is rare *2832*
Blood *Increase* In 27% of 11 patients at initial hospitalization for this disorder *1576*

Hemoglobin *Blood* *Decrease* Anemia is rare *2832*
Blood *Increase* In 45% of 11 patients at initial hospitalization for this disorder *1576*

Heterophile Antibody *Serum* *Increase* Approximately 90% of patients with clinically evident infectious mononucleosis have demonstrable heterophile antibodies *2952* Preset at some stafe of disease in most patients *367* Elevated titers which agglutinate sheep RBCs; 40% have positive tests during 1st week of illness and 80% by the 3rd week *5619* Occurs at some time in most patients *5677* Develop in the 1st week of illness in most patients and ultimately appear in 80 - 90% of patients and persist for 3 - 6 months *1980* Elevated titers may persist longer than a year in 75% of patients. Over 95% of typical cases are heterophile antibody positive if followed long enough *1395*

immunoglobulin A *Serum* *Increase* Reported effect *5677* A modest increase may occur *1971*

Immunoglobulin G *Serum* *Increase* Mean values 50% higher than normal *1971*

Immunoglobulin M *Serum* *Increase* Increase up to 100% over control values in almost all cases, then decline over a period of 2 - 3 months toward normal *1971* Reported effect *5677*

Interferon-γ *Serum* *Increase* In 15 patients with different forms of Epstein-Barr virus-associated diseases: acute self-limiting infectious mononucleosis, chronic active infectious mononucleosis and X-linked lymphoproliferative syndrome. In patients with acute type of infection interferon-γ was elevated in nearly all patients *4686*

Interleukin-6 *Serum* *Increase* In 15 patients with different forms of Epstein-Barr virus-associated diseases: acute self-limiting infectious mononucleosis, chronic active infectious mononucleosis and X-linked lymphoproliferative syndrome. In patients with acute type of infection, interleukin-6 was elevated in nearly all patients *4686*

Isocitrate Dehydrogenase *Serum* *Increase* More than 25 U/L, becomes normal in 2 - 3 weeks *5544*

Lactate Dehydrogenase *Serum* *Increase* Elevations occur in 80 - 100% during acute illness and return to normal in 3 - 5 weeks *5677* 2 to 4 times normal values *1025* In 80% of 10 patients at initial hospitalization for this disorder *1576* All 36 patients showed elevated values, which persisted in 50% of the cases for over 4 months after onset of disease *3692*

Lactate Dehydrogenase Isoenzyme-5 *Serum* *Increase* Mean level in 5 cases was 8.2% of total serum LD. Normal mean activity of 3.0% *3692* Reported effect *1756* Elevated in 35% of the 36 patients with elevated serum LD *3692*

Lactate Dehydrogenase Isoenzymes *Serum* *Increase* Elevated in all 36 patients. Isoenzymes 1, 2, and 3 were most often elevated and remained so for 4 months after onset *3692*

Leucine Aminopeptidase *Serum* *Increase* In 4 patients all had serum levels above the upper limit of normal, ranging from 330-740 U/L *3751*

Leukocytes *Blood* *Decrease* During the first week of illness the count and distribution may be normal; infrequently there is moderate leukopenia *900*
Blood *Increase* Leukocytosis is toward the end of the 1st week or the start of the 2nd week; with counts rising to between 10,000 - 20,000 /μL. Rarely, counts from 30,000 - 80,000 /μL are seen *4061* During the 1st week, WBC count and distribution may be normal; infrequently there is moderate leukopenia. In the 2nd week, total count rises and persists into the 3rd week; then it declines *900*
Blood *No Effect* During the first week of illness the leukocyte count and distribution may be normal; infrequently there is moderate leukopenia *900* Usually within normal limits during the first week or two of disease, but progressively rises *1980* Usual effect observed *2832*

Lymphocytes *Blood* *Increase* Marked lymphocytosis, both relative and absolute. At least 50 - 60% of the WBCs are lymphocytes or monocytes; and at least 10% are atypical lymphocytes *1980* Absolute and relative lymphocytosis are characteristic and requisite for diagnosis *900* An absolute increase in the number of atypical lymphocytes is a characteristic finding during all stages of the disease *2832*

β_2-Microglobulin *Serum* *Increase* In children with infectious mononucleosis mean concentration of 348 μg/dL significantly higher than in controls *2145*

Monocytes *Blood* *Increase* In 54% of 11 patients at initial hospitalization for this disorder *1576* Relative increase *5677*

Neopterin *Serum* *Increase* In 15 patients with different forms of Epstein-Barr virus-associated diseases: acute self-limiting infectious mononucleosis, chronic active infectious mononucleosis and X-linked lymphoproliferative syndrome. In patients with acute type of infection elevated in nearly all patients *4686* Very high concentrations observed in patients with infectious mononuceosis infection due to Epstein virus *121*

Neutrophils *Blood* *Increase* Transient increase with intercurrent bacterial infection *900*

Rheumatoid Factor *Serum* *Increase* Concentration may be increased as in other diseases with chronic inflammation *2952* Rheumatoid factor may be observed in certain patients *2473* Mean concentration increased in patients with infectious mononucleosis *2472*

VDRL *Serum* *Positive* The incidence of false positive reactions is 5% *2304* Occurs occasionally, usually reverts to negative by the 3rd week *2832* Positive tests occur but are unusual *1024* False positive serologic tests for syphilis are sometimes seen *2039*

Weil-Felix Reaction *Serum* *Positive* Positive tests occur but are unusual *1024*

78.50 Cytomegalic Inclusion Disease

Alanine Aminotransferase *Serum* *Increase* Slight increase which becomes more marked with clinical hepatitis in some cases *5545*

Alkaline Phosphatase *Serum* *Increase* Increased in infants *1290*

Aspartate Aminotransferase *Serum* *Increase* Slight increase which becomes more marked with clinical hepatitis in some cases *5545*

Bilirubin *Serum* *Increase* Hemolytic anemia *1557* *5677*

Bilirubin, Direct *Serum* *Increase* Usually > 5% of total concentration and may be 50% *5252*

Bilirubin, Indirect *Serum* *Increase* In hemolytic anemia *2192*

Cells *Cerebrospinal Fluid* *Increase* Pleocytosis in congenital disease *2832*

Complement Fixation *Serum* *Increase* Requires use of multiple serologic types and is too time consuming and not very practical *2832*

C-Reactive Protein *Urine* *No Effect* In 7 patients with cytomegaloviral infection mean concentration of < 6 μg/L not significantly different from < 6 μg/L in 34 renal transplant patients with normal courses *4994*

Erythrocyte Sedimentation Rate *Blood* *Increase* Slightly increased *5545*

α-Fetoprotein *Serum* *Increase* Among 54 patients with verified infection, 8 (15%) had raised levels in sera taken after the onset of infection *1622* In the newborn, the level was abnormal but disappeared by the end of the 1st month *3500*

Haptoglobin *Serum* *Decrease* Hemolytic anemia *2192*

Hematocrit *Blood* *Decrease* Hemolytic anemia *1557* Anemia usually present in congenital disease *2832*

Hemoglobin *Blood* *Decrease* Anemia usually present in congenital disease *2832* Hemolytic anemia *1557*
Plasma *Increase* Reported finding *5677* Hemolytic anemia *1557*

Immunoglobulins *Serum* *Increase* Normal to increased *3731*

Lactate Dehydrogenase *Serum* *Increase* Slight increase which becomes more marked with clinical hepatitis in some cases *5545*

Leukocytes *Blood* *Increase* Increase to 15,000 - 20,000 /μL with 60 - 80% lymphocytes, many of which are Downey cell type *5545*

78.50 Cytomegalic Inclusion Disease *(continued)*

Lymphocytes *Blood* *Increase* Increase in WBC to 15,000 - 20,000 /µL with 60 - 80% lymphocytes, many of which are Downey cell type *5545*

α_2-Macroglobulin *Urine* *No Effect* In 7 patients with cytomegaloviral infection mean concentration of < 180 µg/L not significantly different from < 180 µg/L in 34 renal transplant patients with normal courses *4994*

Myeloperoxidase *Urine* *No Effect* In 7 patients with cytomegaloviral infection mean concentration of < 200 µg/L not significantly different from < 200 µg/L in 34 renal transplant patients with normal courses *4994*

Neopterin *Serum* *Increase* Very high concentrations observed in patients with cytomegalovirus infection *121*

Neutralizing Antibodies *Serum* *Increase* Requires use of multiple serologic types and is too time consuming and not very practical *2832*

Platelets *Blood* *Decrease* Thrombocytopenia usually present in congenital disease *2832* Common manifestation; usually transient and rarely associated with significant bleeding *3731*

Protein *Cerebrospinal Fluid* *Increase* In congenital disease *2832*

78.50 Cytomegalovirus Infection

Neutrophils *Cerebrospinal Fluid* *Increase* In 6 patients with AIDS numerous (> 10 /hpf) neutrophils present and all were associated with cytomegalovirus infection *1847*

78.60 Hemorrhagic Fever with Renal Syndrome

Bleeding Time *Patient* *Increase* Prolonged in hemorrhagic fever caused by dengue viruses *367*

Blood *Urine* *Increase* Hematuria is a characteristic feature of disease *3066*

C-Reactive Protein *Serum* *Increase* In 15 patients the median maximum concentration was 79 mg/L *3066*

Creatinine *Serum* *Increase* Increased concentration is a characteristic feature of disease *3066*

Factor II *Plasma* *Decrease* May be associated with defibrination resulting in platelet and coagulation factor consumption (Korean and Thai fever) *5677*

Factor IV *Plasma* *Decrease* May be associated with defibrination resulting in platelet and coagulation factor consumption (Korean and Thai fever) *5677*

Fibrin Degradation Products *Plasma* *Increase* Indicates occurrence of intravascular coagulation in Dengue hemorrhagic fever patients experiencing shock *509*

Fibrinogen *Plasma* *Decrease* Indicates occurrence of intravascular coagulation in dengue hemorrhagic fever patients experiencing shock *509* May be associated with defibrination resulting in platelet and coagulation factor consumption (Korean and Thai fever) *5677*

Granulocyte-Macrophage Colony Stimulating Factor
Serum *Decrease* In 3 of 7 patients low concentrations were observed *3066*

Hematocrit *Blood* *Increase* Values may reach 70% in the hypotensive phase of epidemic hemorrhagic fever *367*

Immunoglobulin E *Serum* *Increase* 88.2% of patients with dengue hemorrhagic fever had measurable serum IgE, compared to 57.1% of controls. Patient range was 50 - 5,025 U/mL and control was 50 - 2,250 U/mL *4046*

Interferon-γ *Serum* *Increase* In 7 of 15 patients IFN-γ was detected during days 3 - 4 of the acute phase although more than minute amounts were found in only two *3066*

Interleukin-1β *Serum* *Increase* In one of 15 patients IL-1β was detected during the acute phase *3066*

Interleukin-2 *Serum* *Decrease* In 1 of 7 patients low concentrations were observed but since it was also detected at 3 months follow-up, association with disease uncertain *3066*

Interleukin-4 *Serum* *No Effect* Not detected or detected at minute amounts in 7 patients *3066*

Interleukin-6 *Serum* *Increase* In 15 patients the median maximum concentration was 58 ng/L on the first day 3 of hospitalization and rapidly decreased thereafter *3066*

Interleukin-8 *Serum* *Increase* In 6 of 7 patients minute amounts were found with peak levels occurring 2 - 4 days after onset of renal problems *3066*

Interleukin-10 *Serum* *Increase* In 15 patients the median maximum concentration was 25 ng/L on the first day 3 of hospitalization and rapidly decreased thereafter *3066*

Leukocytes *Blood* *Decrease* Almost invariably decreased reaching levels of 1,000 /µL by the 4th day in hemorrhagic fever caused by arenaviruses (Argentine, Bolivian, and Lassa fever) *367*
Blood *Increase* In 15 patients the median maximum leukocyte count was 13.0 x 10^9/L *3066*
Blood *No Effect* Usually normal but may be elevated in severe cases of Dengue fever *367*

Neutrophils *Blood* *Decrease* Leukopenia frequently associated with infectious diseases *2239*

Platelets *Blood* *Decrease* May be associated with defibrination resulting in platelet and coagulation factor consumption (Korean Fever, Thai Fever) *5677* Indicates occurrence of intravascular coagulation in dengue hemorrhagic fever patients experiencing shock *509* Thrombocytopenia is a characteristic feature of disease *3066*

Potassium *Serum* *Increase* Occurs in the oliguric phase of epidemic hemorrhagic fever *367*

Protein *Urine* *Increase* Heavy proteinuria progressing to acute renal failure occurs during the hypotensive phase of epidemic hemorrhagic fever *367* Proteinuria is a characteristic feature of disease *3066*

Prothrombin Consumption *Blood* *Increase* May be associated with defibrination resulting in platelet and coagulation factor consumption (Korean and Thai fever) *5677*

Soluble Tumor Necrosis Factor Receptor-p55
Serum *Increase* In 15 patients the median concentration was significantly increased during the first week of hospitalization *3066*

Soluble Tumor Necrosis Factor Receptor-p75
Serum *Increase* In 15 patients the median concentration was significantly increased during the first week of hospitalization *3066*

Tumor Necrosis Factor-α *Serum* *Increase* In 15 patients the median maximum concentration was 114 ng/L on days 3 - 5 of hospitalization with higher values on day 8 *3066*

79.00 Adenovirus Infections

Amyloid A Protein *Serum* *Increase* In 29 patients mean concentration in acute phase of 2.15 ± 0.65 mg/L *3728*

C-Reactive Protein *Serum* *Increase* In 29 patients mean concentration in acute phase of 1.28 ± 0.61 mg/L *3728*

79.89 California Virus Infection

California Virus LaCrosse Antibodies *Serum* *Increase* Fourfold or greater increase in antibody titer in acute and convalescent sera from patients with California virus LaCrosse indicate recent infection *2952*

79.89 Hantavirus Pulmonary Syndrome

Alanine Aminotransferase *Serum* *No Effect* In 17 patients with hantavirus pulmonary syndrome on admission to hospital mean activity of 55 U/L (range 25 - 148 U/L) compared with reference interval of 35 - 60 U/L *1248*

Albumin *Serum* *No Effect* Mean concentration of 3.0 g/L (range 1.5 - 4.6 g/L) in 17 patients with hantavirus pulmonary syndrome on admission to hospital not significantly different from reference interval *1248*

Aspartate Aminotransferase *Serum* *Increase* In 17 patients with hantavirus pulmonary syndrome on admission to hospital mean activity of 112 U/L (range 28 - 432 U/L) significantly greater than reference interval of 28 - 432 U/L *1248*

Bicarbonate *Serum* *Decrease* Mean concentration in 17 patients with hantavirus pulmonary syndrome on admission to hospital of 18 mmol/L (range 12 - 25 mmol/L) *1248*

Creatine Kinase *Serum* *No Effect* Mean activity in 17 patients with hantavirus pulmonary syndrome on admission to hospital of 46 U/L (range 19 - 1,026 U/L) not significantly different from reference interval of 180 - 269 U/L *1248*

Creatinine *Serum* *No Effect* Mean concentration in 17 patients with hantavirus pulmonary syndrome on admission to hospital of 1.1 mg/dL (range of 0.6 - 2.5 mg/dL) not different from reference interval *1248*

Hematocrit *Blood* *Increase* In patients with hantavirus pulmonary syndrome mean concentration of 51.3% (range 49.9 - 60.0%) in men and 46.4% (range 35.0 - 55.8%) in women on admission of 17 patients to hospital *1248*

Lactate *Plasma* *Increase* Mean concentration in 17 patients with hantavirus pulmonary syndrome on admission to hospital of 4.4 mmol/L (range 2.2 - 11.0 mmol/L) significantly higher than upper reference limit of 2.2 mmol/L *1248*

Lactate Dehydrogenase *Serum* *Increase* Mean activity of 362 U/L (range 209 - 1,525 U/L) in 17 patients with hantavirus pulmonary syndrome on admission to hospital significantly higher than reference interval of 180 - 232 U/L *1248*

Leukocytes *Blood* *Increase* in 17 patients with Hantavirus pulmonary syndrome on admission to hospital mean concentration of 10,400 /µL (range 3,100 - 65,300 /µL) *1248*

Neutrophil Bands *Blood* *Increase* In 17 patients with Hantavirus syndrome on admission to hospital mean concentration of 22% (range 8 - 62%) *1248*

Partial Thromboplastin Time *Plasma* *No Effect* Mean time in 17 patients with hantavirus pulmonary syndrome on admission to hospital of 42.5 s (range 30.0 - 150.0 s) *1248*

Platelets *Blood* *No Effect* In 17 patients with hantavirus pulmonary syndrome on admission to hospital mean concentration of 84,000 /µL (range 26,000 - 320,000 /µL) *1248*

Prothrombin Time *Plasma* *No Effect* In 17 patients with hantavirus pulmonary syndrome on admission to hospital mean time of 13.0 s (range 11.2 - 21.1 s) *1248*

Urea Nitrogen *Serum* *No Effect* Mean concentration of 11 mg/dL (range 3 - 23 mg/dL) in 17 patients with hantavirus pulmonary syndrome on admission to hospital not significantly different from reference interval *1248*

79.89 Parainfluenza Infection

Amyloid A Protein *Serum* *Increase* In 47 patients mean concentration in acute phase of 1.74 ± 0.73 mg/L *3728*

C-Reactive Protein *Serum* *Increase* In 47 patients mean concentration in acute phase 0.78 ± 0.70 mg/L *3728*

79.89 Sabia Virus Infection

Alanine Aminotransferase *Serum* *Increase* In one patient activity reached peak of 128 U/L on 10th day of hospitalization *301*

Leukocytes *Blood* *Decrease* In one patient leukocyte count reached nadir of 1,300 /µL on second day of hospitalization, rising into normal range after day 12 *301*

Neutrophils *Blood* *Decrease* In one patient absolute neutrophil count reached nadir of 560 /µL on second day of hospitalization, rising into normal range after day 12 *301*

Platelets *Blood* *Decrease* In one patient platelet count reached nadir of 98,000 /µL on second day of hospitalization, rising into normal range after day 8 *301*

79.99 Viral Infection

Amyloid A *Serum* *No Effect* Median concentration in patients with viral infection of 5.75 mg/dL not significantly different from approximately 5.75 mg/dL in transplant patients in stable phase *3653*

C-Reactive Protein *Serum* *Increase* In 99 children with viral respiratory infection mean concentration on admission to hospital of 28 mg/L and 36 mg/L in 46 children with mixed viral-bacterial infections significantly different from normal *2773* In 32 patients with viral infection mean concentration of 41 ± 39 mg/L greater than normal concentration of less than 10 mg/L *4038* In 24 patients with acute viral infection mean serum concentration of 36.5 ± 32.6 mg/L *5757*

Granulocyte Colony Stimulating Factor *Serum* *Increase* In 27 patients with viral infection mean concentration of 58 ± 34 ng/L significantly greater than normal concentration of less than 39 ng/L *4038*

Interleukin-6 *Serum* *Increase* In 32 patients with viral infection mean concentration of 32 ± 21 ng/L greater than normal concentration of less than 20 ng/L *4038*

Lactoferrin *Plasma* *No Effect* In 23 patients with viral infection mean concentration of 93 ± 61 µg/L not different from normal concentration of 40 - 215 µg/L *4038*

Leukocytes *Blood* *No Effect* In 32 patients with viral infection mean count of 6,800 ± 4,100 /µL not different from normal count of 4,000 - 9,000 /µL *4038*

Lymphocytes *Blood* *Decrease* In 1,042 hospitalized patients with lymphocytopenia 26 had a viral infection *730*

Monocytes *Blood* *No Effect* In 31 patients with viral infection mean count of 2300 ± 3200 /µL not different from normal count of 2000 - 3000 /µL *4038*

Myeloperoxidase *Serum* *Increase* In 32 patients with viral infection mean concentration of 643 ± 334 µg/L significantly greater than normal concentration of 107 - 678 µg/L *4038*

Neopterin *Serum* *Increase* Activation of T-lymphocytes by viral antigens causes IFN-γ production and release by T-lymphocytes followed by neopterin production in macrophages. During the incubation period, neopterin increases, peaking at the onset of clinical symptoms *121* Median concentration in patients with bacterial infection of approximately 42 nmol/L significantly different from approximately 12 nmol/L in transplant patients in stable phase *3653*

Nerve Growth Factor *Serum* *Increase* Mean concentration of 30.2 ± 44.7 pg/mL in 12 febrile children with URT viral infections significantly higher than 6.5 ± 2.0 pg/mL in 12 healthy control children *1412*

Neutrophil Lipocalcin *Serum* *Increase* In 24 patients with acute viral infection mean serum concentration of 93.78 ± 45.30 µg/L and 47.81 ± 18.18 µg/L in plasma *5757*

Neutrophils *Blood* *No Effect* In 31 patients with viral infection mean count of 4,400 ± 2,900 /µL not different from normal count of 2,000 - 6,000 /µL *4038*

Phospholipase A_2 Type II *Serum* *Increase* Increase in concentration observed of 47 µg/L in patients with viral infections compared with 2 and 4 µg/L in healthy controls *3767*

Procalcitonin *Plasma* *Increase* In 21 children with viral infections concentrations were within the normal range of < 0.1 ng/mL in 21 children without infection with the highest concentration observed of 1.4 ng/mL *203*

Soluble HLA-I *Serum* *Increase* Concentration reportedly increased with viral infection *5306*

Rickettsioses and Arthropodborne Diseases

80.00 Epidemic Typhus

Albumin *Urine* *Increase* During the febrile period *900*

Antibody Titer *Serum* *Increase* Antibodies are demonstrable in significant titers by the 3rd week *900* Acute phase antibodies are of the IgM type *367*

Cells *Cerebrospinal Fluid* *Increase* With severe encephalitis manifestations *900*

Complement Fixation *Serum* *Increase* Antibodies first appear in the serum between 7 and 12 days *367* Antibodies develop which are both group- and species- specific *1980* A demonstration of a 4-fold increase is considered significant *2832*

Creatinine *Serum* *Increase* With varying degrees of renal involvement *900*

Eosinophils *Blood* *Decrease* Absent or rare in the early stages *5252*

Erythrocytes *Urine* *Increase* Microscopic hematuria can be expected *900*

80.00 Epidemic Typhus *(continued)*

γ-Globulin *Serum* *Increase* Often associated with hypergammaglobulinemia *4707*

Hematocrit *Blood* *Decrease* Normal early, falls significantly during the illness *900* May develop in the 2nd or 3rd week *5252*

Hemoglobin *Blood* *Decrease* May develop in the 2nd or 3rd week *5252* Normal early, falls significantly during the illness *900*

Leukocytes *Blood* *Decrease* Leukopenia frequently associated with infectious diseases *2239* In first few days of illness *5252*
Blood *Increase* May signal secondary bacterial infection *900* Only slightly elevated unless complications ensue *5252*

Neutrophils *Blood* *Decrease* Leukopenia frequently associated with infectious diseases *2239*

Oxygen Partial Pressure *Blood* *Decrease* With pulmonary involvement *900*

Protein *Cerebrospinal Fluid* *Increase* With severe encephalitic manifestations *900*
Serum *Decrease* Hypoproteinemia occurs in severe cases *5252*

Sodium *Serum* *Decrease* Chronic illness from Rickettsial disease results in hyponatremia *4707*

Urea Nitrogen *Serum* *Increase* With varying degrees of renal involvement *900* Azotemia is common *5252*

VDRL *Serum* *Positive* In 20% of patients *2192*

Volume *Urine* *Decrease* Oliguria is common *5252*

Weil-Felix Reaction *Serum* *Positive* Serum obtained 5 - 12 days after onset of symptoms usually shows a positive reaction with agglutinating antibody for Proteus Ox 19 and rarely Proteus Ox 2 *900*

81.00 Endemic Typhus

Complement Fixation *Serum* *Increase* Antibodies develop which are both group- and species- specific. Appear during the 2nd week of illness and reach a peak during the 4th week *1980*

Hematocrit *Blood* *No Effect* No significant effect usually observed *900*

Leukocytes *Blood* *Decrease* Normal or slightly low *900* Leukopenia frequently associated with infectious diseases *2239*

Neutrophils *Blood* *Decrease* Leukopenia frequently associated with infectious diseases *2239*

Platelets *Blood* *Decrease* Rarely seen *900*

Protein *Urine* *Increase* During the febrile period *900*

Sodium *Serum* *Decrease* Chronic illness from Rickettsial disease results in hyponatremia *4707*

Weil-Felix Reaction *Serum* *Positive* With Proteus OX-9 and OX-2 *1025* May be superior to complement-fixation procedure in typhus and Rocky Mountain spotted fever *4119* Antibodies to Proteus OX-19 are present in significant titers by the third week *900*

81.10 Brill's Disease

Albumin *Urine* *Increase* Transient albuminuria may occur *900*

Antibody Titer *Serum* *Increase* Acute-phase antibodies are of the IgG class *367*

Complement Fixation *Serum* *Increase* The diagnosis can be made by demonstrating a rising titer of antibodies which fix complement in the presence of epidemic typhus antigen or agglutinate suspensions of washed Rickettsia prowazekii. The antibody occurs earlier (4 - 6th day) and peaks between the 8 - 10th day *900*

Sodium *Serum* *Decrease* Chronic illness from Rickettsial disease results in hyponatremia *4707*

Weil-Felix Reaction *Serum* *Negative* Positive reactions develop in 10 - 20% of cases that occur 10 or more years after the primary attack *2192* A negative test in the presence of rising complement-fixing antibodies distinguishes Brill-Zinsser from primary louse-borne typhus *367*

81.20 Mite-Borne Typhus

Complement Fixation *Serum* *Increase* Available antigens detect complement fixing antibody in only about 50% of the cases *1980* Irregular results *5252*

Leukocytes *Blood* *Decrease* Leukopenia is seen in Rickettsial diseases *5544*
Blood *No Effect* Usually concentration normal *2192*

Sodium *Serum* *Decrease* Chronic illness from Rickettsial disease results in hyponatremia *4707*

Weil-Felix Reaction *Serum* *Positive* Four fold or greater rises in Weil-Felix OX-K titers are found in almost all untreated patients and 75% of those treated with antimicrobial therapy *367* The only rickettsial disease in which OX-K antibody is present *1980* Agglutinins for Proteus OX-K but not for OX-19 or OX-2 are present *5252*

82.00 Rocky Mountain Spotted Fever

Albumin *Serum* *Decrease* Common *900*
Urine *Increase* Varying degrees *900*

Aspartate Aminotransferase *Serum* *Increase* Common *900*

Casts *Urine* *Increase* Varying degrees *900*

Complement Fixation *Serum* *Increase* Antibodies develop which are both group- and species- specific. Appear during the 2nd week of illness and reach a peak during the 4th week *1980* A 4-fold or greater rise is considered confirmatory *367* Significant rise in titer occurs by the 3rd week *2832*

Creatine Kinase MB-Isoenzyme *Serum* *Increase* Observed effect *248*

Factor II *Plasma* *Decrease* May be associated with defibrination resulting in platelet and coagulation factor consumption *5677*

Factor IV *Plasma* *Decrease* May be associated with defibrination resulting in platelet and coagulation factor consumption *5677*

Factor XII *Plasma* *Decrease* Hypofibrinogenemia in 2 of 5 cases with marked reduction of factor XII *5766* May be associated with defibrination resulting in platelet and coagulation factor consumption *5677*

Fibrinogen *Plasma* *Decrease* May be associated with defibrination resulting in platelet and coagulation factor consumption *5677* Hypofibrinogenemia in 2 of 5 cases with marked reduction of factor XII *5766*

Hemagglutination Inhibition *Serum* *Increase* May be superior to complement-fixation procedure in typhus and Rocky Mountain spotted fever *4119*

Hematocrit *Blood* *Decrease* Anemia may develop in the 2nd - 3rd weeks *5252*

Hemoglobin *Blood* *Decrease* Anemia may develop in the 2nd - 3rd weeks *5252*

Leukocytes *Blood* *Decrease* Leukopenia frequently associated with infectious diseases *2239*
Blood *Increase* Common *900*

Monocytes *Blood* *Increase* Increases in some Rickettsial infections *5544*

Neutrophils *Blood* *Decrease* Leukopenia frequently associated with infectious diseases *2239*

Platelets *Blood* *Decrease* Counts below 100,000 /µL were seen in 4 of 5 patients *5766* May be associated with defibrination resulting in platelet and coagulation factor consumption *5677*

Protein *Serum* *Decrease* Hypoproteinemia is common in severe cases *5252*

Prothrombin Consumption *Blood* *Increase* May be associated with defibrination resulting in platelet and coagulation factor consumption *5677*

Sodium *Serum* *Decrease* Chronic illness from Rickettsial disease results in hyponatremia *4707*

Urea Nitrogen *Serum* *Increase* Azotemia is common in severe cases *5252*

Volume *Urine* *Decrease* Oliguria is common *5252*

Weil-Felix Reaction *Serum* *Positive* Agglutinins against Proteus OX-19 and OX-2 develop by the 2nd or 3rd week *2832*

Antibodies first appear between the 8th and 12th day of illness *5619*

83.20 Rickettsialpox

Complement Fixation *Serum Increase* A 4-fold or greater rise in antibody titer in paired sera. Because of cross reactions, the Rocky Mountain spotted fever test will also be positive *2832*

Leukocytes *Blood Decrease* Typify the acute phase *900* Usual *2192*

Lymphocytes *Blood Increase* Typify the acute phase *900*

Sodium *Serum Decrease* Chronic illness from Rickettsial disease results in hyponatremia *4707*

Weil-Felix Reaction *Serum Negative* Negative in Rickettsial Pox, Q fever, and trench fever *5252* With Proteus OX-19, OX-2 and OX-K *2832*
Serum Positive Appears in 2nd - 3rd week of illness. Agglutinins for Proteus OX-19, OX-2, and OX-K do not rise in titer *5252*

84.00 Malaria

Alanine *Plasma Increase* In 4 of 19 patients with cerebral malaria and hypoglycemia mean concentration of 0.63 ± 0.19 mmol/L significantly higher than 0.31 ± 0.17 mmol/L in the 15 normoglycemic patients *4502*

Alanine Aminotransferase *Serum Increase* Mean activity of 44.0 ± 34.8 U/L in 20 patients with complicated falciparum malaria *637* Moderate increase *5545*
Serum No Effect In 50 children with mild malaria median activity of 23.5 U/L and 22.0 U/L in 50 children with severe malaria not significantly different from 17.0 U/L in 50 healthy control children *1017*

Albumin *Serum Decrease* In 50 children with mild malaria mean concentration of 37.0 ± 7.8 g/L and 31.3 ± 7.1 g/L in 50 children with severe malaria significantly different from 45.5 ± 3.1 g/L in 50 healthy control children *1017* Significant decrease observed in patients with cerebral malaria *1016*
Serum No Effect In 8 patients with vivax malaria on admission to hospital mean concentration of 36 (32 - 42) g/L compared with 37 (24 - 45) g/L in 10 patients with falciparum malaria and 46 (42 - 48) g/L in 10 controls *1041*
Urine Increase In uncomplicated infection, mild *900*

Alkaline Phosphatase *Serum Increase* Moderate increase *5545*

Anticardiolipin Antibodies *Serum Increase* Immunoglobulin G-anticardiolipin antibodies measured by enzyme-linked immunosorbent assay occurred significantly more frequently in 62 patients with acute Plasmodium falciparum malaria (33.9%) than in 37 control subjects (2.7%) ($p < 0.0001$) *4537*

Antinuclear Antibodies *Serum Increase* Increased frequency of positivity observed *4551* An unusually high incidence was observed during chronic infection *1864*

Antiphospholipid Antibodies *Serum Increase* The majority (75%) of adult patients with uncomplicated Plasmodium falciparum and P. vivax malaria are positive for anti-phospholipid antibodies (aPLA) as demonstrated by ELISA using a panel of anionic and cationic phospholipids. The highest IgG and IgM binding was to the anionic phospholipids, phosphatidylserine (PS), phosphatidic acid (PA) and cardiolipin (CL), but excluding phosphatidylinositol (PI) to which only low antibody levels were found *1407*

Ascorbic Acid *Serum Decrease* In 50 children with mild malaria median concentration of 27.1 µmol/L (not significant) and 22.8 µmol/L in 50 children with severe malaria significantly different from 33.0 µmol/L in 50 healthy control children *1017*

Aspartate Aminotransferase *Serum Increase* Activity was increased in 11 patients untreated for more than 4 days *4622* Moderate increase *5545* Mean activity on admission to hospital in 10 patients with falciparum malaria of 27 (12 - 112) U/L significantly higher than 18 (7 - 80) U/L in 8 patients with vivax malaria and 18 (11 - 41) U/L in 10 controls *1041* May be elevated *1980* Mean activity of 77.5 ± 52.1 U/L in 20 patients with complicated falciparum malaria *637*

Basic Fibroblast Growth Factor *Serum Increase* Mean concentration peaked at 35.61 pg/mL in 20 patients with complicated falciparum malaria in comparison with 7.87 pg/mL in healthy controls *637*

Bilirubin *Serum Increase* Mean concentration of 4.98 ± 6.51 mg/dL in 20 patients with complicated falciparum malaria *637* Evidence of hemolysis *5545* Mean concentration on admission to hospital in 10 patients with falciparum malaria of 16 (7 - 41) µmol/L significantly higher than 10 (4 - 18) µmol/L in 10 controls and 9 (5 - 53) µmol/L in 8 patients with vivax malaria *1041*

Bilirubin, Indirect *Serum Increase* Evidence of hemolysis *5545*

Calcium *Serum No Effect* In 18 patients with malaria on admission to hospital mean concentration of 2.12 (2.05 - 2.16) mmol/L compared with 2.15 (2.09 - 2.20) mmol/L in 10 healthy controls although mean concentrations in patients with falciparum malaria were generally depressed to 2.11 (1.90 - 2.21) mmol/L *1041*

α-Carotene *Serum Decrease* In 50 children with mild malaria median concentration of 0.019 µmol/L and 0.007 µmol/L in 50 children with severe malaria significantly different from 0.035 µmol/L in 50 healthy control children *1017*

β-Carotene *Serum Decrease* In 50 children with mild malaria median concentration of 0.150 µmol/L and 0.076 µmol/L in 50 children with severe malaria significantly different from 0.310 µmol/L in 50 healthy control children *1017*

Ceruloplasmin *Serum Increase* In 50 children with mild malaria mean activity of 273 ± 57 U/L and 311 ± 68 U/L in 50 children with severe malaria significantly different from 197 ± 44 U/L in 50 healthy control children *1017* In 50 patients with vivax malaria concentration of 440 ± 125 mg/L significantly greater than that in 250 healthy people, mean concentration of 315 ± 119 mg/L *1377*

Ceruloplasmin Ferroxidase *Serum Increase* In 50 patients with vivax malaria mean activity of 740 ± 214 U/L significantly greater than that in 250 healthy people in whom the mean concentration was 537 ± 201 U/L *1377*

Cholesterol *Serum Decrease* In 50 children with mild malaria mean activity of 2.56 ± 0.62 mmol/L and 1.89 ± 0.62 mmol/L in 50 children with severe malaria significantly different from 3.47 ± 0.59 mmol/L in 50 healthy control children *1017*

Cold Agglutinins *Serum Increase* An unusually high incidence was observed during chronic infection *1864*

Complement C_3 *Serum Decrease* Only in patients with defective hemoglobin synthesis *4966*

Complement Fixation *Serum Increase* In natural infections, the complement-fixation and indirect hemagglutination tests detect malarial antibodies equally efficiently for the first 2 months after onset, but titers obtained by complement-fixation rapidly decline within a year, while the indirect hemagglutination titers remain elevated *5688*

Coombs' Test *Serum Positive* Patients occasionally have a Coombs'-positive hemolytic anemia *367*

Copper *Serum Increase* In 50 patients with vivax malaria mean concentration of 25.17 ± 7.19 µmol/L significantly greater than that in 250 healthy people, mean concentration of 15.82 ± 4.15 µmol/L *1377*

Creatine Kinase *Serum Increase* One Nigerian man two weeks after leaving Nigeria was diagnosed with malaria with symptoms including myalgia and muscle tenderness with a serum creatine kinase activity of 32,000 U/L at the time *2720*

Creatinine *Serum Increase* In all patients, independent of the duration of the acute infection, levels were significantly raised *4622* Mean concentration of 1.66 ± 2.08 mg/dL in 20 patients with complicated falciparum malaria *637*
Serum No Effect In the acute phase of vivax malaria in 6 patients mean concentration of 0.83 ± 0.10 mg/dL not significantly different from 0.70 ± 0.14 mg/dL in 7 healthy Japanese controls *3878* Mean concentration of 89 (68 - 121) µmol/L in 8 patients with Vivax malaria and 76 (54 - 102 µmol/L) in 10 with falciparum malaria compared with 85 (55 - 106) µmol/L in 10 controls *1041*

β-Cryptoxanthin *Serum Decrease* In 50 children with mild malaria median concentration of 0.064 µmol/L and 0.042 µmol/L in 50 children with severe malaria significantly different from 0.119 µmol/L in 50 healthy control children *1017*

Eosinophils *Blood Decrease* During acute infections *900*
Blood Increase Depressed during acute infections but may become elevated during convalescence *900*

84.00 **Malaria** *(continued)*

Erythrocytes *Blood* *Decrease* Pancytopenia is a common feature *5677* Anemia with an average of 2.5 million/μL is usually hypochromic; may be macrocytic in severe chronic cases *5545*

Factor II *Plasma* *Decrease* May be associated with defibrination resulting in platelet and coagulation factor consumption (in overwhelming parasitemia) *5677*

Factor IV *Plasma* *Decrease* May be associated with defibrination resulting in platelet and coagulation factor consumption (in overwhelming parasitemia) *5677*

Factor XIII Activity *Plasma* *No Effect* In 45 patients with malaria mean activity of 75% not significantly different from normal values of > 70% *2212*

Factor XIIIa Antigen *Plasma* *No Effect* In 45 patients with malaria mean concentration of 77% not significantly different from normal values of > 70% *2212*

Factor XIIIb Antigen *Plasma* *No Effect* In 45 patients with malaria mean concentration of 90% not significantly different from normal values of > 70% *2212*

Fibrin Degradation Products *Plasma* *Increase* In 25 patients with acute renal failure due to falciparum malaria, marked increase in plasma fibrinogen and elevation of serum fibrin degradation products were observed. The other coagulation parameters were within the normal limits *4878*

Fibrinogen *Plasma* *Decrease* May be associated with defibrination resulting in platelet and coagulation factor consumption (overwhelming parasitemia) *5677*
Plasma *Increase* In 25 patients with acute renal failure due to falciparum malaria, marked increase in fibrinogen and fibrin degradation products were observed. The other coagulation parameters were within the normal limits *4878*

γ-Globulin *Serum* *Increase* Often associated with hypergammaglobulinemia *4707* Especially euglobulin fraction *5545*

Glomerular Filtration Rate *Urine* *Decrease* In acute renal failure due to falciparum malaria *4878*

Glucose *Serum* *Decrease* In 4 of 19 patients with cerebral malaria hypoglycemia with glucose less than 2.0 mmol/L *4502*

Glycated Protein *Serum* *Increase* Serum $alpha_1$-glycoproteins are increased and $alpha_2$-glycoproteins are decreased *367*

Haptoglobin *Serum* *Decrease* Intravascular hemolysis due to parasites *5544*

Hemagglutination Inhibition *Serum* *Increase* In natural infections, the complement-fixation and indirect hemagglutination tests detect malarial antibodies equally efficiently for the first 2 months after onset, but titers obtained by complement-fixation rapidly decline within a year, while the indirect hemagglutination titers remain elevated *5688* Antibody to malarial parasites may be detected by the indirect fluorescent antibody test and by hemagglutination tests *1980*

Hematocrit *Blood* *Decrease* Marked anemia was found only in the patients with defective hemoglobin synthesis *4966* With disease progression a normocytic, normochromic anemia may become apparent *900* Anemia is present in proportion to the severity of the infection *1980*
Blood *No Effect* In 8 patients with vivax malaria mean of 43.0 (31.0 - 48.0)% compared with 43.5 (10.5 - 50.5)% in 10 patients with falciparum malaria and 44.5 (35.5 - 54.0)% in 10 controls *1041*

Hemoglobin *Blood* *Decrease* With disease progression, a normocytic, normochromic anemia may become apparent *900* Anemia is present in proportion to the severity of the infection *1980* In 50 children with mild malaria mean concentration of 97.0 ± 20.2 g/L and 73.3 ± 19.8 g/L in 50 children with severe malaria significantly different from 120.7 ± 18.5 g/L in 50 healthy control children *1017* Marked anemia was found in patients with defective hemoglobin synthesis *4966*
Plasma *Increase* Intravascular hemolysis due to parasites *5544*
Urine *Increase* In severe falciparum infection may be demonstrable *900* Intravascular hemolysis due to parasites *5544*

HIV-1 RNA *Serum* *Increase* Mean concentration in 57 patients with plasmodium falciparum malaria of 15.1 x 10^4 copies/mL approximately 7-fold higher than 2.24 x 10^4 copies/mL in 42 blood donors *2199*

Immunoglobulin E *Serum* *Increase* Significantly increased concentration observed in patients with malaria *4082*

Immunoglobulin G *Serum* *Increase* Mean IgG and IgM were significantly increased. Mean IgG concentration of 179 U/mL, range 119 - 284 U/mL *1720* Marked elevation *367* Despite the considerably increased concentration of immunoglobulins in infected individuals, only 5% of the immune adult IgG combines specifically with P. falciparum antigens *878*

Immunoglobulin M *Serum* *Increase* Marked elevation *367* Reported effect *878* Especially when particulate antigenic material is present in the blood stream *1290* Mean IgG and IgM were significantly increased in malaria patients. Mean IgM = 191 U/mL, range = 87 - 369 *1720*

Immunoglobulins *Serum* *Increase* Despite the considerably increased concentration of immunoglobulins in infected individuals, only 5% of the immune adult IgG combines specifically with P. falciparum antigens *878*

Indirect Fluorescent Antibodies *Serum* *Increase* Antibody to malarial parasites may be detected by the indirect fluorescent antibody test and by hemagglutination tests. Interpretation of antibody titers in a variety of situations has not been clarified *1980*

Intercellular Adhesion Molecule-1 *Serum* *Increase* In the acute phase of vivax malaria in 6 patients mean concentration of 709 ± 397 ng/mL significantly different from 268 ± 105 ng/mL in 7 healthy Japanese controls *3878*

Interferon-γ *Serum* *Increase* In 37 patients with malaria mean concentration on first day of study of 717 ± 260 pg/mL significantly different from 2.2 ± 1.3 pg/mL in 17 healthy controls *5637* In 16 patients with malaria mean concentration of 4.3 ± 6.2 U/L significantly different from 0.5 ± 1.2 U/L in 30 controls *5256*
Serum *No Effect* In 33 Gambian children with severe malaria median concentration of < 5 pg/mL no different from < 5 pg/mL in 32 with mild malaria and 4 with unrelated diseases *2407*

Interleukin-4 *Serum* *Decrease* Median concentration of 10 pg/mL in 33 Gambian children with severe malaria significantly less than median of 80 pg/mL in 8 children with unrelated diseases *2407*
Serum *Increase* Median concentration of 320 pg/mL in 35 Gambian children with mild malaria higher than 10 pg/mL in 33 children with severe malaria and 80 pg/mL in 8 children with unrelated diseases *2407*

Interleukin-4 Receptor *Serum* *Increase* Median concentration of 4,500 pg/mL in 32 Gambian children with mild plasmodium falciparum infection just significantly higher than 3,000 pg/mL in 17 children with severe infection *2407*

Interleukin-6 *Serum* *Increase* In 33 Gambian children with severe malaria median concentration of 150 pg/mL significantly higher than 100 pg/mL in 33 children with mild malaria and in 6 controls with unrelated diseases *2407*

Interleukin-8 *Serum* *Increase* In patients with Plasmodium falciparum malaria mean concentration increased from 87 pg/mL on day of admission to hospital to 212 pg/mL on day 7 and 607 pg/mL on day 14 before decreasing to 374 pg/mL on day 21 and 209 pg/mL on day 28 compared with mean control of 9.25 pg/mL *636*

Interleukin-10 *Serum* *Increase* Fourteen cerebral, 11 severe, and 20 mild malaria cases had mean IL-10 levels of 2,812, 2,882 and 913 pg/mL, respectively, while 98% of healthy individuals had undetectable (less than 100 pg/mL) circulating IL-10. Thirteen of the 25 cerebral/severe cases had concentrations > 2,000 pg/mL *4109* In 37 patients with malaria mean concentration on first day of study of 123 ± 71 pg/mL significantly different from 29 ± 9 pg/mL in 17 healthy controls *5637*

ionized Calcium *Serum* *Decrease* mean concentration on admission to hospital in 10 patients with falciparum malaria of 1.17 (1.12 - 1.23) mmol/L significantly less than 1.20 (1.18 - 1.24) mmol/L in healthy controls *1041*

Iron *Serum* *Decrease* Decreased cellular iron incorporation found in all cases during parasitemia *4966*

Iron-binding Capacity, Total *Serum* *Decrease* Decreased significantly in 11 patients with untreated malaria for more than 4 days *4622*

Lactate *Blood* *Increase* In 4 of 19 patients with cerebral malaria and hypoglycemia mean plasma concentration of 7.95 ± 2.6 mmol/L significantly higher than 4.3 ± 1.7 mmol/L in the 15 normoglycemic patients *4502*

Laminin *Serum* *Increase* Mean concentration of 1,973 ng/mL in 20 patients with complicated falciparum malaria in comparison with 412 ng/mL in healthy controls *637*

Leukocytes *Blood* *Decrease* Pancytopenia is a common feature *5677* Occasionally leukopenia is present *1980*

Lutein *Serum* *Decrease* In 50 children with mild malaria median concentration of 0.267 µmol/L and 0.258 µmol/L in 50 children with severe malaria significantly different from 0.429 µmol/L in 50 healthy control children *1017*

Lycopene *Serum* *Decrease* In 50 children with mild malaria median concentration of 0.038 µmol/L and 0.014 µmol/L in 50 children with severe malaria significantly different from 0.068 µmol/L in 50 healthy control children *1017*

Lymphocytes *Blood* *Increase* Depletion of T cells was found associated with an increased proportion of null cells. K cell activity was also increased and it is likely that some of the increased number of null cells were K cells *1863*

Lymphotoxin *Serum* *Increase* In 36 Gambian children with severe malaria median concentration of 70 pg/mL and 50 pg/mL in 38 with mild malaria significantly higher than < 8 pg/mL in 17 children with unrelated diseases *2407*

Macrophage Inflammatory Protein-1α *Serum* *Increase* In patients with Plasmodium falciparum malaria mean concentration increased from 120 pg/mL on day of admission to hospital to 143 pg/mL on day 7 and 294 pg/mL on day 14 before decreasing to 170 pg/mL on day 21 and 26 pg/mL on day 28 *636*

Malondialdehyde *Cerebrospinal Fluid* *Increase* Concentration increased in patients with cerebral malaria with increase greatest in the patients who are most severely ill *1016*

Monocytes *Blood* *Increase* Increases in many protozoan infections *5544*

Myoglobin *Urine* *Increase* Heme pigment in urine of one patient with malaria due to falciparum malaria with rhabdomyolysis believed to be due to myoglobin *2720*

Neopterin *Serum* *Increase* Increased concentration observed. Concentrations in young children may be extraordinarily high, especially where malaria may be endemic *121*
Urine *Increase* Dramatically increased excretion *4313*

Neutrophil Elastase *Serum* *Increase* In 45 patients with malaria mean concentration of 188 ng/mL significantly different from normal values of < 90 ng/mL *2212*

Neutrophils *Blood* *Decrease* Significant neutropenia may occur *3671*

Nitrate plus Nitrite *Serum* *No Effect* In 16 patients with malaria mean concentration of 30.7 ± 14.9 µmol/L not significantly different from 28.5 ± 5.4 µmol/L in 30 controls *5256*

Parathyroid Hormone *Plasma* *Decrease* In 18 patients with malaria mean concentration of 1.5 (0.8 - 2.3) pmol/L compared with 1.6 (1.1 - 2.6) pmol/L in 10 healthy controls but concentration in 10 patients with falciparum malaria of 1.2 (0.6 - 1.9) pmol/L significantly reduced *1041*

Partial Thromboplastin Time *Plasma* *Increase* Consistent with the diagnosis of disseminated intravascular coagulation *2192*

Phosphate *Serum* *Decrease* Mean concentration in 18 patients with malaria on admission to hospital of 0.9 (0.8 - 1.1) mmol/L significantly less than 1.2 (1.1 - 1.3) mmol/L in 10 controls. Concentration of 0.85 (0.7 - 1.1) mmol/L in 10 patients with falciparum malaria most reduced *1041* Malaria is less common cause of hypophosphatemia *969*

Phospholipase A_2 Type II *Serum* *Increase* Increase in concentration observed of 170 µg/L in malaria compared with 2 and 4 µg/L in healthy controls *3767*

Platelets *Blood* *Decrease* In 2 patients with malaria with cerebral symptoms mean concentration of 30,000 /µL and in 7 without cerebral symptoms 61,500 ± 6,500 /µL compared with 178,000 - 300,000 /µL in 15 healthy controls *497* May be associated with defibrination resulting in platelet and coagulation factor consumption (overwhelming parasitemia) *5677*
Pancytopenia is a common feature *5677* With disease progression may become apparent *900*
Blood *No Effect* Mean concentration of 80,181 ± 11,967 /µL in 20 patients with complicated falciparum malaria *637*

Prealbumin *Serum* *Decrease* Decreased significantly in 11 patients untreated for more than 4 days *4622*

Procalcitonin *Plasma* *Increase* In 35 of 37 patients with acute malaria mean concentrations ranged from 150 pg/mL to 87 ng/mL compared with normal range of less than 50 pg/mL with concentrations higher in patients with P. falciparum than in those with P. vivax infection *202*

Prolactin *Plasma* *Increase* Slightly increased in falciparum malaria *5581*

Protein *Cerebrospinal Fluid* *Increase* Significant increase observed in 73 patients with cerebral malaria compared with 23 control patients with effect greatest in most severely ill patients *1016*
Serum *Decrease* Significantly lower in patients admitted after 5 - 10 days to hospital compared with the control group *4622*

Protein Casts *Urine* *Increase* May be demonstrable in severe falciparum infection *900*

Prothrombin Consumption *Blood* *Increase* May be associated with defibrination resulting in platelet and coagulation factor consumption (in overwhelming parasitemia) *5677*

Prothrombin Time *Plasma* *Increase* Consistent with the diagnosis of disseminated intravascular coagulation *2192*

Renin Activity *Plasma* *Increase* Increased in acute renal failure due to falciparum malaria *4878*

Reticulocytes *Blood* *Increase* Spurious extreme reticulocytosis observed in a patient with falciparum malaria and a high degree of intracellular parasitemia when the reticulocyte count was measured by a Sysmex R analyzer. The spurious increase was attributable to the RNA of the parasites being interpreted as reticulocyte RNA from the reticulocytes *2938* Occurs several days after therapy has begun *367*

Retinol *Serum* *Decrease* In 50 children with mild malaria median concentration of 0.70 µmol/L and 0.43 µmol/L in 50 children with severe malaria significantly different from 1.10 µmol/L in 50 healthy control children *1017*

Retinol-binding Protein *Serum* *Decrease* In 50 children with mild malaria median concentration of 25.5 mg/L and 15.0 mg/L in 50 children with severe malaria significantly different from 40.5 mg/L in 50 healthy control children *1017*

Rheumatoid Factor *Serum* *Increase* Mean concentration increased in patients with malaria *2472* High prevalence of IgM rheumatoid factors showed a positive correlation with malaria antibodies *5491* Rheumatoid factor may be observed in certain patients *2473*

Sodium *Red Blood Cells* *Increase* The content of infected and uninfected erythrocytes is increased as a result of increased permeability *2192*
Serum *Decrease* Caused by salt depletion and water retention *1542* *3492* *2192*

Soluble $CD8^+$ *Serum* *No Effect* Median concentration of 943 U/mL in 37 Gambian children with severe malaria not significantly different from 845 U/mL in 39 with mild malaria and 900 U/mL in 17 with unrelated diseases *2407*

Soluble E-Selectin *Serum* *Increase* In the acute phase of vivax malaria in 6 patients mean concentration of 99 ± 28 ng/mL significantly different from 56 ± 25 ng/mL in 7 healthy Japanese controls *3878*

Soluble Intercellular Adhesion Molecule-1 *Serum* *Increase* In 2 patients with malaria with cerebral symptoms and in 7 without cerebral symptoms maximal concentration of 344 ng/mL compared with 49 ± 6 ng/mL in 15 healthy controls *497*

Soluble Interleukin-2 Receptor *Serum* *Increase* In 2 patients with malaria with cerebral symptoms and in 7 without cerebral symptoms maximal concentration of 92.70 ng/mL compared with 3.29 ± 0.47 ng/mL in 15 healthy controls *497* In 37 Gambian children with severe plasmodium falciparum infection median concentration of 4,700 IU/mL significantly higher than median of 3,200 IU/mL in 39 children with mild malaria and 1,200 IU/mL in 17 controls with other diseases *2407*

Soluble Vascular Cell Adhesion Molecule-1
Serum *Increase* In 2 patients with malaria with cerebral symptoms and in 7 without cerebral symptoms maximal concentration of 4,614 ng/mL compared with 570 ± 25 ng/mL in 15 healthy controls *497* In the acute phase of vivax malaria in 6 patients mean concentration of 2,112 ± 782 ng/mL significantly different from 522 ± 56 ng/mL in 7 healthy Japanese controls *3878*

Thrombin Time *Blood* *Increase* Consistent with the diagnosis of disseminated intravascular coagulation *2192*

84.00 Malaria *(continued)*

Thrombin/Antithrombin III Complex *Plasma* *Increase* In 45 patients with malaria mean concentration of 8 ng/mL significantly different from normal values of < 5 ng/mL *2212*

Thrombomodulin *Plasma* *Increase* In the acute phase of vivax malaria in 6 patients mean concentration of 5.7 ± 1.3 Fujirebio units significantly different from 3.2 ± 0.7 Fujirebio units in 7 healthy Japanese controls *3878* In 2 patients with malaria with cerebral symptoms maximal concentrations of 211 and 332 ng/mL and in 7 without cerebral symptoms mean concentration of 69 ± 6 ng/mL compared with 26 ± 4 ng/mL in 15 healthy controls *497*

Thyroxine Binding Globulin *Serum* *Decrease* In patients with fever *5152*

Thyroxine (T4) *Serum* *Increase* Increased free T4 during fever *5152* Stable or increasing in falciparum malaria *5581*

α-Tocopherol *Serum* *Decrease* In 50 children with mild malaria median concentration of 11.53 μmol/L and 7.33 μmol/L in 50 children with severe malaria significantly different from 17.71 μmol/L in 50 healthy control children *1017*

α-Tocopherol:Cholesterol Ratio *Serum* *Decrease* In 50 children with mild malaria median concentration of 4.3 and 4.61 in 50 children with severe malaria significantly different from 5.15 in 50 healthy control children *1017*

Transforming Growth Factor-α *Serum* *Increase* In 37 patients with acute Plasmodium falciparum malaria mean concentration of 172 ± 108 pg/mL compared with normal value of less than 16 pg/mL *5636*

Transforming Growth Factor-β *Serum* *Decrease* In 37 patients with acute Plasmodium falciparum malaria mean concentration of 14 ± 11 pg/mL compared with 63 ± 15 pg/mL in 17 healthy controls *5636*

Transforming Growth Factor Receptor *Serum* *Increase* In 37 patients with acute Plasmodium falciparum malaria mean concentration of 22 ± 8.7 pg/mL compared with normal value of 1 ± 0.4 pg/mL *5636*

Tri-iodothyronine (T3) *Serum* *Decrease* Patients with fever of infection had significantly lowered levels *5152* Abruptly declined during falciparum malaria infection *5581*

Tumor Necrosis Factor *Serum* *Increase* Significantly increased concentration observed in patients with malaria *4082*

Tumor Necrosis Factor-α *Serum* *Increase* Increased concentration reported *2643* In 45 patients with malaria mean concentration of 39 pg/mL significantly different from normal values of < 15 pg/mL *2212* Concentration increased in children with malaria: outcome least favorable with highest concentrations *1848*
Serum *No Effect* In 36 Gambian children with severe malaria median concentration of < 10 pg/mL not different from < 10 pg/mL in 37 children with mild malaria and 17 with unrelated diseases *2407*

Tumor Necrosis Factor-β *Serum* *Increase* Observed in some patients with malaria *2643*

VDRL *Serum* *Positive* False positive may occur *367* Found in 100% of cases *2192*

Viscosity *Serum* *Increase* Significantly increased in 15 patients with acute renal failure due to falciparum malaria infection *4878*

Volume *Plasma* *Decrease* A rare and serious complication *2192* Initial hypovolemia followed by hypervolemia or normovolemia in acute renal failure due to falciparum malaria *4878*
Plasma *Increase* Initial hypovolemia followed by hypervolemia or normovolemia in acute renal failure due to falciparum malaria *4878* A rare and serious complication *2192*
Plasma *No Effect* A rare and serious complication *2192* Initial hypovolemia followed by hypervolemia or normovolemia in acute renal failure due to falciparum malaria *4878*

85.00 Kala-Azar

Immunoglobulin M *Serum* *Increase* Marked IgM increase in Kala-Azar patients. Mean concentration of 226 U/mL, range of 74 - 509 U/mL *1720*

Rheumatoid Factor *Serum* *Increase* Mean concentration increased in patients with kala-azar *2472* Rheumatoid factor may be observed in certain patients *2473*

85.90 Leishmaniasis

Albumin *Serum* *Decrease* Decreased with reversed A/G ratio *5545*
Serum *Increase* In tropical splenomegaly, increased plasma volume occurs mainly due to raised intravascular pools of albumin IgG and IgM. The variance in plasma volume was attributable to increases in these 3 pools, IgM and IgG accounting for 42% of the total and albumin for 28% *958*

Bilirubin *Serum* *Increase* Hemolytic anemia *5727* *5677*

Bilirubin, Indirect *Serum* *Increase* Hemolytic anemia *5727* *5677*

Clotting Time *Blood* *Increase* Normal early in the disease but later becomes prolonged *367*

Complement Fixation *Serum* *Increase* Positive but is also positive in tuberculosis *5545*

Erythrocyte Sedimentation Rate *Blood* *Increase* Increased due to increased serum globulin *5545*

Erythrocytes *Urine* *Increase* Frequent *5545*

Erythropoietin *Serum* *Increase* In 44 patients with leishmaniasis before treatment mean concentration of 2.12 ± 0.44 (log (U/L serum)) significantly different from 0.80 ± 0.27 (log (U/L serum)) in 44 controls *4501*

Ferritin *Serum* *Increase* In 29 patients with leishmaniasis before treatment mean concentration of 3.02 ± 0.39 μmol/L significantly different from 1.89 ± 0.29 μmol/L in 29 controls *4501*

γ-Globulin *Serum* *Increase* Often associated with hypergammaglobulinemia *4707* Increased with reversed A/G ratio *5545*

Haptoglobin *Serum* *Decrease* Intravascular hemolysis due to parasites *5544* Hemolytic anemia *5727*

Hemagglutination Inhibition *Serum* *Increase* Used for diagnosis but requires fuller development for routine use *1025*

Hematocrit *Blood* *Decrease* Hemolytic anemia *5727* Normochromic, normocytic anemia develops slowly but becomes severe later in the disease *367*

Hemoglobin *Blood* *Decrease* Normocytic, normochromic anemia develops slowly but becomes severe later in the disease *367* In 44 patients with leishmaniasis before treatment mean concentration of 6.4 ± 1.7 g/dL significantly different from 13.1 ± 1.0 g/dL in 44 controls *4501* In 13 patients with leishmaniasis who did not develop post-kala azar dermal leishmaniasis mean concentration of 7.6 ± 2.3 g/dL and 7.4 ± 1.4 g/dL in 16 who did, concentration significantly lower than in healthy individuals *1665* Hemolytic anemia *5727*
Plasma *Increase* Reported observation *5677* Hemolytic anemia *5727*

Immunoglobulin G *Serum* *Increase* Serum protein increases to values > 10 g/dL, almost entirely due to raised IgG levels *367* Marked IgG increase in kala-azar patients. Mean concentration of 591 U/mL, range 305 - 941 U/mL *1720* Increased intravascular pools of albumin, IgG, and IgM in tropical splenomegaly. IgM and IgG accounting for 42% of the total and albumin for 28% *958*

Immunoglobulin M *Serum* *Increase* In tropical splenomegaly; increased intravascular pools of albumin, IgG, and IgM. Variance in plasma volume was attributable to increases in these 3 pools, IgM and IgG accounting for 42% of the total and albumin for 28% *958*

Interleukin-10 *Serum* *Increase* In 13 patients with leishmaniasis who developed post-kala-azar dermal leishmaniasis mean concentration of 46.5 pg/mL significantly higher than in patients who did not develop post-kala-azar dermal leishmaniasis and and even more when compared to healthy individuals *1665*

Iron *Serum* *No Effect* In 30 patients with leishmaniasis before treatment mean concentration of 18.3 ± 6.5 μmol/L not significantly different from 19.3 ± 6.0 μmol/L in 30 controls *4501*

Iron-binding Capacity, Total *Serum* *No Effect* In 30 patients with leishmaniasis before treatment mean concentration of 51.3 ± 25.3 μmol/L not significantly different from 58.2 ± 10.6 μmol/L in 30 controls *4501*

Leukocytes *Blood* *Decrease* In 13 patients with leishmaniasis who did not develop post-kala-azar dermal leishmaniasis mean concentration of 3.4 ± 2.2 x 10^6/mL and 2.6 ± 1.2 x 10^6/mL in 16 who did, concentration significantly lower than in healthy individuals *1665* Characteristic, with counts < 2,000 /µL in 75% of cases *367*

β_2-Microglobulin *Serum* *Increase* In 11 adult patients with active visceral Leishmaniasis mean concentration about 6.0 mg/L significantly higher than 1.6 ± 1 mg/L in 10 healthy controls *5480*

Monocytes *Blood* *Increase* Increases in many protozoan infections *5544*

Neutrophils *Blood* *Decrease* Absolute neutropenia with total WBC count < 2,000 /µL *367* Significant neutropenia may occur *3671*

Partial Thromboplastin Time *Plasma* *Increase* Normal early in the disease but later becomes prolonged *367*

Protein *Serum* *Increase* Elevated to values > 10 g/dL, almost entirely due to increased IgG *367*
Urine *Increase* Frequent *5545*

Prothrombin Time *Plasma* *Increase* Normal early in the disease but later becomes prolonged *367*

Rheumatoid Factor *Serum* *Increase* Parasitic diseases that involve the liver and reticuloendothelial system have a significant incidence of seropositivity, suggesting that these factors may be produced in the tissues locally *1980*

Soluble CD4+ *Serum* *Increase* In 11 adult patients with active visceral Leishmaniasis mean concentration of 61 ± 25 U/mL significantly higher than 25 ± 19 U/mL in 15 healthy controls *5480*

Soluble CD8+ *Serum* *Increase* In 11 adult patients with active visceral Leishmaniasis mean concentration of 1,495 ± 389 U/mL significantly higher than 407 ± 117 U/mL in 15 healthy controls *5480*

Soluble Interleukin-2 Receptor *Serum* *Increase* In 13 patients with leishmaniasis who developed post-kala-azar dermal leishmaniasis mean concentration of 1,703 U/mL significantly higher than in patients who did not develop post-kala-azar dermal leishmaniasis and and even more when compared to healthy individuals *1665*

Soluble Interleukin-4 Receptor-α *Serum* *Increase* In 29 patients with leishmaniasis mean concentration of 121 pg/mL significantly higher than in healthy individuals in whom reference range was 15 - 44 pg/mL *1665*

Uric Acid *Serum* *Increase* In tropical splenomegaly syndrome *2401*

Volume *Plasma* *Increase* In 64 cases of tropical splenomegaly, plasma volumes ranged from 52 - 129 mL/kg. 70% of the increase was attributable to increased intravascular pools of IgG and IgM (42%) and albumin (28%) *958*

86.20 Chagas' Disease

C-Reactive Protein *Serum* *Increase* Mean concentration in children with Chagas' disease 2.5 µg/mL compared with 1.5 µg/L in healthy children *3437*

α_2-Macroglobulin *Serum* *Increase* Mean concentration in children with Chagas' disease 3.70 mg/mL compared with 2.45 mg/L in healthy children *3437*

Neopterin *Serum* *Increase* In 12 patients with intermediate stage Chagas disease concentration of 5.55 ± 1.02 nmol/L not significantly different from 9 normal controls of 5.59 ± 1.20 nmol/L but in 14 patients with cardiac form of disease mean concentration of 8.77 ± 3.24 nmol/L and in 4 with Mega syndrome of 7.37 ± 2.36 nmol/L significantly higher than normal *5853*

Renin Activity *Plasma* *Increase* In 9 patients with Chagas' disease mean activity of 4.11 ± 1.03 ng/mL/h significantly higher than 1.08 ± 0.11 ng/mL/h in 19 asymptomatic patients and 1.65 ± 0.22 ng/mL/h in 9 normal sedentary controls *378*

86.90 Trypanosomiasis

Erythrocyte Survival *Red Blood Cells* *Decrease* Hematological studies indicate the presence of a hemolytic process *5726*

γ-Globulin *Cerebrospinal Fluid* *Increase* In 22% of cases *1738*

Haptoglobin *Serum* *Decrease* Intravascular hemolysis due to parasites *5544*

Hematocrit *Blood* *Decrease* Mild normocytic normochromic anemia associated with reduced marrow activity *2192* Anemia is a characteristic feature *5726*

Hemoglobin *Blood* *Decrease* Anemia is a characteristic feature. Hematological studies indicate the presence of a hemolytic process *5726* Mild normocytic normochromic anemia associated with reduced marrow activity *2192*
Plasma *Increase* Intravascular hemolysis due to parasites *5544*

immunoglobulin A *Serum* *Increase* Reported effect *2192*

Immunoglobulin M *Serum* *Increase* Reported effect *4551* Markedly increased and remains elevated throughout the course of the infection *2192* Marked increase of immunoglobulins, particularly IgM, may be explained by the continuous production of antibodies against new variants *4708*

Immunoglobulins *Serum* *Increase* Marked increase of immunoglobulins, particularly IgM, may be explained by the continuous production of antibodies against new variants *4708*

Interleukin-1β *Serum* *No Effect* In 14 untreated patients with African trypanosomiasis mean concentration of 2.0 ± 0.2 ng/L not significantly different from 0.9 ± 0.2 ng/L in 13 control individuals *4316*

Interleukin-6 *Serum* *Increase* In 14 untreated patients with African trypanosomiasis mean concentration of 19.2 ± 7.3 ng/L significantly increased compared with 1.3 ± 0.2 ng/L in 13 control individuals *4316*

Leukocytes *Blood* *No Effect* Usually normal *2192*

Lymphocytes *Blood* *Increase* Relative lymphocytosis *2192*
Cerebrospinal Fluid *Increase* Up to 2,000 /µL with CNS involvement *2192*

Monocytes *Blood* *Increase* Increased in many protozoan infections *5544*

Rheumatoid Factor *Serum* *Increase* 27% positivity *306* Mean concentration increased in patients with trypanosomiasis *2472* Parasitic diseases that involve the liver and reticuloendothelial system have a significant incidence of seropositivity, suggesting that these factors may be produced in the tissues locally *1980* 27% positivity *874* Rheumatoid factor may be observed in certain patients *2473*

Thyroid Stimulating Hormone *Serum* *Increase* In 14 untreated patients with African trypanosomiasis mean concentration of 2.6 ± 0.4 mU/L significantly increased compared with 1.4 ± 0.2 mU/L in 13 control individuals *4316*

Thyroxine (T4) *Serum* *Decrease* In 14 untreated patients with African trypanosomiasis mean concentration of 10.3 ± 1.2 pmol/L significantly decreased compared with 15.4 ± 0.8 pmol/L in 13 control individuals *4316*

Tri-iodothyronine, Free (fT3) *Serum* *Decrease* In 14 untreated patients with African trypanosomiasis mean concentration of 2.7 ± 0.5 pmol/L significantly decreased compared with 5.8 ± 0.3 pmol/L in 13 control individuals *4316*

Tri-iodothyronine, Reverse (rT3) *Serum* *No Effect* In 14 untreated patients with African trypanosomiasis mean concentration of 2.2 ± 0.3 nmol/L not significantly different from 2.4 ± 0.2 nmol/L in 13 control individuals *4316*

Tumor Necrosis Factor-α *Serum* *Increase* In untreated 14 patients with African trypanosomiasis mean concentration of 16.0 ± 4.1 ng/L significantly increased compared with 2.9 ± 1.4 ng/L in 13 control individuals *4316*

VDRL *Serum* *Positive* False positive in 10% of cases *2192*

87.00 Relapsing Fever

Albumin *Urine* *Increase* Noted occasionally *900*

Bilirubin *Serum* *Increase* Occurs late in the course of the disease *1980*
Urine *Increase* Noted occasionally *900*

Cells *Cerebrospinal Fluid* *Increase* Mononuclear cells sometimes increased *5545*

Complement Fixation *Serum* *Increase* Antibodies develop but antigens are not sufficiently well standardized to be useful *1980*

87.00 Relapsing Fever *(continued)*

Erythrocyte Sedimentation Rate *Blood Increase* Common *900*

Erythrocytes *Urine Increase* There may be blood in urine during the febrile period *1980*

Haptoglobin *Serum Decrease* Intravascular hemolysis due to parasites *5544*

Hematocrit *Blood Decrease* Intravascular hemolysis due to parasites *5544* Moderate anemia may occur later in the disease *1980*

Hemoglobin *Blood Decrease* Moderate anemia may occur later in the disease *1980*
Plasma Increase Intravascular hemolysis due to parasites *5544*

Immunoglobulin G *Serum Increase* Occurs initially after infection, followed by a rise in IgM *367*

Immunoglobulin M *Serum Increase* IgG hyperglobulinemia occurs initially after infection, followed by a rise in IgM *367*

Immunoglobulins *Serum Increase* IgG hyperglobulinemia occurs initially after infection, followed by a rise in IgM *367*

Leukocytes *Blood Decrease* May be elevated or decreased but is usually normal *900*
Blood Increase From the onset, there is marked polymorphonuclear leukocytosis, of 15,000 - 25,000 /μL, with increase in immature forms *367* During the febrile period, with a shift to the left *1980*
Blood No Effect Count may be elevated or decreased but is usually normal *900*
Cerebrospinal Fluid Increase Pleocytosis can occur *900*

Monocytes *Cerebrospinal Fluid Increase* Sometimes increased *900*

Protein *Cerebrospinal Fluid Increase* Sometimes increased in CSF *5545*
Urine Increase Sometimes; during the febrile period *1980*

VDRL *Serum Positive* 30% false positive *2192* 45% false positive *4946*

Weil-Felix Reaction *Serum Positive* Reactive in titers of 1:80 or higher *367* Proteus OX K > 90% positive (> 1:40) *4946*

88.00 Bartonellosis

Haptoglobin *Serum Decrease* Intravascular hemolysis due to parasites *5544*

Hematocrit *Blood Decrease* Intravascular hemolysis due to parasites *5544* Reported effect *4332*

Hemoglobin *Plasma Increase* Observed effect *5677* Reported observation *4332* Intravascular hemolysis due to parasites *5544*
Urine Increase Intravascular hemolysis parasites (Oroya fever); due to Bartonella bacilliformis *5544*

Immunoglobulin M *Serum Increase* Especially when particulate antigenic material is present in the blood stream *1290*

Leukocytes *Blood Decrease* Normal, increased or decreased *2192*
Blood Increase Normal, increased or decreased *2192*
Blood No Effect Normal, increased or decreased *2192*

Platelets *Blood Decrease* Has been reported *2192*

88.81 Lyme Disease

Anticardiolipin Antibodies *Serum Increase* A subset of patients (50%) with neuroborreliosis (Lyme disease) showed IgG reactivity to cardiolipin in solid phase ELISA *1645*

Aspartate Aminotransferase *Serum Increase* May be elevated in Lyme Disease if mild hepatic involvement persists *3461*

Cells *Cerebrospinal Fluid Increase* In 20 patients with Lyme neuroborreliosis mean concentration ranged from 0 - 304 x 10^9/L significantly different from normal reference values of 0 - 5 x 10^9/L, with 16 having counts above upper limit of normal *1226*

Cryoglobulins *Serum Increase* May be detected in Lyme Disease *3461*

Erythrocyte Sedimentation Rate *Blood Increase* Often mildly elevated in Lyme Disease *3461*

Glial Fibrillary Acidic Protein *Cerebrospinal Fluid Increase* In 20 patients with Lyme neuroborreliosis mean concentration of 592 ± 596 pg/mL before antibiotics significantly different from 121 ± 87 pg/mL in 24 healthy controls *1226*

γ-Glutamyltransferase *Serum Increase* With liver involvement *5428*

Immunoglobulin M *Cerebrospinal Fluid Increase* In 46 paired cerebrospinal fluid and serum samples from 32 patients with meningopolyradiculoneuritis due to Borrelia burgdorferi (Lyme borreliosis stage 2); cerebrospinal fluid IgM, IgM index, and cerebrospinal fluid IgM/cerebrospinal fluid IgG ratios were significantly higher than in all other neuroimmunologic disorders evaluated and may be valuable diagnostic indicators for neuroborreliosis *5627*
Serum Increase May be elevated in Lyme Disease *3461*

Interleukin-6 *Cerebrospinal Fluid Decrease* In 7 patients with Lyme disease mean concentration of 27.7 ± 9.7 pg/mL less than 93.6 ± 21.8 pg/mL in 20 control patients with asceptic lumboischiadic syndrome *5872*
Cerebrospinal Fluid Increase In 46 paired cerebrospinal fluid and serum samples from 32 patients with meningopolyradiculoneuritis due to Borrelia burgdorferi (Lyme borreliosis stage 2) cerebrospinal fluid and serum interleukin 6, although not specific for neuroborreliosis, were good indicators of disease activity *5627*
Serum Increase In 46 paired cerebrospinal fluid and serum samples from 32 patients with meningopolyradiculoneuritis due to Borrelia burgdorferi (Lyme borreliosis stage 2) cerebrospinal fluid and serum interleukin 6, although not specific for neuroborreliosis, were good indicators of disease activity *5627*

Lactate Dehydrogenase *Cerebrospinal Fluid No Effect* In 7 patients with Lyme disease mean concentration of 0.26 ± 0.05 μkat/L not significantly different from 0.44 ± 0.12 μkat/L in 20 control patients with asceptic lumboischiadic syndrome *5332*

Lymphocytes *Blood Decrease* Lymphopenia occurs in Lyme Disease *3461*

Oligoclonal Banding *Cerebrospinal Fluid Increase* Observed in 6 patients with positive CSF Lyme disease antibody titers *77*

Protein *Cerebrospinal Fluid Increase* In 20 patients with Lyme neuroborreliosis mean concentration ranged from 0.3 - 3.6 g/L significantly different from normal reference values of < 0.6 g/L, with 9 having counts above upper limit of normal *1226*

Soluble Interleukin-2 Receptor *Serum Increase* In 46 paired cerebrospinal fluid and serum samples from 32 patients with meningopolyradiculoneuritis due to Borrelia burgdorferi (Lyme borreliosis stage 2), serum soluble interleukin 2 receptor level was only mildly elevated *5627*

Tumor Necrosis Factor-α *Cerebrospinal Fluid Decrease* In 7 patients with Lyme disease mean concentration of 0.00 ± 0.00 pg/mL less than 0.94 ± 0.55 pg/mL in 20 patients with asceptic lumboischiadic syndrome *5872*
Cerebrospinal Fluid No Effect In none of 46 paired cerebrospinal fluid and serum samples from 32 patients with meningopolyradiculoneuritis due to Borrelia burgdorferi (Lyme borreliosis stage 2) was tumor necrosis factor-α detected *5627*
Serum No Effect In none of 46 paired cerebrospinal fluid and serum samples from 32 patients with meningopolyradiculoneuritis due to Borrelia burgdorferi (Lyme borreliosis stage 2) tumor necrosis factor-α was detected *5627*

Venereal Disease and Other Spirochetal Diseases

90.90 Congenital Syphilis

α_1-Antichymotrypsin *Serum No Effect* Mean concentration within reference interval of 47.9 ± 8.1 mg/dL in one examined patient with congenital syphilis *3044*

94.90 Neurosyphilis

IgM Index *Cerebrospinal Fluid Increase* In 100% patients with neurosyphilis IgM index increased *5486*

Oligoclonal Banding *Cerebrospinal Fluid Increase* Oligoclonal IgG bands detected in patients with neurosyphilis *3261*

Soluble HLA-I *Cerebrospinal Fluid* *No Effect* In 3 patients with neurosyphilis, mean concentration undetectable in all *216*

Soluble HLA-II *Cerebrospinal Fluid* *No Effect* In 3 patients with neurosyphilis, mean concentration undetectable in all *216*

97.90 Syphilis

Anti-Mitochondrial M1 Antibody *Serum* *Increase* Characteristically present in patients with secondary syphilis *1778*

Anti-Mitochondrial M5 Antibody *Serum* *Increase* May be present in some patients with SLE *1778*

Anticardiolipin Antibodies *Serum* *No Effect* None of the patients with syphilis or healthy controls was positive for any GPI-dependent aPL *3360*

Antiphosphatidic Acid Antibodies *Serum* *No Effect* None of the patients with syphilis or healthy controls was positive for any GPI-dependent aPL *3360*

Antiphosphatidylethanolamine Antibodies *Serum* *No Effect* None of the patients with syphilis or healthy controls was positive for any GPI-dependent aPL *3360*

Antiphosphatidylinositol Antibodies *Serum* *No Effect* None of the patients with syphilis or healthy controls was positive for any GPI-dependent aPL *3360*

Antiphosphatidylserine Antibodies *Serum* *No Effect* None of the patients with syphilis or healthy controls was positive for any GPI-dependent aPL *3360*

Cells *Cerebrospinal Fluid* *Increase* Increased in meningovascular syphilis *2039* First sign of asymptomatic syphilis arising from latency is pleocytosis of > 4 cells /μL, followed by increase in protein. With progress to parenchymatous neurosyphilis, 150 cells /μL and marked increase in protein (globulin) is found *367* Reported effect *1980*

Chloride *Cerebrospinal Fluid* *Decrease* Usually slightly decreased *1980*

Complement Fixation *Serum* *Increase* Kolmer test *2192*

Erythrocyte Sedimentation Rate *Blood* *Increase* Raised in 66.6% of seronegative primary cases, 80% of seropositive cases, 100% secondary cases, 80% early latent cases, and 73.9% of late latent cases. Also raised in 16/17 cases of neurosyphilis and 11/11 cases of cardiovascular syphilis *1540*

γ-Globulin *Cerebrospinal Fluid* *Increase* In active disease *4856* Reflected in an abnormal Lange curve *367*
Serum *Increase* All 3 stages *4707*

Glucose *Cerebrospinal Fluid* *Decrease* 10 - 45 mg/dL *5252* Decreased in 50% of the patients *1980*

Hematocrit *Blood* *Decrease* Secondary anemia *2192*

Hemoglobin *Blood* *Decrease* Secondary anemia *2192*

Immunoglobulin G *Cerebrospinal Fluid* *Increase* Increased with obstruction of the spinal canal, especially in neurosyphilis and tuberculous meningitis *5138*

Leukocytes *Blood* *Increase* In secondary syphilis *2192*
Cerebrospinal Fluid *Increase* Average 500 /μL, usually lymphocytes *367*

Lymphocytes *Blood* *Increase* Absolute increase *2192*
Cerebrospinal Fluid *Increase* CSF count may be elevated, with 5 - 10 or more lymphocytes/μL *1980* Majority of cells are lymphocytes with CNS involvement *5252*

α₂-Macroglobulin *Cerebrospinal Fluid* *No Effect* Neurosyphilis concentrations normal *4641*

Monocytes *Blood* *Increase* In neonatal, primary and secondary syphilis *4426*

Protein *Cerebrospinal Fluid* *Increase* Increased with obstruction of the spinal canal, especially in neurosyphilis and tuberculous meningitis *5138* Over 45 mg/dL in syphilitic meningitis *5252* Usually increased to some degree with CNS involvement *1980*

Rheumatoid Factor *Serum* *Increase* Rheumatoid factor may be observed in certain patients *2473* Concentration may be increased as in other diseases with chronic inflammation *2952* 13% positivity *306* Mean concentration increased in patients with syphilis *2472* 13% positivity *874* The incidence of seropositivity exceeds that of a normal population *4551*

VDRL *Cerebrospinal Fluid* *Positive* In asymptomatic neurosyphilis the blood and spinal fluid VDRL are usually both reactive *1980* Positive as a result of serum or blood leaking into the CSF *2039*
Serum *Positive* Becomes positive in most patients 2 - 3 weeks after the appearance of the chancre or 6 weeks after the initial contact. In the secondary stage, especially when generalized eruptions occur, it is positive in virtually 100% of patients *1980* Negative at the onset of primary syphilis, but within 7 - 14 days it becomes positive in the majority of cases. Almost all sera from patients with secondary syphilis are positive. Asymptomatic or latent syphilis can be diagnosed only by a positive serologic test *2039*

99.10 Lymphogranuloma Venereum

Alanine Aminotransferase *Serum* *Increase* May indicate severe liver impairment *900*

Albumin *Serum* *Decrease* A common finding during active infection. Often reversal of the A/G ratio *1980*

Aspartate Aminotransferase *Serum* *Increase* May indicate severe liver impairment *900*

Bilirubin *Serum* *Increase* May indicate severe liver impairment *900*

Complement Fixation *Serum* *Increase* Much more sensitive than the Frei test, but cross reacts with other chlamydiae infections, such as psittacosis *5252* A rising titer strongly indicates acute disease. May remain positive after antimicrobial therapy and an apparent clinical remission *4891* Early in the course of the disease, in symptomatic and asymptomatic patients, titers of 1:40 - 1:160 will occur. Later stages may produce titers as high as 1:640 in most patients *900* Much more sensitive than the Frei test, but cross reacts with other chlamydiae infections, such as psittacosis *4612* This test is nonspecific and may be positive following infections with other chlamydiae *1980*

Erythrocyte Sedimentation Rate *Blood* *Increase* Is often increased *900*

Frei Test *Skin* *Positive* Diagnostic skin test. A 6 mm nodule with surrounding erythema 48 h after intradermal injection is positive reaction *5252* May be up to 60% false-negative reactions even in established cases *4612*

α₂-Globulin *Serum* *Increase* Elevated with a reversal of the A/G ratio. In such cases, the increase occurs in the α₂- and γ-globulin regions *900*

γ-Globulin *Serum* *Increase* Elevated with a reversal of the A/G ratio. In such cases, the increase occurs in the α₂- and γ-globulin regions *900* Often associated with hypergammaglobulinemia *4707* Are increased with reversed A/G ratio A common finding during active infection. Often reversal of the albumin:globulin ratio *1980*

Glucose *Cerebrospinal Fluid* *Decrease* Characteristically low *2832* In the early stages of infection *900*

Hematocrit *Blood* *Decrease* Anemia and leukopenia are most common when enlargement of the liver and spleen and generalized lymphadenopathy occur *900*

Hemoglobin *Blood* *Decrease* Anemia and leukopenia are most common when enlargement of the liver and spleen and generalized lymphadenopathy occur *900*

immunoglobulin A *Serum* *Increase* Up to 75% of the patients will experience an elevation *900*

Immunoglobulins *Serum* *Increase* Often associated with striking elevations *4707*

Lactate Dehydrogenase *Serum* *Increase* May indicate severe liver impairment *900*

Leukocytes *Blood* *Decrease* Anemia and leukopenia are most common when enlargement of the liver and spleen and generalized lymphadenopathy occur *900*
Blood *Increase* When the nodes suppurate, a leukocytosis of 7,000 - 19,000 /μL and a slight monocytosis may occur *900* Mild leukocytosis with a relative lymphocytosis or monocytosis *4891*
Cerebrospinal Fluid *Increase* Pleocytosis as high as 4,000 /μL may occur *900*
Urine *Increase* Vaginovesical fistulas may cause changes that reflect in the urine as numerous leukocytes or inclusion-filled mononuclear cells *900*

Lymphocytes *Blood* *Increase* Mild leukocytosis with a relative lymphocytosis or monocytosis *4891*

Monocytes *Blood* *Increase* Mild leukocytosis with a relative lymphocytosis or monocytosis *4891*

99.10 Lymphogranuloma Venereum *(continued)*

Monocytes *(continued)*
Urine *Increase* Vaginovesical fistulas may cause changes that reflect in the urine as numerous leukocytes or inclusion-filled mononuclear cells *900*

Protein *Cerebrospinal Fluid* *Increase* High in the early stages of CSF infection, varying from 250 - 3,750 mg/dL *900*
Serum *Increase* Elevated with a reversal of the A/G ratio. In such cases, the increase occurs in the α_2- and γ- globulin regions *900*

VDRL *Serum* *Positive* 20% false positive *2192* Biologic false positive serologic tests are not infrequent *4891*

99.30 Reiter's Disease

Antinuclear Antibodies *Serum* *No Effect* Not usually present *2039*

Cells *Synovial Fluid* *Increase* Reiter's Cells (macrophages with partially digested neutrophils) *413*

Complement, Total *Serum* *Increase* Elevated during active inflammation and subsides with remission *4683* In 14 patients, 64% had increased values *4925*
Synovial Fluid *Increase* Elevated levels appear to be directly related to the severity and duration of joint inflammation *4683* Usually higher than in most other types of effusions in contrast to the very low levels in rheumatoid arthritis *900*

Erythrocyte Sedimentation Rate *Blood* *Increase* The increased ESR parallels clinical course *5545* Common *2039*

α_2-Globulin *Serum* *Increase* Evidence of nonspecific inflammation *900*

γ-Globulin *Serum* *Increase* Increased in long-standing disease *5545*

Glucose *Synovial Fluid* *Decrease* Usually normal but may be decreased when leukocyte count is increased *413*
Synovial Fluid *No Effect* Usually normal but may be decreased when leukocyte count is increased *413*

Hematocrit *Blood* *Decrease* There may be a mild anemia *900*

Hemoglobin *Blood* *Decrease* There may be a mild anemia *900*

HLA Antigens *Blood* *Present* HLA-B27 present in 80% of patients versus 9% of controls *5678* HLA-B27 found in 65% of cases *5428*

Leukocytes *Blood* *Increase* A range of 10,000 - 18,000 /µL *900* Common *2039*
Prostatic Fluid *Increase* Reflects urethritis *413*
Synovial Fluid *Increase* Synovial fluid is typically inflammatory, with cell counts up to 60,000 /µL *2039*
Urine *Increase* Reflects urethritis *413*

Neutrophils *Synovial Fluid* *Increase* Polymorphonuclear leukocytosis in the range of 2,000 - 10,000 /µL *900*

Procollagen Type II Peptide *Serum* *Increase* Reported effect *824*

Rheumatoid Factor *Serum* *No Effect* Concentration usually normal *413*
Synovial Fluid *No Effect* Concentration usually normal *2039*

100.00 Leptospirosis

Agglutination Tests *Serum* *Positive* Antibodies appear during 2nd week of illness *1980* Tests reach peaks in 4 - 7 weeks and may last for many years. An individual titer of 1:300 is suggestive of this disease *5545*

Alanine Aminotransferase *Serum* *Increase* Increased in 50% of the patients but average levels are not as high as in hepatitis *5545*

Albumin *Serum* *Decrease* May occur with jaundice after the 1st week of fever *5252*

Alkaline Phosphatase *Serum* *Increase* Jaundice may appear at the end of the 1st week of fever. Liver tests show hepatic decompensation of the intrahepatic type *5252* Increased in 50% of the patients *5545*

Antibody Titer *Serum* *Increase* The contrast between negative acute-phase and positive convalescent phase sera is diagnostic *5252*

Aspartate Aminotransferase *Serum* *Increase* Values are rarely increased more than 2 - 3 times normal regardless of the degree of hyperbilirubinemia *367* Increased in 50% of the patients but average levels are not as high as in hepatitis *5545* Elevated in patients without clinically evident liver disease *1980*

Bilirubin *Serum* *Increase* May be associated with profound jaundice *3406* May reach 65 mg/dL but is < 20 mg/dL in 66% of patients *367* Jaundice may appear at the end of the 1st week of fever. Liver tests show hepatic decompensation of the intrahepatic type *5252* Increased in 50% of the patients *5545* Elevated values found in patients without clinically evident liver disease *1980*

Bilirubin, Direct *Serum* *Increase* Hyperbilirubinemia, which is predominantly conjugated (direct), may reach 65 mg/dL but is < 20 mg/dL in 66% of patients *367*

Casts *Urine* *Increase* Urine is abnormal in 75% of patients *5545* During the leptospiremic phase *1980*

Cells *Cerebrospinal Fluid* *Increase* Increased up to 500 /µL in about 66% of patients. Indicates meningeal involvement *5545* Pleocytosis of 25 - 500 cells /µL in > 75% of cases *1980*

Cholesterol *Serum* *Decrease* May occur with jaundice *5252*

Complement Fixation *Serum* *Increase* Antibodies appear during second week of illness *1980*

Creatine Kinase *Serum* *Increase* Increased in 33% of patients during the 1st week. Differentiates the condition from hepatitis *5545*

Creatinine *Serum* *Increase* Marked oliguria or anuria develops after the 1st week of disease and is attended by severe azotemia and electrolyte imbalance characteristic of lower nephron nephrosis *5252*

Erythrocyte Sedimentation Rate *Blood* *Increase* Increased in > 50% of the patients but is usually < 50 mm/h *367*

Erythrocytes *Urine* *Increase* In 75% of patients *5545* Hemorrhagic manifestations may occur in the first few days of fever *5252* During the leptospiremic phase *1980* Hematuria, pyuria, and cylindruria in most cases *5252*

α_2-Globulin *Serum* *Increase* May occur with jaundice after the 1st week of fever *5252*

γ-Globulin *Serum* *Increase* May occur with jaundice after the 1st week of fever *5252*

Glucose *Cerebrospinal Fluid* *No Effect* Concentration usually normal *1980* Concentration usually unaffected *2033*

Hematocrit *Blood* *Decrease* With jaundice, anemia may be severe due to intravascular hemolysis. Anemia is unusual in anicteric patients *2033*

Hemoglobin *Blood* *Decrease* With jaundice, anemia may be severe due to intravascular hemolysis. Anemia is unusual in anicteric patients *2033*

Lactate *Blood* *Increase* Increased concentration may be observed *1290*

Leukocytes *Blood* *Decrease* May occur *367*
Blood *Increase* With a preponderance of polymorphonuclears and immature forms *5252* Often normal in mild cases and ranges up to 40,000 /µL in severe cases *1980* Mild elevations in anicteric patients *367* As high as 50,000 /µL in patients with jaundice *2033*
Urine *Increase* During the leptospiremic phase *1980* In 75% of patients *5545*

Lymphocytes *Cerebrospinal Fluid* *Increase* Lymphocytic pleocytosis is common with counts from 100 - 300 /µL *5252*

Neutrophils *Blood* *Increase* Neutrophilia of > 70% is often found regardless of the leukocyte count which may be high or low *367* In a high proportion of cases *5252*

Occult Blood *Feces* *Increase* Hemorrhagic manifestations may occur in the first few days of fever *5252*

Platelets *Blood* *Decrease* Rare *2033*

Potassium *Serum* *Increase* Marked oliguria or anuria develops after the 1st week of disease and is attended by severe azotemia and electrolyte imbalance characteristic of lower nephron nephrosis *5252*

Protein *Cerebrospinal Fluid* *Increase* Increased in about 66% of patients, up to 80 mg/dL, indicating meningeal involvement *5545* Occasionally observed *5252*

Urine *Increase* Heavy proteinuria during the febrile period *5252* In 75% of patients *5545* During the leptospiremic phase *1980*

Prothrombin Time *Plasma* *Increase* May occur with jaundice *5252* In some patients *2033*

Urea Nitrogen *Serum* *Increase* Usually associated with jaundice *2033* During leptospiremic phase, azotemia may be present *1980* Marked oliguria or anuria develops after the 1st week of disease and is attended by severe azotemia and electrolyte imbalance characteristic of lower nephron nephrosis *5252*

Urobilinogen *Urine* *Increase* Jaundice may appear at the end of the 1st week of fever. Liver tests show hepatic decompensation of the intrahepatic type *5252*

VDRL *Serum* *Positive* 10% false positive *2192*

101.00 Neuroborreliosis

Oligoclonal Banding *Cerebrospinal Fluid* *Increase* Oligoclonal IgG bands detected in patients with neuroborreliosis *3261*

102.90 Yaws

Monocytes *Cerebrospinal Fluid* *Increase* Occasionally found but neither symptoms nor signs of neurologic disability have evolved *2192*

Rheumatoid Factor *Serum* *Increase* Rheumatoid factor may be observed in certain patients *2473* Mean concentration increased in patients with yaws *2472*

VDRL *Serum* *Positive* All serological tests for syphilis are positive *2192*

Mycoses

112.90 Candidiasis

Candida Antibody *Serum* *Increase* Positive test indicates the presence of antibodies to candida species *2952*

Mannose *Serum* *Increase* Levels were observed in 20 of 22 patients with invasive candidial infection in a concentration greater than or equal to 60 μmol/L. In 68.2% of them levels were significantly increased. The specificity of the test was 91.8% with a positive predictive value of 58.8% *4252*

112.90 Moniliasis

Agglutination Tests *Serum* *Positive* Serum agglutinin and precipitin titers against Candida are of little value, as many normal individuals harbor the organism without tissue invasion. A low titer probably makes esophageal candidiasis unlikely *4891*

Cells *Cerebrospinal Fluid* *Increase* Pleocytosis in all patients with Candida meningitis, predominantly lymphocytic *338*

Leukocytes *Blood* *Increase* Leukocytosis of 12,000 - 22,000 /μL and neutrophilia of 75 - 90% in Candida meningitis *338*
Cerebrospinal Fluid *Increase* Mean count = 600 /μL in 28 cases of Candida meningitis *338*

Neutrophils *Blood* *Increase* Leukocytosis of 12,000 - 22,000 /μL and neutrophilia of 75 - 90% in Candida meningitis *338*

Precipitins *Serum* *Increase* A low titer probably makes esophageal candidiasis unlikely *4891* Serum agglutinin and precipitin titers against Candida are of little value, as many normal individuals harbor the organism without tissue invasion *4891*

Protein *Cerebrospinal Fluid* *Increase* Mean concentration of 123 mg/dL in 28 cases of Candida meningitis *338*

114.00 Coccidioidomycosis

Angiotensin-converting Enzyme *Serum* *Increase* Decreased *3041*

Cells *Cerebrospinal Fluid* *Increase* CSF cell count and chemistry are indistinguishable from tuberculous meningitis *5252*

Complement Fixation *Cerebrospinal Fluid* *Increase* In 75% of patients with coccidioidal meningitis *5252* Generally the titer is lower than in the serum *4899*
Peritoneal Fluid *Increase* Generally the titer is lower than in the serum *4899*
Pleural Fluid *Increase* Generally the titer is lower than in the serum *4899*
Serum *Increase* Highly specific and has prognostic significance. Positive in about 60% of cases with chronic coccidioidal cavities, but often negative in patients with asymptomatic coccidioidomas *367* Positive 4 - 6 weeks following onset of symptoms with maximum response at 2 - 3 months. Titers > 1:2 may indicate active disease and 80% with disseminated infection have titers > 1:16 *5619* Titer correlates with increasing severity of the disease. A rising titer may indicate spread of the disease to extrapulmonary sites *4746*

Complement-fixing Antibodies *Cerebrospinal Fluid* *Increase* Pleural, joint, and CSF fluids contain complement-fixing antibody but in lower titer than in serum *367*
Pleural Fluid *Increase* Pleural, joint, and CSF fluids contain complement-fixing antibody but in lower titer than in serum *367*
Serum *Increase* Pleural, joint, and CSF fluids contain complement-fixing antibody but in lower titer than in serum *367*
Synovial Fluid *Increase* Pleural, joint, and CSF fluids contain complement-fixing antibody but in lower titer than in serum *367*

Eosinophils *Blood* *Increase* In the initial infection *5252* Occasional eosinophilia during either the primary or the disseminated stages *900*

Erythrocyte Sedimentation Rate *Blood* *Increase* In active infection *5252*

Glucose *Cerebrospinal Fluid* *Decrease* Often an early significant change with CNS involvement *367*
Cerebrospinal Fluid *Increase* CSF cell and chemistry are indistinguishable from tuberculous meningitis *5252*

Interleukin-1 *Cerebrospinal Fluid* *Increase* Concentration in CSF of patients with coccidioidomycosis meningitis concentration relatively low and did not change with time *5172*

Leukocytes *Blood* *Increase* Moderate leukocytosis sometimes with eosinophilia *367* Frequently slightly elevated with a shift to the left *5252*
Cerebrospinal Fluid *Increase* Fewer than 500 /μL with CNS involvement *2192*

Lymphocytes *Cerebrospinal Fluid* *Increase* Fewer than 500 leukocytes/μL, as many as 50% neutrophils initially with lymphocytes predominating later *2192*

Neutrophils *Cerebrospinal Fluid* *Increase* Fewer than 500 leukocytes/μL, as many as 50% neutrophils initially with lymphocytes predominating later *2192*

Oxygen Partial Pressure *Blood* *Decrease* With pulmonary involvement *2192*

Precipitins *Cerebrospinal Fluid* *Increase* Only rarely found in meningitis *4551*
Pleural Fluid *Increase* May be found in the thoracic fluid in pleural effusions *4551*
Serum *Increase* Highly specific and can be detected in 80% of patients within 2 weeks of onset of symptoms; absent in 90% after 6 months *5619* Positive in most patients within a month after onset of symptoms *1980* Present in approximately 80% of patients with primary nondisseminating infection, preceding the development of CF antibodies, and they appear to represent IgM antibodies. Persisting precipitins have been associated with dissemination, and precipitins may reappear when there is systemic reinfection *4551*

Protein *Cerebrospinal Fluid* *Increase* Moderate increase with CNS involvement *2192* CSF cell and chemistry are indistinguishable from tuberculous meningitis *5252*

Tumor Necrosis Factor-α *Cerebrospinal Fluid* *Increase* Concentration in CSF of patients with coccidioidomycosis meningitis concentration relatively low and did not change with time *5172*

VDRL *Serum* *Positive* Low incidence of false positive results *2192*

115.00 Histoplasmosis

Agglutination Tests *Serum* *Positive* Antibodies are demonstrable, but cross reactions with Blastomyces and Coccidioides are seen in these tests *1980*

115.00 Histoplasmosis *(continued)*

Alanine Aminotransferase *Serum Increase* In 5 cases of hepatic granuloma, ALT was elevated to a mean value of 70 U/L (normal = 50 U/L) and a range of 50 - 115 U/L *3161*

Albumin *Serum Decrease* Concentrations of < 3.0 g/dL occur in 60% of patients with disseminated disease *2039*

Alkaline Phosphatase *Serum Increase* Marked elevation in all 5 cases of granuloma of liver. Upper limit of normal of 85 U/L. Average elevated value 425 U/L (range 191 - 700 U/L) *3161* Present in 50% of patients with disseminated disease *2039*

Angiotensin-converting Enzyme *Serum Increase* Increased activities observed in patients with histoplasmosis *2952* Elevated in 25% of 86 patients *4489* Rises acutely in all patients with Histo and then falls gradually towards baseline (n = 44) *1029*

Antibody Titer *Serum Increase* Elevated convalescent phase titer may be the result of skin testing or of active disease *5619*

Aspartate Aminotransferase *Serum Increase* In 5 cases of granuloma of liver, 100% were mildly elevated, showing a mean elevation of 36 U/L over the normal maximum limit of 24 U/L *3161* Present in 70% of patients with disseminated disease *2039*

Bilirubin *Serum Increase* Greater than 1.0 mg/dL in 25% of patients with disseminated disease *2039*

BSP Retention *Serum Increase* Elevated in 70% of patients with disseminated disease *2039*

Cells *Bone Marrow No Effect* Marrow smears reveal no cellular abnormalities *5252*

Complement Fixation *Serum Increase* Of 79 consecutive patients with positive tests 28 (35%) were false positive results. 12 patients (15%) had titers of > 1:32, without cultural or histological evidence of active infection. Using histoplasmin as antigen detected antibodies in the sera of 72.8% of the 70 proven cases, while yeast antigen detected antibodies in 94% *5198* CF antibodies are produced in a high percentage of patients in the acute phase, and fade out as the infection becomes asymptomatic or inactive *5252* In primary pulmonary infection, antibodies to yeast antigen appear 10 - 21 days following fungus exposure. Histoplasmin antibodies are of greater importance in chronic infection, in which antibodies to yeast antigen may be decreased or absent. Titer of > 1:8 is presumed to indicate active infection, most patients have titers > 1:16 *5619* Initially positive in 74% of 228 cases (titers > 1:64) *1817*

γ-Globulin *Serum Increase* Levels > 3.0 g/dL occur in 50% of patients with disseminated disease *2039* Often associated with hypergammaglobulinemia *4707*

γ-Glutamyltransferase *Serum Increase* In 5 patients with liver granulomas, including miliary tuberculosis and sarcoidosis, serum GGT levels were all elevated, mean activity of 303 U/L, range 116 - 740 U/L *3161*

Hematocrit *Blood Decrease* 50% of the patients with disseminated disease may have anemia *2039* A marked to moderate hypochromic anemia occurs in most cases *1980* Usually an iron deficient normochromic normocytic anemia *4891* Normochromic anemia *5252*
Blood No Effect The anemia of chronic disease is conspicuously absent. Normal values found in 91% of patients. Differentiates chronic pulmonary histoplasmosis from pulmonary tuberculosis *1817*

Hemoglobin *Blood Decrease* 50% of the patients may have anemia in disseminated disease *2039* A marked to moderate hypochromic anemia occurs in most cases *1980* Usually an iron deficient normochromic normocytic anemia *4891* Normochromic anemia *5252*
Blood No Effect The anemia of chronic disease is conspicuously absent. Normal values found in 91% of patients differentiate chronic pulmonary histoplasmosis from pulmonary tuberculosis *1817*

Immunoglobulin A *Serum Increase* In patients with chronic cavitary disease, IgM and IgG levels were normal although increased IgA was found *4551* Reported effect *5555*

Iron *Serum Decrease* Usually an iron deficient normochromic normocytic anemia *4891*

Leucine Aminopeptidase *Serum Increase* In 12 patients with granulomatous hepatitis, all showed elevated LAP levels, varying from 380 - 1,000 U/L, with a mean of 622 (normal 322 U/L) *579*

Leukocytes *Blood Decrease* Leukopenia with lymphocytosis is frequently present *5252* In 25% of patients with disseminated disease *2039* Characteristic *1980*
Blood Increase Occurs in 12% of patients with disseminated disease *2039*

Lymphocytes *Blood Increase* Leukopenia with lymphocytosis is frequently present *5252*

MCH *Blood Decrease* A marked to moderate hypochromic anemia occurs in most cases *1980*

MCHC *Blood Decrease* A marked to moderate hypochromic anemia occurs in most cases *1980*

5'-Nucleotidase *Serum Increase* Significantly elevated in 2 of 3 patients with liver granulomata *2803*

Platelets *Blood Decrease* Markedly reduced only in the terminal phases *5252*

Precipitins *Serum Increase* Antibodies are demonstrable, but cross reactions with Blastomyces and Coccidioides are seen in these tests *1980*

Reticulocytes *Blood Increase* 25% of patients with disseminated disease *2039*

116.00 Blastomycosis

Alkaline Phosphatase *Serum Increase* May be increased with bone lesions *5545*

Blastomyces Antibody *Serum Increase* Increased complement fixation titers highly suggest active infection *2952*

Complement Fixation *Serum Increase* Titers of 1:8 or greater may be present in 33 - 50% of the patients. Positive titers of 1:32 or higher are highly suggestive of active disease *900* High titer is correlated with poor prognosis *5545* Reactions are transient and inconsistent with poor sensitivity and high incidence of cross-reactivity *5619*

Erythrocyte Sedimentation Rate *Blood Increase* Most common hematologic abnormality *900*

γ-Globulin *Serum Increase* Slightly increased *5545*

Hematocrit *Blood Decrease* Present in < 50% of patients *900*

Hemoglobin *Blood Decrease* Present in < 50% of patients *900*

Indirect Fluorescent Antibodies *Serum Increase* May be the most useful serodiagnostic technique *5619*

Leukocytes *Blood Increase* Appears in < 50% of patients *900*

117.10 Sporotrichosis

Antinuclear Antibodies *Serum No Effect* Normal in all patients with sporotrichosis arthritis *974*

Complement, Total *Serum No Effect* Concentration usually normal in patients with arthritis *974*

Erythrocyte Sedimentation Rate *Blood Increase* Elevated in all 4 patients studied *3178* Elevated in all patients with Sporotrichosis arthritis (average 55 mm/h) *974*

LE Cells *Blood No Effect* Normal in all patients with Sporotrichosis arthritis *4746*

Leukocytes *Blood No Effect* Near normal (2,000 - 6,150 /μL) *3178*

Rheumatoid Factor *Serum No Effect* Normal in all patients with sporotrichosis arthritis *974*

117.30 Aspergillosis

Bilirubin *Serum Increase* Hemolytic anemia *5677 4379*

Bilirubin, Indirect *Serum Increase* Hemolytic anemia *5677 4379*

Eosinophils *Blood Increase* Mean percentage was 16.2, ranging from 8-29% in 20 cases of allergic bronchopulmonary aspergillosis *4437*

Erythrocyte Survival *Red Blood Cells* *Decrease* Hemolytic anemia *5677 4379*

Erythrocytes *Urine* *Increase* With urinary tract obstruction *2192*

Galactomannan *Serum* *Increase* Measurable amounts detected a mean of 13.4 d before clinical and radiologic evidence of the disease *4408*

Hematocrit *Blood* *Decrease* Hemolytic anemia *5677 4379*

Hemoglobin *Blood* *Decrease* Hemolytic anemia *5677 4379*

Plasma *Increase* Hemolytic anemia *5677 4379*

immunoglobulin A *Serum* *Increase* Elevated in 10 of 15 patients with a mean of 314.6 mg/dL *4437*

Immunoglobulin E *Serum* *Increase* High values are found during the episodes of pulmonary eosinophilia *4551* Markedly elevated in all patients with allergic bronchopulmonary aspergillosis *4437*

Immunoglobulin G *Serum* *Increase* Elevated in 8 of 15 cases with a mean of 1,485 mg/dL *4437*

Immunoglobulin M *Serum* *Increase* Elevated in 10 of 15 cases; mean = 191.6 mg/dL *4437*

Precipitins *Serum* *Increase* Detected in 100% of patients with aspergillomas and 70% with allergic aspergillosis *5619* 48 and 67% having precipitins to Staphylococcus aureus and hemophilus influenzae *4551*

Urea Nitrogen *Serum* *Increase* Either as a result of underlying disease or the infection, azotemia develops rapidly *2192*

117.50 Cryptococcosis

Agglutination Tests *Cerebrospinal Fluid* *Positive* With CNS involvement, about 66% of patients have antigen in their serum, CSF or both *2192*

Serum *Positive* With CNS involvement, about 66% of patients have antigen in their serum, CSF or both *2192*

Antibody Titer *Serum* *Increase* Several serologic tests for anticryptococcal antibody are in use. Although sometimes of value, false positive reactions limit the utility of these tests *2192*

Complement Fixation *Cerebrospinal Fluid* *Increase* With CNS involvement, about 66% of patients have antigen in their serum, CSF or both *2192*

Serum *Increase* With CNS involvement, about 66% of patients have antigen in their serum, CSF or both *2192*

Erythrocyte Sedimentation Rate *Blood* *No Effect* Even in extensive infection, the blood WBC, hematocrit, and ESR remain normal *2192*

Glucose *Cerebrospinal Fluid* *Decrease* In about 50% of cases of symptomatic meningoencephalitis *2192*

Hematocrit *Blood* *No Effect* Even in extensive infection, the blood WBC, hematocrit, and ESR remain normal *2192*

Leukocytes *Blood* *No Effect* Even in extensive infection, the blood WBC, hematocrit, and ESR remain normal *2192*

Cerebrospinal Fluid *Increase* 40 - 400 /µL with meningoencephalitis *2192*

Lymphocytes *Cerebrospinal Fluid* *Increase* Characteristically outnumber neutrophils *2192*

Oxygen Partial Pressure *Blood* *Decrease* With pulmonary involvement *2192*

Protein *Cerebrospinal Fluid* *Increase* Almost always elevated *2192*

117.90 Fungal Meningitis

Oligoclonal Banding *Cerebrospinal Fluid* *Increase* Oligoclonal IgG bands detected in patients with fungal meningitis (Candida, Cryptococcus, Aspergillus) *3261*

117.90 Fungal-type Dysbiosis

Histidine *Urine* *Decrease* In 20 patients with fungal-type dysbiosis median excretion of 376.0 µmol/d significantly different from 371 - 1,771 µmol/d in 25 nonallergic volunteers *1292*

Immunoglobulin E *Serum* *Increase* In 21 patients with fungal-type dysbiosis median concentration of 78 significantly different from normal range *1292*

117.90 Fungus Ball Infection

Aspergillus Antibody *Serum* *Increase* Antibodies are observed in]/- 90% of patients with fungus ball infection *2952*

Helminthiases and Other Parasitic Diseases

120.90 Bilharziasis

β-Chorionic Gonadotropin *Urine* *Increase* In 40 patients with bilharziasis mean excretion of 1.37 ± 0.17 mIU/mL not significantly increased compared with 1.13 ± 0.08 mIU/mL in 31 normal controls *1964*

Endothelin *Plasma* *Increase* Concentrations very high in bilharzial liver disease with presinusoidal portal hypertension *3568*

120.90 Schistosomiasis

Alanine Aminotransferase *Serum* *Increase* Liver disease may develop due to a host immune reaction to the parasite. Laboratory findings may vary from mild to marked depending on the stage of the disease and its severity. Activity may be markedly increased in severe disease *3406* May be mild elevations, but jaundice is uncommon *1980* In 5 cases of hepatic granuloma, ALT was elevated to a mean value of 70 U/L (normal = 50 U/L) and a range of 50 - 115 U/L *3161*

Albumin *Serum* *Decrease* A significant decrease associated with a compensatory increase in globulin throughout the course of the disease. The drop may be due to decreased anabolism or increased catabolism *4526*

Alkaline Phosphatase *Serum* *Increase* Consistently elevated and remains high for 1 month after treatment *4526* Marked elevation in all 5 cases of granuloma of liver. Maximum upper limit of normal is 85 U/L. Average elevated value 425 U/L (range 191 to 700 U/L) *3161* Found in 50% of adult patients but is not useful in children *5545* Liver disease may develop due to a host immune reaction to the parasite. Laboratory findings may vary from mild to marked depending on the stage of the disease and its severity. Activity may be mildly increased *3406*

Aspartate Aminotransferase *Serum* *Increase* Markedly increased without concomitant elevation of ALT. Remains elevated from admission, through nitridazole treatment, and at follow-up 1 month later *4526* May be mild elevations, but jaundice is uncommon *1980* Liver disease may develop due to a host immune reaction to the parasite. Laboratory findings may vary from mild to marked depending on the stage of the disease and its severity. Activity may be markedly increased in severe disease *3406* In 5 cases of granuloma of liver, activities were mildly elevated in 100%, showing a mean elevation of 36 U/L over the normal maximum limit of 24 U/L *3161*

Bilirubin *Serum* *Increase* May be mild elevations, but jaundice is uncommon *1980* Liver disease may develop due to a host immune reaction to the parasite. Laboratory findings may vary from mild to marked depending on the stage of the disease and its severity. Concentration may be markedly increased in severe disease *3406*

BSP Retention *Serum* *Increase* Common *1980* 5% retention upon admission *4526*

Calcium *Urine* *Increase* Increased despite normal serum levels *1952*

Complement Fixation *Serum* *Increase* The best serologic procedure to diagnose chronic disease (100% specific and 95% sensitive) *5545*

Creatinine Clearance *Urine* *Decrease* Significantly decreased in 35 children with hepatic bilharziasis *1952*

Eosinophils *Blood* *Increase* In 2 patients with schistosomiasis and asthma mean concentration of 1,200 x 10^6/L significantly different from upper limit of normal of 440 x 10^6/L in 29 normal

120.90 Schistosomiasis *(continued)*

Eosinophils *(continued)*
individuals *607* Tends to decrease with chronicity *4891* Eosinophilia occurs and may be 20 - 60% of white cell count *5545* In 64 patients (22%) showed eosinophil counts > 1,000 /μL *4530*

Erythrocyte Sedimentation Rate *Blood* *Increase* Increased in acute disease *5545*

γ-Globulin *Serum* *Increase* May be present *4891* Significant increase throughout the course of the disease. The increase in γ-globulin, the main component causing the total elevation may be due to the parasite's presence *4526*

γ-Glutamyltransferase *Serum* *Increase* Liver disease may develop due to a host immune reaction to the parasite. Laboratory findings may vary from mild to marked depending on the stage of the disease and its severity. Activity may be mildly increased *3406* In 5 patients with liver granulomas, including miliary tuberculosis and sarcoidosis, serum GGT levels were all elevated, mean activity of 303 U/L, range 116 - 740 U/L *3161*

Hemagglutination Inhibition *Serum* *Increase* Indirect hemagglutination *2192*

Histamine *Plasma* *Increase* In 2 patients with schistosomiasis and asthma mean concentrations of 13.2 and 18,2 nmol/L significantly different from mean concentration of 4.0 nmol/L in 29 normal individuals *607*

Immunoglobulin A *Serum* *No Effect* Liver disease may develop due to a host immune reaction to the parasite. Laboratory findings may vary from mild to marked depending on the stage of the disease and its severity. Concentration usually normal even in severe disease *3406*

Immunoglobulin E *Serum* *Increase* Increased in bilharziasis *1290* 44% in Egypt and 20% in Brazil were above 24 μg/mL in S. Mansoni infestations *4551*

Immunoglobulin G *Serum* *Increase* Liver disease may develop due to a host immune reaction to the parasite. Laboratory findings may vary from mild to marked depending on the stage of the disease and its severity. Concentration is often increased in severe disease *3406*

Immunoglobulin M *Serum* *Increase* Liver disease may develop due to a host immune reaction to the parasite. Laboratory findings may vary from mild to marked depending on the stage of the disease and its severity. Concentration may be increased in severe disease, but to a lesser extent than IgG *3406*

Lactate Dehydrogenase *Serum* *Increase* Not significantly increased in patients upon the admission, but did increase with nitridazole treatment. LD_4 was the only isoenzyme to increase and had returned to normal at follow-up 1 month later *4526*

Lactate Dehydrogenase Isoenzymes *Serum* *Increase* Total LD was not significantly increased in patients upon admission, but did increase with nitridazole treatment. LD_4 was the only isoenzyme to increase and had returned to normal at follow-up 1 month later *4526*

Leucine Aminopeptidase *Serum* *Increase* In 12 patients with granulomatous hepatitis, all showed elevated LAP levels, varying from 380 - 1,000 U/L, with a mean of 622 (normal 322U/L) *579*

Leukocytes *Blood* *Increase* Tends to decrease with chronicity *4891*

Mucopolysaccharides *Urine* *Increase* Abnormalities of neutral mucopolysaccharides appear in urine in bilharziasis *2658*

Neopterin *Serum* *Increase* Increased concentration observed *121*

5'-Nucleotidase *Serum* *Increase* Significantly elevated in 2 of 3 patients with live granulomata *2803* Elevated above normal upon admission and rose to 2 times normal during treatment *4526*

Oligoclonal Banding *Cerebrospinal Fluid* *Increase* Oligoclonal IgG bands detected in patients with schistosomiasis of CNS *3261*

Ornithine Carbamoyltransferase *Serum* *Increase* Consistently and markedly elevated in patients upon admission, during treatment (highest elevations), and at follow-up 1 month later. Elevated levels may indicate liver cell defect which was not corrected by treatment or by improving the dietary conditions *4526*

Phosphate *Urine* *Increase* Urinary inorganic phosphate was increased in hepatic bilharziasis despite normal serum levels *1952*

Procollagen Type III Peptide *Serum* *Increase* Serum aminoterminal propeptide of type III procollagen levels were elevated in most of patients with active fibrosis but not in those with inactive schistosomiasis *1437*

Rheumatoid Factor *Serum* *Increase* Rheumatoid factor may be observed in certain patients *2473* Mean concentration increased in patients with schistosomiasis *2472* Parasitic diseases that involve the liver and reticuloendothelial system have a significant incidence of seropositivity, suggesting that these factors may be produced in these tissues locally *1980*

Sorbitol Dehydrogenase *Serum* *Increase* Markedly elevated upon admission, during treatment, and at follow-up *4526*

121.10 Clonorchis Infection of Liver

Eosinophils *Blood* *Increase* Liver flukes may colonize the biliary tract and cause biliary tract obstruction and anemia with marked eosinophilia *3406*

Hematocrit *Blood* *Decrease* Liver flukes may colonize the biliary tract and cause biliary tract obstruction and anemia *3406*

Hemoglobin *Blood* *Decrease* Liver flukes may colonize the biliary tract and cause biliary tract obstruction and anemia with the extent of biochemical abnormalities depending on the severity of the disease *3406*

122.80 Liver Hydatid Disease

Acid Ribonuclease *Serum* *Increase* Median activity in 7 patients with liver hydatid disease of 52.0 U/L significantly different from 42.0 U/L in 32 healthy controls *2566*

Alanine Aminotransferase *Serum* *Increase* Median activity in 11 patients with liver hydatid disease of 81 U/L significantly different from 22 U/L in 32 healthy controls *2566*

Albumin *Serum* *Decrease* Median concentration in 11 patients with liver hydatid disease of 3.4 g/dL significantly different from 3.7 g/dL in 32 healthy controls *2566*

Alkaline Phosphatase *Serum* *Increase* Median activity in 11 patients with liver hydatid disease of 119 U/L significantly different from 63 U/L in 32 healthy controls *2566*

Alkaline Ribonuclease *Serum* *Increase* Median activity in 7 patients with liver hydatid disease of 72.1 U/L significantly different from 67.4 U/L in 32 healthy controls *2566*

Bilirubin *Serum* *Increase* Median concentration in 11 patients with liver hydatid disease of 1.1 mg/dL significantly different from 0.7 mg/dL in 32 healthy controls *2566*

Creatinine *Serum* *No Effect* Median concentration in 11 patients with liver hydatid disease of 0.8 mg/dL significantly different from 0.7 mg/dL in 32 healthy controls *2566*

Urea *Serum* *Increase* Median concentration in 11 patients with liver hydatid disease of 41 mg/dL significantly different from 31 mg/dL in 32 healthy controls *2566*

122.90 Hydatidosis

Alanine Aminotransferase *Serum* *Increase* With liver involvement *2192*

Alkaline Phosphatase *Serum* *Increase* May increase with obstruction of biliary system *1642* With bone involvement *2192*

Aspartate Aminotransferase *Serum* *Increase* With liver involvement *2192*

Bilirubin *Serum* *Increase* With liver involvement *2192*

Creatine Kinase *Serum* *Increase* With bone involvement *2192*

Eosinophils *Blood* *Increase* Occurs in parasitic infestation especially with tissue invasion *5544*

γ-Glutamyltransferase *Serum* *Increase* With liver involvement *2192*

Immunoglobulin E *Serum* *Increase* Has been reported *2033* Increased in parasitic diseases *5544*

Lactate Dehydrogenase *Serum* *Increase* With liver involvement *2192*

123.10 Cysticercosis

Dopamine β-Hydroxylase *Cerebrospinal Fluid* *No Effect* In 4 patients with CNS cysticercosis mean concentration of 34.5 ± 9.8 ng/mL did not differ significantly from 31.3 ± 1.4 ng/mL in 32 healthy controls *3855*

Oligoclonal Banding *Cerebrospinal Fluid* *Increase* Oligoclonal IgG bands detected in patients with neurocysticerosis *3261*

123.40 Diphyllobothriasis

Eosinophils *Blood* *Increase* May be a mild eosinophilia, between 5 - 10% *4891*

Hematocrit *Blood* *Decrease* When present, anemia is macrocytic *4891*

Hemoglobin *Blood* *Decrease* When present, anemia is macrocytic *4891*

MCH *Blood* *Increase* When present, anemia is macrocytic *4891*

MCV *Blood* *Increase* When present, anemia is macrocytic *4891*

Vitamin B_{12} *Serum* *Decrease* Loss of ingested vitamin B_{12} *5544*

124.00 Trichinosis

Alanine Aminotransferase *Serum* *Increase* May show a moderate rise *900*

Albumin *Serum* *Decrease* In severe cases there may be hypoalbuminemia *1980* Decrease occurs in severe cases between 2 - 4 weeks and may last for years *5545*
Urine *Increase* In severe cases *5545* Possibly due to capillary leakage *2033*

Aldolase *Serum* *Increase* Activity may be increased in some patients with trichinosis *2952* Moderate rise probably related to myositis *2033*

Aspartate Aminotransferase *Serum* *Increase* Moderate to marked *1025* During the acute stage *1980*

Cholinesterase *Serum* *Decrease* May last up to 6 months *5545*

Complement Fixation *Serum* *Increase* Becomes positive about 2 weeks after occurrence of eosinophilia and may remain positive for 6 months *5545* Using bentonite particles, become positive later in the disease and are most helpful when they exhibit a significant change in titer *1980*

Creatine *Urine* *Increase* Constant finding *900*

Creatine Kinase *Serum* *Increase* During the acute stage *1980* Moderate to marked increase *1025* Is observed as the consequence of muscular necrosis *900*

Eosinophils *Blood* *Increase* May reach 8,000 /µL and persists for several weeks. In fatal cases, it is the only sign of disease *900* Marked; ranging from 15 - 50% of the total WBC. Highest during the active stage of the disease *1980* The most constant finding and one of significance early in the course of disease. Generally appears before the end of the 2nd week *2033* Characteristic *5619*

Erythrocyte Sedimentation Rate *Blood* *Decrease* Characteristically slow *2033*
Blood *Increase* Normal or moderately increased in some patients *900*

γ-Globulin *Serum* *Increase* Often associated with hypergammaglobulinemia *4707* Increase in relative and absolute concentrations parallels titer of serologic tests and of thymol turbidity. The increase occurs between 5 - 8 weeks and may last 6 months or more *5545*

Hemagglutination Inhibition *Serum* *Increase* Tannic acid hemagglutination proved to be very sensitive; antibodies were detected in 6 days *2523*

Hematocrit *Blood* *Decrease* Prolonged infection may result in secondary anemia *5252*

Hemoglobin *Blood* *Decrease* Prolonged infection may result in secondary anemia *5252*

Hyaline Casts *Urine* *Increase* In severe cases *5545*

Immunoglobulin E *Serum* *Increase* The only correlation between trichinosis and an increase in serum IgE was found in patients with a prior history of allergic disease *298*

Immunoglobulin M *Serum* *Increase* In parasitic diseases *1025*

Lactate Dehydrogenase *Serum* *Increase* A consequence of muscular necrosis *900* Moderate to marked elevations *1025*

Leukocytes *Blood* *Increase* Typically, a leukocytosis with a marked hypereosinophilia ranging between 20 - 75% or more *4891* Counts as high as 20,000 - 50,000 /µL are found *5252*

Neutrophils *Blood* *Increase* Neutrophilic leukocytosis is common *5252*

Precipitins *Serum* *Increase* Precipitin test appears to be too nonspecific for general use *2523* Using bentonite particles, become positive later in the disease and are most helpful when they exhibit a significant change in titer *1980*

Protein *Serum* *Decrease* May be marked *900* In severe cases between 2 - 4 weeks and may last for years *5545*

125.00 Filariasis

Rheumatoid Factor *Serum* *Increase* Mean concentration increased in patients with filariasis *2472* Rheumatoid factor may be observed in certain patients *2473*

125.30 Onchocerciasis

Eosinophil Cationic Protein *Serum* *Increase* In 40 Guinean patients with onchocerciasis median concentration of 105 µg/L compared with 9.2 µg/L in 20 healthy Europeans *5235*
Urine *Increase* In 40 Guinean patients with onchocerciasis median concentration of 1.4 µg/g creatinine compared with 0.65 µg/g creatinine in 20 healthy Europeans *5235*

Eosinophil-derived Neurotoxin *Serum* *Increase* In 40 Guinean patients with onchocerciasis median concentration of 175 µg/L compared with 16.5 µg/L in 20 healthy Europeans *5235*
Urine *Increase* In 40 Guinean patients with onchocerciasis median concentration of 2,370 µg/g creatinine compared with 178 µg/g creatinine in 20 healthy Europeans *5235*

Eosinophils *Blood* *Increase* In 4 patients with onchocerciasis and asthma mean concentrations of 980 - 3,663 x 10^6/L significantly different from upper limit of normal of 440 x 10^6/L in 29 normal individuals *607* In 40 Guinean patients with onchocerciasis median concentration of 710 /µL compared with 158.5 /µL in 20 healthy Europeans *5235*

Histamine *Plasma* *Increase* In 4 patients with onchocerciasis and asthma mean concentrations of 3.6 to 10.8 nmol/L significantly different from mean concentration of 4.0 nmol/L in 29 normal individuals *607*

Myeloperoxidase *Serum* *Increase* In 40 Guinean patients with onchocerciasis median concentration of 410 µg/L compared with 350 µg/L in 20 healthy Europeans *5235*

126.00 Ancylostomiasis

Eosinophil Cationic Protein *Serum* *Increase* In 35 Guinean patients with ancyclostomiasis median concentration of 90 µg/L compared with 9 µg/L in 20 healthy Europeans *5235*
Urine *Increase* In 35 Guinean patients with ancyclostomiasis median concentration of 1.6 µg/g creatinine compared with 0.65 µg/g creatinine in 20 healthy Europeans *5235*

Eosinophil-derived Neurotoxin *Serum* *Increase* In 35 Guinean patients with ancyclostomiasis median concentration of 10 µg/L compared with 16.5 µg/L in 20 healthy Europeans *5235*
Urine *Increase* In 35 Guinean patients with ancyclostomiasis median concentration of 1,060 µg/g creatinine compared with 178 µg/g creatinine in 20 healthy Europeans *5235*

Eosinophils *Blood* *Increase* In 35 Guinean patients with ancyclostomiasis median concentration of 896 /µL compared with 159 /µL in 20 healthy Europeans *5235* Generally an eosinophilia of 7 - 15%, and it may exceed 50% in severe cases *4891* Common in hookworm anemia *4340* Very characteristic *900*

Erythrocytes *Blood* *Decrease* May be reduced *5252*

126.00 Ancylostomiasis *(continued)*

Hematocrit *Blood* *Decrease* Anemia occurring in hookworm disease is a classic iron deficiency anemia *4891* A microcytic, hypochromic anemia attributed directly to blood loss; when the patient has severe malnutrition, however, the anemia may be macrocytic hypochromic anemia *900* Development of hypochromic, microcytic anemia depends on the number of worms, recency of infection, and host nutrition *5252*

Hemoglobin *Blood* *Decrease* Anemia occurring in hookworm disease is a classic iron deficiency anemia *4891* Development of hypochromic, microcytic anemia depends on the numbers of worms, recency of infection, and host nutrition *5252* A microcytic, hypochromic anemia attributed directly to blood loss; when the patient has severe malnutrition, however, the anemia may be macrocytic hypochromic anemia *900*

Immunoglobulin E *Serum* *Increase* Increased in parasitic diseases *5544*

Immunoglobulin M *Serum* *Increase* In parasitic diseases *1025*

Iron *Serum* *Decrease* Anemia occurring in hookworm disease is a classic iron deficiency anemia *4891*

Iron-binding Capacity, Total *Serum* *Increase* Classic iron deficiency anemia *4891*

Iron Saturation *Serum* *Decrease* Classic iron deficiency anemia *4891*

Leukocytes *Blood* *Increase* In some early cases may be marked *2033*

MCH *Blood* *Decrease* Anemia occurring in hookworm disease is a classic iron deficiency anemia *4891* Development of hypochromic, microcytic anemia depends on the number of worms, recency of infection, and host nutrition *5252*

MCHC *Blood* *Decrease* Anemia occurring in hookworm disease is a classic iron deficiency anemia *4891* Development of hypochromic, microcytic anemia depends on the number of worms, recency of infection, and host nutrition *5252*

MCV *Blood* *Decrease* Development of hypochromic, microcytic anemia depends on the number of worms, recency of infection, and host nutrition *5252* Anemia occurring in hookworm disease is a classic iron deficiency anemia *4891*

Myeloperoxidase *Serum* *Increase* In 35 Guinean patients with ancyclostomiasismedian concentration of 500 µg/L compared with 350 µg/L in 20 healthy Europeans *5235*

Occult Blood *Feces* *Increase* Occult or frank blood can be demonstrated at all times *5252*

127.00 Ascariasis

Eosinophils *Blood* *Increase* May be a mild eosinophilia ranging between 5 - 10% *4891* Increased during symptomatic phase, especially pulmonary phase *5545* May occur, but this finding is more characteristic of hookworm infection and strongyloidiasis *900* May be a mild eosinophilia ranging between 5 - 10% *2300*

immunoglobulin A *Serum* *Decrease* Immunoglobulin levels, especially IgA, may be depressed owing to enteric protein loss *4891*

Immunoglobulin E *Serum* *Increase* The extent and persistence of elevation is dependent upon several genetically controlled factors *3927* Parasitic disorders may be associated with elevated IgE levels, especially Ascariasis *4891*

Immunoglobulin M *Serum* *Increase* In parasitic diseases *1025*

127.20 Strongyloidiasis

Albumin *Serum* *Decrease* In one patient with strongyloidosis glomerulonephritis and nephrotic syndrome observed with concentration of 0.6 g/dL *5719* Has been observed *4891*

Creatinine *Serum* *No Effect* In one patient with strongyloidosis glomerulonephritis and nephrotic syndrome observed with concentration of 1.2 mg/dL (110 µmol/L) *5719*

Creatinine Clearance *Urine* *Decrease* In one patient with strongyloidosis glomerulonephritis and nephrotic syndrome observed with clearance of 30 mL/min *5719*

Eosinophils *Blood* *Increase* Typically, an eosinophilia between 8 - 10% and in very severe infections, up to 50% *4891* Increase is almost always present, but the number usually decreased with chronicity *5545* In one patient with strongyloidosis glomerulonephritis and nephrotic syndrome observed with concentration of 63% of total leukocytes *5719* 10% eosinophilia is usual and counts of 50% or even higher are occasionally found *900* In 1 patient with strongyloidiasis and asthma mean concentration of 2,457 x 10^6/L significantly different from upper limit of normal of 440 x 10^6/L in 29 normal individuals *607*

γ-Globulin *Serum* *Increase* Has been observed *4891*

Hematocrit *Blood* *Decrease* Anemia, when it occurs, is usually iron deficiency in type *4891*

Hemoglobin *Blood* *Decrease* In one patient with strongyloidosis glomerulonephritis and nephrotic syndrome observed with hemoglobin concentration reduced to 5.0 g/dL *5719* Anemia, when it occurs, is usually iron deficiency in type *4891*

Histamine *Plasma* *Increase* In 1 patient with strongyloidosis and asthma mean concentration of 86.4 nmol/L significantly different from mean concentration of 4.0 nmol/L in 29 normal individuals *607*

Immunoglobulin E *Serum* *Increase* Increased in parasitic diseases *5544*

Immunoglobulin M *Serum* *Increase* In parasitic diseases *1025*

Iron *Serum* *Decrease* Anemia, when it occurs, is usually iron deficiency in type *4891*

Iron-binding Capacity, Total *Serum* *Increase* Classic iron deficiency anemia *4891*

Iron Saturation *Serum* *Decrease* Classic iron deficiency anemia *4891*

Leukocytes *Blood* *Increase* In some patients, there may be a very marked leukocytosis *4891*
Blood *No Effect* In one patient with strongyloidosis glomerulonephritis and nephrotic syndrome observed with leukocyte concentration of 0.8 x 10^9/dL *5719*

MCH *Blood* *Decrease* Anemia, when it occurs, is usually iron deficiency in type *4891*

MCHC *Blood* *Decrease* Anemia, when it occurs, is usually iron deficiency in type *4891*

MCV *Blood* *Decrease* Anemia, when it occurs, is usually iron deficiency in type *4891*

Occult Blood *Feces* *Increase* Stools frequently contain occult blood, mucus, and larvae *4891*

Platelets *Blood* *Decrease* In one patient with strongyloidosis, glomerulonephritis and nephrotic syndrome observed with platelet concentration reduced to 89 x 10^9/L *5719*

Protein *Urine* *Increase* In one patient with strongyloidosis glomerulonephritis and nephrotic syndrome observed with proteinuria of 6.6 g/d *5719*

127.30 Trichuriasis

Eosinophils *Blood* *Increase* May be > 25% *5545*

Erythrocytes *Blood* *Decrease* In children can be accompanied by a microcytic hypochromic anemia *900*

Hematocrit *Blood* *Decrease* In children can be accompanied by a microcytic hypochromic anemia *900*

Hemoglobin *Blood* *Decrease* In children can be accompanied by a microcytic hypochromic anemia *900*

Immunoglobulin E *Serum* *Increase* Increased in parasitic diseases *5544*

Immunoglobulin M *Serum* *Increase* In parasitic diseases *1025*

Leukocytes *Blood* *Increase* May be present *5545*

MCH *Blood* *Decrease* In children can be accompanied by a microcytic hypochromic anemia *900*

MCHC *Blood* *Decrease* In children can be accompanied by a microcytic hypochromic anemia *900*

MCV *Blood* *Decrease* In children can be accompanied by a microcytic hypochromic anemia *900*

Occult Blood *Feces* *Increase* Bloody diarrhea *2192*

128.00 Toxocariasis

Complement Fixation *Serum* *Increase* Positive in 75% of patients *2033*

Eosinophils *Blood* *Increase* Severe eosinophilia, splenomegaly, and lymphadenopathy in several members of the same family were infected from a common environmental source *1214* Highest level of eosinophilia has been described due to Toxocara canis or catis infection in children *4551* Characteristic feature *5252*

γ-Globulin *Serum* *Increase* Often increased *4707* Characteristic feature *5252*

Hemagglutination Inhibition *Serum* *Increase* Tests with Ascaris and Toxocara antigen are helpful, but are rarely diagnostic because cross reactions with other helminths are common *2192*

immunoglobulin A *Serum* *Decrease* Immunoglobulin levels, especially IgA, may be depressed owing to enteric protein loss *4891*

Immunoglobulin E *Serum* *Increase* The extent and persistence of elevation is dependent upon several genetically controlled factors *3927* Parasitic disorders may be associated with elevated IgE levels, especially Ascariasis, and visceral larva migrans *4891*

Immunoglobulin M *Serum* *Increase* In parasitic diseases *1025*

Immunoglobulins *Serum* *Increase* Striking elevations often found with Toxocara cati infection *4707*

Rheumatoid Factor *Serum* *Increase* Parasitic diseases that involve the liver and reticuloendothelial system have a significant incidence of seropositivity, suggesting that these factors may be produced in these tissues locally *1980*

130.90 Toxoplasmosis

Antibody Titer *Cerebrospinal Fluid* *Increase* Congenital infection is indicated when CSF antibody concentration is higher for toxoplasmosis than for rubeola *2951*

Cells *Cerebrospinal Fluid* *Increase* In congenital, both RBC and WBC with a predominance of mononuclear elements. In acquired predominantly mononuclear cells, 30 - 2,000 /μL *2832*

Complement Fixation *Serum* *Increase* Antibody is present within 1 - 2 months of infection and is usually negative within 2 y *4551* CF antibodies appear later than Sabin-Feldman or hemagglutinating antibodies and diminish more rapidly *5252* Becomes positive later than the other serologic tests, and its titer declines earlier *1980* In 26 patients with congenital infection and in 22 of their mothers, tests results were positive on all specimens from the patients younger than 2 y of age and on 69% of specimens collected from older patients *2617*

Complement-fixing Antibodies *Serum* *Increase* Acute infections are characterized by an early and relatively transient IgM and complement-fixing antibody response *4551*

Erythrocytes *Blood* *Decrease* Anemia is present *5545*

α-Fetoprotein *Serum* *Increase* In newborn but disappeared by the end of the 1st month *3500*

Glucose *Cerebrospinal Fluid* *No Effect* In acquired toxoplasmosis, usually normal *2832*

Hemagglutination Inhibition *Serum* *Increase* Specific and sensitive *900* Marked elevations of antibody to toxoplasmosis *5677* Hemagglutinating antibody appears later and rises more slowly than IFA antibody *4551*

Hematocrit *Blood* *Decrease* Anemia is present *5545*

Hemoglobin *Blood* *Decrease* Anemia is present *5545*
Plasma *Increase* Reported effect *992* *5677*

Immunoglobulin M *Serum* *Increase* Acute infections are characterized by an early and relatively transient IgM and complement-fixing antibody response *4551* Reported effect *1570*

Indirect Fluorescent Antibodies *Serum* *Increase* Detects predominantly IgG toxoplasma antibody *4551* Found to be as reliable as the Sabin-Feldman dye test *5252* Marked elevations of antibody to toxoplasmosis *5677* Titers of 1:256 or higher indicate recent infection, and titers of 1:1024 or higher accompany active disease *1980*

Leukocytes *Blood* *Decrease* WBC varies from leukopenia to leukemoid reaction; atypical lymphocytes may be found *5545*
Blood *Increase* WBC varies from leukopenia to leukemoid reaction; atypical lymphocytes may be found *5545*
Cerebrospinal Fluid *Increase* In congenital, both RBC and WBC with a predominance of mononuclear elements. In acquired predominantly mononuclear cells, 30 - 2,000 /μL *2832*

Lymphocytes *Blood* *Increase* Slight *367*
Cerebrospinal Fluid *Increase* In congenital and acquired *2832*

Methylene Blue (Sabin-Feldman) Dye Test *Serum* *Increase* Specific and sensitive *5252* Detects predominantly IgG but also IgM antibodies which appear within 2 - 4 weeks after infection and persist for years. Rising titers in paired sera at least 3 weeks apart are most helpful in the diagnosis of recent infection *4551* Appears within 1 - 2 weeks, rises not less than 1:256 and can be as high as 1:32,000 or more. May persist at high levels for several y then fall slowly to 1:64 or less and tends to persist indefinitely *2832* Titers of 1:16 are considered indicative of past infection or exposure. During active disease, titers of 1:1,000-1:65,000 may be attained *1980*

Monocytes *Blood* *Increase* Slight *367*
Cerebrospinal Fluid *Increase* Moderate number *2192*

Oligoclonal Banding *Cerebrospinal Fluid* *Increase* Oligoclonal IgG bands detected in patients with toxoplasmosis of CNS *3261*

Protein *Cerebrospinal Fluid* *Increase* In congenital, as high as 2,000 mg/dL *2832*
Cerebrospinal Fluid *No Effect* In acquired disease, usually normal *2832*

135.00 Neurosarcoidosis

Angiotensin-converting Enzyme
Cerebrospinal Fluid *Increase* In 2 patients with proved neurosarcoidosis mean concentrations 1.8 μmol/L/min and 5.4 μmol/L/min respectively compared with mean 0.59 ± 0.42 μmol/L/min in 38 control patients *2476*

135.00 Sarcoidosis

Acid Phosphatase, Tartrate Resistant *Serum* *No Effect* No significant increase observed in patients with pulmonary sarcoidosis *2618*

Adenosine Monophosphate *Urine* *Decrease* Reported effect *1197*

Alanine Aminotransferase *Serum* *Increase* In 5 cases of hepatic granuloma, ALT was elevated to a mean value of 70 U/L (normal = 50 U/L) and a range of 50 - 115 U/L *3161*

Albumin *BAL Fluid* *No Effect* In 27 patients mean concentration of 138.5 ± 36.1 μg/mL not significantly different from 52.8 ± 7.8 μg/mL in 13 healthy control volunteers *1595*
Serum *Decrease* Associated with increased globulin in 'sarcoid step' characteristic patterns *5545*
Serum *Increase* Some cases when active *1290*

Alkaline Phosphatase *Serum* *Increase* Marked elevation in all 5 cases of granuloma of liver. Maximum upper limit of normal is 85 U/L. Average elevated value 425 U/L (range 191 to 700 U/L) *3161* Elevated in 40% of cases involving the liver, usually ranging from 25 to 97 U/L, with < 15% presenting with values > 107 U/L *1025*

Alkaline Phosphatase Isoenzymes *Serum* *Increase* Elevated hepatic isoenzyme is characteristically present *2039*

Amino-terminal Propeptide of Type III Procollagen
Serum *Increase* Mean concentration of 18.2 ± 1.09 ng/mL in type I progressive disease and 13.9 ± 1.2 ng/mL in type II/III compared with 9.1 ± 1.09 ng/mL in type I (stable) and 7.6 ± 1.1 ng/mL in type II/III (stable) and 9.4 ± 4 ng/mL in normal volunteers *4162*

Angiotensin-converting Enzyme
Cerebrospinal Fluid *Increase* In 11 of 20 patients with neurosarcoidosis concentration increased, but in systemic sarcoidosis without neurologic abnormality only 1 of 12 had increased CSF ACE *3895*
Serum *Increase* Elevated in 33% of patients with sarcoidosis *1932* Elevated in 75% of patients *4737* Increased levels in 67.2% of 100 patients *4561* Elevated in 60 - 80% of cases *1165* In 37 patients with indications for therapy mean activity of 25.4 ± 2.7 U/L and in 40 without indications for therapy 22.2 ± 2.2 U/L *5858* Increased activities observed in acute sarcoidosis

135.00 **Sarcoidosis** *(continued)*

Angiotensin-converting Enzyme *(continued)*
2952 In 23 patients with active sarcoidosis mean activity of 51.9 ± 23 U/mL compared with 33.4 ± 9.5 U/mL in 24 sarcoidosis patients treated with steroids and 26.1 ± 6.2 U/mL in 32 controls *3042* Most frequently elevated in patients with pulmonary parenchymal involvement *4415* In 8 patients with sarcoidosis mean concentration of 250 ± 34 U/L significantly higher than 108 ± 13 U/L in 85 healthy control individuals *5338* Activity increased in most patients *3045*

Antibody Titer *Serum Increase* Used to differentiate pulmonary sarcoidosis from tuberculosis. Antituberculous antibodies were found in TB in 83%; in sarcoidosis 22% *2786*

Apolipoprotein A-I *Serum Decrease* Mean concentration of 1.18 ± 0.32 g/L in 44 patients with active sarcoidosis significantly different from 1.38 ± 0.27 g/L in 147 control individuals *2842*
Serum No Effect Mean concentration of 1.35 ± 0.35 g/L in 46 patients with inactive sarcoidosis not significantly different from 1.38 ± 0.27 g/L in 147 control individuals *2842*

Apolipoprotein B *Serum No Effect* In 44 patients with active sarcoidosis mean concentration of 0.86 ± 0.25 g/L and 0.82 ± 0.24 g/L in 46 patients with inactive sarcoidosis not significantly different from 0.83 ± 0.24 g/L in 147 control individuals *2842*

Aspartate Aminotransferase *Serum Increase* In 5 cases of granuloma of liver, 100% had mildly elevated activities, showing a mean elevation of 36 U/L over the normal maximum limit of 24 U/L *3161* In 36% of 24 patients at initial hospitalization for this disorder *1576*

Bicarbonate *Serum Increase* In 55% of 20 patients at initial hospitalization for this disorder *1576*

CA 125 *Serum Increase* It may be elevated in conditions characterized by peritoneal inflammation *5281*

Calcium *Feces Decrease* At some stage of disease *2252*
Serum Increase Occurs in approximately 33% of patients at some stage of disease *2252* Much less frequent than hypercalciuria. Found in 6 - 13% of cases *900*
Urine Increase Solitary hypercalciuria without hyperparathyroidism indicates sarcoidosis *900* 30 - 60% of the patients *1025* Solitary hypercalciuria without hyperparathyroidism indicates sarcoidosis *1025* Occurs in approximately 33% of patients at some stage. Urinary levels are high, stool content low, and serum phosphate normal or low *2252*

Carbon Dioxide Partial Pressure *Blood Decrease* Decreased with lung involvement *5545* In 26% of 15 patients at initial hospitalization for this disorder *1576* In 8 patients with sarcoidosis mean of 42 ± 10 mm Hg significantly different from 52 ± 9 mm Hg in 85 healthy control individuals *5338* Impaired gas diffusion in pulmonary sarcoid may cause hyperventilation and reduced pCO_2. In more severe cases, CO_2 retention occurs *4707* Mild hyperventilation is frequent except in advanced disease when ventilatory obstruction occurs *2039*
Blood Increase In more severe cases, CO_2 retention occurs *4707*

$CD4^+$:$CD8^+$ Lymphocyte Ratio *BAL Fluid Increase* Mean ratio in 35 patients with sarcoidosis of 6.07 ± 0.87 *1989* In 16 patients with active sarcoidosis mean ratio of 6.42 ± 4.90 and 6.20 ± 4.57 in 11 patients with inactive sarcoidosis significantly different from mean proportion of 1.52 ± 0.96 in 9 healthy controls *2678* In 24 patients mean ratio of 6.5 ± 1.4 not significantly different from 3.8 ± 0.9 in 13 healthy control volunteers *1595*

CD18 *Lymphocytes Increase* In 16 patients with active sarcoidosis mean expression of 20.6 ± 14.3 and 26.2 ± 17.7 in 11 patients with inactive sarcoidosis significantly different from mean expression of 6.93 ± 6.60 in 9 healthy controls *2678*
Macrophages No Effect In 16 patients with active sarcoidosis mean expression of 5.82 ± 6.59 and 3.32 ± 1.84 in 11 patients with inactive sarcoidosis not significantly different from mean expression of 3.10 ± 3.11 in 9 healthy controls *2678*

Cells *BAL Fluid Increase* In 16 patients with active sarcoidosis mean concentration of 2.49 ± 0.95 x 10^5/L and 2.49 ± 1.61 x 10^5/L in 11 patients with inactive sarcoidosis significantly different from mean concentration of 0.88 ± 0.43 x 10^5/L in 9 healthy controls *2678*
BAL Fluid No Effect In 24 patients mean concentration of 211.0 ± 37.8 x 10^3/mL not significantly different from 147.5 ± 59.3 x 10^3/mL in 13 healthy control volunteers *1595*
Cerebrospinal Fluid Increase In granulomatous basilar meningitis affecting cranial nerves *2033*

Chloride *Serum Decrease* Suggests the presence of sarcoidosis or malignancy in conjunction with other tests *900*

Cholesterol *Serum No Effect* In 44 patients with active sarcoidosis mean concentration of 5.22 ± 0.91 mmol/L and 5.32 ± 0.95 mmol/L in 46 patients with inactive sarcoidosis not significantly different from 5.40 ± 1.1 mmol/L in 147 control individuals *2842*

Complement C_1 *Serum No Effect* Mean concentration typically normal or slightly increased in patients with sarcoidosis *4682*

Complement C_1q *Serum No Effect* Mean concentration typically normal or slightly increased in patients with sarcoidosis *4682*

Complement C_2 *Serum No Effect* Mean concentration typically normal or slightly increased in patients with sarcoidosis *4682*

Complement C_3 *Serum No Effect* Mean concentration typically normal or slightly increased in patients with sarcoidosis *4682*

Complement C_4 *Serum No Effect* Mean concentration typically normal or slightly increased in patients with sarcoidosis *4682*

Complement C_5 *Serum No Effect* Mean concentration typically normal or slightly increased in patients with sarcoidosis *4682*

Complement CH50 *Serum No Effect* Mean concentration typically normal or slightly increased in patients with sarcoidosis *4682*

Complement Fixation *Serum Increase* Used to differentiate pulmonary sarcoidosis from tuberculosis. Antituberculous antibodies were found in TB in 83%; in sarcoidosis 22% *2786*

Copper *Liver Increase* Increased in hepatocytes in 5 patients *4475*

Creatinine *Serum Increase* In 38% of 13 patients at initial hospitalization for this disorder *1576*

1,25-Dihydroxy Vitamin D *Serum Increase* Increased concentrations observed in patients with sarcoidosis *2952*

1,25-Dihydroxy Vitamin D_3 *Serum Increase* Observed effect *126*

Eosinophil Cationic Protein *BAL Fluid Increase* In 24 patients mean concentration of 29.3 ± 9.3 ng/L not significantly different from 12.5 ± 1.7 ng/L in 13 healthy control volunteers *1595*

Eosinophils *BAL Fluid Increase* In 24 patients mean concentration of 2.95 ± 1.30 x 10^3/mL significantly different from 0.03 ± 0.01 x 10^3/mL in 13 healthy control volunteers *1595*
Blood Increase Occurs in 15% of patients *5545* In 44% of 25 patients at initial hospitalization for this disorder *1576*

Erythrocyte Sedimentation Rate *Blood Increase* May reflect raised immunoglobulin levels, or associated erythema nodosum or secondary infection *367*

Erythrocytes *Blood Decrease* Pancytopenia is a common feature *5677*

Fibrinogen *Plasma Increase* Indicates active disease *4407*

α_2-Globulin *Serum Increase* Marked increase is frequent *1290* Stepwise increase of α_2-, β-, and γ- globulin 'sarcoid steps' helps differentiate from other lung diseases *5544*

β-Globulin *Serum Increase* Stepwise increase of α_2-, β-, and γ- globulin. 'sarcoid steps' help differentiate from other lung disease *5544*

γ-Globulin *Serum Increase* Increase of α_2-, and γ- globulins help differentiate from other lung disease *5544* Increased in 75% of patients, producing reduced A/G ratio and increased total protein in 30% of patients *5545* Has been observed in 23.5 - 61% of cases *900*

Glucose *Cerebrospinal Fluid Decrease* Due to involvement of the meninges, in rare cases, involving the central nervous system *1290*

γ-Glutamyltransferase *Serum Increase* In 5 patients with liver granulomas, including miliary tuberculosis and sarcoidosis, serum GGT levels were all elevated, mean activity of 303 U/L, range 116 - 740 U/L *3161*

HDL_2-Cholesterol *Serum* *Decrease* In 44 patients with active sarcoidosis mean concentration of 0.31 ± 0.17 mmol/L and 0.40 ± 0.32 mmol/L in 46 patients with inactive sarcoidosis significantly different from 0.63 ± 0.29 mmol/L in 147 control individuals *2842*

HDL_3-Cholesterol *Serum* *Increase* Mean concentration of 0.99 ± 0.23 mmol/L in 46 patients with inactive sarcoidosis significantly different from 0.87 ± 0.19 mmol/L in 147 control individuals *2842*
Serum *No Effect* In 44 patients with active sarcoidosis mean concentration of 0.84 ± 0.20 mmol/L not significantly different from 0.87 ± 0.19 mmol/L in 147 control individuals *2842*

HDL-Cholesterol *Serum* *Decrease* In 44 patients with active sarcoidosis mean concentration of 1.15 ± 0.27 mmol/L significantly different from 1.40 ± 0.34 mmol/L in 46 patients with inactive sarcoidosis and 1.40 ± 0.34 mmol/L in 147 control individuals *2842*

Hydroxyproline *Plasma* *Increase* No prognostic significance *126*
Urine *Increase* Considerably increased in acute disease, returning to normal as the chest X-ray abnormality resolves. Chronic disease has normal levels *367*

immunoglobulin A *Serum* *Increase* Elevated in 25% of cases *367* Immunoglobulins are frequently elevated and tend to reflect the overall resolution of disease. Falls to normal with resolution *3522*

Immunoglobulin D *Serum* *Increase* Reported effect *1290*

Immunoglobulin E *Serum* *Increase* No prognostic significance *126*

Immunoglobulin G *Serum* *Increase* Consistent increase in 1 or more serum immunoglobulins, noted in 79% of 129 cases studied. IgM and/or IgG are the most frequently increased *900* Elevated in 50% of cases *367* Frequently elevated and tends to reflect the overall resolution of disease. With resolution, falls but tends to remain raised for up to 4 y *3522*

Immunoglobulin M *Serum* *Increase* Serum IgG is elevated in 50%, IgA in 25%, and IgM in 12.5% of cases *367* Consistent increase in 1 or more serum immunoglobulins, noted in 79% of 129 cases studied. IgG and/or IgM are most frequently increased *900* Frequently elevated and tends to reflect the overall resolution of disease. Falls with resolution but remains significantly above normal *3522*

Immunoglobulins *Serum* *Increase* Consistent increase in 1 or more serum immunoglobulins, noted in 79% of 129 cases studied. IgG and/or IgM are most frequently increased *900* Serum IgG is elevated in 50%, IgA in 25%, and IgM in 12.5% of cases *367*

Lactate Dehydrogenase *BAL Fluid* *Increase* In 19 patients mean activity of 60.1 ± 21.5 U/L not significantly different from 22.8 ± 5.4 U/L in 13 healthy control volunteers *1595*
Serum *Increase* In 24% of 25 patients at initial hospitalization for this disorder *1576*

LDL-Cholesterol *Serum* *No Effect* In 44 patients with active sarcoidosis mean concentration of 3.48 ± 0.80 mmol/L and 3.35 ± 0.92 mmol/L in 46 patients with inactive sarcoidosis not significantly different from 3.51 ± 1.02 mmol/L in 147 control individuals *2842*

Leucine Aminopeptidase *Serum* *Increase* In 12 patients with granulomatous hepatitis, all showed elevated LAP levels, varying from 380 - 1,000 U/L, with a mean of 622 (normal 322 U/L) *579*

Leukocytes *Blood* *Decrease* In 30% of patients *5545* Pancytopenia is a common feature *5677*
Cerebrospinal Fluid *Increase* In granulomatous basilar meningitis affecting cranial nerves *2033*

Lymphocytes *BAL Fluid* *Increase* In 16 patients with active sarcoidosis mean proportion of 48.8 ± 17.0% and 34.4 ± 22.8% in 11 patients with inactive sarcoidosis significantly different from mean proportion of 11.0 ± 7.3% in 9 healthy controls *2678* In 16 patients with active sarcoidosis mean concentration of 12.3 ± 6.5 x 10^4/L and 10.7 ± 14.8 x 10^4/L in 11 patients with inactive sarcoidosis significantly different from mean concentration of 1.08 ± 0.96 x 10^4/L in 9 healthy controls *2678* In 24 patients mean concentration of 87.3 ± 23.8 x 10^3/mL significantly different from 7.0 ± 2.4 x 10^3/mL in 13 healthy control volunteers *1595* In 37 patients with indications for therapy mean proportion of lymphocytes 19.1 ± 2.3% and in 40 without indications for therapy 17.1 ± 2.1% *5858* Mean proportion of total cells in 35 patients with sarcoidosis of 46 ± 2.7% significantly different from 12 ± 1% in 21 control individuals *1989*
Blood *Decrease* In 52% of 25 patients at initial hospitalization for this disorder *1576* Absolute lymphopenia occurs in pulmonary sarcoidosis and correlates very closely with prognosis. A steady increase in absolute number indicates good prognosis (with or without treatment). No increase or a very low and unchanged number indicates very poor prognosis *538*

Lysozyme *Serum* *Increase* Most frequently elevated in patients with pulmonary parenchymal involvement *4415* Highest in patients with the most extensive disease and falls progressively in stage II to I. All patients with disease involving the spleen showed increased activity *4021*

β_2-Macroglobulin *Serum* *Increase* Elevated in 63% of patients *4014*

Macrophages *BAL Fluid* *Increase* In 37 patients with indications for therapy mean proportion of macrophages 1.2 ± 0.3% and in 40 without indications for therapy 1.0 ± 0.2% *5858* In 16 patients with active sarcoidosis mean concentration of alveolar macrophages of 11.9 ± 5.7 x 10^4/L and 12.5 ± 5.9 x 10^4/L in 11 patients with inactive sarcoidosis significantly different from mean concentration of 7.79 ± 3.16 x 10^4/L in 9 healthy controls *2678* In 37 patients with indications for therapy mean proportion of macrophages 78.8 ± 2.5% and in 40 without indications for therapy 81.6 ± 2.1% *5858* In 16 patients with active sarcoidosis mean proportion of alveolar macrophages of 48.3 ± 14.9% and 61.8 ± 23.2% in 11 patients with inactive sarcoidosis significantly different from mean proportion of 88.3 ± 7.6% in 9 healthy controls *2678*
BAL Fluid *No Effect* In 24 patients mean concentration of 114.4 ± 22.8 x 10^3/mL not significantly different from 139.0 ± 56.6 x 10^3/mL in 13 healthy control volunteers *1595*

Monocytes *Blood* *Increase* In 72% of 25 patients at initial hospitalization for this disorder *1576*

Neopterin *Serum* *Increase* In 37 patients with indications for therapy mean concentration of 21.0 ± 4.5 nmol/L and in 40 without indications for therapy 9.3 ± 1.0 nmol/L *5858*
Urine *Increase* Concentrations increased with active pulmonary sarcoidosis and may be used to monitor progress of disease *121*

Neutrophils *BAL Fluid* *No Effect* In 16 patients with active sarcoidosis mean proportion of 2.5 ± 5.1% and 1.0 ± 0.8% in 11 patients with inactive sarcoidosis not significantly different from mean proportion of 0.5 ± 0.4% in 9 healthy controls *2678* In 24 patients mean concentration of 2.3 ± 0.7 x 10^3/mL not significantly different from 1.5 ± 0.5 x 10^3/mL in 13 healthy control volunteers *1595*

5'-Nucleotidase *Serum* *Increase* Activities ranging from 14.5 - 91.3 U/L were observed in 5 cases *2803* Significantly elevated in 2 of 3 patients with liver granulomata *2803*

Oligoclonal Banding *Cerebrospinal Fluid* *Increase* Oligoclonal IgG bands detected with neurosarcoidosis *3261*

Oxygen Partial Pressure *Blood* *Decrease* Decreased with lung involvement *5545* Mild hyperventilation is frequent except in advanced disease when ventilatory obstruction occurs *2039* In 71% of 14 patients at initial hospitalization for this disorder *1576*
Blood *No Effect* In 8 patients with sarcoidosis mean of 63 ± 8 mm Hg not significantly different from 69 ± 9 mm Hg in 85 healthy control individuals *5338*

Oxygen Saturation *Blood* *Decrease* Decreased with lung involvement *5545*

Parathyroid Hormone *Plasma* *Decrease* Immeasurably low in most patients, both normo- and hypercalcemic *4318*

pH *Blood* *Increase* In 72% of 15 patients at initial hospitalization for this disorder *1576*
Blood *No Effect* In 8 patients with sarcoidosis mean of 7.40 ± 0.21 not significantly different from 7.40 ± 1.30 in 85 healthy control individuals *5338*

Platelets *Blood* *Decrease* Pancytopenia is a common feature *5677*

Procollagen Type III Peptide *Serum* *Increase* In an overall series of 57 patients the levels were higher (19.18 ± 9.17 ng/mL) than in 25 age and sex-matched controls (11.32 ± 2.15 ng/mL; p less than 0.001). Thus, the usefulness of P-III-P in the treatment of patients with sarcoid may be considered similar to that

135.00 Sarcoidosis *(continued)*

Procollagen Type III Peptide *(continued)*
of S-ACE *3154* Significantly higher levels of S-PCP-III were found in group B (Type I, progressive) (18.2 ± 1.09 ng/mL) and in group D (Type II/III, progressive) (13.9 ± 1.2 ng/mL) compared with those of Group A (Type I, stable) (9.1 ± 1.09 ng/mL) and Group C (Type II/III, stable) (7.6 ± 1.1 ng/mL) or normal volunteers (9.4 ± 4 ng/mL) (p less than 0.001 for all comparisons). Changes in S-PCP-III levels tended to parallel the clinical course *4162*

Properdin Factor B *Plasma* *No Effect* Mean concentration typically normal or slightly increased in patients with sarcoidosis *4682*

Protein *BAL Fluid* *Increase* Mean concentration in 35 patients with sarcoidosis of 250 ± 62 mg/mL significantly different from 82 ± 16 mg/mL in 21 control individuals *1989*
BAL Fluid *No Effect* In 24 patients mean concentration of 34.8 ± 7.3 mg/dL not significantly different from 16.1 ± 1.4 mg/dL in 13 healthy control volunteers *1595*
Cerebrospinal Fluid *Increase* In granulomatous basilar meningitis affecting cranial nerves *2033*

Protein 1 *BAL Fluid* *Positive* Protein 1 detected in fluid from patients with sarcoidosis *2371*

Renin Activity *Plasma* *Increase* In 8 patients with sarcoidosis mean activity of 4.20 ± 1.61 ng/mL/h significantly higher than 2.76 ± 0.64 ng/mL/h in 85 healthy control individuals *5338*

Rheumatoid Factor *Serum* *Increase* 17% positivity *306* The incidence of seropositivity exceeds that of a normal population *4551* 17% positivity *874* High incidence of seropositive tests among those who had the disease for 2 y, especially among those who also had arthritis *1980* Mean concentration increased in patients with sarcoidosis *2472* Rheumatoid factor may be observed in certain patients *2473*

Soluble Intercellular Adhesion Molecule-1
BAL Fluid *Increase* In 16 patients with active sarcoidosis mean concentration of 47.3 ± 19.3 ng/mL and 27.5 ± 19.0 ng/mL in 11 patients with inactive sarcoidosis significantly different from mean concentration of 12.8 ± 6.9 in 9 healthy controls *2678*
Lymphocytes *Increase* In 16 patients with active sarcoidosis mean expression of 3.93 ± 1.33 and 3.18 ± 1.89 in 11 patients with inactive sarcoidosis not significantly different from mean proportion of 2.52 ± 1.40 in 9 healthy controls *2678*
Macrophages *Increase* In 16 patients with active sarcoidosis mean expression of 3.21 ± 1.55 and 1.67 ± 0.66 in 11 patients with inactive sarcoidosis significantly different from mean proportion of 0.94 ± 0.17 in 9 healthy controls *2678*
Serum *Increase* In 16 patients with active sarcoidosis mean concentration of 575 ± 221 ng/mL (significantly) and 263 ± 99 ng/mL in 11 patients with inactive sarcoidosis (not significantly) different from mean concentration of 199 ± 3.89 in 9 healthy controls *2678*

Soluble Interleukin-2 Receptor *Serum* *Increase* In 37 patients with indications for therapy mean concentration of 1,870 ± 263 U/mL and in 40 without indications for therapy 1,274 ± 216 U/mL *5858*

Soluble Interleukin-6 Receptor *BAL Fluid* *No Effect* In 16 patients with active sarcoidosis mean concentration of 7.44 ± 3.19 and 9.23 ± 5.99 in 11 patients with inactive sarcoidosis not significantly different from mean proportion of 8.62 ± 8.88 in 9 healthy controls *2678*

Surfactant Protein A *BAL Fluid* *Increase* Mean concentration in 35 patients with sarcoidosis of 8.0 ± 0.7 µg/mL significantly different from 4.0 ± 0.3 µg/mL in 21 control individuals *1989*

Tissue Polypeptide Antigen *Serum* *No Effect* In 10 patients mean concentration of 62.1 ± 27.5 U/L not significantly different from 72.7 ± 19.2 U/L in 19 healthy controls *5845*

Triglycerides *Serum* *No Effect* In 44 patients with active sarcoidosis mean concentration of 1.21 ± 0.59 mmol/L and 1.14 ± 0.63 mmol/L in 46 patients with inactive sarcoidosis not significantly different from 1.16 ± 0.80 mmol/L in 147 control individuals *2842*

Type III Procollagen Amino-terminal Peptide-related Antigen
BAL Fluid *Increase* In 24 patients mean concentration of 13.4 ± 5.1 ng/L significantly different from 0.5 ± 0.1 ng/L in 13 healthy control volunteers *1595*

Uric Acid *Serum* *Increase* May occur even with normal renal function in up to 50% of patients *5545* In 52% of 25 patients at initial hospitalization for this disorder *1576*

136.10 Behcet's Syndrome

Alkaline Phosphatase *Serum* *Increase* 23 of 213 patients with Behcet's syndrome had activities significantly higher than upper limit of normal of 10.0 U/L *5147*

Amyloid β-Protein *Cerebrospinal Fluid* *No Effect* In 1 patient with neuro-Behcet's disease concentration was 3.45 pmol/mL not significantly different from mean concentration of 4.00 ± 2.92 pmol/mL *3716*

Amyloid β-Protein Precursor *Cerebrospinal Fluid* *Decrease* In 1 patient with neuro-Behcet's disease concentration was 0.22 integrated OD units significantly different from mean concentration of 1.35 ± 0.38 integrated OD units in 25 normal controls *3716*

Anti-Entactin Antibodies *Serum* *Increase* In 5 patients IgM anti-entactin antibodies not observed in any *4604*

Antibodies *Serum* *Increase* Antibodies to human oral mucosa detected *565*

Anticardiolipin Antibodies *Cerebrospinal Fluid* *Increase* Anticardiolipin antibodies, especially the IgM isotype were highly elevated in the cerebrospinal fluid of patients with neuro-Behcet's *5559*

α_1-Antichymotrypsin *Cerebrospinal Fluid* *Increase* In 1 patient with neuro-Behcet's disease concentration was 10.90 µg/mL significantly different from mean concentration of 2.27 ± 1.40 µg/mL in 25 normal controls *3716*

Antithrombin III Activity *Plasma* *No Effect* In 8 patients with deep vein thrombosis and 11 patients without deep vein thrombosis activity not different from reference interval *5313*

Cells *Cerebrospinal Fluid* *Increase* In 1 patient with neuro-Behcet's disease concentration of 16.3 cells/µL significantly different from normal of 3 cells/µL *3716*
Synovial Fluid *Increase* In 2 patients mean concentration of 13,200 ± 7,354 /µL *4343*

Complement C_3 *Serum* *Increase* In 42 patients with Behcet's syndrome mean concentration of 98.4 ± 48.8 mg/dL not significantly different from 86.2 ± 27.3 mg/dL in 40 healthy control individuals *1090*

Complement C_4 *Serum* *Increase* In 42 patients with Behcet's syndrome mean concentration of 45.0 ± 23.3 mg/dL not significantly different from 34 ± 5.0 mg/dL in 40 healthy control individuals *1090*

Copper *Serum* *Increase* In 40 patients with Behcet's disease mean concentration of 1.44 ± 0.32 mg/L as determined by X-ray fluorescence not significantly different from 1.14 ± 0.14 mg/L in 12 control individuals *1196*

C-Reactive Protein *Serum* *Increase* Nonspecific index of inflammation *565* Nonspecific Index of Infection *4636* Concentration increased in 23 of 213 patients with Behcet's syndrome who had alkaline phosphatase activities significantly higher than upper limit of normal of 10.0 U/L *5147*

D-Dimer *Plasma* *No Effect* In 8 patients with deep vein thrombosis median concentration of 0.8 µg/mL and 0.5 µg/mL in 11 patients without deep vein thrombosis not significantly different from reference interval of < 2.5 µg/mL in 11 healthy controls *5313*

Elastase *Neutrophils* *Increase* In 42 patients with Behcet's syndrome mean concentration of 244.2 ± 126.8 µg/L (321.5 ± 117.9 µg/L in acute phase, 158 .9 µg/L in remission) significantly different from 44.3 ± 19.2 µg/L in 40 healthy control individuals *1090*

Elastase-α_1-Proteinase Inhibitor *Serum* *Increase* In 8 patients with deep vein thrombosis mean concentration of granulocyte elastase-α1-proteinase inhibitor complex of 242 ± 73 ng/mL higher than 165 ± 97 ng/mL in 11 patients without deep vein thrombosis and 96 ± 40 ng/mL in 11 healthy controls *5313*

Endothelin-1 *Plasma* *Increase* Mean concentration of 35.99 ± 5.06 fmol/mL in 11 patients with active disease significantly higher than 10.98 ± 0.84 fmol/mL in 20 healthy controls but difference in concentration in patients with inactive disease (12.98 ± 1.14 fmol/mL) and controls not significant *5371*

Erythrocyte Sedimentation Rate *Blood* *Increase* In 2 patients mean rate of 27 ± 11 mm/h *4343* In 42 patients with Behcet's syndrome mean rate of 32.5 ± 15.6 mm/h significantly different from 14.5 ± 3.5 mm/h in 40 healthy control individuals *1090* Nonspecific index of inflammation *565* Nonspecific Index of Infection *4636* Rate increased in 23 of 213 patients with Behcet's syndrome who had alkaline phosphatase activities significantly higher than upper limit of normal of 10.0 U/L *5147*

Fibrinogen *Plasma* *Increase* In 8 patients with deep vein thrombosis median concentration of 376 mg/dL and 328 mg/dL in 11 patients without deep vein thrombosis not significantly different from reference interval of 171 - 289 mg/dL in 11 healthy controls *5313*

Fibrinogen Degradation Products *Plasma* *No Effect* In 8 patients with deep vein thrombosis median concentration of 3.0 μg/mL and 2.3 μg/mL in 11 patients without deep vein thrombosis not significantly different from reference interval of < 5 μg/mL in 11 healthy controls *5313*

α_2-Globulin *Serum* *Increase* In 42 patients with Behcet's syndrome mean concentration of 13.1 ± 1.7% significantly different from 9.0 ± 1.5% in 40 healthy control individuals *1090*

HLA-B_5 *Serum* *Increase* Higher Incidence *4636*

HLA-D_5 Lymphocytes *Blood* *Increase* Higher Incidence *4636*

immunoglobulin A *Serum* *Increase* In 42 patients with Behcet's syndrome mean concentration of 386 ± 163 mg/dL significantly different from 251 ± 66 mg/dL in 40 healthy control individuals *1090*

Immunoglobulin G *Serum* *Increase* In 42 patients with Behcet's syndrome mean concentration of 2,001 ± 1,098 mg/dL significantly different from 1,442 ± 257 mg/dL in 40 healthy control individuals *1090*

Immunoglobulin M *Serum* *Increase* In 42 patients with Behcet's syndrome mean concentration of 251 ± 122 mg/dL significantly different from 145 ± 59 mg/dL in 40 healthy control individuals *1090*

Interleukin-1β *Serum* *Increase* Mean concentration of 639 ± 741 pg/mL in 22 patients significantly higher than 59 ± 53 pg/mL in 20 healthy control volunteers *5821*

Interleukin-6 *Cerebrospinal Fluid* *Increase* IL-6 was highly elevated in the cerebrospinal fluid of patients with neuro-Behcet's *5559*

Interleukin-8 *Serum* *Increase* Mean concentration of 369.3 ± 1,447.8 pg/mL in 20 patients with active disease, 65.6 ± 255.8 pg/mL in 20 patients with inactive disease compared with 13.1 ± 12.3 pg/mL in 25 apparently healthy controls *3965*

Iron *Serum* *No Effect* In 32 patients with Behcet's disease mean concentration of 1.66 ± 0.53 mg/L as determined by X-ray fluorescence not significantly different from 1.56 ± 0.57 mg/L in 12 normal individuals *1196*

Leukocytes *Blood* *Increase* Nonspecific index of inflammation *565* Nonspecific Index of Infection *4636*

Neutrophils *Blood* *Increase* In 42 patients with Behcet's syndrome mean concentration of 4,470 ± 1,212 /μL significantly different from 2,975 ± 1,416 μL in 40 healthy control individuals *1090*

Oligoclonal Banding *Cerebrospinal Fluid* *Increase* Oligoclonal IgG bands detected with Behcet's disease *3261*

Partial Thromboplastin Time *Plasma* *No Effect* In 8 patients with deep vein thrombosis median time of 30.5 s and 28.9 s in 11 patients without deep vein thrombosis not significantly different from reference interval of 27.6 - 38.3 s in 11 healthy controls *5313*

Plasmin-α_2-Plasmin Inhibitor Complex *Plasma* *Increase* In 8 patients with deep vein thrombosis mean concentration of 1.13 ± 0.14 μg/mL higher than 0.68 ± 0.35 μg/mL in 11 patients without deep vein thrombosis and reference interval of < 0.8 μg/mL *5313*

Protein *Cerebrospinal Fluid* *No Effect* In 1 patient with neuro-Behcet's disease concentration of 45 mg/dL not significantly different from normal mean of 29 mg/dL *3716*

Protein C *Plasma* *No Effect* In 8 patients with deep vein thrombosis and 11 patients without deep vein thrombosis activity not different from reference interval *5313*

Protein S *Plasma* *No Effect* In 8 patients with deep vein thrombosis and 11 patients without deep vein thrombosis activity not different from reference interval *5313*

Prothrombin Time *Plasma* *No Effect* In 8 patients with deep vein thrombosis median time of 10.9 s and 9.9 s in 11 patients without deep vein thrombosis not significantly different from reference interval of 11 - 12.5 s in 11 healthy controls *5313* *5313*

Pyridinoline *Synovial Fluid* *Increase* In 2 patients mean concentration of 24.0 ± 8.5 pmol/mL *4343*

Rubidium *Serum* *Decrease* In 34 patients with Behcet's disease mean concentration of 145 ± 29 μg/L as determined by X-ray fluorescence significantly less than 249 ± 43 μg/L in 12 healthy controls *1196*

Selenium *Serum* *Decrease* Mean concentration of 45.8 ± 16.5 μg/L as determined by X-ray fluorescence significantly less than 62.0 ± 17.7 μg/L in 12 healthy controls *1196*

Soluble Interleukin-2 Receptor *Serum* *Increase* Mean concentration of 958 ± 712 U/mL in 25 patients significantly higher than 404 ± 119 U/mL in 20 healthy control volunteers *5821*

Thrombin/Antithrombin III Complex *Plasma* *No Effect* In 8 patients with deep vein thrombosis median concentration of 1.9 μg/L and 1.2 μg/L in 11 patients without deep vein thrombosis not significantly different from reference interval of < 3.0 μg/L in 11 healthy controls *5313*

Thrombomodulin *Plasma* *Increase* Mean concentration of 20 ng/mL in 6 patients with active disease significantly higher than 10 ng/mL in 6 patients with inactive disease and 66 healthy controls *3873*

Zinc *Serum* *Decrease* Mean concentration of 0.92 ± 0.14 mg/L as determined by X-ray fluorescence significantly reduced compared with 1.13 ± 0.20 mg/L in 12 healthy controls *1196*

136.30 Pneumocystis carinii Pneumonitis

Lactate Dehydrogenase *Serum* *Increase* Activity increased in patients with condition and AIDS, higher than in those with AIDS only in whom activity was also increased. Actvity decreased in response to treatment *4840*

136.90 Infections

Alkaline Phosphatase *White Blood Cells* *Increase* Significant increase observed on first day of infection in patients with acute urinary tract or chest infections *1810*

Antithrombin III *Plasma* *Decrease* In 16 of 24 patients significantly decreased concentrations observed *2135*

α_1-Antitrypsin *Serum* *Increase* In 22 patients who had had heart transplants and subsequently developed infections mean concentrations increased to 2,840 ± 560 mg/dL versus baseline of 2,240 ± 650 mg/dL *1868*

C_4b-Binding Protein *Serum* *Increase* Significantly higher mean concentration observed in 24 patients with severe infections (135 ± 43%) but without septic shock *2135*

Carcinoembryonic Antigen *Serum* *Increase* In 4 patients with infectious disease 50.0% had concentrations of 0.0 - 3.0 ng/mL, 25.0% had concentrations from 3.1 - 5.0 ng/mL, 25.0% had concentrations from 5.1 - 10.0 ng/mL and 0.0% had concentrations greater than 10.0 ng/mL when measured by method on Bayer Technicon Immuno 1® system compared with 95.9%, 3.5%, 0.6% and 0.0% respectively in 173 healthy nonsmokers *339*

Chitotriosidase *Serum* *No Effect* Normal activity observed in all of 12 patients with infectious diseases with hepatomegaly *1917*

Cholesterol *Serum* *Decrease* Transient decreases often observed during infectious illnesses *929*

Cholinesterase *Cerebrospinal Fluid* *No Effect* In 12 patients with infective disorders mean concentration of 0.47 ± 0.03 μmol substrate hydrolyzed (0.19 ± 0.02 mg protein/30 min) not significantly different from 0.48 ± 0.01 μmol substrate hydrolyzed (0.18 ± 0.01 mg protein/30 min) in 10 age and sex matched control patients with nonspecific headaches *321*

Complement C_3 *Serum* *Increase* Although normally decreases in response to energy deficiency concentration may increase in infections and in hypermetabolic states when it functions as an acute phase reactant *1959*

136.90 Infections *(continued)*

Complement C_3b *Serum Increase* In patients with acute bacterial infections concentration significantly higher than in patients with acute asthma or healthy controls *4486*

C-Reactive Protein *Serum Increase* With bacterial infection on the first day of pyrexia concentration may be less than 100 mg/L but increases within 48 - 72 hours: concentration decreases with resolution of pyrexia and clinical improvement or may even decrease before pyrexia remits *1834* Mean and median concentrations of 103.0 and 73.0 mg/L respectively during 19 rejection episodes significantly higher than mean and median of 7.0 and 3.0 mg/L respectively in 130 controls *5489* In 36 children followed from birth for 20 days there were 21 episodes of confirmed infection in 16 children each associated with a sustained rise in C-reactive protein concentration *4809* Mean concentration of 35.9 mg/L in patients with proved infections versus 9.0 mg/L in noninfected controls *4772* High concentrations more likely to be observed during bacterial than viral meningitis *4094* Significant increase observed with infections in 20 cardiac transplant patients followed over 9 months *3930* In 22 patients who had had heart transplants and subsequently developed infections mean concentrations increased to 58 ± 49 mg/L versus baseline of 13 ± 14 mg/L *1868*

Creatine Kinase *Serum Increase* High activity observed in serum of patients with severe infections of the CNS, with highest activities observed in patients with bacterial meningitis with cerebral edema and in those with encephalitis *4098*

Creatinine *Amniotic Fluid No Effect* In 15 pregnant women with intra-amniotic infection median concentration of 1.4 mg/dL not significantly different from 1.4 mg/dL in 26 pregnant women without intra-amniotic infection *2260*

CYFRA 21-1 *Serum Increase* In 16 patients with infectious disease median concentration of 2.4 ng/mL significantly different from that in 50 healthy individuals with median concentration of 1.2 ng/mL and range of 0.5 - 2.4 ng/mL *3559*

Di-iodotyrosine *Serum Increase* Mean concentration in patients with severe nonsystemic infections of 3.84 nmol/L (range of 0.24 - 17.2 nmol/L): in patients with moderate infections such as pneumonia 0.44 nmol/L (range of 0.18 - 1.16 nmol/L) compared with normal of 0.02 - 0.55 nmol/L *3443*

Dolichol *Serum No Effect* In patients with bacterial or viral infections concentrations not significantly different from those in healthy individuals *2294* Mean concentration in 3 patients with viral infections 136.4 ± 29.3 ng/mL and in 13 patients with bacterial infections 168.1 ± 12.4 ng/mL not significantly different from 142.1 ± 4.1 ng/mL in healthy controls *2294*

Elastase-α_1-Proteinase Inhibitor Complex *Serum Increase* In capillary blood in infected neonates raised activity (440 - 2,600 µg/L) observed at the outset of infection in each of 24 infectious episodes *4402*

Erythrocyte Sedimentation Rate *Blood Increase* In 138 of 1,480 ESRs in a hospital population rates were greater than 100 mm/h: in a further study of 90 patients with 163 final diagnoses 43 were attributable to infectious diseases *3097*

Ferritin *Serum Increase* Ferritin is an acute phase reactant and inflammation increases serum ferritin concentration 3- to 5-fold *4784*

Fibronectin *Plasma Decrease* Decreases rapidly with onset of infection but responds rapidly with recovery *1959*

Glucose *Amniotic Fluid Decrease* In 15 pregnant women with intra-amniotic infection median concentration of 9 mg/dL significantly different from 29 mg/dL in 26 pregnant women without intra-amniotic infection *2260*

HDL-Cholesterol *Serum Decrease* Transient decreases often observed in patients with infectious diseases *929*

Intercellular Adhesion Molecule-1 *Serum Increase* In 22 patients who had had heart transplants and subsequently developed infections mean concentrations increased to 500 ± 68 µg/L versus baseline of 369 ± 81 µg/L *1868*

Interleukin-1α *Serum Increase* Serum levels increase during infections and other inflammatory conditions *4093*

Interleukin-6 *Amniotic Fluid Increase* In 15 pregnant women with intra-amniotic infection median concentration of 2,005 ng/mg creatinine significantly different from 990 ng/mg creatinine in 26 pregnant women without intra-amniotic infection *2260*
Serum Increase Mean concentration detected in 20% of 23 patients with infections with or without disseminated intravascular coagulation *3890* Increased concentration observed in infection and endotoxemia *4093*

Interleukin-8 *Amniotic Fluid Increase* In 15 pregnant women with intra-amniotic infection median concentration of 4,933 ng/mg creatinine significantly different from 61 ng/mg creatinine in 26 pregnant women without intra-amniotic infection *2260*
Serum Increase Concentration increased markedly above the increase observed with rejection in patients with acute liver transplant rejection *5233*

Iron *Serum Decrease* In patients with intercurrent infections serum iron concentration may be low especially with coexisting severe iron deficiency *4784* Common colds may reduce serum iron concentration to less than 10 µmol/L even in normal individuals. Reduction also occurs with acute infection, inflammation, minor injuries or surgery *745*

17-Ketogenic Steroids *Urine Increase* Excretion may be increased in patients with the stress of infections *2952*

Leukemia Inhibitory Factor *Amniotic Fluid Increase* In 15 pregnant women with intra-amniotic infection median concentration of 5,249 pg/mg creatinine significantly different from 139 pg/mg creatinine in 26 pregnant women without intra-amniotic infection *2260*

Leukocytes *Amniotic Fluid Increase* In 15 pregnant women with intra-amniotic infection median concentration of 100 cells/µL significantly different from 4 cells/µL in 26 pregnant women without intra-amniotic infection *2260*
Blood Increase Median concentration of 10.0 x 10^3 /µL in 22 patients with infectious diseases not significantly different from normal of 8.7 x 10^3 /µL *3203*

Lipoprotein Lp(a) *Serum Increase* In 48 patients with infections mean concentration of 0.262 ± 0.266 g/L significantly greater than 0.118 ± 0.193 g/L in 100 healthy controls *3505*

Magnesium *Granulocyte No Effect* Mean concentration in patients with infection of 3.81 ± 0.61 fmol/cell not significantly different from 4.35 ± 0.62 fmol/cell in healthy controls *3137*
Monocytes No Effect Mean concentration in patients with infection of 4.09 ± 0.86 fmol/cell not significantly different from 3.74 ± 0.66 fmol/cell in healthy controls *3137*

β_2-Microglobulin *Serum Increase* In 22 patients who had had heart transplants and subsequently developed infections mean concentrations increased to 40 ± 26 mg/L versus baseline of 33 ± 18 mg/L *1868*

Myoglobin *Urine Increase* May cause acute muscle necrosis with myoglobinuria *5065*

Neopterin *Serum Increase* Concentrations increased in relation to severity of disease observed with HIV, CMV, and other pathogens. Increase also observed with mycobacterium tuberculosis, mycobacterium leprae, plasmodium falciparum and vivax and bacterial pneumonitis *3651* Mean concentration of 18.3 nmol/L in 12 patients with proved infection compared with 12.6 nmol/L in patients with no clinical symptoms *4772* Mean and median concentrations of 103.9 and 70.0 nmol/L respectively during 19 rejection episodes significantly higher than mean and median of 14.7 and 11.0 nmol/L respectively in 130 controls *5489* Increasing neopterin concentrations observed than observed after organ transplant rejection, with concentrations highest in patients in whom viral infections were complicated by bacterial superinfection *121*
Urine Increase Increased concentration observed in conditions with activated cellular immunity *4093* Increase observed with serious infections *3651*

Nerve Growth Factor *Cerebrospinal Fluid No Effect* Concentrations not increased in any patients with non-CNS infections *5091*

2',5'-Oligoadenylate Synthetase *Serum Increase* In children significant increase of 2'-5'-oligoadenylate synthetase in presence of viral, bacterial and mycoplasmal infections *5074*

Oxidase *Plasma Increase* In 8 patients with infections mean plasma oxidase activity of 214 ± 10 U/L significantly greater than 84 ± 5 U/L in 12 healthy controls *2931*

pH *Amniotic Fluid No Effect* In 15 pregnant women with intra-amniotic infection median pH of 8 not significantly different from 8 in 26 pregnant women without intra-amniotic infection *2260*

Phospholipase A_2 *Serum Increase* Increased concentrations reported *46*

Platelets *Blood Increase* In 732 patients with platelet counts greater than 500,000 /µL, 21.0% had infections *1869*

Blood *No Effect* Median concentration of 26.4 x 10^4 /µL in 22 patients with infectious diseases not significantly different from normal of 32.3 x 10^4 /µL *3203*

Protein S *Plasma* *Decrease* Significantly reduced compared to healthy blood donors to 60 ± 14% *2135*
Plasma *No Effect* In 24 patients with severe infections mean concentration of 119 ± 36.7% compared with normal value of 96 ± 15% *2135*

Protein S, Free *Plasma* *No Effect* In 24 patients with severe infections mean concentration of 27 ± 9.4% compared with normal value of 29 ± 9% *2135*

Selenium *Serum* *Decrease* In 50 hospital patients (mean age 50 years) with injury or infection mean plasma concentration of 0.50 µmol/L (range of 0.1 - 1.0 µmol/L) significantly reduced compared with normals and negatively correlated with plasma C-reactive protein concentration *4595*

Soluble E-Selectin *Serum* *Increase* Mean concentration in 21 patients with infections and disseminated intravascular coagulation of 90.5 ± 71.2 ng/mL significantly different from 51.6 ± 44.4 ng/mL in 12 patients with infections but without DIC *3890*

Soluble Interleukin-2 Receptor *Serum* *Increase* Mean concentration significantly increased in patients with severe infection *5877*

Soluble Vascular Cell Adhesion Molecule-1
Serum *Increase* In 22 patients who had had heart transplants and subsequently developed infections, mean concentrations increased to 1,408 ± 445 µg/L versus baseline of 1,159 ± 440 µg/L *1868*

Specific Gravity *Amniotic Fluid* *No Effect* In 15 pregnant women with intra-amniotic infection median specific gravity of 1.01 not significantly different from 1.01 in 26 pregnant women without intra-amniotic infection *2260*

Tenascin-C *Serum* *Increase* Mean concentration in 16 patients with CRP concentration of 10 - 100 mg/L 2.71 ± 1.63 mg/L, in those with CRP 100 - 200 mg/L 4.52 ± 3.13 mg/L and in those with CRP 200 - 300 mg/L 11.24 ± 8.42 mg/L significantly higher than that in 15 healthy individuals (1.09 ± 0.41 mg/L) *4626*

Thrombin/Antithrombin III Complex *Plasma* *Increase* Increased in 16 of 24 patients with severe infections *2135*

Thyroid Stimulating Hormone *Serum* *Decrease* Typically reduced or normal as with severe non-thyroidal acute illness *3443*
Serum *No Effect* Typically reduced or normal as with severe non-thyroidal acute illness *3443*

Thyroxine (T4) *Serum* *Decrease* Normal or decreased concentration observed as with severe non-thyroidal illness *3443*
Serum *No Effect* Normal or decreased concentration observed as with severe non-thyroidal illness *3443*

Thyroxine (T4), Free *Serum* *No Effect* No significant change observed as with severe non-thyroidal severe illness *3443*

Tissue Polypeptide Antigen *Serum* *Increase* Mean and median concentrations of 213.9 and 158.2 U/L respectively during 19 rejection episodes significantly higher than mean and median of 44.9 and 43.1 U/L respectively in 130 controls *5489*

Tri-iodothyronine, Reverse (rT3) *Serum* *Increase* Typically observed as with severe non-thyroidal illness *3443*

Tri-iodothyronine (T3) *Serum* *Decrease* Reduced concentration typically observed as with severe non-thyroidal illness *3443*

Triglycerides *Serum* *Increase* Transient increases often observed with infections of all types *929*

Tumor Necrosis Factor-α *Serum* *Increase* Mean concentration detected in 12.1% of 23 patients with infections with or without disseminated intravascular coagulation compared with undetectable amounts in patients with liver disease, hematologic disorders and obstetric disorders *3890* Concentrations increase in infections and other inflammatory conditions *4093*

Vascular Endothelial Growth Factor *Serum* *Increase* Median concentration in acute stage of Kawasaki disease in 22 patients with infections of 184.1 pg/mL significantly different from normal of 117.4 pg/mL *3203*

Zinc *Monocytes* *Increase* Concentration increased in all patients studied with infections on first day but declined thereafter *1810*
Neutrophils *No Effect* Concentration remained unchanged during 7 days studied following acute infection *1810*
Serum *Decrease* In patients with acute urinary tract or chest infection concentration decreased on first day in association with reduced serum albumin concentration but returned to normal by seventh day *1810*

136.90 Microbial Infection

α_1-Acid Glycoprotein *Serum* *Decrease* In 22 children hospitalized with urinary tract infection mean concentration decreased from 1.96 g/L on admission to 1.62 g/L after 6 days treatment *717*

NEOPLASMS

Primary Malignant Neoplasms

140.90 Cancer of Lip

Sialic Acid *Serum* *No Effect* Mean concentration in 22 patients with cancer of the lip and skin of 59.24 ± 12.10 mg/dL not significantly different from 55.0 ± 7.2 mg/dL in 80 healthy controls *5755*

141.90 Cancer of Tongue

Sialic Acid *Serum* *Increase* Mean concentration in 20 patients with cancer of the tongue and floor of the mouth of 75.01 ± 12.00 mg/dL significantly different from 55.0 ± 7.2 mg/dL in 80 healthy controls *5755*

142.90 Malignant Disease of the Salivary Glands

Sialic Acid *Serum* *Increase* Mean concentration in 23 patients with salivary gland malignancies of 70.58 ± 12.07 mg/dL significantly different from 55.0 ± 7.2 mg/dL in 80 healthy controls *5755*

145.00 Buccal Cancer

Sialic Acid *Serum* *Increase* Mean concentration in 37 patients with buccal, gingival or palatal cancer of 69.46 ± 11.23 mg/dL significantly different from 55.0 ± 7.2 mg/dL in 80 healthy controls *5755*

145.90 Mouth Cancer

Ceruloplasmin *Serum* *Increase* In 137 men with mouth and gut cancer mean concentration of 90 ± 34 mg/dL significantly different from 71 ± 17 mg/dL in 106 control men and mean of 98 ± 23 mg/dL in 87 women with mouth and gut cancer significantly different from 84 ± 22 mg/dL in 150 control women *2280*

Sialic Acid *Serum* *Increase* Mean concentration in 110 patients with malignant tumors of the mouth of 70.11 ± 13.24 mg/dL significantly different from 55.0 ± 7.2 mg/dL in 80 healthy controls *5755*

Transferrin *Serum* *Decrease* In 137 men with mouth and gut cancer mean concentration of 179 ± 49 mg/dL significantly different from 214 ± 33 mg/dL in 106 control men and in 87 women with skin cancer mean concentration of 187 ± 54 mg/dL not significantly different from 217 ± 39 mg/dL in 150 control women *2280*

147.90 Nasopharyngeal Carcinoma

Epstein Barr Virus Antibodies *Serum* *Increase* The relationship has already been well established *105*

Lactate Dehydrogenase *Serum* *No Effect* In 10 cases with local disease mean activity of 102 ± 32 U/L and in 68 with regional disease activities not higher than reference interval of 40 - 140 U/L *3034*

147.90 Nasopharyngeal Carcinoma *(continued)*

Soluble Interleukin-2 Receptor *Serum Increase* Concentration increased in patients with nasopharyngeal cancer than in matched control patients. Concentration indicative of tumor burden *2326*

Tumor Necrosis Factor-α *Serum Increase* Concentration in patients with nasopharyngeal carcinoma higher than in matched control patients but concentration did not correlate with stage of the disease *2326*

150.90 Cancer of Esophagus

Activated Partial Thrombin Ratio *Plasma No Effect* In 12 patients with stage IV disease mean ratio of 1.09 ± 0.03 not significantly different from normal and 1.47 ± 0.28 in 39 patients with stage III disease, 1.01 ± 0.02 in 15 patients with stage II disease and 1.00 ± 0.04 in 7 patients with stage I disease *5602*

Adenosine Monophosphate *Urine No Effect* In one 59-year old man with squamous cell carcinoma of the esophagus concentration of 0.68 nmol/μmol creatinine (normal < 0.65 nmol/μmol creatinine) *2404*

Albumin *Serum Decrease* In 35% of 40 patients at initial hospitalization for this disorder *1576*

Aldolase *Serum Increase* Significantly elevated in tumors of the gastrointestinal tract. Mean = 4.9 ± 0.8 U/L compared to normal, 1.6 ± 0.21 U/L *2513*

Alkaline Phosphatase *Serum Increase* In 29% of 40 patients at initial hospitalization for this disorder *1576*

Aspartate Aminotransferase *Serum Increase* In 41% of 40 patients at initial hospitalization for this disorder *1576*

CA 15-3 *Serum No Effect* In 4 patients with esophageal cancer mean concentration of 7.5 ± 3 U/mL below cutoff of 22 U/mL *2076*

CA 19-9 *Serum Increase* In 8 of 18 patients (44%) the tumor marker increase was seen prior to other signs of tumor progression *3657* Sensitivity of 8% (n = 24) *2122* CA 19-9 concentration increased in 20% patients with esophageal cirrhosis *1253* In 14 patients with esophageal cancer positive rate of 36% observed using cut-off from normals and 29% at 90% specificity *2594* In 8 of 18 patients (44%) the tumor marker increase was seen prior to other signs of tumor progression *2211*

CA 50 *Serum Increase* In 8 or 18 patients (44%) the tumor marker increase was seen prior to other signs of tumor progression *3657* In 8 of 18 patients (44%) the tumor marker increase was seen prior to other signs of tumor progression *2211*

CA 72-4 *Serum Increase* Sensitivity of 4% (n = 24) *2122*

CA 195 *Serum Increase* Mean concentration of 86.9 ± 431.2 U/mL in 35 patients with esophageal cancer significantly higher than cutoff of 12 U/mL: 9 patients with concentrations greater than 12 U/mL *122*

CA 242 *Serum Increase* In 14 patients with esophageal cancer positive rate of 14% observed using cut-off from normals and 14% at 90% specificity *2594*

Calcium *Serum Increase* In one 59-year old man with squamous cell carcinoma of the esophagus concentration of 4.32 mmol/L (normal < 2.55 mmol/L) observed *2404* In one study of patients with hypercalcemia and low intact PTH concentration, 2 of 42 had carcinoma of esophagus *3280* In 5 of 376 patients with esophageal cancer hypercalcemia detected at time of diagnosis: also observed in 45 patients of 120 with recurrent or unresectable cancer *5119* Neoplasm without evidence of direct bone involvement. Parathyroid hormone-secreting tumors *1025*

Carcinoembryonic Antigen *Ascitic Fluid Increase* CEA > 10 ng/mL ascites indicating cancerous effusion *3102*
Peritoneal Fluid Increase The highest levels (> 1,000 ng/mL) were found in samples from patients with gastrointestinal carcinomas *1295*
Pleural Fluid Increase The highest levels (> 1,000 ng/mL) were found in samples from patients with gastrointestinal carcinomas *1295* 24 (34%) of 70 malignant effusions had levels 12 ng/mL *4369*
Serum Increase Concentration increased in over 60% patients *1601* In 66% of patients with localized upper GI tract malignancy, mean concentration of 4.9 ng/mL *4130* Majority of patients have increased concentrations *4551* Two thirds of patients have increased concentration *5544* Preoperative concentrations above 5 ng/mL observed in 14 of 74 patients with esophageal cancer *857*

Complement C_3 *Serum Increase* Increased in patients with local disease. Very closely linked to the stage of the disease. Patients in remission had normal levels, but further increases were noted in distant metastases. Levels dropped significantly in the terminal phase of the disease *5456*

Complement C_4 *Serum Increase* Increased in patients with local disease. Very closely linked to the stage of the disease. Patients in remission had normal levels, but further increases were noted in distant metastases. Levels dropped significantly in the terminal phase of disease *5456*

Complement, Total *Serum Increase* Found to be very closely linked to the stage of the disease. Patients in remission had normal levels, but further increases were noted in distant metastases. Levels dropped significantly in the terminal phase of the disease *5456*

Copper Zinc Superoxide Dismutase *Serum Increase* Significantly elevated in patients with various digestive cancers *3886*

Creatine Kinase, Mitochondrial *Serum No Effect* Median concentration of 11 U/L in 5 patients not different from normal range of 4 - 15 U/L *3892*

1,25-Dihydroxy Vitamin D *Serum No Effect* In one 59-year old man with squamous cell carcinoma of the esophagus concentration normal *2404*

Epidermal Growth Factor *Urine Increase* Mean concentration in about 6 patients of 28 μg/g creatinine compared with about 10 μg/g creatinine in about 30 controls *5341*

Fibrinogen *Plasma Increase* Mean concentration of 530 mg/L in 73 patients with esophageal cancer significantly higher than 300 mg/L in 30 control patients, with concentration increasing in cancer patients with stage of the disease *5602*

Galactosyltransferase Isoenzyme II *Serum Increase* Sensitivity 0.91 and specificity 0.73 *5348* Sensitivity of 0.91 and specificity of 0.72 *5348*

Gc-Globulin *Serum No Effect* In 6 men and 2 women with brain cancer mean concentrations of 23.0 ± 7.48 mg/dL and 22.5 mg/dL not significantly different from 23.9 ± 3.36 mg/dL in 106 control men and 26.1 ± 4.66 mg/dL in 150 control women *2279*

Hematocrit *Blood Decrease* In 24% of 40 patients at initial hospitalization for this disorder *1576*

Hemoglobin *Blood Decrease* In 27% of 39 patients at initial hospitalization for this disorder *1576*

Hexokinase *Serum Increase* Increased in gastrointestinal tumors. Mean activity of 15.3 ± 3.5 U/L compared to normal of 0.93 ± 0.28 U/L *2513*

25-Hydroxy Vitamin D *Serum No Effect* In one 59-year old man with squamous cell carcinoma of the esophagus concentration normal *2404*

immunoglobulin A *Serum No Effect* In 6 men with cancer of the esophagus mean concentration of 231 ± 97 mg/dL not significantly different from 201 ± 89 mg/dL in 106 healthy controls and mean concentration of 254 mg/dL in 2 women with brain cancer not significantly different from 176 ± 80 mg/dL in 150 healthy control women *2278*

Immunoglobulin G *Serum No Effect* In 6 men with cancer of the esophagus mean concentration of 932 ± 172 mg/dL not significantly different from 1,148 ± 224 mg/dL in 106 healthy controls and mean concentration of 1,407 mg/dL in 2 women with cancer of the esophagus not significantly different from 1,157 ± 271 mg/dL in 150 healthy control women *2278*

Immunoglobulin M *Serum No Effect* In 6 men with cancer of the esophagus mean concentration of 60 ± 39 mg/dL not significantly different from 61 ± 36 mg/dL in 106 healthy controls and in 2 women with cancer of the esophagus mean concentration of 51 mg/dL not significantly different from 77 ± 39 mg/dL in 150 healthy control women *2278*

Laminin *Serum Increase* Median serum level of 1,845 mU/mL (n = 6). Control group median of 1,232 mU/mL (n = 42). Elevated in 6 of 6 patients *4394*

Leukocytes *Blood Increase* In 37% of 40 patients at initial hospitalization for this disorder *1576* Observed effect *126*

Lymphocytes *Blood Decrease* In 55% of 36 patients at initial hospitalization for this disorder *1576*

Metallopanstimulin *Serum* *Increase* In 100% of 3 patients with cancer of the esophagus mean concentration exceeded upper limit of normal of < 10 ng/mL in healthy individuals aged 19 - 88 years *1462*

5-Methyl-2'-Deoxycytidine *Urine* *No Effect* In 4 patients with cancer of the esophagus mean excretion of 0.70 ± 0.19 nmol/μmol creatinine not significantly different from 0.90 ± 0.43 nmol/μmol creatinine in 81 healthy individuals *2368*

Monocytes *Blood* *Increase* In 65% of 37 patients at initial hospitalization for this disorder *1576*

Occult Blood *Feces* *Increase* GI bleeding may occur with malignancies *4891*

Parathyroid Hormone *Plasma* *Decrease* In one study of 42 patients with low intact PTH concentration and hypercalcemia 2 had carcinoma of the esophagus *3280*

Parathyroid Hormone 1-84 *Plasma* *Decrease* In one 59-year old man with squamous cell carcinoma of the esophagus concentration undetectable *2404*

Parathyroid Hormone-related Peptide *Plasma* *Increase* In one 59-year old man with squamous cell carcinoma of the esophagus concentration of 75 pmol/L significantly greater than normal of 0 - 7.5 pmol/L *2404*

Phosphate *Serum* *Decrease* In one 59-year old man with squamous cell carcinoma of the esophagus concentration of 0.76 mmol/L (normal > 0.8 mmol/L) observed *2404*

Platelets *Blood* *No Effect* In 12 patients with stage IV disease mean concentration of 353.8 ± 44.9 x 10^9/L not significantly different from normal and 274.6 ± 16.9 x 10^9/L in 39 patients with stage III disease, 305.9 ± 28.0 x 10^9/L in 15 patients with stage II disease and 251.2 ± 18.3 x 10^9/L in 7 patients with stage I disease *5602*

Sialyltransferase *Serum* *Increase* In 4 patients with cancer of the esophagus mean and median concentrations of 430 and 453 cpm/mg protein/30 min significantly different from 240 and 243 cpm/mg protein/30 min respectively in 20 normal individuals *2111*

Uric Acid *Serum* *Increase* In 46% of 40 patients at initial hospitalization for this disorder *1576*

Urokinase Plasminogen Activator *Tissue* *Increase* Amounts are inversely related to overall survival *1255*

151.90 Adenocarcinoma

Parathyroid Hormone-related Peptide *Plasma* *Increase* In 1 patient with adenocarcinoma of unspecified site with metastases concentration of 8.50 pmol/L significantly greater than upper limit of reference range of 2.6 pmol/L *1200*

151.90 Gastric Cancer

α_1-Acid Glycoprotein *Serum* *Increase* In 60 patients with advanced gastric cancer 8 (13%) had concentrations above the reference range of 50 - 130 mg/L in men and 40 - 120 mg/L in women *5303* In patients with gastric or colorectal cancer mean concentration of 2.04 g/L compared with less than 0.50 g/L in healthy controls *719*

Albumin *Serum* *Decrease* Found occasionally, due to leakage into stomach *2033* In 38% of 47 patients at initial hospitalization for this disorder *1576*

Aldolase *Serum* *Increase* Significantly elevated in tumors of the gastrointestinal tract. Mean = 4.9 ± 0.8 U/L compared to normal, 1.6 ± 0.21 U/L *2513*

Alkaline Phosphatase *Serum* *Increase* In 38% of 45 patients at initial hospitalization for this disorder *1576*
White Blood Cells *Decrease* Low activity is present irrespective of tumor category, activity of disease, or type of therapy. In 11 patients, median activity was 5 U/L (normal 55 U/L) *3110*

Alkaline Phosphatase Isoenzymes *Serum* *Increase* Concentration of Regan isoenzyme was 12.5 - 34.2 U/L *1140*

Amyloid A Protein *Serum* *Increase* In patients with gastric or colorectal cancer mean concentration of 312 mg/L compared with less than 1 mg/L in healthy controls *719*

Androgens *Urine* *Decrease* Both androsterone and etiocholanolone were significantly lower in 18 male patients than in controls and patients with rectal cancer *5180*

Androsterone *Urine* *Decrease* Both androsterone and etiocholanolone were significantly lower in 18 male patients than in controls and patients with rectal cancer *5180*

α_1-Antichymotrypsin *Serum* *Increase* In patients with gastric or colorectal cancer mean concentration of 0.99 g/L compared with less than 0.50 g/L in healthy controls *719*

Arginase *Serum* *Increase* Mean concentration of 117 ± 23 ng/mL in 14 patients with gastric cancer (164 ± 18 ng/mL in 25 patients with recurrences) significantly higher than 51.0 ± 3.3 ng/mL in 143 normal controls *5564*

Arginine *Plasma* *Decrease* In 10 patients with gastric cancer mean concentration decreased *3356*

Aspartate Aminotransferase *Serum* *Increase* In 28% of 47 patients at initial hospitalization for this disorder *1576*

Basic Fibroblast Growth Factor *Serum* *Increase* In 19 of 31 Japanese patients with gastric cancer concentration clearly higher than that in 48 normal blood donors, mean concentration of 190 ± 32 ng/L *2860*

c-erb-B_2 Oncoprotein *Serum* *Increase* Median concentration of 10.3 ng/mL in 9 patients with metastatic cancer. 2 of 9 (22%) of patients with metastases had concentrations exceeding 1.5 ng/mL *3564*

CA 15-3 *Serum* *Increase* In 14 patients with gastric cancer mean concentration of 20.5 ± 30 U/mL below cutoff of 22 U/mL, but 2 having concentrations above 22 U/mL and 1 who had a concentration greater than 40 U/mL *2076*
Serum *No Effect* In 14 patients with gastric cancer mean concentration of 20.5 ± 30 U/mL below cutoff of 22 U/mL, but 2 having concentrations above 22 U/mL and 1 who had a concentration greater than 40 U/mL *2076*

CA 19-9 *Serum* *Increase* Positivity rates of 15.2% in tumor size < 2.0 cm, 30.6% with tumor size 2.1 - 5.0 cm and 50.0% with tumors greater than 5.0 cm *3304* In 106 of 663 patients with gastric cancer concentrations exceeded cutoff value (16.0%), with rate for advanced cancers of 25.9% *2735* In 60 patients with advanced gastric cancer mean concentrations exceeded the upper limit of normal of 30 U/mL in 43 (72%) *5302* In 30 patients with gastric carcinoma 43% had concentrations greater than cut-off value of 37 U/mL *3726* In 66 patients with active gastric cancer concentration increased above 37 U/mL in 39% with median concentration of 35 U/mL in stage IV disease compared with 20 U/mL in stage I disease *1482* In 161 patients with primary or recurrent gastric cancer mean concentration increased above cutoff of 37 U/mL in 52 (32.3%) *1897* Frequently show elevated values *3657* In patients with gastric carcinoma mean positivity rate 30% second to CA 50. Overall positivity rate with CA 19-9 TruQuant 22% *5708* Frequently show elevated values *2026* CA 19-9 concentration increased in 40 - 60% patients with gastric adenocarcinomas *1253* In 107 patients with gastric cancer positive rate of 32% observed using cut-off from normals and 26% at 90% specificity *2594* Median concentration of 12.1 kU/L (range 2.3 - 94.6) in 12 patients with early gastric cancer and 29.8 kU/L (range 2.3 - 2,692) in 40 with late cancer compared with 7 kU/L (range 2.3 - 71.7) in 32 patients with benign lesions *2501* Sensitivity of 52% (n = 27) *2122*

CA 50 *Serum* *Increase* In 60 patients with advanced gastric cancer mean concentrations exceeded the upper limit of normal of 14 U/mL in 25 (41%) *5302* In patients with gastric carcinoma overall positivity 59.5% higher than any other tumor marker followed during this study. CA 50 gave the widest range of increased serum concentrations between the cutoff level and the 90th percentile *5708* Elevated in a high proportion of patients with primary carcinoma *2211*

CA 72-4 *Serum* *Increase* In 60 patients with advanced gastric cancer mean concentrations exceeded the upper limit of normal of 7 U/mL in 42 (70%) *5302* Median concentration of 1.2 kU/L (range of 0.4 - 8.5) in 12 patients with early gastric cancer and 6.8 kU/L (range of 0.6 - 4,396) in 40 with late cancer compared with 1.7 kU/L (range of 1.3 - 4.4) in 32 patients with benign lesions *2501* Positivity rates of 6.1% with tumor size < 2.0 cm, 24.2% with tumor size 2.1 - 5.0 cm and 44.8% with tumors greater than 5.0 cm *3304* In 115 patients with gastric cancer 45 (39%) had a concentration less than 2.5 U/mL, 70 (61%) had a concentration greater than 2.5 U/mL and 30 (26%) had a concentration greater than 10 U/mL *4505* Sensitivity of 59% (n = 27). CA 72-4 has a very high specificity (98%) in benign diseases of the gastrointestinal tract, including inflammatory processes, so that elevated serum levels should always be taken seriously *2122* In patients with gastric carcinoma

151.90 Gastric Cancer *(continued)*

CA 72-4 *(continued)*
overall positivity rate 34% *5708* In 161 patients with primary or recurrent gastric cancer mean concentration increased above cutoff of 6 U/mL in 68 (42.3%) *1897*

CA 125 *Serum* *Increase* A study of 387 patients with gastric cancers revealed elevation in 7.2% of patients. In patients with peritonitis carcinomatosa, positive rate was 42.9% *5135* Mean concentration increased above 35 U/mL with peritoneal dissemination, with sensitivity of 39.4%, specificity of of 95.7% and diagnostic accuracy of 90.8% *3725* In 60 patients with advanced gastric cancer mean concentrations exceeded the upper limit of normal of 38 U/mL in 28 (46%) *5302*

CA 195 *Serum* *Increase* In patients with gastric carcinoma overall positivity rate 29% *5708* Increased concentrations observed in patients with gastric cancer *122*

CA 242 *Serum* *Increase* Less than half of the patients with gastric cancer (44%) had elevated values *2870* In 107 patients with gastric cancer positive rate of 22% observed using cut-off from normals and 26% at 90% specificity *2594*

CA 549 *Serum* *Increase* In 95 patients with gastric cancer, 14 (14.7%) had a concentration greater than the upper limit of normal with BRESMARQ assay *764*

Carcinoembryonic Antigen *Ascitic Fluid* *Increase* CEA > 10 ng/mL ascites indicating cancerous effusion *3102*
Peritoneal Fluid *Increase* The highest levels (> 1,000 ng/mL) were found in samples from patients with gastrointestinal carcinomas *1295*
Pleural Fluid *Increase* 24 (34%) of 70 malignant effusions had levels greater than 12 ng/mL *4369* The highest levels (> 1,000 ng/mL) were found in samples from patients with gastrointestinal carcinomas *1295*
Serum *Increase* In 121 patients with gastric cancer 14 (11.6%) had increased serum CEA *4516* In patients with gastric carcinoma overall positivity rate of 33% *5708* In 66% of patients with localized upper GI tract malignancy, mean concentration of 4.9 ng/mL *4130* In 60 patients with advanced gastric cancer mean concentrations exceeded the upper limit of normal of 5 ng/mL in 31 (52%) *5302* Positivity rates of 0% in tumor size < 2.0 cm, 19.4% with tumor size of 2.1 - 5.0 cm and 34.5% with tumors greater than 5.0 cm *3304* Increase observed in many patients *4551* In 110 of 663 patients with gastric cancer concentrations exceeded cutoff value (16.6%), with rate for advanced cancers of 21.3% *2735* In 56 patients with gastric cancer 44.6% had concentrations up to 3.0 ng/mL, 17.9% had concentrations between 3.1 - 5.0 ng/mL, 17.9% between 5.1 - 10.0 ng/mL and 19.6% had concentrations greater than 10.1 ng/mL in contrast to concentrations in 151 healthy nonsmokers in whom 95.4% had concentrations between 0 and 3.0 ng/mL and 4.6% between 4.1 and 10.0 ng/mL *11* In 161 patients with primary or recurrent gastric cancer mean concentration increased above cutoff of 5 ng/mL in 39 (24.2%) *1897* Increase observed in many patients *1601* Mean concentration increased in 61% of patients with gastric cancer compared with 11% in healthy individuals *3191* In 66 patients with active gastric cancer concentration increased above 5 ng/mL in 33% with median concentration of 5.0 ng/mL in stage IV disease compared with 2 ng/mL in stage I disease *1482* In 30 patients with gastric carcinoma 67% had concentrations greater than cut-off value of 6.5 ng/mL *3726*

Ceruloplasmin *Serum* *Increase* High only in gastric and pulmonary cancer. In 58 cases there was a correlation between copper and ceruloplasmin levels in the same subject; significant only in gastric forms *4610*
Serum *No Effect* In 60 patients with advanced gastric cancer none had concentrations above the reference range of 36 - 71 mg/L *5303*

Chloride *Serum* *Increase* In 34% of 29 patients at initial hospitalization for this disorder *1576*

β-Chorionic Gonadotropin *Plasma* *Increase* Ectopic production *602* *552* *3777* *455*

Colon Specific Antigen *Serum* *No Effect* In patients with gastric cancer 0% had increased concentration compared with 8% in healthy controls *3191*

Complement C_3 *Serum* *Increase* Increased in patients with local disease. Very closely linked to the stage of the disease. Patients in remission had normal levels, but further increases were noted in distant metastases. Levels dropped significantly in the terminal phase of disease *5456*

Complement C_4 *Serum* *Increase* Increased in patients with local disease. Very closely linked to the stage of the disease. Patients in remission had normal levels, but further increases were noted in distant metastases. Levels dropped significantly in the terminal phase of disease *5456*

Complement, Total *Serum* *Increase* CH50, C_1q, C_3, and C_4 were significantly higher in cancer patients than in matched controls. The increase was dependent upon the stage of disease and the therapy *5456*

Copper *Serum* *Increase* A correlation between copper and ceruloplasmin was reported in 58 cases of gastric neoplasm *4610* In 35 cases of primary malignant tumors of the digestive organs, plasma copper was increased (1.24 ± 0.34 ppm) *2341*

Copper Zinc Superoxide Dismutase *Serum* *Increase* Significantly elevated in patients with various digestive cancers *3886*

C-Reactive Protein *Serum* *Increase* In 60 patients with advanced gastric cancer 18 (30%) had concentrations above the reference range of < 5 mg/L *5303* In patients with gastric or colorectal cancer mean concentration of 97 mg/L compared with less than 3 mg/L in healthy controls *719*

Creatine Kinase BB-Isoenzyme *Serum* *Increase* Elevated CK-BB *5884* The highest rate of activity was found in sera of patients with tumors of the stomach (8.1 U/L) *4405*

Creatine Kinase, Mitochondrial *Serum* *No Effect* Median concentration of 12 U/L in 8 patients not different from normal range of 4 - 15 U/L *3892*

Cryofibrinogen *Plasma* *Increase* Reported effect *4551* *3417*

DF3 *Serum* *No Effect* In 12 patients with gastric cancer none had concentration greater than 30 U/mL (concentration in 95% normals) *2076*

Epidermal Growth Factor *Urine* *Increase* Mean concentration in about 6 patients of 22 µg/g creatinine compared with about 10 µg/g creatinine in about 30 controls *5341*

Epidermal Growth Factor Receptor *Serum* *Increase* Mean concentration of 681 ± 226 fmol/mL in 40 patients with gastric carcinoma compared with 440 ± 46 fmol/mL in 29 healthy adults *825*

Erythrocyte Sedimentation Rate *Blood* *Increase* Normal in peptic ulcer, but accelerated in carcinoma of the stomach *1980*

Erythrocytes *Ascitic Fluid* *Increase* > 10,000 cells/µL seen in 20% of cases *233*

Etiocholanolone *Urine* *Decrease* Both androsterone and etiocholanolone were significantly lower in 18 male patients than in controls and patients with rectal cancer *5180*

α-Fetoprotein *Serum* *Increase* In 60 patients with advanced gastric cancer mean concentrations exceeded the upper limit of normal of 15 ng/mL in 5 (8%) *5302* Primary tumors of stomach may secrete AFP regardless of whether they have metastasized to the liver *1778* Elevated in 18% of cases *2913*

Fucose *Serum* *Increase* Total concentration was increased in patients with both malignant and benign tumors of breast, lung and stomach. The glycoprotein-bound fraction was markedly elevated in cases of malignancy and not in benign disease. Mucoprotein fraction was raised in both diseases *5170* Mean value of 13.52 ± 0.65 mg/dL in 35 patients. (normal 6.84 ± 0.13 mg/dL) *2899*

Galactosyltransferase Isoenzyme II *Serum* *Increase* Sensitivity 0.53 and specificity 0.73 *5348*

Gastrin *Serum* *Increase* Found to be normal in 26 patients with gastric cancer. Elevated levels may occur in some patients, due to the accompanying atrophy of the oxyntic glands *2369*
Serum *No Effect* Found to be normal in 26 patients with gastric cancer. Elevated levels may occur in some patients, due to the accompanying atrophy of the oxyntic glands *2369*

Gc-Globulin *Serum* *No Effect* In 28 men and 10 women with cancer of the stomach and duodenum mean concentrations of 24.5 ± 3.87 mg/dL and 25.0 ± 5.39 mg/dL not significantly different from 23.9 ± 3.36 mg/dL in 106 control men and 26.1 ± 5.39 mg/dL in 150 control women *2279*

Glucose *Serum* *Decrease* Observed effect *5544*

β-Glucuronidase *Gastric Material* *Increase* Elevated in gastric cancer. Overlap between noncancer and cancer patients limits usefulness and specificity *2682* Greater than 1 U/mg protein in 90% of subjects with cancer or gastric atrophy *2033* Elevated in gastric cancer. Overlap between noncancer and cancer patients limits usefulness and specificity *4891*

Glutamine *Plasma* *Decrease* In 10 patients with gastric cancer mean concentration reduced *3356*

Gonadotropin, Pituitary *Plasma* *Increase* Can cause the syndrome of ectopic gonadotropin production *1980*

Growth Hormone *Plasma* *Increase* Elevated *1870*

Haptoglobin *Serum* *Increase* Reported effect *2033*

Helicobacter pylori IgA Antibodies *Serum* *Increase* In 60 patients with advanced gastric cancer 15 (35%) had concentrations above the reference range of < 17 IU/mL *5303*

Hematocrit *Blood* *Decrease* The amount of bleeding and the degree of anemia will vary widely. Anemia of more than moderate degree is a late consequence of gastric malignancy *1980* In 43% of 47 patients at initial hospitalization for this disorder *1576* Anemia may be of several types. The most common is iron deficiency anemia caused by chronic occult blood loss *4891*

Hemoglobin *Blood* *Decrease* The amount of bleeding and the degree of anemia will vary widely. Anemia of more than moderate degree is a late consequence of gastric malignancy *1980* In 46% of 46 patients at initial hospitalization for this disorder *1576* Anemia may be of several types. The most common is iron deficiency anemia caused by chronic occult blood loss *4891*

Hexokinase *Serum* *Increase* Increased in gastrointestinal tumors. Mean activity of 15.3 ± 3.5 U/L compared to normal of 0.93 ± 0.28 U/L *2513*

β-Hexosaminidase *Serum* *Increase* Observed effect *3141*

Hydrochloric Acid *Gastric Fluid* *Decrease* Achlorhydria following histamine or betazole stimulation found in 50% of patients and hypochlorhydria in another 25% of patients *5544* Characteristic observation *1980*
Gastric Fluid *Increase* Although rare, does not rule out carcinoma *5544*
Gastric Fluid *No Effect* Normal in 25% of patients *5544*

immunoglobulin A *Serum* *Increase* In 137 men with cancer of the stomach, duodenum and gut mean concentration of 278 ± 156 mg/dL significantly different from 201 ± 89 mg/dL in 106 healthy controls and mean concentration of 228 ± 124 mg/dL in 87 women with cancer of the stomach, duodenum and gut significantly different from 176 ± 80 mg/dL in 150 healthy control women *2278* In 60 patients with advanced gastric cancer 2 had concentrations above the reference range of 60 - 420 ng/mL *5303*
Serum *No Effect* In 28 men with cancer of the stomach or duodenum mean concentration of 240 ± 114 mg/dL not significantly different from 201 ± 89 mg/dL in 106 healthy controls and mean concentration of 226 ± 170 mg/dL in 10 women with cancer of the stomach or duodenum not significantly different from 176 ± 80 mg/dL in 150 healthy control women *2278*

Immunoglobulin E *Serum* *Decrease* In 60 patients with advanced gastric cancer 2 had concentrations below the reference range of 10 - 180 ng/mL *5303*
Serum *Increase* In 60 patients with advanced gastric cancer 3 had concentrations below the reference range of 10 - 180 ng/mL *5303*

Immunoglobulin G *Serum* *Decrease* In 60 patients with advanced gastric cancer 2 had concentrations below the reference range of 700 - 1,540 ng/mL *5303*
Serum *Increase* In 60 patients with advanced gastric cancer 6 had concentrations above the reference range of 700 - 1,540 ng/mL *5303*
Serum *No Effect* In 28 men with cancer of the stomach and duodenum mean concentration of 1,058 ± 366 mg/dL not significantly different from 1,148 ± 224 mg/dL in 106 healthy controls and mean concentration of 1,162 ± 415 mg/dL in 10 women with cancer of the stomach and duodenum not significantly different from 1,157 ± 271 mg/dL in 150 healthy control women *2278*

Immunoglobulin M *Serum* *Decrease* In 60 patients with advanced gastric cancer 3 had concentrations below the reference range of 37 - 205 ng/mL *5303*
Serum *Increase* In 60 patients with advanced gastric cancer 3 had concentrations above the reference range of 37 - 204 ng/mL *5303*
Serum *No Effect* In 28 men with cancer of the stomach or duodenum mean concentration of 56 ± 38 mg/dL not significantly different from 61 ± 36 mg/dL in 106 healthy controls and in 10 women with cancer of the stomach or duodenum mean concentration of 57 ± 33 mg/dL not significantly different from 77 ± 39 mg/dL in 150 healthy control women *2278*

Iron *Serum* *Decrease* Chronic occult blood loss *4891* Repeated small blood losses and consequent iron deficiency fully explain the anemia in most cases of gastric carcinoma. The anemia is of the hypochromic, microcytic type with other features of chronic iron deficiency *1980*

Iron-binding Capacity, Total *Serum* *Increase* Anemia is commonly iron deficient type, due to chronic blood loss *4891*

Iron Saturation *Serum* *Decrease* Anemia is commonly iron deficiency type, due to chronic blood loss *4891*

Islet Amyloid Polypeptide *Serum* *No Effect* In 7 patients with gastric cancer mean concentration of 7.7 ± 4.2 pmol/L not significantly different from 8.0 ± 5.0 pmol/L in 25 healthy controls *4210*

Lactate *Blood* *Increase* In 8 patients with localized tumors, mean concentration was 21.5 ± 5.7 mg/dL compared to normal, 11.7 ± 0.72 mg/dL *2513*
Gastric Material *Increase* Elevated in gastric cancer. Overlap between noncancer and cancer patients limits usefulness and specificity *4142* *4891* Greater than 100 g/L in 50% of patients with carcinoma, but in only 2% of patients with gastric ulcer *2033*

Lactate Dehydrogenase *Gastric Material* *Increase* Elevated in gastric cancer. Overlap between noncancer and cancer patients limits usefulness and specificity *4891* Increase in activity is found in carcinoma, measured as U/mL or U secreted/h *1290* In 18 of 23 patients with gastric carcinoma LD activity greater than 500 U/L, but no LD activity observed in 6 cases of gastric malignancy *2312*
Gastric Material *No Effect* In 6 patients with gastric carcinoma no LD activity detected *2312*
Serum *Increase* Marked elevation in 20 patients with tumors of the gastrointestinal tract. Mean activity of 162.0 ± 23.1 U/L compared to 85.4 ± 1.0 U/L in controls *2513*

Laminin *Serum* *Increase* Median serum level of 1,330 mU/mL (n = 10): in control group median of 1,232 mU/mL (n = 42). Elevated in 4 of 10 patients *4394*

Leukocytes *Ascitic Fluid* *Increase* > 1,000 /µL *233*
Blood *Increase* Complicated by degeneration, infection, or metastasis, there may be an elevation of the count and proportionate increase in the percentage of neutrophils. A marked leukocytosis is rare usually associated with malignant invasion of the bone marrow or large infected tumor tissues *1980* In 26% of 47 patients at initial hospitalization for this disorder *1576*
Blood *No Effect* There are no characteristic early changes in the leukocyte count in large malignant tumors of the stomach *1980*

Lymphocytes *Blood* *Decrease* Relative lymphocytopenia may occur as a result of absolute increase in monocytes and polymorphonuclear cells in inflammatory bowel disease *5205* In 60% of 44 patients at initial hospitalization for this disorder *1576*

MCH *Blood* *Decrease* The amount of bleeding and the degree of anemia will vary widely. Anemia of more than moderate degree is a late consequence of gastric malignancy *1980* Anemia may be of several types. The most common is iron deficiency anemia caused by chronic occult blood loss *4891* Iron deficiency anemia most common form of anemia *5544*

MCHC *Blood* *Decrease* The amount of bleeding and the degree of anemia will vary widely. Anemia of more than moderate degree is a late consequence of gastric malignancy *1980* Anemia may be of several types. The most common is iron deficiency anemia caused by chronic blood loss *4891*

MCV *Blood* *Decrease* The anemia is of the hypochromic, microcytic type with other features of chronic iron deficiency *1980*
Blood *Increase* Macrocytic anemia may be seen in patients with gastric carcinoma and untreated pernicious anemia or folate deficiency *4891*

5-Methyl-2'-Deoxycytidine *Urine* *No Effect* In 23 patients with cancer of the stomach mean excretion of 0.77 ± 0.36 nmol/µmol creatinine not significantly different from 0.90 ± 0.43 nmol/µmol creatinine in 81 healthy individuals *2368*

Monocytes *Blood* *Increase* Relative lymphocytopenia may occur as a result of absolute increase in monocytes and

151.90 **Gastric Cancer** *(continued)*

Monocytes *(continued)* polymorphonuclear cells in inflammatory bowel disease *5205* In 69% of 44 patients at initial hospitalization for this disorder *1576*

N², N²-Dimethylguanosine *Urine* *No Effect* In 3 patients with gastric cancer mean excretion of 12.3 µmol/d compared with 16.9 µmol/d in pooled normal urine *3720*

N-Acetylputrescine *Urine* *Increase* In 13 patients with advanced gastric cancer mean concentration of about 40 mg/L significantly greater than that in 32 healthy adults in whom the mean concentration was approximately 8 mg/L *5075*

N-Acetylspermidine *Urine* *Increase* In 13 patients with advanced gastric cancer mean concentration of about 16 mg/L significantly greater than that in 32 healthy adults in whom the mean concentration was approximately 3 mg/L *5075*

Neopterin *Urine* *Increase* Frequency of increased concentrations in patients with gastric cancer 40% *121* In 4 patients with gastric carcinoma mean excretion of about 200 µmol/mol creatinine compared with 106.6 ± 34.6 µmol/mol creatinine in 31 healthy controls *3632*

Neuron-specific Enolase *Serum* *Increase* Increased in 20% of cases of gastrointestinal carcinoma *5546*

Neutrophils *Blood* *Increase* Neutrophilic leukemoid reactions occur most frequently with gastric, bronchogenic, and pancreatic carcinomas *5677*

Occult Blood *Feces* *Increase* Anemia may be of several types. The most common is iron deficiency anemia caused by chronic occult blood loss *4891* Persistence of occult blood in the stool is strong evidence of malignancy but, does not indicate the location of the lesion *1980*
Gastric Material *Increase* Tests for the presence of blood in the gastric contents are positive in a high percentage of cases. Gross blood in the gastric content is a more important finding; found in nearly 50% of the cases *1980*

Ornithine *Plasma* *Increase* In 10 patients with gastric cancer mean concentration increased *3356*

Parathyroid Hormone *Plasma* *Increase* Lung cancer, hypernephroma, gastrointestinal cancer, and other neoplasms can synthesize and secrete parathyroid hormone *1980*

Pepsinogen *Serum* *Decrease* A level < 200 U/L is conclusive of gastric atrophy, a precursor of gastric cancer *1980*

Pepsinogen I *Serum* *Decrease* In patients with antral gastric cancer of intestinal type significant decrease of chief cell mass and serum pepsinogen I observed *4075* Mean concentration in 107 patients with gastric carcinoma of 46.3 ± 42.9 ng/mL with concentration of 39.0 ± 30.6 ng/mL in 49 patients with well-differentiated carcinoma and 51.5 ± 51.9 ng/mL in 55 with low differentiated adenocarcinoma with concentrations lower in patients with metastases. Ratio of PG-I/II decreased with increasing histologic stage *3199*
Serum *No Effect* In 38 patients with gastric cancer mean concentration of 41.0 ± 25.7 µg/L not significantly different from 49.0 ± 30.8 µg/L in 116 healthy controls *2761*
Urine *Increase* Mean concentration in 15 patients who had undergone successful total gastrectomy at least 5 years previously of 17.5 ± 7.4 ng/mL but in 22 of 74 who had undergone gastrectomy results positive and in 20 of the 22 definite clinical evidence of recurrence observed *5773*

Pepsinogen II *Serum* *Increase* In 107 patients with gastric carcinoma mean concentration of 22.5 ± 33.1 ng/mL, with concentration increased in 49 patients with well-differentiated adenocarcinoma to 26.3 ± 47.4 ng/mL compared with 18.8 ± 11.1 ng/mL in 55 patients with low-differentiated adenocarcinoma and in patients with metastases, especially of the liver *3199*
Serum *No Effect* In 38 patients with gastric cancer mean concentration of 21.7 ± 11.2 µg/L not significantly different from 18.1 ± 13.3 µg/L in 116 healthy controls *2761*

pH *Gastric Material* *Decrease* Observed effect *1980* Achlorhydria following histamine or betazole stimulation found in 50% of patients and hypochlorhydria in another 25% of patients *5544*
Gastric Material *Increase* Although rare, does not rule out carcinoma *5544*
Gastric Material *No Effect* Normal in 25% of patients *5544*

Phenylalanine *Plasma* *Increase* In 10 patients with gastric cancer mean concentration increased *3356*

Platelets *Blood* *Increase* In 39% of 35 patients at initial hospitalization for this disorder *1576*

Polymorphic Epithelial Mucin *Serum* *No Effect* In 12 patients with gastric cancer median concentrations of 17 kU/L by ACS BR, 14 kU/L by Centocor CA 15-3, 14 kU/L by Enzymun-Test CA 15-3 and 13 kU/L by IMx CA 15-3 not significantly different from concentrations in 250 healthy women (mean and 1 SD concentrations of 22 ± 8.8 kU/L by ACS BR, 19 ± 8.8 kU/L by Centocor CA 15-3, 17 ± 7.1 kU/L by Enzymun-Test CA 15-3 and 15 ± 6.4 kU/L by IMx CA 15-3 respectively) *513*

Potassium *Serum* *Increase* In 30% of 29 patients at initial hospitalization for this disorder *1576*

Prealbumin *Serum* *Increase* In 60 patients with advanced gastric cancer 9 (15%) had concentrations above the reference range of 14 - 28 mg/L *5303*

Proline *Plasma* *Decrease* In 10 patients with gastric cancer mean concentration reduced *3356*

ProMetalloproteinase-2 *Serum* *Increase* In 70 patients with gastric cancer mean concentration of 601.9 ± 199.7 µg/L significantly greater than 542.0 ± 79.8 µg/L in 70 healthy controls *1361*

ProMetalloproteinase-9 *Plasma* *Increase* In 70 patients with gastric cancer mean concentration of 118.7 ± 232.0 µg/L significantly greater than 36.9 ± 12.9 µg/L in 70 healthy controls *1361*

Protein *Ascitic Fluid* *Increase* > 2.5 g/dL *233*
Serum *Decrease* Enteric loss of plasma protein *4891*

Pseudouridine *Urine* *Increase* In 4 patients with gastric carcinoma mean excretion of about 24 mmol/mol creatinine significantly higher than 19.6 ± 5.2 mmol/mol creatinine in 31 healthy controls *3632*
Urine *No Effect* In 3 patients with gastric cancer mean excretion of 218 µmol/d not significantly different from 207 µmol/d in pooled normal urine *3720*

Putrescine *Urine* *Increase* In 13 patients with advanced gastric cancer mean concentration of about 13 mg/L significantly greater than that in 32 healthy adults in whom the mean concentration was approximately 2 mg/L *5075*

Pyruvate *Blood* *Increase* Elevated in 8 patients with tumors of the gastrointestinal tract, mean = 1.93 ± 0.18 U/L *2513*

Retinol-binding Protein *Serum* *Increase* In 60 patients with advanced gastric cancer 14 (23%) had concentrations above the reference range of 21 - 56 mg/L *5303*

Sialyl-Tn Antigen *Serum* *Increase* In 30 patients with gastric carcinoma 60% had concentrations greater than cut-off value of 45 U/mL *3726*

Sialyltransferase *Serum* *Increase* In 2 patients with cancer of the stomach mean and median concentrations of 649 and 587 cpm/mg protein/30 min significantly different from 240 and 243 cpm/mg protein/30 min respectively in 20 normal individuals *2111*

Soluble CD44⁺ *Serum* *Increase* In 8 patients with nonmetastatic cancer mean concentration of 13 ± 9.6 nmol/L and in 17 with metastatic gastric cancer of 24.2 ± 9.6 nmol/L compared with 2.7 ± 1.1 nmol/L in 43 age and sex matched controls *1918*

Soluble Interleukin-2 Receptor *Serum* *Increase* In 15 cases of stage I gastric cancer, mean concentration of 466 ± 48 U/mL not significantly different from 370 ± 28 U/mL in 29 normal controls but in 8 cases with stage II disease mean concentration of 763 ± 266 U/mL, in 10 with stage III disease of 757 ± 154 U/mL and in 7 stage IV patients mean concentration of 497 ± 64 U/mL, significantly higher than in controls *3662* In 121 patients with gastric cancer mean preoperative concentration of 482 ± 239 U/mL compared with 413 ± 183 U/mL in 98 healthy controls with higher values observed in patients with greater depth of invasion, lymph node metastases and lymphatic or blood vessel invasion and increased severity (higher stage) *4516*

Spermidine *Urine* *Increase* In 13 patients with advanced gastric cancer mean concentration of about 2.3 mg/L significantly greater than that in 32 healthy adults in whom the mean concentration was approximately 0.6 mg/L *5075*

Spermine *Urine* *Increase* In 13 patients with advanced gastric cancer mean concentration of about 5.0 mg/L significantly greater than that in 32 healthy adults in whom the mean concentration was approximately 1.0 mg/L *5075*

Superoxide Dismutase *Blood* *Decrease* Significantly lower in 11 patients with gastric carcinoma than 30 patients with other gastric diseases *5613*

Tennessee Antigen *Serum* *Increase* In patients with gastric cancer, 74% had increased concentration compared with 7% healthy controls who had increased concentrations *3191*

Tissue Polypeptide Antigen *Serum* *Increase* In patients with gastric carcinoma overall positivity rate 50%. When measured in conjunction with CA 50 overall combined positivity rate increased to 81%. There was no evident correlation with stage of disease and the positive serum levels or the median serum levels *5708*

Transferrin *Serum* *Increase* In 60 patients with advanced gastric cancer 10 (17%) had concentrations above the reference range of 230 - 430 mg/L *5303*

Tumor-associated Glycoprotein-72 *Serum* *Increase* In 66 patients with active gastric cancer, concentration increased above 6 U/mL in 47% with median concentration of 9.5 U/mL in stage IV disease compared with 3 U/mL in stage I disease *1482*

Tumor-associated Trypsin Inhibitor *Serum* *Increase* In 93 patients with gastric cancer 46% had concentrations above 30 µg/L, the upper limit observed in 95% of 45 patients with gastroduodenal ulcers. Increased concentrations more common in patients with advanced disease (68% in stage IVB) and in patients with anaplastic tumors *3109*

Uric Acid *Serum* *Increase* In 36% of 47 patients at initial hospitalization for this disorder *1576*

Urokinase Plasminogen Activator *Tissue* *Increase* uPA is a prognostic marker for gastric cancer. High concentrations have been shown to be significantly associated with decreased survival *1252* Amounts are a significant predictor of overall survival *1255*

Valine *Plasma* *Decrease* In 10 patients with gastric cancer mean concentration reduced *3356*

Vitamin B_{12} *Serum* *Decrease* Inadequate absorption, lack of intrinsic factor, loss of gastric mucosa *5544*

Zinc *Serum* *Decrease* Increased in 35 cases of primary malignant tumors, (1.24 ± 0.34 ppm) and plasma zinc decreased (8.83 ± 0.18 ppm) *2341*

151.90 Gastrointestinal Cancer

Acylcarnitine, Acid-insoluble *Serum* *No Effect* In 4 men with gastrointestinal cancer mean concentration of 3.9 ± 0.5 nmol/mL not significantly different from 3.0 ± 0.4 nmol/mL in 6 healthy control men *1195*

Acylcarnitine, Acid-soluble *Serum* *No Effect* In 4 men with gastrointestinal cancer mean concentration of 17.1 ± 1.9 nmol/mL not significantly different from 15.3 ± 2.6 nmol/mL in 6 healthy control men *1195*

CA 19-9 *Serum* *Increase* In 62 patients with gastrointestinal cancer, sensitivity 32.3%, positive predictive value of 90.9% and negative predictive value of 22.2% *1568* Of 204 patients with CA 19-9 concentrations greater than 60 U/mL, 14 had gastrointestinal malignancies other than colorectal cancer *3423*

CA 125 *Serum* *Increase* Using Boehringer Mannheim Enzymun test in 76 patients with gastrointestinal cancer mean concentration of 87.2 ± 133.2 U/mL with 44.7% having concentrations above 35 U/mL *2636*

Calcium *Serum* *No Effect* None of 3 patients with gastrointestinal cancers had hypercalcemia *1200*

Carcinoembryonic Antigen *Serum* *Increase* In 82 patients with gastrointestinal adenocarcinoma increased CEA concentration observed preoperatively in 41.5% patients *1894* In 62 patients with gastrointestinal cancer sensitivity of 40.3%, positive predictive value of 92.5% and negative predictive value of 24.5% *1568*

Carnitine *Serum* *No Effect* In 4 men with gastrointestinal cancer mean concentration of 66.0 ± 4.2 nmol/mL not significantly different from 72.1 ± 7.0 nmol/mL in 6 healthy control men *1195*

Carnitine, Nonesterified *Serum* *Decrease* In 4 men with gastrointestinal cancer mean concentration of 44.9 ± 3.5 nmol/mL not significantly different from 53.7 ± 4.7 nmol/mL in 6 healthy control men *1195*

Casein *Serum* *Increase* Concentration increased to between 120 and 660 µg/L in 7 of 14 patients with gastrointestinal neoplasms *2113*

Epidermal Growth Factor *Urine* *Increase* In 109 patients with cancer of esophagus, stomach, pancreas, colon or with liver metastases excretion increased significantly to median of 30.2 µg/g creatinine compared with 20.8 µg/g creatinine in 40 healthy controls *844*

α-Fetoprotein *Serum* *Increase* In 83 patients with gastrointestinal cancer 98.8% had concentrations up to 15.0 ng/mL, 0.0% had concentrations between 15.1 - 20.0 ng/mL, 0.0% between 20.1 - 100 ng/mL, 0.0% had concentrations between 100.1 - 350.0 ng/mL and 1.2% had concentrations above 350.0 ng/mL in contrast to concentrations in 400 healthy individuals in whom 99.2% had concentrations between 0 and 15.0 ng/mL, 0.2% between 15.1 and 20.0 ng/mL and 0.5% between 20.1 and 100 ng/mL *11*

Occult Blood *Feces* *Increase* In 124 patients who presented at an ER with gastrointestinal bleeding 3.2% had GI cancer *1383*

Parathyroid Hormone-related Peptide *Plasma* *No Effect* In 3 patients with gastrointestinal cancer and normocalcemia mean concentration of 1.55 pmol/L below upper limit of reference range of 2.6 pmol/L *1200*

Phosphohexoseisomerase *Serum* *Increase* It is 70% specific and 92% sensitive if greater than 20 U/L *2811*

Prostate-specific Antigen *Serum* *Increase* Of 58 patients with gastrointestinal cancer. 93.1% had values below upper limit of normal of 4.0 ng/mL as measured by method on Bayer Technicon Immuno 1®, 5.2% had values between 4.0 and 10.0 ng/mL and 1.7% had values between 10.0 and 40.0 ng/mL *342*

Tissue Factor Pathway Inhibitor *Plasma* *Increase* About half of patients with gastrointestinal tumors had activities greater than median activity of 1.19 U/mL in healthy individuals *2376*

Transforming Growth Factor-α *Urine* *Increase* In 109 patients with cancer of esophagus, stomach, pancreas, colon or with liver metastases excretion increased significantly to median of 27.2 µg/g creatinine compared with 10.3 µg/g creatinine in 40 healthy controls *844*

Tumor-associated Glycoprotein-72 *Serum* *Increase* In 82 patients with gastrointestinal adenocarcinoma increased concentration of TAG-72 observed in 39% patients preoperatively *1894*

152.90 Cancer of Small Intestine

Aldolase *Serum* *Increase* Significantly elevated in tumors of the gastrointestinal tract. Mean = 4.9 ± 0.8 U/L compared to normal, 1.6 ± 0.21 U/L *2513*

Carcinoembryonic Antigen *Ascitic Fluid* *Increase* CEA > 10 ng/mL ascites indicating cancerous effusion *3102*
Peritoneal Fluid *Increase* The highest levels (> 1,000 ng/mL) were found in samples from patients with gastrointestinal carcinomas *1295*
Pleural Fluid *Increase* 24 (34%) of 70 malignant effusions had levels > 12 ng/mL *4369* The highest levels (> 1,000 ng/mL) were found in samples from patients with gastrointestinal carcinomas *1295*
Serum *Increase* Increased concentration observed in two-thirds of patients *4551* Majority of patients has increased concentration *1601* In 66% of patients with localized upper GI tract malignancy, mean concentration of 4.9 ng/mL *4130*

Complement C_3 *Serum* *Increase* Increased in patients with local disease. Very closely linked to the stage of the disease. Patients in remission had normal levels, but further increases were noted in distant metastases. Levels dropped significantly in the terminal phase of the disease *5456*

Complement C_4 *Serum* *Increase* Increased in patients with local disease. Very closely linked to the stage of the disease. Patients in remission had normal levels, but further increases were noted in distant metastases. Levels dropped significantly in the terminal phase of disease *5456*

Erythrocytes *Ascitic Fluid* *Increase* > 10,000 cells/µL seen in 20% of cases *233*

Hematocrit *Blood* *Decrease* Anemia may be of several types. The most common is iron deficiency anemia caused by chronic occult blood loss *4891*

Hemoglobin *Blood* *Decrease* Anemia may be of several types. The most common is iron deficiency anemia caused by chronic occult blood loss *4891*

152.90 Cancer of Small Intestine (continued)

Hexokinase *Serum Increase* Increased in gastrointestinal tumors. Mean activity of 15.3 ± 3.5 U/L compared to normal of 0.93 ± 0.28 U/L *2513*

Iron *Serum Decrease* Anemia is common iron deficiency type, due to chronic blood loss *4891*

Iron-binding Capacity, Total *Serum Increase* Anemia is common iron deficiency type, due to chronic blood loss *4891*

Iron Saturation *Serum Decrease* Anemia is commonly iron deficient type, due to chronic blood loss *4891*

Lactate *Blood Increase* In 8 patients with tumors of the gastrointestinal tract, mean concentration was 21.5 ± 5.7 mg/dL compared to normal, 11.7 ± 0.72 mg/dL *2513*

Lactate Dehydrogenase *Serum Increase* Marked elevation in 20 patients, mean activity of 162.0 - 23.1 U/L compared to 85.4 ± 1.0 U/L in controls *2513*

Leukocytes *Ascitic Fluid Increase* > 1,000 /µL *233*

MCH *Blood Decrease* Iron deficiency anemia is common because of either gross or occult bleeding *4891*

MCHC *Blood Decrease* Iron deficiency anemia is common because of either gross or occult bleeding *4891*

MCV *Blood Decrease* Iron deficiency anemia is common because of either gross or occult bleeding *4891*

N^2, N^2-Dimethylguanosine *Urine No Effect* Mean excretion in 4 patients with intestinal cancer of 13.8 µmol/d compared with 16.9 µmol/d in pooled normal urine *3720*

Occult Blood *Feces Increase* Anemia may be of several types. The most common is iron deficiency anemia caused by chronic occult blood loss *4891* Persistence of occult blood in the stool is strong evidence of malignancy, but does not indicate the location of the lesion *1980*

Parathyroid Hormone *Plasma Increase* Lung cancer, hypernephroma, gastrointestinal cancer, and other neoplasms can synthesize and secrete parathyroid hormone *1980*

Protein *Ascitic Fluid Increase* > 2.5 g/dL *233*
Serum Decrease Enteric loss of plasma protein *4891*

Pseudouridine *Urine No Effect* In 4 patients with intestinal cancer mean excretion of 222 µmol/d not significantly different from 207 µmol/d in pooled normal urine *3720*

Pyruvate *Blood Increase* Moderately elevated in 8 patients, mean = 1.93 ± 0.18 U/L *2513*

153.30 Cancer of Sigmoid Colon

Creatine Kinase, Mitochondrial *Serum No Effect* Median concentration of 11 U/L in 5 patients not different from normal range of 4 - 15 U/L *3892*

153.90 Cancer of Colon

Adenosine Deaminase *Serum Increase* Ninety-one percent of 527 patients with tumors showed activity above normal, whereas eighty-six per cent of 408 nontumorous diseased persons did not *2737 5041*

Albumin *Serum Decrease* In 28% of 149 patients at initial hospitalization for this disorder *1576* Significantly reduced (median of 35.7 g/L compared to controls, 44.0 g/L) *2109*
Urine Increase 24 h excretion and renal clearance were significantly increased in localized tumor patients compared to normals and disseminated cancer cases. Increased high molecular weight protein excretion implies glomerular injury in these patients *2109*

Aldolase *Serum Increase* Significantly elevated in tumors of the gastrointestinal tract. Mean = 4.9 ± 0.8 U/L compared to normal, 1.6 ± 0.21 U/L *2513*

Alkaline Phosphatase *Serum Increase* In 24% of 150 patients at initial hospitalization for this disorder *1576* About 20% of patients have increased activity *2033*
White Blood Cells Decrease Low activity is present irrespective of tumor category, activity of disease, or type of therapy. In 11 patients median value was 18 U/L (normal 55 U/L) *3110*

Alkaline Phosphatase Isoenzymes *Serum Increase* Increased incidence of the Regan (placental) isoenzyme *1497* 13.25% had increased concentration of the Regan isoenzyme, ranging from 7.17 - 24.3 U/L *1140*

Arginase *Serum Increase* Serum levels from 31 patients with colorectal adenocarcinoma were determined by using enzyme immunoassay. The levels (mean 18.96 ng/mL) were significantly higher than levels from control subjects (n = 115; mean 3.09 ng/mL) *3005*

Arylsulfatase *Urine Increase* Urinary arylsulfatase B was observed in high concentrations in patients with colon carcinoma. Increased activity correlated with the extent of disease. Elevations were observed in only 28% of patients with Dukes' A disease. 55% of those with Dukes' B, and in more than 75% of patients with Dukes' C and D lesions *4692*

CA 19-9 *Serum Increase* Frequently show elevated values *2026* Concentration typically increased in patients with colon cancer *2952* Frequently show elevated values *3657*

CA 50 *Serum Increase* Elevated in a high proportion of patients with primary carcinoma *2211*

CA 72-4 *Serum Increase* Sensitivity of 32% (n = 53). CA 72-4 has a very high specificity (98%) in benign diseases of the gastrointestinal tract, including inflammatory processes, so that elevated serum levels should always be taken seriously *2122* In colon carcinomas 30.9% of specimens showed elevated levels *5744*

CA 195 *Serum Increase* A rising level after operation suggested recurrence of the tumor *4508*

CA 242 *Serum Increase* Elevated in 55% of patients with colorectal cancer *2870*

CA 549 *Serum Increase* In 133 patients with cancer of the colon 13 (9.8%) had a concentration greater than the upper limit of normal with BRESMARQ assay *764*

Carcinoembryonic Antigen *Ascitic Fluid Increase* Ascitic fluid assays detected 11 of 13 cases; (CEA > 10 ng/mL ascites indicating cancerous effusion) *3102*
Peritoneal Fluid Increase The highest levels (> 1,000 ng/mL were found in patients with gastrointestinal carcinomas *1295*
Pleural Fluid Increase 24 (34%) of 70 malignant effusions had levels > 12 ng/mL *4369* The highest levels (> 1,000 ng/mL) were found in patients with gastrointestinal carcinomas *1295*
Serum Increase Increase observed in about two-thirds of patients *4551* Increased in about 80% of the patients *5544* Increase observed in majority of patients *1601* 55% of patients had elevated concentrations (mean of 6.3 ng/mL). 91% of patients had positive plasma assays *1714* In 73% of cases *4891* In 66% of patients with localized upper GI tract malignancy, mean concentration of 4.9 ng/mL *4130*
Tissue Increase Using FNA mean concentration of 581.3 ng/mL observed in first drop of aspirated material in 12 patients *4139*

Catalase *Red Blood Cells Increase* In 6 patients with bowel cancer mean activity of 2.05 g hemoglobin/s significantly greater than that in 6 healthy blood donors in whom mean activity was 1.50 g hemoglobin/s *3346*
Red Blood Cells No Effect In 6 patients with gastric cancer mean activity of 1.40 g hemoglobin/s not significantly different from that in 6 healthy blood donors in whom mean activity was 1.50 g hemoglobin/s *3346*

Cholesterol *Feces Increase* Fecal excretion of cholesterol, coprostanol, coprostanone, total bile acids, deoxycholic acid, lithocholic acid was higher in colonic cancer and adenomatous polyps compared to normal controls as well as in patients with other digestive diseases *4301*
Serum Decrease The mean levels were lower (202.2 mg/dL) than controls (219.5 mg/dL). Patients with Duke B stage cancer accounted for most of the difference *3763*

β-Chorionic Gonadotropin *Plasma Increase* Ectopic production *602 552 3777 455*

Complement C_3 *Serum Increase* Increased in patients with local disease. Found to be very closely linked to the stage of the disease. Patients in remission had normal levels, but further increases were noted in distant metastases. Dropped significantly in the terminal phase of disease *5456*

Complement C_4 *Serum Increase* Increased in patients with local disease. Very closely linked to the stage of the disease. Patients in remission had normal levels, but further increases were noted in distant metastases. Levels dropped significantly in the terminal phase of disease *5456*

Complement, Total *Serum Increase* Found to be very closely linked to stage of disease. Patients in remission had normal levels, but further increases were noted in distant metastases. Levels dropped significantly in the terminal phase of disease *5456*

Copper *Serum Increase* Increased in 35 cases of primary malignant tumors of the digestive organs, (mean = 1.24 ± 0.34 ppm) *2341*

Copper Zinc Superoxide Dismutase *Serum Increase* Significantly elevated in patients with various digestive cancers *3886*

Creatine Kinase *Serum Increase* Highest activity of CK-BB in brain and smooth muscle *2912*

Creatine Kinase MB-Isoenzyme *Serum Increase* Ectopic production *768 141*

Creatinine *Serum Increase* In 34% of 63 patients at initial hospitalization for this disorder *1576*

Cryofibrinogen *Plasma Increase* Reported effect *4551 3417*

Deoxycholic Acid *Feces Increase* The fecal excretion of cholesterol, coprostanol, coprostanone, total bile acids, deoxycholic acid, lithocholic acid was higher in colonic cancer and adenomatous polyps compared to normal controls as well as in patients with other digestive diseases *4301*

α-Enolase *Serum No Effect* In 0 of 8 cases of breast cancer mean activity increased *1705*

γ-Enolase *Serum Increase* In 1 of 8 cases of colon cancer mean activity increased *1705*

Erythrocyte Sedimentation Rate *Blood Increase* Increased in significant tissue necrosis. Extreme elevation frequently occurs. Indicates inflammation *5544* Occurs with inflammation *1980*

Erythrocytes *Ascitic Fluid Increase* > 10,000 cells/μL seen in 20% of cases *233*

α-Fetoprotein *Serum Increase* Elevated in 5% of cases *2913*

Fucose *Serum Increase* In 17 patients, mean value was 11.79 ± 0.72 mg/dL (normal = 6.84 ± 0.13 mg/dL) *2899*

Galactosyltransferase Isoenzyme II *Serum Increase* Sensitivity 0.63 and specificity 0.79 *5348*

Gc-Globulin *Serum No Effect* In 66 men and 61 women with cancer of the colon and rectum mean concentrations of 23.4 ± 4.44 mg/dL and 25.2 ± 4.51 mg/dL not significantly different from 23.9 ± 3.36 mg/dL in 106 control men and 26.1 ± 4.66 mg/dL in 150 control women *2279*

α_2-Globulin *Serum Increase* Increased plasma concentrations in primary cancer. Haptoglobin values were especially useful to indicate tumor activity *928*

β-Glucuronidase *Serum Increase* Increased *1498 1777*

Haptoglobin *Serum Increase* Increased in patients (2.2 g/L) compared to normals (1.1 g/L) *2109* Increased in primary cancer, and rises in metastatic cancer especially involving the liver. Values are useful to indicate tumor activity *928*
Urine Increase 24 h excretion and renal clearance were significantly increased in localized tumor patients compared to normals and disseminated cancer cases. Increased high molecular weight protein excretion implies glomerular injury in these patients *2109*

Hematocrit *Blood Decrease* Iron deficiency anemia is common, because of either gross or occult bleeding *4891* Anemia; may be the only symptom of carcinoma of the right side of colon (present in > 50% of these patients, usually hypochromic) *5544* Incidence of anemia between 22 - 74.6% *4891* In 35% of 154 patients at initial hospitalization for this disorder *1576*

Hemoglobin *Blood Decrease* Anemia; may be the only symptom of carcinoma of the right side of colon (present in > 50% of these patients; usually hypochromic *5544* In 45% of 153 patients at initial hospitalization for this disorder *1576* Incidence of anemia between 22 - 74.6%. Iron deficiency anemia is common, because of either gross or occult bleeding *4891*

Hexokinase *Serum Increase* Increased in gastrointestinal tumors. Mean activity of 15.3 ± 3.5 U/L compared to normal of 0.93 ± 0.28 U/L *2513*

β-Hexosaminidase *Serum Increase* Elevated isoenzyme B *4989*

HIV p53 Antigen *Plasma Increase* In 22 cases mean concentration of 0.55 ng/mL with mean in 4 cases with Dukes' stage A 0.60 ng/mL and 0.69 ng/mL with Dules' stages B to D compared with mean of 0.12 ng/mL in 47 healthy controls *3166*

25-Hydroxy Vitamin D *Serum No Effect* Mean concentration of 59.8 ± 3.2 nmol/L not significantly different from 55.8 ± 1.9 nmol/L in 158 healthy control individuals *1749*

immunoglobulin A *Serum Increase* In 66 men with cancer of the colon or rectum mean concentration of 288 ± 190 mg/dL significantly different from 201 ± 89 mg/dL in 106 healthy controls and mean concentration of 215 ± 111 mg/dL in 10 women with cancer of the colon or rectum significantly different from 176 ± 80 mg/dL in 150 healthy control women *2278*
Urine Increase 24 h excretion and renal clearance were significantly increased in localized tumor patients compared to normals and disseminated cancer cases. Increased high molecular weight protein excretion implies glomerular injury in these patients *2109*

Immunoglobulin G *Serum No Effect* In 66 men with cancer of the colon and rectum mean concentration of 1,222 ± 304 mg/dL not significantly different from 1,148 ± 224 mg/dL in 106 healthy controls and mean concentration of 1,249 ± 414 mg/dL in 61 women with cancer of the colon and rectum not significantly different from 1,157 ± 271 mg/dL in 150 healthy control women *2278*
Urine Increase 24 h excretion and renal clearance were significantly increased in localized tumor patients compared to normals and disseminated cancer cases. Increased high molecular weight protein excretion implies glomerular injury in these patients *2109*

Immunoglobulin M *Serum No Effect* In 66 men with cancer of the colon or rectum mean concentration of 74 ± 52 mg/dL not significantly different from 61 ± 36 mg/dL in 106 healthy controls and in 61 women with cancer of the colon or rectum mean concentration of 77 ± 58 mg/dL not significantly different from 77 ± 39 mg/dL in 150 healthy control women *2278*
Urine Increase 24 h excretion and renal clearance were significantly increased in localized tumor patients compared to normals and disseminated cancer cases. Increased high molecular weight protein excretion implies glomerular injury in these patients *2109*

Insulin-like Growth Factor-I *Serum No Effect* In 175 patients with colonic cancer mean concentration of 25.7 ± 0.7 pmol/mL (25.6 ± 0.7 pmol/mL in 146 patients with adenomas and 26.2 ± 1.8 pmol/mL in 29 with carcinomas) compared with 24.0 ± 0.7 pmol/mL in 159 control patients *1750*

Iron *Serum Decrease* Iron deficiency anemia is common, because of either gross or occult bleeding *4891* In 57% of 19 patients at initial hospitalization for this disorder *1576*

Iron-binding Capacity, Total *Serum Decrease* In 10% of 19 patients at initial hospitalization for this disorder *1576* Significantly reduced (median of 2.6 mg/L) compared to controls (3.4 mg/L). 24 h excretion and renal clearance of transferrin were significantly increased in localized tumor patients compared to normals and disseminated cancer cases. Increased high molecular weight protein excretion implies glomerular injury in these patients *2109*

Iron Saturation *Serum Decrease* In 67% of 19 patients at initial hospitalization for this disorder *1576*

Lactate *Blood Increase* In patients with tumors of the gastrointestinal tract, mean concentration was 21.5 ± 5.7 mg/dL compared to normal, 11.7 ± 0.72 mg/dL *2513*

Lactate Dehydrogenase *Serum Increase* Observed effect *2033* Marked elevation in 20 patients, mean activity of 162.0 U/L (compared to 85.4 ± 1.0 U/L in controls) *2513*

Laminin *Serum Increase* Median serum concentration of 14,575 mU/mL (n = 19). Control group median of 1,232 mU/mL (n = 42). Elevated in 10 of 19 patients *4394*

Leukocytes *Ascitic Fluid Increase* > 1,000 /μL *233*
Blood Increase In 25% of 154 patients at initial hospitalization for this disorder *1576* May be noted in patients with inflammatory complications, such as necrosis of tumor, or local colonic perforation *4891*

Lithocholic Acid *Feces Increase* The fecal excretion of cholesterol, coprostanol, coprostanone, total bile acids, deoxycholic acid, lithocholic acid was higher in colonic cancer and adenomatous polyps compared to normal controls as well as in patients with other digestive diseases *4301*

153.90 Cancer of Colon *(continued)*

MCH *Blood* *Decrease* Anemia; may be the only symptom of carcinoma of the right side of the colon (present in > 50% of these patients, usually hypochromic) *5544* Iron deficiency anemia is common because of either gross or occult bleeding *4891*

MCHC *Blood* *Decrease* Anemia; may be the only symptom of carcinoma of the right colon (present in > 50% of these patients, usually hypochromic) *5544* Iron deficiency anemia is common because of either gross or occult bleeding *4891*

MCV *Blood* *Decrease* Many patients have chronic iron deficiency anemia characterized by hypochromic microcytic red cells *4891*

5-Methyl-2'-Deoxycytidine *Urine* *No Effect* In 8 patients with cancer of the colon mean excretion of 1.05 ± 0.32 nmol/μmol creatinine not significantly different from 0.90 ± 0.43 nmol/μmol creatinine in 81 healthy individuals *2368*

Monocytes *Blood* *Increase* In 57% of 150 patients at initial hospitalization for this disorder *1576*

Neopterin *Urine* *Increase* In 7 patients with carcinoma of the colon mean excretion of about 600 μmol/mol creatinine significantly greater than 106.6 ± 34.6 μmol/mol creatinine in 31 healthy controls *3632*

Neuron-specific Enolase *Serum* *Increase* Increased in 20% of cases of gastrointestinal carcinoma *5546*

Occult Blood *Feces* *Increase* GI bleeding may occur with malignancies *4891* The most important screening test for cancer of the large bowel in asymptomatic persons *5694*

p53 Autoantibodies *Serum* *Increase* Presence of p53 antibodies associated with worse prognosis *5640*

Parathyroid Hormone *Plasma* *Increase* Lung cancer, hypernephroma, gastrointestinal cancer, and other neoplasms can synthesize and secrete parathyroid hormone *1980*

Platelets *Blood* *Increase* In 30% of 118 patients at initial hospitalization for this disorder *1576*

Potassium *Serum* *Decrease* Villous tumor of rectum may cause depletion *5544* In 105 patients with adenocarcinoma of the colon or rectum obtained preoperatively showed hypokalemia in 3 patients *4883*

Protein *Ascitic Fluid* *Increase* > 2.5 g/dL *233*
Serum *Decrease* Enteric loss of plasma protein *4891* May be lower than normal in carcinoma of colon *4891*

Pseudouridine *Urine* *No Effect* In 7 patients with carcinoma of the colon mean excretion comparable to that in 31 healthy controls, 19.6 ± 5.2 mmol/mol creatinine *3632*

Putrescine *Urine* *Increase* In 120 patients with colon cancer 46 (26%) had increased excretion above normal *4689*

Pyruvate *Blood* *Increase* Moderately elevated in 8 patients with tumors of the gastrointestinal tract. Mean = 1.93 ± 0.18 U/L *2513*

Sialic Acid, Lipid-associated *Serum* *Increase* In 6 patients with early stage colon cancer mean concentration of 42.3 mg/dL significantly different from 17.7 mg/dL in 50 normal volunteers *1273*

Sialyltransferase *Serum* *Increase* In 18 patients with cancer of the colon mean and median concentrations of 492 and 454 cpm/mg protein/30 min significantly different from 240 and 243 cpm/mg protein/30 min respectively in 20 normal individuals *2111*

Soluble CD44+ *Serum* *Increase* Mean concentration in 10 patients without metastatic disease of 5.6 ± 4.4 nmol/L and of 30.8 ± 11.4 nmol/L in 15 patients with metastatic disease significantly different from 2.7 ± 1.1 nmol/L in 43 age and sex matched controls *1918*

Soluble Urokinase Receptor *Serum* *Increase* In citrated specimens from 10 patients with Duke's stage D cancer concentrations of 1.4 to 4.7 μg/L (10th to 90th percentile range) significantly greater than reference range of 1.2 - 1.9 μg/L in 44 healthy donors *5006*

Spermidine *Urine* *Increase* In 120 patients with colon cancer 59 (49%) had increased excretion above normal *4689*

Spermine *Urine* *Increase* In 109 patients with colon cancer 75 (63%) had increased excretion above normal *4689*

Uric Acid *Serum* *Increase* In 35% of 149 patients at initial hospitalization for this disorder *1576*

Zinc *Serum* *Decrease* In 35 cases of primary malignant tumors of the digestive organs, plasma concentrations were decreased 0.83 ± 0.18 ppm *2341*

154.10 Cancer of Rectum

Aldolase *Serum* *Increase* Significantly elevated in tumors of the gastrointestinal tract. Mean = 4.9 ± 0.8 U/L compared to normal, 1.6 ± 0.21 U/L *2513*

Androgens *Urine* *Decrease* Significantly decreased, 1.86 ± 0.20 mg/g creatinine in 16 male patients *5180*

Androsterone *Urine* *Decrease* Significantly decreased, 1.86 ± 0.20 mg/g creatinine in 16 male patients *5180*

Arginase *Serum* *Increase* Serum levels from 31 patients with colorectal adenocarcinoma were determined by using enzyme immunoassay. The levels (mean 18.96 ng/mL) were significantly higher than levels from control subjects (n = 115; mean 3.09 ng/mL) *3005*

CA 19-9 *Serum* *Increase* Showed a sensitivity of 60.1% and a specificity of 87.9% *294*

Carcinoembryonic Antigen *Ascitic Fluid* *Increase* CEA > 10 ng/mL ascites indicating cancerous effusion *3102*
Peritoneal Fluid *Increase* The highest levels (> 1,000 ng/mL) were found in patients with gastrointestinal carcinomas *1295*
Pleural Fluid *Increase* The highest levels (> 1,000 ng/mL) were found in samples from patients with gastrointestinal carcinomas *1295* 24 (34%) of 70 malignant effusions had levels > 12 ng/mL *4369*
Serum *Increase* In 73% of cases *4891* In 66% of patients with localized upper GI tract malignancy, mean concentration of 4.9 ng/mL *4130* Increases observed in two-thirds patients *4551* Majority of patients have increased concentrations *1601*

Complement C_3 *Serum* *Increase* Increased in patients with local disease. Found to be very closely linked to the stage of the disease. Patients in remission had normal levels, but further increases were noted in distant metastases. Dropped significantly in the terminal phase of disease *5456*

Complement C_4 *Serum* *Increase* Increased in patients with local disease. Very closely linked to the stage of the disease. Patients in remission had normal levels, but further increases were noted in distant metastases. Levels dropped significantly in the terminal phase of disease *5456*

Creatine Kinase, Mitochondrial *Serum* *No Effect* Median concentration of 10 U/L in 4 patients not different from normal range of 4 - 15 U/L *3892*

α-Enolase *Serum* *No Effect* In 1 of 6 cases of rectal cancer mean activity increased *1705*

γ-Enolase *Serum* *Increase* In 1 of 6 cases of rectal cancer mean activity increased *1705*

Galactosyltransferase Isoenzyme II *Serum* *Increase* Sensitivity 0.63 and specificity 0.79 *5348*

α_2-Globulin *Serum* *Increase* alpha$_2$-Globulins, especially haptoglobins, were generally increased in primary colorectal cancer, and the liver. Haptoglobin values were useful to indicate tumor activity *928*

Hematocrit *Blood* *Decrease* Iron deficiency anemia is common, because of either gross or occult bleeding *4891*

Hemoglobin *Blood* *Decrease* Iron deficiency anemia is common, because of either gross or occult bleeding *4891*

Hexokinase *Serum* *Increase* Increased in gastrointestinal tumors. Mean activity of 15.3 ± 3.5 U/L compared to normal of 0.93 ± 0.28 U/L *2513*

β-Hexosaminidase *Serum* *Increase* Elevated isoenzyme B *4989*

Iron *Serum* *Decrease* Iron deficiency anemia is common, because of either gross or occult bleeding *4891*

Iron-binding Capacity, Total *Serum* *Increase* Anemia is commonly iron deficient, due to chronic blood loss *4891*

Iron Saturation *Serum* *Decrease* Anemia is commonly iron deficient type, due to chronic blood loss *4891*

Leukocytes *Blood* *Increase* May be noted in patients with inflammatory complications of their carcinoma, such as necrosis of tumor, or local colonic perforation *4891*

MCH *Blood* *Decrease* Iron deficiency anemia is common because of either gross or occult bleeding *4891*

MCHC *Blood Decrease* Iron deficiency anemia is common because of either gross or occult bleeding *4891*

MCV *Blood Decrease* Many patients have chronic iron deficiency anemia characterized by hypochromic microcytic red cells *4891*

Monocytes *Blood Increase* In 59% of 74 patients at initial hospitalization for this disorder *1576*

Neopterin *Urine Increase* In 10 patients with adenocarcinoma of the rectum mean excretion of 609.1 μmol/mol creatinine significantly greater than 106.6 ± 34.6 μmol/mol creatinine in 31 healthy controls *3632*

Occult Blood *Feces Increase* GI bleeding may occur with malignancies *4891* The most important screening test for cancer of the large bowel in asymptomatic persons *5694*

Protein *Serum Decrease* May be lower than normal in carcinoma of colon *4891*

Pseudouridine *Urine Increase* In 10 patients with adenocarcinoma of the rectum mean excretion of about 25 mmol/mol creatinine compared with 19.6 ± 5.2 mmol/mol creatinine in 31 healthy controls *3632*

Sialyltransferase *Serum Increase* In 5 patients with cancer of the rectum mean and median concentrations of 376 and 300 cpm/mg protein/30 min significantly different from 240 and 243 cpm/mg protein/30 min respectively in 20 normal individuals *2111*

Tissue Plasminogen Activator *Plasma Increase* Showed a sensitivity of 78.8% and a specificity of 60.6% *294*

Uric Acid *Serum Increase* In 43% of 73 patients at initial hospitalization for this disorder *1576*

154.20 Anal Squamous Cell Sarcoma

Calcium *Serum Increase* In one study of 42 patients with hypercalcemia and low intact PTH concentration, 1 had an anal squamous cell carcinoma *3280*

Parathyroid Hormone *Plasma Decrease* In one study of 42 patients with low intact PTH concentration and hypercalcemia 1 patient had anal squamous cell carcinoma *3280*

154.80 Colorectal Cancer

α_1-Acid Glycoprotein *Serum Increase* In patients with colorectal or gastric cancer mean concentration of 2.04 g/L compared with less than 0.50 g/L in healthy controls *719*

Amyloid A Protein *Serum Increase* In patients with gastric or colorectal cancer mean concentration of 312 mg/L compared with less than 1 mg/L in healthy controls *719*

Anti-p53 Antibodies *Serum Increase* Increase observed in 12 of 82 patients (14.6%) *132* Antibodies detected in 32 of 47 (68%) of patients with colorectal cancer. 48% of 33 patients both circulating p53-antibodies and p53 expression in the tumor were observed *4792*

α_1-Antichymotrypsin *Serum Increase* In patients with colorectal or gastric cancer mean concentration of 0.99 g/L compared with less than 0.50 g/L in healthy controls *719*

α_1-Antitrypsin *Feces Increase* 57% of patients with colorectal cancer had results greater than 95% normal dry weight values of a symptomatic control group and 48% had concentrations higher than the wet weight in the control population. Wet weight concentrations in the cancer group were higher in 62% than 95% of an asymptomatic control group *3593* Mean concentration in 20 patients with colorectal cancer 786.8 μg/g (150.82 mg/d) not significantly different from 327.4 μg/g (47.43 mg/d) in 20 healthy controls *4521*

Arginine *Plasma Decrease* In 10 patients with colorectal cancer mean concentration decreased *3356*

Aspartic Acid *Plasma Decrease* In 10 patients with colorectal cancer mean concentration reduced *3356*

c-erb-B_2 Oncoprotein *Serum Increase* Median concentration of < 3 ng/mL in 4 patients with locoregional cancer, and 10 ng/mL in 10 with metastatic cancer. 0 of 4 (0%) of patients with locoregional disease and 3 of 10 (30%) with metastases had concentrations exceeding 1.5 ng/mL *3564*

CA 15-3 *Serum Increase* In 36 patients with colorectal cancer mean concentration of 31.8 ± 25 U/mL higher than cutoff of 22 U/mL, with 22 having concentrations above 22 U/mL, 16 with concentrations above 30 U/mL and 6 with concentrations above 40 U/mL *2076*
Serum No Effect In 36 patients with colorectal cancer average concentration of 13.4 U/mL not significantly higher than in healthy individuals *1683*

CA 19-9 *Serum Increase* In 36 patients with colorectal cancer average concentration of 59.9 U/mL significantly higher than in healthy individuals *1683* Of 204 patients with CA 19-9 concentrations greater than 60 U/mL, 52 had colorectal cancer *3423* Mean concentration of 10,948 ± 5,222 U/mL in 52 patients with advanced colorectal carcinoma significantly different from < 37 U/mL in 25 age- and sex-matched healthy volunteer controls *4043* In 39 patients with colorectal cancer positive rate of 26% observed using cut-off from normals and 18% at 90% specificity *2594* CA 19-9 concentration increased above 37 U/mL in 46% of 164 patients with Dukes C and D stages, but in only 8% of 25 patients with stages A and B disease *1253* In 10% of 10 patients with Dukes' stage A disease concentration increased and in 57% of 30 patients with Dukes' stage D increased *5406*
Tissue Increase In 34 patients with colorectal cancer average concentration in tumor tissue of 86.4 U/g significantly higher than 2.9 U/g in healthy colonic mucosa *1683* In 34 patients with colorectal cancer average concentration in tumor tissue of 123,084 U/g significantly higher than 1,178 U/g in healthy colonic mucosa *1683*

CA 27-29 *Serum Increase* In 13% of 16 patients with cancer of colon concentration increased above 36 U/mL *766*

CA 50 *Serum Increase* In 20 patients with stage 1 disease mean concentration of 7.7 ± 6.6 U/L, in 28 with stage 2 disease 9.6 ± 8.2 U/L, in 14 with stage 3 disease 36.5 U/L and in 25 with stage 4 disease 83.0 ± 142.8 U/L *4103*

CA 72-4 *Serum Increase* In 200 patients with colorectal cancers 86 (43.0%) had concentrations above 6 U/mL *1896* Approximately 40% of patients with colorectal cancer had increased concentrations *1668* In 78 patients with colorectal cancer 43 (55%) had a concentration less than 2.5 U/mL, 35 (41%) had a concentration greater than 2.5 U/mL and 20 (25%) had a concentration greater than 10 U/mL *4505*

CA 125 *Serum No Effect* In 34 patients with colorectal cancer average concentration of 9.2 U/mL not significantly higher than in healthy individuals *1683*
Tissue Increase In 34 patients with colorectal cancer average concentration in tumor tissue of 615 U/g significantly higher than 9.2 U/g in healthy colonic mucosa *1683*

CA 195 *Serum Increase* Increased concentrations observed in patients with colorectal cancer *122*

CA 242 *Serum Increase* Significantly poorer survival observed in patients with concentration greater than 20 U/mL *698* In 20 patients with stage 1 disease mean concentration of 5.3 ± 3.7 U/L, in 28 with stage 2 disease 8.9 ± 8.1 U/L, in 14 with stage 3 disease 54.7 ± 104 U/L and in 25 with stage 4 disease 166 ± 305.5 U/L *4103* In 39 patients with colorectal cancer positive rate of 31% observed using cut-off from normals and 41% at 90% specificity *2594*

CA-M43 *Serum Increase* In none of 10 patients with Dukes stage A disease was a positive result detected but in 77% of 30 patients with Dukes stage D disease results were positive *5406*

Carcinoembryonic Antigen *Bile Increase* 18 patients with local recurrence or extrahepatic metastases had concentrations above 5 ng/mL (range 8 to 848 ng/mL) and less than 5 ng/mL in 11 patients without invasive colorectal cancer *4040* In 30 patients with colorectal cancer and metastases mean concentration of 2,523 μg/L (range 6.0 - 35,760) significantly higher than mean of 1.6 μg/L (range 1.2 - 3.0) in 10 controls *4039*
Serum Increase In 135 patients with colorectal cancer 31.9% had concentrations up to 3.0 ng/mL, 9.6% had concentrations between 3.1 - 5.0 ng/mL, 11.1% between 5.1 - 10.0 ng/mL and 47.4% had concentrations greater than 10.1 ng/mL in contrast to concentrations in 151 healthy nonsmokers in whom 95.4% had concentrations between 0 and 3.0 ng/mL and 4.6% between 4.1 and 10.0 ng/mL *11* Mean concentration of 692 ± 259 ng/mL in 52 patients with advanced colorectal carcinoma significantly different from < 5 ng/mL in 25 age- and sex-matched healthy volunteer controls *4043* In 23 men with advanced colorectal cancer 10 (43.5%) showed an increase significantly different from 1 of 18 men with early colorectal cancer and none of 23 healthy

154.80 **Colorectal Cancer** *(continued)*

Carcinoembryonic Antigen *(continued)*
men without liver dysfunction *2695* In 200 patients with colorectal cancer 86 (43%) had a mean concentration that exceeded the upper limit of normal *1895* In 200 patients with colorectal cancers 86 (43.0%) had concentrations above 5 ng/mL *1896* In 256 patients with colorectal/gastrointestinal malignant disease 46.9% had concentrations of 0.0 - 3.0 ng/mL, 12.5% had concentrations from 3.1 - 5.0 ng/mL, 5.5% had concentrations from 5.1 - 10.0 ng/mL and 35.2% had concentrations greater than 10.0 ng/mL when measured by method on Bayer Technicon Immuno 1® system compared with 95.9%, 3.5%, 0.6% and 0.0% respectively in 173 healthy nonsmokers *339* In 10% of 10 patients with stage A disease and in 77% of 30 patients with stage D disease positive results observed *5406* In 20 patients with stage 1 disease mean concentration of 3.0 ± 2.8 ng/mL, in 28 with stage 2 disease 10.5 ± 17.1 ng/mL, in 14 with stage 3 disease 536.4 ± 1,621 ng/mL and in 25 with stage 4 disease 2,939 ± 1,338 ng/mL *4103* In 30 patients with colorectal cancer and metastases mean concentration of 315 μg/L (range 1.0 - 4,800) significantly higher than mean of 1.6 μg/L (range 1.0 - 2.6) in 10 controls *4039* 14 of 18 patients (78%) with local recurrence or extrahepatic metastases had concentrations above 5 ng/mL and less than 5 ng/mL in 11 patients without invasive colorectal cancer *4040* In 114 patients with colorectal cancer mean concentration of 12.16 ± 1.96 ng/mL significantly higher than mean concentration of 1.44 ± 0.25 ng/mL in 45 healthy controls. CEA concentration increased in 65% of patients with Dukes B or C colorectal cancer *4026* In 6 of 8 cases of colorectal cancer with TNF-α concentrations above detection threshold of 6.8 pg/mL CEA concentrations increased. Of 23 TNF-α negative cases 8 were CEA positive *3664* Mean concentration increased in 72% of patients with colorectal cancer compared with 11% in healthy individuals *3191* In 36 patients with colorectal cancer average concentration of 6.4 ng/mL significantly higher than in healthy individuals *1683*
Tissue *Increase* In 34 patients with colorectal cancer average concentration in tumor tissue of 130.577 ng/g significantly higher than 3,984 ng/g in healthy colonic mucosa *1683*

Cathepsin B *Tissue* *Increase* High amounts of cathepsin B associated with poor prognosis for patients with colorectal cancer *1252*

β-Chorionic Gonadotropin *Plasma* *No Effect* In 36 patients with colorectal cancer average concentration of 1.5 mU/mL not significantly higher than in healthy individuals *1683*
Tissue *Increase* In 34 patients with colorectal cancer average concentration in tumor tissue of 211 mU/g significantly higher than 4 mU/g in healthy colonic mucosa *1683*

Colon Specific Antigen *Serum* *Increase* In patients with colorectal cancer 52% had increased concentration compared with 8% in healthy controls *3191*

C-Reactive Protein *Serum* *Increase* In patients with colorectal or gastric cancer mean concentration of 97 mg/L compared with less than 3 mg/L in healthy controls *719*

CYFRA 21-1 *Serum* *Increase* In 24 patients with colorectal cancer without metastases median concentration of 2.4 ng/mL and in 16 with metastases 4.9 ng/mL significantly different from that in 50 healthy individuals with median concentration of 1.2 ng/mL and range of 0.5 - 2.4 ng/mL *3559*

D-Dimer *Plasma* *Increase* Mean concentration in 40 patients with colorectal cancer 700 μg/L compared with reference range of 0 - 450 μg/L: upper limit of normal exceeded in 71.1% of patients *5402*

DF3 *Serum* *Increase* In 32 patients with colorectal cancer 9% had concentration greater than 25 U/mL (concentration in 90% normals) but none had greater than 30 U/mL (observed in 95% normals) *2076*

Factor VIII Activity *Plasma* *Increase* Although mean activity in 40 patients of 145% and reference range of 61 - 176% activity exceeded upper limit in 29.2% of patients *5402*

Ferritin *Serum* *Decrease* In 23 men with advanced colorectal cancer mean concentration of 48.8 ± 72.8 ng/mL significantly different from mean of 80.5 ± 35.0 ng/mL in 18 men with early colorectal cancer and 117.1 ± 46.8 ng/mL in 23 healthy men without liver dysfunction *2695*

α-Fetoprotein *Serum* *No Effect* In 36 patients with colorectal cancer average concentration of 9.2 U/mL not significantly higher than in healthy individuals *1683*
Tissue *Increase* In 34 patients with colorectal cancer average concentration in tumor tissue of 12.8 ng/g significantly higher than 4 ng/g in healthy colonic mucosa *1683*

Fibrinogen *Plasma* *Increase* Although mean concentration in 40 patients with colorectal cancer was 3.6 g/L (reference range 2.7 - 6.8 g/L) 33% had a concentration that exceeded upper limit *5402*

Folate *Red Blood Cells* *Decrease* In 12 patients with colorectal cancer mean concentration of 298.7 ± 130.9 ng/mL significantly different from 365.1 ± 249.8 ng/mL in 16 control individuals *4178*
Serum *Decrease* In 12 patients with colorectal cancer mean concentration of 6.41 ± 2.74 ng/mL significantly different from 7.93 ± 2.02 ng/mL in 16 control individuals *4178*

Gastrin *Serum* *Increase* In 16 patients with gastric cancer mean concentration of 17.4 ± 3.6 pmol/L higher, but not significantly so, than 12.6 ± 1.9 pmol/L in 14 healthy controls but postprandial increases were significantly and persistently higher than normal in cancer patients *5715*
Serum *No Effect* In 91 patients with colorectal carcinoma mean concentration of 20 pmol/L not significantly different from 21 pmol/L in 101 age-matched controls *5423*

Glucose *Serum* *Increase* Concentrations of 61 - 96 mg/dL in men and 53 - 93 mg/dL in women in first quartile and 116 - 448 mg/dL in men and 111 - 657 mg/dL in women with those in highest quartile having 80% higher risk of developing incident colorectal cancer compared with those in lowest quartile *4658*

Glutamine *Plasma* *Decrease* In 10 patients with colorectal cancer mean concentration reduced *3356*

Glutathione Peroxidase *Serum* *Decrease* Mean activity of 4.27 ± 1.05 nmol/min/mg in 106 patients with colorectal cancer not significantly different from 5.52 ± 1.32 nmol/min/mg in 34 healthy controls *4230*

Haptoglobin *Serum* *Increase* In 25 patients with primary cancer of the colon and/or rectum mean concentration of 2.22 ± 0.62 g/L and 2.29 ± 0.68 g/L in 37 patients with metastatic cancer compared with 1.14 ± 0.34 g/L in 76 healthy controls *928*

HDL-Cholesterol *Serum* *No Effect* Concentrations of 18 - 39 mg/dL in men and 15 - 48 mg/dL in women in first quartile and 55 - 125 mg/dL in men and 66 - 149 mg/dL in women with those in highest quartile not significantly associated with greater risk of developing incident colorectal cancer compared with those in lowest quartile *4658*

Hemoglobin *Blood* *Decrease* In 23 men with advanced colorectal cancer mean concentration of 12.5 ± 2.3 g/dL significantly different from mean of 14.6 ± 0.9 g/dL in 18 men with early colorectal cancer and 14.7 ± 1.5 g/dL in 23 healthy men without liver dysfunction *2695*
Feces *Increase* Mean concentration in 20 patients with colorectal cancer of 480.8 μg/g (70.88 mg/d) significantly different from 1.5 μg/g (0.15 mg/d) in 20 healthy controls *4521*

Immunosuppressive Acidic Protein *Serum* *Increase* In 8 of 9 cases of colorectal cancer with TNF-α concentrations above detection threshold of 6.8 pg/mL concentrations increased above threshold of 500 μg/mL. Of 22 TNF-α negative cases 10 were IAP positive *3664* Progressive increase from 404 ± 80 μg/mL with stage I disease to 802 ± 98 μg/mL with stage IV disease compared with 403 ± 49 μg/mL in 40 normal controls *4593*

Insulin *Plasma* *Increase* Concentrations of 4 - 10 IU/mL in men and 3 - 9 IU/mL in women in first quartile and 19 - 400 IU/mL in men and 19 - 400 IU/mL in women with those in highest quartile having greater risk of developing incident colorectal cancer compared with those in lowest quartile *4658*

Iron *Serum* *Decrease* In 23 men with advanced colorectal cancer mean concentration of 50.5 ± 38.6 μg/dL significantly different from mean of 93.0 ± 32.1 μg/dL in 18 men with early colorectal cancer and 107.1 ± 32.9 μg/dL in 23 healthy men without liver dysfunction *2695*

Islet Amyloid Polypeptide *Serum* *No Effect* Mean concentration in 22 patients with colorectal cancer of 7.6 ± 3.3 pmol/L compared with 8.0 ± 5.0 pmol/L in healthy controls *4210*

LDL-Cholesterol *Serum* *No Effect* Concentrations of 27 - 101 mg/dL in men and 25 - 101 mg/dL in women in first quartile and 144 - 337 mg/dL in men and 158 - 315 mg/dL in women with those in highest quartile not significantly associated with greater risk of developing incident colorectal cancer compared with those in lowest quartile *4658*

Leukocytes *Blood Increase* Progressive increase from 6,320 ± 1,320 /µL with stage I disease to 8,640 ± 1,040 /µL with stage IV disease compared with 5,550 ± 980 /µL in 40 normal controls *4593*

Lymphocytes *Blood Decrease* Progressive decrease from 1,920 ± 420 /µL with stage I disease to 1,360 ± 280 /µL with stage IV disease compared with 1,850 ± 640 /µL in 40 normal controls *4593*

Lysozyme *Feces No Effect* In 23 patients with colorectal cancer mean concentration of 13.3 ± 2.8 µg/g compared with 12.5 ± 2.6 µg/g stool in healthy controls *1247*

Metallopanstimulin *Serum Increase* In 100% of 27 patients with colorectal cancer mean concentration exceeded upper limit of normal of < 10 ng/mL in healthy individuals aged 19 - 88 years *1462*

β_2-Microglobulin *Serum Increase* Mean concentration of 4.4 ± 1.6 mg/L significantly higher than 1.29 ± 0.49 mg/L in age-matched controls *2702*

NCC-ST 439 *Serum Increase* In 121 patients with primary and 36 with recurrent large bowel cancer serum NCC-ST 439 was positive in 27.3% of the former and 66.7% of the latter with a false positive rate of 5.6% in patients with benign disease *5771*

Neopterin *Urine Increase* In 34 patients with colorectal cancer mean excretion of 325 ± 267 µmol/mol creatinine significantly higher than 166 ± 67 µmol/mol creatinine in 15 reference intervals. Concentration significantly higher in stage Dukes D disease 561 ± 372 µmol/mol creatinine than in stage B (188 ± 47 µmol/mol creatinine) and stage C (250 ± 142 µmol/mol creatinine) *3447*

Neutrophil Elastase *Feces Increase* Mean concentration in 20 patients with colorectal cancer of 2.5 µg/g (0.33 mg/d) not significantly different from 0.6 µg/g (0.11 mg/d) in 20 healthy controls *4521*

Neutrophils *Blood Increase* Progressive increase from 3,210 ± 810 /µL with stage I disease to 6,130 ± 1,010 /µL with stage IV disease compared with 2,730 ± 530 /µL in 40 normal controls *4593*

Occult Blood *Feces Increase* In 23 men with advanced colorectal cancer occult blood positive in all compared with 10 of 18 (55.6%) men with early colorectal cancer *2695* In patients with colorectal cancer 69% had increased concentration as measured by Hemoccult II compared with 2% in healthy controls *3191*

Ornithine *Plasma Increase* In 10 patients with colorectal cancer mean concentration increased *3356*

Phenylalanine *Plasma Increase* In 10 patients with colorectal cancer mean concentration increased *3356*

Plasminogen Activator Inhibitor-1 *Plasma Increase* In patients with high concentration increasing severity of disease noted compared with patients in whom concentration was low *3782* Although mean concentration in 40 patients with colorectal cancer was 2.1 x 10^3 AU/L compared with reference range of 0 - 4.6 x 10^3 AU/L, upper limit was exceeded in 12.5% of patients *5402*

Polymorphic Epithelial Mucin *Serum No Effect* In 10 patients with colorectal cancer median concentrations of 22 kU/L by ACS BR, 26 kU/L by Centocor CA 15-3, 21 kU/L by Enzymun-Test CA 15-3 and 19 kU/L by IMx CA 15-3 not significantly different from concentrations in 250 healthy women (mean and 1 SD concentrations of 22 ± 8.8 kU/L by ACS BR, 19 ± 8.8 kU/L by Centocor CA 15-3, 17 ± 7.1 kU/L by Enzymun-Test CA 15-3 and 15 ± 6.4 kU/L by IMx CA 15-3 respectively) *513*

Prolactin *Plasma Increase* In 114 patients with colorectal cancer mean concentration of 34.85 ± 5.42 ng/mL significantly higher than mean 8.89 ± 0.69 ng/mL in 45 healthy controls. In patients with Dukes B or C colorectal cancer 45% had hyperprolactinemia. Concentration significantly higher in patients who had progressive disease than in those who responded to treatment. In patients with concentrations above 20 ng/mL overall survival shorter than in those with lower concentrations *4026*

Proline *Plasma Decrease* In 10 patients with colorectal cancer mean concentration decreased *3356*

Selenium *Serum Decrease* Statistically significant reduced concentration observed in patients with stage T4 colorectal cancer different from 80.5 ± 21.0 µg/L in 34 healthy controls *4230*

Serum No Effect Mean concentration of 80.1 ± 20.1 µg/L in 106 patients with colorectal cancer not significantly different from 80.5 ± 21.0 µg/L in 34 healthy controls *4230*

Serine *Plasma Decrease* In 10 patients with colorectal cancer mean concentration reduced *3356*

Soluble Fibrin Monomer *Plasma Increase* In 40 patients with colorectal cancer mean concentration of 10.7 nmol/L compared with reference range of 8.4 - 13.2 nmol/L but 19.6% of patients had concentrations that exceeded upper limit *5402*

Soluble Interleukin-2 Receptor *Serum Increase* Mean concentration of 1,539 ± 155 U/mL in 52 patients with advanced colorectal carcinoma significantly different from 555 ± 31 U/mL in 25 age- and sex-matched healthy volunteer controls *4043* Progressive increase from 461 ± 17 U/mL in patients with stage I disease to 1,234 ± 198 U/mL with stage IV disease compared with 481 ± 36 U/mL in 40 normal controls *4593* In 12 cases of Dukes A colorectal cancer mean concentration of 443 ± 47 U/mL not significantly different from 481 ± 36 U/mL in 14 normal controls but 3 cases with Dukes B mean concentration of 614 ± 158 U/mL and in 15 Dukes C patients mean concentration of 917 ± 237 U/mL significantly higher than in controls *3663*
Serum No Effect In 12 cases of Dukes A colorectal cancer mean concentration of 443 ± 47 U/mL not significantly different from 481 ± 36 U/mL in 14 normal controls but 3 cases with Dukes B mean concentration of 614 ± 158 U/mL and in 15 Dukes C patients mean concentration of 917 ± 237 U/mL significantly higher than in controls *3663*

Squamous Cell Carcinoma Antigen *Serum No Effect* In 36 patients with colorectal cancer average concentration of 1.5 mU/mL not significantly higher than in healthy individuals *1683*
Tissue Increase In 34 patients with colorectal cancer average concentration in tumor tissue of 58,231 ng/g significantly higher than 43.6 ng/g in healthy colonic mucosa *1683*

Tennessee Antigen *Serum Increase* In patients with colorectal cancer, 89% had increased concentration compared with 7% healthy controls who had increased concentrations *3191*

Threonine *Plasma Decrease* In 10 patients with colorectal cancer mean concentration reduced *3356*

Thrombin/Antithrombin III Complex *Plasma Increase* In 40 patients with colorectal cancer mean concentration of 4.8 µg/L (reference range of 0.7 - 4.3 µg/L) and 52.2% of patients exceeded upper limit *5402*

Tissue Plasminogen Activator *Tissue Increase* High activities of tPA in morphologically normal mucosa remote from tumor are associated with favorable prognosis for colorectal cancer *1252*

Triglycerides *Serum No Effect* Concentrations of 35 - 90 mg/dL in men and 24 - 93 mg/dL in women in first quartile and 163 - 1,323 mg/dL in men and 167 - 1,216 mg/dL in women with those in highest quartile not significantly associated with greater risk of developing incident colorectal cancer compared with those in lowest quartile *4658*

Tumor-associated Glycoprotein-72 *Serum Increase* In 200 patients with colorectal cancer 86 (43%) had a mean concentration that exceeded the upper limit of normal of > 6 U/mL. Only 3% of patients with benign disease had an increased concentration *1895* Only 2 of patients with colorectal cancer had increased concentrations but concentrations correlated with advanced stages of the disease *1668*

Tumor Necrosis Factor-α *Serum Increase* 9 of 34 cases of colorectal cancer had concentrations above detection threshold of 6.8 pg/mL (26.5%). 4 cases with metastases to regional lymph nodes had concentrations above 20 pg/mL *3664*

Urokinase Plasminogen Activator *Tissue Increase* High amounts associated with poor prognosis *1255*

von Willebrand Factor Antigen *Plasma Increase* In 40 patients with colorectal cancer mean antigen concentration of 150% compared with reference range of 52 - 145% and concentration exceeded upper limit in 50% of patients *5402*

155.00 Cancer of Liver

α_1-Acid Glycoprotein *Serum Increase* Sensitivity of 65% and a specificity of 80% with severe liver disease *1439*

Adenosine Deaminase *Serum Increase* Increased in obstructive jaundice seen with neoplastic disease *1340 3926 4956*

155.00 Cancer of Liver *(continued)*

Alanine Aminotransferase *Serum* *Increase* Elevated in only 34% of 32 patients with primary hepatoma (normal = 2.4 - 17 U/L) *90* In all cases of intrahepatic malignant disease, values were above normal, and all but 1 showed higher AST than ALT. ALT values ranged from 31 - 43 U/L *5738*

Albumin *Serum* *Decrease* Reversed A/G ratio in 54% of 51 hepatoma patients *2320* In 42% of 14 patients at initial hospitalization for this disorder *1576* Mean values were found to be highest in the healthy subjects followed by acute viral hepatitis, primary hepatocellular carcinoma and cirrhosis, in that order. Both the mean albumin and mean total globulin of each group of subjects were significantly different from the respective means of the other 3 groups *1459*

Alkaline Phosphatase *Serum* *Increase* Usually moderately elevated; 40 - 50% of patients have activities between 20 - 75 U/L and 15 - 30% are above 81 U/L *762* Elevated in 80.5% of 62 patients with hepatoma *2320* In 90% of 12 patients at initial hospitalization for this disorder *1576* Due to obstruction, elevated in 88% of patients with primary cancer *90* In about 80% of cases *1980* Elevated in 95 - 100% of primary cancers, usually ranging from 80 - 215 U/L, with only 80% having values greater than 107 U/L *1025*

Alkaline Phosphatase Isoenzymes *Serum* *Increase* Of 15 cases all had increased values of isoenzyme-I and 6 had increased isoenzyme-IV as well *2557*

δ-Aminolevulinic Acid *Urine* *Increase* May occur *1025*

Antithrombin III *Plasma* *Decrease* Decreased in parenchymatous liver disease *5220* *3472*

Antithyroglobulin Antibodies *Serum* *Increase* Rare *3925*

α_1-Antitrypsin *Serum* *Increase* In 46 patients with hepatocellular carcinoma mean concentration of 4.8 ± 2.7 mg/mL compared with 1.7 ± 0.7 mg/mL. Sensitivity in 24 patients with high AFP 96% and in 22 with low AFP 64%. Sensitivity for hepatocellular carcinoma using AAT alone 76% *2965* Significant elevation compared with controls (n = 58) *1422*

Aspartate Aminotransferase *Serum* *Increase* In 98% of 12 patients at initial hospitalization for this disorder *1576* Over 10% above normal upper limit in 83.3% of 66 hepatoma patients *2320* Levels may be 10 - 100 times normal and remain elevated for long periods *1642* Elevated from 2 to 5 times the normal level in 66 - 70% of patients with primary carcinoma *90* Elevated in 80% *762*

Bilirubin *Serum* *Increase* In 38% of 13 patients at initial hospitalization for this disorder *1576* Commonly found (60 - 70%), but concentration > 85 mmol/L were found in only 10 - 25% of patients *762* In patients with primary tumors, values ranged from 3.5 - 5.2 mg/dL (normal < 1.0) *5738* Over 10% above upper limit of normal in 43.2% in 67 cases of hepatoma *2320*

Biotin *Serum* *Decrease* Significantly low in hepatoma compared to healthy controls *3703*

BSP Retention *Serum* *Increase* Increased retention in 90% of cases *762*

c-erb-B_2 Oncoprotein *Serum* *Increase* Median concentration of 5 ng/mL in 30 patients with locoregional cancer. 8 of 30 (27%) of patients with locoregional disease had concentrations exceeding 1.5 ng/mL *3564*

CA 15-3 *Serum* *Increase* In 14 patients with hepatocellular-cholangio cancer mean concentration of 44.2 ± 1,247 U/mL significantly different from cutoff of 22 U/mL, of whom 4 had concentrations greater than 25 U/mL and 2 had concentrations greater than 40 U/mL *2076*

CA 19-9 *Serum* *Increase* CA 19-9 concentration increased above 37 U/mL in 44% patients with primary liver cancer *1253* Frequently show elevated values *3657* *2026*

CA 125 *Serum* *Increase* Abnormal results were detected in 67% of patients with primary liver carcinoma *3560*

CA 195 *Serum* *Increase* Mean concentration of 24.6 ± 30.3 U/mL in 16 patients with liver cancer significantly higher than cutoff of 12 U/mL: 10 patients with concentrations greater than 12 U/mL *122* The sensitivity and specificity in hepatocellular carcinoma and metastatic carcinoma were 60% and 22% and 87% and 42% respectively *3228*

CA 549 *Serum* *Increase* In 95 patients with liver cancer, 43 (45.3%) had a concentration greater than the upper limit of normal with BRESMARQ assay *764*

Calcium *Serum* *Increase* A serious complication in many cases of hepatoma *2624* Sometimes present. Occasionally antedate the discovery of the tumor *1980* A serious complication in many cases of hepatoma *3294*

Carcinoembryonic Antigen *Ascitic Fluid* *Increase* In malignant effusions *4891*
Serum *Increase* Increases commonly reported *4551* In 67% of cases *4891* In 29 patients with malignant disease of the liver 72.4% had concentrations of 0.0 - 3.0 ng/mL, 10.3% had concentrations from 3.1 - 5.0 ng/mL, 6.9% had concentrations from 5.1 - 10.0 ng/mL and 10.3% had concentrations greater than 10.0 ng/mL when measured by method on Bayer Technicon Immuno 1® system compared with 95.9%, 3.5%, 0.6% and 0.0% respectively in 173 healthy nonsmokers *339* Increases occur in two-thirds of patients *1601*

Cholesterol *Serum* *Decrease* 20 - 30% incidence *762* The close relationship between serum levels of cholesterol and bile acids has been confirmed in 46 patients with primary hepatoma, serum levels of cholesterol and bile acids are roughly correlated with serum AFP. Because the relationship between serum cholesterol and bile acids did not exist in common hepatocellular diseases, the results suggest a peculiar sterol metabolism occurring in human hepatoma *2172*

β-Chorionic Gonadotropin *Plasma* *Increase* Ectopic production *552* *602* *3777* *455*

Endothelin-1 *Plasma* *Increase* ET-1 levels (3.08 ± 0.93 pg/mL) were significantly higher than those in healthy controls (2.18 ± 0.37 pg/mL) *5339* The mean concentration of plasma ET-IR of 21 hepatocellular carcinoma (HCC) patients (30.3 ± 8.5 pg/mL, n = 21) (mean ± SD) was markedly higher than those in liver cirrhosis (LC) (22.1 ± 4.7 pg/mL, n = 16) ($p < 0.01$), which were also elevated compared with those in normal subjects (9.4 ± 1.6 pg/mL, n = 91) *2174*

Erythrocyte Sedimentation Rate *Blood* *Increase* Sometimes increased *5544*

Erythrocytes *Ascitic Fluid* *Increase* A large number of RBC, especially grossly bloody ascites, suggests a neoplasm, particularly hepatoma or ovarian cancer *4891* Strongly suggests neoplasm, especially hepatoma *367* > 10,000 cells/μL seen in 20% of cases *1417*
Blood *Increase* Erythrocytosis occurs in about 11% of hepatoma patients with increased red cell mass and bone marrow erythroid hyperplasia *3294* In the absence of systemic hypoxia, erythrocytosis may develop in hepatocellular carcinoma as a compensatory response to local liver hypoxia *5304* Erythrocytosis occurs in about 11% of hepatoma patients with increased red cell mass and bone marrow erythroid hyperplasia *603* Occasional erythrocytosis *1980*

Erythropoietin *Serum* *Increase* Increased plasma concentrations are found in patients with erythrocytosis associated with several types of tumor, especially lung, kidney and liver *3084* *3294* *547*

α-Fetoprotein *Pleural Fluid* *Increase* Positive results were most frequently found in samples derived from patients with liver tumors. The highest levels (6 and 30 ng/mL), were determined in samples of two hepatoma patients *1295*
Serum *Increase* Above 30 ng/mL in 69%. Levels declined as age increased. Appeared to be related to the tumor cell type: the relatively immature *4746* Observed effect *799* *75* Detectable in 14 of 19 (76%) patients *90* Observed effect *4734* Incidence of positivity varies with geographical area from 50 - 90%; in this country 50% is a more accurate estimate. Serum concentration > 500 ng/mL indicates hepatoma 97% of the time. Postoperative serial determinations show an exponential fall to normal when the tumor has been completely excised. Recurrence of elevated levels indicates tumor recurrence *5759*

Fibrin Degradation Products *Ascitic Fluid* *Increase* In malignant effusions *4891*

Fucose *Serum* *Increase* Markedly increased *2899*

Fucosidase *Serum* *Increase* In 32 patients with primary hepatic carcinoma mean activity of α-L-fucosidase of 145.5 ± 12 nkat/L compared with 51.4 ± 4.5 nkat/L in 30 controls *1132*

Galactosyltransferase Isoenzyme II *Serum* *Increase* Sensitivity of 0.91 and specificity of 0.72 *5348*

α_2-Globulin *Serum* *Increase* alpha$_2$-Globulins, especially haptoglobins, were generally increased in primary colorectal cancer, and the liver. Haptoglobin values were useful to indicate tumor activity *928*

γ-Globulin *Serum* *Increase* Mean values were found to be lowest in controls followed by acute viral hepatitis, primary hepatocellular carcinoma, and cirrhosis, in that order *1459* Reversed A/G ratio in 54% of 51 hepatoma patients *2320*

Glucose *Serum* *Decrease* Sometimes present. Occasionally antedates the discovery of the tumor *1980* Observed with severe disease *4707* Can occur with various types of liver disease. Hepatic hypoglycemia is a fasting hypoglycemia and often only transiently relieved by food *1980* 5 - 25% incidence *762* Hypoglycemia noted in about 30% of hepatoma patients in some studies *3294*

β-Glucuronidase *Serum* *Increase* Increased *1498* *1777*

γ-Glutamyltransferase *Saliva* *Increase* Significantly higher (10.4 U/L) versus controls (5.12 U/L) *2448*

Hematocrit *Blood* *Decrease* In 35% of 14 patients at initial hospitalization for this disorder *1576*

Hemoglobin *Blood* *Decrease* In 49% of 14 patients at initial hospitalization for this disorder *1576*

Hepatitis B Surface Antigen *Serum* *Increase* Reported incidence varies from 5 - 80% *762* Prevalence of antigen in sera varies with geographic location; 40% incidence was found in an African study and 80% in a study in Taiwan *3294*

^{131}I Uptake *Serum* *Increase* In hepatic disease *4707*

immunoglobulin A *Serum* *No Effect* Concentration usually normal *5544*

Immunoglobulin G *Serum* *No Effect* Concentration usually normal *5544*

Immunoglobulin M *Serum* *Decrease* Reported effect *5544*

Islet Amyloid Polypeptide *Serum* *No Effect* In 6 patients with hepatic cancer mean ± 1 SD was 9.4 ± 5.1 pmol/L not significantly different from 8.0 ± 5.0 pmol/L in 25 normal individuals *4210*

Lactate Dehydrogenase *Ascitic Fluid* *Increase* In malignant effusions *4891*
Serum *Increase* In 83% of 13 patients at initial hospitalization for this disorder *1576* Significant elevation occurred in 66% of patients *90* 70 - 85% incidence of elevation *762* Useful in detecting metastatic or primary liver cancer due to marked sensitivity to carcinomatosis and insensitivity to noncancerous parenchymal hepatic damage *1025*

Lactate Dehydrogenase Isoenzyme-5 *Serum* *Increase* Elevated to a mean of 13% of total LD values (normal = 0 - 6%) *1756*

LDL-Cholesterol *Serum* *Increase* Moderate increase secondary to lack of feedback inhibition of hepatic cholesterol synthesis by dietary cholesterol *126*

Leukocytes *Ascitic Fluid* *Increase* > 1,000 /µL *233*
Blood *Increase* Sometimes increased *5544* In 45% of 13 patients at initial hospitalization for this disorder *1576*

Lipids *Serum* *Increase* Sometimes present. Occasionally antedates the discovery of the tumor *1980*

α_2-Macroglobulin *Serum* *Increase* Moderate elevation *2249*

Malate Dehydrogenase *Serum* *Increase* In neoplastic disease *1025*

5-Methyl-2'-Deoxycytidine *Urine* *No Effect* In 9 patients with cancer of the liver mean excretion of 0.67 ± 0.14 nmol/µmol creatinine not significantly different from 0.90 ± 0.43 nmol/µmol creatinine in 81 healthy individuals *2368*

Monocytes *Blood* *Increase* In 73% of 12 patients at initial hospitalization for this disorder *1576*

5'-Nucleotidase *Serum* *Increase* 88.4% of 51 hepatoma patients had values > 10% above the normal upper limit *2320*

Occult Blood *Feces* *Increase* GI bleeding may occur with malignancies *4891*

Ornithine Carbamoyltransferase *Serum* *Increase* Liver cell damage *5544*

Platelets *Blood* *Increase* In 46% of 13 patients at initial hospitalization for this disorder *1576*

Procollagen Type IV Peptide *Serum* *Increase* The serum concentrations were 4.2 ± 0.9 ng/mL in controls, 14.4 ± 6.9 ng/mL in hepatocellular carcinoma *5765*

Progesterone *Plasma* *Increase* Raised in 36 of 50 men with liver disease compared with 20 healthy male control subjects. Significantly higher in men with nonalcoholic cirrhosis with gynecomastic than those without *1428*

Prolactin *Plasma* *Increase* Found in 14% of men with liver disease. Levels unrelated to presence of gynecomastia *1428*

Proline Hydroxylase *Serum* *Increase* Markedly elevated in hepatoma, and to a lesser extent lymphosarcoma and pheochromocytoma *762*

Prostate-specific Antigen *Serum* *Increase* Of 58 patients with cancer of the liver or pancreas, 90.9% had values below upper limit of normal of 4.0 ng/mL as measured by method on Bayer Technicon Immuno 1® , 4.5% had values between 4.0 and 10.0 ng/mL and 4.5% had values between 10.0 and 40.0 ng/mL *342*

Protein *Ascitic Fluid* *Increase* > 2.5 g/dL *233*

Prothrombin Time *Plasma* *Increase* Abnormal in 21 of 24 hepatoma patients with cirrhosis and 11 of 16 without cirrhosis in tests done within 1 month of death *4037* Prolonged in 26.6% of patients *2320*

Sialyltransferase *Serum* *Increase* In 3 patients with cancer of the liver mean and median concentrations of 555 and 550 cpm/mg protein/30 min significantly different from 240 and 243 cpm/mg protein/30 min respectively in 20 normal individuals *2111*

155.00 Hepatoblastoma

α-Fetoprotein *Serum* *Increase* Increased concentrations are seen in almost all children with hepatoblastoma *1778*

155.00 Hepatocellular Carcinoma

Acid Ribonuclease *Serum* *Increase* Median activity in 8 patients with hepatocellular carcinoma of 49.9 U/L significantly different from 42.0 U/L in 32 healthy controls *2566*

Alanine Aminotransferase *Serum* *Increase* Mean activity of 96 ± 95 U/L in 26 patients with hepatocellular carcinoma significantly different from 28 ± 7 U/L in 29 healthy controls *5316* Mean activity of 87 ± 135 U/L in 61 patients with hepatocellular cirrhosis significantly different from 20 ± 7 U/L in 29 healthy controls *3668* In 12 patients with hepatocellular carcinoma mean activity of 65 ± 24 U/L significantly different from 14 ± 8 U/L in 20 healthy volunteers *2372* Median activity in 8 patients with hepatocellular carcinoma of 218 U/L significantly different from 22 U/L in 32 healthy controls *2566* In one patient with hepatocellular carcinoma mean activity of 66 U/L *108* In 100 patients with hepatocellular carcinoma mean activity of 46 U/L different from reference interval of < 40 U/L *2071* Mean activity of 100 ± 74 U/L in 61 patients with hepatocellular carcinoma significantly different from 24 ± 5 U/L in 29 healthy controls *3668*
Serum *No Effect* In 19 patients with chronic active hepatitis C with hepatocellular carcinoma mean activity of 118 ± 77 U/L not significantly different from normal *2381*

Albumin *Serum* *Decrease* In 100 patients with hepatocellular carcinoma mean concentration of 3.4 ± 0.6 g/L different from reference interval of 3.8 - 5.3 g/L *2071* Median concentration in 8 patients with hepatocellular carcinoma of 3.2 g/dL significantly different from 3.7 g/dL in 32 healthy controls *2566* In 5 patients mean concentration of 35.7 ± 3.3 g/L significantly less than 42.1 ± 4.3 g/L in 30 healthy control individuals *855* Mean concentration of 3.4 ± 0.5 g/dL in 61 patients with hepatocellular carcinoma significantly different from 4.5 ± 0.3 g/dL in 29 healthy controls *3668*
Serum *No Effect* In 19 patients with chronic active hepatitis C with hepatocellular carcinoma mean concentration of 3.5 ± 0.4 g/dL not significantly different from normal *2381* In one patient with hepatocellular carcinoma mean concentration of 3.6 g/dL *108*

Alkaline Phosphatase *Serum* *Increase* Median activity in 8 patients with hepatocellular carcinoma of 224 U/L significantly different from 63 U/L in 32 healthy controls *2566* In 100 patients with hepatocellular carcinoma mean activity of 267 U/L different from reference interval of 90 - 250 U/L *2071* In 25 patients with hepatocellular carcinoma 88% had activities above 112 U/L *1406* Development of hepatocellular carcinoma from cirrhosis may be associated with threefold increase in alkaline phosphatase activity *3625* In 100 patients with hepatocellular carcinoma mean concentration of 1.2 mg/dL different from reference interval of 0.2 - 1.0 mg/dL *2071* In one patient with hepatocellular carcinoma mean activity of 277 U/L *108*

155.00 Hepatocellular Carcinoma *(continued)*

Alkaline Phosphatase *(continued)*
Serum *No Effect* In 19 patients with chronic active hepatitis C with hepatocellular carcinoma mean activity of 196 ± 74 U/L not significantly different from normal *2381*

Alkaline Phosphatase, Kasahara Isoenzyme
Serum *Increase* A variant isoenzyme of alkaline phosphatase has been observed in up to 30% cases of HCC *1778*

Alkaline Ribonuclease *Serum* *Increase* Median activity in 8 patients with hepatocellular carcinoma of 72.8 U/L significantly different from 67.4 U/L in 32 healthy controls *2566*

Antithrombin III *Plasma* *Decrease* In 5 patients mean concentration of 9.2 ± 3.1 U/mL significantly less than 11.8 ± 1.1 U/mL in 30 healthy controls *855*

Aspartate Aminotransferase *Serum* *Increase* In 25 patients with hepatocellular carcinoma 96% had activities above 40 U/L *1406* In one patient with hepatocellular carcinoma mean activity of 66 U/L *108* Mean activity of 135 ± 216 U/L in 26 patients with hepatocellular carcinoma significantly different from 27 ± 5 U/L in 29 healthy controls *5316*
Serum *No Effect* In 19 patients with chronic active hepatitis C with hepatocellular carcinoma mean activity of 90. ± 32 U/L not significantly different from normal *2381*

Aspartate Aminotransferase:Alanine Aminotransferase Ratio
Serum *Increase* Ratio greater than 3.0 with AST activity exceeding 500 U/L (normal < 40 U/L) is suggestive of circulatory disturbances, especially left ventricular failure, or malignant diseases involving the liver *4617*

Basic Fibroblast Growth Factor *Serum* *Increase* Mean concentration of 9.8 pg/mL (range 2.1 - 174 pg/mL) in 39 patients not significantly different from 4.8 pg/mL (range 2.9 - 9.5 pg/mL) in 40 healthy individuals, but with 51.3% abnormal *2262*

Bilirubin *Serum* *Increase* In 12 patients with hepatocellular carcinoma mean concentration of 1.8 ± 0.6 mg/dL significantly different from 0.5 ± 0.3 mg/dL in 20 healthy volunteers *2372* Mean concentration of 1.8 ± 2.0 mg/dL in 61 patients with hepatocellular carcinoma significantly different from 0.6 ± 0.1 mg/dL in 29 healthy controls *3668* Median concentration in 8 patients with hepatocellular carcinoma of 2.1 mg/dL significantly different from 0.7 mg/dL in 32 healthy controls *2566* In 25 patients with hepatocellular carcinoma 76% had concentrations above 26 μmol/L *1406*
Serum *No Effect* In 19 patients with chronic active hepatitis C with hepatocellular carcinoma mean concentration of 1.0. ± 0.2 mg/dL not significantly different from normal *2381* In one patient with hepatocellular carcinoma mean concentration of 0.4 mg/dL *108*

CA 19-9 *Serum* *Increase* In one study 58% patients had concentrations above cutoff value of 60 U/mL *3120* In 13 patients with hepatocellular carcinoma median concentration of 39 kU/L not significantly different from upper limit of normal of 35 kU/L, but 54% of patients had abnormal values *3218* In 25 patients with hepatocellular carcinoma 72% had concentrations above 35 U/mL *1406* Pathological concentrations observed in 12 of 27 (44%) of patients with primary hepatocellular carcinoma *1404*

CA 72-4 *Serum* *Increase* In one study 14% of patients had concentrations above the cutoff value of 4.0 U/mL *3120*

CA 125 *Serum* *Increase* In one study 62% of patients had concentrations above cutoff value of 35 U/mL *3120*

Carbohydrate-deficient Transferrin *Serum* *Increase* Concentration may be increased but specificity is low, making their diagnostic use of little value *5285*

γ-Carboxyglutamic Acid, Free *Plasma* *No Effect* In 10 patients with hepatocellular carcinoma mean concentration of 152 ± 68 pmol/mL not significantly different from that in 19 healthy men and women aged between 35 and 65 years in whom mean concentration was 146 ± 34 pmol/mL *2014*

Carcinoembryonic Antigen *Serum* *Increase* In 13 patients with hepatocellular carcinoma median concentration of 5 μg/L not different from upper limit of normal of 14 μg/L, but 31% of patients had abnormal values *3218* In one study 11% of patients had a concentration above the cutoff value of 5.0 ng/mL *3120*

Cathepsin D *Serum* *Increase* Mean concentration in 51 patients with hepatocellular carcinoma of 40.6 ± 4.2 nmol/L significantly increased compared with 10.0 ± 0.71 nmol/L in 98 healthy controls *3004*

Cholesterol *Ascitic Fluid* *Increase* In 73 specimens from patients with hepatocellular carcinoma or cirrhosis mean concentration of 0.70 ± 0.05 mmol/L but significantly less than 3.14 ± 0.24 mmol/L in 21 specimens from patients with peritoneal neoplasia *728*
Serum *No Effect* In one patient with hepatocellular carcinoma mean concentration of 149 mg/dL *108*

Cholinesterase *Serum* *Decrease* In 25 patients with hepatocellular carcinoma 50% had activities less than 4,000 U/L *1406*

Collagen IV *Serum* *Increase* In 40 patients with hepatocellular carcinoma and liver cirrhosis mean concentration of 389 μg/L significantly higher than 282 μg/L in 60 patients with cirrhosis alone *1405*

C-Reactive Protein *Serum* *Increase* In 25 patients with hepatocellular carcinoma 80% had concentrations above 5 mg/L *1406*

Creatinine *Serum* *Increase* Median concentration in 8 patients with hepatocellular carcinoma of 1.1 mg/dL significantly different from 0.7 mg/dL in 32 healthy controls *2566*

CYFRA 21-1 *Serum* *Increase* In 19 patients with cancer of the liver without metastases median concentration of 3.3 ng/mL significantly different from that in 50 healthy individuals with median concentration of 1.2 ng/mL and range of 0.5 - 2.4 ng/mL *3559*

Descarboxyprothrombin *Serum* *Increase* In 50 - 60% patients with HCC, concentration is increased, but in patients with tumors < 3 cm in size, DCP concentrations are increased n only 15 - 30% *5285* Twenty-four of 60 patients (40%) had a mean concentration that exceeded 40 mAU/mL in 273 normal individuals *3897*

Endothelin *Plasma* *Increase* Concentrations very high when cirrhosis is complicated by hepatocellular carcinoma *3568*

Factor II *Plasma* *No Effect* In one patient with hepatocellular carcinoma mean concentration of 104% *108*

Factor V *Plasma* *No Effect* In one patient with hepatocellular carcinoma mean concentration of 82% *108*

Factor VII *Plasma* *No Effect* In one patient with hepatocellular carcinoma mean concentration of 103% *108*

Factor IX *Plasma* *No Effect* In one patient with hepatocellular carcinoma mean concentration of 120% *108*

Factor X *Plasma* *No Effect* In one patient with hepatocellular carcinoma mean concentration of 96% *108*

Ferritin *Serum* *Increase* In one study 68% had concentrations above cutoff value of 500 ng/mL *3120* In 64 male patients with hepatocellular carcinoma mean concentration of 1,185 ± 1,303 ng/mL significantly different from 165 ± 17 ng/mL in 35 healthy men, and 1,087 ± 2,043 ng/mL in 15 women with hepatocellular hepatocarcinoma significantly greater than 55 ± 37 ng/mL in 35 healthy women *3121*
Serum *No Effect* In 19 patients with chronic active hepatitis C with hepatocellular carcinoma mean concentration of 254 ± 82 ng/mL not significantly different from normal *2381*

α-Fetoprotein *Serum* *Increase* Concentrations increased in 80% patients with symptomatic HCC, but only occasionally increased in patients with metastatic liver disease. Concentrations above 500 μg/L are virtually diagnostic of HCC *1778* Using a cutoff value of 20 ng/mL sensitivity and specificity in European studies for patients with hepatocellular carcinoma are 55 - 69% and 83 - 92% respectively *5285* In 25 patients with hepatocellular carcinoma 73% had concentrations above 30 μg/L *1406* Median concentration of 89.0 ng/mL in 26 patients with hepatocellular carcinoma significantly different from 2.0 ng/mL in 29 healthy controls *5316* Concentration increased in about 70% of patients *2952* Concentration increased at the time of recurrence in 25 of 26 patients with recurrence within 1 year and in 11 of 14 patients with later recurrence *4810* Forty-three of 60 patients (71.7%) had a mean concentration that exceeded 20 ng/mL in 273 normal individuals *3897* 54% of patients in one study had concentrations above 200 ng/mL *3120* Pathological values observed in 23 of 27 (85%) of patients with

primary hepatocellular carcinoma *1404* In 58 patients with hepatocellular carcinoma 32.8% had concentrations up to 15.0 ng/mL, 3.4% had concentrations between 15.1 - 20.0 ng/mL, 10.3% between 20.1 - 100 ng/mL, 10.3% had concentrations between 100.1 - 350.0 ng/mL and 43.1% had concentrations above 350.0 ng/mL in contrast to concentrations in 400 healthy individuals in whom 99.2% had concentrations between 0 and 15.0 ng/mL, 0.2% between 15.1 and 20.0 ng/mL and 0.5%% between 20.1 and 100 ng/mL *11*
Serum No Effect Normal concentrations, i.e., below 20 ng/mL, detected in up to 40% patients with small size HCC and in 15 - 20% of patients with advanced HCC *5285* 47 of 80 patients with hepatocellular carcinoma had concentrations > 200 ng/mL *3121*

α-Fetoprotein mRNA *Serum Increase* In 25 - 33% patients with HCC, AFP mRNA detectable in peripheral blood *5285*

Fibrinogen *Plasma Increase* In one patient with hepatocellular carcinoma mean concentration of 1,324 mg/dL compared with normal of 180 - 380 mg/dL *108*

Fucosidase *Serum Increase* Concentration of α-L-fucosidase may be increased but specificity is low, making their diagnostic use of little value *5285*

γ-Globulin *Serum Increase* In 12 patients with hepatocellular carcinoma mean concentration of 1.8 ± 0.4 g/dL not significantly different from 1.1 ± 0.3 g/dL in 20 healthy volunteers *2372*
Serum No Effect In 19 patients with chronic active hepatitis C with hepatocellular carcinoma mean concentration of 1.8 ± 0.5 g/dL not significantly different from normal *2381*

γ-Glutamyltransferase *Serum Increase* In 25 patients with hepatocellular carcinoma 92% had activities above 55 U/L *1406* In 12 patients with hepatocellular carcinoma mean activity of 76 ± 28 U/L significantly different from 10 ± 3 U/L in 20 healthy volunteers *2372*
Serum No Effect In 19 patients with chronic active hepatitis C with hepatocellular carcinoma mean activity of 74 ± 44 U/L not significantly different from normal *2381*

Hemoglobin *Blood Decrease* In one patient with hepatocellular carcinoma mean concentration of 12.6 g/dL *108*

Hepatitis B Surface Antigen *Serum Positive* In 100 patients with hepatocellular carcinoma 8 were positive for HBsAg *2071*

Hepatitis B Virus-encoded X Antigen *Serum Increase* Concentration of SHBG may be increased but specificity is low, making their diagnostic use of little value *5285*

Hepatitis C Virus Antibodies *Serum Positive* In 100 patients with hepatocellular carcinoma 92 were positive for HCV antibodies *2071*

Hyaluronic Acid *Serum Increase* Mean concentration in patients with hepatocellular carcinoma of 357 ± 316 ng/mL compared with 24.9 ± 12.8 ng/mL in healthy controls *3365*

immunoglobulin A *Serum Increase* Mean concentration in 11 patients with primary hepatocellular carcinoma of about 500 mg/dL significantly higher than 288 ± 121 mg/dL in 18 healthy blood donors *54*
Serum No Effect In 19 patients with chronic active hepatitis C with hepatocellular carcinoma mean concentration of 252 ± 94 mg/dL not significantly different from normal *2381*

Immunoglobulin G *Serum Increase* Mean concentration in 11 patients with primary hepatocellular carcinoma of about 3100 mg/dL significantly higher than 1200 ± 319 mg/dL in 18 healthy blood donors *54*
Serum No Effect In 19 patients with chronic active hepatitis C with hepatocellular carcinoma mean concentration of 1,750 ± 325 mg/dL not significantly different from normal *2381*

Immunoglobulin M *Serum Increase* Mean concentration in 11 patients with primary hepatocellular carcinoma of about 260 mg/dL significantly higher than 80 ± 29 mg/dL in 18 healthy blood donors *54*
Serum No Effect In 19 patients with chronic active hepatitis C with hepatocellular carcinoma mean concentration of 164 ± 94 mg/dL not significantly different from normal *2381*

Indocyanine Green Clearance *Serum Increase* In 20 patients with hepatocellular carcinoma mean retention ratio in 15 minutes 35 ± 8% *2372*

β1-Integrin *Serum Increase* In 12 patients with hepatocellular carcinoma mean concentration of 4.7 ± 0.5 µg/mL significantly higher than 2.1 ± 0.1 µg/mL in 18 healthy adult controls *5785*

β3-Integrin *Serum Increase* In 12 patients with hepatocellular carcinoma mean concentration of 14.1 ± 1.8 µg/mL significantly higher than 5.5 ± 0.5 µg/mL in 18 healthy adult controls *5785*

Lactate Dehydrogenase *Ascitic Fluid Increase* In 73 specimens from patients with hepatocellular carcinoma or cirrhosis mean activity of 103 ± 6 U/L but significantly less than 823 ± 107 U/L in 21 specimens from patients with peritoneal neoplasia. In patients with hepatocellular carcinoma or cirrhosis mean ascitic fluid:serum ratio of 0.41 ± 0.04 significantly less than 3.85 ± 0.96 in 9 specimens from patients with peritoneal neoplasia *728*

Laminin P1 *Serum Increase* Mean concentration significantly increased compared with healthy controls *3670*

Lymphocytes *Blood No Effect* In 19 patients with chronic active hepatitis C with hepatocellular carcinoma mean count of 1,578 ± 720 /µL not significantly different from normal *2381*

Lysyl Oxidase *Serum Increase* Mean activity significantly increased compared with controls but to an extent less than that in cirrhosis *3670*

Macrophage Colony Stimulating Factor *Serum Increase* In 12 patients with hepatocellular carcinoma mean concentration of about 3.4 ng/mL significantly different from 1.95 ± 0.44 ng/mL in 20 healthy volunteers *2372*

β_2-Microglobulin *Serum Increase* In one study 62% of patients had concentrations above cutoff value of 2.0 mg/mL *3120*

Neopterin *Urine Increase* In 3 patients with hepatocellular carcinoma mean excretion of 897.0 µmol/mol creatinine significantly higher than 106.6 ± 34.6 µmol/mol creatinine in 31 healthy controls *3632*

N-terminal Peptide of Type III Procollagen *Serum Increase* In 40 patients with hepatocellular carcinoma and liver cirrhosis mean concentration of 1.64 U/mL significantly higher than 1.54 U/mL in 60 patients with cirrhosis alone *1405*

5'-Nucleotidase *Serum Increase* In 11 patients with liver metastases or hepatocarcinoma mean activity 26 U/L (range 5 - 242 U/L) compared with mean of 3.8 U/L in healthy controls. Isoform % NTP1 45%, NTP2 15% and NTP3 42% compared with 12%, 30% and 58% respectively in healthy controls *3993*

p53 Autoantibodies *Serum Increase* In 20 - 25% European patients with HCC, anti-p53 antibodies are detected *5285*

Parathyroid Hormone-related Peptide *Plasma Increase* In 2 of 3 patients with liver cancer and hypercalcemia concentration increased above upper limit of normal of 1.5 pmol/L (range of concentrations 0.5 to 81.4 pmol/L) *3987*

Partial Thromboplastin Time *Plasma Increase* In one patient with hepatocellular carcinoma mean time of 56.8 s compared with normal range of 34 - 48 s *108*

Plasminogen *Plasma No Effect* In one patient with hepatocellular carcinoma mean concentration of 120% *108*

Platelets *Blood Decrease* In 100 patients with hepatocellular carcinoma mean concentration of 11.3 x 10^9/L different from reference interval of 17 - 39 x 10^9/L *2071*

Prekallikrein *Plasma Increase* Mean concentration in 5 patients of 151.6 ± 36.2% significantly higher than 100.0 ± 23.1% in 30 healthy controls *855*

Pro-Matrix Metalloproteinase 1 *Serum Increase* Mean concentration of 297 ± 119 ng/mL in 61 patients with hepatocellular carcinoma significantly different from 155 ± 17 ng/mL in 29 healthy controls *3668*

Procollagen 1 C-terminal Peptide *Serum Increase* In 40 patients with hepatocellular carcinoma and liver cirrhosis mean concentration of 1,729 µg/L significantly higher than 1,255 µg/L in 60 patients with cirrhosis alone *1405*

Procollagen Type III Peptide *Serum Increase* Increased concentration was useful in assessing extent of hepatic fibrosis *5276*

Proline Hydroxylase *Serum Increase* Mean activity significantly increased compared with healthy controls *3670*

Prolyl Hydroxylase *Serum Increase* In 40 patients with hepatocellular carcinoma and liver cirrhosis mean concentration of 131 µg/L significantly higher than 90 µg/L in 60 patients with cirrhosis alone *1405* Increased activity was useful in assessing extent of hepatic fibrosis *5276*

155.00 Hepatocellular Carcinoma (continued)

Protein *Ascitic Fluid Increase* In 72 specimens from patients with hepatocellular carcinoma or cirrhosis mean concentration of 19.19 ± 1.26 g/L but significantly less than 57.12 ± 3.8 g/L in 17 specimens from patients with peritoneal neoplasia. Ascitic fluid:serum ratio in hepatocellular carcinomatous or cirrhotic patients of 0.29 ± 0.02 but significantly less than 0.75 ± 10 in patients with peritoneal neoplasia *728*
Serum No Effect In 19 patients with chronic active hepatitis C with hepatocellular carcinoma mean concentration of 7.2 ± 0.4 g/dL not significantly different from normal *2381* In one patient with hepatocellular carcinoma mean concentration of 7.3 g/dL *108*

Protein C *Plasma Decrease* In 5 patients mean concentration of 73.9 ± 11.8% significantly less than 105.0 ± 35.0% in 30 healthy controls *855*

Prothrombin Time *Plasma Increase* In one patient with hepatocellular carcinoma mean time of 15.7 s compared with control of 14.3 s, with INR of 1.39 *108*
Plasma No Effect In 19 patients with chronic active hepatitis C with hepatocellular carcinoma mean time of 80 ± 15% not significantly different from normal *2381* In 5 patients mean INR of 1.11 ± 0.16 not significantly different from 1.05 ± 0.11 in 30 healthy controls *855*

Pseudouridine *Ascitic Fluid Increase* Mean concentration in 51 specimens from patients with hepatocellular carcinoma or cirrhosis of 3.78 ± 0.27 µmol/L but significantly less than 7.48 ± 0.72 µmol/L in 10 specimens from patients with peritoneal neoplasia *728*
Urine Increase In 3 patients with hepatocellular carcinoma mean excretion of 37.5 mmol/mol creatinine significantly higher than 19.6 ± 5.2 mmol/mol creatinine in 31 healthy controls *3632*

Putrescine *Urine Increase* Mean excretion in 32 patients with hepatocellular carcinoma of 36.6 ± 10.1 nmol/mg creatinine significantly different from 11.2 ± 1.5 nmol/mg creatinine in 28 healthy controls *152*

Putrescine, Free *Urine Increase* Mean excretion in 32 patients with hepatocellular carcinoma of 4.6 ± 1.2 nmol/mg creatinine significantly different from 0.9 ± 0.4 nmol/mg creatinine in 28 healthy controls *152*

Putrescine, N-monoacetylated *Urine Increase* Mean excretion in 32 patients with hepatocellular carcinoma of 29.8 ± 8.8 nmol/mg creatinine significantly different from 11.2 ± 1.5 nmol/mg creatinine in 28 healthy controls *152*

Sex-Hormone Binding Globulin *Serum Increase* Concentration of SHBG may be increased but specificity is low, making their diagnostic use of little value *5285*

Soluble E-Selectin *Serum Increase* In 25 patients with hepatocellular carcinoma 45% had concentrations greater than 86 µg/L *1406*

Soluble Intercellular Adhesion Molecule-1 *Serum Increase* In 25 patients with hepatocellular carcinoma, 100% had concentrations greater than 286 µg/L *1406*

Soluble Interleukin-2 Receptor *Serum Increase* In 19 patients with chronic active hepatitis C with hepatocellular carcinoma mean concentration of 3,192 ± 1,805 U/mL significantly different from normal *2381*

Soluble Vascular Cell Adhesion Molecule-1
Serum Increase In 25 patients with hepatocellular carcinoma, 100% had concentrations greater than 872 µg/L *1406*

Spermidine *Urine Increase* Mean excretion in 32 patients with hepatocellular carcinoma of 20.1 ± 5.7 nmol/mg creatinine significantly different from 5.9 ± 1.1 nmol/mg creatinine in 28 healthy controls *152*

Spermidine, Free *Urine Increase* Mean excretion in 32 patients with hepatocellular carcinoma of 1.6 ± 0.9 nmol/mg creatinine significantly different from 0.2 ± 0.1 nmol/mg creatinine in 28 healthy controls *152*

Spermidine, N^1-acetylated *Urine Increase* Mean excretion in 32 patients with hepatocellular carcinoma of 13.7 ± 4.3 nmol/mg creatinine significantly different from 3.2 ± 0.8 nmol/mg creatinine in 28 healthy controls *152*

Spermidine, N^1-acetylated:N^8-acetylated Ratio
Urine Increase Mean excretion in 32 patients with hepatocellular carcinoma of 2.8 ± 0.8 significantly different from 1.3 ± 0.2 in 28 healthy controls *152*

Spermidine, N^8-acetylated *Urine Increase* Mean excretion in 32 patients with hepatocellular carcinoma of 4.8 ± 0.4 nmol/mg creatinine significantly different from 2.5 ± 0.4 nmol/mg creatinine in 28 healthy controls *152*

Spermine *Urine Increase* Mean excretion in 32 patients with hepatocellular carcinoma of 2.1 ± 0.8 nmol/mg creatinine significantly different from 0.7 ± 0.5 nmol/mg creatinine in 28 healthy controls *152*

Spermine, Free *Urine Increase* Mean excretion in 32 patients with hepatocellular carcinoma of 1.0 ± 0.2 nmol/mg creatinine significantly different from 0.3 ± 0.3 nmol/mg creatinine in 28 healthy controls *152*

Spermine, N-acetylated *Urine No Effect* Mean excretion in 32 patients with hepatocellular carcinoma of not detectable not different from not detectable in 28 healthy controls *152*

Taurine *Plasma No Effect* Mean concentration of 0.2 mol/mL in patients with liver cancer not significantly different from 0.12 mol/mL in healthy controls *264*

Tissue Inhibitor of Metalloproteinase-1 *Serum Increase* In 45 patients with hepatocellular carcinoma mean concentration of 333.3 ± 182.0 ng/mL significantly higher than 147.8 ± 22.0 ng/mL in 53 normal individuals *3690* Mean concentration of 468 ng/mL in one patient with hepatocellular carcinoma significantly different from 66 ng/mL in the platelet-poor plasma of one healthy individual *3667*

Tissue Inhibitor of Metalloproteinase-2 *Serum Increase* Mean concentration of 88 ± 29 ng/mL in 61 patients with hepatocellular carcinomasignificantly different from 61 ± 13 ng/mL in 29 healthy controls *3668*

Tissue Plasminogen Activator *Plasma Increase* In 67.2% of 64 patients with hepatocellular carcinoma and in 89.3% of 28 patients with advanced hepatocellular carcinoma concentration increased above 8,3 ng/mL *3887*

Tissue Polypeptide Antigen *Serum Increase* Concentration may be increased but specificity is low, making their diagnostic use of little value *5285* Median concentration of 264.1 U/L in 26 patients with hepatocellular carcinoma significantly different from 25.2 U/L in 29 healthy controls *5316*

Transcobalamin I *Serum Increase* Concentrations markedly higher in patients with HCC than in patients with nonmalignant liver disease *1778*

Transcobalamin III *Serum Increase* Concentrations markedly higher in patients with HCC than in patients with nonmalignant liver disease *1778*

Transforming Growth Factor-β *Serum Increase* Mean concentration in 17 patients with hepatocellular carcinoma of 19.2 ± 17.0 ng/mL (range 1.6 - 70.0 ng/mL) significantly higher than in healthy controls *2365*

Transforming Growth Factor-β_1 *Serum Increase* In 94 patients with cirrhotic hepatocellular carcinoma 45 (47.8%) had concentrations greater than 400 ng/mL *5181* Plasma TGF-β_1 concentration increased *5285*
Urine Increase Median concentration of 61.1 µg/g creatinine in 94 patients with cirrhotic hepatocellular carcinoma significantly higher than 12.2 µg/g creatinine in 50 healthy adults *5181* Sensitivity of urine TGF-β_1 was 53% with specificity of 99% *5285*

Urea *Serum Increase* Median concentration in 8 patients with hepatocellular carcinoma of 42 mg/dL significantly different from 31 mg/dL in 32 healthy controls *2566*

Urea Nitrogen *Serum Increase* In 25 patients with hepatocellular carcinoma 44% had concentrations above 8.6 mmol/L *1406*

155.00 Hepatoma

Alcohol Dehydrogenase *Serum Increase* In 105 Nigerians with hepatoma mean activity of 6.4 ± 1.0 U/L significantly different from 0.7 ± 0.1 U/L in 120 healthy controls *3866*

Anti-p53 Antibodies *Serum Increase* Increase observed in 2 of 148 patients (1.4%) *132*

CA 19-9 *Serum Increase* CA 19-9 concentration increased in 50% patients with primary hepatomas *1253* In 122 patients with hepatoma positive rate of 35% observed using cut-off from normals and 28% at 90% specificity *2594*

CA 242 *Serum Increase* In 122 patients with hepatoma positive rate of 7% observed using cut-off from normals and 10% at 90% specificity *2594*

Epidermal Growth Factor *Urine* *No Effect* Mean concentration in about 6 patients of 13 μg/g creatinine not significantly different compared with about 10 μg/g creatinine in about 30 controls *5341*

Gc-Globulin *Serum* *No Effect* In 2 men with hepatoma mean concentration of 19.5 mg/dL not significantly different from 23.9 ± 3.36 mg/dL in 106 control men *2279*

Metallopanstimulin *Serum* *Increase* In 2 patients with hepatoma mean concentration exceeded upper limit of normal of < 10 ng/mL in healthy individuals aged 19 - 88 years *1462*

Neopterin *Serum* *Increase* Mean concentration of 27.4 ± 21.8 nmol/L in 9 patients with hepatoma significantly greater than that in 18 healthy control individuals, 6.4 ± 1.8 nmol/L *3864*

155.00 Primary Hepatocellular Carcinoma

Neopterin *Serum* *Increase* In 17 patients with primary hepatocellular carcinoma mean concentration of 15.5 ± 3.0 nmol/L, with mean in 2 without cirrhosis of 13.0 ± 5.8 nmol/L and 15.8 ± 3.4 nmol/L in 15 with cirrhosis different from 6.0 ± 2.2 nmol/L in healthy controls *5682*

155.10 Cholangiocarcinoma

CA 19-9 *Bile* *Increase* Reported to be useful marker for malignant disease of biliary tract *1057*
Serum *Increase* In 31 patients with biliary tract cancer positive rate of 84% observed using cut-off from normals and 84% at 90% specificity *2594* Concentrations increased in patients with PSC who develop cholangiocarcinoma *1778* Concentration typically increased in patients with cholangiocarcinoma *2952* Reported to be useful marker for malignant disease of biliary tract *1057* Measurement widely used to detect cholangiocarcinoma in patients with primary sclerosing cholangitis. Concentrations greater than 100 U/L (normal < 40 U/L) reported to have sensitivity of 89% and specificity of 86% to detect cholangiocarcinoma in these patients *1057*

CA 50 *Serum* *Increase* Reported to be useful marker for malignant disease of biliary tract *1057*

CA 125 *Bile* *Increase* Reported to be useful marker for malignant disease of biliary tract *1057* *1057*
Serum *Increase* Reported to be useful marker for malignant disease of biliary tract *1057*

CA 195 *Serum* *Increase* Reported to be useful marker for malignant disease of biliary tract *1057*

CA 242 *Serum* *Increase* In 31 patients with biliary tract cancer positive rate of 65% observed using cut-off from normals and 68% at 90% specificity *2594* Reported to be useful marker for malignant disease of biliary tract *1057*

CA-M17.1 *Serum* *Increase* In 5 patients quartile range 19 - 260 U/L compared with 15 - 15 U/L in 75 disease controls with non-malignant non-biliary illness *3772*

Calcium *Serum* *Increase* One patient with cholangiocarcinoma had hypercalcemia *1200*

Carcinoembryonic Antigen *Bile* *Increase* Mean concentration in 25 patients with cholangiocarcinoma of 50.2 ng/mL *3729* Reported to be useful marker for malignant disease of biliary tract *1057*
Serum *Increase* Mean concentration in 10 patients with cholangiocarcinoma of 3.5 ng/mL *3729* Reported to be useful marker for malignant disease of biliary tract *1057* Concentrations increased in patients with PSC who develop cholangiocarcinoma *1778*

Cytokeratin 19 Fragment *Serum* *Increase* Reported to be useful marker for malignant disease of biliary tract *1057*

Dupan-2 *Serum* *Increase* Reported to be useful marker for malignant disease of biliary tract *1057*

Fibronectin *Bile* *Increase* Reported to be useful marker for malignant disease of biliary tract *1057*

Interleukin-6 *Serum* *Increase* Reported to be useful marker for malignant disease of biliary tract *1057*

K-ras Oncogene *Bile* *Increase* Reported to be useful marker for malignant disease of biliary tract *1057*

Lactate *Bile* *Increase* Reported to be useful marker for malignant disease of biliary tract *1057*

Pancreatic Polypeptide *Plasma* *Increase* Reported to be useful marker for malignant disease of biliary tract *1057*

Parathyroid Hormone-related Peptide *Plasma* *Increase* In 1 patient with cholangiocarcinoma concentration of 8.19 pmol/L significantly greater than upper limit of reference range of 2.6 pmol/L *1200*

Sialyl-Tn Antigen *Bile* *Increase* Reported to be useful marker for malignant disease of biliary tract *1057*

Trypsin-2-α_1-Antitrypsin *Serum* *Increase* Reported to be useful marker for malignant disease of biliary tract *1057*

Trypsinogen-2 *Serum* *Increase* Reported to be useful marker for malignant disease of biliary tract *1057*

155.10 Malignant Neoplasm of Intrahepatic Bile Ducts

Alanine Aminotransferase *Serum* *Increase* Found in all cases of malignant disease of biliary tract; ranging from 65.5-87 U/L *5738*

Alkaline Phosphatase *Serum* *Increase* In all cases; elevated from 94 to 263 U/L (normal 25 U/L) due to common duct obstruction *5738*

Alkaline Phosphatase Isoenzymes *Serum* *Increase* Regan isoenzyme concentration was 27.6 U/L *1140*

Aspartate Aminotransferase *Serum* *Increase* May be slightly elevated, but rarely higher than 200 U/L *367*

Bilirubin *Serum* *Increase* Values exceed 10 mg/dL in most cases, with a mean value of about 18 mg/dL *367* Markedly elevated levels, ranging from 16.0 - 23.2 mg/dL *5738*

CA 19-9 *Serum* *Increase* CA 19-9 concentration increased in 60 - 70% patients with bile-duct cancers *1253*

Carcinoembryonic Antigen *Ascitic Fluid* *Increase* In malignant effusions *4891*

Cholesterol *Serum* *Increase* Averages about 400 mg/dL *367*

Fibrin Degradation Products *Ascitic Fluid* *Increase* In malignant effusions *4891*

Occult Blood *Feces* *Increase* Frequently positive *5544*

155.20 Metastatic Neoplasm to Liver

Aspartate Aminotransferase:Alanine Aminotransferase Ratio *Serum* *Increase* Ratio greater than 3.0 with AST activity exceeding 500 U/L (normal < 40 U/L) is suggestive of circulatory disturbances, especially left ventricular failure, or malignant diseases involving the liver *4617*

CA 19-9 *Serum* *Increase* Of 204 patients with CA 19-9 concentrations greater than 60 U/mL, 14 had liver metastases for which the primary site was not found *3423*

Carcinoembryonic Antigen *Bile* *Increase* All of 30 patients with hepatic metastases had concentrations above 5 ng/mL: median ratio of bile:serum concentrations 12.5 *4040*
Serum *Increase* 23 of 30 patients (77%) with hepatic metastases had concentrations above 5 ng/mL *4040*

α-Fetoprotein *Serum* *Increase* Concentrations increased in 80% patients with symptomatic HCC, but only occasionally increased in patients with metastatic liver disease *1778*
Serum *No Effect* Occasionally increased in patients with metastatic liver disease *1778*

156.00 Cancer of Gallbladder

Adenosine Deaminase *Serum* *Increase* Ninety-one percent of 527 patients with tumors showed activity above normal, whereas eighty-six per cent of 408 nontumorous diseased persons did not *5041* *2737*

Alanine Aminotransferase *Serum* *Increase* Cholecystitis and cholestasis due to obstruction of bile flow typically result in mild increases or no change in activity *1057*
Serum *No Effect* Cholecystitis and cholestasis due to obstruction of bile flow typically result in mild increases or no change in activity *1057*

Alkaline Phosphatase *Serum* *Increase* Cholecystitis and cholestasis due to obstruction of bile flow typically result in moderate to marked increases in activity *1057*

156.00 Cancer of Gallbladder *(continued)*

Alkaloids *Serum Increase* Increased *3926 1340*

Aspartate Aminotransferase *Serum Increase* Cholecystitis and cholestasis due to obstruction of bile flow typically result in mild increases or no change in activity *1057*
Serum No Effect Cholecystitis and cholestasis due to obstruction of bile flow typically result in mild increases or no change in activity *1057*

Bile Acids *Serum Increase* Cholecystitis and cholestasis due to obstruction of bile flow typically result in moderate to marked increases in concentration *1057*

Bilirubin *Serum Increase* Cholecystitis and cholestasis due to obstruction of bile flow typically result in moderate to marked increases in concentration *1057*

CA 19-9 *Bile Increase* Reported to be useful marker for malignant disease of biliary tract *1057*
Serum Increase Frequently show elevated values *3657 2026* Sensitivity of 90% (n = 21) *2122* Reported to be useful marker for malignant disease of biliary tract *1057*

CA 50 *Serum Increase* Reported to be useful marker for malignant disease of biliary tract *1057*

CA 72-4 *Serum Increase* Sensitivity of 52% (n = 21). CA 72-4 has a very high specificity (98%) in benign diseases of the gastrointestinal tract, including inflammatory processes, so that elevated serum levels should always be taken seriously *2122*

CA 125 *Bile Increase* Reported to be useful marker for malignant disease of biliary tract *1057*
Serum Increase Reported to be useful marker for malignant disease of biliary tract *1057*

CA 195 *Serum Increase* Reported to be useful marker for malignant disease of biliary tract *1057*

CA 242 *Serum Increase* Reported to be useful marker for malignant disease of biliary tract *1057* High percentages of elevated levels were recorded in patients with pancreatic and biliary cancers (68%). The sensitivity was somewhat lower than CA 19-9 (76%) and CA 50 (73%) *2870*

Carcinoembryonic Antigen *Bile Increase* Reported to be useful marker for malignant disease of biliary tract *1057*
Serum Increase Reported to be useful marker for malignant disease of biliary tract *1057*

Creatine Kinase MM-Isoenzyme *Serum Increase* Elevated CK-MM *919* Elevated CK-MM reported *2427*

Cytokeratin 19 Fragment *Serum Increase* Reported to be useful marker for malignant disease of biliary tract *1057*

Dupan-2 *Serum Increase* Reported to be useful marker for malignant disease of biliary tract *1057*

α-Fetoprotein *Serum Increase* Primary tumors of gall bladder may secrete AFP regardless of whether they have metastasized to the liver *1778*

Fibronectin *Bile Increase* Reported to be useful marker for malignant disease of biliary tract *1057*

γ-Glutamyltransferase *Serum Increase* Cholecystitis and cholestasis due to obstruction of bile flow typically result in moderate to marked increases in activity *1057*

Interleukin-6 *Serum Increase* Reported to be useful marker for malignant disease of biliary tract *1057*

K-ras Oncogene *Bile Increase* Reported to be useful marker for malignant disease of biliary tract *1057*

Lactate *Bile Increase* Reported to be useful marker for malignant disease of biliary tract *1057*

Pancreatic Polypeptide *Plasma Increase* Reported to be useful marker for malignant disease of biliary tract *1057*

Prothrombin Time *Plasma Increase* Prolonged obstruction of bile flow through the common hepatic or common bile duct may lead to deficiency of fat-soluble vitamins and increased prothrombin time *1057*

Sialyl-Tn Antigen *Bile Increase* Reported to be useful marker for malignant disease of biliary tract *1057*

Sialyltransferase *Serum Increase* In 1 patient with cancer of the gall bladder mean and median concentrations of 544 and 560 cpm/mg protein/30 min significantly different from 240 and 243 cpm/mg protein/30 min respectively in 20 normal individuals *2111*

Trypsin-2-α_1-Antitrypsin *Serum Increase* Reported to be useful marker for malignant disease of biliary tract *1057*

Trypsinogen-2 *Serum Increase* Reported to be useful marker for malignant disease of biliary tract *1057*

156.90 Primary Neoplasm of Biliary Tract

CA 19-9 *Serum Increase* Concentrations may be increased markedly with obstruction of bilary tract by primary biliary cancer *1778*

157.40 Non-carcinoid Pancreatic Islet Tumor

5-Hydroxyindoleacetic Acid *Urine Increase* Modest increases observed in patients with non-carcinoid pancreatic islet tumors *2952*

157.40 Pancreatic Islet Cell Tumor

$7B_2$ *Serum Increase* Mean concentration of 1,041 ± 1,786 pmol/L observed in 13 patients with pancreatic islet cell tumors compared with 67 ± 10 pmol/L in 31 healthy controls *2318*

157.80 Gastropancreatic Neoplasm

Chromogranin-A *Serum Increase* In 99 patients with neuroendocrine neoplasms affecting a variety of sites mean concentration of 1,453 μg/L significantly different from 36 ± 18 μg/L in 100 normal individuals *329*

Neuron-specific Enolase *Serum Increase* In 99 patients with neuroendocrine neoplasms affecting a variety of sites mean concentration of 25.5 μg/L significantly different from normal range of < 12.5 μg/L *329*

157.90 Cancer of Pancreas

Adenosine Deaminase *Serum Increase* Ninety-one percent of 527 patients with tumors showed activity above normal, whereas eighty-six per cent of 408 nontumorous diseased persons did not *2737 5041*

Alanine Aminotransferase *Serum Increase* In 40% of 10 patients at initial hospitalization for this disorder *1576* Elevated due to extrahepatic biliary tract obstruction *5738*

Albumin *Serum Decrease* In 44% of 46 patients at initial hospitalization for this disorder *1576*

Alkaline Phosphatase *Serum Increase* Elevated in 85 of 100 patients with histologically proven disease *1900* Elevated without marked abnormalities in all liver function tests *553* In 82% of 46 patients at initial hospitalization for this disorder *1576* Since enzyme is produced by the biliary tract at all levels from the canaliculi to to the mucosa of the gallbladder and the large bile ducts, enzyme, activity may increase with diseases that cause impedance of bile flow such as cancer of the head of the pancreas *4617* Due to biliary tract obstruction values range from 150 to 215 U/L (normal = 21 U/L) *5738*
White Blood Cells Decrease Low activity is present irrespective of tumor category, activity of disease, or type of therapy. In 11 patients, median activity was 5 U/L (normal 55 U/L) *3110*

Alkaline Phosphatase Isoenzymes *Serum Increase* Highest concentrations were found in sera of patients with cancer of the pancreas. Ranges were 11.8 - 81.4 U/L *1140*

Amylase *Pleural Fluid Increase* Carcinoma of the pancreas and other organs *3054*
Serum Decrease Slightly increased in early stages (< 10% of cases). With later destruction of pancreas, normal or decreased *5544*
Serum Increase May be mildly elevated in a few patients as a result of pancreatitis secondary to an obstructing tumor *4891* Activity often increased in patients with advanced pancreatic cancer *4153* In 35% of 14 patients at initial hospitalization for this disorder *1576* Elevated serum and urinary S-amylase has been reported *4802* Hyperamylasemia found in only 9% of 100 histologically proven cases *1900* Early obstruction of the pancreatic duct *367* May be slightly increased in early stages (< 10% of cases). With later destruction of pancreas, normal or decreased *5544*

Serum *No Effect* May be slightly increased in early stages (< 10% of cases). With later destruction of pancreas, normal or decreased *5544*
Urine *Increase* 1 h excretion is increased in up to 30% of patients *2033* May be mildly elevated in a few patients as a result of pancreatitis secondary to an obstructing tumor *4891* Elevated serum and urinary S-amylase has been reported *4802* Activity often increased in patients with advanced pancreatic cancer *4153*

Androstanediol Glucuronide *Plasma* *Decrease* Mean concentration in 13 male patients with cancer of the pancreas of 6.75 ± 5.5 nmol/L significantly different from 9.8 - 43.3 nmol/L in 40 healthy men *2416*

Androstenedione *Plasma* *Increase* Mean concentration in 13 male patients with cancer of the pancreas of 12.9 ± 16.3 nmol/L significantly different from 2.8 - 7.5 nmol/L in 40 healthy men *2416*

Anti-p53 Antibodies *Serum* *Increase* Increase observed in 3 of 46 patients (6.5%) *132*

α_1-Antitrypsin *Serum* *Increase* Only 3 of 16 patients had elevated levels *4221* In patients with pancreatic cancer those with an increase of 100 mg/dL AAT had a 57% higher fatality rate than those with lower concentration *5279* Significantly higher than controls. Pancreatic Ca. patients average 487 mg/dL, Controls average 434 mg/dL *5267* Variations are nonspecific and are of no diagnostic value for pancreatic cancer *4153*

Arylsulfatase *Serum* *Increase* Elevated with metastases to the liver or bones *3833*

Aspartate Aminotransferase *Serum* *Increase* In 74% of 46 patients at initial hospitalization for this disorder *1576* 63% of patients showed elevated values *1900* Slight elevation occurred in 2 of 4 cases. Range of values was 12.5 - 45 U/L, while the maximum upper limit of normal is 24 U/L *3161*

$7B_2$ *Serum* *No Effect* Mean concentration in 11 patients with pancreatic adenocarcinoma remained within normal range of 67 ± 10 pmol/L *2318*

Bicarbonate *Duodenal Contents* *Decrease* Acinar destruction (as in pancreatitis) shows normal volume (20 - 30 mL/10 min collection period) but bicarbonate and enzyme levels may be decreased. In carcinoma, the test result depends on the relative extent and combination of acinar destruction and of duct obstruction *5544*
Duodenal Contents *No Effect* Secretin-pancreozymin stimulation evidences duct obstruction when duodenal intubation shows decreased volume of duodenal contents (< 10 mL/10 min collection period) with usually normal bicarbonate and enzyme levels in duodenal contents *5544*

Bilirubin *Serum* *Increase* Concentration may increase with diseases that cause impedance of bile flow such as cancer of the head of the pancreas *4617* In 39% of 46 patients at initial hospitalization for this disorder *1576* May become significantly elevated with direct fraction greater than the indirect fraction *900* Markedly elevated with values ranging from 4.0 - 17.9 mg/dL *5738* Elevated without marked abnormalities in liver all function tests *553* Increased (12 - 25 mg/dL), mostly direct. Increase is persistent and nonfluctuating *5544*

Bilirubin, Direct *Serum* *Increase* In 91% of 14 patients at initial hospitalization for this disorder *1576*

Bilirubin, Indirect *Serum* *Increase* In 56% of 14 patients at initial hospitalization for this disorder *1576*

CA 15-3 *Serum* *Increase* In 10 patients with pancreatic cancer mean concentration of 51.2 ± 53 U/mL significantly different from cutoff of 22 U/mL, 7 of whom had concentrations greater than 30 U/mL and 5 had concentrations greater than 40 U/mL *2076*

CA 19-9 *Serum* *Decrease* Falsely low concentrations observed in patients with pancreatic cancer negative for the Lewis blood group phenotype *2593*
Serum *Increase* In various studies sensitivity for pancreatic cancer varies from 68 - 93% and specificity also from 68 - 93%, with concentrations highest in patients with metastases *4153* In patients with inoperable cancer mean doubling time 47.1 d, 53.6 d for patients with palliative surgey and 43.4 d during recurrence in patients who had recurrence *3799* Was found in increased concentrations (> 37 U/mL) in 87% of the patients (n = 145) as compared with only 13% in the group with benign disease (n = 1,081) and 29% of those with extrapancreatic malignancies (n = 691) *4506* Majority of concentrations in 13 male patients with cancer of the pancreas higher than 37 U/L *2416* 9 of 9 patients with benign pancreatic disease had concentrations less than 36 U/mL whereas 4 of 5 patients with pancreatic cancer had concentrations greater than 300 U/mL *4265* Values were higher than 40 U/mL in 45 of 54 patients with pancreatic carcinoma and in 18 of 56 patients with other diagnosis (sensitivity of 0.83; specificity of 0.68; positive predictive value of 0.71). High concentrations in patients with diagnosed or suspected exocrine pancreatic carcinoma could strongly indicate metastatic processes *3984* In 14 of 23 cases of pancreatic cancer with tumor sizes of less than 2.0 cm increased concentration observed. In 40 of 51 cases with tumors between 2.1 and 4.0 cm concentration increased. Overall sensitivity for tumors less than 4.0 cm 73% *4587* Of 204 patients with CA 19-9 concentrations greater than 60 U/mL, 34 had pancreatic cancer *3423* In 37 patients with biopsy-proven adenocarcinoma of the pancreas mean concentration of 1,189 ± 2657 U/mL with 33 having concentration increased above cutoff of 37 U/mL and 32 above cutoff of 75 U/mL *4998* Concentration increased in 31 of 40 patients (78%) with ductal adenocarcinomas *411* Values were higher than 40 U/mL in 45 of 54 patients with pancreatic carcinoma and in 18 of 56 patients with other diagnosis (sensitivity of 0.83; specificity of 0.68; positive predictive value of 0.71) *3249* Reported in up to 96% of patients *2026* In 40 patients with stage I pancreatic cancer 68% had concentrations greater than 37 U/mL, 91% of 54 patients with stage II - III disease and 85% of 85 patients with stage IV disease *1957* In 151 patients with pancreatic cancer positive rate of 82% observed using cut-off from normals and 79% at 90% specificity *2594* In 87.2% of 47 patients with pancreatic cancer concentration increased above cut-off of 37 U/mL *2854* Sensitivity of 82% (n = 68) *2122* Concentration typically increased in patients with pancreatic cancer *2952* Concentrations increased so that CA 19-9 measurement is most useful for diagnosis of pancreatic cancer *1778*

CA 27-29 *Serum* *Increase* In 22% of 18 patients with cancer of pancreas concentration increased above 36% *766*

CA 50 *Serum* *Increase* Sensitivity and specificity greater than 80% *3340* Serum pattern in association with pancreatic cancer is quite similar to that of CA 19-9 *4153*

CA 72-4 *Serum* *Increase* Sensitivity of 22% (n = 68). CA 72-4 has a very high specificity (98%) in benign diseases of the gastrointestinal tract, including inflammatory processes, so that elevated serum levels should always be taken seriously *2122* In colon carcinomas 26.5% of specimens showed elevated levels *5744*

CA 125 *Serum* *Increase* Concentration increases with pancreatic cancer as for ovarian cancer, but sensitivity and specificity are not usually high enough for CA 125 to be useful for diagnosing pancreatic cancer *4153* Increased in 61% of cases *5546*

CA 195 *Serum* *Increase* Significantly higher in patients with metastatic disease *4508* Increased concentrations observed in patients with pancreatic cancer *122*

CA 242 *Serum* *Increase* In 151 patients with pancreatic cancer positive rate of 79% observed using cut-off from normals and 81% at 90% specificity *2594* This marker seems to be less sensitive than CEA and CA 50 in detection of pancreatic carcinoma. However it may prove useful because of its high specificity *4020* Sensitivity and specificity greater than 80% *3340* Sensitivity for diagnosing pancreatic cancer varies from 57 - 80% according to different studies. Correlation with serum CA 19-9 concentrations r = 0.962 *4153* In 40 patients with stage I pancreatic cancer 55% had concentrations greater than 20 U/mL, 83% of 54 patients with stage II - III disease and 78% of 85 patients with stage IV disease *1957*

CA-M17.1 *Serum* *Increase* In 23 patients with pancreatic cancer quartile range of 66 - 1,255 U/L compared with 15 - 15 U/L in 75 disease controls with non-malignant non-biliary illness *3772*

Calcium *Serum* *Increase* Without evidence of direct bone involvement. Parathyroid hormone-secreting tumors *1025*
Urine *Decrease* No evidence of direct bone involvement. Parathyroid hormone-secreting tumors *1025*

CAR-3 *Serum* *Increase* Concentration observed to increase in several patients with pancreatic cancer. Has almost 100% specificity in differentiating between pancreatic cancer and chronic pancreatitis *4153*

Carcinoembryonic Antigen *Ascitic Fluid* *Increase* In malignant effusions *4891*

157.90 **Cancer of Pancreas** *(continued)*

Carcinoembryonic Antigen *(continued)*
Serum *Increase* Has low sensitivity and specificity for pancreatic cancer *4153* In 92% of cases *4891* For tumors less than 2.0 cm in diameter sensitivity 30.8% and for tumors between 2.1 and 4.0 cm sensitivity 46.9% *4587* Increase observed in more than 90% of patients *4551* Elevated levels were noted in 33% of the patients with tumors localized to the pancreas. When the carcinoma had extended beyond the pancreas or distant metastases were present, 78% of patients had elevated levels *3983* In 31 patients with biopsy-proven adenocarcinoma of the pancreas mean concentration of 16.1 ± 26.3 ng/mL with 22 having concentration increased above cutoff of 2.5 ng/mL and 15 above 5.0 ng/mL *4998* In 37 patients with malignant disease of the pancreas 43.2% had concentrations of 0.0 - 3.0 ng/mL, 21.6% had concentrations from 3.1 - 5.0 ng/mL, 5.4% had concentrations from 5.1 - 10.0 ng/mL and 29.7% had concentrations greater than 10.0 ng/mL when measured by method on Bayer Technicon Immuno 1® system compared with 95.9%, 3.5%, 0.6% and 0.0% respectively in 173 healthy nonsmokers *339* Concentration increased in 14 of 36 patients (39%) with ductal adenocarcinomas *411* In patients with inoperable cancer mean doubling time not significantly different from that in patients with palliative surgey or during recurrence in patients who had recurrence *3799* In 55.3% of 47 patients with pancreatic cancer concentration increased above cut-off of 37 U/mL *2854* Increase observed in more than 90% of patients *1601* Mean concentration increased in 91% of patients with pancreatic cancer compared with 11% in healthy individuals *3191*
Tissue *Increase* Using FNA mean concentration of 360.5 ng/mL observed in first drop of aspirated material in 17 patients *4139*

Carotene *Serum* *Decrease* Secondary to malabsorption *4891*

Ceruloplasmin *Serum* *Increase* In 3 men with pancreatic cancer mean concentration of 81 mg/dL not significantly different from 71 ± 17 mg/dL in 106 control men and mean of 88 mg/dL in 88 women with pancreatic cancer not significantly different from 84 ± 22 mg/dL in 150 control women *2280*

Cholesterol *Serum* *Decrease* In 27% of 43 patients at initial hospitalization for this disorder *1576*
Serum *Increase* May remain normal until late in the disease *900* Increased (usually > 300 mg/dL) with esters not decreased *5544*

β-Chorionic Gonadotropin *Plasma* *Increase* Elevated immunoreactive hCG was found in 33% of patients *1497*

Colon Specific Antigen *Serum* *Increase* In patients with pancreatic cancer 20% had increased concentration compared with 8% in healthy controls *3191*

Complement C_3 *Serum* *Increase* Increased in patients with local disease. Very closely linked to the stage of the disease, patients in remission had normal levels, but further increases were noted in distant metastases. Dropped significantly in the terminal phase of disease *5456*

Complement C_4 *Serum* *Increase* Increased in patients with local disease. Very closely linked to the stage of the disease. Patients in remission had normal levels, but further increases were noted in distant metastases. Levels dropped significantly in the terminal phase of disease *5456*

Complement, Total *Serum* *Increase* Very closely linked to the stage of the disease. Patients in remission had normal levels, but further increases were noted in distant metastases. Dropped significantly in the terminal phase of disease *5456*

Corticotropin *Plasma* *Increase* Uncommon *3433*

C-Peptide *Plasma* *Decrease* In 34 patients with pancreatic cancer and hyperglycemia C-peptide not detectable (below < 0.15 µg/L) in 26% and reduced (between 0.15 and 0.80 µg/L) in 24%: in 2 of 8 with pancreatic cancer and normoglycemia concentration reduced *1515*
Plasma *Increase* In 11 patients with pancreatic cancer and non-insulin requiring diabetes mean concentration of 1,052 ± 464 pmol/L compared with 497 ± 205 pmol/L in 25 healthy normal individuals with all 11 having concentrations more than 2 SD above the normal mean *4210* In 34 patients with pancreatic cancer and hyperglycemia concentration increased (above 2.0 µg/L) in 29% *1515*
Plasma *No Effect* In 9 patients with pancreatic cancer with normal glucose tolerance mean concentration of 472 ± 144 pmol/L not significantly different from 497 ± 205 pmol/L in 25 healthy controls. In 3 cancer patients with impaired glucose tolerance mean concentration of 452 ± 223 pmol/L and in 7 with pancreatic cancer and who were insulin-requiring diabetics mean of 459 ± 127 pmol/L *4210*

Dehydroepiandrosterone Sulfate *Plasma* *No Effect* Mean concentration in 13 male patients with cancer of the pancreas of 3.5 ± 3.1 µmol/L not significantly different from 2.1 - 11.3 µmol/L in 40 healthy men *2416*

Deoxyribonuclease I *Serum* *Increase* Activity often increased in patients with advanced pancreatic cancer *4153*
Urine *Increase* Activity often increased in patients with advanced pancreatic cancer *4153*

Dihydrotestosterone *Serum* *No Effect* Mean concentration in 13 male patients with cancer of the pancreas of 1.5 ± 0.8 nmol/L not significantly different from 0.9 - 5.8 nmol/L in 40 healthy men *2416*

Dupan-2 *Serum* *Increase* Sensitivity for diagnosing pancreatic cancer varies from 63 - 67% according to different studies *4153* In 22.2% of patients with pancreatic cancer with tumors less than 2.0 cm in diameter increased concentrations observed. In patients with tumors between 2.1 and 4.0 cm in diameter 40.0% had increased concentrations *4587*

EL-1 *Serum* *Increase* In 51.1% of 47 patients with pancreatic cancer concentration increased above cut-off of 37 U/mL *2854*

Elastase 1 *Serum* *Increase* Activity often increased in patients with advanced pancreatic cancer *4153* In patients with pancreatic tumors less than 2.0 cm in diameter 28.9% had increased concentrations. In those with tumors between 2.1 and 4.0 cm 52.6% were positive *4587* Increased concentration seems to be uniquely associated with cancer of the head of the pancreas *2367*
Urine *Increase* Activity often increased in patients with advanced pancreatic cancer *4153*

Epidermal Growth Factor *Serum* *Increase* In 35 patients with pancreatic cancer mean concentration of 28.3 ± 4.8 µg/L significantly different from 17.7 ± 3.8 µg/L in 22 healthy controls *3439*

Erythrocytes *Ascitic Fluid* *Increase* Grossly bloody ascites suggests neoplasm *4891*

Fat *Feces* *Increase* Steatorrhea is found in approximately 10% of the cases as judged by abnormal chemical fat excretion *367* Deficient intraluminal pancreatic enzymes *4891*

Feto-acinar Pancreatic Protein *Serum* *Increase* Observed in the serum of some patients with pancreatic cancer *4153*

α-Fetoprotein *Serum* *Increase* Over 50 ng/mL in 10 - 15% of cases *4734* May be increased in patients with pancreatic cancer, as it is of ductal or acinar origin *4153* In 51 patients with pancreatic carcinoma 96.1% had concentrations up to 15.0 ng/mL, 0.0% had concentrations between 15.1 - 20.0 ng/mL, 2.0% between 20.1 - 100 ng/mL, 0.0% had concentrations between 100.1 - 350.0 ng/mL and 2.0% had concentrations above 350.0 ng/mL in contrast to concentrations in 400 healthy individuals in whom 99.2% had concentrations between 0 and 15.0 ng/mL, 0.2% between 15.1 and 20.0 ng/mL and 0.5%% between 20.1 and 100 ng/mL *11* Primary tumors of pancreas may secrete AFP regardless of whether they have metastasized to the liver *1778*
Serum *No Effect* Not useful as a marker of pancreatic cancer as cncentration fell consistently within normal range *7*

Fibrin Degradation Products *Ascitic Fluid* *Increase* In malignant effusions *4891*
Plasma *Increase* Reported effect *2646*

Fibrinogen Degradation Products *Plasma* *Increase* Sensitive marker for pancreatic cancer but not as good as fibrinopeptide A *7*

Fibrinopeptide A *Plasma* *Increase* In 20 patients with pancreatic cancer fibrinopeptide A most sensitive marker for disease *7*

Fucose *Serum* *Increase* Markedly increased *2899*

Galactosyltransferase Isoenzyme II *Serum* *Increase* Sensitivity 0.69 and specificity 0.46 *5348*

Gastrointestinal Cancer Associated Antigen
Serum *Increase* Sensitive marker for pancreatic cancer but not as good as fibrinopeptide A *7*

Gc-Globulin *Serum* *No Effect* In 3 men and 4 women with cancer of the pancreas mean concentrations of 19.0 ± 7.94 mg/dL and 18.5 ± 6.45 mg/dL not significantly different from 23.9 ± 3.36 mg/dL in 106 control men and 26.1 ± 4.66 mg/dL in 150 control women *2279*

Glucagon *Plasma* *Decrease* Decreased *618* *1038* *1290* Mean concentration reduced in 41% of 34 patients with hyperglycemic pancreatic cancer *1515*
Plasma *Increase* In two patients with pancreatic cancer mean concentrations of immunoreactive glucagon > 574 and 234 fmol/mL compared with reference range of 11 - 40 fmol/mL and of glucagon-like immunoreactivity of 790 and 311 fmol/mL compared with reference interval of 92 - 123 fmol/mL *5168*

Glucagon-like Peptide-1 *Serum* *Increase* In 2 patients with pancreatic endocrine pancreatic cancer concentrations of 3,071 and 825 fmol/mL compared with reference range of 21 - 47 fmol/mL *5168*

Glucose *Serum* *Decrease* In children. Decreased due to excess insulin *1290*
Serum *Increase* 59% of 100 patients had fasting hyperglycemia *1900* In 46% of 46 patients at initial hospitalization for this disorder *1576* Diabetes mellitus occurs in 25 - 50% of cases and is manifest most frequently as an abnormal glucose tolerance test rather than overt glucosuria or fasting hyperglycemia *4891*
Urine *Increase* Diabetes mellitus occurs in 25 - 50% of cases and is manifest most frequently as an abnormal glucose tolerance test rather than overt glucosuria or fasting hyperglycemia *4891*

Glucose Tolerance *Serum* *Decrease* Abnormal in 25 - 50% of patients and is a more frequent abnormality than frank glucosuria or fasting hyperglycemia *4891* Test is abnormal in 25 - 50% of patients and is a more frequent abnormality than frank glycosuria or fasting hyperglycemia *367*

β-Glucuronidase *Serum* *Increase* Increased *1777* *1498*

Glutamic Acid *Plasma* *Increase* High levels of glutamic acid and normal glutamine levels were found in 9 of 10 patients. Mean concentration of 3.40 ± 2.22 mg/dL *734*

Glutamine *Plasma* *No Effect* High levels of glutamic acid and normal glutamine levels were found in 9 of 10 patients. Mean concentration of 3.40 ± 2.22 mg/dL *734*

γ-Glutamyltransferase *Serum* *Increase* Greatest in cases of primary carcinoma of the head of the pancreas and adenocarcinoma of bile duct. In 4 patients range was 264 - 1,040 U/L, mean activity of 590 U/L *3161* In 100% of 10 patients at initial hospitalization for this disorder *1576* Activity reportedly increased in a variety of diseases including diseases of the pancreas, myocardium, kidney and lung as well as in diabetes *4617*

Growth Hormone *Plasma* *No Effect* Concentration within normal range in all of 42 patients with pancreatic cancer *1515*

Hematocrit *Blood* *Decrease* In 33% of 46 patients at initial hospitalization for this disorder *1576* 34% of patients were anemic *1900*

Hemoglobin *Blood* *Decrease* In 41% of 45 patients at initial hospitalization for this disorder *1576*

immunoglobulin A *Serum* *No Effect* In 3 men with cancer of the pancreas mean concentration of 149 mg/dL not significantly different from 201 ± 89 mg/dL in 106 healthy controls and mean concentration of 196 mg/dL in 4 women with cancer of the pancreas not significantly different from 176 ± 80 mg/dL in 150 healthy control women *2278*

Immunoglobulin G *Serum* *No Effect* In 3 men with cancer of the pancreas mean concentration of 1,070 mg/dL not significantly different from 1,148 ± 224 mg/dL in 106 healthy controls and mean concentration of 816 mg/dL in 4 women with cancer of the pancreas not significantly different from 1,157 ± 271 mg/dL in 150 healthy control women *2278*

Immunoglobulin M *Serum* *No Effect* In 3 men with cancer of the pancreas mean concentration of 39 mg/dL not significantly different from 61 ± 36 mg/dL in 106 healthy controls and in 4 women with cancer of the pancreas mean concentration of 49 mg/dL not significantly different from 77 ± 39 mg/dL in 150 healthy control women *2278*

Insulin-like Growth Factor-I *Serum* *No Effect* In 35 patients with pancreatic cancer mean concentration of 93.8 ± 15.9 µg/L not significantly different from 103.3 ± 22.0 µg/L in 22 healthy controls *3439*

Inter-α_1-Antitrypsin *Serum* *Increase* Variations are nonspecific and are of no diagnostic value for pancreatic cancer *4153*

Islet Amyloid Polypeptide *Serum* *Increase* In 30 patients with pancreatic cancer mean concentration ± 1 SD was 22.3 ± 13.6 pmol/L compared with 8.0 ± 5.0 pmol/L in 25 healthy controls. 17 (57%) had concentrations more than 2 SD above normal range *4210*

Lactate Dehydrogenase *Ascitic Fluid* *Increase* In malignant effusions *4891*
Serum *Increase* In 24% of 46 patients at initial hospitalization for this disorder *1576*

Lactate Dehydrogenase Isoenzyme-5 *Serum* *Increase* Mild elevation to a mean of 13% of total LD in patients with carcinoma of the liver, gallbladder and pancreas (normal = 0 - 6%) *1756*

Lactate Dehydrogenase Isoenzymes *Serum* *Increase* Elevated LD_2 and LD_3 *1025*

Leucine Aminopeptidase *Serum* *Increase* Consistently elevated *689* Variable, especially if there is no associated increase in either serum alkaline phosphatase or serum AST *1290* In 3 cases without hepatic metastases, all had markedly elevated values ranging from 430 - 730 U/L *579* When there is an element of obstruction of the common bile duct or metastasis to the liver *367*
Urine *Increase* Marked increase *1290* Over 300 U/L in 60% of patients due to liver metastases or biliary tract obstruction. May also be increased in chronic liver disease *5544*

Leukocytes *Ascitic Fluid* *No Effect* Variable *233*
Blood *Increase* In 32% of 46 patients at initial hospitalization for this disorder *1576* Over 12,000 /µL in 12% of histologically proven cases *1900*

Lipase *Serum* *Decrease* May be slightly increased in early stages (< 10% of cases); with later destruction, they are normal or decreased *5544*
Serum *Increase* Activity often increased in patients with advanced pancreatic cancer *4153* Increased in 38% of 100 histologically proven cases *1900* May be slightly increased in early stages (< 10% of cases); with later destruction, they are normal or decreased *5544* Early obstruction of the pancreatic duct will occasionally elevate *367*
Urine *Increase* Activity often increased in patients with advanced pancreatic cancer *4153*

Lipids *Feces* *Increase* Reduced intraluminal pancreatic enzyme activity with maldigestion of lipid and protein *1980*

α_2-Macroglobulin *Serum* *Increase* Variations are nonspecific and are of no diagnostic value for pancreatic cancer *4153*

Metallopanstimulin *Serum* *Increase* In 1 patient with pancreatic cancer mean concentration exceeded upper limit of normal of < 10 ng/mL in healthy individuals aged 19 - 88 years *1462*

5-Methyl-2'-Deoxycytidine *Urine* *No Effect* In 7 patients with cancer of the pancreas mean excretion of 0.91 ± 0.41 nmol/µmol creatinine not significantly different from 0.90 ± 0.43 nmol/µmol creatinine in 81 healthy individuals *2368*

β_2-Microglobulin *Serum* *Increase* In 40 patitients with pancreatic cancer median concentration of 2.3 mg/L (range 1.2 - 6.0 mg/L) significantly higher than concentration in 40 healthy individuals (median 1.2 mg/L with central 95th percentile range of 0.9 - 1.6 mg/L) *4111*

Monocytes *Blood* *Increase* In 68% of 46 patients at initial hospitalization for this disorder *1576*

Neopterin *Urine* *Increase* Frequency of increased concentrations in patients with pancreatic cancer 65% *121* In 6 patients with adenocarcinoma of the pancreas mean excretion of 632.7 µmol/mol creatinine compared with 106.6 ± 34.6 µmol/mol creatinine in 31 healthy controls *3632* In 6 patients with pancreatic cancer mean excretion of about of 632.7 µmol/mol creatinine significantly greater than 106.6 ± 34.6 ummol/mol creatinine in 31 healthy controls *3632*

Neutrophils *Blood* *Increase* Neutrophilic leukemoid reactions occur most frequently with gastric, bronchogenic, and pancreatic carcinomas *5677*

5'-Nucleotidase *Serum* *Increase* Due to biliary tract obstruction, values range from 28.0 - 40.0 U/L (normal 4.0 U/L) *5738* Values are elevated when there is an element of obstruction of the common bile duct or metastases to the liver *367*

157.90 Cancer of Pancreas *(continued)*

Occult Blood *Feces* *Increase* Often found *2033*
Feces *No Effect* In patients with pancreatic cancer 0% had increased concentration as measured by Hemoccult II compared with 2% in healthy controls *3191*

Pancreatic Oncofetal Antigen *Serum* *Increase* Once thought to be highly sensitive and specific for pancreatic cancer, but later these claims were not substantiated *4153*

Pancreatic Polypeptide *Plasma* *Increase* Fasting concentrations above 330 pg/mL may indicate presence of a pancreatic tumor *2952*

Pancreatic Secretory Trypsin Inhibitor *Serum* *Increase* In 16 of 25 patients with pancreatic carcinoma concentration of PSTI increased to 71.8 ± 17.1 ng/mL *3719*

Parathyroid Hormone-related Peptide *Plasma* *Increase* In all three patients with pancreatic cancer and hypercalcemia concentration increased above upper limit of normal of 1.5 pmol/L (range of concentrations 5.6 to 7.8 pmol/L) *3987*

Phospholipase A_2 *Serum* *Increase* Increased concentrations of PLA2-I observed in sera of patients with pancreatic cancer but release of PLA2-I from the pancreas is caused by the destruction of nonneoplastic pancreatic tissue by the neoplastic process *3766* Activity often increased in patients with advanced pancreatic cancer *4153*
Urine *Increase* Activity often increased in patients with advanced pancreatic cancer *4153*

Polymorphic Epithelial Mucin *Serum* *No Effect* In 11 patients with pancreatic cancer median concentrations of 31 kU/L by ACS BR, 24 kU/L by Centocor CA 15-3, 25 kU/L by Enzymun-Test CA 15-3 and 18 kU/L by IMx CA 15-3 not significantly different from concentrations in 250 healthy women (mean and 1 SD concentrations of 22 ± 8.8 kU/L by ACS BR, 19 ± 8.8 kU/L by Centocor CA 15-3, 17 ± 7.1 kU/L by Enzymun-Test CA 15-3 and 15 ± 6.4 kU/L by IMx CA 15-3 respectively) *513*

Potassium *Serum* *Decrease* In 30% of 33 patients at initial hospitalization for this disorder *1576* Gastrointestinal wasting as a result of pancreatic islet nonbeta cell tumors *3735*

Prostate-specific Antigen *Serum* *Increase* Of 58 patients with cancer of the liver or pancreas, 90.9% had values below upper limit of normal of 4.0 ng/mL as measured by method on Bayer Technicon Immuno 1®, 4.5% had values between 4.0 and 10.0 ng/mL and 4.5% had values between 10.0 and 40.0 ng/mL *342*

Protein *Ascitic Fluid* *Increase* Variable, but often > 2.5 g/dL in ascitic fluid *233*
Feces *Increase* Reduced intraluminal pancreatic enzyme activity with maldigestion of lipid and protein *1980*
Peritoneal Fluid *Increase* Greater than 30 g/L in 70% of cases of pancreatic ascites *1216*

Prothrombin Time *Plasma* *Increase* May be increased but will be correctable with parenterally administered vitamin K *900*

Pseudouridine *Urine* *Increase* In 6 patients with cancer of the pancreas mean excretion of about 30 mmol/mol creatinine significantly greater than 19.6 ± 5.2 mmol/mol creatinine in 31 healthy controls *3632*

Ribonuclease *Serum* *Increase* Activity often increased in patients with advanced pancreatic cancer *4153*
Urine *Increase* Activity often increased in patients with advanced pancreatic cancer *4153*

Scan1 *Serum* *Increase* In 89.4% of 47 patients with pancreatic cancer concentration increased above cut-off of 37 U/mL *2854*

Sialyltransferase *Serum* *Increase* In 6 patients with cancer of the pancreas mean and median concentrations of 388 and 348 cpm/mg protein/30 min significantly different from 240 and 243 cpm/mg protein/30 min respectively in 20 normal individuals *2111*

SLX Antigen *Pancreatic Fluid* *Increase* Possesses a high sensitivity and specificity in discriminating pancreatic cancer from non-neoplastic pancreato-biliary diseases *4153*
Serum *Increase* Possesses a high tumor specificity, although affected by tumors other than pancreatic also *4153*

Soluble Interleukin-2 Receptor *Serum* *Increase* 40 patients with pancreatic cancer had a median concentration of 1,055 U/mL (range 327 - 3,600 U/mL) significantly higher than concentration in 40 healthy individuals (median 260 U/mL with central 95th percentile range of 170 - 388 U/mL) *4111*

Somatostatin *Plasma* *Increase* In 35 patients with pancreatic cancer mean concentration of 53.1 ± 9.0 ng/L significantly different from 29.7 ± 6.3 ng/L in 22 healthy controls *3439*

Span-1 *Serum* *Increase* In 13 of 23 cases of cancers less than 2.0 cm in diameter had concentrations above normal. In 41 of 51 cases of tumors between 2.1 and 4.0 cm concentrations increased above normal. Overall sensitivity of Span-1 for tumors less than 4.0 cm 73% *4587* Sensitivity for pancreatic cancer ranged from 72 - 94% in several stuies and specificity ranged from 59 - 85% *4153*

Tennessee Antigen *Serum* *Increase* In patients with pancreatic cancer, 92% had increased concentration compared with 7% healthy controls who had increased concentrations *3191*

Testosterone *Serum* *No Effect* Mean concentration in 13 male patients with cancer of the pancreas of 10.0 ± 5.6 nmol/L not significantly different from 7.4 - 37 nmol/L in 40 healthy men *2416*

Testosterone:Dehydrotestosterone Ratio *Serum* *Decrease* Mean ratio in 13 male patients with cancer of the pancreas of 6.8 ± 2.2 significantly different from cutoff of 5 in 40 healthy men *2416*

β-Thromboglobulin *Plasma* *Increase* Although useful not as good a marker as fibrinopeptide A for pancreatic cancer *7*

Tissue Factor Pathway Inhibitor *Plasma* *Increase* About half of patients with pancreatic cancer had activities greater than median activity of 1.19 U/mL in healthy individuals *2376*

Tissue Polypeptide Antigen *Serum* *Increase* Sensitivity for pancreatic cancer reported to be up to 100%, but concentration influenced by cholestasis and inflammation, much less specific than CA 19-9 *4153*

Tissue Polypeptide Antigen Epitope M3 *Serum* *Increase* Reported to be effective marker for pancreatic cancer but no more effective than tissue polypeptide antigen *4153*

Transferrin *Serum* *No Effect* In 3 men with pancreatic cancer mean concentration of 213 mg/dL not significantly different from 214 ± 33 mg/dL in 106 control men and in 4 women with pancreatic cancer mean concentration of 165 mg/dL not significantly different from 217 ± 39 mg/dL in 150 control women *2280*

Trypsin *Serum* *Increase* Mean serum concentration in 7 patients was 394 U/L. (normal < 100 U/L) *3734* Activity often increased in patients with advanced pancreatic cancer *4153*
Urine *Increase* Activity often increased in patients with advanced pancreatic cancer *4153*

Tumor-associated Trypsin Inhibitor *Serum* *Increase* Measurement is suggested as a sensitive index of pancreatic cancer but specificity is low, especially in patients with pancreatitis *4153*

Uric Acid *Serum* *Increase* In 29% of 46 patients at initial hospitalization for this disorder *1576*

Urobilinogen *Feces* *Decrease* Absent in cancer of head of pancreas *5544*
Urine *Decrease* Absent in carcinoma of head of pancreas *5544*

Urokinase Plasminogen Activator *Tissue* *Increase* Amounts predictable of overall survival *1255*

157.90 Mucus-producing Pancreatic Tumor

CA 19-9 *Serum* *Increase* In 20% of 10 patients with pancreatic cancer concentration increased above cut-off of 37 U/mL *2854*

Carcinoembryonic Antigen *Serum* *Increase* In 30.0% of 10 patients with mucus-producing pancreatic cancer concentration increased above cut-off of 37 U/mL *2854*

EL-1 *Serum* *Increase* In 20.0% of 10 patients with mucus-producing pancreatic cancer concentration increased above cut-off of 37 U/mL *2854*

Scan1 *Serum* *Increase* In 10.0% of 10 patients with mucus-producing pancreatic cancer concentration increased above cut-off of 37 U/mL *2854*

158.00 Retroperitoneal Sarcoma

Calcium *Serum* *Increase* In one study of 42 patients with hypercalcemia and low intact PTH concentration, 1 had a retroperitoneal sarcoma *3280*

Parathyroid Hormone *Plasma* *Decrease* In one study of 42 patients with low intact PTH concentration and hypercalcemia 1 patient had retroperitoneal sarcoma *3280*

158.80 Mesenteric Tumor

Calcium *Serum* *Increase* In one study of 42 patients with mesenteric tumors and hypercalcemia and low intact PTH concentration, 1 had a mesenteric tumor *3280*

Parathyroid Hormone *Plasma* *Decrease* In one study of 42 patients with low intact PTH concentration and hypercalcemia 1 had a mesenteric tumor *3280*

158.80 Mesothelioma

α_1-Acid Glycoprotein *Serum* *Increase* Median concentration in 25 patients with malignant pleural mesothelioma of 205 mg/dL significantly different from normal values of 32 - 98 mg/dL *3721*

α_1-Antitrypsin *Serum* *Increase* Median concentration in 25 patients with malignant pleural mesothelioma of 402 mg/dL significantly different from normal values of 170 - 274 mg/dL *3721*

C-Reactive Protein *Serum* *Increase* Median concentration in 25 patients with malignant pleural mesothelioma of 7.8 mg/dL significantly different from normal values of < 0.3 mg/dL *3721*

Fibrinogen *Plasma* *Increase* Median concentration in 25 patients with malignant pleural mesothelioma of 522 mg/dL significantly different from normal values of 220 - 470 mg/dL *3721*

Hyaluronic Acid *Ascitic Fluid* *Increase* In 2 patients with mesotheliomas median concentration in ascitic fluid 102 mg uronic acid/L compared with 1.5 mg uronic acid/L in 571 fluids not associated with mesotheliomas *3841*
Pleural Fluid *Increase* In 152 patients with mesothelioma median concentration of 72 mg uronic acid/L compared with 4.9 mg uronic acid/L in 1,039 specimens from patients without mesothelioma *3841*

Interleukin-6 *Serum* *Increase* Median concentration in 25 patients with malignant pleural mesothelioma of 28.7 pg/mL significantly different from normal values of < 4 pg/mL *3721*

Prealbumin *Serum* *Decrease* Median concentration in 25 patients with malignant pleural mesothelioma of 10.4 mg/dL significantly different from normal values of 21 - 43 mg/dL *3721*

161.00 Cancer of Larynx

Gc-Globulin *Serum* *No Effect* In 9 men with cancer of the larynx mean concentration of 19.5 ± 2.85 mg/dL not significantly different from 23.9 ± 3.36 mg/dL in 106 control men *2279*

Hydroxyproline *Urine* *Increase* Significantly raised in 52 patients with this disorder when compared with control group *2701*

immunoglobulin A *Serum* *Increase* In 9 men with cancer of the larynx mean concentration of 273 ± 107 mg/dL significantly different from 201 ± 89 mg/dL in 106 healthy control men *2278*

Immunoglobulin G *Serum* *No Effect* In 9 men with cancer of larynx mean concentration of 1269 ± 451 mg/dL not significantly different from 1148 ± 451 mg/dL in 106 healthy control men *2278*

Immunoglobulin M *Serum* *No Effect* In 9 men with cancer of the larynx mean concentration of 57 ± 23 mg/dL not significantly different from 61 ± 36 mg/dL in 106 healthy controls *2278*

162.80 Adenocarcinoma of Lung

α_1-Acid Glycoprotein *Serum* *Increase* Median concentration in 17 patients with lung adenocarcinoma with cytology-positive pleural effusion of 119 mg/dL different from normal values of 32 - 98 mg/dL *3721*

α_1-Antitrypsin *Serum* *No Effect* Median concentration in 17 patients with lung adenocarcinoma with cytology-positive pleural effusion of 250 mg/dL not different from normal values of 170 - 274 mg/dL *3721*

Carcinoembryonic Antigen *Serum* *Increase* In 38 patients with adenocarcinoma of the lung mean baseline concentration of 7.31 ng/mL compared with upper limit of normal of 3.0 ng/mL *4470*

C-Reactive Protein *Serum* *Increase* Median concentration in 17 patients with lung adenocarcinoma with cytology-positive pleural effusion of 0.6 mg/dL different from normal values of < 0.3 mg/dL *3721*

CYFRA 21-1 *Serum* *Increase* In 6 studies of patients with adenocarcinoma of the lung proportion with increased concentrations ranged from 27 - 60% *1293* In 33 patients with inoperable adenocarcinoma of the lung positive rate 42.4% *5146*

Epidermal Growth Factor *Urine* *No Effect* Mean concentration in about 6 patients of 12 µg/g creatinine not significantly different compared with about 10 µg/g creatinine in about 30 controls *5341*

Fibrinogen *Plasma* *No Effect* Median concentration in 17 patients with lung adenocarcinoma with cytology-positive pleural effusion of 353 mg/dL not different from normal values of 220 - 470 mg/dL *3721*

Interleukin-6 *Serum* *Increase* Median concentration in 17 patients with lung adenocarcinoma with cytology-positive pleural effusion of 6.3 pg/mL different from normal values of < 4 pg/mL *3721*

Prealbumin *Serum* *Decrease* Median concentration in 17 patients with lung adenocarcinoma with cytology-positive pleural effusion of 7.4 mg/dL different from normal values of 21 - 43 mg/dL *3721*

pS2-Protein *Serum* *Increase* In 52 patients with adenocarcinomas of the lung median concentration of 218.0 pg/mL and mean concentration of 266.6 ± 247.9 pg/mL significantly increased compared with median of 148.8 pg/mL and mean of 167.7 ± 134.0 pg/mL in 91 healthy individuals *2152*

Urokinase Plasminogen Activator *Tissue* *Increase* Amounts predictable of overall survival *1255*

162.90 Epidermoid Carcinoma of Lung

Epidermal Growth Factor *Urine* *Increase* Mean concentration in about 10 patients of 19 µg/g creatinine compared with about 10 µg/g creatinine in about 30 controls *5341*

162.90 Large Cell Cancer of Lung

Carcinoembryonic Antigen *Serum* *No Effect* In 15 patients with large cell carcinoma of the lung mean baseline concentration of 2.9 ng/mL compared with upper limit of normal of 3.0 ng/mL *4470*

162.90 Large Cell Carcinoma

CYFRA 21-1 *Serum* *No Effect* In 3 patients with inoperable large-cell cancer of the lung no positive results obtained *5146*

α-Enolase *Serum* *Increase* In 3 of 3 cases of large cell carcinoma of lung mean activity increased *1705*

γ-Enolase *Serum* *Increase* In 1 of 3 cases of large cell carcinoma of lung mean activity increased *1705*

162.90 Lung Cancer

α_1-Acid Glycoprotein *Pleural Fluid* *Increase* Highest levels found in malignant exudates *2597* *4241* *3713*

Acid Phosphatase *Serum* *Increase* In a series of 25 cases of lung cancer 36% had elevated levels. Acid phosphatase is of no value as a marker for lung cancer *3620*

Acylcarnitine, Acid-insoluble *Serum* *Decrease* In 4 men with lung cancer mean concentration of 2.6 ± 0.5 nmol/mL significantly different from 3.0 ± 0.4 nmol/mL in 6 healthy men *1195*

Acylcarnitine, Acid-soluble *Serum* *Decrease* In 4 men with lung cancer mean concentration of 8.1 ± 0.8 nmol/mL significantly different from 15.3 ± 2.6 nmol/mL in 6 healthy men *1195*

Albumin *Serum* *Decrease* Significantly reduced (median of 35.7 g/L) in patients with carcinoma compared to controls (44.0 g/L) *2109*

162.90 **Lung Cancer** *(continued)*

Albumin *(continued)*
Serum *No Effect* In patients with carcinoma of bronchus mean concentration of albumin unaffected *1319*
Urine *Increase* 24 h excretion and renal clearance were significantly increased in localized tumor patients compared to normals and disseminated cancer cases. Increased high molecular weight protein excretion implies glomerular injury in these patients *2109*

Aldolase *Serum* *Increase* Slightly elevated in bronchogenic carcinomas. Mean = 2.8 ± 0.6 U/L compared to normal, 1.6 ± 0.21 U/L *2513*

Alkaline Phosphatase *Serum* *Increase* Elevated shortly before death or with tumor extension. Little diagnostic use but helpful in detecting metastases to bone *1671* In 9 patients, initial values ranged from 43 to 263 U/L (normal < 105 U/L) *5029*
White Blood Cells *Decrease* Low activity is present irrespective of tumor category, activity of disease, or type of therapy. In 12 patients median activity was 8 U/L (normal 55 U/L) *3110*

Amino-terminal Propeptide of Type I Collagen
Serum *Increase* Mean concentration of 45.71 ± 4.22 µg/L observed in 59 patients with lung carcinoma significantly different from 30.01 ± 2.43 µg/L in 18 healthy matched control individuals *2731*

Amylase *Pleural Fluid* *Increase* High pleural fluid concentrations may occur *1360* Elevated in primary or metastatic lung cancer, pancreatitis, or esophageal perforation *4537*
Pleural Fluid *No Effect* Usually less than or equal to serum level *4493*
Serum *Increase* May occur *402* Markedly increased in serum, urine and tumor tissue *5806*
Urine *Increase* Markedly increased in serum, urine and tumor tissue *5806*

Angiotensin-converting Enzyme *Serum* *Decrease* Lower the activity the worse the prognosis *3282* In 141 patients with newly diagnosed primary lung cancer ACE was found to be lower than in the control group. This suggests that low levels may be associated with a poor prognosis in this condition *4414*

Anti-p53 Antibodies *Serum* *Increase* Increased in 6 of 77 (7.8%) patients *132*

α_1-Antichymotrypsin *Serum* *Increase* Mean concentration increased above reference interval of 47.9 ± 8.1 mg/dL in 3 of 4 patients with carcinoma of lung *3044*

Antidiuretic Hormone *Plasma* *Increase* Inappropriate secretion of ADH is associated with hyponatremia, decreased serum osmolality, and inappropriately high sodium concentration in the urine. The entire syndrome resolves following resection of the tumor *1980*

Antithrombin III *Plasma* *Increase* In 286 patients with newly diagnosed primary lung cancer concentration abnormal in 59% *617*

Arylsulfatase A *Serum* *Increase* Sensitivity and specificity for carcinoma of lung 59% and 82% respectively *2895*

Aspartate Aminotransferase *Serum* *Increase* Becomes elevated only shortly before death. In most cases, elevated values indicate the presence of metastases *1671*

c-erb-B_2 Oncoprotein *Serum* *Increase* Median concentration of 7.6 ng/mL in 26 patients with locoregional cancer, < 3 ng/mL in 50 with metastatic cancer and < 3 ng/mL in 10 with no longer detectable disease. 3 of 172 (11.5%) of patients with locoregional disease, 8 of 50 (16%) with metastases and 0 of 10 (0%) without detectable disease had concentrations exceeding 1.5 ng/mL *3564*

CA 15-3 *Serum* *Increase* In 17 patients with lung cancer mean concentration of 63.6 ± 76 U/mL significantly different from cutoff of 22 U/mL with 12 having concentrations above 35 U/mL and 9 having concentrations greater than 40 U/mL *2076*

CA 19-9 *Serum* *Increase* Elevated in 16% of cases *2129* In 32 patients with lung cancer positive rate of 34% observed using cut-off from normals and 34% at 90% specificity *2594* Reported effect *5381*

CA 27-29 *Serum* *Increase* In 24% of 17 patients with cancer of lung concentration increased *766*

CA 50 *Serum* *Increase* Elevated in a high proportion of patients with primary carcinoma *2211*

CA 125 *Serum* *Increase* Elevated in epithelial cancers *5364* In 32 patients with lung cancer using Boehringer Mannheim Enzymun test mean concentration of 108.5 ± 168.8 U/mL with 59.3% having concentrations above 35 U/mL *2636*

CA 242 *Serum* *Increase* In 32 patients with lung cancer positive rate of 25% observed using cut-off from normals and 29% at 90% specificity *2594*

CA 549 *Serum* *Increase* In 137 patients with lung cancer 45 (32.8%) had a concentration greater than the upper limit of normal with BRESMARQ assay *764* Using a value of greater than 11 kU/L as the upper limit of normal, it is increased in 33% of cases *5364* Using a value of greater than 11 kU/L as the upper limits of normal, it is increased in 33% of cases *765*

Calcitonin *Plasma* *Increase* High levels can also be produced ectopically by small cell cancer of the lung *1980* Increase found in both thyroid and bronchogenic carcinomas. Medullary thyroid cancer is characterized by the presence of at least 7 different fractions, ranging from fraction I (> 30,000 molecular weight) to V (2,500 molecular weight). Bronchogenic cancers had a predominance of high molecular weight fractions (I and IIa) *357* Observed effect *3485* Elevated in 75% of patients with oat cell carcinoma *3419* Elevated in 54 (68%) of 79 patients with small cell carcinoma. 20 patients (25%) had levels usually associated with medullary carcinoma of the thyroid *2011* 8 of 11 patients with oat cell carcinoma (including 4 with skeletal metastases) had concentrations > 0.1 ng/mL, ranging up to 5 ng/mL *922*

Calcium *Serum* *Increase* Frequent hypercalcemia in advanced cases *826* Of 42 patients in one study with low intact PTH concentration and hypercalcemia 20 had carcinoma of the bronchus *3280* Hypercalcemia of malignancy common with this type of cancer *3470* In squamous cell neoplasm without evidence of direct bone involvement. Parathyroid hormone- secreting tumors *1025* 2 of 12 patients with lung cancer had hypercalcemia, together with 1 of 1 with cancer of the lung and larynx *1200*
Urine *Decrease* Hypercalcemia of malignancy common with this type of cancer which leads to diminished capacity of renal tubules to concentrate urine which, in turn, decreases the ECF and the kidney's ability to eliminate excess calcium. Renal impairment eventually causes nitrogen retention, acidosis and renal failure and a further decrease in calcium excretion *3470*
Urine *Increase* Hypercalcemia of malignancy common with this type of cancer which is often associated with hypercalciuria occurring with excessive bone reabsorption *3470*

Cancer-associated Serum Antigen *Serum* *Increase* 60 of 258 patients (23%) with lung cancer had concentrations above 9 U/mL *1135*

Carbon Dioxide Partial Pressure *Blood* *Decrease* Impaired gas diffusion and the accompanying hyperventilation results in a low pCO_2, unless the defect is severe and CO_2 retention occurs in bronchiolar cell carcinoma *4707*

Carcinoembryonic Antigen *Pleural Fluid* *Increase* 24 (34%) of 70 malignant effusions had levels > 12 ng/mL *4369*
Serum *Increase* In 12 of 100 patients with localized disease and 22 of 97 with extrathoracic spread concentration increased above upper 95th centile of 40 µg/L *648* Increase observed in more than 50% patients *1601* Found in > 50 % of the patients *1882* In 124 patients with malignant disease of the lung 38.7% had concentrations of 0.0 - 3.0 ng/mL, 20.2% had concentrations from 3.1 - 5.0 ng/mL, 11.3% had concentrations from 5.1 - 10.0 ng/mL and 29.8% had concentrations greater than 10.0 ng/mL when measured by method on Bayer Technicon Immuno 1® system compared with 95.9%, 3.5%, 0.6% and 0.0% respectively in 173 healthy nonsmokers *339* In 228 patients with carcinoma of the lung 49 had concentrations greater than 15 ng/mL with 65% of all patients having a concentration greater than 2.5 ng/mL *5472* Very high titers have been found in 76% of patients *898* 88 of 115 (or 77%) of patients had an initial concentration > 2.5 ng/mL. Of 28 patients with concentration of 15 ng/mL at the time of initial examination, 27 were found to have locally extensive or disseminated disease *5473* Mean concentration significantly increased in patients with lung disease and in healthy controls. Sensitivity at concentration of greater than 5 ng/mL 46.4%. Specificity 88%. Concentration correlated with stage of disease in patients with either small cell lung or nonsmall cell lung cancer *2530* In 72% of cases *4891*

In 57 patients with pulmonary cancer 63.2% had concentrations up to 3.0 ng/mL, 22.8% had concentrations between 3.1 - 5.0 ng/mL, 12.3% between 5.1 - 10.0 ng/mL and 1.8% had concentrations above 10.1 ng/mL in contrast to concentrations in 151 healthy nonsmokers in whom 95.4% had concentrations between 0 and 3.0 ng/mL and 4.6% between 4.1 and 10.0 ng/mL *11* Increase reported in majority of patients *4551* In 92 patients with primary lung cancer mean concentration increased above 5 ng/mL in 51.1% with a greater proportion of patients with extended disease having increased concentrations than in those with limited disease. Patients with adenocarcinomas or small cell carcinomas had highest proportion of increased concentrations *4191* In 121 patients with pulmonary cancer 38.8% had concentrations up to 3.0 ng/mL, 15.7% had concentrations between 3.1 - 5.0 ng/mL, 13.2% between 5.1 - 10.0 ng/mL and 32.2% had concentrations greater than 10.1 ng/mL in contrast to concentrations in 151 healthy nonsmokers in whom 95.4% had concentrations between 0 and 3.0 ng/mL and 4.6% between 4.1 and 10.0 ng/mL *11* Concentrations > 40 μg/L were found in 40.6% of patients with oat cell carcinoma *3419* Mean concentration in 192 patients with carcinoma of the lung 24.21 ± 4.219 ng/mL significantly increased compared with 3.70 ± 0.215 ng/mL in 80 healthy controls *4030*
Serum No Effect In 429 patients with lung cancer median concentration in patients with stage I/II disease 4.7 μg/L, in those with stage IIIa disease 4.1 μg/L and in those with stage IIIb 4.3 μg/L not significantly different compared with threshold value of 4.3 μg/L *4740*
Tissue Increase Using FNA mean concentration of 119.2 - 303.5 ng/mL observed in first drop of aspirated material in 31 patients *4139*

Carnitine *Serum Decrease* In 4 men with lung cancer mean concentration of 60.2 ± 8.5 nmol/mL not significantly different from 72.1 ± 7.0 nmol/mL in 6 healthy men *1195*
Serum No Effect In 4 men with lung cancer mean concentration of 49.6 ± 7.4 nmol/mL not significantly different from 53.7 ± 4.7 nmol/mL in 6 healthy men *1195*

Casein *Serum Increase* In 3 of 24 patients with localized disease and 3 of 18 with extrathoracic spread concentration increased above upper 95th centile of 25 μg/L *648* Casein observed in all 7 patients studied with lung cancer (mean concentration of 342 ± 57 μg/L) *2113*

Cathepsin B *Tissue Increase* High amounts of cathepsin B associated with poor prognosis for patients with lung cancer *1252*

Cells *BAL Fluid Increase* In 38 patients with primary lung cancer mean concentration of 2.4 ± 3.3 x 10^6/L not significantly different from 1.9 ± 1.0 x 10^6/L in 13 healthy controls *961*

Ceruloplasmin *Serum Increase* High in gastric and pulmonary cancer *4610* In 89 men with lung cancer mean concentration of 107 ± 27 mg/dL significantly different from 71 ± 17 mg/dL in 106 control men and mean of 132 ± 40 mg/dL in 8 women with lung cancer significantly different from 84 ± 22 mg/dL in 150 control women *2280*

Cholesterol *Serum No Effect* In patients with carcinoma of bronchus and cachexia mean cholesterol concentration within normal range *1319*

β-Chorionic Gonadotropin *Plasma Increase* Ectopic production *3777 455 1108 602* In 3 of 56 patients with localized disease and 4 of 56 with extrathoracic spread concentration increased above upper 95th centile of 2 μg/L *648* Ectopic production *552*
Plasma No Effect No significant difference observed between β-hCG concentrations in 92 patients with primary lung cancer and 43 controls *4191*

Complement C_3 *Serum Increase* Increased in patients with local disease. Very closely linked to the stage of the disease. Patients in remission had normal levels, but further increases were noted in distant metastases. Levels dropped significantly in the terminal phase of the disease *5456*

Complement C_4 *Serum Increase* Increased in patients with local disease. Very closely linked to the stage of the disease. Patients in remission had normal levels, but further increases were noted in distant metastases. Levels dropped significantly in the terminal phase of disease *5456*

Complement, Total *Serum Increase* Closely linked to the stage of the disease. Patients in remission had normal levels, but further increases were noted in distant metastases. Levels dropped significantly in the terminal phase of disease *5456*

Copper *Serum Increase* Extremely high in 82% of the 34 patients *2748* Increased in stomach, lung and large intestine neoplasm. Serum ceruloplasmin was high in gastric and lung cancer but not in the large intestine *4610*

Copper Zinc Superoxide Dismutase *Serum Increase* Mean value of 16.11 ng/mL compared to 9.51 ng/mL in patients with benign pulmonary disease and 7.22 ng/mL in normal controls *5857*

Corticotropin *Plasma Increase* In 53 patients with cancer of the lung mean morning concentration of 23 pg/mL significantly different from 16 pg/mL in 47 healthy controls. Mean afternoon concentration of 17 pg/mL in 50 patients significantly different from 11 pg/mL in 25 controls *664*

Corticotropin-releasing Hormone *Plasma No Effect* In 30 patients with cancer of the lung mean morning concentration of 7.2 pg/mL not significantly different from 5.1 pg/mL in 15 healthy controls. Mean afternoon concentration of 6.2 pg/mL in 14 patients not significantly different from 7.4 pg/mL in 7 controls *664*

Cortisol *Plasma Increase* In patients with carcinoma of bronchus and cachexia mean concentration increased *1319*
Plasma No Effect In 33 patients with cancer of the lung mean morning concentration of 11.7 μg/dL not significantly different from 10.8 μg/dL in 22 healthy controls. Mean afternoon concentration of 5.6 μg/dL in 41 patients not significantly different from 6.8 μg/dL in 12 controls *664*

Creatine Kinase *Serum Increase* Highest activity of CK-BB in brain and smooth muscle *2912*

Creatine Kinase BB-Isoenzyme *Pleural Fluid Increase* In malignant pleural diseases the serum CK-BB is increased and in malignant pleural effusions the pleural/plasma CK-BB ratio is also increased *4105*
Serum Increase Increased concentrations have been found in adenocarcinoma patients, especially in those with small cell carcinoma *2184 4842* Pathological values in 71% of cases *3761* Detected in 14 of 43 patients (32%) it had a sensitivity of 17% in limited disease and 64% in extensive disease *3058*

Creatinine *Serum Increase* Hypercalcemia of malignancy common with this type of cancer which leads to diminished capacity of renal tubules to concentrate urine which, in turn, decreases the ECF and the kidney's ability to eliminate excess calcium. Renal impairment eventually causes nitrogen retention, acidosis and renal failure and a further decrease in calcium excretion *3470*

C-terminal Telopeptide of Type I Collagen *Serum Increase* Mean concentration of 4.82 ± 0.39 μg/L observed in 59 patients with lung carcinoma significantly different from 2.74 ± 0.15 μg/L in 18 healthy matched control individuals. Concentrations higher in patient with metastases to lung, brain and bone *2731*

CYFRA 21-1 *Serum Increase* Mean concentration in 114 patients with primary lung cancer of 24.0 ± 73.8 ng/mL compared with 1.1 ± 0.3 ng/mL in 29 healthy controls with a positivity rate of 85.1% *3665* In 5 studies of patients with lung cancer proportion with increased concentrations ranged from 46 - 58% *1293* In 87 patients with inoperable cancer of the lung, positive rate of 71.4% in 35 patients with squamous cell cancer, 42.4% in 33 patients with adenocarcinoma and 18.8% in 16 patients with small-cell carcinoma. Concentrations tended to be higher with more advanced stages: 9.2 ± 6.0 ng/mL in stages I and II, 10.2 ± 3.1 ng/mL in stage III and 18.4 ± 5.3 ng/mL in stage IV *5146* In 86 patients with lung cancer without metastases median concentration of 3.0 ng/mL and in 62 with metastases 3.6 ng/mL significantly different from that in 50 healthy individuals with median concentration of 1.2 ng/mL and range of 0.5 - 2.4 ng/mL *3559* In 429 patients with lung cancer median concentration in patients with stage I/II disease of 2.7 μg/L, in those with stage IIIa disease 3.2 μg/L and in those with stage IIIb 6.3 μg/L compared with upper limit of normal of 1.9 μg/L *4740*

D-Dimer *Plasma Increase* In 286 patients with newly diagnosed primary lung cancer concentration abnormal in 59% *617*

DF3 *Serum Increase* In 14 patients with lung cancer 1 had concentration greater than 25 U/mL (concentration in 90% normals) but none had greater than 30 U/mL observed in 95% normals *2076*

2,3-Diphosphoglycerate *Red Blood Cells Increase* Synthesis is increased in response to hypoxia *380*

β-Endorphin *Plasma Increase* In 51 patients with cancer of the lung mean morning concentration of 11.8 pg/mL significantly different from 4.8 pg/mL in 24 healthy controls *664*

162.90 **Lung Cancer** *(continued)*

β-Endorphin *(continued)*
Plasma *No Effect* Mean afternoon concentration of 12.5 pg/mL in 37 patients with cancer of the lung not significantly different from 12.5 pg/mL in 19 controls *664*

Epidermal Growth Factor *Tissue* *Decrease* Median concentration of 0.16 ng/mg tissue protein observed in 30 lung cancer specimens less than 0.2 ng/mg tissue protein in normal tissue *511*

Erythrocytes *Pleural Fluid* *Increase* 1,000 - > 100,000 /μL *1980* *4493*

Erythropoietin *Serum* *Increase* Increased plasma concentrations are found in patients with erythrocytosis associated with several types of tumor, especially lung, kidney and liver *547* *3294* *3084*

Ferritin *Serum* *Increase* In patients with cancer of the lung mean concentration significantly increased compared with normal controls but not increased compared with concentrations in patients with benign lung diseases. Sensitivity at concentration of greater than 300 ng/mL 36%. Specificity 72%. Concentration correlated with stage of disease in small cell lung cancer but not in those with nonsmall cell lung cancer *2530* Increased levels were found in more than 50% of patients *1882* Ferritin proved to be most useful in diagnosing both non-small cell and small cell cancers. It proved useful in monitoring therapy and predicting an impaired prognosis *955* *3112*

α-Fetoprotein *Serum* *Increase* In 0 of 62 patients with localized disease and 2 of 72 with extrathoracic spread concentration increased above upper 95th centile of 10 μg/L *648*
Serum *No Effect* No significant difference observed between concentrations in 92 patients with primary lung cancer and 43 healthy controls *4191*

Fibrinogen *Plasma* *Increase* In 286 patients with newly diagnosed primary lung cancer concentration abnormal in 59% *617*

Fibronectin *BAL Fluid* *Increase* In 38 patients with primary lung cancer median concentration of 847 ng/mL significantly different from 363 ng/mL in 13 healthy controls *961*

Fucose *Serum* *Increase* Increased in patients with both malignant and benign tumors of breast, lung and stomach. The glycoprotein-bound fraction was very markedly elevated in cases of malignancy and not in benign disease. Mucoprotein fraction was raised in both diseases *5170* In 15 patients, mean concentration of 15.98 ± 1.43 mg/dL. Normal range of 6.84 ± 0.13 mg/dL *2899*

Galactosyltransferase Isoenzyme II *Serum* *Increase* Sensitivity 0.55 and specificity 0.75 *5348*

Gastrin *Serum* *Increase* In 35 patients with lung cancer median values of 58 pg/100 U LDH *1231*

Gc-Globulin *Serum* *No Effect* In 80 men and 8 women with cancer of the lung mean concentrations of 25.1 ± 4.84 mg/dL and 28.4 ± 4.07 mg/dL not significantly different from 23.9 ± 3.36 mg/dL in 106 control men and 26.1 ± 4.66 mg/dL in 150 control women *2279*

Gelatinase *Serum* *No Effect* In 37 male patients with lung cancer mean concentration of 344.4 ± 30.8 ng/mL not significantly different from 386.7 ± 33.7 ng/mL in 30 healthy male controls *5878*

α_1-Globulin *Serum* *Increase* Increased in squamous, large and small cell carcinoma and adenocarcinoma of lung. A 2-fold decrease in trypsin inhibitory capacity was also found in association *2027*

γ-Globulin *Serum* *Increase* Good correlation between hypergammaglobulinemia and neoplastic disease, especially bronchogenic carcinoma *4707*

Glucose *Pleural Fluid* *Decrease* Approximately 15% of malignancies have low concentrations in pleural fluids *3052* Markedly reduced, 20 mg/dL or less, is very suggestive and virtually diagnostic of rheumatoid disease. A low level in the range of 40 mg/dL can be found in infectious processes and in malignant pleural effusions *1980*
Serum *Decrease* Occasionally, bronchogenic carcinoma is associated with insulin-like activity which may be reflected by hypoglycemia *1980*
Serum *No Effect* In patients with carcinoma of bronchus and cachexia mean concentration within normal range *1319*

γ-Glutamyltransferase *Serum* *Increase* Activity reportedly increased in a variety of diseases including diseases of the pancreas, myocardium, kidney and lung as well as in diabetes *4617*

Glycated Protein *Serum* *Increase* Increased levels found in > 50% of patients *1882*

Gonadotropin, Pituitary *Plasma* *Increase* All cell types of bronchogenic cancer can cause the syndrome of ectopic gonadotropin production *1980* Gonadotropin activity is clinically manifested by gynecomastia and by elevated gonadotropin blood levels *1980* Anaplastic large cell carcinoma *1611*

Growth Hormone *Plasma* *Increase* Elevated *1870* In patients with cancer and cachexia mean concentration increased *1319*

Haptoglobin *Serum* *Increase* Increased to 2.2 g/L, compared to normals, 1.1 g/L *2109*
Urine *Increase* 24 h excretion and renal clearance were significantly increased in localized tumor patients compared to normals and disseminated cancer cases. Increased high molecular weight protein excretion implies glomerular injury in these patients *2109*

Hexokinase *Serum* *Increase* Significantly increased. Mean activity of 20.4 ± 5.4 U/L compared to normal of 0.93 ± 0.28 U/L *2513*

Hyaluronic Acid *Serum* *Increase* In malignant pleural mesothelioma *1853*

17-Hydroxycorticosteroids *Urine* *Increase* Ectopic ACTH production *1108*

5-Hydroxyindoleacetic Acid *Urine* *Increase* Oat-cell carcinoma of the bronchus and bronchial adenoma of carcinoid type may cause excess secretion *1290* Rarely a carcinoid syndrome is associated with bronchogenic carcinoma with the laboratory manifestation of abnormal urinary levels of 5-HIAA *1980*

5-Hydroxytryptamine *Blood* *Increase* Rarely a carcinoid syndrome is associated with bronchogenic carcinoma with the laboratory manifestation of abnormal urinary levels of 5-HIAA *1980* Oat-cell carcinoma of the bronchus and bronchial adenoma of carcinoid type may cause excessive secretion *1290*

immunoglobulin A *Serum* *Increase* In 89 men with cancer of the lung mean concentration of 280 ± 144 mg/dL significantly different from 201 ± 89 mg/dL in 106 healthy control men *2278*
Serum *No Effect* In 8 women with cancer of the lung mean concentration of 164 ± 63 mg/dL not significantly different from 174 ± 80 mg/dL in 150 healthy control women *2278*
Urine *Increase* 24 h excretion and renal clearance were significantly increased in localized tumor patients compared to normals and disseminated cancer cases. Increased high molecular weight protein excretion implies glomerular injury in these patients *2109*

Immunoglobulin G *Serum* *Increase* In 89 men with cancer of the lung mean concentration of 1,403 ± 417 mg/dL significantly different from 1,148 ± 224 mg/dL in 106 healthy controls and mean concentration of 1,534 ± 359 mg/dL in 8 women with cancer of the lung significantly different from 1,157 ± 271 mg/dL in 150 healthy control women *2278*
Urine *Increase* 24 h excretion and renal clearance were significantly increased in localized tumor patients compared to normals and disseminated cancer cases. Increased high molecular weight protein excretion implies glomerular injury in these patients *2109*

Immunoglobulin M *Serum* *No Effect* In 89 men with cancer of the lung mean concentration of 81 ± 181 mg/dL not significantly different from 61 ± 36 mg/dL in 106 healthy controls and in 8 women with cancer of the lung mean concentration of 61 ± 27 mg/dL not significantly different from 77 ± 39 mg/dL in 150 healthy control women *2278*
Urine *Increase* 24 h excretion and renal clearance were significantly increased in localized tumor patients compared to normals and disseminated cancer cases. Increased high molecular weight protein excretion implies glomerular injury in these patients *2109*

Insulin *Plasma* *No Effect* In patients with carcinoma of bronchus and cachexia mean fasting concentration remains within normal range *1319*

Insulin-like Growth Factor-I *Serum* *Decrease* In patients with cancer and cachexia mean concentration reduced *1319*

Interleukin-6 *Pleural Fluid* *Increase* In 10 patients with lung cancer and carcinomatous pleurisy mean concentration in pleural fluid of 964 ± 176 pg/mL, significantly different from 10.2 ± 1.3 pg/mL in serum *2205*
Serum *Increase* In 10 patients with lung cancer and carcinomatous pleurisy mean concentration of 10.2 ± 1.3 pg/mL, not significantly different from 7.3 ± 1.0 pg/mL in healthy controls *2205*

Interleukin-8 *Pleural Fluid* *No Effect* In 10 patients with lung cancer and carcinomatous pleurisy IL-8 detected at a concentration of 319 ± 85 pg/mL *2205*
Serum *Increase* In 10 patients with lung cancer and carcinomatous pleurisy IL-8 detected in serum of only one patient at 98 pg/mL in contrast to IL-8 being detected in all 10 healthy controls (8.0 ± 1.5 pg/mL) *2205*
Serum *No Effect* In 10 patients with lung cancer and carcinomatous pleurisy IL-8 detected in serum of only one patient at 98 pg/mL in contrast to IL-8 being detected in all 10 healthy controls (8.0 ± 1.5 pg/mL) *2205*

Iron-binding Capacity, Total *Serum* *Decrease* Significantly reduced (median 2.6 mg/L), compared to controls (3.4 mg/L). 24 h excretion and renal clearance were significantly increased in localized tumor patients compared to normals and disseminated cancer cases. Increased high molecular weight protein excretion implies glomerular injury in these patients *2109*

Islet Amyloid Polypeptide *Serum* *No Effect* In 11 patients with cancer of the lung mean ± 1 SD concentration of 9.9 ± 3.6 pmol/L not significantly different from 8.0 ± 5.0 pmol/L in 25 healthy controls *4210*

17-Ketogenic Steroids *Urine* *Increase* Ectopic ACTH production *1108*

Lactate *Blood* *Increase* In 5 patients with bronchogenic tumors, mean concentration was 13.7 ± 3.6 mg/dL compared to normal, 11.7 ± 0.72 mg/dL *2513*

Lactate Dehydrogenase *Pleural Fluid* *Increase* Elevation in pleural fluid without concurrent rise in protein indicates malignancy *3052* In 10 patients with lung cancer and carcinomatous pleurisy mean activity of 555 ± 127 U/L *2205* A markedly elevated pleural LD is consistent with neoplastic involvement of the pleura. Not specific for the diagnosis *1980*
Serum *Increase* Activity was frequently elevated in 30 patients with primary and 4 with secondary neoplasms. Activity increased with tumor extension and often in relation to chemotherapy, but provided little diagnostic or prognostic value, except to indicate metastases *1671* Twice the normal mean in 53 patients with bronchogenic carcinomas. Mean activity of 175.1 ± 10.4 U/L compared to normals, 85.4 ± 1.0 U/L *2513*

Lactate Dehydrogenase Isoenzyme-5 *Pleural Fluid* *Increase* An increase of LD-4 and LD-5 in malignant effusions *4346*

Lactate Dehydrogenase Isoenzymes *Pleural Fluid* *Increase* Pleural effusions with a predominant LD_2 are highly indicative of malignancy *3052* An increase of LD-4 and LD-5 in malignant effusions *4346*

Leukocytes *Pleural Fluid* *Increase* In 10 patients with lung cancer and carcinomatous pleurisy mean concentration of 1,528 ± 695 cells/μL *2205*

Lipoprotein Lp(a) *Serum* *Increase* In 48 patients with carcinoma of the lung median concentration of 241 mg/L significantly different from 43 mg/L in 69 healthy volunteers, with 34% above 95th percentile of 361 mg/L *5417*

Lymphocytes *BAL Fluid* *Increase* In 38 patients with primary lung cancer mean concentration of 6.8 ± 5.5% not significantly different from 5.4 ± 5.7% in 13 healthy controls *961*
Pleural Fluid *Increase* In patients with pulmonary tuberculosis, pulmonary malignancy or nonspecific pleuritis, the percentages and absolute numbers of B lymphocytes were significantly lower in pleural fluid than in peripheral blood *4104* Pleural effusion with > 50% of the WBC as small lymphocytes are highly indicative of malignancy or tuberculosis. Of 96 such effusions, 43 were TB and 47 were cancerous. 47 of 90 patients with lung cancer had predominantly small lymphocytes in effusions *3052* In 10 patients with lung cancer and carcinomatous pleurisy mean concentration of 76 ± 11% of 1,528 ± 695 cells/μL *2205*

Macrophages *BAL Fluid* *Increase* In 38 patients with primary lung cancer mean concentration of 36 ± 36% not significantly different from 81 ± 14% in 13 healthy controls *961*

Metallopanstimulin *Serum* *Increase* In 100% of 27 patients with epithelial lung cancer mean concentration exceeded upper limit of normal of < 10 ng/mL in healthy individuals aged 19 - 88 years *1462*

5-Methyl-2'-Deoxycytidine *Urine* *No Effect* In 7 patients with cancer of the lung mean excretion of 0.81 ± 0.41 nmol/μmol creatinine not significantly different from 0.90 ± 0.43 nmol/μmol creatinine in 81 healthy individuals *2368*

β_2-Microglobulin *Serum* *No Effect* No significant difference observed between concentrations in 92 patients with primary lung cancer and 43 healthy controls *4191*

Monocytes *Pleural Fluid* *Increase* Predominant cell type *4493* In 10 patients with lung cancer and carcinomatous pleurisy mean concentration of 13 ± 6% of 1,528 ± 695 cells/μL *2205*

N^2, N^2-Dimethylguanosine *Urine* *Increase* In 3 patients with bronchogenic carcinoma excretions of 10.3 mg/d in one significantly different from 3.9 ± 2.6 mg/d in 17 healthy controls, but 2.8 and 4.3 mg/d in the others not significantly different *5505*
Urine *No Effect* Mean excretion in 2 patients with lung cancer of 18.7 μmol/d compared with 16.9 μmol/d in pooled normal urine *3720* In 3 patients with bronchogenic carcinoma excretions of 10.3 mg/d in one significantly different from 3.9 ± 2.6 mg/d in 17 healthy controls, but 2.8 and 4.3 mg/d in the others not significantly different *5505*

Neopterin *Serum* *Increase* Mean concentration of 25.8 ± 11.3 nmol/L in 9 patients with lung cancer significantly greater than that in 18 healthy control individuals, 6.4 ± 1.8 nmol/L *3864*
Urine *Increase* In 7 patients with carcinoma of the lung mean excretion of about 400 μmol/mol creatinine significantly greater than 106.6 ± 34.6 μmol/mol creatinine in 31 healthy controls *3632*

Neuron-specific Enolase *Serum* *Increase* Concentration significantly increased in patients with lung cancer compared with healthy controls but not compared with patients with benign liver disease. Sensitivity at concentration of greater than 12.5 ng/mL of 34.5%. Specificity of 58% *2530* The overall sensitivity (value greater than 12.5 ng/mL) was 65% *3058* Found to be of some help in diagnosing small cell lung cancer. Seems to be the best marker for detecting lung cancer patients among subjects with benign lung diseases, diagnosing 63% of the cancers at a specificity of 81% *3112* In 14 of 113 patients (10%) with non-small carcinoma of lung concentration increased above 35.0 ng/mL whereas increased above this in 13 of 15 patients with small cell cancer of lung had increase above 35.0 ng/mL *4794* Concentration increased above 35 ng/mL in 14 of 113 patients with non-small cell cancer of the lung. Reference interval of 5.2 - 17.4 ng/mL *4771*
Serum *No Effect* In 429 patients with lung cancer median concentration in patients with stage I/II disease was 8.4 μg/L, in those with stage IIIa disease 7.8 μg/L, and in those with stage IIIb 9.9 μg/L, not significantly different compared with threshold value of 10 μg/L *4740*

Neutrophils *BAL Fluid* *Increase* In 38 patients with primary lung cancer mean concentration of 52 ± 36% significantly different from 10 ± 11% in 13 healthy controls *961*
Blood *Increase* Neutrophilic leukemoid reactions occur most frequently with gastric, bronchogenic, and pancreatic carcinomas *5677*
Pleural Fluid *Increase* In 10 patients with lung cancer and carcinomatous pleurisy mean concentration of 10 ± 7% of 1,528 ± 695 cells/μL *2205*

Osmolality *Serum* *Decrease* Inappropriate secretion of ADH is associated with hyponatremia, decreased serum osmolality, and inappropriately high sodium concentration in the urine. The entire syndrome resolves following resection of the tumor *1980*

Oxygen Partial Pressure *Blood* *Decrease* Impaired diffusion *4707*

Oxygen Saturation *Blood* *Decrease* Impaired diffusion *4707*

Parathyroid Hormone *Plasma* *Decrease* In one study of 42 patients with low intact PTH concentration and hypercalcemia 20 had carcinoma of the bronchus *3280*
Plasma *Increase* Lung cancer, hypernephroma, gastrointestinal cancer, and other neoplasms can synthesize and secrete parathyroid hormone *1980*

162.90 Lung Cancer *(continued)*

Parathyroid Hormone-related Peptide *Plasma* *No Effect* In 10 patients with cancer of the lung and normocalcemia mean concentration of 1.59 pmol/L below upper limit of reference range of 2.6 pmol/L *1200*

Partial Thromboplastin Time *Plasma* *Decrease* In 286 patients with newly diagnosed primary lung cancer PTT reduced in 8% *617*

pH *Blood* *Decrease* Hypercalcemia of malignancy common with this type of cancer which leads to diminished capacity of renal tubules to concentrate urine which, in turn, decreases the ECF and the kidney's ability to eliminate excess calcium. Renal impairment eventually causes nitrogen retention, acidosis and renal failure and a further decrease in calcium excretion *3470*
Pleural Fluid *Decrease* Exudate (pH < 7.3) *126*
Pleural Fluid *No Effect* pH < 7.40 militates against malignancy, especially in the absence of infection and < 7.30 is rarely encountered in tuberculous pleural disease *1980*

Phosphohexoseisomerase *Serum* *Increase* Serum levels were high in 75.7% of patients. Levels were higher than those of carcinoembryonic antigen in large cell and small cell carcinomas *4568*

Platelets *Blood* *Decrease* In 286 patients with newly diagnosed primary lung cancer thrombocytopenia observed in 4% *617*
Blood *Increase* In 286 patients with newly diagnosed primary lung cancer thrombocytosis of greater than 400,000 /µL observed in 19% *617* In a large proportion of patients *4847* In 1,115 patients with primary lung cancer 32% had platelet counts greater than 400,000 /µL compared with 6% in outpatients with benign lung disorders. The incidence of very high counts was related to disease stage *4057* Reported effect *1098*

Polymorphic Epithelial Mucin *Serum* *No Effect* In 15 patients with lung cancer median concentrations of 25 kU/L by ACS BR, 26 kU/L by Centocor CA 15-3, 23 kU/L by Enzymun-Test CA 15-3 and 21 kU/L by IMx CA 15-3 not significantly different from concentrations in 250 healthy women (mean and 1 SD concentrations of 22 ± 8.8 kU/L by ACS BR, 19 ± 8.8 kU/L by Centocor CA 15-3, 17 ± 7.1 kU/L by Enzymun-Test CA 15-3 and 15 ± 6.4 kU/L by IMx CA 15-3 respectively) *513*

Pregnancy-associated α-Macroglobulin *Serum* *Increase* In 6 of 36 male patients with localized disease and 5 of 39 with extrathoracic spread concentration increased above upper 95th centile of 70 mg/L and in 3 of 11 women with localized spread and 1 of 6 with extrathoracic spread concentration increased above upper 95th centile of 130 mg/L *648*

Pregnancy-specific Glycoprotein *Serum* *No Effect* No significant difference observed between concentrations in 92 patients with primary lung cancer and 43 healthy controls *4191*

Prolactin *Plasma* *Increase* Elevated *1870*

Prostaglandin E_2 *Plasma* *Increase* The mean level was significantly elevated compared to a control group with non-malignant respiratory disorders, but did not correlate with tumor response *2112*

Prostaglandin F_1 *Plasma* *Increase* The mean level of 6-keto-PGF1 alpha, the hydrolysis product of prostacyclin, was significantly elevated compared to a control group with non-malignant respiratory disorders *2112*

Prostaglandin F_2 *Plasma* *No Effect* The mean level was not significantly different compared to a control group with non-malignant respiratory disorders *2112*

Prostate-specific Antigen *Serum* *Increase* Of 26 patients with cancer of the lung, 84.6% had values below upper limit of normal of 4.0 ng/mL as measured by method on Bayer Technicon Immuno 1®, 11.5% had values between 4.0 and 10.0 ng/mL and 3.8% had values between 10.0 and 40.0 ng/mL *342*

Protein *Pleural Fluid* *Increase* More than 3 g/L *5544* Exudate *4493* In 10 patients with lung cancer and carcinomatous pleurisy mean concentration of 46 ± 3 g/L *2205*
Serum *No Effect* In patients with carcinoma of bronchus and cachexia mean concentration of protein not affected *1319*

Prothrombin Time *Plasma* *Decrease* In 286 patients with newly diagnosed primary lung cancer prothrombin time of less than 75% observed in 8% *617*

pS2-Protein *Serum* *No Effect* In 35 patients with cancers of the lung other than adenocarcinoma median concentration of 138.0 pg/mL and mean concentration of 138.1 ± 90.1 pg/mL not significantly different compared with median of 148.8 pg/mL and mean of 167.7 ± 134.0 pg/mL in 91 healthy individuals *2152*

Pseudouridine *Urine* *Increase* In 2 patients with lung cancer mean excretion of 299 µmol/d greater than 207 µmol/d in pooled normal urine *3720* In 3 patients with bronchogenic carcinoma excretions of 102 to 150 mg/d significantly different from 65 ± 31 mg/d in 17 healthy controls *5505* In 7 patients with carcinoma of the lung mean excretion of about 30 mmol/mol creatinine significantly higher than 19.6 ± 5.2 mmol/mol creatinine in 31 healthy controls *3632*

Pyruvate *Blood* *Increase* Mildly elevated in 5 patients with bronchogenic carcinomas. Mean = 0.88 ± 0.13 U/L *2513*

Rheumatoid Factor *Pleural Fluid* *Increase* May be present with rheumatoid disease, but may also be found in other types of pleural effusions (e.g., carcinoma, tuberculosis, bacterial pneumonia) *5544*

Sialic Acid *Serum* *Increase* Mean concentration in 192 patients with carcinoma of the lung 79.72 ± 1.551 mg/dL significantly increased compared with 45.55 ± 0.922 mg/dL in 80 healthy controls *4030* In 150 patients with primary lung cancer mean concentration of 118.7 ± 40.4 mg/dL significantly higher than 64.3 ± 8.5 mg/dL in 84 healthy controls *2530*

Sialic Acid, Lipid-associated *Serum* *Increase* In patients with lung cancer mean concentration increased above 20 mg/dL in 66% of patients *1781* In 148 patients with primary lung cancer mean concentration of 28.6 ± 11.46 mg/dL significantly higher than 15.5 ± 3.4 mg/dL in 207 healthy controls *2530* In 4 patients with early stage lung cancer mean concentration of 41.8 mg/dL significantly different from 17.7 mg/dL in 50 normal volunteers *1273* Mean concentration in 192 patients with carcinoma of the lung of 47.74 ± 1.217 mg/dL significantly increased compared with 15.53 ± 0.516 mg/dL in 80 healthy controls *4030*

Sialyltransferase *Serum* *Increase* In 9 patients with lung cancer mean and median concentrations of 445 and 420 cpm/mg protein/30 min significantly different from 240 and 243 cpm/mg protein/30 min respectively in 20 normal individuals *2111*

Sodium *Serum* *Decrease* Inappropriate secretion of ADH is associated with hyponatremia, decreased serum osmolality, and inappropriately high sodium concentration in the urine. The entire syndrome resolves following resection of the tumor *1980*
Urine *Increase* Excessive excretion due to water retention resulting from abnormally regulated secretion of ADH *367* Inappropriate secretion of ADH is associated with hyponatremia, decreased serum osmolality, and inappropriately high sodium concentration in the urine. The entire syndrome resolves following resection of the tumor *1980*

Soluble Interleukin-2 Receptor *Serum* *Increase* In patients with lung cancer, mean concentration twice as high as in controls *4191*

Soluble Interleukin-6 Receptor *Pleural Fluid* *Increase* In 10 patients with lung cancer and carcinomatous pleurisy mean concentration in serum of 25,698 ± 1,993 pg/mL, significantly different from 9,438 ± 1,407 pg/mL in pleural fluid *2205*
Serum *Increase* In 10 patients with lung cancer and carcinomatous pleurisy mean concentration in serum of 25,698 ± 1,993 pg/mL, significantly different from that in healthy individuals *2205*

Specific Gravity *Pleural Fluid* *Increase* Exudate (> 1.016) *126*

Squamous Cell Carcinoma Antigen *Serum* *No Effect* In 429 patients with lung cancer median concentration in patients with stage I/II disease of 1.1 µg/L, in those with stage IIIa disease of 1.3 µg/L, and in those with stage IIIb of 1.2 µg/L not significantly different compared with threshold value of 1.5 µg/L *4740*

Stromelysin *Plasma* *Increase* In 37 men with lung cancer mean concentration of 196.6 ± 35.1 ng/mL significantly higher than 84.7 ± 11.6 ng/mL in 30 healthy control men *5878*

Thyroid Stimulating Hormone *Serum* *Increase* ACTH producing small cell carcinoma *1108*

Tissue Factor Pathway Inhibitor *Plasma* *Increase* About half of patients with pulmonary cancer had activities greater than median activity of 1.19 U/mL in healthy individuals *2376*

Tissue Polypeptide Antigen *Serum Increase* Mean concentration of 244.3 U/L in 80 patients with bronchogenic carcinoma compared with 72.7 ± 19.2 U/L in 19 healthy controls *5845* In 429 patients with lung cancer median concentration in patients with stage I/II disease of 89.8 IU/mL, in those with stage IIIa disease of 108.5 IU/mL and in those with stage IIIb of 170.7 IU/mL compared with threshold value of 85 IU/mL *4740*

Transferrin *Serum Decrease* In 89 men with lung cancer mean concentration of 157 ± 44 mg/dL significantly different from 214 ± 33 mg/dL in 106 control men and in 8 women with skin cancer mean concentration of 166 ± 70 mg/dL significantly different from 217 ± 39 mg/dL in 150 control women *2280*

Triglycerides *Serum No Effect* In patients with carcinoma of bronchus and cachexia mean triglyceride concentration within normal range *1319*

Urea Nitrogen *Serum Increase* Hypercalcemia of malignancy common with this type of cancer which leads to diminished capacity of renal tubules to concentrate urine which, in turn, decreases the ECF and the kidney's ability to eliminate excess calcium. Renal impairment eventually causes nitrogen retention, acidosis and renal failure and a further decrease in calcium excretion *3470*

Uric Acid *Serum Decrease* Hypouricemia accompanied hyponatremia (< 130 mmol/L) in 75% of patients with the syndrome of inappropriate antidiuretic hormone and small cell carcinoma of the lung *1980 4023*

Urokinase Plasminogen Activator *Tissue Increase* uPA is a prognostic marker for lung cancer *1252*

Volume *Urine Increase* Hypercalcemia of malignancy common with this type of cancer which leads to diminished capacity of renal tubules to concentrate urine which, in turn, decreases the ECF and the kidney's ability to eliminate excess calcium. Renal impairment eventually causes nitrogen retention, acidosis and renal failure and a further decrease in calcium excretion *3470*

162.90 Non-small Cell Cancer of Lung

$5C_7$ *Serum Increase* Of 5 markers tested $5C_7$ most sensitive and accurate for NSCLC: when combined with $5E_8$ and 1F10 more sensitive than SCC plus CEA. Mean sensitivity for squamous cell carcinoma 63% and 64% for adenocarcinoma *3293*

Carcinoembryonic Antigen *Serum Increase* Mean concentration increased above cutoff of 5 ng/mL in 45 of 121 patients with NSCLC (37.2%) compared with 50 of 121 (41.3%) with increased GSH-pi concentrations *2150* In 45 patients with NSCLC concentration increased. Mean sensitivity for squamous cell carcinoma 33% and 64% for adenocarcinoma using cut-off of 3.0 ng/mL *3293* In 94 patients with non-small cell lung carcinoma median concentration in those with adenocarcinoma of 6.2 ng/mL, in those with squamous cell carcinoma 2.9 ng/mL, those with large cell carcinoma 9.7 ng/mL *3809*

CYFRA 21-1 *Serum Increase* In 7 studies of patients with non-small cell cancer of the lung proportion with increased concentrations ranged from 40 - 66% *1293* In 50 patients with non-small cell cancer of the lung concentration increased above cutoff value of 3.3 ng/mL in 46 *5396* In 94 patients with non-small cell lung carcinoma median concentration in those with adenocarcinoma of 1.9 ng/mL, in those with squamous cell carcinoma 3.9 ng/mL, those with large cell carcinoma 4.4 ng/mL *3809*

Cytokeratin 8/18 *Serum Increase* In 9 of 24 patients with NSCLC concentration increased to a mean of 2.62 ng/mL significantly increased compared with healthy controls *4070*

Cytokeratin Polypeptides *Serum Increase* In 24 patients with biopsy proved NSCLC 9 were positive (mean 2.62 ng/mL, range 1.4 - 5.8 ng/mL) with all control specimens being negative *4070*

$5E_8$ *Serum Increase* In 45 patients with NSCLC most specific single marker of 5 tested: when combined with $5C_7$ and 1F10 more sensitive than SCC plus CEA . Mean sensitivity for squamous cell carcinoma 46% and 57% for adenocarcinoma *3293*

1F10 *Serum Increase* of 5 markers tested 1F10 most accurate: when combined with $5C_7$ and $5E_8$ more sensitive than CEA plus SCC. Mean sensitivity for squamous cell carcinoma 67% and 50% for adenocarcinoma *3293*

Gastrin *BAL Fluid Increase* In 26 patients with NSCLC median values of 17.5 pg/100 U LDH *1231*

γ-Glutamyltransferase *Tissue Increase* In tumors from 20 patients with non-small cell cancer of lung mean concentration of 41.9 ± 26.4 U/mg protein significantly different from 22.4 ± 12.3 U/mg protein with normal lung *468*

Glutathione *Tissue Increase* In tumors from 20 patients with non-small cell cancer of lung mean concentration of 20.8 ± 9.4 nmol/mg protein significantly different from 11.6 ± 3.0 nmol/g with normal lung *468*

Glutathione S-Transferase-pi *Serum Increase* In 50 of 121 patients with NCCLC (41.3%) concentrations increased above 34.8 ng/mL. Mean concentration significantly lower in patients with a partial response to chemotherapy (26.9 ± 11.3 ng/mL) significantly less than 38.8 ± 16.7 ng/mL in those with no response to treatment: mean concentration increases with increasing stage of the disease *2150*

Neuron-specific Enolase *Serum Increase* Mean concentration increased above cutoff of 5 ng/mL in 18 of 121 (14.9%) patients compared with 50 of 121 (41.3%) who were positive for GSH-pi *2150*

Progastrin-Releasing Peptide (31-98) *Serum No Effect* Mean concentration in 20 patients with nonsmall cell lung cancer of 16.6 ± 12.0 ng/L not significantly different from that in 247 healthy individuals (12.6 ± 6.9 ng/L) *159*

Squamous Cell Carcinoma Antigen *Serum Increase* Concentration increased in 45 patients with NSCLC. Mean sensitivity for squamous cell carcinoma 25% and 7% for adenocarcinoma using cut-off of 2.5 ng/mL *3293* Mean concentration increased above cutoff of 2.1 ng/mL in 19 of 121 patients with NSCLC (15.7%) compared with 50 of 121 (41.3%) with NSCLC *2150*

Tissue Polypeptide Antigen *Serum Increase* In 50 patients with non-small cell cancer of the lung concentration increased above cutoff value of 170 U/L in 41 *5396* In 94 patients with non-small cell lung carcinoma median concentration in those with adenocarcinoma of 113 U/L, in those with squamous cell carcinoma 112 U/L, those with large cell carcinoma 125 U/L *3809* In 58 patients with stage 3A non-small cell lung cancer median concentration of 116 U/L, 37 with stage 3B disease of 106 U/L and 144 U/L in 108 patients with stage 4 disease *5397*

Tumor Necrosis Factor *Serum No Effect* In 11 patients with non-small cell lung cancer TNF was not detected in plasma *170*

162.90 Small Cell Carcinoma of Lung

Angiotensin-converting Enzyme *Serum Increase* In 14 patients with small cell carcinoma of the lung mean activity of 155 ± 38 U/L significantly higher than 108 ± 13 U/L in 85 healthy control individuals *5338*

Antidiuretic Hormone *Plasma Increase* In 80 patients with small cell carcinoma of the lung concentrations ranged from 0.9 to 116 pmol/L. Concentration was increased (more than 2.4 times) in 37 patients (46%) *3830*

Antineuronal Nuclear Antibody Type 1 (ANNA-1) *Serum Increase* SCLC observed in 84 of 101 seropositive patients with increased ANNA-1 observed in 55% before SCLC diagnosed *2952*

Calcitonin Gene-related Peptide *Serum Increase* In 74 patients with small cell lung carcinoma mean concentration of 55.0 pmol/L compared with 36.6 pmol/L in healthy controls of similar age and sex *2896*

Carbon Dioxide Partial Pressure *Blood No Effect* In 14 patients with small cell carcinoma of the lung mean of 48 ± 17 mm Hg not significantly different from 52 ± 9 mm Hg in 85 healthy control individuals *5338*

Carcinoembryonic Antigen *Serum Increase* In 14 patients with small cell carcinoma of the lung mean baseline concentration of 6.4 ng/mL compared with upper limit of normal of 3.0 ng/mL *4470*

Corticotropin *Plasma Increase* In three patients with medullary carcinoma of the thyroid concentrations ranged from 45 to 805 pg/mL significantly increased compared with normal of less than 60 pg/mL *4262*

CYFRA 21-1 *Serum Increase* In 16 patients with inoperable small-cell carcinoma of the lung positive rate 18.8% *5146* In 6 studies of patients with small cell cancer of the lung proportion with increased concentrations ranged from 16 - 46% *1293*

162.90 Small Cell Carcinoma of Lung *(continued)*

α-Enolase *Serum* *Increase* In 8 of 19 cases of small cell lung carcinoma mean activity increased *1705*

γ-Enolase *Serum* *Increase* In 65 of 75 cases of small cell carcinoma of lung mean activity increased *1705*

Epidermal Growth Factor *Urine* *Increase* Mean concentration in about 8 patients of 20 μg/g creatinine compared with about 10 μg/g creatinine in about 30 controls *5341*

Ferritin *Serum* *Increase* In patients with cancer mean concentration increased *3498*

Gastrin *BAL Fluid* *Increase* In 9 patients with SCLC median values of 22.8 pg/100 U LDH *1231*

Hemoglobin *Blood* *Decrease* When cancer detected in 8 patients mean concentration less than 121 g/L *3498*

Iron *Serum* *Decrease* In patients with cancer mean concentration reduced compared with controls *3498*

Lactate Dehydrogenase *Serum* *Increase* Metastases developed in all 13 patients with pretreatment greater than 240 U/L but in only 31% of patients with lower than this *5027* In 60 patients with small cell lung cancer activity range of 218 - 1,945 U/L (median 396 U/L) increased above cut-off of 450 U/L in a small proportion *2494*

Lipotropic Hormone *Plasma* *Increase* In three patients with medullary carcinoma of the thyroid concentrations ranged from 870 to 8,430 pg/mL significantly increased compared with normal *4262*

Neuron-specific Enolase *Serum* *Increase* In patients with small cell lung cancer mean concentration of 23.54 ± 16.9 ng/mL signifcantly higher than 9.63 ± 4.4 ng/mL in patients with non-small cell lung cancer. Sensitivity in SCLC 74% versus 21.4% in patients with nonsmall cell lung cancer *2234* Serum neuron specific enolase activity increased in 88% of 120 patients with SCLC. Concentrations ranged from 5.2 to 193 ng/mL compared with reference range of 1.5 - 13.5 ng/mL *1500* In 80% of 20 patients with small cell carcinoma of the lung concentration was increased: when the disease was extensive increased concentration observed in 87% *945* Mean concentration increased to above 35.0 ng/mL in 13 of 15 patients (87%) compared with upper limit of 17.4 ng/mL in healthy controls *4794* Increase observed in 5 of 9 patients with recurrent disease but predated a relapse in only one. No increase observed in 9 who remained in complete remission *5419* In 112 patients with SCLC concentration of NSE increased in 71% of patients with limited disease and in 93% with extensive disease: 60% of patients with extensive disease had NSE concentrations above 35 μg/L and 30% of those with limited disease had concentrations above 35 μg/L *4253* In 60 patients with small cell lung cancer concentration range of 6.7 - 150 μg/L (median 26 μg/L) increased above cut-off of 12.5 μg/L *2494* In 265 specimens from patients with SCLC median concentration as determined by RIA 39 μg/L and 39 μg/L as determined by Delfia method compared with upper limit of normal of 12.5 μg/L *1237* Concentration increased above 35.0 ng/mL in 13 of 15 patients with small cell cancer of the lung. Reference interval of 5.2 - 17.4 ng/mL *4771*

Oxygen Partial Pressure *Blood* *Decrease* In 14 patients with small cell carcinoma of the lung mean of 50 ± 2 mm Hg significantly different from 69 ± 9 mm Hg in 85 healthy control individuals *5338*

Oxytocin *Plasma* *Increase* In 72 patients with small cell carcinoma of the lung concentrations ranged from 0.3 to 124 pmol/L with concentrations increased (more than 2.4 times) in 14 (19%) *3830*

pH *Blood* *No Effect* In 14 patients with small cell carcinoma of the lung mean of 7.40 ± 0.25 not significantly different from 7.40 ± 1.30 in 85 healthy control individuals *5338*

Progastrin-Releasing Peptide (31-98) *Serum* *Increase* Mean concentration in 12 patients with small-cell lung cancer (limited disease) of 862 ± 1,203 ng/L and in 13 with extensive disease of 1,645 ± 1491 ng/L significantly different from that in 247 healthy individuals (12.6 ± 6.9 ng/L) *159*

Proopiomelanocortin *Plasma* *Increase* In three patients with medullary carcinoma of the thyroid concentrations ranged from 740 to 8,000 U/mL significantly increased compared with normal of less than 60 U/mL *4262*

Renin Activity *Plasma* *Increase* In 14 patients with small cell carcinoma of the lung mean activity of 3.50 ± 3.11 ng/mL/h significantly higher than 2.76 ± 0.64 ng/mL/h in 85 healthy control individuals *5338*

Soluble Interleukin-2 Receptor *Serum* *Increase* Mean concentration in patients with lung cancer twice as high as in controls with highest concentrations observed in patients with small cell carcinoma *4191*

Striational Antibodies *Serum* *Increase* Approxiately 5% of patients with Lambert-Eaton myesthenic syndrome and/or small-cell lung carcinoma *2952*

Transferrin *Serum* *Decrease* In patients with cancer mean concentration less than in healthy controls *3498*

Transferrin Saturation *Serum* *Decrease* In patients with cancer mean concentration lower than in controls *3498*

Vascular Endothelial Growth Factor *Serum* *Increase* In 68 untreated patients with small cell lung cancer concentrations ranged from 70 to 1,738 pg/mL, with high concentrations associated with poor response to treatment *4540*

162.90 Squamous Cell Carcinoma of Lung

Angiotensin-converting Enzyme *Serum* *No Effect* In 13 patients with squamous cell carcinoma of the lung mean concentration of 97 ± 19 U/L not significantly different from 108 ± 13 U/L in 85 healthy control individuals *5338*

Carbon Dioxide Partial Pressure *Blood* *No Effect* In 13 patients with squamous cell carcinoma of the lung mean of 49 ± 12 mm Hg not significantly different from 52 ± 9 mm Hg in 85 healthy control individuals *5338*

Carcinoembryonic Antigen *Serum* *Increase* In 39 patients with squamous cell carcinoma of the lung mean baseline concentration of 3.7 ng/mL compared with upper limit of normal of 3.0 ng/mL *4470*

CYFRA 21-1 *Serum* *Increase* In 7 studies of patients with squamous cell cancer of the lung proportion with increased concentrations ranged from 52 - 73% *1293* In 35 patients with inoperable squamous cell cancer of the lung positive rate 71.4% *5146* At the time of diagnosis 50 of 91 patients with primary squamous cell lung cancer of the lung had concentrations greater than 3.6 ng/mL *3796*

α-Enolase *Serum* *Increase* In 16 of 16 cases of squamous cell lung carcinoma mean activity increased *1705*

γ-Enolase *Serum* *Increase* In 2 of 16 cases of squamous cell carcinoma of lung mean activity increased *1705*

Oxygen Partial Pressure *Blood* *No Effect* In 13 patients with squamous cell carcinoma of the lung mean of 60 ± 10 mm Hg not significantly different from 69 ± 9 mm Hg in 85 healthy control individuals *5338*

Parathyroid Hormone-related Peptide *Plasma* *Increase* In 3 patients with squamous carcinoma of the lung concentrations of 3.32, 7.29 and 9.51 pmol/L significantly greater than upper limit of reference range of 2.6 pmol/L *1200*

pH *Blood* *No Effect* In 14 patients with squamous cell carcinoma of the lung mean of 7.39 ± 0.12 not significantly different from 7.40 ± 1.30 in 85 healthy control individuals *5338*

Renin Activity *Plasma* *No Effect* In 13 patients with squamous cell carcinoma of the lung mean activity of 2.81 ± 0.95 ng/mL/h not significantly higher than 2.76 ± 0.64 ng/mL/h in 85 healthy control individuals *5338*

170.00 Malignant Fibrous Histiocytoma of Maxilla

Sialic Acid *Serum* *Increase* Mean concentration in 4 patients with malignant fibrous histiocytoma of the maxilla of 85.63 ± 5.45 mg/dL significantly different from 55.0 ± 7.2 mg/dL in 80 healthy controls *5755*

170.00 Maxillary Carcinoma

Epidermal Growth Factor *Urine* *Increase* Mean concentration in about 8 patients with maxillary carcinoma of 20 μg/g creatinine compared with about 10 μg/g creatinine in about 30 controls *5341*

170.10 Cancer of Mandible

Sialic Acid *Serum* *Increase* Concentration in 1 patient with cancer of the mandible of 69.72 mg/dL significantly different from 55.0 ± 7.2 mg/dL in 80 healthy controls *5755*

170.90 Ewing's Sarcoma

Soluble Interleukin-2 Receptor *Serum* *No Effect* In 8 children with localized disease mean concentration of 820 U/mL and in 7 with metastatic disease of 757 U/mL not significantly different from that in healthy controls *4235*

170.90 Malignant Neoplasm of Bone

Acid Phosphatase *Serum* *Increase* The multinucleated giant cells of giant cell tumors are rich in acid phosphatase yet only rarely is this enzyme elevated in the patient's serum *1108*

Adenosine Monophosphate *Urine* *Decrease* Reported effect *1197*

Alkaline Phosphatase *Serum* *Increase* Marked increase up to 40 times normal in osteogenic forms, parallels clinical course *5544* In 39% of 26 patients at initial hospitalization for this disorder *1576* In predominantly osteolytic forms remains normal or only moderately increased *1290* Characteristic observation *1025* All groups of bone tumors showed a significant increase when compared to the norm. Maximum values were found in the group of osteosarcomas and minimum in that of fibrosarcomas *606*
Serum *No Effect* Usually normal in Ewing's sarcoma and other osteolytic tumors *5544*

Aspartate Aminotransferase *Serum* *Increase* In 32% of 25 patients at initial hospitalization for this disorder *1576*

Bence-Jones Protein *Urine* *Present* Uncommon in osteogenic sarcoma *1290*

Calcium *Serum* *Increase* Lytic tumors involving bone can lead to nephrocalcinosis and renal failure. The most frequent cause of hypercalcemia *1025* *1290* *5544*
Serum *No Effect* Usually normal in Ewing's sarcoma and other osteolytic tumors *5544*
Urine *Increase* Lytic tumors *1025*

Ceruloplasmin *Serum* *Increase* A highly significant increase over normal levels in sera from patients with osteosarcoma *4795*

Complement, Total *Serum* *Increase* Levels from sera of 21 patients with bone tumors showed normal or slightly elevated titers *778*

Copper *Serum* *Increase* 12 cases of osteosarcoma at various stages were analyzed. Elevations occurred in primary and metastatic cases. Patients with advanced cases had the highest levels *1494* Significantly elevated in 18 patients with primary untreated osteogenic sarcoma (173 ± 30 µg/dL) *569*

CrossLaps™ *Urine* *Increase* Median excretion in patients with bone metastases of 290 ± 343 µmol/mol creatinine increased in comparison to 134 ± 127 µmol/mol creatinine in patients with malignant disease without metastases *5703*

Eosinophils *Blood* *Increase* Increases in tumors involving the bone *5544*

Hematocrit *Blood* *Decrease* In 24% of 24 patients at initial hospitalization for this disorder *1576*

Hemoglobin *Blood* *Decrease* In 36% of 24 patients at initial hospitalization for this disorder *1576*

Hydroxyproline *Urine* *Increase* Marked elevation *3780*

Lactate Dehydrogenase *Serum* *Increase* In 25% of 26 patients at initial hospitalization for this disorder *1576* In 36 patients with Ewing's sarcoma, pretreatment levels proved an extremely good indicator of which patients would ultimately develop metastases. 3 of 18 patients with levels below the total group median (201 - 214 U/L) developed metastases, while 16 of 18 patients with levels above the median developed metastatic spread ($p < 0.001$) *575*

Monocytes *Blood* *Increase* In 61% of 24 patients at initial hospitalization for this disorder *1576*

Phosphate *Serum* *Increase* Hyperphosphatemia may occur with bone tumors *5204*
Serum *No Effect* Usually normal in Ewing's Sarcoma and other osteolytic tumors *5544*

Pyridinium Crosslinks *Urine* *Increase* Median excretion in patients with bone metastases 120 ± 78 nmol/mmol creatinine increased in comparison to 48 ± 17 nmol/mmol creatinine in patients with malignant disease without metastases *5703*

Type I Collagen Cross-linked N-telopeptide *Urine* *Increase* Median excretion of N-telopeptides in patients with bone metastases of 111 ± 97 µmol/mol creatinine increased in comparison to 42 ± 23 µmol/mol creatinine in patients with malignant disease without metastases *5703*

Uric Acid *Serum* *Increase* In 37% of 26 patients at initial hospitalization for this disorder *1576*

Zinc *Serum* *Increase* Patients with primary osteosarcoma had elevated levels, those with metastases had depressed levels. The ratio of serum copper/serum zinc in metastatic osteosarcoma patients is higher than in patients with primary osteosarcoma. Determination of serum copper and serum zinc in osteosarcoma patients may be of value in prognoses and therapy evaluation. Their ratio may be useful in discriminating between patients with primary and metastatic osteosarcoma *1494*

170.90 Osteosarcoma

Ceruloplasmin *Serum* *Increase* In 7 patients with osteosarcoma mean "concentration" of 80 ± 11.2 sq mm significantly higher than 52 ± 7.3 sq mm in 22 healthy controls *4795*

Copper *Serum* *Increase* In 7 patients with osteosarcoma mean concentration of 161 ± 22.6 µg/dL significantly higher than 105 ± 12.6 µg/dL in 22 healthy controls *4795*

Osteocalcin *Serum* *Decrease* In 11 pediatric patients with osteosarcoma mean concentration of 48 ± 25.4 ng/mL significantly less than 64.8 ± 20.7 ng/mL in 12 age-matched normal children *4741*

Soluble Interleukin-2 Receptor *Serum* *No Effect* In 8 children with localized disease mean concentration of 835 U/mL and in 10 with metastatic disease of 939 U/mL not significantly different from that in healthy controls *4235*

6-Sulfatoxymelatonin *Urine* *Decrease* Mean excretion of 4.98 ± 3.04 µg/d in 8 patients with osteosarcoma significantly less than mean of 14.76 ± 8.38 µg/d in 10 healthy age-matched controls *3995*
Urine *Increase* Mean excretion of 26.94 µg/d in 2 patients with osteosarcoma significantly less than mean of 11.32 µg/d in 10 healthy age-matched controls *3995*

171.90 Lymphatic Tumors

Gc-Globulin *Serum* *No Effect* In 49 men and 42 women with "lymphatic tumors" mean concentrations of 25.6 ± 4.27 mg/dL and 25.1 ± 4.56 mg/dL not significantly different from 23.9 mg/dL in 106 control men and 26.1 mg/dL in 150 control women *2279*

171.90 Rhabdomyosarcoma

Myosin *Serum* *Decrease* In 19 pediatric patients with primary rhabdomyosarcoma mean concentration of 248 ± 606 ng/mL not significantly different from 108.9 ± 70.7 ng/mL in 20 age-matched normal children *4741*

Soluble Interleukin-2 Receptor *Serum* *No Effect* In 10 children with stage II rhabdomyosarcoma mean concentration of 1,190 U/mL and in 8 with stage III disease mean concentration of 805 U/mL not significantly different from that in healthy controls *4235*

171.90 Sarcoma

Carcinoembryonic Antigen *Serum* *Increase* In 5 patients with malignant disease of the prostate 80.0% had concentrations of 0.0 - 3.0 ng/mL, 20.0% had concentrations from 3.1 - 5.0 ng/mL, 0.0% had concentrations from 5.1 - 10.0 ng/mL and 0.0% had concentrations greater than 10.0 ng/mL when measured by method on Bayer Technicon Immuno 1® system compared with 95.9%, 3.5%, 0.6% and 0.0% respectively in 173 healthy nonsmokers *339*

171.90 Sarcoma *(continued)*

Ceruloplasmin *Serum* *Increase* In 21 men with sarcoma mean concentration of 92 ± 31 mg/dL significantly different from 71 ± 17 mg/dL in 106 control men and mean of 88 ± 14 mg/dL in 12 women with sarcoma not significantly different from 84 ± 22 mg/dL in 150 control women *2280*

Complement C_1 *Serum* *Increase* In 13 patients with sarcoma mean concentration of 42.728 ± 11.786 CH50 U/mL not significantly different from 37.251 ± 5.324 CH50 U/mL in 11 controls *3037*

Complement C_2 *Serum* *Increase* In 13 patients with sarcoma mean concentration of 7.871 ± 2.461 CH50 U/mL significantly different from 6.064 ± 1.445 CH50 U/mL in 11 controls *3037*

Complement C_3 *Serum* *Increase* In 13 patients with sarcoma mean concentration of 8.869 ± 2.119 CH50 U/mL not significantly different from 9.720 ± 2.476 CH50 U/mL in 11 controls *3037*

Complement C_4 *Serum* *Increase* In 13 patients with sarcoma mean concentration of 85.310 ± 22.663 CH50 U/mL significantly different from 64.920 ± 10.373 CH50 U/mL in 11 controls *3037*

Complement C_5 *Serum* *Increase* In 13 patients with sarcoma mean concentration of 159.334 ± 44.022 CH50 U/mL significantly different from 118.869 ± 13.547 CH50 U/mL in 11 controls *3037*

Complement C_7 *Serum* *Increase* In 13 patients with sarcoma mean concentration of 102.099 ± 28.356 CH50 U/mL not significantly different from 94.649 ± 22.434 CH50 U/mL in 11 controls *3037*

Complement C_8 *Serum* *Increase* In 13 patients with sarcoma mean concentration of 156.147 ± 28.557 CH50 U/mL significantly different from 79.129 ± 25.316 CH50 U/mL in 11 controls *3037*

Complement C_9 *Serum* *Increase* In 13 patients with sarcoma mean concentration of 135.813 ± 43.341 CH50 U/mL significantly different from 49.401 ± 12.308 CH50 U/mL in 11 controls *3037*

Complement CH50 *Serum* *Increase* In 13 patients with Hodgkin's disease mean concentration of 129.068 ± 30.484 CH50 U/mL significantly different from 104.313 ± 17.058 CH50 U/mL in 11 controls *3037*

Complement, Total *Serum* *Increase* In 13 patients with sarcoma mean concentration of 562 ± 83 CH50 U/mL significantly different from 474 ± 52 CH50 U/mL in 11 controls *3037*

Gc-Globulin *Serum* *No Effect* In 21 men and 12 women with sarcoma mean concentrations of 25.9 ± 4.29 mg/dL and 22.9 ± 4.38 mg/dL not significantly different from 23.9 mg/dL in 106 control men and 26.1 mg/dL in 150 control women *2279*

immunoglobulin A *Serum* *No Effect* In 21 men with sarcoma mean concentration of 193 ± 90 mg/dL not significantly different from 201 ± 89 mg/dL in 106 healthy controls and mean concentration of 132 ± 93 mg/dL in 12 women with sarcoma not significantly different from 176 ± 80 mg/dL in 150 healthy control women *2278*

Immunoglobulin G *Serum* *No Effect* In 21 men with sarcoma mean concentration of 1,246 ± 327 mg/dL not significantly different from 1,148 ± 224 mg/dL in 106 healthy controls and mean concentration of 1,067 ± 325 mg/dL in 12 women with sarcoma not significantly different from 1,157 ± 271 mg/dL in 150 healthy control women *2278*

Immunoglobulin M *Serum* *Increase* In 21 men with sarcoma mean concentration of 87 ± 61 mg/dL significantly different from 61 ± 36 mg/dL in 106 healthy controls *2278*
Serum *No Effect* In 12 women with sarcoma mean concentration of 79 ± 41 mg/dL not significantly different from 77 ± 39 mg/dL in 106 healthy controls *2278*

Sialic Acid *Serum* *Increase* Mean concentration in 20 patients with sarcoma of the mouth of 64.06 ± 5.01 mg/dL significantly different from 55.0 ± 7.2 mg/dL in 80 healthy controls *5755*

Sialyltransferase *Serum* *Increase* In 10 patients with sarcoma mean and median concentrations of 442 and 430 cpm/mg protein/30 min significantly different from 240 and 243 cpm/mg protein/30 min respectively in 20 normal individuals *2111*

Spermidine *Serum* *Increase* In 6 patients with sarcoma concentrations ranged from 0.21 - 0.58 nmol/mL compared with normal mean concentration of 0.33 nmol/mL *3805*

Spermine *Serum* *Increase* In 6 patients with sarcoma concentrations ranged from 0.02 - 0.10 nmol/mL compared with normal mean concentration of 0.04 nmol/mL *3805*

Transferrin *Serum* *No Effect* In 21 men with sarcoma mean concentration of 209 ± 47 mg/dL not significantly different from 214 ± 33 mg/dL in 106 control men and in 12 women with sarcoma mean concentration of 205 ± 69 mg/dL not significantly different from 217 ± 39 mg/dL in 150 control women *2280*

Urokinase Plasminogen Activator *Tissue* *Increase* Amounts in soft tissue sarcoma predictable of overall survival *1255*

171.90 Sarcoma, Synovial

N^2, N^2-Dimethylguanosine *Urine* *Increase* In 1 patient with synovial sarcoma excretion of 10.7 mg/d significantly different from 3.9 ± 2.6 mg/d in 17 healthy controls *5505*

Pseudouridine *Urine* *Increase* In 1 patient with synovial sarcoma excretion of 132 mg/d significantly different from 65 ± 31 mg/d in 17 healthy controls *5505*

172.80 Malignant Melanoma of Skin

Aldolase *Serum* *Increase* Markedly elevated in melanoblastomas. Mean = 9.0 ± 2.9 compared to 1.6 ± 0.21 U/L *2513*

Alkaline Phosphatase *White Blood Cells* *Decrease* Low activity is present irrespective of tumor category, activity of disease, or type of therapy. In 11 patients, median activity was 5 U/L (normal 55 U/L) *3110*

Dopamine *Plasma* *Increase* Significantly increased ($p < 0.001$) in plasma of all 65 patients with active disease (stage II), 2.08 µg/L compared with 32 normal control values of 1.23 µg/L *1417*

Hexokinase *Serum* *Increase* Significantly increased in melanoblastomas. Mean activity of 17.4 ± 3.5 U/L compared to normal of 0.93 ± 0.28 U/L *2513*

Immunoglobulin D *Serum* *Decrease* Malignant melanoma patients with metastases presented significant decreases in IgD and IgM subpopulations *412*

Immunoglobulin M *Serum* *Decrease* Malignant melanoma patients with metastases presented significant decreases in IgD and IgM subpopulations *412*

Lactate Dehydrogenase *Serum* *Increase* Marked elevation in 38 patients with melanoblastomas. Mean activity of 179.7 ± 20.0 U/L compared to normals, 85.4 ± 1.0 U/L *2513*

Lymphocytes *Blood* *Decrease* Active rosettes (T-EA) were decreased only in metastatic patients, while the total T population (T-ET) was decreased in all stages. Patients whose values were constant remained cancer free, while a reduction heralded the appearance of clinical and/or radiological signs of metastases *412*

Melanin *Urine* *Increase* In some patients, when the urine is exposed to air for several h, colorless melanogens are oxidized to melanin and urine becomes deep brown and later black. Melanogenuria occurs in 25% of patients; it is said to be more frequent with extensive liver metastasis. It is not useful for judging completeness of removal or early recurrence *5544*

Phosphate *Serum* *Decrease* In 49% of 67 patients at initial hospitalization for this disorder *1576*

Soluble E-Selectin *Serum* *Increase* In patients with metastatic cutaneous malignant melanoma those with concentrations greater than 60 ng/mL had significantly worse outcomes than those with concentrations less than 60 ng/mL *1558*

Soluble Intercellular Adhesion Molecule-1 *Serum* *Increase* In patients with metastatic cutaneous malignant melanoma those with concentrations greater than 290 ng/mL had significantly worse outcomes than those with concentrations less than 290 ng/mL *1558*

Soluble Vascular Cell Adhesion Molecule-1 *Serum* *Increase* In patients with metastatic cutaneous malignant melanoma those with concentrations greater than 770 ng/mL had significantly worse outcomes than those with concentrations less than 770 ng/mL *1558*

Uric Acid *Serum* *Increase* In 38% of 67 patients at initial hospitalization for this disorder *1576*

172.90 Malignant Melanoma

Anti-p53 Antibodies *Serum* *No Effect* No increase observed in 58 patients with malignant melanoma *132*

Carcinoembryonic Antigen *Serum* *No Effect* In 1 patient with myeloma the concentrationwas between 0.0 - 3.0 ng/mL when measured by method on Bayer Technicon Immuno 1® system compared with 95.9% in 173 healthy nonsmokers *339*

Ceruloplasmin *Serum* *No Effect* In 90 men with malignant melanoma mean concentration of 72 ± 20 mg/dL not significantly different from 71 ± 17 mg/dL in 106 control men and mean of 84 ± 25 mg/dL in 88 women with malignant melanoma not significantly different from 84 ± 22 mg/dL in 150 control women *2280*

Creatine Kinase BB-Isoenzyme *Serum* *Increase* Elevated CK-BB *919* *5884*

Ferritin *Serum* *Increase* Malignant melanoma may increase serum ferritin concentration and ferritin may function as a tumor mrker *4784*

Gc-Globulin *Serum* *No Effect* In 90 men and 88 women with malignant melanoma mean concentrations of 23.6 ± 3.72 mg/dL and 25.8 ± 5.32 mg/dL not significantly different from 23.9 ± 3.36 mg/dL in 106 control men and 26.1 ± 4.66 mg/dL in 150 control women *2279*

immunoglobulin A *Serum* *No Effect* In 90 men with malignant melanoma mean concentration of 198 ± 101 mg/dL not significantly different from 201 ± 89 mg/dL in 106 healthy controls and mean concentration of 176 ± 72 mg/dL in 88 women with malignant melanoma not significantly different from 176 ± 80 mg/dL in 150 healthy control women *2278*

Immunoglobulin M *Serum* *Increase* In 88 women with malignant melanoma mean concentration of 101 ± 66 mg/dL significantly different from 77 ± 39 mg/dL in 106 healthy controls *2278*

Serum *No Effect* In 90 men with malignant melanoma mean concentration of 67 ± 61 mg/dL not significantly different from 61 ± 36 mg/dL in 106 healthy controls *2278*

Interleukin-6 *Serum* *Increase* In 164 patients with melanoma detectable concentrations were observed in 74 (45%) *551*

Melanoma Inhibitory Factor *Serum* *Increase* In 100 patients mean concentration of 18.8 ± 12.5 ng/mL showed significant difference from 3.6 ± 2.8 ng/mL in 120 healthy controls *3655*

N^2, N^2-Dimethylguanosine *Urine* *Increase* In 4 patients with malignant melanoma excretions of 6.0 to 21.0 mg/d in three significantly different from 3.9 ± 2.6 mg/d in 17 healthy controls, but 3.1 mg/d in the fourth not significantly different *5505*

Urine *No Effect* In 4 patients with malignant melanoma excretions of 6.0 to 21.0 mg/d in three significantly different from 3.9 ± 2.6 mg/d in 17 healthy controls, but 3.1 mg/d in the fourth not significantly different *5505*

Neopterin *Serum* *Increase* In 16% of 101 patients with malignant melanoma of the choroid, concentration above mean ± 2 SD (9.1 ± 3.2 nmol/L) observed in 40 healthy controls with greatest number of patients with increased concentrations having untreated tumors *1707*

Urine *Increase* In 101 patients with malignant melanoma of the choroid, 16 had concentrations greater than mean ± 2 SD (410 ± 101) µmol/mol creatinine with 4 of 20 with untreated tumors having increased concentrations, 5 of 34 with partial tumor regression and 7 of 47 with complete tumor regression *1707*

Neuron-specific Enolase *Serum* *Increase* Increased concentrations observed in 30 of 63 patients (48%) during course of the disease *5660* In 24 patients with stage I disease mean concentration of 7.4 µg/L, of 5.8 µg/L in 44 with stage II disease, and 11.0 µg/L in 21 patients with stage III disease *2234*

Pseudouridine *Urine* *Increase* In 4 patients with malignant melanoma excretions of 98 to 232 mg/d significantly different from 65 ± 31 mg/d in 17 healthy controls *5505*

Putrescine *Serum* *Increase* In 5 patients with melanoma concentrations ranged from 0.56 - 1.32 nmol/mL compared with normal mean concentration of 0.23 nmol/mL *3805*

Ribonuclease *Serum* *Increase* In 10 sera from patients with melanoma in Mayo Clinic Serum Bank mean activity of 413 ± 140 U/mL significantly higher than 273 ± 66 U/mL in sera from 21 normal individuals *2793*

S-100 Protein *Serum* *Increase* In 99 patients with metastatic malignant melanoma concentrations greater than 3 µg/L were associated with an unfavorable outcome and median survival of less than 6 mo. In those with concentration less than 3 µg/L median survival of 13 mo *625*

Sialic Acid, Lipid-associated *Serum* *Increase* Mean concentration of 23 mg/dL in 24 patients with low tumor burden and in 22 with intermediate tumor burden and of 34 mg/dL in 24 with high tumor burden significantly higher than 18 mg/dL in 168 individuals with no tumor burden *656*

Sialyltransferase *Serum* *Increase* In 13 patients with melanoma mean and median concentrations of 409 and 375 cpm/mg protein/30 min significantly different from 240 and 243 cpm/mg protein/30 min respectively in 20 normal individuals *2111*

Soluble Interleukin-2 Receptor *Serum* *Increase* In 172 patients with melanoma mean concentration of 424.2 U/mL significantly higher than 336.8 U/mL in 60 healthy controls *551* In 227 patients with melanoma, concentrations significantly higher than in healthy controls *1478*

Spermidine *Serum* *No Effect* In 6 patients with melanoma concentrations ranged from detectable but not quantifiable to 0.44 nmol/mL compared with normal mean concentration of 0.33 nmol/mL *3805*

Spermine *Serum* *No Effect* In 6 patients with melanoma concentrations ranged from detectable but not quantifiable to 0.11 nmol/mL compared with normal mean concentration of 0.04 nmol/mL *3805*

Tissue Factor Pathway Inhibitor *Plasma* *Increase* About half of patients with melanoma had activities greater than median activity of 1.19 U/mL in healthy individuals *2376*

Transferrin *Serum* *Decrease* In 90 men with malignant melanoma mean concentration of 203 ± 40 mg/dL significantly different from 214 ± 33 mg/dL 106 control men but in 88 women with malignant melanoma mean concentration of 214 ± 48 mg/dL not significantly different from 217 ± 39 mg/dL in 150 control women *2280*

173.90 Skin Cancer

Ceruloplasmin *Serum* *Increase* In 32 men with skin cancer mean concentration of 81 ± 19 mg/dL significantly different from 71 ± 17 mg/dL in 106 control men and mean of 83 ± 11 mg/dL in 19 women with skin cancer significantly different from 84 ± 22 mg/dL in 150 control women *2280*

Gc-Globulin *Serum* *No Effect* In 32 men and 19 women with skin cancer mean concentrations of 24.0 ± 3.23 mg/dL and 23.7 ± 3.23 mg/dL not significantly different from 23.9 ± 3.36 mg/dL in 106 control men and 26.1 ± 4.66 mg/dL in 150 control women *2279*

immunoglobulin A *Serum* *Increase* In 32 men with skin cancer mean concentration of 273 ± 105 mg/dL significantly different from 201 ± 89 mg/dL in 106 healthy control men *2278*

Serum *No Effect* In 19 women with skin cancer mean concentration of 204 ± 97 mg/dL not significantly different from 174 ± 80 mg/dL in 150 healthy control women *2278*

Immunoglobulin G *Serum* *Increase* In 32 men with skin cancer mean concentration of 1,344 ± 357 mg/dL not significantly different from 1,148 ± 224 mg/dL in 106 healthy control men *2278*

Serum *No Effect* In 19 women with skin cancer mean concentration of 1,150 ± 241 mg/dL not significantly different from 1,157 ± 271 mg/dL in 150 healthy control women *2278*

Immunoglobulin M *Serum* *No Effect* In 32 men with skin cancer mean concentration of 69 ± 41 mg/dL not significantly different from 61 ± 36 mg/dL in 106 healthy controls and in 19 women with skin cancer mean concentration of 111 ± 184 mg/dL not significantly different from 77 ± 39 mg/dL in 150 healthy control women *2278*

Transferrin *Serum* *Decrease* In 32 men with skin cancer mean concentration of 190 ± 35 mg/dL significantly different from 214 ± 33 mg/dL in 106 control men and in 19 women with skin cancer mean concentration of 181 ± 59 mg/dL not significantly different from 217 ± 39 mg/dL in 150 control women *2280*

174.90 Breast Cancer

α_1-Acid Glycoprotein *Serum Increase* In 9 women with T1, T2 or T3 carcinomas 1 of 10 specimens had concentration above upper limit of normal of 0.88 g/L and 1 of 16 with histological grade III or axillary node involvement and/or a T4 tumor had increased concentrations as did 12 of 16 with overt metastases *924* In patients with metastatic breast cancer mean concentration of 1.43 g/L compared with less than 0.50 g/L in 30 healthy controls *719*

Acid Phosphatase *Serum Increase* Female patients with metastatic breast cancer, selected at random and including both treated and untreated cases, had a mean serum activity which was significantly ($p < 0.001$) above that seen in females with benign disease *4335* Reported effect *1642 2434*

Albumin *Serum Decrease* Significantly reduced (median of 35.7 g/L) in patients with carcinoma compared to controls (44.0 g/L) *2109*
Urine Increase 24 h excretion and renal clearance were significantly increased in localized tumor patients compared to normals and disseminated cancer cases. Increased high molecular weight protein excretion implies glomerular injury in these patients *2109*

Aldolase *Serum Increase* Significantly elevated; mean = 4.8 ± 0.7 U/L compared to normal, 1.6 ± 0.21 U/L *2513*

Alkaline Phosphatase *Serum Increase* Mean level in patients without bone metastases was above the normal range. The mean levels with metastases to bone was even higher, with 56% of all cases above the normal range *5724* In 47 women presenting with metastatic breast cancer concentration abnormal in 15 of 46 (32%) *923* In 19 patients with breast cancer median activity of 155 U/L significantly higher than that in 75 healthy men in whom the median activity was 101 U/L and in 20 premenopausal women, 88 U/L, and in 38 postmenopausal women, 115 U/L *4716* In 9 women with T1, T2 or T3 carcinomas 0 of 10 specimens had concentration above upper limit of normal of 90 U/L and 0 of 15 with histological grade III or axillary node involvement and/or a T4 tumor had increased concentrations but 11 of 17 with overt metastases had increased concentrations *924*
Serum No Effect No significant elevation was found in patients without bone metastases *2803*
White Blood Cells Decrease Low activity is present irrespective of tumor category, activity of disease, or type of therapy. In 21 patients, median value was 25 U/L (normal 55 U/L) *3110*

Alkaline Phosphatase Isoenzymes *Serum Increase* Cancer of the ovary, endometrium, cervix and breast as a group exhibited the highest frequency of Regan isoenzyme (placental) *658*

Alkaline Phosphatase, Placental Isoenzyme
Serum No Effect In 9 women with T1, T2 or T3 carcinomas 0 of 10 specimens had concentration above upper limit of normal of 0.85 U/L and 0 of 16 with histological grade III or axillary node involvement and/or a T4 tumor had increased concentrations as did 0 of 17 with overt metastases *924*

α-Aminohippuric Acid *Urine No Effect* In 12 women with breast cancer and abnormal tryptophan metabolism mean excretion of 25.0 ± 6.6 µmol/d not significantly different from 24.5 ± 6.3 µmol/d in 12 healthy controls *1034*

Amyloid A Protein *Serum Increase* In patients with metastatic breast cancer mean concentration of 123 mg/L compared with less than 1 mg/L in 30 healthy controls *719*

Androgens *Plasma Increase* Plasma testosterone concentrations were measured in sequential samples from 6 women and were compared to concentrations in 6 control women matched for age, menopause, and parity. Concentrations in each cancer patient were significantly higher than in each matched control *3405*
Urine Decrease Significantly decreased in comparison with controls *820*

Androsterone *Urine Decrease* Significantly decreased in comparison with controls *820*
Urine No Effect In 12 women with breast cancer and abnormal tryptophan metabolism mean excretion of 0.846 ± 0.695 mg/d not significantly different from 1.010 ± 0.860 mg/d in 12 healthy controls *1034*

Anthranilic Acid Glucuronide *Urine No Effect* In 12 women with breast cancer and abnormal tryptophan metabolism mean excretion of 5.8 ± 2.8 µmol/d not significantly different from 5.0 ± 1.3 µmol/d in 12 healthy controls *1034*

Anti-p53 Antibodies *Serum Increase* Increased in 16 of 292 patients (5.5%) *132*

α_1-Antichymotrypsin *Serum Increase* Mean concentration in patients with metastatic breast cancer of 0.73 g/L compared with less than 0.50 g/L in 30 healthy controls *719*

α_1-Antitrypsin *Serum Increase* In 9 women with T1, T2 or T3 carcinomas 2 of 9 specimens had concentration above upper limit of normal of 3.2 g/L and 1 of 16 with histological grade III or axillary node involvement and/or a T4 tumor had increased concentrations as did 5 of 16 with overt metastases *924*

Apolipoprotein A-I *Serum No Effect* In 8 women aged over 50 years with malignant disease of the breast mean concentration of 150.3 ± 9.4 mg/dL not significantly different from 156.4 ± 7.8 mg/dL in 24 women with breast masses *2910*

Apolipoprotein A-I:Apolipoprotein B Ratio *Serum No Effect* In 8 women aged over 50 years with malignant disease of the breast mean ratio of 1.74 ± 0.25 not significantly different from 1.93 ± 0.16 in 24 women with breast masses *2910*

Apolipoprotein A-II *Serum No Effect* In 8 women aged over 50 years with malignant disease of the breast mean concentration of 72.1 ± 7.7 mg/dL not significantly different from 76.5 ± 3.5 mg/dL in 24 women with breast masses *2910*

Apolipoprotein B *Serum Increase* In 8 women aged over 50 years with malignant disease of the breast mean concentration of 101.0 ± 15.6 mg/dL not significantly different from 88.4 ± 5.6 mg/dL in 24 women with breast masses *2910*

Apolipoprotein C-III *Serum No Effect* In 8 women aged over 50 years with malignant disease of the breast mean concentration of 10.9 ± 2.6 mg/dL not significantly different from 11.2 ± 0.8 mg/dL in 24 women with breast masses *2910*

Apolipoprotein D *Serum Decrease* In 94 patients with breast cancer and bone metastases mean concentration of about 48 mg/L significantly less than concentration in 28 healthy women 95% confidence interval (50 - 125 mg/L, median 73.5 mg/L) *3944*
Serum No Effect In 8 women aged over 50 years with malignant disease of the breast mean concentration of 13.1 ± 1.1 mg/dL not significantly different from 15.9 ± 1.3 mg/dL in 24 women with breast masses *2910* In 72 patients with early breast cancer mean concentration of about 74 mg/L not significantly different from concentration in 28 healthy women 95% confidence interval (50 - 125 mg/L, median 73.5 mg/L) *3944*

Apolipoprotein E *Serum Decrease* In 8 women aged over 50 years with malignant disease of the breast mean concentration of 13.8 ± 1.7 mg/dL not significantly different from 15.2 ± 0.8 mg/dL in 24 women with breast masses *2910*

Aspartate Aminotransferase *Serum Increase* In 25% of 296 patients at initial hospitalization for this disorder *1576*

Basic Fibroblast Growth Factor *Serum Increase* In 25 of 35 (71%) of women with stage I primary breast cancer concentration increased above normal, as in 10 of 13 (77%) stage II and all 5 (100%) patients with stage III breast cancer *5145*

BCA225 *Serum Increase* In 98 patients with recurrent breast cancer concentration increased above cut-off of 160 U/mL in 43 (43.9%) *2379*

Bone Sialoprotein *Serum Increase* In 19 patients with breast cancer median concentration of 17.8 ng/mL significantly higher than that in 75 healthy men in whom the median concentration was 9.8 ng/mL and in 20 premenopausal women, 8.7 ng/mL, and in 38 postmenopausal women, 11.9 ng/mL *4716*

Breast Antigen BR 27.29 *Serum Increase* In patients with breast cancer cutoff of 38 U/mL differentiated patients with disease from healthy individuals *1188*

c-erb-B_2 Oncoprotein *Serum Decrease* Mean concentration in 67 patients with malignant breast tumors of 3,084 ± 846 HNU/mL significantly different from 3,271 ± 809 HNU/mL in 60 healthy controls *580*
Serum Increase Median concentration of < 3 ng/mL in 172 patients with locoregional cancer, 12 ng/mL in 106 with metastatic cancer and < 3 ng/mL in 10 with no longer detectable disease. 12 of 172 (7%) of patients with locoregional disease, 44 of 106 (41.5%) with metastases and 0 of 35 (0%) without detectable disease had concentrations exceeding 1.5 ng/mL *3564* In 25 patients with primary breast cancer 12% had a serum concentration greater than 12 U/mL, as occurred in 4.9% of 82 patients with non-recurrent breast cancer and 31.4% of 35 patients with recurrent breast cancer *5593* In 186 women with locoregional cancer of the breast 9.1% had concentrations

exceeding 15 U/mL *3562* In 412 patients with breast cancer abnormal concentrations observed in 9.2% with locoregional disease and in 45.4% of patients with advanced disease compared with concentrations of less than 15 U/mL in 50 healthy women *3563* In 33 patients with metastatic breast cancer, 10 of whom were c-erbB$_2$ positive, median concentration of positive values was 63.8 U/mL *4330*
Tissue Increase In breast cancer tissue concentrations greater than 10 U/g protein observed in 25 of 161 (16%) primary breast carcinomas and in 3 of 6 (50%) of breast cancer metastases. High levels were not found in normal breast tissue or benign breast tumors *1256*

CA 15-3 *Serum Increase* In 201 specimens from 32 patients BR-MA concentration as measured on DPC IMMULITE correlated positively with CA 15-3 concentration but IMMULITE measurements were more sensitive in both progressive and stable disease than CA 15-3 *5389* In 40 women with breast cancer sensitivity 67.5%, positive predictive value 90% and negative predictive value 64.9% *1568* In women with breast cancer significant increase in concentration with increase in disease extent from 29 U/mL with a disease score of < 5 to 159 U/mL with a disease score of > 15 *5156* In 298 women with breast cancer probability of 10-year survival of 71.9% when CA 15-3 concentration within normal range, with decreasing concentration of 57.5%, with fluctuating concentration of 24.7% and with increasing concentration of 27.9% *4466* In 98 patients with recurrent breast cancer concentration increased above cut-off of 30 U/mL in 67 (68.4%) *2379* In 31 patients with primary breast cancer mean concentration of 26.9 ± 30 U/mL and in 158 with metastatic breast cancer 175.4 ± 520 U/mL with concentrations in both cases being higher in patients with more advanced disease. Mean concentration in 1,050 normal controls of 13.3 ± 6 U/mL *2076* In 22 patients with metastatic breast cancer median concentration of 43.5 U/mL significantly higher than 22.6 U/mL in 30 women with nonmetastatc breast cancer and in healthy women *223* The median value (43 kU/L) in 26 patients with stage IV disease was significantly higher than the median for 97 patients classified as stage I or II (17 kU/L) *895* *2237* In 186 women with locoregional cancer of the breast, 15.6% had concentrations exceeding 35 U/mL *3562* Using a cutoff of 30.38 U/L probability of disease-free survival for 5 years 44% in patients with high CA 15-3 concentration compared with 65% for patients with low CA 15-3 concentrations *4777*

CA 19-9 *Serum Increase* Reported effect *5381* Elevated in 3% of cases *2129* In 22 patients with metastatic breast cancer concentration increased in 10 (46%) [median concentration of 35.4 U/mL] and in 30 women with breast cancer but without metastases concentration increased in 8 (27%) [median concentration of 23.5 U/mL] *223*

CA 27-29 *Serum Increase* In 40 women with breast cancer sensitivity of 70%, positive predictive value of 93.3% and negative predictive value of 67.5% *1568*

CA 50 *Serum Increase* Elevated in a high proportion of patients with primary carcinoma *2211* *4285*

CA 72-4 *Serum Increase* In colon carcinomas 21% of specimens showed elevated levels *5744*

CA 125 *Serum Increase* In 7 patients with lung metastases and pleural effusion concentration increased *2399* Using Boehringer Mannheim Enzymun test mean concentration of 99.2 ± 581.9 U/mL with 18.7% above 35 U/mL *2636* In 22 patients with metastatic breast cancer concentration increased in 6 (27%) [median concentration of 16.55 U/mL] and in 30 women with breast cancer but without metastases concentration increased in 1 (3%) [median concentration of 12.4 U/mL] *223* Elevated in epithelial cancers *1963*
Serum No Effect In 4 patients with lung metastases but without pleural effusion concentration normal: in most patients with breast cancer and only bone or liver metastases concentration also usually normal *2399*

CA 549 *Serum Increase* In 60 patients with stage I breast cancer 3 (5%) had a concentration greater than the upper limit of normal, as did 9 (14.1%) of 64 with stage II disease, 19 (32.2%) of 59 with stage III disease and 40 (74.1%) of 54 with stage IV disease as measured by the BRESMARQ assay *764* Raised in 83.3% of cases *246* In 117 women with primary breast cancer and tumors less than 2 cm in diameter median concentration of 6.7 U/mL, in 110 with tumors 2 - 5 cm 6.8 U/mL, and in 10 with tumors greater than 5 cm 14.7 U/mL compared with 6.7 ± 3.5 U/mL in 184 healthy control women *1737* Does not appear to be useful in screening patients for the diagnosis of priamry breast cancer *765* Raised in 83.3% of cases *4508* Incidence of positives in patients with breast cancer 0 to 3% in early stages to more than 90% in progressive metastatic disease *5641*

CA-M26 *Serum Increase* Serum values were determined in 125 women: 46 patients with primary breast cancer, 49 patients with benign breast disease, and 30 controls. The mean values in breast cancer patients were higher than in patients with benign breast disease and in control subjects. When we set the cut-off level at 40 kU/L, 33% of all breast cancer patients, 55% of breast cancer patients with axillary node involvement, 8% of patients with benign disease and 23% of controls were above this cut-off level *1390* In patients with breast cancer and stage I or II disease positives infrequent (0 - 15%) but positive in up to 80% of patients with stage III or IV disease but decreases observed treatment and increases with disease progression or relapse *5641*

CA-M29 *Serum Increase* In 6 clinical studies of patients with breast cancer and stage I or II disease positives ranged from 0 to 9% and in those with stage III or IV disease 29% to 80% positive *5641* Serum values were determined in 125 women: 46 patients with primary breast cancer, 49 patients with benign breast disease, and 30 controls. The mean values in breast cancer patients were higher than in patients with benign breast disease and in control subjects. When we set the cu-off level at 10 Ku/L, 65% of all breast cancer patients, 80% of breast cancer patients with axillary node involvement,18% of patients with benign disease and 33% of controls were above this cut-off level *1187*

Calcitonin *Plasma Increase* In 9 women with T1, T2 or T3 carcinomas 2 of 10 specimens had concentration above upper limit of normal of 0.1 µg/L and 2 of 16 with histological grade III or axillary node involvement and/or a T4 tumor had increased concentrations as did 2 of 17 with overt metastases *924*
Plasma No Effect In 107 patients with breast cancer; CEA, ferritin and calcitonin levels were measured. CEA and ferritin but not calcitonin levels were statistically higher in those patients with metastases *431*

Calcium *Serum Decrease* In 19 patients with breast cancer median concentration of 2.19 mmol/L significantly lower than that in 75 healthy men in whom the median concentration was 2.38 mmol/L and in 20 premenopausal women, 2.39 mmol/L, and in 38 postmenopausal women, 2.41 mmol/L *4716*
Serum Increase Frequent hypercalcemia in advanced cases *826* Neoplasm without evidence of direct bone involvement. Parathyroid hormone-secreting tumors. Metastatic or lytic tumors involving bone *1025* In one study of 42 patients with hypercalcemia and low intact PTH concentration, 2 had carcinoma of the breast *3280* Hypercalcemia of malignancy common with this type of cancer *3470*
Serum No Effect None of 13 patients with breast cancer had hypercalcemia *1200*
Urine Decrease Hypercalcemia of malignancy common with this type of cancer which leads to diminished capacity of renal tubules to concentrate urine which, in turn, decreases the ECF and the kidney's ability to eliminate excess calcium. Renal impairment eventually causes nitrogen retention, acidosis and renal failure and a further decrease in calcium excretion *3470*
Urine Increase Hypercalcemia of malignancy common with this type of cancer which is often associated with hypercalciuria occurring with excessive bone reabsorption *3470* Commonly observed with some forms of breast cancer *1025*

Carcinoembryonic Antigen *Ascitic Fluid Increase* 4 of 6 breast cancer patients were detected by CEA estimations in ascitic fluid. Values > 10 ng/mL were considered cancerous effusions *3102*
Pleural Fluid Increase 24 (34%) of 70 malignant effusions had levels > 12 ng/mL *4369*
Serum Increase In 298 women with breast cancer probability of 10-year survival 63% when CEA concentration within normal range, with decreasing concentration of 56.9%, with fluctuating concentration of 40.2% and with increasing concentration of 31.4% *4466* In 158 patients with metastatic breast cancer mean concentration of 24.0 ± 53 ng/mL. In 26 with local metastases mean concentration of 2.9 ± 5 ng/mL, with mean of 11.8 ± 17 ng/mL in those with metastases to bone only and 79 ± 104 ng/mL in 24 with liver metastases only *2076* In 98 patients with recurrent breast cancer concentration increased above cut-off of

174.90 Breast Cancer *(continued)*

Carcinoembryonic Antigen *(continued)* 5.0 ng/mL in 54 (55,1%) *2379* In 206 specimens from 32 patients with breast cancer CEA concentration as measured on DPC IMMULITE correlated positively with CA 19-9 concentration but IMMULITE measurements were generally higher than CA 19-9 results but no clinical discrepancies were found *5389* Increase reported in half of patients *1601* In 186 women with locoregional cancer of the breast 18.3% had concentrations exceeding 5 ng/mL *3562* In 120 patients with breast cancer 62.5% had concentrations up to 3.0 ng/mL, 12.5% had concentrations between 3.1 - 5.0 ng/mL, 9.2% between 5.1 - 10.0 ng/mL and 15.8% had concentrations greater than 10.1 ng/mL in contrast to concentrations in 151 healthy nonsmokers in whom 95.4% had concentrations between 0 and 3.0 ng/mL and 4.6% between 4.1 and 10.0 ng/mL *11* In 40 women with breast cancer sensitivity 40%, positive predictive value of 88.4% and negative predictive value of 27.3% *1568* In 22 patients with metastatic breast cancer concentration increased in 10 (46%) [median concentration of 8.95 ng/mL] and in 30 women with breast cancer but without metastases concentration increased in 11 (37%) [median concentration of 6.8 ng/mL] *223* Increased in 50% patients *4551* In 52% of cases *4891* 12 of 17 patients had initially elevated values. Levels in later stages of the disease were usually higher than those in earlier stages. Referring to the international TNM classification, values were particularly elevated in both the T3 and T4 stages, with axillary node involvement and with the presence of bone metastases *5286* In 9 women with T1, T2 or T3 carcinomas 1 of 10 specimens had concentration above upper limit of normal of 20 μg/L and 2 of 15 with histological grade III or axillary node involvement and/or a T4 tumor had increased concentrations as did 13 of 16 with overt metastases *924* In 47 women presenting with metastatic breast cancer concentration abnormal in 16 of 36 (44%) *923* In specimens from patients with stage IV breast cancer mean concentration approximately 35 ng/mL significantly higher than mean of less than 2 ng/mL in individuals with stages I to III breast cancer and 50 normal individuals *755* In 52% of cases *431* In 122 patients with malignant breast disease, 77.0% had concentrations of 0.0 - 3.0 ng/mL, 11.5% had concentrations from 3.1 - 5.0 ng/mL, 5.7% had concentrations from 5.1 - 10.0 ng/mL and 5.7% had concentrations greater than 10.0 ng/mL when measured by method on Bayer Technicon Immuno 1® system compared with 95.9%, 3.5%, 0.6% and 0.0% respectively in 173 healthy nonsmokers *339*
Serum No Effect In 31 patients with primary breast cancer mean concentration of 1.2 ± 1 ng/mL not significantly different from normal concentration of less than 2.5 ng/mL *2076*

Casein *Serum Increase* In 8 of 11 patients detectable concentrations of casein (mean 500 ± 160 μg/L in positive patients) observed in serum compared with 3 of 36 healthy nonpregnant nonlactating women *2113*

Cathepsin B *Serum Increase* In 17 women with breast cancer mean concentration higher than in serum of 20 healthy control women *1619*
Tissue Increase Significant association reported between cathepsin B amount and a shorter disease-free survival in patients with breast cancer *1252*

Cathepsin D *Tissue Increase* Cathepsin D is an independent prognostic marker for recurrnce-free survival in patients with breast cancer *1252*

Cathepsin L *Tissue Increase* Cathepsin L appears to be a stronger prognostic marker than cathepsin B for survival in patients with breast cancer *1252*

Ceruloplasmin *Serum Increase* In 118 women with breast cancer mean concentration of 98 ± 34 mg/dL significantly different from 84 ± 22 mg/dL in 150 control women *2280* In 9 women with T1, T2 or T3 carcinomas 1 of 9 specimens had concentration above upper limit of normal of 0.45 g/L and 0 of 16 with histological grade III or axillary node involvement and/or a T4 tumor had increased concentrations as did 6 of 16 with overt metastases *924*

Cholesterol *Serum Increase* In 8 women aged over 50 years with malignant disease of the breast mean concentration of 209.6 ± 23.3 mg/dL not significantly different from 184.0 ± 7.2 mg/dL in 24 women with breast masses *2910*

β-Chorionic Gonadotropin *Plasma Increase* In 9 women with T1, T2 or T3 carcinomas, 0 of 10 specimens had concentration above upper limit of normal of 2 μg/L and 1 of 16 with histological grade III or axillary node involvement and/or a T4 tumor had increased concentrations as did 1 of 17 with overt metastases *924* Observed effect *5195* Observed effect in some patients *2740*

Colony Stimulating Factor-1 *Serum No Effect* Mean concentration of 4.2 ± 0.2 ng/mL observed in 118 patients with primary cancer not significantly different from 4.46 ± 1.33 ng/mL in 64 normal volunteers *4665*

Complement C_3 *Serum Increase* Increased in patients with local disease. Very closely linked to the stage of the disease. Patients in remission had normal levels, but further increases were noted in distant metastases. Dropped significantly in the terminal phase of the disease *5456*

Complement C_4 *Serum Increase* Increased in patients with local disease. Very closely linked to the stage of the disease. Patients in remission had normal levels, but further increases were noted in distant metastases. Levels dropped significantly in the terminal phase of the disease *5456*

Complement, Total *Serum Increase* Very closely linked to the stage of the disease. Patients in remission had normal levels, but further increases were noted in distant metastases. Levels dropped significantly in the terminal phase of disease *5456*

Copper *Serum Increase* Mean concentration and mean Cu:Zn ratio in 31 patients with breast cancer significantly higher than in 35 healthy controls *5829* All 23 patients demonstrated elevations (299 ± 34 μg/dL) compared to normal (108 ± 10 μg/dL) *1059* Observed in some patients *4691*

C-Reactive Protein *Serum Increase* Mean concentration in patients with metastatic breast cancer 42 mg/L compared with less than 3 mg/L in 30 healthy controls *719* In 9 women with T1, T2 or T3 carcinomas 0 of 10 specimens had concentration above upper limit of normal of 10 mg/L and 2 of 16 with histological grade III or axillary node involvement and/or a T4 tumor had increased concentrations as did 14 of 16 with overt metastases *924*

Creatinine *Serum Increase* Hypercalcemia of malignancy common with this type of cancer which leads to diminished capacity of renal tubules to concentrate urine which, in turn, decreases the ECF and the kidney's ability to eliminate excess calcium. Renal impairment eventually causes nitrogen retention, acidosis and renal failure and a further decrease in calcium excretion *3470*

CYFRA 21-1 *Serum Increase* In 86 patients with breast cancer without metastases median concentration of 1.4 ng/mL (nonsignificant) and in 58 with metastases 8.2 ng/mL significantly different from that in 50 healthy individuals with median concentration of 1.2 ng/mL and range of 0.5 - 2.4 ng/mL *3559*

Deoxypyridinoline *Urine Increase* In 19 patients with breast cancer median excretion of 24.6 nmol/mmol creatinine significantly higher than that in 75 healthy men in whom the median excretion was 5.0 nmol/mmol creatinine and in 20 premenopausal women, 5.1 nmol/mmol creatinine, and in 38 postmenopausal women, 7.2 nmol/mmol creatinine *4716* In 27 patients with breast cancer mean excretion of 11.52 ± 7.01 nmol/mmol creatinine compared with 5.71 ± 1.59 nmol/mmol creatinine in 79 healthy controls as measured by assay on Ciba Corning ACS:180 system *804*

Deoxypyridinoline, Free *Urine Increase* Mean excretion in 17 patients aged 28 - 78 years of approximately 12 nmol/mol creatinine significantly different from upper limit of normal of up to 7.3 nmol/mol creatinine in healthy controls *4383*

DF3 *Serum Increase* 72 patients with metastatic breast cancer 49 (68%) had concentrations greater than 25 U/mL and 43 (60%) had concentrations greater than 30 U/mL. 95% of normals have concentrations less than 30 U/mL and 90% have concentrations less than 25 U/mL *2076* In 6 patients with primary breast cancer 17% had concentration greater than 25 U/mL (concentration in 90% normals) and 17% greater than 30 U/mL (observed in 95% normals). In 72 patients with metastatic breast cancer the proportions were 68% and 60% respectively *2076*

α-Enolase *Serum Increase* In 4 of 14 cases of breast cancer mean activity increased *1705*

γ-Enolase *Serum Increase* In 4 of 14 cases of breast cancer mean activity increased *1705*

Epidermal Growth Factor *Saliva Increase* Median concentration of 1.85 ng/mL in 20 patients with breast cancer not significantly different from 1.04 ng/mL in a reference population *511*
Serum No Effect Median concentration of 0.97 ng/mL in 20 patients with breast cancer not significantly different from 0.96 ng/mL in a reference population *511*
Tissue Increase Median concentration of 0.19 ng/mg breast tissue protein observed in 21 premenopausal women and 0.12 ng/mg breast tissue in 39 postmenopausal women with breast cancer, compared with about 0.04 ng/mg in healthy breast tissue *511*
Urine Increase Median concentration of 17.4 ng/mg creatinine in 20 patients with breast cancer not significantly different from 10.3 ng/mg creatinine in a reference population *511* Mean concentration in about 5 patients with carcinoma of breast of 24 μg/g creatinine significantly different when compared with about 10 μg/g creatinine in about 30 controls *5341*

Erythrocyte Sedimentation Rate *Blood Increase* In 298 women with breast cancer probability of 10-year survival 85.7% when ESR within normal range, with decreasing ESR 85.7%, with fluctuating ESR 30.9% and with increasing ESR 34.1% *4466* Extreme elevation frequently occurs *5544* In 385 patients, the frequency distribution curve was found to be distorted when compared to controls *4361* In 47 women presenting with metastatic breast cancer, rate abnormal in 5 of 31 (16%) *923* Observed effect *1980*

Etiocholanolone *Urine Decrease* In 12 women with breast cancer and abnormal tryptophan metabolism mean excretion of 0.857 ± 0.518 mg/d significantly different from 1.590 ± 0.640 mg/d in 12 healthy controls *1034*

Ferritin *Serum Increase* In 107 patients with breast cancer; CEA, ferritin and calcitonin levels were measured. CEA and ferritin but not calcitonin levels were statistically higher in those patients with metastases *431* Mean concentration of 96.9 ± 96.8 μg/L in 229 women with untreated early breast cancer significantly higher than 56.6 ± 56.9 μg/L in 250 normal adult women *2387* In 22 patients with metastatic breast cancer median concentration of 115 ng/mL significantly higher than 34 ng/mL in 30 women with nonmetastatc breast cancer and in healthy women *223* In 9 women with T1, T2 or T3 carcinomas 0 of 10 specimens had concentration above upper limit of normal of 150 μg/L and 0 of 15 with histological grade III or axillary node involvement and/or a T4 tumor had increased concentrations but 15 of 17 with overt metastases had increased concentrations *924*

α-Fetoprotein *Serum Increase* Elevated *2913* In 22 patients with metastatic breast cancer concentration increased in 2 (9%) [median concentration of 4.15 IU/mL] and in 30 women with breast cancer but without metastases concentration increased in none (0%) [median concentration of 2.3 IU/mL] *223*

Follicle Stimulating Hormone *Plasma No Effect* In 42 postmenopausal women with biopsy diagnosed breast cancer mean concentration of 47.55 ± 3.18 IU/L not significantly different from reference range of 19 - 130 IU/L *2789*

Fucose *Serum Increase* Increased in patients with both malignant and benign tumors of breast, lung and stomach. The glycoprotein-bound fraction was very markedly elevated in cases of malignancy and not in benign disease. Mucoprotein fraction was raised in both diseases *5170* Mean elevation in 15 cases was 11.12 ± 0.68 mg/dL (normal range 6.84 ± 0.13 mg/dL). Elevation was less significant in early and locally restricted breast cancer *2899*

Galactosyl-Hydroxylysine *Urine Increase* This is a specific marker for bone collagen and provides better productivity for bone metastases then does hydroxyproline: 92% sensitivity and 90% specificity versus 74% and 79% respectively for hydroxyproline *3611*

Galactosyltransferase Isoenzyme II *Serum Increase* Sensitivity 0.50 and specificity 0.85 *5348*

Gc-Globulin *Serum No Effect* In 88 women with breast carcinoma mean concentration of 26.1 ± 5.37 mg/dL not significantly different from 26.1 ± 4.66 mg/dL in 150 control women *2279*

Gelatinase *Serum No Effect* In 28 female patients with breast cancer mean concentration of 492.5 ± 58.9 ng/mL not significantly different from 421.9 ± 53.6 ng/mL in 23 healthy female controls *5878*

α-Glucosidase *Serum Increase* The elevations were observed when the disease was in an early clinical stage *1635*

β-Glucuronidase *Serum Increase* Increased *1777* *1498*

γ-Glutamyltransferase *Serum Increase* In 49% of 41 patients at initial hospitalization for this disorder *1576* In 47 women presenting with metastatic breast cancer concentration abnormal in 9 of 30 (30%) *923*

Glycated Protein *Serum Increase* Significant preoperative elevation of beta$_2$ glycoprotein in cancer patients compared to patients with benign breast tumors *4106*

Haptoglobin *Serum Increase* In 9 women with T1, T2 or T3 carcinomas 1 of 9 specimens had concentration above upper limit of normal of 4.1 g/L and 0 of 16 with histological grade III or axillary node involvement and/or a T4 tumor had increased concentrations as did 6 of 16 with overt metastases *924* Increased to 2.2 g/L compared to normals (1.1 g/L) *2109*
Urine Increase 24 h excretion and renal clearance were significantly increased in localized tumor patients compared to normals and disseminated cancer cases. Increased high molecular weight protein excretion implies glomerular injury in these patients *2109*

Hemopexin *Serum Increase* In 9 women with T1, T2 or T3 carcinomas 1 of 9 specimens had concentration above upper limit of normal of 1.6 g/L and 0 of 16 with histological grade III or axillary node involvement and/or a T4 tumor had increased concentrations as did 3 of 16 with overt metastases *924*

Hexokinase *Serum Increase* Markedly increased. Mean activity of 22.8 ± 3.7 U/L compared to 0.93 ± 0.28 U/L in normals *2513*

Hyaluronic Acid *Serum Increase* Eighty-three women with breast cancer compared to 50 patients with benign diseases of the breast. Hyaluronan was significantly increased in sera of metastatic patients compared to sera of non-metastatic patients ($p < 0.0001$) and also in sera of non-metastatic patients when compared to control sera ($p < 0.01$) *1107*
Serum No Effect The serum hyaluronan (HA) level of 238 women with breast cancer was measured by means of a specific radiometric assay. The results show no significant increase in serum HA when compared to levels in 120 control sera *4173*

17-Hydroxycortisone *Urine No Effect* In 12 women with breast cancer and abnormal tryptophan metabolism mean excretion of 4.10 ± 1.57 mg/d not significantly different from 3.99 ± 1.36 mg/d in 12 healthy controls *1034*

2-Hydroxyestrone *Urine Increase* In 33 postmenopausal women with recently diagnosed breast cancer concentrations ranged from 0.27 to 24.06 μg/g creatinine (median of 1.55) compared with 0.37 to 5.21 μg/g creatinine (median of 0.96) in 14 postmenopausal controls but with considerable overlap of populations *3414*

2-Hydroxyestrone:16α-Hydroxyestrone Ratio
Urine Decrease Mean ratio in postmenopausal women with breast cancer of 1.41 ± 0.73 significantly lower than 1.81 ± 0.71 in healthy postmenopausal controls *2517*
Urine No Effect Mean ratio in both pre- and postmenopausal women with breast cancer of 1.67 ± 0.80 not significantly different from 1.72 ± 0.66 in healthy matched controls *2517*

3-Hydroxykynurenine *Urine No Effect* In 12 women with breast cancer and abnormal tryptophan metabolism mean excretion of 13.7 ± 10.2 μmol/d not significantly different from 16.1 ± 6.8 μmol/d in 12 healthy controls *1034*

Hydroxyproline *Plasma Increase* In 47 women presenting with metastatic breast cancer concentration abnormal in 8 of 32 (25%) *923*
Urine Increase In 9 women with T1, T2 or T3 carcinomas 1 of 10 specimens had hydroxyproline:creatinine ratio above upper limit of normal of 35 and 1 of 16 with histological grade III or axillary node involvement and/or a T4 tumor had increased concentrations as did 11 of 15 with overt metastases *924*

immunoglobulin A *Serum Increase* In 92 patients with breast cancer mean concentration of 262 ± 18 mg/dL (stage I and II), 278 ± 21 mg/dL (stage III) and 262 ± 27 mg/dL (stage IV) significantly different from 189 ± 12 mg/dL in 50 normal individuals *4381*
Serum No Effect In 216 women with breast cancer mean concentration of 191 ± 96 mg/dL not significantly different from 174 ± 80 mg/dL in 150 healthy control women *2278*
Urine Increase 24 h excretion and renal clearance were significantly increased in localized tumor patients compared to normals and disseminated cancer cases. Increased high molecular weight protein excretion implies glomerular injury in these patients *2109*

174.90 **Breast Cancer** *(continued)*

Immunoglobulin G *Serum Decrease* In 92 patients with breast cancer mean concentration of 1,252 ± 59 mg/dL (stage I and II), 1,289 ± 68 mg/dL (stage III) and 1,331 ± 100 mg/dL (stage IV) significantly different from 1,833 ± 110 mg/dL in 50 normal individuals *4381*
Serum No Effect In 216 women with breast cancer mean concentration of 1,270 ± 475 mg/dL not significantly different from 1,157 ± 271 mg/dL in 150 healthy control women *2278*
Urine Increase 24 h excretion and renal clearance were significantly increased in localized tumor patients compared to normals and disseminated cancer cases. Increased high molecular weight protein excretion implies glomerular injury in these patients *2109*

Immunoglobulin M *Serum Decrease* In 92 patients with breast cancer mean concentration of 164 ± 14 mg/dL (stage I and II), 161 ± 11 mg/dL (stage III) and 173 ± 18 mg/dL (stage IV) not significantly different from 196 ± 12 mg/dL in 50 normal individuals *4381*
Serum No Effect In 216 women with breast carcinoma mean concentration of 85 ± 59 mg/dL not significantly different from 77 ± 39 mg/dL in 106 healthy controls *2278*
Urine Increase 24 h excretion and renal clearance were significantly increased in localized tumor patients compared to normals and disseminated cancer cases. Increased high molecular weight protein excretion implies glomerular injury in these patients *2109*

Insulin-like Growth Factor-I *Serum Increase* Median concentration in 76 premenopausal women with breast cancer of 204 ng/mL significantly different from 184 ng/mL in 105 age-matched controls: in 60 premenopausal women aged < 50 y with breast cancer 206 ng/mL significantly different from 175 ng/mL in 78 age-matched controls *2003* Reportedly increased in the plasma of patients with breast cancer *2103*
Serum No Effect Mean concentration of 147 ± 12 ng/mL in 57 women with breast cancer not significantly different from 161 ± 22 ng/mL in 46 women with benign breast disease *2590* Median concentration in 305 postmenopausal women with breast cancer of 142 ng/mL not significantly different from 153 ng/mL in 483 age-matched controls *2003*

Insulin-like Growth Factor-I:Insulin-like Growth Factor Binding Protein-3 Ratio *Serum Increase* Reportedly increased ratio in the plasma of patients with breast cancer *2103*

Insulin-like Growth Factor-II *Serum No Effect* Mean concentration of 667 ± 22 ng/mL in 57 women with breast cancer not significantly different from 668 ± 47 ng/mL in 46 women with benign breast disease *2590*

Insulin-like Growth Factor Binding Protein-1
Serum Decrease Mean concentration of 16 ± 2 ng/mL in 57 women with breast cancer less than 37 ± 4 ng/mL in 46 women with benign breast disease *2590*

Insulin-like Growth Factor Binding Protein-3
Serum Decrease Mean concentration of 1,981 ± 65 ng/mL in 57 women with breast cancer less than 2,603 ± 140 ng/mL in 46 women with benign breast disease *2590*

Insulin-like Growth Factor Binding Protein-3 Protease
Serum Increase Reportedly increased activity in the plasma of two-thirds of patients with breast cancer *2103*

Insulin-like Growth Factor Binding Protein-6
Serum Decrease Mean concentration of 127 ± 16 ng/mL in 57 women with breast cancer less than 157 ± 10 ng/mL in 46 women with benign breast disease *2590*

Interleukin-1α *Serum No Effect* In 123 patients with nonmetastatic breast cancer no significant difference observed between concentration and that in controls *3256*

Interleukin-2 *Serum No Effect* No significant difference observed between concentration in 123 patients with nonmetastatic cancer and that in healthy controls *3256*

Interleukin-6 *Serum Increase* In 21 women with metastatic breast cancer mean concentration prior to treatment of 9.83 ± 2.10 pg/mL significantly greater than 1.24 ± 0.17 pg/mL in healthy controls *5783*

Iron *Serum Decrease* In 37% of 13 patients at initial hospitalization for this disorder *1576*

Iron-binding Capacity, Total *Serum Decrease* Significantly reduced (median of 2.6 mg/L) compared to controls (3.4 mg/L). 24 h excretion and renal clearance were significantly increased in localized tumor patients compared to normal and disseminated cancer cases. Increased high molecular weight protein excretion implies glomerular injury in these patients *2109* In 21% of 14 patients at initial hospitalization for this disorder *1576*

Iron Saturation *Serum Decrease* In 35% of 14 patients at initial hospitalization for this disorder *1576*

17-Ketosteroids *Urine Decrease* Total 17-ketosteroids and the sum of the fractions were significantly decreased in comparison with controls *820*

Kynurenic Acid *Urine No Effect* In 12 women with breast cancer and abnormal tryptophan metabolism mean excretion of 13.5 ± 6.0 μmol/d not significantly different from 12.9 ± 3.1 μmol/d in 12 healthy controls *1034*

Kynurenine *Urine No Effect* In 12 women with breast cancer and abnormal tryptophan metabolism mean excretion of 12.1 ± 4.1 μmol/d not significantly different from 12.2 ± 4.9 μmol/d in 12 healthy controls *1034*

α-Lactalbumin *Serum No Effect* In 9 women with T1, T2 or T3 carcinomas 0 of 10 specimens had concentration above upper limit of normal of 20 μg/L and 0 of 16 with histological grade III or axillary node involvement and/or a T4 tumor had increased concentrations as did 0 of 13 with overt metastases *924*

Lactate *Blood Increase* In 5 cases, mean concentration was 25.8 ± 4.0 mg/dL compared to normal, 11.7 ± 0.72 mg/dL *2513*

Lactate Dehydrogenase *Serum Increase* Marked elevation in 110 patients. Mean activity of 207.2 ± 12.4 U/L, compared to normals, 85.4 ± 1.0 U/L *2513* Observed effect *2434* Highly elevated values (> 300 U/L) may be obtained with or without liver involvement in the presence of bone metastases *2109* Observed effect *5736*

Laminin *Serum Increase* Median serum level of 1,722 mU/mL (n = 22). Control group median concentration of 1,232 mU/mL (n = 42). Elevated in 14 of 22 patients *4394*

LDL-Cholesterol *Serum Increase* In 8 women aged over 50 years with malignant disease of the breast mean concentration of 123.4 ± 20.6 mg/dL not significantly different from 110.8 ± 6.7 mg/dL in 24 women with breast masses *2910*

Lipoprotein Lp(a) *Serum Increase* In 18 women with stage I disease mean concentration of 88.4 ± 28.4 mg/dL and in 21 with stage IV disease mean concentration of 145.0 ± 36.4 mg/dL both significantly higher than 48.9 ± 25.7 mg/dL in 22 healthy women controls *2746*
Serum No Effect In 3 women aged over 50 years with malignant disease of the breast mean concentration of 28.9 ± 8.6 mg/dL not significantly different from 30.0 ± 11.3 in 4 women with breast masses *2910*

Luteinizing Hormone *Plasma No Effect* In 42 postmenopausal women with biopsy diagnosed breast cancer mean concentration of 20.27 ± 1.83 IU/L not significantly different from reference range of 12 - 58 IU/L *2789*

Lymphocytes *Blood Increase* 6 patients with advanced cancer had significantly higher numbers of B lymphocytes than patients with benign breast disease *2977*

Lysophosphatidic Acid *Serum No Effect* In 11 patients with breast cancer median concentration of 0.1 μmol/L not significantly different from 0.1 μmol/L in 48 healthy controls *5758*

Lysozyme *Serum No Effect* In 9 women with T1, T2 or T3 carcinomas 0 of 10 specimens had concentration above upper limit of normal of 9 g/L as did 0 of 16 with histological grade III or axillary node involvement and/or a T4 tumor and 0 of 17 with overt metastases *924*

1-Methyladenosine *Urine Increase* In 72 patients with breast cancer median excretion of 2.14 μmol/mmol creatinine and mean excretion of 2.81 ± 2.49 μmol/mmol creatinine *4585*

5-Methylcytidine *Urine Increase* In 72 patients with breast cancer median excretion of 26.19 μmol/mmol creatinine and mean excretion of 28.62 ± 15.38 μmol/mmol creatinine *4585*

7-Methylguanosine *Urine Increase* In 72 patients with breast cancer median excretion of 0.13 μmol/mmol creatinine and mean excretion of 0.21 ± 0.24 μmol/mmol creatinine *4585*

1-Methylinosine *Urine Increase* In 72 patients with breast cancer median excretion of 1.59 μmol/mmol creatinine and mean excretion of 2.22 ± 2.02 μmol/mmol creatinine *4585*

β_2-Microglobulin *Serum Increase* In 22 patients with metastatic breast cancer median concentration of 3.95 mg/L significantly higher than 2.75 mg/L in 30 women with nonmetastatc breast cancer and in healthy women *223*

Mucin-like Carcinoma Antigen *Serum Increase* In 40 women with breast cancer sensitivity 52.5%, positive predictive value 87.5% and negative predictive value 55.8% *1568* In 25 clinical trials of women with breast cancer in early disease positives ranged from 0 to 20% and in late disease from 33% to 67% *5641*

N^2, N^2-Dimethylguanosine *Urine No Effect* In 2 patients with breast carcinoma excretions of 1.2 and 4.9 mg/d not significantly different from 3.9 ± 2.6 mg/d in 17 healthy controls *5505*

Nα-Acetylkynurenine *Urine No Effect* In 12 women with breast cancer and abnormal tryptophan metabolism mean excretion of 17.4 ± 7.5 µmol/d not significantly different from 10.7 ± 3.9 µmol/d in 12 healthy controls *1034*

Neopterin *Urine Increase* Frequency of increased concentrations in patients with cancer of the breast 14% *121*

Neuron-specific Enolase *Serum Increase* Increased in 20% of cases *5546*

Osteocalcin *Serum Increase* Plasma levels have been studied as a possible means of discriminating between patients with breast cancer with and without bone metastases. The increase in concentration was significant but small relative to controls (15 to 20%) in one study but much larger (42%) in another *884 4135*

p53 Autoantibodies *Serum Increase* Presence of p53 antibodies associated with worse prognosis *5640*

Parathyroid Hormone *Plasma Decrease* In one study of 42 patients with low intact PTH concentration and hypercalcemia 2 had carcinoma of the breast *3280*

Parathyroid Hormone-related Peptide *Plasma Increase* In 12 of 13 hypercalcemic patients with bone metastases mean concentration greater than lower limit of detection of 0.23 pmol/L compared with 10 of 28 normocalcemic patients with bone metastases and 5 of 57 normocalcemic patients without bone metastases *632* In all 7 patients with breast carcinoma and hypercalcemia range of concentrations of 4.0 to 222.4 pmol/L compared with upper limit of normal of 1.5 pmol/L *3987*
Plasma No Effect In 13 patients with cancer of the breast and normocalcemia mean concentration of 1.65 pmol/L below upper limit of reference range of 2.6 pmol/L *1200*

pH *Blood Decrease* Hypercalcemia of malignancy common with this type of cancer which leads to diminished capacity of renal tubules to concentrate urine which, in turn, decreases the ECF and the kidney's ability to eliminate excess calcium. Renal impairment eventually causes nitrogen retention, acidosis and renal failure and a further decrease in calcium excretion *3470*

Phosphohexoseisomerase *Serum Increase* It has a sensitivity of 40% *2811*

Plasminogen Activator Inhibitor-1 *Plasma No Effect* Concentration in women with breast cancer not significantly different from that in controls *846*
Tissue Increase In 657 women with breast cancer median concentration of 15.2 ng/mg cytosolic protein (mean 20.3 ± 20.1 ng/mg cytosolic protein) with concentration positively associated with rate of relapse *1514*

Polymorphic Epithelial Mucin *Serum Increase* In 4 women with stage IV breast cancer median concentrations of 111 kU/L by ACS BR, 126 kU/L by Centocor CA 15-3, 108 kU/L by Enzymun-Test CA 15-3 and 85 kU/L by IMx CA 15-3 significantly different from concentrations in 250 healthy women (mean and 1 SD concentrations of 22 ± 8.8 kU/L by ACS BR, 19 ± 8.8 kU/L by Centocor CA 15-3, 17 ± 7.1 kU/L by Enzymun-Test CA 15-3 and 15 ± 6.4 kU/L by IMx CA 15-3 respectively) *513*
Serum No Effect In 127 women with breast cancer (all stages) median concentrations of 20 kU/L by ACS BR, 24 kU/L by Centocor CA 15-3, 17 kU/L by Enzymun-Test CA 15-3 and 16 kU/L by IMx CA 15-3 not significantly different from concentrations in 250 healthy women (mean and 1 SD concentrations of 22 ± 8.8 kU/L by ACS BR, 19 ± 8.8 kU/L by Centocor CA 15-3, 17 ± 7.1 kU/L by Enzymun-Test CA 15-3 and 15 ± 6.4 kU/L by IMx CA 15-3 respectively) *513*

Prealbumin *Serum Decrease* Mean concentration in 8 patients with clinical stage III disease of 192 ± 25 mg/L and 175 ± 16 mg/L significantly different from 215 ± 15 mg/L in 25 elderly healthy controls *4359*

Pregnancy-associated α-Macroglobulin *Serum Increase* In 9 women with T1, T2 or T3 carcinomas 1 of 10 specimens had concentration above upper limit of normal of 140 g/L and 2 of 16 with histological grade III or axillary node involvement and/or a T4 tumor had increased concentrations as did 6 of 17 with overt metastases *924*

Procollagen Type III Peptide *Serum Increase* Serum P-III-P and IV-C levels were found to be significantly higher in patients who showed postoperative recurrence, with 76.9% of P-III-P-positive cancer bearing patients and 68.0% of IV-C-positive cancer bearing patients having metastases in the bone and/or liver *3738*

Procollagen Type IV Peptide *Serum Increase* Serum P-III-P and IV-C levels were found to be significantly higher in patients who showed postoperative recurrence, with 76.9% of P-III-P-positive cancer bearing patients and 68.0% of IV-C-positive cancer bearing patients having metastases in the bone and/or liver *3738*

Prolactin *Plasma Decrease* In 206 premenopausal women with breast cancer median concentration of 8.15 ng/mL prior to 14.85 ng/mL after mastectomy, in 43 perimenopausal women of 5.80 ng/mL prior to 12.85 ng/mL after mastectomy, and in 223 postmenopausal women with breast cancer of 6.70 ng/mL prior to 12.60 ng/mL after mastectomy *5560*
Plasma Increase Significantly higher concentrations than controls in early breast cancer. In advanced breast cancer elevated levels were only found in postmenopausal patients *4430* Mean concentration was significantly elevated in 148 breast cancer patients. Incidence of elevation was 22% *71*
Plasma No Effect Mean concentration of 6.0 ± 3.7 ng/mL in 115 patients with breast cancer not significantly different from 5.9 ± 2.9 ng/mL in 115 matched controls *2874*

Prostaglandin D Synthase *Tissue Increase* In 12 breast tumor extracts median concentration of 2.0 µg/L and mean concentration of 2.7 ± 2.1 µg/L *3444*

Prostate-specific Antigen *Cyst Fluid Increase* In one case of female breast intracystic carcinoma PSA concentration of 55 µg/L with concentration of 19.52 µg/L in tumor extract *3279*
Serum No Effect Mean concentration of 0.018 ng/mL in 57 women with breast cancer not significantly different from 0.007 ng/mL in 46 women with benign breast disease *2590*

Pseudouridine *Urine Increase* In 72 patients with breast cancer median excretion of 27.27 µmol/mmol creatinine and mean excretion of 36.41 ± 25.88 µmol/mmol creatinine *4585*
Urine No Effect In 2 patients with breast carcinoma excretions of 34 and 67 mg/d not significantly different from 65 ± 31 mg/d in 17 healthy controls *5505*

Putrescine *Serum Increase* In 2 patients with carcinoma of the breast concentrations 0.52 and 1.32 nmol/mL compared with normal mean value of 0.23 nmol/mL *3805*
Urine No Effect In 9 women with T1, T2 or T3 carcinomas 0 of 9 specimens had concentration above upper limit of normal of 9 mg/g creatinine and 0 of 12 with histological grade III or axillary node involvement and/or a T4 tumor had increased concentrations as did 0 of 13 with overt metastases *924*

Pyridinoline *Urine Increase* In 19 patients with breast cancer median excretion of 137 nmol/mmol creatinine significantly higher than that in 75 healthy men in whom the median excretion was 20.8 nmol/mmol creatinine and in 20 premenopausal women, 19.6 nmol/mmol creatinine, and in 38 postmenopausal women, 28.2 nmol/mmol creatinine *4716*

Pyruvate *Blood Increase* Moderately elevated in 6 patients, mean = 1.5 ± 0.35 U/L *2513*

Retinol *Serum Decrease* Mean concentration in 8 patients with clinical stage IV disease of 2.2 ± 0.3 µmol/L significantly different from 3.4 ± 0.3 µmol/L in 25 elderly healthy controls *4359*
Serum No Effect Mean concentration in 9 patients with clinical stage III disease of 3.3 ± 0.7 µmol/L not significantly different from 3.4 ± 0.3 µmol/L in 25 elderly healthy controls *4359*

Retinol-binding Protein *Serum Decrease* Mean concentration in 9 patients with clinical stage III disease of 43.7 ± 5.0 mg/L and in 8 patients with clinical stage IV breast cancer of 37.0 ± 3.2 mg/L significantly reduced compared with 54 ± 2 mg/L in 25 elderly healthy controls *4359*

174.90 Breast Cancer *(continued)*

Rheumatoid Factor *Serum Increase* Treated patients with no evidence of residual tumor had an 89% rate of positive tests. The incidence of seropositivity was low among untreated patients with similar tumors *5336*

Sialic Acid, Lipid-associated *Serum Increase* In patients with breast cancer mean concentration increased above 20 mg/dL in 33% of patients *1781* In 40 patients with early stage breast cancer mean concentration of 79 mg/dL significantly different from 17.7 mg/dL in 50 normal volunteers *1273*

Sialyltransferase *Serum Increase* In 9 women with T1, T2 or T3 carcinomas 0 of 7 specimens had concentration above upper limit of normal of 3400 U/mg protein and 3 of 12 with histological grade III or axillary node involvement and/or a T4 tumor had increased concentrations as did 9 of 16 with overt metastases *924* In 31 patients with breast cancer mean and median concentrations of 395 and 397 cpm/mg protein/30 min significantly different from 240 and 243 cpm/mg protein/30 min respectively in 20 normal individuals *2111*

Soluble Urokinase Receptor *Serum Increase* In citrated specimens from 19 women with stage IV cancer concentrations of 1.9 to 7.1 µg/L (10th to 90th percentile range) significantly greater than reference range of 0.82 - 1.7 µg/L in 42 healthy women *5006*

Spermidine *Serum Increase* In 2 patients with carcinoma of the breast concentrations 0.45 and 0.74 nmol/mL compared with normal mean value of 0.33 nmol/mL *3805*
Urine Increase In 9 women with T1, T2 or T3 carcinomas 0 of 9 specimens had concentration above upper limit of normal of 2.7 mg/g creatinine and 0 of 12 with histological grade III or axillary node involvement and/or a T4 tumor had increased concentrations as did 4 of 13 with overt metastases *924*

Spermine *Serum No Effect* In 2 patients with carcinoma of the breast concentrations detectable but not quantifiable and 0.10 nmol/mL compared with normal mean value of 0.04 nmol/mL *3805*

Stromelysin *Plasma No Effect* In 28 women with breast cancer mean concentration of 36.8 ± 7.8 ng/mL not significantly different from 34.4 ± 6.0 ng/mL in 23 healthy control women *5878*

Stromelysin-3 mRNA *Tissue Increase* Stromelysin-3 mRNA as detected by in situ hybridization correlated with poor outcome in patients with breast cancer *1252*

T3-Uptake *Serum Increase* Slight but significant differences were found, with a higher mean value for thyrotropin, reverse-T3 and T3-resin uptake and a lower mean value for T3 *26*

Tenascin-C *Serum Increase* Mean concentration in 28 patients with breast cancer of 1.57 ± 0.074 mg/L not significantly higher than that in 15 healthy individuals (1.09 ± 0.41 mg/L) *4626*

Testosterone *Serum Increase* Plasma hormone concentrations were measured in sequential samples from 6 women and were compared to concentrations in 6 control women matched for age, years since menopause, and parity. Concentrations in each cancer patient were significantly higher than in each matched control *3405*

Thrombospondin *Plasma Increase* Mean concentration of 2,482 ± 4,095 ng/mL in patients with breast cancer significantly different from 190 ± 42 ng/mL observed in 15 healthy men and 17 women *2074*

Thymidine Kinase *Serum Increase* In 75 women with nonmetastatic breast cancer mean activity of 12.1 ± 1.3 U/L and 39.7 ± 5.1 U/L in 8 with metastatic breast cancer significantly greater than 2.8 ± 0.4 U/L in 30 healthy control women *3284*

Thyroid Stimulating Hormone *Serum Increase* Mean concentrations higher than in normals or other cancers. The difference was statistically significant only in those with advanced disease. 12% of the early cancer and 15% of the advanced had elevated plasma concentrations *4429* Slight but significant differences were found with a higher mean value for thyrotropin, reverse-T3 and T3-resin uptake *26* Elevated in 148 patients (38%) with breast cancer. Mean survival and disease free intervals were shorter for patients with elevated TSH, but not significantly *71*

Thyroxine (T4) *Serum Decrease* Four patients with plasma TSH levels above 85 µU/mL had subnormal plasma T4 levels *4429*

Tissue Factor Pathway Inhibitor *Plasma Increase* About half of patients with breast cancer had activities greater than median activity of 1.19 U/mL in healthy individuals *2376*

Tissue Inhibitor of Metalloproteinase-1 *Serum Increase* Median concentration in 15 patients with nodal metastases of 2.6 ng/mg significantly different from 1.0 ng/mg protein in 15 patients with primary carcinomas *3393* Median concentration in 139 patients with primary breast cancer of 2.71 ng/mg protein significantly different from 1.0 ng/mg protein in 15 patients with primary carcinomas *3393*

Tissue Plasminogen Activator *Tissue Increase* High activities of tPA are associated with favorable prognosis for breast cancer *1252*

Tissue Polypeptide Antigen *Serum Increase* In 20 patients with metastatic breast cancer median concentration of 110 U/L significantly higher than 69 U/L in 30 women with nonmetastatc breast cancer and in healthy women *223* During therapy monitoring tissue polypeptide antigen followed the course of the disease faster than CEA and CA 15-3 *5390* In 75 patients with non-metastatic breast cancer mean activity of 180 ± 16 U/L and 877 ± 206 U/L in 8 patients with metastatic breast cancer significantly greater than 54 ± 5.5 U/L in 30 healthy age-matched control women *3284*

Transferrin *Serum No Effect* In 118 women with breast carcinoma mean concentration of 204 ± 58 mg/dL not significantly different from 217 ± 39 mg/dL in 150 control women *2280*

Transforming Growth Factor-α *Serum Increase* In 83 specimens from patients with breast cancer mean concentration of 353 pg/mL (range 210 - 740 pg/mL) significantly higher than mean of 147 pg/mL (range 120 - 207 pg/mL) in 50 normal individuals *755*

Transforming Growth Factor-β_2 *Serum Increase* In 20 patients with metastatic breast cancer and 7 patients with primary breast cancer without evident metastases concentrations before treatment ranged from 27 to 121 pg/mL *2767*

Tri-iodothyronine (T3) *Serum Decrease* Slight but significant differences were found with a higher mean value for thyrotropin, reverse T3 and T3 resin uptake and a lower mean value for T3 *26*

Triglycerides *Serum No Effect* In 8 women aged over 50 years with malignant disease of the breast mean concentration of 108.6 ± 25.2 mg/dL not significantly different from 89.0 ± 7.8 mg/dL in 24 women with breast masses *2910*

Tumor Necrosis Factor-α *Serum Increase* In 123 patients with nonmetastatic breast cancer concentration significantly increased compared with healthy controls. In patients with progressive disease concentrations higher than in those without recurrences *3256*

Urea Nitrogen *Serum Increase* Hypercalcemia of malignancy common with this type of cancer which leads to diminished capacity of renal tubules to concentrate urine which, in turn, decreases the ECF and the kidney's ability to eliminate excess calcium. Renal impairment eventually causes nitrogen retention, acidosis and renal failure and a further decrease in calcium excretion *3470*

Uric Acid *Serum Increase* In 25% of 300 patients at initial hospitalization for this disorder *1576*

Urokinase Plasminogen Activator *Plasma Decrease* Concentration significantly lower than in healthy women *846*
Tissue Increase High expression associated with either a shortened disease-free interval or overall survival *1255* uPA is one of strongest prognostic markers for breast cancer. It has been shown to be a marker of disease outcome in axillary node-negative patients, but it is also prognostic in node-positive patients, premenopausl patients and ER-positive patients *1252* Median concentration in 141 cases of primary breast cancer of 0.373 ng/mg protein significantly higher than 0.049 ng/mg protein in benign breast tumors *1258*

Urokinase Plasminogen Activator Receptor
Plasma No Effect Concentration in women with breast cancer not significantly different from that in controls *846*
Tissue Increase Median concentration in 141 cases of primary breast cancer of 0.207 ng/mg protein significantly higher than 0.093 ng/mg protein in benign breast tumors *1258*

Vascular Endothelial Growth Factor *Serum* *Increase* In 7 women with carcinoma in situ median concentration of 110 pg/mL (range 32 - 275 pg/mL) not significantly different from that in 18 women with benign breast tumors in whom the median concentration was 57 pg/mL (range 18 - 328 pg/mL) and not significantly different from concentration in healthy control women *4539*

VLDL-Cholesterol *Serum* *No Effect* In 8 women aged over 50 years with malignant disease of the breast mean concentration of 21.7 ± 5.0 mg/dL not significantly different from 17.8 ± 1.6 mg/dL in 24 women with breast masses *2910*

Volume *Urine* *Increase* Hypercalcemia of malignancy common with this type of cancer which leads to diminished capacity of renal tubules to concentrate urine which, in turn, decreases the ECF and the kidney's ability to eliminate excess calcium. Renal impairment eventually causes nitrogen retention, acidosis and renal failure and a further decrease in calcium excretion *3470*

Xanthurenic Acid *Urine* *No Effect* In 12 women with breast cancer and abnormal tryptophan metabolism mean excretion of 6.3 ± 2.7 µmol/d not significantly different from 6.8 ± 2.0 µmol/d in 12 healthy controls *1034*

Zinc *Serum* *Decrease* Mean concentration in 31 patients with breast cancer significantly lower than in 35 healthy controls *5829*

176.90 Kaposi's Sarcoma

Anti-p53 Antibodies *Serum* *No Effect* No increase observed in 11 patients *132*

Antibodies against HHV-8 *Serum* *Increase* In Africans prevalence of antibodies against HHV-8 in patients with Kaposi's sarcoma 83% in 51 patients *4877*

Interleukin-6 *Serum* *Increase* In 14 HIV-1 infected patients with Kaposi's sarcoma mean concentration prior to treatment was 26.2 ± 13.5 pg/mL compared with 8.2 ± 2.8 pg/mL in 10 healthy controls *1080*

179.00 Squamous Cell Carcinoma of Uterus

Squamous Cell Carcinoma Antigen *Serum* *Increase* Increased concentration in 52% of 44 patients with squamous cell carcinoma of the uterus *5457*

180.90 Cancer of Cervix

Aldolase *Serum* *Increase* In 90 women with untreated cervical cancer mean activity of 9.1 ± 7.84 U/L significantly higher than 4.9 ± 2.46 U/L in 84 healthy controls *4031* Mildly elevated in uterine cervix and corpus carcinomas. Mean = 2.9 ± 1.1 U/L compared to normal, 1.6 ± 0.21 U/L *2513*

Alkaline Phosphatase *Serum* *Increase* In 90 women with untreated cervical cancer mean activity of 2.6 ± 0.97 U/L significantly higher than 1.8 ± 0.48 U/L in 84 healthy controls *4031*

Alkaline Phosphatase Isoenzymes *Serum* *Increase* Cancer of the ovary, endometrium, cervix and breast as a group exhibited the highest frequency of Regan isoenzyme (placental) *658*

Alkaline Phosphatase, Placental Isoenzyme *Serum* *Increase* Elevations have been reported in a variety of tumors including cervical and ovarian cancer *3909*

α_1-Antitrypsin *Serum* *Increase* Increased *4241* *4373* *4371* *4763* *83*

CA 125 *Serum* *Increase* Of CA 125 measurements with high concentrations in a hospital 0.9% were due to cervical or vaginal carcinoma *1350* Reported effect *3909*

Carcinoembryonic Antigen *Serum* *Increase* 59% positivity reported. In advanced disease 84% had elevated values *1497* In 42% of cases *1207* Of the 156 patients with carcinoma in situ, 14 (9%) were positive. Progressive increase in the percentage of positive patients as stage increases, from 26% in stage I to 88% in stage IV. 52 of 61 (85%) with recurrent squamous cell carcinoma showed a positive value *1179* Elevated (> 2.5 ng/mL) in 48% of 300 patients, and varied directly with stage of disease and histologic differentiation of the tumor. Rising of concentration indicated recurrence in 29 patients *5410* Elevations found in cervical adenocarcinoma (19%) and squamous cell carcinoma of the uterine cervix (10%) *5326* In 42% of cases *4891*

Ceruloplasmin *Serum* *Increase* Mean concentration of 89 ± 28 mg/dL in 65 women with cervical cancer significantly different from 84 ± 22 mg/dL in 150 control women *2280* Mean concentration of 380 mg/L in 19 women of mean age 55 years significantly higher than mean of 282 mg/L in 19 healthy control women of mean age 30 years *761*

Cholesterol *Urine* *Increase* Nonesterified cholesterol hyperexcretion (values > 1.5 mg/24 h) occurred in 65 of 68 women with active carcinoma including 13 with carcinoma in situ *23*

Cholesterol, Esterified *Urine* *Increase* In 55 patients with active squamous cell carcinoma of the cervix only 3 had normal concentrations with maximum approaching 30.0 mg/d *23*

β-Chorionic Gonadotropin *Plasma* *Increase* CEA, AFP and hCG were measured in 253 patients with gynecologic malignancies and in 317 patients with benign gynecologic diseases. Concentrations of each of these antigens were elevated in a significantly greater number of patients with invasive cancer *1207*

Complement C_3 *Serum* *Increase* Increased in patients with local disease. Closely linked to the stage of the disease. Patients in remission had normal levels, but further increases were noted in distant metastases. Dropped significantly in the terminal phase of the disease *5456*

Complement C_4 *Serum* *Increase* Increased in patients with local disease. Very closely linked to the stage of the disease. Patients in remission had normal levels, but further increases were noted in distant metastases. Levels dropped significantly in the terminal phase of disease *5456*

Complement, Total *Serum* *Increase* Closely linked to the stage of the disease, patients in remission had normal levels, but further increases were noted in distant metastases. Levels dropped significantly in the terminal phase of the disease *5456*

Copper *Serum* *Increase* Mean concentration in 19 women mean age 55 years of 20.3 µmol/L (14.2 - 26.2) significantly higher compared with 14.6 µmol/L (12.2 - 20.8) in 19 healthy controls mean age 30 years *761* Elevations are related to the stage of the disease and decrease in response to treatment *3902*

Copper, Ultrafiltratable *Serum* *No Effect* In 19 women with mean age 55 years mean concentration of 0.183 µmol/L (0.102 - 0.423) not significantly different from 0.174 µmol/L (0.115 - 0.358) in 19 healthy controls of mean age 30 years *761*

CYFRA 21-1 *Serum* *Increase* Mean concentration increased in 17 of 23 patients *515*

Epidermal Growth Factor *Urine* *Increase* Mean concentration in about 25 patients of 18 µg/g creatinine significantly different compared with about 10 µg/g creatinine in about 30 controls *5341*

Ferritin *Serum* *Increase* In 98 patients with untreated disease 51% had elevated serum levels *2364*

α-Fetoprotein *Serum* *Increase* CEA, AFP and hCG were measured in 253 patients with gynecologic malignancies and in 317 patients with benign gynecologic diseases. Concentrations of each of these antigens were elevated in a significantly greater number of patients with invasive cancer *1207*

Fucose *Serum* *Increase* Markedly elevated and correlated with clinical stage of disease. Values ranged from 12.2 - 32.2 mg/dL *1269*

Galactosyltransferase Isoenzyme II *Serum* *Increase* Sensitivity 0.65 and specificity 0.94 *5348*

Gc-Globulin *Serum* *No Effect* In 65 women with cancer of the cervix mean concentration of 25.2 ± 4.19 mg/dL not significantly different from 26.1 ± 4.66 mg/dL in 150 control women *2279*

β-Glucuronidase *Serum* *Increase* Increased *1777* *1498*

Gonadotropin Peptide *Urine* *Increase* In women with cervical cancer mean concentration of 11.9 ± 45.1 fmol/mg creatinine compared with mean value for both pre- and postmenopausal women of 1.51 ± 2.42 fmol/mg creatinine *5538*

Hexokinase *Serum* *Increase* Markedly increased. Mean = 32.0 ± 4.7 U/L *2513*

180.90 Cancer of Cervix *(continued)*

immunoglobulin A *Serum* *No Effect* In 65 women with cancer of the cervix mean concentration of 182 ± 77 mg/dL not significantly different from 174 ± 80 mg/dL in 150 healthy control women *2278*

Immunoglobulin G *Serum* *No Effect* In 65 women with cervical cancer mean concentration of 1,200 ± 312 mg/dL not significantly different from 1,157 ± 271 mg/dL in 150 healthy control women *2278*

Immunoglobulin M *Serum* *No Effect* In 65 women with cancer of the cervix mean concentration of 81 ± 45 mg/dL not significantly different from 77 ± 39 mg/dL in 106 healthy controls *2278*

Lactate Dehydrogenase *Serum* *Increase* Marked elevation in 26 patients with uterine, cervix and corpus carcinomas. Mean activity of 142.5 ± 18.2 U/L compared to normals 85.4 ± 1.0 U/L *2513*

Lymphocytes *Blood* *Increase* In 44% of 146 patients at initial hospitalization for this disorder *1576*

Macrophage Colony Stimulating Factor *Serum* *Decrease* In 60 patients with cervical cancer mean concentration of 948.2 ± 358.9 U/mL significantly lower than baseline normal of 1,056 U/mL *5094*

Neopterin *Urine* *Increase* Frequency of increased concentrations in patients with cervical cancer 56% *121*

Phosphohexoseisomerase *Serum* *Increase* In 90 women with untreated cervical cancer mean concentration of 28.6 ± 15.41 Bodansky units significantly higher than 20.1 ± 3.20 Bodansky units in 84 healthy controls *4031*

Platelets *Blood* *Increase* In 109 of 643 women (17%) with untreated cervical cancer mean concentration exceeded 400,000 /μL *3117*

Polymorphic Epithelial Mucin *Serum* *No Effect* In 9 women with cervical cancer median concentrations of 15 kU/L by ACS BR, 13 kU/L by Centocor CA 15-3, 12 kU/L by Enzymun-Test CA 15-3 and 12 kU/L by IMx CA 15-3 not significantly different from concentrations in 250 healthy women (mean and 1 SD concentrations of 22 ± 8.8 kU/L by ACS BR, 19 ± 8.8 kU/L by Centocor CA 15-3, 17 ± 7.1 kU/L by Enzymun-Test CA 15-3 and 15 ± 6.4 kU/L by IMx CA 15-3 respectively) *513*

Procollagen Type III Peptide *Serum* *Increase* Elevated values of serum PIIINP are also observed in endometrial and cervical malignancies, though less frequently than in ovarian tumours. Very high concentrations of PIIINP are found in ovarian carcinoma ascites *4365*

Prolactin *Plasma* *Increase* In 229 of 743 (30.8%) of patients with uterine cervical carcinoma increased concentrations observed *2261*

Sialic Acid, Lipid-associated *Serum* *Increase* Elevated in 63% of patients *4693*

Sialyltransferase *Serum* *Increase* In 3 patients with carcinoma of the cervix mean and median concentrations of 560 and 553 cpm/mg protein/30 min significantly different from 240 and 243 cpm/mg protein/30 min respectively in 20 normal individuals *2111*

Soluble Interleukin-2 Receptor-α *Serum* *No Effect* In 14 patients with cervical cancer mean concentration of 406.5 ± 32.5 U/mL not significantly different from 367 ± 44.6 U/mL in normal controls *311*

Squamous Cell Carcinoma Antigen *Serum* *Increase* Mean concentration increased in 20 of 23 patients *515* In 157 patients with squamous cell carcinoma of the cervix 96 had increased concentrations. Concentrations tended to increase with stage of the disease *3775* Increased concentration observed in 50% of 50 patients with cervical carcinoma *5457*

Steroid Sulfatase *Serum* *Increase* Mean concentration in 30 patients with cervical carcinoma of 117.8 ± 14.5 ng/mL significantly higher than 75.7 ± 28.3 ng/mL in 57 menstruating control healthy women and 68.8 ± 24.7 ng/mL in 12 postmenopausal women: using a cutoff of 130 ng/mL positive rate of 43.3% observed *5072*

TA-4 *Serum* *Increase* Elevated levels are noted in approximately 55% of patients with squamous cell carcinoma of the cervix *2580*

Tissue Polypeptide Antigen *Serum* *Increase* Mean concentration increased in 8 of 23 patients *515*

Transferrin *Serum* *Decrease* In 65 women with cancer of the cervix mean concentration of 201 ± 39 mg/dL not significantly different from 217 ± 39 mg/dL in 150 control women *2280*

Urokinase Plasminogen Activator *Tissue* *Increase* uPA is a prognostic marker for cancer of the cervix *1252* Amounts predictable of overall survival *1255*

181.00 Malignant Neoplasm of Trophoblast

β-Chorionic Gonadotropin *Plasma* *Increase* In pure choriocarcinomas, human chorionic gonadotropins are always elevated and AFP is absent *5759* In 24 pregnant patients with choriocarcinoma in remission and in 10 with progressive tumors mean concentrations of 584 ± 166 IU/mL and 1,040 ± 180 IU/mL respectively significantly higher than 100 ± 8 IU/mL in 23 healthy pregnant women during the first trimester *4747*
Urine *Increase* Markedly increased with primary chorionepithelioma of ovary *5544*

β-Chorionic Gonadotropin, Free *Plasma* *Increase* In 13 men with choriocarcinoma mean concentration of 10^6 to 10^7 pg/mL which declined with successful treatment *3194*

Estrogens *Plasma* *Increase* May be much increased with primary chorionepithelioma of ovary *5544*

α-Fetoprotein *Serum* *No Effect* In pure choriocarcinomas, human chorionic gonadotropins are always elevated and AFP is absent *5759*

Interleukin-1β *Serum* *Increase* In 24 pregnant patients with choriocarcinoma in remission and in 10 with progressive tumors mean concentrations of 71.2 ± 22.4 pg/mL and 2,144 ± 561 pg/mL respectively significantly higher than 26.2 ± 1.71 pg/mL in 23 healthy pregnant women during the first trimester *4747*

Interleukin-6 *Serum* *Increase* In 24 pregnant patients with choriocarcinoma in remission and in 10 with progressive tumors mean concentrations of 3,301 ± 767 pg/mL and 8,790 ± 1,118 pg/mL, respectively, significantly higher than 30.5 ± 1.31 pg/mL in 23 healthy pregnant women during the first trimester *4747*

Pregnanediol *Urine* *Increase* May be much increased with primary chorionepithelioma of ovary *5544*

Progesterone *Plasma* *Increase* May be much increased with primary chorionepithelioma of ovary *5544*

α-Subunit *Plasma* *Increase* In men with choriocarcinoma mean pretreatment concentration of 10^8 pg/mL with decrease in response to successful treatment *3194*

α-Subunit, Free *Plasma* *Increase* In 13 men with choriocarcinoma mean concentration of 10^5 pg/mL which decreased with successful treatment *3194*

Tumor Necrosis Factor-β *Serum* *Increase* In 14 women with choriocarcinoma in remission and in 12 with progressive disease mean concentrations of 129 ± 30.5 pg/mL and 1,430 ± 198 pg/mL, respectively, significantly different from upper limit of normal in first trimester of 32.6 pg/mL in 23 healthy pregnant women *4747*

182.00 Cancer of Uterus

Albumin *Serum* *Decrease* Significantly reduced (median of 35.7 g/L ± 2.6 g/L) compared to controls (44.0 g/L ± 3.4 g/L) *2109*
Urine *Increase* 24 h excretion and renal clearance were significantly increased in localized tumor patients compared to normals and disseminated cancer cases. Increased high molecular weight protein excretion implies glomerular injury in these patients *2109*

CA 27-29 *Serum* *Increase* In 19% of 21 patients with cancer of uterus concentration increased above 3 U/mL *766*

CA 72-4 *Serum* *Increase* In 48 women with uterine carcinomas 11 (22.9%) had concentrations above 6 U/mL *1896*

CA 125 *Serum* *Increase* In 48 women with uterine carcinomas 8 (16.8%) had concentrations above 65 U/mL *1896* In some cases of invasive serous carcinoma of uterus CA 125 concentration did not precede or predict disease. Sensitivity for advanced disease only 57% *4218* Reported effect *3909*
Serum *No Effect* In some cases of invasive serous carcinoma of uterus CA 125 concentration did not precede or predict disease. Sensitivity for advanced disease only 57% *4218*

CA 549 *Serum Increase* Using a value of greater than 11 kU/L as the upper limits of normal, it is increased in 12% of cases *765*

Carcinoembryonic Antigen *Serum Increase* 67% positivity; incidence rose to 84% in advanced cases *1497* In 27% of the cases *4891* Positive in 25 of 47 patients with adenocarcinoma of the endometrium. A tendency toward higher values in the advanced stages evidenced by 24% incidence in stage I in contrast to a 57% incidence in stage III *1179*

Ceruloplasmin *Serum Increase* Mean concentration of 91 ± 24 mg/dL in 18 women with uterine cancer not significantly different from 84 ± 22 mg/dL in 150 control women *2280*

Cholesterol *Urine Increase* Hyperexcretion in 42 of 45 women with active carcinoma, sequential studies demonstrated an almost perfect correlation between excretion and the clinical status of the patient following surgical and/or radiation therapy *23*

Creatinine *Serum Increase* In 35% of 35 patients at initial hospitalization for this disorder *1576*

Estrogens *Plasma Increase* Mean value was 76.65 ng/dL in 28 patients with endometrial carcinoma. Highest elevations were found in obese patients *72*

Gc-Globulin *Serum No Effect* In 18 women with cancer of the ovary mean concentration of 24.9 ± 4.48 mg/dL not significantly different from 26.1 ± 4.66 mg/dL in 150 control women *2279*

Haptoglobin *Serum Increase* Increased (2.2 g/L) compared to normals (1.1 g/L) *2109*
Urine Increase 24 h excretion and renal clearance were significantly increased in localized tumor patients compared to normals and disseminated cancer cases. Increased high molecular weight protein excretion implies glomerular injury in these patients *2109*

Hematocrit *Blood Decrease* In 25% of 155 patients at initial hospitalization for this disorder *1576*

Hemoglobin *Blood Decrease* In 30% of 154 patients at initial hospitalization for this disorder *1576*

immunoglobulin A *Serum Increase* In 18 women with cancer of the uterus mean concentration of 222 ± 117 mg/dL significantly different from 174 ± 80 mg/dL in 150 healthy control women *2278*
Urine Increase 24 h excretion and renal clearance were significantly increased in localized tumor patients compared to normals and disseminated cancer cases. Increased high molecular weight protein excretion implies glomerular injury in these patients *2109*

Immunoglobulin G *Serum No Effect* In 18 women with uterine cancer mean concentration of 1,111 ± 222 mg/dL not significantly different from 1,157 ± 271 mg/dL in 150 healthy control women *2278*
Urine Increase 24 h excretion and renal clearance were significantly increased in localized tumor patients compared to normals and disseminated cancer cases. Increased high molecular weight protein excretion implies glomerular injury in these patients *2109*

Immunoglobulin M *Urine Increase* 24 h excretion and renal clearance were significantly increased in localized tumor patients compared to normals and disseminated cancer cases. Increased high molecular weight protein excretion implies glomerular injury in these patients *2109*

Iron-binding Capacity, Total *Serum Decrease* Significantly reduced (median of 2.6 mg/L) compared to controls (3.4 mg/L). Significantly increased in localized tumor patients compared to normals and disseminated cancer cases. Increased high molecular weight protein excretion implies glomerular injury in these patients *2109*

Monocytes *Blood Increase* In 51% of 150 patients at initial hospitalization for this disorder *1576*

Polymorphic Epithelial Mucin *Serum No Effect* In 9 women with uterine cancer median concentrations of 17 kU/L by ACS BR, 28 kU/L by Centocor CA 15-3, 16 kU/L by Enzymun-Test CA 15-3 and 14 kU/L by IMx CA 15-3 not significantly different from concentrations in 250 healthy women (mean and 1 SD concentrations of 22 ± 8.8 kU/L by ACS BR, 19 ± 8.8 kU/L by Centocor CA 15-3, 17 ± 7.1 kU/L by Enzymun-Test CA 15-3 and 15 ± 6.4 kU/L by IMx CA 15-3 respectively) *513*

Procollagen Type III Peptide *Serum Increase* A significant serum propeptide was significantly high in the group with gynecologic malignancies and normal in the benign tumor group *12* The serum PIIINP concentration was increased in 35% of the patients and more often (p less than 0.05) so in advanced (63%) than in early disease (31%) *5244* Elevated values of serum PIIINP are also observed in endometrial and cervical malignancies, though less frequently than in ovarian tumours. Very high concentrations of PIIINP are found in ovarian carcinoma ascites *4365*

Sialic Acid, Lipid-associated *Serum Increase* Elevated in 63% of patients *4693*

Squamous Cell Carcinoma Antigen *Serum Increase* In 2 of 6 patients with adenocarcinoma concentration significantly increased *5457*

Tissue Plasminogen Activator *Plasma Increase* Concentrations significantly higher in patients with malignant tumors than in those with benign tumors *4518*

Transferrin *Serum Decrease* In 18 women with uterine cancer mean concentration of 180 ± 47 mg/dL not significantly different from 217 ± 39 mg/dL in 150 control women *2280*

Uric Acid *Serum Increase* In 36% of 151 patients at initial hospitalization for this disorder *1576*

Urokinase *Plasma No Effect* Concentration not significantly different between patients with malignant tumors and healthy controls and those with benign tumors *4518*

182.00 Endometrial Carcinoma

Androstenedione *Plasma Increase* In 128 postmenopausal women with endometrial adenocarcinoma concentration correlated with plasma estrone and estradiol *512*

CA 19-9 *Serum Increase* In 100 women with endometrial carcinoma concentration increased in 33 with median concentration of 83.0 IU/mL *4655*

CA 125 *Serum Increase* In 27 women using Boehringer Mannheim Enzymun test mean concentration of 95.4 ± 287.6 U/mL with 14.8% having concentrations above 35 U/mL *2636* In 19 of 33 patients (58%) with recurrent endometrial carcinoma concentration significantly increased as observed in many cases before treatment *4432* Of CA 125 measurements with high concentrations in a hospital 10.8% were due to endometrial carcinoma *1350* In 63 patients with FIGO stage 1 disease median concentration of 11 U/mL, in 24 with stage II disease of 24 U/mL and in 25 with stage III disease median concentration of 21 U/mL *2764* In 100 women with endometrial carcinoma concentration increased in 33 with median concentration of 49.5 IU/mL *4655*
Tissue Increase Using FNA mean concentration of 39,899 U/mL observed in first drop of aspirated material in patients with metastatic carcinomas of ovary and endometrium *4139*

CA 549 *Serum Increase* In 86 patients with endometrial cancer 13 (15.1%) had a concentration greater than the upper limit of normal with BRESMARQ assay *764*

Cholesterol, Esterified *Urine Increase* In 39 of 44 patients with carcinoma of the endometrium mean excretion increased above 1.50 mg/d *23*

Epidermal Growth Factor *Tissue Increase* Median concentration of 0.2 ng/mg tissue protein observed in 6 endometrial cancer specimens *511*

Estradiol *Plasma Increase* In 128 postmenopausal women concentration correlated with clinical parameters *512*

Estrone *Plasma Increase* In 128 postmenopausal women plasma concentration correlated with clinical parameters *512*

Gonadotropin Peptide *Urine Increase* In women with cervical cancer mean concentration of 3.0 fmol/mg creatinine compared with mean value for both pre- and postmenopausal women of 1.51 ± 2.42 fmol/mg creatinine *5538*

Macrophage Colony Stimulating Factor *Serum Decrease* In 61 patients with endometrial cancer mean concentration of 962.1 ± 335.7 U/mL significantly lower than baseline normal of 1,056 U/mL *5094*

Progesterone *Plasma Increase* Concentration correlated with plasma estrone in 128 postmenopausal women with endometrial adenocarcinoma *512*

182.00 Endometrial Carcinoma *(continued)*

Sialyltransferase *Serum* *Increase* In 3 patients with cancer of the endometrium mean and median concentrations of 514 and 428 cpm/mg protein/30 min significantly different from 240 and 243 cpm/mg protein/30 min respectively in 20 normal individuals *2111*

Steroid Sulfatase *Serum* *Increase* Mean concentration in 17 patients with endometrial carcinoma of 190.8 ± 31.3 ng/mL significantly higher than 75.7 ± 28.3 ng/mL in 57 menstruating control healthy women and 68.8 ± 24.7 ng/mL in 12 postmenopausal women: using a cutoff of 130 ng/mL positive rate of 58.7% observed *5072*

Testosterone *Serum* *Increase* In 128 postmenopausal women with endometrial adenocarcinoma concentration correlated with plasma estrone, estradiol, and androstenedione *512*

183.00 Ovarian Cancer

Albumin *Serum* *Decrease* In patients with epithelial ovarian cancer survival predictable based on serum albumin concentration, with those with best prognosis having albumin over 41 g/L, next best 35 - 40 g/L, and poorest 34 g/L *4010*

Aldolase *Serum* *Increase* Mildly elevated. Mean = 3.8 ± 1.0 U/L compared to normal, 1.6 ± 0.21 U/L *2513*

Alkaline Phosphatase *Serum* *Increase* In 5 cases, the initial value was 45 - 190 U/L (normal < 107 U/L) *658*

Alkaline Phosphatase Isoenzymes *Ascitic Fluid* *Increase* 59% (13 of 22) patients had detectable Regan isoenzyme *5028*
Pleural Fluid *Increase* 59% (13 of 22) patients had detectable Regan isoenzyme in malignant effusions *5028*
Serum *Increase* In 5 cases, the initial value was 44.7 - 191 (normal 106.5 U/L). The Regan isoenzyme was found in all cases and ranged from 99 - 264 U/L placental isoenzyme units *5029* Cancer of the ovary, endometrium, cervix and breast as a group exhibited the highest frequency of Regan isoenzyme (placental) in malignancies *658*

Alkaline Phosphatase, Placental Isoenzyme
Serum *Increase* Although antibodies reactive with placental alkaline phosphatase bind to most ovarian cancers, serum levels are elevated in only 30 to 60 percent of patients *5021* *3909*

Amylase *Ascitic Fluid* *Increase* Rare occurrence of ovarian carcinoma producing amylase-rich ascites and pleural effusions was reported; salivary type amylase was identified in tumor tissue *938*
Pleural Fluid *Increase* Rare occurrence of ovarian carcinoma producing amylase-rich ascites and pleural effusions. Salivary type amylase has been identified in tumor tissue *938*
Serum *Increase* Hyperamylasemia may occur in ovarian papillary cystadenocarcinoma *2983*

Anti-p53 Antibodies *Serum* *Increase* Increase observed in 12 of 86 patients (14.0%) *132*

c-erb-B$_2$ Oncoprotein *Serum* *Increase* Median concentration of 11.15 ng/mL in 14 patients with stage I or II disease and 12.9 ng/mL in 14 patients with stage III or IV disease. 0 of 14 (0%) with stage I or II disease and 9 of 36 (25%) with III or IV disease had concentrations exceeding 1.5 ng/mL *3564*

CA 15-3 *Serum* *Increase* In 44 patients with ovarian cancer mean concentration of 59.0 ± 64 U/mL significantly different from cutoff of 22 U/mL, with 29 having concentrations greater than 22 U/mL and 15 with concentrations above 40 U/mL *2076* In 10 patient with stage 1 disease, 2 with stage 2, 31 with stage 3 disease and 7 with stage 4 disease mean proportion of patients with concentrations greater than 30 U/mL 30%, 50%, 58% and 86% respectively *1133*

CA 19-9 *Serum* *Increase* In 47 specimens from 17 patients with colorectal cancer GI-MA concentration as measured on DPC IMMULITE correlated positively with CA 19-9 concentration but IMMULITE measurements were generally lower than CA 19-9 results but no clinical discrepancies were found *5389* Increased in 18 of 105 (17%) of patients *2770* Elevated in 18 of 105 (17%) of patients *2770*

CA 72-4 *Serum* *Increase* Sensitivity for ovarian carcinoma using cutoff value of 2.9 U/mL 54% and cutoff of 3.0 U/mL sensitivity 54% *2053* In colon carcinomas 16% of specimens showed elevated levels *5744* In 94 women with ovarian cancer 47 (50%) had concentrations above 6 U/mL *1896*

CA 125 *Ascitic Fluid* *Increase* In patients with serous carcinoma 4 out of 4 positive with median concentration of 20,480 U/mL, 7 of 7 with endometrial carcinoma median of 5,200 U/mL, 0 of 1 with mucinous adenocarcinoma median of 3 U/mL, 8 of 8 with undifferentiated carcinoma with median of 3,101 U/mL *2025*
Cyst Fluid *Increase* In patients with serous carcinoma 5 out of 5 positive with median concentration of 13,607 U/mL, 10 of 10 with endometrial carcinoma median 8,890 U/mL, 6 of 6 with mucinous adenocarcinoma median 698 U/mL, 2 of 2 with undifferentiated carcinoma with median of 2,313 U/mL, 6 of 6 with serous cystadenoma with median 7,131 U/mL, 7 of 8 with serous cyst with median 18,688 U/mL and 13 of 13 with mucinous adenoma with median 2,766 U/mL *2025*
Serum *Increase* Concentrations in 5 patients with pure ovarian yolk sac tumors of 51 - 873 U/mL significantly increased, decreasing with successful response to therapy *4727* In 94 women with ovarian cancer 57 (60.6%) had concentrations above 65 U/mL *1896* Using Boehringer Mannheim Enzymun test in 8 women with stage I-II disease mean concentration of 100.1 ± 98.0 U/mL and in 34 with stages III-IV mean 1,530.8 ± 2,469.5 U/mL with proportion above 35 U/mL 62.5% and 91,2% respectively *2636* In patients with serous carcinoma 11 out of 11 positive with median concentration of 760 U/mL, 13 of 14 with endometrial carcinoma median of 564 U/mL, 4 of 7 with mucinous adenocarcinoma median 50 U/mL, 12 of 12 with undifferentiated carcinoma with median of 1,757 U/mL, 1 of 6 with serous cystadenoma with median of 11 U/mL, 2 of 8 with serous cyst with median of 16 U/mL and 3 of 13 with mucinous adenoma with median of 22 U/mL *2025* An increasing concentration has been shown to predict progression of ovarian cancer, often with a lead time of several months *4483* In post-menopausal women with pelvic masses, an elevated level (> 65 U/mL) had a sensitivity of 98% and specificity of 78% *3252* Concentration increased with increasing grade of tumor in 60 patients with primary invasive ovarian carcinoma: 64.5 U/L with grade I tumors, 222.2 U/L with grade II tumors, 408.8 U/L with grade III tumors *651* In 10 patient with stage 1 disease, 2 with stage 2, 31 with stage 3 disease and 7 with stage 4 disease mean proportion of patients with concentrations greater than 35 U/mL 50%, 50%, 94% and 100% respectively *1133* In 309 women with ovarian carcinoma 65% had values greater than 35 U/mL (with concentration typically increasing with increasing severity of disease) compared with 5% in apparently healthy women when measured by second generation Centocor assay *2637* In 30 (65%) of 46 patients with stage I ovarian cancer concentration increased above upper limit of normal of 30 U/mL *5730* In 30 patients with malignant neoplasms of the ovary median concentration of 621 kU/L significantly different from 10.9 kU/L in 39 age-matched controls *1117* In one patient increased concentration observed 10 to 12 months prior to clinical detection of ovarian tumor *231* Sensitivity for ovarian carcinoma using cutoff value of 31 U/mL 85%, cutoff of 65 U/mL sensitivity 69% and cutoff of 160 U/mL sensitivity 52% *2053* Using a cutoff of > 35 U/L sensitivity for stage I disease 55%, stage II 66%, stage III disease 94% and 100% for stage IV disease *1134* In 52 patients with epithelial ovarian cancer mean concentration of 532 ± 129 U/mL significantly higher than cutoff of 35 U/mL in healthy individuals *4044* In 176 specimens from 32 patients OM-MA concentration as measured on DPC IMMULITE correlated positively with CA 15-3 concentration but IMMULITE measurements were generally lower than CA 15-3. results but no clinical discrepancies were found *5389* In 21 patients with histologically proved ovarian cancer concentrations ranged from 51 to 1,939 ku/L conpared with upper limit of normal of 35 ku/L *616* In 48 women with primary ovarian cancer serum concentrations of CA 125 were above the cutoff value of 35 U/mL in 68% of patients. Concentrations were higher in poorly differentiated tumors than in well differentiated tumors and in those with residual tumor after cytoreductive surgery than in those with no residual tumor. Concentrations also higher in stage I and II disease than in more advanced disease *1806* In a population of patients with epithelial ovarian carcinoma using a cutoff of 35 U/mL, 82% were positive for CA 125 compared with 82% for OSA and 73% for CASA *3412* In 56 patients with ovarian cancer median concentration of 210 U/mL significantly increased compared with 17 U/mL in patients with benign ovarian disease *1621* In all 61 patients with epithelial ovarian cancer (FIGO stages III and IV) concentrations increased *3545* Of CA 125 measurements with high concentrations in a hospital 61.3% were due to ovarian and primary peritoneal cancer *1350* Serum from 135 patients with epithelial ovarian cancer were

analyzed and 85% were elevated *5455* In 28 patients with malignant epithelial ovarian tumors median concentration of 160 kU/L (95% confidence limits 75 - 687 kU/L) *462* In 33 patients with ovarian cancer 29 had concentrations greater than 20 U/L *4749* In 65 women with malignant ovarian tumors median concentration of 1688 U/mL significantly higher than 4 U/mL in 458 healthy women *2203* High sensitivity for ovarian carcinoma. However levels are elevated in benign ovarian disease and in other epithelial cancers *5364* Median concentration of 293 μg/L in 37 patients with ovarian cancer *5191* Using a cutoff value of 65 U/mL, 96 of 113 patients with serous cystadenocarcinoma, 17 of 18 with undifferentiated adenocarcinoma, 12 of 21 with mucinous cystadenocarcinoma and in 10 of 18 endometrial carcinoma had abnormal concentrations *4699* In patients with epithelial ovarian cancer survival predictable based on serum log CA 125 concentration *4010* In 37 patients with ovarian cancer median concentration of 293 U/L *2090* In 82 consecutive women with ovarian cancer mean concentration of 1,771 U/mL, with normal upper limit of < 35 U/mL, with no significant correlation between histologic grade and concentration, but increased histologic grade was associated with decreased survival *1684*
Serum *No Effect* In 14 of 25 patients with clinically apparent ovarian cancer (56%) serum CA 125 concentration normal but had increased concentrations of M-CSF *5756*
Tissue *Increase* Using FNA mean concentration of 39,899 U/mL observed in first drop of aspirated material in patients with metastatic carcinomas of ovary and endometrium *4139*

CA 549 *Serum* *Increase* In 125 patients with cancer of the ovaries 48 (38.4%) had a concentration greater than the upper limit of normal with BRESMARQ assay *764* Using a value of greater than 11 kU/L as the upper limits of normal, it is increased in 50% of cases *765*

Calcium *Serum* *No Effect* One patient with ovarian cancer did not have hypercalcemia *1200*

Cancer-associated Serum Antigen *Serum* *Increase* In a population of patients with epithelial ovarian carcinoma using a cutoff of 3.0 U/mL, 76% of patients had increased concentrations *3412* Using a cutoff of > 4 U/L sensitivity for stage I disease 27%, stage II 0%, stage III disease 66% and 75% for stage IV disease *1134* In 10 patient with stage 1 disease, 2 with stage 2, 31 with stage 3 disease and 7 with stage 4 disease mean proportion of patients with concentrations greater than 4 U/mL 20%, 0%, 65% and 71% respectively *1133*

Carcinoembryonic Antigen *Ascitic Fluid* *Increase* In malignant effusions *4891*
Serum *Increase* 77% positivity *1497* Most commonly found in ovarian cancer. Elevated levels occurred in 6 of 30 cases, all at advanced stages III or IV *5326* Of the 132 patients with adenocarcinoma, 73 had positive values. The largest number of patients were in the stage III category where 45 of 77 patients (58%) were positive *1179* Not a very good marker of ovarian cancer since concentration increased in less than 25% of all cases *616* In 30 patients with ovarian cancer 93.3% had concentrations up to 3.0 ng/mL and 6.7% had concentrations between 3.1 - 5.0 ng/mL in contrast to concentrations in 151 healthy nonsmokers in whom 95.4% had concentrations between 0 and 3.0 ng/mL and 4.6% between 4.1 and 10.0 ng/mL *11* In 35% of cases *1207* *4891*

Ceruloplasmin *Serum* *Increase* Mean concentration in 4 women with ovarian carcinoma of mean age 39.5 years 418.5 μmol/L (370 - 515) significantly higher than 283 μmol/L (213 - 385) in 19 healthy control women of mean age 30 years *761* In 27 women with ovarian cancer mean concentration of 101 ± 26 mg/dL significantly different from 84 ± 22 mg/dL in 150 control women *2280*

Cholesterol *Peritoneal Fluid* *Increase* Markedly increased in active cases *3411*
Urine *Increase* Hyperexcretion in 18 of 19 cystadenocarcinomas of the serous and/or mucinous types; 1 of 1 endometrial carcinoma; 4 of 4 malignant granulosa cell tumors; two of two mixed malignant germ cell tumors; and one of one malignant mixed Mullerian tumor. A normal excretion was characteristic of 19 of 21 surviving patients treated by surgery and adjunctive therapy. The 94% correlation between the presence of proven active ovarian carcinomas and urinary hyperexcretion is significant *24*

β-Chorionic Gonadotropin *Ascitic Fluid* *Increase* In 22 patients, 30% had positive serum while 68% had positive pleural and ascites effusions *5028*
Plasma *Increase* In 22 patients, 30% had hCG positive serum *5028* Elevated with invasive carcinoma *1207* The highest incidence was found in patients with carcinoma of testis (61%), adenocarcinoma of ovary (42%), and pancreas (33%) *1497*
Pleural Fluid *Increase* In 22 patients, 30% had positive serum while 68% had positive pleural and ascites effusions *5028*

Complement C_3 *Serum* *Increase* Increased in patients with local disease. Closely linked to the stage of the disease. Patients in remission had normal levels, but further increases were noted in distant metastases. Levels dropped significantly in the terminal phase of disease *5456*

Complement C_4 *Serum* *Increase* Increased in patients with local disease. Very closely linked to the stage of the disease. Patients in remission had normal levels, but further increases were noted in distant metastases. Levels dropped significantly in the terminal phase of the disease *5456*

Complement, Total *Serum* *Increase* Closely linked to the stage of the disease. Patients in remission had normal levels, but further increases were noted in distant metastases. Dropped significantly in the terminal phase of disease *5456*

Copper *Serum* *Increase* In 4 women with ovarian carcinoma and mean age of 39.5 years mean concentration of 21.9 μmol/L (19.2 - 25.9) significantly higher than mean of 14.6 μmol/L (12.2 - 20.8) in 19 healthy control women of mean age 30 years *761* Does not result from a shift of zinc into or release of copper out of malignant tumor tissue *3055*

Copper, Ultrafiltratable *Serum* *No Effect* In 4 women of mean age 39.5 years with carcinoma of ovary mean concentration of 0.214 μmol/L (0.146 - 0.272) not significantly different from 0.174 μmol/L (0.115 - 0.58) in 19 healthy young women of mean age 30 years *761*

Creatine Kinase BB-Isoenzyme *Serum* *Increase* Elevated CK-BB *5884* *4842*

Cryofibrinogen *Plasma* *Increase* Reported effect *3417* *4551*

CYFRA 21-1 *Serum* *Increase* In 15 patients with ovarian cancer stages I and II median concentration of 1.4 ng/mL and in 11 with stage III and IV ovarian cancer 6.1 ng/mL significantly different from that in 50 healthy individuals with median concentration of 1.2 ng/mL and range of 0.5 - 2.4 ng/mL *3559*
Serum *No Effect* Median concentration of 2.4 μg/L in 37 patients with ovarian cancer not different from 1.9 μg/L in 40 healthy controls *5191*

D-Dimer *Plasma* *Increase* In 56 patients with ovarian cancer median concentration of 1,895 ng/mL significantly increased compared with 218 ng/mL in patients with benign ovarian disease *1621* In 30 patients with malignant neoplasms of the ovary median concentration of 5,750 μg/L significantly different from 240 μg/L in 39 age-matched controls *1117*

Dehydroepiandrosterone Sulfate *Plasma* *No Effect* In 28 patients aged 66 - 77 years with malignant epithelial ovarian tumors median concentration not significantly different from that in healthy controls *462*

DF3 *Serum* *Increase* In 40 patients with ovarian cancer 58% had concentration greater than 25 U/mL (concentration in 90% normals) and 43% greater than 30 U/mL (observed in 95% normals) *2076*

Eosinophils *Blood* *Increase* Reported effect *5544*

Erythrocytes *Ascitic Fluid* *Increase* A large number of RBC, especially grossly bloody ascites, suggests a neoplasm, particularly hepatoma or ovarian cancer *4891*

Estradiol *Cyst Fluid* *Increase* In cyst fluid from 19 postmenopausal women patients with ovarian cancer concentration of 980 ± 473 pmol/L higher than in fluid from benign cysts *2565*
Plasma *Increase* In estrogen producing tumors estradiol is the most active estrogen *457* *91* *3935*
Plasma *No Effect* In 24 women with postmenopausal epithelial ovarian tumors mean concentration of 0.04 nmol/L (range of 0.04 - 0.05 nmol/L) compared with 0.06 nmol/L (range of 0.05 - 0.15 nmol/L) in 24 healthy postmenopausal control women *461* In 28 patients aged 66 - 77 years with malignant epithelial ovarian tumors median concentration not significantly different from that in healthy controls *462*

α-Fetoprotein *Serum* *Increase* Concentrations in 5 patients with pure ovarian yolk sac tumors of 1,640 - 324,860 ng/mL significantly increased, decreasing with successful response to therapy *4727* 15 out of 20 cases of teratoblastoma of testis and ovary showed raised levels *14* Over 50 ng/mL in 33% of

183.00 Ovarian Cancer *(continued)*

α-Fetoprotein *(continued)*
cases of gonadal teratoblastoma *4734* *1207* Present in embryonal carcinoma (in 27% of cases) or malignant teratoma (60% of cases) of ovary and testis *5544*
Serum *No Effect* No elevations are seen in conjunction with pure dysgerminomas of the ovary *5759*

Fibrin Degradation Products *Ascitic Fluid* *Increase* In malignant effusions *4891*

Follicle Stimulating Hormone *Plasma* *Decrease* Mean concentration in 24 postmenopausal women with malignant epithelial ovarian tumors of 32.5 IU/L (range 24.0 - 49.0 IU/L) significantly lower than 67.5 IU/L (range 18.0 - 26.0 U/L) in 24 healthy postmenopausal female controls *461* In 28 patients aged 66 - 77 years with malignant epithelial ovarian tumors median concentration of 30.5 IU/L significantly lower than that in healthy controls *462*
Urine *Decrease* Observed effect *456*

Follistatin, Free *Serum* *Increase* Mean concentration in 4 patients with ovarian cancer of 6.1 ± 2.0 μg/L not significantly different from that in patients with other cancers but significantly higher than 3.5 ± 0.2 μg/L in 60 normal individuals *4523*

Galactosyltransferase Isoenzyme II *Serum* *Increase* Sensitivity 0.75 and specificity 0.76 *5348*

Gc-Globulin *Serum* *No Effect* In 27 women with cancer of the ovary mean concentration of 26.3 ± 4.85 mg/dL not significantly different from 26.1 ± 4.66 mg/dL in 150 control women *2279*

Gonadotropin Peptide *Urine* *Increase* In women with ovarian cancer mean concentration of 11.9 ± 45.1 fmol/mg creatinine compared with mean value for both pre- and postmenopausal women of 1.51 ± 2.42 fmol/mg creatinine *5538*

Haptoglobin *Serum* *Increase* In 9 women with ovarian tumors < 6 cm in diameter mean concentration of 144 mg/dL and in 34 with tumors > 6 cm mean concentration of 268 mg/dL compared with mean of 81% in 50 controls *3640*

Hexokinase *Serum* *Increase* Markedly increased. Mean activity of 22.8 ± 4.0 U/L compared to normal of 0.93 ± 0.28 U/L *2513*

17-Hydroxyprogesterone *Plasma* *Increase* The patients with ovarian cancer showed a significantly higher ($p < 0.01$) level than controls *3267*

immunoglobulin A *Serum* *No Effect* In 27 women with cancer of the ovary mean concentration of 182 ± 88 mg/dL not significantly different from 174 ± 80 mg/dL in 150 healthy control women *2278*

Immunoglobulin G *Serum* *No Effect* In 27 women with ovarian cancer mean concentration of 1,233 ± 547 mg/dL not significantly different from 1,157 ± 271 mg/dL in 150 healthy control women *2278*

Immunoglobulin M *Serum* *Decrease* In 27 women with ovarian cancer mean concentration of 51 ± 25 mg/dL significantly different from 77 ± 39 mg/dL in 106 healthy controls *2278*
Serum *No Effect* In 18 women with ovarian cancer mean concentration of 76 ± 42 mg/dL not significantly different from 77 ± 39 mg/dL in 106 healthy controls *2278*

Inhibin *Plasma* *Increase* In 18 of 22 postmenopausal women with mucinous carcinomas of the ovary, 9 of 53 with serous carcinomas and serous borderline cystic tumors, in 2 of 12 with clear cell carcinomas, 4 of 26 with undifferentiated carcinomas, 3 of 3 with granulosa-cell tumors and 5 of 27 with other ovarian cancers concentrations of inhibin increased *2083* In 28 patients with malignant epithelial ovarian tumors median concentration of 0.4 U/L x 10^{-3} (95% confidence limits 0.2 - 0.9 U/L x 10^{-3}) *462* In 24 postmenopausal women with epithelial ovarian cancer mean concentration of 0.4 (range of 0.2 - 0.9) unit/L x10 significantly higher than 0.2 (range of 0.0 - 0.3) unit/L x10 in 24 healthy postmenopausal women *461*

Insulin-like Growth Factor-I *Cyst Fluid* *Increase* Mean concentration of 16.1 ± 2.2 nmol/L in 11 invasive malignant epithelial ovarian tumors compared with 7.3 ± 1.2 nmol/L in 20 simple or benign ovarian cysts *2565*

Insulin-like Growth Factor Binding Protein-2
Cyst Fluid *Increase* In stage III tumors mean concentration of 11.0 ± 6.3 relative units and 3.3 ± 2.2 relative units in stage I tumors compared with almost undetectable concentration in cyst fluid from benign ovarian cysts *2565*
Serum *Increase* Mean concentration in 11 patients with malignant ovarian tumors of 1.32 ± 0.32 relative units compared with 0.53 ± 0.07 relative units in 20 patients with benign ovarian cysts *2565*

Insulin-like Growth Factor Binding Protein-3
Serum *Decrease* In 11 patients with malignant ovarian tumors concentration of 0.39 ± 0.14 relative units significantly less than 0.91 ± 0.11 relative units in patients with benign cysts *2565*

Interleukin-6 *Serum* *Increase* In 18 patients with epithelial ovarian carcinomas mean concentration of 6.3 pg/mL and median concentration of 0.8 pg/mL *4676*

17-Ketosteroids *Urine* *Increase* Excretion may be increased in patients with lutein cell tumors of the ovary *2952*

Lactate Dehydrogenase *Serum* *Increase* In 41.7% of patients with ovarian adenocarcinomas of the common epithelial types and in 29.4% of cases with metastatic ovarian carcinoma activities of serum lactate dehydrogenase increased. All 5 patients with ovarian dysgerminomas had extremely high activities *1591* All 6 cases showed elevation ranging from 150 - 350 U/L with the upper limit of normal at 120 U/L. Marked elevation in 18 patients *221* Mean activity of 158.7 ± 14.9 U/L compared to normals, 85.4 ± 1.0 U/L *2513* In 21 patients with histologically proved ovarian carcinoma, 15 had activities ranging from 445 U/L to 2,567 U/L compared with upper limit of normal of 430 U/L *616*

Lactate Dehydrogenase Isoenzymes *Serum* *Increase* In 21 patients with ovarian carcinoma 13 had increased activity of LD-1 above upper limit of 125 U/L with 5 having increase over 29% of total LD activity *616* In 5 patients with ovarian dysgerminomas activity of 2 fast fractions increased: in all other forms of ovarian cancer activity of slow moving fractions increased *1591*

Luteinizing Hormone *Plasma* *Decrease* In 24 postmenopausal women with malignant epithelial ovarian tumors mean concentration of 15.0 IU/L (range 7.3 - 22.0 IU/L) not significantly less than 21.5 IU/L (range 18.0 - 26.0 IU/L) in 24 healthy control postmenopausal women *461*
Plasma *No Effect* In 28 patients aged 66 - 77 years with malignant epithelial ovarian tumors median concentration not significantly different from that in healthy controls *462*

Lysophosphatidic Acid *Serum* *Increase* In 10 patients with stage I ovarian cancer, stages II, III and IV (24 patients) and recurrent (14 patients), median concentrations were 2.4 μmol/L, 5.2 μmol/L, and 4.1 mol/L. respectively, significantly different from 0.1 μmol/L in 48 healthy controls *5758*

M3/M21 *Serum* *Increase* In 37 patients with ovarian cancer median concentrations for stages I, II and III disease were 145.2, 29.5 and 116 U/L, respectively, compared with that in 40 healthy blood donors in whom the median concentration was 26.3 U/L *2090* In 75 patients with ovarian cancer mean concentration of 111.5 U/mL (range 24.6 ± 1,393.5 U/mL compared with 21.0 U/mL (range of 0 - 52.1 U/mL) observed in50 healthy individuals *5190*

Macrophage Colony Stimulating Factor *Serum* *Increase* In 88 patients with ovarian cancer mean concentration of 1,452.9 ± 916.7 U/mL significantly higher than baseline normal of 1,056 U/mL *5094* In 47 of 68 patients with clinically apparent epithelial ovarian cancer, 47 (68%) had a concentration of at least 2.5 ng/mL compared with only 2 of 80 (2.5%) apparently healthy donors. Circulating concentrations did not correlate with those of CA 125 *5756* In 24 (52%) of 46 patients with stage I ovarian cancer concentration increased above upper limit of normal of 3.1 U/mL *5730*

Manganese Superoxide Dismutase *Serum* *Increase* Thirty-seven of sixty-two patients (59.7%) with epithelial ovarian carcinomas showed high blood levels *2355*

1-Methylinosine *Urine* *Increase* In 3 patients with carcinoma of the ovary, excretions of 6.5 and 7.0 mg/d in two significantly different from 3.9 ± 2.1 mg/d in 17 healthy controls, but 3.4 mg/d in the other within normal range *5505*

N^2, N^2-Dimethylguanosine *Urine* *Increase* In 3 patients with ovarian carcinoma excretions of 11.0 and 22.5 mg/d in two significantly different from 3.9 ± 2.6 mg/d in 17 healthy controls, but excretion of 4.3 mg/d in one not significantly different *5505*

N-Acetylputrescine *Urine* *Increase* In 84 patients with ovarian cancer mean concentration of about 36 mg/L significantly greater than that in 32 healthy adults in whom the mean concentration was approximately 8 mg/L *5075*

N-Acetylspermidine *Urine* *Increase* In 84 patients with ovarian cancer mean concentration of about 23 mg/L significantly greater than that in 32 healthy adults in whom the mean concentration was approximately 3 mg/L *5075*

Neopterin *Serum* *Increase* Mean concentration of 16.2 ± 16.4 nmol/L in 6 patients with ovarian cancer significantly greater than that in 18 healthy control individuals, 6.4 ± 1.8 nmol/L *3864*
Urine *Increase* Frequency of increased concentrations in patients with ovarian cancer 80% *121*

Ovarian Serum Antigen *Serum* *Increase* In a population of patients with epithelial ovarian carcinoma using a cutoff of 2.5 U/mL, 82% had increased concentrations *3412*

OVX1 *Serum* *Increase* In 22 (48%) of 46 patients with stage I ovarian cancer concentration increased above upper limit of normal of 12 U/mL *5730*

Parathyroid Hormone-related Peptide *Plasma* *Increase* In all 3 patients studied with hypercalcemia range of concentrations of 2.6 to 39.9 pmol/L compared with upper limit of normal of 1.5 pmol/L *3987*
Plasma *No Effect* In 1 patient with ovarian cancer and normocalcemia concentration of 1.19 pmol/L below upper limit of reference range of 2.6 pmol/L *1200*

Placental Protein 4 *Serum* *Increase* Concentrations above 3 µg/L were observed in 45 of 52 patients with cancer of ovaries (86.5%): concentration correlated significantly with staging *1768*

Plasminogen Activator Inhibitor-1 *Plasma* *Increase* In 9 premenopausal women with malignant ovarian tumors mean concentration of 13 µg/L and in 69 with benign ovarian tumors mean concentration of 9 µg/L and in 27 postmenopausal women with malignant tumors mean of 25 µg/L and 8 µg/L in 38 postmenopausal women with benign ovarian tumors higher than normals of 3 µg/L in premenopausal women and 11 µg/L in postmenopausal women *727*

Platelets *Blood* *Increase* Counts above 400,000 /µL observed in 24.3% of 82 patients with histologically confirmed ovarian carcinoma *3454*

Polymorphic Epithelial Mucin *Serum* *Increase* In 4 women with ovarian cancer median concentrations of 38 kU/L by ACS BR, 29 kU/L by Centocor CA 15-3, 32 kU/L by Enzymun-Test CA 15-3 and 26 kU/L by IMx CA 15-3 significantly different from concentrations in 250 healthy women (mean and 1 SD concentrations of 22 ± 8.8 kU/L by ACS BR, 19 ± 8.8 kU/L by Centocor CA 15-3, 17 ± 7.1 kU/L by Enzymun-Test CA 15-3 and 15 ± 6.4 kU/L by IMx CA 15-3 respectively) *513*

Procollagen Type III Peptide *Ascitic Fluid* *Increase* Elevated values of serum PIIINP are also observed in endometrial and cervical malignancies, though less frequently than in ovarian tumours. Very high concentrations of PIIINP are found in ovarian carcinoma ascites *4365*
Serum *Increase* Elevated values of serum PIIINP are also observed in endometrial and cervical malignancies, though less frequently than in ovarian tumours. Very high concentrations of PIIINP are found in ovarian carcinoma ascites *4365* A significant serum propeptide was significantly high in the group with gynecologic malignancies and normal in the benign tumor group *12*

Progesterone *Plasma* *Increase* Patients with ovarian cancer showed a significantly higher ($p < 0.01$) level than controls *3267* Mean concentration of 2.28 nmol/L (range 1.0 - 3.6 nmol/L) in 24 women with postmenopausal women with epithelial ovarian tumors not significantly higher than 1.4 nmol/L (range 1.0 - 1.6 nmol/L) in 24 healthy postmenopausal women *461*
Plasma *No Effect* In 28 patients aged 66 - 77 years with malignant epithelial ovarian tumors median concentration not significantly different from that in healthy controls *462*

Pseudouridine *Urine* *Increase* In 3 patients with ovarian carcinoma excretions of 111 and 239 mg/d significantly different from 65 ± 31 mg/d in 17 healthy controls, but 91 mg/d in the other not significantly different from normal *5505*

Putrescine *Urine* *Increase* In 84 patients with ovarian cancer mean concentration of about 7 mg/L significantly greater than that in 32 healthy adults in whom the mean concentration was approximately 2 mg/L *5075*

Sialic Acid, Lipid-associated *Serum* *Increase* In 1 patient with early stage ovarian cancer mean concentration of 33.4 mg/dL significantly different from 17.7 mg/dL in 50 normal volunteers *1273* Elevated in 70% of patients *4693*

Sialyltransferase *Serum* *Increase* In 4 patients with carcinoma of the ovary mean and median concentrations of 423 and 372 cpm/mg protein/30 min significantly different from 240 and 243 cpm/mg protein/30 min respectively in 20 normal individuals *2111*

Soluble Interleukin-2 Receptor *Serum* *Increase* In 52 patients with epithelial ovarian cancer mean concentration of 1,364 ± 120 U/mL significantly higher than 555 ± 31 U/mL in 25 healthy controls *4044*

Soluble Interleukin-2 Receptor-α *Ascitic Fluid* *Increase* In 18 patients with ovarian cancer mean concentration of 2,870 ± 1,870 U/mL *1052*
Cyst Fluid *Increase* In 30 patients with ovarian cancer mean concentration of 1,620 ± 1,350 U/mL significantly greater than that in 31 patients with benign tumors of the ovary in whom the mean concentration was 616 ± 846 U/mL *1052*
Serum *Increase* In 25 patients with ovarian cancer mean concentration of 967.3 ± 205.7 U/mL significantly greater than 367 ± 44.6 U/mL in normal controls *311* In 48 patients with epithelial ovarian tumors mean concentration of 750 ± 450 U/mL significantly different from 390 ± 124 U/mL in 50 healthy female blood donors *1052*

Spermidine *Urine* *Increase* In 84 patients with ovarian cancer mean concentration of about 2.0 mg/L significantly greater than that in 32 healthy adults in whom the mean concentration was approximately 0.6 mg/L *5075*

Spermine *Urine* *Increase* In 84 patients with ovarian cancer mean concentration of about 2.2 mg/L significantly greater than that in 32 healthy adults in whom the mean concentration was approximately 1.0 mg/L *5075*

Steroid Sulfatase *Serum* *Increase* Mean concentration in 13 patients with endometrial carcinoma of 176.1 ± 22.6 ng/mL significantly higher than 75.7 ± 28.3 ng/mL in 57 menstruating control healthy women and 68.8 ± 24.7 ng/mL in 12 postmenopausal women: using a cutoff of 130 ng/mL positive rate of 69.2% observed *5072*

Tenascin-C *Serum* *Increase* Mean concentration in 15 patients with endometrial or ovarian cancer of 1.59 ± 0.92 mg/L not significantly higher than that in 15 healthy individuals (1.09 ± 0.41 mg/L) *4626*

Testosterone *Serum* *No Effect* Mean concentration of 1.10 nmol/L (range of 0.81 - 1.50 nmol/L) in 24 postmenopausal women with epithelial ovarian cancer not significantly different from 1.00 nmol/L (range of 0.76 - 1.50 nmol/L) in 24 healthy postmenopausal women *461*

Testosterone, Free *Serum* *No Effect* Mean concentration of 0.016 nmol/L (range of 0.012 - 0.020 nmol/L) in 24 postmenopausal women with epithelial ovarian cancer not significantly different from 0.013 nmol/L (range of 0.009 - 0.019 nmol/L) in 24 healthy postmenopausal women *461*

Tetranectin *Serum* *Decrease* In 18 women with nonovarian tumors mean concentration of 7.7 ± 2.2 mg/L significantly less than 11.6 ± 2.0 mg/L in 458 healthy women *2203*
Serum *Increase* In 28 patients with malignant epithelial ovarian tumors median concentration of 8.9 mg/L (95% confidence limits 6.8 - 9.2 mg/L) *462*

Tetranectin with A371 Catching Antibody *Serum* *Decrease* In 43 women with ovarian cancer mean concentration of 6.9 ± 2.3 mg/L significantly different from 95% confidence interval of 9.4 - 16.8 mg/L in 43 healthy women *5227*

Tetranectin with Hyb 130-13 Catching Antibody
Serum *Decrease* In 43 women with ovarian cancer mean concentration of 9.0 ± 3.1 mg/L significantly different from 95% confidence interval of 9.8 - 18.0 mg/L in 43 healthy women *5227*

Tetranectin with Hyb 130-14 Catching Antibody
Serum *Decrease* In 43 women with ovarian cancer mean concentration of 9.4 ± 3.0 mg/L significantly different from 95% confidence interval of 8.7 - 16.5 mg/L in 43 healthy women *5227*

Thrombin/Antithrombin III Complex *Plasma* *Increase* In 30 patients with malignant neoplasms of the ovary median concentration of 9.0 µg/L significantly different from 2.3 µg/L in 39 age-matched controls *1117*

Tissue Factor Pathway Inhibitor *Plasma* *Increase* About half of patients with ovarian cancer had activities greater than median activity of 1.19 U/mL in healthy individuals *2376*

183.00 Ovarian Cancer *(continued)*

Tissue Plasminogen Activator *Plasma Increase* In 9 premenopausal women with malignant ovarian tumors and 69 with benign ovarian tumors mean concentration of 5 μg/L and in 27 postmenopausal women with malignant tumors mean of 12 μg/L and 8 μg/L in 38 postmenopausal women with benign ovarian tumors higher than normals of 2.5 μg/L in premenopausal women and of 6 μg/L in postmenopausal women *727* Concentration significantly higher in patients with malignant tumors than in patients with benign tumors *4518*

Tissue Polypeptide Antigen *Serum Increase* In 33 patients with ovarian cancer 23 had concentrations greater than 135 U/L *4749* Using a cutoff of > 80 U/L sensitivity for stage I disease 27%, stage II 33%, stage III disease 63% and 88% for stage IV disease *1134*

TPS *Ascitic Fluid Increase* In patients with serous carcinoma 4 out of 4 positive with median concentration of 3,017 U/L, 7 of 7 with endometrial carcinoma median concentration of 10,520 U/L, 1 of 1 with mucinous adenocarcinoma median of 9,587 U/L, 8 of 8 with undifferentiated carcinoma with median of 14,100 U/L *2025*

Cyst Fluid Increase In patients with serous carcinoma 5 out of 5 positive with median concentration of 53,880 U/L, 10 of 10 with endometrial carcinoma median of 41,240 U/L, 6 of 6 with mucinous adenocarcinoma median of 7,384 U/L, 2 of 2 with undifferentiated carcinoma with median of 3,017 U/L, 6 of 6 with serous cystadenoma with median of 16,785 U/L, 8 of 8 with serous cyst with median 3,039 U/L and 13 of 13 with mucinous adenoma with median of 6,480 U/L *2025*

Serum Increase In patients with serous carcinoma 8 out of 11 positive with median concentration of 215 U/L, 12 of 14 with endometrial carcinoma median of 140 U/L, 5 of 7 with mucinous adenocarcinoma median of 137 U/L, 11 of 12 with undifferentiated carcinoma with median of 430 U/L, 4 of 6 with serous cystadenoma with median of 143 U/L, 2 of 8 with serous cyst with median of 48 U/L and 3 of 13 with mucinous adenoma with median of 60 U/L *2025*

Transferrin *Serum Decrease* In 27 women with ovarian cancer mean concentration of 132 ± 48 mg/dL not significantly different from 217 ± 39 mg/dL in 150 control women *2280*

Tumor-associated Glycoprotein-72 *Serum Increase* In 48 women with primary ovarian cancer serum concentrations of TAG-72 were above the cutoff value of 6 U/mL in 50% of patients. Concentrations were higher in poorly differentiated tumors than in well differentiated tumors and in those with residual tumor after cytoreductive surgery than in those with no residual tumor. Concentrations higher in more advanced disease than in early stages *1806*

Tumor Necrosis Factor-α *Serum Increase* In patients with ovarian cancer concentration increased compared with concentrations in patients with other gynecological cancers and in normal controls *1093*

Urokinase *Plasma No Effect* No significance observed between concentrations in patients with malignant tumors or benign tumors and healthy controls *4518*

Urokinase Plasminogen Activator *Plasma Increase* In 9 premenopausal women with malignant ovarian tumors and 69 with benign ovarian tumors mean concentration of 0.47 μg/L and in 27 postmenopausal women with malignant tumors mean of 0.42 μg/L and 0.48 μg/L in 38 postmenopausal women with benign ovarian tumors higher than normals of 0.33 μg/L in premenopausal women and 0.31 μg/L in postmenopausal women *727*

Tissue Increase uPA is a prognostic marker for cancer of the ovary *1252* Amounts predictable of overall survival *1255*

Zinc *Serum Decrease* Does not result from a shift of zinc into or release of copper out of malignant tumor tissue *3055*

183.20 Fallopian Tube Carcinoma

CA 125 *Serum Increase* Of CA 125 measurements with high concentrations in a hospital 1.3% were due to Fallopian tube carcinoma *1350*

183.90 Malignant Disease of Female Reproductive System

Carcinoembryonic Antigen *Serum Increase* In 124 patients with malignant disease of the female reproductive tract 88.7% had concentrations of 0.0 - 3.0 ng/mL, 5.6% had concentrations from 3.1 - 5.0 ng/mL, 2.4% had concentrations from 5.1 - 10.0 ng/mL and 3.2% had concentrations greater than 10.0 ng/mL when measured by method on Bayer Technicon Immuno 1® system compared with 95.9%, 3.5%, 0.6% and 0.0% respectively in 173 healthy nonsmokers *339*

184.00 Vaginal Cancer

CA 125 *Serum Increase* Of CA 125 measurements with high concentrations in a hospital 0.9% were due to cervical or vaginal carcinoma *1350*

Gonadotropin Peptide *Urine Increase* In women with cervical cancer mean concentration of 4.6 fmol/mg creatinine compared with mean value for both pre- and postmenopausal women of 1.51 ± 2.42 fmol/mg creatinine *5538*

184.90 Malignant Gynecological Tumors

Carcinoembryonic Antigen *Serum Increase* In 19 patients with nonovarian gynecologic cancer 73.7% had concentrations up to 3.0 ng/mL, 5.3% had concentrations between 3.1 - 5.0 ng/mL, 0.0% between 5.1 - 10.0 ng/mL and 21.1% had concentrations greater than 10.1 ng/mL in contrast to concentrations in 151 healthy nonsmokers in whom 95.4% had concentrations between 0 and 3.0 ng/mL and 4.6% between 4.1 and 10.0 ng/mL *11*

D-Dimer *Plasma Increase* In 9 women with malignant tumors and metastases median concentration of 5,000 μg/L significantly higher than 420 μg/L in 23 without metastases and that in 26 patients with benign gynecological tumors (median concentration of 340 μg/L) and of 240 μg/L in 31 age-matched control women *5418*

Prothrombin Fragment 1.2 *Plasma Increase* In 9 women with malignant tumors and metastases median concentration of 2.00 nmol/L and 1.35 nmol/L in 23 without metastases significantly higher than that in 26 patients with benign gynecological tumors (median concentration of 1.00 nmol/L) and 1.10 nmol/L in 31 age-matched control women *5418*

Thrombin/Antithrombin III Complex *Plasma Increase* In 9 women with malignant tumors and metastases median concentration of 8.5 μg/L significantly higher than 2.6 μg/L in 23 without metastases and that in 26 patients with benign gynecological tumors (median concentration of 2.5 μg/L) and 2.3 μg/L in 31 age-matched control women *5418*

185.00 Cancer of Prostate

Acid Phosphatase *Bone Marrow Increase* Significant in detecting unsuspected metastases before they become radiologically apparent. Bone marrow levels elevate at an earlier stage in the disease than serum levels *3307* Of the 25 patients with histologically confirmed malignancy, 18 had an elevation in bone marrow while only 11 had serum elevations *2662*

Serum Increase Characteristic observation *1933* Useful in detecting metastases but is of no value in detecting the presence of resectable carcinoma. 50 - 75% of patients with carcinoma extended beyond the capsule have elevated levels. Patients with carcinoma still confined within the capsule usually have normal serum levels *1642* May be raised, especially if the tumor has extended outside the gland. Anaplastic tumors secrete minimal enzyme *1290* Useful in detecting metastases but is of no value in detecting the presence of resectable carcinoma. 50 - 75% of patients with carcinoma extended beyond the capsule have elevated levels. Patients with carcinoma still confined within the capsule usually have normal serum levels *1025* Normal levels do not exclude possibility of carcinoma. 26% of proved cases had normal concentrations *4746*

Serum No Effect Normal activity may be observed in some patients with advanced cancer *3114* Percentage of patients with normal levels varied from 14 - 96% depending upon the stage of disease *2180* Normal levels do not exclude possibility of this cancer *2465* Some patients with known metastatic carcinoma have low values, possibly due to a recent episode of hyper- or hypothermia, as the enzyme is subject to common serum inhibitors *900*

Acid Phosphatase, Prostatic *Serum* *Increase* In one 67 year old man with poorly differentiated adenocarcinoma of the prostate and bone metastases baseline concentration of 290 ng/mL *3723*

Acid Phosphatase, Tartrate Inhibitable *Serum* *Increase* In 23 specimens from patients with prostatic carcinoma mean activity 6.84 ± 2.09 U/L compared with 1.95 ± 0.89 U/L in 300 specimens from normal men. Ratio of serum tartrate-inhibitable acid phosphatase to total protein in patients with prostatic cancer 94.52 ± 24.39 nU/g compared with 19.14 ± 8.44 nU/g in 300 control specimens *4101*

Acylcarnitine, Acid-insoluble *Serum* *Decrease* In one man with prostatic cancer mean concentration of 2.1 ± 0.2 nmol/mL significantly less than mean of 3.0 ± 0.4 nmol/mL in 6 healthy control men *1195*

Acylcarnitine, Acid-soluble *Serum* *Decrease* In one man with prostatic cancer mean concentration of 5.1 ± 2.4 nmol/mL significantly less than mean of 15.3 ± 2.6 nmol/mL in 6 healthy control men *1195*

Adenosine Deaminase *Serum* *Increase* Increased *1340* *4956* *3926*

Albumin *Serum* *Decrease* In 31% of 86 patients at initial hospitalization for this disorder *1576*

Aldolase *Serum* *Increase* Activity may be slightly increased in patients with prostatic cancer *2952* Cell destruction *5544*

Alkaline Phosphatase *Serum* *Increase* In 18 patients with stage III prostatic cancer mean activity of 82 ± 22 U/L not significantly higher, but 315 ± 287 U/L in 10 patients with stage IV disease significantly higher than 73 ± 26 U/L in 27 patients with benign hypertrophy or stage I or II disease *1158* In 54% of 83 patients at initial hospitalization for this disorder *1576* In one 67 year old man with poorly differentiated adenocarcinoma of the prostate and bone metastases baseline activity of 440 U/L *3723* Levels were elevated above the normal range in cases without bone metastases. With bone metastases, levels were much higher and 90% of patients showed marked elevations *5724*
Serum *No Effect* In 19 patients with prostatic cancer, 12 of whom had bone metastases mean concentration of 30 KAU in those with bone metastases compared with 10 in 11 healthy male volunteers without bone metabolic disease. Mean activity in those with cancer but no bone metastases of 6 KAU *4567*
White Blood Cells *Decrease* Low activity is present irrespective of tumor category, activity of disease, or type of therapy. In 11 patients, median activity was 5 U/L (normal 55 U/L) *3110*

Alkaline Phosphatase, Bone Isoenzyme *Serum* *Increase* In 18 patients with stage III prostatic cancer mean concentration of 17.0 ± 7.5 μg/L and 84.1 ± 76.7 μg/L in 10 patients with stage IV disease significantly higher than 11.0 ± 5.3 μg/L in 27 patients with benign hypertrophy or stage I or II disease *1158* In 14 men with prostate cancer with metastases median activity 82.3 μg/L (25th to 75th percentiles: 61.1 - 186.1 μg/L) significantly increased compared with mean of 13.2 μg/L in 200 healthy adult controls *604*

Amino-terminal Propeptide of Type I Procollagen *Serum* *Increase* In 18 patients with stage III prostatic cancer mean concentration of 80 ± 40 μg/L and 175 ± 105 μg/L in 10 patients with stage IV disease significantly higher than 43 ± 13 μg/L in 27 patients with benign hypertrophy or stage I or II disease *1158*

Amylase *Serum* *Increase* Reported in 95% of patients with benign hypertrophy and 70% of carcinomas. Similar results have not been reported elsewhere *1996*

Androstenedione *Plasma* *No Effect* In 166 patients with cancer of the prostate mean concentration of 8.05 ± 8.8 nmol/L was not significantly different from 8.75 ± 8.0 nmol/L in 220 healthy controls *2095*

Anti-p53 Antibodies *Serum* *Increase* Increase observed in 7 of 65 patients (10.8%) *132*

α_1-Antichymotrypsin *Serum* *Increase* Mean concentration increased above reference interval of 47.9 ± 8.1 mg/dL in 1 of 2 patients (50%) with prostatic cancer *3044*

Apolipoprotein D *Serum* *Increase* In 10 patients with prostatic cancer mean concentration of about 88 mg/L significantly different from concentration in 28 healthy women 95% confidence interval (50 - 125 mg/L, median 73.5 mg/L) *3944*

Aspartate Aminotransferase *Serum* *Increase* In 25% of 86 patients at initial hospitalization for this disorder *1576*

c-erb-B_2 Oncoprotein *Serum* *Increase* Median concentration of 8.6 ng/mL in 36 patients with metastatic cancer. 9 of 36 (25%) of patients had concentrations exceeding 1.5 ng/mL *3564*

CA 15-3 *Serum* *Increase* In 2 patients with prostatic cancer mean concentration of 192.0 ± 233 U/mL significantly different from cutoff of 22 U/mL with both patients having concentrations higher than 25 U/mL and one having a concentration above 40 U/mL *2076*

CA 19-9 *Serum* *Increase* Elevated in 3% of cases *2129* Reported effect *5381*

CA 27-29 *Serum* *Increase* In 6% of 17 patients with cancer of prostate concentration increased above 36 U/mL *766*

CA 549 *Serum* *Increase* In 87 patients with prostatic cancer 17 (19.5%) had a concentration greater than the upper limit of normal with BRESMARQ assay *764* Using a value of greater than 11 kU/L as the upper limits of normal, it is increased in 40% of cases *765*

Calcitonin *Plasma* *Increase* In 9 of 16 patients with small cell carcinoma of the prostate concentrations of 42 - 2,654 pg/mL much higher than reference interval of < 26 pg/mL *4849*

Calcium *Serum* *Decrease* In one 67 year old man with poorly differentiated adenocarcinoma of the prostate and bone metastases baseline activity of 9.1 mg/dL *3723*
Urine *Increase* Increased excretion is seen with metastases from prostatic cancer *2952*

Carcinoembryonic Antigen *Serum* *Increase* 35% of patients *5606* Increased concentrations observed in some patients *1601* *4551* In 40% of cases *4891* 30% of patients with advanced urologic tumors have elevated plasma levels. There is a good correlation between the stage of carcinoma and the degree of elevation. In general, with advanced active disease positive results exceed the normal level of 2.5 ng., whereas levels in inactive disease have been negative or at least below normal *900* In 37 patients with malignant disease of the prostate 78.4% had concentrations of 0.0 - 3.0 ng/mL, 13.8% had concentrations from 3.1 - 5.0 ng/mL, 5.2% had concentrations from 5.1 - 10.0 ng/mL and 2.6% had concentrations greater than 10.0 ng/mL when measured by method on Bayer Technicon Immuno 1® system compared with 95.9%, 3.5%, 0.6% and 0.0% respectively in 173 healthy nonsmokers *339*

Carnitine *Serum* *Decrease* In one man with prostatic cancer mean concentration of 55.9 ± 2.3 nmol/mL significantly less than mean of 72.1 ± 7.0 nmol/mL in 6 healthy control men *1195*

Carnitine, Nonesterified *Serum* *Decrease* In one man with prostatic cancer mean concentration of 38.7 ± 3.7 nmol/mL significantly less than mean of 53.0 ± 3.0 nmol/mL in 6 healthy control men *1195*

Ceruloplasmin *Serum* *Increase* In 6 men with prostatic cancer mean concentration of 159 ± 65 mg/dL significantly different from 71 ± 17 mg/dL in 106 control men *2280*

Cholesterol *Serum* *Decrease* Pretreatment levels (196 ± 1.3 mg/L) (normal 1,093 mg/L) were significantly lower than those reported for age-matched controls *4705*
Serum *Increase* Nonesterified cholesterol hyperexcretion occurred in 44.8% of stage A and B and in 52.6% of stage C and D. Total cholesterol was elevated in 52.2% and 63.2% respectively *2503*
Urine *Increase* In 42 patients, 62% were found to have levels 2.6 mg/24 h *842*

β-Chorionic Gonadotropin *Plasma* *Decrease* Patients with seminomas and teratomas should have a low titer *1108*

Chromogranin-A *Serum* *Increase* Concentration increased in 48% of 25 patients with stage D_2 prostate cancer *2519*
Serum *No Effect* In 22 patients with adenocarcinoma of the prostate mean concentration of 24.5 μg/L not significantly different from upper limit of normal of 23 μg/L *133*

Chromogranin-B *Serum* *No Effect* In 22 patients with adenocarcinoma of the prostate mean concentration of 0.9 nmol/L not significantly different from upper limit of normal of 2.0 nmol/L *133*

185.00 Cancer of Prostate *(continued)*

Complement C_3 *Serum* *Increase* Levels were found to be very closely linked to the stage of the disease. Patients in remission had normal levels, but further increases were noted in distant metastases. Levels dropped significantly in the terminal phase of disease *5456* 26% had raised levels ranging from 208 - 440 mg/dL *16*

Complement C_4 *Serum* *Increase* Increased in patients with local disease. Very closely linked to the stage of the disease. Patients in remission had normal levels, but further increases were noted in distant metastases. Levels dropped significantly in the terminal phase of disease *5456*

Complement, Total *Serum* *Increase* Closely linked to the stage of the disease. Patients in remission had normal levels, but further increases were noted in distant metastases. Dropped significantly in the terminal phase of the disease *5456*

Creatine Kinase *Serum* *Increase* Highest activity of CK-BB in brain and smooth muscle *2912*

Creatine Kinase BB-Isoenzyme *Serum* *Increase* Thirty-two percent had levels higher than 10 ng/mL *2418* *4841*

Creatinine *Serum* *Increase* In 59% of 59 patients at initial hospitalization for this disorder *1576*

CYFRA 21-1 *Serum* *Increase* In 10 patients with prostatic cancer with metastases median concentration of 1.7 ng/mL significantly different from that in 50 healthy individuals with median concentration of 1.2 ng/mL and range of 0.5 - 2.4 ng/mL *3559*

Deoxypyridinoline *Urine* *Increase* In 19 patients with prostatic cancer, 12 of whom had bone metastases mean excretion of 10.8 ± 8.0 nmol/mmol creatinine in those with bone metastases compared with 3.1 ± 2.1 nmol/mmol creatinine in 11 healthy male volunteers without bone metabolic disease. Mean concentration in those with cancer but no bone metastases of 3.5 nmol/mmol creatinine *4567* In 12 patients with prostate cancer and bone metastases mean excretion of 10.8 ± 8.0 nmol/mol creatinine significantly higher than 3.5 ± 1.9 nmol/mol creatinine in 7 patients with prostate cancer but without bone metastases and 3.1 ± 2.1 nmol/mol creatinine in 11 healthy male controls *4567*

α-Enolase *Serum* *Increase* In 4 of 4 cases of prostatic cancer mean activity increased *1705*

γ-Enolase *Serum* *No Effect* In 0 of 4 cases of prostatic cancer mean activity increased *1705*

Erythrocyte Sedimentation Rate *Blood* *Increase* In 299 patients with T > 2 30 mm/h greater than 5 mm/h in 242 patients with T1-2 cancer *533*

Fibrin Degradation Products *Plasma* *Increase* Especially with metastases *2646* Fibrinolysins are found in 12% of patients *5545*

Free Prostate-specific Antigen Percentage *Serum* *Increase* In 18 patients with prostatic cancer range of 1.1 - 30.5% (median 9.04%) *2510*

Free Prostate-specific Antigen:Total Prostate-specific Antigen Ratio *Serum* *Decrease* Median of 0.152 (range of 0.41 - 0.333) in 54 patients with prostatic cancer. At PSA concentrations of < 4 ng/mL median ratio of 0.263, in range of of 4 - 10 ng/mL median of 0.159 and over 10 ng/mL 0.100 *3006* In 74 patients with untreated prostatic cancer mean ratio of 0.100 ± 0.06 significantly lower than cutoff of 0.13 *1481* Ratio significantly lower in patients with prostatic cancer compared with benign prostatic hypertrophy *2510*
Serum *Increase* In 68 men with stages A and B, 13 with stage C and 12 with stage D disease mean ratios of 13.0 ± 7.9, 11.7 ± 8.8 and 12.4 ± 7.1, respectively, significantly different from that in 35 healthy individuals *5451*

Galactosyltransferase Isoenzyme II *Serum* *Increase* Sensitivity 0.65 and specificity 0.75 *5348*

Gc-Globulin *Serum* *No Effect* In 6 men with cancer of the prostate mean concentration of 28.0 ± 10.49 mg/dL not significantly different from 23.9 ± 3.36 mg/dL in 106 control men *2279*

Glucose *Serum* *Increase* In 36% of 86 patients at initial hospitalization for this disorder *1576*

γ-Glutamyltransferase *Serum* *Increase* In 48% of 12 patients at initial hospitalization for this disorder *1576*

Gonadotropin, Pituitary *Plasma* *Decrease* Patients with prostatic carcinoma and benign prostatic hypertrophy showed lower levels of LH when compared with age-matched controls *1992*

Hematocrit *Blood* *Decrease* In 43% of 87 patients at initial hospitalization for this disorder *1576*

Hemoglobin *Blood* *Decrease* In 43% of 87 patients at initial hospitalization for this disorder *1576*

immunoglobulin A *Serum* *Increase* 22% had elevated levels ranging from 365 - 550 mg/dL *16*
Serum *No Effect* In 6 men with cancer of the prostate mean concentration of 268 ± 182 mg/dL not significantly different from 201 ± 89 mg/dL in 106 healthy control men *2278*

Immunoglobulin G *Serum* *No Effect* In 6 men with cancer of the prostate mean concentration of 1,104 ± 620 mg/dL not significantly different from 1,148 ± 224 mg/dL in 106 healthy control men *2278*

Immunoglobulin M *Serum* *No Effect* In 6 men with cancer of the prostate mean concentration of 57 ± 18 mg/dL not significantly different from 61 ± 36 mg/dL in 106 healthy controls *2278*

Insulin-like Growth Factor *Serum* *Increase* Mean concentration in 12 patients with cancer of the prostate of 476 ± 46 µg/L significantly different from 358 ± 50 µg/L in 7 patients with no known prostate abnormality *2181*

Insulin-like Growth Factor-I *Serum* *Increase* Mean concentration in 12 patients with cancer of the prostate of 139 ± 25 µg/L not significantly different from 117 ± 17 µg/L in 7 patients with no known prostate abnormality *2181*

Insulin-like Growth Factor-II *Serum* *Increase* Mean concentration in 12 patients with cancer of the prostate of 337 ± 27 µg/L significantly different from 241 ± 37 µg/L in 7 patients with no known prostate abnormality *2181*

Insulin-like Growth Factor Binding Protein-2
Serum *Increase* Mean concentration in 12 patients with cancer of the prostate of 560 ± 66 µg/L significantly different from 367 ± 44 µg/L in 7 patients with no known prostate abnormality *2181*

Insulin-like Growth Factor Binding Protein-3
Serum *Increase* Mean concentration in 12 patients with cancer of the prostate of 2,434 ± 270 µg/L significantly different from 1,909 ± 364 µg/L in 7 patients with no known prostate abnormality *2181*

Interleukin-8 *Serum* *Increase* In 68 men with stages A and B, 13 with stage C and 12 with stage D disease mean concentrations of 15.0 ± 9.3, 18.4 ± 6.4 and 27.8 ± 16.5 pg/mL, respectively, significantly different from that in 35 healthy individuals in whom the mean concentration was 6.8 ± 3.6 pg/mL *5451*

Lactate Dehydrogenase *Serum* *Increase* In 27% of 83 patients at initial hospitalization for this disorder *1576* In advanced carcinoma following successful stilbestrol therapy and/or orchiectomy *1290* Borderline or elevated in 32 patients, regardless of the status of the disease *1119*
Urine *Increase* Increased in a high proportion of cases; useful for detection of asymptomatic lesions or screening of susceptible population groups. Increased values usually precede clinical symptoms *5544*

Lactate Dehydrogenase Isoenzyme-5 *Serum* *Increase* Consistently elevated in patients with advanced progressive prostatic carcinoma. In patients in remission, at trace levels as found in the control group *1119*

Lactate Dehydrogenase Isoenzymes *Serum* *Increase* LD_4 and LD_5 were consistently elevated in patients with advanced progressive carcinomas. In patients in remission, LD_4 and LD_5 were at trace levels as found in the control group *1119* Some correlation between the LD 5:1 ratio, and the degree of differentiation and the stage of the disease in the patient *900* Rise in LD_4 *4227*

Luteinizing Hormone *Plasma* *Decrease* Patients with prostatic carcinoma and benign prostatic hypertrophy showed lower levels of LH when compared with age-matched controls *1992*

Matrix Metalloproteinase-2 *Serum* *Increase* In 98 patients with prostate cancer mean concentration of 658.7 ± 173.9 ng/mL significantly different from 580.8 ± 162.2 ng/mL in 76 patients with benign prostatic hypertrophy and 538.0 ± 91.2 ng/mL in 70 healthy controls *1772*

Metallopanstimulin *Serum* *Increase* In 98% of 126 patients with prostate cancer mean concentration exceeded upper limit of normal of < 10 ng/mL in healthy individuals aged 19 - 88 years *1462*

Monocytes *Blood* *Increase* In 63% of 81 patients at initial hospitalization for this disorder *1576*

Neopterin *Serum Increase* Mean concentration of 27.8 ± 20.5 nmol/L in 4 patients with prostatic cancer significantly greater than that in 18 healthy control individuals, 6.4 ± 1.8 nmol/L *3864*

Neuron-specific Enolase *Serum Increase* Increased in 20% of cases *5546*
Serum No Effect In 22 patients with adenocarcinoma of the prostate mean concentration of 6.0 µg/L not significantly different from upper limit of normal of 10.0 µg/L *133*

Pancreastatin *Serum Decrease* In 22 patients with adenocarcinoma of the prostate mean concentration of 43 ng/L significantly different from upper limit of normal of 320 ng/L *133*

Pepsinogen C *Serum No Effect* Mean concentration of 2.2 ± 6.2 µg/L in 45 serum specimens from men with prostatic cancer not significantly different from that in 42 specimens from healthy men, 2.0 ± 2.8 µg/L *1151*

Phosphate *Serum Decrease* In 39% of 86 patients at initial hospitalization for this disorder *1576*

Phospholipase A *Serum Increase* With metastases *2200*

Pro-Kallikrein 2 *Serum Increase* In 29 patients with prostatic cancer mean concentration of 0.21 µg/L (range of 0.01-1.51 µg/L) significantly higher than 0.02 µg/L (range of 0.0 - 0.08 µg/L) in 20 healthy men *4500*

Procollagen 1 C-terminal Peptide *Serum Increase* In one 67 year old man with poorly differentiated adenocarcinoma of the prostate and bone metastases baseline concentration of 165 ng/mL *3723*

Prostaglandin D Synthase *Serum No Effect* In 11 men with prostate cancer median concentration of 206 µg/L and mean concentration of 215 ± 60 µg/L not significantly different from that in 33 healthy males in whom the median concentration was 208 µg/L and the mean concentration was 222 ± 72 µg/L *3444*

Prostate-specific Antigen *Serum Increase* In 29 patients with prostatic cancer mean concentration of 8.39 µg/L (range of 0.25 - 43.8 µg/L) compared with mean of 0.43 µg/L (range of 0.03 - 1.73 µg/L) in healthy men *4500* PSA is superior to digital rectal examination and transurethral ultrasound for diagnosis of prostatic cancer, especially for early or localized cancers *1254* Median of 8.8 ng/mL (range of 0.4 - 26) in 54 patients with prostatic cancer *3006* Median concentration in 12 patients with cancer of the prostate of 97.6 µg/L significantly different from 0.6 µg/L in 7 patients with no known prostate abnormality *2181* In 22 patients with adenocarcinoma of the prostate mean concentration of 29.8 µg/L significantly different from upper limit of normal of 4.0 µg/L *133* 76% of 158 patients with newly diagnosed prostatic tumors not metastasizing to bone had PSA concentrations less than 20 ng/mL and 44.5% had concentrations less than 10 ng/mL *5710* In 490 men with newly diagnosed prostatic cancer PSA concentration was directly proportional to to tumor stage and grade with median PSA rising from 6 µg/L with well differentiated tumors to 11 µg/L with moderately differentiated tumors and 29 µg/L with poorly diffentiated tumors: negative bone scans observed in all patients with concentrations less than 10 µg/L but increasing to 40% with concentrations greater than 50 µg/L *1754* In 18 patients with prostatic cancer range of 3.47 - 77.3 µg/L (median 12.4 µg/L) *2510* In 14 patients with prostatic intraepithelial neoplasia mean concentration of 35.1 ng/mL compared with 2.1 ng/mL in 81 men undergoing prostatic resection for bladder outlet obstruction *4181* In 51 patients with prostatectomy proved cancer as determined by Delphia assay mean concentration of 10.0 µg/L (range 2.3 - 37.1) *4211* In 86 patients with malignant prostate disease mean concentration of 11.16 ± 15.15 µg/L significantly increased compared with 4.46 ± 5.90 µg/L in 103 patients with benign prostate disease *80* In one 67 year old man with poorly differentiated adenocarcinoma of the prostate and bone metastases baseline concentration of 1600 ng/mL *3723* In 149 men with stage A disease 44.3% had concentrations less than 4.0 ng/mL: 37.2% of 121 men with stage B disease, 23.7% of 114 men with stage C disease and 20.3% of 74 men with stage D disease had values less than 4.0 ng/mL 30.2%, 15.7%, 18.4% and 8.1% of values respectively were between 4.0 and 10.0 ng/mL, 22.1%, 33.1%, 21.0% and 18.9% of values were respectively between 10.0 and 40 ng/mL and 3.4%, 14.0%, 36.8% and 52.7% values were greater than 40.0 ng/mL as measured by method on Bayer Technicon Immuno 1® *342* Mean concentration increases by about 3 ng/mL with each gram of tissue *4370* In 156 patients with cancer of the prostate mean concentration of 75.14 ± 289.28 µg/L significantly higher than upper limit of normal of 4.0 µg/L *1481* In 65 men with stage A disease 60.0% had concentrations between 0 and 4.0 ng/mL, 30.8% between 4.1 and 10.0 ng/mL, 7.7% between 10.1 and 30.0 ng/mL and 1.5% with concentrations above 60.0 ng/mL. 37.5% of 88 men with stage B disease had concentrations between 0 and 4.0 ng/mL, 26.1% between 4.1 - 10.0 ng/mL, 23.9% between 10.1 - 30.0 ng/mL, 3.4% between 30.1 - 60.0 ng/mL and 9.1% above 60.0 ng/mL. In 152 men with stage C disease 19.7% had concentrations between 0 - 4.1 ng/mL, 23.7% had concentrations between 4.1 - 10.0 ng/mL, 30.3% had concentrations between 10.1 - 30.0 ng/mL, 13.2% had concentrations between, 30.1 - 60.0 ng/mL and 13.2% had concentrations above 60.0 ng/mL. In 136 men with stage D disease 14.7% had concentrations between 0 - 4.0 ng/mL, 18.8% had concentrations between 4.1 - 10.0 ng/mL, 16.2% had concentrations between 10.1 - 30.0 ng/mL, 10.3% had concentrations between 30.1 - 60.0 ng/mL and 47.1% had concentrations exceeding 60.0 ng/mL *11* In patients with localized prostate cancer mean concentration of 0.71 ± 1.70 ng/mL and 5.70 ± 7.77 ng/mL in those with metastatic cancer *4836* Elevated in 122 of 127 patients with newly diagnosed prostatic carcinoma. However, is also elevated with benign prostatic hypertrophy, acute prostatitis and prostatic infarction *5364* Survival related to doubling time: 18 months survival for 53% with doubling time of less than 12 mo, 89% for those with slower doubling time and 97% for those with stable doubling time *2005* Doubling time varied from 1.2 to 36 months with the original grade and stage correlating with the doubling time as did the interval to elevation of prostatic specific antigen *2004* In 18 patients with stage III prostatic cancer mean concentration of 1.26 ± 3.17 µg/L and 551 ± 941 µg/L in 10 patients with stage IV disease significantly higher than 6.5 ± 15.46 µg/L in 27 patients with benign hypertrophy or stage I or II disease *1158* In 8 of 11 patients with adenocarcinoma of the prostate had concentrations of 8.2 - 119 ng/mL much higher than reference interval of < 0.3 - 2.9 ng/mL *4849* Elevated in 56 of 61 patients with prostatic carcinoma at a cut-off value of 2.9 ng/mL *3098* In 68 men with stages A and B, 13 with stage C and 12 with stage D disease mean concentrations of 8.0 ± 5.8, 16.0 ± 8.2 and 204 ± 303 ng/mL, respectively, significantly different from that in 35 healthy individuals *5451*
Serum No Effect In 7 of 8 patients with small cell carcinoma of the prostate concentrations remained within reference interval of < 0.3 - 2.9 ng/mL *4849* In 11 patients with stage 1 prostatic cancer, mean concentration of 2.3 ng/mL (less than mean PSA of 3.8 ng/mL in 111 patients with BPH) *877*

Prostate-specific Antigen, Complexed *Serum Increase* Using a cutoff of 3.4 ng/mL for complexed PSA resulted in 95% sensitivity and 8% specificity for cancer of the prostate *4368*
Serum No Effect In 86 patients with maignant prostate disease mean concentration of 10.59 ± 14.80 µg/L significantly greater than 3.89 ± 5.48 µg/L in 103 patients with benign prostate disease *80*

Prostate-specific Antigen, Free *Serum Increase* Use of 25% free PSA as cutoff detected 98% of cancers at age 50 to 59 y, 94% of cancers in men aged 60 to 69 y and 90% at ages 70 to 75 y when total PSA 4.0 to 10 ng/mL and palpably benign prostate glands *739* In 29 patients with prostatic cancer mean concentration of 1.38 µg/L (range of 0.25 - 8.7 µg/L) *4500* Mean %-free PSA was 9.9 ± 5.5% for cases with organ-confined tumors and 9.5 ± 5.7% for cases in which the tumor had spread beyond the gland, thus rendering the measurement of no value in differentiating extraprostatic spread of tumors from tumors confined within the gland *2116* In 51 patients with prostatectomy proved cancer as determined by Delphia assay mean concentration of 10.0 µg/L (range 2.3 - 37.1) with mean free PSA of 10.0 ± 5.5% (median 8.9%) *4211* In 18 patients with prostatic cancer range of 0.5 - 13.5 µg/L (median 1.26 µg/L) *2510* In 86 patients with malignant prostatic disease mean concentration of 1.41 ± 2.19 µg/L significantly increased compared with 0.85 ± 1.01 µg/L in 103 patients with benign prostate disease *80* Mean %-free PSA was 7.3 ± 4.2% for cases with organ-confined tumors and 12.4 ± 8.4% for cases in which the tumor had spread beyond the gland, but with considerable overlap, thus rendering the measurement of little value in differentiating extraprostatic spread of tumors from tumors confined within the gland *2116*

Protein *Serum No Effect* In 23 specimens from patients with prostatic carcinoma mean concentration of 72.48 ± 8.13 g/L not significantly different from 72.88 ± 8.03 g/L in 300 specimens from healthy men *4101*

185.00 Cancer of Prostate *(continued)*

Pyridinoline *Urine* *Increase* In 12 patients with prostate cancer and bone metastases mean excretion of 73.3 ± 67.1 nmol/mol creatinine significantly higher than 19.5 ± 7.2 nmol/mol creatinine in 11 healthy male controls *4567* In 19 patients with prostatic cancer, 12 of whom had bone metastases mean excretion of 73.3 ± 67.1 nmol/mmol creatinine in those with bone metastases compared with 19.5 ± 7.2 nmol/mmol creatinine in 11 healthy male volunteers without bone metabolic disease. Mean concentration in those with cancer but no bone metastases 24.1 nmol/mmol creatinine *4567*

Sex-Hormone Binding Globulin *Serum* *No Effect* In 166 patients with cancer of the prostate mean concentration of 56.1 ± 24.4 nmol/L was not significantly different from 55.6 ± 20.0 nmol/L in 220 healthy controls *2095*

Sialic Acid, Lipid-associated *Serum* *Increase* In 5 patients with metastatic prostatic cancer mean concentration of 86.2 mg/dL significantly different from 17.7 mg/dL in 50 normal volunteers *1273*

Sialyltransferase *Serum* *Increase* In 4 patients with cancer of the prostate mean and median concentrations of 555 and 570 cpm/mg protein/30 min significantly different from 240 and 243 cpm/mg protein/30 min respectively in 20 normal individuals *2111*

Soluble CD44 Splice Variant 5 *Serum* *Decrease* Mean concentration in 49 patients with prostate cancer of 36 ± 20 μg/L significantly different from 54 ± 23 μg/L in 30 control men *2988* *Serum* *No Effect* Mean concentration in 30 patients with prostatic cancer without metastases and 19 patients with locally advanced prostatic cancer and/or metastatic disease not significantly different from that in healthy men of 54.1 ± 22.7 μg/L *2507*

Soluble CD44 Splice Variant 6 *Serum* *No Effect* Mean concentration in 49 patients with prostate cancer of 173 ± 62 μg/L not significantly different from 179 ± 64 μg/L in 30 control men *2988* Mean concentration in 30 patients with prostatic cancer without metastases and 19 patients with locally advanced prostatic cancer and/or metastatic disease not significantly different from that in healthy men of 179 ± 64 μg/L *2507*

Soluble CD44 Standard *Serum* *Decrease* Mean concentration in 49 patients with prostate cancer of 475 ± 119 μg/L not significantly different from 501 ± 87 μg/L in 30 control men *2988* *Serum* *No Effect* Mean concentration in 30 patients with prostatic cancer without metastases and 19 patients with locally advanced prostatic cancer and/or metastatic disease not significantly different from that in healthy men of 501 ± 87 μg/L *2507*

Tenascin-C *Serum* *Increase* Mean concentration in 16 patients with prostatic cancer of 3.38 ± 2.96 mg/L significantly higher than that in 15 healthy individuals (1.09 ± 0.41 mg/L) *4626*

Testosterone *Serum* *No Effect* In 166 patients with cancer of the prostate mean concentration of 25.4 ± 9.9 nmol/L was not significantly different from 25.0 ± 7.9 nmol/L in 220 healthy controls *2095*

Testosterone:Sex Hormone-binding Globulin Ratio *Serum* *No Effect* In 166 patients with cancer of the prostate mean ratio of 0.484 ± 0.164 was not significantly different from 0.511 ± 0.317 in 220 healthy controls *2095*

Tissue Factor Pathway Inhibitor *Plasma* *Increase* About half of patients with prostatic cancer had activities greater than median activity of 1.19 U/mL in healthy individuals *2376*

Transferrin *Serum* *Decrease* In 6 men with prostatic cancer mean concentration of 195 ± 69 mg/dL not significantly different from 214 ± 33 mg/dL in 106 control men *2280*

Transforming Growth Factor-β_1 *Serum* *No Effect* In 32 patients with prostatic cancer median concentration of 30.7 ng/mL significantly different from value in matched healthy controls: no increase observed with advancing tumor stage *5711*

Uric Acid *Serum* *Increase* In 42% of 86 patients at initial hospitalization for this disorder *1576*

186.00 Cancer of Testis

Albumin *Urine* *No Effect* In 10 men aged 30 - 39 y, mean pretreatment excretion of 4.65 ± 2.54 mg/g creatinine with diuresis and 5.21 ± 2.18 mg/g creatinine without diuresis lower but not significantly different from 9.25 ± 5.86 mg/g in 10 age-matched controls *5143*

Aldolase *Serum* *Increase* Mildly elevated in tumors of the testicle and kidney. Mean = 4.1 ± 0.5 U/L compared to normal, 1.6 ± 0.21 U/L *2513*

Alkaline Phosphatase Isoenzymes *Serum* *Increase* Gonadal neoplasms (ovary and testis) showed the greatest frequency of Regan isoenzymes (placental) in cancers *1497*

Anti-p53 Antibodies *Serum* *No Effect* No increase observed in 4 patients *132*

Carcinoembryonic Antigen *Serum* *Increase* In 6 patients with malignant disease of the testes 83.3% had concentrations of 0.0 - 3.0 ng/mL, 16.7% had concentrations from 3.1 - 5.0 ng/mL, 0.0% had concentrations from 5.1 - 10.0 ng/mL and 0.0% had concentrations greater than 10.0 ng/mL when measured by method on Bayer Technicon Immuno 1® system compared with 95.9%, 3.5%, 0.6% and 0.0% respectively in 173 healthy nonsmokers *339* In 57% of cases *4891*

Ceruloplasmin *Serum* *Increase* In 16 men with testicular cancer mean concentration of 85 ± 28 mg/dL not significantly different from 71 ± 17 mg/dL in 106 control men *2280*

β-Chorionic Gonadotropin *Plasma* *Increase* Elevated in 60% of stage A and B cases and all patients with stage C disease *1538* This is an effective tumor marker in the staging and management of testicular cancer and potentially of non-trophoblastic cancers *2306* The highest incidence of immunoreactive hCG (61%) found in cancers *1497* Elevated marker assay indicates active disease in nonseminomatous testicular germ cell tumors, during and after therapeutic interventions. Normal does not exclude active disease being present *3586* *Urine* *Increase* An elevation of the gonadotropins usually indicates the presence of a tumor containing chorionic tissue and indicates poor prognosis *900* 90% of patients with testicular tumors are positive; useful in gauging efficacy of chemotherapy *5544*

Creatine Kinase BB-Isoenzyme *Serum* *Increase* Elevated CK-BB *5884*

Creatinine *Serum* *Increase* In 53% of 13 patients at initial hospitalization for this disorder *1576*

Endothelin-1 *Urine* *No Effect* In 10 men aged 30 - 39 y mean pretreatment excretion of 61.3 ± 29.8 pg/mg with diuresis and 51.5 ± 33.2 pg/mg without diuresis not significantly different from 70.44 ± 24.55 pg/mg in 10 age-matched controls *5143* In 8 patients with testicular cancer mean concentration of 48.3 ± 29.8 pg/mg creatinine less than 120 pg/mg creatinine in 10 age-matched controls *5142*

Eosinophils *Blood* *Increase* In 46% of 27 patients at initial hospitalization for this disorder *1576*

Estrogens *Urine* *Increase* Observed effect *5544*

α-Fetoprotein *Serum* *Increase* 15 out of 20 cases of teratoblastoma of testis and ovary showed raised levels *14* Elevated in 60% of stage A and B cases and all patients with stage 3 disease *1538* Concentration increased in about 50 - 70% of patients with nonseminiferous testicular carcinoma *2952* Present in embryonal carcinoma (in 27% of cases) or malignant teratoma (in 60% of cases). Concentrations of > 40 g/L are found in 75% of patients with teratocarcinoma *5544* Observed effect *5187* Over 50 ng/mL in 33% of cases of gonadal teratoblastoma *4746* Observed effect *4734* In patients with nonseminomatous testicular germ cell malignant growths during and after therapeutic interventions, an elevated marker assay indicated the presence of active disease. A normal marker assay does not exclude active disease *3586* *Serum* *No Effect* No elevations are found in conjunction with pure seminomas of the testis. In teratoblastoma, both AFP and hCG are usually absent, but may be increased in tumors with small areas of extra-embryonic tumor tissue *5759*

Follicle Stimulating Hormone *Urine* *Increase* Increased with seminoma *1290*

Gc-Globulin *Serum* *No Effect* In 16 men with cancer of the testis mean concentration of 26.5 ± 5.48 mg/dL not significantly different from 23.9 ± 3.36 mg/dL in 106 control men *2279*

Gonadotropin, Pituitary *Urine* *Increase* Increased with seminoma *1290*

Hexokinase *Serum* *Increase* Markedly increased. Mean activity of 12.6 ± 2.8 U/L compared to normal of 0.93 ± 0.28 U/L *2513*

immunoglobulin A *Serum* *No Effect* In 16 men with cancer of the testis mean concentration of 157 ± 48 mg/dL not significantly different from 201 ± 89 mg/dL in 106 healthy control men *2278*

Immunoglobulin G *Serum* *No Effect* In 16 men with cancer of the prostate mean concentration of 1,130 ± 193 mg/dL not significantly different from 1,148 ± 224 mg/dL in 106 healthy control men *2278*

Immunoglobulin M *Serum* *No Effect* In 16 men with cancer of the testis mean concentration of 57 ± 33 mg/dL not significantly different from 61 ± 36 mg/dL in 106 healthy controls *2278*

17-Ketosteroids *Urine* *Increase* Excretion may be increased in patients with interstitial cell tumors of the testes *2952*

Lactate *Blood* *Increase* Mildly elevated in 8 patients with tumors of the testicle mean concentration was 21.5 ± 5.7 mg/dL compared to normal, 11.7 ± 0.72 mg/dL *2513*

Lactate Dehydrogenase *Serum* *Increase* Marked elevation in 47 patients with tumors of the testis and kidney. Mean activity of 168.8 ± 19.5 U/L compared to normals, 85.4 ± 1.0 U/L *2513* In 38% of 23 patients at initial hospitalization for this disorder *1576*

Metallopanstimulin *Serum* *Increase* In 1 patient with testicular cancer mean concentration exceeded upper limit of normal of < 10 ng/mL in healthy individuals aged 19 - 88 years *1462* *1462*

β_2-Microglobulin *Urine* *Increase* In 10 men aged 30 - 39 y mean pretreatment excretion of 0.51 ± 0.21 mg/g with diuresis and 0.4 ± 0.14 mg/g without diuresis significantly different from 0.236 ± 0.046 mg/g in 10 age-matched controls *5143*
Urine *No Effect* In 8 patients with testicular cancer mean concentration of 0.5 ± 0.16 mg/g creatinine not significantly higher than 0.33 mg/g creatinine in 10 age-matched controls *5142*

N^2, N^2-Dimethylguanosine *Urine* *Increase* In 1 patient with testicular carcinoma excretion of 6.2 mg/d significantly different from 3.9 ± 2.6 mg/d in 17 healthy controls *5505*

N-Acetyl-Glucosaminidase *Urine* *No Effect* In 10 men aged 30 - 39 y mean pretreatment excretion of 3.12 ± 1.53 U/g with diuresis and 2.90 ± 1.28 U/g without diuresis higher but not significantly different from 2.25 ± 0.42 U/g in 10 age-matched controls *5143* In 8 patients with testicular cancer mean concentration of 3.21 ± 1.26 U/g creatinine not significantly different from 3.12 Ug/g creatinine in 10 age-matched controls *5142*

Neopterin *Urine* *Increase* In 3 patients with testicular carcinoma mean excretion of about 300 μmol/mol creatinine significantly greater than 10.6 ± 34.6 μmol/mol creatinine in 31 healthy controls *3632*

Platelets *Blood* *Increase* In 34% of 23 patients at initial hospitalization for this disorder *1576*

Pseudouridine *Urine* *Increase* In 1 patient with testicular carcinoma excretion of 114 mg/d significantly different from 65 ± 31 mg/d in 17 healthy controls *5505* In 3 patients with testicular cancer mean excretion of about 25 mmol/mol creatinine significantly greater than 19.6 ± 5.2 mmol/mol creatinine in 31 healthy controls *3632*

Pyruvate *Blood* *Increase* Mildly elevated in 8 patients with tumors of the testicle. Mean = 0.89 ± 0.18 U/L *2513*

Sialyltransferase *Serum* *Increase* In 4 patients with cancer of the testis mean and median concentrations of 588 and 444 cpm/mg protein/30 min significantly different from 240 and 243 cpm/mg protein/30 min respectively in 20 normal individuals *2111*

Transferrin *Serum* *Decrease* In 16 men with testicular cancer mean concentration of 193 ± 50 mg/dL not significantly different from 214 ± 33 mg/dL in 106 control men *2280*

Uric Acid *Serum* *Increase* In 61% of 24 patients at initial hospitalization for this disorder *1576*

186.90 Choriocarcinoma

CA 19-9 *Serum* *No Effect* In 0 of 2 men with a choriocarcinoma concentration was increased above upper limit of normal *5311*

β-Chorionic Gonadotropin *Plasma* *Increase* Median concentration of 30,000 mIU/mL in 9 patients with choriocarcinoma different from 3 mIU/mL in 58 nonpregnant controls *1929*

Major Basic Protein *Serum* *Increase* Median concentration of 174 ng/mL in 9 patients with choriocarcinoma different from 129 ng/mL in 58 nonpregnant controls *1929*

186.90 Embryonal Carcinoma

CA 19-9 *Serum* *Increase* In 5 of 8 men with an embryonal carcinoma concentration increased above upper limit of normal *5311*

186.90 Teratoma

CA 19-9 *Serum* *Increase* In 10 of 10 men with mature teratomas concentration increased above upper limit of normal *5311*
Serum *No Effect* In 0 of 2 men with immature teratomas concentration not increased above upper limit of normal *5311*

186.90 Testicular Seminoma

Alkaline Phosphatase, Liver Isoenzyme *Serum* *Increase* In 10% of stage I patients and in 85% of all stage II and III patients activity increased *2783*

Alkaline Phosphatase, Placental Isoenzyme
Serum *Increase* Activity observed in 50% of stage I seminomas and in all patients with stages II and III *2783*

CA 19-9 *Serum* *Increase* In 6 of 7 men with a testicular seminoma concentration increased above upper limit of normal *5311*

β-Chorionic Gonadotropin *Plasma* *Increase* β-hCG detected in 50 - 60% of all stage I patients *2783*

α-Fetoprotein *Serum* *Increase* In 65 patients with testicular seminoma 92.3% had concentrations up to 15.0 ng/mL, 1.5% had concentrations between 15.1 - 20.0 ng/mL, 6.2% between 20.1 - 100 ng/mL and 0.0% had concentrations above 100.1 ng/mL in contrast to concentrations in 400 healthy individuals in whom 99.2% had concentrations between 0 and 15.0 ng/mL, 0.2% between 15.1 and 20.0 ng/mL and 0.5%% between 20.1 and 100 ng/mL *11*

Lactate Dehydrogenase *Serum* *Increase* Activity increased in 50 - 60% of all patients with stage I disease *2783*

186.90 Yolk Sac Tumor

CA 19-9 *Serum* *No Effect* In 0 of 4 men with a yolk sac tumor concentration not increased above upper limit of normal *5311*

188.00 Bladder Carcinoma

Adenosine Deaminase *Lymphocytes* *Increase* Lymphocyte concentrations were elevated in all patients with transitional cell bladder carcinoma and correlated with stage, activity, clinical course and tumor resection but not with grade. Erythrocyte levels were also elevated in all cases but showed no correlation to disease parameters *5068*
Red Blood Cells *Increase* Lymphocyte concentrations were elevated in all patients with transitional cell bladder carcinoma and correlated with stage, activity, clinical course and tumor resection but not with grade. Erythrocyte levels were also elevated in all cases but showed no correlation to disease parameters *5068*
Serum *Increase* Increased *1340* *4956* *3926*

Albumin *Serum* *Decrease* In 27% of 45 patients at initial hospitalization for this disorder *1576*
Urine *Increase* May be completely negative or may show microscopic evidence of hematuria, pyuria, albumin, and threads of mucus *900*

Alkaline Phosphatase *Urine* *Increase* Elevated in 43% of 35 patients *1670* Elevated in 10 of 26 (38.5%) of active transitional cell carcinomas *4185* Reported effect *1672*

188.00 **Bladder Carcinoma** *(continued)*

4-Aminophenyl Hemoglobin Adduct *Blood* *Increase* In 13 patients with bladder cancer mean concentration of 103 ± 47 significantly higher than 65 ± 44 in controls *1096*

Arylsulfatase *Urine* *Increase* Arylsulfatase A (100%) and B (82.8%) were elevated in 29 cases of active disease *4185* Up to 40-fold increase in urinary activity *1279*

Bladder Tumor Antigen *Urine* *Increase* Sensitivity of 30% in stage Ta grades I and II bladder cancers is better than urine cytology *1142*

BTA TRAK *Urine* *Increase* Mean concentration of 212 U/mL in patients with grade I transitional cell carcinoma, 543 U/mL in patients with grade II and 914 U/mL in grade III transitional cell carcinoma significantly greater than 4.1 U/mL in healthy blood donors *539*

CA 19-9 *Serum* *Increase* Sensitivity in patients with superficial disease 25% and in those with invasive disease 43% *539*
Urine *Increase* Sensitivity in patients with superficial disease 61.5% and in those with invasive disease 69% *539*

Calcium *Serum* *Increase* Neoplasm without evidence of direct bone involvement. Parathyroid hormone-secreting tumors *1025* In one study 1 of 42 patients with hypercalcemia and low intact PTH concentration had carcinoma of bladder *3280* One of 1 patient with bladder and prostate cancer had hypercalcemia *1200*
Urine *Increase* No evidence of bone involvement. Parathyroid hormone-secreting tumors *1025*

Carcinoembryonic Antigen *Ascitic Fluid* *Increase* In malignant effusions *4891*
Serum *Increase* Increase seen in about 50% patients *1601* Sensitivity in patients with invasive disease 39% *539* In 33% of cases *4891* About half patients have increased concentration *4551* Increased in 53% of the patients (without urinary infection). No false positive results *2777*
Urine *Increase* Sensitivity in patients with superficial disease 41% and in those with invasive disease 54% *539*

Cathepsin B *Tissue* *Increase* High amounts of cathepsin B associated with poor prognosis for patients with bladder cancer *1252*

β-Chorionic Gonadotropin *Plasma* *Increase* Observed effect *5195* Observed effect in some patients *2740*
Urine *Increase* In 68 patients with benign urinary tract disorders mean excretion of 9.06 ± 1.94 mIU/mL significantly increased compared with 1.13 ± 0.08 mIU/mL in 31 normal controls with concentration higher in patients with transitional cell carcinoma than squamous cell carcinoma *1964*

Complement C_3 *Serum* *Increase* Increased in patients with local disease. Closely linked to the stage of the disease. Patients in remission had normal levels, but further increases were noted in distant metastases. Dropped significantly in the terminal phase of disease *5456*

Complement C_4 *Serum* *Increase* Increased in patients with local disease. Very closely linked to the stage of the disease. Patients in remission had normal levels, but further increases were noted in distant metastases. Levels dropped significantly in the terminal phase of the disease *5456*

Complement, Total *Serum* *Increase* Closely linked to the stage of the disease. Patients in remission had normal levels, but further increases were noted in distant metastases. Dropped significantly in the terminal phase of disease *5456*

Creatinine *Serum* *Increase* In 70% of 37 patients at initial hospitalization for this disorder *1576*

Cryofibrinogen *Plasma* *Increase* Reported effect *3417* *4551*

CYFRA 21-1 *Serum* *Increase* Sensitivity in patients with superficial disease 17% and in those with invasive disease 56% *539*

Erythrocytes *Urine* *Increase* By far the most common symptom; may be intermittent or persistent, gross or microscopic. The urine can be completely negative or may show microscopic evidence of hematuria, pyuria, albumin, and threads of mucus *900*

α-Fetoprotein *Serum* *Increase* Of 112 cases, 59 (52.8%) showed positive results, and no false positive results occurred *89*

Fibrin Degradation Products *Urine* *Increase* A high degree of accuracy (90%) was found in correlating cytology and urinary fibrinogen degradation products with the activity of the disease *5525*

Galactosyltransferase Isoenzyme II *Serum* *Increase* Sensitivity 0.63 and specificity 0.74 *5348*

Hematocrit *Blood* *Decrease* May show anemia secondary to iron deficiency or secondary to a diffuse metastatic disease *900* In 22% of 46 patients at initial hospitalization for this disorder *1576*

Hemoglobin *Blood* *Decrease* In 26% of 45 patients at initial hospitalization for this disorder *1576* May show anemia secondary to iron deficiency or secondary to a diffuse metastatic disease *900*

immunoglobulin A *Serum* *No Effect* In 16 men with cancer of the urinary tract mean concentration of 242 ± 127 mg/dL not significantly different from 201 ± 89 mg/dL in 106 healthy controls and mean concentration of 93 mg/dL in 5 women with cancer of the urinary tract not significantly different from 176 ± 80 mg/dL in 150 healthy control women *2278*

Immunoglobulin G *Serum* *No Effect* In 16 men with cancer of the bladder or ureter mean concentration of 1,126 ± 474 mg/dL not significantly different from 1,148 ± 224 mg/dL in 106 healthy controls and mean concentration of 815 mg/dL in 2 women with cancer of the bladder or ureter not significantly different from 1,157 ± 271 mg/dL in 150 healthy control women *2278*

Immunoglobulin M *Serum* *No Effect* In 16 men with cancer of the urinary tract mean concentration of 69 ± 49 mg/dL not significantly different from 61 ± 36 mg/dL in 106 healthy controls and in 2 women with cancer of the urinary tract mean concentration of 91 mg/dL not significantly different from 77 ± 39 mg/dL in 150 healthy control women *2278*

Interferon-γ *Urine* *No Effect* Excretion undetectable in 25 patients with untreated bladder cancer, as in healthy controls *2384*

Interleukin-1β *Urine* *No Effect* Excretion undetectable in 14 patients with untreated bladder cancer, as in healthy controls *2384*

Interleukin-2 *Urine* *No Effect* Excretion undetectable in 25 patients with untreated bladder cancer, as in healthy controls *2384*

Interleukin-4 *Urine* *No Effect* Excretion undetectable in 25 patients with untreated bladder cancer, as in healthy controls *2384*

Interleukin-6 *Urine* *No Effect* Excretion undetectable in the majority of 25 patients with untreated bladder cancer, as in healthy controls *2384*

Interleukin-8 *Urine* *No Effect* Excretion undetectable in 25 patients with untreated bladder cancer, as in healthy controls *2384*

Interleukin-10 *Urine* *No Effect* Excretion undetectable in 25 patients with untreated bladder cancer, as in healthy controls *2384*

Iron-binding Capacity, Total *Serum* *Increase* Secondary iron deficiency anemia may develop *900*

Iron Saturation *Serum* *Decrease* Secondary iron deficiency anemia may develop *900*

Lactate Dehydrogenase *Urine* *Increase* Reported effect *1672* Increased in a high proportion of cases; useful for detection of asymptomatic lesions or screening of susceptible population groups, and differential diagnosis of renal cysts. This test is chiefly useful in screening for malignancy of kidney, renal pelvis, and bladder; increased values usually precede clinical symptoms *5544* Reported effect *1670* 60.7% (17 of 28) patients with transitional cell carcinoma showed elevations *4185*

Laminin P1 *Serum* *Increase* Mean concentration of 1.7134 ± 0.053 U/mL in 38 patients with transitional cell carcinoma of the bladder significantly different from 1.3185 ± 0.031 U/mL in 34 healthy controls *3659*

Leukocytes *Urine* *Increase* Pyuria without hematuria is occasionally the only finding associated with widespread epidermoid carcinoma. Urine can be completely negative or may show microscopic evidence of hematuria, pyuria, albumin and threads of mucus *900*

MCH *Blood* *Decrease* May show anemia secondary to iron deficiency or secondary to a diffuse metastatic disease *900*

MCHC *Blood* *Decrease* May show anemia secondary to iron deficiency or secondary to a diffuse metastatic disease *900*

MCV *Blood* *Decrease* May show anemia secondary to iron deficiency or secondary to a diffuse metastatic disease *900*

Metallopanstimulin *Serum* *Increase* In 100% of 6 patients with bladder cancer mean concentration exceeded upper limit of normal of < 10 ng/mL in healthy individuals aged 19 - 88 years *1462*

Monocytes *Blood* *Increase* In 59% of 42 patients at initial hospitalization for this disorder *1576*

Neopterin *Serum* *Increase* Mean concentration of 11.1 ± 6.3 nmol/L in 7 patients with bladder cancer significantly greater than that in 18 healthy control individuals, 6.4 ± 1.8 nmol/L *3864*
Urine *Increase* In 4 patients with bladder cancer mean excretion of about 410 µmol/mol creatinine significantly higher than 106.6 ± 34.6 µmol/mol creatinine in 31 healthy controls *3632*

Neutrophils *Blood* *Increase* A leukoerythroblastic blood picture would indicate marrow metastasis *900*

Nuclear Matrix Protein 22 *Urine* *Increase* Median concentration of 6.0 U/mL superficial transitional cell carcinoma and 30.0 U/mL in invasive transitional cell carcinoma significantly different from 2.9 U/mL in healthy blood donors *539* Mean baseline concentration in 75 patients with 28.88 ± 1.20 U/mL significantly different from 7.42 ± 10.39 U/mL in 30 cancer-free patients *1094*

Parathyroid Hormone *Plasma* *Decrease* In one study of 42 patients with low intact PTH concentration and hypercalcemia 1 had carcinoma of the bladder *3280*

Parathyroid Hormone-related Peptide *Plasma* *Increase* In 1 patient with transitional cell carcinoma of bladder with prostate involvement concentration of 5.37 pmol/L significantly greater than upper limit of reference range of 2.6 pmol/L *1200* In one of two patients with urinary bladder cancer and hypercalcemia concentration increased to 60.7 pmol/L compared with upper limit of normal of 1.5 pmol/L *3987*

Phosphohexoseisomerase *Serum* *Decrease* Observed effect *4636*

Phospholipase A *Serum* *Increase* Reported effect *2200*

Pseudouridine *Urine* *Increase* In 4 patients with bladder cancer mean excretion of 42.8 mmol/mol creatinine significantly greater than 19.6 ± 5.2 mmol/mol creatinine in 31 healthy controls *3632*

Sialyltransferase *Serum* *Increase* In 1 patient with cancer of the bladder mean and median concentrations of 390 and 390 cpm/mg protein/30 min significantly different from 240 and 243 cpm/mg protein/30 min respectively in 20 normal individuals *2111*

Soluble CD44 Splice Variant 5 *Serum* *Decrease* Mean concentration in 19 patients with bladder cancer of 43 ± 24 µg/L not significantly different from 54 ± 23 µg/L in 30 control men *2988*

Soluble CD44 Splice Variant 6 *Serum* *Decrease* Mean concentration in 19 patients with bladder cancer of 151 ± 62 µg/L not significantly different from 179 ± 64 µg/L in 30 control men *2988*

Soluble CD44 Standard *Serum* *Decrease* Mean concentration in 19 patients with bladder cancer of 443 ± 124 µg/L not significantly different from 501 ± 87 µg/L in 30 control men *2988*

Soluble Intercellular Adhesion Molecule-1 *Urine* *No Effect* Excretion undetectable in 25 patients with untreated bladder cancer, as in healthy controls *2384*

Tissue Factor Pathway Inhibitor *Plasma* *Increase* About half of patients with bladder cancer had activities greater than median activity of 1.19 U/mL in healthy individuals *2376*

Tissue Polypeptide Antigen *Serum* *Increase* Sensitivity in patients with superficial disease 19% and in those with invasive disease 66% *539* Concentrations higher than 95 U/L observed in 3% of 61 patients with stage Ta-1 disease, 29% of 7 patients with T1s disease, 20% of 67 patients with stage T2-3 disease, 86% of 7 patients with T4 disease and 50% of 2 patients with N+ disease *5414*
Urine *Increase* Sensitivity in patients with superficial disease 71% and in those with invasive disease of 82% *539*

Tissue Polypeptide Antigen Epitope M3 *Serum* *Increase* In 5 patients with bladder cancer in whom recurrence occurred after transurethral resection of the tumor nonsignificant increase observed from mean baseline of 82.06 ± 51.96 U/mL to 117.46 ± 57.45 U/mL *3435*

Tumor Necrosis Factor *Serum* *No Effect* In 5 patients with bladder cancer in whom recurrence occurred after transurethral resection of the tumor nonsignificant change observed from mean baseline of 5.46 ± 3.32 pg/mL to 2.82 ± 2.58 pg/mL *3435*

Tumor Necrosis Factor-α *Urine* *No Effect* Excretion undetectable in 25 patients with untreated bladder cancer, as in healthy controls *2384*

Urea Nitrogen *Serum* *Increase* In 40% of 45 patients at initial hospitalization for this disorder *1576*

Uric Acid *Serum* *Increase* In 43% of 45 patients at initial hospitalization for this disorder *1576*

Urokinase Plasminogen Activator *Tissue* *Increase* Amounts predictable of overall survival *1255* uPA is a prognostic marker for bladder cancer *1252*

188.90 Vesical Cancer

c-erb-B_2 Oncoprotein *Serum* *Increase* Median concentration of < 3 ng/mL in 9 patients with metastatic cancer. 1 of 9 (11%) of patients had concentrations exceeding 1.5 ng/mL *3564*

189.00 Cancer of Kidney

Adenosine Deaminase *Lymphocytes* *Decrease* Decreased concentration in lymphocyte adenosine deaminase is found in renal cell carcinoma. Progression of disease is associated with a fall in lymphocyte values in all patients. RBC concentrations are low only in blood types B and O *5069*

Albumin *Urine* *Increase* Albuminuria often accompanies hematuria but may occur alone in metastatic renal tumors, especially those of lymphatic or leukemic origin *900*

Aldolase *Serum* *Increase* Mildly elevated in tumors of the testicle and kidney. Mean = 4.1 ± 0.5 U/L compared to normal, 1.6 ± 0.21 U/L *2513*

Alkaline Phosphatase *Urine* *Increase* Elevated in 55% of patients *1670* Occurs mainly when a tumor has extended beyond the renal parenchyma or into bladder muscle *1672*

Alkaline Phosphatase Isoenzymes *Serum* *Increase* Increased incidence of the Regan (placental) isoenzyme *1497*

CA 50 *Serum* *Increase* Elevated in a high proportion of patients with primary carcinoma *2211*

Calcium *Serum* *Increase* 5 - 15% of patients with hypernephroma develop hypercalcemia usually secondary to metastases *1724*

Carcinoembryonic Antigen *Ascitic Fluid* *Increase* In malignant effusions *4891*
Serum *Increase* In 35% of cases *4891*

Ceruloplasmin *Serum* *Increase* In 4 men with kidney cancer mean concentration of 124 mg/dL significantly different from 71 ± 17 mg/dL in 106 control men and mean of 101 ± 25 mg/dL in 5 women with kidney cancer significantly different from 84 ± 22 mg/dL in 150 control women *2280*

β-Chorionic Gonadotropin *Plasma* *Increase* Observed effect *5195* Observed effect in some patients *2740*

Creatine Kinase BB-Isoenzyme *Serum* *Increase* Eighteen of 76 patients with renal cell carcinoma (24%) had positive levels *5139* Elevated CK-BB *5884*

Erythrocyte Sedimentation Rate *Blood* *Increase* Unusually high rates of up to 150 mm/h are characteristic *367* Common *1724* Values over 100 mm/h found in 16 of 34 patients *1820*

Erythrocytes *Ascitic Fluid* *Increase* Grossly bloody ascites suggests neoplasm *4891*
Blood *Increase* Erythrocytosis is common; disappears after nephrectomy if no metastases are present *3035* Erythrocytosis has been associated with hypernephromas *4436* *4450*
Urine *Increase* 95% of patients with this disease will have either gross or microscopic hematuria at some time *900* Intermittent hematuria found in 60%, occasionally causes colic *3035* Urinalysis in malignant tumors usually reveals only painless hematuria *1980*

Erythropoietin *Serum* *Increase* Increased plasma concentrations are found in patients with erythrocytosis associated with several types of tumor, especially lung, kidney, and liver *3294* *3084* Elevated in 63% of patients but did not correlate with

189.00 **Cancer of Kidney** *(continued)*

Erythropoietin *(continued)* tumor grade, type, stage, prognosis *5070* Increased plasma concentrations are found in patients with erythrocytosis associated with several types of tumor, especially lung, kidney, and liver *547* Increased in 49 of 92 patients with renal cell carcinoma or renal cysts. Highest values were found in patients developing metastases after removal of renal carcinoma *3525*

α-Fetoprotein *Serum* *No Effect* Not elevated *2913*

Fibrin Degradation Products *Ascitic Fluid* *Increase* In malignant effusions *4891*

Gc-Globulin *Serum* *No Effect* In 4 men and 5 women with cancer of the kidney mean concentrations of 27.7 ± 5.12 mg/dL and 24.2 ± 2.77 mg/dL not significantly different from 23.9 ± 3.36 mg/dL in 106 control men and 26.1 ± 4.66 mg/dL in 150 control women *2279*

β-Glucuronidase *Urine* *Increase* All 17 patients with renal adenocarcinoma had slightly elevated activity with values ranging from 32-55 U/L (mean 42.8 ± 6.1 U/L). Uncomplicated renal cysts revealed normal urinary enzyme activities (mean concentration of 17.9 ±12.8) *3373*

γ-Glutamyltransferase *Urine* *Decrease* The only renal disorder to demonstrate a decreased value in urine *2068*

Gonadotropin, Pituitary *Plasma* *Increase* Can cause the syndrome of ectopic gonadotropin production *1980*

Haptoglobin *Serum* *Increase* May be elevated without metastases *1724*

Hematocrit *Blood* *Decrease* Anemia occurs in approximately 30% of patients, secondary to bone marrow depression *1724* Anemia is a frequent presenting symptom *3035* 30 of 34 patients with hypernephroma were anemic, due mainly to urinary blood loss. Hemoglobin values varied from 7 to 12 g/dL *1820*
Blood *Increase* Occurs occasionally due to erythropoietin formation by the tumor *413*

Hemoglobin *Blood* *Decrease* A frequent presenting symptom *3035* 30 of 34 patients with hypernephroma were anemic, due mainly to urinary blood loss. Values varied from 7 to 12 g/dL *1820* Anemia occurs in approximately 30% of patients with renal cell carcinoma, secondary to bone marrow depression by tumor *1724*
Blood *Increase* Occurs occasionally due to erythropoietin formation by the tumor *413*

Hexokinase *Serum* *Increase* Markedly increased. Mean activity of 12.6 ± 2.8 U/L compared to 0.93 ± 0.28 U/L in normal controls *2513*

Hyaluronic Acid *Serum* *Increase* In Wilms' tumors *4896*

immunoglobulin A *Serum* *No Effect* In 4 men with cancer of the kidney mean concentration of 173 mg/dL not significantly different from 201 ± 89 mg/dL in 106 healthy controls and mean concentration of 275 ± 251 mg/dL in 5 women with cancer of the kidney not significantly different from 176 ± 80 mg/dL in 150 healthy control women *2278*

Immunoglobulin G *Serum* *No Effect* In 4 men with cancer of the kidney mean concentration of 1,108 mg/dL not significantly different from 1,148 ± 224 mg/dL in 106 healthy controls and mean concentration of 1,009 ± 433 mg/dL in 5 women with cancer of the kidney not significantly different from 1,157 ± 271 mg/dL in 150 healthy control women *2278*

Immunoglobulin M *Serum* *No Effect* In 4 men with cancer of the kidney mean concentration of 54 mg/dL not significantly different from 61 ± 36 mg/dL in 106 healthy controls and in 5 women with cancer of the kidney mean concentration of 62 ± 41 mg/dL not significantly different from 77 ± 39 mg/dL in 150 healthy control women *2278*

Interleukin-6 *Serum* *Increase* In 78 patients with renal cancer mean concentration of 24.2 pg/mL (95% CI 11.1 - 37.3 pg/mL) significantly higher than 11.6 pg/mL (95% CI 10.1 - 13.1 pg/mL) in 39 healthy controls *1225*

Iron *Serum* *Decrease* Found in 30% of patients *1724*

Iron-binding Capacity, Total *Serum* *Decrease* Found in 30% of patients *1724*
Serum *Increase* Anemia due mainly to urinary blood loss *3035* *1820*

Iron Saturation *Serum* *Decrease* Anemia due mainly to urinary blood loss *1820* *3035*

Lactate *Blood* *Increase* Mild elevation in 8 patients, mean = 13.6 - 2.8 mg/dL compared to normal, 11.7 ± 0.72 mg/dL *2513*

Lactate Dehydrogenase *Ascitic Fluid* *Increase* In malignant effusions *4891*
Serum *Increase* Marked elevation in 47 patients with tumors of the testicle and kidney. Mean = 168.8 ± 19.5 U/L compared to normals, 85.4 ± 10.0 U/L *2513*
Urine *Increase* In all 16 cases, urinary activity was increased 10 fold but with no rise in tumor tissue level *2068* Mild elevation occurred in 33% of cases *1672* Elevated in 40% of patients *1670*

Leukocytes *Blood* *Increase* Leukocytosis ranging up to 100,000 /µL may occur *367*

Malate Dehydrogenase *Urine* *Increase* Increased in 75% of patients *2068*

MCH *Blood* *Decrease* 30 of 34 patients with hypernephroma were anemic, due mainly to urinary blood loss. Hemoglobin values varied from 7 - 12 g/dL *1820* Anemia occurs in approximately 30% of patients, secondary to bone marrow depression *1724*

MCHC *Blood* *Decrease* 30 of 34 patients with hypernephroma were anemic, due to urinary blood loss. Hemoglobin values varied from 7 to 12 g/dL *1820* Anemia occurs in approximately 30% of patients, secondary to bone marrow depression *1724*

MCV *Blood* *Decrease* 30 of 34 patients with hypernephroma were anemic, due mainly to urinary blood loss. Hemoglobin values varied from 7 to 12 g/dL *1820* Anemia occurs in approximately 30% of patients, secondary to bone marrow depression *1724*

5-Methyl-2'-Deoxycytidine *Urine* *No Effect* In 9 patients with cancer of the kidney mean excretion of 0.86 ± 0.25 nmol/µmol creatinine not significantly different from 0.90 ± 0.43 nmol/µmol creatinine in 81 healthy individuals *2368*

Neopterin *Urine* *Increase* In 3 patients with carcinoma of the kidney mean excretion of about 300 µmol/mol creatinine significantly greater than 106.6 ± 34.6 µmol/mol in 31 healthy controls *3632*

Neuron-specific Enolase *Serum* *Increase* Wilm's Tumor *5546*

Parathyroid Hormone *Plasma* *Increase* Lung cancer, hypernephroma, gastrointestinal cancer, and other neoplasms can synthesize and secrete parathyroid hormone *1980*

Prolactin *Plasma* *Increase* Elevated *1870*

Prothrombin Time *Plasma* *Increase* Increased in the absence of hepatic metastases *413*

Pseudouridine *Urine* *No Effect* In 3 patients with cancer of the kidney mean excretion of about 22 mmol/mol creatinine not significantly different from 19.6 ± 5.2 mmol/mol creatinine in 31 healthy controls *3632*

Putrescine *Serum* *Increase* In a patient with carcinoma of the kidney mean concentration of 0.87 nmol/mL higher than mean concentration of 0.23 nmol/mL in normal controls *3805*

Pyruvate *Blood* *Increase* Mildly elevated in 8 patients, mean = 0.89 ± 0.18 U/L *2513*

Renin Activity *Plasma* *Increase* Significantly higher in renal vein from affected side and maintains circadian rhythm despite marked elevation with renin-producing renal tumors *5545* Elevation occurred in 37% of cases of renal adenocarcinoma and was associated with high grade, high stage lesions of mixed histologic cell type and predicted poor prognosis *5070*

Sialyltransferase *Serum* *Increase* In 3 patients with cancer of the kidney mean and median concentrations of 545 and 476 cpm/mg protein/30 min significantly different from 240 and 243 cpm/mg protein/30 min respectively in 20 normal individuals *2111*

Soluble CD44 Splice Variant 5 *Serum* *Decrease* Mean concentration in 18 patients with renal cancer of 34 ± 19 µg/L significantly different from 54 ± 23 µg/L in 30 control men *2988*

Soluble CD44 Splice Variant 6 *Serum* *Decrease* Mean concentration in 18 patients with renal cancer of 160 ± 59 µg/L not significantly different from 179 ± 64 µg/L in 30 control men *2988*

Soluble CD44 Standard *Serum* *Decrease* Mean concentration in 18 patients with renal cancer of 399 ± 145 µg/L significantly different from 501 ± 87 µg/L in 30 control men *2988*

Soluble Interleukin-2 Receptor *Serum* *No Effect* In 9 children with stage I disease mean concentration of 1,016 U/mL and in 11 with stage IV disease of 1,107 U/mL not significantly different from that in healthy controls *4235*

Spermidine *Serum* *No Effect* In a patient with carcinoma of the kidney mean concentration of 0.34 nmol/mL not significantly different from mean concentration of 0.33 nmol/mL in normal controls *3805*

Spermine *Serum* *No Effect* In a patient with carcinoma of the kidney mean concentration of 0.04 nmol/mL not significantly different from mean concentration of 0.04 nmol/mL in normal controls *3805*

Transferrin *Serum* *Decrease* In 4 men with kidney cancer mean concentration of 136 mg/dL not significantly different from 214 ± 33 mg/dL in 106 control men and in 5 women with kidney cancer mean concentration of 150 ± 66 mg/dL not significantly different from 217 ± 39 mg/dL in 150 control women *2280*

Tumor Necrosis Factor-α *Serum* *Increase* In 78 patients with renal cancer mean concentration of 9.8 pg/mL (95% CI 7.8 - 11.8 pg/mL) significantly higher than 3.0 pg/mL (95% CI 2.1 - 3.9 pg/mL) in 56 healthy controls *1225*

Volume *Red Blood Cells* *Increase* True polycythemia may occur *3710*

189.00 Genitourinary Cancer

BTA TRAK *Urine* *Increase* Mean concentration of 369 U/mL in patients with genitourinary tract cancer significantly greater than 4.1 U/mL in healthy blood donors *539*

CA 15-3 *Serum* *Increase* In 4 patients with genitourinary cancer mean concentration of 26.2 U/mL higher than cutoff of 22 U/mL, with 3 having concentrations above 22 U/mL and 1 having a concentration between 35 and 40 U/mL *2076*

Prostate-specific Antigen *Serum* *Increase* Of 125 patients with cancer of the genitourinary tract, 90.4% had values below upper limit of normal of 4.0 ng/mL as measured by method on Bayer Technicon Immuno 1®, 8.0% had values between 4.0 and 10.0 ng/mL and 1.6% had values between 10.0 and 40.0 ng/mL *342* In 120 men with genitourinary cancer 88.3% had concentrations between 0 and 4.0 ng/mL, 10.0% between 4.1 and 10.0 ng/mL, 1.7% between 10.1 and 30.0 ng/mL compared with upper limit of normal of 4.0 ng/mL *11*

189.00 Renal Cell Carcinoma

α_1-Acid Glycoprotein *Serum* *Increase* In 170 patients with renal cell carcinoma concentration increased in patients with tumor stages II, III or IV compared to stage I *3095*

Acidic Fibroblast Growth Factor *Serum* *No Effect* Not detectable in the serum of 31 patients with renal cell carcinoma *1594*
Urine *No Effect* Not detectable in the urine of 31 patients with renal cell carcinoma *1594*

Alkaline Phosphatase *Serum* *Increase* Hepatic dysfunction from nonmetastatic renal cell carcinoma is associated with hepatosplenomegaly, increased alkaline phosphatase activity and prolonged prothrombin time *3625* Increased activity observed in 30.2% of 53 patients with metastatic renal cell carcinoma compared with 3.7% of 27 patients with localized renal cell carcinoma *4559* Increased activities observed in 21,1% of 365 consecutive patients withwith patholigally proved renal cell carcinoma *845*

α_1-Antitrypsin *Serum* *Increase* In 170 patients with renal cell carcinoma concentration increased in patients with tumor stages II, III or IV compared to stage I *3095*

Basic Fibroblast Growth Factor *Serum* *Increase* In 16 of 31 patients with renal cell carcinoma concentration was increased above normal of 30 pg/mL. Concentration generally correlated with tumor grade or stage *1594*

CA 15-3 *Serum* *Increase* In 51 patients with renal cell carcinoma 5 had a concentration greater than the cutoff point of 25 µg/L (sensitivity 10%) *3459*

CA 19-9 *Serum* *Increase* In 54 patients with renal cell carcinoma 3 had a concentration greater than the cutoff point of 25 µg/L (sensitivity 5%) *3459*

CA 125 *Serum* *Increase* In 52 patients with renal cell carcinoma 7 had a concentration greater than the cutoff point of 25 µg/L (sensitivity 13%) *3459*

Calcium *Serum* *Increase* Hypercalcemia of malignancy common with this type of cancer *3470* In one study in 3 of 42 patients with hypercalcemia and low intact PTH concentration diagnosis of renal cell carcinoma made *3280*
Urine *Decrease* Hypercalcemia of malignancy common with this type of cancer which leads to diminished capacity of renal tubules to concentrate urine which, in turn, decreases the ECF and the kidney's ability to eliminate excess calcium. Renal impairment eventually causes nitrogen retention, acidosis and renal failure and a further decrease in calcium excretion *3470*
Urine *Increase* Hypercalcemia of malignancy common with this type of cancer which is often associated with hypercalciuria occurring with excessive bone reabsorption *3470*

Carcinoembryonic Antigen *Serum* *Increase* In 53 patients with renal cell carcinoma 3 had a concentration greater than the cutoff point of 25 µg/L (sensitivity 5%) *3459*

C-Reactive Protein *Serum* *Increase* In 132 patients with untreated renal cell carcinoma mean concentration of 17 ± 39 mg/L significantly different from normal with higher concentrations in the presence of metastases *3343* An increase in concentration observed in 18 of 19 patients with metastatic renal cell carcinoma *5208* In 170 patients with renal cell carcinoma concentration increased in patients with tumor stages II, III or IV compared to stage I *3095*

Creatinine *Serum* *Increase* Hypercalcemia of malignancy common with this type of cancer which leads to diminished capacity of renal tubules to concentrate urine which, in turn, decreases the ECF and the kidney's ability to eliminate excess calcium. Renal impairment eventually causes nitrogen retention, acidosis and renal failure and a further decrease in calcium excretion *3470*

Eosinophil Cationic Protein *Serum* *Increase* In 12 patients with renal cell adenocarcinoma median concentration significantly higher than in controls *5293*

Eosinophil Peroxidase *Serum* *Increase* In 12 patients with renal cell adenocarcinoma median concentration significantly higher than in controls *5293*

Eosinophil Protein X *Serum* *Increase* In 12 patients with renal cell adenocarcinoma median concentration significantly higher than in controls *5293*

Erythrocyte Sedimentation Rate *Blood* *Increase* An increase in rate observed in 18 of 19 patients with metastatic renal cell carcinoma *5208* In 170 patients with renal cell carcinoma rate of 54 mm/h or higher was associated with poor prognosis *3095* In 124 patients with untreated renal cell carcinoma mean rate of 28.0 ± 33.3 mm/h significantly different from normal with higher rates in the presence of metastases *3343*

Ferritin *Serum* *Increase* Concentration tended to increase with advancing stage, but not grade and strong correlation between serum ferritin concentration and tumor volume *4017* In 170 patients with renal cell carcinoma concentration increased in patients with tumor stages II, III or IV compared to stage I *3095* In 22 patients with renal cell carcinoma mean concentration in peripheral venous blood of 157.3 ± 18.3 ng/mL (significantly less than in renal vein). In 10 patients with T2 disease mean concentration of 118.9 ± 21.9 ng/mL, in 8 with stage T3 disease of 179.5 ± 27.6 ng/mL and in 4 with stage T4 disease of 208.5 ± 27 ng/mL *2693* In 30 patients with renal cell carcinoma concentration increased. In 3 patients with pathological stage pT1 mean concentration of 113 ± 75 ng/mL, 12 with stage pT2 of 254 ± 270 ng/mL and in 9 with stage pT3 of 425 ± 257 ng/mL *4018* In 49 patients with renal cell carcinoma 17 had a concentration greater than the cutoff point of 25 µg/L (sensitivity 35%) *3459*
Serum *No Effect* Mean concentration in one patient with renal cell cancer remained with reference interval during course of gene therapy *236*

Fibrinogen *Plasma* *Increase* In 121 patients with untreated renal cell carcinoma mean concentration of 3.38 ± 0.98 g/L significantly different from normal with higher concentrations in the presence of metastases *3343*

α_2-Globulin *Serum* *Increase* In 120 patients with untreated renal cell carcinoma mean concentration of 9.8 ± 2.47% significantly different from normal with higher concentration with metastases present *3343*

189.00 Renal Cell Carcinoma *(continued)*

γ-Glutamyltransferase *Serum* *Increase* Increased activity observed in 69.8% of 53 patients with metastatic renal cell carcinoma compared with 3.7% of 27 patients with localized renal cell carcinoma *4559*

Haptoglobin *Serum* *Increase* In 170 patients with renal cell carcinoma concentration increased in patients with tumor stages II, III or IV compared to stage I *3095*

Immunosuppressive Acidic Protein *Serum* *Increase* In 133 patients with untreated renal cell carcinoma mean concentration of 538 ± 295 μg/mL significantly different from the upper limit of normal of 500 μg/mL with higher concentrations present with metastases *3343*

Interleukin-1β *Serum* *No Effect* In 60 patients with renal cellcarcinoma mean concentration of 8.5 pg/mL (95% CI 5.9 - 11.1 pg/mL) not significantly different from 5.4 pg/mL (95% CI 4.0 - 6.8 pg/mL) in 44 healthy controls *1225*

Interleukin-6 *Serum* *Increase* An increase in concentration observed in 12 of 19 patients with metastatic renal cell carcinoma. Lower concentrations associated with longer survival *5208* In the case of rapidly progressive type of bulky metastasis, the concentration of IL-6 in plasma was high *2542*
Serum *No Effect* The plasma level of IL-6 was under the limit of detection in almost all patients with a classification of T2N0M0 or lower *2542* Mean concentration in one patient with renal cell cancer remained with reference interval during course of gene therapy *236*

Macrophage Colony Stimulating Factor *Serum* *Increase* An increase in concentration observed in 9 of 11 patients with metastatic renal cell carcinoma *5208*

Parathyroid Hormone *Plasma* *Decrease* In one study of 42 patients with low intact PTH concentration and hypercalcemia 3 had renal cell carcinoma *3280*

Parathyroid Hormone-related Peptide *Plasma* *Increase* In 6 of 7 patients with renal cell carcinoma and hypercalcemia concentration increased above upper limit of noral of 1.5 pmol/L (range of 0.6 to 5.6 pmol/L) *3987*

pH *Blood* *Decrease* Hypercalcemia of malignancy common with this type of cancer which leads to diminished capacity of renal tubules to concentrate urine which, in turn, decreases the ECF and the kidney's ability to eliminate excess calcium. Renal impairment eventually causes nitrogen retention, acidosis and renal failure and a further decrease in calcium excretion *3470*

Plasminogen Activator Inhibitor-1 *Plasma* *No Effect* In 14 patients with renal cell carcinoma radical resection had no effect on concentraton. Concentration highest when degree of atypia is highest *318*

Prothrombin Time *Plasma* *Increase* Hepatic dysfunction from nonmetastatic renal cell carcinoma is associated with hepatosplenomegaly, increased alkaline phosphatase activity and prolonged prothrombin time *3625*

Soluble Interleukin-2 Receptor *Serum* *Increase* An increase in concentration observed in 12 of 19 patients with metastatic renal cell carcinoma *5208*

Tissue Plasminogen Activator *Plasma* *Increase* Mean concentration preoperatively of 7.7 ng/mL in 14 patients with renal cell carcinoma significantly higher than mean concentration of 4.4 ng/mL 15 days after radical surgery *318*

Tumor-associated Trypsin Inhibitor *Serum* *Increase* In 63 patients with renal cell carcinoma 44 had a concentration greater than the cutoff point of 25 μg/L (sensitivity 69%) and concentration correlated with the stage of the disease. In 15 patients without metastases mean preoperative concentration of 112 μg/L *3459*

Urea Nitrogen *Serum* *Increase* Hypercalcemia of malignancy common with this type of cancer which leads to diminished capacity of renal tubules to concentrate urine which, in turn, decreases the ECF and the kidney's ability to eliminate excess calcium. Renal impairment eventually causes nitrogen retention, acidosis and renal failure and a further decrease in calcium excretion *3470*

Urokinase Plasminogen Activator *Plasma* *Increase* Mean concentration preoperatively of 0.17 ng/mL in 14 patients with renal cell carcinoma significantly higher than mean concentration of 0.11 ng/mL 15 days after radical surgery *318*
Tissue *Increase* Amounts predictable of overall survival *1255*

Vascular Endothelial Growth Factor *Serum* *Increase* Mean concentration in one patient with renal cell cancer of 798 pg/mL *236*

Volume *Urine* *Increase* Hypercalcemia of malignancy common with this type of cancer which leads to diminished capacity of renal tubules to concentrate urine which, in turn, decreases the ECF and the kidney's ability to eliminate excess calcium. Renal impairment eventually causes nitrogen retention, acidosis and renal failure and a further decrease in calcium excretion *3470*

189.10 Carcinoma of Renal Pelvis

Calcium *Serum* *Increase* In one study of 42 patients with hypercalcemia and low intact PTH concentration, 1 had a tumor of the renal pelvis *3280*

Parathyroid Hormone *Plasma* *Decrease* In one study of 42 patients with low intact PTH concentration and hypercalcemia 1 had a tumor of the renal pelvis *3280*

189.80 Transitional Cell Carcinoma

Ferritin *Urine* *Increase* In 58 patients with transitional cell cancer mean excretion of 1.83 ± 0.28 ng/mg creatinine significantly greater than mean excretion of 0.89 ± 0.15 ng/mg creatinine in 58 healthy controls *830*

Nuclear Matrix Protein 22 *Urine* *Increase* Mean concentration of 6.04 U/mL or greater in 175 patients with transitional cell carcinoma of the bladder significantly different from 2.9 U/mL in 175 volunteers *4603*

Plasminogen Activator Inhibitor-1 *Plasma* *Increase* Transitional cell carcinoma of renal tract was associated with increased concentration since concentration decreased significantly after radical resection. Concentration higher when metastases present than in their absence. Concentration also highest with greatest degree of atypia *318*

Tissue Plasminogen Activator *Plasma* *Increase* Mean concentration preoperatively of 8.4 ng/mL in 14 patients with transitional cell carcinoma of urinary tract significantly higher than mean concentration of 5.4 pg/mL15 days after radical surgery *318* In 14 patients with transitional cell carcinoma of renal tract mean concentration significantly higher preoperatively than after radical resection *318*

Transforming Growth Factor-α *Urine* *Increase* In 68 patients with transitional cell carcinoma mean concentration of 116.7 ± 91.9 ng/g creatinine significantly different from mean concentration of 39.1 ± 21.9 ng/g creatinine in 39 healthy controls *831*

Urokinase Plasminogen Activator *Plasma* *Increase* Mean concentration preoperatively of 0.17 ng/mL in 14 patients with transitional cell carcinoma of urinary tract significantly higher than mean concentration of 0.08 ng/mL 15 days after radical surgery *318*

189.90 Cancer of Urinary Tract

Carcinoembryonic Antigen *Serum* *Increase* In 70 patients with malignant disease of the urinary tract 77.1% had concentrations of 0.0 - 3.0 ng/mL, 12.9% had concentrations from 3.1 - 5.0 ng/mL, 2.9% had concentrations from 5.1 - 10.0 ng/mL and 7.1% had concentrations greater than 10.0 ng/mL when measured by method on Bayer Technicon Immuno 1® system compared with 95.9%, 3.5%, 0.6% and 0.0% respectively in 173 healthy nonsmokers *339*

Gc-Globulin *Serum* *No Effect* In 16 men and 2 women with cancer of the urinary tract mean concentrations of 23.1 ± 2.36 mg/dL and 24.5 mg/dL not significantly different from 23.9 mg/dL in 106 control men and 26.1 mg/dL in 150 control women *2279*

191.90 Cerebral Tumor

Aldolase *Serum* *Increase* The serum of cancer patients contains a greater proportion of aldolase A (muscle-type) than serum from normal persons. Gliomas and normal brain tissue contain aldolase C (nerve and brain variant), but in meningiomas or tissue metastatic to brain, only aldolase A (liver and fetal form) is detected *4692*

Antidiuretic Hormone *Plasma* *Increase* Associated with excessive ADH production resulting in sodium loss *4707*

Aspartate Aminotransferase *Serum* *Increase* In 33% of 24 patients at initial hospitalization for this disorder *1576* In occasional cases *5544*

Bicarbonate *Serum* *Increase* In 74% of 21 patients at initial hospitalization for this disorder *1576*

Cells *Cerebrospinal Fluid* *Increase* Mononuclear cells are increased *2039*

Ceruloplasmin *Serum* *No Effect* In 6 men with brain cancer mean concentration of 74 ± 23 mg/dL significantly different from 71 ± 17 mg/dL in 106 control men and mean of 115 ± 89 mg/dL in 5 women with brain cancer significantly different from 84 ± 22 mg/dL in 150 control women *2280*

Creatine Kinase *Cerebrospinal Fluid* *Increase* Of 17 patients with cerebral tumors 10 had increases above upper limit of normal of 10 U/L *4780*
Serum *Increase* Highest activity of CK-BB in brain and smooth muscle *2912* In necrotic glioma *1290*

Creatine Kinase BB-Isoenzyme *Serum* *Increase* Highest activity in CK-BB component *4842*

Eosinophils *Blood* *Increase* In 41% of 23 patients at initial hospitalization for this disorder *1576*

Erythrocytes *Blood* *Increase* Erythrocytosis seen in association with cerebellar hemangioblastomas appears to be due to the secretion of erythropoietin by these lesions *4450*

Erythropoietin *Serum* *Increase* Erythrocytosis seen in association with cerebellar hemangioblastomas appears to be due to the secretion of erythropoietin by these lesions *4450*

β-Galactosidase *Serum* *Decrease* Mean serum concentration in patients with tumors (both benign and malignant) were depressed to 0.065 ± 0.009 mmol/min/L, compared with 0.243 ± 0.038 in controls *2288*

Gc-Globulin *Serum* *No Effect* In 6 men and 5 women with brain cancer mean concentrations of 25.0 ± 2.68 mg/dL and 28.4 ± 8.90 mg/dL not significantly different from 23.9 ± 3.36 mg/dL in 106 control men and 26.1 ± 4.66 mg/dL in 150 control women *2279*

Glomerular Filtration Rate *Urine* *Increase* Associated excess ADH may tend to accelerate GFR *4707*

γ-Glutamyltransferase *Serum* *Increase* Elevated preoperatively in 13 of 23 patients. Those showing elevations included 7 of 13 patients with astrocytomas, grades I-IV, 4 of 6 patients with metastatic brain tumors, and 2 of 4 patients with cerebral meningiomas *1400*

immunoglobulin A *Serum* *Increase* Concentration increased in patients with benign brain tumors but not in those with malignant tumors *3274*
Serum *No Effect* In 6 men with brain cancer mean concentration of 162 ± 56 mg/dL not significantly different from 201 ± 89 mg/dL in 106 healthy controls and mean concentration of 117 ± 65 mg/dL in 5 women with brain cancer not significantly different from 176 ± 80 mg/dL in 150 healthy control women *2278*

Immunoglobulin G *Cerebrospinal Fluid* *Increase* No consistent CSF IgG pattern was found in brain tumors, but highly vascularized tumors had increased concentrations *5138*
Serum *Increase* Concentration increased in presence of both benign and malignant brain tumors *3274*
Serum *No Effect* In 6 men with brain cancer mean concentration of 1,171 ± 455 mg/dL not significantly different from 1,148 ± 224 mg/dL in 106 healthy controls and mean concentration of 1,293 ± 365 mg/dL in 5 women with brain cancer not significantly different from 1,157 ± 271 mg/dL in 150 healthy control women *2278*

Immunoglobulin M *Serum* *Increase* Highly significant correlation observed between presence of any type of brain tumor and concentration of IgM *3274*
Serum *No Effect* In 6 men with brain cancer mean concentration of 60 ± 35 mg/dL not significantly different from 61 ± 36 mg/dL in 106 healthy controls and in 5 women with brain cancer mean concentration of 59 ± 26 mg/dL not significantly different from 77 ± 39 mg/dL in 150 healthy control women *2278*

Isocitrate Dehydrogenase *Cerebrospinal Fluid* *Increase* Increased with primary cerebral tumors *1290*

Lactate Dehydrogenase *Cerebrospinal Fluid* *Increase* In primary and metastatic tumors depending on location, growth rate, etc *5544*

Lead *Cerebrospinal Fluid* *Increase* Markedly increased (ratio 2.1:1 tumor patients/control patients) *1352*

Lymphocytes *Blood* *Decrease* In 38% of 23 patients at initial hospitalization for this disorder *1576* In 19 different groups of neurological diseases, absolute and relative T-lymphocyte populations were significantly decreased only in patients with acute Guillian-Barre Syndrome, active multiple sclerosis, and malignant cerebral tumor *5679*

α_2-Macroglobulin *Cerebrospinal Fluid* *No Effect* In patients with neurotumors concentrations normal *4641*

Monocytes *Blood* *Increase* In 63% of 23 patients at initial hospitalization for this disorder *1576*

Protein *Cerebrospinal Fluid* *Increase* Consistently found with intracranial tumors. Normal value does not exclude the presence of a tumor *900* Typical observation *2288*

Sodium *Serum* *Decrease* Associated with excessive ADH production *4707* Serum sodium usually less than 130 mmol/L *126*
Urine *Increase* Urine is almost always hypertonic to plasma *126* Often observed with decreased serum sodium concentration *4746*

Tenascin-C *Serum* *Increase* Mean concentration in 6 patients with gliomas of 4.58 ± 2.59 mg/L significantly higher than that in 15 healthy individuals (1.09 ± 0.41 mg/L) *4626*

Transferrin *Serum* *Decrease* In 6 men with brain cancer mean concentration of 172 ± 26 mg/dL significantly different from 214 ± 33 mg/dL in 106 control men and in 5 women with brain cancer mean concentration of 179 ± 31 mg/dL not significantly different from 217 ± 39 mg/dL in 150 control women *2280*

Zinc *Cerebrospinal Fluid* *Decrease* Significantly less *1353*

191.90 Malignant Glioma

Amyloid β-Protein *Cerebrospinal Fluid* *No Effect* In 1 patient with glioma concentration was 2.55 pmol/mL not significantly different from mean concentration of 4.00 ± 2.92 pmol/mL *3716*

Amyloid β-Protein Precursor *Cerebrospinal Fluid* *Increase* In 1 patient with glioma concentration was 2.92 integrated OD units significantly different from mean concentration of 1.35 ± 0.38 integrated OD units in 25 normal controls *3716*

α_1-Antichymotrypsin *Cerebrospinal Fluid* *No Effect* In 1 patient with glioma concentration was 3.30 μg/mL not significantly different from mean concentration of 2.27 ± 1.40 μg/mL in 25 normal controls *3716*

Cells *Cerebrospinal Fluid* *No Effect* In 1 patient with glioma concentration of 0.7 cells/μL not significantly different from normal of 3 cells/μL *3716*

Protein *Cerebrospinal Fluid* *Increase* In 1 patient with glioma concentration of 39 mg/dL not significantly different from normal mean of 28 mg/dL *3716*

Soluble CD95 *Cerebrospinal Fluid* *No Effect* Soluble CD95 detected in CSF of 2 of 20 patients with malignant glioma, but concentration not significantly different from that in controls *5044*
Serum *No Effect* Mean concentration of 143 ± 24 U/mL in 20 patients with malignant glioma, not significantly different from healthy controls *5044*

Urokinase Plasminogen Activator *Tissue* *Increase* Amounts predictable of overall survival *1255*

192.90 Central Nervous System Cancer

Angiotensin-converting Enzyme
Cerebrospinal Fluid *Increase* Increased concentrations observed *3895*

192.90 Central Nervous System Cancer *(continued)*

Arylsulfatase A *Serum* *Increase* Sensitivity and specificity of increased concentration for central nervous system cancer 60% and 82% respectively *2895*

Glucose *Cerebrospinal Fluid* *Decrease* Due to multiple tumors in the meninges, but these are rare causes *1290*

Metallopanstimulin *Serum* *Increase* In 1 patient with CNS cancer mean concentration exceeded upper limit of normal of < 10 ng/mL in healthy individuals aged 19 - 88 years *1462*

Metanephrines, Total *Urine* *Increase* Observed effect *3953*

193.00 Cancer of Thyroid

Antibodies against Megalin (gp330) *Serum* *No Effect* In 14 patients with differentiated thyroid cancer mean fluorescence intensity of 18.53 ± 12.90 not significantly different from that in 32 normal individuals in whom mean fluorescence intensity 14.53 ± 12.03 *3299*

Antithyroglobulin Antibodies *Serum* *Increase* In 20% of cases *116*

Carcinoembryonic Antigen *Serum* *Increase* Has been identified as first indicator of medullary carcinoma especially if cervical adenopathy present even no thyroid abnormality present *3542*

Ceruloplasmin *Serum* *No Effect* In 3 men with thyroid cancer mean concentration of 61 mg/dL not significantly different from 71 ± 17 mg/dL in 106 control men and mean of 74 mg/dL in 5 women with thyroid cancer not significantly different from 84 ± 22 mg/dL in 150 control women *2280*

Gc-Globulin *Serum* *No Effect* In 3 men and 5 women with cancer of the thyroid mean concentrations of 22.7 ± 4.73 mg/dL and 24.0 ± 4.47 mg/dL not significantly different from 23.9 ± 3.36 mg/dL in 106 control men and 26.1 ± 4.66 mg/dL in 150 control women *2279*

immunoglobulin A *Serum* *No Effect* In 3 men with cancer of the thyroid mean concentration of 317 mg/dL not significantly different from 201 ± 89 mg/dL in 106 healthy controls and mean concentration of 144 ± 48 mg/dL in 5 women with cancer of the thyroid not significantly different from 176 ± 80 mg/dL in 150 healthy control women *2278*

Immunoglobulin G *Serum* *No Effect* In 3 men with cancer of the thyroid mean concentration of 1,407 mg/dL not significantly different from 1,148 ± 224 mg/dL in 106 healthy controls and mean concentration of 987 ± 105 mg/dL in 5 women with cancer of the thyroid not significantly different from 1,157 ± 271 mg/dL in 150 healthy control women *2278*

Immunoglobulin M *Serum* *Increase* In 3 men with cancer of the thyroid mean concentration of 141 mg/dL different from 61 ± 36 mg/dL in 106 healthy controls and in 5 women with cancer of the thyroid mean concentration of 82 ± 37 mg/dL not significantly different from 77 ± 39 mg/dL in 150 healthy control women *2278*
Serum *No Effect* In 3 men with cancer of the thyroid mean concentration of 141 mg/dL not significantly different from 61 ± 36 mg/dL in 106 healthy controls and in 5 women with cancer of the thyroid mean concentration of 82 ± 37 mg/dL not significantly different from 77 ± 39 mg/dL in 150 healthy control women *2278*

PDN-21 *Serum* *No Effect* In 3 patients with follicular carcinoma and 10 with papillary carcinoma concentrations did not exceed upper limit of normal of 67 pg/mL in 98 healthy controls *5137*

Thyroglobulin *Serum* *Increase* 69 of 70 patients with increased concentration (mean of 16.8 ng/mL) following thyroidectomy had persistent or recurrent disease. Mean concentration in those with lymph node metastases was 45.8 ng/mL and 1,271 ng/mL in those with distant metastases *1266*

Thyroxine Binding Globulin *Serum* *Increase* Elevations > 300 ng/mL were found only in patients with thyroid cancer, with or without irradiation, and in all stages *1091*

Thyroxine (T4) *Serum* *No Effect* Usually euthyroid *2511*

Transferrin *Serum* *Decrease* In 3 men with thyroid cancer mean concentration of 188 mg/dL not significantly different from 214 ± 33 mg/dL in 106 control men and in 5 women with thyroid cancer mean concentration of 190 ± 22 mg/dL not significantly different from 217 ± 39 mg/dL in 150 control women *2280*

Tri-iodothyronine (T3) *Serum* *Increase* Rarely in follicular cancer *2511*
Serum *No Effect* Usually euthyroid *2511*

193.10 Medullary Carcinoma of Thyroid

Aspartate Aminotransferase *Serum* *Increase* In 31% of 22 patients at initial hospitalization for this disorder *1576*

Calcitonin *Plasma* *Increase* In 2 of 2 patients (100%) with medullary thyroid carcinomas and chronic diarrhea was concentration increased above upper limit of normal of 71 pg/mL *4635* Increased in both thyroid and bronchogenic carcinomas. Medullary thyroid cancer is characterized by the presence of at least 7 different fractions, ranging from fraction I to V. Bronchogenic cancers had a predominance of high molecular weight fractions (I and IIa) *357* Increased basal and pentagastrin stimulated concentrations are characteristic of medullary thyroid carcinoma *2952* Observed in 2 patients with medullary cancer of the thyroid *3486* Observed effect *1980* Increased baseline levels or increased level after calcium infusion indicates medullary carcinoma. May be found even in absence of palpable mass in the thyroid *5545*
Urine *Increase* Urinary calcitonin is high in medullary cancer patients *1980*

Calcium *Serum* *No Effect* Usually normal, in spite of very high titers of plasma calcitonin seen in medullary cancer of the thyroid *1980*

Carcinoembryonic Antigen *Serum* *Increase* Over 5 ng/mL in 20% of patients. All patients with medullary carcinoma had considerably elevated levels (> 25 ng/mL) *1297*

Chromogranin-A *Serum* *Increase* In 19 patients with medullary carcinoma of thyroid mean concentration of 228 µg/L significantly different from 36 ± 18 µg/L in 100 normal individuals *329*

Corticotropin *Plasma* *Increase* May occur *2034* In two patients with medullary carcinoma of the thyroid concentrations ranged from 108 to 204 pg/mL significantly increased compared with normal of less than 60 pg/mL *4262*

Fucose *Serum* *Increase* Elevation was less significant in early and locally restricted disease. Mean value was 10.36 ± 0.41 (normal = 6.48 ± 0.13 mg/dL) *2899*

Gastrin-releasing Peptide *Serum* *Increase* In one of 2 patients (50%) with medullary thyroid carcinomas and chronic diarrhea was concentration increased above upper limit of normal of 542 pg/mL *4635*

Histamine *Plasma* *Increase* Abnormally increased activity found in medullary carcinoma, falling after surgical removal, and increasing if residual tumor present *1290*

5-Hydroxytryptamine *Blood* *Increase* In medullary cancer *1980*

Neuron-specific Enolase *Serum* *Increase* In 19 patients with medullary thyroid carcinoma mean concentration of 48.1 µg/L significantly different from normal range of < 12.5 µg/L *329*

Neurotensin *Plasma* *No Effect* In neither of 2 patients with medullary thyroid carcinomas and chronic diarrhea was concentration increased above upper limit of normal of 250 pg/mL *4635*

Pancreatic Polypeptide *Plasma* *No Effect* In neither of 2 patients with medullary thyroid carcinomas and chronic diarrhea was concentration increased above upper limit of normal of 465 pg/mL *4635*

Parathyroid Hormone *Plasma* *Increase* Elevations in about 50% of medullary cancer patients *1980*

PDN-21 *Serum* *Increase* In 25 patients with medullary carcinoma concentrations of PDN-21 (katacalcin) ranged from 110 to 18,300 pg/mL (mean 5,940 pg/mL) significantly higher than upper limit of normal of 67 pg/mL in 98 healthy controls *5137*

Phosphate *Serum* *No Effect* Usually normal, in spite of very high titers of plasma calcitonin seen in medullary cancer of the thyroid *1980*

Potassium *Feces* *Increase* About 33% of patients with medullary carcinoma have watery diarrhea with stools characteristically containing increased sodium and potassium content *4891*

Proopiomelanocortin *Plasma Increase* In two patients with medullary carcinoma of the thyroid concentrations ranged from 399 to 1,741 pg/mL significantly increased compared with normal *4262* In two patients with medullary carcinoma of the thyroid concentrations ranged from 80 to 200 U/mL compared with normal of less than 60 U/mL *4262*

Prostaglandins *Plasma Increase* May occur *2034*

Sodium *Feces Increase* About 33% of patients with medullary carcinoma have watery diarrhea with stools characteristically containing increased sodium and potassium content *4891*

Somatostatin *Plasma No Effect* In neither of 2 patients with medullary thyroid carcinomas and chronic diarrhea was concentration increased above upper limit of normal of 68 pg/mL *4635*

Substance P *Plasma No Effect* In neither of 2 patients with medullary thyroid carcinomas and chronic diarrhea was concentration increased above upper limit of normal of 240 pg/mL *4635*

T3-Uptake *Serum No Effect* Concentration typically normal *5544*

Vasoactive Intestinal Polypeptide *Plasma No Effect* In neither of 2 patients with medullary thyroid carcinomas and chronic diarrhea was concentration increased above upper limit of normal of 84 pg/mL *4635*

194.00 Adrenal Cancer

Aldosterone *Plasma Increase* In tumors of the zona glomerulosa *1108*
Urine Increase In tumors of the zona glomerulosa *1108*

Androgens *Plasma Increase* Excessive androgen secretion in adrenocortical carcinoma *5863*

Corticosterone *Plasma Increase* In tumors of the zona glomerulosa or zona fasciculata *1108*

Corticotropin *Plasma Decrease* Very low or undetectable in Cushing's patients with adrenocortical tumors *5863*

Cortisol *Plasma Increase* Both 9 h and 23 h basal plasma concentrations are very high *5863* In tumors of the zona fasciculata *1108*

Dehydroepiandrosterone *Plasma Increase* Virilizing adrenal tumors *2034*

Dehydroepiandrosterone Sulfate *Plasma Increase* Observed effect *91 3778*

Dehydroisoandrosterone *Urine Increase* Usually increased *5544*

Estrogens *Urine Increase* Principally due to increments in estriol and also to increments in estradiol and estrone *2034*

Follicle Stimulating Hormone *Urine Decrease* Observed effect *456*

Follistatin, Free *Serum Increase* Mean concentration in 4 patients with adrenal cancer of 7.9 ± 3.8 µg/L not significantly different from that in patients with other cancers but significantly higher than 3.5 ± 0.2 µg/L in 60 normal individuals *4523*

Gonadotropin, Pituitary *Plasma Increase* Feminizing adrenal tumor can cause the syndrome of ectopic gonadotropin production *1980*

11-Hydroxycorticosteroids *Urine Increase* Usually very high *5863*

17-Hydroxycorticosteroids *Urine Increase* Excretion typically increased *1025*
Urine No Effect Can be normal to moderately elevated in masculinizing or feminizing tumors *2034*

17-Ketogenic Steroids *Urine Increase* Very high values in Cushing's suggests ectopic ACTH production or adrenocortical carcinoma *5863*
Urine No Effect Can be normal to moderately elevated in masculinizing or feminizing tumors *2034*

17-Ketosteroids *Urine Increase* Often may be greatly increased *5544* Excretion usually increased *1290* Excretion may be increased in patients with adrenal carcinomas *2952* Usually very high *5863*

Pregnanetriol *Urine Increase* Virilizing adrenal tumors *2034*

194.00 Neuroblastoma

Arylsulfatase *Urine Increase* Urine arylsulfatase and homovanillic acid are inversely related in neuroblastomas. In melanotic tumors, HVA is elevated and arylsulfatase normal or slightly elevated. Amelanotic tumors have low-normal HVA and high arylsulfatase *3600*

Carcinoembryonic Antigen *Serum Increase* In 100% of cases *4891*

Catecholamines *Plasma Increase* Catecholamine secretion is as high or higher than in pheochromocytoma *5863*

Chromogranin-A *Serum Increase* Mean concentration in 11 patients with active neuroblastoma significantly higher than that in 21 healthy volunteers in heparin/glutathione plasma (16.3 - 21.5 U/L with upper limit of normal of 30.4 U/L) but with 3 patients (27%) having concentrations below the upper limit of normal *524*

Dopamine *Plasma Increase* Excess secretion in some tumors *5863* Increased production by neuroblastoma cell system *3600*
Urine Increase Elevated levels receded toward normal after treatment *3305*

Homovanillic Acid *Urine Increase* Best diagnostic test for neuroblastoma in 42 patients was homovanillic acid with a sensitivity of 90% *5478* Elevated levels receded toward normal after treatment *3305* Urine arylsulfatase and homovanillic acid are inversely related in neuroblastomas. In melanotic tumors, HVA is elevated and arylsulfatase normal or slightly elevated. Amelanotic tumors have low-normal HVA and high arylsulfatase *3600* increased excretion observed in patients with neuroblastoma *2952*

Neuron-specific Enolase *Serum Increase* In 80 patients with neuroblastoma median concentration of 9.9 ng/mL in stage 1, 45.1 ng/mL in stage 2, 49 ng/mL in stage 3, 93.9 ng/mL in stage 4 and 53.4 ng/mL in stage 4S significantly different from upper limit of normal of 12 ng/mL in 100 healthy children *3336* Reported observation *5546*

Neuropeptide Y *Plasma Increase* Median concentration of 15.2 pmol/L significantly different from reference interval of 1.8 - 2.4 pmol/L *3847*

Polysialylated Neural Cell Adhesion Molecule
Serum No Effect In 14 children with neuroblastoma mean concentrations varied from 30.7 to 1,377.0 kU/L significantly different from mean of 26.8 kU/L in 269 healthy controls *1743*

Vanillylmandelic Acid *Urine Increase* Excretion > 2 times normal is diagnostic providing all dietary restrictions have been followed *5863* False positive results may occur due to certain foods and certain drugs. Detects 75% of neuroblastomas, ganglioneuromas and ganglioblastomas if used alone. In combination with HVA or total catecholamines, 95 - 100% may be detected *5544*

194.30 Malignant Neoplasm of Pituitary Gland

Corticotropin *Cerebrospinal Fluid Increase* 21 of 22 patients with suprasellar extension of a pituitary tumor had elevations of one or more CSF adenohypophyseal hormones *2488*

Follicle Stimulating Hormone *Cerebrospinal Fluid Increase* 21 of 22 patients with suprasellar extension of a pituitary tumor had elevations of one or more CSF adenohypophyseal hormones *2488*

Growth Hormone *Cerebrospinal Fluid Increase* 21 of 22 patients with suprasellar extension of a pituitary tumor had elevations of one or more CSF adenohypophyseal hormones *2488*

Luteinizing Hormone *Cerebrospinal Fluid Increase* 21 of 22 patients with suprasellar extension of a pituitary tumor had elevations of one or more CSF adenohypophyseal hormones *2488*

Prolactin *Cerebrospinal Fluid Increase* 21 of 22 patients with suprasellar extension of a pituitary tumor had elevations of one or more CSF adenohypophyseal hormones *2488*

194.80 Multiple Endocrine Neoplasia Type 2

Epinephrine *Plasma Increase* In 9 patients with MEN-2 and pheochromocytoma mean concentration of 151 pg/mL significantly different from 18 pg/mL in 178 reference individuals *1313*
Urine Increase In 9 patients with MEN-2 and pheochromocytoma mean excretion of 72 µg/d significantly different from 9 µg/d in 178 reference individuals *1313*

Metanephrine *Plasma Increase* In 9 patients with MEN-2 and pheochromocytoma mean concentration of 877 pg/mL significantly different from 27 pg/mL in 178 reference individuals *1313*
Urine Increase In 9 patients with MEN-2 and pheochromocytoma mean excretion of 5.8 µg/d significantly different from 0 - 1.2 µg/d in 178 reference individuals *1313*

Norepinephrine *Plasma Increase* In 9 patients with MEN-2 and pheochromocytoma mean concentration of 723 pg/mL significantly different from 200 pg/mL in 178 reference individuals *1313*
Urine Increase In 9 patients with MEN-2 and pheochromocytoma mean excretion of 137 µg/d significantly different from 38 µg/d in 178 reference individuals *1313*

Normetanephrine *Plasma Increase* In 9 patients with MEN-2 and pheochromocytoma mean concentration of 1,109 pg/mL significantly different from 45 pg/mL in 178 reference individuals *1313*

Vanillylmandelic Acid *Urine Increase* In 9 patients with MEN-2 and pheochromocytoma mean excretion of 19.9 µg/d significantly different from 0 - 7.9 µg/d in 178 reference individuals *1313*

195.00 Head and Neck Cancer

c-erb-B_2 Oncoprotein *Serum No Effect* Median concentration of < 3 ng/mL in 9 patients with locoregional cancer. 0 of 9 (0%) of patients with locoregional disease had concentrations exceeding 1.5 ng/mL *3564*

Calcium *Serum Increase* Hypercalcemia of malignancy common with this type of cancer *3470*
Urine Decrease Hypercalcemia of malignancy common with this type of cancer which leads to diminished capacity of renal tubules to concentrate urine which, in turn, decreases the ECF and the kidney's ability to eliminate excess calcium. Renal impairment eventually causes nitrogen retention, acidosis and renal failure and a further decrease in calcium excretion *3470*
Urine Increase Hypercalcemia of malignancy common with this type of cancer which is often associated with hypercalciuria occurring with excessive bone reabsorption *3470*

Cathepsin D *Serum Increase* Mean concentration of 3.9 pmol/mL or 4.7 pmol/mL, depending on stage of disease (squamous cell carcinoma) significantly different from median concentration of 3.6 pmol/mL in 15 healthy control individuals *5051*

Creatinine *Serum Increase* Hypercalcemia of malignancy common with this type of cancer which leads to diminished capacity of renal tubules to concentrate urine which, in turn, decreases the ECF and the kidney's ability to eliminate excess calcium. Renal impairment eventually causes nitrogen retention, acidosis and renal failure and a further decrease in calcium excretion *3470*

CYFRA 21-1 *Serum Increase* Concentration increased in 60% of new squamous cell carcinoma patients but in only 8% of patients with benign tumors and 3.5% of healthy controls. Concentration tended to increase with increasing severity of the disease and was inversely related to histological grade, i.e. higher in poorly differentiated carcinoma than in well differentiated carcinomas *286* In 42 patients with head and neck cancer without metastases median concentration of 2.0 ng/mL and in 9 with metastases 3.1 ng/mL significantly different from that in 50 healthy individuals with median concentration of 1.2 ng/mL and range of 0.5 - 2.4 ng/mL *3559* In 20 patients with squamous cell carcinoma of head or neck mean concentration of 2.14 ± 1.94 ng/mL significantly higher than 0.79 ± 0.29 ng/mL in 29 healthy controls, although concentration only 0.78 ± 0.35 ng/mL in 16 patients with tumors in remission *1230*

Erythropoietin *Serum Decrease* In 5 of 10 patients with head or neck cancer inappropriately low concentrations were observed and 2 additional patients had a reduced concentration with cisplatin therapy *4901*

Immunosuppressive Acidic Protein *Serum Increase* In patients with advanced disease concentration significantly higher than in early stage disease and control population. Increases also observed in patients with recurrences *3724*

Metallopanstimulin *Serum Increase* In 100% of 6 patients with head and neck cancer mean concentration exceeded upper limit of normal of < 10 ng/mL in healthy individuals aged 19 - 88 years *1462*

Neopterin *Urine Increase* Frequency of increased concentrations in patients with cancer of the neck 20% *121*

p53 Autoantibodies *Serum Increase* In 143 patients with head and neck cancer 39 (27.3%) were seropositive for p53 antibodies, with a prognostic value of p53 antibodies in treatment failures *5640*

pH *Blood Decrease* Hypercalcemia of malignancy common with this type of cancer which leads to diminished capacity of renal tubules to concentrate urine which, in turn, decreases the ECF and the kidney's ability to eliminate excess calcium. Renal impairment eventually causes nitrogen retention, acidosis and renal failure and a further decrease in calcium excretion *3470*

Urea Nitrogen *Serum Increase* Hypercalcemia of malignancy common with this type of cancer which leads to diminished capacity of renal tubules to concentrate urine which, in turn, decreases the ECF and the kidney's ability to eliminate excess calcium. Renal impairment eventually causes nitrogen retention, acidosis and renal failure and a further decrease in calcium excretion *3470*

Volume *Urine Increase* Hypercalcemia of malignancy common with this type of cancer which leads to diminished capacity of renal tubules to concentrate urine which, in turn, decreases the ECF and the kidney's ability to eliminate excess calcium. Renal impairment eventually causes nitrogen retention, acidosis and renal failure and a further decrease in calcium excretion *3470*

195.20 Intra-abdominal Desmoplastic Small Round-Cell Tumors

CA 15-3 *Serum No Effect* In 7 patients with intra-abdominal desmoplastic small round-cell tumors mean concentration within reference interval *1501*

CA 19-9 *Serum No Effect* In 7 patients with intra-abdominal desmoplastic small round-cell tumors mean concentration within reference interval *1501*

CA 125 *Serum Increase* In 7 patients with intra-abdominal desmoplastic small round-cell tumors median concentration increased in six, with median value of 200 U/mL and range of 22 - 735 U/mL *1501*

Carcinoembryonic Antigen *Serum No Effect* In 7 patients with intra-abdominal desmoplastic small round-cell tumors mean concentration within reference interval *1501*

β-Chorionic Gonadotropin *Plasma No Effect* In 7 patients with intra-abdominal desmoplastic small round-cell tumors mean concentration within reference interval *1501*

α-Fetoprotein *Serum No Effect* In 7 patients with intra-abdominal desmoplastic small round-cell tumors mean concentration within reference interval *1501*

Neuron-specific Enolase *Serum Increase* In 5 patients with intra-abdominal desmoplastic small round-cell tumors median concentration increased in three, with median value of 19 ng/mL and range of 6.8 - 37.5 ng/mL *1501*

Secondary Malignant Neoplasms

197.00 Secondary Malignant Neoplasm of Respiratory System

α_1-Acid Glycoprotein *Pleural Fluid Increase* Highest levels found in malignant exudates *3713 2597 4853 4696 4241 4373*
Serum Increase Elevated with metastases and larger tumor mass *4373 4853 2597 3713 4241 4696*

Alanine Aminotransferase *Serum Increase* In 24% of 33 patients at initial hospitalization for this disorder *1576*

Albumin *Serum* *Decrease* In 30% of 601 patients at initial hospitalization for this disorder *1576*

Alkaline Phosphatase *Serum* *Increase* In 49% of 588 patients at initial hospitalization for this disorder *1576*
White Blood Cells *Decrease* Patients with metastases of the lung, bone and skin all showed decreased activity, with median values of 6.4 20.5, and 10.0 U/L respectively (normal 55 U/L) *3110*

Amylase *Pleural Fluid* *No Effect* Usually less than or equal to serum level *4493*

Aspartate Aminotransferase *Serum* *Increase* In 48% of 592 patients at initial hospitalization for this disorder *1576*

Bicarbonate *Serum* *Increase* In 41% of 280 patients at initial hospitalization for this disorder *1576*

Calcium *Serum* *Increase* In 7 cases of bronchogenic metastases, hypercalcemia was recorded (range of 10.6 - 16.4 mg/dL) *4311*

Carcinoembryonic Antigen *Ascitic Fluid* *Increase* In malignant effusions *4891*

Erythrocytes *Pleural Fluid* *Increase* 1,000 - > 100,000 /μL *4493* 1,000 - > 100,000 /μL *1980*

Factor II *Plasma* *Decrease* May be associated with defibrination resulting in platelet and coagulation factor consumption *5677*

Factor IV *Plasma* *Decrease* May be associated with defibrination resulting in platelet and coagulation factor consumption *5677*

Fibrinogen *Plasma* *Decrease* May be associated with defibrination resulting in platelet and coagulation factor consumption *5677*

Glucose *Pleural Fluid* *Decrease* Markedly reduced, 20 mg/dL or less, is very suggestive and virtually diagnostic of rheumatoid disease. A low level in the range of 40 mg/dL can be found in infectious processes and in malignant pleural effusions *1980*

γ-Glutamyltransferase *Serum* *Increase* In 62% of 106 patients at initial hospitalization for this disorder *1576*

Hematocrit *Blood* *Decrease* In 28% of 603 patients at initial hospitalization for this disorder *1576*

Hemoglobin *Blood* *Decrease* In 37% of 597 patients at initial hospitalization for this disorder *1576*

Iron *Serum* *Decrease* In 55% of 43 patients at initial hospitalization for this disorder *1576*

Iron-binding Capacity, Total *Serum* *Decrease* In 39% of 43 patients at initial hospitalization for this disorder *1576*

Iron Saturation *Serum* *Decrease* In 59% of 43 patients at initial hospitalization for this disorder *1576*

Lactate Dehydrogenase *Pleural Fluid* *Increase* A markedly elevated pleural LD is consistent with neoplastic involvement of the pleura. Not specific for the diagnosis *1980*
Serum *Increase* From a study of 50 patients, a semiquantitative relationship appeared with LD, rapidity of tumor growth, and degree of dissemination of the neoplastic process *5736* In 50% of 574 patients at initial hospitalization for this disorder *1576*

Leukocytes *Blood* *Increase* In 25% of 604 patients at initial hospitalization for this disorder *1576*

Lymphocytes *Blood* *Decrease* In 59% of 581 patients at initial hospitalization for this disorder *1576*
Pleural Fluid *Decrease* In patients with pulmonary tuberculosis, pulmonary malignancy or nonspecific pleuritis, the percentages and absolute number of B lymphocytes were significantly lower in pleural fluid than in peripheral blood *4104*

Monocytes *Blood* *Increase* In 61% of 584 patients at initial hospitalization for this disorder *1576*
Pleural Fluid *Increase* Predominant cell type *4493*

Neutrophils *Blood* *Increase* In 55% of 584 patients at initial hospitalization for this disorder *1576*

Oxygen Partial Pressure *Blood* *Decrease* In 65% of 67 patients at initial hospitalization for this disorder *1576*

Oxygen Saturation *Blood* *Decrease* Impaired diffusion *874*

pH *Pleural Fluid* *Decrease* Exudate (pH < 7.3) *126*
Pleural Fluid *No Effect* pH < 7.40 militates against malignancy, especially in the absence of infection and < 7.30 is rarely encountered in tuberculous pleural disease *1980*

Phosphate *Serum* *Decrease* In 26% of 603 patients at initial hospitalization for this disorder *1576*

Platelets *Blood* *Decrease* May be associated with defibrination resulting in platelet and coagulation factor consumption *5677*
Blood *Increase* May be increased in malignancy especially disseminated, advanced or inoperable *5545* In 31% of 508 patients at initial hospitalization for this disorder *1576*

Protein *Pleural Fluid* *Increase* Exudate *4493*

Prothrombin Consumption *Blood* *Increase* May be associated with defibrination resulting in platelet and coagulation factor consumption *5677*

Rheumatoid Factor *Pleural Fluid* *Increase* May be present with rheumatoid disease, but may also be found in other types of pleural effusions (e.g., carcinoma, tuberculosis, bacterial pneumonia) *5544*

Specific Gravity *Pleural Fluid* *Increase* Exudate (> 1.016) *126*

Uric Acid *Serum* *Increase* In 39% of 602 patients at initial hospitalization for this disorder *1576*

197.60 Peritoneal Carcinomatosis

β-Chorionic Gonadotropin *Ascitic Fluid* *Increase* Concentration above 10 mIU/mL observed in 18 of 27 patients with peritoneal carcinomatosis *1702*

197.70 Secondary Cancer of Liver

α_1-Acid Glycoprotein *Serum* *Increase* Sensitivity of 65% and a specificity of 80% with severe liver disease *1439*

Alanine Aminotransferase *Serum* *Increase* Raised in 33% of cases of liver metastases *4692* Modestly elevated (145 U/L). All cases of intrahepatic disease showed elevations. Values ranged from 12.5 - 116 U/L *5738* Generally parallels AST but the increase is less marked *5544* Occasional elevation *5008* 83% of 12 patients showed increase. Mean elevation of 72 U/L (normal = 24 U/L) *3161*

Aldolase *Serum* *Increase* Elevated in 75% of cases of liver metastases *4692*

Alkaline Phosphatase *Serum* *Increase* Closely parallels serum bilirubin *4707* Useful index of partial obstruction of the biliary tree when serum bilirubin is usually normal and urine bilirubin is increased. Increased in 80% of patients with metastatic carcinoma *5544* Degree of elevation may at times be striking with little or no rise in bilirubin. Occurs in 80% of cases, usually ranging from 25 - 375 U/L with 20% of cases showing values > 107 U/L *1025* Consistent elevation with metastases *2803*
White Blood Cells *Increase* Parallel alkaline phosphatase but is not affected by bone disease *5544* Liver metastases appear to be the only metastatic site which tends to increase activity. Patients with liver metastases had a median value of 65 U/L (normal 55 U/L). Other primary and secondary malignancies usually present significantly low levels *3110*

Alkaline Phosphatase Isoenzymes *Serum* *Increase* 23 of 24 patients with metastatic carcinoma of liver had markedly elevated liver alpha$_1$ and alpha$_2$ alkaline phosphatase isoenzyme levels. Mean values were 19 ± 18 U/L and 45 ± 28 U/L respectively *4341*

δ-Aminolevulinic Acid *Urine* *Increase* May occur *1025*

Aspartate Aminotransferase *Serum* *Increase* Approximately 50% of patients with metastatic carcinoma have elevated values, usually in the same range as in patients with cirrhosis and posthepatic jaundice. Usual values < 145 U/L *1025* All 12 cases of liver metastases showed a moderate elevation (mean 106 U/L). Normal upper limit 24 U/L *3161*

Bilirubin *Serum* *Increase* Elevated serum bilirubin values of 2.6 - 12.2 mg/dL were reported in patients with carcinoma metastatic to liver *5738*
Serum *No Effect* Common finding *413*
Urine *Increase* Increased serum alkaline phosphatase is the most useful index of partial obstruction of the biliary tree when serum bilirubin is usually normal and urine bilirubin is increased *5544*

BSP Retention *Serum* *Increase* Increased serum alkaline phosphatase and increased BSP retention is 65% reliable to establish this diagnosis *5544*

197.70 Secondary Cancer of Liver (continued)

CA 195 *Serum* *Increase* The sensitivity and specificity in hepatocellular carcinoma and metastatic carcinoma were 60% and 22% and 87% and 42% respectively *3228*

Carcinoembryonic Antigen *Ascitic Fluid* *Increase* In malignant effusions *4891*
Serum *Increase* Markedly increased (> 25 ng/mL) values are highly suggestive of metastatic cancer, particularly hepatic metastasis *1767*

Cholinesterase *Serum* *Decrease* Some patients *5544*

Copper *Serum* *Increase* High in advanced carcinoma with liver metastases *2341*

Creatine *Urine* *Increase* Increased formation *1290*

Creatine Kinase BB-Isoenzyme *Serum* *Increase* Elevated CK-BB *5884* *4842*

Dopamine *Urine* *Increase* Found to be elevated in the urine of patients with metastatic disease. Excretion appears to be proportional to the tumor burden *3305*

Erythrocytes *Ascitic Fluid* *Increase* > 10,000 cells/µL seen in 20% of cases *233*

α-Fetoprotein *Pleural Fluid* *Increase* Positive results were most frequently found in samples derived from patients with secondary or primary liver tumors. The highest levels (6 and 30 ng/mL) were determined in samples of 2 hepatoma patients *1295*
Serum *Increase* Present in some patients with liver metastases from carcinoma of the stomach or pancreas *5544*

Fibrin Degradation Products *Ascitic Fluid* *Increase* In malignant effusions *4891*

Glucose *Serum* *Decrease* Can occur with various types of liver disease. Hepatic hypoglycemia is a fasting hypoglycemia and often only transiently relieved by food *1980*

β-Glucuronidase *Serum* *Increase* Increased *1777* *1498*

γ-Glutamyltransferase *Serum* *Increase* Marked elevations were observed in 12 patients. Mean activity of 396 U/L was 13.2 times the normal upper limit (range 208 - 820 U/L) *3161* Parallels alkaline phosphatase; elevation precedes positive liver scans *5544*

Glutathione Reductase *Serum* *Increase* Raised in 47% of cases *4692*

Haptoglobin *Serum* *Increase* alpha$_2$-Globulins, especially haptoglobins were generally increased in primary colorectal cancer, and rose in metastatic cancer especially when it involved the liver. Haptoglobin values were useful to indicate tumor activity *928*

Isocitrate Dehydrogenase *Serum* *Increase* Approximately 50% of patients with liver metastases exhibited relatively small elevations. Only those patients with secondary liver involvement had increased concentrations *5008* Raised in 57% of patients *4692*

Lactate Dehydrogenase *Serum* *Increase* Distinctly elevated in most cases *5008* From a study of 50 patients, a semiquantitative relation appeared between serum LD, rapidity of tumor growth, and degree of dissemination of the neoplastic process *5736*

Leucine Aminopeptidase *Serum* *Increase* Of 30 patients with hepatic metastases, 93% had elevated levels, ranging from 305-1,000 U/L with a mean of 572 U/L *579* Moderate increase in serum, which occurs even in the absence of jaundice (especially if steroids given) *1290*

Leukocytes *Ascitic Fluid* *Increase* > 1,000 /µL *233*

Malate Dehydrogenase *Serum* *Increase* Elevated in 62% of patients *4692*

Melanin *Urine* *Increase* Melanogenuria occurs in 25% of patients with malignant melanoma; it is said to be more frequent with extensive liver metastasis. It is not useful for judging completeness of removal or early recurrence. Beware of false positive red-brown or purple suspension due to salicylates *5544*

5'-Nucleotidase *Serum* *Increase* Five patients with carcinoma of head of pancreas metastatic to liver showed elevations ranging from 20 - 118 U/L (normal 2 - 11 U/L) *2803*

Ornithine Carbamoyltransferase *Serum* *Increase* Liver cell damage *5544*

Platelets *Blood* *Increase* May be increased in malignancy especially disseminated, advanced or inoperable *5545*

Protein *Ascitic Fluid* *Increase* > 2.5 g/dL in ascitic fluid *233*

Prothrombin Time *Plasma* *Increase* Prolonged in liver disease *1980*

Zinc *Serum* *Decrease* Low in advanced carcinoma with liver metastases *2341*

197.80 Secondary Malignant Neoplasm of Digestive System

α$_1$-Acid Glycoprotein *Serum* *Increase* Elevated with metastases and larger tumor mass *4696* *4373* *4241* *3713* *4853* *2597*

α$_1$-Antitrypsin *Serum* *Decrease* Increased levels of alpha$_1$-antitrypsin and alpha$_1$-acid glycoprotein are associated with metastases to the large bowel *5572*
Serum *Increase* Increased levels of alpha$_1$-antitrypsin and alpha$_1$-acid glycoprotein are associated with metastases to the large bowel *5572*

Carcinoembryonic Antigen *Serum* *Increase* All but 1 of the patients with metastatic disease of the GI tract had elevated concentrations of CEA. Mean value for upper GI tract disease was 21.8 ± 22.7 ng/mL, and 285.2 ± 441 ng/mL for lower GI tract disease *4130*

Factor II *Plasma* *Decrease* May be associated with defibrination resulting in platelet and coagulation factor consumption *5677*

Factor IV *Plasma* *Decrease* May be associated with defibrination resulting in platelet and coagulation factor consumption *5677*

Fibrinogen *Plasma* *Decrease* May be associated with defibrination resulting in platelet and coagulation factor consumption *5677*

Glycated Protein *Serum* *Increase* Metastases are indicated when levels increase in patients with large intestinal cancer *5572*

Haptoglobin *Serum* *Increase* High levels of haptoglobin may suggest involvement of the bowel wall by recurrent cancer *5572*

Lactate Dehydrogenase *Serum* *Increase* From a study of 50 patients, a semiquantitative relation appeared between serum LD, rapidity of tumor growth, and degree of dissemination of the neoplastic process *5736*

Platelets *Blood* *Decrease* May be associated with defibrination resulting in platelet and coagulation factor consumption *5677*
Blood *Increase* May be increased in malignancy especially disseminated, advanced or inoperable *5544*

Prealbumin *Serum* *Increase* Tends to reflect the nutritional status of patients with primary and metastatic cancer of the large intestine *5572*

198.30 Secondary Malignant Neoplasm of Brain

Aldolase *Serum* *Increase* The serum of cancer patients contains a greater proportion of aldolase A (muscle-type) than serum from normal persons. Gliomas and normal brain tissue contain aldolase C (nerve and brain variant), but in meningiomas or tissue metastatic to brain, only aldolase A (liver and fetal form) is detected *4692*

Antidiuretic Hormone *Plasma* *Increase* Associated with excessive ADH production resulting in sodium loss *4707*

Aspartate Aminotransferase *Cerebrospinal Fluid* *Increase* Elevated activities were associated with metastatic carcinoma of CNS. Patients with primary tumors generally showed normal levels *1030* In all but 2 patients with metastatic tumors of the CNS, the activity was significantly raised. The mean for the group was 20.4 U/L *1030*

Cells *Cerebrospinal Fluid* *Increase* Increased cells which are not usually recognized as blast cells because of poor preservation (meningeal infiltration of leukemic cells) *5544*

Creatine Kinase BB-Isoenzyme
Cerebrospinal Fluid *Increase* Significantly higher in breast cancer patients with CNS metastases than in those without *240*

Glomerular Filtration Rate *Urine* *Increase* Associated excess ADH may tend to accelerate GFR *4707*

Glucose *Cerebrospinal Fluid* *Decrease* Less than 50% of blood level (meningeal infiltration of leukemic cells) *5544*

Isocitrate Dehydrogenase *Serum* *Increase* Increased in CSF with secondary cerebral tumors *1290*

Lactate Dehydrogenase *Cerebrospinal Fluid* *Increase* In group of patients with metastatic tumors of the nervous system showed a highly significant difference in the mean CSF LD activity of 67 U/L. All but 2 patients had significantly elevated individual results *1030*
Serum *Increase* From a study of 50 patients, a semiquantitative relation appeared between LD, rapidity of tumor growth, and degree of dissemination of the neoplastic process *5736* Depending on location, growth rate, etc *5544*

Leukocytes *Blood* *Increase* More frequent when WBC is > 100,000 /μL and with rapid increase in WBC, especially in blastic crises (intracranial hemorrhage) *5544*

α_1-Microglobulin *Cerebrospinal Fluid* *No Effect* Of 8 patients with metastatic brain tumors mean concentration in none greater than that in 15 healthy controls of 34.8 ± 16.0 μg/L *2370*

Phosphohexoseisomerase *Serum* *Increase* With leptomeningeal metastases it is 92% specific and 54% sensitive if greater than 20 U/L *2811*

Platelets *Blood* *Decrease* Platelet count frequently decreased (intracranial hemorrhage) *5544*
Blood *Increase* May be increased in malignancy especially disseminated, advanced or inoperable *5545*

Protein *Cerebrospinal Fluid* *Increase* Increased protein (meningeal infiltration of leukemic cells) *5544*

Sodium *Serum* *Decrease* Associated with excessive ADH production *4707* Serum sodium usually less than 130 mEq/L *126*
Urine *Increase* Urine is almost always hypertonic to plasma *126*

198.40 Neoplastic Meningitis

Adenosine Deaminase *Cerebrospinal Fluid* *Increase* In 8 patients with neoplastic meningitis median concentration of 3.6 U/L significantly different from 1 U/L in 117 individuals without meningitis *3122*

Amyloid β-Protein *Cerebrospinal Fluid* *No Effect* In 1 patient with malignant meningitis concentration was 2.58 pmol/mL not significantly different from mean concentration of 4.00 ± 2.92 pmol/mL *3716*

Amyloid β-Protein Precursor *Cerebrospinal Fluid* *No Effect* In 1 patient with malignant meningitis concentration was 1.72 integrated OD units not significantly different from mean concentration of 1.35 ± 0.38 integrated OD units in 25 normal controls *3716*

α_1-Antichymotrypsin *Cerebrospinal Fluid* *Increase* In 1 patient with malignant menigitis concentration was 12.30 μg/mL significantly different from mean concentration of 2.27 ± 1.40 μg/mL in 25 normal controls *3716*

Carcinoembryonic Antigen *Cerebrospinal Fluid* *Increase* Increased concentrations observed in 62% of patients with meningeal carcinomatosis *2952*

Cells *Cerebrospinal Fluid* *No Effect* In 1 patient with malignant meningitis concentration of 5.0 cells/μL not significantly different from normal of 3 cells/μL *3716*

Glucose *Cerebrospinal Fluid* *No Effect* In 4 patients with neoplastic meningitis mean CSF/glucose ratio of 2 not different from 0 in 15 controls without neurological disorders *3123*

Interleukin-6 *Cerebrospinal Fluid* *No Effect* In 4 patients with neoplastic meningitis mean concentration of < 40 pg/mL not different from < 40 pg/mL in 15 controls without neurological disorders *3123*

Leukocytes *Cerebrospinal Fluid* *Increase* In 4 patients with neoplastic meningitis mean concentration of 566 x 10^9/L significantly greater than < 5 x 10^9/L in 15 controls without neurological disorders *3123* In 8 patients with neoplastic meningitis median concentration of 428 x 10^9/L significantly different from < 5 x 10^9/L in 117 individuals without meningitis *3122*

Oligoclonal Banding *Cerebrospinal Fluid* *Increase* Oligoclonal IgG bands detected in patients with carcinomatous or lymphomatous meningitis *3261*

Protein *Cerebrospinal Fluid* *Increase* In 1 patient with malignant meningitis concentration of 108 mg/dL significantly different from normal mean of 29 mg/dL *3716* In 4 patients with neoplastic meningitis mean concentration of 55 mg/dL different from 16 mg/dL in 15 controls without neurological disorders *3123* In 8 patients with neoplastic meningitis median concentration of 770 mg/L significantly different from 220 mg/L in 117 individuals without meningitis *3122*

198.50 Secondary Bone Cancer

Acid Phosphatase *Bone Marrow* *Increase* Early bone metastases were detected by an increased activity in the bone marrow before any serum elevation or discernible radiographic changes occurred. Bone marrow activity was consistently much higher than in the serum in patients with histologically confirmed bone metastases *843*
Serum *Increase* Occurred in 61% of cases. Normal levels were found in 39% of cases when bone metastases were present *4386* Especially from breast carcinoma; concentrations > 9 U/L indicate active invasion *1290* Often slightly increased, especially in prostatic metastases (osteolytic metastases), and especially in primary tumor of bronchus, breast, kidney, and thyroid *5544*

Alkaline Phosphatase *Serum* *Increase* Usually observed with metastases *1025* Rises in proportion to the formation of new bone cells *1642* Often observed with secondary tumors from breast carcinoma *5724* 23% of patients with bone metastasis showed normal concentrations *4614* Usually increased in osteoblastic metastases (especially from primary tumor in prostate) *5544* Especially secondary metastases to prostate *4386*
White Blood Cells *Decrease* Patients with metastases of the lung, bone and skin all showed decreased activity, with median values of 6.4, 20.5, and 10.0 U/L respectively (normal 55 U/L) *3110*

Alkaline Phosphatase Isoenzymes *Serum* *Increase* 5 of 7 patients with metastatic lesions of bone had elevated isoenzyme-II. Isoenzymes I and IV were elevated in 2 of the 7 cases *2557*

Calcitonin *Plasma* *Increase* 8 patients with skeletal metastases had increased concentrations, ranging from 0.15 - 9.0 ng/mL *922*

Calcium *Serum* *Increase* May be normal or increased in osteolytic metastases (especially from primary tumor of bronchus, breast, kidney, thyroid) *5544* Elevations in patients with carcinoma of prostate metastatic to bone were negligible at first but mild hypercalcemia developed at some time in 9% of patients *5724*
Urine *Decrease* Low in osteoblastic metastases (especially from primary tumor in prostate) *5544*
Urine *Increase* Often increased; marked increase may reflect increased rate of tumor growth *5544* Patients with osteolytic metastatic neoplasms (especially with active or extensive lesions) may display hypercalcemia and hypercalciuria which can be further complicated by nephrocalcinosis and renal failure *1025*

Copper *Serum* *Increase* 12 cases of osteosarcoma at various stages were analyzed for Cu and Zn serum levels. Elevated Cu occurred in primary and metastatic cases, while elevated Zn occurred only in primary osteosarcoma and depressed serum Zn in metastases. Patients with advanced cases had the highest serum Cu:Zn ratios *1494*

Erythrocytes *Blood* *Decrease* Depression of all formed elements of the blood is often seen in disseminated neoplastic disease *2039*

Galactosyl-Hydroxylysine *Urine* *Increase* The excretion rate was increased in all patients with carcinoma metastases in bone *2622*

Glucogalactyosyl-Hydroxylysine *Urine* *Increase* The excretion rate was increased in all patients with carcinoma metastases in bone *2622*

198.50 Secondary Bone Cancer (continued)

γ-Glutamyltransferase *Serum* *Increase* In 4 patients with carcinoma metastatic to bone, 25% one had a slightly elevated concentration (54 U/L) *3161*

Hematocrit *Blood* *Decrease* Depression of all formed elements of the blood is often seen in disseminated neoplastic disease *2039*

Hemoglobin *Blood* *Decrease* Depression of all formed elements of the blood is often seen in disseminated neoplastic disease *2039*

Hydroxyproline *Urine* *Increase* Increased excretion in total hydroxyproline *2622*

Lactate Dehydrogenase *Serum* *Increase* From a study of 50 patients, a semiquantitative relation appeared between LD, rapidity of tumor growth, and degree of dissemination of the neoplastic process *5736*

Leukocytes *Blood* *Decrease* Depression of all formed elements of the blood is often seen in disseminated neoplastic disease *2039*

Neutrophils *Blood* *Decrease* Depression of all formed elements of the blood is often seen in disseminated neoplastic disease *2039*

Osteocalcin *Serum* *Increase* Increased in patients with various bone diseases characterized by increased osteoblastic activity *4219*

Phosphate *Serum* *Increase* May be normal or increased (osteolytic metastases (especially from primary tumor of bronchus, breast, kidney, thyroid)) *5544*

Platelets *Blood* *Decrease* Depression of all formed elements of the blood is often seen in disseminated neoplastic disease *2039*
Blood *Increase* May be increased in malignancy especially disseminated, advanced or inoperable *5545*

Procollagen Type I Peptide *Serum* *Increase* The higher levels of PICP were noted in patients with osteoblastic or mixed metastases *1545*

Reticulocytes *Blood* *Increase* Possibly increased *5544*

Zinc *Serum* *Increase* Serum Cu and Zn concentrations were evaluated in 19 patients with sarcomas, 12 of which were osteosarcomas at various stages. Patients with primary or metastatic osteosarcoma had elevated Cu. Patients with primary osteosarcoma had elevated Zn, those with metastases had depressed Zn. The ratio of Cu:Zn in osteosarcoma. patients may be of value in prognosis and therapy evaluation. The ratio of Cu:Zn may be useful in discriminating between patients with primary and metastatic osteosarcoma *1494*

199.00 Malignant Disease

α_1-Acid Antitrypsin *Cerebrospinal Fluid* *Increase* Mean concentration in 19 malignant intracranial tumors of 2.46 ± 1.23 mg/dL compared with 0.70 ± 0.30 mg/dL in 38 controls *1632*
Serum *Increase* Mean concentration in 19 malignant intracranial tumors of 440.0 ± 213.1 mg/dL compared with 315.8 ± 45.8 mg/dL in 40 controls *1632*

α_1-Acid Glycoprotein *Serum* *Increase* In patients with miscellaneous cancers mean concentration of 1.89 g/L compared with less than 0.50 g/L in healthy controls *719* In 55 patients with solid tumors mean concentration of 0.99 g/L significantly different from 0.59 g/L in 20 controls *3448*

Acid Phosphatase, Tartrate Resistant *Serum* *Increase* In patients with metastatic cancer marked increase observed *4217*

Acylcarnitine, Acid-insoluble *Serum* *Decrease* In 10 men with malignant disease mean concentration of 3.1 ± 0.3 nmol/mL not significantly different from 3.0 ± 0.4 nmol/mL in 6 healthy control men but 2.4 ± 0.2 nmol/mL in 11 women with cancer significantly less than 3.2 ± 0.2 nmol/mL in 7 healthy women *1195*

Acylcarnitine, Acid-soluble *Serum* *Decrease* In 10 men with malignant disease mean concentration of 11.9 ± 1.7 nmol/mL nonsignificantly reduced compared with 15.3 ± 2.6 nmol/mL in 6 healthy control men and 6.7 ± 0.8 nmol/mL in 11 women with cancer significantly less than 10.8 ± 0.7 nmol/mL in 7 healthy women *1195*

Adenosine Monophosphate *Urine* *Increase* Urinary cyclic AMP may be significantly increased in about 50% of patients with humoral hypercalcemia of malignancy *2952* In 72 patients with malignant disease mean excretion 204 nmol/L glomerular filtrate (median 69) significantly greater than reference range of less than 60 nmol/L glomerular filtrate *5552*

Adenosine-N6-diethylthioether-N1-pyridinoximine 5'-phosphate *Serum* *Increase* In patients with various malignancies mean concentration of 601.7 nmol/dL prior to treatment, 497.9 nmol/dL in patients receiving chemotherapy, and 216.5 nmol/dL in cancer patients in remission higher than concentration in healthy individuals in whom the mean concentration was 162.2 nmol/dL *5294*

Albumin *Serum* *Decrease* Concentration may be decreased with hypercatabolism associated with rapidly growing tumors *4617*

Aldolase *Serum* *Increase* Activity may be increased in some patients with carcinomas metastatic to the liver *2952*

Aldosterone *Plasma* *Decrease* In 3 of 82 patients with cancer persistent hyperkalemia and hypoaldosteronemia (< 0.6, 2.0 and < 0.6 ng/dL compared to reference interval of 3 - 10 ng/dL) observed, not attibuable to renal failure, pseudohyperkalemia, or drugs *848*
Pleural Fluid *Increase* In 171 patients with pleural effusions mean concentration of 25.9 ng/mL compared with 4.7 ng/mL in fluids from other causes *3291*

Alkaline Phosphatase *Pleural Fluid* *Increase* In 108 patients with malignant effusions mean activity of 2.2 ± 2.2 µkat/L significantly different from 0.85 ± 1.2 µkat/L in 63 patients with benign effusions *3291*
Serum *Increase* In 68 patients with malignant disease and blastic or mixed metastases median activity of 223 U/L significantly greater than 101 U/L in 68 with lytic metastases and 83 U/L in 62 without identified bone metastases *4140*

Alkaline Phosphatase, Bone Isoenzyme *Serum* *Increase* In 68 patients with malignant disease and blastic or mixed metastases median activity of 197 U/L (51 ng/L) significantly greater than 37 U/L (21.7 ng/L) in 68 with lytic metastases and 25 U/L (11.6 ng/L) in 62 without identified bone metastases *4140* In patients with metastatic carcinoma moderate increase observed *4217*

Amyloid A Protein *Serum* *Increase* In patients with miscellaneous cancer mean concentration of 482 mg/L compared with less than 1 mg/L in healthy controls *719*

Antibodies to Human Leukocyte Interferon *Serum* *Increase* Antibodies to human leukocyte interferon occuring spontaneously without prior treatment observed in certain clinical conditions although their significance is unknown *4392*

α_1-Antichymotrypsin *Serum* *Increase* Mean concentration in patients with miscellaneous cancers 1.15 g/L compared with less tham 0.50 g/L in healthy controls *719*

Antinuclear Antibodies *Pleural Fluid* *No Effect* ANA antibodies observed in 0 of 6 pleural fluid specimens *2665*

Apolipoprotein A *Serum* *Decrease* In 8 children with localized malignant disease mean concentration on diagnosis of 1.00 ± 0.76 g/L significantly different from 1.22 ± 0.18 mmol/L in 15 healthy controls *1981*

Apolipoprotein B *Serum* *Increase* In 8 children with localized malignant disease mean concentration on diagnosis of 0.86 ± 0.26 g/L significantly different from 0.74 ± 0.16 mmol/L in 15 healthy controls *1981*

Basic Fibroblast Growth Factor *Serum* *Increase* In 83 patients with cancer 33 (40%) had concentrations of basic fibroblast growth factor greater than 7.5 pg/mL *1178*

BTA TRAK *Urine* *Increase* Mean concentration of 10.3 U/mL in patients with non-genitourinary tract cancer significantly greater than 4.1 U/mL in healthy blood donors *539*

C_1-Inhibitor Antigen *Serum* *Increase* Concentration significantly higher in patients with malignant disease than in healthy control patients *4982*

CA 19-9 *Serum* *Increase* In 52.8% of 36 patients with cancer other than pancreatic cancer concentration increased above cut-off of 37 U/mL *2854* Of 204 patients with CA 19-9 concentrations greater than 60 U/mL, 130 had malignancies *3423*

CA 72-4 *Serum* *Increase* In 89 patients with malignant disease other than gastric or colorectal cancer 65 (73%) had a concentration less than 2.5 U/mL, 24 (27%) had a concentration greater than 2.5 U/mL and 6 (7%) had a concentration greater than 10 U/mL *4505*

CA 125 *Serum* *Increase* In 18 women with nonovarian malignant tumors median concentration of 655 U/mL significantly higher than 4 U/mL in 458 healthy women *2203*

CA 549 *Serum* *Increase* In patients with cancer (non-breast) combined specificity using cutoffs of 12.5 kU/L in women and 11.9 kU/L in men with BRESMARQ immunoradiometric procedure 75.6% *764*

Calcium *Serum* *Increase* Increased concentrations are seen in metastatic cancer *2952* In 72 patients with malignant disease mean concentration of 3.32 mmol/L (median 3.24 mmol/L) significantly greater than reference range of 2.20 - 2.65 mmol/L *5552*
Urine *Increase* In 72 patients with malignant disease mean excretion of 164 µmol/L glomerular filtrate (median 115) significantly greater than reference range of 8 - 38 µmol/L glomerular filtrate *5552*

Carcinoembryonic Antigen *Ascitic Fluid* *Increase* CEA in 20 malignant ascitic fluids and in 28 nonmalignant fluids had 100% predictive value. Sensitivity of CEA alone for malignant disease 45% *1703*
Pericardial Fluid *Increase* In 36 patients median concentration in malignant effusions 80 ng/mL (range of 0 - 305 ng/mL significantly higher than 1.26 ng/mL (range of 0.2 - 18.4 ng/mL) in nonmalignant effusions *5116*
Pleural Fluid *Increase* Mean concentration of 277 ng/mL in 91 effusions associated with malignant disease, with higher sensitivity of 58% in adenocarcinomas than other malignancies (26%) *1649* In 108 patients with malignant effusions mean concentration of 35.6 ± 56.7 ng/mL significantly different from 4.1 ± 3.0 ng/mL in 63 patients with benign effusions *3291*
Serum *Increase* In 3 patients with unspecified malignant disease two had concentrations of 0.0 - 3.0 ng/mL, none had concentrations from 3.1 - 5.0 ng/mL, none had concentrations from 5.1 - 10.0 ng/mL and one had concentrations greater than 10.0 ng/mL when measured by method on Bayer Technicon Immuno 1® system compared with 95.9%, 3.5%, 0.6% and 0.0% respectively in 173 healthy nonsmokers *339* In 38.9% of 36 patients with cancer other than pancreatic cancer concentration increased above cut-off of 37 U/mL *2854*

Carnitine *Serum* *Decrease* In 10 men with malignant disease mean concentration of 62.7 ± 3.8 nmol/mL nonsignificantly reduced compared with 72.1 ± 7.0 nmol/mL in 6 healthy control men and 51.0 ± 1.4 nmol/mL in 11 women with cancer significantly less than 66.2 ± 4.6 nmol/mL in 7 healthy women *1195*

Carnitine, Nonesterified *Serum* *Decrease* In 10 men with malignant disease mean concentration of 47.6 ± 3.1 nmol/mL nonsignificantly reduced compared with 53.7 ± 3.1 nmol/mL in 6 healthy control men and 41.5 ± 1.5 nmol/mL in 11 women with cancer significantly less than 52.0 ± 4.0 nmol/mL in 7 healthy women *1195*

Cholesterol *Ascitic Fluid* *Decrease* In 28 nonmalignant ascitic fluids and 20 malignant fluids cholesterol had a negative predictive value of 92% using a cutoff concentration of 45 mg/dL *1703*
Ascitic Fluid *Increase* In ascitic fluid from 21 patients with malignant disease mean concentration of 3.14 ± 0.24 mmol/L significantly greater than 0.70 ± 0.05 mmol/L in 73 specimens from patients with cirrhosis or hepatocellular carcinoma *728* In one study all fluids with concentration greater than 1.16 mmol/L (45 mg/dL) were determined to be malignant *2661*
Peritoneal Fluid *Increase* In all fluids in one study in which concentration was greater than 1.16 mmol/L (45 mg/dL) fluids were malignant *2661*
Pleural Fluid *Increase* In one study all fluids with concentration greater than 1.16 mmol/L (45 mg/dL) were determined to be malignant *2661*
Serum *Decrease* Concentrations in the range of 80 - 150 mg/dL may be observed in patients with malnutrition, a variety of serious chronic diseases, cancer, and a variety of anemias *4617*
Serum *No Effect* In 8 children with localized malignant disease mean concentration on diagnosis of 3.71 ± 0.74 mmol/L not significantly different from 3.66 ± 0.74 mmol/L in 15 healthy controls *1981*

Cholinesterase *Cerebrospinal Fluid* *No Effect* In 8 patients with CNS neoplasms mean concentration of 0.47 ± 0.02 µmol substrate hydrolyzed (0.17 ± 0.01 mg protein/30 min) not significantly different from 0.48 ± 0.01 µmol substrate hydrolyzed (0.18 ± 0.01 mg protein/30 min) in 10 age and sex matched control patients with nonspecific headaches *321*

Complement C_3 *Serum* *Increase* In 24 patients with malignant disease mean concentration of 140.3 ± 24 mg/dL significantly different from 107.0 ± 18 mg/dL in 11 normal individuals *1300*

Copper *Serum* *Increase* Hypercupricemia is observed in most patients with carcinomas *5174*

C-Reactive Protein *Serum* *Increase* In patients with miscellaneous cancer mean concentration of 136 mg/L compared with less than 3 mg/L in healthy controls *719* In 55 patients with solid tumors mean concentration of 0.028 g/L significantly different from 0.001 g/L in 20 controls *3448*

C-terminal Propeptide of Type I Procollagen
Serum *Increase* In 68 patients with malignant disease and blastic or mixed metastases median concentration of 218 µg/mL significantly greater than 155 µg/mL in 68 with lytic metastases and 124 µg/mL in 62 without identified bone metastases *4140*

CYFRA 21-1 *Serum* *Increase* Mean concentration in 6 patients with non-lung malignant tumors of 5.3 ± 3.6 ng/mL compared with 1.1 ± 0.3 ng/mL in 29 healthy controls with a positivity rate of 66.6% *3665*

Deoxypyridinoline *Urine* *Increase* In 97 patients with malignant disease mean excretion of 11.7 ± 1.2 µmol/mol creatinine significantly greater than normal with 41 with metastases having a higher excretion of 12.1 ± 1.1 µmol/mol creatinine than in 58 without metastases, 9.1 ± 0.6 µmol/mol creatinine *3085* In 48 patients with hypercalcemia of malignancy 57% had excretions greater than reference interval of 0.4 - 6.4 nmol/mmol creatinine. Mean excretion was 7.3 (range of 0.4 - 15.8) nmol/mmol creatinine *4388* Mean excretion of 120 nmol/L in patients with malignant disease and PTHrP > 2.6 pmol/L: in patients with PTHrP < 2.6 pmol/L but with metastases and in those with hematological malignancies mean excretion of 105 nmol/L, but in those with PTHrP > 2.6 pmol/L but without metastases mean excretion of 37 pmol/L *1560*

1,25-Dihydroxy Vitamin D_3 *Serum* *Decrease* In 6 severely ill patients with malignant disease mean concentration of 49.0 ± 9.1 pmol/L not significantly different from 76.5 ± 11 pmol/L in 10 normal individuals *2397*

Dolichol *Serum* *No Effect* No significant deviation from normal observed in patients with a variety of malignant diseases *2294*

EL-1 *Serum* *Increase* In 27.8% of 36 patients with malignant disease other than pancreatic cancer concentration increased above cut-off of 37 U/mL *2854*

α-Enolase *Serum* *Increase* In 3 of 10 cases of adenocarcinoma of lung mean activity increased *1705*

γ-Enolase *Serum* *Increase* In 3 of 10 cases of adenocarcinoma of lung mean activity increased *1705*

Erythrocyte Sedimentation Rate *Blood* *Increase* In 138 of 1,480 ESRs in a hospital population rates were greater than 100 mm/h: in a further study of 90 patients with 163 final diagnoses 16 were attributable to malignant diseases *3097*

Erythropoietin *Serum* *Increase* In 13 patients with solid tumors and anemia mean concentration of 35.8 ± 19.7 mIU/mL above normal range of 4 - 33 mIU/mL *2654*
Serum *No Effect* In 71 patients with solid tumors without anemia mean concentration of 15.0 ± 5.6 mIU/mL not significantly different from normal range of 4 - 33 mIU/mL *2654*

Estradiol *Plasma* *No Effect* In 27 male post-pubertal survivors of malignant disease mean concentration of 65 ± 24 pmol/L within reference interval of up to 114 pmol/L *2893*

Ferritin *Serum* *Decrease* In 725 patients with serum ferritin concentration of less than 50 ng/mL detected in 15 patients with malignant disease of gastrointestinal tract *2968*
Serum *Increase* Malignancy may increase serum ferritin concentration as some malignant cells contain large amounts of acidic isoferritins *4784* In patients with carcinoma 18 had serum ferritin concentration greater than 150 ng/mL and 10 had concentrations less than 150 ng/mL *3792*

Fibronectin *Ascitic Fluid* *Increase* In 28 nonmalignant fluids and 20 malignant fluids fibronectin had a negative predictive value of 92% *1703*

199.00 **Malignant Disease** *(continued)*

Follicle Stimulating Hormone *Plasma* *No Effect* In 27 male post-pubertal survivors of malignant disease mean concentration of 7.5 ± 6.5 IU/L within reference interval of 1.1 - 10.5 IU/L *2893*

Follistatin, Free *Serum* *Increase* Mean concentration in 39 patients with advanced solid cancer of 8.5 ± 1.0 µg/L significantly different from that in 60 normal adults of 3.5 ± 0.2 µg/L *4523*

Glucose *Pericardial Fluid* *Decrease* In 23 patients median concentration in malignant effusions of 70 mg/dL (range 4 - 129 mg/dL different from 90 mg/dL (range 15 - 125 mg/dL) in nonmalignant effusions *5116*
Pleural Fluid *No Effect* In 108 patients with malignant effusions mean concentration of 101 ± 45 mg/dL not significantly different from 94 ± 49 mg/dL in 63 patients with benign effusions *3291*

α1,4-Glucosidase *Serum* *Increase* In 24 men with malignant disease aged > 50 y mean activity of 4.60 ± 0.74 nmol/h/mg protein (268.6 ± 48.4 nmol/h/mL) significantly increased compared with 2.29 ± 0.13 nmol/h/mg protein (133.5 ± 7.4 nmol/h/mL in 29 healthy male controls and in 30 women 3.56 ± 0.54 nmol/h/mg protein (189.2 ± 22.2 nmol/h/mL) compared with 2.03 ± 0.11 nmol/h/mg protein (123.5 ± 6.2 nmol/h/mL) in 22 healthy female controls *1635*

Glutathione *Plasma* *Decrease* In patients with malignant disease mean concentration of oxidized and reduced glutathione significantly reduced below that in healthy controls, unrelated to chemotherapy or type of neoplasm *426*

Granulocytes *Blood* *Increase* Most probable cause of leukocyte counts greater than 45,000 /µL *4304*

Guanosine Monophosphate *Plasma* *No Effect* In majority of patients concentrations fell within normal range of 3.83 ± 1.27 nmol/L *2406*

Haptoglobin *Serum* *Increase* In 55 patients with solid tumors mean concentration of 2.23 g/L significantly different from 1.23 g/L in 20 controls *3448*

HDL_2-Cholesterol *Serum* *Decrease* In 8 children with localized malignant disease mean concentration on diagnosis of 0.39 ± 0.14 mmol/L significantly different from 0.49 ± 0.25 mmol/L in 15 healthy controls *1981*

HDL_3-Cholesterol *Serum* *No Effect* In 8 children with localized malignant disease mean concentration on diagnosis of 0.23 ± 0.06 mmol/L significantly different from 0.22 ± 0.68 mmol/L in 15 healthy controls *1981*

HDL-Cholesterol *Serum* *Decrease* In 8 children with localized malignant disease mean concentration on diagnosis of 0.96 ± 0.24 mmol/L significantly different from 1.28 ± 0.27 mmol/L in 15 healthy controls *1981*

Hemoglobin *Blood* *Decrease* In 13 patients with solid tumors and anemia mean concentration of 9.7 ± 1.1 g/dL significantly below normal range of 11.8 - 18.0 g/dL *2654*
Blood *No Effect* In 71 patients with solid tumors without anemia mean concentration of 13.7 ± 1.5 g/dL not significantly different from normal range of 11.8 - 18.0 g/dL *2654*

Homocystine *Plasma* *Increase* In some patients with solid tumors concentration is increased *5346*

25-Hydroxy Vitamin D_3 *Serum* *Decrease* In 6 severely ill patients with malignant disease mean concentration of 32.6 ± 7.9 nmol/L not significantly different from 49.9 ± 6.5 nmol/L in 10 normal individuals *2397*

immunoglobulin A *Serum* *No Effect* In 24 patients with malignant disease mean concentration of 223 ± 70 mg/dL not significantly different from 209 ± 92 mg/dL in 11 normal individuals *1300*

Immunoglobulin E *Serum* *No Effect* Mean ± 2 SD in 95 patients with various malignancies of 4 - 780 U/mL not significantly different from 7 - 524 U/mL in 100 healthy blood donors *3422* In 24 patients with malignant disease mean concentration of 74 ± 90 U/mL not significantly different from 61 ± 64 U/mL in 11 normal individuals *1300*

Immunoglobulin G *Serum* *No Effect* In 24 patients with malignant disease mean concentration of 919 ± 240 mg/dL not significantly different from 1,058 ± 185 mg/dL in 11 normal individuals *1300*

Immunoglobulin M *Pleural Fluid* *Decrease* In 108 patients with malignant effusions mean concentration of 77 ± 57 IU/mL significantly different from 119 ± 101 IU/mL in 63 patients with benign effusions *3291*
Serum *No Effect* In 24 patients with malignant disease mean concentration of 116 ± 75 mg/dL not significantly different from 118 ± 52 mg/dL in 11 normal individuals *1300*

Inhibin-B *Plasma* *No Effect* In 27 male post-pubertal survivors of malignant disease mean concentration of 94.1 ± 79.5 pg/mL within reference interval *2893*

Insulin-like Growth Factor Binding Protein-3 Protease *Serum* *Increase* Reportedly increased activity in the plasma in patients with advanced cancer *2103*

Intercellular Adhesion Molecule-1 *Serum* *Increase* Mean concentration in 19 patients with extra-hepatic malignant disease of approximately 1,200 µg/L significantly increased compared with mean concentration in 28 healthy blood donors of 215.5 µg/L (95% confidence limits of mean 198.1 - 232.9 µg/L) *4143*

Interleukin-2 *Serum* *Increase* In 16 patients with non-metastatic malignant disease mean concentration of 0.22 ± 0.01 U/mL significantly higher than that in 24 patients with metastatic malignant disease in whom the mean concentration was 0.14 ± 0.02 U/mL and the reference interval of 0.1 - 0.4 U/mL *3089*

Interleukin-6 *Serum* *Increase* Mean concentration of 20.0 ± 5.4 pg/mL in 29 patients with solid tumors significantly different from barely detectable in 32 healthy controls *2099* In 3 of 82 patients with cancer persistent hyperkalemia and increased serum interleukin-6 concentration (221, 161 and 134 pg/mL compared to reference interval of 13 - 41 pg/mL) observed, not attibuable to renal failure, pseudohyperkalemia, or drugs *848* In 29 patients with untreated malignant disease mean concentration of 20.5 ± 5.4 pg/mL significantly higher than 0.9 ± 0.1 pg/mL in 32 healthy controls *2099*

Interleukin-10 *Serum* *Increase* In 24 patients with metastatic malignant disease mean concentration of 3.4 ± 0.9 pg/mL significantly higher than that in 16 patients with non-metastatic malignant disease in whom the mean concentration was 0.4 ± 0.1 pg/mL and the reference interval of 0.1 - 6 pg/mL *3089*

Interleukin-11 *Serum* *No Effect* In 29 patients with untreated malignant disease mean concentration undetected as in 32 healthy controls *2099* Mean concentration undetectable in 29 patients with solid tumors not different from undetectable amount in 32 healthy controls *2099*

Interleukin-12 *Serum* *Increase* In 24 patients with metastatic malignant disease mean concentration of 105 ± 16 pg/mL significantly higher and in 16 patients with non-metastatic malignant disease mean concentration of 59 ± 7 pg/mL not significantly different from reference interval of 9 - 90 pg/mL *3089*
Serum *No Effect* In 16 patients with non-metastatic malignant solid tumors mean concentration 59 ± 7 pg/mL not significantly different from reference interval of 9 - 89 pg/mL *3088*

ionized Calcium *Serum* *No Effect* In 6 severely ill patients with malignant disease mean concentration of 1.23 ± 0.02 mmol/L not significantly different from 1.26 ± 0.01 mmol/L in 10 normal individuals *2397*

Iron *Serum* *No Effect* In 13 patients with solid tumors and anemia mean concentration of 8.8 ± 12.3 µmol/L towards lower end of normal range of 7 - 24 µmol/L and in 71 without anemia mean concentration of 17.6 ± 9.6 µmol/L at middle of normal range *2654*

Lactate Dehydrogenase *Ascitic Fluid* *Increase* In 21 specimens from patients with malignant disease mean activity of 823 ± 107 U/L significantly greater than 103 ± 6 U/L in 73 specimens from patients with cirrhosis or hepatocellular carcinoma. Ascitic fluid:serum ratio in 9 specimens from patients with malignant disease of 3.85 ± 0.96 significantly greater than 0.41 ± 0.04 in 58 specimens from patients with cirrhosis or hepatocellular carcinoma *728* In one study of 55 patients in whom effusions and malignant cells were present all had LD activity greater than 60 U/L. 38% of control fluids had activity greater than 60 U/L due to presence of erythrocytes *2661*
Peritoneal Fluid *Increase* In 55 patients with effusions and malignant cells were present all fluids had LD activity greater than 60 U/L but 38% of nonmalignant effusions also had LD activity greater than 60 U/L due to leakage from erythrocytes *2661*
Pleural Fluid *Increase* In 41 patients with carcinomatous effusions mean activity of 543.1 ± 468.4 UL significantly higher than 69.5 ± 27.0 U/L in 10 patients with transudative effusions *779*

In 108 patients with malignant effusions mean activity of 16.7 ± 37.3 µkat/L not significantly different from 12.6 ± 28.3 µkat/L in 63 patients with benign effusions *3291* In one study of 55 individuals with effusions and malignant cells LD activity exceeded 60 U/L in all but 38% of nonmalignant effusions also had activity that exceeded 60 U/L due to leakage from erythrocytes *2661*

LDL-Cholesterol *Serum No Effect* In 8 children with localized malignant disease mean concentration on diagnosis of 2.25 ± 0.60 mmol/L not significantly different from 1.98 ± 0.63 mmol/L in 15 healthy controls *1981*

Leukocytes *Blood Increase* Most probable cause of leukocyte counts greater than 45,000 /µL *4304*

Pericardial Fluid No Effect In 23 patients median concentration in malignant effusions of 2.3 x 10^6/L (range of 0.5 - 22 x 10^6/L not significantly different from 2.5 x 10^6/L (range of 0.2 - 45 x 10/L) in nonmalignant effusions *5116*

Pleural Fluid Increase In 41 patients with carcinomatous effusions mean concentration of 2,496 ± 1,524 /µL significantly higher than 574 ± 648 /µL in 10 patients with transudative effusions *779*

Lipase *Serum Increase* Increased serum lipase activity observed in the plasma of 4 patients with different malignant diseases (adenocarcinoma of rectosigmoid, colon adenocarcinoma, hepatocellular carcinoma and laryngeal cancer) but with out increased plasma amylase activity *1155*

Lipoprotein Lp(a) *Serum Decrease* In 8 children with localized malignant disease mean concentration on diagnosis of 0 - 615 mg/L not significantly different from 0 - 476 mg/L in 15 healthy controls *1981*

Serum Increase Reportedly increased concentrations of Lp(a) observed in patients with cancer *2827* In 17 patients with tumors mean concentration of 0.359 ± 0.288 g/L significantly greater than 0.118 ± 0.193 g/L in 100 healthy controls *3505*

Luteinizing Hormone *Plasma No Effect* In 27 male postpubertal survivors of malignant disease mean concentration of 3.9 ± 2.6 IU/L within reference interval of 0.4 - 7.0 IU/L *2893*

Lymphocytes *Blood Decrease* In 1,042 hospitalized patients with lymphocytopenia 180 had malignant disease *730*

Blood Increase In 10 patients with malignant disease and increased mean concentration of IL-12, lymphocyte count of 1,641 ± 123 µL significantly higher than 1,228 ± 114 /µL in 10 patients with notmal concentrations of IL-12 *3089*

Pericardial Fluid Decrease In 23 patients median proportion in malignant effusions of 49% (range of 0 - 100%) significantly different from 90% (range of 17 - 100%) in nonmalignant effusions *5116*

Pleural Fluid Increase In 41 patients with carcinomatous effusions mean concentration of 1,607 ± 1,432 /µL significantly higher than 441 ± 594 /µL in 10 patients with transudative effusions *779*

Macrocytes *Blood Increase* In 75 elderly patients with macrocytosis malignant disease was responsible in 5 *3232*

Magnesium *Serum No Effect* In 6 severely ill patients with malignant disease mean concentration of 0.81 ± 0.09 mmol/L not significantly different from 0.79 ± 0.02 mmol/L in 10 normal individuals *2397*

MCV *Blood Increase* In 100 patients with macrocytosis (MCV greater than 110 fL) 12 had increased MCVs, of whom 8 were receiving or had received recently chemotherapy but 4 were not on chemotherapy *4924*

Metallopanstimulin *Serum Increase* In 100% of 13 patients with malignancies mean concentration exceeded upper limit of normal of < 10 ng/mL in healthy individuals aged 19 - 88 years *1462*

1-Methyladenine *Urine Increase* Mean excretion in 23 patients with malignant disease of 2.80 ± 4.52 mmol/mol creatinine compared with 0.26 ± 0.23 mmol/mol creatinine in 23 healthy controls *5830*

1-Methyladenosine *Urine Increase* Mean excretion in 23 patients with malignant disease of 4.61 ± 4.33 mmol/mol creatinine compared with 2.09 ± 0.42 mmol/mol creatinine in 23 healthy controls *5830*

3-Methylcytosine *Urine Increase* Mean excretion in 23 patients with malignant disease 2.86 ± 5.64 mmol/mol creatinine compared with 0.67 ± 0.81 mmol/mol creatinine in 23 healthy controls *5830*

7-Methylguanine *Urine Increase* Mean excretion in 23 patients with malignant disease of 6.40 ± 3.78 mmol/mol creatinine compared with 2.86 ± 0.50 mmol/mol creatinine in 23 healthy controls *5830*

Neuron-specific Enolase *Pericardial Fluid Increase* In 36 patients median concentration in malignant effusions of 41.8 µg/L (range 2 - 172 µg/mL significantly higher than 5.85 µg/mL (range 1 - 83.9 µg/mL) in nonmalignant effusions *5116*

Neutrophils *Pericardial Fluid Increase* In 23 patients median proportion in malignant effusions of 46% (range of 0 - 100%) significantly different from 17% (range of 0 - 80%) in nonmalignant effusions *5116*

Pleural Fluid Increase In 41 patients with carcinomatous effusions mean concentration of 302 ± 497 /µL significantly higher than 133 ± 81 /µL in 10 patients with transudative effusions *779*

N-Methyladenine *Urine Increase* Mean excretion in 23 patients with malignant disease 2.69 ± 4.80 mmol/mol creatinine compared with 0.29 ± 0.23 mmol/mol creatinine in 23 healthy controls *5830*

Osteocalcin *Serum Increase* In patients with metastatic carcinoma moderate increase observed *4217* In 68 patients with malignant disease and blastic or mixed metastases median activity of 12.3 ng/mL significantly greater than 6.5 ng/mL in 68 with lytic metastases and 7.9 ng/mL in 62 without identified bone metastases *4140*

Parathyroid Hormone *Plasma Increase* In 6 severely ill patients with malignant disease mean concentration of intact parathyroid hormone of 35 ± 7 ng/L not significantly different from 23 ± 3 ng/L in 10 normal individuals *2397*

Parathyroid Hormone-related Peptide *Plasma Increase* Liver metastases occurred in 47% of patients with PTHrP > 2.6 pmol/L and 6 with PTHrP < 2.6 pmol/L. Bone metastases occurred in 58% patients with PTHrP > 2.6 pmol/L and 5 with PTHrP < 2.6 pmol/L *1560* Concentration of PTHrP (middle portion 53-84) increased in 44 of 73 patients with hypercalcemia associated with solid tumors (median 49, range 22 to 333 pmol/L) *483* In 72 patients with malignant disease mean concentration of 3.31 pmol/L (median 1.84 pmol/L) significantly greater than reference range of less than 0.5 pmol/L *5552*

Phosphate *Serum Decrease* Rapidly growing tumors are a less common cause of hypophosphatemia due to shift of phosphate into cells *969*

Serum Increase Lysis of tumors may cause shift of phosphate from cells leads to increased serum concentration *969* Hyperphosphatemia may occur with tumor lysis *5204*

Phospholipase A_2 *Serum Increase* Serum concentrations of PLA2-II increased above normal in more than 50% of patients with various malignant tumors *3766*

Platelets *Blood Increase* Mean concentration of 335 ± 26 /nL in 29 patients with solid tumors significantly different from 254 ± 9 /nL in 32 healthy controls *2099* In 29 patients with untreated malignant disease mean concentration of 335 ± 26 /nL significantly higher than 254 ± 9 /nL in 32 healthy controls *2099* In 732 patients with platelet counts greater than 500,000 /µL, 11.6% had malignancies *1869*

Potassium *Serum Increase* In 3 of 82 patients with cancer persistent hyperkalemia (5.1 - 6.2, 5.1 - 5.8 and 5.1 - 5.8 mmol/L compared to reference interval of 3.5 - 5.0 mmol/L) observed, not attibuable to renal failure, pseudohyperkalemia, or drugs *848*

Urine Decrease In 3 of 82 patients with cancer persistent hyperkalemia and hypokaluria (12 - 23, 29 - 36 and 14 - 27 mmol/d compared to reference interval of 40 - 80 mmol/d) observed, not attibuable to renal failure, pseudohyperkalemia, or drugs *848*

Prealbumin *Serum No Effect* In 55 patients with solid tumors mean concentration of 0.17 g/L not significantly different from 0.23 g/L in 20 controls *3448*

Protein *Ascitic Fluid Increase* In one study in all patients in whom concentration was greater than 25 g/L (2.5 g/dL) malignancy was present *2661* In ascitic fluid from 17 patients with malignant disease mean concentration of 57.12 ± 3.8 g/L significantly greater than 19.19 ± 1.26 g/L in 72 specimens from patients with cirrhosis or hepatocellular carcinoma. Total protein ascitic fluid:serum ratio of 0.75 ± 0.10 in 9 specimens from patients with malignant disease significantly greater than 0.29 ± 0.02 in 58 specimens from patients with cirrhosis or hepatocellular carcinoma *728*

199.00 Malignant Disease *(continued)*

Protein *(continued)*
Pericardial Fluid *No Effect* In 23 patients median concentration in malignant effusions of 4.8 g/dL (range 2.5 - 7.2 g/dL not significantly different from 5.4 g/dL (range 3.2 - 7.3 g/dL) in nonmalignant effusions *5116*
Peritoneal Fluid *Increase* In one study of 55 patients in whom effusions were present all were malignant when protein concentration was greater than 25 g/L (2.5 g/dL) *2661*
Pleural Fluid *Increase* In 41 patients with carcinomatous effusions mean concentration of 39.5 ± 7.7 g/L significantly higher than 16.9 ± 3.4 g/L in 10 patients with transudative effusions *779* In one study in all patients in whom concentration was greater than 25 g/L (2.5 g/dL) fluids were malignant *2661*
Pleural Fluid *No Effect* In 108 patients with malignant effusions mean concentration of 4.59 ± 0.90 g/dL not significantly different from 4.68 ± 1.1 g/dL in 63 patients with benign effusions *3291*

Prothrombin Fragment 1.2 *Plasma* *Increase* Mean concentration of prothrombin fragment 1.2 in platelet-poor plasma from 24 patients with malignant disease of 4.8 ± 3.1 nmol/L significantly higher than 0.51 nmol/L (95% reference interval of 0.21 - 2.78 nmol/L) in 268 healthy individuals less than 44 years of age *1860*

Pseudouridine *Ascitic Fluid* *Increase* In 10 specimens from patients with malignant disease mean concentration of 7.48 ± 0.72 μmol/L significantly greater than 3.78 ± 0.27 μmol/L in 51 specimens from patients with cirrhosis or hepatocellular carcinoma *728*
Pleural Fluid *Increase* In 31 patients with malignant disease median concentration of 53.3 μmol/L markedly different from 40.1 μmol/L in 29 patients with nonmalignant disease-associated pleural fluids *3240*

Putrescine *Urine* *Increase* In 26 patients with localized malignancy mean concentration increased above normal excretion of 0.8 - 6.2 mg/d in 50 healthy men and women aged 18 to 60 years mg/d *3086*

Pyridinoline *Urine* *Increase* Mean excretion of 497 nmol/L observed in patients with malignant disease and PTHrP > 2.6 pmol/L. In patients with metastases and in a subgroup of patients with hematological malignancies but PTHrP < 2.6 pmol/L mean excretion of 478 nmol/L. When patients had no metastases but PTHrP > 2.6 pmol/L mean excretion was 142 pmol/L *1560* In 48 patients with hypercalcemia of malignancy of 91% had excretions greater than reference interval of 5.0 - 21.8 nmol/mmol creatinine. Mean excretion of 53.0 (range 6.0 - 161.6) nmol/mmol creatinine *4388* In 97 patients with malignant disease mean excretion of 39.8 ± 4.9 μmol/mol creatinine compared with 13.8 ± 1.2 μmol/mol creatinine in 65 healthy controls: excretion in 41 patients with metastases of 40.5 ± 4.1 μmol/mol creatinine significantly higher than 30.4 ± 2.2 μmol/mol creatinine in 56 without metastases *3085*

Renin Activity *Plasma* *Increase* In 3 of 82 patients with cancer persistent hyperkalemia and increased basal renin activity (3.7, 7.2 and 3.0 ng/mL/h compared to reference interval of 0.3 - 3.1 ng/mL/h) observed, not attibuable to renal failure, pseudohyperkalemia, or drugs *848*

Ribonuclease *Serum* *Increase* In 47 patients with carcinoma mean activity of of 414 ± 67 U/mL significantly higher than 266 ± 39 U/mL in 15 normal individuals *2793* In 5 patients with malignant diseases other than carcinoma mean activity of 466 ± 69 U/mL significantly higher than 266 ± 39 U/mL in 15 normal individuals *2793*

Scan1 *Serum* *Increase* In 58.3% of 36 patients with malignant disease other than pancreatic cancer concentration increased above cut-off of 37 U/mL *2854*

Selenium *Serum* *Decrease* In 1,096 new cases of cancer from screened population of 39,268 individuals in Finland mean concentration of 59.1 μg/L significantly less than mean of 62.5 μg/L among controls *2717*

Sialyltransferase *Serum* *Increase* Activity increased in 12 of 86 patients with malignancies other than Hodgkin's disease and non-Hodgkin's lymphoma, but associated with liver involvement *1781* In 4 patients with adenocarcinoma with unknown primary mean and median concentrations of 530 and 480 cpm/mg protein/30 min significantly different from 240 and 243 cpm/mg protein/30 min respectively in 20 normal individuals *2111*

Soluble E-Selectin *Serum* *Increase* Mean concentration in 11 patients with solid tumors and disseminated intravascular coagulation of 47.2 ± 41.8 ng/mL significantly different from about 30 ng/mL in 17 patients without DIC *3890*

Soluble Interleukin-2 Receptor *Pleural Fluid* *Increase* In 41 patients with carcinomatous effusions mean concentration of 3.36 ± 0.16 U/mL significantly higher than 2.89 ± 0.12 U/mL in 10 patients with transudative effusions *779*
Serum *Increase* In 16 patients with malignant disease mean concentration of 800 U/mL significantly higher than 320 U/mL in 8 healthy volunteers *3781* In 41 patients with carcinomatous effusions mean plasma concentration of 2.68 ± 0.19 U/mL significantly higher than 2.19 ± 0.09 U/mL in 10 patients with transudative effusions *779* In 11 patients following surgery, treatment with ranitidine caused significant mean increase from mean baseline of 620 U/mL to 700 U/mL on first postoperative day, 830 U/mL on third postoperative day and 950 U/mL on ninth postoperative day significantly higher than control surgical patients on postoperative days 1, 3 and 9 *3781*

Spermidine *Urine* *No Effect* In 26 patients with localized malignant disease mean concentration increased above normal excretion in 50 healthy men and women aged 18 to 60 years to 1.0 - 4.2 mg/d *3086*

Spermine *Urine* *Increase* In 26 patients with localized malignant disease mean excretion increased above normal excretion in 50 healthy men and women aged 18 to 60 years to 1.0 - 4.2 mg/d *3086*

Testosterone *Serum* *No Effect* In 27 male post-pubertal survivors of malignant disease mean concentration of 17.1 ± 8.2 nmol/L within reference interval of 10 - 33 nmol/L *2893*

Tetranectin *Serum* *Decrease* In 18 women with nonovarian tumors mean concentration of 6.9 ± 2.7 mg/L significantly less than 11.6 ± 2.0 mg/L in 458 healthy women *2203*

Thrombopoietin *Plasma* *Increase* Mean concentration of 682 ± 53 pg/mL in 29 patients with solid tumors significantly different from 280 ± 33 pg/mL in 32 healthy controls *2099* In 29 patients with untreated malignant disease mean concentration of 682 ± 53 pg/mL significantly higher than 280 ± 33 pg/mL in 32 healthy controls *2099*

Thymidine-5'-triphosphatase *Serum* *Increase* Activity in 82% of 95 patients with untreated malignant disease showed a significant increase from that in healthy individuals *1781*

Tissue Factor Antigen *Plasma* *Increase* In 13 patients with solid tumors mean concentration of 292 ± 116 pg/mL compared with 126 ± 41 pg/mL in 12 healthy volunteers *5511*

Tissue Polypeptide Antigen *Pleural Fluid* *Increase* In 171 patients with pleural effusions mean concentration significantly higher than in fluids from other causes *3291*
Pleural Fluid *No Effect* In 108 patients with malignant effusions mean concentration of 2,080 ± 1,068 ng/mL not significantly different from 1,726 ± 1,154 ng/mL in 63 patients with benign effusions *3291*

Transferrin *Serum* *No Effect* In 55 patients with solid tumors mean concentration of 2.28 g/L not significantly different from 2.39 g/L in 20 controls *3448* In 13 patients with solid tumors and anemia mean concentration of 208.3 ± 97.2 mg/dL towards lower end of normal range of 170 - 460 mg/dL and in 71 without anemia mean concentration of 261.4 ± 88.9 mg/dL more towards middle of normal range *2654*

Triglycerides *Serum* *Increase* In 8 children with localized malignant disease mean concentration on diagnosis of 1.11 ± 0.76 mmol/L significantly different from 0.88 ± 0.28 mmol/L in 15 healthy controls *1981*

Trypsinogen-2 *Urine* *Increase* Urinary dipstick gave false positive result for acute pancreatitis in 7 patients with abdominal cancers *2633*

Tumor Necrosis Factor-α *Serum* *Increase* Mean concentration detected in 7.6% of 28 patients with solid tumors with or without disseminated intravascular coagulation compared with patients with liver disease, hematologic disorders and obstetric disorders *3890* Mean concentration detected in 23.1% of 28 patients with solid tumors with or without disseminated intravascular coagulation *3890*

Vascular Endothelial Growth Factor *Serum* *Increase* In 88 patients with cancer, 35 (40%) had concentrations of vascular endothelial growth factor greater than 500 pg/mL *1178*

VLDL-Cholesterol *Serum* *Decrease* In 8 children with localized malignant disease mean concentration on diagnosis of 0.15 ± 0.10 mmol/L significantly different from 0.29 ± 0.42 mmol/L in 15 healthy controls *1981*

Zinc *Serum* *Decrease* In patients with malignant disease concentration is typically reduced *2952* Hypozincemia is observed in most patients with carcinomas *5174*
Urine *Increase* In 55 patients with solid tumors mean concentration of 2.33 nmol/mol creatinine significantly different from 0.77 nmol/mol creatinine in 20 controls *3448*

199.10 Metastatic Tumor

α_1-Acid Glycoprotein *Serum* *Increase* Elevated with metastases and larger tumor mass *2597 3713 4373 4241 4853 4696*

Adenosine Deaminase *Serum* *Increase* Ninety-one percent of 527 patients with tumors showed activity above normal, whereas eighty-six per cent of 408 nontumorous diseased persons did not *2737 5041*

Albumin *Serum* *Decrease* Serum concentration of albumin and transferrin were significantly reduced while haptoglobin was increased in disseminated carcinoma compared with localized *2109*

Aldolase *Serum* *Increase* Variable rises in serum levels may be found in carcinomatosis. Serum aldolase and phosphohexose isomerase are roughly parallel *1290*

Alkaline Phosphatase *Serum* *Increase* In a group of patients with malignant disease and lytic metastases median activity of 101 U/L and 223 U/L in patients with osteoblastic or mixed metastases significantly higher than 83 U/L in patients without bone metases *4140*
White Blood Cells *Decrease* Patients with metastases of the lung, bone, and skin all showed decreased activity, with median values of 6.4, 20.5, and 10.0 U/L respectively (normal 55 U/L) *3110*

Alkaline Phosphatase, Bone Isoenzyme *Serum* *Increase* In a group of patients with malignant disease and lytic metastases median activity of 37 U/L (electrophoretic) and 21.7 U/L (immunoradiometric) and 197 U/L (electrophoretic) and 51 U/L (radiometric) in patients with osteoblastic or mixed metastases significantly higher than 25 U/L (electrophoretic) and 11.6 U/L (immunoradiometric) in patients without bone metases *4140* In a group of patients with malignant disease and lytic metastases median activity of 37 U/L and 197 U/L in patients with osteoblastic or mixed metastases significantly higher than 25 U/L in patients without bone metases *4140*

Amylase *Ascitic Fluid* *Increase* With carcinomatous peritonitis 91% of the increased amylase activity was of salivary type and the remainder of pancreatic type *2960* Parallels the degree of metastatic involvement of the peritoneum *4707*

Angiotensin-converting Enzyme *Serum* *Decrease* Most cancer patients present with normal to low levels *3282*
Serum *No Effect* Most cancer patients present with normal to low levels *3282*

α_1-Antichymotrypsin *Serum* *Increase* Reported effect *2628* Increased with any kind of invasive tumor *2663*

Antithrombin III *Plasma* *Decrease* Seen with carcinoma *5220 3472*

α_1-Antitrypsin *Serum* *Increase* Increased *4241 4373 4371 4763 83*

Calcitonin *Plasma* *Increase* Concentration typically increased *1870*

Calcium *Serum* *Increase* In one study of 42 patients with hypercalcemia and low intact PTH concentration, 1 had multiple metastases with unknown primary *3280*

Carcinoembryonic Antigen *Serum* *Increase* High preoperative values had been shown to be associated with an increased risk of metastases or recurrence in patients who apparently had a successful resection of a carcinoma of the large bowel. Measurements after surgery provide an earlier warning of metastases and recurrence often with a lead time of many months *928*

Cholesterol *Pericardial Fluid* *Increase* High levels (2.6 - 5.2 mmol/L; 100 to 200 mg/dL) *566*
Serum *Decrease* Among 150 men who died of cancer, cholesterol level fell 22.7 mg/dL more than in survivors over the equivalent period *4783*

Cortisol *Plasma* *Decrease* Relative hypoadrenalism observed with partial destruction of the adrenal cortex *2901*

C-terminal Propeptide of Type I Procollagen *Serum* *Increase* In a group of patients with malignant disease and lytic metastases median concentration of 155 ng/mL and 218 ng/mL in patients with osteoblastic or mixed metastases significantly higher than 124 ng/mL in patients without bone metastases *4140*

Dopamine *Urine* *Increase* Found to be elevated in the urine of patients with metastatic disease. Excretion appears to be proportional to the tumor burden *3305*

Erythrocyte Sedimentation Rate *Blood* *Increase* ESR > 100 mm in the 1st h indicates serious disease, as in tuberculosis and carcinomatosis *1098*

Factor II *Plasma* *Decrease* May be associated with defibrination resulting in platelet and coagulation factor consumption *5677*

Factor IV *Plasma* *Decrease* May be associated with defibrination resulting in platelet and coagulation factor consumption *5677*

Fibrinogen *Plasma* *Decrease* May be associated with defibrination resulting in platelet and coagulation factor consumption *5677*

Folate *Serum* *Decrease* Decreased with extensive skin disease *602 772 5230*

Fucose *Serum* *Increase* Markedly increased *2899*

Fucosidase *Serum* *No Effect* In 24 patients with secondary metastatic liver carcinoma mean activity of α-L-fucosidase of 58.9 ± 6.4 nkat/L compared with 51.4 ± 4.5 nkat/L in 30 controls *1132*

Glycated Protein *Serum* *Increase* Metastases are indicated when levels increase in patients with large intestinal cancer *5572*

Haptoglobin *Serum* *Increase* Serum concentration of albumin and transferrin were significantly reduced while haptoglobin was increased in disseminated carcinoma compared with localized *2109*

β-Hexosaminidase *Serum* *Increase* Elevated *5229*

Hydroxyproline *Urine* *Increase* The levels of both 3-hydroxyproline and 4-hydroxyproline in cancer patients were significantly higher in 97 patients with cancer than in healthy patients and those with nonmalignant diseases *3893*

Immunoglobulins *Urine* *Increase* 24 h excretion and renal clearance of free lambda and kappa light chains of immunoglobulins were significantly increased in disseminated carcinoma compared with localized *2109*

Interleukin-12 *Serum* *Increase* In 16 patients with metastatic malignant solid tumors mean concentration of 153 ± 24 pg/mL significantly different from reference interval of 9 - 89 pg/mL *3088*

Iron-binding Capacity, Total *Serum* *Decrease* Low serum iron binding capacity (total) due to carcinomatosis *1290*

Iron Saturation *Serum* *Decrease* Serum concentration of albumin and transferrin were significantly reduced while haptoglobin was increased in disseminated carcinoma compared with localized *2109*

Lactate Dehydrogenase *Serum* *Increase* From a study of 50 patients, a semiquantitative relation appeared between serum LD, rapidity of tumor growth, and degree of dissemination of the neoplastic process *5736*

Laminin *Serum* *Increase* Highest levels with metastatic disease *4394*

Leucine Aminopeptidase *Serum* *Increase* Elevated in disseminated malignant disease *4124*

Lymphocyte T-Cells *Blood* *Decrease* Normal *1588*

Lymphocytes *Blood* *Decrease* Active rosettes (T-EA) were decreased only in metastatic patients, while the total T population (T-ET) was decreased in all stages. Patients whose values were constant remained cancer free, while a reduction heralded the appearance of clinical and/or radiological signs of metastases *412*

Lysozyme *Urine* *Increase* 24 h excretion and renal clearance were significantly increased in disseminated carcinoma compared with localized *2109*

α_2-Macroglobulin *Serum* *Increase* Reported effect *3134*

199.10 Metastatic Tumor *(continued)*

β_2-Macroglobulin *Urine* *Increase* 24 h excretion and renal clearance were significantly increased in disseminated carcinoma compared with localized *2109*

Osteocalcin *Serum* *Increase* In a group of patients with malignant disease and lytic metastases median concentration of 12.3 ng/mL in patients with osteoblastic or mixed metastases significantly higher than 7.9 ng/mL in patients without bone metastases *4140*
Serum *No Effect* In a group of patients with malignant disease and lytic metastases median concentration of 6.5 ng/mL not significantly different from 7.9 ng/mL in patients without bone metastases *4140*

Parathyroid Hormone *Plasma* *Decrease* In one study of 42 patients with low intact PTH concentration and hypercalcemia 1 patient had multiple metastases with unknown primary tumor *3280*

Platelets *Blood* *Decrease* May be associated with defibrination resulting in platelet and coagulation factor consumption *5677*
Blood *Increase* May be increased in malignancy especially disseminated, advanced or inoperable *5545*

Porphobilinogen *Urine* *Increase* Elevated porphobilinogen occasionally has been observed in carcinomatosis *367*

Prostate-specific Antigen *Serum* *Increase* 68% of 21 patients with prostatic tumors metastasizing to bone had PSA concentrations greater than 100 ng/mL *5710*

Prothrombin Consumption *Blood* *Increase* May be associated with defibrination resulting in platelet and coagulation factor consumption *5677*

Trypsin Inhibitor *Serum* *Increase* Elevated compared to normal controls or patients with non-neoplastic disorders *3488*

Zinc *Serum* *Decrease* Decreased *5083*

199.10 Squamous Cell Carcinoma

Alanine *Plasma* *Decrease* In 41 patients with previously untreated squamous cell carcinoma of the head or neck mean concentration of 37.0 ± 1.9 µmol/dL significantly different from 43.2 ± 3.6 µmol/dL in 30 healthy controls without a history of cancer *4698*

β-Alanine *Plasma* *No Effect* In 41 patients with previously untreated squamous cell carcinoma of the head or neck mean concentration of 0.1 ± 0.1 µmol/dL not significantly different from 0.3 ± 0.3 µmol/dL in 30 healthy controls without a history of cancer *4698*

α-Amino-n-Butyric Acid *Plasma* *No Effect* In 41 patients with previously untreated squamous cell carcinoma of the head or neck mean concentration of 2.2 ± 0.2 µmol/dL not significantly different from 4.9 ± 1.7 µmol/dL in 30 healthy controls without a history of cancer *4698*

α-Aminoadipic Acid *Plasma* *Decrease* In 41 patients with previously untreated squamous cell carcinoma of the head or neck mean concentration of 0.0 ± 0.0 µmol/dL not significantly different from 3.2 ± 2.1 µmol/dL in 30 healthy controls without a history of cancer *4698*

Arginine *Plasma* *No Effect* In 41 patients with previously untreated squamous cell carcinoma of the head or neck mean concentration of 13.0 ± 0.5 µmol/dL not significantly different from 12.6 ± 0.6 µmol/dL in 30 healthy controls without a history of cancer *4698*

Asparagine *Plasma* *Decrease* In 41 patients with previously untreated squamous cell carcinoma of the head or neck mean concentration of 4.6 ± 0.2 µmol/dL significantly different from 5.6 ± 0.3 µmol/dL in 30 healthy controls without a history of cancer *4698*

Aspartic Acid *Plasma* *Decrease* In 41 patients with previously untreated squamous cell carcinoma of the head or neck mean concentration of 3.0 ± 0.3 µmol/dL significantly different from 4.8 ± 0.2 µmol/dL in 30 healthy controls without a history of cancer *4698*

Citrulline *Plasma* *No Effect* In 41 patients with previously untreated squamous cell carcinoma of the head or neck mean concentration of 3.3 ± 0.2 µmol/dL not significantly different from 5.5 ± 1.5 µmol/dL in 30 healthy controls without a history of cancer *4698*

Cystine *Plasma* *Increase* In 41 patients with previously untreated squamous cell carcinoma of the head or neck mean concentration of 3.4 ± 0.2 µmol/dL significantly different from 2.4 ± 1.0 µmol/dL in 30 healthy controls without a history of cancer *4698*

Glutamic Acid *Plasma* *No Effect* In 41 patients with previously untreated squamous cell carcinoma of the head or neck mean concentration of 13.6 ± 1.4 µmol/dL not significantly different from 16.0 ± 1.8 µmol/dL in 30 healthy controls without a history of cancer *4698*

Glycine *Plasma* *Decrease* In 41 patients with previously untreated squamous cell carcinoma of the head or neck mean concentration of 25.1 ± 1.1 µmol/dL significantly different from 30.1 ± 1.8 µmol/dL in 30 healthy controls without a history of cancer *4698*

Histidine *Plasma* *Decrease* In 41 patients with previously untreated squamous cell carcinoma of the head or neck mean concentration of 7.6 ± 0.2 µmol/dL significantly different from 9.3 ± 0.5 µmol/dL in 30 healthy controls without a history of cancer *4698*

Isoleucine *Plasma* *No Effect* In 41 patients with previously untreated squamous cell carcinoma of the head or neck mean concentration of 7.3 ± 0.3 µmol/dL not significantly different from 9.1 ± 0.7 µmol/dL in 30 healthy controls without a history of cancer *4698*

Leucine *Plasma* *No Effect* In 41 patients with previously untreated squamous cell carcinoma of the head or neck mean concentration of 13.2 ± 0.6 µmol/dL not significantly different from 15.3 ± 1.2 µmol/dL in 30 healthy controls without a history of cancer *4698*

Lysine *Plasma* *No Effect* In 41 patients with previously untreated squamous cell carcinoma of the head or neck mean concentration of 14.9 ± 0.6 µmol/dL not significantly different from 15.8 ± 0.8 µmol/dL in 30 healthy controls without a history of cancer *4698*

Methionine *Plasma* *No Effect* In 41 patients with previously untreated squamous cell carcinoma of the head or neck mean concentration of 3.0 ± 0.1 µmol/dL not significantly different from 3.73 ± 0.7 µmol/dL in 30 healthy controls without a history of cancer *4698*

1-Methylhistidine *Plasma* *Decrease* In 41 patients with previously untreated squamous cell carcinoma of the head or neck mean concentration of 0.1 ± 0.1 µmol/dL significantly different from 0.7 ± 0.2 µmol/dL in 30 healthy controls without a history of cancer *4698*

3-Methylhistidine *Plasma* *Decrease* In 41 patients with previously untreated squamous cell carcinoma of the head or neck mean concentration of 0.3 ± 0.1 µmol/dL significantly different from 1.2 ± 0.3 µmol/dL in 30 healthy controls without a history of cancer *4698*

Ornithine *Plasma* *Decrease* In 41 patients with previously untreated squamous cell carcinoma of the head or neck mean concentration of 6.4 ± 0.4 µmol/dL significantly different from 9.1 ± 0.7 µmol/dL in 30 healthy controls without a history of cancer *4698*

Parathyroid Hormone-related Peptide *Plasma* *Increase* In 20 of 21 patients with hypercalcemia and squamous cell carcinoma concentration increased above upper limit of 1.5 pmol/L (range 1.0 to 30.9 pmol/L) *3987* Significant increase in concentration observed in 17 of 21 (81%) patients with squamous cell carcinoma *483*

Phenylalanine *Plasma* *Decrease* In 41 patients with previously untreated squamous cell carcinoma of the head or neck mean concentration of 6.5 ± 0.4 µmol/dL significantly different from 7.8 ± 0.6 µmol/dL in 30 healthy controls without a history of cancer *4698*

Phosphate *Serum* *Increase* Lysis of squamous cell carcinoma cells even prior to treatment may cause shift of phosphate from cells leading to increased serum concentration, and possible acute renal failure *969*

Proline *Plasma* *No Effect* In 41 patients with previously untreated squamous cell carcinoma of the head or neck mean concentration of 20.4 ± 1.1 µmol/dL not significantly different from 16.0 ± 1.3 µmol/dL in 30 healthy controls without a history of cancer *4698*

Serine *Plasma* *Decrease* In 41 patients with previously untreated squamous cell carcinoma of the head or neck mean concentration of 12.7 ± 0.6 μmol/dL significantly different from 15.6 ± 0.8 μmol/dL in 30 healthy controls without a history of cancer *4698*

Taurine *Plasma* *Decrease* In 41 patients with previously untreated squamous cell carcinoma of the head or neck mean concentration of 9.2 ± 0.6 μmol/dL significantly different from 16.5 ± 1.2 μmol/dL in 30 healthy controls without a history of cancer *4698*

Threonine *Plasma* *Decrease* In 41 patients with previously untreated squamous cell carcinoma of the head or neck mean concentration of 10.8 ± 0.4 μmol/dL significantly different from 13.3 ± 0.5 μmol/dL in 30 healthy controls without a history of cancer *4698*

Tyrosine *Plasma* *No Effect* In 41 patients with previously untreated squamous cell carcinoma of the head or neck mean concentration of 5.7 ± 0.3 μmol/dL not significantly different from 7.3 ± 0.7 μmol/dL in 30 healthy controls without a history of cancer *4698*

Valine *Plasma* *No Effect* In 41 patients with previously untreated squamous cell carcinoma of the head or neck mean concentration of 21.5 ± 0.7 μmol/dL not significantly different from 23.2 ± 2.0 μmol/dL in 30 healthy controls without a history of cancer *4698*

Primary Neoplasms of Lymphatic and Hematopoietic Systems

200.10 Lymphocytic Lymphoma, Poorly-differentiated

immunoglobulin A *Serum* *Decrease* Mean concentration in patients with poorly-differentiated lymphocytic lymphoma significantly reduced *1781*

Immunoglobulin D *Serum* *No Effect* Mean concentration in patients with poorly-differentiated lymphocytic lymphoma not significantly changed *1781*

Immunoglobulin E *Serum* *No Effect* Mean concentration in patients with poorly-differentiated lymphocytic lymphoma not significantly changed *1781*

Immunoglobulin G *Serum* *No Effect* Mean concentration in patients with poorly-differentiated lymphocytic lymphoma not significantly changed *1781*

Immunoglobulin M *Serum* *No Effect* Mean concentration in patients with poorly-differentiated lymphocytic lymphoma not significantly changed *1781*

200.10 Lymphocytic Lymphoma, Well-differentiated

immunoglobulin A *Serum* *Decrease* Mean concentration in patients with well-differentiated lymphocytic lymphoma significantly reduced *1781*

Immunoglobulin D *Serum* *No Effect* Mean concentration in patients with well-differentiated lymphocytic lymphoma not significantly changed *1781*

Immunoglobulin E *Serum* *Decrease* Mean concentration in patients with well-differentiated lymphocytic lymphoma significantly reduced *1781*

Immunoglobulin G *Serum* *Decrease* Mean concentration in patients with well-differentiated lymphocytic lymphoma significantly reduced *1781*

Immunoglobulin M *Serum* *Decrease* Mean concentration in patients with well-differentiated lymphocytic lymphoma significantly reduced *1781*

200.80 Immunocytoma

Lymphocytes *Blood* *Increase* In 41 patients with IC median concentration on entry into study of 2.0 x 10^9/L significantly different from that in healthy controls *1972*

β_2-Microglobulin *Serum* *Increase* In 41 patients with IC progression-free survival substantially greater in patients with serum β_2-microglobulin concentration less than 3.5 μg/L *1972*

Platelets *Blood* *Decrease* In 41 patients with IC progression-free survival substantially greater in patients with platelet count greater than 150 x 10^9/L *1972*

Thymidine Kinase *Serum* *Decrease* In 41 patients with IC progression-free survival substantially greater in patients with serum thymidine kinase activity less than 5 U/L *1972*

201.90 Hodgkin's Disease

α_1-Acid Glycoprotein *Serum* *Increase* Concentration increased in 11 of 15 patients with advanced disease *1781*

Adenosine Deaminase *Lymphocytes* *Decrease* Adenosine deaminase in lymphocytes in 23 patients with Hodgkin's disease had a mean activity significantly less than in 99 controls *1781*
Red Blood Cells *No Effect* Although adenosine deaminase in lymphocytes in 23 patients with Hodgkin's disease had a mean activity significantly less than in 99 controls, activity in erythrocytes normal *1781*
Serum *No Effect* Although adenosine deaminase in lymphocytes in 23 patients with Hodgkin's disease had a mean activity significantly less than in 99 controls, activity in plasma normal *1781*

Alanine Aminotransferase *Serum* *Increase* May be a systemic sign of active disease or may indicate involvement of liver or bone *900* In 30% of 10 patients at initial hospitalization for this disorder *1576*

Albumin *Serum* *Decrease* With active disease *5677* *171* In 22% of 72 patients at initial hospitalization for this disorder *1576*

Aldolase *Serum* *Increase* Markedly elevated in malignant lymphomas. Mean = 5.0 ± 0.4 U/L compared to normal, 1.6 - 0.21 U/L *2513*

Alkaline Phosphatase *Serum* *Increase* Observed with liver and bone involvement *900* Lymphoma associated with hyperbilirubinemia is accompanied by elevations from 43 to 331 U/L. In some cases, reflects osteoblastic lesions as well as metastases *5738* In 20 of 133 patients with Hodgkin's disease and liver involvement activity greater than 210 U/L had a sensitivity of 40%, specificity of of 86% and predictive value of 33% for hepatic involvement *1781* May be a systemic sign of active disease or may indicate involvement of liver or bone *2516* *5677* Progressive increase in patients over 20 y of age with elevated concentrations found with advancing clinical stage. Patients < 20 had frequent (50%) occurrence of elevations but this did not correlate with stage of disease. More sensitive than GGT in following the clinical course *381*
White Blood Cells *Decrease* Activity is low irrespective of tumor category, activity of disease, or type of therapy. In 17 cases of malignant lymphoma, median LAP was 17 U/L (normal 55 U/L) *3110*
White Blood Cells *Increase* Elevated during active phases. Normal during remission *5677* In 4 cases, mean value was 135 U/L, ranging from 92 - 182 U/L. Activities were elevated in patients in spite of good remission with no clinical and radiological sign of disease *3440* 22 of 23 patients with active disease had significant LAP elevations, mean score of 164 ± 51. Of 19 patients with inactive disease, 15 had normal scores, 63 ± 17, and the 4 with elevated scores soon redeveloped symptoms of activity *387*

Alkaline Phosphatase, Bone Isoenzyme *Serum* *Increase* Significant positive correlation observed with stage of disease and general symptoms in 83 patients *1781*

Alkaline Phosphatase, Placental Isoenzyme *Serum* *Increase* Mean activity in 23 patients with Hodgkin's disease significantly greater than the mean in 77 healthy adults but did not correlate with the stage or histology *1781*

Alkaline Phosphatase, Regan Type *Serum* *Increase* Mean activity in 38 patients with Hodgkin's disease (stages I to IV) significantly greater than in 40 age and sex-matched healthy adults, and mean activity increased linearly with the stage of the disease *1781*

Angiotensin-converting Enzyme *Serum* *Decrease* Non-significant reduction observed *4416* No relationship was found between enzyme activity and stage, activity, histopathology, etc. Levels were lower than in healthy controls but not significantly

201.90 Hodgkin's Disease *(continued)*

Angiotensin-converting Enzyme *(continued)*
536 Mean activity normal or reduced in patients with Hodgkin's disease *1781*
Serum *No Effect* Mean activity normal or reduced in patients with Hodgkin's disease *1781*

Aspartate Aminotransferase *Serum* *Increase* May be a systemic sign of active disease or may indicate involvement of liver or bone *900* Minimal elevation was observed in 5 of 11 patients *381*

Bicarbonate *Serum* *Increase* In 60% of 45 patients at initial hospitalization for this disorder *1576*

Bilirubin *Serum* *Increase* May be a systemic sign of active disease or may indicate involvement of liver or bone *900*

Bleeding Time *Patient* *Decrease* Has been reported *5677* *2255* Associated with thrombocytopenia *4979*

BSP Retention *Serum* *Increase* May be a systemic sign of active disease or may indicate involvement of liver or bone *900*

CA 549 *Serum* *Increase* In 14 patients with Hodgkin's disease 1 (7.1%) had a concentration greater than the upper limit of normal with BRESMARQ assay *764*

Calcium *Serum* *Increase* Observed in 6 cases (range 10.6 - 16.4 mg/dL) *4311* In patients with bone and liver disease *5677* Indicates bone involvement *900* In patients with bone and liver disease *2516* Metastatic or lytic tumor involving bone *1025*

Carcinoembryonic Antigen *Serum* *Increase* Concentration correlates with disease stage in patients with Hodgkin's disease *1781* In 22% of cases *4891*
Serum *No Effect* Levels are low in this malignancy, remaining within the normal range or just above it *5286*

$CD3^+$ Lymphocytes *Blood* *Decrease* Concentration in patients with Hodgkin's disease significantly less than in healthy controls with concentration, to some extent, correlated with severity of disease *5321*

$CD4^+$ Lymphocytes *Blood* *Decrease* In patients with Hodgkin's Disease concentration in creased with decrease greatest in patients with stage IV disease *5321*

$CD8^+$ Lymphocytes *Blood* *Decrease* In patients with Hodgkin's disease concentration reduced with reduction most marked in patients with stage IV disease *5321*

Ceruloplasmin *Serum* *Increase* Increased concentration observed in the majority of patients with Hodgkin's disease in relapse with lower concentration in remission. In 54 patients with Hodgkin's disease range of concentrations of 26.3 - 93.2 mg/dL compared with 13.8 - 28.2 mg/dL in 25 healthy controls *1781*

Cholesterol *Serum* *Decrease* In 27% of 72 patients at initial hospitalization for this disorder *1576*

Chylomicrons *Serum* *Increase* Moderate increase due to presence of IgG or IgM that forms complexes with chylomicron remnants and/or VLDL thereby decreasing catabolism *126*

Circulating Immune Complexes *Serum* *Increase* Reported incidence of 19 - 50% in patients with Hodgkin's disease *1781*

Clot Retraction *Blood* *Decrease* With thrombocytopenia *4979*

Complement C_1 *Serum* *Increase* In 10 patients with Hodgkin's disease mean concentration of 45.475 ± 10.411 CH50 U/mL significantly different from 37.251 ± 5.324 CH50 U/mL in 11 controls *3037*

Complement C_2 *Serum* *Increase* In 10 patients with Hodgkin's disease mean concentration of 9.577 ± 2.846 CH50 U/mL significantly different from 6.064 ± 1.445 CH50 U/mL in 11 controls *3037*

Complement C_3 *Serum* *Increase* In 10 patients with Hodgkin's disease mean concentration of 10.516 ± 2.040 CH50 U/mL not significantly different from 9.720 ± 2.476 CH50 U/mL in 11 controls *3037*

Complement C_4 *Serum* *Increase* In 10 patients with Hodgkin's disease mean concentration of 102.318 ± 37.066 CH50 U/mL significantly different from 64.920 ± 10.373 CH50 U/mL in 11 controls *3037*

Complement C_5 *Serum* *Increase* In 10 patients with Hodgkin's disease mean concentration of 153.191 ± 38.071 CH50 U/mL significantly different from 118.869 ± 13.547 CH50 U/mL in 11 controls *3037*

Complement C_7 *Serum* *Increase* In 10 patients with Hodgkin's disease mean concentration of 110.313 ± 40.425 CH50 U/mL not significantly different from 94.649 ± 22.434 CH50 U/mL in 11 controls *3037*

Complement C_8 *Serum* *Increase* In 10 patients with Hodgkin's disease mean concentration of 144.997 ± 29.262 CH50 U/mL significantly different from 79.129 ± 25.316 CH50 U/mL in 11 controls *3037*

Complement C_9 *Serum* *Increase* In 10 patients with Hodgkin's disease mean concentration of 162.341 ± 61.429 CH50 U/mL significantly different from 49.401 ± 12.308 CH50 U/mL in 11 controls *3037*

Complement CH50 *Serum* *Increase* In 10 patients with Hodgkin's disease mean concentration of 133.017 ± 42.210 CH50 U/mL significantly different from 104.313 ± 17.058 CH50 U/mL in 11 controls *3037*

Complement, Total *Serum* *Increase* 58 of 72 patients had elevated total complement levels which were associated with C-reactive protein, ESR and β-globulin levels *4459* A highly significant increase of the mean total serum hemolytic complement activity was found in stages III-A and IV-A and all stages with systemic symptoms in Hodgkin's disease *5518* In 10 patients with Hodgkin's disease mean concentration of 624 ± 106 CH50 U/mL significantly different from 474 ± 52 CH50 U/mL in 11 controls *3037*

Coombs' Test *Serum* *Positive* Usually negative, but on occasion it is positive *1314* *5677*

Copper *Serum* *Increase* Correlates significantly to stage of disease and amount of tumor tissue. Varies with activity of the disease--increases with progression and decreases with improvement *5225* Has been reported *5677* *2255* In all 50 patients with lymphoma, invariably found to be raised. After radiotherapy, the level was significantly lowered *4292* In 54 patients with Hodgkin's disease mean concentration significantly increased almost 3-fold compared with the value in 25 healthy controls *1781*

Copper:Iron Ratio *Serum* *Increase* Ratio in Hodgkin's disease has a sensitivity of 75% as a guide for disease activity *1781*

Corticotropin *Plasma* *No Effect* No change observed in patients with Hodgkin's disease *1781*

Cortisol *Plasma* *No Effect* No change in concentration observed in patients with Hodgkin's disease *1781*

C-Reactive Protein *Serum* *Increase* Increased during active stages; may be normal during remission *5545* Mean concentration increased in 31% of patients with stage I and II disease and 53% of patients with stage III and IV disease. In complete remission the incidence of increased concentrations was 5% at all stages *1781*

Creatine Kinase BB-Isoenzyme *Serum* *Increase* Activities greater than or equal to 2.9 U/L in 15 of 34 (44%) patients with Hodgkin's disease *1781*

Creatinine *Serum* *Increase* In 36% of 37 patients at initial hospitalization for this disorder *1576*

Cryoglobulins *Serum* *Increase* May be associated with cryoglobulinemia *5545*

Eosinophils *Blood* *Increase* Occasionally seen *900* In 29% of 77 patients at initial hospitalization for this disorder *1576* Eosinophilia, usually < 10%, may be seen in 10 - 20% of cases *2039* Tends to occur in patients with severe and longstanding pruritus *367* A striking eosinophilia is the outstanding characteristic *3239*
Liver *Increase* Eosinophilic predominance occurs mainly in the fibrotic types of Hodgkin's disease. The survival time of patients with eosinophilic predominance was significantly shorter than that of the controls *5264*

Epstein Barr Virus Antibodies *Serum* *Increase* Elevated titers were noted and these elevated titers have been shown to precede the disease *2422*

Erythrocyte Sedimentation Rate *Blood* *Increase* Commonly elevated in patients with active disease *367* Increased in significant tissue necrosis, especially neoplasms - most frequently malignant lymphoma, cancer of the colon and breast *5545* Increases with stage of disease *5518*

Erythrocyte Survival *Red Blood Cells* *Decrease* Mild or moderate hemolytic anemia, with a negative Coombs' test, is common in disseminated lymphoma *900*

Erythrocytes *Blood* *Decrease* Pancytopenia is a common feature *5677*

Erythropoietin *Serum* *Decrease* The most frequent finding is a normochromic anemia, most often a result of decreased erythropoiesis *2039*

Ferritin *Serum* *Increase* A high circulating concentration is characteristic *5677* Significant elevation *4970* Serum levels are raised due to increased production by splenic tumor tissue *4576* A high circulating concentration is characteristic *2482* Hodgkin's disease may increase serum ferritin concentration and ferritin may function as a tumor mrker *4784* Increased concentration about three times higher than mean for 300 healthy individuals observed in 20 patients with Hodgkin's disease, with increasing concentration with progression of disease and decline with remission. In one study mean concentration of 210 ng/mL significantly higher than mean of 85 ng/mL in 178 healthy men and 39 ng/mL in 105 healthy women *1781*

Fibrinogen *Plasma* *Increase* Concentration in Hodgkin's disease has a sensitivity of 32% as a guide for disease activity *1781* Increases with stage of disease *5518* The concentration of fibrinogen in 16 patients with Hodgkin's disease significantly higher during acute disease onset and relapse than in 20 healthy controls *1781*

Fucose *Serum* *Increase* Markedly elevated and correlated with clinical stage of disease. Values ranged from 13 mg/dL in stage 1 to 29.5 mg/dL in stage 4 *1269*

α_1-Globulin *Serum* *Increase* Increased alpha$_1$ and alpha$_2$-globulins suggest disease activity *5545* In the presence of fever *5699*

α_2-Globulin *Serum* *Increase* Frequently increased in later stages of disease *5518* With active disease *5677* Often quite high *5699* With active disease *171* Concentration in Hodgkin's disease has a sensitivity of 40% as a guide for disease activity *1781*

β-Globulin *Serum* *Increase* Active disease *171*

γ-Globulin *Serum* *Decrease* Infrequent. Concentrations < 200 mg/dL are rarely documented *2195* Rare occasions *2194* *Serum* *Increase* The concentration of γ-globulin, largely attributable to IgG, is typically increased in patients with Hodgkin's disease *1781* May be increased with macroglobulins present and evidence of autoimmune process *5545* Electrophoretic studies of serum proteins are often normal early in the course of the disease but may show a hyperglobulinemia (commonly alpha$_2$) *2039* With active disease *5677* *171*

γ-Glutamyltransferase *Serum* *Increase* In 73% of 12 patients at initial hospitalization for this disorder *1576* Elevated in 36% (4 of 11) patients *381*

Granulocyte Colony Stimulating Factor *Serum* *No Effect* Concentration below detectable level in 43 patients with untreated Hodgkin's disease *1674*

Granulocyte-Macrophage Colony Stimulating Factor *Serum* *Increase* In 56 patients with untreated disease 22 showed presence of GM-CSF (range 4- 140 pg/mL) *1674*

Growth Hormone *Plasma* *Increase* Concentration increased in 80% patients with Hodgkin's disease at diagnosis *1781*

Haptoglobin *Serum* *Increase* Observed effect *367* Increased in disseminated neoplasms; conditions associated with increased ESR and alpha$_2$-globulin *5544* The concentration of haptoglobin was increased in 32 patients with Hodgkin's disease *1781*

Hematocrit *Blood* *Decrease* Mild or moderate hemolytic anemia, with a negative Coombs' test, is common in disseminated lymphoma *900* In 38% of 76 patients at initial hospitalization for this disorder *1576* Present in 33% of all patients at diagnosis. Develops in nearly every patient who has fever, sweats, or other systemic manifestations. Becomes worse as the disease advances and improves with remission *864* *5677*

Hemoglobin *Blood* *Decrease* In 44% of 76 patients at initial hospitalization for this disorder *1576* Present in 33% of all patients at diagnosis. Develops in nearly every patient who has fever, sweats, or other systemic manifestations. Becomes worse as the disease advances and improves with remission *864* Mild to moderate hemolytic anemia, with a negative Coombs' test, is common in disseminated lymphoma *900* Present in 33% of all patients at diagnosis. Develops in nearly every patient who has fever, sweats, or other systemic manifestations. Becomes worse as the disease advances and improves with remission *5677*

Herpes Simplex Virus Antibodies *Serum* *No Effect* Serial serum samples from 37 patients with Hodgkin's disease and 39 healthy controls were studied for antibodies to human herpes virus-6 using ELISA and indirect immunofluorescent antibody tests and to Epstein Barr virus using a radio complement fixation asssay. Antibodies in the pretreatment sera from patients with this disorder were not significantly different from controls *3013*

Heterophile Antibody *Serum* *Increase* Very rare *1025*

Hexokinase *Serum* *Increase* Markedly increased in malignant lymphomas. Mean activity of 14.6 ± 2.0 U/L compared to normal of 0.93 ± 0.28 U/L *2513*

Hexosamines, Protein-bound *Serum* *Increase* In 30 patients with Hodgkin's syndrome mean concentration of 1,187 ± 232 mg/dm^3 significantly greater than 627 ± 183 mg/dm^3 in 40 healthy controls *1781*

Hexoses, Protein-bound *Serum* *Increase* In 30 patients with Hodgkin's disease mean concentration of 5,400 ± 824 mg/dm^3 significantly greater than 1,530 ± 325 mg/dm^3 in 40 healthy controls *1781*

Hodgkin's Immune Complex-associated Antigen *Serum* *Increase* Reported prevalence of 37% (present in 12 of 33 sera) in patients with Hodgkin's disease *1781*

α_2-HS Glycoprotein *Serum* *Decrease* Significant reduction observed compared with healthy controls probably due to hepatic involvement *2533*

Hydroxyproline *Plasma* *Increase* Observed effect *1228*

immunoglobulin A *Serum* *Increase* The concentration of IgA was increased in patients with untreated Hodgkin's disease especially in patients with nodular sclerosis *1781* *Serum* *No Effect* Concentration usually normal *5544*

Immunoglobulin E *Serum* *Increase* The concentration of IgE was increased in 105 patients with untreated Hodgkin's disease especially in patients with nodular sclerosis: IgE alone increased in lymphocyte-predominant and mixed cellularity forms of the disease *1781* In 19 patients with Hodgkin's disease mean concentration of 945 ng/mL (range 162 - 5,512) significantly higher than mean of 96 ng/mL (range 24 - 386) in 74 healthy controls *2323*

Immunoglobulin G *Serum* *Increase* The concentration of IgG was increased in 105 patients with untreated Hodgkin's disease especially in patients with nodular sclerosis *1781* *Serum* *No Effect* Concentration usually normal *5544*

Immunoglobulin M *Serum* *No Effect* Concentration usually normal *5544*

Insulin *Plasma* *Increase* Concentration increased in patients with Hodgkin's disease in relapse, but low or normal in remission, reciprocal to glucose concentration *1781*

Interferon-γ *Serum* *No Effect* Sixty serum samples from patients with Hodgkin's disease (28 patients) or non-Hodgkin's lymphoma (32 patients), as well as 20 samples from normal volunteers, were collected. The majority of patients had advanced (Stage III or IV) or relapsed disease. There were no statistically significant differences between lymphoma patients and normal subjects *2867*

Interleukin-1 *Serum* *No Effect* Sixty serum samples from patients with Hodgkin's disease (28 patients) or non-Hodgkin's lymphoma (32 patients), as well as 20 samples from normal volunteers, were collected. The majority of patients had advanced (Stage III or IV) or relapsed disease. There were no statistically significant differences between lymphoma patients and normal subjects *2867*

Interleukin-1α *Serum* *Increase* In 7 previously untreated patients with Ann Arbor stage I disease median concentration of 220 (90 - 470) pg/mL, in 12 with stage II disease 210 (< 25 - 500) pg/mL and in 5 stage III - IV disease 190 (45 - 420) pg/mL compared with 43 pg/mL in 24 healthy control volunteers *480*

Interleukin-1β *Serum* *Increase* In 3 of 43 (7%) patients with untreated Hodgkin's disease concentration measurable with range 389 - 1505 pg/mL *1674*

201.90 Hodgkin's Disease *(continued)*

Interleukin-2 *Serum Increase* In 7 previously untreated patients with Ann Arbor stage I disease median concentration of 4 (2.5 - 32) U/mL, in 12 with stage II disease of 2 (< 0.5 - 90) U/mL and in 5 with stage III - IV disease of 4 (< 0.5 - 14) U/mL compared with < 0.5 U/mL in 24 healthy control volunteers *480*

Interleukin-3 *Serum Increase* In 40 patients with untreated Hodgkin's disease presence detected in 5 (40%). Range of concentrations observed 13 - 26 pg/mL *1674*

Interleukin-4 *Serum No Effect* In 24 previously untreated patients with Hodgkin's disease IL-4 not detected as in 24 healthy control volunteers *480*

Interleukin-6 *Serum Increase* Tested the sera of 56 untreated patients with HD by means of a sensitive sandwich ELISA. While IL-6 was only rarely detectable in healthy controls or patients with non-Hodgkin's lymphoma, 32 of 56 patients (57 per cent) had detectable IL-6 levels (range 12 - 32 pg/mL) *1713* In 7 previously untreated patients with Ann Arbor stage I disease mean concentration of < 70 (< 70 - 1,900) pg/mL, in 12 with stage II disease of 75 (< 70 - 690) pg/mL and in 5 stage III - IV disease of 110 (< 70 - 130) pg/mL compared with < 70 pg/mL in 24 healthy control volunteers *480* In patients with Hodgkin's lymphoma concentration higher than in patients with monoclonal gammopathy and healthy controls *4927* Sixty serum samples from patients with Hodgkin's disease (28 patients) or non-Hodgkin's lymphoma (32 patients), as well as 20 samples from normal volunteers, were collected. The majority of patients had advanced (Stage III or IV) or relapsed disease. 20 of 57 patients (35%) with lymphoma as compared with 0 of 19 normal volunteers (0%) had detectable serum IL-6 levels ($p < 0.005$, chi 2 test) *2867* In 12 patients with Hodgkin's lymphoma mean concentration of 26.0 ± 3.5 pg/mL significantly different from 8.8 ± 1.8 pg/mL in 27 healthy control individuals *1120* In 56 patients with untreated Hodgkin's disease, 32 (57%) had detectable concentrations in serum. Range in these patients 12 - 332 pg/mL *1674*

Interleukin-8 *Serum No Effect* In 12 patients with Hodgkin's lymphoma mean concentration of 28.1 ± 7.2 pg/mL not significantly different from 16.2 ± 1.4 pg/mL in 27 healthy control individuals *1120*

Iron *Serum Decrease* Hypoferremia is characteristic and may be associated with excessive uptake of iron by the liver and spleen *5677* In 85 patients with Hodgkin's disease mean concentration significantly decreased by 60% compared to healthy controls but returned to normal with remission *1781* In 77% of 18 patients at initial hospitalization for this disorder *1576*

Iron-binding Capacity, Total *Serum Decrease* In 32% of 18 patients at initial hospitalization for this disorder *1576* Observed effect *367 1228*

Iron Saturation *Serum Decrease* In 94% of 18 patients at initial hospitalization for this disorder *1576*

Lactate *Blood Increase* In 20 patients with malignant lymphomas, mean concentration = 23.2 ± 2.9 mg/dL compared to normal, 11.7 ± 0.72 mg/dL *2513*
Plasma Increase Lactic acidosis may occur in Hodgkin's disease in relapse *1781*

Lactate Dehydrogenase *Serum Increase* Normal or relatively increased; depends on the total mass of the tumor and presence of hemolysis *1025* Marked elevation in 138 patients with malignant lymphomas. Mean activity of 177.7 ± 13.8 U/L compared to normals, 85.4 ± 1.0 U/L *2513* May be a sign of active disease or may indicate involvement of liver or bone *900* In 37% of 72 patients at initial hospitalization for this disorder *1576* Activity increased in most patients with malignant lymphomas *1781*

Lactate Dehydrogenase Isoenzymes *Serum Increase* LD_3 and LD_4 (may even increase LD_2); also useful for following effect of chemotherapy *1642*

Laminin *Serum No Effect* Did not differ from normal controls *4394*

Leukocytes *Blood Decrease* Pancytopenia is a common feature *5677* Variable, maybe normal, decreased, or markedly increased *5545*
Blood Increase In 56% of 77 patients at initial hospitalization for this disorder *1576* In the untreated patient, or if therapy has been minimal, moderate to marked neutrophilic leukocytosis and thrombocytosis are characteristic of active, symptomatic Hodgkin's disease *367* Variable, maybe normal, decreased, or markedly increased *5545* Moderately increased and a granulocytosis and monocytosis may be observed *2039*

Lymphocyte T-Cells *Blood Decrease* Normal *1588*

Lymphocytes *Blood Decrease* Absolute counts tend to be at the lower end of the normal range or slightly below the lower limit. Frequently more severe in the presence of disseminated disease *4551* In 66% of 76 patients at initial hospitalization for this disorder *1576* Lymphopenia is common late in the disease *2039* In patients with stage IV disease concentration lower than in patients with less severe disease and in healthy controls *5321*
Blood Increase Relative lymphocytosis when there is marked neutropenia but not absolute increase *4979*
Pleural Fluid Increase A preponderance of lymphocytes is consistent with tuberculosis, carcinoma, or lymphoma *1980*

Lysozyme *Serum Increase* Significantly higher compared to controls and independent of stage *536* Isolated cases *2012*

β_2-Macroglobulin *Cerebrospinal Fluid Increase* May be increased in lymphomas involving the central nervous system *2586* With Involvement of the CNS *815*
Serum Increase May be increased *2586 815*

Methyl-1-Adenosine *Urine Increase* Excretion increased more than 2 SD above the mean in 85% of 7 patients with Hodgkin's disease *1781*

1-Methylinosine *Urine Increase* In 2 patients with Hodgkin's disease, excretions of 3.7 and 10.8 mg/d, one normal but the other significantly different from 3.9 ± 2.1 mg/d in 17 healthy controls *5505*
Urine No Effect In 2 patients with Hodgkin's disease, excretions of 3.7 and 10.8 mg/d, one normal but the other significantly different from 3.9 ± 2.1 mg/d in 17 healthy controls *5505*

Monocytes *Blood Increase* Appearance of abnormal large mononuclear cells in peripheral blood *900* All varieties of lymphomas have been reported on occasion in association with a monocytosis, sometimes varying with disease activity *2303* 10 - 40% of cases exhibited a monocytosis that did not correlate with prognosis *5355* In 71% of 77 patients at initial hospitalization for this disorder *1576*

N^2, N^2-Dimethylguanosine *Urine Increase* In 2 patients with Hodgkin's disease excretions of 7.2 and 4.9 mg/d significantly different from 3.9 ± 2.6 mg/d in 17 healthy controls *5505*

Neopterin *Urine Increase* In 4 patients with Hodgkin's disease mean excretion increased by 146% over baseline of 106.6 ± 34.6 µmol/mol creatinine in 31 healthy controls *3632* In patients with stage III and IV disease mean concentration of 525 ± 317 µmol/mol creatinine compared with 227 ± 97 µmol/mol creatinine in stage I and II disease and 173 ± 78 µmol/mol creatinine in patients in remission *4128* Urinary excretion in 79 of 112 patients with Hodgkin's disease, non-Hodgkin's lymphoma or other hematologic malignancies greater than mean ± 3 SD in healthy individuals *1781*

Neuron-specific Enolase *Serum Increase* Reported finding *5546*

Neutrophils *Blood Increase* Common *900* In 54% of 77 patients at initial hospitalization for this disorder *1576*

5'-Nucleotidase *Serum Increase* Six patients showed elevations varying from 18.8 - 126.2 U/L (normal 2 - 11 U/L) *2803*

5-Nucleotide Phosphodiesterase Isoenzyme V
Serum Increase Mean activity was increased in the plasma of 54% patients with Hodgkin's disease or other lymphomas without evidence of hepatic metastases *1781*

Osmotic Fragility *Red Blood Cells Increase* A higher degree of light transmission, i.e., osmotic fragility, was found in lymphocytes from Hodgkin's disease patients. After 10 min, light transmission of 70.3 - 5.93% compared to 60 ± 7.33% for normals *4328*

Perchloric Acid Soluble Protein *Serum Increase* In 30 patients with Hodgkin's disease mean concentration of 71.5 ± 12.4 mg tyrosine/dm^3 significantly greater than 43.7 ± 11.8 mg tyrosine/dm^3 in 40 healthy controls *1781*

Phosphohexoseisomerase *Lymphocytes Increase* Activity increased in lymphocytes of patients with Hodgkin's disease *1781*
Monocytes No Effect Activity not affected in monocytes of patients with Hodgkin's disease *1781*

Phospholipase A *Serum Increase* Significantly elevated *2625*

Platelets *Blood Decrease* Pancytopenia is a common feature. May result from hypersplenism *5677*
Blood Increase In 45% of 70 patients at initial hospitalization for this disorder *1576* Thrombocytosis (counts > 400,000 /µL) encountered at times, and large bizarre forms may be observed *2039*

Polyamines *Serum Increase* Mean concentration of 1.2 - 5.7 nmol/mL in 55 patients with Hodgkin's disease significantly increased compared with 0.62 - 0.87 nmol/mL in normal individuals *1781*

Porphobilinogen *Urine Increase* Elevated porphobilinogen occasionally has been observed *367*

Proline Hydroxylase *Serum Increase* Elevated to a lesser degree than that seen in hepatoma *762*

Protein *Pleural Fluid Increase* Pleural effusions are usually exudates *126*
Serum Decrease Occurs commonly *5677* In patients with advanced disease, reduction in serum protein concentration with hypoalbuminemia and hypogammaglobulinemia is frequent *5533* Enteric loss of plasma protein *4891*

Pseudouridine *Urine Increase* Excretion increased more than 2 SD above the mean in 88% of 7 patients with Hodgkin's disease *1781*
Urine No Effect In 4 patients with Hodgkin's disease excretion comparable to that in 31 healthy controls (19.6 ± 5.2 mmol/mol creatinine) *3632* In 2 patients with Hodgkin's disease excretions of 40 and 81 mg/d not significantly different from 65 ± 31 mg/d in 17 healthy controls *5505*

Putrescine *Serum Increase* In two patients with Hodgkins disease concentrations of 1.38 and 2.19 nmol/mL compared with normal mean of 0.23 nmol/mL *3805*
Urine Increase Mean excretion in 20 patients with Hodgkin's disease increased prior to treatment *1781*

Pyruvate *Blood Increase* Moderately elevated in 20 patients with malignant lymphomas. Mean = 1.1 ± 0.15 U/L *2513*

Reticulocytes *Blood Increase* In patients with advanced disease *5677*

Rheumatoid Factor *Serum Increase* Dysproteinemias and paraproteinemias present significant seropositivity *1980* Found in 18% of patients *874*

Ribonuclease *Serum Increase* In 9 patients with Hodgkin's disease mean activity of 437 ± 84 U/mL significantly higher than 266 ± 39 U/mL in 15 normal individuals *2793*

Sialic Acid, Lipid-associated *Serum Increase* In patients with Hodgkin's syndrome mean concentration increased above 20 mg/dL in 94% of patients *1781*

Sialyltransferase *Serum Increase* In 2 patients with Hodgkin's lymphoma mean and median concentrations of 511 and 480 cpm/mg protein/30 min significantly different from 240 and 243 cpm/mg protein/30 min respectively in 20 normal individuals *2111* Activity increased in 4 of 15 patients with Hodgkin's disease but associated with liver involvement *1781*

Soluble CD30 Antigen *Serum Increase* CD30 antigen observed in 24 out of 50 patients (48%) with active Hodgkin's disease. CD30 not detected in healthy controls and in patients in complete remission. In patients with progressive or relapsing disease mean concentration of 458 ± 190 U/mL compared with 116 ± 33 U/mL observed in individuals on presentation. Concentrations highest in stages III and IV 182 ± 60 U/mL, in B' cases 208 ± 73 mU/mL, and in stages I and II 65 ± 30 U/mL or A' patients 64 ± 20 U/mL *4151*

Soluble Interleukin-2 Receptor *Serum Increase* In children with Hodgkin's disease mean concentration in 10 stage 1 patients of 1,738 U/mL, in 33 stage II patients of 2,420 U/mL, in 16 stage III of 3,579 U/mL and in 9 stage IV patients of 9,992 U/mL significantly higher than in controls *4235* In 17 patients with active Hodgkin's disease mean concentration of 2,363 ± 2,876 $\times 10^3$ U/L significantly increased compared with 771 ± 450 $\times 10^3$ U/L in 8 patients in remission *4128*

Spermidine *Serum No Effect* In two patients with Hodgkins disease concentrations of 0.33 and 0.36 nmol/mL compared with normal mean of 0.33 nmol/mL *3805*
Urine Increase Mean excretion in 20 patients with Hodgkin's disease increased prior to treatment *1781*

Spermine *Serum No Effect* In two patients with Hodgkins disease concentrations 0 and 0.07 nmol/mL compared with normal mean of 0.04 nmol/mL *3805*

T23 Protein *Serum Increase* Protein detected in serum of 9 of 19 cases of Hodgkin's disease compared with none in controls *1781*

Thyroxine (T4) *Serum No Effect* No change in concentration observed in patients with Hodgkin's disease *1781*

Tissue Factor *Monocytes Increase* In 14 patients with relapsed Hodgkin's disease activity in both disrupted and intact monocytes significantly greater than in controls with highest values observed typically in men who had undergone splenectomy *1960*

Tissue Polypeptide Antigen *Serum No Effect* No correlation with disease observed in patients with Hodgkin's disease *1781*

Tumor Necrosis Factor *Serum Increase* In 24 previously untreated patients with Hodgkin's disease TNF detectable in 6 (25%) compared with 2 of 24 (8%) healthy controls *480*

Tumor Necrosis Factor-α *Serum Increase* In 3 of 43 patients with untreated Hodgkin's disease (7%) TNF-α detected (range 36 - 66 pg/mL) *1674*
Serum No Effect Sixty serum samples from patients with Hodgkin's disease (28 patients) or non-Hodgkin's lymphoma (32 patients), as well as 20 samples from normal volunteers, were collected. The majority of patients had advanced (Stage III or IV) or relapsed disease. There were no statistically significant differences between lymphoma patients and normal subjects *2867*

Uric Acid *Serum Decrease* Decreased uric acid is seen in occasional cases of neoplasms such as Hodgkin's disease *5544* Hypouricemia associated with markedly elevated clearance has been reported *2605* Rarely reported *1980*
Serum Increase In 31% of 72 patients at initial hospitalization for this disorder *1576* Especially post X-irradiation *5544* Hyperuricemia occurs occasionally *2039*

Uric Acid Clearance *Urine Increase* Hypouricemia associated with markedly elevated clearance has been reported *2605*

Vitamin B_{12} *Serum No Effect* Typical observation *5544*

Vitamin B_{12} Binding Capacity *Serum Increase* Significant elevation; usually correlated with WBC in peripheral blood *4448*

VLDL-Cholesterol *Serum Increase* Moderate increase due to presence of IgG or IgM that forms complexes with chylomicron remnants and/or VLDL thereby decreasing catabolism *126*

Zinc *Hair Decrease* In 51 patients aged 3 - 15 y with Hodgkin's disease mean concentration significantly decreased compared with that in 20 healthy children *1781*
Red Blood Cells Decrease In 51 patients aged 3 - 15 y with Hodgkin's disease mean concentration significantly decreased compared with that in 20 healthy children *1781*
Serum Decrease In 51 patients aged 3 - 15 y with Hodgkin's disease mean concentration significantly decreased compared with that in 20 healthy children *1781*

202.00 Lymphocytic Lymphoma, Nodular

Immunoglobulin A *Serum No Effect* Mean concentration in patients with nodular lymphocytic lymphoma not significantly changed *1781*

Immunoglobulin D *Serum No Effect* Mean concentration in patients with nodular lymphocytic lymphoma not significantly changed *1781*

Immunoglobulin E *Serum Decrease* Mean concentration in patients with nodular lymphocytic lymphoma significantly reduced *1781*

Immunoglobulin G *Serum No Effect* Mean concentration in patients with nodular lymphocytic lymphoma not significantly changed *1781*

Immunoglobulin M *Serum No Effect* Mean concentration in patients with nodular lymphocytic lymphoma not significantly changed *1781*

202.10 Mycosis Fungoides

$CD8^+$ Lymphocytes *Blood Decrease* In patients with mycosis fungoides concentration reduced below normal *4968*

Eosinophils *Blood Increase* Eosinophilia *5678*

202.10 Mycosis Fungoides *(continued)*

immunoglobulin A *Serum* *Increase* May be elevated *5678* No prognostic significance *5678*

Immunoglobulin E *Serum* *Increase* May be elevated *5678*

Lactate Dehydrogenase *Serum* *Increase* Significant correlation between basal levels and malignant gastrinoma but not with benign tumors *5678*

β_2-Macroglobulin *Serum* *Increase* Increased concentration observed compared with healthy controls *2930*

Soluble CD8+ *Serum* *Decrease* Plasma sCD8 concentration was found to be below normal control levels in MF *4968*

Soluble Interleukin-2 Receptor *Serum* *Decrease* In patients with mycosis fungoides in remission mean concentration significantly reduced *4968* Reduced levels of sIL-2R were encountered in HCL patients in remission, in pre-T-ALL, and in mycosis fungoides patients in remission *4968*
Serum *Increase* Elevated sIL-2R levels were found in active MF *4968* In patients with active mycosis fungoides concentration significantly increased *4968*

202.40 Hairy Cell Leukemia

Acid Phosphatase, Tartrate Resistant *Serum* *Increase* In patients with hairy cell leukemia moderate increase observed *4217*

Alkaline Phosphatase *White Blood Cells* *Increase* Mean activity increased in 17 of 23 (74%) patients with hairy cell leukemia *1781*
White Blood Cells *No Effect* Mean activity normal in 6 of 23 (26%) patients with hairy cell leukemia *1781*

Cholesterol *Serum* *Decrease* Mean concentration of 152.8 mg/dL (median 155 mg/dL) observed in 46 patients with hairy cell leukemia significantly less than the mean concentration of 210 mg/dL in the general American population *3988*

Glucose-6-Phosphate Dehydrogenase
Red Blood Cells *Increase* In 6 patients with hairy cell leukemia mean concentration of 15.6 ± 2.4 IU/g hemoglobin not significantly different from 12.0 ± 1.2 IU/g hemoglobin in 50 healthy controls *188*

Soluble CD8+ *Blood* *Decrease* Concentration reduced below normal in patients with HCL with concentration lowest in relapsing cases *4968*
Serum *Decrease* Plasma sCD8 was found to be below normal control levels in HCL, and lowest in relapsing cases *4968*

Soluble Intercellular Adhesion Molecule-1 *Serum* *Increase* Mean concentration of 770 ± 483 ng/mL in 15 patients with HCL significantly different from 333 ± 77 ng/mL in 31 healthy controls *838* In patients with HCL concentration significantly increased *4968*

Soluble Interleukin-2 Receptor *Serum* *Decrease* Reduced concentrations observed in patients in remission *4968* Reduced levels of sIL-2R were encountered in HCL patients in remission, in pre-T-ALL, and in mycosis fungoides patients in remission *4968*
Serum *Increase* Elevated sIL-2R levels were found in HCL patients at initial diagnosis and relapse *4968* In patients at initial diagnosis and in relapse increased concentration observed *4968*

Soluble Transferrin Receptor *Serum* *No Effect* Concentration not changed typically in myeloproliferative diseases *4784* In patients with hairy cell leukemia mean concentration of 7.04 ± 3.69 µg/mL not significantly different from 5.63 ± 1.42 µg/mL in healthy controls *2704*

202.40 Leukemic Reticuloendotheliosis

Anisocytes *Blood* *Increase* Usually normochromic, normocytic anemia; mild anisocytosis and poikilocytosis were common *5330*

Erythrocytes *Blood* *Decrease* Pancytopenia was found in almost 50% of all patients (102) *5330*

Hematocrit *Blood* *Decrease* Usually normochromic, normocytic anemia; mild anisocytosis and poikilocytosis were common *5330*

Hemoglobin *Blood* *Decrease* Usually normochromic, normocytic anemia; mild anisocytosis and poikilocytosis were common *5330*

Leukocytes *Blood* *Decrease* Leukopenia in 63 of 102 patients, while mild leukocytosis was found in 15 *5330*
Blood *Increase* Leukopenia in 63 of 102 patients, while mild leukocytosis was found in 15 *5330*

Lysozyme *Serum* *Decrease* Low, normal or high *1606*
Serum *Increase* Low, normal or high *1606*
Serum *No Effect* Low, normal or high *1606*

Monocytes *Blood* *Decrease* Severe monocytopenia; 299/µL was the highest count and 6 patients had none at all *5330*

Neutrophils *Blood* *Decrease* Severe bone marrow granulocytopenia and poor blood neutrophil response to stimulation are found *5762* Absolute neutropenia observed in 78% of 102 cases; frequently severe *5330*
Bone Marrow *Decrease* Severe bone marrow granulocytopenia and poor neutrophil response to stimulation are found *5762*

Platelets *Blood* *Decrease* Thrombocytopenia found in 84% of patients with counts usually in the 50 - 150,000 /µL range *5330*

Poikilocytes *Blood* *Increase* Usually normochromic, normocytic anemia; mild anisocytosis and poikilocytosis were common *5330*

202.60 Mastocytosis

Alkaline Phosphatase *Serum* *Increase* Hepatic involvement in mastocytosis is rare but increased alkaline phosphatase activity is the most common abnormal liver function test *3625*

Basophils *Blood* *Increase* Occasionally found *5546*

Eosinophils *Blood* *Increase* Observed effect *5546*

Hematocrit *Blood* *Decrease* Observed effect *5546*

Hemoglobin *Blood* *Decrease* Observed effect *5546*

Histamine *Plasma* *Increase* Concentration significantly increased compared with controls *5546*
Urine *Increase* Excretion considerably increased compared with controls *5546*

5-Hydroxyindoleacetic Acid *Plasma* *Increase* Reported effect *5546*

Mast Cells *Blood* *Increase* Observed effect *5546*

N-Methylimidazoleacetic Acid *Urine* *Increase* Excretion of more than 10 mg/d may be observed in patients with mastocytosis *2952*

Platelets *Blood* *Decrease* Observed effect *5546*

Tryptase *Serum* *Increase* In 13 adult patients with systemic manifestations of mastocytosis median concentration measured with B12 mAb-based fluoroimmunoassay of 162 µg/L compared with 2.2 - 8.8 µg/L in healthy individuals *1845*

202.60 Systemic Mast Cell Disease

Calcitonin *Plasma* *Increase* In a patient with aspirin sensitive systemic mast cell disease mean concentration of 40 pg/mL significantly increased compared with upper limit of normal of 19 pg/mL or less *5802*

Gastrin *Serum* *No Effect* In a patient with aspirin sensitive systemic mast cell disease mean concentration of 53 pg/mL not abnormal compared with upper limit of normal of 200 pg/mL or less *5802*

Histamine *Urine* *Increase* In a patient with aspirin sensitive systemic mast cell disease mean excretion of 92 µg/g creatinine significantly increased compared with upper limit of normal of less than < 45 µg/g creatinine *5802* Increased excretion observed in patients with systemic mastocytosis *2952*

5-Hydroxyindoleacetic Acid *Urine* *No Effect* In a patient with aspirin sensitive systemic mast cell disease mean excretion of 3.8 mg/d not abnormal compared with upper limit of normal of 1.3 mg/d or less *5802*

Metanephrine *Urine* *No Effect* In a patient with aspirin sensitive systemic mast cell disease mean excretion of 1.1 mg/d not abnormal compared with upper limit of normal of less than 1.3 mg/d *5802*

N-Methylimidazoleacetic Acid *Urine* *Increase* In a patient with aspirin sensitive systemic mast cell disease mean excretion of 34 mg/d significantly increased compared with upper limit of normal of less than 5 mg/d *5802*

Tryptase *Serum* *No Effect* In a patient with aspirin sensitive systemic mast cell disease mean concentration of 1.3 ng/mL not abnormal compared with upper limit of normal of less than 5 ng/mL *5802*

Vasoactive Intestinal Polypeptide *Plasma* *No Effect* In a patient with aspirin sensitive systemic mast cell disease mean concentration of 17 pg/mL not abnormal compared with upper limit of normal of less than 75 pg/mL *5802*

202.80 B-cell Lymphoma

Adenosine Monophosphate *Urine* *Increase* In one patient with B-cell lymphoma of the kidney admitted to hospital in a terminal state mean excretion of 24.8 µmol/g creatinine significantly different from reference interval of 4.4 - 14.5 µmol/g creatinine *5365*

Alkaline Phosphatase *Serum* *No Effect* In one patient with B-cell lymphoma of the kidney admitted to hospital in a terminal state mean activity of 232 U/L not significantly different from reference interval of 100 - 280 U/L *5365*

Calcium *Serum* *Increase* In one patient with B-cell lymphoma of the kidney admitted to hospital in a terminal state mean concentration of 16.4 mg/dL significantly different from reference interval of 8.4 - 10.4 mg/dL *5365*
Urine *Increase* In one patient with B-cell lymphoma of the kidney admitted to hospital in a terminal state mean excretion of 438.8 mg/d significantly different from reference interval of 100 - 300 mg/d *5365*

C-Reactive Protein *Serum* *Increase* Increased concentrations observed in patients with newly diagnosed lymphomas positively correlated with increased serum IL-6 concentrations *2579*

1,25-Dihydroxy Vitamin D *Serum* *No Effect* In one patient with B-cell lymphoma of the kidney admitted to hospital in a terminal state mean concentration of 20.5 pg/mL not significantly different from reference interval of 20 - 70 pg/mL *5365*

25-Hydroxy Vitamin D *Serum* *Decrease* In one patient with B-cell lymphoma of the kidney admitted to hospital in a terminal state mean concentration of 7.8 ng/mL significantly different from reference interval of 10 - 55 ng/mL *5365*

Hydroxyproline *Urine* *Increase* In one patient with B-cell lymphoma of the kidney admitted to hospital in a terminal state mean excretion of 83.8 mg/g creatinine significantly different from reference interval of 23 - 48 mg/g creatinine *5365*

Interleukin-6 *Serum* *Increase* Increased concentrations observed in patients with newly diagnosed lymphomas; increased concentrations generally associated with poor overall survival rate *2579*

Lactate Dehydrogenase *Serum* *Decrease* In one patient with B-cell lymphoma of the kidney admitted to hospital in a terminal state mean activity of 1,795 U/L significantly different from reference interval of 222 - 401 U/L *5365*

Osteocalcin *Serum* *Decrease* In one patient with B-cell lymphoma of the kidney admitted to hospital in a terminal state mean concentration of < 1 ng/mL significantly different from reference interval of 2.3 - 9.9 ng/mL *5365*

Parathyroid Hormone *Plasma* *Decrease* In one patient with B-cell lymphoma of the kidney admitted to hospital in a terminal state mean concentration of < 5 pg/mL significantly different from reference interval of 23 - 73 pg/mL *5365*

Parathyroid Hormone-related Peptide *Plasma* *Increase* In one patient with B-cell lymphoma of the kidney admitted to hospital in a terminal state mean concentration of 52.0 pg/mL significantly different from reference interval of < 16 pg/mL *5365*

Phosphate *Serum* *Increase* In one patient with B-cell lymphoma of the kidney admitted to hospital in a terminal state mean concentration of 5.0 mg/dL significantly different from reference interval of 2.5 - 4.5 mg/dL *5365*

Tubular Maximum for Phosphate *Urine* *Decrease* In one patient with B-cell lymphoma of the kidney admitted to hospital in a terminal state mean tubular reabsorption of phosphate of 2.9% significantly different from reference interval of 80 - 92% *5365*

202.80 Lymphoma

α_1-Acid Glycoprotein *Serum* *Increase* Concentration increased in 12 of 13 patients with active lymphoma and was normal in 11 of 12 patients with inactive disease *1781*

Adenosine Deaminase *White Blood Cells* *No Effect* Adenosine deaminase activity in peripheral leukocytes in 3 patients with malignant lymphoma normal *1781*

Albumin *Serum* *Decrease* Hypoalbuminemia commonly found in patients with malignant lymphomas, possibly attributable to defective synthesis, intravascular dilution by increased plasma volume or gastrointestinal blood loss. Concentration inversely related to stage of disease *1781*

Alkaline Phosphatase *Serum* *Increase* Significant increase observed in 8 of 9 patients with adult lymphoma and hepatic involvement but in only 1 of 11 who subsequently devloped hepatic disease *1781*

Alkaline Phosphatase, Bone Isoenzyme *Serum* *Increase* Significant increase observed in 8 of 9 patients with adult lymphoma and hepatic involvement but in only 1 of 11 who subsequently developed hepatic disease *1781*

Anti-p53 Antibodies *Serum* *Increase* Increased in 7 of 115 patients (6.1%) *132*

CA 125 *Serum* *Increase* Concentration in one 53-year-old man with Ki-1 lymphoma significantly increased, decreasing with successful response to chemotherapy *2836* In one woman with malignant lymphoma mean concentration of 380 U/mL significantly greater than upper limit of normal of less than 35 U/mL *161*

Calcium *Serum* *Increase* In one study 4 of 42 patients with hypercalcemia and low intact PTH concentration had lymphoma *3280* Hypercalcemia of malignancy common with this type of cancer *3470*
Urine *Decrease* Hypercalcemia of malignancy common with this type of cancer which leads to diminished capacity of renal tubules to concentrate urine which, in turn, decreases the ECF and the kidney's ability to eliminate excess calcium. Renal impairment eventually causes nitrogen retention, acidosis and renal failure and a further decrease in calcium excretion *3470*
Urine *Increase* Hypercalcemia of malignancy common with this type of cancer which is often associated with hypercalciuria occurring with excessive bone reabsorption *3470*

Carcinoembryonic Antigen *Serum* *No Effect* In patients with lymphoma mean baseline concentration of 2.3 ng/mL compared with upper limit of normal of 3.0 ng/mL *4470*

Copper *Serum* *Increase* In patients with malignant lymphoma concentration significantly increased *1781* In 40 children with malignant lymphomas mean concentration of 199.8 ± 29.8 µg/dL significantly higher than 95.8 ± 21.3 µg/dL in 30 healthy controls: with concentration increasing with stage of the disease *1925*

Copper:Zinc Ratio *Serum* *Increase* In patients with malignant lymphoma ratio significantly increased *1781*

Creatinine *Serum* *Increase* Hypercalcemia of malignancy common with this type of cancer which leads to diminished capacity of renal tubules to concentrate urine which, in turn, decreases the ECF and the kidney's ability to eliminate excess calcium. Renal impairment eventually causes nitrogen retention, acidosis and renal failure and a further decrease in calcium excretion *3470*

Epidermal Growth Factor *Urine* *Increase* Mean concentration in about 6 patients of 18 µg/g creatinine significantly different compared with about 10 µg/g creatinine in about 30 controls *5341*

Epstein Barr Virus Antibodies *Serum* *Increase* Elevated levels were associated with satistically significant excess risk *2984*

α_2-Globulin *Serum* *Increase* Increased concentration observed in majority of patients with malignant lymphoma *1781*

Interleukin-6 *Serum* *Increase* Concentration in one 53-year-old man with Ki-1 lymphoma significantly increased, decreasing with successful response to chemotherapy *2836* In 118 untreated patients with diffuse large-cell lymphoma median concentration of 4.6 pg/mL compared with median of undetectable in 45 healthy people *4212* In 29 of 84 patients with newly diagnosed lymphoma concentrations were greater than 20 pg/mL, the lower limit of quantification, with median in these patients of 40 pg/mL *4531*

202.80 Lymphoma *(continued)*

Lactate Dehydrogenase *Serum* *Increase* In 3 patients with occult malignant lymphoma activity ranged from 595 to 615 U/L *4454*

Lactate Dehydrogenase Isoenzymes *Serum* *Increase* In 3 patients with occult malignant lymphoma total LD activity increased to 595 - 615 U/L with predominance of LD isoenzymes 2 and 3 *4454*

Metallopanstimulin *Serum* *Increase* In 100% of 7 patients with leukemia or lymphoma mean concentration exceeded upper limit of normal of < 10 ng/mL in healthy individuals aged 19 - 88 years *1462*

1-Methylinosine *Urine* *Increase* In 2 patients with Burkitt's lymphoma, excretions of 17.0 and 21.8 mg/d significantly different from 3.9 ± 2.1 mg/d in 17 healthy controls *5505*

β_2-Microglobulin *Cerebrospinal Fluid* *Increase* In patients with CNS involvement of lymphoma mean concentration increased *2013*
Serum *Increase* Increased concentration observed in 30 - 40% of untreated patients with malignant lymphoma and is related to the stage of the disease *1781*

N^2, N^2-Dimethylguanosine *Urine* *Increase* In 2 patients with Burkitt's lymphoma excretions of 19.0 and 9.6 mg/d significantly different from 3.9 ± 2.6 mg/d in 17 healthy controls *5505*

Neopterin *Serum* *Increase* Mean concentration of 25.8 ± 26.0 nmol/L in 9 patients with lymphoma significantly greater than that in 18 healthy control individuals, 6.4 ± 1.8 nmol/L *3864*
Urine *Increase* In 12 patients with non-Hodgkin's lymphoma mean excretion increased to 675.7 µmol/mol creatinine (534% above reference interval of 106.6 ± 34.6 µmol/mol creatinine) *3632*

Neuron-specific Enolase *Serum* *Increase* Reported observation *5546*

5'-Nucleotidase *Serum* *Increase* Mean activity was increased in the plasma of 18 of 72 (25%) patients with malignant lymphoma at diagnosis *1781*

5-Nucleotide Phosphodiesterase Isoenzyme V
Serum *Increase* Mean activity was increased in the plasma of 54% patients with Hodgkin's disease or other lymphomas without evidence of hepatic metastases *1781*

Oligoclonal Banding *Cerebrospinal Fluid* *Increase*
Oligoclonal IgG bands detected in patients with primary lymphoma of the CNS *3261*

Parathyroid Hormone *Plasma* *Decrease* In one study of 42 patients with low intact PTH concentration and hypercalcemia 4 had lymphoma *3280*

pH *Blood* *Decrease* Hypercalcemia of malignancy common with this type of cancer which leads to diminished capacity of renal tubules to concentrate urine which, in turn, decreases the ECF and the kidney's ability to eliminate excess calcium. Renal impairment eventually causes nitrogen retention, acidosis and renal failure and a further decrease in calcium excretion *3470*

Phospholipase A *Serum* *Increase* In 18 children with malignant lymphoma 44% had plasma phospholipase A2 activities of greater than 10 U/L *3156*

Pseudouridine *Urine* *Increase* In 2 patients with Burkitt's lymphoma excretions of 291 and 210 mg/d significantly different from 65 ± 31 mg/d in 17 healthy controls *5505* In 12 patients with non-Hodgkin's lymphoma mean excretion 31.8 mmol/mol creatinine significantly higher than 19.6 ± 5.2 mmol/mol creatinine in 31 healthy controls *3632*

Purine Nucleoside Phosphorylase
White Blood Cells *No Effect* Mean activity was normal in the leukocytes of 3 patients with unspecified malignant lymphoma *1781*

Ribonuclease *Serum* *Increase* In 14 patients with lymphoma mean activity of 417 ± 84 U/mL significantly higher than 266 ± 39 U/mL in 15 normal individuals *2793*

Soluble Transferrin Receptor *Serum* *No Effect* In patients with lymphoma mean concentration of 5.73 ± 2.59 µg/mL not significantly different from 5.63 ± 1.42 µg/mL in healthy controls *2704* Concentration not changed typically in myeloproliferative diseases *4784*

Soluble Tumor Necrosis Factor Receptor-p55
Serum *Increase* In 86 patients with newly diagnosed lymphoma concentration ranged from.0.8 to 18.8 ng/mL (median 3.5 ng/mL) significantly different from 1.1 - 2.3 ng/mL in 18 healthy controls *4531*

Thymidine-5'-triphosphatase *Serum* *Increase* Activity in 3 of 5 patients with malignant lymphoma higher than that in 108 healthy blood donors in whom the highest activity was less than 300 mU/L *1781*

Tissue Factor Pathway Inhibitor *Plasma* *No Effect* 15 patients with lymphoma had median activity of 1.16 U/mL not significantly different from median activity of 1.19 U/mL in healthy individuals *2376*

Tissue Factor Pathway Inhibitor Antigen *Plasma* *No Effect* 15 patients with lymphoma had median concentration of 98 ng/mL not significantly different from median concentration of 90 ng/mL in healthy individuals *2376*

Tissue Factor Pathway Inhibitor Antigen, Free
Plasma *No Effect* 15 patients with lymphoma had median concentration of 28 ng/mL not significantly different from median concentration of 15 ng/mL in healthy individuals *2376*

Tissue Factor Pathway Inhibitor, Truncated and Complexed
Plasma *No Effect* 15 patients with lymphoma had median concentration of 65 ng/mL not significantly different from median concentration of 78 ng/mL in healthy individuals *2376*

Tumor Necrosis Factor-α *Serum* *Increase* In 88 patients with newly diagnosed lymphoma concentration ranged from.5 to 380 pg/mL (median 20 pg/mL) significantly different from 4 - 9 pg/mL in 82 healthy controls *4531*
Serum *No Effect* Sixty serum samples from patients with Hodgkin's disease (28 patients) or non-Hodgkin's lymphoma (32 patients), as well as 20 samples from normal volunteers, were collected. The majority of patients had advanced (Stage III or IV) or relapsed disease. There were no statistically significant differences between lymphoma patients and normal subjects *2867*

Urea Nitrogen *Serum* *Increase* Hypercalcemia of malignancy common with this type of cancer which leads to diminished capacity of renal tubules to concentrate urine which, in turn, decreases the ECF and the kidney's ability to eliminate excess calcium. Renal impairment eventually causes nitrogen retention, acidosis and renal failure and a further decrease in calcium excretion *3470*

Volume *Urine* *Increase* Hypercalcemia of malignancy common with this type of cancer which leads to diminished capacity of renal tubules to concentrate urine which, in turn, decreases the ECF and the kidney's ability to eliminate excess calcium. Renal impairment eventually causes nitrogen retention, acidosis and renal failure and a further decrease in calcium excretion *3470*

Zinc *Serum* *Decrease* In patients with malignant lymphoma concentration significantly reduced *1781* In 40 children with malignant lymphomas mean concentration of 86.1 ± 18.9 µg/dL significantly lower than 117.4 ± 18.8 µg/dL in 30 healthy controls: with concentration progressively decreasing with stage of the disease *1925*

202.80 Non-Hodgkins Lymphoma

α_1-Acid Glycoprotein *Serum* *Increase* Mean concentration in stage I and II disease of 1.4 ± 0.7 g/L and in patients with stage III and IV disease of 1.7 ± 0.7 g/L significantly different from normal range of 0.54 - 1.17 g/L *838*

Acid Phosphatase *Serum* *Increase* In a few patients, a striking increase has been noted *5652* A patient with histiocytic medullary reticulosis was found to have up to 60 times the normal upper limit, which then paralleled the activity of disease during temporary responses to therapy *5652*

Alanine Aminotransferase *Serum* *Increase* In 30% of 10 patients at initial hospitalization for this disorder *1576* May be a systemic sign of active disease or may indicate involvement of liver or bone *900*

Albumin *Serum* *Decrease* In 40% of 74 patients at initial hospitalization for this disorder *1576* In patients with advanced disease, reduction in serum protein concentration with hypoalbuminemia and hypogammaglobulinemia is frequent *5533*

Serum *No Effect* Mean concentration in stage I and II disease of 38.8 ± 5.2 g/L and in patients with stage III and IV disease of 37.1 ± 0.8 g/L not significantly different from normal *838*

Aldolase *Serum* *Increase* Markedly elevated in malignant lymphomas. Mean = 5.0 ± 0.4 U/L compared to normal, 1.6 ± 0.21 U/L *2513*

Alkaline Phosphatase *Serum* *Increase* In 10 patients with lymphosarcoma involving the liver, value was 69 ± 28 U/L *2803* Lymphoma associated with hyperbilirubinemia is accompanied by elevations from 43 to 331 U/L. In some cases, reflects osteoblastic lesions as well as metastases *5738* May be a systemic sign of active disease or may indicate involvement of liver or bone *900* May be increased as a result of liver and less frequently bone disease *48* In 10 of 20 patients with non-Hodgkin's lymphoma and initial or late evidence of bone disease alkaline phosphatase activity increased *1781*
White Blood Cells *Decrease* Activity is low irrespective of tumor category, activity of disease, or type of therapy. In 17 cases of malignant lymphoma, median LAP was 17 U/L (normal 55 U/L) *3110*
White Blood Cells *Increase* Usually increased in untreated diseases. Increased in lymphoma (including Hodgkin's disease and reticulum cell sarcoma) *5544*
White Blood Cells *No Effect* In 10 cases, mean activity was found to be in the normal range or slightly below, irrespective of treatment *3440* Typical observation *5544*

Alkaline Phosphatase, Placental Isoenzyme
Serum *Increase* Mean activity in 40 patients with non-Hodgkin's lymphoma significantly greater than the mean in 77 healthy adults but did not correlate with the stage or histology *1781*

Angiotensin-converting Enzyme *Serum* *Decrease* Mean activity normal or reduced in patients with non-Hodgkin's lymphoma *1781* Patients with low values had a poorer prognosis *4746* Correlated with prognosis: lower the concentration the worse the prognosis *4416*
Serum *No Effect* Mean activity normal or reduced in patients with non-Hodgkin's lymphoma *1781*

Anticardiolipin Antibodies *Serum* *Increase* 14 patients with newly-diagnosed NHL were investigated. 5 patients with NHL (35.7%) presented elevated APA at diagnosis, as compared to 3 of 174 persons of the control group ($p < 0.0001$). APA titers became normal in all patients responding to treatment, whereas non-responders retained elevated levels. At presentation, the mean levels of IgG- and IgM-ACA in patients were not significantly different from controls *4984*

α_1-Antitrypsin *Serum* *Increase* Increased *4371* *83* *4373* *4763* *4241*

Aspartate Aminotransferase *Serum* *Increase* May be a systemic sign of active disease or may indicate involvement of liver or bone *900* In 24% of 72 patients at initial hospitalization for this disorder *1576*

Bence-Jones Protein *Urine* *Present* 30 - 40% of patients *5558*

Bilirubin *Serum* *Increase* May be a systemic sign of active disease or may indicate involvement of liver or bone *900*

BSP Retention *Serum* *Increase* May be a systemic sign of active disease or may indicate involvement of liver or bone *900*

CA 125 *Serum* *Increase* Mean concentration of 95 U/mL observed in 157 patients at time of diagnosis with increased concentrations in 40% *2949*

Calcium *Serum* *Increase* Has been observed in the absence of hyperparathyroidism or of skeletal metastases *4861* Metastatic or lytic tumor involving bone *1025*
Urine *Increase* Occurs with metastatic tumors involving the bone *1025*

Carcinoembryonic Antigen *Serum* *Increase* In 22% of cases *4891*

Cells *Bone Marrow* *Increase* Erythrocytic and granulocytic hyperplasia may develop in the bone marrow *5677*

Ceruloplasmin *Serum* *Increase* Increased concentration observed in the majority of patients with non-Hodgkin's lymphoma in relapse with lower concentration in remission *1781*

Cholesterol *Serum* *Decrease* In 24% of 74 patients at initial hospitalization for this disorder *1576*

Chylomicrons *Serum* *Increase* Moderate increase due to presence of IgG or IgM that forms complexes with chylomicron remnants and/or VLDL thereby decreasing catabolism *126*

Coombs' Test *Serum* *Positive* Autoimmune hemolytic anemia, with a positive Coombs' test, occurs in a few patients *2486* May occur *5699*

Copper *Serum* *Increase* Invariably raised in all 50 patients with lymphoma. Significantly lowered after radiotherapy *4292* In 40 untreated patients with non-Hodgkin's lymphoma mean concentration significantly increased almost by 25% compared with the value in 14 matched healthy controls with the concentrations falling during remission *1781*

Corticotropin *Plasma* *No Effect* No change observed in patients with non-Hodgkin's lymphoma *1781*

Cortisol *Plasma* *No Effect* No change in concentration observed in patients with non-Hodgkin's lymphoma *1781*

C-Peptide *Plasma* *Decrease* Concentration normal or low in patients with non-Hodgkin's lymphoma *1781*
Plasma *No Effect* Concentration normal or low in patients with non-Hodgkin's lymphoma *1781*

C-Reactive Protein *Serum* *Increase* Increased concentration observed in 23% patients with stage I and II disease and 40% of patients with stages III and IV disease. In remission the frequencies for the paired subgroups were 7% and 2% respectively. Ratio of precipitable to soluble CRP not more discriminatory than total CRP *1781*

Creatine Kinase BB-Isoenzyme *Serum* *Increase* Activities greater than or equal to 2.9 U/L in 17 of 59 (29%) patients with non-Hodgkin's lymphoma *1781*

Creatinine *Serum* *Increase* In 42% of 47 patients at initial hospitalization for this disorder *1576*

Cryoglobulins *Serum* *Increase* May be associated with cryoglobulinemia *5545*

1,25-Dihydroxy Vitamin D_3 *Serum* *Decrease* In five patients with adult T-Cell Lymphoma all had levels at or below the normal range. These data show that calcitriol levels are not uniformly elevated in this disorder and may not be the usual cause of hypercalcemia *1194*
Serum *Increase* Three patients had elevated levels (56, 72 and 77 pg/mL) compared to normal (< 50 pg/mL) *577*
Serum *No Effect* In five patients with adult T-Cell Lymphoma. All had levels at or below the normal range. These data show that calcitriol levels are not uniformly elevated in this order and may not be the usual cause of hypercalcemia *1194*

Erythrocyte Sedimentation Rate *Blood* *Increase* Mean rate in stage I and II disease of 33 ± 28 mm/h and in patients with stage III and IV disease of 34 ± 30 mm/h significantly different from normal *838* Increased in significant tissue necrosis, especially neoplasms - most frequently malignant lymphoma, cancer of the colon and breast *5544*

Erythrocyte Survival *Red Blood Cells* *Decrease* Characteristically short in patients with bulky lymph nodes or with enlargement of the liver and spleen *2486*

Erythrocytes *Bone Marrow* *Decrease* In histiocytic medullary reticulosis, severe cytopenias may be associated with the abnormal phagocytosis of erythrocytes, platelets or leukocytes seen in the bone marrow *5677*

Ferritin *Serum* *Increase* Increased concentration about three times higher than mean for 300 healthy individuals observed in 18 patients with non-Hodgkin's lymphoma. In 18 patients with NHL mean concentration of 207 ng/mL significantly higher than 85 ng/mL in 178 healthy men and 39 ng/mL in 105 healthy women *1781* Significant elevation *4970*

Fibrinogen *Plasma* *Increase* The concentration of fibrinogen in 14 patients with non-Hodgkin's lymphoma significantly higher during acute disease onset and relapse than in 20 healthy controls *1781*
Plasma *No Effect* The concentration of fibrinogen in 12 patients with non-Hodgkin's lymphoma during remission not significantly different from that in 20 healthy blood donors *1781*

Fucose *Serum* *Increase* Markedly elevated and correlated with clinical stage of disease. Values ranged from 13 mg/dL in stage 1 to 29.5 mg/dL in stage 4 *1269*

α_2-Globulin *Serum* *Increase* Moderate increase *1290*

γ-Globulin *Serum* *Decrease* In patients with advanced disease, reduction in serum protein concentration with hypoalbuminemia and hypogammaglobulinemia is frequent *5533* The concentration of γ-globulin is typically reduced in patients with Hodgkin's disease *1781*

γ-Glutamyltransferase *Serum* *Increase* In 67% of 16 patients at initial hospitalization for this disorder *1576*

202.80 Non-Hodgkins Lymphoma *(continued)*

Granulocyte-Macrophage Colony Stimulating Factor
Serum *No Effect* In 78 patients with aggressive non-Hodgkin's lymphoma mean concentration of 9.9 ± 4.7 pg/mL not significantly different from 8.6 ± 4.3 pg/mL in 54 healthy blood-donor controls *4985*

Growth Hormone *Plasma* *Increase* Concentration increased in 80% patients with non-Hodgkin's lymphoma at diagnosis *1781*

Haptoglobin *Serum* *Increase* The concentration of haptoglobin was increased in all of 18 patients with non-Hodgkin's lymphoma in relapse, as a part of non-specific acute phase reaction *1781* Conditions associated with increased ESR and $alpha_2$-globulin *5544*
Serum *No Effect* The concentration of haptoglobin was normal in all of 18 patients with non-Hodgkin's lymphoma in remission *1781*

HDL-Cholesterol *Serum* *Decrease* In 25 patients with unspecified acute leukemia or non-Hodgkin's lymphoma extremely low concentrations of HDL-cholesterol observed in all, probably related to tumor burden and marrow involvement *1781*

Hematocrit *Blood* *Decrease* Anemia may result from blood loss, hemolysis, or bone marrow infiltration *5677* In 22% of 74 patients at initial hospitalization for this disorder *1576* Present in < 50% of cases and is rarely severe at time of diagnosis *5699*
Blood *No Effect* Anemia is often conspicuously lacking, especially early in the disease *4438*

Hemoglobin *Blood* *Decrease* In 51% of 73 patients at initial hospitalization for this disorder *1576* Present in < 50% of patients and is rarely severe at the time of diagnosis *5699* Anemia occurs frequently and may be due to blood loss, bone marrow infiltration, or hemolysis *5677*
Blood *No Effect* Anemia is often conspicuously lacking, especially early in the disease. Hemoglobin above 12 g/dL found in 90% of 1,269 cases *4438*

Hexokinase *Serum* *Increase* Markedly increased in malignant lymphomas. Mean activity of 14.6 ± 2.0 U/L compared to normal of 0.93 ± 0.28 U/L *2513*

α_2-HS Glycoprotein *Serum* *Decrease* Significant reduction observed compared with healthy controls probably due to hepatic involvement *2533*

5-Hydroxyindoleacetic Acid *Urine* *Decrease* Absent from urine *1290*

immunoglobulin A *Serum* *Decrease* Mean concentration in 80 patients with untreated non-Hodgkin's lymphoma significantly reduced *1781*
Serum *Increase* In 120 patients with non-Hodgkin's lymphoma significantly increased in 19% *1781*

Immunoglobulin G *Serum* *Decrease* Mean concentration in 80 patients with untreated non-Hodgkin's lymphoma significantly reduced *1781*
Serum *Increase* In 120 patients with non-Hodgkin's lymphoma significantly increased in 12% *1781* In a recent survey, 15 of 348 patients (4.6%) with lymphosarcoma and reticulum cell sarcoma had monoclonal serum components. In 10 instances the component was IgM and in 5 IgG *3584*

Immunoglobulin M *Serum* *Decrease* Mean concentration in 80 patients with untreated non-Hodgkin's lymphoma significantly reduced in women but not in men *1781*
Serum *Increase* In a recent survey,15 of 348 patients (4.6%) with lymphosarcoma and reticulum cell sarcoma had monoclonal serum components. In 10 instances the component was IgM and in 5 IgG *3584* In 120 patients with non-Hodgkin's lymphoma significantly increased in 11% *1781*
Serum *No Effect* Mean concentration in 80 patients with untreated non-Hodgkin's lymphoma not significantly changed in men *1781*

Immunoglobulins *Serum* *Decrease* Low levels were present in several patients in one family who developed malignant lymphoma of the small intestine *171*
Serum *Increase* In a recent survey, 15 of 348 patients (4.6%) with lymphosarcoma and reticulum cell sarcoma had monoclonal serum components. In 10 instances the component was IgM and in 5 IgG *3584*

Insulin *Plasma* *Increase* Concentration increased in patients with non-Hodgkin's lymphoma in relapse, but low or normal in remission, reciprocal to glucose concentration *1781*

Interferon-γ *Serum* *No Effect* In 71 patients with aggressive non-Hodgkin's lymphoma mean concentration of 0.17 ± 0.12 U/mL not significantly different from 0.14 ± 0.09 U/mL in 54 healthy blood-donor controls *4985* Sixty serum samples from patients with Hodgkin's disease (28 patients) or non-Hodgkin's lymphoma (32 patients), as well as 20 samples from normal volunteers, were collected. The majority of patients had advanced (Stage III or IV) or relapsed disease. There were no statistically significant differences between lymphoma patients and normal subjects *2867*

Interleukin-1 *Serum* *No Effect* Sixty serum samples from patients with Hodgkin's disease (28 patients) or non-Hodgkin's lymphoma (32 patients), as well as 20 samples from normal volunteers, were collected. The majority of patients had advanced (Stage III or IV) or relapsed disease. There were no statistically significant differences between lymphoma patients and normal subjects *2867*

Interleukin-1β *Serum* *No Effect* In 78 patients with aggressive non-Hodgkin's lymphoma mean concentration of 16.6 ± 12.1 pg/mL not significantly different from 13.4 ± 9.8 pg/mL in 54 healthy blood-donor controls *4985*

Interleukin-2 *Serum* *Increase* In 78 patients with aggressive non-Hodgkin's lymphoma mean concentration of 0.97 ± 0.48 IU/mL significantly different from 0.43 ± 0.17 IU/mL in 54 healthy blood-donor controls *4985* Pretreatment concentrations in three patients significantly elevated compared to controls (p = 0.003, p = 0.009 and p = 0.024 respectively) *4984*

Interleukin-3 *Serum* *No Effect* In 71 patients with aggressive non-Hodgkin's lymphoma mean concentration of 11.6 ± 10.9 pg/mL not significantly different from 10.3 ± 9.4 pg/mL in 54 healthy blood-donor controls *4985*

Interleukin-4 *Serum* *No Effect* In 71 patients with aggressive non-Hodgkin's lymphoma mean concentration of 5.1 ± 3.7 pg/mL not significantly different from 4.6 ± 1.2 pg/mL in 54 healthy blood-donor controls *4985*

Interleukin-6 *Serum* *Increase* Sixty serum samples from patients with Hodgkin's disease (28 patients) or non-Hodgkin's lymphoma (32 patients), as well as 20 samples from normal volunteers, were collected. The majority of patients had advanced (Stage III or IV) or relapsed disease. 20 of 57 patients (35%) with lymphoma as compared with 0 of 19 normal volunteers (0%) had detectable serum IL-6 levels (p < 0.005, chi 2 test) *2867* In 11 cases mean concentration of 0.497 ± 0.692 ng/mL higher than 0.190 ± 0.145 ng/mL in 26 healthy controls *1271* In 25 patients with non-Hodgkin's lymphoma mean concentration of 28.3 ± 6.2 pg/mL significantly different from 8.8 ± 1.8 pg/mL in 27 healthy control individuals *1120* In 78 patients with aggressive non-Hodgkin's lymphoma mean concentration of 25.3 ± 24.5 pg/mL significantly different from 5.4 ± 1.6 pg/mL in 54 healthy blood-donor controls *4985*

Interleukin-7 *Serum* *No Effect* In 73 patients with aggressive non-Hodgkin's lymphoma mean concentration of 12.7 ± 13.1 pg/mL not significantly different from 11.3 ± 10.4 pg/mL in 54 healthy blood-donor controls *4985*

Interleukin-8 *Serum* *Increase* In 25 patients with non-Hodgkin's lymphoma mean concentration of 63.2 ± 16.2 pg/mL significantly different from 16.2 ± 1.4 pg/mL in 27 healthy control individuals *1120* In 78 patients with aggressive non-Hodgkin's lymphoma mean concentration of 92.6 ± 41.4 pg/mL significantly different from 8.4 ± 3.3 pg/mL in 54 healthy blood-donor controls *4985*

Interleukin-10 *Serum* *Increase* In 78 patients with aggressive non-Hodgkin's lymphoma mean concentration of 0.32 ± 0.19 ng/L significantly different from undetectable amount in 54 healthy blood-donor controls *4985*

Iron *Serum* *Decrease* In 58% of 22 patients at initial hospitalization for this disorder *1576*

Iron-binding Capacity, Total *Serum* *Decrease* In 36% of 22 patients at initial hospitalization for this disorder *1576*

Iron Saturation *Serum* *Decrease* In 67% of 22 patients at initial hospitalization for this disorder *1576* Anemia due to blood loss may occur *5677*

Lactate *Blood* *Increase* In 20 patients with malignant lymphomas, mean concentration = 23.2 ± 2.9 mg/dL compared to normal, 11.7 ± 0.72 mg/dL *2513*

Lactate Dehydrogenase *Serum* *Increase* In 55% of 73 patients at initial hospitalization for this disorder *1576*

Increased in about 60% of the patients *1642* *5544* Marked elevation in 138 patients with malignant lymphomas. Mean activity of 177.7 ± 13.8 U/L compared to normals, 85.4 ± 1.0 U/L *2513* May be a sign of active disease or may indicate involvement of liver or bone *900* Activity increased in 46 of 113 patients with non-Hodgkin's lymphoma in stages II through IV. Increased activity associated with lower 2-year survival *1781* Activity increased in patients with non-Hodgkins lymphoma *2949* Mean activity in stage I and II disease of 10.4 ± 9.8 μkat/L and in patients with stage III and IV disease of 14.9 ± 13.4 μkat/L significantly different from normal range of 3.8 - 6.7 μkat/L *838*

Laminin *Serum* *No Effect* Did not differ from normal controls *4394*

Leukocytes *Blood* *Decrease* Uncommon *5699* In 8% of 73 patients at initial hospitalization for this disorder *1576*
Blood *Increase* In 13% of 73 patients at initial hospitalization for this disorder *1576* Uncommon *5699*
Bone Marrow *Decrease* In histiocytic medullary reticulosis, severe cytopenias may be associated with the abnormal phagocytosis of erythrocytes, platelets or leukocytes seen in the bone marrow *5677*

Lymphocytes *Pleural Fluid* *Increase* A preponderance of lymphocytes is consistent with tuberculosis, carcinoma or lymphoma *1980*

β_2-Macroglobulin *Cerebrospinal Fluid* *Increase* May be increased in lymphomas involving the central nervous system *2586* With involvement of the CNS *815*

MCH *Blood* *Decrease* Anemia occurs frequently and may be due to blood loss, bone marrow infiltration, or hemolysis *5677*

MCHC *Blood* *Decrease* Anemia occurs frequently and may be due to blood loss, bone marrow infiltration, or hemolysis *5677*

MCV *Blood* *Decrease* Anemia occurs frequently and may be due to blood loss, bone marrow infiltration, or hemolysis *5677*

Methyl-1-Adenosine *Urine* *Increase* Excretion increased more than 2 SD above the mean in 85% of 8 patients with Hodgkin's disease *1781*

β_2-Microglobulin *Serum* *Increase* Mean concentration in stage I and II disease of 190 ± 115 ng/mL and in patients with stage III and IV disease of 282 ± 231 ng/mL significantly different from normal *838* Increased concentration observed in about 20 - 60% of untreated patients with malignant lymphoma and is related to the stage of the disease *1781* Concentration increased in patients with non-Hodgkins lymphoma *2949* In 11 patients with non-Hodgkin lymphoma mean concentration of 5.98 ± 3.22 mg/L (median 5.02 mg/L) significantly different from mean of 1.71 ± 0.46 mg/L (median 1.55 mg/L) in 81 healthy controls. 91% of patients had increased concentrations *4166*

Monocytes *Blood* *Increase* Peripheral monocytosis is especially likely to occur in circumstances of histiocytic proliferation and increased phagocytosis as strikingly manifested in histiocytic medullary reticulosis *3246* In 57% of 74 patients at initial hospitalization for this disorder *1576* All varieties of lymphomas have been reported on occasion in association with a monocytosis, sometimes varying with disease activity *2303* Appearance of abnormal large mononuclear cells in peripheral blood *900*

Neopterin *Serum* *Increase* In 67 patients with aggressive non-Hodgkin's lymphoma mean concentration of 5.3 ± 2.4 ng/mL significantly different from 1.2 ± 0.7 ng/mL in 54 healthy blood-donor controls *4985*
Urine *Increase* Highest concentrations observed in patients with non-Hodgkin's lymphoma, chronic myelogenous or lymphoblastoid leukemia *121* Urinary excretion in 79 of 112 patients with Hodgkin's disease, non-Hodgkin's lymphoma or other hematologic malignancies greater than mean ± 3 SD in healthy individuals. Excretion correlated well with the tumor stage in NHL *1781* In patients with stage III and IV disease mean excretion of 790 ± 61 μmol/mol creatinine compared with 422 ± 194 μmol/mol creatinine in patients with stage I and II disease and 198 ± 95 μmol/mol creatinine in patients in remission. Significantly higher higher values observed in patients with symptoms (974 ± 752 μmol/mol) than in those without (555 ± 360 μmol/mol creatinine) *4128*

Neutrophils *Blood* *Decrease* Often present in addition to anemia, and almost any combination of cytopenias may be produced by bone marrow infiltration and replacement, by hypersplenism or as the result of therapy *5677*

5'-Nucleotidase *Serum* *Increase* Ten patients with lymphosarcoma, showed 5'-nucleotidase activities ranging from 16 - 59 U/L (normal 2 - 11 U/L) *2803*

Phosphate *Serum* *Increase* Lysis of non-Hodgkins lymphoma cells even prior to treatment may cause shift of phosphate from cells leading to increased serum concentration, and possible acute renal failure *969*

Platelets *Blood* *Decrease* Often present in addition to anemia, and almost any combination of cytopenias may be produced by bone marrow infiltration and replacement, by hypersplenism or as the result of therapy *5677* Unusual *5699*
Bone Marrow *Decrease* In histiocytic medullary reticulosis, severe cytopenias may be associated with the abnormal phagocytosis of erythrocytes, platelets or leukocytes seen in the bone marrow *5677*

Polyamines *Serum* *Increase* Mean concentration of 1.2 - 5.7 nmol/mL in 21 patients with non-Hodgkin's lymphoma significantly increased compared with 0.62 - 0.87 nmol/mL in normal individuals *1781*

Proline Hydroxylase *Serum* *Increase* Elevated to a lesser degree than that seen in hepatoma *762*

Protein *Pleural Fluid* *Increase* Pleural effusions are usually exudates *126*
Serum *Decrease* Occurs commonly *5677* In patients with advanced disease, reduction in serum protein concentration with hypoalbuminemia and hypogammaglobulinemia is frequent *5533* Enteric loss of plasma protein *4891*

Protein Z *Plasma* *No Effect* In 14 patients with non-Hodgkin's lymphoma median baseline concentration of 2.88 ng/mL compared with 2.72 ng/mL in 14 healthy controls *5357*

Pseudouridine *Urine* *Increase* Excretion increased more than 2 SD above the mean in 88% of 8 patients with non-Hodgkin's lymphoma *1781*

Putrescine *Urine* *Increase* Mean excretion in 49 patients with non-Hodgkin's lymphoma increased prior to treatment *1781*

Pyruvate *Blood* *Increase* Moderately elevated in 20 of 20 patients with malignant lymphomas. Mean = 1.1 - 0.15 U/L *2513*

Rheumatoid Factor *Serum* *Increase* Dysproteinemias and paraproteinemias present significant seropositivity *1980*

Sialic Acid, Lipid-associated *Serum* *Increase* In patients with non-Hodgkin's Lymphoma mean concentration increased above 20 mg/dL in 78% of patients *1781*

Sialyltransferase *Serum* *Increase* In 4 patients with non-Hodgkin's lymphoma mean and median concentrations of 453 and 387 cpm/mg protein/30 min significantly different from 240 and 243 cpm/mg protein/30 min respectively in 20 normal individuals *2111* Activity increased in 3 of 9 patients with non-Hodgkin's lymphoma but associated with liver involvement *1781*

Sodium *Serum* *Increase* In 88% of 73 patients at initial hospitalization for this disorder *1576*

Soluble $CD44^+$ *Serum* *Increase* In 194 patients with non-Hodgkin's lymphoma median serum concentration of soluble CD44 prior to treatment was 440 ng/mL (range 13 to 1,220 ng/mL), Patients with lower concentrations had better outcomes to treatment *4364*

Soluble Intercellular Adhesion Molecule-1 *Serum* *Increase* Mean concentration of 692 ± 347 ng/mL in 48 patients with low grade NHL and of 747 ± 388 ng/mL in 79 patients with high grade NHL significantly different from 333 ± 77 ng/mL in 31 healthy controls *838*

Soluble Interleukin-2 Receptor *Serum* *Increase* In 45 patients with active non-Hodgkin's disease mean concentration of 3,634 ± 5,667 x 10^3 U/L significantly greater than 610 ± 586 x 10^3 U/L in 12 patients in remission *4128* In 78 patients with aggressive non-Hodgkin's lymphoma mean concentration of 2,434 ± 992 U/mL significantly different from 219 ± 65 U/mL in 54 healthy blood-donor controls *4985*

Soluble Transferrin Receptor *Serum* *Increase* In 73 patients with aggressive non-Hodgkin's lymphoma mean concentration of 9.8 ± 3.9 mg/mL significantly different from 4.5 ± 2.1 mg/mL in 54 healthy blood-donor controls *4985*

Spermidine *Urine* *Increase* Mean excretion in 49 patients with non-Hodgkin's lymphoma increased prior to treatment *1781*

T23 Protein *Serum* *Increase* Protein detected in serum of 11 of 21 cases of non-Hodgkin's lymphoma compared with none in controls *1781*

Thymidine Kinase *Serum* *Increase* Significant correlation between serum activity and the extent of the disease as well as the malignancy of the tumor in 155 untreated patients *1781*

202.80 Non-Hodgkins Lymphoma *(continued)*

Thymidine Kinase *(continued)*
Mean activity in stage I and II disease of 9 ± 14 U/L and in patients with stage III and IV disease of 24 ± 29 U/L significantly different from normal range of 2.4 ± 1.3 U/L *838*

Thyroxine (T4) *Serum* *No Effect* No change in concentration observed in patients with non-Hodgkin's lymphoma *1781*

Tissue Polypeptide Antigen *Serum* *No Effect* No correlation with disease observed in patients with non-Hodgkin's lymphoma *1781*

Triglycerides *Serum* *Increase* In 25 patients with unspecified acute leukemia or non-Hodgkin's lymphoma increased concentrations of triglycerides observed in all, probably related to tumor burden and marrow involvement *1781*

Tumor Necrosis Factor-α *Serum* *No Effect* In 78 patients with aggressive non-Hodgkin's lymphoma mean concentration of 16.1 ± 12.4 pg/mL not significantly different from 12.7 ± 10.9 pg/mL in 54 healthy blood-donor controls *4985*

Urea Nitrogen *Serum* *Increase* In 26% of 74 patients at initial hospitalization for this disorder *1576*

Uric Acid *Serum* *Increase* May occur, but more often is normal *3627* Especially post X-irradiation *5544* In 39% of 73 patients at initial hospitalization for this disorder *1576*
Serum *No Effect* Usually normal *5699*
Urine *Increase* May occur, but more often is normal *3627*
Urine *No Effect* Usually normal *5699*

Vascular Endothelial Growth Factor *Serum* *Increase* Median concentration in 82 patients with non-Hodgkin's lymphoma of 228 pg/mL (mean 291 pg/mL) with higher concentrations associated with poorer outcome compared with 1 - 177 pg/mL in healthy controls *4541*

Vitamin B_{12} *Serum* *Increase* High levels were found in 15 patients with lymphomas, mean concentration was 1,059 pg/mL compared to normal, 385 pg/mL *4448*
Serum *No Effect* Usually normal *5677*

Vitamin B_{12} Binding Capacity *Serum* *Increase* Significant elevation; usually correlated with WBC in peripheral blood *4448*
Serum *No Effect* Usually normal *5677*

VLDL-Cholesterol *Serum* *Increase* In 25 patients with unspecified acute leukemia or non-Hodgkin's lymphoma increased concentrations of VLDL observed in all, probably related to tumor burden and marrow involvement *1781* Moderate increase due to presence of IgG or IgM that forms complexes with chylomicron remnants and/or VLDL thereby decreasing catabolism *126*

Zinc *Serum* *Decrease* Decreased *5083* In 40 children with NHL concentration significantly reduced *1781*

202.80 T-Cell Lymphoma, Cutaneous

Lactate Dehydrogenase *Serum* *Increase* Strongly correlated with lymph node size *5496*

Soluble Interleukin-2 Receptor *Serum* *Increase* Strongly correlated with lymph node size and severity of skin manifestations in erythrodermic patients *5496*

202.90 Cancer of Lymph Nodes

CA 549 *Serum* *Increase* In 65 patients with cancer of the lymph nodes 10 (15.4%) had a concentration greater than the upper limit of normal with BRESMARQ assay *764*

202.90 Hematologic Malignancies

Calcium *Serum* *Increase* None of 5 patients with hematological malignancies had hypercalcemia *1200*

Ceruloplasmin *Serum* *Increase* In 82 men with hematopoietic cancer mean concentration of 99 ± 31 mg/dL significantly different from 71 ± 17 mg/dL in 106 control men and mean of 113 ± 33 mg/dL in 64 women with hematopoietic cancer significantly different from 84 ± 22 mg/dL in 150 control women *2280*

Ferritin *Serum* *Increase* Some hematological malignancies may increase serum ferritin concentration and ferritin may function as a tumor mrker *4784*

Follistatin, Free *Serum* *Increase* Mean concentration in 18 patients with hematologic malignancies of 6.8 ± 1.0 μg/L significantly different from that in 60 normal adults of 3.5 ± 0.2 μg/L *4523*

Interleukin-6 *Serum* *Increase* Mean concentration not detected in 23.1% of 13 patients with hematologic malignancies with or without disseminated intravascular coagulation *3890*

Neopterin *Urine* *Increase* Urinary excretion in 79 of 112 patients with Hodgkin's disease, non-Hodgkin's lymphoma or other hematologic malignancies greater than mean ± 3 SD in healthy individuals *1781* Concentrations increased in almost all patients with hematological malignancies *121*

Parathyroid Hormone-related Peptide *Plasma* *Increase* In one of five patients with a hematologic malignancy and hypercalcemia concentration increased above upper limit of normal of 1.5 pmol/L to 10.5 pmol/L *3987*
Plasma *No Effect* In 5 patients with hematological malignancies and normocalcemia mean concentration of 1.42 pmol/L below upper limit of reference range of 2.6 pmol/L *1200*

Soluble E-Selectin *Serum* *Increase* Mean concentration in 1 patient with a hematologic tumor and disseminated intravascular coagulation of 36.0 ± 32.8 ng/mL significantly different from about 25 ng/mL in 12 patients without DIC *3890*

Soluble Transferrin Receptor *Serum* *Increase* Concentration significantly increased to 15.47 ± 12.54 μg/mL in patients with myeloproliferative disorders *2704*

Transferrin *Serum* *Decrease* In 82 men with hematopoietic cancer mean concentration of 171 ± 52 mg/dL significantly different from 214 ± 33 mg/dL in 106 control men *2280*

Tumor Necrosis Factor-α *Serum* *No Effect* Mean concentration not detected in 13 patients with hematologic malignancies with or without disseminated intravascular coagulation compared with undetectable amounts in patients with liver disease or obstetric disorders *3890*

203.00 IgA Multiple Myeloma

Albumin *Serum* *Decrease* Mean concentration in 2 patients with IgA myeloma of 4.0 g/dL compared with 4.5 ± 0.1 g/dL in 11 healthy controls *4582*

Albumin:Globulin Ratio *Serum* *Increase* Mean ratio in 2 patients with IgA myeloma of 1.4 *4582*

Erythrocytes *Blood* *Decrease* Mean concentration in 2 patients with IgA myeloma of 297 x 10^4/μL *4582*

immunoglobulin A *Serum* *Increase* Mean concentration in 2 patients with IgA myeloma of 1,317 mg/dL *4582*

Immunoglobulin G *Serum* *No Effect* Mean concentration in 2 patients with IgA myeloma of 415 mg/dL *4582*

Immunoglobulin M *Serum* *No Effect* Mean concentration in 2 patients with IgA myeloma of 46 mg/dL *4582*

Leukocytes *Blood* *No Effect* Mean concentration in 2 patients with IgA myeloma of 5,160 /μL *4582*

β_2-Microglobulin *Serum* *Increase* In 26 patients with IgA multiple myeloma mean concentration of 3.76 ± 3.12 mg/L (median 2.78 mg/L) significantly different from mean of 1.71 ± 0.46 mg/L (median 1.55 mg/L) in 81 healthy controls. 46% of patients in active stage had increased concentration *4166*

Platelets *Blood* *No Effect* Mean concentration in 2 patients with IgA myeloma of 12 x 10^4 /μL *4582*

Protein *Serum* *Increase* Mean concentration in 2 patients with IgA myeloma of 6.7 g/dL *4582*

203.00 IgD Multiple Myeloma

β_2-Microglobulin *Serum* *Increase* In 7 patients with IgD multiple myeloma mean concentration of 12.26 ± 14.06 mg/L (median 9.17 mg/L) significantly different from mean of 1.71 ± 0.46 mg/L (median 1.55 mg/L) in 81 healthy controls *4166*

203.00 IgG Multiple Myeloma

Albumin *Serum* *Decrease* Mean concentration in 10 patients with IgG myeloma of 3.6 ± 0.2 g/dL compared with 4.5 ± 0.1 g/dL in 11 healthy controls *4582*

Albumin:Globulin Ratio *Serum* *Decrease* Mean ratio in 10 patients with IgG myeloma of 0.7 ± 0.1 *4582*

Erythrocytes *Blood* *Decrease* Mean concentration in 10 patients with IgG myeloma of 325 ± 28 x 10^4/µL *4582*

immunoglobulin A *Serum* *No Effect* Mean concentration in 10 patients with IgG myeloma of 36 ± 14 mg/dL *4582*

Immunoglobulin G *Serum* *Increase* Mean concentration in 10 patients with IgG myeloma of 4,043 ± 384 mg/dL *4582*

Immunoglobulin M *Serum* *No Effect* Mean concentration in 10 patients with IgG myeloma of 22 ± 8 mg/dL *4582*

Leukocytes *Blood* *No Effect* Mean concentration in 10 patients with IgG myeloma of 4,079 ± 831 /µL *4582*

β_2-Microglobulin *Serum* *Increase* In 44 patients with IgG multiple myeloma mean concentration of 5.04 ± 6.12 mg/L (median 3.09 mg/L) significantly different from mean of 1.71 ± 0.46 mg/L (median 1.55 mg/L) in 81 healthy controls. 52% of patients in active stage had increased concentration *4166*

Platelets *Blood* *No Effect* Mean concentration in 10 patients with IgG myeloma of 15.7 ± 3.2 x 10^4 /µL *4582*

Protein *Serum* *Increase* Mean concentration in 10 patients with IgG myeloma of 9.4 ± 0.5 g/dL *4582*

203.00 IgM Multiple Myeloma

β_2-Microglobulin *Serum* *Increase* In 14 patients with IgM multiple myeloma mean concentration of 3.06 ± 1.37 mg/L (median 3.12 mg/L) significantly different from mean of 1.71 ± 0.46 mg/L (median 1.55 mg/L) in 81 healthy controls *4166*

203.00 Light Chain Multiple Myeloma

Ammonium Ions *Urine* *Increase* May lead to proximal renal tubular acidosis which is associated with hypokalemia, hyperchloremic metabolic acidosis, urine pH < 5.5, increased urinary ammonium ion excretion, a negative urine anion gap, increased urinary osmol gap, normal urinary citrate, normal urinary calcium excretion and Fanconi syndrome *4071*

Anion Gap *Urine* *Decrease* May lead to proximal renal tubular acidosis which is associated with hypokalemia, hyperchloremic metabolic acidosis, urine pH < 5.5, increased urinary ammonium ion excretion, a negative urine anion gap, increased urinary osmol gap, normal urinary citrate, normal urinary calcium excretion and Fanconi syndrome *4071*

Calcium *Urine* *No Effect* May lead to proximal renal tubular acidosis which is associated with hypokalemia, hyperchloremic metabolic acidosis, urine pH < 5.5, increased urinary ammonium ion excretion, a negative urine anion gap, increased urinary osmol gap, normal urinary citrate, normal urinary calcium excretion and Fanconi syndrome *4071*

Chloride *Serum* *Increase* May lead to proximal renal tubular acidosis which is associated with hypokalemia, hyperchloremic metabolic acidosis, urine pH < 5.5, increased urinary ammonium ion excretion, a negative urine anion gap, increased urinary osmol gap, normal urinary citrate, normal urinary calcium excretion and Fanconi syndrome *4071*

Citrate *Urine* *No Effect* May lead to proximal renal tubular acidosis which is associated with hypokalemia, hyperchloremic metabolic acidosis, urine pH < 5.5, increased urinary ammonium ion excretion, a negative urine anion gap, increased urinary osmol gap, normal urinary citrate, normal urinary calcium excretion and Fanconi syndrome *4071*

Glucose *Urine* *Increase* May lead to proximal renal tubular acidosis which is associated with hypokalemia, hyperchloremic metabolic acidosis, urine pH < 5.5, increased urinary ammonium ion excretion, a negative urine anion gap, increased urinary osmol gap, normal urinary citrate, normal urinary calcium excretion and Fanconi syndrome *4071*

β_2-Microglobulin *Serum* *Increase* In 14 patients with light chain multiple myeloma mean concentration of 6.39 ± 6.89 mg/L (median 3.26 mg/L) significantly different from mean of 1.71 ± 0.46 mg/L (median 1.55 mg/L) in 81 healthy controls. 57% of patients had increased concentrations *4166*

Osmolal Gap *Urine* *Increase* May lead to proximal renal tubular acidosis which is associated with hypokalemia, hyperchloremic metabolic acidosis, urine pH < 5.5, increased urinary ammonium ion excretion, a negative urine anion gap, increased urinary osmol gap, normal urinary citrate, normal urinary calcium excretion and Fanconi syndrome *4071*

pH *Urine* *Decrease* May lead to proximal renal tubular acidosis which is associated with hypokalemia, hyperchloremic metabolic acidosis, urine pH < 5.5, increased urinary ammonium ion excretion, a negative urine anion gap, increased urinary osmol gap, normal urinary citrate, normal urinary calcium excretion and Fanconi syndrome *4071*

Phosphate *Serum* *Decrease* May lead to proximal renal tubular acidosis which is associated with hypokalemia, hyperchloremic metabolic acidosis, urine pH < 5.5, increased urinary ammonium ion excretion, a negative urine anion gap, increased urinary osmol gap, normal urinary citrate, normal urinary calcium excretion and Fanconi syndrome *4071*

Potassium *Serum* *Decrease* May lead to proximal renal tubular acidosis which is associated with hypokalemia, hyperchloremic metabolic acidosis, urine pH < 5.5, increased urinary ammonium ion excretion, a negative urine anion gap, increased urinary osmol gap, normal urinary citrate, normal urinary calcium excretion and Fanconi syndrome *4071*

Uric Acid *Serum* *Decrease* May lead to proximal renal tubular acidosis which is associated with hypokalemia, hyperchloremic metabolic acidosis, urine pH < 5.5, increased urinary ammonium ion excretion, a negative urine anion gap, increased urinary osmol gap, normal urinary citrate, normal urinary calcium excretion and Fanconi syndrome *4071*

203.00 Multiple Myeloma

Acid Phosphatase *Serum* *Increase* 2 patients showed elevated levels of both total and prostatic fraction of the serum acid phosphatase *1569* May be elevated even in the absence of prostatic carcinoma *900*
White Blood Cells *No Effect* Activity usually unchanged *3027*

Acid Phosphatase, Tartrate Resistant *Serum* *Increase* In patients with multiple myeloma slight increase observed *4217*
Serum *No Effect* In 3 men with untreated multiple myeloma mean concentration of 4.2 - 7.9 U/L not significantly different from 5.0 - 9.6 U/L in 8 healthy controls *3747*

Albumin *Serum* *Decrease* In 57% of 33 patients at initial hospitalization for this disorder *1576* In 13 patients with multiple myeloma with amyloidosis mean concentration of 3.3 ± 0.4 g/dL compared with 2.9 ± 0.6 g/dL in 8 patients with multiple myeloma without amyloidosis less than 4.1 ± 0.2 g/dL in 41 healthy controls *5767*
Urine *Increase* Greater than 1.0 g/day *1056* Occurs in 90% of patients *900* Frequent proteinuria due to albumin and globulins *5545*

Alkaline Phosphatase *Serum* *Increase* Normal or slightly elevated, even in patients with extensive bone lesions *5677* In 32 patients with multiple myeloma median activity of 127 U/L not significantly higher than that in 75 healthy men in whom the median activity was 101 U/L and in 20 premenopausal women, 88 U/L, and in 38 postmenopausal women, 115 U/L *4716* In 27% of 31 patients at initial hospitalization for this disorder *1576* In the absence of fracture with callus formation, the level is usually normal, although elevated levels have been reported *900*
Serum *No Effect* Activity typically within normal limits *2033* Usually activity is normal *900*
White Blood Cells *Increase* Over a 13 y period, 60 of 62 patients had consistently elevated levels. One patient had a normal level, and one had an initially normal level which later increased. Elevations could not be correlated with age, hemoglobin, WBC, or BUN *592*

Alkaline Phosphatase, Bone Isoenzyme *Serum* *No Effect* In 3 men with untreated multiple myeloma mean activities of 10.2 - 15.8 U/L not significantly different from 10 8 - 18.7 U/L in 8 healthy controls *3747*

Amino Acids *Urine* *Increase* Aminoaciduria may be nonselective and associated with renal glycosuria and mild renal acidosis *1980*

203.00 **Multiple Myeloma** *(continued)*

Ammonium Ions *Urine* *Increase* May lead to proximal renal tubular acidosis which is associated with hypokalemia, hyperchloremic metabolic acidosis, urine pH < 5.5, increased urinary ammonium ion excretion, a negative urine anion gap, increased urinary osmol gap, normal urinary citrate, normal urinary calcium excretion and Fanconi syndrome *4071*

Angiotensin-converting Enzyme *Serum* *Decrease* Depression of activity. Significant decrease *4416*

Anion Gap *Urine* *Decrease* May lead to proximal renal tubular acidosis which is associated with hypokalemia, hyperchloremic metabolic acidosis, urine pH < 5.5, increased urinary ammonium ion excretion, a negative urine anion gap, increased urinary osmol gap, normal urinary citrate, normal urinary calcium excretion and Fanconi syndrome *4071*

Anti-p53 Antibodies *Serum* *Increase* Increased in 6 of 165 patients (3.6%) *132*

Apolipoprotein A-I *Serum* *Decrease* In 13 patients with multiple myeloma with amyloidosis mean concentration of 114 ± 35 mg/dL compared with 111 ± 39 mg/dL in 8 patients with multiple myeloma without amyloidosis less than 133 ± 29 mg/dL in 41 healthy controls *5767*

Apolipoprotein A-I:Apolipoprotein A-II Ratio *Serum* *Increase* In 13 patients with multiple myeloma with amyloidosis mean ratio of 4.18 compared with 5.26 in 8 patients with multiple myeloma without amyloidosis more than 3.70 in 41 healthy controls *5767*

Apolipoprotein A-II *Serum* *Decrease* In 13 patients with multiple myeloma with amyloidosis mean concentration of 27 ± 8 mg/dL compared with 21 ± 8 mg/dL in 8 patients with multiple myeloma without amyloidosis less than 35 ± 6 mg/dL in 41 healthy controls *5767*

Apolipoprotein D *Serum* *Increase* In 20 patients with multiple myeloma mean concentration of about 92 mg/L significantly different from concentration in 28 healthy women 95% confidence interval (50 - 125 mg/L, median 73.5 mg/L) *3944*

Aspartate Aminotransferase *Serum* *Increase* In 45% of 33 patients at initial hospitalization for this disorder *1576*

Bence-Jones Protein *Serum* *Present* Demonstrable in the serum or urine, or both, of over 90% of cases of overt, symptomatic myeloma, it is only the rare case in which there is not an abnormal serum or urinary protein *4551* Electrophoresis of sera reveals a double spike *5485*
Urine *Present* The amount excreted varies from a few mg to 25 - 40 g/d. Found in the urine of 70 - 80% of patients *2877* Demonstrable in the serum or urine, or both, of over 90% of cases of overt, symptomatic myeloma, it is only the rare case in which there is not an abnormal serum or urinary protein *4551* Highly indicative *4919* Kappa or lambda light chains with no heavy chains attached found in 26 of 35 patients. 11 excreted large amounts (> 1 g/day) *1056*

Bicarbonate *Serum* *Decrease* May lead to proximal renal tubular acidosis which is associated with hypokalemia, hyperchloremic metabolic acidosis, urine pH < 5.5, increased urinary ammonium ion excretion, a negative urine anion gap, increased urinary osmol gap, normal urinary citrate, normal urinary calcium excretion and Fanconi syndrome *4071*

Bone Sialoprotein *Serum* *Increase* In 32 patients with multiple myeloma median concentration of 39.6 ng/mL significantly higher than that in 75 healthy men in whom the median concentration was 9.8 ng/mL and in 20 premenopausal women, 8.7 ng/mL, and in 38 postmenopausal women, 11.9 ng/mL *4716*

Calcium *Serum* *Decrease* In 32 patients with multiple myeloma median concentration of 2.29 mmol/L significantly lower than that in 75 healthy men in whom the median concentration was 2.38 mmol/L and in 20 premenopausal women, 2.39 mmol/L, and in 38 postmenopausal women, 2.41 mmol/L *4716*
Serum *Increase* Found in about 21% of patients *5724* In 91 patients with creatinine concentration > 177 µmol/L 35 (38%) had calcium concentrations greater than 2.88 mmol/L compared with 33 of 307 (10.7%) with creatinine concentrations less than 177 µmol/L *466* Frequent hypercalcemia in advanced cases *826* If the renal excretory capacity for calcium is exceeded *4551* Increased concentrations are seen in multiple myeloma *2952* Elevated above 11.0 mg/dL in about 30% of patients at the time of diagnosis, and rises above this level in an additional 30% during the course of the disease *400* In one study 42 patients with hypercalcemia and low intact PTH concentration, 5 had myeloma *3280* Hypercalcemia of malignancy common with this type of cancer *3470*
Urine *Decrease* Hypercalcemia of malignancy common with this type of cancer which leads to diminished capacity of renal tubules to concentrate urine which, in turn, decreases the ECF and the kidney's ability to eliminate excess calcium. Renal impairment eventually causes nitrogen retention, acidosis and renal failure and a further decrease in calcium excretion *3470*
Urine *Increase* Increased excretion is seen with diseases that destroy bone such as multiple myeloma *2952* Skeletal destruction results in hypercalciuria in virtually all cases *4551* Hypercalcemia of malignancy common with this type of cancer which is often associated with hypercalciuria occurring with excessive bone reabsorption *3470*
Urine *No Effect* In 3 men with untreated multiple myeloma mean concentration of 0.10 - 1.62 mmol/mmol creatinine not significantly different from 0.16 - 0.90 mmol/mmol creatinine in 8 healthy controls *3747* May lead to proximal renal tubular acidosis which is associated with hypokalemia, hyperchloremic metabolic acidosis, urine pH < 5.5, increased urinary ammonium ion excretion, a negative urine anion gap, increased urinary osmol gap, normal urinary citrate, normal urinary calcium excretion and Fanconi syndrome *4071*

Chloride *Serum* *Increase* Typical hyperchloremic acidosis with respiratory compensation in 9 of 35 patients *1056* May lead to proximal renal tubular acidosis which is associated with hypokalemia, hyperchloremic metabolic acidosis, urine pH < 5.5, increased urinary ammonium ion excretion, a negative urine anion gap, increased urinary osmol gap, normal urinary citrate, normal urinary calcium excretion and Fanconi syndrome *4071*

Cholesterol *Serum* *Decrease* In 27% of 31 patients at initial hospitalization for this disorder *1576* 150 mg/dL in 25% of patients while only 5% have a level > 300 mg/dL *900*
Serum *Increase* 150 mg/dL in 25% of patients while only 5% have a level > 300 mg/dL *900*

Chylomicrons *Serum* *Increase* Moderate increase due to presence of IgG or IgM that forms complexes with chylomicron remnants and/or VLDL thereby decreasing catabolism *126*

Citrate *Urine* *No Effect* May lead to proximal renal tubular acidosis which is associated with hypokalemia, hyperchloremic metabolic acidosis, urine pH < 5.5, increased urinary ammonium ion excretion, a negative urine anion gap, increased urinary osmol gap, normal urinary citrate, normal urinary calcium excretion and Fanconi syndrome *4071*

Cold Agglutinins *Serum* *Increase* Cold agglutinin or cryoglobulins with lymphocytes *5545*

Complement C_1b *Serum* *Increase* 7 out of 10 patients had increased concentrations *3152*

Complement C_1r *Serum* *Decrease* 9 out of 10 patients had decreased concentrations *3152*

Complement C_1s *Serum* *Decrease* 9 out of 10 patients had decreased concentrations *3152*

Complement C_2 *Serum* *Decrease* 9 out of 10 patients had decreased concentrations *3152*

Complement C_4d *Serum* *Increase* 8 out of 10 patients had increased concentrations *3152*

Coombs' Test *Serum* *Negative* Usually *5677*

C-Reactive Protein *Serum* *Increase* In 30 patients with multiple myeloma median concentration at time of diagnosis of 2 mg/L (range < 2 - 140 mg/L) higher than in healthy control population with prognosis worse in those individuals with concentrations greater than 20 mg/L *4238* In 16 patients with IIIA myeloma mean concentration of 13.0 mg/L, in 6 with IIIB 31.0 mg/L, 11 with IIA 15.0 mg/L and 9 with IA 8.0 mg/L *1506* In 23 patients with multiple myeloma, 14 patients had concentrations in peripheral blood of less than 8 mg/L, the upper limit of normal, and in 9 concentrations were the same as or greater than 8 mg/L *2828*

Creatinine *Serum* *Increase* In 68% of 28 patients at initial hospitalization for this disorder *1576* Hypercalcemia of malignancy common with this type of cancer which leads to diminished capacity of renal tubules to concentrate urine which, in turn, decreases the ECF and the kidney's ability to eliminate excess calcium. Renal impairment eventually causes nitrogen retention, acidosis and renal failure and a further decrease in calcium excretion *3470* Not uncommon *900* Ranged from 53.0 - 981 µmol/L in 35 patients *1056*

Creatinine Clearance *Urine* *Decrease* Clearance ranged from 0.03 - 2.02 mL/s (2 - 121 mL/min) in 35 cases. 19 had rates > 0.83 mL/s. Mean clearance was significantly lower in the patients with Bence-Jones proteinuria *1056*

Cryoglobulins *Serum* *Increase* Associated cryoglobulinemia *5545*

C-terminal Propeptide of Type I Procollagen *Serum* *No Effect* In 3 men with untreated multiple myeloma mean concentration of 50.9 - 93.2 ng/mL not significantly different from 69.4 - 108.6 ng/mL in 8 healthy controls *3747*

Deoxypyridinoline *Urine* *Increase* In 32 patients with multiple myeloma median excretion of 21.3 nmol/mmol creatinine significantly higher than that in 75 healthy men in whom the median excretion was 5.0 nmol/mmol creatinine and in 20 premenopausal women, 5.1 nmol/mmol creatinine, and in 38 postmenopausal women, 7.2 nmol/mmol creatinine *4716*

Dipyridinoline *Urine* *Increase* In 3 men with untreated multiple myeloma mean concentration of 8.4 - 12.3 nmol/mmol creatinine significantly different from 3.8 - 7.1 nmol/mmol creatinine in 8 healthy controls *3747*

Epidermal Growth Factor *Urine* *Increase* Mean concentration in about 9 patients of 18 μg/g creatinine significantly different compared with about 10 μg/g creatinine in about 30 controls *5341*

Erythrocyte Sedimentation Rate *Blood* *Increase* Over 100 mm/h in almost 50% of patients *4434* A result of hyperglobulinemia *5677* Typically increased but a normal or modestly elevated rate does not exclude the diagnosis. Approximately 25% of patients have a ESR > 50 mm/h (Westergren) *900*

Erythrocytes *Blood* *Decrease* Overgrowth of plasma cells may produce pancytopenia, or may evoke a leukoerythroblastic reaction *5677*
Blood *Increase* Has been found in a small number of patients *2942*

Ferritin *Serum* *Increase* In 14 patients with multiple myeloma mean concentration of 285 ng/mL significantly higher than 85 ng/mL in 178 healthy men and 39 ng/mL in 105 healthy women *1781* Significant elevation *4970*

Fructosamine *Serum* *Increase* In patients with IgA myeloma mean fructosamine concentration significantly increased *3575*
Serum *No Effect* In patients with IgG myeloma mean concentration not significantly different from normal *3575*

Fucosyltransferase *Serum* *Increase* In 19 patients with untreated multiple myeloma activity significantly increased but did not decline with treatment with alkylating agents and and prednisolone. No difference observed in activities between those patients with stage III disease and stage I and II disease *1582*

Gc-Globulin *Serum* *No Effect* In 15 men and 7 women with multiple myeloma mean concentrations of 23.9 ± 4.65 mg/dL and 28.3 ± 2.81 mg/dL not significantly different from 23.9 mg/dL in 106 control men and 26.1 mg/dL in 150 control women *2279*

α_2-Globulin *Serum* *Increase* Homogeneous component seen in some patients *2033* Marked increase *1290*

β-Globulin *Serum* *Increase* Markedly increased *1290*

γ-Globulin *Cerebrospinal Fluid* *Increase* Increased in about 66% of patients, with corresponding colloidal gold curve *367*
Serum *Increase* Over 80 g/L in 60% of patients *4434* Greater than 32 g/L in 27 of 35 patients and reduced to 20 g/L in 1 case *1056* Plasma cell dyscrasias are among the most common causes of serum elevations, which may exceed 5 g/dL *2039* Very elevated serum total protein is due to increase in globulins (with decreased A/G ratio) in 50 - 66% of the patients *5545* A homogeneous protein component ranging from slow γ to alpha$_2$-globulin is seen in 60% of patients *2033*

Glomerular Filtration Rate *Urine* *Decrease* Marked reduction in PAH clearance in patients with Bence-Jones proteinuria 3.22 ± 0.65 mL/s. Diminished out of proportion to the GFR *1056* Renal function is decreased. There is no correlation between the degree of Bence-Jones proteinuria and renal functional impairment *1980*

Glucose *Urine* *Increase* Aminoaciduria may be nonselective and associated with renal glycosuria and mild renal acidosis *1980* May lead to proximal renal tubular acidosis which is associated with hypokalemia, hyperchloremic metabolic acidosis, urine pH < 5.5, increased urinary ammonium ion excretion, a negative urine anion gap, increased urinary osmol gap, normal urinary citrate, normal urinary calcium excretion and Fanconi syndrome *4071*

Hematocrit *Blood* *Decrease* A normocytic, normochromic anemia is present in 66% of patients at the time of diagnosis *900* Virtually all patients exhibit anemia of varying severity, either at the time of diagnosis or subsequently with disease progression *4551* In 69% of 33 patients at initial hospitalization for this disorder *1576*

Hemoglobin *Blood* *Decrease* In 78% of 33 patients at initial hospitalization for this disorder *1576* High tumor mass is indicated if hemoglobin < 8.5 g/dL, low tumor mass is present in hemoglobin > 10.5 g/dL *5544* In 94 patients with creatinine concentration > 177 μmol/L 49 (53%) had hemoglobin concentrations less than 90 g/L compared with 84 of 329 (26.0%) with creatinine concentrations less than 177 μmol/L *466* A normocytic, normochromic anemia is present in 66% of patients at the time of diagnosis *900* Virtually all patients exhibit anemia of varying severity, either at the time of diagnosis or subsequently with disease progression *4551* Reduced to < 12.0 g/dL in 62% of the patients *2877*

Hemoglobin F *Blood* *Increase* Observed effect *5544*

β-Hexosaminidase *Serum* *Increase* Elevated *5229*

α_2-HS Glycoprotein *Serum* *Decrease* Significant reduction observed compared with healthy controls probably due to hepatic involvement *2533*

immunoglobulin A *Serum* *Decrease* May occur in IgG form *5677*
Serum *Increase* Peak of > 5 g/dL indicates high tumor mass. A peak of < 3 g/dL indicates low tumor mass *5544* In 94 patients with creatinine concentration > 177 μmol/L 23 (24%) had increased IgA concentrations compared with 98 of 329 (29.8%) with creatinine concentrations less than 177 μmol/L *466* The abnormal serum M component was IgG in 20 of 35 patients and IgA in 7. There was no correlation between type of M component and presence of renal failure *1056*

Immunoglobulin D *Serum* *Increase* Rare *2033*

Immunoglobulin E *Serum* *Increase* Only 5 cases of IgE myeloma have been reported *2033*
Serum *No Effect* In 51 patients with IgA myeloma mean concentration of 2 - 576 U/mL not significantly different from 7 - 524 U/mL in 100 healthy blood donors *3422*

Immunoglobulin G *Serum* *Decrease* May occur in IgA form *5677*
Serum *Increase* Most common *2033* The abnormal serum M component was IgG in 20 of 35 patients and IgA in 7. There was no correlation between type of M component and presence of renal failure *1056* In 94 patients with creatinine concentration > 177 μmol/L 35 (38%) had increased IgG concentrations compared with 185 of 329 (56.2%) with creatinine concentrations less than 177 μmol/L *466*

Immunoglobulin Light Chains *Serum* *Increase* In 94 patients with creatinine concentration of > 177 μmol/L 30 (32%) had increased light chains only concentrations compared with 29 of 329 (8.8%) with creatinine concentrations less than 177 μmol/L *466*

Immunoglobulin M *Serum* *Decrease* May occur *5677*
Serum *No Effect* Concentration usually normal *2033*

Immunoglobulins *Serum* *Decrease* The amount of normal immunoglobulin is usually low, but does not correlate with the increased concentration of anomalous protein *5677*

Interleukin-2 *Serum* *Decrease* Concentration of 21 ± 68 pg/mL observed in 23 patients with multiple myeloma compared with reference interval of 153 ± 277 pg/mL *2828*

Interleukin-4 *Serum* *No Effect* Concentration in peripheral blood and bone marrow of 0 ± 0 pg/mL observed in 23 patients with multiple myeloma compared with reference interval of 0.3 ± 0.7 pg/mL *2828*

Interleukin-6 *Serum* *Increase* Concentration of 1.7 ± 3.3 pg/mL observed in 23 patients with multiple myeloma compared with reference interval of 0.0 ± 0.61 pg/mL *2828* In patients with multiple myeloma mean concentration significantly higher than in healthy control population *4927* In 66 cases mean concentration of 0.290 ± 0.151 ng/mL higher than 0.190 ± 0.145

203.00 Multiple Myeloma *(continued)*

Interleukin-6 *(continued)*
ng/mL in 26 healthy controls *1271* In 30 patients with multiple myeloma median concentration of 1.8 ng/L with range from less than 0.4 to 43.9 ng/L at time of diagnosis compared with median concentration of 1.4 ng/L (range < 0.4 - 3.2 ng/L) in the reference population *4238* In 16 patients with IIIA myeloma mean concentration of 14.0 mg/L, in 6 with IIIB 14.0 mg/L, 11 with IIA 11.0 mg/L and 9 with IA 24.5 mg/L *1506*

Interleukin-7 *Serum Increase* Concentration of 24 ± 27 pg/mL observed in 23 patients with multiple myeloma compared with reference interval of 8.2 ± 6.5 pg/mL *2828*

Interleukin-13 *Serum No Effect* Concentration in peripheral blood and bone marrow of 0 ± 0 pg/mL observed in 23 patients with multiple myeloma compared with reference interval of < 0.1 pg/mL *2828*

Kappa Light Chains *Serum Increase* In 94 patients with creatinine concentration > 177 μmol/L 38 (40%) had increased kappa light chain concentrations compared with 165 of 329 (50.2%) with creatinine concentrations less than 177 μmol/L *466*

Lactate Dehydrogenase *Serum Increase* In 391 patients with multiple myeloma 11% had increased activity of more than 5 μkat/L. Increase observed in 26% with high tumor mass. Only 20% patients with high LD responded to chemotherapy compared with 57% of patients with low LD *1175* In 74 patients with creatinine concentration > 177 μmol/L 25 (34%) had increased LD activity compared with 37 of 240 (15.4%) with creatinine concentrations less than 177 μmol/L *466*

Lambda Light Chains *Serum Increase* In 94 patients with creatinine concentration > 177 μmol/L 48 (51%) had increased kappa light chain concentrations compared with 137 of 329 (41.6%) with creatinine concentrations less than 177 μmol/L *466*

Latent Tumor Growth Factor-β1 *Serum Increase* Concentration in peripheral blood and bone marrow of 9.5 ± 7.4 ng/mL observed in 23 patients with multiple myeloma compared with reference interval of 3.5 ± 1.6 ng/mL *2828*

Leukocytes *Blood Decrease* Progressive plasma cell proliferation in the marrow may result in leukopenia *2039* Leukopenia and thrombocytopenia were present in 16 and 13% of the patients, respectively. The degree of disease in untreated patients is usually mild *2877* Occasionally, moderate to severe leukopenia or thrombocytopenia, or both, may be observed prior to treatment *4551* About 33% have leukopenia with diminished granulocytes and decreased platelets *4434*
Blood No Effect Usually within normal limits prior to cytotoxic therapy *4551*

Lymphocytes *Blood Increase* 40 - 55% lymphocytosis frequently present on differential count, with variable number of immature lymphocytic and plasmacytic forms *5545* Relative lymphocytosis of 40 - 55% with a variable proportion of immature lymphocytic and plasmacytic forms *4551*

Lysozyme *Serum Increase* Isolated cases *2012*

α_2-Macroglobulin *Serum Decrease* Mild *2411*

β_2-Macroglobulin *Serum Increase* Showed the best correlation with survival. May be increased *2586*

M Component *Serum Increase* In 23 patients with multiple myeloma 7 patients had concentrations in peripheral blood of less than 17 g/L, the upper limit of normal, and in 16 concentrations were the same as or greater than 17 g/L *2828*

MCV *Blood Increase* Anemia may be macrocytic *5677*

β_2-Microglobulin *Serum Increase* In 16 patients with IIIA myeloma mean concentration of 6.3 mg/L, in 6 with IIIB 6.3 mg/L, 11 with IIA 4.2 mg/L and 9 with IA 4.4 mg/L *1506* In patients with concentration greater than 4 μg/mL median survival 43 months whereas survival in those with concentration less than 4 μg/mL only 12 months *2952* Patients with concentrations greater than 4 mg/L survived a median of 15 months versus 46 months for those with a concentration less than 4 mg/L *3827* In 23 patients with multiple myeloma 18 patients had concentration in peripheral blood of less than 2.4 mg/L, the upper limit of normal, and in 5 concentrations were the same as or greater than 2.4 mg/L *2828*

Neopterin *Serum Increase* Mean concentration of 32.1 ± 33.6 nmol/L in 10 patients with myeloma significantly greater than that in 18 healthy control individuals, 6.4 ± 1.8 nmol/L *3864*
Urine Increase In 7 patients with multiple myeloma mean excretion of about 420 μmol/mol creatinine significantly greater than 106.6 ± 34.6 μmol/mol creatinine in 31 healthy controls *3632*

Neutrophils *Blood Decrease* About 33% have leukopenia with diminished granulocytes and decreased platelets *4434* Total WBC is often reduced to 3,000 - 4,000 /μL, largely because of neutropenia *5677*

Osmolal Gap *Urine Increase* May lead to proximal renal tubular acidosis which is associated with hypokalemia, hyperchloremic metabolic acidosis, urine pH < 5.5, increased urinary ammonium ion excretion, a negative urine anion gap, increased urinary osmol gap, normal urinary citrate, normal urinary calcium excretion and Fanconi syndrome *4071*

Osmolality *Urine Decrease* Mean for the group following overnight dehydration was 444 ± 26 mOsm/kg; patients with Bence-Jones proteinuria had further reduced concentrating ability *1056*

Osteocalcin *Serum Decrease* Significant negative correlation observed between concentration and stage of disease with lowest concentrations being observed with most advanced disease. Significant correlation observed between initial concentration and patient survival *692*
Serum Increase In 3 men with untreated multiple myeloma mean concentrations of 7.0 - > 32.0 ng/mL significantly different from 5.4 - 8.8 ng/mL in 8 healthy controls *3747* High values were found in 5 of 26 (19%) patients at presentation *5676*

Parathyroid Hormone *Plasma Decrease* In one study of 42 patients with low intact PTH concentration and hypercalcemia 5 had myeloma *3280*

pH *Blood Decrease* Hypercalcemia of malignancy common with this type of cancer which leads to diminished capacity of renal tubules to concentrate urine which, in turn, decreases the ECF and the kidney's ability to eliminate excess calcium. Renal impairment eventually causes nitrogen retention, acidosis and renal failure and a further decrease in calcium excretion *3470*
Urine Decrease May lead to proximal renal tubular acidosis which is associated with hypokalemia, hyperchloremic metabolic acidosis, urine pH < 5.5, increased urinary ammonium ion excretion, a negative urine anion gap, increased urinary osmol gap, normal urinary citrate, normal urinary calcium excretion and Fanconi syndrome *4071*

Phosphate *Serum Decrease* May lead to proximal renal tubular acidosis which is associated with hypokalemia, hyperchloremic metabolic acidosis, urine pH < 5.5, increased urinary ammonium ion excretion, a negative urine anion gap, increased urinary osmol gap, normal urinary citrate, normal urinary calcium excretion and Fanconi syndrome *4071* In 21% of 32 patients at initial hospitalization for this disorder *1576* Due to renal loss of phosphate *5545* Common *1980*
Serum Increase In 27% of 32 patients at initial hospitalization for this disorder *1576* Multiple myeloma proteins may cause interference with the formation of phosphomolybdate complexes *969* In vitro artefactual cause of hyperphosphatemia reported *5204* Some cases *5544*
Urine Increase Renal loss *5545*

Plasma Cells *Blood Increase* A small number may be found in the circulating blood of many patients, and if the absolute number of plasma cells exceeds 2,000 /μL, the diagnosis of plasma cell leukemia may be made *5677*
Bone Marrow Increase Increased numbers and abnormal forms have been found in all cases, although more than one attempt may be necessary *4551* In average patients with moderately advanced disease, 20 - 95% of the nucleated cells in the bone marrow are mature or immature plasma cells. The percent varies with the sample and is not a reliable measure of the total amount of disease present *5677* Bone marrow infiltrated with over 20% plasma cells in clusters or sheets *4434* Marked bone marrow plasmacytosis. Many patients had cytoplasmic abnormalities of cells, including size and contour of nucleus, mitochondria and rough ER *1837*

Platelets *Blood Decrease* Occasionally, moderate to severe leukopenia or thrombocytopenia, or both, may be observed prior to treatment *4551* Leukopenia and thrombocytopenia were present in 16 and 13% of the patients, respectively. The degree in untreated patients is usually mild *2877* About 33% have leukopenia with diminished granulocytes and decreased platelets *4434* In 31% of 31 patients at initial hospitalization for this disorder *1576*

Blood *No Effect* Usually within normal limits prior to cytotoxic therapy *4551*

Potassium *Serum* *Decrease* May lead to proximal renal tubular acidosis which is associated with hypokalemia, hyperchloremic metabolic acidosis, urine pH < 5.5, increased urinary ammonium ion excretion, a negative urine anion gap, increased urinary osmol gap, normal urinary citrate, normal urinary calcium excretion and Fanconi syndrome *4071* Common *1980*
Urine *Increase* Due to myeloma nephropathy *413*

Protein *Cerebrospinal Fluid* *Increase* Usually normal or slightly elevated to values of 50 - 100 mg/dL *367*
Pleural Fluid *Increase* With pleural involvement increased total protein with a sharp spike in the γ-globulin region *4504*
Serum *Increase* Over 80 g/L in 18 of 35 patients, all of whom had total globulin concentration > 52 g/L *1056* Very elevated serum total protein is due to increase in globulins (with decreased A/G ratio) in 50 - 66% of the patients *5545*
Urine *Increase* Unexplained, persistent proteinuria may last for years *5545* Minimal elevation (0.15 - 0.5 g/L) in 7, mild-moderate (0.5 - 3 g/L) in 17 and heavy (> 3 g/L) in 9 of 35 patients *1056*

Pseudouridine *Urine* *Increase* In 7 patients with multiple myeloma mean excretion of about 26 mmol/mol creatinine significantly greater than 19.6 ± 5.2 mmol/mol creatinine in 31 healthy controls *3632*

Pyridinoline *Urine* *Increase* In 32 patients with multiple myeloma median excretion of 66.9 nmol/mmol creatinine significantly higher than that in 75 healthy men in whom the median excretion was 20.8 nmol/mmol creatinine and in 20 premenopausal women, 19.6 nmol/mmol creatinine, and in 38 postmenopausal women, 28.2 nmol/mmol creatinine *4716*

Rheumatoid Factor *Serum* *Increase* Dysproteinemias and paraproteinemias may present significant seropositivity *1980*

Sialyltransferase *Serum* *Increase* In 19 untreated patients activity significantly increased, but decline observed during treatment with alkylating drugs and prednisolone. Activity higher in stage III disease than in stage I and II disease *1582*

Sodium *Serum* *Decrease* In 31% of 28 patients at initial hospitalization for this disorder *1576*

Soluble CD16 *Serum* *Decrease* In 35 patients with multiple myeloma median concentration of 0.7 μg/mL significantly different from median concentration of 2.7 μg/mL in 29 healthy controls *3349* In 10 patients with early myeloma mean concentration of 1.1 ± 0.5 μg/mL not significantly different from 2.7 ± 1.4 μg/mL in 29 healthy volunteer controls. Mean concentration of 0.7 ± 1.2 μg/mL in 35 patients with multiple myeloma significantly less than in controls *3350*

Soluble Interleukin-2 Receptor *Serum* *Decrease* Concentration of 874 ± 308 U/mL observed in 23 patients with multiple myeloma compared with reference interval of 1,079 ± 331 U/mL *2828*

Soluble Interleukin-6 Receptor *Serum* *Decrease* In 10 patients with early myeloma mean concentration of 80.5 ± 23 ng/mL not significantly different from 70.3 ± 13.4 μg/mL in 24 healthy volunteer controls. Mean concentration of 78.4 ± 20.1 ng/mL in 30 patients with multiple myeloma significantly less than in controls *3350*
Serum *Increase* Concentration of 102 ± 93 ng/mL observed in 23 patients with multiple myeloma compared with reference interval of 80 ± 42 ng/mL *2828*

Soluble Transferrin Receptor *Serum* *No Effect* Concentration not changed typically in myeloproliferative diseases *4784* In patients with multiple myeloma mean concentration of 5.47 ± 1.31 μg/mL not significantly different from 5.63 ± 1.42 μg/mL in healthy controls *2704*

Urea Nitrogen *Serum* *Increase* In 51% of 33 patients at initial hospitalization for this disorder *1576* Impaired renal function in > 50%, decreasing concentrating ability and azotemia *5545* Ranged from 5.0 - 92.1 mmol/L in 35 patients *1056* Hypercalcemia of malignancy common with this type of cancer which leads to diminished capacity of renal tubules to concentrate urine which, in turn, decreases the ECF and the kidney's ability to eliminate excess calcium. Renal impairment eventually causes nitrogen retention, acidosis and renal failure and a further decrease in calcium excretion *3470* Observed with renal involvement *900*

Uric Acid *Serum* *Decrease* May lead to proximal renal tubular acidosis which is associated with hypokalemia, hyperchloremic metabolic acidosis, urine pH < 5.5, increased urinary ammonium ion excretion, a negative urine anion gap, increased urinary osmol gap, normal urinary citrate, normal urinary calcium excretion and Fanconi syndrome *4071* Common *1980* Occasionally decreased due to altered renal tubular function *5545*
Serum *Increase* May accompany renal failure or may occur in the absence of azotemia *5677* Seen in about 33% of patients *900* 10 of 35 patients had hyperuricemia (> 416 mmol/L). 8 of these had only mild elevations, consistent with the severity of renal insufficiency *1056* In 63% of 33 patients at initial hospitalization for this disorder *1576*

Viscosity *Serum* *Increase* Occurs in only 2 - 4% of patients *4932* An increase of IgM is the most common clinical situation producing hyperviscosity of serum *1980*

Vitamin B_{12} *Serum* *No Effect* Usual observation *5544*

Vitamin B_{12} Binding Capacity *Serum* *Increase* Significant elevation; usually correlated with WBC in peripheral blood *4448*

VLDL-Cholesterol *Serum* *Increase* Moderate increase due to presence of IgG or IgM that forms complexes with chylomicron remnants and/or VLDL thereby decreasing catabolism *126*

Volume *Plasma* *Increase* Often expands as the amount of myeloma protein increases in the serum, and the resulting hemodilution may be great enough to produce a significant reduction in hemoglobin concentration with little or no change in total red cell mass *2769*

203.00 Myelomatosis

Tissue Factor Pathway Inhibitor *Plasma* *No Effect* 11 patients with myelomatosis had median activity of 1.07 U/mL not significantly different from median activity of 1.19 U/mL in healthy individuals *2376*

Tissue Factor Pathway Inhibitor Antigen *Plasma* *No Effect* 11 patients with myelomatosis had median concentration of 112 ng/mL not significantly different from median concentration of 90 ng/mL in healthy individuals *2376*

Tissue Factor Pathway Inhibitor Antigen, Free
Plasma *No Effect* 11 patients with myelomatosis had median concentration of 31 ng/mL not significantly different from median concentration of 15 ng/mL in healthy individuals *2376*

Tissue Factor Pathway Inhibitor, Truncated and Complexed
Plasma *No Effect* 11 patients with myelomatosis had median concentration of 83 ng/mL not significantly different from median concentration of 78 ng/mL in healthy individuals *2376*

204.00 Acute Lymphatic Leukemia

Acetylspermidine *Urine* *Increase* Mean excretion increased in 8 of 10 children with ALL *1781*

Adenosine *Serum* *Increase* Concentration increased in 19 patients with ALL in remission or receiving chemotherapy compared with 19 healthy individuals *1781*

Adenosine Deaminase *Lymphocytes* *Decrease* Mean adenosine deaminase activity in the lymphocytes of 17 patients with uncharacterized acute lymphatic leukemia was significantly reduced compared with 23 healthy controls *1781*

Hypoxanthine *Serum* *Increase* Concentration increased in 19 patients with ALL in remission or receiving chemotherapy compared with 19 healthy individuals *1781*

Inosine *Serum* *Increase* Concentration increased in 19 patients with ALL in remission or receiving chemotherapy compared with 19 healthy individuals, with high concentrations associated with a poor prognosis *1781*

1-Methylinosine *Urine* *Increase* Excretion at initial diagnosis or in relapse was significantly increased compared with normal individuals *1781*

Myelin Basic Protein *Cerebrospinal Fluid* *Increase* Possible CSF marker of CNS spread in ALL *1781*

N^2, N^2-Dimethylguanosine *Urine* *Increase* Excretion at initial diagnosis or in relapse was significantly increased compared with normal individuals *1781*

N-Acetylputrescine *Urine* *Increase* Mean excretion increased in 8 of 10 children with ALL *1781*

204.00 Acute Lymphatic Leukemia *(continued)*

Neopterin *Urine* *Increase* Urinary excretion increased in patients with ALL, decreasing with response to treatment and remission *1781*

Purine Nucleoside Phosphorylase *Lymphocytes* *Decrease* Mean activity reported in the lymphocytes of 17 patients with acute lymphatic leukemia to be very low *1781*
Lymphocytes *Increase* Activity in the lymphocytes of 8 patients with acute lymphatic leukemia reported to be slightly increased *1781*

Spermidine *Cerebrospinal Fluid* *Increase* Mean concentration in 11 children with ALL generally higher in those without CNS involvement *1781*

204.00 Acute Lymphoblastic Leukemia

Adenosine Deaminase *Lymphocytes* *Increase* Mean adenosine deaminase activity in the lymphocytes of 50 patients with acute lymphoblastic leukemia was generally increased *1781*
Serum *Increase* Mean adenosine deaminase activity was increased in the plasma of patients with this disease *1781*

Amino-terminal Propeptide of Type III Collagen
Cerebrospinal Fluid *No Effect* In 44 children with acute lymphoblastic leukemia mean concentration at diagnosis 5.8 ± 2.8 µg/L not significantly different from 6.7 ± 3.2 µg/L in age-matched controls *5380*

Apolipoprotein A *Serum* *No Effect* In 11 children with ALL mean concentration on diagnosis of 0.79 ± 0.21 g/L *1981*

Apolipoprotein A-I *Serum* *Decrease* In 11 patients with ALL mean concentration at diagnosis of 0.79 ± 0.21 g/L significantly different from normal *1981* In 10 patients with newly diagnosed acute lymphoblastic leukemia moderate hypertriglyceridemia observed with decreased plasma apolipoprotein A-I *1781*

Apolipoprotein B *Serum* *Increase* In 10 patients with newly diagnosed acute lymphoblastic leukemia moderate hypertriglyceridemia observed with increased plasma apolipoprotein B *1781*
Serum *No Effect* In 11 patients with ALL mean concentration at diagnosis of 1.87 ± 0.98 g/L not significantly different from normal *1981*

Apolipoprotein Lp(a) *Serum* *No Effect* In 11 patients with ALL median concentration at diagnosis of 112 (range of 0 - 914) mg/L not significantly different from normal *1981*

CD8+ Lymphocytes *Blood* *Increase* Elevated levels of sCD8 were observed *4968*

Cholesterol *Serum* *Increase* In 11 patients with ALL mean concentration at diagnosis of 3.72 ± 0.63 mmol/L not significantly different from normal *1981*
Serum *No Effect* In 11 children with ALL mean concentration on diagnosis of 3.72 ± 0.63 mmol/L *1981*

Ferritin *Serum* *Increase* In 4 patients with acute lymphoblastic leukemia mean concentration of 522 ng/mL significantly higher than 85 ng/mL in 178 healthy men and 39 ng/mL in 105 healthy women *1781*

Granulocyte Colony Stimulating Factor *Serum* *Decrease* In children with ALL and 9 episodes of neutropenia mean concentration of 13.3 ± 11.7 pg/mL *5324*

Granulocyte-Macrophage Colony Stimulating Factor
Serum *Decrease* In children with ALL and 9 episodes of neutropenia mean concentration of 12.2 ± 10.9 pg/mL *5324*

HDL_2-Cholesterol *Serum* *Decrease* In 11 patients with ALL mean concentration at diagnosis of 0.19 ± 0.11 mmol/L significantly different from normal *1981*
Serum *No Effect* In 11 children with ALL mean concentration on diagnosis of 0.19 ± 0.11 mmol/L *1981*

HDL_3-Cholesterol *Serum* *Increase* In 11 patients with ALL mean concentration at diagnosis of 0.19 ± 0.11 mmol/L not significantly different from normal *1981*
Serum *No Effect* In 11 children with ALL mean concentration on diagnosis of 0.19 ± 0.11 mmol/L *1981*

HDL-Cholesterol *Serum* *Decrease* In 11 patients with ALL mean concentration at diagnosis of 0.57 ± 0.22 mmol/L significantly different from normal *1981*
Serum *No Effect* In 11 children with ALL mean concentration on diagnosis of 0.57 ± 0.22 mmol/L *1981*

Hepatocyte Growth Factor *Serum* *Increase* In 3 of 8 patients with ALL concentration increased above 0.4 ng/mL *3714*

Immunoglobulin G *Serum* *Decrease* In 880 untreated children with acute lymphoblastic leukemia a low concentration was associated with an adverse outcome *1781*

Interferon-γ *Serum* *Increase* In children with ALL and 9 episodes of neutropenia mean concentration of 204.1 ± 210.3 pg/mL *5324*

LDL-Cholesterol *Serum* *No Effect* In 11 patients with ALL mean concentration at diagnosis of 1.87 ± 0.98 mmol/L not significantly different from normal *1981* In 11 children with ALL mean concentration on diagnosis of 1.87 ± 0.98 mmol/L *1981*

Leukocytes *Blood* *Increase* In 13 patients mean concentration of 12.9 x 10^9/L with range 1.2 - 40.7 x 10^9/L *3685*

Lysozyme *Serum* *Decrease* Activity decreased in patients with acute lymphoblastic leukemia *1781*

β_2-Microglobulin *Cerebrospinal Fluid* *Increase* In patients with CNS involvement mean concentration significantly increased *2013*

Neutrophils *Blood* *Decrease* In children with ALL and 9 episodes of neutropenia mean absolute neutrophil count 427.5 ± 395.6 /µL *5324*

Nitrate plus Nitrite *Cerebrospinal Fluid* *Increase* In 11 patients with ALL median concentration of 21.0 µmol/L significantly different from median of reference interval of 9.2 (interval 7.2 - 13.0) µmol/L *5086*

Phosphate *Serum* *Increase* Lysis of ALL cells even prior to treatment may cause shift of phosphate from cells leads to increased serum concentration, and possible acute renal failure *969*

Plasminogen Activator Inhibitor-1
Cerebrospinal Fluid *Increase* In 7 patients with acute lymphoblastic leukemia mean concentration of 1.53 ± 0.42 ng/mL significantly different from 0.31 ± 0.06 ng/mL in 20 reference individuals *56*

Protein Z *Plasma* *Increase* In 5 patients with acute lymphoblastic leukemia median baseline concentration of 3.49 ng/mL compared with 2.72 ng/mL in 14 healthy controls *5357*

Soluble CD8+ *Serum* *Decrease* Plasma sCD8 was found to be below normal control levels in pre-T-ALL *4968*

Soluble Interleukin-2 Receptor *Serum* *Increase* Elevated sIL-2R levels were found in non-T/non-B acute lymphoblastic leukemia, in B-acute lymphoblastic leukemia, in mixed lineage acute lymphoblastic leukemia, in T-chronic lymphocytic leukemia, in T-acute lymphoblastic leukemia, and in active MF *4968* In patients with non-T/non-B ALL, B-ALL, mixed lineage ALL, and T-ALL significant increase in concentration observed *4968*

Soluble L-Selectin *Serum* *Increase* Patients with untreated acute lymphoblastic leukemia have increased serum concentration *613*

Soluble Urokinase Receptor *Serum* *Increase* In 13 patients mean concentration of 2.31 ng/mL with range of 0.79 - 3.52 ng/mL compared with mean of 1.14 ng/mL and range of 0.79 - 1.72 in 21 healthy controls *3685*

Spermidine *Red Blood Cells* *Increase* Median concentration in 63 children with acute lymphoblastic leukemia of 9.5 nmol/8 x 10^9 RBC significantly different from 8.4 ± 0.5 nmol/8 x 10^9 RBC in 12 healthy children *398*

Spermine *Red Blood Cells* *Increase* Median concentration in 63 children with acute lymphoblastic leukemia of 9.9 nmol/8 x 10^9 RBC significantly different from 4.3 ± 0.4 nmol/8 x 10^9 RBC in 12 healthy children *398*

Thymidine Kinase *Serum* *Increase* Activity increased in all of 12 patients with acute lymphoblastic leukemia *1781*

Tissue Factor Antigen *Plasma* *Increase* In 13 patients with ALL and disseminated intravascular coagulation mean concentration of 252 ± 60 pg/mL compared with 126 ± 41 pg/mL in 12 healthy volunteers *5511*

Triglycerides *Serum* *Increase* In 10 patients with newly diagnosed acute lymphoblastic leukemia moderate hypertriglyceridemia observed *1781* In 11 patients with ALL mean concentration at diagnosis of 2.45 ± 1.52 mmol/L significantly different from normal *1981*

Serum *No Effect* In 11 children with ALL mean concentration on diagnosis of 2.45 ± 1.52 mmol/L *1981*

Tumor Necrosis Factor-α *Serum* *Increase* In children with ALL and 9 episodes of neutropenia mean concentration of 93.5 ± 161 pg/mL *5324*

Urokinase Plasminogen Activator *Plasma* *Increase* In 13 patients mean concentration of 0.62 ng/mL with range of 0.25 - 1.37 ng/mL compared with mean of 0.32 ng/mL and range of 0.14 - 0.60 in 21 healthy controls *3685*

VLDL-Cholesterol *Serum* *Increase* In 11 patients with ALL mean concentration at diagnosis of 0.54 ± 0.34 mmol/L not significantly different from normal *1981*
Serum *No Effect* In 11 children with ALL mean concentration on diagnosis of 0.54 ± 0.34 mmol/L *1981*

204.00 Acute Lymphocytic Leukemia

α_1-Acid Glycoprotein *Serum* *Increase* Elevated levels in states associated with cell proliferation *3713 4241 4373 4696 4853 2597*

Adenosine Deaminase *Serum* *Increase* Mean adenosine deaminase activity was increased in the plasma of patients with this disease *1781 1781*

Adenylate Cyclase *Lymphocytes* *Decrease* Activity depressed in cells from patients with acute lymphocytic leukemia *1781*

Albumin *Serum* *Decrease* In 30% of 44 patients at initial hospitalization for this disorder *1576* Normal at diagnosis and declines as disease advances *1409 5699*

Alkaline Phosphatase *Serum* *Increase* In 56% of 42 patients at initial hospitalization for this disorder *1576* Infiltration of the liver may result in obstruction of biliary system *5545* Elevations > 95 U/L *2848*
White Blood Cells *Increase* The mean activity score was 159.4 ranging from 83 - 308 (12 cases) *3440* Tend to be high, in contrast to acute myelogenous leukemia *2077*

Alkaline Phosphatase Isoenzymes *Serum* *Increase* In all 6 patients, an electrophoretically distinct isoenzyme (phosphatase N) was present in the serum. The range of phosphatase N was 26-100% of the total alkaline phosphatase activity *3765*

Alkaline Phosphatase, Placental Isoenzyme
Serum *Increase* In 33 patients with ALL mean activity of 0.578 ± 0.112 U/L significantly higher than 0.311 ± 0.012 in 15 healthy controls *4027*

Antinuclear Antibodies *Serum* *Increase* Positive in 25% of patients *4068*

Aspartate Aminotransferase *Serum* *Increase* Infiltration of the liver *1290* Moderately elevated levels are observed in lymphomas and leukemia but less frequently than in other hepatic disease *1025* In 71% of 43 patients at initial hospitalization for this disorder *1576*

Calcium *Serum* *Decrease* Hypocalcemia with values of 6.6 - 8.3 mg/dL was observed within 24 - 48 h after initiation of chemotherapy *5881*
Serum *Increase* May be increased in some cases *1025* Has been observed but is uncommon *5699* Elevated levels (> 11.0 mg/dL) may occur with leukemic infiltration of bone *2848*
Urine *Increase* May be increased in some cases *1025*

Carcinoembryonic Antigen *Serum* *Increase* Above 2.5 ng/mL in 38% of patients with acute and chronic leukemia *456*

$CD8^+$ Lymphocytes *Blood* *Increase* Mean concentration in patients with non-T/non-B ALL, B-ALL, mixed lineage ALL, and T-ALL significantly increased *4968*

Cells *Bone Marrow* *Increase* Almost always hypercellular and heavily infiltrated or replaced by abnormal lymphoid elements *5677*
Cerebrospinal Fluid *Increase* Pleocytosis with meningeal infiltration *5677*

Cholesterol *Serum* *Decrease* In 37% of 42 patients at initial hospitalization for this disorder *1576*

Cold Agglutinins *Serum* *Increase* Tends to rise *3953*

Copper *Serum* *Increase* Significant increase observed in 16 children with acute leukemias. Drop in concentration occurs in cases who respond to quadruple chemotherapy while those who failed to respond showed persistently high serum levels *1321*

Creatine *Serum* *Increase* Increased formation *1290*
Urine *Increase* Pronounced increase in children and adult males with acute leukemias *4707* Extremely variable *5523*

Creatinine *Serum* *Increase* In 49% of 16 patients at initial hospitalization for this disorder *1576*

Erythropoietin *Serum* *Increase* Found to be increased and negatively correlated with hemoglobin concentration *4045*
Urine *Increase* Urine levels are usually increased in lymphoblastic but not myeloblastic leukemia *4045*

Ferritin *Serum* *Increase* Significant elevation *4970*

Fibrinogen *Plasma* *Increase* Nonspecific increase in concentration may be observed *1781* Frequently elevated when the disease is in relapse. The absolute levels vary considerably from individual to individual *557*

α_1-Globulin *Serum* *Increase* Often reflects the presence of fever or infection *5699 1409*

α_2-Globulin *Serum* *Increase* Often reflects the presence of fever or infection *5699 1409*

β-Globulin *Serum* *Decrease* Common *1409 5699*

γ-Globulin *Serum* *No Effect* Most often normal in contrast to acute myelogenous leukemia *1409 5699*

Glucose *Cerebrospinal Fluid* *Decrease* With meningeal infiltration *5677*

Guanylate Cyclase *Lymphocytes* *Increase* Activity increased in cells from patients with acute lymphocytic leukemia *1781*

Hematocrit *Blood* *Decrease* Often severe, usually normochromic, normocytic *5699* Most patients will have anemia *900* In 81% of 36 patients at initial hospitalization for this disorder *1576*

Hemoglobin *Blood* *Decrease* Often severe, usually normochromic, normocytic *5699* Most patients will have anemia *900* In 82% of 37 patients at initial hospitalization for this disorder *1576*

Heterophile Antibody *Serum* *Decrease* Positive presumptive test but negative differential test if Forsman antigen is used *3953*
Serum *Increase* Positive presumptive test but negative differential test if Forsman antigen is used *3953*

α_2-HS Glycoprotein *Serum* *Decrease* In patients with ALL significant reduction observed probably due to hepatic involvement *2533*

immunoglobulin A *Serum* *Decrease* Reported effect *5544*

Immunoglobulin G *Serum* *No Effect* Concentration usually normal *5544*

Immunoglobulin M *Serum* *No Effect* Concentration usually normal *5544*

Interleukin-6 *Serum* *Increase* In comparison with normal subjects, IL-6 activity was significantly elevated in patients with ALL and ANLL ($p < 0.01$) *3167*

Iron *Serum* *Increase* Increased in acute leukemias *1290*

Lactate Dehydrogenase *Serum* *Increase* Increased in acute, but not in chronic lymphocytic leukemia. Usually reflected changes in the course of the disease-falling during remission and rising during relapses, occasionally indicating the onset before the WBC had begun to change *469* Mean value of 54 patients was 2 times normal adult value. 47 of 54 patients had significantly increased activities *447* Activity increased above 900 U/L in 15 of 19 patients with ALL *1781* In 91% of 39 patients at initial hospitalization for this disorder *1576* Frequently elevated when the disease is in relapse. The absolute levels vary considerably from individual to individual *1916* May be large increase in activity observed *1980* In 51 patients with ALL mean activity of 668.7 ± 121.5 U/L *4027*

Laminin *Serum* *Increase* No difference in concentrations between different leukemias. Median concentration of all leukemias was 1,609 mU/mL (n = 12), versus control concentration of 1,232 mU/mL (n = 41) *3786*

Leukocytes *Blood* *Decrease* Variable and can be very high (> 100,000 /μL), moderately elevated (20,000 - 100,000 /μL), normal, or low *900*
Blood *Increase* Elevated in slightly over 50% of patients *5699* Variable and can be very high (> 100,000 /μL), moderately elevated (20,000 - 100,000 /μL), normal, or low *900* Initial counts above 100,000 /μL indicate significantly poor prognosis *4858*
Blood *No Effect* Variable and can be very high (> 100,000 /μL), moderately elevated (20,000 - 100,000 /μL), normal, or low *900*

204.00 Acute Lymphocytic Leukemia *(continued)*

Lysozyme *Serum* *Decrease* Low or normal *1606*
Serum *No Effect* Activity normal in most patients with acute lymphocytic leukemia *1781* Low or normal *1606*

β_2-Macroglobulin *Serum* *Increase* May be increased in leukemia of B-lymphocyte lineage *2586*

β_2-Microglobulin *Serum* *Increase* In 6 children with ALL mean concentration of 2.3 mg/L significantly higher than in controls *2145* In children with ALL mean concentration of 2.9 mg/L significantly higher than in controls *2145*

Monocytes *Blood* *Decrease* In 64% of 34 patients at initial hospitalization for this disorder *1576*
Blood *Increase* On occasion associated with a monocytosis of relatively minor proportions *3246*

Naphthol-As-D-Chloroacetate Esterase
Granulocyte *Increase* Mean density of 496 ± 17 in 2 patients with acute lymphocytic leukemia significantly different from 478 ± 52 in 32 normal controls *1303*

Neopterin *Serum* *No Effect* Concentration of 6.7 nmol/L in one patient with ALL not significantly different from that in 18 healthy control individuals, 6.4 ± 1.8 nmol/L *3864*

Neutrophils *Blood* *Decrease* The absolute number is almost always decreased, and usually to a greater extent than in acute myelogenous leukemia *5677* In 92% of 34 patients at initial hospitalization for this disorder *1576*

Phosphate *Serum* *Increase* Hyperphosphatemia with values of 5.7 - 9.4 mg/dL was observed within 24 - 48 h after initiation of chemotherapy *5881* In 40% of 44 patients at initial hospitalization for this disorder *1576*
Urine *Increase* Marked hyperphosphaturia was observed within 24 - 48 h after initiation of chemotherapy *5881*

Phosphoglucomutase *Serum* *Increase* Increases in some cases *1290*

Platelets *Blood* *Decrease* The absolute number is almost always decreased, and usually to a greater extent than in acute myelogenous leukemia *5677* Pronounced at diagnosis *5699* In 78% of 29 patients at initial hospitalization for this disorder *1576* Most patients will have thrombocytopenia *900*
Blood *Increase* On very rare occasions *177*

Protein *Cerebrospinal Fluid* *Increase* With meningeal infiltration *5677*
Pleural Fluid *Increase* Pleural effusions are usually exudates *126*

Reticulocytes *Blood* *Decrease* Usually low *900* Reflects decreased cell production *5699*

Rheumatoid Factor *Serum* *Increase* Dysproteinemias and paraproteinemias present significant seropositivity *1980*

Sodium *Serum* *Increase* In 94% of 39 patients at initial hospitalization for this disorder *1576*

Soluble Intercellular Adhesion Molecule-1 *Serum* *Increase* Mean concentration increased in patients with non-T/non-B ALL, B-ALL, mixed lineage ALL and in T-ALL *4968*

Soluble Interleukin-2 Receptor *Serum* *Decrease* Reduced levels of sIL-2R were encountered in HCL patients in remission, in pre-T-ALL, and in mycosis fungoides patients in remission *4968*

Terminal Deoxynucleotidyl Transferase
Lymphocytes *Increase* Enzyme found in immature cells *1781*

Tumor Necrosis Factor-α *Serum* *No Effect* TNF-α level increased in patients with ALL ($p < 0.05$) *3167*

Urea Nitrogen *Serum* *Increase* Can be elevated in kidney infiltration and should be followed especially if nephrotoxic antibiotics are used *900*

Uric Acid *Serum* *Increase* In 39% of 46 patients at initial hospitalization for this disorder *1576* Observed with increased catabolism of cells *5677* Nonspecific increase in concentration may be observed *1781* Frequently elevated when the disease is in relapse. The absolute levels vary considerably from individual to individual *557* In 50% of patients *2146* Frequent biochemical abnormality. Secondary to the increased cell turnover *900*
Urine *Increase* Almost invariably *2146* Secondary to the increased cell turnover *900*

Vitamin B_{12} *Serum* *No Effect* Usually normal, in contrast to acute myelogenous leukemia *350* Concentration typically normal in contrast to that in CML in which it may be strikingly increased *1781*

Vitamin B_{12} Binding Capacity *Serum* *Increase* Significant elevation; usually correlated with WBC in peripheral blood *4448*

Zinc *Serum* *Decrease* Decreased *5083*

204.00 Acute Lymphoid Leukemia

Manganese Superoxide Dismutase *Serum* *Increase* The level for normal subjects was 94.1 ng/mL versus 154.4 ng/mL for ALL patients *3806*

Soluble c-kit Molecule *Serum* *Decrease* Median concentration of 106.0 AU/mL in patients with ALL significantly different from that in 51 healthy volunteers of 199.0 AU/mL *2598*

204.00 Chronic Lymphoblastoid Leukemia

Neopterin *Urine* *Increase* Highest concentrations observed in patients with non-Hodgkin's lymphoma, chronic myelogenous or lymphoblastoid leukemia with highest concentrations predictive of a shorter survival *121*

204.00 Lymphatic Leukemia

Gc-Globulin *Serum* *No Effect* In 23 men and 15 women with lymphatic leukemia mean concentrations of 22.6 ± 5.02 mg/dL and 23.7 ± 4.86 mg/dL not significantly different from 23.9 mg/dL in 106 control men and 26.1 mg/dL in 150 control women *2279*

204.00 Lymphocytic Leukemia

Magnesium *Monocytes* *Decrease* Mean concentration in patients with lymphocytic leukemia of 2.31 ± 0.63 fmol/cell different from 3.74 ± 0.66 fmol/cell in healthy controls *3137*

Tissue Factor Pathway Inhibitor, Truncated and Complexed
Plasma *No Effect* 6 patients with CLL had median concentration of 77 ng/mL not significantly different from median concentration of 78 ng/mL in healthy individuals *2376*

204.00 Pre-acute T-lymphocytic Leukemia

$CD8^+$ Lymphocytes *Blood* *Decrease* Concentration below normal control concentrations in pre-T-ALL *4968*

Soluble Interleukin-2 Receptor *Serum* *Decrease* In patients with pre-acute T-ALL mean concentration significantly reduced *4968*

204.00 Prolymphocytic Leukemia

$CD8^+$ Lymphocytes *Blood* *Increase* Elevated levels of sCD8 were observed *4968* In patients with PLL mean concentration significantly increased *4968*

Interleukin-2 *Serum* *Increase* Elevated levels *4968*

Soluble Interleukin-2 Receptor *Serum* *Increase* In patients with promyelocytic leukemia significant increase in concentration observed *4968*

204.00 T-Cell Leukemia

$CD2^+$ Lymphocytes *Blood* *Increase* T cell lymphoblastic leukemia *4968*

$CD5^+$ Lymphocytes *Blood* *Increase* T cell lymphoblastic leukemia *4968*

$CD7^+$ Lymphocytes *Blood* *Increase* T cell lymphoblastic leukemia *4968*

$CD8^+$ Lymphocytes *Blood* *Increase* Elevated concentrations of CD8 lymphocytes were observed *4968* Mean concentration increased in patients with adult T-cell leukemia *4968*

Dehydroepiandrosterone *Plasma Decrease* Mean concentration of 1.34 ± 0.59 ng/mL in 7 men aged 40 - 49 y decreased significantly compared with 4.39 ± 1.69 ng/mL in 10 healthy men of the same age: comparable difference seen in women and in men of other ages *5369*

Dehydroepiandrosterone Sulfate *Plasma Decrease* Mean concentration of 421.4 ± 255.4 ng/mL in 7 men aged 40 - 49 y decreased significantly compared with 703.6 ± 396.2 ng/mL in 10 healthy men of the same age: comparable difference seen in women and in men of other ages *5369*

Interleukin-2 *Serum Increase* Elevated levels in T-chronic lymphocytic and T-acute lymphoblastic leukemia *4968*

Interleukin-4 *Cerebrospinal Fluid No Effect* In 50 patients with adult T-cell leukemia and meningeal infiltration no IL-4 detectable *5367*

Interleukin-6 *Cerebrospinal Fluid Increase* In 3 of 10 patients with adult T-cell leukemia with meningeal infiltration and in 1 of 19 without CSF pleocytosis IL-4 detectable *5367*
Serum Increase In 59 adults with T-cell leukemia/Lymphoma median concentration of 8.2 (range < 1.0 - 185.7) pg/mL significantly higher than concentrations in 30 healthy adults of < 1.0 to 3.5 pg/mL with median < 1.0 pg/mL *5779*

Lactate Dehydrogenase *Serum Increase* In 38 patients with adult T-cell leukemia close correlation between pretreatment serum LD activity and leukocyte count, absolute number of abnormal lymphocytes, platelet count, length of survival, serum thymidine kinase activity, PTHrP and β_2-microglobulin *4497*

Macrophage Colony Stimulating Factor *Serum Increase* In 35 patients with ATL mean concentration of 4.62 ± 2.2 ng/mL significantly higher than 2.0 ± 0.5 ng/mL in 133 healthy controls. Mean concentration in acute ATL patients of 5.4 ± 1.9 ng/mL compared with 2.2 ± 0.8 ng/mL in smouldering and chronic ATL forms *5769*

β_2-Microglobulin *Serum Increase* In 38 patients with adult T-cell leukemia close correlation between pretreatment serum LD activity and leukocyte count, absolute number of abnormal lymphocytes, platelet count, length of survival, serum thymidine kinase activity, calcium and length of survival *4497*

Parathyroid Hormone-related Peptide *Plasma Increase* In 38 patients with adult T-cell leukemia close correlation between pretreatment serum LD activity and leukocyte count, absolute number of abnormal lymphocytes, platelet count, length of survival, serum calcium, LD activity, thymidine kinase activity and β_2-microglobulin *4497*

Phosphate *Serum Increase* Lysis of T-cell leukemia cells even prior to treatment may cause shift of phosphate from cells leading to increased serum concentration, and possible acute renal failure *969*

Soluble c-kit Molecule *Serum Decrease* Median concentration of 106.0 AU/mL in patients with adult ATL significantly different from that in 51 healthy volunteers of 199.0 AU/mL *2598*

Soluble CD4+ *Cerebrospinal Fluid Increase* All 8 patients with adult T-cell leukemia and pleocytosis had increased concentrations and In 14 of 23 patients without CSF pleocytosis soluble CD4 concentration increased *5367* In patients with adult T-cell leukemia and meningeal leukemia mean concentration markedly increased to 53.7 ± 34.9 U/mL and ATL patients without CSF pleocytosis had mean concentration increased to 15.1 ± 9.2 U/mL. Non-ATL patients with CSF pleocytosis had mean concentration increased to 23.3 ± 12.2 U/mL and those without CSF pleocytosis concentration was increased to 16.8 ± 9.3 U/mL compared undetectable concentration in healthy individuals *5368*

Soluble CD25+ *Cerebrospinal Fluid Increase* In 13 of 18 patients with adult T-cell leukemia and pleocytosis concentrations increased higher than in patients with ATL but without CSF pleocytosis and in non-ATL patients *5367*

Thymidine Kinase *Serum Increase* In 38 patients with adult T-cell leukemia close correlation between pretreatment serum LD activity and leukocyte count, absolute number of abnormal lymphocytes, platelet count, length of survival, serum calcium, LD activity, PTHrP and β_2-microglobulin *4497*

204.10 Chronic B-lymphocytic Leukemia

CD8+ Lymphocytes *Blood Increase* Significant increase observed in patients with accelerated stage B-CLL *4968*
Blood No Effect Concentration in the non-accelerated phase of B-CLL approximately the same as that in healthy controls *4968*

204.10 Chronic Lymphatic Leukemia

Adenosine Kinase *Lymphocytes No Effect* Activity in 25 patients with CLL showed no significant difference from that in 23 control individuals *1781*

Adenosine Phosphoribosyltransferase *Lymphocytes No Effect* Activity in 25 patients with CLL showed no significant difference from that in 23 control individuals *1781*

Hexosamines, Protein-bound *Serum Increase* In 20 patients with chronic lymphatic leukemia mean concentration of 1,185 ± 264 mg/dm³ significantly greater than 627 ± 183 mg/dm³ in 40 healthy controls *1781*

Hexoses, Protein-bound *Serum Increase* In 20 patients with chronic lymphatic leukemia mean concentration of 5,262 ± 562 mg/dm³ significantly greater than 1,530 ± 325 mg/dm³ in 40 healthy controls *1781*

Hypoxanthine Guanosine Phosphoribosyltransferase *Lymphocytes No Effect* Activity in 25 patients with CLL showed no significant difference from that in 23 control individuals *1781*

Myeloperoxidase *Granulocyte No Effect* Mean density of 502 ± 78 in 13 patients with chronic lymphatic leukemia not significantly different from 478 ± 52 in 32 normal controls *1303*

Naphthol-As-D-Chloroacetate Esterase *Granulocyte Increase* Mean density of 529 ± 49 in 8 patients with chronic lymphatic leukemia significantly different from 478 ± 52 in 32 normal controls *1303*

Perchloric Acid Soluble Protein *Serum Increase* In 20 patients with chronic lymphatic leukemia mean concentration of 68.3 ± 10.2 mg tyrosine/dm³ significantly greater than 43.7 ± 11.8 mg tyrosine/dm³ in 40 healthy controls *1781*

Purine Nucleoside Phosphorylase *Lymphocytes Decrease* Mean activity was somewhat reduced in the lymphocytes of 75 patients with chronic lymphatic leukemia *1781*
Lymphocytes No Effect Normal activity reported in the lymphocytes of 9 patients with chronic lymphatic leukemia *1781*

Thymidine-5'-triphosphatase *Serum Increase* Activity in all of 12 patients with CLL showed a significant increase from that in healthy individuals *1781*

204.10 Chronic Lymphocytic Leukemia

α_1-Acid Glycoprotein *Serum Increase* Elevated levels in states associated with cell proliferation *3713 2597 4696 4373 4241 4853*

Adenosine Deaminase *Lymphocytes Decrease* Mean adenosine deaminase activity was decreased in the lymphocytes of 25 patients with chronic lymphocytic leukemia compared with 23 healthy controls *1781*
Serum Increase Astonishingly high values *3003* Adenosine deaminase activity was increased in the plasma of 4 of 6 patients with chronic lymphocytic leukemia *1781* Astonishingly high values *2737*

Adenylate Cyclase *Lymphocytes Decrease* Activity depressed in cells from patients with chronic lymphocytic leukemia *1781*

Albumin *Serum Decrease* In 47% of 27 patients at initial hospitalization for this disorder *1576*
Serum No Effect Concentration usually normal *5699* Usually within normal limits *504*

Alkaline Phosphatase *Serum Increase* Elevations > 95 U/L *2848* In 42% of 27 patients at initial hospitalization for this disorder *1576* Infiltration of the liver may result in obstruction of the biliary system *5545*
White Blood Cells Increase Mean score of 139.4 with a range of 73 - 180 *3440* The range of actual enzyme levels per 10^{10} leukocytes was 2.5 - 68.2 with a mean of 20.8. Only 3 determinations were higher than 26.5. Normal = 25.8, ranging from 13.4 - 58.0 *354*

Alkaline Phosphatase Isoenzymes *Serum Increase* A distinct isoenzyme (phosphatase N) was found in the serum of 5 patients. Values ranged from 35 - 39% of the total activity *3765*

204.10 Chronic Lymphocytic Leukemia *(continued)*

Angiotensin-converting Enzyme *Serum* *Decrease* Significant decrease. Depression of activity *4416*

Antinuclear Antibodies *Serum* *Increase* Positive in 20% of patients *4068*

Aspartate Aminotransferase *Serum* *Increase* Moderately elevated levels are observed in lymphomas and leukemia but less frequently than in other hepatic disease *1025* In 27% of 27 patients at initial hospitalization for this disorder *1576*

Bilirubin *Serum* *Increase* 20% of patients develop severe hemolysis *2033*

Bilirubin, Indirect *Serum* *Increase* 20% of patients develop severe hemolysis *2033*

Calcium *Serum* *Increase* Elevations > 11 mg/dL may occur with leukemic infiltration of bone *2848* Hypercalcemia observed sporadically in CLL *1781*
Urine *Increase* Frequent observation *1025*

Carcinoembryonic Antigen *Serum* *Increase* Above 2.5 ng/mL in 38% of patients with acute and chronic leukemia *456*

$CD8^+$ Lymphocytes *Blood* *No Effect* Levels in the non-accelerated phase of B-CLL approximated those of controls *4968*

Cholesterol *Serum* *Decrease* In 43% of 27 patients at initial hospitalization for this disorder *1576*

Cold Agglutinins *Serum* *Increase* Tends to rise *3953*

Complement C_3 *Serum* *No Effect* In one study of 15 patients with chronic lymphocytic leukemia mean concentration normal *1781*

Complement C_4 *Serum* *No Effect* In one study of 15 patients with chronic lymphocytic leukemia mean concentration normal *1781*

Complement CH50 *Serum* *No Effect* In one study of 15 patients with chronic lymphocytic leukemia mean concentration normal *1781*

Coombs' Test *Serum* *Positive* 20% of patients develop severe hemolysis *2033*

Copper *Serum* *Increase* In acute and chronic leukemias *5545*

C-Reactive Protein *Serum* *No Effect* In one study of 15 patients with chronic lymphocytic leukemia mean concentration normal *1781*

Creatine *Urine* *Increase* Increased breakdown *5545*

Creatinine *Serum* *Increase* In 49% of 24 patients at initial hospitalization for this disorder *1576*

Cryoglobulins *Serum* *Increase* May be associated with cryoglobulinemia *5545*

Erythrocyte Survival *Red Blood Cells* *Decrease* Characteristically short even when there is no evidence of autoimmunity *5584*

Erythrocytes *Blood* *Decrease* Reduced production plus shortened survival *5677*

Factor B *Serum* *No Effect* In one study of 15 patients with chronic lymphocytic leukemia mean concentration normal *1781*

α_1-Globulin *Serum* *No Effect* Usually within normal limits *504*

α_2-Globulin *Serum* *No Effect* Usually within normal limits *504* Typically no change observed *5699*

β-Globulin *Serum* *No Effect* Usually within normal limits *504* Concentration usually normal *5699*

γ-Globulin *Serum* *Decrease* Concentrations of 0.7 - 0.8 g/dL are common in early and uncomplicated disease. As disease advances, may fall to 0.3 - 0.4 g/dL, at which time patients become vulnerable to infections *5356*

β-Glucuronidase *Lymphocytes* *Decrease* Lymphocytes from patients with CLL had decreased activity of enzyme *1781*

Guanylate Cyclase *Lymphocytes* *Increase* Activity increased in cells from patients with chronic lymphocytic leukemia *1781*

Haptoglobin *Serum* *Decrease* 20% of patients develop severe hemolysis *2033*

Hematocrit *Blood* *Decrease* Anemia is not a feature of early disease; it may begin to develop when 50% or more of the bone marrow is usurped by lymphoid tissue *5584* Characteristically normochromic normocytic anemia *900* In 76% of 27 patients at initial hospitalization for this disorder *1576* Anemia, usually mild, was present at diagnosis in 50% of patients *5699*

Hemoglobin *Blood* *Decrease* Anemia is not a feature of early disease; it may begin to develop when 50% or more of the bone marrow is usurped by lymphoid tissue *5584* Characteristically normochromic normocytic anemia *900* In 76% of 27 patients at initial hospitalization for this disorder *1576* Anemia, usually mild, was present at diagnosis in 50% of patients *5699*
Plasma *Increase* Observed effect *5699* On occasion, severe hemolytic anemia is present at diagnosis *226* *5001*

α_2-HS Glycoprotein *Serum* *Decrease* No significant effect observed in patients with CLL compared with healthy controls probably due to hepatic involvement *2533*

Immunoglobulin A *Serum* *Decrease* Reported effect *5544* In 70 patients with chronic lymphocytic leukemia concentration decreased progressively as disease progressed *1781*

Immunoglobulin E *Serum* *Decrease* In 32 patients with chronic lymphatic leukemia mean concentration of 4.4 ng/mL (range 3.4 - 6.0) significantly less than mean of 96 ng/mL (range 24 - 386) in 74 healthy controls *2323*

Immunoglobulin G *Serum* *Decrease* In patients with chronic lymphocytic leukemia at the time of diagnosis concentration was decreased in 18.7% and after 6 years a low concentration was observed in 50% *1781* In 70 patients with chronic lymphocytic leukemia concentration decreased progressively as disease progressed *1781*

Immunoglobulin M *Serum* *Decrease* Reported effect *5544* In patients with chronic lymphocytic leukemia at the time of diagnosis concentration was decreased but in 43% increased during follow-up *1781*
Serum *Increase* In patients with chronic lymphocytic leukemia at the time of diagnosis concentration was decreased but in 43% increased during follow-up *1781*

Immunoglobulins *Serum* *Decrease* All classes of immunoglobulins tend to be reduced either early in the course or later as marrow, spleen, and liver infiltration develops *4479*

Interleukin-6 *Serum* *Increase* In 7 cases mean concentration of 0.229 ± 0.065 ng/mL higher than 0.190 ± 0.145 ng/mL in 26 healthy controls *1271*
Serum *No Effect* In 6 patients with chronic lymphocytic leukemia mean concentration of 8.3 ± 1.6 pg/mL not significantly different from 8.8 ± 1.8 pg/mL in 27 healthy control individuals *1120*

Interleukin-8 *Serum* *No Effect* In 6 patients with chronic lymphocytic leukemia mean concentration of 20.4 ± 14.0 pg/mL not significantly different from 16.2 ± 1.4 pg/mL in 27 healthy control individuals *1120*

Lactate Dehydrogenase *Serum* *Increase* 84 of 91 patients with leukemias had values elevated above the normal upper limit *447* Increased in all 15 patients, mean of 104.3 U/L *3335* In 64% of 27 patients at initial hospitalization for this disorder *1576*

Lactate Dehydrogenase Isoenzymes *Serum* *Increase* Isoenzyme 2 was usually the most intensive, LD_1 was also increased, and LD_5 was only detectable in a few cases *3335*

Leukocytes *Blood* *Increase* Usually 50,000 - 250,000 /µL with 90% lymphocytes *5545*

Lymphocytes *Blood* *Increase* In 113 patients with CLL median concentration on entry into study of 17.1 x 10^9/L significantly different from that in healthy controls *1972* In 24 treated patients, the origin of malignant cells was found to be the B lymphocyte population. On the basis of a reactive T lymphocyte proliferation in patients with chronic lymphatic leukemia, a coefficient of active T lymphocytes has been deduced which proved to be a rapid indicator of a short-term prognosis *4746* Generally, lymphocytosis consisting of mature lymphocytes with counts > 100,000 /µL in a patient over 50 y of age is diagnostic *900*

Lysozyme *Serum* *Decrease* Low or normal *1606*
Serum *Increase* Activity slightly increased in patients with chronic lymphocytic leukemia but much less than in acute disease *1781*
Serum *No Effect* Low or normal *1606*

β_2-Macroglobulin *Serum* *Increase* With leukemia of B-lymphocyte lineage *4952* May be increased in leukemia of B-lymphocyte lineage *2586*

β_2-Microglobulin *Serum* *Increase* Increased concentration observed in the majority of untreated patients with CLL *1781* In 113 patients with CLL progression-free survival substantially greater in patients with serum β_2-microglobulin concentration less than 3.5 µg/L *1972*

Monocytes *Blood* *Decrease* In 66% of 27 patients at initial hospitalization for this disorder *1576*

N-Acetyl-Glucosaminidase *Lymphocytes* *Decrease* Activity decreased in lymphocytes of 19 patients with chronic B-cell lymphocytic leukemia *1781*
Lymphocytes *No Effect* Activity unchanged in lymphocytes of 1 patient with chronic T-cell lymphocytic leukemia *1781*

Neopterin *Urine* *Increase* Mean excretion in 15 patients with CLL of 438.4 µmol/mol creatinine compared with 106.6 ± 34.6 µmol/mol creatinine in 31 healthy controls *3632* Urinary excretion increased above mean + 3 SD in patients with CLL, and correlated well with tumor stage and and the presence of hepatosplenomegaly *1781*

Neutrophils *Blood* *Decrease* Neutropenia and thrombocytopenia, ranging in severity from mild to catastrophic, are characteristically present in patients with marrow replacement in the late stages *5677* In 95% of 27 patients at initial hospitalization for this disorder *1576*
Blood *Increase* The percentage is often reduced, but the absolute number may be somewhat increased in early stages of the disease *503*
Blood *No Effect* Usually normal, mean concentration of 6,000 /µL *503*

5'-Nucleotidase *Lymphocytes* *Decrease* Reduced or absent in the lymphocytes of most patients *3118*

Osmotic Fragility *Red Blood Cells* *Increase* Degree of light transmission is used as a measure of lysis of lymphocytes, (i.e., as a measure of osmotic fragility). After 10 min, light transmission of lymphocytes was 78.5 ± 4.65%, compared to 60 ± 7.33% *4328*

Phosphoglucomutase *Serum* *Increase* Increases in some cases *1290*

Phospholipase A *Serum* *Increase* Reported effect *2200*

Platelets *Blood* *Decrease* Neutropenia and thrombocytopenia, ranging in severity from mild to catastrophic, are characteristically present in patient with marrow replacement in the late stages *5677* With thrombocytopenia, and associated bleeding diathesis, a microcytic hypochromic picture could be present *900* In 113 patients with CLL progression-free survival substantially greater in patients with platelet count greater than 150 x 10^9/L *1972* In 47% of 27 patients at initial hospitalization for this disorder *1576* Mild thrombocytopenia may occur in < 50% of cases *5699* Anemia and thrombocytopenia develop as the disorder progresses *2039*
Blood *No Effect* Normal counts in > 50% of patients *5699*

Protein *Pleural Fluid* *Increase* Pleural effusions are usually exudates *126*
Serum *Decrease* Reduction in serum protein concentration is a feature of advanced disease and one which carries a poor prognosis *5677*

Pseudouridine *Urine* *Increase* In 15 patients with CLL mean excretion of 29.5 mmol/mol compared with 19.6 ± 5.2 mmol/mol creatinine in 31 healthy controls *3632*

Reticulocytes *Blood* *Increase* Secondary to hemolysis *5677*
Blood *No Effect* Normal or slightly decreased *374*

Sodium *Serum* *Increase* In 99% of 27 patients at initial hospitalization for this disorder *1576*

Soluble c-kit Molecule *Serum* *Decrease* Median concentration of 106.0 AU/mL in patients with CLL significantly different from that in 51 healthy volunteers of 199.0 AU/mL *2598*

Soluble CD40L *Serum* *Increase* Mean concentration of 0.80 ng/mL in 51 patients with CLL significantly different from mean concentration of 0.29 ng/mL in 55 healthy donors controls *5823*

Soluble Intercellular Adhesion Molecule-1 *Serum* *Increase* Mean concentration increased in patients with CLL but did not appear to be related to disease activity *4968*

Soluble Interleukin-2 Receptor *Serum* *Increase* Elevated sIL-2R levels were found in B-chronic lymphocytic leukemia *4968* In the accelerated and non-accelerated phases of B-CLL significant increase in concentration observed: in non-accelerated CLL concentration less increased than in later stages of the disease *4968*

Soluble Transferrin Receptor *Serum* *Increase* In patients with chronic lymphocytic leukemia mean concentration of 14.17 ± 12.29 µg/mL significantly increased compared with 5.63 ± 1.42 µg/mL in healthy controls *2704*
Serum *No Effect* Concentration not changed typically in myeloproliferative diseases *4784*

Terminal Deoxynucleotidyl Transferase
Lymphocytes *No Effect* Enzyme not found in mature T-cells. Absent or present in very low concentration in lymphocytes of most patients with CLL *1781*

Thymidine Kinase *Serum* *Decrease* In 113 patients with CLL progression-free survival substantially greater in patients with serum thymidine kinase activity less than 5 U/L *1972*

Tissue Factor Pathway Inhibitor *Plasma* *No Effect* 6 patients with CLL had median activity of 1.06 U/mL not significantly different from median activity of 1.19 U/mL in healthy individuals *2376*

Tissue Factor Pathway Inhibitor Antigen *Plasma* *No Effect* 6 patients with CLL had median concentration of 104 ng/mL not significantly different from median concentration of 90 ng/mL in healthy individuals *2376*

Tissue Factor Pathway Inhibitor Antigen, Free
Plasma *No Effect* 6 patients with CLL had median concentration of 27 ng/mL not significantly different from median concentration of 15 ng/mL in healthy individuals *2376*

Urea Nitrogen *Serum* *Increase* Can be elevated in kidney infiltration and should be followed especially if nephrotoxic antibiotics are used *900* In 54% of 27 patients at initial hospitalization for this disorder *1576*

Uric Acid *Serum* *Increase* A frequent association of the treated condition *900* Not as frequent as in other leukemias *2033*
Serum *No Effect* Usually normal *4556* Concentration typically normal and not increased with chemotherapy *1781*
Urine *Increase* Not as frequent as in other leukemias *2033*
Urine *No Effect* Often normal *4556*

Vitamin B_{12} *Serum* *Increase* About 33% of cases *5544* Significant increase in 19 patients, mean concentration of 1,223 pg/mL compared to normal, 385 pg/mL *4448*
Serum *No Effect* Concentration may be normal *5545* *350* Concentration typically normal in contrast to that iin CML in which it may be strikingly increased *1781*

Vitamin B_{12} Binding Capacity *Serum* *Increase* Significant elevation; usually correlated with WBC in peripheral blood *4448*

Zinc *Lymphocytes* *Decrease* In 17 patients with chronic lymphocytic leukemia mean concentration significantly decreased by 40% compared with the value in 20 healthy controls *1781*
Serum *Decrease* Decreased *5083*

204.10 Chronic T-lymphocytic Leukemia

CD8+ Lymphocytes *Blood* *Increase* Significant increase observed in patients with T-CLL *4968*

Soluble Interleukin-2 Receptor *Serum* *Increase* Increase in concentration observed in patients with T-CLL but not very marked *4968*

204.90 Lymphoid Leukemia

Alkaline Phosphatase *White Blood Cells* *Decrease* Mean activity not decreased in any of 26 patients with lymphoid leukemia *1781*
White Blood Cells *Increase* Mean activity increased in 54% patients with lymphoid leukemia *1781*

β-Galactosidase *White Blood Cells* *Decrease* Leukemic cells from patients with lymphogenous leukemia had decreased activity of enzyme *1781*

205.00 Acute Granulocytic Leukemia

Myeloperoxidase *Granulocyte* *Increase* Mean density of 625 ± 45 in 17 patients with acute granulocytic leukemia significantly different from 478 ± 52 in 32 normal controls *1303*

205.00 Acute Granulocytic Leukemia (continued)

Naphthol-As-D-Chloroacetate Esterase *Granulocyte* *Increase* Mean density of 840 ± 91 in 16 patients with acute granulocytic leukemia significantly different from 478 ± 52 in 32 normal controls *1303*

205.00 Acute Myeloblastic Leukemia

Adenosine Deaminase *Serum* *Increase* Adenosine deaminase activity in plasma of patients with acute myeloblastic leukemia frequently increased *1781*
White Blood Cells *Increase* Adenosine deaminase activity in leukocytes of patients with acute myeloblastic leukemia frequently increased *1781*

Creatine Kinase *Serum* *Increase* High percentage of CK-BB *5809*

Creatine Kinase BB-Isoenzyme *Serum* *Increase* High percentage of CK-BB *5809*

Ferritin *Serum* *Increase* In 10 patients with acute myeloblastic leukemia mean concentration of 883 ng/mL significantly higher than 85 ng/mL in 178 healthy men and 39 ng/mL in 105 healthy women *1781*

Hepatocyte Growth Factor *Serum* *Increase* In 21 of 31 patients with AML concentration increased above 0.4 ng/mL, and 11 had concentrations greater than 1.0 ng/mL. Average concentration in AML patients 2.03 ng/mL compared with 0.25 ± 0.06 ng/mL in 10 normal individuals *3714*

β_2-Microglobulin *Cerebrospinal Fluid* *Increase* Mean concentration increased in patients with CNS involvement *2013*

Protein Z *Plasma* *Decrease* In 11 patients with acute myeloblastic leukemia median baseline concentration of 2.49 ng/mL compared with 2.72 ng/mL in 14 healthy controls *5357*

Purine Nucleoside Phosphorylase *Lymphocytes* *Decrease* Activity in the lymphocytes of 44% of 43 patients with acute myeloblastic leukemia reported to be more than 1 SD below mean in healthy patients *1781*
Lymphocytes *No Effect* Activity in the lymphocytes of 20 patients with acute myeloblastic leukemia reported to be normal *1781*

Thymidine Kinase *Serum* *Increase* Activity increased in all but 3 of 54 patients with acute myelooblastic leukemia *1781*

205.00 Acute Myelocytic Leukemia

α_1-Acid Glycoprotein *Serum* *Increase* Elevated levels in states associated with cell proliferation *4696* *4373* *2597* *3713* *4241* *4853*

Alanine Aminotransferase *Serum* *Increase* Moderate elevation observed in lymphomas and leukemia but less frequently than in other hepatic disease *1025* Infiltration of the liver *1290*

Albumin *Serum* *Decrease* Normal at diagnosis, but falls as disease progresses *1409* *5699* In 34% of 36 patients at initial hospitalization for this disorder *1576*

Aldolase *Serum* *Increase* Slight elevation in 50% of patients *5545*

Alkaline Phosphatase *Serum* *Increase* Elevations > 95 U/L *2848* Infiltration of the liver may result in obstruction of the biliary system *5545*
White Blood Cells *Decrease* Leukemia *4374* *3440* The range of activity per 10^{10} leukocytes was 0.0 - 6.2 U/L, the mean being 1.6 U/L. The tendency toward low levels for both alkaline and acid phosphatase activity suggests that the blast form is poor in phosphatase; the activity being attributable chiefly to the more mature cells in acute leukemia *354*
White Blood Cells *Increase* Slightly elevated in > 50% of cases *5699*

Angiotensin-converting Enzyme *Serum* *Decrease* Observed effect *4416* Mean value for group of 19.9 U/L compared with 24.4 U/L for control group *4746*

α_1-Antichymotrypsin *Serum* *Increase* Increased 24 - 48 hours after chemotherapy in patients with or without DIC *2663* Reported effect *1634*

Antinuclear Antibodies *Serum* *Increase* Positive in 25% of patients *4068*

Arylsulfatase *Serum* *Increase* 30 - 50% increase in serum activity *1279*

Aspartate Aminotransferase *Serum* *Increase* Moderately elevated levels are observed in lymphomas and leukemia but less frequently than in other hepatic disease *1025* In 37% of 36 patients at initial hospitalization for this disorder *1576*

Basophils *Blood* *Increase* Occasionally *2033*

Calcium *Serum* *Increase* Has been observed, but is uncommon *5699* Elevation > 11 mg/dL may occur with leukemic infiltration of bone *2848*
Urine *Increase* Frequent observation *1025*

Carcinoembryonic Antigen *Serum* *Increase* Above 2.5 ng/mL in 38% of patients with acute and chronic leukemia *456*

CD8+ Lymphocytes *Blood* *Increase* Mean concentration significantly increased in patients with AML *4968* Elevated levels of sCD8 were observed in AML *4968*

Cells *Bone Marrow* *Increase* Marked occurrence of either sea-blue histiocytes or Gaucher like cells, or of both, was observed in bone marrow smears and the hematopoietic tissues of 23 patients with chronic disease and in acute, but with lower frequency and degree *5128* Blast cells are present even when none are found in the peripheral blood *5545*
Cerebrospinal Fluid *Increase* Pleocytosis with meningeal infiltration *5677*

Cholesterol *Serum* *Decrease* In 51% of 36 patients at initial hospitalization for this disorder *1576*

Copper *Serum* *Increase* Significant increase observed in 16 cases of acute leukemia. Drop occurs in cases who respond to quadruple chemotherapy while those who failed to respond showed persistently high levels *1321*

Creatine *Urine* *Increase* Extremely variable *5523* Pronounced increase in children and adult males with acute leukemias *4707*

Creatinine *Serum* *Increase* In 55% of 27 patients at initial hospitalization for this disorder *1576*

Eosinophils *Blood* *Increase* Occasionally *2033*

Erythropoietin *Serum* *Increase* Increased and negatively correlated with hemoglobin concentration *4045*

Factor V *Plasma* *Decrease* Intravascular clotting has been documented in occasional patients *1815*

Factor VIII *Plasma* *Decrease* Intravascular clotting has been documented in occasional patients *1815*

Ferritin *Serum* *Increase* Significant elevation *4970*

Fibrin Degradation Products *Plasma* *Increase* Intravascular clotting has been documented in occasional patients *1815*

Fibrinogen *Plasma* *Decrease* Moderate depression occurs *1290* Intravascular clotting has been documented in occasional patients *1815*

α_1-Globulin *Serum* *Increase* Often reflects the presence of fever or infection *1409* *5699*

α_2-Globulin *Serum* *Increase* Often reflects the presence of fever or infection *5699* *1409*

β-Globulin *Serum* *Increase* Common *1409* *5699*

γ-Globulin *Serum* *Increase* Diffuse hypergammaglobulinemia is common *5699* *1409*

Glucose *Cerebrospinal Fluid* *Decrease* With meningeal infiltration *5677*

Hematocrit *Blood* *Decrease* In 90% of 35 patients at initial hospitalization for this disorder *1576* Most patients will have anemia *900* Often severe, may be macrocytic *5699*

Hemoglobin *Blood* *Decrease* Most patients will have anemia *900* In 90% of 35 patients at initial hospitalization for this disorder *1576* Often severe, may be macrocytic *5699*

Hemoglobin F *Blood* *Increase* Increased in some leukemias (especially juvenile myeloid leukemia); with Hb F of 30 - 60%, absence of Philadelphia chromosome, rapid fatal course, more pronounced thrombocytopenia, and lower total WBC count *5545*

Hepatocyte Growth Factor *Serum* *Increase* Median concentration of 0.70 ng/mL in 60 patients with acute myelocytic leukemia significantly different from 0.39 ng/mL in 33 healthy controls *2178*

Heterophile Antibody *Serum* *Decrease* Positive presumptive test but negative differential test if Forsman antigen is used *3953*
Serum *Increase* Positive presumptive test but negative differential test if Forsman antigen is used *3953*

Hexosamines, Protein-bound *Serum* *Increase* In 10 patients with acute myelocytic leukemia mean concentration of 1,138 ± 276 mg/dm³ significantly greater than 627 ± 183 mg/dm³ in 40 healthy controls *1781*

Hexoses, Protein-bound *Serum* *Increase* In 10 patients with acute myelocytic leukemia mean concentration of 4,622 ± 516 mg/dm³ significantly greater than 1,530 ± 325 mg/dm³ in 40 healthy controls *1781*

immunoglobulin A *Serum* *No Effect* Concentration usually normal *5544*

Immunoglobulin G *Serum* *Increase* In 2 of 15 patients with acute myelocytic leukemia monoclonal IgG gammopathy observed *1781*
Serum *No Effect* Concentration usually normal *5544*

Immunoglobulin M *Serum* *No Effect* Concentration usually normal *5544*

Iron *Serum* *Increase* Increased in acute leukemias *1290*

Lactate Dehydrogenase *Serum* *Increase* 2 to 4 times normal values *1025* In 87% of 34 patients at initial hospitalization for this disorder *1576* Markedly elevated levels in untreated acute leukemia *1642* Increased in about 90% of the patients. The degree of increase is not correlated with the level of WBC *5544* 84 of 91 patients with leukemias had values elevated above the normal upper limit *447* Increased activity observed *1980*

Laminin *Serum* *Increase* No difference in concentrations between different leukemias. Median level of all leukemias was 1,609 mU/mL (n = 12) versus control concentration of 1,232 mU/mL (n = 41) *4394*

Leukocytes *Blood* *Decrease* In 26% of 34 patients at initial hospitalization for this disorder *1576* Variable and can be very high (> 100,000 /µL), moderately elevated (20,000 - 100,000 /µL), normal, or low *900*
Blood *Increase* Variable and can be very high (> 100,000 /µL), moderately elevated (20,000 - 100,000 /µL), normal, or low *900* Number of blasts can range from 0 to 1 million. Not increased in approximately 40% at time of diagnosis. Normal blood leukocytes are almost always decreased *2033* Slightly elevated in > 50% of cases *5699* In 46% of 34 patients at initial hospitalization for this disorder *1576*
Blood *No Effect* Variable and can be very high, moderately elevated, normal or low *900* Variable and can be very high (> 100,000 /µL), moderately elevated (20,000 - 100,000 /µL), normal, or low *900*

Lysozyme *Serum* *Decrease* Low, normal or moderately increased *1606*
Serum *Increase* Activity increased in most patients (90%) with acute myelocytic leukemia *1781* Low, normal, or moderately increased *1606* During the transition from a variety of myeloproliferative disorders to acute myeloblastic or acute myelomonocytic leukemia, there is a striking elevation in serum and urine muramidase activity *4692*
Serum *No Effect* Low, normal, or moderately increased *1606*
Urine *Increase* Activity increased in most patients (90%) with acute myelocytic leukemia but only when serum activity greater than 4 times the upper limit of normal *1781* During the transition from a variety of myeloproliferative disorders to acute myeloblastic or acute myelomonocytic leukemia, there is a striking elevation in serum and urine muramidase activity *4692* Elevated only in patients who do not have the Philadelphia chromosome. No correlation is apparent between urine and serum levels *4692*

MCH *Blood* *Increase* Often severe anemia, may be macrocytic *5699*

MCV *Blood* *Increase* Often severe anemia, may be macrocytic *5699*

Monocytes *Blood* *Increase* On occasion associated with a monocytosis of relatively minor proportions *3246*

Neopterin *Serum* *Increase* Mean concentration of 15.5 ± 7.2 nmol/L in 4 patients with AML significantly greater than that in 18 healthy control individuals, 6.4 ± 1.8 nmol/L *3864*

Neutrophils *Blood* *Increase* The number of blasts can range from 0 to 1 million. Not increased in approximately 40% at time of diagnosis. Normal blood leukocytes are almost always decreased *2033*

Partial Thromboplastin Time *Plasma* *Increase* Intravascular clotting has been documented in occasional patients *1815*

Perchloric Acid Soluble Protein *Serum* *Increase* In 10 patients with acute myelocytic leukemia mean concentration of 66.4 ± 9.3 mg tyrosine/dm³ significantly greater than 43.7 ± 11.8 mg tyrosine/dm³ in 40 healthy controls *1781*

Phosphoglucomutase *Serum* *Increase* In some cases *1290*

Plasminogen Activator Inhibitor-1
Cerebrospinal Fluid *No Effect* In 2 patients with acute myelocytic leukemia mean concentration of 0.42 ± 0.05 ng/mL not significantly different from 0.31 ± 0.06 ng/mL in 20 reference individuals *56*

Platelets *Blood* *Decrease* Common; frequently pronounced at diagnosis *5699* In 85% of 35 patients at initial hospitalization for this disorder *1576* Intravascular clotting has been documented in occasional patients *1815* Most patients will have thrombocytopenia *900*
Blood *Increase* On very rare occasions *177*

Potassium *Serum* *Decrease* Below 3.5 mmol/L in 19 (59%) of 32 patients *3509*
Urine *Increase* Inappropriately large quantities of potassium were excreted in relation to the low serum content. 12 of 32 patients excreted more than the mean potassium intake *3509*

Protein *Cerebrospinal Fluid* *Increase* With meningeal infiltration *5677*
Pleural Fluid *Increase* Pleural effusions are usually exudates *126*

Prothrombin Time *Plasma* *Increase* Intravascular clotting has been documented in occasional patients *1815*

Reticulocytes *Blood* *Decrease* Reflects decreased cell production *5699* Usually low, however, if RBC morphology is bizarre, and nucleated RBCs and an increased reticulocyte count are present, erythroleukemia should be suspected *900*

Rheumatoid Factor *Serum* *Increase* Dysproteinemias and paraproteinemias present significant seropositivity *1980*

Sodium *Serum* *Increase* In 98% of 34 patients at initial hospitalization for this disorder *1576*

Soluble Intercellular Adhesion Molecule-1 *Serum* *Increase* Mean concentration increased in patients with AML *4968*

Soluble Interleukin-2 Receptor *Serum* *Increase* Increased concentrations observed in patients with AML *4968*

Thrombin Time *Blood* *Increase* Intravascular clotting has been demonstrated in occasional patients *1815*

Urea Nitrogen *Serum* *Increase* Can be elevated in kidney infiltration and should be followed especially if nephrotic antibiotics are used *900* In 33% of 37 patients at initial hospitalization for this disorder *1576*

Uric Acid *Serum* *Increase* Frequent biochemical abnormality. Secondary to the increased cell turnover *900* In 44% of 35 patients at initial hospitalization for this disorder *1576* Observed with increased turnover of cells *1980* Due to excessive excretion of urate, but no correlation was found between serum and urinary levels in myeloid patients, contrary to normal controls (r = 0.85). Serum levels tends to fall in relapse *3508* In approximately 50% of patients *5699* *2146*
Urine *Increase* Almost invariable *5699* Mean urate excretion was 0.774 ± 0.057 mg/min, significantly higher than normal, 0.595 ± 0.035 *3508* Almost invariable *2146*

Vitamin B_{12} *Serum* *Increase* Usually high, in contrast to acute lymphocytic leukemia *350* Acute myelocytic leukemic cells may secrete a vitamin B_{12} binding protein in large quantity, accounting for high serum levels of B_{12} *367*

Vitamin B_{12} Binding Capacity *Serum* *Increase* Significant elevation; usually correlated with WBC in peripheral blood *4448*

Zinc *Serum* *Decrease* Decreased *5083*

205.00 Acute Myelogenous Leukemia

Acetylspermidine *Urine* *Increase* Mean excretion increased in 2 children with AML *1781*

Alkaline Phosphatase *White Blood Cells* *Decrease* Mean activity decreased in 6 of 41 (15%) patients with AML *1781*
White Blood Cells *Increase* Mean activity increased in 63% patients with AML *1781*

205.00 Acute Myelogenous Leukemia *(continued)*

Anticardiolipin Antibodies *Serum* *Increase* Nineteen patients with de novo AML. Five patients with AML (26.3%) presented elevated APA at diagnosis, as compared to 3 of 174 persons of the control group ($p < 0.0001$). APA titers became normal in all patients responding to treatment, whereas non-responders retained elevated levels. At presentation, the mean levels of IgG- and IgM-ACA in patients were not significantly different from controls *4984*

6-Hydroxymethylpterin *Urine* *Increase* Urinary excretion reflects total tumor burden and response to chemotherapy *1781*

Interleukin-6 *Serum* *Increase* Pretreatment concentrations of IL-6 and TNF-α in AML were found significantly elevated compared to controls ($p = 0.003$, $p = 0.009$ and $p = 0.024$ respectively) *4984* In comparison with normal subjects, IL-6 activity was significantly elevated in patients with ALL and ANLL ($p < 0.01$) *3167*

Lactate Dehydrogenase *Serum* *Increase* In 72 elderly patients with acute myelogenous leukemia LD activity greater than 400 U/L at the time of diagnosis was associated with poor outcome *1467*

Leukocytes *Blood* *Increase* In 72 elderly patients with acute myelogenous leukemia LD activity greater than 400 U/L at the time of diagnosis and leukocyte count among these patients was significantly higher *1467*

Lysozyme *Serum* *Increase* Activity markedly increased in patients with acute myelogenous leukemia *1781*

1-Methylinosine *Urine* *No Effect* Excretion remained normal in patients with AML compared with normal individuals *1781*

N^2, N^2-Dimethylguanosine *Urine* *No Effect* Excretion remained normal in patients with AML compared with normal individuals *1781*

N-Acetylputrescine *Urine* *Increase* Mean excretion increased in 2 children with AML *1781*

Neopterin *Urine* *Increase* Urinary excretion increased in patients with AML, decreasing with response to treatment and remission *1781*

Soluble HLA-I *Cerebrospinal Fluid* *No Effect* In 2 patients with acute myelogenous leukemia, mean concentration undetectable in both *216*

Soluble HLA-II *Cerebrospinal Fluid* *No Effect* In 2 patients with acute myelogenous leukemia, mean concentration undetectable in both *216*

Soluble L-Selectin *Serum* *Increase* Patients with untreated acute myelogenous leukemia have increased serum concentration *613*

Tumor Necrosis Factor-α *Serum* *Increase* Pretreatment concentrations of TNF-α in AML were found significantly elevated compared to controls ($p = 0.024$) *4984* TNF-α level increased in patients with AMLL ($p < 0.05$) *3167* Concentration increased in patients with either acute or chronic leukemia especially those with advanced disease *4968*

205.00 Acute Myeloid Leukemia

Acetyl-N-Ser-Asp-Lys-Pro *Serum* *Increase* In 20 patients with acute myeloid leukemia mean concentration of 3.19 ± 0.73 pmol/mL not significantly higher than 1.66 ± 0.15 pmol/mL in 21 healthy controls *3081*

Alkaline Phosphatase *Serum* *Increase* In 33 patients with AML mean activity 2.42 ± 0.157 U/L significantly higher than 1.94 ± 0.054 in 15 healthy controls *4027*

Alkaline Phosphatase, Placental Isoenzyme *Serum* *Increase* In 51 patients with AML mean activity of 0.620 ± 0.070 U/L significantly higher than 0.311 ± 0.012 in 15 healthy controls *4027*

α_1-Antichymotrypsin *Serum* *Increase* In 16 patients with acute myeloid leukemia concentration increased with further increase with chemotherapy *1781*

α_2-Antiplasmin *Plasma* *No Effect* In 28 adult patients with AML mean concentration of 96% (range 88 - 102) compared with normal range of 80 - 120% *753*

Antithrombin III *Plasma* *No Effect* In 28 adult patients with AML mean concentration of 89% (range 83 - 94) compared with normal range of 80 - 120% *753*

α_1-Antitrypsin *Serum* *Increase* In 16 patients with acute myeloid leukemia concentration increased with further increase with chemotherapy *1781*

C-Reactive Protein *Serum* *No Effect* In 28 adult patients with AML mean concentration of 6 mg/L (range 1 - 10) compared with normal range of < 10 mg/L *753*

Fibrinogen *Plasma* *No Effect* In 28 adult patients with AML mean concentration of 2.5 g/L (range 2.0 - 3.1) compared with normal range of 2 - 4 g/L *753*

Fibrinopeptide A *Plasma* *Increase* In 28 adult patients with AML mean concentration of 4.8 ng/mL (range 1.3 - 12.1) compared with normal range of 2 - 4 ng/mL *753*

Glycosyltransferase A Enzyme *Serum* *No Effect* Activity normal at diagnosis *1781*

Glycosyltransferase H Enzyme *Serum* *Decrease* Abnormaly low values (1 - 3%) observed at diagnosis, returning to normal of 3 - 15% on remission, becoming low again on relapse *1781*

Interleukin-6 *Serum* *Increase* In 12 patients with acute myeloid leukemia mean concentration of 44.1 ± 14.3 pg/mL significantly different from 8.8 ± 1.8 pg/mL in 27 healthy control individuals *1120*

Interleukin-8 *Serum* *Increase* In 8 patients with AML who had 14 episodes of fever IL-8 was detected in 18 of 25 specimens during bacterial infections, 2 of 3 clinically defined infections, and 3 of 7 specimens during unexplained infection: IL-8 detected in 22 of 90 specimens when no infection present. Median concentration of IL-8 during febrile episodes 194 ng/mL and 0 on days without fever *5504* In 12 patients with acute myeloid leukemia mean concentration of 57.4 ± 12.2 pg/mL significantly different from 16.2 ± 1.4 pg/mL in 27 healthy control individuals *1120*

Lactate Dehydrogenase *Serum* *Increase* In 51 patients with AML mean activity 500.0 ± 48.54 U/L *4027*

Leukocytes *Blood* *Increase* In 36 patients mean concentration of 32.9 x 10^9/L with range of 0.5 - 173.0 x 10^9/L *3685*

α_2-Macroglobulin *Serum* *Decrease* In 16 patients with acute myeloid leukemia concentration decreased in most patients *1781*

Manganese Superoxide Dismutase *Serum* *Increase* The level for normal subjects was 94.1 ng/mL versus 159.6 ng/mL for AML patients *3806*

α-Mannosidase *White Blood Cells* *Increase* Leukemic cells from children with acute myeloid leukemia had very high activity of enzyme *1781*

N-Acetyl-Glucosaminidase *White Blood Cells* *Increase* Leukemic cells from children with acute myeloid leukemia had greater activity of enzyme than those of non-T, non-B ALL cells *1781*

N-Acetyl-Glucosaminidase B *White Blood Cells* *Decrease* Leukemic cells from children with acute myeloid leukemia had a relative reduction of the B-isoenzyme *1781*

Plasminogen *Plasma* *No Effect* In 28 adult patients with AML mean concentration of 101% (range 92 - 109) compared with normal range of 75 - 140% *753*

Plasminogen Activator Inhibitor *Plasma* *No Effect* In 28 adult patients with AML mean concentration of 9.3 U/mL (range 5.2 - 12.6) compared with normal range of 0.5 - 10.5 U/mL *753*

Platelets *Blood* *Decrease* In 28 adult patients with AML mean concentration of 86 x 10^9/L (range 37 - 272) *753*

Protein C *Plasma* *No Effect* In 28 adult patients with AML mean concentration of 94% (range 86 - 102) compared with normal range of 70 - 140% *753*

Soluble c-kit Molecule *Serum* *Increase* Median concentration of 361.0 AU/mL in patients with AML phenotypes M0 or M1, 233.5 AU/mL, 196.5 for phenotype M2, 233.5 AU/mL for phenotype M3, 210.0 AU/mL for phenotype M4, 255.0 AU/mL for phenotype M6 and 222.0 AU/mL for phenotype M7 significantly different from that in 51 healthy volunteers of 199.0 AU/mL *2598*

Soluble Intercellular Adhesion Molecule-1 *Serum* *Increase* In 10 patients with AML mean concentrations ranged from 188 ± 56 ng/mL to 567 ± 77 ng/mL before bone marrow transplantation with 4 having means greater than the normal range of 200 to 260 ng/mL *3202*

Soluble Urokinase Receptor *Serum* *Increase* In 36 patients mean concentration of 2.92 ng/mL with range of 0.68 - 11.28 ng/mL compared with mean of 1.14 ng/mL and range of 0.79 - 1.72 in 21 healthy controls *3685*

Tissue Plasminogen Activator Antigen *Plasma* *Decrease* In 28 adult patients with AML mean concentration of 3.2 ng/mL (range 1.2 - 4.3) compared with normal range of 4 - 10 ng/mL *753*

Urokinase Plasminogen Activator *Plasma* *Increase* In 36 patients mean concentration of 0.55 ng/mL with range of 0.09 - 2.37 ng/mL compared with mean of 0.32 ng/mL and range of 0.14 - 0.60 in 21 healthy controls *3685*

205.00 Acute Myelomonocytic Leukemia

CD8+ Lymphocytes *Blood* *Increase* Increased concentration observed in patients with acute myelomonocytic leukemia *4968*

Lysozyme *Serum* *Increase* Activity markedly increased in patients with acute myelomonocytic leukemia *1781*

Soluble Intercellular Adhesion Molecule-1 *Serum* *Increase* Mean concentration increased in patients with acute myelomonocytic leukemia *4968*

Soluble Interleukin-2 Receptor *Serum* *Increase* Elevated sIL-2R levels were found in acute myelomonocytic leukemia *4968*

Soluble Interleukin-3 Receptor *Serum* *Increase* Increased concentrations observed in patients with AMMoL *4968*

205.00 Acute Promyelocytic Leukemia

Antithrombin III *Plasma* *No Effect* Concentration usually normal *3456*

α_2-Plasmin Inhibitor *Plasma* *Decrease* Hemorrhagic complications of disease may be due to increased fibrinolysis. Concentration of plasminogen may be low *3456*

Plasminogen *Plasma* *Decrease* Hemorrhagic complications of disease may be due to increased fibrinolysis. Concentration of plasminogen may be low *3456*

Plasminogen Activator Inhibitor-1 *Plasma* *Decrease* Hemorrhagic complications of disease may be due to increased fibrinolysis. Concentration of plasminogen may be low *3456*

Protein C *Plasma* *No Effect* Concentration usually normal *3456*

Thrombomodulin *Plasma* *No Effect* No significant change observed in patients with acute promyelocytic leukemia *193*

Tissue Factor Antigen *Plasma* *Increase* In 11 patients with APL and disseminated intravascular coagulation mean concentration of 279 ± 64 pg/mL compared with 126 ± 41 pg/mL in 12 healthy volunteers *5511*

205.00 Myeloblastic Leukemia

Adenosine Deaminase *Serum* *Increase* Adenosine deaminase activity in plasma of patients with chronic myeloblastic leukemia invariably increased *1781*
White Blood Cells *Increase* Adenosine deaminase activity in buffy coat of 69 patients with chronic myeloblastic leukemia increased in 89% *1781*

Granulocyte Colony Stimulating Factor *Serum* *Decrease* In children with AML and 6 episodes of neutropenia mean concentration of 6.6 ± 12.1 pg/mL *5324*

Granulocyte-Macrophage Colony Stimulating Factor *Serum* *Decrease* In children with AML and 6 episodes of neutropenia mean concentration of 13.3 ± 4 pg/mL *5324*

Interferon-γ *Serum* *Increase* In children with AML and 6 episodes of neutropenia mean concentration of 139.8 ± 138.3 pg/mL *5324*

Neutrophils *Blood* *Decrease* In children with AML and 6 episodes of neutropenia mean absolute neutrophil count 611 ± 335.6 /µL *5324*

Tumor Necrosis Factor-α *Serum* *Increase* In children with AML and 6 episodes of neutropenia mean concentration of 78.3 ± 61.4 pg/mL *5324*

205.00 Promyelocytic Leukemia

Soluble Intercellular Adhesion Molecule-1 *Serum* *Increase* Mean concentration increased in patients with PLL *4968*

205.10 Chronic Granulocytic Leukemia

Acid Ribonuclease *Serum* *Increase* Mean activity in 26 patients with chronic granulocytic leukemia three times greater than in healthy subjects *1781*

Alkaline Ribonuclease *Serum* *Increase* Mean activity in 26 patients with chronic granulocytic leukemia twice that in healthy subjects *1781*

Fucosyltransferase *Serum* *Increase* Activity generally increased in untreated patients and in patients with stable disease, with further increase 30 - 60 days before development of a blast cycle *1781*

α_2-HS Glycoprotein *Serum* *No Effect* Concentration significantly reduced compared with healthy controls probably due to hepatic involvement *2533*

Myeloperoxidase *Granulocyte* *Increase* Mean density of 844 ± 57 in 21 patients with chronic granulocytic leukemia significantly different from 478 ± 52 in 32 normal controls *1303*

Naphthol-As-D-Chloroacetate Esterase *Granulocyte* *Increase* Mean density of 649 ± 72 in 10 patients with chronic granulocytic leukemia significantly different from 511 ± 46 in 40 normal controls *1303*

Neopterin *Urine* *Increase* In 4 patients with CGL mean excretion of about 300 µmol/mol creatinine significantly greater than 106.6 ± 34.6 µmol/mol creatinine in 31 healthy controls *3632*

Pseudouridine *Urine* *Increase* In 4 patients with CGL mean excretion of about 30 mmol/mol creatinine significantly greater than 19.6 ± 5.2 mmol/mol creatinine in 31 healthy controls *3632*

Soluble Transferrin Receptor *Serum* *No Effect* No significant difference in concentration (7.89 ± 3.56 µg/mL) compared with normal controls (5.63 ± 1.42 µg/mL) *2704*

205.10 Chronic Myelocytic Leukemia

Acid Phosphatase *Serum* *Increase* 9 of 16 patients with myeloid metaplasia or chronic granulocytic leukemia were found to have slight but significant elevations *317*

Alanine Aminotransferase *Serum* *Increase* Less elevation than in acute leukemia *5545*

Albumin *Serum* *Decrease* In 46% of 21 patients at initial hospitalization for this disorder *1576* Electrophoresis shows decrease *5545*
Serum *No Effect* Usually normal *5699*

Aldolase *Serum* *Increase* Less elevation than in acute leukemia *5545*

Alkaline Phosphatase *Serum* *Increase* Infiltration of the liver may result in obstruction of the biliary system *5545* In 54% of 21 patients at initial hospitalization for this disorder *1576* 21 of 54 patients had levels > 95 U/L *2848*
White Blood Cells *Decrease* Abnormally low and may actually be absent *4746* A striking decrease can be demonstrated; about 20% of normal mature granulocytes give a positive reaction *5677* In 60 patients, mean activity of 33 U/L, ranging from 0 - 294 U/L. In untreated cases, the mean score was 6.6 U/L, ranging from 0 - 28 U/L. Mean in 19 treated cases was 45.15 U/L with a range of 3 - 294 U/L. Leukopenic cases showed the average score as 104 U/L, ranging from 52 - 208 U/L *3440* 25% of 38 patients who achieved remission had normal activity *4447*
White Blood Cells *Increase* Occasionally can be elevated if some complicating condition (ulcerative colitis, a second neoplasm, or an acute infection) is present *900*

Antithrombin III *Plasma* *Decrease* Below normal in some patients *5127*

Arylsulfatase *Serum* *Increase* 30 - 50% increase in serum activity *1279*

Aspartate Aminotransferase *Serum* *Increase* In 54% of 21 patients at initial hospitalization for this disorder *1576* Less elevation than in acute leukemia *5545* Infiltration of the liver *1290* Moderately elevated levels are observed in lymphomas and leukemia but less frequently than in other hepatic disease *1025*

205.10 Chronic Myelocytic Leukemia *(continued)*

Basophils *Blood* *Increase* Slight to moderate persistent basophilia may occur. Often regarded as a poor prognostic sign *5677* Particularly in the stage preceding acute blastic crisis *900* High absolute number in almost all patients *5699*
Bone Marrow *Increase* May be considerably increased; usually in proportion to their number in the circulating blood *5677*

Calcium *Serum* *Increase* Has been described occasionally *271* *3036* Elevation > 11 mg/dL may occur with leukemic infiltration of bone *2848*
Urine *Increase* Frequently observed *1025*

Carcinoembryonic Antigen *Serum* *Increase* Above 2.5 ng/mL in 38% of patients with acute and chronic leukemia *456*

Cells *Bone Marrow* *Increase* Bone marrow aspirated from almost any site usually yields a grossly hypercellular specimen in which the fat is practically absent *5677* Occurrence of either sea-blue histiocytes or Gaucher like cells, or of both, was observed in bone marrow smears of 23 patients and in the hematopoietic tissues of 44 of the examined cases; particularly marked in chronic disease and in acute forms, though less in frequency or degree *5128*

Cholesterol *Serum* *Increase* In 65% of 21 patients at initial hospitalization for this disorder *1576*

Complement C_4 *Serum* *Decrease* Occasionally occurs *2332*

Complement, Total *Serum* *Decrease* Occasionally occurs *2332*

Coombs' Test *Serum* *Positive* Positive in 33% of patients *5545*

Creatine *Urine* *Increase* Increased breakdown *5544*

Creatinine *Serum* *Increase* In 83% of 13 patients at initial hospitalization for this disorder *1576*

Eosinophils *Blood* *Increase* Increased in percentage, which means a striking absolute increase *367* Absolute increase in almost all cases *5699* Characteristic shift toward immaturity of the granulocytes and the increase in eosinophils and basophils *367* Often regarded as a poor prognostic sign *5677*
Bone Marrow *Increase* Particularly in the stage preceding acute blastic crisis *900* May be considerably increased; usually in proportion to their number in the circulating blood *5677*

Erythrocyte Survival *Red Blood Cells* *Decrease* Some shortening of survival occurs in the presence of gross splenomegaly and hepatomegaly *5677*

Factor II *Plasma* *Decrease* Low levels found *5127*

Factor V *Plasma* *Decrease* Low levels found *5127* Intravascular clotting has been documented for rare patients *1815*

Factor VIII *Plasma* *Decrease* Intravascular clotting has been documented for rare patients *1815*

Fat *Bone Marrow* *Decrease* Bone marrow aspirated from almost any site usually yields a grossly hypercellular specimen in which the fat is practically absent *5677*

Ferritin *Serum* *Increase* Significant elevation *4970*

Fibrin Degradation Products *Plasma* *Increase* Intravascular clotting has been documented for rare patients *1815*

Fibrinogen *Plasma* *Decrease* Intravascular clotting has been documented for rare patients *1815* Moderate depression *1290*
Plasma *Increase* Either elevated or normal *5127*

α_1-Globulin *Serum* *Increase* Increased α- and γ- globulins *5545*

α_2-Globulin *Serum* *Increase* Increased α- and γ- globulins *5545*

γ-Globulin *Serum* *Increase* Increased α- and γ- globulins *5545* Often moderately elevated *5699*

Glucose *Serum* *Decrease* Artifactual hypoglycemia may be due to leukocyte glucose utilization in vitro *1477*
Serum *Increase* In 49% of 21 patients at initial hospitalization for this disorder *1576*

Hematocrit *Blood* *Decrease* In 75% of 20 patients at initial hospitalization for this disorder *1576* Anemia, when present, is characteristically normochromic normocytic *900* Anemia is almost always a feature of active disease, and generally increases in severity as the disease advances. Usually normocytic and normochromic with little evidence of iron deficiency, accelerated RBC hemolysis, or erythrocyte abnormality *5677*
Blood *Increase* In a small percentage of patients there may be a mild elevation *900*

Hemoglobin *Blood* *Decrease* Anemia, when present, is characteristically normochromic normocytic *900* In 85% of 22 patients at initial hospitalization for this disorder *1576* Anemia is almost always a feature of active disease, and generally increases in severity as the disease advances. Usually normocytic and normochromic with little evidence of iron deficiency, accelerated RBC hemolysis, or erythrocyte abnormality *5677*
Blood *Increase* In a small percentage of patients there may be a mild elevation *900*

Hexosamines, Protein-bound *Serum* *Increase* In 20 patients with chronic myelocytic leukemia mean concentration of 1,150 ± 259 mg/dm³ significantly greater than 627 ± 183 mg/dm³ in 40 healthy controls *1781*

Hexoses, Protein-bound *Serum* *Increase* In 20 patients with chronic myelocytic leukemia mean concentration of 5,085 ± 677 mg/dm³ significantly greater than 1,530 ± 325 mg/dm³ in 40 healthy controls *1781*

Histamine *Plasma* *Increase* In a group of patients with no symptoms attributable to histamine, mean plasma concentration was greater than three times normal. Tends to reflect the number of basophils *5095* Reported effect *5699* Histamine and histamine metabolites are raised in plasma and WBC in most patients *393*

immunoglobulin A *Serum* *Decrease* Reported effect *5544*

Immunoglobulin G *Serum* *Increase* In 5 of 40 patients with chronic myelocytic leukemia monoclonal IgG gammopathy observed *1781*
Serum *No Effect* Concentration usually normal *5544*

Immunoglobulin M *Serum* *No Effect* Concentration usually normal *5544*

α-Ketoglutarate *Serum* *Increase* Increased in the vast majority of patients with myeloproliferative disorders, reflective of the WBC pool size *678*

Lactate Dehydrogenase *Serum* *Increase* Considerably elevated, but appears to be a nonspecific abnormality *3220* In 95% of 20 patients at initial hospitalization for this disorder *1576* Elevated in all 20 patients, mean activity of 197.5 U/L *3335* Elevated above the normal upper limit in 84 of 91 patients with leukemias *447* Usually reflects changes in the course of the disease - falling during remission and rising during relapses, occasionally indicating the onset before the WBC had begun to change *5545*
Serum *No Effect* Frequently normal *5545*

Lactate Dehydrogenase Isoenzyme-5
Red Blood Cells *Increase* Increase observed in hemolysates. In 5 cases values ranged from 5 - 16% activity while normal activity of 2% *4983*
Serum *Decrease* Observed effect *4995* Isoenzyme 2 and 3 were the most intense and 5 was decreased *3335*

Lactate Dehydrogenase Isoenzymes *Serum* *Increase* Fractions 2 and 3 were increased and fraction 5 was decreased *4995*

Leukocytes *Blood* *Increase* In 94% of 22 patients at initial hospitalization for this disorder *1576* Over 100,000 /µL in 62 - 90% at diagnosis *3306* Characteristically > 75,000 /µL, and may exceed 500,000 /µL *2039* Increase due to increase in myeloid series is earliest change. In earlier stages the more mature forms predominate with sequentially fewer cells of the younger forms; in the later, more advanced stages the younger cells become predominant *5545* Over 100,000 /µL in 62 - 90% at diagnosis *5706*

Lymphocytes *Blood* *Decrease* In 85% of 21 patients at initial hospitalization for this disorder *1576*
Blood *No Effect* Absolute count is usually within normal limits *5699*

Lysozyme *Serum* *Increase* Elevated only in patients who do not have the Philadelphia chromosome. No correlation is apparent between urine and serum levels *4692*

Malate Dehydrogenase *Serum* *Increase* Less elevation than in acute leukemia *5545*

Metamyelocytes *Blood* *Increase* In the great majority of patients *5677*

1-Methylinosine *Urine* *Increase* In 2 patients with chronic myelocytic leukemia, excretions of 15.2 and 19.4 mg/d significantly different from 3.9 ± 2.1 mg/d in 17 healthy controls *5505*

Monocytes *Blood* *Increase* May be normal or increased *2033* Increase in absolute number in almost all cases *5699* On occasion associated with a monocytosis of relatively minor proportions *3246*

Myelocytes *Blood* *Increase* In the great majority of patients *5677*

N^2, N^2-Dimethylguanosine *Urine* *Increase* In 2 patients with chronic myelocytic leukemia excretions of 13.9 and 14.8 mg/d significantly different from 3.9 ± 2.6 mg/d in 17 healthy controls *5505*

Neutrophils *Blood* *Increase* Granulocytes in all stages of development occur in profusion in the peripheral blood and for the most part appear to be normal in morphology. The most mature elements are ordinarily present in greatest number and the less mature in diminishing frequency *5677* 80 - 90% of the cells are granulocytes. The distribution shows only a slight shift toward immaturity *367* Most patients have > 100,000 /μL granulocytes at time of diagnosis and the count may exceed 1 million *2033*
Bone Marrow *Increase* Resemble those in the peripheral blood, but on the average they are about 1 stage less mature *5677* Granulocytic and sometimes megakaryocytic hyperplasia in bone marrow *678*

Partial Thromboplastin Time *Plasma* *Increase* Intravascular clotting has been documented for rare patients *1815*

Perchloric Acid Soluble Protein *Serum* *Increase* In 20 patients with chronic myelocytic leukemia mean concentration of 64.2 ± 8.7 mg tyrosine/dm^3 significantly greater than 43.7 ± 11.8 mg tyrosine/dm^3 in 40 healthy controls *1781*

Phosphoglucomutase *Serum* *Increase* In some cases *1290*

Plasminogen Antigen *Plasma* *Decrease* Below normal in some patients *5127*

Platelets *Blood* *Decrease* Intravascular clotting has been documented in rare patients *1815* Severe thrombocytopenia is rare at diagnosis *5699* In 56% of 21 patients at initial hospitalization for this disorder *1576* Rarely develops spontaneously in the absence of blastic crisis *2033* Decreased in terminal stages with findings of thrombocytopenic purpura *5545*
Blood *Increase* In 23% of 21 patients at initial hospitalization for this disorder *1576* High in approximately 50% of patients *3306* 33% or more of patients have pronounced thrombocytosis *3334* High in approximately 50% of patients *5706* Elevated in a small percentage of patients, with counts reaching 1 - 2 million/μL. Occasionally precedes the increase in WBC and a diagnosis of essential or primary thrombocythemia may be made *900*

Potassium *Serum* *Increase* Artifactual hyperkalemia may occur *5699* Pseudohyperkalemia due to the release of potassium from white cells during clotting has been reported *591*

Protein *Pleural Fluid* *Increase* Pleural effusions are usually exudates *126*

Prothrombin Time *Plasma* *Increase* Intravascular clotting has been documented for rare patients *1815*

Pseudouridine *Urine* *Increase* In 2 patients with chronic myelocytic leukemia excretions of 300 and 302 mg/d significantly different from 65 ± 31 mg/d in 17 healthy controls *5505*

Reticulocytes *Blood* *Increase* Generally normal or slightly increased *5677*
Blood *No Effect* Normal or slightly increased *374*

Sodium *Serum* *Increase* In 100% of 20 patients at initial hospitalization for this disorder *1576*

Thrombin Time *Blood* *Increase* Intravascular clotting has been documented for rare patients *1815*

Urea Nitrogen *Serum* *Increase* Can be elevated in kidney infiltration and should be followed especially if nephrotoxic antibiotics are used *900* In 23% of 21 patients at initial hospitalization for this disorder *1576*

Uric Acid *Serum* *Increase* In 80% of 21 patients at initial hospitalization for this disorder *1576* Frequent biochemical abnormality *900* Especially with high WBC and antileukemic therapy. Urinary obstruction may develop on account of intrarenal and extrarenal crystallization *5545* Often moderately elevated; increased production *5699*
Urine *Increase* Almost invariably increased; gout may occur *5699* Often 2 - 3 times normal in patients with active disease, and if aggressive therapy leads to rapid cell lysis, excretion of the additional purine load may produce urinary tract blockage *2816*

Vitamin B_{12} *Serum* *Increase* Increased to an average of approximately 15 times the normal mean concentration, generally proportional to the height of the leukocyte count in untreated patients, but still 4 times normal in patients who have normal WBC counts during remissions *5677* Significant increase found in 27 patients, mean concentration for the group of 675 pg/mL, compared to normal, 385 pg/mL *4448*

Vitamin B_{12} Binding Capacity *Serum* *Increase* Despite the increased amount of vitamin B_{12}, there is considerable additional unsaturated binding capacity *4148* Increased in the vast majority of patients with myeloproliferative disorders, reflective of the WBC pool size *678*

Vitamin B_{12} Binding Capacity, Unsaturated *Serum* *Increase* Increased concentrations observed during chronic myelocytic leukemia *2952*

Zinc *Serum* *Decrease* Decreased *5083*

205.10 Chronic Myelogenous Leukemia

Adenosine Deaminase *Serum* *Increase* Astonishingly high values *2737* *3003*

Alkaline Phosphatase *Neutrophils* *Decrease* Striking decrease in activity may be observed *1781*
White Blood Cells *Decrease* Decreased activity observed in the majority of patients with the disease *443* Mean activity decreased in 17 of 22 (77%) patients with CML *1781*
White Blood Cells *Increase* Mean activity increased in 9% patients with CML *1781*

α_2-Antiplasmin/Plasmin Complex *Plasma* *No Effect* In 15 patients at the time of their diagnosis concentration observed to be almost normal *3609*

Arylsulfatase *White Blood Cells* *Increase* Leukemic cells from patients with chronic myelogenous leukemia had increased activity of enzyme *1781*

Arylsulfatase A *White Blood Cells* *Increase* Leukemic cells from patients with chronic myelogenous leukemia had increased activity of enzyme *1781*

Arylsulfatase B *White Blood Cells* *Increase* Leukemic cells from patients with chronic myelogenous leukemia had increased activity of enzyme *1781*

Calcium *Serum* *Increase* Hypercalcemia occasionally observed, occurring most often in blast crisis and is accompanied by PTH suppression *1781*

Elastase-α_1-Proteinase Inhibitor Complex *Serum* *Increase* Significant increase observed at the time of diagnosis in 15 patients *3609*

Ferritin *Serum* *Increase* In 3 patients with chronic myelogenous leukemia mean concentration increased 8-fold in blast phase, although concentration not significantly altered in chronic phase *1781*

Fibrin Degradation Products (D-Dimer) *Plasma* *No Effect* Insignificant increase observed in 15 patients at the time of their diagnosis *3609*

Granulocyte Colony Stimulating Factor *Serum* *Increase* 9 of 17 patients with CML (52%) demonstrated detectable levels of G-CSF, i.e., greater than 50 pg/mL (range 150 - 2,830 pg/mL) compared with detectable amount in none of 15 healthy volunteer controls *272*

Granulocyte-Macrophage Colony Stimulating Factor *Serum* *Increase* 8 of 17 patients with CML (44%) demonstrated detectable levels of GM-CSF, i.e., greater than 3 pg/mL (range 3.9 - 55 pg/mL), compared with detectable amount in only one of 15 healthy volunteer controls *272*

Hemoglobin *Blood* *Decrease* Anemia observed in the majority of patients with the disease *443*

Interleukin-1α *Serum* *No Effect* In 15 patients with CML, concentration not detectable as in 14 healthy controls *545*

Interleukin-1β *Serum* *No Effect* In 15 patients with CML, concentration not detectable as in 14 healthy controls *545*

205.10 Chronic Myelogenous Leukemia *(continued)*

Interleukin-2 *Serum* *Increase* In 15 patients with CML mean concentration of 181 ± 72 pg/mL significantly higher than undetectable amount in 14 healthy controls *545* In 15 patients with CML mean concentration of 993 ± 322 U/mL significantly higher than 582 ± 164 U/mL in 14 healthy controls *545*

Interleukin-6 *Serum* *No Effect* In 15 patients with CML concentration not different from that in 14 healthy controls *545*

Interleukin-10 *Serum* *No Effect* In 15 patients with CML concentration not different from that in 14 healthy controls *545*

Lactate Dehydrogenase *Serum* *Increase* In 9 patients with CML before institution of treatment mean activity of 184 ± 41 U/L only slightly higher than 62 ± 30 U/L in healthy controls *1721* Activity may be substantially increased due to release from white cells *1781* Increased activity observed in the majority of patients *443*

Lactate Dehydrogenase Isoenzyme-5 *Serum* *No Effect* No increase observed in 9 patients with CML prior to treatment *1721*

Lactate Dehydrogenase Isoenzymes *Serum* *Increase* In CML nonsignificant increases of LD_1, LD_2 and LD_3 of 64.4 ± 13.5 U/L, 76.7 ± 20 U/L, and 37.6 ± 16.2 U/L respectively compared with normal of 20 ± 11.6 U/L, 24 ± 14.5 U/L, and 21.6 ± 10 U/L *1721*

Leukocytes *Blood* *Increase* Leukocytosis characteristic of the disease *443*

Lysozyme *Serum* *Increase* Activity markedly increased in patients with chronic myelogenous leukemia *1781*

α-Mannosidase *White Blood Cells* *Increase* Leukemic cells from patients with myelogenous leukemia had higher activity of enzyme than in patients with lymphogenous forms of leukemia *1781*

β_2-Microglobulin *Serum* *Increase* In 15 patients with chronic myelogenous leukemia mean concentration of 2,718 ± 481 μg/L significantly higher than 1,721 ± 673 μg/L in 14 healthy controls *545*

Neopterin *Urine* *Increase* Highest concentrations observed in patients with non-Hodgkin's lymphoma, chronic myelogenous or lymphoblastoid leukemia *121*

Platelets *Blood* *Decrease* In more than 50% of patients with the disease concentration increased *443*
Blood *Increase* Thrombocytosis observed in 30% of all patients with the disease *443*

Potassium *Serum* *Increase* Increased concentration observed in the majority of patients *443* Concentration may be substantially increased due to release from white cells *1781*

Thrombin/Antithrombin III Complex *Plasma* *No Effect* Insignificant increase observed in 15 patients observed at the time of their diagnosis *3609*

Thrombomodulin *Plasma* *Increase* In 15 patients at diagnosis mean concentration of 19.5 ± 6.2 ng/mL significantly higher than 8.0 ± 1.9 ng/mL in 20 normal controls *3609*

Tumor Necrosis Factor-α *Serum* *Increase* In 15 patients with chronic myelogenous leukemia mean concentration of 10 ± 2.5 pg/mL different from 0 pg/mL in 14 healthy controls *545*

Uric Acid *Serum* *Increase* Increase observed in the majority of patients with the disease *443* Concentration may be substantially increased due to release from white cells *1781*

Vitamin B_{12} *Serum* *Increase* Increased concentration observed in the majority of patients with the disease *443* Concentration may be increased as much as 15 times normal *1781*

205.10 Chronic Myeloid Leukemia

Alkaline Phosphatase *Serum* *Increase* In 46 patients with CML mean activity of 3.19 ± 0.252 U/L significantly higher than 1.94 ± 0.054 in 15 healthy controls *4027*

Alkaline Phosphatase, Placental Isoenzyme *Serum* *Increase* In 46 patients with CML mean activity of 0.786 ± 0.101 U/L significantly higher than 0.311 ± 0.012 in 15 healthy controls *4027*

Anti-Neutrophil Cytoplasm Antibodies *Serum* *No Effect* In a group of patients with chronic myeloid leukemia and myelodysplasia in none were ANCA demonstrated *4602* *4602*

C-Reactive Protein *Serum* *Increase* In 22 patients with myelodysplastic syndromes mean concentration increased to 1.43 mg/dL *1822*

Fibrinogen *Plasma* *No Effect* In 22 patients with myelodysplastic syndromes mean concentration of 280.7 ± 48.0 mg/dL within normal range *1822*

Lactate Dehydrogenase *Serum* *Increase* In 51 patients with CML mean activity of 621.0 ± 48.47 U/L *4027*

Lactoferrin *Plasma* *Increase* Mean concentration in 8 patients with chronic myeloid leukemia in relapse varied from 12.1 - 22.0 μg/mL significantly higher than in normal women (1.62 μg/mL) and in healthy men (1.62 μg/mL) *388*

α_2-Macroglobulin *Serum* *No Effect* In 22 patients with myelodysplastic syndromes mean concentration of 215.3 ± 884.8 mg/dL within normal range *1822*

β_2-Microglobulin *Serum* *Increase* Increased concentration observed in about 20 - 30% of untreated patients with malignant lymphoma and is higher in patients with blast crisis *1781*

Platelets *Blood* *Increase* In 732 patients with platelet counts greater than 500,000 /μL, 3.3% had CML *1869*
Blood *No Effect* Of 250 patients with platelet counts of more than 250,000 /μL, 6 had chronic myeloid leukemia *3939*

Soluble c-kit Molecule *Serum* *No Effect* Median concentration of 189.5 AU/mL in patients with CML not significantly different from that in 51 healthy volunteers of 199.0 AU/mL *2598*

Transferrin *Serum* *No Effect* In 22 patients with myelodysplastic syndromes mean concentration of 220.8 ± 49.2 mg/dL within normal range *1822*

Triglycerides *Serum* *Increase* In 50% of 22 patients with chronic myeloid leukemia serum triglyceride concentration increased before treatment *4069*

205.10 Chronic Myelomonocytic Leukemia

Anti-Neutrophil Cytoplasm Antibodies *Serum* *Increase* In 2 patients with chronic myelomonocytic leukemia ANCA were demonstrated *4602*

α_2-HS Glycoprotein *Serum* *Decrease* Significant reduction observed compared with healthy controls probably due to hepatic involvement *2533*

205.10 Myelocytic Leukemia

Lysozyme *Serum* *Increase* Activity increased in patients with myelocytic leukemia *1781*
Urine *Increase* Activity increased in patients with myelocytic leukemia *1781*

Magnesium *Granulocyte* *Decrease* Mean concentration in patients with myeloocytic leukemia of 3.43 ± 0.48 fmol/cell significantly different from 4.35 ± 0.62 fmol/cell in healthy controls *3137*
Monocytes *Decrease* Mean concentration in patients with myeloocytic leukemia of 3.31 ± 0.54 fmol/cell not significantly different from 3.74 ± 0.66 fmol/cell in healthy controls *3137*

205.90 Myeloid Leukemia

Gc-Globulin *Serum* *No Effect* In 13 men and 12 women with myeloid leukemia mean concentrations of 22.8 ± 4.45 mg/dL and 24.8 ± 4.39 mg/dL not significantly different from 23.9 mg/dL in 106 control men and 26.1 mg/dL in 150 control women *2279*

206.00 Acute Monocytic Leukemia

Lysozyme *Serum* *Increase* Activity increased in most patients (90%) with acute monocytic leukemia *1781*
Urine *Increase* Activity increased in most patients (90%) with acute monocytic leukemia but only when serum activity greater than 4 times the upper limit of normal *1781*

α-Mannosidase *White Blood Cells* *Increase* Leukemic cells from children with acute myeloid leukemia had very high activity of enzyme *1781*

N-Acetyl-Glucosaminidase *White Blood Cells* *Increase* Leukemic cells from children with acute monocytic leukemia had greater activity of enzyme than those of non-T, non-B ALL cells *1781*

Phospholipase A *Serum* *Increase* Significantly elevated *2625*

206.90 Monocytic Leukemia

Albumin *Serum* *Decrease* In 33% of 23 patients at initial hospitalization for this disorder *1576*

Alkaline Phosphatase *Serum* *Increase* In 34% of 21 patients at initial hospitalization for this disorder *1576*
White Blood Cells *Increase* Mean value in 13 cases of acute monomyelocytic leukemia was 103.4 with a range of 12 - 208 *3440*

Aspartate Aminotransferase *Serum* *Increase* In 63% of 23 patients at initial hospitalization for this disorder *1576*

Cholesterol *Serum* *Decrease* In 51% of 23 patients at initial hospitalization for this disorder *1576*

Creatinine *Serum* *Increase* In 49% of 22 patients at initial hospitalization for this disorder *1576*

Factor V *Plasma* *Decrease* With disseminated intravascular clotting *3418*

Factor VIII *Plasma* *Decrease* With disseminated intravascular clotting *3418*

Fibrin Degradation Products *Plasma* *Increase* With disseminated intravascular clotting *3418*

Fibrinogen *Plasma* *Decrease* With disseminated intravascular clotting *3418*

γ-Globulin *Serum* *Increase* An increased concentration of heterogeneous or polyclonal γ-globulin in the plasma occurs frequently *5677* *5544*

Hematocrit *Blood* *Decrease* In 90% of 24 patients at initial hospitalization for this disorder *1576* Anemia is often quite severe, usually normochromic and normocytic *5699*

Hemoglobin *Blood* *Decrease* In 91% of 24 patients at initial hospitalization for this disorder *1576* Anemia is often quite severe, usually normochromic and normocytic *5699*

Iron *Serum* *Increase* Increased in acute leukemias *1290*

Lactate Dehydrogenase *Serum* *Increase* In 80% of 22 patients at initial hospitalization for this disorder *1576*

Leukocytes *Blood* *Decrease* Variable percentage of abnormal monocytes in about 33% of all patients initially. Usually present *5677* Patients are usually leukopenic *5699*
Blood *Increase* The majority have a moderate to pronounced leukocytosis, with some 50 - 75% of the WBC being monocytes, promonocytes, or monoblasts *5677* In 58% of 24 patients at initial hospitalization for this disorder *1576*

Lysozyme *Serum* *Increase* Markedly increased *1606* During the transition from a variety of myeloproliferative disorders to acute myeloblastic or acute myelomonocytic leukemia, there is a striking elevation in serum and urine muramidase activity *4692* Elevated in serum and urine in some patients with acute monocytic and myelomonocytic leukemia *900* Activity increased in patients with monocytic leukemia *1781*
Urine *Increase* During the transition from a variety of myeloproliferative disorders to acute myeloblastic or acute myelomonocytic leukemia, there is a striking elevation in serum and urine muramidase activity *4692* Elevated in serum and urine in some patients with acute monocytic and myelomonocytic leukemia *900* Patients with heavy lysozymuria develop an apparently unique type of glomerular-tubular dysfunction, with hypokalemia, hyperkaluria, and azotemia *3642* Activity increased in patients with monocytic leukemia *1781*

Monocytes *Blood* *Increase* In 38% of 23 patients at initial hospitalization for this disorder *1576* Occurs in monocytic and other leukemias *5544*

Neutrophils *Blood* *Decrease* In 94% of 24 patients at initial hospitalization for this disorder *1576*

Partial Thromboplastin Time *Plasma* *Increase* With disseminated intravascular clotting *3418*

Platelets *Blood* *Decrease* With disseminated intravascular clotting *3418* Usually present *5677* In 83% of 24 patients at initial hospitalization for this disorder *1576*

Protein *Pleural Fluid* *Increase* Pleural effusions are usually exudates *126*
Urine *Increase* A unique type of proteinuria develops in about 50% of patients. In addition to ordinary plasma components, the low molecular weight enzyme lysozyme is excreted in amounts up to 0.6 - 2.4 g/d *3941*

Prothrombin Time *Plasma* *Increase* With disseminated intravascular clotting *3418*

Reticulocytes *Blood* *Increase* Usually modest in degree, considering the severity of the anemia *5677*

Thrombin Time *Blood* *Increase* With disseminated intravascular clotting *3418*

Urea Nitrogen *Serum* *Increase* In 36% of 24 patients at initial hospitalization for this disorder *1576*

Uric Acid *Serum* *Increase* In 55% of 23 patients at initial hospitalization for this disorder *1576*

Vitamin B_{12} *Serum* *Increase* Increases in some cases *5544*

Zinc *Serum* *Decrease* Decreased *5083*

207.00 Erythroleukemia

Alkaline Phosphatase *White Blood Cells* *Increase* In 2 cases of erythroleukemia, the scores from polymorphonuclears were 24 and 78. Normal mean 61.9 *3440*

Bilirubin *Serum* *Increase* Evidence of a mild or moderate increase in hemolysis is commonly observed, but the erythrokinetic findings are those of ineffective erythropoiesis *5677*

Cells *Bone Marrow* *Increase* Marrow is nearly always hypercellular and characteristically shows a selective hyperplasia of the erythroid cells, with a myeloid/erythroid ratio of 1.0 or even lower *5677*

Coombs' Test *Serum* *Negative* Typical observation *5677*

Erythrocyte Survival *Red Blood Cells* *Decrease* Evidence of a mild or moderate increase in hemolysis is commonly observed, but the erythrokinetic findings are those of ineffective erythropoiesis *5677*

Haptoglobin *Serum* *Decrease* Evidence of a mild or moderate increase in hemolysis is commonly observed, but the erythrokinetic findings are those of ineffective erythropoiesis *5677*

Hematocrit *Blood* *Decrease* Anemia is nearly always present, but its severity is variable. Usually normocytic and normochromic *5677*

Hemoglobin *Blood* *Decrease* Anemia is nearly always present, but its severity is variable. Usually normocytic and normochromic *5677*

Lactate Dehydrogenase *Serum* *Increase* Normal or high levels *5677*

Leukocytes *Blood* *Increase* Count varies from subnormal to frankly leukemic levels but tends to rise as the disease progresses *5677*

MCV *Blood* *Increase* A mild macrocytosis is sometimes present *5677*

Platelets *Blood* *Decrease* In about 50% of the cases *5677*

Reticulocytes *Blood* *Increase* Occasionally *1916*

Uric Acid *Serum* *Increase* Normal or high levels *5677*

Urobilinogen *Feces* *Increase* Evidence of a mild or moderate increase in hemolysis is commonly observed, but the erythrokinetic findings are those of ineffective erythropoiesis *5677*

Vitamin B_{12} *Serum* *Increase* In many, but not all patients *5677*

208.00 Acute Leukemia

Alanine *Urine* *Increase* Mean excretion of 0.798 ± 2.18 mmol/d in 52 patients with acute leukemia higher than 0.184 ± 0.579 mmol/d in 29 healthy controls of both sexes *5700*

Amino Acids *Urine* *Increase* Mean excretion of 33.7 ± 23.9 mmol/d in 30 patients with active disease significantly higher than 19.8 ± 10.4 mmol/d in 29 healthy controls of both sexes *5700*

208.00 Acute Leukemia *(continued)*

Amino Acids *(continued)*
Urine *No Effect* Mean excretion of 21.7 ± 14.4 mmol/d in 14 patients in complete remission not significantly different from 19.8 ± 10.4 mmol/d in 29 healthy controls of both sexes *5700*

Anti-Lactoferrin Antibodies *Serum* *Decrease* In 10 patients with acute leukemia in remission anti-lactoferrin antibodies detected in three which persisted after intensive chemotherapy *613*

Aspartic Acid *Urine* *Increase* Mean excretion of 2.22 ± 2.29 mmol/d in 52 patients with acute leukemia higher than 1.34 ± 0.799 mmol/d in 29 healthy controls of both sexes *5700*

Complement C_1 *Serum* *Increase* In 19 patients with acute leukemia mean concentration of 43.624 ± 18.501 CH50 U/mL not significantly different from 37.251 ± 5.324 CH50 U/mL in 11 controls *3037*

Complement C_2 *Serum* *Increase* In 19 patients with acute leukemia mean concentration of 7.468 ± 4.443 CH50 U/mL not significantly different from 6.064 ± 1.445 CH50 U/mL in 11 controls *3037*

Complement C_3 *Serum* *Increase* In 19 patients with acute leukemia mean concentration of 8.294 ± 3.141 CH50 U/mL not significantly different from 9.720 ± 2.476 CH50 U/mL in 11 controls *3037*

Complement C_4 *Serum* *Increase* In 19 patients with acute leukemia mean concentration of 77.744 ± 36.625 CH50 U/mL significantly different from 64.920 ± 10.373 CH50 U/mL in 11 controls *3037*

Complement C_5 *Serum* *Increase* In 19 patients with acute leukemia mean concentration of 143.160 ± 41.704 CH50 U/mL significantly different from 118.869 ± 13.547 CH50 U/mL in 11 controls *3037*

Complement C_7 *Serum* *Increase* In 19 patients with acute leukemia mean concentration of 114.030 ± 3.493 CH50 U/mL significantly different from 94.649 ± 22.434 CH50 U/mL in 11 controls *3037*

Complement C_8 *Serum* *Increase* In 19 patients with acute leukemia mean concentration of 107.116 ± 34.059 CH50 U/mL significantly different from 79.129 ± 25.316 CH50 U/mL in 11 controls *3037*

Complement C_9 *Serum* *Increase* In 19 patients with acute leukemia mean concentration of 120.039 ± 39.727 CH50 U/mL significantly different from 49.401 ± 12.308 CH50 U/mL in 11 controls *3037*

Complement CH50 *Serum* *Increase* In 19 patients with acute leukemia mean concentration of 109.996 ± 29.023 CH50 U/mL not significantly different from 104.313 ± 17.058 CH50 U/mL in 11 controls *3037*

Complement, Total *Serum* *Increase* In 19 patients with acute leukemia mean concentration of 543 ± 119 CH50 U/mL significantly different from 474 ± 52 CH50 U/mL in 11 controls *3037*

C-Reactive Protein *Serum* *Increase* Increased concentration above 100 mg/L observed in 29 episodes of infection in 22 neutropenic patients with unspecified acute leukemia *1781*

Cysteine *Urine* *Increase* Mean excretion of 0.331 mmol/d in 52 patients with acute leukemia higher than 0.109 ± 0.237 mmol/d in 29 healthy controls of both sexes *5700*

Fibronectin *Plasma* *No Effect* The concentration of fibronectin in patients with acute leukemia on admission was normal in the presence of infection *1781* The concentration of fibronectin in patients with acute leukemia on admission was normal in the absence of infection *1781*

Glutamic Acid *Urine* *Decrease* Mean excretion of 3.49 ± 2.61 mmol/d in 52 patients with acute leukemia lower than 4.08 ± 4.18 mmol/d in 29 healthy controls of both sexes *5700*

Glycine *Urine* *Increase* Mean excretion of 13.9 ± 11.7 mmol/d in 52 patients with acute leukemia significantly higher than 10.54 ± 8.78 mmol/d in 29 healthy controls of both sexes *5700*

HDL-Cholesterol *Serum* *Decrease* In 25 patients with unspecified acute leukemia or non-Hodgkin's lymphoma extremely low concentrations of HDL-cholesterol observed in all, possibly related to tumor burden and marrow involvement *1781*

Interleukin-6 *Serum* *Increase* In 10 acute leukemics prior to institution of chemotherapy serum concentrations were increaseded significantly (median 5.9 pg/mL) compared with concentrations in 11 normal controls (median 1.05 pg/mL) *611* In patients with acute leukemia mean concentration higher than in patients with multiple myeloma and in healthy controls *4927*

Isoleucine *Urine* *Increase* Mean excretion of 0.383 ± 1.27 mmol/d in 52 patients with acute leukemia higher than 0 mmol/d in 29 healthy controls of both sexes *5700*

Lactoferrin *Plasma* *Increase* In 8 patients with untreated acute leukemia concentration was positively correlated with the peripheral neutrophil count *1781*

Leucine *Urine* *Increase* Mean excretion of 1.09 ± 2.95 mmol/d in 52 patients with acute leukemia higher than 0.300 ± 0.347 mmol/d in 29 healthy controls of both sexes *5700*

Lysine *Urine* *Increase* Mean excretion of 0.290 ± 1.01 mmol/d in 52 patients with acute leukemia higher than 0 mmol/d in 29 healthy controls of both sexes *5700*

Methionine *Urine* *Increase* Mean excretion of 2.14 ± 2.10 mmol/d in 52 patients with acute leukemia higher than 1.83 ± 2.22 mmol/d in 29 healthy controls of both sexes *5700*

1-Methylinosine *Urine* *Increase* In 2 patients with acute leukemia, excretions of 5.0 and 6.4 mg/d significantly different from 3.9 ± 2.1 mg/d in 17 healthy controls *5505*

N^2, N^2-Dimethylguanosine *Urine* *Increase* In 2 patients with acute leukemia excretions of 7.6 and 4.7 mg/d significantly different from 3.9 ± 2.6 mg/d in 17 healthy controls *5505*

Phenylalanine *Urine* *Increase* Mean excretion of 0.331 ± 0.496 mmol/d in 52 patients with acute leukemia higher than 0.223 ± 0.365 mmol/d in 29 healthy controls of both sexes *5700*

Phospholipase A_2 *Serum* *Increase* In 16 children with acute leukemia 44% had activities greater than 10 U/L *3156*

Proline *Urine* *Increase* Mean excretion of 0.668 ± 0.832 mmol/d in 52 patients with acute leukemia higher than 0.535 ± 0.434 mmol/d in 29 healthy controls of both sexes *5700*

Protein Z *Plasma* *No Effect* In 16 patients with acute leukemia median baseline concentration of 2.55 ng/mL compared with 2.72 ng/mL in 14 healthy controls *5357*

Pseudouridine *Urine* *Increase* In 2 patients with acute leukemia excretions of 88 and 299 mg/d significantly different from 65 ± 31 mg/d in 17 healthy controls *5505*

Serine *Urine* *Increase* Mean excretion of 1.46 ± 2.32 mmol/d in 52 patients with acute leukemia higher than 0.308 ± 0.454 mmol/d in 29 healthy controls of both sexes *5700*

Sialyltransferase *Serum* *Increase* In 2 patients with acute leukemia mean and median concentrations of 426 and 426 cpm/mg protein/30 min significantly different from 240 and 243 cpm/mg protein/30 min respectively in 20 normal individuals *2111*

Soluble E-Selectin *Serum* *Decrease* In 10 acute leukemics before chemotherapy serum concentrations were reduced significantly compared with concentrations in 11 normal controls *611*

Soluble Intercellular Adhesion Molecule-1 *Serum* *Increase* Increased concentration detected in patients with untreated acute leukemia which may reflect the leukemia cell burden *613*

Soluble P-Selectin *Serum* *No Effect* In 10 acute leukemics before chemotherapy serum concentrations were not significantly different when compared with concentrations in 11 normal controls *611*

Threonine *Urine* *Increase* Mean excretion of 2.58 ± 2.21 mmol/d in 52 patients with acute leukemia higher than 0.316 ± 0.549 mmol/d in 29 healthy controls of both sexes *5700*

Triglycerides *Serum* *Increase* In 25 patients with unspecified acute leukemia or non-Hodgkin's lymphoma increased concentrations of triglycerides observed in all, probably related to tumor burden and marrow involvement *1781*

Tumor Necrosis Factor-α *Serum* *Decrease* In acute leukemic patients with bacterial infections concentration significantly decreased to 1.6 pg/mL compared with 2.7 pg/mL in heathy controls *612*

Tyrosine *Urine* *Increase* Mean excretion of 0.676 ± 2.79 mmol/d in 52 patients with acute leukemia higher than 0.078 ± 0.307 mmol/d in 29 healthy controls of both sexes *5700*

Valine *Urine* *Increase* Mean excretion of 0.263 ± 0.881 mmol/d in 52 patients with acute leukemia higher than 0 mmol/d in 29 healthy controls of both sexes *5700*

VLDL-Cholesterol *Serum* *Increase* In 25 patients with unspecified acute leukemia or non-Hodgkin's lymphoma increased concentrations of VLDL observed in all, probably related to tumor burden and marrow involvement *1781*

208.00 Acute Nonlymphoblastic Leukemia

Albumin *Serum* *Decrease* Hypoalbuminemia commonly found but not useful predictor of response to treatment or length of remission *1781*

Tissue Factor Antigen *Plasma* *Increase* In 12 patients with ANLL other than acute promyelocytic leukemia mean concentration of 326 ± 85 pg/mL compared with 126 ± 41 pg/mL in 12 healthy volunteers *5511*

208.00 Acute Nonlymphocytic Leukemia

Antithrombin *Plasma* *No Effect* 12 patients with ANLL had median concentration of 1.05 U/mL not significantly different from median concentration of 0.98 U/mL in healthy individuals *2376*

D-Dimer *Plasma* *No Effect* 12 patients with ANLL had median concentration of 3.3 μg/L not significantly different from median concentration of 0.3 μg/L in healthy individuals *2376*

Lactate Dehydrogenase Isoenzymes *Serum* *Increase* In 57 patients with active ANLL increased LD-3 activity observed in 44 (77%) but not observed in patients in complete remission or in 3 patients in preleukemic phase of disease *3092*

Protein C *Plasma* *No Effect* 12 patients with ANLL had median concentration of 0.92 U/mL not significantly different from median concentration of 1.01 U/mL in healthy individuals *2376*

Soluble Fibrin Monomer *Plasma* *No Effect* 12 patients with ANLL had median concentration of 30 mg/L not significantly different from median concentration of 1.4 mg/L in healthy individuals *2376*

Soluble Transferrin Receptor *Serum* *No Effect* In patients with acute nonlymphocytic leukemia mean concentration of 3.85 ± 3.50 μg/mL compared with 5.63 ± 1.42 μg/mL in healthy controls *2704*

Tissue Factor Pathway Inhibitor *Plasma* *No Effect* 12 patients with ANLL had median activity of 0.94 U/mL not significantly different from median activity of 1.19 U/mL in healthy individuals *2376*

Tissue Factor Pathway Inhibitor Antigen *Plasma* *No Effect* 12 patients with ANLL had median concentration of 89 ng/mL not significantly different from median concentration of 90 ng/mL in healthy individuals *2376*

Tissue Factor Pathway Inhibitor Antigen, Free *Plasma* *No Effect* 6 patients with ANLL had median concentration of 7 ng/mL not significantly different from median concentration of 15 ng/mL in healthy individuals *2376*

Tissue Factor Pathway Inhibitor, Truncated and Complexed *Plasma* *No Effect* 12 patients with ANLL had median concentration of 83 ng/mL not significantly different from median concentration of 78 ng/mL in healthy individuals *2376*

208.00 Non-T non-B Acute Lymphoblastic Leukemia

β_2-Microglobulin *Cerebrospinal Fluid* *Increase* Increased concentration observed in 9 patients with overt CNS relapse but because of large individual variations of little value in determining whether lymphoblasts present in CSF *1781*

208.10 Chronic Leukemia

Aldolase *Serum* *Increase* Activity may be increased in some patients with chronic leukemias *2952*

208.10 Leukemia

α_1-Acid Glycoprotein *Serum* *Increase* Increased concentration observed in 14 of 16 patients with various forms of active disease and was normal in all but 2 of 16 patients with inactive disease *1781*

Angiotensin-converting Enzyme *Serum* *Decrease* Mean activity normal or reduced in patients with leukemia *1781*
Serum *No Effect* Mean activity normal or reduced in patients with leukemia *1781*

Anti-p53 Antibodies *Serum* *Increase* Increase observed in 2 of 107 patients (1.9%) *132*

Cadaverine *Urine* *Increase* In 12 patients with initial stage of a variety of leukemias mean concentration of 9.91 μmol/g creatinine and 15.60 μmol/g creatinine significantly different from 2.17 μmol/g creatinine in 32 healthy controls *2973*

Carcinoembryonic Antigen *Serum* *Increase* In 6 patients with leukemia 83.3% had concentrations of 0.0 - 3.0 ng/mL, 16.7% had concentrations from 3.1 - 5.0 ng/mL, 0.0% had concentrations from 5.1 - 10.0 ng/mL and 0.0% had concentrations greater than 10.0 ng/mL when measured by method on Bayer Technicon Immuno 1® system compared with 95.9%, 3.5%, 0.6% and 0.0% respectively in 173 healthy nonsmokers *339*

Circulating Immune Complexes *Serum* *Increase* Incidence increased compared with healthy controls. Higher concentrations found in patients in blast crises *1781*

Complement C_3 *Serum* *Increase* Increased concentration reported in some patients with advanced Hodgkin's disease *1781*

Complement C_4 *Serum* *Increase* Increased concentration reported in some patients with advanced Hodgkin's disease *1781*

Deoxycytidine Kinase *Serum* *Increase* Activity correlated with the peripheral white blood cell count *1781*

1,3-Diacetylpropane *Urine* *No Effect* In 12 patients with initial stage of a variety of leukemias mean concentration of 0.96 μmol/g creatinine and 2.94 μmol/g creatinine not significantly different from 2.55 μmol/g creatinine in 32 healthy controls *2973*

Epidermal Growth Factor *Urine* *Increase* Mean concentration in about 5 patients with leukemia of 25 μg/g creatinine significantly different compared with about 10 μg/g creatinine in about 30 controls *5341*

Epstein Barr Virus Antibodies *Serum* *Increase* Elevated levels were associated with satistically significant excess risk *2984*

Ferritin *Cerebrospinal Fluid* *Increase* The concentration of ferritin in CSF tended to be more increased in patients with CNS infitration than in those without CNS involvement *1781*
Serum *Increase* In 10 patients with leukemia or myeloma concentration increased above 150 ng/mL in 9 patients *3792*

Fucosidase *White Blood Cells* *Increase* Leukemic cells from 6 of 19 patients with leukemia had increased activity of α-fucosidase *1781*

β-Galactosidase *White Blood Cells* *Increase* Leukemic cells from 6 of 19 patients with leukemia had increased activity of enzyme *1781*

Glucose *Serum* *Decrease* Rate of decrease of blood glucose concentration increased in 12 leukemic patients 0.23 mmol/L/h compared with 0.17 mmol/L/h in 10 controls *205*

γ-Glutamyltransferase *Urine* *Increase* Activity increased in urine of leukemic patients *1781*
White Blood Cells *Decrease* Activity reduced in leukemic lymphocytes *1781*

Hexose *Serum* *Increase* Mean concentration in 145 patients with leukemia of 45.1 ± 1.80 mg/dL significantly higher than 9.9 ± 0.29 mg/dL in 150 healthy controls *4029*

Homocystine *Plasma* *Increase* Moderate increase observed in some patients with leukemia *5346*

Lactate Dehydrogenase *Serum* *Increase* In 145 patients with leukemia mean activity of 584.5 ± 40.50 U/L significantly different from 115.3 ± 3.25 U/L in 150 healthy controls *4028*
Activity increased in most patients with leukemia *1781*

Lactate Dehydrogenase Isoenzyme-1 *Serum* *Increase* In 145 patients with leukemia mean activity of 161.0 ± 10.81 U/L significantly different from 35.5 ± 1.29 U/L in 150 healthy controls *4028*

208.10 Leukemia *(continued)*

Lactate Dehydrogenase Isoenzyme-2 *Serum Increase* In 145 patients with leukemia mean activity of 232.9 ± 16.17 U/L significantly different from 43.2 ± 1.32 U/L in 150 healthy controls *4028*

Lactate Dehydrogenase Isoenzyme-3 *Serum Increase* In 145 patients with leukemia mean activity of 144.6 ± 13.38 U/L significantly different from 26.6 ± 0.74 U/L in 150 healthy controls *4028*

Lactate Dehydrogenase Isoenzyme-4 *Serum Increase* In 145 patients with leukemia mean activity of 30.7 ± 4.35 U/L significantly different from 6.3 ± 0.26 U/L in 150 healthy controls *4028*

Lactate Dehydrogenase Isoenzyme-5 *Serum Increase* In 145 patients with leukemia mean activity of 9.2 ± 4.17 U/L not significantly different from 3.6 ± 0.16 U/L in 150 healthy controls *4028*

Lysophosphatidic Acid *Serum No Effect* In 5 patients with leukemia median concentration of 0.1 μmol/L not significantly different from 0.1 μmol/L in 48 healthy controls *5758*

α-Mannosidase *White Blood Cells Increase* Leukemic cells from 5 of 19 patients with leukemia had increased activity of enzyme *1781*

Metallopanstimulin *Serum Increase* In 100% of 7 patients with leukemia or lymphoma mean concentration exceeded upper limit of normal of < 10 ng/mL in healthy individuals aged 19 - 88 years *1462*

5-Methyl-2'-Deoxycytidine *Urine Increase* In 35 patients with active leukemia mean excretion of 1.69 ± 0.96 nmol/μmol creatinine significantly different from 0.90 ± 0.43 nmol/μmol creatinine in 81 healthy individuals, but mean of 1.40 ± 1.14 nmol/μmol/creatinine not significantly different *2368*

β_2-Microglobulin *Cerebrospinal Fluid Increase* In 17 patients with CNS leukemia or non-Hodgkins lymphoma mean concentration of 5.29 mg/L (range of 0.18 - 16.0) significantly higher than mean ± 2 SD of 1.01 ± 0.14 mg/L in control patients *5421*

Mucoprotein *Serum Increase* Mean concentration in 145 patients with leukemia of 233.5 ± 8.57 mg/dL significantly higher than 87.0 ± 1.83 mg/dL in 150 healthy controls *4029*

N^1-Acetylspermidine *Urine Increase* In 12 patients with initial stage of a variety of leukemias mean concentration of 10.30 μmol/g creatinine and 20.00 μmol/g creatinine significantly different from 1.99 μmol/g creatinine in 32 healthy controls *2973*

N^1-Acetylspermine *Urine Increase* In 12 patients with initial stage of a variety of leukemias mean concentration of 2.39 μmol/g creatinine and 2.12 μmol/g creatinine significantly different from 0.10 μmol/g creatinine in 32 healthy controls *2973*

N^1,N^{12}-Diacetylspermine *Urine Increase* In 12 patients with initial stage of a variety of leukemias mean concentration of 2.68 μmol/g creatinine and 4.76 μmol/g creatinine significantly different from 0.08 μmol/g creatinine in 32 healthy controls *2973*

N^8-Acetylspermidine *Urine Increase* In 12 patients with initial stage of a variety of leukemias mean concentration of 3.94 μmol/g creatinine and 6.68 μmol/g creatinine significantly different from 2.71 μmol/g creatinine in 32 healthy controls *2973*

N-Acetyl-Glucosaminidase *White Blood Cells Increase* Activity increased in leukocyte homogenates from 6 of 19 patients with unspecified leukemia and correlated with monocyte count *1781*

N-Acetylcadaverine *Urine No Effect* In 12 patients with initial stage of a variety of leukemias mean concentration of 4.60 μmol/g creatinine and 3.92 μmol/g creatinine not significantly different from 2.79 μmol/g creatinine in 32 healthy controls *2973*

N-Acetylputrescine *Urine Increase* In 12 patients with initial stage of a variety of leukemias mean concentration of 26.60 μmol/g creatinine and 37.40 μmol/g creatinine significantly different from 8.27 μmol/g creatinine in 32 healthy controls *2973* In 13 patients with acute or chronic leukemia mean concentration of about 60 mg/L significantly greater than that in 32 healthy adults in whom the mean concentration was approximately 8 mg/L *5075*

N-Acetylspermidine *Urine Increase* In 13 patients with acute or chronic leukemia mean concentration of about 21 mg/L significantly greater than that in 32 healthy adults in whom the mean concentration was approximately 3 mg/L *5075*

5-Nucleotide Phosphodiesterase Isoenzyme V
Serum Increase Mean activity was increased in the plasma of 2 of 3 patients with no initial evidence of liver metastases but in whom these were confirmed 3 to 6 months later *1781*

Phosphate *Serum Decrease* Low concentrations may occur in various forms of leukemia, usually secondary to hypercalcemia, but also be due to excessive uptake or retention of phosphate by leukemic cells *1781*
Serum Increase Hyperphosphatemia may occur *5204*

Phosphohexoseisomerase *Serum Increase* Activity increased in plasma of 87 - 91% of patients with all forms of leukemia *1781*

Phospholipase A_2 Type I *Serum Increase* Concentration reported as high as 194 μg/L in febrile leukemia compared with 2 and 4 μg/L in healthy controls *3767*

Plasminogen Activator Inhibitor-1
Cerebrospinal Fluid Increase In 9 patients with leukemia mean concentration of 1.28 ± 0.36 ng/mL significantly different from 0.31 ± 0.06 ng/mL in 20 reference individuals *56*

Putrescine *Urine Increase* In 12 patients with initial stage of a variety of leukemias mean concentration of 3.50 μmol/g creatinine and 5.26 μmol/g creatinine significantly different from 0.98 μmol/g creatinine in 32 healthy controls *2973* In 13 patients with acute or chronic leukemia mean concentration of about 18 mg/L significantly greater than that in 32 healthy adults in whom the mean concentration was approximately 2 mg/L *5075*

Ribonuclease *Serum Increase* In 13 patients with leukemia mean activity of 376 ± 85 U/mL significantly higher than 266 ± 39 U/mL in 15 normal individuals *2793*

Sialic Acid, Lipid-associated *Serum Increase* Mean concentration in 145 patients with leukemia of 39.4 ± 1.12 mg/dL significantly higher than 19.4 ± 0.38 mg/dL in 150 healthy controls *4029* In patients with leukemia mean concentration increased above 20 mg/dL in 90% of patients *1781*

Soluble L-Selectin *Cerebrospinal Fluid Increase* Increased concentration detected with meningeal leukemia but not in those without meningeal involvement *613*

Spermidine *Urine Increase* In 12 patients with initial stage of a variety of leukemias mean concentration of 3.47 μmol/g creatinine and 4.68 μmol/g creatinine significantly different from 0.50 μmol/g creatinine in 32 healthy controls *2973* In 13 patients with acute or chronic leukemia mean concentration of about 3.3 mg/L significantly greater than that in 32 healthy adults in whom the mean concentration was approximately 0.6 mg/L *5075*

Spermine *Urine Increase* In 13 patients with acute or chronic leukemia mean concentration of about 1.8 mg/L significantly greater than that in 32 healthy adults in whom the mean concentration was approximately 1.0 mg/L *5075* In 12 patients with initial stage of a variety of leukemias mean concentration of 4.63 μmol/g creatinine and 6.41 μmol/g creatinine significantly different from 0.58 μmol/g creatinine in 32 healthy controls *2973*

Zinc *Serum Decrease* In 17 patients with various forms of leukemia mean concentration significantly decreased by 7.2% in whole blood *1781*

Benign Neoplasms

210.40 Benign Tumor of the Mouth

Sialic Acid *Serum No Effect* Mean concentration in 60 patients with benign tumors of the mouth of 58.3 ± 8.3 mg/dL not significantly different from 55.0 ± 7.2 mg/dL in 80 healthy controls *5755*

211.10 Benign Neoplasm of Stomach

Albumin *Serum Decrease* Secondary to protein-losing enteropathy in adenocarcinoma *4707*

Fucose *Serum Increase* Total concentration was increased in patients with both malignant and benign tumors. The glycoprotein-bound fraction was very markedly elevated in cases of malignancy and not in benign disease. Mucoprotein fraction was raised in both diseases *5170*

Hematocrit *Blood Decrease* With occult bleeding, iron deficiency anemia may be present, in which case the bone marrow will not contain iron *4891*

Hemoglobin *Blood Decrease* With occult bleeding, iron deficiency anemia may be present, in which case the bone marrow will not contain iron *4891*

β-Hexosaminidase *Serum Increase* Elevated *5229*

Iron *Bone Marrow Decrease* With occult bleeding, iron deficiency anemia may be present, in which case the bone marrow will not contain iron *4891*
Serum Decrease With occult bleeding, iron deficiency anemia may be present *4891*

Iron-binding Capacity, Total *Serum Increase* Anemia is commonly iron deficient type, due to chronic blood loss *4891*

Iron Saturation *Serum Decrease* Anemia is commonly iron deficient type, due to chronic blood loss *4891*

MCH *Blood Decrease* With occult bleeding, iron deficiency anemia may be present *4891*

MCHC *Blood Decrease* With occult bleeding, iron deficiency anemia may be present *4891*

MCV *Blood Decrease* With occult bleeding, iron deficiency anemia may be present *4891*

Occult Blood *Feces Increase* Adenomatous and villous polyps may result in GI bleeding *4891*

211.10 Gastric Polyps

Pepsinogen I *Serum No Effect* In 18 patients with gastric polyps mean concentration of 36.3 ± 18.9 μg/L not significantly different from 49.0 ± 30.8 μg/L in 116 healthy controls *2761*

Pepsinogen II *Serum No Effect* In 18 patients with gastric polyps mean concentration of 19.9 ± 12.2 μg/L not significantly different from 18.1 ± 13.3 μg/L in 116 healthy controls *2761*

211.30 Adenoma of Colon

Ferritin *Serum Decrease* Serum ferritin concentration of 84.5 ± 4.4 ng/mL in 92 patients with colorectal adenomas greater than 1 cm in diameter significantly different from 101.4 ± 4.3 ng/mL in 92 healthy controls *2696*
Serum No Effect Serum ferritin concentration of 100.8 ± 6.0 ng/mL in 92 patients with colorectal adenomas less than 1 cm in diameter not significantly different from 101.4 ± 4.3 ng/mL in 92 healthy controls *2696*

HIV p53 Antigen *Plasma Increase* In 54 cases mean concentration of 0.44 ng/mL with concentration greater with increasing size of adenoma compared with mean of 0.12 ng/mL in 47 normal controls *3166*

25-Hydroxy Vitamin D *Serum No Effect* In 146 patients with colonic adenoma mean concentration of 56.4 ± 2.0 nmol/L not significantly different from 55.8 ± 1.9 nmol/L in 158 healthy controls *1749*

Iron *Serum Decrease* Serum iron concentration of 93.4 ± 3.4 μg/dL in 92 patients with colorectal adenomas greater than 1 cm in diameter significantly different from 103.6 ± 3.1 μg/dL in 92 healthy controls *2696*
Serum No Effect Serum iron concentration of 96.3 ± 3.3 μg/dL in 92 patients with colorectal adenomas less than 1 cm in diameter not significantly different from 103.6 ± 3.1 μg/dL in 92 healthy controls *2696*

211.30 Colonic Polyps

α_1-Antitrypsin *Feces No Effect* Mean concentration in 19 patients with colonic polyps of 623.8 μg/g (100.37 mg/d) not significantly different from 327.4 μg/g (47.43 mg/d) in 20 healthy controls *4521*

Hemoglobin *Feces No Effect* Mean concentration in 19 patients with colonic polyps of 3.4 μg/g (0.60 mg/d) not significantly different from 1.5 μg/g (0.15 mg/d) in 20 healthy controls *4521*

Neutrophil Elastase *Feces No Effect* Mean concentration in 19 patients with colonic polyps of 0.8 μg/g (0.13 mg/d) not significantly different from 0.6 μg/g (0.11 mg/d) in 20 healthy controls *4521*

211.40 Benign Neoplasm of Rectum and Anus

Carcinoembryonic Antigen *Serum Increase* 14 (15%) of 93 adult patients with sporadic colorectal adenomata had concentration > 2.5 ng/mL. No associations were found with age, polyp volume, or villous histology *1218* 19% of patients had values > 2.5 ng/mL *4891*

Chenocholic Acid *Serum No Effect* Mean concentration in 10 men with colorectal adenoma of 1.89 ± 1.37 nmol/L not significantly different from 1.23 ± 0.74 nmol/L in 12 healthy controls. In 8 women with adenomas mean concentration of 1.23 ± 0.74 nmol/L not significantly different from 1.07 ± 0.46 nmol/L in 9 healthy controls *344*

Cholesterol *Feces Increase* Although the total fecal neutral sterol concentrations were not different between the groups, the patients with familial polyposis excreted a high amount of cholesterol and low levels of coprostanol and coprostanone compared with other groups. Increased cholesterol and decreased lithocholic acid is excreted in patients with familial polyposis *4300* The fecal excretion of cholesterol, coprostanol, coprostanone, total bile acids, deoxycholic acid, lithocholic acid was higher in patients with colon cancer and patients with adenomatous polyps compared to normal American and Japanese controls as well as in patients with other digestive diseases *4301*

Cholic Acid *Serum No Effect* In 10 men with colorectal adenoma mean concentration of 0.49 ± 0.24 nmol/L not significantly different from 0.59 ± 0.50 nmol/L in 12 healthy controls. In 8 women with adenoma mean concentration of 0.42 ± 0.21 nmol/L not significantly different from 0.44 ± 0.23 nmol/L in 9 healthy controls *344*

Deoxycholic Acid *Feces Increase* The fecal excretion was higher in patients with colon cancer and patients with adenomatous polyps compared to normal American and Japanese controls as well as patients with other digestive diseases *4301*
Serum Increase Mean concentration in 10 men of 1.62 ± 0.62 nmol/L with colorectal adenoma significantly higher than 0.87 ± 0.45 nmol/L in 12 healthy controls, and in 8 women with colorectal adenomas mean of 1.19 ± 0.53 nmol/L higher than 0.89 ± 0.46 nmol/L in 9 healthy controls *344*

Lithocholic Acid *Feces Decrease* Increased cholesterol and decreased lithocholic acid is excreted in patients with familial polyposis *4300*
Feces Increase The fecal excretion of cholesterol, coprostanol, coprostanone, total bile acids, deoxycholic acid, lithocholic acid was higher in patients with colon cancer and patients with adenomatous polyps compared to normal American and Japanese controls as well as in patients with other digestive diseases *4301*
Serum No Effect Mean concentration of 0.44 ± 0.23 nmol/L in 10 men with colorectal adenoma not significantly different from 0.36 ± 0.14 nmol/L in 12 healthy controls. Mean concentration of 0.45 ± 0.13 nmol/L in 8 women with colorectal adenoma not significantly different from 0.41 ± 0.24 nmol/L in 9 healthy control women *344*

Occult Blood *Feces Increase* Adenomatous and villous polyps may result in GI bleeding *4891* Large amount of mucus tinged with blood; frequent watery diarrhea *5544*

Potassium *Serum Decrease* Sometimes decreased *5544*

Ursodeoxycholic Acid *Serum No Effect* In 10 men with colorectal adenoma mean concentration of 0.34 ± 0.13 nmol/L not significantly different from 0.37 ± 0.11 nmol/L in 12 healthy controls. In 8 women with colorectal adenoma mean concentration of 0.55 ± 0.25 nmol/L not significantly different from 0.35 ± 0.25 nmol/L in 9 healthy controls *344*

211.40 Colorectal Adenoma

Ferritin *Serum Decrease* In 184 patients with colorectal adenomas mean concentration in patients with adenomas > 1 cm of 85.4 ng/mL less than 100.8 ng/mL in patients with adenomas < 1 cm and 101.4 ng/mL in 92 control men *2696*

Iron *Serum Decrease* In 184 patients with colorectal adenomas mean concentration in patients with adenomas > 1 cm of 93.4 μg/dL less than 96.3 μg/dL in patients with adenomas < 1 cm and 103.6 μg/dL in 92 control men *2696*

211.40 Colorectal Polyps

α_1-Antitrypsin *Feces* *No Effect* In 10 patients with colorectal polyps concentrations no different than in 95% normal dry weight values of a symptomatic control group *3593*

CA 72-4 *Serum* *Increase* In 77 patients with colorectal polyps 4 (5%) had a concentration greater than cut-off of 2.5 U/mL with median concentration of 1.5 U/mL *4505*

Carcinoembryonic Antigen *Serum* *Increase* In 77 patients with colorectal polyps 4 (13%) had a concentration greater than cut-off of 3 ng/mL with median value of 1.9 ng/mL *4505* In 14 nonsmokers with colorectal polyps concentration of 0.73 µg/L (Roche) and 1.48 µg/L (Hybritech) compared with 0.41 µg/L (Roche) and 1.69 µg/L (Hybritech) in 20 nonsmoking controls and 2.33 µg/L (Roche) and 4.00 (Hybritech) in 14 smokers with colorectal polyps compared with 1.72 µg/L (Roche) and 3.71 µg/L (Hybritech) in 9 healthy smoking controls *4751* In 58 patients with rectal polyps 77.6% had concentrations up to 3.0 ng/mL, 13.8% had concentrations between 3.1 - 5.0 ng/mL, 5.2% between 5.1 - 10.0 ng/mL and 3.4% had concentrations above 10.1 ng/mL in contrast to concentrations in 151 healthy nonsmokers in whom 95.4% had concentrations between 0 and 3.0 ng/mL and 4.6% between 4.1 and 10.0 ng/mL *11* In 90 patients with rectal polyps 81% had concentrations less than 2.5 ng/mL, 15% had concentrations between 2.6 and 5.0 ng/mL, 3% had concentrations between 5.1 and 10.0 ng/mL and 1% had concentrations greater than 10.0 ng/mL *2010* In 93 patients with colorectal polyps 15% of patients had concentrations greater than 2.5 ng/mL, two-thirds of whom had concentrations between 2.5 ng/mL and 4.0 ng/mL *1218*

Gastrin *Serum* *No Effect* In 89 patients with colorectal polyps mean concentration of 20 pmol/L not significantly different from 21 pmol/L in 101 age-matched controls *5423*

Metallopanstimulin *Serum* *Increase* In all of 4 patients with colorectal polyps mean concentration exceeded upper limit of normal of < 10 ng/mL in healthy individuals aged 19 - 88 years *1462*

211.60 Benign Neoplasm of Pancreas

Glucose *Serum* *Decrease* Decreased glucose due to excess insulin in pancreatic islet cell *1290*

Glucose Tolerance *Serum* *Increase* Flat peak. Late hypoglycemia *5544*

Insulin *Plasma* *Increase* Elevated levels of plasma insulin following an overnight fast, as well as increased concentrations of C-peptide or proinsulin, strongly suggest the presence of insulinoma *2039* Characteristic finding *245* Fasting blood insulin level over 50 µU/mL in presence of low or normal blood glucose level. Intravenous tolbutamide or administration of leucine causes rapid rise to very high levels within a few minutes with rapid return to normal *5544*

Insulin Tolerance *Plasma* *Decrease* An excessive fall in the blood sugar may occur in pancreatic islet cell hyperplasia *1290*

Phosphate *Serum* *Decrease* Hyperinsulinism; during successful treatment of diabetic ketosis, insulin causes phosphate ions to enter the cells with glucose and potassium *1290* *5544*

Potassium *Serum* *Decrease* Gastrointestinal wasting as a result of pancreatic islet nonbeta cell tumors *3735*

Proinsulin *Plasma* *Increase* Elevated levels of plasma insulin following an overnight fast, as well as increased concentrations of C-peptide or proinsulin, strongly suggest the presence of insulinoma *2039*

211.70 Glucagonoma

Glucagon *Plasma* *Increase* Increased concentrations may occur with glucagonoma *2952*

211.70 Insulinoma

C-Peptide *Plasma* *Increase* In hypoglycemic patients with increased plasma C-peptide concentration may have an insulinoma *2952*

Glucose *Serum* *Decrease* In 2 patients with insulinoma mean concentrations of 1.9 mmol/L and 1.7 mmol/L significantly different from normal range of 4.0 - 6.2 mmol/L *3332*

Growth Hormone *Plasma* *No Effect* In 2 patients with insulinoma mean concentrations of 0.3 and 2.7 µg/L within normal range of 0 - 20 µg/L *3332*

Insulin-like Growth Factor-I *Serum* *No Effect* In 2 patients with insulinoma mean concentrations of 76 and 86 µg/L within normal range of 90 - 360 µg/L *3332*

Insulin-like Growth Factor-II *Serum* *No Effect* In 2 patients with insulinoma mean concentrations of 640 and 825 µg/L within normal range of 490 - 1,056 µg/L *3332*

Insulin-like Growth Factor Binding Protein-3 *Serum* *No Effect* In 2 patients with insulinoma mean concentrations of 2.1 and 3.5 µg/mL within normal range of 1.7 - 4.0 µg/mL *3332*

211.90 Adenomatous Polyp of Alimentary Tract

Ferritin *Serum* *Decrease* In 725 patients with serum ferritin concentration of less than 50 ng/mL detected in 6 patients with adenomatous polyps > 1.0 cm *2968*

Hydrochloric Acid *Gastric Fluid* *Decrease* Gastric analysis - achlorhydria in 85% of patients. Polyps occur in 5% of patients with pernicious anemia and 2% of patients with achlorhydria *5544*

pH *Gastric Material* *Increase* Gastric analysis - achlorhydria in 85% of patients. Polyps occur in 5% of patients with pernicious anemia and 2% of patients with achlorhydria *5544*

212.30 Nonmalignant Pulmonary Disease

Progastrin-Releasing Peptide (31-98) *Serum* *No Effect* Mean concentration in 20 patients with nonmalignant pulmonary disease of 15.2 ± 6.7 ng/L not significantly different from that in 247 healthy individuals (12.6 ± 6.9 ng/L) *159*

212.60 Thymoma

Acetylcholine Receptor Modulating Antibodies *Serum* *Increase* Detectable in most patients with thymoma with myesthenia gravis *2952*

Immunoglobulin E *Serum* *Decrease* In 9 patients with thymoma and hypogammaglobulinemia mean concentration of 4.4 ng/mL (range 3.4 - 6.0) significantly less than mean of 96 ng/mL (range 24 - 386) in 74 healthy controls *2323*

212.70 Benign Neoplasm of Cardiovascular Tissue

Aspartate Aminotransferase *Serum* *Increase* May reflect many small emboli to striated muscle *5544*

C-Reactive Protein *Serum* *Increase* May be increased in myxoma of left atrium *5544*

Erythrocyte Sedimentation Rate *Blood* *Increase* Reflection of abnormal serum proteins *5544* Occurs with myxoma, possibly reflecting tumor emboli or tumor breakdown products *2304*

Erythrocyte Survival *Red Blood Cells* *Decrease* Occurs with myxoma, possibly reflecting tumor emboli or tumor breakdown products *2304* Hemolytic anemia of mechanical origin (due to local turbulence of blood) may occur and may be severe. The anemia is recognized in about 50% of the patients *5544*

γ-Globulin *Serum* *Increase* Recognized to be increased in about 50% of patients *5544* Occurs with myxoma, possibly reflecting tumor emboli or tumor breakdown products *2304*

Hematocrit *Blood* *Decrease* Occurs with myxoma, possibly reflecting tumor emboli or tumor breakdown products *2304* Hemolytic anemia of mechanical origin (due to local turbulence of blood) may occur and may be severe. The anemia is recognized in about 50% of patients *5544*

Hemoglobin *Blood* *Decrease* Occurs with myxoma, possibly reflecting tumor emboli or tumor breakdown products *2304* Hemolytic anemia of mechanical origin (due to local turbulence of blood) is usual and may be severe. The anemia is recognized in about 50% of patients with this tumor *5544*
Blood *Increase* Often elevated without arterial hypoxemia in right atrial myxoma *2304*

Lactate Dehydrogenase *Serum* *Increase* Reflects hemolysis *5544*

Leukocytes *Blood* *Increase* Occurs with myxoma, possibly reflecting tumor emboli or tumor breakdown products *2304* *Urine* *Increase* Occasionally *5544*

Platelets *Blood* *Decrease* May be decreased (possibly mechanical) with resultant findings due to thrombocytopenia *5544*

Reticulocytes *Blood* *Increase* Hemolytic anemia of mechanical origin (due to local turbulence of blood) is usual and may be severe. The anemia is recognized in about 50% of patients with this tumor *5544*

217.00 Benign Breast Disease

α_1-Acid Glycoprotein *Serum* *No Effect* In 9 patients with benign breast disease (fibroadenoma or fibroadenosis) mean concentration below upper limit of reference range of 0.88 g/L *924*

Alkaline Phosphatase *Serum* *No Effect* In 9 patients with benign breast disease (fibroadenoma or fibroadenosis) mean concentration below upper limit of reference range of 90 U/L *924*

Alkaline Phosphatase, Placental Isoenzyme *Serum* *No Effect* In 9 patients with benign breast disease (fibroadenoma or fibroadenosis) mean concentration below upper limit of reference range of 0.85 U/L *924*

α_1-Antitrypsin *Serum* *No Effect* In 9 patients with benign breast disease (fibroadenoma or fibroadenosis) mean concentration below upper limit of reference range of 3.2 g/L *924*

Apolipoprotein D *Serum* *No Effect* In 26 patients with benign breast disease mean concentration not significantly different from concentration in 28 healthy women 95% confidence interval (50 - 125 mg/L, median 73.5 mg/L) *3944*

Bicarbonate *Serum* *Increase* In 42% of 14 patients at initial hospitalization for this disorder *1576*

c-erb-B_2 Oncoprotein *Serum* *No Effect* In 56 women with benign breast disease (28 fibroadenomas and 28 with fibrocystic disease) all had concentrations less than 15 U/mL. Of the 56, 55% had undetectable concentrations *3563* In 56 women with benign breast disease none had concentrations exceeding 15 U/mL (in 50 healthy women concentrations ranged from < 3 to 14.9 U/mL) *3562*

CA 15-3 *Serum* *No Effect* In 42 women with benign breast disease using a cutoff of 32 U/mL only 1 (3%) had an increased concentration *1071* In 25 patients with benign breast disease (fibrocystic disease, fibroadenoma, cysts, mastalgia, mastitis etc) mean concentration of 15.5 ± 9 U/mL not significantly different from cutoff of 22 U/mL *2076* In 56 women with benign breast disease none had concentrations exceeding cutoff of 35 U/mL *3562*

CA 27-29 *Serum* *No Effect* In 42 women with breast cancer using a cutoff of 46.5 U/mL none had an increased concentration *1071*

CA 549 *Serum* *No Effect* In women with benign breast disease using a cutoff of 12.5 kU/L specificity of 94.8% obtained *764* In 173 patients with benign disease of the breast none had a concentration greater than 30.0 kU/L with BRESMARQ assay *764* None of 54 patients with benign breast disease had a concentration above 11 U/mL *5260* None of 10 patients with benign breast disease had a concentration above 11 U/mL *5260*

Calcitonin *Plasma* *No Effect* In 9 patients with benign breast disease (fibroadenoma or fibroadenosis) mean concentration below upper limit of reference range of < 0.1 µg/L *924*

Carcinoembryonic Antigen *Serum* *Increase* 15% of patients had values > 2.5 ng/mL *4891* In 115 patients with benign breast disease 85% had concentrations less than 2.5 ng/mL, 11% had concentrations between 2.6 and 5.0 ng/mL, 4% had concentrations between 5.1 and 10.0 ng/mL and 0% had concentrations greater than 10.0 ng/mL *2010* In 43 women with benign breast disease 88.4% had concentrations of 0.0 - 3.0 ng/mL, 7.0% had concentrations from 3.1 - 5.0 ng/mL, 4.6% had concentrations from 5.1 - 10.0 ng/mL and 0.0% had concentrations greater than 10.0 ng/mL when measured by method on Bayer Technicon Immuno 1® system compared with 95.9%, 3.5%, 0.6% and 0.0% respectively in 173 healthy nonsmokers *339* *Serum* *No Effect* In 56 women with benign breast disease none had concentrations exceeding cutoff of 5 ng/mL *3562* In 9 patients with benign breast disease (fibroadenoma or fibroadenosis) mean concentration below upper limit of reference range of 20 µg/L *924* In 42 women with breast cancer using a cutoff of 4 ng/mL only 1 (3%) had an increased concentration *1071*

Casein *Serum* *No Effect* In one of 7 patients with benign breast disease casein detectable at a concentration of 350 µg/L *2113*

Ceruloplasmin *Serum* *No Effect* In 9 patients with benign breast disease (fibroadenoma or fibroadenosis) mean concentration below upper limit of reference range of 0.45 g/L *924*

β-Chorionic Gonadotropin *Plasma* *No Effect* In 9 patients with benign breast disease (fibroadenoma or fibroadenosis) mean concentration below upper limit of reference range of < 2 µg/L *924*

C-Reactive Protein *Serum* *No Effect* In 9 patients with benign breast disease (fibroadenoma or fibroadenosis) mean concentration below upper limit of reference range of 10 mg/L *924*

CYFRA 21-1 *Serum* *No Effect* In 25 patients with benign breast disease median concentration of 1.1 ng/mL not significantly different from that in 50 healthy individuals with median concentration of 1.2 ng/mL and range of 0.5 - 2.4 ng/mL *3559*

Ferritin *Serum* *No Effect* In 9 patients with benign breast disease (fibroadenoma or fibroadenosis) mean concentration below upper limit of reference range of 150 µg/L *924*

Fucose *Serum* *Increase* Total concentration was increased in patients with both malignant and benign tumors. The glycoprotein-bound fraction was very markedly elevated in cases of malignancy and not in benign disease. Mucoprotein fraction was raised in both diseases *5170*

Growth Hormone *Plasma* *Increase* Elevated *1870*

Haptoglobin *Serum* *No Effect* In 9 patients with benign breast disease (fibroadenoma or fibroadenosis) mean concentration below upper limit of reference range of 4.1 g/L *924*

Hemopexin *Serum* *No Effect* In 9 patients with benign breast disease (fibroadenoma or fibroadenosis) mean concentration below upper limit of reference range of 3.6 g/L *924*

Hydroxyproline *Urine* *No Effect* In 9 patients with benign breast disease (fibroadenoma or fibroadenosis) mean hydroxyproline:creatinine ratio below upper limit of reference range of 35 *924*

α-Lactalbumin *Serum* *No Effect* In 9 patients with benign breast disease (fibroadenoma or fibroadenosis) mean concentration below upper limit of reference range of 20 µg/L *924*

Lysozyme *Serum* *No Effect* In 9 patients with benign breast disease (fibroadenoma or fibroadenosis) mean concentration below upper limit of reference range of 9 g/L *924*

Phosphate *Serum* *Decrease* In 43% of 32 patients at initial hospitalization for this disorder *1576*

Polymorphic Epithelial Mucin *Serum* *No Effect* In 60 women with benign breast disease median concentrations of 19 kU/L by ACS BR, 18 kU/L by Centocor CA 15-3, 17 kU/L by Enzynmun-Test CA 15-3 and 15 kU/L by IMx CA 15-3 not significantly different from concentrations in 250 healthy women (mean and 1 SD concentrations of 22 ± 8.8 kU/L by ACS BR, 19 ± 8.8 kU/L by Centocor CA 15-3, 17 ± 7.1 kU/L by Enzymun-Test CA 15-3 and 15 ± 6.4 kU/L by IMx CA 15-3 respectively) *513*

Prealbumin *Serum* *Increase* Mean concentration in 28 patients with benign breast disease 230 ± 10 mg/L significantly different from 215 ± 15 mg/L in 25 elderly healthy controls *4359*

Pregnancy-associated α-Macroglobulin *Serum* *No Effect* In 9 patients with benign breast disease (fibroadenoma or fibroadenosis) mean concentration below upper limit of reference range of 140 g/L *924*

Pregnanediol *Urine* *Decrease* Average daily values were lower in 109 women with benign disease than normal women. No change was found in plasma estradiol *3381*

Progesterone *Plasma* *Decrease* Average daily values were lower in 109 women with benign disease than normal women. No change was found in plasma estradiol *3381*

Putrescine *Urine* *No Effect* In 9 patients with benign breast disease (fibroadenoma or fibroadenosis) mean concentration below upper limit of reference range of 9 mg/g creatinine *924*

217.00 Benign Breast Disease *(continued)*

Retinol *Serum* *Decrease* Mean concentration in 28 patients with benign breast disease 2.5 ± 0.2 μmol/L significantly reduced compared with 3.4 ± 0.3 μmol/L in 25 elderly healthy controls *4359*

Retinol-binding Protein *Serum* *Decrease* Mean concentration in 28 patients with benign breast disease of 44 ± 1 mg/L significantly reduced compared with 54 ± 2 mg/L in 25 elderly healthy controls *4359*

Sialyltransferase *Serum* *No Effect* In 9 patients with benign breast disease (fibroadenoma or fibroadenosis) mean concentration below upper limit of reference range of 90 U/L *924*

SP2 *Serum* *No Effect* Eight of 54 patients with benign breast disease had a concentration of 14 U/mL and 6 had a concentration of 15 U/mL when the upper limit of normal was 14 U/mL *5260*

Spermidine *Urine* *No Effect* In 9 patients with benign breast disease (fibroadenoma or fibroadenosis) mean concentration below upper limit of reference range of 2.7 mg/g creatinine *924*

Thrombospondin *Plasma* *Increase* Mean concentration of 691 ± 702 ng/mL in 10 patients with benign breast disease significantly different from 190 ± 42 ng/mL observed in 15 healthy men and 17 women *2074*

Thymidine Kinase *Serum* *No Effect* In 18 women with benign breast disease mean activity of 2.7 ± 0.6 U/L not significantly different from 2.8 ± 0.4 U/L in 30 age-matched healthy control women *3284*

Tissue Polypeptide Antigen *Serum* *No Effect* In 18 women with benign breast disease mean activity of 58 ± 6.2 U/L not significantly different from 54 ± 5.5 U/L in 30 healthy age-matched control women *3284*

217.00 Benign Breast Tumor

c-erb-B_2 Oncoprotein *Serum* *No Effect* Mean concentration in 51 patients with benign breast tumors of 3,211 ± 737 HNU/mL not significantly different from 3,271 ± 809 HNU/mL in 60 healthy controls *580*

Urokinase Plasminogen Activator *Tissue* *No Effect* Median concentration in 21 cases of benign breast tumors of 0.049 ng/mg protein *1258*

Urokinase Plasminogen Activator Receptor *Tissue* *No Effect* Median concentration in 21 cases of benign breast tumors of 0.093 ng/mg protein *1258*

Vascular Endothelial Growth Factor *Serum* *No Effect* In 18 women with benign breast tumors median concentration of 57 pg/mL (range 18 - 328 pg/mL) not significantly different from concentration in healthy control women *4539*

217.00 Fibroadenoma of Breast

c-erb-B_2 Oncoprotein *Serum* *No Effect* In 28 women with fibroadenoma of the breast none had concentrations exceeding 15 U/mL *3562*

CA 15-3 *Serum* *No Effect* In 28 women with fibroadenoma of the breast none had concentrations exceeding 35 U/mL *3562*

Carcinoembryonic Antigen *Serum* *No Effect* In 28 women with fibroadenoma of the breast none had concentrations exceeding 5 ng/mL *3562*

Tissue Inhibitor of Metalloproteinase-1 *Serum* *Increase* Median concentration of 1.0 ng/mg protein in 15 patients with primary carcinomas *3393*

218.90 Uterine Leiomyoma

CA 125 *Serum* *Increase* False positive result *3909*
Serum *No Effect* In 51 premenopausal women with uterine myomas > 14 weeks mean concentrations in follicular and luteal phases of 18.8 ± 2.4 U/mL and 21.5 ± 3.7 U/mL respectively compared with 15.9 ± 1.5 U/mL and 15.8 ± 1.3 U/mL respectively in 30 normal women *1042*

Estradiol *Plasma* *No Effect* In 51 premenopausal women with uterine myoma of > 14 weeks gestation mean concentration in follicular phase of 94.6 ± 19.0 pg/mL and 128.7 ± 24.8 pg/mL in luteal phase not significantly different from normal *1042*

Estrone *Plasma* *No Effect* Mean concentration in 51 premenopausal women with uterine myomas > 14 weeks gestation of 91.9 ± 11.5 pg/mL in follicular phase and 105.8 ± 11.2 pg/mL in luteal phase not significantly different from normal *1042*

Insulin-like Growth Factor-I *Serum* *Increase* In 51 premenopausal women with uterine leiomyomas mean concentration in follicular and luteal phases of 2,006 ± 185 mU/mL and 2,335 ± 287 mU/mL compared with 1,702 ± 120 mU/mL and 1,774 ± 239 mU/mL respectively in 30 normal women (not significantly different) *1042*

Progesterone *Plasma* *No Effect* In 51 premenopausal women with uterine myomas > 14 weeks mean concentration in follicular phase 1.5 ± 0.4 ng/mL and 9.6 ± 1.6 ng/mL in luteal phase not significantly different from normal *1042*

220.00 Benign Neoplasm of Ovary

Androgens *Plasma* *Increase* Observed effect *900*

CA 125 *Serum* *Increase* In 30 patients with benign neoplasms of the ovary median concentration of 18.2 kU/L not significantly different from 10.9 kU/L in 39 age-matched controls *1117* In 211 women with benign ovarian tumors median concentration of 21 U/mL significantly higher than 4 U/mL in 458 healthy women *2203*

D-Dimer *Plasma* *Increase* In 30 patients with benign neoplasms of the ovary median concentration of 325 μg/L not significantly different from 240 μg/L in 39 age-matched controls *1117*

Estradiol *Plasma* *Increase* In estrogen producing tumors estradiol is the most active estrogen *91* *457* *3935*

Estrogens *Urine* *Increase* Observed effect *5544*

Follicle Stimulating Hormone *Urine* *Decrease* Inhibited by increased estrogen *5544*

Gonadotropin, Pituitary *Urine* *Decrease* Inhibited by increased estrogen *5544*

Interleukin-6 *Serum* *No Effect* In 49 patients with benign ovarian tumors mean concentration of 0.5 pg/mL and median concentration of 0.0 pg/mL *4676*

17-Ketosteroids *Urine* *Increase* May be slightly increased in arrhenoblastoma. May be moderately increased in Leydig cell tumors in masculinizing ovarian tumors *5544*

Lactate Dehydrogenase *Serum* *No Effect* In 11 cases of benign solid ovarian tumors activity normal *1591*

Macrophage Colony Stimulating Factor *Serum* *No Effect* In 72 patients with benign ovarian tumors mean concentration of 742.2 ± 256.6 U/mL not significantly lower than baseline normal of 1,056 U/mL *5094*

Pregnanediol *Urine* *Decrease* Absent in ovarian tumors *5545*

Progesterone *Plasma* *Decrease* Absent in ovarian tumors *5545*

Soluble Interleukin-2 Receptor-α *Cyst Fluid* *Increase* In 31 patients with benign tumors of the ovary mean concentration of 616 ± 846 U/mL *1052*
Serum *No Effect* In 28 patients with benign tumors of the ovary mean concentration of 469 ± 144 U/mL not significantly different from 390 ± 124 U/mL in 50 healthy female blood donors *1052*

Steroid Sulfatase *Serum* *Increase* Using a cutoff of 130 ng/mL positive rate of 22.2% observed compared with 69.2% for patients with ovarian carcinomas *5072*

Testosterone *Serum* *Increase* Plasma testosterone levels are elevated and confirmatory *900*

Tetranectin *Serum* *Decrease* In 211 women with benign ovarian tumors mean concentration of 10.0 ± 1.9 mg/L significantly less than 11.6 ± 2.0 mg/L in 458 healthy women *2203*

Thrombin/Antithrombin III Complex *Plasma* *No Effect* In 30 patients with benign neoplasms of the ovary median concentration of 2.25 μg/L not significantly different from 2.3 μg/L in 39 age-matched controls *1117*

220.00 Teratoma (Dermoid)

α-Fetoprotein *Serum* *No Effect* Typical observation *5545*

220.92 Granulosa Cell Tumor of Ovary

Estrogens *Plasma* *Increase* Estrogens are increased in granulosa cell tumor of ovary *5545*
Urine *Increase* Normal urinary excretion of total estrogens will be below 10 µg/d. Values > 20 µg/d are suggestive of a granulosa cell tumor *900*

Follicle Stimulating Hormone *Urine* *Decrease* Inhibited by increased estrogen *5544*

17-Ketosteroids *Plasma* *Increase* Ketosteroids are increased in virilizing ovarian tumors (e.g., adrenal rest tumor, granulosa cell tumor, hilar cell tumor, Brenner tumor, and most frequently, arrhenoblastoma) increased in 50% of patients and normal in 50% of the patients *5544*
Urine *Increase* Urine 17-KS may be slightly increased in arrhenoblastoma. May be markedly increased in adrenal tumors of ovary. May be moderately increased in Leydig cell tumors in masculinizing ovarian tumors *5544*

Pregnanediol *Urine* *Decrease* Absent in ovarian tumors *5545*

Progesterone *Plasma* *Decrease* Absent in ovarian tumors *5545*

220.93 Lutein Cell Tumor of Ovary

Estrogens *Plasma* *Increase* Estrogens are increased in luteoma of ovary *5544*
Urine *Increase* Observed effect *5544*

Follicle Stimulating Hormone *Urine* *Decrease* Inhibited by increased estrogen *5544*

17-Ketogenic Steroids *Urine* *Increase* Increased in lutein cell tumor of the ovary if androgenic *5544*

17-Ketosteroids *Plasma* *Increase* Ketosteroids are increased in virilizing ovarian tumors (e.g., adrenal rest tumor, granulosa cell tumor, hilar cell tumor, Brenner tumor, and most frequently, arrhenoblastoma) increased in 50% of the patients and normal in 50% of the patients *5544*
Urine *Increase* Urine 17-KS may be slightly increased in arrhenoblastoma. May be markedly increased in adrenal tumors of ovary. May be moderately increased in Leydig cell tumors in masculinizing ovarian tumors *5544*

Pregnanediol *Urine* *Decrease* Absent in ovarian tumors *5545*

Progesterone *Plasma* *Decrease* Absent in ovarian tumors *5545*

220.94 Theca Cell Tumor of Ovary

Estrogens *Plasma* *Increase* Estrogens are increased in theca-cell tumor of ovary *5544*
Urine *Increase* Observed effect *1290*

Follicle Stimulating Hormone *Urine* *Decrease* Inhibited by increased estrogen *5544*

17-Ketosteroids *Plasma* *Increase* Ketosteroids are increased in virilizing ovarian tumors (e.g., adrenal rest tumor, granulosa cell tumor, hilar cell tumor, Brenner tumor, and most frequently, arrhenoblastoma) increased in 50% of the patients and normal in 50% of the patients *5544*
Urine *Increase* Urinary 17-KS may be slightly increased in arrhenoblastoma. May be markedly increased in adrenal tumors of ovary. May be moderately increased in Leydig cell tumors in masculinizing ovarian tumors *5544*

Pregnanediol *Urine* *Decrease* Absent in ovarian tumors *5545*

Progesterone *Plasma* *Decrease* Absent in ovarian tumors *5545*

220.95 Androgenic Arrhenoblastoma

17-Ketosteroids *Urine* *Increase* Excretion may be increased in patients with androgenic arrhenoblastoma *2952*

220.95 Arrhenoblastoma

17-Ketosteroids *Urine* *Increase* May be slightly increased in arrhenoblastoma. May be moderately increased in Leydig cell tumors in masculinizing ovarian tumors *5544*

Pregnanediol *Urine* *Increase* In arrhenoblastoma of ovary *5545*

Progesterone *Plasma* *Increase* In arrhenoblastoma of ovary *5545*

221.80 Benign Gynecological Tumors

D-Dimer *Plasma* *No Effect* In 26 patients with benign gynecological tumors median concentration of 340 µg/L compared with 240 µg/L in 31 age-matched control women *5418*

Prothrombin Fragment 1.2 *Plasma* *No Effect* In 26 patients with benign gynecological tumors median concentration of 1.00 nmol/L compared with 1.10 nmol/L in 31 age-matched control women *5418*

Thrombin/Antithrombin III Complex *Plasma* *No Effect* In 26 patients with benign gynecological tumors median concentration of 2.5 µg/L compared with 2.3 µg/L in 31 age-matched control women *5418*

222.00 Benign Neoplasm of Testis

Estrogens *Urine* *Increase* Observed effect *1290*

17-Ketogenic Steroids *Urine* *Increase* The 17-ketosteroids occasionally are elevated when a Leydig cell tumor is present *900*

225.20 Meningioma

α_1-Antichymotrypsin *Serum* *No Effect* Mean concentration within reference interval of 47.9 ± 8.1 mg/dL in one examined patient with meningioma *3044*

225.90 Benign Neoplasm of Brain and CNS

α_1-Acid Antitrypsin *Cerebrospinal Fluid* *Increase* Mean concentration in 21 patients with benign intracranial tumors of 1.78 ± 1.13 mg/dL compared with 0.70 ± 0.30 mg/dL in 38 controls *1632*
Serum *Increase* Mean concentration in 21 patients with benign intracranial tumors of 358.6 ± 156.2 mg/dL compared with 315.8 ± 45.8 mg/dL in 40 controls *1632*

Aldolase *Serum* *Increase* The serum of cancer patients contains a greater proportion of aldolase A (muscle-type) than serum from normal persons. Gliomas and normal brain tissue contain aldolase C (nerve and brain variant), but in meningiomas or tissue metastatic to brain, only aldolase A (liver and fetal form) is detected *4692*

Antidiuretic Hormone *Plasma* *Increase* Associated with excessive ADH production resulting in sodium loss *4707*

Aspartate Aminotransferase *Serum* *Increase* In 31% of 22 patients at initial hospitalization for this disorder *1576*

Bicarbonate *Serum* *Increase* In 74% of 16 patients at initial hospitalization for this disorder *1576*

Carcinoembryonic Antigen *Serum* *Increase* In 14 patients with nonmalignant CNS disease 85.7% had concentrations of 0.0 - 3.0 ng/mL, 14.3% had concentrations from 3.1 - 5.0 ng/mL, 0.0% had concentrations from 5.1 - 10.0 ng/mL and 0.0% had concentrations greater than 10.0 ng/mL when measured by method on Bayer Technicon Immuno 1® system compared with 95.9%, 3.5%, 0.6% and 0.0% respectively in 173 healthy non-smokers *339*

Cells *Cerebrospinal Fluid* *Increase* Reported effect *1980* Elevated from 5 - 100 /µL in 33% of cases. May exceed 1,000 /µL, particularly if the tumor involves the ventricular wall and has undergone necrosis *367*

β-Galactosidase *Serum* *Decrease* Mean serum concentration in patients with tumors (both benign and malignant) were depressed to 0.065 ± 0.009 mmol/min/L, compared to 0.243 ± 0.038 in normals *2288*

225.90 Benign Neoplasm of Brain and CNS (continued)

Glomerular Filtration Rate *Urine* *Increase* Associated excess ADH may tend to accelerate GFR *4707*

Glucose *Cerebrospinal Fluid* *Decrease* Values are characteristically < 40 mg/dL in patients with diffuse neoplastic involvement of the meninges, but are normal in other tumors of the brain *367*

Hematocrit *Blood* *Increase* In 22% of 22 patients at initial hospitalization for this disorder *1576*

Hemoglobin *Blood* *Increase* In 31% of 22 patients at initial hospitalization for this disorder *1576*

Immunoglobulin G *Cerebrospinal Fluid* *Increase* No consistent CSF IgG pattern was found in brain tumors, but highly vascularized tumors had increased concentrations *5138*

Protein *Cerebrospinal Fluid* *Increase* Total CSF protein is increased. Individual increase of proteins depended on the degree of blood/CSF barrier damage *2288* Protein content > 100 mg/dL is associated with rapidly growing tumors near the ventricles or subarachnoid space. Slowly growing tumors may have only slightly elevated or normal values *367* In acoustic neuromas nearly always high (100 - 500 mg/dL). Cerebellar tumors usually have normal or only moderately increased protein (20 - 100 mg/dL) *1980*

Sodium *Serum* *Decrease* Serum sodium usually less than 130 mEq/L *126* Associated with excessive ADH production *4707*
Urine *Increase* Urine is almost always hypertonic to plasma *126*

Uric Acid *Serum* *Increase* In 31% of 22 patients at initial hospitalization for this disorder *1576*

Zinc *Cerebrospinal Fluid* *Decrease* Significantly less *1353*

226.00 Thyroid Adenoma

PDN-21 *Serum* *No Effect* In 5 patients with follicular thyroid adenomas concentrations did not exceed upper limit of normal of 67 pg/mL in 98 healthy controls *5137*

227.00 Adrenal Adenoma

Aldosterone *Plasma* *No Effect* Mean concentration of 0.24 nmol/L in 4 patients with adrenal adenomas not significantly different from reference range of 0.14 - 0.42 nmol/L *5350*

Corticotropin *Plasma* *Decrease* Mean concentration in 2 patients with primary adrenal insufficiency of 2.1 pmol/L less than range in 50 healthy Caucasian volunteers of 4.4 - 18 pmol/L *3605*
Plasma *No Effect* Mean concentration of about 2.8 pmol/L in 4 patients with adrenal adenomas not significantly different from reference range of 1.94 - 11.2 pmol/L *5350*

Cortisol *Plasma* *Increase* Mean concentration of 630 nmol/d in 4 female patients with adrenal adenomas significantly different from reference range of 138 - 331 nmol/L *5350* Mean concentration of 973 ± 266 nmol/L in 10 patients with adrenal adenoma significantly greater than that in 50 healthy Caucasian volunteers, 344 ± 81 nmol/L *3605*
Urine *Increase* Mean concentration in 10 patients with adrenal adenoma of 717 ± 537 nmol/d significantly greater than that in 50 healthy Caucasian volunteers, 130 ± 104 nmol/d *3605* Mean concentration in 2 patients with Cushing's disease of 687 nmol/d significantly greater than that in 50 healthy Caucasian volunteers, 130 ± 104 nmol/d *3605*

Cortisone *Plasma* *Increase* Mean concentration in 10 patients with adrenal adenoma of 125 ± 50.3 nmol/L significantly greater than that in 50 healthy Caucasian volunteers, 51.4 ± 16.7 nmol/L *3605*
Urine *Increase* Mean concentration in 10 patients with adrenal adenoma of 1.55 ± 0.39 nmol/d greater than that in 50 healthy Caucasian volunteers, 0.52 ± 0.29 nmol/d *3605* Mean concentration in 2 patients with Cushing's disease of 1.05 nmol/d greater than that in 50 healthy Caucasian volunteers, 0.52 ± 0.29 nmol/d *3605*

17-Hydroxycorticosteroids *Urine* *Increase* Mean concentration of 52.2 µmol/d in 4 patients with adrenal adenomas significantly different from reference range of 11.0 - 22.1 µmol/d *5350*

18-Hydroxycortisol *Serum* *Increase* Mean concentration of 7.95 ± 6.02 nmol/L in 4 female patients with adrenal adenomas significantly different from reference range of 2.44 ± 0.39 nmol/L in women *5350*
Urine *Increase* Mean excretion of 487 ± 339 nmol/d in 4 female patients with adrenal adenomas significantly different from reference range of 173 ± 27 nmol/d in women *5350*

18-Oxycortisol *Serum* *Increase* Mean concentration of 0.27 ± 0.14 nmol/L in 4 female patients with adrenal adenomas significantly different from reference range of 0.16 ± 0.04 nmol/L in women *5350*
Urine *Increase* Mean excretion of 9.04 ± 6.16 nmol/d in 4 female patients with adrenal adenomas significantly different from reference range of 3.59 ± 0.66 nmol/d in women *5350*

Renin Activity *Plasma* *No Effect* Mean concentration of 2.2 ng/L/s in 4 patients with adrenal adenomas not significantly different from reference range of 1.1 - 4.1 ng/L/s *5350*

227.00 Benign Neoplasm of Adrenal Cortex

Cortisol *Plasma* *Increase* Basal plasma concentrations may be normal or raised at 9 h and raised at 23 h *5863*

Dehydroepiandrosterone Sulfate *Plasma* *Increase* Observed effect *91* *3778*

11-Hydroxycorticosteroids *Urine* *Increase* In Cushingoid patients *5863*

17-Ketogenic Steroids *Urine* *Increase* May be normal or raised *5863*

17-Ketosteroids *Urine* *Increase* In Cushing's patients with adrenocortical adenoma *5863*

227.30 Nonfunctioning Pituitary Adenoma

β-Chorionic Gonadotropin *Plasma* *Increase* In 77 patients with a nonfunctioning pituitary adenoma mean baseline concentration undetectable in all except 7 patients in whom concentrations 0.05 to 0.72 U/L *1732*
Plasma *No Effect* In 7 patients in whom concentrations of β-subunit of chorionic gonadotropin exceeded 0.04 U/L, concentrations of chorionic gonadotropin were within reference interval of < 5 U/L *1732* In 77 patients with a nonfunctioning pituitary adenoma mean baseline concentration undetectable in all except 7 patients in whom concentrations 0.05 to 0.72 U/L *1732*

Follicle Stimulating Hormone *Plasma* *Increase* In 7 patients in whom concentrations of β-subunit of chorionic gonadotropin exceeded 0.04 U/L, concentrations of follicle stimulating hormone were within reference interval of 0.25 - 8 U/L except for two patients in whom the concentrations were 13.3 and 21.0 U/L *1732*
Plasma *No Effect* In 7 patients in whom concentrations of β-subunit of chorionic gonadotropin exceeded 0.04 IU/L, concentrations of follicle stimulating hormone were within reference interval of 0.25 - 8 IU/L except for two patients in whom the concentrations were 13.3 and 21.0 IU/L *1732*

Luteinizing Hormone *Plasma* *No Effect* In 7 patients in whom concentrations of β-subunit of chorionic gonadotropin exceeded 0.04 U/L, concentrations of luteinizing hormone were within reference interval of 0.2 - 6.5 U/L except for one patient in whom the concentration was 9.5 U/L *1732*

α-Subunit *Plasma* *Increase* In 7 patients in whom concentrations of β-subunit of chorionic gonadotropin exceeded 0.04 U/L, concentrations of α-subunit were within reference interval of < 0.1- 0.9 µg/L except for two patients in whom the concentrations were 4.3 and 4.8 µg/L *1732*
Plasma *No Effect* In 7 patients in whom concentrations of β-subunit of chorionic gonadotropin exceeded 0.04 U/L, concentrations of α-subunit were within reference interval of < 0.1- 0.9 µg/L except for two patients in whom the concentrations were 4.3 and 4.8 µg/L *1732*

Thyroid Stimulating Hormone *Serum* *No Effect* In 7 patients in whom concentrations of β-subunit of chorionic gonadotropin exceeded 0.04 U/L, concentrations of thyroid stimulating hormone were within reference interval of 0.26 - 5 U/L except for one patient in whom the concentration was 0.1 mU/L *1732*

227.30 Pituitary Adenoma

Calcitonin *Plasma* *No Effect* In one patient with acromegaly and hyperthyroidism due to a growth hormone-, thyrotropin- and α-subunit-secreting pituitary adenoma mean concentration normal at 28 ng/L *3078*

Calcium *Serum* *No Effect* In one patient with acromegaly and hyperthyroidism due to a growth hormone-, thyrotropin- and α-subunit-secreting pituitary adenoma mean concentration normal at 2.50 mmol/L *3078*

β-Chorionic Gonadotropin *Plasma* *No Effect* In 20 patients with a growth hormone secreting adenoma mean baseline concentration undetectable as in healthy controls *1732*

C-terminal Telopeptide of Type I Collagen *Serum* *Increase* Mean concentration of 8.7 ± 5.0 µg/L in 10 patients with TSH-secreting pituitary adenomas significantly different compared with 3.8 ± 1.6 µg/L in 61 healthy control adults *4089*

Follistatin, Free *Serum* *No Effect* Mean concentration in 5 patients with pituitary adrenomas not significantly different from 3.5 ± 0.2 µg/L in 60 normal individuals *4523*

Gastrin *Serum* *No Effect* In one patient with acromegaly and hyperthyroidism due to a growth hormone-, thyrotropin- and α-subunit-secreting pituitary adenoma mean concentration normal at 47 ng/L *3078*

Glucose *Serum* *No Effect* In one patient with acromegaly and hyperthyroidism due to a growth hormone-, thyrotropin- and α-subunit-secreting pituitary adenoma mean concentration within normal limits *3078*

Growth Hormone *Plasma* *Increase* In one patient with acromegaly and hyperthyroidism due to a growth hormone-, thyrotropin- and α-subunit-secreting pituitary adenoma mean concentration significantly increased to 14.3 µg/L *3078*

Insulin-like Growth Factor-I *Serum* *Increase* In one patient with acromegaly and hyperthyroidism due to a growth hormone-, thyrotropin- and α-subunit-secreting pituitary adenoma mean concentration significantly increased to 7.3 kU/L *3078*

Parathyroid Hormone *Plasma* *No Effect* In one patient with acromegaly and hyperthyroidism due to a growth hormone-, thyrotropin- and α-subunit-secreting pituitary adenoma mean concentration normal at 0.7 pmol/L *3078*

α-Subunit of Glycoprotein Hormones *Plasma* *Increase* Fourteen of 63 patients with nonfunctioning pituitary tumors (22%) had increased concentration with monoclonal assay *3923*

Thyroid Stimulating Hormone *Serum* *Increase* Mean concentration of 3.8 ± 2.8 mU/L in 10 patients with TSH-secreting pituitary adenomas significantly different compared with 1.2 ± 0.4 mU/L in 61 healthy control adults *4089* In one patient with acromegaly and hyperthyroidism due to a growth hormone-, thyrotropin- and α-subunit-secreting pituitary adenoma mean concentration significantly increased to 2.9 mU/L *3078*

Thyroxine (T4), Free *Serum* *Increase* In one patient with acromegaly and hyperthyroidism due to a growth hormone-, thyrotropin- and α-subunit-secreting pituitary adenoma mean concentration significantly increased to 38 pmol/L *3078* Mean concentration of 38.9 ± 18.2 pmol/L in 10 patients with TSH-secreting pituitary adenomas significantly different compared with 14.3 ± 1.8 pmol/L in 61 healthy control adults *4089*

Tri-iodothyronine, Free (fT3) *Serum* *Increase* Mean concentration of 13.0 ± 5.2 pmol/L in 10 patients with TSH-secreting pituitary adenomas significantly different compared with 6.0 ± 1.1 pmol/L in 61 healthy control adults *4089* In one patient with acromegaly and hyperthyroidism due to a growth hormone-, thyrotropin- and α-subunit-secreting pituitary adenoma mean concentration significantly increased to 13 pmol/L *3078*

227.91 Chromaffin Cell Tumors

Catecholamines *Urine* *Increase* In 6 patients with pheochromocytomas or paragangliomas excretions ranged from 145 µg/d to 560 µg/d compared with less than 120 µg/d in healthy individuals *2343*

Epinephrine *Plasma* *Increase* In 6 patients with paragangliomas or pheochromocytomas concentrations ranged from 12 to 1,340 pg/mL compared with less than 60 pg/mL in healthy controls *2343*

Norepinephrine *Plasma* *Increase* Concentrations in 6 patients with paragangliomas or pheochromocytomas ranged from 786 pg/mL to 7,518 pg/mL compared with less than 300 pg/mL in healthy controls *2343*

227.91 Pheochromocytoma

Albumin *Urine* *Increase* In 6 patients with adrenal pheochromocytoma mean excretion of 47.68 ± 31.11 mg/d significantly greater than 9.08 ± 3.92 mg/d in 39 healthy controls *3087*

α_1-Antitrypsin *Urine* *Increase* In 6 patients with adrenal pheochromocytoma mean excretion of 1.58 ± 1.64 mg/d significantly greater than 0.12 ± 0.44 mg/d in 39 healthy controls *3087*

Calcitonin *Plasma* *Increase* Observed effect *3485*

Calcium *Serum* *Increase* May be caused by ectopic parathyroid hormone production in a few patients but usually results from associated parathyroid hyperplasia in the familial cases *900* Can occur, disappearing after removal of the tumor *1980* Hypercalcemia can occur independently or in association with coexistent hyperparathyroidism *1980*

Catecholamines *Plasma* *Increase* Usually very high, there is significant overlap with values that may be obtained with excitement, emotional disturbance, essential hypertension and depression *367* Twice upper limit of normal *2039* In pediatric cases, venous catheterization showed a great increase in catecholamine efflux from the left adrenal vein, while dopamine-β-hydroxylase (DBH) was only slightly elevated. Circulating catecholamines fluctuated greatly during removal of tumors, but DBH decreased gradually *2102*
Urine *Increase* Of the 3 different types of catecholamines present in the urine - the metanephrine test is positive in more than 97% of patients with the disease and is rarely falsely positive in hypertensive subjects who do not have the disease *2559* Most excrete > 300 µg/d *2304*

Cholesterol *Serum* *No Effect* No characteristic changes *2304*

Chromogranin-A *Serum* *Increase* Mean concentration in 45 patients with pheochromocytoma significantly higher than that in 21 healthy volunteers in heparin/glutathione plasma (16.3 - 21.5 U/L with upper limit of normal of 30.4 U/L) but with 13 patients (29%) having concentrations below the upper limit of normal *524* In 10 patients with pheochromocytoma mean concentration of 4,435 µg/L significantly different from 36 ± 18 µg/L in 100 normal individuals *329*

Dopamine *Urine* *Increase* Increased concentration observed in 9 of 18 patients with proved pheochromocytoma, always in association with increased epinephrine or norepinephrine excretion *3430*

Dopamine β-Hydroxylase *Serum* *Increase* In pediatric cases, venous catheterization showed a great increase in catecholamine efflux from the left adrenal vein, while dopamine-β-hydroxylase (DBH) was only slightly elevated. Circulating catecholamines fluctuated greatly during removal of tumors, but DBH decreased gradually *2102*

Epinephrine *Plasma* *Increase* In 44 patients with pheochromocytoma plasma concentration greater than 0.54 nmol/L and/or epinephrine concentration of less than 3.0 mmol/L *2994* In 90 - 95% of patients with pheochromocytomas plasma concentrations greater than 110 pg/mL *2952* In 5 patients with pure epinephrine secreting tumors plasma concentration increased 2- to 4- fold *1710*
Urine *Increase* In 19 patients with pheochromocytoma excretion normal in 4 (21%), moderately increased in 3 (16%) and markedly increased in 12 (63%) *1710* Increased concentration observed in 8 of 18 patients with proved pheochromocytoma, typically more than twice the upper limit of normal *3430* Among hypertensive patients a pheochromocytoma is highly likely when

227.91 Pheochromocytoma *(continued)*

Epinephrine *(continued)*
the urinary excretion is greater than 35 µg/d *2952* In almost all patients, analysis of any 24 h urine collection will reveal increased excretion *367*

Erythrocytes *Blood Increase* Erythrocytosis associated with pheochromocytoma *5534*
Urine Increase Gross or microscopic hematuria may occur early *900*

Erythropoietin *Serum Increase* Large amounts *4450*

Fatty Acids (FFA), Free *Serum Increase* Plasma insulin levels are inappropriately low and free fatty acids are correspondingly high *900* May be elevated *1980*

Gastrin *Serum Increase* In a few patients, elevated concentrations have become normal after tumor resection *4891*

Glucose *Serum Increase* Attacks may be accompanied by hyperglycemia and glucosuria *5863* Fasting level is elevated in about 50% the patients, usually only slightly above normal values *2304* May be elevated *1980*
Urine Increase Usually intermittent *2304* Attacks may be accompanied by hyperglycemia and glucosuria *5863*

Glucose Tolerance *Serum Decrease* Impaired glucose tolerance which may be misdiagnosed as diabetes mellitus *367* May be decreased because of suppressed insulin release and catecholamine-induced insulin resistance *1980*

Hematocrit *Blood Increase* Occasionally found and may be due to a decreased plasma volume, a true increase in RBC mass, or both *900* Hemoconcentration is not uncommon *1980* Hemoconcentration can cause increased hematocrit and plasma proteins *1980*

Hemoglobin *Blood Increase* Hemoconcentration is not uncommon *1980*

Homovanillic Acid *Urine Increase* Increased in neuroblastomas, benign ganglioneuromas, and pheochromocytomas *3600* increased excretion observed in patients with pheochromocytoma *2952*
Urine No Effect Patients with pheochromocytoma excrete normal amounts *4091*

Hydroxy-Methoxymandelic Acid *Urine Increase* Increased concentration observed in 13 of 16 patients with proved pheochromocytoma, all of whom had increased excretion of at least one catecholamine *3430*

Insulin *Plasma Decrease* May be a decreased glucose tolerance because of suppressed insulin release and catecholamine-induced insulin resistance *1980* Plasma levels are inappropriately low for the simultaneous blood glucose *900*

Isocitrate Dehydrogenase *Serum No Effect* No effect on activity observed *5008*

Metanephrine *Plasma Increase* In one patient with pheochromocytoma who did not have an increased plasma normetanephrine concentration plasma metanephrine concentration was significantly increased *2994*
Urine Increase In 41 of 52 patients with pheochromocytoma showed increased excretions of greater than 6.8 µmol/d *2994* In 20 patients with active pheochromocytoma mean excretion of 16.4 µmol/d compared with 1.8 ± 1.3 µmol/d in 16 patients with cured pheochromocytoma *2131* In 8 patients with pheochromocytoma mean excretion of 13.0 ± 11.3 µmol/d compared with 0.93 ± 0.51 µmol/d in hypertensive men aged over 35 years *2529* In 19 patients excretion moderately increased in 3 (17%) and markedly increased in 15 (83%) *1710*

Metanephrines, Total *Plasma Increase* Values should be twice upper limit of normal *2039*
Urine Increase In almost all patients, analysis of any 24 h urine collection will reveal increased excretion *367* Of the 3 different types of catecholamines present in the urine - the metanephrine test is positive in more than 97% of patients with the disease and is rarely falsely positive in hypertensive subjects who do not have the disease *2559*

Neuron-specific Enolase *Serum Increase* In 10 patients with pheochromocytoma mean concentration of 22.6 µg/L significantly different from normal range of < 12.5 µg/L *329*

Norepinephrine *Plasma Increase* In 11 of 13 patients with pheochromocytoma concentrations were 7.1 - 110 nmol/L significantly different from 0.47 - 4.12 nmol/L in healthy individuals *4449* In 90 - 95% of patients with pheochromocytomas plasma concentrations greater than 750 pg/mL *2952* Blood levels of norepinephrine and to a lesser extent, epinephrine are increased, usually even when patient is asymptomatic and normotensive; rarely are increases found only following a paroxysm *5544*
Plasma No Effect In 44 patients with pheochromocytoma plasma concentration less than 3.0 nmol/L and/or increased plasma epinephrine concentration *2994*
Urine Increase In almost all patients with pheochromocytoma, analysis of any 24 h urine collection will reveal increased excretion of norepinephrine *367* In 11 of 13 patients with pheochromocytoma concentrations were 867 - 33,000 nmol/d significantly different from 50 - 571 nmol/d in healthy individuals *4449* Urine levels of norepinephrine and, to a lesser extent, epinephrine are increased, usually even when patient is asymptomatic and normotensive; rarely are increases found only following a paroxysm *5544* In 19 patients concentration normal in 6 (32%), moderately increased in 2 (11%) and markedly increased in 11 (58%) *1710* Increased concentration observed in 16 of 18 patients with proved pheochromocytoma, typically more than twice the upper limit of normal *3430* Among hypertensive patients a pheochromocytoma is highly likely when the urinary excretion is greater than 170 µg/d *2952*

Normetanephrine *Plasma Increase* In 52 patients with pheochromocytoma plasma concentration increased above 0.66 mmol/L in 51 *2994*
Urine Increase In 19 patients with pheochromocytoma excretion normal in 3 (17%), moderately increased in 3 (17%) and markedly increased in 12 (67%) *1710* In 8 patients with pheochromocytoma mean excretion of 23.3 ± 35.0 µmol/d compared with reference interval of 2.10 ± 1.10 µmol/d in hypertensive men aged over 35 years *2529*

Phosphate *Serum Decrease* May be caused by ectopic parathyroid hormone production in a few patients but usually results from associated parathyroid hyperplasia in the familial cases *900*

Potassium *Serum Decrease* High plasma renin activity has been noted and may result in mild hypokalemia *900*

Proline Hydroxylase *Serum Increase* Elevated to a lesser degree than that seen in hepatoma *762*

Protein *Serum Increase* Hemoconcentration can cause increased hematocrit and plasma proteins *1980*

Vanillylmandelic Acid *Serum Increase* Values should be twice upper limit of normal (normal < 6.8 mg/day) *2039*
Urine Increase Phenolic acids of dietary origin may yield many false positive tests *2304* In almost all patients analysis of any 24 h urine collection will reveal increased excretion *367* In 19 patients excretion normal in 3 (16%), moderately increased in 3 (16%) and increased in 13 (66%) *1710* False positive results may occur due to certain foods and certain drugs. Monamine oxidase inhibitors may increase metanephrine and decrease VMA. Excretion is considerably increased *5544* Excretion > 2 times normal is diagnostic providing all dietary restrictions have been followed *5863* In 8 patients with pheochromocytoma mean excretion of 108.5 ± 88.3 µmol/d compared with reference interval of 10 to 54 µmol/d in hypertensive men *2529* Reported effect *3600*

Volume *Plasma Decrease* Low in < 33% of patients *900*
Red Blood Cells Decrease Decreased in the hypertension resulting from pheochromocytoma *3710*

228.09 Hemangioendothelioma

Endothelin-1 *Plasma Increase* In 2 patients with hemangioendothelioma mean concentration of 12.5 ± 1.8 pg/mL increased by 12-fold above normal range *328*

229.80 Benign Head and Neck Disease

CYFRA 21-1 *Serum Increase* In 10 patients with benign head and neck disease median concentration of 2.5 ng/mL significantly different from that in 50 healthy individuals with median concentration of 1.2 ng/mL and range of 0.5 - 2.4 ng/mL *3559*
Serum No Effect In 37 patients with benign tumors of the head or neck mean concentration of 0.74 ± 0.42 ng/mL not significantly different from 0.79 ± 0.29 ng/mL in 29 healthy controls *1230*

229.90 Benign Tumors

Carcinoembryonic Antigen *Serum* *No Effect* In 16 patients with unspecified benign tumors 100.0% had concentrations of 0.0 - 3.0 ng/mL, 0.0% had concentrations from 3.1 - 5.0 ng/mL, 0.0% had concentrations from 5.1 - 10.0 ng/mL and 0.0% had concentrations greater than 10.0 ng/mL when measured by method on Bayer Technicon Immuno 1® system compared with 95.9%, 3.5%, 0.6% and 0.0% respectively in 173 healthy non-smokers *339*

immunoglobulin A *Serum* *No Effect* In 57 women with benign tumors mean concentration of 181 ± 90 mg/dL not significantly different from 174 ± 80 mg/dL in 150 healthy control women *2278*

Immunoglobulin G *Serum* *No Effect* In 57 women with benign tumors mean concentration of 1,114 ± 226 mg/dL not significantly different from 1,157 ± 271 mg/dL in 150 healthy control women *2278*

Immunoglobulin M *Serum* *No Effect* In 57 women with benign tumors mean concentration of 89 ± 46 mg/dL not significantly different from 77 ± 39 mg/dL in 106 healthy controls *2278*

Ribonuclease *Serum* *Increase* In 29 sera from patients with benign tumors in Mayo Clinic Serum Bank mean activity of 376 ± 149 U/mL significantly higher than 273 ± 66 U/mL in sera from 21 normal individuals *2793*

233.00 Metastatic Breast Cancer

CA 15-3 *Serum* *Increase* 80% of all patients with metastases from breast cancer had increased marker concentrations several months before or at the time of the development of distant metastases *1556* *2400*

Carcinoembryonic Antigen *Serum* *Increase* 80% of all patients with metastases from breast cancer had increased marker concentrations several months before or at the time of the development of distant metastases *2400*

Colony Stimulating Factor-1 *Serum* *Increase* Mean concentration of 9.7 ± 0.8 ng/mL in 75 patients wih metastatic breast cancer significantly higher than 4.2 ± 0.2 ng/mL in 118 patients with primary cancer *4665*

Epidermal Growth Factor *Saliva* *No Effect* Median concentration of 1.16 ng/mL in 20 patients with breast cancer not significantly different from 1.85 ng/mL in a reference population *511*
Serum *No Effect* Median concentration of 1.41 ng/mL in 20 patients with breast cancer not significantly different from 0.96 ng/mL in a reference population *511*
Urine *No Effect* Median concentration of 15.5 ng/mg creatinine in 20 patients with breast cancer not significantly different from 11.9 ng/mg creatinine in a reference population *511*

Sialic Acid, Lipid-associated *Serum* *Increase* In 14 patients with metastatic breast cancer mean concentration of 66.4 mg/dL significantly different from 17.7 mg/dL in 50 normal volunteers *1273*

Urokinase Plasminogen Activator *Tissue* *Increase* Median concentration in 14 cases of metastatic breast cancer of 0.233 ng/mg protein significantly higher than 0.049 ng/mg protein in benign breast tumors *1258*

Urokinase Plasminogen Activator Receptor
Tissue *No Effect* Median concentration in 14 cases of metastatic breast cancer of 0.118 ng/mg protein not significantly higher than 0.093 ng/mg protein in benign breast tumors *1258*

Vascular Endothelial Growth Factor *Serum* *Increase* In 32 women with metastatic breast cancer median concentration of 186 pg/mL (range 7 - 1,347 pg/mL) not significantly different from that in 7 women with carcinoma in situ in whom the median concentration was 110 pg/mL (range 32 - 273 pg/mL) and not significantly different from concentration in healthy control women *4539*

235.20 Metastatic Cancer of Colon

α_1-Antichymotrypsin *Serum* *Increase* Mean concentration increased above reference interval of 47.9 ± 8.1 mg/dL in 2 of 2 patients (100%) with metastatic cancer of the colon *3044*

Sialic Acid, Lipid-associated *Serum* *Increase* In 9 patients with metastatic colon cancer mean concentration of 96.2 mg/dL significantly different from 17.7 mg/dL in 50 normal volunteers *1273*

235.70 Metastatic Lung Cancer

Carcinoembryonic Antigen *Serum* *No Effect* In patients with solitary metastatic carcinoma of the lung mean baseline concentration of 2.3 ng/mL compared with upper limit of normal of 3.0 ng/mL *4470*

Sialic Acid, Lipid-associated *Serum* *Increase* In 13 patients with metastatic lung cancer mean concentration of 108.9 mg/dL significantly different from 17.7 mg/dL in 50 normal volunteers *1273*

236.20 Metastatic Ovarian Cancer

Sialic Acid, Lipid-associated *Serum* *Increase* In 6 patients with metastatic ovarian cancer mean concentration of 82.3 mg/dL significantly different from 17.7 mg/dL in 50 normal volunteers *1273*

238.40 Polycythemia Rubra Vera

Alanine Aminotransferase *Serum* *No Effect* Normal in uncomplicated cases *3016* Activity typically normal *5677*

Albumin *Urine* *Increase* Occasionally *5699*

Alkaline Phosphatase *White Blood Cells* *Increase* Strikingly increased *3527* Three polycythemic patients showed elevations the mean of 82, compared with the mean of the normal group (25.8) and that of the group with chronic myelocytic leukemia (4.0) *354* Increase observed in 80% of patients *443* 70 - 90% of patients have above the upper limits of normal, while a small number of patients have normal values. No clinical or hematologic differences are apparent in patients with normal activity as compared with those with increased activity *147*

Anisocytes *Blood* *Increase* Mild anisocytosis and poikilocytosis may be seen in the peripheral blood *5677*

Antithrombin III *Plasma* *Decrease* Below normal in some patients *5127*

Antithrombin III Activity *Plasma* *Decrease* Mean activity in patients with polycythemia vera or essential thrombocythemia with thrombosis of 96.4 ± 18.5% significantly different from 105 .5 ± 16.2% in patients without thrombosis *663*

Aspartate Aminotransferase *Serum* *No Effect* Normal in uncomplicated cases *3016* Usually normal in typical case *5677*

Basophilic Stippling *Blood* *Increase* May be found *5699*

Basophils *Blood* *Increase* Slight to moderate persistent basophilia may occur *5677* Usually a mild basophilia *900* Increase in the absolute count (above 65 /µL) is observed in about 66% of cases *1728*
Bone Marrow *Increase* An unusually high number may be found *5699*

Bence-Jones Protein *Urine* *Present* Appears in the urine uncommonly *1290*

Bilirubin *Serum* *Increase* Rarely *2034* Increase observed in 56% of patients with the disease *443* Slightly elevated *405*

Bleeding Time *Patient* *No Effect* Usually no effect observed *5545*

Calcium *Serum* *Increase* Slight rise, cause unknown *1290*

Casts *Urine* *Increase* Occasionally *5699*

Cells *Bone Marrow* *Increase* Hyperplasia of erythroid, myeloid and megakaryocytic elements within those areas of the skeleton that normally contain active marrow. Marrow differential count may be normal or may reveal a reduction in the myeloid/erythroid ratio, reflecting a predominant normoblastic hyperplasia *5677*

Clot Retraction *Blood* *Decrease* A common defect has been the excessive number of untrapped RBCs after clot retraction (the escape phenomenon of excessive red cell fallout). An increased rate of retraction has also been observed *5677* A common defect has been the excessive number of untrapped RBCs after clot retraction (the escape phenomenon of excessive red cell fallout). An increased rate of retraction has also been

238.40 Polycythemia Rubra Vera *(continued)*

Clot Retraction *(continued)* observed *4286* *4443* Bleeding time and coagulation time are normal but clot retraction may be poor *5545*

Clotting Time *Blood* *No Effect* Usually no effect *5545*

Cryoglobulins *Serum* *Increase* Variable elevation of cryoglobulins *4707*

Eosinophils *Blood* *Increase* Sometimes eosinophilia *900*
Bone Marrow *Increase* An unusually high number may be found *5699*

Erythrocyte Sedimentation Rate *Blood* *Decrease* Characteristically decreased and may be 0 mm/h *5677*

Erythrocyte Survival *Red Blood Cells* *Decrease* As the disease progresses, there are increasing degrees of extramedullary ineffective hematopoiesis with progressive shortening of the red cell life-span secondary to increasing splenic sequestration *5677* *4169*
Red Blood Cells *No Effect* Red cell life span is normal as is arterial oxygen saturation *2039*

Erythrocytes *Blood* *Increase* RBC count is 7 - 12 million/μL; may increase to > 15 million/μL *5545* RBC > 6.5 million/μL in men and 5.6 million in women *1098*

Erythropoietin *Serum* *Decrease* Usually lower than normal or undetectable *2039* In 21 proved cases, concentrations were all < 5 mIU/mL (the limit of sensitivity) whereas 35 control subjects had a mean of 7.8 mIU/mL *1384* In 43 patients with polycythemia rubra vera mean concentration of 2.2 ± 2.6 IU/L compared with 9 ± 4 IU/L in 79 reference controls *4320*
Urine *Decrease* Poor sensitivity of the assay techniques prevents a reliable method to differentiate secondary polycythemia from polycythemia vera *900*

Factor V *Plasma* *Decrease* Low levels found *5127*

Fibrinogen *Plasma* *Decrease* Usually normal although a moderate decrease (115 - 200 mg/dL) was found in one study *5588*
Plasma *No Effect* Mean concentration in patients with polycythemia vera or essential thrombocythemia with thrombosis of 3.2 g/L not significantly different from 3.0 g/L in patients without thrombosis *663*

Glomerular Filtration Rate *Urine* *No Effect* GFR is kept to almost normal levels by an increased renal blood flow *5575* No obvious effect usually observed *5699*

Hematocrit *Blood* *Increase* Over 60% in males and 55% in females *900* Before treatment, hematocrit values range between 55 - 80% *2039* Increase observed in 100% of patients *443*
Blood *No Effect* Mean value in patients with polycythemia vera or essential thrombocythemia with thrombosis of 44.2% not significantly different from 44.2% in patients without thrombosis *663*

Hemoglobin *Blood* *Increase* In 43 patients with polycythemia rubra vera mean concentration of 185 ± 12.9 g/dL compared with 14.0 ± 1.1 g/dL in 79 reference controls *4320* Increase observed in 100% of patients *443*

Heterophile Antibody *Serum* *Decrease* Positive presumptive test but negative differential test if Forsman antigen is used *3953*
Serum *Increase* Positive presumptive test but negative differential test if Forsman antigen is used *3953*

Histamine *Plasma* *Increase* Present in the majority of patients with uncontrolled disease *5677* *1728*
Urine *Increase* Present in the majority of patients with uncontrolled disease *1728* *5677*

α_2-HS Glycoprotein *Serum* *No Effect* No significant change observed compared with healthy controls *2533*

Immunoglobulin G *Serum* *Increase* Significant diffuse increases in IgG and IgM have been noted *5677*

Immunoglobulin M *Serum* *Increase* Significant diffuse increases in IgG and IgM have been noted *5677*

Interleukin-1α *Serum* *No Effect* In 10 patients with polycythemia rubra vera, concentration not detectable as in 14 healthy controls *545*

Interleukin-1β *Serum* *No Effect* In 10 patients with polycythemia rubra vera, concentration not detectable as in 14 healthy controls *545*

Interleukin-2 *Serum* *Increase* In 10 patients with polycythemia rubra vera mean concentration of 207 ± 53 pg/mL significantly higher than undetectable amount in 14 healthy controls *545*

Interleukin-6 *Serum* *No Effect* In 10 patients with polycythemia rubra vera concentration not different from that in 14 healthy controls *545*

Interleukin-10 *Serum* *No Effect* In 10 patients with polycythemia rubra vera concentration not different from that in 14 healthy controls *545*

Iron *Bone Marrow* *Decrease* Decreased or absent bone marrow iron stores that are characteristic of this disease *5677* *1342*
Serum *Decrease* Decrease observed in 52% of all patients with the disease *443* Frequently decreased, reflecting therapeutic or spontaneous blood loss *5677*

Lactate Dehydrogenase *Serum* *No Effect* Normal in uncomplicated cases *5677*

Leukocytes *Blood* *Increase* Elevated in a majority of cases *1098* Increase observed in 50% of all patients with the disease *443* A peripheral leukocytosis, with an absolute granulocytosis, occurs in about 66% of cases *5677*
Blood *No Effect* Mean concentration in patients with polycythemia vera or essential thrombocythemia with thrombosis of 9.4 x 10^9/L not significantly different from 9.0 x 10^9/L in patients without thrombosis *663*

Lysozyme *Serum* *Increase* Significantly elevated, reflecting participation of the granulocyte in the proliferative process *5677* *453*

β_2-Microglobulin *Serum* *Increase* In 10 patients with polycythemia rubra vera mean concentration of 2,130 ± 562 μg/L significantly higher than 1,721 ± 673 μg/L in 14 healthy controls *545*

Myeloperoxidase *Granulocyte* *Increase* Mean density of 658 ± 72 in 11 patients with polycythemia rubra vera significantly different from 478 ± 52 in 32 normal controls *1303*

Naphthol-As-D-Chloroacetate Esterase
Granulocyte *No Effect* Mean density of 546 ± 83 in 13 patients with polycythemia rubra vera not significantly different from 478 ± 52 in 32 normal controls *1303*

Neopterin *Urine* *Increase* In patients with polycythemia vera mean excretion of about 300 μmol/mol creatinine significantly greater than 106.6 ± 34.6 μmol/mol in 31 healthy controls *3632*

Neutrophils *Blood* *Increase* An absolute granulocytosis is seen in the majority of patients with a circulatory count of 15,000 - 30,000 /μL *900* Occurs in about 66% of cases. Usually of moderate degree but extreme degrees are sometimes observed late in the course. A moderate shift to the left in the granulocyte series frequently accompanies the increase *5677*

Oxygen Saturation *Blood* *Decrease* Mild degrees of unsaturation may occur in patients with otherwise well-documented cases, uncomplicated by independent cardiac or pulmonary disease *3679* Arterial oxygen saturation is normal in early cases but mild desaturation is not unusual later in the course of the disease due to the complication of pulmonary emboli *900*
Blood *No Effect* Usually normal *5677* Nearly all patients with true polycythemia vera have a near normal arterial oxygen saturation *5587*

Phospholipase A *Serum* *Increase* Significantly elevated *2625*

Plasminogen Antigen *Plasma* *Decrease* Below normal in some patients *5127*

Platelets *Blood* *Increase* In 732 patients with platelet counts greater than 500,000 /μL, 2.5% had CML *1869* In about 50% of patients at time of diagnosis. Degree is usually modest, with counts in the range of 450,000 - 800,000 /μL *5677* Usually increased in number and counts as high as 3 million have been reported *367* Elevated in a majority of cases *1098* Increase observed in 62% of patients with the disease *443*
Blood *No Effect* Of 250 patients with platelet counts of more than 250,000 /μL, 22 had polycythemia rubra vera *3939* Mean concentration in patients with polycythemia vera or essential thrombocythemia with thrombosis of 635.8 x 10^9/L not significantly different from 688.8 x 10^9/L in patients without thrombosis *663*

Poikilocytes *Blood* *Increase* Mild anisocytosis and poikilocytosis may be seen in the peripheral blood *5677*

Potassium *Serum* *Increase* Has been reported in myeloproliferative disorders associated with thrombocytosis. May be spurious and related to K release from the increased number of platelets during the process of blood coagulation *3691* Associated with polycythemia *5677*

Procollagen Type III Peptide *Serum* *Increase* High values are observed in primary and post-polycythemia vera (PV) myelofibrosis, but excessive PC III levels in active PV are not predictive of evolution toward myelofibrosis *3711*

Protein C Activity *Plasma* *No Effect* Mean activity in patients with polycythemia vera or essential thrombocythemia with thrombosis of 78.7 ± 19.7% not significantly different from 85.6 ± 16.9% in patients without thrombosis *663*

Protein S Antigen *Plasma* *Decrease* Mean activity in patients with polycythemia vera or essential thrombocythemia with thrombosis of 111.7 ± 26.7% significantly different from 121.6 ± 24.5% in patients without thrombosis *663*

Prothrombin Time *Plasma* *No Effect* No effect observed *5588*

Pseudouridine *Urine* *No Effect* In patients with polycythemia vera mean excretion comparable to that in 31 healthy controls of 19.6 ± 5.2 mmol/mol creatinine *3632*

Reticulocytes *Blood* *Increase* Increase observed in 44% of all patients with the disease *443* Possibly increased *5544*

Soluble c-kit Molecule *Serum* *No Effect* Median concentration in patients with polycythemia rubra vera not significantly different from that in 51 healthy volunteers of 199.0 AU/mL *2598*

Soluble Interleukin-2 Receptor *Serum* *Decrease* In 10 patients with polycythemia rubra vera mean concentration of 172 ± 97 U/mL significantly lower than 582 ± 164 U/mL in 14 healthy controls *545*

Thromboplastin Generation *Blood* *No Effect* Conventional coagulation tests are usually normal *20* Usually unaffected by disease *5677*

Thrombopoietin *Plasma* *Increase* Mean plasma concentration in 34 patients with polycythemia rubra vera of 407 pg/mL significantly higher than the mean of 133 pg/mL in healthy individuals *3565*

Tumor Necrosis Factor-α *Serum* *Increase* In 10 patients with polycythemia rubra vera mean concentration of 10 ± 2.5 pg/mL different from 0 pg/mL in 14 healthy controls *545*

Uric Acid *Serum* *Increase* Increased RBC formation produces hyperuricemia and hyperuricosuria in 30 - 50% of patients at the time of diagnosis. Both tend to increase in frequency and severity as the disease progresses and may remain asymptomatic but approximately 5 - 10% of patients develop symptoms and signs of gout *5826* Increase observed in 54% of patients with the disease *443* Increased RBC formation produces hyperuricemia and hyperuricosuria in 30 - 50% of patients at the time of diagnosis. Both tend to increase in frequency and severity as the disease progresses and may remain asymptomatic but approximately 5 - 10% of patients develop symptoms and signs of gout *1729* *5677* High in a significant proportion of patients *2039*
Urine *Increase* Increased formation produces hyperuricemia and hyperuricosuria in 30 - 50% of patients at the time of diagnosis. Both tend to increase in frequency and severity as the disease progresses and may remain asymptomatic, but approximately 5 - 10% of patients develop symptoms and signs of gout *5677* *1729* *5826*

Urobilinogen *Urine* *Increase* Rarely *2034*

Viscosity *Serum* *Increase* Clinical manifestations may be related to increased blood viscosity *2039*

Vitamin B_{12} *Serum* *Increase* Marked increase; mean concentration was 741 pg/mL in 40 patients (normal 385 pg/mL) *4448* Above 900 pg/mL found in about 33% of patients before treatment or during relapse *5677* Usually increased *2039*

Vitamin B_{12} Binding Capacity *Serum* *Increase* Increased to values > 2,200 pg/mL in about 75% of these patients. Found to be related directly to disease activity *5677* *1730* Significant elevation; usually correlated with WBC in peripheral blood *4448*

Vitamin B_{12} Binding Capacity, Unsaturated *Serum* *Increase* Increased concentrations observed during polycythemia vera *2952*

Vitamin B_{12} Binding Protein *Serum* *Increase* Increase observed in 36% of all patients with the disease *443*

Volume *Plasma* *Decrease* Most often *2034*
Plasma *Increase* The greatest increase occurs in patients with a significant degree of hepatosplenomegaly *4169* *5677*
Plasma *No Effect* Within the normal range in the majority of patients, reduced in some, and increased in others *5677* *2296*
Red Blood Cells *Increase* Unless the RBC volume is > 38 mL/kg for males and 36 mL/kg for females, the diagnosis of polycythemia vera cannot be considered established *367*

238.40 Primary Proliferative Polycythemia

Anti-Neutrophil Cytoplasm Antibodies *Serum* *No Effect* In a group of patients with primary proliferative polycythemia and myelodysplasia in none were ANCA demonstrated *4602*

Erythropoietin *Serum* *Decrease* Mean concentration below 3.7 IU/L in 26 of 36 patients with primary polycythemia *3462*

238.60 Plasmacytoma

C-Reactive Protein *Serum* *Increase* In 5 patients with plasmacytoma mean concentration of 50 mg/L *1506*

Interleukin-6 *Serum* *Increase* In 5 patients with plasmacytoma mean concentration of 13.5 pg/L *1506*

β_2-Microglobulin *Serum* *Increase* In 5 patients with plasmacytoma mean concentration of 3.7 mg/L *1506*

238.70 Myelodysplastic Syndrome

Glycocalicin *Plasma* *Decrease* Mean plasma concentration in 5 patients with myelodysplasic syndrome of 0.18 ± 0.12 µg/mL significantly decreased compared with that in 36 healthy individuals of 1.40 ± 0.25 µg/mL *2853*

Interleukin-1β *Serum* *Increase* In 26 patients with myelodysplastic syndrome mean concentration of 114 ± 58.5 pg/mL significantly higher than 36.1 ± 21.7 pg/mL in 42 healthy controls *3688*

MCV *Blood* *Increase* In 100 patients with macrocytosis (MCV greater than 110 fL) 2 had myelodysplastic syndrome *4924*

Soluble c-kit Molecule *Serum* *No Effect* Median concentration in patients with myelodysplastic syndrome not significantly different from that in 51 healthy volunteers of 199.0 AU/mL *2598*

Soluble Interleukin-2 Receptor *Serum* *Increase* In 19 high-risk patients with myelodysplastic syndrome mean concentration of 1,394 ± 1,112 U/mL compared with 651 ± 299 U/mL in 21 low-risk MDS patients and 495 ± 137 U/mL in 13 normal individuals *5803* In 15 patients with MDS mean concentration of 439 ± 36 U/mL (median 405 U/mL) compared with less than 55 U/mL in healthy controls *4722*

Thrombopoietin *Plasma* *Increase* Mean serum concentration in 5 patients with myelodysplastic syndrome of 16.9 ± 8.2 fmol/mL significantly higher than that in 49 healthy individuals of 0.76 ± 0.32 fmol/mL *2853*

Tumor Necrosis Factor-α *Serum* *Increase* In 26 patients with myelodysplastic syndrome mean concentration of 54.2 ± 93 pg/mL significantly higher than 4.2 ± 7.9 pg/mL in 42 healthy controls *3688* In 15 patients with myelodysplastic syndrome mean concentration of 14.2 ± 2.4 pg/mL compared with 9.1 ± 1.1 pg/mL in healthy controls *4723*

238.70 Myeloproliferative Disorders

Erythropoietin *Serum* *No Effect* Mean serum concentration of 7.2 ± 1.1 mIU/L in patients with myeloproliferative disease not significantly different from 0.0 - 16.9 mIU/mL in 21 healthy controls *5370*

Uric Acid *Serum* *Increase* May cause sustained hyperuricemia *1357*

239.00 Cancer of Ampulla of Vater

CA 195 *Serum* *Increase* Mean concentration of 9 ± 17.6 U/mL in 6 patients with cancer of the ampulla of Vater significantly higher than cutoff of 12 U/mL: 1 patient with concentration greater than 12 U/mL *122*

239.00 Cancer of Biliary Tract

CA 195 *Serum* *Increase* Mean concentration of 153.4 ± 295.5 U/mL in 6 patients with cancer of the biliary tract significantly higher than cutoff of 12 U/mL: 12 patients with concentrations greater than 12 U/mL *122*

239.00 Peritoneal Cancer

Interleukin-1β *Serum* *No Effect* Mean concentration undetectable in 6 patients with peritoneal cancer not different from undetectable amount in 17 healthy controls *4228*

Interleukin-6 *Ascitic Fluid* *Increase* Mean concentration in 26 patients with peritoneal cancer of 24 ± 5.7 ng/mL *4228*
Serum *Increase* Mean concentration in 6 patients with peritoneal cancer of 420 ± 215 pg/mL significantly different from undetectable amount in 17 healthy controls *4228* Mean concentration in 6 patients with peritoneal cancer of 420 ± 215 pg/mL significantly different from 228 ± 24 ng/mL in 17 healthy controls *4228*

6-Keto-Prostaglandin $F_{1\alpha}$ *Ascitic Fluid* *Increase* Mean concentration in 26 patients with peritoneal cancer of 359 ± 110 pg/mL *4228*
Plasma *No Effect* Mean concentration in 6 patients with peritoneal cancer of 14 ± 14.3 pg/mL not significantly different from 8.8 ± 1.4 pg/mL in 16 healthy controls *4228*

Leukotriene B_4 *Ascitic Fluid* *Increase* Mean concentration in 26 patients with peritoneal cancer of 193 ± 67 pg/mL *4228*

Prostaglandin E_2 *Ascitic Fluid* *Increase* Mean concentration in 26 patients with peritoneal cancer of 122 ± 27 pg/mL *4228*
Plasma *No Effect* Mean concentration in 6 patients with peritoneal cancer of 68 ± 32.1 pg/mL not significantly different from 70 ± 13 pg/mL in 17 healthy controls *4228*

Protein *Ascitic Fluid* *Increase* Mean concentration in 26 patients with peritoneal cancer of 44 ± 2.6 mg/mL *4228*

Soluble Intercellular Adhesion Molecule-1
Ascitic Fluid *Increase* Mean concentration in 26 patients with peritoneal cancer of 385 ± 66 ng/mL *4228*
Serum *Increase* Mean concentration in 5 patients with peritoneal cancer of 781 ± 367 ng/mL significantly different from 228 ± 24 ng/mL in 17 healthy controls *4228*

Thromboxane B_2 *Ascitic Fluid* *Increase* Mean concentration in 26 patients with peritoneal cancer of 70 ± 9.4 pg/mL *4228*
Plasma *Increase* Mean concentration in 6 patients with peritoneal cancer of 14 ± 14.1 pg/mL significantly different from undetectable amount in 17 healthy controls *4228*
Plasma *No Effect* Mean concentration in 6 patients with peritoneal cancer of 141 ± 51 pg/mL not significantly different from 153 ± 67 pg/mL in 16 healthy controls *4228*

Tumor Necrosis Factor-α *Serum* *No Effect* Mean concentration undetectable in 6 patients with peritoneal cancer not different from undetectable amount in 17 healthy controls *4228*

239.50 Malignant Disease of Female Genital Tract

CA 125 *Serum* *No Effect* In 17 women with malignancies of the genital tract (10 squamous carcinoma, 2 cancer of the vulva and 5 with endometrial carcinoma) median concentration of 15.3 U/mL (range 3.0 - 1,590 U/mL) not significantly different from median of 8.3 U/mL (range 3.0 - 23.5 U/mL) in 15 healthy controls *4575*
Vaginal Fluid *No Effect* In 17 women with malignancies of the genital tract (10 squamous carcinoma, 2 cancer of the vulva and 5 with endometrial carcinoma) median concentration of 15.3 U/mL (range 3.0 - 1,590 U/mL) not significantly different from median of 8.3 U/mL (range 3.0 - 23.5 U/mL) in 15 healthy controls *4575*

Carcinoembryonic Antigen *Serum* *No Effect* In 17 women with malignancies of the genital tract (10 squamous carcinoma, 2 cancer of the vulva and 5 with endometrial carcinoma) median concentration of 1.5 ng/mL (range of 0.7 - 8.6 ng/mL) not significantly different from median of 1.0 ng/mL (range of 0.5 - 2.5 ng/mL) in 15 healthy controls *4575*
Vaginal Fluid *Decrease* In 17 women with malignancies of the genital tract (10 squamous carcinoma, 2 cancer of the vulva and 5 with endometrial carcinoma) median concentration of 50 ng/mL (range 12 - 186 ng/mL) significantly different from median of 171 ng/mL (range 13 - 672 ng/mL) in 15 healthy controls *4575*

Squamous Cell Carcinoma Antigen *Serum* *No Effect* In 17 women with malignancies of the genital tract (10 squamous carcinoma, 2 cancer of the vulva and 5 with endometrial carcinoma) median concentration of 1.5 ng/mL (range of 0.7 - 19 ng/mL) not significantly different from median of 0.8 ng/mL (range of 0.3 - 2.7 ng/mL) in 15 healthy controls *4575*
Vaginal Fluid *No Effect* In 17 women with malignancies of the genital tract (10 squamous carcinoma, 2 cancer of the vulva and 5 with endometrial carcinoma) median concentration of 710 ng/mL (range 107 - 7,000 ng/mL) not significantly different from median of 1,340 ng/mL (range 27 - 5,430 ng/mL) in 15 healthy controls *4575*

239.50 Testicular Nonseminoma Tumor

β-Chorionic Gonadotropin *Plasma* *Increase* Concentrations increased initially in 58% patients *1081*

α-Fetoprotein *Serum* *Increase* Concentrations increased initially in 51% patients *1081* In 150 patients with testicular nonseminoma 46.7% had concentrations up to 15.0 ng/mL, 3.3% had concentrations between 15.1 - 20.0 ng/mL, 10.7% between 20.1 - 100 ng/mL, 7.3% had concentrations between 100.1 - 350.0 ng/mL and 32.0% had concentrations above 350.0 ng/mL in contrast to concentrations in 400 healthy individuals in whom 99.2% had concentrations between 0 and 15.0 ng/mL, 0.2% between 15.1 and 20.0 ng/mL and 0.5%% between 20.1 and 100 ng/mL *11*

239.60 Neoplasm of Brain

3,3'-Di-iodothyronine *Serum* *Increase* In 22 patients with liver disease mean concentration of 72.6 ± 56.7 pmol/L not significantly different from that in 22 healthy age and sex-matched controls in whom the mean plasma concentration was 45.5 ± 16.3 pmol/L *4138*

α_1-Microglobulin *Cerebrospinal Fluid* *Increase* Of 6 patients with primary brain tumors mean concentration in 1 greater than that in 15 healthy controls of 34.8 ± 16.0 μg/L *2370*

239.70 Adrenal Incidentaloma

Alkaline Phosphatase *Serum* *No Effect* In 8 women with adrenal incidentalomas and subclinical hypercortisolism mean activity of 207 ± 104 U/L and in 24 without subclinical hypercortisolism of 190 ± 70 U/L not significantly different from 167 ± 43 U/L in 64 matched controls *5254*

Corticotropin *Plasma* *Decrease* In 8 women with adrenal incidentalomas and subclinical hypercortisolism mean morning concentration of 5.9 ± 2.7 pg/mL significantly different from mean concentration in 24 without subclinical hypercortisolism of 12.1 ± 8.5 pg/mL and not significantly different from reference value of greater than 10 pg/mL *5254*

Cortisol *Plasma* *No Effect* In 8 women with adrenal incidentalomas and subclinical hypercortisolism mean concentration of 14.7 ± 5.4 μg/dL not significantly different from mean concentration in 24 without subclinical hypercortisolism of 15.3 ± 7.6 μg/dL and not significantly different from reference interval of 7 - 25 μg/dL *5254*

Cortisol, Free *Urine* *No Effect* In 8 women with adrenal incidentalomas and subclinical hypercortisolism mean excretion of 120.6 ± 80.6 μg/d significantly different from mean excretion in 24 without subclinical hypercortisolism of 40.6 ± 17.4 μg/d and significantly different from reference value of less than 70 μg/d *5254*

Cortisol response to Dexamethasone *Plasma* *No Effect* In 8 women with adrenal incidentalomas and subclinical hypercortisolism mean morning concentration after 1 mg dexamethasone overnight of 4.8 ± 4.8 μg/dL not significantly different from mean concentration in 24 without subclinical hypercortisolism of 2.0 ± 0.9 μg/dL and not significantly different from reference value of less than 5 μg/dL *5254*

Cross-linked C-terminal Telopeptide of Type I Collagen
Serum *No Effect* In 8 women with adrenal incidentalomas and subclinical hypercortisolism mean concentration of 4.08 ± 1.29 µg/mL not significantly different from mean concentration in 24 without subclinical hypercortisolism of 3.90 ± 2.39 µg/mL and not significantly different from 4.01 ± 1.57 µg/mL in 64 matched controls *5254*

C-terminal Telopeptide of Type I Collagen *Serum* *Decrease* In 35 patients with adrenal incidentaloma mean concentration of 2..9 - 0.2 ng/mL significantly less than mean concentration of 3.9 ± 0.2 ng/mL in 28 control individuals *4579*

Deoxypyridinoline *Urine* *No Effect* In 8 women with adrenal incidentalomas and subclinical hypercortisolism mean excretion of 28.6 ± 12.8 pmol/pmoL creatinine not significantly different from mean excretion in 24 without subclinical hypercortisolism of 24.6 ± 7.9 pmol/pmoL creatinine and not significantly different from 24.6 ± 6.8 pmol/pmoL creatinine in 64 matched controls *5254*

N-terminal Propeptide of Type III Procollagen
Serum *No Effect* In 35 patients with adrenal incidentaloma mean concentration of 3.6 - 0.2 ng/mL not significantly different from mean concentration of 3.2 ± 0.2 ng/mL in 28 control individuals *4579*

Osteocalcin *Serum* *Decrease* In 8 women with adrenal incidentalomas and subclinical hypercortisolism mean concentration of 3.8 ± 2.3 ng/mL significantly different from mean concentration in 24 without subclinical hypercortisolism of 7.5 ± 3.1 ng/mL and not significantly different from 8.8 ± 3.2 ng/mL in 64 matched controls *5254* In 35 patients with adrenal incidentaloma mean concentration of 4.2 - 0.5 ng/mL significantly less than mean concentration of 5.5 ± 0.2 ng/mL in 28 control individuals *4579*

Parathyroid Hormone *Plasma* *Increase* In 8 women with adrenal incidentalomas and subclinical hypercortisolism mean concentration of 57.1 ± 13.6 pg/mL and in 24 without subclinical hypercortisolism of 46.0 ± 14.8 pg/mL significantly higher than 37.2 ± 10.9 pg/mL in 64 matched controls *5254*

239.70 Adrenal Tumor

Amino-terminal Propeptide of Type III Collagen
Serum *Decrease* In 11 patients with asymptomatic incidentally discovered adrenal tumors mean basal concentration of 2.2 ± 0.15 µg/L significantly different from 3.3 ± 0.2 µg/L in healthy controls *106*

Androstenedione *Plasma* *Decrease* In 30 patients with asymptomatic incidentally discovered adrenal tumors mean basal concentration of 4.27 ± 0.47 nmol/L significantly different from 7.43 ± 0.75 nmol/L in 14 healthy controls *106*

Corticotropin *Plasma* *Decrease* Very low or undetectable in Cushing's patients with adrenocortical tumor *5863*
Plasma *No Effect* In 32 patients with asymptomatic incidentally discovered adrenal tumors mean basal concentration ranged from 0.4 - 8.9 pmol/L not significantly different from 0.7 - 13.2 pmol/L in 14 healthy controls *106*

Cortisol *Plasma* *No Effect* In 30 patients with asymptomatic incidentally discovered adrenal tumors mean basal concentration of 442 ± 31 nmol/L not significantly different from 421 ± 50 nmol/L in 14 healthy controls *106*

Cortisol, Free *Urine* *No Effect* In 32 patients with asymptomatic incidentally discovered adrenal tumors mean basal excretion ranged from 32 - 690 nmol/d not significantly different from 55 - 275 nmol/d in 14 healthy controls *106*

Dehydroepiandrosterone Sulfate *Plasma* *Decrease* Mean concentration reduced below normal in 21 of 24 patients (87.5%) *1502*
Plasma *Increase* Increased concentrations may indicate hyperandrogenism from an adrenal source *2952*

17-Hydroxyprogesterone *Plasma* *No Effect* In 30 patients with asymptomatic incidentally discovered adrenal tumors mean basal concentration of 2.14 ± 0.49 nmol/L not significantly different from 2.23 ± 0.54 nmol/L in 14 healthy controls *106*

17-Ketogenic Steroids *Urine* *Increase* Excretion increased with hyperfunction of the zona fasciculata and reticullaris *2952*

Osteocalcin *Serum* *Decrease* In 11 patients with asymptomatic incidentally discovered adrenal tumors mean basal concentration of 3.9 ± 0.6 µg/L significantly different from 5.4 ± 0.15 µg/L in healthy controls *106*

Progesterone *Plasma* *No Effect* In 32 patients with asymptomatic incidentally discovered adrenal tumors mean basal concentration in men of 2.72 ± 0.93 nmol/L and 3.28 ± 1.16 nmol/L not significantly different from 2.00 ± 0.50 nmol/L and 2.17 ± 0.58 nmol/L in healthy men and women respectively *106*

Pyridinoline Cross-linked Telopeptide of Type I Collagen
Serum *Decrease* In 11 patients with asymptomatic incidentally discovered adrenal tumors mean basal concentration of 2.4 ± 0.1 µmol/L significantly different from 4.1 ± 0.3 µg/L in healthy controls *106*

239.70 Pituitary Tumor

α-Subunit of Glycoprotein Hormones *Plasma* *Increase* Median concentration in 18 patients with non-secreting pituitary tumors of 278 ng/L (range 73 - 3,850 ng/L) higher than median in 24 healthy adult men [250 ng/L (range 120 - 790 ng/L)] and 291 ng/mL (range 88 - 604 ng/mL) in 22 adult premenopausal women: in 3 patients concentrations abnormally high *5468*

239.90 Prolactinoma

5-Androstene-3α,16β,17β-triol *Urine* *No Effect* In 27 women with prolactinoma mean excretion of 4.30 ± 1.25 nmol/g creatinine not significantly different from 2.02 ± 0.57 nmol/g creatinine in 31 healthy women *2972*

5-Androstenediol *Urine* *Increase* In 27 women with prolactinoma mean excretion of 3.93 ± 0.25 nmol/g creatinine significantly different from 0.54 ± 0.11 nmol/g creatinine in 31 healthy women *2972*

δ^4-Androstenedione *Urine* *Increase* In 27 women with prolactinoma mean excretion of 3.61 ± 0.12 nmol/g creatinine significantly different from 0.78 ± 0.13 nmol/g creatinine in 31 healthy women *2972*

Androsterone *Urine* *Increase* In 27 women with prolactinoma mean excretion of 20.58 ± 5.07 nmol/g creatinine significantly different from 6.69 ± 1.65 nmol/g creatinine in 31 healthy women *2972*

Cholesterol *Urine* *Increase* In 27 women with prolactinoma mean excretion of 13.43 ± 5.48 nmol/g creatinine significantly different from 3.79 ± 0.59 nmol/g creatinine in 31 healthy women *2972*

β-Chorionic Gonadotropin *Plasma* *Increase* In 23 patients with a prolactinoma mean baseline concentration undetectable in all except 4 patients in whom concentrations 0.05 to 0.18 U/L *1732*
Plasma *No Effect* In 23 patients with a prolactinoma mean baseline concentration undetectable in all except 4 patients in whom concentrations 0.05 to 0.18 U/L *1732* In 4 patients with a prolactinoma mean baseline concentration in whom β-subunit of chorionic gonadotropin was detectable concentrations of CG were within the reference interval of < 5 U/L *1732*

α-Cortol *Urine* *No Effect* In 27 women with prolactinoma mean excretion of 2.58 ± 0.14 nmol/g creatinine not significantly different from 1.61 ± 0.77 nmol/g creatinine in 31 healthy women *2972*

β-Cortol *Urine* *No Effect* In 27 women with prolactinoma mean excretion of 3.46 ± 1.54 nmol/g creatinine not significantly different from 1.46 ± 0.57 nmol/g creatinine in 31 healthy women *2972*

α-Cortolone *Urine* *No Effect* In 27 women with prolactinoma mean excretion of 12.9 ± 3.60 nmol/g creatinine not significantly different from 6.44 ± 1.78 nmol/g creatinine in 31 healthy women *2972*

β-Cortolone *Urine* *No Effect* In 27 women with prolactinoma mean excretion of 2.01 ± 0.11 nmol/g creatinine not significantly different from 1.71 ± 1.01 nmol/g creatinine in 31 healthy women *2972*

Dehydroepiandrosterone *Urine* *Increase* In 27 women with prolactinoma mean excretion of 32.82 ± 5.56 nmol/g creatinine significantly different from 3.05 ± 0.62 nmol/g creatinine in 31 healthy women *2972*

6-Dehydroestrone *Urine* *Increase* In 27 women with prolactinoma mean excretion of 28.15 ± 78.41 nmol/g creatinine significantly different from 5.46 ± 0.58 nmol/g creatinine in 31 healthy women *2972*

239.90 **Prolactinoma** *(continued)*

2,3-Dimethoxyestradiol *Urine* *Increase* In 27 women with prolactinoma mean excretion of 149.8 ± 34.0 nmol/g creatinine significantly different from 27.7 ± 12.3 nmol/g creatinine in 31 healthy women *2972*

16-Epiestriol *Urine* *Increase* In 27 women with prolactinoma mean excretion of 67.2 ± 16.0 nmol/g creatinine significantly different from 22.6 ± 6.8 nmol/g creatinine in 31 healthy women *2972*

16,17-Epiestriol *Urine* *Increase* In 27 women with prolactinoma mean excretion of 9.79 ± 1.64 nmol/g creatinine significantly different from 3.35 ± 0.48 nmol/g creatinine in 31 healthy women *2972*

17-Epiestriol *Urine* *Increase* In 27 women with prolactinoma mean excretion of 34.6 ± 10.5 nmol/g creatinine significantly different from 7.6 ± 1.5 nmol/g creatinine in 31 healthy women *2972*

17α-Estradiol *Urine* *Increase* In 27 women with prolactinoma mean excretion of 5.78 ± 0.97 nmol/g creatinine significantly different from 2.62 ± 0.65 nmol/g creatinine in 31 healthy women *2972*

17β-Estradiol *Urine* *Increase* In 27 women with prolactinoma mean excretion of 138.0 ± 33.8 nmol/g creatinine significantly different from 47.0 ± 10.2 nmol/g creatinine in 31 healthy women *2972*

Estriol *Urine* *Increase* In 27 women with prolactinoma mean excretion of 127.0 ± 27.7 nmol/g creatinine significantly different from 53.0 ± 17.2 nmol/g creatinine in 31 healthy women *2972*

Estrone *Urine* *Increase* In 27 women with prolactinoma mean excretion of 227.2 ± 35.2 nmol/g creatinine significantly different from 82.1 ± 20.1 nmol/g creatinine in 31 healthy women *2972*

Etiocholanolone *Urine* *Increase* In 27 women with prolactinoma mean excretion of 45.36 ± 10.76 nmol/g creatinine significantly different from 4.89 ± 1.01 nmol/g creatinine in 31 healthy women *2972*

Follicle Stimulating Hormone *Plasma* *No Effect* In 4 patients with a prolactinoma mean baseline concentration in whom β-subunit of chorionic gonadotropin was detectable concentrations of FSH were within the reference interval of 0.5 - 8 U/L *1732*

11β-Hydroxy Androstanediol *Urine* *Increase* In 27 women with prolactinoma mean excretion of 9.68 ± 1.87 nmol/g creatinine significantly different from 2.51 ± 0.38 nmol/g creatinine in 31 healthy women *2972*

16α-Hydroxy Dehydroepiandrosterone *Urine* *Increase* In 27 women with prolactinoma mean excretion of 16.28 ± 5.05 nmol/g creatinine significantly different from 3.72 ± 0.60 nmol/g creatinine in 31 healthy women *2972*

11β-Hydroxy Etiocholanolone *Urine* *Increase* In 27 women with prolactinoma mean excretion of 6.83 ± 1.69 nmol/g creatinine significantly different from 0.78 ± 0.13 nmol/g creatinine in 31 healthy women *2972*

6α-Hydroxycortisol *Urine* *Increase* In 27 women with prolactinoma mean excretion of 70.2 ± 15.4 nmol/g creatinine significantly different from 20.2 ± 7.1 nmol/g creatinine in 31 healthy women *2972*

2-Hydroxyestradiol-3-Methylether *Urine* *Increase* In 27 women with prolactinoma mean excretion of 65.1 ± 14.0 nmol/g creatinine significantly different from 20.8 ± 7.7 nmol/g creatinine in 31 healthy women *2972*

6α-Hydroxyestriol *Urine* *Increase* In 27 women with prolactinoma mean excretion of 8.4 ± 2.5 nmol/g creatinine significantly different from 1.2 ± 0.3 nmol/g creatinine in 31 healthy women *2972*

2-Hydroxyestrone *Urine* *Increase* In 27 women with prolactinoma mean excretion of 1,738.5 ± 306.6 nmol/g creatinine significantly different from 259.0 ± 17.8 nmol/g creatinine in 31 healthy women *2972*

16α-Hydroxyestrone *Urine* *Increase* In 27 women with prolactinoma mean excretion of 358.1 ± 60.5 nmol/g creatinine significantly different from 39.0 ± 8.5 nmol/g creatinine in 31 healthy women *2972*

6-Ketoestradiol *Urine* *Increase* In 27 women with prolactinoma mean excretion of 18.4 ± 3.9 nmol/g creatinine significantly different from 5.1 ± 0.9 nmol/g creatinine in 31 healthy women *2972*

16-Ketoestradiol *Urine* *Increase* In 27 women with prolactinoma mean excretion of 24.7 ± 4.5 nmol/g creatinine significantly different from 6.9 ± 1.4 nmol/g creatinine in 31 healthy women *2972*

6-Ketoestriol *Urine* *Increase* In 27 women with prolactinoma mean excretion of 9.3 ± 1.2 nmol/g creatinine significantly different from 1.7 ± 0.5 nmol/g creatinine in 31 healthy women *2972*

Luteinizing Hormone *Plasma* *No Effect* In 4 patients with a prolactinoma mean baseline concentration in whom β-subunit of chorionic gonadotropin was detectable concentrations of LH were within the reference interval of 0.2 - 6.5 U/L *1732*

2-Methoxyestradiol *Urine* *Increase* In 27 women with prolactinoma mean excretion of 127.7 ± 26.5 nmol/g creatinine significantly different from 35.5 ± 8.0 nmol/g creatinine in 31 healthy women *2972*

4-Methoxyestradiol *Urine* *Increase* In 27 women with prolactinoma mean excretion of 64.9 ± 12.8 nmol/g creatinine significantly different from 30.3 ± 10.0 nmol/g creatinine in 31 healthy women *2972*

2-Methoxyestrone *Urine* *Increase* In 27 women with prolactinoma mean excretion of 210.9 ± 39.1 nmol/g creatinine significantly different from 44.5 ± 11.1 nmol/g creatinine in 31 healthy women *2972*

Prolactin *Plasma* *Increase* In 4 patients with a prolactinoma mean baseline concentration in whom β-subunit of chorionic gonadotropin was detectable concentrations of prolactin were 73, 80, 120, and 340 µg/L greatly exceeding the reference interval of 5 - 25 µg/L *1732* In 27 women with prolactinoma mean concentration of 689.7 ± 214 ng/mL significantly different from 18.8 ± 3.1 ng/mL in 31 healthy women *2972* Concentrations above 200 ng/mL usually indicate prolactinoma *2952*

α-Subunit *Serum* *No Effect* In 4 patients with a prolactinoma mean baseline concentration in whom β-subunit of chorionic gonadotropin was detectable concentrations of α-subunit were within the reference interval of < 0.1 - 0.8 µg/L, except for one patient in whom the concentration was 1.2 µg/L *1732*

α-Subunit of Glycoprotein Hormones *Plasma* *Increase* Median concentration in 13 patients of 226 ng/L (range 93 - 5,600 ng/L) higher than median in 24 healthy adult men [250 ng/L (range 120 - 790 ng/L)] and 291 ng/mL (range 88 - 604 ng/mL) in 22 adult premenopausal women: in 4 patients concentrations abnormally high *5468*

Testosterone *Urine* *No Effect* In 27 women with prolactinoma mean excretion of 1.27 ± 0.79 nmol/g creatinine not significantly different from 1.07 ± 0.19 nmol/g creatinine in 31 healthy women *2972*

Tetrahydro-11-deoxycortisol *Urine* *No Effect* In 27 women with prolactinoma mean excretion of 1.22 ± 0.84 nmol/g creatinine not significantly different from 0.37 ± 0.03 nmol/g creatinine in 31 healthy women *2972*

5α-Tetrahydrocorticosterone *Urine* *No Effect* In 27 women with prolactinoma mean excretion of 2.37 ± 0.64 nmol/g creatinine not significantly different from 2.11 ± 0.16 nmol/g creatinine in 31 healthy women *2972*

5β-Tetrahydrocorticosterone *Urine* *No Effect* In 27 women with prolactinoma mean excretion of 6.91 ± 1.04 nmol/g creatinine not significantly different from 2.13 ± 0.25 nmol/g creatinine in 31 healthy women *2972*

5α-Tetrahydrocortisol *Urine* *No Effect* In 27 women with prolactinoma mean excretion of 8.66 ± 1.13 nmol/g creatinine not significantly different from 5.85 ± 1.43 nmol/g creatinine in 31 healthy women *2972*

5β-Tetrahydrocortisol *Urine* *Increase* In 27 women with prolactinoma mean excretion of 45.11 ± 8.33 nmol/g creatinine not significantly different from 8.68 ± 0.24 nmol/g creatinine in 31 healthy women *2972*

Tetrahydrocortisone *Urine* *No Effect* In 27 women with prolactinoma mean excretion of 22.9 ± 5.00 nmol/g creatinine not significantly different from 17.0 ± 5.77 nmol/g creatinine in 31 healthy women *2972*

Thyroid Stimulating Hormone *Serum* *No Effect* In 4 patients with a prolactinoma mean baseline concentration in whom β-subunit of chorionic gonadotropin was detectable concentrations of TSH were within the reference interval of 0.26 - 5 mU/L, except for one patient in whom the concentration was 6.4 mU/L *1732*

239.90 VIPoma

Calcitonin *Plasma* *No Effect* In a patient with a VIPoma and chronic diarrhea concentration was not increased above upper limit of normal of 71 pg/mL *4635*

Gastrin-releasing Peptide *Serum* *No Effect* In neither of 2 patients with a VIPoma and chronic diarrhea was concentration increased above upper limit of normal of 542 pg/mL *4635*

Neurotensin *Plasma* *No Effect* In neither of 2 patients with a VIPoma and chronic diarrhea was concentration increased above upper limit of normal of 250 pg/mL *4635*

Pancreatic Polypeptide *Plasma* *No Effect* In neither of 2 patients with a VIPoma and chronic diarrhea was concentration increased above upper limit of normal of 465 pg/mL *4635*

Somatostatin *Plasma* *No Effect* In neither of 2 patients with a VIPoma and chronic diarrhea was concentration increased above upper limit of normal of 68 pg/mL *4635*

Substance P *Plasma* *No Effect* In neither of 2 patients with a VIPoma and chronic diarrhea was concentration increased above upper limit of normal of 240 pg/mL *4635*

Vasoactive Intestinal Polypeptide *Plasma* *Increase* In both of 2 patients (100%) with a VIPoma and chronic diarrhea concentration was increased above upper limit of normal of 240 pg/mL *4635*

ENDOCRINE, NUTRITIONAL AND METABOLIC DISEASES, AND IMMUNITY DISORDERS

Diseases of the Endocrine Glands

240.00 Simple Goiter

Eosinophils *Blood* *Increase* In 50% of 19 patients at initial hospitalization for this disorder *1576*

Fibronectin *Plasma* *No Effect* Mean fasting concentration in 9 patients with simple goiter of 29.1 ± 8.0 mg/dL not significantly different from that in 28 normal men, 32.5 ± 7.1 mg/dL, and 31.6 ± 5.7 mg/dL in 34 normal women *4811*

^{131}I Uptake *Serum* *Increase* In some patients, elevated to the 70-95% range *367*
Serum *No Effect* Usually normal *5679*

T3-Uptake *Serum* *No Effect* Concentration typically normal *5544*

Thyroid Stimulating Hormone *Serum* *Increase* Normal or slightly increased *1980*
Serum *No Effect* Usually normal *5679* Normal in nontoxic goiter without autoimmune thyroiditis *1966* Normal or slightly low *1980*

Thyroxine (T4) *Serum* *Decrease* Normal or slightly low *1980*
Serum *No Effect* Usually normal *5679* Normal or slightly low *1980*

Tri-iodothyronine (T3) *Serum* *Increase* Normal or increased *1980*
Serum *No Effect* Usually normal *5679* Normal or slightly low *1980*

241.00 Nontoxic Goiter

Anti-TSH Receptor Antibodies *Serum* *No Effect* In 24 individuals with nontoxic goiter mean concentration < 5 U/L not different from healthy controls *5521*

Antibodies against Megalin (gp330) *Serum* *Increase* In 19 patients with nontoxic goiter mean fluorescence intensity of 24.06 ± 15.54 significantly different from that in 32 normal individuals in whom mean fluorescence intensity 14.53 ± 12.03 *3299*

Interleukin-6 *Serum* *No Effect* In 20 individuals with nontoxic goiter mean concentration of 47.3 ± 7.1 fmol/L not significantly higher than 37.8 ± 6.2 fmol/L in healthy controls *303*

Sex-Hormone Binding Globulin *Serum* *Increase* Patients with non-toxic goiter have reduced concentrations of TSH with which concentration of SHBG is inversely correlated *4234*

Thyroid Stimulating Hormone *Serum* *Decrease* Patients with non-toxic goiter have reduced concentrations *4234*
Serum *No Effect* In 24 patients with nontoxic goiter mean concentration of 0.9 ± 0.7 mU/L not significantly different from 0.9 ± 0.4 mU/L in 24 healthy controls *5521*

Thyroxine (T4) *Serum* *No Effect* Mean concentration of 9.8 ± 2.1 nmol/L not significantly different from 10.2 ± 2.3 nmol/L in 24 normal controls *5521*

Thyroxine (T4), Free *Serum* *No Effect* In 24 patients with nontoxic goiter mean concentration of 1.4 ± 0.3 pmol/L not significantly different from 1.2 ± 0.3 pmol/L in 24 normal controls *5521*

Tri-iodothyronine (T3) *Serum* *No Effect* Mean concentration of 143 ± 24 nmol/L not significantly different from 157 ± 39 nmol/L in 24 normal controls *5521*

241.00 Thyroid Nodule

Calcitonin *Plasma* *Increase* Mean concentration increased above 6 pg/mL in 55 of 1,062 consecutive patients with thyroid nodular disease, with concentrations above 100 pg/mL in three of them *5470*

Sex-Hormone Binding Globulin *Serum* *Increase* Patients with thyroid nodules may have suppressed TSH concentrations and high SHBG in relation to degree of increase of thyroid hormone concentrations *4234*

Thyroid Stimulating Hormone *Serum* *Decrease* Patients with thyroid nodules may have suppressed TSH concentrations *4234*

Thyroxine (T4) *Serum* *No Effect* Patients with thyroid nodules may have suppressed TSH concentrations and high SHBG in relation to degree of increase of thyroid hormone concentrations, but in some caes thyroxine concentration is nomal *4234*

241.10 Nontoxic Diffuse Goiter

Interleukin-6 *Serum* *No Effect* In 15 patients with nontoxic diffuse goiter mean concentration of 5.7 pg/mL not significantly different from 6.0 pg/mL in 15 healthy controls *5364*

Thyroxine (T4) *Serum* *No Effect* In 15 patients with nontoxic diffuse goiter mean concentration of 101.6 ± 14 nmol/L not significantly different from 122.8 ± 26 nmol/L in 15 healthy controls *5364*

Tri-iodothyronine (T3) *Serum* *No Effect* In 15 patients with nontoxic diffuse goiter mean concentration of 2.28 ± 0.38 nmol/L not significantly different from 2.12 ± 0.38 nmol/L in 15 healthy controls *747*

Tumor Necrosis Factor-α *Serum* *No Effect* In 15 patients with nontoxic diffuse goiter mean concentration of 5.4 pg/mL not significantly different from 5.0 pg/mL in 15 healthy controls *5364*

241.90 Nodular Goiter

Interleukin-6 *Serum* *Increase* In 20 individuals with toxic adenoma/nodular goiter mean concentration of 97.6 ± 10.3 fmol/L significantly greater than 37.8 ± 6.2 fmol/L in healthy controls *303*

242.00 Basedow's Disease

Osteocalcin *Serum* *No Effect* With ExtrAvidin® -biotin system method the mean concentration in patients with Basedow disease of 2.1 ± 1.0 nmol/L not significantly different from that in healthy adults, 1.4 ± 0.8 nmol/L *2417*

242.00 Toxic Goiter

Anti-TSH Receptor Antibodies *Serum* *No Effect* In 13 patients with toxic goiter/toxic adenoma mean concentration < 5 U/L not different from normal *5521*

242.00 Toxic Goiter *(continued)*

Neopterin *Serum* *Increase* In 13 patients with toxic goiter/toxic adenoma mean concentration of 5.8 ± 2.0 nmol/L not significantly greater than 3.9 ± 0.9 nmol/L in 24 normal controls *5521*

Thyroid Stimulating Hormone *Serum* *Decrease* Mean concentration of < 0.16 mU/L in 13 patients with toxic goiter/toxic adenoma significantly less than 0.9 ± 0.4 mU/L in 24 normal controls *5521*

Thyroxine (T4) *Serum* *Increase* In 13 patients with toxic goiter/toxic adenoma mean concentration of 18.1 ± 6.3 nmol/L higher than 10.2 ± 2.3 nmol/L in 24 normal controls *5521*

Thyroxine (T4), Free *Serum* *Increase* In 13 patients with toxic goiter/toxic adenoma mean concentration of 2.8 ± 0.4 pmol/L higher than 1.2 ± 0.3 pmol/L in 24 normal controls *5521*

Tri-iodothyronine (T3) *Serum* *Increase* In 13 patients with toxic goiter/toxic adenoma mean concentration of 276 ± 78 nmol/L significantly increased above 157 ± 39 nmol/L in 24 normal controls *5521*

242.20 Toxic Multinodular Goiter

Interleukin-6 *Serum* *Increase* In 9 patients with toxic multinodular goiter mean concentration of 26.5 pg/mL significantly different from 6.0 pg/mL in 15 healthy controls *5364*

Thyroxine (T4) *Serum* *Increase* In 9 patients with toxic multinodular goiter mean concentration of 230.6 ± 67 nmol/L significantly different from 122.8 ± 26 nmol/L in 15 healthy controls *747*

Tumor Necrosis Factor-α *Serum* *No Effect* In 9 patients with toxic multinodular goiter mean concentration of 5.0 pg/mL not significantly different from 5.0 pg/mL in 15 healthy controls *5364*

242.30 Toxic Nodular Goiter

Antithyroglobulin Antibodies *Serum* *No Effect* In 31 patients with toxic nodular goiter prior to treatment mean concentration of 55.4 ± 21.2 U/mL not significantly different from 48.5 ± 18.3 U/mL in 34 healthy controls *5633* In 24 patients with untreated toxic nodular goiter mean concentration of 54.8 U/mL (range 24.4 - 83.4) not significantly different from mean of 47.4 U/mL (range 22.5 - 78.3) in 26 healthy controls *5635*

Antithyroid Peroxidase Antibodies *Serum* *No Effect* In 31 patients with toxic nodular goiter prior to treatment mean concentration of 53.4 ± 13.7 U/mL not significantly different from 51.2 ± 23.3 U/mL in 34 healthy controls *5633* In 24 patients with untreated toxic nodular goiter mean concentration of 51.2 U/mL (range 13.6 - 69.8) not significantly higher than mean of 49.8 U/mL (range 10.6 - 67.9) in 26 healthy controls *5635*

Antithyroid Receptor Antibodies *Serum* *No Effect* In 24 patients with untreated toxic nodular goiter mean concentration of 2.9 U/mL (range of 0.8 - 7.4) not significantly different from mean of 2.7 U/mL (range of 0.7 - 6.6) in 26 healthy controls *5635* In 31 patients with toxic nodular goiter prior to treatment mean concentration of 3.0 ± 0.4 U/mL not significantly different from 2.8 ± 0.8 U/mL in 34 healthy controls *5633*

C-terminal Propeptide of Type I Procollagen *Serum* *No Effect* In 31 patients with toxic nodular goiter prior to treatment mean concentration of 167 ± 89 ng/mL not significantly different from 144 ± 57 ng/mL in 34 healthy controls *5633*

Laminin *Serum* *No Effect* In 24 patients with untreated toxic nodular goiter mean concentration of 471 ng/mL (range 284 - 891) not significantly different from mean of 493 ng/mL (range 235 - 675) in 26 healthy controls *5635* In 31 patients with toxic nodular goiter prior to treatment mean concentration of 167 ± 89 ng/mL not significantly different from 492 ± 112 ng/mL in 34 healthy controls *5633*

Pyridinoline Cross-linked Telopeptide of Type I Collagen *Serum* *Increase* In 31 patients with toxic nodular goiter prior to treatment mean concentration of 8.6 ± 35 ng/mL not significantly different from 4.2 ± 1.5 ng/mL in 34 healthy controls *5633*

Thyroid Stimulating Hormone *Serum* *Decrease* In 24 patients with untreated toxic nodular goiter mean concentration of < 0.01 µU/mL significantly less than mean of 2.1 µU/mL (range of 0.5 - 3.7) in 26 healthy controls *5635* In 31 patients with toxic nodular goiter prior to treatment mean concentration of < 0.01 µIU/mL significantly different from 2.0 ± 1.1 µIU/mL in 34 healthy controls *5633*

Thyroxine (T4), Free *Serum* *Increase* In 24 patients with untreated toxic nodular goiter mean concentration of 49.1 pg/mL (range 19.2 - 93.3) significantly higher than mean 11.2 pg/mL (range 7.5 - 8.9) in 26 healthy controls *5635* In 31 patients with toxic nodular goiter prior to treatment mean concentration of 49.4 ± 20.1 pg/mL significantly higher than 12.0 ± 5.6 pg/mL in 34 healthy controls *5633*

Tri-iodothyronine, Free (fT3) *Serum* *Increase* In 31 patients with toxic nodular goiter prior to treatment mean concentration of 13.7 ± 4.8 pg/mL significantly higher than 2.9 ± 1.6 pg/mL in 34 healthy controls *5633*

242.90 Hyperthyroidism

Acid Phosphatase, Tartrate Resistant *Serum* *Increase* In 3 premenopausal hyperthyroid women mean concentration of 291 (range 213 - 351) µg/L, 6.5 (5.5 - 17.2) U/L and 379 (367 - 391) µg/L, 23.3 (20.9 - 26.3) U/L in 3 postmenopausal women significantly greater than mean concentration and range of 178 (41 - 288) µg/L, 5.6 (1.8 - 10.3) U/L in 29 healthy premenopausal women and 302 (range 129 - 348) µg/L, 7.5 (range 4.2 - 12.9) U/L in 12 healthy postmenopausal women *812* In patients with hyperthyroidism slight increase observed *4217*

Alanine Aminotransferase *Serum* *Increase* Slight rise (mean = 12.1 U/L, normal = 8.1). The differences between hyper- and euthyroid groups were statistically significant but individually, minor changes would be of little positive diagnostic significance *2833* Hyperthyroidism, independent of congestive heart failure or concomitant unrelated liver disease, may cause abnormal liver tests but activity less than 250 U/L *3625*

Albumin *Serum* *Decrease* Possibly due to rapid turnover in severe thyrotoxicosis *1290* In 18 patients with hyperthyroidism mean concentration of 31 ± 0.5 g/L significantly different from 34 ± 0.4 g/L in 20 controls *4273*

Aldosterone *Plasma* *No Effect* Typical finding *3151*

Alkaline Phosphatase *Serum* *Increase* Hyperthyroidism, independent of congestive heart failure or concomitant unrelated liver disease, may cause abnormal liver tests but activity less than 250 U/L *3625* Mean activity in 15 women with active Graves' thyrotoxicosis of 2.18 ± 0.2 µkat/L significantly higher than 1.14 ± 0.1 µkat/L in healthy controls *1154* Mean level was 42.5 U/L or 55% higher in the hyperthyroid than in the euthyroid group *2833*

Alkaline Phosphatase, Bone Isoenzyme *Serum* *Increase* Mean activity of 21.5 ± 16.8 U/L observed in 27 patients with hyperthyroidism significantly higher than 10.0 ± 5.0 U/L in 30 healthy controls *1658* In patients with hyperthyroidism slight increase observed *4217*

Amino Acids *Plasma* *Increase* Slight increase *1290*

Amylase *Serum* *Decrease* When accompanied by severe liver damage *5544* Severe thyrotoxicosis *1290*

Angiotensin-converting Enzyme *Serum* *Increase* Consistently elevated in untreated patients compared with controls *3717* Significantly higher than hypothyroid or normal subjects. Higher than all other groups but fell from 30.8 to 17.4 U/mL with therapy in 35 patients studied *4894* Significantly elevated in 21 patients with hyperthyroidism (mean 65 U/mL) compared with healthy control subjects (mean 30 U/mL) *5822* Significantly higher than hypothyroid or normal subjects. Higher than all other groups but fell from 30.8 to 17.4 U/mL with therapy in 35 patients studied *1831* Consistently elevated in untreated patients compared with controls *4845* Mean levels were significantly increased in patients with this disorder (32.06 ± 10.3 nmol/mL/min) in respect to control subjects (14.66 ± 3.88 nmol/mL/min). There was a significant linear correlation between SACE and thyroxine *3002* Consistently elevated in untreated patients compared with controls *574*

Anti-TSH Receptor Antibodies *Serum* *Increase* In 33 patients with Graves' disease mean concentration before therapy of 51 ± 42 IU/L compared with 3 ± 1.3 IU/L in 38 healthy controls *5634* In 24 hyperthyroid patients with Graves' disease mean concentration of 74 ± 93 U/L significantly higher than < 5 U/L in 24 normal controls. Treatment caused reduction to 15 ± 15 U/L in 24 patients in remission *5521*

Antibodies against Megalin (gp330) *Serum* *Increase* In 19 patients with Graves' disease mean fluorescence intensity of 27.47 ± 33.05 significantly higher than that in 32 normal individuals in whom mean fluorescence intensity 14.53 ± 12.03 *3299*

α_1-Antichymotrypsin *Serum* *No Effect* Mean concentration within reference interval of 47.9 ± 8.1 mg/dL in one examined patient with hyperthyroidism *3044*

Antithyroglobulin Antibodies *Serum* *Increase* In 27 patients with Graves' disease prior to treatment mean concentration of 197.8 ± 78.4 U/mL significantly different from 48.5 ± 18.3 U/mL in 34 healthy controls *5633* Patients with Graves' disease often have some or all of the thyroid autoantibodies of Hashimoto's disease *4551* High incidence reflects focal toxicity in the gland and correlates with the development of postoperative hypothyroidism *5863* In 23 patients with untreated Graves' disease mean concentration of 191.5 U/mL (range 22.0 - 1196.0) significantly higher than mean of 47.4 U/mL (range 22.5 - 78.3) in 26 healthy controls *5635*

Antithyroid Peroxidase Antibodies *Serum* *Increase* In 27 patients with Graves' disease prior to treatment mean concentration of 2402 ± 687 U/mL significantly different from 51.2 ± 23.3 U/mL in 34 healthy controls *5633* In 33 patients with Graves' disease mean concentration before therapy of 2,018 ± 1,047 IU/L compared with 50 ± 11 IU/L in 38 healthy controls *5634* In 23 patients with untreated Graves' disease mean concentration of 2,348 U/mL (range 230 - 9,996) significantly higher than mean of 49.8 U/mL (range 10.6 - 67.9) in 26 healthy controls *5635* In 14 patients with Graves' hyperthyroidism before treatment mean concentration of 23 ± 10 U/mL significantly higher than 6.3 ± 10 U/mL in 6 healthy controls *3676*

Antithyroid Receptor Antibodies *Serum* *Increase* In 27 patients with Graves' disease prior to treatment mean concentration of 46.3 ± 17.4 U/mL significantly different from 2.8 ± 0.8 U/mL in 34 healthy controls *5633* In 23 patients with untreated Graves' disease mean concentration of 45.1 U/mL (range of 14.4 - 173.1) significantly higher than mean of 2.7 U/mL (range of 0.7 - 6.6) in 26 healthy controls *5635*

Apolipoprotein A-I *Serum* *Increase* In 40 hyperthyroid patients 95% range concentration of 1.84 - 2.3 g/L significantly different from 1.41 - 1.51 g/L in 119 healthy controls *2852*
Serum *No Effect* In 30 patients with untreated hyperthyroidism mean concentration of 1.49 ± 0.25 g/L towards the lower limit of normal but significantly increasing to 1.66 ± 0.28 g/L during and after treatment *1368*

Apolipoprotein B *Serum* *Decrease* In 13 hyperthyroid patients mean concentration of 63.1 ± 15.8 mg/dL compared with 106.4 ± 30.0 mg/dL in euthyroid state *5777* In 30 patients with untreated hyperthyroidism mean concentration of 0.91 ± 0.27 g/L significantly lower than in treated patients (1.17 - 0.36 g/L) *1368* Mean concentration in 40 women with untreated Graves' disease of 0.80 ± 0.03 g/L significantly different from 1.09 ± 0.04 g/L in 35 healthy adult women of comparable age and life style *4357* Mean concentration of 61.1 ± 12.5 mg/dL in 7 hyperthyroid patients significantly different from post-treatment concentration of 99.7 ± 36.4 mg/dL *2072* In 40 hyperthyroid patients 95% range concentration of 0.59 - 0.73 g/L significantly different from 1.06 - 1.19 g/L in 119 healthy controls *2852*

Apolipoprotein C-II *Serum* *No Effect* Mean concentration of 3.5 ± 1.9 mg/dL in 7 hyperthyroid patients not significantly different from post-treatment concentration of 3.6 ± 2.0 mg/dL *2072*

Apolipoprotein Lp(a) *Serum* *Decrease* In 40 hyperthyroid patients 95% range concentration of 90 - 170 IU/L significantly lower than 244 - 366 IU/L in 119 healthy controls *2852*

Ascorbic Acid *Serum* *Decrease* Secondary to increased metabolic processes *5679*

Aspartate Aminotransferase *Serum* *Increase* Hyperthyroidism, independent of congestive heart failure or concomitant unrelated liver disease, may cause abnormal liver tests, but activity typically less than 250 U/L *3625* A slight rise in mean activity over the normal with hepatic dysfunction (mean 13.5 U/L, normal 11.1 U/L) *2833*

Atrial Natriuretic Peptide *Plasma* *Increase* In 20 untreated patients with hyperthyroidism mean concentration (± 1 SD) of 18.31 ± 6.38 pmol/L significantly increased compared with 11.89 ± 7.82 in 18 healthy controls *5661* In 5 women aged 40 - 59 years with thyrotoxicosis caused by toxic nodular goiter and sinus cardiac rhythm median concentration of 20.0 pmol/L significantly higher than 8.3 pmol/L in 8 healthy control women aged 39 - 56 years *990*

Bicarbonate *Serum* *Decrease* Respiratory alkalosis may occur *1980*

Bilirubin *Serum* *Increase* Due to hemolysis *367* Hyperthyroidism, independent of congestive heart failure or concomitant unrelated liver disease, may cause abnormal liver tests *3625*

Bleeding Time *Patient* *No Effect* In 10 untreated patients median template bleeding time of 3.5 minutes not significantly different from 4.0 minutes in 38 healthy controls *3694*

BSP Retention *Serum* *Increase* Mild retention *5679*

Calcium *Feces* *Increase* Excess of thyroid hormone induces a marked increase in fecal and urinary excretion *2252*
Serum *Increase* Found in rare occasions with severe thyrotoxicosis due to increased turnover of bone *5863* Usually normal but may occur in as many as 20% of patients *5679* Ionized and total calcium levels were elevated in 21 of 45 (47%) and in 12 of 45 (27%) thyrotoxic patients, respectively. Mean ionized and total calcium levels were higher in these 45 patients than in normal persons *640* An incidental finding and an uncommon complication *2039* Mean concentration in 15 women with active Graves' thyrotoxicosis of 2.42 ± 0.04 mmol/L significantly higher than 2.31 ± 0.02 mmol/L in healthy controls *1154*
Serum *No Effect* Significant hypercalcemia did not occur in patients over 60 years of age *1039*
Urine *Increase* Urinary excretion was increased and correlated positively to degree of hyperthyroidism *3624*

Carbon Dioxide Partial Pressure *Blood* *Decrease* Respiratory alkalosis may occur *1980*

Carbonic Anhydrase I *Red Blood Cells* *Decrease* In patients with hyperthyroidism mean concentration reduced *5813*

Catecholamines *Plasma* *Decrease* Decreased plasma levels correlate inversely with total T4 *4774*
Plasma *No Effect* Concentration usually unaffected by disease *5679*
Urine *No Effect* Usually concentration unaffected by disease *5679*

Cholesterol *Serum* *Decrease* In 40 hyperthyroid patients 95% range concentration of 3.80 - 4.34 mmol/L significantly different from 5.03 - 5.39 mmol/L in 119 healthy controls *2852* Mean concentration of 125.6 ± 20.6 mg/dL in 7 hyperthyroid patients significantly different from post-treatment concentration of 199.3 ± 34.4 mg/dL *2072* In 14 hyperthyroid patients mean concentration of 148 ± 49 mg/dL *4951* In 25 patients mean concentration of 194.8 ± 54.2 mg/dL significantly different from 226.9 ± 68.0 mg/dL during treatment *2228* Mean concentration in 40 women with untreated Graves' disease of 4.26 ± 0.14 mmol/L significantly different from 5.12 ± 0.11 mmol/L in 35 healthy adult women of comparable age and life style *4357* Falls, but not in simple relation to the associated rise in the BMR. Diet has a variable effect on the blood level *1642* In 13 hyperthyroid patients mean concentration of 118.3 ± 16.4 mg/dL compared with 168.2 ± 35.5 mg/dL in euthyroid state *5777* Direct stimulation of synthesis and metabolism *5679*
Serum *No Effect* In 30 patients with untreated hyperthyroidism mean concentration of 4.5 ± 1.0 mmol/L towards lower limit of normal significantly increasing to 5.9 ± 1.4 mmol/L during and after treatment *1368*

Cholesterol Esters *Serum* *Increase* Reported effect *2886*

Cholinesterase *Serum* *Increase* In some cases of thyrotoxicosis. Not a useful measure of thyroid activity, because of the wide overlap with normal cases *1290*

C-Peptide *Plasma* *Increase* In 9 patients with Graves' disease mean total integrated C-peptide AUC of 269 ± 37 nmol/min not significantly different from 241 ± 47 nmol/min in 9 healthy controls *353*

Creatine *Serum* *Increase* Excess T4 or TSH stimulates creatinuria *4707*
Urine *Increase* Increased excretion when the muscle mass is reduced, or is unable to take up creatine due to muscle catabolism *1290* Urinary creatine may be significantly increased in patients with hyperthyroidism *2952*

Creatine Kinase *Serum* *Decrease* Below normal but increased after treatment *1193*

Creatine Kinase MB-Isoenzyme *Serum* *Increase* May be due to change in clearance *200* *768*

Creatinine *Serum* *Decrease* In 77 untreated patients with hyperthyroidism mean concentration significantly depressed compared with healthy controls: since urea nitrogen increased,

242.90 **Hyperthyroidism** *(continued)*

Creatinine *(continued)*
urea N:creatinine ratio markedly increased *4813* In 66 women with Graves' disease before treatment mean concentration of 0.64 ± 0.01 mg/dL not significantly different from 0.87 ± 0.01 mg/dL in 49 healthy women and 0.74 ± 0.02 mg/dL in 26 men with untreated Graves' disease not significantly different from 0.92 ± 0.02 mg/dL in 21 healthy control men *4589*
Urine Decrease With associated rise in urine creatine *1290*

C-terminal Propeptide of Type I Procollagen
Serum Increase Concentration significantly higher in patients with thyrotoxicosis on presentation than in age and sex matched controls *5670* In 27 patients with Graves' disease prior to treatment mean concentration of 198 ± 79 ng/mL not significantly different from 144 ± 57 ng/mL in 34 healthy controls *5633*

C-terminal Telopeptide of Type I Collagen *Serum Increase* Mean concentration of 9.4 ± 4.7 µg/L in 28 adult patients with primary hyperthyroidism significantly different compared with 3.8 ± 1.6 µg/L in 61 healthy control adults *4089*

3,3'-Di-iodothyronine *Serum Increase* In 9 patients with hyperthyroidism mean concentration of 85.4 ± 43.0 pmol/L significantly higher than that in 14 healthy age and sex-matched controls in whom the mean plasma concentration was 50.5 ± 9.3 pmol/L *4138*

2,3-Diphosphoglycerate *Red Blood Cells Increase* Results in reduced oxygen affinity *3496*

Eosinophils *Blood Increase* Often occurs *5679*

Erythrocyte Sedimentation Rate *Blood Increase* Raised in 12% of patients over 60 *1039*

Erythrocyte Survival *Red Blood Cells Decrease* In patients with thyrotoxicosis, a moderate shortening *5677 3397*

Estradiol *Plasma Increase* In 7 male patients with hyperthyroidism concentration significantly increased compared with that n healthy controls *2275*

Estrogens *Plasma No Effect* Estradiol is normal *3905*

Factor VIII *Plasma Increase* Increased activity in hyperthyroid states *1308* May reflect increased adrenergic activity *5679*

Fatty Acids (FFA), Free *Serum Increase* Hyperthyroidism is frequently associated with high concentrations of free fatty acids due to increased thyroid hormone-enhancing lipoplysis *2963* Increased lipid degradation *5679*

Ferritin *Serum Increase* Increased concentration (89.5 ± 60.4 µg/L) observed in 13 patients with hyperthyroidism possibly related to direct action of thyroid hormones on its synthesis *2837*

Fibrinogen *Plasma Increase* In 8 untreated patients median concentration of 5.2 g/L significantly different from 4.1 g/L during treatment in 4 individuals *3694*

Fibronectin *Plasma Increase* Mean fasting concentration in 25 patients with untreated hyperthyroidism of 62.6 ± 16.1 mg/dL significantly higher than that in 28 normal men, 32.5 ± 7.1 mg/dL, and 31.6 ± 5.7 mg/dL in 34 normal women *4811*
Plasma No Effect In 8 untreated patients median concentration of 0.40 g/L not significantly different from 0.41 g/L during treatment in 4 individuals *3694*

Follicle Stimulating Hormone *Plasma Increase* In 7 men with hyperthyroidism aged 36 - 46 years mean concentration significantly increased compared with healthy controls *2275*

Gastrin *Serum Increase* Mean fasting levels in untreated hyperthyroid patients was 356 ± 26 pg/mL, (normal = 89 ± 4 pg/mL). No correlation was apparent between gastrin level and any parameter of thyroid function *4720*

GH response to GHRH *Plasma Decrease* In 38 hyperthyroid patients response of 19.6 ± 2.2 mU/L at 90 min to GHRH significantly less than 34.0 ± 4.6 mU/L at 30 min in 30 normal controls *5383*

γ-Globulin *Serum No Effect* Concentration usually within normal limits *5544*

Glucose *Serum Increase* Possibly due to increased circulating epinephrine in thyrotoxicosis. Increased rate of absorption from intestine *1290* Significantly elevated in 42 untreated patients, mean concentration was 92 ± 8 mg/dL *114*

Glucose Tolerance *Serum Decrease* Early high peak due to increased intestinal absorption (normal IV curve) with normal return to fasting level. Decreased formation of glycogen with low fasting levels and subsequent hypoglycemia *5544* Oral test resulted in significantly increased responses in 20 untreated patients *114*

Glutathione S-Transferase *Serum Increase* In 10 of 14 hyperthyroid patients activity increased *361*

Glycerol *Serum Increase* Increased lipid degradation *5679*

Growth Hormone *Plasma No Effect* In 38 hyperthyroid patients mean concentration of 4.2 ± 0.6 mU/L not signficantly different from 4.4 ± 1.4 mU/L in 30 normal individuals *5383*

Guanosine Monophosphate *Plasma Increase* In 5 women aged 40 - 59 years with thyrotoxicosis caused by toxic nodular goiter and sinus cardiac rhythm median concentration of 6.5 nmol/L significantly higher than 4.3 nmol/L in 8 healthy control women aged 39 - 56 years *990*

HDL-Cholesterol *Serum Decrease* In 25 patients mean concentration of 42.7 ± 9.04 mg/dL significantly different from 51.6 ± 21.2 mg/dL during treatment *2228* In 40 hyperthyroid patients 95% range concentration of 0.96 - 1.16 mmol/L significantly different from 1.18 - 1.31 mmol/L in 119 healthy controls *2852* Mean concentration of 40.1 ± 11.5 mg/dL in 7 hyperthyroid patients significantly different from post-treatment concentration of 52.4 ± 12.8 mg/dL *2072* In 14 hyperthyroid patients mean concentration of 39 ± 9 mg/dL *4951* In 13 hyperthyroid patients mean concentration of 36.8 ± 5.5 mg/dL compared with 45.5 ± 8.0 mg/dL in euthyroid state *5777* Mean concentration in 40 women with untreated Graves' disease of 1.22 ± 0.05 mmol/L significantly different from 1.45 ± 0.06 mmol/L in 35 healthy adult women of comparable age and life style *4357*
Serum No Effect In 30 patients with untreated hyperthyroidism mean concentration of 1.3 ± 0.3 mmol/L falls within normal range but increased to 1.4 ± 0.4 mmol/L during and after treatment *1368*

Hematocrit *Blood Decrease* Patients occasionally develop a mild hypochromic anemia *5679*

Hemoglobin *Blood Decrease* In 239 patients with uncomplicated disease, the concentration was < 12.0 g/dL in 37 of 207 women and < 13.0 g/dL in 9 of 32 men. A small fall is usual and it may sometimes be sufficient to cause a mild degree of anemia *3789* Often patients develop a normochromic and normocytic anemia with 9 - 11 g/dL *367*

HLA-A_1 *Serum Increase* In 105 patients with Graves' disease frequency of HLA B8 of 31.47% significantly increased compared with 23.28% in 6,682 controls *260*

HLA Antigens *Blood Present* HLA-DR3 present in 53% of patients with Graves' Disease versus 18% of controls *5678*

HLA-B_8 *Serum Increase* In 105 patients with Graves' disease frequency of HLA B8 of 23.80% significantly increased compared with 12.01% in 6,682 controls *260*

HLA-Cw7 *Serum Increase* In 105 patients with Graves' disease frequency of HLA B8 of 38.10% significantly increased compared with 26.73% in 6,682 controls *260*

HLA-D_5 *Serum Increase* In 105 patients with Graves' disease frequency of HLA B8 of 31.43% significantly increased compared with 18.00% in 6,682 controls *260*

Homocystine *Plasma Decrease* Concentration reduced in most patients with hyperthyroidism *5346*

Hyaluronic Acid *Serum No Effect* Serum concentration was measured by radiometric assay in patients with pretibial myxedema (PTM) and Graves' ophthalmopathy (GO). The mean HA concentration in the patients (n = 8) was 21.2 ± 15.3 (mean ± SD) µg/L, while that of Graves' disease without skin or eye involvement (n = 7) was 23.5 ± 11.0 (mean ± SD) µg/L and that of the controls (n = 8) was 25.5 ± 16.4 (mean ± SD) µg/L *2329*

11-Hydroxycorticosteroids *Urine No Effect* Excretion usually normal *5679*

17-Hydroxycorticosteroids *Urine Increase* Normal or slightly increased *5679*

Hydroxyproline *Plasma Increase* Observed effect *367*
Urine Decrease Reduced excretion in 22 of 33 patients *5484*
Urine Increase Because of excess bone resorption *1980* Elevated in 107 of 111 patients, aged 18-61 y and 10 of 14 patients over 65 *5484*

^{131}I Uptake *Serum Increase* Uptake is > 30% in 6 h, > 40% in 12 h, and > 55% in 24 h, with rapid release *1290* Thyroid uptake is increased. It is relatively more affected at 1, 2, or 6 h than at 24 h. It may be normal in presence of recent iodine ingestion *5544* May be present *1980* Mean uptake of 63.6% in patients over 60 y of age *1039*

Immunoglobulins *Serum* *Decrease* Possibly due to LATS effect *4707*

Insulin *Plasma* *Increase* Significantly elevated in 42 untreated patients, mean concentration was 23 ± 13 µU/mL *114* In 9 patients with Graves' disease mean total integrated immunoreactive insulin AUC of 67 ± 7 nmol/min significantly different from 44 ± 7 nmol/min in 9 healthy controls *353*

Insulin-like Growth Factor-I *Serum* *Decrease* In 18 patients with hyperthyroidism mean concentration of 131 ± 10 µg/L significantly different from 201 ± 16 µg/L in 20 controls *4273*
Serum *Increase* In 38 patients with hyperthyroidism mean concentration of 1,410 ± 200 U/L compared with 1,100 ± 50 U/L in 30 healthy controls *5383*

Interferon-γ *Serum* *No Effect* Median concentration of 0.0 pg/mL in patients with Graves' disease not different when compared with 0.0 pg/mL in normal controls *2307*

Interleukin-1α *Serum* *No Effect* Median concentration of 84 pg/mL in patients with Graves' disease not significantly different when compared with 100 pg/mL in normal controls *2307*

Interleukin-1β *Serum* *No Effect* Concentration not detectable in patients with Graves' disease or controls *2307*

Interleukin-2 *Serum* *Increase* Median concentration of 6.3% in patients with Graves' disease significantly increased when compared with 3.6% in normal controls *2307*

Interleukin-4 *Serum* *No Effect* Median concentration of 0 pg/mL in patients with Graves' disease not significantly different when compared with 0 pg/mL in normal controls *2307*

Interleukin-6 *Serum* *Increase* In 56 patients with spontaneous hypertjyroidism due to Graves' disease 108.2 ± 18.2 fmol/L significantly higher than 37.8 ± 6.2 fmol/L in healthy controls *303* In 16 patients with Graves' disease mean concentration of 23.0 pg/mL significantly different from 6.0 pg/mL in 15 healthy controls *5364*
Serum *No Effect* In 33 patients with Graves' disease mean concentration before therapy of 0.5 ± 0.3 ng/L compared with 1.0 ± 0.5 ng/L in 38 healthy controls *5634*

Interleukin-10 *Serum* *No Effect* Median concentration of 0 pg/mL in patients with Graves' disease not significantly different when compared with 0 pg/mL in normal controls *2307*

ionized Calcium *Serum* *Increase* Ionized and total calcium levels were elevated in 21 of 45 (47%) and in 12 of 45 (27%) thyrotoxic patients, respectively. Mean ionized and total calcium levels were higher in these 45 patients than in normal persons *640*

Isocitrate Dehydrogenase *Serum* *No Effect* Activity unaffected *5008*

17-Ketogenic Steroids *Urine* *Decrease* May be moderately reduced *5679*
Urine *Increase* Normal or slightly increased *5679*

Ketones *Serum* *Increase* Due to increased carbohydrate requirement in thyrotoxicosis *1290*
Urine *Increase* Children are more liable to develop ketosis than adults with thyrotoxicosis *1290*

17-Ketosteroids *Urine* *Decrease* Excretion may be slightly decreased in patients with thyrotoxicosis *2952*

Laminin *Serum* *Increase* In 23 patients with untreated Graves' disease mean concentration of 1,376 ng/mL (range 712 - 2,402) significantly higher than mean of 493 ng/mL (range 235 - 675) in 26 healthy controls *5635* In 27 patients with Graves' disease prior to treatment mean concentration of 1,444 ± 404 ng/mL significantly different from 492 ± 112 ng/mL in 34 healthy controls *5633*

LDL-Cholesterol *Serum* *Decrease* In 14 hyperthyroid patients mean concentration of 87 ± 38 mg/dL *4951* In 13 hyperthyroid patients mean concentration of 55.9 ± 11.9 mg/dL compared with 82.5 ± 24.6 mg/dL in euthyroid state *5777* In 40 hyperthyroid patients 95% range concentration of 2.19 - 2.75 mmol/L significantly different from 3.24 - 3.57 mmol/L in 119 healthy controls *2852* In 25 patients mean concentration of 122.1 ± 48.6 mg/dL significantly different from 146.8 ± 56.0 mg/dL during treatment *2228* Mean concentration in 40 women with untreated Graves' disease of 2.42 ± 0.11 mmol/L significantly different from 3.20 ± 0.12 mmol/L in 35 healthy adult women of comparable age and life style *4357* Mean concentration of 67.9 ± 13.8 mg/dL in 7 hyperthyroid patients significantly different from post-treatment concentration of 115.6 ± 15.7 mg/dL *2072*
Serum *No Effect* In 30 untreated patients with hyperthyroidism mean concentration of 2.6 ± 0.8 mmol/L towards lower limit of normal significantly increasing to 3.7 ± 1.2 mmol/L during and after treatment *1368*

Leptin *Serum* *Decrease* Conflicting results observed. Some studies suggest no change, others decreased concentrations with hyperthyroidism *713*
Serum *No Effect* Conflicting results observed. Some studies suggest no change, others decreased concentrations with hyperthyroidism *713*

Leukocytes *Blood* *Decrease* About 10% of patients develop low count due to decreased neutrophils *5679*

Lipids *Serum* *Decrease* Total lipids are usually decreased *5544*

Lipoprotein Lp(a) *Serum* *Decrease* Mean concentration of 9.7 ± 5.3 mg/dL in 7 hyperthyroid patients significantly different from post-treatment concentration of 17.9 ± 6.5 mg/dL *2072* In 13 hyperthyroid patients mean concentration of 9.4 ± 13.9 mg/dL compared with 15.5 ± 16.4 mg/dL in euthyroid state *5777* Mean concentration of 75 ± 28 mg/L significantly reduced in 27 hyperthyroid individuals compared with 150 ± 36 mg/L in 54 euthyroid individuals and 155 ± 31 mg/L in 114 blood bank donors *1053* In 30 patients with untreated hyperthyroidism mean concentration of 73 mg/L (range 46 - 117) significantly less than when the patients were undergoing treatment (102 mg/L, range 62 - 168) *1368*
Serum *No Effect* In 25 patients mean concentration of 7.60 ± 7.66 mg/dL not significantly different from 7.73 ± 7.13 mg/dL during treatment *2228* No significant difference observed between concentrations in hyperthyroid patients and healthy controls *3637*

Long Acting Thyroid Stimulating Hormone *Serum* *Increase* Found in at most 80% of patients with Graves' disease, and its presence or level does not correlate uniformly with thyroid hyperactivity *367* Present in most patients with Graves' disease *4778* Detected in about 50% of patients with hyperthyroidism of Graves' disease and in many patients who are euthyroid or hypothyroid *3083*

Low Density Lipoprotein Receptor Activity *Serum* *Increase* Mean activity of 88.3 ± 23.4% in 7 hyperthyroid patients significantly different from post-treatment activity of 75.9 ± 17.7% *2072*

Luteinizing Hormone *Plasma* *Increase* In 7 men aged 36 - 46 years wth hyperthyroidism mean concentration significantly increased compared with healthy controls *2275* Observed effect *3905*

Lymphocytes *Blood* *Increase* Relative lymphocytosis *5679* Although a peripheral blood lymphocytosis has been noted in the past, a recent study of the distribution of T and B lymphocytes showed a slightly decreased number of T cells, and consequently of total lymphocytes *5372*

α_2-Macroglobulin *Serum* *No Effect* In 8 untreated patients median concentration of 2.4 g/L not significantly different from 2.5 g/L during treatment in 4 individuals *3694*

Magnesium *Serum* *Decrease* Concentration is reduced in association with hyperthyroidism *2952*

MCH *Blood* *Decrease* Patients occasionally develop a mild hypochromic anemia *5679*

MCHC *Blood* *Decrease* Patients occasionally develop a mild hypochromic anemia *5679*

MCV *Blood* *Decrease* Decreased in hyperthyroid patients with neither anemia nor a reduced transferrin saturation. After treatment, it rose by an average of 6 fL. A diminution, even within the normal range, is an invariable concomitant of hyperthyroidism *3789*

Mean Platelet Volume *Blood* *No Effect* In 15 patients with hyperthyroidism mean of 10.4 fL compared with normal range of 9 - 13 fL *5020*

Monocytes *Blood* *Increase* May occur *5679*

N-Acetyl-Glucosaminidase *Urine* *No Effect* No significant difference observed between mean excretion of 5.85 mg/d in 41 patients with active Graves' ophthalmopathy and 4.63 mg/d in healthy controls *3321*

Neopterin *Serum* *Increase* In 24 patients with hyperthyroid Graves' disease mean concentration of 5.6 ± 1.7 nmol/L not significantly increased over 3.9 ± 0.9 nmol/L in 24 normal controls *5521*

242.90 Hyperthyroidism *(continued)*

Neutrophil Elastase *Plasma Increase* In 13 hyperthyroid patients mean concentration of 1,086.5 ± 12,30.0 µg/L compared with 160.3 ± 47.2 µg/L in 11 euthyroid controls *2018*

Neutrophils *Blood Decrease* About 10% of patients develop low count due to decreased neutrophils *5679*

Osteocalcin *Serum Decrease* In hyperthyroidism decreased serum concentrations have been reported. Serum osteocalcin levels have been found *4850 5808*
Serum Increase In hyperthyroidism T3 and T4 increase the rate of bone turnover and cause a new loss of bone matrix. Increased bone loss and increased serum osteocalcin levels have been found *3157* Levels were significantly increased (5.94 ± 2.55 ng/mL) than in control subjects (2.89 ± 1.58 ng/mL) ($p = 5.66^{-4}$). There was a significant linear correlation between osteocalcin and thyroxine *3002* In patients with hyperthyroidism slight increase observed *4217* Mean concentration in 15 women with active Graves' thyrotoxicosis of 7.5 ± 0.8 ng/mL significantly higher than 4.3 ± 0.5 ng/mL in healthy controls *1154* In hyperthyroidism T3 and T4 increase the rate of bone turnover and cause a new loss of bone matrix. Increased bone loss and increased serum osteocalcin levels have been found *1660* In 27 patients with hyperthyroidism mean concentration of 54.7 ± 23.0 µg/L significantly higher than 22.5 ± 7.4 µg/L in 30 healthy controls *1658* In 27 patients with hyperthyroidism mean concentration of 44 ± 16 µg/L (7.6 nmol/L) significantly different from that in healthy adults (men 25 ± 5 µg/L, women 20 ± 6 µg/L) *541*

Oxygen Partial Pressure *Blood Decrease* Dyspnea *4891*

Oxygen Saturation *Blood Decrease* Dyspnea *4891*

Parathyroid Hormone *Plasma Decrease* Subnormal levels were found in 28.9% of cases. Parathyroid hormone correlated inversely to serum calcium and degree of hyperthyroidism *3624*

PDN-21 *Serum No Effect* In 3 patients with hyperthyroidism concentrations did not exceed upper limit of normal of 67 pg/mL in 98 healthy controls *5137*

pH *Blood Increase* Respiratory alkalosis may occur *1980*

Phosphate *Feces Increase* Poorly understood *5679*
Serum Increase Serum phosphate concentration may be increased with hyperthyroidism *5204* Hyperphosphatemia may occur, partially attributable to relative suppression of parathyroid hormone by hypercalcemia *5204*
Urine Increase Poorly understood *5679* Urinary excretion was increased and correlated positively to degree of hyperthyroidism *3624*

Phospholipids *Serum Decrease* Falls, but not in simple relation to the associated rise in the BMR. Diet has a variable effect on the blood level *1642*
Serum Increase Reported effect *1290*

Platelet Aggregation response to ADP *Blood No Effect* In 10 untreated patients median % with 1 µmol/L at 5 min of 8% not significantly different from 8% in 15 control individuals *3694*

Platelet Aggregation response to Collagen *Blood No Effect* In 10 untreated patients median % with 1 mg/L at 5 min of 72% not significantly different from 68% in 15 control individuals *3694*

Platelets *Blood No Effect* In 15 patients with hyperthyroidism mean concentration of 239 x 10^9/L compared with normal range of 150 - 350 x 10^9/L *5020* No effect typically observed *5679* In 10 untreated patients median concentration of 219 x 10^9/L not significantly different from 233 x 10^9/L in 38 healthy controls *3694*

Potassium *Serum Increase* In 20 patients with untreated hyperthyroidism mean concentration of 4.4 ± 0.3 mmol/L significantly higher than 4.2 ± 0.4 mmol/L in 18 healthy controls *5661*

Procollagen Type III Peptide *Serum Increase* Increased in 66% of patients *1402* Concentration typically increased in patients with hyperthyroidism but with normal liver function *2339*

Prothrombin Time *Plasma Increase* Hyperthyroidism, independent of congestive heart failure or concomitant unrelated liver disease, may cause abnormal liver tests *3625*

Pyridinoline *Urine Increase* In 29 patients with hyperthyroidism mean excretion of 126.5 ± 84.2 nmol/mmol creatinine significantly greater than 25.7 ± 10.4 and 33.1 ± 14.7 nmol/mol creatinine in healthy men and women respectively *167* Mean excretion of 246.3 ± 180.6 nmol/mmol creatinine significantly higher than 39.5 ± 11.6 nmol/mmol creatinine in 30 healthy controls *1658*

Pyridinoline Cross-linked Telopeptide of Type I Collagen
Serum Increase Concentration significantly higher in patients with thyrotoxicosis on presentation than in age and sex matched controls *5670* In 27 patients with Graves' disease prior to treatment mean concentration of 8.6 ± 35 ng/mL significantly different from 3.1 ± 1.3 ng/mL in 34 healthy controls *5633*

Pyridinoline, Free *Urine Increase* Mean excretion in women with thyroid disease significantly greater than 16 - 32 nmol/mmol creatinine in healthy premenopausal women *1798*

Reticulated Platelets *Blood Increase* In 15 patients with hyperthyroidism mean of 6.5 x 10^9/L (3.3% of total platelets) compared with normal of 1.75 x 10^9/L (0.9% of total) *5020*

Rheumatoid Factor *Serum Increase* Titers > 1:160 are more common in Graves' disease patients than in controls. In patients under 40, titers > 1:80 are more frequent than in control subjects *4838*

Riboflavin *Serum Decrease* Secondary to increased metabolic processes *5679*

Ristocetin Agglutination *Blood Increase* In 10 untreated patients median threshold of 1.25 g/L significantly different from 1.00 g/L in 38 healthy controls *3694*

Sex-Hormone Binding Globulin *Serum Increase* Patients who are clinically hyperthyroid usually have increased concentrations *2952* Concentration significantly increased in patients with hyperthyroidism (thyrotoxicosis) *1424* In 7 men aged 36 - 46 years with hyperthyroidism mean concentration significantly increased compared with healthy controls *2275* Concentration increased in patients with hyperthyroidism *4234*

Sodium *Serum Decrease* In 20 patients with untreated hyperthyroidism mean concentration of 136 ± 2 mmol/L compared with 141 ± 3 mmol/L in 18 healthy controls *5661*

Soluble CD8+ *Serum Increase* In 14 patients with Graves' hyperthyroidism before treatment mean concentration of 464 ± 91 U/mL significantly higher than 341 ± 97 U/mL in 20 healthy controls *3676*

Soluble CD23 *Serum Increase* In 14 patients with Graves' hyperthyroidism before treatment mean concentration of 345 ± 310 U/mL significantly higher than 189 ± 188 U/mL in 22 healthy controls *3676*

Soluble CD25+ *Serum Increase* In 14 patients with Graves' hyperthyroidism before treatment mean concentration of 1,574 ± 1,154 U/mL significantly higher than 385 ± 159 U/mL in 20 healthy controls *3676*

Soluble E-Selectin *Serum Increase* In 33 patients with Graves' disease mean concentration before therapy of 112 ± 48 µg/L compared with 26 ± 11 µg/L in 38 healthy controls *5634*

Soluble Intercellular Adhesion Molecule-1 *Serum Increase* In 33 patients with Graves' disease mean concentration before therapy of 556 ± 131 µg/L compared with 184 ± 88 µg/L in 38 healthy controls *5634* Positive results (concentrations greater than 337 ng/mL) observed in 56.4% of 45 patients with Graves' disease *3337*

Soluble Interleukin-2 Receptor *Serum Increase* Concentration significantly increased in all patients with hyperthyroidism (in Graves' disease of 3,276 ± 1,273 U/mL, in toxic nodular goiter of 4,183 ± 1,832 U/mL and in toxic adenoma of 1,671 ± 648 U/mL compared with normal range of 535 ± 240 U/mL) *2794* In 46 patients with hyperthyroid Graves' disease mean concentration of 1,683 ± 1,016 U/mL compared with 461 ± 186 U/mL in 20 normal controls and 1,111 ± 617 U/mL in 21 patients with untreated toxic adenoma *3300*

Soluble L-Selectin *Serum Increase* In 33 patients with Graves' disease mean concentration before therapy of 1,118 ± 238 µg/L compared with 580 ± 154 µg/L in 38 healthy controls *5634*

Soluble P-Selectin *Serum Increase* In 33 patients with Graves' disease mean concentration before therapy of 244 ± 102 µg/L compared with 214 ± 68 µg/L in 38 healthy controls *5634*

Soluble Vascular Cell Adhesion Molecule-1
Serum Increase In 33 patients with Graves' disease mean concentration before therapy of 52 ± 16 µg/L compared with 15 ± 7 µg/L in 38 healthy controls *5634*

T3-Uptake *Serum Increase* In 10 untreated patients median concentration of 1.30 arbitrary units significantly different from 1.00 arbitrary units in 38 healthy controls *3694* May be present

1980 Elevated in 57% of 21 patients in an elderly population. 9 of the patients with normal T3 uptakes had elevated PBI. T3 uptake was not a useful indicator of metabolic status *1039*

Testosterone *Serum* *Increase* In 7 men with hyperthyroidism aged 36 - 46 years concentration significantly increased compared with that in healthy controls *2275* Concentration increased in patients with hyperthyroidism *4234*

Theophylline *Serum* *Decrease* Mean half life of 4.5 h and mean total body clearance 0.8 mL/kg/min compared with 8.7 h and 0.65 mL/kg/min in healthy controls *2656*

Thiamine *Serum* *Decrease* Secondary to increased metabolic processes *5679*

Thyroglobulin Antibody *Serum* *Increase* In 33 patients with Graves' disease mean concentration before therapy of 192 ± 89 IU/L compared with 46 ± 22 IU/L in 38 healthy controls *5634*

Thyroid Stimulating Antibodies *Serum* *Increase* Positive antibodies (> 125%) observed in 93.3% of patients with Graves' disease, mean activity being 379% of normal values *3337*

Thyroid Stimulating Hormone *Serum* *Decrease* Classic picture of Graves' disease *1965* In 40 hyperthyroid patients mean concentration of < 0.05 mIU/L significantly lower than 0.23 - 3.7 mIU/L in 119 healthy controls *2852* In 30 patients with hyperthyroidism prior to treatment mean concentration of 0.05 ± 0.04 mIU/L significantly increased to 5.36 ± 11.2 mIU/L during and after treatment *1368* In 27 hyperthyroid individuals mean concentration of < 0.1 mU/L significantly less than 1.2 ± 0.6 mU/L in 54 euthyroid individuals and 0.3 - 5.0 mU/L in reference population of 114 blood donors *1053* In 5 women aged 40 - 59 years with thyrotoxicosis caused by toxic nodular goiter and sinus cardiac rhythm median concentration of 0.15 mU/L significantly lower than 2.0 ± mU/L in 8 healthy control women aged 39 - 56 years *990* Significantly reduced, but may occasionally fall in the normal range *1966* In 13 hyperthyroid patients mean concentration of < 0.1 µU/mL significantly less than 1.1 ± 1.5 /µU/mL in 11 euthyroid controls *2018* In 10 untreated patients median concentration of 0.07 µU/mL significantly different from 1.3 µU/mL in 38 healthy controls *3694* Mean concentration of 0.17 ± 0.29 µU/mL in 7 hyperthyroid patients significantly different from post-treatment concentration of 6.81 ± 9.43 µU/mL *2072* Mean concentration in 14 patients with Graves' disease prior to treatment of 0.14 ± 0.08 µU/mL significantly lower than 2.70 ± 0.15 µUm/L in 15 healthy controls *3676* In 13 hyperthyroid patients mean concentration of 0.077 ± 0.066 µU/mL compared with higher concentration in euthyroid state *5777* Plasma TSH levels are actually subnormal in Graves' disease in its hyperthyroid stage, normal in its euthyroid stage, and supranormal if the patient becomes hypothyroid *4551* Mean concentration of < 0.1 mU/L in 28 adult patients with primary hyperthyroidism significantly different compared with 1.2 ± 0.4 mU/L in 61 healthy control adults *4089* In 33 patients with Graves' disease mean concentration before therapy of < 0.01 mU/L compared with 2..4 ± 1.2 mU/L in 38 healthy controls *5634* In 23 patients with untreated Graves' disease mean concentration of < 0.01 µU/mL significantly lower than mean of 2.1 µU/mL (range of 0.5 - 3.7) in 26 healthy controls *5635* In 66 women with Graves' disease before treatment mean undetectable concentration significantly different from 2.0 ± 0.2 µU/mL in 49 healthy women and undetectable concentration in 26 men with untreated Graves' disease significantly different from 1.31 ± 0.14 µU/mL in 21 healthy control men *4589* In 27 patients with Graves' disease prior to treatment mean concentration of < 0.01 µIE/mL significantly different from 2.0 ± 1.1 µIE/mL in 34 healthy controls *5633* Mean concentration of < 0.16 mU/L in 24 hyperthyroid patients with Graves' disease significantly less than 0.9 ± 0.4 mU/L in 24 normal controls, with concentration rising in patients to 1.4 ± 1 mU/L in remission after first treatment *5521* In 9 patients with Graves' disease mean concentration of 0.07 ± 0.01 mU/L significantly different from 2.05 ± 1.13 mU/L in 9 healthy controls *353* In 20 patients with untreated hyperthyroidism mean concentration of 0.22 ± 0.16 mU/L significantly lower than 2.92 ± 1.38 mIU/L in18 healthy controls *5661* Mean concentration in 14 untreated patients with hyperthyroidism of < 0.1 µU/mL significantly less than normal range of < 4 µU/mL *4951* *Serum* *Increase* In 15 patients with hyperthyroidism mean concentration not detectable compared with normal of < 4.0 nmol/L *5020* Plasma TSH levels are actually subnormal in Graves' disease in its hyperthyroid stages, normal in its euthyroid stage, and supranormal if the patient becomes hypothyroid *4551* In pituitary hyperthyroidism associated with increased free thyroxine and TSH concentrations. Increased α-subunit confirms thyrotropinoma *1965*
Serum *No Effect* In 150 patients mean concentration of 0.8 ± 0.6 mIU/L not significantly different from 0.4 - 3.7 mIU/L in healthy individuals *304*

Thyroid Stimulating Hormone Binding Inhibiting Antibody *Serum* *No Effect* In 13 hyperthyroid patients mean concentration of 36.3 ± 24.6% not significantly different from 33.6 ± 30.6% in 11 euthyroid controls *2018*

Thyroid Stimulating Hormone Receptor Antibodies *Serum* *Increase* In 14 patients with Graves' hyperthyroidism before treatment mean concentration of 58 ± 70 U/L significantly higher than 0.4 ± 1.0 U/L in 6 healthy controls *3676* In 150 patients mean concentration of 49 ± 56 IU/L significantly different from < 5 IU/L in healthy individuals *304* Mean concentration in 40 women with untreated Graves' disease of 2.1 ± 1.4% significantly different from < 7% in 35 healthy adult women of comparable age and life style *4357*

Thyroid Stimulating Immunoglobulins *Serum* *Increase* In more than 90% specimens from patients with Graves' disease stimulating activity observed *2952*

Thyrotropin-Receptor Antibodies *Serum* *Increase* Positive antibodies (25%) observed in 60% of 45 patients with Graves' disease *3337*

Thyroxine Binding Globulin *Serum* *Increase* Elevated in all patients and fell to normal with therapy; patients whose illness recurred after cessation of drug therapy had higher pretreatment thyroglobulin values and no fall during treatment *598*

Thyroxine (T4) *Serum* *Increase* Hyperthyroidism diagnosed in six men aged 24 to 30 years because of mean concentration of 282.5 ± 11.0 nmol/L (reference range 64.4 ± 148.0 nmol/L) *2963* May be present *1980* In 20 patients with hyperthyroidism mean concentration of 314 ± 78 nmol/L significantly increased compared with 159 ± 45 nmol/L in 18 healthy controls *5661* In 24 patients with hyperthyroid Graves' disease mean concentration of 15.7 ± 4.5 nmol/L higher than 10.2 ± 2.3 nmol/L in 24 normal controls *5521* In 5 women aged 40 - 59 years with thyrotoxicosis caused by toxic nodular goiter and sinus cardiac rhythm median concentration of 232.8 ng/mL significantly higher than 105.0 ng/mL in 8 healthy control women aged 39 - 56 years *990* Mean concentration in 15 women with active Graves' thyrotoxicosis of 218 ± 12 nmol/L significantly higher than 112 ± 7 nmol/L in healthy controls *1154* Classic finding as seen in Graves' disease *1965* In 13 newly diagnosed patients mean concentration of 264 ± 46 nmol/L compared with reference interval of 51 - 142 nmol/L *2837* In 66 women with Graves' disease before treatment mean concentration of 22.53 ± 0.78 µg/dL significantly different from 8.47 ± 0.23 µg/dL in 49 healthy women and 21.60 ± 1.12 µg/dL in 26 men with untreated Graves' disease significantly different from 8.31 ± 0.31 µg/dL in 21 healthy control men *4589* In 10 untreated patients median concentration of 206 nmol/L significantly different from 100 nmol/L in 38 healthy controls *3694* Mean concentration in 14 patients with Graves' disease prior to treatment of 196 ± 63 nmol/L significantly higher than 100 ± 10 nmol/L in 15 healthy controls *3676* In 15 patients with hyperthyroidism mean concentration of 136.4 nmol/L compared with normal of 64.4 - 144.1 nmol/L *5020* In 40 hyperthyroid patients mean concentration of 254 ± 59 nmol/L significantly higher than 62 - 154 nmol/L in 119 healthy controls *2852* In 16 patients with Graves' disease mean concentration of 274.9 ± 46 nmol/L significantly different from 122.8 ± 26 nmol/L in 15 healthy controls *747*

Thyroxine (T4), Free *Serum* *Increase* Mean concentration in 40 women with untreated Graves' disease of 55.8 ± 3.3 pmol/L significantly different from 14.2 ± 1.3 pmol/L in 35 healthy adult women of comparable age and life style *4357* Mean concentration of 46.4 ± 31.6 pmol/L in 28 adult patients with primary hyperthyroidism significantly different compared with 14.3 ± 1.8 pmol/L in 61 healthy control adults *4089* Hyperthyroidism diagnosed in six men aged 24 to 30 years because of mean concentration of 84.8 ± 11.6 pmol/L (reference range of 10.3 ± 25.8 pmol/L) *2963* In 30 patients with untreated hyperthyroidism mean concentration of 42.0 ± 12.2 pmol/L significantly decreasing to 16.4 ± 8.4 pmol/L during or after treatment *1368* In 33 patients with Graves' disease mean concentration before therapy of 76.3 ± 11.1 pmol/L compared with 14.3 ± 5.5 pmol/L in 38 healthy controls *5634* In 13 hyperthyroid patients mean concentration of 6.2 ± 1.9 ng/dL compared with euthyroid state

242.90 Hyperthyroidism *(continued)*

Thyroxine (T4), Free *(continued)*
of 1.3 ± 0.6 pg/mL *5777* In 23 patients with untreated Graves' disease mean concentration of 58.2 pg/mL (range 24.3 - 92.2) significantly higher than mean 11.2 pg/mL (range 7.5 - 8.9) in 26 healthy controls *5635* Mean concentration of 5.29 ± 0.97 ng/dL in 7 hyperthyroid patients significantly different from post-treatment concentration of 0.95 ± 0.32 ng/dL *2072* Mean concentration of 63.5 ± 33.1 pmol/L in 27 patients with hyperthyroidism significantly higher than 14.4 ± 1.9 pmol/L in 30 healthy controls *1658* In 27 patients with Graves' disease prior to treatment mean concentration of 58.5 ± 24.3 pg/mL significantly higher than 12.0 ± 5.6 pg/mL in 34 healthy controls *5633* Classic picture of Graves' disease *1965* Mean concentration of 7.1 ± 6.5 ng/dL in 13 hyperthyroid patients significantly higher than 1.1 ± 0.4 ng/dL in 11 euthyroid controls *2018* Mean concentration of 3.3 ± 1.8 pmol/L in 24 patients with hyperthyroid Graves' disease significantly higher than 1.2 ± 0.3 pmol/L in 24 healthy controls *5521* In 25 patients mean concentration of 60.10 ± 30.19 U/L significantly higher than 18.37 ± 10.39 U/L during treatment *2228* In 14 hyperthyroid patients mean concentration of 35 ± 15 pg/mL compared with normal range of 8 - 18 pg/mL *4951* Observed effect *413*
Serum *No Effect* In 150 patients mean concentration of 1.2 ± 0.1 ng/dL not significantly different from 0.6 - 1.8 ng/dL in healthy individuals *304*

Thyroxine (T4) Index, Free *Serum* *Increase* In 27 hyperthyroid patients mean index 86.2 ± 33.2 significantly higher than 41.9 ± 6.9 in 54 euthyroid individuals and 25 - 65 in reference population derived from 114 healthy blood donors *1053* In 10 untreated patients median concentration of 283 arbitrary units significantly different from 95 arbitrary units in 38 healthy controls *3694* In 9 patients with Graves' disease mean index of 349 ± 29 significantly different from 92 ± 6 in 9 healthy controls *353* In 40 hyperthyroid patients mean concentration of 302 ± 80 significantly higher than 76 - 152 in 119 healthy controls *2852*

Tri-iodothyronine, Free (fT3) *Serum* *Increase* Mean concentration of 23.12 ± 9.10 pg/mL in 7 hyperthyroid patients significantly different from post-treatment concentration of 4.85 ± 2.03 pg/mL *2072* Mean concentration of 27.5 ± 25.3 pmol/L in 28 adult patients with primary hyperthyroidism significantly different compared with 6.0 ± 1.1 pmol/L in 61 healthy control adults *4089* In 33 patients with Graves' disease mean concentration before therapy of 25.2 ± 9.7 pmol/L compared with 4.3 ± 1.7 pmol/L in 38 healthy controls *5634* Mean concentration of 15 ± 9 pg/mL in 14 hyperthyroid patients significantly greater than normal range of 3 - 5.6 pg/mL *4951* Classic picture of Graves' disease *1965* In 13 hyperthyroid patients mean concentration of 20.0 ± 4.8 pg/mL compared with euthyroid state of 4.4 ± 1.8 pg/mL *5777* In 27 patients with Graves' disease prior to treatment mean concentration of 16.3 ± 5.2 pg/mL significantly higher than 2.9 ± 1.6 pg/mL in 34 healthy controls *5633* In 23 patients with untreated Graves' disease mean concentration of 16.1 pg/mL (range 5.4 - 32.6) significantly higher than mean of 2.8 pg/mL (range 1.9 - 3.8) in 26 healthy controls *5635* Mean concentration of 12.3 ± 6.0 pg/mL in 13 hyperthyroid patients significantly higher than 3.8 ± 0.8 pg/mL in 11 euthyroid controls *2018*
Serum *No Effect* In 150 patients mean concentration of 0.4 ± 0.4 ng/dL not significantly different from 0.25 - 0.6 ng/dL in healthy individuals *304*

Tri-iodothyronine (T3) *Serum* *Decrease* Mean concentration in 15 women with active Graves' thyrotoxicosis of 5.1 ± 0.4 nmol/L significantly reduced to 1.8 ± 0.2 nmol/L with antithyroid therapy *1154*
Serum *Increase* In 13 newly diagnosed patients mean concentration of 9.1 ± 2.6 nmol/L compared with reference interval of 1.2 - 3.4 nmol/L *2837* In 15 patients with hyperthyroidism mean concentration of 3.74 nmol/L compared with normal of 1.39 - 2.70 nmol/L *5020* In 40 hyperthyroid patients mean concentration of 5.0 ± 2.0 pmol/L significantly higher than 0.8 - 3.0 pmol/L in 119 healthy controls *2852* A small group of patients whose hypermetabolism is due to T3 excess alone has been identified. These patients are clinically hyperthyroid but have normal levels of total serum T4 and free T4. Their radioiodine uptakes are variable, but are usually in the upper normal range. Total serum T3 values are high *2039* In 30 patients with untreated hyperthyroidism mean concentration of 4.5 ± 2.0 nmol/L significantly declining to 2.1 ± 0.6 nmol/L during and after treatment *1368* Mean concentration in 14 patients with Graves' disease prior to treatment of 6.1 ± 2.1 nmol/L significantly higher than 4.1 ± 0.9 nmol/L in 15 healthy controls *3676* In 66 women with Graves' disease before treatment mean concentration of 405.0 ± 22.1 ng/dL significantly different from 112.0 ± 5.2 ng/dL in 49 healthy women and 470.7 ± 33.2 ng/dL in 26 men with untreated Graves' disease significantly different from 108.1 ± 5.9 ng/dL in 21 healthy control men *4589* Increased before overt hyperthyroidism is apparent and before serum T4 levels have increased *1290* Mean concentration of 23.6 ± 12.8 pmol/L in 27 patients with hyperthyroidism significantly higher than 5.3 ± 1.7 pmol/L in 30 healthy controls *1658* Mean concentration in 15 women with active Graves' thyrotoxicosis of 5.1 ± 0.4 nmol/L significantly higher than 2.1 ± 0.1 nmol/L in healthy controls *1154* May be present *1980* In 5 women aged 40 - 59 years with thyrotoxicosis caused by toxic nodular goiter and sinus cardiac rhythm median concentration of 4.0 ng/mL significantly higher than 1.5 ng/mL in 8 healthy control women aged 39 - 56 years *990* Classic picture of Graves' disease *1965* In 16 patients with Graves' disease mean concentration of 7.83 ± 2.9 nmol/L significantly different from 2.12 ± 0.38 nmol/L in 15 healthy controls *747* Hyperthyroidism diagnosed in six men aged 24 to 30 years because of mean concentration of 6.01 ± 0.45 nmol/L (reference range 1.23 ± 2.46 nmol/L) *2963* In 20 patients with hyperthyroidism mean concentration of 6.1 ± 1.9 nmol/L significantly higher than 2.4 ± 0.9 nmol/L in 18 healthy controls *5661* In 10 untreated patients median concentration of 5.4 nmol/L significantly different from 1.74 nmol/L in 38 healthy controls *3694* In 24 patients with hyperthyroid Graves' disease mean concentration of 369 ± 146 nmol/L significantly greater than 157 ± 39 nmol/L in 24 normal controls, but concentration fell to 154 ± 37 nmol/L during remission after first treatment *5521*

Tri-iodothyronine (T3) Index, Free *Serum* *Increase* In 10 untreated patients median concentration of 8.5 arbitrary units significantly different from 1.8 arbitrary units in 38 healthy controls *3694* In 9 patients with Graves' disease mean index of 10.9 ± 1.0 significantly different from 1.6 ± 0.1 in 9 healthy controls *353*

Triglycerides *Serum* *Decrease* In 13 hyperthyroid patients mean concentration of 126.3 ± 16.4 mg/dL compared with 185.4 ± 35.5 mg/dL in euthyroid state *5777* Falls, but not in simple relation to the associated rise in the BMR. Diet has a variable effect on the blood level *1642* In 25 patients mean concentration of 118.0 ± 62.4 mg/dL significantly different from 144.6 ± 83.6 mg/dL during treatment *2228* Mean concentration of 89.1 ± 44.2 mg/dL in 7 hyperthyroid patients not significantly different from post-treatment concentration of 156.1 ± 164.3 mg/dL *2072*
Serum *Increase* Mean concentration in 40 women with untreated Graves' disease of 0.96 ± 0.04 mmol/L significantly different from 0.83 ± 0.04 mmol/L in 35 healthy adult women of comparable age and life style *4357*
Serum *No Effect* In 40 hyperthyroid patients 95% range concentration of 1.05 - 1.33 mmol/L not significantly different from 1.10 - 1.38 mmol/L in 119 healthy controls *2852*

Tumor Necrosis Factor *Serum* *Increase* In 33 patients with Graves' disease mean concentration before therapy of 1.5 ± 0.6 ng/L compared with 1.1 ± 0.8 ng/L in 38 healthy controls *5634*

Tumor Necrosis Factor-α *Serum* *Increase* In 16 patients with Graves' disease mean concentration of 20.0 pg/mL significantly different from 5.0 pg/mL in 15 healthy controls *5364*
Serum *No Effect* Median concentration in patients with Graves' disease not significantly different from that in normal controls *2307*

Type IV Collagen 7S Domain *Serum* *Increase* In patients with hyperthyroidism concentration increased in the presence of normal liver function *2339*

Type IV Collagen Peptide *Serum* *Increase* Increased concentration observed in patients with hyperthyroidism in the presence of normal liver function *2339*

Urea Nitrogen *Serum* *Increase* Excessive protein catabolism *1025* In 77 untreated patients with hyperthyroidism mean concentration significantly increased compared with healthy controls *4813*
Serum *No Effect* In 66 women with Graves' disease before treatment mean concentration of 14.3 ± 0.5 mg/dL not significantly different from 13.0 ± 0.5 mg/dL in 49 healthy women and 12.6 ± 0.4 mg/dL in 26 men with untreated Graves' disease not significantly different from 13.8 ± 0.8 mg/dL in 21 healthy control men *4589*

Uric Acid *Serum* *Increase* In 66 women with Graves' disease before treatment mean concentration of 6.1 ± 0.2 mg/dL significantly different from 4.2 ± 0.1 mg/dL in 49 healthy women and 6.6 ± 0.2 mg/dL in 26 men with untreated Graves' disease significantly different from 4.5 ± 0.2 mg/dL in 21 healthy control men *4589*

Urobilin *Feces* *Increase* May be secondary to erythroid hyperplasia *5679*

Vitamin B_{12} *Serum* *Decrease* Secondary to increased metabolic processes *5679*

Volume *Plasma* *Increase* Corpuscular and total hypervolemia may occur to facilitate oxygen delivery to tissues *3710* Increase in plasma volume keeps the hemoglobin concentration from reaching polycythemic values *3648* *5677*
Urine *Increase* Mild polyuria *4891*

von Willebrand Factor Antigen *Plasma* *Increase* In 8 untreated patients median concentration of 2.8 IU/mL significantly different from 1.7 IU/mL during treatment in 4 individuals *3694*

Zinc *Urine* *Increase* Excretion enhanced as a consequence of rapid cellular turnover in thyrotoxicosis resulting in moderate zincuria *5174*

242.90 Thyrotoxicosis

Bilirubin, Indirect *Serum* *Increase* Concentration may be increased in patients with thyrotoxicosis because oxidative phosphorylation of bilirubin is inhibited *4617*

C-terminal Propeptide of Type I Collagen *Serum* *Increase* In 22 thyrotoxic patients mean concentration of 134 µg/L significantly higher than in controls *5669*

C-terminal Telopeptide of Type I Collagen *Serum* *Increase* In 22 thyrotoxic patients mean concentration of 4.1 - 17.7 µg/L significantly higher than reference interval of 2.0 - 4.4 µg/L *5669*

Phosphate *Serum* *Increase* Thyrotoxicosis may increase the serum phosphate concentration *969*

Tri-iodothyronine, Free (fT3) *Serum* *Increase* In 22 thyrotoxic patients mean concentration of 8 - > 43 pmol/L significantly higher than reference interval of 3.5 - 7.3 pmol/L *5669*

242.90 Tri-iodothyronine Toxicosis

Thyroid Stimulating Hormone *Serum* *Decrease* Concentration typically reduced in patients with tri-iodothyronine toxicosis *1965*

Thyroxine (T4) *Serum* *No Effect* Concentration usually normal in patients with tri-iodothyronine toxicosis *1965*

Thyroxine (T4), Free *Serum* *No Effect* Concentration usually normal in patients with tri-iodothyronine toxicosis *1208* Mean concentration usually normal in patients with tri-iodothyronine toxicosis *1965*

Tri-iodothyronine, Free (fT3) *Serum* *Increase* Mean concentration increased in patients with tri-iodothyronine toxicosis *1965*

Tri-iodothyronine (T3) *Serum* *Increase* Concentration increased typically in patients with tri-iodothyronine toxicosis *1965*

243.00 Congenital Hypothyroidism

Sex-Hormone Binding Globulin *Serum* *Decrease* Low concentrations reported in patients with congenital hypothyroidism, due to lack of rise in SHBG as seen in normal infants in the first two weeks of life *4234*

243.00 Cretinism

17-Ketogenic Steroids *Urine* *Decrease* Excretion reduced in cretinism *2952*

244.80 Central Hypothyroidism

C-terminal Telopeptide of Type I Collagen *Serum* *Decrease* Mean concentration of 1.8 ± 0.7 µg/L in 23 adult patients with primary hypothyroidism significantly different compared with 3.8 ± 1.6 µg/L in 61 healthy control adults *4089*

Thyroid Stimulating Hormone *Serum* *Increase* Mean concentration of 2.1 ± 2.2 mU/L in 23 adult patients with primary hypothyroidism not significantly different compared with 1.2 ± 0.4 mU/L in 61 healthy control adults *4089*

Thyroxine (T4), Free *Serum* *Decrease* Mean concentration of 4.0 ± 2.3 pmol/L in 23 adult patients with primary hypothyroidism significantly different compared with 14.3 ± 1.8 pmol/L in 61 healthy control adults *4089*

Tri-iodothyronine, Free (fT3) *Serum* *Decrease* Mean concentration of 3.2 ± 1.2 pmol/L in 23 adult patients with primary hypothyroidism significantly different compared with 6.0 ± 1.1 pmol/L in 61 healthy control adults *4089*

244.90 Hypothyroidism

Acid Phosphatase, Tartrate Resistant *Serum* *Decrease* In patients with hypothyroidism slight decrease observed *4217*

Adenosine Monophosphate *Urine* *Decrease* Lack of primary messenger necessary to activate adenyl cyclase system resulting in decreased levels. No hormonal effect noted *5229*

Albumin *Serum* *Increase* Increase in total pool may occur *5679* In 37% of 13 patients at initial hospitalization for this disorder *1576*
Urine *Increase* Urinalysis commonly demonstrates mild proteinuria without significant formed elements, and there is preservation of normal concentrating ability *900*

Aldolase *Serum* *Increase* May be elevated *900*

Aldosterone *Plasma* *No Effect* Typical finding *3151*

Alkaline Phosphatase *Serum* *Decrease* Reported effect. In one study represented 9.2% of all cases of low alkaline phosphatase activity *3160* Characteristically low in infantile and juvenile cases *5679*
Serum *Increase* Excess enzyme originates from the bone *5545* In 24% of 12 patients at initial hospitalization for this disorder *1576*

Alkaline Phosphatase, Bone Isoenzyme *Serum* *Decrease* In patients with hypothyroidism slight decrease observed *4217*

Angiotensin-converting Enzyme *Serum* *Decrease* Levels of 13.9 U/mL in hypothyroid patients versus 17.0 U/mL in controls. In 12 hypothyroid patients levels rose from 11.6 to 15.8 U/mL after thyroid replacement therapy. Patients with thyroxine index less than 5.0 had significantly lower levels than normal controls *574* Positive correlation with degree of hypothyroidism *4894*
Serum *No Effect* Patients had concentrations within normal range *3717*

Anisocytes *Blood* *Increase* A minor degree of anisocytosis and also acanthocytosis (32 of 172) was demonstrated *2241*

Anti-Endothelial Cell Antibodies *Serum* *Increase* Patients with hypothyroidism as defined by high levels of TSH have AECA significantly more often than patients with low or normal TSH (22.2% versus 2.8% and 5.8%) *5566*

Antibody Titer *Serum* *Increase* Antiparietal cell antibodies present in up to 40% of cases *413*

Antithyroglobulin Antibodies *Serum* *Increase* Found in 50% of cases of myxedema *116* May be detected in high titer if due to thyroiditis *5863*

Apolipoprotein A-I *Serum* *Increase* In 12 patients with hypothyroidism mean concentration of 1.38 ± 0.09 g/L significantly increased compared with concentration of 1.25 ± 0.08 g/L after one month's treatment with levothyroxine *4049*
Serum *No Effect* In 19 hypothyroid individuals with initial FTI of 0 - 15 mean baseline concentration of apolipoprotein A-I 1.72 ± 0.37 g/L *1053* In 32 patients with untreated hypothyroidism mean concentration of 1.60 ± 0.34 g/L unaffected by treatment *1368*

Apolipoprotein B *Serum* *Increase* In 32 patients with untreated hypothyroidism mean concentration of 1.51 ± 0.36 g/L decreased significantly to 1.20 ± 0.24 g/L during and after treatment *1368* In 19 hypothyroid individuals mean baseline concentration of 1,174 ± 268 mg/L significantly higher than in euthy-

244.90 Hypothyroidism *(continued)*

Apolipoprotein B *(continued)*
roid individuals *1053* In 12 patients with hypothyroidism mean concentration of 1.89 ± 0.02 g/L significantly increased compared with concentration of 1.52 ± 0.17 g/L after one month's treatment with levothyroxine *4049*

Aspartate Aminotransferase *Serum Increase* Hypothyroidism sometimes asociated with increased activity secondary to release from muscle *3625* The muscle involvement of this disease appears to be responsible for the elevation *1025* May be elevated *900* In 58% of 13 patients at initial hospitalization for this disorder *1576*

Bicarbonate *Serum Increase* Significant CO_2 retention can occur *900* In 60% of 13 patients at initial hospitalization for this disorder *1576*

Bleeding Time *Patient Increase* In 9 untreated patients median template bleeding time of 9.3 minutes significantly different from 4.0 minutes in 38 healthy controls *3694*

Calcium *Serum Increase* Sometimes increased *5545*
Serum No Effect Usually normal *5679*
Urine Decrease In general *5679*

Carcinoembryonic Antigen *Serum Increase* In 47 patients with hypothyroidism 68% had concentrations less than 2.5 ng/mL, 28% had concentrations between 2.6 and 5.0 ng/mL, 4% had concentrations between 5.1 and 10.0 ng/mL and 0% had concentrations greater than 10.0 ng/mL *2010*

Catecholamines *Plasma No Effect* Usually normal *5679*

Cholesterol *Pericardial Fluid Increase* High levels (2.6 - 5.2 mmol/L; 100 to 200 mg/dL) *566*
Serum Increase In true myxedema, level is usually > 200 mg/dL, but may be normal if there is also associated malnutrition *1290* A moderate elevation that may reflect depression in overall metabolism is almost always demonstrable *1025* Values ranged from 143 - 556 mg/dL in 10 patients *1839* In 58% of 12 patients at initial hospitalization for this disorder *1576* In patients with suspected hypothyroidism significantly increased only in patients with TSH greater than 20 mU/L *2469* In 70 patients with primary hypothyroidism median concentration of 272 mg/dL *3851* In 12 patients with hypothyroidism mean concentration of 8.04 ± 0.67 mmol/L significantly increased compared with concentration of 6.43 ± 0.41 mmol/L after one month's treatment with levothyroxine *4049* In pituitary hypothyroidism, may be normal or low *5679* In 29 thyroidectomized patients mean concentration increased to 342 ± 78 mg/dL *4951* Mean concentration of 317 mg/dL in patients with TSH of 5.0 to 9.9 mIU/L, 356 mg/dL with TSH of 10.0 to 39.9 mIU/L and 410 mg/dL i patients with TSH > 40 mIU/L *1163*
Serum No Effect In 32 patients with untreated hypothyroidism mean concentration of 6.8 ± 1.5 mmol/L decreased significantly to 5.9 ± 1.4 mmol/L during and after treatment *1368*

Cholesterol Esters *Serum Decrease* No significant difference in rate of esterification between hypo-, hyper- and euthyroid subjects. The fractional rates were highly significant, decreased in hypo- and increased in hyperthyroid patients *2886*

Chylomicrons *Serum Increase* Increased *4358 3017 4372*

Cortisol *Plasma No Effect* Concentration usually unaffected by disease *5679*

Creatine Kinase *Serum Increase* Often raised, but of no diagnostic value *5863* Slight increase *1980* Abnormally high serum levels found *1290* Significantly higher than in normal controls in patients with primary hypothyroidism *1193* Muscle involvement appears to be responsible for the elevation *1025* Found in 66% of 15 patients. Values returned to normal after restoration of thyroid function *1839*

Creatine Kinase MB-Isoenzyme *Serum Increase* May be due to accompanying myopathy. May be due to change in clearance *768* May be due to accompanying myopathy. May be due to change in clearance *1794*

Creatinine *Serum Increase* In 6 patients with hypothyroidism mean concentration of 1.05 ± 0.04 mg/dL significantly different from 0.87 ± 0.01 mg/dL in 49 healthy women and 0.92 ± 0.02 mg/dL in 21 healthy control men *4589* In 29 paired prior euthyroid and hypothyroid serum creatinine values the hypothyroid value was greater in 26 (89.7%) and equal in 3 (10.3%) *2820*
Urine Increase Usually normal *5679* Occasionally increased *1290*
Urine No Effect Usually normal *5679*

C-terminal Telopeptide of Type I Collagen *Serum Decrease* Mean concentration of 2.6 ± 1.0 µg/L in 28 adult patients with primary hypothyroidism significantly different compared with 3.8 ± 1.6 µg/L in 61 healthy control adults *4089*

3,3'-Di-iodothyronine *Serum Decrease* In 12 patients with hypothyroidism mean concentration of 14.9 ± 9.2 pmol/L significantly different from that in 14 healthy age and sex-matched controls in whom the mean plasma concentration was 50.5 ± 9.3 pmol/L *4138*

Epinephrine *Plasma No Effect* In 9 women with primary hypothyroidism mean concentration of 180 ± 49 pmol/L not significantly different from 229 ± 54 pmol/L in 7 healthy female controls *5444*

Estrogens *Plasma Increase* Increased estradiol *3905*

Factor VIII *Plasma Decrease* May occur *4857*

Factor IX *Plasma Decrease* May occur *4857*

Fibrinogen *Plasma Decrease* In 7 untreated patients median concentration of 4.0 g/L significantly different from 4.9 g/L during treatment in 5 individuals *3694*

Fibronectin *Plasma Decrease* In 7 untreated patients median concentration of 0.17 g/L significantly different from 0.31 g/L during treatment in 5 individuals *3694* Mean fasting concentration in 9 patients with untreated hyperthyroidism of 19.2 ± 8.0 mg/dL significantly lower than that in 28 normal men, 32.5 ± 7.1 mg/dL, and 31.6 ± 5.7 mg/dL in 34 normal women *4811*

Folate *Serum Decrease* May occur *5679*

Follicle Stimulating Hormone *Plasma Increase* Mean concentration of 6.3 ± 2.0 IU/L observed in 8 hypothyroid men compared with normal range of 1.2 - 5.0 IU/L *2849*

Follistatin, Free *Serum No Effect* Mean concentration in about 25 patients with hypothyroidism not significantly different from 3.5 ± 0.2 µg/L in 60 normal individuals *4523* Mean concentration in about 30 patients with hyperthyroidism not significantly different from 3.5 ± 0.2 µg/L in 60 normal individuals *4523*

Gastrin *Serum Decrease* Mean fasting plasma level was 64 ± 5 pg/mL compared to normal, 89 ± 4 pg/mL. No correlation was found between gastrin and any other parameters of thyroid function *4743*

GH response to Vasoactive Inhibitory Peptide
Plasma No Effect Infusion of 75 µg VIP over 12 min had no significant effect in 6 hypothyroid women before and after treatment with thyroid hormone *5383*

Glomerular Filtration Rate *Urine Decrease* Observed effect *5679*

Glucose *Serum Decrease* Fasting blood sugar is decreased *5545*
Serum Increase In 35% of 14 patients at initial hospitalization for this disorder *1576*

Glucose Tolerance *Serum Increase* Curve may be flat *5863*

Glutathione S-Transferase *Serum No Effect* Activity normal in 8 patients with hypothyroidism *361*

HDL_2-Cholesterol *Serum Increase* In 12 patients with hypothyroidism mean concentration of 0.65 ± 0.09 mmol/L significantly increased compared with concentration of 0.52 ± 0.07 mmol/L after one month's treatment with levothyroxine *4049*

HDL_2-Phospholipids *Serum Increase* In 12 patients with hypothyroidism mean concentration of 0.67 ± 0.08 mmol/L significantly increased compared with concentration of 0.59 ± 0.08 mmol/L after one month's treatment with levothyroxine *4049*

HDL_2-Triglycerides *Serum No Effect* In 12 patients with hypothyroidism mean concentration of 0.07 ± 0.01 mmol/L not significantly increased compared with concentration of 0.05 ± 0.01 mmol/L after one month's treatment with levothyroxine *4049*

HDL_3-Cholesterol *Serum No Effect* In 12 patients with hypothyroidism mean concentration of 0.81 ± 0.04 mmol/L not significantly increased compared with concentration of 0.80 ± 0.06 mmol/L after one month's treatment with levothyroxine *4049*

HDL_3-Phospholipids *Serum No Effect* In 12 patients with hypothyroidism mean concentration of 0.90 ± 0.07 mmol/L not significantly different compared with concentration of 0.91 ± 0.07 mmol/L after one month's treatment with levothyroxine *4049*

HDL_3-Triglycerides *Serum* *No Effect* In 12 patients with hypothyroidism mean concentration of 0.26 ± 0.03 mmol/L not significantly increased compared with concentration of 0.26 ± 0.03 mmol/L after one month's treatment with levothyroxine *4049*

HDL-Cholesterol *Serum* *Increase* In 29 thyroidectomized patients mean concentration of 75 ± 22 mg/dL *4951*
Serum *No Effect* In 32 patients with hypothyroidism mean concentration of 1.4 ± 0.4 mmol/L decreased nonsignificantly to 1.3 ± 0.3 mmol/L during and after treatment *1368* In 19 hypothyroid patients with FTI 0 - 15 mean concentration of 1.12 ± 0.28 mmol/L not significantly different from euthyroid controls *5364* In 12 patients with hypothyroidism mean concentration of 1.46 ± 0.13 mmol/L not significantly increased compared with concentration of 1.32 ± 0.10 mmol/L after one month's treatment with levothyroxine *4049* Median concentration in 42 patients with primary hypothyroidism of 58 mg/dL *3851*

HDL-Phospholipids *Serum* *No Effect* In 12 patients with hypothyroidism mean concentration of 1.57 ± 0.14 mmol/L not significantly increased compared with concentration of 1.50 ± 0.13 mmol/L after one month's treatment with levothyroxine *4049*

HDL-Triglycerides *Serum* *No Effect* In 12 patients with hypothyroidism mean concentration of 0.33 ± 0.03 mmol/L not significantly increased compared with concentration of 0.30 ± 0.03 mmol/L after one month's treatment with levothyroxine *4049*

Hematocrit *Blood* *Decrease* Many patients have a hypoplastic anemia which is unresponsive to therapy with iron, vitamin B_{12}, or folic acid. The degree is mild to moderate *5677* Anemia observed in 21 - 60% of patients *5699* Seldom < 30% *900* Mild to moderate normochromic, normocytic, or slightly macrocytic anemia with normal leukocyte and platelet counts *900* Of 202 patients, anemia was present on diagnosis in 39 of 172 women and 14 of 30 men. Microcytic anemia was present in only 9 patients in the entire series *2241*

Hemoglobin *Blood* *Decrease* Anemia observed in 21-60% of patients *5699* Many patients have a hypoplastic anemia which is unresponsive to therapy with iron, vitamin B_{12}, or folic acid. The degree is mild to moderate, with concentration rarely < 8 - 9 g/dL *5677* Anemia may occur, hemoglobin < 13 g/dL *1098* In 42% of 14 patients at initial hospitalization for this disorder *1576* Seldom < 9 g/dL. Of 202 patients, anemia was present on diagnosis in 39 of 172 women and in 14 of 30 men. Microcytic anemia was present in only 9 patients in the entire series *2241*

Hyaluronic Acid *Serum* *Increase* Reported finding *1401*

11-Hydroxycorticosteroids *Plasma* *Increase* Due to slow disposal of circulating cortisol *1290*

17-Hydroxycorticosteroids *Urine* *Decrease* Low in untreated disease. Does not necessarily indicate pituitary origin *5863* As a result of decreased rate of turnover of cortisol *5679*

^{131}I Uptake *Serum* *Decrease* Usually low but may be normal or in a rare patient slightly elevated at 2 or 4 h *2039*

Immunoglobulins *Cerebrospinal Fluid* *Increase* Disproportionate rise in immunoglobulin fraction of CSF protein in myxedema. Rise is not seen in plasma *4707*

Insulin-like Growth Factor-I *Serum* *Decrease* Observed effect *2166*

Interleukin-1 *Serum* *No Effect* A normal level of IL-1β (23 ± 15 fmol/mL) was shown in hypothyroid patients versus controls (IL-1β, 24 ± 5 fmol/mL) *2755*

Interleukin-2 *Serum* *Increase* An increased IL-2 level (82 ± 56 fmol/mL) has been shown in hypothyroid patients versus controls (33 ± 13 fmol/mL) *2755*

Iodide *Serum* *Decrease* The degree of iodine deficiency dictates the severity of the hypothyroidism *2039*

Iron *Serum* *Decrease* Of 202 patients, anemia was present on diagnosis in 39 of 172 women and 14 of 30 men *2241* Low in 50% of patients *2241* The most frequent type of anemia observed is a microcytic, hypochromic anemia caused by iron deficiency *2929* Concentration was < 50 µg/dL *1098* The most frequent type of anemia observed is a microcytic, hypochromic anemia caused by iron deficiency *5677*

Iron-binding Capacity, Total *Serum* *Decrease* Total IBC < 200 - 300 µg/dL *1098*
Serum *Increase* The serum iron concentration was < 12 µmol/L in 60 out of 118 patients. The TIBC was increased in only 21 of these 60 patients *2241*

Iron Saturation *Serum* *Decrease* Transferrin saturation < 20% *1098*

17-Ketogenic Steroids *Urine* *Decrease* Low in untreated disease. Does not necessarily indicate pituitary origin *5863* As a result of decreased rate of turnover of cortisol *5679*

17-Ketosteroids *Urine* *Decrease* Low in untreated disease. Does not necessarily indicate pituitary origin *5863* Excretion may be decreased in patients with myxedema *2952*

Lactate Dehydrogenase *Serum* *Increase* LD and CK activity are elevated, while AST, ALT, and alkaline phosphatase were within normal limits *2833* The muscle involvement of this disease appears to be responsible for the elevated levels seen in this condition *1025* In 60% of 13 patients at initial hospitalization for this disorder *1576* Regularly elevated *1025*

LDL-Cholesterol *Serum* *Increase* Mean concentration in 29 thyroidectomized patients mean concentration significantly increased to 225 ± 72 mg/dL *4951* Marked elevation secondary to decreased catabolism *126* Mean concentration of 225 mg/dL in patients with TSH of 5.0 to 9.9 mIU/L, 267 mg/dL with TSH of 10.0 to 39.9 mIU/L and 321 mg/dL i patients with TSH > 40 mIU/L *1163* Marked elevation secondary to decreased catabolism *5864* Median concentration in 42 patients with primary hypothyroidism 195 mg/dL *3851* In 12 patients with hypothyroidism mean concentration of 5.71 ± 0.62 mmol/L compared with concentration of 4.37 ± 0.44 mmol/L after one month's treatment with levothyroxine *4049* In 19 hypothyroid individuals with FTI 0 - 15 mean concentration of 6.45 ± 1.13 mmol/L *1053*
Serum *No Effect* In 32 patients with untreated hypothyroidism mean concentration of 4.6 ± 1.3 mmol/L, while still within normal range, decreased significantly to 3.9 ± 1.2 mmol/L during and after treatment *1368*

Leptin *Serum* *Increase* Conflicting results observed. Some studies suggest no change, others increased concentrations with hypothyroidism *713*
Serum *No Effect* Conflicting results observed. Some studies suggest no change, others decreased concentrations with hypothyroidism *713*

Lipids *Serum* *Increase* Thyroid hormone insufficiency results in abnormal lipid metabolism with minimal to marked increases in circulating levels of cholesterol and triglycerides *2039*

Lipoprotein Lp(a) *Serum* *Increase* In 32 patients with untreated hypothyroidism mean concentration of 136 mg/L (range 88 - 217) decreased significantly to 114 mg/L (range 69 - 191) during and after treatment *1368* Mean concentration of 255 ± 28 mg/L significantly higher in 19 overtly hypothyroid individuals than 150 ± 36 mg/L in 54 euthyroid individuals and 155 ± 31 mg/L in 114 blood bank donors *1053*
Serum *No Effect* In 12 patients with hypothyroidism mean concentration of 496 ± 123 mg/L not significantly increased compared with concentration of 464 ± 128 mg/L after one month's treatment with levothyroxine *4049* No significant difference observed between mean concentration of 278 mg/L in 30 hypothyroid patients and 272 mg/L in 30 euthyroid age and sex matched controls *277* No significant difference observed between concentrations in hypothyroid patients and healthy controls *3637*

Luteinizing Hormone *Plasma* *Increase* In 8 men with hypothyroidism mean concentration of 18.7 ± 7.3 IU/L compared with normal range of 2.5 - 9.8 IU/L *2849*

Macrocytes *Blood* *Increase* In 75 elderly patients with macrocytosis hypothyroidism was responsible in 15 *3232*

α_2-Macroglobulin *Serum* *No Effect* In 7 untreated patients median concentration of 2.1 g/L not significantly different from 2.4 g/L during treatment in 5 individuals *3694*

MCH *Blood* *Decrease* Microcytic hypochromic anemia may occur due to blood loss, increased demand or dietary inadequacy. MCH < 27 pg, MCV < 80 fL *1098*
Blood *Increase* Mild to moderate normochromic, normocytic, or slightly macrocytic anemia with normal leukocyte and platelet counts *900*

MCV *Blood* *Decrease* Microcytic hypochromic anemia may occur due to blood loss, increased demand or dietary inadequacy. MCH < 27 pg, MCV < 80 fL *1098*

244.90 **Hypothyroidism** *(continued)*

MCV *(continued)*
Blood *Increase* Mean MCV exceeded 90 fL in 29 of 53 patients with normal vitamin B_{12}, folic acid and iron levels. MCV invariably fell with T4 treatment even if initial levels were within the normal range. 9 of 53 patients with normal folic acid, vitamin B_{12} and iron had anemia and increased MCV -- the macrocytic anemia of hypothyroidism *2241* In 100 patients with macrocytosis (MCV greater than 110 fL) 2 had hypothyroidism *4924* Mild to moderate normochromic, normocytic, or slightly macrocytic anemia with normal leukocyte platelet counts *900*
Blood *No Effect* A true increase occurs in < 10% of the patients, and in these cases it is usually caused by a megaloblastic erythropoiesis due to vitamin B_{12} or folic acid deficiency *5318* *5677*

Myoglobin *Serum* *Increase* Significantly higher than normal in patients with primary hypothyroidism *1193*

Norepinephrine *Plasma* *Increase* In 9 women with primary hypothyroidism mean basal concentration of 1.48 ± 0.15 nmol/L significantly different from 0.79 ± 0.06 nmol/L in 7 healthy female controls *5444* Circulating levels are elevated and hypertension is not uncommon *2039*

Osteocalcin *Serum* *Decrease* In patients with hypothyroidism slight decrease observed *4217* Reported effect *4850*

Oxygen Partial Pressure *Blood* *Decrease* Rare dyspnea secondary to pleural effusion *5679*

Oxygen Saturation *Blood* *Decrease* Rare dyspnea secondary to pleural effusion *5679*

pH *Gastric Material* *Increase* True achlorhydria after maximum histamine stimulation occurs in 50% of patients with primary hypothyroidism *5679* Achlorhydria present in up to 40% of cases *4746*
Pleural Fluid *Decrease* Exudate (pH < 7.3) *126*

Phospholipids *Serum* *Increase* Reported effect *1290*

Platelet Aggregation response to ADP *Blood* *Increase* In 9 untreated patients median % with 1 µmol/L at 5 min of 40% significantly different from 8% in 15 control individuals *3694*

Platelet Aggregation response to Collagen *Blood* *No Effect* In 9 untreated patients median % with 1 mg/L at 5 min of 53% not significantly different from 68% in 15 control individuals *3694*

Platelets *Blood* *No Effect* In 9 untreated patients median concentration of 206 x 10^9/L not significantly different from 233 x 10^9/L in 38 healthy controls *3694*

Procollagen Type III Peptide *Serum* *Decrease* Concentration typically decreased in patients with hypothyroidism and normal liver function *2339*

Prolactin *Plasma* *Increase* In 8 hypothyroid men mean concentration of 582.3 ± 396.3 mIU/L compared with normal range of 436.3 ± 564.9 mIU/L *2849* Can trigger a mild to moderate increase (20 - 300 ng/mL) *3391* Over 14.0 ng/mL in 39% of patients with untreated primary disease. Mean concentration of 14.3 ± 1.1, range 4.7 - 42.0 ng/mL in 49 subjects. Normal range of 8.2 ± 0.5. Significant differences occurred only between female patients and controls, not with male patients and controls *2218* Associated with amenorrhea and pituitary enlargement secondary to primary hypothyroidism *2657* Can trigger a mild to moderate increase (20 - 300 ng/mL) *3394*

Prolactin response to Vasoactive Inhibitory Peptide
Plasma *Increase* In 6 hypothyroid women VIP infusion increased serum prolactin concentration with peak concentrations of 28.8 ± 3.4 µg/L being reached at 15 minutes with response unchanged from this once hypothyroidism treated *5383*

Protein *Cerebrospinal Fluid* *Increase* Perhaps due to increased capillary permeability *5679*
Pleural Fluid *Increase* Exudate (> 3 g/dL) *126*
Urine *Increase* May occur to a mild degree *1180*

Pyrophosphate *Synovial Fluid* *Increase* Has been identified *4681*

Ristocetin Agglutination *Blood* *Increase* In 9 untreated patients median threshold of 1.25 g/L significantly different from 1.00 g/L in 38 healthy controls *3694*

Sex-Hormone Binding Globulin *Serum* *Decrease* Hypothyroid patients have low or normal SHBG concentrations *4234* Significantly reduced concentrations observed in women with myxedema but not in men *1424* In 19 hypothyroid individuals with initial FTI of 0 - 15 mean SHBG concentration of 15.4 ± 12.6 nmol/L *1053* In 8 hypothyroid men mean concentration of 13.3 ± 3.0 nmol/L compared with normal range of 20 - 55 nmol/L *2849*
Serum *No Effect* Hypothyroid patients have low or normal SHBG concentrations *4234*

Sodium *Serum* *Decrease* Significant hyponatremia can occur *900*

Soluble Interleukin-2 Receptor *Serum* *Decrease* Concentration significantly reduced below normal in patients with hypothyroidism *2794*

Specific Gravity *Pleural Fluid* *Increase* Exudate (> 1.016) *126*
Urine *Decrease* May occur to a mild degree *1180*

T3-Uptake *Serum* *Decrease* Mean T3 was 76.7 ± 76 ng/mL, ranging from 20 - 600 ng/mL. 72 of 100 patients had subnormal values. No correlation with TSH concentration was found *2850* In 9 untreated patients median concentration of 0.68 arbitrary units significantly different from 1.00 arbitrary units in 38 healthy controls *3694*

Testosterone *Serum* *Decrease* In 8 hypothyroid men mean concentration of 6.1 ± 2.8 nmol/L compared with normal range of 13 - 33 nmol/L *2849*

Testosterone response to hCG *Serum* *Decrease* In 8 hypothyroid men hCG stimulation produced only 30% increase in serum testosterone concentration compared with normal doubling in euthyroid normal controls *2849*

Theophylline *Serum* *Increase* Mean half life of 11.6 h and mean total body clearance of 0.38 mL/kg/min compared with 8.7 h and 0.65 mL/kg/min in healthy controls *2656*

Thyroid Stimulating Hormone *Serum* *Decrease* Not increased in pituitary hypothyroidism and does not respond to TRH administration *5679*
Serum *Increase* In 32 patients with untreated hypothyroidism mean concentration of 51.6 ± 51.5 mIU/L significantly higher than when undergoing or after treatment (5.5 ± 5.7 mIU/L) *1368* In 62 patients with primary hypothyroidism median concentration of 43 mIU/L *5364* In mild hypothyroidism concentration slightly raised. In subclinical hypothyroidism mean concentration slightly raised. In pituitary hypothyroidism mean concentration can be low, normal or slightly raised *1208* In 6 patients with hypothyroidism mean concentration of 40.0 ± 2.3 µU/mL different from 2.0 ± 0.2 µU/mL in 49 healthy women and 1.31 ± 0.14 µU/mL in 21 healthy control men *4589* In 29 hypothyroid patients mean concentration of 48 ± 15 µU/mL significantly increased compared with normal range of < 4 µU/mL *4951* In 9 women with primary hypothyroidism mean concentration of 82 ± 19 mU/L significantly different from 1.9 ± 0.5 mU/L in 7 healthy female controls *5444* Elevated in all patients, mean of 76.7 ± 55 µU/mL, range of 11 - 240 µU/mL. Mean values for patients < 20 y old was significantly higher than for older patients *2850* Raised in all cases due to primary thyroid disease *1966* Concentration typicaaly increased in patients with myxedema *1965* Not increased in pituitary hypothyroidism and does not respond to TRH administration *5679* Mean concentration of 49 ± 49 mU/L in 28 adult patients with primary hypothyroidism significantly different compared with 1.2 ± 0.4 mU/L in 61 healthy control adults *4089* In 19 hypothyroid individuals mean concentration of 91.7 ± 11.5 mU/L significantly higher than 1.2 ± 0.6 mU/L in 54 euthyroid individuals and range of 0.3 - 5.0 mU/L in 114 blood donors *1053*

Thyroxine Binding Globulin *Serum* *Increase* Marked elevations found in the vast majority of patients with chronic lymphocytic thyroiditis, though an occasional patient will have low or nonmeasurable titers *2039*
Serum *No Effect* In some cases *5544*

Thyroxine (T4) *Serum* *Decrease* In 6 patients with hypothyroidism mean concentration of 1.79 ± 0.23 µg/dL different from 8.47 ± 0.23 µg/dL in 49 healthy women and 8.31 ± 0.31 µg/dL in 21 healthy control men *4589* Median concentration in 65 patients with primary hypothyroidism of 4.1 mg/dL *3851* In mild hypothyroidism concentration low or low normal. In subclinical hypothyroidism mean concentration normal. In pituitary hypothyroidism mean concentration concentration low or low normal *1965* Average T4 was 1.8 ± 1.5 µg/dL, range of 0.2 to 7.0 µg/dL. An inverse correlation was found with TSH and T4, r = 0.73 *2850* In 9 untreated patients median concentration of less than 6 nmol/L significantly different from 100 nmol/L in 38 healthy controls *3694* Concentration typically reduced in patients with myxedema *1965*

Thyroxine (T4), Free *Serum* *Decrease* In 32 patients with untreated hypothyroidism mean concentration of 7.6 ± 4.4 pmol/L significantly increased to 18.7 ± 5.7 pmol/L during and after treatment *1368* Concentration in myxedema typically reduced *1965* In 9 women with primary hypothyroidism mean concentration of 4.1 ± 1.1 pmol/L significantly different from 14.8 ± 0.8 pmol/L in 7 healthy female controls *5444* In mild hypothyroidism mean concentration low or low normal. In pituitary hypothyroidism concentration also low or low normal. In subclinical hypothyroidism concentration normal *1965* In 29 hypothyroid patients mean concentration of 2.4 ± 0.4 pg/mL compared with normal range of 8 - 18 pg/mL *4951* Mean concentration of 4.5 ± 2.7 pmol/L in 28 adult patients with primary hypothyroidism significantly different compared with 14.3 ± 1.8 pmol/L in 61 healthy control adults *4089* Significant efect observed *413*

Thyroxine (T4) Index, Free *Serum* *Decrease* In 19 hypothyroid patients mean index of 12.8 ± 6.4 significantly less than 41.9 ± 6.9 in 54 euthyroid individuals and range of 25 to 65 in reference population of 114 blood donors *1053* In 9 untreated patients median concentration of 8 arbitrary units significantly different from 95 arbitrary units in 38 healthy controls *3694*

Tri-iodothyronine, Free (fT3) *Serum* *Decrease* In 9 women with primary hypothyroidism mean concentration of 1.6 ± 0.2 pmol/L significantly different from 6.8 ± 1.4 pmol/L in 7 healthy female controls *5444* Concentration typically reduced in patients with myxedema *1965* In 29 hypothyroid patients mean concentration of 1.2 ± 3.0 pg/mL compared with normal range of 3 - 5.6 pg/mL *4951* Mean concentration of 3.2 ± 1.4 pmol/L in 28 adult patients with primary hypothyroidism significantly different compared with 6.0 ± 1.1 pmol/L in 61 healthy control adults *4089*
Serum *No Effect* In mild hypothyroidism concentration normal. In subclinical hypothyroidism mean concentration normal. In pituitary hypothyroidism concentration normal *1965*

Tri-iodothyronine, Reverse (rT3) *Serum* *Decrease* Serum thyroglobulin was elevated in 92% of 38 patients in the early stage of this disorder. After two months of corticosteroid treatment the levels were significantly decreased in 25 patients who could be rechecked *3582*

Tri-iodothyronine (T3) *Serum* *Decrease* Usually decreased but may be normal in approximately 20% of patients *5545* In 6 patients with hypothyroidism mean concentration of 57.3 ± 9.8 ng/dL different from 112.0 ± 5.2 ng/dL in 49 healthy women and 108.1 ± 5.9 ng/dL in 21 healthy control men *4589* In 9 untreated patients median concentration of less than 0.7 nmol/L significantly different from 1.74 nmol/L in 38 healthy controls *3694* In 32 patients with untreated hypothyroidism mean concentration of 1.3 ± 0.7 nmol/L nonsignificantly increased to 1.7 ± 0.5 nmol/L during and after treatment *1368* Concentration typically reduced in patients with myxedema *1965*

Tri-iodothyronine (T3) Index, Free *Serum* *Decrease* In 9 untreated patients median concentration of 0.5 arbitrary units significantly different from 1.8 arbitrary units in 38 healthy controls *3694*

Triglycerides *Serum* *Increase* Median concentration in 69 patients with primary hypothyroidism of 108 mg/dL *3851* In 12 patients with hypothyroidism mean concentration of 1.91 ± 0.38 mmol/L compared with concentration of 1.60 ± 0.21 mmol/L after one month's treatment with levothyroxine *4049* In 29 hypothyroid patients mean concentration of 182 ± 87 mg/dL *4951* In 19 overtly hypothyroid patients mean concentration of 3.03 ± 1.61 mmol/L significantly higher than in euthyroid individuals of about 1.33 mmol/L *1053* Thyroid hormone insufficiency results in abnormal lipid metabolism with minimal to marked increases in circulating levels of cholesterol and triglycerides *2039*

Type IV Collagen 7S Domain *Serum* *Decrease* In patients with hypothyroidism and normal liver function concentration typically decreased *2339*

Type IV Collagen Peptide *Serum* *Decrease* Concentration decreased in patients with hypothyroidism in the presence of normal liver function *2339*

Urea Nitrogen *Serum* *Increase* May be slightly elevated but returns to normal with replacement therapy *900* Usually normal *5679*
Serum *No Effect* Usually normal *5679*

Uric Acid *Serum* *Decrease* In 6 patients with hypothyroidism mean concentration of 3.2 ± 0.1 mg/dL significantly different from 4.2 ± 0.1 mg/dL in 49 healthy women and 4.5 ± 0.2 mg/dL in 21 healthy control men *4589*
Serum *Increase* In 45% of 13 patients at initial hospitalization for this disorder *1576* May be slightly elevated but returns to normal with replacement therapy *900*

Vitamin B_{12} *Serum* *Decrease* Almost 50% of patients have achlorhydria with intrinsic factor failure and low vitamin B_{12}; rarely megaloblastic anemia develops *5544*

VLDL-Cholesterol *Serum* *Decrease* In 19 hypothyroid individuals with FTI of 0 - 15 treatment to bring FTI to 55 - 65 caused VLDL-cholesterol concentration to decrease from 2.45 ± 1.32 mmol/L to 0.56 ± 0.23 mmol/L *1053*
Serum *Increase* Observed effect *5864*

Volume *Plasma* *Decrease* Total volume is reduced by 25% on the average *3710*

von Willebrand Factor Antigen *Plasma* *Decrease* In 7 untreated patients median concentration of 1.1 IU/mL significantly different from 2.1 IU/mL during treatment in 5 individuals *3694*

245.10 Subacute Thyroiditis

Alkaline Phosphatase *Serum* *Increase* Elevated in 3 of 10 patients; no apparent relation to degree of T4 elevation and of unknown origin *1001*

Antithyroglobulin Antibodies *Serum* *Increase* Circulating thyroid antibodies are present in low titer in a minority of cases and disappear when disease subsides *5679*

Antithyroid Peroxidase Antibodies *Serum* *No Effect* In 5 patients with subacute thyroiditis in hyperthyroid phase mean concentration of 0 U/L not significantly different from 0.4 ± 1.0 U/L in 6 healthy controls *3676*

α_1-Antitrypsin *Serum* *Decrease* These conditions reduce activity *2091*

Cholesterol *Serum* *Increase* If hypothyroid *367*

Complement C_3 *Serum* *Increase* Increased serum C_3, IgM, alpha$_1$-acid glycoprotein and alpha$_1$-antitrypsin levels in 40 patients *3846*

Creatine Kinase *Serum* *Increase* If hypothyroid *367*

Creatinine *Serum* *No Effect* In 8 patients with subacute thyroiditis mean concentration of 0.70 ± 0.03 mg/dL not significantly different from 0.87 ± 0.01 mg/dL in 49 healthy women and 0.92 ± 0.02 mg/dL in 21 healthy control men *4589*

Erythrocyte Sedimentation Rate *Blood* *Increase* Frequently greatly elevated *1980* Invariably elevated in the 1st month, reaching very high levels that appear out of proportion to the degree of inflammation and remain so long after symptoms disappear *2302* Consistently increased, normal rate mitigates against the diagnosis *900*

Glucose *Serum* *Decrease* Severe hyponatremia and hypoglycemia may occur as a manifestation of primary or secondary thyroid failure *367*

γ-Glutamyltransferase *Serum* *Increase* Elevated in 3 patients, suggesting hepatic origin of the enzymes *1001*

Glycated Protein *Serum* *Increase* Increased serum C_3, alpha$_1$-acid glycoprotein and alpha$_1$-antitrypsin levels found in 40 patients *3846*

^{131}I Uptake *Serum* *Decrease* The association of a very low uptake with a normal or high serum T4 concentration is characteristic of the early phase of disease. Subnormal values for thyroid ^{131}I uptake are usually found *5679* Extremely low *1980*

immunoglobulin A *Serum* *Decrease* In 40 patients, levels were decreased in those who were BW-35 negative but were normal in the patients who were BW-35 positive *3846*

Immunoglobulin D *Serum* *Increase* Reported effect *1290*

Immunoglobulin M *Serum* *Increase* In 40 patients, there was an increase in serum C_3, IgM, alpha$_1$-acid glycoprotein and alpha$_1$-antitrypsin levels *3846*

Leukocytes *Blood* *Increase* May be moderately elevated to 15,000 - 20,000 /µL *2302* A slight leukocytosis may or may not be present *900*

Lymphocytes *Blood* *No Effect* T-lymphocytes may increase with a concomitant decrease in B-lymphocytes *367* Usually normal *5679*

PDN-21 *Serum* *No Effect* In 6 patients with subacute thyroiditis concentrations did not exceed upper limit of normal of 67 pg/mL in 98 healthy controls *5137*

245.10 Subacute Thyroiditis *(continued)*

Sodium *Serum Decrease* Severe hyponatremia and hypoglycemia may occur as a manifestation of primary or secondary thyroid failure *367*

Soluble CD8+ *Serum No Effect* In 5 patients with subacute thyroiditis in hyperthyroid phase mean concentration of 346 ± 34 U/mL not significantly different from 341 ± 97 U/mL in 20 healthy controls *3676*

Soluble CD23 *Serum No Effect* In 5 patients with subacute thyroiditis in hyperthyroid phase mean concentration of 97 ± 37 U/mL not significantly different from 189 ± 188 U/mL in 22 healthy controls *3676*

Soluble CD25+ *Serum Increase* In 5 patients with subacute thyroiditis in hyperthyroid phase mean concentration of 696 ± 127 U/mL significantly different from 385 ± 159 U/mL in 22 healthy controls *3676*

Thyroid Stimulating Hormone *Serum Decrease* Mean concentration in 5 patients with subacute thyroiditis in hyperthyroid phase of 0.27 ± 0.3218 µU/L significantly lower than 2.70 ± 0.15 µU/L in 15 healthy controls *3676* In 8 patients with subacute thyroiditis mean concentration of 0.67 ± 0.15 µU/mL different from 2.0 ± 0.2 µU/mL in 49 healthy women and 1.31 ± 0.14 µU/mL in 21 healthy control men *4589*
Serum Increase Defective hormonal synthesis causes increased secretion of TSH *2039* During recovery the TSH may be transiently elevated while T4 is depressed, and then over a period of 2 - 3 months all tests return to normal *367*

Thyroid Stimulating Hormone Receptor Antibodies *Serum No Effect* In 5 patients with subacute thyroiditis in hyperthyroid phase mean concentration of 0.4 ± 0.3 U/L not significantly different from 0.4 ± 1.0 U/L in 6 healthy controls *3676*

Thyroxine Binding Globulin *Serum Increase* Elevated during acute stage *2302* Serum thyroglobulin was elevated in 92% of 38 patients in the early stage of this disorder. After two months of corticosteroid treatment the levels were significantly decreased in 25 patients who could be rechecked *3193*

Thyroxine (T4) *Serum Decrease* May be subnormal late in the disease *5679*
Serum Increase The association of a very low iodine uptake with an elevated T4 is characteristic of the early phase of disease *5679* Elevated in 50% of patients *2302* Mean concentration in 5 patients with subacute thyroiditis in hyperthyroid phase of 130 ± 30 nmol/L not significantly higher than 100 ± 10 nmol/L in 15 healthy controls *3676* In 8 patients with subacute thyroiditis mean concentration of 12.67 ± 0.93 µg/dL different from 8.47 ± 0.23 µg/dL in 49 healthy women and 8.31 ± 0.31 µg/dL in 21 healthy control men *4589*
Serum No Effect May be normal with acute thyroiditis *367*

Tri-iodothyronine (T3) *Serum Increase* In 5 patients with subacute thyroiditis in hyperthyroid phase mean concentration of 4.1 ± 0.9 nmol/L significantly higher than 2.4 ± 0.4 nmol/L in 15 healthy controls *3676* In 8 patients with subacute thyroiditis mean concentration of 151.0 ± 11.1 ng/dL different from 112.0 ± 5.2 ng/dL in 49 healthy women and 108.1 ± 5.9 ng/dL in 21 healthy control men *4589* Invariably elevated at some time during acute stage *2302*

Urea Nitrogen *Serum No Effect* In 8 patients with subacute thyroiditis mean concentration of 14.5 ± 1.2 mg/dL not significantly different from 13.0 ± 0.5 mg/dL in 49 healthy women and 13.8 ± 0.8 mg/dL in 21 healthy control men *4589*

Uric Acid *Serum No Effect* In 8 patients with subacute thyroiditis mean concentration of 4.5 ± 0.4 mg/dL not significantly different from 4.2 ± 0.1 mg/dL in 49 healthy women and 4.5 ± 0.2 mg/dL in 21 healthy control men *4589*

245.20 Autoimmune Thyroiditis

Ammonium Ions *Urine Increase* May be associated with classic distal renal tubular acidosis which is associated with hyokalemia, hyperchloremic metabolic acidosis, urine pH > 5.5, increased urinary ammonium ion excretion, a negative urine anion gap, increased urinary osmol gap, decreased urinary citrate and increased urinary calcium in some patients *4071*

Anion Gap *Urine Decrease* May be associated with classic distal renal tubular acidosis which is associated with hyokalemia, hyperchloremic metabolic acidosis, urine pH > 5.5, increased urinary ammonium ion excretion, a negative urine anion gap, increased urinary osmol gap, decreased urinary citrate and increased urinary calcium in some patients *4071*

Anti-TSH Receptor Antibodies *Serum No Effect* In 17 patients mean concentration of < 5 U/L not different from normal *5521*

Antibodies against Megalin (gp330) *Serum Increase* In 26 patients with autoimmune thyroiditis mean fluorescence intensity of 65.72 ± 67.11 significantly higher than that in 32 normal individuals in whom mean fluorescence intensity 14.53 ± 12.03 *3299*

Calcium *Urine Increase* May be associated with classic distal renal tubular acidosis which is associated with hyokalemia, hyperchloremic metabolic acidosis, urine pH > 5.5, increased urinary ammonium ion excretion, a negative urine anion gap, increased urinary osmol gap, decreased urinary citrate and increased urinary calcium in some patients *4071*

Chloride *Serum Increase* May be associated with classic distal renal tubular acidosis which is associated with hyokalemia, hyperchloremic metabolic acidosis, urine pH > 5.5, increased urinary ammonium ion excretion, a negative urine anion gap, increased urinary osmol gap, decreased urinary citrate and increased urinary calcium in some patients *4071*

Citrate *Urine Decrease* May be associated with classic distal renal tubular acidosis which is associated with hyokalemia, hyperchloremic metabolic acidosis, urine pH > 5.5, increased urinary ammonium ion excretion, a negative urine anion gap, increased urinary osmol gap, decreased urinary citrate and increased urinary calcium in some patients *4071*

Glutamic Acid Decarboxylase Antibodies *Serum Increase* In only 3 of 85 patients with autoimmune thyroid disease GAD antibodies detected significantly greater than in healthy controls *3880*

Neopterin *Serum No Effect* In 17 patients with autoimmune thyroiditis mean concentration of 4.6 ± 1.5 nmol/L not significantly increased over 3.9 ± 0.9 nmol/L in 24 normal controls *5521*
Urine Increase Concentrations increased in autoimmune autothyroiditis and may be used to differentiate it from nonautoimmune thyroid disease *121*

Net Acid Excretion *Urine Increase* May be associated with classic distal renal tubular acidosis which is associated with hyokalemia, hyperchloremic metabolic acidosis, urine pH > 5.5, increased urinary ammonium ion excretion, a negative urine anion gap, increased urinary osmol gap, decreased urinary citrate and increased urinary calcium in some patients *4071*

Osmolal Gap *Urine Increase* May be associated with classic distal renal tubular acidosis which is associated with hyokalemia, hyperchloremic metabolic acidosis, urine pH > 5.5, increased urinary ammonium ion excretion, a negative urine anion gap, increased urinary osmol gap, decreased urinary citrate and increased urinary calcium in some patients *4071*

pH *Urine Increase* May be associated with classic distal renal tubular acidosis which is associated with hyokalemia, hyperchloremic metabolic acidosis, urine pH > 5.5, increased urinary ammonium ion excretion, a negative urine anion gap, increased urinary osmol gap, decreased urinary citrate and increased urinary calcium in some patients *4071*

Potassium *Serum Decrease* May be associated with classic distal renal tubular acidosis which is associated with hyokalemia, hyperchloremic metabolic acidosis, urine pH > 5.5, increased urinary ammonium ion excretion, a negative urine anion gap, increased urinary osmol gap, decreased urinary citrate and increased urinary calcium in some patients *4071*

Soluble Interleukin-2 Receptor *Serum Decrease* In 22 patients with hypothyroid autoimmune thyroiditis mean concentration of 48.6 pmol/L significantly less than 86.4 pmol/L in 21 age and sex-matched controls *3140*

Thyroid Stimulating Hormone *Serum No Effect* Mean concentration of 1.2 ± 1 mU/L in 17 patients with autoimmune thyroiditis not significantly different from 0.9 ± 0.4 mU/L in 24 normal controls *5521*

Thyroxine (T4) *Serum No Effect* Mean concentration of 10.3 ± 2.0 nmol/L not significantly different from 102 ± 2.3 nmol/L in 24 normal controls *5521*

Thyroxine (T4), Free *Serum* *No Effect* In 17 patients with autoimmune thyroiditis mean concentration of 1.3 ± 0.4 pmol/L not significantly different from 1.2 ± 0.3 pmol/L in 24 normal controls *5521*

Tri-iodothyronine (T3) *Serum* *No Effect* In 17 patients with autoimmune thyroiditis mean concentration of 142 ± 29 nmol/L not significantly different from 157 ± 39 nmol/L in 24 normal controls *5521*

245.20 Hashimoto's Disease

Alkaline Phosphatase *Serum* *Increase* Elevated in 3 patients, suggesting hepatic origin of the enzymes *1001*

Anti-Mitochondrial Antibodies *Serum* *Increase* Presence correlates with degree of lymphocytic infiltration of the gland *413*

Antibody Titer *Serum* *Increase* Almost all patients have thyroid autoantibodies in their serum, and extremely high titers of any of the autoantibodies are inconsistent with most other diagnoses *4551* Antimicrosomal antibodies present in 78% of patients *2033* Characteristically present in high titer during the active phase of chronic thyroiditis *2039* Virtually all patients with this disease have circulating autoantibodies *5679*

Antinuclear Antibodies *Serum* *Increase* Present in 1 - 8% of cases *2034*

Antithyroglobulin Antibodies *Serum* *Increase* May be detected in high titer *5863* Almost all patients have thyroid autoantibodies in their serum, and extremely high titers of any of the autoantibodies are inconsistent with most other diagnoses *4551* Characteristically present in high titer during the active phase of chronic thyroiditis *2039* In most patients present in high titers (> 1:25,000 in tanned red cell test). Young patients may have low titers of autoantibodies *5679* In over 80% of cases *116*

α_1-Antitrypsin *Serum* *Decrease* Reduced activity *2091*
Serum *Increase* Increased *4373* There was an increase in serum C_3, IgM, alpha$_1$-acid glycoprotein and alpha$_1$-antitrypsin levels found in 40 patients *3846* Increased *4241* *83* *4763* *4371*

Complement C_3 *Serum* *Increase* There was an increase in serum C_3, IgM, alpha$_1$-acid glycoprotein and alpha$_1$-antitrypsin levels found in 40 patients *3846*

Complement Fixation *Serum* *Increase* Antimicrosomal antibodies present in 78% of patients *2033* Positive for cytoplasmic microsomal antigen in > 80% of cases. High titers of 1:256 usually occur in chronic thyroiditis *2039* Virtually all patients with this disease have circulating autoantibodies *5679*

Erythrocyte Sedimentation Rate *Blood* *Increase* In 50% of chronic thyroiditis patients *2039* May be mildly elevated *1980*

γ-Globulin *Serum* *Increase* Occurs in approximately 50% of chronic patients, and may reflect the degree of thyroiditis or autoantibody production *2039* May be present *1980*

Gonadotropin, Pituitary *Plasma* *Increase* In the far advanced stage of thyroid destruction, all tests show the results of hypothyroidism *4551*

^{131}I Uptake *Serum* *Decrease* May be normal, elevated, or low *1980* Subnormal values are usually found early in the disease *5679* Markedly depressed *2033* In the far advanced stage of thyroid destruction, all tests show the results of hypothyroidism: radioiodide uptake is low normal to low *4551*
Serum *Increase* May be slightly elevated in chronic patients *2039* May be normal or elevated in euthyroid patients *2302* An early abnormality is a relative impairment of the process of organification of iodide trapped by the thyroid cell. Radioiodide uptake studies from 20 min to 6 h after administration may be relatively high, compared to the 24 h uptake *4551* May be normal, elevated, or low *1980*
Serum *No Effect* Uptake usually normal *1980*

Immunoglobulin G *Serum* *Increase* Often slightly raised *4551*

Immunoglobulin M *Serum* *Increase* There was an increase in serum C_3, IgM, alpha$_1$-acid glycoprotein and alpha$_1$-antitrypsin levels found in 40 patients *3846*

Long Acting Thyroid Stimulating Hormone *Serum* *Increase* Occasionally *5679*

β_2-Microglobulin *Serum* *No Effect* In 22 patients with Hashimoto's disease treated conservatively for 2 - 14 years mean concentration of 4.20 ± 2.77 mg/L significantly higher than 1.24 ± 0.09 mg/L in 30 controls *2734*

Precipitins *Serum* *Increase* Unusual but, when present, seem to be pathognomonic of Hashimoto's disease *4551* Precipitin test for thyroglobulin is positive in 60% of chronic thyroiditis cases. The least sensitive test for thyroid antibodies but the most specific *2039*

T3-Uptake *Serum* *Decrease* Mean value was 76.7 ± 76 ng/dL, ranging from 20 - 600 ng/dL. 72 of 100 patients had subnormal values. No correlation was found with TSH concentration *2850* In the far advanced stage of thyroid destruction, all tests show the results of hypothyroidism *4551*

Thyroid Microsomal Antibodies *Serum* *No Effect* In 22 patients with Hashimoto's disease treated conservatively for 2 - 14 years mean concentration of 197 ± 5.17 kU/L *2734*

Thyroid Stimulating Hormone *Serum* *Increase* May occur as disease progresses *5679* Elevated in all patients, mean of 76.7 ± 55 µU/mL, range of 11 - 240 µU/mL. Mean values for patients < 20 years old was significantly higher than for older patients *2850* Endogenous serum TSH may be normal or moderately elevated *1980*
Serum *No Effect* Usually normal at time of diagnosis *5679* In 22 patients with Hashimoto's disease treated conservatively for 2 - 14 years mean concentration of 1.91 ± 14.22 mU/L not significantly different from 2.47 ± 1.21 mU/L in 30 controls *2734*

Thyroxine Binding Globulin *Serum* *Increase* Elevated and fell to normal with therapy; patients whose illness recurred after cessation of drug therapy had higher pretreatment thyroglobulin values and no fall during treatment *598*

Thyroxine (T4) *Serum* *Decrease* Average T4 was 1.8 ± 1.5 µg/dL, range of 0.2 to 7.0 µg/dL. An inverse correlation was found with TSH and T4, r = 0.73 *2850* In 119 patients with rheumatoid arthritis 6 had Hashimoto's thyroiditis confirmed *4812* Normal in 25 euthyroid, reduced in 22 hypothyroid and increased in 4 hyperthyroid patients with Hashimoto's thyroiditis. No specific abnormalities in serum concentrations of thyroid hormones were found *1716* May be depressed, depending on the stage of development of the process *367* In the far advanced stage of thyroid destruction, all tests show the results of hypothyroidism *4551*
Serum *Increase* Normal in 25 euthyroid, reduced in 22 hypothyroid and increased in 4 hyperthyroid patients with Hashimoto's thyroiditis. No specific abnormalities in serum concentrations of thyroid hormones were found *1716*
Serum *No Effect* In 22 patients with Hashimoto's disease treated conservatively for 2 - 14 years mean concentration of 97.00 ± 59.8 nmol/L not significantly different from 83.27 ± 28.1 nmol/L in 30 controls *2734* Normal in 25 euthyroid, reduced in 22 hypothyroid and increased in 4 hyperthyroid patients with Hashimoto's thyroiditis. No specific abnormalities in serum concentrations of thyroid hormones were found *1716* The majority of patients are euthyroid at diagnosis with normal T3, T4, free hormones and TSH *2302* Concentrations typically normal *1980*

Tri-iodothyronine (T3) *Serum* *Decrease* Normal in 25 euthyroid, reduced in 22 hypothyroid and increased in 4 hyperthyroid patients with Hashimoto's thyroiditis. No specific abnormalities in serum concentrations of thyroid hormones were found *1716*
Serum *Increase* Normal in 25 euthyroid, reduced in 22 hypothyroid and increased in 4 hyperthyroid patients with Hashimoto's thyroiditis. No specific abnormalities in serum concentrations of thyroid hormones were found *1716* May occur as disease progresses *5679*
Serum *No Effect* Concentration typically normal at presentation *1980* The majority of patients are euthyroid at diagnosis with normal T3, T4, free hormones and TSH *2302* In 22 patients with Hashimoto's disease treated conservatively for 2 - 14 years mean concentration of 1.84 ± 0.77 nmol/L not significantly different from 2.07 ± 0.54 nmol/L in 30 controls *2734* Normal in 25 euthyroid, reduced in 22 hypothyroid and increased in 4 hyperthyroid patients with Hashimoto's thyroiditis. No specific abnormalities in serum concentrations of thyroid hormones were found *1716*

VDRL *Serum* *Positive* Persistent false positive reactions are seen *2039* A false positive serologic test may occur *1980*

245.80 Chronic Thyroiditis

PDN-21 *Serum* *No Effect* In 2 patients with chronic thyroiditis concentrations did not exceed upper limit of normal of 67 pg/mL in 98 healthy controls *5137*

245.90 Resistance to Thyroid Hormone in Adults

C-terminal Telopeptide of Type I Collagen *Serum* *Decrease* Mean concentration of 3.0 ± 1.0 µg/L in 31 adult patients with resistance to thyroid hormone significantly different compared with 3.8 ± 1.6 µg/L in 61 healthy control adults *4089*

Thyroid Stimulating Hormone *Serum* *No Effect* Mean concentration of 1.8 ± 0.9 mU/L in 31 adult patients with resistance to thyroid hormone compared with 1.2 ± 0.4 mU/L in 61 healthy control adults *4089*

Thyroxine (T4), Free *Serum* *Increase* Mean concentration of 29.3 ± 7.4 pmol/L in 31 adult patients with resistance to thyroid hormone significantly different compared with 14.3 ± 1.8 pmol/L in 61 healthy control adults *4089*

Tri-iodothyronine, Free (fT3) *Serum* *Increase* Mean concentration of 13.4 ± 2.3 pmol/L in 31 adult patients with resistance to thyroid hormone significantly different compared with 6.0 ± 1.1 pmol/L in 61 healthy control adults *4089*

245.90 Resistance to Thyroid Hormone in Pre- or Peri-pubertal children

C-terminal Telopeptide of Type I Collagen *Serum* *No Effect* Mean concentration of 13.2 ± 5.1 µg/L in 9 pre- or peripubertal patients with resistance to thyroid hormone not significantly different compared with 14.4 ± 3.1 µg/L in 32 healthy matched controls *4089*

Thyroid Stimulating Hormone *Serum* *Increase* Mean concentration of 1.7 ± 0.7 mU/L in 9 pubertal or peripubertal patients with resistance to thyroid hormone compared with 1.2 ± 0.4 mU/L in 61 healthy control adults *4089*

Thyroxine (T4), Free *Serum* *Increase* Mean concentration of 27.6 ± 6.2 pmol/L in 9 pre- or peripubertal patients with resistance to thyroid hormone significantly different compared with 16.0 ± 1.0 pmol/L in 32 healthy matched controls *4089*

Tri-iodothyronine, Free (fT3) *Serum* *Increase* Mean concentration of 12.7 ± 2.9 pmol/L in 9 pre- or peripubertal patients with resistance to thyroid hormone significantly different compared with 7.1 ± 0.8 pmol/L in 32 healthy matched controls *4089*

246.90 Benign Thyroid Disease

CA 72-4 *Serum* *Increase* In 69 patients with benign thyroid disease 6 (9%) had a concentration greater than cut-off of 2.5 U/mL with median concentration of 1.6 U/mL *4505*

Carcinoembryonic Antigen *Serum* *Increase* In 69 patients with benign thyroid disease 5 (7%) had a concentration greater than cut-off of 3 ng/mL with median concentration of 1.9 ng/mL *4505*

246.90 Nonthyroidal Illness

Bilirubin *Serum* *Increase* In 100 consecutive hospital patients with nonthyroidal illness 13 patients had subnormal T3 and T4 concentrations but with median bilirubin concentration of 25 µmol/L compared with normal range of 3 - 17 µmol/L *498*
Serum *No Effect* In 100 consecutive hospital patients with nonthyroidal illness, 41 had normal T4 and T3 concentrations with median bilirubin concentration of 8 µmol/L, 46 had subnormal T3 but normal T4 with bilirubin concentration of 8 µmol/L compared with normal range of 3 - 17 µmol/L *498*

C-Reactive Protein *Serum* *Increase* In 100 consecutive hospital patients with nonthyroidal illness, 41 had normal T4 and T3 concentrations with median CRP of 11 mg/L, 46 had subnormal T3 but normal T4 with CRP concentration of 61 mg/L and another 13 patients had subnormal T3 and T4 concentrations but with median concentration of 43 mg/L compared with normal range of < 8 mg/L *498*

Creatinine *Serum* *No Effect* In 100 consecutive hospital patients with nonthyroidal illness, 41 had normal T4 and T3 concentrations with median creatinine concentration of 76 µmol/L, 46 had subnormal T3 but normal T4 with creatinine concentration of 87 µmol/L and another 13 patients had subnormal T3 and T4 concentrations but with median creatinine concentration of 108 µmol/L compared with normal range of 55 - 110 µmol/L *498*

Fatty Acids (FFA), Free *Serum* *No Effect* In 100 consecutive hospital patients with nonthyroidal illness, 41 had normal T4 and T3 concentrations with median FFA concentration of 0.54 mmol/L, 46 had subnormal T3 and normal T4 with median FFA concentration of 0.53 mmol/L and another 13 patients had subnormal T3 and T4 concentrations but with median FFA concentration of 0.60 mmol/L compared with normal range of 0.10 - 0.70 mmol/L *498*

Interleukin-6 *Serum* *Increase* In 100 consecutive hospital patients with nonthyroidal illness, 46 had subnormal T3 but normal T4 with median IL-6 concentration of 39 U/mL and another 13 patients had subnormal T3 and T4 concentrations but with median IL-6 concentration of 59 U/mL compared with normal range of < 10 U/mL *498*
Serum *No Effect* In 100 consecutive hospital patients with nonthyroidal illness, 41 had normal T4 and T3 concentrations with median IL-6 concentration of 9 U/mL compared with normal range of < 10 U/mL *498*

T3-Uptake *Serum* *No Effect* In 100 consecutive hospital patients with nonthyroidal illness, 41 had normal T4 and T3 concentrations with median T3-uptake of 0.92 and another 46 patients had subnormal T3 concentrations but with normal T4 mean uptake of 0.98 and in 13 patients with subnormal T3 and T4 concentrations of 1.07 compared with normal range of 0.84 - 1.11 *498*

Thyroid Stimulating Hormone *Serum* *Increase* Whereas nocturnal surge (mean nighttime concentration greater than mean daytime concentration) was present in all 11 of 11 controls it was only present in 11 of 26 patients with nonthyroidal illness with both absolute and relative concentrations less *4420*
Serum *No Effect* No significant difference observed between mean concentrations in 26 patients with nonthyroidal illness and 11 healthy controls *4420* In 100 consecutive hospital patients with nonthyroidal illness, 41 had normal T4 and T3 concentrations with median TSH of 1.6 mU/L, 46 had subnormal T3 but normal T4 with TSH concentration of 1.4 mU/L and another 13 patients had subnormal T3 and T4 concentrations but with median TSH concentration of 2.3 mU/L compared with normal range of 0.4 - 4.0 mU/L *498* Mean concentration in 120 patients with NTI 1.143 ± 1.234 mU/L not significantly different from 0.881 ± 0.540 mU/L in 66 controls when measured by Amerlite MAB procedure *1403*

Thyroxine (T4) *Serum* *Decrease* In 100 consecutive hospital patients with nonthyroidal illness 13 had subnormal T4 and T3 concentrations with median FTI of 66 compared with normal range of 70 - 130 *498*
Serum *No Effect* In 100 consecutive hospital patients with nonthyroidal illness, 41 had normal T4 and T3 concentrations with median T4 of 100 nmol/L and another 46 patients had subnormal T3 concentrations but with normal T4 mean concentration of 100 nmol/L compared with normal range of 75 - 135 nmol/L *498* No significant difference observed between mean concentrations in 26 patients with nonthyroidal illness and 11 healthy controls *4420* Mean concentration in 120 patients with NTI 89.5 ± 28.1 nmol/L not significantly different from 89.8 ± 16.1 nmol/L in 66 controls when measured by Amerlite MAB procedure *1403*

Thyroxine (T4), Free *Serum* *No Effect* In 100 consecutive hospital patients with nonthyroidal illness, 41 had normal T4 and T3 concentrations with median FT4 of 14.3 pmol/L, 46 had subnormal T3 but normal T4 with FT4 concentration of 15.5 pmol/L and another 13 patients had subnormal T3 and T4 concentrations but with median FT4 concentration of 11.1 pmol/L compared with normal range of 10 - 20 pmol/L *498* No significant difference observed between mean concentrations in 26 patients with nonthyroidal illness and 11 healthy controls *4420*

Thyroxine (T4) Index, Free *Serum* *No Effect* In 100 consecutive hospital patients with nonthyroidal illness, 41 had normal T4 and T3 concentrations with median FTI of 103 and another 46 patients had subnormal T3 concentrations but with normal T4 mean FTI of 96 compared with normal range of 70 - 130 *498* *498*

Tri-iodothyronine, Free (fT3) *Serum Decrease* Mean concentration in 120 patients with NTI of 6.99 ± 1.54 pmol/L significantly different from 7.60 ± 1.28 pmol/L in 66 controls when measured by ultrafiltration procedure *1403*
Serum No Effect Mean concentration in 120 patients with NTI of 5.47 ± 1.29 pmol/L not significantly different from 5.32 ± 0.71 pmol/L in 66 controls when measured by Amerlite MAB procedure *1403*

Tri-iodothyronine, Reverse (rT3) *Serum Increase* In 26 patients with nonthyroidal illness mean concentration significantly higher than in 11 healthy controls (0.81 ± 0.24 nmol/L versus 0.23 ± 0.01 nmol/L) *4420* In 100 consecutive hospital patients with nonthyroidal illness, 46 had normal T4 and but subnormal T3 concentrations with median rT3 of 0.42 nmol/L compared with normal range of 0.14 - 0.38 nmol/L *498*
Serum No Effect In 100 consecutive hospital patients with nonthyroidal illness, 41 had normal T4 and T3 concentrations with median rT3 of 0.26 nmol/L and another 13 patients had subnormal T3 and T4 concentrations mean rT3 concentration of 0.37 nmol/L compared with normal range of 0.14 - 0.38 nmol/L *498*

Tri-iodothyronine (T3) *Serum Decrease* In 100 consecutive hospital patients with nonthyroidal illness, 46 had subnormal T3 concentrations with normal T4 concentrations with median of 0.98 nmol/L and 13 had subnormal concentrations of T4 and T3 with mean T3 concentration of 0.80 nmol/L compared with normal range of 1.30 - 2.45 nmol/L *498* In 26 patients with nonthyroidal illness mean concentrations significantly less than in healthy controls (1.11 ± 0.08 nmol/L versus 18.4 ± 0.11 nmol/L) *4420*
Serum No Effect In 100 consecutive hospital patients with nonthyroidal illness, 41 had normal T3 concentrations with median of 1.55 nmol/L compared with normal range of 1.30 - 2.45 nmol/L *498*

248.90 Thyrotoxic Periodic Paralysis

Phosphate *Serum Decrease* Thyrotoxic periodic paralysis is less common cause of hypophosphatemia due to shift of phosphate into cells *969*

250.00 Diabetes Mellitus

Acid Phosphatase *Serum Increase* Increased activity correlated with blood sugar concentration *372* In 90 diabetics, an increased activity of 137%, $p < 0.001$) was found. The increase was moderate (55%) in uncomplicated diabetics with slightly elevated glycemia (148 ± 24 mg/dL), and about twice normal levels in diabetics with either vasculopathies or marked hyperglycemia (343 ± 108 mg/dL) *371*

Acylcarnitine, Long Chain *Serum Increase* In diabetic patients concentration increased in comparison with control individuals *2809*

Acylcarnitine, Short Chain *Serum Increase* In diabetic patients concentration increased in comparison with control individuals, greatest in patients with ketoacidosis and correlated with plasma β-butyrate concentration *2809*

Adenosine-N6-diethylthioether-N1-pyridinoximine 5'-phosphate *Serum No Effect* In 3 patients with diabetes mellitus concentrations ranged from 112.0 - 368.0 nmol/dL not significantly different from concentration in healthy individuals in whom the mean concentration was 162.2 nmol/dL *5294*

Advanced Glycation End-products *Serum Increase* In 21 diabetics without diabetes-related complications mean content 18.0 ± 6.2%, in 25 diabetics with complications 24.1 ± 15.4% and 92.2 ± 30.1% significantly greater than that in 10 healthy individuals in whom mean content was 10.1 ± 1.0% as measured by method of Wröbel et al *5739*

Alanine *Plasma Decrease* Decreased *4798 237* Decreased concentration observed frequently *555*

Albumin *Serum Decrease* Mean concentration of 31.9 ± 1.1 g/L in 15 patients with diabetic nephropathy significantly less than 35 - 50 g/L in 91 healthy controls *5570* Tends to be low with increased alpha$_2$-globulins, particularly with vascular complications *4707* In 29% of 105 patients at initial hospitalization for this disorder *1576*
Serum No Effect In 61 patients with diabetes mellitus (11 with IDDM and 50 with NIDDM) mean concentration of 46 ± 3 g/L not significantly different from 42 ± 8 g/L in 57 heathy volunteers *4399*
Urine Increase In 250 diabetics mean concentration of 22.30 ± 3.50 mg/dL compared with 9.25 ± 1.11 mg/dL in 125 healthy controls *166* An early sign of diabetic nephropathy *4707* In 69 Albustix negative diabetic patients mean excretion 2.6 - 47.1 mg/dL or 0.6 - 46.4 mg/g creatinine compared with 0.3 - 30.1 mg/dL or 0.2 - 59.8 mg/g creatinine in 120 nondiabetic Albustix negative normal blood donors *4569*

Aldosterone *Plasma Decrease* Commonly found, a result of reduced renin secretion or a specific defect in synthesis are common *4214*
Urine Decrease Commonly found, a result of reduced renin secretion or a specific defect in synthesis are common *4214*

Alkaline Phosphatase *Serum Increase* Elevated by 40% in 44% of 166 untreated patients. Activity did not correlate with blood sugar concentration *372* In 24% of 105 patients at initial hospitalization for this disorder *1576* Occurred in 11 - 17% of the patients. Ketoacidosis and death occurred more often among patients with elevated serum enzymes than those with normal levels *1782*
Serum No Effect In 27 poorly controlled diabetic men (both IDDM and NIDDM) mean activity of 79.8 ± 26.9 U/L compared with normal range of 41 - 133 U/L *4607*

Amino Acids *Plasma Increase* Found with ketosis, probably associated with gluconeogenesis *1290*
Urine Increase In severe diabetic ketosis *1290*

Ammonia *Urine Increase* Reflects severity of acidosis and parallels the degree of ketonuria *1290*

Amylase *Serum Decrease* Both abnormally high and low values have been observed *4707*
Serum Increase High incidence of pancreatic abnormality in patients with no clinical evidence of pancreatic acinar disease *5378* Increased activity correlated with blood sugar concentration *372*
Urine Increase High incidence of pancreatic abnormality in patients with no clinical evidence of pancreatic acinar disease *5378*

Angiotensin-converting Enzyme *Serum Increase* Elevated levels were detected in 24% of 265 patients with this disease *3043* Elevated in 32% of 81 patients *4628*

1,5-Anhydroglucitol *Serum Decrease* In 25 diabetics mean concentration as measured by LC/MS 50.0 ± 8.5 μmol/L and 56.7 ± 8.5 μmol/L measured enzymatically compared with 151.8 ± 11.6 μmol/L and 159.8 ± 9.8 μmol/L respectively in healthy controls *3812*

Anti-Endothelial Cell Antibodies *Serum Increase* AECA became progressively more frequent with the duration of diabetes, being 4% in diabetics tested within 2 weeks of diagnosis and reaching 34% after an average disease duration of 11.2 years *5567*

Anti-Platelet Factor 4-heparin Antibodies *Serum Increase* In 46 patients with diabetes (type unspecified) positive titer (more than 2 SD above mean in 140 healthy men or women) observed in 4 (8.7%) *5536*

α_2-Antiplasmin *Plasma Increase* High fast-antiplasmin levels and low or missing slow-antiplasmin levels *107*

Antithrombin III *Plasma Decrease* Reports of increased and decreased levels *5220 3472*
Plasma Increase Reports of increased and decreased levels *3472 5220*
Plasma No Effect Normal levels seen with diabetic nephropathy *771*

Apolipoprotein B *Serum Increase* In 15 patients with diabetic nephropathy mean concentration of 175 ± 13 mg/dL significantly higher than 113 ± 3 mg/dL in 91 healthy controls *5570*

Apolipoproteins *Serum Decrease* Apolipoprotein A-1 markedly decreased in Type I and Type II diabetes *1692*
Serum Increase Compared to non-diabetic control subjects apolipoprotein A-I and B were significantly higher *1083* Apolipoprotein B was markedly increased. Apolipoprotein C-III was significantly elevated in Type II diabetes but not in Type I *86*
Serum No Effect Apolipoproteins C-II and A-II were not significantly different from controls in either Type I and Type II diabetes *1692*

Aspartate Aminotransferase *Serum Increase* Of 200 untreated diabetics, 12% had unexplainable elevations *1782*

250.00 Diabetes Mellitus *(continued)*

Basophils *Blood* *Increase* Reported effect *5677*

Bicarbonate *Serum* *Decrease* Frequently observed abnormality in diabetic patients *5544*

Brain Natriuretic Peptide *Urine* *Increase* In 19 patients with diabetes mellitus mean excretion of 6.09 ± 0.79 pmol/d significantly different from that in 11 healthy individuals in whom the mean excretion was 3.82 ± 0.62 pmol/d *5265*

CA 19-9 *Serum* *Increase* The biosynthesis of CA 19-9 seems to be accelerated in hyperglycemic diabetic patients, especially in females *158* CA 19-9 concentration increased in some patients with diabetes mellitus *1253* Simple regression shows a significant correlation between CA 19-9 and fasting blood glucose. CA 19-9 in diabetic patients is raised in acute metabolic situations and correlated very well with blood glucose concentration *2026*

Calcium *Serum* *Decrease* Osmotic diuresis secondary to hyperglycemia *5679*
Serum *No Effect* In 27 poorly controlled diabetic men (both IDDM and NIDDM) mean concentration of 2.4 ± 0.1 mmol/L compared with normal range of 2.2 - 2.6 mmol/L *4607*
Urine *Increase* Osmotic diuresis secondary to hyperglycemia *5679*

Carbon Dioxide Partial Pressure *Blood* *Decrease* Observed effect *4214*

Carboxymethyllysine *Serum* *Increase* Concentration is increased in diabetic children and adolescents compared to healthy controls *995*

Carcinoembryonic Antigen *Serum* *Increase* In 230 patients with diabetes mellitus 62% had concentrations less than 2.5 ng/mL, 34% had concentrations between 2.6 and 5.0 ng/mL, 3% had concentrations between 5.1 and 10.0 ng/mL and 1% had concentrations greater than 10.0 ng/mL *2010* 38% of patients had values > 2.5 ng/mL *4891*

Carnitine *Serum* *Increase* In patients with chronic renal failure mean concentration of 55.4 mmol/L higher than 41.7 mmol/L in nondiabetics *3976*

Carnitine, Free *Serum* *Decrease* In diabetic patients concentration decreased in comparison with control individuals *2809*
Serum *No Effect* In patients with chronic renal failure no significant difference observed between mean concentration in diabetics (19.2 mmol/L) and in nondiabetics (19.7 mmol/L) *3976*

Carotene *Serum* *Increase* Reported effect *5544*

α-Carotene *Serum* *Decrease* Mean concentration in 143 newly dicovered diabetics of 0.070 ± 0.006 μmol/L significantly different from 0.098 ± 0.005 μmol/L in population with normal glucose tolerance *1527*

β-Carotene *Serum* *Decrease* Mean concentration in 143 newly dicovered diabetics of 0.262 ± 0.022 μmol/L significantly different from 0.425 ± 0.018 μmol/L in population with normal glucose tolerance *1527*

Catecholamines *Plasma* *Decrease* Commonly observed abnormality *4214* Long-term diabetics with neuropathy showed significant reductions. Diabetics without neuropathy had normal concentrations *835*
Plasma *No Effect* Long-term diabetics with neuropathy showed significant reductions. Diabetics without neuropathy had normal concentrations *835*
Urine *Decrease* Long-term diabetics with neuropathy showed significant reductions. Diabetics without neuropathy had normal concentrations *835* Commonly observed abnormality *4214*

Chloride *Serum* *Decrease* Osmotic diuresis secondary to hyperglycemia *5679*
Urine *Increase* Osmotic diuresis secondary to hyperglycemia *5679*

Cholesterol *Serum* *Increase* Mean concentration of 9.8 ± 0.5 mmol/L in 15 patients with diabetic nephropathy significantly greater than 4.6 ± 0.1 mmol/L in 91 healthy controls *5570* In 50 patients with diabetes mellitus (both IDDM and NIDDM) mean concentration of 5.5 ± 2.2 mmol/L not significantly different from 5.1 ± 1.4 mmol/L in 19 healthy controls *3403* Moderate increase *1025*
Serum *No Effect* Mean concentration in 143 newly dicovered diabetics of 223.1 ± 3.7 mg/dL not significantly different from other populations *1527* In one patient with lipoatrophic diabetes mean concentration of 5.8 mmol/L at upper limit of reference range of < 6.0 mmol/L *3994*

Cholinesterase *Serum* *Increase* Obese type *1290*

Chondrex *Serum* *No Effect* Mean concentration of 66.5 ± 38.6 μg/L in 35 patients with diabetes not significantly different from 50.7 ± 38.6 μg/L in 329 apparently healthy controls *2040*

Chylomicrons *Serum* *Increase* Increased *4358* Minimal elevation secondary to decreased catabolism due to reduced lipoprotein lipase activity *126* Increased *4372* *3017*

Collagen IV *Serum* *Decrease* Median concentration in type I and type II diabetics significantly reduced compared to that in healthy controls (300 μg/L), 55 μg/L in diabetics excreting less than 30 μg/min albumin, 50 μg/L in those excreting 30 - 200 μg/min and 65 μg/L in those excreting more than 200 μg/min *2383*
Urine *Increase* In healthy controls collagen IV not detected whereas 2% of normoalbuminuric diabetics had detectable amounts, 45% of microalbuminuric diabetics and 50% of macroalbuminurics had detectable collagen IV in their urine *2383*

C-Peptide *Plasma* *Increase* In 27 poorly controlled diabetic men (both IDDM and NIDDM) mean concentration of 2.33 μg/L compared with normal range of 0.80 - 4.00 μg/L *4607* In one patient with lipoatrophic diabetes mean concentration of 1.5 nmol/L significantly greater than reference range of 0.3 - 1.0 nmol/L *3994*

Creatine *Serum* *Increase* Increased formation and decreased renal absorption *1290*
Urine *Increase* Creatinuria occurs with gonadal dysfunction in males and females *4707*

Creatinine *Serum* *Increase* In 49% of 102 patients at initial hospitalization for this disorder *1576* In 15 patients with diabetic neuropathy mean concentration of 368 ± 51 μmol/L significantly higher than range of 45 - 120 μg/L in 91 healthy controls *5570* High levels may be the result of interference by the high levels of glucose and acetone present *2064*
Serum *No Effect* In 27 poorly controlled diabetic men (both IDDM and NIDDM) mean concentration of 74.2 ± 19.4 μmol/L compared with normal range of 45 - 96 μmol/L *4607* In 61 patients with diabetes mellitus (11 with IDDM and 50 with NIDDM) mean concentration of 84.9 ± 30.0 μmol/L not significantly different from 77.8 ± 13.3 μmol/L in 57 heathy volunteers *4399*

Creatinine Clearance *Urine* *Decrease* In 18 patients with diabetes mellitus mean clearance of 67.4 ± 14.7 mL/min significantly different from that in 11 healthy individuals *5265*

Cryofibrinogen *Plasma* *Increase* Reported effect *1763* *4573* *4551* *3417*

β-Cryptoxanthin *Serum* *Decrease* Mean concentration in 143 newly dicovered diabetics of 0.122 ± 0.012 μmol/L significantly different from 0.156 ± 0.006 μmol/L in population with normal glucose tolerance *1527*

C-terminal Propeptide of Type I Procollagen
Serum *No Effect* Concentration of 103.4 ± 33.3 μg/L in 22 patients with diabetes mellitus not significantly different from 132.1 ± 41.3 μg/L in 8 healthy controls *2839*

5-D-Lactosylglutathione *Blood* *Increase* In 24 patients with diabetes mellitus mean concentration of 4.76 ± 1.95 pmol/10^6 erythrocytes compared with 3.37 ± 0.85 pmol/10^6 erythrocytes in 8 healthy controls *3425*

2,3-Diphosphoglycerate *Red Blood Cells* *Increase* Increased to 15.0 μmol/g (normal concentration of 13.7 μmol/g). Concentrations vary in response to plasma inorganic phosphate levels *1183*
Urine *Increase* Reported effect *1025*

Endothelin-1 *Plasma* *Increase* We found that 60% of patients with type 1 diabetes mellitus and elevated endothelin levels higher than 2.5 pg/mL (highest value in a control person) had had diabetes for more than 20 years (p less than 0.05 vs patients with normal endothelin levels). In type 2 diabetes mellitus the relation between elevated endothelin levels and diabetes duration was reversed *1941*

Factor VIII *Plasma* *Increase* Increased activity has been reported *1309*

Fat *Feces* *Increase* Defects of multiple stages of digestion-absorption *4891*

Fatty Acids (FFA), Free *Serum* *Increase* In one patient with lipoatrophic diabetes mean concentration of 2.3 mmol/L significantly higher than reference range of 0.3 - 0.8 mmol/L *3994*

Marked elevation in circulating concentration due to release of fatty acids from fat stores *4707*

Fibrin Degradation Products *Urine Increase* With diabetic nephropathy the greater the degree of proteinuria the greater the loss of fibrinogen degradation product in the urine *771*

Fibrinogen *Plasma Increase* Mean concentration in diabetic individuals younger than 30 years 12 mg/dL higher (significant) than in nondiabetic individuals of the same age. In individuals younger than 30 years those with parental history of diabetes mellitus had mean concentration of 5 mg/dL significantly higher than in controls *1519* Significantly higher in both juvenile and maturity onset diabetics *364*

Fibronectin *Plasma Increase* Median concentration in type I and type II diabetics significantly increased compared to that in healthy controls (400 mg/L), 900 mg/L in diabetics excreting less than 30 µg/min albumin, 800 mg/L in those excreting 30 - 200 µg/min and 750 mg/L in those excreting more than 200 µg/min *2383*
Urine Increase Median excretion in type I and type II diabetics significantly increased compared to that in healthy controls (20 µg/12 h), 120 µg/12 h in diabetics excreting less than 30 µg/min albumin, 120 µg/12 h in those excreting 30 - 200 µg/min and 200 µg/12 h in those excreting more than 200 µg/min *2383*

Follistatin, Free *Serum No Effect* Mean concentration in about 20 patients with diabetes mellitus not significantly different from 3.5 ± 0.2 µg/L in 60 normal individuals *4523*

Fructosamine *Serum Increase* Marked increase compared to controls *86* In 25 diabetics mean concentration of 429 ± 29 µmol/L significantly increased compared with 261 ± 5 µmol/L in 20 healthy controls *3812* In 61 patients with diabetes mellitus (11 with IDDM and 50 with NIDDM) mean concentration of 441 ± 82 mmol/L significantly different from 258 ± 23 mmol/L in 57 heathy volunteers *4399* Good sensitivity (97%) but poor specificity (19%). Does not seem suitable for diagnosis of mild abnormalities of glucose tolerance *1909*

α_2-Globulin *Serum Increase* Reported effect *5544*

β-Globulin *Serum Increase* Reported effect *5544*

β-Glucosaminidase *Serum Increase* Increased activity correlated with blood sugar concentration *372*

Glucose *Serum Increase* In one patient with lipoatrophic diabetes mean concentration of 14.0 mmol/L significantly greater than reference range of 3.4 - 7.2 mmol/L *3994* In 61 patients with diabetes mellitus (11 with IDDM and 50 with NIDDM) mean concentration of 11.3 ± 3.6 mmol/L significantly different from 5.2 ± 0.5 mmol/L in 57 heathy volunteers *4399* Characteristic finding in diabetic patients *900* Diagnosis can be readily made when there is an unequivocal and persistent elevation of the fasting plasma glucose. For venous plasma, the fasting glucose is normally between 60 - 100 mg/dL and values consistently > 120 mg/dL should be considered diagnostic of diabetes *2039* In 27 poorly controlled diabetic men (both IDDM and NIDDM) fasting glucose of 12.8 ± 4.2 mmol/L compared with normal range of 3.3 - 5.1 mmol/L *4607* In 23 Japanese American men who developed diabetes mean concentration of 5.7 ± 0.4 mmol/L compared with 5.3 ± 0.6 mmol/L in 212 who did not. In 17 women who developed diabetes mean concentration of 5.3 ± 0.4 mmol/L compared to 4.9 ± 0.5 mmol/L in 158 who did not *3429* Characteristic of diabetes *1642*
Serum No Effect May be normal in mild diabetes *1642* A large percentage of patients with early diabetes have perfectly normal fasting blood glucose levels. When elevated this test is very helpful, but when normal it is of little consequence. This is a poor screening test for diabetes *900*
Urine Increase Glycosuria is characteristic of the diabetic state, but its presence is neither necessary nor sufficient for the diagnosis *4333* Urine testing as a preliminary screening procedure for diabetes is the cheapest method available, however, it is not very productive *900*

Glucose Tolerance *Serum Decrease* The responses in nondiabetic and diabetic population do not describe a bimodal distribution, but constitute a single curve skewed in the direction of higher blood sugar values *2039* Decreased tolerance; decreased utilization with slow fall to fasting level *5544*

β-Glucuronidase *Serum Increase* Increased activity correlated with blood sugar concentration *372*

γ-Glutamyltransferase *Serum Increase* Increased activity reported with diabetes mellitus *3625* Frequently observed abnormality in patients with diabetes mellitus *1787* Activity reportedly increased in a variety of diseases including diseases of the pancreas, myocardium, kidney and lung as well as in diabetes mellitus *4617* A study of 228 patients has shown a significant positive association between serum GGT and triglyceride levels. Both fall with treatment, the most marked reduction occurring in patients on insulin. This association may reflect hepatic triglyceride levels in new diabetics may reflect hepatic microsomal enzyme induction of the rate-limiting enzymes of triglyceride synthesis. Serum GGT does not seem to correlate with hepatomegaly in diabetes mellitus *3313* In 50% of 20 patients at initial hospitalization for this disorder *1576*

Glycated Hemoglobin *Blood No Effect* In one patient with lipoatrophic diabetes mean concentration of 8.0% at upper limit of reference range of 5 - 8% *3994*

Glycated Protein *Serum Increase* Mean concentrations of 610 µmol/L in 14 patients with urinary albumin less than 15 µg/min, 840 µmol/L in 9 patients with urinary albumin between 15 and 150 µg/min and 680 µmol/L in 7 patients with urinary albumin above 150 µg/min compared with 370 µmol/L in 15 normal individuals *5354*
Urine Increase In 14 patients with urinary albumin less than 15 µg/min mean of 7.1 (SE 0.8) µmol/L, in 9 with albumin between 15 and 150 µg/min mean of 12 (SE 2) µmol/L and in 7 with albumin greater than 150 µg/min mean of 44 (SE 10) µmol/L compared with 6.1 (SE 0.6) µmol/L in 15 healthy individuals *5354*

Granular Casts *Urine Increase* With diabetic nephropathy *413*

Growth Hormone *Plasma Increase* Often abnormally high *4707*
Urine Increase Mean nocturnal excretion in 12 diabetic children of 5.6 ± 5.1 ng/g creatinine higher than in controls and correlated positively with blood glucose concentration at 07:00 h and with the increment of blood glucose between 24:00 h and 07:00 h *2953*

HDL-Cholesterol *Serum Decrease* Decreased *5707 325 3327* In one patient with lipoatrophic diabetes mean concentration of 0.3 mmol/L below reference range of > 0.9 mmol/L *3994*
Serum No Effect In 15 patients with diabetic nephropathy mean concentration of 1.2 ± 0.1 mmol/L not different from 1.2 ± 0.05 mmol/L in 91 healthy controls *5570*

Hemoglobin A_{1c} *Blood Increase* 2 - 3 fold increase in the red cells of diabetic patients. By providing an integrated measurement of blood glucose, Hb A_{1c} is useful in assessing the *4746* All patients classified as diabetic were found to have values greater than 9.9% *2462* In 27 poorly controlled diabetic men (both IDDM and NIDDM) mean concentration of 10.1% compared with normal range of 5.8 - 7.8% *4607*

Hepatocyte Growth Factor *Serum No Effect* In 14 patients with peripheral arterial disease and diabetes mellitus mean concentration of 0.44 ± 0.03 ng/mL not significantly different from 0.38 ± 0.03 ng/mL in 23 nondiabetic patients with peripheral arterial disease *5817*

β-Hexosaminidase *Serum Increase* Increase in total concentration (hexosaminidase A and B) *3850* Activity increased in patients with diabetes mellitus *2291*

β-Hexosaminidase Isoenzyme P *Serum Increase* Activity substantially increased in patients with diabetes mellitus *2291*

HLA Antigens *Blood Present* HLA-DR4 present in 38% of patients with insulin dependent disease versus 13% of controls. HLA-DR3 present in 50% of insulin dependent disease versus 21% of controls *5678* HLA-B_8 and HLA-Bw15 also associated with this disease *4879*

Homocysteine *Plasma Increase* The levels of total homocysteine in plasma were significantly higher in diabetic patients with macroangiopathy (10.8 ± 3.8 nmol/mL) than in those without macroangiopathy (8.3 ± 3.1 mmol/mL, $p < 0.001$) or non-diabetic subjects (7.5 ± 2.1 nmol/mL, $p < 0.001$) *165*
Plasma No Effect In 27 patients with diabetes mellitus aged 2 months to 10 years median concentration of 5.3 µmol/L, in 65 children aged 11 - 15 y 6.5 µmol/L and in 43 aged 16 - 18 y 7.8 µmol/L compared with 5.8 µmol/L, 6.6 µmol/L and 8.1 µmol/L in healthy children in the same age groups *5471*

Hyaline Casts *Urine Increase* With diabetic nephropathy *413*

25-Hydroxy Vitamin D *Serum Decrease* Of 290 medical patients, 63 had diabetes mellitus which had a correlation of p = 0.04 with hypovitaminosis *5212*

250.00 **Diabetes Mellitus** *(continued)*

17-Hydroxycorticosteroids *Urine* *Decrease* Observed effect *1025*

Hydroxyproline *Urine* *No Effect* In 27 poorly controlled diabetic men (both IDDM and NIDDM) mean concentration of 20.8 mg/m²/d compared with normal range of 6.0 - 22.0 mg/m²/d *4607*

Immunoglobulin G *Serum* *Increase* The levels of glycosylated IgG were significantly higher *4823*

Insulin *Plasma* *Decrease* A critical amount of insulin secretory reserve distinguishes between 2 qualitatively distinct clinical syndromes: true diabetes mellitus (the development of signs and symptoms of insulin deficiency) and the syndrome of pure resistance to insulin (signs and symptoms of hyperglycemia in the setting of adequate or excessive insulin secretion, frequently with obesity, but without diabetic complication) *5328* Absent in severe diabetes mellitus with ketosis and weight loss. In less severe cases, insulin is frequently present but only at lower glucose concentrations *5544*
Plasma *Increase* Increased in mild cases of untreated obese diabetics; fasting level is often increased *5544* In one patient with lipoatrophic diabetes mean concentration of 164 pmol/L significantly greater than reference range of < 120 pmol/L *3994* In 23 Japanese American men who developed diabetes mean concentration of 94 ± 52 pmol/L compared with 74 ± 41 pmol/L in 212 who did not. In 17 women who developed diabetes mean concentration of 89 ± 46 pmol/L compared to 82 ± 42 pmol/L in 158 who did not *3429*

Insulin-like Growth Factor-I *Serum* *Increase* In 22 patients with IDDM or NIDDM mean concentration in patients with proliferative retinopathy of 216 ± 22 ng/mL, in those with non-proliferative retinopathy 126 ± 15 ng/mL and in those without retinopathy 136 ± 37 ng/mL *1325*

Interleukin-1β *Urine* *Decrease* In 21 patients with diabetic nephropathy mean excretion of 39.9 ± 3.0 pg/mg creatinine significantly decreased compared with 172 ± 27 pg/mg creatinine in 13 healthy controls *2985*

Iron *Serum* *Decrease* In those patients with marked urinary loss serum concentration reduced to 592 ± 189 µg/L compared with 979 ± 394 µg/L in control population *2251*
Urine *Increase* Increased excretion observed early in the course of diabetic renal disease, being increased in 3 of 11 patients without proteinuria and in 8 of 10 patients with mild proteinuria. In those with nephrotic range proteinuria markedly increased urinary iron excretion observed *2251*

Isocitrate Dehydrogenase *Serum* *No Effect* Reported effect *5008*

17-Ketogenic Steroids *Urine* *Decrease* Reported effect *1025*

Ketones *Serum* *Increase* Increased as a result of disturbed fat and carbohydrate metabolism *4214* Up to 300 - 400 mg/dL or more *1290*
Urine *Increase* Children are more liable to develop ketosis than adults *1290*

Lactate *Blood* *Increase* Moderately elevated in 11 of 28 diabetics *1603*

Lactate Dehydrogenase *Serum* *Increase* Of 200 untreated diabetics, 21% had an unexplainable elevation *1782*

Laminin P1 *Serum* *No Effect* Median concentration in type I and type II diabetics comparable to that in healthy controls (1.2 kU/L) regardless of the extent of renal involvement *2383*
Urine *No Effect* Median concentration in type I and type II diabetics comparable to that in healthy controls (220 ng/12 h) regardless of the extent of renal involvement *2383*

LDL-Cholesterol *Serum* *Increase* In 15 patients with diabetic nephropathy mean concentration of 6.2 ± 0.5 mmol/L significantly greater than 2.9 ± 0.08 mmol/L in 91 healthy controls *5570*

Leptin *Serum* *Increase* In 23 Japanese American men who developed diabetes mean concentration of 6.0 ± 4.4 ng/mL compared with 3.8 ± 2.3 ng/mL in 212 who did not. In 17 women who developed diabetes mean concentration of 12.3 ± 5.4 ng/mL compared to 11.6 ± 7.5 ng/mL in 158 who did not *3429*

Lipids *Urine* *Increase* Lipids in the urine include all fractions. Double refractile (cholesterol) bodies can be seen *5544*

β-Lipoprotein *Serum* *Increase* Observed effect *1565* *1566* *1564*

Lipoprotein Lp(a) *Serum* *Increase* In diabetic patients who become proteinuric or nephrotic with progression of the disease plasma concentrations of Lp(a) may increase *2827* In 15 patients with diabetic nephropathy mean concentration of 50 ± 13 mg/dL significantly greater than 18 ± 2 mg/dL in 91 healthy controls *5570*
Serum *No Effect* In 45 patients with unspecified form of diabetes mellitus mean and median concentrations of 160 and 73 mg/L not significantly different from 174 and 106 mg/L in 766 nondiabetic controls *4892*

Lutein/Zeaxanthin *Serum* *Decrease* Mean concentration in 143 newly dicovered diabetics of 0.380 ± 0.033 µmol/L significantly different from 0.413 ± 0.016 µmol/L in population with normal glucose tolerance *1527*

Lycopene *Serum* *Decrease* Mean concentration in 143 newly dicovered diabetics of 0.377 ± 0.028 µmol/L significantly different from 0.415 ± 0.013 µmol/L in population with normal glucose tolerance *1527*

Lysozyme *Urine* *Increase* Lysozymuria *1425*

α_2-Macroglobulin *Serum* *Increase* Extent of elevation is usually found to directly correlate with duration of disease and presence of vascular complications *266* *760* *2515* All age groups *2412*

Magnesium *Platelets* *Increase* Mean concentration in 22 patients with diabetes mellitus of 51.0 ± 22.4 µmol/g protein higher than 35.2 ± 22.5 µmol/g protein in 22 age and sex matched controls *943*
Red Blood Cells *No Effect* Mean concentration of 0.18 ± 0.024 /10¹⁰ cells in 22 patients with diabetes mellitus not significantly different from 0.19 ± 0.024 /10¹⁰ cells in 22 age and sex matched controls *943*
Serum *Decrease* In 29 of 191 female diabetics (14.7%) mean serum magnesium concentration less than 0.73 mmol/L. Mean concentration of 0.82 ± 0.10 mmol/L observed in diabetic women compared with 0.87 ± 0.07 mmol/L in healthy women *818* Osmotic diuresis secondary to hyperglycemia *5679* Mean concentration of 0.67 ± 0.07 mmol/L in 22 patients with diabetes mellitus lower than 0.72 ± 0.06 mmol/L in 22 age and sex matched controls *943*
Serum *Increase* In diabetic coma before treatment and in controlled diabetes in older age groups *5544* Observed effect *5060*
Urine *Increase* Osmotic diuresis secondary to hyperglycemia *5679*

Magnesium, Ultrafiltrable *Serum* *Decrease* Mean concentration of 0.43 ± 0.04 mmol/L in 22 patients with diabetes mellitus lower than 0.47 ± 0.05 mmol/L in 22 age and sex matched controls *943*

Monocyte Chemotactic Protein-1 *Serum* *Decrease* Mean concentration undetectable in 1 patient with diabetes mellitus compared with 101 ± 24 pg/mL in 16 healthy women and men *4460*
Urine *Increase* In 4 patients with diabetes mellitus mean concentration of 642 ± 74 pg/mg creatinine significantly different when compared with mean concentration of 130 ± 30 pg/mg creatinine in 30 healthy women and 32 healthy men *4460*

myo-Inositol *Serum* *Increase* In 25 diabetics mean concentration of 52 ± 5 µmol/L not significantly increased compared with 37 ± 7 µmol/L in 20 healthy controls *3812*

Myoglobin *Urine* *Increase* Sporadic; metabolic myoglobinuria *5544* In 250 diabetics mean concentration of 0.82 ± 0.09 µg/dL compared with 0.45 ± 0.07 µg/dL in 125 healthy controls *166*

Na/K-ATPase *Platelets* *Decrease* Activity is reduced in diabetic patients *767*

N-Acetyl-Galactosidase *Urine* *Increase* In 69 Albustix negative diabetic patients mean concentration of 0.5 - 51.0 U/L or 0.2 - 49.8 U/g creatinine compared with 0.02 - 9.0 U/L or 0.05 - 2.88 U/g creatinine *4569*

N-Acetyl-Glucosaminidase *Urine* *Increase* The diabetic patients had higher concentrations than did the control subjects ($p < 0.01$). The results indicate that concentrations of urinary NAG are positively correlated to the degree of nephropathy, whereas *39* The diabetic patients had higher concentrations than did the control subjects ($p < 0.01$). The results indicate that concentrations of urinary NAG are positively correlated to the degree of nephropathy *5656*

Norepinephrine *Plasma* *Decrease* Long-term diabetics with neuropathy showed significant reductions. Diabetics without neuropathy had normal concentrations *835*
Plasma *No Effect* Long-term diabetics with neuropathy showed significant reductions. Diabetics without neuropathy had normal concentrations *835*

Osteocalcin *Serum* *Decrease* Patients were divided in 3 groups: 17 IDDM, 62 NIDDM treated with oral hypoglycaemic agents and 19 NIIDM patients treated with insulin. Results were compared with 2 different control groups. In IDDM patients the levels were significantly lower if compared to either the control group or to NIIDM patients *684*
Serum *Increase* Patients were divided in 3 groups: 17 IDDM, 62 NIDDM treated with oral hypoglycaemic agents and 19 NIIDM patients treated with insulin. Results were compared with 2 different control groups. The 2 groups of NIIDM patients showed significantly higher values than controls *684*
Serum *No Effect* In 27 poorly controlled diabetic men (both IDDM and NIDDM) mean concentration of 3.99 ± 1.46 μg/L compared with normal range of 2.00 - 12.00 μg/L *4607*

Oval Fat Bodies *Urine* *Increase* With diabetic nephropathy *413*

Oxygen Saturation *Blood* *Increase* Diabetics with pronounced hyperlipidemia due to accumulation of chylomicrons showed markedly increased hemoglobin-oxygen affinity (21.1 vs 26.6 mm Hg) *1184*

Parietal Cell Antibodies *Serum* *Increase* Parietal cell antibodies observed in some patients with diabetes mellitus *2952*

Pentosidine *Serum* *Increase* No significant difference between concentrations in uremic diabetic patients (1,199 ± 584 nmol/L) and nondiabetic uremics (1,273 ± 706 nmol/L) but both considerably increased compared with healthy controls (77 ± 40 nmol/L) *5130* In 35 individuals with diabetes mellitus mean concentration of 1,620 ± 1,940 μmol/L significantly higher than 151 ± 55 μmol/L in 19 healthy individuals *5160* In 61 patients with diabetes mellitus (11 with IDDM and 50 with NIDDM) mean concentration of 69.6 ± 42.4 nmol/L significantly different from 48.3 ± 11.5 nmol/L in 57 heathy volunteers *4399*

pH *Blood* *Decrease* Observed effect *4214* From an accumulation of acetoacetate and β-hydroxybutyric acid *5679*
Urine *Decrease* From an accumulation of acetoacetate and β-hydroxybutyric acid *5679*
Urine *Increase* Osmotic diuresis secondary to hyperglycemia *5679*

Phosphate *Serum* *Decrease* Osmotic diuresis secondary to hyperglycemia *5679*
Serum *Increase* Reported effect *1290*
Serum *No Effect* In 27 poorly controlled diabetic men (both IDDM and NIDDM) mean concentration of 1.0 ± 0.1 mmol/L compared with normal range of 0.8 - 1.5 mmol/L *4607*
Urine *Increase* Osmotic diuresis secondary to hyperglycemia *5679*

Phospholipase A *Serum* *Increase* Severe diabetes mellitus *2200*

Phospholipids *Serum* *Increase* Reported effect *1290*

Platelets *Blood* *Increase* In 23% of 21 patients at initial hospitalization for this disorder *1576*

Potassium *Serum* *Decrease* Osmotic diuresis secondary to hyperglycemia *5679*
Serum *Increase* hyperkalemia may occur due to low insulin levels, which normally would cause a net influx of K^+ into cells, and low aldosterone levels, which would stimulate K^+ excretion in a normal state *4214* In 29% of 107 patients at initial hospitalization for this disorder *1576*
Serum *No Effect* Normal or increased *5544*
Urine *Increase* Osmotic diuresis secondary to hyperglycemia *5679*

Proinsulin *Plasma* *Increase* Increased percentage in 11 of 59 maturity-onset cases and correlated with plasma glucose but not to total insulin *3241*
Plasma *No Effect* No consistent abnormality has been found. Patients with mild diabetes have repeatedly shown normal proportions. Severe cases may have an elevated proinsulin:insulin ratio *2243*

Prorenin *Plasma* *Increase* In 22 patients with IDDM or NIDDM mean concentration in patients with proliferative retinopathy 1,870 ± 785 mU/L, in those with nonproliferative retinopathy 326 ± 73 mU/L and in those without retinopathy 319 ± 47 mU/L *1325*

Prostacyclin *Plasma* *Decrease* In platelet poor plasma, the levels were significantly decreased *3928*

Protein *Cerebrospinal Fluid* *Increase* Approximately 70% of patients with neuropathy have unusual spinal fluid protein (50 - 100 mg/dL) *5679*
Serum *Decrease* With diabetic nephropathy *413*
Serum *No Effect* In 61 patients with diabetes mellitus (11 with IDDM and 50 with NIDDM) mean concentration of 73 ± 4 g/L not significantly different from 72 ± 4 g/L in 57 heathy volunteers *4399*
Urine *Increase* With diabetic nephropathy; often > 5 g/24 h *413* Mean excretion of 8.2 ± 1.2 g/d in 15 patients with diabetic nephropathy significantly greater than range of 0.04 - 0.15 g/d in 91 healthy controls *5570*

Protein 1 *Urine* *Increase* Excretion in diabetics typically increased and correlated with excretion of albumin *408*

Prothrombin Fragment 1.2 *Plasma* *Increase* Mean concentration of prothrombin fragment 1.2 in platelet-poor plasma from 21 patients with diabetes mellitus of 3.2 ± 2.6 nmol/L significantly higher than 0.51 nmol/L (95% reference interval of 0.21 - 2.78 nmol/L) in 268 healthy individuals less than 44 years of age *1860*

Pyridinoline Cross-linked Telopeptide of Type I Collagen *Serum* *No Effect* Concentration of 3.8 ± 1.9 μg/L in 22 patients with diabetes mellitus not significantly higher than 3.2 ± 0.48 μg/L in 8 healthy controls *2839*

Renin *Plasma* *Increase* Mean concentration in diabetics of 134.4 ± 14.8 pg/mL compared with 105.3 ± 8.6 pg/mL in healthy controls *5073*

Renin Activity *Plasma* *Decrease* Decreased catecholamine levels, which reduce renin secretion, are common *4214*

Sodium *Serum* *Decrease* Osmotic diuresis secondary to hyperglycemia *5679* In 22% of 104 patients at initial hospitalization for this disorder *1576*
Urine *Increase* Osmotic diuresis secondary to hyperglycemia *5679*

Sulfisoxazole, Free *Serum* *Decrease* In patients with diabetes mellitus concentration is increased in proportion to the extent of albumin glycosylation *5869*

Superoxide Dismutase *Red Blood Cells* *Decrease* In 119 patients with diabetes mellitus mean activity of 759.9 ± 101 U/g hemoglobin significantly reduced compared with 862.4 ± 122 U/g hemoglobin in 135 healthy control individuals with no significant difference between patients with IDDM and NIDDM. Reduction in diabetics probably due to inactivation of ESOD by glycation *251*

T3-Uptake *Serum* *No Effect* Reported effect *5544*

Thrombomodulin Antigen *Urine* *No Effect* In 47 diabetics mean excretion of 57.3 ± 45.9 ng/mL (35.5 ± 9.4 ng/mg creatinine) not significantly different from that in 87 healthy individuals not receiving any medication in whom the mean excretion was 48.6 ± 20.7 ng/mL (35.5 ± 9.4 ng/mg creatinine) *4245*

Thromboxane A_2 *Plasma* *No Effect* In platelet poor plasma, the levels remained unchanged *3928*

Thyro-Binding Index *Serum* *No Effect* Serum T4, T3RU, free T4 and TSH in patients prior to therapy was not significantly different from normal subjects *2515*

Thyroid Stimulating Hormone *Serum* *No Effect* Serum T4, T3RU, free T4 and TSH in patients prior to therapy was not significantly elevated compared to normals *2515*

Thyroxine Binding Globulin *Serum* *Decrease* In 171 diabetic pubertal children TBG concentrations were below the 50th percentile for the normal range, with 20% below the 95% CI for both sexes *902*

Thyroxine (T4) *Serum* *Decrease* In 171 diabetic pubertal children in 80% of girls and 63% of boys T4 concentrations were below the 50th percentile for the normal range, with higher concentrations in girls with the lowest HbA1c concentrations *902*
Serum *No Effect* Serum T4, T3RU, free T4 and TSH in patients prior to therapy was not significantly different from controls *2515*

Thyroxine (T4), Free *Serum* *No Effect* Serum T4, T3RU, free T4 and TSH in patients prior to therapy was not significantly

250.00 Diabetes Mellitus *(continued)*

Thyroxine (T4), Free *(continued)* different from controls *2515* In 171 diabetic pubertal children FT4 concentrations were within the normal range, with higher concentrations in girl with the lowest HbA1c concentrations *902*

Tissue Factor Antigen *Urine Decrease* In 43 patients with diabetes mellitus mean excretion of 204.5 ± 169.5 pg/mL (187.9 ± 88.0 pg/mg creatinine) significantly less than that in 87 healthy individuals not receiving any medication in whom the mean excretion was 363.1 ± 174.4 pg/mL (187.9 ± 88.0 pg/mg creatinine) *4245*

Trehalase *Serum Increase* Increased but does not correlate with blood sugar concentration *372*

Tri-iodothyronine, Reverse (rT3) *Serum Increase* Prior to treatment serum rT3 was significantly higher than in normal controls *2515*

Tri-iodothyronine (T3) *Serum Increase* Prior to treatment serum T3 was significantly lower than in normal controls *2515*

Triglycerides *Serum Increase* In 50 patients with diabetes mellitus (both IDDM and NIDDM) mean concentration of 2.13 ± 2.48 mmol/L not significantly different from 1.20 ± 1.40 mmol/L in 19 healthy controls *3403* Higher values correlate with hyperglycemia and poorer control of diabetes; reduced by insulin therapy *5544* In 15 patients with diabetic nephropathy mean concentration of 4.9 ± 0.6 mmol/L significantly greater than 1.2 ± 0.08 mmol/L in 91 healthy controls *5570* In 228 patients, a significant positive association between GGT and triglyceride concentration was found. May reflect hepatic microsomal effect *4746* Mean concentration in 143 newly dicovered diabetics of 227.9 ± 14.0 mg/dL significantly different from 136.0 ± 4.7 mg/dL in population with normal glucose tolerance *1527* Mean levels for children were elevated to 120 ± 63 mg/dL vs 85 ± 23 mg/dL for controls. 8 had hypercholesterolemia, 5 had hypertriglyceridemia, and 9 had combined hypercholesterolemia and hypertriglyceridemia *792* In one patient with lipoatrophic diabetes mean concentration of 11.1 mmol/L significantly higher than reference range of < 1.7 mmol/L *3994* Observed effect *3313*

Trypsin *Serum Increase* High incidence of pancreatic abnormality in patients with no clinical evidence of pancreatic acinar disease *5378*

Tumor Necrosis Factor-α *Urine No Effect* In 21 patients with diabetic nephropathy mean excretion of 18.3 ± 3.0 pg/mg creatinine not significantly different from 13.5 ± 1.5 pg/mg creatinine in 13 healthy controls *2985*

Ubiquinol:Cholesterol Ratio *Serum Decrease* In 50 patients with diabetes mellitus (both IDDM and NIDDM) mean ratio of 0.18 ± 0.06 µmol/mmol significantly different from 0.22 ± 0.05 µmol/mmol in 19 healthy controls *3403*

Urea Nitrogen *Serum Increase* In 61 patients with diabetes mellitus (11 with IDDM and 50 with NIDDM) mean concentration of 8.2 ± 3.0 mmol/L different from 6.1 ± 1.5 mmol/L in 57 heathy volunteers *4399* Uncontrolled diabetes mellitus may be associated with excessive protein catabolism *1025* In 29% of 117 patients at initial hospitalization for this disorder *1576*

Uric Acid *Serum Increase* In 28% of 104 patients at initial hospitalization for this disorder *1576* Increased occurrence of hyperuricemia has been reported *3484*

VLDL-Cholesterol *Serum Increase* Marked elevation due to increased secretion and decreased catabolism secondary to reduced lipoprotein lipase activity *126 5864*

Volume *Plasma Decrease* Reported effect *5544*
Urine Increase As the urine sugar content rises, glucose acts as a diuretic, i.e., the renal tubules are reabsorbing glucose at their maximum rate and the excess glucose prevents further water reabsorption *1290*

Xylose Tolerance Test *Urine Abnormal* Defects of multiple stages of digestion-absorption *4891*

250.00 Noninsulin-dependent Diabetes Mellitus

Adenosine Deaminase *Serum Increase* In 52 patients with NIDDM mean activity of 20.6 ± 7.5 U/L significantly higher than that in 52 healthy blood donors (mean activity of 13.4 ± 7.5 U/L) *2245*

Adenosine Deaminase 1 *Serum Increase* In 52 patients with NIDDM mean activity of 9.5 ± 3.5 U/L significantly higher than that in 52 healthy blood donors (mean activity of 6.5 ± 1.9 U/L) *2245*

Adenosine Deaminase 2 *Serum Increase* In 52 patients with NIDDM mean activity of 11.2 ± 4.5 U/L significantly higher than that in 52 healthy blood donors (mean activity of 7.0 ± 1.7 U/L) *2245*

Advanced Glycation End-products *Serum Increase* Mean concentration in 125 patients with NIDDM of 7.2 ± 14.8 mU/mL significantly different from 3.3 ± 1.0 mU/mL in 63 healthy controls *3920*

Albumin *Serum Decrease* Mean concentration of 4.03 ± 0.03 g/dL in 212 Japanese patients with NIDDM significantly different from 4.18 ± 0.02 g/dL in 76 healthy controls *2616*
Urine Increase In 92 patients with NIDDM median excretion rate of 247.01 µg/min significantly higher than 1.83 µg/min in 23 healthy controls *2366* In 539 patients with NIDDM at time of diagnosis albumin excretion increased above 25 g/L in 32% compared with 11% of reference population of 250 normoglycemic controls *3276* In about 16 patients with NIDDM mean excretion of 38 ± 7 µg/min significantly different from 11 ± 1 µg/min in non-diabetic controls *2842* In 13 patients with NIDDM and microalbuminuria mean albumin excretion rate of 46.04 ± 6.84 µg/min significantly higher than 3.31 ± 0.55 µg/min in 13 comparable normoalbuminuric NIDDM patients *1888* In 36 patients with NIDDM and microalbuminuria mean excretion of 73.4 ± 9.4 µg/min and 7.3 ± 0.9 µg/min in 36 with normoalbuminuria increased when compared with healthy individuals *1889* Mean excretion in 16 NIDDM patients with microalbuminuria of 40.3 ± 8.3 µg/min significantly different from 7.5 ± 0.5 µg/min in 31 normoalbuminuric NIDDM patients anf significantly different from that in 30 healthy controls *5713* In 26 normoalbuminuric type II diabetics mean excretion rate of 16.5 ± 6.6 µg/min and in 52 microalbuminuric type II diabetics 78.1 ± 23.2 µg/min significantly greater than 1.1 ± 0.8 µg/min in 28 controls *3959*

Albumin:Creatinine Ratio *Urine Increase* In 34 patients with NIDDM mean ratio of 1.24 ± 0.88 mg/mmol not significantly different from 1.04 ± 0.53 mg/mmol in 32 healthy controls *5500*
Urine No Effect In patients with newly diagnosed NIDDM median values fell within normal range of < 2.5 g/mol but 90th percentile above twice the upper limit of normal *3277*

Amylin *Plasma Increase* Reported effect *2987*

Androstenedione *Plasma No Effect* Mean concentration in 39 patients with NIDDM 71.6 ± 4.9 ng/dL not significantly different compared with 85.7 ± 9.7 ng/dL in 17 healthy controls *115*

Angiotensin-converting Enzyme *Serum Increase* In 53 patients with NIDDM mean activity of 334.0 ± 97.0 U/L compared with 250.5 ± 85.5 U/L in 33 healthy nondiabetic individuals. Activities highest in 20 patients with background retinopathy (344.6 ± 96.8 U/L) and 8 with proliferative retinopathy (357.3 ± 93.2 U/L) *3481*

1,5-Anhydroglucitol *Serum Increase* In 71 patients with NIDDM mean concentration of 3.23 ± 3.15 µg/mL significantly higher than concentration in 132 age-matched control individuals *199*

Anion Gap *Serum No Effect* In about 16 patients with NIDDM mean 13 ± 4 mmol/L not significantly different from 13 ± 2 mmol/L in non-diabetic controls *2842*

Antioxidant Capacity *Serum No Effect* In 34 patients with NIDDM mean total oxidant status of 1.79 ± 0.20 mmol/L not significantly different from 1.81 ± 0.12 mmol/L in 32 healthy controls *5500*

Antiphospholipid Antibodies *Serum Increase* In 0 of 26 patients with mild NIDDM, 8 of 22 with moderate NIDDM and 6 of 20 patients with severe NIDDM with diabetic neuropathy antibodies detected *4796*

Antisulfatide Antibodies *Serum Increase* In 1 of 26 patients with mild NIDDM, 4 of 22 with moderate NIDDM and 8 of 20 patients with severe NIDDM with diabetic neuropathy antibodies detected *4796*

Antithrombin III *Plasma No Effect* In 19 patients with NIDDM and nephropathy mean concentration of 102 U/dL compared with reference interval of 80 - 120 U/dL *4640*

Apolipoprotein A *Serum No Effect* In 80 patients with untreated NIDDM mean concentration of 138.9 ± 24.1 mg/dL *5201*

Apolipoprotein A-I *Serum Decrease* In 92 patients with NIDDM mean concentration of 123.6 ± 34.9 mg/dL significantly different from 159.0 ± 26.6 mg/dL in 82 healthy controls *10*
Serum No Effect In 16 patients with NIDDM median concentration of 1.22 g/L not significantly different from 1.23 g/L in 16 healthy controls *4353*

Apolipoprotein A-IV *Serum Increase* In 43 men and 40 women with NIDDM mean concentrations of 17.1 ± 7.9 mg/dL and 18.9 ± 9.9 mg/dL respectively significantly different from 12.3 ± 3.6 mg/dL in 50 healthy control men and 11.9 ± 3.5 mg/dL in 50 control women *5454*

Apolipoprotein B *Serum Increase* In patients with NIDDM mean concentration increased in well controlled patients *3853* In 16 patients with NIDDM median concentration of 0.99 g/L significantly different from 0.73 g/L in 16 healthy controls *4353* Mean concentration of 135 ± 27 mg/dL in 60 patients with IDDM significantly increased compared with concentration in 45 apparently healthy controls *2284* In 92 patients with NIDDM mean concentration of 106.7 ± 31.7 mg/dL significantly different from 91.6 ± 26.6 mg/dL in 82 healthy controls *10*
Serum No Effect Mean concentration of 1.27 ± 0.05 g/L in 70 patients with NIDDM significantly higher than 1.05 ± 0.02 g/L in 142 patients with IDDM but not significantly different from normal range *470* In 80 patients with untreated NIDDM mean concentration of 143.2 ± 30.6 mg/dL *5201*

Apolipoprotein H *Serum No Effect* In 127 patients with NIDDM mean concentration of 30.1 ± 9.9 mg/dL not significantly different from 22.5 ± 7.7 mg/dL in 286 healthy controls *725*

Atrial Natriuretic Peptide *Plasma Increase* Mean concentration in 16 NIDDM patients with microalbuminuria of 13.8 ± 2.5 pg/mL not significantly different from 10.8 ± 1.1 pg/mL in 31 normoalbuminuric NIDDM patients but significantly different from 8.2 ± 0.7 pg/mL in 30 healthy controls *5713*

Basic Fibroblast Growth Factor *Serum Increase* In 12 male patients with NIDDM with micro- or macroalbuminuria mean growth promoting activity significantly increased to 151 ± 30% compared with 114 ± 19% in 12 normoalbuminuric patients with NIDDM *5865*

Calcium *Serum Decrease* In 20 patients with NIDDM and nephropathy mean concentration decreased to 9.26 ± 0.72 mg/dL *2167*

Ceruloplasmin *Serum Increase* Mean concentrations of 190.8, 200.1 and 184.6 µg/mL observed in patients with 141.8 µg/mL in healthy controls in patients with NIDDM and normoalbuminria, microalbuminuria and macroalbuminuria respectively *5786*
Urine Increase Median excretions of 1.43, 15.6 and 161.2 ng/min observed in patients with 0.4 ng/min in healthy controls in patients with NIDDM and normoalbuminria, microalbuminuria and macroalbuminuria respectively *5786*

Cholest-5, 3β-ol, 7-one *Serum No Effect* In 10 type II diabetics mean concentration of 166 ± 120 nmol/L not significantly different from mean concentration of 121 ± 38 nmol/L in 13 healthy controls *3556*

Cholest-5 ene 3β 7β-diol *Serum No Effect* In 10 type II diabetics mean concentration of 47.1 ± 24.9 nmol/L not significantly different from mean concentration of 38.4 ± 12.3 nmol/L in 13 healthy controls *3556*

Cholest-5 ene 3β, 25-diol *Serum No Effect* In 10 type II diabetics mean concentration of 22.5 ± 5.7 nmol/L not significantly different from mean concentration of 25.6 ± 7.9 nmol/L in 13 healthy controls *3556*

5α-Cholestan-3β,5,6-triol *Serum No Effect* In 10 type II diabetics mean concentration of 36.6 ± 38.6 nmol/L not significantly different from mean concentration of 29.3 ± 7.3 nmol/L in 13 healthy controls *3556*

Cholesterol *Serum Increase* In 14 patients with NIDDM mean concentration of 6.29 ± 0.42 mmol/L *2119* In 20 patients with NIDDM and nephropathy mean concentration increased to 189 ± 43 mg/dL *2167* In 8 patients with NIDDM mean concentration of 5.76 ± 1.50 mmol/L significantly greater than 5.10 ± 0.89 mmol/L in 29 healthy controls *4719* In 80 patients with untreated NIDDM mean concentration of 211.5 ± 35.0 mg/dL *5201* In 36 patients with NIDDM and microalbuminuria mean concentration of 205.4 ± 7.8 mg/dL and 189.7 ± 8.1 mg/dL in 36 with normoalbuminuria increased compared with healthy individuals *1889* In 67 patients with type II diabetes mean concentration of 6.38 ± 2.19 mmol/L *2943* In 13 patients with NIDDM and microalbuminuria mean concentration of 5.07 ± 0.36 mmol/L significantly higher than 4.16 ± 0.18 mmol/L in 13 comparable normoalbuminuric NIDDM patients *1888* In 2,425 newly diagnosed NIDDM men and 1,752 NIDDM women mean concentrations of 5.5 ± 1.1 mmol/L and 5.9 ± 1.2 mmol/L respectively significantly higher than 5.2 ± 0.9 mmol/L and 5.5 ± 1.1 mmol/L in 195 age matched male and female controls *3275* In 17 patients with NIDDM mean concentration of 5.5 ± 2.2 mmol/L not significantly different from 5.1 ± 1.4 mmol/L in 19 healthy controls *3403* Mean concentration in 43 patients with NIDDM of 5.54 ± 1.57 mmol/L different from 4.64 ± 0.89 mmol/L in 235 healthy control individuals *3884* In 26 normoalbuminuric type II diabetics mean concentration of 5.2 ± 1.0 mmol/L and in 52 microalbuminuric type II diabetics 5.8 ± 1.9 mmol/L significantly greater than 4.2 ± 0.9 mmol/L in 28 controls *3959* In patients with NIDDM mean concentration increased in poorly controlled patients *3853* In 26 patients with NIDDM mean concentration of 5.60 ± 0.99 mmol/L significantly different from 4.51 ± 0.74 mmol/L in 10 healthy control subjects *5090* In 40 women with NIDDM mean concentration of 215 ± 45 mg/dL significantly different from 181 ± 32 mg/dL in 50 healthy control women *5454* In 17 men with NIDDM mean concentration of 5.42 ± 0.86 mmol/L compared with 4.07 ± 1.04 mmol/L in 25 normal controls: in 30 women with NIDDM mean concentration of 6.00 ± 1.03 mmol/L compared with 5.51 ± 1.13 mmol/L in 35 control women *4025*
Serum No Effect In 100 patients with NIDDM mean concentration of 210.9 ± 45.5 mg/dL not significantly different from 203.9 ± 38.7 mg/dL in 854 normoglycemic controls *2330* In 43 men with NIDDM mean concentration of 202 ± 43 mg/dL not significantly different from 189 ± 29 mg/dL in 50 healthy control men *5454* In 127 patients with NIDDM mean concentration of 5.28 ± 1.06 mmol/L not significantly different from 5.74 ± 1.11 mmol/L in 286 healthy controls *725* Mean concentration of 5.3 ± 0.2 mmol/L in 46 men with NIDDM not significantly different from 5.8 ± 0.3 mmol/L in 11 normal men *115* In 12 type II diabetics mean concentration of 4.99 ± 0.83 mmol/L not significantly higher than 4.91 ± 0.62 mmol/L in 17 nondiabetic control individuals *2471* In patients with NIDDM mean concentration normal in well controlled patients *3853* Mean concentration of 5.77 ± 1.32 mmol/L in 16 NIDDM patients not significantly different from mean of 6.33 ± 1.25 mmol/L in 16 healthy controls *5014* In 92 patients with NIDDM mean concentration of 6.07 ± 1.33 mmol/L not significantly different from 5.69 ± 1.30 mmol/L in 82 healthy controls *10* In 11 patients with NIDDM treated with oral hypoglycemics or insulin mean concentration of 5.2 ± 0.8 mmol/L not significantly different from 5.3 ± 0.8 mmol/L in 14 healthy controls *3556* Mean concentration of 5.78 ± 0.15 mmol/L in 70 patients with IDDM not significantly different from normal range *470* In 37 NIDDM patients with normoalbuminuria mean concentration of 5.84 ± 1.63 mmol/L, in 11 with microalbuminuria 5.65 ± 1.52 mmol/L and in 7 with macroalbuminuria 6.50 ± 1.71 mmol/L not significantly different from 5.40 ± 1.21 mmol/L in 55 healthy controls *4329* In 82 patients with type II diabetes mellitus mean concentration of 5.8 ± 1.6 mmol/L not significantly higher than 5.7 ± 1.4 mmol/L in 48 healthy controls *5795* In 16 patients with NIDDM median concentration of 5.03 mmol/L not significantly different from 4.80 mmol/L in 16 healthy controls *4353* Mean concentration of 6.05 ± 0.21 mmol/L in 44 patients with NIDDM not significantly different from 6.21 ± 0.31 mmol/L in 28 healthy controls *4117* In 20 patients with NIDDM mean concentration the same as in 20 age and sex matched controls (5.7 ± 0.2 mmol/L) *970* Mean concentration of 4.88 ± 0.08 mmol/L in 212 Japanese patients with NIDDM not significantly different from 4.88 ± 0.08 mmol/L in 76 healthy controls *2616* In 39 patients with NIDDM mean concentration of 5.32 ± 1.28 mmol/L not significantly different from 5.45 ± 1.37 mmol/L in 24 healthy controls *4713* In about 16 patients with NIDDM mean concentration of 197 ± 9 mg/dL not significantly different from 173 ± 10 mg/dL in non-diabetic controls *2842* In 12 male patients with NIDDM mean concentration of 5.53 ± 0.41 mmol/L not significantly different from 5.22 ± 0.17 mmol/L in 16 healthy control men *2581* In 539 patients at time of diagnosis of NIDDM mean concentration of 5.7 ± 1.2 mmol/L not significantly different from 5.6 ± 1.1 mmol/L in 250 normoglycemic controls *3276* In 81 patients with NIDDM median concentration of 5.72 mmol/L compared with 5.72 mmol/L in 62 healthy controls *1867* Mean concentration in 16 NIDDM patients with microalbuminuria of 5.23 ± 0.25 mmol/L not significantly different from 5.27 ± 0.16 mmol/L in 31 normoalbuminuric NIDDM patients nor significantly different from 5.17 ± 0.14

250.00 Noninsulin-dependent Diabetes Mellitus *(continued)*

Cholesterol *(continued)*
mmol/L in 30 healthy controls *5713* Mean concentration in 225 patients with NIDDM 5.14 ± 1.02 mmol/L not significantly different from 5.04 ± 0.99 mmol/L in 163 healthy controls *3852*

Cholesterol Ester Transfer *Serum* *Increase* In 16 patients with NIDDM median transfer of 28.5 nmol/mL/h significantly different from 19.2 nmol/mL/h in 16 healthy controls *4353*

Cholesterol Ester Transfer Protein *Serum* *No Effect* In 16 patients with NIDDM median activity of 72 AU not significantly different from 76 AU in 16 healthy controls *4353*

Cholesterol Ester Transfer Rate *Serum* *Increase* In 16 patients with NIDDM median transfer of 76.7 nmol/mL/h significantly different from 61.2 nmol/mL/h in 16 healthy controls *4353*

Copper *Serum* *Increase* Mean concentration in 43 patients with uncontrolled NIDDM of 17.67 ± 5.25 µmol/L and of 16.02 ± 3.97 µmol/L in 40 patients with controlled NIDDM different from 13.91 ± 3.02 µmol/L in 30 healthy controls *5844*

Copper Zinc Superoxide Dismutase *Lymphocytes* *Decrease* In 34 patients with NIDDM mean concentration of 1.61 ± 0.48 U/mg total protein significantly different from 2.06 ± 0.58 U/mg protein in 32 healthy controls *5499*
Neutrophils *Decrease* In 34 patients with NIDDM mean concentration of 0.51 ± 0.24 U/mg total protein significantly different from 1.06 ± 0.43 U/mg protein in 32 healthy controls *5499*

Corticotropin *Plasma* *Increase* In 17 patients with NIDDM mean baseline concentration of pg/mL significantly higher than 16 pg/mL in 12 healthy controls *2047*

Corticotropin-releasing Hormone *Plasma* *Decrease* Mean baseline concentration in 17 patients with NIDDM 4.0 pg/mL significantly less than 8.0 pg/mL in 12 healthy controls *2047*

Cortisol *Plasma* *Increase* Mean basal concentration in 17 patients with NIDDM 13 µg/dL significantly higher than 9 µg/dL in 12 healthy controls *2047*

C-Peptide *Plasma* *Increase* In about 16 patients with NIDDM mean concentration of 2.93 ± 1.26 ng/mL significantly different from 1.48 ± 0.51 ng/mL in non-diabetic controls *2842* In 12 type II diabetics mean concentration of 1.03 ± 0.30 nmol/L significantly higher than 0.73 ± 0.26 nmol/L in 17 nondiabetic control individuals *2471* In 59 patients with type 2 diabetes mean concentration of 4.71 ± 0.69 ng/mL significantly different from 1.46 ± 0.25 ng/mL in 35 controls *5695*

Creatinine *Serum* *Increase* In 20 patients with NIDDM and nephropathy mean concentration increased to 1.5 ± 0.8 mg/dL *2167* Mean concentration in 125 patients with NIDDM of 2.3 ± 2.6 mg/dL significantly different from 0.9 ± 0.2 mg/dL in 63 healthy controls *3920* Mean concentration of 82.2 ± 1.8 mg/dL in 212 Japanese patients with NIDDM significantly different from 75.1 ± 1.8 mg/dL in 76 healthy controls *2616* In 12 male patients with NIDDM with micro- or macroalbuminuria mean concentration of 106 ± 35 µmol/L increased but not significantly different from 88 ± 9 µmol/L in 12 normoalbuminuric patients with NIDDM *5865* In patients with NIDDM, 28 with renal insufficiency had a mean concentration of 153.7 ± 78.0 µmol/L increased above normal but also higher than 61.2 ± 14.7 µmol/L in 45 patients with macroalbuminuria, 54.6 ± 17.6 µmol/L in 98 patients with microalbuminuria and 54.6 ± 17.6 µmol/L in 127 patients with normoalbuminuria *5760*
Serum *No Effect* In 34 patients with NIDDM mean concentration of 78.4 ± 12.2 µmol/L not significantly different from 80.3 ± 12.9 µmol/L in 32 healthy controls *5500* Mean concentration of 100 ± 4.4 µmol/L in 44 patients with NIDDM not significantly different from 104 ± 6 µmol/L in 28 healthy controls *4117* In 26 normoalbuminuric type II diabetics mean concentration of 79.6 ± 17.7 µmol/L and in 52 microalbuminuric type II diabetics 97.2 ± 35.4 µmol/L not significantly different from 88.4 ± 17.7 µmol/L in 28 controls *3959* In 8 patients with NIDDM with microalbuminuria mean concentration in men of 1.1 ± 0.2 mg/dL compared with 1.0 ± 0.2 mg/dL in 22 patients with normal UAE *1294*

Creatinine Clearance *Urine* *Decrease* In 36 patients with NIDDM and microalbuminuria mean clearance of 102 ± 10 mL/min/1.73 sq m and 113 ± 8 mL/min/1.73 sq m in 36 with normoalbuminuria reduced compared with healthy individuals *1889*
Urine *No Effect* Mean value in 16 NIDDM patients with microalbuminuria of 1.56 ± 0.04 mL/s not significantly different from 1.60 ± 1.56 mL/s in 31 normoalbuminuric NIDDM patients and 30 healthy controls *5713*

D-Dimer *Plasma* *Increase* In 10 patients with NIDDM and hyperlipidemia mean concentration of 67 µg/mL significantly higher than 46 µg/mL in 10 healthy male controls *5815*

Dehydroepiandrosterone *Plasma* *Decrease* Mean concentration in 39 women with NIDDM 229 ± 28 ng/dL significantly less than 378 ± 30 ng/dL in 17 healthy controls *115*

Dehydroepiandrosterone Sulfate *Plasma* *No Effect* Mean concentration of 53 ± 4 pg/dL in 39 women with NIDDM not significantly different from 68 ± 12 pg/dL in 17 healthy controls *115* In 12 male patients with NIDDM mean concentration of 3.03 ± 0.44 pmol/L not significantly different from 3.30 ± 0.24 pmol/L in 16 healthy control men *2581*

IV-EIA *Serum* *Increase* Mean concentration increased from 71.3 ± 13.0 ng/mL in 26 patients without retinopathy to 98.0 ± 25.5 ng/mL in 11 patients with proliferative retinopathy *3894*

Endothelin-1 *Plasma* *Increase* In NIDDM patients with angiopathy mean concentration of 1.73 ± 0.29 pg/mL and in those without 1.68 ± 0.20 pg/mL increased above concentrations in healthy individuals *2553* In 2 studies of patients with type II diabetes mellitus mean concentration increased to 4.4 ± 0.3 pg/mL, 3.4-fold above normal in one (n = 84) and to 1.2 pg/mL, 0.9-fold of normal in the other (n = 10) *328*
Plasma *No Effect* In 44 patients with NIDDM mean concentration of 6.29 ± 0.47 pg/mL not significantly different from 8.23 ± 1.68 pg/mL in 30 normal individuals *418* In 13 patients with NIDDM and microalbuminuria mean concentration of 5.37 ± 0.3 pg/mL not significantly different from 4.71 ± 0.42 pg/mL in 13 comparable normoalbuminuric NIDDM patients *1888*
Urine *Increase* Mean excretion in 28 albuminuric NIDDM patients of 174.4 ± 12.9 ng/d and 154.9 ± 13.5 ng/d in patients with normoalbuminuria higher than 111.8 ± 7.9 ng/d in 40 normal control individuals *2976*

Endothelin-1, Big *Plasma* *Increase* In 10 patients with type II diabetes mellitus mean concentration of 4.3 ± 0.2 pg/mL, 1.3-fold above appropriate normals *328*

5,6α-Epoxy-5α cholestan-3α-ol *Serum* *No Effect* In 10 type II diabetics mean concentration of 49.1 ± 14.1 nmol/L not significantly different from mean concentration of 51.0 ± 18.6 nmol/L in 13 healthy controls *3556*

Estradiol *Plasma* *No Effect* In 39 women with NIDDM mean concentration of 1.50 ± 0.10 ng/dL not significantly different from 1.72 ± 0.17 ng/dL in 17 healthy controls *115* In 12 male patients with NIDDM mean concentration of 87.66 ± 12.55 pmol/L not significantly different from 76.06 ± 11.09 pmol/L in 16 healthy control men *2581*

Estrone *Plasma* *Increase* Mean concentration of 39 women with NIDDM 5.82 ± 0.56 ng/dL sigificantly higher than 3.92 ± 0.39 ng/dL in 17 control individuals *115*

Factor VII *Plasma* *Increase* In 13 patients with NIDDM and microalbuminuria mean concentration of 87.85 ± 4.94% significantly higher than 76.54 ± 2.31% in 13 comparable normoalbuminuric NIDDM patients *1888*
Plasma *No Effect* In 1,121 men with NIDDM mean concentration of 2.7 ± 1.0 ng/mL comparable to 2.6 ± 1.0 ng/mL in 1,480 women with NIDDM *2336*

Fatty Acids (FFA), Free *Serum* *Increase* In 43 men and 40 women with NIDDM mean concentrations of 0.675 ± 0.410 mmol/L and 0.805 ± 0.349 mmol/L respectively significantly different from 0.278 ± 0.197 mmol/L in 50 healthy control men and 0.334 ± 0.150 mmol/L in 50 control women *5454* In 20 patients with NIDDM and nephropathy mean concentration increased to 312 ± 58 mg/dL *2167* In 16 patients with NIDDM median concentration of 0.64 mmol/L significantly different from 0.46 mmol/L in 16 healthy controls *4353* In 8 obese individuals with NIDDM mean concentration of 787 ± 60 µmol/L significantly different from 488 ± 43 µmol/L in 9 lean controls and 690 ± 70 µmol/L in 9 obese nondiabetics *320*

Fibrinogen *Plasma* *Increase* In 36 patients with NIDDM and microalbuminuria mean concentration of 344 ± 19 mg/dL and 309 ± 11 mg/dL in 36 with normoalbuminuria increased when compared with healthy individuals *1889* In 1,525 patients mean concentration of 3.6 ± 0.9 g/L with concentrations exceeding 3.5 g/L in 50.3% of patients compared with2.5 ± 0.5 g/L in 200 healthy controls *610* In 19 patients with NIDDM and nephropathy mean concentration of 5.85 g/L compared with reference

interval of 1.50 - 3.85 g/L *4640* In 67 patients with type II diabetes mean concentration of 3.37 ± 0.60 g/L *2943* In 13 patients with NIDDM and microalbuminuria mean concentration of 3.38 ± 0.21 g/L significantly higher than 2.65 ± 0.13 g/L in 13 comparable normoalbuminuric NIDDM patients *1888* In 10 patients with NIDDM and hyperlipidemia concentration of 333 ± 50 mg/dL significantly higher than 228 ± 4 mg/dL in 8 patients with NIDDM but without hyperlipidemia and 223 ± 65 mg/dL in 10 healthy male controls *5815*
Plasma No Effect In 1,121 men with NIDDM mean concentration of 2.4 ± 0.5 g/L comparable to 2.5 ± 0.5 g/L in 1,480 women with NIDDM *2336*

Fibrinopeptide A *Plasma Increase* In patients with NIDDM mean concentration significantly but reversibly increased compared with that in healthy controls *2484*
Urine Increase In patients with NIDDM mean excretion significantly but reversibly increased compared with healthy controls *2484*

Fructosamine *Serum Increase* In 80 patients with untreated NIDDM mean concentration of 300.4 ± 55.9 µmol/L *5201* In 82 patients with type II diabetes mellitus mean concentration of 365 ± 60 µmol/L significantly higher than 265 ± 30 µmol/L in 48 healthy controls with concentration higher in those with complications than those without *5795* In 40 patients with type II diabetes mellitus mean concentration of 1.7 ± 0.4 mmol/L significantly higher than 0.9 ± 0.3 mmol/L in control patients *4887* In 26 normoalbuminuric type II diabetics mean concentration of 350.6 ± 12.8 µmol/L and in 52 microalbuminuric type II diabetics 379.9 ± 11.3 µmol/L significantly greater than 272.5 ± 13.8 µmol/L in 28 controls *3959* Mean concentration in 43 patients with uncontrolled NIDDM of 407 ± 95.2 µmol/L and of 225 ± 34.8 µmol/L in 40 patients with controlled NIDDM different from 178 ± 43 µmol/L in 30 healthy controls *5844*

Galanin *Plasma Increase* Mean concentration of 50.0 ± 8.0 pg/mL in 7 diabetic overweight women with BMI of 31 - 40 kg/m^2 not significantly different from 54.0 ± 7.1 pg/mL in 22 nondiabetic women with a similar degree of obesity but significantly different from 21.6 ± 7.0 pg/mL observed in 19 lean healthy women *287*

Glucagon *Plasma Increase* In 14 patients with NIDDM mean concentration of 250 ± 20 ng/L *2119* In 59 patients with type 2 diabetes mean concentration of 105.4 ± 17.3 pg/mL significantly different from 65.6 ± 12.7 pg/mL in 35 controls *5695*

Glucose *Serum Increase* Mean concentration in 16 NIDDM patients with microalbuminuria of 6.9 ± 0.4 mmol/L not significantly different from 6.3 ± 0.3 pmol/L in 31 normoalbuminuric NIDDM patients but significantly different from 4.9 ± 0.1 pmol/L in 30 healthy controls *5713* In 12 type II diabetics mean concentration of 12.0 ± 5 mmol/L significantly higher than 5.2 ± 0.5 mmol/L in 17 nondiabetic control individuals *2471* Mean concentration in 125 patients with NIDDM of 156 ± 52 mg/dL significantly different from 91 ± 9 mg/dL in 63 healthy controls *3920* In 71 patients with NIDDM mean concentration of 10.5 ± 3.4 mmol/L significantly higher than concentration in 132 age-matched control individuals *199* In 12 obese patients with NIDDM mean concentration of 8.92 ± 0.52 mmol/L and in 12 nonobese patients with NIDDM 8.97 ± 0.37 mmol/L significantly higher than 4.96 ± 0.14 mmol/L in 12 normal individuals *2582* In patients with NIDDM, 28 with renal insufficiency had a mean concentration of 8.18 ± 2.12 mmol/L increased above normal but lower than 9.78 ± 3.74 mmol/L in 45 patients with macroalbuminuria, 10.23 ± 4.35 mmol/L in 98 patients with microalbuminuria and 9.00 ± 3.08 mmol/L in 127 patients with normoalbuminuria *5760* In about 16 patients with NIDDM mean concentration of 192 ± 11 mg/dL not significantly different from 97 ± 4 mg/dL in non-diabetic controls *2842* Mean fasting concentration of 7.94 ± 0.17 mmol/L in 212 Japanese patients with NIDDM significantly higher than 5.39 ± 0.06 mmol/L in 76 healthy controls *2616* In 11 patients with NIDDM treated with oral hypoglycemics or insulin mean concentration of 11.7 ± 3.0 mmol/L significantly different from 4.9 ± 0.5 mmol/L in 14 healthy controls *3556* Mean concentration in 10 obese NIDDM patients of 12.2 ± 1.1 mmol/L significantly greater than 4.8 ± 0.1 mmol/L in 10 healthy lean controls *806* In 13 patients with NIDDM mean concentration of 160 ± 23 mg/dL significantly greater than 91 ± 8 mg/dL in 13 healthy controls *4457* In 34 patients with NIDDM mean concentration of 11.1 ± 3.9 mmol/L significantly higher than 4.7 ± 1.8 mmol/L in 32 healthy controls *5500* In 34 patients with NIDDM mean concentration of 11.1 ± 3.9 mmol/L significantly different from 4.7 ± 1.8 mmol/L in 32 healthy controls *5499* In 8 obese individuals with NIDDM mean concentration of 10.9 ± 1.2 mmol/L significantly different from 5.2 ± 0.2 mmol/L in 9 lean controls and 5.4 ± 0.2 mmol/L in 9 obese nondiabetics *320* In 539 patients at time of diagnosis of NIDDM mean concentration of 12.3 ± 3.8 mmol/L compared with 5.0 ± 0.5 in 250 controls *3276* In 106 patients with NIDDM mean concentration of 13.60 ± 6.77 mmol/L significantly increased compared with 5.22 ± 0.65 mmol/L in 20 healthy controls *3425* In 40 patients with type II diabetes mellitus mean concentration of 11.0 ± 4.3 mmol/L significantly higher than 4.9 ± 0.8 mmol/L in control patients *4887* Mean concentration in 46 men with NIDDM 9.1 ± 0.7 mmol/L significantly higher than 4.9 ± 0.6 mmol/L in 11 healthy control men *115* In 29 obese patients with NIDDM mean concentration of 241 ± 32 mg/dL significantly different from 105 ± 2 mg/dL in 21 healthy obese individuals and 91 ± 3 mg/dL in 19 lean controls *4192* In 26 normoalbuminuric type II diabetics mean concentration of 9.2 ± 4.2 mmol/L and in 52 microalbuminuric type II diabetics 11.5 ± 4.7 mmol/L significantly greater than 4.6 ± 0.5 mmol/L in 28 controls *3959* In 12 male patients with NIDDM mean concentration of 9.00 ± 1.10 mmol/L significantly different from 5.29 ± 0.13 mmol/L in 16 healthy control men *2581* In 14 patients with NIDDM mean fasting concentration of 15.7 ± 0.7 mmol/L *2119* In 82 patients with type II diabetes mellitus mean concentration of 10.2 ± 4.2 mmol/L significantly higher than 5.1 ± 0.6 mmol/L in 48 healthy controls with concentration significantly higher in those with complications than those without *5795* In 26 patients with NIDDM mean concentration of 9.4 ± 2.6 mmol/L significantly different from 4.9 ± 0.5 mmol/L in 10 healthy control subjects *5090* Mean concentration in 43 patients with uncontrolled NIDDM of 10.72 ± 3.92 mmol/L and of 5.9 ± 1.02 mmol/L in 40 patients with controlled NIDDM different from 4.46 ± 0.83 mmol/L in 30 healthy controls *5844*
Serum No Effect In 80 patients with untreated NIDDM mean concentration of 129.1 ± 10.2 mg/dL *5201* In 1,121 men with NIDDM mean concentration of 5.4 ± 1.2 mmol/L comparable to 5.2 ± 1.0 mmol/L in 1,480 women with NIDDM *2336*
Urine Increase In 14 patients with NIDDM mean excretion 600 ± 126 mmol/d *2119*

Glutamic Acid Decarboxylase Antibodies *Serum Increase* Antibodies were detected in 4 of 27 (11%) patients with newly diagnosed NIDDM *2307* In 9 of 106 patients with NIDDM GAD antibodies detected significantly greater than in healthy controls *3880*
Serum No Effect In 6 of 125 nonobese patients with noninsulin-dependent diabetes GAD antibodies detected, with 5 of the patients subsequently progressing to require insulin *274*

Glutathione, Reduced *Red Blood Cells No Effect* In 101 patients with NIDDM mean concentration of 0.212 ± 0.0417 nmol/10^6 erythrocytes compared with 0.217 ± 0.0419 nmol/10^6 erythrocytes in 21 healthy controls *3425*

Glycated Albumin *Serum Increase* In 82 patients with type II diabetes mellitus mean concentration of 163 ± 54 µmol/L significantly higher than 124 ± 34 µmol/L in 48 healthy controls, with concentration in those with complications not significantly different from that in than those without *5795*

Glycated Apolipoprotein B *Serum Increase* Mean proportion of 5.9 ± 1.1% in 60 patients with IDDM compared with 4.3 ± 1.0% in 45 apparently healthy controls *2284*

Glycated Hemoglobin *Blood Increase* In 26 patients with NIDDM mean proportion of 8.7 ± 2.0% significantly different from that in 10 healthy control subjects *5090* In 82 patients with type II diabetes mellitus mean concentration of 10.7 ± 2.9% significantly higher than 6.5 ± 0.5% in 48 healthy controls *5795* Mean concentration of 13.7 ± 1.2% in 10 obese NIDDM patients significantly greater than 5.8 ± 0.3% in 10 lean controls *806* In 8 patients with NIDDM with microalbuminuria mean concentration in men of 8.4 ± 1.2% compared with 8.2 ± 1.0% in males of 22 patients with normal UAE *1294*

Glycated Hemoglobin A_{1c} *Blood Increase* In 127 patients with NIDDM mean proportion 8.3 ± 1.6% *725* In 71 patients with NIDDM mean concentration of 9.6 ± 2.0% significantly higher than concentration in 132 age-matched control individuals *199*

Glycated High Density Lipoprotein *Serum Increase* In 82 patients with type II diabetes mellitus mean concentration of 35 ± 16 µmol/L significantly higher than 27 ± 12 µmol/L in 48 healthy controls with concentration in those with complications not significantly different from that in than those without *5795*

250.00 Noninsulin-dependent Diabetes Mellitus *(continued)*

Glycated Low Density Lipoprotein *Serum* *Increase* In 82 patients with type II diabetes mellitus mean concentration of 83 ± 26 μmol/L significantly higher than 58 ± 23 μmol/L in 48 healthy controls with concentration in those with complications not significantly different from that in than those without *5795*

Glycated Very Low Density Lipoprotein *Serum* *Increase* In 82 patients with type II diabetes mellitus mean concentration of 86 ± 37 μmol/L significantly higher than 54 ± 21 μmol/L in 48 healthy controls with concentration in those with complications significantly higher than that in than those without *5795*

Glycosaminoglycans *Urine* *Increase* In 108 type II diabetics median excretion was 3.80 mg/mmol creatinine (range 1.2 - 13.0) higher than median 2.45 mg/mmol creatinine (range 1.67 - 3.60) in controls *1872*
Urine *No Effect* In 26 normoalbuminuric type II diabetics mean excretion of 7.0 ± 0.5 CPC U/mmol creatinine and in 52 microalbuminuric type II diabetics 6.9 ± 0.4 CPC U/mmol creatinine not significantly greater than 6.0 ± 0.8 CPC U/mmol creatinine in 28 controls *3959*

Glyoxalase I *Blood* *Increase* In 100 patients with NIDDM mean activity of 4.61 ± 1.79 mU/10^6 erythrocytes significantly increased compared with 3.21 ± 1.81 mU/10^6 erythrocytes in 21 healthy controls *3425*

Glyoxalase II *Blood* *Increase* In 101 patients with NIDDM mean activity of 2.10 ± 0.46 mU/10^6 erythrocytes significantly increased compared with 1.83 ± 0.27 mU/10^6 erythrocytes in 21 healthy controls *3425*

HDL_2-Cholesterol *Serum* *Decrease* In 43 men and 40 women with NIDDM mean concentrations of 11 ± 10 mg/dL and 18 ± 15 mg/dL respectively significantly different from 21 ± 11 mg/dL in 50 healthy control men and 31 ± 13 mg/dL in 50 control women *5454*

HDL_3-Cholesterol *Serum* *No Effect* In 43 men and 40 women with NIDDM mean concentrations of 32 ± 9 mg/dL and 31 ± 10 mg/dL respectively not significantly different from 33 ± 8 mg/dL in 50 healthy control men and 32 ± 7 mg/dL in 50 control women *5454*

HDL-Cholesterol *Serum* *Decrease* In 12 type II diabetics mean concentration of 0.91 ± 0.21 mmol/L not significantly lower than 1.11 ± 0.34 mmol/L in 17 nondiabetic control individuals *2471* In patients with NIDDM mean concentration decreased in poorly controlled patients *3853* In patients with NIDDM mean concentration decreased in well controlled patients *3853* In 43 men and 40 women with NIDDM mean concentrations of 42 ± 14 mg/dL and 48 ± 16 mg/dL respectively significantly different from 53 ± 10 mg/dL in 50 healthy control men and 62 ± 12 mg/dL in 50 control women *5454* In 12 male patients with NIDDM mean concentration of 1.04 ± 0.10 mmol/L significantly different from 1.22 ± 0.11 mmol/L in 16 healthy control men *2581* In 16 patients with NIDDM median concentration of 1.00 mmol/L significantly different from 1.20 mmol/L in 16 healthy controls *4353* In 2,425 newly diagnosed NIDDM men and 1,752 NIDDM women mean concentrations of 1.01 ± 0.24 mmol/L and 1.09 ± 0.25 mmol/L respectively significantly lower than 1.11 ± 0.22 mmol/L and 1.42 ± 0.33 mmol/L in 195 age matched male and female controls *3275* In 127 patients with NIDDM mean concentration of 1.14 ± 0.33 mmol/L not significantly different from 1.49 ± 0.33 mmol/L in 286 healthy controls *725* In 17 men with NIDDM mean concentration of 1.15 ± 0.27 mmol/L less than 1.28 ± 0.32 mmol/L in 25 control men: in 30 women with NIDDM mean concentration of 1.13 ± 0.32 mmol/L significantly less than 1.51 ± 0.37 mmol/L in 35 control women *4025* In 26 normoalbuminuric type II diabetics mean concentration of 0.6 ± 0.2 mmol/L and in 52 microalbuminuric type II diabetics 0.7 ± 0.3 mmol/L significantly less than 1.0 ± 0.3 mmol/L in 28 controls *3959* Mean concentration in 43 patients with NIDDM of 1.19 ± 0.42 mmol/L different from 1.43 ± 0.35 mmol/L in 235 healthy control individuals *3884* In 92 patients with NIDDM mean concentration of 1.25 ± 0.30 mmol/L significantly different from 1.51 ± 0.44 mmol/L in 82 healthy controls *10* Mean concentration of 0.92 ± 0.28 mmol/L in 220 patients with NIDDM significantly less than 1.21 ± 0.39 mmol/L in 163 healthy controls *3852* In 539 patients with NIDDM at time of diagnosis mean concentration of 1.0 mmol/L (range of 0.8 - 1.3) significantly lower than 1.3 mmol/L (range of 1.0 - 1.6) in 250 normoglycemic controls *3276* Mean concentration of 1.03 ± 0.09 mmol/L in 44 patients with NIDDM significantly different from 1.40 ± 0.17 mmol/L in 28 healthy controls *4117* Mean concentration of 1.05 ± 0.02 mmol/L in 212 Japanese patients with NIDDM significantly different from 1.21 ± 0.04 mmol/L in 76 healthy controls *2616*
Serum *Increase* In 13 patients with NIDDM mean concentration of 17 ± 1 mg/dL not significantly greater than 13 ± 1 mg/dL in 13 healthy controls *4457*
Serum *No Effect* In 82 patients with type II diabetes mellitus mean concentration of 1.1 ± 0.3 mmol/L not significantly different from 1.1 ± 0.4 mmol/L in 48 healthy controls *5795* In 26 patients with NIDDM mean concentration of 1.03 ± 0.20 mmol/L not significantly different from 1.25 ± 0.16 mmol/L in 10 healthy control subjects *5090* In 14 patients with NIDDM mean concentration of 0.97 ± 0.08 mmol/L not significantly different from normal *2119* In 100 patients with NIDDM mean concentration of 41.9 ± 14.2 mg/dL not significantly different from 45.0 ± 13.3 mg/dL in 854 normoglycemic controls *2330* In 11 patients with NIDDM treated with oral hypoglycemics or insulin mean concentration of 1.35 ± 0.32 mmol/L not significantly different from 1.47 ± 0.33 mmol/L in 14 healthy controls *3556* In 37 patients with NIDDM and normoalbuminuria mean concentration of 1.28 ± 0.44 mmol/L, in 11 with microalbuminuria 1.05 ± 0.21 mmol/L and in 7 with macroalbuminuria 0.97 ± 0.13 mmol/L not significantly different from 1.18 ± 0.37 mmol/L in 55 healthy controls *4329* In 36 patients with NIDDM and microalbuminuria mean concentration of 40.4 ± 1.8 mg/dL and 43.9 ± 1.6 mg/dL in 36 with normoalbuminuria not different when compared with healthy individuals *1889* In about 16 patients with NIDDM mean concentration of 39 ± 2 mg/dL not significantly different from 44 ± 3 mg/dL in non-diabetic controls *2842* In 80 patients with untreated NIDDM mean concentration of 49.4 ± 12.1 mg/dL *5201* In 39 patients with NIDDM mean concentration of 1.35 ± 0.48 mmol/L not significantly different from 1.33 ± 0.41 mmol/L in 24 healthy controls *4713* In 16 patients with NIDDM mean concentration of 1.00 ± 0.37 mmol/L not significantly different from 1.16 ± 0.27 mmol/L in 16 healthy controls *5014* Mean concentration of 1.35 ± 0.05 mmol/L in 70 patients with NIDDM significantly less than 1.63 ± 0.03 mmol/L in 142 patients with IDDM but not significantly different from normal range *470* In 1,121 men with NIDDM mean concentration of 1.3 ± 0.3 mmol/L comparable to 1.3 ± 0.3 mmol/L in 1,480 women with NIDDM *2336*

HDL-Cholesterol Esters *Serum* *Decrease* In 16 patients with NIDDM median concentration of 0.82 mmol/L significantly different from 1.04 mmol/L in 16 healthy controls *4353*

HDL-Protein *Serum* *No Effect* In 37 patients with NIDDM and normoalbuminuria mean concentration of 1.22 ± 0.28 mmol/L, in 11 with microalbuminuria 1.18 ± 0.11 mmol/L and in 7 with macroalbuminuria 1.10 ± 0.19 mmol/L, compared with 1.16 ± 0.21 mmol/L in 55 healthy controls *4329*

HDL-Triglycerides *Serum* *Increase* In 37 patients with NIDDM and normoalbuminuria mean concentration of 0.17 ± 0.07 mmol/L, in 11 with microalbuminuria 0.13 ± 0.04 mmol/L and in 7 with macroalbuminuria 0.28 ± 0.14 mmol/L significantly greater than 0.07 ± 0.06 mmol/L in 55 healthy controls *4329* In 16 patients with NIDDM median concentration of 0.21 mmol/L significantly different from 0.15 mmol/L in 16 healthy controls *4353*

Hematocrit *Blood* *No Effect* In 25 newly diagnosed untreated patients with NIDDM mean of 42.3 ± 5.8% compared with 43 ± 1.3% in 15 normal controls *3264* Mean value in 16 NIDDM patients with microalbuminuria of 43.0 ± 1.0% not significantly different from 43.6 ± 0.8% in 31 normoalbuminuric NIDDM patients and 30 healthy controls *5713*

Hemoglobin *Blood* *No Effect* In 25 newly diagnosed untreated patients with diabetes mellitus mean concentration of 140.2 ± 19 g/L compared with 140.8 ± 13 g/L in 15 normal controls *3264*

Hemoglobin A_1 *Blood* *Increase* Mean concentration of 8.4 ± 0.1% in 212 Japanese patients with NIDDM significantly higher than that in 76 healthy controls *2616* In 12 male patients with NIDDM with micro- or macroalbuminuria mean concentration of 9.1 ± 2.2% increased but not significantly different from 8.5 ± 2.1% in 12 normoalbuminuric patients with NIDDM *5865*

Hemoglobin A_{1c} *Blood* *Increase* In 539 patients with NIDDM concentration at time of diagnosis of 9.3 ± 2.3% compared with

5.4 ± 0.5% in 250 normoglycemic controls *3276* In patients with NIDDM, 28 with renal insufficiency had a mean concentration of 7.9 ± 1.2% increased above normal but lower than 8.8 ± 1.9% in 45 patients with macroalbuminuria, 8.8 ± 1.6% in 98 patients with microalbuminuria and 8.2 ± 1.9% in 127 patients with normoalbuminuria *5760* In 12 obese patients with NIDDM mean concentration of 8.62 ± 0.56% and in 12 nonobese patients with NIDDM 9.05 ± 0.48% *2582* In 67 patients with type II diabetes mean concentration of 10.84 ± 2.14% compared with 5.85 - 8.85% in healthy controls *2943* In 34 patients with NIDDM mean concentration of 7.8 ± 1.9% significantly different from 4.3 ± 0.9% in 32 healthy controls *5499* Mean concentration of 9.02 ± 0.32% in 70 patients with NIDDM not significantly different from 9.07 ± 0.15% in 142 patients with IDDM but significantly different from normal range *470* In 12 type II diabetics mean concentration of 7.5 ± 2.3% significantly higher than 5.0 ± 0.8% in 17 nondiabetic control individuals *2471* In 14 patients with NIDDM mean concentration of 7.7 ± 0.3% *2119* In 29 obese patients with NIDDM mean concentration of 13 ± 1% significantly different from 6 ± 1% in 21 healthy obese individuals and 19 lean controls *4192* In 34 patients with NIDDM mean proportion of 7.6 ± 1.9% not significantly different from 4.2 ± 0.9% in 32 healthy controls *5500* In 100 patients with NIDDM mean concentration of 7.93 ± 2.40% significantly increased compared with 4.33 ± 1.70% in 8 healthy controls *3425* In 80 patients with untreated NIDDM mean concentration of 7.8 ± 1.7% *5201* In 13 patients with NIDDM mean proportion of 11.1 ± 1.7% significantly greater than 6.3 ± 1.1% in 13 healthy controls *4457* In 81 patients with NIDDM median concentration of 9.0% compared with 3.8% in 62 healthy controls *1867* In 92 patients with NIDDM mean concentration of 7.5 ± 1.6% significantly higher than 4.7 ± 0.4% in 23 healthy controls *2366* Mean concentration in 125 patients with NIDDM of 6.8 ± 1.0% significantly different from 5.1 ± 0.4% in 63 healthy controls *3920* Mean proportion in 16 NIDDM patients with microalbuminuria of 7.7 ± 0.5% not significantly different from 7.5 ± 0.4% in 31 normoalbuminuric NIDDM patients but significantly higher than in 30 healthy controls *5713* In 40 patients with type II diabetes mellitus mean concentration of 8.1 ± 1.7% significantly higher than 5.2 ± 0.5% in control patients *4887* In about 16 patients with NIDDM mean proportion of 10.3 ± 0.7% significantly different from 5.6 ± 0.3% in non-diabetic controls *2842*

High Molecular Weight Kininogen *Plasma* *Increase* In 13 patients with NIDDM mean concentration of 1.25 ± 0.19 μg BK eq/mL significantly different from 0.72 ± 0.10 μg BK eq/mL in 13 healthy controls *4457*

Homocysteine *Plasma* *Decrease* Median concentration in 163 patients with NIDDM and normal renal function of 6.9 μmol/L, 7.7 μmol/L in 34 patients with mildly impaired renal function and 13.6 μmol/L in 6 patients with moderately to severely impaired renal function *4993*

β-Hydroxyisovaleric Acid *Urine* *Increase* In 21 non-proteinuric type II diabetic patients with and without ketosis excretion higher in patients with ketosis than in those without and in controls although excretion in nonketotic diabetics higher than in controls *5828*

IDL-Cholesterol *Serum* *Increase* In 7 patients with NIDDM and macroalbuminuria mean concentration of 0.39 ± 0.32 mmol/L significantly greater than 0.19 ± 0.12 mmol/L in 55 healthy controls *4329*
Serum *No Effect* In 37 patients with NIDDM and normoalbuminuria mean concentration of 0.22 ± 0.15 mmol/L and in 11 with microalbuminuria 0.16 ± 0.03 mmol/L not significantly different from 0.10 ± 0.12 mmol/L in 55 healthy controls *4329*

IDL-Protein *Serum* *Increase* In patients with NIDDM mean concentration increased in well controlled patients *3853* In 7 patients with NIDDM and macroalbuminuria mean concentration of 0.14 ± 0.09 g/L significantly higher than 0.06 ± 0.05 g/L in 55 healthy controls *4329*
Serum *No Effect* In 37 patients with NIDDM and normoalbuminuria mean concentration of 0.09 ± 0.09 g/L and in 11 with microalbuminuria mean concentration of 0.07 ± 0.03 mmol/L not significantly different from 0.06 ± 0.05 mmol/L in 55 healthy controls *4329*

IDL-Triglycerides *Serum* *Increase* In 37 patients with NIDDM and normoalbuminuria mean concentration of 0.23 ± 0.17 mmol/L, in 11 with microalbuminuria of 0.22 ± 0.14 mmol/L, and in 7 with macroalbuminuria of 0.49 ± 0.29 mmol/L significantly greater than 0.15 ± 0.11 mmol/L in 55 healthy controls *4329*

Insulin *Plasma* *Decrease* In 14 patients with NIDDM mean concentration of 308 ± 80 pmol/L *2119* In 34 patients with NIDDM mean concentration of 13.8 ± 6.4 mU/L not significantly different from 16.8 ± 4.7 mU/L in 32 healthy controls *5500*
Plasma *Increase* In 1,121 men with NIDDM mean concentration of 35.9 ± 40.0 pmol/L less than 41.1 ± 36.2 pmol/L in 1,480 women with NIDDM *2336* In 8 obese individuals with NIDDM mean concentration of 20 ± 3 mIU/L significantly different from 6 ± 1 mIU/L in 9 lean controls and 11 ± 2 mIU/L in 9 obese nondiabetics *320* In 12 obese patients with NIDDM mean concentration of 46.14 ± 6.00 pmol/L significantly higher and in 12 nonobese patients with NIDDM 35.52 ± 5.28 pmol/L not significantly higher than 28.62 ± 4.68 pmol/L in 12 normal individuals *2582* In 12 male patients with NIDDM mean concentration of 55.98 ± 6.00 pmol/L significantly different from 36.90 ± 4.32 pmol/L in 16 healthy control men *2581* In 29 obese patients with NIDDM mean concentration of 52 ± 9 μU/mL significantly different from 31 ± 3 μU/mL in 21 healthy obese individuals and 6 ± 1 μU/mL in 19 lean controls *4192* In about 16 patients with NIDDM mean concentration of 20.9 ± 2.4 μU/mL significantly different from 12.3 ± 1.6 μU/mL in non-diabetic controls *2842* In 19 obese type II diabetic patients median fasting concentration of 14.2 μU/L significantly different from median concentration of 5.1 μU/L in 28 lean controls *2067* In 10 obese patients with NIDDM mean concentration of 111 ± 7 pmol/L significantly greater than 54 ± 5 pmol/L in 10 healthy lean controls *806* Mean concentration of 18.5 ± 1.8 mU/L in 46 men with NIDDM significantly higher than 6.5 ± 0.4 mU/L in 11 healthy normal men *115* In 539 patients with NIDDM at time of diagnosis mean concentration of 13.4 mU/L (range 7.7 - 23.1) compared with 7.0 mU/L (range 4.5 - 11.0) in 250 normoglycemic controls *3276*
Plasma *No Effect* Mean concentration in 16 NIDDM patients with microalbuminuria of 25.6 ± 4.4 pmol/L not significantly different from 25.2 ± 3.7 pmol/L in 31 normoalbuminuric NIDDM patients and 27.0 ± 2.6 pmol/L in 30 healthy controls *5713* In 26 patients with NIDDM mean concentration of 18.2 ± 14.3 mU/L not significantly different from 11.4 ± 9.0 mU/L in 10 healthy control subjects *5090*

Insulin-like Growth Factor-I *Serum* *Decrease* In 29 obese patients with NIDDM mean concentration of 105 ± 11 ng/dL significantly different from 143 ± 11 ng/dL in 21 healthy obese individuals and 177 ± 14 ng/dL in 19 lean controls *4192*

Insulin, Nonspecific *Plasma* *Increase* In 12 type II diabetics mean concentration of 151 ± 66 pmol/L significantly higher than 95 ± 43 pmol/L in 17 nondiabetic control individuals *2471*

Insulin, Specific *Plasma* *Increase* In 12 type II diabetics mean concentration of 110 ± 55 pmol/L significantly higher than 87 ± 33 pmol/L in 17 nondiabetic control individuals *2471*

Intercellular Adhesion Molecule-1 *Serum* *Increase* In patients with NIDDM mean serum concentration about 36% higher than in controls *5519*

Interferon-γ *Serum* *No Effect* Median concentration of 0.0 pg/mL in patients with NIDDM not different when compared with 0.0 pg/mL in normal controls *2307*

Interleukin-1 Receptor Antagonist *Serum* *No Effect* In 11 type II diabetics mean concentration of 0.13 ± 0.07 pmol/L not significantly different from that in 14 healthy controls, in whom mean concentration was 0.10 ± 0.04 pmol/L *3556*

Interleukin-1α *Serum* *No Effect* Median concentration of 105 pg/mL in patients with NIDDM not significantly different when compared with 100 pg/mL in normal controls *2307*

Interleukin-1β *Serum* *No Effect* In 11 type II diabetics mean concentration of 0.048 ± 0.008 pmol/L not significantly different from that in 14 healthy controls, in whom mean concentration was 0.052 ± 0.009 pmol/L *3556* Concentration not detectable in patients with NIDDM or controls *2307*

Interleukin-2 *Serum* *Increase* Median concentration of 6.4% in patients with NIDDM significantly increased when compared with 3.6% in normal controls *2307*

Interleukin-4 *Serum* *No Effect* Median concentration of 0 pg/mL in patients with NIDDM not significantly different when compared with 0 pg/mL in normal controls *2307*

250.00 Noninsulin-dependent Diabetes Mellitus *(continued)*

Interleukin-10 *Serum* *No Effect* Median concentration of 0 pg/mL in patients with NIDDM not significantly different when compared with 0 pg/mL in normal controls *2307*

Islet Amyloid Polypeptide *Serum* *Increase* In 12 patients with NIDDM concentrations ranged from non-detectable to 14.5 pmol/L compared with normal range of 6.0 ± 4.0 pmol/L *5404*
Serum *No Effect* In 7 insulin-treated NIDDM patients mean concentration of 3.6 ± 2.9 pmol/L and in 11 drug-treated patients with NIDDM mean concentration of 7.2 ± 4.3 pmol/L compared with 8.0 ± 5.0 pmol/L in 25 normal individuals *4210* In 12 patients with NIDDM concentrations ranged from not detectable to 14.5 pmol/L compared with 6.0 ± 4.0 pmol/L in healthy individuals *5404*

Islet Cell Antibodies *Serum* *Increase* No antibodies were detected in any patients with newly diagnosed NIDDM *2307*

Lactate *Blood* *Increase* In 105 patients with NIDDM mean concentration of 20.0 nmol/g blood compared with 9.7 ± 4.3 nmol/g blood in 21 healthy controls *3425*

Laminin *Serum* *Increase* Mean concentration increased from 1.23 ± 0.21 U/mL in 25 patients without retinopathy to 1.51 ± 0.34 U/mL in 11 patients with proliferative retinopathy *3894*
Urine *Increase* In 33 patients with NIDDM and macroalbuminuria mean excretion of 174.0 ± 23.2 µg/g creatinine significantly greater than that in 85 patients with NIDDM and normoalbuminuria in whom mean excretion was 54.3 ± 4.6 µg/g creatinine, not greater than upper limit of normal of 70.6 µg/g creatinine *283*
Urine *No Effect* In 85 patients with NIDDM and normoalbuminuria mean excretion of 54.3 ± 4.6 µg/g creatinine not greater than upper limit of normal of 70.6 µg/g creatinine *283*

LDL-Cholesterol *Serum* *Increase* In 26 patients with NIDDM mean concentration of 3.76 ± 0.92 mmol/L significantly different from 2.99 ± 0.59 mmol/L in 10 healthy control subjects *5090* In patients with NIDDM mean concentration increased in poorly controlled patients *3853* In 26 normoalbuminuric type II diabetics mean concentration of 3.8 ± 0.9 mmol/L and in 52 microalbuminuric type II diabetics of 3.7 ± 1.4 mmol/L significantly greater than 2.6 ± 0.8 mmol/L in 28 controls *3959* In 17 men with NIDDM mean concentration of 3.36 ± 0.74 mmol/L compared with 3.11 ± 0.91 mmol/L in 25 control men: in 30 women with NIDDM mean concentration of 3.98 ± 0.98 mmol/L significantly greater than 3.47 ± 0.93 mmolL in 35 controls *4025* In 13 patients with NIDDM mean concentration of 35 ± 3 mg/dL not significantly greater than 33 ± 2 mg/dL in 13 healthy controls *4457*
Serum *No Effect* In 82 patients with type II diabetes mellitus mean concentration of 3.7 ± 0.6 mmol/L not significantly different from 3.8 ± 0.4 mmol/L in 48 healthy controls *5795* In 100 patients with NIDDM mean concentration of 121.7 ± 51.0 mg/dL not significantly different from 128.4 ± 39.3 mg/dL in 854 normoglycemic controls *2330* In 36 patients with NIDDM and microalbuminuria mean concentration of 123.9 ± 7.1 mg/dL and 115.8 ± 6.7 mg/dL in 36 with normoalbuminuria not different when compared with healthy individuals *1889* In 1,121 men with NIDDM mean concentration of 2.9 ± 0.8 mmol/L comparable to 3.3 ± 0.8 mmol/L in 1,480 women with NIDDM *2336* In 16 patients with NIDDM mean concentration of 3.82 ± 0.98 mmol/L not significantly different from mean of 4.64 ± 1.15 mmol/L in 16 healthy controls *5014* In patients with NIDDM mean concentration normal in well controlled patients *3853* In about 16 patients with NIDDM mean concentration of 124 ± 7 mg/dL not significantly different from 103 ± 9 mg/dL in non-diabetic controls *2842* In 12 type II diabetics mean concentration of 3.26 ± 0.96 mmol/L not significantly higher than 3.13 ± 0.67 mmol/L in 17 nondiabetic control individuals *2471* In 14 patients with NIDDM mean concentration of 2.98 ± 0.31 mmol/L not significantly different from normal *2119* In 11 patients with NIDDM treated with oral hypoglycemics or insulin mean concentration of 3.4 ± 0.8 mmol/L not significantly different from 3.6 ± 0.7 mmol/L in 14 healthy controls *3556* In 37 patients with NIDDM and normoalbuminuria mean concentration of 3.28 ± 1.34 mmol/L, in 11 with microalbuminuria 3.23 ± 1.18 mmol/L and in 7 with macroalbuminuria 3.63 ± 1.05 mmol/L not significantly different from 3.26 ± 0.86 mmol/L in 55 healthy controls *4329* Mean concentration of 3.24 ± 0.88 mmol/L in 184 patients with NIDDM not significantly different from 3.21 ± 0.93 mmol/L in 160 healthy controls *3852*

LDL-Protein *Serum* *No Effect* In 37 patients with NIDDM and normoalbuminuria mean concentration of 0.53 ± 0.14 g/L, in 11 with microalbuminuria 0.59 ± 0.16 g/L and in 7 with macroalbuminuria 0.57 ± 0.16 g/L, not significantly different from 0.52 ± 0.15 g/L in 55 healthy controls *4329*

LDL-Triglycerides *Serum* *Increase* In 37 patients with NIDDM and normoalbuminuria mean concentration of 0.28 ± 0.11 mmol/L, in 11 with microalbuminuria 0.30 ± 0.10 mmol/L and in 7 with macroalbuminuria 0.50 ± 0.22 mmol/L significantly greater than 0.20 ± 0.08 mmol/L in 55 healthy controls *4329*

Lecithin:Cholesterol Acyltransferase *Serum* *Increase* In 16 patients with NIDDM median activity of 95 AU/L significantly different from 86 AU/L in 16 healthy controls *4353*

Leptin *Serum* *Increase* Mean concentration of 63.1 ± 4.1 ng/mL in 7 diabetic overweight women with BMI of 31 - 40 kg/m^2 significantly different from 31.7 ± 2.4 ng/mL observed in 19 lean healthy women *287*

Leucine *Plasma* *Increase* In type II diabetic ketotic patients serum concentration higher than in nonketotic diabetic patients and normal controls *5828*

Leukocytes *Blood* *No Effect* Mean concentration of 8.3 ± 0.4 /nL in 44 patients with NIDDM not significantly different from 8.3 ± 0.3 /nL in 28 healthy controls *4117* In 25 untreated newly diagnosed patients with NIDDM mean concentration of 7,800 ± 2,400 /µL compared with 7,800 ± 1,100 /µL in 15 normal controls *3264*

Lipase, Hepatic *Serum* *No Effect* In 16 patients with NIDDM median activity of 436 U/L not significantly different from 425 U/L in 16 healthy controls *4353*

Lipid Peroxide *Serum* *Increase* In 16 men and 15 women with NIDDM but without complications mean concentration of 5.4 nmol/mL compared with normals of 4.1 and 4.4 nmol/mL respectively *822*
Serum *No Effect* In 67 patients with type II diabetes mean concentration of 1.06 ± 0.51 µg/L *2943*

Lipoprotein Lp(a) *Serum* *Decrease* Mean concentration of 14.4 mg/dL in 212 Japanese patients with NIDDM significantly different from 10.8 mg/dL in 76 healthy controls *2616* In 17 men with NIDDM mean concentration of 6.06 ± 7.87 mmol/L less than 8.65 ± 10.03 mmol/L in 25 control men *4025*
Serum *Increase* In 19 patients with NIDDM and nephropathy mean concentration of 43 mg/dL compared with reference interval of < 25 mg/dL *4640* In 90 patients with NIDDM median concentration of 0.11 g/L not significantly different from median of 0.12 g/L, although concentrations above 0.25 g/L were observed in 22% of patients with poor glycemic control *5644* Mean concentration of 17.5 ± 19.4 mg/dL in 227 patients with NIDDM significantly higher than 13.7 ± 14.5 mg/dL in 163 healthy controls *3852* In 46 insulin-treated NIDDM patients mean concentration of 26.7 ± 25.0 mg/dL compared with 21.1 ± 30.4 mg/dL in 142 nondiabetic controls *2104* Mean concentration in 43 patients with NIDDM of 206 ± 213 mg/L different from 125 ± 111 mg/L in 235 healthy control individuals *3884* In 11 patients with NIDDM treated with oral hypoglycemics or insulin mean concentration of 260 mg/L (range 122 - 840) not significantly different from 185 mg/L (range 16 - 1050) in 14 healthy controls *3556* In 30 women with NIDDM mean concentration of 12.82 ± 11.29 mmol/L significantly greater than 7.78 ± 10.10 mmol/L in 35 control women *4025*
Serum *No Effect* No significant difference between the median concentration of 24.0 mg/dL in 103 African-American patients with NIDDM and 25.5 mg/dL in 38 non-NIDDM patients *4616* In 65 patients with NIDDM median concentration of 63 mg/L not significantly different from 43 mg/L in 69 healthy volunteers, but with 7.4% above 95th percentile of 361 mg/L *5417* In 90 patients with NIDDM median concentration of 0.11 g/L not significantly different from median of 0.12 g/L, although concentrations above 0.25 g/L were observed in 22% of patients with poor glycemic control *5644* In 1,121 men with NIDDM mean concentration of 18.5 ± 17.9 mg/dL less than 21.4 ± 20.1 mg/dL in 1,480 women with NIDDM *2336* Diabetes appears to have no significant effect on plasma concentrations of Lp(a) *2827* In 37 patients with NIDDM and normoalbuminuria mean concentration of 0.12 ± 0.11 g/L, in 11 with microalbuminuria 0.17 ± 0.13 g/L and in 7 with macroalbuminuria 0.23 ± 0.1 g/L not significantly different from 0.12 ± 0.12 g/L in 55 healthy controls *4329* In 577 patients with NIDDM mean concentration of 27.2 ± 19.3 mg/dL not significantly different from 27.1 ± 18.2 mg/dL in 261 relatives and 23.1 ± 15.1 mg/dL in 49 unrelated healthy individuals *5450*

Urine *No Effect* Mean excretion in 43 patients with NIDDM of 1,008 ± 855 μg/d not significantly different from 1,527 ± 896 μg/d in 23 healthy control individuals *3884*

Low Molecular Weight Kininogen *Serum* *Increase* In 13 patients with NIDDM mean concentration of 3.65 ± 0.25 μg BK eq/mL significantly different from 2.31 ± 0.21 μg BK eq/mL in 13 healthy controls *4457*

Malondialdehyde *Serum* *Increase* In 40 patients with type II diabetes mellitus mean concentration of 2.3 ± 0.4 μmol/L significantly different from 2.1 ± 0.3 μmol/L in control patients *4887*

α-Mannosidase *Serum* *Increase* Mean activity of 0.484 ± 0.162 mU/L in 12 individuals with NIDDM significantly different from 0.321 ± 0.132 mU/L in 35 healthy controls *939*

Metalloproteinase-9 *Serum* *Increase* In 8 patients with NIDDM with microalbuminuria mean concentration of 34 μg/L initially increased to 56 μg/L after 12 months, 88 μg/L after 24 months and 117 μg/L after 48 months compared with 32 μg/L initially, 36 μg/L after 12 months, 39 μg/L after 24 months and 44 μg/L in 22 patients with normal UAE *1294*

Methylglyoxal *Blood* *Increase* In 105 patients with NIDDM mean concentration of 268.8 pmol/g blood compared with 79.8 pmol/g blood in 21 healthy controls *3425*

α_1-Microglobulin *Urine* *Increase* In 33 patients with NIDDM and macroalbuminuria mean excretion of 17.7 ± 2.8 mg/g creatinine significantly greater than that in 85 patients with NIDDM and normoalbuminuria in whom mean excretion was 4.2 ± 0.4 mg/g creatinine, not greater than upper limit of normal of 7.0 mg/g creatinine *283*

Urine *No Effect* In 85 patients with NIDDM and normoalbuminuria mean excretion of 4.2 ± 0.4 mg/g creatinine not greater than upper limit of normal of 7.0 mg/g creatinine *283*

β_2-Microglobulin *Serum* *Increase* Mean concentration in 125 patients with NIDDM of 5.4 ± 7.0 mg/L significantly different from that in 63 healthy controls *3920*

N-Acetyl-Glucosaminidase *Serum* *Increase* In 539 patients with NIDDM at time of diagnosis mean activity of 664 μmol/h/L (range 506 - 874) not significantly different from 619 μmol/h/L (range 490 - 783) in 250 normoglycemic controls *3276* In 40 patients with type II diabetes mellitus mean activity of 20.8 U/L significantly higher than 16.9 U/L in control patients *4887* In type II patients mean concentration of 657 (481 - 898) μmol/h/L compared with 587 (443 - 780) μmol/h/L in 48 normal controls *644* Mean activity of 12.19 ± 2.95 mU/L in 12 individuals with NIDDM significantly different from 10.45 ± 2.19 mU/L in 35 healthy controls *939*

Urine *Increase* In 539 patients with NIDDM at time of diagnosis excretion greater than 300 μmol/h/L in 70% compared with 15% in 250 normoglycemic controls *3276* In patients with NIDDM, 28 with renal insufficiency had a mean activity of 1.09 ± 0.21 log[U]/L increased above normal but also higher than 0.91 ± 0.31 log[U]/L in 45 patients with macroalbuminuria, 0.68 ± 0.39 log[U]/L in 98 patients with microalbuminuria, 0.55 ± 0.38 log[U]/L in 127 patients with normoalbuminuria and 0.40 ± 0.43 log[U]/L in 80 healthy controls *5760* In 33 patients with NIDDM and macroalbuminuria mean excretion of 14.4 ± 1.4 U/g creatinine significantly greater than that in 85 patients with NIDDM and normoalbuminuria in whom mean excretion was 5.8 ± 0.4 U/g creatinine, not greater than upper limit of normal of 6.5 U/g creatinine *283*

Urine *No Effect* In 85 patients with NIDDM and normoalbuminuria mean excretion of 5.8 ± 0.4 U/g creatinine not greater than upper limit of normal of 6.5 U/g creatinine *283*

N-Acetyl-Glucosaminidase:Creatinine Ratio *Urine* *Increase* In patients with newly diagnosed NIDDM median ratio outside normal range of > 500 U:mol with 75th percentile above twice the upper limit of normal *3277*

Neuropeptide Y *Plasma* *Increase* Mean concentration of 41.0 ± 3.5 pg/mL in 7 diabetic overweight women with BMI of 31 - 40 kg/m^2 significantly greater than 21.2 ± 5.1 pg/mL in 22 nondiabetic women with a similar degree of obesity and 8.1 ± 1.7 pg/mL observed in 19 lean healthy women *287*

Non-HDL-Cholesterol *Serum* *No Effect* Mean concentration of 4.38 ± 0.15 mmol/L in 70 patients with NIDDM significantly higher than 3.95 ± 0.09 mmol/L in 142 patients with IDDM but not significantly different from normal range *470*

N-terminal Peptide of Type III Procollagen *Serum* *Increase* In 11 nonproteinuric patients mean concentration of 0.66 ± 0.09 U/mL, in 15 patients with microalbuminuria of 0.82 ± 0.07 U/mL and 1.14 ± 0.21 U/mL in 7 patients with proteinuria different from reference range of 0.38 - 0.80 U/mL *2357*

Osmolality *Serum* *No Effect* In about 16 patients with NIDDM mean osmolality of 271 ± 8 mOsm/kg not significantly different from 267 ± 4 mOsm/kg in non-diabetic controls *2842*

Oubain-like Substance *Serum* *Increase* In 98 hypertensive NIDDM patients serum mean concentrations of 0.918 ± 0.212 nmol/L significantly higher than 0.589 ± 0.162 nmol/L in 60 normotensive NIDDM patients *767*

Oxysterols, Total *Serum* *No Effect* In 10 type II diabetics mean concentration of 321 ± 191 nmol/L not significantly different from mean concentration of 265 ± 66 nmol/L in 13 healthy controls *3556*

Paraoxonase *Serum* *No Effect* In 92 patients with NIDDM mean concentration of 54.0 ± 3.1 μg/mL not significantly different from 42.5 ± 2.2 μg/mL in 82 healthy controls *10*

Phosphate *Serum* *Increase* In 20 patients with NIDDM and nephropathy mean concentration increased to 3.85 ± 0.60 mg/dL *2167*

Phospholipid Transfer Protein *Serum* *Increase* In 16 patients with NIDDM median activity of 96 AU/L significantly different from 76 AU/L in 16 healthy controls *4353*

Plasminogen Activator Inhibitor *Plasma* *No Effect* In 15 type II diabetics mean activity not different from that in controls *1023*

Plasminogen Activator Inhibitor-1 *Plasma* *Increase* In 12 NIDDM patients mean specific activity 0.42 AU/mL compared with 0.31 AU/mL in 12 normal volunteer controls *5255* In 12 NIDDM patients mean activity of 13 AU/mL compared with 7 AU/mL in 12 normal volunteer controls *5255* In 13 patients with NIDDM and microalbuminuria mean concentration of 5.65 ± 1.92 IU/mL significantly higher than 0.85 ± 0.58 IU/mL in 13 comparable normoalbuminuric NIDDM patients *1888* In 10 patients with NIDDM and hyperlipidemia mean PAI-1 concentration of 73 ng/L and 46 ng/L in 8 patients with NIDDM but without hyperlipidemia significantly higher than 21 ng/mL in 10 healthy male controls *5815*

Plasma *No Effect* In 19 patients with NIDDM and nephropathy mean concentration of 7.5 U/mL compared with reference interval of 0 - 24 U/mL *4640*

Platelets *Increase* In 12 type II diabetics mean concentration of 264 ± 83 ng/5 x 10^8 platelets significantly higher than 202 ± 71 ng/5 x 10^8 platelets *2471* In 12 NIDDM patients mean activity of 0.017 AU/mL compared with 0.011 AU/mL in 12 normal volunteer controls *5255* In 12 NIDDM patients mean specific activity of 0.07 AU/ng compared with 0.03 AU/ng in 12 normal volunteer controls *5255*

Plasminogen Activator Inhibitor-1 Antigen
Plasma *Increase* In 12 NIDDM patients mean concentration of 38 ng/mL compared with 22 ng/mL in 12 normal volunteer controls *5255*

Platelets *Decrease* In 12 NIDDM patients mean concentration of 0.25 ng/10^6 platelets compared with 0.50 ng/10^6 platelets in 12 normal volunteer controls *5255*

Plasminogen Activator Inhibitor Antigen *Plasma* *Increase* In 18 patients with type II diabetes and CAD mean concentration significantly higher than in controls *1023*

Platelet Activating Factor *Urine* *Increase* In about 16 patients with NIDDM mean excretion of 2,606 ± 513 ng/d (1,706 ± 421 pg/mL) significantly different from 78 ± 14 ng/d (85 ± 18 pg/mL) in non-diabetic controls *2842*

Platelet Aggregation *Blood* *Increase* In 23 patients with uncontrolled NIDDM maximum response to 10 μmol/L ADP of 15.4 ± 5.2 ohm compared with 8.1 ± 2.4 ohm in 15 controls. In response to 20 μmol/L ADP patients with NIDDM had a maxmum response of 16.4 ± 4.5 ohm and 10.0 ± 3.9 ohm in controls. 25 mmol/L arachdonic acid caused maximum response of 15.9 ± 5.7 ohm in 25 NIDDM patients compared with 9.3 ± 6.5 ohm in 13 controls. In response to 50 mmol/L maximum response in 18 patients with NIDDM 15.8 ± 4.4 ohm compared with 14.1 ± 2.3 ohm in 15 normal controls *3264*

Platelet-derived Growth Factor *Plasma* *No Effect* In 42 patients with NIDDM mean concentration not significantly different from 4,980 - 15,070 pg/mL in 18 healthy controls *2030*

250.00 **Noninsulin-dependent Diabetes Mellitus** *(continued)*

Platelets *Blood* *No Effect* Mean concentration of 286 ± 15 n/nL in 44 patients with NIDDM not significantly different from 255 ± 14 n/nL in 28 healthy controls *4117*

Postheparin Lipoprotein Lipase *Plasma* *No Effect* In 16 patients with NIDDM median activity of 142 U/L not significantly different from 109 U/L in 16 healthy controls *4353*

Potassium *Serum* *No Effect* Mean value in 16 NIDDM patients with microalbuminuria of 4.1 ± 0.1 mmol/L not significantly different from 4.2 ± 0.1 mmol/L in 31 normoalbuminuric NIDDM patients and 30 healthy controls *5713*

Protein *Serum* *Decrease* In 13 patients with NIDDM mean concentration of 60.9 ± 2.6 g/L not significantly different from 65.5 ± 2.6 g/L in 13 healthy controls *4457*

Protein C *Plasma* *No Effect* In 19 patients with NIDDM and nephropathy mean concentration of 123 U/dL compared with reference interval of 65 - 140 U/dL *4640*

Prothrombin Time *Plasma* *Increase* In 10 patients with NIDDM and hyperlipidemia fluorescent prothrombin time of 137 ± 36% significantly higher than 101 ± 21% in 8 patients with NIDDM but without hyperlipidemia and 105 ± 11% in 10 healthy male controls *5815*

Retinol *Serum* *Increase* In 20 patients with NIDDM and nephropathy mean concentration increased to 101.0 ± 45.9 µg/dL *2167*

Sex-Hormone Binding Globulin *Serum* *Decrease* A low SHBG concentration has been shown to be predictive of NIDDM in women but not men *4234* Mean concentration of 5.59 ± 0.46 mol x 10^8 in 39 women with NIDDM significantly reduced compared with 13.1 ± 1.82 mol x 10^8 in 17 healthy female controls: mean concentration of 25.0 ± 2.4 nmol/L in 46 men with NIDDM significantly less than 41.3 ± 5.9 nmol/L in 11 healthy men *115* In 12 male patients with NIDDM mean concentration of 37.54 ± 4.87 nmol/L significantly different from 57.38 ± 3.89 pmol/L in 16 healthy control men *2581*

Sialic Acid *Serum* *Increase* NIDDM patients with hypertension and retinopathy have significantly increased concentrations *213* In 20 patients with NIDDM mean concentration of 0.74 ± 0.11 g/L compared with 0.60 ± 0.22 g/L in 20 age and sex matched controls *970* In 26 normoalbuminuric type II diabetics mean concentration of 1.9 ± 0.4 mmol/L and in 52 microalbuminuric type II diabetics 2.0 ± 0.4 mmol/L significantly greater than 1.6 ± 0.1 mmol/L in 28 controls *3959*
Urine *Increase* In 26 normoalbuminuric type II diabetics mean excretion of 0.08 ± 0.01 mmol/mmol creatinine and in 52 microalbuminuric type II diabetics 0.08 ± 0.01 mmol/mmol creatinine significantly greater than 0.04 ± 0.01 mmol/mmol creatinine in 28 controls *3959*

Sialic Acid, Lipid-associated *Serum* *Increase* In 20 patients with NIDDM mean concentration of 0.18 ± 0.04 g/L higher than 0.12 ± 0.04 g/L in 20 age and sex matched controls *970*
Serum *No Effect* In 26 normoalbuminuric type II diabetics mean concentration of 0.5 ± 0.2 mmol/L and in 52 microalbuminuric type II diabetics 0.6 ± 0.2 mmol/L not significantly different from 0.5 ± 0.1 mmol/L in 28 controls *3959*

Sodium *Serum* *No Effect* Mean value in 16 NIDDM patients with microalbuminuria of 141.2 ± 0.6 mmol/L not significantly different from 141.8 ± 0.4 mmol/L in 31 normoalbuminuric NIDDM patients and 30 healthy controls *5713*
Urine *No Effect* Mean 24 h excretion in 16 NIDDM patients with microalbuminuria of 132 ± 9 mmoL/d not significantly different from 125 ± 6 mmoL/d in 31 normoalbuminuric NIDDM patients and 30 healthy controls *5713*

Soluble E-Selectin *Serum* *Increase* In patients with NIDDM mean serum concentration about 70% higher than in controls *5519*

Soluble Interleukin-2 Receptor-α *Serum* *Increase* In 39 patients with NIDDM mean concentration of 9.8 ± 2.8 mmol/L significantly higher than 4.7 ± 0.7 mmol/L in 24 healthy controls *4713*

Soluble Tumor Necrosis Factor Receptor-p60
Serum *Increase* In 19 obese type II diabetic patients median concentration of about 1,300 pg/mL significantly different from median concentration of about 1,000 pg/mL in 28 lean controls *2067*

Soluble Tumor Necrosis Factor Receptor-p80
Serum *Increase* In 19 obese type II diabetic patients median concentration of about 2,750 pg/mL significantly different from median concentration of about 2,000 pg/mL in 28 lean controls *2067*

Soluble Vascular Cell Adhesion Molecule-1
Serum *Increase* In 40 patients with NIDDM and no retinopathy mean concentration of 979 ± 49 ng/mL, of 1,035 ± 104 ng/mL in 17 patients with background retinopathy and 1,282 ± 166 ng/mL in 11 with proliferative retinopathy *5819* In patients with NIDDM mean serum concentration about 14% higher than in controls *5519*

Spermidine *Red Blood Cells* *No Effect* In 39 patients with NIDDM mean concentration of 15 (range 6 - 35.9) nmol/mL packed erythrocytes not significantly different from 14.7 (range 10 - 23.9) nmol/mL packed erythrocytes in 24 healthy controls, although concentration increased with increasing albuminuria and the presence of macroangiopathy and retinopathy *4713*

Spermidine:Spermine Ratio *Red Blood Cells* *No Effect* In 39 patients with NIDDM mean concentration of 1.9 ± 0.9 not significantly different from 1.8 ± 0.7 in 24 healthy controls, not significantly affected by albumin excretion rate, with significant increase with retinopathy but not of macroangiopathy *4713*

Spermine *Red Blood Cells* *No Effect* In 39 patients with NIDDM mean concentration of 9 (range 3.5 - 25) nmol/mL packed erythrocytes not significantly different from 8.2 (range 4.9 - 14.2) nmol/mL packed erythrocytes in 24 healthy controls, although concentration increased significantly with increasing albuminuria and macroangiopathy but not of retinopathy *4713*

Superoxide Dismutase *Red Blood Cells* *No Effect* In 40 patients with type II diabetes mellitus mean concentration of 1.2 ± 0.3 units not significantly different from 1.3 ± 0.3 units in control patients *4887*

Testosterone *Serum* *Decrease* In 12 male patients with NIDDM mean concentration of 15.46 ± 0.94 nmol/L significantly different from 21.05 ± 1.47 nmol/L in 16 healthy control men *2581* In 46 men with NIDDM mean concentration of 16.0 ± 1.1 nmol/L significantly less than 22.6 ± 3.2 nmol/L in 11 healthy normal men *115*
Serum *No Effect* Mean concentration of 24.7 ± 2.5 ng/dL in 39 women with NIDDM not significantly different from 26.0 ± 2.7 ng/dL in 17 healthy controls *115*

Testosterone, Free *Serum* *Increase* Mean concentration of 5.86 ± 0.76 (molar ratio of total testosterone:SHBG) in 39 women with NIDDM significantly higher than 3.14 ± 0.76 in 17 healthy controls *115*
Serum *No Effect* Mean concentration of 0.712 ± 0.07 (molar ratio of total testosterone:SHBG) in 46 men with NIDDM not significantly different from 0.644 ± 0.05 in 11 healthy normal men *115*

Testosterone Index, Free *Serum* *No Effect* In 12 male patients with NIDDM mean concentration of 46.45 ± 4.97 not significantly different from 41.90 ± 3.87 in 16 healthy control men *2581*

Thiobarbituric Acid-reacting Substances *Serum* *Increase* In 11 type II diabetics mean concentration of 0.77 ± 0.22 µmol MDA equivalents/L significantly different from 0.62 ± 0.10 µmpl/MDA equivalents/L in 14 healthy controls *3556* In 81 patients with NIDDM median concentration of 11.88 µmol/L compared with 5.39 µmol/L in 62 healthy controls *1867*

Thrombin/Antithrombin III Complex *Plasma* *Increase* In 18 type II diabetic patients with coronary artery disease concentration higher than in controls *1023*

Thrombomodulin *Plasma* *Increase* In 71 patients with NIDDM mean concentration of 24.9 ± 13.2 U/mL significantly higher than 16.9 ± 8.0 U/mL in 132 age-matched control individuals *199*
Urine *Increase* In 71 patients with NIDDM mean concentration of 41.5 ± 15.2 U/mg creatinine significantly higher than 34.2 ± 5.7 U/mg creatinine in 132 age-matched control individuals *199*

Tissue Plasminogen Activator *Plasma* *Increase* In 9 obese individuals with NIDDM mean concentration of 11 ± 1 ng/mL (as in 9 obese nondiabetics) significantly different from 4 ± 1 ng/mL in 9 lean controls *320*

Plasma No Effect In 13 patients with NIDDM and microalbuminuria mean concentrations of 0.12 ± 0.03 IU/mL (basal) and 0.16 ± 0.03 IU/mL (after stasis) not significantly different from 0.17 ± 0.04 IU/mL (basal) and 0.19 ± 0.14 IU/mL (after stasis) in 13 comparable normoalbuminuric NIDDM patients *1888*

Tissue Plasminogen Activator Antigen *Plasma No Effect* In 15 type II diabetics with coronary artery disease mean concentration not different from controls *1023*

Tissue Plasminogen Activator Inhibitor-1 *Plasma Increase* In 8 obese individuals with NIDDM mean concentration of 57 ± 10 ng/mL and 48 ± 9 ng/mL in 9 obese nondiabetics significantly different from 4 ± 1 ng/mL in 9 lean controls *320*

α-Tocopherol *Serum Increase* In 67 patients with type II diabetes mean concentration of 39.64 ± 16.74 μmol/L *2943*

Transferrin *Urine Increase* In patients with NIDDM, 28 with renal insufficiency had a mean concentration of 0.90 ± 0.45 log[mg/mmol] creatinine increased above normal but also higher than 0.451 ± 0.69 log[mg/mmol] creatinine in 45 patients with macroalbuminuria, -0.69 ± 0.50 log[mg/mmol] creatinine in 98 patients with microalbuminuria, -1.41 ± 0.52 log[mg/mmol] creatinine in 127 patients with normoalbuminuria and -1.54 ± 0.30 log[mg/mmol] creatinine in 80 healthy controls *5760*

Transforming Growth Factor-β_1 *Serum Increase* Mean concentration of 7.9 ± 1.0 ng/mL in 44 patients with NIDDM not significantly different from 3.1 ± 0.4 ng/mL in 28 healthy controls *4117*

Triglycerides *Serum Increase* In 16 patients with NIDDM median concentration of 1.66 mmol/L significantly different from 0.90 mmol/L in 16 healthy controls *4353* In 11 patients with NIDDM treated with oral hypoglycemics or insulin mean concentration of 1.5 ± 0.7 mmol/L significantly different from 0.9 ± 0.3 mmol/L in 14 healthy controls *3556* In 37 NIDDM patients with normoalbuminuria mean concentration of 1.37 ± 0.72 mmol/L (nonsignificantly different), in 11 with microalbuminuria 1.48 ± 0.29 mmol/L (nonsignificantly different) and 2.46 ± 1.10 mmol/L in those with macroalbuminuria significantly different from 1.22 ± 0.40 mmol/L in 55 healthy controls *4329* In 13 patients with NIDDM mean concentration of 248 ± 50 mg/dL not significantly greater than 125 ± 10 mg/dL in 13 healthy controls *4457* In 17 men with NIDDM mean concentration of 2.00 ± 0.89 mmol/L significantly greater than 1.35 ± 0.70 mmol/L in 25 control men: in 30 women mean concentration of 1.98 ± 1.12 mmol/L significantly increased compared with 1.16 ± 0.27 mmol/L in 35 healthy control women *4025* In 43 men and 40 women with NIDDM mean concentrations of 201 ± 190 mg/dL and 184 ± 126 mg/dL respectively significantly different from 63 ± 24 mg/dL in 50 healthy control men and 55 ± 19 mg/dL in 50 control women *5454* In 92 patients with NIDDM median concentration of 1.91 mmol/L significantly different from 1.03 mmol/L in 82 healthy controls *10* In 36 patients with NIDDM and microalbuminuria mean concentration of 173.8 ± 13.9 mg/dL and 123.8 ± 9.7 mg/dL in 36 with normoalbuminuria increased compared with healthy individuals *1889* In patients with NIDDM mean concentration markedly increased in poorly controlled patients *3853* In patients with NIDDM mean concentration increased in well controlled patients *3853* Mean concentration of 1.56 ± 0.08 mmol/L in 212 Japanese patients with NIDDM significantly different from 1.16 ± 0.06 mmol/L in 76 healthy controls *2616* In 100 patients with NIDDM mean concentration of 196.7 ± 112.5 mg/dL significantly different from 142.7 ± 76.6 mg/dL in 854 normoglycemic controls *2330* Mean concentration in 20 NIDDM patients 2.9 ± 0.8 mmol/L significantly higher than 1.6 ± 0.1 mmol/L in 20 age and sex matched controls *970* Mean concentration of 2.3 ± 0.3 mmol/L in 46 men with NIDDM significantly higher than 1.5 ± 0.2 mmol/L in 11 healthy normal men *115* In 2,425 newly diagnosed NIDDM men and 1,752 NIDDM women concentrations of 1.0 - 3.2 mmol/L and 1.1 - 3.0 mmol/L respectively significantly higher than 0.7 - 1.8 mmol/L and 0.6 - 1.7 mmol/L in 195 age matched male and female controls *3275* In 12 type II diabetics mean concentration of 1.98 ± 1.02 mmol/L not significantly higher than 1.65 ± 1.36 mmol/L in 17 nondiabetic control individuals *2471* In 81 patients with NIDDM median concentration of 1.68 mmol/L compared with 1.16 mmol/L in 62 healthy controls *1867* In 26 patients with NIDDM mean concentration of 2.14 ± 1.30 mmol/L significantly different from 0.82 ± 0.30 mmol/L in 10 healthy control subjects *5090* In 20 patients with NIDDM and nephropathy mean concentration increased to 120 ± 45 mg/dL *2167* In 13 patients with NIDDM and microalbuminuria mean concentration of 1.44 ± 0.27 mmol/L significantly higher than 0.69 ± 0.07 mmol/L in 13 comparable normoalbuminuric NIDDM patients *1888* Mean concentration in 43 patients with NIDDM of 2.08 ± 3.24 mmol/L different from 0.89 ± 0.56 mmol/L in 235 healthy control individuals *3884* In 33 NIDDM patients mean concentration of 1.90 ± 2.32 mmol/L not significantly different from 1.20 ± 1.40 mmol/L in 19 healthy controls *3403* In 14 patients with NIDDM mean concentration of 5.02 ± 1.22 mmol/L *2119* In 539 NIDDM patients at time of diagnosis mean concentration of 1.8 mmol/L (range of 1.1 - 2.9) significantly higher than 1.1 mmol/L (range of 0.7 - 1.9) in 250 normoglycemic controls *3276* In 8 patients with NIDDM mean concentration of 2.30 ± 1.30 mmol/L significantly greater than 0.90 ± 0.64 mmol/L in 29 healthy controls *4719* In 19 obese type II diabetic patients median fasting concentration of 210 μmol/L significantly different from median concentration of 77 μmol/L in 28 lean controls *2067* Mean concentration in 225 patients with NIDDM of 2.47 ± 1.83 mmol/L significantly higher than 1.34 ± 0.89 mmol/L in 163 healthy controls *3852* In 26 normoalbuminuric type II diabetics mean concentration of 1.7 ± 0.7 mmol/L (nonsignificant) and in 52 microalbuminuric type II diabetics 2.2 ± 0.7 mmol/L significantly greater than 1.1 ± 0.5 mmol/L in 28 controls *3959*

Serum No Effect Mean concentration of 1.99 ± 0.17 mmol/L in 70 patients with NIDDM significantly higher than 1.14 ± 0.05 mmol/L in 142 patients with IDDM but not significantly different from normal range *470* Mean concentration of 2.35 ± 1.40 mmol/L in 16 patients with NIDDM not significantly different from mean of 1.70 ± 1.14 mmol/L in 16 healthy controls *5014* Mean concentration of 1.68 ± 0.12 mmol/L in 44 patients with NIDDM not significantly different from 1.34 ± 0.09 mmol/L in 28 healthy controls *4117* In about 16 patients with NIDDM mean concentration of 147 ± 17 mg/dL not significantly different from 127 ± 19 mg/dL in non-diabetic controls *2842* In 80 patients with untreated NIDDM mean concentration of 174.7 ± 123.4 mg/dL *5201* In 82 patients with type II diabetes mellitus mean concentration of 2.3 ± 1.6 mmol/L not significantly higher than 1.7 ± 0.9 mmol/L in 48 healthy controls *5795* In 1,121 men with NIDDM mean concentration of 1.3 ± 1.0 mmol/L comparable to 1.1 ± 0.6 mmol/L in 1,480 women with NIDDM *2336* Mean concentration in 16 NIDDM patients with microalbuminuria of 1.56 ± 0.13 mmol/L not significantly different from 1.50 ± 0.16 mmol/L in 31 normoalbuminuric NIDDM patients nor significantly different from 1.41 ± 0.15 mmol/L in 30 healthy controls *5713* In 39 patients with NIDDM mean concentration of 1.88 ± 1.63 mmol/L not significantly different from 1.96 ± 1.76 mmol/L in 24 healthy controls *4713* In 127 patients with NIDDM mean concentration of 1.63 ± 1.04 mmol/L not significantly different from 1.50 ± 1.15 mmol/L in 286 healthy controls *725*

Tumor Necrosis Factor-α *Serum Increase* In 12 obese patients with NIDDM mean concentration of approximately 1.8 pmol/L significantly higher than 0.70 pmol/L in 12 normal individuals *2582* Median concentration of 7 pg/mL in patients with NIDDM significantly increased when compared with 0.0 pg/mL in normal controls *2307* In 59 patients with type 2 diabetes mean activity of 3.60 ± 0.40 U/mL significantly greater than 0.88 ± 0.08 U/mL in 35 controls and mean concentration of 10.51 ± 0.84 pg/mL significantly different from 6.32 ± 0.26 pg/mL in 35 controls *5695*

Serum No Effect In 12 nonobese patients with NIDDM mean concentration of 0.75 pmol/L not significantly higher than 0.70 pmol/L in 12 normal individuals *2582* In 10 obese type II diabetics, median concentration of 2.7 pg/mL not significantly different from 1.8 pg/mL in 23 lean controls *2067* In 11 type II diabetics mean concentration of 0.068 ± 0.017 pmol/L not significantly different from that in 14 healthy controls, in whom mean concentration was 0.075 ± 0.025 pmol/L *3556*

Type IV Collagen 7S Domain *Serum Increase* Mean concentration increased from 3.17 ± 0.71 ng/mL in 26 patients without retinopathy to 4.24 ± 1.50 ng/mL in 10 patients with proliferative retinopathy *3894* In 11 nonproteinuric patients mean concentration of 4.08 ± 0.24 ng/mL, in 15 patients with microalbuminuria of 5.22 ± 0.20 ng/mL and 5.86 ± 0.47 ng/mL in 7 patients with proteinuria different from reference range of 1.0 - 5.0 ng/mL *2357*

Type IV Collagen Peptide *Serum Increase* In patients with NIDDM, 28 with renal insufficiency had a mean concentration of 161 ± 51 μg/L increased above normal but also higher than 134 ± 66 μg/L in 45 patients with macroalbuminuria, 115 ± 48 μg/L in 98 patients with microalbuminuria, 100 ± 34 μg/L in 127 patients with normoalbuminuria and 98 ± 23 μg/L in 80 healthy controls *5760*

250.00 Noninsulin-dependent Diabetes Mellitus *(continued)*

Type IV Collagen Peptide *(continued)*
Urine Increase In 33 patients with NIDDM and macroalbuminuria mean excretion of 201.5 ± 31.5 µg/g creatinine significantly greater than that in 85 patients with NIDDM and normoalbuminuria in whom mean excretion was 59.2 ± 6.2 µg/g creatinine, not greater than upper limit of normal of 71.7 µg/g creatinine *283* In patients with NIDDM, 28 with renal insufficiency had a mean concentration of 2.85 ± 2.07 µg/mmol creatinine increased above normal but also higher than 1.26 ± 0.70 µg/mmol creatinine in 45 patients with macroalbuminuria, 0.79 ± 0.61 µg/mmol creatinine in 98 patients with microalbuminuria, 0.42 ± 0.37 µg/mmol creatinine in 127 patients with normoalbuminuria and 0.29 ± 0.09 µg/mmol creatinine in 80 healthy controls *5760*
Urine No Effect In 85 patients with NIDDM and normoalbuminuria mean excretion of 59.2 ± 6.2 µg/g creatinine not greater than upper limit of normal of 71.7 µg/g creatinine *283*

Ubiquinol:Cholesterol Ratio *Serum No Effect* In 17 patients with NIDDM mean ratio of 0.21 ± 0.07 µmol/mmol not significantly different from 0.22 ± 0.05 µmol/mmol in 19 healthy controls *3403*

Urea *Serum No Effect* In 26 normoalbuminuric type II diabetics mean concentration of 6.7 ± 1.9 mmol/L and in 52 microalbuminuric type II diabetics of 8.5 ± 3.4 mmol/L not significantly different from 5.7 ± 1.7 mmol/L in 28 controls *3959*

Urea Nitrogen *Serum Increase* Mean concentration in 125 patients with NIDDM of 29.3 ± 18.5 mg/dL significantly different from 16.7 ± 3.6 mg/dL in 63 healthy controls *3920* In 20 patients with NIDDM and nephropathy mean concentration increased to 24 ± 14 mg/dL *2167*

Uric Acid *Serum Increase* In 81 patients with NIDDM median concentration of 321 µmol/L compared with 266 µmol/L in 62 healthy controls *1867*
Serum No Effect In 34 patients with NIDDM mean concentration of 322 ± 86 µmol/L in men and 251 ± 93 µmol/L in women not significantly different from 346 ± 47 µmol/L in male and 256 ± 58 µmol/L in healthy female controls *5500*

Vitamin E *Serum No Effect* In 11 type II diabetics mean concentration of 29 ± 8 mg/L not significantly different from 26 ± 6 mg/L in 14 healthy controls *3556* Mean concentration of 24.8 ± 1.3 µmol/Lin 70 patients with IDDM not significantly different from normal range *470* In 81 patients with NIDDM median concentration of 21.4 µmol/L compared with 26.5 µmol/L in 62 healthy controls *1867*

VLDL + LDL-Cholesterol *Serum No Effect* In 16 patients with NIDDM median concentration of 4.00 mmol/L not significantly different from 3.60 mmol/L in 16 healthy controls *4353*

VLDL-Cholesterol *Serum Decrease* In 37 patients with NIDDM and normoalbuminuria mean concentration of 0.25 ± 0.13 mmol/L and in 11 with microalbuminuria 0.28 ± 0.19 mmol/L significantly less than 0.41 ± 0.40 mmol/L in 55 healthy controls *4329*
Serum Increase Mean concentration of 0.99 ± 0.68 mmol/L in 16 patients with NIDDM significantly higher than mean of 0.52 ± 0.48 mmol/L in 16 healthy controls *5014* In 26 patients with NIDDM mean concentration of 0.75 ± 0.49 mmol/L significantly different from 0.23 ± 0.10 mmol/L in 10 healthy control subjects *5090* In 26 normoalbuminuric type II diabetics mean concentration of 0.8 ± 0.3 mmol/L (nonsignificant) and in 52 microalbuminuric type II diabetics 1.5 ± 0.2 mmol/L significantly greater than 0.5 ± 0.2 mmol/L in 28 controls *3959* In 13 patients with NIDDM mean concentration of 209 ± 38 mg/dL significantly greater than 71 ± 7 mg/dL in 13 healthy controls *4457* In 12 type II diabetics mean concentration of 0.83 ± 0.36 mmol/L not significantly higher than 0.65 ± 0.36 mmol/L in 17 nondiabetic control individuals *2471*
Serum No Effect In 7 patients with NIDDM and macroalbuminuria mean concentration of 0.61 ± 0.65 mmol/L not significantly different from 0.41 ± 0.40 mmol/L in 55 healthy controls *4329* In 82 patients with type II diabetes mellitus mean concentration of 1.0 ± 0.7 mmol/L not significantly different from 0.8 ± 0.4 mmol/L in 48 healthy controls *5795*

VLDL-Protein *Serum No Effect* In 30 patients with NIDDM and normoalbuminuria mean concentration of 0.17 ± 0.14 g/L, in 11 with microalbuminuria of 0.23 ± 0.21 g/L and in 7 with macroalbuminuria of 0.29 ± 0.12 g/L not significantly different from 0.13 ± 0.11 g/L in 55 healthy controls *4329*

VLDL-Triglycerides *Serum Increase* In 7 patients with NIDDM and macroalbuminuria mean concentration of 1.08 ± 0.65 mmol/L significantly greater than 0.55 ± 0.34 mmol/L in 55 healthy controls *4329*
Serum No Effect In 37 patients with NIDDM and normoalbuminuria mean concentration of 0.52 ± 0.47 mmol/L and in 11 with microalbuminuria 0.58 ± 0.22 mmol/L not significantly different from 0.55 ± 0.34 mmol/L in 55 healthy controls *4329*

Volume *Urine Increase* In about 16 patients with NIDDM mean excretion of 1,950 mL/d significantly different from 1,020 mL/d in non-diabetic controls *2842*

von Willebrand Factor Antigen *Plasma Increase* In 539 patients with NIDDM at time of diagnosis mean concentration of 169 IU/dL (range 110- 2 59) compared with 117 IU/dL (range 77 - 178) in 250 normoglycemic controls *3276* In type II patients mean concentration of 155 (102 - 237) IU/dL compared with 120 (82 - 177) IU/dL in 45 healthy controls *649*

Zinc *Serum Increase* Mean concentration in 43 patients with uncontrolled NIDDM of 17.31 ± 4.58 µmol/L and of 16.20 ± 3.22 µmol/L in 40 patients with controlled NIDDM different from 15.80 ± 4.12 µmol/L in 30 healthy controls *5844*

250.01 Insulin-dependent Diabetes Mellitus

Adenosine Deaminase *Serum Increase* In 53 patients with IDDM mean activity of 23.1 ± 6.5 U/L significantly higher than that in 52 healthy blood donors (mean activity of 7.0 ± 1.7 U/L) *2245*

Adenosine Deaminase 1 *Serum Increase* In 53 patients with IDDM mean activity of 8.1 ± 1.6 U/L not significantly higher than that in 52 healthy blood donors (mean activity of 6.5 ± 1.6 U/L) *2245*

Adenosine Deaminase 2 *Serum Increase* In 53 patients with IDDM mean activity of 14.9 ± 5.7 U/L significantly higher than that in 52 healthy blood donors (mean activity of 7.0 ± 1.7 U/L) *2245*

Adenosine Monophosphate *Plasma Increase* Mean concentration of 8.8 ± 2.0 nmol/L in 46 IDDM patients without complications, 9.4 ± 2.6 nmol/L in 24 patients with IDDM and retinopathy only, 9.8 ± 2.3 nmol/L in 14 patients with IDDM and microalbuminuria and 12.2 ± 3.1 nmol/L in 19 IDDM patients with renal insufficiency compared with 9.4 ± 1.7 nmol/L in 41 healthy adults *1651*

Adrenomedullin *Plasma Increase* Mean concentration of 78.1 ± 28.1 pg/mL in 46 IDDM patients without complications, 101.4 ± 40 pg/mL in 24 patients with IDDM and retinopathy only, 96.4 ± 44.5 pg/mL in 14 patients with IDDM and microalbuminuria and 235.7 ± 138.8 pg/mL in 19 IDDM patients with renal insufficiency compared with 82.7 ± 40.8 pg/mL in 41 healthy adults *1651*

Albumin *Serum No Effect* In 28 male patients with IDDM mean concentration of 46.4 ± 3.9 g/L and 44.1 ± 4.1 g/L in 26 women with IDDM *1842* In 28 men with IDDM and 26 women with IDDM mean concentrations of 46.4 ± 3.9 g/L and 44.1 ± 4.1 g/L respectively *1842*
Urine Increase In IDDM patients with HbA_{1C} greater than 8% mean excretion of 21 ± 9 mg/d significantly greater than 15 ± 7 mg/d in patients with HbA_{1C} less than 8% and in healthy controls *1334* In 13 IDDM patients without retinopathy mean excretion of 0.66 g/mol creatinine, in 12 with new retinopathy 0.9 g/mol creatinine and in 17 with established retinopathy 1.15 g/mol creatinine significantly higher than 0.47 g/mol creatinine in 20 controls *4888* In 52 patients with IDDM median excretion of 10 µg/min significantly different from that in 52 healthy controls in whom the mean excretion was undetectable *866* Mean excretion of 8.9 ± 6.9 mg/g creatinine in 46 IDDM patients without complications, 7.5 ± 3.7 mg/g creatinine in 24 patients with IDDM and retinopathy only and 144.3 ± 97 mg/g creatinine in 14 patients with IDDM and microalbuminuria compared with unde-

tectable amounts in 41 healthy adults *1651* Mean excretion in 18 normoalbuminuric patients of 5.43 μg/min, in 13 IDDM patients with microalbuminuria of 39.95 μg/min and of 1,142 μg/min compared with that in 16 nondiabetic healthy normotensive individuals, 2.29 - 9.68 μg/min or 3.06 - 10.00 mg/g *1339* In 41 normotensive, normoalbuminuric patients with IDDM mean overnight excretion of 3.4 μg/min significantly different from 1.9 μg/min in 11 control individuals *737* In 10 diabetic patients with microalbuminuria mean excretion of 54.17 ± 33.9 mg/L significantly different from 6.92 ± 2.3 mg/L in 10 healthy controls *937* In 45 pairs of identical twins with IDDM mean excretion rate of 20.1 ± 96.4 μg/min compared with 4.7 ± 2.6 μg/min in 45 pairs of nondiabetic twins and 3.8 ± 1.8 μg/min in 45 nondiabetic controls *1246*

Urine No Effect In 10 diabetic patients with normoalbuminuria mean excretion of 6.43 ± 6.85 mg/L not significantly different from 6.92 ± 2.3 mg/L in 10 healthy controls *937*

Albumin:Creatinine Ratio *Urine Increase* In 33 patients with IDDM mean ratio of 1.56 ± 1.05 mg/mmol not significantly different from 1.04 ± 0.53 mg/mmol in 32 healthy controls *5500*

Alkaline Phosphatase *Serum Increase* In 6 adult patients with IDDM mean activity of 298.0 ± 10.5 U/L significantly different from 57.4 ± 1.5 U/L in 122 healthy control adults, and of 224.1 ± 10.6 U/L in 69 children with IDDM significantly different from 160.0 ± 10.6 U/L in 18 healthy control children *2006*

Alkaline Phosphatase Band-10 Isoenzyme *Serum Increase* In 69 children with IDDM mean activity of 28.2 ± 3.30 U/L significantly different from 10.13 ± 1.93 U/L in 18 healthy control children *2006*

Serum No Effect In 6 adult patients with IDDM mean activity of 6.61 ± 1.59 U/L not significantly different from 10.0 ± 0.69 U/L in 122 healthy control adults *2006*

Amylin *Plasma No Effect* Basal serum concentration in healthy individuals of 1.5 - 2.5 pmol/L, but concentrations reduced in patients with IDDM *4495*

δ^4-Androstenedione *Plasma No Effect* In 20 male patients with IDDM mean concentration of 3.8 nmol/L not significantly different from 3.9 nmol/L in 20 healthy controls *834*

Angiogenin *Serum Increase* In 40 diabetic children and adolescents mean concentration of 353.3 ± 20.0 ng/mL significantly different from 244.7 ± 9.6 ng/mL in 30 healthy control people *3243*

Anti-Islet Cell Cytoplasmic Antibodies *Serum Increase* Positive results occur in about 30% patients with type I diabetes mellitus with polyendocrine autoimmunity and about 20% of patients with simple diabetes mellitus *2952*

Antibody Titer *Serum Increase* Antibodies to Islet cells present in 60% of juvenile onset diabetics of less than 1 years duration. Such antibodies tend to disappear rapidly after the disease is recognized clinically *3712*

Antioxidant Capacity *Serum Decrease* In 33 patients with IDDM mean total oxidant status of 1.68 ± 0.17 mmol/L significantly different from 1.81 ± 0.12 mmol/L in 32 healthy controls *5500*

Antithrombin III *Plasma No Effect* In 17 patients with IDDM and urinary excretion of albumin of less than 30 mg/d mean AT-III activity of 117%, in 20 with albumin excretion of 30 - 300 mg/d 120% and in 25 with excretion greater than 300 mg/d, 116% not significantly increased compared with 116% in 14 healthy controls *3695*

Antithyroid Peroxidase Antibodies *Serum Increase* Anti-TPO titers > 500 AU/mL in 3.3%, 200 - 500 AU/mL in 5.0%, 100 - 200 AU/mL in 5.3% of patients with IDDM compared with 0 in controls, and 8.2% with titers of 11.4 - 200 AU/mL versus 2.9% in controls *775*

Apolipoprotein A-I *Serum Decrease* In 170 pubertal children with IDDM mean concentration of 1.04 g/L (0.94 - 1.17) significantly less than 1.21 g/L (1.10 - 1.31) in 233 healthy Caucasian pubertal children *947* In children with IDDM regardless of whether control was good, fair or poor concentration significantly reduced *63*

Serum No Effect In 78 patients with IDDM mean concentration of 146.6 ± 48.5 mg/dL not significantly different from 159.0 ± 26.6 mg/dL in 82 healthy controls *10* In 45 pairs of identical twins with IDDM mean concentration of 145.2 ± 23.3 mg/dL compared with 139.4 ± 22.5 mg/dL in 45 pairs of nondiabetic twins and 154.2 ± 24.4 mg/dL in 45 nondiabetic controls *1246* In 51 men with IDDM mean concentration of 1.46 ± 0.21 g/L not significantly different from 1.43 ± 0.34 g/L in 48 control men and in 35 women with IDDM mean concentration of 1.56 ± 0.16 g/L not significantly different from 1.50 ± 0.25 g/L in 26 control women *2528*

Apolipoprotein A-II *Serum Decrease* In 51 men with IDDM mean concentration of 0.35 ± 0.08 g/L not significantly different from 0.38 ± 0.08 g/L in 48 control men and in 35 women with IDDM mean concentration of 0.35 ± 0.08 g/L significantly different from 0.45 ± 0.08 g/L in 26 control women *2528*

Serum No Effect In children with IDDM regardless of whether the control is good, fair or poor concentration unaffected *5364*

Apolipoprotein B *Serum Increase* In patients with IDDM mean concentration increased in well controlled patients, but less commonly than in patients with IDDM *3853* Concentration significantly increased in children with IDDM with poor or fair control in comparison with healthy children *63* Mean concentration of 99 ± 24 mg/dL in 17 patients with IDDM significantly increased compared with concentration in 45 apparently healthy controls *2284*

Serum No Effect In 78 patients with IDDM mean concentration of 96.2 ± 28.4 mg/dL not significantly different from 91.6 ± 26.6 mg/dL in 82 healthy controls *10* In 45 pairs of identical twins with IDDM mean concentration of 81.4 ± 20.6 mg/dL compared with 84.5 ± 21.6 mg/dL in 45 pairs of nondiabetic twins and 83.0 ± 24.9 mg/dL in 45 nondiabetic controls *1246* Mean concentration of 1.05 ± 0.02 g/L in 142 patients with IDDM significantly lower than 1.27 ± 0.05 g/L in 70 patients with NIDDM but not significantly different from normal range *470*

Apolipoprotein B-100 *Serum No Effect* In pubertal children with IDDM mean concentration of 0.53 g/L (0.45 - 0.61) not significantly different from 0.53 g/L (0.46 - 0.62) in healthy Caucasian children *947*

Apolipoprotein C-II *Serum No Effect* In children with IDDM regardless of whether the control was good, fair or poor concentration unaffected *63*

Apolipoprotein C-III *Serum Increase* In children with IDDM with fair or poor control concentration significantly increased in comparison with healthy controls *63*

Apolipoprotein H *Serum No Effect* In 118 patients with IDDM mean concentration of 31.3 ± 9.9 mg/dL not significantly different from 22.5 ± 7.7 mg/dL in 286 healthy controls *725*

Apolipoprotein Lp(a) *Urine Increase* In 52 patients with IDDM median concentration of 25.7 μg/dL significantly different from that in 52 healthy controls in whom the median concentration was 16.0 μg/dL *866*

Atrial Natriuretic Peptide *Plasma Decrease* In uncontrolled diabetic patients mean concentrations observed to fall below 10 pg/mL in several patients in whom concentration reverted to 40 - 50 pg/mL once glycemic control obtained *4770*

Plasma Increase In 83 patients with IDDM mean concentration of 30.7 ± 5.1 pg/mL compared with 11.5 ± 0.9 pg/mL 45 healthy controls *2512*

Plasma No Effect In 10 men with IDDM mean concentration of 9.2 pmol/L (range 1.3 - 23.4 pmol/L) not significantly different from 7.6 pmol/L (range 1.9 - 15.6 pmol/L) in 10 nondiabetic controls *4916*

Basic Fibroblast Growth Factor *Serum No Effect* In 40 children with IDDM mean concentration of 3.95 ± 0.88 pg/mL not significantly different from 3.78 ± 0.59 pg/mL in 30 healthy pediatric controls *3258*

Bile Salt-dependent Lipase, Bile Salt Activated

Serum Increase Mean activity in 5 type I diabetics of 95 ± 13 U/g BSDL x 10^6 significantly greater than that in 5 healthy individuals of 54 ± 28 U/g BSDL x 10^6 *661*

Bile Salt-dependent Lipase, DFP-inhibited *Serum Increase* Mean activity in 5 type I diabetics of 94 ± 23 U/g BSDL x 10^6 significantly greater than that in 5 healthy individuals of 46 ± 22 U/g BSDL x 10^6 *661*

Bile Salt-dependent Lipase, Immunprecipitated

Serum Increase Mean activity in 5 type I diabetics of 76 ± 23 U/g BSDL x 10^6 significantly greater than that in 5 healthy individuals of 24 ± 16 U/g BSDL x 10^6 *661*

Brush-border Antigen *Urine Increase* In insulin-dependent diabetic patients with nephropathy increased excretion observed in conjunction with tubulopathy *3689*

250.01 Insulin-dependent Diabetes Mellitus *(continued)*

Carbamylated Hemoglobin *Blood Increase* In 24 patients with IDDM mean concentration of 38 ± 10.8 µg carbamylated valine/g hemoglobin not significantly less than 41 ± 11.5 µg carbamylated valine/g hemoglobin *2875*

Carnitine *Serum Decrease* The plasma levels of carnitine were significantly diminished in type I diabetic patients compared to controls. Carnitine concentrations in erythrocytes and 24 hour urine did not differ from controls *4207*
Urine No Effect Carnitine concentrations in erythrocytes and 24 hour urine in type I diabetes mellitus did not differ from controls *4207*

α-Carotene *Serum Increase* In 28 male patients with IDDM 95% CI of 0.05 - 0.07 µmol/L not significantly different from 0.06 - 0.09 µmol/L in 113 nonrelative healthy controls. In 26 women with IDDM 95% CI 0.07 - 0.12 µmol/L compared with 0.08 - 0.10 µmol/L in 123 nonrelative healthy controls *1842*
Serum No Effect In 60 male IDDM patients 5th to 95th percentile of concentrations of 0.008 - 0.153 µmol/L not significantly different from range in 210 healthy men (5th to 95th percentile 0.016 - 0.146 µmol/L) and 0.014 - 0.271 µmol/L in 63 women with IDDM not significantly different from 0.018 - 0.225 µmol/L in 240 healthy women *3906* In 28 men with IDDM median concentration of 0.06 µmol/L not significantly different when compared with 0.06 µmol/L in 113 male controls and 0.08 µmol/L in 26 women with IDDM not significantly different when compared with 0.07 µmol/L female controls *1842*

β-Carotene *Serum Increase* In 28 male patients with IDDM 95% CI of 0.25 - 0.37 µmol/L not significantly different from 0.24 - 0.31 µmol/L in 113 nonrelative healthy controls. In 26 women with IDDM 95% CI 0.34 - 0.55 µmol/L compared with 0.33 - 0.42 µmol/L in 123 nonrelative healthy controls *1842* In 28 men with IDDM median concentration of 0.29 µmol/L significantly different when compared with 0.24 µmol/L in 113 male controls and 0.41 µmol/L in 26 women with IDDM significantly different when compared with 0.31 µmol/L female controls *1842*
Serum No Effect In 60 male IDDM patients 5th to 95th percentile of concentrations of 0.045 - 0.640 µmol/L not significantly different from range in 210 healthy men (5th to 95th percentile of 0.067 - 0.553 µmol/L) and of 0.124 - 0.988 µmol/L in 63 women with IDDM not significantly different from 0.087 - 0.818 µmol/L in 240 healthy women *3906*

Cholesterol *Serum Increase* In patients with IDDM mean concentration increased in poorly controlled patients *3853* In 12 patients with IDDM mean concentration of 5.27 ± 0.90 mmol/L not significantly greater than 5.10 ± 0.89 mmol/L in 29 healthy controls *4719* Concentration significantly increased in children with poor or fair diabetic control *63* In 33 patients with IDDM mean concentration of 5.5 ± 2.0 mmol/L not significantly different from 5.1 ± 1.4 mmol/L in 19 healthy controls *3403* Mean levels in children (205 ± 78 mg/dL) were significantly higher than for controls (155 ± 27 mg/dL), as were mean triglyceride levels. 8 with diabetes had hypercholesterolemia, 5 had hypertriglyceridemia, and 9 had combined hypercholesterolemia and hypertriglyceridemia *792* In 40 patients with IDDM and nephropathy mean concentration of 6.2 ± 1.3 mmol/L significantly different from 5.2 ± 0.94 mmol/L in 49 patients with IDDM but without nephropathy for 5 - 10 years *5010*
Serum No Effect In 52 patients with IDDM mean concentration of 5.3 ± 0.9 mmol/L not significantly different from that in 52 healthy controls in whom the mean concentration was 4.9 ± 1.2 mmol/L *866* In 28 men with IDDM and 26 women with IDDM mean concentrations of 4.80 ± 1.5 mmol/L and 5.42 ± 1.2 mmol/L respectively *1842* In 78 patients with IDDM mean concentration of 6.20 ± 2.30 mmol/L not significantly different from 5.69 ± 1.30 mmol/L in 82 healthy controls *10* In 44 patients aged under 45 years with IDDM mean concentration of 4.97 ± 0.86 mmol/L compared with 5.23 ± 0.67 mmol/L in 18 controls aged under 45 years: in 16 patients older than 45 years mean concentration of 6.36 ± 1.36 mmol/L compared with 5.72 ± 1.26 mmol/L in 8 healthy controls aged over 45 years *3324* Mean concentration of 5.58 ± 0.08 mmol/L in 142 patients with IDDM not significantly different from normal range *470* In 10 patients with uncontrolled IDDM on admission to hospital mean concentration of 4.74 ± 1.29 mmol/L not significantly different from 4.44 ± 0.55 mmol/L in 10 healthy normolipidemic controls *5614* Median concentration in 42 patients with IDDM of 212 mg/dL not significantly different from 203 mg/dL in 42 healthy controls *2446* In 10 diabetic patients with normoalbuminuria and in 10 with microalbuminuria mean concentrations of 180.7 ± 26.8 mg/dL and 182.5 ± 35.4 mg/dL respectively not significantly different from 174.6 ± 21.3 mg/dL in 10 healthy controls *937* In 70 patients with IDDM mean concentration of 5.28 ± 1.01 mmol/L not significantly different from 5.17 ± 0.83 mmol/L in 70 age-matched healthy controls *1429* Mean concentration in 45 pairs of diabetic identical twins of 5.1 ± 1.0 mmol/L compared with 5.3 ± 1.1 mmol/L in 45 pairs of nondiabetic twins and 5.4 ± 1.2 mmol/L in 45 nondiabetic controls *1246* In 50 patients with IDDM mean concentration of 200 ± 38 mg/dL compared with 205 ± 38 mg/dL in 50 healthy controls *1334* In 77 patients with IDDM median concentration of 5.05 mmol/L compared with 5.72 mmol/L in 62 healthy controls *1867* In 51 men with IDDM mean concentration of 5.03 ± 1.20 mmol/L not significantly different from 5.23 ± 0.91 mmol/L in 48 control men and in 35 women with IDDM mean concentration of 4.86 ± 0.79 mmol/L not significantly different from 5.10 ± 1.1 mmol/L in 26 control women *2528* In 28 male patients with IDDM mean concentration of 4.80 ± 1.5 mmol/L and 5.42 ± 1.2 mmol/L in 26 women with IDDM *1842* In 28 male patients with IDDM mean concentration of 1.37 ± 0.51 mmol/L and 1.66 ± 0.57 mmol/L in 26 women with IDDM *1842* In 118 patients with IDDM mean concentration of 4.93 ± 1.11 mmol/L not significantly different from 5.74 ± 1.11 mmol/L in 286 healthy controls *725* In patients with IDDM mean concentration normal in well controlled patients *3853*
Urine Increase Mean concentration of 175 ± 28 mg/dL in 46 IDDM patients without complications, 193 ± 40 mg/dL in 24 patients with IDDM and retinopathy only and 180 ± 48 mg/dL in 14 patients with IDDM and microalbuminuria compared with 189 ± 37 mg/dL in 41 healthy adults *1651*

Cholesterol Esters *Serum No Effect* In 10 patients with uncontrolled IDDM on admission to hospital mean concentration of 3.40 ± 0.28 mmol/L not significantly different from 3.46 ± 0.14 mmol/L in 10 healthy normolipidemic controls *5614*

Cholesterol, Free *Serum Increase* In 10 patients with uncontrolled IDDM on admission to hospital mean concentration of 1.34 ± 0.13 mmol/L significantly different from 0.98 ± 0.06 mmol/L in 10 healthy normolipidemic controls *5614*

Complement C_3 *Serum No Effect* In 10 patients with newly diagnosed IDDM mean concentration of 1.09 ± 0.22 g/L compared with 1.09 ± 0.14 g/L in controls *3903*

Complement C_4 *Serum No Effect* In 10 newly diagnosed IDDM patients mean concentration of 0.24 ± 0.09 g/L not significantly different from 0.22 ± 0.06 g/L in controls *3903*

Copper *Lymphocytes No Effect* In 45 children with IDDM mean concentration of 0.13 ± 0.016 µmol/10^{10} cells not significantly different from 0.19 ± 0.036 µmol/10^{10} cells in 12 healthy children *3049*
Neutrophils No Effect In 45 children with IDDM mean concentration of 0.11 ± 0.016 µmol/10^{10} cells not different from 0.076 ± 0.013 µmol/10^{10} cells in 12 healthy children *3049*
Red Blood Cells No Effect Copper not detected in the erythrocytes of either 45 children with IDDM or in 12 healthy control children *4406*
Serum Increase In 16 stabilized diabetics mean concentration of 17.43 ± 2.70 µmol/L not significantly increased compared with 16.55 ± 3.51 µmol/L in healthy reference population *1434*
Serum No Effect In 43 children with IDDM mean concentration of 18.8 ± 0.79 µmol/L not significantly different from 19.3 ± 1.88 µmol/L in 12 healthy control children *4406*

Copper Zinc Superoxide Dismutase *Lymphocytes Decrease* In 33 patients with IDDM mean concentration of 1.69 ± 0.45 U/mg total protein significantly different from 2.06 ± 0.58 U/mg protein in 32 healthy controls *5499*
Neutrophils Decrease In 33 patients with IDDM mean concentration of 0.62 ± 0.39 U/mg total protein significantly different from 1.06 ± 0.43 U/mg protein in 32 healthy controls *5499*
Red Blood Cells Increase Increased in erythrocytes of patients with insulin dependent diabetes mellitus *2602*
Red Blood Cells No Effect In patients with IDDM and no vascular complications activities of 527 ± 136, 555 ± 139 and 498 ± 118 U/g hemoglobin in patients with Hb A_{1c} concentrations of < 7.3, 7.3 - 9.4, and > 9.4% respectively and in IDDM patients with vascular complications of 508 ± 146, 527 ± 111, 490 ± 111 U/g hemoglobin at the same Hb A_{1c} concentrations compared with 544 ± 120 U/g hemoglobin in healthy controls *4476*

C-Peptide *Plasma* *Decrease* In 70 patients with IDDM mean concentration of 0.07 ± 0.07 nmol/L significantly different from 0.78 ± 0.37 nmol/L in 70 age-matched healthy controls *1429* Compared with fasting and postprandial concentrations of 1.56 ± 0.33 pmol/L and 4.26 ± 0.46 pmol/L respectively concentrations in IDDM patients with HbA_{1C} greater than 8% were 0.07 ± 0.12 pmol/L and 0.16 ± 0.30 pmol/L respectvely and in those with HbA_{1C} above 8% 0.02 ± 0.07 pmol/L and 0.08 ± 0.14 pmol/L respectively *1334*

Creatinine *Serum* *Increase* Mean concentration in 45 pairs of identical diabetic twins of 87.9 ± 11.0 μmol/L compared with 87.1 ± 12.2 μmol/L in 45 pairs of nondiabetic twins and 88.4 ± 11.0 μmol/L in 45 nondiabetic controls *1246* In 40 patients with IDDM and nephropathy mean concentration of 123 ± 59 μmol/L significantly different from 84 ± 12 μmol/L in 49 patients with IDDM but without nephropathy for 5 - 10 years *5010* In 28 male patients with IDDM mean concentration of 90 ± 10 μmol/L and 73 ± 8 μmol/L in 26 women with IDDM *1842* In 17 patients with IDDM and macroalbuminuria mean concentration of 95 ± 26 μmol/L and in 20 with microalbuminuria 82 ± 15 μmol/L significantly higher than that in 37 patients with IDDM and normoalbuminuria in whom mean concentration was 79 ± 12 μmol/L *5805*
Serum *No Effect* In 13 IDDM patients without retinopathy mean concentration of 94 ± 9 μmol/L, in 12 with new retinopathy 88 ± 8 μmol/L, and in 17 with established retinopathy 91 ± 10 μmol/L, not significantly higher than 83 ± 10 μmol/L in 20 controls *4888* In 50 patients with IDDM mean concentration of 0.9 ± 0.1 mg/dL not significantly different from 0.8 ± 0.1 mg/dL in 50 healthy controls *1334* In 28 men with IDDM and 26 women with IDDM mean concentrations of 89.9 ± 9.9 μmol/L and 73.3 ± 7.9 μmol/L respectively *1842* In 33 patients with IDDM mean concentration of 76.8 ± 13.4 μmol/L not significantly different from 80.3 ± 12.9 μmol/L in 32 healthy controls *5500* Mean concentration of 1.01 ± 0.12 mg/dL in 46 IDDM patients without complications, 1.00 ± 0.14 mg/dL in 24 patients with IDDM and retinopathy only and 1.02 ± 0.12 mg/dL in 14 patients with IDDM and microalbuminuria compared with 0.99 ± 0.11 mg/dL in 41 healthy adults *1651*

Creatinine Clearance *Urine* *Decrease* In 8 patients with IDDM and hyporeninemia mean clearance of 63 ± 12 mL/min/1.73 sq m significantly different when compared with 123 ± 9 mL/min/1.73 sq m in 11 controls *1212*
Urine *No Effect* In 13 well-controlled patients with IDDM median clearance of 137.4 ± 26.6 mL/min/ 1.73 m^2 not significantly different from 132.7 ± 35.1 mL/min/1.73 m^2 creatinine in 11 matched healthy controls *3501* Mean concentration of 86.6 ± 10.4 mL/min/m^2 in 46 IDDM patients without complications, 86.2 ± 14.3 mL/min/m^2 in 24 patients with IDDM and retinopathy only and 84.7 ± 11.2 mL/min/m^2 in 14 patients with IDDM and microalbuminuria compared with 85.1 ± 10.5 mL/min/m^2 in 41 healthy adults *1651* In 52 patients with IDDM mean clearance of 86 ± 22 mL/min not significantly different from that in 52 healthy controls *866*

β-Cryptoxanthin *Serum* *Increase* In 28 male patients with IDDM 95% CI of 0.41 - 0.70 μmol/L not significantly different from 0.34 - 0.44 μmol/L in 113 nonrelative healthy controls. In 26 women with IDDM 95% CI 0.42 - 0.70 μmol/L compared with 0.46 - 0.68 μmol/L in 123 nonrelative healthy controls *1842* In 28 men with IDDM median concentration of 0.47 μmol/L significantly different when compared with 0.32 μmol/L in 113 male controls and 0.50 μmol/L in 26 women with IDDM significantly different when compared with 0.45 μmol/L female controls *1842*
Serum *No Effect* In 60 male IDDM patients 5th to 95th percentile of concentrations of 0.059 - 1.569 μmol/L not significantly different from range in 210 healthy men (5th to 95th percentile 0.067 - 1.005 μmol/L) and 0.118 - 1.519 μmol/L in 63 women with IDDM not significantly different from 0.096 - 1.443 μmol/L in 240 healthy women *3906*

D-Dimer *Plasma* *Increase* In 40 normoalbuminuric IDDM patients mean concentration of 174.2 ± 99.3 ng/mL significantly greater than 130.0 ± 54.0 ng/mL in healthy controls *750*

Dehydroepiandrosterone Sulfate *Plasma* *No Effect* In 20 male patients with IDDM mean concentration of 8.0 μmol/L not significantly different from 8.4 μmol/L in 20 healthy controls *834*

Dihydrotestosterone *Serum* *Increase* In 20 male patients with IDDM mean concentration of 4.2 nmol/L significantly different from 1.7 nmol/L in 20 healthy controls *834*

Endothelin *Plasma* *Decrease* In 10 men with IDDM mean concentration of 1.7 ± 0.5 pmol/L significantly lower than 2.1 ± 0.4 pmol/L in 10 nondiabetic controls *4916*
Plasma *Increase* Mean concentration in 7 patients with uncomplicated IDDM of 0.88 ± 0.17 pg/mL not significantly higher than 0.62 ± 0.08 pg/mL in 7 healthy controls but significantly increased to 0.92 ± 0.06 pg/mL in 6 patients with IDDM and complications *2692*
Urine *Increase* In 11 children with IDDM mean excretion of 95 ng/d significantly greater than 36 ng/d in 24 healthy children *3375*

Endothelin-1 *Plasma* *Increase* In 2 studies of patients with IDDM mean concentrations increased 4.7 ± 0.2 pg/mL (n = 10) and 5.0 ± 0.7 pg/mL (n = 16), 0.9-fold and 3.9-fold respectively of appropriate normal values *328*

Erythrocyte Sedimentation Rate *Blood* *Increase* In 17 patients with IDDM and macroalbuminuria mean rate of 14 mm/h and in 20 with microalbuminuria 7 mm/h significantly higher than that in 37 patients with IDDM and normoalbuminuria in whom mean rate 6 mm/h *5805*

Erythropoietin *Serum* *Decrease* In 8 patients with IDDM and hyporeninemia mean concentration of 26% significantly different when compared with 93% in 11 controls *1212*

Estradiol *Plasma* *Increase* In 20 male patients with IDDM mean concentration of 0.12 nmol/L significantly different from 0.08 nmol/L in 20 healthy controls *834*

Estrone *Plasma* *Increase* In 20 male patients with IDDM mean concentration of 0.29 nmol/L significantly different from 0.16 nmol/L in 20 healthy controls *834*

Euglobulin Lysis Time *Blood* *No Effect* In 50 patients with IDDM mean time of 224 ± 187 min before ischemia and 122 ± 110 min after ischemia not significantly different from 221 ± 167 min and 92 ± 98 min respectively in 50 healthy controls *1334*

Factor VIII Coagulant *Plasma* *Increase* In 50 patients with IDDM mean concentration of 107 ± 31% not significantly greater than 96 ± 14% in 50 healthy controls *1334*

Factor VIII Coagulant:Factor: VIII Antigen Ratio *Plasma* *Decrease* In 50 patients with IDDM mean ratio of 0.96 ± 0.18 significantly less than 1.06 ± 0.14 in 50 healthy controls *1334*

Factor VIIIR Antigen *Plasma* *Increase* In 50 patients with IDDM mean concentration of 114 ± 37% significantly greater than 91 ± 13% in 50 healthy controls *1334*

Factor VIIIR:VW *Plasma* *Increase* In 50 patients with IDDM mean concentration of 117 ± 33% significantly greater than 91 ± 13% in 50 healthy controls *1334*

Fatty Acids (FFA), Free *Serum* *Increase* Abnormally high concentrations observed in patients with uncontrolled diabetes mellitus *2952*

Ferritin *Red Blood Cells* *Increase* Mean concentration in 23 poorly controlled patients with IDDM of 29 ± 11.4 ag/cell significantly higher than 15.7 ± 10.6 ag/cell in 23 healthy male controls *1629*
Serum *Increase* Mean concentration in 23 patients with poorly controlled IDDM and no obvious cause of hyperferritinemia 141.1 ± 80.7 μg/L significantly higher than 67.9 ± 44.3 μg/L in 23 healthy male controls *1629*

Fibrinogen *Plasma* *Increase* In 40 normoalbuminuric IDDM patients mean concentration of 261.0 ± 46.0 mg/dL significantly greater than 190.3 ± 30.4 mg/dL in healthy controls *750* In 17 patients with IDDM and urinary excretion of albumin of less than 30 mg/d mean concentration of 6.8 μmol/L, in 20 with albumin excretion of 30 - 300 mg/d 7.8 μmol/L and in 25 with excretion greater than 300 mg/d 9.0 μmol/L compared with 7.0 μmol/L in 14 healthy controls *3695* In 17 patients with IDDM and macroalbuminuria mean concentration of 9.6 μmol/L, and in 20 with microalbuminuria 8.7 μmol/L, significantly higher than that in 37 patients with IDDM and normoalbuminuria in whom mean concentration was 7.6 μmol/L *5805*
Plasma *No Effect* In 50 patients with IDDM mean concentration of 304 ± 67 mg/dL not significantly increased compared with 285 ± 54 mg/dL in 50 healthy controls *1334*

Fibrinopeptide A *Plasma* *Increase* In 50 patients with IDDM mean concentration of 2.1 ± 0.6 ng/mL significantly greater than 1.5 ± 0.5 ng/mL in 50 healthy controls *1334* In patients with IDDM mean concentration reversibly increased compared with healthy individuals: concentration correlated with duration of diabetes *2484*

250.01 Insulin-dependent Diabetes Mellitus *(continued)*

Fibrinopeptide A *(continued)*
Plasma No Effect In 62 patients with IDDM mean concentration of about 3 ng/mL regardless of urinary excretion of albumin not significantly different from the concentration in 14 healthy controls *3695*
Urine Increase Mean excretion reversibly increased in patients with IDDM compared with healthy individuals: concentration correlated with duration of diabetes *2484* In 50 patients with IDDM mean excretion of 2.37 ± 0.78 ng/mg creatinine compared with 1.75 ± 0.48 ng/mg creatinine in 50 healthy controls *1334*

Fractional Excretion of Sodium *Urine No Effect* In 13 well-controlled patients with IDDM median fractional water clearance of 2.9 ± 1.2% significantly different from 0.8 ± 0.3.% in 11 matched healthy controls *3501*

Fractional Reabsorption of Sodium *Urine No Effect* In 8 patients with IDDM and hyporeninemia mean fractional reabsorption of 98.7 ± 0.3 mL% not significantly different when compared with 99.4 ± 9% in 11 controls *1212*

Fractional Water Clearance *Urine No Effect* In 13 well-controlled patients with IDDM median fractional water clearance of 15.7 ± 4.7% significantly different from 9.3 ± 2.9% in 11 matched healthy controls *3501*

Fructosamine *Serum Increase* In 28 male patients with IDDM mean concentration of 3.61 ± 0.69 mmol/L and 3.84 ± 0.56 mmol/L in 26 women with IDDM *1842* In 13 IDDM patients without retinopathy mean concentration of 1.36 ± 0.20 mmol/L, in 12 with new retinopathy of 1.44 ± 0.22 mmol/L and in 17 with established retinopathy of 1.62 ± 0.48 mmol/L significantly higher than 0.80 ± 0.25 mmol/L in 20 controls *4888* Mean concentration in 5 type I diabetics of 542 ± 101 µmol/L significantly greater than that in 5 healthy individuals of 263 ± 17 µmol/L *661* In 40 patients with type I diabetes mellitus mean concentration of 2.0 ± 0.5 mmol/L significantly higher than 1.1 ± 0.2 mmol/L in control patients *4887* In 20 patients with IDDM and albumin excretion rate of less than 20 µg/min mean concentration of 386 µmol/L, in 29 with AER between 20 and 200 µg/min 365 µmol/L, and in 11 with AER greater than 200 µg/min mean concentration of 379 µmol/L, all greater than 247 µmol/L in 20 healthy controls *2475* In 28 men with IDDM and 26 women with IDDM mean concentration of 3.61 ± 0.69 mmol/L and 3.84 ± 0.56 mmol/L respectively *1842*

Fructosamine:Glycated Albumin Ratio *Serum Increase* Mean ratio in 5 type I diabetics of 0.47 ± 0.07 mol/mol significantly greater than that in 5 healthy individuals of 0.24 ± 0.01 mol/mol *661*

α-Galactosidase *Serum Decrease* In 11 diabetics aged 20 - 37 y mean plasma concentration of 6.26 (1.76 - 12) U/h/mL significantly different from 9.66 (6.23 - 15) U/h/mL in 14 comparable controls *4418*
Urine No Effect In 11 diabetics aged 20 - 37 y mean urine concentration of 16.9 (11.4 - 156) U/mg creatinine not significantly different from 26.2 (1.5 - 68.4) U/mg creatinine in 14 comparable controls *4418*

Glucagon *Plasma No Effect* Baseline concentration in 13 patients with IDDM and no residual B-cell function 27 ± 4.7 pmol/L compared with 36 ± 5.0 pmol/L in 13 age and sex matched controls *4882*

Glucagon response to Arginine *Plasma Increase* In 13 patients with IDDM and no residual B-cell function 10 minutes after arginine infusion concentration increased from mean baseline of 27 ± 4.7 pmol/L to 176 ± 23.1 pmol/L compared with increase from 36 ± 5.0 pmol/L to 302 ± 31.9 pmol/L in 13 age and sex matched controls *4882*

Glucose *Serum Decrease* In 8 patients with IDDM and hyporeninemia mean concentration of 126 ± 24 mmol/L significantly different when compared with 200 ± 23 mmol/L in 11 controls *1212*
Serum Increase In 33 patients with IDDM mean concentration of 10.3 ± 3.8 mmol/L significantly different from 4.7 ± 1.8 mmol/L in 32 healthy controls *5499* In 18 newly diagnosed patients with IDDM mean concentration of 409 ± 163 mg/dL compared with normal values in 18 controls *2768* In 70 patients with IDDM mean concentration of 6.67 ± 3.47 mmol/L significantly different from 4.70 ± 0.67 mmol/L in 70 age-matched healthy controls *1429* Median concentration in 77 patients with IDDM of 10.9 mmol/L significantly different from 4.5 mmol/L in 46 controls *2388* In 13 IDDM patients without retinopathy mean concentration of 10.0 ± 4.7 mmol/L, in 12 with new retinopathy 8.9 ± 2.8 mmol/L and in 17 with established retinopathy 10.2 ± 3.6 mmol/L significantly higher than 4.0 ± 0.9 mmol/L in 20 controls *4888* Mean concentration of 167 ± 80 mg/dL in 46 IDDM patients without complications, 168 ± 88 mg/dL in 24 patients with IDDM and retinopathy only and 192 ± 97 mg/dL in 14 patients with IDDM and microalbuminuria compared with 90 ± 12 mg/dL in 41 healthy adults *1651* In 44 patients under age 45 years with IDDM mean concentration of 9.5 ± 3.9 mmol/L compared with 4.7 ± 0.7 mmol/L in 18 patients aged under 45 years. In 16 patients aged over 45 years mean concentration of 10.3 ± 4.1 mmol/L compared with 5.2 ± 0.8 mol/L in 8 controls aged over 45 years *3324* In 45 pairs of identical twins with IDDM mean concentration of 9.7 ± 5.4 mmol/L compared with 5.2 ± 0.9 mmol/L in 45 pairs of nondiabetic twins and 5.2 ± 0.7 mmol/L in 45 healthy controls *1246* Median concentration in 42 patients with IDDM of 116 mg/dL significantly different from 87 mg/dL in 42 healthy controls *2446* In 33 patients with IDDM mean concentration of 10.3 ± 3.8 mmol/L significantly higher than 4.7 ± 1.8 mmol/L in 32 healthy controls *5500* In 43 patients with IDDM mean concentration of 14.24 ± 8.22 mmol/L significantly increased compared with 5.22 ± 0.65 mmol/L in 20 healthy controls *3425* In 40 patients with type I diabetes mellitus mean concentration of 10.9 ± 4.0 mmol/L significantly higher than 4.0 ± 0.9 mmol/L in control patients *4887* Mean concentration in 5 type I diabetics of 9.4 ± 2.2 mmol/L significantly greater than that in 5 healthy individuals of 4.4 ± 1.1 mmol/L *661*

β-Glucuronidase *Serum No Effect* In 11 diabetics aged 20 - 37 y mean plasma concentration of 46.8 (16.8 - 103) U/h/mL not significantly different from 43.4 (16 - 119) U/h/mL in 14 comparable controls *4418*
Urine No Effect In 11 diabetics aged 20 - 37 y mean urine concentration of 54.0 (11.4 - 156) U/mg creatinine not significantly different from 34.7 (6.18 - 425) U/mg creatinine in 14 comparable controls *4418*

Glutamic Acid Decarboxylase 65 Antibodies
Serum Increase In 100 children with IDDM, IA2-antibodies detected with GADA and ICA in 46 children, with ICA only in 21, with GADA only in one and by themselves in 2, with all three antibodies only being detected in one control child *530*

Glutamic Acid Decarboxylase Antibodies *Serum Increase* Frequency of 45.6% observed in a population of Taiwanese with IDDM *775* In 65 of 94 patients with IDDM GAD antibodies detected significantly greater than in healthy controls *3880* In 140 young Chinese diabetics prevalence of GAD antibodies observed in 12.1% *2725* Antibodies detected in 12 of 31 (39%) patients with newly diagnosed IDDM and in 4 of 32 (13%) patients with long standing IDDM *2307*

γ-Glutamyltransferase *Urine Increase* In 11 patients with IDDM in coma median excretion of 9.68 µg/min/m² significantly different from 2.72 µg/min/m² in 18 matched healthy controls *3501*
Urine No Effect In 13 well-controlled patients with IDDM median excretion of 3.31 µg/min/m² not significantly different from 2.72 µg/min/m² in 18 matched healthy controls *3501*

Glutathione Peroxidase *Red Blood Cells Decrease* In patients with IDDM and no vascular complications activities of 73.9 ± 13.7, 65.1 ± 10.7 and 50.6 ± 12.3 U/g hemoglobin in patients with Hb A_{1c} concentrations of < 7.3, 7.3 - 9.4, and > 9.4% respectively and in IDDM patients with vascular complications of 70.1 ± 13.1, 66.2 ± 11.6, 50.2 ± 11.6 U/g hemoglobin at the same Hb A_{1c} concentrations compared with 72.9 ± 12.6 U/g hemoglobin in healthy controls *4476* In 16 stabilized diabetics mean activity of 31 ± 6 U/g hemoglobin significantly less than 49 ± 5 U/g hemoglobin in 20 healthy adult controls *1434*
Red Blood Cells No Effect In 16 stabilized diabetics mean activity of 220 ± 25 U/g hemoglobin compared with 235 ± 13 U/g hemoglobin in 20 healthy adult controls *1434*
Serum Decrease In 16 stabilized diabetics mean concentration of 323 ± 71.0 U/L not significantly reduced below 400 ± 68 U/L in 20 healthy adult controls *1434*

Glutathione, Reduced *Red Blood Cells No Effect* In 41 patients with IDDM mean concentration of 0.215 ± 0.0405 nmol/10⁶ erythrocytes compared with 0.217 ± 0.0419 nmol/10⁶ erythrocytes in 21 healthy controls *3425*

Glycated Apolipoprotein B *Serum Increase* Mean proportion of 5.3 ± 0.7% in 17 patients with IDDM compared with 4.3 ± 1.0% in 45 apparently healthy controls *2284*

Glycated Hemoglobin A_{1c} *Blood Increase* In 18 newly diagnosed patients with IDDM mean concentration of 12 ± 3% compared with normal values in 18 controls *2768* In 118 patients with IDDM mean proportion 9.1 ± 1.9% *725*
Blood No Effect In 8 patients with IDDM and hyporeninemia mean concentration of 8.5 ± 0.4% not significantly different when compared with 8.9 ± 0.2% in 11 controls *1212*

Glycosaminoglycans *Urine Increase* In 156 type I diabetics median excretion was 3.35 mg/mmol creatinine (range 1.0 - 16.2) higher than median of 2.45 mg/mmol creatinine (range 1.67 - 3.60) in controls *1872* In 96 patients with IDDM mean excretion of 19.0, 12.4, 35.6 mg/d for median, 25th and 75th percentile compared with 15.8, 10.4 and 21.5 mg/d in 103 non-diabetic controls *2009*

Glyoxalase I *Blood Increase* In 41 patients with IDDM mean activity of 4.35 ± 1.34 mU/10^6 erythrocytes significantly increased compared with 3.21 ± 1.81 mU/10^6 erythrocytes in 21 healthy controls *3425*

Glyoxalase II *Blood Increase* In 41 patients with IDDM mean activity of 1.97 ± 0.36 mU/10^6 erythrocytes significantly increased compared with 1.83 ± 0.27 mU/10^6 erythrocytes in 21 healthy controls *3425*

Growth Hormone *Plasma Increase* Median concentration in 77 patients with IDDM of 8.0 mU/L significantly different from 3.0 mU/L in 46 controls *2388* In insulin-dependent diabetics high values are usually observed *1766*
Urine Decrease In prepubertal and pubertal children significantly reduced excretion per kilogram body weight compared with control children *4249*
Urine Increase In 21 diabetics mean excretion of 73 - 422 /µU/h and in 13 with poor glycemic control excretion of 10 - 5,283 /µU/h significantly increased compared with mean of 0.4 /µU/h in 10 healthy controls *5331*

Growth Hormone Binding Protein *Serum Decrease* Mean concentration significantly reduced in both prepubertal and postpubertal children with IDDM compared with matched healthy control groups *3660*
Serum Increase In 25 prepubertal and 29 pubertal patients with IDDM concentration was significantly higher than in controls *4260*

Guanosine Monophosphate *Plasma No Effect* In 10 men with IDDM mean concentration of 4.2 ± 1.6 nmol/L not significantly different from 4.8 ± 2.1 nmol/L in 10 nondiabetic controls *4916*

HDL_2-Apolipoprotein A-I *Serum Decrease* In 10 patients with uncontrolled IDDM on admission to hospital mean concentration of 10.86 ± 3.91 mg/dL significantly different from 26.98 ± 5.77 mg/dL in 10 healthy normolipidemic controls *5614*

HDL_2-Apolipoprotein A-II *Serum No Effect* In 10 patients with uncontrolled IDDM on admission to hospital mean concentration of 3.65 ± 0.90 mg/dL not significantly different from 3.72 ± 0.96 mg/dL in 10 healthy normolipidemic controls *5614*

HDL_2-Cholesterol *Serum Decrease* In children with IDDM regardless of whether control was good, fair or poor concentration reduced *63*
Serum Increase In 51 men with IDDM mean concentration of 0.90 ± 0.35 mmol/L significantly different from 0.79 ± 0.47 mmol/L in 48 control men and in 35 women with IDDM mean concentration of 1.05 ± 0.27 mmol/L significantly different from 0.86 ± 0.23 mmol/L in 26 control women *2528*

HDL_2-Cholesterol Esters *Serum Decrease* In 10 patients with uncontrolled IDDM on admission to hospital mean concentration of 0.10 ± 0.04 mmol/L significantly different from 0.34 ± 0.06 mmol/L in 10 healthy normolipidemic controls *5614*

HDL_2-Cholesterol, Free *Serum Decrease* In 10 patients with uncontrolled IDDM on admission to hospital mean concentration of 0.05 ± 0.01 mmol/L significantly different from 0.13 ± 0.03 mmol/L in 10 healthy normolipidemic controls *5614*

HDL_2-Phosphatidylcholine *Serum Decrease* In 10 patients with uncontrolled IDDM on admission to hospital mean concentration of 0.10 ± 0.03 mmol/L significantly different from 0.24 ± 0.04 mmol/L in 10 healthy normolipidemic controls *5614*

HDL_2-Phospholipids *Serum Decrease* In 10 patients with uncontrolled IDDM on admission to hospital mean concentration of 0.12 ± 0.05 mmol/L significantly different from 0.34 ± 0.08 mmol/L in 10 healthy normolipidemic controls *5614*

HDL_2-Triglycerides *Serum No Effect* In 10 patients with uncontrolled IDDM on admission to hospital mean concentration of 0.03 ± 0.01 mmol/L not significantly different from 0.02 ± 0.01 mmol/L in 10 healthy normolipidemic controls *5614*

HDL_3-Apolipoprotein A-I *Serum Decrease* In 10 patients with uncontrolled IDDM on admission to hospital mean concentration of 91.27 ± 7.24 mg/dL significantly different from 118.20 ± 6.57 mg/dL in 10 healthy normolipidemic controls *5614*

HDL_3-Apolipoprotein A-II *Serum No Effect* In 10 patients with uncontrolled IDDM on admission to hospital mean concentration of 3.18 ± 0.17 mg/dL not significantly different from 3.13 ± 0.12 mg/dL in 10 healthy normolipidemic controls *5614*

HDL_3-Cholesterol *Serum Decrease* In children with IDDM regardless of whether control was good, fair or poor concentration significantly reduced *63*
Serum No Effect In 51 men with IDDM mean concentration of 0.65 ± 0.16 mmol/L not significantly different from 0.66 ± 0.19 mmol/L in 48 control men and in 35 women with IDDM mean concentration of 0.69 ± 0.11 mmol/L not significantly different from 0.70 ± 0.12 mmol/L in 26 control women *2528*

HDL_3-Cholesterol Esters *Serum No Effect* In 10 patients with uncontrolled IDDM on admission to hospital mean concentration of 0.73 ± 0.04 mmol/L not significantly different from 0.82 ± 0.04 mmol/L in 10 healthy normolipidemic controls *5614*

HDL_3-Cholesterol, Free *Serum No Effect* In 10 patients with uncontrolled IDDM on admission to hospital mean concentration of 0.22 ± 0.02 mmol/L not significantly different from 0.23 ± 0.01 mmol/L in 10 healthy normolipidemic controls *5614*

HDL_3-Phosphatidylcholine *Serum No Effect* In 10 patients with uncontrolled IDDM on admission to hospital mean concentration of 0.56 ± 0.05 mmol/L not significantly different from 0.62 ± 0.05 mmol/L in 10 healthy normolipidemic controls *5614*

HDL_3-Phospholipids *Serum No Effect* In 10 patients with uncontrolled IDDM on admission to hospital mean concentration of 0.86 ± 0.07 mmol/L not significantly different from 0.90 ± 0.07 mmol/L in 10 healthy normolipidemic controls *5614*

HDL_3-Triglycerides *Serum No Effect* In 10 patients with uncontrolled IDDM on admission to hospital mean concentration of 0.08 ± 0.02 mmol/L not significantly different from 0.08 ± 0.01 mmol/L in 10 healthy normolipidemic controls *5614*

HDL-Cholesterol *Serum Decrease* In patients with IDDM mean concentration decreased in poorly controlled patients *3853* Concentration decreased significantly in diabetic children regardless of whether the control of their condition was good, fair or poor in comparison with healthy children *63*
Serum Increase In 51 men with IDDM mean concentration of 1.54 ± 0.38 mmol/L not significantly different from 1.45 ± 0.50 mmol/L in 48 control men and in 35 women with IDDM mean concentration of 1.74 ± 0.28 mmol/L significantly different from 1.56 ± 0.28 mmol/L in 26 control women *2528* In patients with IDDM mean concentration increased or normal in well controlled patients *3853* In 44 patients with IDDM aged under 45 years mean concentration of 1.57 ± 0.35 mmol/L compared with 1.45 ± 0.34 mmol/L in 18 healthy age-matched controls: in 16 patients with IDDM older than 45 years mean concentration of 1.60 ± 0.47 mmol/L compared with 1.20 ± 0.22 mmol/L in 8 age-matched healthy controls *3324*
Serum No Effect In 118 patients with IDDM mean concentration of 1.49 ± 0.39 mmol/L not significantly different from 1.49 ± 0.33 mmol/L in 286 healthy controls *725* In 28 men with IDDM and 26 women with IDDM mean concentrations of 1.37 ± 0.51 mmol/L and 1.66 ± 0.57 mmol/L respectively *1842* In 52 patients with IDDM mean concentration of 1.5 ± 0.4 mmol/L not significantly different from that in 52 healthy controls in whom the mean concentration was 1.2 ± 0.4 mmol/L *866* Mean concentration in 50 IDDM patients (regardless of HbA_{1C} concentration) of 56 ± 17 mg/dL compared with 57 ± 16 mg/dL in 50 healthy controls *1334* Mean concentration in 45 pairs of identical twins with IDDM 1.36 ± 0.31 mmol/L compared with 1.25 ± 0.29 mmol/L in 45 pairs of nondiabetic twins and 1.33 mmol/L in 45 nondiabetic controls *1246* In 70 patients with IDDM mean concentration of 1.40 ± 0.39 mmol/L not significantly different from 1.30 ± 0.34 mmol/L in 70 age-matched healthy controls *1429* In patients with IDDM mean concentration increased or normal in well controlled patients *3853* Mean concentration of 1.63 ± 0.03 mmol/L in 142 patients with IDDM significantly higher than 1.35 ± 0.05 mmol/L in 70 patients with NIDDM but

250.01 Insulin-dependent Diabetes Mellitus *(continued)*

HDL-Cholesterol *(continued)* not significantly different from normal range *470* In 78 patients with IDDM mean concentration of 1.53 ± 0.53 mmol/L not significantly different from 1.51 ± 0.44 mmol/L in 82 healthy controls *10*

HDL-Triglycerides *Serum* *Increase* In children whose control of diabetes mellitus was poor or fair, concentration was significantly increased *63*

Hemoglobin *Blood* *Decrease* In 8 patients with IDDM and hyporeninemia mean concentration of 100 g/L significantly different when compared with 135 g/L in 11 controls *1212*

Hemoglobin A_1 *Blood* *Increase* In 45 pairs of identical twins with IDDM mean concentration of 9.6 ± 1.9% compared with 7.1 ± 1.8% in 45 pairs of nondiabetic twins and 6.9 ± 1.2% in 45 nondiabetic controls *1246*

Hemoglobin A_{1c} *Blood* *Increase* In 70 patients with IDDM mean concentration of 7.0 ± 1.3% significantly different from 5.3 ± 0.3% in 70 age-matched healthy controls *1429* Mean concentration of 8.2 ± 1.4% in 46 IDDM patients without complications, 8.2 ± 1.1% in 24 patients with IDDM and retinopathy only and 9.4 ± 1.3% in 14 patients with IDDM and microalbuminuria compared with 5.3 ± 0.3% in 41 healthy adults *1651* In 17 patients with IDDM and macroalbuminuria mean concentration of 9.4 ± 1.5% and in 20 with microalbuminuria 8.9 ± 1.9% significantly higher than that in 37 patients with IDDM and normoalbuminuria in whom mean concentration of 8.0 ± 1.2% *5805* In 13 IDDM patients without retinopathy mean concentration of 8.0 ± 0.7%, in 12 with new retinopathy 7.7 ± 1.3% and in 17 with established retinopathy 7.9 ± 2.3% significantly higher than 4.8 ± 0.4% in 20 controls *4888* In 33 patients with IDDM mean proportion of 8.7 ± 2.7% not significantly different from 4.2 ± 0.9% in 32 healthy controls *5500* Mean concentration of 9.07 ± 0.15% in 142 patients with IDDM not significantly different from 9.02 ± 0.32% in 70 patients with NIDDM but significantly different from normal range *470* In 33 patients with IDDM mean concentration of 8.6 ± 2.7% significantly different from 4.3 ± 0.9% in 32 healthy controls *5499* In 10 diabetic patients with normoalbuminuria and in 10 with microalbuminuria mean concentrations of 8.5 ± 1.4% and 8.2 ± 2.8% respectively significantly higher than 4.3 ± 0.7% in 10 healthy controls *937* In 40 diabetic children and adolescents mean concentration of 9.6 ± 1.8% *3243* Median concentration in 42 patients with IDDM of 7.3% significantly different from 5.3% in 42 healthy controls *2446* In 44 patients aged less than 45 years with IDDM mean concentration of 7.7 ± 1.5% compared with 5.3 ± 0.7% in 18 healthy controls: in 16 IDDM patients aged over 45 years mean 8.4 ± 1.8% compared with 5.5 ± 0.8% in 8 healthy controls *3324* Mean concentration in 50 IDDM patients 8.2 ± 1.2% compared with 4.1 ± 0.7% in 50 nondiabetic controls *1334* In 52 patients with IDDM mean concentration of 7.7 ± 0.9% significantly different from that in 52 healthy controls in whom the mean concentration was 4.3 ± 1.2% *866* In 28 men with IDDM and 26 women with IDDM mean concentrations of 9.81 ± 2.72% and 10.42 ± 2.14% respectively *1842* In 77 patients with IDDM median concentration of 8.9% compared with 3.8% in 62 healthy controls *1867* In 43 patients with IDDM mean concentration of 8.06 ± 1.70% significantly increased compared with 4.33 ± 1.70% in 8 healthy controls *3425* In 40 patients with type I diabetes mellitus mean concentration of 7.7 ± 1.3% significantly higher than 4.8 ± 0.4% in control patients *4887* In 28 male patients with IDDM mean concentration of 9.81 ± 2.72% and 10.42 ± 2.14% in 26 women with IDDM *1842* Mean concentration of 10.6% significantly higher in 11 iron-deficient children with IDDM compared with control children with iron-deficiency but without diabetes (7.7%) *5165* In 40 patients with IDDM and nephropathy mean concentration of 9.0 ± 1.9% significantly different from 8.2 ± 1.8% in 49 patients with IDDM but without nephropathy for 5 - 10 years *5010*

Heparan Sulfate Proteoglycan *Urine* *Increase* In 10 patients with IDDM and microalbuminuria and 20 without microalbuminuria mean excretion of 8.3 HSPG/creatinine ratio (range 4.8 - 19.7) and 8.2 (range 2.2 - 27) respectively significantly greater than 3.3 (range 1.6 - 6.4) in 10 healthy controls *4793*

β-Hexosaminidase *Serum* *Increase* In 11 diabetics aged 20 - 37 y mean plasma concentration of 630 (412 - 922) U/h/mL significantly different from 485 (279 - 901) U/h/mL in 14 comparable controls *4418*
Urine *No Effect* In 11 diabetics aged 20 - 37 y mean urine concentration of 256 (52.1 - 696) U/mg creatinine not significantly different from 170 (33.7 - 425) U/mg creatinine in 14 comparable controls *4418*

IDL + VLDL-Triglycerides *Serum* *Increase* In 10 patients with uncontrolled IDDM on admission to hospital mean concentration of 0.92 ± 0.24 mmol/L increased but not significantly different from 0.54 ± 0.09 mmol/L in 10 healthy normolipidemic controls *5614*

IDL-Protein *Serum* *Increase* In patients with IDDM mean concentration increased in well controlled patients, but less commonly than in patients with IDDM *3853*

Insulin *Plasma* *Decrease* In 33 patients with IDDM mean concentration of 6.9 ± 2.1 mU/L significantly different from 16.8 ± 4.7 mU/L in 32 healthy controls *5500*
Plasma *Increase* In 70 patients with IDDM mean concentration of 141 ± 172 pmol/L significantly different from 76 ± 65 pmol/L in 70 age-matched healthy controls *1429*

Insulin-like Growth Factor-I *Serum* *Decrease* In 51 treated patients with IDDM mean and median concentrations of 174 ± 98 μg/L and 140 μg/L significantly reduced compared with healthy controls *5040* Median concentration in 77 patients with IDDM of 17.0 nmol/L significantly different from 24.6 nmol/L in 46 controls *2388* In 25 prepubertal and 29 pubertal patients with IDDM concentration was significantly less than in controls *4260* Mean concentration of 197 ± 17 ng/mL in 49 prepubertal children with IDDM compared with 242 ± 9 ng/mL in 252 matched controls and 328 ± 34 ng/mL in 9 patients after complete puberty with IDDM compared with 660 ± 32 ng/mL in 79 matched controls *3660*
Serum *Increase* Concentration increased during pregnancy as in nondiabetics but comparable: in first trimester mean 163 versus 167 ng/mL; in second trimester 252 versus 277 ng/mL and in third 505 versus 455 ng/mL *1686*
Urine *Decrease* In prepubertal and pubertal children significantly reduced excretion per kilogram body weight observed when compared with control subjects *4249*

Insulin-like Growth Factor-II *Serum* *Decrease* In 51 treated patients with IDDM mean and median concentrations of 489 ± 120 μg/L and 479 μg/L significantly reduced compared with healthy controls *5040*
Serum *Increase* Mean concentrations increased during pregnancy but changes in diabetics and nondiabetics comparable; in first trimester 411 versus 425 ng/mL; in second 506 versus 418 ng/mL and in third 603 versus 559 ng/mL *1686*

Insulin-like Growth Factor Binding Protein-1
Serum *Decrease* In 51 treated patients with IDDM mean and median concentrations of 30.6 ± 16.7 μg/L and 25 μg/L not significantly reduced compared with healthy controls *5040*
Serum *Increase* Mean concentration of 26.1 ± 3.1 ng/L in 49 prepubertal children with IDDM compared with 11.9 ± 1.1 ng/L in 252 matched controls and 8.9 ± 3.1 ng/L in 9 patients after complete puberty with IDDM compared with 2.3 ± 0.3 ng/L in 79 matched controls *3660* In 25 prepubertal and 29 pubertal patients with IDDM concentration was significantly higher than in controls *4260*

Insulin-like Growth Factor Binding Protein-2
Serum *Increase* In 51 treated patients with IDDM mean and median concentrations of 381 ± 141 μg/L and 356 μg/L not significantly increased compared with healthy controls *5040* In 25 prepubertal and 29 pubertal patients with IDDM concentration was significantly higher than in controls *4260*

Insulin-like Growth Factor Binding Protein-3
Serum *Increase* In 51 treated patients with IDDM mean and median concentrations of 3,868 ± 882 μg/L and 3,694 μg/L significantly increased compared with healthy controls *5040*
Serum *No Effect* Mean concentration of 3.4 ± 0.1 mg/L in 49 prepubertal children with IDDM compared with 3.2 ± 0.1 mg/L in 252 matched controls and 4.2 ± 0.2 mg/L in 9 patients after complete puberty with IDDM compared with 4.1 ± 0.9 mg/L in 79 matched controls *3660* In 25 prepubertal and 29 pubertal patients with IDDM concentrations were not significantly significantly different from that in controls *4260*

Insulin-like Growth Factor Binding Protein-4
Serum *Increase* In 25 prepubertal patients with IDDM concentration was significantly higher than in controls *4260*

Intercellular Adhesion Molecule-1 *Serum* *Increase* In patients with IDDM mean serum concentration about 30% higher than in controls *5519*

Interferon-γ *Serum* *Increase* Median concentration of 225 pg/mL in patients with newly diagnosed IDDM significantly increased when compared with 0.0 pg/mL in normal controls *2307*
Serum *No Effect* Median concentration of 0.0 pg/mL in patients with long standing IDDM not different when compared with 0.0 pg/mL in normal controls *2307*

Interleukin-1 Receptor Antagonist *Serum* *No Effect* In 18 patients with recent onset IDDM mean concentration of 471 ± 39 ng/L and of 416 ± 56 ng/L in 10 patients with long-standing IDDM not significantly different from 472 ± 29 ng/L in 35 healthy controls *3266*

Interleukin-1α *Serum* *Increase* Median concentration of 260 pg/mL in patients with newly diagnosed IDDM and 129 pg/mL in patients with long standing IDDM significantly increased when compared with 100 pg/mL in normal controls *2307*

Interleukin-1β *Serum* *No Effect* Concentration not detectable in patients with IDDM or controls *2307*

Interleukin-2 *Serum* *Increase* Median concentration of 12% in patients with newly diagnosed IDDM and 8% in patients with long standing IDDM significantly increased when compared with 3.6% in normal controls *2307*

Interleukin-4 *Serum* *No Effect* Median concentration of 0 pg/mL in patients with newly diagnosed IDDM and 0 pg/mL in patients with long standing IDDM not significantly different when compared with 0 pg/mL in normal controls *2307*

Interleukin-10 *Serum* *No Effect* Median concentration of 0 pg/mL in patients with newly diagnosed IDDM and 0 pg/mL in patients with long standing IDDM not significantly different when compared with 0 pg/mL in normal controls *2307*

Islet Amyloid Polypeptide *Serum* *Decrease* In 5 patients with IDDM mean concentration of 0.5 ± 0.2 pmol/L significantly less than 8.0 ± 5.0 pmol/L in 25 healthy controls *4210* In 5 patients with IDDM IAPP was not detectable in the plasma whereas the concentration of IAPP was 6.0 ± 4.0 pmol/L in 10 healthy individuals *5404*

Islet Cell Antibodies *Serum* *Increase* In 100 children with IDDM, ICA detected with IA2-Ab and GADA 65 antibodies in 46 children, with IA2-Ab only in 21, with GADA 65 antibodies only in 16 and by themselves in 5, with all three antibodies only being detected in one control child *530* Antibodies detected in 24 of 31 (78%) patients with newly diagnosed IDDM and in 6 of 32 (19%) patients with long-standing IDDM *2307* In 5 of 8 children and adolescents with IDDM islet cell antibodies identified *1662*

Lactate *Blood* *Increase* In 42 patients with IDDM mean concentration of 18.3 nmol/g blood compared with 9.7 ± 4.3 nmol/g blood in 21 healthy controls *3425*

Laminin *Serum* *Increase* Observed effect in type I diabetes mellitus *2056*

LDL-Cholesterol *Serum* *Increase* In patients with IDDM mean concentration increased or normal in poorly controlled patients *3853* Calculated LDL-cholesterol using Friedewald formula versus measured LDL-cholesterol had greater than 10% false increase in 39% patients with diabetes mellitus and falsely low by more than 10% in 13% and falsely high in 26% control individuals and falsely low in 1% *4467* In children with fair or poor control of their diabetes concentration significantly increased *63*
Serum *No Effect* In 70 patients with IDDM mean concentration of 3.35 ± 0.96 mmol/L not significantly different from 3.22 ± 0.83 mmol/L in 70 age-matched healthy controls *1429* In 50 patients with IDDM (regardless of HbA_{1C} concentration) mean concentration of 123 ± 34 mg/dL compared with 125 ± 34 mg/dL in 50 healthy controls *1334* Median concentration in 42 patients with IDDM of 124 mg/dL not significantly different from 129 mg/dL in 42 healthy controls *2446* In 51 men with IDDM mean concentration of 2.95 ± 0.99 mmol/L not significantly different from 3.31 ± 0.87 mmol/L in 48 control men and in 35 women with IDDM mean concentration of 2.73 ± 0.65 mmol/L not significantly different from 3.02 ± 0.82 mmol/L in 26 control women *2528* In 52 patients with IDDM mean concentration of 3.2 ± 0.8 mmol/L not significantly different from that in 52 healthy controls in whom the mean concentration was 3.2 ± 0.8 mmol/L *866* In 45 pairs of identical twins with IDDM mean concentration of 3.16 ± 0.80 mmol/L compared with 3.27 ± 0.93 mmol/L in 45 pairs of nondiabetic twins and 3.45 ± 1.04 mmol/L in 45 nondiabetic controls *1246* In patients with IDDM mean concentration increased or normal in poorly controlled patients *3853* In patients with IDDM mean concentration normal in well controlled patients *3853*

LDL-Triglycerides *Serum* *Increase* In children in whom control of diabetes was poor or fair concentration significantly increased *63*

Lecithin:Cholesterol Acyltransferase *Serum* *No Effect* In 10 patients with uncontrolled IDDM on admission to hospital mean activity of 74.47 ± 7.30 nmol/mL/h not significantly different from 78.84 ± 12.78 nmol/mL/h in 10 healthy normolipidemic controls *5614*

Leucine Aminopeptidase *Urine* *Increase* In 11 patients with IDDM in coma median excretion of 0.321 μg/mmol creatinine significantly different from 0.14 μg/mmol creatinine in 18 matched healthy controls *3501*
Urine *No Effect* In 13 well-controlled patients with IDDM median excretion of 0.192 μg/mmol creatinine not significantly different from 0.14 μg/mmol creatinine in 18 matched healthy controls *3501*

Leukocytes *Blood* *Increase* Median concentration in 42 patients with IDDM of 6.5 G/L significantly different from 6.0 G/L in 42 healthy controls *2446*

Lipase, Hepatic *Serum* *Decrease* In 10 patients with uncontrolled IDDM on admission to hospital mean activity of 49.00 ± 25.15 nmol oleic acid/min decreased but not significantly different from 81.98 ± 48.03 nmol oleic acid/min in 10 healthy normolipidemic controls *5614*

Lipid Peroxide *Serum* *No Effect* In 16 men with IDDM but without complications mean concentration of 4.2 nmol/mL and of 4.7 nmol/mL in 16 women with IDDM without complications compared with normals of 4.1 and 4.4 nmol/mL respectively *822*

Lipoprotein A-I *Serum* *Increase* In 51 men with IDDM mean concentration of 0.91 ± 0.16 g/L not significantly different from 0.52 ± 0.16 g/L in 48 control men and in 35 women with IDDM mean concentration of 0.71 ± 0.16 g/L significantly different from 0.54 ± 0.14 g/L in 26 control women *2528*

Lipoprotein Lp(a) *Serum* *Increase* Concentration increased in patients with IDDM but less in those with normoalbuminuria (mean 90 U/L) than in those with micro- or macro- albuminuria (mean 137 U/L). The prevalence of patients with Lp(a) greater than 200 U/L greater (45% versus 24%) in patients with albuminuria than in controls *5697* In children with IDDM mean concentration at Tanner stage 1 of 193 mg/L compared with 178 mg/L in controls at same stage, 252 mg/L versus 170 mg/L in stages 2 - 4, and 286 mg/L versus 181 mg/L in Tanner stage 5 *947* In 80 patients with IDDM median concentration of 0.11 g/L not significantly different from median of 0.12 g/L, although concentrations above 0.25 g/L were observed in 33% of patients with poor glycemic control *5644*
Serum *No Effect* In 80 patients with IDDM median concentration of 0.11 g/L not significantly different from median of 0.12 g/L in healthy controls, although concentrations above 0.25 g/L were observed in 33% of patients with poor glycemic control *5644* In 52 patients with IDDM median concentration of 11.4 mg/dL not significantly different from that in 52 healthy controls in whom the median concentration was 12.0 mg/dL *866* In 148 patients with IDDM median concentration of 56 mg/L not significantly different from 43 mg/L in 69 healthy volunteers, but with 9.8% above 95th percentile of 361 mg/L *5417* Diabetes appears to have no significant effect on plasma concentrations of Lp(a) *2827* In 45 pairs of identical twins with IDDM mean concentration of 20.6 ± 22.9 mg/dL compared with 19.6 ± 19.7 mg/dL in 45 pairs of nondiabetic twins and 19.6 ± 24.0 mg/dL in 45 nondiabetic controls *1246*

Lutein *Serum* *No Effect* In 60 male IDDM patients 5th to 95th percentile of concentrations of 0.054 - 0.313 μmol/L not significantly different from range in 210 healthy men (5th to 95th percentile 0.078 - 0.438 μmol/L) and 0.081 - 0.472 μmol/L in 63 women with IDDM not significantly different from 0.094 - 0.442 μmol/L in 240 healthy women *3906* In 28 male patients with IDDM 95% CI of 0.16 - 0.22 μmol/L not significantly different from 0.21 - 0.26 μmol/L in 113 nonrelative healthy controls. In 26 women with IDDM 95% CI 0.17 - 0.27 μmol/L compared with 0.22 - 0.27 μmol/L in 123 nonrelative healthy controls *1842*

250.01 Insulin-dependent Diabetes Mellitus *(continued)*

Lycopene *Serum Increase* In 60 male IDDM patients 5th to 95th percentile of concentrations of 0.077 - 1.403 µmol/L significantly different from range in 210 healthy men (5th to 95th percentile of 0.112 - 0.877 µmol/L) but 0.147 - 0.929 µmol/L in 63 women with IDDM not significantly different from 0.107 - 0.922 µmol/L in 240 healthy women *3906*
Serum No Effect In 28 male patients with IDDM 95% CI of 0.34 - 0.50 µmol/L not significantly different from 0.37 - 0.47 µmol/L in 113 nonrelative healthy controls. In 26 women with IDDM 95% CI 0.32 - 0.49 µmol/L compared with 0.41 - 0.51 µmol/L in 123 nonrelative healthy controls *1842* In 28 men with IDDM median concentration of 0.44 µmol/L not significantly different when compared with 0.35 µmol/L in 113 male controls and 0.39 µmol/L in 26 women with IDDM not significantly different when compared with 0.41 µmol/L female controls *1842* Concentration range of 0.147 - 0.929 µmol/L in 63 women with IDDM not significantly different from 0.107 - 0.922 µmol/L in 240 healthy women *3906*

Lymphocytes *Blood Decrease* The percentage and absolute number of peripheral T-lymphocytes were significantly lower (38.1% and 833 /µL) in juvenile-onset diabetics than in normal subjects or maternity-onset diabetics. There was no significant difference between normals and maternity-onset cases *740*

Magnesium *Lymphocytes Decrease* Mean concentration in 45 children with IDDM of 21.4 ± 1.4 µmol/10^{10} cells significantly reduced compared with 36.5 ± 3.5 µmol/10^{10} cells *3049*
Neutrophils No Effect Mean concentration of 30.7 ± 3.7 µmol/10^{10} cells not significantly different from 25.6 ± 3.3 µmol/10^{10} cells in 12 healthy control children *3049*
Platelets Decrease In 10 diabetic patients with normoalbuminuria and in 10 with microalbuminuria mean concentrations of 2.340 ± 0.46 µmol/10^8 cells and 1.859 ± 0.47 µmol/10^8 cells respectively significantly different from 2.836 ± 0.12 µmol/10^8 cells in 10 healthy controls *937*
Red Blood Cells Decrease In 10 diabetic patients with normoalbuminuria and in 10 with microalbuminuria mean concentrations of 2.065 ± 0.62 mmol/L and 1.871 ± 0.64 mmol/L respectively significantly different from 2.586 ± 0.20 mmol/L in 10 healthy controls *937*
Red Blood Cells No Effect In 45 children with IDDM mean concentration of 6.13 ± 0.21 µmol/g hemoglobin not significantly different from 6.67 ± 0.58 µmol/g hemoglobin in 12 healthy children *4406*
Serum Decrease In 45 children with IDDM mean concentration of 780 ± 16 µmol/L significantly less than 860 ± 29 µmol/L in 12 normal children *4406* In 10 diabetic patients with microalbuminuria mean concentration of 0.502 ± 0.20 mmol/L significantly different from 0.778 ± 0.09 mmol/L in 10 healthy controls *937*
Serum No Effect In 10 diabetic patients with normoalbuminuria mean concentration of 0.673 ± 0.16 mmol/L not significantly different from 0.778 ± 0.09 mmol/L in 10 healthy controls *937*

Malondialdehyde *Serum No Effect* In 16 stabilized diabetics mean concentration of 2.42 ± 0.25 µmol/L compared with 2.51 ± 0.25 µmol/L in 31 adult controls but concentration significantly less than in ketoacidotic state *1434* In 40 patients with type I diabetes mellitus mean concentration of 1.8 ± 0.3 µmol/L not significantly different from 1.8 ± 0.3 µmol/L in control patients *4887*

Mean Platelet Volume *Blood No Effect* In 18 newly diagnosed patients with IDDM mean volume of 9.2 ± 0.8 fL compared with 8.4 ± 1.5 fL in 18 controls *2768*

Methylglyoxal *Blood Increase* In 42 patients with IDDM mean concentration of 470.7 pmol/g blood compared with 79.8 pmol/g blood in 21 healthy controls *3425*

β_2-Microglobulin *Urine Increase* In patients with insulin-dependent diabetes mellitus and nephropathy excretion increased in association with tubulopathy *3689* In 11 patients with IDDM in coma median excretion of 3.89 µg/min/m^2 significantly different from 0.08 µg/min/m^2 in 18 matched healthy controls *3501*
Urine No Effect In 13 well controlled patients with IDDM median excretion of 0.09 µg/min/m^2 not significantly different from 0.08 µg/min/m^2 in 18 matched healthy controls *3501*

N-Acetyl-Glucosaminidase *Serum Increase* In 12 patients with IDDM and new retinopathy mean activity of 17.0 U/L and in 17 with established retinopathy 16.9 U/L significantly higher than 15.3 U/L in 20 controls *4888* In 40 patients with type I diabetes mellitus mean activity of 18.6 U/L significantly higher than 15.3 U/L in control patients *4887*
Serum No Effect In 13 IDDM patients without retinopathy mean activity of 15.0 U/L not significantly different from 15.3 U/L in 20 controls *4888*
Urine Increase In 20 patients with IDDM and albumin excretion rate less than 20 µg/min mean excretion of 0.34 U/mmol creatinine, in 29 with AER between 20 and 200 µg/min 0.40 U/mmol creatinine and in 11 with AER greater than 200 µg/min mean excretion of 0.78 U/mmol creatinine, all greater than 0.08 U/mmol creatinine in 20 healthy controls *2475* In 13 patients with well-controlled IDDM median excretion of 0.19 µg/mmol creatinine and in 11 IDDM in coma median excretion of 0.32 µg/mmol creatinine significantly different from 0.26 µg/mmol creatinine in 18 matched healthy controls *3501*

Non-HDL-Cholesterol *Serum No Effect* Mean concentration of 3.95 ± 0.09 mmol/L in 142 patients with IDDM significantly lower than 4.38 ± 0.15 mmol/L in 70 patients with NIDDM but not significantly different from normal range *470*

Organic Hydroperoxides *Serum Increase* In patients with IDDM and no vascular complications activities of 71.6 ± 16.7, 72.3 ± 12.8 and 95.8 ± 12.7 µmol/L in patients with Hb A_{1c} concentrations of < 7.3, 7.3 - 9.4, and > 9.4% respectively and in IDDM patients with vascular complications of 79.7 ± 18.3, 100.8 ± 14.7, 110.0 ± 15.4 µmol/L at the same Hb A_{1c} concentrations compared with 67.9 ± 15.0 µmol/L in healthy controls *4476*
Serum No Effect In 16 stabilized diabetics mean concentration of 132.3 ± 34.0 µmol/L not significantly different from 127.8 ± 14 µmol/L in 20 healthy adult controls *1434*

Paraoxonase *Serum No Effect* In 78 patients with IDDM mean concentration of 52.0 ± 3.2 µg/mL not significantly different from 42.5 ± 2.2 µg/mL in 82 healthy controls *10*

Platelet Aggregation *Blood Increase* In response to ADP mean maximal aggregation of 74 ± 138 % in 50 patients with IDDM compared with 68 ± 11% in 50 control individuals. In response to collagen mean maximal response in IDDM patients 81 ± 11% significantly greater than 75 ± 9% in controls. In IDDM patients maximal spontaneous response 5 ± 6% significantly greater than 1 ± 2% in healthy controls *1334*

Platelet-derived Growth Factor *Plasma No Effect* In 18 patients with IDDM mean concentration not significantly different from 4,980 - 15,070 pg/mL in 18 healthy controls *2030*

Platelet Factor 4 *Plasma Increase* In 50 patients with IDDM mean concentration of 5.5 ± 2.6 ng/mL significantly greater than 3.4 ± 1.2 ng/mL in 50 healthy controls *1334*

Platelets *Blood Increase* In 50 patients with IDDM mean concentration of 26,3000 ± 49,000 /µL significantly increased compared with 232,000 ± 38,000 /µL in 50 healthy controls *1334* Median concentration in 42 patients with IDDM of 286 G/L significantly different from 232 G/L in 42 healthy controls *2446* In 34 patients with IDDM mean concentration of 283 ± 8.3 x 10^9/L significantly different from 198 ± 51 x 10^9/L in 36 nondiabetic patients *5010*
Blood No Effect In 18 newly diagnosed patients with IDDM mean concentration of 219 ± 52 x 10^3 /µL compared with 236 ± 59 x 10^3 /µL in 18 controls *2768*

Postheparin Lipoprotein Lipase *Plasma No Effect* In 10 patients with uncontrolled IDDM on admission to hospital mean activity of 49.14 ± 2.58 nmol oleic acid/min not significantly different from 52.41 ± 5.18 nmol oleic acid/min in 10 healthy normolipidemic controls *5614*

Prolactin *Plasma No Effect* In 20 male patients with IDDM mean concentration of 200 mIU/L not significantly different from 192 mIU/L in 20 healthy controls *834*

Prorenin *Plasma Increase* In 50 patients with IDDM mean concentration of 1,97.5 ± 9.3 pg/mL significantly higher than 134.0 ± 7.9 pg/mL in 39 non-diabetic siblings. Mean concentration in 5 patients with microalbuminuria of 226.4 ± 13.6 pg/mL and in 25 without microalbuminuria 168.5 ± 10.1 pg/mL *1007*

Prostaglandins *Plasma Increase* Prostaglandin E_2 and $F_{2\alpha}$ were significantly elevated in children at all times measured *791*

Protein C *Plasma Increase* In 50 patients with IDDM mean concentration of 99 ± 19% significantly increased compared with 90 ± 13% in 50 healthy controls *1334*

Protein S *Plasma* *Increase* In 50 patients with IDDM mean concentration of 95 ± 21% significantly greater than 86 ± 15% in 50 healthy controls *1334*

Prothrombin Fragment 1.2 *Plasma* *Increase* In 62 patients with IDDM mean concentration about 1 nmol/L regardless of urinary excretion of albumin significantly higher than 0.6 nmol/L in 14 healthy controls *3695* In 40 normoalbuminuric IDDM patients mean concentration of 0.92 ± 0.26 nmol/L significantly greater than 0.60 ± 0.12 nmol/L in healthy controls *750*

P-Selectin *Serum* *Increase* Median concentration in 42 patients with IDDM of 285 ng/mL significantly different from 236 ng/mL in 42 healthy controls *2446*

Pyrraline *Urine* *Increase* Mean concentration in 15 IDDM patients of 1.37 ± 0.6 µg pyrraline/mg creatinine (1.47 ± 0.7 µg pyrraline/mL creatinine) significantly higher than that in 15 healthy adults aged 17 - 35 y, 1.21 ± 0.40 µg pyrraline/mg creatinine (0.98 ± 0.36 µg pyrraline/mL urine *4183*

Pyruvate *Blood* *Increase* Raised levels have been reported in unstable diabetes (insulin sensitive) *1290*

Red Cell Mass *Blood* *Decrease* In 8 patients with IDDM and hyporeninemia mean concentration of 14.8 mL/kg significantly different when compared with 21 mL/kg in 11 controls *1212*

Renin *Plasma* *No Effect* In 50 patients with IDDM mean concentration of 36.8 ± 3.3 pg/mL not significantly higher than 35.6 ± 1.9 pg/mL in 39 non-diabetic siblings. Mean concentration in 5 patients with microalbuminuria of 40.0 ± 4.6 pg/mL and in 25 without microalbuminuria of 33.6 ± 4.7 pg/mL *1007*

Renin Activity *Plasma* *Decrease* In 8 patients with IDDM and hyporeninemia mean stimulated activity of 1.3 ± 0.3 ng/mL/h significantly decreased compared with 2.9 ± 0.3 ng/mL/h in 11 controls *1212*

Retinol *Serum* *Decrease* In 28 male patients with IDDM 95% CI of 1.34 - 1.6.9 µmol/L significantly different from 1.84 - 1.99 µmol/L in 113 nonrelative healthy controls. In 26 women with IDDM 95% CI 1.16 - 1.36 µmol/L compared with 1.60 - 1.75 µmol/L in 123 nonrelative healthy controls *1842* In 28 men with IDDM median concentration of 1.40 µmol/L significantly reduced compared with 1.92 µmol/L in 113 male controls and 1.27 µmol/L in 26 women with IDDM significantly reduced compared with 123 µmol/L female controls *1842* In 60 male IDDM patients 5th to 95th percentile of concentrations of 0.82 - 2.21 µmol/L significantly lower than range in 210 healthy men (5th to 95th percentile 1.13 - 2.63 µmol/L) and 0.85 - 1.85 µmol/L in 63 women with IDDM significantly less than 1.01 - 2.44 µmol/L in 240 healthy women *3906* In 44 patients with IDDM aged under 45 years mean concentration of 1.45 ± 0.3 µmol/L significantly less than mean 1.82 ± 0.45 µmol/L in 18 age-matched controls: in 16 patients aged over 45 years mean concentration of 1.85 ± 0.54 µmol/L not significantly different from 1.84 ± 0.36 µmol/L in 8 age-matched controls *3324*

Retinol-binding Protein *Urine* *Increase* In 109 patients with insulin-dependent diabetes mellitus with nephropathy excretion higher than in 44 controls. 30 and 40% of patients with and without microalbuminuria, respectively, exhibited signs of tubulopathy *3689* Mean excretion in 18 normoalbuminuric patients of 89.4 ng/min, in 13 IDDM patients with microalbuminuria 113 ng/min, and 509 ng/min in 15 patients compared with that in 16 nondiabetic healthy normotensive individuals, 25.5 - 72.8 ng/min or 34.2 - 79.5 µg/g *1339*

Selenium *Serum* *Decrease* In 16 stabilized diabetics mean concentration of 0.87 ± 0.16 µmol/L compared with 1.08 ± 0.20 µmol/L in reference population *1434*

Semicarbazide-sensitive Amine Oxidase *Serum* *Increase* In 104 patients with IDDM mean activity of 555 ± 172 mU/L significantly higher than 352 ± 102 mU/L in 67 controls, with concentration higher in patients with retinopathy or nephropathy or both than in those without *525*

Sex-Hormone Binding Globulin *Serum* *Increase* In 20 male patients with IDDM mean concentration of 42.4 nmol/L significantly different from 33.8 nmol/L in 20 healthy controls *834*

Sialic Acid *Serum* *Increase* In 17 patients with IDDM and macroalbuminuria mean concentration of 2.13 ± 0.33 mmol/L and in 20 with microalbuminuria 2.02 ± 0.37 mmol/L significantly higher than that in 37 patients with IDDM and normoalbuminuria in whom the mean concentration was 1.90 ± 0.21 mmol/L and 1.67 ± 0.26 mmol/L in 26 healthy controls *5805* IDDM patients following the onset of complications have significantly increased concentrations *213* In 23 patients with IDDM and microalbuminuria mean concentration of 1.93 ± 0.26 mmol/L significantly greater than 1.76 ± 0.27 mmol/L in 23 patients with IDDM and normoalbuminuria *971*

Sodium *Urine* *No Effect* In 8 patients with IDDM and hyporeninemia meanexcretion of 129 ± 17 mmol/d not significantly different when compared with 128 ± 13 mmol/d in 11 controls *1212*

Soluble E-Selectin *Serum* *Increase* In 70 patients with IDDM mean concentration of 50 ± 25 ng/mL not significantly different from 46 ± 23 ng/mL in 70 age-matched healthy controls *1429*

Serum *No Effect* In 18 newly diagnosed patients with IDDM mean concentration of 42 ± 17 ng/mL, with concentration unchanged at 43 ± 19 ng/mL 2 years later, compared with 41 ± 14 ng/mL in 18 controls *2768* In patients with IDDM mean serum concentration not significantly different from that in controls *5519*

Soluble Intercellular Adhesion Molecule-1 *Serum* *Increase* In 10 diabetic patients with normoalbuminuria and in 10 with microalbuminuria mean concentrations of 192.7 ± 19.0 ngl/mL and 190.0 ± 20.9 ng/mL respectively significantly different from 162.8 ± 21.8 ng/mL in 10 healthy controls *937* In 70 patients with IDDM mean concentration of 276 ± 71 ng/mL significantly different from 212 ± 57 ng/mL in 70 age-matched healthy controls *1429*

Urine *Increase* In 10 diabetic patients with microalbuminuria mean excretion of 2.226 ± 0.92 ng/mL significantly different from 1.347 ± 0.52 ng/mL in 10 healthy controls *937*

Urine *No Effect* In 10 diabetic patients with normoalbuminuria mean excretion of 1.392 ± 0.68 ngl/mL not significantly different from 1.347 ± 0.52 ng/mL in 10 healthy controls *937*

Soluble Interleukin-2 Receptor *Serum* *No Effect* In 38 children and adolescents with IDDM mean concentration of 1,106 ± 105 U/mL not significantly different from 1,067 ± 99 U/mL in 39 nondiabetic age-matched controls *1662*

Soluble P-Selectin *Serum* *Increase* In 18 newly diagnosed patients with IDDM mean concentration of 210 ± 120 ng/mL, although concentration declined to 127 ± 75 ng/mL 2 years later, compared with 110 ± 31 ng/mL in 18 controls *2768*

Soluble Tumor Necrosis Factor Receptor-p55
Serum *Decrease* In 10 patients with long-standing IDDM mean concentration of 3.58 ± 0.17 µg/L not significantly different from 4.72 ± 0.24 µg/L in 35 healthy controls *3266*

Serum *No Effect* In 18 patients with recent onset IDDM mean concentration of 4.10 ± 0.32 µg/L not significantly different from 4.72 ± 0.24 µg/L in 35 healthy controls *3266*

Soluble Vascular Cell Adhesion Molecule-1
Serum *Increase* In 70 patients with IDDM mean concentration of 781 ± 245 ng/mL significantly different from 615 ± 151 ng/mL in 70 age-matched healthy controls *1429* In patients with IDDM mean serum concentration about 30% higher than in controls *5519*

Somatostatin *Plasma* *Increase* In 13 patients with IDDM without B-cell function baseline concentration of 24.2 ± 2.5 pmol/L compared with 19.7 ± 1.7 pmol/L in 13 age and sex matched controls *4882*

Somatostatin response to Arginine *Plasma* *Increase* In 13 patients with IDDM without residual B-cell function 10 minutes after infusion of arginine caused increase from mean baseline of 24.2 ± 2.5 pmol/L to 31.1 ± 31.1 ± 3.9 pmol/L compared with increase from 19.7 ± 1.7 pmol/L to 23.9 ± 3.4 pmol/L in 13 age and sex matched controls *4882*

Sorbitol *Red Blood Cells* *Increase* In 9 young adults aged 19 - 34 years with IDDM mean concentration of 22.0 ± 3.8 nmol sorbitol/g hemoglobin significantly increased compared with 11.7 ± 1.5 nmol sorbitol/g hemoglobin in 11 healthy controls *982*

Superoxide Dismutase *Red Blood Cells* *Increase* In 13 IDDM patients without retinopathy mean activity of Cu,Zn-SOD 0.70 ± 0.08 units, in 12 with new retinopathy 0.75 ± 0.10 units and in 17 with established retinopathy 0.74 ± 0.13 units significantly higher than 0.64 ± 0.07 units in 20 controls *4888*

Red Blood Cells *No Effect* In 40 patients with type I diabetes mellitus mean concentration of 1.3 ± 0.3 units not significantly different from 1.3 ± 0.3 units in control patients *4887*

Tamm-Horsfall Glycoprotein *Urine* *No Effect* In 41 normotensive, normoalbuminuric patients with IDDM mean overnight excretion of 26.1 µg/mL not significantly different from 23.5 µg/mL in 11 control individuals *737*

250.01 Insulin-dependent Diabetes Mellitus *(continued)*

Taurine *Plasma Decrease* Mean concentration of 65.6 ± 3.1 μmol/L in 35 patients with IDDM significantly less than 93.3 ± 6.3 μmol/L in 34 healthy controls *1553*
Platelets Decrease Mean concentration of 0.66 ± 0.01 mol/g protein in 35 patients with IDDM significantly less than 0.99 ± 0.16 mol/g protein in 34 healthy controls *1553*

Testosterone *Serum Increase* In 20 male patients with IDDM mean concentration of 20.7 nmol/L significantly different from 17.8 nmol/L in 20 healthy controls *834*

Testosterone, Free *Serum No Effect* In 20 male patients with IDDM mean concentration of 0.34 nmol/L not significantly different from 0.40 nmol/L in 20 healthy controls *834*

Theophylline, Free *Serum Increase* In 8 patients with IDDM mean free fraction of 0.61 ± 0.04 versus 0.56 ± 0.02 in 8 healthy controls *2774*

Thiobarbituric Acid-reacting Substances *Serum Increase* In 77 patients with IDDM median concentration of 9.18 μmol/Lcompared with 5.39 μmol/L in 62 healthy controls *1867* In 6 patients with IDDM mean concentration of thiobarbituric acid-reactive substances of 1.74 ± 0.70 μmol/L compared with 1.01 ± 0.21 μmol/L in 47 healthy individuals *5585* In patients with IDDM and no vascular complications concentrations of 1.60 ± 0.24, 2.06 ± 0.27 and 2.50 ± 0.38 μmol/L in patients with HbA_{1c} concentrations of < 7.3, 7.3 - 9.4, and > 9.4% respectively and in IDDM patients with vascular complications of 1.91 ± 0.26, 2.17 ± 0.24, 2.55 ± 0.31 μmol/L at the same HbA_{1c} concentrations compared with 1.41 ± 0.24 μmol/L in healthy controls *4476*

Thrombin/Antithrombin III Complex *Plasma Increase* In 17 patients with IDDM and urinary excretion of albumin of less than 30 mg/d mean concentration of 3.8 μg/L, in 20 with albumin excretion of 30 - 300 mg/d 3.3 μg/L and in 25 with excretion greater than 300 mg/d 3.3 μg/L not significantly increased compared with 3.3 μg/L in 14 healthy controls *3695*

β-Thromboglobulin *Plasma Increase* In 50 patients with IDDM mean concentration of 41 ± 19 ng/mL significantly greater than 27 ± 7 ng/mL in 50 healthy controls *1334*

Tissue Plasminogen Activator *Urine Increase* In 13 IDDM patients without retinopathy mean excretion of 2.65 ± 1.17 U/mL, in 12 with new retinopathy 2.24 ± 1.13 U/mL and in 17 with established retinopathy 2.31 ± 1.28 U/mL significantly higher than 1.19 ± 0.56 U/mL in 20 controls *4888*

Tocopherol *Serum Decrease* In 60 male IDDM patients 5th to 95th percentile of concentrations of 13.23 - 40.54 μmol/L significantly lower than range in 210 healthy men (5th to 95th percentile 18.34 - 45.97 μmol/L) and 18.34 - 42.03 μmol/L in 63 women with IDDM not significantly different from 17.65 - 41.33 μmol/L in 240 healthy women *3906*

α-Tocopherol *Serum Decrease* In 28 men with IDDM median concentrations of 25.5 μmol/L significantly reduced compared with 29.5 μmol/L in 113 male controls *1842*
Serum No Effect Median concentrations of 29.0 μmol/L in 26 women with IDDM not significantly reduced compared with 30.0 μmol/L female controls *1842* In 44 patients with IDDM aged under 45 years mean concentration of 22.43 ± 5.09 μmol/L compared with 22.76 ± 5.96 μmol/L in 18 healthy controls: in 16 patients aged over 45 years mean concentration of 30.78 ± 5.28 μmol/L compared with 29.40 ± 6.89 μmol/L in 8 healthy age-matched controls *3324* In 28 male patients with IDDM 95% CI of 23.8 - 30.1 μmol/L not significantly different from 29.7 - 32.8 μmol/L in 113 nonrelative healthy controls. In 26 women with IDDM 95% CI 26.0 - 31.7 μmol/L compared with 29.4 - 31.9 μmol/L in 123 nonrelative healthy controls *1842*

γ-Tocopherol *Serum Increase* Median concentrations of 1.20 μmol/L in 26 women with IDDM significantly increased compared with 0.78 μmol/L female controls *1842*
Serum No Effect In 28 male patients with IDDM 95% CI of 1.03 - 1.62 μmol/L not significantly different from 0.89 - 1.17 μmol/L in 113 nonrelative healthy controls. In 26 women with IDDM 95% CI 1.10 - 1.57 μmol/L compared with 0.63 - 0.95 μmol/L in 123 nonrelative healthy controls *1842* In 28 men with IDDM median concentrations of 1.27 μmol/L not significantly increased compared with 0.86 μmol/L in 113 male controls *1842*

Tocopherol:Retinol Ratio *Serum No Effect* In 60 male IDDM patients 5th to 95th percentile of concentrations of 4.13 - 8.84 not significantly different from range in 210 healthy men (5th to 95th percentile 3.85 - 7.56) and 3.60 - 7.32 in 63 women with IDDM not significantly different from 4.06 - 7.13 in 240 healthy women *3906*

Transferrin *Serum Decrease* Mean concentration in 23 patients with poorly controlled IDDM of 2.31 ± 0.41 g/L significantly lower than 2.85 ± 0.29 g/L in 23 healthy control men *1629*

Transforming Growth Factor-β *Urine Increase* Mean excretion in 18 normoalbuminuric patients of 5.43 pg/min, in 13 IDDM patients with microalbuminuria 39.95 pg/min and 13.22 pg/min in 15 patients compared with that in 16 nondiabetic healthy normotensive individuals, 3.01 - 32.10 pg/min or 2.55 - 36.30 ng/g *1339*

Triglycerides *Serum Increase* In patients with IDDM mean concentration increased in poorly controlled patients *3853* In 40 patients with IDDM and nephropathy mean concentration of 1.6 ± 1.2 mmol/L significantly different from 1.0 ± 0.55 mmol/L in 49 patients with IDDM but without nephropathy for 5 - 10 years *5010* In children whose diabetes was poorly or fairly controlled significantly increased *63* In 78 patients with IDDM median concentration of 1.57 mmol/L significantly different from 1.03 mmol/L in 82 healthy controls *10* In 12 patients with IDDM mean concentration of 1.77 ± 1.96 mmol/L significantly greater than 0.90 ± 0.64 mmol/L in 29 healthy controls *4719* In 33 NIDDM patients mean concentration of 2.57 ± 2.56 mmol/L not significantly different from 1.20 ± 1.40 mmol/L in 19 healthy controls *3403*
Serum No Effect In 51 men with IDDM mean concentration of 0.97 ± 0.34 mmol/L not significantly different from 1.17 ± 0.56 mmol/L in 48 control men and in 35 women with IDDM mean concentration of 1.01 ± 0.75 mmol/L not significantly different from 1.05 ± 0.61 mmol/L in 26 control women *2528* Median concentration in 42 patients with IDDM of 92 mg/dL not significantly different from 104 mg/dL in 42 healthy controls *2446* In 77 patients with IDDM median concentration of 1.11 mmol/L compared with 1.16 mmol/L in 62 healthy controls *1867* In 70 patients with IDDM mean concentration of 1.23 ± 0.58 mmol/L not significantly different from 1.44 ± 0.57 mmol/L in 70 age-matched healthy controls *1429* In 50 IDDM patients mean concentration of 119 ± 64 mg/dL (regardless of HbA_{1C} concentration) not significantly different from 109 ± 74 mg/dL in 50 healthy controls *1334* In 52 patients with IDDM mean concentration of 1.2 ± 0.9 mmol/L not significantly different from that in 52 healthy controls in whom the mean concentration was 1.2 ± 0.6 mmol/L *866* In 45 pairs of identical diabetic twins mean concentration of 1.36 ± 1.00 mmol/L compared with 1.67 ± 1.05 mmol/L in 45 pairs of nondiabetic twins and 1.38 ± 0.79 mmol/L in 45 nondibetic controls *1246* Mean concentration of 1.14 ± 0.05 mmol/L in 142 patients with IDDM significantly lower than 1.99 ± 0.17 mmol/L in 70 patients with NIDDM but not significantly different from normal range *470* In 44 patients with IDDM aged under 45 years mean concentration of 0.92 ± 0.55 mmol/L compared with 1.0 ± 0.39 mmol/L in 18 healthy controls aged under 45 years: in 16 patients aged over 45 years with IDDM mean concentration of 1.28 ± 0.60 mmol/L compared with 1.38 ± 0.79 mmol/L in 8 healthy controls *3324* In patients with IDDM mean concentration increased in well controlled patients *3853* In 118 patients with IDDM mean concentration of 1.04 ± 0.59 mmol/L not significantly different from 1.50 ± 1.15 mmol/L in 286 healthy controls *725*

Tumor Necrosis Factor-α *Serum Increase* Median concentration of 29 pg/mL in patients with newly diagnosed IDDM and 17 pg/mL in patients with long standing IDDM significantly increased when compared with 0.0 pg/mL in normal controls *2307*

Type III Collagen *Urine Increase* Mean excretion in 18 normoalbuminuric patients of 9.30 ng/min, in 13 IDDM patients with microalbuminuria of 26.89 ng/min, and 18.42 ng/min in 15 patients compared with that in 16 nondiabetic healthy normotensive individuals, 0.96 - 6.58 ng/min or 1.38 - 9.37 μg/g *1339*

Tyrosine Phosphatase-like Protein IA2-Antibodies
Serum Increase In 100 children with IDDM, GADA 65 antibodies detected with IA2-Ab and ICA in 46 children, with ICA only in 16, with IA2-Ab only in one and by themselves in 4, with all three antibodies only being detected in one control child *530*

Ubiquinol:Cholesterol Ratio *Serum* *Decrease* In 33 patients with IDDM mean ratio of 0.17 ± 0.05 µmol/mmol significantly different from 0.22 ± 0.05 µmol/mmol in 19 healthy controls *3403*

Urea *Serum* *Increase* In 28 men with IDDM and 26 women with IDDM mean concentrations of 12.9 ± 2.4 mmol/L and 12.2 ± 2.4 mmol/L respectively *1842*
Serum *No Effect* In 28 male patients with IDDM mean concentration of 12.9 ± 2.4 µmol/L and 12.2 ± 2.4 µmol/L in 26 women with IDDM *1842*

Uric Acid *Serum* *Decrease* In 33 patients with IDDM mean concentration of 256 ± 78 µmol/L in men and 151 ± 33 µmol/L in women significantly different from 346 ± 47 µmol/L in male and 256 ± 58 µmol/L in healthy female controls *5500*
Serum *Increase* In 28 men with IDDM and 26 women with IDDM mean concentrations of 246.1 ± 49.4 µmol/L and 194.5 ± 68.5 µmol/L respectively *1842* In 28 male patients with IDDM mean concentration of 246 ± 49 µmol/L and 195 ± 69 µmol/L in 26 women with IDDM *1842* In 77 patients with IDDM median concentration of 291 µmol/L compared with 266 µmol/L in 62 healthy controls *1867*

Vascular Endothelial Growth Factor *Serum* *No Effect* In 40 children with IDDM mean concentration of 138.3 ± 16.0 pg/mL not significantly different from 183.9 ± 31.7 pg/mL in 30 healthy pediatric controls *3258*

Viscosity *Plasma* *Increase* In 50 patients with IDDM mean viscosity of 1.9 ± 0.1 centipoises significantly increased compared with 1.7 ± 0.1 centipoises in 50 healthy controls *1334*

Vitamin E *Serum* *No Effect* In 77 patients with IDDM median concentration of 22.7 µmol/L compared with 26.5 µmol/L in 62 healthy controls *1867* Mean concentration of 25.9 ± 0.5 µmol/Lin 142 patients with IDDM not significantly different from normal range *470*

VLDL-Cholesterol *Serum* *Increase* In children with poor or fair control concentration significantly increased *63*

VLDL-Triglycerides *Serum* *Decrease* In 51 men with IDDM mean concentration of 0.44 ± 0.23 mmol/L significantly different from 0.67 ± 0.47 mmol/L in 48 control men and in 35 women with IDDM mean concentration of 0.46 ± 0.58 mmol/L not significantly different from 0.51 ± 0.49 mmol/L in 26 control women *2528*
Serum *Increase* In children with diabetes mellitus in whom control was poor or fair, concentration significantly increased *63*

von Willebrand Factor Antigen *Plasma* *Increase* Median concentration in 42 patients with IDDM of 96 U/dL significantly different from 87 U/dL in 42 healthy controls *2446* In 17 patients with IDDM and urinary excretion of albumin of less than 30 mg/d mean concentration of 1.18 mU/L, in 20 patients with albumin excretion of 30 - 300 mg/d 1.16 mU/L, and in 25 with albumin excretion greater than 300 mg/d 1.24 mU/L compared with 0.95 mU/L in 14 healthy controls *3695*

Water Clearance *Urine* *Increase* In 13 well-controlled patients with IDDM median clearance of 14.1 ± 5.3 significantly different from 8.9 ± 2.6 in 11 matched healthy controls *3501*

Zeaxanthin *Serum* *No Effect* In 28 men with IDDM median concentration of 0.06 µmol/L not significantly different when compared with 0.06 µmol/L in 113 male controls and 0.07 µmol/L in 26 women with IDDM not significantly different when compared with 0.06 µmol/L female controls *1842* In 60 male IDDM patients 5th to 95th percentile of concentrations of 0.014 - 0.123 µmol/L not significantly different from range in 210 healthy men (5th to 95th percentile of 0.020 - 0.132 µmol/L) and 0.022 - 0.122 µmol/L in 63 women with IDDM not significantly different from 0.020 - 0.132 µmol/L in 240 healthy women *3906* In 28 male patients with IDDM 95% CI of 0.05 - 0.07 µmol/L not significantly different from 0.06 - 0.08 µmol/L in 113 nonrelative healthy controls. In 26 women with IDDM 95% CI 0.05 - 0.08 µmol/L compared with 0.06 - 0.08 µmol/L in 123 nonrelative healthy controls *1842*

Zinc *Lymphocytes* *No Effect* In 45 children with IDDM mean concentration of 1.4 ± 0.11 µmol/10^{10} cells compared with 1.5 ± 0.23 µmol/10^{10} cells in 12 healthy children *3049*
Neutrophils *No Effect* In 45 children with IDDM mean concentration of 1.1 ± 0.093 µmol/10^{10} cells not significantly different from 1.2 ± 0.24 µmol/10^{10} cells in 12 healthy children *4406*
Red Blood Cells *Decrease* In 45 children with IDDM mean concentration of 0.48 ± 0.12 µmol/g hemoglobin significantly less than 0.57 ± 0.046 µmol/g hemoglobin in 12 healthy control children *4406*
Serum *Increase* In 16 patients with stabilized diabetes mean concentration of 16.62 ± 2.55 µmol/L compared with 15.24 ± 2.22 µmol/L in reference population *1434*
Serum *No Effect* In 45 children with IDDM mean concentration of 14.4 ± 0.52 µmol/L not significantly different from 15.0 ± 0.86 µmol/L in 12 healthy children *4406*

250.01 Juvenile-onset Diabetes

6-Keto-Prostaglandin $F_{1\alpha}$ *Urine* *Decrease* In urine from individuals with juvenile-onset diabetes excretion reduced compared with that in normal individuals *4187*

250.10 Diabetic Acidosis

Alanine Aminotransferase *Serum* *Increase* In some instances, mostly in severe cases, especially with severe circulatory failure and liver enlargement *372*

Amylase *Serum* *Increase* Occurs frequently; 21 of 35 patients (60%) had elevated concentrations. Occurs most often when blood sugar > 500 mg/dL *1783* Raised in ketoacidosis *5579* Elevated levels *5618* 21 of 35 patients were hyperamylasemic, with 6 showing values > 1,000 Somogyi U. No relation was found between degree of elevation and morbidity and mortality or acidosis or azotemia. Relation was found with degrees of hyperglycemia *2718*

Aspartate Aminotransferase *Serum* *Increase* In some instances, mostly in severe cases, especially with severe circulatory failure and liver enlargement *372* Mild-moderate abnormalities may occur in 20 - 65% of patients but bears no relation to degree of abdominal pain or prognosis *2819*

Bicarbonate *Serum* *Decrease* May be < 2 mmol/L in profound cases and 15 mmol/L in severe cases *5679* Metabolic acidosis may occur *1980*

Carbon Dioxide Partial Pressure *Blood* *Decrease* Metabolic acidosis may occur *1980* Hyperventilation *5679*

Cholinesterase *Serum* *Decrease* Decreases 2 - 3 days after episodes of ketoacidosis *372*

Copper *Serum* *No Effect* In 16 patients with diabetic ketoacidosis on admission to hospital mean concentration of 17.22 ± 3.91 µmol/L not significantly increased compared with 16.55 ± 3.51 µmol/L in reference population *1434*

Creatine *Urine* *Increase* Urinary creatine may be significantly increased in patients with diabetic acidosis *2952*

Creatine Kinase *Serum* *Increase* Mild-moderate abnormalities may occur in 20 - 65% of patients but bears no relation to degree of abdominal pain or prognosis *2819*

Eosinophils *Blood* *Decrease* Often a polymorphonucleocytosis with a lymphopenia and eosinopenia *1980*

Glucagon *Plasma* *Increase* Frequently observed *3654*

Glucose *Serum* *Increase* Seldom in excess of 800 mg/dL *2819* Increased, usually > 300 mg/dL *5544*

Glutamate Dehydrogenase *Serum* *Increase* In some instances, mostly in severe cases, especially with severe circulatory failure and liver enlargement *372*

γ-Glutamyltransferase *Saliva* *Increase* Significantly higher (11.6 U/L) versus controls (5.12 U/L) *2448*

Glutathione Peroxidase *Serum* *Decrease* In 16 patients with diabetic ketoacidosis on admission to hospital mean activity of 337 ± 84.0 U/L not significantly less than 400 ± 68 U/L in 20 adult control patients *1434*

Growth Hormone *Plasma* *Increase* Reported effect *5679*

Hematocrit *Blood* *Increase* Secondary to dehydration *2039* May be moderately increased because of hemoconcentration *1980*

Isocitrate Dehydrogenase *Serum* *Increase* In some instances, mostly in severe cases, especially with severe circulatory failure and liver enlargement *372*

Ketones *Serum* *Increase* β-hydroxybutyrate accumulates and is one of the major causes of acidosis as a result of disturbed carbohydrate and fat metabolism *4214* Initial values range from 11.3 - 15 mmol/L in several studies. Target ketone concentration was reached in 4 - 7 h *2819*
Urine *Increase* Accumulates and is one of the major causes of acidosis as a result of disturbed carbohydrate and fat metabolism *4214*

250.10 Diabetic Acidosis *(continued)*

Lactate *Blood* *Increase* Coexistent and biochemically significant lactic acidosis is a relatively infrequent complication of ketoacidosis; usually due to underlying disorders associated with poor tissue perfusion *2819* Accumulates and is one of the major causes of acidosis as a result of disturbed carbohydrate and fat metabolism *4214*

Lactate Dehydrogenase *Serum* *Increase* In some instances, mostly severe cases, especially with severe circulatory failure and liver enlargement *372*

Leukocytes *Blood* *Increase* Often a polymorphonucleocytosis with a lymphopenia and eosinopenia *1980* Leukocytosis is common (15,000 - 30,000 /μL) *5679*

Lipase *Serum* *Increase* In patients with diabetic ketoacidosis activity may be increased *5231*
Serum *No Effect* Normal levels *4289*

Lipids *Serum* *Increase* Level of serum sodium depends on degree of increased plasma lipids *2039* Often found *1980*

Lymphocytes *Blood* *Decrease* Often a polymorphonucleocytosis with a lymphopenia and eosinopenia *1980*

Magnesium *Serum* *Increase* In the early phase *1980*

Malate Dehydrogenase *Serum* *Increase* In some instances, mostly severe cases, especially with severe circulatory failure and liver enlargement *372*

Malondialdehyde *Serum* *Increase* In 16 patients with diabetic ketoacidosis on admission to hospital mean concentration of 3.03 ± 0.27 μmol/L significantly increased compared with 2.51 ± 0.25 μmol/L in 31 healthy adult controls *1434*

Neutrophils *Blood* *Increase* May be associated with a moderate to severe neutrophilia *5677*

Norepinephrine *Plasma* *Increase* With fasting, profound exercise and orthostatic changes, norepinephrine secretion is enhanced *5679*
Plasma *No Effect* Following insulin-induced hypoglycemia, there is no change *5452*

Organic Hydroperoxides *Serum* *Increase* In 16 patients with diabetic ketoacidosis mean concentration of 150.7 ± 19.1 μmol/L significantly greater than 127.8 ± 14 μmol/L in 20 healthy adult controls *1434*

pH *Blood* *Decrease* Acidosis with low plasma pH and bicarbonate (usually < 10 mmol/L) is seen *2039* Metabolic acidosis may occur *1980*

Phosphate *Serum* *Decrease* Common in patients recovering from severe diabetic ketoacidosis *2719* Common; usually becomes manifest in 4 - 12 h of institution of therapy *2819* During successful treatment of diabetic ketosis insulin causes phosphate ions to enter the cells with glucose and potassium *1290*

Potassium *Serum* *Decrease* Renal wasting leads to hypokalemic state *3735* Total body deficit. Only 4 - 10% have decreased plasma concentrations and these patients are at high risk for developing life-threatening hypokalemia during early hours of treatment *3312* Despite the markedly negative K^+ balance, hyperkalemia is often present because the acidosis causes the K^+ to shift from inside the cells into the extracellular space *5679*
Serum *Increase* Despite the markedly negative K^+ balance, hyperkalemia is often present because the acidosis causes the K^+ to shift from inside the cells into the extracellular space *5679* Usually normal or elevated, despite total body deficit. Only 4 - 10% have decreased plasma concentrations and these patients are at high risk for developing life-threatening hypokalemia during early hours of treatment *3312* Impaired uptake by the cells secondary to acidosis and increased liberation of cell potassium following protein breakdown and gluconeogenesis *1290*

Prolactin *Plasma* *Increase* Elevated in 8 patients, (24.8 ± 10.2 ng/mL). After correction of the ketoacidosis, levels decreased to 10.9 ± 6.4 ng/mL (normal range: men 4.9 ± 0.8, women 5.1 ± 1.6 ng/mL) *2016*

Protein *Serum* *Increase* Secondary to dehydration *2039*

Pyruvate *Blood* *Increase* Can be demonstrated after removal of acetoacetic acid *1290*

Selenium *Serum* *Decrease* In 16 patients with ketoacidosis on admission to hospital mean concentration of 0.89 ± 0.18 μmol/L not significantly reduced compared with 1.08 ± 0.20 μmol/L in healthy reference population *1434*

Sodium *Serum* *Decrease* Despite the markedly negative sodium balance, the plasma concentration may be hypernormal, normal or subnormal *5679*
Serum *Increase* Despite the markedly negative sodium balance, the plasma concentration may be hypernormal, normal or subnormal *5679* May be normal or elevated depending on the relative losses of sodium and water and the degree of increased plasma lipids. Because of the increase in plasma lipids a sodium concentration of 150 mmol/L of plasma may represent 170 mmol/L of water *2039*

Sorbitol Dehydrogenase *Serum* *Increase* In some instances, mostly in severe cases, especially with severe circulatory failure and liver enlargement *372*

Thyroxine (T4) *Serum* *Decrease* In 19 euthyroid patients with severe ketoacidosis, a 'low T3 syndrome' was found, with lowered serum concentrations of T3, increased reverse T3, slightly low T4 (T4) and normal thyrotropin *3701*

Tri-iodothyronine (T3) *Serum* *Decrease* In 19 euthyroid patients with severe ketoacidosis a 'low T3 syndrome' was found, with lowered serum concentrations of T3, increased reverse T3, slightly low T4, and normal thyrotropin *3701*

Urea Nitrogen *Serum* *Increase* May reflect prerenal azotemia or diabetic nephropathy *1980*

Uric Acid *Serum* *Increase* Frequently increased *2039* Often found *1980* Elevated in 50% of patients; parallels the degree of ketoacidosis and returns to normal when diabetes is controlled *3969*

Zinc *Serum* *Decrease* In 16 patients hospitalized with diabetic ketoacidosis mean concentration of 12.11 ± 2.02 μmol/L significantly reduced compared with 15.24 ± 2.22 μmol/L in reference population *1434*

250.40 Diabetic Nephropathy

Ammonium Ions *Urine* *Decrease* May cause distal renal tubular acidosis (type IV) is associated with hyperkalemia, hyperchloremic metabolic acidosis, urine pH < 5.5, decreased urinary ammonium ion excretion, a positive urine anion gap, normal urinary citrate and urinary calcium excretion *4071*

Anion Gap *Urine* *Increase* May cause distal renal tubular acidosis (type IV) is associated with hyperkalemia, hyperchloremic metabolic acidosis, urine pH < 5.5, decreased urinary ammonium ion excretion, a positive urine anion gap, normal urinary citrate and urinary calcium excretion *4071*

Arginine *Plasma* *No Effect* In 6 patients with diabetic nephropathy without dialysis concentrations of 143 - 362 ng/mL not different from 63 - 508 ng/mL in 10 normal controls *2331*

Calcium *Urine* *No Effect* May cause distal renal tubular acidosis (type IV) is associated with hyperkalemia, hyperchloremic metabolic acidosis, urine pH < 5.5, decreased urinary ammonium ion excretion, a positive urine anion gap, normal urinary citrate and urinary calcium excretion *4071*

Chloride *Serum* *Increase* May cause distal renal tubular acidosis (type IV) is associated with hyperkalemia, hyperchloremic metabolic acidosis, urine pH < 5.5, decreased urinary ammonium ion excretion, a positive urine anion gap, normal urinary citrate and urinary calcium excretion *4071*

Citrate *Urine* *No Effect* May cause distal renal tubular acidosis (type IV) is associated with hyperkalemia, hyperchloremic metabolic acidosis, urine pH < 5.5, decreased urinary ammonium ion excretion, a positive urine anion gap, normal urinary citrate and urinary calcium excretion *4071*

Creatine *Serum* *No Effect* In 6 patients with diabetic nephropathy concentrations of 27 - 85 ng/mL not different from 7 - 128 ng/mL in 10 normal controls *2331*

Creatinine *Serum* *Increase* In 6 patients with diabetic nephropathy concentrations of 58 - 500 ng/mL higher than 17 - 103 ng/mL in 10 normal controls *2331*

D-Dimer *Urine* *Increase* In 8 patients with diabetic nephropathy median concentration of 16.9 ng/mL significantly different from that in normal controls in whom the mean concentration was 0.69 ± 0.60 ng/mL *4789*

Fibrin/Fibrinogen Degradation Product E *Urine* *Increase* In 10 patients with diabetic nephropathy mean excretion of 93.8 ± 146.3 ng/mL significantly different from 1.68 ± 1.05 ng/mL in 30 controls *4790*

Guanidine *Serum* *Increase* In 6 patients with diabetic nephropathy concentrations of 0 - 0.33 ng/mL higher than undetectable amounts in 10 normal controls *2331*

Guanidinoacetic Acid *Serum* *Increase* In 6 patients with diabetic nephropathy concentrations of 1.29 - 3.97 ng/mL higher than 0.58 - 2.03 ng/mL in 10 normal controls *2331*

γ-Guanidinobutyric Acid *Serum* *No Effect* In 6 patients with diabetic nephropathy concentrations of 0 ng/mL not different from undetectable amounts in 10 normal controls *2331*

β-Guanidinopropionic Acid *Serum* *Increase* In 6 patients with diabetic nephropathy concentrations of 0 - 0.20 ng/mL higher than undetectable amounts in 10 normal controls *2331*

Guanidinosuccinic Acid *Serum* *Increase* In 6 patients with diabetic nephropathy concentrations of 0.94 - 13.20 ng/mL higher than undetectable amounts in 10 normal controls *2331*

Methylguanidine *Serum* *Increase* In 6 patients with diabetic nephropathy concentrations of 0 - 1.05 ng/mL higher than undetectable amounts in 10 normal controls *2331*

pH *Urine* *Decrease* May cause distal renal tubular acidosis (type IV) is associated with hyperkalemia, hyperchloremic metabolic acidosis, urine pH < 5.5, decreased urinary ammonium ion excretion, a positive urine anion gap, normal urinary citrate and urinary calcium excretion *4071*

Potassium *Serum* *Increase* May cause distal renal tubular acidosis (type IV) which is associated with hyperkalemia, hyperchloremic metabolic acidosis, urine pH < 5.5, decreased urinary ammonium ion excretion, a positive urine anion gap, normal urinary citrate and urinary calcium excretion *4071*

Renin *Plasma* *Increase* Mean concentration in 12 diabetics with microalbuminuria of 316 ± 128 ng/L significantly different from 236 ± 110 ng/L in 43 diabetics with normoalbuminuria *3354*

Taurocyamine *Serum* *Increase* In 6 patients with diabetic nephropathy concentrations of 0 - 0.59 ng/mL different from undetectable amounts in 10 normal controls *2331*

250.50 Diabetic Retinopathy, Proliferative

Hepatocyte Growth Factor *Vitreous Fluid* *Increase* Median concentration in fluids from 73 patients with proliferative diabetic retinopathy of 6.00 ng/mL significantly different from 2.86 ng/mL in fluids from 17 nondiabetic controls *2583*

Protein *Vitreous Fluid* *No Effect* Mean concentration in fluids from 73 patients with proliferative diabetic retinopathy of 6.00 ± 2.98 mg/mL not different from 7.43 ± 0.05 mg/mL in fluids from 17 nondiabetic controls *2583*

Vascular Endothelial Growth Factor *Vitreous Fluid* *Increase* Median concentration in fluids from 73 patients with proliferative diabetic retinopathy of 1.62 ng/mL significantly different from 0.16 ng/mL in fluids from 17 nondiabetic controls *2583*

251.20 Functional Hypoglycemia

Dopamine *Plasma* *Increase* Type 1 functional hypoglycemia, according to OGTT, associated with high conceration prior to glucose administration *2955*

Epinephrine:Norepinephrine Ratio *Plasma* *Decrease* Type 3 functional hypoglycemia, according to OGTT, associated with low ratio prior to glucose administration *2955*
Plasma *Increase* Type I functional hypoglycemia, according to OGTT, associated with high ratio prior to glucose administration *2955*

5-Hydroxytryptamine, Free *Plasma* *Increase* Type 2 functional hypoglycemia, according to OGTT, associated with high ratio prior to glucose administration *2955*

3-Methoxy-4-hydroxyphenylglycol *Plasma* *Increase* Type 3 functional hypoglycemia, according to OGTT, associated with high concentration prior to glucose administration *2955*

Norepinephrine *Plasma* *Increase* Type 3 functional hypoglycemia, according to OGTT, associated with high concentration prior to glucose administration *2955*

251.20 Hypoglycemia, Unspecified

Glucose *Serum* *Decrease* In 3 patients with hypoglycemia of uncertain cause mean concentrations of 1.8 - 2.1 mmol/L significantly different from normal range of 4.0 - 6.2 mmol/L *3332* Insulin excess probably due to excessively rapid absorption as in postgastrectomy. This may occur particularly in: underweight, poorly nourished babies; twins; premature infants. A low birth-weight baby with a proportionally large head is very prone to hypoglycemia. Infants of diabetic mothers (fetal blood glucose is controlled by the maternal blood glucose level, but at term the newborn infant's pancreas may respond to maternal hyperglycemia by secretion of insulin and hence hypoglycemia) *1290*

Glycine *Plasma* *Increase* Persistently elevated and is generally higher than in secondary hyperglycinemias *900*
Urine *Increase* Persistently elevated and are generally higher than in secondary hyperglycinemias *900*

Growth Hormone *Plasma* *Increase* Reported effect *1290*

Insulin *Plasma* *Increase* Increased in reactive hypoglycemia after glucose ingestion, particularly when a diabetic type of glucose tolerance curve is present *5544*
Plasma *No Effect* Normal in hypoglycemia associated with nonpancreatic tumors. Normal in idiopathic hypoglycemia of childhood except after administration of leucine *5544*

Insulin-like Growth Factor-I *Serum* *Decrease* In 3 patients with hypoglycemia of uncertain cause mean concentrations of 36 - 103 μg/L different from normal range of 90 - 360 μg/L *3332*

Insulin-like Growth Factor-II *Serum* *Decrease* In 3 patients with hypoglycemia of uncertain cause mean concentrations of 94 - 494 μg/L different from normal range of 490 - 1,056 μg/L *3332*

Insulin-like Growth Factor Binding Protein-3
Serum *Decrease* In 3 patients with hypoglycemia of uncertain cause mean concentration of 0.2 - 1.2 μg/mL significantly different from normal range of 1.7 - 4.0 μg/mL *3332*

Prolactin *Plasma* *Increase* Increased levels *4289* Can trigger a mild to moderate increase (20 - 300 ng/mL) *3391*

251.50 Zollinger-Ellison Syndrome

Albumin *Serum* *Decrease* Serum concentration in 20 patients with proved or presumed ZE syndrome (4.1 ± 0.8 g/dL) were significantly lower than observed in 40 normal controls (5.1 ± 0.3). 40 duodenal ulcer patients (5.1 ± 0.4 g/dL). Total gastrectomy induced a rise in serum albumin in 8 patients studied *2904* A low serum albumin will reflect possible malabsorption of protein or protein-losing enteropathy *1980*

Alkaline Phosphatase *Serum* *Decrease* An indication of vitamin D and calcium malabsorption *1980*

Calcitonin *Plasma* *Increase* In some cases *2144*

Calcium *Serum* *Decrease* An indication of vitamin D and calcium malabsorption *1980*

Carotene *Serum* *Decrease* A useful indication of fat malabsorption, low levels are found in as many as 80% of patients with steatorrhea *1980*

β-Chorionic Gonadotropin *Plasma* *Increase* Significant correlation between basal levels and malignant gastrinoma but not with benign tumors *4970*

Fat *Feces* *Increase* Hyperacidity in duodenum inactivates pancreatic enzymes *1980*

Gastrin *Serum* *Increase* Concentrations reach 2,800 - 300,000 pg/mL associated with non- insulin producing pancreatic tumors *1290* Patients with gastrinoma (Zollinger-Ellison syndrome) may have increased serum concentrations *2952* Significant correlation between basal levels and malignant gastrinoma but not with benign tumors *4970*

Lipids *Feces* *Increase* Hyperacidity in duodenum inactivates pancreatic enzymes *1980*

Lymphocytes *Blood* *Decrease* Often an absolute lymphopenia due to loss of lymphocytes into the small intestine *1980*

pH *Gastric Material* *Increase* Gastric secretion > 100 mmol/12 h is strongly indicative of this disorder *1733* Markedly elevated levels of gastric acid secretion *5679*

Phosphate *Serum* *Decrease* An indication of vitamin D and calcium malabsorption *1980*

Potassium *Serum* *Decrease* Hypokalemia; frequently associated with chronic severe diarrhea *5545*

Prolactin *Plasma* *Increase* Observed effect *4746* Levels were measured in 36 patients with ZES, eight patients had elevated levels *4971*

251.50 Zollinger-Ellison Syndrome (continued)

Protein *Feces* *Increase* Hyperacidity in duodenum inactivates pancreatic enzymes *1980*

Prothrombin Time *Plasma* *Increase* An indication of vitamin K malabsorption *1980*

Triolein ^{131}I Test *Feces* *Positive* Positive test for lipid droplets in the stool, but results are inconsistent *1980*

252.00 Hyperparathyroidism

Acid Phosphatase *Serum* *Increase* Observed in some patients *1642* Found in 28 cases with definite skeletal changes. Activity was increased in every instance from 1.4-16 times the normal maximum *1935*

Acid Phosphatase, Tartrate Resistant *Serum* *Increase* In patients with primary hyperparathyroidism moderate increase observed *4217* In 3 premenopausal hyperparathyroid women mean concentration of 321 (range 268 - 371) µg/L, 19.5 (8.1 - 26.3) U/L and 352 (340 - 388) µg/L, 16.1 (11.7 - 21.8) U/L in 3 postmenopausal women significantly greater than mean concentration and range of 178 (41 - 288) µg/L, 5.6 (1.8 - 10.3) U/L in 29 healthy premenopausal women and 302 (range 129 - 348) µg/L, 7.5 (range 4.2 - 12.9) U/L in 12 healthy postmenopausal women *812* In 15 patients with primary hyperparathyroidism mean activity of 10.8 ± 2.5 U/L significantly higher than 7.4 ± 1.8 U/L in 26 healthy controls *1063* In 17 patients with primary hyperparathyroidism mean activity of 18.0 ± 1.0 U/L compared with normal values of 12.9 ± 2.4 U/L *3506*
Serum *No Effect* In 17 patients with secondary hyperparathyroidism mean activity of 7.5 ± 4.5 U/L not significantly different from 7.4 ± 1.8 U/L in 26 healthy controls *1063*

Adenosine Monophosphate *Urine* *Increase* Urinary cyclic AMP may be significantly increased in about 85% of patients with hyperparathyroidism *2952* In 39 patients with hyperparathyroidism mean excretion 88 nmol/L glomerular filtrate (median 62) significantly greater than reference range of less than 60 nmol/L glomerular filtrate *5552* Parathyroid hormone action on the kidney leads to increased cAMP excretion. Mean urinary concentration was almost twice that of normals *3255*
Urine *No Effect* In 21 patients, mean urinary excretion of cAMP/24h was 5.0 ± 1.9 µmol uncorrected. When correlated to albumin-corrected serum calcium, this overlap between hyperparathyroidism and normality disappears completely. Excretion is influenced to a considerable degree by the biological activity of circulating parathyroid hormone *3196* Urinary excretion usually normal *3255*

Alkaline Phosphatase *Serum* *Increase* In 17 patients with primary hyperparathyroidism mean activity of 192.5 ± 38 U/L compared with normal values of 75 ± 18 U/L *3506* In 11 patients with primary hyperparathyroidism median activity of 145 U/L not significantly higher than 125 U/L in 90 healthy controls *2572* Found to be elevated in only 30%, and each of these showed normal results for other liver function tests. Correlated well with serum calcium, but only significant in female patients *3255* In 77 postmenopausal women with asymptomatic primary hyperparathyroidism median activity of 126 U/L not significantly different from reference interval of 93 - 250 U/L *27* Following the removal of the parathyroid tumor, the increased serum concentration persists and may even rise temporarily, falling gradually over a period of months as bone repair is completed *1290* In 62 untreated patients with primary hyperparathyroidism mean activity of 2.0 ± 0.1 µkat/L compared with 1.5 ± 0.1 µkat/L in 25 postoperative patients and reference interval of < 1.7 µkat/L *4826*

Alkaline Phosphatase, Bone Isoenzyme *Serum* *Increase* In patients with primary hyperparathyroidism moderate increase observed *4217*
Serum *No Effect* Mean activity of 29.3 U/L in 20 patients with primary hyperparathyroidism not significantly different from reference intervals of 15.0 - 41.3 U/L in men and 11.6 - 30.6 U/L in premenopausal women *1799*

Amino Acids *Urine* *Increase* Quite common *5679*

Ammonium Ions *Urine* *Increase* Primary hyperparathyroidism may be associated with classic distal renal tubular acidosis which is asociated with hyokalemia, hyperchloremic metabolic acidosis, urine pH > 5.5, increased urinary ammonium ion excretion, a negative urine anion gap, increased urinary osmol gap, decreased urinary citrate and increased urinary calcium in some patients *4071*

Anion Gap *Urine* *Decrease* Primary hyperparathyroidism may be associated with classic distal renal tubular acidosis which is asociated with hyokalemia, hyperchloremic metabolic acidosis, urine pH > 5.5, increased urinary ammonium ion excretion, a negative urine anion gap, increased urinary osmol gap, decreased urinary citrate and increased urinary calcium in some patients *4071*

Antibody Titer *Serum* *Increase* Parathyroid antibodies *3712*

Bicarbonate *Serum* *Decrease* Decreased bicarbonate in 24% of cases *3255*

Bone Sialoprotein *Serum* *Increase* In 26 patients with primary hyperparathyroidism median concentration of 17.8 ng/mL significantly higher than that in 75 healthy men in whom the median concentration was 9.8 ng/mL and in 20 premenopausal women, 8.7 ng/mL, and in 38 postmenopausal women, 11.9 ng/mL *4716* In 11 patients with primary hyperparathyroidism mean concentration of 24.7 ± 13.5 µg/L significantly higher than that in 90 healthy controls in whom the mean concentration was 12.1 ± 5.0 µg/L *2572*

Calcitonin *Plasma* *Decrease* Observed effect *1290* *1069*

Calcium *Cerebrospinal Fluid* *Increase* In 22 patients with primary hyperparathyroidism mean concentration of 1.21 ± 0.08 mmol/L significantly higher than in 11 normocalcemic controls *2451*
Serum *Increase* Increased concentrations are seen in primary hyperparathyroidism (concentrations may double in severe cases) *2952* In 17 patients with primary hyperparathyroidism mean concentration increased to 2.87 ± 0.03 mmol/L *3506* In 26 patients with primary hyperparathyroidism median concentration of 2.80 mmol/L significantly higher than that in 75 healthy men in whom the median concentration was 2.38 mmol/L and in 20 premenopausal women, 2.39 mmol/L, and in 38 postmenopausal women, 2.41 mmol/L *4716* Of 50 primary cases, 47 had increased concentration (> 10.3 mg/dL) *4393* In 11 patients with primary hyperparathyroidism median concentration of 2.83 mmol/L significantly higher than 2.35 mmol/L in 90 healthy controls *2572* In 77 postmenopausal women with asymptomatic primary hyperparathyroidism median concentration of 2.94 mmol/L significantly different from reference interval of 2.12 - 2.60 mmol/L *27* In 149 samples, 0.7% of serum ionized calcium and 7.5% of total calcium determinations were within the normal range. All patients exhibited abnormally elevated values upon repeated testing *1298* Hyperparathyroidism associated with pathologic lesions, shows hypercalcemia of 10.5 mg/dL. Probably the single most important diagnostic aid *1025* In 39 patients with hyperparathyroidism mean concentration of 2.92 mmol/L (median 2.78 mmol/L) significantly greater than reference range of 2.20 - 2.65 mmol/L *5552* In 62 untreated patients with primary hyperparathyroidism mean concentration of 2.77 ± 0.1 mmol/L compared with 2.35 ± 0.1 mmol/L in 25 postoperative patients and reference interval of 2.17 - 2.67 mmol/L *4826*
Serum *No Effect* In 13 of 50 patients with primary hyperparathyroidism serum total corrected calcium was normal *1755*
Urine *Decrease* Although they may have hypercalciuria, compared with normal controls, they have very low rates for their serum calcium *5679*
Urine *Increase* Most patients are hypercalcemic and hypercalciuric *3255* 24 h excretion is high because of significant hypercalcemia, even though the renal clearance of calcium is relatively reduced *367* In 17 patients with primary hyperparathyroidism mean excretion of 255 ± 21 mg/g creatinine compared with normal values of 113 ± 62 mg/g creatinine *3506* Increased excretion is seen in hyperparathyroidism *2952* In 39 patients with hyperparathyroidism mean excretion of 110 µmol/L glomerular filtrate (median 83) significantly greater than reference range of 8 - 38 µmol/L glomerular filtrate *5552* 39 of 54 patients had elevations above the normal upper limit of normal (250 - 300 mg/24 h) *4834* Found in about 50% of primary

cases *4393* Primary hyperparathyroidism may be associated with classic distal renal tubular acidosis which is asociated with hyokalemia, hyperchloremic metabolic acidosis, urine pH > 5.5, increased urinary ammonium ion excretion, a negative urine anion gap, increased urinary osmol gap, decreased urinary citrate and increased urinary calcium in some patients *4071*
Urine No Effect In 62 untreated patients with untreated primary hyperparathyroidism mean excretion 0.6 ± 0.1 mmol/mmol creatinine compared with 0.4 ± 0.1 mmol/mmol creatinine in 25 postoperative patients and reference interval of < 0.7 mmol/mmol creatinine *4826*

Chloride *Serum Increase* Hyperchloremic acidosis occurs as a result of renal effects *4746* Primary hyperparathyroidism may be associated with classic distal renal tubular acidosis which is asociated with hyokalemia, hyperchloremic metabolic acidosis, urine pH > 5.5, increased urinary ammonium ion excretion, a negative urine anion gap, increased urinary osmol gap, decreased urinary citrate and increased urinary calcium in some patients *4071* Increases and phosphate decreases resulting in a Cl/PO_4 ratio > 33 *4393* The chloride values were higher (mean 107 mmol/L) and phosphate, lower (mean 2.6 mg/dL) in the 25 hyperparathyroid patients, whereas the chloride concentrations were lower (mean 98 mmol/L) and phosphate, higher (mean 4.5 mg/dL) in the 27 patients with hypercalcemia from other causes. The chloride to phosphate ratio ranged from 31.8 - 80 in hyperparathyroidism, with 96% more than 33, and from 17.1 - 32.3 in those with hypercalcemia from other causes, with 92% < 30 *3982*
Serum No Effect Appears to be more reliable than inorganic phosphate for differentiating hyperparathyroidism from other causes of hypercalcemia *5681*

Cholesterol *Serum Decrease* Hypercalcemia due to hyperparathyroidism is linked with low cholesterol levels and high parathyroid hormone and calcitonin production. An average increase of 41 µg/dL occurred after corrective surgery *1069* About 8 - 10% lower in both females and males compared with corresponding control cases *836*

Citrate *Plasma Increase* Elevated in the high normal range *5679*
Urine Decrease Primary hyperparathyroidism may be associated with classic distal renal tubular acidosis which is asociated with hyokalemia, hyperchloremic metabolic acidosis, urine pH > 5.5, increased urinary ammonium ion excretion, a negative urine anion gap, increased urinary osmol gap, decreased urinary citrate and increased urinary calcium in some patients *4071*
Urine Increase High or in high normal range *5679* Often elevated *2033*

Copper *Serum Increase* Slightly > normal mean *3250*
Urine Increase Mean 24 h urinary excretion was greater than normal in 17 patients with untreated disease *3250*

Creatinine *Serum Increase* In 45% of 11 patients at initial hospitalization for this disorder *1576* Mean concentration was 4.8 ± 1.8 mg/dL *3196*
Serum No Effect In 77 postmenopausal women with asymptomatic primary hyperparathyroidism median concentration of 96 µmol/L not significantly different from reference interval of 50 - 115 µmol/L *27*

Creatinine Clearance *Urine Decrease* Strong negative correlation between creatinine clearance and serum calcium *3255*

C-terminal Propeptide of Type I Procollagen
Serum Increase In 17 patients with primary hyperparathyroidism mean concentration of 194.5 ± 27 µg/L compared with normal values of 135 ± 40 µg/L *3506*

Deoxypyridinoline *Urine Increase* In 26 patients with primary hyperparathyroidism median excretion of 12.9 nmol/mmol creatinine significantly higher than that in 75 healthy men in whom the median excretion was 5.0 nmol/mmol creatinine and in 20 premenopausal women, 5.1 nmol/mmol creatinine, and in 38 postmenopausal women, 7.2 nmol/mmol creatinine *4716* In 87 patients with primary hyperparathyroidism mean excretion of deoxypyridinoline crosslinks of 17.6 ± 1.3 nmol/mmol creatinine compared with less than 14.6 nmol/mmol creatinine in 84 healthy age and sex matched controls *4826* In 18 patients with primary hyperparathyroidism 11% had excretions greater than reference interval of 0.4 - 6.4 nmol/mmol creatinine. Mean excretion was 4.3 (range 1.7 - 8.1) nmol/mmol creatinine *4388*

Deoxypyridinoline, Free *Urine Increase* In 17 patients with primary hyperparathyroidism mean excretion of 9.4 ± 4.9 µmol/mol creatinine significantly different from 1.7 - 5.9 µmol/mol creatinine in healthy men and 3.1 - 8.1 µmol/mol creatinine in healthy women when measured by CLIA technique *4427* Mean excretion in 23 patients aged 17 - 73 years of approximately 8.0 nmol/mol creatinine significantly different from upper limit of approximately 7.3 nmol/mol creatinine in normal individuals *4383*

1,25-Dihydroxy Vitamin D *Serum Increase* Increased concentrations observed in patients with primary hyperparathyroidism *2952*

1,25-Dihydroxy Vitamin D_3 *Serum Increase* Observed effect *126*

Erythrocyte Sedimentation Rate *Blood Increase* Raised in 48%, without apparent explanation *3255*

Gastrin *Serum Increase* Mean preoperative concentration in 18 uncomplicated patients was 122 ± 39 pg/mL *1123* Patients may be hypergastrinemic. Some of these patients also have gastric hypersecretion. In these the hypergastrinemia can be consider pathologic *4891* Elevated in patients without ulcer and fell to normal after parathyroidectomy *5045* Gastrin levels above normal occurred in 22% of patients with primary hyperparathyroidism *5841*

α_2-Globulin *Serum Increase* Slightly increased but return to normal after parathyroidectomy *5544*

Hematocrit *Blood Decrease* Unexplained anemia found in 21% of 57 patients *3255*

Hemoglobin *Blood Decrease* Unexplained anemia found in 21% of 57 patients *3255*

Homovanillic Acid *Cerebrospinal Fluid Decrease* In 22 patients with primary hyperparathyroidism mean concentration significantly less than in 11 normocalcemic controls *2451*

5-Hydroxyindoleacetic Acid *Cerebrospinal Fluid Decrease* Concentration significantly less in 22 patients with primary hyperparathyroidism than in 11 normocalcemic controls *2451*

Hydroxyproline *Urine Increase* Tends to parallel the extent and severity of bone involvement. Also seen in the secondary hyperparathyroidism of chronic renal disease *1980* Normal or increased. Increased with significant bone involvement *5679* In 17 patients with primary hyperparathyroidism mean excretion of 92.5 ± 20.6 mg/g creatinine compared with normal values of 30 ± 10 mg/g creatinine *3506*
Urine No Effect In 62 untreated patients with primary hyperparathyroidism mean excretion of 297 ± 23 µmol/d compared with 279 ± 23 µmol/d in 25 postoperative patients and reference interval of less than 305 µmol/d *4826* In 77 postmenopausal women with asymptomatic primary hyperparathyroidism median of 37 mmol/mol creatinine not significantly different from reference interval of 24 - 50 mmol/mol creatinine *27*

Hypoxanthine *Cerebrospinal Fluid No Effect* In 22 patients with primary hyperparathyroidism mean concentration no consistent difference from concentration in 11 normocalcemic controls *2451*

Insulin *Plasma Increase* Fasting concentrations and response were significantly increased in primary disease *2679*

ionized Calcium *Cerebrospinal Fluid Increase* In 22 patients with primary hyperparathyroidism mean concentration of 1.09 mmol/L significantly higher than in 11 normocalcemic controls *2451*
Serum Increase In 149 samples, 0.7% of serum ionized calcium and 7.5% of total calcium determinations were within the normal range. All patients exhibited abnormally elevated values upon repeated testing *1298*

Leukocytes *Blood Decrease* Frequently found *5544*

Magnesium *Serum Decrease* Normal or low *5679* May occur *5507* Found in 14% *3255*

Net Acid Excretion *Urine Increase* Primary hyperparathyroidism may be associated with classic distal renal tubular acidosis which is asociated with hyokalemia, hyperchloremic metabolic acidosis, urine pH > 5.5, increased urinary ammonium ion excretion, a negative urine anion gap, increased urinary osmol gap, decreased urinary citrate and increased urinary calcium in some patients *4071*

Osmolal Gap *Urine Increase* Primary hyperparathyroidism may be associated with classic distal renal tubular acidosis which is asociated with hyokalemia, hyperchloremic metabolic acidosis, urine pH > 5.5, increased urinary ammonium ion excretion, a negative urine anion gap, increased urinary osmol gap, decreased urinary citrate and increased urinary calcium in some patients *4071*

Osteocalcin *Serum Increase* In 40 patients with untreated primary hyperparathyroidism mean concentration of 21 ± 24

252.00 **Hyperparathyroidism** *(continued)*

Osteocalcin *(continued)*
μg/L higher than 12.2 ± 4.5 μg/L in normal women *2556* In 15 patients with primary hyperparathyroidism mean concentrations by sandwich EIA and RIA of 14.3 ± 16.8 μg/L and 11.6 ± 10.3 μg/L compared with mean concentrations of 4.2 ± 1.2 μg/L and 6.6 ± 1.4 μg/L by sandwich EIA and RIA methods respectively in 20 healthy individuals *2246* Using the Diagnostic Systems Laboratories' method mean concentration of 21.7 ± 15.9 μg/L in 11 patients with primary hyperparathyroidism significantly higher than that in 68 healthy adults (4 ± 3.6 μg/L) *1149* Reported effect *1103* In 24 patients with hyperparathyroidism mean concentration of 54 ± 33 μg/L (9.3 nmol/L) significantly different from that in healthy adults (men 25 ± 5 μg/L, women 20 ± 6 μg/L) *541* In 17 patients with primary hyperparathyroidism mean concentration of 9.7 ± 1.4 μg/L compared with normal values of 3.3 ± 1.0 μg/L *3506* In patients with primary hyperparathyroidism moderate increase observed *4217*

Parathyroid Hormone *Cerebrospinal Fluid Increase* In 22 patients with primary hyperparathyroidism mean concentration significantly higher than in 11 normocalcemic controls *2451*
Plasma Increase In 17 patients with primary hyperparathyroidism mean concentration increased to 130 ± 7.3 ng/L *3506* Raised serum calcium levels fail to depress hormone secretion *1290* Mean concentration in 15 patients with primary hyperparathyroidism of 159 ± 63 ng/L and 46 ± 37 ng/L in 17 patients with secondary hyperparathyroidism significantly greater than 30 ± 15 ng/L in 26 healthy controls *1063* Concentration rises above baseline level after neck massage only on the side of the adenoma, thereby aiding preoperative localization of the adenoma *5544* In 11 patients with primary hyperparathyroidism mean concentration of 341 ± 374 ng/L compared with 29.8 ± 13.8 ng/L in 57 healthy adults *1150* In over 90% of cases *126* In 62 untreated patients with primary hyperparathyroidism mean concentration of midmolecule of 735 ± 66 ng/L, compared with 266 ± 16 ng/L in 25 postoperative patients and reference interval of 50 - 330 ng/L. By IRMA assay mean concentration in untreated patients of 120 ± 9 ng/L, 48 ± 4 ng/L in postoperative patients and reference interval of 10 - 65 ng/L *4826*

Parathyroid Hormone 1-84 *Plasma Increase* Mean concentration in 27 patients with primary hyperparathyroidism of 21.0 pmol/L (range 5.8 - 100 pmol/L) significantly different from mean of 2.21 pmol/L (range 1.0 - 5.0 pmol/L) in 57 healthy laboratory staff *3105*

Parathyroid Hormone, Intact *Plasma Increase* In 77 postmenopausal women with asymptomatic primary hyperparathyroidism median concentration of 133 pg/mL significantly different from reference interval of < 65 pg/mL *27* In 11 patients with primary hyperparathyroidism median concentration of 123 μg/L significantly higher than 35.2 μg/L in 90 healthy controls *2572*
Plasma No Effect In 4 of 50 patients with primary hyperparathyroidism serum intact parathyroid concentration was normal *1755*

Parathyroid Hormone-related Peptide *Plasma Increase* In 5 patients with hyperparathyroidism range of concentrations of 0.57 - 1.54 pmol/L significantly greater than reference range of less than 0.5 pmol/L *5552*
Plasma No Effect Concentration normal in 30 of 32 patients with primary hyperparathyroidism *483*

pH *Urine Increase* Primary hyperparathyroidism may be associated with classic distal renal tubular acidosis which is associated with hyokalemia, hyperchloremic metabolic acidosis, urine pH > 5.5, increased urinary ammonium ion excretion, a negative urine anion gap, increased urinary osmol gap, decreased urinary citrate and increased urinary calcium in some patients *4071*

Phosphate *Saliva Increase* Increased inorganic phosphate in saliva *1290*
Serum Decrease In 77 postmenopausal women with asymptomatic primary hyperparathyroidism median concentration of 0.77 mmol/L significantly different from reference interval of 0.78 - 1.40 mmol/L *27* Occurs in 50% of patients *2039* Range of concentration in 34 patients was 1.2 - 3.4 mg/dL, mean concentration of 4.35 mg/dL *4311* In 83% of 19 patients at initial hospitalization for this disorder *1576* Severe burns are common cause of severe hypophosphatemia due to increased renal loss of phosphate *969*
Serum No Effect In 62 untreated patients with primary hyperparathyroidism mean concentration of 0.90 ± 0.1 mmol/L compared with 1.07 ± 0.1 mmol/L in 25 postoperative patients and reference interval of 0.81 - 1.45 mmol/L *4826*
Urine Increase Marked phosphaturia due to parathyroid hormones *1290* Increased unless there is a renal insufficiency or phosphate depletion (especially due to commonly used antacids containing aluminum) *5545*
Urine No Effect In 62 untreated patients with primary hyperparathyroidism mean excretion of 24.9 ± 2.9 mmol/d and 22.70 ± 1.8 mmol/d in 25 postoperative patients *4826*

Potassium *Serum Decrease* Primary hyperparathyroidism may be associated with classic distal renal tubular acidosis which is asociated with hyokalemia, hyperchloremic metabolic acidosis, urine pH > 5.5, increased urinary ammonium ion excretion, a negative urine anion gap, increased urinary osmol gap, decreased urinary citrate and increased urinary calcium in some patients *4071* Occasionally observed; attributed to decreased distal tubular reabsorption *367* Rare (3%) *2039* Related to the hypercalcemia and does not aid in differential diagnosis *900*
Serum Increase Incidence of 40% (7 of 17 cases) was reported. Other studies indicate a lower frequency *3255* *5862*
Urine Increase May occur *5679*

Pyridinoline *Urine Increase* In 18 patients with primary hyperparathyroidism 22% had excretions greater than reference interval of 5.0 - 21.8 nmol/mmol creatinine. Mean excretion of 16.9 (range 10.3 - 27.1) nmol/mmol creatinine *4388* In 87 patients with untreated primary hyperparathyroidism mean excretion of pyridinoline crosslinks of 46.8 ± 2.7 nmol/mmol creatinine compared with less than 51.8 nmol/mmol creatinine in 84 healthy age and sex matched controls *4826* In 10 patients with hyperparathyroidism mean excretion of 57.4 ± 23.9 nmol/mmol creatinine significantly greater than 25.7 ± 10.4 and 33.1 ± 14.7 nmol/mol creatinine in healthy men and women respectively *167* In 26 patients with primary hyperparathyroidism median excretion of 64.3 nmol/mmol creatinine significantly higher than that in 75 healthy men in whom the median excretion was 20.8 nmol/mmol creatinine and in 20 premenopausal women, 19.6 nmol/mmol creatinine, and in 38 postmenopausal women, 28.2 nmol/mmol creatinine *4716*

Pyridinoline Cross-linked Telopeptide of Type I Collagen
Serum Increase In 15 patients with primary hyperparathyroidism mean concentration of 3.5 ± 3.5 μg/L and in 17 with secondary hyperparathyroidism of 46 ± 37 μg/L significantly higher than 2.07 ± 0.58 μg/L in 26 healthy controls *1063*

Pyrophosphate *Synovial Fluid Increase* Has been identified *4681*

Specific Gravity *Urine Decrease* Polyuria due to the inability to concentrate the urine. Related to the hypercalcemia and does not aid in differential diagnosis *900*

Thyroid Stimulating Hormone *Serum No Effect* Serum thyroglobulin was elevated in 92% of 38 patients in the early stage of this disorder. After two months of corticosteroid treatment the levels were significantly decreased in 25 patients who could be rechecked *2563*

Thyroxine (T4) *Serum No Effect* Serum thyroglobulin was elevated in 92% of 38 patients in the early stage of this disorder. After two months of corticosteroid treatment the levels were significantly decreased in 25 patients who could be rechecked *2563*

Thyroxine (T4), Free *Serum No Effect* Serum thyroglobulin was elevated in 92% of 38 patients in the early stage of this disorder. After two months of corticosteroid treatment the levels were significantly decreased in 25 patients who could be rechecked *2563*

Tri-iodothyronine, Reverse (rT3) *Serum No Effect* Despite the low serum total T3 levels *2563*

Tri-iodothyronine (T3) *Serum Decrease* Significantly lower in patients with primary hyperparathyroidism (118 ng/dL) than in normal controls (147 ng/dL). There was a significant inverse correlation between serum levels of total T3 and PTH *2563*

Triglycerides *Serum Decrease* Levels were about 22% in females and 60% lower in males compared to controls. After operation levels normalized *836*

Tubular Maximum for Phosphate *Urine Decrease* In 77 postmenopausal women with asymptomatic primary hyperparathyroidism median of 0.60 mmol/L GFR significantly different from reference interval of > 0.80 mmol/L GFR *27*

Urea Nitrogen *Serum Increase* May occur *5679*

Uric Acid *Cerebrospinal Fluid* *Increase* Mean concentration in 22 primary hyperparathyroid patients significantly higher than in 11 normocalcemic reference individuals *2451*
Serum *Increase* Over 6.8 mg/dL in 62% of patients *2039* In 54% of 18 patients at initial hospitalization for this disorder *1576* Increased frequency of hyperuricemia and gout. 66% of the patients showed elevations, with no difference of frequency among males or females or with type of disease *3255*

Volume *Urine* *Increase* Polyuria due to the inability to concentrate the urine. Related to the hypercalcemia and does not aid in differential diagnosis *900*

Xanthine *Cerebrospinal Fluid* *No Effect* In 22 patients with primary hyperparathyroidism mean concentration not consistently different from that in 11 normocalcemic reference individuals *2451*

Zinc *Urine* *Increase* Mean 24 h excretion was above normal in 17 patients with untreated primary disease *3250*

252.10 Hypoparathyroidism

Alkaline Phosphatase *Serum* *Decrease* Normal or slightly low *5679* Reported effect *3160*
Serum *No Effect* Normal or slightly low *5679*

Amyloid β-Protein *Cerebrospinal Fluid* *No Effect* In 1 patient with hypoparathyroidism concentration was 1.26 pmol/mL not significantly different from mean concentration of 4.00 ± 2.92 pmol/mL *3716*

Amyloid β-Protein Precursor *Cerebrospinal Fluid* *Decrease* In 1 patient with hypoparathyroidism concentration was 0.92 integrated OD units significantly different from mean concentration of 1.35 ± 0.38 integrated OD units in 25 normal controls in one but normal in the other *3716*

α_1-Antichymotrypsin *Cerebrospinal Fluid* *Increase* In 1 patient with hypoparathyroidism concentration was 9.40 µg/mL significantly different from mean concentration of 2.27 ± 1.40 µg/mL in 25 normal controls *3716*

Bicarbonate *Serum* *Increase* Normal or decreased *2889*

Calcium *Serum* *Decrease* Rapidly reduced to a stable low level following removal of gland *4707* In a study involving 28 patients with hypocalcemia and low intact PTH concentration, 11 had idiopathic hypoparathyroidism and 13 had other causes following parathyroidectomy or thyroidectomy for a variety of causes *3280* Decreased PTH causes increased serum phosphate and reduced serum calcium *1025*
Urine *Decrease* Rises acutely, then falls to low levels as plasma calcium falls *5679*
Urine *Increase* Rises acutely, then falls to low levels as plasma calcium falls *5679*

Cells *Cerebrospinal Fluid* *No Effect* In 1 patient with hypoparathyroidism concentration of 0.3 cells/µL not significantly different from normal of 3 cells/µL *3716*

Chloride *Urine* *Decrease* May occur *5679*
Urine *No Effect* Usually normal *5679*

1,25-Dihydroxy Vitamin D *Serum* *Decrease* Decreased concentrations observed in patients with hypoparathyroidism *2952*

1,25-Dihydroxy Vitamin D_3 *Serum* *Decrease* Observed effect *126*

Glucose Tolerance *Serum* *Increase* Flat peak. Poor absorption from the GI tract (normal IV GTT curve) *5544*

Hydroxyproline *Urine* *Decrease* May occur *5679*

Magnesium *Red Blood Cells* *Increase* In 5 of 8 patients, the RBC concentration was at or above the normal upper limit. For the group the mean was 6.3 µmol/L packed cells, significantly over the normal ($p < 0.001$) *5547*
Serum *Decrease* Concentration is reduced in association with hypoparathyroidism *2952* Hypomagnesemia may occur *5507*
Serum *No Effect* Initial diuresis without significant change in serum concentrations *5679*
Urine *Decrease* Initial diuresis without significant change in serum concentrations *5679*

Osteocalcin *Serum* *Decrease* Reported effect *1089*

Parathyroid Hormone *Plasma* *Decrease* In a study involving 28 patients with hypocalcemia and low intact PTH concentration, 11 had idiopathic hypoparathyroidism and 13 had reduced concentrations following thyroidectomy or parathyroidectomy for variety of problems *3280*

Parathyroid Hormone 1-84 *Plasma* *Decrease* Mean concentration in 6 patients with hypoparathyroidism of < 0.5 pmol/L significantly different from mean 2.21 pmol/L (range 1.0 - 5.0 pmol/L) in 57 healthy laboratory staff *3105*

pH *Blood* *Increase* Normal or decreased *2889*

Phosphate *Serum* *Decrease* Initial fall followed by a rise *5679*
Serum *Increase* Hypoparathyroidism may increase the serum phosphate concentration *969* Hyperphosphatemia may occur with hypoparathyroidism *5204* Initial fall followed by a rise. May range from 6 to 16 mg/dL *5679* Increased (usually 5 - 6 mg/dL; as high as 12 mg/dL) *5544*
Urine *Decrease* Urine phosphate and phosphate clearance is decreased *5545*

Protein *Cerebrospinal Fluid* *No Effect* In 1 patient with hypoparathyroidism concentration of 39 mg/dL not significantly different from normal of 28 mg/dL in 25 healthy controls *3716*

Urea Nitrogen *Serum* *No Effect* Concentration usually normal *5679*

Uric Acid *Serum* *Increase* In primary cases *1242*

253.00 Acromegaly

Acetoacetate *Serum* *Increase* Elevated levels *5229*

Albumin *Urine* *Increase* In 14 adult acromegalics mean albumin excretion rate of 8.4 µg/min compared with 3.3 µg/min in 20 healthy controls *2224*

Alkaline Phosphatase *Serum* *Increase* Increased bone turnover found in this condition may result in elevation *1980* May indicate secretory activity of tumor *5544*

Amino-terminal Propeptide of Type III Collagen
Serum *Increase* In 15 adult patients with active acromegaly mean concentration of 4.8 ± 1.4 µg/L significantly increased compared with 3.1 ± 0.7 µg/L in healthy volunteer controls *4141*

Androgens *Plasma* *Decrease* Testosterone has been reported to be low in the presence of normal gonadotropin levels *900*

Basal Metabolic Rate *Patient* *Increase* Increase observed in patients with acromegaly *4937*

Calcium *Serum* *Increase* Often noted, because of increased GI absorption *1980* In 10 patients with active acromegaly mean concentration of 9.48 ± 0.12 mg/dL significantly increased compared with 9.08 ± 0.40 mg/dL in 25 healthy controls *2980* In 20 patients with active disease, gut absorption was greater than normal and positively correlated with both the elevated serum and urine concentration *4834*
Urine *Increase* In 20 patients with active disease, gut absorption was greater than normal and positively correlated with both the elevated serum and urine concentrations *4834*

C-Peptide *Plasma* *Increase* Fasting concentration increased *4937*

Creatine *Serum* *Increase* Accelerated rate of synthesis may result in high serum and urine concentrations *4707*
Urine *Increase* Accelerated rate of synthesis may result in high serum and urine concentrations *4707*

Creatinine *Serum* *Increase* Increased rate of formation *5544*

Creatinine Clearance *Urine* *Increase* In 14 adult acromegalic patients mean clearance of 125 mL/min/1.73 sq m significantly greater than 100 mL/min/1.73 sq m in 20 healthy controls *2224*

C-terminal Propeptide of Type III Procollagen
Serum *No Effect* In 15 adult patients with active acromegaly mean concentration of 152 ± 55 µg/L not significantly different when compared with 120 ± 55 µg/L in healthy volunteer controls *4141*

Fatty Acids (FFA), Free *Serum* *Increase* May be elevated because of decreased lipogenesis *1980*

Glomerular Filtration Rate *Urine* *Increase* GFR often increased in acromegaly *900* May be abnormally high *1980*

Glucose *Serum* *Increase* Overt diabetes is found manifested by fasting hyperglycemia *1980* Plasma concentration increased *4937*
Urine *Increase* Increase in glucose tolerance because of glycosuria *1290*

253.00 **Acromegaly** *(continued)*

Glucose Tolerance *Serum* *Decrease* In 50% of these patients, the oral administration of glucose will demonstrate decreased tolerance *1980* Impaired in most patients with acromegaly and gigantism *5545*

Gonadotropins *Plasma* *Decrease* Serum and urinary gonadotropins may be diminished; azoospermia and amenorrhea may ensue *1980*
Urine *Decrease* Serum and urinary gonadotropins may be diminished; azoospermia and amenorrhea may ensue *1980*

Growth Hormone *Plasma* *Increase* In 14 adult acromegalics mean concentration of 16.8 μg/L significantly higher than in healthy adult controls *2224* In patients with clinically active acromegaly mean concentration of 4.4 μg/L (range of 0.16 - 55.0 μg/L) *3233* Hypersecretion causes acromegaly in adults *2952* Conversely hypersecretion causes dwarfism in children *2952* In 14 patients integrated mean concentrations ranged from 11 to 118 mU/L significantly different from normal *3934* Usually basal levels > 20 ng/mL. High basal growth hormone levels and failure of suppression by glucose at 1 or 2 h are the definitive criteria for the diagnosis *1980* In 8 patients with active acromegaly mean baseline concentration of 23.2 mU/L higher than 2.8 mU/L in 14 normal individuals *852* Characteristic of disease *367* The definitive test for diagnosis is an increase of 10 ng/mL, which is not suppressible by glucose *900* In 8 acromegalics mean daytime serum growth hormone concentration was increased and ranged from 5.8 to 48.4 μg/L *2344*
Urine *Increase* In 15 acromegalic patients mean daily excretion of 190 ± 100 pg/min compared with 3.89 ± 0.56 pg/min in healthy controls *3377* Excretion was correlated significantly with clinical activity ($r = 0.53$). Median excretion in clinically inactive patients of 3.7 ng/d not significantly different from controls, with mild clinical activity median of 7.38 ng/d and in patients with strong activity median of 74.0 ng/d. 95% prediction interval in healthy controls 0.6 - 20.9 ng/d *3233*

Growth Hormone Binding Protein *Serum* *Decrease* Mean concentration of 1.05 ± 0.18 μg/L in 9 patients with active disease and 1.46 ± 0.18 μg/L in 9 patients with moderately active disease significantly lower than 1.71 ± 0.32 μg/L in 11 patients with inactive disease *2814*

Growth Hormone Binding Protein-II *Serum* *Decrease* In 28 patients with active acromegaly mean concentration of 628 ± 220 fmol/L compared with means of 1,340 fmol/L in 40 healthy women and 999 fmol/L in 31 healthy men *4404*

Hydroxyproline *Urine* *Increase* Indicates secretory activity of tumor *5544* Increased bone turnover found in this condition may result in elevation *1980*

Insulin *Plasma* *Increase* Fasting plasma concentration increased *4937* In 8 acromegalics mean basal serum insulin concentration was increased to 22.3 ± 6.32 mU/L *2344* Large amounts of growth hormone have a diabetogenic effect. As a result, the basal plasma insulin values may be higher than normal, and their insulin response to a glucose load may be increased *1980*

Insulin-like Growth Factor-I *Serum* *Increase* Observed effect *2166* In 8 patients with active acromegaly mean baseline concentration of 1016 μg/L higher than 229.5 μg/L in 14 normal individuals *852* Mean concentration of 4.8 kU/L in 14 adult acromegalics higher than reference interval of 0.34 - 2.2 kU/L *2224* Mean concentration correlated significantly with urinary growth hormone excretion ($r = 0.56$ to $5 = 0.64$) and to clinical state *3233* In patients with active acromegaly mean concentration significantly increased to about 700 ng/mL compared with upper limit of about 230 ng/mL in healthy normals, with lower concentrations observed in patients with weak active and inactive acromegaly *2813* In 8 acromegalics mean daytime serum IGF-I concentration was increased and ranged from 514 to 1,116 μg/L *2344* Mean concentration in 14 patients with acromegaly of about 800 ng/mL significantly different from mean of about 180 ng/mL in healthy adults *2971* Concentration increased in patients with acromegaly *2952* In 10 patients with acromegaly mean concentration of about 530 μg/L significantly different from normal concentration of 90 - 360 μg/L *3332*

Insulin-like Growth Factor-II *Serum* *No Effect* In 10 patients with acromegaly mean concentration of about 700 μg/L not significantly different from normal concentration of 490 - 1,056 μg/L *3332*

Insulin-like Growth Factor Binding Protein-3
Serum *Increase* In 10 patients with acromegaly mean concentration of about 4.2 mg/L significantly different from normal range of 1.7 - 4.0 mg/L *3332* In 8 acromegalics mean daytime serum IGFBP-3 concentration was increased to 5.7 ± 0.5 mg/L *2344*

Insulin Tolerance *Plasma* *Decrease* The blood sugar falls by < 25% of its initial value and rapidly returns to the fasting level *1290*

Ketones *Serum* *No Effect* The overt diabetes associated with acromegaly is frequently insulin-resistant and not associated with elevated ketones in the blood or urine *1980*

17-Ketosteroids *Urine* *Decrease* Varies from low, normal to high *1025*
Urine *Increase* Varies from low, normal to high *1025*
Urine *No Effect* Varies from low, normal to high *1025*

Osteocalcin *Serum* *Increase* In 9 acromegalic patients concentration highly significantly increased *4825* Concentrations recorded in the acromegalic patients were significantly elevated (14.2 ± 4.2 μg/L versus 8.0 ± 3.3 μg/L, $p < 0.001$) *5199* Reported effect *1062* In 15 adult patients with active acromegaly mean concentration of 14.3 ± 2.1 ng/mL compared with 8.3 ± 2.1 ng/mL in healthy volunteer controls *4141* Mean concentration of 11.78 ± 2.84 μg/L in 10 patients with active acromegaly significantly higher than 8.00 ± 2.00 μg/L in 25 healthy controls *2980*

Parathyroid Hormone *Plasma* *No Effect* In 10 patients with active acromegaly mean concentration of 30.50 ± 11.02 mg/L not significantly different from 34.20 ± 11.20 mg/L in 25 healthy controls *2980*

Phosphate *Serum* *Increase* There may be a mild hyperphosphatemia, a reversal of the diurnal rhythmicity of urinary phosphate excretion, and an increased tubular reabsorption of phosphate *1980* Hyperphosphatemia may occur with growth hormone excess or administration *5204* In 10 patients with active acromegaly mean concentration of 3.90 ± 0.41 mg/dL significantly greater than 3.40 ± 0.38 mg/dL in 25 healthy controls *2980* Acromegaly may increase the serum phosphate concentration *969*

Procollagen Type I Peptide *Serum* *No Effect* PICP levels recorded in the acromegalics did not differ from control subjects (146 ± 46 μg/L versus 127 ± 44 μg/L, NS) *5199*

Prolactin *Plasma* *Increase* In 14 patients mean concentrations ranged from 101 to 98,000 mU/L significantly different from normal *3934* Can trigger a mild to moderate increase (20 - 300 ng/mL) *3391* Measured in 73 untreated patients and found to be elevated in 32% *1070* In 8 patients with active acromegaly mean baseline concentration of 132 mU/L higher than 98 mU/L in 14 normal individuals *852*

Protein *Cerebrospinal Fluid* *Increase* Occasionally seen; reflects the intracranial lesion *1980*

Pyrophosphate *Synovial Fluid* *Increase* Has been identified *4681*

Somatomedin *Plasma* *Increase* Observed effect *3141*

Specific Gravity *Urine* *Decrease* Usually 1.001-1.005 *367*

α-Subunit *Plasma* *Increase* In 19 patients with acromegaly 7 (37%) had increased concentration as measured with monoclonal assay *3923*

α-Subunit of Glycoprotein Hormones *Plasma* *Increase* Median concentration in 25 patients of 219 ng/L (range 94 - 1,038 ng/L) higher than median in 24 healthy adult men [250 ng/L (range 120 - 790 ng/L)] and 291 ng/mL (range 88 - 604 ng/mL) in 22 adult premenopausal women: in 3 patients concentrations abnormally high *5468*

T3-Uptake *Serum* *No Effect* Thyroid functions were all found to be normal in active disease, contrary to several earlier reports *940*

Testosterone *Serum* *Decrease* Have been reported to be low in the presence of normal gonadotropin levels *900*

Thyroid Stimulating Hormone *Serum* *Decrease* The expanding tumor within the pituitary fossa may cause a diminution of secretion of other pituitary hormones. Loss of thyroid-stimulating hormone will cause hypothyroidism *1980*
Serum *No Effect* Normal, even with thyroid enlargement *1966*

Thyroxine Binding Globulin *Serum* *Decrease* Decreased concentration observed *206* Typically associated with low concentration of TBG *1965*

Serum *Increase* Elevated in 38% of 26 females with acne between ages of 27 and 42 y *126*

Thyroxine (T4) *Serum* *Decrease* Decreased concentration observed due to reduced concentration of TBG *206* Low concentration of TBG typically observed *1965*
Serum *No Effect* Thyroid functions were all found to be normal in active disease, contrary to several earlier reports *940*

Tri-iodothyronine (T3) *Serum* *Decrease* Typically associated with decreased TBG concentration *1965*
Serum *No Effect* Thyroid functions were all found to be normal in active disease, contrary to several reports *940*

Urea Nitrogen *Serum* *Decrease* In some patients, because of the high uptake of amino acids required for enhanced protein synthesis *1980*

Uric Acid *Serum* *Decrease* Some patients *5544*
Serum *Increase* Increased in some patients *5544*

VLDL-Cholesterol *Serum* *Increase* Minimal elevation due to increased secretion *126*

Zinc *Serum* *Decrease* Decreased *5083* *2785*

253.10 Hyperprolactinemia

Growth Hormone *Plasma* *No Effect* In 6 women with hyperprolactinemia mean baseline concentration of 0.4 mU/L not significantly different from 2.8 mU/L in 14 normal individuals *852*

Insulin-like Growth Factor-I *Serum* *No Effect* In 6 women with hyperprolactinemia mean baseline concentration of 166.5 µg/L not significantly different from that in 14 normal individuals *852*

Prolactin *Plasma* *Increase* In 6 women with pathological hyperprolactinemia mean baseline concentration of 1,300 mU/L significantly higher than 98 mU/L in 14 normal individuals *852*

253.20 Anterior Pituitary Hypofunction

Androgens *Plasma* *Decrease* Decreased testosterone in hypopituitarism and hypogonadism *1290*

Angiotensin *Plasma* *Decrease* Both plasma renin substrate and angiotensin are low and unresponsive to adequate stimulation *254*

Basal Metabolic Rate *Patient* *Decrease* In patients with hypopitiutarism mean rate decreased when expressed per kg body weight but increased when expressed per kg lean body mass *4937*

Chloride *Urine* *Increase* Diminished tubular sodium reabsorption because of adrenal cortical steroid deficiency. The urine volume is increased, with loss of the normal diurnal variation, and an increased sodium and chloride concentration *1290*

Cholesterol *Serum* *Increase* In some cases due to secondary hypothyroidism *900*

Chylomicrons *Serum* *Increase* Increased *4372* *3017* *4358*

Corticotropin *Plasma* *Decrease* Observed effect *2034* May be deficient and lead to secondary adrenocortical hypofunction *5863*

Cortisol *Plasma* *Decrease* Low or low normal levels are suggestive but not diagnostic *5863*

C-Peptide *Plasma* *Increase* Mean fasting concentration increased *4937*

Eosinophils *Blood* *Increase* With reduced adrenal cortical or pituitary function eosinophilia may be seen *900*

Follicle Stimulating Hormone *Plasma* *Decrease* Characterized by absent or reduced production and release *2304* Compatible with stage of sexual development, not with age *835*

Glucose *Serum* *Decrease* In children with hypopituitarism fasting hypoglycemia may be observed *1324* May result from growth hormone and cortisol deficiency *5863*

Glucose Tolerance *Serum* *Increase* Late hypoglycemia *5544*

Gonadotropin, Pituitary *Plasma* *Decrease* Decreased in secondary hypogonadism *5544*
Urine *Decrease* Deficiency leads to amenorrhea and genital atrophy *5863*

Growth Hormone *Plasma* *Decrease* Deficiency may lead to dwarfism in children and contribute to hypoglycemia in children and adults *5863* Reported effect *2034* Characterized by absent or reduced production and release *2304*

Hematocrit *Blood* *Decrease* In some cases slight anemia is seen *900* Reduced thyroid, adrenal cortical, pituitary or testicular function can produce anemia. The hematocrit is seldom < 30%. The RBC is normochromic and normocytic *900*

Hemoglobin *Blood* *Decrease* Reduced thyroid, adrenal cortical, pituitary or testicular function can produce anemia. The hemoglobin is seldom < 9 g/dL. The RBC is normochromic and normocytic *900* In some cases slight anemia is seen *900*

17-Hydroxycorticosteroids *Urine* *No Effect* Usual observation *5544*

^{131}I Uptake *Serum* *No Effect* The thyroidal uptake is often inexplicably normal even when the patient is clinically hypothyroid *367*

Insulin *Plasma* *Increase* Mean fasting concentration increased and positive association with fat mass *4937*

17-Ketogenic Steroids *Urine* *Decrease* Excretion reduced in hypopituitarism *2952* Low or low normal levels are suggestive but not diagnostic *5863*
Urine *No Effect* No significant effect observed *5544*

17-Ketosteroids *Urine* *Decrease* Low or low normal levels are suggestive but not diagnostic *5863* Excretion may be decreased in patients with panhypopituitarism *2952*

Leukocytes *Blood* *Decrease* With reduced adrenal cortical or pituitary function leukopenia may be seen *900*

Luteinizing Hormone *Plasma* *Decrease* Compatible with stage of sexual development, not with age *835* Characterized by absent or reduced production and release *2304* Decreased to values seen during follicular phase rather than luteal phase of menstrual cycle with galactorrhea amenorrhea syndromes *5545*

Lymphocytes *Blood* *Increase* Marked *900* Relative lymphocytosis *2034*

Osteocalcin *Serum* *Decrease* Levels decreased in patients with growth hormone deficiency, but increased to normal values after treatment with human growth hormone from human pituitaries *1102*

Phosphate *Serum* *Decrease* Hypopituitarism with growth hormone deficiency in children *1290*

Potassium *Serum* *No Effect* Usually *2034*

Pregnanetriol *Urine* *Decrease* Decreased to values seen during follicular phase rather than luteal phase of menstrual cycle with galactorrhea amenorrhea syndromes *5545*

Progesterone *Plasma* *Decrease* Decreased to values seen during follicular phase rather than luteal phase of menstrual cycle with galactorrhea amenorrhea syndromes *5545*

Prolactin *Plasma* *Decrease* Characterized by absent or reduced production and release *2304* Patients with pituitary tumors or postpartum pituitary necrosis will be found to have impaired prolactin and growth hormone reserve *2039*

Renin Activity *Plasma* *Decrease* Both plasma renin substrate and angiotensin are low and unresponsive to adequate stimulation *254*

Reticulocytes *Blood* *Decrease* Absolute count is decreased *900*

Sodium *Serum* *Decrease* May be 120 mmol/L or lower without symptoms of adrenal insufficiency *367*
Urine *Increase* Increased output in Addison's Disease and hypopituitarism *1290* There is diminished tubular sodium reabsorption because of adrenal cortical steroid deficiency. The urine volume is increased, with loss of the normal diurnal variation, and an increased sodium and chloride concentration *1290*

Somatomedin *Plasma* *Decrease* Dwarfism *3141*

Testosterone *Serum* *Decrease* Decreased in hypopituitarism and hypogonadism *1290*

Thyroid Stimulating Hormone *Serum* *Decrease* Characterized by absent or reduced production and release *2304* May be deficient and lead to secondary hypothyroidism *5863*

Thyroxine (T4) *Serum* *Decrease* Low or low normal levels are suggestive but not diagnostic *5863*

Urea Nitrogen *Serum* *No Effect* Usually *2034*

Volume *Urine* *Increase* Diminished tubular sodium reabsorption because of adrenal cortical steroid deficiency. The urine volume is increased, with loss of the normal diurnal variation, and an increased sodium and chloride concentration *1290*

253.20 Corticotropin Deficiency

Amyloid β-Protein *Cerebrospinal Fluid No Effect* In 1 patient with corticotropin deficiency concentration was 3.54 pmol/mL not significantly different from mean concentration of 4.00 ± 2.92 pmol/mL *3716*

Amyloid β-Protein Precursor *Cerebrospinal Fluid Decrease* In 1 patient with corticotropin deficiency concentration was 0.88 integrated OD units significantly different from mean concentration of 1.35 ± 0.38 integrated OD units in 25 normal controls in one but normal in the other *3716*

α_1-Antichymotrypsin *Cerebrospinal Fluid No Effect* In 1 patient with corticotropin deficiency concentration was 0.60 µg/mL not significantly different from mean concentration of 2.27 ± 1.40 µg/mL in 25 normal controls *3716*

Cells *Cerebrospinal Fluid No Effect* In 1 patient with corticotropin deficiency concentration of 0.0 cells/µL not significantly different from normal of 3 cells/µL *3716*

Protein *Cerebrospinal Fluid No Effect* In 1 patient with corticotropin deficiency concentration of 23 mg/dL not significantly different from normal of 28 mg/dL in 25 healthy controls *3716*

253.20 Hypopituitarism

Apolipoprotein A-I *Serum No Effect* Mean concentration of 154 ± 14 mg/dL in 12 hypopituitary patients with growth hormone-deficiency not significantly different from 152 ± 9 mg/dL in 14 matched healthy control adults *93*

Apolipoprotein B *Serum Increase* Mean concentration of 132 ± 6 mg/dL in 12 hypopituitary patients with growth hormone-deficiency significantly different from 114 ± 8 mg/dL in 14 matched healthy control adults *93*

Cholesterol *Serum Increase* Mean concentration of 6.44 ± 0.19 mmol/L in 12 hypopituitary patients with growth hormone-deficiency significantly different from 5.73 ± 0.16 mmol/L in 14 matched healthy control adults *93* Mean concentration of 5.95 ± 0.37 mmol/L in 15 hypopituitary patients with growth hormone-deficiency not significantly different from 5.33 ± 0.16 mmol/L in 21 healthy control adults *92*

Glucose *Serum Decrease* Mean concentration of 4.2 ± 0.1 mmol/L in 15 hypopituitary patients with growth hormone-deficiency significantly less than 5.3 ± 0.1 mmol/L in 21 healthy control adults *92*

HDL-Cholesterol *Serum Decrease* Mean concentration of 1.10 ± 0.11 mmol/L in 15 hypopituitary patients with growth hormone-deficiency not significantly different from 1.26 ± 0.12 mmol/L in 21 healthy control adults *92* Mean concentration of 1.20 ± 0.05 mmol/L in 12 hypopituitary patients with growth hormone-deficiency not significantly different from 1.26 ± 0.07 mmol/L in 14 matched healthy control adults *93*
Serum Increase Mean concentration of 1.75 ± 0.15 mmol/L in 12 hypopituitary patients with growth hormone-deficiency significantly different from 1.39 ± 0.09 mmol/L in 14 matched healthy control adults *93*

Insulin *Plasma Decrease* Mean concentration of intact insulin of 20.3 pmol/L in 15 hypopituitary patients with growth hormone-deficiency significantly less than 47.5 pmol/L in 21 healthy control adults *92*

Insulin-like Growth Factor-I *Serum Decrease* In 10 patients with hypopituitarism mean concentration of about 50 µg/L significantly different from normal concentration of 90 - 360 µg/L *3332*

Insulin-like Growth Factor-II *Serum Decrease* In 10 patients with hypopituitarism mean concentration of about 470 µg/L significantly different from normal concentration of 490 - 1,056 µg/L *3332*

Insulin-like Growth Factor Binding Protein-3
Serum Decrease In 10 patients with hypopituitarism mean concentration of about 1.4 µg/mL significantly different from normal range of 1.7 - 4.0 µg/mL *3332*

LDL-Cholesterol *Serum Increase* Mean concentration of 4.21 ± 0.21 mmol/L in 15 hypopuitary patients with growth hormone-deficiency significantly different from 3.41 ± 0.19 mmol/L in 21 healthy control adults *92* Mean concentration of 4.53 ± 0.19 mmol/L in 12 hypopituitary patients with growth hormone-deficiency significantly different from 3.89 ± 0.15 mmol/L in 14 matched healthy control adults *93*

Leptin *Serum Decrease* Mean concentration of 4.2 ± 0.1 mmol/L in 15 hypopituitary patients with growth hormone-deficiency significantly less than 5.3 ± 0.1 mmol/L in 21 healthy control adults *92*

Lipoprotein Lp(a) *Serum Decrease* Mean concentration of 9 mg/dL in 12 hypopituitary patients with growth hormone-deficiency not significantly different from 17 mg/dL in 14 matched healthy control adults *93*

Proinsulin *Plasma Decrease* Mean concentration of intact proinsulin of 4.2 pmol/L in 15 hypopituitary patients with growth hormone-deficiency not significantly less than 6.7 pmol/L in 21 healthy control adults *92*

Triglycerides *Serum Increase* Mean concentration of 1.85 ± 0.40 mmol/L in 15 hypopituitary patients with growth hormone-deficiency not significantly different from 1.45 ± 0.19 mmol/L in 21 healthy control adults *92*

253.30 Growth Hormone Deficiency

Acid-labile Subunit *Serum Decrease* In 20 patients with growth hormone deficiency mean concentration about 8 mg/L significantly less than range of 15 - 34 mg/L in healthy individuals *5224*

Albumin *Urine Decrease* In 8 GH-deficient adults mean excretion rate of 2.0 µg/min reduced below 3.3 µg/min in 20 healthy controls *2224*

Alkaline Phosphatase *Serum Decrease* In 66 children with growth hormone deficiency mean activity of 175.3 ± 9.2 U/L significantly different from 202.6 ± 7.9 U/L in a control group of children with short stature not associated with GH deficiency *1748*
Serum No Effect In 8 adults with GH deficiency mean total alkaline phosphatase activity of 119.5 ± 14.8 U/L not significantly different from 116.2 ± 3.6 U/L in healthy normals *4580* In 16 growth hormone deficient children mean baseline of 210 ± 48 U/L not different from normal range of 70 - 450 U/L *151*

Alkaline Phosphatase, Bone Isoenzyme *Serum Decrease* Considerable overlap observed between concentrations in patients with GH-deficiency and normal children *5240* Mean activity of 44.9 ± 6.9 U/L in 8 adults with GH deficiency significantly lower than 61.8 ± 1.9 U/L in healthy normal controls *4580*
Serum Increase Considerable overlap observed between concentrations in patients with GH-deficiency and normal children *5240*
Serum No Effect Considerable overlap observed between concentrations in patients with GH-deficiency and normal children *5240*

Amino-terminal Propeptide of Type III Collagen
Serum No Effect Mean concentration of 3.7 ± 0.6 ng/mL in 8 adults with GH deficiency similar to 3.2 ± 0.2 ng/mL in healthy controls *4580*

Anion Gap *Serum Increase* In 66 children with growth hormone deficiency mean concentration of 9.3 ± 0.6 mmol/L significantly different from 7.3 ± 0.4 mmol/L in a control group of children with short stature not associated with GH deficiency *1748*

Apolipoprotein A-I *Serum Decrease* In 64 adult patients with childhood onset of growth hormone deficiency mean concentration of 1.26 ± 0.23 mmol/L decreased compared with 1.35 ± 0.18 mmol/L in 45 healthy controls *1047*

Apolipoprotein A-II *Serum Increase* In 64 adults with childhood onset growth hormone deficiency mean concentration of 0.42 ± 0.07 mmol/L significantly higher than 0.37 ± 0.07 mmol/L in 45 healthy controls *1047*

Apolipoprotein B *Serum Increase* In 64 adults with childhood onset of growth hormone deficiency mean concentration of 1.25 ± 0.30 mmol/L significantly higher than 1.04 ± 0.22 mmol/L in 45 healthy controls *1047*

Aspartate Aminotransferase *Serum No Effect* In 21 young adult patients mean activity not significantly different from normal *2514*

Bicarbonate *Serum Decrease* In 66 children with growth hormone deficiency mean concentration of 23.9 ± 0.4 mmol/L significantly different from 25.2 ± 0.3 mmol/L in a control group of children with short stature not associated with GH deficiency *1748*

Bilirubin *Serum No Effect* In 21 young adult patients mean concentration not significantly different from normal *2514*

Calcium *Serum* *No Effect* In 66 children with growth hormone deficiency mean concentration of 9.7 ± 0.1 mg/dL not significantly different from 9.8 ± 0.1 mg/dL in a control group of children with short stature not associated with GH deficiency *1748* In 16 growth hormone deficient children mean concentration of 9.66 ± 0.41 mg/dL not different from normal range of 9.16 - 10.88 mg/dL *151*

Cholesterol *Serum* *Increase* In 64 adults with childhood onset of growth hormone deficiency mean concentration of 5.54 ± 1.06 mmol/L significantly higher than 1.17 ± 0.21 mmol/L in 45 healthy controls *1047*

Creatinine Clearance *Urine* *Decrease* In 8 GH-deficient adults mean clearance 86 mL/min/1.73 sq m significantly reduced compared with 100 mL/min/1.73 sq m in 20 healthy controls *2224*

Deoxypyridinoline *Urine* *Decrease* In 17 growth hormone deficient children mean excretion significanly less than in healthy children of the same age. Mean Z score - 0.67 *1596*

Growth Hormone *Plasma* *Decrease* In children with growth hormone deficiency mean 12 h concentration of 1.4 µg/L (1 SD range of 0.9 - 2.1 µg/L) in 79 males and 1.2 µg/L (1 SD range of 0.7 - 2.0 µg/L) in 26 females significantly lower than 2.1 µg/L (1 SD range of 1.2 - 3.5 µg/L) in 47 male and 2.7 µg/L (1 SD range of 1.4 - 5.1 µg/L) in 35 female controls *694* In 8 adult patients mean concentration less than detectable threshold of 0.5 µg/L *2224* In 64 adults with childhood onset of growth hormone deficiency mean concentration of 3.0 ± 2.5 µg/L *1047* In 44 adult patients peak GH concentration < 2mU/L in response to insulin stress *323* In 20 patients with growth hormone deficiency, all had serum growth hormone concentrations below 2 µg/L *5224* *Urine* *Decrease* In 11 patients with severe growth hormone deficiency mean excretion of 3.69 ± 2.9 ng/L (0.53 ± 0.43 ng/mmol creatinine) markedly different and in 24 with partial growth hormone deficiency of 13.6 ± 6.38 ng/L (1.60 ± 1.01 ng/mmol creatinine) not significantly different from those in healthy individuals *1698*

Growth Hormone Binding Protein *Serum* *Decrease* In children with growth hormone deficiency (GH less than 10 µg/L) mean concentration of 146 pmol/L (1 SD range 86 - 250 pmol/L) in 80 males and 182 pmol/L (1 SD range 89 - 372 pmol/L) in 27 females lower than 183 pmol/L (1 SD range 103 - 326 pmol/L) in 407 male and 228 pmol/L (1 SD 133 - 394 range pmol/L) in 228 female controls *694*

HDL-Cholesterol *Serum* *No Effect* Mean concentration of 1.13 ± 0.28 mmol/L in 64 adult patients with childhood onset growth hormone deficiency not significantly different from 1.17 ± 0.21 mmol/L in 45 healthy controls *1047*

Insulin *Plasma* *Decrease* In 20 patients with growth hormone deficiency mean concentration of 95 pmol/L not significantly different from upper limit of normal of 132 pmol/L in healthy individuals *5224*

Insulin-like Growth Factor-I *Serum* *Decrease* Concentration decreased in patients with growth hormone deficiency *2952* In 20 patients with growth hormone deficiency all had serum IGF-I concentrations below -2 SD for age. Mean concentration was of the order of 37 ± 7 µg/L *5224* Mean concentration in 135 adult patients with growth hormone deficiency of 77.8 ± 4.9 µg/L significantly different from 170.2 ± 4.7 µg/L in 336 healthy controls *47* In 8 GH-deficient adults mean concentration of 0.13 kU/L reduced below reference interval of 0.34 - 2.2 kU/L *2224* In 16 growth hormone-deficient children mean baseline concentration of 61 ± 11 ng/mL compared with normal range of 315 ± 64 ng/mL *151* In 21 prepubertal children with GH-deficiency concentration paralleled that of free IGF-1 which ranged from -3.30 to 0.30 (mean -1.59) below that in age-matched normal subjects *2596* In children with growth hormone deficiency mean concentration of 99 µg/L (1 SD range 41 - 238 µg/L) in 80 males and 84 µg/L (1 SD range 36 - 195 µg/L) in 27 females significantly lower than 217 µg/L (1 SD range 130 - 363 µg/L) in 47 male and 308 µg/L (1 SD range 178 - 531 µg/L) in 35 female controls *694* In 66 children with growth hormone deficiency mean concentration of 88.0 ± 16.7 ng/mL significantly different from 147.8 ± 19.4 ng/mL in a control group of children with short stature not associated with GH deficiency *1748* In 64 adults with childhood onset of growth hormone deficiency mean concentration of 8.6 ± 3.5 nmol/L significantly reduced compared with 26.7 ± 4.7 nmol/L in 45 healthy controls *1047* In 21 young adult patients mean concentration of 104 ± 10 µg/L significantly less than normal range of 163 - 395 µg/L *2514*

Urine *Decrease* Excretion reduced in many adult patients with growth homone deficiency *323*

Insulin-like Growth Factor-I, Free *Serum* *Decrease* In 21 prepubertal children with GH-deficiency concentration ranged from -3.30 to 0.30 (mean -1.59) below that in age-matched normal subjects *2596*

Insulin-like Growth Factor-II *Urine* *Decrease* In 15 growth hormone deficient children mean excretion of 0.9 ± 0.1 pmol/kg body weight (12.9 ± 2.0 nmol/mol creatinine) compared with 2.4 ± 0.2 pmol/kg body weight (33.2 ± 3.8 nmol/mol creatinine) in healthy controls *4250*

Insulin-like Growth Factor Binding Protein-1 *Serum* *No Effect* In 20 patients with growth hormone deficiency mean concentration of 35 µg/L not significantly different from mean of 34 µg/L in healthy individuals *5224*

Insulin-like Growth Factor Binding Protein-3 *Serum* *Decrease* In 21 prepubertal children with GH-deficiency concentration paralleled that of free IGF-1 which ranged from -3.30 to 0.30 (mean -1.59) below that in age-matched normal subjects *2596* In 66 children with growth hormone deficiency mean concentration of 1.46 ± 0.28 mg/L significantly different from 2.56 ± 0.24 mg/L in a control group of children with short stature not associated with GH deficiency *1748* In 21 young adult patients mean concentration of 1,930 ± 163 µg/L significantly less than normal range of 2,735 - 3,954 µg/L *2514* In 20 patients with growth hormone deficiency all had reduced serum concentrations with mean concentration about 1.6 mg/L significantly less than mean of 3.6 mg/L in men and 3.8 mg/L in women *5224*

Lactate Dehydrogenase *Serum* *No Effect* In 21 young adult patients mean activity not significantly different from normal *2514*

LDL-Cholesterol *Serum* *Increase* In 64 adult patients with childhood onset growth hormone deficiency mean concentration of 3.87 ± 0.95 mmol/L significantly higher than 3.16 ± 0.82 mmol/L in 45 healthy controls *1047*

LDL-Cholesterol:HDL-Cholesterol Ratio *Serum* *Increase* In 64 adults with childhood onset growth hormone deficiency mean ratio of 3.62 ± 1.21 significantly higher than 2.75 ± 0.91 in 45 healthy controls *1047*

Leptin *Serum* *Increase* Mean concentration of 12.0 ± 1.8 µg/L observed in 15 growth hormone-deficient patients with hypopituitarism significantly higher than 8.0 ± 1.5 µg/L observed in 21 healthy control adults, with increase more marked in obese patients and in obese controls *92*

Osteocalcin *Serum* *Decrease* Mean concentration in 8 adults with GH deficiency mean concentration of bone Gla protein 3.8 ± 0.5 ng/mL significantly lower than 5.4 ± 0.1 ng/mL in healthy normals *4580* In 16 growth hormone-deficient children mean baseline concentration of 9.39 ± 3.19 ng/mL compared with normal range of 18.20 ± 4.1 ng/mL *151*

Serum *No Effect* In patients with growth hormone deficiency bone Gla concentration normal *4825*

Phosphate *Serum* *No Effect* In 66 children with growth hormone deficiency mean concentration of 4.9 ± 0.2 mg/dL not significantly different from 4.8 ± 0.1 mg/dL in a control group of children with short stature not associated with GH deficiency *1748* In 16 growth hormone deficient children mean baseline concentration of 4.98 ± 0.37 mg/dL not different from normal range of 3.26 - 5.17 mg/dL *151*

Pyridinoline *Urine* *Decrease* In 17 growth hormone deficient children mean excretion significanly less than in healthy children of the same age. Mean Z score - 1.39 *1596*

Pyridinoline Cross-linked Telopeptide of Type I Collagen *Serum* *No Effect* In 8 adults with GH deficiency mean concentration of 4.7 ± 0.8 ng/mL similar to 4.1 ± 0.3 ng/mL in healthy controls *4580*

Thyroxine (T4), Free *Serum* *No Effect* In 64 adults with childhood onset growth hormone deficiency mean concentration of 17.9 ± 5.6 pmol/L not significantly different from 17.3 ± 2.9 pmol/L in 45 healthy controls *1047*

Tri-iodothyronine, Free (fT3) *Serum* *Decrease* In 64 adult patients with childhood onset growth hormone deficiency mean concentration of 5.4 ± 1.4 pmol/L significantly less than 6.4 ± 1.0 pmol/L in 45 healthy controls *1047*

253.30 Growth Hormone Deficiency (continued)

Triglycerides *Serum* *No Effect* In 64 adult patients with childhood onset of growth hormone deficiency mean concentration of 1.15 ± 0.60 mmol/L not significantly different from 0.99 ± 0.49 mmol/L in 45 healthy controls *1047*

253.30 Growth Hormone Receptor Deficiency

Insulin-like Growth Factor-I *Serum* *Increase* Mean concentration barely detectable in 18 children with growth hormone receptor deficiency significantly different from mean of about 180 ng/mL in healthy adults *2971*

253.40 Gonadotroponin Releasing Hormone Deficiency

Follicle Stimulating Hormone *Plasma* *Decrease* Median concentration in 24 male patients with GnRH deficiency of 2.4 ± 1.2 IU/L significantly different from 1.6 - 15.7 IU/L in controls *3699*

Inhibin-B *Plasma* *Decrease* Median concentration in 24 male patients with GnRH deficiency of 60 ± 21 pg/mL significantly different from 87 - 361 pg/mL in controls *3699*

Luteinizing Hormone *Plasma* *Decrease* Median concentration in 24 male patients with GnRH deficiency of 1.6 ± 1.2 IU/L significantly different from 4.7 - 18.4 IU/L in controls *3699*

Sperm Count *Semen* *Decrease* Median concentration in 24 male patients with GnRH deficiency of 0.0 x 10^6/mL significantly different from 25 - 70 x 10^6/mL in controls *3699*

Testosterone *Serum* *Decrease* Median concentration in 24 male patients with GnRH deficiency of 49 ± 20 ng/dL significantly different from 318 - 739 ng/dL in controls *3699*

253.40 Idiopathic Hypogonadotropic Hypogonadism

Dehydroepiandrosterone Sulfate *Plasma* *No Effect* Mean concentration of 0.53 ± 0.27 µmol/L observed in 21 men with IHH not significantly different from 0.71 ± 0.38 µmol/L in 11 healthy controls *3956*

Estradiol *Plasma* *Increase* Mean concentration of 241 ± 112 pmol/L observed in 21 men with IHH significantly different from 155 ± 79 pmol/L in 11 healthy controls *3956*

Follicle Stimulating Hormone *Plasma* *Decrease* Mean concentration of 0.73 ± 0.49 IU/L observed in 21 men with IHH significantly different from 8.6 ± 3.7 IU/L in 11 healthy controls *3956* Median concentration in 10 male patients with idiopathic hypogonadotropic hypogonadism of 2.9 ± 1.7 IU/L significantly different from 1.6 - 15.7 IU/L in controls *3699*

Inhibin-A *Plasma* *No Effect* Concentration undetectable in 7 men with IHH, as in 16 healthy men aged 19 - 45 y *113*

Inhibin-B *Plasma* *Decrease* Mean concentration of 45 ± 11 pg/mL in 7 men with IHH significantly less than 187 ± 28 pg/mL in 16 healthy men aged 19 - 45 y *113*
Plasma *No Effect* Median concentration in 10 male patients with idiopathic hypogonadotropic hypogonadism of 119 ± 59 pg/mL not significantly different from 87 - 361 pg/mL in controls *3699*

Luteinizing Hormone *Plasma* *Decrease* Mean concentration of 1.60 ± 1.74 IU/L observed in 21 men with IHH significantly different from 5.8 ± 2.1 IU/L in 11 healthy controls *3956* Median concentration in 10 male patients with idiopathic hypogonadotropic hypogonadism of 1.5 ± 1.2 IU/L significantly different from 4.7 - 18.4 IU/L in controls *3699*

Melatonin *Plasma* *Increase* Mean morning concentration of 41.8 ± 24.4 pmol/L observed in 21 men with IHH significantly different from 21.7 ± 10.8 pmol/L in 11 healthy controls *3956*

Prolactin *Plasma* *No Effect* Mean concentration of 2.39 ± 0.44 µg/L observed in 21 men with IHH not significantly different from 3.8 ± 3.3 µg/L in 11 healthy controls *3956*

Sex-Hormone Binding Globulin *Serum* *Increase* Mean concentration of 60.9 ± 34.2 nmol/L observed in 21 men with IHH significantly different from 28.2 ± 16.2 nmol/L in 11 healthy controls *3956*

Sperm Count *Semen* *Decrease* Median concentration in 10 male patients with idiopathic hypogonadotropic hypogonadism of 0.0 x 10^6/mL significantly different from 25 - 70 x 10^6/mL in controls *3699*

Testosterone *Serum* *Decrease* Median concentration in 10 male patients with idiopathic hypogonadotropic hypogonadism of 78 ± 34 ng/dL significantly different from 318 - 739 ng/dL in controls *3699* Mean concentration of 2.14 ± 1.8 nmol/L observed in 21 men with IHH significantly different from 17.6 ± 6.5 nmol/L in 11 healthy controls *3956*

Testosterone, Free *Serum* *Decrease* Mean concentration of 7.80 ± 10.15 pmol/L observed in 21 men with IHH significantly different from 81.8 ± 18.1 pmol/L in 11 healthy controls *3956*

253.40 Juvenile Hypogonadism

Phosphate *Serum* *Increase* Serum phosphate concentration may be increased with juvenile hypogonadism *5204*

253.40 Kallmann's Syndrome

Pro-α-C-related Peptide *Plasma* *No Effect* Mean concentration of approximately 870 pg/mL in 7 men with Kallmann's syndrome not significantly different from 880 pg/mL in 16 healthy men aged 19 - 45 y *113*

253.50 Diabetes Insipidus

Aldosterone *Plasma* *Decrease* Under basal conditions mean concentration in 9 patients approximately 300 pmol/L compared with 325 pmol/L in 11 healthy controls *148*
Plasma *No Effect* In 4 children with nephrogenic diabetes insipidus baseline concentrations of aldosterone of about 370 pmol/L within normal range *2408*

Antidiuretic Hormone *Plasma* *Decrease* Posterior pituitary insufficiency is signaled by the deficiency of ADH *2304*

Aquaporin-2 *Urine* *Increase* In 6 individuals with nephrogenic diabetes insipidus, excretion after overnight dehydration of 0.4 ± 0.05 pmol/mg creatinine significantly less than 11.2 ± 2.2 pmol/mg creatinine in 5 normal indviduals under same conditions *2554*

Bicarbonate *Serum* *No Effect* Usually concentration unchanged from normal *5544*

Chloride *Urine* *Decrease* Urine chloride concentration is very low, but because of the large urine volume, the daily output is normal *1290*

Cortisol *Plasma* *No Effect* Under basal conditions mean concentration approximately 500 nmol/L in 9 patients with diabetes insipidus and 11 healthy controls *148*

Effective Renal Plasma Flow *Patient* *No Effect* In 4 children with nephrogenic diabetes insipidus mean ERPF within normal range *2408*

Glomerular Filtration Rate *Urine* *No Effect* In 4 children with nephrogenic diabetes insipidus mean GFR within normal range *2408*

Osmolality *Serum* *Increase* Mean basal concentration of 303.4 ± 4.1 mmol/kg significantly greater than 292.4 ± 2.1 mmol/kg in 11 healthy controls *148* If the water intake does not keep pace with the urinary output, there may be mild hypernatremia and a tendency toward serum hyperosmolality *1980*
Urine *Decrease* In 9 patients studied under basal conditions mean concentration of 98.6 ± 15.3 mmol/kg significantly less than 546.0 ± 116.7 mmol/kg in 11 healthy controls *148* Usually < 200 mOsm/kg *1980*

pH *Urine* *No Effect* Usually within normal limits *5544*

Potassium *Serum* *No Effect* In 9 patients studied under basal conditions mean concentration of 4.5 ± 0.1 mmol/L not significantly different from 4.6 ± 0.1 mmol/L in healthy controls *148*
Urine *No Effect* Usualy excretion remains normal *5544*

Renin Activity *Plasma Increase* Under basal conditions in 9 patients mean concentration of 23 ng/L/min compared with 8 ng/L/min in 11 healthy controls *148*
Plasma No Effect In 4 children with nephrogenic diabetes insipidus baseline concentrations of renin activity of about 5 µg/L/h within normal range *2408*

Sodium *Serum Increase* If the water intake does not keep pace with the urinary output, there may be mild hypernatremia and a tendency toward serum hyperosmolality *1980* In 9 patients with diabetes insipidus studied under basal conditions mean concentration of 150.4 ± 1.3 mmol/L significantly increased compared with 147.9 ± 1.4 mmol/L in 11 healthy controls *148*
Serum No Effect Normal or increased *5544*
Urine No Effect Concentration usually unaffected *5544*

Specific Gravity *Urine Decrease* Polyuria and hyposthenuria *4979* Always abnormal *900*

Uric Acid *Serum Increase* Occasionally *1819*

Vasopressin *Plasma Decrease* In 9 patients under basal conditions mean concentration of 1.35 ± 0.42 pmol/L significantly reduced compared with 3.35 ± 0.33 pmol/L in 11 healthy controls *148*
Plasma No Effect In 2 children with nephrogenic diabetes insipidus baseline concentrations of arginine vasopressin of 20 and 43 pmol/L significantly increased whereas concentrations of 2 and 5 pmol/L in 2 children with partial diabetes insipidus within normal range *2408*

Volume *Urine Increase* Polyuria and hyposthenuria *4979* Large volume (4 - 15 L/24 h) is characteristic *5545* Usually > 3 L/day *1980* After ingestion of 1,000 mL of 1% sodium chloride the urine volume in normal subjects and in pathological polydipsia is 25% of the ingested fluid. In diabetes insipidus the excretion rate is unchanged *1290*

253.50 Diabetes Insipidus, Central

Creatinine *Serum Increase* Mean concentration of 1.0 ± 0.3 mg/dL in 13 patients with central diabetes insipidus significantly different from 0.7 ± 0.2 mg/dL in 27 healthy controls *1084*

Creatinine Clearance *Urine No Effect* Mean clearance of 95 ± 22 mL/min in 13 patients with central diabetes insipidus not significantly different from 108 ± 10 mL/min in 27 healthy controls *1084*

Fractional Excretion of Sodium *Urine No Effect* Mean excretion of 0.9 ± 0.6% in 13 patients with central diabetes insipidus not significantly different from 0.5 ± 0.2% in 27 healthy controls *1084*

Fractional Excretion of Urea *Urine Increase* Mean excretion of 64 ± 16% in 13 patients with central diabetes insipidus significantly different from 45 ± 7.5% in 27 healthy controls *1084*

Fractional Excretion of Uric Acid *Urine Decrease* Mean excretion of 4.9 ± 0.8% in 13 patients with central diabetes insipidus significantly different from 8.2 ± 2.0% in 27 healthy controls *1084*

Osmolality *Urine No Effect* Mean excretion of 106 ± 40 mOsm/kg in 13 patients with central diabetes insipidus not significantly different from 50 - 1,000 mOsm/kg in 27 healthy controls *1084*

Protein *Serum No Effect* Mean concentration of 7.2 ± 0.7 g/dL in 13 patients with central diabetes insipidus not significantly different from 7.2 ± 0.7 g/dL in 27 healthy controls *1084*

Renin Activity *Plasma Increase* Mean activity of 4.0 ± 2.0 ng/mL/h in 13 patients with central diabetes insipidus significantly different from 1.5 ± 0.6 ng/mL/h in 27 healthy controls *1084*

Sodium *Serum No Effect* Mean concentration of 142.5 ± 3 mmol/L in 13 patients with central diabetes insipidus not significantly different from 140 ± 2.5 mmol/L in 27 healthy controls *1084*

Urea *Serum Decrease* Mean concentration of 21 ± 7 mg/dL in 13 patients with central diabetes insipidus significantly different from 32 ± 7 mg/dL in 27 healthy controls *1084*

Uric Acid *Serum Increase* Mean concentration of 7.1 ± 2.2 mg/dL in 13 patients with central diabetes insipidus significantly different from 4.3 ± 0.9 mg/dL in 27 healthy controls *1084*
Urine No Effect Mean excretion of 480 ± 120 mg/d in 13 patients with central diabetes insipidus not significantly different from 548 ± 100 mg/d in 27 healthy controls *1084*

255.00 Adrenal Cortical Hyperfunction (Glucocorticoid Excess)

Alanine *Plasma Increase* Increased *237 555 4798*

Alkaline Phosphatase *Serum Increase* Presumably due to excess ACTH *1290*

Amino Acids *Plasma Decrease* Cortisol accelerates the catabolism of protein and stimulates the hepatic uptake and deamination of amino acids *367*

Androgens *Plasma Increase* Secretion may be increased and may be a factor in hirsutism, but virilization is rare *5863*

Angiotensin-II *Plasma Decrease* In 4 patients with Cushing's Syndrome values were extremely low in renal venous blood *2873*

Bicarbonate *Serum Increase* Metabolic alkalosis may occur with potassium loss *1980*

Calcium *Serum Increase* Some cases with osteoporosis *1290*
Urine Increase Observed effect *1025*

Carbon Dioxide Partial Pressure *Blood Increase* Metabolic alkalosis may occur with potassium loss *1980*

Cholesterol *Serum Increase* Slight elevations *1025*

Corticotropin *Plasma Decrease* Very low or undetectable in Cushing's patients with primary adrenocortical tumor *5863*
Plasma Increase Loss of the diurnal rhythm, with 6 p.m. levels abnormally raised in spite of increased cortisol concentration. Secondary disease (pituitary) *1290*

Cortisol *Plasma Increase* Increased due to adrenal hyperplasia and adrenal neoplasia *3155* Untreated patients almost always have concentrations in excess of 15 µg/dL at all times *367* Elevated night values or the lack of significant day-night variation is a consistent feature *2002* All forms demonstrate some degree of autonomous secretion of excessive amounts of cortisol *2039*

Creatine *Serum Increase* Increased formation *1290*
Urine Increase Increased formation *5545*

Dehydroepiandrosterone Sulfate *Plasma Increase* Observed effect *3778 91*

Eosinophils *Blood Decrease* Eosinopenia is frequent (usually < 100 /µL) *5545* Patients with hypercortisolism often have neutrophilia, lymphopenia, and eosinopenia *1980* Below 100 /µL in 90% of cases *2034*

Erythrocytes *Blood Increase* Mild erythrocytosis in some patients *5677*

α_2-Globulin *Serum Increase* May be moderately increased *5544*

γ-Globulin *Serum Decrease* May be decreased *5545*

Glucocorticoids *Plasma Increase* In most cases of hypercortisolism, the baseline plasma and urinary corticosteroids are elevated. Loss of the normal diurnal rhythm is usually noted *1980* Diagnosed by demonstrating an excessive secretion of glucocorticoid hormone *2304*
Urine Increase In most cases of hypercortisolism, the baseline plasma and urinary corticosteroids are elevated. Loss of the normal diurnal rhythm is usually noted *1980*

Glucose *Serum Increase* Abnormally high amounts of cortisol tend to raise the blood glucose *367* Frequently complicated by an insulin resistant diabetes *5544*
Urine Increase Glycosuria appears in 50% of patients *5545*

Glucose Tolerance *Serum Decrease* Frequently abnormal *1980* Decreased in < 50% of patients *5544*

Growth Hormone *Plasma Decrease* Basal levels are often low and respond poorly to stimuli *1980*

Hematocrit *Blood Decrease* Normal or occasionally slightly elevated unless a malignancy is present in which case it may be depressed *900* Patients with ectopic ACTH syndrome may be anemic *1980*
Blood Increase Normal or occasionally slightly elevated unless a malignancy is present in which case it may be depressed *900*
Blood No Effect Normal or occasionally slightly elevated unless a malignancy is present in which case it may be depressed *900*

Hemoglobin *Blood Decrease* Normal or occasionally slightly elevated unless a malignancy is present in which case it may be depressed *900* Patients with ectopic ACTH syndrome may be anemic *1980*

255.00 Adrenal Cortical Hyperfunction (Glucocorticoid Excess) *(continued)*

Hemoglobin *(continued)*
Blood Increase Normal or occasionally slightly elevated unless a malignancy is present in which case it may be depressed *900*
Blood No Effect Normal or occasionally slightly elevated unless a malignancy is present in which case it may be depressed *900*

11-Hydroxycorticosteroids *Plasma Increase* Cortisol-binding globulin becomes saturated at the upper limit of normal for plasma cortisol, resulting in a disproportionately high unbound cortisol concentration *2039* Increased free plasma concentration and failure to reduce secretion with dexamethasone *5863*
Urine Increase Raised and relatively constant urinary excretions usually occur, but values may fluctuate from normal to elevated over a period of days *2002* Increased in all forms of the syndrome *5863*

17-Hydroxycorticosteroids *Urine Increase* Elevated values at a time when the patient is not under acute exogenous stress strongly favor the diagnosis. Confirmed by demonstrating nonsuppressibility of urinary 17-OHCS to low-dose dexamethasone *2304* Increased excretion of 17-OHCS and 17-KS is characteristic *1731*

17-Hydroxyprogesterone *Plasma Increase* Increased 17 OH-progesterone in recurring and cancerous patients *3155*

Insulin *Plasma Increase* Typically observed with adrenal cortical hyperfunction *1290*

Insulin Tolerance *Plasma Increase* The blood sugar falls by < 25% of its initial value and rapidly returns to the fasting level *1290*

Isocitrate Dehydrogenase *Serum No Effect* No effect on activity observed *5008*

17-Ketogenic Steroids *Urine Increase* Very high values suggest ectopic ACTH production or adrenocortical carcinoma *5863* Diagnosis is confirmed by demonstrating nonsuppressibility of 17-KS to low-dose dexamethasone *2304* Over 4 times normal in 50% of adrenal carcinomas, 15% of extrapituitary tumors that secrete ACTH, 3% of adrenal hyperplasias without tumors with Cushing's Syndrome *5544*
Urine No Effect May be normal in pituitary-dependent Cushing's syndrome *5863*

17-Ketosteroids *Urine Increase* Characteristic *1731* May be very high in Cushing's syndrome with adrenocortical carcinoma *5863*
Urine No Effect Usually normal in hyperplasia and adenoma of adrenal cortex *5863*

LDL-Cholesterol *Serum Increase* Moderate elevation secondary to increased conversion of VLDL to LDL *126*

Leukocytes *Blood Increase* May be elevated as a result of the ability of glucocorticoids to increase circulating polymorphonuclear neutrophils *900* Mild neutrophilic leukocytosis *2034*

Lymphocytes *Blood Decrease* Relative lymphopenia is frequent (differential is usually < 15%) *5545* Patients with hypercortisolism often have neutrophilia, lymphopenia, and eosinopenia *1980*

Neutrophils *Blood Increase* In many cases *2304* If hypokalemia is severe *2034* Some patients have granulocytosis, lymphopenia, and eosinopenia *367*

pH *Blood Increase* Metabolic alkalosis may occur with potassium loss *1980*

Phosphate *Serum Decrease* Occasional hypophosphatemia as a result of high corticosteroid concentrations *2719*

Potassium *Serum Decrease* Characterized by low serum concentration and hypertension *2304* Severe hypokalemia and weakness are best explained by the enormous quantities of cortisol secreted by the hyperplastic adrenals *367*
Urine Increase There is excessive endogenous adrenocortical activity with increased potassium loss in the urine *1290*

Pregnanetriol *Urine Increase* Increased in recurring and cancerous patients *3155*

Prolactin *Plasma Increase* Can trigger a mild to moderate increase (20 - 300 ng/mL) *3391*

Prostaglandins *Plasma Decrease* In 4 patients with Cushing's Syndrome values were extremely low in renal venous blood *2873*

Protein *Serum Decrease* Cortisol accelerates the catabolism of protein and stimulates the hepatic uptake and deamination of amino acids *367*

Renin Activity *Plasma Decrease* In 4 patients with Cushing's Syndrome values were extremely low in renal venous blood *2873*

Sodium *Serum Increase* Sodium retention and elevated blood pressure can occur *367*
Serum No Effect Sodium retention leads to increased total body concentration, but serum concentration is normal due to water retention *5863*

Testosterone *Serum Decrease* Decreased in male patients *3155*

Thyroid Stimulating Hormone *Serum No Effect* Concentration typically normal *5544*

Urea Nitrogen *Serum Increase* A condition that may be associated with excessive protein catabolism *1025*

VLDL-Cholesterol *Serum Increase* Minimal elevation due to increased secretion *126*

Volume *Plasma Decrease* Polycythemia occurs in 10 - 20% of patients, due either to an increase in red cell volume or decrease in plasma volume *3710*
Red Blood Cells Increase Polycythemia occurs in 10 - 20% of patients, due either to an increase in red cell volume or decrease in plasma volume *3710*
Urine Increase Polyuria *2034*

Zinc *Serum Decrease* Mean concentration of 5.2 µg/L (n = 33) compared with mean in controls of 2.6 µg/L (n = 42) *1589*

255.00 Cushing's Disease

Aldosterone *Plasma No Effect* Mean concentration of 191.4 ± 44.9 pmol/L in 11 patients with Cushing's disease not significantly different from 203.3 ± 13.7 pmol/L in 47 healthy controls *5775*

Androstenedione *Plasma Increase* In 2 of 14 patients with Cushing's disease concentration increased (range 4.1 - 11.3 nmol/L) compared with normal ranges of 2.1 - 7.7 nmol/L in men and 3.3 - 9.9 nmol/L in women *984*

Arginine Vasopressin *Plasma No Effect* Mean concentration of 9.5 ± 0.9 pmol/L observed in 18 patients, similar to that in healthy individuals *880*

Corticotropin *Plasma Increase* Increased concentration observed in about 50% of patients but in other 50% concentration within normal range *2952*
Plasma No Effect Mean concentration of 15.5 ± 2.8 pmol/L observed in 18 patients compared with normal range of 2.3 - 20.7 pmol/L *880* Mean concentration in 2 patients with Cushing's disease of 18.5 pmol/L not significantly different from range in 50 healthy Caucasian volunteers of 4.4 - 18 pmol/L *3605*

Cortisol *Plasma Increase* In 13 patients with Cushing's disease mean concentration of 832.0 ± 136.7 nmol/L significantly higher than 344.6 ± 16.2 nmol/L in 47 healthy controls *5775* In 9 of 14 patients with Cushing's disease mean concentration was increased *984*
Plasma No Effect Mean concentration of 392 nmol/L in 2 patients with Cushing's disease not significantly different from that in 50 healthy Caucasian volunteers, 344 ± 81 nmol/L *3605*

Cortisone *Plasma No Effect* Mean concentration of 45 nmol/L in 2 patients with Cushing's disease not significantly different from that in 50 healthy Caucasian volunteers, 51.4 ± 16.7 nmol/L *3605*

Dehydroepiandrosterone *Plasma Decrease* In all 14 adult patients with Cushing's disease concentration normal or low *984*

Dehydroepiandrosterone Sulfate *Plasma Increase* In 3 of 14 adult patients with Cushing's disease concentration increased *984*

Galanin *Plasma No Effect* Mean concentration in 15 patients with Cushing's disease of 15.8 ± 1.60 pmol/L not significantly different from 14.8 ± 1.6 pmol/L in 33 healthy controls *2345*

Growth Hormone *Plasma Decrease* In children with Cushing's disease mean 24 hour concentration significantly reduced compared with sex and pubertal stage matched controls *3219*

Plasma *Increase* Mean 24 h concentration in 11 patients with Cushing's disease of 3.6 µg/L significantly greater than in healthy individuals *3219*

Growth Hormone Binding Protein *Serum* *Increase* Concentration in 14 patients with Cushing's disease of 1,229.4 ± 93.9 pmol/L significantly greater than 983.5 ± 120.8 pmol/L 6 - 12 months after surgery to remove tumor *3219*
Serum *No Effect* In 14 children with Cushing's disease mean concentration not significantly different from concentration in sex and pubertal stage matched controls *3219*

Insulin-like Growth Factor-I *Serum* *Increase* Concentration in 14 patients with Cushing's disease of 353.4 ± 48.3 ng/mL significantly greater than 276.2 ± 37.0 ng/mL 6 - 12 months after surgery to remove tumor *3219*
Serum *No Effect* Mean concentration in 14 children with Cushing's disease mean concentration not significantly different from concentration in sex and pubertal stage matched controls *3219*

Insulin-like Growth Factor Binding Protein-3
Serum *Increase* Concentration in 14 patients with Cushing's disease of 3.3 ± 0.3 mg/L significantly greater than 2.4 ± 0.2 mg/L 6 - 12 months after surgery to remove tumor *3219*
Serum *No Effect* In 14 children with Cushing's disease mean concentration not significantly different from sex and pubertal stage matched controls *3219*

18-Oxycortisol *Plasma* *Increase* Mean concentration in 13 patients with Cushing's disease of 2.921 ± 0.431 nmol/L significantly higher than 0.827 ± 0.40 nmol/L in 47 healthy controls *5775*

Sex-Hormone Binding Globulin *Serum* *Decrease* In women with Cushing's disease very low concentrations of SHBG have been observed *1424*

255.00 Cushing's Syndrome

Aldosterone *Plasma* *No Effect* In 10 patients with Cushing's syndrome due to adrenocortical adenoma mean concentration of 131.9 ± 26.3 pmol/L not significantly different from 203.3 ± 13.7 pmol/L in 47 healthy controls *5775*

Alkaline Phosphatase, Bone Isoenzyme *Serum* *Increase* In patients with Cushing's syndrome slight increase observed *4217*

Amino-terminal Propeptide of Type III Collagen
Serum *Decrease* In 12 patients with active Cushing's syndrome mean concentration of 2.8 ± 0.8 µg/L significantly less than 3.7 ± 0.8 µg/L in 27 healthy volunteer controls *4141*

Corticotropin *Plasma* *Increase* In 8 patients with pituitary corticotroph macroadenomas concentrations ranged from 77 to 5,730 pg/mL compared with normal of less than 60 pg/mL *4262* In 6 patients with active Cushing's syndrome concentrations ranged from 7.0 - 20.0 pmol/L significantly different from 5.4 ± 0.8 pmol/L in age and sex-matched controls *4578*

Cortisol *Plasma* *Increase* In 14 patients with Cushing's syndrome mean concentration of 774 ± 193 nmol/L compared with reference interval of 165 - 689 nmol/L *520* 150 patients with Cushing's syndrome had detectable midnight sleeping concentrations of cortisol (70 - 2,000 pmol/L) compared with undetectable amounts in healthy controls *3771* Mean concentration in 10 patients with Cushing's syndrome due to adrenocortical adenoma of 585.9 ± 43.4 nmol/L significantly higher than 344.6 ± 16.2 nmol/L in 47 healthy controls *5775* In 6 patients with active Cushing's syndrome concentrations ranged from 469 - 1,217 nmol/L significantly different from 403 ± 20 nmol/L in age and sex-matched controls *4578*
Saliva *Increase* In 14 patients with Cushing's syndrome mean concentration of 161 ± 400 nmol/L compared with reference interval of 6.9 - 30 nmol/L *520*
Urine *Increase* In 14 patients with Cushing's syndrome mean concentration of 2,634 ± 1,140 nmol/L compared with reference interval of 207 - 745 nmol/L *520*

Cortisol, Free *Urine* *Increase* Mean concentration in 26 patients with Cushing's syndrome of 180 ± 26 µg/d different from 23 ± 8 µg/d in 60 healthy controls *3062* In 6 patients with active Cushing's syndrome excretions ranged from 316 - 1,475 nmol/d significantly different from 120 ± 8.8 nmol/d in age and sex-matched controls *4578*

Cortisone, Free *Urine* *Increase* Mean concentration in 26 patients with Cushing's syndrome of 258 ± 152 µg/d different from 73 ± 22 µg/d in 60 healthy controls *3062*

Cross-linked C-terminal Telopeptide of Type I Collagen
Serum *Decrease* In 8 patients with active Cushing's syndrome mean concentration of 3.0 ± 0.4 ng/mL not significantly different from 4.1 ± 0.3 ng/mL in age and sex-matched controls *4578*

C-terminal Propeptide of Type III Procollagen
Serum *No Effect* In 12 adult patients with active Cushing's syndrome mean concentration of 128 ± 46 µg/L not significantly different when compared with 117 ± 44 µg/L in healthy volunteer controls *4141*

C-terminal Telopeptide of Type I Collagen *Serum* *Decrease* In 12 patients with active Cushing's syndrome mean concentration of 2..7 - 0.2 ng/mL significantly less than mean concentration of 3.9 ± 0.2 ng/mL in 28 control individuals *4579*

Free Cortisone:Free Cortisol Ratio *Urine* *Decrease* Mean ratio in 26 patients with Cushing's syndrome of 2.35 ± 1.20 different from 3.35 ± 1.28 in 60 healthy controls *3062*

17-Ketogenic Steroids *Urine* *Increase* Excretion may be increased in patients with Cushing's syndrome *2952*

17-Ketosteroids *Urine* *Increase* Excretion may be increased in patients with Cushing's syndrome *2952*

Lipotropic Hormone *Plasma* *Increase* In 6 patients with pituitary corticotroph macroadenomas concentrations ranged from 517 to 13,3600 pg/mL compared with normal of less than 60 pg/mL *4262*

N-terminal Propeptide of Type III Procollagen
Serum *Decrease* In 12 patients with active Cushing's syndrome mean concentration of 1.9 - 0.2 ng/mL significantly less than mean concentration of 3.2 ± 0.2 ng/mL in 28 control individuals *4579*

Osteocalcin *Serum* *Decrease* In 12 patients with active Cushing's syndrome mean concentration of 0.9 - 0.2 ng/mL significantly less than mean concentration of 5.5 ± 0.2 ng/mL in 28 control individuals *4579* In 12 patients with active Cushing's syndrome mean concentration of 3.6 ± 2.4 ng/mL significantly less than 8.2 ± 3.2 ng/mL in 27 healthy volunteer controls *4141* In 8 patients with active Cushing's syndrome mean concentration of 1.0 ± 0.35 ng/mL significantly reduced compared with 5.4 ± 0.15 ng/mL in age and sex-matched controls *4578*
Serum *Increase* In patients with Cushing's syndrome slight increase observed *4217*

18-Oxycortisol *Plasma* *Increase* In 10 patients with Cushing's syndrome due to adrenocortical adenoma mean concentration of 1.752 ± 0.358 nmol/L significantly higher than 0.827 ± 0.40 nmol/L in 47 healthy controls *5775*

Proopiomelanocortin *Plasma* *Increase* In 8 patients with pituitary corticotroph macroadenomas concentrations ranged from < 60 to 4,200 U/mL compared with undetectable concentrations in 17 healthy individuals *4262*

255.00 Ectopic ACTH Secretion

Corticotropin *Plasma* *Increase* Mean concentration in 5 patients with ectopic ACTH secretion of 84 ± 62 pmol/L significantly different from range in 50 healthy Caucasian volunteers of 4.4 - 18 pmol/L *3605*

Cortisol *Plasma* *Increase* Mean concentration of 2,959 ± 3,874 nmol/L in 5 patients with ectopic adrenocorticotropin secretion significantly different from that in 50 healthy Caucasian volunteers, 344 ± 81 nmol/L *3605*
Urine *Increase* Concentrations in 3 patients with ectopic ACTH secretion of 490, 607 and 2662 nmol/d significantly greater than that in 50 healthy Caucasian volunteers, 130 ± 104 nmol/d *3605*

Cortisone *Plasma* *No Effect* Mean concentration of 79.7 ± 34.0 nmol/L in 5 patients with ectopic ACTH secretion not significantly different from that in 50 healthy Caucasian volunteers, 51.4 ± 16.7 nmol/L *3605*
Urine *Increase* Concentrations in 3 patients with ectopic ACTH secretion of 3.1, 7.1 and 68.2 nmol/d greater than that in 50 healthy Caucasian volunteers, 0.52 ± 0.29 nmol/d *3605*

255.00 Nelson's Syndrome

Chloride *Serum* *Decrease* In one patient with Nelson's syndrome serum sodium concentration was slightly decreased at 91 mmol/L *2621*

Corticotropin *Plasma* *Increase* In one patient with Nelson's syndrome plasma ACTH concentration was increased at 56 pmol/L (reference interval 0.0 - 8.1 pmol/L) *2621*

Creatinine *Serum* *No Effect* In one patient with Nelson's syndrome serum urea nitrogen concentration was normal at 88 µmol/L *2621*

Follicle Stimulating Hormone *Plasma* *No Effect* In one patient with Nelson's syndrome plasma FSH concentration was normal at 5.6 IU/L (reference interval 4 - 10 IU/L) *2621*

Glucose *Serum* *Decrease* In one patient with Nelson's syndrome fasting blood glucose concentration was slightly reduced at 3.9 mmol/L *2621*
Serum *No Effect* In one patient with Nelson's syndrome fasting blood glucose concentration was normal at 3.9 mmol/L *2621*

Luteinizing Hormone *Plasma* *No Effect* In one patient with Nelson's syndrome plasma LH concentration was normal at 3.0 IU/L (reference interval 1 - 8 IU/L) *2621*

Potassium *Serum* *Increase* In one patient with Nelson's syndrome serum sodium concentration was slightly increased at 6.3 mmol/L *2621*

Prolactin *Plasma* *No Effect* In one patient with Nelson's syndrome plasma prolactin concentration was normal at 4.5 µg/L (reference interval 3.3 - 10 µg/L) *2621*

Sodium *Serum* *Decrease* In one patient with Nelson's syndrome serum sodium concentration was slightly reduced at 125 mmol/L *2621*

Thyroxine (T4), Free *Serum* *No Effect* In one patient with Nelson's syndrome plasma TSH concentration was normal at 2.3 mIU/L (reference interval 0.6 - 4.6 mIU/L) *2621* In one patient with Nelson's syndrome plasma free T4 concentration was normal at 17.2 nmol/L (reference interval 10 - 25 nmol/L) *2621*

Tri-iodothyronine, Free (fT3) *Serum* *No Effect* In one patient with Nelson's syndrome plasma free T3 concentration was low normal at 2.2 pmol/L (reference interval 2.1 - 6.1 IU/L) *2621*

Urea Nitrogen *Serum* *No Effect* In one patient with Nelson's syndrome serum urea nitrogen concentration was normal at 4.9 mmol/L *2621*

255.10 Adrenal Cortical Hyperfunction (Mineralocorticoid Excess)

Aldosterone *Plasma* *Increase* If the secretion rate is elevated, it may be assumed that the patient has either primary or secondary aldosteronism *367*
Urine *Increase* Increased on normal salt diet (not detectable on all days); cannot be reduced by high sodium intake and DOCA administration. Increased in primary and secondary hyperaldosteronism due to adrenal adenoma and adrenal carcinoma *5545*

Ammonia *Urine* *Increase* Exaggerated ammonia production results in a tendency to a persistently alkaline urine *2304* In primary hyperaldosteronism, possibly due to hormone action on the renal tubule cells or to the associated potassium depletion *1290*

Angiotensin-II *Plasma* *Decrease* In 8 patients with primary aldosteronism values were extremely low in renal venous blood *2873*

Bicarbonate *Serum* *Increase* Most patients exhibit a CO_2 content in the range of 32 - 38 mmol/L *2304* Reported effect *5544* Metabolic alkalosis may occur with potassium loss *1980*

Carbon Dioxide Partial Pressure *Blood* *Increase* Metabolic alkalosis may occur with potassium loss *1980*

Chloride *Serum* *Decrease* Depressed reciprocally with the bicarbonate elevation *2304* May be seen *1980*
Serum *Increase* The electrolyte pumps respond to mineralocorticoids by conserving sodium and chloride and by wasting bodily potassium *5679*

Chylomicrons *Serum* *Increase* Increased *3017* *4372* *4358*

Cortisol *Plasma* *Increase* Untreated patients almost always have concentration in excess of 15 µg/dL at all times *367* Increased due to adrenal hyperplasia and adrenal carcinoma *3155* Elevated night values or the lack of significant day-night variation is a consistent feature *2002* All forms demonstrate some degree of autonomous secretion of excessive amounts of cortisol *2039*

Dehydroepiandrosterone Sulfate *Plasma* *Increase* Observed effect *91* *3778*

Hematocrit *Blood* *Decrease* An increased volume, with slight decrease of the hematocrit value, is usual *2304*

Hemoglobin *Blood* *Decrease* An increased volume, with slight decrease of the hematocrit value, is usual *2304*

17-Hydroxycorticosteroids *Urine* *Increase* Urine 17-hydroxycorticosteroids and 17-KS excretion levels are always within normal range in patients with aldosteronomas but may occasionally be elevated in more rare instances of primary aldosteronism due to adrenal carcinoma *2034* May cause high excretion with feminization and no Cushing's syndrome involved *2039*
Urine *No Effect* Urine 17-hydroxycorticosteroids and 17-KS excretion levels are always within normal range in patients with aldosteronomas but may occasionally be elevated in more rare instances of primary aldosteronism due to adrenal carcinoma *2034*

17-Hydroxyprogesterone *Plasma* *Increase* Congenital adrenal hyperplasia *5799*

Insulin-like Growth Factor-I *Serum* *Increase* Observed effect *2166*

17-Ketosteroids *Urine* *Increase* Urine 17-hydroxycorticosteroids and 17-KS excretion levels are always within normal range in patients with aldosteronomas but may occasionally be elevated in more rare instances of primary aldosteronism due to adrenal carcinoma *2034*

Leukocytes *Urine* *Increase* Pyuria due to the predilection of potassium depleted kidneys for infection *2034*

Magnesium *Serum* *Decrease* In many cases *2304* If hypokalemia is severe *2034*

pH *Blood* *Increase* Metabolic alkalosis *2034* Metabolic alkalosis may occur with potassium loss *1980*
Urine *Increase* Exaggerated ammonia production results in a tendency to a persistently alkaline urine *2304* An alkaline urine implies the presence of alkalosis, a characteristic finding in primary aldosteronism *2304* Usually 7.0 or higher *2039*
Urine *No Effect* Normal or alkaline *5544*

Potassium *Serum* *Decrease* Characterized by low serum concentration and hypertension. Mean concentration < 3.0 mmol/L and is usually persistently in this range *2304* Renal wasting leads to hypokalemic state *3735* Progressive weakness and lack of stamina due to potassium depletion are frequent complaints *900*
Urine *Increase* Significant urinary potassium loss may be encountered despite hypokalemia *2039*
Urine *No Effect* Usually within normal limits in spite of hypokalemia and tissue potassium depletion *2304*

Prostaglandins *Plasma* *Decrease* In 8 patients with primary aldosteronism values were extremely low in renal venous blood *2873*

Protein *Urine* *Increase* Negative to trace amounts *2034* In the majority of patients *2039*

Renin Activity *Plasma* *Decrease* Low value is essential for the diagnosis of primary aldosteronism *2304* In 8 patients with primary aldosteronism values were extremely low in renal venous blood *4746* Markedly decreased (normal or increased in secondary aldosteronism). It cannot be stimulated by use of salt restriction and upright posture to deplete plasma volume *1470*

Sodium *Saliva* *Decrease* Low sweat and salivary concentration while total body exchangeable sodium is high *2304*
Serum *Increase* May be seen *1980* Frequent, although not constant *2304*
Sweat *Decrease* Low sweat and salivary concentration while total body exchangeable sodium is high *2304*

Specific Gravity *Urine* *Decrease* Less than 1.015 due to impaired ability to concentrate urine *2034*

Tetrahydroaldosterone *Urine* *Increase* Patients with primary aldosteronism can be shown at some time to have increased urinary excretion of aldosterone and/or tetrahydroaldosterone *2304*

Uric Acid *Serum* *No Effect* In the absence of azotemia *2034*

Volume *Plasma* *Increase* An increased volume, with slight decrease of the hematocrit value, is usual *2304*

255.10 Bartter's Syndrome

Aldosterone *Plasma* *Increase* Mean concentration in 7 patients with Bartter's syndrome of 0.73 ± 0.17 nmol/L significantly different from 0.18 ± 0.015 nmol/L in 7 healthy controls *663*

Calcium *Urine* *Decrease* Mean concentration in 7 patients with Bartter's syndrome of 3.8 ± 0.74 mmol/d significantly different from 4.53 ± 0.57 mmol/d in 7 healthy controls *663*

Chloride *Serum* *No Effect* Mean concentration in 7 patients with Bartter's syndrome of 97 ± 1.1 mmol/L not significantly different from 99 ± 0.8 mmol/L in 7 healthy controls *663*

Guanosine Monophosphate *Urine* *Increase* Mean concentration of cyclic guanosine monophosphate in 7 patients with Bartter's syndrome of 0.057 ± 0.028 μmol/μmol creatinine significantly different from 0.022 ± 0.01 μmol/μmol creatinine in 7 healthy controls *663*

Nitrate plus Nitrite *Urine* *Increase* Mean concentration in 7 patients with Bartter's syndrome of 0.45 ± 0.14 μmol/μmol creatinine significantly different from 0.25 ± 0.04 μmol/μmol creatinine in 7 healthy controls *663*

Potassium *Serum* *Decrease* Mean concentration in 7 patients with Bartter's syndrome of 2.6 ± 0.5 mmol/L significantly different from 4.03 ± 0.14 mmol/L in 7 healthy controls *663*

Renin Activity *Plasma* *Increase* Mean concentration in 7 patients with Bartter's syndrome of 10.86 ± 6.20 ng/h/mL significantly different from 0.96 ± 0.09 ng/h/mL in 7 healthy controls *663*

Sodium *Serum* *No Effect* Mean concentration in 7 patients with Bartter's syndrome of 138 ± 0.8 mmol/L not significantly different from 138 ± 0.9 mmol/L in 7 healthy controls *663*

255.10 Gitelman's Syndrome

Aldosterone *Plasma* *Increase* Median value of 18.5 ng/mL/h observed in one boy with Gitelman's syndrome aged 10 years different from reference interval of < 5.9 ng/mL/h *2724* In 10 patients with Gitelman's disease (hypocalciuric variant of Bartter's disease) concentrations varied from 16 to 60 ng/dL compared with an upright normal range of 7 - 24 ng/dL with 6 having concentrations higher than the upper limit of normal *896*

Bicarbonate *Serum* *Increase* In 10 patients with Gitelman's disease (hypocalciuric variant of Bartter's disease) concentrations varied from 27.0 to 33.0 mmol/L compared with a normal range of 20 - 26.5 mmol/L *896*
Serum *No Effect* Median value of 32 mmol/L observed in one boy with Gitelman's syndrome aged 10 years not different from reference interval of 21 - 29 mmol/L *2724*

Calcium *Serum* *No Effect* In 10 patients with Gitelman's disease (hypocalciuric variant of Bartter's disease) concentrations varied from 9.2 to 10.5 mg/dL compared with a normal range of 8.6 - 10.2 mg/dL with 2 at concentrations of 10.3 and 10.5 mg/dL exceeding the upper limit of normal *896* Median concentration of 9.8 mg/dL observed in one boy with Gitelman's syndrome aged 10 years not different from reference interval of 8.8 - 10.8 mg/dL *2724*
Urine *Decrease* In 10 patients with Gitelman's disease (hypocalciuric variant of Bartter's disease) excretions varied from 11 to 159 mg/d compared with a normal range of 60 - 320 mg/d with 6 having concentrations lower than the lower limit of normal and only one having a concentration in the middle of the normal range *896*

Carbon Dioxide Partial Pressure *Blood* *No Effect* Median value of 43 mm Hg observed in one boy with Gitelman's syndrome aged 10 years not different from reference interval of 32 - 46 mm Hg *2724*

Chloride *Serum* *Increase* Median concentration of 193 mmol/L observed in one boy with Gitelman's syndrome aged 10 years different from reference interval of 100 - 108 mmol/L *2724*

Creatinine Clearance *Urine* *Decrease* In 21 patients with Gitelman's syndrome mean clearance of 92.6 ± 17.0 mL/min not significantly different from 96.7 ± 23.1 mL/min in 16 controls *896*

Fractional Potassium Clearance *Urine* *Increase* In 17 patients with Gitelman's syndrome mean clearance of 20.2 ± 13.1% significantly increased compared with 13.1 ± 4.9% in 14 controls *896*

ionized Calcium *Serum* *No Effect* In 10 patients with Gitelman's disease (hypocalciuric variant of Bartter's disease) concentrations varied from 4.56 to 5.20 mg/dL compared with a normal range of 4.6 - 5.4 mg/dL, with 2 at concentrations of 10.3 and 10.5 mg/dL exceeding the upper limit of normal *896*

Magnesium *Serum* *Decrease* In 10 patients with Gitelman's disease (hypocalciuric variant of Bartter's disease) concentrations varied from 1.06 to 2.12 mg/dL compared with a normal range of 1.56 - 2.18 mg/dL, with 7 having concentrations below lower limit of normal *896* Median concentration of 1.3 mEq/L observed in one boy with Gitelman's syndrome aged 10 years different from reference interval of 1.8 - 2.4 mEq/L *2724*
Urine *Decrease* In 10 patients with Gitelman's disease (hypocalciuric variant of Bartter's disease) excretions varied from 57 to 122 mg/d compared with a normal range of 25 - 170 mg/d *896*

Oxygen Partial Pressure *Blood* *No Effect* Median value of 95 mm Hg observed in one boy with Gitelman's syndrome aged 10 years not different from reference interval of 74 - 108 mm Hg *2724*

Parathyroid Hormone *Plasma* *No Effect* Median value of 25 pg/mL observed in one boy with Gitelman's syndrome aged 10 years not different from reference interval of 1 - 43 pg/mL *2724*

pH *Blood* *Increase* In 17 patients with Gitelman's syndrome mean 7.46 ± 0.02 significantly increased compared with 7.40 ± 0.02 in 12 controls *896* Median value of 7.53 observed in one boy with Gitelman's syndrome aged 10 years different from reference interval of 7.38 - 7.46 *2724*

Phosphate *Serum* *Decrease* Median concentration of 2.5 mg/dL observed in one boy with Gitelman's syndrome aged 10 years different from reference interval of 2.9 - 5.4 mg/dL *2724*

Potassium *Serum* *Decrease* Median concentration of 1.7 mmol/L observed in one boy with Gitelman's syndrome aged 10 years different from reference interval of 3.5 - 5.2 mmol/L *2724* In 10 patients with Gitelman's disease (hypocalciuric variant of Bartter's disease) concentrations varied from 2.3 to 3.1 mmol/L compared with a normal range of 3.5 - 4.7 mmol/L *896*

Prostaglandin E_2 *Urine* *Increase* Median value of 37 ng/h/1.73 m^2 observed in one boy with Gitelman's syndrome aged 10 years not different from reference interval of > 27 ng/h/1.73 M^2 *2724*

Renin Activity *Plasma* *Increase* Median value of 68.3 pg/mL observed in one boy with Gitelman's syndrome aged 10 years different from reference interval of 3 - 35 pg/mL *2724* In 10 patients with Gitelman's disease (hypocalciuric variant of Bartter's disease) concentrations varied from 5.5 to 25.8 ng/mL/h compared with a normal range of 1 - 5 ng/mL/h *896*

Sodium *Serum* *Decrease* Median concentration of 126 mmol/L observed in one boy with Gitelman's syndrome aged 10 years different from reference interval of 140 - 148 mmol/L *2724*

255.10 Hyperaldosteronism

Aldosterone *Plasma* *Increase* Mean supine concentratration of 606 ± 70 pg/mL in 5 cases with adrenal adenoma and 585 ± 73 pg/mL in 7 with primary adrenal hyperplasia significantly different from 150 ± 10 pg/mL in 15 normal individuals *5443* Concentration typically increased in patients with primary aldosteronism *2952* Mean concentration of 902.2 ± 94.7 pmol/L in 21 patients with aldosterone producing adenoma significantly increased compared with 203.3 ± 13.7 pmol/L in 47 healthy controls *5775*
Plasma *No Effect* Concentration may be normal in 3% of patients with primary aldosteronism *2952*
Urine *Increase* Excretion typically increased in patients with primary aldosteronism *2952*

Cortisol *Plasma* *No Effect* Mean concentration in 20 patients with aldosterone secreting adenoma of 292.3 ± 25.9 nmol/L not significantly different from 344.6 ± 16.2 nmol/L in 47 healthy controls *5775*

255.10 Hyperaldosteronism *(continued)*

Endothelin-1 *Plasma* *No Effect* Mean concentratration of 6.2 ± 1.4 pg/mL in 5 cases with adrenal adenoma and 6.5 ± 1.0 pg/mL in 7 with primary adrenal hyperplasia not significantly different from 8.8 ± 1.6 pg/mL in 15 normal individuals *5443*

Magnesium *Serum* *Decrease* Concentration is reduced in association with hyperaldosteronism *2952*
Urine *Increase* Excretion is increased in association with aldosteronism *2952*

18-Oxycortisol *Plasma* *Increase* In 20 patients with primary hyperaldosteronism due to aldosterone producing adenoma mean concentration of 3.223 ± 0.466 nmol/L significantly increased compared with 0.827 ± 0.40 nmol/L in 47 healthy controls *5775*

Potassium *Serum* *Decrease* Concentration typically decreased in patients with primary aldosteronism *2952*
Serum *No Effect* Concentration may be normal in 7 to 30% of patients with primary aldosteronism *2952*

Renin Activity *Plasma* *Decrease* Mean supine concentration of < 0.2 ng AI/mL/h in 5 cases with adrenal adenoma and < 0.2 ng AI/mL/h in 7 with primary adrenal hyperplasia significantly different from 1.2 ± 0.5 ng AI/mL/h in 15 normal individuals *5443* Concentration typically decreased below 3.0 ng/mL/h, 4 hour upright on sodium restricted diet or diuretic therapy in patients with primary aldosteronism *2952*

255.10 Pseudo-Bartter's Syndrome

Guanosine Monophosphate *Urine* *No Effect* Mean concentration of cyclic guanosine phosphate in 7 patients with pseudo-Bartter's syndrome of 0.024 ± 0.004 µmol/µmol creatinine not significantly different from 0.022 ± 0.01 µmol/µmol creatinine in 7 healthy controls *663*

Nitrate plus Nitrite *Urine* *No Effect* Mean concentration in 7 patients with pseudo-Bartter's syndrome of 0.28 ± 0.05 µmol/µmol creatinine not significantly different from 0.25 ± 0.04 µmol/µmol creatinine in 7 healthy controls *663*

255.20 Adrenogenital Syndrome

17-Ketogenic Steroids *Urine* *Increase* Excretion may be increased in patients with adrenogenital syndrome *2952*

17-Ketosteroids *Urine* *Increase* Excretion may be increased in patients with the adrenogenital syndrome associated with adrenal hyperplasia *2952*

Pregnanetriol *Urine* *Increase* Increased excretion is consistent finding in patients with adrenogenital syndrome due to a defect in 21-hydroxylation *2952*

255.20 Congenital Adrenal Hyperplasia

Androgens *Plasma* *Increase* Concentration significantly increased compared with controls *3008*

3α-Androstanediol Glucuronide *Plasma* *Increase* Increased concentrations observed *1148*

Androstenedione *Plasma* *Increase* Concentration greatly increased: test is commonly used to detect 21-hydroxylase deficiency *5541*

Dehydroepiandrosterone Sulfate *Plasma* *Increase* Increased concentrations may indicate hyperandrogenism from an adrenal source *2952*

21-Deoxycortisol *Plasma* *Increase* In 27 individuals with late onset congenital adrenal hyperplasia mean concentration of 6.00 ± 6.58 nmol/L, with concentration in 18 heterozygotes of 0.77 ± 0.52 nmol/L and in 30 heterozygotes with classical congenital adrenal hyperplasia of 0.69 ± 0.49 nmol/L *1480*

Estradiol, Free *Plasma* *Increase* Significant increase observed in patients with congenital adrenal hyperplasia *3008*

Estrone *Plasma* *No Effect* No difference from normal observed in 9 newly diagnosed patients with congenital adrenal hyperplasia *3008*

17-Hydroxyprogesterone *Plasma* *Increase* Concentration increased: test is most commonly used to detect 21-hydroxylase deficiency: in most pediatric cases concentrations increased above 100 nmol/L although only at upper limit of normal in late-onset or non-classical cases *5541* Increased concentrations observed in patients with congenital adrenal hyperplasia (11- and 21-hydroxylase deficiencies) *2952*

Luteinizing Hormone *Plasma* *Increase* Mean concentration increased above normal *3008*

Mullerian Inhibiting Substance *Serum* *No Effect* In 5 girls with mean age 0.2 y but with 46,XX congenital adrenal hyperplasia or mild idiopathic clitoromegaly (46,XX) mean concentrations were at lower limit of sensitivity of 0.5 ng/mL compared with mean of 0.6 ng/mL in healthy girls of the same age *2970*

255.20 Desmolase Deficiency

Ammonium Ions *Urine* *Decrease* May cause distal renal tubular acidosis (type IV) is associated with hyperkalemia, hyperchloremic metabolic acidosis, urine pH < 5.5, decreased urinary ammonium ion excretion, a positive urine anion gap, normal urinary citrate and urinary calcium excretion *4071*

Anion Gap *Urine* *Increase* May cause distal renal tubular acidosis (type IV) is associated with hyperkalemia, hyperchloremic metabolic acidosis, urine pH < 5.5, decreased urinary ammonium ion excretion, a positive urine anion gap, normal urinary citrate and urinary calcium excretion *4071*

Calcium *Urine* *No Effect* May cause distal renal tubular acidosis (type IV) is associated with hyperkalemia, hyperchloremic metabolic acidosis, urine pH < 5.5, decreased urinary ammonium ion excretion, a positive urine anion gap, normal urinary citrate and urinary calcium excretion *4071*

Chloride *Serum* *Increase* May cause distal renal tubular acidosis (type IV) is associated with hyperkalemia, hyperchloremic metabolic acidosis, urine pH < 5.5, decreased urinary ammonium ion excretion, a positive urine anion gap, normal urinary citrate and urinary calcium excretion *4071*

Citrate *Urine* *No Effect* May cause distal renal tubular acidosis (type IV) is associated with hyperkalemia, hyperchloremic metabolic acidosis, urine pH < 5.5, decreased urinary ammonium ion excretion, a positive urine anion gap, normal urinary citrate and urinary calcium excretion *4071*

pH *Urine* *Decrease* May cause distal renal tubular acidosis (type IV) is associated with hyperkalemia, hyperchloremic metabolic acidosis, urine pH < 5.5, decreased urinary ammonium ion excretion, a positive urine anion gap, normal urinary citrate and urinary calcium excretion *4071*

Potassium *Serum* *Increase* May cause distal renal tubular acidosis (type IV) which is associated with hyperkalemia, hyperchloremic metabolic acidosis, urine pH < 5.5, decreased urinary ammonium ion excretion, a positive urine anion gap, normal urinary citrate and urinary calcium excretion *4071*

255.20 Female Virilization

Androstenedione *Plasma* *Increase* Concentration often increased in female virilization *2952*

255.20 21-Hydroxylase Deficiency

Ammonium Ions *Urine* *Decrease* May cause distal renal tubular acidosis (type IV) is associated with hyperkalemia, hyperchloremic metabolic acidosis, urine pH < 5.5, decreased urinary ammonium ion excretion, a positive urine anion gap, normal urinary citrate and urinary calcium excretion *4071*

Anion Gap *Urine* *Increase* May cause distal renal tubular acidosis (type IV) is associated with hyperkalemia, hyperchloremic metabolic acidosis, urine pH < 5.5, decreased urinary ammonium ion excretion, a positive urine anion gap, normal urinary citrate and urinary calcium excretion *4071*

Calcium *Urine* *No Effect* May cause distal renal tubular acidosis (type IV) is associated with hyperkalemia, hyperchloremic metabolic acidosis, urine pH < 5.5, decreased urinary ammonium ion excretion, a positive urine anion gap, normal urinary citrate and urinary calcium excretion *4071*

Chloride *Serum* *Increase* May cause distal renal tubular acidosis (type IV) is associated with hyperkalemia, hyperchloremic metabolic acidosis, urine pH < 5.5, decreased urinary ammonium ion excretion, a positive urine anion gap, normal urinary citrate and urinary calcium excretion *4071*

Citrate *Urine No Effect* May cause distal renal tubular acidosis (type IV) is associated with hyperkalemia, hyperchloremic metabolic acidosis, urine pH < 5.5, decreased urinary ammonium ion excretion, a positive urine anion gap, normal urinary citrate and urinary calcium excretion *4071*

Follicle Stimulating Hormone *Plasma Decrease* In 9 girls with 21-hydroxylase deficiency aged 20 to 90 days mean concentration of about 2.19 ± 3.25 IU/L significantly less than about 6.7 IU/L in 16 control girls aged 27 to 90 days *373*

Luteinizing Hormone *Plasma Increase* In 9 girls with 21-hydroxylase deficiency aged 20 to 90 days mean concentration of about 1.4 IU/L significantly greater than 0.47 ± 0.38 IU/L in 16 control girls aged 27 to 90 days *373*

pH *Urine Decrease* May cause distal renal tubular acidosis (type IV) is associated with hyperkalemia, hyperchloremic metabolic acidosis, urine pH < 5.5, decreased urinary ammonium ion excretion, a positive urine anion gap, normal urinary citrate and urinary calcium excretion *4071*

Potassium *Serum Increase* May cause distal renal tubular acidosis (type IV) which is associated with hyperkalemia, hyperchloremic metabolic acidosis, urine pH < 5.5, decreased urinary ammonium ion excretion, a positive urine anion gap, normal urinary citrate and urinary calcium excretion *4071*

255.20 11β-Hydroxysteroid Dehydrogenase Deficiency Type 2

Corticotropin *Plasma Decrease* Concentrations of 6.9 and 8.7 pmol/L in 3 patients with 11β-steroid dehydrogenase deficiency type-2 significantly different from that in 50 healthy Caucasian volunteers, 4.4 - 18 pmol/L *3605*

Saliva Decrease Concentrations of 2.4, 8.0 and 8.2 pmol/L in 3 patients with 11β-steroid dehydrogenase deficiency type-2 significantly different in one patient from that in 50 healthy Caucasian volunteers, 9.3 ± 4.0 pmol/L *3605*

Saliva No Effect Concentrations of 2.4, 8.0 and 8.2 pmol/L in 3 patients with 11β-steroid dehydrogenase deficiency type-2 not significantly different in two patients from that in 50 healthy Caucasian volunteers, 9.3 ± 4.0 pmol/L *3605*

Cortisol *Plasma Decrease* Concentrations of 146, 193 and 215 nmol/L in 3 patients with 11β-hydroxysteroid deficiency type-2 significantly different from that in 50 healthy Caucasian volunteers, 344 ± 81 nmol/L *3605*

Saliva Decrease Concentrations of 2.2, 7.2 and 8.6 nmol/L in 3 patients with 11β-steroid dehydrogenase deficiency type-2 significantly different from that in 50 healthy Caucasian volunteers, 17.9 ± 7.6 nmol/L *3605*

Urine Decrease Concentrations of 8.5, 34 and 44 nmol/d in 3 patients with 11β-steroid dehydrogenase deficiency type-2 significantly different from that in 50 healthy Caucasian volunteers, 130 ± 104 nmol/d *3605*

Cortisone *Plasma Decrease* Concentrations of 34, 47 and 52 nmol/L in 3 patients with 11β-steroid dehydrogenase deficiency type-2 significantly different from that in 50 healthy Caucasian volunteers, 51.4 ± 16.7 nmol/L *3605*

Saliva Increase Concentrations of 0.95, 1.10 and 1.11 nmol/L in 3 patients with 11β-steroid dehydrogenase deficiency type-2 significantly different from that in 50 healthy Caucasian volunteers, 0.50 ± 0.19 nmol/L *3605*

Urine Increase Concentrations of 4.56, 5.26 and 6.25 nmol/d in 3 patients with 11β-steroid dehydrogenase deficiency type-2 significantly different from that in 50 healthy Caucasian volunteers, 0.52 ± 0.29 nmol/d *3605*

255.30 Adrenal Hyperandrogenism

Androgen Index, Free (FAI) *Plasma Increase* In 8 women with adrenal hyperandrogenism mean index of 10.8 ± 4.0 significantly different from 2.4 ± 1.8 in 17 healthy control women *1388*

Androstenedione *Plasma Increase* In 8 women with adrenal hyperandrogenism mean concentration of 4.1 ± 1.4 ng/mL significantly different from 2.5 ± 0.8 ng/mL in 17 healthy control women *1388*

Cortisol *Plasma No Effect* In 8 women with adrenal hyperandrogenism mean concentration of 18.3 ± 6.0 μg/dL not significantly different from 15.3 ± 4.6 μg/dL in 17 healthy control women *1388*

Dehydroepiandrosterone Sulfate *Plasma Increase* In 8 women with adrenal hyperandrogenism mean concentration of 5,512 ± 3,226 ng/mL significantly different from 1,902 ± 705 ng/mL in 17 healthy control women *1388*

11-Deoxycortisol *Plasma No Effect* In 8 women with adrenal hyperandrogenism mean concentration of 3.7 ± 1.2 ng/mL not significantly different from 3.2 ± 2.1 ng/mL in 17 healthy control women *1388*

Growth Hormone *Plasma Increase* In 8 women with adrenal hyperandrogenism mean concentration of 7.5 ± 8.6 ng/mL not significantly different from 2.9 ± 3.9 ng/mL in 15 women with ovarian hyperadrenalism and 3.3 ± 4.1 ng/mL in 17 women with idiopathic hirsutism *1388*

17-Hydroxyprogesterone *Plasma No Effect* In 8 women with adrenal hyperandrogenism mean concentration of 1.4 ± 0.7 ng/mL not significantly different from 0.8 ± 0.3 ng/mL in 17 healthy control women *1388*

Insulin-like Growth Factor-I *Serum Increase* In 8 women with adrenal hyperandrogenism mean concentration of 401 ± 175 ng/mL significantly different from 227 ± 72 ng/mL in 15 women with ovarian hyperadrenalism and 197 ± 79 ng/mL in 17 women with idiopathic hirsutism and in healthy control women *1388*

Insulin-like Growth Factor Binding Protein-3
Serum No Effect In 8 women with adrenal hyperandrogenism mean concentration of 3.5 ± 1.0 μg/mL not significantly different from 2.7 ± 0.6 μg/mL in 15 women with ovarian hyperadrenalism and 2.9 ± 0.7 μg/mL in 17 women with idiopathic hirsutism and in healthy control women *1388*

Progesterone *Plasma No Effect* In 8 women with adrenal hyperandrogenism mean concentration of 1.0 ± 0.4 ng/mL not significantly different from 0.7 ± 0.2 ng/mL in 17 healthy control women *1388*

Prostate-specific Antigen *Serum Increase* In 7 women with functional adrenal hyperandrogenism median concentration of 7 pg/mL compared with 0 pg/mL in 11 healthy controls *1387*

Sex-Hormone Binding Globulin *Serum Decrease* In 8 women with adrenal hyperandrogenism mean concentration of 169 ± 90 μg/dL significantly different from 351 ± 138 μg/dL in 17 healthy control women *1388*

Testosterone *Serum Increase* In 8 women with adrenal hyperandrogenism mean concentration of 91 ± 21 ng/dL significantly different from 40 ± 14 ng/dL in 17 healthy control women *1388*

255.30 Hyperandrogenital Activity

3α-Androstanediol *Plasma Increase* In 20 premenopausal hyperandrogenic women without alopecia mean concentration of 0.67 ± 0.07 nmol/L significantly higher than 0.41 ± 0.03 nmol/L in 10 female controls *2981*

3α-Androstanediol Glucuronide *Plasma Increase* In 20 premenopausal hyperandrogenic women without alopecia mean concentration of 13.2 ± 1.3 nmol/L significantly higher than 6.2 ± 0.47 nmol/L in 10 female controls *2981*

3α-Androstanediol Sulfate *Plasma Increase* In 20 premenopausal hyperandrogenic women without alopecia mean concentration of 125.5 ± 15.9 nmol/L significantly higher than 67.2 ± 4.2 nmol/L in 10 female controls *2981*

Androstenedione *Plasma Increase* In 20 premenopausal hyperandrogenic women without alopecia mean concentration of 14.7 ± 0.7 nmol/L significantly higher than 5.3 ± 0.7 nmol/L in 10 female controls *2981*

Androsterone Glucuronide *Plasma Increase* In 20 premenopausal hyperandrogenic women without alopecia mean concentration of 151.1 ± 15.4 nmol/L significantly higher than 73 ± 4.6 nmol/L in 10 female controls *2981*

Androsterone Sulfate *Plasma Increase* In 20 premenopausal hyperandrogenic women without alopecia mean concentration of 2,724 ± 297 nmol/L significantly higher than 2,038 ± 200 nmol/L in 10 female controls *2981*

Dehydroepiandrosterone Sulfate *Plasma Increase* In 20 premenopausal hyperandrogenic women without alopecia mean concentration of 6.9 ± 0.5 μmol/L significantly higher than 4.5 ± 0.5 μmol/L in 10 female controls *2981*

255.30 Hyperandrogenital Activity *(continued)*

Testosterone *Serum* *Increase* In 20 premenopausal hyperandrogenic women without alopecia mean concentration of 2.74 ± 0.2 nmol/L significantly higher than 1.03 ± 0.1 nmol/L in 10 female controls *2981*

255.40 Addison's Disease

Alanine Aminotransferase *Serum* *Increase* Addison's disease may be associated with moderately increased activity and vague constitutional symptoms *3625*

Ammonium Ions *Urine* *Decrease* May cause distal renal tubular acidosis (type IV) is associated with hyperkalemia, hyperchloremic metabolic acidosis, urine pH < 5.5, decreased urinary ammonium ion excretion, a positive urine anion gap, normal urinary citrate and urinary calcium excretion *4071*

Anion Gap *Urine* *Increase* May cause distal renal tubular acidosis (type IV) is associated with hyperkalemia, hyperchloremic metabolic acidosis, urine pH < 5.5, decreased urinary ammonium ion excretion, a positive urine anion gap, normal urinary citrate and urinary calcium excretion *4071*

Aspartate Aminotransferase *Serum* *Increase* Addison's disease may be associated with moderately increased activity and vague constitutional symptoms *3625*

Calcium *Urine* *No Effect* May cause distal renal tubular acidosis (type IV) is associated with hyperkalemia, hyperchloremic metabolic acidosis, urine pH < 5.5, decreased urinary ammonium ion excretion, a positive urine anion gap, normal urinary citrate and urinary calcium excretion *4071*

Citrate *Urine* *No Effect* May cause distal renal tubular acidosis (type IV) is associated with hyperkalemia, hyperchloremic metabolic acidosis, urine pH < 5.5, decreased urinary ammonium ion excretion, a positive urine anion gap, normal urinary citrate and urinary calcium excretion *4071*

Corticotropin *Plasma* *Increase* In 4 patients with Addison's disease concentrations ranged from 362 to 1,058 pg/mL compared with normal of less than 60 pg/mL *4262*

Potassium *Serum* *Increase* May cause distal renal tubular acidosis (type IV) which is associated with hyperkalemia, hyperchloremic metabolic acidosis, urine pH < 5.5, decreased urinary ammonium ion excretion, a positive urine anion gap, normal urinary citrate and urinary calcium excretion *4071*

Proopiomelanocortin *Plasma* *No Effect* Concentration undetectable in 4 patients as in 17 healthy individuals *4262*

255.40 Adrenal Cortical Hypofunction

Aldosterone *Plasma* *Decrease* Adrenal cortex destruction results in deficiency of glucocorticoids, androgens, and mineralocorticoids *5863* In 7 patients with adrenal insufficiency concentrations ranged from 28 to 114 pmol/L compared with normal range of 220 - 430 pmol/L *2545*
Urine *Decrease* Decreased as a result of the progressive destruction of the adrenal cortex *1290*

Alkaline Phosphatase *Serum* *No Effect* In 30 patients with Addison's disease 23 without osteoporosis had mean activity of 92.5 ± 40.3 U/L and in 7 with osteoporosis mean activity of 101.3 ± 39.2 U/L compared with normal range of 30 - 115 U/L *5385*

Androgens *Plasma* *Decrease* Adrenal cortex destruction results in deficiency of glucocorticoids, androgens, and mineralocorticoids *5863*
Plasma *No Effect* No significant effect observed *5863*

Antibody Titer *Serum* *Increase* Antibodies to adrenocortical cell in primary Addison's Disease *3712*

Anticardiolipin Antibodies *Serum* *Increase* Reported effect *1532*

Arginine Vasopressin *Plasma* *Increase* In 7 patients with adrenal insufficiency concentrations ranged from 0.49 to 3.91 pmol/L, increased in relation to their osmolality *2545*

Bicarbonate *Serum* *Decrease* Normal or decreased *5544* Dehydration and hypotension lead to prerenal impairment of renal function *900*
Serum *No Effect* Normal or decreased *5544*

Calcium *Serum* *Increase* In most instances the clinical picture is not altered by the hypercalcemia. It is not clear in all cases that the hypercalcemia reflects an increase in ionized calcium since hemoconcentration may contribute to the elevation if nausea, vomiting, and dehydration are prominent. Hypercalcemia may appear, however, with acute withdrawal of exogenous corticosteroids. It usually vanishes promptly with small doses of steroids *2039* Reported effect *1025*
Serum *No Effect* In 30 patients with Addison's disease 23 without osteoporosis had mean concentration of 10.0 ± 0.5 mg/dL and in 7 with osteoporosis mean concentration of 9.7 ± 0.3 mg/dL compared with normal range of 8.5 - 10.5 mg/dL *5385*
Urine *No Effect* In 30 patients with Addison's disease 23 without osteoporosis had mean excretion of 105.8 ± 13.4 mg/d and in 7 with osteoporosis mean excretion of 105.3 ± 8.4 mg/d compared with normal range of < 250 mg/d *5385*

Chloride *Serum* *Decrease* Observed effect *5544*
Urine *Decrease* Inability of the renal tubules to reabsorb sodium chloride and water and relative inability to excrete potassium *1290*

Corticosterone *Plasma* *Decrease* Adrenal cortex destruction results in deficiency of glucocorticoids, androgens, and mineralocorticoids *5863*

Corticotropin *Plasma* *Decrease* In 7 patients with adrenal insufficiency concentrations ranged from < 2 to 42 pmol/L compared with normal range of 4 - 22 pmol/L *2545*
Plasma *Increase* Results from the lack of cortisol-suppression feedback mechanism *5863*

Cortisol *Plasma* *Decrease* Adrenal cortex destruction results in deficiency of glucocorticoids, androgens, and mineralocorticoids *5863* In 7 patients with adrenal insufficiency concentrations ranged from < 28 to 69 nmol/L compared with normal range of 110 - 520 nmol/L *2545* Markedly decreased (< 5 µg/dL) and fails to rise to more than twice this level 1 h after injection of ACTH. This is a reliable easy screening test to establish primary adrenocortical insufficiency *5544*

Creatinine *Serum* *Decrease* In 7 patients with adrenal insufficiency concentrations ranged from 35 to 80 µmol/L compared with normal range of 50 - 110 µmol/L *2545*
Serum *Increase* Dehydration and hypotension lead to prerenal impairment of renal function *900*
Serum *No Effect* In 7 patients with adrenal insufficiency concentrations ranged from 35 to 80 µmol/L compared with normal range of 50 - 110 µmol/L *2545*

Dehydroepiandrosterone Sulfate *Plasma* *Decrease* Observed effect *3778* *91*

Eosinophils *Blood* *Increase* May be a relative lymphocytosis and moderate eosinophilia *1980* A total count of 50/µL is evidence against severe adrenocortical hypofunction *5545* With reduced adrenal cortical or pituitary function *900*

Glomerular Filtration Rate *Urine* *Decrease* Fluid depletion leads to reduced circulating blood volume and renal circulatory insufficiency *5863* Dehydration may result in hemoconcentration *1980*

Glucocorticoids *Plasma* *Decrease* Baseline plasma and urinary corticosteroids will be low in Addison's disease *1980* Adrenal cortex destruction results in deficiency of glucocorticoids, androgens, and mineralocorticoids *5863*
Urine *Decrease* Baseline plasma and urinary corticosteroids will be low in Addison's disease *1980*

Glucose *Serum* *Decrease* In 7 patients with adrenal insufficiency concentrations ranged from 2.7 to 6.8 mmol/L compared with normal range of 3.5 - 6.1 mmol/L *2545* Patients with diminished glucocorticoid secretion commonly manifest low levels of blood glucose, and symptomatic hypoglycemia may follow a period of fasting. Occasionally, patients with glucocorticoid deficiency exhibit hypoglycemic symptoms late in the postprandial period *2039* Fasting blood sugar may be low, and the glucose tolerance test may be flat *1980* May occur due to insulin hypersensitivity in the hypoadrenal state *5863*
Serum *Increase* In 7 patients with adrenal insufficiency concentrations ranged from 2.7 to 6.8 mmol/L compared with normal range of 3.5 - 6.1 mmol/L *2545*
Serum *No Effect* In 7 patients with adrenal insufficiency concentrations ranged from 2.7 to 6.8 mmol/L compared with normal range of 3.5 - 6.1 mmol/L *2545*

Glucose Tolerance *Serum* *Increase* Fasting blood sugar may be low, and the glucose tolerance test may be flat *1980*

Flat peak. Poor absorption from the GI tract (normal IV GTT curve) *5544* Curve is flat in adrenal hypofunction *5863*

Hematocrit *Blood* *Decrease* Reduced thyroid, adrenal cortical, pituitary or testicular function can produce anemia. Hematocrit is seldom < 30%. The RBC is normochromic and normocytic *900*
Blood *Increase* Dehydration and hemoconcentration due to severe renal sodium loss *5863*

Hemoglobin *Blood* *Decrease* Reduced thyroid, adrenal cortical, pituitary or testicular function can produce anemia. Hemoglobin is seldom < 9 g/dL *900*

HLA Antigens *Blood* *Present* HLA-DR3 present in 70% of patients versus 21% of controls *5678*

25-Hydroxy Vitamin D *Serum* *No Effect* In 30 patients with Addison's disease, 23 without osteoporosis had mean concentration of 27.6 ± 8.9 ng/mL and in 7 with osteoporosis mean concentration of 29.8 ± 1.0 ng/mL compared with normal range of 17 - 40 ng/mL *5385*

17-Hydroxycorticosteroids *Urine* *Decrease* Low for males in the diagnosis of Addison's Disease *2039*
Urine *No Effect* Usual observation *5544*

17-Ketogenic Steroids *Urine* *Decrease* Excretion reduced in Addison's disease *2952* Markedly decreased *5545*

17-Ketosteroids *Urine* *Decrease* Markedly decreased *5544* Excretion may be decreased in patients with Addison's disease *2952*

Leukocytes *Blood* *Decrease* With reduced adrenal cortical or pituitary function leukopenia may be seen *900*
Blood *Increase* With relative or absolute lymphocytosis and eosinophilia in Addison's disease *2039* May be normal or increased with a tendency to lymphocytosis and eosinophilia *900*

Lymphocytes *Blood* *Increase* WBC may be normal or increased with a tendency to lymphocytosis and eosinophilia *900* May be a relative lymphocytosis and moderate eosinophilia *1980*

Magnesium *Serum* *Increase* Concentration is increased in association with Addison's disease *2952*

Neutrophils *Blood* *Decrease* Neutropenia and relative lymphocytosis are common *5544*

Osmolality *Serum* *Decrease* In 7 patients with adrenal insufficiency concentrations ranged from 220 to 236 mOsm/kg compared with normal range of 280 - 300 mOsm/kg *2545*

Osteocalcin *Serum* *No Effect* In 30 patients with Addison's disease 23 without osteoporosis had mean concentration of 6.0 ± 1.6 ng/mL and in 7 with osteoporosis mean concentration of 4.5 ± 1.6 ng/mL compared with normal range of 4.5 - 6.5 ng/mL *5385*

Parathyroid Hormone *Plasma* *No Effect* In 30 patients with Addison's disease, 23 without osteoporosis had mean concentration of 33.5 ± 9.2 pg/mL and in 7 with osteoporosis mean concentration of 47.0 ± 5.4 pg/mL compared with normal range of 3 - 50 pg/mL *5385*

pH *Blood* *Decrease* Raised potassium concentration and metabolic acidosis usually occur *5863*
Urine *Increase* Normal or increased *5544*
Urine *No Effect* Normal or increased *5544*

Phosphate *Serum* *Decrease* Acute adrenal insufficiency may be accompanied by hypophosphatemia (and hypercalcemia) *2039*
Serum *Increase* Reported effect *5544*

Potassium *Serum* *Increase* Raised potassium concentration and metabolism acidosis usually occur *5863* Normal in mild insufficiency, but in severe insufficiency, particularly of aldosterone, there are hyponatremia and hyperkalemia *900*
Serum *No Effect* In 7 patients with adrenal insufficiency concentrations ranged from 3.8 to 4.5 mmol/L compared with normal range of 3.5 - 5.0 mmol/L *2545*
Urine *Decrease* Inability of the renal tubules to reabsorb sodium chloride and water and relative inability to excrete potassium *1290*
Urine *No Effect* Normal or decreased *5544*

Procollagen Type I Peptide *Serum* *No Effect* Of 30 patients with Addison's disease, 23 without osteoporosis had a mean concentration of 114.5 ± 33.8 μg/L and 7 with osteoporosis had a mean concentration of 123.2 ± 74.1 μg/L compared with normal range of 40 - 166 μg/L *5385*

Prolactin *Plasma* *Increase* Increased levels *4289*

Protein *Serum* *Increase* Dehydration and hemoconcentration due to severe renal sodium loss *5863*

Renin Activity *Plasma* *Increase* Due to reduced plasma volume *5544*
Plasma *No Effect* In 7 patients with adrenal insufficiency concentrations ranged from 0.06 to 0.97 ng/L/s compared with normal range of 0.30 - 1.14 ng/L/s *2545*

Reticulocytes *Blood* *Decrease* Absolute count is decreased *900*

Sodium *Serum* *Decrease* In 7 patients with adrenal insufficiency concentrations ranged from 106 to 118 mmol/L compared with normal range of 138 - 146 mmol/L *2545* Serum concentration may remain normal until a crisis, when sodium loss exceeds water loss *5863* Often occurs *1980* Normal in mild insufficiency, but in severe insufficiency, particularly of aldosterone, there are hyponatremia and hyperkalemia *900*
Serum *No Effect* Normal in mild insufficiency, but in severe insufficiency, particularly of aldosterone, there are hyponatremia and hyperkalemia *900*
Urine *Increase* Inability of the renal tubules to reabsorb sodium and water and relative inability to excrete potassium *1290*

T3-Uptake *Serum* *No Effect* Concentration typically normal *5544*

Testosterone *Serum* *No Effect* Androgen deficiency is not clinically evident because testosterone production is unimpaired *5863*

Urea Nitrogen *Serum* *Decrease* In 7 patients with adrenal insufficiency concentrations ranged from 2.0 to 4.5 mmol/L compared with normal range of 3.5 - 6.5 mmol/L *2545*
Serum *Increase* Dehydration may result in hemoconcentration *1980* Dehydration and hypotension lead to prerenal impairment of renal function *900* Fluid depletion leads to reduced circulating blood volume and renal circulatory insufficiency *5863*
Serum *No Effect* In 7 patients with adrenal insufficiency concentrations ranged from 2.0 to 4.5 mmol/L compared with normal range of 3.5 - 6.5 mmol/L *2545*

Volume *Plasma* *Decrease* Fluid depletion leads to reduced circulating blood volume and renal circulatory insufficiency *5863*
Urine *Decrease* Normal or decreased *5544*
Urine *No Effect* Normal or decreased *5544*

255.40 Adrenal Hemorrhage

Cortisol *Plasma* *Decrease* Relative hypoadrenalism observed with acute partial destruction of the adrenal cortex due to massive retroperitoneal bleeding, thrombocytopenia or anticoagulant therapy *2901*

255.40 Primary Adrenal Insufficiency

Corticotropin *Plasma* *Increase* Mean concentration in 2 patients with primary adrenal insufficiency of 39 pmol/L greater than range in 50 healthy Caucasian volunteers of 4.4 - 18 pmol/L *3605*

Cortisol *Plasma* *Decrease* Mean concentration of 7.5 nmol/L in 2 patients with primary adrenal insufficiency (Addison's disease) significantly less than that in 50 healthy Caucasian volunteers, 344 ± 81 nmol/L *3605*
Urine *Decrease* Mean concentration in 2 patients with primary adrenal insufficiency (Addison's disease) of 51 nmol/d significantly less than that in 50 healthy Caucasian volunteers, 130 ± 104 nmol/d *3605*

Cortisone *Plasma* *Decrease* Mean concentration in 2 patients with primary adrenal insufficiency (Addison's disease) < 2 nmol/L significantly less than that in 50 healthy Caucasian volunteers, 51.4 ± 16.7 nmol/L *3605*
Urine *Decrease* Mean concentration in 2 patients with primary adrenal insufficiency (Addison's disease) of 0.30 nmol/d less than that in 50 healthy Caucasian volunteers, 0.52 ± 0.29 nmol/d *3605*

255.40 Secondary Adrenal Insufficiency

Corticotropin *Plasma* *Decrease* Mean concentration in 2 patients with primary adrenal insufficiency of 1.3 pmol/L less than range in 50 healthy Caucasian volunteers of 4.4 - 18 pmol/L *3605*

Cortisol *Plasma* *Decrease* Mean concentration of 25 nmol/L in 2 patients with secondary adrenal insufficiency (Addison's disease) significantly less than that in 50 healthy Caucasian volunteers, 344 ± 81 nmol/L *3605*

Cortisone *Plasma* *Decrease* Mean concentration in 2 patients with secondary adrenal insufficiency (Addison's disease) of 3.7 mol/L significantly less than that in 50 healthy Caucasian volunteers, 51.4 ± 16.7 nmol/L *3605*

255.80 Acquired Adrenal Insensitivity

Ammonium Ions *Urine* *Decrease* May cause distal renal tubular acidosis (type IV) is associated with hyperkalemia, hyperchloremic metabolic acidosis, urine pH < 5.5, decreased urinary ammonium ion excretion, a positive urine anion gap, normal urinary citrate and urinary calcium excretion *4071*

Anion Gap *Urine* *Increase* May cause distal renal tubular acidosis (type IV) is associated with hyperkalemia, hyperchloremic metabolic acidosis, urine pH < 5.5, decreased urinary ammonium ion excretion, a positive urine anion gap, normal urinary citrate and urinary calcium excretion *4071*

Calcium *Urine* *No Effect* May cause distal renal tubular acidosis (type IV) is associated with hyperkalemia, hyperchloremic metabolic acidosis, urine pH < 5.5, decreased urinary ammonium ion excretion, a positive urine anion gap, normal urinary citrate and urinary calcium excretion *4071*

Chloride *Serum* *Increase* May cause distal renal tubular acidosis (type IV) is associated with hyperkalemia, hyperchloremic metabolic acidosis, urine pH < 5.5, decreased urinary ammonium ion excretion, a positive urine anion gap, normal urinary citrate and urinary calcium excretion *4071*

Citrate *Urine* *No Effect* May cause distal renal tubular acidosis (type IV) is associated with hyperkalemia, hyperchloremic metabolic acidosis, urine pH < 5.5, decreased urinary ammonium ion excretion, a positive urine anion gap, normal urinary citrate and urinary calcium excretion *4071*

pH *Urine* *Decrease* May cause distal renal tubular acidosis (type IV) is associated with hyperkalemia, hyperchloremic metabolic acidosis, urine pH < 5.5, decreased urinary ammonium ion excretion, a positive urine anion gap, normal urinary citrate and urinary calcium excretion *4071*

Potassium *Serum* *Increase* May cause distal renal tubular acidosis (type IV) which is associated with hyperkalemia, hyperchloremic metabolic acidosis, urine pH < 5.5, decreased urinary ammonium ion excretion, a positive urine anion gap, normal urinary citrate and urinary calcium excretion *4071*

255.80 Adrenal Hyperplasia

Aldosterone *Plasma* *No Effect* Mean concentration of 0.22 nmol/L in 4 patients with adrenal hyperplasia not significantly different from reference range of 0.14 - 0.42 nmol/L *5350*

Androstenedione *Plasma* *Increase* Concentration often increased in congenital adrenal hyperplasia *2952* In 53 women with adrenal hyperplasia due to 21-hydoxylase deficiency mean concentration of δ4-androstenedione 13.65 ± 5.60 nmol/L significantly higher than in normals *1454*

Corticotropin *Plasma* *Increase* Mean concentration of 18.14 pmol/L in 4 patients with adrenal hyperplasia significantly different from reference range of 1.94 - 11.2 pmol/L *5350*

Cortisol *Plasma* *Increase* Mean concentration of 710 nmol/d in 4 patients with adrenal hyperplasia significantly different from reference range of 138 - 331 nmol/L *5350*

Follicle Stimulating Hormone *Plasma* *No Effect* In 53 women with adrenal hyperplasia due to 21-hydroxylase deficiency mean concentration normal *1454*

FSH response to LHRH *Plasma* *No Effect* In 53 women with adrenal hyperplasia due to 21-hydroxylase deficiency normal response observed *1454*

17-Hydroxycorticosteroids *Urine* *Increase* Mean concentration of 53.7 µmol/d in 4 patients with adrenal hyperplasia significantly different from reference range of 11.0 - 22.1 µmol/d *5350*

18-Hydroxycortisol *Serum* *No Effect* Mean concentration of 2.27 ± 0.31 nmol/L in 3 female patients and 1 male patient with adrenal hyperplasia not different from reference range of 2.44 ± 0.39 nmol/L in 30 women and 2.60 ± 0.62 nmol/L in 30 men *5350*

Urine *No Effect* Mean excretion of 176 ± 47 nmol/d in 3 female patients and 1 male patient with adrenal hyperplasia not significantly different from reference range of 173 ± 27 nmol/d in 30 women and 172 ± 24 nmol/d in 30 men *5350*

17-Hydroxyprogesterone *Plasma* *Increase* In 53 women with late-onset adrenal hyperplasia due to 21-hydroxylase deficiency mean concentration of 26.8 ± 18.9 nmol/L significantly higher than normal *1454*

17-Ketogenic Steroids *Urine* *Increase* Excretion increased with hyperfunction of the zona fasciculata and reticullaris *2952*

LH response to LHRH *Plasma* *Increase* In 53 women with adrenal hyperplasia due to 21-hydroxylase deficiency mean concentration increased *1454*

Luteinizing Hormone *Plasma* *Increase* In 53 women with adrenal hyperplasia due to 21-hydroxylase deficiency mean basal concentration increased *1454*

18-Oxycortisol *Serum* *No Effect* Mean concentration of 0.15 ± 0.01 nmol/L in 3 female patients and 1 male patient with adrenal hyperplasia not different from reference range of 0.16 ± 0.04 nmol/L in 30 women and in 30 men *5350*

Urine *No Effect* Mean excretion of 3.51 ± 1.14 nmol/d in 3 female patients and 1 male patient with adrenal hyperplasia not significantly different from reference range of 3.59 ± 0.66 nmol/d in 30 women and 3.75 ± 1.00 nmol/d in 30 men *5350*

Prolactin *Plasma* *No Effect* In 53 women with adrenal hyperplasia due to 21-hydroxylase deficiency mean basal concentration normal *1454*

Prolactin response to TRH *Plasma* *No Effect* TRH stimulated prolactin concentration normal in 53 women with adrenal hyperplasia due to 21-hydroxylase deficiency *1454*

Renin Activity *Plasma* *No Effect* Mean concentration of 2.7 ng/L/s in 4 patients with adrenal hyperplasia not significantly different from reference range of 1.1 - 4.1 ng/L/s *5350*

Testosterone *Serum* *Increase* In 53 women with adrenal hyperplasia due to 21-hydroxylase deficiency mean concentration of 3.25 ± 2.03 nmol/L significantly higher than in normals *1454*

255.80 Autoimmune Adrenalitis

Cortisol *Plasma* *Decrease* Relative hypoadrenalism observed with partial destruction of the adrenal cortex *2901*

255.80 Pseudohypoaldosteronism

Ammonium Ions *Urine* *Decrease* May cause distal renal tubular acidosis (type IV) is associated with hyperkalemia, hyperchloremic metabolic acidosis, urine pH < 5.5, decreased urinary ammonium ion excretion, a positive urine anion gap, normal urinary citrate and urinary calcium excretion *4071*

Anion Gap *Urine* *Increase* May cause distal renal tubular acidosis (type IV) is associated with hyperkalemia, hyperchloremic metabolic acidosis, urine pH < 5.5, decreased urinary ammonium ion excretion, a positive urine anion gap, normal urinary citrate and urinary calcium excretion *4071*

Calcium *Urine* *No Effect* May cause distal renal tubular acidosis (type IV) is associated with hyperkalemia, hyperchloremic metabolic acidosis, urine pH < 5.5, decreased urinary ammonium ion excretion, a positive urine anion gap, normal urinary citrate and urinary calcium excretion *4071*

Chloride *Serum* *Increase* May cause distal renal tubular acidosis (type IV) is associated with hyperkalemia, hyperchloremic metabolic acidosis, urine pH < 5.5, decreased urinary ammonium ion excretion, a positive urine anion gap, normal urinary citrate and urinary calcium excretion *4071*

Citrate *Urine* *No Effect* May cause distal renal tubular acidosis (type IV) is associated with hyperkalemia, hyperchloremic metabolic acidosis, urine pH < 5.5, decreased urinary ammonium ion excretion, a positive urine anion gap, normal urinary citrate and urinary calcium excretion *4071*

pH *Urine* *Decrease* May cause distal renal tubular acidosis (type IV) is associated with hyperkalemia, hyperchloremic metabolic acidosis, urine pH < 5.5, decreased urinary ammonium ion excretion, a positive urine anion gap, normal urinary citrate and urinary calcium excretion *4071*

Potassium *Serum* *Increase* May cause distal renal tubular acidosis (type IV) which is associated with hyperkalemia, hyperchloremic metabolic acidosis, urine pH < 5.5, decreased urinary ammonium ion excretion, a positive urine anion gap, normal urinary citrate and urinary calcium excretion *4071*

256.00 Ovarian Hyperfunction

Apolipoprotein A-I *Serum* *Increase* Estrogen effect *2034*

Calcium *Serum* *Increase* Estrogen effect *2034*

Ceruloplasmin *Serum* *Increase* Estrogen effect *2034*

Chloride *Serum* *Decrease* Progesterone effect *2034*

Cholesterol *Serum* *Decrease* Estrogen effect *2034*

Copper *Serum* *Increase* Estrogen effect *2034*

Corticosteroid-Binding Globulin *Serum* *Increase* Estrogen effect *2034*

Factor II *Plasma* *Increase* Estrogen effect *2034*

β-Lipoprotein *Serum* *Increase* Estrogen effect *2034*

Luteinizing Hormone *Urine* *Decrease* Decreased excretion typically observed in women with primary ovarian hyperfunction *2952*

pH *Blood* *Increase* Progesterone effect *2034*

Phosphate *Serum* *Increase* Estrogen effect *2034*

Sodium *Serum* *Decrease* Progesterone effect *2034*

Thyroxine Binding Globulin *Serum* *Increase* Estrogen effect *2034*

Volume *Plasma* *Decrease* Progesterone effect *2034*

256.10 Ovarian Hyperandrogenism

Androgen Index, Free (FAI) *Plasma* *Increase* In 15 women with ovarian hyperandrogenism mean index of 10.7 ± 9.8 significantly different from 2.4 ± 1.8 in 17 healthy control women *1388*

Androstenedione *Plasma* *No Effect* In 15 women with ovarian hyperandrogenism mean concentration of 3.1 ± 1.1 ng/mL not significantly different from 2.5 ± 0.8 ng/mL in 17 healthy control women *1388*

Cortisol *Plasma* *No Effect* In 15 women with ovarian hyperandrogenism mean concentration of 14.4 ± 5.0 μg/dL not significantly different from 15.3 ± 4.6 μg/dL in 17 healthy control women *1388*

Dehydroepiandrosterone Sulfate *Plasma* *Increase* In 15 women with ovarian hyperandrogenism mean concentration of 3,464 ± 1,520 ng/mL significantly different from 1,902 ± 705 ng/mL in 17 healthy control women *1388*

11-Deoxycortisol *Plasma* *No Effect* In 15 women with ovarian hyperandrogenism mean concentration of 2.5 ± 1.6 ng/mL not significantly different from 3.2 ± 2.1 ng/mL in 17 healthy control women *1388*

Growth Hormone *Plasma* *No Effect* Mean concentration of 2.9 ± 3.9 ng/mL in 15 women with ovarian hyperadrenalism not significantly different from 3.3 ± 4.1 ng/mL in 17 women with idiopathic hirsutism and in healthy control women *1388*

17-Hydroxyprogesterone *Plasma* *No Effect* In 15 women with ovarian hyperandrogenism mean concentration of 1.1 ± 0.5 ng/mL not significantly different from 0.8 ± 0.3 ng/mL in 17 healthy control women *1388*

Insulin-like Growth Factor-I *Serum* *No Effect* Mean concentration of 227 ± 72 ng/mL in 15 women with ovarian hyperadrenalism not significantly different from 197 ± 79 ng/mL in 17 women with idiopathic hirsutism and in healthy control women *1388*

Insulin-like Growth Factor Binding Protein-3
Serum *No Effect* Mean concentration of 2.7 ± 0.6 μg/mL in 15 women with ovarian hyperadrenalism not significantly different from 2.9 ± 0.7 μg/mL in 17 women with idiopathic hirsutism and in healthy control women *1388*

Progesterone *Plasma* *No Effect* In 15 women with ovarian hyperandrogenism mean concentration of 0.8 ± 0.3 ng/mL not significantly different from 0.7 ± 0.2 ng/mL in 17 healthy control women *1388*

Prostate-specific Antigen *Serum* *Increase* In 15 women with functional ovarian hyperandrogenism median concentration of 7 pg/mL compared with 0 pg/mL in 11 healthy controls *1387*

Sex-Hormone Binding Globulin *Serum* *Decrease* In 15 women with ovarian hyperandrogenism mean concentration of 221 ± 132 μg/dL significantly different from 351 ± 138 μg/dL in 17 healthy control women *1388*

Testosterone *Serum* *Increase* In 15 women with ovarian hyperandrogenism mean concentration of 86 ± 22 ng/dL significantly different from 40 ± 14 ng/dL in 17 healthy control women *1388*

256.10 Ovarian Hyperstimulation Syndrome

Aldosterone *Plasma* *Increase* In 16 patients with ovarian hyperstimulation syndrome mean concentration of 190.6 ± 28.4 ng/dL compared with 14.8 ± 1.5 ng/dL 4 to 5 weeks after recovery *256*

Angiogenin *Ascitic Fluid* *Increase* Mean concentration in 10 patients with severe OHSS of 2,794 ± 1,024 ng/mL significantly different from 254 ± 105 ng/mL with long term treatment with GnRH *18*
Serum *Increase* Mean concentration in 10 patients with severe OHSS of 8,390 ± 6,837 μg/mL significantly different from 234 ± 91 μg/mL with long term treatment with GnRH *18*

Antidiuretic Hormone *Plasma* *Increase* In 16 patients with ovarian hyperstimulation syndrome mean concentration of 4.1 ± 0.7 pg/mL compared with 1.0 ± 0.1 pg/mL 4 to 5 weeks after recovery *256*

Atrial Natriuretic Peptide *Plasma* *Increase* In 16 patients with ovarian hyperstimulation syndrome mean concentration of 10.9 ± 1.6 fmol/mL compared with 4.7 ± 0.2 fmol/mL 4 to 5 weeks after recovery *256*

Creatinine *Serum* *Increase* In 16 patients with ovarian hyperstimulation syndrome mean concentration of 0.8 ± 0.05 mg/dL compared with 0.5 ± 0.3 mg/dL 4 to 5 weeks after recovery *256*

Endothelin *Plasma* *Increase* In 16 patients with ovarian hyperstimulation syndrome mean concentration of 8.9 ± 0.9 pg/mL compared with 3.9 ± 0.2 pg/mL 4 to 5 weeks after recovery *256*

Hematocrit *Blood* *Increase* In 16 patients with ovarian hyperstimulation syndrome mean value of 45.5 ± 1.1% compared with 38.1 ± 0.4% 4 to 5 weeks after recovery *256*

Norepinephrine *Plasma* *Increase* In 16 patients with ovarian hyperstimulation syndrome mean concentration of 602.1 ± 91.0 pg/mL compared with 220.5 ± 12.1 pg/mL 4 to 5 weeks after recovery *256*

Renin Activity *Plasma* *Increase* In 16 patients with ovarian hyperstimulation syndrome mean activity of 36.0 ± 9.1 ng/mL/h compared with 1.2 ± 0.08 ng/mL/h 4 to 5 weeks after recovery *256*

Vascular Endothelial Growth Factor *Serum* *Increase* In 10 patients with ovarian hyperstimulation syndrome mean concentration of 50 ± 780 pg/mL *3150*

Volume *Urine* *Decrease* In 16 patients with ovarian hyperstimulation syndrome mean excretion of 630.6 ± 40.7 mL/d compared with 1,306.2 ± 43.9 mL/d 4 to 5 weeks after recovery *256*

256.30 Ovarian Failure

Calcium *Serum* *No Effect* In 113 women who desired fertility and had premature ovarian failure normal concentration observed *2680*

256.30 Ovarian Failure *(continued)*

Thyroxine (T4) *Serum* *Decrease* In 119 women who desired fertility and had premature ovarian failure hypothyroidism was found in 32 (27%) *2680*

Thyroxine (T4), Free *Serum* *Decrease* In 119 women who desired fertility and had premature ovarian failure hypothyroidism was found in 32 (27%) *2680*

Vitamin B_{12} *Serum* *No Effect* In 113 women who desired fertility and had premature ovarian failure normal concentration observed *2680*

256.30 Ovarian Hypofunction

Apolipoprotein A-I *Serum* *Decrease* Estrogen effect *2034*

Calcium *Serum* *Decrease* Estrogen effect *2034*

Ceruloplasmin *Serum* *Decrease* Estrogen effect *2034*

Chloride *Serum* *Increase* Estrogen effect *2034*

Cholesterol *Serum* *Increase* Estrogen effect *2034*

Copper *Serum* *Decrease* Estrogen effect *2034*

Corticosteroid-Binding Globulin *Serum* *Decrease* Estrogen effect *2034*

Creatine *Urine* *Increase* Creatinuria occurs with gonadal dysfunction in males and females *4707*

Estrogens *Plasma* *Decrease* Decreased in primary and secondary hypofunction of ovary *5544*
Urine *Decrease* Observed effect *1290* *5544*

Factor II *Plasma* *Decrease* Estrogen effect *2034*

Gonadotropin, Pituitary *Urine* *Decrease* Increased or decreased depending on whether it is primary or secondary failure *5679*
Urine *Increase* Increased or decreased depending on whether it is primary or secondary failure *5679*

β-Lipoprotein *Serum* *Decrease* Estrogen effect *2034*

Luteinizing Hormone *Urine* *Increase* Increased excretion typically observed in women with primary ovarian hyperfunction *2952*

pH *Blood* *Decrease* Progesterone effect *2034*

Phosphate *Serum* *Decrease* Estrogen effect *2034*

Pregnanediol *Urine* *Decrease* Decreased in amenorrhea *5545*

Progesterone *Plasma* *Decrease* Decreased in amenorrhea *5545*

Sodium *Serum* *Increase* Estrogen effect *2034*

Thyroxine Binding Globulin *Serum* *Decrease* Estrogen effect *2034*

Volume *Plasma* *Increase* Estrogen effect *2034*

256.40 Polycystic Ovary Disease

Androgen Index, Free (FAI) *Plasma* *Increase* Mean index in 16 patients of 10.3 ± 5.7 significantly different from 3.1 ± 1.0 in 8 healthy women during during the early follicular phase of their menstrual cycle *4638*
Serum *Increase* In 7 female patients with PCOS mean index of 6.4 ± 0.9 was significantly different from 2.2 ± 0.1 in 8 healthy controls *1633*

Androgens *Plasma* *Increase* Women with polycystic ovary had significantly higher plasma androgen levels than women with 'simple' amenorrhea both before treatment and during induction of ovulation *2941* Concentration significantly increased compared with controls *3008*

3α-Androstanediol Glucuronide *Plasma* *Increase* Mean concentration typically increased in women with PCOS *1148*

Androstenedione *Plasma* *Increase* In 11 women with PCOS mean concentration of 3.7 ± 0.3 ng/mL significantly greater than 1.5 ± 0.2 ng/mL in 6 healthy controls *3616* In women with PCOS mean concentration nonsignificantly higher in those with enlarged ovaries than in others *4242* Concentration often increased in polycystic ovary disease *2952* In 12 obese women with polycystic ovary syndrome mean fasting concentration of 10.21 ± 1.77 nmol/L not significantly different from 10.07 ± 1.57 nmol/L in 11 healthy obese women *2410* In 9 anovulatory women with PCOS mean concentration of 1.98 ± 0.35 ng/mL compared with 0.54 ± 0.03 ng/mL in 5 control women *4524* Mean concentration of 186 ± 14 ng/dL in 25 women with PCOS significantly higher than 125 ± 14 ng/dL in 20 healthy controls *655* In 6 women with PCOS mean concentration of 15.9 ± 2.2 nmol/L significantly greater than normal range of 0.5 - 10.2 nmol/L *4175* Mean concentration in 5 nonobese women with PCOS of 14.0 ± 1.0 nmol/L significantly different from 7.3 ± 0.1 nmol/L in 4 non-obese control women *1681* In 13 patients with PCOS mean concentration of 2.3 ± 0.3 ng/mL significantly higher when compared with 1.6 ± 0.1 ng/mL in 15 healthy control women *3606* In 7 female patients with PCOS mean concentration of 12.0 ± 0.9 nmol/L was significantly different from 6.9 ± 0.8 nmol/L in 8 healthy controls *1633* In 44 patients with PCOS mean concentration of 361.0 ± 120.3 ng/dL significantly greater than 177.7 ± 65.9 ng/dL in 25 healthy controls *2382* Mean concentration in 16 patients of 23.9 ± 9.8 nmol/L significantly different from 10.5 ± 3.2 nmol/L in 8 healthy women during during the early follicular phase of their menstrual cycle *4638*
Saliva *Increase* Maximum concentration in women with polycystic ovary disease of 400 pmol/L slightly higher than mean concentration in healthy control individuals of 210 ±50 pmol/L *5155*

Angiotensin-II *Plasma* *No Effect* In 13 patients with PCOS mean concentration of 53.5 ± 7 pg/mL not significantly different when compared with 38 ± 5 pg/mL in 15 healthy control women *3606*

Cholesterol *Serum* *No Effect* In patients with POS no significant difference between insulin-resistant group (4.76 ± 0.26 mmol/L) and nonresistant group of 4.61 ± 0.18 mmol/L *2896*

Cortisol *Plasma* *No Effect* In 25 women with PCOS mean concentration of 7.4 ± 0.7 μg/dL not significantly different from 8.4 ± 1.0 μg/dL in 20 healthy controls *655*
Urine *Decrease* In 65 women with PCOS mean excretion of 22.9 μg/g creatinine (95% range 20.9 - 25.1) compared with 28.8 μg/g creatinine (95% range 25.2 - 33.0) in 45 control women *4397*

Dehydroepiandrosterone *Plasma* *Increase* In 25 women with PCOS mean concentration of 470 ± 61 ng/dL not significantly increased compared with 421 ± 49 ng/dL in 20 healthy controls *655*

Dehydroepiandrosterone Sulfate *Plasma* *Increase* Mean concentration nonsignificantly higher in women with PCOS with enlarged ovaries than in those with ovaries of normal size *4242* Increased concentrations may be associated with polycystic ovary disease in women *2952* In 12 obese women with polycystic ovary syndrome mean fasting concentration of 7.03 ± 1.28 μmol/L not significantly different from 4.21 ± 0.35 μmol/L in 11 healthy obese women *2410* In 11 women with PCOS mean concentration of 2.4 ± 0.3 μg/mL not significantly greater than 1.7 ± 0.3 μg/mL in 6 healthy controls *3616* In 13 patients with PCOS mean concentration of 2.6 ± 0.3 μg/mL significantly higher when compared with 1.5 ± 0.2 μg/mL in 15 healthy control women *3606*
Plasma *No Effect* Mean concentration in 5 nonobese women with PCOS of 5.5 ± 1.0 μmol/L not significantly different from 6.0 ± 1.2 μmol/L in 4 non-obese control women *1681* In 26 women with PCOS mean concentration of 250 ± 112 μg/mL not significantly different from 223 ± 89 μg/mL in normal women *5446* In 6 women with PCOS mean concentration of 6.7 ± 0.8 nmol/L not significantly different from normal range of 3.2 - 9.7 nmol/L *4175*

Estradiol *Plasma* *Decrease* Mean concentration of 45.3 ± 18 pg/mL in 26 women with PCOS markedly reduced below 70 ± 9.4 pg/mL in normal women *5446* In 6 women with PCOS mean concentration of 214 ± 60 pmol/L significantly different from normal range of 300 - 1211 pmol/L *4175*
Plasma *No Effect* Mean concentration in 5 nonobese women with PCOS of 256 ± 45 pmol/L not significantly different from 189 ± 37 pmol/L in 4 non-obese control women *1681* In 25 women with PCOS mean concentration of 84 ± 13 pg/mL not significantly different from 75 ± 16 pg/mL in 20 healthy controls *655*

17β-Estradiol *Plasma* *Decrease* In 12 obese women with polycystic ovary syndrome mean fasting concentration of 159 ± 34 pmol/L not significantly different from 259 ± 79 pmol/L in 11 healthy obese women *2410*

Estradiol, Free *Plasma* *Increase* Significant increase observed in patients with polycystic ovary syndrome *3008*

Estrone *Plasma* *Increase* Mean concentration increased compared with healthy controls *3008* Mean concentration of 77 ± 9 pg/mL in 25 women with PCOS significantly higher than 56 ± 5 pg/mL in 20 healthy controls *655*

Plasma *No Effect* In 18 women aged 26 - 35 years with PCOS 95% range of 190 - 730 pmol/L not significantly higher than that in 42 premenopausal women aged 20 - 44 years (95% range 93 - 710 pmol/L) *3170*

Follicle Stimulating Hormone *Plasma* *Decrease* In 44 patients with PCOS mean concentration of 4.3 ± 1.8 IU/L significantly less than 6.4 ± 2.3 IU/L in 25 healthy controls *2382* In 26 women with PCOS mean concentration of 7.9 ± 4.4 mIU/mL reduced below 10.4 ± 0.8 mIU/mL in normal women *5446* In 13 patients with PCOS mean concentration of 6.0 ± 0.5 mIU/mL significantly lower when compared with 9 ± 1 mIU/mL in 15 healthy control women *3606*
Plasma *Increase* Mean concentration in 65 women with PCOS of 5.0 mIU/mL (95% range 4.6 - 5.5) compared with 6.0 mIU/mL (95% range 5.5 - 6.6) in 45 control women *4397*
Plasma *No Effect* In 7 female patients with PCOS mean concentration of 5.9 ± 0.7 IU/L was not significantly different from 6.4 ± 0.9 IU/L in 8 healthy controls *1633* In 6 women with PCOS mean concentration of 4.3 ± 0.5 IU/L not significantly different from normal range of 3 - 11 IU/L *4175* Mean concentration in 5 nonobese women with PCOS of 6.0 ± 0.6 IU/L not significantly different from 6.2 ± 0.4 IU/L in 4 non-obese control women *1681* Mean concentration in 16 patients of 4.8 ± 0.8 IU/L not significantly different from 5.4 ± 1.2 IU/L in 8 healthy women during during the early follicular phase of their menstrual cycle *4638*

Glucose *Serum* *Decrease* In 12 obese women with polycystic ovary syndrome mean fasting concentration of 4.0 ± 0.1 mmol/L significantly less than 4.7 ± 0.2 mmol/L in 11 healthy obese women *2410*
Serum *No Effect* Mean concentration in 25 women with PCOS of 90.1 ± 1.8 mg/dL not significantly different from 88.3 ± 1.8 mg/dL in 20 healthy controls *655* In 7 female patients with PCOS mean concentration of 5.2 ± 0.3 mmol/L was not significantly different from 4.9 ± 0.2 mmol/L in 8 healthy controls *1633*

Glucose Tolerance *Serum* *Decrease* After oral GTT mean area under the concentration curve for glucose of 16,488 ± 647 mg x min/dL in 25 women with PCOS compared with 14,144 ± 483 mg x min/dL in 20 healthy controls *655*

Gonadotropin, Pituitary *Plasma* *Increase* Elevated in polycystic ovary disease *1791*

Growth Hormone *Plasma* *No Effect* Mean concentration in 5 nonobese women with PCOS of 2.8 ± 1.0 mU/L not significantly different from 2.0 ± 0.6 mU/L in 4 non-obese control women *1681*

HDL-Cholesterol *Serum* *Decrease* In patients with insulin-resistant POS mean concentration of 0.71 ± 0.071 mmol/L below normal range and significantly lower than 1.02 ± 0.08 mmol/L in 17 noninsulin-resistant POS patients *2896*

17-Hydroxyprogesterone *Plasma* *Increase* In 25 women with PCOS mean concentration of 93 ± 10 ng/dL not significantly different from 73 ± 10 ng/dL in 20 healthy controls *655*

17α-Hydroxyprogesterone *Plasma* *Increase* In 12 obese women with polycystic ovary syndrome mean fasting concentration of 2.8 ± 0.4 nmol/L not significantly different from 2.2 ± 0.2 nmol/L in 11 healthy obese women *2410*

Insulin *Plasma* *Increase* In 25 women with PCOS mean basal concentration of 17 ± 2 μU/mL significantly higher than 10 ± 1 μU/mL in 20 healthy controls *655* In 12 obese women with polycystic ovary syndrome mean fasting concentration of 231 ± 84 pmol/L not significantly greater than 196 ± 28 pmol/L in 11 healthy obese women *2410* In 11 women with PCOS mean concentration of 16 ± 1.4 μU/mL significantly greater than 10 ± 1.6 μU/mL in 6 healthy controls *3616* In 11 lean PCOS patients mean fasting insulin concentration of 58 (40 - 137) pmol/L compared with 30 (20 - 60) pmol/L in 11 normal controls *858*
Plasma *No Effect* Mean concentration in 5 nonobese women with PCOS of 118 ± 23 pmol/L not significantly different from 122 ± 12 pmol/L in 4 non-obese control women *1681* In 44 patients with PCOS mean concentration of 21.0 ± 18.0 mU/L not significantly different from 25.5 ± 15.9 mU/L in 25 healthy controls *2382*

Insulin-like Growth Factor-I *Serum* *No Effect* In 11 women with PCOS mean concentration of 271 ± 38 ng/mL not significantly different from 280 ± 16 ng/mL in 6 healthy controls *3616* Mean concentration in 5 nonobese women with PCOS of 32.5 ± 3.6 nmol/L not significantly different from 30.5 ± 1.6 nmol/L in 4 non-obese control women *1681*

Insulin-like Growth Factor-I Receptor
Red Blood Cells *Increase* Mean concentration in 5 nonobese women with PCOS of 2.56 ± 0.49 sites/cell not significantly different from 1.30 ± 0.38 sites/cell in 4 non-obese control women *1681*

Insulin-like Growth Factor Binding Protein-3
Serum *No Effect* In 11 women with PCOS mean concentration of 4.7 ± 0.4 mg/L not significantly different from 4.8 ± 1.3 mg/L in 6 healthy controls *3616*

Luteinizing Hormone *Plasma* *Increase* In 7 female patients with PCOS mean concentration of 14.9 ± 2.1 IU/L was significantly different from 4.9 ± 0.9 IU/L in 8 healthy controls *1633* In 9 anovulatory women with PCOS mean bioactive LH and immunoreactive LH concentrations of 51.4 ± 8.6 mIU/mL and 36.0 ± 4.5 mIU/mL respectively compared with 19.2 ± 1.6 mIU/mL and 21.4 ± 1.2 mIU/mL respectively in 5 control women *4524* Mean concentration in 16 patients of 10.5 ± 1.2 IU/L significantly different from 3.5 ± 1.3 IU/L in 8 healthy women during during the early follicular phase of their menstrual cycle *4638* Mean concentration significantly incresed to an extent greater than in congenital adrenal hyperplasia *3008* In 11 women with PCOS mean concentration of 14.6 ± 1.3 mIU/mL significantly greater than 8.5 ± 0.5 mIU/mL in 6 healthy controls *3616* In 6 women with PCOS mean concentration of 9.1 ± 0.6 IU/L significantly different from normal range of 5.5 ± 0.3 IU/L *4175* Elevated in polycystic ovary disease *1791* Mean concentration in 65 women with PCOS of 5.4 mIU/mL (95% range 4.5 - 6.4) compared with 3.2 mIU/mL (95% range 2.8 - 3.7) in 45 control women *4397* In 44 patients with PCOS mean concentration of 11.4 ± 6.3 IU/L significantly greater than 4.3 ± 1.8 IU/L in 25 healthy controls *2382* In 26 women with PCOS mean concentration of 17.3 ± 8.3 mIU/mL compared with 8.4 ± 0.9 mIU/mL in normal women *5446*
Plasma *No Effect* In 13 patients with PCOS mean concentration of 10 ± 1 mIU/mL not significantly different when compared with 9 ± 2 mIU/mL in 15 healthy control women *3606* Mean concentration in 5 nonobese women with PCOS of 9.3 ± 2.4 IU/L not significantly different from 5.9 ± 1.0 IU/L in 4 non-obese control women *1681*
Urine *Increase* Increased excretion typically observed *2952*

Luteinizing Hormone:Follicle Stimulating Hormone Ratio
Plasma *Increase* In 13 patients with PCOS mean ratio of 2.0 ± 0.4 significantly higher when compared with 1.1 ± 0.2 in 15 healthy control women *3606*

Platelets *Blood* *Increase* Count above 400,000 /μL observed in 2.9% of 35 patients with benign ovarian cysts *3454*

Progesterone *Plasma* *No Effect* Mean concentration in 5 nonobese women with PCOS of 1.0 ± 0.0 nmol/L not significantly different from 0.9 ± 0.1 nmol/L in 4 non-obese control women *1681*

Prolactin *Plasma* *Increase* Increased levels *4289*
Plasma *No Effect* In 6 women with PCOS mean concentration of 203 ± 81 mU/L not significantly different from normal range of 53 - 520 mU/L *4175*

Prorenin *Plasma* *Increase* In 13 patients with PCOS mean concentration of 122 ± 15 pg/mL significantly higher when compared with 75 ± 8 pg/mL in 15 healthy control women *3606*

Renin *Plasma* *Increase* In 44 patients with PCOS mean concentration of 236 ± 96 ng/L significantly greater than 143 ± 61 ng/L in 25 healthy controls *2382*

Renin, Active *Plasma* *No Effect* In 13 patients with PCOS mean concentration of 13.4 ± 1 pg/mL not significantly different when compared with 11 ± 1 pg/mL in 15 healthy control women *3606*

Sex-Hormone Binding Globulin *Serum* *Decrease* In 7 female patients with PCOS mean concentration of 57.0 ± 7.7 nmol/L was significantly different from 84.5 ± 6.8 nmol/L in 8 healthy controls *1633* In 6 women with PCOS mean concentration of 32 ± 6.3 nmol/L significantly less than normal range of 35 - 118 nmol/L *4175* In 12 obese women with polycystic ovary syndrome mean fasting concentration of 17.37 ± 1.83 nmol/L not significantly different from 20.94 ± 2.17 nmol/L in 11 healthy obese women *2410* Mean concentration of 31.5 ± 3.3 nmol/L in 25 women with PCOS significantly less than 43.0 ± 3.5 nmol/L in 20 healthy controls *655*
Serum *No Effect* In 44 patients with PCOS mean concentration of 1.3 ± 0.7 μg/dL not significantly different from 1.4 ± 0.8 μg/dL in 25 healthy controls *2382*

256.40 Polycystic Ovary Disease *(continued)*

Testosterone *Saliva Increase* Maximum concentration in women with polycystic ovary disease of 156 pmol/L slightly higher than mean concentration in 10 healthy control individuals *5155*
Serum Increase In 12 obese women with polycystic ovary syndrome mean fasting concentration of 2.47 ± 0.52 nmol/L not significantly different from 1.45 ± 0.24 nmol/L in 11 healthy obese women *2410* Mean concentration nonsignificantly increased in women with PCOS with enlarged ovaries compared with those with ovaries of normal size *4242* In 25 women with PCOS mean concentration of 440 ± 36 pg/mL significantly greater than 294 ± 23 pg/mL in 20 healthy controls *655* In 9 patients with anovulatory polycystic ovarian syndrome (PCOS) mean concentration of 1.18 ± 0.13 ng/mL significantly higher than 0.28 ± 0.03 ng/mL in 5 control women *4524* In 44 patients with PCOS mean concentration of 86.5 ± 25.9 ng/dL significantly greater than 46.1 ± 14.4 ng/dL in 25 healthy controls *2382* In 7 female patients with PCOS mean concentration of 3.3 ± 0.11 nmol/L was significantly different from 1.86 ± 0.12 nmol/L in 8 healthy controls *1633* In 13 patients with PCOS mean concentration of 68 ± 7 ng/dL significantly higher when compared with 28 ± 4 ng/dL in 15 healthy control women *3606* In 6 women with PCOS mean concentration of 5.6 ± 1.0 nmol/L significantly greater than normal range of up to 3 nmol/L *4175* Mean concentration in 5 nonobese women with PCOS of 2.2 ± 0.3 nmol/L significantly different from 1.4 ± 0.2 nmol/L in 4 non-obese control women *1681* Mean concentration of 0.6 ± 0.3 ng/mL in 26 women with PCOS significantly higher than 0.26 ± 0.16 ng/mL in normal women *5446* Mean concentration in 65 women with PCOS of 55 ng/dL (95% range 49 - 58) compared with 37 ng/dL (95% range 35 - 40) in 45 control women *4397* In 11 women with PCOS mean concentration of 94 ± 4 ng/dL significantly greater than 26 ± 4 ng/dL in 6 healthy controls *3616* Mean concentration in 16 patients of 3.1 ± 1.2 nmol/L significantly different from 1.8 ± 0.5 nmol/L in 8 healthy women during during the early follicular phase of their menstrual cycle *4638*

Testosterone, Free *Serum Increase* In 12 obese women with polycystic ovary syndrome mean fasting concentration of 9.03 ± 1.39 pmol/L significantly different from 5.99 ± 0.51 pmol/L in 11 healthy obese women *2410* Mean concentration of 11.3 ± 6.97 pg/mL in 26 women with PCOS significantly higher than 5.4 ± 2.7 pg/mL in normal women *5446* Mean concentration of 9.1 ± 0.9 pg/mL in 25 women with PCOS significantly higher than 4.9 ± 0.5 pg/mL in 20 healthy controls *655* Mean concentration in 5 nonobese women with PCOS of 15.4 ± 0.4 pmol/L significantly different from 4.9 ± 0.5 pmol/L in 4 non-obese control women *1681*

Triglycerides *Serum No Effect* Although within normal range mean concentration higher in 10 insulin-resistant patients (1.39 ± 0.18 mmol/L) than in 17 noninsulin-resistant patients (0.91 ± 0.09 mmol/L) *2896*

256.41 Stein-Leventhal Syndrome

Androgens *Plasma Increase* Plasma levels of androstenedione and dehydroepiandosterone are elevated *2034*

Androstenedione *Plasma Increase* Concentration often increased in Stein-Leventhal syndrome *2952* Plasma levels of androstenedione and dehydroepiandosterone are elevated *2034*

Dehydroepiandrosterone *Plasma Increase* Plasma levels of androstenedione and dehydroepiandosterone are elevated *2034*

Dehydroepiandrosterone Sulfate *Plasma Increase* Observed effect *91 3778*

Follicle Stimulating Hormone *Plasma Decrease* Observed effect *367*

Gonadotropin, Pituitary *Plasma Increase* Slightly elevated levels of LH in Stein-Leventhal syndrome *367*

Luteinizing Hormone *Plasma Increase* Slightly elevated levels *367* Slightly elevated levels of LH in Stein-Leventhal syndrome *367*

pH *Blood Decrease* Normal or decreased *2889*

Testosterone *Serum Increase* On occasion *2034*

257.20 Primary Male Hypogonadism

Dehydroepiandrosterone Sulfate *Plasma No Effect* Mean concentration of 0.66 ± 0.46 µmol/L observed in 10 men not significantly different from 0.71 ± 0.38 µmol/L in 11 healthy controls *3956*

Estradiol *Plasma Increase* Mean concentration of 363 ± 116 pmol/L observed in 10 men significantly different from 155 ± 79 pmol/L in 11 healthy controls *3956*

Follicle Stimulating Hormone *Plasma Increase* Mean concentration of 47.5 ± 10.7 IU/L observed in 10 men significantly different from 8.6 ± 3.7 IU/L in 11 healthy controls *3956*

Luteinizing Hormone *Plasma Increase* Mean concentration of 22.6 ± 5.9 IU/L observed in 10 men significantly different from 5.8 ± 2.1 IU/L in 11 healthy controls *3956*

Melatonin *Plasma Increase* Mean morning concentration of 34.2 ± 21.1 pmol/L observed in 10 men slightly but not significantly different from 21.7 ± 10.8 pmol/L in 11 healthy controls *3956*

Prolactin *Plasma No Effect* Mean concentration of 3.42 ± 2.62 µg/L observed in 10 men not significantly different from 3.8 ± 3.3 µg/L in 11 healthy controls *3956*

Sex-Hormone Binding Globulin *Serum Increase* Mean concentration of 56.2 ± 27.1 nmol/L observed in 10 men significantly different from 28.2 ± 16.2 nmol/L in 11 healthy controls *3956*

Testosterone *Serum Decrease* Mean concentration of 3.15 ± 1.6 nmol/L observed in 10 men significantly different from 17.6 ± 6.5 nmol/L in 11 healthy controls *3956*

Testosterone, Free *Serum Decrease* Mean concentration of 19.1 ± 16.6 pmol/L observed in 10 men significantly different from 81.8 ± 18.1 pmol/L in 11 healthy controls *3956*

257.20 Testicular Hypofunction

Androgens *Plasma Decrease* Decreased testosterone in primary and secondary hypogonadism *5544*

Creatine *Urine Increase* Increased formation *5544*

Estrogens *Plasma Increase* The average daily production of estrogen is increased and the circulating levels of estrogen are relatively constant *367*

Gonadotropin, Pituitary *Urine Decrease* Decreased in secondary hypogonadism *5545*
Urine Increase Increased in primary hypogonadism *5545*

Hematocrit *Blood Decrease* Reduced testicular function can produce anemia. Hematocrit is seldom < 30%. The RBC is normochromic and normocytic *900*

Hemoglobin *Blood Decrease* Reduced testicular function can produce anemia. The hemoglobin is seldom < 9 g/dL. The RBC is normocytic and normochromic *900*

17-Hydroxycorticosteroids *Urine Decrease* Decreased with castration in men *5544*

17-Ketogenic Steroids *Urine Decrease* Decreased with castration in men *5544*

17-Ketosteroids *Urine Decrease* Excretion may be slightly decreased in patients with eunuchism or castration in the male *2952* Decreased in primary and secondary hypogonadism *5544*

Luteinizing Hormone *Urine Decrease* Decreased excretion typically observed in primary hypergonadism in men *2952*
Urine Increase Increased excretion typically observed in primary hypogonadism in men *2952*

Prostate-specific Antigen *Serum Decrease* In 31 men aged 17 to 65 y with hypogonadism concentrations ranged from 0.05 - 2.22 ng/mL compared with 0.11 - 3.74 ng/mL in normal men *679*

Reticulocytes *Blood Decrease* The absolute count is decreased *900*

Sex-Hormone Binding Globulin *Serum Increase* In men with hypogonadism or gynecomastia increased SHBG concentrations have been observed *1424*

Testosterone *Serum Decrease* Observed effect *5545* Decreased in primary and secondary hypogonadism *5544* In 31 men with hypogonadism aged 17 to 65 years range of 88 - 521 ng/dL significantly less than 695 ± 202 ng/dL in normal men *5469*

259.10 Precocious Puberty

Estradiol *Plasma Increase* In 21 girls with precocious puberty mean concentration of 69 pmol/L significantly greater than normal for age of < 30 pmol/L *1655*
Plasma No Effect In 6 girls with premature adrenarche mean concentration of 21 ± 2 pmol/L not significantly different from normal for age of < 30 pmol/L *1655* In 7 girls with exaggerated thelarche mean concentration of 20 ± 1.2 pmol/L not different from normal range for age of < 30 pmol/L *1655*

Follicle Stimulating Hormone *Plasma No Effect* In 21 girls with precocious puberty mean concentration of 4.2 ± 0.4 IU/L within normal range of 0.5 - 5 IU/L for age *1655* In 7 girls with exaggerated thelarche mean concentration of 3.2 ± 0.9 IU/L not different from normal for age of < 0.5 - 5 IU/L *1655* Mean concentration of 1.4 ± 0.3 IU/L in 6 girls with premature adrenarche compared with normal for age of < 0.5 - 5 IU/L *1655*

Luteinizing Hormone *Plasma Increase* In 21 girls with precocious puberty mean concentration of 3.6 ± 0.8 IU/L significantly increased compared with normal for age of < 0.5 IU/L *1655*
Plasma No Effect In 6 girls with premature adrenarche mean concentration of 0.27 ± 0.02 IU/L compared with normal for age of < 0.5 IU/L *1655* In 7 girls with exaggerated thelarche mean concentration of 0.36 ± 0.1 IU/L not different from < 0.5 IU/L (normal for age) *1655*

Melatonin *Plasma Decrease* In 56 children with central precocious puberty mean concentration significantly less than in age-matched prepubertal children *5530*

259.20 Carcinoid Syndrome

Albumin *Serum Decrease* Commonly observed in patients with carcinoid tumor *3297*

Amino Acids *Plasma Decrease* Decreased tryptophan, valine, isoleucine, lysine and ornithine were found. All others were normal except methionine, which was elevated. The low plasma levels were not due to hyperexcretion, as urinary levels were normal *1452*

Bilirubin *Serum Increase* Rare until extensive hepatic metastases occur *5679*

Bradykinin *Plasma No Effect* The concentrations of bradykinin-like immunoreactivity in extracts of peripheral blood was compared in patients with carcinoid syndrome (n = 11) and healthy subjects (n = 6). In the fasted state the levels were not significantly different *265*

BSP Retention *Serum Increase* May be seen in later course of disease *5679*

Calcitonin *Plasma Increase* In one of 4 patients (25%) with carcinoid tumors and chronic diarrhea was concentration increased above upper limit of normal of 71 pg/mL *4635* Secreted in bronchial and intestinal carcinoid tumors *3485*

Carbon Dioxide Partial Pressure *Blood Decrease* Hyperventilation may occur during the flush *5679*

Carotene *Serum Decrease* Secondary to malabsorption or steatorrhea *5679*

Catecholamines *Urine Increase* Catecholamines and their metabolites have been elevated in the urine of some patients. This abnormality is unusual and to date has not been correlated with specific symptoms or origins of the tumors *4891 3452*

Cholesterol *Serum Decrease* Secondary to malabsorption or steatorrhea *5679*

Corticotropin *Plasma Increase* In some patients with bronchial carcinoid concentrations ranged from 251 to 9,265 pg/mL compared with normal of less than 60 pg/mL *4262*

CYFRA 21-1 *Serum Increase* In 3 patients with carcinoid tumors median concentration of 2.6 ng/mL significantly different from that in 50 healthy individuals with median concentration of 1.2 ng/mL and range of 0.5 - 2.4 ng/mL *3559*

Fat *Feces Increase* Secondary to malabsorption or steatorrhea *5679*

Gastrin-releasing Peptide *Serum No Effect* In none of 4 patients with carcinoid tumors and chronic diarrhea was concentration increased above upper limit of normal of 542 pg/mL *4635*

Glucose Tolerance *Serum No Effect* No significant effect observed *5679*

Growth Hormone *Plasma Increase* Elevated *1870*

Histamine *Urine Increase* Some patients with gastric carcinoids have been shown to have frequent and consistent elevations of histamine, which is inconsistently elevated in those with ileal tumors. Often seen in patients with gastric and bronchial carcinoids *4891* Persistently elevated in gastric carcinoid tumors *5373*

17-Hydroxycorticosteroids *Urine Increase* May be increased to 10 times normal *367*

5-Hydroxyindoleacetic Acid *Urine Increase* Usually associated with 5-HIAA urinary concentrations of 25 mg/d *5373* 75% of 75 patients with this disorder had elevated levels *1453* Normally there are 2 - 9 mg/d while levels up to 1 g/d may occur in the carcinoid syndrome *1980* Diagnostic of a carcinoid tumor *2304* Observed effect *5545* Excretion > 130 mmol/24 h is diagnostic provided walnuts and bananas have been excluded from the diet for 24 h *5863* Carcinoid tumors produce 5-hydroxytryptamine in excess with increased urinary 5-HIAA *2952* Increased, usually when tumor is far advanced, but may not be increased despite massive metastases. Useful in confirming diagnosis in only 5 - 7% *4746*
Urine No Effect Hyperserotoninemia with normal urinary 5-HIAA in ileal carcinoid tumors *5373*

5-Hydroxytryptamine *Blood Increase* Systemic symptoms appear only after metastasis to the liver; the serotonin released from the metastasis passes directly to the systemic circulation, avoiding hepatic metabolism *1980* Serotonin and related products are the biochemical markers of this disorder *5373* Usually associated with an excess of circulating 5-HT *5863* Carcinoid tumors differ widely in their ability to produce or store 5-HT. Excessive production remains their most characteristic chemical abnormality *4891*
Platelets Increase Platelet serotonin is more sensitive than urinary 5-HIAA for detecting carcinoids that secrete only small amounts of serotonin *2630*
Urine Increase Usually associated with an excess of circulating 5-HT *5863* Systemic symptoms appear only after metastasis to the liver; the serotonin released from the metastasis passes directly to the systemic circulation, avoiding hepatic metabolism *1980* Carcinoid tumors differ widely in their ability to produce or store 5-HT. Excessive production remains their most characteristic chemical abnormality *4891*

Isoleucine *Plasma Decrease* Decreased plasma concentration, but normal urinary excretion was found *1452*

Leukocytes *Blood Increase* In abdominal crises leukocytosis and thrombocytosis are usual *900*

Lipotropic Hormone *Plasma Increase* In some patients with bronchial carcinoid concentrations ranged from 1,487 to 750,000 pg/mL compared with normal of less than 60 pg/mL *4262*

Lysine *Plasma Decrease* Decreased plasma concentration, but normal urinary excretion was found *1452*

Methionine *Plasma Increase* The only amino acid found to be increased, all others were decreased or normal *1452*

Motilin *Plasma No Effect* In none of two patients with carcinoid tumors and chronic diarrhea was concentration increased above upper limit of normal of 125 pg/mL *4635*

Neurotensin *Plasma No Effect* In none of 4 patients with carcinoid tumors and chronic diarrhea was concentration increased above upper limit of normal of 250 pg/mL *4635*

Pancreatic Polypeptide *Plasma Increase* In 2 of 4 patients (50%) with carcinoid tumors and chronic diarrhea was concentration increased above upper limit of normal of 465 pg/mL *4635*

pH *Blood Increase* Hyperventilation may occur during the flush *5679*

Platelets *Blood Increase* In abdominal crises leukocytosis and thrombocytosis are usual *900*

Potassium *Serum Decrease* Severe hypokalemia and weakness are common, due to the enormous quantities or cortisol secreted by the hyperplastic adrenals *367*

Proopiomelanocortin *Plasma Increase* In some patients with bronchial carcinoid concentrations ranged from < 60 to 2,088 U/mL compared with normal of less than 60 U/mL *4262*

Prostaglandins *Plasma Increase* During a flush *4558*

Protein *Serum Increase* Common and may add to the peripheral manifestations of cardiac failure *2304*

Somatostatin *Plasma No Effect* In none of 4 patients with carcinoid tumors and chronic diarrhea was concentration increased above upper limit of normal of 68 pg/mL *4635*

259.20 Carcinoid Syndrome *(continued)*

Substance P *Plasma* *Increase* In 1 of 4 patients (25%) with carcinoid tumors and chronic diarrhea was concentration increased above upper limit of normal of 240 pg/mL *4635*

Tryptophan *Plasma* *Decrease* Due to increased production of serotonin by the tumor; may result in clinical pellagra *1452*

Valine *Plasma* *Decrease* Decreased plasma concentration, but normal urinary excretion was found *1452*

Vasoactive Intestinal Polypeptide *Plasma* *No Effect* In none of 4 patients with carcinoid tumors and chronic diarrhea was concentration increased above upper limit of normal of 84 pg/mL *4635*

Vitamin A *Serum* *Decrease* Secondary to malabsorption or steatorrhea *5679*

259.40 Dwarfism

Growth Hormone *Plasma* *Decrease* Hyposecretion causes dwarfism in children *2952*

259.40 Laron Dwarfism

Growth Hormone *Urine* *Increase* In 5 patients with idiopathic short stature mean excretion of 35.3 ± 12.1 ng/L (7.39 ± 3.43 ng/mmol creatinine) significantly different from that in healthy individuals *1698*

Insulin-like Growth Factor-I *Serum* *Decrease* Mean concentration of 4.3 ± 1.1 nmol/L in 5 children with Laron syndrome and of 3.4 ± 8 nmol/L significantly decreased compared with reference interval *2925* Concentration decreased in patients with Laron dwarfism *2952*

Lipoprotein Lp(a) *Serum* *Increase* Mean concentration of 76 ± 45 mg/L observed in 10 patients with Laron syndrome significantly increased compared with reference interval *2925*

259.80 Progeria

Hyaluronic Acid *Urine* *Increase* Increase in HA excretion seen in progeria *5105*

Nutritional Deficiency States

260.00 Kwashiorkor

Antidiuretic Hormone *Plasma* *Increase* Typical observation in children with kwashiorkor *355*
Urine *Increase* Typical observation in children with kwashiorkor *355*

Cholesterol *Serum* *Decrease* In 21 children with kwashiorkor mean concentration significantly reduced *1143*

Cholesterol, Esterified *Serum* *Decrease* In 21 children with kwashiorkor mean concentration significantly reduced compared with concentration following treatment *1143*

Epinephrine *Urine* *Increase* Marasmic and normal weight infants excreted proportionally 3 - 4 times less epinephrine than norepinephrine (ratio: 0.20 - 0.38). Children with kwashiorkor excreted nearly similar amounts of epinephrine and norepinephrine (ratio: 0.88). In marasmus, norepinephrine may predominate and in kwashiorkor epinephrine may predominate, in the regulation of the metabolic adaptations to assure survival *4271*

immunoglobulin A *Saliva* *No Effect* Nonsignificant reduction to mean of 2.8 mg/dL in 10 children with kwashiorkor increased nonsignificantly to 3.3 mg/dL with refeeding *5601*
Serum *Increase* In 21 children with kwashiorkor mean concentration of 215 mg/dL decreased to 135 mg/dL with renutrition *5601*
Tears *No Effect* Nonsignificant increase to 19.9 mg/dL in 21 children with marasmus which decreased to 17.4 mg/dL with renourishment *5601*

Immunoglobulin G *Serum* *Decrease* In 21 children with kwashiorkor mean concentration of 1,046 mg/dL significantly increased to 1,763 mg/dL with renutrition *5601*
Tears *No Effect* Nonsignificant increase to 20.9 mg/dL in 21 children with marasmus decreasing to 16.1 mg/dL with renourishment *5601*

Immunoglobulin M *Serum* *No Effect* In 21 children with kwashiorkor mean concentration of 173 mg/dL not significantly different from mean concentration of 187 mg/dL once they were renourished *5601*

Lecithin:Cholesterol Acyltransferase *Serum* *Decrease* In 21 children with kwashiorkor mean activity before treatment of 78.2 µmol/L/h compared with 139.2 µmol/L/h after 10 days treatment and 108.0 µmol/L/h after treatment *1143*

Lysozyme *Saliva* *Increase* Nonsignificant increase to 0.32 mg/dL in 10 children with kwashiorkor decreased to mean concentration of 0.257 mg/dL with refeeding *5601*
Tears *Decrease* Significant decrease to 107 mg/dL in 21 children with kwashiorkor which increased to 210 mg/dL with renourishment *5601*

Thyroxine (T4), Free *Serum* *No Effect* Normal or increased concentrations observed *355*

Tri-iodothyronine (T3) *Serum* *Decrease* Effect on Wien Laboratory test possibly related to decrease protein *5398*

260.00 Protein Malnutrition

Albumin *Serum* *Decrease* Usually 1.5 - 2.5 g/dL but may be < l g/dL. Correlates with the degree of fatty liver and of edema; becomes normal after 3 weeks of normal diet; standard test for diagnosis of kwashiorkor and to monitor response to treatment *5545* Albumin, prealbumin and transferrin concentrations were found to be lower in cases of protein-energy malnutrition associated with infection than the corresponding values for a group of healthy preschool children *4623*

Alkaline Phosphatase *Serum* *Decrease* Marked reductions are recognized characteristics *367* Decreased unless dehydration is present with marasmus *5545*

Amino Acids *Plasma* *No Effect* In starvation, the amino acid level in the blood does not usually fall below the normal fasting level. Protein concentration is maintained at the expense of body protein *1290* Severe protein deficiency alters the qualitative pattern, not the total amount *4707*

α-Amino-Nitrogen *Plasma* *Decrease* Abnormally low *367*

β-Aminoisobutyric Acid *Plasma* *Increase* In Kwashiorkor, there is an increase in β-aminoisobutyric acid. During recovery ethanolamine is elevated *1290*
Urine *Increase* Increased β-aminoisobutyric acid and ethanolamine in urine of patients with kwashiorkor *1290*

Amylase *Gastric Material* *Decrease* Activity is lowered almost to zero in kwashiorkor *367*
Serum *Decrease* Marked reductions are recognized characteristics *367* Circulating concentration appears consistent with the amount of structural damage to the pancreas, characteristic of kwashiorkor *4707*

α_1-Antichymotrypsin *Serum* *Increase* Elevated in children with clinical protein malnutrition *4624*

α_1-Antitrypsin *Serum* *Decrease* Decreased *4241* *4373* *4371* *4763* *83* These conditions reduce activity *2091*

Calcium *Serum* *Decrease* Decreased in hypoproteinemia *1025*

Carotene *Serum* *Decrease* Extremely low in children with kwashiorkor *367*

Cells *Bone Marrow* *Decrease* Normally cellular or slightly hypocellular, and the erythroid/myeloid ratio was decreased *5677*

Ceruloplasmin *Serum* *Decrease* Moderate transient deficiencies in patients with nephrosis *5544*

Chloride *Serum* *No Effect* Concentration usually unaffected *5544*

Cholesterol *Serum* *Decrease* With protein malnutrition *5545* In kwashiorkor *367*

Cholinesterase *Serum* *Decrease* May be decreased in some conditions in which albumin is low *5544* In Kwashiorkor *367*

Complement C_1q *Serum* *Decrease* Observed effect *3910*

Complement C_1s *Serum* *Decrease* Observed effect *3910*

Complement C_2 *Serum* *Decrease* Observed effect *4746*

Complement C_3 *Serum* *Decrease* C_3 was the only fraction which is significantly diminished in marasmic infants *1951* All complement components except C_4 and C_5 were significantly lower in children with protein-calorie malnutrition: C_3 and C_9 were the most severely depressed. C_5 was the only complement that was significantly higher in malnourished children than in normal children *3910*

Complement C_4 *Serum* *No Effect* All complement components except C_4 and C_5 were significantly lower in children with protein-calorie malnutrition. C_3 and C_9 were the most severely depressed. C_5 was the only complement that was significantly higher in malnourished children than in normal children *3910*

Complement, Total *Serum* *Decrease* Individual components of the complement system were significantly lower in kwashiorkor than in normal controls *1951* Mean activity in children with kwashiorkor was significantly less on hospital days 1 and 4 than in control subjects. On day 8 it rose to normal, and by day 50 it was significantly higher than the controls. 11 (40%) evidence anticomplementary activity in their serum on either day 1 or day 4 *5089* All complement components except C_4 and C_5 were significantly lower in children with protein-calorie malnutrition: C_3 and C_9 were the most severely depressed. C_5 was the only complement that was significantly higher in malnourished children than in normal children *3910*

Copper *Red Blood Cells* *Decrease* Serum, erythrocyte, and urinary copper levels showed decline in marasmic malnutrition and kwashiorkor. Marked fall of serum and erythrocyte copper level in children suffering from kwashiorkor *2403*
Serum *Decrease* Serum, erythrocyte and urinary copper levels showed decline in marasmic malnutrition and kwashiorkor. Marked fall of serum and erythrocyte copper level in children suffering from kwashiorkor *2403*
Urine *Decrease* Serum, erythrocyte, and urinary copper levels showed decline in marasmic malnutrition and kwashiorkor *2403*

Creatinine *Urine* *Decrease* Decreased 24 hour urinary creatinine *413*

Cystine *Plasma* *Decrease* Observed effect *367*

Epinephrine *Plasma* *Increase* Marasmic and normal weight infants excreted proportionally 3 - 4 times less epinephrine than norepinephrine (ratio: 0.20 - 0.38). Children with kwashiorkor excreted nearly similar amounts of epinephrine and norepinephrine (ratio: 0.88). In marasmus, norepinephrine may predominate and in kwashiorkor epinephrine may predominate, in the regulation of the metabolic adaptations to assure survival *4271*
Urine *Increase* Marasmic and normal weight infants excreted proportionally 3 - 4 times less epinephrine than norepinephrine (ratio: 0.20 - 0.38). Children with kwashiorkor excreted nearly similar amounts of epinephrine and norepinephrine (ratio: 0.88). In marasmus, norepinephrine may predominate and in kwashiorkor epinephrine may predominate, in the regulation of the metabolic adaptations to assure survival *4271*

Erythrocyte Sedimentation Rate *Blood* *Decrease* Observed with cachexia *4949*

Factor VIII *Plasma* *Decrease* During 10 days of total fasting in healthy normal weight males, a reduction of plasma activity with a concomitant decrease in factor VIII antigen was found, without other laboratory evidence for a disseminated intravascular coagulation *1306*

Factor B *Plasma* *Decrease* Found in 50% of patients *5229* *4431*

Fatty Acids (FFA), Free *Serum* *Increase* Reported effect *1290*

Folate *Serum* *Decrease* Observed effect *5545*

β-Globulin *Serum* *Decrease* Tends to be both relatively and absolutely decreased *367*

γ-Globulin *Serum* *Decrease* Minimal reduction *2034*
Serum *Increase* Relatively high as a result of concurrent infectious process *367* Slightly increased with marasmus *5545*

Glucose *Serum* *Decrease* Decreased due to excess insulin resulting from deficiency in available glycogen *1290* In kwashiorkor *367*

Glucose Tolerance *Serum* *Increase* In kwashiorkor *367*

Growth Hormone *Plasma* *Increase* Elevated fasting plasma concentrations in all groups of malnourished children *4387*

Hematocrit *Blood* *Decrease* There may be moderate anemia *900* Mild or moderate normocytic normochromic anemia occurs after 24 weeks of controlled semistarvation *5677*

Hemoglobin *Blood* *Decrease* Mild or moderate normocytic normochromic anemia occurs after 24 weeks of controlled semistarvation. Fall was to 11 g/dL in males and 9.5 g/dL in females *5677* Mild anemia *900* In infants and children, may fall to 8 - 10 g/dL of blood, but some children are admitted with normal levels, probably due to a shrunken plasma volume *5677*

immunoglobulin A *Serum* *Decrease* Reported effect *1025*

Immunoglobulin M *Serum* *Decrease* Reported effect *5544*

Immunoglobulins *Serum* *Increase* Usually normal or increased despite protein deficiency in kwashiorkor *4707*

Insulin *Plasma* *Decrease* Decreased fasting plasma levels found in both marasmus and kwashiorkor but no significant difference was found between types of severe protein-energy malnutrition *4387*

Insulin-like Growth Factor-I *Serum* *Decrease* Decreased *2166*

Iron *Serum* *Decrease* With kwashiorkor *5545* Usually low because of decreased transferrin concentration or actual iron deficiency *5677*

Iron-binding Capacity, Total *Serum* *Decrease* Albumin, prealbumin and transferrin concentrations were found to be low in cases of protein-energy malnutrition associated with preschool children *4623*

Ketones *Urine* *Increase* 50 mg/dL; more common in children than adults *1290* *5544*

Leukocytes *Blood* *Decrease* Leukopenia with a mean count diminishing from 6,346 to 4,129 /μL *2034*

Lipase *Gastric Material* *Decrease* In kwashiorkor *367*
Serum *Decrease* Decreased with protein malnutrition. In kwashiorkor *367* Circulating concentration appears consistent with the amount of structural damage to the pancreas, characteristic of kwashiorkor *4707*

Lymphocyte T-Cells *Blood* *Decrease* Normal *1588*

Lymphocytes *Blood* *Decrease* Decreased total count of < 1,500 /μL *413*

α_2-Macroglobulin *Serum* *Decrease* Found to be lower in cases of protein-energy malnutrition associated with preschool children *4623*

Magnesium *Red Blood Cells* *Decrease* RBC concentration was decreased in 2 of 4 patients with prolonged malnutrition *5547*
Serum *Decrease* Hypomagnesemia may occur *5507*

Methionine *Plasma* *Decrease* Observed effect *367*

N-Formiminoglutamic Acid *Urine* *Increase* Increased in some cases of marasmus *5544*

Nitrogen *Liver* *Decrease* The level of nitrogen in the liver of children with kwashiorkor is markedly decreased over that for children of the same age *367*

pH *Blood* *Decrease* The plasma pH tends to fall *1290*

Phosphate *Serum* *Decrease* Serum concentration generally remains normal but may decline to or slightly below the lower range of normal *2719*

Phospholipids *Serum* *Decrease* Reported observation *367*

Potassium *Serum* *Decrease* Potassium depletion is a major biochemical characteristic of kwashiorkor *367*
Urine *Increase* Increased breakdown of the body cells, occurs with release of intracellular potassium. Carbohydrate intake (glucose 100 g/d) greatly reduces the rate of cell breakdown *1290*
Urine *No Effect* Increased or normal *5544*

Prealbumin *Serum* *Decrease* Albumin, prealbumin and transferrin concentrations, as well as alpha$_2$-macroglobulin were found to be lower in cases of protein-energy malnutrition associated with preschool children *4623*

Protein *Serum* *Decrease* Albumin, prealbumin and transferrin concentrations, as well as alpha$_2$-macroglobulin were found to be lower in cases of protein-energy malnutrition associated with infection than the corresponding values for a group of healthy preschool children *4623*

Reticulocytes *Blood* *Decrease* Normal or slightly decreased *5677*

Sodium *Serum* *No Effect* Usual observation *5544*
Urine *Increase* Normal or increased *5544*

Somatomedin *Plasma* *Decrease* Observed effect *3141*

260.00 **Protein Malnutrition** *(continued)*

T3-Uptake *Serum* *Increase* T3 resin uptake is significantly elevated in the acute stage of kwashiorkor and returns to normal after 2 weeks of appropriate refeeding *2334*

Thyroid Stimulating Hormone *Serum* *No Effect* In frank kwashiorkor, concentrations were within the normal range throughout the entire course of dietary therapy, indicating that the children remained euthyroid *2335*

Thyroxine Binding Globulin *Serum* *Decrease* In hypoproteinemias *4707* Decreased in nephrosis and other causes of marked hypoproteinemia *5544*

Thyroxine (T4) *Serum* *Decrease* Decreased T4 with hypoproteinemia *5544*

Tri-iodothyronine, Reverse (rT3) *Serum* *Increase* Mean serum reverse T3 was elevated in patients with severe protein calorie malnutrition to 53 ng/dL. In the same patients after feeding treatment the value dropped to 22 ng/dL *827*

Tri-iodothyronine (T3) *Serum* *Decrease* Protein-calorie malnutrition in a group of 43 children aged 18 - 30 months was characterized by a sharp fall in T3 concentration to 25 - 30% of the mean value in controls. This decrease was significantly more pronounced in kwashiorkor of recent onset than in long-term *2335*

Trypsin *Gastric Material* *Decrease* In kwashiorkor *367*

Tryptophan *Plasma* *Decrease* Reported effect *367*

Tyrosine *Plasma* *Decrease* Observed effect *367*

Urea Nitrogen *Serum* *Decrease* Indicates decreased protein metabolism *30* *413*

Uric Acid *Serum* *Increase* High in starvation, ketosis, and high fat diets *3969*

Valine *Plasma* *Decrease* Observed effect *367*

Vitamin A *Serum* *Decrease* Extremely low *367*

Vitamin B_{12} *Serum* *Increase* Usually increased with kwashiorkor *5545*

Volume *Plasma* *Decrease* Normal or decreased *5544*
Plasma *Increase* Plasma volume expressed in mL/kg of body weight was increased. Dilution was a major factor responsible for the reduction in hemoglobin concentration *5677*
Urine *Decrease* In total colonic starvation *2034*
Urine *Increase* In semistarvation, polyuria of 2 - 3 L/day and nocturia *2034*

Xylose Tolerance Test *Urine* *No Effect* No change in xylose absorption observed *5544*

Zinc *Serum* *Decrease* Decreased *5083* *4562*

261.00 **Marasmus**

Alanine Aminotransferase *Serum* *No Effect* In 20 children with protein energy malnutrition aged 13.5 ± 6.1 months mean activity of 35 ± 15 U/L not significantly different from 32 ± 7 U/L after refeeding and 33 ± 5 U/L in age matched controls *3619*

Albumin *Serum* *No Effect* With calorie deficiency but without protein deficiency plasma albumin concentration unaffected *1959*

Ammonia *Plasma* *Increase* In 20 children with protein energy malnutrition aged 13.5 ± 6.1 months mean concentration of 177 ± 66 µg/dL significantly higher than 38 ± 18 µg/dL after refeeding and 61 ± 24 µg/dL in 10 age-matched controls *3619*

Antidiuretic Hormone *Plasma* *No Effect* Near normal concentrations observed in children *355*
Urine *No Effect* Near normal excretion observed in children *355*

Arginine *Plasma* *Decrease* In 20 children with protein energy malnutrition aged 13.5 ± 6.1 months mean concentration of 106 ± 56 µmol/L not significantly less than 161 ± 45 µmol/L after refeeding and 175 ± 49 µmol/L in 10 age-matched controls *3619*

Aspartate Aminotransferase *Serum* *No Effect* In 20 children with protein energy malnutrition aged 13.5 ± 6.1 months mean activity of 40 ± 18 U/L not significantly increased above 35 ± 5 U/L after refeeding and 32 ± 8 U/L in 10 controls *3619*

Citrulline *Plasma* *Decrease* In 20 children with protein energy malnutrition aged 13.5 ± 6.1 months nonsignificant decrease to 105 ± 52 µmol/L compared with 166 ± 61 µmol/L after refeeding and 135 ± 72 µmol/L in 10 age-matched controls *3619*

Cortisol *Plasma* *Increase* In 32 children with grade II-III marasmus baseline concentration significantly increased to mean of 480 nmol/L compared with 234 nmol/L after caloric rehabilitation *3260*

Epinephrine *Urine* *Increase* Marasmic and normal weight infants excreted proportionally 3 - 4 times less epinephrine than norepinephrine (ratio: 0.20 - 0.38). Children with kwashiorkor excreted nearly similar amounts of epinephrine and norepinephrine (ratio: 0.88). In marasmus, norepinephrine may predominate and in kwashiorkor epinephrine may predominate, in the regulation of the metabolic adaptations to assure survival *4271*

17-Hydroxysteroids *Urine* *No Effect* In children with marasmus excretion normal or increased *355*

immunoglobulin A *Saliva* *No Effect* In 10 children with marasmus mean concentration of 4.4 mg/dL increased non-significantly to 5.2 mg/dL with refeeding *5601*
Serum *Increase* In 11 children with marasmus mean concentration significantly increased to 120 mg/dL before refeeding at which time it decreased to 83 mg/dL *5601*
Tears *Decrease* Significant decrease to 21.5 mg/dL in 11 children with marasmus which increased to 38.7 mg/dL with refeeding *5601*

Immunoglobulin G *Serum* *No Effect* In 11 children with marasmus no significant difference in mean concentration before (1,241 mg/dL) and after (1,329 mg/dL) refeeding *5601*
Tears *No Effect* Nonsignificant reduction to 13.2 mg/dL observed in 11 children with marasmus which increased to 23.0 mg/dL with refeeding *5601*

Immunoglobulin M *Serum* *No Effect* In 11 children with marasmus no significant difference in mean concentration before (202 mg/dL) and after (198 mg/dL) refeeding *5601*

Lysozyme *Saliva* *No Effect* Concentration of 0.32 mg/dL in 10 children with marasmus unaffected by refeeding *5601*
Tears *Decrease* In 11 children with marasmus reduction to 80 mg/dL observed in 11 children with marasmus which increased significantly to 168 mg/dL with refeeding *5601*

Ornithine *Plasma* *Decrease* In 20 children with protein energy malnutrition aged 13.5 ± 6.1 months mean concentration of 105 ± 92 µmol/L not significantly different from 190 ± 167 µmol/L after refeeding and 155 ± 105 µmol/L in 10 age-matched controls *3619*

Protein *Serum* *Decrease* In 20 children with protein energy malnutrition aged 13.5 ± 6.1 months mean concentration of 50 ± 5 g/L significantly less than 66 ± 5 g/L after refeeding and of 73 ± 4 g/L in 20 age-matched controls *3619*

Thyroid Stimulating Hormone *Serum* *No Effect* Normal or sometimes decreased concentrations observed *355*

Urea Nitrogen *Serum* *No Effect* In 20 children with protein energy malnutrition aged 13.5 ± 6.1 months mean concentration of 20 ± 7 mg/dL not significantly different from 25 ± 6 mg/dL after refeeding and 21 ± 6 mg/dL in healthy age-matched controls *3619*

264.90 **Vitamin A Deficiency**

Retinol-binding Protein *Serum* *Decrease* Concentration declines in vitamin A deficiency, frequently present in protein-calorie deficiency, and responds quickly when patients given vitamin A *1959*

265.10 **Thiamine Deficiency**

Bicarbonate *Serum* *Decrease* Respiratory alkalosis may occur *1980*

Carbon Dioxide Partial Pressure *Blood* *Decrease* Respiratory alkalosis may occur *1980*

Hematocrit *Blood* *Decrease* Characteristic *2304*

Hemoglobin *Blood* *Decrease* Characteristic *2304*

pH *Blood* *Increase* Respiratory alkalosis may occur *1980*

Protein *Serum* *Decrease* Characteristic *2304*

Pyrophosphate *Serum Increase* Thiamine pyrophosphate is elevated prior to thiamine administration but falls rapidly after therapy *2304*

Pyruvate *Blood Increase* In 16 of 17 untreated cases *5215* Acute advanced beriberi (vitamin B_1 deficiency). Many cases of alcoholic polyneuritis are due to vitamin B_1 deficiency *1290*

Thiamine *Urine Decrease* Urinary excretion of thiamine of 0 - 14 mg in 24 h has been reported in beriberi, and early signs have been observed with excretions of < 40 mg/24 h *367*

266.10 Vitamin B_6 Deficiency

Alanine Aminotransferase *Serum Decrease* More affected than AST *346*

Aspartate Aminotransferase *Serum Decrease* Effect observed at once, less marked then SGPT *346*

Cholesterol *Serum No Effect* No effect observed with 25 d poor diet *346*

Cystathionine *Urine Increase* Direct correlation between increased excretion and decreased diet *163*

Pyridoxal Phosphate *Serum Decrease* No change for 15 d then marked fall *346*

4-Pyridoxic Acid *Urine Decrease* Zero detectable after 25 d deprivation *346*

Pyridoxine *Serum Decrease* 20% control value after 5 d, zero after 25 d *346*
Urine Decrease Marked decrease within few days *346*

Quinolinic Acid *Urine Increase* Observed with experimental dietary deficiency *4428*

266.10 Vitamin B_6 Deficiency Anemia

Acetylcholinesterase *Red Blood Cells Decrease* Megaloblastic anemia may occur during relapse *3141*

Alkaline Phosphatase *White Blood Cells Decrease* Score is reduced in about 50% of the patients *2868*

Anisocytes *Blood Increase* Blood smear shows anisocytosis with many bizarre forms, target cells, hypochromia with pyridoxine-responsive anemia *5544* Prominent findings on blood smear *5699*

Basophilic Stippling *Blood Increase* Prominent findings on blood smear *5699*

Bilirubin *Serum No Effect* Rarely elevated despite the mild hemolytic anemia *900*

Cells *Bone Marrow Increase* Bone marrow is characterized by intense erythroid hyperplasia, often associated with a shift to younger forms, particularly polychromatophilic normoblasts, some of which show megaloblastic nuclear changes *5677*

Erythrocytes *Blood Decrease* Reported to be low in about 80% of patients *900*

Folate *Serum Decrease* Observed effect *5677* Reported to be low in about 80% of patients *3181*

Haptoglobin *Serum Decrease* Decreased in hemoglobinemias (related to the duration and severity of hemolysis) due to extravascular hemolysis *5544*

Hematocrit *Blood Decrease* The anemia is normocytic or slightly macrocytic *5677*

Hemoglobin *Blood Increase* The degree of anemia is variable, ranging from concentrations as low as 5 g/dL, severely affected boys with sex-linked sideroblastic anemia to almost normal levels in the milder cases. Older people with idiopathic or secondary forms of this disease usually have moderate anemias with concentration ranging from 7 - 10 g/dL *900* Anemia may be normocytic or slightly macrocytic *367* Normocytic or slightly macrocytic *5677*

Iron *Bone Marrow Increase* Increased in the marrow fragments and in the developing erythroblasts *367* Bone marrow is hyperplastic and contains increased amounts of normoblastic iron, often forming ringed sideroblasts *5677*
Serum Increase Increased serum iron and reduced iron-binding capacity in > 50% of cases *1098* Increased with pyridoxine-responsive anemia *5544*
Serum No Effect Characteristically normal to elevated *900*

Iron-binding Capacity, Total *Serum Decrease* Normal to low *900* Somewhat decreased with pyridoxine-responsive anemia *5544* Associated increased serum iron and reduced iron-binding capacity in > 50% of cases *1098*
Serum No Effect Binding capacity typically normal to low *900*

Iron Saturation *Serum Increase* Invariably increased saturation *5699*

Leukocytes *Blood Decrease* Count varies from normal to leukopenic levels; when present, leukopenia is accompanied by neutropenia *5677*

MCH *Blood Decrease* Microcytic hypochromic anemia may occur due to blood loss, increased demand, or dietary inadequacy: MCH < 27 pg, MCV < 80 fL *1098*

MCHC *Blood Decrease* Degree of anemia may vary but is usually in the range of 7 - 8 g/dL of hemoglobin, with a lowered MCHC *367*

MCV *Blood Decrease* Microcytic hypochromic anemia may occur due to blood loss, increased demand, or dietary inadequacy: MCH < 27 pg, MCV < 80 fL *1098*

Monocytes *Blood Increase* Morphologically normal, but the proportion may be moderately increased *5677*

Neutrophils *Blood Decrease* Leukopenia is accompanied by neutropenia *5677*

Osmotic Fragility *Red Blood Cells Decrease* Tends to be decreased *5677*

Platelets *Blood Decrease* Usually normal, but thrombocytopenia and thrombocytosis occur in a minority of patients *5677*
Blood Increase Usually normal, but thrombocytopenia and thrombocytosis occur in a minority of patients *5677*
Blood No Effect Usually normal, but thrombocytopenia and thrombocytosis occur in a minority of patients *5677*

Poikilocytes *Blood Increase* Prominent findings on blood smear *5699* Blood smear shows poikilocytosis with many bizarre forms, target cells, hypochromia with pyridoxine-responsive anemia *5544*

Protoporphyrin *Red Blood Cells Increase* Elevated (40 - 300 mg/dL compared to normal levels of 15 - 35 mg/dL) reflecting a functional block to hemoglobin synthesis *900* Almost always moderately increased, and rarely it is markedly so *2868* Marked increase often observed *5677*

Reticulocytes *Blood Decrease* Absolute count is usually reduced *367*
Blood Increase Count is usually normal but may be slightly increased *5677*

Target Cells *Blood Increase* Blood smear shows anisocytosis with many bizarre forms, target cells, hypochromia with pyridoxine-responsive anemia *5544*

Xanthurenic Acid *Urine Increase* Detects pyridoxine (B_6) deficiency *5677* Abnormal tryptophan metabolism indicated by excessive excretion of xanthurenic acid following TRP load has been found in 33% of cases *5699*

266.20 Vitamin B_{12} Deficiency

Cobalamin *Serum No Effect* Concentrations in 15 patients with cobalamin deficiency ranged from 31 - 180 pmol/L not significantly different from that in 44 healthy individuals with mean age 48 years, 261 pmol/L (mean ± 1.96 SD range 32 - 490 pmol/L) *4654*

Homocysteine *Plasma Increase* Concentration increased more than 3 SD above mean in 97.8% of 313 episodes in patients with anemia (mean concentration of 14,663 ± 30,698 nmol/L) and 90.9% of 121 without anemia (mean concentration of 8,599 ± 25,554 nmol/L) *4598* Concentrations in 15 patients with cobalamin deficiency ranged from 28.9 - 144.3 μmol/L significantly higher than mean concentration in 44 healthy individuals with mean age 48 years, 10.9 μmol/L (mean ± 1.96 SD range 3.7 - 18 μmol/L) *4654* Increased concentration observed in patients with abnormal vitamin B_{12} metabolism and deficiency *2952* Of 62 patients with normal histology and Schilling's tests concentration was increased above 13 μmol/L in 15% *3068* Concentrations increased in most patients with cobalamin deficiency with increase most marked when cobalamin concentration decreases below 130 pmol/L *5364*
Urine Increase Increased excretion observed in patients with abnormal vitamin B_{12} metabolism and deficiency *2952*

Macrocytes *Blood Increase* In 75 elderly patients with macrocytosis vitamin B_{12} deficiency was responsible in 15 *3232*

266.20 Vitamin B_{12} Deficiency *(continued)*

MCV *Blood* *Increase* Of 100 patients with macrocytosis (MCV greater than 110 fL) 4 had vitamin B_{12} deficiency *4924*

Methylmalonate *Serum* *Increase* Concentration increased by more than 3 SD above mean in 98.4% of 313 episodes in patients with anemia (mean concentration of 89.4 ± 55.0 μmol/L) and 98.3% of 121 without anemia (significantly lower mean concentration of 60.2 ± 41.3 μmol/L) *4598* Concentrations in 15 patients with cobalamin deficiency ranged from 0.40 - 77.37 μmol/L significantly higher than mean concentration in 44 healthy individuals with mean age 48 years, 0.19 μmol/L (mean ± 1.96 SD range of 0.02 - 0.35 μmol/L) *4654* In patients with low normal vitamin B_{12} concentrations due to vitamin B_{12} deficiency serum methylmalonate is usually > 0.4 μmol/L in the fasting state (normals less than or equal to 0.40 μmol/L) *2952* Of 62 patients with normal histology and Schilling's tests concentration was increased above 0.4 μmol/L in 31% *3068*
Urine *Increase* In patients with low normal vitamin B_{12} concentrations due to vitamin B_{12} deficiency urinary methylmalonate excretion is usually > 3.6 μmol/mol creatinine in the fasting state (normals < 3.60 μmol/mol creatinine) *2952*

Vitamin B_{12} *Serum* *Decrease* Of 62 patients with normal histology and Schilling's tests concentration was decreased below 200 pmol/L in 23% *3068*

267.00 Scurvy

Ascorbic Acid *Serum* *Decrease* Mean concentration less than 6 μmol/L compared with reference interval of 28 - 114 μmol/L *2467*

267.00 Vitamin C Deficiency

Albumin *Serum* *Decrease* Decreased in scurvy *1290*

Alkaline Phosphatase *Serum* *Decrease* Reported effect *3160*

Ascorbic Acid *Serum* *Decrease* Not reliable for diagnostic purposes because tissue levels vary widely. Ascorbic acid assay of the buffy coat for the WBC and platelet count of this vitamin is more helpful, the normal level being 20 - 30 mg/dL. In latent or overt deficiency, this level falls to 0 - 2 mg/dL *900* Plasma level of ascorbic acid is decreased, usually to 0 in frank scurvy. Normal is 0.5 - 1.5 mg/dL but lower level does not prove diagnosis *5545* In 22 individuals with subnormal vitamin C mean concentration of 13.3 ± 4.0 μmol/L compared with reference interval of 28 - 114 μmol/L *2467*
Urine *Decrease* In 22 individuals with subnormal vitamin C mean concentration of 2.80 ± 1.06 μmol/mg creatinine during first week of repletion with 10 mg/d vitamin C *2467*

Bleeding Time *Patient* *No Effect* Usual finding *5544*

Carnitine, Free *Plasma* *Decrease* In 22 individuals with subnormal vitamin C mean concentration of 61.7 ± 15.8 μmol/L during first week of repletion with 10 mg/d vitamin C *2467*
Urine *No Effect* In 22 individuals with subnormal vitamin C mean concentration of 2.87 ± 1.47 μmol/mg creatinine during first week of repletion with 10 mg/d vitamin C *2467*

Cells *Bone Marrow* *Increase* Normoblastic hyperplasia in the bone marrow *5677*

Erythrocytes *Urine* *Increase* Microscopic hematuria is present is 33% of patients with scurvy *5545*

Fibrinogen *Plasma* *Decrease* Moderate depression occurs in scurvy *1290*

Folate *Serum* *Decrease* Decreased *5230 602 772*

Haptoglobin *Serum* *Increase* Conditions associated with increased ESR and α_2-globulin; increases in collagen diseases *5544*

Hematocrit *Blood* *Decrease* Associated with anemia of normocytic, macrocytic, or hypochromic variety in about 80% of cases *5677*

Hemoglobin *Blood* *Decrease* Associated with anemia of normocytic, macrocytic, or hypochromic variety in about 80% of cases *5677*

Histamine *Blood* *Increase* In 22 individuals with subnormal vitamin C mean concentration of 667 ± 171 μmol/L during first week of repletion with 10 mg/d vitamin C *2467*

Iron *Serum* *Decrease* Dietary iron deficiency is common *5677*

Iron-binding Capacity, Total *Serum* *Decrease* In scurvy *1290*

MCH *Blood* *Decrease* Associated with anemia of normocytic, macrocytic, or hypochromic variety in about 80% of cases *5677*

MCHC *Blood* *Decrease* Associated with anemia of normocytic, macrocytic, or hypochromic variety in about 80% of cases *5677*

MCV *Blood* *Increase* Associated with anemia of normocytic, macrocytic, or hypochromic variety in about 80% of cases *5677*

Occult Blood *Feces* *Increase* May be positive in scurvy *5545*

Reticulocytes *Blood* *Increase* Normocytic, normochromic anemia with a reticulocytosis of 5 - 10% *5677*

268.00 Rickets

Calcium *Serum* *Decrease* Decreased concentrations are seen in rickets *2952*

268.00 Vitamin D Deficiency

Ammonium Ions *Urine* *Increase* May lead to proximal renal tubular acidosis which is associated with hypokalemia, hyperchloremic metabolic acidosis, urine pH < 5.5, increased urinary ammonium ion excretion, a negative urine anion gap, increased urinary osmol gap, normal urinary citrate, normal urinary calcium excretion and Fanconi syndrome *4071*

Anion Gap *Urine* *Decrease* May lead to proximal renal tubular acidosis which is associated with hypokalemia, hyperchloremic metabolic acidosis, urine pH < 5.5, increased urinary ammonium ion excretion, a negative urine anion gap, increased urinary osmol gap, normal urinary citrate, normal urinary calcium excretion and Fanconi syndrome *4071*

Bicarbonate *Serum* *Decrease* May lead to proximal renal tubular acidosis which is associated with hypokalemia, hyperchloremic metabolic acidosis, urine pH < 5.5, increased urinary ammonium ion excretion, a negative urine anion gap, increased urinary osmol gap, normal urinary citrate, normal urinary calcium excretion and Fanconi syndrome *4071*

Calcium *Urine* *No Effect* May lead to proximal renal tubular acidosis which is associated with hypokalemia, hyperchloremic metabolic acidosis, urine pH < 5.5, increased urinary ammonium ion excretion, a negative urine anion gap, increased urinary osmol gap, normal urinary citrate, normal urinary calcium excretion and Fanconi syndrome *4071*

Chloride *Serum* *Increase* May lead to proximal renal tubular acidosis which is associated with hypokalemia, hyperchloremic metabolic acidosis, urine pH < 5.5, increased urinary ammonium ion excretion, a negative urine anion gap, increased urinary osmol gap, normal urinary citrate, normal urinary calcium excretion and Fanconi syndrome *4071*

Citrate *Urine* *No Effect* May lead to proximal renal tubular acidosis which is associated with hypokalemia, hyperchloremic metabolic acidosis, urine pH < 5.5, increased urinary ammonium ion excretion, a negative urine anion gap, increased urinary osmol gap, normal urinary citrate, normal urinary calcium excretion and Fanconi syndrome *4071*

Glucose *Urine* *Increase* May lead to proximal renal tubular acidosis which is associated with hypokalemia, hyperchloremic metabolic acidosis, urine pH < 5.5, increased urinary ammonium ion excretion, a negative urine anion gap, increased urinary osmol gap, normal urinary citrate, normal urinary calcium excretion and Fanconi syndrome *4071*

Hydroxylysylpyridinoline *Urine* *Increase* In 36 elderly patients with secondary hyperparathyroidism and vitamin D deficiency mean concentration of 109.5 ± 50.7 nmol/mmol creatinine significantly higher than that in 30 healthy men (mean excretion of 32.3 ± 9.4 nmol/mmol creatinine) and 37.6 ± 6.8 nmol/mmol creatinine in 14 healthy women *2541*

Lysylpyridinoline *Urine* *Increase* In 36 elderly patients with secondary hyperparathyroidism and vitamin D deficiency mean concentration of 17.4 ± 7.6 nmol/mmol creatinine significantly higher than that in 30 healthy men (mean excretion of 5.6 ± 2.0 nmol/mmol creatinine) and 6.0 ± 1.4 nmol/mmol creatinine in 14 healthy women *2541*

Osmolal Gap *Urine* *Increase* May lead to proximal renal tubular acidosis which is associated with hypokalemia, hyperchloremic metabolic acidosis, urine pH < 5.5, increased urinary ammonium ion excretion, a negative urine anion gap, increased urinary osmol gap, normal urinary citrate, normal urinary calcium excretion and Fanconi syndrome *4071*

Osteocalcin *Serum* *Decrease* In 65 patients with biochemical vitamin D deficiency mean concentration of 18 ± 8 µg/L (3.1 nmol/L) significantly different from that in healthy adults (men 25 ± 5 µg/L, women 20 ± 6 µg/L) *541*

pH *Urine* *Decrease* May lead to proximal renal tubular acidosis which is associated with hypokalemia, hyperchloremic metabolic acidosis, urine pH < 5.5, increased urinary ammonium ion excretion, a negative urine anion gap, increased urinary osmol gap, normal urinary citrate, normal urinary calcium excretion and Fanconi syndrome *4071*

Phosphate *Serum* *Decrease* May lead to proximal renal tubular acidosis which is associated with hypokalemia, hyperchloremic metabolic acidosis, urine pH < 5.5, increased urinary ammonium ion excretion, a negative urine anion gap, increased urinary osmol gap, normal urinary citrate, normal urinary calcium excretion and Fanconi syndrome *4071*

Potassium *Serum* *Decrease* May lead to proximal renal tubular acidosis which is associated with hypokalemia, hyperchloremic metabolic acidosis, urine pH < 5.5, increased urinary ammonium ion excretion, a negative urine anion gap, increased urinary osmol gap, normal urinary citrate, normal urinary calcium excretion and Fanconi syndrome *4071*

Pyridinoline *Urine* *Increase* In 36 elderly patients with secondary hyperparathyroidism and vitamin D deficiency mean concentration of 102.9 ± 63.4 nmol/mmol creatinine significantly higher than that in 30 healthy men (mean excretion 30.4 ± 8.6 nmol/mmol creatinine) and 37.7 ± 7.3 nmol/mmol creatinine in 14 healthy women *2541*

Uric Acid *Serum* *Decrease* May lead to proximal renal tubular acidosis which is associated with hypokalemia, hyperchloremic metabolic acidosis, urine pH < 5.5, increased urinary ammonium ion excretion, a negative urine anion gap, increased urinary osmol gap, normal urinary citrate, normal urinary calcium excretion and Fanconi syndrome *4071*

268.20 Oncogenic Osteomalacia

Phosphate *Serum* *Decrease* Oncogenic osteomalacia is less common cause of hypophosphatemia due to increased renal loss of phosphate *969*

268.20 Osteomalacia

Acid Phosphatase, Tartrate Resistant *Serum* *Increase* In patients with osteomalacia marked increase observed *4217*

Alkaline Phosphatase *Serum* *Increase* Typically *4891* Persistently raised concentration despite evident relief of symptoms *916* In adults this test represents the single most sensitive indicator of active disease. The earliest biochemical alteration *5544*

Alkaline Phosphatase, Bone Isoenzyme *Serum* *Increase* In patients with osteomalacia and rickets moderate increase observed *4217* Mean activity of 61.7 U/L in 20 patients with primary hyperparathyroidism significantly different from reference intervals of 15.0 - 41.3 U/L in men and 11.6 - 30.6 U/L in premenopausal women *1799*

Amino Acids *Urine* *Increase* Aminoaciduria secondary to PTH excess is seen *2039*

Calcium *Serum* *Decrease* Advanced and sustained vitamin D deficiency. Renal tubular acidosis, hypophosphatasia, and dietary deficiency or a failure of absorption of calcium and vitamin D as well as other causes of increased loss of calcium must be considered in patients with osteomalacia *5544* *1025* Advanced disease *4891*

Serum *No Effect* In early stages, stimulation of skeletal mobilization of calcium compensates for the high renal loss or the low intestinal absorption. Serum concentration is therefore normal or low normal *4891*

Urine *Increase* Other factors than vitamin D in adults *1025*

Deoxypyridinoline, Free *Urine* *Increase* In 21 patients with osteomalacia mean excretion of 12.4 ± 8.5 µmol/mol creatinine significantly different from 1.7 - 5.9 µmol/mol creatinine in healthy men and 3.1 - 8.1 µmol/mol creatinine in healthy women when measured by CLIA technique *4427*

Glucose *Urine* *Increase* Reflects variable degree of disturbance of proximal tubular function *2034*

25-Hydroxy Vitamin D_3 *Serum* *Decrease* Vitamin D deficiency *2034*

Hydroxyproline *Urine* *Increase* Increased formation of osteoid tissue results in hydroxyprolinuria, values will decrease with adequate therapy with vitamin D *1980*

Osteocalcin *Serum* *Increase* Increased in patients with various bone diseases characterized by increased osteoblastic activity *4219* In patients with osteomalacia and rickets slight increase observed *4217*

pH *Blood* *Decrease* In systemic acidosis *2034*

Phosphate *Serum* *Decrease* Osteomalacia resulting from PO_3 or Ca deficiencies may be associated with moderate hypophosphatemia *2719* Invariably low. May be the only demonstrable abnormality *367*

Uric Acid *Urine* *Increase* Reflects variable degree of disturbance of proximal tubular function *2034*

268.30 Molybdenum Cofactor Deficiency

Chitotriosidase *Serum* *No Effect* Normal activity observed in one patient with condition *1917*

269.00 Vitamin K Deficiency

Factor VII *Plasma* *Decrease* Synthesized in the liver by a process that requires vitamin K *2033*

Factor IX *Plasma* *Decrease* Synthesized in the liver by a process that requires vitamin K *2033*

Factor X *Plasma* *Decrease* Synthesized in the liver by a process that requires vitamin K *2033*

269.30 Iodine Deficiency

Iodine *Urine* *Decrease* In 95 specimens from iodine deficient area of Ukraine mean excretion of 0.12 - 1.28 µmol/L compared with 1.09 - 46.60 µmol/L in 84 specimens from an iodine-rich area of Japan *5307* Excretions of less than 100 µg/24 h suggest dietary iodine deficiency *2952*

269.30 Zinc Deficiency

Alkaline Phosphatase *Serum* *Decrease* Reported effect *3160*

Zinc *Serum* *Decrease* Mean concentration in patients with zinc deficiency significantly reduced *3696*

269.80 Biotinidase Deficiency

Biotinidase *Serum* *Decrease* Most values below 3.5 U/L suggest biotinidase deficiency *2952*

269.80 Carnitine Deficiency

Carnitine *Serum* *Decrease* Reduced concentrations observed in patients with primary systemic carnitine deficiency *2952*

269.80 Multiple Sulfatase Deficiency

Lysosome-associated Membrane Protein-2 *Serum* *Increase* Concentration of 1.55 mg/L in 1 patient with multiple sulfatase deficiency with age 5 y compared with 1.21 mg/L in 202 healthy controls aged 0 - 66 y (median 7 years) *2265*

Lysosome-associated Membrane Protein-2:Lysosome-associated Membrane Protein-1 Ratio *Serum* *No Effect* Mean ratio of 3.47 in 3 patients with multiple sulfatase deficiency with aged 5 y not significantly different when compared with 4.74 in 202 healthy controls aged 0 - 66 y (median 7 years) *2265*

269.80 Steroid Sulfatase Deficiency

β-Glucuronidase *Mononuclear Cells* *No Effect* In 7 heterozygotes mean activity of 22.4 ± 6.4 nmol methyl umbelliferone/1 x 10^6 cells/h compared with activities in 86 normal women and 92 normal men of 21.4 ± 4.0 and 26.6 ± 5.0 nmol methyl umbelliferone/1 x 10^6 cells/h, respectively *3143*
White Blood Cells *No Effect* In 13 heterozygotes mean activity of 18.0 ± 3.5 nmol methyl umbelliferone/1 x 10^6 cells/h compared with activities in 100 normal women and 100 normal men of 19.86 ± 5.08 and 22.03 ± 5.14 nmol methyl umbelliferone/1 x 10^6 cells/h, respectively *3143*

17α-Hydroxyprogesterone *Saliva* *Increase* In steroid C_{21}-deficiency concentration of 26,300 pmol/L reported compared with maximum prepubertal concentration of 490 pmol/L *5155*

Steroid Sulfatase *Mononuclear Cells* *Decrease* In 7 heterozygotes mean activity of 4.34 ± 1.86 fmol DHA/pmol $DHASO_4$/1 x 10^6 cells/h compared with activities in 86 normal women and 92 normal men of 6.63 ± 2.24 and 5.2 ± 1.93 fmol DHA/pmol $DHASO_4$/1 x 10^6 cells/h, respectively *3143*
White Blood Cells *Decrease* In 18 heterozygotes mean activity of 2.63 ± 0.98 and 0.15 ± 0 0.8 fmol DHA/pmol $DHASO_4$/1 x 10^6 cells/h in 11 deficient individuals compared with activities in 100 normal women and 100 normal men of 5.98 ± 1.57 and 4.89 ± 1.45 fmol DHA/pmol $DHASO_4$/1 x 10^6 cells/h, respectively *3143*

269.80 Tyrosine Hydroxylase Deficiency

Biopterin *Cerebrospinal Fluid* *No Effect* Concentrations in 4 patients within reference interval *614*
Urine *No Effect* Concentrations in 4 patients within reference interval *614*

Biopterin:Neopterin Ratio *Cerebrospinal Fluid* *No Effect* Ratio in 4 patients within reference interval *614*
Urine *No Effect* Ratio in 4 patients within reference interval *614*

Dopamine *Urine* *Decrease* Excretion in 1 patient of 14 nmol/mmol creatinine significantly less than the reference interval 70 - 825 nmol/mmol creatinine *614*
Urine *No Effect* Excretions in 3 patients of 70, 195 and 293 nmol/mmol creatinine within the respective reference intervals of 50 - 700, 70 - 795 and 70 - 825 nmol/mmol creatinine *614*

Epinephrine *Urine* *Increase* Excretion in 1 patient of 50.9 nmol/mmol creatinine significantly greater than the reference interval 1 - 20 nmol/mmol creatinine *614*
Urine *No Effect* Excretions in 3 patients of 21.2, 4.5 and 10.6 nmol/mmol creatinine within the reference interval 1.5 - 30 nmol/mmol creatinine *614*

Epinephrine:Norepinephrine Ratio *Urine* *Increase* Excretion ratios in 4 patients of 5.4, 1.6, 1.2 and 1.0 greater than the reference value of < 1.0 *614*

Homovanillic Acid *Cerebrospinal Fluid* *Decrease* Concentrations in 4 patients of 117, 111, 76 and 31 nmol/L, significantly less than 2.5 percentile of 384 nmol/L *614*
Urine *Decrease* Excretions in 2 patients of 2.5 and 4.1 μmol/mmol creatinine significantly less than the reference interval of 5 - 15 μmol/mmol creatinine and in two other affected children with excretions of 1.4 and 5.3 μmol/mmol creatinine, one within reference interval of 2 - 10 μmol/mmol creatinine and the other below *614*

Homovanillic Acid:5-Hydroxyindoleacetic Acid Ratio *Cerebrospinal Fluid* *Decrease* Ratios in 4 patients of 0.77, 0.48, 0.28 and 0.13, significantly less than 2.5 percentile of 1.8 *614*

4-Hydroxy-3-Methoxy-Phenylglycol *Cerebrospinal Fluid* *Decrease* Concentrations in 4 patients of 13, 6, 12 and 2 nmol/L, all below the 2.5 percentile of 35 nmol/L *614*

5-Hydroxyindoleacetic Acid *Cerebrospinal Fluid* *Increase* Concentrations in 4 patients of 151, 233, 268 and 234 nmol/L, all above the 2.5 percentile of 110 nmol/L *614*
Urine *No Effect* Excretions in 2 patients of 4.1 and 7.5 μmol/mmol creatinine within the reference interval of 3 - 12 μmol/mmol creatinine and in two other affected children with excretions of 3.4 and 10.0 μmol/mmol creatinine also within reference interval of 1 - 10 μmol/mmol creatinine *614*

Neopterin *Cerebrospinal Fluid* *No Effect* Concentrations in 4 patients within reference interval *614*
Urine *No Effect* Concentrations in 4 patients within reference interval *614*

Norepinephrine *Urine* *Decrease* Excretion in 1 patient of 3.8 nmol/mmol creatinine below the reference interval of 7 - 85 nmol/mmol creatinine *614*
Urine *No Effect* Excretions in 3 patients of 9.5, 13.5 and 10.6 nmol/mmol creatinine within the respective reference intervals of 8 - 70, 10 - 100 and 7 - 85 nmol/mmol creatinine *614*

Phenylalanine *Cerebrospinal Fluid* *No Effect* Concentrations in 4 patients with tyrosine hydroxylase deficiency within the reference interval *614*
Plasma *No Effect* Concentrations in 4 patients with tyrosine hydroxylase deficiency within the reference interval *614*
Urine *No Effect* Concentrations in 4 patients with tyrosine hydroxylase deficiency within the reference interval *614*

Tyrosine *Cerebrospinal Fluid* *No Effect* Concentrations in 4 patients of 14, 13, 10 and 12 μmol/L, all within reference interval of 6 - 19 μmol/L *614* Concentrations in 4 patients with tyrosine hydroxylase deficiency within the reference interval *614*
Plasma *No Effect* Concentrations in 4 patients within reference interval *614*
Urine *No Effect* Concentrations in 4 patients within reference interval *614*

Vanillylactic Acid *Cerebrospinal Fluid* *No Effect* Concentrations in 4 patients within the reference interval *614*

Vanillylmandelic Acid *Urine* *Decrease* Excretions in 2 patients of 1.1 and 1.2 μmol/mmol creatinine below the reference interval of 2 - 15 μmol/mmol creatinine and in two other affected children with excretions of 1.0 and 1.2 μmol/mmol creatinine also below reference interval of 2 - 10 μmol/mmol creatinine *614*

269.90 Deficiency State (Unspecified)

Albumin *Serum* *Decrease* Serum concentration falls before other indicators change *1290*

Alkaline Phosphatase *Serum* *Decrease* Decreased in malnutrition *5544*

Cholinesterase *Serum* *Decrease* Low in malnourished patients (from starvation, anorexia, or debilitating disease) reflecting protein depletion and hepatic function impairment. The rise to normal levels parallels nutritional improvement and weight gain *5498*

MCV *Blood* *Increase* Macrocytic anemia may occur due to vitamin B_{12} or folate deficiency. MCV > 100 fL *1098*

N-Formiminoglutamic Acid *Urine* *Increase* Some patients *5544*

Xylose Tolerance Test *Urine* *No Effect* Typical observation *5544*

269.90 Glutathione Synthetase Deficiency

5-Oxoproline *Red Blood Cells* *Decrease* Mean values of approximately 0.51, 0.43 and 0.29 mmol/L in 3 patients with glutathione synthetase deficiency significantly decreased compared with 2.36 ± 0.37 mmol/L in 100 healthy controls *3384*
Urine *Increase* Mean values of approximately 6,230, 3,315 and 5,010 mmol/mol creatinine in 3 patients with glutathione synthetase deficiency significantly increased compared with < 50 mmol/mol creatinine in 100 healthy controls *3384*

269.90 Hypothyroxine-binding Globulinemia

Thyroxine Binding Globulin *Serum* *Decrease* Observed as consequence of natural deficiency of thyroxine binding globulin occurring in approximately 1 in 9,000 individuals *206*

Thyroxine (T4) *Serum* *Decrease* Observed as consequence of natural deficiency of thyroxine binding globulin occurring in approximately 1 in 9,000 individuals *206*

269.90 Lipoamide Deficiency

Acetoacetate *Serum* *Increase* In one Ashkenazi-Jewish patient concentration on admission to hospital increased to 0.28 mmol/L significantly higher than reference interval of 0.02 - 0.15 mmol/L *1345*

Alanine Aminotransferase *Serum* *Increase* In one Ashkenazi-Jewish patient activity increased on admission to hospital to 757 U/L significantly higher than reference interval of 5 - 50 U/L *1345*

Amino Acids, Branched-chain *Plasma* *Increase* In one Ashkenazi-Jewish patient concentration on admission to hospital increased 1.5 - 2.5 times the upper limit of normal *1345*

Aspartate Aminotransferase *Serum* *Increase* In one Ashkenazi-Jewish patient activity increased to 400 U/L significantly higher than reference interval of 7 - 56 U/L *1345*

Carbon Dioxide Partial Pressure *Blood* *Decrease* In one Ashkenazi-Jewish patient decreased with metabolic acidosis to 14 mm Hg *1345*

Carnitine *Serum* *Increase* In one Ashkenazi-Jewish patient concentration on admission to hospital increased to 167 µmol/L significantly higher than reference interval of 30 - 60 µmol/L *1345*

Creatine Kinase *Serum* *Increase* In one Ashkenazi-Jewish patient activity on admission to hospital increased to 11,277 U/L significantly higher than reference interval of 30 - 150 U/L *1345*

β-Hydroxybutyrate *Serum* *Increase* In one Ashkenazi-Jewish patient concentration on admission to hospital increased to 2.77 mmol/L significantly higher than reference interval of 0.05 - 0.2 mmol/L *1345*

Lactate *Plasma* *Increase* In one Ashkenazi-Jewish patient concentration on admission to hospital increased to 29.7 mmol/L significantly higher than reference interval of 0.9 - 2.1 mmol/L *1345*

Myoglobin *Urine* *Increase* In one Ashkenazi-Jewish patient recurrent myoglobinuria observed *1345*

pH *Blood* *Decrease* In one Ashkenazi-Jewish patient decreased with metabolic acidosis to 6.8 *1345*

Prothrombin Time *Plasma* *Increase* In one Ashkenazi-Jewish patient on admission to hospital prothrombin time increased *1345*

269.90 Lipoprotein Lipase Deficiency

Lipoprotein Lp(a) *Serum* *Decrease* Patients with condition have extremely low concentrations of Lp(a) *2827*

269.90 5-Oxoprolinase Deficiency

5-Oxoproline *Red Blood Cells* *Increase* Value of 3.12 mmol/L in a patient with 5-oxoprolinase deficiency significantly increased compared with 2.36 ± 0.37 mmol/L in 100 healthy controls *3384*
Urine *Increase* Values of 1,980 - 6,040 mmol/mol creatinine in a patient with 5-oxoprolinase deficiency significantly increased compared with < 50 mmol/mol creatinine in 100 healthy controls *3384*

Disorders of Amino Acid Transport and Metabolism

270.00 Cystinosis

Alanine *Urine* *Increase* Nonspecific pattern of aminoaciduria with Fanconi's syndrome *2034*

Alkaline Phosphatase *Serum* *Increase* With the appearance of rickets *4979*

Amino Acids *Urine* *Increase* Aminoaciduria with increased cystine *1290* May be masked by severely reduced GFR, so that total urinary amino acids are in the normal range *4979*
Urine *No Effect* Aminoaciduria with increased cystine *1290* May be masked by severely reduced GFR, so that total urinary amino acids are in the normal range *4979*

Ammonia *Urine* *Increase* Increased ammonium ion *4979*

Ammonium Ions *Urine* *Increase* May lead to proximal renal tubular acidosis which is associated with hypokalemia, hyperchloremic metabolic acidosis, urine pH < 5.5, increased urinary ammonium ion excretion, a negative urine anion gap, increased urinary osmol gap, normal urinary citrate, normal urinary calcium excretion and Fanconi syndrome *4071*

Anion Gap *Urine* *Decrease* May lead to proximal renal tubular acidosis which is associated with hypokalemia, hyperchloremic metabolic acidosis, urine pH < 5.5, increased urinary ammonium ion excretion, a negative urine anion gap, increased urinary osmol gap, normal urinary citrate, normal urinary calcium excretion and Fanconi syndrome *4071*

Arginine *Urine* *Increase* Nonspecific pattern of aminoaciduria with Fanconi's syndrome *2034*

Asparagine *Urine* *Increase* Nonspecific pattern of aminoaciduria with Fanconi's syndrome *2034*

Bicarbonate *Serum* *Decrease* Metabolic, hyperchloremic acidosis *900* May lead to proximal renal tubular acidosis which is associated with hypokalemia, hyperchloremic metabolic acidosis, urine pH < 5.5, increased urinary ammonium ion excretion, a negative urine anion gap, increased urinary osmol gap, normal urinary citrate, normal urinary calcium excretion and Fanconi syndrome *4071* Reflects renal bicarbonate loss *4979*

Calcium *Serum* *Decrease* Hypocalcemic, hypophosphatemic rickets resistant to the usual doses of vitamin D *900*
Urine *Increase* Secondary from acidosis *2034*
Urine *No Effect* May lead to proximal renal tubular acidosis which is associated with hypokalemia, hyperchloremic metabolic acidosis, urine pH < 5.5, increased urinary ammonium ion excretion, a negative urine anion gap, increased urinary osmol gap, normal urinary citrate, normal urinary calcium excretion and Fanconi syndrome *4071*

Chloride *Serum* *Increase* May lead to proximal renal tubular acidosis which is associated with hypokalemia, hyperchloremic metabolic acidosis, urine pH < 5.5, increased urinary ammonium ion excretion, a negative urine anion gap, increased urinary osmol gap, normal urinary citrate, normal urinary calcium excretion and Fanconi syndrome *4071* Metabolic, hyperchloremic acidosis *900*

Citrate *Urine* *No Effect* May lead to proximal renal tubular acidosis which is associated with hypokalemia, hyperchloremic metabolic acidosis, urine pH < 5.5, increased urinary ammonium ion excretion, a negative urine anion gap, increased urinary osmol gap, normal urinary citrate, normal urinary calcium excretion and Fanconi syndrome *4071*

Creatinine *Serum* *Increase* Elevated with advanced renal disease as early as 2 y of age in some patients *4979*

Cystathionine *Urine* *Increase* Nonspecific pattern of aminoaciduria with Fanconi's syndrome *2034*

Cysteine *Urine* *Increase* Nonspecific pattern of aminoaciduria with Fanconi's syndrome *2034*

Cystine *Urine* *Increase* Nonspecific pattern of aminoaciduria with Fanconi's syndrome *2034* Generally increased in the same proportion as other amino acids *4979*

Erythrocyte Sedimentation Rate *Blood* *Increase* Usually *4979*

Erythrocytes *Urine* *Increase* As glomerular damage progresses *4979*

270.00 Cystinosis *(continued)*

γ-Globulin *Urine Increase* Over 50 times the normal excretion of light chain γ-globulin *5531*

Glomerular Filtration Rate *Urine Decrease* Diminishes with advancing renal disease *4979*

Glucose *Serum No Effect* In most cases concentration unaffected *2034*
Urine Increase May be scanty and intermittent or profuse and constant *2034* May lead to proximal renal tubular acidosis which is associated with hypokalemia, hyperchloremic metabolic acidosis, urine pH < 5.5, increased urinary ammonium ion excretion, a negative urine anion gap, increased urinary osmol gap, normal urinary citrate, normal urinary calcium excretion and Fanconi syndrome *4071* Up to 5 g/dL *4979*

Glutamic Acid *Urine Increase* Nonspecific pattern of aminoaciduria with Fanconi's syndrome *2034*

Granular Casts *Urine Increase* As glomerular damage progresses *4979*

Growth Hormone *Plasma No Effect* Growth failure is characteristic even though growth hormone concentrations are normal *4979*

Hematocrit *Blood Decrease* Often significant anemia before renal failure is substantial *4979*

Hemoglobin *Blood Decrease* Often significant anemia before renal failure is substantial *4979*

Histidine *Urine Increase* Nonspecific pattern of aminoaciduria with Fanconi's syndrome *2034*

Homocystine *Urine Increase* Nonspecific pattern of aminoaciduria with Fanconi's syndrome *2034*

Hydroxyproline *Urine Increase* Nonspecific pattern of aminoaciduria with Fanconi's syndrome *2034*

Isoleucine *Urine Increase* Nonspecific pattern of aminoaciduria with Fanconi's syndrome *2034*

Leucine *Urine Increase* Nonspecific pattern of aminoaciduria with Fanconi's syndrome *2034*

Lysine *Urine Increase* Nonspecific pattern of aminoaciduria with Fanconi's syndrome *2034*

Methionine *Urine Increase* Nonspecific pattern of aminoaciduria with Fanconi's syndrome *2034*

Ornithine *Urine Increase* Nonspecific pattern of aminoaciduria with Fanconi's syndrome *2034*

Osmolal Gap *Urine Increase* May lead to proximal renal tubular acidosis which is associated with hypokalemia, hyperchloremic metabolic acidosis, urine pH < 5.5, increased urinary ammonium ion excretion, a negative urine anion gap, increased urinary osmol gap, normal urinary citrate, normal urinary calcium excretion and Fanconi syndrome *4071*

pH *Blood Decrease* Marked acidosis *4979* Metabolic, hyperchloremic acidosis *900*
Urine Decrease May lead to proximal renal tubular acidosis which is associated with hypokalemia, hyperchloremic metabolic acidosis, urine pH < 5.5, increased urinary ammonium ion excretion, a negative urine anion gap, increased urinary osmol gap, normal urinary citrate, normal urinary calcium excretion and Fanconi syndrome *4071*
Urine Increase Tends to remain alkaline despite systemic acidosis *4979*

Phenylalanine *Urine Increase* Nonspecific pattern of aminoaciduria with Fanconi's syndrome *2034*

Phosphate *Feces Increase* Decreased intestinal absorption *444*
Serum Decrease May lead to proximal renal tubular acidosis which is associated with hypokalemia, hyperchloremic metabolic acidosis, urine pH < 5.5, increased urinary ammonium ion excretion, a negative urine anion gap, increased urinary osmol gap, normal urinary citrate, normal urinary calcium excretion and Fanconi syndrome *4071* Decreased serum concentrations will become normal and then elevated as renal deterioration progress *4979*
Serum Increase Decreased serum concentrations will become normal and then elevated as renal deterioration progress *4979*
Urine Increase Usually increased excretion before renal disease is advanced *2031* Failure of tubular reabsorption *2034*

Potassium *Serum Decrease* Hypokalemia and severe intracellular potassium depletion can be most difficult problems, causing severe muscle weakness *900* Decreased serum concentrations will become normal and then elevated as renal deterioration progress *4979* May lead to proximal renal tubular acidosis which is associated with hypokalemia, hyperchloremic metabolic acidosis, urine pH < 5.5, increased urinary ammonium ion excretion, a negative urine anion gap, increased urinary osmol gap, normal urinary citrate, normal urinary calcium excretion and Fanconi syndrome *4071* Due to high urine potassium *5545*
Serum Increase Decreased serum concentrations will become normal and then elevated as renal deterioration progress *4979*

Proline *Urine Increase* Nonspecific pattern of aminoaciduria with Fanconi's syndrome *2034*

Protein *Urine Increase* Frequent *4979*

Pyruvate *Blood Increase* In some but not all patients *4979*

Serine *Urine Increase* Nonspecific pattern of aminoaciduria with Fanconi's syndrome *2034*

Threonine *Urine Increase* Nonspecific pattern of aminoaciduria with Fanconi's syndrome *2034*

Tryptophan *Urine Increase* Nonspecific pattern of aminoaciduria with Fanconi's syndrome *2034*

Tyrosine *Urine Increase* Nonspecific pattern of aminoaciduria with Fanconi's syndrome *2034*

Urea Nitrogen *Serum Increase* Elevated with advanced renal disease as early as 2 y of age in some patients *4979*

Uric Acid *Serum Decrease* May lead to proximal renal tubular acidosis which is associated with hypokalemia, hyperchloremic metabolic acidosis, urine pH < 5.5, increased urinary ammonium ion excretion, a negative urine anion gap, increased urinary osmol gap, normal urinary citrate, normal urinary calcium excretion and Fanconi syndrome *4071* Failure of reabsorption *2034*
Urine Increase Failure of reabsorption *2034*

Valine *Urine Increase* Nonspecific pattern of aminoaciduria with Fanconi's syndrome *2034*

270.00 Cystinuria

Amino Acids *Urine Increase* Cystine, lysine, arginine, and ornithine are increased in urine *1290*

Arginine *Urine Increase* Characteristic *4979*

Cystathionine *Urine Increase* Has been reported *4979* *1581*

Cystine *Urine Increase* Characteristic *4979* Increased (20 - 30 times normal) with cystinuria *5545*

Lysine *Urine Increase* Characteristic *4979*

Methionine *Urine Increase* Has been reported *4979* *2688*

Occult Blood *Urine Increase* Reported effect *2034*

Ornithine *Urine Increase* Characteristic *4979*

270.00 Fanconi Syndrome

Carnitine *Serum Decrease* Reduced concentrations observed in patients with secondary carnitine deficiency which may be associated with some forms of renal Fanconi syndrome *2952*

270.00 Hartnup Disease

Alanine *Urine Increase* 5 - 20 times normal values *4979*

Amino Acids *Feces Increase* Closely mirrors the pattern in urine *4979*
Plasma Decrease Reduced about 30% due to increased excretion and reduced absorption *4979*
Saliva No Effect Concentrations usually normal *4979*
Sweat No Effect Concentrations usually normal *4979*
Urine Increase Aminoaciduria is the single most important diagnostic finding; it is constantly present, even between episodes of symptoms. An increased urinary excretion of the monoamino-monocarboxylic amino acids with neutral or aromatic side chains, i.e., alanine, serine, threonine, valine, leucine, isoleucine, phenylalanine, tyrosine, histidine, asparagine, glutamine, and tryptophan is characteristic *900* Usually at least a 10-fold increase *4979*

Asparagine *Urine* *Increase* 5 - 20 times normal values *4979*

Citrulline *Urine* *Increase* 5 - 20 times normal values *4979*

Glutamine *Urine* *Increase* Urine chromatography shows greatly increased amount of glutamine *5545* 5 - 20 times normal values *4979*

Glycine *Urine* *Increase* 5 - 20 times normal values *4979*
Urine *No Effect* No significant effect observed *1304*

Histidine *Urine* *Increase* 5 - 20 times normal values *4979*

5-Hydroxyindoleacetic Acid *Urine* *Decrease* Low; may represent a slight diversion of tryptophan from serotonin formation *4979*

5-Hydroxytryptamine *Blood* *Decrease* Low; may represent a slight diversion of tryptophan from serotonin formation *4979*

Indican *Urine* *Increase* Large, but variable amounts excreted, almost entirely as indoxyl sulfate *4979*

Indoleacetic Acid *Urine* *Increase* Urine chromatography shows greatly increased amounts *5545* Almost all patients have an elevated excretion of indolic acids on some occasion *4979*

Isoleucine *Urine* *Increase* 5 - 20 times normal values *4979*

Leucine *Urine* *Increase* 5 - 20 times normal values observed *4979* Considerable increase observed *2034*

Nicotinamide *Serum* *Decrease* From loss of precursor tryptophan *2034*

Phenylalanine *Urine* *Increase* 5 - 20 times normal values *4979*

Porphyrin, Total *Feces* *No Effect* Excretion usually normal *4979*
Urine *No Effect* Excretion usually normal *4979*

Serine *Urine* *Increase* 5 - 20 times normal values *4979* Reported effect *2034*

Threonine *Urine* *Increase* 5 - 20 times normal values *4979*

Tryptophan *Plasma* *Decrease* Reduced blood levels of tryptophan metabolites *367*
Urine *Increase* 5 - 20 times normal values *4979* Urine chromatography shows greatly increased amount *5545*

Tyrosine *Urine* *Increase* 5 - 20 times normal values *4979*

Uric Acid *Serum* *Decrease* There is possibly a congenital tubular defect resulting in decreased reabsorption *1290*

Valine *Urine* *Increase* 5 - 20 times normal values *4979*

270.10 Atypical Phenylketonuria

Biopterin *Serum* *Decrease* Pyruvoyl-tetrahydropterin synthase deficiency is associated with decreased concentrations *121*
Serum *Increase* Dihydropteridine reductase deficiency is associated with markedly increased concentrations *121*

Dihydrobiopterin *Serum* *Increase* Dihydropteridine reductase deficiency is associated with markedly increased concentrations *121*

Neopterin *Serum* *Increase* Pyruvoyl-tetrahydropterin synthase deficiency is associated with increased concentrations *121*

270.10 Phenylketonuria

Amino Acids *Plasma* *Increase* Phenylalanine is increased *1290*
Urine *Increase* Phenylalanine and ketoderivatives are increased *1290*

Carnitine *Serum* *Decrease* Although total, free and esterified carnitine blood levels were found to be low (less than 0.001) in these patients under dietary treatment compared to controls, no clinical signs of deficiency were noticed *4678*

5-Hydroxyindoleacetic Acid *Urine* *Decrease* Observed effect *5545*

Molybdenum *Serum* *No Effect* In 15 children with phenylketonuria mean concentration of 1.33 ± 0.5 μg/L did not differ significantly from 1.75 ± 0.8 μg/L in 14 control children *5364*

Phenylalanine *Plasma* *Increase* Patients are clinically normal at birth, distinguishable only by hyperphenylalaninemia, which is established in the 1st postnatal week *367* Early diagnosis can only be made by determining the blood concentration. Rises to abnormal levels after the infant has received protein-containing feedings *4979*
Saliva *No Effect* In 10 children with PKU mean concentration of 61 μmol/L compared with plasma concentration of 432 μmol/L *1967*
Urine *Increase* Early diagnosis can only be made by determining the blood concentration. Rises to abnormal levels after the infant has received protein-containing feedings *4979*

Tyrosine *Plasma* *Decrease* Characteristic of disease *413* With normal phenylalanine intake *4746*

270.20 Alkaptonuria

Homogentisic Acid *Urine* *Increase* Excessive amounts are excreted in the urine. The output is proportional to the amount of protein in the diet *1290* increased excretion indicates the presence of alkaptonuria *2952* All diagnostic tests are based on the presence of homogentisic acid in the urine *4979*

270.20 Tyrosinemia

Ammonium Ions *Urine* *Increase* May lead to proximal renal tubular acidosis which is associated with hypokalemia, hyperchloremic metabolic acidosis, urine pH < 5.5, increased urinary ammonium ion excretion, a negative urine anion gap, increased urinary osmol gap, normal urinary citrate, normal urinary calcium excretion and Fanconi syndrome *4071*

Anion Gap *Urine* *Decrease* May lead to proximal renal tubular acidosis which is associated with hypokalemia, hyperchloremic metabolic acidosis, urine pH < 5.5, increased urinary ammonium ion excretion, a negative urine anion gap, increased urinary osmol gap, normal urinary citrate, normal urinary calcium excretion and Fanconi syndrome *4071*

Bicarbonate *Serum* *Decrease* May lead to proximal renal tubular acidosis which is associated with hypokalemia, hyperchloremic metabolic acidosis, urine pH < 5.5, increased urinary ammonium ion excretion, a negative urine anion gap, increased urinary osmol gap, normal urinary citrate, normal urinary calcium excretion and Fanconi syndrome *4071*

Calcium *Urine* *No Effect* May lead to proximal renal tubular acidosis which is associated with hypokalemia, hyperchloremic metabolic acidosis, urine pH < 5.5, increased urinary ammonium ion excretion, a negative urine anion gap, increased urinary osmol gap, normal urinary citrate, normal urinary calcium excretion and Fanconi syndrome *4071*

Chloride *Serum* *Increase* May lead to proximal renal tubular acidosis which is associated with hypokalemia, hyperchloremic metabolic acidosis, urine pH < 5.5, increased urinary ammonium ion excretion, a negative urine anion gap, increased urinary osmol gap, normal urinary citrate, normal urinary calcium excretion and Fanconi syndrome *4071*

Citrate *Urine* *No Effect* May lead to proximal renal tubular acidosis which is associated with hypokalemia, hyperchloremic metabolic acidosis, urine pH < 5.5, increased urinary ammonium ion excretion, a negative urine anion gap, increased urinary osmol gap, normal urinary citrate, normal urinary calcium excretion and Fanconi syndrome *4071*

Glucose *Urine* *Increase* May lead to proximal renal tubular acidosis which is associated with hypokalemia, hyperchloremic metabolic acidosis, urine pH < 5.5, increased urinary ammonium ion excretion, a negative urine anion gap, increased urinary osmol gap, normal urinary citrate, normal urinary calcium excretion and Fanconi syndrome *4071*

Osmolal Gap *Urine* *Increase* May lead to proximal renal tubular acidosis which is associated with hypokalemia, hyperchloremic metabolic acidosis, urine pH < 5.5, increased urinary ammonium ion excretion, a negative urine anion gap, increased urinary osmol gap, normal urinary citrate, normal urinary calcium excretion and Fanconi syndrome *4071*

pH *Urine* *Decrease* May lead to proximal renal tubular acidosis which is associated with hypokalemia, hyperchloremic metabolic acidosis, urine pH < 5.5, increased urinary ammonium ion excretion, a negative urine anion gap, increased urinary osmol gap, normal urinary citrate, normal urinary calcium excretion and Fanconi syndrome *4071*

270.20 Tyrosinemia *(continued)*

Phosphate *Serum* *Decrease* May lead to proximal renal tubular acidosis which is associated with hypokalemia, hyperchloremic metabolic acidosis, urine pH < 5.5, increased urinary ammonium ion excretion, a negative urine anion gap, increased urinary osmol gap, normal urinary citrate, normal urinary calcium excretion and Fanconi syndrome *4071*

Potassium *Serum* *Decrease* May lead to proximal renal tubular acidosis which is associated with hypokalemia, hyperchloremic metabolic acidosis, urine pH < 5.5, increased urinary ammonium ion excretion, a negative urine anion gap, increased urinary osmol gap, normal urinary citrate, normal urinary calcium excretion and Fanconi syndrome *4071*

Uric Acid *Serum* *Decrease* May lead to proximal renal tubular acidosis which is associated with hypokalemia, hyperchloremic metabolic acidosis, urine pH < 5.5, increased urinary ammonium ion excretion, a negative urine anion gap, increased urinary osmol gap, normal urinary citrate, normal urinary calcium excretion and Fanconi syndrome *4071*

270.20 Tyrosinemia Type I

Alanine Aminotransferase *Serum* *Increase* Moderate to severe derangement of liver function tests observed *3406*

Alkaline Phosphatase *Serum* *Increase* Moderate to severe derangement of liver function tests observed *3406*

Amino Acids *Urine* *Increase* Characteristically, a marked amino aciduria with tyrosine, phenylalanine and methionine most affected *3406* Renal tubular dysfunction and hypophosphatemic rickets may be observed *3406*

δ-Aminolevulinic Acid *Urine* *Increase* High excretion due to inhibition of porphobilinogen synthase by succinylacetone *3406*

Aspartate Aminotransferase *Serum* *Increase* Moderate to severe derangement of liver function tests observed *3406*

Bilirubin *Serum* *Increase* Moderate to severe derangement of liver function tests observed *3406*

Copper *Serum* *Decrease* In 4 patients with tyrosinemia type I less than 2 months of age plasma concentrations of 1.6 - 2.9 μmol/L compared with reference range of 7 - 25 μmol/L. In 5 patients older than 2 years of age concentrations were between 7.5 and 12.3 μmol/L (reference interval 12 - 26 μmol/L) *4206*

α-Fetoprotein *Serum* *Increase* AFP concentration may be increased 100-fold even in the absence of liver cancer *3406*

Glucose *Urine* *Increase* Renal tubular dysfunction and hypophosphatemic rickets may be observed *3406*

γ-Glutamyltransferase *Serum* *Increase* Moderate to severe derangement of liver function tests observed *3406*

International Normalized Ratio *Plasma* *Increase* Moderate to severe derangement of liver function tests observed, but markedly increased INR *3406*

Methionine *Urine* *Increase* Characteristically, a marked amino aciduria with tyrosine, phenylalanine and methionine most affected *3406*

5-Oxoproline *Red Blood Cells* *Decrease* Value of 1.69 mmol/L observed in one patient with tyrosinemia type I significantly decreased compared with 2.36 ± 0.37 mmol/L in 100 healthy controls *3384*
Urine *Increase* Value of 150 mmol/mol creatinine observed in one patient with tyrosinemia type I significantly increased compared with < 50 mmol/mol creatinine in 100 healthy controls *3384*

Phenylalanine *Urine* *Increase* Characteristically, a marked amino aciduria with tyrosine, phenylalanine and methionine most affected *3406*

Phosphate *Serum* *Decrease* Renal tubular dysfunction and hypophosphatemic rickets may be observed *3406*

Succinylacetone *Urine* *Increase* Diagnostic feature of condition: succinylacetone formed from maleylacetate and fumarylacetoacetate *3406*

Tyrosine *Plasma* *Increase* Increased concentration characteristic of tyrosinemia type I *4206*
Urine *Increase* Characteristically, a marked amino aciduria with tyrosine, phenylalanine and methionine most affected *3406*

270.30 Maple Syrup Urine Disease

Alloisoleucine *Serum* *Increase* Alloisoleucine, an amino acid not normally present in plasma, is elevated *900*

Amino Acids *Plasma* *Increase* Large excess of branched-chain amino acids and keto acids in blood and urine in the untreated patient *4979* The branched-chain amino acids valine, leucine, and isoleucine, are increased to 10 - 30 times above normal levels *900*
Urine *Increase* Large excess of branched-chain amino acids and keto acids in blood and urine in the untreated patient *4979* Valine, leucine, and isoleucine are present in the urine *1290*

Glucose *Serum* *Decrease* Hypoglycemic episodes are probably caused by the high concentrations of leucine *4979* *4066*

Isoleucine *Plasma* *Increase* Excessively high *4979* *4066*
Urine *Increase* Greatly increased *5545*

Leucine *Plasma* *Increase* Excessively high *4979* *4066*
Urine *Increase* Greatly increased *5545*

Valine *Plasma* *Increase* Excessively high *4979* *4066*
Urine *Increase* Greatly increased urinary excretion *5545*

270.40 Cystathioninuria

Amino Acids *Urine* *Increase* Elevated cystathionine *1304* *4979*

Methionine *Plasma* *Increase* Reported effect *4979*

270.40 Homocystinuria

Amino Acids *Urine* *Increase* Increased homocystine *1304*

Copper *Urine* *Increase* Excretion enhanced as a consequence of disease *5174*

Cystathionine *Plasma* *Decrease* In patients in whom homocysyinuria is due to cystathionine β-synthase deficiency concentration is low or low-normal *5346*
Plasma *Increase* In patients whose homocystinuria is due to 5,10-methylenetetrahydrofolate reductase deficiency or impaired methylcobalamin synthesis concentration is increased *5346*

Homocysteine *Plasma* *Increase* Increased concentration observed in patients with homocystinuria *2952*
Urine *Increase* Increased excretion observed in patients with homocystinuria *2952*

Homocystine *Plasma* *Increase* Decreased rate of metabolism results in excessive concentration *4979* When caused by cystathionine β-synthase deficiency increase of concentration up to 500 μmol/L observed. Concentration also increased in patients with 5,10-methylenetetrahydrofolate reductase deficiency and when methylcobalamin synthesis is impaired *5346*
Urine *Increase* Excretion increased in urine when homocystinuria caused by cystathioneine β-synthase deficiency and by 5,10-methylenetetrahydrofolate reductase deficiency and impaired methylcobalamin synthesis *5346* Reported effect *2034* Decreased rate of metabolism results in excessive concentration *4979*

Iron *Urine* *Increase* Excretion enhanced as a consequence of disease *5174*

Isocitrate Dehydrogenase *Serum* *Increase* Reported effect *1290*

Methionine *Cerebrospinal Fluid* *Increase* Observed effect *5545*
Plasma *Decrease* Low or low normal in homocystinuria caused by deficient 5-methyltetrahydrofolate-dependent homocysteine methylation *4979* Concentration normal or low-normal when homocystinuria due to 5,10-methylenetetrahydrofolate reductase deficiency or impaired methylcobalamin synthesis *5346*
Plasma *Increase* In homocystinuria caused by cystathionine β-synthetase deficiency *4979* In patients with cystathionine β-synthase deficiency plasma concentration considerably increased *5346*
Urine *Increase* Reported effect *367*

2-Methylcitric Acid *Serum* *Increase* In patients whose homocystinuria is due to defects in cobalamin metabolism concentration increased *5346*
Urine *Increase* In patients whose homocystinuria is due to defects in cobalamin metabolism concentration increased *5346*

Methylmalonate *Serum* *Increase* In patients whose homocystinuria is due to defects in cobalamin metabolism concentration is increased *5346*
Urine *Increase* In patients whose homocystinuria is due to defects in cobalamin metabolism concentration is increased *5346*

5-Oxoproline *Red Blood Cells* *Decrease* Value of 1.85 mmol/L observed in one patient with homocystinuria significantly decreased compared with 2.36 ± 0.37 mmol/L in 100 healthy controls *3384*
Urine *Increase* Value of 150 mmol/mol creatinine observed in one patient with homocystinuria significantly increased compared with < 50 mmol/mol creatinine in 100 healthy controls *3384*

Zinc *Urine* *Increase* Excretion enhanced as a consequence of disease *5174*

270.50 Histidinemia

Alanine *Plasma* *Decrease* Reported effect *2034*
Urine *Increase* Moderate increase *1715* *4979*

Amino Acids *Urine* *Increase* Slight increase in several amino acids other than histidine *4979* *1715*

Ammonia *Blood* *Increase* Postprandial elevation *2034*

Glutamic Acid *Cerebrospinal Fluid* *Decrease* In some reports *4979* *2214* *1715*
Plasma *Decrease* Reported effect *2034*

Glutamine *Cerebrospinal Fluid* *Increase* In some reports *1715* *2214* *4979*

Histidine *Cerebrospinal Fluid* *Increase* Frequently elevated. Values of 2 to 10 times normal have been noted *5516* *4979* Frequently elevated. Values of 2 - 10 times normal have been noted *1715*
Plasma *Increase* Quantitative amino acid analysis demonstrate plasma levels of histidine from 5 - 17 mg/dL (normal 1 - 3 mg/dL) *900* A marked elevation is the most consistent and characteristic finding *4979*
Urine *Increase* Characteristic, but not as specific an indicator as the serum concentration *4979* Quantitative amino acid analysis will demonstrate urinary excretion which usually exceeds 300 mg/24 h *900*

5-Hydroxytryptamine *Blood* *Decrease* In the 3 cases in which serotonin concentration has been determined, values were found to be 50% of the normal concentration *4979*

Imidazolepyruvic Acid *Urine* *Increase* Excreted in substantial quantities in the urine but no significant concentration was found in the blood *4979* Chromatography of the urinary metabolites of histidine will reveal the presence of imidazole pyruvic acid *900*

Urocanic Acid *Urine* *Decrease* Reported to be absent from urine in several studies, but normal concentrations are low and methods of detection lack specificity *2214* *5729* *4979* Chromatography of the urinary metabolites of histidine will reveal an absence of urocanic acid *900*

270.60 Arginosuccinic Acid Synthetase Deficiency

Alanine Aminotransferase *Serum* *Increase* Indicates hepatic involvement in condition *3406*

Ammonia *Plasma* *Increase* Hyperammonemia is characteristic of disease *3406*

Aspartate Aminotransferase *Serum* *Increase* Indicates hepatic involvement in condition *3406*

Glutamine *Plasma* *Increase* Concentration markedly increased in patients with hyperammonemic coma *3406*

Orotic Acid *Urine* *Increase* Orotic acid, formed from diversion of carbamoyl phosphate to pyrimidine, detected in urine *3406*

270.60 Arginosuccinicate Lyase Deficiency

Alanine Aminotransferase *Serum* *Increase* Indicates hepatic involvement in condition *3406*

Ammonia *Plasma* *Increase* Hyperammonemia is characteristic of disease *3406*

Aspartate Aminotransferase *Serum* *Increase* Indicates hepatic involvement in condition *3406*

Glutamine *Plasma* *Increase* Concentration markedly increased in patients with hyperammonemic coma *3406*

Orotic Acid *Urine* *Increase* Orotic acid, formed from diversion of carbamoyl phosphate to pyrimidine, detected in urine *3406*

270.60 Carbamyl Phosphate Synthetase Deficiency

Alanine Aminotransferase *Serum* *Increase* Indicates hepatic involvement in condition *3406*

Ammonia *Plasma* *Increase* Hyperammonemia is characteristic of disease *3406*

Aspartate Aminotransferase *Serum* *Increase* Indicates hepatic involvement in condition *3406*

Glutamine *Plasma* *Increase* Concentration markedly increased in patients with hyperammonemic coma *3406*

5-Oxoproline *Red Blood Cells* *Decrease* Values of 1.43, 1.28 and 1.39 mmol/L in 3 patients with carbamyl phosphate synthetase deficiency significantly decreased compared with 2.36 ± 0.37 mmol/L in 100 healthy controls *3384*
Urine *Increase* Values of 520, 1,260 and 830 mmol/mol creatinine in 3 patients with carbamyl phosphate synthetase deficiency significantly increased compared with < 50 mmol/mol creatinine in 100 healthy controls *3384*

270.60 Citrullinemia

Adipate *Urine* *Decrease* In two patients with adult-type citrullinemia excretions of 1.2 and 1.0 μg/mg creatinine compared with 4.0 ± 1.2 μg/mg creatinine in 4 healthy controls *2340*

Alanine *Plasma* *Increase* Mild elevations have been found *4979*
Plasma *No Effect* In two patients with adult-type citrullinemia concentrations of 453 and 200 nmol/mL compared with normal range of 218 - 553 nmol/mL *2340*

Amino Acids *Urine* *Increase* Generalized hyperaminoaciduria may be found in severely affected infants *4979*

Ammonia *Blood* *Increase* Characteristic elevation. May rise to 400-1,000 mg/dL postprandial *4979*
Plasma *Increase* In two patients with adult-type citrullinemia concentrations of 108 and 450 μg/dL compared with normal range of 18 - 48 μg/dL *2340*

Arginine *Plasma* *Increase* In two patients with adult-type citrullinemia concentrations of 574 and 150 nmol/mL compared with normal range of 61 - 144 nmol/mL *2340*

Asparagine *Plasma* *Increase* In two patients with adult-type citrullinemia, concentrations of 62 and 73 nmol/mL compared with normal range of 48 - 90 nmol/mL *2340*

Aspartic Acid *Plasma* *Increase* In two patients with adult-type citrullinemia, concentrations of 40 and 16 nmol/mL compared with normal range of 10 - 21 nmol/mL *2340*

Citrulline *Cerebrospinal Fluid* *Increase* Greatly increased. Ranges between 0.1 - 0.3 μmol/L (normal < 0.003). CSF concentrations are lower than in blood *4979*
Plasma *Increase* Marked accumulation. Increased to 1 - 4.5 μmol/L, at least 40 times normal. Concentration does not correlate with severity of symptoms *4979* In two patients with adult-type citrullinemia concentrations of 1,700 and 470 nmol/mL compared with normal range of 29 - 47 nmol/mL *2340*
Urine *Increase* Ranges from several hundred mg/d in infants to several g/d in adults *4979*

2-Deoxytetronic Acid *Urine* *Increase* In one patient with adult-type citrullinemia excretion of 3.4 μg/mg creatinine compared with 0.8 ± 0.0 μg/mg creatinine in 4 healthy controls *2340*

Glutamic Acid *Plasma* *Increase* In two patients with adult-type citrullinemia concentrations of 81 and 12 nmol/mL compared with normal range of 14 - 47 nmol/mL *2340*

Glutamine *Plasma* *Decrease* In two patients with adult-type citrullinemia concentrations of 484 and 342 nmol/mL compared with normal range of 436 - 713 nmol/mL *2340*
Plasma *Increase* Mild elevations have been found *4979*

270.60 Citrullinemia *(continued)*

Glycine *Plasma Decrease* In two patients with adult-type citrullinemia concentrations of 107 and 138 nmol/mL compared with normal range of 146 - 337 nmol/mL *2340*

3-Hydroxyisobutyrate *Urine Increase* In two patients with adult-type citrullinemia excretions of 6.4 and 32.4 μg/mg creatinine compared with 92 ± 2.0 μg/mg creatinine in 4 healthy controls *2340*

Isoleucine *Plasma Decrease* In two patients with adult-type citrullinemia concentrations of 1 and 49 nmol/mL compared with normal range of 35 - 96 nmol/mL *2340*

Lactate *Urine Increase* In two patients with adult-type citrullinemia excretions of 9.6 and 1,39.6 μg/mg creatinine compared with 17.2 ± 7.6 μg/mg creatinine in 4 healthy controls *2340*

Leucine *Plasma Decrease* In two patients with adult-type citrullinemia, concentrations of 36 and 100 nmol/mL compared with normal range of 70 - 167 nmol/mL *2340*

Methionine *Plasma No Effect* In two patients with adult-type citrullinemia concentrations of 13 and 28 nmol/mL compared with normal range of 19 - 39 nmol/mL *2340*

Ornithine *Plasma Increase* In two patients with adult-type citrullinemia concentrations of 585 and 110 nmol/mL compared with normal range of 33 - 83 nmol/mL *2340*

Phenylalanine *Plasma Decrease* In two patients with adult-type citrullinemia concentrations of 38 and 55 nmol/mL compared with normal range of 56 - 86 nmol/mL *2340*

Suberate *Urine Decrease* In one patient with adult-type citrullinemia excretion of 2.0 μg/mg creatinine compared with 4.0 ± 1.2 μg/mg creatinine in 4 healthy controls *2340*
Urine Increase In one patient with adult-type citrullinemia excretion of 8.4 μg/mg creatinine compared with 4.0 ± 1.2 μg/mg creatinine in 4 healthy controls *2340*

Tryptophan *Plasma No Effect* In two patients with adult-type citrullinemia concentrations of 46 and 60 nmol/mL compared with normal range of 34 - 73 nmol/mL *2340*

Tyrosine *Plasma Decrease* In two patients with adult-type citrullinemia concentrations of 21 and 81 nmol/mL compared with normal range of 51 - 91 nmol/mL *2340*

Valine *Plasma No Effect* In two patients with adult-type citrullinemia concentrations of 90 and 179 nmol/mL compared with normal range of 132 - 302 nmol/mL *2340*

270.60 Ornithine Transcarbamylase Deficiency

Alanine Aminotransferase *Serum Increase* Indicates hepatic involvement in condition *3406*

Ammonia *Plasma Increase* Hyperammonemia is characteristic of disease *3406*

Aspartate Aminotransferase *Serum Increase* Indicates hepatic involvement in condition *3406*

Glutamine *Plasma Increase* Concentration markedly increased in patients with hyperammonemic coma *3406*

Orotic Acid *Urine Increase* Orotic acid, formed from diversion of carbamoyl phosphate to pyrimidine, detected in urine *3406*

5-Oxoproline *Red Blood Cells Decrease* Values of 1.25 and 1.44 mmol/L in 2 patients with ornithine transcarbamylase deficiency significantly decreased compared with 2.36 ± 0.37 mmol/L in 100 healthy controls *3384*
Urine Increase Values of 650 and 730 mmol/mol creatinine in 2 patients with ornithine transcarbamylase deficiency significantly increased compared with < 50 mmol/mol creatinine in 100 healthy controls *3384*

270.70 Cow's Milk Protein Intolerance

Soluble Interleukin-2 Receptor *Serum Increase* In 13 children receiving milk-containing diet, mean concentration of 2,076 U/mL not significantly different from 1,805 U/mL in age-matched controls. In 17 on milk free diet mean 1,672 U/mL not significantly different from 1,259 U/mL in age-matched controls *769*

270.80 Aspartylglycosaminuria

Chitotriosidase *Serum No Effect* No abnormal activities observed in 3 patients *1917*

Glycosylasparaginase *Lymphocytes Decrease* Mean activity of 59.3 ± 65 mU/g protein in 21 carriers and 6.0 ± 4.6 mU/g protein in 7 patients with aspartylglycosaminuria compared with 242 ± 108 mU/g protein in 17 normal controls *3574*
Serum Decrease Mean activity in 10 patients with aspartylglycosaminuria of 0.7 ± 0.4 mU/L compared with 20.2 ± 5.0 mU/L in 24 normal adult controls. In 29 carriers mean activity of 15.3 ± 4.5 mU/L *3574*

270.80 Hydroxyprolinemia

Amino Acids *Plasma Increase* Other amino acids (excluding hydroxyproline) are normal *4979*

Hydroxyproline *Cerebrospinal Fluid No Effect* Concentration usually normal *4979*
Plasma Increase Elevated > 15-fold above normal concentration *4979*
Urine Increase Greatly increased. Excretion rates of 285-550 mg/24 h have been reported in patients aged 12-31 y *1302* *4066*

Hydroxyproline, Free *Urine Increase* Increased excretion reported in patients with hydroxyprolinemia *2952*

270.80 Hyperprolinemia

Amino Acids *Urine Increase* Hyperaminoaciduria of proline, glycine and hydroxyproline is specific *4979*

Glycine *Urine Increase* Hyperaminoaciduria of proline, glycine and hydroxyproline is specific *4979*

Hydroxyproline *Urine Increase* Hyperaminoaciduria of proline, glycine and hydroxyproline is specific *4979*

Proline *Plasma Increase* Higher in type II than in type I *4979* Characteristic of disease *2034*
Urine Increase Hyperaminoaciduria of proline, glycine and hydroxyproline is specific *4979* Observed effect *2034*

270.80 Lowe's Syndrome

Ammonium Ions *Urine Increase* May lead to proximal renal tubular acidosis which is associated with hypokalemia, hyperchloremic metabolic acidosis, urine pH < 5.5, increased urinary ammonium ion excretion, a negative urine anion gap, increased urinary osmol gap, normal urinary citrate, normal urinary calcium excretion and Fanconi syndrome *4071*

Anion Gap *Urine Decrease* May lead to proximal renal tubular acidosis which is associated with hypokalemia, hyperchloremic metabolic acidosis, urine pH < 5.5, increased urinary ammonium ion excretion, a negative urine anion gap, increased urinary osmol gap, normal urinary citrate, normal urinary calcium excretion and Fanconi syndrome *4071*

Bicarbonate *Serum Decrease* May lead to proximal renal tubular acidosis which is associated with hypokalemia, hyperchloremic metabolic acidosis, urine pH < 5.5, increased urinary ammonium ion excretion, a negative urine anion gap, increased urinary osmol gap, normal urinary citrate, normal urinary calcium excretion and Fanconi syndrome *4071*

Calcium *Urine No Effect* May lead to proximal renal tubular acidosis which is associated with hypokalemia, hyperchloremic metabolic acidosis, urine pH < 5.5, increased urinary ammonium ion excretion, a negative urine anion gap, increased urinary osmol gap, normal urinary citrate, normal urinary calcium excretion and Fanconi syndrome *4071*

Chloride *Serum Increase* May lead to proximal renal tubular acidosis which is associated with hypokalemia, hyperchloremic metabolic acidosis, urine pH < 5.5, increased urinary ammonium ion excretion, a negative urine anion gap, increased urinary osmol gap, normal urinary citrate, normal urinary calcium excretion and Fanconi syndrome *4071*

Citrate *Urine* *No Effect* May lead to proximal renal tubular acidosis which is associated with hypokalemia, hyperchloremic metabolic acidosis, urine pH < 5.5, increased urinary ammonium ion excretion, a negative urine anion gap, increased urinary osmol gap, normal urinary citrate, normal urinary calcium excretion and Fanconi syndrome *4071*

Glucose *Urine* *Increase* May lead to proximal renal tubular acidosis which is associated with hypokalemia, hyperchloremic metabolic acidosis, urine pH < 5.5, increased urinary ammonium ion excretion, a negative urine anion gap, increased urinary osmol gap, normal urinary citrate, normal urinary calcium excretion and Fanconi syndrome *4071*

Osmolal Gap *Urine* *Increase* May lead to proximal renal tubular acidosis which is associated with hypokalemia, hyperchloremic metabolic acidosis, urine pH < 5.5, increased urinary ammonium ion excretion, a negative urine anion gap, increased urinary osmol gap, normal urinary citrate, normal urinary calcium excretion and Fanconi syndrome *4071*

pH *Urine* *Decrease* May lead to proximal renal tubular acidosis which is associated with hypokalemia, hyperchloremic metabolic acidosis, urine pH < 5.5, increased urinary ammonium ion excretion, a negative urine anion gap, increased urinary osmol gap, normal urinary citrate, normal urinary calcium excretion and Fanconi syndrome *4071*

Phosphate *Serum* *Decrease* May lead to proximal renal tubular acidosis which is associated with hypokalemia, hyperchloremic metabolic acidosis, urine pH < 5.5, increased urinary ammonium ion excretion, a negative urine anion gap, increased urinary osmol gap, normal urinary citrate, normal urinary calcium excretion and Fanconi syndrome *4071*

Potassium *Serum* *Decrease* May lead to proximal renal tubular acidosis which is associated with hypokalemia, hyperchloremic metabolic acidosis, urine pH < 5.5, increased urinary ammonium ion excretion, a negative urine anion gap, increased urinary osmol gap, normal urinary citrate, normal urinary calcium excretion and Fanconi syndrome *4071*

Uric Acid *Serum* *Decrease* May lead to proximal renal tubular acidosis which is associated with hypokalemia, hyperchloremic metabolic acidosis, urine pH < 5.5, increased urinary ammonium ion excretion, a negative urine anion gap, increased urinary osmol gap, normal urinary citrate, normal urinary calcium excretion and Fanconi syndrome *4071*

Disorders of Carbohydrate Transport and Metabolism

271.00 Amylopectinosis

Alanine Aminotransferase *Serum* *Increase* Mild cholestasis may be observed until late stages of disease when hepatic failure occurs *3406*

Alkaline Phosphatase *Serum* *Increase* Mild cholestasis observed until late stages when hepatic failure occurs *3406*

Aspartate Aminotransferase *Serum* *Increase* Mild cholestasis may be observed until late stages of disease when hepatic failure occurs *3406*

Bilirubin *Serum* *Increase* Mild cholestasis may be observed until late stages of disease when hepatic failure occurs *3406*

Cholesterol *Serum* *Increase* Mild cholestasis may be observed until late stages of disease when hepatic failure occurs *3406*

Glucose *Serum* *Decrease* One of most prominent features of condition *3406*

γ-Glutamyltransferase *Serum* *Increase* Mild cholestasis may be observed until late stages of disease when hepatic failure occurs *3406*

pH *Blood* *Decrease* Mild cholestasis may be observed until late stages of disease when hepatic failure occurs *3406*

Triglycerides *Serum* *Increase* Mild cholestasis may be observed until late stages of disease when hepatic failure occurs *3406*

Uric Acid *Serum* *Increase* Mild cholestasis may be observed until late stages of disease when hepatic failure occurs *3406*

271.00 Andersen Disease

Alanine Aminotransferase *Serum* *Increase* Mild cholestasis may be observed until late stages of disease when hepatic failure occurs *3406*

Alkaline Phosphatase *Serum* *Increase* Mild cholestasis observed until late stages when hepatic failure occurs *3406*

Aspartate Aminotransferase *Serum* *Increase* Mild cholestasis may be observed until late stages of disease when hepatic failure occurs *3406*

Bilirubin *Serum* *Increase* Mild cholestasis may be observed until late stages of disease when hepatic failure occurs *3406*

Cholesterol *Serum* *Increase* Mild cholestasis may be observed until late stages of disease when hepatic failure occurs *3406*

Glucose *Serum* *Decrease* One of most prominent features of condition *3406*

γ-Glutamyltransferase *Serum* *Increase* Mild cholestasis may be observed until late stages of disease when hepatic failure occurs *3406*

pH *Blood* *Decrease* Mild cholestasis may be observed until late stages of disease when hepatic failure occurs *3406*

Triglycerides *Serum* *Increase* Mild cholestasis may be observed until late stages of disease when hepatic failure occurs *3406*

Uric Acid *Serum* *Increase* Mild cholestasis may be observed until late stages of disease when hepatic failure occurs *3406*

271.00 Cori Disease

Alanine Aminotransferase *Serum* *Increase* Mild cholestasis may be observed until late stages of disease when hepatic failure occurs *3406*

Alkaline Phosphatase *Serum* *Increase* Mild cholestasis observed until late stages when hepatic failure occurs *3406*

Aspartate Aminotransferase *Serum* *Increase* Mild cholestasis may be observed until late stages of disease when hepatic failure occurs *3406*

Bilirubin *Serum* *Increase* Mild cholestasis may be observed until late stages of disease when hepatic failure occurs *3406*

Cholesterol *Serum* *Increase* Mild cholestasis may be observed until late stages of disease when hepatic failure occurs *3406*

Glucose *Serum* *Decrease* One of most prominent features of condition *3406*

γ-Glutamyltransferase *Serum* *Increase* Mild cholestasis may be observed until late stages of disease when hepatic failure occurs *3406*

Triglycerides *Serum* *Increase* Mild cholestasis may be observed until late stages of disease when hepatic failure occurs *3406*

Uric Acid *Serum* *Increase* Mild cholestasis may be observed until late stages of disease when hepatic failure occurs *3406*

271.00 Glycogen Storage Disease

Albumin *Serum* *No Effect* In 22 patients with type I hepatic glycogen storage disease mean concentration of 40.3 ± 5.65 g/L, in 15 with type III disease 40.2 ± 4.44 g/L and in 18 with types VI and IX disease 41 ± 4.5 g/L not significantly different from normal of 33 - 39 g/L *2884*

C-Reactive Protein *Serum* *Increase* In 22 patients with type I hepatic glycogen storage disease mean concentration of 48 ± 17.5 mg/L significantly higher than upper limit of normal of less than 10 mg/L *2884*

Serum *No Effect* In 15 patients with type III hepatic glycogen storage disease mean concentration of 11.8 ± 3 mg/L and < 10 in 18 patients with types VI and IX disease mean concentration not significantly different from normal of less than 10 mg/L *2884*

Fibrinogen *Plasma* *Increase* In 22 patients with type I disease mean concentration of 5.65 ± 3.13 g/L significantly higher than normal range of 2 - 4 g/L *2884*

271.00 Glycogen Storage Disease *(continued)*

Fibrinogen *(continued)*
Plasma *No Effect* Mean concentration of 3.66 ± 0.49 g/L in 15 patients with type III hepatic glycogen storage disease and 3 ± 1.0 g/L in 18 patients with types VI and IX disease not significantly different from normal of 2 - 4 g/L *2884*

Fibronectin *Plasma* *No Effect* In 22 patients with type I disease mean concentration of 315 ± 120 mg/L, in 15 with type III disease 240 ± 80 mg/L and in 18 with types VI and IX 190 ± 57 mg/L not significantly different from normal range of 204 - 391 mg/L *2884*

α_2-Macroglobulin *Serum* *Increase* Mean concentrations of 5.54 ± 2.02 g/L in 22 patients with type I hepatic glycogen storage disease, 4.2 ± 1.25 g/L in 15 type III patients and 4.6 ± 1.64 g/L in 18 types VI and IX patients significantly greater than normal of 1 - 3 g/L *2884*

Prealbumin *Serum* *No Effect* In 22 patients with type I disease mean concentration of 260 ± 130 mg/L, in 15 with type III disease 204 ± 95 mg/L and 220 ± 55 mg/L in 18 patients with types VI and IX disease not significantly different from normal range of 239 - 437 mg/L *2884*

Retinol-binding Protein *Serum* *Decrease* In 22 patients with type I disease mean concentration of 26 ± 10 mg/L, in 15 with type III disease 25 ± 9 mg/L and 29 ± 10 mg/L in 18 with types VI and IX disease significantly lower than normal range of 55 - 69 mg/L *2884*

Transferrin *Serum* *Increase* In 22 patients with type I disease mean concentration of 4.24 ± 1.14 g/L significantly greater than normal range of 2.5 - 3.1 g/L *2884*
Serum *No Effect* Mean concentration of 3.5 ± 0.70 g/L in 15 type I patients and 3.0 ± 0.55 g/L in 18 patients with types VI and IX disease not significantly different from normal range of 2.5 - 3.1 g/L *2884*

271.00 Glycogen Storage Disease I

Ammonium Ions *Urine* *Increase* May lead to proximal renal tubular acidosis which is associated with hypokalemia, hyperchloremic metabolic acidosis, urine pH < 5.5, increased urinary ammonium ion excretion, a negative urine anion gap, increased urinary osmol gap, normal urinary citrate, normal urinary calcium excretion and Fanconi syndrome *4071*

Anion Gap *Urine* *Decrease* May lead to proximal renal tubular acidosis which is associated with hypokalemia, hyperchloremic metabolic acidosis, urine pH < 5.5, increased urinary ammonium ion excretion, a negative urine anion gap, increased urinary osmol gap, normal urinary citrate, normal urinary calcium excretion and Fanconi syndrome *4071*

Bicarbonate *Serum* *Decrease* May lead to proximal renal tubular acidosis which is associated with hypokalemia, hyperchloremic metabolic acidosis, urine pH < 5.5, increased urinary ammonium ion excretion, a negative urine anion gap, increased urinary osmol gap, normal urinary citrate, normal urinary calcium excretion and Fanconi syndrome *4071*

Calcium *Urine* *No Effect* May lead to proximal renal tubular acidosis which is associated with hypokalemia, hyperchloremic metabolic acidosis, urine pH < 5.5, increased urinary ammonium ion excretion, a negative urine anion gap, increased urinary osmol gap, normal urinary citrate, normal urinary calcium excretion and Fanconi syndrome *4071*

Chloride *Serum* *Increase* May lead to proximal renal tubular acidosis which is associated with hypokalemia, hyperchloremic metabolic acidosis, urine pH < 5.5, increased urinary ammonium ion excretion, a negative urine anion gap, increased urinary osmol gap, normal urinary citrate, normal urinary calcium excretion and Fanconi syndrome *4071*

Citrate *Urine* *No Effect* May lead to proximal renal tubular acidosis which is associated with hypokalemia, hyperchloremic metabolic acidosis, urine pH < 5.5, increased urinary ammonium ion excretion, a negative urine anion gap, increased urinary osmol gap, normal urinary citrate, normal urinary calcium excretion and Fanconi syndrome *4071*

Glucose *Urine* *Increase* May lead to proximal renal tubular acidosis which is associated with hypokalemia, hyperchloremic metabolic acidosis, urine pH < 5.5, increased urinary ammonium ion excretion, a negative urine anion gap, increased urinary osmol gap, normal urinary citrate, normal urinary calcium excretion and Fanconi syndrome *4071*

Osmolal Gap *Urine* *Increase* May lead to proximal renal tubular acidosis which is associated with hypokalemia, hyperchloremic metabolic acidosis, urine pH < 5.5, increased urinary ammonium ion excretion, a negative urine anion gap, increased urinary osmol gap, normal urinary citrate, normal urinary calcium excretion and Fanconi syndrome *4071*

pH *Urine* *Decrease* May lead to proximal renal tubular acidosis which is associated with hypokalemia, hyperchloremic metabolic acidosis, urine pH < 5.5, increased urinary ammonium ion excretion, a negative urine anion gap, increased urinary osmol gap, normal urinary citrate, normal urinary calcium excretion and Fanconi syndrome *4071*

Phosphate *Serum* *Decrease* May lead to proximal renal tubular acidosis which is associated with hypokalemia, hyperchloremic metabolic acidosis, urine pH < 5.5, increased urinary ammonium ion excretion, a negative urine anion gap, increased urinary osmol gap, normal urinary citrate, normal urinary calcium excretion and Fanconi syndrome *4071*

Potassium *Serum* *Decrease* May lead to proximal renal tubular acidosis which is associated with hypokalemia, hyperchloremic metabolic acidosis, urine pH < 5.5, increased urinary ammonium ion excretion, a negative urine anion gap, increased urinary osmol gap, normal urinary citrate, normal urinary calcium excretion and Fanconi syndrome *4071*

Uric Acid *Serum* *Decrease* May lead to proximal renal tubular acidosis which is associated with hypokalemia, hyperchloremic metabolic acidosis, urine pH < 5.5, increased urinary ammonium ion excretion, a negative urine anion gap, increased urinary osmol gap, normal urinary citrate, normal urinary calcium excretion and Fanconi syndrome *4071*

271.00 Glycogen Storage Disease II

Chitotriosidase *Serum* *Increase* Abnormal activities observed in 2 of 8 patients, with activities of 360 and 420 nmol/h/mL *1917*

271.00 Glycogen Storage Disease III

Chitotriosidase *Serum* *No Effect* Normal activity observed in none of three patients with condition *1917*

271.00 Glycogen Storage Disease IV

Chitotriosidase *Serum* *No Effect* Normal activity observed in one patient with condition *1917*

271.00 Glycogen Storage Disease V

Chitotriosidase *Serum* *No Effect* Normal activity observed in none of two patients with condition *1917*

271.00 Glycogen Storage Disease VI

Chitotriosidase *Serum* *No Effect* Normal activity observed in none of two patients with condition *1917*

271.00 Glycogen Storage Disease VIII

Chitotriosidase *Serum* *No Effect* Normal activity observed in none of five patients with condition *1917*

271.00 Hers Disease

Alanine Aminotransferase *Serum* *Increase* Mild cholestasis may be observed until late stages of disease when hepatic failure occurs *3406*

Alkaline Phosphatase *Serum* *Increase* Mild cholestasis observed until late stages when hepatic failure occurs *3406*

Aspartate Aminotransferase *Serum* *Increase* Mild cholestasis may be observed until late stages of disease when hepatic failure occurs *3406*

Bilirubin *Serum* *Increase* Mild cholestasis may be observed until late stages of disease when hepatic failure occurs *3406*

Cholesterol *Serum* *Increase* Mild cholestasis may be observed until late stages of disease when hepatic failure occurs *3406*

Glucose *Serum* *Decrease* One of most prominent features of condition *3406*

γ-Glutamyltransferase *Serum* *Increase* Mild cholestasis may be observed until late stages of disease when hepatic failure occurs *3406*

pH *Blood* *Decrease* Mild cholestasis may be observed until late stages of disease when hepatic failure occurs *3406*

Triglycerides *Serum* *Increase* Mild cholestasis may be observed until late stages of disease when hepatic failure occurs *3406*

Uric Acid *Serum* *Increase* Mild cholestasis may be observed until late stages of disease when hepatic failure occurs *3406*

271.00 Limit Dextrinosis

Alanine Aminotransferase *Serum* *Increase* Mild cholestasis may be observed until late stages of disease when hepatic failure occurs *3406*

Alkaline Phosphatase *Serum* *Increase* Mild cholestasis observed until late stages when hepatic failure occurs *3406*

Aspartate Aminotransferase *Serum* *Increase* Mild cholestasis may be observed until late stages of disease when hepatic failure occurs *3406*

Bilirubin *Serum* *Increase* Mild cholestasis may be observed until late stages of disease when hepatic failure occurs *3406*

Cholesterol *Serum* *Increase* Mild cholestasis may be observed until late stages of disease when hepatic failure occurs *3406*

Glucose *Serum* *Decrease* One of most prominent features of condition *3406*

γ-Glutamyltransferase *Serum* *Increase* Mild cholestasis may be observed until late stages of disease when hepatic failure occurs *3406*

pH *Blood* *Decrease* Mild cholestasis may be observed until late stages of disease when hepatic failure occurs *3406*

Triglycerides *Serum* *Increase* Mild cholestasis may be observed until late stages of disease when hepatic failure occurs *3406*

Uric Acid *Serum* *Increase* Mild cholestasis may be observed until late stages of disease when hepatic failure occurs *3406*

271.00 Tauri Disease

Alanine Aminotransferase *Serum* *Increase* Mild cholestasis may be observed until late stages of disease when hepatic failure occurs *3406*

Alkaline Phosphatase *Serum* *Increase* Mild cholestasis observed until late stages when hepatic failure occurs *3406*

Aspartate Aminotransferase *Serum* *Increase* Mild cholestasis may be observed until late stages of disease when hepatic failure occurs *3406*

Bilirubin *Serum* *Increase* Mild cholestasis may be observed until late stages of disease when hepatic failure occurs *3406*

Cholesterol *Serum* *Increase* Mild cholestasis may be observed until late stages of disease when hepatic failure occurs *3406*

Glucose *Serum* *Decrease* One of most prominent features of condition *3406*

γ-Glutamyltransferase *Serum* *Increase* Mild cholestasis may be observed until late stages of disease when hepatic failure occurs *3406*

pH *Blood* *Decrease* Mild cholestasis may be observed until late stages of disease when hepatic failure occurs *3406* *3406*

Triglycerides *Serum* *Increase* Mild cholestasis may be observed until late stages of disease when hepatic failure occurs *3406*

Uric Acid *Serum* *Increase* Mild cholestasis may be observed until late stages of disease when hepatic failure occurs *3406*

271.01 Von Gierke's Disease

Alanine Aminotransferase *Serum* *Increase* Mild cholestasis may be observed until late stages of disease when hepatic failure occurs *3406*
Serum *No Effect* Liver may be massively enlarged but liver function tests are normal *4979*

Aspartate Aminotransferase *Serum* *Increase* Mild cholestasis may be observed until late stages of disease when hepatic failure occurs *3406*
Serum *No Effect* Liver may be massively enlarged but liver function tests are normal *4979*

Bilirubin *Serum* *Increase* Jaundice is rare *3406*

Bleeding Time *Patient* *Increase* Prolonged bleeding is a major clinical problem, probably due to impaired platelet function *4979*

BSP Retention *Serum* *No Effect* Liver may be massively enlarged but liver function tests are normal *4979*

Cholesterol *Serum* *Increase* Significant elevations generally occur in the glycogen storage diseases *4707* Striking elevation *4979* Mild cholestasis may be observed until late stages of disease when hepatic failure occurs *3406* Striking elevation *2253*

Chylomicrons *Serum* *Increase* Minimal elevation secondary to decreased catabolism due to reduced lipoprotein lipase activity *126*

Fatty Acids (FFA), Free *Serum* *Increase* Due to hypoglycemia *4979* *2253*

Glucose *Serum* *Decrease* Degree of hypoglycemia is variable *4979* Usually low *4707* One of most prominent features of condition *3406* Decreased glucose due to excess insulin as a result of deficiency in available glycogen *1290*

Glucose-6-Phosphatase *Liver* *Decrease* Deficient enzyme in the liver *4979*

Glucose Tolerance *Serum* *Decrease* Decreased because of inability to form glycogen from administered glucose *1290* Decreased tolerance:excessive peak decreased formation of glycogen with low fasting levels and subsequent hypoglycemia *5544* Characteristically diabetic *2253*

γ-Glutamyltransferase *Serum* *Increase* Mild cholestasis may be observed until late stages of disease when hepatic failure occurs *3406*

Glycerol *Serum* *Increase* Has been observed *3854*

Haptoglobin *Serum* *Decrease* Reflects chronic hemolysis *413*

Insulin *Plasma* *Decrease* Basal plasma concentrations were found to be 50 - 60% of normal in 5 older patients with type I *3101* *4979*

Insulin Tolerance *Plasma* *Decrease* Increased insulin sensitivity may result in an excessive fall in the blood sugar in some cases *1290*

Ketones *Serum* *Increase* Increased, especially after fasting *1290* Ketosis is characteristic *2253*
Urine *Increase* Children are more liable to develop ketosis than adults, especially after fasting *1290*

Lactate *Blood* *Increase* Striking elevation *4979* Significant elevations generally occur in the glycogen storage diseases *4707* Striking elevation *2253*

Lipids *Serum* *Increase* Rarely is there an increase, which is associated with impaired carbohydrate metabolism and associated ketosis *1290* Hyperlipidemia is a dominant feature *2253* Total lipids are significantly elevated *4707*

pH *Blood* *Decrease* Acidosis *1980*
Blood *Increase* Mild cholestasis may be observed until late stages of disease when hepatic failure occurs *3406*

271.01 Von Gierke's Disease *(continued)*

Phosphate *Serum* *Decrease* Mean fasting inorganic phosphate level was significantly decreased to 3.9 ± 0.3 mg/dL, (normal range of 4.8 ± 0.3). Concentrations were further diminished by fructose and glucagon administration *4403*

Phospholipids *Serum* *Increase* Striking elevation *2253* *4979*

Pyruvate *Blood* *Increase* Striking elevation *2253* *4979*

Triglycerides *Serum* *Increase* Types I and VI glycogen storage disease *1290* Striking elevation *4979* *2253* Mild cholestasis may be observed until late stages of disease when hepatic failure occurs *3406*

Uric Acid *Serum* *Increase* Significant elevations generally occur in the glycogen storage diseases *4707* Mild cholestasis may be observed until late stages of disease when hepatic failure occurs *3406* Hyperuricemia appears in early infancy, but rarely becomes symptomatic before age 10. May become a major problem in the adult *4979* Fasting blood levels were > 2 times normal mean; further significant increases occurred after fructose and glucagon administration in children *4403* Hyperuricemia appears in early infancy, but rarely becomes symptomatic before age 10. May become a major problem in the adult *2253*
Urine *Increase* Mean excretion was 1.5 ± 0.6 mg/mg creatinine, slightly elevated compared to 0.6 ± 0.1 mg/mg creatinine in normal children *4403*

VLDL-Cholesterol *Serum* *Increase* Marked elevation due to increased secretion and decreased catabolism due to reduced lipoprotein lipase activity *126*

271.02 McArdle's Disease

Alanine Aminotransferase *Serum* *Increase* Mild cholestasis may be observed until late stages of disease when hepatic failure occurs *3406*

Aldolase *Serum* *Increase* Increases dramatically within 1 h after strenuous exercise *1991* *4979*

Alkaline Phosphatase *Serum* *Increase* Mild cholestasis observed until late stages when hepatic failure occurs *3406*

Aspartate Aminotransferase *Serum* *Increase* Slight to moderate increase *1025* Mild cholestasis may be observed until late stages of disease when hepatic failure occurs *3406*

Bilirubin *Serum* *Increase* Mild cholestasis may be observed until late stages of disease when hepatic failure occurs *3406*

Cholesterol *Serum* *Increase* Mild cholestasis may be observed until late stages of disease when hepatic failure occurs *3406* Significant elevations generally occur in the glycogen storage diseases *4707*

Creatine Kinase *Serum* *Increase* During myoglobinuric attacks *1290* Increases dramatically within 1 h after strenuous exercise *4979* *1991*

Glucose *Serum* *Decrease* Usually low *4707* One of most prominent features of condition *3406*
Serum *No Effect* The blood sugar level, glucose tolerance, and galactose tolerance are normal, as is the response to injected glucagon and epinephrine *2304* Type V patients are not hypoglycemic *4979*

Glucose Tolerance *Serum* *No Effect* The blood sugar level, glucose tolerance, and galactose tolerance are normal, as is the response to injected glucagon and epinephrine *2304*

α-Glucosidase *Serum* *Decrease* Absence of activity in skeletal muscle or liver biopsy tissue or in the blood leukocytes *2304*

γ-Glutamyltransferase *Serum* *Increase* Mild cholestasis may be observed until late stages of disease when hepatic failure occurs *3406*

Lactate *Blood* *Increase* Significant elevations generally occur in the glycogen storage diseases *4707*

Lactate Dehydrogenase *Serum* *Increase* Increases dramatically within 1 h after strenuous exercise *1991* Slight to moderate increase *1025* Increases dramatically within 1 h after strenuous exercise *4979*

Lipids *Serum* *Increase* Total lipids are significantly elevated *4707*

Myoglobin *Urine* *Increase* Myoglobinuria appeared in > 50% of patients following episodes of exercise *4979* Transient attacks of myoglobinuria *1290*

pH *Blood* *Decrease* Mild cholestasis may be observed until late stages of disease when hepatic failure occurs *3406*

Triglycerides *Serum* *Increase* Mild cholestasis may be observed until late stages of disease when hepatic failure occurs *3406*

Uric Acid *Serum* *Increase* Mild cholestasis may be observed until late stages of disease when hepatic failure occurs *3406* Significant elevations generally occur in the glycogen storage diseases *4707*

271.03 Forbes' Disease

Alanine Aminotransferase *Serum* *Increase* Mild cholestasis may be observed until late stages of disease when hepatic failure occurs *3406* There may be some mild abnormalities of liver function. Elevations of AST and ALT are common, especially in Type III *900*

Alkaline Phosphatase *Serum* *Increase* Mild cholestasis observed until late stages when hepatic failure occurs *3406*

Aspartate Aminotransferase *Serum* *Increase* Mild cholestasis may be observed until late stages of disease when hepatic failure occurs *3406* There may be some mild abnormalities of liver function. Elevations of AST and ALT are common, especially in Type III *900*

Bilirubin *Serum* *Increase* Mild cholestasis may be observed until late stages of disease when hepatic failure occurs *3406*

Cholesterol *Serum* *Increase* Mild cholestasis may be observed until late stages of disease when hepatic failure occurs *3406* Significant elevations generally occur in the glycogen storage diseases *4707* Increased in all 49 cases *3602* Concentrations vary from 200 to > 1,400 mg/dL. Extreme variability of cholesterol and triglyceride concentration is a diagnostic feature and in distinct contrast to the steady elevations in Type II *1566*

Glucose *Serum* *Decrease* Usually low *4707* One of most prominent features of condition *3406*

γ-Glutamyltransferase *Serum* *Increase* Mild cholestasis may be observed until late stages of disease when hepatic failure occurs *3406*

Lactate *Blood* *Increase* Significant elevations generally occur in the glycogen storage diseases *4707*

Lipids *Serum* *Increase* Total lipids are significantly elevated *4707*

pH *Blood* *Decrease* Mild cholestasis may be observed until late stages of disease when hepatic failure occurs *3406* Acidosis *1980*

Triglycerides *Serum* *Increase* Mild cholestasis may be observed until late stages of disease when hepatic failure occurs *3406*

Uric Acid *Serum* *Increase* Usually but not always *4979* Mild cholestasis may be observed until late stages of disease when hepatic failure occurs *3406*

271.04 Pompe's Disease

Alanine Aminotransferase *Serum* *Increase* Mild cholestasis may be observed until late stages of disease when hepatic failure occurs *3406*

Alkaline Phosphatase *Serum* *Increase* Mild cholestasis observed until late stages when hepatic failure occurs *3406*

Aspartate Aminotransferase *Serum* *Increase* Mild cholestasis may be observed until late stages of disease when hepatic failure occurs *3406*

Bilirubin *Serum* *Increase* Mild cholestasis may be observed until late stages of disease when hepatic failure occurs *3406*

Cholesterol *Serum* *Increase* Mild cholestasis may be observed until late stages of disease when hepatic failure occurs *3406* *3406*

Glucose *Serum* *Decrease* One of most prominent features of condition *3406*

α-Glucosidase *Fibroblasts* *Decrease* Low activity suggests type II glycogen storage disease (Pompe's disease) *2952*

γ-Glutamyltransferase *Serum* *Increase* Mild cholestasis may be observed until late stages of disease when hepatic failure occurs *3406*

Lysosome-associated Membrane Protein-2 *Serum* *No Effect* Median concentration of 1.27 mg/L in 4 patients with Pompe's disease with median age 0.4 y compared with 1.21 mg/L in 202 healthy controls aged 0 - 66 y (median 7 years) *2265*

Lysosome-associated Membrane Protein-2:Lysosome-associated Membrane Protein-1 Ratio *Serum* *Decrease* Mean ratio of 3.02 in 10 patients with Pompe's disease with median age 0.4 y significantly different when compared with 4.74 in 202 healthy controls aged 0 - 66 y (median 7 years) *2265*

pH *Blood* *Increase* Mild cholestasis may be observed until late stages of disease when hepatic failure occurs *3406*

Triglycerides *Serum* *Increase* Mild cholestasis may be observed until late stages of disease when hepatic failure occurs *3406*

Uric Acid *Serum* *Increase* Mild cholestasis may be observed until late stages of disease when hepatic failure occurs *3406*

271.10 Galactosemia

Alanine Aminotransferase *Serum* *Increase* Deranged liver function *4979* Grossly abnormal liver function tests observed with a predominantly cholestatic pattern, although transaminases may also be raised indicating hepatocellular necrosis *3406*

Albumin *Urine* *Increase* Manifestation of a renal toxicity syndrome *2217*

Alkaline Phosphatase *Serum* *Increase* Grossly abnormal liver function tests observed with a predominantly cholestatic pattern, although transaminases may also be raised indicating hepatocellular necrosis *3406*

Amino Acids *Plasma* *Increase* Frequent in patients receiving a milk diet *4707*
Urine *Increase* Manifestation of a renal toxicity syndrome *2216* General aminoaciduria - identified by chromatography *5545* Aminoaciduria may be observed associated with grossly abnormal liver function tests observed with a predominantly cholestatic pattern, although transaminases may also be raised indicating hepatocellular necrosis *3406*

Ammonium Ions *Urine* *Increase* May lead to proximal renal tubular acidosis which is associated with hypokalemia, hyperchloremic metabolic acidosis, urine pH < 5.5, increased urinary ammonium ion excretion, a negative urine anion gap, increased urinary osmol gap, normal urinary citrate, normal urinary calcium excretion and Fanconi syndrome *4071*

Anion Gap *Urine* *Decrease* May lead to proximal renal tubular acidosis which is associated with hypokalemia, hyperchloremic metabolic acidosis, urine pH < 5.5, increased urinary ammonium ion excretion, a negative urine anion gap, increased urinary osmol gap, normal urinary citrate, normal urinary calcium excretion and Fanconi syndrome *4071*

Aspartate Aminotransferase *Serum* *Increase* Grossly abnormal liver function tests observed with a predominantly cholestatic pattern, although transaminases may also be raised indicating hepatocellular necrosis *3406* Deranged liver function *4979*

Bicarbonate *Serum* *Decrease* May lead to proximal renal tubular acidosis which is associated with hypokalemia, hyperchloremic metabolic acidosis, urine pH < 5.5, increased urinary ammonium ion excretion, a negative urine anion gap, increased urinary osmol gap, normal urinary citrate, normal urinary calcium excretion and Fanconi syndrome *4071*

Bilirubin *Serum* *Increase* Grossly abnormal liver function tests observed with a predominantly cholestatic pattern, although transaminases may also be raised indicating hepatocellular necrosis *3406*

BSP Retention *Serum* *Increase* Deranged liver function *4979*

Calcium *Urine* *No Effect* May lead to proximal renal tubular acidosis which is associated with hypokalemia, hyperchloremic metabolic acidosis, urine pH < 5.5, increased urinary ammonium ion excretion, a negative urine anion gap, increased urinary osmol gap, normal urinary citrate, normal urinary calcium excretion and Fanconi syndrome *4071*

Chitotriosidase *Serum* *No Effect* Normal activity observed in none of four patients with condition *1917*

Chloride *Serum* *Increase* Hyperchloremic acidosis. May be secondary to GI disturbance, poor food intake, or renal tubular dysfunction *4066* May lead to proximal renal tubular acidosis which is associated with hypokalemia, hyperchloremic metabolic acidosis, urine pH < 5.5, increased urinary ammonium ion excretion, a negative urine anion gap, increased urinary osmol gap, normal urinary citrate, normal urinary calcium excretion and Fanconi syndrome *4071* Hyperchloremic acidosis. May be secondary to GI disturbance, poor food intake, or renal tubular dysfunction *4979*

Citrate *Urine* *No Effect* May lead to proximal renal tubular acidosis which is associated with hypokalemia, hyperchloremic metabolic acidosis, urine pH < 5.5, increased urinary ammonium ion excretion, a negative urine anion gap, increased urinary osmol gap, normal urinary citrate, normal urinary calcium excretion and Fanconi syndrome *4071*

Galactitol *Urine* *Increase* In 32 patients mean concentration decreased from baseline concentration to 388 ± 1.69 µmol/mmol creatinine with treatment over 2 - 3 months *2309*

Galactose *Serum* *Increase* Concentration increased in 9 untreated patients (range of 0 ± 12.0 mmol/L) *5018* Galactosemia (equal to total reducing sugar minus glucose oxidase sugar) with galactosemia *5545*
Urine *Increase* May be intermittent *4979* Increase above 30 mg/dL characteristic of galactosemia *2952* May be intermittent *2217* Galactosuria--detected by nonspecific reducing tests; identified by chromatography with galactosemia *5545*

Galactose-1-Phosphate *Red Blood Cells* *Increase* In 32 patients mean concentration decreased from baseline concentration to 225 ± 1.69 µmol/L with treatment over 2 - 3 months *2309* On galactose restricted diet diagnosis of galactosemia made at 80 - 125 µg/g hemoglobin and on unrestricted diet at concentration of more than 125 µg/g hemoglobin *2952*
Serum *Increase* Concentration increased in 9 untreated patients (range of 0 ± 5.4 mmol/L) *5018*

Galactose-1-Phosphate Uridyltransferase *Blood* *Decrease* Reduction below normal range of 18.5 - 28.5 U/g hemoglobin is characteristic of one form of galactosemia *2952*

Glucose *Serum* *Decrease* In children; following ingestion of galactose blood glucose falls (as blood galactose rises) to dangerously low levels *5544* *1290* Replacement or destruction of functioning hepatic tissue may evoke hypoglycemia *4707* On rare occasions *4979*
Urine *Increase* May lead to proximal renal tubular acidosis which is associated with hypokalemia, hyperchloremic metabolic acidosis, urine pH < 5.5, increased urinary ammonium ion excretion, a negative urine anion gap, increased urinary osmol gap, normal urinary citrate, normal urinary calcium excretion and Fanconi syndrome *4071*

γ-Glutamyltransferase *Serum* *Increase* Grossly abnormal liver function tests observed with a predominantly cholestatic pattern, although transaminases may also be raised indicating hepatocellular necrosis *3406*

Hematocrit *Blood* *Decrease* Hemolytic anemia may be observed associated with grossly abnormal liver function tests observed with a predominantly cholestatic pattern, although transaminases may also be raised indicating hepatocellular necrosis *3406*

Hemoglobin *Blood* *Decrease* Hemolytic anemia may be observed associated with grossly abnormal liver function tests observed with a predominantly cholestatic pattern, although transaminases may also be raised indicating hepatocellular necrosis *3406*

International Normalized Ratio *Plasma* *Increase* Grossly abnormal liver function tests observed with a predominantly cholestatic pattern, although transaminases may also be raised indicating hepatocellular necrosis *3406*

Osmolal Gap *Urine* *Increase* May lead to proximal renal tubular acidosis which is associated with hypokalemia, hyperchloremic metabolic acidosis, urine pH < 5.5, increased urinary ammonium ion excretion, a negative urine anion gap, increased urinary osmol gap, normal urinary citrate, normal urinary calcium excretion and Fanconi syndrome *4071*

pH *Blood* *Decrease* Hyperchloremic acidosis. May be secondary to GI disturbance, poor food intake, or renal tubular dysfunction *4979* *4066*

271.10 Galactosemia *(continued)*

pH *(continued)*
Urine *Decrease* May lead to proximal renal tubular acidosis which is associated with hypokalemia hyperchloremic metabolic acidosis, urine pH < 5.5, increased urinary ammonium ion excretion, a negative urine anion gap, increased urinary osmol gap, normal urinary citrate, normal urinary calcium excretion and Fanconi syndrome *4071*

Phosphate *Serum* *Decrease* May lead to proximal renal tubular acidosis which is associated with hypokalemia, hyperchloremic metabolic acidosis, urine pH < 5.5, increased urinary ammonium ion excretion, a negative urine anion gap, increased urinary osmol gap, normal urinary citrate, normal urinary calcium excretion and Fanconi syndrome *4071*

Potassium *Serum* *Decrease* May lead to proximal renal tubular acidosis which is associated with hypokalemia, hyperchloremic metabolic acidosis, urine pH < 5.5, increased urinary ammonium ion excretion, a negative urine anion gap, increased urinary osmol gap, normal urinary citrate, normal urinary calcium excretion and Fanconi syndrome *4071*

Protein *Urine* *Increase* Proteinuria, indicating renal involvement, may be observed associated with grossly abnormal liver function tests observed with a predominantly cholestatic pattern, although transaminases may also be raised indicating hepatocellular necrosis *3406*

Tyrosine *Urine* *Increase* General aminoaciduria - identified by chromatography *5545* Manifestation of a renal toxicity syndrome *2216*

Uric Acid *Serum* *Decrease* May lead to proximal renal tubular acidosis which is associated with hypokalemia, hyperchloremic metabolic acidosis, urine pH < 5.5, increased urinary ammonium ion excretion, a negative urine anion gap, increased urinary osmol gap, normal urinary citrate, normal urinary calcium excretion and Fanconi syndrome *4071*

271.20 Fructose-1,6-Bisphosphatase Deficiency

Alanine *Plasma* *Increase* One of most prominent features of condition *3406*

Alanine Aminotransferase *Serum* *Increase* Usually has less severe effects on liver than fructosemia: aminotransferases mildly to moderately affected *3406*

Amino Acids *Plasma* *Increase* One of most prominent features of condition *3406*

Aspartate Aminotransferase *Serum* *Increase* Usually has less severe effects on liver than fructosemia: aminotransferases mildly to moderately affected *3406*

Bilirubin *Serum* *Increase* Usually has less severe effects on liver than fructosemia: bilirubin concentrations, at most, mildly increased *3406*

Chitotriosidase *Serum* *No Effect* Normal activity observed in both of two patients with deficiency *1917*

Glucose *Serum* *Decrease* One of most prominent features of condition *3406*

Glutamine *Plasma* *Increase* One of most prominent features of condition *3406*

Ketones *Serum* *Increase* One of most prominent features of condition *3406*

Lactate *Plasma* *Increase* One of most prominent features of condition *3406*

271.20 Fructosemia

Alanine Aminotransferase *Serum* *Increase* May be observed associated with grossly abnormal liver function tests including transaminases which may be markedly raised indicating hepatocellular necrosis *3406*

Albumin *Serum* *Decrease* May be observed associated with grossly abnormal liver function tests including transaminases which may be markedly raised indicating hepatocellular necrosis with many other abnormalities *3406*

Aspartate Aminotransferase *Serum* *Increase* May be observed associated with grossly abnormal liver function tests including transaminases which may be markedly raised indicating hepatocellular necrosis *3406*

Bilirubin *Serum* *Increase* May be observed associated with grossly abnormal liver function tests including transaminases which may be markedly raised indicating hepatocellular necrosis *3406*

Bilirubin, Conjugated *Serum* *Increase* May be observed associated with grossly abnormal liver function tests including transaminases which may be markedly raised indicating hepatocellular necrosis *3406*

Glucose *Serum* *Decrease* May be observed associated with grossly abnormal liver function tests including transaminases which may be markedly raised indicating hepatocellular necrosis with many other abnormalities *3406*

International Normalized Ratio *Plasma* *Increase* May be observed associated with grossly abnormal liver function tests including transaminases which may be markedly raised indicating hepatocellular necrosis with many other abnormalities *3406*

Phosphate *Serum* *Decrease* May be observed associated with grossly abnormal liver function tests including transaminases which may be markedly raised indicating hepatocellular necrosis with many other abnormalities *3406*

Platelets *Blood* *Decrease* May be observed associated with grossly abnormal liver function tests including transaminases which may be markedly raised indicating hepatocellular necrosis with many other abnormalities *3406*

Potassium *Serum* *Decrease* May be observed associated with grossly abnormal liver function tests including transaminases which may be markedly raised indicating hepatocellular necrosis with many other abnormalities *3406*

271.20 Hereditary Fructose Intolerance

Alanine Aminotransferase *Serum* *Increase* Marked rise was noted within 1.5 h after a single large dose of fructose *4979*

Albumin *Urine* *Increase* Develops rapidly after ingestion *4979* Characteristic symptom in small children *401*

Aldolase *Serum* *Increase* Marked rise was noted within 1.5 h after a single large dose of fructose *4979*

Amino Acids *Plasma* *Increase* Excess amino acids in serum and urine *367*
Urine *Increase* During acute intoxication, signs of a proximal tubular syndrome and of liver failure are common *900* Characteristic symptom in small children *401* Develops rapidly after ingestion *4979*

Ammonium Ions *Urine* *Increase* May lead to proximal renal tubular acidosis which is associated with hypokalemia, hyperchloremic metabolic acidosis, urine pH < 5.5, increased urinary ammonium ion excretion, a negative urine anion gap, increased urinary osmol gap, normal urinary citrate, normal urinary calcium excretion and Fanconi syndrome *4071*

Anion Gap *Urine* *Decrease* May lead to proximal renal tubular acidosis which is associated with hypokalemia, hyperchloremic metabolic acidosis, urine pH < 5.5, increased urinary ammonium ion excretion, a negative urine anion gap, increased urinary osmol gap, normal urinary citrate, normal urinary calcium excretion and Fanconi syndrome *4071*

Aspartate Aminotransferase *Serum* *Increase* Marked rise was noted within 1.5 h after a single large dose of fructose *4979*

Bicarbonate *Serum* *Decrease* May lead to proximal renal tubular acidosis which is associated with hypokalemia, hyperchloremic metabolic acidosis, urine pH < 5.5, increased urinary ammonium ion excretion, a negative urine anion gap, increased urinary osmol gap, normal urinary citrate, normal urinary calcium excretion and Fanconi syndrome *4071*

Bilirubin *Serum* *Increase* Noted with the chronic syndrome found in young children and after fructose administration in adults *4979*

Calcium *Urine* *No Effect* May lead to proximal renal tubular acidosis which is associated with hypokalemia, hyperchloremic metabolic acidosis, urine pH < 5.5, increased urinary ammonium ion excretion, a negative urine anion gap, increased urinary osmol gap, normal urinary citrate, normal urinary calcium excretion and Fanconi syndrome *4071*

Chloride *Serum* *Increase* May lead to proximal renal tubular acidosis which is associated with hypokalemia, hyperchloremic metabolic acidosis, urine pH < 5.5, increased urinary ammonium ion excretion, a negative urine anion gap, increased urinary osmol gap, normal urinary citrate, normal urinary calcium excretion and Fanconi syndrome *4071*

Citrate *Urine* *No Effect* May lead to proximal renal tubular acidosis which is associated with hypokalemia, hyperchloremic metabolic acidosis, urine pH < 5.5, increased urinary ammonium ion excretion, a negative urine anion gap, increased urinary osmol gap, normal urinary citrate, normal urinary calcium excretion and Fanconi syndrome *4071*

Fructose *Serum* *Increase* Noted with the chronic syndrome found in young children and after fructose administration in adults *4979*
Urine *Increase* Noted with the chronic syndrome found in young children and after fructose administration in adults *4979*

Glucose *Serum* *Decrease* Frequent severe attacks of hypoglycemia *4979* The causes of hypoglycemia are complex and include impairment of glycogenolysis *900*
Urine *Increase* May lead to proximal renal tubular acidosis which is associated with hypokalemia, hyperchloremic metabolic acidosis, urine pH < 5.5, increased urinary ammonium ion excretion, a negative urine anion gap, increased urinary osmol gap, normal urinary citrate, normal urinary calcium excretion and Fanconi syndrome *4071* During acute intoxication, signs of a proximal tubular syndrome and of liver failure are common *900*

Methionine *Plasma* *Increase* During acute intoxication, signs of proximal tubular syndrome and of liver failure are common *900*

Nitrogen *Serum* *Increase* Amino acid nitrogen increases as a result of deranged hepatic function after administration *4979*

Osmolal Gap *Urine* *Increase* May lead to proximal renal tubular acidosis which is associated with hypokalemia, hyperchloremic metabolic acidosis, urine pH < 5.5, increased urinary ammonium ion excretion, a negative urine anion gap, increased urinary osmol gap, normal urinary citrate, normal urinary calcium excretion and Fanconi syndrome *4071*

pH *Urine* *Decrease* May lead to proximal renal tubular acidosis which is associated with hypokalemia, hyperchloremic metabolic acidosis, urine pH < 5.5, increased urinary ammonium ion excretion, a negative urine anion gap, increased urinary osmol gap, normal urinary citrate, normal urinary calcium excretion and Fanconi syndrome *4071*
Urine *Increase* Abrupt loss of the ability to acidify urine after ingestion of fructose *4979*

Phosphate *Serum* *Decrease* May lead to proximal renal tubular acidosis which is associated with hypokalemia, hyperchloremic metabolic acidosis, urine pH < 5.5, increased urinary ammonium ion excretion, a negative urine anion gap, increased urinary osmol gap, normal urinary citrate, normal urinary calcium excretion and Fanconi syndrome *4071* Noted with the chronic syndrome found in young children and after fructose administration in adults *4979*
Urine *Increase* Phosphate reabsorption is impaired *4979*

Potassium *Serum* *Decrease* May lead to proximal renal tubular acidosis which is associated with hypokalemia, hyperchloremic metabolic acidosis, urine pH < 5.5, increased urinary ammonium ion excretion, a negative urine anion gap, increased urinary osmol gap, normal urinary citrate, normal urinary calcium excretion and Fanconi syndrome *4071*

Tyrosine *Plasma* *Increase* During acute intoxication, signs of proximal tubular syndrome and of liver failure are common *900*

Uric Acid *Serum* *Decrease* May lead to proximal renal tubular acidosis which is associated with hypokalemia, hyperchloremic metabolic acidosis, urine pH < 5.5, increased urinary ammonium ion excretion, a negative urine anion gap, increased urinary osmol gap, normal urinary citrate, normal urinary calcium excretion and Fanconi syndrome *4071*

271.30 Lactosuria

Albumin *Serum* *Decrease* A low serum albumin will reflect possible malabsorption of protein or protein-losing enteropathy *1980*

Alkaline Phosphatase *Serum* *Decrease* An indication of vitamin D and calcium malabsorption *1980*

Calcium *Serum* *Decrease* An indication of vitamin D and calcium malabsorption *1980*

Carotene *Serum* *Decrease* A useful indication of fat malabsorption, low levels are found in as many as 80% of patients with steatorrhea *1980*

Lactose *Intestinal Contents* *Increase* Deficiency of intestinal lactase results in high concentration of intraluminal lactose with osmotic diarrhea *1980*
Urine *Increase* Lactose intolerance in children and infants without lactase deficiency:lactosuria usually exists *900*

Lymphocytes *Blood* *Decrease* Often an absolute lymphopenia due to loss of lymphocytes into the small intestine *1980*

pH *Urine* *Decrease* Lactose intolerance in children and infants without lactase deficiency:renal acidosis usually exists *900*

Phosphate *Serum* *Decrease* An indication of vitamin D and calcium malabsorption *1980*

Prothrombin Time *Plasma* *Increase* An indication of vitamin K malabsorption *1980*

Triglycerides *Serum* *Decrease* Significantly decreased in the lactose malabsorption group (after taking into account the effects of other variables). Other lipids and proteins were not different from the control group *4514*

Triolein ^{131}I Test *Feces* *Positive* Positive test for lipid droplets in the stool, but results are inconsistent *1980*

271.80 Fucosidosis

Fucosidase *Fibroblasts* *Decrease* Low activity suggests fucosidosis *2952*
White Blood Cells *Decrease* Low activity suggests fucosidosis *2952*

271.80 Infantile Sialic Acid Storage Disease

Sialic Acid, Free *Urine* *Increase* Free sialic acid concentration in urine reported to be increased 10 - 200 times *5594*

271.80 Kanzaki Disease

Sialic Acid, Lipid-associated *Urine* *Increase* Bound sialic acid concentration in urine reported to be increased up to 20 times *5594*

271.80 Mannosidosis

α-Mannosidase *Fibroblasts* *Decrease* Low activity suggests α-mannosidosis *2952*
White Blood Cells *Decrease* Low activity suggests α-mannosidosis *2952*

271.80 α-Mannosidosis

Chitotriosidase *Serum* *Increase* Abnormal activity observed in 1 of 3 patients, with activity of 300 nmol/h/mL *1917*

Lysosome-associated Membrane Protein-2 *Serum* *Increase* Median concentration of 3.29 mg/L in 4 patients with α-mannosidosis with median age 4 y compared with 1.21 mg/L in 202 healthy controls aged 0 - 66 y (median 7 years) *2265*

Lysosome-associated Membrane Protein-2:Lysosome-associated Membrane Protein-1 Ratio *Serum* *Decrease* Mean ratio of 2.83 in 4 patients with α-mannosidosis with median age 4 y significantly reduced compared with 1.21 mg/L in 202 healthy controls aged 0 - 66 y (median 7 years) *2265*

271.80 β-Mannosidosis

Chitotriosidase *Serum* *No Effect* Abnormal activity observed in none of 2 patients *1917*

271.80 Primary Hyperoxaluria

Alanine:Glyoxylate Aminotransferase *Liver* *Decrease* In 30 of 39 patients with primary hyperoxaluria type 1 activity varied from 0.8 to 9.5 µmol/h/mg protein compared with activity in nine normal livers in which mean activity was 27.9 ± 7.9 µmol/h/mg protein *4478*

Ammonium *Urine* *Increase* Mean excretion in 12 patients with primary hyperoxaluria of 0.64 ± 0.39 mg/mg creatinine significantly different from 0.38 ± 0.13 mg/mg creatinine in 16 normal subjects *3497*

Bicarbonate *Urine* *No Effect* Mean excretion in 12 patients with primary hyperoxaluria 0.26 ± 0.14 mg/mg creatinine not significantly different from 0.43 ± 0.31 mg/mg creatinine in 16 normal subjects *3497*

Calcium *Urine* *No Effect* Mean excretion in 12 patients with primary hyperoxaluria of 0.11 ± 0.07 mg/mg creatinine not different from 0.11 ± 0.04 mg/mg creatinine in 16 normal subjects *3497*

Citrate *Urine* *No Effect* Mean excretion in 12 patients with primary hyperoxaluria of 0.47 ± 0.41 mg/mg creatinine not different from 0.49 ± 0.20 mg/mg creatinine in 16 normal subjects *3497*

Glycerate *Urine* *Increase* In 2 patients with primary hyperoxaluria type II mean excretion of 314 and 1,359 µg/mg creatinine substantially different from that in 58 healthy children of all ages and adults excretion (19 - 115 µg/mg creatinine) *1168*
Urine *No Effect* In 5 patients with primary hyperoxaluria type I mean excretion of < 5 to 71 µg/mg creatinine typically not different from that in 58 healthy children of all ages and adults excretion (19 - 115 µg/mg creatinine) *1168*

Glycolate *Urine* *Increase* In 5 patients with primary hyperoxaluria type I mean excretion of 53 to 281 µg/mg creatinine typically different from that in 58 healthy children of all ages and adults in whom excretion was 14 - 72 µg/mg creatinine *1168*
Urine *No Effect* In 2 patients with primary hyperoxaluria type II mean excretion of 18 and 23 µg/mg creatinine not different from that in 58 healthy children of all ages and adults in whom excretion was 14 - 72 µg/mg creatinine *1168*

Magnesium *Urine* *No Effect* Mean excretion in 12 patients with primary hyperoxaluria of 0.12 ± 0.04 mg/mg creatinine not different from 0.11 ± 0.02 mg/mg creatinine in 16 normal subjects *3497*

Oxalate *Urine* *Increase* Mean excretion in 12 patients with primary hyperoxaluria of 0.18 ± 0.13 mg/mg creatinine significantly higher than 0.02 ± 0.01 mg/mg creatinine in 16 normal subjects *3497*

Phosphate *Urine* *No Effect* Mean excretion in 12 patients with primary hyperoxaluria of 0.82 ± 0.28 mg/mg creatinine not different from 0.73 ± 0.32 mg/mg creatinine in 16 normal subjects *3497*

Pyrophosphate *Urine* *No Effect* Mean excretion in 12 patients with primary hyperoxaluria of 0.0058 ± 0.0053 mg/mg creatinine not different from 0.0050 ± 0.0030 mg/mg creatinine in 16 normal subjects *3497*

271.80 Salla Disease

N-Acetylneuraminic Acid, Free *Urine* *Increase* Excretion in 10 patients of 34.2 to 272 µmol/mmol creatinine compared with that in about 200 healthy adults aged 27 to 53 years (mean excretion of 11.8 ± 9.7 µmol/mmol creatinine) *4421*

Sialic Acid, Free *Urine* *Increase* Free sialic acid concentration in urine reported to be increased 2 - 16 times *5594*

271.80 Sialic Acid Storage Disease

Chitotriosidase *Serum* *No Effect* Normal activity observed in one patient with sialic acid storage disorder *1917*

Lysosome-associated Membrane Protein-2 *Serum* *Increase* Median concentration of 2.89 mg/L in 2 patients with sialic acid storage disease with median age 2 y compared with 1.21 mg/L in 202 healthy controls aged 0 - 66 y (median 7 years) *2265*

Lysosome-associated Membrane Protein-2:Lysosome-associated Membrane Protein-1 Ratio *Serum* *Decrease* Mean ratio of 2.80 in 2 patients with Sandhoff disease with median age 2 y significantly different when compared with 4.74 in 202 healthy controls aged 0 - 66 y (median 7 years) *2265*

271.80 Sialidosis

Chitotriosidase *Serum* *No Effect* Normal activity observed in one patient with sialidosis *1917*

Sialic Acid, Lipid-associated *Urine* *Increase* Bound sialic acid concentration in urine reported to increase 3 to 20 times *5594*

271.80 Sialuria

Sialic Acid, Free *Urine* *Increase* Free sialic acid concentration in urine reported to be increased 200 - 1500 times *5594*

271.90 Carbohydrate-Deficient Glycoprotein Syndrome

Activated Partial Thrombin Ratio *Plasma* *Increase* 9 of 23 patients had prolonged times *5824*

Antithrombin III Activity *Plasma* *Decrease* 28 of 32 patients had reduced concentrations *5824*

Antithrombin III Antigen *Plasma* *Decrease* 22 of 24 patients had reduced concentrations *5824*

Factor II *Plasma* *Decrease* 10 of 30 patients had reduced concentrations but none less than 50% *5824*

Factor V *Plasma* *Decrease* 7 of 32 patients had reduced concentrations with 6 less than 50% *5824*

Factor VII *Plasma* *Decrease* 3 of 28 patients had reduced concentrations with 1 less than 50% *5824*

Factor VIII *Plasma* *Decrease* 4 of 15 patients had reduced concentrations with 3 less than 50% *5824*

Factor IX *Plasma* *Decrease* 5 of 31 patients had reduced concentrations with 4 less than 50% *5824*

Factor X *Plasma* *Decrease* 11 of 30 patients had reduced concentrations with 3 less than 50% *5824*

Factor XI *Plasma* *Decrease* 23 of 29 patients had reduced concentrations *5824*

Factor XII *Plasma* *Decrease* 2 of 15 patients had reduced concentrations *5824*

Factor XIII *Plasma* *Decrease* None of 15 patients had reduced concentrations *5824*

Fibrinogen *Plasma* *No Effect* None of 20 patients had prolonged times *5824*

Heparin-Cofactor II *Plasma* *Decrease* 5 of 9 patients had reduced concentrations *5824*

Plasminogen *Plasma* *No Effect* None of 20 patients had reduced concentrations *5824*

α-2 Plasminogen Inhibitor Activity *Plasma* *Decrease* 3 of 16 patients had reduced concentrations *5824*

α-2 Plasminogen Inhibitor Antigen *Plasma* *Decrease* 3 of 3 patients had reduced concentrations *5824*

Protein C Activity *Plasma* *Decrease* 22 of 31 patients had reduced activity *5824*

Protein C Antigen *Plasma* *Decrease* 6 of 9 patients had reduced concentrations *5824*

Protein S Antigen *Plasma* *Decrease* 3 of 3 patients had reduced concentrations *5824*

Protein S Antigen, Free *Plasma* *Decrease* 13 of 16 patients had reduced concentrations *5824*

Protein S, Functional *Plasma* *Decrease* 2 of 3 patients had reduced activity *5824*

Prothrombin Time *Plasma* *Increase* 4 of 9 patients had prolonged times *5824*

von Willebrand Factor *Plasma* *Decrease* 1 of 12 patients had reduced concentrations *5824*

271.90 Carbohydrate-Deficient Glycoprotein Syndrome-1

Carbohydrate-deficient Transferrin *Serum Increase* Concentration increased in untreated patients (mean 219 ± 76 mg/L) compared with reference interval of 18 ± 6 mg/L *5018*

Chitotriosidase *Serum No Effect* Normal activity observed in three patients with carbohydrate-deficient glycoprotein syndrome *1917*

271.90 Galactosialidosis

Lysosome-associated Membrane Protein-2 *Serum Increase* Concentration of 8.77 mg/L in one patient with galactosialidosis with age 16 years compared with 1.21 mg/L in 202 healthy controls aged 0 - 66 y (median 7 years) *2265*

Lysosome-associated Membrane Protein-2:Lysosome-associated Membrane Protein-1 Ratio *Serum Decrease* Ratio of 5.31 in one patient with gangliosialidosis aged 16 years not significantly higher compared with 4.74 in 202 healthy controls aged 0 - 66 y (median 7 years) *2265*

Sialic Acid, Lipid-associated *Urine Increase* Bound sialic acid concentration in urine reported to increase 3 to 5 times *5594*

271.90 Glutaricacidemia I

Chitotriosidase *Serum No Effect* Normal activity observed in none of three patients with condition *1917*

Disorders of Lipid Metabolism

272.00 Familial Hypercholesterolemia

Antibodies to LDL-Cholesterol, Oxidized *Serum Decrease* In 26 patients homozygous for familial hypercholesterolemia (9 with CAD) median antibody titer of 325.5 significantly different from 854.5 in 10 healthy controls *3974*

Ascorbic Acid *Serum No Effect* In 25 patients with familial hypercholesterolemia mean concentration of 49.29 ± 11.24 µmol/L not significantly different from reference interval of 22.88 - 100.89 µmol/L *2295*

Cholesterol *Serum Increase* In 25 patients with familial hypercholesterolemia mean concentration of 8.78 ± 1.66 mmol/L significantly greater than reference interval of 4.1 - 6.2 mmol/L *2295* In five patients with familial hypercholesterolemia geographically dispersed throughout the UK mean concentration of 11.5 mmol/L significantly higher than in healthy individuals *5632* In 63 children with untreated familial hypercholesterolemia mean concentration of 8.6 ± 1.5 mmol/L significantly higher than 4.6 ± 0.8 mmol/L in 30 healthy control children *5251* In 26 patients homozygous for familial hypercholesterolemia (9 with CAD) mean concentration of 16.4 ± 3.54 mmol/L significantly different from 4.59 ± 0.89 mmol/L in 10 healthy controls *3974*

Coenzyme Q_{10} *Serum Increase* In 25 patients with familial hypercholesterolemia mean concentration of 1,519 ± 503 nmol/L significantly different from reference interval of 9 - 85 nmol/L *2295*

Epinephrine *Plasma No Effect* Concentration in both untreated and treated patients not significantly different from controls *422*
Platelets No Effect Concentration in both untreated and untreated patients not significantly different from that in controls *422*

HDL-Cholesterol *Serum Decrease* In 26 patients homozygous for familial hypercholesterolemia (9 with CAD) mean concentration of 0.72 ± 0.28 mmol/L significantly different from 1.41 ± 0.53 mmol/L in 10 healthy controls *3974*
Serum No Effect In 25 patients with familial hypercholesterolemia, mean concentration of 1.15 ± 0.34 mmol/L not significantly different from reference interval of 0.9 - 1.6 mmol/L *2295*

LDL-Cholesterol *Serum Increase* In 25 patients with familial hypercholesterolemia mean concentration of 7.09 ± 1.59 mmol/L significantly greater than reference interval of 2.6 - 3.14 mmol/L *2295* In 26 patients homozygous for familial hypercholesterolemia (9 with CAD) mean concentration of 14.92 ± 3.54 mmol/L significantly different from 2.62 ± 0.78 mmol/L in 10 healthy controls *3974* In five patients with familial hypercholesterolemia geographically dispersed throughout the UK mean concentration of 9.4 mmol/L significantly higher than in healthy individuals *5632*

Lipoprotein Lp(a) *Serum Increase* Patients with condition have increased concentrations of Lp(a) *2827*

Norepinephrine *Plasma Increase* Plasma concentrations 36% higher in treated patients and 116% higher in untreated patients compared with controls *422* In untreated patients concentration 40% higher than in controls: concentration in treated patients no different from controls *422*

Retinol *Serum No Effect* In 25 patients with familial hypercholesterolemia mean concentration of 2.69 ± 0.63 µmol/L not significantly different from reference interval of 0.8 - 3.5 µmol/L *2295*

α-Tocopherol *Serum No Effect* In 63 children with untreated familial hypercholesterolemia mean concentration of 34 µmol/L not significantly higher than 30 µmol/L in 30 healthy control children *5251* In 25 patients with familial hypercholesterolemia mean concentration of 43.0 ± 6.2 µmol/L not significantly different from reference interval of 12.0 - 42.0 µmol/L *2295*

α-Tocopherol:Lipids Ratio *Serum Decrease* In 63 children with untreated familial hypercholesterolemia mean ratio of 3.3 significantly different from 5.1 in 30 healthy control children *5251*

Triglycerides *Serum Increase* In 26 patients homozygous for familial hypercholesterolemia (9 with CAD) mean concentration of 1.52 ± 1.82 mmol/L not significantly different from 1.10 ± 0.32 mmol/L in 10 healthy controls *3974* In 63 children with untreated familial hypercholesterolemia mean concentration of 1.1 ± 0.6 mmol/L significantly higher than 0.8 ± 0.4 mmol/L in 30 healthy control children *5251*

272.00 Familial Hypercholesterolemia (Heterozygous)

Antibodies to LDL-Cholesterol, Oxidized *Serum No Effect* In 20 patients heterozygous for familial hypercholesterolemia and without CAD median antibody titer of 684 not significantly different from 854.5 in 10 healthy controls *3974*

Apolipoprotein A-I *Serum Decrease* In 82 Greek patients with familial heterozygous hypercholesterolemia mean concentration of 133 ± 34 mg/dL significantly different from 149 ± 28 mg/dL in 82 healthy controls *1331*

Apolipoprotein B *Serum Increase* In 82 Greek patients with familial heterozygous hypercholesterolemia mean concentration of 247 ± 70 mg/dL significantly different from 126 ± 38 mg/dL in 82 healthy controls *1331*

Cholesterol *Serum Increase* In 3 women aged 62.6 ± 11.3 years mean concentration of 356.0 ± 28.7 mg/dL *2219* In 82 Greek patients with familial heterozygous hypercholesterolemia mean concentration of 363 ± 86 mg/dL significantly different from 180 ± 45 mg/dL in 82 healthy controls *1331* In 20 patients heterozygous for familial hypercholesterolemia and without CAD mean concentration of 9.93 ± 1.29 mmol/L significantly different from 4.59 ± 0.89 mmol/L in 10 healthy controls *3974*

HDL-Cholesterol *Serum Decrease* In 82 Greek patients with familial heterozygous hypercholesterolemia mean concentration of 50 ± 15 mg/dL significantly different from 57 ± 13 mg/dL in 82 healthy controls *1331*
Serum No Effect In 20 patients heterozygous for familial hypercholesterolemia and without CAD mean concentration of 1.23 ± 0.34 mmol/L not significantly different from 1.41 ± 0.53 mmol/L in 10 healthy controls *3974*

LDL-Cholesterol *Serum Increase* In 20 patients heterozygous for familial hypercholesterolemia and without CAD mean concentration of 7.98 ± 1.27 mmol/L not significantly different from 2.62 ± 0.78 mmol/L in 10 healthy controls *3974* In 82 Greek patients with familial heterozygous hypercholesterolemia mean concentration of 278 ± 83 mg/dL significantly different from 118 ± 46 mg/dL in 82 healthy controls *1331*

Lipoprotein Lp(a) *Serum Increase* In 82 Greek patients with familial heterozygous hypercholesterolemia mean concentration of 14.5 mg/dL significantly different from 0.8 - 34.5 mg/dL in 82 healthy controls *1331*

272.00 Familial Hypercholesterolemia (Heterozygous) *(continued)*

Triglycerides *Serum* *Increase* In 20 patients heterozygous for familial hypercholesterolemia and without CAD mean concentration of 1.58 ± 0.76 mmol/L not significantly different from 1.10 ± 0.32 mmol/L in 10 healthy controls *3974*
Serum *No Effect* In 82 Greek patients with familial heterozygous hypercholesterolemia mean concentration of 130 ± 102 mmol/L not significantly different from 110 ± 70 mg/dL in 82 healthy controls *1331*

272.00 Familial Hyperlipoproteinemia (Heterozygous)

Cholesterol Ester Transfer Protein *Serum* *Increase* In 3 women aged 62.6 ± 11.3 years mean activity of 166.0 ± 48.0 units *2219*

HDL-Cholesterol *Serum* *No Effect* In 3 women aged 62.6 ± 11.3 years mean concentration of 50.3 ± 11.0 mg/dL *2219*

Triglycerides *Serum* *Increase* In 3 women aged 62.6 ± 11.3 years mean concentration of 131.6 ± 82.5 mg/dL *2219*

272.00 Hypercholesterolemia

Activated Natural Killer Cells *Blood* *No Effect* Mean concentration of 30 ± 25 /µL in 19 men with hypocholesterolemia not significantly different from 38 ± 25 /µL in 39 men with hypercholesterolemia *3647*

Antithyroid Antibodies *Serum* *Increase* In 87 hypercholesterolemic patients 22 (25%) had positive antithyroid antibodies compared to 5 (6%) controls *3980*

Apolipoprotein A-I *Serum* *No Effect* In 19 patients with primary hypercholesterolemia mean concentration of 1.51 ± 0.27 g/L not different from normal range *906*

Apolipoprotein B *Serum* *Increase* In 19 patients with primary hypercholesterolemia mean concentration of 1.50 ± 0.11 g/L different from normal range *906*

Ascorbic Acid *Serum* *No Effect* In 21 patients with familial hypercholesterolemia mean concentration of 53.83 ± 17.37 µmol/L not significantly different from reference interval of 22.88 - 100.89 µmol/L *2295*

Calprotectin *Plasma* *No Effect* In 1 patient mean concentration of 450 µg/L not significantly different from normal range of 80 - 880 µg/L in women and 150 - 910 µg/L in men *2169*

Carnitine *Serum* *Increase* In 71 women with mean plasma cholesterol concentration greater than 6.5 mmol/L, median carnitine concentration of 42 µmol/L significantly higher than 38 µmol/L in 147 women with cholesterol concentration less than 6.5 mmol/L. In 59 men with cholesterol concentration greater than 6.5 mmol/L median total carnitine concentration of 47 µmol/L significantly greater than 43 µmol/L in 138 men with cholesterol less than 6.5 mmol/L *542*

Carnitine, Free *Serum* *Increase* Median concentration of 35 µmol/L in 71 women with plasma cholesterol concentrations greater than 6.5 mmol/L significantly greater than 31 µmol/L in 147 women with cholesterol concentrations less than 6.5 mmol/L *542*

CD16+ Lymphocytes *Blood* *No Effect* Mean concentration of 220 ± 115 /µL in 19 men with hypocholesterolemia not significantly different from 199 ± 90 /µL in 39 men with hypercholesterolemia *3647*

Cholesterol *Neutrophils* *Decrease* In 12 hypercholesterolemic patients mean concentration of 4.19 fmol/cell significantly higher than 3.10 fmol/cell in 20 normolipidemic healthy controls *1043*
Serum *Decrease* Mean concentration of 261.2 ± 35.0 mg/dL in 39 men with hypercholesterolemia *3647*
Serum *Increase* In 19 patients with primary hypercholesterolemia mean concentration of 6.7 ± 0.5 mmol/L significantly different from normal range *906* Mean concentration in 11 individuals with hypercholesterolemia 7.89 ± 0.94 mmol/L significantly greater than 5.3 ± 0.9 mmol/L in 20 healthy controls *4257* Mean concentration in 57 hypercholesterolemic men of 7.16 ± 0.75 mmol/L significantly different from 5.23 ± 0.64 mmol/L in 56 normocholesterolemic healthy controls *4854* In 21 patients with nonfamilial hypercholesterolemia mean concentration of 7.97 ± 1.41 mmol/L significantly greater than reference interval of 4.1 - 6.2 mmol/L *2295* In 39 patients with hypercholesterolemia but asymptomatic for peripheral artery disease mean concentration of 7.3 ± 1.2 mmol/L significantly different from 5.5 ± 1.0 mmol/L in 132 age and sex matched asymptomatic controls *477*

Cholesterol Ester Transfer *Serum* *Increase* In 19 patients with primary hypercholesterolemia mean rate of 251 ± 125 nmol/mL/6 h different from normal range *906*

Cholesterol Ester Transfer Protein *Serum* *Increase* In 19 patients with primary hypercholesterolemia mean activity of 37.9 ± 12.2 nmol/mL plasma/ h different from normal range *906*

Coenzyme Q_{10} *Serum* *Increase* In 21 patients with nonfamilial hypercholesterolemia mean concentration of 1,409 ± 347 nmol/L significantly different from reference interval of 9 - 85 nmol/L *2295*

Cytotoxic Suppressor T-Cells *Blood* *Increase* Mean concentration of 320 ± 133 /µL in 19 men with hypocholesterolemia significantly different from 425 ± 132 /µL in 39 men with hypercholesterolemia *3647*

Endothelin-1 *Plasma* *Increase* In one study of 13 patients with hypercholesterolemia mean concentration increased 1.8 times above normal *328*

Fibrinogen *Plasma* *Increase* In 39 patients with hypercholesterolemia but asymptomatic for peripheral artery disease mean concentration of 3.3 ± 0.6 g/L significantly different from 3.0 ± 0.5 g/L in 132 age and sex matched asymptomatic controls *477*

HDL-Cholesterol *Serum* *Decrease* In 39 patients with hypercholesterolemia but asymptomatic for peripheral artery disease mean concentration of 1.39 ± 0.36 mmol/L significantly different from 1.45 ± 0.34 mmol/L in 132 age and sex matched asymptomatic controls *477*
Serum *Increase* In a hypercholesterolemic man mean concentration of 2.33 mmol/L artecactually increased when serum cholesterol concentration was 47.4 mmol/L *2726* In 19 patients with primary hypercholesterolemia mean concentration of 1.18 ± 0.31 mmol/L significantly different from normal range *906*
Serum *No Effect* Mean concentration of 45.0 ± 10.2 mg/dL in 39 men with hypercholesterolemia *3647* In 21 patients with nonfamilial hypercholesterolemia mean concentration of 1.38 ± 0.39 mmol/L not significantly different from reference interval of 0.9 - 1.6 mmol/L *2295*

Hepatocyte Growth Factor *Serum* *No Effect* In 16 patients with peripheral arterial disease and hypercholesterolemia mean concentration of 0.37 ± 0.03 ng/mL not significantly different from 0.43 ± 0.03 ng/mL in 21 normocholesterolemic patients with peripheral arterial disease *5817*

Homocysteine *Plasma* *No Effect* Mean concentration in individuals being screened for cardiac risk factors showed mean concentration of 9.4 ± 1.3 µmol/L in 134 hypercholesterolemics not significantly different from mean of 9.4 ± 1.3 µmol/L in 126 normocholesterolemics *3251*

Insulin *Plasma* *No Effect* In 11 patients with hypercholesterolemia mean concentration of 10.1 ± 3.8 µU/mL not significantly greater than 9.2 ± 2.8 µU/mL in 20 healthy controls *4257*

Interleukin-2 *Serum* *Increase* Mean concentration of 868 ± 616 pg/mL in 19 men with hypocholesterolemia significantly different from 1212 ± 747 pg/mL in 39 men with hypercholesterolemia *3647*

LDL-Cholesterol *Serum* *Increase* In 21 patients with nonfamilial hypercholesterolemia mean concentration of 6.01 ± 1.03 mmol/L significantly greater than reference interval of 2.6 - 3.14 mmol/L *2295* Mean concentration in 57 hypercholesterolemic men of 5.18 ± 0.76 mmol/L significantly different from 3.50 ± 0.56 mmol/L in 56 normocholesterolemic healthy controls *4854* In 19 patients with primary hypercholesterolemia mean concentration of 4.8 ± 0.5 mmol/L significantly different from normal range *906* Mean concentration of 185.5 ± 31.9 mg/dL in 39 men with hypercholesterolemia *3647* In 39 patients with hypercholesterolemia but asymptomatic for peripheral artery disease mean concentration of 5.1 ± 0.7 mmol/L significantly different from 3.4 ± 0.9 mmol/L in 132 age and sex matched asymptomatic controls *477*

Lymphocyte B-Cells *Blood* *No Effect* Mean concentration of 174 ± 148 /µL in 19 men with hypocholesterolemia not significantly different from 228 ± 130 /µL in 39 men with hypercholesterolemia *3647*

Lymphocyte T-Cells *Blood* *Increase* Mean concentration of 1,051 ± 298 /μL in 19 men with hypocholesterolemia significantly different from 1,303 ± 393 /μL in 39 men with hypercholesterolemia *3647*

Lymphocyte T-Helper Cells *Blood* *Increase* Mean concentration of 662 ± 244 /μL in 19 men with hypocholesterolemia significantly different from 831 ± 339 /μL in 39 men with hypercholesterolemia *3647*

Lymphocytes *Blood* *Increase* Mean concentration of 1,483 ± 402 /μL in 19 men with hypocholesterolemia significantly different from 1,771 ± 488 /μL in 39 men with hypercholesterolemia *3647*

Plasminogen Activator Inhibitor *Plasma* *No Effect* In 11 patients with hypercholesterolemia mean activity of 13.4 ± 8 U/mL not significantly greater than 9.76 ± 5.38 U/mL in 20 healthy controls *4257*

Retinol *Serum* *No Effect* In 102 patients with primary hypercholesterolemia mean concentration of 3.46 ± 0.08 μmol/L not significantly different from 3.32 ± 0.09 μmol/L in 70 normocholesterolemic controls *3641* In 21 patients with nonfamilial hypercholesterolemia mean concentration of 2.98 ± 0.83 μmol/L not significantly different from reference interval of 0.8 - 3.5 μmol/L *2295*

Sodium *Serum* *Decrease* In a hypercholesterolemic man mean concentration of 110 mmol/L as measured by indirect potentiometric method at a time when serum cholesterol concentration was 47.4 mmol/L *2726*

Soluble Intercellular Adhesion Molecule-1 *Serum* *No Effect* In 39 patients with hypercholesterolemia but asymptomatic for peripheral artery disease, mean concentration of 281 ± 95 ng/mL not significantly different from 298 ± 103 ng/mL in 132 age and sex matched asymptomatic controls *477*

Soluble Vascular Cell Adhesion Molecule-1 *Serum* *No Effect* In 39 patients with hypercholesterolemia but asymptomatic for peripheral artery disease mean concentration of 546 ± 94 ng/mL not significantly different from 595 ± 159 ng/mL in 132 age and sex matched asymptomatic controls *477*

Thyroid Stimulating Hormone *Serum* *Increase* In 8 of 87 hypercholesterolemic patients plasma TSH concentration above 5 mU/L, i.e. they had subclinical hypothyroidism whereas all normocholesterolemic patients had normal thyroid function. Hypercholesterolemic patients had on average a significantly higher TSH than the controls *3980*

α-Tocopherol *Serum* *No Effect* In 21 patients with nonfamilial hypercholesterolemia mean concentration of 47.7 ± 11.7 μmol/L not significantly different from reference interval of 12.0 - 42.0 μmol/L *2295*

Triglycerides *Serum* *Increase* Mean concentration of 161.9 ± 80.4 mg/dL in 39 men with hypercholesterolemia *3647* In 19 patients with primary hypercholesterolemia mean concentration of 2.0 ± 0.7 mmol/L significantly different from normal range *906* Mean concentration in 57 hypercholesterolemic men of 1.35 ± 0.44 mmol/L significantly different from 0.98 ± 0.46 mmol/L in 56 normocholesterolemic healthy controls *4854* In 39 patients with hypercholesterolemia but asymptomatic for peripheral artery disease mean concentration of 1.8 mmol/L significantly different from 1.4 mmol/L in 132 age and sex matched asymptomatic controls *477*
Serum *No Effect* In 11 hypercholesterolemic patients mean concentration of 1.33 ± 0.38 mmol/L not significantly different from 1.23 ± 0.21 mmol/L in 20 healthy controls *4257*

Ubiquinone *Serum* *Increase* In 20 hypercholesterolemic men range of concentrations varied from 1.1 - 3.0 mg/L compared with mean concentration of 1.36 mg/L in healthy individuals with concentrations ranging from 0.57 - 3.03 mg/L. 95% confidence interval of 1.21 - 1.50 mg/L *2881*

Vitamin E *Red Blood Cells* *Decrease* Mean erythrocyte concentration in 57 hypercholesterolemic men of 3.27 ± 0.70 μmol/L significantly different from 3.78 ± 1.10 μmol/L in 56 normocholesterolemic healthy controls *4854*
Serum *Increase* Mean plasma concentration in 57 hypercholesterolemic men of 42.49 ± 10.02 μmol/L significantly different from 33.06 ± 7.48 μmol/L in 56 normocholesterolemic healthy controls *4854*

272.00 Hypercholesterolemia Type II

Endothelin-1 *Plasma* *Increase* In 12 with type II hypercholesterolemia mean concentrations increased 1.1-fold above appropriate normal range *328*

272.00 Hyperlipoproteinemia Type IIa

Albumin *Serum* *Decrease* Reduced, while the serum γ-globulin fraction is increased *5544* *1290*

Calcium *Serum* *Increase* The greatest increment being in the protein-bound calcium form *1025*

Carotene *Serum* *Increase* Increased concentration carried in β-lipoproteins is easily visible *2033*

Cholesterol *Serum* *Increase* In 10 healthy hyperlipoproteinemic type IIa individuals (3 men, 7 women) aged 62.5 ± 6.3 years mean concentration of 288.9 ± 29.1 mg/dL *2219* Manifested by high cholesterol concentration in low density lipoproteins. Generally 2 times normal mean for heterozygotes and 6 times normal in homozygotes *4979* The plasma is clear even with extremely elevated cholesterol *1980*

Cholesterol Ester Transfer Protein *Serum* *Increase* In 10 individuals (3 men, 7 women) aged 62.5 ± 6.3 years mean activity of 128.1 ± 51.2 units *2219*

Dehydroepiandrosterone *Plasma* *Decrease* Observed effect *602* *5679* *5229*

β-Globulin *Serum* *Increase* Marked increase due to primary xanthomatosis *1290*

γ-Globulin *Serum* *Increase* Serum albumin is reduced, while the serum γ-globulin fraction is increased *1290* *5544*

Glucose Tolerance *Serum* *No Effect* Usually not affected by disease *1980* Tolerance usually unaffected by disease *2033*

HDL-Cholesterol *Serum* *No Effect* Observed effect *5864* In 10 individuals (3 men, 7 women) aged 62.5 ± 6.3 years mean concentration of 57.3 ± 10.3 mg/dL *2219*

LDL-Cholesterol *Serum* *Increase* Observed effect *5864*

β-Lipoprotein *Serum* *Increase* Observed response *367* Marked increase *5544* Characterized by an increase in β-lipoproteins clearly visible on electrophoresis *2304*

Lipoproteins, Pre-β *Serum* *No Effect* No significant effect observed *1025*

Phospholipids *Serum* *Increase* Moderate elevation in heterozygotes and marked in homozygotes *4979* Elevated, but not as high as cholesterol *2033*

Triglycerides *Serum* *Increase* Occasionally. Usually normal in heterozygotes but may at times be > 250 mg/dL *4979* Normal to elevated at 100 - 400 mg/dL *1980* Usually a marked elevation of plasma cholesterol and a modest elevation of plasma triglyceride *2304* In 10 individuals (3 men, 7 women) aged 62.5 ± 6.3 years mean concentration of 127.3 ± 21.1 mg/dL *2219*

Uric Acid *Serum* *Increase* Common *2033*
Serum *No Effect* Not affected by disease *1980*

VLDL-Cholesterol *Serum* *No Effect* Observed effect *5864*

272.00 Hyperproteinemia Type II

Albumin *Serum* *No Effect* In 16 patients with type II hyperproteinemia mean value of 41 ± 3 g/L not significantly different from 41 ± 3 g/L in 16 normal controls *5308*

Cholesterol *Serum* *Increase* In 16 patients with type II hyperproteinemia mean concentration of 270 mg/dL significantly greater than the upper limit of normal *5308*

Fibrinogen *Plasma* *Increase* In 16 patients with type II hyperproteinemia mean concentration of 270 mg/dL significantly greater than the mean of 259 mg/dL in 16 normal controls *5308*

Hematocrit *Blood* *No Effect* In 16 patients with type II hyperproteinemia mean value of 42.6 ± 3.3% not significantly different from 39.9 ± 3.1% in 16 normal controls *5308*

Protein *Serum* *No Effect* In 16 patients with type II hyperproteinemia mean value of 72 ± 3 g/L not significantly different from 70 ± 6 g/L in 16 normal controls *5308*

Triglycerides *Serum* *Increase* In 16 patients with type II hyperproteinemia mean concentration of 251 mg/dL significantly greater than the upper limit of normal *5308*

272.00 Hyperproteinemia Type II (continued)

Triglycerides *(continued)*
Serum *No Effect* In 16 patients with type II hyperproteinemia mean concentration of 44 mg/dL within the limits of normal *5308*

Viscosity *Plasma* *Increase* In 16 patients with type II hyperproteinemia mean viscosity of 1.39 mPa/s significantly greater than the mean of 1.28 mPa/s in 16 normal controls *5308*

272.10 Familial Hypertriglyceridemia

Apolipoprotein A-I *Serum* *Decrease* Mean concentration of 70.4 ± 2.7 mg/dL in 6 lean patients significantly less than 106.9 ± 7.0 mg/dL in healthy controls *4525*

Apolipoprotein A-II *Serum* *Decrease* In 6 lean patients with familial hypertriglyceridemia mean concentration of 24.2 ± 1.6 mg/dL significantly lower than 39.2 ± 0.9 mg/dL *4525*

Apolipoprotein B-48 in Triglyceride-rich Lipoproteins
Serum *Increase* In 10 patients with familial hypertriglyceridemia mean concentration of 3.4 ± 1.0 mg/dL significantly different from normal *3950*

Apolipoprotein B-100 in Triglyceride-rich Lipoproteins
Serum *Increase* In 10 patients with familial hypertriglyceridemia mean concentration of 15.6 ± 6.8 mg/dL significantly different from normal *3950*

Apolipoprotein B in Triglyceride-rich Lipoproteins
Serum *Increase* In 10 patients with familial hypertriglyceridemia mean concentration of 19.0 ± 7.6 mg/dL significantly different from normal *3950*

Cholesterol *Serum* *Increase* In 10 patients with familial hypertriglyceridemia mean concentration of 6.71 ± 0.41 mmol/L moderately increased but significantly different from normal *3950*

Erythrocyte Aggregation *Blood* *No Effect* In 10 patients with familial hypertriglyceridemia mean aggregation was within reference range of 3.5 - 5.0 at stasis and 8.0 - 11.0 at shear rate 3/s *3950*

Fibrinogen *Plasma* *No Effect* In 10 patients with familial hypertriglyceridemia mean concentration was within reference range of 1.5 - 4.0 g/L *3950*

HDL_2-Cholesterol *Serum* *Decrease* In 10 patients with familial hypertriglyceridemia mean concentration of 0.13 ± 0.02 mmol/L significantly different from normal *3950*

HDL_3-Cholesterol *Serum* *Decrease* In 10 patients with familial hypertriglyceridemia mean concentration of 0.55 ± 0.03 mmol/L significantly different from normal *3950*

HDL-Cholesterol *Serum* *Decrease* In 10 patients with familial hypertriglyceridemia mean concentration of 0.67 ± 0.04 mmol/L significantly different from normal *3950*

LDL-Cholesterol *Serum* *Decrease* In 10 patients with familial hypertriglyceridemia mean concentration of 2.34 ± 0.28 mmol/L significantly different from normal *3950*

Triglyceride-rich Lipoprotein Cholesterol *Serum* *Increase* In 10 patients with familial hypertriglyceridemia mean concentration of 3.69 ± 0.59 mmol/L significantly different from normal *3950*

Triglyceride-rich Lipoprotein Triglycerides *Serum* *Increase* In 10 patients with familial hypertriglyceridemia mean concentration of 8.21 ± 1.53 mmol/L significantly different from normal *3950*

Triglycerides *Serum* *Increase* In 10 patients with familial hypertriglyceridemia mean concentration of 9.53 ± 1.72 mmol/L significantly different from normal *3950*

Viscosity *Blood* *No Effect* In 10 patients with familial hypertriglyceridemia mean concentration was within upper-reference range of 3.5 - 5.0 mPa *3950*
Plasma *No Effect* In 10 patients with familial hypertriglyceridemia mean concentration was within upper-reference range of 1.20 - 1.40 mPa *3950*

272.10 Hyperlipoproteinemia Type IV

Apolipoprotein B *Serum* *Increase* Mean concentration in 8 patients with type IV hyperlipoproteinemia of 150 ± 10 mg/dL significantly different from 104 ± 6 mg/dL in 8 normolipidemic controls *1561*

Apolipoprotein C-III *Serum* *Increase* Mean concentration in 8 patients with type IV hyperlipoproteinemia of 37.6 ± 4.4 mg/dL significantly different from 10.0 ± 1.0 mg/dL in 8 normolipidemic controls *1561*

Apolipoprotein E *Serum* *Increase* Mean concentration in 8 patients with type IV hyperlipoproteinemia of 7.3 ± 1.0 mg/dL significantly different from 3.7 ± 0.3 mg/dL in 8 normolipidemic controls *1561*

Cholesterol *Serum* *Increase* Mean concentration in 8 patients with type IV hyperlipoproteinemia of 5.76 ± 0.40 mmol/L significantly different from 4.37 ± 0.21 mmol/L in 8 normolipidemic controls *1561* The percentage of esterified cholesterol in plasma and the esterification rate were always reduced when the triglyceride concentration exceeded 600 mg/dL and the rate of esterification rose significantly with appropriate triglyceride-lowering therapy in patients with hypertriglyceridemia *1824* An increase in cholesterol of about 1 mg/dL for each 5 mg/dL increase in triglyceride concentration *1564*
Serum *No Effect* Concentration normal or only slightly increased *367* Usually found to be normal or only moderately elevated *2304*

Cholinesterase *Serum* *Increase* Both GGT and pseudocholinesterase were increased in hypertriglyceridemic subjects. Both strongly correlated with the logarithm of serum triglyceride and the prebeta electrophoretic fraction. Increase of GGT was rather characteristic for gross hypertriglyceridemia *978*

Dehydroepiandrosterone *Plasma* *Decrease* Observed effect *5679* *5229* *602*

Glucose *Serum* *Increase* Hyperglycemia is only occasionally severe enough to produce symptoms of diabetes *367*

Glucose Tolerance *Serum* *Decrease* Present in 19 of 36 patients (52%) *1761* Occurs in most patients but not with sufficient constancy to indicate a role in causing the disorder *4979*

γ-Glutamyltransferase *Serum* *Increase* Both GGT and pseudocholinesterase were increased in hypertriglyceridemic subjects. Both strongly correlated with the logarithm of serum triglyceride and the prebeta electrophoretic fraction. Increase of GGT was rather characteristic for gross hypertriglyceridemia *978*

HDL-Cholesterol *Serum* *Decrease* Decreased *4746* Mean concentration in 8 patients with type IV hyperlipoproteinemia of 0.67 ± 0.03 mmol/L significantly different from 1.13 ± 0.10 mmol/L in 8 normolipidemic controls *1561*

Hemoglobin A_{1c} *Blood* *Increase* Triglyceride concentrations greater than 1,750 mg/dL would falsely raise the HbA1 levels *3278*

Insulin *Plasma* *Increase* Occurs in most patients but not with sufficient constancy to indicate a role in causing the disorder *4979*

LDL-Cholesterol *Serum* *No Effect* Observed effect *5864*

Lipoproteins, Pre-β *Serum* *Increase* Type IV hyperlipemia is manifested as hyper-preβ-lipoproteinemia. This is associated with an increase in triglycerides above normal limits and is commonly accompanied by a rise in cholesterol of about 1 mg/dL for each 5 mg/dL increase in triglyceride concentration *1564* Characteristic lipid abnormality is an increase in plasma triglyceride and VLDL cholesterol levels *2304* Preβ-lipoproteins alone are generally increased *367*

Triglycerides *Serum* *Increase* Mean concentration in 8 patients with type IV hyperlipoproteinemia of 5.55 ± 0.45 mmol/L significantly different from 0.84 ± 0.10 mmol/L in 8 normolipidemic controls *1561* Elevated, sometimes to an extreme degree *1980* Characteristic increase in plasma triglyceride and VLDL cholesterol levels *2304* Seldom exceeds 1,000 mg/dL. Cholesterol is usually < half when triglyceride exceeds 500 mg/dL *900* Values of 200 - 500 mg/dL are common *4979*

Uric Acid *Serum* *Increase* Occurs in most patients but not with sufficient constancy to indicate a role in causing the disorder *4979* Hyperuricemia is common *367* 9 of 22 patients *4979*

VLDL-Cholesterol *Serum* *Increase* Observed effect *5864*

272.20 Hyperlipoproteinemia Type III

Apolipoprotein A-I *Serum* *Decrease* Decreased concentration of both low and high density lipoproteins *3602* There is generally a decrease in α- and β-lipoproteins *1565* An excess of lipoproteins with beta mobility but abnormally low density *1566* Slight to moderately decreased *4979*

Apolipoprotein B *Serum Increase* Mean concentration in 8 patients with type III hyperlipoproteinemia of 130 ± 8 mg/dL significantly different from 104 ± 6 mg/dL in 8 normolipidemic controls *1561*

Apolipoprotein C-III *Serum Increase* Mean concentration in 8 patients with type III hyperlipoproteinemia of 33.1 ± 3.4 mg/dL significantly different from 10.0 ± 1.0 mg/dL in 8 normolipidemic controls *1561*

Apolipoprotein E *Serum Increase* Mean concentration in 8 patients with type III hyperlipoproteinemia of 27.1 ± 2.5 mg/dL significantly different from 3.7 ± 0.3 mg/dL in 8 normolipidemic controls *1561*

Cholesterol *Serum Increase* Usually > 300 mg/dL *4979* Mean concentration in 8 patients with type III hyperlipoproteinemia of 8.08 ± 0.66 mmol/L significantly different from 4.37 ± 0.21 mmol/L in 8 normolipidemic controls *1561*

Dehydroepiandrosterone *Plasma Decrease* Observed effect *5679 5229 602*

β-Globulin *Serum Increase* Marked increase due to essential hyperlipemia *1290*

Glucose *Serum Increase* Fasting hyperglycemia and ketosis are uncommon *4979*

Glucose Tolerance *Serum Decrease* In roughly 55% of cases *4979*

HDL-Cholesterol *Serum Decrease* Mean concentration in 8 patients with type III hyperlipoproteinemia of 0.80 ± 0.07 mmol/L significantly different from 1.13 ± 0.10 mmol/L in 8 normolipidemic controls *1561*
Serum No Effect Observed effect *5864*

Ketones *Serum Increase* Fasting hyperglycemia and ketosis are uncommon *4979*

LDL-Cholesterol *Serum Increase* Observed effect *5864*

Lipids *Serum Increase* Diagnosis of abnormal lipoproteins can be done when the lipids are at normal concentration, but most patients are hyperlipidemic before they are diagnosed *4979*

β-Lipoprotein *Serum Decrease* There is generally a decrease in α- and β-lipoproteins *1565* Slight to moderately decreased *4979*

Lipoprotein Lp(a) *Serum No Effect* Mean concentration of 14.1 ± 19.1 mg/dL in 76 patients not significantly different from 13.3 ± 16.2 mg/dL in 76 healthy age- and sex-matched controls *1473*

α-Lipoproteins *Serum Decrease* There is generally a decrease in α- and β-lipoproteins *1565*

Lipoproteins, Pre-β *Serum Increase* VLDL defined as including all lipoproteins of density < 1.006 *4979* An increase in very low density lipoproteins of abnormal composition is the basis for type III diagnosis *3602*

Triglycerides *Serum Increase* Increased in all 49 cases of type III *3602* Cholesterol and triglycerides are usually elevated to a similar extent; levels often exceed 400 mg/dL *900* Mean concentration in 8 patients with type III hyperlipoproteinemia of 5.76 ± 0.62 mmol/L significantly different from 0.84 ± 0.10 mmol/L in 8 normolipidemic controls *1561* Usually concentrations range from 200 - 800 mg/dL, and tend to exceed cholesterol concentration *4979*

Uric Acid *Serum Increase* In 40% of patients *4979* Occurs in 15 - 20% of patients *1290*

VLDL-Cholesterol *Serum Increase* Observed effect *5864*

272.20 Hyperlipoproteinemia Type IIb

Albumin *Serum Decrease* Reduced, while the serum γ-globulin fraction is increased *5544 1290*

Calcium *Serum Increase* The greatest increment being in the protein-bound calcium form *1025*

Carotene *Serum Increase* Increased concentration carried in β-lipoproteins is easily visible *2033*

Cholesterol *Serum Increase* In 9 individuals (4 men, 5 women) aged 57.3 ± 7.6 years mean concentration of 273.3 ± 25.9 mg/dL *2219* Median concentration of 3.10 ± 0.47 g/L in 12 patients with hyperlipidemia type IIb significantly increased above 2.25 ± 0.32 g/L after 8 weeks treatment with simvastatin *2890* Manifested by high cholesterol concentration in low density lipoproteins. Generally 2 times normal mean for heterozygotes and 6 times normal in homozygotes *4979* The plasma is clear even with extremely elevated cholesterol *1980*

Cholesterol Ester Transfer Protein *Serum Increase* Median concentration of CETP of 2.46 ± 0.79 mg/L in 12 patients with hyperlipidemia type IIb significantly different from 2.07 ± 0.58 mg/L after 8 weeks treatment with simvastatin *2890*
Serum No Effect In 9 individuals (4 men, 5 women) aged 57.3 ± 7.6 years mean concentration of 100.8 ± 43.8 units *2219*

Dehydroepiandrosterone *Plasma Decrease* Observed effect *5229 602 5679*

β-Globulin *Serum Increase* Marked increase due to primary xanthomatosis *1290*

γ-Globulin *Serum Increase* Serum albumin is reduced, while the serum γ-globulin fraction is increased *1290 5544*

Glucose Tolerance *Serum No Effect* No significant effect observed *2033 1980*

HDL-Cholesterol *Serum Decrease* In 9 individuals (4 men, 5 women) aged 57.3 ± 7.6 years mean concentration of 41.7 ± 12.3 mg/dL *2219*
Serum No Effect Observed effect *5864* Median concentration of 0.42 ± 0.09 g/L in 12 patients with hyperlipidemia type IIb significantly increased above 0.44 ± 0.10 g/L after 8 weeks treatment with simvastatin *2890*

HDL-Cholesterol Esters *Serum No Effect* Median concentration of HDL-cholesterol esters of 0.48 ± 0.12 g/L in 12 patients with hyperlipidemia type IIb not significantly different from 0.51 ± 0.13 g/L after 8 weeks treatment with simvastatin *2890*

HDL-Cholesterol, Free *Serum No Effect* Median concentration of HDL-unesterified cholesterol of 0.10 ± 0.02 g/L in 12 patients with hyperlipidemia type IIb not significantly different from 0.10 ± 0.02 g/L after 8 weeks treatment with simvastatin *2890*

HDL-Phospholipids *Serum No Effect* Median concentration of HDL-phospholipids of 0.92 ± 0.21 g/L in 12 patients with hyperlipidemia type IIb not significantly different from 0.94 ± 0.16 g/L after 8 weeks treatment with simvastatin *2890*

HDL-Triglycerides *Serum No Effect* Median concentration of HDL-triglycerides of 0.25 ± 0.08 g/L in 12 patients with hyperlipidemia type IIb not significantly different from 0.23 ± 0.05 g/L after 8 weeks treatment with simvastatin *2890*

LDL-Cholesterol *Serum Increase* Median concentration of 2.23 ± 0.54 g/L in 12 patients with hyperlipidemia type IIb significantly increased above 1.36 ± 0.33 g/L after 8 weeks treatment with simvastatin *2890* Serum cholesterol level is elevated, equal to, or greater than the triglyceride level; both LDL and VLDL are increased *367 5864*

β-Lipoprotein *Serum Increase* Characterized by an increase in β-lipoproteins clearly visible on electrophoresis *2304* Serum cholesterol level is elevated, equal to or > triglyceride level, both LDL and VLDL are increased *367* Marked increase *5544*

Lipoproteins, Pre-β *Serum Increase* May be elevated *2033*

Phospholipids *Serum Increase* Moderate elevation in heterozygotes and marked in homozygotes *4979* Elevated, but not as high as cholesterol *2033*

Triglycerides *Serum Increase* Serum cholesterol and triglycerides are usually elevated to a similar extent. Neither generally exceeds 400 mg/dL and triglyceride levels are not more than 100 mg/dL higher than cholesterol levels *900* Median concentration of 2.41 ± 0.34 g/L in 12 patients with hyperlipidemia type IIb significantly increased above 2.33 ± 1.15 g/L after 8 weeks treatment with simvastatin *2890* In 9 individuals (4 men, 5 women) aged 57.3 ± 7.6 years mean concentration of 236.1 ± 38.0 mg/dL *2219*
Serum No Effect Usually normal in heterozygotes but may at times be > 250 mg/dL *4979* Normal to elevated at 100 - 400 mg/dL *1980* Occasionally normal *2034*

Uric Acid *Serum Increase* Common *2033*
Serum No Effect Usually concentration normal *1980*

VLDL-Cholesterol *Serum Increase* Serum cholesterol level is elevated, equal to, or greater than triglyceride level. Both LDL and VLDL are increased *5864 367*

272.30 Hyperlipoproteinemia Type I

Alanine Aminotransferase *Serum* *No Effect* Usually unaffected by disease *4979*

Amylase *Serum* *Increase* During bouts of abdominal pain *4979*

Apolipoprotein A-I *Serum* *Decrease* Decreased concentration of both low and high density lipoproteins *3602* There is generally a decrease in α- and β-lipoproteins in hyperlipoproteinemia *1565* Characteristic observation *1566*

Aspartate Aminotransferase *Serum* *No Effect* Usually unaffected by disease *4979*

Cholesterol *Serum* *Increase* Moderate elevation *900*

Cholesterol, Free *Serum* *Increase* The unesterified cholesterol proportion may be as high as 50% *4979* The proportion of free cholesterol is elevated to about 50% instead of 30% *1565*

Chylomicrons *Serum* *Increase* Chylomicronemia develops as soon as fat is ingested, and the disorder has been diagnosed during the 1st week of life *367* Characterized by the presence of chylomicrons in high concentration in plasma 14 h or more after the last meal of normal diet *1565* Heavy chylomicronemia and subnormal concentrations of all other lipoproteins. A qualitative abnormality which is not a specific marker for a single genetic disease. Occurs in familial lipoprotein lipase deficiency *4979*

Dehydroepiandrosterone *Plasma* *Decrease* Observed effect *5229* *5679* *602*

β-Globulin *Serum* *Increase* Marked increase due to essential hyperlipemia *1290*

Glucose Tolerance *Serum* *Decrease* May follow pancreatitis, but is not a feature of uncomplicated disease *4979*

HDL-Cholesterol *Serum* *Decrease* Observed effect *5864*

Hematocrit *Blood* *No Effect* Usually unaffected by disease *4979*

Hemoglobin *Blood* *No Effect* Usually unaffected by disease *4979*

Hemoglobin A_{1c} *Blood* *Increase* Triglyceride concentrations greater than 1,750 mg/dL would falsely raise the HbA1 levels *3278*

Lactate Dehydrogenase *Serum* *No Effect* Usually unaffected by disease *4979*

LDL-Cholesterol *Serum* *No Effect* Observed effect *5864*

Lipase *Serum* *Increase* During bouts of abdominal pain *4979*

β-Lipoprotein *Serum* *Decrease* There is generally a decrease in α- and β-lipoproteins *1565*

Lipoproteins *Serum* *Decrease* Heavy chylomicronemia and subnormal concentrations of all other lipoproteins. (Type I hyperlipoproteinemia) is a qualitative abnormality which is not a specific marker for a single genetic disease. Occurs in familial lipoprotein lipase deficiency *4979*

α-Lipoproteins *Serum* *Decrease* There is generally a decrease in α- and β-lipoproteins *1565*

Lipoproteins, Pre-β *Serum* *Decrease* Normal or decreased *1025*
Serum *Increase* May be raised *2034*

Oxygen Saturation *Blood* *Increase* Hemoglobin-oxygen affinity is increased *1184*

Triglycerides *Serum* *Increase* Often exceed 1,000 mg/dL with only moderate elevation of cholesterol *900* Grossly elevated, range from 2,500 - 12,000 mg/dL in lipoprotein lipase deficiency *4979*

VLDL-Cholesterol *Serum* *No Effect* Observed effect *5864*

272.30 Hyperlipoproteinemia Type V

Amylase *Serum* *Increase* During bouts of abdominal pain *4979*

Apolipoprotein A-I *Serum* *Decrease* In severely affected patients *4979* Reduced pools of α- and β-lipoproteins *4859*

Cholesterol *Serum* *Increase* Usually abnormally high, although initial normal values are frequently found *4979* In 11 patients with Type V hyperlipoproteinemia, concentration ranged from 212 - 1,512 mg/dL *4859*

Chylomicrons *Serum* *Increase* Chylomicronemia and hyperpreβ-lipoproteinemia *4859* In severely affected patients *4979*

Dehydroepiandrosterone *Plasma* *Decrease* Observed effect *5229* *5679* *602*

Glucose Tolerance *Serum* *Decrease* More than 75% of patients *1761* Abnormal in 80% *4979*

HDL-Cholesterol *Serum* *Decrease* Observed effect *5864*

Hemoglobin A_{1c} *Blood* *Increase* Triglyceride concentrations greater than 1,750 mg/dL would falsely raise the HbA1 levels *3278*

LDL-Cholesterol *Serum* *No Effect* Observed effect *5864*

Lipase *Serum* *Increase* During bouts of abdominal pain *4979*

β-Lipoprotein *Serum* *Decrease* In severely affected patients *4979* Chylomicronemia and hyperpreβ-lipoproteinemia were accompanied by reduction in pools of β- and α-lipoproteins *4859*

α-Lipoproteins *Serum* *Decrease* Hyperpreβ-lipoproteinemia accompanied by low α- and β-lipoproteins *4859*

Lipoproteins, Pre-β *Serum* *Increase* In severely affected patients *4979* Hyperpreβ-lipoproteinemia accompanied by low α- and β-lipoproteinemia *4859*

Sodium *Serum* *Decrease* Lipemia was associated with significant hyponatremia *4859*

Triglycerides *Serum* *Increase* Averages 10 - 20 times normal *4979* In 11 patients with type V hyperlipoproteinemia *4859*

Uric Acid *Serum* *Increase* Common in type V *1859* In 40% of patients *4979*

VLDL-Cholesterol *Serum* *Increase* Observed effect *5864*

272.40 Familial Combined Hyperlipidemia

Apolipoprotein A-I *Serum* *No Effect* In 30 individuals with familial combined hyperlipidemia mean concentration of 1,223 ± 263 mg/L not significantly different from 1,219 ± 204 mg/L in 56 clinically healthy controls *4342*

Apolipoprotein B *Serum* *Increase* In 30 individuals with familial combined hyperlipidemia mean concentration of 1,221 ± 226 mg/L significantly different from 837 ± 213 mg/L in 56 clinically healthy controls *4342*

Apolipoprotein C-II *Serum* *Increase* In 30 individuals with familial combined hyperlipidemia mean concentration of 66 ± 13 mg/L significantly different from 47 ± 5 mg/L in 56 clinically healthy controls *4342*

Apolipoprotein C-III *Serum* *Increase* In 30 individuals with familial combined hyperlipidemia mean concentration of 145 ± 30 mg/L significantly different from 109 ± 20 mg/L in 56 clinically healthy controls *4342*

Cholesterol *Serum* *Increase* In 30 individuals with familial combined hyperlipidemia mean concentration of 6.47 ± 0.93 mmol/L significantly greater than 4.92 ± 0.91 mmol/L in 56 clinically healthy controls *4342* Mean concentration in 53 patients with FCHL of 282 ± 48 mg/dL significantly increased compared with 226 ± 44 mg/dL in 347 healthy controls *1521*

HDL_2-Cholesterol *Serum* *Decrease* In 30 individuals with familial combined hyperlipidemia mean concentration of 0.17 ± 0.09 mmol/L not significantly lower than 0.27 ± 0.15 mmol/L in 56 clinically healthy controls *4342*

HDL_3-Cholesterol *Serum* *Decrease* In 30 individuals with familial combined hyperlipidemia mean concentration of 0.92 ± 0.28 mmol/L not significantly lower than 1.05 ± 0.26 mmol/L in 56 clinically healthy controls *4342*

HDL-Cholesterol *Serum* *Decrease* In 53 patients with FCHL mean concentration of 39 ± 8 mg/dL significantly less than 57 ± 16 mg/dL in 347 healthy controls *1521* In 30 individuals with familial combined hyperlipidemia mean concentration of 1.09 ± 0.33 mmol/L not significantly lower than 1.32 ± 0.35 mmol/L in 56 clinically healthy controls *4342*

IDL-Cholesterol *Serum* *Increase* In 30 individuals with familial combined hyperlipidemia mean concentration of 0.38 ± 0.27 mmol/L significantly greater than 0.15 ± 0.09 mmol/L in 56 clinically healthy controls *4342*

IDL-Triglycerides *Serum* *Increase* In 30 individuals with familial combined hyperlipidemia mean concentration of 0.24 ± 0.12 mmol/L significantly greater than 0.12 ± 0.05 mmol/L in 56 clinically healthy controls *4342*

LDL-Cholesterol *Serum* *Increase* In 30 individuals with familial combined hyperlipidemia mean concentration of 4.34 ± 0.87 mmol/L significantly greater than 3.27 ± 0.76 mmol/L in 56 clinically healthy controls *4342* Mean concentration of 181 ± 43 mg/dL in 53 patients with FCHL significantly higher than 142 ± 40 mg/dL in 347 healthy controls *1521*

LDL-Triglycerides *Serum* *Increase* In 30 individuals with familial combined hyperlipidemia mean concentration of 0.36 ± 0.13 mmol/L significantly greater than 0.25 ± 0.08 mmol/L in 56 clinically healthy controls *4342*

Lipoprotein Lp(a) *Serum* *Decrease* In 30 individuals with familial combined hyperlipidemia mean concentration of 208 ± 179 mg/L not significantly lower than 230 ± 140 mg/L in 56 clinically healthy controls *4342*
Serum *No Effect* Mean concentration in 53 patients not significantly different from that in 347 healthy control individuals, although distribution markedly shifted towards right (median 17 mg/dL). In controls distribution shifted towards left (median 11 mg/dL). Concentration not significantly different between patients with and without coronary artery disease *1521*

Retinol *Serum* *Decrease* In 30 individuals with familial combined hyperlipidemia mean concentration of 1.96 ± 0.83 μmol/L significantly different from 2.91 ± 1.23 μmol/L in 56 clinically healthy controls *4342*

Triglycerides *Serum* *Increase* In 30 individuals with familial combined hyperlipidemia mean concentration of 1.82 ± 0.83 mmol/L significantly greater than 0.99 ± 0.53 mmol/L in 56 clinically healthy controls *4342* Mean concentration in 53 patients with FCHL of 311 ± 99 mg/dL significantly higher than 126 ± 76 mg/dL in 347 healthy controls *1521*

VLDL-Cholesterol *Serum* *Increase* In 30 individuals with familial combined hyperlipidemia mean concentration of 0.65 ± 0.47 mmol/L significantly greater than 0.20 ± 0.17 mmol/L in 56 clinically healthy controls *4342*

VLDL-Triglycerides *Serum* *Increase* In 30 individuals with familial combined hyperlipidemia mean concentration of 1.11 ± 0.67 mmol/L significantly greater than 0.46 ± 0.42 mmol/L in 56 clinically healthy controls *4342*

272.40 Hyperlipidemia

α_1-Acid Glycoprotein *Serum* *No Effect* Mean concentration in 35 patients with hyperlipidemia of 0.85 ± 0.20 g/L not significantly different from mean of 0.75 ± 0.20 g/L in 32 normolipidemic controls *5631*

Adenosine-N6-diethylthioether-N1-pyridinoximine 5'-phosphate *Serum* *No Effect* In 3 patients with hyperlipidemia concentrations ranged from 98.3 - 223.8 nmol/dL not significantly different from concentration in healthy individuals in whom the mean concentration was 162.2 nmol/dL *5294*

Albumin *Serum* *No Effect* Mean concentration in 35 patients with hyperlipidemia of 45 ± 3 g/L not significantly different from mean of 46 ± 2 g/L in 32 normolipidemic controls *5631*

α_1-Antitrypsin *Serum* *Decrease* Mean concentration in 35 patients with hyperlipidemia of 1.9 ± 0.3 g/L significantly different from mean of 2.1 ± 0.3 g/L in 32 normolipidemic controls *5631*

Apolipoprotein A-I *Serum* *Decrease* Mean concentration in 103 patients with hyperlipidemia of 1.58 ± 0.32 g/L different from 1.85 ± 0.27 g/L in 110 healthy controls *4002*
Serum *No Effect* In 61 patients with serum cholesterol concentration greater than 2.5 g/L mean concentration of 1.41 ± 0.04 g/L not significantly different from 1.41 ± 0.05 g/L in 50 healthy individuals *1942*

Apolipoprotein B *Serum* *Increase* In 61 patients with serum cholesterol concentration greater than 2.5 g/L mean concentration of 1.68 ± 0.05 g/L significantly greater than 0.99 ± 0.04 g/L in 50 healthy individuals *1942* Mean concentration in 103 patients with hyperlipidemia of 1.63 ± 0.72 g/L different from 1.11 ± 0.31 g/L in 110 healthy controls *4002*

CA 549 *Serum* *Increase* In 11 patients with hyperlipidemia 2 had a concentration of 11 U/mL, 2 with a concentration of 12 U/mL and 1 with a concentration of 13 U/mL with an upper limit of normal of 11 U/mL *5260*

Ceruloplasmin *Serum* *No Effect* Mean concentration in 35 patients with hyperlipidemia of 0.27 ± 0.05 g/L not significantly different from mean of 0.29 ± 0.13 g/L in 32 normolipidemic controls *5631*

Cholesterol *Serum* *Increase* Mean concentration in 35 patients with hyperlipidemia of 7.0 ± 0.8 mmol/L significantly different from mean of 5.1 ± 0.8 mmol/L in 32 normolipidemic controls *5631* In 26 patients with hyperlipidemia mean concentration of 6.6 ± 2.4 mmol/L not significantly different from 5.1 ± 1.4 mmol/L in 19 healthy controls *3403* In 61 patients with serum cholesterol concentration greater than 2.5 g/L mean concentration of 3.07 ± 0.06 g/L significantly greater than 2.12 ± 0.06 g/L in 50 healthy individuals *1942* Mean concentration in 103 patients with hyperlipidemia of 7.15 ± 1.63 mmol/L significantly different from 4.71 ± 0.89 mmol/L in 110 healthy controls *4002*

Endothelin *Plasma* *Increase* In 61 patients with serum cholesterol concentration greater than 2.5 g/L mean concentration of 1.75 ± 0.16 ng/L significantly greater than 0.86 ± 0.08 ng/L in 50 healthy individuals *1942*

Fibrinogen *Plasma* *Increase* Mean concentration in 35 patients with hyperlipidemia of 3.0 ± 0.5 g/L significantly different from mean 2.7 ± 0.3 g/L in 32 normolipidemic controls *5631*

Haptoglobin *Serum* *No Effect* Mean concentration in 35 patients with hyperlipidemia of 1.9 ± 0.7 g/L not significantly different from mean of 1.5 ± 0.8 g/L in 32 normolipidemic controls *5631*

HDL-Cholesterol *Serum* *Decrease* Mean concentration in 35 patients with hyperlipidemia of 1.1 ± 0.3 mmol/L significantly different from mean of 1.4 ± 0.4 mmol/L in 32 normolipidemic controls *5631*
Serum *No Effect* Mean concentration in 103 patients with hyperlipidemia of 1.36 ± 0.44 mmol/L not different from 1.43 ± 0.31 mmol/L in 110 healthy controls *4002* In 61 patients with serum cholesterol concentration greater than 2.5 g/L mean concentration of 0.57 ± 0.03 g/L not significantly greater than 0.43 ± 0.02 g/L in 50 healthy individuals *1942*

Immunoglobulin G *Serum* *No Effect* Mean concentration in 35 patients with hyperlipidemia of 11 ± 2 g/L not significantly different from mean of 12 ± 3 g/L in 32 normolipidemic controls *5631*

LDL-Cholesterol *Serum* *Increase* Mean concentration in 117 patients with uremia of 4.62 ± 1.54 mmol/L different from 2.6 ± 0.6 mmol/L in 110 healthy controls *4002* In 61 patients with serum cholesterol concentration greater than 2.5 g/L mean concentration of 2.10 ± 0.08 g/L significantly greater than 1.45 ± 0.07 g/L in 50 healthy individuals *1942* Mean concentration in 35 patients with hyperlipidemia of 4.8 ± 0.6 mmol/L significantly different from mean of 3.2 ± 0.6 mmol/L in 32 normolipidemic controls *5631*

Lipoprotein Lp(a) *Serum* *Increase* In 61 patients with serum cholesterol concentration greater than 2.5 g/L mean concentration of 503 ± 70 U/L significantly greater than 234 ± 36 U/L in 50 healthy individuals *1942*

Paraoxonase *Serum* *Decrease* Mean concentration in 103 patients with hyperlipidemia of about 163 U/mL different from about 190 U/mL in 110 healthy controls *4002*

Phosphate *Serum* *Increase* In vitro artefactual cause of hyperphosphatemia if colorimetric methods used *5204*

SP2 *Serum* *No Effect* 2 of 11 patients with hyperlipidemia had a concentration of 14 U/mL when the upper limit of normal was 14 U/mL with 9 having lower concentrations *5260*

Triglycerides *Serum* *Increase* Mean concentration in 103 patients with hyperlipidemia of 2.53 ± 1.81 mmol/L different from 1.06 ± 0.52 mmol/L in 110 healthy controls *4002* In 61 patients with hyperlipidemia with serum cholesterol concentration greater than 2.5 g/L mean concentration of 2.70 ± 0.34 g/L significantly greater than 1.17 ± 0.12 g/L in 50 healthy individuals *1942* Mean concentration in 35 patients with hyperlipidemia of 2.7 ± 2.3 mmol/L significantly different from mean of 1.1 ± 0.6 mmol/L in 32 normolipidemic controls *5631*

Ubiquinol:Cholesterol Ratio *Serum* *No Effect* In 26 patients with hyperlipidemia mean ratio of 0.21 ± 0.07 μmol/mmol not significantly different from 0.22 ± 0.05 μmol/mmol in 19 healthy controls *3403*

272.50 A-β-lipoproteinemia

Alanine Aminotransferase *Serum* *Increase* Two subjects *4979*

272.50 A-β-lipoproteinemia *(continued)*

Apolipoprotein A *Serum* *Decrease* In 3 patients with a-β-lipoproteinemia concentrations of 63, 76 and 56 mg/dL significantly reduced compared with normal values of 115 - 190 mg/dL *5278*

Apolipoprotein A-I *Serum* *Increase* Highly variable *4979* *Serum* *No Effect* No significant abnormality observed *1790*

Apolipoprotein B *Serum* *Decrease* In 3 patients with a-β-lipoproteinemia concentrations of 20, 20 and 20 mg/dL significantly reduced compared with normal values of 70 - 160 mg/dL *5278* Urine is almost always hypertonic to plasma *126* Individuals with abetalipoproteinemia have no detectable apo B. People who are heterozygous for hypolipoproteinemia have concentrations that are approximately 50% of those of unaffected first degree relatives *2952*

Bilirubin *Serum* *Increase* Reflects increased RBC turnover *3479*

Carotene *Serum* *Decrease* Very low *1790*

Cholesterol *Serum* *Decrease* Diagnosis is established by finding very low cholesterol concentration (about 50 mg/dL): the lowest serum cholesterol level in any disease *1290* In 3 patients with a-β-lipoproteinemia concentrations of 46, 65 and 43 mg/dL significantly reduced compared with normal values of < 270 mg/dL *5278* Markedly reduced. Average < 50 mg/dL *392* *4979*

Chylomicrons *Serum* *Decrease* None present *1790* Complete absence of chylomicrons *367* Totally absent *4979*

Coombs' Test *Serum* *Negative* Reported observation *319*

Erythrocyte Sedimentation Rate *Blood* *Decrease* High percentage of acanthocytes results in low ESR *4979*

Erythrocyte Survival *Red Blood Cells* *Decrease* Usually shortened, but may be normal *5603* *4979* *4688*

Fat *Feces* *Increase* Marked impairment of GI fat absorption *5544* By 4th or 5th year of life, steatorrhea becomes less marked *4979*

Fatty Acids (FFA), Free *Serum* *Decrease* Slightly diminished or at low normal concentrations *239* *3479*

Folate *Serum* *Decrease* Secondary to malabsorption of fat *4536*

Haptoglobin *Serum* *Decrease* Reflects increased red cell turnover *4855*

HDL-Cholesterol *Serum* *No Effect* In 3 patients with a-β-lipoproteinemia concentrations of 43, 61 and 41 mg/dL not significantly different when compared with normal values of 41 - 58 mg/dL in men and 48 - 75 mg/dL in women *5278*

Hematocrit *Blood* *Decrease* Anemia has been described *4979* Severe anemia with hemoglobin as low as 4 - 8 g/dL is common in children. Most adult patients do not have significant anemia *4979* *3479*

Hemoglobin *Blood* *Decrease* Severe anemia with hemoglobin as low as 4 - 8 g/dL is common in children. Most adult patients do not have significant anemia *4979* *3479*

Iron *Serum* *No Effect* Concentration usually normal *5603*

LDL-Cholesterol *Serum* *Decrease* Absent *126* In 3 patients with a-β-lipoproteinemia concentrations of 0, 2 and 1 mg/dL significantly reduced compared with normal values of 108 - 188 mg/dL *5278*

Lipids *Serum* *Decrease* Concentration of all major lipids reduced to 50% of normal *4979* In 3 patients with a-β-lipoproteinemia total lipid concentrations of 35, 204 and 147 mg/dL significantly reduced compared with normal values of 500 - 700 mg/dL *5278*

β-Lipoprotein *Serum* *Decrease* Complete absence of LDL *367* None present *1790*

Lipoproteins *Serum* *Decrease* Only alpha lipoproteins are present *367*

Lipoproteins, Pre-β *Serum* *Decrease* Absent or below standard measuring capabilities *4979* None present *1790*

Phospholipids *Serum* *Decrease* Wide range of variation. Reduced by approximately 75% *4979* *2478*

Phytanic Acid *Serum* *Increase* Characteristic *2034*

Poikilocytes *Blood* *Increase* Acanthocytosis of 50 - 70% *4979*

Protein *Urine* *Increase* Proteinuria is an early finding and patients ultimately develop renal failure *2039*

Prothrombin Time *Plasma* *Increase* Abnormal bleeding is rare *239* Frequently prolonged, secondary to vitamin K malabsorption *1181*

Reticulocytes *Blood* *Increase* Reflects increased RBC turnover *3479*

Triglycerides *Serum* *Decrease* Usually below accurate measuring capabilities of conventional laboratory methods *4979* In 3 patients with a-β-lipoproteinemia concentrations of 0, 0 and 0 mg/dL significantly reduced compared with normal values of 60 - 165 mg/dL in men and 40 - 140 mg/dL in women *5278*

Vitamin A *Serum* *Decrease* Very low *1790*

Vitamin B_{12} *Serum* *No Effect* Concentration usually normal *3479*

Vitamin B_{12} Binding Capacity *Serum* *No Effect* Concentration usually normal *3479*

Vitamin E *Serum* *Decrease* Very low concentration *2547* In 3 patients with a-β-lipoproteinemia concentrations of 0, 0 and 0.28 mg/L significantly reduced compared with normal values of 0.5 - 15 mg/L *5278*

VLDL-Cholesterol *Serum* *Decrease* In 3 patients with a-β-lipoproteinemia concentrations of 3, 2 and 1 mg/dL significantly reduced compared with normal values of < 60 mg/dL *5278* Absent *126*

272.50 Abetalipoproteinemia

Lipoprotein Lp(a) *Serum* *Decrease* Patients with condition have extremely low concentrations of Lp(a) *2827*

272.50 Hypoalphalipoproteinemia

Apolipoprotein A-I *Serum* *Decrease* In 5 patients with primary hypoalphalipoproteinemia mean concentration of 112.2 ± 4.9 mg/dL lower than 156.6 ± 8.7 mg/dL in 5 healthy controls *1544*

Apolipoprotein A-II *Serum* *Decrease* In 5 patients with primary hypoalphalipoproteinemia mean concentration of 29.8 ± 1.9 mg/dL lower than 40.8 ± 2.5 mg/dL in 5 healthy controls *1544*

Cholesterol *Serum* *Increase* In 5 patients with primary hypoalphalipoproteinemia mean concentration of 232.0 ± 15.7 mg/dL higher than 209.7 ± 52.4 mg/dL in 5 healthy controls *1544*

HDL_2-Cholesterol *Serum* *Decrease* In 5 patients with primary hypoalphalipoproteinemia mean concentration of 6.7 ± 1.3 mg/dL lower than 16.7 ± 3.9 mg/dL in 5 healthy controls *1544*

HDL_3-Cholesterol *Serum* *Decrease* In 5 patients with primary hypoalphalipoproteinemia mean concentration of 26.5 ± 2.2 mg/dL lower than 36.3 ± 6.3 mg/dL in 5 healthy controls *1544*

HDL-Cholesterol *Serum* *Decrease* In 5 patients with primary hypoalphalipoproteinemia mean concentration of 33.2 ± 2.1 mg/dL lower than 53.0 ± 5.2 mg/dL in 5 healthy controls *1544*

LDL-Cholesterol *Serum* *Increase* In 5 patients with primary hypoalphalipoproteinemia mean concentration of 170.4 ± 14.6 mg/dL higher than 136.7 ± 40.5 mg/dL in 5 healthy controls *1544*

Triglycerides *Serum* *Increase* In 5 patients with primary hypoalphalipoproteinemia mean concentration of 142.0 ± 17.0 mg/dL higher than 100.0 ± 28.5 mg/dL in 5 healthy controls *1544*

272.50 Hypocholesterolemia

Activated Natural Killer Cells *Blood* *No Effect* Mean concentration of 30 ± 25 /µL in 19 men with hypocholesterolemia not significantly different from 38 ± 25 /µL in 39 men with hypercholesterolemia *3647*

$CD16^+$ Lymphocytes *Blood* *No Effect* Mean concentration of 220 ± 115 /µL in 19 men with hypocholesterolemia not significantly different from 199 ± 90 /µL in 39 men with hypercholesterolemia *3647*

Cholesterol *Serum* *Decrease* Mean concentration of 151.1 ± 16.5 mg/dL in 19 men with hypocholesterolemia *3647*

Cytotoxic Suppressor T-Cells *Blood* *Decrease* Mean concentration of 320 ± 133 /µL in 19 men with hypocholesterolemia significantly different from 425 ± 132 /µL in 39 men with hypercholesterolemia *3647*

HDL-Cholesterol *Serum* *No Effect* Mean concentration of 42.7 ± 10.3 mg/dL in 19 men with hypocholesterolemia *3647*

Interleukin-2 *Serum* *Decrease* Mean concentration of 868 ± 616 pg/mL in 19 men with hypocholesterolemia significantly different from 1,212 ± 747 pg/mL in 39 men with hypercholesterolemia *3647*

LDL-Cholesterol *Serum* *Decrease* Mean concentration of 88.3 ± 10.3 mg/dL in 19 men with hypocholesterolemia *3647* *Serum* *No Effect* Mean concentration of 103.9 ± 67.0 mg/dL in 19 men with hypocholesterolemia *3647*

Lymphocyte B-Cells *Blood* *No Effect* Mean concentration of 174 ± 148 /µL in 19 men with hypocholesterolemia not significantly different from 228 ± 130 /µL in 39 men with hypercholesterolemia *3647*

Lymphocyte T-Cells *Blood* *Decrease* Mean concentration of 1,051 ± 298 /µL in 19 men with hypocholesterolemia significantly different from 1,303 ± 393 /µL in 39 men with hypercholesterolemia *3647*

Lymphocyte T-Helper Cells *Blood* *Decrease* Mean concentration of 662 ± 244 /µL in 19 men with hypocholesterolemia significantly different from 831 ± 339 /µL in 39 men with hypercholesterolemia *3647*

Lymphocytes *Blood* *Decrease* Mean concentration of 1,483 ± 402 /µL in 19 men with hypocholesterolemia significantly different from 1,771 ± 488 /µL in 39 men with hypercholesterolemia *3647*

Natural Killer Cell Activity *Blood* *No Effect* Mean activity of 71.8 ± 30.3 cytoxicity units in 19 men with hypocholesterolemia not significantly different from 66.1 ± 23.4 cytoxicity units in 39 men with hypercholesterolemia *3647*

272.50 Lecithin Acyl Transferase Deficiency

Chitotriosidase *Serum* *No Effect* Normal activity observed in one patient with LCAD-deficiency *1917*

Lipoprotein Lp(a) *Serum* *Decrease* Patients with condition have no detectable concentrations of Lp(a) *2827*

272.50 Long-chain Acyl CoA Dehydrogenase Deficiency

Leukotriene B_4 *Urine* *No Effect* Median excretion in 4 patients with LCAD deficiency of < 5 nmol/mol creatinine not different from < 5 nmol/mol creatinine in 25 normal individuals *3385*

w-Carboxy-Leukotriene B_4 *Urine* *No Effect* Median excretion in 4 patients with LCAD deficiency of < 5 nmol/mol creatinine not different from < 5 nmol/mol creatinine in 25 normal individuals *3385*

w-Carboxy-Tetranor-Leukotriene B_4 *Urine* *No Effect* Median excretion in 4 patients with LCAD deficiency of < 5 nmol/mol creatinine not different from < 5 nmol/mol creatinine in 25 normal individuals *3385*

272.50 Tangier Disease

Apolipoprotein A-I *Serum* *Decrease* Congenital absence or gross reduction *5544* Electrophoretically absent, irrespective of the medium used *4979* Congenital absence or gross reduction *1290* Almost none *367* Individuals with Tangier disease have less than 1% of the normal amounts of HDL and apolipoprotein A-I *2952*

Carotene *Serum* *Decrease* Tends to be low, probably due to the absence of high and low density lipoproteins, not malabsorption *4979* Occasionally low *1790*

Cholesterol *Red Blood Cells* *No Effect* Typically observed *4979*
Serum *Decrease* Unique combination of low cholesterol and high triglycerides is indicative. Ranges from 40 - 125 mg/dL *4746* Ranges from 30 - 125 mg/dL *4979*

Chylomicrons *Serum* *Increase* Frequently *4979*

β-Lipoprotein *Serum* *Decrease* Levels tend to be reduced *367*

Partial Thromboplastin Time *Plasma* *Increase* Occasionally prolonged PTT, with normal prothrombin time *4979*

Phospholipids *Red Blood Cells* *No Effect* Typically observed *4979*
Serum *Decrease* Typically 30 - 50% below normal *4979* Observed effect *2733*

Prothrombin Time *Plasma* *No Effect* Occasionally prolonged PTT, with normal prothrombin time *4979*

Triglycerides *Serum* *Increase* Unique combination of low cholesterol and high triglycerides is indicative *4979* Concentrations range from 150 - 330 mg/dL *4979* Slight increase in homozygotes *367*
Serum *No Effect* May be normal in the postabsorptive state *4979* Observed in some patients *4979*

Vitamin A *Serum* *Decrease* Occasionally low *1790*
Serum *No Effect* Concentration usually normal *4979*

Vitamin E *Serum* *Decrease* One subject *4979*

272.50 Zellweger Syndrome

Chitotriosidase *Serum* *No Effect* Normal activity observed in one patient with condition *1917*

Leukotriene B_4 *Urine* *Increase* Median excretion in 10 patients with Zellweger syndrome of 97 nmol/mol creatinine significantly greater than < 5 nmol/mol creatinine in 25 normal individuals *3385*

w-Carboxy-Leukotriene B_4 *Urine* *Increase* Median excretion in 10 patients with Zellweger syndrome of 898 nmol/mol creatinine significantly greater than < 5 nmol/mol creatinine in 25 normal individuals *3385*

w-Carboxy-Tetranor-Leukotriene B_4 *Urine* *Increase* Median excretion in 10 patients with Zellweger syndrome of < 5 nmol/mol creatinine not significantly greater than < 5 nmol/mol creatinine in 25 normal individuals *3385*

272.70 Anderson's Disease

Alanine Aminotransferase *Serum* *Increase* Liver involvement *4979*

Aspartate Aminotransferase *Serum* *Increase* Liver involvement *4979*

Cholesterol *Serum* *Increase* Significant elevations generally occur in the glycogen storage diseases *4707*

Glucose *Serum* *Decrease* Usually low *4707*

Lactate *Blood* *Increase* Significant elevations generally occur in the glycogen storage diseases *4707*

Lipids *Serum* *Increase* Total lipids are significantly elevated *4707*

Uric Acid *Serum* *Increase* Significant elevations generally occur in the glycogen storage diseases *4707*

272.70 Fabry's Disease

Ammonium Ions *Urine* *Increase* May be associated with classic distal renal tubular acidosis which is associated with hyokalemia, hyperchloremic metabolic acidosis, urine pH > 5.5, increased urinary ammonium ion excretion, a negative urine anion gap, increased urinary osmol gap, decreased urinary citrate and increased urinary calcium in some patients *4071*

Anion Gap *Urine* *Decrease* May be associated with classic distal renal tubular acidosis which is associated with hyokalemia, hyperchloremic metabolic acidosis, urine pH > 5.5, increased urinary ammonium ion excretion, a negative urine anion gap, increased urinary osmol gap, decreased urinary citrate and increased urinary calcium in some patients *4071*

Calcium *Urine* *Increase* May be associated with classic distal renal tubular acidosis which is associated with hyokalemia, hyperchloremic metabolic acidosis, urine pH > 5.5, increased urinary ammonium ion excretion, a negative urine anion gap, increased urinary osmol gap, decreased urinary citrate and increased urinary calcium in some patients *4071*

272.70 Fabry's Disease *(continued)*

Chitotriosidase *Serum* *No Effect* No abnormal activities observed in 8 patients *1917*

Chloride *Serum* *Increase* May be associated with classic distal renal tubular acidosis which is associated with hyokalemia, hyperchloremic metabolic acidosis, urine pH > 5.5, increased urinary ammonium ion excretion, a negative urine anion gap, increased urinary osmol gap, decreased urinary citrate and increased urinary calcium in some patients *4071*

Citrate *Urine* *Decrease* May be associated with classic distal renal tubular acidosis which is associated with hyokalemia, hyperchloremic metabolic acidosis, urine pH > 5.5, increased urinary ammonium ion excretion, a negative urine anion gap, increased urinary osmol gap, decreased urinary citrate and increased urinary calcium in some patients *4071*

α-Galactosidase *Fibroblasts* *Decrease* Low activity suggests Fabry's disease *2952*
Serum *Decrease* Low activity suggests Fabry's disease *2952*
White Blood Cells *Decrease* Low activity suggests Fabry's disease *2952*

Lysosome-associated Membrane Protein-2
Serum *Decrease* Median concentration of 0.98 mg/L in 23 patients with Fabry's disease with median age 27 years compared with 1.21 mg/L in 202 healthy controls aged 0 - 66 y (median 7 years) *2265*

Lysosome-associated Membrane Protein-2:Lysosome-associated Membrane Protein-1 Ratio *Serum* *Decrease* Mean ratio of 3.05 in 23 patients with Fabry's disease with median age of 27 years significantly lower compared with 4.74 in 202 healthy controls aged 0 - 66 y (median 7 years) *2265*

Monocyte Chemotactic Protein-1 *Serum* *Decrease* Mean concentration undetectable in 1 patient with Fabry's disease compared with 101 ± 24 pg/mL in 16 healthy women and men *4460*
Urine *Increase* In 1 patient with Fabry's disease mean concentration of 196 pg/mg creatinine significantly different when compared with mean concentration of 130 ± 30 pg/mg creatinine in 30 healthy women and 32 healthy men *4460*

Net Acid Excretion *Urine* *Increase* May be associated with classic distal renal tubular acidosis which is associated with hyokalemia, hyperchloremic metabolic acidosis, urine pH > 5.5, increased urinary ammonium ion excretion, a negative urine anion gap, increased urinary osmol gap, decreased urinary citrate and increased urinary calcium in some patients *4071*

Osmolal Gap *Urine* *Increase* May be associated with classic distal renal tubular acidosis which is associated with hyokalemia, hyperchloremic metabolic acidosis, urine pH > 5.5, increased urinary ammonium ion excretion, a negative urine anion gap, increased urinary osmol gap, decreased urinary citrate and increased urinary calcium in some patients *4071*

pH *Urine* *Increase* May be associated with classic distal renal tubular acidosis which is associated with hyokalemia, hyperchloremic metabolic acidosis, urine pH > 5.5, increased urinary ammonium ion excretion, a negative urine anion gap, increased urinary osmol gap, decreased urinary citrate and increased urinary calcium in some patients *4071*

Potassium *Serum* *Decrease* May be associated with classic distal renal tubular acidosis which is associated with hyokalemia, hyperchloremic metabolic acidosis, urine pH > 5.5, increased urinary ammonium ion excretion, a negative urine anion gap, increased urinary osmol gap, decreased urinary citrate and increased urinary calcium in some patients *4071*

272.70 Gaucher's Disease

Acid Phosphatase *Serum* *Increase* In 12 proved cases, there was a range of 12 - 25 U/L, with a mean of 16.8 U/L, (normal range = 7 - 9 U/L) *5317* Characteristically increased *3458* Commonly elevated or high normal serum concentrations, irrespective of the patient's clinical status. The excess is caused by spillage from tissue accumulations, primarily from the spleen *966* A 5 - 50 fold elevation in serum activity in 8 patients with the adult, non-neuropathic form of Gaucher's disease was found *758*

Acid Phosphatase, Tartrate Resistant *Serum* *Increase* In patients with Gaucher's disease moderate increase observed *4217*

Alanine Aminotransferase *Serum* *Increase* May be abnormal with liver involvement *2034*

Alkaline Phosphatase *Serum* *Increase* With bone resorption *1642* *1290*

Alkaline Phosphatase, Bone Isoenzyme *Serum* *Increase* In patients with Gaucher's disease slight increase observed *4217*

Angiotensin-converting Enzyme *Serum* *Increase* Elevated *3041* Increased activities observed in patients with Gaucher's disease *2952*

Anisocytes *Blood* *Increase* If splenectomy has been carried out, severe anisocytosis and poikilocytosis occur, with many target cells, some nucleated red cells, and Howell-Jolly bodies usually present *5677*

Cerebroside β-Glucosidase *Liver* *Increase* Many times the normal concentration *4979*
Red Blood Cells *Increase* Frequently increased, with highly variable range of values *4979*
Serum *Increase* Frequently increased, with highly variable range of values *4979*

Chitotriosidase *Serum* *Increase* Mean activity in 504 patients of 1,980 - 69,900 nmol/h/mL significantly different from that in 86 healthy male blood donors of 4 - 157 nmol/h/mL and in 88 female blood donors of 6 - 142 nmol/h/mL *1917*

Erythrocytes *Blood* *Decrease* Pancytopenia is a common feature *5677*

Factor IX *Plasma* *Decrease* Clotting factor abnormalities may be present. Factor IX deficiency seems to be particularly common, and it does not appear to be related to liver disease *5677*

β-Glucosidase *Fibroblasts* *Decrease* Activities of less than 2.0 U/g of cellular protein associated with Gaucher's disease *2952*
Serum *Decrease* At pH 4.0, individuals demonstrate a marked reduction. However, little or no reduction is found at the optimum pH, 5.5 *4097*
White Blood Cells *Decrease* Activities of less than 0.05 U/10^{10} cells associated with Gaucher's disease *2952*

γ-Glutamyltransferase *Serum* *Increase* May be abnormal with liver involvement *2034*

Hematocrit *Blood* *Decrease* A normocytic, normochromic anemia is frequently present, but Hb levels rarely fall below 8 g/dL *5677* Unexplained splenomegaly with mild-moderate anemia and thrombocytopenia *4097*

Hemoglobin *Blood* *Decrease* A normocytic, normochromic anemia is frequently present, but concentrations rarely fall below 8 g/dL *5677* Unexplained splenomegaly with mild-moderate anemia and thrombocytopenia *4097*

β-Hexosaminidase A *Serum* *Decrease* Although absolute amount increased, proportion of 51.0 ± 15.5% reduced compared with 67.8 ± 4.0% in normal controls *3742*

β-Hexosaminidase *Serum* *Increase* In 55 patients mean activity of 2,067 ± 1491 nmol/mL/h compared to 1,086 ± 260 nmol/mL/h in normal controls *3742*

Iron *Serum* *Decrease* Iron is diverted from the plasma and stored within Gaucher cells *3128*
Serum *Increase* Increase in concentration to above 150 µg/dL observed in Gaucher's disease *2952*

Lactate Dehydrogenase *Serum* *Increase* May be abnormal with liver involvement *2034*

Leukocytes *Blood* *Decrease* Pancytopenia is a common feature. May be decreased to levels as low as 1,000 /µL, although milder degrees of leukopenia are much more common *5677*

Lysosome-associated Membrane Protein-2 *Serum* *Increase* Median concentration of 3.31 mg/L in 51 patients with Gaucher's disease with median age 12 years compared with 1.21 mg/L in 202 healthy controls aged 0 - 66 y (median 7 years) *2265*

Lysosome-associated Membrane Protein-2:Lysosome-associated Membrane Protein-1 Ratio *Serum* *Decrease* Mean ratio of 4.12 in 51 patients with Gaucher's disease with median age 12 years significantly increased compared with 4.74 in 202 healthy controls aged 0 - 66 y (median 7 years) *2265*

Lysozyme *Serum* *Increase* Increased (15.6 ± 3.37 g/L) in 80% of adult chronic non-neuropathic type I Gaucher's Disease *4844*

Monocytes *Blood* *Increase* Lipid storage diseases *5544*

5'-Nucleotidase *Serum* *Increase* May be abnormal with liver involvement *2034*

Osteocalcin *Serum* *Increase* In patients with Gaucher's disease slight increase observed *4217*

Oxygen Partial Pressure *Blood* *Decrease* With lung involvement *4979*

Oxygen Saturation *Blood* *Decrease* With lung involvement *4979*

Platelets *Blood* *Decrease* Pancytopenia is a common feature. May become quite severe *5677* Unexplained splenomegaly with mild-moderate anemia and thrombocytopenia *4097*

Poikilocytes *Blood* *Increase* If splenectomy has been carried out, severe anisocytosis and poikilocytosis occur, with many target cells, some nucleated red cells, and Howell-Jolly bodies usually present *5677*

Reticulocytes *Blood* *Increase* A modest reticulocytosis is often present in anemic patients *5677*

Tumor Necrosis Factor-α *Serum* *Increase* Mean concentration of about 50 pg/mL in 25 patients with type I disease significantly different from mean concentration of about 10 pg/mL in 11 healthy controls *3475*

272.70 Gaucher's Type I Disease

Chitotriosidase *Serum* *Increase* Abnormal activities observed in 20 of 21 patients, ranging from 5,580 - 51,800 nmol/h/mL *1917*

272.70 Gaucher's Type II and III Disease

Tumor Necrosis Factor-α *Serum* *Increase* Mean concentration of about 120 pg/mL in 5 patients with type II or III disease significantly different from mean concentration of about 10 pg/mL in 11 healthy controls *3475*

272.70 Mucolipidosis II

Chitotriosidase *Serum* *No Effect* Abnormal activities observed in 0 of 3 patients with mucolipidosls types II and III *1917*

β-Glucuronidase *Serum* *Increase* In 2 patients activity of 77,655 and 69,305 mU/L significantly greater than 701 ± 317 mU/L in 100 normal controls *3743*

β-Hexosaminidase A and B *Plasma* *Increase* In 2 patients activities of 295,273 and 580,743 mU/L significantly greater than 19,823 ± 6,229 mU/L in 100 normal controls *3743*

β-Hexosaminidase B *Plasma* *Increase* In 2 patients percentage of A and B hexosaminidase activity of 57.4% and 57.0% significantly greater than 32.7 ± 4.2% in 100 normal controls *3743*

Hyaluronidase *Plasma* *Decrease* In 2 patients, activity of 2,572 and 1,453 mU/L significantly less than 4,476 ± 1,144 mU/L in 100 normal controls *3743*

α-Mannosidase *Serum* *Increase* In 2 patients activity of 35,070 and 13,360 mU/L significantly greater than 200 ± 67 mU/L in 100 normal controls *3743*

Sialic Acid, Lipid-associated *Urine* *Increase* Bound sialic acid concentration in urine reported to increase 4 to 10 times *5594*

Tumor Necrosis Factor-α *Serum* *No Effect* Mean concentration of about 15 pg/mL in 4 patients with mucolipidosis types II or III not significantly different from mean concentration of about 10 pg/mL in 11 healthy controls *3475*

272.70 Mucolipidosis III

β-Glucuronidase *Serum* *Increase* In 3 patients activity of 40,247, 30,895 and 41,416 mU/L significantly greater than 701 ± 317 mU/L in 100 normal controls *3743*

β-Hexosaminidase A and B *Plasma* *Increase* In 3 patients activities of 538,809, 638,191 and 205,577 mU/L significantly greater than 19,823 ± 6,229 mU/L in 100 normal controls *3743*

β-Hexosaminidase B *Plasma* *Increase* In 3 patients percentage of A and B hexosaminidase activity of 61.9%, 62.6% and 59.0% significantly greater than 32.7 ± 4.2% in 100 normal controls *3743*

Hyaluronidase *Plasma* *Decrease* In 3 patients activity of 3,874, 3,624 and 2,839 mU/L not significantly less than 4,476 ± 1,144 mU/L in 100 normal controls *3743*

α-Mannosidase *Serum* *Increase* In 3 patients activity of 77,321, 55,611 and 37,241 mU/L significantly greater than 200 ± 67 mU/L in 100 normal controls *3743*

Sialic Acid, Lipid-associated *Urine* *No Effect* Bound sialic acid concentration in urine reported to be normal to slightly increased *5594*

272.70 Niemann-Pick Disease

Acid Phosphatase *Serum* *Increase* Ranging from 35 - 45 U/L over a 4 month period in a patient with this disease *2058* Increased levels have been documented in only a few cases *965*
Serum *No Effect* Normal activity typically observed *2058* Eleven measurements on 6 different patients all fell within the normal range for their respective age groups. Observations of increased concentration have not been able to be confirmed *965* Typically normal activity observed *966*

Alanine Aminotransferase *Serum* *Increase* Seen in type B disease *4979*

Alkaline Phosphatase *Serum* *Increase* Seen in type B disease *4979*

Aspartate Aminotransferase *Serum* *Increase* Seen in type B disease *4979*

Cells *Bone Marrow* *Increase* Bone marrow contains typical foam cells, containing small droplets throughout the cytoplasm *5677*

Cholesterol *Liver* *Increase* Usually elevated, may be more prominent than sphingomyelin in type D *4979*

Erythrocytes *Blood* *Decrease* Pancytopenia is a common feature *5677*

Hematocrit *Blood* *Decrease* May be normal or mild anemia may be present *5677*

Hemoglobin *Blood* *Decrease* May be normal, or mild anemia may be present *5677*

Leukocytes *Blood* *Decrease* Pancytopenia is a common feature *5677*

Platelets *Blood* *Decrease* Pancytopenia is a common feature *5677* May be severe *2034*

Sphingomyelinase *Fibroblasts* *Decrease* Typical values in patients with Niemann-Pick disease are < 1.0 U/g cellular protein *2952*

Tumor Necrosis Factor-α *Serum* *Increase* Mean concentration of about 50 pg/mL in 3 patients with Niemann-Pick disease significantly different from mean concentration of about 10 pg/mL in 11 healthy controls *3475*

272.70 Niemann-Pick Disease (A & B)

Chitotriosidase *Serum* *Increase* Abnormal activities observed in 13 of 15 patients with Niemann-Pick A/B disease of 250 and 602 - 2,800 nmol/h/mL significantly different from normal *1917*

Lysosome-associated Membrane Protein-2
Serum *No Effect* Median concentration of 1.36 mg/L in 10 patients with Niemann-Pick (A & B) disease with median age 22 y compared with 1.21 mg/L in 202 healthy controls aged 0 - 66 y (median 7 years) *2265*

Lysosome-associated Membrane Protein-2:Lysosome-associated Membrane Protein-1 Ratio *Serum* *Decrease* Mean ratio of 3.86 in 10 patients with Nemann-Pick (A & B) disease with median age 22 y significantly different when compared with 4.74 in 202 healthy controls aged 0 - 66 y (median 7 years) *2265*

272.70 Niemann-Pick Disease (C)

Chitotriosidase *Serum Increase* Abnormal activities observed in 6 of 11 patients with Niemann-Pick C disease of 263 and 304 - 940 nmol/h/mL significantly different from normal *1917*

Lysosome-associated Membrane Protein-2 *Serum No Effect* Median concentration of 1.32 mg/L in 10 patients with Niemann-Pick (C) disease with median age 12 y compared with 1.21 mg/L in 202 healthy controls aged 0 - 66 y (median 7 years) *2265*

Lysosome-associated Membrane Protein-2:Lysosome-associated Membrane Protein-1 Ratio *Serum Decrease* Mean ratio of 3.61 in 10 patients with Niemann-Pick (C) disease with median age 12 y significantly different when compared with 4.74 in 202 healthy controls aged 0 - 66 y (median 7 years) *2265*

272.70 Wolman's Disease

Lysosome-associated Membrane Protein-2 *Serum Increase* Median concentration of 1.41 mg/L in 2 patients with Wolman's disease with median age 1 y compared with 1.21 mg/L in 202 healthy controls aged 0 - 66 y (median 7 years) *2265*

Lysosome-associated Membrane Protein-2:Lysosome-associated Membrane Protein-1 Ratio *Serum Decrease* Mean ratio of 3.075 in 2 patients with Wolman's disease with median age 1 y not significantly different when compared with 4.74 in 202 healthy controls aged 0 - 66 y (median 7 years) *2265*

272.80 Multiple Symmetric Lipomatosis

Apolipoprotein A-I *Serum Increase* Mean concentration in 4 males with multiple symmetric lipomatosis of 164.8 ± 43.9 mg/dL higher, but not significantly so because of small population size, than 122.0 ± 20.9 mg/dL in 20 controls *1099*

Apolipoprotein B *Serum Decrease* Mean concentration of 71.3 ± 36.9 mg/dL in 4 males with multiple symmetric lipomatosis lower but not significantly so because of small population size than 92.6 ± 28.5 mg/dL in 20 controls *1099*

Cholesterol *Serum No Effect* In 4 males with multiple symmetric lipomatosis mean concentration of 215.3 ± 18.6 mg/dL not significantly different from 212.4 ± 44 mg/dL in 20 controls *1099*

HDL-Cholesterol *Serum No Effect* Mean concentration in 4 males with multiple symmetric lipomatosis of 77.3 ± 45.0 mg/dL not significantly different from 53.2 ± 10.4 mg/dL in 20 controls *1099*

Lipoprotein Lp(a) *Serum No Effect* Mean concentration in 4 males with multiple symmetric lipomatosis of 15.1 ± 5.2 mg/dL compared with 18.9 ± 15.7 mg/dL in 20 controls *1099*

Triglycerides *Serum Increase* Mean concentration in 4 males with multiple symmetric lipomatosis of 199.8 ± 151.0 mg/dL higher, but not significantly so because of small size of population, than 109.9 ± 47.6 mg/dL in 20 controls *1099*

Disorders of Plasma Protein Metabolism

273.10 Monoclonal Gammopathy

Osteocalcin *Serum No Effect* Normal levels found in 6 patients *5676*

273.10 Monoclonal Gammopathy of Undetermined Significance

Anticardiolipin Antibodies *Serum Increase* In 93 patients with MGUS of mean age 70 ± 21 years mean incidence of IgG antibodies 9%, IgM antibodies 5% and IgA antibodies 50% *5009*

Antiphosphatidic Acid Antibodies *Serum Increase* In 93 patients with MGUS of mean age 70 ± 21 years mean incidence of IgG antibodies 9%, IgM antibodies 45% and IgA antibodies 25% *5009* In 93 patients with MGUS of mean age 70 ± 21 years mean incidence of IgG antibodies 15% and IgM antibodies 25% *5009*

Antiphosphatidylcholine Antibodies *Serum Increase* In 93 patients with MGUS of mean age 70 ± 21 years mean incidence of IgG antibodies 9% and IgM antibodies 25% *5009*

Antiphosphatidylethanolamine Antibodies *Serum Increase* In 93 patients with MGUS of mean age 70 ± 21 years mean incidence of IgG antibodies 13%, IgM antibodies 10% but 0% IgA antibodies *5009*

Antiphosphatidylglycerol Antibodies *Serum Increase* In 93 patients with MGUS of mean age 70 ± 21 years mean incidence of IgG antibodies 12% and IgM antibodies 10% *5009*

Antiphosphatidylinositol Antibodies *Serum Increase* In 93 patients with MGUS of mean age 70 ± 21 years mean incidence of IgG antibodies 32% and IgM antibodies 35% *5009*

C-Reactive Protein *Serum Increase* In 14 patients with MGUS mean concentration of 2.4 mg/L *1506*

Interleukin-6 *Serum Increase* In 128 cases mean concentration of 0.246 ± 0.166 ng/mL higher than 0.190 ± 0.145 ng/mL in 26 healthy controls *1271* In 14 patients with MGUS mean concentration of 9.25 pg/L *1506*

β_2-Microglobulin *Serum Increase* In 14 patients with MGUS mean concentration of 3.05 mg/L *1506* In 3 patients with MGUS mean concentration of 2.91 ± 0.30 mg/L (median 3.07 mg/L) significantly different from mean of 1.71 ± 0.46 mg/L (median 1.55 mg/L) in 81 healthy controls. 50% of patients had increased concentrations *4166*

Soluble CD16 *Serum Decrease* In 35 patients with MGUS median concentration of 2.3 μg/mL not significantly different from median concentration of 2.7 μg/mL in 29 healthy controls *3349* In 39 patients with MGUS mean concentration of 2.3 ± 1.1 μg/mL not significantly different from 2.7 ± 1.4 μg/mL in 29 healthy volunteer controls *3350*

Soluble Interleukin-6 Receptor *Serum Decrease* In 44 patients with MGUS mean concentration of 71.1 ± 19.4 ng/mL not significantly different from 70.3 ± 13.4 μg/mL in 24 healthy volunteer controls *3350*

Thymidine Kinase *Serum Decrease* In patients with MGUS mean concentration less than in those with stage I multiple myeloma: in those patients with MGUS higher concentrations were associated with decreased survival *3168*

273.20 Cryoglobulinemia

Ammonium Ions *Urine Increase* May be associated with classic distal renal tubular acidosis which is associated with hyokalemia, hyperchloremic metabolic acidosis, urine pH > 5.5, increased urinary ammonium ion excretion, a negative urine anion gap, increased urinary osmol gap, decreased urinary citrate and increased urinary calcium in some patients *4071*

Anion Gap *Urine Decrease* May be associated with classic distal renal tubular acidosis which is associated with hyokalemia, hyperchloremic metabolic acidosis, urine pH > 5.5, increased urinary ammonium ion excretion, a negative urine anion gap, increased urinary osmol gap, decreased urinary citrate and increased urinary calcium in some patients *4071*

Calcium *Urine Increase* May be associated with classic distal renal tubular acidosis which is asociated with hyokalemia, hyperchloremic metabolic acidosis, urine pH > 5.5, increased urinary ammonium ion excretion, a negative urine anion gap, increased urinary osmol gap, decreased urinary citrate and increased urinary calcium in some patients *4071*

Chloride *Serum Increase* May be associated with classic distal renal tubular acidosis which is associated with hyokalemia, hyperchloremic metabolic acidosis, urine pH > 5.5, increased urinary ammonium ion excretion, a negative urine anion gap, increased urinary osmol gap, decreased urinary citrate and increased urinary calcium in some patients *4071*

Citrate *Urine Decrease* May be associated with classic distal renal tubular acidosis which is associated with hyokalemia, hyperchloremic metabolic acidosis, urine pH > 5.5, increased urinary ammonium ion excretion, a negative urine anion gap, increased urinary osmol gap, decreased urinary citrate and increased urinary calcium in some patients *4071*

Complement C_1 *Serum Decrease* Mean concentration typically slightly reduced in patients with cryoglobulinemia or vasculitis *4682*

Complement C_1q *Serum* *Decrease* Mean concentration typically slightly reduced in patients with cryoglobulinemia or vasculitis *4682*

Complement C_2 *Serum* *Decrease* Mean concentration typically slightly reduced or normal in patients with cryoglobulinemia or vasculitis *4682*

Complement C_3 *Serum* *Decrease* Mean concentration typically slightly reduced or normal in patients with cryoglobulinemia or vasculitis *4682*

Complement C_4 *Serum* *Decrease* Mean concentration typically slightly reduced in patients with cryoglobulinemia or vasculitis *4682*

Complement C_5 *Serum* *No Effect* Mean concentration typically normal in patients with cryoglobulinemia or vasculitis *4682*

Complement CH50 *Serum* *Decrease* Mean concentration typically slightly reduced in patients with cryoglobulinemia or vasculitis *4682*

Net Acid Excretion *Urine* *Increase* May be associated with classic distal renal tubular acidosis which is asociated with hyokalemia, hyperchloremic metabolic acidosis, urine pH > 5.5, increased urinary ammonium ion excretion, a negative urine anion gap, increased urinary osmol gap, decreased urinary citrate and increased urinary calcium in some patients *4071*

Osmolal Gap *Urine* *Increase* May be associated with classic distal renal tubular acidosis which is asociated with hyokalemia, hyperchloremic metabolic acidosis, urine pH > 5.5, increased urinary ammonium ion excretion, a negative urine anion gap, increased urinary osmol gap, decreased urinary citrate and increased urinary calcium in some patients *4071*

pH *Urine* *Increase* May be associated with classic distal renal tubular acidosis which is asociated with hyokalemia, hyperchloremic metabolic acidosis, urine pH > 5.5, increased urinary ammonium ion excretion, a negative urine anion gap, increased urinary osmol gap, decreased urinary citrate and increased urinary calcium in some patients *4071*

Potassium *Serum* *Decrease* May be associated with classic distal renal tubular acidosis which is asociated with hyokalemia, hyperchloremic metabolic acidosis, urine pH > 5.5, increased urinary ammonium ion excretion, a negative urine anion gap, increased urinary osmol gap, decreased urinary citrate and increased urinary calcium in some patients *4071*

Properdin Factor B *Plasma* *No Effect* Mean concentration typically normal in patients with cryoglobulinemia or vasculitis *4682*

Rheumatoid Factor *Serum* *Increase* Mean concentration increased in patients with cryoglobulinemia *2472* Rheumatoid factor may be observed in certain patients *2473*

273.20 Cryoglobulinemia (Essential Mixed)

Albumin *Urine* *Increase* Common *900*

Complement C_1q *Serum* *Decrease* Low levels of early components (C_1q, C_1s, and C_4) *5163*

Complement C_3 *Serum* *No Effect* In 26 patients affected by essential cryoglobulinemia, a peculiar pattern was observed which was characterized by: low levels of early components (C_1q, C_1s and C_4), normal levels of C_3 and high concentrations of late components (C_5 and C_9) and CH50 values significantly lower than normal *5163* May be normal in mixed cryoglobulinemia *5651*

Complement C_4 *Serum* *Decrease* C_1q, C_2, and C_4 are especially decreased whereas C_3 may be normal in mixed cryoglobulinemia *5651* In 26 patients affected by essential cryoglobulinemia, a peculiar pattern was observed which was characterized by: low levels of early components (C_1q, C_1s and C_4), normal levels of C_3 and high concentrations of late components (C_5, C_9) and CH50 values significantly lower than normal *5163*

Complement, Total *Serum* *Decrease* In 26 patients affected by essential cryoglobulinemia, peculiar pattern was observed which was characterized by: low levels of early components (C_1q, C_1s and C_4), normal levels of C_3 and high concentrations of late components (C_5,C_9) and CH50 values significantly lower than normal *5163*

Serum *Increase* In 26 patients affected by essential cryoglobulinemia, a peculiar pattern was observed which was characterized by: low levels of early components (C_1q, C_1s and C_4), normal levels of C_3 and high concentrations of late components (C_5,C_9) and CH50 values significantly lower than normal *5163*

Erythrocyte Sedimentation Rate *Blood* *Decrease* Rare finding of a rate approaching 0 mm/h (in the absence of marked hypofibrinogenemia) *4551*

Blood *Increase* May be increased at 37 °C *5545*

Blood *No Effect* Normal at room temperature *5545*

Erythrocytes *Urine* *Increase* Urinary sediment contains erythrocytes and finely granular casts *900*

Fibronectin *Plasma* *Decrease* In 21 patients with EMC concentration reduced *5262*

Granular Casts *Urine* *Increase* Urinary sediment contains erythrocytes and finely granular casts *900*

Immunoglobulin G *Serum* *Increase* Monoclonal spike may occur *4551*

Immunoglobulin M *Serum* *Increase* Monoclonal spike may occur *4551*

Rheumatoid Factor *Serum* *Increase* High titer when tested at 37 °C *4551*

Thrombin/Antithrombin III Complex *Plasma* *Increase* In patients with EMC concentration typically increased *5262*

Tissue Polypeptide Antigen *Serum* *Increase* In patients with EMC concentration typically increased suggesting endothelial cell damage *5262*

von Willebrand Factor *Plasma* *Increase* In patients with EMC concentration usually increased *5262*

273.20 Heavy Chain Disease (Alpha)

Albumin *Serum* *Decrease* Usually reduced with reversed A/G ratio *5677*

Bence-Jones Protein *Urine* *No Effect* Not detected *5545*

Calcium *Serum* *Decrease* Patients usually present with chronic diarrhea, hypocalcemia, and excessive fecal losses of water and electrolytes *5677*

Chloride *Feces* *Increase* Patients usually present with chronic diarrhea, hypocalcemia, and excessive fecal losses of water and electrolytes *5677*

α_2-Globulin *Serum* *Increase* Markedly elevated broad peak *4551*

β-Globulin *Serum* *Increase* Markedly elevated broad peak *4551*

immunoglobulin A *Serum* *Increase* Distinctive increase in IgA heavy chains (alpha chains) *4551*

Potassium *Feces* *Increase* Patients usually present with chronic diarrhea, hypocalcemia, and excessive fecal losses of water and electrolytes *5677*

Sodium *Feces* *Increase* Patients usually present with chronic diarrhea, hypocalcemia, and excessive fecal losses of water and electrolytes *5677*

Vitamin B_{12} *Serum* *Decrease* Impaired absorption *4551*

273.20 Heavy Chain Disease (Gamma)

Albumin *Serum* *Decrease* Usually reduced with reversed A/G ratio *5677*

Bence-Jones Protein *Urine* *No Effect* Not observed *5545*

Calcium *Serum* *Decrease* Patients usually present with chronic diarrhea, hypocalcemia, and excessive fecal losses of water and electrolytes *5677*

Chloride *Feces* *Increase* Patients usually present with chronic diarrhea, hypocalcemia, and excessive fecal losses of water and electrolytes *5677*

Eosinophils *Blood* *Increase* Often associated with mild to marked leukopenia and eosinophilia *5677* Eosinophilia sometimes marked with relative lymphocytosis *5545*

Bone Marrow *Increase* Bone marrow may be normal, but usually there is an increased proportion of plasma cells or lympho-

273.20 Heavy Chain Disease (Gamma) *(continued)*

Eosinophils *(continued)*
cytes or both, often accompanied by eosinophilia *5677* Bone marrow aspirations and lymph node biopsies have demonstrated a proliferation of plasmacytic and lymphocytic forms, along with eosinophils and large reticulum or reticuloendothelial cells, (the pattern of a pleomorphic reticular neoplasm) *4551*

γ-Globulin *Serum* *Decrease* In 50% of patients the concentration of the anomalous protein is > 2.0 g/dL and marked hypogammaglobulinemia is present *5677* Almost absent on electrophoresis *5544*

Hematocrit *Blood* *Decrease* Normochromic, normocytic anemia present in all cases *2039* Presumably related to hypersplenism *4551* All patients have mild to moderate anemia *5677*

Hemoglobin *Blood* *Decrease* Normochromic, normocytic anemia present in all cases of γ heavy chain disease *2039* All patients have mild to moderate anemia *5677* Presumably related to hypersplenism *4551*

immunoglobulin A *Serum* *Decrease* Marked decrease *5545*

Immunoglobulin G *Serum* *Decrease* Marked decrease in IgG *5545* Excessive quantities of the Fe fragment of the heavy chain of IgG *4551*

Immunoglobulin M *Serum* *Decrease* Marked decrease *5544*

Immunoglobulins *Serum* *Decrease* Marked decrease in IgG, IgA, and IgM *5545*

Leukocytes *Blood* *Decrease* Often associated with mild to marked leukopenia and eosinophilia *5677* Presumably related to hypersplenism *4551*

Lymphocytes *Blood* *Increase* Relative lymphocytosis *5545* Atypical lymphocytes *413*
Bone Marrow *Increase* Bone marrow aspirations and lymph node biopsies have demonstrated a proliferation of plasmacytic and lymphocytic forms, along with eosinophils and large reticulum or reticuloendothelial cells, (the pattern of a pleomorphic reticular neoplasm) *4551* Bone marrow may be normal, but usually there is an increased proportion of plasma cells or lymphocytes or both, often accompanied by eosinophilia *5677*

Plasma Cells *Blood* *Increase* Presence of atypical lymphocytes or plasma cells in the blood *5677*
Bone Marrow *Increase* Bone marrow may be normal, but usually there is an increased proportion of plasma cells or lymphocytes or both, often accompanied by eosinophilia *5677* Bone marrow aspirations and lymph node biopsies have demonstrated a proliferation of plasmacytic and lymphocytic forms, along with eosinophils and large reticulum or reticuloendothelial cells, (the pattern of a pleomorphic reticular neoplasm) *4551*

Platelets *Blood* *Decrease* Mild to marked thrombocytopenia *5677* Presumably related to hypersplenism *4551*

Potassium *Feces* *Increase* Patients usually present with chronic diarrhea, hypocalcemia, and excessive fecal losses of water and electrolytes *5677*

Protein *Urine* *Increase* Up to 1 gram/day *413*

Sodium *Feces* *Increase* Patients usually present with chronic diarrhea, hypocalcemia, and excessive fecal losses of water and electrolytes *5677*

Urea Nitrogen *Serum* *Increase* Increased (30 - 50 mg/dL) *5545*

Uric Acid *Serum* *Increase* Increased, (> 8.5 mg/dL) *5545*

273.30 Waldenström's Macroglobulinemia

Acid Phosphatase *White Blood Cells* *Increase* Reported finding *3027*

Albumin *Serum* *Decrease* Usually associated with increased globulin concentration *5544*

Antinuclear Antibodies *Serum* *Increase* Positive in 16% *4068*

Antithyroglobulin Antibodies *Serum* *Increase* Rare *5280*

α_1-Antitrypsin *Serum* *No Effect* Concentration typically normal *5544*

Basophils *Bone Marrow* *Increase* Characteristic presence of large numbers of basophils and tissue mast cells interspersed among the other cells *5699*

Bence-Jones Protein *Urine* *Present* Reported to occur in 25% of patients *5677* Present in approximately 10% of cases, but renal functional impairment is much less common than in myeloma *4551*

Bleeding Time *Patient* *Increase* Evidence of impaired platelet function *5677*

Calprotectin *Plasma* *Increase* In 3 patients mean concentration of 1,031 μg/L significantly higher than normal range of 80 - 880 μg/L in women and 150 - 910 μg/L in men *2169*

Cells *Bone Marrow* *Increase* Bone marrow sections are always hypercellular and show extensive infiltration with atypical lymphocytes and also plasma cells, with macroglobulinemia *5545* Bone marrow punctures may result in dry tap due to great cellularity of the marrow combined with increased viscosity of the tissue fluid *2562*

Chylomicrons *Serum* *Increase* Moderate increase due to presence of IgG or IgM that forms complexes with chylomicron remnants and/or VLDL thereby decreasing catabolism *126*

Clot Retraction *Blood* *Decrease* Evidence of impaired platelet function *5677*

Cold Agglutinins *Serum* *Increase* Reported observation *4551*

Complement C_3 *Serum* *No Effect* Concentration typically normal *5544*

Complement, Total *Serum* *Decrease* In some cases *38*

Coombs' Test *Serum* *Negative* Almost always negative *5677*

Creatinine *Serum* *No Effect* Urine is almost always hypertonic to plasma *126*

Cryofibrinogen *Plasma* *Increase* Reported observation *413*

Cryoglobulins *Serum* *Increase* Demonstrated in the sera of 37% of the tested patients *5677* Marked elevation of cryoglobulins *4707*

Eosinophils *Blood* *Increase* Reported effect *4551* Reported observation *315*

Erythrocyte Sedimentation Rate *Blood* *Increase* Usually markedly increased *4551* Markedly increased *5699* The presence of cryomacroglobulins may give the appearance of a normal ESR *900*
Blood *No Effect* The presence of cryomacroglobulins may give the appearance of a normal ESR *5544*

Erythrocyte Survival *Red Blood Cells* *Decrease* Observed in the majority of patients *5677* Found in 6 of 8 patients *863*

Factor II *Plasma* *Decrease* A number of patients have reduced activity of one or more coagulation factors *5677*

Factor V *Plasma* *Decrease* A number of patients have reduced activity of one or more coagulation factors *5677*

Factor VII *Plasma* *Decrease* A number of patients have reduced activity of 1 or more coagulation factors *5677*

Factor VIII *Plasma* *Decrease* A number of patients have reduced activity of one or more coagulation factors *5677*

Factor X *Plasma* *Decrease* A number of patients have reduced activity of one or more coagulation factors *5677*

Fibrinogen *Plasma* *Decrease* A number of patients have reduced activity of one or more coagulation factors *5677*

γ-Globulin *Serum* *Increase* Electrophoresis shows an intense sharp peak in globulin fraction, usually in the γ zone, and takes PAS stain. Total serum protein and globulin are markedly increased. Immunoelectrophoresis identifies IgM as a component of increased globulin *5545*

Haptoglobin *Serum* *No Effect* Concentration typically normal *5544*

Hematocrit *Blood* *Decrease* Anemia is the most common presenting manifestation and is frequently profound. Usually due to a combination of factors including accelerated RBC destruction, blood loss, and especially decreased erythropoiesis *4551* A normochromic, normocytic anemia is usually present *5677*

Hemoglobin *Blood* *Decrease* A normochromic, normocytic anemia is usually present *5677* Anemia is the most common presenting manifestation and is frequently profound, with hemoglobin levels in the range of 6 - 9 g/dL. Usually due to a combination of factors including accelerated RBC destruction, blood loss, and especially decreased erythropoiesis *4551*

immunoglobulin A *Serum* *Decrease* Reported effect *5544*

Immunoglobulin E *Serum* *Decrease* In 56 patients with Waldenstrom's macroglobulinemia mean concentration of 67.3 ng/mL (range 15 - 305) not significantly less than mean of 96 ng/mL (range 24 - 386) in 74 healthy controls *2323*

Immunoglobulin G *Serum* *Decrease* Reported observation *5544*

Immunoglobulin M *Serum* *Increase* Immunoelectrophoresis identified IgM as a component of increased globulin *5545* IgM > 15% of total serum protein and/or 1,000 mg/dL *2039*

Interleukin-6 *Serum* *Increase* In 27 cases with macroglobulinemia mean concentration of 0.263 ± 0.148 ng/mL higher than 0.190 ± 0.145 ng/mL in 26 healthy controls *1271*

Iron-binding Capacity, Total *Serum* *No Effect* Concentration typically normal *5544*

Leukocytes *Blood* *Decrease* WBC count is decreased with relative lymphocytosis *5545* Reported observation *4551*
Blood *No Effect* Leukocytosis and thrombocytopenia are uncommon *5677*

Lymphocytes *Blood* *Increase* Relative lymphocytosis *5545* Absolute lymphocytosis with atypical, immature, and plasmacytic forms in many cases, and occasionally reaching leukemic proportions *4551*
Bone Marrow *Increase* Proliferation of lymphocytic and plasmacytic forms with many intermediate and apparently transitional cell types *4551* Many intermediate and transitional forms observed *419*

β_2-Macroglobulin *Serum* *Increase* Marked increase *5544*

Monocytes *Blood* *Increase* Has been observed *315*

Neutrophils *Blood* *Decrease* In some patients, neutropenia, as part of general pancytopenia, has been observed *315* *5699*

Osteocalcin *Serum* *No Effect* Normal levels found in 7 patients *5676*

Plasma Cells *Bone Marrow* *Increase* Increased number observed in bone marrow *419* Proliferation of lymphocytic and plasmacytic forms with many intermediate and apparently transitional cell types *4551*

Platelets *Blood* *Decrease* Leukocytosis and thrombocytopenia are uncommon *5677* Observed in about 50% patients with bleeding tendency but otherwise usually normal *4551* Found in about 50% of patients suffering from bleeding diathesis *5699*
Blood *No Effect* Count is usually normal, but abnormalities of platelet function appear to be important causes of bleeding in these patients *5677*

Protein *Serum* *Increase* Total serum proteins are increased owing to elevation of γ-globulins *900*
Urine *Increase* 5 of 16 patients excreted 2.0 g or more of protein/24 h *3598* Excretion increased in about one quarter of patients with disease *5677*

Prothrombin Consumption *Blood* *Decrease* Evidence of impaired platelet function *5677*

Rheumatoid Factor *Serum* *Increase* Dysproteinemias and paraproteinemias present significant seropositivity *1980* In some cases *38* Occasionally observed *4551*

Thrombin Time *Blood* *Increase* Coagulation defect detected most frequently is prolongation of the thrombin time *5677*

Thromboplastin Generation *Blood* *Increase* Evidence of impaired platelet function *5677*

Urea Nitrogen *Serum* *Increase* Reported to occur in about one quarter of patients *5677* Elevated in 5 of 16 patients *3598*
Serum *No Effect* Renal insufficiency is reported to be uncommon *3187* Renal damage is rare *5677*

Uric Acid *Serum* *Increase* May occur *5699* Reported finding *1980*

VDRL *Serum* *Positive* Biologic false positive found in some cases *38*

Viscosity *Serum* *Increase* A great increase in serum viscosity. This is usually associated with the presence of macroglobulins *5677* The relative serum viscosity was elevated above 4 in 41% of patients and 36% of these patients developed symptoms of hyperviscosity sometime in the course of their disease *3187* Common observation *1980* Some increase in serum viscosity is found in about 66% of patients tested, but only 50% of these will manifest symptoms of the hyperviscosity syndrome *5699*

VLDL-Cholesterol *Serum* *Increase* Moderate increase due to presence of IgG or IgM that forms complexes with chylomicron remnants and/or VLDL thereby decreasing catabolism *126*

Volume *Plasma* *Increase* Reported finding *413*

273.80 Analbuminemia

Albumin *Serum* *Decrease* Marked decrease due to impaired synthesis *4707* Cannot be detected by routine laboratory methods *900*

α_1-Antitrypsin *Serum* *No Effect* Concentration usually normal *5544*

Calcium *Serum* *Decrease* Lower limits of normal *900*

Cholesterol *Serum* *Increase* Often elevated *900*

Complement C_3 *Serum* *No Effect* Concentration usually normal *5544*

Erythrocyte Sedimentation Rate *Blood* *Increase* Usually elevated owing to the increased globulin level *900*

α_1-Globulin *Serum* *No Effect* Concentration usually normal *5544*

γ-Globulin *Serum* *Increase* Usually present in increased concentration *900*

Haptoglobin *Serum* *No Effect* Concentration usually normal *5544*

Iron-binding Capacity, Total *Serum* *No Effect* Concentration usually normal *5544*

Protein *Serum* *Decrease* Marked decrease *5544*

273.80 Haptoglobin Deficiency

Haptoglobin *Serum* *Decrease* Deficiency observed in approximately 0.9% of the population *5816*

274.00 Gout

Adenosine Deaminase *Serum* *Increase* Increased *1340* *4956* *3926*

Alanine *Plasma* *Increase* Increased *237* *4798* *555*

Alanine Aminotransferase *Serum* *No Effect* In 175 male patients with primary gout mean activity of 23.5 ± 0.8 U/L not significantly different from 23.3 ± 0.8 U/L in 172 control men *5133*

Apolipoprotein A-I *Serum* *No Effect* In 175 male patients with primary gout mean concentration of 131.8 ± 1.9 mg/dL not significantly different from 130.0 ± 1.7 mg/dL in 172 control men *5133*

Apolipoprotein A-II *Serum* *Increase* In 175 male patients with primary gout mean concentration of 37.0 ± 0.7 mg/dL significantly different from 33.1 ± 0.4 mg/dL in 172 control men *5133*

Apolipoprotein B *Serum* *Increase* In 175 male patients with primary gout mean concentration of 108.5 ± 1.8 mg/dL significantly different from 99.6 ± 1.9 mg/dL in 172 control men *5133*

Apolipoprotein C-II *Serum* *Increase* In 175 male patients with primary gout mean concentration of 5.6 ± 0.2 mg/dL significantly different from 4.3 ± 0.2 mg/dL in 172 control men *5133*

Apolipoprotein C-III *Serum* *Increase* In 175 male patients with primary gout mean concentration of 15.1 ± 0.6 mg/dL significantly different from 11.6 ± 0.5 mg/dL in 172 control men *5133*

Apolipoprotein E *Serum* *Increase* In 175 male patients with primary gout mean concentration of 6.8 ± 0.2 mg/dL significantly different from 5.1 ± 0.2 mg/dL in 172 control men *5133*

Aspartate Aminotransferase *Serum* *Increase* Increased levels have been reported in acute stages *1290*
Serum *No Effect* In 175 male patients with primary gout mean activity of 22.9 ± 0.5 U/L not significantly different from 22.7 ± 0.6 U/L in 172 control men *5133*

Calcium *Serum* *No Effect* Mean concentration in 114 male patients with gout of 9.8 ± 0.3 mg/dL not significantly different from 9.8 ± 0.2 mg/dL observed in 51 healthy male controls *5132*

274.00 Gout *(continued)*

Cholesterol *Serum* *Increase* Many patients *2029* Frequently elevated in individual patients; no correlation has been shown between urate and cholesterol *4979*
Serum *No Effect* In 175 male patients with primary gout mean concentration of 209.7 ± 2.8 mg/dL not significantly different from 207.4 ± 2.9 mg/dL in 172 control men *5133*

Complement C_1 *Serum* *No Effect* Mean concentration typically normal or slightly increased in patients with gout *4682*

Complement C_1q *Serum* *No Effect* Mean concentration typically normal or slightly increased in patients with gout *4682*

Complement C_2 *Serum* *No Effect* Mean concentration typically normal or slightly increased in patients with gout *4682*

Complement C_3 *Serum* *No Effect* Mean concentration typically normal or slightly increased in patients with gout *4682*

Complement C_4 *Serum* *No Effect* Mean concentration typically normal or slightly increased in patients with gout *4682*

Complement C_5 *Serum* *No Effect* Mean concentration typically normal or slightly increased in patients with gout *4682*

Complement CH50 *Serum* *No Effect* Mean concentration typically normal or slightly increased in patients with gout *4682*

Complement, Total *Serum* *Decrease* Depleted in serum by urate crystals *3702*
Serum *Increase* Elevated during active inflammation and subsides with remission *4683*
Synovial Fluid *Increase* Frequently occurs *4683*

C-Reactive Protein *Serum* *Increase* In 14 patients median concentration of 60 µg/mL *5287*

Creatinine *Serum* *Increase* In 80 patients with pure gout mean concentration of 1.56 ± 0.64 mg/dL significantly higher than 0.90 ± 0.16 mg/dL in 72 healthy controls *5166* Rises with renal failure, but these changes may be subtle and slow *900*
Serum *No Effect* In 175 male patients with primary gout mean concentration of 1.0 ± 0.0 mg/dL not significantly different from 1.0 ± 0.0 mg/dL in 172 control men *5133* Mean concentration in 114 male patients with gout of 0.86 ± 0.18 mg/dL not significantly different from 0.86 ± 0.11 mg/dL observed in 51 healthy male controls *5132*

Creatinine Clearance *Urine* *Decrease* In 80 patients with pure gout mean clearance of 59.91 ± 30.90 mL/min significantly lower than 97.10 ± 27.19 mL/min in 72 healthy controls *5166*

1,25-Dihydroxy Vitamin D_3 *Serum* *Decrease* Mean concentration in 114 male patients with gout of 38.4 ± 11.9 pg/mL significantly different from 44.4 ± 11.0 pg/mL observed in 51 healthy male controls *5132*

Erythrocyte Sedimentation Rate *Blood* *Increase* In 14 patients median rate of 65 mm/h *5287* Increased in gouty arthritis *1980* Frequently elevated with acute gout *900*

Gelatinase *Serum* *Increase* In 5 male patients with gout mean concentration of 437.0 ± 108.1 ng/mL significantly higher than 386.7 ± 33.7 ng/mL in 30 healthy male controls *5878*

α_1-Globulin *Serum* *Decrease* alpha$_1$ and alpha$_2$-Globulins reduced in many gouty patients *103*

α_2-Globulin *Serum* *Decrease* alpha$_1$ and alpha$_2$-globulins reduced in many gouty patients *103*

Glomerular Filtration Rate *Urine* *Decrease* Moderate but significant reduction in all age groups *1934*

Glucose *Serum* *No Effect* In 175 male patients with primary gout mean concentration of 98.0 ± 1.2 mg/dL not significantly different from 98.5 ± 0.8 mg/dL in 172 control men *5133*
Synovial Fluid *Decrease* Typical of inflammatory reactions sometimes showing a slight reduction in glucose *2039*

Glutamic Acid *Plasma* *Increase* Remains elevated even after casein loading. Fasting values range from 68 - 72 µmol/L (45 - 51 µmol/L in controls) *3970*
Red Blood Cells *Increase* Average values range from 214 to 243 µmol/L compared to 216 µmol/L in controls *3970*

Glutamine *Plasma* *No Effect* Concentration usually normal *4979*

γ-Glutamyltransferase *Serum* *No Effect* In 175 male patients with primary gout mean activity of 46.1 ± 2.2 U/L not significantly different from 44.5 ± 2.4 U/L in 172 control men *5133*

Glycine *Plasma* *Decrease* Distinct reduction *5827*

HDL-Cholesterol *Serum* *Decrease* In 175 male patients with primary gout mean concentration of 47.8 ± 0.9 mg/dL significantly different from 51.1 ± 1.1 mg/dL in 172 control men *5133*

25-Hydroxy Vitamin D_3 *Serum* *No Effect* Mean concentration in 114 male patients with gout of 25.5 ± 6.2 ng/mL not significantly different from 23.6 ± 8.8 ng/mL observed in 51 healthy male controls *5132*

Interleukin-6 *Serum* *Increase* Mean concentration of 116.8 ± 105.4 pg/mL in 10 patients with gout significantly different from 11.4 ± 1.9 pg/mL in healthy blood donors *1130*
Synovial Fluid *Increase* Mean concentration of 137.1 ± 86.8 ng/L in 10 patients with gout *1130* High concentrations observed in patients with gout *605*

Interleukin-10 *Serum* *No Effect* In 6 patients with gout mean concentration of 3.3 ± 1.7 U/mL not significantly different from 8.8 ± 1.9 U/mL in 22 healthy controls *986*
Synovial Fluid *No Effect* In 6 patients with gout mean concentration of 13.0 ± 7.8 U/mL not significantly different from 8.8 ± 1.9 U/mL in serum of 22 healthy controls *986*

Interleukin-11 *Serum* *No Effect* In 14 patients median concentration of 156.5 pg/mL *5287*
Synovial Fluid *Increase* In 14 patients median concentration of 196 pg/mL *5287*

Inulin Clearance *Urine* *Decrease* The lowest values are found in older patients or those with hypertension *1934* Below 90 mL/min in 33% of patients *925*

17-Ketosteroids *Urine* *Decrease* Moderate decrease *1025* Excretion may be slightly decreased in patients with gout *2952*

Leukocytes *Blood* *Increase* Occurs during acute attacks *5544* Usually accompanied by leukocytosis *2039*
Blood *No Effect* In 14 patients median concentration of 8.9 x 10^3/L *5287*
Synovial Fluid *Increase* Counts between 750 - 45,000 /µL in acute attacks *1980* The synovial fluid is typical of inflammatory reactions showing polymorphonuclear leukocytosis (5,000 - 50,000 /µL) *2039* In 14 patients median concentration of 11.6 x 10^3/L *5287*

Lipoprotein Lp(a) *Serum* *Increase* In 175 male patients with primary gout median concentration of 15.5 mg/dL significantly higher than 8.6 mg/dL in 172 control men *5133* Primary gout is associated with increased Lp(a) concentrations *2827*

Melanoma Inhibitory Factor *Serum* *No Effect* In 12 patients mean concentration of 2.6 ± 1.0 ng/mL showed no significant difference from 3.6 ± 2.8 ng/mL in 120 healthy controls *3655*

Neutrophils *Blood* *Increase* May be associated with a moderate to severe neutrophilia *5677*
Synovial Fluid *Increase* Increase in percentage of neutrophils in acute attacks; range of 48-94% (normal less than 5%) *5544*

Parathyroid Hormone *Plasma* *No Effect* Mean concentration in 114 male patients with gout of 361.3 ± 117.6 pg/mL not significantly different from 39.2 ± 110.5 pg/mL observed in 51 healthy male controls *5132*

pH *Urine* *Decrease* Often low: 5.0 - 5.5 *900* Tends to be low throughout the day, with decreased diurnal variations *1726*

Phosphate *Serum* *Decrease* Hypophosphatemia has been observed in association with acute attacks *2719* Gout is less common cause of hypophosphatemia due to shift of phosphate into the cells and increased renal loss of phosphate *969*
Serum *No Effect* Mean concentration in 114 male patients with gout of 3.0 ± 0.4 mg/dL not significantly different from 3.0 ± 0.5 mg/dL observed in 51 healthy male controls *5132*

Phospholipids *Serum* *No Effect* In 175 male patients with primary gout mean concentration of 237.7 ± 3.7 mg/dL not significantly different from 233.8 ± 3.2 mg/dL in 172 control men *5133*

Properdin Factor B *Plasma* *No Effect* Mean concentration typically normal or slightly increased in patients with gout *4682*

Prostaglandin E_2 *Synovial Fluid* *Increase* Mean concentration in 3 patients of 0.73 nmol/L *3366*

Protein *Synovial Fluid* *Increase* The synovial fluid is typical of inflammatory reactions showing an increase in protein content *2039*
Urine *Increase* Low-grade proteinuria occurs in 20 - 80% of gouty persons for many years before further evidence of renal disease appears *5545* Incidence varies from 20 - 40%. May be intermittent and rarely heavy *4979*

Pyrophosphate *Synovial Fluid* *Increase* Moderately elevated levels *2386*

Rheumatoid Factor *Serum* *Increase* In 14 patients rheumatoid factor present in 12 and absent in 2 patients with gout *5287*
Serum *No Effect* Concentration usually normal *5544*

Serine *Plasma* *Decrease* Reported effect *5827*

Soluble Interleukin-6 Receptor-α *Synovial Fluid* *Increase* Mean concentration of 23.2 ± 9.1 ng/mL in 10 patients with gout *1130*

Stromelysin *Plasma* *Increase* In 5 men with gout mean concentration of 196.6 ± 35.1 ng/mL significantly higher than 58.7 ± 5.7 ng/mL in 30 healthy control men *5878*

Thyroid Stimulating Hormone *Serum* *Increase* In 54 patients with crystal proven gouty arthritis mean concentration of 5.2 ± 1.2 μU/mL significantly greater than 1.8 ± 1.1 μU/mL in 55 age, sex, race and weight matched control patients *1378*

Tissue Plasminogen Activator *Urine* *Increase* In one patient with gout t-PA detectable *2139*

Triglycerides *Serum* *Increase* Observed in 75 - 84% of patients *295* 75 - 84% of patients *4979* In 175 male patients with primary gout mean concentration of 197.5 ± 11.1 mg/dL significantly different from 154.5 ± 10.9 mg/dL in 172 control men *5133* 75 - 84% of patients *1451*

Urea Nitrogen *Serum* *Increase* Rises with renal failure, but these changes may be subtle and slow *900*

Uric Acid *Cerebrospinal Fluid* *No Effect* Very low in normal and gouty patients. Probably explains the absence of tophaceous deposits in the CNS *5753*
Serum *Increase* Mean concentration in 114 male patients with gout of 8.8 ± 1.3 mg/dL significantly different from 5.7 ± 1.0 mg/dL observed in 51 healthy male controls *5132* In 80 patients with pure gout mean concentration of 10.15 ± 1.99 mg/dL significantly higher than 5.08 ± 1.14 mg/dL in 72 healthy controls *5166* May rise above 6.0 mg/dL in men, or 5.5 mg/dL in women. Possibly the rise is due to increased renal tubular reabsorption. 25% of patients' relatives have raised serum concentration also, but without symptoms of gout (possibly the effect of a single autosomal dominant gene) *1290* In 175 male patients with primary gout mean concentration of 8.8 ± 0.1 mg/dL significantly higher than 5.5 ± 0.1 mg/dL in 172 control men *5133* More than 95% of patients eventually have an elevated serum concentration *900*
Synovial Fluid *Increase* Many patients have a concentration which is greater than in serum *4310*
Urine *Increase* May occur during acute attack *225*

274.11 Uric Acid Nephrolithiasis

Calcium *Serum* *No Effect* Mean concentration of 4.7 ± 0.2 mEq/L observed in 33 patients compared with 4.7 ± 0.2 mEq/L in 14 healthy controls *2363*
Urine *Decrease* Mean excretion of 116.1 ± 74.1 mg/g creatinine observed in 26 patients with uric acid nephrolithiasis compared with 153.0 ± 135.5 mg/g creatinine in 14 healthy controls *2363*

Citrate *Urine* *No Effect* Mean excretion of 358.9 ± 235.4 mg/g creatinine observed in 26 patients with uric acid nephrolithiasis compared with 425.4 ± 268.9 mg/g creatinine in 14 healthy controls *2363*

Oxalate *Urine* *Increase* Mean excretion of 23.4 ± 12.3 mg/g creatinine observed in 26 patients with uric acid nephrolithiasis compared with 17.6 ± 8.3 mg/g creatinine in 14 healthy controls *2363*

Uric Acid *Serum* *Increase* Mean concentration of 7.3 ± 1.6 mg/dL observed in 33 patients compared with 6.7 ± 0.9 mg/dL in 14 healthy controls *2363*
Urine *No Effect* Mean excretion of 426.8 ± 136.0 mg/g creatinine observed in 26 patients with uric acid nephrolithiasis compared with 447.8 ± 101.6 mg/g creatinine in 14 healthy controls *2363*

Metabolic Disorders (Others)

275.00 Hemochromatosis

Adenosine Deaminase *Serum* *Increase* Increased *4956* *1340* *3926*

Alanine Aminopeptidase *Serum* *Increase* Activity may be mildly abnormal in asyptomatic patients with hereditary hemochromatosis *3406*

Aldosterone *Plasma* *Decrease* In 10 patients with idiopathic hemochromatosis mean concentration of 294 ± 126 pmol/L not significantly less than 357 ± 116 pmol/L in age matched controls in the upright position *5554*

Alkaline Phosphatase *Serum* *Increase* Activity may be mildly abnormal in asyptomatic patients with hereditary hemochromatosis *3406* With liver involvement *1980*
Serum *No Effect* Over 50% of patients have no laboratory evidence of liver dysfunction *2034* In about 175 patients with genetic hemochromatosis mean activity of 83.9 ± 28.9 U/L not significantly different from normal range of 37 - 110 U/L *4047*

Androgens *Plasma* *Decrease* Decreased testosterone found in 12 of 12 patients *432*

Aspartate Aminotransferase *Serum* *Increase* With liver involvement *1980* Activity may be mildly abnormal in asyptomatic patients with hereditary hemochromatosis *3406*
Serum *No Effect* Over 50% of patients have no laboratory evidence of liver dysfunction *2034*

Bilirubin *Serum* *Increase* Concentration may be mildly abnormal in asyptomatic patients with hereditary hemochromatosis *3406* With liver involvement *1980*
Serum *No Effect* Over 50% of patients have no laboratory evidence of liver dysfunction *2034*

BSP Retention *Serum* *Increase* With liver involvement *1980*
Serum *No Effect* Over 50% of patients have no laboratory evidence of liver dysfunction *2034*

Calcium *Serum* *No Effect* In about 175 patients with genetic hemochromatosis mean concentration of 2.34 ± 0.08 mmol/L not significantly different from normal range of 2.0 - 2.6 mmol/L *4047*

Cholesterol *Serum* *Decrease* In 5 patients with high iron overload mean concentration of 161 ± 42 mg/dL less than 191 ± 33 mg/dL in 23 healthy controls *5493*
Serum *No Effect* In 12 patients with no iron overload hemochromatosis mean concentration of 192 ± 41 mg/dL not significantly different from 191 ± 33 mg/dL in 23 healthy controls *5493*

Corticotropin *Plasma* *Decrease* 9 of 15 patients had pituitary dysfunction *5025* A frequent complication *4979*

Creatinine *Serum* *No Effect* In about 175 patients with genetic hemochromatosis mean concentration of 90.8 ± 12.5 μmol/L not significantly different from normal range of 45 - 115 μmol/L *4047*

Ferritin *Serum* *Increase* In about 175 patients with genetic hemochromatosis mean concentration of 1,410 ± 1,337 μg/L significantly different from normal range of 30 - 400 μg/L *4047* Concentration typically greater than 1,000 μg/L in symptomatic patients but may be only slightly increased (300 - 500 μg/L) in asyptomatic patients with hereditary hemochromatosis *3406* In 44 patients who were homozygous for hereditary hemochromatosis mean concentration of 442.4 ± 108.8 ng/mL and 123.2 ± 15.7 ng/mL in 19 heterozygotes compared with 89.1 ± 14.3 ng/mL in 33 normal controls *312* In 8 patients with transfusion iron overload mean concentration of 5,376.0 ± 1,784.6 ng/mL compared with 89.1 ± 14.3 ng/mL in 33 normal controls *312* Markedly increased due to gross increase in iron stores *349* Concentration was grossly raised in all 41 patients, ranging from 670 - 4,100 μg/L *4200* Plasma concentration of > 1,000 ng/mL is indicative of increased body iron stores, although it does not differentiate between reticuloendothelial and parenchymal storage. Correlates well with iron stores in cirrhotic patients with primary disease *4979* In 210 male heterozygous for hemochromatosis aged 1 - 30 y geometric and arithmetic mean concentrations of 49/82 μg/L, in 209 aged 31 - 60 y 131/181 μg/L and in 86 aged 61 - 90 y 130/204 μg/L significantly higher than 37/59, 60/83 and 116/162 μg/L in corresponding control groups respectively. Similar differences seen in women heterozygous for hemochromatosis *627* In patients with genetic hemochromatosis serum ferritin concentration may increase above 700 μg/L *4784* Increased plasma concentrations have been effectively used as a screening test for hemochromatosis *1301* Increased concentration is sensitive indicator of disease *3625* Mean concentration of 1,828 μg/L in 26 patients with hemochromatosis significantly greater than 736 μg/L in 42 patients who also had had liver iron analyses performed *1697* Plasma concentration may be increased 15-fold *5276*

275.00 Hemochromatosis *(continued)*

Ferritin *(continued)*
Serum *No Effect* Normal or marginal elevation in the precirrhotic stage *4979* Concentrations normal although transferrin saturation increased in patients heterozygous for hemochromatosis *3421*

Follicle Stimulating Hormone *Plasma* *Decrease* Frequently occurs in idiopathic hemochromatosis *5553*

Glucose *Serum* *Increase* About 82% of all patients with this disorder develop diabetes mellitus *2034*

Glucose Tolerance *Serum* *Decrease* Decreased tolerance:excessive peak decreased utilization with slow fall to fasting level *5544*

γ-Glutamyltransferase *Serum* *Increase* With liver involvement *1980*
Serum *No Effect* Over 50% of patients have no laboratory evidence of liver dysfunction *2034*

Gonadotropin, Pituitary *Plasma* *Decrease* Basal gonadotropin levels and/or their response to LHRH were low in 9 of 12 patients *432*
Urine *Decrease* A frequent complication *4979* 9 of 15 patients had pituitary dysfunction *5025*

Growth Hormone *Plasma* *Decrease* A frequent complication *4979* 9 of 15 patients had pituitary dysfunction *5025*
Urine *Increase* Marked elevation *3144*

Hematocrit *Blood* *No Effect* Anemia is not usually present with primary hemochromatosis; when present, anemia suggests secondary causes such as alcoholic cirrhosis, transfusion-induced iron overload, sideroblastic anemia, or thalassemia *900*

Hemoglobin *Blood* *No Effect* Anemia is not usually present with primary hemochromatosis; when present, anemia suggests secondary causes such as alcoholic cirrhosis, transfusion-induced iron overload, sideroblastic anemia, or thalassemia *900*

HLA Antigens *Blood* *Present* HLA-A3 present in 72% of patients versus 21% of controls *5678*

25-Hydroxy Vitamin D_3 *Serum* *No Effect* In about 175 patients with genetic hemochromatosis mean concentration of 21.7 ± 12.7 ng/mL not significantly different from normal range of 10 - 40 ng/mL *4047*

Iron *Liver* *Increase* Increased serum and hepatic iron concentrations *4200* Increased iron deposition principally in the parenchymal cells of the liver *1980* Large amounts of stainable iron, predominantly within the parenchymal cells *5863* Increased concentration is sensitive indicator of disease, with hepatic iron index of greater than 2 diagnostic of hemochromatosis *3625* Hemochromatosis present if amount of iron greater than 2.0 µmol/g dry tissue *1697* In 10 patients with hemochromatosis and cirrhosis mean hepatic iron index of 7.6 in tissue compared with 4.3 in 45 patients without cirrhosis *33*
Serum *Increase* Diagnosis established when concentration > 220 µg/dL *2039* In about 175 patients with genetic hemochromatosis mean concentration of 34.2 ± 8 µmol/L significantly different from normal range of 12.5 - 25 µmol/L *4047* Increased serum and hepatic iron concentration *4200* Increase in concentration to above 150 µg/dL observed in hereditary hemochromatosis *2952* In the absence of infection, inflammation, neoplasia, or recent blood loss, concentrations usually range from 175 - 275 µg/dL *4979* In 210 men heterozygous for hemochromatosis aged 1 - 30 y mean concentration of 132 ± 47 µg/dL, in 209 aged 31 - 60 y 124 ± 41 µg/dL and in 86 aged 61 - 90 y 117 ± 38 µg/dL significantly higher than 111 ± 46 µg/dL, 108 ± 35 µg/dL and 99 ± 27 µg/dL in corresponding control groups respectively. Similar differences seen in women heterozygous for hemochromatosis *627* Average level is 250 µg/dL, with a range of from 225 - 325 µg/dL *5677*
Serum *No Effect* Up to one quarter of patients with hereditary hemochromatosis have plasma iron concentrations within the reference range of 10 - 30 µmol/L *3406*

Iron-binding Capacity, Total *Serum* *Decrease* Reduced transferrin as shown by a low TIBC *5863* Occurs early in the course of the disease *4200* Usually < 300 µg/dL *4979*
Serum *Increase* Concentration usually normal in patients with hereditary hemochromatosis *3406*
Serum *No Effect* No significant effect observed *2034*

Iron Saturation *Serum* *Increase* Mean saturation of 71% in 26 patients with hemochromatosis significantly greater than 30% in 42 patients who also had had liver iron analyses performed *1697* Usually > 80% and often 100% *5863* Usually 75% *4979*

Lactate Dehydrogenase *Serum* *Increase* With liver involvement *1980*
Serum *No Effect* Over 50% of patients have no laboratory evidence of liver dysfunction *2034*

Lead *Blood* *Increase* In 44 patients who were homozygous for hereditary hemochromatosis mean concentration of 5.6 ± 0.5 µg/dL and 4.1 ± 0.5 µg/dL in 19 heterozygotes compared with 3.6 ± 0.5 µg/dL in 33 normal controls *312*

Leucine Aminopeptidase *Serum* *Increase* With liver involvement *1980*
Serum *No Effect* Over 50% of patients have no laboratory evidence of liver dysfunction *2034*

Luteinizing Hormone *Plasma* *Decrease* Hypogonadism frequently occurs in idiopathic hemochromatosis *5553* Depressed in 44% of 32 patients; generalized depression of pituitary function *5026*

Magnesium *Red Blood Cells* *No Effect* In about 175 patients with genetic hemochromatosis mean concentration of 2.09 ± 0.28 mmol/L not significantly different from normal range of 1.85 - 2.27 mmol/L *4047*
Serum *No Effect* In about 175 patients with genetic hemochromatosis mean concentration of 0.83 ± 0.07 mmol/L not significantly different from normal range of 0.65 - 1.05 mmol/L *4047*

Neopterin *Serum* *Increase* In 14 patients with genetic hemochromatosis mean concentration of 9.0 ± 1.7 nmol/L, with mean in 8 without cirrhosis of 7.8 ± 1.0 nmol/L and 11.0 ± 4.3 nmol/L in 6 with cirrhosis different from 6.0 ± 2.2 nmol/L in healthy controls *5682*

5'-Nucleotidase *Serum* *Increase* With liver involvement *1980*
Serum *No Effect* Over 50% of patients have no laboratory evidence of liver dysfunction *2034*

Parathyroid Hormone 1-84 *Plasma* *No Effect* In about 175 patients with genetic hemochromatosis mean concentration of 25.1 ± 11.7 pg/mL not significantly different from normal range of 10 - 55 pg/mL *4047*

Parathyroid Hormone 44-68 *Plasma* *No Effect* In about 175 patients with genetic hemochromatosis mean concentration of 301 ± 117 pg/mL not significantly different from normal range of 80 - 340 pg/mL *4047*

Phosphate *Serum* *No Effect* In about 175 patients with genetic hemochromatosis mean concentration of 1.01 ± 0.2 mmol/L not significantly different from normal range of 0.8 - 1..65 mmol/L *4047*

Phospholipids *Serum* *No Effect* In 5 patients with high iron overload and 12 with no iron overload mean concentrations of 228 ± 36 mg/dL and 218 ± 38 mg/dL respectively not significantly different from 214 ± 42 mg/dL in 23 healthy controls *5493*

Pyrophosphate *Synovial Fluid* *Increase* Has been identified *4681*

Renin Activity *Plasma* *Decrease* In 10 patients with idiopathic hemochromatosis mean activity of 1.44 ± 1.41 µg/L/h not significantly less than 2.6 ± 1.8 µg/L/h in age matched controls in the upright position *5554*

Testosterone *Serum* *Decrease* Found in 12 of 12 patients *432*

Transferrin Saturation *Serum* *Increase* In about 175 patients with genetic hemochromatosis mean saturation of 69.2 ± 19% significantly different from normal range of 25 - 50% *4047* In 210 men heterozygous for hemochromatosis aged 1 - 30 y mean concentration of 38 ± 14%, in 209 aged 31 - 60 y 37 ± 12% and in 86 aged 61 - 90 y 38 ± 14% significantly higher than 29 ± 11%, 30 ± 9% and 30 ± 8% in corresponding control groups respectively. Similar differences seen in women heterozygous for hemochromatosis *627* A transferrin saturation of more than 60% correctly classified 96% of 174 Danish patients who were homozygous for hemochromatosis *1301* Mean saturations of 37.3% for men and 37.6% for women with heterozygous hemochromatosis significantly higher than 24.1% and 22.5% in healthy men and women respectively, with means of 82.7% and 75.3% in homozygous men and women respectively *3421* % Transferrin saturation of greater than 50% is sensitive indicator of disease *3625* Saturation almost always above the reference range (20 - 50%) in hereditary hemochromatosis *3406*

Triglycerides *Serum* *Increase* In 5 patients with high iron overload and 12 with no high iron overload mean concentrations of 115 ± 39 mg/dL and 168 ± 89 mg/dL respectively higher than 87 ± 23 mg/dL in 23 healthy controls *5493*

Vitamin E *Serum* *Decrease* In 5 patients with high iron overload mean concentration of 17.6 ± 3.9 µmol/L and 3.49 ± 0.35 µmol/g lipids significantly less than 26.0 ± 4.4 µmol/L and 5.28 ± 0.49 µmol/g lipids respectively in 23 healthy controls *5493*
Serum *No Effect* Mean concentrations of 28.0 ± 9.1 µmol/L and 4.84 ± 0.88 µmol/g lipids not significantly different from 26.0 ± 4.4 µmol/L and 5.28 ± 0.49 µmol/g lipids respectively in 23 healthy controls *5493*

275.00 Iron Overload

Ferritin Iron *Serum* *Increase* Concentration in 22 of 22 patients with iron overload greater than 35 ng/mL (with 17 having values greater than 100 ng/mL) compared with range in healthy controls of 10 - 35 ng Fe/mL *2125*

Ferritin Protein *Serum* *Increase* Concentration in 22 patients with iron overload of 917.9 ± 112.0 ng/mL compared with concentration in 17 healthy controls of 136.6 ± 11.9 ng/mL *2125*

Iron *Serum* *Increase* Concentration in 22 patients with iron overload of 260 ± 113 µg/dL compared with concentration in 17 healthy controls of 103.9 ± 66 µg/dL *2125*

Transferrin Saturation *Serum* *Increase* Mean saturation in 16 patients with iron overload of 93.0 ± 10.6% compared with 16.4 ± 3.0% in 10 normal volunteers *88* Saturation in 22 patients with iron overload of 88.5 ± 2.1% compared with saturation in 17 healthy controls of 30.3 ± 2.6% *2125*

275.10 Hepatolenticular Degeneration

Alanine *Urine* *Increase* Observed with renal damage *1025*

Alanine Aminotransferase *Serum* *Increase* Minimal elevation in 14% (5 of 37 patients). Mean = 30 U/L *5047*

Albumin *Serum* *Decrease* Reduced in 27% or 10 of 37 patients *5047*

Alkaline Phosphatase *Serum* *Increase* With liver involvement *2034*

Amino Acids *Urine* *Increase* 77% of patients tested before penicillamine therapy had hyperaminoaciduria. Urinary excretion of amino acids decreased after therapy *5047*

α-Amino-Nitrogen *Urine* *Increase* Increased in 79% of patients *5047*

Aspartate Aminotransferase *Serum* *Increase* Minimally elevated in 36% (14 of 39) patients. Mean activity of 30 U/L *5047*

Bicarbonate *Serum* *Decrease* Decreased serum CO_2 in 12 of 27 patients (44%) *5047*

Bilirubin *Serum* *Increase* Elevated in 13 of 38 (34%) patients; mean of 1.45 mg/dL. Direct bilirubin was increased in 9 of 36 (25%) patients *5047*

Bilirubin, Direct *Serum* *Increase* Increased in 9 of 36 (25%) patients *5047*

BSP Retention *Serum* *Increase* Excretion was delayed in 76% of cases. Mean retention in 29 patients tested was 15%, and 9 patients had values > 20% *5047*

Calcium *Serum* *Decrease* Related to decreased albumin *5047*
Urine *Increase* Slightly increased clearance in 19% of patients *5047*

Ceruloplasmin *Serum* *Decrease* Most patients are deficient; concentration is usually 15 mg/dL, but patients are seen with concentration within the normal range (25 - 45 mg/dL). This is particularly likely to be the case when liver damage predominates *900* Values less than 14 mg/dL are expected in patients with Wilson's disease *2952* Concentration typically reduced in patients with Wilson's disease *3499* Low ceruloplasmin and elevated copper are characteristic. This is the result of an impaired ability to incorporate copper into protein, particularly ceruloplasmin, which causes unbound copper to be deposited in tissues and fluids throughout the body *2039*
Serum *No Effect* Normal in 5% of patients with overt disease *5544*

Chloride *Serum* *Increase* Frequent hyperchloremia; occurred in 13 of 31 patients (42%) *5047*

Cholesterol *Serum* *Decrease* Related to liver disease *5047*
Serum *No Effect* Mean concentration of 183 ± 18 mg/dL in 3 patients with Wilson's disease and serum free copper concentration of greater than 10 mg/dL and of 170 ± 64 mg/dL in 9 with serum free copper of less than 10 mg/dL not significantly different from 191 ± 33 mg/dL in 23 healthy controls *5493*

Copper *Liver* *Increase* Hepatic copper concentration is the most exact criterion in the diagnosis. In the course of the penicillamine therapy the copper content in the liver decreases, but normal values are achieved only after 5 or more y of treatment. The urinary copper excretion is a good indicator of the copper concentration in the liver *3290* Liver biopsy shows high copper concentration (250 µg/g of dry liver) *5544*
Serum *Decrease* The serum concentration is directly related to that of the ceruloplasmin, for the protein binds the majority of the metal. Estimation of the serum copper seldom gives additional diagnostic information unless there is a discrepancy indicating a higher level of serum copper than can be accounted for by that present in ceruloplasmin. The normal serum concentration is between 90 - 140 µg/dL; in untreated disease it is commonly between 40 - 60 µg/dL but the range of variation is enormous *900* Characteristic finding of disease *5544*
Urine *Increase* In untreated disease the amount is usually > 200 µg/d but occasionally much lower, particularly in young presymptomatic siblings *900* A good indirect indicator of the copper concentration in the liver *3290* The ceruloplasmin fraction is defective. Copper is excreted in the urine, bound to amino acids which act as chelating agents *1290*

Copper, Nonceruloplasmin *Serum* *Increase* There is a complete absence of ceruloplasmin in this condition, and copper is deposited in the liver, brain, and renal tubules. The copper-carrying protein present is abnormal *1290* Heterozygotes and treated homozygotes had nonceruloplasmin copper concentration of 5.9 and 9.8 µg/dL, respectively) which did not differ significantly from normal (10.1 ± 1.6 µg/dL). Untreated patients had very significantly raised free copper concentration (22.9 ± 4.5 µg/dL) *2748*

Creatine Kinase *Serum* *No Effect* Normal *5047*

Creatinine *Serum* *Decrease* Definitely elevated in 4 of 30 (13%) but decreased in 3 others *5047*
Serum *Increase* Definitely elevated in 4 of 30 (13%) but decreased in 3 others *5047*

Creatinine Clearance *Urine* *Decrease* Reduced in 7 of 24 patients (29%) *5047*

Erythrocyte Sedimentation Rate *Blood* *Increase* May be increased, particularly if liver damage is present *900*

Erythrocyte Survival *Red Blood Cells* *Decrease* Reduced and found to correlate with splenic enlargement *5046*

Erythrocytes *Urine* *Increase* Microscopic hematuria may occur *5047*

Glomerular Filtration Rate *Urine* *Decrease* Significantly reduced *351*

Glucose *Serum* *Decrease* In 5% of patients related to malnutrition *5047*
Serum *Increase* Fasting glucose consistently elevated *5047*
Urine *Increase* Tubular reabsorption of glucose is frequently impaired *351*

Glucose Tolerance *Serum* *Decrease* Abnormal in some patients. Fasting blood sugar levels are consistently increased *5047*

γ-Glutamyltransferase *Serum* *Increase* With liver involvement *2034*

Haptoglobin *Serum* *Decrease* Hemolytic anemia *2034*

Hematocrit *Blood* *Decrease* Pancytopenia occurred frequently; hematocrit, platelets, WBC were often decreased *5047* Mild normochromic anemia with anisocytosis and poikilocytosis *900*

Hemoglobin *Blood* *Decrease* Mild normochromic anemia with anisocytosis and poikilocytosis *900* Reported observation *1092*
Plasma *Increase* Hemolytic episodes frequently occur several years prior to onset of other symptoms; due to increased oxidative stress on RBC from excess copper *1092*

275.10 Hepatolenticular Degeneration *(continued)*

Homocystine *Urine* *Increase* Observed with renal damage *1025*

immunoglobulin A *Serum* *Decrease* Decreased in 6 and elevated in 2 of 16 patients *5047*
Serum *Increase* Decreased in 6 and elevated in 2 of 16 patients *5047*

Immunoglobulin G *Serum* *Increase* Elevated in over 50% of patients *5047*

Immunoglobulin M *Serum* *Increase* Found to be increased in 5 out of 16 patients *5047*

Inulin Clearance *Urine* *Decrease* Reduced clearance in 8 of 9 patients; although none had elevated BUN *351*

Isoleucine *Urine* *Increase* Observed effect with renal damage *1025*

Lactate Dehydrogenase *Serum* *Increase* With liver involvement *2034*

Leucine *Urine* *Increase* Observed effect with renal damage *1025*

Leucine Aminopeptidase *Serum* *Increase* With liver involvement *2034*

Leukocytes *Blood* *Decrease* Reported observation *900* Pancytopenia occurred frequently; Hematocrit, platelets, WBC were often decreased *5047*

Neopterin *Serum* *No Effect* In 9 patients with Wilson's disease mean concentration of 5.4 ± 0.8 nmol/L, with mean in 6 without cirrhosis of 6.3 ± 1.0 nmol/L and 3.6 ± 0.6 nmol/L in 3 with cirrhosis different from 6.0 ± 2.2 nmol/L in healthy controls *5682*

5'-Nucleotidase *Serum* *Increase* With liver involvement *2034*

pH *Urine* *Increase* Value in 50% of patients was > 6.5 with multiple specimens. 9 of 22 patients were unable to adequately acidify their urine during acid loading tests (pH > 5.3) *5047*

Phenylalanine *Urine* *Increase* Observed effect with renal damage *1025*

Phosphate *Serum* *Decrease* Decreased in 18 of 30 (60%), mean concentration of 3.0 mg/dL *5047*
Urine *Increase* Marked increase in clearance in 36% (8 of 22) *5047*

Phospholipids *Serum* *Decrease* Mean concentration of 182 ± 14 mg/dL in 3 patients with Wilson's disease and serum free copper concentrations greater than 10 µg/dL less than 214 ± 42 µg/dL in 23 healthy controls *5493*
Serum *No Effect* Mean concentration of 217 ± 31 µg/dL in 9 patients with Wilson's disease and serum free copper concentrations less than 10 µg/dL not significantly different from 214 ± 42 µg/dL in 23 healthy controls *5493*

Platelets *Blood* *Decrease* Count often reduced *900* Frequently decreased; 13 of 32 patients had counts < 100,000 /µL *5047*

Potassium *Serum* *Decrease* Found in 9 of 31 patients (29%) *5047*

Proline *Urine* *Increase* Observed with renal damage *1025*

Protein *Serum* *Decrease* Reduced to 6.0 mg/dL or less in 29% of patients (9 of 31) *5047*
Urine *Increase* Present in 33% of patients; always minimal and decreases with penicillamine therapy. Probably due to tubular reabsorption than increased GFR of protein *5047*

Prothrombin Time *Plasma* *Increase* Mean time = 17.3 sec, abnormally prolonged in 79% (26 of 33) patients *5047*

Pyrophosphate *Synovial Fluid* *Increase* Has been identified *4681*

Pyruvate *Blood* *Increase* Reverts to normal after treatment with copper-chelating agent *1290*

Specific Gravity *Urine* *Decrease* Reduced concentrating ability; 20% had maximum specific gravities of < 1.015 on overnight specimens *5047*

Threonine *Urine* *Increase* Observed with renal damage *1025*

Triglycerides *Serum* *No Effect* Mean concentrations of 82 ± 12 mg/dL in 3 patients with Wilson's disease and serum free copper concentrations of greater than 10 µg/dL and 94 ± 44 mg/dL in 9 with copper concentrations less than 10 µg/dL not significantly different from 87 ± 23 mg/dL in 23 healthy controls *5493*

Tryptophan *Urine* *Increase* Observed with renal damage *1025*

Tyrosine *Urine* *Increase* Observed with renal damage *1025*

Urea Nitrogen *Serum* *Decrease* Mildly elevated between 20 - 25 mg/dL in 6 of 35 (17%) and decreased < 10 mg/dL in 4 cases *5047*
Serum *Increase* Mildly elevated between 20 - 25 mg/dL in 6 of 35 (17%) and decreased < 10 mg/dL in 4 cases *5047*

Uric Acid *Serum* *Decrease* Occurs in most patients with untreated disease *5687* Decreased urate, mean concentration of 2.5 mg/dL in 25 of 32 (78%). One patient had an elevated concentration *5047* Renal tubular reabsorption of uric acid is reduced, possibly as a result of damage to the tubule cells by excess unbound copper *1290* Common observation *4707*
Urine *Increase* Due to decreased renal tubular reabsorption *1290*

Uric Acid Clearance *Urine* *Increase* Consistently high renal clearance even though some patients have total excretion values within the normal range *5687* Mean clearance is 17.1 mL/min/1.73 m^2. 87% of 24 patients had elevated clearance *5047* Observed effect *4707*

Valine *Urine* *Increase* Observed effect with renal damage *1025*

Vitamin E *Serum* *Decrease* In 3 patients with Wilson's disease and serum free copper concentration of more than 10 µg/dL mean concentrations of 14.9 ± 4.2 µmol/L and 3.33 ± 0.57 µmol/g lipids significantly reduced compared with 26.0 ± 4.4 µmol/L and 5.28 ± 0.49 µmol/g lipids respectively in 23 healthy controls *5493*
Serum *No Effect* Mean concentrations of 22.8 ± 5.2 µmol/L and 4.74 ± 0.93 µmol/g lipids in 9 patients with Wilson's disease and serum free copper concentrations less than 10 µg/dL not significantly different from 26.0 ± 4.4 µmol/L and 5.28 ± 0.49 µmol/g lipids respectively in 23 healthy controls *5493*

275.10 Wilson's Disease

Alanine Aminotransferase *Serum* *Increase* Activity usually normal in asymptomatic patients, abnormal but variable in symptomatic patients with insidious onset of the disease and severely deranged in patients with acute onset *3406* Activity may be normal or mildly increased *3625*
Serum *No Effect* Activity may be normal or mildly increased *3625*

Alkaline Phosphatase *Serum* *Decrease* Activity decreased in patients with severe liver disease and acute hemolytic anemia *3625*
Serum *Increase* Activity usually normal in asymptomatic patients, abnormal but variable in symptomatic patients with insidious onset of the disease and severely deranged in patients with acute onset *3406*

Alkaline Phosphatase:Bilirubin Ratio *Serum* *Decrease* Ratio of less than 2.0 has been proposed to differentiate fulminant Wilson's disease from other causes of fulminant hepatic failure *3625*

Ammonium Ions *Urine* *Increase* May lead to proximal renal tubular acidosis which is associated with hypokalemia, hyperchloremic metabolic acidosis, urine pH < 5.5, increased urinary ammonium ion excretion, a negative urine anion gap, increased urinary osmol gap, normal urinary citrate, normal urinary calcium excretion and Fanconi syndrome *4071* May be associated with classic distal renal tubular acidosis which is asociated with hyokalemia, hyperchloremic metabolic acidosis, urine pH > 5.5, increased urinary ammonium ion excretion, a negative urine anion gap, increased urinary osmol gap, decreased urinary citrate and increased urinary calcium in some patients *4071*

Anion Gap *Urine* *Decrease* May lead to proximal renal tubular acidosis which is associated with hypokalemia, hyperchloremic metabolic acidosis, urine pH < 5.5, increased urinary ammonium ion excretion, a negative urine anion gap, increased urinary osmol gap, normal urinary citrate, normal urinary calcium excretion and Fanconi syndrome *4071* May be associated with classic distal renal tubular acidosis which is asociated with hyokalemia, hyperchloremic metabolic acidosis, urine pH > 5.5, increased urinary ammonium ion excretion, a negative urine anion gap, increased urinary osmol gap, decreased urinary citrate and increased urinary calcium in some patients *4071*

Aspartate Aminotransferase *Serum* *Increase* Activity may be normal or mildly increased *3625* Activity usually normal in asymptomatic patients, abnormal but variable in symptomatic patients with insidious onset of the disease and severely deranged in patients with acute onset *3406*
Serum *No Effect* Activity may be normal or mildly increased *3625*

Aspartate Aminotransferase:Alanine Aminotransferase Ratio *Serum* *Increase* Ratio of greater than 4.0 has been proposed to differentiate fulminant Wilson's disease from other causes of fulminant hepatic failure *3625*

Bicarbonate *Serum* *Decrease* May lead to proximal renal tubular acidosis which is associated with hypokalemia, hyperchloremic metabolic acidosis, urine pH < 5.5, increased urinary ammonium ion excretion, a negative urine anion gap, increased urinary osmol gap, normal urinary citrate, normal urinary calcium excretion and Fanconi syndrome *4071*

Bilirubin *Serum* *Increase* Concentration usually normal in asymptomatic patients, abnormal but variable in symptomatic patients with insidious onset of the disease and severely deranged in patients with acute onset *3406*

Calcium *Urine* *Increase* May be associated with classic distal renal tubular acidosis which is asociated with hyokalemia, hyperchloremic metabolic acidosis, urine pH > 5.5, increased urinary ammonium ion excretion, a negative urine anion gap, increased urinary osmol gap, decreased urinary citrate and increased urinary calcium in some patients *4071*
Urine *No Effect* May lead to proximal renal tubular acidosis which is associated with hypokalemia, hyperchloremic metabolic acidosis, urine pH < 5.5, increased urinary ammonium ion excretion, a negative urine anion gap, increased urinary osmol gap, normal urinary citrate, normal urinary calcium excretion and Fanconi syndrome *4071*

Calculi *Urine* *Decrease* Renal calculi and nephrocalcinosis may follow primary and distal renal renal tubular dysfunction which are common in Wilson's disease *3625*

Ceruloplasmin *Serum* *Decrease* Concentration decreased *3625* In 1 patient with Wilson's disease concentration of 17 mg/L significantly less than that in 250 healthy people, mean concentration of 315 ± 119 mg/L *1377* A low concentration is typically observed in most patients *5174*
Serum *Increase* Plasma concentration increased *5276* Concentration < 300 mgmol/L in asymptomatic patients, and < 200 mg/L in symptomatic patients with insidious onset of the disease and < 200 mg/L in patients with acute onset, compared with reference interval of 160 - 350 mg/L *3406*

Ceruloplasmin Ferroxidase *Serum* *Decrease* In 1 patient with Wilson's disease mean activity of 25 U/L significantly less than that in 250 healthy people in whom the mean concentration was 537 ± 201 U/L *1377*

Chloride *Serum* *Increase* May be associated with classic distal renal tubular acidosis which is asociated with hyokalemia, hyperchloremic metabolic acidosis, urine pH > 5.5, increased urinary ammonium ion excretion, a negative urine anion gap, increased urinary osmol gap, decreased urinary citrate and increased urinary calcium in some patients *4071* May lead to proximal renal tubular acidosis which is associated with hypokalemia, hyperchloremic metabolic acidosis, urine pH < 5.5, increased urinary ammonium ion excretion, a negative urine anion gap, increased urinary osmol gap, normal urinary citrate, normal urinary calcium excretion and Fanconi syndrome *4071*

Citrate *Urine* *Decrease* May be associated with classic distal renal tubular acidosis which is asociated with hyokalemia, hyperchloremic metabolic acidosis, urine pH > 5.5, increased urinary ammonium ion excretion, a negative urine anion gap, increased urinary osmol gap, decreased urinary citrate and increased urinary calcium in some patients *4071*
Urine *No Effect* May lead to proximal renal tubular acidosis which is associated with hypokalemia, hyperchloremic metabolic acidosis, urine pH < 5.5, increased urinary ammonium ion excretion, a negative urine anion gap, increased urinary osmol gap, normal urinary citrate, normal urinary calcium excretion and Fanconi syndrome *4071*

Copper *Liver* *Increase* Concentration of 1 - 4 µmol/g dry weight in asymptomatic patients, and > 4 µmol/g dry weight in symptomatic patients with insidious onset of the disease and > 4 µmol/g dry weight in patients with acute onset, compared with reference interval of < 1 µmol/g dry weight *3406* Concentration increased in liver biopsies is diagnostic of disease *3625*
Serum *Decrease* In 1 patient with Wilson's disease concentration of 2.63 µmol/L significantly less than that in 250 healthy people, mean concentration of 15.82 ± 4.15 µmol/L *1377* Hypocupricemia is typically observed in most patients *5174*
Serum *Increase* Concentration variable in asymptomatic patients, and variable in symptomatic patients with insidious onset of the disease and above 30 µmol/L in patients with acute onset, compared with reference interval of 10 - 30 µmol/L *3406* Plasma concentration increased *5276*
Urine *Increase* Concentration > 1 µmol/d in asymptomatic patients, and > 2 µmol/d in symptomatic patients with insidious onset of the disease and > 15 µmol/d in patients with acute onset, compared with reference interval of 0.25 - 0.75 µmol/d *3406* Concentration increased *3625* Concentration increased after penicillamine challenge *5276*

Copper, Free *Serum* *Increase* Concentration > 2 µmol/L in asymptomatic patients, and > 10 µmol/L in symptomatic patients with insidious onset of the disease and above 10 µmol/L in patients with acute onset, compared with reference interval of < 2 µmol/L *3406*

Copper, Nonceruloplasmin *Serum* *Increase* Concentration increased *3625*

Glucose *Urine* *Increase* May lead to proximal renal tubular acidosis which is associated with hypokalemia, hyperchloremic metabolic acidosis, urine pH < 5.5, increased urinary ammonium ion excretion, a negative urine anion gap, increased urinary osmol gap, normal urinary citrate, normal urinary calcium excretion and Fanconi syndrome *4071*

Net Acid Excretion *Urine* *Increase* May be associated with classic distal renal tubular acidosis which is asociated with hyokalemia, hyperchloremic metabolic acidosis, urine pH > 5.5, increased urinary ammonium ion excretion, a negative urine anion gap, increased urinary osmol gap, decreased urinary citrate and increased urinary calcium in some patients *4071*

Osmolal Gap *Urine* *Increase* May be associated with classic distal renal tubular acidosis which is asociated with hyokalemia, hyperchloremic metabolic acidosis, urine pH > 5.5, increased urinary ammonium ion excretion, a negative urine anion gap, increased urinary osmol gap, decreased urinary citrate and increased urinary calcium in some patients *4071* May lead to proximal renal tubular acidosis which is associated with hypokalemia, hyperchloremic metabolic acidosis, urine pH < 5.5, increased urinary ammonium ion excretion, a negative urine anion gap, increased urinary osmol gap, normal urinary citrate, normal urinary calcium excretion and Fanconi syndrome *4071*

pH *Urine* *Decrease* May lead to proximal renal tubular acidosis which is associated with hypokalemia, hyperchloremic metabolic acidosis, urine pH < 5.5, increased urinary ammonium ion excretion, a negative urine anion gap, increased urinary osmol gap, normal urinary citrate, normal urinary calcium excretion and Fanconi syndrome *4071*
Urine *Increase* May be associated with classic distal renal tubular acidosis which is asociated with hyokalemia, hyperchloremic metabolic acidosis, urine pH > 5.5, increased urinary ammonium ion excretion, a negative urine anion gap, increased urinary osmol gap, decreased urinary citrate and increased urinary calcium in some patients *4071*

Phosphate *Serum* *Decrease* Hypophosphatemia may follow primary and distal renal renal tubular dysfunction which are common in Wilson's disease *3625* May lead to proximal renal tubular acidosis which is associated with hypokalemia, hyperchloremic metabolic acidosis, urine pH < 5.5, increased urinary ammonium ion excretion, a negative urine anion gap, increased urinary osmol gap, normal urinary citrate, normal urinary calcium excretion and Fanconi syndrome *4071*

Potassium *Serum* *Decrease* May be associated with classic distal renal tubular acidosis which is asociated with hyokalemia, hyperchloremic metabolic acidosis, urine pH > 5.5, increased urinary ammonium ion excretion, a negative urine anion gap, increased urinary osmol gap, decreased urinary citrate and

275.10 Wilson's Disease *(continued)*

Potassium *(continued)*
increased urinary calcium in some patients *4071* May lead to proximal renal tubular acidosis which is associated with hypokalemia, hyperchloremic metabolic acidosis, urine pH < 5.5, increased urinary ammonium ion excretion, a negative urine anion gap, increased urinary osmol gap, normal urinary citrate, normal urinary calcium excretion and Fanconi syndrome *4071*

Uric Acid *Serum* *Decrease* May lead to proximal renal tubular acidosis which is associated with hypokalemia, hyperchloremic metabolic acidosis, urine pH < 5.5, increased urinary ammonium ion excretion, a negative urine anion gap, increased urinary osmol gap, normal urinary citrate, normal urinary calcium excretion and Fanconi syndrome *4071* Hypouricemia may follow may follow primary and distal renal renal tubular dysfunction which are common in Wilson's disease *3625*

275.20 Hypermagnesemia

Aluminum *Serum* *No Effect* In 24 patients on regular hemodialysis with hypermagnesemia mean concentration of 25 ± 17 µg/mL compared with 25 ± 17 µg/mL in 17 without hypermagnesemia *3745*

Bicarbonate *Serum* *No Effect* In 24 patients on regular hemodialysis with hypermagnesemia mean concentration of 23.3 ± 3.7 mmol/L compared with 22.7 ± 3.3 mmol/L in 17 without hypermagnesemia *3745*

Ferritin *Serum* *No Effect* In 24 patients with hypermagnesemia on regular hemodialysis mean concentration of 239 ± 125 µg/L compared with 187 ± 150 µg/L in 17 without hypermagnesemia *3745*

Phosphate *Serum* *Increase* Serum phosphate concentration may be increased with hypermagnesemia *5204*
Serum *No Effect* In 24 patients on regular hemodialysis with hypermagnesemia mean concentration of 1.6 ± 0.5 mmol/L compared with 1.9 ± 0.6 mmol/L in 17 without hypermagnesemia *3745*

Vitamin D *Serum* *No Effect* In 24 patients on regular hemodialysis with hypermagnesemia mean concentration of 51.4 ± 11 ng/L compared with 53.7 ± 12 ng/L in 17 without hypermagnesemia *3745*

275.20 Hypomagnesemia

Creatinine *Serum* *Decrease* In 33 patients with hypomagnesemia of extrarenal origin mean concentration of 0.95 ± 0.2 mg/dL and 1.2 ± 0.3 mg/dL in 41 patients with hypomagnesemia of renal origin not significantly different from mean concentration of 1.00 ± 0.23 mg/dL in 142 healthy controls *1332*

Fractional Excretion of Magnesium *Urine* *Increase* In 41 patients with hypomagnesemia of renal origin mean FEMg of 15 ± 12% significantly different from mean FEMg of 1.8 ± 0.8% in 142 healthy controls *1332*
Urine *No Effect* In 33 patients with hypomagnesemia of extrarenal origin mean FEMg of 1.4 ± 0.7% not significantly different from mean FEMg of 1.8 ± 0.8% in 142 healthy controls *1332*

ionized Calcium *Serum* *Decrease* Plasma ionized calcium is reduced in patients with hypomagnesemia *1290*

Magnesium *Serum* *Decrease* Urine is almost always hypertonic to plasma *126* In 33 patients with hypomagnesemia of extrarenal origin mean concentration of 0.55 ± 0.05 mmol/L and 0.52 ± 0.06 mmol/L in 41 patients with hypomagnesemia of renal origin significantly different from mean concentration of 0.88 ± 0.1 mmol/L in 142 healthy controls *1332*

Magnesium:Creatinine Ratio *Serum* *Increase* In 41 patients with hypomagnesemia of renal origin mean molar ratio of 0.64 ± 0.48 in 41 patients with hypomagnesemia of renal origin significantly different from mean concentration of 0.16 ± 0.08 in 142 healthy controls *1332*
Serum *No Effect* In 33 patients with hypomagnesemia of extrarenal origin mean molar ratio of 0.14 ± 0.06 not significantly different from mean concentration of 0.16 ± 0.08 in 142 healthy controls *1332*

Parathyroid Hormone *Plasma* *Decrease* In 59 patients with hypomagnesemia in one study with low intact PTH and normocalcemia 1 had idiopathic hypomagnesemia *3280*

Phosphate *Serum* *Increase* Serum phosphate concentration may be increased with hypomagnesemia *5204*

275.20 Idiopathic Hypomagnesemia

Calcium *Serum* *No Effect* In a study of 59 patients with normocalcemia and low intact PTH concentration, 1 had idiopathic hypomagnesemia *3280*

275.20 Magnesium Deficiency

Alkaline Phosphatase *Serum* *Decrease* Reported effect. In one study represented 0.3% of all cases of low alkaline phosphatase activity *3160*

Calcium *Serum* *Decrease* In 26 healthy individuals a magnesium deficient diet for 3 weeks caused decrease in mean concentration from 2.36 ± 0.02 mmol/L to 2.31 ± 0.03 mmol/L *1431*

1,25-Dihydroxy Vitamin D *Serum* *Decrease* In 26 healthy individuals a magnesium-deficient diet for 3 weeks caused significant decrease from mean baseline of 55 ± 4 pmol/L to 43 ± 3 pmol/L *1431*

Magnesium *Serum* *Decrease* In 26 healthy individuals feeding a magnesium deficient diet for 3 weeks caused magnesium concentration to decrease from 0.80 ± 0.01 mmol/L to 0.61 ± 0.02 mmol/L *1431*

Magnesium, Free *Red Blood Cells* *Decrease* In 26 healthy individuals feeding a magnesium-deficient diet for 3 weeks caused significant decrease from a mean of 205 ± 10 µmol/L to 162 ± 7 µmol/L *1431*

275.30 Familial Hyperphosphatasemia

Acid Phosphatase *Serum* *Increase* Increased in this uncommon inherited disorder showing painful swelling of the periosteal soft tissue and spontaneous fractures *5544* The lesions show pronounced increases in the amount of alkaline and acid phosphatase, aminopeptidase and lactic dehydrogenase, acid mucopolysaccharides and reticulin *5002*

Alanine Aminopeptidase *Serum* *Increase* Increased in the uncommon inherited disorder showing painful swelling of the periosteal soft tissue and spontaneous fractures *5544* Pronounced increase *5002*

Alkaline Phosphatase *Serum* *Increase* Pronounced increase *5002*

Alkaline Phosphatase, Bone Isoenzyme *Serum* *Increase* In patients with familial hyperphosphatasemia slight increase observed *4217*

Lactate Dehydrogenase *Serum* *Increase* Pronounced increase *5002*

Mucopolysaccharides *Serum* *Increase* Pronounced increase *5002*

275.30 Hypophosphatasia

Alkaline Phosphatase *Serum* *Decrease* Reported effect *3160* Marked reduction in activity is one of the cardinal features of hypophosphatasia. Reduced to 25% of the lower limit of normal, the mean levels varying widely with individual cases between almost no activity to 40% activity. There is no correlation between the degree of serum depression and the severity of the clinical manifestations *1559*
White Blood Cells *Decrease* In untreated hereditary hypophosphatasia *5544*

Alkaline Phosphatase, Bone Isoenzyme *Serum* *Decrease* In patients with hypophosphatasia slight decrease observed *4217*

Alkaline Phosphatase, Tissue Unspecific *Serum* *No Effect* In 11 members of 4 families with hypophosphatasia mean activity of 32 ± 20 U/L compared with reference interval of 40 -130 U/L *2349*

Calcium *Serum* *Increase* Total serum concentration was elevated in 10 patients and normal or undetermined in 6. Individual readings tended to vary widely and hypercalcemic patients had normal readings occasionally *1559* Intermittent hypercalcemia may be observed in these patients, who also demonstrate an increase in phosphoethanolamine in their blood and urine *1025*
Serum *No Effect* In a study of 59 patients with normocalcemia and low intact PTH concentrations, 2 had hypophosphatasia *3280*

Creatine Kinase *Serum* *No Effect* In 2 patients with X-linked hypophosphatemia with osteosclerosis mean activities of 50 U/L and 117 U/L compared with upper limit of normal of 195 U/L *5659*

Creatine Kinase BB-Isoenzyme *Serum* *No Effect* In 2 patients with X-linked hypophosphatemia with osteosclerosis mean activities of < 5 U/L and < 10 U/L (not detected %) compared with normal of 0 - 1% *5659*

Hydroxyproline *Urine* *Decrease* Extremely low *1365* May be extremely low, reflecting bone destruction *5196* *4979*

Parathyroid Hormone *Plasma* *Decrease* In a study of 59 patients with normocalcemia and low intact PTH concentration, 2 had hypophosphatasia *3280*

Phosphate *Serum* *No Effect* No significant effect observed *1290*

Phosphoethanolamine *Plasma* *Increase* Two times normal concentration reported *4283*
Urine *Increase* 3 - 8 times normal *4283*

Pyridoxal Phosphate *Serum* *Increase* In 11 members of 4 families with hypophosphatasia mean concentration of 428.8 ± 692.0 nmol/L compared with reference interval of 12 - 97 nmol/L *2349*

275.30 Infantile Hyperphosphatemia

Phosphate *Serum* *Increase* Serum phosphate concentration may be increased in patients with infantile hyperphosphatemia *5204*

275.30 Vitamin D Deficiency Rickets

Alkaline Phosphatase *Serum* *Increase* The earliest and most reliable biochemical abnormality; until bone healing is complete *5544* Consistently elevated *4979* Increased in active rickets, the degree of elevation corresponding to the severity of the disease. The average phosphatase in 9 cases of uncomplicated rickets was 0.75, with a range of 0.3 - 1.4 (units not stated) *4908*

Amino Acids *Urine* *Increase* Decreased net reabsorption, probably due to increased circulating parathyroid hormone *4979*

Calcium *Feces* *Increase* Urine and serum concentration is low with high stool content *4979*
Serum *Decrease* Concentrations < 8 mg/dL are common *4979* Decreased absorption in the gut leads to overproduction of parathyroid hormone and the resulting phosphaturia and hypophosphatemia *2719*
Serum *No Effect* Usually normal or slightly decreased *5544* concentration usually little changed *900*
Urine *Decrease* Low in the untreated state *4979*
Urine *Increase* In young persons *367*

Chloride *Serum* *Increase* Mild acidosis and hyperchloremia may be observed *4979*

Hydroxyproline *Urine* *Increase* Increased formation of osteoid tissue results in hydroxyprolinuria, values will decrease with adequate therapy with vitamin D *1980*

Parathyroid Hormone *Plasma* *Increase* Decreased calcium absorption in the gut leads to overproduction of parathyroid hormone and the resulting phosphaturia and hypophosphatemia *2719* Increased in nutritional rickets *4318*

pH *Blood* *Decrease* Mild acidosis and hyperchloremia may be observed *4979*

Phosphate *Serum* *Decrease* Decreased calcium absorption in the gut leads to overproduction of parathyroid hormone and the resulting phosphaturia and hypophosphatemia *2719* May be low, but usually not as severe as in vitamin D resistant rickets *4979*
Serum *No Effect* Concentration usually within normal limits *900* Concentration usually normal or low *4979* In some individuals, serum calcium and phosphate may be normal *5544*
Urine *Increase* Decreased calcium absorption in the gut leads to overproduction of parathyroid hormone and the resulting phosphaturia and hypophosphatemia *2719*

275.30 Vitamin D Resistant Rickets

Adenosine Monophosphate *Urine* *No Effect* Reported to be normal in untreated heterozygotes and homozygotes, with normal response to PTH infusion *4979* *1757*

Alkaline Phosphatase *Serum* *Increase* In older infants or children *1025* As skeletal changes develop *4979* Many children and patients continued to show persistently raised concentration, despite evident relief of symptoms in those with rickets or osteomalacia and increased growth rate in the school children *916*
Serum *No Effect* Normal in most patients without radiologic signs of rickets *4979*

Amino Acids *Urine* *Increase* Generalized aminoaciduria is present *900*
Urine *No Effect* Normal, in contrast to Vitamin D deficient rickets *4979*

Bicarbonate *Serum* *No Effect* Concentration usually normal *4979*

Calcium *Feces* *Increase* Diminished intestinal absorption *4979*
Serum *No Effect* Usually normal *4979*
Urine *Decrease* In children, urinary excretion is 10 - 20 mg/24 h whereas in adults urinary excretion ranges between 50 - 120 mg/24 h *367* Usually low in untreated cases *4979*

1,25-Dihydroxy Vitamin D_3 *Serum* *Decrease* Observed effect *126*

Glomerular Filtration Rate *Urine* *Decrease* Characteristic of the first few months of life. May result in a normal phosphate concentration even if the tubular defect is already present *2032*

Glucose *Serum* *No Effect* Found in excess quantities in the urine but not in the plasma *900*
Urine *Increase* Found in excess quantities in the urine but not in the plasma *900* Mild renal glycosuria has been reported in a few cases *4979*

Glycine *Plasma* *No Effect* Found in excess quantities in the urine but not in the plasma *900*
Urine *Increase* Found in excess quantities in the urine but not in the plasma *900*

Hydroxyproline *Urine* *Increase* Some patients *1980*

Parathyroid Hormone *Plasma* *Increase* Normal or only slight elevations *4979*

pH *Blood* *No Effect* Usually no change observed *4979*

Phosphate *Feces* *Increase* Diminished intestinal absorption *4979*
Serum *Decrease* May be present at birth or develop within the 1st y *4979* Familial hypophosphatemic rickets; with impaired transport of phosphate ion in both kidney and gut. Usually decreased *5544*
Urine *Increase* High in untreated patients *4979*

Urea Nitrogen *Serum* *No Effect* Concentration usually normal *4979*

275.40 Calcium Pyrophosphate Crystal Deposition Disease

Leukocytes *Synovial Fluid* *Increase* Mean concentration of 780 ± 150 /µL in 9 patients *1161*

Nerve Growth Factor *Serum* *Increase* Mean concentration of 36.9 ± 86 pg/mL in 11 patients *1161*
Synovial Fluid *Increase* Mean concentration of 20 ± 54 pg/mL in 9 patients *1161*

Nerve Growth Factor Autoantibodies *Serum* *Increase* Mean value of 0.55 ± 0.24 in 11 patients significantly different from 0.42 ± 0.13 in 30 healthy controls *1161*
Synovial Fluid *Increase* Mean value of 0.61 ± 0.37 in 11 patients *1161*

275.40 Calcium Pyrophosphate Crystal Deposition Disease *(continued)*

Nucleotide Pyrophosphohydrolase, Soluble
Serum *Increase* Mean activity in 37 patients with CPPD crystal deposition disease of 1410 ± 38 pmol nitrophenol/h/mL significantly different from that in 85 healthy individuals 1141 ± 22 pmol nitrophenol/h/mL *691*

275.40 Chondrocalcinosis

Interleukin-6 *Serum* *Increase* Mean concentration of 105.3 ± 117.6 pg/mL in 18 patients with chondrocalcinosis significantly different from 11.4 ± 1.9 pg/mL in healthy blood donors *1130*
Synovial Fluid *Increase* Mean concentration of 95.9 ± 95 ng/L in 18 patients with chondrocalcinosis *1130*

Soluble Interleukin-6 Receptor-α *Synovial Fluid* *Increase* Mean concentration of 19.5 ± 7.4 ng/mL in 18 patients with chondrocalcinosis *1130*

275.40 Crystal-associated Arthritis

Phospholipase A_2 Type II *Synovial Fluid* *Increase* Considerable increase in catalytic activity observed in patients with crystal-associated arthritis *3767*

Prostaglandin E_2 *Synovial Fluid* *Increase* Mean concentration in 3 patients of about 2.9 nmol/L *3366*

275.40 Familial Tumoral Calcinosis

Phosphate *Serum* *Increase* Familial tumoral calcinosis may increase the serum phosphate concentration *969*

275.40 Hypercalcemia

Parathyroid Hormone 1-84 *Plasma* *Decrease* Mean concentration in 14 of 18 patients with hypercalcemia of malignancy of < 0.5 pmol/L significantly different from mean 2.21 pmol/L (range 1.0 - 5.0 pmol/L) in 57 healthy laboratory staff *3105*

275.40 Hypercalciuria, Idiopathic

Ammonium Ions *Urine* *Increase* May be associated with classic distal renal tubular acidosis which is associated with hyokalemia, hyperchloremic metabolic acidosis, urine pH > 5.5, increased urinary ammonium ion excretion, a negative urine anion gap, increased urinary osmol gap, decreased urinary citrate and increased urinary calcium in some patients *4071*

Anion Gap *Urine* *Decrease* May be associated with classic distal renal tubular acidosis which is asociated with hyokalemia, hyperchloremic metabolic acidosis, urine pH > 5.5, increased urinary ammonium ion excretion, a negative urine anion gap, increased urinary osmol gap, decreased urinary citrate and increased urinary calcium in some patients *4071*

Calcium *Serum* *No Effect* In a study of 59 patients with normocalcemia and low intact PTH concentrations 4 had idiopathic hypercalciuria *3280*
Urine *Increase* May be associated with classic distal renal tubular acidosis which is associated with hyokalemia, hyperchloremic metabolic acidosis, urine pH > 5.5, increased urinary ammonium ion excretion, a negative urine anion gap, increased urinary osmol gap, decreased urinary citrate and increased urinary calcium in some patients *4071*

Chloride *Serum* *Increase* May be associated with classic distal renal tubular acidosis which is asociated with hyokalemia, hyperchloremic metabolic acidosis, urine pH > 5.5, increased urinary ammonium ion excretion, a negative urine anion gap, increased urinary osmol gap, decreased urinary citrate and increased urinary calcium in some patients *4071*

Citrate *Urine* *Decrease* May be associated with classic distal renal tubular acidosis which is asociated with hyokalemia, hyperchloremic metabolic acidosis, urine pH > 5.5, increased urinary ammonium ion excretion, a negative urine anion gap, increased urinary osmol gap, decreased urinary citrate and increased urinary calcium in some patients *4071*

Endothelin-1 *Urine* *Increase* In 9 children with idiopathic hypercalciuria mean excretion of 31.3 pmol/sq m/d significantly different from 12.9 (lower and upper quartiles 10.0 - 15.2 pmol/sq m/d) in 60 healthy children *5733*

Net Acid Excretion *Urine* *Increase* May be associated with classic distal renal tubular acidosis which is associated with hyokalemia, hyperchloremic metabolic acidosis, urine pH > 5.5, increased urinary ammonium ion excretion, a negative urine anion gap, increased urinary osmol gap, decreased urinary citrate and increased urinary calcium in some patients *4071*

Osmolal Gap *Urine* *Increase* May be associated with classic distal renal tubular acidosis which is asociated with hyokalemia, hyperchloremic metabolic acidosis, urine pH > 5.5, increased urinary ammonium ion excretion, a negative urine anion gap, increased urinary osmol gap, decreased urinary citrate and increased urinary calcium in some patients *4071*

Parathyroid Hormone *Plasma* *Decrease* In a study of 59 patients with low intact PTH concentrations and normocalcemia 4 had idiopathic hypercalciuria *3280*

pH *Urine* *Increase* May be associated with classic distal renal tubular acidosis which is asociated with hyokalemia, hyperchloremic metabolic acidosis, urine pH > 5.5, increased urinary ammonium ion excretion, a negative urine anion gap, increased urinary osmol gap, decreased urinary citrate and increased urinary calcium in some patients *4071*

Potassium *Serum* *Decrease* May be associated with classic distal renal tubular acidosis which is associated with hyokalemia, hyperchloremic metabolic acidosis, urine pH > 5.5, increased urinary ammonium ion excretion, a negative urine anion gap, increased urinary osmol gap, decreased urinary citrate and increased urinary calcium in some patients *4071*

275.40 Pseudohypoparathyroidism

Calcitonin *Plasma* *Increase* Observed effect *1290*

Calcium *Serum* *Decrease* End organ failure, a rare cause of hypocalcemia, must be considered in osteomalacia *1025*

1,25-Dihydroxy Vitamin D_3 *Serum* *Decrease* Observed effect *126*

Parathyroid Hormone *Plasma* *Increase* Normally high and can be used to distinguish from true hypoparathyroidism *5679* Deficient end organ response *126*

Phosphate *Serum* *Increase* Normal excretory mechanisms are impaired *2039* Hyperphosphatemia may occur with pseudohypoparathyroidism types I and II *5204* Pseudohypoparathyroidism may increase the serum phosphate concentration *969*
Urine *Decrease* Normal excretory mechanisms are impaired *2039*

276.20 Acidosis

Phosphate *Serum* *Increase* Shift of phosphate from cells leading to increased serum concentration *969*

Urea Nitrogen *Serum* *Decrease* Much lower concentration by Azostix® than diacetyl value *1968*

276.20 Metabolic Acidosis

Aspartate Aminotransferase *Serum* *Increase* In type II-B, with lactic acidosis *5545*

Bicarbonate *Serum* *Decrease* Serum bicarbonate falls as hydrogen ions accumulate *1980* Total plasma CO_2 content is decreased; < 15 mmol/L almost certainly rules out respiratory alkalosis *5545*

Carbon Dioxide Partial Pressure *Blood* *Decrease* Tends to fall below normal range as the blood pH and bicarbonate fall *1290* Ventilation is stimulated and pCO_2 falls *1980*

2,3-Diphosphoglycerate *Red Blood Cells* *Decrease* Concentration will be low *379*

ionized Calcium *Serum* *Increase* Increase in ionized calcium *1587*

Lactate *Blood* *Increase* Increased blood lactate with lactate-pyruvate ratio greater than 10:1 in type II-B, with lactic acidosis *5545*

Lactate Dehydrogenase *Serum* *Increase* Increased in type II-B, with lactic acidosis *5545*

Leukocytes *Blood* *Increase* Intoxications due to metabolic causes can cause leukocytosis *5544* Increased WBC in Type II-B, with lactic acidosis *5545*

pH *Blood* *Decrease* Low, usually 6.98 - 7.25 in type II-B, with lactic acidosis *5545*
Urine *Decrease* Urine is strongly acid (pH of 4.5 - 5.2) if renal function is normal *5545*

Phosphate *Serum* *Increase* Increased in type II-B, with lactic acidosis *5545* Hyperphosphatemia may occur with lactic acidosis before therapy and diabetic and/or alcoholic ketoacidosis before therapy *5204*

Potassium *Serum* *Increase* Frequently increased. Often 6-7 mmol/L in type II-B, with lactic acidosis *5545*

276.30 Metabolic Alkalosis

Bicarbonate *Serum* *Increase* Total plasma CO_2 is increased (bicarbonate > 30 mmol/L) *5545*

Carbon Dioxide Partial Pressure *Blood* *Increase* Normal or slightly elevated *1980*

Chloride *Serum* *Decrease* Is relatively lower than sodium *5545*

ionized Calcium *Serum* *Decrease* Decrease in ionized calcium *1587*

pH *Blood* *Increase* Deficit of hydrogen ion due to loss or alkali administration *1980*
Urine *Increase* Urine pH > 7.0 (< 7.9) if potassium depletion and concomitant sodium are not severe *5545*

Potassium *Serum* *Decrease* Usually decreased, which is the chief danger in alkalosis *5545*

Urea Nitrogen *Serum* *Increase* May be increased *5545*

276.30 Respiratory Alkalosis

Phosphate *Serum* *Decrease* Common cause of hypophosphatemia due to shift of phosphate into the cells *969*
Serum *Increase* Hyperphosphatemia may occur with acute respiratory alkalosis *5204*

276.80 Hypokalemia

Creatine Kinase *Serum* *Increase* Patients with severe hypokalemia such as that occurring in hyperaldosteronism with muscle weakness may have elevated CK directly related to their hypokalemia. In other patients with hypokalemia, 10% may have increased CK but this is related to other disease processes *959*

Myoglobin *Urine* *Increase* Sporadic; metabolic myoglobinuria *5544*

Potassium *Serum* *Decrease* Urine is almost always hypertonic to plasma *126*

276.90 Familial Intermittent Hyperphosphatemia

Calcium *Serum* *Decrease* Hyperphosphatemia may occur with hypocalcemia, polyuria and seizures *5204*

Phosphate *Serum* *Increase* Hyperphosphatemia may occur with hypocalcemia, polyuria and seizures *5204*

277.00 Cystic Fibrosis

Alanine Aminotransferase *Serum* *Increase* In 5 of 34 patients with acute exacerbation of cystic fibrosis mean activity greater than 30 U/L *1257*

Albumin *Duodenal Contents* *Increase* In excess of that found in the duodenal fluid of controls *823*
Serum *Decrease* With advanced lung disease the development of hypoalbuminemia suggests expansion of plasma volume secondary to cor pulmonale *900* May be found before cardiac involvement is clinically apparent *5544* In 56% of 12 patients at initial hospitalization for this disorder *1576* Occasionally a prolonged conjugated hyperbilirubinemia may be observed due to extrahepatic biliary obstruction, in association with marked hypoalbuminemia *3406*
Serum *No Effect* In only 1 of 30 patients with acute exacerbation of cystic fibrosis mean concentration less than 30 g/L *1257* In 8 patients with serum 25-hydroxyvitamin D concentrations less than 10 ng/mL mean concentration of 3.9 ± 0.2 g/dL and in 12 with 25-hydroxyvitamin D concentrations greater than 10 ng/mL mean concentration of 4.2 ± 0.1 g/dL, within normal range of 3.9 - 4.8 g/dL *1215*

Alkaline Phosphatase *Serum* *Increase* Noted in 40% of 36 children. Serum activity as a whole is fairly insensitive to occurrence and degree of disease because of high upper limits for normal children *1202* In 8 patients with serum 25-hydroxyvitamin D concentrations less than 10 ng/mL mean activity of 124 ± 10 U/L and in 12 with 25-hydroxyvitamin D concentrations greater than 10 ng/mL mean activity of 123 ± 12 U/L just outside normal range of 30 - 117 U/L *1215* In 7 of 32 patients with acute exacerbation of cystic fibrosis mean activity greater than upper limit of normal *1257* In 65% of 12 patients at initial hospitalization for this disorder *1576*

Alkaline Phosphatase, Bone Isoenzyme *Serum* *No Effect* In 8 patients with serum 25-hydroxyvitamin D concentrations less than 10 ng/mL mean concentration of 13.3 ± 2.0 ng/mL and in 12 with 25-hydroxyvitamin D concentrations greater than 10 ng/mL mean concentration of 11.4 ± 2.9 ng/mL within normal range of 4.3 - 19 ng/mL (men) and < 15.0 ng/mL (women) *1215*

Alkaline Phosphatase Isoenzymes *Serum* *Increase* Liver fraction *4979*

Amylase *Saliva* *Increase* In healthy adults and children the value for pancreatic:salivary amylase is > 1. In 80% of gene carriers, the P:S is < 1 with a mean of 0.68 ± 0.13. In addition to the higher total amylase activity, in homozygotes P:S is < 0.1, and even 0.001. The phenomenon is explained by a compensatory enhancement of salivary activity *5123* Submaxillary saliva is turbid, with increased calcium, total protein, and amylase. These changes are not generally found in parotid saliva *5544*

α_1-Antichymotrypsin *Serum* *Increase* Increase compared to matched controls *5607*

Ascorbic Acid *Serum* *No Effect* In 122 cystic fibrosis patients taking vitamin C supplements mean concentration of 63.6 ± 18.8 μmol/L not significantly different from 69.5 ± 16.6 μmol/L in 34 healthy controls not taking vitamin C *5696*

Asialo-Transferrin *Serum* *No Effect* In cystic fibrosis patients mean proportion of 0.0% not significantly different from reference interval 0.0% *2927*

Aspartate Aminotransferase *Serum* *Increase* In 56% of 12 patients at initial hospitalization for this disorder *1576* With liver involvement *2584*

Benzoylcholinesterase *Serum* *Decrease* Mean activity in 29 patients with cystic fibrosis before treatment of 917 ± 274 nmol/mL/min significantly less than that in 27 healthy volunteers of 1191 ± 298 nmol/mL/min, with increase to 1013 ± 237 nmol/mL/min after treatment *17*

Bile Acids *Serum* *Increase* Serum bile acid determination seems to be of no value in evaluating the extent of liver disease in cystic fibrosis. Chenodeoxycholic acids are more frequent and more elevated than cholic acid *5039*

Bilirubin *Serum* *Increase* Occasionally a prolonged conjugated hyperbilirubinemia may be observed due to extrahepatic biliary obstruction *3406*

Bilirubin, Conjugated *Serum* *Increase* Occasionally a prolonged conjugated hyperbilirubinemia may be observed due to extrahepatic biliary obstruction *3406*

Bleeding Time *Patient* *Increase* Secondary to vitamin K deficiency *1147*

Butyrylcholinesterase *Serum* *Decrease* Mean activity in 29 patients with cystic fibrosis before treatment of 5.54 ± 1.64 μmol/mL/min significantly less than that in 27 healthy volunteers of 7.01 ± 1.79 μmol/mL/min, with increase to 6.31 ± 1.58 μmol/mL/min after treatment *17*

CA 19-9 *Serum* *Increase* CA 19-9 concentration increased in some patients with cystic fibrosis *1253* Both CA 19-9 and CA 195 can be used as sensitive markers for the early detection of exacerbation in cystic fibrosis patients *5745*

277.00 Cystic Fibrosis *(continued)*

CA 195 *Serum* *Increase* Both CA 19-9 and CA 195 can be used as sensitive markers for the early detection of exacerbations in cystic fibrosis patients *3249*

Calcium *Saliva* *Increase* Submaxillary saliva is turbid, with increased calcium, total protein, and amylase. These changes are not generally found in parotid saliva *5544*
Serum *Decrease* Hypoalbuminemia *5544*
Serum *No Effect* In 8 patients with serum 25-hydroxyvitamin D concentrations less than 10 ng/mL mean concentration of 8.8 ± 0.2 mg/dL and in 12 with 25-hydroxyvitamin D concentrations greater than 10 ng/mL mean concentration of 9.1 ± 0.3 mg/dL within normal range of 8.4 - 10.2 mg/dL *1215* Normal unless complications occur (e.g., chronic pulmonary disease with accumulation of CO_2, massive salt loss due to sweating) *5544*
Urine *No Effect* In 8 patients with serum 25-hydroxyvitamin D concentrations less than 10 ng/mL mean excretion of 116 ± 17 mg/g creatinine and in 12 with 25-hydroxyvitamin D concentrations greater than 10 ng/mL mean excretion of 249 ± 43 mg/g creatinine within normal range of 100 - 300 mg/g creatinine *1215*

Carbon Dioxide Partial Pressure *Blood* *Increase* Salt loss may lead to metabolic alkalosis *2189*

Carnitine *Serum* *No Effect* Total and free carnitine concentrations were not significantly different from controls. Levels of acylcarnitine were significantly lower *3096*

β-Carotene *Serum* *Decrease* In 122 cystic fibrosis patients taking vitamin C supplements mean concentration of 0.35 ± 0.60 µmol/L significantly different from 0.92 ± 0.47 µmol/L in 34 healthy controls not taking vitamin C *5696*

Carotenoids *Serum* *Decrease* In 243 females and 307 males with cystic fibrosis mean concentration significantly less than in reference population *3387*

Chenodeoxycholic Acid *Serum* *Increase* Fifteen patients had elevated levels not correlated to liver morphology *4746*

Chloride *Saliva* *Increase* Submaxillary saliva has slightly increased chloride and sodium but not potassium; however, considerable overlap with normal individuals prevents diagnostic usage *5544*
Serum *No Effect* Serum electrolytes are normal unless complications occur (e.g., chronic pulmonary disease with accumulation of CO_2, massive salt loss due to sweating) *5544* In 13 patients with cystic fibrosis mean concentration of 100 mmol/L not significantly different from 103 mmol/L in 16 healthy controls *881*
Sweat *Increase* A value > 60 mmol/L is consistent with the diagnosis *900* In 13 patients with cystic fibrosis mean concentration increased to 105 ± 2 mmol/L compared with 21 ± 1 mmol/L in 16 healthy controls *881* Striking increase in sweat sodium and chloride 60 mmol/L) and to a lesser extent potassium is present in virtually all homozygous patients. It is present throughout life from time of birth and is not related to severity of disease or organ involvement *5544*

Cholesterol *Serum* *Increase* In 91% of 12 patients at initial hospitalization for this disorder *1576*

Cholic Acid *Serum* *Increase* Eight patients had elevated levels not correlated with liver pathology *4746* Of cystic fibrosis patients with steatorrhea, 38% had fasting levels greater than 3 standard deviation above mean fasting control levels *1027*

Chymotrypsin *Feces* *Decrease* Fecal concentrations may be related to the severity of pancreatic insufficiency *290*

Complement C_3 *Serum* *Increase* Found in 13 patients *4168*
Serum *No Effect* No significant effect observed *3040*

C-Reactive Protein *Serum* *Increase* In 12 untreated patients mean concentration of 21.32 µg/mL significantly higher than 0.33 µg/mL in 12 control subjects *3815* Mean activity in 29 patients with cystic fibrosis before treatment of 19.5 µg/mL significantly greater than that in 27 healthy volunteers of 0.5 µg/mL, with decrease to 3.3 µg/mL after treatment *17* In 30 patients with acute exacerbation of cystic fibrosis mean concentration of 25.7 ± 26 mg/L significantly increased compared with 9.8 ± 9 mg/L on discharge and above reference range of < 10 mg/L *1257*

Deoxypyridinoline *Urine* *No Effect* In 8 patients with serum 25-hydroxyvitamin D concentrations less than 10 ng/mL mean excretion of 14.9 ± 1.6 nmol/mmol creatinine and in 12 with 25-hydroxyvitamin D concentrations greater than 10 ng/mL mean excretion of 19.5 ± 2.6 nmol/mmol creatinine within normal range of 4 - 19 nmol/mmol creatinine (men) and 6 - 23 nmol/mmol creatinine (women) *1215*

1,25-Dihydroxy Vitamin D *Serum* *No Effect* In 8 patients with serum 25-hydroxyvitamin D concentrations less than 10 ng/mL mean concentration of 47 ± 7 pg/mL and in 12 with 25-hydroxyvitamin D concentrations greater than 10 ng/mL mean concentration of 34 ± 4 pg/mL within normal range of 15 - 60 pg/mL *1215*

3,4-Dihydroxyphenylalanine *Plasma* *Increase* Total concentration of 3,4-dopa significantly increased to 35.4 ± 16.9 nmol/L in newly diagnosed cystic fibrosis *4666*

3,4-Dihydroxyphenylalanine, Free *Plasma* *Increase* Significant increase to 27.0 ± 6.1 nmol/L observed in 11 newly diagnosed infants compared with 19.1 ± 5.0 nmol/L in controls. In heterozygotes concentrations lowest at 11.5 ± 5.8 nmol/L *4666*

2,3-Diphosphoglycerate *Red Blood Cells* *Increase* A study of 35 patients demonstrated that increasing severity of pulmonary involvement was associated with a mild but definite increase in erythrocyte 2,3-DPG and a decrease in hemoglobin affinity for oxygen *4442*

Disialo-Transferrin *Serum* *Increase* In cystic fibrosis patients mean proportion of 0.954% significantly different from reference interval 0.735 ± 0.238% *2927*

Elastase *Sputum* *Increase* In 12 patients with cystic fibrosis mean baseline concentration of 18.8 µg/g sputum *3815*

Erythrocytes *Blood* *Increase* Slight, in older children *685*

Fat *Feces* *Increase* In this study of 12 patients, average was 41 g/day, compared to < 7 g/day for controls *4979* Deficient intraluminal pancreatic enzymes *4891*

Fatty Acids (FFA), Free *Serum* *Decrease* Analyses of children with this disease have indicated a deficiency in essential fatty acids. Arachidonic acid was found only in trace amounts or was absent *4441* The oleate fatty acids increase while the linoleatic portion decreases. The basis for this seems to be that oleic and linoleic acid differ in changes in oxygen pressure. The oxygen complex of linoleic acid dissociates at relatively high pressures, whereas that of oleic dissociates only at low pressures *672*

α-Fetoprotein *Serum* *No Effect* In CF patients 97.5% and in normal children 95% of the values were within the normal range for healthy adults (1 - 9 ng/mL) *2721* In 30 patients, the highest value obtained was 10.2 ng/mL and in a control 10.8 ng/mL. These are within published normal limits. Previously reported large increases in CF patients and in heterozygote carriers have not been confirmed *587*

γ-Globulin *Duodenal Contents* *Increase* In excess of that found in the duodenal fluid of controls *823*
Serum *Increase* Rises with progressive pulmonary disease, mainly due to IgG and IgA; IgM and IgD are not appreciably increased *5544*

Glucagon *Plasma* *Decrease* Both alpha and beta cell function is disrupted resulting in low insulin and glucagon concentration in contrast to diabetes mellitus *3614*

Glucose *Serum* *Increase* Fasting hyperglycemia and glycosuria occurred in only 8% of patients *3614* In 45% of 13 patients at initial hospitalization for this disorder *1576*
Urine *Increase* Fasting hyperglycemia and glycosuria occurred in only 8% of patients *3614* Urinalysis reveals glycosuria due to chemical diabetes *900*

Glucose Tolerance *Serum* *Decrease* Found in 36% of 31 patients *1999* Up to 40% of patients are known to have varying degrees of intolerance. Probably secondary to strangulation of the islets by fibrosis. More common with advancing age *3614*

α-Glucosidase *Serum* *Increase* Acutely ill patients with cystic fibrosis demonstrated significant increases compared with cystic fibrosis outpatients *4182*

γ-Glutamyltransferase *Serum* *Increase* In 5 of 16 patients with acute exacerbation of cystic fibrosis mean activity greater than 32 U/L *1257*

Growth Hormone *Plasma* *Decrease* Reported effect *1858*

Plasma *Increase* In 10 patients with normal glucose tolerance 12 h mean concentration of 2.99 mU/L and in 10 with diabetes mellitus mean concentration of 4.53 mU/L significantly different from 2.66 mU/L in 20 controls *2939*

Hematocrit *Blood* *Decrease* In late stages of chronic lung disease, decreased serum electrolytes, hemoglobin, hematocrit, etc. may reflect hemodilution *5544*

Hemoglobin *Blood* *Decrease* In late stages of chronic lung disease, decreased serum electrolytes, hemoglobin, hematocrit, etc., may reflect hemodilution *5544*

25-Hydroxy Vitamin D_3 *Serum* *Decrease* Patients supplemented with multivitamins still presented a 36% decrease in 25-OH vitamin D concentration *1958*

25-Hydroxy Vitamin D *Serum* *Decrease* In 20 patients with advanced cystic fibrosis lung disease mean serum 25-hydroxyvitamin D concentrations of 16 ± 2 ng/mL at low end of normal range of 10 - 52 ng/mL, with 8 patients having concentrations less than 10 ng/mL *1215*

immunoglobulin A *Serum* *Increase* Rises with progressive pulmonary disease *5544* Reported effect *1290*

Immunoglobulin D *Serum* *No Effect* Not appreciably increased *5544*

Immunoglobulin G *Serum* *Increase* Rises with progressive pulmonary disease *5544*

Immunoglobulin M *Serum* *No Effect* Not appreciably increased *5544*

Insulin *Plasma* *Decrease* Both alpha and beta cell function is disrupted resulting in low insulin and glucagon concentration in contrast to diabetes mellitus *3614*

Insulin-like Growth Factor-I *Serum* *Decrease* In 27 patients with cystic fibrosis mean concentration of 1.13 ± 0.41 ng/mL significantly different from 6.72 ± 3.62 ng/mL in 12 matched healthy controls *191* In 10 patients with normal glucose tolerance mean concentration of 154 ng/mL and in 10 with diabetes mellitus mean concentration of 163 ng/mL significantly different from 228 ng/mL in 20 controls *2939*

Insulin-like Growth Factor Binding Protein-3
Serum *Decrease* In 10 patients with normal glucose tolerance mean concentration of 2,896 ng/mL and in 10 with diabetes mellitus mean concentration of 2,860 ng/mL significantly different from 3,754 ng/mL in 20 controls *2939*

Interleukin-6 *Serum* *Increase* In 12 untreated patients mean concentration of 7.28 pg/mL significantly higher than 0.65 pg/mL in 12 control subjects *3815*
Sputum *Increase* In 12 patients with cystic fibrosis mean baseline concentration of 5.76 pg/g sputum *3815*

Interleukin-8 *Feces* *Increase* In 9 patients with cystic fibrosis mean concentration in wet stool of 32,113 pg/g significantly increased compared with < 43.5 pg/g in 9 healthycontrols *583*

Iron *Serum* *Increase* Intestinal absorption increased *685*

Leptin *Serum* *No Effect* In 27 patients with cystic fibrosis mean concentration of 5.3 ± 4.1 ng/mL not significantly different from 4.4 ± 3.6 ng/mL in 12 matched healthy controls *191*

Leukocytes *Blood* *Increase* In 79% of 16 patients at initial hospitalization for this disorder *1576*

Lipase, Pancreatic *Serum* *Decrease* In individuals aged 10 years or older with pancreatic insufficiency activity markedly reduced below normal *510*
Serum *Increase* In infants concentration of pancreatic lipase markedly increased. In individuals aged 11 years or older without pancreatic insufficiency activity within the normal range or increased *510*

Lipids *Feces* *Increase* Reduced intraluminal pancreatic enzyme activity with maldigestion of lipid and protein *1980*

Malondialdehyde *Serum* *Decrease* In 122 cystic fibrosis patients taking vitamin C supplements mean concentration of 0.69 ± 0.26 µmol/L not significantly different from 0.72 ± 0.28 µmol/L in 34 healthy controls not taking vitamin C *5696*

Mucin *Serum* *Increase* Concentration reportedly increased in patients with cystic fibrosis *4797*

Mucin-associated Antigen *Serum* *Increase* Concentration reportedly increased in patients with cystic fibrosis *4797*

Neutrophil Elastase-α_1-Antiproteinase Complex
Serum *Increase* In 12 untreated patients mean concentration of 29.27 ng/mL significantly higher than 17.29 ng/mL in 12 control subjects *3815* Mean activity in 29 patients with cystic fibrosis before treatment of 49.0 ng/mL significantly greater than that in 27 healthy volunteers of 21.4 ng/mL, with decrease to 36.3 ng/mL after treatment *17*

Neutrophils *Blood* *Increase* In 12 untreated patients mean concentration of 8.4 x 10^9/L significantly higher than 2.9 x 10^9/L in 12 control subjects *3815*

Nitrate plus Nitrite *Sputum* *Increase* Mean concentration increased to 774 ± 307 µmol/L in 13 patients with acute cystic fibrosis compared with 387 ± 203 µmol/L in 25 patients and 421 ± 261 µmol/L in 9 control individuals *3079*

Nitric Oxide *Breath* *Decrease* Mean exhaled concentration decreased to 3.8 ± 3.9 ppb in 13 patients with acute cystic fibrosis compared with 5.0 ± 2.5 ppb in 25 patients and 8.8 ± 4.9 ppb in 9 control individuals *3079*

Osteocalcin *Serum* *No Effect* In 8 patients with serum 25-hydroxyvitamin D concentrations less than 10 ng/mL mean phosphate concentration of 4.6 ± 1.9 ng/mL and in 12 with 25-hydroxyvitamin D concentrations greater than 10 ng/mL mean concentration of 3.7 ± 0.9 ng/mL within normal range of 3 - 13 ng/mL (men) and 0.4 - 8.7 ng/mL (women) *1215*

Oxygen Partial Pressure *Blood* *Decrease* Pulmonary involvement *913*

Oxygen Saturation *Blood* *Decrease* Pulmonary involvement *913*

Pentasialo-Transferrin *Serum* *Increase* In cystic fibrosis patients mean proportion of 12.347% significantly different from reference interval 9.794 ± 1.760% *2927*

pH *Blood* *Increase* Salt loss may lead to metabolic alkalosis *2189*

Phosphate *Saliva* *Increase* Increased *2944*
Serum *No Effect* Normal unless complications occur (e.g., chronic pulmonary disease with accumulation of CO_2, massive salt loss due to sweating) *5544* In 8 patients with serum 25-hydroxyvitamin D concentrations less than 10 ng/mL mean phosphate concentration of 3.2 ± 0.3 mg/dL and in 12 with 25-hydroxyvitamin D concentrations greater than 10 ng/mL mean concentration of 3.7 ± 0.3 mg/dL within normal range of 2.7 - 4.5 mg/dL *1215*

Potassium *Saliva* *No Effect* Submaxillary saliva has slightly increased chloride and sodium but not potassium *5544*
Serum *No Effect* Normal unless complications occur (e.g., chronic pulmonary disease with accumulation of CO_2, massive salt loss due to sweating) *5544* Concentration usually within normal limits *261*
Sweat *Increase* Striking increase in sweat sodium and chloride and to a lesser extent potassium is present in virtually all homozygous patients. It is present throughout life from time of birth and is not related to severity of disease or organ involvement *5544*

Protein *Duodenal Contents* *Increase* In excess of that found in the duodenal fluid of controls *823*
Feces *Increase* Reduced intraluminal pancreatic enzyme activity with maldigestion of lipid and protein *1980*
Saliva *Increase* Submaxillary saliva is more turbid, with increased calcium, total protein, and amylase. These changes are not generally found in parotid saliva *5544*
Sputum *Increase* In 12 patients with cystic fibrosis mean baseline concentration of 14.7 mg/g sputum *3815*

Prothrombin Time *Plasma* *Increase* Secondary to vitamin K deficiency *1147*

Retinol *Serum* *Decrease* In 243 females with cystic fibrosis mean concentration of 1.28 ± 0.57 µmol/L compared with reference range of 1.78 ± 0.49 µmol/L *3387*

Retinol-binding Protein *Serum* *Decrease* In 30 patients with acute exacerbation of cystic fibrosis mean concentration of 1.46 ± 0.6 µmol/L significantly reduced compared with 2.24 ± 0.7 µmol/L on discharge but still within reference range of 1.43 - 2.86 µmol/L *1257*

Selenium *Serum* *Decrease* Low concentrations may occur due to reduced absorption *5174*

Sodium *Saliva* *Increase* Submaxillary saliva has slightly increased chloride and sodium but not potassium; however, considerable overlap with normal individuals prevents diagnostic usage *5544*
Serum *Decrease* Normal unless complications occur (e.g., chronic pulmonary disease with accumulation of CO_2, massive salt loss due to sweating) *5544*

277.00 Cystic Fibrosis *(continued)*

Sodium *(continued)*
Serum *No Effect* Concentration usually within normal range 261 Normal unless complications occur (e.g., chronic pulmonary disease with accumulation of CO_2, massive salt loss due to sweating) 5544
Sweat *Increase* Sweat sodium and T3 normalized after 1 y of oral essential fatty acid therapy 4441 A sweat sodium value of above 70 mmol/L is consistent with the diagnosis 900 Striking increase in sweat sodium and chloride is present in virtually all homozygous patients. Present throughout life from time of birth and is not related to severity of disease or organ involvement 5544

Sulfate *Serum* *No Effect* In 13 patients with cystic fibrosis mean concentration of 302 ± 22 µmol/L not significantly different from 298 ± 9 µmol/L in 22 healthy controls 881
Sweat *Decrease* In 13 patients with cystic fibrosis mean concentration reduced to 58 ± 7 µmol/L (38 ± 24% of control values) compared with 88 µmol/L in healthy controls 881

Tetrasialo-Transferrin *Serum* *No Effect* In cystic fibrosis patients mean proportion of 84.118% not significantly different from reference interval 84.886 ± 1.717% 2927

α-Tocopherol *Serum* *No Effect* In 122 cystic fibrosis patients taking vitamin C supplements mean concentration of 26.9 ± 9.2 µmol/L not significantly different from 28.0 ± 5.6 µmol/L in 34 healthy controls not taking vitamin C 5696

Trisialo-Transferrin *Serum* *Decrease* In cystic fibrosis patients mean proportion of 2.584% significantly different from reference interval 4.575 ± 1.315% 2927

Trypsin *Serum* *Decrease* In individuals aged 10 years or older with pancreatic insufficiency concetration of immunorective trypsin markedly reduced below normal 510
Serum *Increase* In infants with cystic fibrosis serum immunoreactive trypsin concentration markedly increased. In individuals aged over 11 years without pancreatic insufficiency concentration also increased or in the normal range 510

Tumor Necrosis Factor-α *Feces* *Increase* In 9 patients with cystic fibrosis mean concentration in wet stool of 3,187 pg/g significantly increased compared with 99 pg/g in 9 healthy controls 583
Serum *Increase* In 12 untreated patients mean concentration of 1.23 pg/mL significantly higher than 0.80 pg/mL in 12 control subjects 3815
Sputum *Increase* In 12 patients with cystic fibrosis mean baseline concentration of 14.5 pg/g sputum 3815

Urea Nitrogen *Saliva* *Increase* Increased 2944
Serum *Decrease* In 46% of 13 patients at initial hospitalization for this disorder 1576

Uric Acid *Saliva* *Increase* Increased 2944

Vitamin A *Serum* *Decrease* In 30 patients with acute exacerbation of cystic fibrosis mean concentration of 1.14 ± 0.5 µmol/L significantly reduced compared with 1.70 ± 0.6 µmol/L on discharge but still within reference range of 0.70 - 2.79 µmol/L 1257

Vitamin E *Serum* *Decrease* Reported effect 1821
Serum *No Effect* In 30 patients with acute exacerbation of cystic fibrosis mean concentration of 18.3 ± 7 µmol/L not significantly reduced compared with 23.0 ± 11 µmol/L on discharge but still within reference range of 11.6 - 46.4 µmol/L 1257

Vitamin K *Serum* *Decrease* Occasionally occurs 1147

Xylose Tolerance Test *Blood* *Abnormal* 48 children had 1 h blood xylose levels within the normal range, but the means at 90, 120, and 180 min after load exceeded significantly those of controls 653
Blood *No Effect* 48 children had 1 h blood xylose levels within the normal range, but the means at 90, 120, and 180 min after load exceeded significantly those of controls 653

Zinc *Serum* *Decrease* Decreased 5083

277.10 Acute Hepatic Porphyria

α-Fetoprotein *Serum* *No Effect* None of 44 patients in remission had a concentration greater than the upper limit of normal with 32 having a concentration of less than 2 kU/L. In most cases during attacks concentrations remained normal 1229

277.10 Acute Intermittent Porphyria

δ-Aminolevulinic Acid *Serum* *Increase* Observed during severe attacks 4979
Urine *Increase* Concentration increased 3406 May contain as much as 180 mg/24 h 3382 A reduction in the activity of the enzyme uroporphyrinogen I synthetase appears to explain the accumulation in body fluids and increased amounts in the urine. Excessive accumulation is further aggravated by an increased ALA synthetase activity 5037 Observed effect 5699 In one patient with acute intermittent porphyria mean excretion of 402 µmol/d significantly different from reference range of 2 - 49 µmol/d 1877 One of most effective diagnostic tests 2592 In the hereditary hepatic porphyrias 356 In 21 symptomatic patients, an average of 43 mg ALA/24 h was excreted. Tends to decrease somewhat during remission 4996 Observed effect 1980

δ-Aminolevulinic Acid Dehydratase
Red Blood Cells *Decrease* Activities of less than 3.5 nmol/s/L are diagnostic of AIP 2952

Antidiuretic Hormone *Plasma* *Increase* Syndrome of inappropriate ADH secretion has been documented in a number of cases 5699

BSP Retention *Serum* *Increase* Normal liver function tests except for BSP. Over10% BSP retained in 79% of symptomatic patients and in 55% of those in remission 4996

Chloride *Serum* *Decrease* Hyponatremia, hypochloremia, hypokalemia, hypomagnesemia, and alkalosis associated with azotemia of variable degree are often present on admission but may also develop acutely during the course of the attack. The electrolyte disorders are attributable in many patients to electrolyte depletion with inappropriate and injudicious overhydration 900

Coproporphyrin *Feces* *Increase* Slight to moderate increase 5598 Mean excretion of 42.2 nmol/g in 23 patients with acute intermittent porphyria greater than 11.0 nmol/g (range 8.0 - 35.0) in 20 healthy control individuals 2844 Small increases may be found 4979
Liver *Increase* Has been isolated from hepatic tissue in some cases 4645 4979
Red Blood Cells *No Effect* No significant effect 2034
Urine *Increase* Mean excretion of 835 nmol/d in 30 patients with acute intermittent porphyria significantly different from 106 nmol/d (range 61.0 - 119) in 20 healthy control individuals 2844 Excessive amounts 2034 In one patient with acute intermittent porphyria mean excretion of 1,166 nmol/d significantly different from reference range of 37 - 159 nmol/d 1877

Coproporphyrin I *Feces* *No Effect* Mean proportion of coproporphyrin I excretion 72.1 ± 8.3% in 23 patients with acute intermittent porphyria greater than 69.6 ± 6.2% of 11.0 nmol/g (range 8.0 - 35.0) in 20 healthy control individuals 2844
Urine *Decrease* Mean proportion of 13.4 ± 5.7% of total coproporphyrin excreted in 30 patients with acute intermittent porphyria different from 25.3 ± 4.7% of 106 nmol/d (range 61.0 - 119) in 20 healthy control individuals 2844

Coproporphyrin II *Feces* *No Effect* Mean proportion of coproporphyrin II excretion of 1.0 ± 0.5% in 23 patients with acute intermittent porphyria not significantly different from 0.9 ± 0.3% of 11.0 nmol/g (range 8.0 - 35.0) in 20 healthy control individuals 2844
Urine *No Effect* Mean proportion of 1.6 ± 0.9% of total coproporphyrin excreted in 30 patients with acute intermittent porphyria not significantly different from 1.8 ± 0.8% of 106 nmol/d (range 61.0 - 119) in 20 healthy control individuals 2844

Coproporphyrin II + IV *Feces* *No Effect* Mean proportion of coproporphyrin II + IV excretion 2.6 ± 1.2% in 23 patients with acute intermittent porphyria not significantly different from 2.5 ± 1.2% of 11.0 nmol/g (range 8.0 - 35.0) in 20 healthy control individuals 2844
Urine *No Effect* Mean proportion of 4.9 ± 2.7% of total coproporphyrin excreted in 30 patients with acute intermittent porphyria not significantly different from 4.6 ± 2.3% of 106 nmol/d (range 61.0 - 119) in 20 healthy control individuals 2844

Coproporphyrin III *Feces* *No Effect* Mean proportion of coproporphyrin III excretion of 35.7 ± 10.6% in 31 patients with acute intermittent porphyria not significantly different from 27.5 ± 5.9% of 11.0 nmol/g (range 8.0 - 35.0) in 20 healthy control individuals 2844

Urine *Increase* Mean proportion of 81.7 ± 6.1% of total coproporphyrin excreted in 30 patients with acute intermittent porphyria not significantly different from 69.0 ± 6.2% of 106 nmol/d (range 61.0 - 119) in 20 healthy control individuals *2844*

Coproporphyrin III:Coproporphyrin I Ratio *Feces* *No Effect* Mean proportion of coproporphyrin III:I excretion of 0.5 ± 0.4% in 23 patients with acute intermittent porphyria not significantly different from 0.4 ± 0.1% of 11.0 nmol/g (range 8.0 - 35.0) in 20 healthy control individuals *2844*
Urine *Increase* Mean proportion of 5.9 ± 3.3% of total coproporphyrin excreted in 30 patients with acute intermittent porphyria significantly different from 2.7 ± 0.8% of 106 nmol/d (range 61.0 - 119) in 20 healthy control individuals *2844*

Coproporphyrin IV *Urine* *No Effect* Mean proportion of 3.3 ± 1.5% of total coproporphyrin excreted in 30 patients with acute intermittent porphyria not significantly different from 3.9 ± 1.8% of 106 nmol/d (range 61.0 - 119) in 20 healthy control individuals *2844*

Erythrocyte Survival *Red Blood Cells* *No Effect* Suggests that the decreased RBC mass results from reduced effective erythropoiesis *488*

γ-Globulin *Serum* *Increase* Constant finding *900*

Hematocrit *Blood* *Decrease* Microcytic hypochromic anemia may occur due to blood loss or increased demand *1098*

Hemoglobin *Blood* *Decrease* Microcytic hypochromic anemia may occur due to blood loss or increased demand *1098*

17-Hydroxycorticosteroids *Urine* *Increase* In acute attacks *4979*

Iron *Serum* *Increase* Frequently markedly elevated *900*

Isocitrate Dehydrogenase *Serum* *No Effect* No effect on activity observed *5008*

17-Ketogenic Steroids *Urine* *Increase* In acute attacks *4979*

LDL-Cholesterol *Serum* *Increase* Moderate elevation *126*

Leukocytes *Blood* *Increase* Occasionally during acute attacks *4996*

Magnesium *Serum* *Decrease* Electrolyte depletion and alkalosis associated with azotemia of variable degree are often present on admission but may also develop acutely during the course of the attack. The electrolyte disorders are attributable in many patients to electrolyte depletion with inappropriate and injudicious overhydration *900*

MCH *Blood* *Decrease* Microcytic hypochromic anemia may occur due to blood loss or increased demand. MCH < 27 pg *1098*

MCV *Blood* *Decrease* Microcytic hypochromic anemia may occur due to blood loss or increased demand. MCV < 80 fL *1098*

pH *Blood* *Increase* Electrolyte depletion and alkalosis associated with azotemia of variable degree are often present on admission but may also develop acutely during the course of the attack *900*

Porphobilinogen *Cerebrospinal Fluid* *Increase* In patients with severe attacks *5106*
Liver *Increase* Liver and kidney regularly contain large amounts *4979* *4645* Large amounts *1849*
Serum *Increase* Increased production of the porphyrin precursors *356* In patients with severe attacks *5106*
Urine *Increase* In a patient with probable acute porphyria excretion of 20 µmol/L significantly greater than reference upper limit of normal of less than 8.8 µg/L: In a patient with proved acute intermittent porphyria excretion of 98 µmol/L *81* In one patient with acute intermittent porphyria mean excretion of 409 µmol/d significantly different from reference range of 1 - 8 µmol/d *1877* During relapse the presence of this compound is a constant feature. During remission it is usually present but the absence does not exclude the diagnosis *5528* Concentration increased *3406* One of most effective diagnostic tests *2592* Occurs fairly specifically in acute idiopathic porphyria *5599* During relapse the presence of this compound is a constant feature. During remission it is usually present but the absence does not exclude the diagnosis *5677* Characteristic *4979* In 21 symptomatic patients, an average of 83 mg porphobilinogen/24 h was excreted. Tends to decrease somewhat during remission *4996*

Porphobilinogen Deaminase *Red Blood Cells* *Decrease* Activities of less than 6.0 nmol/s/L are diagnostic of AIP *2952*

Porphyrin, Total *Urine* *Increase* In 27 patients with AIP median concentration of 641 (88 - 14,834) µg/L in nonoxidized specimens and 815 (102 - 15,211) µg/L in oxidized specimens significantly greater than 68 (20 -121) µg/L and 94 (23 - 184) µg/L respectively in 30 healthy controls *2130* In one patient with acute intermittent porphyria mean excretion of 9581 nmol/d significantly different from reference range of 63 - 205 nmol/d *1877* In a patient with probable acute porphyria excretion of 383 µmol/L greater than reference upper limit of normal of less than 320 µg/L. In a patient with proved acute intermittent porphyria excretion 3154 µmol/L *81*

Porphyrinogens *Urine* *Decrease* In 27 patients with PCT mean proportion of total porphyrins of 20 ± 15% significantly less than38 ± 15% in 30 healthy controls *2130*

Potassium *Serum* *Decrease* Electrolyte depletion and alkalosis associated with azotemia of variable degree are often present on admission but may also develop acutely during the course of the attack. The electrolyte disorders are attributable in many patients to electrolyte depletion with inappropriate and injudicious overhydration *900*

Protoporphyrin *Feces* *Increase* Small increases may be found *4979* Slight or moderate elevation *5598*
Red Blood Cells *No Effect* No significant effect observed *2034*

Sodium *Serum* *Decrease* Electrolyte depletion and alkalosis associated with azotemia of variable degree are often present on admission but may also develop acutely during the course of the attack. The severity of the hyponatremia is a particularly striking feature, and although it may by symptomless, it is often associated with the encephalopathic manifestations of the acute attack. Attributable in many patients to electrolyte depletion with inappropriate and injudicious overhydration *900*

Urea Nitrogen *Serum* *Increase* During an attack *900* Frequent *4996*

Uroporphyrin *Feces* *Increase* In some patients *5598* Small increases may be found *4979*
Liver *Increase* Has been isolated from hepatic tissue in some cases *4645* *4979*
Red Blood Cells *No Effect* No significant effect observed *2034*
Urine *Increase* May contain little if any increase *917* May develop in urine on standing *4979* Excessive amounts *2034* In one patient with acute intermittent porphyria mean excretion of 7,605 nmol/d significantly different from reference range of 4 - 29 nmol/d *1877*

Volume *Plasma* *Decrease* Frequently observed during attacks *4996*
Urine *Decrease* Prolonged vomiting may cause dehydration, oliguria, and azotemia *367*

277.10 5-Aminolevulinic Acid Deficiency Protoporphyria

δ-Aminolevulinic Acid *Urine* *Increase* One of most effective diagnostic tests *2592*

277.10 Erythropoietic Coproporphyria

δ-Aminolevulinic Acid *Urine* *No Effect* No significant effect observed *3222* *2034*

Coproporphyrin *Feces* *No Effect* No significant effect observed *5677*
Red Blood Cells *Increase* Large amounts *1290*
Urine *No Effect* No significant effect observed *1290*

Hematocrit *Blood* *Decrease* Microcytic hypochromic anemia may occur due to blood loss or increased demand *1098*

Hemoglobin *Blood* *Decrease* Microcytic hypochromic anemia may occur due to blood loss or increased demand *1098*

MCH *Blood* *Decrease* Microcytic hypochromic anemia may occur due to blood loss or increased demand. MCH < 27 pg *1098*

MCV *Blood* *Decrease* Microcytic hypochromic anemia may occur due to blood loss or increased demand. MCV < 80 fL *1098*

Porphobilinogen *Urine* *Increase* Slight increase *4979*
Urine *No Effect* Excretion usually normal *2034*

Protoporphyrin *Feces* *No Effect* No significant effect typically observed *2034*

277.10 Erythropoietic Coproporphyria (continued)

Protoporphyrin *(continued)*
Red Blood Cells *Increase* Small increase *4979*

Uroporphyrin *Feces* *No Effect* No significant effect observed *2034*
Red Blood Cells *Increase* Moderate concentrations *2034*
Urine *No Effect* No significant effect seen *3382*

277.10 Erythropoietic Porphyria, Congenital

δ-Aminolevulinic Acid *Urine* *No Effect* With chromatographic methods, within normal limits *1779* No significant effect observed *5453* *2034*

Coproporphyrin *Feces* *Increase* Mean excretion of 2,009 nmol/g in 12 patients with congenital erythropoietic porphyria significantly greater than 11.0 nmol/g (range 8.0 - 35.0) in 20 healthy control individuals *2844* Large amounts *4644*
Red Blood Cells *Increase* Variable *4979* *4645* Elevated, but lower than uroporphyrins *4979*
Urine *Increase* Large amounts but less than the uroporphyrin *4645* Mean excretion of 5,681 nmol/d in 12 patients with congenital erythropoietic porphyria significantly different from 106 nmol/d (range 61.0 - 119) in 20 healthy control individuals *2844*

Coproporphyrin I *Feces* *Increase* Mean proportion of coproporphyrin I excretion 89.0 ± 4.0% in 12 patients with congenital erythropoietic porphyria significantly greater than 69.6 ± 6.2% of 11.0 nmol/g (range 8.0 - 35.0) in 20 healthy control individuals *2844*
Urine *Increase* Mean proportion of 92.0 ± 3.3% of total coproporphyrin excreted in 12 patients with congenital erythropoietic porphyria significantly different from 25.3 ± 4.7% of 106 nmol/d (range 61.0 - 119) in 20 healthy control individuals *2844*

Coproporphyrin II *Feces* *Decrease* Mean proportion of coproporphyrin II excretion 0.4 ± 0.2% in 12 patients with congenital erythropoietic porphyria significantly different from 0.9 ± 0.3% of 11.0 nmol/g (range 8.0 - 35.0) in 20 healthy control individuals *2844*
Urine *Decrease* Mean proportion of 0.3 ± 0.2% of total coproporphyrin excreted in 12 patients with congenital erythropoietic porphyria significantly different from 1.8 ± 0.8% of 106 nmol/d (range 61.0 - 119) in 20 healthy control individuals *2844*

Coproporphyrin II + IV *Feces* *No Effect* Mean proportion of coproporphyrin II + IV excretion of 1.2 ± 0.8% in 12 patients with congenital erythropoietic porphyria not significantly different from 2.5 ± 1.2% of 11.0 nmol/g (range 8.0 - 35.0) in 20 healthy control individuals *2844*
Urine *Decrease* Mean proportion of 0.7 ± 0.6% of total coproporphyrin excreted in 12 patients with congenital erythropoietic porphyria significantly different from 4.6 ± 2.3% of 106 nmol/d (range 61.0 - 119) in 20 healthy control individuals *2844*

Coproporphyrin III *Feces* *Decrease* Mean proportion of coproporphyrin III excretion of 9.5 ± 3.2% in 12 patients with congenital erythropoietic porphyria significantly different from 27.5 ± 5.9% of 11.0 nmol/g (range 8.0 - 35.0) in 20 healthy control individuals *2844*
Urine *Decrease* Mean proportion of 6.9 ± 2.9% of total coproporphyrin excreted in 12 patients with congenital erythropoietic porphyria significantly different from 69.0 ± 6.2% of 106 nmol/d (range 61.0 - 119) in 20 healthy control individuals *2844*

Coproporphyrin III:Coproporphyrin I Ratio *Feces* *Decrease* Mean proportion of coproporphyrin III:I excretion of 0.1 ± 0.03% in 12 patients with congenital erythropoietic porphyria significantly different from 0.4 ± 0.1% of 11.0 nmol/g (range 8.0 - 35.0) in 20 healthy control individuals *2844*
Urine *Decrease* Mean proportion of 0.08 ± 0.03% of total coproporphyrin excreted in 12 patients with congenital erythropoietic porphyria significantly different from 2.7 ± 0.8% of 106 nmol/d (range 61.0 - 119) in 20 healthy control individuals *2844*

Coproporphyrin IV *Urine* *Decrease* Mean proportion of 0.8 ± 0.5% of total coproporphyrin excreted in 12 patients with congenital erythropoietic porphyria significantly different from 3.9 ± 1.8% of 106 nmol/d (range 61.0 - 119) in 20 healthy control individuals *2844*

Erythrocyte Survival *Red Blood Cells* *Decrease* Hemolysis occurs in most patients *4979* *4644* With moderate to severe anemia *5699*

Hematocrit *Blood* *Decrease* Normochromic anemia, only rarely severe *4644* Anemia is normohromic and normocytic and tends to be mild in degree *5699*

Hemoglobin *Blood* *Decrease* In most patients, reduction was only slight and hemolysis was compensated by increased RBC production *4979* Anemia is normochromic and normocytic and tends to be mild in degree *5699* In most patients, reduction was only slight and hemolysis was compensated by increased RBC production *4644*

MCH *Blood* *Decrease* Microcytic hypochromic anemia may occur due to blood loss or increased demand. MCH < 27 pg *1098*

MCV *Blood* *Decrease* Microcytic hypochromic anemia may occur due to blood loss or increased demand. MCV < 80 fL *1098*

Osmotic Fragility *Red Blood Cells* *No Effect* Usually no effect observed *1779*

Porphobilinogen *Urine* *No Effect* With chromatographic methods, within normal limits *1779* Excretion usually normal *5453*

Protoporphyrin *Feces* *Increase* Variable although not significantly elevated *4979*
Feces *No Effect* Variable although not significantly elevated *4979*
Red Blood Cells *Increase* As in other hemolytic conditions *5597*

Reticulocytes *Blood* *Increase* With moderate to severe anemia *5699* Secondary to increased hemolytic activity *4644*

Uroporphyrin *Bone Marrow* *Increase* Bone marrow is studded with red cell precursors containing uroporphyrin in the nucleus and showing intense fluorescence when examined under ultraviolet light *4644*
Feces *Increase* Usually large amounts *4979*
Red Blood Cells *Increase* High concentrations *4645* High RBC concentration of uroporphyrin I *4645* *4979*
Serum *Increase* Variable *4645* *4979*
Urine *Increase* Daily excretion of 500 µg/d has been reported *1915* Most characteristic metabolic abnormality *5699* Up to 500 µg/d has been reported *4979* Large amounts *5677*

Uroporphyrin I *Red Blood Cells* *Increase* One of most effective diagnostic tests *2592*
Urine *Increase* One of most effective diagnostic tests *2592*

277.10 Erythropoietic Protoporphyria

δ-Aminolevulinic Acid *Urine* *No Effect* No significant effect observed *3222* *2034*

Coproporphyrin *Feces* *Increase* In some carriers, elevated even with normal RBC porphyrins. Fluctuates markedly from one time period to another in the same patient *1206* At times *5677*
Feces *No Effect* No significant effect usually seen *5677*
Urine *No Effect* No significant effect observed *3222*

Hematocrit *Blood* *Decrease* A moderate hypochromic or normochromic anemia is frequently observed *5677*
Blood *No Effect* In most reported patients, there have been no quantitative blood abnormalities *5699*

Hemoglobin *Blood* *Decrease* A moderate hypochromic or normochromic anemia is frequently observed *5677*
Blood *No Effect* In most reported patients, there have been no quantitative blood abnormalities *5699*

Iron *Serum* *No Effect* No significant effect observed *5677*

MCH *Blood* *Decrease* Microcytic hypochromic anemia may occur due to blood loss or increased demand. MCH < 27 pg *1098* A moderate hypochromic or normochromic anemia is frequently observed *5677*

MCHC *Blood* *Decrease* A moderate hypochromic or normochromic anemia is frequently observed *5677*

MCV *Blood* *Decrease* A moderate hypo- or normochromic anemia is frequently observed *5677* Microcytic hypochromic anemia may occur due to blood loss or increased demand. MCV < 80 fL *1098*

Porphobilinogen *Urine* *No Effect* Excretion usually normal *3222*

Protoporphyrin *Feces* *Increase* In some carriers, elevated even with normal RBC porphyrins. Fluctuates markedly from one time period to another in the same patient *1206* Contains only increased protoporphyrin, a unique finding among porphyrias *5677* Usually but not always increased in symptomatic patients, from 30 - 300 µg/g dry weight and occasionally higher *3177*
Red Blood Cells *Increase* Increased 5 - 30 times *3222* Reported values range from 300 - 4,500 mg/dL (normal < 50 mg/dL) *5699* May be up to 100-fold *3221* The red cells hemolyze if blood in thin layers is exposed to ultraviolet light *2028* Marked increase *4979* The red cells hemolyze if blood in thin layers is exposed to ultraviolet light *5677* Excess does not occur in all cells, from 7 - 60% were found to contain excess *2561* In 30 patients with erythropoietic protoporphyria mean concentration of 1,300 ± 758 nmol protoporphyrin/dL significantly different from 50 ± 25 nmol protoporphyrin/dL in 50 healthy controls *1771*
Serum *Increase* Frequently elevated *3222* Most striking finding is the elevation in RBC, feces, and plasma *4979*

Uroporphyrin *Feces* *No Effect* Excretion usually normal *4979*
Red Blood Cells *Increase* Moderate concentrations *2034*
Urine *Increase* Only in patients with hepatic complications *4979*
Urine *No Effect* No significant effect observed *4979* Typically unchanged by disease *3222*

Zinc Chelatase *Lymphocytes* *Decrease* In 30 patients with erythropoietic protoporphyria mean concentration of 0.45 ± 0.10 nmol zinc protoporphyrin/h/mg protein significantly different from 0.84 ± 0.27 nmol zinc protoporphyrin/h/mg in 50 healthy controls *1771*

277.10 Erythropoietic Protoporphyria Carrier

Protoporphyrin *Red Blood Cells* *No Effect* In 14 carriers of erythropoietic protoporphyria mean concentration of 60 ± 24 nmol protoporphyrin/dL not significantly different from 50 ± 25 nmol protoporphyrin/dL in 50 healthy controls *1771*

Zinc Chelatase *Lymphocytes* *Decrease* In 14 carriers of erythropoietic protoporphyria mean concentration of 0.42 ± 0.09 nmol zinc protoporphyrin/h/mg protein significantly different from 0.84 ± 0.27 nmol zinc protoporphyrin/h/mg in 50 healthy controls *1771*

277.10 Hepatic Porphyria, Congenital

Levulinic Acid *Urine* *Increase* Urinary excretion may be increased in patients with congenital hepatic porphyria *2952*

277.10 Porphobilinogen Synthase Deficiency Porphyria

Coproporphyrin *Feces* *No Effect* Mean excretion of 18.8 nmol/g in 3 patients with porphobilinogen synthase deficiency porphyria not significantly greater than 11.0 nmol/g (range 8.0 - 35.0) in 20 healthy control individuals *2844*
Urine *Increase* Mean excretion of 4,533 nmol/d in 3 patients with porphobilinogen synthase deficiency porphyria significantly different from 106 nmol/d (range 61.0 - 119) in 20 healthy control individuals *2844*

Coproporphyrin I *Feces* *No Effect* Mean proportion of coproporphyrin I excretion of 54.0 ± 9.5% in 3 patients with porphobilinogen synthase deficiency porphyria not significantly different from 69.6 ± 6.2% of 11.0 nmol/g (range 8.0 - 35.0) in 20 healthy control individuals *2844*
Urine *Decrease* Mean proportion of 5.0 ± 0.5% of total coproporphyrin excreted in 3 patients with porphobilinogen synthase deficiency porphyria significantly different from 25.3 ± 4.7% of 106 nmol/d (range 61.0 - 119) in 20 healthy control individuals *2844*

Coproporphyrin II *Feces* *No Effect* Mean proportion of coproporphyrin II excretion 0.7 ± 0.3% in 3 patients with porphobilinogen synthase deficiency porphyria significantly different from 0.9 ± 0.3% of 11.0 nmol/g (range 8.0 - 35.0) in 20 healthy control individuals *2844*
Urine *Increase* Mean proportion of 4.2 ± 1.7% of total coproporphyrin excreted in 3 patients with porphobilinogen synthase deficiency porphyria significantly different from 1.8 ± 0.8% of 106 nmol/d (range 61.0 - 119) in 20 healthy control individuals *2844*

Coproporphyrin II + IV *Feces* *No Effect* Mean proportion of coproporphyrin II + IV excretion 2.4 ± 1.1% in 3 patients with porphobilinogen synthase deficiency porphyria not significantly different from 2.5 ± 1.2% of 11.0 nmol/g (range 8.0 - 35.0) in 20 healthy control individuals *2844*
Urine *Increase* Mean proportion of 11.2 ± 4.2% of total coproporphyrin excreted in 3 patients with porphobilinogen synthase deficiency porphyria significantly different from 4.6 ± 2.3% of 106 nmol/d (range 61.0 - 119) in 20 healthy control individuals *2844*

Coproporphyrin III *Feces* *Increase* Mean proportion of coproporphyrin III excretion of 43.7 ± 8.5% in 3 patients with porphobilinogen synthase deficiency porphyria significantly different from 27.5 ± 5.9% of 11.0 nmol/g (range 8.0 - 35.0) in 20 healthy control individuals *2844*
Urine *Increase* Mean proportion of 84.0 ± 1.7% of total coproporphyrin excreted in 3 patients with porphobilinogen synthase deficiency porphyria not significantly different from 69.0 ± 6.2% of 106 nmol/d (range 61.0 - 119) in 20 healthy control individuals *2844*

Coproporphyrin III:Coproporphyrin I Ratio *Feces* *Increase* Mean proportion of coproporphyrin III:I excretion of 0.8 ± 0.3% in 3 patients with porphobilinogen synthase deficiency porphyria not significantly different from 0.4 ± 0.1% of 11.0 nmol/g (range 8.0 - 35.0) in 20 healthy control individuals *2844*
Urine *Increase* Mean proportion of 16.3 ± 1.9% of total coproporphyrin excreted in 3 patients with porphobilinogen synthase deficiency porphyria significantly different from 2.7 ± 0.8% of 106 nmol/d (range 61.0 - 119) in 20 healthy control individuals *2844*

Coproporphyrin IV *Urine* *Increase* Mean proportion of 8.7 ± 2.5% of total coproporphyrin excreted in 3 patients with porphobilinogen synthase deficiency porphyria significantly different from 3.9 ± 1.8% of 106 nmol/d (range 61.0 - 119) in 20 healthy control individuals *2844*

277.10 Porphyria

Thyroxine Binding Globulin *Serum* *Increase* May increase TBG concentration *1965*

Thyroxine (T4) *Serum* *Increase* May increase TBG concentration *1965*

Tri-iodothyronine (T3) *Serum* *Increase* May increase TBG concentration *1965*

277.10 Porphyria Variegata

δ-Aminolevulinic Acid *Urine* *Increase* Observed effect *2034* May appear during acute attacks *5699* Normal or moderate increase in asymptomatic patients. Sharp rise with acute attacks *1281* Concentration increased *3406*

Coproporphyrin *Feces* *Increase* Large amounts *1082* Even when clinical manifestations are minimal *1887* Mean excretion of 259 nmol/g in 13 patients with porphyria variegata significantly greater than 11.0 nmol/g (range 8.0 - 35.0) in 20 healthy control individuals *2844* Ranges from 70 - > 1,000 µg/g dry weight (normal < 100 µg/g) *5699* The most characteristic and consistent abnormality *4996*
Red Blood Cells *No Effect* No significant effect *2034* *4979*
Urine *Increase* During acute attacks *4979* Sharp rise in acute attacks *1281* Characteristic finding in urine and feces *4362* Mean excretion of 931 nmol/d in 10 patients with porphyria variegata significantly different from 106 nmol/d (range 61.0 - 119) in 20 healthy control individuals *2844*

Coproporphyrin I *Feces* *Decrease* Mean proportion of coproporphyrin I excretion of 17.8 ± 6.7% in 13 patients with porphyria variegata significantly different from 69.6 ± 6.2% of 11.0 nmol/g (range 8.0 - 35.0) in 20 healthy control individuals *2844*
Urine *Decrease* Mean proportion of 11.0 ± 7.4% of total coproporphyrin excreted in 10 patients with porphyria variegata significantly different from 25.3 ± 4.7% of 106 nmol/d (range 61.0 - 119) in 20 healthy control individuals *2844*

277.10 Porphyria Variegata *(continued)*

Coproporphyrin II *Feces Increase* Mean proportion of coproporphyrin II excretion 2.0 ± 0.6% in 13 patients with porphyria variegata significantly different from 0.9 ± 0.3% of 11.0 nmol/g (range 8.0 - 35.0) in 20 healthy control individuals *2844*
Urine No Effect Mean proportion of 2.1 ± 0.9% of total coproporphyrin excreted in 10 patients with porphyria variegata not significantly different from 1.8 ± 0.8% of 106 nmol/d (range 61.0 - 119) in 20 healthy control individuals *2844*

Coproporphyrin II + IV *Feces Increase* Mean proportion of coproporphyrin II + IV excretion 6.3 ± 1.6% in 13 patients with porphyria variegata significantly different from 2.5 ± 1.2% of 11.0 nmol/g (range 8.0 - 35.0) in 20 healthy control individuals *2844*
Urine Increase Mean proportion of 7.2 ± 3.1% of total coproporphyrin excreted in 10 patients with porphyria variegata different from 4.6 ± 2.3% of 106 nmol/d (range 61.0 - 119) in 20 healthy control individuals *2844*

Coproporphyrin III *Feces Increase* Mean proportion of coproporphyrin III excretion of 75.7 ± 5.8% in 13 patients with porphyria variegata significantly different from 27.5 ± 5.9% of 11.0 nmol/g (range 8.0 - 35.0) in 20 healthy control individuals *2844*
Urine Increase Mean proportion of 81.8 ± 8.4% of total coproporphyrin excreted in 10 patients with porphyria variegata not significantly different from 69.0 ± 6.2% of 106 nmol/d (range 61.0 - 119) in 20 healthy control individuals *2844*

Coproporphyrin III:Coproporphyrin I Ratio *Feces Increase* Mean proportion of coproporphyrin III I excretion of 4.8 ± 2.0% in 13 patients with porphyria variegata significantly different from 0.4 ± 0.1% of 11.0 nmol/g (range 8.0 - 35.0) in 20 healthy control individuals *2844*
Urine Increase Mean proportion of 12.3 ± 5.3% of total coproporphyrin excreted in 10 patients with porphyria variegata significantly different from 2.7 ± 0.8% of 106 nmol/d (range 61.0 - 119) in 20 healthy control individuals *2844*

Coproporphyrin IV *Urine Increase* Mean proportion of 5.0 ± 2.2% of total coproporphyrin excreted in 10 patients with porphyria variegata significantly different from 3.9 ± 1.8% of 106 nmol/d (range 61.0 - 119) in 20 healthy control individuals *2844*

γ-Globulin *Serum Increase* Constant finding *900*

β-Hexosaminidase *Serum Increase* Observed effect *3141*

Iron *Serum Increase* Frequently markedly elevated *900*

MCH *Blood Decrease* Microcytic hypochromic anemia may occur due to blood loss or increased demand. MCH < 27 pg *1098*

MCV *Blood Decrease* Microcytic hypochromic anemia may occur due to blood loss or increased demand. MCV < 80 fL *1098*

Porphobilinogen *Serum Increase* Increased production of the porphyrin precursors *356*
Urine Increase May appear during acute attacks *5699* May be as high as levels in acute intermittent porphyria *1082* Concentration increased *3406*

Protoporphyrin *Feces Increase* Even when clinical manifestations are minimal *1887* Concentration increased *3406* The most characteristic and consistent abnormality *4996* One of most effective diagnostic tests *2592* Large amounts *1082*
Red Blood Cells No Effect No significant effect observed *4979 2034*

Uroporphyrin *Feces Increase* Variable *1780* May be increased *5104*
Red Blood Cells No Effect No significant effect observed *4979 2034*
Urine Increase Sharp rise in acute attacks *1281* Characteristic finding in urine and feces *4362* During acute attacks *2034*

277.10 Protoporphyria

Coproporphyrin *Blood Increase* Concentration increased *3406*
Feces Increase Mean excretion of 32.9 nmol/g in 12 patients with protoporphyria greater than 11.0 nmol/g (range 8.0 - 35.0) in 20 healthy control individuals *2844* Concentration increased *3406*
Urine Increase Mean excretion of 312 nmol/d in 12 patients with protoporphyria significantly different from 106 nmol/d (range 61.0 - 119) in 20 healthy control individuals *2844*

Coproporphyrin I *Feces Increase* Mean proportion of coproporphyrin I excretion 77.5 ± 6.7% in 12 patients with protoporphyria greater than 69.6 ± 6.2% of 11.0 nmol/g (range 8.0 - 35.0) in 20 healthy control individuals *2844*
Urine Increase Mean proportion of 57.0 ± 22.7% of total coproporphyrin excreted in 12 patients with protoporphyria significantly different from 25.3 ± 4.7% of 106 nmol/d (range 61.0 - 119) in 20 healthy control individuals *2844*

Coproporphyrin II *Feces Decrease* Mean proportion of coproporphyrin II excretion 0.4 ± 0.2% in 12 patients with protoporphyria significantly different from 0.9 ± 0.3% of 11.0 nmol/g (range 8.0 - 35.0) in 20 healthy control individuals *2844*
Urine No Effect Mean proportion of 1.7 ± 1.5% of total coproporphyrin excreted in 12 patients with protoporphyria not significantly different from 1.8 ± 0.8% of 106 nmol/d (range 61.0 - 119) in 20 healthy control individuals *2844*

Coproporphyrin II + IV *Feces No Effect* Mean proportion of coproporphyrin II + IV excretion of 1.4 ± 0.7% in 12 patients with protoporphyria not significantly different from 2.5 ± 1.2% of 11.0 nmol/g (range 8.0 - 35.0) in 20 healthy control individuals *2844*
Urine No Effect Mean proportion of 4.1 ± 2.7% of total coproporphyrin excreted in 12 patients with protoporphyria not significantly different from 4.6 ± 2.3% of 106 nmol/d (range 61.0 - 119) in 20 healthy control individuals *2844*

Coproporphyrin III *Feces No Effect* Mean proportion of coproporphyrin III excretion of 21.0 ± 6.4% in 12 patients with protoporphyria not significantly different from 27.5 ± 5.9% of 11.0 nmol/g (range 8.0 - 35.0) in 20 healthy control individuals *2844*
Urine Decrease Mean proportion of 43.0 ± 22.7% of total coproporphyrin excreted in 12 patients with protoporphyria significantly different from 69.0 ± 6.2% of 106 nmol/d (range 61.0 - 119) in 20 healthy control individuals *2844*

Coproporphyrin III:Coproporphyrin I Ratio *Feces No Effect* Mean proportion of coproporphyrin III:I excretion of 0.1 ± 0.03% in 12 patients with protoporphyria not significantly different from 0.4 ± 0.1% of 11.0 nmol/g (range 8.0 - 35.0) in 20 healthy control individuals *2844*
Urine Decrease Mean proportion of 0.8 ± 0.3% of total coproporphyrin excreted in 12 patients with protoporphyria significantly different from 2.7 ± 0.8% of 106 nmol/d (range 61.0 - 119) in 20 healthy control individuals *2844*

Coproporphyrin IV *Urine No Effect* Mean proportion of 3.3 ± 2.4% of total coproporphyrin excreted in 12 patients with protoporphyria not significantly different from 3.9 ± 1.8% of 106 nmol/d (range 61.0 - 119) in 20 healthy control individuals *2844*

Porphyrin, Total *Urine No Effect* Concentration normal *3406*

Protoporphyrin *Blood Increase* Concentration increased *3406*
Feces Increase Concentration increased *3406*
Red Blood Cells Increase One of most effective diagnostic tests *2592*

277.11 Erythropoietic Uroporphyria

Uroporphyrinogen III Synthase *Red Blood Cells Decrease* In patients with erythropoietic uroporphyria concentrations typically < 10 relative units compared with > 40 relative units in healthy individuals *2952*

277.16 Porphyria Cutanea Tarda

Alanine Aminotransferase *Serum Increase* Liver function is highly variable. May be mildly elevated *5699*

δ-Aminolevulinic Acid *Urine Increase* Rarely occurs *1281 4979* During acute stage *2034*
Urine No Effect Concentration normal *3406* No significant effect observed *2903*

Aspartate Aminotransferase *Serum Increase* Liver function is highly variable. May be mildly elevated *5699*

BSP Retention *Serum Increase* Usually abnormal *5529*

Coproporphyrin *Feces Increase* Highly variable, but never as high as in variegata porphyria *5120* Mean excretion of 44.0 nmol/g in 31 patients with porphyria cutanea tarda greater than 11.0 nmol/g (range 8.0 - 35.0) in 20 healthy control individuals *2844* Large amounts *2034*

Feces *No Effect* No significant abnormality in excretion of total coproporphyrin observed in patients with either familial or sporadic familial porphyria cutanea tarda *243*
Red Blood Cells *No Effect* No significant effect *2034*
Urine *Increase* Mean excretion of 299 nmol/d in 30 patients with porphyria cutanea tarda significantly different from 106 nmol/d (range 61.0 - 119) in 20 healthy control individuals *2844* Average in 66 patients was 560 µg/d (normal < 200 µg/d) *1282*

Coproporphyrin I *Feces* *Increase* Significant increase to 79 ± 46 µmol/kg dry weight observed in excretion in patients with sporadic porphyria cutanea tarda *243*
Feces *No Effect* Mean proportion of coproporphyrin I excretion 72.1 ± 8.3% in 31 patients with porphyria cutanea tarda greater than 69.6 ± 6.2% of 11.0 nmol/g (range 8.0 - 35.0) in 20 healthy control individuals *2844* No significant change to 36 ± 26 µmol/kg dry weight observed in excretion in patients with familial porphyria cutanea tarda *243*
Urine *Increase* Concentration increased *3406* Mean proportion of 36.6 ± 17.2% of total coproporphyrin excreted in 30 patients with porphyria cutanea tarda different from 25.3 ± 4.7% of 106 nmol/d (range 61.0 - 119) in 20 healthy control individuals *2844*

Coproporphyrin II *Feces* *Decrease* Mean proportion of coproporphyrin II excretion 0.7 ± 0.3% in 31 patients with porphyria cutanea tarda significantly different from 0.9 ± 0.3% of 11.0 nmol/g (range 8.0 - 35.0) in 20 healthy control individuals *2844*
Urine *No Effect* Mean proportion of 2.2 ± 1.1% of total coproporphyrin excreted in 30 patients with porphyria cutanea tarda not significantly different from 1.8 ± 0.8% of 106 nmol/d (range 61.0 - 119) in 20 healthy control individuals *2844*

Coproporphyrin II + IV *Feces* *No Effect* Mean proportion of coproporphyrin II + IV excretion of 1.8 ± 1.1% in 31 patients with porphyria cutanea tarda not significantly different from 2.5 ± 1.2% of 11.0 nmol/g (range 8.0 - 35.0) in 20 healthy control individuals *2844*
Urine *Increase* Mean proportion of 7.0 ± 2.2% of total coproporphyrin excreted in 30 patients with porphyria cutanea tarda significantly different from 4.6 ± 2.3% of 106 nmol/d (range 61.0 - 119) in 20 healthy control individuals *2844*

Coproporphyrin III *Feces* *No Effect* Mean proportion of coproporphyrin III excretion of 25.8 ± 7.6% in 12 patients with porphyria cutanea tarda not significantly different from 27.5 ± 5.9% of 11.0 nmol/g (range 8.0 - 35.0) in 20 healthy control individuals *2844* Mean proportion of coproporphyrin III excretion of 25.8 ± 7.6% in 31 patients with porphyria cutanea tarda not significantly different from 27.5 ± 5.9% of 11.0 nmol/g (range 8.0 - 35.0) in 20 healthy control individuals *2844* No significant abnormality in excretion of coproporphyrin III observed in patients with either familial or sporadic familial porphyria cutanea tarda *243*
Urine *Decrease* Mean proportion of 57.0 ± 16.6% of total coproporphyrin excreted in 30 patients with porphyria cutanea tarda not significantly different from 69.0 ± 6.2% of 106 nmol/d (range 61.0 - 119) in 20 healthy control individuals *2844*

Coproporphyrin III:Coproporphyrin I Ratio *Feces* *No Effect* Mean proportion of coproporphyrin III:I excretion of 0.3 ± 0.2% in 31 patients with porphyria cutanea tarda not significantly different from 0.4 ± 0.1% of 11.0 nmol/g (range 8.0 - 35.0) in 20 healthy control individuals *2844*
Urine *No Effect* Mean proportion of 2.0 ± 1.2% of total coproporphyrin excreted in 30 patients with porphyria cutanea tarda not significantly different from 2.7 ± 0.8% of 106 nmol/d (range 61.0 - 119) in 20 healthy control individuals *2844*

Coproporphyrin IV *Urine* *No Effect* Mean proportion of 4.2 ± 1.9% of total coproporphyrin excreted in 30 patients with porphyria cutanea tarda not significantly different from 3.9 ± 1.8% of 106 nmol/d (range 61.0 - 119) in 20 healthy control individuals *2844*

Ferritin *Serum* *Increase* Concentration increased *3406*

γ-Glutamyltransferase *Serum* *Increase* Greater than 3.5-fold increase above upper reference limit observed in patients with sporadic porphyria cutanea tarda *243*
Serum *No Effect* Consistently normal activity observed in patients with familial porphyria cutanea tarda in contrast to patients with sporadic porphyria cutanea tarda in whom activity was increased more than 3.5-fold *243*

Hematocrit *Blood* *Decrease* Microcytic hypochromic anemia may occur due to blood low or increased demand *1098*

Hemoglobin *Blood* *Decrease* Microcytic hypochromic anemia may occur due to blood low or increased demand *1098*

β-Hexosaminidase *Serum* *Increase* Observed effect *3141*

Iron *Bone Marrow* *Increase* General increase in body iron stores, in liver, marrow and plasma *5329*
Liver *Increase* General increase in body iron stores, in liver, marrow and plasma *5329*
Serum *Increase* Often increased *5699* Concentration increased *3406*

Iron Saturation *Serum* *Increase* Over 70% saturation in 4 of 20 patients *1374*

Isocoproporphyrin *Feces* *Increase* One of most effective diagnostic tests *2592*

MCH *Blood* *Decrease* Microcytic hypochromic anemia may occur due to blood loss or increased demand. MCH < 27 pg *1098*

MCV *Blood* *Decrease* Microcytic hypochromic anemia may occur due to blood loss or increased demand. MCV < 80 fL *1098*

Porphobilinogen *Urine* *Increase* Rarely occurs *1281* *4979*
Urine *No Effect* Not present *5677* Concentration normal *3406* In a patient with porphyria cutanea tarda excretion of 1.2 µmol/L below reference upper limit of normal of less than 8.8 µg/L *81* Not present *2903*

Porphyrin, Total *Bone Marrow* *No Effect* Usually unaffected by disease *4645*
Feces *No Effect* Highly variable *4979* Normal or only slightly increased in the stool *5699*
Liver *Increase* May precede clinical manifestations and persist after remission *4645*
Urine *Increase* In a patient with porphyria cutanea tarda excretion of 856 µmol/L significantly greater than reference upper limit of normal of less than 8.8 µg/L *81* Usually enough to produce a pinkish or brown color *4979* In 30 patients with PCT median concentration of 1,059 (49 - 4,477) µg/L in nonoxidized specimens and 1,338 (77 - 4,851) µg/L in oxidized specimens significantly greater than 68 (20 - 121) µg/L and 94 (23 - 184) µg/L respectively in 30 healthy controls *2130*

Porphyrinogens *Urine* *Decrease* In 30 patients with PCT mean proportion of total porphyrins of 17 ± 11% significantly less than 38 ± 15% in 30 healthy controls *2130*

Protoporphyrin *Feces* *Increase* Highly variable *5120* Large amounts *2034*
Red Blood Cells *No Effect* No significant effect observed *2034*

Urobilinogen *Urine* *Increase* May be increased because of liver disease *5529*

Uroporphyrin *Feces* *Increase* Highly variable *5120*
Red Blood Cells *No Effect* No significant effect observed *2034*
Urine *Increase* Usually 1 - 10 mg/24 h *1281* In 66 patients, average was 2,819 µg/L and exceeded 1,000 µg/L in 70% of the group (normal < 40 mg/24 h) *1282* During acute attacks *2034* One of most effective diagnostic tests *2592*

Uroporphyrin I *Urine* *Increase* Concentration increased *3406*

Uroporphyrinogen Decarboxylase *Red Blood Cells* *Increase* Mean activity of 2.1 ± 0.4 U/L at 37 °C observed in patients with sporadic porphyria cutanea tarda in contrast to 0.8 ± 0.2 U/L in normal individuals *243*
Red Blood Cells *No Effect* Mean activity of 0.8 ± 0.2 U/L at 37 °C observed in patients with familial porphyria cutanea tarda in contrast to 0.8 ± 0.2 U/L in normal individuals *243*

277.17 Hereditary Coproporphyria

δ-Aminolevulinic Acid *Urine* *Increase* Concentration increased *3406* Mild increase during latent and acute stage *2034* In one patient with hereditary coproporphyria mean excretion of 727 µmol/d significantly different from reference range of 2 - 49 µmol/d *1877* Observed effect *4979* Only during acute attacks *5699*

Coproporphyrin *Feces* *Increase* One of most effective diagnostic tests *2592* Between 100 - 3,000 µg/g dry weight (normal < 40 µg/g dry weight) *5699* In one patient with hereditary coproporphyria mean excretion of 15,450 nmol/g dry weight significantly different from reference range of 5 - 37 nmol/g dry weight *1877* Concentration increased *3406* Unremitting excretion of large amounts *5677* Mean excretion of 3,904 nmol/g in 12 patients with hereditary coproporphyria significantly greater than 11.0 nmol/g (range 8.0 - 35.0) in 20 healthy control

277.17 Hereditary Coproporphyria *(continued)*

Coproporphyrin *(continued)* individuals *2844* Striking abnormality, large excess of coproporphyrin III *4979*
Red Blood Cells *No Effect* No increase demonstrable *1780* No significant effect *2034* No increase demonstrable *4979*
Urine *Increase* Mean excretion of 3,298 nmol/d in 13 patients with hereditary coproporphyria significantly different from 106 nmol/d (range 61.0 - 119) in 20 healthy control individuals *2844* In one patient with hereditary coproporphyria mean excretion of 297 ± 15 nmol/d significantly different from reference range of 37 - 159 nmol/d *1877* One of most effective diagnostic tests *2592* May occur during symptomatic periods but is usually normal during remission *5699*

Coproporphyrin I *Feces* *Decrease* Mean proportion of coproporphyrin I excretion of 17.8 ± 6.7% in 13 patients with hereditary coproporphyria significantly different from 69.6 ± 6.2% of 11.0 nmol/g (range 8.0 - 35.0) in 20 healthy control individuals *2844*
Urine *Decrease* Mean proportion of 12.6 ± 4.8% of total coproporphyrin excreted in 13 patients with hereitary coproporphyria significantly different from 25.3 ± 4.7% of 106 nmol/d (range 61.0 - 119) in 20 healthy control individuals *2844*

Coproporphyrin II *Feces* *Increase* Mean proportion of coproporphyrin II excretion 2.4 ± 0.4% in 12 patients with hereditary coproporphyria significantly different from 0.9 ± 0.3% of 11.0 nmol/g (range 8.0 - 35.0) in 20 healthy control individuals *2844*
Urine *No Effect* Mean proportion of 2.4 ± 1.3% of total coproporphyrin excreted in 13 patients with hereditary coproporphyria not significantly different from 1.8 ± 0.8% of 106 nmol/d (range 61.0 - 119) in 20 healthy control individuals *2844*

Coproporphyrin II + IV *Feces* *Increase* Mean proportion of coproporphyrin II + IV excretion 7.9 ± 1.4% in 12 patients with hereditary coproporphyria significantly different from 2.5 ± 1.2% of 11.0 nmol/g (range 8.0 - 35.0) in 20 healthy control individuals *2844*
Urine *Increase* Mean proportion of 8.1 ± 1.9% of total coproporphyrin excreted in 13 patients with hereditary coproporphyria different from 4.6 ± 2.3% of 106 nmol/d (range 61.0 - 119) in 20 healthy control individuals *2844*

Coproporphyrin III *Feces* *Increase* Mean proportion of coproporphyrin III excretion of 87.0 ± 1.8% in 12 patients with hereditary coproporphyria significantly different from 27.5 ± 5.9% of 11.0 nmol/g (range 8.0 - 35.0) in 20 healthy control individuals *2844*
Urine *Increase* Mean proportion of 79.8 ± 5.8% of total coproporphyrin excreted in 13 patients with hereditary coproporphyria not significantly different from 69.0 ± 6.2% of 106 nmol/d (range 61.0 - 119) in 20 healthy control individuals *2844*

Coproporphyrin III:Coproporphyrin I Ratio *Feces* *Increase* Mean proportion of coproporphyrin III:I excretion of 17.0 ± 4.2% in 12 patients with hereditary coproporphyria significantly different from 0.4 ± 0.1% of 11.0 nmol/g (range 8.0 - 35.0) in 20 healthy control individuals *2844*
Urine *Increase* Mean proportion of 6.1 ± 3.4% of total coproporphyrin excreted in 13 patients with hereditary coproporphyria significantly different from 2.7 ± 0.8% of 106 nmol/d (range 61.0 - 119) in 20 healthy control individuals *2844*

Coproporphyrin IV *Urine* *Increase* Mean proportion of 5.3 ± 2.9% of total coproporphyrin excreted in 13 patients with hereditary porphyria significantly different from 3.9 ± 1.8% of 106 nmol/d (range 61.0 - 119) in 20 healthy control individuals *2844*

γ-Globulin *Serum* *Increase* Constant finding *900*

Hematocrit *Blood* *Decrease* Microcytic hypochromic anemia may occur due to blood loss or increased demand *1098*

Hemoglobin *Blood* *Decrease* Microcytic hypochromic anemia may occur due to blood loss or increased demand *1098*

17-Hydroxycorticosteroids *Urine* *Increase* In acute attacks *4979*

Iron *Serum* *Increase* Frequently markedly elevated *900*

17-Ketogenic Steroids *Urine* *Increase* In acute attacks *4979*

MCH *Blood* *Decrease* Microcytic hypochromic anemia may occur due to blood loss or increased demand. MCH < 27 pg *1098*

MCV *Blood* *Decrease* Microcytic hypochromic anemia may occur due to blood loss or increased demand. MCV < 80 fL *1098*

Porphobilinogen *Serum* *Increase* Increased production of the porphyrin precursors *356*
Urine *Increase* Only during acute attacks *5699* Concentration increased *3406* In one patient with acute hereditary coproporphyria mean excretion of 370 µmol/d significantly different from reference range of 1 - 8 µmol/d *1877* In a patient with hereditary coproporphyria excretion of 30 µmol/L significantly greater than reference upper limit of normal of less than 8.8 µg/L *81*

Porphyrin, Total *Bone Marrow* *No Effect* No increase demonstrable *4979* *1780*
Feces *Increase* In one patient with hereditary coproporphyria mean excretion of 17,186 nmol/g dry weight significantly different from reference range of 27 - 224 nmol/g dry weight *1877*
Urine *Increase* In a patient with hereditary coproporphyria excretion of 405 µmol/L significantly greater than reference upper limit of normal of less than 320 µg/L *81* In one patient with hereditary coproporphyria mean excretion of 35,598 nmol/d significantly different from reference range of 63 - 205 nmol/d *1877*

Protoporphyrin *Feces* *Increase* Increased but not to the same extent as coproporphyrin *5677* In one patient with hereditary coproporphyria mean excretion of 742 nmol/g dry weight significantly different from reference range of 21 - 151 nmol/g dry weight *1877*
Feces *No Effect* Normal or only slightly increased *5699*
Red Blood Cells *No Effect* No significant effect observed *2034* No increase demonstrable *1780* *4979*

Uroporphyrin *Red Blood Cells* *No Effect* No increase demonstrable *1780* *4979* Typically normal *2034*
Urine *Increase* In one patient with hereditary coproporphyria mean excretion of 822 nmol/d significantly different from reference range of 4 - 29 nmol/d *1877*

277.20 Lesch-Nyhan Syndrome

Chitotriosidase *Serum* *No Effect* Normal activity observed in all of five patients with condition *1917*

Dopamine β-Hydroxylase *Serum* *Decrease* Decreased although norepinephrine is normal *2765*

Erythrocytes *Urine* *Increase* Hematuria often occurs *4979*

Folate *Serum* *Decrease* Decreased *602* *772* *5230*

Hematocrit *Blood* *Decrease* Many patients are anemic prior to the occurrence of renal insufficiency *4979*

Hemoglobin *Blood* *Decrease* Many patients are anemic prior to the occurrence of renal insufficiency *4979*

Uric Acid *Serum* *Increase* Ranges from 7 - 18 mg/dL in the absence of renal insufficiency. Occasionally a normal value may occur *4979* *406*
Urine *Increase* Markedly increased. Ranges from 25 - 143 mg/kg/d compared to 18 mg/kg/d as the normal upper limit in children *3478* *4979*

277.20 Xanthinuria

Hypoxanthine *Urine* *Increase* Characterized by the replacement of uric acid by xanthine and hypoxanthine in urine *4979*

Uric Acid *Serum* *Decrease* Characterized by the replacement of uric acid by xanthine and hypoxanthine in urine *4979* Concentrations below level of detection have been documented as well as elevations *4707*
Serum *Increase* Concentrations below level of detection have been documented as well as elevations *4707*
Urine *Decrease* Characterized by the replacement of uric acid by xanthine and hypoxanthine in urine *4979*

Xanthine *Urine* *Increase* Characterized by the replacement of uric acid by xanthine and hypoxanthine in urine *4979*

277.30 Amyloidosis

Acid Phosphatase *Serum* *Increase* Increased in 66% of 14 patients tested. The tartrate inhibition (< 20%) was within normal limits *2878*

Alanine Aminotransferase *Serum* *No Effect* Usually normal *308*

Albumin *Serum* *Decrease* Has been observed. No correlation with severity or duration of disease *299* *4979* Found to be < 3.0 g/dL in 76% of patients *2878* Frequently found with liver involvement *1980*
Urine *Increase* Frequently seen. Massive proteinuria (over 10 g/d) and other manifestations of the nephrotic syndrome may also be present *900*

Alkaline Phosphatase *Serum* *Increase* Hepatic involvement in systemic amyloidosis is rare but increased alkaline phosphatase activity is the most common abnormal liver function test *3625* Frequently elevated, usually ranging from 25 - 535 U/L. No jaundice. In patients with space-occupying lesions such as amyloidosis the degree of elevation at times may be striking with little or no rise in the serum bilirubin values *338* *347* Increased in almost 50% of patients with primary disease, mean value = 108 U/L *2878* With hepatic involvement *308* Frequently elevated, usually ranging from 25 - 535 U/L. No jaundice. In patients with space-occupying lesions such as amyloidosis the degree of elevation at times may be striking with little or no rise in the serum bilirubin values *5544* Frequently found with liver involvement *1980*

Amino Acids *Plasma* *No Effect* No significant effect observed *4979*

Ammonium Ions *Urine* *Increase* May lead to proximal renal tubular acidosis which is associated with hypokalemia, hyperchloremic metabolic acidosis, urine pH < 5.5, increased urinary ammonium ion excretion, a negative urine anion gap, increased urinary osmol gap, normal urinary citrate, normal urinary calcium excretion and Fanconi syndrome *4071* May be associated with classic distal renal tubular acidosis which is associated with hyokalemia, hyperchloremic metabolic acidosis, urine pH > 5.5, increased urinary ammonium ion excretion, a negative urine anion gap, increased urinary osmol gap, decreased urinary citrate and increased urinary calcium in some patients *4071*

Angiotensin-converting Enzyme *Serum* *Increase* Increased activities observed in adults with amyloidosis *2952*

Anion Gap *Urine* *Decrease* May lead to proximal renal tubular acidosis which is associated with hypokalemia, hyperchloremic metabolic acidosis, urine pH < 5.5, increased urinary ammonium ion excretion, a negative urine anion gap, increased urinary osmol gap, normal urinary citrate, normal urinary calcium excretion and Fanconi syndrome *4071* May be associated with classic distal renal tubular acidosis which is associated with hyokalemia, hyperchloremic metabolic acidosis, urine pH > 5.5, increased urinary ammonium ion excretion, a negative urine anion gap, increased urinary osmol gap, decreased urinary citrate and increased urinary calcium in some patients *4071*

α_1-Antitrypsin *Serum* *Increase* In patients with rheumatoid arthritis complicated by amyloidosis *3378*

Aspartate Aminotransferase *Serum* *Increase* Elevated in > 33% of patients with primary disease *2878*
Serum *No Effect* Usually normal *308*

Bence-Jones Protein *Serum* *Present* Found in 21 of 22 patients with primary disease *3940* May occur *2039*
Urine *Present* Detected in 6 of 15 cases; excretion was < 1 g/d in all patients *308* Found in 57% of secondary and only 8% of primary cases *2878*

Bicarbonate *Serum* *Decrease* May lead to proximal renal tubular acidosis which is associated with hypokalemia, hyperchloremic metabolic acidosis, urine pH < 5.5, increased urinary ammonium ion excretion, a negative urine anion gap, increased urinary osmol gap, normal urinary citrate, normal urinary calcium excretion and Fanconi syndrome *4071*

Bilirubin *Serum* *Increase* 10% of patients had increased direct bilirubin and 5% had high indirect bilirubin *2878*

Bilirubin, Direct *Serum* *Increase* 10% of patients had increased direct bilirubin and 5% had high indirect bilirubin *2878*

Bilirubin, Indirect *Serum* *Increase* 10% of patients had increased direct bilirubin and 5% had high indirect bilirubin *2878*

BSP Retention *Serum* *Increase* Found to be elevated in over 50% of patients 5% in 1 h), contrary to the suggestion that hepatomegaly with normal or only slightly abnormal liver function is characteristic *2878* With hepatic involvement *308* Retention is increased in 75% of patients with liver involvement *5545*

Calcium *Serum* *No Effect* Rarely elevated in primary disease *2878*
Urine *Increase* May be associated with classic distal renal tubular acidosis which is associated with hyokalemia, hyperchloremic metabolic acidosis, urine pH > 5.5, increased urinary ammonium ion excretion, a negative urine anion gap, increased urinary osmol gap, decreased urinary citrate and increased urinary calcium in some patients *4071*
Urine *No Effect* May lead to proximal renal tubular acidosis which is associated with hypokalemia, hyperchloremic metabolic acidosis, urine pH < 5.5, increased urinary ammonium ion excretion, a negative urine anion gap, increased urinary osmol gap, normal urinary citrate, normal urinary calcium excretion and Fanconi syndrome *4071*

CD45 Leukocytes *Tissue* *Increase* In 1 patient with amyloidosis number of positive cells 1,130 cells/mm^2 in renal tissue *3026*

Chloride *Serum* *Increase* May be associated with classic distal renal tubular acidosis which is associated with hyokalemia, hyperchloremic metabolic acidosis, urine pH > 5.5, increased urinary ammonium ion excretion, a negative urine anion gap, increased urinary osmol gap, decreased urinary citrate and increased urinary calcium in some patients *4071* May lead to proximal renal tubular acidosis which is associated with hypokalemia, hyperchloremic metabolic acidosis, urine pH < 5.5, increased urinary ammonium ion excretion, a negative urine anion gap, increased urinary osmol gap, normal urinary citrate, normal urinary calcium excretion and Fanconi syndrome *4071*

Cholesterol *Serum* *Increase* High concentrations found in 33% of primary cases and < 20% of secondary cases *2878*

Citrate *Urine* *Decrease* May be associated with classic distal renal tubular acidosis which is associated with hyokalemia, hyperchloremic metabolic acidosis, urine pH > 5.5, increased urinary ammonium ion excretion, a negative urine anion gap, increased urinary osmol gap, decreased urinary citrate and increased urinary calcium in some patients *4071*
Urine *No Effect* May lead to proximal renal tubular acidosis which is associated with hypokalemia, hyperchloremic metabolic acidosis, urine pH < 5.5, increased urinary ammonium ion excretion, a negative urine anion gap, increased urinary osmol gap, normal urinary citrate, normal urinary calcium excretion and Fanconi syndrome *4071*

Complement C_3 *Serum* *Increase* Found mostly in the recovery phase *2694* *1033* *931* *1588*

Congo Red Test *Blood* *Positive* Positive in up to 50% of patients with cardiac amyloidosis *367* Of 20 patients with amyloidosis, only 9 had > 60% disappearance of congo red from blood in 1 h. False-negative tests may be expected in > 50% of cases *689* Positive in 33% of patients with primary and in 66% of patients with secondary amyloidosis *5545*

Cortisol *Plasma* *No Effect* In 10 patients with renal amyloidosis concentration ranged from 113 to 365 nmol/L compared with reference range of 160 - 1000 nmol/L *1346*

Creatinine *Serum* *Increase* In 1 patient with amyloidosis concentration of 1.50 mg/dL different from 0.88 ± 0.17 mg/dL in 20 healthy controls *3026* Increased in > 50% of patients at time of diagnosis due to renal insufficiency *2878*

Erythrocyte Sedimentation Rate *Blood* *Increase* Over 55 mm/h (Westergren) in 50% of patients *2878*

Erythrocytes *Urine* *Increase* Microscopic hematuria is frequently seen *900*

Estradiol *Plasma* *No Effect* In 4 female patients with renal amyloidosis concentration ranged from 34 to 140 pmol/L compared with reference range of 70 - 620 pmol/L *1346*

Fat *Feces* *Increase* In small intestinal disease *4891*

α_2-Globulin *Serum* *Increase* Hyperglobulinemia occurs in 15% of cases of cardiac amyloidosis; α_2- and γ- fractions moderately increased *367*

γ-Globulin *Serum* *Decrease* Hypogammaglobulinemia was found in patients with Bence-Jones proteinuria but not in any other patients *308* In 25% of patients *2878* A low albumin and globulin profile may be observed *900*
Serum *Increase* Hyperglobulinemia occurs in 15% of cases of cardiac amyloidosis; α_2- and γ- fractions moderately increased *367* Has been observed. No correlation with severity or duration of disease *4979* Increased concentration with reversed A/G ratio is frequent *5545* Has been observed. No correlation with severity or duration of disease *299*

Glomerular Filtration Rate *Urine* *Decrease* Decreased due to reduced filtration surface (fewer functioning glomeruli) *1290*

277.30 Amyloidosis *(continued)*

Glucose *Urine Increase* May lead to proximal renal tubular acidosis which is associated with hypokalemia, hyperchloremic metabolic acidosis, urine pH < 5.5, increased urinary ammonium ion excretion, a negative urine anion gap, increased urinary osmol gap, normal urinary citrate, normal urinary calcium excretion and Fanconi syndrome *4071*

Haptoglobin *Serum Increase* Conditions associated with increased ESR and alpha$_2$-globulin *5544*

Hematocrit *Blood Decrease* Mild anemia present in < 50% of patients *2878*

Hemoglobin *Blood Decrease* Mild anemia present in < 50% of patients *2878*

Hexosamine *Serum No Effect* No significant effect observed *4979* Usually no significant effect *299*

immunoglobulin A *Serum Decrease* Mean concentration (0.61 g/L) was significantly decreased in patients with Bence-Jones proteinuria *307*

Immunoglobulin G *Serum Decrease* Mean concentration (540 mg/dL) was significantly decreased in patients with Bence-Jones proteinuria *307* Decreased in 50% of primary and 66% of secondary disease *2878*

Immunoglobulin M *Serum Decrease* Mean concentration (0.46 g/L) was significantly decreased in patients with Bence-Jones proteinuria *307* The most significant finding. All 14 patients without macroglobulinemia had reduced concentration, mean concentration of 0.5 g/L, only 34% of the control value *307*

Immunoglobulins *Serum Decrease* Mean serum concentration of all 3 classes of immunoglobulins, IgA, IgM and IgG, were significantly reduced in patients with increased Bence-Jones protein excretion *307*

Insulin *Plasma No Effect* In 10 patients with renal amyloidosis concentration of free insulin ranged from 3 to 10 µU/L compared with reference range of < 30 µU/L *1346*

Intercellular Adhesion Molecule-1 *Tissue Increase* In 1 patient with amyloidosis percentage of ICAM-1 positive renal tubuli 8.0% *3026*

Leukocytes *Blood Decrease* Leukopenia, if present, suggests multiple myeloma as the cause for amyloidosis *900*
Blood Increase Frequently increased (> 12,000 /µL) *5545*

Lipoproteins *Serum Increase* Has been observed. No correlation with severity or duration of the disease *4979* May be present *2304* Has been observed. No correlation with severity or duration of the disease *299*

α_2-Macroglobulin *Serum Increase* Has been observed. No correlation with severity or duration of disease *299* *4979*

Net Acid Excretion *Urine Increase* May be associated with classic distal renal tubular acidosis which is associated with hyokalemia, hyperchloremic metabolic acidosis, urine pH > 5.5, increased urinary ammonium ion excretion, a negative urine anion gap, increased urinary osmol gap, decreased urinary citrate and increased urinary calcium in some patients *4071*

Osmolal Gap *Urine Increase* May be associated with classic distal renal tubular acidosis which is asociated with hyokalemia, hyperchloremic metabolic acidosis, urine pH > 5.5, increased urinary ammonium ion excretion, a negative urine anion gap, increased urinary osmol gap, decreased urinary citrate and increased urinary calcium in some patients *4071* May lead to proximal renal tubular acidosis which is associated with hypokalemia, hyperchloremic metabolic acidosis, urine pH < 5.5, increased urinary ammonium ion excretion, a negative urine anion gap, increased urinary osmol gap, normal urinary citrate, normal urinary calcium excretion and Fanconi syndrome *4071*

pH *Urine Decrease* May lead to proximal renal tubular acidosis which is associated with hypokalemia, hyperchloremic metabolic acidosis, urine pH < 5.5, increased urinary ammonium ion excretion, a negative urine anion gap, increased urinary osmol gap, normal urinary citrate, normal urinary calcium excretion and Fanconi syndrome *4071*
Urine Increase May be associated with classic distal renal tubular acidosis which is asociated with hyokalemia, hyperchloremic metabolic acidosis, urine pH > 5.5, increased urinary ammonium ion excretion, a negative urine anion gap, increased urinary osmol gap, decreased urinary citrate and increased urinary calcium in some patients *4071*

Phosphate *Serum Decrease* May lead to proximal renal tubular acidosis which is associated with hypokalemia, hyperchloremic metabolic acidosis, urine pH < 5.5, increased urinary ammonium ion excretion, a negative urine anion gap, increased urinary osmol gap, normal urinary citrate, normal urinary calcium excretion and Fanconi syndrome *4071*

Plasma Cells *Bone Marrow Increase* None of the patients with primary disease had > 15% plasma cells, whereas over 50% of the secondary cases did. Mean percentage of cells was 4 in primary and 23 in secondary *2878* Many patients can be shown to have homogeneous immunoglobulins in the serum and/or urine, and plasmacytosis in the marrow, and ultimately to develop morphologic and clinical evidence of a plasma cell dyscrasia *2358* A bone marrow plasmacytosis is found in a high proportion of cases *2304*

Platelets *Blood Increase* Mild thrombocytosis in primary disease *2878*

Potassium *Serum Decrease* May be associated with classic distal renal tubular acidosis which is asociated with hyokalemia, hyperchloremic metabolic acidosis, urine pH > 5.5, increased urinary ammonium ion excretion, a negative urine anion gap, increased urinary osmol gap, decreased urinary citrate and increased urinary calcium in some patients *4071* May lead to proximal renal tubular acidosis which is associated with hypokalemia, hyperchloremic metabolic acidosis, urine pH < 5.5, increased urinary ammonium ion excretion, a negative urine anion gap, increased urinary osmol gap, normal urinary citrate, normal urinary calcium excretion and Fanconi syndrome *4071*

Progesterone *Plasma No Effect* In 4 female patients with renal amyloidosis concentration ranged from 0.1 to 4 nmol/L compared with reference range of 0.3 - 5 nmol/L *1346*

Protein *Cerebrospinal Fluid Increase* Usually elevated *4979*
Serum Decrease Hypoproteinemia occurs in 15% of cases of cardiac amyloidosis *367*
Urine Increase Proteinuria is usually the first sign of renal amyloid, may persist for years or temporarily disappear *367* In 1 patient with amyloidosis excretion of 6.18 mg/mg creatinine *3026* Frequently massive, with up to 20 g/d excreted in patients with renal amyloid *308* Found in 90% of primary and 98% of secondary cases *2878*

Soluble Intercellular Adhesion Molecule-1 *Serum No Effect* In 1 patient with amyloidosis concentration of soluble ICAM-1 of 340 ng/mL compared with 306 ± 52 ng/mL in 20 healthy controls *3026*
Urine Increase In 1 patient with amyloidosis excretion of soluble ICAM-1 of 34.0 ng/mL or 24.7 ng/mg creatinine compared with 2.6 ± 1.7 ng/mL or 2.5 ± 3.0 ng/mg creatinine in 20 healthy controls *3026*

Testosterone *Serum No Effect* In 6 male patients with renal amyloidosis concentration ranged from 3 to 76 nmol/L compared with reference range of 9 - 88 nmol/L *1346*

Thyroid Stimulating Hormone *Serum Increase* In 4 of 10 patients with renal amyloidosis concentration ranged from 7 to 15 mIU/mL compared with reference range of 0.6 - 5 mIU/mL *1346*

Thyroxine (T4), Free *Serum No Effect* In 10 patients with renal amyloidosis concentration ranged from 2 to 16 pmol/L compared with reference range of 9 - 22 pmol/L *1346*

Uric Acid *Serum Decrease* May lead to proximal renal tubular acidosis which is associated with hypokalemia, hyperchloremic metabolic acidosis, urine pH < 5.5, increased urinary ammonium ion excretion, a negative urine anion gap, increased urinary osmol gap, normal urinary citrate, normal urinary calcium excretion and Fanconi syndrome *4071*
Serum Increase Increased in 22% of primary and 31% of secondary cases *2878*

277.31 Familial Mediterranean Fever

Alanine Aminotransferase *Serum No Effect* No consistent abnormalities of liver or renal function *565*

Alkaline Phosphatase *Serum No Effect* No consistent abnormalities of liver or renal function *565*

Aspartate Aminotransferase *Serum No Effect* No consistent abnormalities of liver or renal function *565*

Ceruloplasmin *Serum Increase* Increased during episodes *565*

Cholesterol *Serum No Effect* No effect observed *565*

C-Reactive Protein *Serum* *Increase* Increased during episodes *565*

Creatinine *Serum* *No Effect* No consistent abnormalities of liver or renal function *565*

Erythrocyte Sedimentation Rate *Blood* *Increase* Elevated during attacks but returns to normal between attacks *565*

Fibrinogen *Plasma* *Increase* Increased during episodes *565*

γ-Glutamyltransferase *Serum* *No Effect* No consistent abnormalities of liver or renal function *565*

Haptoglobin *Serum* *Increase* Increased during episodes *565*

Lactate Dehydrogenase *Serum* *No Effect* No consistent abnormalities of liver or renal function *565*

Leukocytes *Blood* *Increase* Polymorphonuclear leukocytosis ranging from 15,000 to 20,000 /µL is almost invariable during acute attacks *565*

β_2-Microglobulin *Serum* *Decrease* In 20 patients during attacks of familial Mediterranean fever mean concentration decreased to 1.5 ± 0.2 mg/L compared with 2.3 ± 0.4 mg/L in controls *4491*
Urine *Increase* In 20 patients with familial Mediterranean fever mean β_2-microglobulin:creatinine ratio during attacks of 0.009 ± 0.002 compared with 0.006 ± 0.002 in healthy controls *4491*

Triglycerides *Serum* *No Effect* No effect observed *565*

Urea Nitrogen *Serum* *No Effect* No consistent abnormalities of liver or renal function *565*

277.31 Mediterranean Spotted Fever

Fibrinogen *Plasma* *Increase* In 28 patients with Mediterranean spotted fever mean concentration of 4.6 ± 1.6 g/L significantly increased compared with 2.8 ± 0.5 g/L in 30 normal individuals *5465*

Plasminogen Activator Inhibitor *Plasma* *Increase* In 28 patients with Mediterranean spotted fever mean concentration of 7 U/mL (median 7 U/mL) not significantly increased compared with mean and median of 3 U/mL in 30 normal individuals *5465*

Plasminogen Activator Inhibitor-1 Antigen *Plasma* *Increase* In 28 patients with Mediterranean spotted fever mean concentration of 55 ± 30 ng/mL significantly increased compared with 11 ± 4 ng/mL in 30 normal individuals *5465*

Platelets *Blood* *Decrease* In 28 patients with Mediterranean spotted fever mean concentration of 185,000 ± 89,000 /µL significantly decreased compared with 301,000 ± 61,000 /µL in 30 normal individuals *5465*

Tissue Plasminogen Activator Antigen *Plasma* *Increase* In 28 patients with Mediterranean spotted fever mean concentration of 30 ± 20 ng/mL significantly increased compared with 9 ± 4 in 30 normal individuals *5465*

Tumor Necrosis Factor-α *Serum* *No Effect* In 28 patients with Mediterranean spotted fever mean concentration of 84 ± 19 pg/mL not significantly increased compared with 86 ± 15 pg/mL in 30 normal individuals *5465*

von Willebrand Factor Antigen *Plasma* *Increase* In 28 patients with Mediterranean spotted fever mean concentration of 551 ± 315% significantly increased compared with 106 ± 20% in 30 normal individuals *5465*

277.40 Crigler-Najjar Syndrome

Alanine Aminotransferase *Serum* *No Effect* Liver function tests were uniformly normal *4979* Liver function usually normal *962*

Alkaline Phosphatase *Serum* *No Effect* Liver function unaffected by disease *962*

Aspartate Aminotransferase *Serum* *No Effect* Liver function tests were uniformly normal *4979* Liver function usually normal *962*

Bilirubin *Serum* *Increase* Almost invariably in the range of 15 - 48 mg/dL with virtually all giving an indirect van den Bergh reaction. Fluctuations are frequent, with higher values in winter and incidental illness *4646* Patients with apparent autosomal recessive pattern of inheritance with severe hyperbilirubinemia (20 - 31 mg/dL) *2039*
Urine *No Effect* None detectable *4979*

Bilirubin, Indirect *Serum* *Increase* Familial unconjugated hyperbilirubinemia due to low or absent hepatic glucuronyl-transferase activity *1980* Increased; it appears on 1st or 2nd day of life, rises to 12 - 45 mg/dL, and persists for life *5544*

Bilirubin, Unconjugated *Serum* *Increase* Crigler-Najjar syndrome is associated with unconjugated hyperbilirubinemia *3625*

BSP Retention *Serum* *No Effect* Liver function tests were uniformly normal *4979*

Hematocrit *Blood* *No Effect* No evidence of hemolytic anemia or splenomegaly *4979* No anemia observed typically *962*

Hemoglobin *Blood* *No Effect* No significant effect observed typically *962* No evidence of hemolytic anemia or splenomegaly *4979*

Lactate Dehydrogenase *Serum* *No Effect* Liver function usually normal. Anemia rarely present *962*

Reticulocytes *Blood* *No Effect* No anemia usually observed *962* No evidence of hemolytic anemia or splenomegaly *4979*

Urobilinogen *Feces* *Decrease* Usually very low but stool is of normal color *4979*
Urine *Decrease* Normal or decreased *5544*

277.40 Dubin-Johnson Syndrome

Alanine Aminotransferase *Serum* *Increase* May be normal or moderately increased *1243*
Serum *No Effect* Routine liver function tests are normal *1980* Activity typically normal *3406*

Alkaline Phosphatase *Serum* *Increase* May be normal or moderately increased *1243*
Serum *No Effect* Routine liver function tests are normal *1980* Activity typically normal *3406*

Aspartate Aminotransferase *Serum* *Increase* May be normal or moderately increased *1243*
Serum *No Effect* Activity typically normal *3406* Routine liver function tests are normal *1980*

Bilirubin *Serum* *Increase* Slight to marked in degree with marked fluctuations in intensity *4979* Concentration increased intermittently *3406* Characterized by chronic nonhemolytic, predominantly conjugated hyperbilirubinemia *404* The total serum bilirubin ranges between 2 - 10 mg/dL *1980* Slight to marked in degree with marked fluctuations in intensity *1243*
Urine *Increase* Patient presents with intermittent jaundice and bilirubinuria *1980* May be seen *404*

Bilirubin, Conjugated *Serum* *Increase* Concentration increased intermittently *3406*

Bilirubin, Direct *Serum* *Increase* Familial, conjugated hyperbilirubinemia due to a defect in the excretion of bilirubin from the liver *1980* Characterized by chronic nonhemolytic, predominantly conjugated hyperbilirubinemia associated with jaundice *404*

Bilirubin, Unconjugated *Serum* *Increase* Concentration increased intermittently *3406*

BSP Retention *Serum* *Increase* Normal decrease in serum concentration 45 min after injection, followed by a rise at 2 h, due to difficulty in its excretion from the liver with leakage back into the bloodstream *1980* Normal or slightly impaired excretion *4979* Higher at 90 min than at 45 min after IV administration *404*

Coproporphyrin *Red Blood Cells* *No Effect* Total concentration is normal but the isomer percentages are different. Normally, coproporphyrin III constitutes 75%, while in homozygous patients it is over 80% of the total *404*
Urine *Increase* Increases in the urinary excretion of coproporphyrin I have been found not only in patients with this syndrome but also in close relatives *1980* Total excretion is normal or slightly increased, but 84 - 90% is type I isomer, strikingly different from normal *4979* Mean excretion is 3 - 4 times that of normal subjects *5714*
Urine *No Effect* Total excretion is normal or slightly increased, but 84 - 90% is type I isomer, strikingly different from normal *4979*

Coproporphyrin I *Urine* *Increase* Excretion increased *3406*

Coproporphyrin III *Urine* *Decrease* Excretion decreased *3406*

Lactate Dehydrogenase *Serum* *Increase* May be normal or moderately increased *1243*

277.40 Dubin-Johnson Syndrome *(continued)*

Urobilinogen *Urine* *Increase* Excretion increased *3406* Urine contains bile and urobilinogen *5544*

277.40 Gilbert's Syndrome

Alanine Aminotransferase *Serum* *No Effect* Liver function usually normal *2034* Activity normal *3406*

Alkaline Phosphatase *Serum* *No Effect* No effect of disease observed *2034* Activity normal *3406*

Aspartate Aminotransferase *Serum* *No Effect* Activity normal *3406* No liver damage observed *2034*

Bile Acids *Serum* *No Effect* An elevated bilirubin coexisting with a normal bile acid level suggests Gilbert's disease *4891* Fasting and postprandial levels were normal with reduced and normal caloric loads *584*

Bilirubin *Serum* *Increase* Concentration may be increased in patients with Gilbert's syndrome associated with decreased transfer of bilirubin from albumin to the Y protein (ligandin) in the liver *4617* Mild increase in unconjugated serum bilirubin reduced by phenobarbital and increased within 24 h of a reduced calorie diet *1290* Degree of elevation does not correlate with symptoms *404* Usually in range of 1.2 - 3 mg/dL, rarely > 5 mg/dL *2034* Highest after fasting and rarely exceeds 3 mg/dL *1980* Concentration increased during asymptomatic episodes up to 80 - 100 µmol/L *3406*
Urine *No Effect* Typical observation *4979*

Bilirubin, Direct *Serum* *No Effect* 20% of total bilirubin *2034*

Bilirubin, Indirect *Serum* *Increase* Mild asymptomatic increase of indirect serum bilirubin, usually discovered on routine laboratory testing. May rise to 18 mg/dL but usually is < 4 mg/dL *5544* Unexplained, mild, chronic elevation *4979* Concentration may be increased in patients with Gilbert's syndrome associated with decreased transfer of bilirubin from albumin to the Y protein(ligandin) in the liver *4617*

Bilirubin, Unconjugated *Serum* *Increase* Gilbert's syndrome is associated with unconjugated hyperbilirubinemia *3625*

BSP Retention *Serum* *Increase* In a significant number of patients *403* Mild 45 min retention has been observed in 20% of patients *404*

Chenodeoxycholic Acid *Serum* *No Effect* Normal levels in hyperbilirubinemic patients *4396 1513*

Cholic Acid *Serum* *Decrease* Significantly reduced in hyperbilirubinemic patients *4396*
Serum *No Effect* Fasting levels were normal in all 24 patients studied *4396*

Erythrocyte Survival *Red Blood Cells* *Decrease* Mild, but fully compensated hemolysis in a significant number of patients *1536*

Hemoglobin *Plasma* *Increase* Mild, but fully compensated hemolysis in a significant number of patients *1536*

Lactate Dehydrogenase *Serum* *No Effect* No significant change observed with disease *2034*

Urobilinogen *Feces* *Decrease* Normal or decreased *5544*
Urine *Decrease* Normal or decreased *5544*

277.40 Rotor's Syndrome

Alanine Aminotransferase *Serum* *No Effect* Routine liver function tests are normal *1980* Activity typically normal *3406*

Alkaline Phosphatase *Serum* *No Effect* Routine liver function tests are normal *1980* Activity typically normal *3406*

Aspartate Aminotransferase *Serum* *No Effect* Activity typically normal *3406* Routine liver function tests are normal *1980*

Bilirubin *Serum* *Increase* The total serum bilirubin ranges between 2 - 10 mg/dL *1980* Slight to moderate direct bilirubinemia *4979* Concentration increased intermittently *3406*
Urine *Increase* Patient presents with intermittent jaundice and bilirubinuria *1980*
Urine *No Effect* Excretion usually within normal limits *4979*

Bilirubin, Conjugated *Serum* *Increase* Concentration increased intermittently and higher than unconjugated *3406*

Bilirubin, Direct *Serum* *Increase* Familial, conjugated hyperbilirubinemia due to a defect in the excretion of bilirubin from the liver *1980*

Bilirubin, Unconjugated *Serum* *Increase* Concentration increased intermittently but to less extent than conjugated *3406*

BSP Retention *Serum* *Increase* Marked retention *4979* Defects in the excretion of BSP and of gallbladder dye may reveal a normal decrease in its serum concentration 45 min after injection, followed by a rise at 2 h, due to difficulty in its excretion from the liver with leakage back into the bloodstream *1980*

Coproporphyrin *Urine* *Increase* Excretion increased due to increased excretion of both coproporphyrins I and III *3406* Marked increase in some patients *5539* Increases in the urinary excretion of coproporphyrin I have been found not only in patients with this syndrome but also in close relatives *1980*

Coproporphyrin I *Urine* *Increase* Excretion increased *3406*

Coproporphyrin III *Urine* *Increase* Excretion increased *3406*

Urobilinogen *Urine* *Increase* Normal or increased *5544*

277.50 Hurler's Disease

α-L-Iduronidase *Fibroblasts* *Decrease* Low activity suggests mucopolysaccharidoses I H or I S for diagnosis of Hurler's and Scheie's syndromes *2952*
White Blood Cells *Decrease* Low activity suggests mucopolysaccharidoses I H or I S for diagnosis of Hurler's and Scheie's syndromes *2952*

277.50 Maroteaux-Lamy Disease

Arylsulfatase B *Fibroblasts* *Decrease* Absence observed in patients with mucopolysaccharidosis (MPS) type VI *2952*

277.50 Morquio's Disease

β-Galactosidase *Fibroblasts* *Decrease* Deficient β-galactosidase is associated with generalized gangliosidosis (GM1 gangliosidosis or Morquio's disease) depending on clinical presentation *2952*
White Blood Cells *Decrease* Deficient β-galactosidase is associated with generalized gangliosidosis (GM1 gangliosidosis or Morquio's disease) depending on clinical presentation *2952*

277.50 Mucopolysaccharidosis Type I

Chitotriosidase *Serum* *Increase* Abnormal activities observed in 2 of 63 patients with mucopolysaccharidoses types I, II, IIIA, B, C, IVA and B, with activities of 400 and 600 nmol/h/mL *1917*

Lysosome-associated Membrane Protein-2 *Serum* *Increase* Median concentration of 4.34 mg/L in 18 patients with mucopolysaccharidosis type I with median age 1 y compared with 1.21 mg/L in 202 healthy controls aged 0 - 66 y (median 7 years) *2265*

Lysosome-associated Membrane Protein-2:Lysosome-associated Membrane Protein-1 Ratio *Serum* *Decrease* Mean ratio of 3.13 in 18 patients with mucopolysaccharidosis type I with median age 1 y significantly decreased when compared with 4.74 in 202 healthy controls aged 0 - 66 y (median 7 years) *2265*

277.50 Mucopolysaccharidosis Type II

Lysosome-associated Membrane Protein-2 *Serum* *Increase* Median concentration of 4.65 mg/L in 23 patients with mucopolysaccharidosis type II with median age 1 y compared with 1.21 mg/L in 202 healthy controls aged 0 - 66 y (median 7 years) *2265*

Lysosome-associated Membrane Protein-2:Lysosome-associated Membrane Protein-1 Ratio *Serum* *Decrease* Mean ratio of 3.40 in 23 patients with mucopolysaccharidosis type II with median age 1 y significantly decreased when compared with 4.74 in 202 healthy controls aged 0 - 66 y (median 7 years) *2265*

277.50 Mucopolysaccharidosis Type VI

Lysosome-associated Membrane Protein-2 *Serum Increase* Median concentration of 2.72 mg/L in 10 patients with mucopolysaccharidosis type VI with median age 4 y compared with 1.21 mg/L in 202 healthy controls aged 0 - 66 y (median 7 years) *2265*

Lysosome-associated Membrane Protein-2:Lysosome-associated Membrane Protein-1 Ratio *Serum Decrease* Mean ratio of 2.54 in 3 patients with mucopolysaccharidosis type VI with median age 4 y significantly different when compared with 4.74 in 202 healthy controls aged 0 - 66 y (median 7 years) *2265*

277.50 Mucopolysaccharidosis Type VII

β-Glucuronidase *Fibroblasts Decrease* Values less than 0.34 U/g cellular protein characteristic of type VII mucopolysaccharidosis *2952*

277.50 Mucopolysaccharidosis Type IIIA

Lysosome-associated Membrane Protein-2 *Serum Increase* Median concentration of 4.19 mg/L in 19 patients with mucopolysaccharidosis type IIIA with median age 4 y compared with 1.21 mg/L in 202 healthy controls aged 0 - 66 y (median 7 years) *2265*

Lysosome-associated Membrane Protein-2:Lysosome-associated Membrane Protein-1 Ratio *Serum Decrease* Mean ratio of 4.03 in 19 patients with mucopolysaccharidosis type IIIA with median age 1 y significantly decreased when compared with 4.74 in 202 healthy controls aged 0 - 66 y (median 7 years) *2265*

277.50 Mucopolysaccharidosis Type IIIB

Lysosome-associated Membrane Protein-2 *Serum Increase* Median concentration of 3.75 mg/L in 16 patients with mucopolysaccharidosis type IIIB with median age 3 y compared with 1.21 mg/L in 202 healthy controls aged 0 - 66 y (median 7 years) *2265*

Lysosome-associated Membrane Protein-2:Lysosome-associated Membrane Protein-1 Ratio *Serum Decrease* Mean ratio of 4.12 in 16 patients with mucopolysaccharidosis type IIIB with median age 1 y significantly decreased when compared with 4.74 in 202 healthy controls aged 0 - 66 y (median 7 years) *2265*

Tumor Necrosis Factor-α *Serum No Effect* Mean concentration of about 15 pg/mL in 7 patients with mucopolysaccharidosis type IIIB not significantly different from mean concentration of about 10 pg/mL in 11 healthy controls *3475*

277.50 Mucopolysaccharidosis Type IIIC

Lysosome-associated Membrane Protein-2 *Serum Increase* Median concentration of 3.10 mg/L in 3 patients with mucopolysaccharidosis type IIIC with median age 11 y compared with 1.21 mg/L in 202 healthy controls aged 0 - 66 y (median 7 years) *2265*

Lysosome-associated Membrane Protein-2:Lysosome-associated Membrane Protein-1 Ratio *Serum Decrease* Mean ratio of 4.36 in 3 patients with mucopolysaccharidosis type IIIC with median age 11 y significantly decreased when compared with 4.74 in 202 healthy controls aged 0 - 66 y (median 7 years) *2265*

277.50 Mucopolysaccharidosis Type IIID

Lysosome-associated Membrane Protein-2 *Serum Increase* Median concentration of 3.69 mg/L in 3 patients with mucopolysaccharidosis type IIID with median age 11 y compared with 1.21 mg/L in 202 healthy controls aged 0 - 66 y (median 7 years) *2265*

Lysosome-associated Membrane Protein-2:Lysosome-associated Membrane Protein-1 Ratio *Serum Decrease* Mean ratio of 3.27 in 3 patients with mucopolysaccharidosis type IIID with median age 3 y significantly decreased when compared with 4.74 in 202 healthy controls aged 0 - 66 y (median 7 years) *2265*

277.50 Mucopolysaccharidosis Type IVA

Lysosome-associated Membrane Protein-2 *Serum Increase* Median concentration of 2.88 mg/L in 17 patients with mucopolysaccharidosis type IVA with median age 3 y compared with 1.21 mg/L in 202 healthy controls aged 0 - 66 y (median 7 years) *2265*

Lysosome-associated Membrane Protein-2:Lysosome-associated Membrane Protein-1 Ratio *Serum No Effect* Mean ratio of 4.74 in 3 patients with mucopolysaccharidosis type IVA with median age 3 y not different when compared with 4.74 in 202 healthy controls aged 0 - 66 y (median 7 years) *2265*

277.50 Sanfilippo Type B Disease

N-Acetyl-Glucosaminidase *Fibroblasts Decrease* Deficiency is diagnostic of Type B Sanfilippo disease *2952*
Serum Decrease Deficiency is diagnostic of Type B Sanfilippo disease *2952*

277.50 Scheie's Syndrome

α-L-Iduronidase *Fibroblasts Decrease* Low activity suggests mucopolysaccharidoses I H or I S for diagnosis of Hurler's and Scheie's syndromes *2952*
White Blood Cells Decrease Low activity suggests mucopolysaccharidoses I H or I S for diagnosis of Hurler's and Scheie's syndromes *2952*

277.60 α_1-Antitrypsin Deficiency

Alanine Aminotransferase *Serum Increase* Related to liver disease *3618*

Albumin *Serum Decrease* Related to liver disease *3618*
Serum No Effect Concentration usually normal *5544*

Alkaline Phosphatase *Serum Increase* Related to liver disease *3618*

α_1-Antitrypsin *Serum Decrease* Characteristic feature of disease is reduction of α-AT concentration to 10 - 15% of normal *4083* Disease presence confirmed by detection of absent or reduced concentration *3625*

Apolipoprotein A-I *Serum Increase* In patients with liver disease all apolipoproteins were elevated *1172*

Apolipoprotein A-II *Serum Increase* In patients with liver disease all apolipoproteins were elevated *1172*

Apolipoprotein B *Serum Increase* In patients with liver disease all apolipoproteins were elevated *1172*

Aspartate Aminotransferase *Serum Increase* Related to liver disease *3618*

Bicarbonate *Serum Decrease* Associated COPD *3618*

Bile Acids *Feces Increase* Excretion was increased *1172*
Serum Increase In 34 patients with this disease all patients with morphological cirrhosis *3760*
Urine Increase Excretion was increased *1172*

Bilirubin *Serum Increase* Related to liver disease *3618*

Calcium *Serum Decrease* Related to decreased albumin *3618*

Chenodeoxycholic Acid *Serum Increase* In 34 patients with this disease all patients with morphological cirrhosis *3760*

Chloride *Serum Decrease* Seen with associated hyperventilation *3618*

Cholesterol *Serum Decrease* Related to liver disease *3618*
Serum Increase Average 604 mg/dL *1172*

Cholesterol Esters *Serum Decrease* Greatly depressed as was cholesterol absorption *1172*

Cholic Acid *Serum Increase* In 34 patients with this disease all patients with morphological cirrhosis *3760*

Complement C_3 *Serum No Effect* Concentration usually normal *5544*

277.60 α_1-Antitrypsin Deficiency *(continued)*

Euglobulin Lysis Time *Blood* *Increase* Increased *597* *5220*

Fatty Acids (FFA), Free *Serum* *No Effect* Normal concentration usually observed *1172*

α_1-Globulin *Serum* *Decrease* Disease often initially detected by finding of reduced α_1-globulin band on electrophoresis *5276* Low alpha$_1$-globulin fraction in a patient with cirrhosis of the liver suggests the diagnosis *1980* Disease presence supported by absence of α_1-globulin peak *3625*

γ-Glutamyltransferase *Serum* *Increase* Related to liver disease *3618*

Haptoglobin *Serum* *No Effect* Concentration usually normal *5544*

Hematocrit *Blood* *Decrease* With associated hypersplenism *3618*
Blood *Increase* With associated polycythemia secondary to hypoxemia *3618*

Hemoglobin *Blood* *Decrease* With associated hypersplenism *3618*
Blood *Increase* With associated polycythemia secondary to hypoxemia *3618*

Hyaluronic Acid *Serum* *Increase* Measured serum levels at presentation and 1 year follow-up in 37 infants who presented with hepatobiliary disease in the first 6 months of life. In patients at presentation, the hyaluronic acid concentration was raised in 6 of 11 with α-1 antitrypsin deficiency. One year later, the 9 patients who developed progressive liver disease showed 2 - 6-fold increases in hyaluronic acid concentration while no increase was observed in the 28 with undetectable or mild disease *5283*

Iron-binding Capacity, Total *Serum* *No Effect* Concentration usually normal *5544*

Lactate Dehydrogenase *Serum* *Increase* Related to liver disease *3618*

Leukocytes *Blood* *Decrease* With associated hypersplenism *3618*

Lipoprotein X *Serum* *Increase* Lipoprotein X was increased to an average of 855 mg/dL *1172*

Lipoproteins *Serum* *Increase* Lipoprotein X was increased to an average of 855 mg/dL *1172*

α_2-Macroglobulin *Serum* *Increase* Patients with all types of this disorder were found to have significantly elevated levels *585*

Neopterin *Serum* *Increase* In 16 patients with α_1-antitrypsin deficiency mean concentration of 14.1 ± 3.9 nmol/L, with mean in 10 without cirrhosis of 8.3 ± 1.4 nmol/L and 23.8 ± 9.1 nmol/L in 6 with cirrhosis different from 6.0 ± 2.2 nmol/L in healthy controls *5682*

Platelets *Blood* *Decrease* With associated hypersplenism *3618*

Potassium *Serum* *Increase* Seen with acidosis *3618*

Triglycerides *Serum* *Increase* Average concentration of 336 mg/dL *1172*

277.60 Carbonic Anhydrase II Deficiency

Ammonium Ions *Urine* *Increase* Carbonic anhydrase isoform deficiency with osteoporosis may lead to proximal renal tubular acidosis which is associated with hypokalemia, hyperchloremic metabolic acidosis, urine pH < 5.5, increased urinary ammonium ion excretion, a negative urine anion gap, increased urinary osmol gap, normal urinary citrate, normal urinary calcium excretion and Fanconi syndrome *4071*

Anion Gap *Urine* *Decrease* Carbonic anhydrase isoform II deficiency with osteoporosis may lead to proximal renal tubular acidosis which is associated with hypokalemia, hyperchloremic metabolic acidosis, urine pH < 5.5, increased urinary ammonium ion excretion, a negative urine anion gap, increased urinary osmol gap, normal urinary citrate, normal urinary calcium excretion and Fanconi syndrome *4071*

Calcium *Urine* *No Effect* Carbonic anhydrase isoform II deficiency with osteoporosis may lead to proximal renal tubular acidosis which is associated with hypokalemia, hyperchloremic metabolic acidosis, urine pH < 5.5, increased urinary ammonium ion excretion, a negative urine anion gap, increased urinary osmol gap, normal urinary citrate, normal urinary calcium excretion and Fanconi syndrome *4071*

Chloride *Serum* *Increase* Carbonic anhydrase isoform II deficiency with osteoporosis may lead to proximal renal tubular acidosis which is associated with hypokalemia, hyperchloremic metabolic acidosis, urine pH < 5.5, increased urinary ammonium ion excretion, a negative urine anion gap, increased urinary osmol gap, normal urinary citrate and normal urinary calcium excretion *4071*

Citrate *Urine* *No Effect* Carbonic anhydrase isoform II deficiency with osteoporosis may lead to proximal renal tubular acidosis which is associated with hypokalemia, hyperchloremic metabolic acidosis, urine pH < 5.5, increased urinary ammonium ion excretion, a negative urine anion gap, increased urinary osmol gap, normal urinary citrate, normal urinary calcium excretion and Fanconi syndrome *4071*

Creatine Kinase *Serum* *No Effect* In 3 patients mean activities of 78 U/L, 52 U/L and 48 U/L *5659*

Creatine Kinase BB-Isoenzyme *Serum* *Increase* In 3 patients mean activities of 10 U/L, 5 U/L and 17 U/L (13%, 10% and 35%, respectively, of total CK) compared with normal of 0 - 1% *5659*

Glucose *Urine* *Increase* Carbonic anhydrase isoform II deficiency with osteoporosis may lead to proximal renal tubular acidosis which is associated with hypokalemia, hyperchloremic metabolic acidosis, urine pH < 5.5, increased urinary ammonium ion excretion, a negative urine anion gap, increased urinary osmol gap, normal urinary citrate, normal urinary calcium excretion and Fanconi syndrome *4071*

Osmolal Gap *Urine* *Increase* Carbonic anhydrase isoform II deficiency with osteoporosis may lead to proximal renal tubular acidosis which is associated with hypokalemia, hyperchloremic metabolic acidosis, urine pH < 5.5, increased urinary ammonium ion excretion, a negative urine anion gap, increased urinary osmol gap, normal urinary citrate, normal urinary calcium excretion and Fanconi syndrome *4071*

pH *Urine* *Decrease* Deficiency of isoform II with osteoporosis may lead to proximal renal tubular acidosis which is associated with hypokalemia, hyperchloremic metabolic acidosis, urine pH < 5.5, increased urinary ammonium ion excretion, a negative urine anion gap, increased urinary osmol gap, normal urinary citrate, normal urinary calcium excretion and Fanconi syndrome *4071*

Phosphate *Serum* *Decrease* Deficiency of isoform II with osteoporosis may lead to proximal renal tubular acidosis which is associated with hypokalemia, hyperchloremic metabolic acidosis, urine pH < 5.5, increased urinary ammonium ion excretion, a negative urine anion gap, increased urinary osmol gap, normal urinary citrate, normal urinary calcium excretion and Fanconi syndrome *4071*

Potassium *Serum* *Decrease* May lead to proximal renal tubular acidosis which is associated with hypokalemia, hyperchloremic metabolic acidosis, urine pH < 5.5, increased urinary ammonium ion excretion, a negative urine anion gap, increased urinary osmol gap, normal urinary citrate, normal urinary calcium excretion and Fanconi syndrome *4071*

Uric Acid *Serum* *Decrease* May lead to proximal renal tubular acidosis which is associated with hypokalemia, hyperchloremic metabolic acidosis, urine pH < 5.5, increased urinary ammonium ion excretion, a negative urine anion gap, increased urinary osmol gap, normal urinary citrate, normal urinary calcium excretion and Fanconi syndrome *4071*

277.60 Congenital Dopamine-β-Hydroxylase Deficiency

Dopamine β-Hydroxylase *Cerebrospinal Fluid* *Decrease* In 2 individuals with congenital dopamine-β-hydroxylase deficiency activity not detectable *3855*
Serum *Decrease* In 2 individuals with congenital dopamine-β-hydroxylase deficiency immunoreactive DBH not detectable in plasma *3855*

277.60 Familial Methyl Oxidase Deficiency

Ammonium Ions *Urine* *Decrease* May cause distal renal tubular acidosis (type IV) is associated with hyperkalemia, hyperchloremic metabolic acidosis, urine pH < 5.5, decreased urinary ammonium ion excretion, a positive urine anion gap, normal urinary citrate and urinary calcium excretion *4071*

Anion Gap *Urine* *Increase* May cause distal renal tubular acidosis (type IV) is associated with hyperkalemia, hyperchloremic metabolic acidosis, urine pH < 5.5, decreased urinary ammonium ion excretion, a positive urine anion gap, normal urinary citrate and urinary calcium excretion *4071*

Calcium *Urine* *No Effect* May cause distal renal tubular acidosis (type IV) is associated with hyperkalemia, hyperchloremic metabolic acidosis, urine pH < 5.5, decreased urinary ammonium ion excretion, a positive urine anion gap, normal urinary citrate and urinary calcium excretion *4071*

Chloride *Serum* *Increase* May cause distal renal tubular acidosis (type IV) is associated with hyperkalemia, hyperchloremic metabolic acidosis, urine pH < 5.5, decreased urinary ammonium ion excretion, a positive urine anion gap, normal urinary citrate and urinary calcium excretion *4071*

Citrate *Urine* *No Effect* May cause distal renal tubular acidosis (type IV) is associated with hyperkalemia, hyperchloremic metabolic acidosis, urine pH < 5.5, decreased urinary ammonium ion excretion, a positive urine anion gap, normal urinary citrate and urinary calcium excretion *4071*

pH *Urine* *Decrease* May cause distal renal tubular acidosis (type IV) is associated with hyperkalemia, hyperchloremic metabolic acidosis, urine pH < 5.5, decreased urinary ammonium ion excretion, a positive urine anion gap, normal urinary citrate and urinary calcium excretion *4071*

Potassium *Serum* *Increase* Distal renal tubular acidosis (type IV) is associated with hyperkalemia, hyperchloremic metabolic acidosis, urine pH < 5.5, decreased urinary ammonium ion excretion, a positive urine anion gap, normal urinary citrate and urinary calcium excretion *4071*

277.60 Hereditary Angioedema

C_1-Esterase Inhibitor *Serum* *Decrease* Low concentration is characteristic of C_1-esterase inhibitor deficiency which results in hereditary angioedema *2952*

Complement C_1 *Serum* *No Effect* Mean concentration typically normal in patients with hereditary angiodema *4682*

Complement C_1q *Serum* *No Effect* Mean concentration typically normal in patients with hereditary angiodema *4682*

Complement C_2 *Serum* *Decrease* Mean concentration typically slightly decreased in patients with hereditary angiodema *4682*

Complement C_3 *Serum* *No Effect* Mean concentration typically normal in patients with hereditary angiodema *4682*

Complement C_4 *Serum* *Decrease* Mean concentration typically slightly decreased in patients with hereditary angiodema *4682*

Complement C_5 *Serum* *No Effect* Mean concentration typically normal in patients with hereditary angiodema *4682*

Complement CH50 *Serum* *Decrease* Mean concentration typically markedly reduced in patients with hereditary angiodema *4682*

Properdin Factor B *Plasma* *No Effect* Mean concentration typically normal in patients with hereditary angiodema *4682*

277.60 Heriditary Angioneurotic Edema

β-Endorphin *White Blood Cells* *Increase* Concentration increased in patients with heriditary angioneurotic edema *633*

277.60 3-β-Hydroxydehydrogenase Deficiency

Ammonium Ions *Urine* *Decrease* May cause distal renal tubular acidosis (type IV) is associated with hyperkalemia, hyperchloremic metabolic acidosis, urine pH < 5.5, decreased urinary ammonium ion excretion, a positive urine anion gap, normal urinary citrate and urinary calcium excretion *4071*

Anion Gap *Urine* *Increase* May cause distal renal tubular acidosis (type IV) is associated with hyperkalemia, hyperchloremic metabolic acidosis, urine pH < 5.5, decreased urinary ammonium ion excretion, a positive urine anion gap, normal urinary citrate and urinary calcium excretion *4071*

Calcium *Urine* *No Effect* May cause distal renal tubular acidosis (type IV) is associated with hyperkalemia, hyperchloremic metabolic acidosis, urine pH < 5.5, decreased urinary ammonium ion excretion, a positive urine anion gap, normal urinary citrate and urinary calcium excretion *4071*

Chloride *Serum* *Increase* May cause distal renal tubular acidosis (type IV) is associated with hyperkalemia, hyperchloremic metabolic acidosis, urine pH < 5.5, decreased urinary ammonium ion excretion, a positive urine anion gap, normal urinary citrate and urinary calcium excretion *4071*

Citrate *Urine* *No Effect* May cause distal renal tubular acidosis (type IV) is associated with hyperkalemia, hyperchloremic metabolic acidosis, urine pH < 5.5, decreased urinary ammonium ion excretion, a positive urine anion gap, normal urinary citrate and urinary calcium excretion *4071*

pH *Urine* *Decrease* May cause distal renal tubular acidosis (type IV) is associated with hyperkalemia, hyperchloremic metabolic acidosis, urine pH < 5.5, decreased urinary ammonium ion excretion, a positive urine anion gap, normal urinary citrate and urinary calcium excretion *4071*

Potassium *Serum* *Increase* May cause distal renal tubular acidosis (type IV) which is associated with hyperkalemia, hyperchloremic metabolic acidosis, urine pH < 5.5, decreased urinary ammonium ion excretion, a positive urine anion gap, normal urinary citrate and urinary calcium excretion *4071*

277.60 N-Acetylgalactosaminidase Deficiency

N-Acetyl-Galactosaminidase *Fibroblasts* *Decrease* In one patient with α-N-acetylgalactosaminidase deficiency mean activity of 3.3 nmol/h/mg protein compared with reference interval of 44 - 128 nmol/h/mg protein *1058*
Plasma *Decrease* In one patient with α-N-acetylgalactosaminidase deficiency mean activity of 0.4 nmol/h/mL compared with reference interval of 10 - 55 nmol/h/mL *1058*
White Blood Cells *Decrease* In one patient with α-N-acetylgalactosaminidase deficiency mean activity of 0.8 nmol/h/mg protein compared with reference interval of 10 - 55 nmol/h/mg protein *1058*

277.80 Histiocytosis X

Bilirubin *Serum* *Increase* May occur in the presence of extensive liver involvement *900*

Carbon Dioxide Partial Pressure *Blood* *Decrease* With lung involvement, impaired gas diffusion *4707*

Eosinophils *Blood* *No Effect* No associated eosinophilia *5699*

Erythrocyte Sedimentation Rate *Blood* *Increase* Correlates with the prognosis and extent of disease *5214*

Hematocrit *Blood* *Decrease* A normocytic, normochromic anemia, sometimes severe and sometimes hemolytic in nature, may be present, especially in patients with disseminated disease. Aplastic anemia has also been described *900*

Hemoglobin *Blood* *Decrease* A normocytic, normochromic anemia, sometimes severe and sometimes hemolytic in nature, may be present, especially in patients with disseminated disease. Aplastic anemia has also been described *900*

Leukocytes *Blood* *Decrease* May be normal, decreased, or increased *900*
Blood *Increase* May be normal, decreased, or increased *900*

Monocytes *Blood* *Increase* Monocytes, sometimes morphologically quite immature, may be noted in increased numbers in the peripheral blood *900*

Oxygen Partial Pressure *Blood* *Decrease* With lung involvement, impaired gas diffusion *4707*

Platelets *Blood* *Decrease* With involvement of the spleen *5677* Thrombocytopenia may occur in patients with the so-called Letterer-Siwe Syndrome and if associated with hemorrhage manifestations constitutes a grave prognostic sign *900*

277.80 Histiocytosis X (continued)

Protein *Serum Decrease* May occur in the presence of extensive liver involvement *900*

Specific Gravity *Urine Decrease* Low, fixed specific gravity of urine is characteristic in patients with hypothalamic involvement *900*

277.80 Methylmalonic Aciduria

5-Oxoproline *Red Blood Cells Decrease* Value of 1.61 mmol/L observed in one patient with methylmalonic aciduria significantly decreased compared with 2.36 ± 0.37 mmol/L in 100 healthy controls *3384*
Urine Increase Value of 170 mmol/mol creatinine observed in one patient with methylmalonic aciduria significantly increased compared with < 50 mmol/mol creatinine in 100 healthy controls *3384*

277.80 Propionic Acidemia

Chitotriosidase *Serum No Effect* Normal activity observed in one patient with condition *1917*

5-Oxoproline *Red Blood Cells Decrease* Values of 1.46 and 1.52 mmol/L observed in two patients with propionic acidemia significantly decreased compared with 2.36 ± 0.37 mmol/L in 100 healthy controls *3384*
Urine Increase Values of 170 and 180 mmol/mol creatinine observed in two patients with propionic acidemia significantly increased compared with < 50 mmol/mol creatinine in 100 healthy controls *3384*

277.90 I-cell Disease

Lysosome-associated Membrane Protein-2 *Serum Increase* Median concentration of 5.33 mg/L in 15 patients with I-cell disease with median age 3 y compared with 1.21 mg/L in 202 healthy controls aged 0 - 66 y (median 7 years) *2265*

Lysosome-associated Membrane Protein-2:Lysosome-associated Membrane Protein-1 Ratio *Serum Decrease* Mean ratio of 2.83 mg/L in 15 patients with I-cell disease with median age 3 y compared with 4.74 in 202 healthy controls aged 0 - 66 y (median 7 years) *2265*

278.40 Hypervitaminosis D

Alkaline Phosphatase *Serum Decrease* Observed effect *1025*

Calcium *Feces Decrease* Decreased in stool. More calcium is absorbed from the diet than normal *1290*
Serum Increase Especially with added calcium in the diet; hypercalcemia corrected by steroids *1290* Increased concentrations are seen in vitamin D overdose *2952* 4 cases with hypercalcemia (range 10.6 - 16.4 mg/dL) *4311* In 7 patients with vitamin D intoxication mean concentration of 3.30 ± 0.25 mmol/L significantly higher than normal range of 2.25 - 2.62 mmol/L *4375* Observed effect *4891*
Urine Increase Observed effect *4891* In 7 patients with vitamin D intoxication mean excretion of 0.192 ± 0.067 mmol/L GFR significantly different from normal range of 0.010 - 0.045 mmol/L GFR *4375* Increased excretion is seen in vitamin D intoxication *2952*

Creatinine *Serum Increase* In 7 patients with vitamin D intoxication mean concentration of 202 ± 42 µmol/L significantly higher than normal range of 55 - 115 µmol/L *4375*

1,25-Dihydroxy Vitamin D *Serum No Effect* In 7 patients with vitamin D intoxication mean concentration of 90 ± 26 pmol/L not significantly different from normal range of 38 - 170 pmol/L *4375*

25-Hydroxy Vitamin D *Serum Increase* In 7 patients with vitamin D intoxication mean concentration of 710 ± 179 nmol/L significantly different from normal range of 20 - 90 nmol/L *4375*

Phosphate *Serum Decrease* Normal to decreased values *1025*
Serum Increase Observed effect *1642* Usually increased with increased urinary phosphate *5544* Observed effect *1025*
Serum No Effect In 7 patients with vitamin D intoxication mean concentration of 1.10 ± 0.07 mmol/L not significantly different from normal range of 0.80 - 1.30 mmol/L *4375*
Urine Increase In large doses vitamin D causes increased renal excretion of phosphate; to this extent its renal effect resembles parathyroid hormone *1642* *1025*

Immune Disorders

279.00 C1-Inhibitor Deficiency

Kallistatin *Plasma No Effect* Mean concentration in 5 patients with C1-inhibitor deficiency of 21.1 ± 3.8 µg/mL not significantly different from 21.2 ± 3.5 µg/mL in 30 healthy controls *781*

279.00 Transient Mineralocorticoid Deficiency of Infancy

Ammonium Ions *Urine Decrease* May cause distal renal tubular acidosis (type IV) is associated with hyperkalemia, hyperchloremic metabolic acidosis, urine pH < 5.5, decreased urinary ammonium ion excretion, a positive urine anion gap, normal urinary citrate and urinary calcium excretion *4071*

Anion Gap *Urine Increase* May cause distal renal tubular acidosis (type IV) is associated with hyperkalemia, hyperchloremic metabolic acidosis, urine pH < 5.5, decreased urinary ammonium ion excretion, a positive urine anion gap, normal urinary citrate and urinary calcium excretion *4071* *4071*

Calcium *Urine No Effect* May cause distal renal tubular acidosis (type IV) is associated with hyperkalemia, hyperchloremic metabolic acidosis, urine pH < 5.5, decreased urinary ammonium ion excretion, a positive urine anion gap, normal urinary citrate and urinary calcium excretion *4071*

Chloride *Serum Increase* May cause distal renal tubular acidosis (type IV) is associated with hyperkalemia, hyperchloremic metabolic acidosis, urine pH < 5.5, decreased urinary ammonium ion excretion, a positive urine anion gap, normal urinary citrate and urinary calcium excretion *4071*

Citrate *Urine No Effect* May cause distal renal tubular acidosis (type IV) is associated with hyperkalemia, hyperchloremic metabolic acidosis, urine pH < 5.5, decreased urinary ammonium ion excretion, a positive urine anion gap, normal urinary citrate and urinary calcium excretion *4071*

pH *Urine Decrease* May cause distal renal tubular acidosis (type IV) is associated with hyperkalemia, hyperchloremic metabolic acidosis, urine pH < 5.5, decreased urinary ammonium ion excretion, a positive urine anion gap, normal urinary citrate and urinary calcium excretion *4071*

Potassium *Serum Increase* May cause distal renal tubular acidosis (type IV) which is associated with hyperkalemia, hyperchloremic metabolic acidosis, urine pH < 5.5, decreased urinary ammonium ion excretion, a positive urine anion gap, normal urinary citrate and urinary calcium excretion *4071*

279.01 IgA Deficiency

$CD3^+$ Lymphocytes *Blood No Effect* In 17 patients with IgA deficiency median concentration of 1,240 x 10^6/L (25 - 75 percentiles 810 - 1,510) not significantly reduced compared with median of 1,190 x 10^6/L (25 - 75 percentiles 1,045 - 1,375) in 20 healthy blood donor controls *3649*

$CD4^+$ Lymphocytes *Blood No Effect* In 17 patients with IgA deficiency median concentration of 510 x 10^6/L (25 - 75 percentiles 475 - 630) not significantly reduced compared with median of 615 x 10^6/L (25 - 75 percentiles 500 - 880) in 20 healthy blood donor controls *3649*

$CD8^+$ Lymphocytes *Blood No Effect* In 17 patients with IgA deficiency median concentration of 300 x 10^6/L (25 - 75 percentiles 275 - 560) not significantly reduced compared with median of 420 x 10^6/L (25 - 75 percentiles 310 - 570) in 20 healthy blood donor controls *3649*

CD19+ Lymphocytes *Blood* *No Effect* In 17 patients with IgA deficiency median concentration of 215 x 10^6/L (25 - 75 percentiles 120 - 300) compared with median of 225 x 10^6/L (25 - 75 percentiles 155 - 350) in 20 healthy blood donor controls *3649*

Interleukin-4 *Serum* *Decrease* In 17 patients with IgA deficiency measurable concentrations observed in 4 and median concentration of 9 pg/mL (range 8 - 10) in these *3649*

Interleukin-6 *Serum* *Decrease* In 17 patients with IgA deficiency measurable concentrations observed in 4, and median concentration of 19 pg/mL (range 5 - 108) in these *3649*

Interleukin-7 *Serum* *No Effect* In 17 patients with IgA deficiency measurable concentrations observed in 7 and median concentration of 9 pg/mL (range 6 - 20) in these *3649*

Transforming Growth Factor-β *Serum* *Decrease* In 17 patients with IgA deficiency median concentration of 360 pg/mL (in 9 with infections of 330 pg/mL and in 8 without 380 pg/mL) compared with 425 pg/mL in 20 healthy blood donors *3649*

279.01 Selective IgA Deficiency

α_1-Antitrypsin *Serum* *No Effect* No deficiency was found in children with this disorder *3943*

immunoglobulin A *Serum* *Decrease* Less than 5 mg/dL *1588*

Immunoglobulin D *Serum* *No Effect* No prognostic significance *1588*

Immunoglobulin E *Serum* *Decrease* In 25 patients with selective IgA deficiency mean concentration of 35 ng/mL (range 5.6 - 214) not significantly less than mean of 96 ng/mL (range 24 - 386) in 74 healthy controls *2323*
Serum *No Effect* No prognostic significance *1588*

Immunoglobulin G *Serum* *No Effect* No prognostic significance *1588*

Immunoglobulin M *Serum* *No Effect* No prognostic significance *1588*

Lymphocyte B-Cells *Blood* *No Effect* No prognostic significance *1588*

Lymphocyte T-Cells *Blood* *No Effect* No prognostic significance *1588*

279.04 Agammaglobulinemia (Congenital Sex-linked)

Albumin *Serum* *No Effect* Concentration usually normal *5544*

Antibody Titer *Serum* *Decrease* Very low levels of antibody to certain animal viruses can be demonstrated *4551*

α_1-Antitrypsin *Serum* *No Effect* Concentration usually normal *5544*

Complement C_3 *Serum* *No Effect* Concentration typically normal *5544*

Complement, Total *Serum* *No Effect* Usually concentration is normal *5678* Other serum constituents involved in resistance to infection are normal *4979* Concentration typically normal *4551*

Erythrocyte Survival *Red Blood Cells* *Decrease* Hemolytic anemia *4551*

α_1-Globulin *Serum* *No Effect* Typical observation *5677*

α_2-Globulin *Serum* *No Effect* Typical observation *5677*

β-Globulin *Serum* *No Effect* Typical observation *5677*

γ-Globulin *Serum* *Decrease* The total serum globulins are decreased (100 - 200 mg/dL). Paper electrophoresis of serum shows complete absence of γ-globulins *900* Serum contains < 100 mg γ- G globulin/dL. γA- and M- globulins are present in concentrations < 1% of normal *4979*

Haptoglobin *Serum* *No Effect* Concentration typically normal *5544*

Hematocrit *Blood* *Decrease* Hemolytic anemia *4551* Hemolytic anemia frequently occurs *4979*

Hemoglobin *Blood* *Decrease* Hemolytic anemia frequently occurs *4979* Hemolytic anemia *4551*
Plasma *Increase* Hemolytic anemia frequently occurs *4979*

immunoglobulin A *Serum* *Decrease* Undetectable *5677* Usually < 1% of normal adult values *4551*

Immunoglobulin D *Serum* *Decrease* Undetectable *5677*

Immunoglobulin E *Serum* *Decrease* Undetectable *5677*

Immunoglobulin G *Serum* *Decrease* Minute amounts of IgG and sometimes IgM are identifiable by sensitive methods, functional levels of antibody are absent *2039* In primary acquired form, the serum levels may be as high as 500 mg/dL *2220* 100 mg/dL *4551*

Immunoglobulin M *Serum* *Decrease* Usually < 1% of normal adult values *4551* Undetectable *5677*

Immunoglobulins *Serum* *Decrease* All classes are deficient, including the secretory immunoglobulins *5699*

Iron-binding Capacity, Total *Serum* *No Effect* Concentration typically normal *5544*

Leukocytes *Blood* *Decrease* Not uncommon to observe either leukopenia or striking leukocytosis in these patients at the time of severe pyogenic infections *4551*
Blood *Increase* Not uncommon to observe either leukopenia or striking leukocytosis in these patients at the time of severe pyogenic infections *4551*

Lymphocyte B-Cells *Blood* *Decrease* Complete absence *5678*

Lymphocyte T-Cells *Blood* *No Effect* Normal to increased *5678*

Lymphocytes *Blood* *Decrease* There is a decreased number of lymphocytes in the congenital forms *900*
Blood *No Effect* Counts are normal (> 2,000 /μL) *4551*

Lysozyme *Serum* *No Effect* Other serum constituents involved in resistance to infection are normal *4979* *5678*

Plasma Cells *Bone Marrow* *Decrease* The basic deficiency is an absence of plasma cells from the lymph nodes, spleen, intestine, and bone marrow *5677*

Properdin *Plasma* *No Effect* Other serum constituents involved in resistance to infection are normal *4979* Normal concentration usually observed *5678*

279.06 Common Variable Immunodeficiency

Adenosine Deaminase *Serum* *Decrease* Decreased in Severe Combined Immunodeficiency Disease *4956* *3926* *1340*

Albumin *Serum* *No Effect* Concentration usually within normal limits *5544*

Antibody Titer *Serum* *Decrease* Antibody responses to most antigens are low or absent *5699*

Fat *Feces* *Increase* In small intestinal disease *4891*

α_1-Globulin *Serum* *No Effect* Concentration usually within normal limits *5544*

α_2-Globulin *Serum* *No Effect* Concentration usually within normal limits *5544*

β-Globulin *Serum* *No Effect* Concentration usually normal *5544*

γ-Globulin *Serum* *Decrease* Observed effect *5544*

Hematocrit *Blood* *Decrease* High incidence of pernicious anemia *5677*

Hemoglobin *Blood* *Decrease* High incidence of pernicious anemia *5677*

immunoglobulin A *Serum* *Decrease* Most common *1290* *5678*

Immunoglobulin E *Serum* *Decrease* Observed effect *4551*

Immunoglobulin G *Serum* *Decrease* Usually < 500 mg/dL *4551* Usually under 500 mg/dL but may not exhibit normal heterogeneity *5678*

Immunoglobulin M *Serum* *Decrease* Normal *1290* *5678* *5545*

Immunoglobulins *Serum* *Decrease* IgG primarily deficient, but other immunoglobulins may also be low *5699* *5678*

279.06 Common Variable Immunodeficiency *(continued)*

Interleukin-1 *Serum* *No Effect* Measured in 42 patients with primary hypogammaglobulinemia, 25 with common variable immunodeficiency (CVI), 10 congenital hypogammaglobulinemia (CH), 7 X-linked agammaglobulinemia (XLA), and in 21 healthy controls. IL-1α was detected in only a few serum samples with no significant differences between patients and controls *214*

Interleukin-4 *Serum* *Increase* Measured in 42 patients with primary hypogammaglobulinemia (25 common variable immunodeficiency (CVI), 10 congenital hypogammaglobulinemia (CH), 7 X-linked agammaglobulinemia (XLA), and in 21 healthy controls. IL-4 was detectable in 36% of the CVI patients, but in none of the controls *214*

Interleukin-6 *Serum* *Increase* Measured in 42 patients with primary hypogammaglobulinemia (25 common variable immunodeficiency (CVI), 10 congenital hypogammaglobulinemia (CH), 7 X-linked agammaglobulinemia (XLA), and in 21 healthy controls. IL-6 was detectable in 48% of the CVI patients, but in none of the controls *214*

Isocitrate Dehydrogenase *Serum* *No Effect* No effect on activity observed *5008*

Lymphocyte B-Cells *Blood* *Decrease* Normal or decreased *5678*

Lymphocyte T-Cells *Blood* *Decrease* Normal or decreased *5678*

Lymphocytes *Blood* *Decrease* Observed effect *2035* Reported observation *5545* Significant deficiency of T and B Lymphocytes. Clinical findings are usually associated with abnormal T-Lymphocyte function *5678*

MCV *Blood* *Increase* High incidence of pernicious anemia *5677*

Plasma Cells *Bone Marrow* *Decrease* Ordinarily, sparse in infancy, are absent with disease *5699* Decreased in transient hypogammaglobulinemia of infancy *5545*

Platelets *Blood* *Decrease* Observed effect *4551* Count is decreased, with bleeding tendency *5545*

Protein *Serum* *Decrease* Observed effect *5544*

Tumor Necrosis Factor-α *Serum* *Increase* Measured in 42 patients with primary hypogammaglobulinemia (25 common variable immunodeficiency (CVI), 10 congenital hypogammaglobulinemia (CH), 7 X-linked agammaglobulinemia (XLA), and in 21 healthy controls. TNF-α was detected in only a few serum samples with no significant differences between patients and controls *214*

279.06 Hypogammaglobulinemia (Common Variable)

Immunoglobulin E *Serum* *Decrease* In 36 patients with common variable hypogammaglobulinemia mean concentration of 11 ng/mL (range 3.24 - 38.9) significantly less than mean of 96 ng/mL (range 24 - 386) in 74 healthy controls *2323*

279.07 Dysgammaglobulinemia (Selective Immunoglobulin Deficiency)

Hematocrit *Blood* *Decrease* Not uncommon *900*

Hemoglobin *Blood* *Decrease* Not uncommon *900*

immunoglobulin A *Serum* *Decrease* Types I, II, and IV; 1 in 500 of the population have IgA deficiency *1290* In type III *5545* Reported effect *1793* *900* One of the common partial immunoglobulin defects is characterized by a deficiency of IgA and IgG and increased amounts of IgM in the serum *4551*

Immunoglobulin G *Serum* *Decrease* Type I, II, III, IV *1290* One of the common partial immunoglobulin defects is characterized by a deficiency of IgA and IgG and increased amounts of IgM in the serum *4551*
Serum *No Effect* In type I and II dysgammaglobulinemias *5545*

Immunoglobulin M *Serum* *Decrease* In type II *5545* Types I, V, VII *1290*
Serum *Increase* Type I *5544* Reported effect *900* *1793* One of the common partial immunoglobulin defects is characterized by a deficiency of IgA and IgG and increased amounts of IgM in the serum *4551*
Serum *No Effect* Normal or increased *5544*

Neutrophils *Blood* *Decrease* Not uncommon *900*

Rheumatoid Factor *Serum* *Increase* Dysproteinemias and paraproteinemias present significant seropositivity *1980*

279.11 DiGeorge's Syndrome

Calcium *Serum* *Decrease* Atypical lymphocytes *5203*

immunoglobulin A *Serum* *No Effect* Frequently normal *2035*

Immunoglobulin E *Serum* *No Effect* Frequently normal *2035*

Immunoglobulin G *Serum* *No Effect* Frequently normal *5203* *2035*

Immunoglobulin M *Serum* *No Effect* Frequently normal *2035*

Lymphocyte B-Cells *Blood* *No Effect* No prognostic significance *1588*

Lymphocyte T-Cells *Blood* *Decrease* Usually low but may be normal or increased *1588*

Lymphocytes *Blood* *Decrease* Profound lymphopenia and T5+/T8+ cells are relatively more deficient than T4+ cells *5678*
Blood *No Effect* May be normal but virtually all are B-cells *2035* Patients have partial or complete T cell immunodeficiency with normal or near normal B cell immune function *5678*

Parathyroid Hormone *Plasma* *Decrease* No prognostic significance *1588*

279.12 Wiskott-Aldrich Syndrome

Creatinine *Serum* *Increase* Increased incidence of renal failure *1588*

immunoglobulin A *Serum* *Increase* Elevated levels *5678* *5203*
Serum *No Effect* Normal *2035*

Immunoglobulin E *Serum* *Increase* In 12 patients with Wiskott-Aldrich syndrome mean concentration of 3,475 ng/mL (range 499 - 24,257) significantly higher than mean of 96 ng/mL (range 24 - 386) in 74 healthy controls *2323* Frequently elevated *2035*

Immunoglobulin G *Serum* *Increase* Elevated levels *5678*
Serum *No Effect* Normal *2035*

Immunoglobulin M *Platelets* *Increase* Platelet associated immunoglobulins were increased presplenectomy *934*
Serum *Decrease* Low levels *5678* Usually decreased *5203* *2035*

Lymphocyte B-Cells *Blood* *No Effect* Normal concentration usually observed *5678*

Lymphocyte T-Cells *Blood* *Decrease* Normal immunity initially but may decline with advancing years *5678*

Lymphocytes *Blood* *Decrease* Diminished T-Lymphocytes in some patients *2035* *5203*

Platelets *Blood* *Decrease* Thrombocytopenia *934* *5678*

Protein *Urine* *Increase* Increased incidence of renal failure *1588*

Urea Nitrogen *Serum* *Increase* Increased incidence of renal failure *1588*

Volume *Platelets* *Decrease* Mean platelet volume was markedly decreased but returned to normal post-splenectomy *934*

279.13 Nezelof's Syndrome

Granulocytes *Blood* *Decrease* Atypical lymphocytes *5203*

immunoglobulin A *Serum* *Decrease* 50% of patients *5203*

Immunoglobulin G *Serum* *Decrease* 50% of patients *5203*

Lymphocyte B-Cells *Blood* *No Effect* Normal concentration usually observed *1588*

Lymphocyte T-Cells *Blood* *Decrease* Studies of T cell immunity are abnormal but the degree of deficiency may vary *1588*

279.20 Adenosine Deaminase Deficiency

Adenosine Deaminase *Lymphocytes* *Decrease* In 2 adult patients with adenosine deaminase deficiency, activities of 68 and 55 nmol/h/mg protein observed compared with 1,162 - 4,500 nmol/h/mg protein in healthy controls *4820*
Red Blood Cells *Decrease* In 2 adult cases with adenosine deaminase deficiency activities of less than 1 nmol/h/mg hemoglobin compared with 40 - 100 nmol/h/mg hemoglobin in normal individuals *4820*

$CD4^+$ Lymphocytes *Blood* *Decrease* In 2 adult cases with adenosine deaminase deficiency proportion of total count of 14% and 6% compared with normal range of 26 - 46% *4820*

$CD8^+$ Lymphocytes *Blood* *Increase* In 2 adult cases with adenosine deaminase deficiency proportion of total count of 58% and 60% compared with normal range of 13 - 33% *4820*

$CD19^+$ Lymphocytes *Blood* *Decrease* In 2 adult cases with adenosine deaminase deficiency proportion of total lymphocytes 0% compared with normal of 7 - 23% *4820*

Deoxyadenosine *Urine* *Increase* In 2 adult cases with adenosine deaminase deficiency excretion of 86 and 45 μmol/d observed compared with undetectable amounts in controls *4820*

Deoxyadenosine Triphosphate *Red Blood Cells* *Increase* Concentrations of 234 and 105 μmol/L observed in 2 adult patients with adenosine deaminase deficiency compared with undetectable amounts in normal controls *4820*

immunoglobulin A *Serum* *Decrease* In 2 adult cases with adenosine deaminase deficiency concentrations of 0.96 and 0.4 g/L compared with normal of 1.2 - 4.2 g/L *4820*

Immunoglobulin E *Serum* *Increase* In 2 adult cases with adenosine deaminase deficiency concentrations of 100 and 888 IU/mL compared with normal range of 0 - 81 IU/mL *4820*

Immunoglobulin G *Serum* *No Effect* In 2 adult cases with adenosine deaminase deficiency concentrations of 15.2 and 14.4 g/L compared with 5 - 16 g/L in normals *4820*

Immunoglobulin G_1 *Serum* *Increase* In 2 adult cases with adenosine deaminase deficiency concentrations of > 5.89 and 14.6 g/L compared with normal range of 3.2 - 10.2 g/L *4820*

Immunoglobulin G_2 *Serum* *Decrease* In 2 adult cases with adenosine deaminase deficiency concentrations of 0.73 and 0.5 g/L compared with normal range of 1.2 - 6.6 g/L *4820*

Immunoglobulin M *Serum* *Decrease* In 2 adult cases with adenosine deaminase deficiency concentrations of 0.3 and 0.56 g/L observed compared with normal range of 0.5 - 4.25 g/L *4820*

Lymphocyte T-Cells *Blood* *No Effect* In 2 adult cases with adenosine deaminase deficiency proportion of total lmphocyte count 60 and 75% compared with normal of 60 - 85% *4820*

Lymphocytes *Blood* *Decrease* In 2 adult cases with adenosine deaminase deficiency concentrations of 100 and 1,200 /μL compared with normal range of 1,500 - 3,500 /μL *4820*

279.20 Immunodeficiency (Severe Combined)

Adenosine Deaminase *Serum* *No Effect* Normal levels *1588*

Eosinophils *Blood* *Increase* Commonly elevated *5678*

HLA Antigens *Blood* *Present* HLA-B_8 and DRw3 are found *1588*

Lymphocyte B-Cells *Blood* *Decrease* Absent or markedly reduced *1588*

Lymphocyte T-Cells *Blood* *Decrease* Deficient immunity *1588*

279.40 Autoimmune Disorders

Alkaline Phosphatase *Serum* *No Effect* In 8 patients with various autoimmune disorders mean activity of 141 ± 27 U/L not significantly different from 116 ± 4 U/L in 40 healthy age and sex matched controls *907*

Amino-terminal Propeptide of Type III Procollagen *Serum* *Decrease* In 8 patients with various autoimmune disorders mean concentration of 2.2 ± 0.3 ng/mL significantly less than 3.3 ± 0.2 ng/mL in 40 healthy age and sex matched controls *907*

Complement C_5 *Serum* *Increase* Increased concentrations are consistent with chronic infections and autoimmune disorders *2952*

Osteocalcin *Serum* *No Effect* In 6 patients with various autoimmune disorders mean concentration of 5.3 ± 0.4 ng/mL not significantly different from 5.4 ± 0.1 ng/mL in 40 healthy age and sex matched controls *907*

279.40 Reproductive Autoimmune Failure Syndrome

Anticardiolipin Antibodies *Serum* *Increase* Incidence of 12.4% in 259 patients suspected of having RAF not significantly higher than 5.2% in 97 healthy controls *156*

Antiphosphatidic Acid Antibodies *Serum* *Increase* Incidence of 2.7% in 259 patients suspected of having RAF not significantly higher than 0.0% in 97 healthy controls *156*

Antiphosphatidylethanolamine Antibodies *Serum* *No Effect* Incidence of 6.2% in 259 patients not significantly different from 0.0% in 97 healthy controls *156*

Antiphosphatidylglycerol Antibodies *Serum* *No Effect* Incidence of 1.9% in 259 patients not significantly different from 0.0% in 97 healthy controls *156*

Antiphosphatidylinositol Antibodies *Serum* *Increase* Incidence of 5.0% in 259 patients suspected of having RAF not significantly higher than 2.1% in 97 healthy controls *156*

Antiphosphatidylserine Antibodies *Serum* *Increase* Incidence of 12.4% in 259 patients suspected of having RAF not significantly higher than 5.2% in 97 healthy controls *156*

β_2-Glycoprotein I-dependent Anticardiolipin Antibodies *Serum* *Increase* Incidence of 5.4% in 259 patients suspected of having RAF significantly higher than 0.0% in 97 healthy controls *156*

279.80 Complement C_2 Deficiency

Complement C_1 *Serum* *No Effect* Mean concentration typically normal in patients with complement C_2 deficiency *4682*

Complement C_1q *Serum* *No Effect* Mean concentration typically normal in patients with complement C_2 deficiency *4682*

Complement C_2 *Serum* *Decrease* Mean concentration typically undetectable in patients with complement C_2 deficiency *4682*

Complement C_3 *Serum* *No Effect* Mean concentration typically normal in patients with complement C_2 deficiency *4682*

Complement C_4 *Serum* *No Effect* Mean concentration typically normal in patients with complement C_2 deficiency *4682*

Complement C_5 *Serum* *No Effect* Mean concentration typically normal in patients with complement C_2 deficiency *4682*

Complement CH50 *Serum* *Decrease* Mean concentration typically undetectable in patients with complement C_2 deficiency *4682*

Properdin Factor B *Plasma* *No Effect* Mean concentration typically normal in patients with complement C_2 deficiency *4682*

DISEASES OF THE BLOOD

Deficiency Anemias

280.81 Plummer-Vinson Syndrome

Hematocrit *Blood* *Decrease* Hypochromic anemia associated with dysphagia and cardiospasm in women *5544*

Hemoglobin *Blood* *Decrease* Hypochromic anemia associated with dysphagia and cardiospasm in women *5544*

MCH *Blood* *Decrease* Microcytic anemia *2034*

280.81 Plummer-Vinson Syndrome *(continued)*

MCHC *Blood* *Decrease* Hypochromic anemia associated with dysphagia and cardiospasm in women *5544*

MCV *Blood* *Decrease* Hypochromic anemia associated with dysphagia and cardiospasm in women *5544*

280.90 Iron Deficiency Anemia

Albumin *Serum* *No Effect* Concentration usually normal *5544*

Anisocytes *Blood* *Increase* Usually there is moderate to marked anisocytosis and poikilocytosis *2039* Characteristic of well-developed iron deficiency *1980*

α_1-Antitrypsin *Serum* *No Effect* Concentration usually normal *5544*

Atrial Natriuretic Peptide *Plasma* *Increase* Mean concentration in 11 aged patients with iron deficiency anemia of 58.3 ± 23.5 pg/mL *2676*

Bilirubin *Serum* *Decrease* A test of minor or incidental importance *900*

Catalase *Red Blood Cells* *Decrease* Has been demonstrated to be decreased in RBCs *258*

Cells *Bone Marrow* *Increase* Characterized by erythroid hyperplasia of mild-moderate degree *5699*

Chylomicrons *Serum* *Increase* Increased *4358* *4372* *3017*

Complement C_3 *Serum* *No Effect* Concentration usually normal *5544*

Copper *Serum* *Decrease* Decreases in some iron-deficiency anemias of childhood (that require copper as well as iron therapy) *5544* Ceruloplasmin lost in urine *5544*

2,3-Diphosphoglycerate *Red Blood Cells* *Increase* Synthesis is increased in response to hypoxia *380*

Erythrocyte Survival *Red Blood Cells* *Decrease* Slight to moderate shortening *5677* Somewhat shortened. High correlation with the number of morphologically abnormal cells. Only severe changes can be detected by the ^{53}Cr method *1170* *5699* Slight to moderate shortening *3131*

Erythrocytes *Blood* *Decrease* Mean concentration in 42 aged patients with iron deficiency anemia of 3.82 ± 0.55 x $10^6/\mu L$ *2676*
Blood *Increase* In infants and children, hypochromia may occur earlier in the course of iron deficiency and counts > 5.5 million/µL are sometimes encountered with iron-deficiency anemia *5677*

Ferritin *Bone Marrow* *Decrease* The amount is not as important diagnostically as presence or absence. The presence is strong evidence against the diagnosis of clinically significant iron deficiency *1980*
Serum *Decrease* Invariably reduced *2039* In one 39-year old woman with iron deficiency anemia with generalized weakness and increased vaginal bleeding concentration low *854* In 19 women with iron deficient anemia mean concentration of 12.1 ± 4.4 µg/L significantly less than reference interval of 25 - 210 µg/L in women: in 72 women with severe iron deficiency mean concentration of 5.1 ± 3.0 µg/L *2057* In 19 patients with iron deficiency mean concentration of 9 ± 6 µg/L significantly less than 72 ± 89 µg/L in 19 healthy controls *4239* Concentration < 10 ng/mL is characteristic. The usefulness of the assay is limited by the fact that when iron deficiency and inflammatory disease coexist, concentration may be within the normal range *5677*
Serum *No Effect* Concentration < 10 ng/mL is characteristic. The usefulness of the assay is limited by the fact that when iron deficiency and inflammatory disease coexist, concentration may be within the normal range *5677*

Ferritin Iron *Serum* *Decrease* Concentration in 4 of 4 patients with iron deficiency and in 5 of 6 with negative iron balance of less than 10 ng/mL compared with range in healthy controls of 10 - 35 ng Fe/mL *2125*

Ferritin Protein *Serum* *Decrease* Concentration in 4 patients with iron deficiency of 9.0 ± 0.7 ng/mL compared with concentration in 17 healthy controls of 136.6 ± 11.9 ng/mL *2125*

Glutamic Acid *Red Blood Cells* *Increase* Raised RBC L-glutamate levels occur in iron deficiency anemias in the presence of a large population of young cells *5394*

Haptoglobin *Serum* *No Effect* Concentration usually normal *5544*

Hematocrit *Blood* *Decrease* Mean value in 42 aged patients with iron deficiency anemia of 35.8 ± 4.8% *2676*

Hemoglobin *Blood* *Decrease* In one 39-year old woman with iron deficiency anemia with generalized weakness and increased vaginal bleeding concentration of 89 g/L *854* Mean concentration in 42 aged patients with iron deficiency anemia of 11.6 ± 1.8 g/dL *2676* Mean concentration of 89 ± 19 g/L in 19 patients with iron deficiency less than 138 ± 13 g/L in 19 controls *4239* Reduced to a mean of 7.6 g/dL in 371 patients *427* Concentration significantly reduced in 72 women with severe iron deficiency to 81 ± 14 g/L compared with upper limit of reference interval of 120 g/L *2057*
Blood *No Effect* Mean concentration in 19 women of 132 ± 9 g/L, within normal range (upper limit of 130 g/L in men and 120 g/L in women) *2057*

Hemoglobin A_{1c} *Blood* *Increase* Mean concentration of 10.3% significantly higher in a group of iron-deficient children compared with control children (5.9%) *5165*

Hydrochloric Acid *Gastric Fluid* *Decrease* The augmented histamine test has shown true achlorhydria in 16% of cases *2034*

Iron *Bone Marrow* *Decrease* Reticuloendothelial stores are severely reduced or absent in marrow and liver *296* The amount is not as important diagnostically as presence or absence. The presence is strong evidence against the diagnosis of clinically significant iron deficiency *1980* Depleted of stainable iron *5677* Reticuloendothelial stores are severely reduced or absent in marrow and liver *5699*
Liver *Decrease* Reticuloendothelial stores are severely reduced or absent in marrow and liver *296* *5699*
Serum *Decrease* Nearly all patients will have serum values < 50 µg/dL *900* Reduced to an average of 28 µg/dL in adults *296* Concentration in 4 patients with iron deficiency of 35.0 ± 8.2 µg/dL compared with concentration in 17 healthy controls of 103.9 ± 6.6 µg/dL *2125* Mean concentration of 3.9 ± 2.0 µmol/L in 72 women with severe iron deficiency less than 6.4 ± 2.8 µmol/L in 11 women with mild iron deficiency and reference interval of 10.7 ± 32.2 µmol/L *2057* Decrease in concentration observed in patients with iron deficiency anemia *2952* Usually < 80 µg/dL, associated with a total plasma iron-binding capacity of > 400 µg/dL *367* In one 39-year old woman with iron deficiency anemia with generalized weakness and increased vaginal bleeding concentration low *854* As deficiency intensifies, serum concentration falls *2039* In well-developed deficiency often below 30 µg/dL *1980* In 19 patients with iron deficient anemia mean concentration of 4.3 ± 2.5 µmol/L compared with 17.3 ± 6.3 µmol/L in 19 healthy controls *4239*
Serum *No Effect* Usually low in untreated anemia; however, it may be normal *1341* Concentration sometimes normal *5677* Mild deficiency is often accompanied by a normal serum level, and sometimes the deficiency may be symptomatic without measurably depressing the level *1980* Mean concentration in 19 women with iron deficient anemia of 13.2 ± 4.9 µmol/L compared with normal range of 10.7 - 32.2 µmol/L *2057*

Iron-binding Capacity, Total *Serum* *Decrease* Often increased, but may be normal or low *5699* Mean concentration of 346 µg/dL, ranging from 170 - 460 µg/dL. Patients with reduced capacity also have hypoalbuminemia *296*
Serum *Increase* Often increased, but may be normal or low *5699* In well-developed iron deficiency, the percentage of saturation of transferrin is usually very low, 16%. Low saturation from other causes is rare *1980* Observed effect *5677*

Iron Crystals *Urine* *Increase* If the spun sediment of the morning's first-voided specimen is stained for iron, it may frequently be seen to contain hemosiderin crystals *900*

Iron Saturation *Serum* *Decrease* Saturation of 15% or less is often found *5677* 16% and averages 7% *5699* In 92% of 15 patients at initial hospitalization for this disorder *1576* Transferrin saturation is almost always under 15% and, in severe deficiency, under 10% *2039* In well-developed iron deficiency, the percentage of saturation of transferrin is usually very low, < 16%. Low saturation from other causes is rare *1980*

Lactate Dehydrogenase *Serum* *No Effect* Normal, even in severe iron-deficiency *5545*

Lactate Dehydrogenase Isoenzymes *Serum Increase* LD_3 was elevated to 31% in serum of patients with hypochromic microcytic anemia *1756*

Leukocytes *Blood Decrease* Observed response to anemia *5677* 14% were found to have counts between 3,000 - 4,000 /µL. Leukopenia was unrelated to severity of anemia and could not be ascribed to any other condition. Differential counts were normal *2576*

MCH *Blood Decrease* Microcytic hypochromic anemia may occur due to blood loss, increased demand or dietary inadequacy. MCH < 27 pg, MCV < 80 fL *1098* Morphologic changes are paralleled by decreases in the MCV, MCH, and MCHC. The decline in MCHC is the more consistent *1980* Mean in 42 aged patients with iron deficiency anemia 30.5 ± 2.5 pg *2676* In 72 women with severe iron deficiency mean value 19.5 ± 2.3 pg compared with 28.5 ± 0.5 pg in 11 women with mild iron deficiency and reference interval of 28 - 34 pg *2057* Average is 20 pg, range = 14-29 *296*
Blood No Effect Red cell indices are related to the duration and severity of anemia. Mild cases or those of short duration may have normal values *425* Mean MCH in 19 female patients with iron deficient anemia 30.0 ± 1.9 pg, within normal range of 28 - 34 pg *2057*

MCHC *Blood Decrease* Of little diagnostic value except when anemia is severe *5677* Morphologic changes are paralleled by decreases in the MCV, MCH, and MCHC. The decline in MCHC is the more consistent *1980* Mean in 42 aged patients with iron deficiency anemia of 32.3 ± 1.2 *2676* Average is 28, ranging from 22 - 31 *296*
Blood No Effect Red cell indices are related to the duration and severity of anemia. Mild cases or those of short duration may have normal values *425*

MCV *Blood Decrease* Hypochromic microcytosis parallels severity of anemia with marked variation in size and shape *367* Mean in 42 aged patients with iron deficiency anemia 94.1 ± 6 fL *2676* Mean volume of 73 ± 9 fL in 19 patients with iron deficient anemia compared with 91 ± 4 fL in 19 healthy controls *4239* Mean concentration of 67 ± 7 fL in 69 patients with iron deficiency anemia significantly different from normal *2037* Average is 74 fL, range - 53 - 93 fL *296* In 72 women with severe iron deficiency mean volume 69.7 ± 5.9 fL compared with 85.9 ± 3.1 fL in 11 with mild deficiency and reference interval of 80 - 96 fL *2057* In severe uncomplicated anemia, erythrocytes are hypochromic and microcytic *5677* Characteristic of well-developed iron deficiency *1980* Microcytic hypochromic anemia may occur due to blood loss, increased demand or dietary inadequacy. MCH < 27 pg, MCV < 80 fL *1098*
Blood No Effect Red cell indices are related to the duration and severity of anemia. Mild cases or those of short duration may have normal values *425* In 19 iron deficient women mean MCV of 90.5 ± 3.6 fL, within normal range of 80 - 96 fL *2057*

Neutrophils *Blood Decrease* WBC is usually normal in number, but slight granulocytopenia may occur in long standing cases *5490*

Osmotic Fragility *Red Blood Cells Decrease* May be within the normal range, but often there is increased resistance to destruction in hypotonic salt solution. Extreme resistance is unusual *5699* Decreased, reflecting the diminished hemoglobin concentration *367*

Parietal Cell Antibodies *Serum Increase* Parietal cell antibodies observed in some patients with iron deficiency anemia *2952*

Platelets *Blood Decrease* In infants and children, thrombocytopenia occurred almost as frequently (28%) as did thrombocytosis (35%). Associated with more severe anemia *1883*
Blood Increase Reported in 50 - 75% of adults with classic hypochromic anemia due to chronic blood loss. May be found only in those patients who are actively bleeding *2576* Usually twice the normal level *4642* In infants and children, thrombocytopenia occurred almost as frequently (28%) as did thrombocytosis (35%). Associated with more severe anemia *1883* In one 39-year old woman with iron deficiency anemia with generalized weakness and increased vaginal bleeding initial concentration of 380 x 10^9/L *854*

Poikilocytes *Blood Increase* Usually there is moderate to marked anisocytosis and poikilocytosis *2039* Characteristic of well-developed iron deficiency *1980* A moderate number, especially tailed and elongated forms, are found *5699*

Protoporphyrin *Red Blood Cells Increase* Defective heme synthesis is associated with raised RBC protoporphyrin *5677*

Reticulocytes *Blood Decrease* Usually normal or decreased *5677* Rarely reduced *5699*
Blood Increase Occasionally a count of 2 - 3% may be noted *5677* Both the percentage and absolute number tend to be normal or slightly increased *296*
Blood No Effect Usually normal or decreased *5677* Usually normal *2034*

Selenium *Serum Decrease* In 27 normally developed iron-deficient children mean concentration of 63.98 ± 11.02 µg/L and mean concentration of 53.58 ± 8.16 µg/L in 13 malnourished children with iron-deficiency anemia significantly less than 73.90 ± 12.60 µg/L in 40 age and sex matched control children *5800*

Sideroblasts *Blood Decrease* Mean concentration in 72 women with severe iron deficiency of 2.8 ± 2.3% and 5 ± 2% in 11 with mild iron deficiency compared reference interval of 30 - 50% of erythroblasts *2057*

Soluble Transferrin Receptor *Serum Increase* In iron deficiency concentration may rise to three times the mean concentration of 5 - 8.3 mg/L in health. In the case of defective erythropoiesis the concentration may rise 10-fold *4784* Mean concentration of 10.9 mg/L (range 3.4 - 29.0 mg/L) observed in 45 patients with iron-deficient anemia significantly greater than 2.1 mg/L (95% interval 1.3 - 3.3 mg/L) in 119 apparently healthy nonanemic men and 96 women aged 24 - 69 years *5085* In 19 patients with iron deficiency mean concentration of 5.3 ± 1.8 mg/L compared with 1.7 ± 0.5 mg/L in 19 healthy controls *4239*

Transferrin *Serum Increase* In 19 women with iron deficiency mean concentration of 3.3 ± 0.5 g/L higher than 2.5 ± 0.4 g/L in 19 healthy controls *4239* Concentrations as high as 700 mg/dL observed in patients with severe iron deficiecy *2952*

Transferrin Receptor:Ferritin Ratio *Serum No Effect* Ratio may increase to over 1,000 in iron-deficient anemics compared with 200 in healthy individuals *4784*

Transferrin Saturation *Serum Decrease* In 72 women with severe iron deficiency mean saturation of 7.5 ± 2.9% and in 11 with mild iron deficiency of 10.1 ± 2.8% compared with reference interval of 25 - 50% *2057* Saturation in 4 patients with iron deficiency of 8.3 ± 2.4% compared with saturation in 17 healthy controls of 30.3 ± 2.6% *2125*
Serum No Effect Mean saturation in 19 women with mild iron deficient anemia of 35.6 ± 4.6% compared with reference interval of 25 - 50% *2057*

Uropepsinogen *Urine Decrease* With achlorhydria *1290*

Vitamin B_{12} *Serum Increase* Slight increase; mean concentration of 466 pg/mL in 118 patients (normal 385 pg/mL) *4448*

Zinc Protoporphyrin *Red Blood Cells Increase* In 72 women with severe iron deficiency mean zinc protoporphyrin concentration of 265 ± 100 µmol/mol heme significantly greater than 100 ± 16 µmol/mol heme in 19 women with mild iron deficiency and 19 - 39 µmol/mol heme in healthy controls *2057* Mean concentration of 0.79 ± 0.47 mmol/mol hemoglobin in 69 patients with iron deficiency anemia significantly greater than 0.06 - 0.22 mmol/mol hemoglobin in healthy controls *2037* In iron-deficient individuals concentration typically greater than 100 µmol/mol heme compared with the range reported range in healthy adults of 30 - 70 µmol/mol heme. Concentrations between 70 and 100 µmol/mol heme may also be observed in iron-deficiency anemia *4784*
Red Blood Cells No Effect In 19 women with mild iron deficiency mean concentration in washed erythrocytes of 30 ± 6 µmol/mol heme, within normal range of 19 - 39 µmol/mol heme *2057*

281.00 Pernicious Anemia

Aldolase *Serum Increase* Increased less consistently and to a lesser degree than LD *1337* *5699*

Alkaline Phosphatase *Serum Decrease* Decreased activity *5392* Observed in 33% of patients *5544* Reported effect *3160*

Amino Acids *Urine Increase* Amino aciduria with an excess excretion of taurine, especially if there is associated subacute combined degeneration of the spinal cord. Amino aciduria does not occur in other megaloblastic anemias *5545* May be slight excess of urinary amino acids, especially taurine *5241* *1537*

Antibody Titer *Serum Increase* Antibodies against parietal cells are found in 75% of all patients. Antibodies against intrinsic factor are seen in 50% of these patients *1980*

281.00 Pernicious Anemia *(continued)*

Antithyroglobulin Antibodies *Serum* *Increase* In 25% of cases *116*

Bilirubin *Serum* *Increase* Mild due to increase in indirect fraction *2034*

Bilirubin, Indirect *Serum* *Increase* Slight indirect hyperbilirubinemia as a result of increased production of bile pigment. Normal values are common and values > 2 mg/dL are unusual *5699* Mild unconjugated hyperbilirubinemia *367*

Bleeding Time *Patient* *Increase* May be prolonged *5699*

Calcitonin *Plasma* *Increase* In some cases *2144*

Cholesterol *Serum* *Decrease* In relapse, increased fatty acid and triglyceride concentrations but decreased concentrations of total cholesterol, unesterified cholesterol and all examined phospholipid fractions *5550* Decreases in relapse; during remission, or following treatment the serum cholesterol increases as the reticulocyte count rises *1642*

Cholesterol, Free *Serum* *Decrease* In relapse, increased free fatty acid and triglyceride concentrations but decreased concentrations of total cholesterol, unesterified cholesterol and all examined phospholipid fractions *5550*

Clot Retraction *Blood* *Decrease* May be poor *5699*

Complement C_3 *Serum* *Decrease* Significantly reduced in patients with vitamin B_{12} deficiency. Levels correlate with the degree of anemia but not with serum vitamin B_{12} levels at diagnosis *2242*

Creatine Kinase *Serum* *No Effect* Activity usually normal *5544*

2,3-Diphosphoglycerate *Red Blood Cells* *Increase* Synthesis is increased in response to hypoxia *380*

Eosinophils *Blood* *Increase* Occurs in some hematopoietic diseases *5544* In 1 patient with pernicious anemia and asthma mean concentration of 550 x 10^6/L significantly different from upper limit of normal of 440 x 10^6/L in 29 normal individuals *607*

Erythrocyte Survival *Red Blood Cells* *Decrease* Ranged from 27 - 75 days in 5 patients (normal 120 days) *3138* Moderately reduced *5699* Ranged from 27 - 75 days in 5 patients (normal 120 days) *4862*

Fatty Acids (FFA), Free *Serum* *Increase* In relapse, increased free fatty acid and triglyceride concentrations but decreased concentrations of total cholesterol, unesterified cholesterol and all examined phospholipid fractions *5550*

Fibrinogen *Plasma* *Decrease* Moderate depression of fibrinogen formation occurs *1290*

Folate *Serum* *Increase* Normal or high *2039*

Gastrin *Serum* *Increase* May be due to G cell hyperplasia in the pyloric antral mucosa *3020* Concentration in the serum is high, probably because of the high pH within the lumen of the stomach *2039* High level may approach that in the Zollinger-Ellison syndrome *5544*

Glucose-6-Phosphate Dehydrogenase *Red Blood Cells* *Increase* Increased to about the same extent as LD *5699* *1337*

Haptoglobin *Serum* *Decrease* Associated with hemolysis *900* Probably due at least partly to impaired formation *1290*

Hematocrit *Blood* *Decrease* Classical anemia, leukopenia (primarily granulopenia) and thrombocytopenia. Occasionally, the primary reduction may be in only 1 of these 3 major formed elements of the blood. Although patients usually present primarily with anemia they may occasionally present initially with infection associated with granulocytopenia or with bleeding associated with thrombocytopenia *900* In 5 cases, hematocrit varied from 12 - 20% (normal = 37 - 54%) *4995* Anemia may be very severe or very mild *5699*

Hemoglobin *Blood* *Decrease* Classical anemia, leukopenia (primarily granulocytopenia) and thrombocytopenia. Occasionally, the primary reduction may be in only 1 of these 3 major formed elements of the blood. Although patients usually present primarily with anemia they may occasionally present initially with infection associated with granulocytopenia or with bleeding associated with thrombocytopenia *900* Concentration ranges from very severe to near normal. Usually 7 - 8 g/dL at presentation *5699*

Hemoglobin F *Blood* *Increase* In 50% of untreated patients; increases after treatment and then gradually decreases during next 6 months; some patients still have slight elevation thereafter *5544*

Histamine *Plasma* *No Effect* In 1 patient with pernicious anemia and asthma mean concentration of < 1.8 nmol/L not significantly different from mean concentration of 4.0 nmol/L in 29 normal individuals *607*

Hydrochloric Acid *Gastric Fluid* *Decrease* Gastric parietal cells lose ability to secrete HCl as well as intrinsic factor. Achlorhydria is therefore characteristic of intrinsic factor deficiency but not diagnostic *1980*

Intrinsic Factor Blocking Antibody *Serum* *Increase* Test for intrinsic factor blocking antibody is positive in the sera of 50% of patients with proved pernicious anemia *2952*

Iron *Bone Marrow* *Increase* Marrow sideroblasts and reticuloendothelial stores tend to be increased *5699*
Serum *Increase* Moderately increased unless there is associated iron deficiency *773*

Iron-binding Capacity, Total *Serum* *Decrease* Total plasma capacity tends to be slightly reduced *5699* In relapse *1290*

Isocitrate Dehydrogenase *Serum* *Increase* Increased less consistently and to a lesser degree than LD *5699* *1337*
Serum *No Effect* Activity unaffected by disease *5008*

Lactate Dehydrogenase *Serum* *Increase* Mean value in 16 patients was 2,335 U/L (normal 116 U/L) *118* Magnitude of increase is related to the degree of anemia *5699* Total LD (chiefly LD_1) is markedly increased especially with hemoglobin < 8 g/dL *5544* In 5 cases, levels ranged from 310 U/L (in relapse) - 4,820 U/L (normal concentration of 50 - 220 U/L) *4995*

Lactate Dehydrogenase Isoenzyme-5 *Serum* *Increase* Increased to about the same extent as LD *1337* *5699*

Lactate Dehydrogenase Isoenzymes *Serum* *Increase* LD_1 and LD_2 account for the increase in total LD *5699* Predominantly LD_1, in untreated cases *5544*

Leukocytes *Blood* *Decrease* Anemia, leukopenia (primarily granulopenia) and thrombocytopenia. Occasionally, the primary reduction may be in only 1 of these 3 major formed elements of the blood *900* Hematopoietic diseases *5544* Varies with degree of anemia from normal to very low. Usually due to absolute neutropenia *5699*

Lipids *Red Blood Cells* *Decrease* Decreased in serum and the red cell membrane *1290*
Serum *Decrease* Decreased in serum and the red cell membrane *1290*

Malate Dehydrogenase *Serum* *Increase* Increased to about the same extent as LD *1337* *5699*

MCH *Blood* *Increase* Generally 33 - 38 pg in moderate anemia, and 33 - 56 pg, with severe cases (normal amount 27 - 31 pg) *5699*

MCHC *Blood* *No Effect* Usually unchanged by disease *2034* When not complicated by iron deficiency, anemia is normochromic and macrocytic *5699*

MCV *Blood* *Increase* Usually macrocytic anemia. Rise in MCV is largely proportional to the degree of anemia. Usual values are 95 - 110 fL, but may be 110 - 160 fL with severe anemia *5699* Macrocytic anemia may occur due to vitamin B_{12} or folate deficiency. MCV > 100 fL *1098*

Methylmalonate *Urine* *Increase* Relatively specific for vitamin B_{12} deficiency *900*

Monoamine Oxidase *Platelets* *Increase* Increased in patients with megaloblastic anemia *4312*

N-Formiminoglutamic Acid *Urine* *Increase* Increased urinary formiminoglutamate after an oral histidine load *900*

Parietal Cell Antibodies *Serum* *Increase* Approximately 90% of patients with pernicious anemia have antibodies to gastric parietal cells *2952*

Pepsinogen I *Serum* *Decrease* Decreased in 90% of patients. Values less than 30 μg/L were found in 92% of patients *696*

Phosphate *Serum* *Decrease* Treatment of pernicious anemia is a less common cause of severe hypophosphatemia due to shift of phosphate into cells *969*

Phospholipids *Red Blood Cells* *Decrease* Decreased concentration in red cells *1290*

Serum *Decrease* All phospholipid fractions decreased in relapse *5550*

Platelets *Blood* *Decrease* Anemia, leukopenia (primarily granulopenia) and thrombocytopenia. Occasionally, the primary reduction may be in only 1 of these 3 major formed elements of the blood. May present initially with bleeding associated with thrombocytopenia *900* Generally reduced, may be < 100,000 /µL *5699* *3968*

Poikilocytes *Blood* *Increase* Many bizarre-shaped corpuscles are found *2034*

Potassium *Serum* *Decrease* Slightly reduced *5699* 17 of 34 patients had a concentration of < 4 mmol/L, the lower limit of normal *2945*

Reticulocytes *Blood* *Decrease* Inappropriately low corrected count due to marrow failure *2039*
Blood *No Effect* Usually within normal limits in untreated patients *2034*

Taurine *Urine* *Increase* May be slight excess of urinary amino acids, especially taurine *5241* Amino aciduria with an excess excretion of taurine, especially if there is associated subacute combined degeneration of the spinal cord. Amino aciduria does not occur in other megaloblastic anemias *5545* May be slight excess of urinary amino acids, especially taurine *1537*

Triglycerides *Serum* *Increase* In relapse, increased free fatty acid and triglyceride concentrations but decreased concentrations of total cholesterol, unesterified cholesterol and all examined phospholipid fractions *5550*

Uric Acid *Serum* *Decrease* Decreased in some patients in relapse *5544* Rarely reported *1980*
Serum *Increase* Especially after treatment *1290*

Urobilinogen *Feces* *Increase* Possibly in some cases *1290*
Urine *Increase* Possibly in some cases *1290*

Uropepsinogen *Urine* *Decrease* With achlorhydria *1290*

Vitamin B_{12} *Serum* *Decrease* In 20 patients with pernicious anemia concentrations ranged from 20 to 40 pg/mL compared with 145 to 914 pg/mL in 75 healthy individuals when concentrations measure on Sanofi Access analyzer *3047* Markedly decreased, mean value in 39 patients was 34 pg/mL compared to 385 pg/mL in normals *4448*

Vitamin B_{12} Binding Capacity *Serum* *Increase* Increased binding capacity, mean concentration of 1,682 (normal 1,208 pg/mL) and decreased serum concentration *4448*

Zinc *Serum* *Decrease* Decreased *4464* *5083*

281.20 Folic Acid Deficiency

Acetylcholinesterase *Red Blood Cells* *Decrease* Megaloblastic anemia during relapse *3141*

Aldolase *Serum* *Increase* 12 of 16 patients had levels elevated from 2 - 20 times the normal mean *2105* Increased less consistently and to a lesser degree than LD *5699* *1337*

Alkaline Phosphatase *Serum* *Decrease* Reported effect *5392* Observed effect *5677*

Amino Acids *Urine* *Increase* May be slight excess of urinary amino acids, especially taurine *5241* *1537* Aminoaciduria reportedly occurs, but observers differ on its frequency and significance *5677*

Bilirubin *Serum* *Increase* Observed effect *367* Slightly to moderately increased *5677*

Bilirubin, Indirect *Serum* *Increase* Slight indirect hyperbilirubinemia as a result of increased production of bile pigment. Normal values are common and values 2 mg/dL are unusual *5699*

Bleeding Time *Patient* *Increase* May be prolonged *5699*

Cells *Bone Marrow* *Increase* Aspirated bone marrow is cellular and often hyperplastic *5677* Bone marrow shows megaloblastic dysplasia that varies from mild to marked in megaloblastic anemia of infancy *5544*

Cholesterol *Serum* *Decrease* Reported effect *347* Hypocholesterolemia occurred consistently in 10 patients with anemia. Values ranged from 80 - 180 mg/dL *5645*

Cholinesterase *Serum* *Decrease* Observed effect *5677* Reported effect *3466*

Clot Retraction *Blood* *Decrease* May be poor *5699*

Complement C_3 *Serum* *Decrease* Significantly reduced in patients with vitamin B_{12} deficiency. Levels correlate with the degree of anemia but not with serum vitamin B_{12} levels at diagnosis *2242*

Copper *Serum* *Increase* Due to intramedullary hemolysis found in megaloblastic anemias *5544* A secondary finding *367*

Erythrocyte Survival *Red Blood Cells* *Decrease* Ranged from 27 - 75 days in 5 patients (normal of 120 days) *4862* Moderately reduced *5699* Ranged from 27 - 75 days in 5 patients (normal of 120 days) *3138*

Erythrocytes *Blood* *Decrease* Pancytopenia is a common feature in vitamin B_{12} and folic acid deficiency *5677* Depressed to a greater degree than other parameters *1980*

Folate *Red Blood Cells* *Decrease* A better measure of tissue folate and is less dependent on recent intake than serum *1980*
Serum *Decrease* When intake is reduced, the serum level falls promptly and precedes evidence of tissue deficiency *1980* Low; < 4 ng/mL *2039*

Glucose-6-Phosphate Dehydrogenase
Red Blood Cells *Increase* Elevated in 5 of 9 patients. Upper limit of normal 4.6 units *2105*
Serum *Increase* Increased to about the same extent as LD *1337* Elevated in 12 of 12 patients from 2.5 - 20 times the normal mean *2105* Increased to about the same extent as LD *5699* Reported effect *5677* *2106*

Hematocrit *Blood* *Decrease* Anemia is normochromic (unless iron deficiency coexists) and macrocytic, with MCV ranging from 100 to 150 fL *5677* Anemia may be very severe or very mild *5699* Anemia ranges from absent to severe *1980* Hematocrit levels ranged from 12 - 25% in 10 patients *5645*

Hemoglobin *Blood* *Decrease* Concentration ranges from very severe to near normal. Usually < 7 - 8 g/dL at presentation *5699* Anemia is normochromic (unless iron deficiency coexists) and macrocytic, with MCV ranging from 100 to > 150 fL *5677* Anemia ranges from absent to severe *1980*

Hemoglobin F *Blood* *Increase* Minimal elevation occurs in about 15% of patients with megaloblastic anemia *5544*

Homocysteine *Plasma* *Increase* Concentration increased by more than 3 SD above mean in 89.8% of episodes in patients with folate deficiency and anemia *4598* In 19 patients with folate concentrations less than 2 µg/L, 137 with low-normal concentrations of 2 - 3.9 µg/L and 44 subjects with normal concentrations of 4 - 17.9 µg/L serum concentration of homocysteine negatively correlated with serum folate concentration *5346* Increased concentration observed in patients with folic acid deficiency *2952*
Urine *Increase* Increased excretion observed in patients with folic acid deficiency *2952*

Iron *Bone Marrow* *Increase* Marrow sideroblasts and reticuloendothelial stores tend to be increased *5699*
Serum *Increase* Slightly to moderately increased *5677* Moderately increased unless there is associated iron deficiency *773*

Iron-binding Capacity, Total *Serum* *Decrease* Total plasma capacity tends to be slightly reduced *5699*

Isocitrate Dehydrogenase *Red Blood Cells* *Increase* 6 out of 8 patients had elevated concentration. The highest elevation was 7.3 U/L and the normal upper limit was 2.5 U/L *2105*
Serum *Increase* Increased less consistently and to a lesser degree than LD *1337* Serum levels 5 times the upper limit of normal *1290* In 5 of 9 patients, the plasma level was elevated above the maximum normal limit *2105* Increased less consistently and to a lesser degree than LD *5699*

Lactate *Blood* *Increase* Reported effect *367*

Lactate Dehydrogenase *Red Blood Cells* *Increase* 5 of 15 patients had RBC concentrations above the normal upper limit of 96 U/L *2105*
Serum *Increase* Mean value in 16 patients was 2,335 U/L (normal 116 U/L) *118* Magnitude of increase is related to the degree of anemia *5699* Observed effect *2105* More sensitive reflection of this disease state than other tests. 2 - 40 fold elevations. Almost all patients have increased concentrations, often marked *1025* In some cases; LD activity and red cell count inversely related in folic acid and/or vitamin B_{12} deficiency *1290* More sensitive reflection of this disease state than other tests. 2 - 40 fold elevations. Almost all patients have increased concentrations, often marked *1642* Observed effect *1980* In 13 patients ranged from normal to 40 fold elevation *4995*

281.20 Folic Acid Deficiency *(continued)*

Lactate Dehydrogenase Isoenzyme-5 *Serum* *Increase* Increased to about the same extent as total LD *5699* *1337*

Lactate Dehydrogenase Isoenzymes
Red Blood Cells *Increase* In normal erythrocytes, LD_2 activity exceeds that of LD_1. In megaloblastic anemia, LD_1 exceeds LD_2 *5698* Reported effect *5677*
Serum *Increase* Isozymes 1 and 2 are markedly elevated in rough proportion to the severity of the anemia *1355* Observed effect *5677* LD_1 and LD_2 account for the increase in total LD *5699*

Leukocytes *Blood* *Decrease* Pancytopenia is a common feature in vitamin B_{12} and folic acid deficiency *5677* Varies with degree of anemia from normal to very low. Usually due to absolute neutropenia *5699*

Lysozyme *Serum* *Increase* Observed effect *4079* *5677*

Macrocytes *Blood* *Increase* In 75 elderly patients with macrocytosis folic acid deficiency was responsible in 15 *3232*

Malate Dehydrogenase *Red Blood Cells* *Increase* 10 of 16 patients had red cell activity elevated significantly above the normal upper limit of 96 *2105*
Serum *Increase* Increased to about the same extent as total LD *5677* In 17 patients, the plasma content was consistently and markedly elevated *2105* Increased to about the same extent as LD *1337* Serum levels rise to up to 40 times normal value *1290* Increased to about the same extent as LD *5699*

MCH *Blood* *Increase* Erythrocytes are increased in diameter and thickness. Abnormalities are reflected in the increased MCV and MCH *1980* Generally 33 - 38 pg in moderate anemia, and 33 - 56 pg, with severe cases (normal = 27 - 31 pg) *5699*

MCHC *Blood* *No Effect* When not complicated by iron deficiency, anemia is normochromic and macrocytic *5699*

MCV *Blood* *Increase* Erythrocytes are increased in diameter and thickness. Abnormalities are reflected in the increased MCV and MCH *1980* In 100 patients with macrocytosis (MCV greater than 110 fL) 3 had folate deficiency *4924* Usually macrocytic anemia. Rise in MCV is largely proportional to the degree of anemia. Usual values are 95 - 110 fL, but may be 110 - 160 fL with severe anemia *5699* Anemia is normochromic (unless iron deficiency coexists) and macrocytic, with MCV ranging from 100 to > 150 fL *5677* Macrocytic anemia may occur due to vitamin B_{12} or folate deficiency with MCV > 100 fL *1098*

Methylmalonate *Serum* *Increase* Concentration increased more than 3 SD above the mean in 4.1% of 98 episodes in patients with folate deficiency and anemia *4598*
Urine *No Effect* Excretion unaffected with pure folate deficiency *5677*

Neutrophils *Blood* *Decrease* Neutropenia and thrombocytopenia are less frequent but still common. Rarely severe *1980*

N-Formiminoglutamic Acid *Urine* *Increase* Urine FIGLU is increased; disappears after folic acid treatment in megaloblastic anemia of infancy *5544* Increased excretion is a consistent feature of folate deficiency but is not confined to that situation *1980* Less specific than the serum folate assay. It becomes abnormal later and thus gives a better measure of tissue coenzyme levels *5677*

Osmotic Fragility *Red Blood Cells* *Decrease* Observed effect *5544*

Platelets *Blood* *Decrease* Neutropenia and thrombocytopenia are less frequent but still common. Rarely severe *1980* Generally reduced, may be < 100,000 /μL *5699* *3968* Pancytopenia is a common feature in vitamin B_{12} and folic acid deficiency *5677*

Potassium *Serum* *Decrease* 17 of 34 patients had a concentration of < 4 mmol/L, the lower limit of normal *2945* Slightly reduced *5699*

Reticulocytes *Blood* *Decrease* Tends to be low or at the low extreme of the normal range *1980* Lower than normal, both in absolute and in percentage terms *5677*

Taurine *Urine* *Increase* May be slight excess of urinary amino acids, especially taurine *1537* *5241*

Uric Acid *Serum* *Decrease* Often depressed *5677*
Urine *Decrease* Often depressed *5677*

Vitamin B_{12} *Serum* *No Effect* Concentration unaffected with pure folate deficiency *5677*

Vitamin B_{12} Binding Capacity *Serum* *Increase* Significant elevation; usually correlated with WBC in peripheral blood *4448*

Hemolytic Disorders

282.00 Hereditary Spherocytosis

Alanine Aminotransferase *Serum* *Increase* Observed effect *1980*

Aldolase *Serum* *Increase* Observed effect *1980*

Anisocytes *Blood* *Increase* Anisocytosis is marked *5545*

Aspartate Aminotransferase *Serum* *Increase* Observed effect *1980*

Basophils *Blood* *Increase* During the chronic stage of anemia *5699* *1640*

Bilirubin *Serum* *Increase* Primarily indirect *5677*

Bilirubin, Indirect *Serum* *Increase* Typical observation *5677* Mean 1.6 ± 1.1 mg/dL *3188*

Calcium *Red Blood Cells* *Increase* A marked increase in calcium uptake was observed in the ATP depleted red cells of the unsplenectomized patients *4801* RBC content of Ca^{++} is increased *1441* In 18 cases of congenital hemolytic anemias, increased erythrocytic Ca^{++} level was observed in 10 cases *410*

Cholesterol *Serum* *Decrease* Low serum values correlated well with hemoglobin concentration *4721* Observed in 8 patients. Values ranged from 110 - 170 mg/dL *4363*

Coombs' Test *Serum* *Negative* Usually negative *5699*

Coproporphyrin *Urine* *Increase* Associated with increased hemopoiesis *367* Increased hemopoiesis *1290*

Creatine Kinase *Serum* *Decrease* Reported effect *5677*
Serum *No Effect* Usually no effect observed *1980*

Erythrocyte Sedimentation Rate *Blood* *Decrease* Very low rate typically observed *4949*

Erythrocytes *Blood* *Decrease* Anemia may be absent, moderate or severe. The RBC count is reduced proportionately to the hemoglobin concentration *900* Reductions in RBC count may not be proportional to hemoglobin *5699*

Haptoglobin *Serum* *Decrease* Decreased in hemoglobinemia (related to the duration and severity of hemolysis) due to extravascular hemolysis. Seen in hereditary spherocytosis with marked hemolysis. Becomes normal in 4 - 6 days after treatment with splenectomy *5544*

Hematocrit *Blood* *Decrease* In 91% of 12 patients at initial hospitalization for this disorder *3053* Anemia may be absent, moderate or severe. RBC is reduced proportionately to the hemoglobin concentration *900* Observed effect *1576* Hematocrit values ranged from 21 - 36% in 8 patients *5645* Hematocrit typically reduced *5677*

Hemoglobin *Blood* *Decrease* In 91% of 12 patients at initial hospitalization for this disorder *1576* The mean value of the hemoglobin concentration in a large series is usually 11.5 g/dL rarely as low as 7 g/dL *900* Concentrations between 9 - 12 g/dL are most common. Rapid fall to 3 - 4 g/dL may occur during a crisis *5699* Anemia typically observed *5677*
Blood *No Effect* In approximately 10 - 20% of patients, particularly young men *4979*
Plasma *No Effect* Very little or none. Hemoglobin released during hemolysis is catabolized at the site of destruction *4979*

Iron *Serum* *Increase* May occur *5699* Due to increased rate of blood destruction *1290*

Iron-binding Capacity, Total *Serum* *Increase* Hemolytic anemia, with raised serum iron concentration (i.e., the total transferrin concentration is increased, but the unsaturated iron binding capacity is reduced) *1290*

Lactate Dehydrogenase *Serum* *Increase* Occurs as a result of hemolysis *1980* In hemolytic anemia *1290*

Leukocytes *Blood* *Decrease* Normal except during aplastic crises *900*
Blood *Increase* In 40% of 12 patients at initial hospitalization for this disorder *1576* Generally slightly increased. Marked increase and shift to the left after a crisis *5699*
Blood *No Effect* Normal except during aplastic crises *900*

Lipids *Serum* *Decrease* Generalized hypolipidemia; with reduced phospholipids and total lipids occurs in children as well as adults with uncomplicated cases *4721*

Lipoproteins *Serum* *Decrease* All classes of lipoproteins were reduced in children as well as adults with uncomplicated cases of congenital hemolytic anemia and spherocytosis *4721*

Lymphocytes *Blood* *Increase* During the chronic stage of anemia *1640* *5699*

MCH *Blood* *Increase* Variations usually correspond to changes in volume *5699*

MCHC *Blood* *Increase* Very high *2039* Usually elevated, often as high as 37% *1385* Concentration typically of the order of 37 - 39 g/dL *5677* The mean MCHC is usually increased (36 - 39%) reflecting the loss of membrane surface in relation to cell volume *900* Characteristically high, 37 - 39 g/dL *5699*

MCV *Blood* *Decrease* Small, dense, round, red cells (microspherocytes) seen in large numbers *2039* May be normal, high, or very low *5699* Mean value in 76 affected patients was 83 ± 8.5 fL; ranging from 62 - 125 fL *3188*
Blood *Increase* May be normal, high, or very low *5699*

N-Formiminoglutamic Acid *Urine* *Increase* Reported effect *5544*

Osmotic Fragility *Red Blood Cells* *Increase* Usual finding *5677* Typically increased. Hemolysis may be complete at the concentration where it normally commences *5699* Typical observation with associated hemolysis *367* Almost always increased; in cases in which the cell defect is minor, incubation will bring out the abnormal fragility *1980*

Phosphate *Serum* *Increase* Reported effect *1980*

Phospholipids *Serum* *Decrease* Generalized hypolipidemia; with reduced phospholipids and total lipids occurs in children as well as adults with uncomplicated cases *4721*

Plasma Cells *Blood* *Increase* During the chronic stage of anemia *5699* *1640*

Platelets *Blood* *Decrease* Rarely moderately reduced *5699*
Blood *Increase* Increased during aplastic crises *900* Usually within the normal to high range or slight increase *5699*
Blood *No Effect* Normal except during aplastic crises *900*

Poikilocytes *Blood* *Increase* Slight poikilocytosis *5545*

Pyruvate Kinase *Red Blood Cells* *Increase* Mean activity in 5 patients with hereditary spherocytosis of 20 U/g hemoglobin compared with that in 48 healthy men, 14.6 ± 2.0 U/g hemoglobin and in 41 healthy women 17.5 ± 2.4 U/g hemoglobin *3623*

Reticulocytes *Blood* *Increase* Is increased 5 - 20% *900* Characteristic increase *5699* Concentration typically increased above 5% *5677* Common chronic hemolytic finding *4979*

Soluble Transferrin Receptor *Serum* *Increase* Concentration increases with disease *4784*

Triglycerides *Serum* *Decrease* The majority of values were low (15/18 children) but there was a greater scatter of triglyceride than cholesterol concentrations *4721*

Uric Acid *Serum* *Increase* Occurs with hemolysis *1980* Associated with hemolysis *2707*

Urobilinogen *Feces* *Increase* As much as 5 - 20 times normal *5699* Occurs as a result of hemolysis *5677*
Urine *Increase* Hemolysis observed *2034* Associated with hemolysis *5677*

282.10 Hereditary Elliptocytosis

Bilirubin *Serum* *Increase* In patients with more severe forms of this disease there may be a compensated hemolytic anemia with raised serum bilirubin *900* Hemolysis and hyperbilirubinemia have been observed in the newborn period *218* Primarily indirect *2034*

Coombs' Test *Serum* *Negative* In uncomplicated cases *5699*

Haptoglobin *Serum* *Decrease* In patients with more severe forms of this disease there may be a compensated hemolytic anemia with reduced serum haptoglobin *900* Effect observed with hemolysis *5677*

Hematocrit *Blood* *Decrease* In severe cases *5677*

Hemoglobin *Blood* *Decrease* In severe cases, levels rarely fall below 9 - 10 g/dL *5677*
Plasma *Increase* In 10 - 15% of patients the rate of hemolysis is substantially increased with red cell half-life times as short as 5 days *5677* Hemolysis and hyperbilirubinemia have been observed in the newborn period *218*

Hemoglobin A_{1c} *Blood* *Decrease* Significantly lower ($p < 0.0005$) in patients with hemolytic anemia (n = 20) compared to patients with nonhemolytic anemia and normal controls *3996*

Lactate Dehydrogenase *Serum* *Increase* In severe cases *900*

Osmotic Fragility *Red Blood Cells* *Increase* Usually normal but may be increased in patients with overt hemolysis *5677*
Red Blood Cells *No Effect* Usually normal even after incubation *5699*

Reticulocytes *Blood* *Increase* The great majority of these patients manifest only mild hemolysis with hemoglobin > 12 g/dL, reticulocytes < 4%. In 10 - 15% of patients the rate of hemolysis is increased and reticulocytosis ranging to 20% *5677* In patients with more severe forms of this disease there may be a compensated hemolytic anemia with raised reticulocyte count *900*

Urobilinogen *Feces* *Increase* In severe cases *900*
Urine *Increase* In severe cases *900*

282.20 Anemias Due To Disorders of Glutathione Metabolism

Albumin *Serum* *No Effect* Concentration usually normal *5544*

Alkaline Phosphatase *White Blood Cells* *No Effect* Typical observation *5544*

α_1-Antitrypsin *Serum* *No Effect* Concentration usually normal *5544*

Bilirubin *Serum* *Increase* Varying degrees may be evident *5677*

Bilirubin, Indirect *Serum* *Increase* Indirect laboratory evidence that hemolysis is present *900*

Complement C_3 *Serum* *No Effect* Concentration usually normal *5544*

Folate *Serum* *Decrease* Excessive utilization due to marked cellular proliferation *5544*

Haptoglobin *Serum* *Decrease* Effect observed with hemolysis *5544*

Hemoglobin *Blood* *Decrease* As the hemoglobin level falls, reticulocytosis occurs and polychromasia is seen *5677*
Plasma *Increase* Indirect laboratory evidence that hemolysis is present *900*
Urine *Increase* Intravascular hemolysis due to antibodies *5544* Indirect laboratory evidence that hemolysis is present *900*

Hemoglobin A_{1c} *Blood* *Decrease* Significantly lower ($p < 0.0005$) in patients with hemolytic anemia (n = 20) compared to patients with nonhemolytic anemia and normal controls *3996*

Iron *Serum* *Increase* Elevated serum iron and transferrin saturation. Indirect laboratory evidence that hemolysis is present *900*

Iron Saturation *Serum* *Increase* Elevated serum iron and transferrin saturation. Indirect laboratory evidence that hemolysis is present *900* May be completely saturated *5699*

Lactate Dehydrogenase *Serum* *Increase* 2 to 4 times normal values *1025* Especially if intravascular; derived from RBCs *1290*

Reticulocytes *Blood* *Increase* As the hemoglobin level falls, reticulocytosis occurs, and polychromasia is seen *5677* Laboratory clue that hemolysis may be present *900*

Urobilinogen *Urine* *Increase* Increased hemolysis *5544*

282.20 Glucose-6-Phosphate Dehydrogenase Deficiency

Chitotriosidase *Serum* *No Effect* Normal activity observed in one patient with condition *1917*

Glucose-6-Phosphate Dehydrogenase
Red Blood Cells *Decrease* Mean concentration in 7 African-Americans of 1.5 ± 0.52 U/g hemoglobin significantly different from 7.4 ± 1.21 U/g hemoglobin in 65 healthy matched controls *2402*

Glutathione *Red Blood Cells* *Decrease* Mean concentration in 7 African-Americans of 4.2 ± 0.83 µmol/g hemoglobin significantly different from 6.2 ± 1.33 µmol/g hemoglobin in 65 healthy matched controls *2402*

282.20 Glucose-6-Phosphate Dehydrogenase Deficiency *(continued)*

Glutathione, Oxidized *Red Blood Cells* *Increase* Mean concentration in 7 African-Americans of 1.32 ± 0.41 µmol/g hemoglobin significantly different from 0.81 ± 0.24 µmol/g hemoglobin in 65 healthy matched controls *2402*

Malondialdehyde *Red Blood Cells* *Increase* Mean concentration in 7 African-Americans of 1.46 ± 0.11 µmol/mL cells significantly different from 1.31 ± 0.16 µmol/mL cells in 65 healthy matched controls *2402*

Serum *Increase* Mean concentration in 7 African-Americans of 0.51 ± 0.08 nmol/mL significantly different from 0.41 ± 0.12 nmol/mL in 65 healthy matched controls *2402*

282.31 Hereditary Nonspherocytic Hemolytic Anemia

Bilirubin, Indirect *Serum* *Increase* In some cases *5677*

Cells *Bone Marrow* *Increase* Erythroid hyperplasia *5677*

Haptoglobin *Serum* *Decrease* Reflects chronic hemolysis *413*

Hematocrit *Blood* *Decrease* Anemia *5677*

Hemoglobin *Blood* *Decrease* In most subjects, the range is 5 - 11.5 g/dL *5677*

Plasma *Increase* During acute hemolysis *900*

Urine *Increase* During acute hemolysis *900* Hemosiderinuria and hemoglobinuria, particularly when oxidative stresses have been induced by drugs or other environmental factors *5677*

Hexokinase *Red Blood Cells* *Decrease* Deficient in erythrocytes in congenital nonspherocytic hemolytic anemia *1290*

Iron *Bone Marrow* *Increase* Marrow iron content is normal to increased *900*

Lactate Dehydrogenase *Serum* *Increase* In hemolytic anemias *5863*

Leukocytes *Blood* *Increase* Tends to be normal or elevated with some increase in the immature granulocytes *900*

Blood *No Effect* Tends to be normal or elevated with some increase in the immature granulocytes *900*

MCV *Blood* *Increase* Mild to moderate macrocytosis *5677*

Osmotic Fragility *Red Blood Cells* *No Effect* The osmotic fragility of fresh erythrocytes is usually normal *5677*

Platelets *Blood* *Increase* Normal or slightly increased *900*

Pyruvate Kinase *Red Blood Cells* *Decrease* PK deficiency is limited to the red cell; the leukocyte does not share the deficiency *5677*

Reticulocytes *Blood* *Increase* Increase in count is marked, even with mild anemia with hereditary nonspherocytic hemolytic anemias *5545*

282.40 α-Thalassemia

Hematocrit *Blood* *No Effect* In 84 patients with α-thalassemia mean value of 37 ± 5.0% not significantly different from 41 ± 3.8% in 64 normal individuals *1836*

MCH *Blood* *Decrease* In 84 patients with α-thalassemia trait mean value of 23 ± 2.2 pg significantly different from 30 ± 1.8 pg in 64 normal individuals *1836*

MCHC *Blood* *Decrease* In 84 patients with α-thalassemia trait mean value of 32 ± 0.9 significantly different from 34 ± 0.7 in 64 normal individuals *1836*

MCV *Blood* *Decrease* In 84 patients with α-thalassemia mean value of 70 ± 5.4 fL significantly different from 88 ± 4.8 fL in 64 normal individuals *1836*

Zinc Protoporphyrin:Heme Ratio *Blood* *Increase* In 84 patients with α-thalassemia trait mean ratio of 73 ± 37 µmol/mol not significantly different from 60 ± 8 µmol/mol in 64 normal individuals, with 17 (20%) of affected individuals having ratios greater than 80 µmol/mol *1836*

282.40 Thalassemia Intermedia

Erythropoietin *Serum* *Increase* In 45 patients with thalassemia intermedia, mean concentration of 195 ± 191 mIU/mL significantly increased when compared with 12.8 ± 2.6 mIU/mL *1220*

Ferritin *Serum* *Increase* In 18 untransfused patients with thalassemia intermedia mean concentration of 639 ± 500 ng/mL significantly different from normal *1221*

Hemoglobin *Blood* *Decrease* In 18 untransfused patients with thalassemia intermedia mean concentration of 9.6 ± 0.78 g/dL significantly different from normal *1221*

Interleukin-8 *Serum* *Increase* In 18 untransfused patients with thalassemia intermedia mean concentration of 366 ± 294 pg/mL significantly different from 34.2 ± 32 pg/mL in 15 healthy normal controls *1221*

282.40 Thalassemia Minor

Adenosine Diphosphate *Red Blood Cells* *Decrease* ATP and ADP levels are decreased in erythrocytes from individuals with β-thalassemia minor *5852*

Adenosine Triphosphate *Red Blood Cells* *Decrease* ATP and ADP levels are decreased in erythrocytes from individuals with β-thalassemia minor *5852*

Anisocytes *Blood* *Increase* Defective globin synthesis *1980* Aniso- and poikilocytosis may be very striking and far out of proportion to the degree of anemia *5699*

Basophilic Stippling *Blood* *Increase* Mild anemia, usually with microcytosis, hypochromia, stippling, and target cells usually occurs in heterozygous beta thalassemia *367*

Cells *Bone Marrow* *Increase* Bone marrow is cellular and shows erythroid hyperplasia and contains stainable iron with thalassemias *5545*

Copper *Serum* *Increase* May be increased on occasion *709* In 42 patients (age 3 mo to 22 y) with homozygous β-thalassemia and thalassemia intermedia, serum zinc was significantly decreased while Cu and Fe were increased *168*

Erythrocyte Survival *Red Blood Cells* *Decrease* Normal or slightly shortened *4052*

Erythrocytes *Blood* *Decrease* With the more severe expression of the disease, homozygote or heterozygote, all parameters of erythrocyte numbers are depressed *1980*

Blood *Increase* Typically, the RBC are increased in number but are microcytic hypochromic and show prominent poikilocytosis and targeting *900* In many heterozygotes the hematocrit and hemoglobin are slightly depressed but the erythrocyte number is normal or increased *1980* Over 5.7 million/µL and MCV is < 75 fL are most often due to thalassemia trait *5545*

Blood *No Effect* In many heterozygotes the hematocrit and hemoglobin are slightly depressed but the erythrocyte number is normal or increased *1980*

Ferritin *Serum* *No Effect* No significant effect observed *413*

Folate *Serum* *Decrease* Reflects increased marrow utilization of folate *413*

Hematocrit *Blood* *Decrease* In periods of stress such as pregnancy or during severe infection, a moderate degree of anemia may be present *5677* Mild anemia, usually with microcytosis, hypochromia, stippling, and target cells usually occurs in heterozygous beta thalassemia *367*

Hemoglobin *Blood* *Decrease* Tends to be 1 - 2 g/dL lower than in normal subjects *900* In periods of stress such as pregnancy or during severe infection, a moderate degree of anemia may be present in these patients *5677* Mild anemia, usually with microcytosis, hypochromia, stippling, and target cells usually occurs *367* Hypochromic microcytic anemia in thalassemia minor can be distinguished from iron deficiency by a normal or even elevated serum iron concentration and by the failure of the anemia to respond to iron *2039*

Hemoglobin F *Blood* *Increase* Elevated in about 50% of patients, usually to 1 - 3% and rarely to more than 5% *5677*

Iron *Serum* *Increase* Hypochromic microcytic anemia in these patients can be distinguished from iron deficiency anemia by a normal or even elevated serum iron concentration and by

the failure of the anemia to respond to iron *2039* In 42 patients (age 3 mo to 22 y) with homozygous β-thalassemia and thalassemia intermedia serum zinc was significantly decreased while Cu and Fe were increased *168*
Serum *No Effect* Normal concentration usually observed *2034*

Iron-binding Capacity, Total *Serum* *Increase* Total capacity is increased *5545*

MCH *Blood* *Decrease* The most striking and consistent finding is that of small, poorly hemoglobinized red cells, MCH values of 20 - 22 pg and MCV values of 50 - 70 fL *5677* Mean in 45 cases was 20.26 ± 2.23 pg *4053*

MCHC *Blood* *Decrease* Slightly reduced. Mean in 45 cases was 31.22 ± 0.96 % *4053*

MCV *Blood* *Decrease* Unusually low for the mild degree of anemia *5699* In 45 cases, the range was 52-75, with a mean of 64.7 fL *4053* The most striking and consistent finding is that of small, poorly hemoglobinized red cells, MCH values of 20 - 22 pg and MCV values of 50 - 70 fL *5677* Mean concentration of 68 ± 6 fL in 44 patients with α-thalassemia minor significantly different from that in healthy controls *2037*

Osmotic Fragility *Red Blood Cells* *Decrease* Decreased osmotic fragility is a method for identifying the heterozygote *2039*

Phosphate *Serum* *Decrease* 24 h excretion level was higher than net absorption, indicating normal phosphate absorption and high renal phosphaturia, leading to deficiency *2920*
Urine *Increase* 24 h excretion level was higher than net absorption, indicating normal phosphate absorption and high renal phosphaturia, leading to deficiency *2920*

Poikilocytes *Blood* *Increase* Defective globin synthesis *1980* Aniso- and poikilocytosis may be very striking and far out of proportion to the degree of anemia *5699*

Protoporphyrin *Red Blood Cells* *Increase* May be increased on occasion *709*

Reticulocytes *Blood* *Increase* Normal or slightly increased *4015* Count is increased (2 - 10%) with thalassemias *5545*

Target Cells *Blood* *Increase* Mild anemia, usually with microcytosis, hypochromia, stippling, and target cells usually occurs in heterozygous beta thalassemia *367*

Zinc Protoporphyrin *Red Blood Cells* *No Effect* Mean concentration of 0.18 ± 0.05 mmol/mol hemoglobin in 44 patients with α-thalassemia minor not significantly different from 0.06 - 0.22 mmol/mol hemoglobin in healthy controls *2037*

282.41 Thalassemia Major

Adenosine Deaminase *Serum* *Increase* Significantly elevated and related to the transfusion schedule of the patient *4264*

Amino Acids *Urine* *Increase* Found to be markedly increased in children *828*

Anisocytes *Blood* *Increase* The red cells show marked anisopoikilocytosis, with hypochromia, target-cell formation, and a variable degree of basophilic stippling *5677*

Aspartate Aminotransferase *Serum* *Increase* Usually elevated *5699*

Basophilic Stippling *Blood* *Increase* The red cells show marked anisopoikilocytosiss, with hypochromia, target-cell formation, and a variable degree of basophilic stippling *5677*

Bilirubin *Serum* *Increase* Usually increased *2039*

Bilirubin, Indirect *Serum* *Increase* Unconjugated bilirubinemia (1 - 3 mg/dL) and slightly increased icterus index *5699*

Cells *Bone Marrow* *Increase* Bone marrow is cellular and shows erythroid hyperplasia *5545*

Copper *Serum* *Increase* May be increased *5699* In 42 patients (age 3 mo to 22 y) with homozygous β-thalassemia and thalassemia intermedia, serum zinc was significantly decreased while Cu and Fe were increased *168*

Erythrocyte Survival *Red Blood Cells* *Decrease* Usually shortened *5677* Generally ranges from 7 to 22 days as measured by ^{51}Chromium-labeling *5057*

Erythrocytes *Blood* *Decrease* With the more severe expression of the disease, homozygote or heterozygote, all parameters of erythrocyte numbers are depressed *1980* Count is often between 2 - 3 million/µL, with great variation in size and shape of cells *5699*

Ferritin *Serum* *Increase* In 48 patients with thalassemia major without cirrhosis median concentration before phlebotomy of 1,498 ng/mL *134*

Glucose Tolerance *Serum* *Decrease* 50% of patients had some abnormality in their oral test, 5 falling into the diabetic category. Intolerance correlated with number of transfusions received and age *4597*

Gonadotropin, Pituitary *Plasma* *Decrease* Markedly impaired gonadotropin response to LH releasing hormones in β-thalassemia *2905*

Haptoglobin *Serum* *Decrease* Decreased in hemoglobinemias (related to the duration and severity of hemolysis) due to extravascular hemolysis *5544*

Hematocrit *Blood* *Decrease* Anemia is severe, microcytic and hypochromic *2034*

Hemoglobin *Blood* *Decrease* May be in the 2 - 3 g/dL range or even lower *5677* Severe hemolytic anemia, hypochromic and microcytic in type, is found *2039* Common very low in untransfused patients usually below 7 g/dL *900*
Plasma *Increase* Moderate increase *5544*

Hemoglobin F *Blood* *Increase* The proportion is usually between 20 - 60%, but values as high as 90% may occur *367* Increased, ranging from 10 - 90% is characteristic and there may be a total deficiency of hemoglobin A synthesis *5677*

Iron *Bone Marrow* *Increase* Abundance of iron in the reticuloendothelial cells *5699*
Liver *Increase* In 48 patients with thalassemia major without cirrhosis mean concentration before phlebotomy 10.8 ± 6.3 mg/g dry weight *134*
Serum *Increase* In 42 patients (age 3 mo to 22 y) with homozygous β-thalassemia and thalassemia intermedia, serum zinc was significantly decreased while Cu and Fe were increased *168* Serum concentration is elevated with increased saturation of iron-binding protein *367* In contrast to the thin cells of iron deficiency, the serum iron is normal or increased *1980*

Iron-binding Capacity, Total *Serum* *Increase* Total capacity is increased *5545*

Iron Saturation *Serum* *Increase* Serum concentration is elevated with increased saturation of iron-binding protein *367* Often totally saturated *4900*

Lactate Dehydrogenase *Serum* *Increase* May be markedly elevated in the serum presumably due to marrow hyperplasia and ineffective erythropoiesis *900* Usually elevated *5699*

Leukocytes *Blood* *Decrease* With the gross splenomegaly which may occur, a secondary thrombocytopenia and leukopenia frequently develop, leading to a further tendency to infection and bleeding *5677*
Blood *Increase* Slightly elevated unless there is secondary hypersplenism *5677* Leukocytosis may be marked and persistent *367* Normoblasts, reticulocytes, and leukocytosis (about 20,000 /µL) with a shift to the left in the peripheral blood reflect the bone marrow hyperplasia *2039*

Lipids *Red Blood Cells* *Decrease* In 20 cases of thalassemia there was reduction in red cell lipids and their fractions, plasma lipids and their fractions, and derangement of liver functions compared to controls *2660*
Serum *Decrease* Serum total lipid levels were found to be low in children with β-thalassemia. The difference between the mean total lipid level in patients (365 ± 75 mg/dL) as compared to that of the controls (581 ± 94 mg/dL) was highly significant *5842* In 20 cases of thalassemia, there was reduction in red cell lipids and their fractions, plasma lipids and their fraction, and derangement of liver functions compared to controls *2660*

Lipoproteins, Pre-β *Serum* *Increase* Mean concentration in 50 children was significantly elevated *1128*

Lymphocytes *Blood* *Increase* Especially in infants *5699*

MCH *Blood* *Decrease* Defective globin synthesis *1980* Microcytic hypochromic anemia may occur due to blood loss, increased demand or dietary inadequacy. MCH < 27 pg, MCV < 80 fL *1098*

MCHC *Blood* *Decrease* Normal or slightly decreased *5545* Hypochromic anemia with MCHC between 23 - 32% *5699*

MCV *Blood* *Decrease* MCV < 75 fL are most often due to thalassemia trait *5545* Microcytic, hypochromic anemia may occur due to blood loss, increased demand or dietary inadequacy. MCH < 27 pg, MCV < 80 fL *1098* Hypochromic micro-

282.41 Thalassemia Major *(continued)*

MCV *(continued)*
cytic anemia with MCV between 28 - 43 fL *5699* In nonsplenectomized patients, large poikilocytes are common, whereas after splenectomy large flat macrocytes and small deformed microcytes are frequently seen *5677*

Monocytes *Blood Increase* May be somewhat increased *5699*

Osmotic Fragility *Red Blood Cells Decrease* Osmotic fragility is reduced; the red cells are usually resistant to hemolysis in hypotonic saline *2039*

Phosphate *Serum Decrease* 24 h excretion level was higher than net absorption, indicating normal phosphate absorption and high renal phosphaturia, leading to deficiency *2920*
Urine Increase 24 h excretion level was higher than net absorption, indicating normal phosphate absorption and high renal phosphaturia, leading to deficiency *2920*

Platelets *Blood Decrease* With the gross splenomegaly which may occur, a secondary thrombocytopenia and leukopenia frequently develop, leading to a further tendency to infection and bleeding *5677*
Blood Increase The white cell and platelet counts are slightly elevated unless there is secondary hypersplenism *5677*

Poikilocytes *Blood Increase* The red cells show marked anisopoikilocytosis, with hypochromia, target-cell formation, and a variable degree of basophilic stippling *5677*

Reticulocytes *Blood Increase* Only slightly increased *1980* Moderate increase (19,000 - 25,000 /µL) *2034* Moderately elevated *5677*
Blood No Effect Reticulocyte index normal or slightly increased *2039*

Target Cells *Blood Increase* The red cells show marked anisopoikilocytosiss, with hypochromia, target-cell formation, and a variable degree of basophilic stippling *5677*

Transferrin Saturation *Serum Increase* In 48 patients with thalassemia major without cirrhosis median saturation before phlebotomy 87% *134*

Triglycerides *Serum Increase* Significantly elevated mean concentrations were found in 50 children *1128*

Urobilinogen *Urine Increase* Increased in urine without bile *5545*

Zinc *Serum Decrease* In 42 patients ranging in age from 3 months to 22 years with homozygous β-thalassemia and thalassemia intermedia. Mean serum concentration was significantly decreased *168*

282.42 β-Thalassemia

Erythropoietin *Serum Increase* Concentrations are inversely related to the mean pre-transfusion hemoglobin concentration *5720*

Hematocrit *Blood No Effect* In 142 patients with β-thalassemia trait mean value of 37 ± 4.0% not significantly different from 41 ± 3.8% in 64 normal individuals *1836*

Hemoglobin *Blood Decrease* Baseline hemoglobin typically varies from 7.0 - 11 g/dL *5720*

Hemoglobin A_2 *Blood Increase* Values of 3.5 - 9% are found in patients with β-thalassemia trait *2952*

Hemoglobin F *Blood Increase* Concentration significantly higher than in hemoglobin S heterozygotes and in healthy controls *1322*

Interleukin-8 *Serum Increase* Patients with β-thalassemia had higher IL-8 concentrations than did normal controls, patients with liver disease, and patients on chronic transfusion. β-Thalassemic patients with severe liver siderosis and fibrosis had the highest IL-8 concentrations *5352*

MCH *Blood Decrease* In 12 patients with homozygous hemoglobin E mean value of 22 ± 2.8 pg significantly different from 30 ± 1.8 pg in 64 normal individuals *1836* In 142 patients with β-thalassemia trait mean value of 21 ± 1.8 pg significantly different from 30 ± 1.8 pg in 64 normal individuals *1836*

MCHC *Blood Decrease* In 142 patients with β-thalassemia trait mean value of 32 ± 0.8 significantly different from 34 ± 0.7 in 64 normal individuals *1836*

MCV *Blood Decrease* In 142 patients with β-thalassemia trait mean value of 65 ± 4.8 fL significantly different from 88 ± 4.8 fL in 64 normal individuals *1836* Mean concentration of 63 ± 4 fL in 57 patients with β-thalassemia significantly different from that in healthy controls *2037*

Soluble Intercellular Adhesion Molecule-1 *Serum Increase* Patients with β-thalassemia who had sustained bone marrow engraftment had significantly higher pretransplant mean concentration of 400 ng/mL than the mean of 312 ng/mL in a control marow donors group *748* Patients with β-thalassemia who had sustained bone marrow engraftment had significantly higher concentration of 400 ng/mL than 312 ng/mL in a control marow donors group *748*

Soluble Transferrin Receptor *Serum Increase* Concentration 1 - 2 times normal for the mean hemoglobin concentration between 10 and 11 g/dL, 1 - 4 times for hemoglobin levels from 9 to 10 g/dL and 2 - 6 times for hemoglobin levels from 8.6 to 10 g/dL *5720*

Zinc Protoporphyrin *Red Blood Cells Increase* Mean concentration of 0.25 ± 0.07 mmol/mol hemoglobin in 57 patients with β-thalassemia significantly different from 0.06 - 0.22 mmol/mol hemoglobin in healthy controls *2037*

Zinc Protoporphyrin:Heme Ratio *Blood Increase* In 142 patients with β-thalassemia trait mean ratio of 87 ± 32 µmol/mol significantly different from 60 ± 8 µmol/mol in 64 normal individuals, with 73 (51%) of affected individuals having ratios greater than 80 µmol/mol *1836*

282.50 Sickle Cell Trait

Circulating Endothelial Cells *Blood No Effect* In 3 blood donors with sickle cell trait mean concentration of 3.0 ± 2.6 cells/mL not significantly different from that in 14 healthy individuals in whom mean concentration was 2.6 ± 1.6 cells/mL *4930*

Hemoglobin A *Blood Decrease* In 37 African American adults reference range of 54.1 ± 2.6% of total hemoglobin significantly less than 93.6 ± 1.3% in 200 healthy controls *4376*

Hemoglobin A_2 *Blood Increase* In 37 African American adults reference range of 2.2 ± 1.1% of total hemoglobin compared with 1.2 ± 0.4% in 200 healthy controls *4376*

Hemoglobin F *Blood Decrease* In 37 African American adults reference range of 2.7 ± 1.5% of total hemoglobin less than 3.2 ± 0.7% in 200 healthy controls *4376*

Hemoglobin S *Blood Increase* In 37 African American adults reference range of 39.5 ± 0.2% of total hemoglobin *4376*

282.60 Sickle Cell Disease

Acid Phosphatase *Serum Increase* Marked rise may occur during a severe hemolytic episode *4707*

Albumin *Serum No Effect* In 18 black patients in Curacao with sickle cell disease mean concentration of 48 ± 1.8 g/L not significantly different from 47 ± 2.5 g/L in 15 controls without neurological disorders *5395*
Urine Increase May develop *900* Urine microalbumin/creatinine ratios of > 20 mg/g creatinine reported in 39 - 43% adults with HbSS *1144*

Aldolase *Red Blood Cells Increase* Mean red cell concentrations were slightly elevated in 15 patients. Mean of 2.2 U/L (normal 1.2 U/L) and range of 0.9 to 3.9 U/L *2105*
Serum Increase Slightly elevated in a group of 15 patients. The range was 1.0 to 7.3 U/L with a mean of 2.7 U/L (normal 1.8 U/L) *2105*

Alkaline Phosphatase *Serum Increase* Serum concentration and the isoenzyme pattern appear to be in concordance with severity of sickle cell crisis. Bone isoenzyme is the principal enzyme fraction that increases during symptomatic crises. Serum concentration may be an additional indicator of degree, frequency, and persistence of tissue injuries. Increased during crisis, representing vaso-occlusive bone injury as well as liver damage with sickle cell disease *5544* In 20 young adult sickle cell patients total alkaline phosphatase was higher than in 58 matching normal controls. Heat inactivation and isoenzyme electrophoresis indicated that bone is the predominant isoenzyme in the patients *3552*
White Blood Cells Decrease Decreased activity *5545* Low activities found *5524*

Alkaline Phosphatase Isoenzymes *Serum Increase* Serum concentration and the isoenzyme pattern appear to be in concordance with severity of sickle cell crisis. Bone isoenzyme is the principal enzyme fraction that increases during symptomatic crises *5544*

Ammonium Ions *Urine Increase* May be associated with voltage-dependent distal renal tubular acidosis which is associated with hyerkalemia, hyperchloremic metabolic acidosis, urine pH > 5.5, increased urinary ammonium ion excretion, a positive urine anion gap, increased urinary osmol gap, low urinary citrate and high or normal urinary calcium excretion *4071*

Androgens *Plasma Decrease* Deficient as a result of primary rather than secondary hypogonadism in 29 of 32 adult male patients *8*

Androstenedione *Plasma Decrease* Basal serum testosterone, dihydrotestosterone, and androstenedione were lower in 32 adult male patients. Secondary sex characteristics were abnormal in 29 of 32 patients *8*

Anion Gap *Urine Decrease* May be associated with voltage-dependent distal renal tubular acidosis which is associated with hyerkalemia, hyperchloremic metabolic acidosis, urine pH > 5.5, increased urinary ammonium ion excretion, a positive urine anion gap, increased urinary osmol gap, low urinary citrate and high or normal urinary calcium excretion *4071*

Anisocytes *Blood Increase* Blood film reveals marked poikilocytosis and anisocytosis, target cells, some macrocytes, and occasional sickled erythrocytes. Nucleated red cells are frequently seen, particularly in children *2039*

Bilirubin *Serum Increase* Intrahepatic cholestasis with extremely high circulating levels also appears to be characteristic *5677*

Bilirubin, Indirect *Serum Increase* Laboratory signs of hemolysis with increased indirect-reacting serum bilirubin *5677* Elevation is always seen but late in the course true liver function abnormalities also develop *900*

Calcium *Serum Decrease* In 20 Saudis aged 16 - 25 y with sickle cell disease mean concentration of 2.31 ± 0.12 mmol/L significantly different from 2.48 ± 0.16 mmol/L in 41 healthy controls. Similar observation in younger age groups *3551* In 18 black patients in Curacao with sickle cell disease mean concentration of 2.32 ± 0.07 mmol/L significantly different from 2.44 ± 0.14 mmol/L in 15 controls without neurological disorders *5395*
Urine Increase May be associated with voltage-dependent distal renal tubular acidosis which is associated with hyerkalemia, hyperchloremic metabolic acidosis, urine pH > 5.5, increased urinary ammonium ion excretion, a positive urine anion gap, increased urinary osmol gap, low urinary citrate and high or normal urinary calcium excretion *4071*

Chloride *Serum Increase* May be associated with voltage-dependent distal renal tubular acidosis which is associated with hyerkalemia, hyperchloremic metabolic acidosis, urine pH > 5.5, increased urinary ammonium ion excretion, a positive urine anion gap, increased urinary osmol gap, low urinary citrate and high or normal urinary calcium excretion *4071*

Cholesterol *Red Blood Cells Increase* Plasma lipids are significantly reduced and RBC cholesterol is higher in sickle cell patients than in normal subjects *60*
Serum Decrease Hypocholesterolemia was found in 8 cases. Values ranged from 2.6 - 4.3 mmol/L *5645* Plasma lipids are significantly reduced *60*

Circulating Endothelial Cells *Blood Increase* In 18 patients with sickle cell anemia in acute painful crisis mean concentration of 22.8 ± 18.2 cells/mL significantly different from that in 14 healthy individuals in whom mean concentration was 2.6 ± 1.6 cells/mL. In 33 patients not in crisis mean concentration was 13.2 ± 11.8 cells/mL *4930*

Citrate *Urine Decrease* May be associated with voltage-dependent distal renal tubular acidosis which is associated with hyerkalemia, hyperchloremic metabolic acidosis, urine pH > 5.5, increased urinary ammonium ion excretion, a positive urine anion gap, increased urinary osmol gap, low urinary citrate and high or normal urinary calcium excretion *4071*

Complement, Total *Synovial Fluid No Effect* Total hemolytic complement ranged from 22 - 80 U/L, usually at the upper limit of normal *1392*

Copper *Serum Increase* Significantly increased in patients with SS compared to controls p < 0.001 Increased *3900 4586*

Creatinine Clearance *Urine No Effect* Creatinine clearance in patients with urine microalbumin/creatinine ratios of > 20 mg/g creatinine of 204 mL/min/1.73 sq m compared with 173 mL/min/sq m in those with normal U albumin/creatinine *1144*

1,25-Dihydroxy Vitamin D *Serum Increase* In 30 Saudis aged 11 - 15 y with sickle cell disease mean concentration of 34.6 ± 8.0 pg/mL significantly different from 28.6 ± 6.7 pg/mL in 34 healthy controls *3551*
Serum No Effect In 18 black patients in Curacao with sickle cell disease mean concentration of 112 ± 30 pmol/L not significantly different from 127 ± 35 pmol/L in 15 controls without neurological disorders *5395* In 20 Saudis aged 16 - 25 y with sickle cell disease mean concentration of 34.1 ± 8.4 pg/mL not significantly different from 31.0 ± 8.7 pg/mL in 41 healthy controls. Similar observation in paients aged 5 - 10 years *3551*

2,3-Dinor-Thromboxane B_2 *Plasma Increase* In 15 adult patients with hemoglobin SS disease mean concentration of 21.53 ± 5.10 ng/mL significantly greater than 2.75 ± 0.83 ng/mL in 12 healthy hemoglobin AA controls *2857*
Urine Increase In 15 adult patients with hemoglobin SS disease mean excretion 317.6 ± 15.0 pg/mmol creatinine significantly greater than 191.8 ± 3.60 pg/mmol creatinine in 12 healthy hemoglobin AA controls *2857*

Endothelin-1 *Plasma Increase* In 13 patients aged about 21 years with sickle cell anemia mean concentration of 10.9 ± 1.9 pmol/L significantly different from 3.0 ± 1.3 pmol/L in 12 healthy age-matched African-American controls *5639*

Erythrocyte Sedimentation Rate *Blood Decrease* Consistently decreased *5699* Decreased ESR becomes normal after blood is aerated *5544*
Blood Increase Elevated in 6 of 18 patients *1392*

Erythrocyte Survival *Red Blood Cells Decrease* Mean red cell life span was 17.32 ± 4.51 days and half-life was 10.11 ± 2.82 days. Mean life span was inversely correlated with number of sickled cells *3402* Shortened in all the varieties of sickle cell disease *5677*

Erythrocytes *Blood Decrease* Usually count between 2.0 - 3.5 million/µL *5677*
Urine Increase Hematuria is frequent *5544*

Factor VIII *Plasma Increase* May be increased *5699 4347*

Factor IX *Plasma No Effect* No significant effect usually seen *5699* No significant effect usually observed *4347*

Factor XI *Plasma No Effect* No significant effect usually observed *5699 4347*

Factor XII *Plasma No Effect* Concentration typically normal *4347 5699*

Factor B *Plasma Decrease* Found in 50% of patients *5229 4431*

Ferritin *Serum Increase* Concentration in patients with urine microalbumin/creatinine ratios of > 20 mg/g creatinine of 2,256 ng/mLnot significantly different from 317 ng/mL in those with normal U albumin/creatinine *1144*

Fibrinogen *Plasma Increase* In 9 patients with homozygous sickle cell disease during vaso-occlusive crisis concentration rose significantly to a maximum on approximately the second day of the onset of pain crisis and after treatment was instituted *1414*

Follicle Stimulating Hormone *Plasma Decrease* Consistent with primary testicular failure in all 14 adult male patients tested *8*

α-Galactosidase *Serum Decrease* In 11 patients with sickle cell anemia mean activity of 13.4 ± 7.5 U/L significantly different from 17.5 ± 4.9 U/L in 11 healthy controls *5794*
Urine Decrease In 11 patients with sickle cell anemia mean activity of 15.7 ± 11.7 U/mg creatinine significantly different from 43.2 ± 37.9 U/L in 11 healthy controls *5794*

β-Galactosidase *Serum No Effect* In 11 patients with sickle cell anemia mean activity of 16.1 ± 7.2 U/L not significantly different from 12.5 ± 5.3 U/L in 11 healthy controls *5794*
Urine No Effect In 11 patients with sickle cell anemia mean activity of 28.8 ± 33.4 U/L not significantly different from 43.3 ± 51.1 U/L in 11 healthy controls *5794*

Glucose-6-Phosphate Dehydrogenase
Red Blood Cells Increase Mean activities in red cells were slightly increased to a mean of 5.4 units (range = 1.5 - 9.8) *2105*
Serum Increase Elevated in 15 cases. Values ranged from 1 - 14 with a mean of 4.8 (normal 1.6 units) *2105*

282.60 **Sickle Cell Disease** *(continued)*

β-Glucuronidase *Serum* *No Effect* In 11 patients with sickle cell anemia mean activity of 85.8 ± 27.6 U/L not significantly different from 100.0 ± 52.4 U/L in 11 healthy controls *5794*
Urine *Decrease* In 11 patients with sickle cell anemia mean activity of 6.5 ± 5.9 U/mg creatinine significantly different from 59.3 ± 76.4 U/mg creatinine in 11 healthy controls *5794*

Glutamic Acid *Plasma* *Increase* Mean concentration of 867 ± 196 µmol/L in 11 patients with sickle cell disease significantly different from 660 ± 124 µmol/L in 7 normal individuals *3790*
Red Blood Cells *Increase* Mean concentration of 549 ± 127 µmol/L in 11 patients with sickle cell disease significantly different from 288 ± 70 µmol/L in 7 normal individuals *3790*

Glutamine *Plasma* *Increase* Mean concentration in 11 patients with sickle cell disease of 697 ± 101 µmol/L not significantly different from 625 ± 98 µmol/L in 7 normal individuals *3790*
Red Blood Cells *Increase* Mean concentration of 867 ± 196 µmol/L in 11 patients with sickle cell disease significantly different from 660 ± 124 µmol/L in 7 normal individuals *3790*

Gonadotropin, Pituitary *Plasma* *Decrease* Serum LH and FSH before and after stimulation with gonadotropin releasing hormone were consistent with primary testicular failure in all 14 adult male patients tested *8*

Granulocyte-Macrophage Colony Stimulating Factor
Serum *Increase* In 23 homozygote patients mean concentration in those patients with Hb F < 9% of 9.4 ± 4.6 pg/mL significantly higher than 1.1 ± 3.1 pg/mL in patients with Hb F > 9% and nondetectable amounts in 10 normal individuals *967*

Haptoglobin *Serum* *Decrease* RBC destruction is partially intravascular, producing elevated plasma heme proteins and decreased haptoglobin concentration *5699* Observed effect *5677* RBC destruction is partially intravascular, producing elevated plasma heme proteins and decreased haptoglobin concentration *973*

Hematocrit *Blood* *Decrease* In 13 patients aged about 21 years with sickle cell anemia mean value of 27 ± 1% significantly different from 42 ± 1% in 12 healthy age-matched African-American controls *5639* Decreased in 7 cases, ranging from 17-24% *5645*

Hemoglobin *Blood* *Decrease* Mild anemia *900* In 13 patients aged about 21 years with sickle cell anemia mean concentration of 8.5 ± 0.3 g/dL significantly different from 13.2 ± 0.3 g/dL in 12 healthy age-matched African-American controls *5639* Steady-state is usually between 5 - 11 g/dL. The anemia is normochromic *5677*
Plasma *Increase* Seen between as well as during crises, and no consistent increase in this value occurs in crises *900*

Hemoglobin A_{1c} *Blood* *Decrease* Due to increased RBC turnover *4746*
Blood *Increase* Significantly elevated in children with this disease (13.1% n = 36) compared with normal children (6.25% n = 27) *2506*

Hemoglobin F *Blood* *Increase* Increased in various hemoglobinopathies; Hb F over 30% protects the cell from sickling; therefore, infants with homozygous S have few problems before age of 3 months *5542* Electrophoresis of the hemoglobin confirms the diagnosis by showing the typical pattern of homozygous sickle inheritance: Hb S with variable amounts of Hb F and no Hb A *2039* Concentration significantly higher in patients with sickle cell disease compared with hemoglobin S heterozygotes and normal individuals *1322*

β-Hexosaminidase *Serum* *No Effect* In 11 patients with sickle cell anemia mean activity of 170.9 ± 46.2 U/L not significantly different from 341.5 ± 261.8 U/L in 11 healthy controls *5794*
Urine *No Effect* In 11 patients with sickle cell anemia mean activity of 134.9 ± 79.3 U/L not significantly different from 247.8 ± 134.9 U/L in 11 healthy controls *5794*

25-Hydroxy Vitamin D *Serum* *Decrease* In 20 Saudis aged 16 - 25 y with sickle cell disease mean concentration of 14.6 ± 4.1 ng/mL significantly different from 19.2 ± 4.4 ng/mL in 41 healthy controls. Similar observation in younger age groups *3551*
Serum *No Effect* In 18 black patients in Curacao with sickle cell disease mean concentration of 87 ± 27 nmol/L not significantly different from 86 ± 15 nmol/L in 15 controls without neurological disorders *5395*

Hydroxyproline *Urine* *Increase* Excretion significantly higher in sickle cell patients than in controls and correlated well with serum alkaline phosphatase activity (r = 0.73). Both increased with age in sickle cell patients *3552*

Immunoglobulin G *Serum* *Increase* Markedly elevated in both Black and Caucasian patients *4724*

Interleukin-1α *Serum* *Increase* Measured using enzyme-linked immunosorbent assay in 59 plasma samples from 34 adult subjects with Hb SS or Hb SC who did not have documented infections. Interleukin-1 was elevated on at least one occasion in 6 subjects, including 3 subjects in the steady state and 3 subjects in crisis *1548*

Interleukin-3 *Serum* *Increase* In 39 homozygote patients mean concentration in those patients with Hb F < 9% of 8.6 ± 20 pg/mL and 84.8 ± 57 pg/mL in patients with Hb F > 9% significantly higher than nondetectable amounts in 3 normal individuals *967*

Interleukin-6 *Serum* *Increase* In 36 homozygote patients 11 were positive for IL-6 compared with negative concentrations in other SS patients and 3 normal individuals *967* Mean concentration in 27 patients at steady state with sickle cell disease of 60 ± 7 pg/mL 5-fold higher than 12 ± 5 pg/mL in 19 healthy normal controls *5179*

Interleukin-8 *Serum* *Increase* In 48 children with sickle cell disease mean concentration and that during vaso-occlusive crisis significantly different from that in 20 healthy children *3473*
Serum *No Effect* In 13 asymptomatic patients with sickle cell disease (9 Hb-SS and 4 Hb-SC) mean concentration of 10 ± 0.2 pg/mL not significantly different from 6 ± 7 pg/mL in 38 healthy blood donors *1259*

Isocitrate Dehydrogenase *Red Blood Cells* *Increase* Mean RBC concentration was elevated to 2.8 U/L in 15 patients *2105*
Serum *Increase* Elevated in 15 patients. Values ranged from 1.5 - 13.0 U/L and the mean was 5.2 U/L (normal 2.5 U/L) *2105*

6-Keto-Prostaglandin $F_{1\alpha}$ *Plasma* *Increase* In 15 adult patients with hemoglobin SS disease mean concentration of 4.718 ± 0.562 ng/mL significantly greater than 0.078 ± 0.011 ng/mL in 12 healthy hemoglobin AA controls *2857*
Urine *Increase* In 15 adult patients with hemoglobin SS disease mean excretion of 1,546.6 ± 204.8 pg/mmol creatinine significantly greater than less than 0.005 pg/mmol creatinine in 12 healthy hemoglobin AA controls *2857*

Lactate Dehydrogenase *Red Blood Cells* *Increase* Mean concentration elevated to 180 U/L (3 times the normal mean) in 15 patients. Values ranged from 83 to 388 U/L *2105*
Serum *Increase* Usually elevated to about twice normal in the steady state *3751*

Lactate Dehydrogenase Isoenzymes *Serum* *Increase* LD_1 and LD_2 *5544* *1642*

Leukocytes *Blood* *Increase* Polymorphonuclear leukocytosis with a left shift is common even in the steady state and may be due in part to redistribution of leukocytes from the marginal to the circulating granulocyte pool *502* Leukocytosis, even after correction for nucleated red blood cells, is the rule *900* Tends to persist and increase during crises, when counts > 20,000 /µL are common *367*
Synovial Fluid *Increase* Ranged from 600 - 270,000 /µL in 13 patients. Polymorphonuclear cells predominate *1392*

Leukotriene B_4 *Plasma* *Decrease* Mean concentration in 15 patients of 6.15 ± 0.42 ng/mL significantly less than 8.95 ± 0.26 ng/mL in age-matched healthy controls *2311*
Urine *Increase* Mean excretion in 15 patients 27.50 ± 3.33 ng/mmol creatinine in 15 patients significantly greater than 10.60 ± 0.35 ng/mmol creatinine in age-matched healthy controls *2311*

Leukotriene C_4 *Plasma* *Increase* Mean concentration in 15 patients of 13.61 ± 1.45 ng/mL significantly increased compared with 7.24 ± 0.21 ng/mL in age-matched healthy controls *2311*
Urine *No Effect* In 15 patients mean excretion of 356.0 ± 17.87 ng/mmol creatinine not significantly different from 360.0 ± 9.82 ng/mmol creatinine in age-matched healthy controls *2311*

Leukotriene D_4 *Plasma* *Decrease* Mean concentration of 6.44 ± 0.51 ng/mL in 15 patients significantly less than 11.42 ± 0.40 ng/mL in age-matched healthy controls *2311*
Urine *Increase* In 15 patients with sickle cell disease mean excretion of 69.90 ± 14.51 ng/mmol creatinine compared with undetectable amounts in age-matched healthy controls *2311*

Leukotriene E_4 *Plasma* *Decrease* Mean concentration of 4.97 ± 0.37 ng/mL in 15 patients significantly less than 14.51 ± 0.50 ng/mL in age-matched healthy controls *2311*

Lipids *Serum Decrease* Plasma lipids are significantly reduced and RBC cholesterol is higher in patients than in normal subjects *60*

Luteinizing Hormone *Plasma Decrease* Serum LH and FSH before and after stimulation with gonadotropin releasing hormone were consistent with primary testicular failure in all 14 adult male patients tested *8*

Malate Dehydrogenase *Red Blood Cells Increase* Mean RBC concentration was elevated to 245 ± 93 U/L in 15 patients. Levels ranged from 80 to 460 U/L (normal 160 U/L) *2105*
Serum Increase Elevated to a median of 193 U/L (normal 52 U/L) with a range of 87 to 337 U/L in 15 patients *2105*

α-Mannosidase *Serum Decrease* In 11 patients with sickle cell anemia mean activity of 73.8 ± 41.0 U/L significantly different from 97.8 ± 32.6 U/L in 11 healthy controls *5794*
Urine No Effect In 11 patients with sickle cell anemia mean activity of 8.6 ± 9.5 U/mg creatinine not significantly different from 30.2 ± 47.9 U/mg in 11 healthy controls *5794*

MCV *Blood Decrease* Red cell indices are usually normal, but the MCV may be increased or decreased *5699*
Blood Increase Red cell indices are usually normal, but the MCV may be increased or decreased *5699* In 100 patients with macrocytosis (MCV greater than 110 fL) one had sickle cell anemia *4924*

Monocytes *Blood Increase* Leukocytosis with monocytosis (5 - 25%) *5677*

Net Acid Excretion *Urine Increase* May be associated with voltage-dependent distal renal tubular acidosis which is associated with hyerkalemia, hyperchloremic metabolic acidosis, urine pH > 5.5, increased urinary ammonium ion excretion, a positive urine anion gap, increased urinary osmol gap, low urinary citrate and high or normal urinary calcium excretion *4071*

5'-Nucleotidase *Serum Increase* In 59 patients with homozygous sickle cell anemia significantly increased activity observed compared with healthy controls, but not significantly greater than in heterozygous sicklers *3549*

Osmolal Gap *Urine Increase* May be associated with voltage-dependent distal renal tubular acidosis which is associated with hyerkalemia, hyperchloremic metabolic acidosis, urine pH > 5.5, increased urinary ammonium ion excretion, a positive urine anion gap, increased urinary osmol gap, low urinary citrate and high or normal urinary calcium excretion *4071*

Osmolality *Urine Decrease* Chronic defect in renal concentrating ability frequently present *2059*

Osmotic Fragility *Red Blood Cells Decrease* Decreased (more resistant RBCs) *5544*

Oxygen Partial Pressure *Blood Decrease* Decreased oxygenation and increased acidosis lead to further sickling and further vaso-occlusion *1785* The partial pressure of oxygen in arterial blood is usually diminished as a result of shunting within the lung *900*

Oxygen Saturation *Blood Decrease* The partial pressure of oxygen in arterial blood is usually diminished as a result of shunting within the lung *900* Decreased oxygenation and increased acidosis and pO_2 lead to further sickling and further vaso-occlusion *1785* In 13 patients aged about 21 years with sickle cell anemia mean saturation of 94 ± 1% significantly different from 97 ± 0.2% in 12 healthy age-matched African-American controls *5639*

Parathyroid Hormone *Plasma Increase* In 20 Saudis aged 16 - 25 y with sickle cell disease mean concentration of 96.0 ± 18.4 pmol/L significantly different from 78.1 ± 10.9 pmol/L in 41 healthy controls. Similar observation in younger age groups *3551*
Plasma No Effect In 18 black patients in Curacao with sickle cell disease mean concentration of 2.6 ± 1.2 pmol/L not significantly different from 3.2 ± 1.8 pmol/L in 15 controls without neurological disorders *5395*

pH *Blood Decrease* Decreased oxygenation and increased acidosis develop and lead to further sickling and further vaso-occlusion *1785*
Urine Increase May be associated with voltage-dependent distal renal tubular acidosis which is associated with hyerkalemia, hyperchloremic metabolic acidosis, urine pH > 5.5, increased urinary ammonium ion excretion, a positive urine anion gap, increased urinary osmol gap, low urinary citrate and high or normal urinary calcium excretion *4071*

Phosphate *Serum Increase* Sickle cell anemia may increase the serum phosphate concentration *969* Serum phosphate concentration may be increased in patients with sickle cell disease *5204*
Serum No Effect In 18 black patients in Curacao with sickle cell disease mean concentration of 1.56 ± 0.14 mmol/L not significantly different from 1.60 ± 0.17 mmol/L in 15 controls without neurological disorders *5395*

Phospholipids *Serum Decrease* Plasma lipids are significantly reduced and RBC cholesterol is higher in patients than in normal subjects *60*

Platelets *Blood Decrease* Decreased with folate deficiency or during an aplastic crisis *5699*
Blood Increase Common, but the count may fall during infarctive crisis *5677* Thrombocytosis often accompanies the leukocytosis *900* Increased (300,000 - 500,000 /µL) with abnormal forms *5544*

Poikilocytes *Blood Increase* Blood film reveals marked poikilocytosis and anisocytosis, target cells, some macrocytes, and occasional sickled erythrocytes. Nucleated red cells are frequently seen, particularly in children *2039*

Potassium *Serum Increase* May be associated with voltage-dependent distal renal tubular acidosis which is associated with hyerkalemia, hyperchloremic metabolic acidosis, urine pH > 5.5, increased urinary ammonium ion excretion, a positive urine anion gap, increased urinary osmol gap, low urinary citrate and high or normal urinary calcium excretion *4071*

Prostaglandin E_2 *Plasma Increase* In 15 adult patients with hemoglobin SS disease mean concentration of 0.560 ± 0.105 ng/mL significantly greater than less than 0.005 ng/mL in 12 healthy hemoglobin AA controls *2857*
Urine Increase In 15 adult patients with hemoglobin SS disease mean excretion of 234.2 ± 63.1 pg/mmol creatinine significantly greater than 22.4 ± 3.90 pg/mmol creatinine in 12 healthy hemoglobin AA controls *2857*

Protein *Serum No Effect* In 18 black patients in Curacao with sickle cell disease mean concentration of 77 ± 5.3 g/L significantly different from 75 ± 4.2 g/L in 15 controls without neurological disorders *5395*
Synovial Fluid Increase Elevated in 6 of 13 patients *1392*

Protein C *Plasma Decrease* In 100 patients with sickle cell disease significant reduction in concentration observed with lowest concentrations in patients with most severe disease and frequent episodes of crisis, but concentration did not change with crises *1323*

Protein S *Plasma Decrease* In 100 patients with sickle cell disease concentration significantly reduced with lowest concentrations in patients with most severe disease and most frequent episodes of crisis. Concentration unchanged during crises *1323*

Prothrombin Fragment 1.2 *Plasma Increase* Mean concentration of prothrombin fragment 1.2 in platelet-poor plasma from 21 patients with sickle cell disease of 5.6 ± 4.2 nmol/L significantly higher than 0.51 nmol/L (95% reference interval 0.21 - 2.78 nmol/L) in 268 healthy individuals less than 44 years of age *1860*

Reticulocytes *Blood Increase* In 15 cases, mean count was 345,000/µL with a range of 62,000 - 750,000 /µL, markedly increased over the normal value of 50,000 /µL *2105* Mean concentration in 11 patients with sickle cell disease of 11.4 ± 4.2% significantly different from 1.6 ± 0.3% in 7 normal individuals *3790* Reticulocytosis (5 - 20%) with circulating nucleated red cells. Count is diminished during aplastic crises *5677*

Sickle Cells *Blood Increase* Mean number of irreversibly sickled cells was 9 ± 5.06 in 25 patients. Number of cells correlated inversely with RBC life span *3402* Sickled erythrocytes may not be numerous in the blood smear, but in blood deoxygenated with sodium metabisulfite virtually all the red cells are sickled *367*
Synovial Fluid Increase Sickled erythrocytes were found in 7 of 13 joint fluid specimens *1392*

Soluble Transferrin Receptor *Serum Increase* Concentration increases with disease *4784*

Specific Gravity *Urine Decrease* Despite the relative benignity of sickle cell trait, adults with this condition are unable to concentrate their urine and characteristically have a urine specific gravity around 1.010 *900* Specific gravity is low reflecting the loss of renal concentrating ability due to repeated microinfarcts in the medulla of the kidneys *2039*

282.60 Sickle Cell Disease *(continued)*

Substance P *Plasma Increase* In 48 children with sickle cell disease mean concentration of about 40 pg/mL, rising to about 90 pg/mL during vaso-occlusive crisis significantly different from less than 5 pg/mL in 20 healthy children *3473*

Target Cells *Blood Increase* Blood film reveals marked poikilocytosis and anisocytosis, target cells, some macrocytes, and occasional sickled erythrocytes. Nucleated red cells are frequently seen, particularly in children *2039*

Testosterone *Serum Decrease* Basal serum testosterone, dihydrotestosterone, and androstenedione were lower in 32 adult male patients. Secondary sex characteristics were abnormal in 29 of 32 patients *8 8*

Thromboxane B_2 *Plasma Increase* In 15 adult patients with hemoglobin SS disease mean concentration of 0.543 ± 0.101 ng/mL significantly greater than less than 0.005 ng/mL in 12 healthy hemoglobin AA controls *2857*
Urine Increase In 15 adult patients with hemoglobin SS disease mean excretion of 103.2 ± 28.20 pg/mmol creatinine significantly greater than 46.0 ± 34.0 pg/mmol creatinine in 12 healthy hemoglobin AA controls *2857*

Tumor Necrosis Factor-α *Serum Increase* TNF-α was measured using enzyme-linked immunosorbent assay in 59 plasma samples from 34 adult subjects with Hb SS or Hb SC who did not have documented infections. Tumor necrosis factor was elevated on at least one occasion in 27 subjects, including 18 of 21 subjects in the steady state and 13 of 19 subjects during painful crisis *565*
Serum No Effect In 48 children with sickle cell disease mean concentration and that during vaso-occlusive crisis not significantly different from that in 20 healthy children *3473*

Uric Acid *Serum Increase* May be increased *5544*
Serum No Effect Patients have normal serum levels as a result of increased clearance *1152*
Urine Increase Increased tubular secretion of urate; patients have normal serum levels as a result of increased clearance *1152*

Uric Acid Clearance *Urine Increase* Increased tubular secretion of urate; patients have normal serum levels as a result of increased clearance *1152*

Urobilinogen *Urine Increase* Urine contains increased urobilinogen but is negative for bile *5544*

Viscosity *Serum Increase* Increased viscosity of circulating whole blood may contribute to vaso-occlusion *1785*

Zinc *Red Blood Cells Decrease* RBC and hair zinc concentrations were decreased in adult male patients. RBC zinc correlated (r = 0.61) with serum testosterone, which was low (primary testicular failure) in all patients tested *8*
Serum Decrease Decreased *5083 4742*
Urine Increase Excretion enhanced as a consequence of increased red cell fragility resulting in moderate zincuria *5174*

282.61 Sickle Cell Hb-S Disease

Interleukin-8 *Serum Increase* In 9 patients with painful vaso-occlusive crises mean concentration of 287 ± 630 pg/mL significantly higher than 6 ± 7 pg/mL in 38 healthy blood donors *1259*

Soluble Transferrin Receptor *Serum Increase* In 100 male patients aged 8 y with SS-disease mean concentration of 40.4 mg/L significantly different from 5.9 mg/L in 16 age-matched healthy male AA controls, and 35.9 mg/L in 82 girls aged 8 y compared with 7.2 mg/L in 25 healthy female age-matched AA controls *4868*

282.63 Sickle Cell Hb-C Disease

Interleukin-8 *Serum Increase* In 4 patients with painful vaso-occlusive crises mean concentration of 516 ± 917 pg/mL significantly higher than 6 ± 7 pg/mL in 38 healthy blood donors *1259*

Soluble Transferrin Receptor *Serum Increase* In 25 male patients aged 8 y with SS-disease mean concentration of 26.1 mg/L significantly different from 5.9 mg/L in 16 age-matched healthy male AA controls, and 20.5 mg/L in 22 girls aged 8 y compared with 7.2 mg/L in 25 healthy female age-matched AA controls *4868*

282.71 Hemoglobin C Disease

Bilirubin *Serum Increase* Increase is minimal *5545*

Bilirubin, Indirect *Serum Increase* Manifested by a hemolytic state *1980*

Erythrocyte Survival *Red Blood Cells Decrease* Mean life span of 30 to 55 days *5210*

Erythrocytes *Blood Increase* Seen in large numbers in Hemoglobin C disease *2039*

Haptoglobin *Serum Decrease* Substantially reduced or even absent *5677*

Hematocrit *Blood Decrease* Mild anemia, hematocrit usually between 30 - 35% *900*

Hemoglobin *Blood Decrease* Hemoglobin concentration of 8 - 12 g/dL *5677* Mild anemia *900*
Plasma Increase Slight to moderate increase *5544* Manifested by a hemolytic state *1980*

Hemoglobin F *Blood Increase* Slightly increased *5545*

Lactate Dehydrogenase *Serum Increase* Due to slight hemolysis *413*

Leukocytes *Blood Decrease* May be low due to hypersplenism *900*

Osmotic Fragility *Red Blood Cells Decrease* Biphasic, with both increased and decreased fragility *1025* Osmotic fragility curves are abnormal, indicating the presence of populations of fragile cells (microspherocytes) and resistant in homozygotes *5545*
Red Blood Cells Increase Biphasic, with both increased and decreased fragility *1025*

Oxygen Saturation *Blood Decrease* Low oxygen affinity *3678*

Platelets *Blood Decrease* May be low due to hypersplenism *900*

Reticulocytes *Blood Increase* Manifested by a hemolytic state *1980* Count is increased (2 - 10%) *5545*

Sickle Cells *Blood Increase* Sickling produces prominent clinical manifestations *5677*

Target Cells *Blood Increase* One of the most striking features of homozygous disease is the marked increase in the number of target cells in the peripheral blood *5677*

Viscosity *Red Blood Cells Increase* A tendency to increased intracellular viscosity with decreased cell deformability *5699*
Serum Increase Blood viscosity is increased *1980*

282.72 Hemoglobin E Disease

Haptoglobin *Serum Decrease* Substantially reduced or even absent *5677*

Hematocrit *Blood Decrease* Exhibits mild or no anemia *900* Homozygotes for hemoglobin E have a relatively mild anemia characterized by microcytosis and targeting of the red cells *810*

Hemoglobin *Blood Decrease* Homozygotes for hemoglobin E have a relatively mild anemia characterized by microcytosis and targeting of the red cells *810* Exhibits mild or no anemia *900*

Hemoglobin F *Blood Increase* Sometimes slightly increased *5545*

MCV *Blood Decrease* Homozygotes for hemoglobin E have a relatively mild anemia characterized by microcytosis and targeting of the red cells *810* Definite microcytosis *900*

Oxygen Saturation *Blood Decrease* RBC oxygen affinity has been found to be decreased, possibly accounting for the anemia *900*

Zinc Protoporphyrin:Heme Ratio *Blood Increase* In 36 patients with α-thalassemia trait mean ratio of 73 ± 24 μmol/mol not significantly different from 60 ± 8 μmol/mol in 64 normal individuals, with 8 (22%) of affected individuals having ratios greater than 80 μmol/mol *1836*

282.72 Hemoglobin E (Homozygous)

Hematocrit *Blood No Effect* In 12 patients with homozygous hemoglobin E mean value of 36 ± 3.2% not significantly different from 41 ± 3.8% in 64 normal individuals *1836*

MCHC *Blood* *Decrease* In 12 patients with homozygous hemoglobin E mean value of 32 ± 0.7 significantly different from 34 ± 0.7 in 64 normal individuals *1836*

MCV *Blood* *Decrease* In 12 patients with homozygous hemoglobin E mean value of 65 ± 1.7 fL significantly different from 88 ± 4.8 fL in 64 normal individuals *1836*

282.72 Hemoglobin E Trait

Hematocrit *Blood* *No Effect* In 24 patients with hemoglobin E trait mean value of 37 ± 4.7% not significantly different from 41 ± 3.8% in 64 normal individuals *1836*

MCH *Blood* *Decrease* In 24 patients with hemoglobin E trait mean value of 26 ± 1.9 pg significantly different from 30 ± 1.8 pg in 64 normal individuals *1836*

MCHC *Blood* *Decrease* In 24 patients with hemoglobin E trait mean value of 33 ± 0.7 significantly different from 34 ± 0.7 in 64 normal individuals *1836*

MCV *Blood* *Decrease* In 24 patients with hemoglobin E trait mean value of 78 ± 5.1 fL significantly different from 88 ± 4.8 fL in 64 normal individuals *1836*

282.73 Hemoglobin H Disease

Anisocytes *Blood* *Increase* Anisopoikilocytosis of RBC *4979*

Ferritin *Serum* *Increase* In 14 patients with hemoglobin H disease mean concentration of 137 ± 61 pg/mL significantly different from 34.2 ± 32 pg/mL in 15 healthy normal controls *1221*
Serum *No Effect* In 14 patients withhemoglobin H disease mean concentration of 178 ± 154 ng/mL not significantly different from normal *1221*

Haptoglobin *Serum* *Decrease* Substantially reduced or even absent *5677*

Hematocrit *Blood* *Decrease* Life-long anemia with variable splenomegaly and bone changes *5677* Variable degree of anemia *4979*

Hemoglobin *Blood* *Decrease* In 14 patients withhemoglobin H disease mean concentration of 9.4 ± 0.68 g/dL significantly different from normal *1221* Life-long anemia with variable splenomegaly and bone changes *5677* Concentration in these patients usually range from about 7 - 10 g/dL. Both higher and lower levels have been observed *900* Variable degree of anemia. Hb A constitutes the majority and Hb H varies from 5 - 30% *4979*

Poikilocytes *Blood* *Increase* Anisopoikilocytosis of RBC *4979*

Reticulocytes *Blood* *Increase* Usually in the 5% range *5677* Observed with anemia *4979*

283.00 Acquired Hemolytic Anemia (Autoimmune)

Adenosine Deaminase *Serum* *Increase* Increased in hemolytic anemia *3926* *1340* *4956*

Antinuclear Antibodies *Serum* *Increase* Found in a significant number of patients without other features of SLE or other rheumatic disease *4551*

Basophils *Blood* *Increase* Punctate basophilia and normoblastemia are common in severe cases *4551*

Bilirubin *Serum* *Increase* Increase depends on liver function and amount of hemolysis. With normal liver function, it is increased 1 mg/dL in 1 - 6 h to maximum in 3 - 12 h following hemolysis of 100 mL of blood, with hemolytic anemias *5545* Although clinical jaundice is present in < 50% of patients, elevated serum bilirubin, particularly of the unconjugated fraction, is common *5677*

Bilirubin, Direct *Serum* *Increase* Elevated if the total serum bilirubin exceeds 4 mg/dL; attributed to an associated hepatic injury permitting conjugated bilirubin to regurgitate into the general circulation *5237*

Bilirubin, Indirect *Serum* *Increase* Although clinical jaundice is present in < 50% of patients, elevated serum bilirubin, particularly of the unconjugated fraction, are common *5677* There is increased indirect serum bilirubin (< 6 mg/dL because of compensatory excretory capacity of liver) *5545*

Calcium *Red Blood Cells* *Increase* In 19 cases of acquired autoimmune hemolysis, increased erythrocytic Ca^{++} level was observed in 6 cases *410*

Cold Agglutinins *Serum* *Increase* In hemolytic anemias *5545*

Complement C_3 *Red Blood Cells* *Increase* Only fractions of the complement system of proteins, principally C_3 and C_4 components, are detected on the red cells by antiglobulin sera having anti-C specificity *991*
Serum *Decrease* Caused by hypercatabolism *2694* *1033* *1588* *785*

Complement C_4 *Red Blood Cells* *Increase* Only fractions of the complement system of proteins, principally C_3 and C_4 components, are detected on the red cells by antiglobulin sera having anti-C specificity *991*

Complement, Total *Serum* *Decrease* Low serum titers have been reported in patients with warm antibody hemolytic disease *4087*

Coombs' Test *Serum* *Positive* May or may not be positive, depending on the total amount of autoantibody present and its binding affinity for the red cell mass *5677*

Creatine Kinase *Serum* *No Effect* Not affected by disease *1980*

Creatinine *Serum* *Increase* In 72% of 11 patients hospitalized for this disorder *1576*

Cryoglobulins *Serum* *Increase* Variable elevation of cryoglobulins *4707*

2,3-Diphosphoglycerate *Red Blood Cells* *Increase* Synthesis is increased in response to hypoxia *380*

Erythrocyte Survival *Red Blood Cells* *Decrease* Shortened survival of both the patient's own red cell population and normal donor cells *3569*

Folate *Serum* *Decrease* Decreased with extensive skin disease *5230* *772* *602*

Haptoglobin *Serum* *Decrease* Usually depleted; the return to normal is a valuable indicator of remission *5677* Decreased in hemoglobinemia (related to the duration and severity of hemolysis) due to extravascular hemolysis *5544*

Hematocrit *Blood* *Decrease* In cases with more active hemolysis, anemia may be moderate to severe (with hematocrits in the 10 - 25% range) and the reticulocyte count markedly elevated to 50% or more *4551*

Hemoglobin *Blood* *Decrease* In cases with more active hemolysis, anemia may be moderate to severe and the reticulocyte count markedly elevated to 50% or more *4551*
Plasma *Increase* Common *4551* Moderate increase when hemolysis is very rapid *5545*
Urine *Increase* Rarely encountered, although it is seen in occasional cases with intense hemolysis *4551* In those patients with hyperacute hemolysis *5677*

Hemoglobin A_{1c} *Blood* *Decrease* Significantly lower ($p < 0.0005$) in patients with hemolytic anemia ($n = 20$) compared to patients with nonhemolytic anemia and normal controls *3996*

Immunoglobulin G *Red Blood Cells* *Increase* May be detected on the red cell surface in up to 80% of patients *991*

Immunoglobulins *Serum* *Decrease* Immunoglobulin deficiency, in the form of generalized hypogammaglobulinemia or selective deficiency of one immunoglobulin, has been observed in a minority of patients, with or without associated lymphoproliferative disease *4551*

Iron *Urine* *Increase* Hemosiderinuria and increased urinary iron excretion indicate recent hemoglobinemia. May occur several days after an acute intravascular hemolytic episode and persist for some time *1983* *5699*

Lactate Dehydrogenase *Serum* *Increase* Often increased, although not as high as in megaloblastic anemia *5699*

Lactate Dehydrogenase Isoenzymes *Serum* *Increase* LD_2 predominates in hemolytic, whereas LD_1 predominates in megaloblastic anemia *5699*

Leukocytes *Blood* *Decrease* Varies widely, from slight leukopenia and neutropenia to moderately elevated total WBC counts, in the range of 20,000 /µL *4551* A minority of patients will have persistent leukopenia and neutropenia *1396*

283.00 Acquired Hemolytic Anemia (Autoimmune) *(continued)*

Leukocytes *(continued)*
Blood Increase Most patients have modestly elevated counts with neutrophilia *5677* Varies widely, from slight leukopenia and neutropenia to moderately elevated total WBC counts, in the range of 20,000 /µL *4551*

MCV *Blood Increase* Reflects increased number of reticulocytes *413*

Methemalbumin *Serum Increase* Low levels of hemoglobinemia and methemalbuminemia are common *4551*

Neutrophils *Blood Decrease* A minority of patients will have persistent leukopenia and neutropenia *1396*
Blood Increase Most patients have modestly elevated counts *5677*

Osmotic Fragility *Red Blood Cells Increase* May be normal with mild hemolysis. With more rapid rates of hemolysis, the cumulative curve shows increasing populations of fragile cells correlated with the appearance of spherocytosis in the peripheral blood smear *5825*
Red Blood Cells No Effect Increased in some cases of secondary hemolytic anemia but it is usually normal *5544*

Platelets *Blood Decrease* Commonly normal or slightly depressed. Severe thrombocytopenia with bleeding is encountered occasionally and has been termed the Evans' Syndrome *1398*

Reticulocytes *Blood Increase* Increased polychromasia, reflecting reticulocytosis in patients with slightly or moderately increased erythrocyte destruction *5677* In cases with more active hemolysis, anemia may be moderate to severe (with hematocrits in the 10 - 25% range) and the reticulocyte count markedly elevated to 50% or more *4551*

Urea Nitrogen *Serum Increase* In 32% of 12 patients hospitalized for this disorder *1576*

Uric Acid *Serum Increase* In 63% of 11 patients hospitalized for this disorder *1576*

Urobilinogen *Feces Increase* Uniformly increased, but seldom necessary or useful for clinical purposes at present *5677*
Urine Increase Commonly increased *5677*

283.00 Autoimmune Hemolytic Anemia

Adenosine-N6-diethylthioether-N1-pyridinoximine 5'-phosphate *Serum No Effect* In one patient with autoimmune hemolytic anemia concentration of 213.0 nmol/dL not significantly different from concentration in healthy individuals in whom the mean concentration was 162.2 nmol/dL *5294*

Antithyroid Antibodies *Serum Increase* Antithyroid antibodies observed in 5 (11.4%) of 44 patients with autoimmune hemolytic anemia *3080*

MCV *Blood Increase* Of 100 patients with macrocytosis (MCV greater than 110 fL) 3 had autoimmune hemolytic anemia *4924*

Soluble Transferrin Receptor *Serum Increase* Concentration increases with disease *4784*

Thyroid Stimulating Hormone *Serum Increase* Increased concentration observed in 9 (20.4%) of 44 patients with auoimmune hemolytic anemia *3080*

283.11 Anemia of Chronic Renal Failure

MCV *Blood No Effect* Mean concentration in 17 patients of 90 ± 7 fL compared with 91 ± 4 fL in 19 healthy controls *4239*

283.11 Hemolytic Uremic Syndrome

Albumin *Serum Decrease* In 122 patients with HUS on admission to hospital mean concentration in those with diarrhea 3.03 g/dL and 3.35 g/dL in those without which increased to 4.25 g/dL and 4.10 g/dL respectively after 6 months treatment *1818*

Amino-terminal Propeptide of Type III Procollagen
Serum Decrease In 13 children with HUS concentrations ranged from 3.7 to 9.5 mmol/L *5391*

Anti-Endothelial Cell Antibodies *Serum Increase* AECA have been detected in systemic lupus erythematosus, scleroderma and dermatomyositis but are also found in systemic vasculitis, Kawasaki disease, hemolytic uremic syndrome, thrombotic thrombocytopenic purpura and renal allograft recipients at the time of rejection *1174 5604*

Antibodies to O_{157} Lipopolysaccharide *Serum Increase* In 14 of 16 pediatric patients with HUS on admission to hospital antibodies detected indicating prior infection with VT-producing E. coli O_{157} *5416*

Anticardiolipin-specific IgA Antibodies *Serum Increase* In 17 pediatric patients with hemolytic uremic syndrome concentrations ranged from 0 to 11 APLU/mL with eight having concentrations greater than 10, the upper limit of normal *169*

Anticardiolipin-specific IgG Antibodies *Serum Increase* In 17 pediatric patients with hemolytic uremic syndrome concentrations ranged from 0 to 18 GPLU/mL with eight having concentrations greater than 7, the upper limit of normal *169*

Anticardiolipin-specific IgM Antibodies *Serum Increase* In 17 pediatric patients with hemolytic uremic syndrome concentrations ranged from 0 to 22 MPLU/mL with two having concentrations greater than 16, the upper limit of normal *169*

α_1-Antitrypsin *Feces Increase* In 122 patients with HUS on admission to hospital mean concentration of 3.3 mg/g compared with 1.85 mg/g in healthy controls *1818*

Blood *Urine Increase* In 16 pediatric patients with HUS on admission to hospital, 3 had hematuria *5416*

Burr Cells *Blood Increase* In 16 pediatric patients with HUS on admission to hospital Burr cells present in all *5416*

Creatinine *Serum Increase* In 13 children with HUS concentrations ranged from 54 to 1,020 µmol/L compared with normal range of 30 - 90 µmol/L *5391* In 19 children with hemolytic uremic syndrome median concentration of 416 mol/L significantly different from 52 mmol/L in 10 healthy children *2347* In 17 pediatric patients with hemolytic uremic syndrome concentrations ranged from 1.45 mg/dL to 9.00 mg/dL *169* In 20 children with acute HUS with diarrhoea median concentration of 416 µmol/L significantly different from 52 µmol/L in 8 healthy pediatric controls *2346* In 16 pediatric patients with HUS on admission to hospital mean concentration of 319.3 ± 138.2 µmol/L *5416*

Endothelin *Urine Increase* Urinary excretion in individuals with acute hemolytic uremic syndrome reported to be significantly higher than in healthy individuals *6*

Endothelin-1 *Urine Increase* In 4 children with hemolytic uremic syndrome mean excretion of 25.5 pmol/sq m/d not significantly different from 12.9 (lower and upper quartiles 10.0 - 15.2 pmol/sq m/d) in 60 normal children *5733*

Erythrocytes *Blood Decrease* In 16 pediatric patients with HUS on admission to hospital hemolytic anemia observed *5416*

α_1-Globulin *Serum Increase* In 122 patients with HUS on admission to hospital mean concentration in those with diarrhea of 0.36 g/dL, and 0.31 g/dL in those without, which decreased to 0.22 g/dL and 0.27 g/dL respectively after 6 months treatment *1818*

α_2-Globulin *Serum Decrease* In 122 patients with HUS on admission to hospital mean concentration in those with diarrhea of 0.55 g/dL and 0.57 g/dL in those without which increased to 0.72 g/dL and 0.68 g/dL respectively after 6 months treatment *1818*

β-Globulin *Serum No Effect* In 122 patients with HUS on admission to hospital mean concentration in those with diarrhea of 0.63 g/dL and 0.64 g/dL in those without which changed to 0.65 g/dL and 0.65 g/dL respectively after 6 months treatment *1818*

γ-Globulin *Serum Decrease* In 122 patients with HUS on admission to hospital mean concentration in those with diarrhea of 0.59 g/dL and of 0.72 g/dL in those without, which changed to 0.77 g/dL and 0.92 g/dL respectively after 6 months treatment *1818*

Glomerular Filtration Rate *Urine Decrease* In 16 pediatric patients with HUS on admission to hospital mean clearance of 84 ± 19 mL/min/1.73 m^2 *5416*

Hemoglobin *Blood Decrease* In 16 pediatric patients with HUS on admission to hospital mean concentration of 5.3 ± 1.5 mmol/L *5416*

Interleukin-1β *Serum Increase* In 8 of 19 children with hemolytic uremic syndrome was IL-1β detected in serum (median 2,250 pg/mL, range 1,200-10,900 pg/mL) *2347*
Serum No Effect In 13 children with HUS mean concentration of < 0.085 ng/mL compared with 0.07 ± 0.02 ng/mL in 8 controls *5391*
Urine No Effect In none of 19 children with hemolytic uremic syndrome was IL-β detected in urine *2347*

Interleukin-6 *Serum Increase* In 1 of 19 children with hemolytic uremic syndrome IL-6 was detected in serum, at a concentration of 650 pg/mL *2347*
Serum No Effect In 13 children with HUS mean concentration of < 30 ng/mL compared with < 20 ng/mL in 8 controls *5391*
Urine Increase In 2 of 19 children with hemolytic uremic syndrome IL-6 was detected in urine, at concentrations of 1,560 and 2,550 pg/mL *2347*

Interleukin-8 *Serum Increase* In 8 of 19 children with hemolytic uremic syndrome IL-8 was detected in serum (median 1,070 pg/mL, range 625 - 80,000 pg/mL) *2347* In 14 pediatric patients with HUS on admission to hospital median concentration of 145 pg/mL and mean concentration of 1,852 ± 5,657 pg/mL significantly increased compared with undetectable concentrations in 11 of 14 healthy control children *5416*
Urine Increase In 16 pediatric patients with HUS on admission to hospital mean concentration of 120 ± 170 ng/mmol creatinine significantly increased compared with < 4 ± 2 ng/mmol creatinine in 17 healthy control children. Excretion increased in all patients with HUS *5416* In 7 of 19 children with hemolytic uremic syndrome IL-8 was detected in urine (median 2,440 pg/mL, range 850 - 8,270 pg/mL) *2347*

Leukocytes *Blood Increase* In 16 pediatric patients with HUS on admission to hospital mean concentration of 18.1 ± 9.7 x 10^9/L. Concentration increased in 63% children *5416* In 19 children with hemolytic uremic syndrome median concentration of 14.5 x 10^{-9}/L significantly different from 8.9 x 10^9/L in 10 healthy children *2347* In 13 children with HUS concentrations ranged from 8.8 to 53.6 x 10^9/L compared with normal range of 140 - 440 x 10^9/L *5391* In 20 children with acute HUS with diarrhea median concentration of 14.5 x 10^9/L significantly different from 8.9 x 10^9/L in 8 healthy pediatric controls *2346*

Monocyte Chemotactic Protein-1 *Serum Increase* In 16 pediatric patients with HUS on admission to hospital median concentration of 270 pg/mL and mean concentration of 342 ± 331 pg/mL significantly increased compared with median of 200 pg/mL and mean of 342 ± 331 pg/mL in 14 healthy control children *5416*
Urine Increase In 16 pediatric patients with HUS on admission to hospital mean concentration of 2,570 ± 1,705 ng/mmol creatinine significantly increased compared with < 45 ± 20 ng/mmol creatinine in 17 healthy control children. Excretion increased in all patients with HUS *5416*

Monocytes *Blood Increase* In 16 pediatric patients with HUS on admission to hospital mean concentration of 1.3 ± 1.6 x 10^9/L. Concentration increased in 31% of all patients *5416*

Neutrophils *Blood Increase* In 16 pediatric patients with HUS on admission to hospital mean concentration of 11.2 ± 6.9 x 10^9/L. Concentration increased in 56% of all patients *5416* In 19 children with hemolytic uremic syndrome median concentration of 10.1 x 10^{-9}/L significantly different from 4.3 x 10^9/L in 10 healthy children *2347* In 20 children with acute HUS with diarrhea median concentration of 10.1 x 10^9/L significantly different from 4.3 x 10^9/L in 8 healthy pediatric controls *2346*

Platelet Activating Factor *Urine Increase* In 10 children with acute-phase hemolytic uremic syndrome excretion significantly increased to mean of 2.04 ± 1.66 ng/mg creatinine compared with 0.72 ± 0.43 ng/mg creatinine in 10 healthy age-matched controls *386*

Platelets *Blood Decrease* In 16 pediatric patients with HUS on admission to hospital mean concentration of 43.5 ± 16.0 x 10^9/L *5416* In 17 pediatric patients with hemolytic uremic syndrome concentrations ranged from 10,000 to 150,000 /μL with seven having concentrations less than 50,000 /μL *169* In 17 pediatric patients with hemolytic uremic syndrome concentrations ranged from 3.1 to 8.8 g/dL with all having concentrations less than the lower limit of normal *169* In 13 children with HUS concentrations ranged from 11 to 304 x 10^9/L compared with normal range of 140 - 440 x 10^9/L *5391*
Blood Increase In 17 pediatric patients with hemolytic uremic syndrome concentrations ranged from 4,600 to 50,200 /μL with 15 having concentrations greater than 10,000 /μL *169*

Protein *Serum Decrease* In 122 patients with HUS on admission to hospital mean concentration in those with diarrhea of 5.20 g/dL and 5.75 g/dL in those without, which changed to 6.75 g/dL and 6.65 g/dL respectively after 6 months treatment *1818*
Urine Increase In 16 pediatric patients with HUS on admission to hospital 4 had excretions greater than 150 mg/d *5416*

Soluble E-Selectin *Serum Increase* In 20 children with acute diarrhoea and HUS median concentration of 80 ng/mL not significantly different from 55 ng/mL in 8 healthy pediatric controls *2346*

Soluble Fas Antigen *Serum Increase* In 24 patients with thrombotic thrombocytopenic purpura and 9 with hemolytic uremic syndrome mean concentration of 2.39 ± 1.62 ng/mL significantly higher than 1.01 ± 0.24 ng/mL in 25 healthy individuals *2229*

Soluble Fas Ligand Antigen *Serum Increase* In 24 patients with thrombotic thrombocytopenic purpura and 9 with hemolytic uremic syndrome mean serum concentration of 0.307 ± 0.230 ng/mL significantly higher than 0.057 ± 0.039 ng/mL in 25 healthy individuals *2229*

Soluble Tumor Necrosis Factor Receptor-p55
Serum Increase In 13 children with HUS concentrations ranged from 20 ± 16 ng/mL compared with 1.4 ± 1 ng/mL in 8 controls *5391*

Soluble Tumor Necrosis Factor Receptor-p75
Serum Increase In 13 children with HUS concentrations ranged from 17 ± 14 ng/mL compared with 4.2 ± 1 ng/mL in 8 controls *5391*

Soluble Vascular Cell Adhesion Molecule-1
Serum Increase In 20 children with acute HUS with diarrhoea median concentration of 1,875 ng/mL significantly different from 1,200 ng/mL in 8 healthy pediatric controls *2346*

Thrombomodulin *Plasma Increase* In 24 patients with thrombotic thrombocytopenic purpura and in 9 with hemolytic uremic syndrome mean serum concentration of 46.6 ± 26.6 ng/mL significantly higher than 10.5 ± 1.9 ng/mL in 25 healthy individuals *2229*

Tumor Necrosis Factor-α *Serum Increase* In 25 children with HUS mean concentration of 44.2 ± 23.8 pg/mL significantly different from 17.9 ± 14.2 pg/mL in 39 healthy children *3119* In 2 of 19 children with hemolytic uremic syndrome TNF-α detected in serum *2347*
Serum No Effect In 13 children with HUS concentrations ranged from 0.13 ± 0.02 ng/mL compared with 0.12 ± 0.02 ng/mL in 8 controls *5391*
Urine No Effect In none of 19 children with hemolytic uremic syndrome was TNF-α detected in urine *2347*

Urea *Serum Increase* In 13 children with HUS concentrations ranged from 6.8 to 68.2 mmol/L compared with normal range of 3 - 7 mmol/L *5391* In 16 pediatric patients with HUS on admission to hospital mean concentration of 34.8 ± 14.0 mmol/L *5416*

von Willebrand Factor *Plasma Increase* In 20 children with acute HUS with diarrhoea median concentration of 1.9 U/mL significantly different from 0.55 U/mL in 8 healthy pediatric controls *2346*

283.19 Hemolytic Anemia

Circulating Endothelial Cells *Blood No Effect* In 4 patients with hemolytic anemia not due to sickle cell disease mean concentration of 2.0 ± 0.8 cells/mL not significantly different from that in 14 healthy individuals in whom mean concentration was 2.6 ± 1.6 cells/mL *4930*

Pyruvate Kinase *Red Blood Cells Increase* Mean activity in 8 patients with hemolytic anemia from various causes of 42 U/g hemoglobin compared with that in 48 healthy men, 14.6 ± 2.0 U/g hemoglobin and in 41 healthy women 17.5 ± 2.4 U/g hemoglobin *3623*

Soluble Transferrin Receptor *Serum Increase* In 21 patients with hemolytic or iron-deficiency anemia mean concentration of 2.73 ± 2.58 mg/L significantly different from 2.19 ± 0.40 mg/L in nonanemic controls *4673*

Urobilinogen *Urine Increase* In patients with hemolytic anemia excretion may exceed 8 mg/d compared with upper limit of normal of 4 mg/d *2952*

283.21 Paroxysmal Nocturnal Hemoglobinuria

Acetylcholinesterase *Red Blood Cells* *Decrease* Observed effect *3141*

Albumin *Urine* *Increase* Has been demonstrated immediately before and after an episode of hemoglobinuria, but usually there is none between attacks *972* *5699*

Alkaline Phosphatase *White Blood Cells* *Decrease* Often very low or absent *3023* Usually decreased *5677*

Bilirubin, Indirect *Serum* *Increase* Reflects hemolysis *5699*

Cells *Bone Marrow* *Decrease* The cellularity of the marrow may be decreased and may even appear aplastic *5677*

Complement C_3 *Serum* *Decrease* Caused by hypercatabolism *785* *2694* *1033* *1588*
Serum *Increase* May, on occasion, be detected in the direct Coombs' test *5677*

Coombs' Test *Serum* *Negative* Usually negative *5677*

Erythrocytes *Blood* *Decrease* Pancytopenia is a common feature *5677*

Haptoglobin *Serum* *Decrease* Associated with hemolysis *84* Absent during a hemolytic episode *5545*

Hematocrit *Blood* *Decrease* Degree of anemia may vary from none to very severe *5677* May be moderate or severe *900*

Hemoglobin *Blood* *Decrease* Degree of anemia may vary from none to very severe *5677* May be moderate or severe *900*
Plasma *Increase* At times of active hemolysis *900* Increases during sleep *5545*
Urine *Increase* Worse at night and remits during the day; probably observed initially in < 25% of all patients. Parallels changes in pH, circadian variation in cortisol excretion, complement levels, activation of the alternative pathway of complement, and other variable components of plasma *3610* Observed with hemolysis *5677*

Hemoglobin Casts *Urine* *Increase* May be present *5677*

Hemoglobin F *Blood* *Increase* Reported effect *5677* Elevated levels have been reported *4286*

Iron *Bone Marrow* *Decrease* Often absent *5677*
Serum *Decrease* A remarkable amount is often lost in the urine, even in the absence of observable hemoglobinuria *5677*
Urine *Increase* A remarkable amount is often lost in the urine, even in the absence of observable hemoglobinuria *5677* The excretion of iron in the urine continues between hemolytic episodes and is a simple and valuable indication of chronic hemoglobinuria *900*

Lactate Dehydrogenase *Serum* *Increase* Very high during active hemolysis *5699*

Leukocytes *Blood* *Decrease* Leukopenia, especially granulocytopenia, is present at some time in about 60% of patients *993* Pancytopenia is a common feature *5677*

MCV *Blood* *Decrease* Occasional microcytosis, when urinary iron loss has occurred *5699*
Blood *Increase* RBC are usually macrocytic but there may be great variation in size *5699*

Methemalbumin *Serum* *Increase* May be detected at times of active hemolysis *900*

Neutrophils *Blood* *Decrease* In 44 of 80 patients at time of diagnosis (55%) had a neutrophil count of less than 1500 /μL *2163* Leukopenia, especially granulocytopenia, is present at some time in about 60% of patients *993* Common *900*

Osmotic Fragility *Red Blood Cells* *Increase* Increased in symptomatic hemolytic anemia *5544*
Red Blood Cells *No Effect* Typically unaffected by disease *5699*

Platelets *Blood* *Decrease* In 64 of 80 patients at time of diagnosis (80%) had platelet count of less than 150,000 /μL and 48% had a count of less than 50,000 /μL *2163* Usually decreased but shows thrombotic rather than hemorrhagic complications *5545* Moderate thrombocytopenia is common *1652* Occurs at some stage in the disease in about 66% of patients *993* Pancytopenia is a common feature *5677*
Blood *No Effect* Moderate thrombocytopenia, but life span and function are normal *1652* May be normal or reduced *900*

Reticulocytes *Blood* *Increase* May be greatly increased from 20 - 24% depending on the severity of the hemolysis and the degree of marrow response *900* Count may be elevated above the level usually seen in iron deficiency *5677* There may be relative reticulocytosis but the absolute count is often inappropriately low in relation to the severity of the anemia *5699*

Soluble c-kit Molecule *Serum* *No Effect* Median concentration in patients with PNH not significantly different from that in 51 healthy volunteers of 199.0 AU/mL *2598*

Urobilinogen *Urine* *Increase* Increased blood destruction *5699*

283.90 Reactive Hemophagocytic Syndrome

Ferritin *Serum* *Increase* In 4 patients mean concentrations ranged from 34,976 to 425,984 ng/mL *2736*

Fibrinogen *Plasma* *Decrease* In 4 patients mean concentrations ranged from 100 to 119 mg/dL *2736*

Hemoglobin *Blood* *Decrease* In 4 patients mean concentrations ranged from 6.3 to 8.0 g/dL *2736*

Lactate Dehydrogenase *Serum* *Increase* In 4 patients mean activities ranged from 2,383 to > 5,000 U/L *2736*

Leukocytes *Blood* *No Effect* In 4 patients mean concentrations ranged from 0.3 to 6.0 x 10^9/L *2736*

Platelets *Blood* *Decrease* In 4 patients mean concentrations ranged from 12 to 26 x 10^{12}/L *2736*

Other Anemias

284.00 Aplastic Anemia, Congenital

Cells *Bone Marrow* *Decrease* Marrow is described as fatty and hypocellular or normocellular *1415*

Erythrocyte Survival *Red Blood Cells* *No Effect* Shortened survival has been described in some cases but earlier reports indicate no evidence of a hemolytic process *5699*

Fat *Bone Marrow* *Increase* Marrow is described as fatty and hypocellular or normocellular *1415*

Hematocrit *Blood* *Decrease* The anemia is normochromic or slightly macrocytic, and macrocytes and target cells may be seen in the blood *5699*

Hemoglobin *Blood* *Decrease* The anemia is normochromic or slightly macrocytic, and macrocytes and target cells may be seen in the blood *5699*

Leukocytes *Blood* *Decrease* In most patients, leukopenia has been due to neutropenia, but frequently all types of WBC are affected *5699*

MCH *Blood* *Increase* The anemia is normochromic or slightly macrocytic, and macrocytes and target cells may be seen in the blood *5699*

MCHC *Blood* *Increase* The anemia is normochromic or slightly macrocytic, and macrocytes and target cells may be seen in the blood *5699*

MCV *Blood* *Increase* The anemia is normochromic or slightly macrocytic, and macrocytes and target cells may be seen in the blood *5699*

Neutrophils *Blood* *Decrease* In most patients, leukopenia has been due to neutropenia, but frequently all types of WBC are affected *5699*

Plasma Cells *Bone Marrow* *Increase* There may be many plasma cells and mastocytes *1415*

Reticulocytes *Blood* *Decrease* May be slightly increased relatively but the absolute count is reduced *5699*

Target Cells *Blood* *Increase* The anemia is normochromic or slightly macrocytic, and macrocytes and target cells may be seen in the blood *5699*

284.00 Joseph Disease

β-Endorphin *Cerebrospinal Fluid* *Decrease* In 7 patients with Joseph disease mean concentration of 3.87 ± 2.09 pmol/L significantly less than 9.60 ± 1.64 pmol/L in 5 controls with other diseases *3364*

284.90 Aplastic Anemia

Alkaline Phosphatase *White Blood Cells* *Increase* Usually increased in untreated disease *5544*

Bleeding Time *Patient* *Increase* Reflects low platelet count *5677* Usually moderately prolonged *5699*

Capillary Fragility *Blood* *Increase* Reflects low platelet count *5677*

Cells *Bone Marrow* *Decrease* Marked hypocellularity of the marrow fragments with a predominance of reticulum cells, mast cells, lymphocytoid cells, and plasma cells. Cells of the myeloid series are often grossly reduced in numbers *367* Observed effect *865*

Clot Retraction *Blood* *Decrease* Observed effect *5699* Reflects low platelet count *5677*

2,3-Diphosphoglycerate *Red Blood Cells* *Increase* Synthesis is increased in response to hypoxia *380*

Erythrocyte Survival *Red Blood Cells* *Decrease* May be somewhat shortened but evidence of blood destruction is lacking *5699* There may be evidence of premature red cell destruction *3022*
Red Blood Cells *No Effect* Red cell survival is normal or only slightly reduced *2039*

Erythrocytes *Blood* *Decrease* Peripheral pancytopenia associated with hypocellular bone marrow *865* Invariable finding *5677* RBC and all cellular elements are decreased *367*
Bone Marrow *Decrease* Nucleated red cells are decreased in number, but may be the most numerous cell type *5677*

Erythropoietin *Serum* *Increase* Titers in plasma and the 24 h urinary excretion rates usually exceed those found in most other types of anemia at the same hemoglobin concentration *5677* In 74 patients with aplastic anemia mean concentration of 2418 ± 415 mIU/mL significantly higher than 286 ± 488 mIU/mL in 39 anemic controls and 9.4 ± 3.7 mIU/mL in nonanemic controls *4673* Activity of erythropoietin is high, in fact, higher than observed in patients with anemia of comparable severity due to other causes *2039*
Urine *Increase* Titers in plasma and the 24 h urinary excretion rates usually exceed those found in most other types of anemia at the same hemoglobin concentration *5677* Activity is high, in fact higher than observed in patients with anemia of comparable severity due to other causes *2039*

Glycocalicin *Plasma* *Decrease* Mean plasma concentration in 2 patients with aplastic anemia of 0.08 μg/mL significantly decreased compared with that in 36 healthy individuals of 1.40 ± 0.25 μg/mL *2853*

Hematocrit *Blood* *Decrease* Peripheral pancytopenia associated with hypocellular bone marrow *865* A severe anemia may be found at the time of presentation. The RBC are usually normocytic or slightly macrocytic *900* In 100% of 20 patients hospitalized for this disorder *1576*

Hemoglobin *Blood* *Decrease* A severe anemia may be found at the time of presentation. The RBC are usually normocytic or slightly macrocytic *900* Usually > 7 g/dL *5699* In 100% of 20 patients hospitalized for this disorder *1576*

Hemoglobin F *Blood* *Increase* In adults, substantial increases are rare, but in children the concentration has been reported to be as high as 1.5 g/dL *4753* Observed effect *5677* Returns to normal only after complete remission, and therefore is reliable indicator of complete recovery. Better prognosis in patients with higher initial level 400 mg/dL) *5544*

Interferon-γ *Serum* *Increase* In 4 of 27 perirpheral blood plasma specimens from patients with aplastic anemia interferon-γ detected *4679*

Iron *Serum* *Increase* Often > 200 μg/dL with 100% saturation of the iron-binding capacity. Decreased number of normal marrow cells *900* Increased with an almost complete saturation of iron-binding capacity. May be the first sign of erythroid suppression and is of considerable screening value in patients receiving potentially toxic drugs *5677*

Iron-binding Capacity, Total *Serum* *Decrease* Serum iron concentration is elevated and total capacity is reduced *367*

Iron Saturation *Serum* *Increase* Percent saturation of transferrin is increased *2039* Almost 100% saturation *5677*

Lactate Dehydrogenase *Serum* *Increase* In 42% of 21 patients hospitalized for this disorder *1576*

Leukocytes *Blood* *Decrease* An invariable finding *5677* Peripheral pancytopenia associated with hypocellular bone marrow *865* Counts as low as 1,000 /μL are common with 70 - 90% lymphocytes *900*

Lymphocytes *Blood* *Decrease* The absolute count is often decreased *5677*
Blood *No Effect* Production is not considered impaired *5677*
Bone Marrow *Increase* 60 - 100% of the nucleated cells are lymphocytes *5699*

MCV *Blood* *Increase* Occasional macrocytosis *900*

Monocytes *Blood* *Decrease* Absolute monocytopenia and reduction in total circulating white cells usually occurs *367*

Neutrophils *Blood* *Decrease* Absolute granulocytopenia invariably occurs. Counts of 200 /μL indicate high risk of infection *367* Absolute granulocytopenia is always present and is responsible for the leukopenic part of pancytopenia *5677* Abnormal granulation of the polymorphonuclear cells has been described. Decreased number of normal marrow cells *900*

Osmotic Fragility *Red Blood Cells* *No Effect* RBC fragility is normal *5699*

Platelets *Blood* *Decrease* Peripheral pancytopenia associated with hypocellular bone marrow *865* Often markedly decreased *900* Invariable finding. Many patients continue to have decreased counts for years after other abnormalities have disappeared *5677*

Reticulocytes *Blood* *Decrease* Percentage ranges from 0 to as high as 5%, but the absolute number is usually subnormal. Many are large and immature, possibly reflecting an increased concentration of erythropoietin and a short bone marrow transit time *2162*

Soluble c-kit Molecule *Serum* *No Effect* Median concentration in patients with aplastic anemia not significantly different from that in 51 healthy volunteers of 199.0 AU/mL *2598*

Soluble Transferrin Receptor *Serum* *Decrease* Concentration decreases with disease *4784* In 39 patients with aplastic anemia at diagnosis mean concentration of 1.77 ± 0.87 mg/L not significantly different from 2.19 ± 0.40 mg/L in nonanemic controls *4673*
Serum *Increase* In 17 patients with aplastic anemia in remission mean concentration of 2.73 ± 2.58 mg/L significantly different from 2.19 ± 0.40 mg/L in nonanemic controls *4673*

Thrombopoietin *Plasma* *Increase* Mean serum concentration in 2 patients with aplastic anemia of 40.7 ± 7.4 fmol/mL significantly higher than that in 49 healthy individuals of 0.76 ± 0.32 fmol/mL *2853*

Tumor Necrosis Factor-α *Serum* *Increase* 11 of 24 patients with aplastic anemia had increased amounts of TNF-α in peripheral plasma with mean concentration of 27.1 ± 17.2 pg/mL and median of 18 pg/mL: mean concentration of 21.0 ± 10.8 pg/mL in bone marrow plasma *4679*

285.00 Ineffective Erythropoiesis

Bilirubin, Unconjugated *Serum* *Increase* Ineffective erythropoiesis is associated with unconjugated hyperbilirubinemia *3625*

285.00 Refactory Anemia with excess of Blasts

Interleukin-6 *Serum* *No Effect* In 8 patients with refractory anemia with excess of blasts mean concentration of 12.1 ± 2.3 pg/mL not significantly different from 8.8 ± 1.8 pg/mL in 27 healthy control individuals *1120*

Interleukin-8 *Serum* *Increase* In 8 patients with refractory anemia with excess of blasts mean concentration of 38.7 ± 7.5 pg/mL significantly different from 16.2 ± 1.4 pg/mL in 27 healthy control individuals *1120*

285.00 Sideroblastic Anemia

Alkaline Phosphatase *White Blood Cells* *Decrease* Score is reduced in about 50% of the patients *2868*

Anisocytes *Blood* *Increase* Prominent findings on blood smear. In hereditary X-linked sideroblastic anemia *5699* Blood smear shows anisocytosis with many bizarre forms, target cells, hypochromia with pyridoxine-responsive anemia *5544*

285.00 Sideroblastic Anemia *(continued)*

Basophilic Stippling *Blood Increase* Prominent findings on blood smear *5699*

Bilirubin *Serum No Effect* Concentration usually within normal limits *2868* Rarely elevated despite the mild hemolytic anemia *900*

Cells *Bone Marrow Increase* Bone marrow is characterized by intense erythroid hyperplasia, often associated with a shift to younger forms, particularly polychromatophilic normoblasts, some of which show megaloblastic nuclear changes *5677*

Coproporphyrin *Red Blood Cells Increase* Conflicting reports from marked elevation to normal *2868*

Erythrocytes *Blood Decrease* Reported to be low in about 80% of patients *900*

Folate *Serum Decrease* Reported to be low in about 80% of patients *3181* Observed effect *5677*

Hematocrit *Blood Decrease* The anemia is normocytic or slightly macrocytic *5677*

Hemoglobin *Blood Decrease* The degree of anemia is variable, ranging from concentrations as low as 5 g/dL, in severely affected boys with sex-linked sideroblastic anemia to almost normal levels in the milder cases. Older people with idiopathic or secondary forms of this disease usually have moderate anemias with concentrations ranging from 7 - 10 g/dL *900* The anemia is normocytic or slightly macrocytic *5677*

Iron *Bone Marrow Increase* Increased in the marrow fragments and in the developing erythroblasts *367* Bone marrow is hyperplastic and contains increased amounts of normoblastic iron, often forming ringed sideroblasts *5677*
Serum Increase Increased serum iron and reduced iron-binding capacity in > 50% of cases *1098* Characteristically normal to elevated *900* Increased with primary inherited sex-linked sideroblastic anemia *1290*
Serum No Effect Characteristically normal to elevated *900*

Iron-binding Capacity, Total *Serum Decrease* Associated increased serum iron and reduced iron-binding capacity in > 50% of cases *1098* Somewhat decreased with pyridoxine-responsive anemia *5544* Normal to low *900*
Serum No Effect Concentration usually normal to low *900*

Iron Saturation *Serum Increase* High degree of saturation *5677*

Leukocytes *Blood Decrease* Count varies from normal to leukopenic levels; when present, leukopenia is accompanied by neutropenia. Values below 2,000 /µL are rare *5677*

MCH *Blood Decrease* Reduced hemoglobin synthesis. Microcytic hypochromic anemia *5699* Microcytic hypochromic anemia may occur due to blood loss, increased demand or dietary inadequacy. MCH < 27 pg, MCV < 80 fL *1098*
Blood Increase The anemia is normocytic or slightly macrocytic *5677*

MCHC *Blood Decrease* Degree of anemia may vary but is usually in the range of 7 - 8 g/dL of hemoglobin, with a lowered MCHC *367* Reduced hemoglobin synthesis. Microcytic hypochromic anemia *5699*

MCV *Blood Decrease* Microcytic hypochromic anemia may occur due to blood loss, increased demand or dietary inadequacy. MCH < 27 pg, MCV < 80 fL *1098* Reduced hemoglobin synthesis. Microcytic hypochromic anemia *5699*
Blood Increase The anemia is normocytic or slightly macrocytic *5677*

Monocytes *Blood Increase* Morphologically normal, but the proportion may be moderately increased *5677*

Neutrophils *Blood Decrease* Leukopenia is accompanied by neutropenia *5677*

Osmotic Fragility *Red Blood Cells Decrease* Tends to be decreased *5677*

Platelets *Blood Decrease* Usually normal, but thrombocytopenia and thrombocytosis occurs in a minority of patients *5677*
Blood Increase Usually normal, but thrombocytopenia and thrombocytosis occurs in a minority of patients *5677*
Blood No Effect Usual effect observed *900* Usually normal, but thrombocytopenia and thrombocytosis occurs in a minority of patients *5677*

Poikilocytes *Blood Increase* Blood smear shows poikilocytosis with many bizarre forms, target cells, hypochromia with pyridoxine-responsive anemia *5544* Prominent findings on blood smear. In hereditary X-linked sideroblastic anemia *5699*

Protoporphyrin *Red Blood Cells Decrease* May be characteristically high or very low, depending upon the type of sideroblastic anemia. Usually high in idiopathic and low in hereditary *5699*
Red Blood Cells Increase Almost always moderately increased, and rarely it is markedly so *2868* Elevated (40 - 300 mg/dL compared to normal levels of 15 - 35 mg/dL) reflecting a functional block to hemoglobin synthesis *900* May be characteristically high or very low, depending upon the type of sideroblastic anemia. Usually high in idiopathic and low in hereditary *5699*

Reticulocytes *Blood Decrease* Absolute count is usually reduced *367* Inappropriately low *5677*
Blood Increase Count is usually normal but may be slightly increased *5677*

Target Cells *Blood Increase* Blood smear shows anisocytosis with many bizarre forms, target cells, hypochromia with pyridoxine-responsive anemia *5544*

Volume *Red Blood Cells Decrease* Erythrocytes are formed in normal numbers but are reduced in size *5699*

Xanthurenic Acid *Urine Increase* Abnormal tryptophan metabolism indicated by excessive excretion in response to loading dose of L-tryptophan has been found in pyridoxine responsive cases *5699*

285.80 Anemia of Chronic Disease

Cholesterol *Serum Decrease* Concentrations in the range of 80 - 150 mg/dL may be observed in patients with malnutrition, a variety of serious chronic diseases, cancer, and a variety of anemias *4617*

Erythropoietin *Serum Increase* In 16 of 39 patients with anemia of chronic disease mean concentration exceeded upper limit of normal of 19 mIU/mL compared with 0 in 41 healthy controls *1862*

Ferritin *Serum Increase* Mean concentration in 17 patients of 288 ± 274 µg/L compared with 72 ± 89 µg/L in 19 healthy controls *4239* In 39 patients with anemia of chronic disease mean concentration of 197 ± 226 mg/mL compared with 126 ± 79 mg/mL in 41 healthy controls *1862* Observed effect *2811*

Granulocyte Colony Stimulating Factor *Serum Increase* In 4 of 39 patients with anemia of chronic disease concentration increased above upper limit of normal of 39 pg/mL compared with 0 in 41 healthy controls *1862*

Granulocyte-Macrophage Colony Stimulating Factor *Serum Increase* In 2 of 39 patients with anemia of chronic disease concentration increased above upper limit of normal (not detectable) compared with 1 of 41 healthy controls *1862*

Hematocrit *Blood Decrease* Observed effect *2811*

Hemoglobin *Blood Decrease* In 17 patients mean concentration of 103 ± 13 g/L compared with 138 ± 13 g/L in 19 healthy controls *4239* In 39 patients with anemia of chronic disease mean hemoglobin concentration of 10.6 ± 1.0 g/dL compared with 13.8 ± 1.0 g/dL in 41 controls *1862* Observed effect *2811*

Interleukin-1 *Serum Increase* In 1 of 39 patients with anemia of chronic renal failure concentration increased above upper limit of normal of 3.9 pg/mL compared with 0 of 41 healthy controls *1862*

Interleukin-3 *Serum Increase* In 4 of 39 patients with anemia of chronic disease concentration increased above upper limit of normal in 4 compared with 0 in 41 healthy controls *1862*

Iron *Serum Decrease* In 39 patients with anemia of chronic disease mean concentration of 43.6 ± 34.0 µg/dL (7.8 ± 6.1 µmol/L) compared with 68.7 ± 50.5 µg/dL (12.3 ± 9.0 µmol/L) in 41 healthy controls *1862* Observed effect *2811* In 19 patients mean concentration of 7.1 ± 4.0 µmol/L signficantly less than 17.3 ± 6.3 µmol/L in 19 healthy controls *4239*

Iron-binding Capacity, Total *Serum Decrease* Observed effect with chronic diseases *2811*

MCHC *Blood Decrease* Usually about 32 g/dL RBC *565*

MCV *Blood No Effect* Usually normal *2811*

Protoporphyrin *Red Blood Cells Increase* Protoporphyrin IX accumulates in the red cell because there is insufficient iron to convert it to heme *565*

Reticulocytes *Blood Increase* In 39 patients with anemia of chronic disease mean concentration of 1.1 ± 0.5% compared with 0.8 ± 0.3% in 41 healthy controls *1862*

Blood *No Effect* Usually not strikingly increased or decreased *1220 5228*

Soluble Transferrin Receptor *Serum* *Increase* Concentration may be slightly, but not significantly, higher than in normal individuals *4784*

Serum *No Effect* Mean concentration of 2.4 mg/L (range 1.2 - 4.2 mg/L) observed in 36 patients with anemia of chronic disease not significantly greater than 2.1 mg/L (95% interval 1.3 - 3.3 mg/L) in 119 apparently healthy nonanemic men and 96 women aged 24 - 69 years *5085* Mean concentration of 1.6 ± 0.4 mg/L in 17 patients with anemia of chronic disease compared with 1.7 ± 0.5 mg/L in 19 healthy controls *4239*

Transferrin *Serum* *Decrease* In 17 patients mean concentration of 1.9 ± 0.5 g/L compared with 2.5 ± g/L in 19 healthy controls *4239*

Tumor Necrosis Factor-β *Serum* *Increase* In 1 of 25 patients with anemia of chronic disease concentration increased above upper limit of normal (not detectable) compared with 0 of 39 healthy controls *1862*

Zinc Protoporphyrin *Red Blood Cells* *Increase* In individuals with anemia of chronic iron-deficiency concentration may be between 70 and 100 μmol/mol heme compared with the range reported range in healthy adults of 30 - 70 μmol/mol heme *4784*

285.80 Congenital Dyserythropoietic Anemia Type III

Cobalamin *Serum* *No Effect* In 20 patients with congenital dyserythropoietic anemia type III median concentration normal as in 10 of their healthy siblings *4563*

Hemoglobin *Blood* *Decrease* In 20 patients with congenital dyserythropoietic anemia type III median concentration of 118 g/L significantly lower than in 10 of their healthy siblings *4563*

Lactate Dehydrogenase *Serum* *Increase* In 20 patients with congenital dyserythropoietic anemia type III median activity of 16.6 mkat/L (range 11.6 - 29.6 mkat/L) significantly higher than in 10 of their healthy siblings *4563*

Thymidine Kinase *Serum* *Increase* In 20 patients with congenital dyserythropoietic anemia type III median activity of 56.2 U/L (range 18.1 - 250 U/L) significantly higher than 2.65 U/L (range 1 - 6.4 U/L) in 10 of their healthy siblings *4563* In 20 patients significant positive correlation of activity of r = 0.83 with serum lactate dehydrogenase activity *4563*

285.90 Anemia

Alkaline Phosphatase *Serum* *Decrease* Reported effect with severe anemia. In one case represented 32.4% of all cases of low alkaline phosphatase activity *3160*

Carcinoembryonic Antigen *Serum* *Increase* In 70 patients with anemia 57% had concentrations less than 2.5 ng/mL, 34% had concentrations between 2.6 and 5.0 ng/mL, 8% had concentrations between 5.1 and 10.0 ng/mL and 1% had concentrations greater than 10.0 ng/mL *2010*

Cholesterol *Serum* *Decrease* Concentrations in the range of 80 - 150 mg/dL may be observed in patients with malnutrition, a variety of serious chronic diseases, cancer, and a variety of anemias *4617*

Cortisol *Plasma* *No Effect* No effect observed on basal concentration in 11 patients with severe anemia compared with 15 healthy controls *4490*

Cortisol response to ACTH *Plasma* *Decrease* Significantly lower response observed in 11 patients with severe iron deficiency compared with 15 healthy controls at 30, 60 and 120 minutes after 25 units of ACTH administered intravenously *4490*

2,3-Diphosphoglycerate *Red Blood Cells* *Increase* Increased concentrations observed with nearly all anemias *2952*

Erythropoietin *Serum* *Increase* In elderly individuals aged 70 - 89 years similar response to anemia observed as in younger individuals with inverse correlation with hemoglobin concentration *3603* In 20 patients with anemia from chronic inflammatory disease mean concentration of 69 ± 11 mIU/mL higher than in 15 patients with malignant disease, 43 ± 5 mIU/mL, and in 15 patients with chronic infectious disease, 27 ± 4 mIU/mL *667*

Ferritin *Serum* *Increase* Mean concentration of 647 μg/L (range 8 - 14,904 μg/L) observed in 99 patients with hemoglobin monomer concentration of < 7.0 mmol/L for at least 3 months compared with reference interval of 25 - 300 μg/L *5413*

Hemoglobin *Blood* *Decrease* Anemia defined as blood hemoglobin concentration less than 140 g/L in one study of boys aged 13 - 15 years *3512*

Hexose *Serum* *Increase* Mean concentration in 77 patients with anemia of 33.4 ± 1.90 mg/dL significantly higher than 9.9 ± 0.29 mg/dL in 150 healthy controls *4029*

Iron *Serum* *Decrease* Mean concentration of 10.2 μmol/L (range 1.4 - 39.2 μmol/L) observed in 99 patients with hemoglobin monomer concentration of < 7.0 mmol/L for at least 3 months compared with reference interval of 10 - 32 μmol/L *5413*

Lactate Dehydrogenase *Serum* *Increase* In 77 patients with anemia mean activity of 380.7 ± 70.41 U/L significantly different from 115.3 ± 3.25 U/L in 150 healthy controls *4028*

Lactate Dehydrogenase Isoenzyme-1 *Serum* *Increase* In 77 patients with anemia mean activity of 146.9 ± 24.95 U/L significantly different from 35.5 ± 1.29 U/L in 150 healthy controls *4028*

Lactate Dehydrogenase Isoenzyme-2 *Serum* *Increase* In 77 patients with anemia mean activity of 158.8 ± 29.74 U/L significantly different from 43.2 ± 1.32 U/L in 150 healthy controls *4028*

Lactate Dehydrogenase Isoenzyme-3 *Serum* *Increase* In 77 patients with anemia mean activity of 71.2 ± 17.18 U/L significantly different from 26.6 ± 0.74 U/L in 150 healthy controls *4028*

Lactate Dehydrogenase Isoenzyme-4 *Serum* *No Effect* In 77 patients with anemia mean activity of 9.7± 2.43 U/L not significantly different from 6.3 ± 0.26 U/L in 150 healthy controls *4028*

Lactate Dehydrogenase Isoenzyme-5 *Serum* *Increase* In 77 patients with anemia mean activity of 7.4 ± 2.71 U/L not significantly different from 3.6 ± 0.16 U/L in 150 healthy controls *4028*

Mucoprotein *Serum* *Increase* Mean concentration in 77 patients with anemia of 195.5 ± 11.43 mg/dL significantly higher than 87.0 ± 1.83 mg/dL in 150 healthy controls *4029*

Partial Thromboplastin Time *Plasma* *No Effect* In patients with severe anemia no significant effect of hematocrit observed *4829*

Pepsinogen Antibodies *Serum* *Positive* More common in patients with pernicious anemia than intrinsic factor antibodies. Found in about 50% patients with active duodenal ulcers *4093*

Prothrombin Time *Plasma* *No Effect* In patients with severe anemia no significant effect of hematocrit observed *4829*

Sialic Acid, Lipid-associated *Serum* *Increase* Mean concentration in 77 patients with anemia of 29.7 ± 1.28 mg/dL significantly higher than 19.4 ± 0.38 mg/dL in 150 healthy controls *4029*

Transferrin *Serum* *Decrease* Mean concentration of 2.26 g/L (range of 0.36 - 4.39 g/L) observed in 99 patients with hemoglobin monomer concentration of < 7.0 mmol/L for at least 3 months compared with reference interval of 1.84 - 3.50 g/L *5413*

Viscosity *Plasma* *No Effect* No effect of anemia observed *4093*

285.90 Hemophagocytic Syndrome

Interferon-γ *Serum* *Increase* In children with HPS mean concentration of 89.5 U/mL significantly higher than in controls *2145*

Interleukin-6 *Serum* *Increase* In children with HPS mean concentration of 104 pg/mL significantly higher than in controls *2145*

β_2-Microglobulin *Serum* *Increase* In 6 children with HPS mean concentration of 7.5 mg/L significantly higher than in controls *2145*

Urine *Increase* In 6 children with HPS mean concentration of greater than 31,650 μg/g creatinine significantly higher than in controls *2145*

Soluble Interleukin-2 Receptor *Serum* *Increase* In children with HPS mean concentration of 14,650 U/mL significantly higher than in controls *2145*

285.90 **Hemophagocytic Syndrome** *(continued)*

Soluble Interleukin-2 Receptor *(continued)*

Coagulation Defects

286.00 Hemophilia

AHF-Like Antigen *Plasma Increase* Plasma contains normal or even elevated amounts of antigenic material detected by heterologous antiserum *5867*

Antibody Titer *Serum Increase* Titers of antibodies to cytomegalovirus were generally higher in hemophiliac patients than in a control group of healthy volunteers *3009*

Bleeding Time *Patient Increase* In severe cases *2034* *Patient No Effect* Not usually abnormal *4979* Bleeding time and prothrombin time are not significantly prolonged *5677*

Capillary Fragility *Blood Increase* Occasional patients may have positive tourniquet tests *5699*

Cholesterol *Serum Decrease* May be below normal in this condition *1290*

Clotting Time *Blood Increase* May be 24 h or longer and show spontaneous irregular variations *5699* In severe cases *5699* Typical observation *2034*

Creatine Kinase *Serum Increase* Increases when bleeding occurs into the muscles. Serum activity returns to normal after 10 days following treatment with cryoprecipitate. The test is useful in distinguishing between hemorrhage into the psoas muscle (raised levels) and into the hip joint only (no increase) *1290*

Erythrocytes *Urine Increase* Bleeding from the kidneys is often caused by trauma, but usually the cause cannot be determined. May occasionally be due to infection. Occurs in approximately 20% of the moderate and severe cases and in 5% of the mild cases *5677* Hematuria may persist for weeks or months *2039*

Factor VIII *Plasma Decrease* May be due to decreased or absent synthesis of factor VIII or to the synthesis of a functionally inactive factor VII molecule *3465* The basic defect appears to be a failure to synthesize functional AHF *4979* Varies from 0% of normal in severe to 25% in mild cases *5699*

Hematocrit *Blood Decrease* Presence or absence of anemia depends on the severity and frequency of bleeding *5699*

Hemoglobin *Blood Decrease* Presence or absence of anemia depends on the severity and frequency of bleeding *5699*

Iron-binding Capacity, Total *Serum Increase* Depending upon the severity and frequency of bleeding *5699*

Iron Saturation *Serum Decrease* Depending upon the severity and frequency of bleeding *5699*

Lee-White Clotting Time *Blood Increase* Deficient factor VIII (AHG) *900*

β_2-Macroglobulin *Serum Increase* Significantly higher *2821*

MCH *Blood Decrease* Presence or absence of anemia depends on the severity and frequency of bleeding *5699*

MCHC *Blood Decrease* Presence or absence of anemia depends on the severity and frequency of bleeding *5699*

MCV *Blood Decrease* Presence or absence of anemia depends on the severity and frequency of bleeding *5699*

Partial Thromboplastin Time *Plasma Increase* Observed effect *4979* The most sensitive screening test, usually prolonged if AHG levels are < 20% of normal *2039* Observed effect *1980* Always significantly prolonged in patients with 20% factor VIII. Individuals with levels ranging between 20 - 30% may have a PTT value either just outside or at the upper end of the normal range *5677*

Platelets *Blood Increase* Usually normal or elevated *5699*

Prothrombin Time *Plasma No Effect* No significant effect usually observed *4979* Bleeding time and prothrombin time are not significantly prolonged *5677*

Recalcification Time *Plasma Increase* Greatly prolonged *5699*

Thrombin Time *Blood No Effect* Not affected *4979* Usually unaffected by disease *1980* Unaffected by disease *2034*

Thromboplastin Generation *Blood Increase* Due to deficient function of the adsorbed plasma reagent *5699*

286.01 Hemophilia A

Cholesterol *Serum No Effect* Mean concentration of 190.7 ± 13.6 mg/dL not significantly different from 204.2 ± 8.8 mg/dL in 19 female controls and 200.2 ± 11.0 mg/dL in 20 male controls *370*

HDL-Cholesterol *Serum No Effect* Mean concentration in 17 patients of 50.5 ± 2.8 mg/dL not significantly different from 56.2 ± 4.5 mg/dL in 19 female controls and 46.0 ± 2.9 mg/dL in 20 male controls *370*

Thromboxane A_2 Generation *Blood Decrease* In 17 patients mean generation in spontaneously clotting blood at 60 minutes of 157.31 ± 24.24 ng/mL compared with 194.19 ± 28.86 ng/mL at 60 minutes in 20 male controls *370*

286.10 Christmas Disease

Bleeding Time *Patient Increase* In severe cases *5545* *Patient No Effect* Usually unaffected by disease *4979* *5677*

Clotting Time *Blood Increase* In severe cases *5545* In severe deficiencies *5677*

Creatine Kinase *Serum Increase* Increases when bleeding occurs into the muscles. Serum activity returns to normal after 10 days following treatment with cryoprecipitate. The test is useful in distinguishing between hemorrhage into the psoas muscle (raised levels) and into the hip joint only (no increase) *1290*

Erythrocytes *Urine Increase* Bleeding from the kidneys is often caused by trauma, but usually the cause cannot be determined. May occasionally be due to infection. Occurs in approximately 20% of the moderate and severe cases and in 5% of the mild cases *5677* Hematuria may persist for weeks or months *2039*

Factor IX *Plasma Decrease* Titers < 5% of normal are usual, and may be undetectable in severe cases. In mildly affected patients, values may be > 30% *300* Present in carriers in approximately half the concentration of that found in patients *5677*

Fibrinogen *Plasma No Effect* Concentration usually normal *413*

Lee-White Clotting Time *Blood Increase* Deficient factor IX (PCT) *900*

Partial Thromboplastin Time *Plasma Increase* Reported effect *4979* In contrast to hemophilia A, the abnormality is corrected by serum but not by adsorbed plasma *5677* Reported effect *1980*

Prothrombin Consumption *Blood Increase* In severe cases *5544*

Prothrombin Time *Plasma No Effect* All patients have a normal test using human brain tissue factor (thromboplastin), but when ox-brain tissue factor is used, the prothrombin time is prolonged in approximately 6% of cases *5337* No significant abnormality usually observed *5677* No significant usually observed *4979*

Thrombin Time *Blood No Effect* No significant effect observed with disease *4979*

Thromboplastin Generation *Blood Increase* In contrast to hemophilia A, the abnormality resides in the serum rather than in the adsorbed plasma *5677* In mild deficiency, may be the only abnormal test *5544*

286.10 Hemophilia B

Cholesterol *Serum No Effect* Mean concentration of 191.6 ± 18.0 mg/dL not significantly different from 204.2 ± 8.8 mg/dL in 19 female controls and 200.2 ± 11.0 mg/dL in 20 male controls *370*

Thromboxane A_2 Generation *Blood Decrease* In 9 patients in spontaneously clotting blood mean concentration increased to 122.78 ± 24.79 ng/mL after 60 minutes compared with 194.19 ± 26.86 ng/mL in 20 healthy male controls *370*

286.20 Factor XI Deficiency

Bleeding Time *Patient Increase* Variable *4979* In severe cases *2034*

Patient *No Effect* Usually normal *5677*

Clotting Time *Blood* *Increase* Observed effect *5545* Typical observation *4979*

Factor XI *Plasma* *Decrease* Definitive diagnosis is by a factor XI assay using blood from a patient with established factor XI deficiency *5677* Plasma thromboplastin antecedent (factor XI) deficiency *4979*

Partial Thromboplastin Time *Plasma* *Increase* PTT or activated PTT test is prolonged and the prothrombin time normal *5677* Reported effect *4979*

Prothrombin Time *Plasma* *No Effect* PTT or activated PTT test is prolonged and the prothrombin time normal *5677* No significant effect usually observed *4979*

Thrombin Time *Blood* *No Effect* No significant effect usually observed *4979*

Thromboplastin Generation *Blood* *Increase* The most marked abnormality is found when the patient's adsorbed plasma and serum are incubated together *5677*

286.31 Congenital Dysfibrinogenemia

Bleeding Time *Patient* *Increase* Usually prolonged, but in some cases no clot forms at all *5677*

Clot Retraction *Blood* *Decrease* Reported effect *5677*

Clotting Time *Blood* *Increase* The clotting time of whole blood or the recalcification time of platelet-poor plasma has usually been normal or prolonged *5677*
Blood *No Effect* The clotting time of whole blood or the recalcification time of platelet-poor plasma has usually been normal or prolonged *5677*

Estrogens *Plasma* *No Effect* Usually unaffected by disease *5677*

Factor II *Plasma* *No Effect* Usually unaffected by disease *5677*

Factor V *Plasma* *No Effect* Usually unaffected by disease *5677*

Factor VII *Plasma* *No Effect* Usually unaffected by disease *5677*

Factor VIII *Plasma* *No Effect* Usually unaffected by disease *5677*

Factor IX *Plasma* *No Effect* Usually unaffected by disease *5677*

Factor X *Plasma* *No Effect* Usually unaffected by disease *5677*

Factor XIII *Plasma* *No Effect* Concentration usually normal *5677*

Fibrinogen *Plasma* *Decrease* Reduced level by any technique. The discordant values suggest that abnormal fibrinogen molecules are inhibitory to coagulation of the normal fibrinogen or have a markedly delayed clotting time and are present in sufficient concentration to give a falsely low level of fibrinogen *5677* Concentration is usually normal or only slightly depressed, but is functionally defective *4979*
Plasma *No Effect* In most cases determined by immunologic assays, fibrin tyrosine content, or gravimetric methods have been normal *413* *5677*

Partial Thromboplastin Time *Plasma* *Increase* Variable. Even when abnormal, rarely as prolonged as the prothrombin time or the thrombin time *5677*

Plasminogen Antigen *Plasma* *No Effect* Invariably normal *5677*

Platelets *Blood* *No Effect* Usually unaffected by disease *5677*

Prothrombin Time *Plasma* *Increase* Usually prolonged, but in some cases no clot forms at all *5677* In many cases *4979*

Recalcification Time *Plasma* *No Effect* The clotting time of whole blood or the recalcification time of platelet-poor plasma has usually been normal *5677*

Reptilase® Time *Blood* *Increase* Usually prolonged, but in some cases no clot forms at all *5677*

Thrombin Time *Blood* *Increase* Usually prolonged, but in some cases no clot forms at all *5677* Abnormally long *4979*

Thromboplastin Generation *Blood* *No Effect* Typically unaffected by disease *5677*

286.32 Factor XII Deficiency

Bleeding Time *Patient* *No Effect* Usually unaffected by disease *4979* Prothrombin and bleeding times are normal *5677*

Clotting Time *Blood* *Increase* Observed effect *5545* In severe deficiencies *2034*

Factor XII *Plasma* *Decrease* Nondetectable *4287* Definitive diagnosis is made by testing against plasma from an established case *5677*

Partial Thromboplastin Time *Plasma* *Increase* Activated partial thromboplastin time is prolonged *5677* Reported effect *4979*

Prothrombin Time *Plasma* *No Effect* No significant effect usually observed *4979* Prothrombin and bleeding times are normal *5677*

Thrombin Time *Blood* *No Effect* No significant effect usually observed *4979* *900*

286.33 Factor XIII Deficiency

Bleeding Time *Patient* *No Effect* Time usually normal *5677* Time usually unaffected *4979*

Clot Solubility *Blood* *Poor* Observed effect *900*

Clotting Time *Blood* *No Effect* No significant change observed *4979*

Partial Thromboplastin Time *Plasma* *No Effect* No significant effect usually observed *4979*

Platelets *Blood* *No Effect* Concentration usually unaffected *5677*

Prothrombin Time *Plasma* *No Effect* No significant effect usually observed *4979*

Thrombin Time *Blood* *No Effect* No significant effect usually observed *900* No significant effect observed *4979*

286.34 Congenital Afibrinogenemia

Bleeding Time *Patient* *Increase* Prolonged bleeding times, unrelated to thrombocytopenia, are found in some patients *5770* Typical finding observed *5677* Often increased (33% of patients) *5545* Variable *4979*

Clotting Time *Blood* *Increase* Corrected by the addition of normal plasma or normal fibrinogen to the patient's plasma *5677* Infinite *4979*

Fibrinogen *Plasma* *Decrease* Undetectable by almost all physicochemical measurements or functional assays *5677*

Partial Thromboplastin Time *Plasma* *Increase* Corrected by the addition of normal plasma or normal fibrinogen to the patient's plasma *5677* Infinite *4979*

Platelets *Blood* *Decrease* Mild to moderate thrombocytopenia occurs occasionally. Count is rarely below 100,000 /µL *5770*

Prothrombin Time *Plasma* *Increase* Infinite *4979* Corrected by the addition of normal plasma or normal fibrinogen to the patient's plasma *5677*

Recalcification Time *Plasma* *Increase* Corrected by the addition of normal plasma or normal fibrinogen to the patient's plasma *5677*

Reptilase® Time *Blood* *Increase* Corrected by the addition of normal plasma or normal fibrinogen to the patient's plasma *5677*

Thrombin Time *Blood* *Increase* Infinite *4979* Corrected by the addition of normal plasma or normal fibrinogen to the patient's plasma *5677*

286.35 Factor V Deficiency

Bleeding Time *Patient* *Increase* Slightly prolonged in approximately 33% of cases *5677*
Patient *No Effect* Usually unaffected by disease *4979* Slightly prolonged in 33% of cases and normal in the remainder *5677*

Clotting Time *Blood* *Increase* Observed finding *5677* Increase in coagulation time is not corrected by administration of vitamin K *5545*

286.35 Factor V Deficiency *(continued)*

Erythrocyte Sedimentation Rate *Blood Decrease* Nearly 0; RBC remain suspended even after 24 h *4979*

Partial Thromboplastin Time *Plasma Increase* Prothrombin time and partial thromboplastin time, activated or unactivated, are all prolonged *5677* Reported effect *4979*

Prothrombin Consumption *Blood Increase* Increase in prothrombin consumption is not corrected by administration of vitamin K, with factor V deficiency *5545*

Prothrombin Time *Plasma Increase* Deficient factor V (labile) *900* Not corrected by administration of vitamin K *5545* Prothrombin time and partial thromboplastin time, activated or unactivated, are all prolonged *5677*

Thrombin Time *Blood No Effect* No change from normal usually observed *900* No significant effect usually observed *2034* No significant deviation from normal usually observed *4979*

Thromboplastin Generation *Blood Increase* Abnormal when the reaction mixture contains adsorbed plasma from the patient, but is normal when serum from the patient is used *2034* Abnormal when the reaction mixture contains adsorbed plasma from the patient but is normal when serum from the patient is used *5677* Abnormal results *4979*

286.36 Factor X Deficiency

Bleeding Time *Patient No Effect* Usually unaffected by disease *2034* No significant effect usually observed *4979*

Clotting Time *Blood Increase* Observed finding *2034*

Factor X *Plasma Decrease* True deficiency in some patients and deficiency of functional factor X in others *4979*

Partial Thromboplastin Time *Plasma Increase* Prolonged *5677* Observed effect *4979* Reported effect *900*

Prothrombin Consumption *Blood Increase* Abnormal results *4979*

Prothrombin Time *Plasma Increase* Not corrected by administration of vitamin K. Prolonged *5677*

Thrombin Time *Blood No Effect* No significant effect usually observed *2034 4979 900*

286.37 Factor VII Deficiency

Bleeding Time *Patient Increase* May be abnormally long *4979*
Patient No Effect No significant effect usually observed *2034 4979*

Clotting Time *Blood No Effect* Clotting time of recalcified plasma is normal, distinguishing this from Stuart factor deficiency *4979* No significant effect usually observed *5677*

Erythrocytes *Urine Increase* Hematuria has been observed *4979*

Factor VII *Plasma Decrease* Some patients appear to synthesize a nonfunctional variant, and other patients are truly deficient *4979*

Partial Thromboplastin Time *Plasma No Effect* Usually no effect of disease seen *4979* Typically no influence of disease observed *5677*

Prothrombin Time *Plasma Increase* Usually greatly prolonged *74*

Thrombin Time *Blood No Effect* No significant effect usually observed *4979 2034*

Thromboplastin Generation *Blood No Effect* No change usually observed *4979*

286.38 Factor II Deficiency

Bleeding Time *Patient No Effect* Typical observation *4979*

Clotting Time *Blood Increase* Typical observation *4979*

Partial Thromboplastin Time *Plasma Increase* Variable *4979*

Thrombin Time *Blood No Effect* No change usually observed with disease *4979* No significant effect usually seen *900*

286.40 von Willebrand's Disease

Bleeding Time *Patient Increase* Usually prolonged 2 h after dose of 10 grains of aspirin; bleeding time is variable without this aspirin tolerance test *5544* May be detected by Dukes' method or the standard Ivy procedure *5677* In one patient with type I von Willebrand's disease bleeding time of 4.0 min compared with normal range of less than 7.5 min *2298* Prolonged *485* Commonly occurs in homozygotes and heterozygotes *3032* Bleeding time typically increased *4979*

Cholesterol *Serum No Effect* Mean concentration in 17 patients of 196.0 ± 12.8 mg/dL not significantly different from 204.2 ± 8.8 mg/dL in 19 female controls and 200.2 ± 11.0 mg/dL in 20 male controls *370*

Clot Retraction *Blood No Effect* Usually no effect observed *5677*

Clotting Time *Blood Increase* Variable *4979*

Factor VIII *Plasma Decrease* Characteristically reduced, usually from 20 - 40%. A wide range may be seen and a normal concentration is not incompatible with the diagnosis *900* A true decrease in amount of AHF protein accompanied by a proportional or even more severe decrease in AHF-like antigens *5867* Activity is usually higher than in classic hemophilia, but values of 1 - 5% of normal may sometimes be found. May show wide fluctuation in the same person on repeated testing *5677* A true decrease in amount of AHF protein accompanied by a proportional or even more severe decrease in AHF-like antigens *4979* Commonly occurs in both homozygotes and heterozygotes *3032*

Factor VIII Activity *Plasma No Effect* In one patient activity of 66 U/dL compared with normal range of 45 - 145 U/dL *2298*

Fibrinogen *Plasma No Effect* Concentration usually normal *486*

HDL-Cholesterol *Serum Increase* In 17 patients mean concentration of 59.6 ± 6.7 mg/dL higher than 56.2 ± 4.5 mg/dL in 19 female controls and 46.0 ± 2.9 mg/dL in 20 male controls *370*

Lee-White Clotting Time *Blood No Effect* Usually normal *5544*

Partial Thromboplastin Time *Plasma Increase* May be prolonged and is related to the decreased factor VIII AHF activity *5677* Observed effect *1980* Variable *4979*

Platelets *Blood Decrease* Usually normal, but thrombocytopenia has been reported in some families *936*
Blood No Effect Concentration usually unaffected *5677* Usually normal, but thrombocytopenia has been reported in some families *936*

Protein Z *Plasma Decrease* Mean protein Z concentration in patients with von Willebrand syndrome < 1,500 µg/L compared with 2,680 ± 490 µg/L in healthy controls *2645*

Prothrombin Consumption *Blood Decrease* May be present and is related to the decreased factor VIII AHF activity *5677*

Prothrombin Time *Plasma No Effect* PT usually normal *4979* No significant effect observed *1980*

Ristocetin Cofactor Activity *Plasma Decrease* In one patient with von Willebrand's disease activity of 13 U/dL significantly less than lower limit of normal range of 47 - 196 U/dL *2298*

Thrombin Time *Blood No Effect* Usually unaffected by disease *1980 4979*

Thromboxane A_2 Generation *Blood Decrease* In 17 patients with spontaneous clotting concentration increased to 120 ng/mL at 60 minutes compared with 228 ng/mL in 17 healthy female controls *370*

von Willebrand Factor Antigen *Plasma No Effect* In one patient activity of 53 U/dL close to lower limit of normal range of 49 - 192 U/dL *2298*

286.60 Disseminated Intravascular Coagulation

α_2-Antiplasmin *Plasma Decrease* Measured values in 9 patients with DIC. Subnormal values in 6, normal in 2 and increased in 1 *5187* Significantly decreased levels in 25 patients with acute, subacute and chronic compensated and uncompensated DIC *4543*

Antithrombin *Plasma Decrease* In 126 patients with conditions other than leukemia activity on day that they developed DIC of 65.0 ± 25.6% significantly different from 77.4 ± 24.0% 7 days before the onset of DIC *5512*
Plasma No Effect In 114 leukemics who developed DIC mean activity of 81.9 ± 24.2% on day that they developed DIC not significantly different from 87.2 ± 26.3% from activity 7 days before the onset of DIC *5512*

Antithrombin III *Plasma Decrease* Early and significant decreases occur and therefore this may serve as a useful diagnostic test *5220 442*

γ-Carboxyglutamic Acid, Free *Plasma Increase* In 11 hospitalized patients with deep venous thrombosis mean concentration of 559 ± 361 pmol/mL significantly higher than that in 19 healthy men and women aged between 35 and 65 years in whom mean concentration was 146 ± 34 pmol/mL *2014*

D-Dimer *Plasma Increase* In 18 trauma patients with DIC mean concentration of 7,126 ± 1,411 ng/mL significantly different from 2,643 ± 688 ng/mL in 24 without DIC. In 15 patients with sepsis and DIC mean concentration of 3,728 ± 1,066 ng/mL significantly different from 507 ± 97 ng/mL in 5 without DIC *1636* In 40 patients with pre-DIC mean concentration of 1,524 ± 233 μg/mL and 3,501 ± 526 μg/mL in 80 patients with DIC concentration higher than 621 ± 58 ng/mL in 50 healthy controls *5509* In 55 patients with DIC mean concentration of 3,205 ± 514 ng/mL, in 15 with pre-DIC of 1,428 ± 284 ng/mL and in 10 with non-DIC of 657 ± 47 ng/mL *5511* In 114 leukemics who developed DIC mean concentration of 4,439 ± 2,297 ng/mL and 4,677 ± 2,847 ng/mL in 126 patients with other conditions, respectively, on day that they developed DIC, significantly higher than 1,387 ± 999 ng/mL and 1,759 ± 1,015 ng/mL in the respective populations 7 days before the onset of DIC *5512*

Endothelin-1 *Plasma Increase* A significant elevation of plasma levels of ET-1 was observed in some cases of DIC *2174* In two studies patients had 2.1 and 5.2-fold increases *328* In 4 patients with gastric cancer, colon cancer, malignant lymphoma or acute pyelonephritis mean concentration of 3.1 ± 0.6 pg/mL, 2.1-fold above appropriate normal values *328*

Endothelin-1, Big *Plasma Increase* In 4 patients with gastric cancer, colon cancer, malignant lymphoma or acute pyelonephritis mean concentration of 30.4 ± 14.4 pg/mL, 5.2-fold above normal values *328*

Factor V *Plasma Decrease* Reported effect *5677*

Factor VIII *Plasma Decrease* Reported effect *5677*

Factor XIII *Plasma Decrease* Substantial depression of factor XIII concentrations developed with concomitant significant increases in the proportion and concentration of plasma high molecular weight fibrinogen complexes (HMWFC). An inverse correlation between factor XIII and percentage of HMWFC was demonstrated in the early stages of the illness *3253*

Fibrin Degradation Products *Plasma Decrease* Deposition of fibrin usually stimulates local secondary fibrinolysis producing reduced circulating plasminogen level due to consumption and a decrease in systemic fibrinolytic activity *5677*
Plasma Increase If large amounts are present, the thrombin time will be markedly prolonged; latex agglutination test for fibrin degradation products will be positive *5677*

Fibrinogen *Plasma Decrease* Reported effect *5677* In 18 trauma patients with DIC mean concentration of 1.4 ± 0.1 g/L significantly lower than 1.8 ± 0.1 g/L in 24 without DIC. In 15 patients with sepsis and DIC mean concentration of 3.9 ± 0.5 g/L significantly different from 5.4 ± 0.1 g/L in 5 without DIC *1636* In 114 leukemics who developed DIC mean concentration of 206 ± 133 mg/dL and 253 ± 170 mg/dL in 126 patients with other conditions, respectively, on day that they developed DIC, significantly lower than 326 ± 165 mg/dL and 321 ± 164 mg/dL in the respective populations 7 days before the onset of DIC *5512* Low or falling levels *900*
Plasma Increase Substantial depression of factor XIII concentrations developed together with concomitant significant increases in the proportion and concentration of plasma high molecular weight fibrinogen complexes (HMWFC). An inverse correlation between factor XIII and percentage of HMWFC was demonstrated in the of the illness *3253*

Fibrinogen Degradation Products *Plasma Increase* In 18 trauma patients with DIC mean concentration of 34 ± 7 mg/L significantly different from 10 ± 1 mg/L in 24 without DIC. In 15 patients with sepsis and DIC mean concentration of 31 ± 9 mg/L significantly different from 6 ± 2 mg/L in 5 without DIC *1636* In 114 leukemics who developed DIC mean concentration of 41.0 ± 34.7 μg/mL and 41.0 ± 34.7 μg/mL in 126 patients with other conditions, respectively, on day that they developed DIC, significantly higher than 11.1 ± 7.0 μg/mL and 29.0 ± 34.0 μg/mL in the respective populations 7 days before the onset of DIC *5512*

Fibrinopeptide A *Plasma Increase* In 18 trauma patients with DIC mean concentration of 61 ± 14 ng/mL significantly different from 19 ± 7 ng/mL in 24 without DIC. In 15 patients with sepsis and DIC mean concentration of 22 ± 4 ng/mL not significantly different from 9 ± 1 ng/mL in 5 without DIC *1636*

Fibronectin *Plasma Decrease* Mean fasting concentration in 5 of 10 patients with DIC was low at 21.5 ± 11.2 mg/dL, significantly lower than that in 28 normal men, 32.5 ± 7.1 mg/dL, and 31.6 ± 5.7 mg/dL in 34 normal women *4811*

Granulocyte Elastase-α_1-Proteinase Inhibitor Complex *Plasma Increase* In 41 patients with DIC mean concentration of 421.0 ± 45.6 ng/mL significantly higher than 246.1 ± 41.9 ng/mL in 27 patients with similar underlying conditions but without DIC *3889*

Haptoglobin *Serum Decrease* Decreases in 6 - 10 h and lasts for 2 - 3 days after lysis of 20 - 30 mL of blood. Determination is relatively reliable and very sensitive *5545*

Hemoglobin *Plasma Increase* Increases transiently with return to normal in 8 h *5545*
Urine Increase Occurs 1 - 2 h after severe hemolysis and lasts 24 h. It is a transient finding and is relatively insensitive. False positive is due to myoglobinuria or to lysis of RBCs in urine with intravascular hemolysis *5545*

Interleukin-1 *Serum Increase* Levels of IL-1β were also significantly higher in patients with DIC *5513*

Interleukin-6 *Serum Increase* Plasma interleukin-6 (IL-6) was higher in patients with disseminated intravascular coagulation (DIC) than in those without DIC. Plasma IL-6 was highest in patients with underlying sepsis and was also high in those with advanced solid cancer *5513*

International Normalized Ratio *Plasma Increase* In 114 leukemics who developed DIC mean ratio of 1.10 ± 0.12 and in 126 patients with other conditions on day that DIC developed mean ratios of 1.31 ± 0.30 and 1.39 ± 0.42 respectively, significantly higher than 1.10 ± 0.12 and 1.16 ± 0.17 in the respective populations 7 days before the onset of DIC *5512*

Partial Thromboplastin Time *Plasma Increase* Prolonged because of consumption of clotting factors and the anticoagulant effects of fibrin degradation products *5677*

Plasmin-α_2-Plasmin Inhibitor Complex *Plasma Increase* In 55 patients with DIC mean concentration of 3.67 ± 0.44 μg/mL, in 15 with pre-DIC of 2.65 ± 0.51 μg/mL and in 10 with non-DIC 1.35 ± 0.33 μg/mL *5511* Mean concentration in 40 patients with pre-DIC of 2.95 ± 0.53 μg/mL and 3.78 ± 0.35 μg/mL in 80 patients with DIC higher than 1.45 ± 0.36 μg/mL in 50 healthy controls *5509*

Plasmin-Plasmin Inhibitor Complex *Plasma Increase* In 114 leukemics who developed DIC mean concentration of 4.6 ± 5.2 μg/mL on day that they developed DIC significantly higher than 1.3 ± 1.2 μg/mL 7 days before the onset of DIC *5512*
Plasma No Effect In 126 patients with conditions other than leukemia on day that they developed DIC mean concentration of 2.9 ± 2.8 μg/mL not significantly different from 3.6 ± 3.6 μg/mL 7 days before the onset of DIC *5512*

Plasminogen Activator Inhibitor-1 *Plasma Increase* Concentrations increased and highest in patients with disseminated intravascular coagulation and multiple organ failure *193* In 80 patients with DIC mean concentration of 93.6 ± 5.7 ng/mL higher than 30.0 ± 5.6 ng/mL in 40 patients with pre-DIC and 50 healthy controls with mean concentration of 28.1 ± 7.2 ng/mL *5509* Mean concentration in 55 patients with DIC of 91.5 ± 7.3 ng/mL, in 15 with pre-DIC of 28.4 ± 6.2 ng/mL and in 10 with non-DIC of 24.5 ± 7.9 ng/mL *5511* In 114 leukemics and 126 patients with other conditions who developed DIC mean concentration of 70.2 ± 66.7 ng/mL significantly different from 20.9 ± 16.6 ng/mL 7 days before the onset of DIC *5512*

Plasminogen Antigen *Plasma Decrease* Deposition of fibrin usually stimulates local secondary fibrinolysis producing reduced circulating plasminogen level due to consumption and a decrease in systemic fibrinolytic activity *5677*

286.60 Disseminated Intravascular Coagulation *(continued)*

Platelets *Blood Decrease* Reported effect *5677* Low or falling platelet counts *900* In 18 trauma patients with DIC mean concentration of 100 ± 16 x 10^6/L significantly lower than 185 ± 12 x 10/L in 24 without DIC. In 15 patients with sepsis and DIC mean concentration of 40 ± 6 x 10^6/L significantly different from 98 ± 19 x 10^6/L in 5 without DIC *1636* In 126 patients with conditions other leukemia, mean concentration on day that they developed DIC, of 7.9 ± 6.3 x 10^4/µL significantly lower than 17.7 ± 10.6 x 10^4/µL 7 days before the onset of DIC *5512*
Blood No Effect In 114 leukemics who developed DIC mean concentration of 5.2 ± 5.3 x 10^4/µL on day that they developed DIC, not significantly different from 5.5 ± 4.8 x 10^4/µL 7 days before the onset of DIC *5512*

Prothrombin Fragment 1.2 *Plasma Increase* Mean concentration of prothrombin fragment 1.2 in platelet-poor plasma from 11 patients with DIC of 4.6 ± 3.7 nmol/L significantly higher than 0.51 nmol/L (95% reference interval of 0.21 - 2.78 nmol/L) in 268 healthy individuals less than 44 years of age *1860* In 18 trauma patients with DIC mean concentration of 12.2 ± 3.1 nmol/L not significantly different from 9.0 ± 1.7 nmol/L in 24 without DIC. In 15 patients with sepsis and DIC mean concentration of 3.8 ± 1.3 nmol/L not significantly different from 3.1 ± 0.3 nmol/L in 5 without DIC *1636*

Prothrombin Time *Plasma Decrease* In 18 trauma patients with DIC mean time of 58 ± 5% significantly lower than 73 ± 4% in 24 without DIC. In 15 patients with sepsis and DIC mean time of 56 ± 9% significantly different from 70 ± 7% in 5 without DIC *1636*
Plasma Increase Reported effect *900* Prolonged because of consumption of clotting factors and the anticoagulant effects of fibrin degradation products *5677*

Soluble E-Selectin *Serum Increase* Mean concentration in 96 patients with disseminated intravascular coagulation of 68.0 ± 61.8 ng/mL significantly different from 42.0 ± 30.9 ng/mL in 33 patients without DIC *3890*

Soluble Fas Antigen *Serum Increase* In 19 patients with thrombotic thrombocytopenic purpura mean concentration of 4.82 ± 3.01 ng/mL significantly higher than 1.01 ± 0.24 ng/mL in 25 healthy individuals *2229*

Soluble Fas Ligand Antigen *Serum Increase* In 19 patients with disseminated intravascular coagulation mean serum concentration of 0.321 ± 0.245 ng/mL significantly higher than 0.057 ± 0.039 ng/mL in 25 healthy individuals *2229*

Soluble Fibrin Monomer *Plasma Increase* In 114 leukemics who developed DIC mean concentration of soluble fibrin monomer of 311 ± 196 µg/mL and 340 ± 252 µg/mL in 126 patients with other conditions, respectively, on day that they developed DIC, significantly higher than 44.7 ± 57.7 µg/mL and 118 ± 27.3 µg/mL in the respective populations 7 days before the onset of DIC *5512* In 74 patients with DIC mean concentration of 363 ± 314 µg/mL significantly different from 181 ± 132 µg/mL in 28 patients with pre-DIC and 5.9 ± 1.4 µg/mL in 20 healthy controls *5514*

Thrombin Time *Blood Increase* Prolonged because of consumption of clotting factors and the anticoagulant effects of fibrin degradation products *5677*

Thrombin/Antithrombin III Complex *Plasma Increase* In 18 trauma patients with DIC mean concentration of 665 ± 147 ng/mL significantly different from 201 ± 39 ng/mL in 24 without DIC. In 15 patients with sepsis and DIC mean concentration of 74 ± 25 ng/mL not significantly different from 32 ± 24 ng/mL in 5 without DIC *1636* In 114 leukemics who developed DIC mean concentration of 39.6 ± 19.0 ng/mL and 39.6 ± 27.5 ng/mL in 126 patients with other conditions, respectively, on day that they developed DIC, significantly higher than 9.9 ± 6.1 ng/mL and 22.6 ± 12.9 ng/mL in the respective populations 7 days before the onset of DIC *5512* Mean concentration in 40 patients with pre-DIC of 31.4 ± 7.2 ng/mL and 54.6 ± 9.3 ng/mL in 80 patients with DIC compared with 18.5 ± 9.0 ng/mL in 50 controls *5509* In 55 patients with DIC mean concentration of 51.6 ± 9.7 ng/mL, in 15 with pre-DIC of 28.9 ± 9.2 ng/mL and in 10 patients with non-DIC of 11.5 ± 10.1 ng/mL *5511*

Thrombomodulin *Plasma Increase* Significant increase observed in most of 66 cases of DIC, especially in those with sepsis. Concentration higher in patients with DIC and multiple organ failure than in those with multiple organ failure alone. Concentration in patients with DIC decreased with clinical improvement in most cases of DIC but increased or remained constant in patients who showed no improvement of DIC *193* In 40 patients with pre-DIC mean concentration of 6.77 ± 0.87 ng/mL and 11.9 ± 1.9 ng/mL in 80 patients with DIC higher than 5.4 ± 1.4 ng/mL in 50 healthy controls *5509* In 114 leukemics and 126 patients with other conditions who developed DIC, mean concentration of 13.1 ± 9.6 ng/mL significantly different from 3.5 ± 1.5 ng/mL 7 days before the onset of DIC *5512* In 19 patients with mean serum concentration of 59.4 ± 27.3 ng/mL significantly higher than 10.5 ± 1.9 ng/mL in 25 healthy individuals *2229*

Tissue Factor *Plasma Increase* In 79 patients with DIC mean concentration of 274 ± 90 pg/mL significantly increased compared with 117 ± 19 pg/mL in 10 healthy volunteers *4807* In 18 trauma patients with DIC mean concentration of 242 ± 39 pg/mL significantly different from 178 ± 25 pg/mL in 24 without DIC. In 15 patients with sepsis and DIC mean concentration of 658 ± 226 mg/L significantly different from 307 ± 95 mg/L in 5 without DIC *1636*
Plasma No Effect In 114 leukemics and 126 patients with other conditions who developed DIC mean concentration of 252 ± 82 pg/mL not significantly different from 220 ± 54 pg/mL 7 days before the onset of DIC *5512*

Tissue Factor Antigen *Plasma Increase* Concentration significantly higher in DIC patients than in non-DIC patients (126 ± 41 pg/mL) although concentration in some within the normal range. In patients with DIC and ALL mean concentration of 252 ± 60 pg/mL, with APL of 279 ± 64 pg/mL, ANLL other than APL of 326 ± 85 pg/mL, solid cancer of 292 ± 116 pg/mL, sepsis of 288 ± 87 pg/mL and other diseases of 208 ± 69 pg/mL *5511*

Tissue Factor Pathway Inhibitor *Plasma Increase* High concentrations observed in fulmitant DIC complicating sepsis *2376* In 79 patients with DIC mean concentration of 252 ± 125 ng/mL significantly increased compared with 102 ± 19 ng/mL in 10 healthy volunteers *4807*

Tissue Plasminogen Activator *Plasma Increase* In 40 patients with pre-DIC mean concentration of 25.8 ± 3.9 ng/mL and 27.7 ± 2.2 ng/mL in 80 patients with DIC higher than 19.3 ± 3.2 ng/mL in 50 healthy controls *5509*

Tissue Polypeptide Antigen *Serum Increase* In 55 patients with DIC mean concentration of 29.6 ± 4.6 ng/mL, in 15 with pre-DIC of 24.6 ± 4.6 ng/mL and in 10 non-DIC of 17.3 ± 4.6 ng/mL *5511*

Tumor Necrosis Factor-α *Serum Increase* TNF-α were also significantly higher in patients with DIC *5513*

von Willebrand Factor *Plasma Increase* In 40 patients with pre-DIC mean concentration of 170 ± 12% and in 80 with DIC mean concentration of 173 ± 12% higher than 152 ± 14% in 50 healthy controls *5509*

286.60 HELLP Syndrome

Alanine Aminotransferase *Serum Increase* In 54 women who had HELLP syndrome during their pregnancies on follow-up median activity of 6 U/L compared with reference range of < 30 U/L, but with 1 (2%) having abnormal activity *2711* Plasma liver enzyme activities are increased but rarely rise above 1,000 U/L *1778* In 34 women with HELLP syndrome mean activity of 173 U/L significantly different from 7 U/L in 41 women with normotensive pregnancies *2714* In 1 patient with HELLP syndrome activity of 420 U/L compared with reference interval of 0 - 35 U/L *5030* In 21 patients mean activity increased to about 100 U/L *5248* In 79 pregnant women with HELLP syndrome median activity of 191 U/L significantly greater than that in 87 normotensive pregnant women in whom the median activity was 4 U/L *2712*

Albumin *Serum Decrease* In 54 women who had HELLP syndrome during their pregnancies on follow-up median concentration of 45 g/L compared with reference range of 40 - 50 g/L, but with 1 (2%) having an abnormally decreased concentration *2711*

Serum *Increase* In 54 women who had HELLP syndrome during their pregnancies on follow-up median concentration of 45 g/L compared with reference range of 40 - 50 g/L, but with 4 (7%) having abnormally increased concentrations *2711*

Alkaline Phosphatase *Serum* *Increase* Plasma liver enzyme activities are increased but rarely rise above 1,000 U/L *1778*
Serum *No Effect* In 54 women who had HELLP syndrome during their pregnancies on follow-up median activity of 42 U/L compared with reference range of < 120 U/L, but with none (0%) having abnormal activity *2711*

Ammonia *Plasma* *No Effect* Concentration characteristically normal *1778*

Antithrombin III *Plasma* *Decrease* Plasma concentrations usually reduced *1778*

Aspartate Aminotransferase *Serum* *Increase* In 21 patients mean activity increased to about 100 U/L *5248* In 1 patient with HELLP syndrome activity of 512 U/L compared with reference interval of 0 - 35 U/L *5030* Plasma liver enzyme activities are increased but rarely rise above 1,000 U/L *1778* In 34 women with HELLP syndrome mean activity of 206 U/L significantly different from 9 U/L in 41 women with normotensive pregnancies *2714* In 54 women who had HELLP syndrome during their pregnancies on follow-up median activity of 11 U/L compared with reference range of < 25 U/L, but with 2 (4%) having abnormal activities *2711* In 23 women with pregnancies complicated by preeclampsia or HELLP syndrome median activity of 125 U/L *2713*

Bilirubin *Serum* *Increase* In 54 women who had HELLP syndrome during their pregnancies on follow-up median concentration of 6 μmol/L compared with reference range of < 10 μmol/L, but with 11 (20%) having abnormal concentrations *2711* Hyperbilirubinemia is usually moderate and predominantly involves the unconjugated fraction, reflecting intravascular hemolysis *1778* In 1 patient with HELLP syndrome concentration of 55 μmol/L compared with reference interval of 5 - 21 μmol/L *5030*

Bilirubin, Conjugated *Serum* *Increase* In 54 women who had HELLP syndrome during their pregnancies on follow-up median concentration of 1 μmol/L compared with reference range of < 3 μmol/L, but with (4%) having abnormal concentrations *2711*

Bilirubin, Indirect *Serum* *Increase* In 1 patient with HELLP syndrome total bilirubin concentration of 55 μmol/L, of which the majority was indirect, compared with reference interval of 5 - 21 μmol/L *5030*

Bilirubin, Unconjugated *Serum* *Increase* Hyperbilirubinemia is usually moderate and predominantly involves the unconjugated fraction *1778*

Creatinine *Serum* *No Effect* In 23 women with pregnancies complicated by preeclampsia or HELLP syndrome median concentration of 82 μmol/L *2713*

Fibrin Degradation Products *Plasma* *Increase* Plasma concentrations usually increased *1778*

Fibrinogen *Plasma* *Decrease* Plasma concentrations usually reduced *1778*

γ-Glutamyltransferase *Serum* *Increase* Plasma liver enzyme activities are increased but rarely rise above 1,000 U/L *1778* In 54 women who had HELLP syndrome during their pregnancies on follow-up median activity of 10 U/L compared with reference range of < 35 U/L, but with 1 (2%) having abnormal activity *2711*

Glutathione *Blood* *Decrease* In 15 women with pregnancies complicated by HELLP syndrome median concentration of 679 μmol/L compared with 750 μmol/L in 22 normotensive pregnant women *2713*

Glutathione S-Transferase Alpha 1-1 *Serum* *Increase* In 79 pregnant women with HELLP syndrome median concentration of 131.7 μg/L significantly greater than that in 87 normotensive pregnant women in whom the median concentration was 1.0 μg/L *2712*

Glutathione S-Transferase-pi 1-1 *Serum* *Increase* In 34 women with HELLP syndrome median concentration of 34.5 μg/L significantly different from 7.9 μg/L in 81 healthy nonpregnant female volunteers *2714*

Glutathione:Hemoglobin Ratio *Blood* *Decrease* In 15 women with pregnancies complicated by HELLP syndrome median ratio of 0.091 compared with 0.101 in 22 normotensive pregnant women *2713*

Haptoglobin *Serum* *Decrease* In 34 women with HELLP syndrome median concentration of < 0.02 g/L significantly different from 0.92 g/L in 81 healthy nonpregnant female volunteers *2714*

Hematocrit *Blood* *Decrease* Iintravascular hemolysis ultimately leads to anemia *1778* In 1 patient with HELLP syndrome hematocrit 0.26, low even in pregnancy *5030*

Hemoglobin *Blood* *Decrease* Iintravascular hemolysis ultimately leads to anemia *1778*
Blood *No Effect* In 23 women with pregnancies complicated by the HELLP syndrome or preeclampsia median concentration of 7.9 mmol/L not different from 7.45 mmol/L in 22 women wih normal pregnancies *2713*

Interleukin-12 (p40 Subunit) *Serum* *Increase* Concentrations increased in women with HELLP syndrome *1250*

Interleukin-12 p75 Dimer *Serum* *Increase* Concentrations increased in women with HELLP syndrome *1250*

International Normalized Ratio *Plasma* *Increase* INR usually prolonged *1778*

Lactate Dehydrogenase *Serum* *Increase* In 1 patient with HELLP syndrome activity of 718 U/L compared with reference interval of 122 - 220 U/L *5030* In 34 women with HELLP syndrome median activity of 825 U/L significantly different from 147 U/L in 10 healthy volunteers *2714* In 23 women with pregnancies complicated by preeclampsia or HELLP syndrome median activity of 807 U/L *2713*
Serum *No Effect* In 54 women who had HELLP syndrome during their pregnancies on follow-up median activity of 209 U/L compared with reference range of < 330 U/L, but with none (0%) having abnormal activity *2711*

Leukocytes *Blood* *No Effect* Leukocyte count characteristically normal *1778*

Matrix Metalloproteinase-8 *Serum* *Increase* Mean concentration of 43 ± 30 ng/mL in 18 women with HELLP syndrome not significantly different from 29 ± 19 ng/mL in 18 healthy pregnant controls *2749*

Matrix Metalloproteinase-9 *Serum* *No Effect* Mean concentration of 505 ± 253 ng/mL in 18 women with HELLP syndrome not significantly different from 487 ± 306 ng/mL in 18 healthy pregnant controls *2749*

Plasminogen Activator Inhibitor-1 *Plasma* *Increase* Mean concentration of 442 ± 378 ng/mL in 18 women with HELLP syndrome significantly different from 159 ± 122 ng/mL in 18 healthy pregnant controls *2749*

Platelets *Blood* *Decrease* In 1 patient with HELLP syndrome concentration of 69,000 x 10^9/L significantly reduced compared with normal *5030* In 34 women with HELLP syndrome mean concentration of < 100 x 10^9 /L *2714* In 23 women with pregnancies complicated by HELLP syndrome or preeclampsia median concentration of 88 x 10^9/L low *2713* Concentration usually reduced below 100 x 10^9/L *1778* In 21 patients mean concentration decreased to about 100,000 /μL *5248*

Protein *Urine* *Increase* In 1 patient with HELLP syndrome 3+ proteinuria detected *5030* In 23 women with pregnancies complicated by preeclampsia or HELLP syndrome median excretion of 1 g/L *2713*

Tissue Inhibitor of Metalloproteinase-1 *Serum* *Increase* Mean concentration of 251 ± 124 ng/mL in 18 women with HELLP syndrome significantly different from 170 ± 55 ng/mL in 18 healthy pregnant controls *2749*

Tissue Plasminogen Activator *Plasma* *Increase* Mean concentration of 13.3 ± 10.4 ng/mL in 18 women with HELLP syndrome significantly different from 6.6 ± 3.9 ng/mL in 18 healthy pregnant controls *2749*

Uric Acid *Serum* *No Effect* In 23 women with pregnancies complicated by preeclampsia or HELLP syndrome median concentration of 0.42 mmol/L *2713*

Urokinase Plasminogen Activator *Plasma* *Increase* Mean concentration of 3.9 ± 4.9 ng/mL in 18 women with HELLP syndrome not significantly different from 2.2 ± 1.1 ng/mL in 18 healthy pregnant controls *2749* *2749*

286.60 HELLP Syndrome *(continued)*

Urokinase Plasminogen Activator Receptor
Plasma *No Effect* Mean concentration of 1.0 ± 0.9 ng/mL in 18 women with HELLP syndrome not significantly different from 1.0 ± 0.9 ng/mL in 18 healthy pregnant controls *2749*

Disorders of the Platelets, Leukocytes, and Blood-forming Organs

287.00 Allergic Purpura

Albumin *Serum* *Decrease* Hypoalbuminemia occurs in patients with gastrointestinal involvement *2481*
Urine *Increase* Mild proteinuria associated with normal Addis count signifies renal involvement *900*

Anti-Streptolysin-O Titer *Serum* *Increase* A hemolytic streptococci can be implicated both by culture and by antistreptolysin O titers. This is an inconstant finding *1980*

Bleeding Time *Patient* *No Effect* Tourniquet test may be positive, but other tests of hemostasis are usually normal *5699*

Capillary Fragility *Blood* *Increase* Tourniquet tests are, at times, positive *5677*

Complement, Total *Serum* *No Effect* Usually normal *1980*

Creatinine *Serum* *Increase* Elevated in the presence of renal failure *5677* Increase is mild and transitory *900*

Eosinophils *Blood* *Increase* May be a polymorphonuclear leukocytosis and an increase in eosinophils *5677* Slight leukocytosis and occasional eosinophilia may be seen *1980*

Erythrocyte Casts *Urine* *Increase* Indicate active glomerulitis *1980* Common but often transient *5699*

Erythrocyte Sedimentation Rate *Blood* *Increase* During the acute illness *900* Usually elevated *5677*
Blood *No Effect* Unlike with other necrotizing angiitis, the ESR is often normal *1980*

Erythrocytes *Blood* *Decrease* The RBC is generally within normal limits except if severe gastrointestinal blood loss has occurred *900*
Blood *No Effect* The RBC count is generally within normal limits except if severe gastrointestinal blood loss has occurred *900*
Urine *Increase* In varying degrees signify renal involvement *900* An early feature of urinalysis is macroscopic hematuria *1980*

Granular Casts *Urine* *Increase* May be seen *5677*

Hematocrit *Blood* *Decrease* Anemia is not usually present unless the hemorrhagic manifestations have been severe *5677*
Blood *No Effect* Anemia is unusual with disease *1980* Unusual for anemia to be present *5699* Anemia is not usually present unless the hemorrhagic manifestations have been severe *5677*

Hemoglobin *Blood* *Decrease* Anemia is not usually present unless the hemorrhagic manifestations have been severe *5677*
Blood *No Effect* Anemia not usually present *5699* Anemia is not usually present unless the hemorrhagic manifestations have been severe *5677* Anemia not typically present *1980*

Immunoglobulin A *Serum* *Increase* Found in 50% of patients *5699*

Immunoglobulins *Serum* *No Effect* Except for IgA, the immunoglobulins remain normal *1980*

Iron-binding Capacity, Total *Serum* *Increase* Anemia from blood loss may be present *5677*

Iron Saturation *Serum* *Decrease* Anemia from blood loss may be present *5677*

Leukocytes *Blood* *Increase* A mild leukocytosis, mainly of polymorphonuclear cells, with WBC counts of 10,000 - 20,000 /μL is common *900* WBC, neutrophils, and eosinophils may be increased *5544*

MCH *Blood* *Decrease* Anemia is not usually present unless the hemorrhagic manifestations have been severe *5677*

MCHC *Blood* *Decrease* Anemia is not usually present unless the hemorrhagic manifestations have been severe *5677*

MCV *Blood* *Decrease* Anemia is not usually present unless the hemorrhagic manifestations have been severe *5677*

Neutrophils *Blood* *Increase* A mild leukocytosis, mainly of polymorphonuclear cells, with WBC counts of 10,000 - 20,000 /μL common *900* Modest neutrophilia *5699*

Occult Blood *Feces* *Increase* Reported effect *5699* Stool may show blood *5545*

Platelets *Blood* *Decrease* Defect in hemostasis in drug-sensitivity allergic purpura *1980*
Blood *No Effect* Tourniquet test may be positive but other tests of hemostasis are usually normal *5699* Count is normal *5677*

Protein *Urine* *Increase* Proteinuria is manifest and moderate in quantity *1980* Urine may show hematuria and proteinuria *5677*

Urea Nitrogen *Serum* *Increase* Azotemia is a common but transient finding *5699* Elevated in the presence of renal failure *5677*

287.00 Anaphylactoid Purpura

Interleukin-6 *Serum* *No Effect* Determined in 8 patients with anaphylactoid purpura (AP) and in healthy children. IL-6 activity in the sera of patients did not increase during the active stage *3357*

Tumor Necrosis Factor-α *Serum* *Increase* Determined in 8 with anaphylactoid purpura (AP), and in healthy children. Levels in patients increased during the acute stage *3357*

287.00 Henoch-Schönlein Purpura

Anti-Neutrophil Cytoplasm Antibodies *Serum* *No Effect* Antibodies not detected in any of 19 patients *162*

Copper Zinc Superoxide Dismutase
Red Blood Cells *No Effect* In 16 children with acute HSP aged 3 to 13 y mean activity of 3,982 ± 181 U/g hemoglobin not significantly different from 4,035 ± 142 U/g hemoglobin in 17 healthy control children *1111*

C-Reactive Protein *Serum* *Increase* Mean concentration of 19 mg/L in 16 patients with active disease significantly greater than in healthy controls *208* Mean concentration of 55 ± 11 mg/L in 20 patients with active disease significantly different and 12 ± 3 mg/L in 20 patients with inactive disease not significantly different from 7 ± 2 mg/L observed in 12 healthy controls *4950*

Creatinine *Serum* *No Effect* Mean concentration in 20 patients with active disease and in 20 patients with inactive disease not significantly different from that observed in 12 healthy controls *4950*

Elastase Antineutrophil Cytoplasmic Autoantibodies
Serum *No Effect* Antibodies not detected in any of 19 patients *162*

Erythrocyte Sedimentation Rate *Blood* *Increase* Mean of 33 mm/h in 33 patients significantly greater than in healthy controls *208*

Fibrinogen *Plasma* *No Effect* Mean concentration of 3.8 g/L in 18 patients significantly greater than in healthy controls *208*

Hepatocyte Growth Factor *Serum* *Increase* In 14 patients with Henoch-Schönlein purpura and coronary atherosclerosis patients mean concentration in acute phase of 0.36 ng/mL significantly different from 0.12 ng/mL in 19 patients in remission and 0.03 ng/mL in 17 healthy controls *3803*

Immune Complexes *Serum* *Increase* Mean concentration of 167 μg/mL in 14 patients with active disease significantly greater than in healthy controls *208*

Intercellular Adhesion Molecule-1 *Serum* *Increase* Mean concentration of 432 ± 35 ng/mL in 20 patients with active disease significantly greater than 307 ± 33 ng/mL observed in 12 healthy controls *4950*
Serum *No Effect* Mean concentration of 295 ± 3 ng/mL in 20 patients with inactive disease not significantly different from 307 ± 33 ng/mL observed in 12 healthy controls *4950*

Interleukin-1β *Serum* *No Effect* In 16 patients with IgA nephropathy and Schonlein-Henoch purpura IL-1β not detected in any as in none of 16 patients with other nephropathies or who were normal *5747*

Urine *Increase* In 16 patients with IgA nephropathy and Schonlein-Henoch purpura IL-1β detected in 10 at a mean concentration of 144.10 ± 45.14 pg/mL compared with 2 of 16 patients with other nephropathies or who were normal in whom the concentration was 8.67 ± 2.39 pg/mL *5747*

Interleukin-2 *Serum* *No Effect* In 16 patients with IgA nephropathy and Schonlein-Henoch purpura IL-2 not detected in any as in none of 16 patients with other nephropathies or who were normal *5747*

Urine *No Effect* In 16 patients with IgA nephropathy and Schonlein-Henoch purpura IL-2 detected in 3 at a mean concentration of 64.77 ± 8.74 pg/mL compared with 5 of 16 patients with other nephropathies or who were normal in whom the concentration was 47.60 ± 19.26 pg/mL *5747*

Interleukin-4 *Serum* *No Effect* In 16 patients with IgA nephropathy and Schonlein-Henoch purpura IL-4 not detected in any as in none of 16 patients with other nephropathies or who were normal *5747*

Urine *No Effect* In 16 patients with IgA nephropathy and Schonlein-Henoch purpura IL-4 detected in 10 at a mean concentration of 22.49 ± 6.63 pg/mL compared with 13 of 16 patients with other nephropathies or who were normal in whom the concentration was 24.01 ± 5.59 pg/mL *5747*

Interleukin-6 *Urine* *No Effect* In 16 patients with IgA nephropathy and Schonlein-Henoch purpura IL-6 detected in 5 at a mean concentration of 87.47 ± 94.83 pg/mL compared with 6 of 16 patients with other nephropathies or who were normal in whom the concentration was 104.00 ± 90.88 pg/mL *5747*

Interleukin-12 *Serum* *No Effect* In 16 patients with IgA nephropathy and Schonlein-Henoch purpura IL-12 not detected in any as in none of 16 patients with other nephropathies or who were normal *5747*

Urine *No Effect* In 16 patients with IgA nephropathy and Schonlein-Henoch purpura IL-12 not detected in any compared with none of 16 patients with other nephropathies or who were normal *5747*

Malondialdehyde *Serum* *Increase* In 16 children with acute HSP aged 3 to 13 y mean concentration of 5.03 ± 0.18 nmol/mL significantly different from 3.15 ± 0.25 nmol/mL in 17 healthy control children *1111*

Myeloperoxidase Antineutrophil Cytoplasmic Autoantibodies *Serum* *Increase* Antibodies detected in 10.5% of 19 patients *162*

Perinuclear Antineutrophil Cytoplasmic Autoantibodies *Serum* *Increase* Antibodies detected in 10.5% of 19 patients *162*

Proteinase 3-Antineutrophil Cytoplasmic Autoantibodies *Serum* *No Effect* Antibodies not detected in any of 19 patients *162*

Ristocetin Cofactor *Plasma* *Increase* Mean concentration of 367 ± 179% of normal in 18 patients with active disease significantly greater than 103 ± 20% in 20 healthy controls *208*

Soluble E-Selectin *Serum* *Increase* Concentration increased in 12 of 41 children (29%) with Henoch-Schönlein purpura *5680*

Serum *No Effect* Mean concentration of 46.9 ± 3 ng/mL in 20 patients with active disease and 43 ± 3 ng/mL in 20 patients with inactive disease not significantly different from 46 ± 3 ng/mL observed in 12 healthy controls *4950*

Soluble Intercellular Adhesion Molecule-1 *Serum* *No Effect* Concentration increased in only one of 41 children (29%) with Henoch-Schönlein purpura *5680*

Tumor Necrosis Factor-α *Urine* *Increase* In 16 patients with IgA nephropathy and Schonlein-Henoch purpura TNF-α detected in 11 at a mean concentration of 84.76 ± 46.63 pg/mL compared with 1 of 16 patients with other nephropathies or who were normal in whom the concentration was 30.37 pg/mL *5747*

Urea Nitrogen *Serum* *No Effect* Mean concentration in 20 patients with active disease and in 20 patients with inactive disease not significantly different from that observed in 12 healthy controls *4950*

von Willebrand Factor *Plasma* *Increase* Mean concentration of 206 ± 17% in 20 patients with active disease significantly different and 127 ± 10% in 20 patients with inactive disease not significantly different from 107 ± 9% observed in 12 healthy controls *4950*

von Willebrand Factor Antigen *Plasma* *Increase* Mean concentration of 251 ± 155% normal in 18 patients with active disease significantly greater than 72 ± 21% in 20 healthy controls *208*

287.10 Thrombasthenia (Glanzmann's)

Bleeding Time *Patient* *Increase* Often marked *4979* Deficient platelet factor III *900* Typical observation *5699* Bleeding time is usually prolonged and aggregation of platelets by collagen or thrombin is abnormal *2039*

Clot Retraction *Blood* *Decrease* Due to platelet function abnormalities *4979*

Clotting Time *Blood* *No Effect* No significant effect observed *4979*

Factor IX *Plasma* *Decrease* Deficient platelet factor III *900*

Partial Thromboplastin Time *Plasma* *No Effect* Usually normal *4979*

Platelets *Blood* *Decrease* Count is usually normal, but mild reduction may occur *659*

Blood *No Effect* Typical observation *900* *5677* Present in normal numbers and are morphologically normal. Deficient platelet aggregation is the most significant abnormality *5699*

Prothrombin Consumption *Blood* *No Effect* Usually unaffected by disease *4979*

Prothrombin Time *Plasma* *No Effect* PT usually normal *4979*

Thrombin Time *Blood* *No Effect* Time usually normal *4979*

Thromboplastin Generation *Blood* *Increase* Contact activation is abnormal, resulting in abnormal TGT test *5699*

Blood *No Effect* Usually normal *4979*

287.20 Purpura

Rheumatoid Factor *Serum* *Increase* Mean concentration increased in patients with hypergammaglobulinemic purpura *2472*

287.30 Congenital Thrombocytopenia

Interleukin-6 *Serum* *No Effect* In 5 patients with congenital thrombocytopenia with absent radii concentrations were less than the upper limit of normal of 8 pg/mL *273*

Interleukin-11 *Serum* *No Effect* In 5 patients with congenital thrombocytopenia with absent radii concentrations were less than the upper limit of normal of 30 pg/mL *273*

Platelets *Blood* *Decrease* In 5 patients with congenital thrombocytopenia with absent radii concentrations ranged from 10,000 to 72,000 cells/μL *273*

Thrombopoietin *Plasma* *Increase* In 5 patients with congenital thrombocytopenia with absent radii concentrations on 7 of 8 occasions were greater than upper limit of normal of < 100 pg/mL *273*

287.30 Essential Thrombocythemia

Alkaline Phosphatase *Serum* *Increase* Increased activity observed in the majority of patients with the disease *443*

White Blood Cells *Increase* Increased or normal activity observed in patients with the disease *443*

Anti-Neutrophil Cytoplasm Antibodies *Serum* *No Effect* In a group of patients with essential thrombocythemia and myelodysplasia in none were ANCA demonstrated *4602*

Antithrombin III Activity *Plasma* *Decrease* Mean activity in patients with polycythemia vera or essential thrombocythemia with thrombosis of 96.4 ± 18.5% significantly different from 105 .5 ± 16.2% in patients without thrombosis *663*

Fibrinogen *Plasma* *No Effect* Mean concentration in patients with polycythemia vera or essential thrombocythemia with thrombosis of 3.2 g/L not significantly different from 3.0 g/L in patients without thrombosis *663*

287.30 Essential Thrombocythemia *(continued)*

Hematocrit *Blood* *No Effect* Mean value in patients with polycythemia vera or essential thrombocythemia with thrombosis of 44.2% not significantly different from 44.2% in patients without thrombosis *663*

Interleukin-1α *Serum* *No Effect* In 20 patients with essential thrombocytopenia, concentration not detectable as in 14 healthy controls *545*

Interleukin-1β *Serum* *No Effect* In 20 patients with essential thrombocytopenia, concentration not detectable as in 14 healthy controls *545*

Interleukin-2 *Serum* *Increase* In 10 patients with essential thrombocytopenia mean concentration of 263 ± 220 pg/mL significantly higher than undetectable amount in 14 healthy controls *545* In 20 patients with essential thrombocytopenia mean concentration of 783 ± 207 U/mL significantly higher than 582 ± 164 U/mL in 14 healthy controls *545*

Interleukin-6 *Serum* *No Effect* In 20 patients with essential thrombocytopenia concentration not different from that in 14 healthy controls *545*

Interleukin-10 *Serum* *No Effect* In 20 patients with essential thrombocytopenia concentration not different from that in 14 healthy controls *545*

Iron *Serum* *Decrease* Iron deficiency observed in the majority of patients with the disease *443*

Lactate Dehydrogenase *Serum* *Increase* Increased activity observed in the majority of patients with the disease *443*

Leukocytes *Blood* *Increase* Mild leukemia characteristic of the disease *443*
Blood *No Effect* Mean concentration in patients with polycythemia vera or essential thrombocythemia with thrombosis of 9.4 x 10^9/L not significantly different from 9.0 x 10^9/L in patients without thrombosis *663*

Lysozyme *Serum* *Increase* Increased activity observed in the majority of patients with the disease *443*

β_2-Microglobulin *Serum* *Increase* In 20 patients with essential thrombocytopenia mean concentration of 2,323 ± 2,441 µg/L significantly higher than 1,721 ± 673 µg/L in 14 healthy controls *545*

Platelets *Blood* *Decrease* Thrombocythemia observed characteristically in patients with the disease *443*
Blood *No Effect* Mean concentration in patients with polycythemia vera or essential thrombocythemia with thrombosis of 635.8 x 10^9/L not significantly different from 688.8 x 10^9/L in patients without thrombosis *663* Of 250 patients with platelet counts of more than 250,000 /µL, 12 had essential thrombocytopenia *3939*

Protein C Activity *Plasma* *No Effect* Mean activity in patients with polycythemia vera or essential thrombocythemia with thrombosis of 78.7 ± 19.7% not significantly different from 85.6 ± 16.9% in patients without thrombosis *663*

Protein S Antigen *Plasma* *Decrease* Mean activity in patients with polycythemia vera or essential thrombocythemia with thrombosis of 111.7 ± 26.7% significantly different from 121.6 ± 24.5% in patients without thrombosis *663*

Soluble c-kit Molecule *Serum* *No Effect* Median concentration in patients with essential thrombocythemia not significantly different from that in 51 healthy volunteers of 199.0 AU/mL *2598*

Tumor Necrosis Factor-α *Serum* *Increase* In 20 patients with essential thrombocytopenia mean concentration of 10 ± 2.5 pg/mL different from 0 pg/mL in 14 healthy controls *545*

Uric Acid *Serum* *Increase* Hyperuricemia observed in the majority of patients with the disease *443*

287.30 Thrombocytopenic Purpura, Idiopathic

Acid Phosphatase *Serum* *Increase* Plasma β-glycerol acid phosphatase may be elevated in any form of thrombocytopenia due to accelerated plasma destruction *5699* 13 of 15 patients had elevations. In 15 of 16 patients, serum gave higher values than plasma *3937* Only 2 out of 9 cases showed plasma levels to be of diagnostic value. Results of previous studies could not be reproduced successfully *920*

Bleeding Time *Patient* *Increase* Bleeding time typically increased *5699* Time increased *4979*

Capillary Fragility *Blood* *Increase* Positive tourniquet test *5699*

Cells *Bone Marrow* *Increase* Normal or increased numbers of megakaryocytes, many of which are smooth in contour, are found in the bone marrow *5677*

Clot Retraction *Blood* *Decrease* observed effect *900* Absent or deficient due to thrombocytopenia *5699*

Clotting Time *Blood* *No Effect* No significant effect observed *4979* Time usually normal *5699*

Complement C_3 *Serum* *No Effect* In one series *2659*

Coombs' Test *Serum* *Positive* In chronic ITP when autoimmune hemolytic anemia and ITP occur together (Evans' syndrome) *1397*

Eosinophils *Blood* *Increase* Originally thought to be common, has not been a constant finding *3399* Described in many patients, but has not been confirmed as a prognostic indicator *5699*

Fibrin Degradation Products *Plasma* *Increase* During the acute stage in this series *3704*

Glycocalicin *Plasma* *No Effect* Mean plasma concentration in 6 patients with ITP of 0.93 ± 0.24 µg/mL within normal range compared with that in 36 healthy individuals of 1.40 ± 0.25 µg/mL *2853*

Hematocrit *Blood* *Decrease* An anemia from blood loss may be present, but the red blood cell morphology is normal *900*

Hemoglobin *Blood* *Decrease* An anemia from blood loss may be present, but the RBC morphology is normal *900*

Immunoglobulin G *Serum* *Decrease* Mean IgG levels were subnormal *2659*
Serum *Increase* Children with both acute and chronic disease had significantly greater levels than normal or thrombocytopenic controls. Acute cases were elevated more than chronic *3056*

Iron-binding Capacity, Total *Serum* *Decrease* Anemia from blood loss may be present *5677*

Iron Saturation *Serum* *Increase* Anemia from blood loss may be present *5677*

LE Cells *Blood* *Positive* Occurs in 1 - 2% of patients *1189*

Lee-White Clotting Time *Blood* *No Effect* Usually normal *5544*

Leukocytes *Blood* *Increase* Occasionally, as a result of severe bleeding *5699* Normal or slightly elevated *900*
Blood *No Effect* Normal or slightly elevated *900*

Lymphocytes *Blood* *Increase* In chronic cases *2034* Lymphocytosis with abnormal cells resembling those found in infectious mononucleosis *5699*

MCH *Blood* *No Effect* An anemia from blood loss may be present, but the RBC morphology is normal *900*

MCHC *Blood* *No Effect* An anemia from blood loss may be present, but the RBC morphology is normal *900*

MCV *Blood* *Increase* Occasional moderate macrocytosis, if there has been a recent severe hemorrhage *5699*
Blood *No Effect* An anemia from blood loss may be present, but the RBC morphology is normal *900*

Neutrophils *Blood* *Increase* Shift to the left *2034* Usually normal, but moderate neutrophilia may occur due to severe bleeding *5699*

Partial Thromboplastin Time *Plasma* *No Effect* No significant effect usually observed *4979* *5699*

Platelet Survival *Blood* *Decrease* Markedly shortened *900* The life-span of transfused normal platelets is extremely short, sometimes only a few h *5677*

Platelets *Blood* *Decrease* Usually severe at the onset; in most cases platelets are < 20,000 /µL *5677* There is a marked decrease with values under 10,000 /µL in the acute form. In the chronic form a moderate thrombocytopenia with counts of 30,000 - 100,000 /µL is present *900* May be totally absent or only slightly decreased *5699*

Prothrombin Consumption *Blood* *Decrease* Defect phase I or II blood coagulation *5544*

Prothrombin Time *Plasma* *No Effect* No change in PTT usually observed *4979* No significant effect usually observed *5699* *900*

Reticulocytes *Blood* *Increase* Occasionally, if there has been a recent severe hemorrhage *5699*

Thrombin Time *Blood* *No Effect* Time usually normal *4979*

Thrombopoietin *Plasma* *Increase* Mean serum concentration in 6 patients with ITP of 1.7 ± 1.1 fmol/mL not significantly higher (still within reference interval) than that in 49 healthy individuals of 0.76 ± 0.32 fmol/mL *2853*

Thyroid Stimulating Hormone *Serum* *Increase* Increased concentration observed in 1 (5.0%) of 20 patients with idiopathic thrombocytopenic purpura *3080*

287.50 Thrombocytopenia

D-Dimer *Plasma* *Increase* Concentration significantly higher in patients with chronic idiopathic thrombocytopenic purpura and in those with central thrombocytopenia compared with healthy volunteers *2015*

Euglobulin Fibrinolytic Activity *Plasma* *No Effect* No significant difference observed between activities in patients with chronic idiopathic thrombocytopenia and central thrombocytopenia compared with healthy control volunteers *2015*

Osteonectin *Serum* *No Effect* No significant difference observed between plasma of individuals with low and normal platelet counts *3245*

Plasminogen Activator Inhibitor Activity *Plasma* *No Effect* No significant difference observed between activities in patients with chronic idiopathic thrombocytopenia and central thrombocytopenia compared with healthy control volunteers *2015*

Tissue Plasminogen Activator *Plasma* *Increase* Concentration significantly increased both in patients with chronic idiopathic thrombocytopenic purpura and chronic central thrombocytopenia compared with healthy volunteers *2015*

von Willebrand Factor Antigen *Plasma* *Increase* Concentration significantly higher in patients with chronic idiopathic thrombocytopenic purpura and chronic central thrombocytopenia compared with healthy controls *2015*

288.00 Agranulocytosis

Albumin *Urine* *Increase* Urine may contain traces of albumin but is otherwise normal *5699*

Alkaline Phosphatase *White Blood Cells* *Increase* Usually increased in untreated disease *5544*

Bleeding Time *Patient* *No Effect* Normal in most typical cases *5699*

Clotting Time *Blood* *No Effect* Normal in most typical cases *5699*

Eosinophils *Blood* *Increase* May occur *2033*

Erythrocyte Sedimentation Rate *Blood* *Increase* Greatly accelerated *5699*

γ-Globulin *Serum* *Increase* In some patients *2033*

Hematocrit *Blood* *Decrease* Depending on the underlying process the patient may also manifest moderate to severe anemia *900*
Blood *No Effect* Typically normal; some cases have had anemia but this was most often pre-existing *5699*

Hemoglobin *Blood* *Decrease* Depending on the underlying process the patient may also manifest moderate to severe anemia *900*
Blood *No Effect* Typically normal; some cases have had anemia but this was most often pre-existing *5699*

Leukocytes *Blood* *Decrease* In acute fulminant form, WBC is decreased to < 2,000 /μL *5545* Absolute concentration of circulating neutrophils is reduced. In acute cases these cells may be virtually absent. The remaining cells may show toxic changes such as increased granulation or cytoplasmic vacuolization *900* Leukopenia exists when a reduction below about 4,000 /μL occurs *367*

Lymphocytes *Blood* *Decrease* The lymphocytes number below about 1,400 /μL in children or 1,000 /μL in adults *367* Variable *2033*
Blood *Increase* Variable and may be decreased, normal or increased *2033*
Blood *No Effect* Variable and may be decreased, normal or increased *2033*

Metamyelocytes *Bone Marrow* *Decrease* Characteristic lack of granulocytes, including polymorphonuclears, metamyelocytes, and myelocytes *5699*

Monocytes *Blood* *Increase* Sometimes occurs. Increases in the recovery *5544* May be relatively and absolutely increased *5699*

Neutrophils *Blood* *Decrease* Counts of 500 - 1,000 /μL have moderately increased risks, whereas below this the invasion of mucous membranes, skin and blood by microorganisms becomes increasingly frequent and severe *367* 0 - 2%. May show pyknosis or vacuolization with agranulocytosis *5545* Marked decrease or complete absence of mature granulocytes *900*
Bone Marrow *Decrease* Bone marrow shows absence of cells in granulocytic series but normal erythroid and megakaryocytic series *5545* Cells not observed *5699*

Plasma Cells *Bone Marrow* *Increase* Plasma cells, lymphocytes and reticulum cells may be increased *5699*

Platelets *Blood* *Decrease* Depending on the underlying process the patient may manifest a reduced platelet count *900*

288.00 Neutropenia

Granulocyte Colony Stimulating Factor *Serum* *No Effect* In 63 patients with antibody-induced neutropenia including neonatal immune neutropenia, autoimmune neutropenia and drug-induced immune neutropenia concentration not increased unless infectious disease also present *654*

Soluble E-Selectin *Serum* *No Effect* In 12 neutropenic patients with hematological malignancies mean concentration of 51 ± 20 ng/mL not significantly different compared with 33 ± 4 ng/mL in 15 healthy control individuals *3879*

Soluble L-Selectin *Serum* *Decrease* In 12 neutropenic patients with hematological malignancies mean concentration of 514 ± 56 ng/mL compared with 916 ± 61 ng/mL in 15 healthy control individuals *3879*

Soluble P-Selectin *Serum* *Increase* In 12 neutropenic patients with hematological malignancies mean concentration of 638 ± 115 ng/mL compared with 238 ± 27 ng/mL in 15 healthy control individuals *3879*

288.30 Eosinophilia

Myelin Basic Protein *Serum* *Increase* Mean concentration in 64 patients with eosinophilia of 281 ± 408 ng/mL significantly higher than 41 ± 19 ng/mL in 100 normal individuals *5776*

288.30 Hypereosinophilic Syndrome

Eosinophils *Blood* *Increase* In 6 patients with hypereosinophilic syndrome and eosinophilia mean concentration of 8,060 ± 3,940 /μL compared with less than 500 /μL in 100 normal individuals and 3 patients with hypereosinophilic syndrome but without eosinophilia *5776*

Granulocyte-Macrophage Colony Stimulating Factor
Serum *No Effect* Not detected in the serum of any of 13 patients with condition *2744*

Interleukin-3 *Serum* *No Effect* Not detected in the serum of any of 13 patients with condition *2744*

Interleukin-5 *Serum* *Increase* Detected in the serum of 4 of 13 patients with hypereosinophilic syndrome *2744*

Myelin Basic Protein *Serum* *Increase* In 6 patients with hypereosinophilic syndrome and eosinophilia mean concentration of 655 ± 446 ng/mL and in patients with hypereosinophilic syndrome but without eosinophilia mean concentration of 2,110 ± 2,750 ng/mL significantly increased compared with mean of 41 ± 19 ng/mL in 100 normal individuals *5776*

288.80 Reactive Neutrophilia

Myeloperoxidase *Granulocyte* *Increase* Mean density of 823 ± 77 in 8 patients with reactive neutrophilia significantly different from 478 ± 52 in 32 normal controls *1303*

288.80 Reactive Neutrophilia *(continued)*

Naphthol-As-D-Chloroacetate Esterase *Granulocyte* *No Effect* Mean density of 519 ± 71 in 12 patients with reactive neutrophilia not significantly different from 511 ± 46 in 40 normal controls *1303*

289.00 Polycythemia, Relative

Erythropoietin *Serum* *No Effect* In 20 patients with relative polycythemia mean concentration of 10 ± 4 U/L compared with 9 ± 4 U/L in 79 reference controls *4320*

Hemoglobin *Blood* *Increase* In 20 patients with relative polycythemia mean concentration of 17.5 ± 0.34 g/dL compared with 14.0 ± 1.1 g/dL in 79 reference controls *4320*

289.00 Polycythemia, Secondary

Alkaline Phosphatase *White Blood Cells* *No Effect* Typical observation *5544*

Basophils *Blood* *No Effect* Number usually unaffected by disease *5677*

Bilirubin *Serum* *Increase* Increased slightly *367*

Coproporphyrin *Urine* *Increase* Increased hemopoiesis *1290*

Eosinophils *Blood* *No Effect* Usually no efect observed *2034*

Erythrocyte Sedimentation Rate *Blood* *Decrease* An elevated bilirubin coexisting with a norma bile acid bilirubin concentration suggests Gilbert's Disease *4949*

Erythrocytes *Blood* *Increase* Absolute erythrocytosis caused by an enhanced stimulation of RBC production *5677* Frequently counts are 7 - 10 million or more/µL when patients are first seen *367*

Erythropoietin *Serum* *Increase* Secondary polycythemia caused by excessive release of erythropoietin *5677* In 127 patients with secondary polycythemia mean concentration of 47 ± 111 U/L compared with 9 ± 4 U/L in 79 reference controls *4320*

Hemoglobin *Blood* *Increase* May be increased less, in proportion, than the erythrocyte level because of a low MCV and MCH *367* In 127 patients with secondary polycythemia mean concentration of 18.4 ± 1.1 g/dL compared with 14.0 ± 1.1 g/dL in 79 reference controls *4320*

Histamine *Plasma* *No Effect* Usually no effect observed *5677*

Iron *Serum* *No Effect* Usually normal concentration *4331*

Iron-binding Capacity, Total *Serum* *No Effect* Usually concentration normal *4331*

Leukocytes *Blood* *No Effect* Usually no effect observed *5677*

MCHC *Blood* *Decrease* Low MCHC in addition to microcytosis, especially after large hemorrhages or repeated phlebotomies *367*

MCV *Blood* *Decrease* Decreased resulting in a smaller increase in hemoglobin than usually would occur with the increased RBC count. Low MCHC and MCV, especially after large hemorrhages or repeated phlebotomies *367*

Metamyelocytes *Blood* *Increase* Are seen *367*

Myelocytes *Blood* *Increase* Occasionally seen *367*

Oxygen Partial Pressure *Blood* *No Effect* Usually normal *5677*

Platelets *Blood* *No Effect* Count may be normal *5677*

Reticulocytes *Blood* *Increase* Percentage is usually normal, but the absolute number is increased *367*

Urobilin *Feces* *Increase* Increased slightly *367*

Urobilinogen *Urine* *Increase* Increased slightly *367*

Vitamin B_{12} *Serum* *No Effect* Concentration typically unchanged *5677*

Vitamin B_{12} Binding Capacity *Serum* *No Effect* Usually unaffected by disease *5677*

Volume *Plasma* *Increase* Red cell mass increased *1290*

289.30 Necrotizing Lymphadenitis

Interferon-α *Serum* *No Effect* In 4 patients mean concentration in acute phase was within the normal range *2838*

Interferon-γ *Serum* *Increase* In 4 patients mean concentration in acute phasewas significantly higher than in controls *2838*

Interleukin-2 *Serum* *No Effect* In 4 patients mean concentration in acute phase was within the normal range *2838*

Interleukin-6 *Serum* *Increase* In 4 patients mean concentration in acute phase was significantly higher than in controls *2838*

Tumor Necrosis Factor-α *Serum* *No Effect* In 4 patients mean concentration in acute phase was within the normal range *2838*

289.40 Hypersplenism

Erythrocyte Survival *Red Blood Cells* *Decrease* May or may not be reduced *4979* *4147*

Erythrocytes *Blood* *Decrease* Pancytopenia is a common feature *5677* As much as 38% may be trapped in the enlarged spleen *4147*

Hematocrit *Blood* *Decrease* Apparent anemia is often due to expansion of plasma volume in the presence of normal RBC volume *4147*

Hemoglobin *Blood* *Decrease* Apparent anemia is often due to expansion of plasma volume in the presence of normal RBC volume *4147*

Leukocytes *Blood* *Decrease* Pancytopenia is a common feature *5677* Due to increased destruction and sequestration *459* *4979* Hematopoietic diseases *5544*

MCV *Blood* *No Effect* Apparent anemia is often due to expansion of plasma volume in the presence of normal RBC volume *4147*

Neutrophils *Blood* *Decrease* Count may be low, even in the range of 1%, but the patient can make pus and usually is not subject to septic disease *5677* Due to increased destruction and sequestration *459* *4979*

Platelets *Blood* *Decrease* Pancytopenia is a common feature *5677* As much as 50 - 90% of the total plasma mass may be sequestered *204*

Volume *Plasma* *Increase* Apparent anemia is often due to expansion of plasma volume in the presence of normal RBC volume *4147* When the spleen is greatly enlarged, the plasma volume and total blood volume are significantly expanded *5677*

289.80 Agnogenic Myeloid Metaplasia

Alanine Aminotransferase *Serum* *Increase* Abnormal liver function or increased activity of enzymes observed in 30% of all patients with the disease *443*

Prothrombin Time *Plasma* *Increase* Observed in 75% of all patients with the disease *443*

Uric Acid *Serum* *Increase* Increase obsered in 37% of all patients with the disease *443*

289.80 Hypergammaglobulinemia

Ammonium Ions *Urine* *Increase* May be associated with classic distal renal tubular acidosis which is associated with hyokalemia, hyperchloremic metabolic acidosis, urine pH > 5.5, increased urinary ammonium ion excretion, a negative urine anion gap, increased urinary osmol gap, decreased urinary citrate and increased urinary calcium in some patients *4071*

Anion Gap *Urine* *Decrease* May be associated with classic distal renal tubular acidosis which is asociated with hyokalemia, hyperchloremic metabolic acidosis, urine pH > 5.5, increased urinary ammonium ion excretion, a negative urine anion gap, increased urinary osmol gap, decreased urinary citrate and increased urinary calcium in some patients *4071*

Calcium *Urine* *Increase* May be associated with classic distal renal tubular acidosis which is asociated with hyokalemia, hyperchloremic metabolic acidosis, urine pH > 5.5, increased urinary ammonium ion excretion, a negative urine anion gap, increased urinary osmol gap, decreased urinary citrate and increased urinary calcium in some patients *4071*

Chloride *Serum* *Increase* May be associated with classic distal renal tubular acidosis which is associated with hyokalemia, hyperchloremic metabolic acidosis, urine pH > 5.5, increased urinary ammonium ion excretion, a negative urine anion gap, increased urinary osmol gap, decreased urinary citrate and increased urinary calcium in some patients *4071*

Citrate *Urine* *Decrease* May be associated with classic distal renal tubular acidosis which is associated with hyokalemia, hyperchloremic metabolic acidosis, urine pH > 5.5, increased urinary ammonium ion excretion, a negative urine anion gap, increased urinary osmol gap, decreased urinary citrate and increased urinary calcium in some patients *4071*

Net Acid Excretion *Urine* *Increase* May be associated with classic distal renal tubular acidosis which is asociated with hyokalemia, hyperchloremic metabolic acidosis, urine pH > 5.5, increased urinary ammonium ion excretion, a negative urine anion gap, increased urinary osmol gap, decreased urinary citrate and increased urinary calcium in some patients *4071*

Osmolal Gap *Urine* *Increase* May be associated with classic distal renal tubular acidosis which is asociated with hyokalemia, hyperchloremic metabolic acidosis, urine pH > 5.5, increased urinary ammonium ion excretion, a negative urine anion gap, increased urinary osmol gap, decreased urinary citrate and increased urinary calcium in some patients *4071*

pH *Urine* *Increase* May be associated with classic distal renal tubular acidosis which is asociated with hyokalemia, hyperchloremic metabolic acidosis, urine pH > 5.5, increased urinary ammonium ion excretion, a negative urine anion gap, increased urinary osmol gap, decreased urinary citrate and increased urinary calcium in some patients *4071*

Potassium *Serum* *Decrease* May be associated with classic distal renal tubular acidosis which is associated with hyokalemia, hyperchloremic metabolic acidosis, urine pH > 5.5, increased urinary ammonium ion excretion, a negative urine anion gap, increased urinary osmol gap, decreased urinary citrate and increased urinary calcium in some patients *4071*

289.80 Myelodysplasia

Anti-Neutrophil Cytoplasm Antibodies *Serum* *Decrease* Found in other vasculitides, but not associated with the vasculitis of myelodysplasia *4600*

Tissue Factor Pathway Inhibitor *Plasma* *No Effect* 8 patients with myelodysplasia had median activity of 0.94 U/mL not significantly different from median activity of 1.19 U/mL in healthy individuals *2376*

Tissue Factor Pathway Inhibitor Antigen *Plasma* *No Effect* 8 patients with myelodysplasia had median concentration of 65 ng/mL not significantly different from median concentration of 90 ng/mL in healthy individuals *2376*

Tissue Factor Pathway Inhibitor Antigen, Free *Plasma* *No Effect* 6 patients with myelodysplasia had median concentration of 12 ng/mL not significantly different from median concentration of 15 ng/mL in healthy individuals *2376*

Tissue Factor Pathway Inhibitor, Truncated and Complexed *Plasma* *No Effect* 6 patients with myelodysplasia had median concentration of 55 ng/mL not significantly different from median concentration of 78 ng/mL in healthy individuals *2376*

Tumor Necrosis Factor-α *Bone Marrow* *Increase* On a scale of 0 - 8, median of 3.0 in 18 patients with myelodysplasia responding to treatment and 25 who failed to respond *4339*
Serum *Increase* Median concentration of 6.9 pg/mL observed in 18 patients with myelodysplasia responding to treatment and 25 who failed to respond *4339*

289.80 Myelofibrosis

Acid Phosphatase *Serum* *Increase* 9 of 16 patients with myeloid metaplasia or chronic granulocytic leukemia were found to have slight but significant elevations of serum acid phosphatase *317* A patient with histiocytic medullary reticulosis was found to have up to 60 times the normal upper limit, which then paralleled the activity of disease during temporary responses to therapy *5652*

Alkaline Phosphatase *Serum* *Increase* Observed in some patients *367*
White Blood Cells *Decrease* In myelofibrosis, variable with normal, high, and low figures being found. Level tends to fall as the disease progresses *5677* Significantly elevated in most cases but in 10% of the cases in myelofibrosis the levels were in the CML range (markedly decreased or absent) *900*
White Blood Cells *Increase* Variable; tends to fall as the disease progresses *5677* In agnogenic myeloid metaplasia, 41 of 78 patients had scores > 1.00. A significant negative correlation was found between LAP and absolute percentage of immature cells *4846* Findings tend to be inconsistent. Generally elevated in the majority of patients *5124* Usually high but in 10% of cases, scores were in the CML range (markedly decreased or absent) *900*

Anisocytes *Blood* *Increase* In myelofibrosis is usually pronounced *5677*

Basophils *Blood* *Decrease* Observed effect in some patients *1098*
Blood *Increase* Reported effect *1098* Eosinophilia and basophilia occur in 10 - 30% of myelofibrosis patients *5124* Reported effect *5677*

Calmodulin *Urine* *Increase* In 13 patients with idiopathic myelofibrosis mean excretion of 0.34 ± 0.05 μg/mmol creatinine compared with 0.10 ± 0.02 μg/mmol creatinine in 12 controls *1289*

Coombs' Test *Serum* *Positive* Positive in 6 of 29 myelofibrosis patients. Positivity tends to develop in later stages of disease *5124*

Creatine Kinase *Serum* *No Effect* In 1 patient with idiopathic myelofibrosis mean activity of 23 U/L compared with upper limit of normal of 195 U/L *5659*

Creatine Kinase BB-Isoenzyme *Serum* *No Effect* In 1 patient with idiopathic myelofibrosis mean activity of < 3 U/L compared with normal of 0 - 1% *5659*

Cryofibrinogen *Plasma* *Increase* Reported effect in myelofibrosis *3417*

Eosinophils *Blood* *Increase* Eosinophils and basophils may be increased in agnogenic myeloid metaplasia *5545* Eosinophilia and basophilia occur in 10 - 30% of myelofibrosis patients *5124*

Erythrocytes *Blood* *Decrease* Pancytopenia is a common feature *5677*

Extracellular Growth Factor *Urine* *Decrease* In 13 patients with idiopathic myelofibrosis mean excretion of 3.23 ± 0.35 μg/mmol creatinine compared with 4.74 ± 0.35 μg/mmol creatinine in 12 controls *1289*

Folate *Serum* *Decrease* Decrease with extensive skin disease *5230* Macrocytic anemia was reported in over 50% of the patients, the probable cause was folic acid deficiency secondary to chronic excessive cell proliferation (in myelofibrosis) *2193* Reported effect *5677* Decrease with extensive skin disease *772* *602*

Glutathione *Red Blood Cells* *Increase* In myelofibrosis, usually increased *1830*

Glutathione, Reduced *Red Blood Cells* *Increase* In myelofibrosis, usually increased *1830* RBC reduced glutathione occurred in 16 of 17 myelofibrosis patients *5124*

Hematocrit *Blood* *Decrease* Anemia is present in 66% of all patients when they are first seen. Usually normochromic and moderate in degree but may become severe in advanced disease in myelofibrosis *5677* Anemia mostly normochromic is found in a majority of cases. Hemoglobin < 12 g/dL occurred in 73% of cases *5124* Usually there is a mild to moderate anemia with a mean hematocrit of 32% *900*

Hemoglobin *Blood* *Decrease* Anemia mostly normochromic is found in a majority of cases. 12 g/dL occurred in 73% of cases *5124* Usually there is a mild to moderate anemia *900* Anemia is present in 66% of all patients when they are first seen. Usually normochromic and moderate in degree but may become severe in advanced disease in myelofibrosis *5677*

α_2-HS Glycoprotein *Serum* *Decrease* Significant reduction observed compared with healthy controls probably due to hepatic involvement *2533*

Hyaluronic Acid *Serum* *Increase* The serum concentration of hyaluronan (HYA) was determined in 59 patients with various myeloproliferative disorders, including 33 patients with idiopathic myelofibrosis. Raised serum HYA levels were seen in patients with active disease compared with age-matched healthy subjects, whereas no significant difference in serum HYA was seen between patients with stable disease and age-matched controls *2055*

289.80 Myelofibrosis *(continued)*

Interleukin-1α *Serum No Effect* In 10 patients with myelofibrosis, concentration not detectable as in 14 healthy controls *545*

Interleukin-1β *Serum No Effect* In 10 patients with myelofibrosis, concentration not detectable as in 14 healthy controls *545*

Interleukin-2 *Serum Increase* In 10 patients with myelofibrosis mean concentration of 1,064 ± 369 pg/mL significantly higher than undetectable amount in 14 healthy controls *545*
Serum No Effect In 10 patients with myelofibrosis mean concentration of 538 ± 1,221 U/mL not significantly different from 582 ± 164 U/mL in 14 healthy controls *545*

Interleukin-6 *Serum No Effect* In 10 patients with myelofibrosis concentration not different from that in 14 healthy controls *545*

Interleukin-10 *Serum No Effect* In 10 patients with myelofibrosis concentration not different from that in 14 healthy controls *545*

Lactate Dehydrogenase *Serum Increase* Increased in every patient irrespective of the disease. The maximum rise was observed in cases of myelosclerosis, the smallest in lymphatic leukemia *3335* May be elevated usually correlating with the degree of myelofibrosis or WBC elevation *900* Reported effect *5677*

Lactate Dehydrogenase Isoenzyme-5
Red Blood Cells Increase A slight mean increase was observed in hemolysates from 12 cases of agnogenic myeloid metaplasia *4983*

Leukocytes *Blood Decrease* The WBC averages 20,000 /µL, but may be as high as 100,000 /µL or as low as 1,000 /µL with slight granulocytic immaturity *900* Pancytopenia is a common feature *5677*
Blood Increase Nearly always present in myelofibrosis. The most numerous cells are mature neutrophils *5677* Initial count was normal in 42%, increased in 47% and decreased in 12% of myelofibrosis patients. Leukopenia occurred with anemia and leukocytosis with high RBC count *5124* The WBC averages 20,000 /µL, but may be as high as 100,000 /µL or as low as 1,000 /µL with slight granulocytic immaturity *900* Elevated in about 50%, normal in 33%, and low in the remainder due to agnogenic myeloid metaplasia *367*
Blood No Effect The WBC averages 20,000 /µL, but may be as high as 100,000 /µL or as low as 1,000 /µL with slight granulocytic immaturity *900*

Lysozyme *Serum Increase* During the transition from a variety of myeloproliferative disorders to acute myeloblastic or acute myelomonocytic leukemia, there is a striking elevation in serum and urine muramidase activity *4692*
Urine Increase During the transition from a variety of myeloproliferative disorders to acute myeloblastic or acute myelomonocytic leukemia, there is a striking elevation in serum and urine muramidase activity *4692*

Metamyelocytes *Blood Increase* Can generally be found in myelofibrosis *5677*

β_2-Microglobulin *Serum Increase* In 10 patients with myelofibrosis mean concentration of 2,919 ± 455 µg/L significantly higher than 1,721 ± 673 µg/L in 14 healthy controls *545*

Monocytes *Blood Increase* Peripheral monocytosis is especially likely to occur in circumstances of histiocytic proliferation and increased phagocytosis as strikingly manifested in histiocytic medullary reticulosis *3246*

Myelocytes *Blood Increase* Can generally be found in myelofibrosis *5677*

Myeloperoxidase *Granulocyte No Effect* Mean density of 575 ± 98 in 21 patients with myelofibrosis not significantly different from 478 ± 52 in 32 normal controls *1303*

Naphthol-As-D-Chloroacetate Esterase
Granulocyte Increase Mean density of 721 ± 58 in 88 patients with myelofibrosis significantly different from 478 ± 52 in 32 normal controls *1303*

Neopterin *Urine Increase* In 4 patients with myelofibrosis mean excretion of about 430 µmol/mol creatinine significantly increased compared with 106.6 ± 34.6 µmol/mol creatinine in 31 healthy controls *3632*

Osmotic Fragility *Red Blood Cells Decrease* Red cell osmotic fragility was decreased in 63% of myelofibrosis patients *5124*

Phospholipase A *Serum Increase* Elevated with myeloid metaplasia *2625*

Platelets *Blood Decrease* Count ranges from 30,000 - 3,200,000 /µL with an average of 400,000 /µL *900* Pancytopenia is a common feature *5677* Thrombocytopenia occurred in 48% of myelofibrosis patients, mostly in the later stages. Counts > 400,000 /µL occurred in 16% in the early stages *5124* In myelofibrosis as the disease progresses, may be aggravated by therapy *5677*
Blood Increase Significant increase frequently observed *1098* Count ranges from 30,000 - 3,200,000 /µL with an average of 400,000 /µL *900* May appear large and bizarre with agnogenic myeloid metaplasia *367* In myelofibrosis, occurs in about 33% of cases, especially in the earlier stages, and may at times reach levels of 1,000,000 /µL or higher *5677*
Blood No Effect Of 250 patients with platelet counts of more than 250,000 /µL, 2 had myelofibrosis *3939*

Procollagen Type III Peptide *Serum Increase* High values are observed in primary and post-polycythemia vera (PV) myelofibrosis, but excessive PC III levels in active PV are not predictive of evolution toward myelofibrosis *3711*

Prothrombin Time *Plasma Increase* Prolonged in 75% of patients with agnogenic myeloid metaplasia *5545*

Pseudouridine *Urine Increase* In 4 patients with myelofibrosis mean excretion about 30 mmol/mol creatinine compared with 19.6 ± 5.2 mmol/mol creatinine in 31 healthy controls *3632*

Thrombopoietin *Plasma Increase* Mean plasma concentration in 14 patients with idiopathic myelofibrosis of 292 pg/mL significantly higher than the mean of 133 pg/mL in healthy individuals *3565*

Tumor Necrosis Factor-α *Serum Increase* In 10 patients with myelofibrosis mean concentration of 10 ± 2.5 pg/mL different from 0 pg/mL in 14 healthy controls *545*

Uric Acid *Serum Increase* May be elevated usually correlating with the degree of myelofibrosis or WBC elevation *900* Associated with increased cellular production *1980* In myelofibrosis, secondary gout and the formation of urinary uric acid calculi are frequent consequences of the hyperuricosuria *5677*
Urine Increase In myelofibrosis, secondary and the formation of urinary uric acid calculi are frequent consequences of the hyperuricemia and hyperuricosuria *5677*

Vitamin B_{12} *Serum Increase* Significantly increased in 7 cases of myelofibrosis, mean concentration of 1,525 pg/mLcompared to normal, 385 pg/mL *4448* Normal or elevated in myelofibrosis *5124* Serum concentration is generally raised, as is the binding power, but neither of them is as high as in chronic granulocytic leukemia (in myelofibrosis) *1730* Observed effect *350*

Vitamin B_{12} Binding Capacity *Serum Increase* In myelofibrosis, serum concentration is generally raised as is the binding power, but neither of them is as high as in chronic granulocytic leukemia *1730* Significant elevation; usually correlated with WBC in peripheral blood *4448*

289.90 Myeloplastic Disorders

Soluble Transferrin Receptor *Serum No Effect* No significant change observed from controls (5.63 ± 1.42 µg/mL) in patients with myeloplastic disorders (9.25 ± 4.73 µg/mL) *2704*

289.90 Thrombocytosis

C-Reactive Protein *Serum Increase* Mean serum concentration in 45 patients with reactive thrombocytosis of 46 ± 10 mg/L significantly higher than 3 ± 1 mg/L in 37 patients with myeloproliferative thrombocytosis and 1 ± 0.7 mg/L in 21 healthy controls *5370* In 64 patients with reactive thrombocytosis median concentration of 4.67 mg/dL significantly different from less than 1.0 mg/dL in healthy controls *5186*
Serum No Effect In 20 patients with clonal thrombocytosis median concentration of 0.62 mg/dL not different from less than 1.0 mg/dL in healthy controls *5186*

Erythropoietin *Serum* *Increase* Mean serum concentration of 19.5 ± 2.2 mIU/mL in patients with reactive thrombocytosis significantly different from 0.0 - 16.9 mIU/mL in 21 healthy controls *5370*

Interleukin-6 *Serum* *Increase* In 64 patients with reactive thrombocytosis median concentration of 16.5 pg/mL significantly different from undetectable concentration in healthy controls *5186* Mean serum concentration in 45 patients with reactive thrombocytosis of 26.3 ± 25.3 pg/mL significantly higher than 1.6 ± 0.4 pg/mL in 37 patients with myeloproliferative thrombocytosis and 0.2 ± 0.1 in 21 pg/mL healthy controls *5370*
Serum *No Effect* In 20 patients with clonal thrombocytosis median concentration of less than 2.0 pg/mL not significantly different from undetectable concentration in healthy controls *5186*

Phosphate *Serum* *Increase* Artefactual cause of hyperphosphatemia *5204* In 111 patients with thrombocytosis mean serum - plasma difference increased when the platelet count was significantly increased compared with difference in 20 healthy controls with normal platelet counts *3173*

Platelets *Blood* *Increase* Mean concentration in 45 patients with reactive thrombocytosis of 552.4 ± 19.1 x 10^9/L and of 607.3 ± 23.9 x 10^9/L in 37 patients with myeloproliferative thrombocytosis significantly higher than 268.0 ± 9.3 x 10^9/L in 21 healthy controls *5370* In 732 patients with platelet counts greater than 500,000 /µL, 5.5% had essential thrombocytosis *1869*

Potassium *Serum* *Increase* In 111 patients with thrombocytosis mean serum - plasma difference of 0.6 to 0.8 mmol/L when the platelet count reached approximately 600,000 /µL compared with 0.43 mmol/L in 20 healthy controls with normal platelet counts *3173*

Thrombopoietin *Plasma* *Increase* Mean serum concentration in 45 patients with reactive thrombocytosis of 560.7 ± 110.1 pg/mL and of 271.4 ± 50.4 pg/mL in 37 patients with myeloproliferative thrombocytosis significantly higher than 159.9 ± 18.2 pg/mL in 21 healthy controls *5370*

MENTAL DISORDERS

290.00 Dementia, Unspecified

Arginine Vasopressin *Cerebrospinal Fluid* *No Effect* In 10 hospitalized patients with dementia mean 08:00 concentration of 1.16 ± 0.07 ng/L not significantly different from 1.13 ± 0.06 ng/L in 11 healthy elderly controls and 1.01 ± 0.03 ng/L in 9 young healthy volunteers *3700*
Plasma *Increase* In 10 hospitalized patients with dementia mean 08:00 concentration of 3.09 ± 0.49 ng/L significantly different from 1.61 ± 0.29 ng/L in 11 healthy elderly controls and 1.56 ± 0.24 ng/L in 9 young healthy volunteers *3700*

Carbonic Anhydrase II *Cerebrospinal Fluid* *Increase* In 19 patients with dementia median concentration of 45.6 µg/L significantly different from median of 7.8 µg/L in 97 controls *4012*

Cholesterol *Serum* *No Effect* In 19 patients with unspecified dementia mean concentration of 6.9 ± 1.6 mmol/L not significantly different from concentration in patients with other forms of dementia and in the general population of the same age *2908*

Cortisol *Plasma* *No Effect* In 19 patients with unspecified disease mean concentration of 493 ± 107 nmol/L not significantly different from that in patients with other dementias and in the general age-matched population *2908*

Erythrocytes *Cerebrospinal Fluid* *No Effect* In 19 patients with dementia median concentration of 2 x 10^6/L not significantly different from median of 1 x 10^6 /L in 97 controls *4012*

Leukocytes *Cerebrospinal Fluid* *No Effect* In 19 patients with dementia median concentration of 1 x 10^6/L not significantly different from median of 1 x 10^6 /L in 97 controls *4012*

Monoamine Oxidase-B *Platelets* *Increase* Concentration observed to increase significantly in demented patients *1832*

Osmolality *Serum* *Increase* In 10 patients with dementia mean osmolality of 291 ± 1 mOsm/kg within the reference interval but significantly different from 289 ± 1 mOsm/kg in 11 healthy elderly and also significantly higher than 288 ± 2 mOsm/kg in 9 young healthy volunteers *3700*

Protein *Cerebrospinal Fluid* *No Effect* In 19 patients with dementia median concentration of 441 mg/L not significantly different from median of 400 mg/L in 97 controls *4012*

Sodium:Arginine Vasopressin Ratio *Serum* *Decrease* In 10 patients with dementia mean 08:00 ratio of 119 ± 29 significantly different from 241 ± 35 in 11 healthy elderly but not significantly different from 134 ± 24 in 9 young healthy volunteers *3700*

Triglycerides *Serum* *No Effect* In 19 patients with unspecified dementia mean concentration of 1.5 ± 0.9 mmol/L not significantly different from that in the general population of the same age *2908*

290.00 HIV-associated Dementia

Interleukin-8 *Cerebrospinal Fluid* *No Effect* Detected in 66 of 67 HIV+ patients with dementia with median concentration of 17.0 pg/mL not significantly different from detctable amount in 20 of 20 patients without HIV infection and median concentration of 22.5 pg/mL *2620*

Macrophage Inflammatory Protein-1α
Cerebrospinal Fluid *No Effect* Detected in 10 of 35 HIV+ patients with dementia with median concentration of 0.0 pg/mL not significantly different from undetctable amount in all 6 of 23 patients without HIV infection *2620*

Macrophage Inflammatory Protein-1β
Cerebrospinal Fluid *No Effect* Detected in 3 of 28 HIV+ patients with dementia with median concentration of 0.0 pg/mL not significantly different from undetctable amount in 3 of 17 patients without HIV infection *2620*

Monocyte Chemotactic Protein-1
Cerebrospinal Fluid *Increase* Detected in 18 of 181 HIV+ patients with dementia with median concentration of 711 pg/mL significantly different from detctable amount in all 59 patients without HIV infection and median concentration of 409 pg/mL *2620*

Monocyte Chemotactic Protein-3
Cerebrospinal Fluid *No Effect* Detected in 11 of 20 HIV+ patients with dementia with median concentration of 1.6 pg/mL not significantly different from detctable amount in 9 of 15 patients without HIV infection and median concentration of 0.6 pg/mL *2620*

RANTES *Cerebrospinal Fluid* *No Effect* Detected in 78 of 130 HIV+ patients with dementia with median concentration of 2.5 pg/mL not significantly different from detctable amount in 24 of 41 patients without HIV infection and median concentration of 1.9 pg/mL *2620*

290.00 Multi-Infarct Dementia

α_1-Antichymotrypsin *Serum* *Increase* Mean concentration increased above reference interval of 47.9 ± 8.1 mg/dL in 2 of 10 patients (20%) with multi-infarct dementia *3044*

Tumor Necrosis Factor-α *Serum* *Decrease* In patients with multi-infarct dementia mean concentration of 1.64 ± 1.17 pg/mL significantly less than 10.66 ± 8.92 pg/mL in healthy controls *657*

290.00 Vascular Dementia

Acetylcholinesterase G4 Isoenzyme *Serum* *Increase* In 19 patients with vascular dementia mean concentration of 3.2 nmol/min/mL significantly increased compared with mean of 2.7 nmol/min/mL in 20 age-matched controls *5778*

Arginine Aminopeptidase *Cerebrospinal Fluid* *No Effect* In 10 patients mean concentration of 0.063 ± 0.033 nmol/min/mL not significantly different from 0.096 ± 0.016 nmol/min/mL in 21 healthy controls *160*

Cathepsin B *Cerebrospinal Fluid* *No Effect* In 10 patients with vascular dementia mean concentration of 0.036 ± 0.013 nmol/min/mL nonsignificantly increased compared with 0.003 ± 0.002 nmol/min/mL in 21 healthy controls *160*

Cholesterol *Serum* *No Effect* In 14 patients with vascular dementia mean concentration of 6.7 ± 1.9 mmol/L not significantly different from that in patients with other forms of dementia and in the general population of the same age *2908*

290.00 Vascular Dementia *(continued)*

Cortisol *Plasma No Effect* Mean concentration of 509 ± 132 nmol/L in 14 patients with vascular disease not significantly different from that in patients with other dementias and in the general population of the same age *2908*

Dipeptidyl Peptidase II *Cerebrospinal Fluid No Effect* In 10 patients mean concentration of 0.913 ± 0.094 nmol/min/mL not significantly different from 0.715 ± 0.073 nmol/min/mL in 21 healthy controls *160*

Dipeptidyl Peptidase III *Cerebrospinal Fluid Decrease* In 10 patients mean concentration of 0.030 ± 0.014 nmol/min/mL significantly less than 0.118 ± 0.015 nmol/min/mL in 21 healthy controls *160*

Dipeptidyl Peptidase IV *Cerebrospinal Fluid No Effect* In 10 patients with vascular dementia mean concentration of 0.071 ± 0.022 nmol/min/mL not significantly different from 0.27 ± 0.012 nmol/min/mL in 21 healthy controls *160*

Interleukin-6 *Cerebrospinal Fluid Increase* In 8 patients with vascular dementia mean concentration of 3.20 ± 1.08 pg/mL significantly greater than 2.67 ± 0.34 pg/mL in 7 age-matched controls *5763*

Lactate *Cerebrospinal Fluid No Effect* In 49 patients with vascular dementia mean concentration of 1.78 ± 0.28 mmol/L not significantly different from 1.85 ± 0.06 mmol/L in 20 healthy controls *3823*

Leucine Aminopeptidase *Cerebrospinal Fluid Increase* In 10 individuals with vascular dementia mean concentration of 0.203 ± 0.023 nmol/min/mL significantly higher than 0.058 ± 0.013 nmol/min/mL in 21 healthy controls *5364*

Lymphoid Serine Protease *Cerebrospinal Fluid No Effect* In 10 patients with vascular dementia mean concentration of 0.026 ± 0.004 nmol/min/mL not significantly different from 0.035 ± 0.005 nmol/min/mL in 21 healthy controls *160*

Myelin Basic Protein *Cerebrospinal Fluid Increase* In 46 patients with vascular dementia mean concentration of 1.3 ± 1.8 µg/L not significantly different from 0.8 ± 0.6 µg/L in 20 healthy controls *3823*

Neuron-specific Enolase *Cerebrospinal Fluid No Effect* In 41 patients with vascular dementia mean concentration of 8.2 ± 3.1 µg/L not significantly different from 8.8 ± 2.6 µg/L in 20 healthy controls *3823*

Proline Iminopeptidase *Cerebrospinal Fluid No Effect* In 10 patients with vascular dementia mean concentration of 0.010 ± 0.009 nmol/min/mL not significantly different from 0.009 ± 0.003 nmol/min/mL in 21 healthy controls *160*

S-100 Protein *Cerebrospinal Fluid No Effect* In 40 patients with vascular dementia mean concentration of 3.1 ± 1.2 µg/L not significantly different from 3.4 ± 1.3 µg/L in 20 healthy controls *3823*

Sulfatide *Cerebrospinal Fluid Increase* In 20 patients with vascular dementia mean concentration of 307 ± 118 nmol/L significantly higher than in 20 age-matched controls *1563*

Tau Protein *Cerebrospinal Fluid No Effect* In 10 patients with vascular dementia mean concentration of 229.1 ± 39.7 pg/mL not significantly different compared with 212.1 ± 41.6 pg/mL 23 controls *3434*

α-Thrombin *Cerebrospinal Fluid No Effect* In 10 patients with vascular disease mean concentration of 0.016 ± 0.006 nmol/min/mL not significantly different from 0.013 ± 0.004 nmol/min/mL in 21 healthy controls *160*

Tissue Kallikrein *Cerebrospinal Fluid No Effect* In 10 patients mean concentration of 0.199 ± 0.025 nmol/min/mL not significantly different from 0.160 ± 0.014 nmol/min/mL in 21 healthy controls *160*

Triglycerides *Serum Increase* In 14 patients with vascular dementia mean concentration of 1.9 ± 0.8 mmol/L significantly higher than in other forms of dementia and in the general population *2908*

290.10 Alzheimer-Type Dementia

γ-Aminobutyric Acid *Cerebrospinal Fluid Decrease* In 16 female patients with senile dementia of Alzheimer's type concentration significantly reduced compared with that in 8 matched healthy controls *5866*

α_1-Antichymotrypsin *Serum Increase* Mean concentration in 57 patients with presumed Alzheimer-type dementia of 73.1 ± 22 mg/dL significantly different from 47.9 ± 8.1 mg/dL in 110 healthy controls *3044*

Arginine Aminopeptidase *Cerebrospinal Fluid No Effect* In 10 patients mean concentration of 0.104 ± 0.023 nmol/min/mL not significantly different from 0.096 ± 0.016 nmol/min/mL in 21 healthy controls *160*

Calcium *Serum No Effect* In 12 patients with dementia of the Alzheimer type mean concentration of 2.39 ± 0.07 mmol/L not significantly different from 2.44 ± 0.12 mmol/L in 12 healthy controls *2992*

Cathepsin B *Cerebrospinal Fluid Increase* Reported effect *160* In 10 patients with Alzheimer-type dementia mean concentration of 0.054 ± 0.016 nmol/min/mL significantly higher than 0.003 ± 0.002 nmol/min/mL in 21 healthy controls *160*

Ceruloplasmin *Serum No Effect* In 44 patients with probable Alzheimer's dementia mean concentration of 382 mg/L not significantly different from 383 mg/L in age and gendered matched controls *4917*

Ceruloplasmin Ferroxidase *Serum Decrease* In 44 patients with probable Alzheimer's dementia mean activity of 89 U/L significantly different from 136 U/L in age and gendered matched controls *4917*

Copper *Serum No Effect* In 44 patients with probable Alzheimer's dementia mean concentration of 19.1 µmol/L not significantly different from 19.4 µmol/L in age and gendered matched controls *4917*

Creatinine *Urine Decrease* Progressive decrease observed in elderly with increasing severity of disease: in healthy aged controls mean 109 ± 13 mg/dL decreasing to 88 ± 9 mg/dL in patients with severe dementia and 57 ± 11 mg/dL in demented patients in a vegetative state *3070*

Dipeptidyl Peptidase II *Cerebrospinal Fluid No Effect* In 10 patients mean concentration of 0.938 ± 0.114 nmol/min/mL not significantly different from 0.715 ± 0.073 nmol/min/mL in 21 healthy controls *160*

Dipeptidyl Peptidase III *Cerebrospinal Fluid Increase* In 10 patients mean concentration of 0.125 ± 0.034 nmol/min/mL significantly higher than 0.118 ± 0.015 nmol/min/mL in 21 healthy controls *160*

Dipeptidyl Peptidase IV *Cerebrospinal Fluid Increase* In 10 patients mean concentration of 0.191 ± 0.091 nmol/min/mL significantly higher than 0.027 ± 0.012 nmol/min/mL in 21 healthy controls *160*

Ferritin *Serum No Effect* In 41 patients with Alzheimer-type dementia mean concentration of 185 ± 138 ng/mL not significantly different from 147 ± 110 ng/mL in 19 age-matched controls *1490*

Homovanillic Acid *Cerebrospinal Fluid No Effect* In 23 patients with Alzheimer's dementia concentration normal and relatively stable over 2 weeks *4710* In 16 female patients with senile dementia of Alzheimer's type concentration not significantly different from that in 8 matched controls *5866*
Plasma Increase In 21 patients with Alzheimer's type dementia mean concentration of 96 ± 57 pmol/mL prior to drug treatment, with significant positive correlation between baseline concentration and Parkinsonian rigidity *5107*

4-Hydroxy-3-Methoxy-Phenylglycol
Cerebrospinal Fluid No Effect In 23 patients with Alzheimer's dementia concentration normal and stable over two weeks *4710*

5-Hydroxyindoleacetic Acid *Cerebrospinal Fluid No Effect* Concentration normal and stable over two weeks in patients with Alzheimer's dementia *4710*

Interleukin-1β *Cerebrospinal Fluid No Effect* No difference observed between concentrations between patients with condition and healthy controls *3248*

Interleukin-6 *Cerebrospinal Fluid Decrease* In 12 patients with Alzheimer's dementia mean concentration of 1.17 ± 0.26 pg/mL significantly less than 2.67 ± 0.34 pg/mL in 7 age-matched controls (mean in 6 patients with early onset disease of 0.57 ± 0.14 pg/mL and 1.78 ± 0.36 pg/mL in 6 late onset patients) *5763*
Serum No Effect No difference observed between concentrations between patients with condition and healthy controls, although measurements were made by bioassay *3248*

Lactate *Cerebrospinal Fluid* *No Effect* Mean concentration of 1,777 ± 262 μmol/L in 36 patients with Alzheimer's disease not significantly different from 1,850 ± 63 μmol/L in 20 controls without dementia *3823*

Leucine Aminopeptidase *Cerebrospinal Fluid* *No Effect* In 10 patients with Alzheimer-type dementia mean concentration of 0.097 ± 0.043 nmol/min/mL not significantly different from 0.058 ± 0.013 nmol/min/mL in 21 healthy controls *160*

Lymphoid Serine Protease *Cerebrospinal Fluid* *No Effect* In 10 patients mean concentration of 0.043 ± 0.013 nmol/min/mL not significantly different from 0.035 ± 0.005 nmol/min/mL in 21 healthy controls *160*

Magnesium *Serum* *Decrease* In 12 patients with dementia of the Alzheimer type mean concentration of 0.58 ± 0.07 mmol/L significantly different from 0.7 ± 0.08 mmol/L in 12 controls *2992*

Monoamine Oxidase-B *Platelets* *Increase* In 20 patients with Alzheimer-type dementia without depression mean concentration of 2.6 ± 0.9 nmol/mg protein/min and 2.2 ± 1.0 nmol/mg protein/min in 19 with depression significantly higher than 1.7 ± 0.8 nmol/mg protein/min in 9 controls *1491* Concentration observed to increase significantly in patients with Alzheimer type dementia *1832*

Myelin Basic Protein *Cerebrospinal Fluid* *No Effect* In 32 patients with Alzheimer's dementia mean concentration of 0.8 ± 0.5 μg/L not significantly different from 0.8 ± 0.6 μg/L in 20 healthy controls *3823*

Neuron-specific Enolase *Cerebrospinal Fluid* *No Effect* In 28 patients with Alzheimer's dementia mean concentration of 8.8 ± 2.3 μg/L not significantly different from 8.8 ± 2.6 μg/L in 20 healthy controls *3823*

Potassium *Serum* *No Effect* In 12 patients with dementia of the Alzheimer type mean concentration of 3.95 ± 0.37 mmol/L not significantly different from 4.19 ± 0.29 mmol/L in 12 healthy controls *2992*

Proline Iminopeptidase *Cerebrospinal Fluid* *No Effect* In 10 patients mean concentration of 0.019 ± 0.0.012 nmol/min/mL not significantly different from 0.009 ± 0.003 nmol/min/mL in 21 healthy controls *160*

S-100 Protein *Cerebrospinal Fluid* *No Effect* Mean concentration of 3.6 ± 1.5 μg/L in 28 patients with Alzheimer's disease not significantly different from 3.4 ± 1.3 μg/L in 20 controls without dementia *3823*

Sodium *Serum* *No Effect* In 12 patients with dementia of the Alzheimer type mean concentration of 134 ± 3.5 mmol/L not significantly different from 136.3 ± 3.3 mmol/L in 12 healthy controls *2992*

Superoxide Dismutase *Red Blood Cells* *Decrease* In 44 patients with probable Alzheimer's dementia mean activity of 269 - 525 SOD units significantly different from 287 - 525 SOD units in age and gendered matched controls *4917*

Tau Protein *Cerebrospinal Fluid* *Increase* Median concentration in 11 patients with mild to moderate disease of 714 ng/L significantly different from 160 ng/L in 19 controls *4354*

α-Thrombin *Cerebrospinal Fluid* *No Effect* In 10 patients mean concentration of 0.015 ± 0.007 nmol/min/mL compared with 0.013 ± 0.004 nmol/min/mL in 21 healthy controls *160*

Tissue Kallikrein *Cerebrospinal Fluid* *No Effect* In 10 patients with Alzheimer-type dementia mean concentration of 0.219 ± 0.034 nmol/min/mL not significantly different from 0.160 ± 0.014 nmol/min/mL in 21 healthy controls *160*

Transferrin *Serum* *Decrease* In 41 patients with Alzheimer-type dementia mean concentration of 74.3 ± 21.1 g/L significantly different from 83.2 ± 15.9 g/L in 19 age-matched controls *1490*

Truncated Nerve Growth Factor Receptor *Urine* *Decrease* With increasing dementia progressive reduction in excretion to less than 0.1 ng/μL compared with 0.9 ng/μL in healthy aged controls *3070*
Urine *Increase* In elderly patients with mild or very mild dementia mean excretion increased to 2.2 - 2.3 ng/μL compared with 0.9 ng/μL in healthy aged controls *3070*

Tumor Necrosis Factor-α *Serum* *Decrease* Both increased and decreased concentrations have been reported with condition *3248*
Serum *Increase* Both increased and decreased concentrations have been reported with condition *3248*

Vitamin B_{12} *Serum* *Decrease* In 20 patients with Alzheimer-type dementia without depression mean concentration of 255 ± 155 pg/mL and 246 ± 177 pg/mL in 19 with depression not significantly lower than 326 ± 249 pg/mL in 9 controls *1491*

290.10 Creutzfeldt-Jakob Disease with Dementia

Myelin Basic Protein *Cerebrospinal Fluid* *Increase* In 2 patients with Creutzfeldt-Jakob's disease with dementia mean concentration of 1.4 ± 0.9 μg/L not significantly different from 0.8 ± 0.6 μg/L in 20 healthy controls *3823*

Neuron-specific Enolase *Cerebrospinal Fluid* *Increase* In 2 patients with Creutzfeldt-Jakob's disease with dementia mean concentration of 32.6 ± 0.9 μg/L significantly different from 8.8 ± 2.6 μg/L in 20 healthy controls *3823*

S-100 Protein *Cerebrospinal Fluid* *Increase* Mean concentration of 10.8 ± 3.6 μg/L in 2 patients with Creutzfeld-Jakob disease significantly different from 3.4 ± 1.3 μg/L in 20 controls without dementia *3823*

290.10 Pick's Dementia

α_1-Antichymotrypsin *Serum* *No Effect* Mean concentration within reference interval of 47.9 ± 8.1 mg/dL in one patient with Pick's disease *3044*

Lactate *Cerebrospinal Fluid* *No Effect* Mean concentration of 1,646 ± 185 μmol/L in 7 patients with Pick's dementia not significantly different from 1,850 ± 63 μmol/L in 20 controls without dementia *3823*

Myelin Basic Protein *Cerebrospinal Fluid* *No Effect* Mean concentration of 1.2 ± 0.8 μg/L in 6 patients with Pick's dementia not significantly different from 0.8 ± 0.6 μg/L in 20 controls without dementia *3823*

Neuron-specific Enolase *Cerebrospinal Fluid* *Decrease* In 5 patients with dementia and Pick's disease mean concentration of 8.1 ± 1.9 μg/L not significantly different from 8.8 ± 2.6 μg/L in 20 healthy controls *3823*

S-100 Protein *Cerebrospinal Fluid* *Increase* Mean concentration of 4.3 ± 3.6 μg/L in 5 patients with Pick's dementia not significantly different from 3.4 ± 1.3 μg/L in 20 controls without dementia *3823*

291.00 Delirium Tremens

Aldolase *Serum* *Increase* Activity may be increased in some patients with delirium tremens *2952*

Aspartate Aminotransferase *Serum* *Increase* Irrespective of associated hepatic disease and may arise in muscle *1025*

Bicarbonate *Serum* *Decrease* Respiratory alkalosis may occur *3124*

Carbon Dioxide Partial Pressure *Blood* *Decrease* Respiratory alkalosis may occur *1980*

Creatine Kinase *Serum* *Increase* High elevations irrespective of associated hepatic disease and may arise in muscle *1642 1025*

Lactate Dehydrogenase *Serum* *Increase* Relatively slight elevations found in almost all patients. Perhaps of skeletal muscle origin since, like the elevated LD values of progressive muscular dystrophy, they are accompanied by increased CK. High elevations irrespective of associated hepatic disease and may arise in muscle *1025*

Nickel *Serum* *No Effect* Mean concentration of 2.3 μg/L (n = 35) compared with mean in controls of 2.6 μg/L (n = 42) *3428*

Ornithine Carbamoyltransferase *Serum* *Increase* Liver cell damage *5544*

pH *Blood* *Increase* Respiratory alkalosis may occur *1980*

Selenium *Serum* *Decrease* In patients with delirium tremens concentration in both serum and whole blood reduced *73*

Uric Acid *Cerebrospinal Fluid* *Increase* High CSF levels of 0.9 - 1.3 mg/dL, with normal serum levels *2892*

291.20 Alcoholic Dementia

α_1-Antichymotrypsin *Serum* *No Effect* Mean concentration within reference interval of 47.9 ± 8.1 mg/dL in two examined patients with alcoholic dementia *3044*

294.80 Melancholic Psychotic Depression

Albumin *Serum* *Decrease* Mean concentration of 42.3 ± 3.5 g/L in 12 patients with major depression and melancholia significantly different from 46.7 ± 2.3 g/L in 18 healthy controls *3216*

Cortisol *Plasma* *Increase* In 21 patients with melancholic psychotic depression mean concentration of 456 ± 33 nmol/L not significantly different from 374 ± 25 nmol/L in 20 healthy controls *2627*

Plasma *No Effect* In 22 patients with melancholia and depression mean concentration of 23.4 ± 7.9 μg/dL not significantly different fom normal *3198*

Urine *No Effect* In 22 patients with melancholia and depression mean excretion of 219 μg/d not significantly different fom normal *3198*

α_1-Globulin *Serum* *Increase* Mean concentration of 2.5 ± 0.4 g/L in 12 patients with major depression and melancholia not different from 2.2 ± 0.3 g/L in 18 healthy controls, although as proportion of total protein increased to 3.5 ± 0.8% compared with 3.0 ± 0.4% in healthy controls *3216*

α_2-Globulin *Serum* *Increase* Mean concentration of 6.8 ± 0.9 g/L in 12 patients with major depression and melancholia not different from 6.1 ± 0.8 g/L in 18 healthy controls, although as proportion of total protein increased to 10.0 ± 1.5% compared with 8.3 ± 1.1% in healthy controls *3216*

β-Globulin *Serum* *No Effect* Mean concentration of 8.1 ± 1.0 g/L in 12 patients with major depression and melancholia not different from 9.2 ± 1.2 g/L in 18 healthy controls, and as proportion of total protein unchanged at 12.0 ± 1.6% compared with 12.4 ± 1.4% in healthy controls *3216*

γ-Globulin *Serum* *No Effect* Mean concentration of 8.2 ± 2.3 g/L in 12 patients with major depression and melancholia not different from 9.4 ± 1.6 g/L in 18 healthy controls, and as proportion of total protein decreased at 12.0 ± 2.8% compared with 12.8 ± 2.0% in healthy controls *3216*

Interleukin-1 Receptor Antagonist *Serum* *Increase* In 22 patients with melancholic depression mean concentration of 0.186 ng/mL and 0.186 ng/mL in 25 patients with simple major depression compared with 0.110 ng/mL in 22 healthy controls *3198*

Neopterin *Serum* *Increase* In patients with melancholia significant positive correlation with serum IL-2R concentration *3206*

Norepinephrine *Plasma* *Increase* In 21 patients with melancholic psychotic depression mean concentration of 462 ± 98 ng/mL significantly different from 221 ± 41 ng/mL in 20 healthy controls *2627*

Protein *Serum* *Decrease* Mean concentration of 67.7 ± 4.4 g/L in 12 patients with major depression and melancholia significantly different from 73.6 ± 2.9 g/L in 18 healthy controls *3216*

Soluble Interleukin-2 Receptor *Serum* *Increase* In patients with melancholia mean concentration of 369 ± 82 U/mL significantly different from 224 ± 107 U/mL in 19 normal controls *3206*

294.80 Non-Alzheimer's Dementia

Tau Protein *Cerebrospinal Fluid* *No Effect* In 25 patients with non-Alzheimer's dementia mean concentration of 235 ± 104 pg/mL not significantly different from 190 ± 80 pg/mL in 26 controls *4065* In 10 patients with frontal lobe dementia mean concentration of 179.1 ± 22.7 pg/mL not significantly different compared with 212.1 ± 41.6 pg/mL 23 controls *3434*

295.90 Schizoaffective Disorder

Phenylacetic Acid *Cerebrospinal Fluid* *No Effect* Mean concentration in 12 patients with schizoaffective disorder of 19.5 ± 8.8 ng/mL not significantly different from that in 30 healthy volunteers in whom the mean concentration was 26.6 ± 15.2 ng/mL *4761*

Phenylacetic Acid, Conjugated
Cerebrospinal Fluid *No Effect* Mean concentration in 13 patients with schizoaffective disorder of 6.5 ± 4.3 ng/mL not significantly different from that in 30 healthy volunteers in whom the mean concentration was 11.7 ± 5.5 ng/mL *4761*

Phenylacetic Acid, Unconjugated
Cerebrospinal Fluid *No Effect* Mean concentration in 13 patients with schizoaffective disorder of 12.9 ± 6.4 ng/mL not significantly different from that in 30 healthy volunteers in whom the mean concentration was 14.8 ± 12.8 ng/mL *4761*

295.90 Schizophrenia

Acetylcholinesterase *Cerebrospinal Fluid* *No Effect* The AChE levels were unrelated to the degree of cognitive decline and they were in the same range as in the control group *2766*

α_1-Acid Glycoprotein *Serum* *Increase* In 27 unmedicated schizophrenic patients mean concentration of 80 ± 17 mg/dL significantly greater than 58 ± 13 mg/dL in 21 normal controls *3208*

Angiotensin-converting Enzyme
Cerebrospinal Fluid *Decrease* In both drug-treated and untreated schizophrenics concentration significantly less than in normal controls but no correlation existed with the scores of Brief Psychiatric Rating Scale *363*

α_1-Antichymotrypsin *Serum* *Increase* Mean concentration increased above reference interval of 47.9 ± 8.1 mg/dL in 2 of 9 patients (22%) with schizophrenia *3044*

α_1-Antitrypsin *Serum* *Increase* In 27 unmedicated schizophrenic patients mean concentration of 206 ± 43 mg/dL not significantly greater than 187 ± 50 mg/dL in 21 normal controls *3208*

Cadmium *Hair* *No Effect* In 12 schizophrenic patients mean concentration of 1.0 ± 0.2 μg/g not significantly different from mean concentration in 30 healthy control individuals of 1.1 ± 0.2 μg/g *2614*

Nails *No Effect* In 30 schizophrenic patients mean concentration of 1.8 ± 0.2 μg/g not significantly different from mean concentration in 30 healthy control individuals of 1.6 ± 0.1 μg/g *2614*

Calcium *Cerebrospinal Fluid* *No Effect* In 8 acute schizophrenics mean concentration of 2.66 ± 0.4 mEq/L not significantly different from 2.46 ± 0.3 mEq/L in 8 schizophrenics in remission *3012*

Hair *Decrease* In 12 schizophrenic patients mean concentration of 1779.0 ± 4.6 μg/g significantly different from mean concentration in 30 healthy control individuals of 2015.1 ± 96.4 μg/g *2614*

Nails *Decrease* In 30 schizophrenic patients mean concentration of 975.9 ± 13.5 μg/g significantly different from mean concentration in 30 healthy control individuals of 1250.4 ± 15.5 μg/g *2614*

Serum *No Effect* In 8 acute schizophrenics mean concentration of 4.83 ± 0.1 mEq/L not significantly different from 4.91 ± 0.2 mEq/L in 8 schizophrenics in remission *3012*

Chromium *Hair* *No Effect* In 12 schizophrenic patients mean concentration of 4.1 ± 0.8 μg/g not significantly different from mean concentration in 30 healthy control individuals of 4.9 ± 0.7 μg/g *2614*

Nails *No Effect* In 30 schizophrenic patients mean concentration of 9.4 ± 0.9 μg/g not significantly different from mean concentration in 30 healthy control individuals of 9.7 ± 0.5 μg/g *2614*

Clara Cell Protein *Serum* *Decrease* In 17 patients with schizophrenia mean concentration of 37 ± 16 ng/mL significantly different from 51 ± 19 ng/mL in 23 normal volunteers *3204* In 14 untreated schizophrenics mean concentration of 19.0 ± 4.0 ng/mL significantly less than that in 30 healthy study controls in whom mean concentration was 23.0 ± 4.1 ng/mL *3205*

Complement C_3 *Serum* *Increase* In 27 unmedicated schizophrenic patients mean concentration of 92 ± 19 mg/dL significantly greater than 74 ± 17 mg/dL in 21 normal controls *3208*

Complement C_4 *Serum* *Increase* In 27 unmedicated schizophrenic patients mean concentration of 41 ± 14 mg/dL significantly greater than 29 ± 12 mg/dL in 21 normal controls *3208*

Copper *Hair* *Decrease* In 10 female schizophrenics mean concentration of 9.23 µg/g significantly less than 12.4 µg/g in 12 female controls but mean concentration of 9.46 µg/g in 12 male schizophrenics not significantly less than 9.97 µg/g in 16 male controls *5096*
Hair *No Effect* In 12 schizophrenic patients mean concentration of 13.9 ± 3.1 µg/g not significantly different from mean concentration in 30 healthy control individuals of 12.7 ± 2.7 µg/g *2614*
Nails *No Effect* In 30 schizophrenic patients mean concentration of 7.4 ± 0.5 µg/g not significantly different from mean concentration in 30 healthy control individuals of 7.2 ± 0.7 µg/g *2614*

Corticotropin-releasing Hormone
Cerebrospinal Fluid *No Effect* No significant difference between concentration in treated chronic schizophrenics and healthy controls *1528*

Cortisol *Plasma* *Increase* In 7 patients with schizophrenia mean concentration of 411 ± 57 mmol/L significantly increased compared with 321 ± 32 mmol/L in 22 healthy age- and sex-matched controls *3226* Concentration increased in patients with schizophrenia compared with that in controls *5649*
Plasma *No Effect* In 7 men with paranoid schizophrenia normal circadian variation persists in spite of absent variation of melatonin *3578*

Cyclo(His-Pro) *Cerebrospinal Fluid* *Increase* In a group of unmedicated schizophrenics 53% increase observed in never-medicated schizophrenics and 25% increase in medicated schizophrenics compared with controls *4205*

3,4-Dihydroxyphenylacetic Acid
Cerebrospinal Fluid *No Effect* In 36 patients with chronic schizophrenia the mean concentration was 5.97 ± 0.90 pmol/mL not significantly different from 6.70 ± 0.92 pmol/mL in 8 controls *4209*

3,4-Dihydroxyphenylacetic Acid, Conjugated
Cerebrospinal Fluid *Decrease* In 36 patients with chronic schizophrenia the mean concentration was 3.99 ± 0.42 pmol/mL not significantly different from 5.97 ± 1.35 pmol/mL in 8 controls *4209*

3,4-Dihydroxyphenylacetic Acid, Free
Cerebrospinal Fluid *No Effect* In 36 patients with chronic schizophrenia the mean concentration was 2.75 ± 0.28 pmol/mL not significantly different from 2.97 ± 0.67 pmol/mL in 8 controls *4209*

Dopamine *Plasma* *Increase* MESOR is higher in schizophrenics than in healthy controls *4277*

Dopamine Sulfate *Cerebrospinal Fluid* *No Effect* In 36 patients with chronic schizophrenia the mean concentration was 3.35 ± 0.24 pmol/mL not significantly different from 4.33 ± 0.82 pmol/mL in 8 controls *4209*

β-Endorphin *Plasma* *Increase* In 37 patients with chronic schizophrenia, not medicated for at least 10 days, mean concentration significantly higher than in 21 age and sex matched controls *559*

Fibrinogen *Plasma* *Increase* In 27 unmedicated schizophrenic patients mean concentration of 198 ± 48 mg/dL significantly greater than 131 ± 47 mg/dL in 21 normal controls *3208*

α1,3-Fucosyltransferase *Serum* *Decrease* In 44 schizophrenics mean activity of 139.5 ± 83.5 pmol/mL/h significantly different from 178.2 ± 76.4 pmol/mL/h in 50 healthy controls *5793*

Glutamic Acid *Cerebrospinal Fluid* *Increase* In 19 untreated patients mean concentration of 0.138 ± 0.06 µg/mL with significant positive association with severity of condition *1435*
Plasma *Increase* Significantly higher concentration observed in schizophrenia *3179*

Glycine *Plasma* *Increase* Significantly higher concentration observed in patients with paranoid or undifferentiated schizophrenia but not in disorganized patients *3179*

Growth Hormone *Plasma* *Decrease* In drug-free schizophrenics mean nocturnal concentration of 2.5 ng/mL compared with 7.5 ng/mL in healthy controls *2527*

Haptoglobin *Serum* *Increase* In 27 unmedicated schizophrenic patients mean concentration of 214 ± 91 mg/dL significantly greater than 102 ± 38 mg/dL in 21 normal controls *3208*

Hemopexin *Serum* *Increase* In 27 unmedicated schizophrenic patients mean concentration of 81 ± 16 mg/dL significantly greater than 63 ± 10 mg/dL in 21 normal controls *3208*

Homovanillic Acid *Cerebrospinal Fluid* *Increase* In 19 untreated patients mean concentration of 35.90 ± 13.44 ng/mL without significant positive association or severity of condition *1435*
Cerebrospinal Fluid *No Effect* In 36 patients with chronic schizophrenia the mean concentration was 207.5 ± 20.8 pmol/mL not significantly different from 193.8 ± 15.8 pmol/mL in 8 controls *4209* In 12 drug-free patients with childhood-onset of schizophrenia mean concentration of 163.8 ± 50.8 pmol/mL not significantly different from 189.8 ± 45.3 pmol/mL in 12 schizophrenic patients treated with clozapine for 12 weeks or 228.7 ± 86.5 pmol/mL in 10 treated for 10 weeks with haloperidol *2392*
Plasma *Decrease* Concentrations lower in schizophrenics at all times throughout day including during sleep, but within schizophrenics the more symptomatic patients had higher concentrations than the less severely ill patients *1028*
Plasma *Increase* Plasma total homovanillic acid significantly increased in schizophrenics although conjugated homovanillic acid concentration significantly reduced *1643* Mean concentration significantly correlated with severity of disease (r = 0.66 when correlated with CGI scores) *1036*

Homovanillic Acid, Conjugated *Plasma* *Decrease* Significant decrease observed in schizophrenia patients *1643*

Homovanillic Acid, Free *Plasma* *Increase* Substantial and significant increase observed in patients with schizophrenia *1643*

Homovanillic Acid:3-Methoxy-4-hydroxyl-phenylglycol Ratio
Cerebrospinal Fluid *No Effect* In 12 drug-free patients with childhood-onset of schizophrenia mean ratio of 3.6 ± 1.1 not significantly different from 4.3 ± 0.9 in 12 schizophrenic patients treated with clozapine for 12 weeks or 5.3 ± 2.0 in 10 treated for 10 weeks with haloperidol *2392*

Homovanillic Acid:5-Hydroxyindoleacetic Acid Ratio
Cerebrospinal Fluid *No Effect* In 12 drug-free patients with childhood-onset of schizophrenia mean ratio of 2.3 ± 1.0 not significantly different from 2.4 ± 0.7 in 12 schizophrenic patients treated with clozapine for 12 weeks or 3.2 ± 1.4 in 10 treated for 10 weeks with haloperidol *2392*

5-Hydroxyindoleacetic Acid *Cerebrospinal Fluid* *No Effect* In 36 patients with chronic schizophrenia the mean concentration was 102.9 ± 6.8 pmol/mL not significantly different from 92.5 ± 6.4 pmol/mL in 8 controls *4209* In 12 drug-free patients with childhood-onset of schizophrenia mean concentration of 81.4 ± 31.2 pmol/mL not significantly different from 85.2 ± 28.9 pmol/mL in 12 schizophrenic patients treated with clozapine for 12 weeks or 275.8 ± 22.7 pmol/mL in 10 treated for 10 weeks with haloperidol *2392*

5-Hydroxytryptamine *Platelets* *Increase* Mean concentration in 117 schizophrenic male patients of 1.51 ± 0.47 nmol/mg protein significantly higher than that in 90 healthy individuals, 1.26 ± 0.26 nmol/mg protein *2409*

Immunoglobulin G *Serum* *Increase* In 27 unmedicated schizophrenic patients mean concentration of 1,000 ± 264 mg/dL but not significantly greater than 866 ± 255 mg/dL in 21 normal controls *3208*

Immunoglobulin M *Serum* *Increase* In 27 unmedicated schizophrenic patients mean concentration of 203 ± 88 mg/dL but not significantly greater than 177 ± 93 mg/dL in 21 normal controls *3208*

Inosine Monophosphate *Red Blood Cells* *Increase* In 40 chronic schizophrenic patients mean concentration of 0.65 $\mu mol/10^{10}$ cells/h about 35% greater than 0.48 $\mu mol/10^{10}$ cells/h in 30 normal controls *5861*

Interferon-α *Serum* *No Effect* No IFN-α detected in sera of either 16 schizophrenics or 15 healthy matched controls *1666*

Interferon-γ *Serum* *No Effect* No difference observed in concentrations in 16 schizophrenics or in 15 healthy matched controls *1666*

Interleukin-1 Receptor Antagonist *Serum* *Increase* In 14 patients with untreated schizophrenia mean concentration of 342.7 ± 229.2 pg/mL significantly different from 242.3 ± 82.5 pg/mL in 26 controls *61* In 14 untreated schizophrenics mean concentration of 0.34 ± 0.23 U/mL significantly greater than that in 30 healthy study controls in whom mean concentration was 0.16 ± 0.06 U/mL *3205* In 17 patients with schizophrenia mean concentration of 0.30 ± 0.33 ng/mL significantly different from 0.16 ± 0.12 ng/mL in 23 normal volunteers *3204*

Interleukin-1β *Serum* *Increase* In 59% of 34 schizophrenics detectable amounts (above 15.6 pg/mL) of IL-1β observed com-

295.90 **Schizophrenia** *(continued)*

Interleukin-1β *(continued)*
pared with 38% of controls *2578* In 16 Korean patients with schizophrenia IL-1β detectable in 6 of 16 patients and in 4 of 16 healthy controls *2681*

Interleukin-2 *Lymphocytes* *Increase* In 13 neuroleptic-free schizophrenics mean concentration in phytohemagglutin stimulated lymphocytes of 23.7 ± 25.5 IU/mL significantly greater than 2.6 ± 3.8 IU/mL in 13 healthy control individuals *3857*
Serum *Increase* In 16 Korean patients with schizophrenia IL-2 production decreased but serum concentration increased above 4.5 pg/mL in 16 patients and 8 healthy controls: mean concentration in schizophrenics of 184.8 ± 49.6 pg/mL compared with 104.2 ± 96.4 pg/mL in normal controls *2681*
Serum *No Effect* No significant difference observed in concentrations between 16 patients and 15 matched healthy controls *1666*

Interleukin-6 *Serum* *Decrease* Mean concentration of 1.05 ± 1.11 pg/mL in 128 schizophrenic patients significantly increased compared with 0.68 ± 1.03 pg/mL in 110 healthy controls. Concentration correlated with duration of illness (r = 0.32) *1637*
Serum *Increase* In 17 patients with schizophrenia 25th to 75th quartiles of 3.7 to 9.7 pg/mL significantly different from 2.6 to 5.0 in 23 normal volunteers *3204* Mean concentration of 37 ± 5 pg/mL in 20 patients with schizophrenia significantly different from 12 ± 7 pg/mL in 15 healthy controls *3744* In 14 patients with untreated schizophrenia mean concentration of 2,165 ± 2,029 fg/mL significantly different from 999 ± 495 fg/mL in 26 controls *61*
Serum *No Effect* In Korean patients with schizophrenia IL-6 not detectable in any of 16 patients or 16 healthy controls *2681* In none of 34 patients with schizophrenia was concentration observed above detection limit of 3.9 pg/mL *2578*

Iron *Hair* *Increase* In 12 schizophrenic patients mean concentration of 41.9 ± 3.9 µg/g significantly different from mean concentration in 30 healthy control individuals of 32.0 ± 5.5 µg/g *2614*
Nails *Increase* In 30 schizophrenic patients mean concentration of 573.6 ± 52.8 µg/g significantly different from mean concentration in 30 healthy control individuals of 387.2 ± 57.1 µg/g *2614*

Lead *Hair* *No Effect* In 12 schizophrenic patients mean concentration of 11.5 ± 1.2 µg/g not significantly different from mean concentration in 30 healthy control individuals of 15.4 ± 1.7 µg/g *2614*
Nails *No Effect* In 30 schizophrenic patients mean concentration of 11.2 ± 1.5 µg/g not significantly different from mean concentration in 30 healthy control individuals of 13.5 ± 1.8 µg/g *2614*

β-Lipotropin *Plasma* *Increase* In 37 chronic schizophrenics, not medicated for at least 10 days, mean concentration significantly higher than in 21 age and sex matched controls *559*

Magnesium *Cerebrospinal Fluid* *Decrease* In 8 acute schizophrenics mean concentration of 2.12 ± 0.1 mEq/L significantly different from 2.46 ± 0.3 mEq/L in 8 schizophrenics in remission *3012*
Hair *Decrease* In 12 schizophrenic men mean concentration of 69 µg/g not significantly less than 30 µg/g in 16 healthy control men and 104 µg/g in 10 schizophrenic men compared with 109 µg/g in 12 healthy control women *5096* In 12 schizophrenic patients mean concentration of 201.6 ± 3.9 µg/g significantly different from mean concentration in 30 healthy control individuals of 211.2 ± 1.7 µg/g *2614*
Nails *Decrease* In 30 schizophrenic patients mean concentration of 436.3 ± 2.4 µg/g significantly different from mean concentration in 30 healthy control individuals of 441.7 ± 11.4 µg/g *2614*
Serum *No Effect* In 8 acute schizophrenics mean concentration of 1.89 ± 0.3 mEq/L not significantly different from 1.89 ± 0.4 mEq/L in 8 schizophrenics in remission *3012*

Manganese *Hair* *No Effect* In 12 schizophrenic patients mean concentration of 2.3 ± 0.9 µg/g not significantly different from mean concentration in 30 healthy control individuals of 2.4 ± 0.6 µg/g *2614*
Nails *No Effect* In 30 schizophrenic patients mean concentration of 4.7 ± 0.5 µg/g not significantly different from mean concentration in 30 healthy control individuals of 4.7 ± 1.1 µg/g *2614*

Melatonin *Plasma* *Decrease* In 7 men with paranoid schizophrenia circadian rhythm absent *3578*

Methionine *Plasma* *No Effect* In 18 schizophrenic patients mean concentration of 28 ± 5 µmol/L not significantly different from 26 ± 4 µmol/L in 22 healthy controls *1450*

3-Methoxy-4-hydroxyphenylglycol
Cerebrospinal Fluid *No Effect* In 36 patients with chronic schizophrenia the mean concentration was 23.2 ± 1.9 pmol/mL not significantly different from 24.9 ± 4.3 pmol/mL in 8 controls *4209* In 12 drug-free patients with childhood-onset of schizophrenia mean concentration of 45.5 ± 5.3 pmol/mL not significantly different from 44.5 ± 3.9 pmol/mL in 12 schizophrenic patients treated with clozapine for 12 weeks or 43.6 ± 4.0 pmol/mL in 10 treated for 10 weeks with haloperidol *2392*

Neurotensin *Cerebrospinal Fluid* *No Effect* In 27 patients, either drug-free or undergoing treatment, mean concentration of 51.7 ± 12.7 pg/mL not significantly different from 56.2 ± 16.2 pg/mL in 10 controls *578*

Nickel *Hair* *No Effect* In 12 schizophrenic patients mean concentration of 3.0 ± 0.5 µg/g not significantly different from mean concentration in 30 healthy control individuals of 3.5 ± 0.6 µg/g *2614*
Nails *No Effect* In 30 schizophrenic patients mean concentration of 4.2 ± 0.2 µg/g not significantly different from mean concentration in 30 healthy control individuals of 4.5 ± 0.4 µg/g *2614*

Norepinephrine *Cerebrospinal Fluid* *Increase* Concentration significantly increased compared with concentration in individuals without a personal or family history of major psychoses *2631* In 30 patients the concentration in those with polyuria of 1.47 ± 0.37 pmol/mL greater than twice 0.72 ± 0.06 pmol/mL in those without polyuria *4208*
Cerebrospinal Fluid *No Effect* In 36 patients with chronic schizophrenia the mean concentration was 0.93 ± 0.11 pmol/mL not significantly different from 0.91 ± 0.15 pmol/mL in 8 controls *4209*

Oxytocin *Cerebrospinal Fluid* *No Effect* In 31 patients who were neuroleptic free mean concentration of 8.05 ± 4.46 pg/mL not significantly different from mean of 8.92 ± 3.01 pg/mL in 15 healthy volunteers *1758*

p-Methylimidazoleacetic Acid *Cerebrospinal Fluid* *No Effect* In 36 patients with chronic schizophrenia the mean concentration was 36.9 ± 3.7 pmol/mL not significantly different from 44.6 ± 8.5 pmol/mL in 8 controls *4209*

Phenylacetic Acid *Cerebrospinal Fluid* *No Effect* Mean concentration in 29 patients with schizophrenia of 27.9 ± 14.1 ng/mL not significantly different from that in 30 healthy volunteers in whom the mean concentration was 26.6 ± 15.2 ng/mL *4761*
Urine *No Effect* No significant difference observed in excretions between normals and schizophrenics *5814*

Phenylacetic Acid, Conjugated
Cerebrospinal Fluid *No Effect* Mean concentration in 29 patients with schizophrenia of 8.14 ± 7.9 ng/mL not significantly different from that in 30 healthy volunteers in whom the mean concentration was 11.7 ± 5.5 ng/mL *4761*

Phenylacetic Acid, Unconjugated
Cerebrospinal Fluid *No Effect* Mean concentration in 29 patients with schizophrenia of 19.8 ± 12.3 ng/mL not significantly different from that in 30 healthy volunteers in whom the mean concentration was 14.8 ± 12.8 ng/mL *4761*

Phenylalanine *Plasma* *No Effect* In 11 patients with early-onset schizophrenia without neuroleptics mean concentration of 10.4 ± 2.4 µg/mL and 12 patients with late-onset schizophrenia without neuroleptics mean concentration of 9.5 ± 1.3 µg/mL not significantly different from 10.0 ± 1.3 µg/mL in 28 healthy controls *5612*

Phenylethylamine *Urine* *Increase* Increased urinary excretion of β-phenylethylamine observed in paranoid schizophrenics *5814*

Phosphatidylinositol Biphosphate *Platelets* *Increase* Mean concentration of 9.8 ± 0.6 nmol/10^9 platelets in 7 treated schizophrenics significantly higher than 3.7 ± 0.3 nmol/10^9 platelets in controls *1018*

Phospholipase A_2 *Platelets* *Increase* In 31 schizophrenics mean concentration of 28.4 ± 10.3 pmol/mg protein/min significantly higher than 24.1 ± 10.9 pmol/mg protein/min in healthy controls *1667*

Potassium *Hair* *No Effect* In 12 schizophrenic patients mean concentration of 109.4 ± 1.3 µg/g not significantly different from mean concentration in 30 healthy control individuals of 108.0 ± 3.1 µg/g *2614*
Nails *No Effect* In 30 schizophrenic patients mean concentration of 1,159.7 ± 13.4 µg/g not significantly different from mean concentration in 30 healthy control individuals of 1,190.4 ± 13.6 µg/g *2614*

Prolactin *Plasma* *Decrease* MESOR in drug-free schizophrenics lower with lower amplitude *4277*
Plasma *Increase* Concentration increased compared with that in controls *5649*
Plasma *No Effect* In 12 drug-free patients with childhood-onset of schizophrenia mean concentration of 9.0 ± 5.7 µg/L not significantly different from 4.3 ± 0.9 µg/L in 12 schizophrenic patients treated with clozapine for 12 weeks *2392* In 67 male and 42 female patients mean concentrations of 8.29 ± 5.1 µg/L and 10.74 ± 8.1 µg/L respectively not significantly different from 9.81 ± 6.4 µg/L and 11.10 ± 7.0 µg/L in 78 male and 42 female controls *2865* Mean concentration of 9.05 ± 5.13 ng/mL in 39 patients with positive symptoms, 9.00 ± 5.32 ng/mL in 30 patients with negative syndromes, 7.24 ± 4.51 ng/mL in 37 patients with mixed symptoms not significantly different from 10.26 ± 6.66 ng/mL in 120 healthy controls *2866*

Properdin Factor B *Plasma* *Decrease* In patients with a family history of schizophrenia significant decrease of FS type observed *4471*

Protein *Cerebrospinal Fluid* *No Effect* Mean concentration in postmortem ventricular CSF in 12 patients of 62.0 ± 9.1 mg/dL not significantly different from 60.9 ± 5.8 mg/dL in 16 normal controls *5435*

Selenium *Serum* *No Effect* No significant change from normal observed *73*

Serine *Plasma* *Increase* Significantly higher concentration observed in patients with schizophrenia *3179*
Plasma *No Effect* In 18 schizophrenic patients with mean concentration of 124 ± 26 µmol/L not significantly different from 125 ± 16 µmol/L in 22 healthy controls *1450*

Sialyltransferase *Serum* *No Effect* In 7 patients with schizophrenia mean activity of 1.01 pmol NeuNAc/mg protein/h not significantly different from 1.06 pmol NeuNAc/mg protein/h in 22 healthy age- and sex-matched controls *3226*

Sodium *Hair* *No Effect* In 12 schizophrenic patients mean concentration of 1,118.2 ± 22.5 µg/g not significantly different from mean concentration in 30 healthy control individuals of 1,099.3 ± 32.7 µg/g *2614*
Nails *No Effect* In 30 schizophrenic patients mean concentration of 3390.8 ± 36.1 µg/g not significantly different from mean concentration in 30 healthy control individuals of 3426.9 ± 43.1 µg/g *2614*

Soluble CD8$^+$ *Serum* *No Effect* In 17 patients with schizophrenia mean concentration of 489 ± 184 U/mL not significantly different from 440 ± 159 U/mL in 23 normal volunteers *3204* In 14 untreated schizophrenics mean concentration of 392 ± 105 U/mL not significantly different from that in 30 healthy study controls in whom mean concentration was 439 ± 175 U/mL *3205*

Soluble Interleukin-2 Receptor *Lymphocytes* *Increase* In 13 neuroleptic-free schizophrenics mean concentration in phytohemagglutin stimulated lymphocytes 2,152 ± 744 IU/mL significantly less than 2,327 ± 1,121 IU/mL in 13 healthy control individuals *3857*
Serum *Increase* In 14 untreated schizophrenics mean concentration of 82 ± 82 U/mL not significantly different from that in 30 healthy study controls in whom mean concentration was 45 ± 44 U/mL *3205* In 37 Caucasian schizophrenics mean concentration of 763 ± 347 U/mL significantly higher than 567 ± 231 U/mL in 37 normal controls *4279*

Soluble Interleukin-2 Receptor-α *Serum* *Increase* In 14 patients with untreated schizophrenia mean concentration of 739.3 ± 217.2 pg/mL significantly different from 520.9 ± 162.4 pg/mL in 26 controls *61* In 27 patients with schizophrenia concentrations of 749 - 5673 pg/mL (median 1010 pg/mL) were significantly higher than 400 - 1480 pg/mL (median 792 pg/mL) in 32 healthy controls *1669*

Soluble Interleukin-6 Receptor *Serum* *Increase* In 17 patients with schizophrenia mean concentration of 172 ± 62 ng/mL significantly different from 136 ± 41 ng/mL in 23 normal volunteers *3204*

Soluble Transferrin Receptor *Serum* *Decrease* In 17 patients with schizophrenia mean concentration of 564 ± 158 U/mL not significantly different from 627 ± 246 U/mL in 23 normal volunteers *3204*

Taurine *Plasma* *No Effect* In 18 schizophrenic patients mean concentration of 91 ± 30 µmol/L not significantly different from 90 ± 16 µmol/L in 22 healthy controls *1450*

Taurine:Product of Serine and Methionine Ratio
Plasma *No Effect* In 18 schizophrenic patients mean TSM ratio of 2.77 ± 0.99 not significantly different from 2.90 ± 0.54 in 22 healthy controls *1450*

tele-Methylhistamine *Cerebrospinal Fluid* *Increase* In 36 patients with chronic schizophrenia the mean concentration was 2.90 ± 0.27 pmol/mL significantly different from 1.12 ± 0.22 pmol/mL in 8 controls *4209*
Cerebrospinal Fluid *No Effect* In 30 patients the concentration in those with polyuria of 3.47 ± 0.43 pmol/mL not significantly different from 2.78 ± 0.38 pmol/mL in those without polyuria *4208*

tele-Methylhistamine + tele-Methylimidazoleacetic Acid
Cerebrospinal Fluid *No Effect* In 36 patients with chronic schizophrenia the mean concentration was 9.70 ± 0.62 pmol/mL not significantly different from 8.25 ± 1.29 pmol/mL in 8 controls *4209*

Transforming Growth Factor-β *Cerebrospinal Fluid* *No Effect* Mean concentration in 20 inpatient schizophrenics of 29.9 ± 2.1 pg/mL not significantly different from 26.0 ± 2.7 pg/mL in 44 healthy controls *5434*

Transforming Growth Factor-β_1
Cerebrospinal Fluid *No Effect* Mean concentration in postmortem ventricular CSF in 12 patients of 12.3 ± 1.8 pg/mL not significantly different from 23.7 ± 4.6 pg/mL in 16 normal controls *5435* Mean concentration in CSF in 20 patients of 29.9 ± 2.1 pg/mL not significantly different from 26.0 ± 2.7 pg/mL in 20 normal controls *5434*

Transforming Growth Factor-β_1, Free
Cerebrospinal Fluid *Decrease* Mean concentration in 20 inpatient schizophrenics of 7.1 ± 1.2 pg/mL not significantly different from 9.4 ± 1.2 pg/mL in 44 healthy controls *5434*

Transforming Growth Factor-β_2
Cerebrospinal Fluid *No Effect* Mean concentration in CSF in 20 patients of 267.1 ± 16.3 pg/mL not significantly different from 341.8 ± 25.4 pg/mL in 20 normal controls *5434* Mean concentration in postmortem ventricular CSF in 12 patients of 29.8 ± 2.4 pg/mL not significantly different from 80.6 ± 21.9 pg/mL in 16 normal controls *5435*

Tryptophan *Plasma* *No Effect* In 11 patients with early-onset schizophrenia without neuroleptics mean concentration of 9.1 ± 1.5 µg/mL and 12 patients with late-onset schizophrenia without neuroleptics mean concentration of 9.6 ± 1.2 µg.mL not significantly different from 9.9 ± 1.6 µg/mL in 28 healthy controls *5612*

Tumor Necrosis Factor-α *Serum* *Increase* Mean concentration of 21 ± 6 pg/mL in 20 patients with schizophrenia not significantly different from 15 ± 5 pg/mL in 15 healthy controls *3744*

Tyrosine *Plasma* *Decrease* In 11 patients with early-onset schizophrenia without neuroleptics mean concentration of 10.9 ± 1.1 µg.mL significantly different from 11.9 ± 1.8 µg/mL in 28 healthy controls *5612*
Plasma *No Effect* In 12 patients with late-onset schizophrenia without neuroleptics mean concentration of 12.0 ± 2.5 µg.mL not significantly different from 11.9 ± 1.8 µg/mL in 28 healthy controls *5612*

Volume *Urine* *Increase* In medication-free chronic schizophrenic patients volume of 2,319 ± 2,052 mL/d compared with 1,054 ± 471 mL/d for nonschizophrenic patients and 1,265 ± 613 mL/d in normal individuals *2948*

Zinc *Hair* *Decrease* In 12 schizophrenic men mean concentration of 139 µg/g significantly less than 172 µg/g in 16 male controls but mean concentration of 151 µg/g in 10 schizophrenic women not significantly less than 160 µg/g in 12 healthy female controls *5096*
Hair *No Effect* In 12 schizophrenic patients mean concentration of 191.2 ± 7.9 µg/g not significantly different from mean concentration in 30 healthy control individuals of 183.5 ± 4.7 µg/g *2614*

295.90 Schizophrenia *(continued)*

Zinc *(continued)*
Nails *No Effect* In 30 schizophrenic patients mean concentration of 201.6 ± 9.5 μg/g not significantly different from mean concentration in 30 healthy control individuals of 209.0 ± 12.0 μg/g *2614*

296.00 Mania

α_1-Acid Glycoprotein *Serum* *Increase* In 23 unmedicated patients with major depression mean concentration of 67 ± 17 mg/dL significantly different from 58 ± 13 mg/dL in 21 normal controls *3208*

α_1-Antitrypsin *Serum* *No Effect* In 23 unmedicated patients with major depression mean concentration of 195 ± 50 mg/dL not significantly different from 187 ± 50 mg/dL in 21 normal controls *3208*

Aspartate Aminotransferase *Serum* *Increase* In patients with mania activity increased as is activity of lactate dehydrogenase (correlation coefficient in manic patients r = 0.70) *5102*

Cholesterol *Serum* *Decrease* Mean concentration in patients with mania 10% less than in non-psychiatric controls *5101*

Complement C_3 *Serum* *Increase* In 23 unmedicated patients with major depression mean concentration of 88 ± 23 mg/dL significantly different from 74 ± 17 mg/dL in 21 normal controls *3208*

Complement C_4 *Serum* *Increase* In 23 unmedicated patients with major depression mean concentration of 37 ± 15 mg/dL significantly different from 29 ± 12 mg/dL in 21 normal controls *3208*

Cortisol *Plasma* *Increase* Concentration increased in patients with mania compared with concentration in controls *5649* Concentration significantly increased in majority of patients with mania *918*

Fibrinogen *Plasma* *Increase* In 23 unmedicated patients with major depression mean concentration of 171 ± 65 mg/dL significantly different from 131 ± 47 mg/dL in 21 normal controls *3208*

Haptoglobin *Serum* *Increase* In 23 unmedicated patients with major depression mean concentration of 152 ± 36 mg/dL significantly different from 102 ± 38 mg/dL in 21 normal controls *3208*

Hemopexin *Serum* *Increase* In 23 unmedicated patients with major depression mean concentration of 74 ± 17 mg/dL significantly different from 63 ± 10 mg/dL in 21 normal controls *3208*

5-Hydroxytryptamine Receptor *Platelets* *No Effect* In 29 manic individuals mean concentration of 3.14 ± 3.44 fmol/mg protein not significantly different from 3.51 - 3.04 fmol/mg protein in 29 normal controls *5445*

Immunoglobulin G *Serum* *No Effect* In 23 unmedicated patients with major depression mean concentration of 834 ± 231 mg/dL not significantly different from 866 ± 255 mg/dL in 21 normal controls *3208*

Immunoglobulin M *Serum* *Increase* In 23 unmedicated patients with major depression mean concentration of 200 ± 70 mg/dL not significantly different from 177 ± 93 mg/dL in 21 normal controls *3208*

Lactate Dehydrogenase *Serum* *Increase* In 100 otherwise healthy patients with mania mean concentration of 229 ± 106 U/L significantly higher than in 90 nonpsychiatric inpatients. Incidence of abnormal activities 14% compared with 1% in controls *5102*

Luteinizing Hormone *Plasma* *Increase* Significant increase compared with controls observed at all times of the day *5649*

Phenylacetic Acid *Cerebrospinal Fluid* *No Effect* Mean concentration in 7 patients with mania of 34.3 ± 26.0 ng/mL not significantly different from that in 30 healthy volunteers in whom the mean concentration was 26.6 ± 15.2 ng/mL *4761*

Phenylacetic Acid, Conjugated
Cerebrospinal Fluid *No Effect* Mean concentration in 7 patients with mania of 7.0 ± 5.5 ng/mL not significantly different from that in 30 healthy volunteers in whom the mean concentration was 11.7 ± 5.5 ng/mL *4761*

Phenylacetic Acid, Unconjugated
Cerebrospinal Fluid *No Effect* Mean concentration in 8 patients with mania of 25.7 ± 26.1 ng/mL not significantly different from that in 30 healthy volunteers in whom the mean concentration was 14.8 ± 12.8 ng/mL *4761*

Prolactin *Plasma* *Increase* Concentration increased in patients with mania compared with controls *5649*

Thyroid Stimulating Hormone *Serum* *No Effect* In 23 patients with bipolar mania mean concentration of 1.61 ± 1.34 mU/L within the normal range of 0.4 - 5.0 mU/L *777*

Thyroxine (T4) *Serum* *No Effect* In 23 patients with bipolar mania mean concentration of 8.64 ± 2.45 nmol/L within the normal range of 4.2 - 11.3 nmol/L *777*

Tri-iodothyronine (T3) *Serum* *No Effect* In 23 patients with bipolar mania mean concentration of 131 ± 27 nmol/L within the normal range of 65 - 155 nmol/L *777*

296.00 Mixed Mania

Thyroid Stimulating Hormone *Serum* *Increase* In 14 patients with bipolar mixed mania mean concentration of 3.14 ± 2.70 mU/mL just above the normal range of 0.4 - 5.0 mU/mL *777*

Thyroxine (T4) *Serum* *No Effect* In 23 patients with bipolar mania mean concentration of 7.03 ± 1.40 nmol/L within the normal range of 4.2 - 11.3 nmol/L *777*

Tri-iodothyronine (T3) *Serum* *No Effect* In 23 patients with bipolar mania mean concentration of 119 ± 22 nmol/L within the normal range of 65 - 155 nmol/L *777*

296.20 Major Depressive Disorder

Activated Natural Killer Cells *Blood* *Increase* In 27 patients with major depressive disorder mean concentration of 150 ± 11 /μL significantly different from 92 ± 8 /μL in 44 healthy controls *4291*

$CD3^+$ Lymphocytes *Blood* *No Effect* In 27 patients with major depressive disorder mean concentration of 1,268 ± 73 /μL not significantly different from 1,175 ± 57 /μL in 44 healthy controls *4291*

$CD4^+$:$CD8^+$ Lymphocyte Ratio *Blood* *No Effect* In 27 patients with major depressive disorder mean ratio of 2.078 ± 0.115 not significantly different from 2.242 ± 0.132 in 44 healthy controls *4291*

$CD4^+$ Lymphocytes *Blood* *No Effect* In 27 patients with major depressive disorder mean concentration of 822 ± 45 /μL not significantly different from 796 ± 36 /μL in 44 healthy controls *4291*

$CD8^+$ Lymphocytes *Blood* *No Effect* In 27 patients with major depressive disorder mean concentration of 437 ± 35 /μL not significantly different from 389 ± 20 /μL in 44 healthy controls *4291*

$CD19^+$ Lymphocytes *Blood* *No Effect* In 27 patients with major depressive disorder mean concentration of 237 ± 20 /μL not significantly different from 194 ± 14 /μL in 44 healthy controls *4291*

Corticotropin *Plasma* *Decrease* In 35 patients with unmedicated major depression median concentration of 4.21 ng/L significantly different from median concentration of 7.07 ng/L in 35 healthy controls *3947*

Cortisol *Plasma* *Increase* In 35 patients with unmedicated major depression median concentration of 62.8 μg/L significantly different from median concentration of 51.6 μg/L in 35 healthy controls *3947*

Creatinine *Serum* *No Effect* In 35 patients with unmedicated major depression mean concentration of 0.78 ± 0.20 mg/dL not significantly different from mean concentration of 0.73 ± 0.26 mg/dL in 35 healthy controls *3947*

Lymphocytes *Blood* *No Effect* In 27 patients with major depressive disorder mean concentration of 1,714 ± 90 /μL not significantly different from 1,522 ± 58 /μL in 44 healthy controls *4291*

Neopterin *Serum* *No Effect* In 35 patients with unmedicated major depression median concentration of 1.58 μg/L not significantly different from median concentration of 1.66 μg/L in 35 healthy controls *3947*

296.20 Nonmelancholic Psychotic Depression

Cortisol *Plasma Increase* In 17 patients with nonmelancholic psychotic depression mean concentration of 467 ± 37 nmol/L not significantly different from 374 ± 25 nmol/L in 20 healthy controls *2627*

Norepinephrine *Plasma Increase* In 17 patients with nonmelancholic psychotic depression mean concentration of 381 ± 92 ng/mL significantly different from 221 ± 41 ng/mL in 20 healthy controls *2627*

296.80 Manic Depressive Disorder

Catecholamines *Plasma Increase* Patients with a 6 month or longer history of anxiety and depression had total plasma catecholamine concentration significantly above normal *2765*
Urine Increase Patients with a 6 month or longer history of anxiety and depression had total plasma catecholamine concentration significantly above normal *2765*

Creatine Kinase *Serum Increase* Return towards normal following successful lithium therapy *1290*

Norepinephrine *Plasma Decrease* Usually high in patients with a 6 month or longer history of depression and anxiety, but individual patients may have a markedly low value *2765*
Plasma Increase Usually high in patients with a 6 month or longer history of depression and anxiety, but individual patients may have a markedly low value *2765*

Renin Activity *Plasma Increase* High resting renin activity was found in a group of manic depressives, but no relation to mood was observed. Aldosterone production rates were inappropriate for the renin activity found *2285*

Taurine *Plasma Decrease* Mean concentration in depressed patients free of any drugs and under drug therapy was 29 ± 2 and 25 ± 3 nmol/mL platelet-free plasma respectively. Normal mean was 45 ± 4 nmol/mL *5118*

Uric Acid *Cerebrospinal Fluid Increase* Markedly increased with decreased CSF:blood ratio, possibly due to cellular breakdown and nucleoprotein catabolism *5100*
Serum Increase Increased in both blood and CSF with a lowered CSF:blood ratio, possibly due to cellular breakdown and nucleoprotein catabolism *5100*
Urine Increase Increased excretion in neurological and psychiatric disorders; progressive rise in urinary level following slight rise in blood, due to disturbed purine metabolism *5100*

296.81 Affective Disorders

Cholesterol *Serum Decrease* In 66 men with affective disorders mean concentration of 194 ± 45 mg/dL significantly reduced compared with 228 ± 40 mg/dL in 66 healthy urban supermarket-screened men: in 134 women with affective disorders mean concentration of 201 ± 42 mg/dL significantly less than 222 ± 47 mg/dL in 134 healthy urban supermarket-screened women *5364* Patients with affective disorders were 4 - 10 times more likely to have low plasma cholesterol concentrations than a supermarket screening population *1762*

HDL-Cholesterol *Serum Decrease* In 66 men with affective disorders mean concentration of 37 ± 10 mg/dL significantly reduced compared with 46 ± 10 mg/dL in 66 healthy urban supermarket-screened men: in 134 women with affective disorders mean concentration of 45 ± 12 mg/dL significantly less than 54 ± 15 mg/dL in 134 healthy urban supermarket-screened women *5364*

Interleukin-1β *Serum Increase* In 9 of 17 patients with affective disorders detectable amounts of IL-1β observed (above 15.6 pg/mL) compared with 41% of controls, but mean plasma concentrations not significantly different *2578*

Interleukin-6 *Serum No Effect* In none of 17 patients with affective disorders was concentration above detectable amount of 3.9 pg/mL *2578*

LDL-Cholesterol *Serum Decrease* In 66 men with affective disorders mean concentration of 123 ± 39 mg/dL significantly reduced compared with 153 ± 34 mg/dL in 66 healthy urban supermarket-screened men: in 134 women with affective disorders mean concentration of 126 ± 37 mg/dL significantly less than 142 ± 40 mg/dL in 134 healthy urban supermarket-screened women *5364*

Magnesium *Cerebrospinal Fluid No Effect* Mean concentration of 1.13 ± 0.10 mmol/L not significantly different from 1.13 ± 0.07 mmol/L in 59 healthy controls *1696*

Melatonin *Plasma Increase* In 9 patients with bipolar affective disorder mean concentration significantly lower than in 12 healthy controls, in manic, depressed and euthymic states *2640*

Methionine *Plasma No Effect* In 15 patients with bipolar affective disorder mean concentration of 23 ± 3 µmol/L not significantly different from 26 ± 4 µmol/L in 22 healthy controls *1450*

Radioactive Iodine Uptake *Serum Decrease* In 11 patients with affective disorders mean uptake of 3.9 ± 1.9% at 4 h, 9.3 ± 5.3% at 24 h and 10.7 ± 5.0% at 48 h significantly less than 6.3 ± 2.5%, 14.4 ± 5.4% and 15.2 ± 5.8% at 4, 24 and 48 h respectively in 24 healthy controls *1124*

Serine *Plasma Decrease* In 15 patients with bipolar affective disorder mean concentration of 101 ± 16 µmol/L significantly different from 125 ± 16 µmol/L in 22 healthy controls *1450*

6-Sulfatoxymelatonin *Urine No Effect* In 9 patients with bipolar affective disorder mean excretion not significantly different from that in 12 healthy controls, in manic, depressed and euthymic states *2640*

Taurine *Plasma No Effect* In 15 patients with bipolar affective disorder mean concentration of 94 ± 29 µmol/L not significantly different from 90 ± 16 µmol/L in 22 healthy controls *1450*

Taurine:Product of Serine and Methionine Ratio
Plasma Increase In 15 patients with bipolar affective disorder mean TSM ratio of 4.11 ± 1.30 significantly different from 2.90 ± 0.54 in 22 healthy controls *1450*

Thyroid Stimulating Hormone *Serum Increase* In 11 patients with affective disorders mean concentration of 3.0 ± 1.8 µIU/mL significantly different from 2.31 ± 0.54 µIU/mL in 24 healthy controls *1124*

Thyroxine (T4) *Serum Increase* In 11 patients with affective disorders mean concentration of 10.2 ± 4.0 µg/dL not significantly different from 8.2 ± 2.6 µg/dL in 24 healthy controls *1124*

Tri-iodothyronine (T3) *Serum Increase* In 11 patients with affective disorders mean concentration of 1.62 ± 0.8 ng/mL significantly different from 1.43 ± 0.36 ng/mL in 24 healthy controls *1124*

Triglycerides *Serum Increase* In 66 men with affective disorders mean concentration of 169 ± 88 mg/dL significantly increased compared with 148 ± 108 mg/dL in 66 healthy urban supermarket-screened men: in 134 women with affective disorders mean concentration of 154 ± 80 mg/dL significantly greater than 131 ± 74 mg/dL in 134 healthy urban supermarket-screened women *5364*

296.82 Atypical Major Depressive Disorder

Activated Natural Killer Cells *Blood Increase* In 32 patients with atypical major depressive disorder mean concentration of 113 ± 14 /µL significantly different from 92 ± 8 /µL in 44 healthy controls *4291*

CD3+ Lymphocytes *Blood No Effect* In 32 patients with atypical major depressive disorder mean concentration of 1,231 ± 80 /µL not significantly different from 1,175 ± 57 /µL in 44 healthy controls *4291*

CD4+:CD8+ Lymphocyte Ratio *Blood No Effect* In 32 patients with atypical major depressive disorder mean ratio of 2.060 ± 0.148 not significantly different from 2.242 ± 0.132 in 44 healthy controls *4291*

CD4+ Lymphocytes *Blood No Effect* In 32 patients with atypical major depressive disorder mean concentration of 803 ± 53 /µL not significantly different from 796 ± 36 /µL in 44 healthy controls *4291*

CD8+ Lymphocytes *Blood No Effect* In 32 patients with atypical major depressive disorder mean concentration of 431 ± 35 /µL not significantly different from 389 ± 20 /µL in 44 healthy controls *4291*

CD19+ Lymphocytes *Blood No Effect* In 32 patients with atypical major depressive disorder mean concentration of 230 ± 17 /µL not significantly different from 194 ± 14 /µL in 44 healthy controls *4291*

296.82 Atypical Major Depressive Disorder *(continued)*

Lymphocytes *Blood* *No Effect* In 32 patients with atypical major depressive disorder mean concentration of 1,638 ± 92 /µL not significantly different from 1,522 ± 58 /µL in 44 healthy controls *4291*

296.90 Seasonal Affective Disorder

Cortisol *Plasma* *Increase* In 10 untreated patients mean concentration in winter of 8.73 ± 1.28 µg/mL significantly higher than 6.02 ± 1.03 µg/mL in 10 healthy controls *1648*
Plasma *No Effect* In 10 untreated patients mean concentration in winter of 9.09 ± 1.05 µg/mL not significantly different from 9.36 ± 0.67 µg/mL in 10 healthy controls *1648*

Melatonin *Plasma* *No Effect* In 10 patients with seasonal affective disorder mean concentration similar throughout 24-hour day to that in healthy controls *816*

Prolactin *Plasma* *Decrease* In 10 untreated patients mean concentration in winter of 7.35 ± 0.67 µg/mL significantly less than 8.41 ± 0.87 µg/mL in 10 healthy controls and 6.51 ± 1.52 µg/mL in patients in summer slightly less than 6.63 ± 0.80 µg/mL in healthy controls *1648*

297.90 Paranoid States and Other Psychoses

Aldolase *Serum* *Increase* The increased activity of CK or aldolase or both, was generally present at the onset of a psychotic episode in acute patients and lasted about 5 - 10 days. Increased activities ranged from 5 - 50 fold above control limits *3453*

Angiotensin-converting Enzyme
Cerebrospinal Fluid *Decrease* Both treated and drug free patients had low activity when compared with controls *363*

α_1-Antichymotrypsin *Cerebrospinal Fluid* *Increase* Detected in the CSF of patients suffering from various psychotic and neurological disorders *494*
Serum *Increase* Schizophrenic patients do exhibit a marked and rapid increase during acute phase reaction *494* *495*
Serum *No Effect* Serum and plasma levels in acutely psychotic patients and schizophrenic patients are comparable to normals *495* *494*

Arylsulfatase *White Blood Cells* *Increase* In a population of 22 adult psychotic in-patients who filled the criteria of DSM III of schizophrenic disorders, none of these patients showed a level different from 27 adult healthy controls *2990*

Aspartate Aminotransferase *Serum* *Increase* In 39% of 33 patients hospitalized for this disorder *1576*

Ceruloplasmin *Serum* *Increase* Elevated serum copper and ceruloplasmin blood levels were reported. It is postulated that this may be an important pathognomonic feature *129* *58*

Cholecystokinin *Cerebrospinal Fluid* *Decrease* Significant decrease in cholecystokinin in untreated schizophrenics (1.4 pmol/L) compared with controls (4.0 pmol/L) *3136*

Copper *Serum* *Increase* Elevated serum copper and ceruloplasmin blood levels were reported. It is postulated that this may be an important pathognomonic feature *58* *129*

Creatine Kinase *Serum* *Increase* Increased in 24 of 37 acutely psychotic patients, some of whom had had repeated admissions. Activity was 20 times the upper limits of normal in some specimens. There were no increases in nonpsychotic psychiatric patients, but patients with toxic psychoses and with some acute brain diseases, such as brain trauma, had increased activity *3453*

Dehydroepiandrosterone *Plasma* *Decrease* Observed effect *5229* *5679* *602*

Fucokinase *Blood* *No Effect* Enzyme activity in schizophrenics was no different from that found in the blood of a control group *2223*

Prolactin *Plasma* *Decrease* Concentrations in 17 drug-free chronic schizophrenic patients correlated inversely with ratings of their psychopathology *4746* Reported effect *2703*

Prostaglandins *Plasma* *Increase* Increased synthesis in schizophrenia *2238*

Pyridoxine *Serum* *Decrease* Has been noted in schizophrenia *4707*

Quinolinic Acid *Cerebrospinal Fluid* *No Effect* The concentrations were highly variable but mean levels were not significant different from controls *4687*

Uric Acid *Cerebrospinal Fluid* *Increase* Markedly increased with decreased CSF:blood ratio, possibly due to cellular breakdown and nucleoprotein catabolism *5100*
Serum *Increase* Increased in both blood and CSF with a lowered CSF:blood ratio, possibly due to cellular breakdown and nucleoprotein catabolism *5100* In 34% of 36 patients hospitalized for this disorder *1576*
Urine *Increase* Increased excretion in neurological and psychiatric disorders; progressive rise in urinary level following slight rise in blood, due to disturbed purine metabolism *5100*

Xanthurenic Acid *Urine* *Increase* Has been noted in schizophrenia *4707*

297.90 Psychosis

Copper Zinc Superoxide Dismutase *Serum* *Increase* The overall blood content of Cu Zn superoxide dismutase in patients with schizophrenia was significantly higher than that of controls *5562*

Interleukin-1β *Serum* *Increase* In 8 of 9 patients with psychoses other than schizophrenia detectable amounts of IL-1β (above 15.6 pg/mL) compared with detectable amount only observed in 4 of 13 controls *2578*

Interleukin-6 *Serum* *Increase* In only one patient with an acute atypical psychosis was a detectable and abnormal concentration detected (488 pg/mL) compared with detection limit of 3.9 pg/mL, but undetectable amount observed in all other psychotic patients and in controls *2578*

297.90 Psychosis, Acute

Serine *Plasma* *Decrease* Concentration in patients with transient acute polymorphic psychoses significantly reduced compared with normal individuals *1450*

297.90 Psychosis, Acute Polymorphic

Methionine *Plasma* *No Effect* In 28 patients with transient acute polymorphic psychosis mean concentration of 23 ± 5 µmol/L not significantly different from 26 ± 4 µmol/L in 22 healthy controls *0*

Serine *Plasma* *Decrease* In 28 patients with transient acute polymorphic psychosis mean concentration of 102 ± 16 µmol/L significantly different from 125 ± 16 µmol/L in 22 healthy controls *1450*

Taurine *Plasma* *No Effect* In 28 patients with transient acute polymorphic psychosis mean concentration of 108 ± 37 µmol/L not significantly different from 90 ± 16 µmol/L in 22 healthy controls *1450*

Taurine:Product of Serine and Methionine Ratio
Plasma *Increase* In 28 patients with transient acute polymorphic psychosis mean TSM ratio of 4.80 ± 1.49 significantly different from 2.90 ± 0.54 in 22 healthy controls *1450*

298.90 Catatonic Psychosis

Iron *Serum* *Decrease* Concentrations reduced below 50 µg/dL in 35% of 40 patients with catatonic psychosis *4074*

298.90 Cognitive Impairment

Soluble β-Amyloid Peptide 40 *Serum* *Decrease* In 6 patients with mild cognitive impairment mean concentration of 1,936 ± 596 pmol/L significantly different from 2,311 ± 546 pmol/L in 24 age and sex matched controls *2440*

Soluble β-Amyloid Peptide 42 *Serum* *Increase* In 15 patients with mild cognitive impairment mean concentration of 166 ± 84 pmol/L significantly different from 74 ± 30 pmol/L in 24 age and sex matched controls *2440*

298.90 Noncatatonic Psychosis

Iron *Serum* *Decrease* Concentrations reduced below 50 µg/dL in 7.5% of 40 patients with noncatatonic psychosis *4074*

298.90 Psychosis, Atypical

Methionine *Plasma* *No Effect* In 12 patients with atypical psychosis mean concentration of 26 ± 4 µmol/L not significantly different from 26 ± 4 µmol/L in 22 healthy controls *1450*

Serine *Plasma* *No Effect* In 12 patients with atypical psychosis mean concentration of 125 ± 30 µmol/L not significantly different from 125 ± 16 µmol/L in 22 healthy controls *1450*

Taurine *Plasma* *No Effect* In 12 patients with atypical psychosis mean concentration of 78 ± 29 µmol/L not significantly different from 90 ± 16 µmol/L in 22 healthy controls *1450*

Taurine:Product of Serine and Methionine Ratio *Plasma* *No Effect* In 12 patients with atypical psychosis mean TSM ratio of 2.57 ± 1.20 not significantly different from 2.90 ± 0.54 in 22 healthy controls *1450*

299.00 Autism

5-Hydroxytryptamine, Free *Plasma* *Increase* In 45 of 69 patients with mean age of 5.7 years concentration exceeded 1.12 µmol/L with mean value of 1.80 µmol/L compared with 0.75 µmol/L in healthy controls *1449*

Oxytocin *Plasma* *Decrease* In 29 prepubertal autistic children mean concentration of 0.64 ± 0.58 pg/mL significantly different from 1.16 ± 0.77 pg/mL in 30 age-matched normal children *3540*

Prolactin *Plasma* *No Effect* No significant difference in concentrations observed between boys with autism, minimal brain dysfunction and healthy controls *2052*

Prolactin response to TRH *Plasma* *No Effect* No significant difference in response observed between boys with autism, minimal brain dysfunction and in healthy controls *2052*

Thyroid Stimulating Hormone *Serum* *Decrease* Mean concentration significantly less in boys with autism than in those with mental retardation, minimal brain dysfunction and in controls *2052*

TSH response to TRH *Serum* *Decrease* Response to TRH significantly less in boys with autism compared with controls *2052*

300.00 Anxiety

Cortisol *Plasma* *Increase* Significant direct correlation observed between degree of preoperative anxiety and plasma concentration. Mean cortisol concentration of 472 nmol/L (median 434 nmol/L, range up to 1,220 nmol/L) *594* In 17 patients with anxiety mean concentration of 412 ± 46 nmol/L not significantly different from 374 ± 25 nmol/L in 20 healthy controls *2627*

Cortisol, Free *Urine* *Increase* Higher excretion observed in individuals who responded poorly to bereavement within the past month than in those who adjusted rapidly to the situation *2389*

Growth Hormone *Plasma* *Increase* Significant increase to mean of 5.0 mU/L (median 1.8 mU/L, range up to 26.5 mU/L) observed in over 100 patients prior to elective surgery *594*

4-Hydroxy-3-Methoxy-Phenylglycol *Plasma* *No Effect* In 70 depressed patients mean concentration of 16.1 ± 0.9 ng/mL in 34 with high anxiety not significantly different from 15.7 ± 1.0 ng/mL in 36 with low anxiety *2923*

Norepinephrine *Plasma* *Increase* In 17 patients with anxiety mean concentration of 309 ± 62 ng/mL significantly different from 221 ± 41 ng/mL in 20 healthy controls *2627*

pH *Blood* *Increase* Anxiety prior to venipuncture reported to increase blood pH due to decreased partial pressure of carbon dioxide *4986*

Prolactin *Plasma* *No Effect* No correlation observed between extent of preoperative anxiety and plasma concentration *594*

Tribulin *Urine* *Increase* Increased excretion observed in patients with general anxiety disorder compared with controls *2997*

300.01 Panic Attack

Cortisol *Plasma* *Increase* Concentration increased during some panic attacks *670*

Epinephrine *Plasma* *No Effect* No significant change observed during panic attacks *670*

Growth Hormone *Plasma* *No Effect* Increase observed in some panic attacks although not increased at other times *670*

4-Hydroxy-3-Methoxy-Phenylglycol *Plasma* *No Effect* No significant change observed during panic attacks *670*

Norepinephrine *Plasma* *Increase* Small increase observed during panic attacks although not at other times when compared with controls *670*

Prolactin *Plasma* *Increase* Although concentration no different from that in control individuals between panic attacks increased at the peak of most attacks and correlated with attack severity *670*

300.01 Panic Disorder

γ-Aminobutyric Acid *Plasma* *Increase* In 10 patients with panic disorder mean concentration of 132 ± 33 pmol/mL not significantly different from 120 ± 19 pmol/mL in 10 healthy controls *1769*

$CD3^+$ Lymphocytes *Blood* *No Effect* In 20 medication-free patients with panic disorder 95% confidence interval of 1,219 - 1,815 /µL not significantly different from 1,207 - 1,459 /µL in 32 healthy volunteers *4278*

$CD4^+$ Lymphocytes *Blood* *No Effect* In 20 medication-free patients with panic disorder 95% confidence interval of 786 - 1,162 /µL not significantly different from 750 - 928 /µL in 32 healthy volunteers *4278*

$CD8^+$ Lymphocytes *Blood* *No Effect* In 20 medication-free patients with panic disorder 95% confidence interval of 467 - 712 /µL not significantly different from 460 - 581 /µL in 32 healthy volunteers *4278*

$CD16^+$ Lymphocytes *Blood* *Increase* In 20 medication-free patients with panic disorder 95% confidence interval of 229 - 339 /µL significantly different from 165 - 239 /µL in 32 healthy volunteers *4278*

$CD19^+$/$CD5^+$ Lymphocytes *Blood* *No Effect* In 20 medication-free patients with panic disorder 95% confidence interval of 40 - 78 /µL not significantly different from 23 - 47 /µL in 32 healthy volunteers *4278*

$CD19^+$/HLA-DR Lymphocytes *Blood* *Increase* In 20 medication-free patients with panic disorder 95% confidence interval of 186 - 313 /µL significantly different from 100 - 162 /µL in 32 healthy volunteers *4278*

$CD19^+$ Lymphocytes *Blood* *Increase* In 20 medication-free patients with panic disorder 95% confidence interval of 108 - 328 /µL significantly different from 124 - 195 /µL in 32 healthy volunteers *4278*

$CD25^+$ Lymphocytes *Blood* *No Effect* In 20 medication-free patients with panic disorder 95% confidence interval of 88 - 161 /µL not significantly different from 79 - 126 /µL in 32 healthy volunteers *4278*

$CD29^+$/$CD4^+$ Lymphocytes *Blood* *No Effect* In 20 medication-free patients with panic disorder 95% confidence interval of 401 - 654 /µL not significantly different from 398 - 505 /µL in 32 healthy volunteers *4278*

Cholecystokinin *Cerebrospinal Fluid* *Decrease* In 25 patients with panic disorder mean concentration of CCK-8 16.2 ± 5.9 pg/mL compared with 20.6 ± 7.7 pg/mL in healthy controls *3174*

Corticotropin-releasing Hormone *Cerebrospinal Fluid* *No Effect* In 23 patients with panic disorder mean concentration of 44.5 ± 9.1 pg/mL not significantly different from 46.1 ± 9.5 pg/mL in 14 healthy controls *1534*

Growth Hormone *Plasma* *No Effect* In 10 patients with panic disorder mean baseline concentration of 0.8 µg/L not significantly different from 1.5 µg/L in 14 age and sex matched controls *15*

HLA-DR Lymphocytes *Blood* *Increase* In 20 medication-free patients with panic disorder 95% confidence interval of 278 - 437 /µL significantly different from 207 - 285 /µL in 32 healthy volunteers *4278*

300.01 Panic Disorder *(continued)*

4-Hydroxy-3-Methoxy-Phenylglycol *Plasma* *Increase* In 10 patients with panic disorder mean baseline concentration of 4.0 µg/L significantly greater than mean of 3.3 µg/L in 14 age and sex matched controls *15*

Interleukin-1β *Serum* *Increase* In 10 outpatients with panic disorder mean concentration of 38.1 ± 12.4 pg/mL significantly higher than 13.1 ± 9.1 pg/mL in 10 age-matched controls *558*

Neuropeptide Y *Plasma* *Increase* 12 patients with panic disorder had mean concentration of 129 ± 12 pg/mL significantly higher than 58.75 ± 15.41 pg/mL in 22 healthy controls *543*

Pyridoxal Phosphate *Serum* *No Effect* In 81 patients mean concentration of 40.6 ± 16.8 nmol/L not significantly different from 42.6 ± 27.2 nmol/L in 26 healthy controls *1356*

Thyroid Stimulating Hormone *Serum* *No Effect* No significant difference observed between concentrations in 26 patients with panic disorder and 26 matched controls *4997*

Thyroxine Binding Globulin *Serum* *No Effect* No significant difference observed between concentrations in 26 patients with panic disorder and 26 matched controls *4997*

Thyroxine (T4) *Serum* *No Effect* No significant difference observed between concentrations in 26 patients with panic disorder and 26 matched controls *4997*

Thyroxine (T4), Free *Serum* *No Effect* No significant difference observed between concentrations in 26 patients with panic disorder and 26 matched controls *4997*

Tri-iodothyronine (T3) *Serum* *No Effect* No significant difference observed between concentrations in 26 patients with panic disorder and 26 matched controls *4997*

300.20 Anxiety Neurosis

Lactate *Blood* *Increase* Patients manifested an excessive rise in blood lactate and a lower oxygen consumption when compared with normal controls in a standard exercise test *2479* Reported effect *2304*

T3-Uptake *Serum* *No Effect* Concentration typically normal *5544*

300.20 Generalized Anxiety Disorder

Corticotropin-releasing Hormone
Cerebrospinal Fluid *No Effect* In 11 patients with general anxiety disorder mean concentration of 38.9 ± 10.6 pg/mL not significantly different from 46.1 ± 9.5 pg/mL in 14 healthy controls *1534*

Pyridoxal Phosphate *Serum* *No Effect* In 31 patients mean concentration of 43 ± 22.5 nmol/L not significantly different from 42.6 ± 27.2 nmol/L in 26 healthy controls *1356*

300.23 Generalized Social Phobia

CD3⁺ Lymphocytes *Blood* *No Effect* In 33 medication-free patients with generalized social phobia 95% confidence interval of 1,229 - 1,591 /µL not significantly different from 1,207 - 1,459 /µL in 32 healthy volunteers *4278*

CD4⁺ Lymphocytes *Blood* *No Effect* In 33 medication-free patients with generalized social phobia 95% confidence interval of 755 - 1,003 /µL not significantly different from 750 - 928 /µL in 32 healthy volunteers *4278*

CD8⁺ Lymphocytes *Blood* *No Effect* In 33 medication-free patients with generalized social phobia 95% confidence interval of 479 - 615 /µL not significantly different from 460 - 581 /µL in 32 healthy volunteers *4278*

CD16⁺ Lymphocytes *Blood* *Increase* In 33 medication-free patients with generalized social phobia 95% confidence interval of 221 - 321 /µL significantly different from 165 - 239 /µL in 32 healthy volunteers *4278*

CD19⁺/CD5⁺ Lymphocytes *Blood* *No Effect* In 33 medication-free patients with generalized social phobia 95% confidence interval of 14 - 108 /µL not significantly different from 23 - 47 /µL in 32 healthy volunteers *4278*

CD19⁺/HLA-DR Lymphocytes *Blood* *No Effect* In 33 medication-free patients with generalized social phobia 95% confidence interval of 130 - 227 /µL not significantly different from 100 - 162 /µL in 32 healthy volunteers *4278*

CD25⁺ Lymphocytes *Blood* *No Effect* In 33 medication-free patients with generalized social phobia 95% confidence interval of 83 - 193 /µL not significantly different from 79 - 126 /µL in 32 healthy volunteers *4278*

CD29⁺/CD4⁺ Lymphocytes *Blood* *No Effect* In 33 medication-free patients with generalized social phobia 95% confidence interval of 391 - 5,528 /µL not significantly different from 398 - 505 /µL in 32 healthy volunteers *4278*

HLA-DR Lymphocytes *Blood* *No Effect* In 33 medication-free patients with generalized social phobia 95% confidence interval of 225 - 366 /µL not significantly different from 207 - 285 /µL in 32 healthy volunteers *4278*

300.30 Obsessive-Compulsive Disorder

Antidiuretic Hormone *Cerebrospinal Fluid* *Increase* Significantly increased basal arginine vasopressin concentration observed in patients with obsessive-compulsive disorder *95*

Cholinesterase *Serum* *No Effect* No significant difference in activities observed between obsessive-compulsive patients and normal individuals *1386*

Corticotropin-releasing Hormone
Cerebrospinal Fluid *No Effect* In 20 patients with obsessive compulsive disorder mean concentration of 5.1 fmol/mL significantly diffferent from 5.3 fmol/mL in 29 healthy controls *787* In 9 patients with obsessive-compulsive disorder mean concentration of 49.3 ± 11.5 pg/mL not significantly different from 46.1 ± 9.5 pg/mL in 14 healthy controls *1534*

GH response to TRH *Plasma* *No Effect* No significant difference between 10 patients with obsessive-compulsive disorder and 10 healthy controls *52*

Neuropeptide Y *Cerebrospinal Fluid* *No Effect* In 14 patients with obsessive-compulsive disorder mean concentration of 257 ± 23 pg/mL not significantly different from 233 ± 10 pg/mL in 26 healthy normal volunteers *94*

Oxytocin *Cerebrospinal Fluid* *Increase* In 29 patients with obsessive-compulsive disorder mean concentration of 13.7 pmol/L significantly higher than 7.7 pmol/L in 31 normal controls *2958*
Cerebrospinal Fluid *No Effect* In 14 patients with obsessive-compulsive disorder mean concentration of 4.1 ± 0.3 pg/mL not significantly different from 3.7 ± 0.2 pg/mL in 26 healthy normal volunteers *94*

Prolactin response to TRH *Plasma* *No Effect* No significant difference between 10 patients with obsessive-compulsive disorder and 10 healthy controls *52*

Pyridoxal Phosphate *Serum* *No Effect* In 27 patients mean concentration of 43.3 ± 21.1 nmol/L not significantly different from 42.6 ± 27.2 nmol/L in 26 healthy controls *1356*

Thyroid Stimulating Hormone *Serum* *No Effect* In 16 individuals with obsessive-compulsive disorder mean concentration within normal range *2017*

Thyroxine (T4) *Serum* *No Effect* In 16 individuals with obsessive-compulsive disorder mean concentration within normal range *2017*

Tri-iodothyronine (T3) *Serum* *No Effect* In 16 individuals with obsessive-compulsive disorder mean concentration normal *2017*

Tryptophan *Plasma* *No Effect* In 13 patients with obsessive compulsive disorder mean concentration of 68 µmol/L not significantly less than 75 µmol/L in 29 healthy controls *3148*

TSH response to TRH *Serum* *Decrease* Response significantly blunted in 10 patients with obsessive-compulsive disorder compared with 10 healthy controls *52*

Vasopressin *Cerebrospinal Fluid* *No Effect* In 29 patients with obsessive-compulsive disorder mean concentration of 12.8 pmol/L not significantly different from 11.6 pmol/L in 31 normal controls *2958*

300.40 Atypical Dysthymia

Activated Natural Killer Cells *Blood* *Increase* In 38 patients with atypical dysthymia mean concentration of 109 ± 10 /µL significantly different from 92 ± 8 /µL in 44 healthy controls *4291*

CD4+:CD8+ Lymphocyte Ratio *Blood* *No Effect* In 38 patients with atypical dysthymia mean ratio of 2.234 ± 0.159 not significantly different from 2.242 ± 0.132 in 44 healthy controls *4291*

CD4+ Lymphocytes *Blood* *No Effect* In 38 patients with atypical dysthymia mean concentration of 789 ± 44 /µL not significantly different from 796 ± 36 /µL in 44 healthy controls *4291*

CD8+ Lymphocytes *Blood* *No Effect* In 38 patients with atypical dysthymia mean concentration of 391 ± 27 /µL not significantly different from 389 ± 20 /µL in 44 healthy controls *4291*

CD19+ Lymphocytes *Blood* *No Effect* In 38 patients with atypical dysthymia mean concentration of 221 ± 15 /µL not significantly different from 194 ± 14 /µL in 44 healthy controls *4291*

Lymphocytes *Blood* *No Effect* In 38 patients with atypical dysthymia mean concentration of 1,571 ± 68 /µL not significantly different from 1,522 ± 58 /µL in 44 healthy controls *4291*

300.40 Depressive Neurosis

Adenosine Monophosphate *Urine* *Decrease* Lack of primary messenger necessary to activate adenyl cyclase system resulting in decreased levels. No hormonal effect noted *5229*

Catecholamines *Plasma* *Increase* Patients with a 6 month or longer history of anxiety and depression had total plasma catecholamine concentration significantly above normal *2765*
Urine *Decrease* Documented decrease in urinary excretion of catecholamine and indolamine metabolites reported in depressed patients. Not used as a clinical tool at this time *900*
Urine *Increase* Patients with a 6 month or longer history of anxiety and depression had total plasma catecholamine concentration significantly above normal *2765*

Hematocrit *Blood* *Decrease* Anemia is often present *900*

Hemoglobin *Blood* *Decrease* Anemia is often present *900*

Indoleamine *Urine* *Decrease* Documented decrease in urinary excretion of catecholamine and indolamine metabolites reported in depressed patients. Not used as a clinical tool at this time *900*

Norepinephrine *Plasma* *Decrease* Usually high in patients with a 6 month or longer history of depression and anxiety, but individual patients may have a markedly low value *2765*
Plasma *Increase* Usually high in patients with a 6 month or longer history of depression and anxiety, but individual patients may have a markedly low value *2765*

Prostaglandins *Plasma* *Increase* Increased synthesis in schizophrenia and depression *2238*

Somatostatin *Cerebrospinal Fluid* *Decrease* Low levels appear to be a marker for episodes of depression *43*

Taurine *Plasma* *Decrease* Mean concentration in depressed patients free of any drugs and under drug therapy was 29 ± 2 and 25 ± 3 nmol/mL platelet-free plasma respectively. Normal mean was 45 ± 4 nmol/mL *5118*

Uric Acid *Cerebrospinal Fluid* *Increase* Markedly increased with decreased CSF:blood ratio, possibly due to cellular breakdown and nucleoprotein catabolism *5100*
Serum *Increase* Increased in both blood and CSF with a lowered CSF:blood ratio, possibly due to cellular breakdown and nucleoprotein catabolism *5100*
Urine *Increase* Increased excretion in neurological and psychiatric disorders; progressive rise in urinary level following slight rise in blood, due to disturbed purine metabolism *5100*

300.40 Dysthymia

Activated Natural Killer Cells *Blood* *Increase* In 46 patients with dysthymia mean concentration of 113 ± 9 /µL significantly different from 92 ± 8 /µL in 44 healthy controls *4291*

CD3+ Lymphocytes *Blood* *No Effect* In 38 patients with atypical dysthymia mean concentration of 1,169 ± 58 /µL not significantly different from 1,175 ± 57 /µL in 44 healthy controls *4291* In 46 patients with dysthymia mean concentration of 1,084 ± 44 /µL not significantly different from 1,175 ± 57 /µL in 44 healthy controls *4291*

CD4+:CD8+ Lymphocyte Ratio *Blood* *No Effect* In 46 patients with dysthymia mean ratio of 2.605 ± 0.263 not significantly different from 2.242 ± 0.132 in 44 healthy controls *4291*

CD4+ Lymphocytes *Blood* *No Effect* In 46 patients with dysthymia mean concentration of 749 ± 33 /µL not significantly different from 796 ± 36 /µL in 44 healthy controls *4291*

CD8+ Lymphocytes *Blood* *No Effect* In 46 patients with dysthymia mean concentration of 338 ± 21 /µL not significantly different from 389 ± 20 /µL in 44 healthy controls *4291*

CD19+ Lymphocytes *Blood* *No Effect* In 46 patients with dysthymia mean concentration of 197 ± 15 /µL not significantly different from 194 ± 14 /µL in 44 healthy controls *4291*

Lymphocytes *Blood* *No Effect* In 46 patients with dysthymia mean concentration of 1,475 ± 52 /µL not significantly different from 1,522 ± 58 /µL in 44 healthy controls *4291*

300.90 Acute Psychiatric Illness

Thyroid Stimulating Hormone *Serum* *No Effect* No effect observed in acute psychiatric illness *1965*

Thyroxine (T4) *Serum* *Increase* Observed with acute psychiatric illness but concentration returns to normal as disease process settles *1965*

Thyroxine (T4), Free *Serum* *Increase* Probable increase observed in patients with acute psychiatric illness although concentration reverts to normal as disease process settles *1965*

Tri-iodothyronine, Free (fT3) *Serum* *No Effect* No effect observed in acute psychiatric illness *1965*

Tri-iodothyronine, Reverse (rT3) *Serum* *No Effect* No abnormality noted with acute psychiatric illnesses *1965*

Tri-iodothyronine (T3) *Serum* *No Effect* No abnormality observed in patients with acute psychiatric illness *1965*

TSH response to TRH *Serum* *Decrease* Although TSH concentration normal its response to TRH was impaired *1965*

300.90 Psychoneurosis

Creatine Kinase *Cerebrospinal Fluid* *No Effect* Of 3 patients with psychoneurosis 0 had increases above upper limit of normal of 10 U/L *4780*

302.90 Paraphilia

Follicle Stimulating Hormone *Plasma* *No Effect* In 30 untreated men with paraphilia mean concentration of 7.1 ± 6.8 mIU/mL not significantly different from reference interval of 2 - 10 mIU/mL *4446*

Luteinizing Hormone *Plasma* *No Effect* In 30 untreated men with paraphilia mean concentration of 10.6 ± 5.3 mIU/mL not significantly different from reference interval of 3 - 15 mIU/mL *4446*

Testosterone *Serum* *No Effect* In 30 untreated men with paraphilia mean concentration of 545 ± 196 ng/dL not significantly different from reference interval of 280 - 870 ng/dL *4446*

303.00 Acute Alcoholic Intoxication

Aldosterone *Plasma* *Decrease* Decreased during ethanol intoxication, but increased greatly during hangover *3075*

Amylase *Serum* *Increase* Increased in serum and urine in 8.5% of 129 patients after acute intoxication, due to changes in salivary isoenzyme, not as a result of pancreatic damage *402* Common as a result of vomiting and increased peptic stimulation of the pancreas *4707*
Urine *Increase* Increased in serum and urine in 8.5% of 129 patients after acute intoxication, due to changes in salivary isoenzyme, not as a result of pancreatic damage *402*

Bicarbonate *Serum* *Decrease* Plasma bicarbonate ranged from 2 - 10 mmol/L in acidosis following alcoholic binge *3493*

Calcium *Serum* *Decrease* Hypocalcemia is common in alcoholic subjects *3039*

303.00 Acute Alcoholic Intoxication (continued)

Calcium *(continued)*
Serum *Increase* Increased following alcoholic binge of several days duration *3493*

Cortisol *Plasma* *Increase* Increased following alcoholic binge of several days duration *3493*

Fat *Urine* *Increase* Significant lipuria occurred in a group of acutely intoxicated patients with neurological symptoms *589*

Fatty Acids (FFA), Free *Serum* *Increase* Increased following alcoholic binge of several days duration *3493*

Growth Hormone *Plasma* *Increase* Increased following alcoholic binge of several days duration *3493*

β-Hexosaminidase *Serum* *Increase* Elevated in 94% of cases *2453*

11-Hydroxycorticosteroids *Plasma* *Increase* Alcohol excess in nonalcoholics. No rise in chronic alcoholics *1290*

Iron *Bone Marrow* *Increase* Iron overload shown by plasma cells containing iron in bone marrow may occur *3493*

Lactate *Blood* *Increase* Acidosis due to lactate and ketoacid accumulation following alcoholic binge of several days duration *3493*

Osteocalcin *Serum* *Decrease* Reported effect *2883*

Parathyroid Hormone *Plasma* *Increase* Increased following alcoholic binge of several days duration *3493*

pH *Blood* *Decrease* Severe metabolic acidosis with pH ranging between 6.96 - 7.28 occurred after alcoholic binge of several days duration *3493*

Phosphate *Serum* *Decrease* Observed in some patients *1290*
Serum *Increase* Increased following alcoholic binge of several days duration *3493*

Pyridoxine *Serum* *Decrease* Has been noted in acute alcoholism *4707*

Renin Activity *Plasma* *Increase* Increased more than 100%, when 1.5 - 2.3 g ethanol/kg body weight was ingested over a 3 h period. During hangover the increase even exceed 200% *3075*

Xanthurenic Acid *Urine* *Increase* Has been noted in acute alcoholism *4707*

303.00 Acute Alcoholism

Bilirubin *Serum* *Increase* In 3 patients with acute alcoholic intoxication and liver disease mean concentration of 15.6 ± 4.2 mg/dL compared with 0.6 ± 0.3 mg/dL in 23 healthy controls *5493*

Cholesterol *Serum* *No Effect* Mean concentration of 211 ± 80 mg/dL in 3 patients with acute alcoholic intoxication and liver disease not significantly greater than 191 ± 33 mg/dL in 23 healthy controls *5493*

Phenytoin *Serum* *Increase* Acute administration of alcohol with phenytoin may increase plasma phenytoin concentration *4008*

Phospholipids *Serum* *Increase* In 3 patients with acute alcoholic intoxication and liver disease mean concentration of 248 ± 13 mg/dL greater than 214 ± 42 mg/dL in 23 healthy controls *5493*

Prothrombin Time *Plasma* *Decrease* In 3 patients with acute alcoholic liver damage mean prothrombin time reduced below 50% of normal *5493*

Triglycerides *Serum* *Increase* In 3 patients with acute alcoholic intoxication and liver disease mean concentration of 294 ± 148 mg/dL significantly greater than 87 ± 23 mg/dL in 23 healthy controls *5493*

Vitamin E *Serum* *Increase* In 3 patients with acute alcoholic intoxication and liver disease mean concentration of 3.34 ± 0.91 μmol/g lipids significantly greater than 5.28 ± 0.49 μmol/g lipids in 23 healthy controls *5493*
Serum *No Effect* Mean concentration of 25.2 ± 11.4 μmol/L in 3 patients with acute alcoholic intoxication and liver disease not significantly different from 26.0 ± 4.4 μmol/L in 23 healthy controls *5493*

303.90 Alcoholism

Acetaldehyde Adduct Antibodies *Serum* *Positive* Observed in 73% alcoholics and 39% people with nonalcoholic liver disease *4093*

Acetate *Blood* *Increase* Mean blood concentration in alcoholics about 0.75 mmol/L and 0.7 mmol/L in heavy drinkers significantly higher than 0.4 mmol/L in healthy controls *2775*

Acetylcholinesterase *Cerebrospinal Fluid* *No Effect* The AChE levels were unrelated to the degree of cognitive decline and they were in the same range as in the control group *2766*
Red Blood Cells *Decrease* Mean activity in 36 alcoholic individuals (69.0 ± 14.4 U/g hemoglobin) significantly lower than in 41 healthy non-alcoholic control subjects (144.6 ± 48.0 U/g hemoglobin) *1948*

α_1-Acid Glycoprotein *Serum* *No Effect* In 18 male alcoholics following recent debauche mean concentration of 0.99 g/L compared with reference interval of 0.6 - 1.2 g/L *2824*

Acylcarnitine, Long Chain *Serum* *Increase* In 20 male chronic alcoholic patients long chain acylcarnitine concentration increased in comparison with healthy controls *2809*

Adenosine Monophosphate *Plasma* *Decrease* In 8 chronic alcoholic men mean concentration of 12 ± 3 nmol/L significantly less than 16 ± 2 nmol/L in reference range *450*
Urine *Increase* In 8 long-term alcoholic men mean excretion of 2.7 ± 1.9 nmol/dL glomerular filtrate significantly increased compared with reference range of 1.5 ± 0.4 nmol/dL glomerular filtrate *450* In 27 men with a history of at least 10 years alcoholism mean excretion of 4 ± 2 nmol/100 mL glomerular filtrate tended to be increased compared with normal range of 3.1 ± 0.7 nmol/100 mL glomerular filtrate *451*

Alanine Aminotransferase *Serum* *Increase* Mean activity of 1.06 μkat/L in 6 alcoholic men versus 0.26 μkat/L in 14 nonalcoholic men, and 0.81 μkat/L in 6 alcoholic women versus 0.28 μkat/L in 17 nonalcoholic women *1571* Mean activity of 13.1 ± 8.2 U/L higher than 8.8 ± 4.3 U/L in 16 social drinkers but lower than 16.5 ± 6.0 U/L in 27 teetotallers *2571* 50% of 182 male chronic alcoholics had raised values. Highest values were found after 5 - 20 y of confirmed alcoholism. Patients with > 20 y duration displayed a tendency to normalization of enzyme activity *4889* In 18 male alcoholics mean activity of 0.77 μkat/L compared with reference interval of < 0.65 μkat/L *2824* In 19 alcoholic women mean activity of 50 U/L (9 - 383) significantly greater than 12 U/L (6 - 29) in 14 healthy controls *2897* In 23 chronic alcoholics mean concentration of 46 U/L significantly higher than 26 U/L in 36 social drinkers *839* Only moderately increased activity observed in patients with alcoholic liver disease *4528* Mean activity of 61 ± 82 U/L in 104 alcoholic men significantly higher than 24 ± 13 U/L in 37 teetotalers. Mean activity of 27 ± 15 U/L in 137 moderate drinkers and 36 ± 28 U/L in 90 heavy drinkers *4837* In about 21,000 men positive correlation observed between enzyme activity and amount of alcohol consumed *4385* Mean activity in 52 alcoholics of 58 ± 47 U/L significantly different from 26 ± 21 U/L in 38 healthy controls *2008* In 23 actively drinking alcohol-habituated individuals mean activity of 36 ± 32 U/L significantly different from 13 ± 10 U/L in 10 alcohol-naive control individuals *2176* In 26 chronic alcoholics on admission to hospital activity increased above normal range of 0 to 0.27 μkat/L in 18 *786* Above the normal limit (18 U/L) in 30% of 67 alcoholics, during or immediately after a heavy bout of drinking *4032*

Albumin *Serum* *Decrease* In 27 individuals with a history of at least 10 years of alcoholism mean concentration (39 ± 4 g/L) slightly reduced *451* In 18 chronic alcoholics mean concentration of 626 (range 234 - 751) μmol/L significantly less than 677 (623 - 750) μmol/L in 10 abstinent controls *3069* In 159 alcoholic patients (119 men and 40 women) admitted to a detoxification center median concentration of 44 g/L (range 32 - 53) significantly lower than 45 g/L (range 37 - 57) in an age and sex matched control group *1526* In 127 patients with chronic alcoholism mean concentration below 40 g/L in 16 (12.5%) *1330*
Serum *No Effect* In 19 alcoholic women mean concentration of 38 g/L (23 - 44) not significantly different from 41 g/L (37 - 42) in 14 healthy controls *2897* In 101 postmenopausal women who ingested moderate amounts of alcohol mean concentration of 45 ± 1 g/L not significantly different from 47 ± 1 g/L in 27 alcohol abstaining postmenopausal women *1675* In 18 male alcoholics mean concentration of 0.58 mmol/L at lower limit of reference interval of 0.56 - 0.82 mmol/L *2824*

Aldehyde Dehydrogenase *Red Blood Cells* *Decrease* Activity significantly less in 40 alcoholics (mean 128 mU/g hemoglobin) than in 145 teetotalers (mean 219 mU/g hemoglobin) *2466* In 44 chronic alcoholic patients, activity determined 18 - 36 h after discontinuation of chronic alcohol intake was 4.98 ± 0.52 mU/mg protein compared with activity of 8.25 ± 1.29 mU/mg protein in controls *3061*

Aldolase *Serum* *Decrease* There was a high correlation between systolic and diastolic BP and cadmium levels *310*

Aldosterone *Plasma* *Increase* In 23 actively drinking alcohol-habituated individuals mean concentration of 358 ± 179 pmol/L significantly increased above normal *2176*
Plasma *No Effect* Concentration normal in chronic alcoholics although serum osmolality normal *889*

Alkaline Phosphatase *Serum* *Increase* Mild elevation occurred in 80% of 5 cases with range of 75-140 U/L. Maximum upper limit for normal individuals of 84 U/L *3161* In 28% of 14 patients hospitalized for this disorder *1576* Mean activity of 175 ± 40 U/L in 104 alcoholic men significantly higher than 146 ± 34 U/L in 37 teetotaler controls. Mean activity of 137 ± 38 U/L observed in 137 moderate drinkers and 141 ± 40 U/L in 90 heavy drinkers *4837* In 7 of 24 chronic alcoholics on admission to hospital activity increased above normal range of 0.40 to 1.33 µkat/L *786* In 19 alcoholic women mean activity of 219 U/L (68 - 630) significantly greater than mean of 126 U/L (85 - 158) in 14 healthy controls *2897* In 27 individuals with a history of at least 10 years of alcoholism mean concentration slightly increased (110 ± 46 U/L versus normal range of 30 - 115 U/L) with 10 individuals having activities above normal range *451* Elevation occurred in 10.4% of cases *4032*
Serum *No Effect* In 18 chronic alcoholics mean activity of 233 (range 117 - 921) U/L not significantly different from 203 (136 - 379) U/L in 10 abstinent controls *3069* No significant difference observed between activities in 34 hospitalized male alcoholics and 35 healthy age matched controls *460*

Alkaline Phosphatase Isoenzymes *Serum* *Increase* In 19 chronic alcoholic women mean activities of 205 U/L (total), 144 U/L (liver) and 39 U/L (bone) higher than 126 U/L (total), 81 U/L (liver) and 39 U/L (bone) in 14 healthy controls *2897*

Amino-terminal Propeptide of Type III Procollagen
Serum *Increase* Increased plasma concentrations observed in patients with alcoholic cirrhosis *4093*

5-Aminolevulinate Dehydrogenase
Red Blood Cells *Decrease* Test provides highest efficiency in distinguishing patients with alcoholic liver damage from those with nonalcohol related chronic liver damage *1503*

Amylase *Serum* *Decrease* 20% of 182 male chronic alcoholics had decreased activity of serum pancreatic isoamylase, whereas only 6% had low total serum amylase activity *4889*
Serum *Increase* Increased activity observed in 25 of 300 drunken drivers *3779* Increased activity observed in 7 of 202 alcoholics without abdominal symptoms *1912* Rises after gross ethanol intake (in the chronic alcoholic) *1290*
Serum *No Effect* In 14 alcoholics in relapse mean activity of 38.3 ± 2.8 U/L not significantly different from 37.0 ± 3.0 U/L in 21 healthy controls. In 8 alcoholics in remission mean activity of 38.6 ± 4.2 U/L *1086*

Amylase, Pancreatic Isoenzyme *Serum* *Decrease* In 8 alcoholics in remission mean activity of 12.8 ± 1.7 U/L significantly less than 19.0 ± 1.7 U/L in 21 healthy controls *1086*
Serum *No Effect* In 14 alcoholics in relapse mean activity of 19.0 ± 1.7 U/L not significantly different from 19.0 ± 1.7 U/L in 21 healthy controls *1086*

Amylase, Salivary Isoenzyme *Serum* *No Effect* In 14 alcoholics in relapse mean activity of 22.6 ± 2.5 U/L not significantly different from 17.9 ± 2.0 U/L in 21 healthy controls. In 8 alcoholics in remission mean activity of 25.9 ± 3.2 U/L not significantly different from controls *1086*

Angiotensin-II *Plasma* *No Effect* Concentration normal in chronic alcoholics although serum osmolality increased *889*

Angiotensin-converting Enzyme *Serum* *Increase* Activity strongly correlated with alcohol consumption and γ-glutamyltransferase activity in hypertensive middle-aged drinkers: probably not caused by induction of γ-glutamyltransferase but due to hepatic damage caused by alcohol *5768*

Antidiuretic Hormone *Plasma* *Decrease* In 23 actively drinking alcohol-habituated individuals mean concentration of 0.8 ± 0.7 pg/mL significantly reduced below normal range *2176*
Plasma *No Effect* In chronic alcoholics mean basal concentration normal although serum osmolality increased *889*

Apolipoprotein A-I *Serum* *Decrease* In 59 male alcoholics mean concentration of 146 ± 27 mg/L significantly less than 160 ± 25 mg/dL in 140 controls. In 13 alcoholic women mean concentration of 168 ± 50 mg/dL not significantly different from 158 ± 36 mg/dL in 145 controls *2305* Although just within normal range mean concentration in 84 chronic alcoholics with increased plasma immunoreactive trypsin concentration of 1.15 ± 0.27 g/L compared with 1.74 ± 0.35 g/L in 62 with normal trypsin concentration *2474*
Serum *Increase* Mean concentration significantly increased in intemperate drinkers compared with control individuals *4231*

Apolipoprotein A-I:Apolipoprotein B Ratio
Serum *Decrease* In 84 chronic alcoholics with increased plasma immunoreactive trypsin concentration mean ratio of 0.91 ± 0.44 reduced below normal of > 1, compared with normal of 1.63 ± 0.77 in 62 patients with normal trypsin concentration *2474*

Apolipoprotein A-II *Serum* *Increase* Mean concentration significantly increased by 45% in 78 intemperate drinkers compared with control individuals *4231* In 13 alcoholic women mean concentration of 68 ± 24 mg/dL significantly higher than 56 ± 13 mg/dL in 145 controls *2305*
Serum *No Effect* In 59 male alcoholics mean concentration of 56 ± 20 mg/dL not significantly different from 53 ± 14 mg/dL in 140 controls *2305*

Apolipoprotein B *Serum* *Increase* In 84 chronic alcoholics with increased immunoreactive trypsin concentration mean concentration of 1.35 ± 0.38 g/L compared with 1.15 ± 0.36 g/L in 62 with normal trypsin concentration *2474*

Arylsulfatase A *White Blood Cells* *Increase* 21% of 56 patients with alcoholism have a variant enzyme *2293*

Ascorbic Acid *White Blood Cells* *Decrease* Abnormally reduced in 32 of 35 cases (91%) *250*

Aspartate Aminotransferase *Serum* *Decrease* In 27 chronic alcoholics on admission to hospital activity reduced below normal range of 0.28 to 0.90 µkat/L in 3 *786*
Serum *Increase* Mean activity in 52 alcoholics of 66 ± 49 U/L significantly different from 30 ± 19 U/L in 30 healthy controls *2008* In 26 alcohol-dependent patients mean activity of 63 ± 33 U/L significantly different from 17 ± 6 U/L in 34 healthy controls *3867* In about 21,000 men positive correlation observed between enzyme activity and amount of alcohol consumed *4385* 73% of 182 male chronic alcoholics had raised activities. Highest values were found after 5 - 20 y of confirmed alcoholism. Patients with 20 y duration displayed a tendency to normalization of activities *4889* In 5 of 27 chronic alcoholics on admission to hospital activity increased above normal range of 0.28 to 0.90 µkat/L *786* In 23 actively drinking alcohol-habituated individuals mean activity of 38 ± 35 U/L significantly different from 12 ± 5 U/L in 10 alcohol-naive control individuals *2176* In 104 alcoholic men mean activity of 60 ± 61 U/L significantly higher than 25 ± 21 U/L in 37 teetotaler controls. Mean activity of 23 ± 7 U/L in 137 moderate drinkers and 32 ± 20 U/L in 90 heavy drinkers *4837* Mean activity in 25 drunken arrestees 37.9 ± 19.3 U/L significantly higher than 13.1 ± 4.7 U/L in 16 social drinkers and 22.2 ± 5.1 U/L in 27 teetotallers *2571* In 66% of 13 patients hospitalized for this disorder *1576* In 159 alcoholic patients (119 men and 40 women) admitted to a detoxification center median activity of 42 U/L (range 9 - 428) significantly greater than 18 U/L (range 6 - 40) in an age and sex matched control group *1526* Mean activity of 1.13 µkat/L in 6 alcoholic men versus 0.32 µkat/L in 14 nonalcoholic men, and 0.89 µkat/L in 6 alcoholic women versus 0.35 µkat/L in 17 nonalcoholic women *1571* In various studies, increased activity reported in 18 - 100% of chronic alcoholics or heavy drinkers *4528* 60% of 5 cases showed mild elevation, with a mean of 16 times the normal upper limit *3161* In 19 alcoholic women mean activity of 98 U/L (19 - 570) significantly greater than 22 U/L (15 - 37) in 14 healthy controls *2897* Activity increased in 49 of 300 drunken drivers *3779* In 18 male alcoholics following recent debauche mean activity of 0.81 µkat/L compared with reference interval of < 0.65 µkat/L *2824*
Serum *No Effect* In 101 postmenopausal women who ingested moderate amounts of alcohol mean activity of 32.0 ± 0.8 U/L not significantly different from 28.6 ± 2.3 U/L in 27 alcohol abstaining postmenopausal women *1675*

303.90 Alcoholism *(continued)*

Aspartate Aminotransferase Isoenzymes *Serum Increase* In 30 alcoholics with liver disease mean activity of mitochondrial isoenzyme of AST of 10.4 U/L, in 16 without liver disease 1.95 U/L than in healthy controls (0.43 U/L) *3730*

Aspartate Aminotransferase, Mitochondrial *Serum Increase* In 46 chronic alcoholics mean activity higher with or without obvious alcoholic liver disease than in controls *4528*

Aspartate Aminotransferase (Pyridoxine Activation) *Red Blood Cells No Effect* No significant effect observed in 35 alcoholics reflecting no cases of vitamin B_6 deficiency *250*

Atrial Natriuretic Peptide *Plasma Increase* In a group of 54 patients in whom alcohol withdrawal produced delirium tremens initial concentration of ANP increased *2796*

Bilirubin *Serum Increase* In 19 alcoholic women mean concentration of 17 µmol/L (range 3 - 39) significantly greater than 9 µmol/L (range 4 - 14) in 14 healthy controls *2897* 12% of 182 male chronic alcoholics had increased concentrations. Highest values were found after 5 - 20 y of confirmed alcoholism *4889* In 23 actively drinking alcohol-habituated individuals mean concentration of 1.6 ± 1.3 mg/dL significantly different from 0.4 ± 0.2 mg/dL in 10 alcohol-naive control individuals *2176*
Serum No Effect In 21 individuals with alcoholic liver disease but without cirrhosis mean concentration of 15 (SD 3) µmol/L, close to upper limit of normal, but in patients with cirrhosis mean concentration about 60 µmol/L *1709*

Bilirubin, Conjugated *Serum Increase* In 18 male alcoholics following recent debauche mean concentration of 3.6 µmol/L compared with reference interval of 0 - 3.4 µmol/L *2824*

Bilirubin, Indirect *Serum No Effect* In 21 patients with alcoholic liver disease but without cirrhosis mean concentration of 10 (SD 3) µmol/L although mean concentration increased to 36 µmol/L in patients with moderate cirrhosis and 48 µmol/L in those with advanced cirrhosis *1709*

Bilirubin, Unconjugated *Serum No Effect* In 18 male alcoholics following recent debauche mean concentration of 6.3 µmol/L compared with reference interval of 3.4 - 18.6 µmol/L *2824*

Cadmium *Hair No Effect* In 23 alcoholic patients mean concentration of 1.1 ± 0.3 µg/g not significantly different from mean concentration in 30 healthy control individuals of 1.1 ± 0.2 µg/g *2614*
Nails No Effect In 22 alcoholic patients mean concentration of 1.9 ± 0.2 µg/g not significantly different from mean concentration in 30 healthy control individuals of 1.6 ± 0.1 µg/g *2614*
Serum Increase There was a high correlation between systolic and diastolic BP and cadmium levels *310*

Calcifediol *Serum Increase* In 8 long-term chronic alcoholic men mean concentration of 21 ± 6 ng/mL not significantly increased compared with reference range of 18 ± 8 ng/mL *450*

Calcitonin *Plasma No Effect* No significant difference observed between concentrations in 34 hospitalized male alcoholics and 35 healthy age matched controls *460*

Calcium *Hair Decrease* In 23 alcoholic patients mean concentration of 1,801.0 ± 5.6 µg/g significantly different from mean concentration in 30 healthy control individuals of 2,015.1 ± 96.4 µg/g *2614*
Nails Decrease In 22 alcoholic patients mean concentration of 975.9 ± 13.5 µg/g significantly different from mean concentration in 30 healthy control individuals of 1250.4 ± 15.5 µg/g *2614*
Serum Decrease Mean concentration reduced below lower reference limit in 9 of 34 hospitalized male alcoholics *460* In 8 white males who had abused alcohol for at least 10 years mean concentration of 9.2 ± 0.2 mg/dL significantly less than reference range of 9.5 ± 0.3 mg/dL *450* Hypocalcemia is common in alcoholic subjects *3039*
Serum Increase Increased following alcoholic binge of several days duration *3493*
Serum No Effect Normal concentration observed in chronic alcoholics *1265* In 27 individuals with a history of at least 10 years of alcoholism mean concentration normal *451* In 18 chronic alcoholics mean concentration of 2.26 (range 1.81 - 2.43) mmol/L not significantly different from 2.22 (2.02 - 2.46) mmol/L in 10 abstinent controls *3069*
Urine Increase In 27 men with a history of at least 10 years of alcoholism mean excretion of 5.0 ± 3.4 mmol/d but with 4 individuals excreting more than 7.5 mmol/d *451* Increase observed, with hypermagnesuria, in patients with chronic alcoholism *4348* Increased excretion observed in chronic alcoholics *2535*
Urine No Effect No significant difference between excretion in 8 long-term alcoholic men of 181 ± 95 mg/d compared with reference range of 200 ± 100 mg/d *450* In 19 chronic alcoholic women mean concentration of 3.2 mmol/d not significantly different from 3.1 mmol/d in 14 healthy controls *5447*

Carbohydrate-deficient Transferrin *Serum Increase* In 14 alcoholic patients with mean blood alcohol concentration of 65 mmol/L with median intake of alcohol of 250 g/d for 1 - 3 weeks, demonstrated an increased concentration observed in serum *5017* In 90 alcoholic men mean concentration of 107 ± 61.4 mg/L significantly different from that in 74 healthy men in whom the mean conentration was 46 ± 16.6 mg/L *4621* In individuals with heavy alcohol consumption (greater than 60 g/d) specificity 94% and sensitivity 64% for increased enzyme activity. In men sensitivity 75% using 17 U/L as cutoff and in women sensitivity 38% using 25 U/L as cutoff *150* Detected in 19 of 22 (86%) self-confessed alcohol abusers but in none of 47 patients with non-alcoholic liver disease and in one of 38 (3%) controls *2564* Sensitivity and specificity for excess drinking as reported in several studies 20 - 91% (typically over 70%) and 71 - 100% (typically over 90%), respectively *3090* In 81% of patients consuming more than 60 g ethanol daily abnormal transferrin identified *4528* Increased amounts of transferrin with pI 5.7 and in some cases pI 5.8 and especially pI 5.9 observed. Transferrin from alcoholics contains significantly less sialic acid, neutral galactose and N-acetylglucosamine than normal *4093* Mean activity in 15 alcoholics of 55 ± 37 U/L significantly different from 18 ± 11 U/L in 7 healthy controls *2008*

Carcinoembryonic Antigen *Serum Increase* In 37 patients with alcohol addiction 35% had concentrations less than 2.5 ng/mL, 40% had concentrations between 2.6 and 5.0 ng/mL, 13% had concentrations between 5.1 and 10.0 ng/mL and 12% had concentrations greater than 10.0 ng/mL *2010*

Carnitine *Serum Increase* Elevated levels in patients with alcoholic liver disease compared to healthy control subjects *1602* Total concentration significantly increased in 11 of 14 patients with severe alcohol dependence *1751*
Serum No Effect In 20 male chronic alcoholic patients carnitine concentration unchanged in comparison with 12 healthy controls *2809*
Urine No Effect In 20 male chronic alcoholic patients carnitine excretion unchanged in comparison with 12 healthy controls *2809*

Carnitine, Free *Serum Increase* Significant increase observed in 11 of 14 patients with severe alcohol dependence *1751*

Carnitine, Long Chain *Serum Increase* In 20 alcoholic patients significantly higher concentration observed than in 32 healthy men of identical age *1602*

Carnitine, Short Chain *Serum Decrease* Significantly lower concentration observed in 20 chronic alcoholics compared with concentration in 28 men with alcoholic liver disease *1602*

Catalase *Red Blood Cells No Effect* No significant difference observed between activity in healthy controls (410 ± 42 kat/g hemoglobin), (mean ± 1 SD) and in patients with alcoholic liver disease but without cirrhosis (408 ± 66 kat/g hemoglobin) but decrease with advanced cirrhosis *1709*

Catecholamines *Plasma No Effect* In chronic alcoholics concentration normal although serum osmolality increased *889*

Ceruloplasmin *Serum Increase* Mean concentration in male alcoholics increased but not significantly above that in controls *5742*
Serum No Effect No significant difference observed between 21 patients with alcoholic liver disease in whom the concentration was 368 ± 74 mg/L (mean ± 1 SD) and in 50 healthy controls, in whom the concentration was 368 ± 88 mg/L or in patients with different degrees of alcoholic cirrhosis *1709*

Cholesterol *Serum Increase* Mean concentration of 6.85 ± 2.58 mmol/L in 11 alcoholic individuals significantly greater than 5.3 ± 0.9 mmol/L in 20 healthy controls *4257* Significant increase observed in women regardless of degree of obesity with alcohol intakes of greater than 10 g/d *1572* In 59 male alcoholics mean concentration of 226 ± 54 mg/dL significantly higher than 204 ± 49 mg/dL in 140 healthy controls. In 13 alcoholic women mean concentration of 222 ± 52 mg/dL not significantly increased compared with 198 ± 46 mg/dL in 145 controls *2305*

Serum *No Effect* In 62 chronic alcoholics with normal plasma trypsin activity mean concentration of 6.14 ± 1.04 mmol/L not significantly different from 6.24 ± 1.97 mmol/L in 84 individuals with high trypsin activity and from healthy individuals *2474* No significant difference observed between mean concentration in 26 male alcoholics (5.66 mmol/L) compared with 17 healthy controls (5.47 mmol/L) *2650*

Cholesterol Ester Transfer Protein *Serum* *Decrease* Mean concentration in 52 alcoholics of 100 ± 20 nmol/h/mL significantly different from 134 ± 29 nmol/h/mL in 38 healthy controls *2008*

Cholesterol:HDL-Cholesterol Ratio *Serum* *Increase* In 62 chronic alcoholics with normal plasma immunoreactive trypsin concentration mean concentration of 3.57 ± 1.15 and of 6.73 ± 3.66 in 84 chronic alcoholics with increased plasma immunoreactive trypsin concentration *2474*

Cholinesterase *Serum* *Increase* There was a high correlation between systolic and diastolic BP and cadmium levels *1290* *310*

Chromium *Hair* *No Effect* In 23 alcoholic patients mean concentration of 4.5 ± 1.1 µg/g not significantly different from mean concentration in 30 healthy control individuals of 4.9 ± 0.7 µg/g *2614*
Nails *No Effect* In 22 alcoholic patients mean concentration of 9.4 ± 0.9 µg/g not significantly different from mean concentration in 30 healthy control individuals of 9.7 ± 0.5 µg/g *2614*

Chylomicrons *Serum* *Increase* Increased *4372* *4358* *3017*

Citrate Lyase *Serum* *Increase* In 32 chronic alcoholics mean activity 56.4 ± 17.3 U/L versus 29.4 ± 5.7 U/L in 37 controls *1376*

Copper *Hair* *No Effect* In 23 alcoholic patients mean concentration of 14.9 ± 4.1 µg/g not significantly different from mean concentration in 30 healthy control individuals of 12.7 ± 2.7 µg/g *2614*
Nails *No Effect* In 22 alcoholic patients mean concentration of 7.1 ± 0.4 µg/g not significantly different from mean concentration in 30 healthy control individuals of 7.2 ± 0.7 µg/g *2614*
Serum *Increase* Mean concentration in male alcoholics higher than in controls but not significantly so *5742* Nonsignificant increase to 16.8 ± 3.4 µmol/L (93 ± 22 µg/dL) in 21 patients with alcoholic liver disease without cirrhosis and significant increase to 18.9 ± 5.3 µmol/L (120 ± 34 µg/dL) in those with mild alcoholic liver cirrhosis *1709*

Coproporphyrin *Urine* *Increase* In chronic alcoholics after acute ingestion excretion increased to 373 nmol/d compared with upper limit of normal of 119 nmol/d: in nonalcoholics following acute ingestion, excretion of 140 nmol/d *4828*

Corticotropin *Cerebrospinal Fluid* *Decrease* Mean concentration of 23 pg/mL in 23 alcoholic patients with antisocial personality disorder significantly less than 34 pg/mL in 21 healthy control individuals *5479*
Plasma *No Effect* In 5 chronically alcoholic men mean fasting concentration not significantly different from that in 6 healthy controls *1700*

Corticotropin-releasing Hormone
Cerebrospinal Fluid *Decrease* In 5 chronically alcoholic men mean concentration of 26 ± 15 pg/mL significantly less than 60 ± 30 pg/mL in 6 healthy controls *1700*
Cerebrospinal Fluid *No Effect* Mean concentration in 23 alcoholics with antisocial behavior not significantly different from that in 21 healthy control individuals *5479*

Cortisol *Plasma* *Increase* In 11 current alcohol abusers mean concentration of 12.1 ± 1.1 mg/dL compared with 7.7 ± 1.1 mg/dL in 11 lifelong abstainers *5600* Enhanced secretion observed in chronic alcoholics *4348* Mean concentration of 545 ± 203 nmol/L in 19 chronic alcoholic women not significantly increased compared with 500 ± 143 nmol/L in 14 healthy controls *2897* Secretion enhanced in chronic alcoholics *4035* In 93 male chronic alcoholics mean concentration of 791 ± 5 nmol/L observed *2795* Increased following alcoholic binge of several days duration *3493*
Plasma *No Effect* In 5 chronically alcoholic men mean fasting concentration of 5.93 ± 2.50 µg/dL not significantly different from 7.83 ± 2.66 µg/dL in 6 healthy controls *1700*
Urine *Increase* In 18 chronic alcoholics mean excretion of 196 (range 23 - 590) nmol/d not significantly greater than 161 (92 - 324) nmol/d in 10 abstinent controls *3069* Mean excretion of 174 ± 81 nmol/d in 19 chronic alcoholic women significantly increased compared with 127 ± 23 nmol/d in 14 healthy controls *2897*

Creatine Kinase *Serum* *Increase* In 21 alcoholic patients, mean values were found to be elevated to 35.1 U/L (normal value 7.0 U/L) *4081*

Creatinine *Serum* *Decrease* In 18 chronic alcoholics mean concentration of 76 (range 50 - 143) µmol/L not significantly less than 81 (63 - 94) µmol/L in 10 abstainers *3069* In 19 alcoholic women mean concentration of 70 ± 9 µmol/L significantly less than 80 ± 9 µmol/L in 14 healthy controls *2897*
Serum *No Effect* In 27 individuals with a history of at least 10 years alcoholism mean concentration normal *451* In 23 actively drinking alcohol-habituated individuals mean concentration of 0.8 ± 0.2 mg/dL not significantly different from 0.9 ± 0.1 mg/dL in 10 alcohol-naive control individuals *2176*
Urine *Decrease* In 19 alcoholic women mean excretion of 8.3 ± 1.5 mmol/d significantly less than 10.1 ± 2.0 mmol/d in 14 healthy controls *2897*
Urine *No Effect* In 27 men with a history of at least 10 years alcoholism mean concentration of 12.7 ± 3.4 mmol/d not significantly different from normal range of 8.8 - 17.6 mmol/d *451*

C-terminal Propeptide of Type I Procollagen
Serum *Increase* In 19 chronic alcoholic women mean concentration of 109 µg/L not significantly increased compared with 97 µg/L in 14 healthy controls *2897*

Dehydroepiandrosterone Sulfate *Plasma* *Decrease* Compared with controls of similar age non-cirrhotic alcoholic women had significantly reduced concentrations of DHEA-S *360*

Diazepam Binding Inhibitor *Cerebrospinal Fluid* *No Effect* Mean concentration in 23 alcoholics with antisocial behavior not significantly different from that in 21 healthy control individuals *5479*

Dihydrotestosterone *Serum* *Decrease* Compared with controls of comparable age more alcoholic cirrhotic women had reduced concentrations *360*

1,25-Dihydroxy Vitamin D *Serum* *Decrease* In 18 chronic alcoholics mean concentration of 56 (range 24 -118) pmol/L significantly less than 112 (72 - 166) pmol/L in 10 abstinent controls *3069*
Serum *No Effect* in 27 individuals with a history of at least 10 years alcoholism mean concentration of 96 ± 25 pmol/L not significantly different from normal range of 84 ± 24 pmol/L *451* In 8 long-term chronic alcoholic men mean concentration of 35 pg/mL not significantly different from reference range of 34 pg/mL *450*

1,25-Dihydroxy Vitamin D_3 *Serum* *Decrease* In 34 hospitalized male alcoholics mean concentration reduced by 24% compared with concentration in 35 age matched controls *460* Mean concentration of 111 ± 54 pmol/L in 19 chronic alcoholic women not significantly less than 132 ± 26 pmol/L observed in 14 healthy controls *2897*
Serum *Increase* High concentration observed possibly in association with high parathyroid hormone concentration *1446*
Serum *No Effect* No significant effect of chronic alcoholism observed *4348* No significant changes observed in alcoholic patients *450*

Dolichol *Urine* *Increase* In chronic alcoholics urinary excretion 2.5 to 4 times excretion in nonalcoholic controls *4528* Slight increase observed in 21 alcohol-dependent in-patients compared with 21 healthy controls *5011* In alcoholics mean excretion significantly increased compared with controls: Sensitivity for detecting alcoholism 68% compared with 44% for serum γ-glutamyltransferase. 3.9% false positives in control group *4410*
Urine *No Effect* In chronic alcoholics when excretion related to creatinine excretion no significant difference from normals observed *5011*

Dopamine Sulfate *Plasma* *Increase* In 40 chronic alcoholics with mean concentration of 3,896 ± 438 pg/mL significantly higher than 2,124 ± 104 pg/mL in 29 healthy controls *1419*

β-Endorphin *Plasma* *Decrease* Significant reduction observed in individuals with chronic alcoholism *44*
Plasma *Increase* Mean concentration in 11 current alcohol abusers of 14.64 ± 2.73 pg/mL compared with 11.85 ± 2.48 pg/mL in 11 lifelong abstainers *5600* In 93 chronic alcoholic men mean concentration increased to 8.91 ± 1.03 pmol/L *2795*

303.90 Alcoholism *(continued)*

Erythrocyte Sedimentation Rate *Blood Increase* In 18 male chronic alcoholics mean rate of 10.5 mm/h immediately following alcoholic debauche *2824*

Erythrocytes *Blood Decrease* Significant reduction from concentration in 184 controls of 4.7 x 10^{12}/L to 4.4 x 10^{12}/L in 106 alcoholics *4732* In 73 female alcoholics mean concentration of 4.0 ± 0.5 x10^{12}/L significantly reduced compared with 4.2 ± 0.2 x10^{12}/L in 138 healthy control women *4733*
Blood No Effect No significant difference in concentrations in 184 controls and 88 heavy drinkers 4.7 ± 0.0 10^9/L (mean and SEM) *4732*

Erythropoietin *Serum Increase* In infants born to alcoholic mothers significant increase of plasma erythropoietin observed at birth in those in whom mothers drank more than 300 g alcohol per week (median 37 mIU/mL) compared with infants of control women (32 mIU/mL, range 11-73 mIU/mL) *1979*

Estradiol *Plasma Decrease* Tendency for concentration to decrease with increasing alcohol intake in postmenopausal women with increasing alcohol consumption *743* In pregnant alcoholics concentration observed to be reduced *1978*
Plasma Increase In 101 postmenopausal women who ingested moderate amounts of alcohol mean concentration of 44.3 ± 3.0 pg/mL significantly higher than 27.5 ± 3.3 pg/mL in 27 alcohol abstaining postmenopausal women *1675* Compared with controls of comparable age more alcoholic cirrhotic women had detectable serum estradiol concentrations *360* In 18 chronic alcoholics mean concentration of 120 (range 55 - 420) pmol/L not significantly greater than 100 (60 - 140) pmol/L in 10 abstinent controls *3069*
Plasma No Effect In 21 women with amenorrhea who were noncirrhotic alcoholics mean concentration of 0.09 ± 0.06 nmol/L not significantly different from reference interval of 0.08 - 0.11 nmol/L *375*

Estrone *Plasma Decrease* In pregnant alcoholics concentration observed to be reduced *1978* Concentration tended to decline in postmenopausal women with increasing alcohol consumption *743*
Plasma Increase Compared with controls of comparable age more alcoholic cirrhotic women had increased plasma estrone concentrations *360* In 18 chronic alcoholics mean concentration of 215 (range 68 - 660) pmol/L not significantly greater than 160 (120 - 310) pmol/L in 10 abstinent controls *3069*

Ethanol *Serum Increase* Blood alcohol exceeding 1.5 mill without gross evidence of intoxication, over 3 mill at any time and over 1 mill in routine examinations are first level criteria of alcoholism according to National Council on Alcoholism *4528*

Fat *Urine Increase* Significant lipuria occurred in a group of acutely intoxicated patients with neurological symptoms *589*

Fatty Acids (FFA), Free *Serum Increase* Rises only after the acute ingestion of large doses of alcohol *1980* Increased following alcoholic binge of several days duration *3493*

Ferritin *Serum Increase* In 159 alcoholic patients (119 men and 40 women) admitted to a detoxification center median concentration of 188 µg/L (range 5 - 1,900) significantly greater than 66 µg/L (range 4 - 409) in an age and sex matched control group *1526* Increased concentrations observed in 40% to 70% of chronic alcoholics. Both free and concanavalin A bound ferritin were increased in equal proportions. Both concentrations increased with the severity of liver disease *3553* In 67% heavy drinkers with increased GGT activity but no signs of liver disease or obvious blood, gastrointestinal or inflammatory disorder have increased serum ferritin concentrations *4528* In 23 of 30 alcoholic individuals concentration increased *3463*

α-Fetoprotein *Serum Decrease* In 409 male alcoholics with liver injury values below normal observed in 78% patients and were undetectable in 42%: concentrations lowest in the more severely ill patients with the poorest one year survival *3455*
Serum Increase In 23 chronic alcoholics median concentration of 4.1 kIU/L compared with 3.0 kIU/L in 36 normal healthy adults *839*

Fibrinogen *Plasma Decrease* Low plasma fibrinogen concentration observed in patients with chronic alcoholism *1146*

Folate *Blood No Effect* In 18 male alcoholics following recent debauche mean concentration of 248 nmol/L compared with reference interval of 100 - 450 nmol/L *2824*
Serum No Effect In 18 male alcoholics following recent debauche mean concentration of 7.7 nmol/L compared with reference interval of 4 - 35 nmol/L *2824*

Follicle Stimulating Hormone *Plasma Increase* In 21 women with amenorrhea who were noncirrhotic alcoholics mean concentration of 47 ± 39 IU/L significantly different from upper limit of reference interval of less than 12 IU/L *375* 48 male chronic alcoholics classified in 2 groups according to the presence (22) or absence (26) of clinically evident sexual disorders. The level was significantly higher in the group with sexual disorders *4851*
Plasma No Effect In 101 postmenopausal women who ingested moderate amounts of alcohol mean concentration of 63.2 ± 2.1 mIU/mL not significantly different from 63.3 ± 5.5 mIU/mL in 27 alcohol abstaining postmenopausal women *1675*

Fractional Excretion of Phosphate *Urine Increase* In 27 men with a history of at least 10 years of alcoholism mean FEP 0.165 ± 0.047 tending to the high side of the normal range of 0.005 - 0.18 *451*

Galactosyltransferase *Serum Decrease* In 14 alcoholic patients with mean blood alcohol of 65 mmol/L, with mean intake of 250 g/d for 1 - 3 weeks, demonstrated reduced activity by 35 - 55% compared with controls *5017*

Glucaric Acid *Urine Increase* In 33 noncirrhotic male alcoholics excretion was significantly increased when compared with excretion in 30 healthy controls exceeding the upper limit of normal in 38% of alcoholics *5334*

Glucose *Serum Decrease* Due to depletion of glycogen stores, and an inhibitory effect of alcohol on gluconeogenesis *1980*
Serum No Effect In 23 actively drinking alcohol-habituated individuals mean concentration of 5.9 ± 1.9 mmol/L not significantly different from 6.4 ± 0.9 mmol/L in 10 alcohol-naive control individuals *2176*

Glucose Tolerance *Serum Decrease* Decrease in glucose tolerance because of inability of tissues to utilize glucose *1290*

Glutamate Dehydrogenase *Serum Increase* In patients an increase of activity of glutamate dehydrogenase exceeding 2.5 times the upper limit of normal indicative of alcoholic hepatitis *4528*

γ-Glutamyltransferase *Serum Increase* 69% of 182 male chronic alcoholics had increased GGT activities. Highest values were found in patients with 5 - 20 y of alcoholism. Patients with > 20 y duration had a tendency toward normalization of enzyme activity *4889* In 7 of 16 chronic alcoholics on admission to hospital activity increased above normal range of 0 to 0.75 µkat/L *786* In 104 alcoholic men mean activity of 140 ± 172 U/L significantly higher than 23 ± 12 U/L in 37 teetotaler controls. In 137 moderate drinkers mean activity of 33 ± 22 U/L and 65 ± 72 U/L in 90 heavy drinkers *4837* Increased activity found in man after chronic alcohol consumption before development of alcohol-related liver injury *4528* Sensitivity and specificity for excess drinking as reported in several studies 19 - 100% (typically over 60%) and 9 - 95% (typically over 70%), respectively *3090* In about 21,000 men positive correlation observed between amount of alcohol ingested and activity *4385* Activity increased in 54 - 88% chronic alcoholics and declines slowly during abstention *4093* Activity increased in 49 of 300 drunken drivers *3779* In 5 cases of chronic alcoholism, range 27-850 U/L. The highest activities were seen in the patients with the most extensive hepatic damage *3161* In 19 alcoholic women mean activity of 127 ± 15 U/L significantly greater than 13 U/L (4 - 29) in 14 healthy controls *2897* In 26 alcohol-dependent patients mean activity of 229 ± 162 U/L significantly different from 20 ± 8 U/L in 34 healthy controls *3867* In 18 male alcoholics following recent debauche mean activity of 2.70 µkat/L compared with reference interval of < 0.60 µkat/L *2824* Activity increased in 88% of 33 noncirrhotic male alcoholics *5334* Using cutoff of enzyme activity of 50 U/L specificity for heavy drinking 100% and sensitivity in men 72% and in women 54% *150* Mean activity of 2.30 µkat/L in 6 alcoholic men versus 0.30 µkat/L in 14 nonalcoholic men, 1.72 µkat/L in 6 alcoholic women and 0.31 µkat/L in 17 nonalcoholic women *1571* Mean activity in 52 alcoholics of 162 ± 214 U/L significantly different from 25 ± 18 U/L in 38 healthy controls *2008* In 84 chronic alcoholics with increased plasma immunoreactive trypsin concentration mean activity of 83.0 ± 230.5 U/L compared with 99.9 ± 153.6 U/L in 62 with normal concentration and less than 28 U/L in healthy individuals *2474* In 159 alcoholic patients (119 men and 40 women) admitted to a detoxification center, median activity of 98 U/L (range 11 - 2,480 U/L) significantly greater than 20 U/L (range 7 - 131 U/L) in an age and sex

matched control group *1526* In 25 drunken arrestees mean activity of 77.3 ± 81.8 U/L compared with 24.4 ± 10.7 U/L in 16 social drinkers and 27.1 ± 20.9 U/L in 27 teetotallers *2571*
Serum *No Effect* In 101 postmenopausal women who ingested moderate amounts of alcohol mean activity of 27.6 ± 1.3 U/L not significantly different from 25.7 ± 2.7 U/L in 27 alcohol abstaining postmenopausal women *1675*

Glutathione Peroxidase *Red Blood Cells* *Decrease* Mean concentration in 25 chronic alcoholics 68% of that in 25 age and sex matched controls *1741*
Serum *Decrease* In 25 alcoholics mean concentration 80% of that in 25 age and sex matched controls *1741*

Glutathione, Reduced *Red Blood Cells* *No Effect* No significant difference between concentrations in 21 patients with alcoholic liver disease but without cirrhosis of 2,243 ± 354 µmol/L RBC (mean ± 1 SD) compared with 2,391 ± 411 µmol/L RBC in 50 healthy controls although decreased in cirrhotics *1709*

Glutathione Reductase *Red Blood Cells* *No Effect* No significant difference observed in 21 patients with alcoholic liver disease without cirrhosis 24.12 ± 6.47 U/g hemoglobin, (mean ± 1 SD) compared with 50 healthy controls (22.06 ± 4.67 U/g hemoglobin) but decreased in advanced cirrhosis *1709*

Glutathione Reductase (Flavin Activation)
Red Blood Cells *Increase* In 8 of 35 cases (23%) activation increased by flavin reflecting vitamin B_2 deficiency *250*

Gonadotropin, Pituitary *Plasma* *Increase* 48 male chronic alcoholics classified in 2 groups according to the presence (22) or absence (26) of clinically evident sexual disorders. The level was significantly higher in the group with sexual disorders *4851*

Granulocytes *Blood* *No Effect* No significant difference observed between 74 chronic alcoholics after a period of excessive drinking and 18 alcoholic subjects who had not been drinking for at least 6 months *5250*

Growth Hormone *Plasma* *Increase* Increased following alcoholic binge of several days duration *3493* Mean basal concentration of 3.23 ± 0.91 ng/mL in 12 alcoholic men after 4 weeks of abstinence significantly higher than in normal controls (1 ± 0.17 ng/mL) *3288*

Haptoglobin *Serum* *Increase* Mean concentration of 99.85 mg/dL in alcoholics. Normal value was 71.66 mg/dL *1077*
Serum *No Effect* In 18 male alcoholics following recent debauche mean concentration of 1.4 g/L compared with reference interval of 0.3 - 1.8 g/L *2824*

HDL_2-Cholesterol *Serum* *Increase* In 104 male alcoholics mean concentration of 0.45 ± 0.37 mmol/L significantly higher than 0.21 ± 0.15 mmol/L in 37 teetotaler controls. Mean concentration in 137 moderate drinkers of 0.22 ± 0.17 mmol/L and in 90 heavy drinkers 0.22 ± 0.20 mmol/L *4837*

HDL_3-Cholesterol *Serum* *Increase* In 104 male alcoholics mean concentration of 1.16 ± 0.26 mmol/L significantly higher than 0.95 ± 0.15 mmol/L in 37 teetotaler controls. In 137 moderate drinkers mean concentration of 0.97 ± 0.16 mmol/L and 1.03 ± 0.24 mmol/L in 90 heavy drinkers *4837*

HDL-Cholesterol *Serum* *Decrease* In 146 chronic alcoholics in the 84 with high plasma trypsin activity mean concentration of 0.95 ± 0.23 mmol/L significantly reduced compared with mean of 1.86 ± 0.60 mmol/L in 62 patients with normal trypsin immunoreactivity although still within normal range *2474* In alcoholics with severe hepatic damage HDL-cholesterol concentrations are markedly decreased *5169*
Serum *Increase* Mean concentration significantly increased in intemperate drinkers compared with control individuals *4231* Increased *325* Mean concentration of 1.61 ± 0.54 mmol/L in 104 alcoholic men significantly greater than 1.16 ± 0.25 mmol/L in 37 teetotaler controls. In 137 moderate drinkers mean concentration of 1.19 ± 0.29 mmol/L and in 90 heavy drinkers mean concentration of 1.25 ± 0.40 mmol/L *4837* Increased *3327* Concentration increased in chronic alcoholics but only when no signs of hepatic insufficiency *5169* Significantly increased after period of alcohol abuse but fell after withdrawal of alcohol *5611* Increased *5707* In a population of industrial workers positive correlation of r = 0.127 between alcohol consumption and plasma HDL-cholesterol concentration *2497* In chronic alcoholic men mean concentration increased *929* Long-term alcohol intake associated with increased HDL-cholesterol concentration *929* In 26 male alcoholics immediately following a drinking binge mean concentration of 2.19 mmol/L significantly higher than in 17 healthy controls (1.15 mmol/L) *2650* Mean concentration in 52 alcoholics of 1.9 ± 0.8 mmol/L significantly different from 1.4 ± 0.3 mmol/L in 38 healthy controls *2008*
Serum *No Effect* In 59 male alcoholics mean concentration of 44 ± 19 mg/dL not significantly different from 42 ± 12 mg/dL in 140 controls. In 13 alcoholic women mean 65 ± 32 mg/dL not significantly different from 54 ± 14 mg/dL in 145 healthy controls *2305*

HDL-Phospholipids *Serum* *Increase* Mean concentration significantly increased in intemperate drinkers compared with control individuals *4231*

Hematocrit *Blood* *Decrease* Concentration in 18 chronic alcoholics after alcoholic debauche at lower limit of reference interval *2824*
Blood *No Effect* No significant difference observed between 184 controls, 88 heavy drinkers and 106 alcoholics *4732* In 104 alcoholic men mean value of 0.42 ± 0.04 not significantly different from 0.43 ± 0.03 in 37 teetotalers *4837* In 73 female alcoholics mean 0.39 ± 0.05 not significantly different from 0.38 ± 0.03 in 138 healthy control women *4733*

Hemoglobin *Blood* *No Effect* In 21 patients with alcoholic liver disease without cirrhosis mean concentration of 139 (SD 18) g/L but in patients with severe cirrhosis mean concentration reduced to 106 (SD 32) g/L *1709* No significant deviation from the reference interval observed in 18 male chronic alcoholics after alcoholic debauche *2824* In 19 alcoholic women mean concentration of 134 ± 14 g/L not significantly different from 138 ± 9 g/L in 14 healthy controls *2897*

Hemopexin *Serum* *No Effect* In 18 male alcoholics following recent debauche mean concentration of 0.71 g/L at lower end of reference interval of 0.7 - 1.2 g/L *2824*

β-Hexosaminidase *Serum* *Increase* Activity increased in 94.4% alcoholics. Sensitivity for heavy drinking 72% *4528* In 38 alcoholics all had increased activity of β-hexosaminidase B isoenzyme although only 35 had increased activity of total hexosaminidase. Only one abstinent individual had increased activities of total hexosaminidase and isoenzymes A and B *2289* Marked increases observed in intoxicated individuals. Activity increase mainly due to thermostable component of enzyme *5610* Mean 2 times higher in drunken arrestees than among social drinkers. Average daily alcohol intake correlated positively (r = 0.69) with β-Hexosaminidase. Sensitivity of β-Hexosaminidase in detection of heavy drinking 85.7% versus 47.6% for GGT. Specificity 97.6% *2571*

Homocysteine *Plasma* *Increase* A significantly higher concentration of plasma homocysteine compared with controls was noted in a group of alcoholics (n = 42) hospitalized for detoxication *2287*

Homovanillic Acid *Cerebrospinal Fluid* *Decrease* In 43 alcoholic impulsive offenders mean concentration of 143 pmol/mL less than 160 pmol/mL in 21 healthy controls *5479*
Cerebrospinal Fluid *Increase* Mean concentration of 180 pmol/mL in 15 nonimpulsive alcoholic offenders higher than 160 pmol/mL in 21 healthy control individuals *5479*

Hyaluronic Acid *Serum* *No Effect* The median level in patients with alcoholic liver disease (53 µg/L) did not differ significantly from the corresponding value in the control group (36 µg/L) *1371*

4-Hydroxy-3-Methoxy-Phenylglycol
Cerebrospinal Fluid *No Effect* In 5 chronically alcoholic men mean concentration of 42 ± 7 pmol/mL not significantly less than 46 ± 2 pmol/mL in 6 healthy controls *1700* Mean concentration in alcoholic impulsive and nonimpulsive offenders not significantly different from that in healthy controls *5479*

25-Hydroxy Vitamin D_3 *Serum* *Decrease* In 34 hospitalized male alcoholics mean concentration reduced by 28% compared with 35 age-matched controls *460* Lower mean value (15.0 ± 7.6 ng/mL) was found in 13 chronic alcoholics with no evidence of cirrhosis on biopsy. Normal concentration of 23.6 ± 9.8 ng/mL *5449* Deficient absorption of vitamin D observed in alcoholism. Impaired synthesis in liver also partially responsible, especially with cirrhosis *1446* In patients with chronic alcoholism and liver disease concentrations reduced *4348* Concentration low in alcoholics when liver disease is present *2490* Reduced concentration observed in chronic alcoholics due to deficient intestinal absorption of vitamin D or due to impaired liver synthesis *4348* In 19 chronic alcoholic women mean concentration of 42 ± 23 nmol/L significantly reduced compared with 74 ± 21 nmol/L in 14 healthy controls *2897*

303.90 Alcoholism *(continued)*

25-Hydroxy Vitamin D *Serum* *Decrease* In 18 chronic alcoholics mean concentration of 40 (18-102) nmol/L not significantly less than 54 (23-87) nmol/L in 10 abstinent controls *3069* *Serum* *No Effect* No significant change observed in chronic alcoholics *4348* In 27 individuals with a history of at least 10 years alcoholism mean concentration of 52 ± 26 nmol/L not significantly different from normal range of 45 ± 20 nmol/L *451* No significant change observed in alcoholic patients *450*

5-Hydroxyindoleacetic Acid *Cerebrospinal Fluid* *Decrease* Mean concentration of 53 pmol/mL in 43 alcoholic impulsive offenders lower than 90 pmol/mL in 15 alcoholic nonimpulsive offenders and 65 pmol/mL in 21 control individuals *5479* *Cerebrospinal Fluid* *No Effect* In 5 chronically alcoholic men mean concentration of 146 ± 53 pmol/mL not significantly different from 133 ± 19 pmol/mL in 6 healthy controls *1700*

Hydroxyproline *Urine* *Decrease* In 18 chronic alcoholics mean excretion of 233 (range 43-597) nmol/d not significantly less than 256 (98-596) nmol/d in 10 abstinent controls *3069* *Urine* *No Effect* Mean excretion of 67 μmol/sq m/d in 19 chronic alcoholic women not significantly different from 68 μmol/sq m/d in 14 healthy controls *2897*

5-Hydroxytryptamine *Platelets* *Decrease* In 108 chronic alcoholics mean concentration on admission to hospital of 312 ± 167 ng/10^9 platelets compared with 475 ± 217 ng/10^9 platelets in healthy controls *249*

5-Hydroxytryptophol *Urine* *Increase* Excretion increases as much as 100-fold even after moderate alcohol consumption and does not normalize until several hours after the ethanol has been eliminated from the body *531*

IDL-Cholesterol *Serum* *No Effect* In 13 male alcoholics mean concentration of 0.11 mmol/L not significantly different from 0.17 mmol/L in 8 healthy controls *2650*

IDL-Phospholipids *Serum* *No Effect* In 13 male alcoholics mean concentration of 0.06 mmol/L not significantly different from mean concentration of 0.10 mmol/L in 8 healthy controls *2650*

IDL-Triglycerides *Serum* *No Effect* In 13 male alcoholics mean concentration of 0.05 mmol/L no different from concentration in 8 healthy controls *2650*

Immunoglobulin A *Serum* *No Effect* In 18 male alcoholics following recent debauche mean concentration of 3.4 g/L at upper limit of reference interval of 1.2 - 3.5 g/L *2824*

Immunoglobulin A_1 *Serum* *Increase* Significant increase to 6.05 ± 4.98 g/L observed in alcoholic liver cirrhosis *3442*

Immunoglobulin A_2 *Serum* *Increase* Significantly increased to 0.56 ± 0.51 g/L in heavy drinkers and to 1.15 ± 1.10 g/L in alcoholic liver cirrhosis *3442*

Immunoglobulin G *Serum* *No Effect* In 18 male alcoholics following recent debauche mean concentration of 10.1 g/L compared with reference interval of 7.0 - 14.0 g/L *2824*

Insulin *Plasma* *Increase* In 11 alcoholics mean concentration of 11.9 ± 4.7 μU/mL not significantly greater than 9.2 ± 2.8 μU/mL in 20 healthy controls *4257*

Interferon-α *Serum* *Decrease* In 40 patients with alcoholic cirrhosis concentration significantly decreased *5466*

Interferon-γ *Serum* *Decrease* Significant reduction observed in individuals with alcoholic cirrhosis but concentration not correlated with severity *5466*

Interleukin-1 *Serum* *Increase* Concentration increased in patients with chronic alcoholism *2667*

Interleukin-2 *Serum* *Decrease* Significant reduction observed in patients with alcoholic cirrhosis although not correlated with degree of hepatic damage *5466*

Interleukin-6 *Serum* *Increase* High serum IL-6 concentrations (60 ± 38 ng/L) correlated with IgA_1 and IgA_2 concentrations in heavy alcohol drinkers *3442* Concentration increased in patients with chronic alcoholism *2667* Increased concentration observed in alcoholic liver cirrhosis *4093* Concentration significantly increased in patients with alcoholic hepatitis compared with control groups of patients (normal, or alcoholics without liver disease, inactive alcoholic cirrhotics, chronic liver disease and chronic renal failure) *4779*

Ionized Calcium *Serum* *No Effect* In 18 chronic alcoholics mean concentration of 1.25 (range 1.05-1.35) mmol/L not significantly different from 1.22 (1.17-1.30) mmol/L in 10 abstinent controls *3069* In 19 chronic alcoholic women mean concentration of 1.20 mmol/L not significantly different from 1.21 mmol/L in 14 healthy controls *2897*

Iron *Bone Marrow* *Increase* Iron overload shown by plasma cells containing iron in bone marrow may occur *3493* *Hair* *Increase* In 23 alcoholic patients mean concentration of 43.9 ± 4.9 μg/g significantly different from mean concentration in 30 healthy control individuals of 32.0 ± 5.5 μg/g *2614* *Nails* *Increase* In 22 alcoholic patients mean concentration of 573.6 ± 52.8 μg/g significantly different from mean concentration in 30 healthy control individuals of 387.2 ± 57.1 μg/g *2614* *Serum* *Increase* In 159 alcoholic patients (119 men and 40 women) admitted to a detoxification center median concentration of 20 μmol/L (range 3 - 53) significantly greater than 16 μmol/L (range 4 - 33) in an age and sex matched control group *1526* Nonsignificant increase to 21.6 ± 7.2 μmol/L (121 ± 40 μg/dL) in 21 patients with alcoholic liver disease without cirrhosis with comparable concentrations observed in patients with mild or moderate alcoholic cirrhosis *1709* *Serum* *No Effect* In 18 male alcoholics mean concentration of 21.8 μmol/L compared with reference interval of 10 - 35 μmol/L *2824*

Iron-binding Capacity, Total *Serum* *Decrease* In 159 alcoholic patients (119 men and 40 women) admitted to a detoxification center median concentration of 55 μmol/L (range 32 - 91) significantly lower than 58 μmol/L (range 36 - 90) in an age and sex matched control group *1526* *Serum* *No Effect* In 18 male alcoholics following recent debauche mean concentration of 54 μmol/L compared with reference interval of 43 - 90 μmol/L *2824*

Lactate *Blood* *Increase* Increased in serum lactate produced from pyruvate in the presence of the increased NADH/NAD ratio *1980* Acidosis due to lactate and ketoacid accumulation following alcoholic binge of several days duration *3493*

Lactate Dehydrogenase *Serum* *Increase* In 42% of 14 patients hospitalized for this disorder *1576*

Laminin *Serum* *Increase* In patients with alcohol abuse without cirrhosis levels were significantly higher (mean 1.57 U/mL) compared with healthy controls (mean 1.28 U/mL) *5420*

LDL-Cholesterol *Serum* *Decrease* Mean concentration of 2.65 mmol/L in 26 male alcoholics significantly less than mean of 3.66 mmol/L in 15 healthy controls *2650* In chronic alcoholic men mean concentration reduced *929* In chronic alcoholics in the 59 with normal plasma trypsin activity mean concentration of 4.04 ± 1.05 mmol/L compared with 4.84 ± 2.09 mmol/L in 78 with increased plasma trypsin activity (significantly different) *2474* Long-term alcohol intake associated with decreased serum concentration *929*

LDL-Phospholipids *Serum* *Decrease* Mean concentration of 0.95 mmol/L in 26 male alcoholics significantly less than mean of 1.31 mmol/L in 15 healthy controls *2650*

LDL-Triglycerides *Serum* *No Effect* Mean concentration of 0.20 mmol/L the same in 26 male alcoholics and in 15 healthy controls *2650*

Lead *Blood* *Increase* In 161 chronic alcoholic patients in France mean concentration of 280 μg/L with blood lead concentration being positively correlated with hypertension *1000* *Hair* *No Effect* In 23 alcoholic patients mean concentration of 12.5 ± 1.5 μg/g not significantly different from mean concentration in 30 healthy control individuals of 15.4 ± 1.7 μg/g *2614* *Nails* *No Effect* In 22 alcoholic patients mean concentration of 14.2 ± 1.8 μg/g not significantly different from mean concentration in 30 healthy control individuals of 13.5 ± 1.8 μg/g *2614*

Leukocytes *Blood* *Increase* Significant increase to 6.7 ± 0.2 10^{12}/L (mean ± SEM) in 88 heavy drinkers, 7.6 ± 0.3 10^{12}/L in 106 alcoholics from 6.1 ± 0.1 10^{12}/L in 184 controls *4732* *Blood* *No Effect* No significant difference observed between concentrations in 74 addictive alcoholics after a period of excessive drinking and 18 alcoholics who had not been drinking for 6 months *5250* Mean concentration of 5,300 /μL observed in 18 male alcoholics following recent debauche compared with reference interval of 3,500 - 9,000 /μL *2824*

Lipase *Serum* *Increase* Increased activity observed in 66 of 202 chronic alcoholics without abdominal symptoms *1912* In patients with alcoholism activity may be increased *5231* In 202 asymptomatic alcoholics admitted to hospital for detoxification, 66 had serum lipase activities above the normal range (0 - 213 U/L) of which 85% had activities that were 1 - 2 times normal while the remainder had activities 2 - 3 times normal *1914*

Lipids *Serum* *Increase* Rise after ingestion of moderate amounts of alcohol due to increased hepatic production and release of lipoproteins *1980*

Lipoprotein Lp(a) *Serum* *Decrease* Since Lp(a) is synthesized in the liver concentration may be reduced with impaired liver function *2827*

Liver-specific Membrane Lipoprotein Antibodies *Serum* *Positive* Observed in patients with alcoholic liver disease *4093*

Luteinizing Hormone *Plasma* *Increase* The basal level of LH was significantly elevated in alcoholics with and without clinically evident sexual disorders *4851* In 21 women with amenorrhea who were noncirrhotic alcoholics mean concentration of 24 ± 19 IU/L significantly different from upper limit of reference interval of less than 12 IU/L *375*
Plasma *No Effect* In 101 postmenopausal women who ingested moderate amounts of alcohol mean concentration of 23.6 ± 0.9 mIU/mL not significantly different from 24.0 ± 2.8 mIU/mL in 27 alcohol abstaining postmenopausal women *1675*

Lymphocytes *Blood* *Decrease* In chronic alcoholics mean concentration reduced in relation to recency of drinking: mean of 1,920 /µL at 1 day, 2,020 /µL at 3 days, 2,430 /µL at 7 days, 2,950 /µL at 10 days, 3,160 /µL at 30 days and 2,670 /µL at more than 6 months *5250*

Macrocytes *Blood* *Increase* Percentage of macrocytes increased in individuals both with and without liver damage *3932*

Magnesium *Hair* *Decrease* In 23 alcoholic patients mean concentration of 168.6 ± 4.9 µg/g significantly different from mean concentration in 30 healthy control individuals of 211.2 ± 1.7 µg/g *2614*
Nails *Decrease* In 22 alcoholic patients mean concentration of 426.3 ± 2.4 µg/g significantly different from mean concentration in 30 healthy control individuals of 441.7 ± 11.4 µg/g *2614*
Serum *Decrease* Significant reduction to 1.8 ± 0.2 mg/dL in 8 chronic alcohol abusing men from reference range concentration of 2.1 ± 0.1 mg/dL *450* Concentration observed to be decreased in patients with chronic alcoholism *4348* In 9 of 81 patients with serum magnesium concentration of less than 0.72 mmol/L patients had chronic alcoholism *3159* Observed in chronic alcoholics but with normal serum calcium and phosphate *1265* In 127 patients with chronic alcoholism mean concentration of 0.7 ± 0.2 mmol/L significantly different from 0.9 ± 0.3 mmol/L in 203 normal controls, but when corrected for hypoalbuminemia mean magnesium concentration rose to 0.73 mmol/L *1330*
Serum *No Effect* In 27 individuals with a history of at least 10 years of alcoholism mean concentration normal *451* In 19 chronic alcoholic women mean concentration of 0.78 mmol/L not significantly different from 0.83 mmol/L in 14 healthy controls *2897* In 18 chronic alcoholics mean concentration of 0.76 mmol/L (range of 0.50 - 0.90) not significantly different from 0.81 mmol/L (0.71 - 0.90) in 10 abstinent controls *3069* No significant difference observed between concentrations in 35 male hospitalized alcoholics and 34 age matched controls *460*
Urine *Decrease* Mean excretion of 2.6 ± 1.7 mmol/d in 19 chronic alcoholic women significantly less than 4.4 ± 1.0 mmol/d in 14 healthy controls *2897*
Urine *Increase* In chronic alcoholics urinary excretion may be 167 - 260% of control values *1510* Excretion increased in patients with chronic alcoholism and with acute alcohol intake *4348*
Urine *No Effect* In 8 long-term alcoholic men mean excretion of 70 ± 31 mg/d not significantly different from 137 ± 87 mg/d of reference range *450*

Manganese *Hair* *No Effect* In 23 alcoholic patients mean concentration of 2.6 ± 0.9 µg/g not significantly different from mean concentration in 30 healthy control individuals of 2.4 ± 0.6 µg/g *2614*
Nails *No Effect* In 22 alcoholic patients mean concentration of 4.7 ± 0.5 µg/g not significantly different from mean concentration in 30 healthy control individuals of 4.7 ± 1.1 µg/g *2614*

α-Mannosidase *Serum* *Increase* Increase less pronounced in alcoholics than increase of α-hexosaminidase *5610*

MCH *Blood* *No Effect* In 23 actively drinking alcohol-habituated individuals mean concentration of 32 ± 2 pg not significantly different from 32 ± 11 pg in 10 alcohol-naive control individuals *2176*

MCV *Blood* *Increase* Observed in individuals with and without liver damage *3932* Mean in 52 alcoholics of 96 ± 4 fL significantly different from 90 ± 4 fL in 37 healthy controls *2008* In 73 female alcoholics mean volume 96.7 ± 7.0 fL not significantly different from 91.8 ± 4.3 fL in 138 healthy control women *4733* In several different studies increased values observed in 31 - 96% alcoholic patients *4528* In 19 alcoholic women mean concentration of 96 ± fL significantly higher than 89 ± 2 fL in 14 healthy controls *2897* In 23 actively drinking alcohol-habituated individuals mean concentration of 97 ± 5 fL significantly different from 89 ± 10 fL in 10 alcohol-naive control individuals *2176* Increase observed in 80% of subjects with an alcohol problem *4093* In 62 chronic alcoholics with normal plasma immunoreactive concentration mean volume 99.1 fL, compared with 96.4 fL in 84 with increased plasma immunoreactive trypsin concentration and < 98.0 fL in healthy individuals *2474* In 12 of 25 chronic alcoholics on admission to hospital mean increased above normal range of 80 to 94 fL *786* In 100 patients with macrocytosis (MCV greater than 110 fL) 19 were chronic alcoholics *4924* Observed in both individuals with and without documented liver damage *3932* In 21 patients with alcoholic liver disease but without cirrhosis mean volume 102 (SD 10) fL as in patients with advanced alcoholic cirrhosis *1709* In 88 heavy drinkers mean ± SEM was 92.7 ± 0.5 fL compared with 95.9 ± 0.5 fL in 106 alcoholics and 90.0 ± 0.3 fL in 184 controls *4732*
Blood *No Effect* In 18 male alcoholics immediately after debauche mean volume of 95 fL compared with reference interval of 82 - 102 fL *2824*

Melatonin *Urine* *Increase* In patients, during alcohol intake, 24 h excretion significantly greater than in controls. Normally night excretion greater than day excretion but reverse observed in drinking alcoholics. In drinking alcoholics mean day excretion higher than in controls *3672*

Methanol *Blood* *Increase* Ethanol inhibits oxidation of methanol so high blood methanol concentrations observed after prolonged drinking, especially in chronic alcoholics *4528*

Monoamine Oxidase *Platelets* *Decrease* The activity was found to lower in type 2 alcoholics when compared both with healthy controls and with type 1 alcoholics. Also, the type 1 alcoholics had lower activity than the controls *3986* In 14 male chronic alcoholics mean of 4.22 ± 0.70 nmol product formed/mg protein/h significantly less than 13.66 ± 0.60 nmol product formed/mg protein/h in 52 male controls: mean concentration of 5.85 ± 1.43 nmol product formed/mg protein/h in 12 female chronic alcoholics significantly less than 16.12 ± 1.70 nmol product formed/mg protein/h in 15 healthy control women *1418* The activity was found to lower in type 2 alcoholics when compared both with healthy controls and with type 1 alcoholics. Also, the type 1 alcoholics had lower activity than the controls *5494* The alcoholic female was found to have slightly lower platelet MAO activity than the controls *1977* The activity was found to lower in type 2 alcoholics when compared both with healthy controls and with type 1 alcoholics. Also, the type 1 alcoholics had lower activity than the controls *3643* *197*

Myoglobin *Urine* *Increase* Sporadic; metabolic myoglobinuria *5544*

N-Acetyl-Glucosaminidase *Serum* *Increase* In 25 drunken arrestees mean activity (35.0 ± 11.6 U/L) two times higher than in 16 social drinkers (16.8 ± 4.6 U/L) or 27 teetotallers (19.8 ± 3.3 U/L) *2571* In 32 alcoholic men prior to detoxification mean activity of 34.9 ± 12.1 U/L compared with 19.8 ± 3.3 U/L in 27 control non-drinking men *2570*
Urine *Increase* In 32 alcoholic men prior to detoxification mean activity of 1.53 ± 1.22 U/L compared with 0.45 ± 0.18 U/L in 27 control men *2570*

N-Acetylglucosaminyltransferase *Serum* *Decrease* In 14 alcoholic individuals with mean blood alcohol concentration of 65 mmol/L, with a mean intake 250 g/d for 1 - 3 weeks, decreased activity observed of from 35 - 55% *5017*

Neopterin *Serum* *Decrease* In 26 alcohol-dependent patients mean concentration of 4.3 ± 1.6 nmol/L significantly different from 5.5 ± 1.6 nmol/L in 34 healthy controls *3867*

303.90 Alcoholism *(continued)*

Neopterin *(continued)*
Serum *Increase* Mean concentration in 105 chronic alcoholics of 6.63 nmol/L significantly higher than 2.91 nmol/L in 12 healthy controls with concentrations highest in patients with cirrhosis, ascites, jaundice and in those with alcoholic hepatitis *1808*

Nickel *Hair* *No Effect* In 23 alcoholic patients mean concentration of 3.1 ± 0.3 µg/g not significantly different from mean concentration in 30 healthy control individuals of 3.5 ± 0.6 µg/g *2614*
Nails *No Effect* In 22 alcoholic patients mean concentration of 4.2 ± 0.2 µg/g not significantly different from mean concentration in 30 healthy control individuals of 4.5 ± 0.4 µg/g *2614*

Norepinephrine *Cerebrospinal Fluid* *Decrease* In 5 chronically alcoholic men mean concentration of 0.33 ± 0.09 pmol/mL significantly less than 1.15 ± 0.51 pmol/mL in 6 healthy controls *1700*
Plasma *No Effect* In 5 chronically alcoholic men mean concentration of 1.2 ± 0.69 pmol/mL not significantly different from 1.0 ± 0.13 pmol/mL in 6 healthy controls *1700*

Ornithine Carbamoyltransferase *Serum* *Increase* Liver cell damage *5544*

Osmolality *Serum* *Increase* In 23 actively drinking alcohol-habituated individuals mean concentration of 309 mOsmkg significantly increased above normal *2176* Basal concentration in alcoholics significantly higher than in controls *889*

Osteocalcin *Serum* *Decrease* Mean concentration of 0.92 (0.26 - 2.55) nmol/L in 18 chronic alcoholics significantly less than 1.43 (0.91 - 2.02) nmol/L in 10 abstinent controls *3069* In 40 alcoholics mean concentration of 3.0 ± 2.6 µg/L significantly less than healthy controls (3.0 ± 2.6 µg/L) *2419* In 19 chronic alcoholic women mean concentration of 0.5 µg/L significantly less than 2.3 µg/L in 14 healthy controls *2897* Observed effect *2883*

Parathyroid Hormone *Plasma* *Decrease* In 18 chronic alcoholics mean concentration of 1.95 (range of 0.9 - 4.4) pmol/L significantly less than 3.95 (range of 1.8 - 6.8) pmol/L in 10 abstinent controls *3069*
Plasma *Increase* Increased following alcoholic binge of several days duration *3493* High concentration observed in chronic alcoholics when middle fragment measured but carboxy terminal fragment measurement normal. Note since hormone metabolized in liver abnormal concentration might be related to liver lesions *1446* In 27 individuals with a history of at least 10 years alcoholism mean concentration of 36 ± 26 µL/Eq/mL compared with upper limit of normal of < 40 µL/Eq/mL but with 8 individuals having values above the upper limit of normal *451* Concentration reported to be increased in chronic alcoholics *2490* In 8 long-term alcoholic men mean concentration of 33 ± 5 µLEq/mL significantly increased compared with reference range of 23 ± 5 µLEq/mL *450*
Plasma *No Effect* Concentration reported to be normal in chronic alcoholics *4348* Mean concentration of 27 ± 16 ng/L in 19 chronic alcoholic women not significantly different from 31 ± 9 ng/L in 14 healthy control women *2897* No significant difference observed between concentrations in 34 hospitalized male alcoholics and 35 age matched controls *460*

pH *Blood* *Decrease* Severe metabolic acidosis with pH ranging between 6.96 - 7.28 occurred after alcoholic binge of several days duration *3493*

Phenytoin *Serum* *Decrease* Metabolism stimulated in long term alcohol abusers and effect continues for several days to weeks after abuse ended *3038* Chronic administration of alcohol with phenytoin may decrease plasma phenytoin concentration *4008*
Serum *No Effect* No significant effect of alcohol use in relation to dose observed on plasma concentration *1065*

Phosphate *Serum* *Decrease* Concentration reduced in alcoholics *130* Alcoholism is common cause of severe hypophosphatemia due to shift of phosphate into the cells, reduced absorption of phosphate from the intestinal tract and increased renal loss of phosphate *969* An association of hypophosphatemia with chronic alcoholism was found in 11 patients studied. The hypophosphatemia was associated with low levels of RBC ATP, abnormal erythrocyte filtration, and, in at least 1 patient, with hemolytic anemia *5197* Occurs in about 50% of hospitalized alcoholics *2719*
Serum *Increase* Increased following alcoholic binge of several days duration *3493*
Serum *No Effect* In 27 individuals with a history of at least 10 years of alcoholism mean concentration normal *451* No significant difference observed in mean concentration of 3.1 ± 0.4 mg/dL in 8 men who had abused alcohol for 10 years and reference range of 2.9 ± 0.5 mg/dL *450* No significant difference observed in concentrations of 34 hospitalized male alcoholics and 35 healthy age matched controls *460* Mean concentration of 1.12 ± 0.20 mmol/L in 19 chronic alcoholic women not significantly different from 1.05 ± 0.22 mmol/L in 14 healthy controls *2897* Normal concentration observed in chronic alcoholics *1265* In 18 chronic alcoholics mean concentration of 1.0 (range of 0.9 - 1.8) mmol/L not significantly different from 1.2 (0.9 - 1.4) mmol/L in 10 abstinent controls *3069*
Urine *Decrease* In 19 chronic alcoholic women mean excretion of 15.3 ± 9.1 mmol/d significantly less than 26.9 ± 5.9 mmol/d in 14 healthy controls *2897*
Urine *Increase* Increase observed in chronic alcoholics *130*
Urine *No Effect* In 8 long-term chronic alcoholic men mean excretion of 640 ± 227 mg/d not significantly different from reference range of 750 ± 250 mg/d *450*

Phospholipids *Serum* *Increase* Fasting serum lipid values were have been analyzed in 85 male and 10 female alcoholics of various ages in connection with an acute drinking bout and compared to control subjects. The most prominent finding was an increase in the mean concentration of triglycerides and phospholipids, most marked in the younger age groups. The elevations were moderate and most alcoholics had the same serum total lipid values as the controls *540*

Plasminogen Activator Inhibitor-1 *Plasma* *Increase* Significant increase observed in patients with mild and severe liver cirrhosis *5442*

Plasminogen Activator Inhibitor-1 Antigen
Plasma *Increase* Significant increase observed in chronic alcoholics without abnormal liver function, in those with abnormal liver function and in those with cirrhosis *5442*

Plasminogen Activator Inhibitor Activity *Plasma* *Increase* In 11 alcoholics mean activity of 21 ± 9.7 U/mL significantly greater than 9.76 ± 5.38 U/mL in 20 healthy controls *4257*

Platelets *Blood* *Decrease* Counts as low as 20,000 /µL have been recorded. Recovery to a normal count occurs within 1 week of abstinence *1980* In 106 alcoholics mean concentration of 215 ± 7 x 10^9/L significantly reduced below that in 184 controls (231 ± 4 x 10^9/L) *4732*
Blood *No Effect* In 184 controls mean concentration of 231 ± 4 10^9/L (mean ± SEM) compared with 224 ± 5 10^9/L in 88 heavy drinkers *4732* No significant deviation from reference interval of 150,000 - 400,000 /µL in 18 male alcoholics immediately after alcoholic debauche (mean concentration of 176,000 /µL) *2824*

Potassium *Hair* *No Effect* In 23 alcoholic patients mean concentration of 107.2 ± 1.5 µg/g not significantly different from mean concentration in 30 healthy control individuals of 108.0 ± 3.1 µg/g *2614*
Nails *No Effect* In 22 alcoholic patients mean concentration of 1,149.7 ± 12.4 µg/g not significantly different from mean concentration in 30 healthy control individuals of 1,190.4 ± 13.6 µg/g *2614*
Serum *Decrease* In alcoholics episodes of hypokalemia observed accompanied by normal or increased serum concentrations of sodium *1203* In 26 patients in whom delirium tremens developed, a continuing decrease led to hypokalemia, (mean 2.9 mmol/L) when delirium tremens started *5517*
Serum *No Effect* In 23 actively drinking alcohol-habituated individuals mean concentration of 3.9 ± 0.38 mmol/L not significantly different from 3.6 ± 0.35 mmol/L in 10 alcohol-naive control individuals *2176*

Prealbumin *Serum* *No Effect* In 19 alcoholic women mean concentration of 320 ± 107 mg/L not significantly different from 291 ± 39 mg/L in 14 healthy controls *2897*

Prolactin *Plasma* *Increase* In 38% of 93 chronic alcoholic men mean concentration of 621 ± 46 IU/L observed reflecting severe hyperprolactinemia *2795* In 18 chronic alcoholics mean concentration of 7.4 (4.6 - 17.8) µg/L significantly higher than 5.0 (4.5 - 10.1) µg/L in 10 abstinent controls *3069* In some heavy drinking women (greater than 5 drinks per day) serum prolactin concentration may be increased *37* In pregnant alcoholics concentration observed to be increased *1978*

Plasma *No Effect* In 62% of 93 chronic alcoholic men mean concentration within normal range (154 ± 13 IU/L) *2795* In 101 postmenopausal women who ingested moderate amounts of alcohol mean concentration of 5.9 ± 0.2 ng/mL not significantly different from 5.7 ± 0.4 ng/mL in 27 alcohol abstaining postmenopausal women *1675* In 21 women with amenorrhea who were noncirrhotic alcoholics mean concentration of 428 ± 311 mIU/L not significantly different from reference interval of 50 - 700 mIU/L *375*

Propranolol *Serum* *Decrease* In long term alcohol abusers drug metabolism is stimulated and effect continues for several days to weeks after abuse ended *3038*

Prothrombin Index *Plasma* *Increase* In 19 alcoholic women mean index of 1.20 (0.41 - 1.52) not significantly greater than 1.09 (0.87 - 1.61) in 14 healthy controls *2897*

Prothrombin Time *Plasma* *No Effect* In 23 actively drinking alcohol-habituated individuals mean time of 12 ± 5 s not significantly different from 10 ± 3 s in 10 alcohol-naive control individuals *2176*

Red Cell Distribution Width *Blood* *Increase* In 73 female alcoholics mean RDW of 15.1 ± 2.4% significantly different from 12.7 ± 1.1% in 138 healthy control women *4733*
Blood *No Effect* In 73 female alcoholics mean RDW of 23.5 ± 4.0 g/L not significantly different from 23.3 ± 2.0 g/L in 138 healthy control women *4733*

Renin Activity *Plasma* *Increase* In patients with alcoholic liver disease activity increased in 14 of 57 studies *4297*
Plasma *No Effect* Basal concentration normal in chronic alcoholics although serum osmolality increased *889* In 23 actively drinking alcohol-habituated individuals mean concentration of 3.1 ± 1.7 ng/mL/h not significantly different from normal *2176*

Reticulocytes *Blood* *Increase* In 73 female alcoholics mean proportion of 1.6 ± 0.6% significantly different from 1.3 ± 0.5% in 138 healthy control women *4733* Significant increase from mean concentration in 184 controls (1.3%) to 1.4% in 88 heavy drinkers and 1.5 ± 0.1% in 106 alcoholics *4732* In patients with alcoholic liver disease but without cirrhosis mean count 105 (SD 81) 10^9/L increasing to 128 10^9/L in patients with advanced alcoholic liver cirrhosis *1709*
Blood *No Effect* In 18 male alcoholics following recent debauche mean concentration of 0.9% compared with reference interval of 0.2 - 1.0% *2824*

Retinol *Serum* *Decrease* In 16 of 28 chronic alcoholics (57.1%) on admission to hospital concentration below normal of 1.57 to 2.09 μmol/L *786*

Retinol-binding Protein *Serum* *Decrease* In 28 chronic alcoholics on admission to hospital concentration reduced below normal range of 63.0 to 126.0 mg/dL in 7 (25%) *2652*

Rifampin *Serum* *Decrease* In long term alcohol abusers drug metabolism is stimulated and effect continues for several days to weeks after abuse has ended *3038*

Salsolinol Sulfate *Serum* *Increase* In 40 chronic alcoholics mean concentration of 627 ± 195 pg/mL significantly higher than 99.5 ± 7.5 pg/mL in 29 healthy controls *1419*

Selenium *Blood* *Decrease* In 30 chronic alcoholics mean concentration of 0.076 ± 0.011 μg/mL compared with 0.114 ± 0.015 μg/mL in 20 healthy controls *1275*
Red Blood Cells *Decrease* In 30 chronic alcoholics mean concentration of 0.092 ± 0.016 μg/mL compared with 0.130 ± 0.025 μg/mL in 20 normal controls *1275* Mean concentration in 25 chronic alcoholics 70% of that in 25 age and sex matched healthy controls *1741*
Serum *Decrease* Mean concentration of 0.065 ± 0.012 μg/mL in 30 patients with history of chronic heavy alcohol ingestion compared with 0.100 ± 0.016 μg/mL in 20 healthy control individuals *1275* In 25 chronic alcoholics mean concentration of 71% of that in 25 age and sex matched controls *1741* In 21 patients with alcoholic liver disease without cirrhosis nonsignificant reduction to 0.85 ± 0.23 μmol/L (6.7 ± 1.8 μg/dL) with significant reductions observed in patients with alcoholic liver cirrhosis *1709* Mean concentration in 30 asymptomatic alcoholics 65 ± 12 μg/L compared with 95 ± 16 μg/L in 27 normal controls and 38 ± 7 μg/L in 16 alcoholics with severe liver disease *1274*

Sex-Hormone Binding Globulin *Serum* *Decrease* In 18 chronic alcoholics mean concentration of 49 (21 - 186) nmol/L not significantly less than 58 (30 - 83) nmol/L in 10 abstinent controls *3069*
Serum *Increase* Compared with controls of comparable age more alcoholic cirrhotic women had increased concentration *360* Increase observed in alcoholic men leading to a decrease in free testosterone concentration *37*
Serum *No Effect* In 21 women with amenorrhea who were noncirrhotic alcoholics mean concentration of 66 ± 34 nmol/L not significantly different from reference interval of 30 - 90 nmol/L *375*

Sialyltransferase *Serum* *No Effect* No significant effect observed in chronic alcoholics *5017*

Sodium *Hair* *No Effect* In 23 alcoholic patients mean concentration of 1120.2 ± 18.5 μg/g not significantly different from mean concentration in 30 healthy control individuals of 1099.3 ± 32.7 μg/g *2614*
Nails *No Effect* In 22 alcoholic patients mean concentration of 3,290.8 ± 36.1 μg/g not significantly different from mean concentration in 30 healthy control individuals of 3,426.9 ± 43.1 μg/g *2614*
Serum *No Effect* In 23 actively drinking alcohol-habituated individuals mean concentration of 142 ± 5 mmol/L not significantly different from 142 ± 4 mmol/L in 10 alcohol-naive control individuals *2176*

Superoxide Dismutase *Red Blood Cells* *No Effect* In 21 patients with alcoholic liver disease of 2,196 ± 552 U/g hemoglobin (mean ± 1 SD) but in patients with advanced liver cirrhosis no significant difference from concentrations in either healthy controls or in those without cirrhosis *1709*

Testosterone *Serum* *Decrease* In 18 chronic alcoholics mean concentration of 18.6 (range 3.0 - 46.6) nmol/L not significantly less than 24.6 (18.0 - 31.9) nmol/L in 10 abstinent controls *3069* Deleterious effect observed on hypothalamic-hypophyseal-gonadal axis described but probably also direct effect on testosterone secreting cells *1764* After abstaining from alcohol and cigarettes for one week, the testosterone levels in 30 alcoholics allowed alcohol during the second week dropped rapidly and significantly, but did not correlate with amount of alcohol ingested *4090* Lower concentration observed due to direct effect of alcohol on testosterone-secreting cells *4348* Decrease observed in alcoholic men due to toxic effect on testes and by metabolites formed by alcohol dehydrogenase. Testicular LH receptors also depleted and testosterone clearance increased *37*
Serum *No Effect* In 101 postmenopausal women who ingested moderate amounts of alcohol mean concentration of 0.63 ± 0.03 ng/mL not significantly different from 0.74 ± 0.06 ng/mL in 27 alcohol abstaining postmenopausal women *1675* In a study of alcoholics with osteopenia no effect on circulating concentration observed *963* In 27 men with a history of at least 10 years alcoholism mean concentration of 21 ± 6 nmol/L not significantly different from normal (upper limit > 10.4 nmol/L) *451* In 21 women with amenorrhea who were noncirrhotic alcoholics mean concentration of 1.7 ± 1.3 nmol/L not significantly different from reference interval of 0.3 - 2.8 nmol/L *375*

Testosterone, Free *Cerebrospinal Fluid* *Increase* Mean concentration of 370 pg/mL in 23 alcoholics with antisocial personality disorder significantly higher than 270 pg/mL in 21 healthy control individuals *5479*
Serum *Decrease* Effect observed in chronic alcoholics probably due to effects on both hypothalamic-hypophyseal-gonadal axis and direct effect on testosterone secreting cells *1764* Observed effect due to direct effect on testosterone secreting cells *4348* In 18 chronic alcoholics mean concentration of 0.40 (range of 0.06 - 0.95) nmol/L not significantly less than 0.46 (0.17 - 0.69) nmol/L in 10 abstinent controls *3069* Decrease observed in alcoholic men *37*

Thiamine *Serum* *Decrease* Concentration significantly reduced in heavy drinkers but free thiamine concentration unchanged *4193*

Tissue Plasminogen Activator *Plasma* *Increase* Increase observed in patients with mild and severe liver cirrhosis *5442*

Tissue Plasminogen Activator Antigen *Plasma* *No Effect* In chronic alcoholics with normal liver function concentration remains within normal range *5442*

Tissue Plasminogen Activator Inhibitor *Plasma* *Increase* In chronic alcoholics with abnormal liver function tests but without evidence of cirrhosis antigen concentrations about twice as high as in controls and in those with cirrhosis antigen concentration increased about 6-fold *5442*

Tolbutamide *Serum* *Decrease* Metabolism stimulated in long term alcohol abusers and effect continues for several days to weeks after abuse ended *3038*

303.90 Alcoholism *(continued)*

Transferrin Saturation *Serum* *Increase* In 159 alcoholic patients (119 men and 40 women) admitted to a detoxification center median saturation of 38% (range 5 - 100) significantly greater than 29% (range 6 - 59) in an age and sex matched control group *1526*

Transketolase (Thiamine Activation)
Red Blood Cells *Increase* Increased activation (reflecting vitamin B_1 deficiency) observed in 11 of 35 patients (31%) *250*

Triglycerides *Serum* *Increase* In 26 male alcoholics immediately following a drinking binge mean concentration of 1.33 mmol/L significantly increased compared with 0.97 mmol/L in 17 healthy controls *2650* In 84 chronic alcoholic patients with increased plasma immunoreactive trypsin concentration mean concentration of 1.94 ± 1.15 mmol/L compared with 1.12 ± 0.66 mmol/L in 62 with normal plasma immunoreactive trypsin concentration *2474* In 59 male alcoholics mean concentration of 164 ± 33 mg/dL significantly higher than 126 ± 31 mg/dL in 140 controls. In 13 alcoholic women mean concentration of 103 ± 29 mg/dL not significantly different from 93 ± 41 mg/dL in 145 healthy controls *2305* Rise after ingestion of moderate amounts of alcohol due to increased hepatic production and release of lipoproteins *1980* Significant increase observed in 653 women regardless of degree of obesity with alcohol intakes of more than 10 g/d *1572* With long term alcohol intake serum triglyceride concentration greatly increased *929* In 9 of 28 chronic alcoholics (33%) on admission to hospital mean concentration increased above normal range of 0.28 to 1.81 µmol/L *786* 38% of the patients had a type IV hyperlipoproteinemia with elevated serum triglycerides still after 17 days of abstinence *5551* In 104 alcohloic men mean concentration of 2.21 ± 1.51 mmol/L significantly higher than 1.35 ± 0.60 mmol/L in 37 teetotalers. Mean concentration of 1.55 ± 0.94 mmol/L in 137 moderate drinkers and 1.95 ± 1.55 mmol/L in 90 heavy drinkers *4837* Mean concentration in 11 alcoholics of 3.64 ± 1.8 mmol/L significantly greater than 1.23 ± 0.21 mmol/L in 20 healthy controls *4257* In alcoholics may be both fatty liver and increased serum triglycerides due to increased triglyceride synthesis *37* 19 (26%) of these male patients had serum concentrations > 150 mg/dL *3051*

Trypsin *Serum* *Increase* In 43 of 300 drunken drivers activity increased *3779* In 146 male chronic alcoholics 84 showed high trypsin-like activity (47.0 ± 23.1 mmol/min/L) and 62 showed normal activity (10.9 ± 7.1 mmol/min/L) *2474*

Tryptophan *Cerebrospinal Fluid* *No Effect* In 5 chronically alcoholic men mean concentration of 1,967 ± 544 pmol/mL not significantly different from 2,148 ± 595 pmol/mL in 6 healthy controls *1700*

Tubular Maximum for Phosphate *Urine* *No Effect* In 8 long-term alcoholic men mean of 2.7 ± 0.7 mg/dL glomerular filtrate not significantly different from reference range of 3.2 ± 1.1 mg/dL glomerular filtrate *450*

Tumor Necrosis Factor *Serum* *Increase* Concentration increased in chronic alcoholics *2667*

Urea Nitrogen *Serum* *No Effect* In 23 actively drinking alcohol-habituated individuals mean concentration of 9 ± 4 mg/dL not significantly different from 12 ± 4 mg/dL in 10 alcohol-naive control individuals *2176*

Uric Acid *Serum* *Increase* Increased lactic acid concentration inhibits uric acid excretion in the distal renal tubule. Usually decreases to normal within 1 week after abstinence *1980*

Urokinase Plasminogen Activator *Plasma* *Increase* Significant increase observed in chronic alcoholics without abnormal liver function tests and in those with abnormal liver function and in those with cirrhosis *5442*

Vasopressin *Cerebrospinal Fluid* *No Effect* Mean concentration in 23 alcoholic patients with antisocial behavior not significantly different from that in 21 healthy control individuals *5479*

Vitamin B_{12} *Serum* *No Effect* In 18 male alcoholics following recent debauche mean concentration of 338 nmol/L compared with reference interval of 135 - 735 nmol/L *2824*

Vitamin D Binding Protein *Serum* *No Effect* No significant difference observed between concentrations in 35 hospitalized male alcoholics and 35 healthy age matched controls *460*

Vitamin E *Red Blood Cells* *Decrease* Mean concentration in 25 chronic alcoholics 83% of value in 25 age and sex matched healthy controls *1741*
Serum *Decrease* In 25 chronic alcoholics mean concentration 89% of that in 25 age and sex matched healthy controls *1741*

VLDL-Cholesterol *Serum* *No Effect* Mean concentration in 26 male alcoholics 0.28 mmol/L not significantly different from that in 17 healthy controls (0.26 mmol/L) *2650*

VLDL-Phospholipids *Serum* *No Effect* No significant difference observed between mean concentration in 26 male alcoholics, 0.26 mmol/L, and 0.19 mmol/L in 17 healthy controls *2650*

VLDL-Triglycerides *Serum* *Increase* Mean concentration of 0.83 mmol/L in 26 male alcoholics significantly increased compared with mean of 0.48 mmol/L in 17 healthy controls *2650*
Serum *No Effect* In chronic alcoholic men with normal liver function normal VLDL-triglyceride concentration observed *929*

Zinc *Hair* *Increase* In 23 alcoholic patients mean concentration of 205.2 ± 4.9 µg/g not significantly different from mean concentration in 30 healthy control individuals of 183.5 ± 4.7 µg/g *2614*
Nails *No Effect* In 22 alcoholic patients mean concentration of 201.6 ± 9.5 µg/g not significantly different from mean concentration in 30 healthy control individuals of 209.0 ± 12.0 µg/g *2614*
Serum *Decrease* Statistically significant *310* In chronic alcoholism zinc deficiency observed *4348* Statistically significant *4871* Mean concentration in male alcoholics significantly less than in control patients *5742* Serum concentration reduced below normal range of 11.48 to 21.42 µmol/L in 3 of 27 chronic alcoholics on admission to hospital *786* Elevated in alcoholics with normal or fatty liver and low in those with alcoholic hepatitis or cirrhosis *2038*
Serum *Increase* Elevated in alcoholics with normal or fatty liver and low in those with alcoholic hepatitis or cirrhosis *2038* Nonsignificant increase to 12.8 ± 3.4 µmol/L (84 ± 22 µg/dL) in patients with alcoholic liver disease without cirrhosis but with significant reductions observed in those with moderate or severe alcoholic cirrhosis *1709*

303.90 Chronic Alcoholism

Alanine Aminotransferase *Serum* *No Effect* Median activity of 34 U/L in 13 patients with alcoholism compared with 26 U/L in 8 healthy controls *4146*

Albumin *Serum* *Decrease* In 12 detoxified alcohol-dependent patients mean concentration of 39.67 ± 3.45 g/dL significantly different from 46.72 ± 3.38 g/dL in 12 controls *1078* Median concentration of 4.1 g/dL in 13 patients with alcoholism and 4.7 g/dL in 8 healthy controls *4146*
Serum *No Effect* In 14 alcoholic patients without liver disease mean concentration of 44 ± 5 g/L not significantly different from normal range of 35 - 50 g/L *2932*

Aspartate Aminotransferase *Serum* *No Effect* Median activity of 29 U/L in 13 patients with alcoholism compared with 26 U/L in 8 healthy controls *4146* In 14 alcoholic patients without liver disease mean activity of 32 ± 3 U/L not significantly different from normal range of 10 - 40 U/L *2932*

Bilirubin *Serum* *Increase* In 8 patients with chronic alcoholism and liver disease mean concentration of 4.0 ± 3.2 mg/dL significantly greater than 0.6 ± 0.3 mg/dL in 23 healthy controls *5493*
Serum *No Effect* In 14 alcoholic patients without liver disease mean concentration of 0.9 ± 0.1 mg/dL not significantly different from normal range of 0.1 - 1.0 mg/dL *2932*

Cholesterol *Serum* *Decrease* In 8 patients with chronic alcoholic intoxication and liver disease mean concentration of 161 ± 61 mg/dL nonsignificantly reduced compared with 191 ± 33 mg/dL in 23 healthy controls *5493*
Serum *No Effect* Median concentration of 5.2 mmol/L in 13 patients with alcoholism compared with 4.9 mmol/L in 8 healthy controls *4146*

Cortisol *Plasma* *Increase* Patients with a history of chronic alcohol abuse may have classical clinical and biochemical features of Cushing's syndrome with raised midnight serum cortisol *5723*
Urine *Increase* Patients with a history of chronic alcohol abuse may have classical clinical and biochemical features of Cushing's syndrome with raised urinary excretion of cortisol *5723*

Creatine Kinase Isoenzymes *Serum* *Increase* Increased release of non-myocardial CK *768*

Dexamethasone Suppression *Patient Abnormal* Patients with a history of chronic alcohol abuse may have classical clinical and biochemical features of Cushing's syndrome. In such patients may be a lack of suppression of cortisol concentration with dexamethasone suppression test *5723*

Dihydrotestosterone *Serum No Effect* In 13 chronic alcoholics mean bioavailable concentration not significantly different from that in healthy controls *4629*

Erythrocytes *Blood No Effect* In 13 patients with alcoholism median concentration of 4.7 x $10^6/\mu L$ and 4.6 x $10^6/\mu L$ in 8 healthy controls *4146*

α_1-Globulin *Serum No Effect* In 12 detoxified alcohol-dependent patients mean concentration of 2.32 ± 0.35 g/L not significantly different from 2.37 ± 0.35 g/L in 12 controls *1078*

α_2-Globulin *Serum No Effect* In 12 detoxified alcohol-dependent patients mean concentration of 6.68 ± 0.70 g/L not significantly different from 6.43 ± 1.47 g/L in 12 controls *1078*

β-Globulin *Serum Decrease* In 12 detoxified alcohol-dependent patients mean concentration of 7.98 ± 0.89 g/L significantly different from 9.05 ± 1.11 g/L in 12 controls *1078*

γ-Globulin *Serum No Effect* In 14 alcoholic patients without liver disease mean concentration of 9.0 ± 0.2 g/L not significantly different from normal range of 6 - 16 g/L *2932* In 12 detoxified alcohol-dependent patients mean concentration of 8.88 ± 2.21 g/dL not significantly different from 10.03 ± 2.28 g/dL in 12 controls *1078*

γ-Glutamyltransferase *Serum Increase* In 14 alcoholic patients without liver disease mean activity of 113 ± 30 U/L significantly different from normal range of 4 - 60 U/L *2932* Median activity of 66 U/L in 13 patients with alcoholism compared with 23 U/L in 8 healthy controls *4146*

HDL-Cholesterol *Serum Increase* Increased mortality observed in heavy drinkers with HDL-cholesterol concentration greater than 0.90 mmol/L *4042*

Hemoglobin *Blood No Effect* In 14 alcoholic patients without liver disease mean concentration of 13 ± 0.1 g/dL not significantly different from normal range of 13 - 17 g/dL *2932*

β-Hexosaminidase *Serum Increase* Activity increased in patients with chronic alcoholism *2291*

β-Hexosaminidase Isoenzyme P *Serum Increase* Activity substantially increased in patients with chronic alcoholism *2291*

Interleukin-6 *Serum Increase* In 12 detoxified alcohol-dependent patients mean concentration of 16.09 ± 25.43 pg/mL significantly different from 4.09 ± 5.16 pg/mL in 12 controls *1078*

Interleukin-8 *Serum Increase* In 12 detoxified alcohol-dependent patients mean concentration of 300 ± 303 pg/mL significantly different from 70 ± 111 pg/mL in 12 controls *1078*

6-Keto-Prostaglandin $F_{1\alpha}$ *Plasma No Effect* Median concentration of 71.2 pg/mL in 13 patients with alcoholism compared with 67.0 pg/mL in 8 healthy controls *4146*

Leukocytes *Blood No Effect* In 14 alcoholic patients without liver disease mean concentration of 8,077 ± 1,022 x 10^6/L not significantly different from normal range of 4,500 - 10,000 x 10^6/L *2932*

Luteinizing Hormone *Plasma No Effect* In 13 chronic alcoholics mean concentration not significantly different from that in healthy controls, although alcoholics tended to have higher concentration in morning *4629*

Lymphocytes *Blood No Effect* In 14 alcoholic patients without liver disease mean concentration of 3,332 ± 601 x 10^6/L not significantly different from normal range of 1,300 - 4,000 x 10^6/L *2932*

Magnesium *Serum Decrease* Concentration is reduced in association with malabsorption of chronic alcoholism *2952*

MCV *Blood No Effect* In 13 patients with alcoholism median MCV of 92 fL compared with 91 fL in 8 healthy controls *4146*

Osteocalcin *Serum No Effect* With ExtrAvidin® -biotin system method the mean concentration in patients with chronic alcoholism of 0.6 ± 0.3 nmol/L not significantly different from that in healthy adults, 1.4 ± 0.8 nmol/L *2417*

Phenytoin *Serum Decrease* In patients who abuse alcohol treated with fosphenytoin, concentration of phenytoin may be decreased *4007*

Phospholipids *Serum No Effect* In 8 patients with chronic alcoholic intoxication and liver disease mean concentration of 223 ± 21 mg/dL not significantly different from 214 ± 42 mg/dL in 23 healthy controls *5493*

Platelets *Blood No Effect* Median count of 250 x $10^3/\mu L$ in 13 patients with alcoholism and 255 x $10^3/\mu L$ in 8 healthy controls *4146*

Prolactin *Plasma No Effect* In 13 chronic alcoholics mean concentration not significantly different from that in healthy controls *4629*

Protein *Serum Decrease* In 12 detoxified alcohol-dependent patients mean concentration of 65.50 ± 6.05 mg/dL significantly different from 74.58 ± 4.10 mg/dL in 12 controls *1078*

Prothrombin Time *Plasma No Effect* In 14 alcoholic patients without liver disease mean time of 97 ± 3% not significantly different from normal range of 80 - 100% *2932*

Testosterone *Serum No Effect* In 13 chronic alcoholics mean bioavailable concentration not significantly different from that in healthy controls *4629*

Thiamine *Red Blood Cells Decrease* In 85 chronic alcoholics ingesting more than 50 g alcohol/d for at least one year mean concentration of 2.9 ± 2.7 nmol/L significantly different when compared with 4.0 ± 2.0 nmol/L in 28 healthy women and 24 healthy men *2133*

Thiamine Diphosphate *Red Blood Cells Decrease* In 85 chronic alcoholics ingesting more than 50 g alcohol/d for at least one year mean concentration of 148 ± 54.7 nmol/L significantly different when compared with 176 ± 28.0 nmol/L in 28 healthy women and 24 healthy men *2133*

Thiamine Phosphate *Red Blood Cells No Effect* In 85 chronic alcoholics ingesting more than 50 g alcohol/d for at least one year mean concentration of < 2 nmol/L not significantly different when compared with < 2 nmol/L in 28 healthy women and 24 healthy men *2133*

Thiamine Triphosphate *Red Blood Cells Decrease* In 85 chronic alcoholics ingesting more than 50 g alcohol/d for at least one year mean concentration of 4.9 ± 3.9 nmol/L significantly different when compared with 7.0 ± 6.0 nmol/L in 28 healthy women and 24 healthy men *2133*

Transketolase *Red Blood Cells Decrease* In 85 chronic alcoholics ingesting more than 50 g alcohol/d for at least one year mean concentration of 153 ± 51.1 U/L significantly different when compared with 165 ± 20.6 U/L in 28 healthy women and 24 healthy men *2133*

Triglycerides *Serum Increase* In 8 patients with chronic alcoholic intoxication and liver disease mean concentration of 129 ± 45 mg/dL not significantly increased compared with 87 ± 23 mg/dL in 23 healthy controls *5493*

Vitamin E *Serum Decrease* In 8 patients with chronic alcoholic intoxication and liver disease mean concentrations of 17.2 ± 0.6 µmol/L and 3.35 ± 0.69 µmol/g lipids significantly reduced compared with 26.0 ± 4.4 µmol/L and 5.28 ± 0.49 µmol/g lipids respectively in 23 healthy controls *5493*

Zinc *Serum Decrease* In 12 detoxified alcohol-dependent patients mean concentration of 111.2 ± 16.9 µg/L significantly different from 124.2 ± 16.9 µg/L in 12 controls *1078*

304.00 Drug Dependence (Opium and Derivatives)

Adenosine Monophosphate *Plasma Decrease* Significantly decreased in heroin addiction *2182*

Alanine Aminotransferase *Serum Increase* This and other liver function tests are increased in 75% of patients *5545*

Amylase *Serum Increase* Large doses of morphine or codeine will provoke a sharp rise *4707* Increased levels were found in 19% of 91 addicts admitted after overdose. The rise was due to elevated salivary-type isoenzyme *402*

Aspartate Aminotransferase *Serum Increase* This and other liver function tests are usually increased in 75% of patients *5545*

Cholesterol *Serum Decrease* Significantly decreased in heroin addiction *2182*

Creatine Kinase *Serum Increase* Following intravenous adulterated heroin associated with myopathy and myoglobinuria *1290* Concentrations up to 14,000 U/L were recorded in heroin addicts *4345*

Eosinophils *Blood Increase* Eosinophilia occurs in 25% of drug addicts *5545*

304.00 Drug Dependence (Opium and Derivatives) *(continued)*

Hepatitis B Surface Antigen *Serum* *Increase* Found in 10% of drug patients *5545*

Lactate Dehydrogenase *Serum* *Increase* Markedly elevated in 4 heroin addicts after admission. Acute skeletal muscle necrosis in all 4 cases, and acute renal failure in 2 of the 4 occurred as a result of intravenous use of heroin-adulterant mixtures *4345*

Lymphocytes *Blood* *Increase* Persistent absolute and relative lymphocytosis occurs with often bizarre and atypical cells that may resemble Downey cells *5545*

Myoglobin *Serum* *Increase* Serum concentrations as high as 0.310 g/L were found in heroin addicts *4345*
Urine *Increase* Acute myoglobinuria up to 3.25 g/L in heroin addicts *4345*

Oxygen Partial Pressure *Blood* *Decrease* Overdose *2034*

Oxygen Saturation *Blood* *Decrease* Overdose *2034*

Thyroxine (T4) *Serum* *Increase* Significantly raised in heroin addiction *2182*

VDRL *Serum* *Positive* Incidence of false positive reactions is 20% in narcotic addicts *2304*

306.10 Hyperventilation Syndrome

Carbon Dioxide Partial Pressure *Blood* *Decrease* Respiratory alkalosis *4706* Characteristically the pCO_2 is reduced to 20 - 30 mm Hg *900*

Ionized Calcium *Serum* *Decrease* Respiratory alkalosis reduces ionized Ca concentration *4706*

pH *Blood* *Increase* The arterial pH is raised to 7.5 - 7.65 *900* Respiratory alkalosis *4706*

Phosphate *Serum* *Decrease* Respiratory alkalosis *4706* Often decreased during prolonged hyperventilation *900*

307.10 Anorexia Nervosa

α_1-Acid Glycoprotein *Serum* *No Effect* In 15 subjects concentration same as that in age and sex matched controls *2082*

Albumin *Serum* *Decrease* Observed effect *565*
Serum *No Effect* In 12 patients with anorexia nervosa serum concentrations of calcium, phosphate, albumin, alkaline phosphatase, parathyroid hormone, calcitonin, osteocalcin, and 24-hour calcium excretion were normal *3907* In 9 Japanese women mean concentration of 44 ± 1 g/L on admission to hospital not significantly different from 44 ± 1 g/L once they had gained 10 kg body weight *2754*

Alkaline Phosphatase *Serum* *No Effect* In 12 patients with anorexia nervosa serum concentrations of calcium, phosphate, albumin, alkaline phosphatase, parathyroid hormone, calcitonin, osteocalcin, and 24-hour calcium excretion were normal *3907* Median activity in 15 previously treated anorexic patients 5.7 ng/mL not different from that in an age-matched control population *4990*

γ-Aminobutyric Acid *Cerebrospinal Fluid* *No Effect* No significant difference observed between concentrations in 33 women with schizophrenia and 14 normal women *1711*

Amylase *Serum* *Increase* May be increased in the absence of signs or symptoms of pancreatitis *565* Measured in 34 patients (average age 28.5 (18 - 64) years) with anorexia nervosa (9 patients) and bulimia (25 patients), hyperamylasaemia was demonstrated in 13 of the 34 patients (38%) *2110*

Androstenediol *Plasma* *Increase* Mean concentration significantly higher in 10 women with anorexia nervosa than in 8 normal women *4874*

Androstenediol Sulfate *Plasma* *No Effect* Mean concentration in 10 women with anorexia nervosa similar to that in 8 normal women *4874*

Angiotensin-converting Enzyme *Serum* *Decrease* In 10 patients with anorexia nervosa mean activity significantly reduced at 9.8 ± 2.2 U/L compared with activity of 13.4 ± 3.5 U/L in normal individuals *3358*
Serum *No Effect* In 9 Japanese women mean concentration of about 12 U/L on admission to hospital significantly different from 17 U/L after 10 kg weight gain but not different from normal range in healthy controls with upper limit of normal of about 11 U/L *2754*

Apolipoprotein B *Serum* *Increase* Concentration tended to be higher in acute phase of illness in 29 young women although tended to normalize as disease became chronic *4554*

Aspartate Aminotransferase *Serum* *Increase* Assocated with muscle dysfunction *2847*

Atrial Natriuretic Peptide *Plasma* *Increase* In patients with anorexia nervosa mean concentration of 55.4 ± 9.0 pg/mL compared with 11.4 ± 6.1 pg/mL in healthy controls but no response to saline infusion in contrast to the 3-fold increase observed in young healthy individuals *3869*

Basal Metabolic Rate *Patient* *Decrease* In 6 women (mean 67% of ideal body weight) mean BMR 4.17 MJ/d compared with 5.52 MJ/d in control individuals *723*

Basophils *Blood* *Decrease* In 67 patients with anorexia nervosa mean concentration of 37 ± 30 /µL significantly less than 48 ± 20 /µL in 67 age and sex matched controls *1139*

Calcitonin *Plasma* *No Effect* In 12 patients with anorexia nervosa serum concentrations of calcium, phosphate, albumin, alkaline phosphatase, parathyroid hormone, calcitonin, osteocalcin, and 24-hour calcium excretion were normal *3907*

Calcium *Cerebrospinal Fluid* *No Effect* No significant difference observed between concentrations in 34 women with anorexia and 14 normal women *1711*
Serum *No Effect* Median concentration in 15 previously treated anorexic patients 5.7 ng/mL not different from that in an age-matched control population *4990* In 12 patients with anorexia nervosa serum concentrations of calcium, phosphate, albumin, alkaline phosphatase, parathyroid hormone, calcitonin, osteocalcin, and 24-hour calcium excretion were normal *3907*
Urine *No Effect* In 12 patients with anorexia nervosa serum concentrations of calcium, phosphate, albumin, alkaline phosphatase, parathyroid hormone, calcitonin, osteocalcin, and 24-hour calcium excretion were normal *3907*

Carotene *Serum* *Increase* Well documented association described with anorexia nervosa but mechanism causing this not known *2642*

β-Carotene *Serum* *Increase* Tend to be elevated *565*

Catecholamines *Urine* *Decrease* Typical observation in adults *355*

Ceruloplasmin *Serum* *No Effect* Observed effect *565* Mean concentration of 230 ± 20 mg/L in 12 anorectic women was the same as in 12 healthy controls although increased significantly to 320 ± 40 mg/L with weight gain in anorectics *289*

Cholecystokinin *Plasma* *Increase* Significantly increased in the anorectic group (1.8 ± 0.4 pmol/L) (p less than or equal to 0.005) *4122*

Cholesterol *Serum* *Increase* Occasionally increased *565* In 29 young female patients concentration tended to be higher at acute phase of illness although tended to normalize during chronic phase *4554*

Choline *Cerebrospinal Fluid* *No Effect* No significant difference observed between concentrations of 33 women with anorexia nervosa and 14 normal women although choline concentration negatively correlated with anorexia severity *1711*

Complement C_2 *Serum* *Decrease* Low levels *565*

Complement C_3 *Serum* *Decrease* Characteristically reduced in patients with anorexia nervosa *2642* Low levels *565*

Complement C_4 *Serum* *No Effect* No apparent effect observed in patients with anorexia nervosa *2642*

Complement CH50 *Serum* *Decrease* Low levels *565*

Copper *Hair* *No Effect* No significant change noted *565*
Serum *Decrease* Observed effect *565*

Corticosteroid-Binding Globulin *Serum* *No Effect* Concentrations typically normal *4234*

Corticotropin *Plasma* *No Effect* No significant difference observed in 6 women with anorexia nervosa compared with healthy controls *723*

Corticotropin-releasing Hormone
Cerebrospinal Fluid *Increase* In underweight patients with anorexia nervosa hypercortisolism observed with significantly increased CRF concentrations *2611*

Cortisol *Plasma Decrease* Decreased despite normal production rates *565*
Plasma Increase In 24 patients with anorexia nervosa before weight gain mean concentration of 20.1 ± 11.1 µg/dL not significantly different from 15.4 ± 4.2 µg/dL in 11 healthy control individuals *1296* Malnourished patients with anorexia nervosa had higher concentrations than in age- and sex-matched controls *2955* Concentration significantly increased in patients when emaciated (at 9, 10, 11, and 12 p.m. and at 6 a.m.) compared with concentrations in refed state and in control population *2639* In both men and women with anorexia nervosa concentration increased with loss of circadian rhythm and slight inhibition by dexamethasone *1074* High despite normal production rates. This is due to decreased metabolism and prolongation of plasma half-life *565* Has been observed *2888* In patients with anorexia nervosa morning and mean 24-hour concentration with either normal or abnormal diurnal rhythm observed *355* In 15 patients with this disorder (one male and 14 female) aged 14 - 26 y high midnight concentrations *4788* Mean concentration significantly higher in 10 patients with anorexia nervosa than in 8 normal women *4874*
Plasma No Effect No significant difference observed in 6 women with anorexia nervosa compared with healthy controls *723*

Cortisol, Free *Urine Increase* Excretion typically higher than in controls *355*

C-Peptide *Plasma Decrease* Undetectable in plasma in one woman with long-standing anorexia nervosa with severe emaciation during hypoglycemic episode *1522*

Creatine Kinase *Serum Increase* Assocated with muscle dysfunction *2847*

Creatinine *Serum Decrease* Concentration significantly reduced in patients with anorexia nervosa but increased with refeeding *493*
Serum No Effect In 9 Japanese women mean concentration of 62.8 ± 3.4 µmol/L on admission to hospital not significantly different from 60.7 ± 3.5 µmol/L once they had gained 10 kg body weight *2754*
Urine Decrease Excretion diminished in all patients with anorexia nervosa compared with situation after refeeding *493*

Creatinine Clearance *Urine Decrease* Significantly reduced in patients with anorexia nervosa but increased with refeeding *493* Clearance improves by a mean of 80% following treatment *4048*

C-terminal Propeptide of Type I Collagen *Serum Increase* Median concentration in 15 previously treated anorexic patients of 163 ± 219 ng/mL significantly increased compared with 112 ± 79 ng/mL in an age-matched control population *4990*
Serum No Effect Median concentration in 28 previously untreated anorexic patients of 112 ± 29 ng/mL compared with 112 ± 79 ng/mL in an age-matched control population *4990*

C-terminal Propeptide of Type I Procollagen *Serum Increase* In 36 patients with anorexia nervosa aged 17 - 46 years mean concentration of 6.5 ± 4.2 µg/L increased by about 70% compared with 16 age-matched controls *3190*

C-terminal Telopeptide of Type I Collagen *Serum Increase* Median concentration in 15 previously treated anorexic patients 5.7 ng/mL significantly increased compared with 3.9 ng/mL in an age-matched control population *4990*

Dehydroepiandrosterone *Plasma Increase* In 10 women with anorexia nervosa mean concentration significantly higher than in 8 normal women *4874*

Dehydroepiandrosterone Sulfate *Plasma Decrease* Mean concentration significantly lower in 10 women with anorexia nervosa than in 8 normal women *4874*

Deoxypyridinoline *Urine Increase* In 36 patients with anorexia nervosa aged 17 - 46 years mean excretion of 19.3 ± 14.3 nmol/mmol creatinine increased by about 90% compared with 16 age-matched controls *3190* Median concentration in 28 previously untreated anorexic patients of 17.8 ± 15.2 nmol/mmol creatinine compared with 9.2 ± 4.0 nmol/mmol creatinine in an age-matched control population *4990*

Dexamethasone Suppression *Patient Abnormal* Two patients showed minor abnormal false positive result with 1 mg overnight dose of dexamethasone and lack of suppression of cortisol concentration with dexamethasone suppression test *5723*

1,25-Dihydroxy Vitamin D *Serum Decrease* In 2 of 17 patients with anorexia nervosa mean concentration reduced below normal *1523* In 12 patients with anorexia nervosa, the 1,25-dihydroxyvitamin D (1,25 (OH)2D) concentrations were significantly reduced in patients (62 ± 17 pmol/L vs 82 ± 17 pmol/L); p less than 0.05) *3907*

3,3'-Dityrosine *Serum Increase* Typically observed in patients with anorexia nervosa *355*

β-Endorphin *Cerebrospinal Fluid Decrease* Women with bulimia had significantly lower concentrations *582*
Plasma Increase The morning levels of immunoreactive-β-endorphin and 17β-estradiol were assessed in 25 adolescents with this disorder and compared with 24 healthy controls. The mean level was significantly higher (84%) when compared to the control group *5195*

Eosinophils *Blood Decrease* In 67 patients mean concentration of 97 ± 110 /µL significantly less than 140 ± 120 /µL in 67 age and sex matched controls *1139*

Epinephrine *Plasma Increase* Malnourished patients with anorexia nervosa had higher concentrations than in age- and sex-matched controls *2955*

Estradiol *Plasma Decrease* In 12 anorectic women mean concentration of 73.4 ± 1.1 pmol/L significantly decreased compared with 176.2 ± 22.0 pmol/L in 12 healthy controls and little change to 77.0 ± 0.7 pmol/L with weight gain in anoretics *289* In 24 women with anorexia nervosa mean concentration of 0.07 ± 0.03 nmol/L significantly different from 0.20 ± 0.10 nmoll/L in 10 healthy control women *5033* In 22 women aged 23 ± 4 y mean concentration of 46 ± 31 pg/mL low and consistent with concentrations seen in the early follicular phase *1876*
Urine Decrease Reduced excretion observed in 20 women with anorexia nervosa *1074*

Estrogens *Plasma Decrease* In 20 patients with anorexia nervosa before weight gain mean concentration of total estrogens of 126.7 ± 71.0 pg/mL not significantly different from 196.3 ± 129.6 pg/mL in 12 healthy control individuals *1296* Significantly lower *819*

Factor VIII Antigen *Plasma Increase* In 9 Japanese women mean concentration of 129.2 ± 14.1% on admission to hospital significantly different from 88.2 ± 9.7% after 10 kg weight gain and normal range in healthy controls of 50 - 155% *2754*

Fatty Acids (FFA), Free *Serum Increase* In the majority of a group of patients with anorexia nervosa concentration increased *4145*

Fibronectin *Plasma Decrease* In 9 Japanese women mean concentration of 211.5 ± 14.9 µg/mL on admission to hospital significantly different from 274.7 ± 16.6 µg/mL after 10 kg weight gain and normal range in healthy controls of 250 - 460 µg/mL *2754*

Follicle Stimulating Hormone *Plasma Decrease* In 22 patients with anorexia nervosa before weight gain mean concentration of 3.9 ± 7.1 IU/L not significantly different from 5.3 ± 2.8 IU/L in 12 healthy control individuals *1296* Usual finding in both adults and children *355* In 15 patients with this disorder (one male and 14 females) aged 14 - 26 years *4788* Basal levels are low when weight loss is severe. Response to LHRH is normal *565* Effect observed in extreme cases *2148* In 24 women with anorexia nervosa mean concentration of 2.2 ± 0.4 IE/L significantly different from 5.1 ± 1.0 IE/L in 10 healthy control women *5033*

Galanin *Plasma No Effect* Mean concentration in 15 women with anorexia nervosa not significantly different from 21.6 ± 7.0 pg/mL observed in 19 lean healthy women *287*

Glucose *Serum Decrease* Effect observed in extreme cases *2148* In one woman with severe emaciation due to long-standing anorexia nervosa recurrent hypoglycemia observed *1522* Mean concentration in 10 patients with anorexia nervosa significantly less than in 15 healthy controls *4670* In both men and women with anorexia nervosa basal concentration reduced with flat glucose tolerance curve *1074*
Serum Increase Glucose tolerance is abnormal as in other forms of starvation *565*
Serum No Effect In 24 women with anorexia nervosa mean concentration of 4.1 ± 0.1 mmol/L not significantly different from 3.9 ± 0.7 mmoll/L in 10 healthy control women *5033*

Growth Hormone *Plasma Decrease* In 18 patients with anorexia nervosa before weight gain mean concentration of 5.6 ± 6.9 µg/L not significantly different from 3.6 ± 5.1 µg/L in 11 healthy control individuals *1296*
Plasma Increase May be normal or increased in the basal state. A rise in GH occurs after injection of thyrotropin-releasing

307.10 **Anorexia Nervosa** *(continued)*

Growth Hormone *(continued)*
hormone *565* In 15 patients with this disorder (one male and 14 female) aged 14 - 26 y high basal levels *4788* Fasting levels were significantly increased *946* Basal concentration increased in both men and women with anorexia nervosa *1074* In 24 women with anorexia nervosa mean concentration of 15.7 ± 3.2 mU/L significantly different from 2.9 ± 0.8 mU/L in 10 healthy control women *5033*
Plasma No Effect May be normal or increased in the basal state. A rise in GH occurs after injection of thyrotropin-releasing hormone *565*

Growth Hormone Binding Protein *Serum Decrease* In 24 women with anorexia nervosa mean concentration of 0.63 ± 0.086 nmol/L significantly different from 1.02 ± 0.16 nmol/L in 10 healthy control women *5033*

Hematocrit *Blood Decrease* Effect observed in extreme cases *2148* Anemia *565* In 25 patients with this disorder between the ages of 12 and 38 the mean value was 36%. The anemia was normocytic in 7, hypochromic in 7 and megaloblastic in 2 *2926*

Hemoglobin *Blood Decrease* Effect observed in extreme cases *2148* Anemia *565* In 67 patients with anorexia nervosa mean concentration of 131 ± 19 g/L reduced, although still within normal range, compared with 137 ± 1‑ g/L in 67 age and sex matched controls *1139*

Homocysteine *Plasma Increase* In 27 patients with anorexia nervosa aged 11 to 10 years median concentration of 9.5 µmol/L and in 16 aged 16 - 18 y 11.2 µmol/L significantly increased compared with 6.6 µmol/L and 8.1 µmol/L in healthy children in the same age groups *5471*

Homovanillic Acid *Cerebrospinal Fluid Decrease* Significantly lower concentration in bulemic patients *2449*
Cerebrospinal Fluid No Effect No significant difference observed between concentrations in 33 women with anorexia and 14 normal women *1711*
Plasma Increase In 9 patients with anorexia nervosa mean concentration of 21.8 ± 8.1 ng/mL significantly higher than 13.4 ± 3.7 ng/mL in 29 healthy controls *549*

4-Hydroxy-3-Methoxy-Phenylglycol
Cerebrospinal Fluid No Effect Nonsignificant increase observed in concentration in 33 anorexic women compared with 14 normal women *1711*
Plasma Increase In 9 patients with anorexia nervosa mean concentration of 4.1 ± 1.3 ng/mL significantly higher than 3.0 ± 0.5 ng/mL in 29 healthy controls *549*
Urine No Effect No significant difference from excretion in normal individuals unless complicating depression in which case excretion significantly reduced *445*

25-Hydroxy Vitamin D *Serum Decrease* Concentrations below normal were observed in 88% of 17 patients *1523*
Serum No Effect In 12 patients with anorexia nervosa serum 25-hydroxyvitamin D (25-OHD) concentration was similar in patients and normal subjects *3907*

β-Hydroxybutyrate *Serum Increase* In majority of a group of patients with anorexia nervosa concentration increased *4145*

17-Hydroxycorticosteroids *Urine Decrease* Either normal or reduced excretion typically observed *355*

5-Hydroxyindoleacetic Acid *Cerebrospinal Fluid Decrease* In 9 low weight anorectics mean concentration of 107.2 ± 31.4 nmol/L significantly different from 146.3 ± 30.2 nmol/L in 8 healthy normals *1114* Significantly lower concentration in bulemic patients *2449*
Cerebrospinal Fluid No Effect No significant difference observed between concentrations in 33 women with anorexia and 14 normal women *1711*

5-Hydroxytryptamine *Blood No Effect* Mean whole blood concentration of 429 ± 27 nmol/mL in 10 anorexic patients with bulimic attitudes and 395 ± 243 nmol/mL in 9 patients with anorexia but without bulimic attitudes not significantly different from 372 ± 98 nmol/mL observed in 12 healthy controls *198*

Immunoglobulin G *Serum Decrease* Low levels *565*

Immunoglobulin M *Serum Decrease* Low levels *565*

Insulin *Plasma Decrease* Undetectable amount in plasma of one woman with severe emaciation due to anorexia nervosa during an episode of hypoglycemia *1522* Mean concentration of 3.6 ± 0.42 µU/mL in 11 anorectic women significantly different from 6.4 ± 0.64 µU/mL in 35 normal weight control women *2342* Reduced concentration observed with slight increase after glucose administration in both men and women with anorexia nervosa *1074* Mean concentration in 10 patients with anorexia nervosa significantly less than in 15 healthy controls *4670* In 24 women with anorexia nervosa mean concentration of 19 ± 3 pmol/L significantly different from 41 ± 6 pmoll/L in 10 healthy control women *5033*

Insulin-like Growth Factor-I *Serum Decrease* In 24 women with anorexia nervosa mean concentration of 166.5 ± 19.8 µg/L significantly different from 244.1 ± 17.6 µg/L in 10 healthy control women *5033* In 29 patients with anorexia nervosa before weight gain mean concentration of 186.6 ± 69.7 µg/L significantly different from 326.4 ± 81.8 µg/L in 14 healthy control individuals *1296* In 14 patients on admission to hospital mean concentration of 20.8 ± 3.5 nmol/L which increased to 31.0 ± 2.2 nmol/L after 4 weeks. Admission concentration low compared with healthy controls *2160* In 22 women aged 23 ± 4 y mean concentration of 202 ± 93 ng/mL significantly reduced compared with 310 ± 72 ng/mL with 23 age-matched healthy women *1876*

Insulin-like Growth Factor-I, Free *Serum Decrease* In 24 women with anorexia nervosa mean concentration of 410.1 ± 83.4 ng/L significantly different from 1,333 ± 188.3 ng/L in 10 healthy control women *5033*

Insulin-like Growth Factor-II *Serum Decrease* In 24 women with anorexia nervosa mean concentration of 820.6 ± 49.5 µg/L significantly different from 929.9 ± 37.0 µg/L in 10 healthy control women *5033* Insulin-like growth factor-I, growth hormone binding protein and insulin-like growth factor binding protein-3 were all significantly decreased in low weight patients with this disorder and returned to nearly normal with refeeding. Insulin-like growth factor-II was 27% lower in the low weight group than in normal subjects *946*

Insulin-like Growth Factor-II, Free *Serum Decrease* In 24 women with anorexia nervosa mean concentration of 578.6 ± 88.9 ng/L significantly different from 1259 ± 130.1 ng/L in 10 healthy control women *5033*

Insulin-like Growth Factor Binding Protein-1
Serum Increase In 24 women with anorexia nervosa mean concentration of 27.1 ± 7.9 µg/L significantly different from 4.24 ± 0.71 µg/L in 10 healthy control women *5033*

Insulin-like Growth Factor Binding Protein-2
Serum Increase In 24 women with anorexia nervosa mean concentration of 852.6 ± 108 µg/L not significantly different from 543.3 ± 63.1 µg/L in 10 healthy control women *5033*

Insulin-like Growth Factor Binding Protein-3
Serum Decrease In 24 women with anorexia nervosa mean concentration of 2,958 ± 217 µg/L significantly different from 3,656 ± 199 µg/L in 10 healthy control women *5033*

Insulin-like Growth Factor Binding Protein-4
Serum No Effect In 24 women with anorexia nervosa mean concentration of 106.7 ± 5.9 AU/mm³ not significantly different from 104.4 ± 7.9 AU/mm³ in 10 healthy control women *5033*

Interleukin-6 *Serum Increase* Serum IL-6 and TGF-β concentrations were both significantly elevated during starvation and returned to levels comparable to those of normal-weight controls by the end of therapy *4172*

Iron *Serum No Effect* Observed effect *565*

Iron-binding Capacity, Total *Serum Decrease* Observed effect with prolonged disease *565*

Kynurenic Acid *Cerebrospinal Fluid Decrease* Measured in medication-free female patients meeting DSM-III-R criteria for either anorexia nervosa (n = 10) or normal-weight bulimia nervosa (n = 22), studied at varying stages of nutritional recovery. Eight healthy, normal-weight females served as a comparison group. Cerebrospinal fluid levels of kynurenic acid were significantly reduced in underweight anorectics, compared to normal females, but returned to normal values with restoration of normal body weight *1114* In 9 low weight anorectics mean concentration of 1.5 ± 0.5 nmol/L significantly different from 2.8 ± 1.2 nmol/L in 8 healthy normals *1114*

Kynurenine *Cerebrospinal Fluid No Effect* In 9 low weight anorectics mean concentration of 25.6 ± 9.9 nmol/L not significantly different from 34.4 ± 12.3 nmol/L in 8 healthy normals *1114*

Lactate Dehydrogenase *Serum Increase* Assocated with muscle dysfunction *2847*

Leptin *Serum* *Decrease* Mean concentration in 15 women with anorexia nervosa of 18.8 ± 1.5 ng/mL significantly different from 31.7 ± 2.4 ng/mL observed in 19 lean healthy women *287* Using ELISA procedure of Imagawa et al mean concentration of 0.343 ± 0.266 μg/L in 16 anorexic women significantly less than 8.48 ± 5.84 μg/L in 15 healthy women *2327* In 29 patients with anorexia nervosa before weight gain mean concentration of 3.6 ± 1.6 ng/mL significantly different from 12.0 ± 6.9 ng/mL in 14 healthy control individuals *1296* In 24 female patients with anorexia nervosa best predictor for serum leptin concentration is percentage body fat *3347* In 22 women aged 23 ± 4 y mean concentration of 5.6 ± 3.7 ng/mL significantly reduced compared with 19.1 ± 8.1 ng/mL with 23 age-matched healthy women *1876*

Leukocytes *Blood* *Decrease* Leukopenia *565* In 67 patients with anorexia nervosa mean concentration of 4,940 ± 1,900 /μL significantly less than 6,780 ± 2,400 /μL in 67 age and sex matched controls *1139* Effect observed in extreme cases *2148*

Lipase *Serum* *Increase* Measured in 34 patients (average age 28.5 (18 - 64) years) anorexia nervosa (9 patients) and bulimia (25 patients). In only two of them was there an elevated concentration of lipase and human pancreatic lipase *2110*

Lipase, Pancreatic *Serum* *Increase* Measured in 34 patients (average age 28.5 (18 - 64) years) anorexia nervosa (9 patients) and bulimia (25 patients). In only two of them was there an elevated concentration of lipase and human pancreatic lipase *2110*

Luteinizing Hormone *Plasma* *Decrease* Effect observed in extreme cases *2148* In 24 women with anorexia nervosa mean concentration of 0.7 ± 0.2 IE/L significantly different from 0.7 ± 0.2 IE/L in 10 healthy control women *5033* Basal levels are low when weight loss is severe. Response to LHRH is impaired *565* In 22 patients with anorexia nervosa before weight gain mean concentration of 1.0 ± 2.1 IU/L significantly different from 6.1 ± 6.1 IU/L in 13 healthy control individuals *1296* In 15 patients with this disorder (one male and 14 female) aged 14 - 26 y *4788* Usual observation in both adults and children with protein calorie malnutrition *355*

Lymphocytes *Blood* *Decrease* In 67 patients with anorexia nervosa mean concentration of 1,740 ± 730 /μL significantly less than 2,010 ± 630 /μL in 67 age and sex matched controls *1139*

Melatonin *Plasma* *Increase* Plasma melatonin levels were measured at three-hourly intervals over 24 hours in 11 women with untreated anorexia nervosa, and in nine healthy women of normal weight. The circadian rhythm was unaltered but the nocturnal secretion of melatonin was significantly greater in anorectics *172*
Plasma *No Effect* No significant difference observed in patients when emaciated, when refed, and in comparison with control population *2639* Mean daily peak concentration in 7 women with anorexia nervosa of 325 ± 43 pmol/L not significantly different from 334 ± 30 pmol/L in 21 normal cycling control women *3621*

Monocytes *Blood* *Decrease* Mean concentration of 240 ± 150 /μL in 67 patients with anorexia nervosa significantly less than 350 ± 130 /μL in 67 age and sex matched controls *1139*

Neopterin *Cerebrospinal Fluid* *No Effect* In 9 low weight anorectics mean concentration of 13.1 ± 5.1 nmol/L not significantly different from 13.7 ± 4.5 nmol/L in 8 healthy normals *1114*

Neuropeptide Y *Cerebrospinal Fluid* *Increase* In underweight anorectic patients and in many studied at intervals after weight restoration concentration significantly increased *2609*
Plasma *No Effect* Mean concentration in 15 women with anorexia nervosa not significantly different from 3.1 ± 0.3 pg/mL observed in 19 lean healthy women *287*

Neutrophils *Blood* *Decrease* In 67 patients with anorexia nervosa mean concentration of 2,790 ± 1,520 /μL to 4,090 ± 1,900 /μL in 67 age and sex matched controls *1139*

Norepinephrine *Plasma* *Decrease* Concentrations are depressed *565* Malnourished patients with anorexia nervosa had significantly lower concentrations than in age- and sex-matched controls *2955* In adults typical observation *355*
Urine *Decrease* In both men and women with anorexia nervosa concentration reduced *1074*

Osteocalcin *Serum* *Decrease* In 7 of 14 patients with anorexia nervosa mean concentration reduced below normal range *1523* Reported effect *1523*
Serum *No Effect* In 12 patients with anorexia nervosa serum concentrations of calcium, phosphate, albumin, alkaline phosphatase, parathyroid hormone, calcitonin, osteocalcin, and 24-hour calcium excretion were normal *3907*

Oxytocin *Cerebrospinal Fluid* *Decrease* Decreased in five underweight women with restricting anorexia compared with 11 control subjects *1115*

Parathyroid Hormone *Plasma* *Decrease* In 2 of 17 patients mean concentration reduced below normal range *1523*
Plasma *No Effect* In 12 patients with anorexia nervosa serum concentrations of calcium, phosphate, albumin, alkaline phosphatase, parathyroid hormone, calcitonin, osteocalcin, and 24-hour calcium excretion were normal *3907*

Phosphate *Serum* *Decrease* Severe hypophosphataemia that had been precipitated during binge eating *2612* Hypophosphatemia may play a role in the development of cardiac arrhythmia and delirium *141*

Phospholipase A *Serum* *No Effect* Measured in 34 patients (average age 28.5 (18 - 64) years), anorexia nervosa (9 patients) and bulimia (25 patients). Normal in all patients *2110*

Platelet Aggregation *Blood* *Increase* Malnourished patients with anorexia nervosa had significantly increased aggregability compared with age- and sex-matched controls *2955*

Platelets *Blood* *Decrease* Mean concentration of 241000 ± 86000 /μL in 67 patients with anorexia less than 261000 ± 50000 /μL in 67 age and sex matched controls *1139*

Potassium *Serum* *Decrease* Observed effect *565*

Prealbumin *Serum* *Decrease* Effect observed in extreme cases *2148*
Serum *No Effect* In 9 Japanese women mean concentration of 0.27 ± 0.02 g/L on admission to hospital not significantly different from 0.29 ± 0.01 g/L once they had gained 10 kg body weight *2754* In 12 anorectic women mean concentration of 250 ± 20 mg/L not significantly different from 270 ± 10 mg/L in 12 healthy controls although increased significantly to 300 ± 10 mg/L with weight gain *289* Mean concentration of about 25 mg/dL not different from normal range of 10 - 40 mg/dL *2160*

Prolactin *Plasma* *Decrease* Basal concentration significantly reduced in patients with anorexia nervosa compared with controls *1788*
Plasma *No Effect* No significant change observed in basal concentration in both men and women with anorexia nervosa *1074*

Prolactin response to TRH *Plasma* *Increase* Exaggerated response observed in men with anorexia nervosa *1074*

Protein *Serum* *No Effect* In 9 Japanese women mean concentration of 70 ± 2 g/L on admission to hospital not significantly different from 74 ± 2 g/L once they had gained 10 kg body weight *2754*

Quinolinic Acid *Cerebrospinal Fluid* *No Effect* Measured in medication-free female patients meeting DSM-III-R criteria for either anorexia nervosa (n = 10) or normal-weight bulimia nervosa (n = 22), studied at varying stages of nutritional recovery. Eight healthy, normal-weight females served as a comparison group. Levels were not different from controls *1114* In 9 low weight anorectics mean concentration of 13.4 ± 5.4 nmol/L not significantly different from 13.8 ± 4.3 nmol/L in 8 healthy normals *1114*

Retinol-binding Protein *Serum* *No Effect* In 14 patients with anorexia nervosa mean concentration of about 3.7 mg/dL not different from normal range of 3 - 6 mg/dL *2160* In 12 anorectic women mean concentration of 39 ± 4 mg/L not significantly different from 35 ± 2 mg/L in 12 healthy controls although increased significantly to 50 ± 4 mg/L with weight gain *289*

Sex-Hormone Binding Globulin *Serum* *Increase* In 12 anorectic women before weight gain mean concentration of 7.0 ± 0.7 mg/L significantly higher than 3.1 ± 0.4 mg/L in 12 healthy controls but decreased to 3.8 ± 0.3 mg/L with weight gain *289* Patients have high concentrations *4234*

Somatomedin *Plasma* *Decrease* Concentrations are low *565*

Somatostatin *Plasma* *Increase* Measured before and after a standardized fat and protein-rich fluid test meal. Significantly elevated after the test meals *4144*

Testosterone *Serum* *Decrease* Basal concentration reduced in 3 men with anorexia nervosa when compared with

307.10 Anorexia Nervosa *(continued)*

Testosterone *(continued)*
normals *1074* In 12 anorectic women mean concentration of 1.25 ± 0.14 nmol/L significantly less than 1.66 ± 0.14 nmol/L in 12 healthy controls: with weight gain in anoretics mean concentration declined to 1.18 ± 0.14 nmol/L *289*
Serum Increase Increased concentration observed in 20 women with anorexia nervosa *1074*
Serum No Effect Concentration typically normal in patients with anorexia nervosa *355* Mean concentration in 10 women with anorexia nervosa similar to that in 8 normal women *4874*

Thyroid Stimulating Hormone *Serum No Effect* Concentration reported to be normal in both adults and children *355* Basal concentration normal in both men and women with anorexia nervosa *1074* In 9 Japanese women mean concentration of 2.3 ± 0.50 mU/L on admission to hospital not significantly different from 2.17 ± 0.31 mU/L once they had gained 10 kg body weight and 2.91 ± 0.47 mU/L in healthy controls *2754* No significant difference observed in 6 women with anorexia nervosa compared with healthy controls *723* Basal levels are normal. Response to TRH is intact *565*

Thyrotropin Releasing Hormone
Cerebrospinal Fluid Decrease In 19 female underweight patients mean concentration of 2.7 ± 8 pg/mL before and in 16 after they had attained goal weight mean concentration of 2.4 ± 1.0 pg/mL significantly reduced compared with 3.6 ± 1.2 pg/mL in 17 healthy control women *3000*

Thyroxine Binding Globulin *Serum No Effect* In 9 Japanese women mean concentration of 244.5 ± 16.8 nmol/L on admission to hospital not significantly different from 260.6 ± 10.2 nmol/L once they had gained 10 kg body weight *2754*

Thyroxine (T4) *Serum Decrease* Slight reduction in concentration observed compared with healthy controls *723* Effect observed in extreme cases *2148* In adults low concentrations observed *355*
Serum No Effect In 9 Japanese women mean concentration of 79.9 ± 8.0 nmol/L on admission to hospital not significantly different from 91.0 ± 5.1 nmol/L once they had gained 10 kg body weight and 99.5 ± 5.9 nmol/L in healthy controls *2754* No significant difference observed in 20 patients with anorexia nervosa *1075* No significant change observed in either men or women with anorexia nervosa *1074*

Thyroxine (T4), Free *Serum Increase* Slight increase observed in both men and women with anorexia nervosa *1074* Slight increase observed in 20 patients with anorexia nervosa *1075*
Serum No Effect In 12 anorectic women mean concentration of 10.5 ± 0.6 pmol/L, declining to 9.8 ± 1.7 pmol/L with weight gain, compared with 12.1 ± 1.2 pmol/L in healthy controls *289* Despite low total thyroxine concentrations free thyroxine concentration unaffected *355* Normal levels *565* In 9 Japanese women mean concentration of 13.7 ± 1.0 pmol/L on admission to hospital not significantly different from 13.4 ± 0.7 pmol/L once they had gained 10 kg body weight and 14.8 ± 0.7 nmol/L in healthy controls *2754* No significant difference in 6 women with anorexia nervosa compared with healthy controls *723*

Tissue Plasminogen Activator *Plasma No Effect* In 9 Japanese women mean concentration of about 17 ng/L on admission to hospital not significantly different from 19 ng/L after 10 kg weight gain and not different from normal range in healthy controls with upper limit of normal of about 21 ng/L *2754*

Transferrin *Serum Decrease* In 24 patients with anorexia nervosa before weight gain mean concentration of 271.3 ± 76.4 mg/dL not significantly different from 313.7 ± 50.2 mg/dL in 13 healthy control individuals *1296* Effect observed in extreme cases *189*
Serum No Effect In 12 anorectic women mean concentration of 2.16 ± 0.21 g/L not significantly different from 2.55 ± 0.11 g/L in 12 healthy controls although increased significantly to 3.26 ± 0.26 g/L with weight gain *289*

Transforming Growth Factor-β *Serum Increase* Serum IL-6 and TGF-β concentrations were both significantly elevated during starvation and returned to levels comparable to those of normal-weight controls by the end of therapy *4172*

Tri-iodothyronine, Free (fT3) *Serum Decrease* Reduced concentration observed in both men and women with anorexia nervosa *1074* In 9 Japanese women mean concentration of 2.57 ± 0.23 pmol/L on admission to hospital significantly different from 5.18 ± 0.40 pmol/L once they had gained 10 kg body weight and 5.31 ± 0.34 pmol/L in healthy controls *2754* Significant reduction observed in 20 patients with anorexia nervosa *1075*

Tri-iodothyronine, Reverse (rT3) *Serum Decrease* Reduced concentration observed in both men and women with anorexia nervosa *1074*
Serum Increase Typical observation in patients with anorexia nervosa *355* Concentrations are increased *565* Significant increase observed in 20 patients with anorexia nervosa *1075*
Serum No Effect No significant difference observed in 6 women with anorexia nervosa compared with healthy controls *723*

Tri-iodothyronine (T3) *Serum Decrease* Associated with muscle dysfunction *2847* Significant reduction observed in 20 patients with anorexia nervosa *1075* In 9 Japanese women mean concentration of 0.85 ± 0.07 nmol/L on admission to hospital significantly different from 1.51 ± 0.11 nmol/L once they had gained 10 kg body weight and 1.53 ± 0.08 nmol/L in healthy controls *2754* In adults low concentrations observed *355* In 24 women with anorexia nervosa mean concentration of 0.7 ± 0.1 nmol/L significantly different from 1.6 ± 0.4 nmoll/L in 10 healthy control women *5033* Low concentrations observed in 10 patients with anorexia nervosa compared with concentrations in 15 healthy controls *4670* In 12 anorectic women mean concentration of 1.6 ± 0.1 nmol/L significantly less than 2.1 ± 0.1 nmol/L in 12 healthy controls and increased to 2.2 ± 0.2 nmol/L with weight gain in the anoretics *289* Concentrations are decreased *565* Effect observed in extreme cases *2148* In 6 women (mean 67% of ideal body weight) mean concentration of 1.20 nmol/L compared with 2.04 nmol/L in healthy controls *723* Marked reduction observed in both men and women with anorexia nervosa *1074*

Triglycerides *Serum Increase* Concentration tended to be higher in acute phase of illness in 29 young women although tended to normalize in chronic phase *4554*
Serum No Effect Not increased despite low activities of hepatic and lipoprotein lipases *565*

Tryptophan *Cerebrospinal Fluid No Effect* No significant difference between concentrations in 33 anorexic women and in 14 normal women *1711* In 9 low weight anorectics mean concentration of 1.9 ± 0.5 nmol/L not significantly different from 2.1 ± 0.3 nmol/L in 8 healthy normals *1114*
Plasma Decrease Mean whole blood concentration of 52.8 ± 10.8 nmol/mL in 10 anorexic patients with bulimic attitudes and 53.0 ± 13.7 nmol/mL in 9 patients with anorexia but without bulimic attitudes significantly different from 64.3 ± 11.2 nmol/mL observed in 12 healthy controls *198*

Tryptophan, Free *Plasma Decrease* Mean whole blood concentration of 2.4 ± 1.2 nmol/mL in 10 anorexic patients with bulimic attitudes and 2.7 ± 1.0 nmol/mL in 9 patients with anorexia but without bulimic attitudes significantly different from 4.0 ± 1.4 nmol/mL observed in 12 healthy controls *198*

TSH response to TRH *Serum Decrease* Delayed peak observed after TRH in both men and women with anorexia nervosa *1074* In 20 patients with anorexia nervosa response delayed (30 minutes compared with 20 minutes in normal individuals) *1075*
Serum Increase Normal response observed in both children and adults with anorexia nervosa although peak response may be delayed *355*

Tumor Necrosis Factor-α *Serum No Effect* Serum TNF-α levels were undetectable in all patients and controls *4172*

Tyrosine *Cerebrospinal Fluid Decrease* In 33 anorexic women concentration significantly reduced compared with concentration in 14 normal women *1711*

Urea Nitrogen *Serum Decrease* Effect observed in extreme cases *2148*
Serum Increase Prerenal azotemia may occur if vomiting or laxative use are prominent. The levels may be as high as 60 - 70 mg/dL *565*
Serum No Effect In 9 Japanese women mean concentration of 5.19 ± 0.38 mmol/L on admission to hospital not significantly different from 5.04 ± 0.37 mmol/L once they had gained 10 kg body weight *2754*

Vanillylmandelic Acid *Urine Decrease* In both men and women with anorexia nervosa concentration reduced *1074*

Vitamin A *Serum Decrease* Plasma levels were determined following an oral bolus in normal women and in women suffering from this disorder. Circulating levels were lower *5381*

Vitamin E *Serum* *Decrease* Plasma levels were determine following an oral bolus in normal women and in women suffering from this disorder. Circulating levels were lower *5381*

Zinc *Hair* *No Effect* No significant effect observed *565*
Serum *Decrease* Observed effect *565* In patients with anorexia nervosa concentration is typically reduced *2952*
Serum *No Effect* Studied in 18 patients in the age range of 11 to 25 years. There were no significant abnormalities *4409*

307.23 Tourette's Syndrome

Corticotropin-releasing Hormone
Cerebrospinal Fluid *Increase* In 21 medication-free out-patients with Tourette's syndrome mean concentration of 6.7 fmol/mL significantly higher than 5.3 fmol/mL in 29 healthy controls *787*

Oxytocin *Cerebrospinal Fluid* *No Effect* In 23 patients with Tourette's syndrome mean concentration of 6.7 pmol/L not significantly different from 7.7 pmol/L in 31 normal controls *2958*

Vasopressin *Cerebrospinal Fluid* *No Effect* In 23 patients with Tourette's syndrome mean concentration of 12.0 pmol/L not significantly different from 11.6 pmol/L in 31 normal controls *2958*

307.52 Geophagia

Zinc *Serum* *Decrease* Zinc concentrations tend to be at the low because ingested clay adsorbs dietary zinc rendering it unavailable for absorption from the gastrointestinal tract *5174*

307.81 Tension Headache

Dopamine *Plasma* *Increase* Significant increase observed in patients with tension headaches during attacks, normalizing during remissions *2955*

5-Hydroxytryptamine *Plasma* *Decrease* Significant reduction observed in patients with tension headaches *2955*

Interleukin-2 *Serum* *Decrease* Forty six subjects (20 males and 26 females, mean age: 39.7 years) with tension-type headache (TH) were selected for this study. Forty-three normal healthy volunteers composed the control group (15 males and 28 females, average age 41.6 years). The IL-2 levels in serum were 3.18 ± 1.8 U/mL (mean ± SD) in the healthy controls, and 1.59 ± 1.0 U/mL in the patients with TH. The serum level of IL-2 in the patients with TH was significantly lower than in the controls *4806*

309.81 Posttraumatic Stress

α_1-Antichymotrypsin *Serum* *No Effect* Mean concentration within reference interval of 47.9 ± 8.1 mg/dL in one examined patient with post-traumatic stress disorder *3044*

CC16 *Serum* *No Effect* In 13 patients with posttraumatic stress disorder mean concentration of 36 ± 16 ng/mL not significantly different from 37 ± 21 ng/mL in 32 healthy normal volunteers *3210*

Cholesterol *Serum* *Increase* Mean concentration of 237 ± 64 mg/dL in 73 male Vietnam veterans with posttraumatic stress disorder significantly higher than 200 mg/dL in Vietnam veterans overall and 212 mg/dL in the general male population *2522*

Corticotropin-releasing Hormone
Cerebrospinal Fluid *Increase* In 11 patients with post-traumatic stress mean concentration of 29.0 ± 7.8 pg/mL significantly higher than 21.9 ± 6.0 pg/mL in 19 comparison individuals *571*

Cortisol *Plasma* *Decrease* In 15 combat veterans mesor concentration of 7.45 ± 1.69 µg/dL significantly reduced compared with 9.06 ± 1.92 µg/dL in 15 healthy controls *5797*
Urine *Decrease* Mean excretion of 32.6 ± 17.0 µg/d in 22 post-Holocaust patients with posttraumatic stress disorder compared with 62.7 ± 25.3 µg/d in 25 Holocaust-survivors without posttraumatic stress disorder *5796* *5796*

Dexamethasone Suppression *Patient* *Abnormal* Following psychological, surgical or traumatic stress a lack of suppression of cortisol concentration with dexamethasone suppression test may occur *5723*

Dopamine *Urine* *Increase* In 17 male out-patients with combat-related posttraumatic stress disorder mean excretion of 265.6 ± 130.0 µg/d significantly higher than 158.5 ± 81.3 µg/d in 10 healthy normal controls *4961*

HDL-Cholesterol *Serum* *Decrease* Mean concentration of 42 ± 13 mg/dL in 73 male Vietnam veterans with posttraumatic stress disorder significantly less than concentrations in Vietnam veterans overall, a group of substance abusing Vietnam veterans and the general male population *2522*

Homovanillic Acid *Urine* *Increase* In 17 male out-patients with combat-related posttraumatic stress disorder mean excretion of 7.0 ± 5.1 mg/d significantly higher than 4.3 ± 2.2 mg/d in 10 healthy normal controls *4961*

5-Hydroxytryptamine *Plasma* *Decrease* In 17 male out-patients with combat-related posttraumatic stress disorder mean concentration in platelet-poor plasma of 10.9 ± 7.7 ng/mL significantly lower than 28.4 ± 17.8 ng/mL in 10 healthy normal controls *4961*

Interleukin-1 Receptor Antagonist *Serum* *No Effect* In 13 patients with posttraumatic stress disorder mean concentration of 0.46 ± 0.72 ng/mL not significantly different from 0.26 ± 0.26 ng/mL in 32 healthy normal volunteers *3210*

Interleukin-6 *Serum* *Increase* In 13 patients with posttraumatic stress disorder mean concentration of 71 ± 65 pg/mL significantly greater than 7 ± 9 pg/mL in 32 healthy normal volunteers *3210*

LDL-Cholesterol *Serum* *Increase* Mean concentration of 151 ± 45 mg/dL in 73 male Vietnam veterans with posttraumatic stress disorder significantly higher than concentrations in Vietnam veterans overall, a group of substance abusing Vietnam veterans and the general male population *2522*

Norepinephrine *Plasma* *Increase* In 17 male out-patients with combat-related posttraumatic stress disorder mean concentration in platelet-poor plasma of 435.2 ± 270.4 ng/mL significantly higher than 188.3 ± 102.1 ng/mL in 10 healthy normal controls *4961*
Urine *Increase* In 17 male out-patients with combat-related posttraumatic stress disorder mean excretion of 43.7 ± 27.3 µg/d significantly higher than 28.6 ± 17.8 µg/d in 10 healthy normal controls *4961*

Norepinephrine:5-Hydroxytryptamine Ratio
Plasma *Increase* In 17 male out-patients with combat-related posttraumatic stress disorder mean ratio in platelet-poor plasma of 44.7 ± 37.3 (pg/mL:ng/mL) significantly higher than 15.2 ± 16.5 in 10 healthy normal controls *4961*

Soluble $CD8^+$ *Serum* *No Effect* In 13 patients with posttraumatic stress disorder mean concentration of 349 ± 94 U/mL not significantly different from 416 ± 124 U/mL in 32 healthy normal volunteers *3210*

Soluble gp130 *Serum* *No Effect* In 13 patients with posttraumatic stress disorder mean concentration of 1,149 ± 183 ng/mL not significantly different from 1,112 ± 199 ng/mL in 32 healthy normal volunteers *3210*

Soluble Interleukin-6 Receptor *Serum* *Increase* In 13 patients with posttraumatic stress disorder mean concentration of 262 ± 69 ng/mL significantly greater than 190 ± 58 ng/mL in 32 healthy normal volunteers *3210*

Thyroxine Binding Globulin *Serum* *Increase* Mean concentration of 376 ± 13 nmol/L in 96 patients with posttraumatic stress significantly higher than 252 ± 13 nmol/L in 24 healthy controls *3333*

Thyroxine (T4) *Serum* *Increase* Mean concentration of 110 ± 2.4 nmol/L in 96 patients with posttraumatic stress significantly higher than 87 ± 3.6 nmol/L in 24 healthy controls *3333*

Thyroxine (T4), Free *Serum* *No Effect* Mean concentration of 20 ± 0.4 pmol/L in 96 patients with posttraumatic stress not different from 20 ± 1.0 pmol/L in 24 healthy controls *3333*

Tri-iodothyronine, Free (fT3) *Serum* *Increase* Mean concentration of 5.11 ± 0.11 pmol/L in 96 patients with posttraumatic stress significantly higher than 4.06 ± 0.15 pmol/L in 24 healthy controls *3333*

Tri-iodothyronine, Reverse (rT3) *Serum* *No Effect* In 20 patients with posttraumatic stress disorder mean concentration of 0.40 ± 0.02 nmol/L not significantly different from 0.41 ± 0.02 nmol/L in 20 healthy controls *3333*

309.81 Posttraumatic Stress *(continued)*

Tri-iodothyronine (T3) *Serum Increase* Mean concentration of 2.7 ± 0.06 nmol/L in 96 patients with posttraumatic stress significantly higher than 2.0 ± 0.08 nmol/L in 24 healthy controls *3333*

Triglycerides *Serum Increase* Mean concentration of 194 ± 129 mg/dL in 73 male Vietnam veterans with posttraumatic stress disorder significantly higher than concentrations in Vietnam veterans overall, a group of substance abusing Vietnam veterans and the general male population *2522*

311.00 Depression

α_1-Acid Glycoprotein *Serum Increase* In 49 subjects with major depressive disorder compared with age and sex matched controls *2082* Significant positive correlation of positive acute phase reactant protein concentrations in patients with major depression compared with normal controls *3216*

Albumin *Serum Decrease* In 31 patients with major depression mean concentration of 40.7 ± 3.5 g/L significantly different from 44.1 ± 3.6 g/L in 15 healthy controls *3215* Significant negative correlation of negative acute phase reactant protein concentrations in patients with major depression compared with normal controls *3216* Mean concentration of 47.4 ± 4.3 g/L in 23 patients with simple major depression significantly different from 46.7 ± 2.3 g/L in 18 healthy controls *3216* In patients with depression mean concentration 5.4% lower than in non-psychiatric controls *5101* In 37 patients with major depression mean serum concentration of 41.2 ± 4.1 g/L compared with 46.1 ± 4.4 g/L in 29 normal male volunteers *5405*
Serum Increase Concentration tended to be higher in 81 depressed in-patients than in 82 psychiatric controls *798*
Serum No Effect In 42 patients with major depression mean concentration of 47.7 ± 4.6 g/L not significantly different from 46.4 ± 2.7 g/L in 24 healthy controls *3217* Mean concentration of 47.4 ± 4.3 g/L in 14 patients with minor depression not different from 46.7 ± 2.3 g/L in 18 healthy controls *3216*

γ-Aminobutyric Acid *Plasma No Effect* In 46 patients with primary unipolar depression mean concentration of 106 ± 24 pmol/mL not significantly different from that in 71 healthy individuals, mean 123 ± 20 pmol/mL *4107*

Amyloid β-Protein *Cerebrospinal Fluid No Effect* Mean concentration in patients with major depression and Alzheimer's disease similar and similar to 9.8 ± 1.1 ng/mL in 17 control individuals *2190*

Amyloid Precursor Protein *Cerebrospinal Fluid No Effect* Mean concentration in patients with major depression and patients with Alzheimer's disease not significantly different from 1,490 ± 74 ng/mL in 15 control individuals *2190*

α_1-Antichymotrypsin *Serum Increase* Mean concentration increased above reference interval of 47.9 ± 8.1 mg/dL in 2 of 8 patients (25%) with depression *3044* Significant positive correlation of positive acute phase reactant protein concentrations in patients with major depression compared with normal controls *3216*

Antidiuretic Hormone *Cerebrospinal Fluid Decrease* In patients with either endogenous or nonendogenous depression concentration of vasopressin significantly reduced compared with controls *1744*
Plasma No Effect No significant difference observed in patients with either endogenous or nonendogenous depression compared with controls *1744*

Antithyroid Antibodies *Serum Increase* In 20% of 45 psychiatric patients with depression significantly higher than in the 5 - 10% observed in the normal population *3759*

α_1-Antitrypsin *Serum Increase* Significant positive correlation of positive acute phase reactant protein concentrations in patients with major depression compared with normal controls *3216* Significant increase observed in patients with major depression with lesser increase observed in those with minor depression *3213*

Arginine *Plasma Increase* Mean concentration increased in 59 depressed patients compared with concentration in healthy controls *3351*

Arginine Vasopressin *Cerebrospinal Fluid No Effect* Mean concencentration of 21.2 ± 4.5 pg/mL in 19 patients with major depression not significantly different from 22.5 ± 9.1 pg/mL in 18 healthy controls *4150*
Plasma Increase Mean 8:00 a.m. concentration in 52 patients with major depression of 8.94 ± 7.25 pg/mL significantly different from 5.32 ± 4.00 pg/mL observed in 37 healthy controls *5409*

Biopterin *Serum Increase* In 10 patients with monopolar depression mean concentration in depressive phase of 36 6 ± 5.0 pmol/mL significantly greater than 21.5 ± 4.8 pmol/mL in healthy controls, but in remission phase mean concentration of 24.6 ± 5.5 pmol/mL not significantly different from controls *2048* Concentration significantly increased in 12 depressed patients compared with normal controls but during remission concentrations similar to that in normal controls *2049*
Urine No Effect No significant difference between excretion in 26 patients with depression (635 ± 281 nmol/mmol creatinine) and 45 control individuals (614 ± 267 nmol/mmol creatinine) *2236*

Ceruloplasmin *Serum Increase* Significant increase observed in patients with major depression and lesser increase observed in patients with minor depression *3213* Significant positive correlation of positive acute phase reactant protein concentrations in patients with major depression compared with normal controls *3216*

Chloride *Serum Decrease* In 81 depressed in-patients mean concentration tended to be lower than in 82 psychiatric controls *798*

Cholesterol *Serum Decrease* In men aged 70 years or older depression 3 times more common in those with low plasma cholesterol concentration (< 4.14 mmol/L) than in those with higher concentrations (16% versus 6%) *3601*

Complement C_3c *Serum Increase* Significant positive correlation of positive acute phase reactant protein concentrations in patients with major depression compared with normal controls *3216*

Complement C_4 *Serum Increase* Significant positive correlation of positive acute phase reactant protein concentrations in patients with major depression compared with normal controls *3216*

Copper *Serum Increase* In 19 patients with unipolar depression mean concentration of 1.15 ± 0.17 mg/L significantly different from 0.95 ± 0.09 mg/L in 16 healthy controls *4639*
Serum No Effect In 31 patients with major depression mean concentration of 118 ± 28 µg/dL not significantly different from 119 ± 12 µg/dL in 15 healthy controls *3215*

Corticosteroid-Binding Globulin *Serum Decrease* Clear cut decrease of binding activity observed in 10 severely depressed inpatients *2835*

Corticotropin *Plasma Increase* In 26 severely depressed patients mean 24 h concentration of 7.14 ± 2.06 pmol/L significantly different from 5.72 ± 1.36 pmol/L in 33 healthy controls *2138*
Plasma No Effect No significant difference observed between 24-hour mean concentration in depressed men and control men *3077*

Corticotropin-releasing Hormone
Cerebrospinal Fluid No Effect Mean concencentration of 38.6 ± 10.0 pg/mL in 19 patients with major depression not significantly different from 43.3 ± 8.1 pg/mL in 18 healthy controls *4150*
Plasma No Effect No significant difference observed between concentrations in 22 depressed patients and 18 normal controls *4463*

Cortisol *Plasma Increase* Mean concentration of plasma cortisol significantly higher in men and women depressives compared with age and sex matched controls: significant increase with age observed in both sexes *1962* Marked increase observed in total concentration in association with reduction in transcortin binding capacity *2835* Significant increase observed in 27 depressed patients compared with 14 normal individuals *3524* In 12 patients with unipolar major depression mean concentration of 17.5 ± 4.4 µg/dL significantly different from 12.7 ± 5.5 µg/dL in 11 healthy controls *5141* In 32 patients with major depression none had morning concentrations greater than 280 ng/mL (upper limit of normal) although the patients fell into classes of 143.4 ± 39.8 ng/mL and 66.7 ± 20.6 ng/mL *4129* In 15 patients with unipolar depression mean concentration of 469 ± 37 mmol/L significantly increased compared with 321 ± 32 mmol/L in 22 healthy age- and sex-matched controls *3226* In 26 severely depressed patients mean 24 h concentration of 286 ± 65 nmol/L significantly different from 184 ± 29 nmol/L in 33 healthy controls *2138*

Plasma No Effect In 14 patients with depression mesor concentration of 10.27 ± 3.04 μg/dL not significantly different from 9.06 ± 1.92 μg/dL in 15 healthy controls *5797* Mean 8:00 a.m. concentration in 52 patients with major depression of 0.59 ± 0.19 pg/mL not different from 0.49 ± 0.17 pg/mL observed in 37 healthy controls *5409* In 21 patients with minor depression mean concentration of 21.8 ± 4.2 μg/dL and 21.3 μg/dL in 25 patients with simple major depression not significantly different fom normal *3198*
Saliva Decrease Concentration significantly less in depressed in prepubertal children than in healthy age-matched controls *4078*
Saliva No Effect Mean evening and morning concentrations in 26 female patients with community depression of 1.5 ± 2.1 nmol/L and 6.0 ± 6.1 nmol/L, respectively, not significantly reduced in comparison with 1.5 ± 1.5 nmol/L and 7.0 ± 3.5 nmol/L in 131 matched controls *5048*
Urine No Effect In 21 patients with minor depression mean excretion of 202 μg/d and 168 μg/d in 25 patients with simple major depression not significantly different fom normal *3198*

Cortisol, Free *Plasma Increase* Significant increase observed in 10 severely depressed in-patients in association with reduced transcortin binding capacity *2835*
Urine Increase In 10 patients with melancholic depression mean excretion of 252.7 ± 33.3 nmol/d significantly different from 181.3 ± 42.9 nmol/d in 15 healthy control individuals *4700*

C-Reactive Protein *Serum Increase* In 39 patients on first day after mitogen stimulation mean concentration of 0.45 ± 0.31 mg/dL in serum significantly increased compared with 0.31 ± 0.11 mg/dL in 39 healthy controls *4717* Significant positive correlation of positive acute phase reactant protein concentrations in patients with major depression compared with normal controls *3216*

Cystine *Plasma Increase* Mean concentration increased in 59 depressed patients compared with concentration in healthy controls *3351*

Dehydroepiandrosterone *Plasma Increase* In 26 severely depressed patients mean 24 h concentration of 5.8 ± 3.6 nmol/L significantly different from 3.4 ± 1.9 nmol/L in 33 healthy controls *2138*

Dehydroepiandrosterone Sulfate *Plasma Increase* In 12 patients with unipolar major depression mean concentration of 262.9 ± 79.9 μg/mL significantly different from 201.2 ± 47.7 μg/mL in 11 healthy controls *5141*

Dexamethasone Suppression *Patient Abnormal* 30 - 50% patients with depression, especially unipolar depression, demonstrate a lack of suppression of cortisol concentration with dexamethasone suppression test *5723*

Dipeptidyl Peptidase IV *Serum Decrease* Significantly lower activity observed in depressed patients compared with healthy controls. Lower in melancholics than in minor depressives *3207*

Dopamine *Cerebrospinal Fluid Increase* Statistically significantly increased concentration observed in 24 depressed patients *1746*

Erythropoietin *Cerebrospinal Fluid Increase* In 13 patients with depression, mean concentration of 3.21 ± 0.46 mIU/mL significantly different from 0.98 ± 0.26 mIU/mL in 15 healthy control individuals *3715*
Serum No Effect In 13 patients with depression mean concentration not significantly different from that in 15 healthy control individuals *3715*

Folate *Red Blood Cells No Effect* Concentration typically normal as measured by Corning Magic Lite method *3477*
Serum No Effect No significant difference observed between concentrations in depressed patients and age and sex matched controls *2715* Concentration typically normal in depressed patients as measured by Corning Magic Lite method *3477*

GH response to Clonidine *Plasma Decrease* In 45 acute and remitted depressed patients response blunted (change of less than 4 ng/mL) compared with healthy controls *4833*

α_1-Globulin *Serum Increase* Mean concentration of 2.5 ± 0.4 g/L in 23 patients with major depression not different from 2.2 ± 0.3 g/L in 18 healthy controls, although as proportion of total protein increased to 3.6 ± 0.6% compared with 3.0 ± 0.4% in healthy controls *3216*
Serum No Effect Mean concentration of 2.3 ± 0.5 g/L in 14 patients with minor depression and 2.5 ± 0.4 g/L in 23 patients with major depression not different from 2.2 ± 0.3 g/L in 18 healthy controls, although as proportion of total protein increased to 3.6 ± 0.6% compared with 3.0 ± 0.4% in healthy controls *3216* In 37 patients with major depression mean serum concentration of 2.35 ± 0.40 g/L compared with 2.33 ± 0.44 g/L in 29 normal male volunteers *5405*

α_2-Globulin *Serum Increase* Mean concentration of 7.1 ± 1.2 g/L in 14 patients with minor depression and 6.7 ± 1.2 g/L in 23 patients with major depression not different from 6.1 ± 0.8 g/L in 18 healthy controls, although as proportion of total protein increased to 9.7 ± 1.4% and 9.6 ± 1.5%, respectively, compared with 8.3 ± 1.1% in healthy controls *3216* In 42 patients with major depression mean concentration of 6.9 ± 1.0 g/L significantly different from 6.1 ± 0.8 g/L in 24 healthy controls *3217*
Serum No Effect In 37 patients with major depression mean serum concentration of 6.55 ± 1.21 g/L compared with 6.56 ± 1.14 g/L in 29 normal male volunteers *5405*

β-Globulin *Serum Decrease* In 37 patients with major depression mean serum concentration of 7.97 ± 1.18 g/L compared with 9.68 ± 1.31 g/L in 29 normal male volunteers *5405*
Serum No Effect Mean concentration of 8.5 ± 2.0 g/L in 14 patients with minor depression and 8.2 ± 1.4 g/L in 23 patients with major depression not different from 9.2 ± 1.2 g/L in 18 healthy controls, and as proportion of total protein unchanged at 11.6 ± 2.3% and 11.7 ± 1.4%, respectively, compared with 12.4 ± 1.4% in healthy controls *3216*

γ-Globulin *Serum Decrease* Mean concentration of 7.8 ± 1.9 g/L in 14 patients with minor depression and 7.2 ± 1.9 g/L in 23 patients with major depression significantly different from 9.4 ± 1.6 g/L in 18 healthy controls, and as proportion of total protein decreased at 10.7 ± 2.4% and 10.3 ± 2.2%, respectively, compared with 12.8 ± 2.0% in healthy controls *3216* In 37 patients with major depression mean serum concentration of 7.72 ± 1.79 g/L compared with 9.66 ± 2.09 g/L in 29 normal male volunteers *5405*

Glutamine *Plasma Increase* Mean concentration increased in 59 depressed patients compared with that in healthy controls *3351*

Guanosine Monophosphate *Plasma Increase* In 5 depressed patients mean concentration about 25 pmol/mL versus 10 pmol/mL in healthy controls *2524*

Haptoglobin *Serum Increase* In patients with major depression significant increase observed compared with controls but with a lesser increase observed in patients with minor depression *3213* Significant positive correlation of positive acute phase reactant protein concentrations in patients with major depression compared with normal controls *3216* In 39 patients on first day after mitogen stimulation mean concentration of 227.7 ± 91.9 mg/dL in serum significantly increased compared with 181.7 ± 57.1 mg/dL in 39 healthy controls *4717*

Homocysteine *Plasma Increase* Twenty-seven depressed elderly acute inpatients by DSM-III-R criteria had significantly higher plasma homocysteine levels and lower cognitive screening test scores than did 15 depressed young adult in-patients *376*

Homovanillic Acid *Cerebrospinal Fluid Decrease* In 9 non-medicated patients with major depression mean concentration of 182.9 ± 49.7 pmol/mL nonsignificantly reduced compared with 219.5 ± 109.9 pmol/mL in healthy individuals *1045* Significant reduction observed in depressed patients who had attempted suicide compared with the concentration in those who had not attempted suicide and in normal control individuals *4462*
Cerebrospinal Fluid No Effect No significant difference observed between concentrations in 24 depressed patients and 10 controls *1746*

4-Hydroxy-3-Methoxy-Phenylglycol
Cerebrospinal Fluid No Effect No significant difference observed between concentrations in 24 depressed patients and 10 controls *1746* In 9 patients with non-medicated major depression mean concentration of 46.7 ± 14.2 pmol/mL not significantly different from 48.0 ± 9.5 pmol/mL in healthy control individuals *1045*
Plasma Decrease Mean concentration of 15.4 ± 1.0 ng/mL in 70 depressed patients significantly different from 17.6 ± 1.2 ng/mL in 24 healthy controls *2567*

311.00 **Depression** *(continued)*

5-Hydroxyindoleacetic Acid *Cerebrospinal Fluid Decrease* In 9 patients with non-medicated major depression mean concentration of 95.9 ± 24.6 pmol/mL not significantly reduced compared with 111.2 ± 44.5 pmol/L in healthy control individuals *1045*
Cerebrospinal Fluid No Effect No significant difference observed between concentrations in depressed and control individuals *4462*

5-Hydroxytryptamine *Cerebrospinal Fluid Increase* Concentration significantly higher than in controls, with highest concentration observed in endogenous group compared with non-endogenous group *1745*
Platelets Decrease Mean concentration in 49 nonpsychotic depressive patients of 1.05 ± 0.41 nmol/mg protein significantly different from that in 90 healthy individuals, 1.26 ± 0.26 nmol/mg protein *2409*
Platelets Increase Low platelet serotonin uptake rate has been connected to unipolar depression and the rate of efflux *1976*
Platelets No Effect In 30 drug-free depressed patients mean concentration of 1.405 ng/10^9 platelets not significantly different from 1.307 ng/10^9 platelets in 20 healthy controls *2568* Mean concentration in 88 depressed patients of 1.26 ± 0.26 nmol/mg protein not significantly different from that in 90 healthy individuals, 1.26 ± 0.26 nmol/mg protein *2409*

Immunoglobulin G *Serum Increase* Significant positive correlation of positive acute phase reactant protein concentrations in patients with major depression compared with normal controls *3216*

Immunoglobulin M *Serum Increase* Significant positive correlation of positive acute phase reactant protein concentrations in patients with major depression compared with normal controls *3216*

Interferon-α *Serum Increase* In 5 depressed patients mean concentration almost 10^2 pg/mL versus 1 pg/mL in healthy controls *2524*

Interferon-γ *Serum Increase* In 16 patients with major depression mean concentration of interferon-γ of 710 ± 775 IU/mL statistically different when compared with 206 ± 244 IU/mL in 30 controls *3212* In 39 patients on first day after mitogen stimulation mean concentration of about 3,200 pg/mL in whole blood significantly increased compared with about 2,200 pg/mL in 39 healthy controls *4717*

Interleukin-1 Receptor Antagonist *Serum Increase* In 21 patients with minor depression mean concentration of 0.201 ng/mL and 0.186 ng/mL in 25 patients with simple major depression compared with 0.110 ng/mL in 22 healthy controls *3198*

Interleukin-1β *Serum Increase* In 39 patients on first day after mitogen stimulation mean concentration of 537.3 ± 397.9 pg/mL in whole blood compared with 460.0 ± 300.0 pg/mL in 39 healthy controls *4717*

Interleukin-2 *Serum Increase* In 39 patients on first day after mitogen stimulation mean concentration of about 420 pg/mL in whole blood not significantly increased compared with about 300 pg/mL in 39 healthy controls *4717*

Interleukin-6 *Serum Increase* In 61 patients with major depression mean concentration of 5.52 ± 1.00 pg/mL significantly greater than 2.50 ± 0.55 pg/mL in 38 normal controls *3211* In 39 patients on first day after mitogen stimulation mean concentration of 1,909.5 ± 935.2 pg/mL in whole blood compared with 1,609.2 ± 710.1 pg/mL in 39 healthy controls *4717*

Interleukin-10 *Serum Increase* In 39 patients on first day after mitogen stimulation mean concentration of about 340 pg/mL in whole blood not significantly increased compared with about 220 pg/mL in 39 healthy controls *4717*

Isoleucine *Plasma Increase* Mean concentration increased in 59 depressed patients compared with concentration in healthy controls *3351*

Leucine *Plasma Increase* Mean concentration increased in 59 depressed patients compared with that in healthy controls *3351*

Lysine *Plasma Increase* Mean concentration increased in 59 depressed patients compared with concentration in healthy controls *3351*

α_2-Macroglobulin *Serum Increase* In 39 patients on first day after mitogen stimulation mean concentration of 1.895 ± 0.50 g in serum significantly increased compared with 1.576 ± 0.34 g in 39 healthy controls *4717*

Melanin *Plasma No Effect* No circannual variation observed in 5 manic-depressive patients *1416*

Monoamine Oxidase-B *Platelets No Effect* In 9 depressed patients mean concentration of 1.8 ± 0.5 nmol/mg protein/min not significantly different from 1.7 ± 0.8 nmol/mg protein/min in 9 controls *1491*

Neopterin *Serum Increase* In patients with minor depression and in patients with simple major depression significant positive correlation with sIL-2R concentration *3206* In 16 patients with major depression mean concentration of 6.4 nmol/L statistically different when compared with 5.3 nmol/L in 30 controls *3212*
Urine Decrease Significant reduction observed in 26 patients with acute depression (441 ± 261 nmol/mmol creatinine) compared with control individuals (604 ± 318 nmol/mmol creatinine) and excretion tended to revert to normal as active symptoms lessened *2236*

Neuropeptide Y *Plasma Decrease* In 6 patients with major depression mean concentration in platelet-poor plasma of 155 ± 22 pmol/L significantly different from 186 ± 14 pmol/L in 6 healthy control individuals *3798*
Platelets Increase In 6 patients with major depression mean concentration of 77 ± 17 pmol/μg protein significantly different from 51 ± 13 pmol/μg protein in 6 healthy control individuals *3798*

Norepinephrine *Cerebrospinal Fluid Increase* In 8 studies mean concentration in depressed patients of 146 ng/L compared with 91 ng/L in healthy controls *4189*
Cerebrospinal Fluid No Effect No significant difference observed between 24 depressed patients and 10 controls *1746*
Plasma Increase In 8 studies mean supine concentration of 2.32 nmol/L and upright concentration of 3.94 nmol/L in depressed patients compared with 1.42 nmol/L and 2.81 nmol/L respectively in healthy controls *4189*
Urine Increase In depressed patients baseline concentration significantly increased in comparison with normal individuals *998*

Osmolality *Cerebrospinal Fluid No Effect* No significant difference observed between concentrations in patients with either endogenous or nonendogenous depression and controls *1744*
Serum No Effect Mean 8:00 a.m. concentration in 52 patients with major depression of 291.3 ± 5.3 mOsm/kg not different from 293.0 ± 7.6 mOsm/kg observed in 37 healthy controls *5409* No significant difference observed in concentrations in patients with endogenous or nonendogenous depression compared with controls *1744*

Oxytocin *Cerebrospinal Fluid No Effect* Mean concencentration of 7.1 ± 3.2 μU/mL in 19 patients with major depression not significantly different from 8.1 ± 3.5 μU/mL in 18 healthy controls *4150*
Plasma Increase Mean 8:00 a.m. concentration in 52 patients with major depression of 1.51 ± 0.75 pg/mL different from 1.28 ± 0.57 pg/mL observed in 37 healthy controls *5409*

Partial Thromboplastin Time *Plasma No Effect* In 16 patients with minor depression mean time of 33.5 ± 2.1 s, 40 patients with simple minor depression mean time of 33.4 ± 3.4 s and in 13 with melancholia 32.9 ± 3.8 s not significantly different from 33.5 ± 2.1 s in 16 healthy controls *3214*

Phenylacetic Acid *Cerebrospinal Fluid No Effect* Mean concentration in 19 patients with depression of 28.0 ± 10.9 ng/mL not significantly different from that in 30 healthy volunteers in whom the mean concentration was 26.6 ± 15.2 ng/mL *4761*

Phenylacetic Acid, Conjugated
Cerebrospinal Fluid No Effect Mean concentration in 19 patients with depression of 10.1 ± 4.2 ng/mL not significantly different from that in 30 healthy volunteers in whom the mean concentration was 11.7 ± 5.5 ng/mL *4761*

Phenylacetic Acid, Unconjugated
Cerebrospinal Fluid No Effect Mean concentration in 19 patients with depression of 17.9 ± 8.2 ng/mL not significantly different from that in 30 healthy volunteers in whom the mean concentration was 14.8 ± 12.8 ng/mL *4761*

Phenylethylamine *Urine Increase* 7 of 53 patients had concentrations exceeding 3 times the highest value found in 16 normal controls *1173*

Platelet Aggregation response to ADP *Blood* *No Effect* In 16 patients with minor depression mean, 40 patients with simple minor depression and in 13 with melancholia platelet aggregability with 2, 6.7 and 4 µmol/L ADP not significantly different from that in 16 healthy controls *3214*

Platelet Aggregation response to Collagen *Blood* *No Effect* In 16 patients with minor depression mean, 40 patients with simple minor depression and in 13 with melancholia platelet aggregability with 2 µ/mL collagen not significantly different from that in 16 healthy controls *3214*

Platelets *Blood* *Decrease* In 30 drug-free depressed patients mean concentration of 369,000 ± 19,000 /µL significantly different from 429,000 ± 15,000 /µL in 20 healthy controls *2568*

Prolactin *Plasma* *Decrease* In 27 depressed patients mean concentration significantly reduced compared with concentration in 14 normal individuals *3524*
Plasma *No Effect* Basal concentrations similar in 27 depressed patients and 64 age and sex matched healthy controls *336*

Prostaglandin 2α *Saliva* *Increase* Significant increase in 32 patients with major depressive disorder to 444 ± 100 pg/mL compared with 164 ± 17 pg/mL in 28 healthy controls *3875*

Prostaglandin D_2 *Saliva* *Increase* Concentration in 37 patients with major depressive disorder of 385 ± 71 pg/mL compared with 129 ± 18 pg/mL in 28 healthy controls *3875*

Prostaglandin E_2 *Saliva* *Increase* In 32 patients with major depressive disorder mean concentration of 498 ± 105 pg/mL significantly higher than the mean of 207 ± 25 pg/mL in 28 healthy controls *3875*

Protein *Serum* *Decrease* In 37 patients with major depression mean serum concentration of 65.8 ± 5.6 g/L compared with 74.3 ± 4.8 g/L in 29 normal male volunteers *5405* Mean concentration of 69.6 ± 6.0 g/L in 23 patients with simple major depression significantly different from 73.6 ± 2.9 g/L in 18 healthy controls *3216* In 31 patients with major depression mean concentration of 65.1 ± 5.1 g/L significantly different from 73.9 ± 5.0 g/L in 15 healthy controls *3215*
Serum *No Effect* Mean concentration of 73.1 ± 6.7 g/L in 14 patients with minor depression not different from 73.6 ± 2.9 g/L in 18 healthy controls *3216* In 42 patients with major depression mean concentration of 73.1 ± 7.3 g/L not significantly different from 73.6 ± 3.4 g/L in 24 healthy controls *3217*

Prothrombin Time *Plasma* *Decrease* In 13 patients with melancholia 86.6 ± 18.6% not significantly different from 97.3 ± 5.6% in 16 healthy controls *3214*
Plasma *No Effect* In 16 patients with minor depression mean time of 91.7 ± 11.2% and in 40 patients with simple minor depression mean time of 91.5 ± 10.5% not significantly different from 97.3 ± 5.6% in 16 healthy controls *3214*

Retinol-binding Protein *Serum* *Decrease* Significant decrease observed in patients with both major and minor depression *3213*

Serine *Plasma* *Increase* Significant increase observed in 59 depressed patients compared with a healthy control population *3351*

Sodium *Serum* *No Effect* Mean 8:00 a.m. concentration in 52 patients with major depression of 140.5 ± 2.4 mmol/L not different from 141.1 ± 2.1 mmol/L observed in 37 healthy controls *5409*

Soluble β-Amyloid Peptide 40 *Serum* *Decrease* In 15 reference patients with depression mean concentration of 1,895 ± 662 pmol/L significantly different from 2,311 ± 546 pmol/L in 24 age and sex matched controls *2440*

Soluble β-Amyloid Peptide 42 *Serum* *Increase* In 15 reference depressed patients mean concentration of 180 ± 95 pmol/L significantly different from 74 ± 30 pmol/L in 24 age and sex matched controls *2440*

Soluble Interleukin-2 Receptor *Serum* *Increase* In 5 depressed patients mean concentration about 1,700 pmol/mL versus 1,450 pg/mL in healthy controls *2524* In patients with minor depression mean concentration of 364 ± 72 U/mL and in patients with simple major depression 371 ± 83 U/mL significantly different from 224 ± 107 U/mL in 19 normal controls *3206* In 39 patients on first day after mitogen stimulation mean concentration of about 640 pg/mL in serum not significantly increased compared with about 560 pg/mL in 39 healthy controls although significantly increased in supernatant *4717* In 61 patients with major depression mean concentration of 292 ± 9 U/mL significantly greater than 236 ± 16 U/mL in 38 normal controls *3211*

Soluble Interleukin-6 Receptor *Serum* *Increase* In 61 patients with major depression mean concentration of 85.2 ± 4.2 ng/mL significantly greater than 69.9 ± 3.6 ng/mL in 38 normal controls *3211*

Soluble Transferrin Receptor *Serum* *Increase* In 61 patients with major depression mean concentration of 642 ± 29 U/mL significantly greater than 499 ± 36 U/mL in 38 normal controls *3211*

Tetrahydrobiopterin *Plasma* *Increase* Mean concentration significantly increased in depressed patients to about 150% of the concentration in age and sex matched controls *2715*
Plasma *No Effect* In 10 patients with monopolar depression mean concentration in depressive phase of 13.0 ± 6.2 pmol/mL not significantly different from 14.0 ± 6.6 pmol/mL in healthy controls. In remission phase mean concentration of 13.7 ± 4.8 pmol/mL also not significantly different from controls *2048*

Thromboxane B_2 *Plasma* *No Effect* Mean concentration in 32 patients with depression fell into two classes 36.1 ± 18.4 pg/0.1 mL and 15.0 ± 11.2 pg/0.1 mL similar to two classes of cortisol *4129*

Thyroid Stimulating Hormone *Serum* *Decrease* Significant reduction in nocturnal serum concentration *4469*
Serum *Increase* Mean concentration significantly higher in 27 men with unipolar depression compared with concentration in 38 healthy controls *5522*

Thyrotropin Releasing Hormone
Cerebrospinal Fluid *No Effect* No difference in concentrations observed between patients with endogenous and non-endogenous depression and controls *1744*

Thyroxine (T4) *Serum* *Increase* In 81 depressed in-patients mean concentration significantly higher than in 82 psychiatric controls *798*
Serum *No Effect* No significant differences observed between concentrations in depressed patients and controls *4469* No significant difference observed in concentrations between 27 men with unipolar depression and 38 healthy controls *5522*

Thyroxine (T4), Free *Serum* *No Effect* No significant difference observed in concentrations between 27 men with unipolar depression and 38 healthy controls *5522*

Thyroxine (T4) Index, Free *Serum* *Increase* In 81 depressed patients mean measurement significantly higher than in 82 psychiatric controls *798*

Transferrin *Serum* *Decrease* Significant negative correlation of negative acute phase reactant protein concentrations in patients with major depression compared with normal controls *3216* In 31 patients with major depression mean concentration of 248 ± 31 µg/dL significantly different from 290 ± 26 µg/dL in 15 healthy controls *3215*

Tri-iodothyronine (T3) *Serum* *Decrease* Mean concentration reduced in 27 men with unipolar depression in comparison with 38 healthy controls *5522* Significant reduction in nocturnal concentration observed in depressed patients *4469*

Tryptophan *Plasma* *Decrease* Significantly decreased concentration observed in 12 depressed patients compared with 12 healthy controls: ratio of plasma total tryptophan to neutral aminoacids was also decreased *952* In 3 patients with bipolar depression concentration moderately depressed and blunted circadian rhythm observed during depressive phase *677* In 30 drug-free depressed patients mean concentration of 8.52 ± 0.4 µg/mL significantly different from 11.84 ± 0.3 µg/mL in 20 healthy controls *2568* In 28 depressed patients mean concentration of 50 µmol/L compared with 75 µmol/L in 29 healthy controls. Ratio of tryptophan to large neutral amino acids also markedly reduced *3148*
Plasma *No Effect* In 16 patients with major depression mean concentration of L-tryptophan of 68.8 nmol/L not statistically different when compared with 69.1 nmol/L in 30 controls *3212* In 42 patients with major depression mean concentration of 74.7 ± 17.4 µmol/L not significantly different from 76.4 ± 11.2 µmol/L in 24 healthy controls *3217*

TSH response to TRH *Serum* *No Effect* No significant difference observed between depressed patients and controls *4469*

Valine *Plasma* *Increase* Mean concentration increased in 59 depressed patients compared with concentration in healthy controls *3351*

311.00 Depression *(continued)*

Vitamin B_{12} *Serum* *No Effect* In 9 patients with depression mean concentration of 325 ± 134 pg/mL not significantly different from 326 ± 249 pg/mL in 9 controls *1491*

Zinc *Serum* *Decrease* In 19 patients with unipolar depression mean concentration of 0.79 ± 0.11 mg/L significantly different from 0.90 ± 0.09 mg/L in 16 healthy controls *3836* In 31 patients with major depression mean concentration of 95 ± 11 µg/dL significantly lower than 115 ± 12 µg/dL in 15 healthy controls *3215* Concentration in 18 major depressed patients with melancholia 1.78 ± 0.22 mg/L and in 14 major depressed patients without melancholia 1.77 ± 0.25 mg/L and in 16 with minor depression 1.89 ± 0.34 mg/L significantly less than 2.02 ± 0.20 mg/L in 32 normal volunteers *3209*

311.00 Depressive Spectrum Disease

3-Methoxy-4-hydroxyphenylglycol *Urine* *No Effect* In 38 patients with depressive spectrum disease mean excretion of 1,655 ± 90 mg/d *1663*

311.00 Nondepressive Spectrum Disease

3-Methoxy-4-hydroxyphenylglycol *Urine* *No Effect* In 24 patients with nondepressive spectrum disease mean excretion of 1,965 ± 174 mg/d *1663*

311.00 Postpartum Depression

Cholesterol *Serum* *Decrease* Mean concentration in 20 patients with postpartum depression decreased from 6.52 ± 1.19 mmol/L 14 days before delivery to 5.40 ± 0.88 mmol/L on first day after delivery and 5.92 ± 1.58 mmol/L on third day post-delivery correlating well with mood score *4159*

HDL-Cholesterol *Serum* *Decrease* Mean concentration in 20 patients with postpartum depression decreased from 1.50 ± 0.26 mmol/L 14 days before delivery to 1.29 ± 0.28 mmol/L on first day after delivery and 1.34 ± 0.31 mmol/L on third day post-delivery correlating well with mood score *4159*

LDL-Cholesterol *Serum* *Decrease* Mean concentration in 20 patients with postpartum depression decreased from 4.11 ± 1.14 mmol/L 14 days before delivery to 3.28 ± 0.80 mmol/L on first day after delivery and 3.52 ± 1.24 mmol/L on third day post-delivery correlating well with mood score *4159*

Progesterone *Plasma* *Decrease* Mean concentration in 20 patients with postpartum depression decreased from 614 ± 417 nmol/L 14 days before delivery to 54 ± 35 nmol/L on first day after delivery and 32 ± 19 nmol/L on third day post-delivery correlating well with mood score *4159*

Triglycerides *Serum* *Decrease* Mean concentration in 20 patients with postpartum depression decreased from 2.96 ± 0.78 mmol/L 14 days before delivery to 2.35 ± 0.98 mmol/L on first day after delivery and 2.27 ± 0.79 mmol/L on third day post-delivery correlating well with mood score *4159*

312.30 Impulsive Disorder

Albumin *Serum* *No Effect* In 8 untreated adolescent patients with impulsive behavior mean concentration of 40.4 ± 1.9 g/L not significantly different from 38.6 ± 1.2 g/L in 8 hospitalized controls of the same age *676*

Testosterone *Cerebrospinal Fluid* *Increase* In 43 alcoholic, impulsive offenders with antisocial personality disorder high mean concentration observed *5479*

Tryptophan *Plasma* *No Effect* In 8 untreated adolescent patients with impulsive behavior mean concentration of 52.1 ± 13.7 µmol/L not significantly different from 58.2 ± 5.5 µmol/L in 8 hospitalized controls of the same age *676*

Tryptophan, Free *Plasma* *Decrease* In 8 untreated adolescent patients with impulsive behavior mean concentration of 1.92 µmol/L significantly different from 2.30 µmol/L in 8 hospitalized controls of the same age *676*

Tyrosine *Plasma* *No Effect* In 8 untreated adolescent patients with impulsive behavior mean concentration of 62.4 µmol/L not significantly different from 60 ± 13 µmol/L in 8 hospitalized controls of the same age *676*

314.01 Attention Deficit Disorder with Hyperactivity

Calcium *Urine* *Decrease* In 14 children with attention deficit disorder with hyperactivity mean excretion per kg body weight significantly less than that in 9 healthy children *3847*

Creatinine *Urine* *No Effect* In 14 children with attention deficit disorder with hyperactivity mean excretion of 1.12 g/L not significantly different from 1.14 g/L in 9 healthy children *3847*

3,4-Dihydroxyphenylacetic Acid *Urine* *No Effect* In 15 boys with ADHD mean excretion of 93.9 ± 45.6 pmol/min/m^2 surface area not significantly different from 77.4 ± 24.4 pmol/min/m^2 surface area in 16 healthy controls *2007*

3,4-Dihydroxyphenylalanine *Urine* *No Effect* In 15 boys with ADHD mean excretion of 2.4 ± 1.0 pmol/min/m^2 surface area not significantly different from 2.8 ± 1.2 pmol/min/m^2 surface area in 16 healthy controls *2007*

3,4-Dihydroxyphenylglycol *Urine* *Decrease* In 15 boys with ADHD mean excretion of 5.3 ± 1.2 pmol/min/m^2 surface area significantly different from 6.9 ± 1.9 pmol/min/m^2 surface area in 16 healthy controls *2007*

Dopamine *Urine* *No Effect* In 15 boys with ADHD mean excretion of 19.7 ± 7.1 pmol/min/m^2 surface area not significantly different from 24.6 ± 9.0 pmol/min/m^2 surface area in 16 healthy controls *2007*

Epinephrine *Plasma* *Increase* In 14 children with attention deficit disorder with hyperactivity mean concentration of 111.9 ± 86.4 pg/mL not significantly different from 81.7 ± 86.4 pg/mL in 9 healthy children *3847*
Urine *No Effect* In 15 boys with ADHD mean excretion of 0.7 ± 0.3 pmol/min/m^2 surface area not significantly different from 1.0 ± 0.5 pmol/min/m^2 surface area in 16 healthy controls *2007*

Neuropeptide Y *Plasma* *Increase* In 14 children with attention deficit disorder with hyperactivity mean concentration of 4.15 ± 1.81 fmol/mL significantly different from 2.71 ± 0.79 fmol/mL in 9 healthy children *3847*

Norepinephrine *Plasma* *Increase* In 14 children with attention deficit disorder with hyperactivity mean concentration of 735.5 ± 446.7 pg/mL not significantly different from 481.9 ± 246.6 pg/mL in 9 healthy children *3847*
Urine *No Effect* In 15 boys with ADHD mean excretion of 2.3 ± 0.9 pmol/min/m^2 surface area not significantly different from 2.8 ± 1.1 pmol/min/m^2 surface area in 16 healthy controls *2007*

Phosphate *Urine* *Decrease* In 14 children with attention deficit disorder with hyperactivity mean excretion per kg body weight significantly less than that in 9 healthy children *3847*

Sodium *Urine* *Decrease* In 14 children with attention deficit disorder with hyperactivity mean excretion per kg body weight significantly less than that in 9 healthy children *3847*

Volume *Urine* *Decrease* In 14 children with attention deficit disorder with hyperactivity mean excretion of 612 mL/d significantly different from 870 mL/d in 9 healthy children *3847*

319.00 Cohen Syndrome

Hematocrit *Blood* *No Effect* Hematocrit normal in patients with Cohen's syndrome *2700*

Hemoglobin *Blood* *No Effect* Hemoglobin normal in patients with Cohen's syndrome *2700*

Leukocytes *Blood* *Decrease* White blood cell count typically reduced, below 4.0 x 10^9/L on at least one occasion in 12 of 18 patients *2700*

Metamyelocytes *Bone Marrow* *Increase* Mean concentration of 151 per 1,000 polychromatic erythroblasts in 16 patients with Cohen's syndrome significantly higher than 118 in 16 age-matched controls *2700*

Myelocytes *Bone Marrow* *Increase* Mean concentration of 108 per 1,000 polychromatic erythroblasts in 16 patients with Cohen's syndrome higher than 90 in 16 age-matched controls *2700*

Neutrophil Bands *Bone Marrow* *Increase* Mean concentration of 95 per 1,000 polychromatic erythroblasts in 16 patients with Cohen's syndrome not significantly different from 94 in 16 age-matched controls *2700*

Neutrophils *Blood* *Decrease* Neutrophil count reduced below 1.0 x 10^9/L in patients with Cohen syndrome on at least one occasion in all infants, below 1.5 x 10^9/L in other infants and below 1.8 x 10^9/L in 18 patients *2700*

Platelets *Blood* *No Effect* Platelet count normal in patients with Cohen's syndrome *2700*

Promyelocytes *Bone Marrow* *Increase* Mean concentration of 45 per 1,000 polychromatic erythroblasts in 16 patients with Cohen's syndrome significantly higher than 26 in 16 age-matched controls *2700*

Segmented Neutrophils *Bone Marrow* *Decrease* Mean concentration of 101 per 1,000 polychromatic erythroblasts in 16 patients with Cohen's syndrome not significantly different from 125 in 16 age-matched controls *2700*

319.00 Mental Retardation

γ-Aminobutyric Acid *Plasma* *Increase* In 13 children with mental retardation mean concentration of 340.1 ± 126.5 nmol/L compared with about 120 nmol/L in normals *5879*

Cholesterol *Serum* *Decrease* Serum values from over 1,400 patients were significantly lower than corresponding results from normal subjects. Male patients had significantly lower results than the female patients. There appeared to be no significant correlation between serum cholesterol values and IQ, systolic or diastolic blood pressures, drugs used in treatment, presence or absence of epilepsy *1288*

Glutamic Acid *Plasma* *Increase* Increased glutamic acid with associated decrease in glutamine may occur in De Lange Syndrome and other mental retardation syndromes *1010*

Glutamine *Plasma* *Decrease* Increased glutamic acid with associated decrease in glutamine may occur in De Lange Syndrome and other mental retardation syndromes *1010*

Soluble β-Amyloid Peptide 40 *Serum* *Increase* In 19 mentally retarded patients median concentration of 109 pg/mL significantly different from 53 pg/mL in 43 age-matched normal controls *3441*

Soluble β-Amyloid Peptide 42 *Serum* *No Effect* In 19 mentally retarded patients median concentration of 25 pg/mL significantly different from 25 pg/mL in 43 age-matched normal controls *3441*

DISEASES OF THE NERVOUS SYSTEM

320.00 Hemophilus influenzae B Meningitis

Anti-ribosylphosphate IgG *Serum* *Decrease* Concentrations significantly reduced in acute phase of the disease *2352*

Anti-Ribosylphosphate IgG_2 *Serum* *Decrease* Concentrations significantly reduced in acute phase of the disease *2352*

Immunoglobulin G_1 *Serum* *Increase* In children aged less than 1 y median concentration of 505 mg/dL compared with 331 mg/dL in controls, 518 mg/dL in children aged 1 - 2 y versus 487 mg/dL in controls and 566 mg/dL in children aged 2 - 5 y versus 575 mg/dL in controls *2352*

Immunoglobulin G_2 *Serum* *Decrease* In children aged less than 1 y median concentration of 35 mg/dL compared with 46 mg/dL in controls, 40 mg/dL in children aged 1 - 2 y versus 82 mg/dL in controls and 67 mg/dL in children aged 2 - 5 y versus 130 mg/dL in controls *2352*

Immunoglobulin G_3 *Serum* *Increase* In children aged less than 1 y median concentration of 64 mg/dL compared with 29 mg/dL in controls, 40 mg/dL in children aged 1 - 2 y versus 29 mg/dL in controls and 37 mg/dL in children aged 2 - 5 y versus 45 mg/dL in controls *2352*

Immunoglobulin G_4 *Serum* *Decrease* In children aged less than 1 y median concentration of 4.87 mg/dL compared with 6.17 mg/dL in controls, 4.25 mg/dL in children aged 1 - 2 y versus 9.1 mg/dL in controls and 11.77 mg/dL in children aged 2 - 5 y versus 15.48 mg/dL in controls *2352*

320.90 Bacterial Meningitis

α_1-Acid Glycoprotein *Cerebrospinal Fluid* *Increase* In 30 patients with bacterial meningitis median concentration on first day of admission 40.0 mg/L *4001*
Serum *Increase* In 30 patients with bacterial meningitis median concentration on first day of admission of 1,325 mg/L significantly different from 702 mg/L in 60 healthy controls *4001*

Albumin *Cerebrospinal Fluid* *Increase* Often 100 - 200 mg/dL *900* In 23 children with bacterial meningitis mean concentration of 2,200 mg/L *1690* CSF IgG and albumin are increased due to defect in the blood-CSF barrier *1639* In 30 patients with bacterial meningitis median concentration on first day of admission 956 mg/L *4001*

Albumin Index *Cerebrospinal Fluid* *Increase* Range in 31 patients with bacterial meningitis of 6.5 - 165.0 significantly different from mean of 4.0 in 33 normal controls *3019*

Angiotensin-converting Enzyme
Cerebrospinal Fluid *Increase* Increased concentrations observed *3895*

α_1-Antichymotrypsin *Cerebrospinal Fluid* *Increase* Increased in patients with meningitis or mild hemorrhage, but equal to normal in patients with encephalitis, epilepsy, degenerative disorders or diseases of the CNS *187*

Antidiuretic Hormone *Plasma* *Increase* Associated with excessive ADH production resulting in sodium loss *4707*

α_1-Antitrypsin *Cerebrospinal Fluid* *Increase* In 30 patients with bacterial meningitis median concentration on first day of admission 65.1 mg/L *4001*
Serum *Increase* In 30 patients with bacterial meningitis median concentration on first day of admission of 3,585 mg/L significantly different from 1,630 mg/L in 60 healthy controls *4001*

Aspartate Aminotransferase *Serum* *Increase* In 70% of 14 patients hospitalized for this disorder *1576*

Cells *Cerebrospinal Fluid* *Increase* Increased polymorphonuclear cells are found in CSF. Mononuclear cells appear later in the disease *2039* In 123 patients concentration of 125 to > 2,000 /μL significantly higher than < 1 to 262 /μL in 111 controls *2045* CSF cells are always elevated, ranging from 100 - 100,000 /μL initially polymorphonuclear leukocytes predominate; these are replaced by lymphocytes as the inflammatory process progresses *367* In 23 children with bacterial meningitis mean concentration of 4,710 /μL *1690*
Cerebrospinal Fluid *No Effect* In 12 patients concentration of < 1 to 210 /μL not significantly different from < 1 to 262 /μL in 111 controls *2045*

α_2-Ceruloplasmin *Cerebrospinal Fluid* *Increase* In 30 patients with bacterial meningitis median concentration on first day of admission of 16.8 mg/L *4001*
Serum *Increase* In 30 patients with bacterial meningitis median concentration on first day of admission of 475 mg/L significantly different from 254 mg/L in 60 healthy controls *4001*

Chloride *Cerebrospinal Fluid* *Decrease* Characteristically reduced *5252*
Serum *Decrease* The chloride content is reduced but not as dramatically as in tubercular meningitis *900* In 33% of 18 patients hospitalized for this disorder *1576* Slight decrease *1025*

C-Reactive Protein *Cerebrospinal Fluid* *Increase* Concentration significantly increased in most cases of acute bacterial meningitis with a concentration of 100 ng/mL being useful to separate acute bacterial from acute viral infections. Using this a sensitivity of 80% would be attained for acute bacterial meningitis *4988* Mean and median concentration (1,768 and 289 ng/mL respectively) in 15 patients with bacterial meningitis significantly higher than in those with viral meningitis and healthy controls (median 34 ng/mL, normal range < 20 - 100 ng/mL) *4987* Concentration increased in 95% of patients with bacterial meningitis *3929* In 30 patients with bacterial meningitis median concentration on first day of admission 5.15 mg/L *4001* CRP detectable in 73 of 79 patients with bacterial meningitis *3929*
Serum *Increase* Markedly elevated *2889* In 30 patients with bacterial meningitis median concentration on first day of admission of 146 mg/L significantly different from 14.8 mg/L in 60 healthy controls *4001* In 23 children with bacterial meningitis mean concentration of 143.3 mg/L *1690*

Creatine Kinase *Serum* *Increase* Reported effect *1980*

320.90 Bacterial Meningitis *(continued)*

Creatinine *Serum Increase* Dehydration may be observed *2034*

Cryofibrinogen *Plasma Increase* May be observed *4551*

Culture *Blood Positive* Positive culture observed in 80% of patients with bacterial meningitis *3929*
Cerebrospinal Fluid Positive Positive culture observed in 95% of patients with bacterial meningitis *3929*

Erythrocyte Sedimentation Rate *Blood Increase* Observed effect *900*

α_2-Globulin *Serum Increase* Observed effect *5544*

γ-Globulin *Cerebrospinal Fluid Increase* Elevated in all forms of meningeal inflammation *5252*

Glomerular Filtration Rate *Urine Increase* Associated excess ADH may tend to accelerate GFR *4707*

Glucose *Cerebrospinal Fluid Decrease* Concentration decreased below 2.5 mmol/L in 69% of patients with bacterial meningitis *3929* Usual values < 40 mg/dL, and may be close to 0 mg/dL. Low CSF sugar distinguishes bacterial from viral meningitides *367* CSF/blood sugar ratios were of diagnostic and prognostic value, especially in suboptimally treated cases *4298* In 105 patients median concentration of 0.5 mmol/L (0.1 - 4.9) significantly lower than 3.6 mmol/L (1.7 - 13.3) in 84 controls *2045* Usually well below 50% of the blood sugar and may be entirely absent *1980* CSF glucose is < 50% blood sugar *2039* Mean concentration in 79 patients with bacterial meningitis of 2.18 mmol/L *3929* Decreased in children with transverse myelitis and mycoplasma pneumoniae meningoencephalitis *2706*
Serum Increase In 32% of 18 patients hospitalized for this disorder *1576*

Gram Stain *Cerebrospinal Fluid Positive* Positive reaction observed in 83% of patients with bacterial meningitis *3929*

Granulocyte-Macrophage Colony Stimulating Factor
Cerebrospinal Fluid No Effect In none of 5 patients with bacterial meningitis was GM-CSF detected *4804*

α_2-Haptoglobin *Cerebrospinal Fluid Increase* In 30 patients with bacterial meningitis median concentration on first day of admission 22.6 mg/L *4001*
Serum Increase In 30 patients with bacterial meningitis median concentration on first day of admission 2,095 mg/L significantly different from 767 mg/L in 60 healthy controls *4001*

Hematocrit *Blood Decrease* In 54% of 18 patients hospitalized for this disorder *1576*

Hemoglobin *Blood Decrease* In 66% of 18 patients hospitalized for this disorder *1576*

Immunoglobulin G *Cerebrospinal Fluid Increase* Characteristic of brucella meningitis. Increased in acute meningitis due to impairment of blood:CSF barrier. Increases in absolute not relative amount of individual proteins are found in CSF. Little or no IgG was found to be synthesized intrathecally. A high correlation (r = 0.95) was found between plasma and CSF IgG and albumin concentrations *1639* Observed effect *1157* Increased with obstruction of the spinal canal, especially in neurosyphilis and tuberculous meningitis *5138*

Immunoglobulins *Cerebrospinal Fluid Increase* Early rise in CSF *1290*

Insulin-like Growth Factor Binding Protein-3
Cerebrospinal Fluid Increase Mean concentration in 79 patients with bacterial meningitis of 118.3 mg/dL *3929*

Interleukin-1β *Cerebrospinal Fluid Increase* Median concentration often increased in patients with bacterial meningitis *2314*

Interleukin-6 *Cerebrospinal Fluid Increase* In 11 patients mean concentration ranged from less than 3 to 3,520 pg/mL with median of 470 pg/mL compared with median of less than 3 pg/mL in controls *4987* In 16 patients with bacterial meningitis mean concentration of 2,528.0 ± 403.3 pg/mL compared with 93.6 ± 21.8 pg/mL in control population with asceptic lumboischiadic syndrome *5872* Median concentration often increased in patients with bacterial meningitis *2314* In 9 patients with CSF bacterial meningitis mean concentration of 49,017 ± 44,730 pg/mL significantly higher than upper limit of normal of 5 pg/mL in 21 control patients *3372* In 5 patients with proved bacterial meningitis concentrations ranged from 10.7 to 28.4 ng/mL compared with 0.04 to 2.65 ng/mL in controls *2054* In 123 patients median concentration of 99.2 ng/mL (0.04 - 707.9) significantly higher than 0.37 ng/mL (0.04 - 12.5) in 111 controls *2045*
Serum Increase In 23 children with bacterial meningitis mean concentration of 1,340.9 pg/mL *1690*

Interleukin-8 *Cerebrospinal Fluid Increase* The IL-8 concentration was markedly higher in the CSF of patients with bacterial meningitis (224 ± 2.57 pg/mL; mean ± SD) than in the CSF of patients with aseptic meningitis (less than 30 pg/mL) *4726*

Isocitrate Dehydrogenase *Cerebrospinal Fluid Increase* Observed effect *1290*

Lactate *Cerebrospinal Fluid Increase* CSF specimens from 60 of 62 patients with bacterial or mycoplasma etiology showed levels > 20 mg/dL *910* In 28 patients median concentration of 18.25 mmol/L (8.95 - 35.75) significantly higher than 1.75 mmol/L (1.15 - 6.62) in 42 controls *2045*

Lactate Dehydrogenase *Cerebrospinal Fluid Increase* 234 specimens from 183 different children were analyzed. Activity was elevated in patients with meningitis, especially bacterial infections, and CNS leukemia. The isoenzyme pattern generally reflected the number and distribution of lymphocytes and granulocytes in the CSF *3757* In 16 patients with bacterial meningitis mean concentration of 2.32 ± 0.50 µkat/L compared with 0.44 ± 0.12 µkat/L in 20 controls with asceptic lumboischiadic syndrome *5872* Elevations varied from 2 - 100 times the normal values in 23 cases. Significantly lower levels were found in patients with viral meningitis and in CNS infection *1455*
Serum Increase LD and its isoenzymes are elevated, mostly due to a rise in the leukocyte fraction. Patients with increased brain LD isoenzyme usually develop neurologic sequelae or die *367* In 64% of 12 patients hospitalized for this disorder *1576*

Lactate Dehydrogenase Isoenzyme-5
Cerebrospinal Fluid Increase LD activity varies widely from 2 - 100 times the normal CSF concentration. Invariably the most prominent isoenzyme *3757*

Lactate Dehydrogenase Isoenzymes
Cerebrospinal Fluid Increase Slightly elevated but rise sharply in patients who die or develop neurologic sequelae *2034*
Serum Increase LD isoenzymes are elevated, mostly due to a rise in the leukocyte fraction. Patients with increased brain isoenzyme usually develop neurologic sequelae or die *367*

Leukocytes *Blood Increase* Generally elevated with a shift to the left *2034* In 72% of 19 patients hospitalized for this disorder *1576*
Cerebrospinal Fluid Increase Mean concentration in 79 patients with bacterial meningitis of 1,326 /µL *3929* In 13 of 15 patients count abnormal with counts in all 15 patients ranging from 2 to 9,000 /µL compared with < 5 /µL in healthy controls *4987* Mean concentration of 10,833 ± 16,510 /µL in 7 patients with bacterial meningitis with poor outcome different from 7,179 ± 8,845 /µL in 23 patients with good outcome *4963* Ranges between 500 - 20,000 /µL, with about 90% polymorphonuclears. Counts > 25,000 /µL suggest a ruptured brain abscess *1980* Typical response to infection *2039* In 30 patients with bacterial meningitis median concentration on first day of admission 2,008 /µL *4001* Several hundred to 60,000 /µL with predominantly polymorphonuclear cells present *367* Concentration increased above 500 /µL in 43% of patients with bacterial meningitis *3929* Normal response to infection *5358*

Lymphocytes *Cerebrospinal Fluid Increase* Lymphocytes will be more prevalent in the CSF if the disease moves into the subacute or chronic stage. Polymorphonuclear neutrophils may predominate in the early phase of an aseptic or viral meningitis *900*

Lysozyme *Cerebrospinal Fluid Increase* May be increased but clinical significance is unknown *2034*

α_2-Macroglobulin *Cerebrospinal Fluid Increase* All age groups *4641*

α_1-Microglobulin *Cerebrospinal Fluid Increase* Of 2 patients with bacterial meningitis mean concentration in one greater than that in 15 healthy controls of 34.8 ± 16.0 µg/L *2370*

β-Microglobulin *Cerebrospinal Fluid Increase* In 6 neonates with CNS infection mean concentration of 6.98 ± 2.5 mg/L significantly higher than 1.86 ± 0.6 mg/L in 16 without CNS infection *1647*
Serum Increase In 6 neonates with CNS infection mean concentration of 3.2 ± 0.25 mg/L significantly higher than 2.9 ± 0.57 mg/L in 16 without CNS infection *1647*

Nerve Growth Factor *Cerebrospinal Fluid Increase* Concentration increased (mean of 7.3 ± 1.9 pg/mL) in 2 of 7 patients with bacterial meningitis *5091*

Neutrophils *Blood Increase* Typical response *900* In 55% of 20 patients hospitalized for this disorder *1576*
Cerebrospinal Fluid Increase Response to infection *2039* Ranges between 500 - 20,000 /µL, with about 90% polymorphonuclears. Counts > 25,000 suggest a ruptured brain abscess *1980* Mean concentration in 79 patients with bacterial meningitis of 1,098 /µL *3929* Typical response to infection *5358* Several hundred to 60,000 /µL with predominantly polymorphonuclear cells present *367* Concentration increased above 200 /µL in 67% of patients with bacterial meningitis *3929*

Nitroblue Tetrazolium Test *Blood Increase* Mean percentage of positive neutrophils was 21.5% in 30 patients. Useful in differential diagnosis of bacterial and tubercular meningitis (all tubercular meningitis NBT scores were normal) *821*

Procalcitonin *Plasma Increase* In 23 children with bacterial meningitis mean concentration of 60.9 µg/L *1690*

Protein *Cerebrospinal Fluid Increase* Observed effect *367* Concentration increased above 100 mg/dL in 35% of patients with bacterial meningitis *3929* In 13 of 15 patients concentration increased up to 4.9 g/L although 2 patients had normal concentrations of less than 0.4 g/L *4987* In 30 patients with bacterial meningitis median concentration on first day of admission 3,500 mg/L *4001* Nearly always elevated above 50 mg/dL *5358* In 109 patients median concentration of 2.75 g/L (0.1 - 10.95) significantly higher than 0.37 g/L (0.15 - 1.33) in 93 controls *2045* Observed effect *2039* Ranges between 50 - 500 mg/dL, with an average of 200 - 300 mg/dL *1980* Increased with obstruction of the spinal canal, especially in neurosyphilis and tuberculous meningitis *5138*

Rheumatoid Factor *Cerebrospinal Fluid Increase* In 18 samples of CSF from patients with pneumococcal meningitis, 11 were found to be positive by the latex fixation test *927*

Sodium *Serum Decrease* Frequently observed *126* Associated with excessive ADH production *4707* Serum concentrations below 135 mmol/L were noted on admission in 72 of 124 (58.1%) of patients. Low initial concentration and prolonged depression despite fluid restriction correlated significantly with the presence of neurologic sequelae of the disease *1443*
Urine Increase Urine is almost always hypertonic to plasma *126*

Soluble Intercellular Adhesion Molecule-1
Cerebrospinal Fluid Increase Range in 31 patients with bacterial meningitis of 4.36 - 107.2 ng/mL significantly different from mean of 1.51 ng/mL in 33 normal controls *3019*
Serum Increase Range in 31 patients with bacterial meningitis of 256.3 - 1,134.0 ng/mL significantly different from mean of 285.1 ng/mL in 33 normal controls *3019*

Thromboplastin Generation *Cerebrospinal Fluid Increase* Increased thromboplastic activity is about 145 fold more common in bacterial meningitis than in viral meningitis *5335*

β-Trace Protein *Cerebrospinal Fluid Decrease* In 41 patients with bacterial meningitis mean concentration of 8.7 ± 3.9 mg/L significantly reduced compared with 16.6 ± 3.6 mg/L in 27 normal controls *5323*

Tumor Necrosis Factor *Cerebrospinal Fluid Increase* Concentrations significantly increased in patients with acute bacterial meningitis *4988*

Tumor Necrosis Factor-α *Cerebrospinal Fluid Increase* In 14 of 15 patients TNF-α detected with values ranging from 20 U/mL to 1,000 U/mL with median of 836 U/mL compared with less than 10 U/mL in 22 of 24 controls *4987* In 16 patients with bacterial meningitis mean concentration of 18.60 ± 8.60 pg/mL compared with 0.94 ± 0.55 pg/mL in 20 controls with asceptic lumboischiadic syndrome *5872* Median concentration often increased in patients with bacterial meningitis *2314* Observed effect *5503*

Urea Nitrogen *Serum Increase* Dehydration may be observed *2034*

Uric Acid *Cerebrospinal Fluid Increase* Markedly increased with decreased blood:CSF ratio, possibly due to cellular breakdown and nucleoprotein catabolism *5100* High CSF levels of 0.9 - 1.3 mg/dL, with normal serum levels *2892*
Serum Increase In 36% of 11 patients hospitalized for this disorder *1576* Increased in both blood and CSF with a lowered blood:CSF ratio, possibly due to cellular breakdown and nucleoprotein catabolism *5100*
Serum No Effect High CSF levels of 0.9 - 1.3 mg/dL, with normal serum levels *2892*
Urine Increase Increased excretion in neurological and psychiatric disorders; progressive rise in urinary level following slight rise in blood, due to disturbed purine metabolism *5100*

320.90 Meningitis

α₁-Acid Glycoprotein *Serum Increase* In 17 hospitalized adults mean concentration on admission of 1.97 ± 0.32 g/L compared with less than 0.50 g/L in 30 healthy controls *721*

Albumin *Cerebrospinal Fluid Increase* In 11 patients with meningitis mean concentration of 1,249 ± 1,384 mg/L significantly higher than 179 ± 53 mg/L in 5 controls *429*

Amyloid A Protein *Serum Increase* In 17 adults with meningitis mean concentration on admission to hospital of 752 ± 48 mg/L compared with less than 1.5 mg/L in 30 healthy controls *721*

Anti-Neutrophil Cytoplasm Antibodies *Serum No Effect* In 0 of 4 patients (0%) with meningitis/encephalitis pANCA detected *3722*

α₁-Antichymotrypsin *Serum Increase* Mean concentration in 17 adults on admission to hospital of 0.95 ± 0.25 g/L compared with less than 0.50 g/L in 30 healthy controls *721*

Antinuclear Antibodies *Serum No Effect* In 1 of 4 patients (25%) with meningitis/encephalitis ANA detected *3722*

Apolipoprotein A-I *Cerebrospinal Fluid Increase* In 10 patients with acute meningitis mean concentration of 7.74 ± 1.78 mg/L in the active stage significantly greater than 2.72 ± 0.38 mg/L in the convalescent stage *4936*

Apolipoprotein E *Cerebrospinal Fluid Increase* In 24 patients with acute meningitis mean concentration of 6.80 ± 0.65 mg/L in the active stage significantly greater than 4.16 ± 0.35 mg/L in a control population *4936*

C-Reactive Protein *Serum Increase* Mean concentration in 17 adult patients on admission to hospital of 138 ± 28 mg/L compared with less than 3 mg/L in 30 healthy controls *721*

Creatine Kinase BB-Isoenzyme
Cerebrospinal Fluid Increase Proved to be increased. Due to liberation from the brain tissue and penetration into the intercellular fluid and then into CSF related to structural changes in the cellular membrane *4898*

Growth-related Protein-α *Cerebrospinal Fluid Increase* Detected in CSF of patients with meningitis, with concentration highest in patients with bacterial meningitis *5172*

Immunoglobulin G *Cerebrospinal Fluid Increase* Mean concentration in 17 patients with CNS infection of 4.65 ± 3.09 mg/dL higher than 2.11 ± 1.03 mg/dL in 20 patients with CNS non-inflammation (controls) *5295* In 11 patients with meningitis mean concentration of 519 ± 726 mg/L significantly higher than 21 ± 4.6 mg/L in 5 controls *429*

Interferon-α *Cerebrospinal Fluid No Effect* In 17 patients with CNS infections IFN-α not detectable *5295*

Interleukin-1 *Cerebrospinal Fluid Increase* Detected in CSF of patients with meningitis *5172*

Interleukin-1β *Cerebrospinal Fluid No Effect* In 17 patients with CNS infections IL-1β not detectable *5295*

Interleukin-6 *Cerebrospinal Fluid Increase* Detected in CSF of patients with meningitis *5172* IL-6 detected in 11 of 17 patients with CNS infections (mean concentration of 374.24 ± 92.61 pg/mL) whereas it was present in only 2 of 20 controls *5295*

Interleukin-8 *Cerebrospinal Fluid Increase* Detected in CSF of patients with meningitis, with concentration highest in patients with bacterial meningitis *5172*

Macrophage Inflammatory Protein-1α
Cerebrospinal Fluid Increase Detected in CSF of patients with meningitis, with concentration highest in patients with bacterial meningitis *5172*

Macrophage Inflammatory Protein-1β
Cerebrospinal Fluid Increase Detected in CSF of patients with meningitis, with concentration highest in patients with bacterial meningitis *5172*

Monocyte Chemotactic Protein-1
Cerebrospinal Fluid Increase Detected in CSF of patients with meningitis, with concentration highest in patients with bacterial meningitis *5172*

320.90 Meningitis *(continued)*

Neuropeptide Y *Cerebrospinal Fluid* *No Effect* In 10 patients mean concentration of 96.3 ± 25.9 pg/mL not significantly different from 87.5 ± 40.3 pg/mL in 11 controls less than 60 years *3201*

Plasminogen Activator Inhibitor-1 *Cerebrospinal Fluid* *No Effect* In 3 patients with meningits mean concentration of 0.39 ± 0.11 ng/mL not significantly different from 0.31 ± 0.06 ng/mL in 20 reference individuals *56*

Prostaglandin E_2 *Cerebrospinal Fluid* *Increase* Mean concentration of 49.58 ± 42.51 pg/mL in 17 patients with CNS infection significantly higher than 0.20 ± 0.07 pg/mL in 20 patients with CNS non-inflammation (controls) *5295*

Protein *Cerebrospinal Fluid* *Increase* In 12 patients with meningitis mean concentration of 1.89 ± 2.26 g/L significantly higher than 0.21 ± 0.06 g/L in 7 controls *429*

Soluble E-Selectin *Serum* *Increase* In 10 patients with meningococcal disease serum concentrations were significantly increased when compared with concentrations in 11 normal controls *611*

Soluble P-Selectin *Serum* *No Effect* In 10 patients with meningococcal disease serum concentrations were not significantly different when compared with concentrations in 11 normal controls *611*

Somatostatin *Cerebrospinal Fluid* *Decrease* In 10 patients mean concentration of 21.3 ± 10.1 pg/mL significantly less than 38.8 ± 12.3 pg/mL in 11 controls less 60 years *3201*

Tumor Necrosis Factor-α *Cerebrospinal Fluid* *Increase* Detected in CSF of patients with meningitis *5172* *Cerebrospinal Fluid* *No Effect* In 17 patients with CNS infection TNF-α not detected *5295*

320.90 Pyogenic Meningitis

Adenosine Deaminase *Cerebrospinal Fluid* *Increase* In 30 patients with pyogenic meningitis median concentration of 6.2 U/L significantly different from 1 U/L in 117 individuals without meningitis *3122*

Glucose *Cerebrospinal Fluid* *Increase* In 15 patients with pyogenic meningitis mean CSF/serum ratio of 11 significantly greater than 0 in 15 controls without neurological disorders *3123*

Interleukin-6 *Cerebrospinal Fluid* *Increase* In 15 patients with pyogenic meningitis mean concentration of 44,695 pg/mL significantly greater than < 40 pg/mL in 15 controls without neurological disorders *3123*

Leukocytes *Cerebrospinal Fluid* *Increase* In 30 patients with pyogenic meningitis median concentration of 4,966 x 10^9/L significantly different from < 5 x 10^9/L in 117 individuals without meningitis *3122* In 15 patients with pyogenic meningitis mean concentration of 6,778 x 10^9/L significantly greater than < 5 x 10^9/L in 15 controls without neurological disorders *3123*

Neutrophils *Cerebrospinal Fluid* *Increase* In 15 patients with pyogenic meningitis mean proportion of 14% significantly greater than 0 in 15 controls without neurological disorders *3123*

Oligoclonal Banding *Cerebrospinal Fluid* *Increase* Oligoclonal IgG bands detected in late phase of pyogenic meningitis *3261*

Protein *Cerebrospinal Fluid* *Increase* In 15 patients with pyogenic meningitis mean concentration of 246 mg/dL significantly greater than 16 mg/dL in 15 controls without neurological disorders *3123* In 30 patients with pyogenic meningitis median concentration of 2,640 mg/L significantly different from 220 mg/L in 117 individuals without meningitis *3122*

322.90 Meningeal Leukemia

α_1-Microglobulin *Cerebrospinal Fluid* *No Effect* Of 6 patients with meningeal leukemia mean concentration in none greater than that in 15 healthy controls of 34.8 ± 16.0 μg/L *2370*

322.90 Varicella Meningitis

Soluble HLA-I *Cerebrospinal Fluid* *Increase* Known to be present in CSF of people with AIDS with concentration correlating with the stage of the disease *216*

323.90 Central Nervous System Infection

Carbonic Anhydrase II *Cerebrospinal Fluid* *No Effect* In 20 patients with brain infarction median concentration of 39.1 μg/L not significantly different from median of 7.9 μg/L in 97 controls *4012*

Erythrocytes *Cerebrospinal Fluid* *No Effect* In 20 patients with brain infarction median concentration of 4 x 10^6/L not significantly different from median of 1 x 10^6/L in 97 controls *4012*

Leukocytes *Cerebrospinal Fluid* *Increase* In 20 patients with brain infarction median concentration of 43 x 10^6/L significantly different from median of 1 x 10^6/L in 97 controls *4012*

Protein *Cerebrospinal Fluid* *Increase* In 20 patients with brain infarction median concentration of 770 mg/L significantly different from median of 400 mg/L in 97 controls *4012*

323.90 Encephalitis

Interleukin-1β *Cerebrospinal Fluid* *Increase* In 8 children with acute encephalitis/encephalopathy concentrations ranged from < 4 - 11 pg/mL different from normal concentration of < 4 pg/mL *2314*

Interleukin-6 *Cerebrospinal Fluid* *Increase* In 9 patients with encephalitis mean concentration of 409 ± 835 pg/mL significantly higher than upper limit of normal of 5 pg/mL in 21 control patients *3372* In 8 children with acute encephalitis/encephalopathy concentrations ranged from < 31.2 - 626 pg/mL different from normal concentration of < 31.2 pg/mL *2314*

Nerve Growth Factor *Cerebrospinal Fluid* *Increase* Concentration increased (mean 8.5 ± 6.8 pg/mL) in 7 of 14 patients with viral meningitis or encephalitis *5091*

Neuron-specific Enolase *Serum* *No Effect* In 4 patients with encephalitis concentrations ranged from 4.4 - 6.9 μg/L compared with 8.11 ± 3.17 μg/L in 35 control individuals *983*

Plasminogen Activator Inhibitor-1 *Cerebrospinal Fluid* *Increase* In 20 patients with encephalitis mean concentration of 1.19 ± 0.20 ng/mL significantly different from 0.31 ± 0.06 ng/mL in 20 reference individuals *56*

Tumor Necrosis Factor-α *Cerebrospinal Fluid* *Increase* In 8 children with acute encephalitis/encephalopathy concentrations ranged from < 15 - 543 pg/mL different from normal concentration of < 15 pg/mL *2314*

323.90 Encephalitis, Limbic

Oligoclonal Banding *Cerebrospinal Fluid* *Increase* Oligoclonal IgG bands detected with limbic encephalitis *3261*

323.90 Encephalomyelitis

Amylase *Serum* *Increase* If amylase levels are elevated, mumps or Coxsackie virus may be indicated *900*

α_1-Antichymotrypsin *Cerebrospinal Fluid* *No Effect* Increased in patients with meningitis or mild hemorrhage, but equal to normal in patients with encephalitis, epilepsy, degenerative disorders or diseases of the CNS *187*

Antidiuretic Hormone *Plasma* *Increase* Associated with excessive ADH production resulting in sodium loss *4707*

Cells *Cerebrospinal Fluid* *Increase* Usually increased (< 100 /μL), mostly polymorphonuclear leukocytes. After the third day cell count is > 90% lymphocytes *5545*

Chloride *Cerebrospinal Fluid* *Increase* Usually normal or increased *900*

Creatine Kinase *Serum* *Increase* Enzyme studies may help suggest certain causes, (e.g., CK is elevated with myopathy, particularly in Coxsackie A infections and leptospirosis) *900*

Erythrocytes *Urine* *Increase* Hematuria may occur with viremia but is transient *900*

Glomerular Filtration Rate *Urine* *Increase* Associated excess ADH may tend to accelerate GFR *4707*

Immunoglobulin G *Cerebrospinal Fluid* *Increase* Total protein and IgG concentration were increased *5138*

Leukocytes *Blood* *Decrease* The peripheral WBC reveals leukopenia at the onset of most viral infections *900*

Cerebrospinal Fluid *Increase* Pleocytosis ranges from 10 - 500 /µL. In most infections, and these are predominantly lymphocytes; however, granulocytes may prevail for 1 - 2 days after onset. Counts may exceed 100 /µL especially in lymphocytic choriomeningitis and eastern equine encephalomyelitis *900*

Lymphocytes *Cerebrospinal Fluid* *Increase* Approximately 66% of the patients show a lymphocytic pleocytosis in the spinal fluid, but in the remaining 33%, the CSF is normal *900*

Neutrophils *Cerebrospinal Fluid* *Increase* Pleocytosis ranges from 10 - 500 /µL. Granulocytes may prevail for 1 - 2 days after onset. Counts may exceed 100 /µL especially in lymphocytic choriomeningitis and eastern equine encephalomyelitis *900*

Protein *Cerebrospinal Fluid* *Increase* The protein concentration is elevated but rarely exceeds 150 mg/dL. A slight elevation is common *900* Total protein and IgG concentration were increased *5138*

Sodium *Serum* *Decrease* Associated with excessive ADH production *4707* Serum sodium is usually less than 130 mEq/L *126*
Urine *Increase* Urine is almost always hypertonic to plasma *126*

Uric Acid *Cerebrospinal Fluid* *Increase* High CSF levels of 0.9 - 1.3 mg/dL, with normal serum levels are seen in acute encephalitis *2892* Markedly increased with decreased blood:CSF ratio, possibly due to cellular breakdown and nucleoprotein catabolism *5100*
Serum *Increase* Increased in both blood and CSF with a lowered blood:CSF ratio, possibly due to cellular breakdown and nucleoprotein catabolism *5100*
Serum *No Effect* High CSF levels of 0.9 -1.3 mg/dL, with normal serum levels are seen in acute encephalitis *2892*
Urine *Increase* Increased excretion in neurological and psychiatric disorders; progressive rise in urinary level following slight rise in blood, due to disturbed purine metabolism *5100*

323.90 Leukoencephalopathy

Amyloid β-Protein *Cerebrospinal Fluid* *No Effect* In 1 patient with encephalopathy concentration was 2.37 pmol/mL not significantly different from mean concentration of 4.00 ± 2.92 pmol/mL *3716*

Amyloid β-Protein Precursor *Cerebrospinal Fluid* *Decrease* In 1 patient with leukoencephalopathy concentration was 0.86 integrated OD units significantly different from mean concentration of 1.35 ± 0.38 integrated OD units in 25 normal controls *3716*

α_1-Antichymotrypsin *Cerebrospinal Fluid* *Increase* In 1 patient with leukoencephalopathy concentration was 7.60 µg/mL significantly different from mean concentration of 2.27 ± 1.40 µg/mL in 25 normal controls *3716*

Cells *Cerebrospinal Fluid* *No Effect* In 1 patient with leukoencephalopathy concentration of 0.3 cells/µL not significantly different from normal of 3 cells/µL *3716*

Protein *Cerebrospinal Fluid* *No Effect* In 1 patient with leukoencephalopathy concentration of 37 mgL not significantly different from normal of 28 mg/dL in 25 healthy controls *3716*

323.91 Myelitis

Anti-Neutrophil Cytoplasm Antibodies *Serum* *Increase* In 2 of 17 patients (11.8%) with myelitis pANCA detected *3722*

Antinuclear Antibodies *Serum* *Increase* In 3 of 17 patients (17.6%) with myelitis ANA detected *3722*

Cells *Cerebrospinal Fluid* *Increase* Spinal fluid may be normal or may show increased protein and cells (20 - 1,000 /µL - lymphocytes and mononuclear cells) *5544* Increased WBCs, mononuclear, and polymorphonuclear cells are found *2039*

Glucose *Cerebrospinal Fluid* *Decrease* Decreased in children with transverse myelitis and mycoplasma pneumoniae meningoencephalitis *2706*

Leukocytes *Cerebrospinal Fluid* *Increase* Spinal fluid may be normal or may show increased protein and cells (20 - 1,000 /µL- lymphocytes and mononuclear cells) *5544* Increased WBCs, mononuclear, and polymorphonuclear cells are found *2039*

Lymphocytes *Cerebrospinal Fluid* *Increase* Spinal fluid may be normal or may show increased protein and cells (20 - 1,000 /µL -- lymphocytes and mononuclear cells) *5544*

Monocytes *Cerebrospinal Fluid* *Increase* Spinal fluid may be normal or may show increased protein and cells (20 - 1,000 /µL - lymphocytes and mononuclear cells) *5544*

Oligoclonal Banding *Cerebrospinal Fluid* *Increase* Oligoclonal IgG bands detected with myelitis (HTLV-1) *3261*

Protein *Cerebrospinal Fluid* *Increase* Increased to 45 - 200 mg/dL in encephalitis and myelitis *2039*

324.00 Intracranial Abscess

Cells *Cerebrospinal Fluid* *Increase* May vary from 0 to many thousands /µL, depending on the degree of meningitic involvement, and may be particularly high if the abscess has ruptured into the ventricles. In most chronic abscesses, the cell count is usually > 100 /µL, and the cells are usually mononuclear *900* Usually < 500 /µL with polymorphonuclears predominating in chronic encapsulating infections *2039*

Chloride *Cerebrospinal Fluid* *Decrease* 600 - 750 mg/dL *1980*

Erythrocyte Sedimentation Rate *Blood* *Increase* Usually elevated, as in other chronic infections, and when present with symptoms and signs of an intracranial mass lesion one should consider the possibility of brain abscess *900*

Glucose *Cerebrospinal Fluid* *Increase* Elevated in lumbar CSF in all patients with subdural empyema. Moderate-marked elevation in lumbar CSF in 14 of 17 patients *2588*
Cerebrospinal Fluid *No Effect* Usually normal until the process extends to actively involve the meninges *1980* Usually normal; however, in the meningitic phase it may be low *900* Concentration usually normal *2034*

Leukocytes *Blood* *Increase* May be normal or slightly elevated in the range of 12,000 - 15,000 /µL. In the acute phase it may be markedly elevated with an increase in the polymorphonuclears *900*
Blood *No Effect* May be normal or slightly elevated in the range of 12,000 - 15,000 /µL. In the acute phase it may be markedly elevated with an increase in the polymorphonuclears *900*
Cerebrospinal Fluid *Increase* In the range of 50 - 1,000 /µL *2034* Usually ranges from 50 - 300 /µL and consists predominantly of lymphocytes. With intraventricular rupture, counts may exceed 50,000 /µL *1980* Counts may be < 100 to several thousand /µL in subdural empyema *367*

Lymphocytes *Cerebrospinal Fluid* *Increase* In the range of 50 - 1,000 /µL *2034* Count usually ranges from 50 - 300 /µL and consists predominantly of lymphocytes *1980*

Neutrophils *Blood* *Increase* In the acute phase WBC may be markedly elevated with an increase in the polymorphonuclear leukocytes *900* Slight increase in neutrophils and lymphocytes (20 - 100 /µL) *5544*

Protein *Cerebrospinal Fluid* *Increase* Usually elevated, varying between 60 - 200 mg/dL *900* Raised, particularly if the abscess is near to the surface, 75 - 300 mg/dL *2034*
Cerebrospinal Fluid *No Effect* Normal or increased *2034*

324.10 Intraspinal Abscess

Leukocytes *Cerebrospinal Fluid* *Increase* Usually 10 - 100 WBC/µL with predominantly lymphocytes present in spinal epidural abscess *367*

Lymphocytes *Cerebrospinal Fluid* *Increase* Usually 1 - 100 WBC/µL with predominantly lymphocytes present in spinal epidural abscess *367*

Protein *Cerebrospinal Fluid* *Increase* Increased (usually 100 - 400 mg/dL), and WBCs (lymphocytes and neutrophils) are relatively few in number *5544*

330.00 Adrenoleukodystrophy

Chitotriosidase *Serum* *No Effect* Normal activity observed in one patient with adrenoleukodystrophy *1917*

330.00 Canavan Disease

Chitotriosidase *Serum* *No Effect* Normal activity observed in one patient with adrenoleukodystrophy *1917*

330.00 Krabbe's Disease

Chitotriosidase *Serum* *Increase* Abnormal activities observed in 7 of 11 patients, with activities ranging from 610 - 1,670 nmol/h/mL *1917*

Galactosylceramide β-Galactosidase *Fibroblasts* *Decrease* Deficiency of enzyme causes Krabbe's disease (globoid cell leukodystrophy) *2952*
White Blood Cells *Decrease* Deficiency of enzyme causes Krabbe's disease (globoid cell leukodystrophy) *2952*

Lysosome-associated Membrane Protein-2
Serum *No Effect* Median concentration of 1.33 mg/L in 12 patients with Krabbe's disease with median age 0.4 y compared with 1.21 mg/L in 202 healthy controls aged 0 - 66 y (median 7 years) *2265*

Lysosome-associated Membrane Protein-2:Lysosome-associated Membrane Protein-1 Ratio *Serum* *Decrease* Mean ratio of 3.45 in 12 patients with Krabbe's disease with median age of 0.4 y significantly lower compared with 4.74 in 202 healthy controls aged 0 - 66 y (median 7 years) *2265*

Tumor Necrosis Factor-α *Serum* *Increase* Mean concentration of about 30 pg/mL in 5 patients with Krabbe's disease significantly different from mean concentration of about 10 pg/mL in 11 healthy controls *3475*

330.00 Metachromatic Leukodystrophy

Aldolase *Cerebrospinal Fluid* *Increase* Increased initially, then diminishes *184*

Ammonium Ions *Urine* *Increase* May lead to proximal renal tubular acidosis which is associated with hypokalemia, hyperchloremic metabolic acidosis, urine pH < 5.5, increased urinary ammonium ion excretion, a negative urine anion gap, increased urinary osmol gap, normal urinary citrate, normal urinary calcium excretion and Fanconi syndrome *4071*

Anion Gap *Urine* *Decrease* May lead to proximal renal tubular acidosis which is associated with hypokalemia, hyperchloremic metabolic acidosis, urine pH < 5.5, increased urinary ammonium ion excretion, a negative urine anion gap, increased urinary osmol gap, normal urinary citrate, normal urinary calcium excretion and Fanconi syndrome *4071*

Arylsulfatase *Liver* *Decrease* Just at the limit of detection in 8 patients with metachromatic leukodystrophy *4979*
Serum *Decrease* Heterozygote carriers for metachromatic leukodystrophy have leukocyte arylsulfatase A concentrations of 40 - 60% of normal range. Patients with disease showed levels only 20% of normal value *2489* Most types of leukodystrophy are associated with a basic deficiency in arylsulfatase A *4979*

Arylsulfatase A *Fibroblasts* *Decrease* Marked reduction observed in patients with MLD *2952*
Serum *Decrease* Marked reduction observed in patients with MLD *2952*
Urine *Decrease* Marked reduction observed in patients with MLD *2952*
White Blood Cells *Decrease* Marked reduction observed in patients with MLD *2952*

Aspartate Aminotransferase *Cerebrospinal Fluid* *Increase* Increased initially, then diminishes *184*
Serum *Increase* Invariable in initial phases of disease. Diminishes to normal range by 4th year *185*

Bicarbonate *Serum* *Decrease* May lead to proximal renal tubular acidosis which is associated with hypokalemia, hyperchloremic metabolic acidosis, urine pH < 5.5, increased urinary ammonium ion excretion, a negative urine anion gap, increased urinary osmol gap, normal urinary citrate, normal urinary calcium excretion and Fanconi syndrome *4071*

Calcium *Urine* *No Effect* May lead to proximal renal tubular acidosis which is associated with hypokalemia, hyperchloremic metabolic acidosis, urine pH < 5.5, increased urinary ammonium ion excretion, a negative urine anion gap, increased urinary osmol gap, normal urinary citrate, normal urinary calcium excretion and Fanconi syndrome *4071*

Chitotriosidase *Serum* *Increase* Abnormal activity observed in 1 of 29 patients, with activity of 550 nmol/h/mL *1917*

Chloride *Serum* *Increase* May lead to proximal renal tubular acidosis which is associated with hypokalemia, hyperchloremic metabolic acidosis, urine pH < 5.5, increased urinary ammonium ion excretion, a negative urine anion gap, increased urinary osmol gap, normal urinary citrate, normal urinary calcium excretion and Fanconi syndrome *4071*

Citrate *Urine* *No Effect* May lead to proximal renal tubular acidosis which is associated with hypokalemia, hyperchloremic metabolic acidosis, urine pH < 5.5, increased urinary ammonium ion excretion, a negative urine anion gap, increased urinary osmol gap, normal urinary citrate, normal urinary calcium excretion and Fanconi syndrome *4071*

Glucose *Urine* *Increase* May lead to proximal renal tubular acidosis which is associated with hypokalemia, hyperchloremic metabolic acidosis, urine pH < 5.5, increased urinary ammonium ion excretion, a negative urine anion gap, increased urinary osmol gap, normal urinary citrate, normal urinary calcium excretion and Fanconi syndrome *4071*

Lactate *Blood* *Increase* Invariable in initial phases of disease. Diminishes to normal range by 4th year *185*

Lactate Dehydrogenase *Cerebrospinal Fluid* *Increase* Increases initially, then diminishes *184*

Lysosome-associated Membrane Protein-2 *Serum* *Increase* Median concentration of 1.48 mg/L in 31 patients with metachromatic leukodystrophy with median age 3 y compared with 1.21 mg/L in 202 healthy controls aged 0 - 66 y (median 7 years) *2265*

Lysosome-associated Membrane Protein-2:Lysosome-associated Membrane Protein-1 Ratio *Serum* *Decrease* Mean ratio of 4.00 in 31 patients with metachromatic leukodystrophy with median age 3 y significantly reduced compared with 1.21 mg/L in 202 healthy controls aged 0 - 66 y (median 7 years) *2265*

Osmolal Gap *Urine* *Increase* May lead to proximal renal tubular acidosis which is associated with hypokalemia, hyperchloremic metabolic acidosis, urine pH < 5.5, increased urinary ammonium ion excretion, a negative urine anion gap, increased urinary osmol gap, normal urinary citrate, normal urinary calcium excretion and Fanconi syndrome *4071*

pH *Urine* *Decrease* May lead to proximal renal tubular acidosis which is associated with hypokalemia, hyperchloremic metabolic acidosis, urine pH < 5.5, increased urinary ammonium ion excretion, a negative urine anion gap, increased urinary osmol gap, normal urinary citrate, normal urinary calcium excretion and Fanconi syndrome *4071*

Phosphate *Serum* *Decrease* May lead to proximal renal tubular acidosis which is associated with hypokalemia, hyperchloremic metabolic acidosis, urine pH < 5.5, increased urinary ammonium ion excretion, a negative urine anion gap, increased urinary osmol gap, normal urinary citrate, normal urinary calcium excretion and Fanconi syndrome *4071*

Potassium *Serum* *Decrease* May lead to proximal renal tubular acidosis which is associated with hypokalemia, hyperchloremic metabolic acidosis, urine pH < 5.5, increased urinary ammonium ion excretion, a negative urine anion gap, increased urinary osmol gap, normal urinary citrate, normal urinary calcium excretion and Fanconi syndrome *4071*

Protein *Cerebrospinal Fluid* *Increase* Common *900*

Tumor Necrosis Factor-α *Serum* *Increase* Mean concentration of about 30 pg/mL in 5 patients with metachromatic leukodystrophy significantly different from mean concentration of about 10 pg/mL in 11 healthy controls *3475*

Uric Acid *Serum* *Decrease* May lead to proximal renal tubular acidosis which is associated with hypokalemia, hyperchloremic metabolic acidosis, urine pH < 5.5, increased urinary ammonium ion excretion, a negative urine anion gap, increased urinary osmol gap, normal urinary citrate, normal urinary calcium excretion and Fanconi syndrome *4071*

330.10 Gangliosidosis

β-Galactosidase *Fibroblasts* *Decrease* Deficient β-galactosidase is associated with generalized gangliosidosis (GM1 gangliosidosis or Morquio's disease) depending on clinical presentation *2952*

White Blood Cells *Decrease* Deficient β-galactosidase is associated with generalized gangliosidosis (GM1 gangliosidosis or Morquio's disease) depending on clinical presentation *2952*

330.10 GM_1-Gangliosidosis

Chitotriosidase *Serum* *Increase* Abnormal activities observed in 7 of 13 patients, with activities of 380 and 720 - 1,420 nmol/h/mL *1917*

Lysosome-associated Membrane Protein-2 *Serum* *Increase* Median concentration of 2.85 mg/L in 12 patients with GM_1-gangliosidosis with median age 1 year compared with 1.21 mg/L in 202 healthy controls aged 0 - 66 y (median 7 years) *2265*

Lysosome-associated Membrane Protein-2:Lysosome-associated Membrane Protein-1 Ratio *Serum* *Decrease* Mean ratio of 2.72 in 12 patients with GM_1-gangliosidosis with median age 1 year significantly less when compared with 4.74 in 202 healthy controls aged 0 - 66 y (median 7 years) *2265*

Tumor Necrosis Factor-α *Serum* *Increase* Mean concentration of about 25 pg/mL in 6 patients with GM_1-gangliosidosis significantly different from mean concentration of about 10 pg/mL in 11 healthy controls *3475*

330.10 GM_2-Gangliosidosis

Chitotriosidase *Serum* *No Effect* Abnormal activities observed in none of 11 patients *1917*

5-Oxoproline *Red Blood Cells* *No Effect* Value of 2.16 mmol/L observed in one patient with GM_2 gangliosidosis not significantly decreased compared with 2.36 ± 0.37 mmol/L in 100 healthy controls *3384*
Urine *Increase* Value of 150 - 250 mmol/mol creatinine observed in one patient with GM_2 gangliosidosis significantly increased compared with < 50 mmol/mol creatinine in 100 healthy controls *3384*

Tumor Necrosis Factor-α *Serum* *Increase* Mean concentration of about 25 pg/mL in 3 patients with GM_2-gangliosidosis significantly different from mean concentration of about 10 pg/mL in 11 healthy controls *3475*

330.10 Sandhoff Disease

Lysosome-associated Membrane Protein-2
Serum *No Effect* Median concentration of 1.25 mg/L in 6 patients with Sandhoff disease with median age 1 y compared with 1.21 mg/L in 202 healthy controls aged 0 - 66 y (median 7 years) *2265*

Lysosome-associated Membrane Protein-2:Lysosome-associated Membrane Protein-1 Ratio *Serum* *Decrease* Mean ratio of 2.21 in 6 patients with Sandhoff disease with median age 1 y significantly different when compared with 4.74 in 202 healthy controls aged 0 - 66 y (median 7 years) *2265*

330.10 Sanhoff's Disease

β-Hexosaminidase *Amniotic Fluid Cells* *Decrease* Deficiency of both A and B isoenzymes is diagnostic for Sandhoff's disease *2952*
Fibroblasts *Decrease* Deficiency of both A and B isoenzymes is diagnostic for Sandhoff's disease *2952*
White Blood Cells *Decrease* Deficiency of both A and B isoenzymes is diagnostic for Sandhoff's disease *2952*

330.10 Tay-Sachs (AB) Disease

Lysosome-associated Membrane Protein-2 *Serum* *Increase* Median concentration of 1.06 mg/L in 2 patients with Tay-Sachs (AB) disease with median age 7 y compared with 1.21 mg/L in 202 healthy controls aged 0 - 66 y (median 7 years) *2265*

Lysosome-associated Membrane Protein-2:Lysosome-associated Membrane Protein-1 Ratio *Serum* *Decrease* Mean ratio of 1.82 in 2 patients with Tay-Sachs (AB) disease with median age 7 y significantly different when compared with 4.74 in 202 healthy controls aged 0 - 66 y (median 7 years) *2265*

330.10 Tay-Sachs Disease

Hexosaminidase A *Amniotic Fluid* *Decrease* Deficiency of enzyme is diagnostic for Tay-Sachs disease *2952*
Fibroblasts *Decrease* Deficiency of enzyme is diagnostic for Tay-Sachs disease *2952*
White Blood Cells *Decrease* Deficiency of enzyme is diagnostic for Tay-Sachs disease *2952*

β-Hexosaminidase A *Serum* *Decrease* Although activity of β-hexoseaminidase similar to that in healthy controls proportion of hexoseaminidase A reduced to 43.6 ± 5.5% from 67.8 ± 4.0% in healthy controls *3742*

β-Hexosaminidase *Serum* *Decrease* Hexosaminidase A (possessing both acetylglucosaminidase and acetyl-galactosaminidase activities) is nearly absent in fetal Tay-Sach's serum. Heterozygotes have intermediate reductions in serum, leukocytes, and cultured fibroblasts *4979*
Serum *No Effect* Mean concentration in Tay-Sachs patients of 965 ± 261 nmol/mL/h not significantly different from 1,086 ± 260 nmol/mL/h in healthy controls *3742*

Lysosome-associated Membrane Protein-2 *Serum* *Increase* Median concentration of 0.90 mg/L in 17 patients with Tay-Sachs disease with median age 1 y compared with 1.21 mg/L in 202 healthy controls aged 0 - 66 y (median 7 years) *2265*

Lysosome-associated Membrane Protein-2:Lysosome-associated Membrane Protein-1 Ratio *Serum* *Decrease* Mean ratio of 2.77 in 17 patients with Tay-Sachs disease with median age 1 y significantly different when compared with 4.74 in 202 healthy controls aged 0 - 66 y (median 7 years) *2265*

330.80 Rett's Syndrome

Nerve Growth Factor *Cerebrospinal Fluid* *Decrease* Mean concentration in 11 pediatric patients with Rett's syndrome of 1.8 ± 2.6 pg/mL compared with 10.0 ± 8.1 pg/mL in 24 control children with unrelated diseases *2921*

331.00 Alzheimer's Disease

Aβ1-40 Protein *Serum* *No Effect* Mean concentration of 70.6 ± 42.1 pmol/L in 28 patients with Alzheimer's disease not significantly different from 68.6 ± 21.1 pmol/L in 25 healthy controls *5154*

Aβ1-42(43) Protein *Serum* *No Effect* Mean concentration of 61.3 ± 40.5 pmol/L in 28 patients with Alzheimer's disease not significantly different from 43.1 ± 25.5 pmol/L in 25 healthy controls *5154*

Acetylcholinesterase G4 Isoenzyme *Serum* *Decrease* In 11 patients with Alzheimer-type dementia mean concentration of 2.2 nmol/min/mL significantly less than mean of 2.7 nmol/min/mL in age-matched controls *5778*

AD7c-NTP *Cerebrospinal Fluid* *Increase* In 89 patients with early Alzheimer's disease mean concentration of 4.6 ± 3.4 ng/mL significantly higher than that in 18 controls in whom mean concentration was 1.7 ± 0.7 ng/mL *1061*

Albumin *Cerebrospinal Fluid* *No Effect* No significant effect observed *782* No significant difference in levels compared with controls *4746*
Serum *Decrease* Mean concentration of 31.67 ± 5.12 g/L in 20 patients with Alzheimer's disease significantly different from 38.05 ± 3.93 g/L in 40 age-matched healthy controls *415*
Serum *No Effect* In 16 patients with Alzheimer's disease mean concentration of 4.14 ± 0.31 g/dL not significantly different from 4.28 ± 0.51 g/dL in 16 healthy controls *3808*

Ammonia *Blood* *Increase* Postprandial blood ammonia levels were significantly higher in 22 patients with Alzheimer's than in 37 control subjects *4746*

Amyloid β-Protein *Cerebrospinal Fluid* *No Effect* Mean concentration in 28 patients with Alzheimer's disease of 10.0 ± 1.3 ng/mL similar to 9.8 ± 1.1 ng/mL in 17 control individuals *2190* Mean concentration in 14 patients with early onset disease of 4.14 ± 1.37 pmol/mL and 3.17 ± 1.15 pmol/mL in 24 patients with late-onset disease compared with concentration in 25 healthy controls of 4.00 ± 2.92 pmol/mL, but significant increase in concentration in early onset group versus older controls *3716* In 19 patients mean concentration of 11.9 ± 4.55 ng/mL not significantly different from controls *3810*

331.00 Alzheimer's Disease *(continued)*

Amyloid β-Protein Precursor *Cerebrospinal Fluid* *Decrease* Concentration markedly lower (by about 3.5 fold) in patients with probable Alzheimer's disease than in demented non-Alzheimer-type patients and healthy controls *5411*
Cerebrospinal Fluid *No Effect* Mean concentration in 38 Alzheimer's disease patients with either early or late onset disease of about 1.4 integrated OD units not significantly different from that in 25 healthy controls in whom the concentration was 1.35 ± 0.38 integrated OD units *3716*

Amyloid P *Serum* *Decrease* In 16 patients with Alzheimer's disease mean concentration of 22.4 ± 7.0 µg/mL significantly different from 34.4 ± 6.6 µg/mL in 16 healthy controls *3808*

Amyloid Precursor Protein *Cerebrospinal Fluid* *No Effect* Mean concentration of 1,357 ± 97 ng/mL in 15 patients with Alzheimer's disease not significantly different from 1,490 ± 74 ng/mL in 15 control individuals *2190*

Angiotensin-converting Enzyme
Cerebrospinal Fluid *Decrease* Decreased in 41% of cases compared to age and sex matched controls *5876*
Cerebrospinal Fluid *No Effect* In 17 patients with probable Alzheimer's disease mean activity of 0.95 ± 0.29 U/L (2.30 ± 0.84 U/g) not significantly different from 5.4 ± 0.98 U/L (2.27 ± 0.68 U/g) in 19 healthy controls *2760*

α_1-Antichymotrypsin *Cerebrospinal Fluid* *No Effect* Mean concentration in 38 patients with Alzheimer's disease of 4.98 ± 4.35 µg/mL with concentration of 3.12 ± 2.18 µg/mL in 14 patients with early onset disease and 5.92 ± 4.98 µg/mL in 24 patients with late onset disease compared with concentrations in 25 healthy controls of 2.27 ± 1.40 µg/mL, with concentration in 12 younger individuals of 2.33 ± 1.29 µg/mL not different from 2.21 ± 1.56 µg/mL in 13 older individuals *3716*
Serum *Increase* Mean concentration in 36 patients with Alzheimer's disease of 738.5 ± 284.1 mg/L higher than 603.1 ± 112.9 mg/L in 36 sex and age matched controls *2165* In 77 patients with Alzheimer's disease mean concentration of 93 ± 48 mg/dL and 77 ± 47 mg/dL in 56 nondemented first degree relatives of Alzheimer's disease patients concentration significantly higher than 44 ± 18 mg/dL in 48 age-matched controls *98*
Serum *No Effect* Not useful as a marker for disease as concentration unaffected *2845*

Antioxidant Capacity *Serum* *Decrease* Mean total oxidant capacity of 234 ± 16 µmol/L in 18 patients with probable Alzheimer's disease significantly different (24%) from 308 ± 34 µmol/L in 18 healthy controls *4326*

Apolipoprotein A *Serum* *No Effect* In 51 patients with Alzheimer's disease mean concentration of 137.1 mg/dL not significantly different from 135.8 mg/dL in 40 patients without Alzheimer's disease *1807*

Apolipoprotein A:Apolipoprotein B Ratio *Serum* *No Effect* In 51 patients with Alzheimer's disease mean ratio of 1.28 not significantly different from 1.15 in 40 patients without Alzheimer's disease *1807*

Apolipoprotein B *Serum* *Increase* Concentration increases with increase in allele number from e2 to e3 to e4 *4163*
Serum *No Effect* In 51 patients with Alzheimer's disease mean concentration of 111.0 mg/dL not significantly different from 119.5 mg/dL in 40 patients without Alzheimer's disease *1807*

Apolipoprotein E *Serum* *Decrease* Concentration decreases with increase in allele number from e2 to e3 to e4 *4163*

Apolipoprotein E4 *Cerebrospinal Fluid* *No Effect* In 27 patients with Alzheimer's disease mean concentration of 63 ± 55 µg/dL not significantly different from 82 ± 62 µg/dL in 31 matched controls *3645* In 30 patients with Alzheimer's disease mean concentration of 86.6 ± 50.8 mg/dL not significantly different from 105.7 ± 61.9 mg/dL in 30 matched controls *3645*

Ascorbic Acid *Cerebrospinal Fluid* *Decrease* Mean concentration of 17.9 ± 5.7 µmol/L in 12 patients with Alzheimer's dementia significantly less than mean concentration in 15 healthy young adults (mean age 35 ± 5 years) of 49.2 ± 9.3 µmol/L *285*

Basophils *Blood* *No Effect* In 15 patients with Alzheimer's disease aged over 70 y mean proportion of 1.14 ± 0.31% not significantly different from 0.85 ± 0.35% in 16 age-matched healthy normal volunteers *4934*

Calcium *Cerebrospinal Fluid* *Decrease* A significant decrease in both Ca and P in CSF was observed in Alzheimer's type dementia (p less than 0.01) and multi-infarct dementia cases (p less than 0.01) *5062*
Serum *Decrease* In patients with Alzheimer's disease concentration typically slightly reduced by more than 1 SD from the control group mean *2906*

Catalase *Red Blood Cells* *Increase* Mean concentration of 4.46 ± 0.47 pmol/mg protein in 18 patients with probable Alzheimer's disease significantly different (75%) from 2.55 ± 0.39 pmol/mg protein in 18 healthy controls *4326*

Cells *Cerebrospinal Fluid* *No Effect* In 14 patients with early onset disease mean count 2 /µL and in 24 with late onset 4 cells /µL not significantly different from 3 µL in 25 healthy controls *3716*

Cholesterol *Serum* *Increase* Concentration increases with increase in allele number from e2 to e3 to e4 *4163*
Serum *No Effect* In 8 patients with Alzheimer's disease mean concentration of 197 ± 30 mg/dL not significantly different from 193 ± 37 mg/dL in 8 age matched controls *2716* In 51 patients with Alzheimer's disease mean concentration of 216.9 mg/dL not significantly different from 216.4 mg/dL in 40 patients without Alzheimer's disease *1807* Mean concentration in 38 patients with Alzheimer's disease 6.7 ± 1.3 mmol/L not significantly different from general population of same age *2908*

Cholesterol Ester Transfer Protein *Serum* *No Effect* In 8 patients with senile dementia of Alzheimer's type mean concentration of 1.76 ± 0.19 µg/mL not significantly different from 1.55 ± 0.30 µg/mL in 8 age-matched controls *2716*

Cholesterol Esters *Serum* *No Effect* Mean proportion of 73.9 ± 2.3% of total cholesterol in 8 patients with senile dementia of Alzheimer's type not significantly different from 73.6 ± 4.0 mg/dL in 8 age-matched controls *2716*

Cholesterol, Free *Serum* *No Effect* Mean concentration of 50.3 ± 5.1 mg/dL in 8 patients with senile dementia of Alzheimer's type not significantly different from 50.1 ± 17.4 mg/dL in 8 age-matched controls *2716*

Copper *Serum* *No Effect* In 51 patients with Alzheimer's disease mean concentration of 105.7 µg/dL not significantly different from 97.7 µg/dL in 40 patients without Alzheimer's disease *1807*

Copper Zinc Superoxide Dismutase
Red Blood Cells *Increase* A significant increase was observed compared to controls *4088*

Corticotropin-releasing Hormone
Cerebrospinal Fluid *Increase* Measured in 77 female inpatients with moderate to extreme dementia and in 17 elderly female controls. They had elevated corticotropin-releasing hormone (CRH), thyrotropin-releasing hormone (TRH) but not somatostatin (SRIF) levels as compared with the controls. This elevation was, however, not seen in patients with simple dementia while it was most prominent in those exhibiting marked depressive symptoms *2766*

Cortisol *Plasma* *Increase* With deterioration over one year mean midnight concentration increased from 17.32 ± 1.59 µg/dL to 25.10 ± 2.63 µg/dL *5630* In 11 women with Alzheimer's disease with mean age of 78.8 y mean concentration of 24.4 ± 6.0 µg/mL significantly higher than 17.1 ± 4.6 µg/mL in 10 controls with mean age 75.3 y: in men of same age group mean concentration of 18.6 ± 4.1 µg/mL in 13 men with Alzheimer's disease compared with 16.5 ± 4.5 µg/mL in age-matched controls *2954*
Plasma *No Effect* In 38 patients with Alzheimer's disease mean concentration of 484 ± 140 nmol/L not significantly different from that in patients with other dementias and in the general population of the same age *2908*

Creatine Kinase BB-Isoenzyme *Serum* *Increase* No relationship was found between levels and degree of dementia with the specific clinical diagnosis *567*

Dehydroascorbic Acid *Cerebrospinal Fluid* *Decrease* Mean concentration of 2.6 ± 0.9 µmol/L in 12 patients with Alzheimer's dementia significantly less than mean concentration in 15 healthy young adults (mean age 35 ± 5 years) of 12.4 ± 2.7 µmol/L *285*

Dehydroascorbic Acid:Ascorbic Acid Ratio
Cerebrospinal Fluid *Decrease* Mean ratio of 0.14 ± 0.05 in 12 patients with Alzheimer's dementia significantly less than mean ratio in 15 healthy young adults (mean age 35 ± 5 years) of 0.25 ± 0.07 *285*

Dehydroepiandrosterone Sulfate *Plasma* *Decrease* Concentration significantly less in 45 patients with Alzheimer's disease compared with 86 patients with dementia and 41 with multi-infarct dementia and an elderly control group *3740* In 11 women with mean age 78.8 y and Alzheimer's disease, mean concentration of 430 ± 272 ng/mL less than 735 ± 634 ng/mL in age matched controls: in men with Alzheimer's disease mean concentration of 847 ± 711 ng/mL compared with 796 ± 583 ng/mL in age matched controls *2954*

1,25-Dihydroxy Vitamin D *Serum* *Decrease* In 40 elderly female patients with Alzheimer's disease mean concentration of 27.4 ± 15.6 pg/mL significantly different from 49.6 ± 9.1 pg/mL in 140 age-matched healthy women *4591*

β-Endorphin *Cerebrospinal Fluid* *No Effect* Cerebrospinal fluid of 13 patients with dementia of the Alzheimer type (DAT), 13 patients with multi-infarct dementia (MID) and 15 age-matched control subjects. Neuropeptide Y, β-endorphin and IL-1β showed similar concentrations in the three groups studied *3318* No difference from controls *4282*

Endothelin-1 *Cerebrospinal Fluid* *Decrease* We have measured the endothelin-1 concentrations in the cerebrospinal fluid samples from 5 patients with Alzheimer's disease (AD), and 7 patients with other diseases without dementia (disease control: DC). The cerebrospinal fluid endothelin-1 level was significantly lower in AD than in DC *5820*

Eosinophils *Blood* *No Effect* In 15 patients with Alzheimer's disease aged over 70 y mean proportion of 1.55 ± 0.82% not significantly different from 1.87 ± 1.65% in 16 age-matched healthy normal volunteers *4934*

Epinephrine *Cerebrospinal Fluid* *Increase* In 74 patients with Alzheimer's disease mean concentration of 170 ± 100 pmol/L in patients with advanced disease, compared with 130 ± 60 pmol/L in those with mild or moderate disease and 110 ± 70 pmol/L in 42 cognitively normal healthy old people and about 95 pmol/L in 54 healthy young people *4092*
Plasma *Increase* In 74 patients with Alzheimer's disease mean concentration of 340 ± 200 pmol/L compared with 240 ± 160 pmol/L in 42 cognitively normal healthy old people and 270 ± 130 pmol/L in 54 healthy young people *4092*

F_2-Isoprostane *Cerebrospinal Fluid* *Increase* In 11 patients with Alzheimer's disease mean concentration in lateral ventricular CSF of 72 ± 7 pg/mL significantly different from 46 ± 4 pg/mL in 11 control patients *3579*

Glucose *Serum* *Decrease* In 38 patients with Alzheimer's disease mean concentration of 4.3 ± 0.5 mmol/L significantly less than 5.6 ± 1.6 mmol/L in age-matched controls *2908*
Serum *No Effect* In 51 patients with Alzheimer's disease mean concentration of 93.0 mg/dL not significantly different from 89.0 mg/dL in 40 patients without Alzheimer's disease *1807*

GM1-Ganglioside *Cerebrospinal Fluid* *Increase* In 43 patients with probable type I Alzheimer's disease concentration significantly higher than in type II patients and 19 age-matched healthy controls *482*

Growth Hormone *Plasma* *No Effect* Mean basal concentration of 0.9 ± 0.2 µg/L in 15 patients aged 61 - 78 years not signficantly different from 0.8 ± 0.2 µg/L in 14 healthy individuals aged 65 - 75 years *1718*

Haptoglobin *Serum* *Increase* Mean concentration of 1.61 ± 0.53 g/L in 20 patients with Alzheimer's disease not significantly different from 1.32 ± 0.60 g/L in 40 age-matched healthy controls *415*

HDL-Cholesterol *Serum* *No Effect* Mean concentration of 61 ± 11 mg/dL in 8 patients with Alzheimer's disease not significantly increased over mean of 51 ± 14 mg/dL in 8 age-matched controls *2716*

HDL-Cholesterol:LDL-Cholesterol Ratio *Serum* *No Effect* In 8 patients with Alzheimer's disease mean value of 0.56 ± 0.15 not significantly different from 0.50 ± 0.20 in 8 age-matched controls *2716*

Hexokinase *White Blood Cells* *No Effect* In 28 individuals with either familial or sporadic Alzheimer's disease mean activity of 48.2 ± 17 nmol/min/prot not significantly different from that in 13 healthy elderly with mean age 76 years, mean activity of 45.8 ± 17 nmol/min/prot, but significantly higher when compared with 23.1 ± 5 nmol/min/prot in 11 healthy individuals with mean age 31 years *153*

Homovanillic Acid *Cerebrospinal Fluid* *Decrease* Reported effect *3981* Lower than in an aged matched control group *4746*
Cerebrospinal Fluid *No Effect* Level was unchanged from normal controls *4746* Concentration usually normal *5866*

25-Hydroxy Vitamin D *Serum* *Decrease* In 40 elderly female patients with Alzheimer's disease mean concentration of 7.1 ± 3.9 ng/mL significantly different from 21.6 ± 3.1 ng/mL in 140 age-matched healthy women *4591*

7α-Hydroxydehydroepiandrosterone Fatty Acid Esters *Serum* *Increase* In 10 patients with probable Alzheimer's disease mean concentration of 66 ± 7 pg/mL significantly different from 41 ± 9 pg/mL in 8 age matched control individuals *210*

7α-Hydroxydehydroepiandrosterone, Free *Serum* *Increase* In 10 patients with probable Alzheimer's disease mean concentration of 240 ± 37 pg/mL not significantly different from 207 ± 22 pg/mL in 8 age matched control individuals *210*

7α-Hydroxydehydroepiandrosterone Sulfate *Serum* *Increase* In 10 patients with probable Alzheimer's disease mean concentration of 262 ± 28 pg/mL significantly different from 145 ± 28 pg/mL in 8 age matched control individuals *210*

7α-Hydroxydehydroepiandrosterone, Total *Serum* *Increase* In 10 patients with probable Alzheimer's disease mean concentration of 568 ± 59 pg/mL significantly different from 393 ± 27 pg/mL in 8 age matched control individuals *210*

5-Hydroxyindoleacetic Acid *Cerebrospinal Fluid* *Decrease* Lower than in an aged matched control group *4746* Observed effect *3981*

4-Hydroxynonenal *Cerebrospinal Fluid* *No Effect* In 36 patients with Alzheimer's disease mean concentration of 0.51 ± 0.14 ng/mL not significantly different from 0.51 ± 0.05 ng/mL in 236 patients with other neurological diagnoses *4909*

Hydroxyproline *Urine* *Increase* In 40 elderly female patients with Alzheimer's disease mean concentration of 147.7 ± 83.8 µmol/d significantly different from 99.9 ± 54.1 µmol/d in 140 age-matched healthy women *4591*

immunoglobulin A *Serum* *Increase* Mean concentration of 3.55 ± 1.26 g/L in 20 patients with Alzheimer's disease not significantly different from 2.98 ± 1.63 g/L in 40 age-matched healthy controls *415*

Immunoglobulin G *Cerebrospinal Fluid* *No Effect* Concentration usually normal *782* No significant difference in levels compared with controls *4746*
Serum *Increase* Mean concentration of 15.41 ± 4.22 g/L in 20 patients with Alzheimer's disease significantly different from 11.18 ± 3.35 g/L in 40 age-matched healthy controls *415*

Immunoglobulin M *Serum* *Increase* Mean concentration of 1.73 ± 0.91 g/L in 20 patients with Alzheimer's disease significantly different from 1.05 ± 0.67 g/L in 40 age-matched healthy controls *415*

Insulin *Plasma* *No Effect* In 51 patients with Alzheimer's disease mean concentration of 7.20 µU/dL not significantly different from 5.50 µU/dL in 40 patients without Alzheimer's disease *1807*

Insulin-like Growth Factor-I *Serum* *Decrease* Mean concentration of 108.0 ± 5.9 µg/L in 15 patients aged 61 - 78 years significantly less than 288.7 ± 22.1 µg/L in 22 healthy young volunteers aged 20 - 35 years but slightly higher than 73.9 ± 8.2 µg/L in 14 healthy elderly individuals aged 65 - 75 years *1718*

Interleukin-1 *Cerebrospinal Fluid* *No Effect* Studied cerebrospinal fluid of 13 patients with dementia of the Alzheimer type (DAT), 13 patients with multi-infarct dementia (MID) and 15 age-matched control subjects. Neuropeptide Y, β-endorphin and IL-1β showed similar concentrations in the three groups studied *3318*

Interleukin-6 *Cerebrospinal Fluid* *No Effect* In 17 patients with Alzheimer's disease mean concentration of 1.6 ± 0.93 pg/mL not significantly different from mean of 1.7 ± 1.01 pg/mL in 18 normal controls *3328* Mean concentration in 25 patients with Alzheimer's disease of 2.90 ± 1.60 pg/mL similar to 2.90 ± 1.29 pg/mL observed in 19 healthy controls *1994*

ionized Calcium *Serum* *Decrease* In 40 elderly female patients with Alzheimer's disease mean concentration of 2.448 ± 0.168 mEq/L significantly different from 2.516 ±0.113 mEq/L in 140 age-matched healthy women *4591*

Large Unstained Cells *Blood* *Decrease* In 15 patients with Alzheimer's disease aged over 70 y mean proportion of 1.33 ± 0.35% significantly different from 1.79 ± 0.58% in 16 age-matched healthy normal volunteers *4934*

331.00 Alzheimer's Disease *(continued)*

LDL-Cholesterol *Serum* *Increase* Concentration increases with increase in allele number from e2 to e3 to e4 *4163*
Serum *No Effect* Mean calculated concentration of 114 ± 28 mg/dL in 8 patients with Alzheimer's disease not significantly different from 113 ± 34 mg/dL in 8 age-matched controls *2716*

Leukocytes *Blood* *No Effect* In 15 patients with Alzheimer's disease aged over 70 y mean concentration of 6.9 ± 1.6 x 10^3 cells/μL not significantly different from 6.7 ± 1.5 x 10^3 cells/mL in 16 age-matched healthy normal volunteers *4934*

Lipoprotein Lp(a) *Serum* *No Effect* Mean concentration of 12 ± 17 mg/dL in 8 patients with Alzheimer's disease not significantly different from 13 ± 15 mg/dL in 8 age-matched controls *2716*

Lymphocyte response to Concanavalin A *Blood* *No Effect* In 15 patients with Alzheimer's disease aged over 70 y mean response of 99 ± 41 cpm x 10^3 not significantly different from 89 ± 54 cpm x 10^3 in 16 age-matched healthy normal volunteers *4934*

Lymphocyte response to Phytohemagglutinin
Blood *Increase* In 15 patients with Alzheimer's disease aged over 70 y mean response of 95 ± 27 cpm x 10^3 significantly different from 68 ± 32 cpm x 10^3 in 16 age-matched healthy normal volunteers *4934*

Lymphocyte response to Pokeweed Mitogen
Blood *No Effect* In 15 patients with Alzheimer's disease aged over 70 y mean response of 43 ± 18 cpm x 10^3 not significantly different from 31 ± 22 cpm x 10^3 in 16 age-matched healthy normal volunteers *4934*

Lymphocytes *Blood* *No Effect* In 15 patients with Alzheimer's disease aged over 70 y mean proportion of 25.6 ± 9.9% not significantly different from 28.5 ± 6.8% in 16 age-matched healthy normal volunteers *4934*

Mercury *Blood* *Decrease* Mean concentration of 0.4 ± 0.1 ng/mL in 18 patients with Alzheimer's disease not significantly reduced compared with 0.76 ± 0.1 ng/mL in 18 control individuals *1605*

β_2-Microglobulin *Cerebrospinal Fluid* *Increase* Studied cerebrospinal fluid of 13 patients with dementia of the Alzheimer type (DAT), 13 patients with multi-infarct dementia (MID) and 15 age-matched control subjects. β_2-Microglobulin was higher in DAT patients than in controls ($p < 0.01$) *3318*

Monoamine Oxidase *Platelets* *Increase* Increased in patients with senile dementia of Alzheimer type *4312*

Monocytes *Blood* *No Effect* In 15 patients with Alzheimer's disease aged over 70 y mean proportion of 8.6 ± 2.6% not significantly different from 7.3 ± 1.8% in 16 age-matched healthy normal volunteers *4934*

Neuropeptide Y *Cerebrospinal Fluid* *No Effect* Studied cerebrospinal fluid of 13 patients with dementia of the Alzheimer type (DAT), 13 patients with multi-infarct dementia (MID) and 15 age-matched control subjects. Neuropeptide Y, β-endorphin and IL-1β showed similar concentrations in the three groups studied *3318*

Neutrophils *Blood* *No Effect* In 15 patients with Alzheimer's disease aged over 70 y mean proporion of 61.1 ± 9.2% not significantly different from 58.9 ± 7.12% in 16 age-matched healthy normal volunteers *4934*

Norepinephrine *Cerebrospinal Fluid* *Increase* In 18 patients with advanced Alzheimer's disease mean concentration of 279 ± 122 pg/L significantly different from 219 ± 88 pg/L in 32 healthy older individuals *1347*
Cerebrospinal Fluid *No Effect* In 33 patients with mild Alzheimer's disease mean concentration of 198 ± 89 pg/L not significantly different from 219 ± 88 pg/L in 32 healthy older individuals *1347*
Plasma *Increase* In 18 patients with advanced Alzheimer's disease mean concentration of 405 ± 206 pg/L not significantly different from 327 ± 149 pg/L in 32 healthy older individuals *1347*
Plasma *No Effect* In 33 patients with mild Alzheimer's disease mean concentration of 332 ± 222 pg/mL not significantly different from 327 ± 149 pg/mL in 32 healthy older individuals *1347*

N-terminal Amyloid β-Protein Precursor
Cerebrospinal Fluid *No Effect* In 19 patients mean concentration of 1.62 ± 0.41 μg/mL not significantly different from controls *3810*

Osteocalcin *Serum* *Increase* In 40 elderly female patients with Alzheimer's disease mean concentration of 11.515 ± 3.994 ng/mL significantly different from 7.657 ± 4.463 ng/mL in 140 age-matched healthy women *4591*

Oxytocin *Cerebrospinal Fluid* *No Effect* No difference from controls *4282*

Parathyroid Hormone *Plasma* *Increase* In 40 elderly female patients with Alzheimer's disease mean concentration of 51.8 ± 25.1 pg/mL significantly different from 35.0 ± 11.4 pg/mL in 140 age-matched healthy women *4591* *4591*

Phagocytosis *Blood* *No Effect* In 15 patients with Alzheimer's disease aged over 70 y mean effect of 82 ± 9% not significantly different from 82 ± 8% in 16 age-matched healthy normal volunteers *4934*

Phosphate *Cerebrospinal Fluid* *Decrease* A significant decrease in both Ca and P in CSF was observed in Alzheimer's type dementia (p less than 0.01) and multi-infarct dementia cases (p less than 0.01) *5062*
Serum *Decrease* In patients with Alzheimer's disease characteristically low serum phosphate concentration observed (below 1 SD of control group mean) *2906*

Prealbumin *Serum* *Decrease* Mean concentration of 0.169 ± 0.055 g/L in 20 patients with Alzheimer's disease significantly different from 0.224 ± 0.067 g/L in 40 age-matched healthy controls *415*

Prostaglandin E_2 *Plasma* *No Effect* In 15 patients with Alzheimer's disease aged over 70 y mean concentration of 157 ± 142 pg/mL not significantly different from 169 ± 110 pg/mL in 16 age-matched healthy normal volunteers *4934*

Protein *Cerebrospinal Fluid* *Decrease* Mean concentration in postmortem ventricular CSF in 30 patients of 26.6 ± 4.8 mg/dL significantly different from 60.9 ± 5.8 mg/dL in 16 normal controls *5435*
Cerebrospinal Fluid *No Effect* In 14 patients with early onset disease mean concentration of 34 mg/dL and in 24 with late onset 38 mg/dL not significantly different from 29 mg/dL in 25 healthy controls *3716* In 17 patients with probable Alzheimer's disease mean concentration of 0.43 ± 0.11 g/L not significantly different from 0.38 ± 0.09 g/L in 19 healthy controls *2760* In 24 patients with Alzheimer's disease mean concentration of 40.1 ± 13.0 mg/dL not significantly different from 42.0 ± 17.8 mg/dL in 26 neurological controls and 40.8 ± 19.0 mg/dL in 14 normal controls *3661*
Serum *No Effect* In 16 patients with Alzheimer's disease mean concentration of 6.86 ± 0.49 g/dL not significantly different from 7.25 ± 0.74 g/dL in 16 healthy controls *3808*

Protein Kinase C *Platelets* *Increase* In 10 patients with Alzheimer's disease mean concentration of cytosolic type II PKC of 1250 ng/mg protein significantly higher than 980 ng/mg protein in 10 healthy controls, but no significant difference between mean concentrations of about 300 ng/mg protein in membranous type II PKC *3370*

Quinolinic Acid *Cerebrospinal Fluid* *No Effect* No difference between Alzheimer patients and age-matched control subjects *3634*

Selenium *Blood* *Decrease* Mean concentration of 189.7 ± 10.5 ng/mL in 18 patients with Alzheimer's disease not significantly reduced compared with 209.6 ± 13.5 ng/mL in 18 control individuals *1605*

α2,3-Sialoglycoprotein *Serum* *Decrease* In 12 patients aged 77 ± 7 years mean concentration of 400 Abs units significantly less than 485 Abs units in 12 controls of similar age and gender *3225*

α2,6-Sialoglycoprotein *Serum* *No Effect* In 12 patients aged 77 ± 7 years mean concentration of 320 Abs units not significantly different from 340 Abs units in 12 controls of similar age and gender *3225*

Sialyltransferase *Serum* *Decrease* In a group of elderly patients (aged over 60 years) significant decrease of the soluble form of sialyltransferase (352 ± 24 cpm/mg protein/h) observed compared with age matched controls (641 ± 57 cpm/mg protein/h) *3224*

α2,3-Sialyltransferase *Serum* *Decrease* In 12 patients aged 77 ± 7 years mean concentration of 80 Abs units significantly less than 110 Abs units (30% reduction) in 12 controls of similar age and gender *3225*

α2,6-Sialyltransferase *Serum* *No Effect* In 12 patients aged 77 ± 7 years mean concentration of 120 Abs units not significantly different from 100 Abs units in 12 controls of similar age and gender *3225*

Soluble β-Amyloid Peptide 40 *Serum* *Decrease* In 80 patients with Alzheimer's disease mean concentration of 1,922 ± 547 pmol/L (mild 2,015 pmol/L, moderate 1,834 pmol/L and severe 1,890 pmol/L) significantly different from 2,311 ± 546 pmol/L in 24 age and sex matched controls *2440*

Soluble β-Amyloid Peptide 42 *Serum* *Increase* In 80 patients with Alzheimer's disease mean concentration of 119 ± 63 pmol/L (mild 129 pmol/L, moderate 124 pmol/L and severe 81 pmol/L) significantly different from 74 ± 30 pmol/L in 24 age and sex matched controls *2440*

Soluble gp130 *Cerebrospinal Fluid* *No Effect* In 17 patients with Alzheimer's disease mean concentration of 108.4 ± 45.28 ng/mL not significantly different from mean of 91.8 ± 47.28 ng/mL in 18 age-matched nondemented normal controls *3328*

Soluble Interleukin-6 Receptor
Cerebrospinal Fluid *Decrease* In 41 patients with Alzheimer's disease mean concentration of 1,069 ± 384 pg/mL significantly less than 1,298 ± 381 pg/mL in 20 age-matched healthy controls *1995*
Cerebrospinal Fluid *No Effect* In 17 patients with Alzheimer's disease mean concentration of 1.51 ± 0.63 ng/mL not significantly different from mean of 1.51 ± 0.726 ng/mL in 18 normal controls *3328*

Somatostatin *Cerebrospinal Fluid* *Decrease* The CSF concentration was also significantly reduced in patients with AD *5665* Significant difference from elderly normal subjects but did not differ from normal younger subjects *4282* Studied cerebrospinal fluid of 13 patients with dementia of the Alzheimer type (DAT), 13 patients with multi-infarct dementia (MID) and 15 age-matched control subjects. Somatostatin was significantly lower in DAT patients than in controls ($p < 0.05$) *3318* Significantly lower mean CSF levels than in other neurological patients. All 11 patients with Alzheimer's disease or Parkinsons disease dementia had levels well below 21.8 ng/mL *4739*
Cerebrospinal Fluid *No Effect* Measured in 77 female inpatients with moderate to extreme dementia and in 17 elderly female controls. They had elevated corticotropin-releasing hormone (CRH), thyrotropin-releasing hormone (TRH) but not somatostatin (SRIF) levels as compared with the controls. This elevation was, however, not seen in patients with simple dementia while it was most prominent in those exhibiting marked depressive symptoms *279*

Substance P *Cerebrospinal Fluid* *Decrease* Studied cerebrospinal fluid of 13 patients with dementia of the Alzheimer type (DAT), 13 patients with multi-infarct dementia (MID) and 15 age-matched control subjects. Substance P was significantly lower in DAT patients than in controls ($p < 0.05$) *3318*

Sulfatide *Cerebrospinal Fluid* *Increase* In 43 patients with Alzheimer's disease mean concentration of 178 ± 79 nmol/L not significantly higher than 145 ± 86 nmol/L in 20 age-matched controls *1563*

Superoxide Dismutase Release *Blood* *No Effect* In 15 patients with Alzheimer's disease aged over 70 y mean response of 39.1 ± 9.1 nmol/L not significantly different from 39.8 nmol/L in 16 age-matched healthy normal volunteers *4934*

Tau Protein *Cerebrospinal Fluid* *Increase* Median concentration in 11 patients with very mild disease of 454 ng/L significantly different from 160 ng/L in 19 controls *4354* In 71 patients with Alzheimer's disease mean concentration of 361 ± 166 pg/mL significantly different from 190 ± 80 pg/mL in 26 controls *4065* In 14 patients with late onset Alzheimer's disease mean concentration of 576.0 ± 112.0 pg/mL significantly different compared with 212.1 ± 41.6 pg/mL 23 controls *3434* Mean concentration of 251.4 ± 36.0 ng/L in 31 patients with Alzheimer's disease significantly higher than that in healthy controls, 51.1 ± 7.3 ng/L *1546* In 24 patients with Alzheimer's disease mean concentration of 1430 ± 739 pg/mL significantly greater than 790 ± 579 pg/mL in 26 neurological controls and 816 ± 355 pg/mL in 14 normal controls *3661*
Cerebrospinal Fluid *No Effect* In 14 patients with early onset Alzheimer's disease mean concentration of 285.0 ± 44.7 pg/mL not significantly different compared with 212.1 ± 41.6 pg/mL 23 controls *3434* In 19 patients mean concentration of 274 ± 118 pg/mL not significantly different from controls *3810*

tert-Butyl Hydroperoxide-initiated Chemiluminescence
Red Blood Cells *Increase* Mean chemiluminescence of 177,600 ± 702 cps/mg hemoglobin in 18 patients with probable Alzheimer's disease significantly different (52%) from 116,700 ± 6690 cps/mg hemoglobin in 18 healthy controls *4326*

Thyrotropin Releasing Hormone
Cerebrospinal Fluid *Increase* Measured in 77 female inpatients with moderate to extreme dementia and in 17 elderly female controls. They had elevated corticotropin-releasing hormone (CRH), thyrotropin-releasing hormone (TRH) but not somatostatin (SRIF) levels as compared with the controls. This elevation was, however, not seen in patients with simple dementia while it was most prominent in those exhibiting marked depressive symptoms *2766*

Transferrin *Serum* *Decrease* Mean concentration of 2.33 ± 0.60 g/L in 20 patients with Alzheimer's disease not significantly different from 2.59 ± 0.59 g/L in 40 age-matched healthy controls *415*

Transforming Growth Factor-β_1
Cerebrospinal Fluid *No Effect* Mean concentration in postmortem ventricular CSF in 30 patients of 19.2 ± 3.3 pg/mL not significantly different from 23.7 ± 4.6 pg/mL in 16 normal controls *5435*

Transforming Growth Factor-β_2 *Cerebrospinal Fluid* *Increase* Mean concentration in postmortem ventricular CSF in 30 patients of 173.9 ± 38.8 pg/mL not significantly different from 80.6 ± 21.9 pg/mL in 16 normal controls *5435*

Triglycerides *Serum* *Decrease* In 8 patients with Alzheimer's disease mean concentration of 112 ± 48 mg/dL not significantly less than 147 ± 103 mg/dL in 8 age-matched controls *2716*
Serum *No Effect* In 51 patients with Alzheimer's disease mean concentration of 110.0 mg/dL not significantly different from 99.5 mg/dL in 40 patients without Alzheimer's disease *1807* In 38 patients with Alzheimer's disease mean concentration of 1.4 ± 1.1 mmol/L not significantly different from that in 19 patients with unspecified dementia and the general population of the same age *2908*

Tumor Necrosis Factor-α *Serum* *Decrease* In patients with Alzheimer's disease mean concentration of 2.5 ± 1.25 pg/mL significantly less than 10.66 ± 8.92 pg/mL in age-matched controls *657*
Serum *Increase* In patients with Alzheimer's disease concentration significantly increased compared with controls *1483*

Ubiquitin *Cerebrospinal Fluid* *Increase* In 17 patients with Alzheimer's disease mean concentration of 34 ± 20% in postmortem ventricular CSF significantly higher than 16 ± 15% in 12 non-neurological controls but not different from 28 ± 17% in 17 neurological controls *2841*

Vasoactive Intestinal Polypeptide
Cerebrospinal Fluid *No Effect* Reported effect *5665*

Vasopressin *Cerebrospinal Fluid* *Decrease* Significant decrease in arginine vasopressin compared to elderly and younger normal control subjects *4282*

Vitamin B_{12} *Serum* *No Effect* A low B_{12} level may not be a risk factor for dementia in general or Alzheimer's disease in particular *976* Mean concentration in demented individuals, those with Alzheimer's disease and in those who were non-demented not significantly different *322*

VLDL-Cholesterol *Serum* *No Effect* Mean calculated concentration of 22 ± 10 mg/dL in 8 patients with Alzheimer's disease not significantly different from 29 ± 20 mg/dL in 8 age-matched controls *2716*

331.00 Alzheimer's Disease ε4 Allele Carrier

Apolipoprotein A *Serum* *No Effect* In 34 η4 carrier patients with Alzheimer's disease mean concentration of 136.3 mg/dL not significantly different from 139.7 mg/dL in 9 patients without Alzheimer's disease *1807*

Apolipoprotein A:Apolipoprotein B Ratio *Serum* *No Effect* In 34 η4 carrier patients with Alzheimer's disease mean ratio of 1.21 not significantly different from 1.23 in 9 patients without Alzheimer's disease *1807*

331.00 Alzheimer's Disease ε4 Allele Carrier *(continued)*

Apolipoprotein B *Serum* *No Effect* In 34 η4 carrier patients with Alzheimer's disease mean concentration of 116.0 mg/dL not different from 116.0 mg/dL in 9 patients without Alzheimer's disease *1807*

Apolipoprotein E *Serum* *Increase* In patients with Alzheimer's disease frequency of 0.17 in 15 patients aged 45 - 54 y, 0.43 in 36 patients aged 55 - 64 y, 0.42 in 54 patients aged 65 - 74 y and 0.19 in 18 patients aged 75 to 87 years *3673*

Cholesterol *Serum* *No Effect* In 34 η4 carrier patients with Alzheimer's disease mean concentration of 222.7 mg/dL not significantly different from 219.3 mg/dL in 9 patients without Alzheimer's disease *1807*

Copper *Serum* *Increase* In 34 η4 carrier patients with Alzheimer's disease mean concentration of 107.5 µg/dL significantly different from 91.7 µg/dL in 9 patients without Alzheimer's disease *1807*

Glucose *Serum* *No Effect* In 34 η4 carrier patients with Alzheimer's disease mean concentration of 93.0 mg/dL not significantly different from 84.0 mg/dL in 9 patients without Alzheimer's disease *1807*

Insulin *Plasma* *Increase* In 34 η4 carrier patients with Alzheimer's disease mean concentration of 6.40 µU/dL significantly different from 4.10 µU/dL in 9 patients without Alzheimer's disease *1807*

Insulin:Glucose Ratio *Plasma* *Increase* In 34 η4 carrier patients with Alzheimer's disease mean ratio of 0.07 significantly different from 0.04 in 9 patients without Alzheimer's disease *1807*

Triglycerides *Serum* *No Effect* In 34 η4 carrier patients with Alzheimer's disease mean concentration of 102.5 mg/dL not significantly different from 96.0 mg/dL in 9 patients without Alzheimer's disease *1807*

Zinc *Serum* *Increase* In 34 η4 carrier patients with Alzheimer's disease mean concentration of 70.4 µg/dL significantly different from 61.5 µg/dL in 9 patients without Alzheimer's disease *1807*

331.40 Acquired Hydrocephalus

Amyloid β-Protein *Cerebrospinal Fluid* *Decrease* In 1 patient with hydrocephalus concentration was 0.93 pmol/mL significantly different from mean concentration of 4.00 ± 2.92 pmol/mL *3716*

Amyloid β-Protein Precursor *Cerebrospinal Fluid* *Increase* In 1 patient with hydrocephalus concentration was 2.04 integrated OD units significantly different from mean concentration of 1.35 ± 0.38 integrated OD units in 25 normal controls *3716*

α_1-Antichymotrypsin *Cerebrospinal Fluid* *Increase* In 1 patient with hydrocephalus concentration was 8.00 µg/mL significantly different from mean concentration of 2.27 ± 1.40 µg/mL in 25 normal controls *3716*

Cells *Cerebrospinal Fluid* *No Effect* In 1 patient with hydrocephalus concentration of 0.7 cells/µL not significantly different from normal of 3 cells/µL *3716*

Lactate Dehydrogenase *Cerebrospinal Fluid* *Increase* Range of LD activity in 9 patients with hydrocephalus for shunt insertion or revision was 17 - 53 U/L, with normal CSF values from 3 - 17 U/L *3757*

Leukocytes *Cerebrospinal Fluid* *No Effect* No increase usually observed *3757*

Protein *Cerebrospinal Fluid* *No Effect* In 1 patient with hydrocephalus concentration of 39 mg/dL not significantly different from normal of 28 mg/dL in 25 healthy controls *3716*

331.40 Normal Pressure Hydrocephalus Syndrome

Lactate *Cerebrospinal Fluid* *Increase* Mean concentration of 2,029 ± 389 µmol/L in 52 patients with normal pressure hydrocephalus significantly different from 1,850 ± 63 µmol/L in 20 controls without dementia *3823*

Myelin Basic Protein *Cerebrospinal Fluid* *No Effect* In 46 patients with normal pressure hydrocephalus mean concentration of 1.0 ± 0.8 µg/L not significantly different from 0.8 ± 0.6 µg/L in 20 healthy controls *3823*

Neuron-specific Enolase *Cerebrospinal Fluid* *Decrease* In 43 patients with normal pressure hydrocephalus mean concentration of 7.5 ± 3.1 µg/L not significantly different from 8.8 ± 2.6 µg/L in 20 healthy controls *3823*

Neuropeptide Y *Cerebrospinal Fluid* *Decrease* Mean concentration in 7 patients with normal pressure hydrocephalus syndrome of 64.6 ± 25.1 pg/mL significantly less than 117.3 ± 33.4 pg/mL in 10 controls *736*

S-100 Protein *Cerebrospinal Fluid* *No Effect* In 44 patients with normal pressure hydrocephalus mean concentration of 3.6 ± 1.5 µg/L not significantly different from 3.4 ± 1.3 µg/L in 20 healthy controls *3823*

Tau Protein *Cerebrospinal Fluid* *Increase* Median concentration in 11 patients with dementia associated with normal pressure hydrocephalus or frontal lobe degeneration of 401 ng/L significantly different from 160 ng/L in 19 controls *4354*

331.40 Obstructive Hydrocephalus

Interleukin-6 *Cerebrospinal Fluid* *No Effect* In 6 patients with obstructive hydrocephalus mean concentration of 91.1 ± 38.0 pg/mL compared with 93.6 ± 21.8 pg/mL in 20 control patients with asceptic lumboischiadic syndrome *5872*

Lactate Dehydrogenase *Cerebrospinal Fluid* *Increase* Mean concentration in 6 patients with obstructive hydrocephalus of 2.04 ± 0.76 µkat/L significantly higher than 0.44 ± 0.12 µkat/L in 20 control patients with asceptic lumboischiadic syndrome *5872*

Tumor Necrosis Factor-α *Cerebrospinal Fluid* *Increase* In 6 patients with obstructive hydrocephalus mean concentration of 12.07 ± 5.96 pg/mL compared with 0.94 ± 0.55 pg/mL in 20 control patients with asceptic lumboischiadic syndrome *5872*

331.40 Shunted Hydrocephalus

Growth Hormone *Plasma* *Decrease* In 6 prepubertal children with spinal bifida and shunted hydrocephalus mean concentration of 1.0 µg/L significantly less than 2.1 µg/L in 32 control prepubertal children and in 11 postpubertal affected children mean concentration of 2.7 µg/L less than 8.5 µg/L in 41 postpubertal children *3125*

Insulin-like Growth Factor-I *Serum* *Decrease* In 6 prepubertal children with spinal bifida and shunted hydrocephalus mean concentration of 5.2 nmol/L significantly less than 12.4 nmol/L in 32 control prepubertal children and in 11 postpubertal affected children mean concentration of 15.9 nmol/L less than 21.3 nmol/L in 41 postpubertal children *3125*

Insulin-like Growth Factor Binding Protein-3 *Serum* *Decrease* In 6 prepubertal children with spinal bifida and shunted hydrocephalus mean concentration of 1.9 mg/L significantly less than 3.7 mg/L in 32 control prepubertal children and in 11 postpubertal affected children mean concentration of 4.1 mg/L not significantly less than 4.3 mg/L in 41 postpubertal children *3125*

331.81 Reye's Syndrome

Alanine Aminotransferase *Serum* *Increase* Reflects hepatic damage *367* High serum transaminases *1980*

Amino Acids *Plasma* *Increase* Markedly elevated reflecting hepatic injury *904*

Ammonia *Blood* *Increase* Reflects hepatic damage *367* Increased ammonia may reflect accumulation of octopamine *686* Elevated in most patients *3192* Hyperammonemia results from excess waste nitrogen that overwhelms the ability of reduced ornithine transcarbamylase to detoxify the ammonia load *4922*

Aspartate Aminotransferase *Serum* *Increase* 2 - 300 times normal values *867* High serum transaminases *1980* Reflects hepatic damage *367*

Bicarbonate *Serum* *Decrease* Due to impaired oxidative metabolism *904*

Bilirubin *Serum* *Increase* Normal or mildly elevated *1980* Usually remains below 3 mg/dL *867*

Carbon Dioxide Partial Pressure *Blood* *Decrease* Hypocapnia is common in children with this syndrome *367*

Carnitine *Serum* *Decrease* Reduced concentrations observed in patients with secondary carnitine deficiency which may be associated with Reye syndrome and Reye syndrome-like attacks associated with some organic acidurias *2952*

Creatine Kinase *Serum* *Increase* Especially muscle (CK-MM) fraction in severely affected children *904* Markedly abnormal *4289*

Creatine Kinase MB-Isoenzyme *Serum* *Increase* Observed effect *248*

Creatinine *Serum* *Increase* Markedly elevated reflecting renal injury *904*

Fatty Acids (FFA), Free *Serum* *Increase* Commonly elevated *367*

Glucose *Cerebrospinal Fluid* *Decrease* Hypoglycemia with decreased CSF glucose is common in patients < 5 years of age, but is rare in older children *367* Low levels of glucose and protein found in the CSF *867*
Serum *Decrease* Hypoglycemia with decreased CSF glucose is common in patients < 5 years of age, but is rare in older children *367* Occasionally hypoglycemia *1980* Replacement or destruction of functioning hepatic tissue may evoke hypoglycemia *4707*

Lactate *Blood* *Increase* Due to impaired oxidative metabolism *904*

Lactate Dehydrogenase *Serum* *Increase* Markedly elevated reflecting hepatic injury *904*

pH *Blood* *Decrease* Later in disease along with decreased pCO_2 reflecting respiratory acidosis *904* Due to impaired oxidative metabolism *904*

Phosphate *Serum* *Increase* Indicates muscle involvement *4289*

Potassium *Serum* *Decrease* Hypokalemia and hyponatremia are common *367*

Protein *Cerebrospinal Fluid* *Decrease* Low levels of glucose and protein found in the CSF *4746* With involvement of the CNS *867*

Prothrombin Time *Plasma* *Increase* Reflects hepatic damage *367* May be prolonged *867*

Sodium *Serum* *Decrease* Hyponatremia is common in children *367*

Urea Nitrogen *Serum* *Increase* Markedly elevated reflecting renal injury *904*

331.90 Cerebral and Cortical Atrophy

Acid Phosphatase *Cerebrospinal Fluid* *Increase* Increased in lumbar CSF in relation to the degree of cerebral atrophy and duration of dementia *5792*

Cholesterol *Cerebrospinal Fluid* *Decrease* Significantly low CSF values for cholesterol and total lipids were found in a group of patients with brain atrophy in comparison with a control group. It is possible that these changes are a function of reduced brain mass or of defect in brain lipid metabolism in brain atrophy patients *2128*

Creatine Kinase *Cerebrospinal Fluid* *Increase* Of 9 patients with cerebral infarction 3 had increases above upper limit of normal of 10 U/L *4780*

β-Galactosidase *Serum* *Decrease* In cerebral atrophy due to presenile dementia and/or cerebrovascular disease *5792*

Immunoglobulin G *Cerebrospinal Fluid* *No Effect* Within the normal range *5138*

Lipids *Cerebrospinal Fluid* *Decrease* Significantly low CSF values for cholesterol and total lipids were found in a group of patients with brain atrophy in comparison with a control group. It is possible that these changes are a function of reduced brain mass or of defect in brain lipid metabolism *2128*

Uric Acid *Cerebrospinal Fluid* *Decrease* Very low CSF levels of 0.02 - 0.04 mg/dL, with normal serum levels found in the chronic stage of disease *2892*
Serum *No Effect* In the chronic stage *2892*

331.90 Olivopontocerebellar Atrophy

Amyloid β-Protein *Cerebrospinal Fluid* *No Effect* In 2 patients with olivopontocerebellar atrophy concentrations were 2.96 and 4.21 pmol/mL not significantly different from mean concentration of 4.00 ± 2.92 pmol/mL *3716*

Amyloid β-Protein Precursor *Cerebrospinal Fluid* *Increase* In 2 patients with olivopontocerebellar atrophy concentrations were 1.16 and 2.12 integrated OD units significantly different in one from mean concentration of 1.35 ± 0.38 integrated OD units in 25 normal controls *3716*
Cerebrospinal Fluid *No Effect* In 2 patients with olivopontocerebellar atrophy concentrations were 1.16 and 2.12 integrated OD units not significantly different in one from mean concentration of 1.35 ± 0.38 integrated OD units in 25 normal controls *3716*

α_1-Antichymotrypsin *Cerebrospinal Fluid* *Increase* In 2 patients with olivopontocerebellar atrophy concentrations were 2.50 and 4.80 µg/mL significantly different from mean concentration of 2.27 ± 1.40 µg/mL in 25 normal controls in one and normal in the other *3716*
Cerebrospinal Fluid *No Effect* In 2 patients with olivopontocerebellar atrophy concentrations were 2.50 and 4.80 µg/mL significantly different from mean concentration of 2.27 ± 1.40 µg/mL in 25 normal controls in one and normal in the other *3716*

Cells *Cerebrospinal Fluid* *No Effect* In 2 patients with olivopontocerebellar atrophy concentrations of 0.3 and 0.0 cells/µL not significantly different from normal of 3 cells/µL *3716*

Protein *Cerebrospinal Fluid* *Increase* In 2 patients with olivopontocerebellar atrophy concentrations of 33 and 60 mg/dL significantly different from normal mean of 29 mg/dL in one and normal in the other *3716*
Cerebrospinal Fluid *No Effect* In 2 patients with olivopontocerebellar atrophy concentrations of 33 and 60 mg/dL significantly different from normal mean of 29 mg/dL in one and normal in the other *3716*

332.00 Parkinson's Disease

Acetylcholinesterase *Cerebrospinal Fluid* *Decrease* In 18 patients with Parkinson's disease and dementia mean activity of 17.6 ± 1.41 U/L significantly different from 20.7 ± 1.03 U/L in 20 healthy controls and 26.3 ± 1.92 immunoreactive arbitrary U/L significantly different from 35.0 ± 2.31 immunoreactive arbitrary U/L in 20 healthy controls *2759*
Cerebrospinal Fluid *No Effect* No significant difference observed between concentrations in untreated Parkinson's disease compared with control individuals *3286* In 85 patients with Parkinson's disease mean activity of 21.4 ± 0.62 immunoreactive arbitrary U/L not significantly different from 20.7 ± 1.03 immunoreactive arbitrary U/L in 20 healthy controls and 33.2 ± 1.18 immunoreactive arbitrary U/L not significantly different from 35.0 ± 2.31 immunoreactive arbitrary U/L in 20 healthy controls *2759*

AD7c-NTP *Cerebrospinal Fluid* *No Effect* In 32 patients with Parkinson's disease mean concentration of 1.8 ± 1.1 ng/mL not significantly different from that in 18 controls in whom mean concentration was 1.7 ± 0.7 ng/mL *1061*

Amyloid β-Protein *Cerebrospinal Fluid* *No Effect* In 1 patient with Parkinson's disease concentration was 1.83 pmol/mL not significantly different from mean concentration of 4.00 ± 2.92 pmol/mL *3716*

Amyloid β-Protein Precursor *Cerebrospinal Fluid* *No Effect* In 1 patient with Parkinson's disease concentration was 1.15 integrated OD units not significantly different from mean concentration of 1.35 ± 0.38 integrated OD units in 25 normal controls *3716*

Angiotensin-converting Enzyme
Cerebrospinal Fluid *Decrease* Decreased in 27% of cases compared with an age and sex matched control group *5876*
Cerebrospinal Fluid *No Effect* In 35 patients with untreated Parkinson's disease mean concentration of 0.83 ± 0.26 U/L not significantly different from 0.81 ± 0.18 U/L in 20 healthy controls *2758*

α_1-Antichymotrypsin *Cerebrospinal Fluid* *No Effect* In 1 patient with Parkinson's disease concentration was 3.20 µg/mL not significantly different from mean concentration of 2.27 ± 1.40 µg/mL in 25 normal controls *3716*

332.00 Parkinson's Disease *(continued)*

α_1-Antichymotrypsin *(continued)*
Serum *Increase* Mean concentration increased above reference interval of 47.9 ± 8.1 mg/dL in 1 of 4 patients (25%) with Parkinson's disease *3044*
Serum *No Effect* Not useful as a marker as concentration unaffected by disease *2845*

Ascorbic Acid *Serum* *No Effect* In 63 patients with Parkinson's disease mean concentration of 47.13 ± 0.89 µg/mL not significantly different from 47.60 ± 0.60 µg/mL in spouses serving as controls *1461*
White Blood Cells *No Effect* Concentration in leukocytes of 27 patients with Parkinson's disease 150 ± 35 not significantly different from 101 ± 25 in matched elderly population *4382*

Caffeine *Saliva* *No Effect* Mean concentration in patients with both treated or untreated Parkinson's disease not significantly different from that in healthy controls *1531*

Carnosinase *Serum* *Decrease* Mean activity of 109 ± 11 nmol/mL/min in 17 patients significantly less than 161 ± 7 nmol/mL/min in 16 healthy controls *5590*

Cells *Cerebrospinal Fluid* *No Effect* In 1 patient with Parkinson's disease concentration of 2.7 cel s/µL not significantly different from normal of 3 cells/µL *3716*

Cholecystokinin *Cerebrospinal Fluid* *Decrease* Significantly decreased cholecystokinin (1.9 pmol/L) versus control (4.0 pmol/L) *3136*

Choline *Cerebrospinal Fluid* *Decrease* In 8 untreated patients with Parkinson's disease mean concentration of 1.31 ± 0.29 nmol/mL markedly less than 2.97 ± 0.79 nmol/mL in 9 control individuals *3286*

Cholinesterase (True) *Cerebrospinal Fluid* *No Effect* In 85 patients with Parkinson's disease without dementia mean activity of 21.4 ± 0.62 U/L (33.2 ± 1.18 arb U/L immunologically) not significantly different from 20.7 ± 1.03 U/L (35.0 ± 2.31 arb U/L immunologicallly) in 20 healthy controls *2759*

Citrate Synthase *Platelets* *No Effect* In 18 patients with early Parkinson's disease mean activity of 442 ± 105 nmol/min/mg mitochondrial protein not significantly different from 443 ± 93 nmol/min/mg mitochondrial protein in 18 age- and sex-matched controls *1946*

Copper *Cerebrospinal Fluid* *Increase* Although there was considerable overlap between the 24 Parkinsonian and 34 control subjects, the former had significantly higher levels ($p < 0.001$) *3978*

Cysteine *Plasma* *Increase* Levels are high *5675*

Dopamine *Plasma* *No Effect* Mean concentration of 5,877.2 ± 2,488.2 pg/mL in 25 "de novo" Parkinsonian patients not significantly different from 5,247.2 ± 2,345.1 pg/mL in 25 age- and sex-matched control individuals *3652*

Dopamine β-Hydroxylase *Cerebrospinal Fluid* *Decrease* In 7 patients with Parkinson's disease mean concentration of 16.3 ± 2.9 ng/mL significantly less than 31.3 ± 1.4 ng/mL in 32 healthy individuals *3855*

Homovanillic Acid *Plasma* *No Effect* Mean concentration of 9.8 ng/mL in 17 patients with Parkinson's disease not significantly different from 8.2 ng/mL in young healthy volunteers *4433*

4-Hydroxynonenal *Cerebrospinal Fluid* *No Effect* In 31 patients with Parkinson's disease mean concentration of 0.55 ± 0.14 ng/mL not significantly different from 0.51 ± 0.05 ng/mL in 236 patients with other neurological diagnoses *4909*

Iron *Cerebrospinal Fluid* *No Effect* Moderate elevation *3978*

Malondialdehyde *Serum* *No Effect* In 37 patients with Parkinson's disease mean concentration of 8.7 ± 0.51 nmol/mL not significantly different from 8.8 ± 0.48 nmol/mL in controls *3558*

Manganese *Cerebrospinal Fluid* *No Effect* Moderate elevation *3978*

Mitochondrial Complex I *Platelets* *Decrease* In 18 patients with early Parkinson's disease mean activity of 15.1 ± 3.5 nmol/min/mg mitochondrial protein significantly different from 20.1 ± 4.6 nmol/min/mg mitochondrial protein in 18 age- and sex-matched controls *1946*

Mitochondrial Complex II/III *Platelets* *Decrease* In 18 patients with early Parkinson's disease mean activity of 110.3 ± 35.9 nmol/min/mg mitochondrial protein significantly different from 138.3 ± 36.7 nmol/min/mg mitochondrial protein in 18 age- and sex-matched controls *1946*

Mitochondrial Complex IV *Platelets* *No Effect* In 18 patients with early Parkinson's disease mean activity of -0.21 ± 0.08 nmol/min/mg mitochondrial protein not significantly different from -0.19 ± 0.07 nmol/min/mg mitochondrial protein in 18 age- and sex-matched controls *1946*

Monoamine Oxidase *Platelets* *Increase* Increased monoamine oxidase B activity in platelets *523*

Protein *Cerebrospinal Fluid* *No Effect* In 1 patient with Parkinson's disease concentration of 44 mgL not significantly different from normal of 28 mg/dL in 25 healthy controls *3716* Mean concentration in postmortem ventricular CSF in 30 patients of 57.5 ± 6.0 mg/dL not significantly different from 60.9 ± 5.8 mg/dL in 16 normal controls *5435* In 35 patients with untreated Parkinson's mean concentration of 0.45 ± 0.17 g/L not significantly different from 0.38 ± 0.09 g/L in 20 healthy controls *2758*

R-Salsolinol *Plasma* *No Effect* Mean concentration of 496.4 ± 470.7 pg/mL in 25 "de novo" Parkinsonian patients not significantly different from 612.2 ± 685.5 pg/mL in 25 age- and sex-matched control individuals *3652*

Somatostatin *Cerebrospinal Fluid* *Decrease* Significantly lower mean CSF levels than in other neurological patients. All 11 patients with Alzheimer's disease or Parkinson's disease dementia had levels well below 21.8 ng/mL *4739*

S-Salsolinol *Plasma* *No Effect* Mean concentration of 443.6 ± 347.3 pg/mL in 25 "de novo" Parkinsonian patients not significantly different from 512.9 ± 344.0 pg/mL in 25 age- and sex-matched control individuals *3652*

Sulfate *Serum* *Decrease* Levels are low. Enzymes involved with sulfur oxidation and methylation are under-active *5675*

Transforming Growth Factor-β_1 *Cerebrospinal Fluid* *Increase* Mean concentration in postmortem ventricular CSF in 30 patients of 53.8 ± 11.8 pg/mL significantly different from 23.7 ± 4.6 pg/mL in 16 normal controls *5435*

Transforming Growth Factor-β_2 *Cerebrospinal Fluid* *Increase* Mean concentration in postmortem ventricular CSF in 30 patients of 320.4 ± 53.1 pg/mL significantly different from 80.6 ± 21.9 pg/mL in 16 normal controls *5435*

Tumor Necrosis Factor-α *Cerebrospinal Fluid* *Increase* In 15 patients with Parkinson's disease mean concentration of 96.3 ± 9.1 pg/mL compared with 22.3 ± 9.5 pg/mL in 16 control patients without neurological disease *3548*

Uric Acid *Serum* *Decrease* In patients with uric acid concentrations above the median 40% reduction in incidence of idiopathic Parkinson's disease *1035*

Vitamin A *Serum* *No Effect* No significant difference observed between mean concentration of 530 ± 60 µg/L in 27 elderly women with Parkinson's disease and 500 ± 100 µg/L in a matched control group *4382*

Vitamin E *Serum* *No Effect* No significant difference observed between mean concentration of 11.1 ± 1.5 mg/L in 27 elderly patients with Parkinson's disease and 11.1 ± 2.0 mg/L in a matched control group *4382*

332.00 Parkinson's Disease with Dementia

Angiotensin-converting Enzyme
Cerebrospinal Fluid *No Effect* In 18 patients with Parkinson's disease with dementia mean concentration of 0.78 ± 0.23 U/L not significantly different from 0.81 ± 0.18 U/L in 20 healthy controls *2758*

Cholinesterase (True) *Cerebrospinal Fluid* *Decrease* In 18 patients with Parkinson's disease with dementia mean activity of 17.6 ± 1.41 U/L (26.3 ± 1.92 arb U/L immunologically) significantly different from 20.7 ± 1.03 U/L (35.0 ± 2.31 arb U/L immunologicallly) in 20 healthy controls *2759*

Protein *Cerebrospinal Fluid* *No Effect* In 18 patients with Parkinson's disease with dementia mean concentration of 0.46 ± 0.19 g/L not significantly different from 0.38 ± 0.09 g/L in 20 healthy controls *2758*

333.20 Opsoclonus-Myoclonus Syndrome

Homovanillic Acid *Cerebrospinal Fluid* *Decrease* In 17 children with opsoclonus-myoclonus syndrome mean concentration of 52.8 ± 3.7 ng/mL significantly different from 80.1 ± 6.2 ng/mL in 15 matched controls *4204*

5-Hydroxyindoleacetic Acid *Cerebrospinal Fluid* *Decrease* In 17 children with opsoclonus-myoclonus syndrome mean concentration of 25.7 ± 2.1 ng/mL significantly different from 41.5 ± 5.0 ng/mL in 15 matched controls *4204*

333.40 Huntington's Chorea

Alanine *Plasma* *Decrease* 19 patients showed a significantly lower concentration of proline, alanine, valine, leucine, isoleucine, and tyrosine compared to 38 normal controls *1101*

Alanine Aminotransferase *Serum* *No Effect* No abnormalities in 8 patients *1101*

Amino Acids *Plasma* *Decrease* 19 patients showed a significantly lower concentration of proline, alanine, valine, leucine, isoleucine, and tyrosine compared to 38 normal controls *1101*

Aspartate Aminotransferase *Serum* *No Effect* No abnormalities in 8 patients *1101*

Calcium *Serum* *No Effect* No significant effect observed *2641*

Copper *Serum* *Increase* Some studies show elevated levels while others did not *1790*
Serum *No Effect* Some studies show elevated levels while others did not *1790*

Creatine Kinase *Serum* *No Effect* No abnormalities in 8 patients *1101*

Fatty Acids (FFA), Free *Serum* *Increase* High fasting concentrations. The elevation was maintained under hypoglycemic conditions, but not in hyperglycemic states *4125*

γ-Globulin *Serum* *Increase* In 23 of 27 patients *615*

Homovanillic Acid *Cerebrospinal Fluid* *Decrease* Reported effect *1790*

Isocitrate Dehydrogenase *Serum* *No Effect* No abnormalities in 8 patients *1101*

Isoleucine *Plasma* *Decrease* 19 patients showed a significantly lower concentration of proline, aminolevulinic acid, valine, leucine, isoleucine, and tyrosine compared to 38 normal controls *1101* Reduced fasting plasma concentrations of leucine, isoleucine and valine *4125*

Lactate Dehydrogenase *Serum* *No Effect* No abnormalities in 8 patients *1101*

Leucine *Plasma* *Decrease* 19 patients showed a significantly lower concentration of proline, aminolevulinic acid, valine, leucine, isoleucine, and tyrosine compared to 38 normal controls *1101* Reduced fasting plasma concentrations of leucine, isoleucine and valine *4125*

Magnesium *Red Blood Cells* *No Effect* No significant effect observed *1505*
Serum *No Effect* No significant effect observed *2641*

Malate Dehydrogenase *Serum* *No Effect* No abnormalities in 8 patients *1101*

Norepinephrine *Urine* *No Effect* No significant effect observed *3698*

Proline *Plasma* *Decrease* 19 patients showed a significantly lower concentration of proline, alanine, valine, leucine, isoleucine, and tyrosine compared to 38 normal controls *1101*

Protein *Serum* *Increase* In 23 of 27 patients *615*

Quinolinic Acid *Cerebrospinal Fluid* *Decrease* The concentrations were slightly lower in patients with this disorder, however the changes were not significant *2142*
Cerebrospinal Fluid *No Effect* The concentrations were highly variable but mean levels were not significantly different from controls *4687*

Tryptophan *Cerebrospinal Fluid* *No Effect* In 7 patients *5791*

Tryptophan, Free *Plasma* *Decrease* Markedly reduced as a result of the increased concentrations of nonesterified fatty acids. In induced hypoglycemia, the difference in free tryptophan between control and diseased groups was much less severe *4125*

Tyrosine *Cerebrospinal Fluid* *No Effect* In 7 patients *5791*
Plasma *Decrease* 19 patients showed a significantly lower concentration of proline, alanine, valine, leucine, isoleucine, and tyrosine compared to 38 normal controls *1101*

Valine *Plasma* *Decrease* 19 patients showed a significantly lower concentration of proline, aminolevulinic acid, valine, leucine, isoleucine, and tyrosine compared to 38 normal controls *1101* Reduced fasting plasma concentrations of leucine, isoleucine and valine *4125*

333.70 Vogt-Koyanagi-Harada's Disease

Anti-Neutrophil Cytoplasm Antibodies *Serum* *No Effect* In 0 of 6 patients (0%) pANCA detected *3722*

Antinuclear Antibodies *Serum* *Increase* In 2 of 6 patients (33.3%) ANA detected *3722*

333.91 Stiff-man Syndrome

Anti-Islet Cell Cytoplasmic Antibodies *Serum* *Increase* Positive results occur in about 90% patients with stiff-man syndrome with values high *2952*

333.92 Neuroleptic Malignant Syndrome

Phosphate *Serum* *Decrease* Neuroleptic malignant syndrome is less common cause of severe hypophosphatemia due to reduced absorption of phosphate from intestinal tract *969*

334.00 Friedreich's Ataxia

Acid Phosphatase *Serum* *Increase* One pair of siblings displayed a slight elevation *4389*

Aldolase *Serum* *Increase* Elevated in 11 cases but markedly so in only 5 of 23 cases *4389*

Alkaline Phosphatase *Serum* *Increase* One pair of siblings displayed a slight elevation *4389*

Cholesterol *Serum* *Increase* In Friedreich's patients, the relative proportion of cholesterol and triglycerides was increased while the relative protein content was greatly reduced *2270*

Cholinesterase *Serum* *Increase* Altered or increased in 7 of 23 patients. However, the elevation was considered to be significant in only 3 *4389*

Ferritin *Serum* *No Effect* In 6 premenopausal women with Friedreich's ataxia mean concentration of 34 ng/mL not different from reference range of 15 - 95 ng/mL. In 4 men mean concentration of 109 ng/mL within male reference interval of 30 - 370 ng/mL *5690*

Iron *Serum* *No Effect* In 6 premenopausal women and 3 men with Friedreich's ataxia mean concentration of 86 µg/dL not different from reference range of 40 - 175 µg/dL *5690*

β-Lipoprotein *Serum* *Decrease* Total amount of high density lipoprotein reduced in Friedreich's and familial spastic ataxia *2270*

Lipoproteins *Serum* *Decrease* Their total amount of high density lipoprotein was reduced and the composition was abnormal in both Friedreich's and familial spastic ataxia *2270*

Protein *Serum* *Decrease* In Friedreich's patients, the relative proportion of cholesterol and triglycerides was increased while the relative protein content was greatly reduced *2270*

Triglycerides *Serum* *No Effect* Significantly higher in Friedreich's ataxia, but remained within the normal limit *2270*

334.80 Ataxia-Telangiectasia

Cholesterol *Serum* *No Effect* In 5 patients with ataxia telangectasia mean concentration of 44.1 ± 7.1 µmol/L not significantly different from 42.2 ± 6.9 µmol/L in 165 age matched controls *327*

α-Fetoprotein *Serum* *Increase* In 5 patients with ataxia telangectasia mean concentration of 211 ± 104 ng/mL significantly different from 9.2 ± 5.6 ng/mL in 165 age matched controls *327* Present in inordinately high concentration in a majority of patients *367* Ataxia telangiectasia in children may be associated with an increased concentration *1778* Has been reported *5532*

γ-Globulin *Serum* *Decrease* May be decreased, resulting in increased susceptibility to infection *2039*

immunoglobulin A *Serum* *Decrease* Deficient in 66% of patients *4170* About 80% of patients lack both serum and secretory IgA *4551* Reported effect *5677*

334.80 Ataxia-Telangiectasia *(continued)*

Immunoglobulin A, Secretory *Serum Decrease* About 80% of patients lack both serum and secretory IgA *4551*

Immunoglobulin E *Serum Decrease* Deficient in 80% of patients *4170* In 44 patients with ataxia telangiectasia mean concentration of 12 ng/mL (range 3.6 - 40) not significantly less than mean of 96 ng/mL (range 24 - 336) in 74 healthy controls *2323* Decreased or absent serum IgA and IgE causing recurrent pulmonary infections *5544*

Immunoglobulin G *Serum No Effect* Concentration usually normal *5544*

Immunoglobulin M *Serum Decrease* Low levels have been reported *367*
Serum No Effect Concentration usually normal *5544*

Immunoglobulins *Serum Decrease* Deficiency appears to contribute to the frequent severe infections associated with the syndrome *4707*

Lymphocytes *Blood Decrease* T-lymphocytes and T-cell functions are regularly grossly deficient *367* Variable; below 1,000 /µL in 33% of patients *5699*

Vitamin E *Serum No Effect* In 5 patients with ataxia telangectasia mean concentration of 17.2 ± 6.0 µmol/L not significantly different from 18.0 ± 5.3 µmol/L in 165 age matched controls *327*

Vitamin E:Cholesterol Ratio *Serum No Effect* In 5 patients with ataxia telangectasia mean ratio of 0.39 not significantly different from 0.42. in 165 age matched controls *327*

334.90 Cerebellar Degeneration

Oligoclonal Banding *Cerebrospinal Fluid Increase* Oligoclonal IgG bands detected with cerebellar degeneration *3261*

334.90 Spinocerebellar Degeneration

α_1-Microglobulin *Cerebrospinal Fluid Increase* Of 15 patients with degenerative diseases of brain including spinocerebellar degeneration mean concentration in none exceeded that in 15 healthy controls of 34.8 ± 16.0 µg/L *2370*

Neuropeptide Y *Cerebrospinal Fluid No Effect* In 7 patients mean concentration of 92.1 ± 21.4 pg/mL not significantly different from 80.2 ± 35.3 pg/mL in 11 controls older than 60 years *3201*

Somatostatin *Cerebrospinal Fluid No Effect* In 7 patients mean concentration of 15.6 ± 9.0 pg/mL not significantly different from 16.0 ± 11.8 pg/mL in 7 controls older than 60 years *3201*

335.11 Familial Progressive Spinal Muscular Atrophy

Alanine Aminotransferase *Serum Increase* Elevations of serum enzymes are frequently encountered but never reach the magnitude seen in Duchenne muscular dystrophy *900*

Aldolase *Serum Increase* Elevations of serum enzymes are frequently encountered but never reach the magnitude seen in Duchenne muscular dystrophy *900*

Aspartate Aminotransferase *Serum Increase* Elevations of serum enzymes are frequently encountered but never reach the magnitude seen in Duchenne muscular dystrophy *900*

Creatine Kinase *Serum Increase* Elevations of CK and other serum enzymes are frequently encountered but never reach the magnitude seen in Duchenne muscular dystrophy *900*

Lactate Dehydrogenase *Serum Increase* Elevations of serum enzymes are frequently encountered but never reach the magnitude seen in Duchenne muscular dystrophy *900*

Lactate Dehydrogenase Isoenzyme-5 *Serum Increase* In rapidly destructive neurogenic atrophies such as Werdnig-Hoffmann disease a rise was noted, reflecting a temporary leakage of cytoplasmic LD_5 from muscle to peripheral blood *2225*

335.20 Amyotrophic Lateral Sclerosis

Acetylcholine Receptor Binding Antibodies
Serum Increase Unexplained positive results are observed in about 5% of patients with amyotropic lateral sclerosis *2952*

Acetylcholinesterase G4 Isoenzyme *Serum No Effect* No significant deviation from normal observed in a small number of patients *5778*

Alanine *Cerebrospinal Fluid No Effect* Mean concentration in 16 patients with ALS 50.5 ± 4.4 µmol/L not significantly different from 44.5 ± 3 µmol/L in 19 age-matched controls *674*
Plasma Decrease In 22 patients with ALS mean concentration of 355 ± 26 µmol/L significantly different from 457 ± 19 µmol/L in 44 age-matched controls *674*

Albumin *Serum No Effect* No significant effect observed *1366*

Aldolase *Serum Increase* Rises in the early stages, falling to normal later. This pattern occurs in any primary neurogenic muscular dystrophy *1290* Normal or slightly increased *1980*

Amino Acids *Urine No Effect* No significant change observed *1366*

Amyloid β-Protein *Cerebrospinal Fluid No Effect* In 1 patient with ALS concentration was 3.94 pmol/mL not significantly different from mean concentration of 4.00 ± 2.92 pmol/mL *3716*

Amyloid β-Protein Precursor *Cerebrospinal Fluid Increase* In 1 patient with ALS concentration was 1.91 integrated OD units significantly different from mean concentration of 1.35 ± 0.38 integrated OD units in 25 normal controls *3716*

Antibody Titer *Serum Increase* IgA and IgM antibodies to myelin of rabbit spinal cord. Found in 70% of patients. When IgG antimyelin antibody is present in titers greater than 1:8 it is suggestive, but not diagnostic *3712*

α_1-Antichymotrypsin *Cerebrospinal Fluid No Effect* In 1 patient with ALS concentration was 3.20 µg/mL not significantly different from mean concentration of 2.27 ± 1.40 µg/mL in 25 normal controls *3716*

Arginine *Cerebrospinal Fluid No Effect* Mean concentration in 16 patients with ALS 39.7 ± 3.0 µmol/L not significantly different from 33.9 ± 1.7 µmol/L in 19 age-matched controls *674*
Plasma No Effect In 22 patients with ALS mean concentration of 171 ± 8 µmol/L not significantly different from 195 ± 7 µmol/L in 44 age-matched controls *674*

Asparagine *Cerebrospinal Fluid No Effect* Mean concentration in 16 patients with ALS of 12.5 ± 2.1 µmol/L not significantly different from 9.6 ± 1.3 µmol/L in 19 age-matched controls *674*
Plasma No Effect In 22 patients with ALS mean concentration of 59 ± 2 µmol/L not significantly different from 70 ± 2.6 µmol/L in 44 age-matched controls *674*

Aspartic Acid *Plasma Increase* In 10 patients with ALS mean concentration significantly increased compared with age and sex matched controls *2378*
Plasma No Effect In 22 patients with ALS mean concentration of 2.3 ± 0.3 µmol/L not significantly different from 2.3 ± 0.3 µmol/L in 44 age-matched controls *674*

Calcium *Urine Increase* Disuse atrophy with a major portion of the body immobilized *1025*

Cells *Cerebrospinal Fluid No Effect* In 1 patient with ALS concentration of 1.0 cells/µL not significantly different from normal of 3 cells/µL *3716*

Ceruloplasmin *Serum No Effect* No significant effect observed *1366*

Creatine *Urine Increase* Urinary creatine may be significantly increased in patients with amyotrophic lateral sclerosis *2952*

Creatine Kinase *Serum No Effect* No significant effect observed *1980*

Creatine Kinase BB-Isoenzyme *Serum Increase* Mean activity in patients with ALS 1.22 times normal *1456*

Creatine Kinase MM-Isoenzyme *Serum Increase* Mean activity in patients with ALS 1.34 times normal *1456*

Creatinine *Serum Increase* Severe muscle disease *1025*
Urine Decrease Roughly in proportion to loss of muscle mass *1366*

Cystine *Plasma No Effect* In 22 patients with ALS mean concentration of 61 ± 3 µmol/L not significantly different from 72 ± 4 µmol/L in 44 age-matched controls *674*

Fibrinogen *Plasma* *No Effect* No significant effect observed *1366*

Glucose Tolerance *Serum* *Decrease* In 30% of patients with the disease and is related to decreased muscle mass *1366*

Glutamic Acid *Cerebrospinal Fluid* *No Effect* Mean concentration in 16 patients with ALS of 4.1 ± 0.5 µmol/L not significantly different from 3.5 ± 0.3 µmol/L in 19 age-matched controls *674*
Plasma *Increase* In 10 patients with ALS mean concentration significantly increased compared with age and sex matched controls *2378*
Plasma *No Effect* In 22 patients with ALS mean concentration of 41 ± 3 µmol/L not significantly different from 40 ± 2 µmol/L in 44 age-matched controls *674*

Glutamic Acid Decarboxylase Antibodies *Serum* *No Effect* In none of 23 patients with amyotrophic lateral sclerosis were GAD antibodies detected *3880*

Glutamine *Cerebrospinal Fluid* *No Effect* Mean concentration in 16 patients with ALS of 704 ± 55 µmol/L not significantly different from 566 ± 41 µmol/L in 19 age-matched controls *674*
Plasma *No Effect* In 22 patients with ALS mean concentration of 641 ± 26 µmol/L not significantly different from 644 ± 13 µmol/L in 44 age-matched controls *674*

Glycine *Cerebrospinal Fluid* *No Effect* Mean concentration in 16 patients with ALS of 34.7 ± 6.4 µmol/L not significantly different from 21.5 ± 5.5 µmol/L in 19 age-matched controls *674*
Plasma *Increase* In 10 patients with ALS mean concentration significantly higher than in age and sex matched controls *2378*
Plasma *No Effect* In 22 patients with ALS mean concentration of 378 ± 50 µmol/L not significantly different from 331 ± 19 µmol/L in 44 age-matched controls *674*

Histidine *Cerebrospinal Fluid* *No Effect* Mean concentration in 16 patients with ALS of 20.7 ± 2.2 µmol/L not significantly different from 18.4 ± 2.5 µmol/L in 19 age-matched controls *674*
Plasma *No Effect* In 22 patients with ALS mean concentration of 89 ± 4 µmol/L not significantly different from 96 ± 4 µmol/L in 44 age-matched controls *674*

Homovanillic Acid *Cerebrospinal Fluid* *Decrease* Reported effect *3265*

5-Hydroxyindoleacetic Acid *Cerebrospinal Fluid* *No Effect* No significant change observed *3265*

4-Hydroxynonenal *Cerebrospinal Fluid* *Increase* In 186 patients with sporadic ALS mean concentration of 1.82 ± 0.15 ng/mL significantly different from 0.51 ± 0.05 ng/mL in 236 patients with other neurological diagnoses *4909*

immunoglobulin A *Serum* *No Effect* No significant effect observed *1366*

Immunoglobulin G *Serum* *No Effect* No significant effect observed *1366*

Immunoglobulin M *Serum* *No Effect* No significant effect observed *1366*

Immunoglobulins *Serum* *No Effect* No significant effect observed *1366*

Interleukin-6 *Serum* *No Effect* Cerebrospinal fluid (CSF) IL-6 levels were measured in patients with ALS and compared with those in psychiatric and neurodegenerative disorders not believed to be due to immune disorders of the central nervous system. No significant differences in CSF IL-6 levels were found between these groups *2823*

Isoleucine *Cerebrospinal Fluid* *No Effect* Mean concentration in 16 patients with ALS of 9.8 ± 0.9 µmol/L not significantly different from 8.7 ± 0.7 µmol/L in 19 age-matched controls *674*
Plasma *Decrease* In 22 patients with ALS mean concentration of 84 ± 4 µmol/L significantly different from 102 ± 4 µmol/L in 44 age-matched controls *674*

Lactate Dehydrogenase *Serum* *Increase* Slight elevations of LD are common in adults, but it is unclear whether muscular atrophy or hepatic disease is the cause *5430* Especially in the early stages *1290*

Lactate Dehydrogenase Isoenzyme-5 *Serum* *Increase* In rapidly destructive progressive muscular atrophies, such as amyotrophic lateral sclerosis and Werdnig-Hoffmann disease, a rise was noted reflecting leakage of cytoplasmic LD_5 from muscle to peripheral blood *2225*

Leucine *Cerebrospinal Fluid* *No Effect* Mean concentration in 16 patients with ALS of 26.4 ± 2.1 µmol/L not significantly different from 23.4 ± 1.7 µmol/L in 19 age-matched controls *674*
Plasma *Decrease* In 22 patients with ALS mean concentration of 160 ± 7 µmol/L significantly different from 185 ± 7 µmol/L in 44 age-matched controls *674*

Lipids *Serum* *No Effect* No significant effect observed *1366*

Lipoproteins *Serum* *No Effect* No significant effect observed *1366*

Lysine *Cerebrospinal Fluid* *No Effect* Mean concentration in 16 patients with ALS of 47.3 ± 3.8 µmol/L not significantly different from 39 ± 2.3 µmol/L in 19 age-matched controls *674*
Plasma *No Effect* In 22 patients with ALS mean concentration of 263 ± 15 µmol/L not significantly different from 293 ± 11 µmol/L in 44 age-matched controls *674*

Methionine *Cerebrospinal Fluid* *No Effect* Mean concentration in 16 patients with ALS of 4.1 ± 0.4 µmol/L not significantly different from 4.0 ± 0.6 µmol/L in 19 age-matched controls *674*
Plasma *Decrease* In 22 patients with ALS mean concentration of 25 ± 1 µmol/L significantly different from 30 ± 1 µmol/L in 44 age-matched controls *674*

Neuropeptide Y *Cerebrospinal Fluid* *No Effect* In 5 patients mean concentration of 75.8 ± 37.2 pg/mL not significantly different from 80.2 ± 35.3 pg/mL in 11 controls older than 60 years *3201*

Ornithine *Cerebrospinal Fluid* *No Effect* Mean concentration in 16 patients with ALS 21.4 ± 2.6 µmol/L not significantly different from 25.4 ± 2.3 µmol/L in 19 age-matched controls *674*
Plasma *No Effect* In 22 patients with ALS mean concentration of 152 ± 10 µmol/L not significantly different from 191 ± 12 µmol/L in 44 age-matched controls *674*

Phenylalanine *Cerebrospinal Fluid* *No Effect* Mean concentration in 16 patients with ALS of 17 ± 1.7 µmol/L not significantly different from 12.9 ± 1.5 µmol/L in 19 age-matched controls *674*
Plasma *No Effect* In 22 patients with ALS mean concentration of 77 ± 4 µmol/L not significantly different from 85 ± 3 µmol/L in 44 age-matched controls *674*

Phytanic Acid *Serum* *No Effect* No significant effect observed *1366*

Protein *Cerebrospinal Fluid* *No Effect* In 1 patient with ALS concentration of 42 mg/dL not significantly different from normal of 28 mg/dL in 25 healthy controls *3716*

Serine *Cerebrospinal Fluid* *No Effect* Mean concentration in 16 patients with ALS of 36.6 ± 2.2 µmol/L not significantly different from 31.4 ± 1.8 µmol/L in 19 age-matched controls *674*
Plasma *No Effect* In 22 patients with ALS mean concentration of 127 ± 5 µmol/L not significantly different from 129 ± 5 µmol/L in 44 age-matched controls *674*

Soluble E-Selectin *Serum* *No Effect* Mean concentration of 37 ± 17 ng/mL in 15 patients with ALS not significantly different from 30 ± 9 ng/mL in 12 healthy control individuals *3885*

Somatostatin *Cerebrospinal Fluid* *No Effect* In 5 patients mean concentration of 12.3 ± 4.0 pg/mL not significantly different from 16.0 ± 11.8 pg/mL in 7 controls older than 60 years *3201*

Threonine *Cerebrospinal Fluid* *No Effect* Mean concentration in 16 patients with ALS of 43.6 ± 3.4 µmol/L not significantly different from 39.3 ± 3.1 µmol/L in 19 age-matched controls *674*
Plasma *No Effect* In 22 patients with ALS mean concentration of 155 ± 6 µmol/L not significantly different from 176 ± 7 µmol/L in 44 age-matched controls *674*

Transglutaminase *Cerebrospinal Fluid* *Decrease* In 8 patients with sporadic amyotrophic lateral sclerosis mean concentration of 23.3 ± 2.6 pmol/100 µL/h significantly different from 28.8 ± 4.8 pmol/100 µL/h in 19 control patients *1599*
Serum *No Effect* In 8 patients with sporadic amyotrophic lateral sclerosis mean concentration of 20.5 ± 12.2 pmol/100 µL/h not significantly different from 19.8 ± 4.2 pmol/100 µL/h in 19 control patients *1599*

Tryptophan *Cerebrospinal Fluid* *No Effect* Mean concentration in 16 patients with ALS of 3.9 ± 0.4 µmol/L not significantly different from 4.8 ± 1.9 µmol/L in 19 age-matched controls *674*
Plasma *No Effect* In 22 patients with ALS mean concentration of 57 ± 2 µmol/L not significantly different from 63 ± 3 µmol/L in 44 age-matched controls *674*

Tyrosine *Cerebrospinal Fluid* *No Effect* Mean concentration in 16 patients with ALS of 12.5 ± 1 µmol/L not significantly different from 10.4 ± 1 µmol/L in 19 age-matched controls *674*

335.20 Amyotrophic Lateral Sclerosis (continued)

Tyrosine *(continued)*
Plasma *Decrease* In 22 patients with ALS mean concentration of 70 ± 3 µmol/L significantly different from 84 ± 4 µmol/L in 44 age-matched controls *674*

Valine *Cerebrospinal Fluid* *No Effect* Mean concentration in 16 patients with ALS of 25.5 ± 2.3 µmol/L not significantly different from 23.8 ± 2.2 µmol/L in 19 age-matched controls *674*
Plasma *No Effect* In 22 patients with ALS mean concentration of 278 ± 15 µmol/L not significantly different from 279 ± 10 µmol/L in 44 age-matched controls *674*

Vanillylmandelic Acid *Urine* *No Effect* No significant change observed *1366*

335.20 Motor Neuron Disease

Alanine *Cerebrospinal Fluid* *No Effect* In 31 patients median concentration of 29.55 ± 2.07 µmol/L not significantly different from 32.47 ± 2.77 µmol/L in 30 healthy controls *4765*
Plasma *No Effect* In 37 patients median concentration of 315.92 ± 18.07 µmol/L not significantly different from 348.97 ± 12.29 µmol/L in 35 healthy controls *4765*

α-Amino-n-Butyric Acid *Cerebrospinal Fluid* *No Effect* In 31 patients median concentration of 3.16 ± 0.37 µmol/L not significantly different from 2.97 ± 0.46 µmol/L in 30 healthy controls *4765*
Plasma *No Effect* In 37 patients median concentration of 18.34 ± 1.54 µmol/L not significantly different from 16.97 ± 1.34 µmol/L in 35 healthy controls *4765*

Anti-Neutrophil Cytoplasm Antibodies *Serum* *No Effect* In 0 of 2 patients (0%) with motor neuron disease pANCA detected *3722*

Antinuclear Antibodies *Serum* *No Effect* In 0 of 2 patients (0%) with motor neuron disease ANA detected *3722*

Arginine *Cerebrospinal Fluid* *No Effect* In 31 patients median concentration of 16.55 ± 1.23 µmol/L not significantly different from 16.30 ± 1.67 µmol/L in 30 healthy controls *4765*
Plasma *No Effect* In 37 patients median concentration of 59.53 ± 8.23 µmol/L not significantly different from 73.44 ± 5.39 µmol/L in 35 healthy controls *4765*

Asparagine *Cerebrospinal Fluid* *No Effect* In 31 patients median concentration of 5.61 ± 0.57 µmol/L not significantly different from 6.57 ± 0.44 µmol/L in 30 healthy controls *4765*
Plasma *No Effect* In 37 patients median concentration of 42.63 ± 1.67 µmol/L not significantly different from 46.38 ± 3.23 µmol/L in 35 healthy controls *4765*

Aspartic Acid *Cerebrospinal Fluid* *No Effect* In 31 patients median concentration of 7.42 ± 0.24 µmol/L not significantly different from 7.87 ± 0.55 µmol/L in 30 healthy controls *4765*
Plasma *No Effect* In 37 patients median concentration of 27.37 ± 1.26 µmol/L not significantly different from 25.74 ± 0.87 µmol/L in 35 healthy controls *4765*

Carnosinase *Serum* *No Effect* In 14 patients with motor neurone disease mean activity of 155 ± 15 nmol/mL/min not significantly different from 161 ± 7 nmol/mL/min in 16 healthy controls *5590*

Citrulline *Cerebrospinal Fluid* *No Effect* In 31 patients median concentration of 0.58 ± 0.21 µmol/L not significantly different from 1.00 ± 0.49 µmol/L in 30 healthy controls *4765*
Plasma *No Effect* In 37 patients median concentration of 33.11 ± 3.17 µmol/L not significantly different from 31.71 ± 3.20 µmol/L in 35 healthy controls *4765*

Cystine *Plasma* *Increase* In 37 patients median concentration of 92.42 ± 6.72 µmol/L different from 74.71 ± 6.31 µmol/L in 35 healthy controls *4765*

Glucose *Serum* *No Effect* Mean fasting concentration of 4.8 ± 0.2 mmol/L in 8 patients with motor neuron disease not significantly different from 5.2 ± 0.2 mmol/L in 8 healthy controls *2822*

Glucose Tolerance *Serum* *Decrease* 6 of 8 patients with motor neuron disease had impaired glucose tolerance although fasting glucose concentration normal *2822*

Glutamic Acid *Cerebrospinal Fluid* *Increase* In 31 patients median concentration of 9.23 ± 2.38 µmol/L significantly different from 3.53 ± 1.13 µmol/L in 30 healthy controls *4765*
Plasma *No Effect* In 37 patients median concentration of 50.50 ± 3.56 µmol/L not significantly different from 58.15 ± 3.81 µmol/L in 35 healthy controls *4765*

Glutamine *Cerebrospinal Fluid* *No Effect* In 31 patients median concentration of 563.90 ± 14.05 µmol/L not significantly different from 549.27 ± 15.29 µmol/L in 30 healthy controls *4765*
Plasma *No Effect* In 37 patients median concentration of 635.13 ± 22.76 µmol/L not significantly different from 620.29 ± 20.07 µmol/L in 35 healthy controls *4765*

Glycine *Cerebrospinal Fluid* *No Effect* In 31 patients median concentration of 10.06 ± 0.61 µmol/L not significantly different from 11.70 ± 1.30 µmol/L in 30 healthy controls *4765*
Plasma *No Effect* In 37 patients median concentration of 242.89 ± 11.35 µmol/L not significantly different from 237.71 ± 13.00 µmol/L in 35 healthy controls *4765*

Histidine *Cerebrospinal Fluid* *No Effect* In 31 patients median concentration of 14.42 ± 0.66 µmol/L not significantly different from 15.13 ± 0.78 µmol/L in 30 healthy controls *4765*
Plasma *No Effect* In 37 patients median concentration of 77.42 ± 2.39 µmol/L not significantly different from 76.76 ± 2.18 µmol/L in 35 healthy controls *4765*

4-Hydroxynonenal *Cerebrospinal Fluid* *No Effect* In 13 patients with motor neuron disease mean concentration of 0.42 ± 0.17 ng/mL not significantly different from 0.51 ± 0.05 ng/mL in 236 patients with other neurological diagnoses *4909*

Insulin *Plasma* *No Effect* Mean concentration of 54 pmol/L in 8 patients with motor neuron disease not significantly different from 44 pmol/L in 8 healthy matched controls *2822*

Isoleucine *Cerebrospinal Fluid* *No Effect* In 31 patients median concentration of 5.19 ± 0.26 µmol/L not significantly different from 6.03 ± 0.82 µmol/L in 30 healthy controls *4765*
Plasma *No Effect* In 37 patients median concentration of 59.26 ± 3.35 µmol/L not significantly different from 63.26 ± 2.61 µmol/L in 35 healthy controls *4765*

Leucine *Cerebrospinal Fluid* *No Effect* In 31 patients median concentration of 13.71 ± 0.67 µmol/L not significantly different from 15.55 ± 1.34 µmol/L in 30 healthy controls *4765*
Plasma *No Effect* In 37 patients median concentration of 122.97 ± 5.62 µmol/L not significantly different from 128.03 ± 4.81 µmol/L in 35 healthy controls *4765*

Lysine *Cerebrospinal Fluid* *No Effect* In 31 patients median concentration of 28.16 ± 0.99 µmol/L not significantly different from 28.20 ± 1.35 µmol/L in 30 healthy controls *4765*
Plasma *No Effect* In 37 patients median concentration of 191.29 ± 8.31 µmol/L not significantly different from 195.97 ± 6.52 µmol/L in 35 healthy controls *4765*

Methionine *Cerebrospinal Fluid* *No Effect* In 31 patients median concentration of 2.61 ± 0.35 µmol/L not significantly different from 2.83 ± 0.46 µmol/L in 30 healthy controls *4765*
Plasma *No Effect* In 37 patients median concentration of 16.79 ± 1.64 µmol/L not significantly different from 20.21 ± 1.31 µmol/L in 35 healthy controls *4765*

Multiubiquitin Chains *Serum* *Decrease* In 29 patients with motor neuron disease mean concentration of 2.76 ± 0.975 µg/cells in 1 L blood significantly different from that in 45 healthy men and 51 healthy women in whom the mean concentration was 3.86 ± 1.55 µg/cells from 1 liter of blood *5125*

Ornithine *Cerebrospinal Fluid* *No Effect* In 31 patients median concentration of 6.26 ± 0.37 µmol/L not significantly different from 5.63 ± 0.33 µmol/L in 30 healthy controls *4765*
Plasma *No Effect* In 37 patients median concentration of 101.24 ± 6.35 µmol/L not significantly different from 89.03 ± 4.50 µmol/L in 35 healthy controls *4765*

Phenylalanine *Cerebrospinal Fluid* *No Effect* In 31 patients median concentration of 10.26 ± 0.56 µmol/L not significantly different from 10.53 ± 0.79 µmol/L in 30 healthy controls *4765*
Plasma *No Effect* In 37 patients median concentration of 61.92 ± 2.42 µmol/L not significantly different from 61.85 ± 2.00 µmol/L in 35 healthy controls *4765*

Proinsulin *Plasma* *No Effect* Mean concentration of 1.7 pmol/L in 8 patients with motor neuron disease not significantly different from 1.3 pmol/L in 8 healthy matched controls *2822*

Serine *Cerebrospinal Fluid* *No Effect* In 31 patients median concentration of 25.35 ± 0.87 µmol/L not significantly different from 27.03 ± 1.33 µmol/L in 30 healthy controls *4765*
Plasma *No Effect* In 37 patients median concentration of 113.00 ± 3.29 µmol/L not significantly different from 105.29 ± 4.07 µmol/L in 35 healthy controls *4765*

32-33 Split Proinsulin *Plasma* *Increase* Mean concentration of 5.8 pmol/L in 8 patients with motor neuron disease significantly different from 3.6 pmol/L in 8 healthy matched controls *2822*

Threonine *Cerebrospinal Fluid* *No Effect* In 31 patients median concentration of 31.67 ± 1.25 μmol/L not significantly different from 33.10 ± 2.36 μmol/L in 30 healthy controls *4765*
Plasma *No Effect* In 37 patients median concentration of 118.37 ± 4.52 μmol/L not significantly different from 121.68 ± 4.69 μmol/L in 35 healthy controls *4765*

Tryptophan *Plasma* *No Effect* In 37 patients median concentration of 49.76 ± 2.40 μmol/L not significantly different from 51.97 ± 3.62 μmol/L in 35 healthy controls *4765*

Tyrosine *Cerebrospinal Fluid* *No Effect* In 31 patients median concentration of 10.74 ± 1.00 μmol/L not significantly different from 12.27 ± 1.04 μmol/L in 30 healthy controls *4765*
Plasma *No Effect* In 37 patients median concentration of 61.18 ± 2.72 μmol/L not significantly different from 67.21 ± 2.44 μmol/L in 35 healthy controls *4765*

Ubiquitin, Free *Blood* *Decrease* In 29 patients with motor neuron disease mean concentration of 76.5 ± 38.4 μg/cells in 1 liter blood less than that in 45 healthy men and 51 healthy women in whom the mean concentration was 126 ± 24.4 μg/cells from 1 liter of blood *5125*

Valine *Cerebrospinal Fluid* *No Effect* In 31 patients median concentration of 17.13 ± 0.96 μmol/L not significantly different from 19.27 ± 1.98 μmol/L in 30 healthy controls *4765*
Plasma *No Effect* In 37 patients median concentration of 208.16 ± 6.88 μmol/L not significantly different from 219.88 ± 6.54 μmol/L in 35 healthy controls *4765*

336.00 Syringomyelia and Syringobulbia

Anti-Neutrophil Cytoplasm Antibodies *Serum* *No Effect* In 0 of 2 patients (0%) with syringomyelia pANCA detected *3722*

Antinuclear Antibodies *Serum* *No Effect* In 0 of 2 patients (0%) with syringomyelia ANA detected *3722*

Protein *Cerebrospinal Fluid* *Increase* In a minority of cases the lumbar CSF protein content is elevated in the range of 40 - 100 mg/dL *900*
Cerebrospinal Fluid *No Effect* In a minority of cases the lumbar CSF protein content is elevated in the range of 40 - 100 mg/dL *900*

336.90 Adrenomyeloneuropathy

Anti-Neutrophil Cytoplasm Antibodies *Serum* *No Effect* In 0 of 2 patients (0%) with adrenomyelopathy pANCA detected *3722*

Antinuclear Antibodies *Serum* *No Effect* In 0 of 2 patients (0%) with adrenomyelopathy ANA detected *3722*

336.90 Chronic Progressive Idiopathic Myelopathy

Cobalamin *Serum* *Increase* In 9 patients mean concentration of 618.3 ± 221.5 pg/mL and median of 592 pg/mL significantly more than mean of 445.5 ± 286.1 pg/mL and median of 381 pg/mL in 67 healthy controls *1811*

340.00 Multiple Sclerosis

Acetylcholinesterase G4 Isoenzyme *Serum* *No Effect* No significant deviation from normal observed in a small number of patients *5778*

AD7c-NTP *Cerebrospinal Fluid* *No Effect* In 41 patients with multiple sclerosis mean concentration of 1.0 ± 0.9 ng/mL not significantly different from that in 18 controls in whom mean concentration was 1.7 ± 0.7 ng/mL *1061*

Albumin *Cerebrospinal Fluid* *Decrease* 18.7% of patients had concentrations < 45% of total proteins; 7.8% had values > 65% of total proteins *2747*
Cerebrospinal Fluid *Increase* In 24 patients with relapsing-remitting multiple sclerosis mean concentration of 17 ± 8 ng/mL not significantly increased compared with 10 ng/mL in 6 healthy controls *1222* 18.7% of patients had concentrations < 45% of total proteins; 7.8% had > 65% of total proteins *2747* In 12 patients with multiple scerosis mean concentration of 311 ± 175 mg/L not significantly higher than 179 ± 53 mg/L in 5 controls *429* In 12 patients with multiple sclerosis mean concentration of 311 ± 157 mg/L not significantly higher than 179 ± 53 mg/L in 5 controls *429*
Serum *Decrease* 12.5% of 64 patients had concentrations < 45% of total protein. 10.9% had concentrations > 65% of total proteins *2747*
Serum *Increase* 12.5% of 64 patients had concentrations < 45% of total protein. 10.9% had concentrations > 65% of total proteins *2747*

Albumin Index *Cerebrospinal Fluid* *Increase* Range in 15 patients with multiple sclerosis of 2.0 - 24.2 significantly different from mean of 4.0 in 33 normal controls *3019*

Aldolase *Serum* *No Effect* Normal activities usually observed in patients with multiple sclerosis *2952*

Alkaline Phosphatase *Serum* *Increase* In 9 adult patients with multiple sclerosis mean activity of 78.0 ± 8.5 U/L significantly different from 57.4 ± 1.5 U/L in 122 healthy control adults *2006*

Alkaline Phosphatase Band-10 Isoenzyme *Serum* *No Effect* In 9 adult patients with multiple sclerosis mean activity of 5.74 ± 1.11 U/L not significantly different from 10.0 ± 0.69 U/L in 122 healthy control adults *2006*

Alkaline Phosphatase Isoenzymes *Serum* *Decrease* Preliminary studies indicate a depression of serum alkaline phosphatase of intestinal origin (serum type PP2) especially in blood group O. Comparisons were made with normal sera after matching blood groups, a factor not previously taken into account *3971*

Angiotensin-converting Enzyme *Serum* *Increase* 17 of 75 patients with multiple sclerosis had activities greater than the upper limit of 50 U/L *905*

1,5-Anhydroglucitol *Cerebrospinal Fluid* *Increase* In 7 patients with multiple sclerosis mean concentration of 44 ± 12 mg/L compared with 37.1 ± 16.5 mg/L in 6 healthy controls *4913*

Anti-Interferon-γ Autoantibodies
Cerebrospinal Fluid *Increase* Mean concentration of 3.56 ± 0.068 ng/mL in 15 patients with multiple sclerosis compared with 0.0044 ± 0.004 ng/mL in 15 healthy adults *1333*
Serum *Increase* Mean concentration of 3.92 ± 0.034 ng/mL in 15 patients with multiple sclerosis compared with 0.006 ± 0.005 ng/mL in 15 healthy adults *1333*

Anti-Interleukin-4 Autoantibodies
Cerebrospinal Fluid *Increase* Mean concentration of 0.318 ± 0.01 ng/mL in 15 patients with multiple sclerosis compared with 0.005 ± 0.001 ng/mL in 15 healthy adults *1333*
Serum *Increase* Mean concentration of 2.4 ± 0.023 ng/mL in 15 patients with multiple sclerosis compared with 0.013 ± 0.007 ng/mL in 15 healthy adults *1333*

Anti-Interleukin-10 Autoantibodies
Cerebrospinal Fluid *Increase* Mean concentration of 1.5 ± 0.023 ng/mL in 15 patients with multiple sclerosis compared with 0.0018 ± 0.001 ng/mL in 15 healthy adults *1333*
Serum *Increase* Mean concentration of 226.1 ± 0.131 ng/mL in 15 patients with multiple sclerosis compared with 0.01 ± 0.006 ng/mL in 15 healthy adults *1333*

Anti-Neutrophil Cytoplasm Antibodies *Serum* *Increase* In 3 of 58 patients (5.2%) with multiple sclerosis pANCA detected *3722*

Anti-Tumor Necrosis Factor-α Autoantibodies
Cerebrospinal Fluid *Increase* Mean concentration of 4.61 ± 0.07 ng/mL in 15 patients with multiple sclerosis compared with 0.0046 ± 0.001 ng/mL in 15 healthy adults *1333*
Serum *Increase* Mean concentration of 103.8 ± 0.024 ng/mL in 15 patients with multiple sclerosis compared with 0.0042 ± 0.004 ng/mL in 15 healthy adults *1333*

Antibody Titer *Serum* *Increase* Serum IgE and measles antibodies were increased more frequently in hypocomplementemic patients than in normal populations *5291* IgA and IgM antibodies to myelin of rabbit spinal cord. Found in 70% of patients. When IgG antimyelin antibody is present in titers greater than 1:8 it is suggestive, but not diagnostic *3712*

α_1-Antichymotrypsin *Serum* *Increase* Mean concentration increased above reference interval of 47.9 ± 8.1 mg/dL in 2 of 4 patients (50%) with multiple sclerosis *3044*

340.00 Multiple Sclerosis *(continued)*

Antinuclear Antibodies *Serum* *Increase* In 12 of 58 patients (20.7%) with multiple sclerosis ANA detected *3722*

α_2-Antiplasmin *Cerebrospinal Fluid* *No Effect* In 34 patients with multiple sclerosis mean concentration of 7.37 ± 0.31% not significantly different from 7.08 ± 0.16% in 24 reference individuals *55*
Plasma *No Effect* In 34 patients with multiple sclerosis mean concentration of 117.7 ± 4.5% not significantly different from 132 ± 3.1% in 24 reference individuals *55*

α_1-Antitrypsin *Cerebrospinal Fluid* *No Effect* In 34 patients with multiple sclerosis mean concentration of 4.95 ± 0.04% not significantly different from 5.04 ± 0.07% in 24 reference individuals *55*
Serum *No Effect* In 34 patients with multiple sclerosis mean concentration of 89.3 ± 7.3% not significantly different from 100 ± 5.3% in 24 reference individuals *55*

Carbonic Anhydrase II *Cerebrospinal Fluid* *No Effect* In 18 patients with multiple sclerosis median concentration of 14.7 µg/L not significantly different from median of 7.8 µg/L in 97 controls *4012*

Carnosinase *Serum* *Decrease* In 11 patients with multiple sclerosis mean activity of 82.5 ± 10.0 significantly different from 161 ± 7 nmol/mL/min in 16 healthy controls *5590*

Cells *Cerebrospinal Fluid* *Increase* About 50% of patients have mononuclear cells in the CSF during an acute episode in the range of 10 - 50 cells/µL *2039*

Ceruloplasmin *Serum* *Decrease* Slight elevation of serum copper with significant reduction of serum ceruloplasmin *4161*

Cholesterol *Cerebrospinal Fluid* *Increase* Raised in several neurologic diseases including multiple sclerosis *1857*

Cholesterol Esters *Cerebrospinal Fluid* *Increase* Significantly higher *1857*

Cobalamin *Serum* *Increase* In 156 patients mean concentration of 525.0 ± 292.5 pg/mL and median of 441 pg/mL significantly more than mean of 445.5 ± 286.1 pg/mL and median of 381 pg/mL in 67 healthy controls *1811*

Complement C_3 *Cerebrospinal Fluid* *No Effect* Mean concentrations in 8 patients with MS of 2.0 ± 0.6 mg/L by TR-IFMA and 3.0 ± 0.7 mg/L by EID compared with mean concentrations in 30 normal individuals of 2.4 ± 0.9 mg/L by TR-IFMA and 3.6 ± 1.0 mg/L by EID *1623*
Serum *Decrease* Mean level was slightly lower than normal *146* Hypocomplementemia (fall in factor C_3 related to a fall in total hemolytic activity) was found in 29.5% of the patients not on corticotherapy at the first assay, and in 36% of the patients when repeated assays were carried out. Hypocomplementemia is significantly more frequent in MS than in the normal population (0%) and in neurological patients (9.6%) *5291*

Complement, Total *Cerebrospinal Fluid* *Decrease* Significantly lower *2872*
Serum *Decrease* Hypocomplementemia was found in 29.5% of the patients not on corticotherapy at the first assay, and in 36% of the patients when repeated assays were carried out. Hypocomplementemia is significantly more frequent than in the normal population (0%) and in neurological patients (9.6%) *5291*

Copper *Serum* *Increase* Slight elevation of serum copper with significant reduction of serum ceruloplasmin *4161*

Dopamine β-Hydroxylase *Serum* *No Effect* No significant difference observed between concentrations in patients with multiple sclerosis and healthy controls *3301*

Erythrocytes *Blood* *Decrease* In 156 patients mean count of 4.611 ± 0.494 x 10^{12}/L and median count of 4.65 x 10^{12}/L significantly less than mean of 88.56 ± 5.17 x 10^{12}/L and median of 88.8 x 10^{12}/L in 67 healthy controls *1811*
Cerebrospinal Fluid *No Effect* In 18 patients with multiple sclerosis median concentration of 0 x 10^6/L not significantly different from median of 1 x 10^6/L in 97 controls *4012*

Fat *Feces* *Increase* Malabsorption tests were studied in 52 patients. Fat and undigested meat fibers content were found to be abnormal in 41.6 and 40.9% respectively *1920*

Fructose *Cerebrospinal Fluid* *Increase* In 7 patients with multiple sclerosis mean concentration of 31.2 ± 11.5 mg/L significantly increased compared with 7.6 ± 3.6 mg/L in 6 healthy controls *4913*

β-Galactosidase *Serum* *Decrease* In 10 patients, mean activity was 0.163 ± 0.025 U/L at pH = 4.5, normal = 0.243 ± 0.038 *2288*

α_1-Globulin *Cerebrospinal Fluid* *Increase* Concentrations > 79% of total proteins found in 10.9% of cases *2747*
Serum *Increase* 7.8% of 64 patients had concentration of 8% of total proteins *2747*

α_2-Globulin *Cerebrospinal Fluid* *Increase* Values of > 8% of total proteins found in 26.5% of patients *2747*
Serum *Increase* Concentrations > 14% of total protein occurred in 14% of patients *2747*

β-Globulin *Serum* *Increase* Concentration > 15% of total protein was observed in 9.3% of patients *2747*

γ-Globulin *Cerebrospinal Fluid* *Increase* An increase, particularly the IgG fraction, may develop. An elevation to over 15% of the total protein and an abnormal colloidal gold curve are found in more than 75% of the patients. No relationship has been drawn with degree, type or duration of disease, or any other clinical criteria *4650* 4.5-23.8% of total protein in 13 patients *4830* 79.3% of patients had concentrations > 12% of total protein. Over 50% had concentrations > 16%, and 9.5% of cases were > 30% *2747*
Serum *Increase* Increased to > 20% of total protein in 14% of 64 patients *2747*

Glucose *Cerebrospinal Fluid* *Increase* In 7 patients with multiple sclerosis mean concentration of 838 ± 204 mg/L compared with 789 ± 275 mg/L in 6 healthy controls *4913*

Glucose-6-Phosphate Dehydrogenase
Red Blood Cells *No Effect* In 20 patients with MS mean activity of 8.07 ± 2.44 U/g hemoglobin, 0.18 ± 0.04 U/U LDH not significantly different from that in 20 healthy individuals, mean activity of 7.98 ± 1.57 U/g hemoglobin, 0.18 ± 0.05 U/U LDH *2325*

Glucose Tolerance *Serum* *Decrease* Many patients have impaired carbohydrate metabolism exhibited by abnormal curves *4707*

Glutamic Acid Decarboxylase Antibodies *Serum* *No Effect* In none of 29 patients with multiple sclerosis were GAD antibodies detected *3880*

γ-Glutamyltransferase *Serum* *Increase* 6 of 33 patients had concentrations elevated above normal (40 U/L) *1400*

Glutathione Peroxidase *Red Blood Cells* *No Effect* Mean activity in 20 patients with MS of 9.85 ± 3.3 U/g hemoglobin and 0.18 ± 0.04 U/U LDH not significantly that in 20 healthy individuals, mean activity 9.01 ± 4.35 U/g hemoglobin, 0.20 ± 0.08 U/U LDH *2325*

Glutathione Reductase *Red Blood Cells* *No Effect* In 20 patients with MS mean activity of 3.95 ± 1.25 U/g hemoglobin, 0.09 ± 0.03 U/U LDH not significantly different from that in 20 healthy individuals, mean activity of 3.96 ± 1.54 U/g hemoglobin, 0.08 ± 0.02 U/U LDH *2325*

Histamine *Cerebrospinal Fluid* *No Effect* In 55 patients with multiple sclerosis mean concentration of 0.04 ± 0.08 ng/mL not significantly different from 0.04 ± 0.04 ng/mL in 39 healthy controls *4465*

HLA Antigens *Blood* *Present* HLA-DR2 present in 55% of patients versus 23% of control *5678* HLA antigen Dw2 found in 36% of patients with this disease compared to 0% of controls *4584* Increased incidence of HLA-DR2 *5428*

Homocysteine *Plasma* *Increase* Multiple sclerosis (MS) is occasionally associated with vitamin B_{12} deficiency. Recent studies have shown an increased risk of macrocytosis, low serum and/or CSF vitamin B_{12} levels, raised plasma homocysteine and raised unsaturated R-binder capacity in MS *4334*

IgG Index *Cerebrospinal Fluid* *Increase* Index increased in approximately 80% of patients with multiple sclerosis *2952* In 85% patients with multiple sclerosis IgG index increased *5486*

Immunoglobulin A *Cerebrospinal Fluid* *Increase* 35.9% of patients had CSF values > 0.6 mg/dL *2747* In patients with multiple sclerosis 27% had increased concentration of IgA *5486* Found in 5 of 45 patients *4349*
Serum *Increase* Levels > 388 mg/dL in 13.8% of 64 patients *2747*

Immunoglobulin D *Serum* *Increase* 6.4% of patients had concentrations > 29 mg/dL *2747*

Immunoglobulin E *Serum* *Decrease* Median level was slightly lower than in controls. All other serum immunoglobulins were normal *146*

Serum *Increase* Serum IgE and measles antibodies were increased more frequently in hypocomplementemic patients than in normal populations *5291*

Immunoglobulin G *Cerebrospinal Fluid* *Increase* Total IgG is often increased > 15 mg/dL in CSF in all forms of multiple sclerosis *2039* In 62% of cases *4349* Increased due to intrathecal synthesis not blood:CSF barrier damage *2288* In one study all patients with multiple sclerosis had increased concentrations *5486* Concentrations > 4 mg/dL in 77.7% of patients *2747* In patients with multiple sclerosis 83% had increased concentration *5486* In 12 patients with multiple sclerosis mean concentration of 62 ± 40 mg/L not significantly higher than 21 ± 4.6 mg/L in 5 controls *429*
Serum *Increase* Levels > 1,871 mg/dL in 12.3% of 64 patients *2747*

Immunoglobulin M *Cerebrospinal Fluid* *Increase* In one study all patients with multiple sclerosis had increased concentrations *5486* In 33% patients with multiple sclerosis concentration increased *5486* Detected in CSF samples from 26.9% of patients *2747*
Serum *Increase* Levels > 161 mg/dL in 7.8% of cases; 3.1% had values 34 mg/dL *2747*

Inositol *Cerebrospinal Fluid* *No Effect* In 7 patients with multiple sclerosis mean concentration of 49 ± 11 mg/L compared with 54 ± 12 mg/L in 6 healthy controls *4913*

Interferon-γ *Serum* *Increase* In 21 patients with multiple sclerosis mean concentration of 971 ± 520 pg/mL significantly higher than 113 ± 91 pg/mL in 12 healthy controls *2206*

Interleukin-1 *Cerebrospinal Fluid* *No Effect* In 31 cases of MS no IL-1α (or IL-1β) was detected *5309*
Serum *Increase* Increased levels of TNF were also detected in 35.5% of the MS sera, and especially in those with acute relapsing MS in exacerbation *5309*
Serum *No Effect* In 31 cases of MS no IL-1α (or IL-1β) was detected *5309* Serum levels of the cytokines interleukin-1α (IL-1α), IL-1β, were measured in chronic progressive multiple sclerosis patients (CPMS) and normal, inflammatory, and noninflammatory disease controls. No significance in statistical group analyses *5288*

Interleukin-2 *Serum* *Increase* In patients with active disease significantly increased concentration observed. Initial concentration varied inversely with the duration of the disease and predicted subsequent worsening in chronic progressive patients *5289* Measured in chronic progressive multiple sclerosis patients (CPMS) and normal, inflammatory, and noninflammatory disease controls. Serum IL-2 levels displayed the most consistent abnormalities in the group of tests for the CPMS group, and were the only cytokine levels to achieve significance in statistical group analyses. However, several patients with CPMS had normal serum IL-2 levels *5288*

Interleukin-4 *Serum* *Increase* In 21 patients with multiple sclerosis mean concentration of 452 ± 297 pg/mL significantly higher than 97 ± 35 pg/mL in 12 healthy controls *2206*
Serum *No Effect* Measured in chronic progressive multiple sclerosis patients (CPMS) and normal, inflammatory, and noninflammatory disease controls. No significance in statistical group analyses *5288*

Interleukin-6 *Cerebrospinal Fluid* *Increase* The upper limit of IL-6 levels in the CSF of normal controls was 6.5 pg/mL. A significant elevation of IL-6 levels was observed in the CSF of patients with MS (131 ± 307 pg/mL) ($p < 0.05$) *4800*
Serum *Increase* Significant elevations of IL-6 levels were observed in the sera of patients with multiple sclerosis (MS) (212 ± 320 pg/mL) when compared to those of controls ($p < 0.05$) *4800* Levels were measured in cerebrospinal fluid (CSF) and plasma of patients with multiple sclerosis (MS), acute meningo-encephalitis (AM) and muscular tension headache (TH). MS patients had in repeated samples higher levels of IL-6 in plasma compared to patients with AM and TH *1567*
Serum *No Effect* No significance in statistical group analyses *5288*

Interleukin-10 *Serum* *Increase* In 21 patients with multiple sclerosis mean concentration of 965 ± 1,040 pg/mL significantly not higher than 706 ± 236 pg/mL in 12 healthy controls *2206*

α-Ketoglutarate *Serum* *Increase* High concentrations noted in these patients imply a defect in carbohydrate metabolism *4707*

Lactate *Blood* *Increase* High concentrations noted in these patients imply a defect in carbohydrate metabolism *4707*

Leukocytes *Cerebrospinal Fluid* *Increase* A pleocytosis of usually not more than 25 mononuclear cells/μL can be found *900*
Cerebrospinal Fluid *No Effect* In 18 patients with multiple sclerosis median concentration of 4 - 5 x 10^6/L not significantly different from median of 1 x 10^6/L in 97 controls *4012*

Lipoprotein Lp(a) *Cerebrospinal Fluid* *Decrease* Mean concentration in 39 patients with multiple sclerosis of 63 ± 9 μg/L not significantly less than 70 ± 16 μg/L in 24 individuals free of neurological and inflammatory disease and dyslipoproteinemia *1624*
Serum *No Effect* Mean concentration in 39 patients with multiple sclerosis of 0.23 ± 0.20 g/L not significantly different from 0.24 ± 0.19 g/L in 24 individuals free of neurological and inflammatory disease and dyslipoproteinemia *1624*

Lymphocytes *Blood* *Decrease* In 19 different groups of neurological diseases, absolute and relative T-lymphocyte populations were significantly decreased only in patients with acute Guillain-Barre Syndrome, active multiple sclerosis and malignant cerebral tumor *5679*
Cerebrospinal Fluid *Increase* Significant increase in T-lymphocytes *2544*

α_2-Macroglobulin *Cerebrospinal Fluid* *No Effect* Concentration normal in all age groups *4641* In 34 patients with multiple sclerosis mean concentration of 0.42 ± 0.01% not significantly different from 0.44 ± 0.01% in 24 reference individuals *55*
Serum *No Effect* In 34 patients with multiple sclerosis mean concentration of 90.4 ± 4.2% not significantly different from 100 ± 2.1% in 24 reference individuals *55*

Mannose *Cerebrospinal Fluid* *Increase* In 7 patients with multiple sclerosis mean concentration of 12 ± 8 mg/L compared with 8.5 ± 5.5 mg/L in 6 healthy controls *4913*

MCV *Blood* *Increase* In 156 patients mean concentration of 90.34 ± 5.06 fL and median of 90.3 fL significantly more than mean of 88.56 ± 5.17 fL and median of 88.8 fL in 67 healthy controls *1811*

Methylhistamine *Cerebrospinal Fluid* *No Effect* In 55 patients with multiple sclerosis mean concentration of 0.19 ± 0.17 ng/mL not significantly different from 0.30 ± 0.53 ng/mL in 39 healthy controls *4465*

β_2-Microglobulin *Cerebrospinal Fluid* *Increase* In 148 patients with multiple sclerosis mean concentration of 2.13 mg/L compared with 1.01 mg/L in control patients *5421*

Monoamine Oxidase *Platelets* *No Effect* No significant difference observed between concentrations in patients with multiple sclerosis and healthy controls *3301*

Monocytes *Cerebrospinal Fluid* *Increase* CSF shows a slight increase in mononuclear cells and normal or slightly increased protein (50% of cases) *5544*

Multiubiquitin Chains *Serum* *Decrease* In 10 patients with multiple sclerosis mean concentration of 2.57 ± 0.740 μg/cells in 1 L blood significantly different from that in 45 healthy men and 51 healthy women in whom the mean concentration was 3.86 ± 1.55 μg/cells from 1 liter of blood *5125*

Myelin Basic Protein *Cerebrospinal Fluid* *Increase* Increased concentration associated with demyelinating disorders *2952*

Neopterin *Urine* *Increase* Mean excretion of 187 μmol/mol creatinine in 10 patients with primary progressive disease and 187 μmol/mol creatinine in 10 patients with relapsing remitting disease greater than 134 μ/mol observed in 14 healthy controls *1739*

Nerve Growth Factor *Cerebrospinal Fluid* *Increase* Concentration increased (mean 8.8 pg/mL) in one patient with multiple sclerosis *5091*

Neuron-specific Enolase *Serum* *No Effect* In 21 patients with multiple sclerosis all concentrations were less than 14.45 μg/L compared with 8.11 ± 3.17 μg/L in 35 control individuals *983*

Neuropeptide Y *Cerebrospinal Fluid* *Decrease* In 10 patients mean concentration of 43.5 ± 24.0 pg/mL significantly less than 87.5 ± 40.3 pg/mL in 11 controls aged less 60 years *3201*

Oligoclonal Banding *Cerebrospinal Fluid* *Increase* Observed in 11 patients with clinical evidence of multiple sclerosis *77* Oligoclonal IgG bands detected *3261*

340.00 **Multiple Sclerosis** *(continued)*

Phospholipids *Cerebrospinal Fluid Increase* Raised in patients with high total CSF proteins but lowered in chronic multiple sclerosis *5268*
Serum Decrease Particularly in patients with evidence of recent progression *1790*

Plasmin *Cerebrospinal Fluid No Effect* In 34 patients with multiple sclerosis mean concentration undetectable not significantly different from undetectable in 24 reference individuals *55*
Plasma No Effect In 34 patients with multiple sclerosis mean concentration undetectable not significantly different from undetectable in 24 reference individuals *55*

Plasmin-α_2Antiplasmin Complex
Cerebrospinal Fluid Increase In 34 patients with multiple sclerosis mean concentration of 58 ± 7.5 ng/mL significantly different from 29 ± 8 ng/mL in 24 reference individuals *55*
Plasma Increase In 34 patients with multiple sclerosis mean concentration of 628 ± 60 ng/mL not significantly different from 574 ± 70 ng/mL in 24 reference individuals *55*

Plasminogen *Cerebrospinal Fluid Increase* In 34 patients with multiple sclerosis mean concentration of 0.40 ± 0.03% significantly different from 0.67 ± 0.12% in 24 reference individuals *55*
Plasma Increase In 34 patients with multiple sclerosis mean concentration of 146 ± 4% not significantly different from 134 ± 8% in 24 reference individuals *55*

Plasminogen Activator Inhibitor-1
Cerebrospinal Fluid Increase In 19 patients with multiple sclerosis mean concentration of 0.65 ± 0.05 ng/mL significantly different from 0.31 ± 0.06 ng/mL in 20 reference individuals *56* In 19 patients with multiple sclerosis mean concentration of 0.65 ± 0.1 ng/mL significantly different from 0.31 ± 0.1 ng/mL in 20 reference individuals *57*
Plasma Increase In 8 patients with multiple sclerosis mean concentration of 11.3 ± 2.4 ng/mL significantly different from 4.5 ± 0.7 ng/mL in 9 reference individuals *57*

Protein *Cerebrospinal Fluid Increase* Increased total protein and IgG concentration *5138* A slight increase in mononuclear cells and normal or slightly increased protein (50% of cases). Diagnosis is probable if more than 20% is γ-globulin *5544* In all forms of MS approximately 70% of patients have abnormalities of CSF proteins *2039*
Cerebrospinal Fluid No Effect In 18 patients with multiple sclerosis median concentration of 385 mg/L not significantly different from median of 400 mg/L in 97 controls *4012* Mean concentration in postmortem ventricular CSF in 15 patients of 66.6 ± 11.6 mg/dL not significantly different from 60.9 ± 5.8 mg/dL in 16 normal controls *5435*

Prothrombin *Cerebrospinal Fluid No Effect* Mean concentration of 0.40 mg/L in 4 patients with multiple sclerosis not significantly different from 0.55 mg/L in 18 normal control patients *3018*
Plasma No Effect Mean concentration of 122.1 mg/L in 4 patients with multiple sclerosis not significantly different from 121.8 mg/L in 18 normal control patients *3018*

Pyruvate *Blood Increase* High concentrations noted in these patients imply a defect in carbohydrate metabolism *4707* Raised levels have been reported in some cases. The cause for this has not been discovered *1290*

Ribitol *Cerebrospinal Fluid No Effect* In 7 patients with multiple sclerosis mean concentration of 2.6 ± 3.8 mg/L compared with 3.4 ± 2.0 mg/L in 6 healthy controls *4913*

Soluble CD95 *Serum Increase* Mean concentration in 71 patients with relapsing-remitting multiple sclerosis of 194 ± 45 U/mL significantly increased compared with 87 ± 15 U/mL in 66 healthy controls *5870*

Soluble E-Selectin *Cerebrospinal Fluid Increase* In 22 patients with multiple sclerosis mean concentration of 0.07 ± 0.03 ng/mL significantly different from 0.04 ± 0.03 ng/mL in 6 healthy controls *1222*
Serum Increase In 56 patients with multiple sclerosis mean concentration of 10.3 ± 9 ng/mL significantly different from 7.4 ± 8 ng/mL in 33 healthy controls *1222*
Serum No Effect In 18 patients with active MS mean concentration of 34.8 ± 11.2 ng/mL not significantly different from 30.2 ± 12.8 ng/mL in 11 patients with stable MS and 28.9 ± 8.8 ng/mL in 10 normal controls *4351*

Soluble Endothelial Leukocyte Adhesion Molecule
Cerebrospinal Fluid Increase In 22 patients with relapsing-remitting multiple sclerosis mean concentration of serum endothelial leukocyte adhesion molecule of 0.07 ± 0.03 ng/mL significantly different from 0.04 ± 0.01 ng/mL in 6 healthy controls *1222*
Serum Increase In 35 patients with relapsing-remitting multiple sclerosis mean concentration of serum endothelial leukocyte adhesion molecule of 10.3 ± 9 ng/mL significantly different from 7.4 ± 8 ng/mL in 24 healthy controls *1222*

Soluble Intercellular Adhesion Molecule-1
Cerebrospinal Fluid Increase Range in 15 patients with multiple sclerosis of 1.2 - 7.2 ng/mL significantly different from mean of 1.51 ng/mL in 33 normal controls *3019*
Cerebrospinal Fluid No Effect In 10 patients with relapsing-remitting multiple sclerosis mean concentration of < 8.0 ng/mL significantly increased compared with < 8.0 ng/mL in 5 healthy controls *1222*
Serum Increase In 18 patients with active MS mean concentration of 502 ± 218 ng/mL significantly higher than 225 ± 82 ng/mL in 11 patients with stable MS and 218 ± 68 ng/mL in 10 normal controls *4351* In 56 patients with multiple sclerosis mean concentration of 239 ± 138 ng/mL significantly increased compared with 146 ± 41 ng/mL in 33 healthy controls *1222*
Serum No Effect Range in 15 patients with multiple sclerosis of 153.9 - 467.4 ng/mL not significantly different from mean of 285.1 ng/mL in 33 normal controls *3019*

Soluble Interleukin-2 Receptor *Serum Increase* Concentration significantly increased in chronic progressive MS but concentration normalizes when patients treated with steroids *282*

Soluble Vascular Cell Adhesion Molecule-1
Cerebrospinal Fluid Increase In 22 patients with relapsing-remitting multiple sclerosis mean concentration of 6 ± 3 ng/mL significantly different from 1.1 ± 0.7 ng/mL in 6 healthy controls *1222*
Serum No Effect In 56 patients with multiple sclerosis mean concentration of 406 ± 130 ng/mL not significantly different from 428 ± 84 ng/mL in 33 healthy controls *1222* In 35 patients with relapsing-remitting multiple sclerosis mean concentration of 406 ± 130 ng/mL not significantly different from 428 ± 84 ng/mL in 24 healthy controls *1222*

Somatostatin *Cerebrospinal Fluid Decrease* In 10 patients mean concentration of 5.5 ± 2.5 pg/mL significantly less than 38.8 ± 12.3 pg/mL in 11 controls less 60 years *3201*

Sorbitol *Cerebrospinal Fluid Increase* In 7 patients with multiple sclerosis mean concentration of sorbitol (glucitol) of 9.4 ± 3.2 mg/L compared with 4.8 ± 3.0 mg/L in 6 healthy controls *4913*

Superoxide Dismutase *Red Blood Cells Decrease* The study included 34 patients aged 19 to 54 years. The control group comprised 64 healthy subjects. A significant reduction was found of SOD-1 activity in the erythrocytes of patients which may suggest a lower enzymatic defense mechanism against oxidative stress *5834*
Red Blood Cells Increase The activities were higher than those of normal healthy individuals *2540*

Tissue Plasminogen Activator *Cerebrospinal Fluid Increase* In 19 patients with multiple sclerosis mean concentration of 360 ± 24 mIU/mL significantly different from 43.7 ± 6 mIU/mL in 20 reference individuals *57*
Plasma No Effect In 8 patients with multiple sclerosis mean concentration of 19.1 ± 5.9 mIU/mL not significantly different from 23.6 ± 8 mIU/mL in 9 reference individuals *57*

β-Trace Protein *Cerebrospinal Fluid No Effect* In 14 patients with multiple sclerosis mean concentration of 17.9 ± 4.3 mg/L not significantly different from 16.6 ± 3.6 mg/L in 27 normal controls *5323*

Transforming Growth Factor-β_1 *Cerebrospinal Fluid Increase* Mean concentration in postmortem ventricular CSF in 15 patients of 54.2 ± 8.0 pg/mL significantly different from 23.7 ± 4.6 pg/mL in 16 normal controls *5435*

Transforming Growth Factor-β_2 *Cerebrospinal Fluid Increase* Mean concentration in postmortem ventricular CSF in 15 patients of 244.5 ± 39.3 pg/mL not significantly different from 80.6 ± 21.9 pg/mL in 16 normal controls *5435*

Tryptase *Cerebrospinal Fluid Increase* In 55 patients with multiple sclerosis mean concentration of 0.74 ± 0.62 ng/mL significantly different from 0.40 ± 0.39 ng/mL in 39 healthy controls *4465*

Tumor Necrosis Factor-α *Cerebrospinal Fluid* *Increase* Concentrations correlated in patients with active, progressive disease and high concentrations were predictive of poor outcome *4757* In 31 patients, TNF was detected in 29 (93.5%) of CSF from 31 cases of MS. TNF was also detectable in 100% of CSF from patients with acute relapsing MS in exacerbation. Patients with acute relapsing MS in exacerbation showed significantly higher CSF levels of TNF as compared with either those in remission or the controls (p less than 0.001 and p less than 0.0001, respectively) *5309*
Serum *Increase* In patients with active multiple sclerosis concentration significantly higher than in patients with inactive MS or in controls *4757* In 21 patients with multiple sclerosis mean concentration of 362 ± 235 pg/mL significantly higher than 161 ± 69 pg/mL in 12 healthy controls *2206*
Serum *No Effect* Measured in chronic progressive multiple sclerosis patients (CPMS) and normal, inflammatory, and noninflammatory disease controls. No significance in statistical group analyses *5288*

Tumor Necrosis Factor Receptor p60 *Serum* *Increase* In 18 patients with active MS mean concentration of 1.5 ± 0.6 ng/mL significantly lower than 2.3 ± 0.5 ng/mL in 11 patients with stable MS and 1.9 ± 0.4 ng/mL in 10 normal controls *4351*

Ubiquitin, Free *Blood* *No Effect* In 10 patients with multiple sclerosis mean concentration of 86.6 ± 36.8 μg/cells in 1 L blood not significantly different from that in 45 healthy men and 51 healthy women in whom the mean concentration was 126 ± 24.4 μg/cells from 1 liter of blood *5125*

Uric Acid *Cerebrospinal Fluid* *Decrease* Very low CSF levels of 0.02 - 0.04 mg/dL, with normal serum levels found in the chronic stage of disease *2892*
Serum *No Effect* Very low CSF levels of 0.02 - 0.04 mg/dL, with normal serum levels found in the chronic stage of disease *2892*

Urokinase *Cerebrospinal Fluid* *Increase* In 19 patients with multiple sclerosis mean concentration of 5.6 ± 1.6 mIU/mL significantly different from < 0.01 mIU/mL in 20 reference individuals *57*
Plasma *Increase* In 8 patients with multiple sclerosis mean concentration of 19.2 ± 6.7 mIU/mL significantly different from < 0.01 mIU/mL in 9 reference individuals *57*

Vitamin B_{12} *Cerebrospinal Fluid* *Decrease* Multiple sclerosis (MS) is occasionally associated with vitamin B_{12} deficiency. Recent studies have shown an increased risk of macrocytosis, low serum and/or CSF vitamin B_{12} levels, raised plasma homocysteine and raised unsaturated R-binder capacity in MS *4334*
Feces *Increase* Malabsorption of vitamin B_{12} was found in 11.9% of 52 patients *1920*
Serum *Decrease* Malabsorption of vitamin B_{12} was found in 11.9% of 52 patients *1920*

341.90 Demyelinating Disease

Creatine Kinase *Cerebrospinal Fluid* *Increase* Of 11 patients with demyelinating disease, 7 had increases above upper limit of normal of 10 U/L *4780*

343.90 Cerebral Palsy

Antithrombin III *Plasma* *No Effect* In 31 children with cerebral palsy mean concentration of 22.0 ± 7.6 mg/dL not significantly different from 20.6 ± 5.0 mg/dL in 65 control children *3756*

Calcitonin Gene-related Peptide *Serum* *Increase* In 31 children with cerebral palsy mean concentration of 29.2 ± 32.5 pg/mL significantly different from 12.7 ± 8.9 pg/mL in 65 control children *3756*

Complement C_1 *Serum* *Decrease* In 31 children with cerebral palsy mean concentration of 143.0 ± 24.9 μg/mL significantly different from 156.9 ± 23.1 μg/mL in 65 control children *3756*

Complement C_1 Inhibitor *Serum* *No Effect* In 31 children with cerebral palsy mean concentration of 16.2 ± 7.1 mg/dL not significantly different from 13.7 ± 4.3 mg/dL in 65 control children *3756*

Complement C_2 *Serum* *Decrease* In 31 children with cerebral palsy mean concentration of 25.6 ± 4.4 μg/mL significantly different from 28.4 ± 4.7 μg/mL in 65 control children *3756*

Complement C_3 *Serum* *Decrease* In 31 children with cerebral palsy mean concentration of 1,067.6 ± 499.1 μg/mL significantly different from 1,562.8 ± 434.5 μg/mL in 65 control children *3756*

Complement C_3b Inhibitor *Serum* *Increase* In 31 children with cerebral palsy mean concentration of 14.4 ± 6.0 mg/dL significantly different from 10.9 ± 4.3 mg/dL in 65 control children *3756*

Complement C_4 *Serum* *Decrease* In 31 children with cerebral palsy mean concentration of 310.5 ± 170.6 μg/mL significantly different from 447.3 ± 136.4 μg/mL in 65 control children *3756*

Complement C_5 *Serum* *No Effect* In 31 children with cerebral palsy mean concentration of 79.7 ± 3.8 μg/mL not significantly different from 76.2 ± 8.3 μg/mL in 65 control children *3756*

Complement C_6 *Serum* *No Effect* In 31 children with cerebral palsy mean concentration of 69.6 ± 4.9 μg/mL not significantly different from 67.1 ± 7.1 μg/mL in 65 control children *3756*

Complement C_7 *Serum* *No Effect* In 31 children with cerebral palsy mean concentration of 65.9 ± 7.4 μg/mL not significantly different from 66.7 ± 9.1 μg/mL in 65 control children *3756*

Complement C_8 *Serum* *Increase* In 31 children with cerebral palsy mean concentration of 67.3 ± 9.6 μg/mL significantly different from 58.0 ± 11.7 μg/mL in 65 control children *3756*

Complement C_9 *Serum* *Decrease* In 31 children with cerebral palsy mean concentration of 126.0 ± 45.7 μg/mL significantly different from 155.6 ± 46.9 μg/mL in 65 control children *3756*

Factor V Leiden Mutation Product *Plasma* *No Effect* In 31 children with cerebral palsy mean concentration of 7.7 ± 5.3 μg/mL not significantly different from 5.6 ± 2.8 μg/mL in 65 control children *3756*

Granulocyte Colony Stimulating Factor *Serum* *Increase* In 31 children with cerebral palsy mean concentration of 31.3 ± 24.5 pg/mL significantly different from 8.7 ± 4.7 pg/mL in 65 control children *3756*

Granulocyte-Macrophage Colony Stimulating Factor *Serum* *Increase* In 31 children with cerebral palsy mean concentration of 23.4 ± 18.7 pg/mL significantly different from 9.6 ± 4.1 pg/mL in 65 control children *3756*

Immunoglobulin A *Serum* *Decrease* In 31 children with cerebral palsy mean concentration of 199.6 ± 25.8 mg/dL significantly different from 236.9 ± 37.1 mg/dL in 65 control children *3756*

Immunoglobulin E *Serum* *No Effect* In 31 children with cerebral palsy mean concentration of 89.6 ± 68.4 IU/mL not significantly different from 103.8 ± 81.5 IU/mL in 65 control children *3756*

Immunoglobulin G *Serum* *Decrease* In 31 children with cerebral palsy mean concentration of 808.7 ± 114.8 mg/dL significantly different from 1,268.7 ± 286.3 mg/dL in 65 control children *3756*

Immunoglobulin M *Serum* *Decrease* In 31 children with cerebral palsy mean concentration of 79.6 ± 9.9 mg/dL significantly different from 130.7 ± 33.2 mg/dL in 65 control children *3756*

Interleukin-1 *Serum* *Increase* In 31 children with cerebral palsy mean concentration of 56.6 ± 50.5 pg/mL significantly different from 10.3 ± 3.9 pg/mL in 65 control children *3756*

Interleukin-2 *Serum* *Decrease* In 31 children with cerebral palsy mean concentration of 23.7 ± 6.9 pg/mL significantly different from 28.4 ± 4.4 pg/mL in 65 control children *3756*

Interleukin-3 *Serum* *Decrease* In 31 children with cerebral palsy mean concentration of 18.4 ± 6.3 pg/mL significantly different from 24.1 ± 4.5 pg/mL in 65 control children *3756*

Interleukin-4 *Serum* *No Effect* In 31 children with cerebral palsy mean concentration of 15.9 ± 4.5 pg/mL not significantly different from 14.6 ± 3.0 pg/mL in 65 control children *3756*

Interleukin-5 *Serum* *No Effect* In 31 children with cerebral palsy mean concentration of 14.6 ± 4.4 pg/mL not significantly different from 15.7 ± 4.0 pg/mL in 65 control children *3756*

Interleukin-6 *Serum* *Increase* In 31 children with cerebral palsy mean concentration of 54.3 ± 49.1 pg/mL significantly different from 13.1 ± 4.2 pg/mL in 65 control children *3756*

343.90 Cerebral Palsy *(continued)*

Interleukin-7 *Serum* *Increase* In 31 children with cerebral palsy mean concentration of 12.1 ± 2.9 pg/mL significantly different from 8.7 ± 2.7 pg/mL in 65 control children *3756*

Interleukin-8 *Serum* *Increase* In 31 children with cerebral palsy mean concentration of 35.8 ± 20.9 pg/mL significantly different from 6.2 ± 2.5 pg/mL in 65 control children *3756*

Interleukin-9 *Serum* *Increase* In 31 children with cerebral palsy mean concentration of 17.1 ± 5.4 pg/mL significantly different from 4.1 ± 1.7 pg/mL in 65 control children *3756*

Interleukin-10 *Serum* *No Effect* In 31 children with cerebral palsy mean concentration of 17.8 ± 5.3 pg/mL not significantly different from 16.7 ± 2.9 pg/mL in 65 control children *3756*

Interleukin-11 *Serum* *Increase* In 31 children with cerebral palsy mean concentration of 17.5 ± 5.7 pg/mL significantly different from 5.5 ± 2.7 pg/mL in 65 control children *3756*

Interleukin-12 *Serum* *Increase* In 31 children with cerebral palsy mean concentration of 19.3 ± 6.5 pg/mL significantly different from 9.1 ± 3.7 pg/mL in 65 control children *3756*

Interleukin-13 *Serum* *Increase* In 31 children with cerebral palsy mean concentration of 31.2 ± 17.5 pg/mL significantly different from 6.1 ± 3.6 pg/mL in 65 control children *3756*

Macrophage Colony Stimulating Factor *Serum* *Increase* In 31 children with cerebral palsy mean concentration of 29.3 ± 29.7 ng/mL significantly different from 9.3 ± 4.7 ng/mL in 65 control children *3756*

Macrophage Inflammatory Protein-1α *Serum* *Increase* In 31 children with cerebral palsy mean concentration of 35.5 ± 34.7 pg/mL significantly different from 5.2 ± 2.1 pg/mL in 65 control children *3756*

Macrophage Inflammatory Protein-1β *Serum* *Increase* In 31 children with cerebral palsy mean concentration of 45.9 ± 49.8 pg/mL significantly different from 4.6 ± 1.8 pg/mL in 65 control children *3756*

Macrophage Inflammatory Protein-2 *Serum* *Increase* In 31 children with cerebral palsy mean concentration of 37.4 ± 34.2 pg/mL significantly different from 4.7 ± 1.7 pg/mL in 65 control children *3756*

Monocyte Chemotactic Protein-1 *Serum* *Increase* In 31 children with cerebral palsy mean concentration of 37.5 ± 39.1 pg/mL significantly different from 5.1 ± 2.1 pg/mL in 65 control children *3756*

Monocyte Chemotactic Protein-2 *Serum* *Increase* In 31 children with cerebral palsy mean concentration of 34.4 ± 32.8 pg/mL significantly different from 5.5 ± 2.1 pg/mL in 65 control children *3756*

Properdin *Plasma* *Increase* In 31 children with cerebral palsy mean concentration of 31.7 ± 20.7 mg/dL significantly different from 13.8 ± 4.9 mg/dL in 65 control children *3756*

Protein C *Plasma* *Increase* In 31 children with cerebral palsy mean concentration of 1.1 ± 0.3% significantly different from 0.7 ± 0.3% in 65 control children *3756*

Protein S *Plasma* *Increase* In 31 children with cerebral palsy mean concentration of 1.1 ± 0.3% significantly different from 0.8 ± 0.2% in 65 control children *3756*

RANTES *Serum* *Increase* In 31 children with cerebral palsy mean concentration of 32.2 ± 29.3 ng/mL significantly different from 5.4 ± 2.1 ng/mL in 65 control children *3756*

Substance P *Plasma* *Increase* In 31 children with cerebral palsy mean concentration of 46.8 ± 53.8 pg/mL significantly different from 14.8 ± 7.0 pg/mL in 65 control children *3756*

Thyroid Stimulating Hormone *Serum* *Increase* In 31 children with cerebral palsy mean concentration of 26.1 ± 17.6 mU/mL significantly different from 8.1 ± 2.2 mU/mL in 65 control children *3756*

Thyroxine (T4) *Serum* *No Effect* In 31 children with cerebral palsy mean concentration of 12.9 ± 10.0 µg/dL not significantly different from 9.8 ± 3.7 µg/dL in 65 control children *3756*

Thyroxine (T4), Free *Serum* *No Effect* In 31 children with cerebral palsy mean concentration of 4.3 ± 3.9 µg/dL not significantly different from 4.6 ± 3.0 µg/dL in 65 control children *3756*

Transforming Growth Factor-β *Serum* *Increase* In 31 children with cerebral palsy mean concentration of 29.9 ± 31.9 pg/mL significantly different from 10.3 ± 5.0 pg/mL in 65 control children *3756*

Tri-iodothyronine (T3) *Serum* *No Effect* In 31 children with cerebral palsy mean concentration of 20.7 ± 9.2 mg/dL not significantly different from 25.2 ± 3.6 mg/dL in 65 control children *3756*

Tumor Necrosis Factor-α *Serum* *Increase* In 31 children with cerebral palsy mean concentration of 58.4 ± 47.7 pg/mL significantly different from 11.2 ± 2.6 pg/mL in 65 control children *3756*

Vasoactive Intestinal Polypeptide *Plasma* *Increase* In 31 children with cerebral palsy mean concentration of 24.9 ± 36.0 pg/mL significantly different from 9.9 ± 6.2 pg/mL in 65 control children *3756*

344.00 Quadriplegia

Cholesterol *Serum* *Decrease* In 21 quadriplegic men aged 24 to 47 years significantly lower concentration than in 20 age-matched healthy control men *4786*
Serum *No Effect* Mean concentration of 185 ± 4 mg/dL in 94 quadriplegic patients *5856*

Glucose *Serum* *No Effect* Mean peak concentration of 188 ± 5 mg/dL in 94 quadriplegic patients *5856*

HDL_2-Cholesterol *Serum* *Decrease* In 21 quadriplegic men significantly lower concentration observed than in 20 age-matched control men *4786*

HDL_3-Cholesterol *Serum* *Decrease* In 21 quadriplegic men aged 24 to 47 years concentration significant lower than in 20 age-matched control men *4786*

HDL-Cholesterol *Serum* *Decrease* In 21 quadriplegic men aged 24 to 47 years significantly lower concentration observed than in 20 healthy control men *4786*
Serum *No Effect* Mean concentration of 39 ± 1 mg/dL in 94 quadriplegic patients *5856*

Insulin *Plasma* *No Effect* Mean peak concentration of 175 ± 14 µU/mL in 94 quadriplegic patients *5856*

LDL-Cholesterol *Serum* *No Effect* Mean concentration of 123 ± 4 mg/dL in 94 quadriplegic patients *5856*

Melatonin *Plasma* *Decrease* In quadriplegics mean concentration at 07:00 h of 26 pg/mL significantly less than 54 pg/mL in healthy controls: at 01:00 h concentrations of 30 pg/mL and 105 pg/mL respectively. In paraplegics concentrations intermediate between those of quadriplegics and healthy controls *5412*

Nucleotide Pyrophosphohydrolase, Soluble
Serum *No Effect* Mean activity in 12 patients with quadriplegia or paraplegia of 1,192 ± 81 pmol nitrophenol/h/mL not significantly different from that in 85 healthy individuals 1,141 ± 22 pmol nitrophenol/h/mL *691*

Triglycerides *Serum* *No Effect* Mean concentration of 114 ± 8 mg/dL in 94 quadriplegic patients *5856*

Uric Acid *Serum* *No Effect* Mean concentration of 5.8 ± 0.2 mg/dL in 94 quadriplegic patients *5856*

344.10 Paraplegia

Cholesterol *Serum* *No Effect* Mean concentration of 191 ± 4 mg/dL in 103 paraplegic patients *5856*

Estradiol *Plasma* *No Effect* No significant difference observed between concentrations in 30 male paraplegics aged 20 - 47 years and healthy male controls *4080*

Follicle Stimulating Hormone *Plasma* *No Effect* No significant difference observed between concentrations in 30 paraplegic men and healthy male volunteer controls *4080*

Glucose *Serum* *No Effect* Mean peak concentration of 184 ± 6 mg/dL in 103 paraplegic patients *5856*

HDL-Cholesterol *Serum* *No Effect* Mean concentration of 39 ± 1 mg/dL in 103 paraplegic patients *5856*

Insulin *Plasma* *No Effect* Mean peak concentration of 143 ± 13 µU/mL in 103 paraplegic patients *5856*

LDL-Cholesterol *Serum* *No Effect* Mean concentration of 125 ± 3 mg/dL in 103 paraplegic patients *5856*

Luteinizing Hormone *Plasma* *Increase* In 30 male paraplegics aged 20 - 47 years mean concentration significantly higher than in intact male volunteers of the same age *4080*

Nucleotide Pyrophosphohydrolase, Soluble *Serum* *No Effect* Mean activity in 12 patients with quadriplegia or paraplegia of 1,192 ± 81 pmol nitrophenol/h/mL not significantly different from that in 85 healthy individuals 1,141 ± 22 pmol nitrophenol/h/mL *691*

Osteocalcin *Serum* *Increase* Significantly increased in patients with spinal cord injury ($p < 0.02$) *4132*

Prolactin *Plasma* *No Effect* No significant difference observed between concentrations in 30 paraplegic men aged 20 - 47 years and healthy male volunteer controls *4080*

Testosterone *Serum* *Increase* Mean concentration significantly higher in 30 male paraplegic patients aged 20 - 47 years than among intact male volunteers of the same age *4080*

Triglycerides *Serum* *No Effect* Mean concentration of 130 ± 9 mg/dL in 103 paraplegic patients *5856*

Uric Acid *Serum* *No Effect* Mean concentration of 5.4 ± 0.2 mg/dL in 103 paraplegic patients *5856*

344.90 Spastic Paraparesis

Anti-Neutrophil Cytoplasm Antibodies *Serum* *No Effect* In 0 of 3 patients (0%) with spastic parararesis pANCA detected *3722*

Antinuclear Antibodies *Serum* *No Effect* In 0 of 3 patients (0%) with spastic parararesis ANA detected *3722*

345.30 Status Epilepticus

Prolactin *Plasma* *No Effect* In 15 patients with status epilepticus concentration unaffected by seizures *5249*

345.60 Infantile Spasm

Aspartic Acid *Cerebrospinal Fluid* *Increase* Mean concentration in 13 children aged 4 - 38 months 968 ± 416 nmol/L significantly different from 426 ± 272 nmol/L in comparable control group *2333*

Glutamic Acid *Cerebrospinal Fluid* *No Effect* Mean concentration in 13 children aged 4 - 38 months of 966 ± 395 nmol/L not significantly different from 1135 ± 594 nmol/L in comparable control group *2333*

345.90 Epilepsy

Acylcarnitine *Serum* *No Effect* Mean concentration of 9.29 ± 5.81 µg/mL in 17 epileptic children before treatment not significantly different from 6.30 ± 2.50 µg/mL in 71 healthy control children *735*

Adenosine Monophosphate *Cerebrospinal Fluid* *Increase* CSF concentration was measured in 62 neurological patients, 46 of whom were epileptics and 16 with CNS damage. In epileptic patients the CSF concentration was significantly elevated for 3 days after an attack when compared with those free from attacks for at least 2 weeks *3693*

Alanine *Cerebrospinal Fluid* *Increase* In 25 patients with epilepsy mean concentration of 53.7 ± 23 (no units given) in postictal state following generalized tonic-clonic seizures not significantly different from 73.8 ± 20 (no units given) in 11 healthy controls *1136*

Albumin *Cerebrospinal Fluid* *Decrease* Slightly decreased in CSF of patients with grand mal epilepsy *3590*

Amino Acids *Urine* *Increase* Transient rise due to disturbed renal function during grand mal seizure *4707*

γ-Aminobutyric Acid *Cerebrospinal Fluid* *Increase* In 25 patients with epilepsy mean concentration of 8.8 ± 4.2 (no units given) in postictal state following generalized tonic-clonic seizures not significantly different from 9.4 ± 2.0 (no units given) in 11 healthy controls *1136*

Androgen Index, Free (FAI) *Plasma* *No Effect* In 11 untreated epileptic patients mean concentration of 98.3 ± 47.4 not significantly increased compared with 86.5 ± 21.8 in 18 control subjects *2361*

α_1-Antichymotrypsin *Cerebrospinal Fluid* *No Effect* Increased in patients with meningitis or mild hemorrhage, but equal to normal in patients with encephalitis, epilepsy, degenerative disorders or diseases of the CNS *187*
Serum *No Effect* Mean concentration within reference interval of 47.9 ± 8.1 mg/dL in one examined patient with epilepsy *3044*

Aspartic Acid *Cerebrospinal Fluid* *No Effect* In 25 patients with epilepsy mean concentration of 9.8 ± 2.5 (no units given) in postictal state following generalized tonic-clonic seizures not significantly different from 9.8 ± 2.2 (no units given) in 11 healthy controls *1136*

Atrial Natriuretic Peptide *Cerebrospinal Fluid* *Increase* In 25 patients with epilepsy mean concentration of 2,903 ± 716 (no units given) in postictal state following generalized tonic-clonic seizures not significantly different from 1,994 ± 383 (no units given) in 11 healthy controls *1136*

Basophils *Blood* *No Effect* In 12 children with atopic asthma mean concentration of 0.04 x 10^9/L compared with 0.05 x 10^9/L in 9 control children *2825*

Calcium *Cerebrospinal Fluid* *No Effect* Normal concentrations usually observed *234*
Serum *Decrease* Up to 33% of epileptic children on long-term anticonvulsant therapy *1290*
Serum *Increase* High in cases of idiopathic grand mal epilepsy. CSF calcium remained normal. This increase in serum calcium may be due to hyperparathyroidism because of low magnesium concentration *234*

Carbonic Anhydrase II *Cerebrospinal Fluid* *Increase* In 17 patients with epilepsy median concentration of 20.3 µg/L not significantly different from median of 7.8 µg/L in 97 controls *4012*

Carnitine *Serum* *Decrease* Mean concentration of 44.2 ± 5.75 µg/mL in 17 epileptic children before treatment significantly different from 55.37 ± 9.40 µg/mL in 71 healthy control children *735*

Carnitine, Free *Serum* *Decrease* Mean concentration of 34.35 ± 8.46 µg/mL in 17 epileptic children before treatment significantly different from 49.00 ± 5.92 µg/mL in 71 healthy control children *735*

Carnosinase *Serum* *No Effect* In 23 patients with idiopathic epilepsy mean activity of 148 ± 11 nmol/mL/min not significantly different from 161 ± 7 nmol/mL/min in 16 healthy controls *5590*

Ceruloplasmin *Cerebrospinal Fluid* *Decrease* Slightly decreased in grand mal epilepsy *3590*
Serum *Increase* Slightly elevated (62.30 ± 6.62 mg/dL) in patients with grand mal epilepsy *3590*

Cholecystokinin *Cerebrospinal Fluid* *Increase* In 25 patients with epilepsy mean concentration of 177 ± 74 (no units given) in postictal state following generalized tonic-clonic seizures not significantly different from 160 ± 33 (no units given) in 11 healthy controls *1136*

Copper *Serum* *Increase* Hypercupricemia observed in some epileptics prior to treatment *5174*
Serum *No Effect* In 12 untreated female epileptics mean concentration of 106 ± 19 µg/dL not significantly different from 98 ± 17 µg/dL in 20 healthy controls *3091*

Copper Zinc Superoxide Dismutase *Serum* *No Effect* In 12 untreated female epileptics mean activity of 122 ± 47 U/dL not significantly different from 97 ± 36 U/dL in 20 healthy controls *3091*

Corticotropin *Cerebrospinal Fluid* *Decrease* In 25 patients with epilepsy mean concentration of 721 ± 199 (no units given) in postictal state following generalized tonic-clonic seizures not significantly different from 990 ± 139 (no units given) in 11 healthy controls *1136*

Corticotropin-releasing Hormone
Cerebrospinal Fluid *Decrease* In 25 patients with epilepsy mean concentration of 80.7 ± 36 (no units given) in postictal state following generalized tonic-clonic seizures not significantly different from 157 ± 38 (no units given) in 11 healthy controls *1136*

Cortisol *Cerebrospinal Fluid* *Decrease* In 25 patients with epilepsy mean concentration of 0.49 ± 0.09 (no units given) in postictal state following generalized tonic-clonic seizures not significantly different from 0.81 ± 0.13 (no units given) in 11 healthy controls *1136*

345.90 Epilepsy *(continued)*

C-Reactive Protein *Serum* *Increase* In 12 children with atopic asthma mean concentration of 6.0 mg/L compared with < 5.0 mg/L in 9 control children *2825*

Creatine Kinase *Cerebrospinal Fluid* *Increase* In 43 patients, 14 had increases above upper limit of normal of 10 U/L *4780*
Serum *Increase* Increases in necrosis or acute atrophy of striated muscle in status epilepticus *5544* In 50% of 10 patients hospitalized for this disorder *1576* Especially after status epilepticus *1290*

Creatine Kinase MB-Isoenzyme *Serum* *Increase* With seizures *768*

β-Endorphin *Cerebrospinal Fluid* *Decrease* In 25 patients with epilepsy mean concentration of 267 ± 57 (no units given) in postictal state following generalized tonic-clonic seizures not significantly different from 617 ± 153 (no units given) in 11 healthy controls *1136*

Eosinophil Cationic Protein *Serum* *Increase* In 12 children with atopic asthma mean concentration of 37.0 µg/L significantly increased compared with 14.8 µg/L in 9 control children *2825*

Eosinophils *Blood* *Increase* In 12 children with atopic asthma mean concentration of 0.34 x 10^9/L compared with 0.14 x 10^9/L in 9 control children *2825*

Erythrocytes *Cerebrospinal Fluid* *No Effect* In 17 patients with epilepsy median concentration of 2 x10^6/L not significantly different from median of 1 x 10^6/L in 97 controls *4012*

Folate *Red Blood Cells* *Decrease* In about 25% epileptic patients concentration as measured with Corning Magic Lite method below lower limit of reference interval (271.8 - 973.95 nmol/L) *3477*
Serum *Decrease* Reduced in 33 of 68 institutionalized patients with severe epilepsy *1040* In about 25% patients concentration as measured by Corning Magic Lite method below lower limit of reference interval (7.61 - 25.0 nmol/L) *3477*

Glutamic Acid *Cerebrospinal Fluid* *Increase* In 25 patients with epilepsy mean concentration of 145 ± 34 (no units given) in postictal state following generalized tonic-clonic seizures not significantly different from 110 ± 16 (no units given) in 11 healthy controls *1136*

Glutamic Acid Decarboxylase Antibodies *Serum* *No Effect* In none of 36 patients with epilepsy were GAD antibodies detected *3880*

γ-Glutamyltransferase *Serum* *Increase* Elevated in the sera of 64 of 75 patients (85.4%) with epilepsy. Enzyme activity usually remains at a constant level, characteristic of the patients, with some peaks and depressions in activity *1400*

Glutathione, Reduced *Plasma* *No Effect* In 12 untreated female epileptics mean concentration of 30 ± 6 µmol/L not significantly different from 32 ± 6 µmol/L in 20 healthy controls *3091*

Glycine *Cerebrospinal Fluid* *Increase* In 25 patients with epilepsy mean concentration of 125 ± 41 (no units given) in postictal state following generalized tonic-clonic seizures not significantly different from 90.0 ± 20.3 (no units given) in 11 healthy controls *1136*

Immunoglobulin A *Cerebrospinal Fluid* *Decrease* Slightly decreased in grand mal epilepsy *3590*

Immunoglobulin E *Serum* *Increase* In 12 children with atopic asthma mean concentration of 238 kU/L compared with 23 kU/L in 9 control children *2825*

Immunoglobulin G *Cerebrospinal Fluid* *Decrease* Absolute concentration and percent of total CSF protein were low *5138* Slightly decreased in grand mal epilepsy *3590*

Iron-binding Capacity, Total *Serum* *Decrease* Mean concentration was 123.66 ± 8.31 µg/dL in grand mal epileptic patients *3590*

Leukocytes *Cerebrospinal Fluid* *No Effect* In 17 patients with epilepsy median concentration of 1 x10^6/L not significantly different from median of 1 x 10^6/L in 97 controls *4012*

Magnesium *Cerebrospinal Fluid* *Decrease* In idiopathic grand mal epilepsy the concentrations both in serum and CSF were significantly low just after the seizure *234*
Serum *Decrease* In idiopathic grand mal epilepsy the concentrations both in serum and CSF were significantly low just after the seizure. During interseizure period (more than 24 h) the levels increased both in the serum and CSF but in serum it still remained significantly low *234*

Malondialdehyde *Serum* *No Effect* In 12 untreated female epileptics mean concentration of 1.7 ± 0.7 µmol/L not significantly different from 1.8 ± 0.6 µmol/L in 20 healthy controls *3091*

Met-Enkephalin *Cerebrospinal Fluid* *Increase* In 25 patients with epilepsy mean concentration of 1,155 ± 146 (no units given) in postictal state following generalized tonic-clonic seizures not significantly different from 710 ± 111 (no units given) in 11 healthy controls *1136*

Myeloperoxidase *Serum* *Increase* In 12 children with atopic asthma mean concentration of 633.9 µg/L compared with 345.5 µg/L in 9 control children *2825*

Nerve Growth Factor *Cerebrospinal Fluid* *No Effect* Mean concentration in 6 pediatric patients with epilepsy of 7.6 ± 3.1 pg/mL compared with 10.0 ± 8.1 pg/mL in 24 control children with unrelated diseases *2921*

Neuron-specific Enolase *Serum* *Increase* In two patients with nonconvulsive status epilepticus concentration increased to about 16 ng/mLcompared with upper limit of normal of about 1 ng/mL *4255*

Neuropeptide Y *Cerebrospinal Fluid* *Increase* In 25 patients with epilepsy mean concentration of 162 ± 42 (no units given) in postictal state following generalized tonic-clonic seizures not significantly different from 103 ± 25 (no units given) in 11 healthy controls *1136*

Neurotensin *Cerebrospinal Fluid* *Increase* In 25 patients with epilepsy mean concentration of 247 ± 67 (no units given) in postictal state following generalized tonic-clonic seizures not significantly different from 155 ± 30 (no units given) in 11 healthy controls *1136*

Prealbumin *Cerebrospinal Fluid* *Increase* Only protein to increase in CSF of epileptics. Mean concentration was 1.50 ± 0.11 mg/dL *3590*

Prolactin *Cerebrospinal Fluid* *Increase* In 25 patients with epilepsy mean concentration of 11.9 ± 5.4 (no units given) in postictal state following generalized tonic-clonic seizures not significantly different from 7.84 ± 2.6 (no units given) in 11 healthy controls *1136*
Plasma *Increase* In three men with treatment-resistant complex-partial and/or grand mal seizures of frontal lobe origin prolactin concentration increased by over 700 /µU/mL following seizures *331*

Protein *Cerebrospinal Fluid* *Increase* In 17 patients with epilepsy median concentration of 470 mg/L not significantly different from median of 400 mg/L in 97 controls *4012*

Pyridoxine *Serum* *Decrease* Has been noted in epilepsy *4707*

Sex-Hormone Binding Globulin *Serum* *No Effect* In 11 untreated epileptic patients mean concentration of 28.0 ± 9.3 nmol/L compared with 26.9 ± 8.2 nmol/L in 18 control subjects *2361*

Somatostatin *Cerebrospinal Fluid* *No Effect* In 25 patients with epilepsy mean concentration of 22.2 ± 9.4 (no units given) in postictal state following generalized tonic-clonic seizures not significantly different from 24.6 ± 2.5 (no units given) in 11 healthy controls *1136*

Taurine *Cerebrospinal Fluid* *Increase* In 25 patients with epilepsy mean concentration of 139 ± 49 (no units given) in postictal state following generalized tonic-clonic seizures not significantly different from 167 ± 28 (no units given) in 11 healthy controls *1136*

Testosterone *Serum* *No Effect* In 11 untreated epileptic patients mean concentration of 24.6 ± 6.6 nmol/L compared with 23.2 ± 8.3 nmol/L in 18 control subjects *2361*

Vasoactive Inhibitory Peptide *Cerebrospinal Fluid* *No Effect* In 25 patients with epilepsy mean concentration of 316 ± 67.6 (no units given) in postictal state following generalized tonic-clonic seizures not significantly different from 277 ± 31 (no units given) in 11 healthy controls *1136*

Xanthurenic Acid *Urine* *Increase* Has been noted in epilepsy *4707*

Zinc *Serum* *No Effect* In 12 untreated female epileptics mean concentration of 88 ± 15 µg/dL not significantly different from 87 ± 12 µg/dL in 20 healthy controls *3091*

346.20 Cluster Headaches

β-Endorphin *White Blood Cells* *Decrease* Concentration decreased in patients with cluster headache *633*

Interleukin-1 *Serum* *Increase* In 24 episodic cluster headache (CH) patients and 45 normal controls using a specific ELISA method, there was an increase in IL-1β in all CH patients compared to controls. IL-1β was further increased during the ictal phase of CH compared to patients between attacks and normal individuals. Between attacks, IL-1β was also significantly increased compared to controls *3308*

346.90 Migraine

Adenosine *Plasma* *Increase* In 10 patients with migraine, during attacks mean concentration of 330 ± 189 nmol/L significantly different from 195 ± 128 nmol/L between attacks and 198 ± 78 nmol/L in 8 healthy controls *1908*
Plasma *No Effect* In 10 patients with migraine between attacks mean concentration of 195 ± 128 nmol/L not significantly different from 198 ± 78 nmol/L in 8 healthy controls *1908*

Anticardiolipin Antibodies *Serum* *Increase* Studied the prevalence of lupus anticoagulant, anticardiolipin antibodies (aCL) and various hemostatic parameters in 71 patients with migraine and compared the results with a control group of 32 subjects with back pain never having experienced migraine. No difference in aCL positivity was noted between migrainous patients and controls and between common migraine and complicated migraine patients *5298*
Serum *No Effect* No difference was noted between migrainous patients and controls and between common migraine and complicated migraine patients *5298*

Corticotropin *Plasma* *No Effect* Plasma cortisol and adrenocorticotropic hormone responses were similar to those found with experimentally-induced pain in normal subjects, i.e. elevated cortisol and unchanged adrenocorticotropic hormone levels *5403*

Cortisol *Plasma* *Increase* Plasma cortisol and adrenocorticotropic hormone responses were similar to those found to experimentally-induced pain in normal subjects, i.e. elevated cortisol and unchanged adrenocorticotropic hormone levels *5403*

Creatine Kinase *Cerebrospinal Fluid* *No Effect* Of 5 patients with migraine 0 had increases above upper limit of normal of 10 U/L *4780*

Dopamine *Plasma* *Decrease* Significant decrease observed during migraine attacks *2955*

β-Endorphin *Cerebrospinal Fluid* *Decrease* Closely correlated with severity of disease. Decreased significantly in patients with common migraine (38.5 fmol/mL) compared with healthy controls (86.1 fmol/mL) *1689*

Endothelin-1 *Plasma* *Increase* The mean ET-1 values were elevated in all migraine patients above the range of normal subjects, and were 10.6 (range of 6.0 - 16.0) pg/mL in migraine patients and 3.8 (range of 0.7 - 5.8) pg/mL in controls *1423*

Epinephrine *Plasma* *Increase* Significant increase observed during migraine attacks *2955*

Epinephrine:Norepinephrine Ratio *Plasma* *Increase* Significant increase in ratio observed during migraine attacks *2955*

Histamine *Plasma* *Increase* Levels are increased during acute attacks *2035*
White Blood Cells *Increase* Mean spontaneous histamine release was increased 33.7% compared to controls *4729*

5-Hydroxyindoleacetic Acid *Urine* *Increase* Levels are increased during acute attacks *2035*

5-Hydroxytryptamine *Platelets* *Decrease* Marked decrease observed at the onset of migraine attacks *2955*

5-Hydroxytryptamine, Free *Plasma* *Increase* Significant increase observed during migraine attacks *2955* Significant increase observed at the onset of migraine attacks *2955*

Interleukin-1 *Serum* *No Effect* No evidence of systemic rise of cytokines found during migraine attacks *5403*

Interleukin-2 *Serum* *Decrease* Thirteen subjects suffering from migraine without aura (5 males and 8 females, mean age: 32.8 years). Forty-three normal healthy volunteers composed the control group (15 males and 28 females, average age 41.6 years). The IL-2 levels of sera were 3.18 ± 1.8 U/mL (mean ± SD) in the healthy controls, 2.29 ± 2.6 U/mL in the patients with migraine. The serum level of IL-2 in the patients with migraine was significantly lower than in the controls *4806*

β-Lipoprotein *Cerebrospinal Fluid* *Decrease* Significantly lower ($p < 0.005$) *1689*

Met-Enkephalin *Plasma* *Increase* In migraine patients, either during an attack or when pain-free, significantly higher platelet-rich and platelet-poor plasma methionine-enkephalin than healthy race and sex-matched and age comparable controls *3630*

Monoamine Oxidase *Platelets* *Decrease* Significantly reduced when compared with normal patients *688*
Platelets *Increase* Platelet levels are increased during acute attacks *2035*

Norepinephrine *Plasma* *Decrease* Decrease observed at the onset of migraine attacks *2955*
Plasma *Increase* Increase observed during migraine attacks *2955* Levels are increased during acute attacks *2035*

Platelet Aggregation response to ADP *Blood* *Increase* Increased response observed during migraine attacks, possibly attributable to stress *2955*

Platelet Aggregation response to Epinephrine *Blood* *Increase* Increased response to catecholamines observed during migraine attacks, possibly attributable to stress *2955*

Platelet Aggregation response to Serotonin *Blood* *Increase* Increased response observed during migraine attacks, possibly attributable to stress *2955*

Platelets *Blood* *Increase* Increased number but depleted of their serotonin concentration *2035*

Thromboxane B_2 *Plasma* *Decrease* The patients ability to produce thromboxane B_2 was reduced in both children and adults with migraine *2619*

Tumor Necrosis Factor-α *Serum* *No Effect* No evidence of systemic rise of cytokines during migraine attacks *5403*

Vanillylmandelic Acid *Urine* *Increase* Increased excretion observed during migraine attacks *2955* Levels are increased during acute attacks *2035*

347.00 Narcolepsy

Interleukin-1β *Serum* *Decrease* Mean concentration of 0.50 ± 0.23 pg/mL (detected in 72.7% patients) in 11 patients with narcolepsy not significantly different from 0.60 ± 0.29 pg/mL (detected in 50.0% individuals) in 10 healthy controls *5463*

Interleukin-6 *Serum* *Increase* Mean concentration of 1.72 ± 0.58 pg/mL in 11 patients with narcolepsy not significantly different from 1.02 ± 0.42 pg/mL in 10 healthy controls *5463*

Tumor Necrosis Factor-α *Serum* *Increase* Mean concentration of 2.09 ± 0.25 pg/mL in 11 patients with narcolepsy significantly different from 1.17 ± 0.10 pg/mL in 10 healthy controls *5463*

348.10 Hypoxic Ischemic Encephalopathy

Interleukin-6 *Cerebrospinal Fluid* *Increase* In 6 neonates with stage 3 hypoxic ischemic encephalopathy concentrations ranged from 65 - 2,250 pg/mL compared with < 2 pg/mL in 12 neonates with stage 0 - 2 disease *3316*

348.30 West Syndrome

Corticotropin *Cerebrospinal Fluid* *Increase* In 3 patients with cryptogenic West syndrome mean concentration of 17 ± 4.4 pg/mL *2098*

β-Endorphin *Cerebrospinal Fluid* *Increase* In 3 patients with cryptogenic West syndrome mean concentration of 69 ± 22 pg/mL *2098*

348.30 West Syndrome *(continued)*

Nerve Growth Factor *Cerebrospinal Fluid Decrease* In 22 children with noninfectious etiology of disease mean concentration of 0.77 ng/mL compared with 6.29 ± 1.14 pg/mL in controls *4360*
Cerebrospinal Fluid No Effect In 6 children with cryptogenic etiology of disease mean concentration of 6.3 ± 0.9 ng/mL compared with 6.29 ± 1.14 pg/mL in controls *4360*

348.90 Cerebrovascular Disease

Erythropoietin *Cerebrospinal Fluid Increase* In 10 patients with old cerebrovascular disease, mean concentration of 1.80 ± 0.32 mIU/mL significantly different from 0.98 ± 0.26 mIU/mL in 15 healthy control individuals *3715*
Serum No Effect In 10 patients with old cerebrovascular disease mean concentration not significantly different from that in 15 healthy control individuals *3715*

349.89 Nonimmune Neurological Disease

4-Hydroxynonenal *Cerebrospinal Fluid No Effect* In 92 patients with nonimmune neurological disease mean concentration of 0.41 ± 0.06 ng/mL not significantly different from 0.51 ± 0.05 ng/mL in 236 patients with other neurological diagnoses *4909*

Soluble Intercellular Adhesion Molecule-1 *Serum No Effect* In 40 patients with non-immune neurological disorders mean concentration of 285.1 ± 115.6 ng/mL not significantly different from that in 26 healthy laboratory workers, mean concentration of 268.0 ± 70.9 ng/mL *2092*

349.90 Immune Neurological Disease

4-Hydroxynonenal *Cerebrospinal Fluid No Effect* In 64 patients with immune neurological disease mean concentration of 0.60 ± 0.12 ng/mL not significantly different from 0.51 ± 0.05 ng/mL in 236 patients with other neurological diagnoses *4909*

350.10 Trigeminal Neuralgia

Carbonic Anhydrase II *Cerebrospinal Fluid Increase* In 6 patients with trigeminal neuralgia median concentration of 44.0 µg/L significantly different from median of 7.8 µg/L in 97 controls *4012*

Catecholamines *Plasma Increase* Significant increase observed in patients with trigeminal neuralgia during relapse, normalizing during remission periods *2955*

Cortisol *Plasma Increase* Significant increase observed in patients with trigeminal neuralgia during relapse, normalizing during remission periods *2955*

Erythrocytes *Cerebrospinal Fluid No Effect* In 6 patients with trigeminal neuralgia median concentration of 3 x 10^6/L not significantly different from median of 1 x 10^6/L in 97 controls *4012*

5-Hydroxytryptamine, Free *Plasma Increase* Significant increase observed in patients with trigeminal neuralgia during relapse, normalizing during remission periods *2955*

Leukocytes *Cerebrospinal Fluid No Effect* In 6 patients with trigeminal neuralgia median concentration of 1 x 10^6/L not significantly different from median of 1 x 10^6/L in 97 controls *4012*

Platelet Aggregation *Blood Increase* Significant increase observed in patients with trigeminal neuralgia during relapse, normalizing during remission periods *2955*

Protein *Cerebrospinal Fluid Increase* In 6 patients with trigeminal neuralgia median concentration of 484 mg/L not significantly different from median of 400 mg/L in 97 controls *4012*

356.30 Refsum's Disease

Cells *Cerebrospinal Fluid No Effect* High CSF protein concentration in the absence of pleocytosis has been found in all cases *4979*

Phytanic Acid *Serum Increase* Patients with untreated Refsum's disease usually have concentrations exceeding 250 mg/L *4738* Concentration of > 0.5% strongly suggests Refsum's disease *2952*

Protein *Cerebrospinal Fluid Increase* Elevated in 20 patients, ranging from 55 - 732 mg/dL. Mean concentration of 275 mg/dL, and mode of 165 mg/dL *1790* High CSF protein concentration in the absence of pleocytosis has been found in all cases *4979*

356.90 Chronic Inflammatory Demyelinating Polyneuropathy

4-Hydroxynonenal *Cerebrospinal Fluid Increase* In 19 patients with Guillain-Barre syndrome or chronic inflammatory demyelinating polyneuropathy mean concentration of 1.49 ± 0.25 ng/mL not significantly different from that in patients with amyotrophic lateral sclerosis but significantly different from 0.51 ± 0.05 ng/mL in 236 patients with other neurological diagnoses *4909*

356.90 Peripheral Neuropathy

Albumin *Cerebrospinal Fluid Increase* In 8 patients with peripheral neuropathy mean concentration of 426 ± 308 mg/L not significantly higher than 179 ± 53 mg/L in 5 controls *429*

Fibronectin *Plasma Increase* In 13 patients with peripheral neuropathies significant increase in concentration observed *1712*

Immunoglobulin G *Cerebrospinal Fluid Increase* In 8 patients with peripheral neuropathy mean concentration of 78 ± 69 mg/L not significantly higher than 21 ± 4.6 mg/L in 5 controls *429*

Protein *Cerebrospinal Fluid Increase* In 10 patients with peripheral neuropathy mean concentration of 0.89 ± 0.46 g/L not significantly higher than 0.21 ± 0.06 g/L in 7 controls *429*

356.90 Polyneuropathy

Creatine Kinase *Cerebrospinal Fluid Increase* Of 6 patients with neuropathy 3 had increases above upper limit of normal of 10 U/L *4780*

Glutamic Acid Decarboxylase Antibodies *Serum No Effect* In none of 17 patients with polyneuropathy were GAD antibodies detected *3880*

Soluble HLA-I *Cerebrospinal Fluid No Effect* In 2 patients with polyneuropathy, mean concentration undetectable in all *216*

Soluble HLA-II *Cerebrospinal Fluid No Effect* In 2 patients with polyneuropathy, mean concentration undetectable in both *216*

357.00 Fisher-Evans Syndrome

Antithyroid Antibodies *Serum Increase* Antithyroid antibodies observed in 5 (25.0%) of 20 patients with Fisher-Evans syndrome *3080*

Thyroid Stimulating Hormone *Serum Increase* Increased concentration observed in 4 (20.0%) of 20 patients with Fisher-Evans syndrome *3080*

357.00 Guillain-Barre Syndrome

Acetylcholinesterase G4 Isoenzyme *Serum No Effect* No significant deviation from normal observed in a small number of patients *5778*

Albumin *Cerebrospinal Fluid Increase* Usually elevated between 65 and 1000 mg/dL but may not peak until four to six weeks after onset of neurologic signs. Elevation may persist for several months. Elevation is primarily albumin *2784* IgG and Albumin increased probably result from blood/CSF barrier damage *2288*

Albumin Index *Cerebrospinal Fluid Increase* Range in 8 patients with Guillain-Barre syndrome of 11.7 - 55.1 significantly different from mean of 4.0 in 33 normal controls *3019*

Amyloid β-Protein *Cerebrospinal Fluid No Effect* In 2 patients with Guillain-Barre syndrome concentrations were 5.72 and 2.13 pmol/mL not significantly different from mean concentration of 4.00 ± 2.92 pmol/mL *3716*

Amyloid β-Protein Precursor *Cerebrospinal Fluid Increase* In 2 patients with Guillain-Barre syndrome concentrations were 2.40 and 2.84 integrated OD units significantly different from mean concentration of 1.35 ± 0.38 integrated OD units in 25 normal controls *3716*

Anti-Neutrophil Cytoplasm Antibodies *Serum No Effect* In 0 of 4 patients (0%) with Guillain-Barre syndrome pANCA detected *3722*

α_1-Antichymotrypsin *Cerebrospinal Fluid Increase* In 2 patients with Guillain-Barre syndrome concentrations were 7.70 and 9.60 μg/mL significantly different from mean concentration of 2.27 ± 1.40 μg/mL in 25 normal controls *3716*

Antinuclear Antibodies *Serum No Effect* In 0 of 4 patients (0%) with Guillain-Barre syndrome ANA detected *3722*

Bicarbonate *Serum Increase* Respiratory acidosis may occur *1980*

Calprotectin *Plasma Increase* In 6 patients mean concentration of 6,957 μg/L significantly higher than normal range of 80 - 880 μg/L in women and 150 - 910 μg/L in men *2169*

Carbon Dioxide Partial Pressure *Blood Increase* Respiratory acidosis may occur *1980*

Cells *Cerebrospinal Fluid No Effect* In 2 patients with Guillain-Barre syndrome concentrations of 2.3 and 3.0 cells/μL not significantly different from normal of 3 cells/μL *3716* Characteristic findings are elevated protein concentration but no increase in number of cells in CSF *367*

Complement-fixing Antibodies *Serum Increase* 30 patients (33%) had markedly elevated levels of complement-fixing antibody to cytomegalovirus and in 21, a 4-fold or more alteration in titer was demonstrated *1232*

Complement, Total *Cerebrospinal Fluid Increase* Oligoclonal IgG bands, specific elevation of IgM and complement activation products have been reported during the acute phase of the disease *2784*

Cortisol *Plasma Increase* In 15 patients with Guillain-Barre syndrome on admission to hospital concentrations were above neurological control values of 162.8 ± 19.3 ng/mL in 7 of 15 patients on admission *960*

Erythrocyte Sedimentation Rate *Blood Increase* Moderately elevated *1790*

β-Galactosidase *Serum Decrease* In 10 patients, mean activity was 0.163 ± 0.025 mmol/min at pH = 4.5, normal = 0.243 ± 0.038 *2288*

Helicobacter pylori IgA Antibodies *Serum Increase* Four of 7 patients with GBS had antibodies *814*

4-Hydroxynonenal *Cerebrospinal Fluid Increase* In 19 patients with Guillain-Barre syndrome or chronic inflammatory demyelinating polyneuropathy mean concentration of 1.49 ± 0.25 ng/mL not significantly different from that in patients with amyotrophic lateral sclerosis but significantly different from 0.51 ± 0.05 ng/mL in 236 patients with other neurological diagnoses *4909*

Immunoglobulin A *Cerebrospinal Fluid Increase* Early in disease *1790*

Immunoglobulin G *Cerebrospinal Fluid Increase* IgG and albumin increased, probably resulting from blood: CSF barrier damage *2288* Oligoclonal IgG bands, specific elevation of IgM and complement activation products have been reported during the acute phase of the disease *2784*

Immunoglobulin M *Cerebrospinal Fluid Increase* Oligoclonal IgG bands, specific elevation of IgM and complement activation products have been reported during the acute phase of the disease *2784*

Interferon-γ *Serum Increase* In 14 patients with Guillain-Barre syndrome mean concentration of 1,081 ± 362 pg/mL significantly higher than 113 ± 91 pg/mL in 12 healthy controls *2206*

Interleukin-1β *Serum Increase* In 15 patients with Guillain-Barre syndrome on admission to hospital, IL-1β was detected in one patient *960*

Interleukin-4 *Serum Increase* In 15 patients with Guillain-Barre syndrome on admission to hospital IL-4 detected in two patients *960* In 14 patients with Guillain-Barre Syndrome mean concentration of 345 ± 156 pg/mL significantly higher than 97 ± 35 pg/mL in 12 healthy controls *2206*

Interleukin-6 *Cerebrospinal Fluid No Effect* The upper limit of IL-6 levels in the CSF of normal controls was 6.5 pg/mL. No significant elevation of IL-6 levels was observed in the CSF of patients with GBS *4800*
Serum Increase Significant elevations of IL-6 levels were observed in the sera of patients with Guillain-Barre syndrome (GBS) (90 ± 62 pg/mL), when compared to those of controls ($p < 0.05$) *4800* In 15 patients with Guillain-Barre syndrome on admission to hospital IL-6 detected in five patients *960*

Interleukin-7 *Serum No Effect* In 15 patients with Guillain-Barre syndrome on admission to hospital IL-7 not detected in any *960*

Interleukin-10 *Serum Increase* In 15 patients with Guillain-Barre syndrome on admission to hospital IL-10 detected in two patients *960* In 14 patients with Guillain-Barre Syndrome mean concentration of 1,040 ± 895 pg/mL not significantly higher than 706 ± 236 pg/mL in 12 healthy controls *2206*

Leukocytes *Blood Increase* A moderate polymorphonuclear leukocytosis *1790*
Cerebrospinal Fluid No Effect Normal cell count; usually below 10 monocytes /μL. The presence of more than 50 mononuclear cells /μL or the presence of any polymorphonuclear cells should suggest another disease *2784*

Lymphocytes *Blood Decrease* During active phase of disease *1790* In 19 different groups of neurological diseases, absolute and relative T-lymphocyte populations were significantly decreased only in patients with acute Guillain-Barre Syndrome, active multiple sclerosis and malignant cerebral tumor *5679*
Cerebrospinal Fluid Increase While it is true most cases show few, if any, lymphocytes, a few show up to 20 - 30 cells/μL *1790*

α_1-Microglobulin *Cerebrospinal Fluid Increase* Of 3 patients with Guillain-Barre syndrome mean concentration in none exceeded that in 15 healthy controls of 34.8 ± 16.0 μg/L *2370*

Neuron-specific Enolase *Serum No Effect* In 4 patients with Guillain-Barre syndrome concentrations ranged from 3.8 - 6.4 μg/L compared with 8.11 ± 3.17 μg/L in 35 control individuals *983*

Neuropeptide Y *Cerebrospinal Fluid Decrease* In 8 patients mean concentration of 65.0 ± 13.5 pg/mL not significantly less than 87.5 ± 40.3 pg/mL in 11 controls less than 60 years *3201*

Neutrophils *Blood Increase* A moderate polymorphonuclear leukocytosis *1790*

pH *Blood Decrease* Respiratory acidosis may occur *1980*

Protein *Cerebrospinal Fluid Increase* Increased total protein (1.21 ± 0.274 g/L) *2288* May reach as high as 2 g/dL *1790* CSF shows albuminocytologic dissociation with normal cell count and increased protein (average, 50 - 100 mg/dL). Protein increase parallels increasing clinical severity; may be prolonged *5544* Usually elevated between 65 and 1,000 mg/dL but may not peak until 4 to 6 weeks after onset of neurological sign. Elevation may persist for several months. Primarily albumin contributing to the increased concentration *2784* In 2 patients with Guillain-Barre syndrome concentrations 60 and 102 mg/dL significantly different from normal mean of 29 mg/dL *3716*

Soluble E-Selectin *Serum Increase* Mean concentration of 59 ± 23 ng/mL in 17 patients with GBS in the acute stage significantly higher than 30 ± 9 ng/mL in 12 healthy control individuals *3885*

Soluble Intercellular Adhesion Molecule-1
Cerebrospinal Fluid Increase Range in 8 patients with Guillain-Barre syndrome of 2.8 - 9.2 ng/mL significantly different from mean of 1.51 ng/mL in 33 normal controls *3019*
Serum No Effect Range in 8 patients with Guillain-Barre syndrome of 179.6 - 507.9 ng/mL not significantly different from mean of 285.1 ng/mL in 33 normal controls *3019*

Somatostatin *Cerebrospinal Fluid Decrease* In 8 patients mean concentration of 10.8 ± 6.1 pg/mL significantly less than 38.8 ± 12.3 pg/mL in 11 controls less 60 years *3201*

β-Trace Protein *Cerebrospinal Fluid No Effect* In 13 patients with Guillain-Barre syndrome mean concentration of 16.1 ± 6.2 mg/L not significantly different from 16.6 ± 3.6 mg/L in 27 normal controls *5323*

357.00 Guillain-Barre Syndrome *(continued)*

Transforming Growth Factor-β_1 *Serum* *Decrease* In 15 patients with Guillain-Barre syndrome on admission to hospital median concentration of 31.2 ± 7.7 ng/mL less than in controls. 13 of the 15 patients had concentrations less than controls. Concentrations tended to decrease to day 3 then remain stable to day 10 then rise to control values on day 15 *960*

Tumor Necrosis Factor *Cerebrospinal Fluid* *Increase* Increased TNF levels were also frequent in the CSF and serum of patients with Guillain-Barre syndrome (GBS), which is also a demyelinating disease *5309*
Serum *Increase* Increased TNF levels were also frequent in the CSF and serum of patients with Guillain-Barre syndrome (GBS), which is also a demyelinating disease *5309*

Tumor Necrosis Factor-α *Serum* *Increase* In 14 patients with Guillain-Barre syndrome mean concentration of 215 ± 103 pg/mL not significantly higher than 161 ± 69 pg/mL in 12 healthy controls *2206* In 15 patients with Guillain-Barre syndrome on admission to hospital median concentration of 15.9 ± 5.3 ng/mL higher than in controls in 9 patients. Concentrations tended to decrease to day 15 when they were 10.9 ± 5 ng/mL *960*

357.00 Miller-Fisher Syndrome

Interferon-γ *Serum* *Increase* In 7 patients with Miller-Fisher syndrome mean concentration of 684 ± 330 pg/mL significantly higher than 113 ± 91 pg/mL in 12 healthy controls *2206*

Interleukin-4 *Serum* *Increase* In 7 patients with Miller-Fisher syndrome mean concentration of 375 ± 114 pg/mL significantly higher than 97 ± 35 pg/mL in 12 healthy controls *2206*

Interleukin-10 *Serum* *No Effect* In 7 patients with Miller-Fisher syndrome mean concentration of 690 ± 364 pg/mL not significantly different from 706 ± 236 pg/mL in 12 healthy controls *2206*

Tumor Necrosis Factor-α *Serum* *Increase* In 7 patients with Miller-Fisher syndrome mean concentration of 219 ± 127 pg/mL not significantly higher than 161 ± 69 pg/mL in 12 healthy controls *2206*

357.90 Polyneuritis

Albumin *Cerebrospinal Fluid* *Increase* CSF shows a gradual increase in protein, almost all of which is albumin in postinfectious polyneuritis, without a concomitant rise in cells *2039*

Cells *Cerebrospinal Fluid* *Increase* Characteristically, fewer than 10 cells/µL usually lymphocytes, are present in the CSF, and the presence of > 40 /µL raises other diagnostic considerations, such as herpes simplex myelitis and poliomyelitis *900*

γ-Globulin *Cerebrospinal Fluid* *Increase* Rarely elevated *900*
Cerebrospinal Fluid *No Effect* Rarely elevated *900*

Immunoglobulin A *Cerebrospinal Fluid* *Increase* Increased amounts of immunoglobulins particularly IgA and IgM have been demonstrated *900*

Immunoglobulin M *Cerebrospinal Fluid* *Increase* Increased amounts of immunoglobulins particularly IgA and IgM have been demonstrated *900*

Leukocytes *Blood* *Increase* In 35% of 14 patients hospitalized for this disorder *1576* A mild increase in peripheral leukocytes may occur in the early stages of the illness *900*

Lymphocytes *Cerebrospinal Fluid* *Increase* CSF shows increased protein and up to several hundred mononuclear cells in polyneuritis due to infectious mononucleosis *5544*

Neutrophils *Blood* *Increase* In 53% of 13 patients hospitalized for this disorder *1576*

Protein *Cerebrospinal Fluid* *Increase* From day 3 - 7 of the illness, over 50% of the patients will have high concentrations, frequently > 100 mg/dL. From the 2 - 7th week, almost all patients will have high CSF protein values *900*

358.00 Lambert-Eaton Myesthenic Syndrome

Acetylcholine Receptor Binding Antibodies
Serum *Increase* Unexplained positive results are observed in about 5% of patients with Lambert-Eaton myesthenic syndrome *2952*

Striational Antibodies *Serum* *Increase* Approxiately 5% of patients with Lambert-Eaton myesthenic syndrome and/or small-cell lung carcinoma *2952*

358.00 Myasthenia Gravis

Acetylcholine Receptor Binding Antibodies
Serum *Increase* Values greater than 0.03 nmol/L are consistent with a diagnosis of acquired myesthenia gravis. In generalized myesthenia gravis approximately 90% of patients have increased concentration *2952* AChR blocking antibodies observed in 90% of patients with generalized myesthenia gravis, 71% of patients with ocular myesthenia gravis and 81% of patients in remission *2952*

Acetylcholine Receptor Blocking Antibodies
Serum *Increase* Detectable in 52% of patients with myesthenia gravis and 30% with ocular myesthenia gravis *2952*

Acetylcholine Receptor Modulating Antibodies
Serum *Increase* AChR modulating antibodies observed in 94% of patients with generalized myesthenia gravis *2952*

Aldolase *Serum* *No Effect* Normal activities usually observed in patients with myesthenia gravis *2952* Activity usually normal including muscle fraction in severely affected children *4608*

Anti-Mitochondrial Antibodies *Serum* *Increase* There is an increased incidence of this compared to the population as a whole *4551*

Antibody Titer *Serum* *Increase* 50% of patients with this disease, usually those with thymoma, have antibodies to striated muscle. At times there is an increasing titer in severe disease. Generally a titer greater than 1:60 is diagnostic *3712*

Antinuclear Antibodies *Serum* *Increase* There is an increased incidence of this compared to the population as a whole *4551* Approximately 20% contain antinuclear factor which can occur in IgA, IgG, or IgM *3408*

Antithyroglobulin Antibodies *Serum* *Increase* Serum contains at least one form of antithyroid antibody *4551*

Aspartate Aminotransferase *Serum* *No Effect* Activity usually normal including muscle fraction in severely affected children *4608*

Bicarbonate *Serum* *Increase* Associated respiratory insufficiency *2034*

Carbon Dioxide Partial Pressure *Blood* *Increase* Associated respiratory insufficiency *2034*

Carcinoembryonic Antigen *Serum* *Increase* 18% of patients had values > 2.5 ng/mL *4891* In 183 patients with myasthenia gravis, 82% had concentrations less than 2.5 ng/mL, 17% had concentrations between 2.6 and 5.0 ng/mL, 1% had concentrations between 5.1 and 10.0 ng/mL and 0% had concentrations greater than 10.0 ng/mL *2010*

Catecholamines *Urine* *Increase* Some cases *5544*

CD5+ Lymphocytes *Blood* *No Effect* In 20 patients with myasthenia gravis mean proportion of 67.86 ± 6.51% not significantly different from 67.45 ± 9.02% in 21 healthy controls *164*

CD20+ Lymphocytes *Blood* *No Effect* In 20 patients with myasthenia gravis mean proportion of 11.84 ± 6.12% not significantly different from 13.30 ± 6.02% in 21 healthy controls *164*

Complement, Total *Serum* *Decrease* 40 of 68 patients had activity below normal at some time in the course of disease. On the basis of clinical correlations, 15 patients with subnormal levels were judged to be in exacerbation *3741*

Creatine *Urine* *Increase* Increased formation; myopathy *5544* Urinary creatine may be significantly increased in patients with myesthenia gravis *2952*

Creatine Kinase *Serum* *No Effect* Activity usually normal including muscle (CPK-MM) fraction. In severely affected children *4608*

Erythrocyte Sedimentation Rate *Blood* *No Effect* Complete blood count and ESR are normal *5544*

Glutamic Acid Decarboxylase Antibodies *Serum* *No Effect* In none of 29 patients with myasthenia gravis were GAD antibodies detected *3880*

Hematocrit *Blood* *Decrease* Occasional cases of macrocytic anemia *5544*

Hemoglobin *Blood* *Decrease* Occasional cases of macrocytic anemia *5544*

HLA Antigens *Blood* *Present* HLA-DR3 present in 30% of patients versus 17% of controls *5678*

Interleukin-6 *Serum* *Increase* Significant elevations of IL-6 levels were observed in the sera of patients with myasthenia gravis (41 ± 22 pg/mL), when compared to those of controls ($p < 0.05$) *4800*

Lactate Dehydrogenase *Serum* *No Effect* Activity usually normal including muscle fraction in severely affected children *4608*

LE Cells *Blood* *Positive* Lupus erythematosus may occur in conjunction *2034*

Lymphocytes *Blood* *Decrease* 17 of 32 patients had counts < 1,500 /µL and 18 of the 32 did not develop sensitivity to dinitrochlorobenzene *3* Observed effect *4551*

MCH *Blood* *Increase* Occasional cases of macrocytic anemia *5544*

MCV *Blood* *Increase* Occasional cases of macrocytic anemia *5544*

α_1-Microglobulin *Cerebrospinal Fluid* *No Effect* Of 2 patients with rheumatoid arthritis mean concentration in neither greater than that in 15 healthy controls of 34.8 ± 16.0 µg/L *2370*

Oxygen Partial Pressure *Blood* *Decrease* Associated respiratory insufficiency *2034*

Oxygen Saturation *Blood* *Decrease* Associated respiratory insufficiency *2034*

Rheumatoid Factor *Serum* *Increase* Somewhat elevated compared to the population at large. Demonstrated in a small percentage of patients *4551*

T3-Uptake *Serum* *Increase* Thyrotoxicosis may occur in conjunction with this disease *2034*

Thyroxine (T4) *Serum* *Increase* Thyrotoxicosis may occur in conjunction with this disease *2034*

Tri-iodothyronine (T3) *Serum* *Increase* Thyrotoxicosis may occur in conjunction with this disease *2034*

358.80 Amyotonia Congenita

Creatine *Urine* *Increase* Increased formation; myopathy *5544* Urinary creatine may be significantly increased in patients with amyotonia congenita *2952*

358.90 Neuromuscular Disease

Carbonic Anhydrase III *Serum* *Increase* In 14 patients with neuromuscular diseases mean concentration significantly increased to approximately 100 µg/L *5377*

Creatine Kinase *Serum* *Increase* In 5 of 14 patients with neuromuscular diseases mean concentration of 150 U/L significantly higher than in healthy controls *5377*

Myoglobin *Serum* *Increase* In 14 patients with neuromuscular diseases mean concentration of 270 µg/L compared with upper limit of normal of 80 µg/L in men and 70 µg/L in women *5377*

359.11 Duchenne Muscular Dystrophy

Aldolase *Serum* *Increase* Highest activities observed in patients with Duchenne muscular dystrophy *2952*

Basic Fibroblast Growth Factor *Serum* *Increase* Concentration increased from 40 to 165 pg/mL in 11 of 18 patients with DMD whereas concentration less than 30 pg/mL in 200 control individuals: concentration poorly correlated with serum creatine kinase activity *1006*

Creatine Kinase *Serum* *Increase* Mean activity in 11 patients with basal fibroblast growth factor concentration greater than 30 pg/mL of 10,141 ± 6,642 U/L compared with 2,985 ± 1,867 U/L in 7 with concentrations of bFGF less than 30 pg/mL *1006*

Troponin T *Serum* *Increase* Slightly increased concentrations observed in 8 of 33 patients with Duchenne's muscular dystrophy *333*

359.11 Limb-girdle Dystrophy

Aldolase *Serum* *Increase* Increased activities observed in patients with limb-girdle dystrophy *2952*

359.11 Muscular Dystrophy

Amyloid β-Protein *Cerebrospinal Fluid* *Decrease* In 2 patients with muscular dystrophy concentrations were 0.90 and 1.82 pmol/mL significantly different from mean concentration of 4.00 ± 2.92 pmol/mL in one and within reference limits in the other *3716*
Cerebrospinal Fluid *No Effect* In 2 patients with muscular dystrophy concentrations were 0.90 and 1.82 pmol/mL significantly different from mean concentration of 4.00 ± 2.92 pmol/mL in one and within reference limits in the other *3716*

Amyloid β-Protein Precursor *Cerebrospinal Fluid* *Increase* In 2 patients with muscular dystrophy concentrations were 1.76 and 2.40 integrated OD units significantly different from mean concentration of 1.35 ± 0.38 integrated OD units in 25 normal controls in one but normal in the other *3716*
Cerebrospinal Fluid *No Effect* In 2 patients with muscular dystrophy concentrations were 1.76 and 2.40 integrated OD units significantly different from mean concentration of 1.35 ± 0.38 integrated OD units in 25 normal controls in one but normal in the other *3716*

α_1-Antichymotrypsin *Cerebrospinal Fluid* *No Effect* In 2 patients with muscular dystrophy concentrations were 0.40 and 4.55 µg/mL not significantly different from mean concentration of 2.27 ± 1.40 µg/mL in 25 normal controls *3716*

Cells *Cerebrospinal Fluid* *Increase* In 2 patients with muscular dystrophy concentrations of 2.0 and 7.0 cells/µL significantly different from normal of 3 cells/µL in one and normal in the other *3716*
Cerebrospinal Fluid *No Effect* In 2 patients with muscular dystrophy concentrations of 2.0 and 7.0 cells/µL significantly different from normal of 3 cells/µL in one and normal in the other *3716*

Creatine *Urine* *Increase* Urinary creatine may be significantly increased in patients with rapidly progressing muscular dystrophies *2952*

Creatinine *Urine* *Decrease* In 9 patients with muscular dystrophy mean excretion of 1.15 ± 0.08 g/d compared with 1.80 ± 0.17 g/d in 4 healthy controls *5626*

Protein *Cerebrospinal Fluid* *No Effect* In 2 patients with muscular dystrophy concentrations of 13 and 17 mg/dL not significantly different from normal mean of 29 mg/dL *3716*

359.11 Progressive Muscular Dystrophy

Alanine Aminotransferase *Serum* *Increase* Particularly during the early and middle stages of the disease. In the late stage of the disease when the muscle mass has been severely reduced, serum enzyme levels may be only minimally elevated *900*

Aldolase *Serum* *Increase* Strikingly elevated *1980* Increases in the early stages to 10 - 15 times normal in 90% of cases. Levels are normal in the later and terminal stages *1290* Serum enzymes reach extremely high levels, particularly during the early and middle stages of the disease. In the late stage of the disease when the muscle mass has been severely reduced, serum enzyme levels may be only minimally elevated *900*

Aldosterone *Urine* *No Effect* The differences between the patient group and the control group for sodium and potassium in serum and urine and for urinary aldosterone were not significant. The pathologically elevated sodium:potassium ratio in skeletal muscle is not due to increased aldosterone or other causes of renal wastage of potassium *1661*

359.11 Progressive Muscular Dystrophy *(continued)*

Alkaline Phosphatase *White Blood Cells Decrease* Untreated disease *5544*

Aspartate Aminotransferase *Serum Increase* A marked increase in CK, LD, and AST was noted. 21 of 23 cases showed moderate to high activities of AST ranging from 24 to 105 U/L *3733* Released from breaking down muscle. Levels tend to be increased in affected young children *1025 900* May have elevated levels. Usual values 145 U/L *1025*

Carbonic Anhydrase III *Serum Increase* Plasma levels were found to be up to 39 times greater than levels in a control group *2084 3554* Raised in a majority of patients with Duchenne dystrophy *3555* In Duchenne muscular dystrophy, elevation of plasma levels to at least 10 times normal levels have been found *2085* Duchenne dystrophy (age < 6 y) mean concentration of 2,092 ng/L: Duchenne dystrophy (age > 6 y) mean concentration of 1,230 ng/L. Controls (aged 5 - 12 y) mean concentration of 140 ng/L *708*

Cholic Acid *Serum Decrease* In 15 patients with this disorder the serum values were usually low (0.16 µmol/L) compared with controls (1.47 µmol/L) *5159*

Creatine *Serum Increase* Decreased transport into muscle and leakage out of muscle occur in muscular dystrophies *4979*
Urine Increase Excessive concentrations appearing in urine are newly synthesized and do not originate from muscle cells *4707* Urine creatine is increased; urine creatinine is decreased. These changes are less marked in limb-girdle and fascioscapulohumeral types than in the Duchenne type. May occur irregularly *5544* Decreased transport into muscle and leakage out of muscle occur in muscular dystrophies *4979*

Creatine Kinase *Serum Increase* Range of values up to 50 times normal upper limit with higher results in the younger patients. Abnormal results are accentuated if vasoconstriction is applied for 10 min before venesection. (Muscular atrophy of neurogenic origin shows no such increase in serum levels) *1290* Especially Duchenne type. The most sensitive reflection of certain types of muscular dystrophy *1025* Observed with muscle wasting *900* Especially Duchenne type. The most sensitive reflection of certain types of muscular dystrophy *1642* Extremely high concentrations, particularly during the early and middle stages of the disease. In the late stage of the disease when the muscle mass has been severely reduced, may be only *4746*

Creatine Kinase MB-Isoenzyme *Serum Increase* The single best test for carrier detection *5754 2653*

Creatinine *Urine Decrease* Reduced excretion in any myopathic or neurogenic condition which decreases muscle mass *4979* Urine creatine is increased; urine creatinine is decreased. These changes are less marked in limb-girdle and fascioscapulohumeral types than in the Duchenne type *5544*

HDL-Cholesterol *Serum No Effect* Within normal limits in 15 patients with this disorder *5159*

Hydroxyproline *Urine Decrease* In boys with Duchenne type *1790*

Lactate Dehydrogenase *Serum Increase* Particularly during the early and middle stages of the disease. In the late stage of the disease when the muscle mass has been severely reduced, may be only minimally elevated *900* Observed with muscle wasting *3733*

Lactate Dehydrogenase Isoenzyme-5 *Serum Decrease* In 76 cases of Duchenne MD, was markedly depressed and remained low until the final stages of the disease. Abnormal isoenzyme patterns persisted over time even though the total LD value fell to normal with increasing age of patient *2225*

Lactate Dehydrogenase Isoenzymes *Serum Increase* In Duchenne dystrophy combined LD-1 and 2 values are 72% of total LD. Abnormal isoenzyme patterns persist with age of patient although total LD falls to normal *2225* Isoenzyme patterns revealed an increase in 1 (38%) and 2 (47.5%), with concomitant decrease or absence of 3, 4, 5 *2226*

Malate Dehydrogenase *Serum Increase* In Duchenne type *1790*

Manganese Superoxide Dismutase *Serum Decrease* Patients with Duchenne dystrophy had a significantly lower concentration than control serum *5761*

Myoglobin *Urine Increase* Sporadic *5544*

Nickel *Serum No Effect* Mean concentration of 2.3 µg/L (n = 10) compared with mean in controls of 2.6 µg/L (n = 42) *3428*

Potassium *Serum No Effect* The differences between the patients and the control group of normal boys for sodium and potassium in serum and urine were not significant. The pathologically elevated sodium:potassium ratio in skeletal muscle is not due to increased aldosterone or other causes of renal wastage of potassium *1661*
Urine No Effect The differences between the patients and the control group of normal boys for sodium and potassium in serum and urine were not significant. The pathologically elevated sodium:potassium ratio in skeletal muscle is not due to increased aldosterone or other causes of renal wastage of potassium *1661*

Ribose *Urine Increase* Probably derived from the nucleoprotein of breaking down muscle cells *1290*

Sodium *Serum No Effect* The differences between the patient group and the group of normal boys for sodium and potassium in serum and urine were not significant. The pathologically elevated sodium:potassium ratio in skeletal muscle is not due to increased aldosterone or other causes of renal wastage of potassium *1661*
Urine No Effect The differences between the patient group and the control group for sodium and potassium in serum and urine were significant. The pathologically elevated sodium potassium ratio in skeletal muscle is not due to increased aldosterone or other causes of renal wastage of potassium *1661*

359.21 Myotonia Atrophica

Alanine Aminotransferase *Serum Increase* Usually normal or minimally elevated *900*

Aldolase *Serum Increase* Usually normal or minimally elevated *900* Due to cell destruction. Increased in about 20% of the patients *5544*
Serum No Effect Usually normal or minimally elevated *900*

Aspartate Aminotransferase *Serum Increase* Slight to moderate increase *1025* Increased in about 15% of the patients *5544* Usually normal or minimally elevated *900*
Serum No Effect Usually normal in myotonic dystrophy *4979*

Calcium *Red Blood Cells Increase* Erythrocytes from these patients accumulate calcium at a significantly higher rate than normals do. This increased rate of net accumulation appears related to an enhanced permeability of the membrane, rather than to an impairment in its active outward transport *4158*

Carbon Dioxide Partial Pressure *Blood Increase* Respiratory muscle weakness may develop *742*

Carbonic Anhydrase III *Serum Increase* Reported effect *3555*

Cortisol *Plasma Decrease* Abnormal diurnal variation with decreased 8 a.m. values in 4 of 7 patients *2117*

Creatine *Serum Increase* Decreased transport into muscle and leakage out of muscle occur in muscular dystrophies *4979*
Urine Increase Decreased transport into muscle and leakage out of muscle occur in muscular dystrophies *4979*

Creatine Kinase *Serum Increase* Increased in about 50% of the patients *5544* Slight to moderate increase *1025*

Creatinine *Serum Increase* In severe muscle disease *1025*
Urine Decrease Reduced excretion in any myopathic or neurogenic condition which decreases muscle mass *4979*

Erythrocyte Sedimentation Rate *Blood No Effect* Usually normal *5544*

Glucose Tolerance *Serum Increase* Biphasic response was found in 19 patients (49%) compared with 12 of the control population (24%). In 9 patients (23%), the height of the 2nd peak was 20 mg/dL *4480*

Immunoglobulin G *Serum Decrease* In 4 of 8 cases studied *2437*

Insulin *Plasma Increase* In response to glucose load, in myotonic dystrophy *4979* Found in 7 of 7 patients *2117* 80% of patients had insulin values > 2 S.D. above the normal mean during oral glucose tolerance test and 42% had high fasting plasma values *292*

17-Ketosteroids *Urine Decrease* Primary testicular failure in males *1790*

Lactate Dehydrogenase *Serum Increase* Slightly or moderately increased *1025* In about 10% of the patients *5544*

Serum *No Effect* Usually normal *4979*

Lactate Dehydrogenase Isoenzyme-5 *Serum* *Increase* Elevation of fast moving LD in serum *5544*

Myoglobin *Urine* *Increase* Metabolic defect, hereditary *5544*

Oxygen Partial Pressure *Blood* *Decrease* Respiratory muscle weakness may develop *742*

Oxygen Saturation *Blood* *Decrease* Respiratory muscle weakness may develop *742*

Prolactin *Plasma* *Increase* Basal levels elevated in 3 of 7 patients *2117*

359.21 Myotonic Dystrophy

C-Peptide *Plasma* *No Effect* Mean basal concentration in 12 patients of 0.75 nmol/24 h not significantly different from 0.7 nmol/24 h in healthy controls *1800*
Urine *No Effect* Mean basal concentration in 12 patients of 0.7 nmol/L not significantly different from 0.6 nmol/L in healthy controls *1800*

Growth Hormone *Plasma* *No Effect* Mean basal concentration in 12 patients 0.85 µg/L not significantly different from 0.9 µg/L in healthy controls *1800*

Insulin *Plasma* *No Effect* Mean basal concentration in 12 patients of 146 pmol/L not significantly different from 110 pmol/L in healthy controls *1800*

359.22 Myotonia Congenita

Aspartate Aminotransferase *Serum* *Increase* Slight to moderate increase *1025*

Creatine *Urine* *Increase* May be increased in some patients (Thomsen's disease) *5544*

Creatine Kinase *Serum* *Increase* Slight to moderate increase *1025*

Lactate Dehydrogenase *Serum* *Increase* Slightly or moderately increased *1025*

359.30 Familial Periodic Paralysis

Aldolase *Serum* *Increase* Occasional patients with paramyotonia congenita *1541*

Aldosterone *Urine* *Increase* Striking change noted prior to attack *4979*

Aspartate Aminotransferase *Serum* *Increase* Occasional patients with paramyotonia congenita *1541*

Chloride *Urine* *Decrease* Precedes attack *4979*

Eosinophils *Blood* *Decrease* Occasionally during attacks *4979*

Follicle Stimulating Hormone *Urine* *Increase* During attack *752*

Glucose *Urine* *Increase* Occasional patients *4979*

Gonadotropin, Pituitary *Urine* *Increase* During attack *752*

Ketones *Serum* *Increase* Occasional patients *4979*

17-Ketosteroids *Urine* *Increase* In the most severe attacks *4979* *1835*

Lactate *Blood* *Increase* Observed effect *3390*

Leukocytes *Blood* *Increase* Occasionally during attacks *4979*

Neutrophils *Blood* *Increase* Occasionally during attacks *4979*

Phosphate *Serum* *Decrease* During attacks *85*

Potassium *Cerebrospinal Fluid* *Decrease* Rarely found to be quite low during attack *1280*
Cerebrospinal Fluid *No Effect* Only a slight drop during attacks *4232*
Serum *Decrease* Ranges from 2.5 - 3.5 mmol/L in hypokalemic attacks. May be normal between attacks *367* Rarely, may shift from extra- to intracellular sites. There is no evidence of GI or renal wasting, volume depletion or total body K depletion *3735* Marked fall *2463*
Serum *No Effect* Normal between attacks *4979*
Urine *Decrease* Excretion decreases at the time of attack *5544*

Protein *Urine* *Increase* Occasional patients *4979*

Sodium *Serum* *Increase* Precedes attack *4979*
Urine *Decrease* Precedes attack *4979*

Thyroxine (T4) *Serum* *No Effect* No abnormality usually observed *4979*

Tri-iodothyronine (T3) *Serum* *No Effect* No abnormality usually observed *4979*

Uric Acid *Urine* *Increase* Uricosuria accompanies attacks *4707*

359.80 Chronic Inflammatory Demyelinating Myopathy

Soluble E-Selectin *Serum* *Increase* Mean concentration of 56 ± 29 ng/mL in 14 patients with chronic inflammatory demyelinating myopathy significantly higher than 30 ± 9 ng/mL in 12 healthy control individuals *3885*

359.80 Hypertrophic Non-obstructive Myopathy

Adrenomedullin *Plasma* *Increase* In 26 patients with hypertrophic nonobstructive myopathy mean concentration of 7.8 ± 1.9 pmol/L significantly different from mean concentration of 5.2 ± 0.4 pmol/L in 14 control individuals *1986*

Atrial Natriuretic Peptide *Plasma* *Increase* In 26 patients with hypertrophic nonobstructive myopathy mean concentration of 39.9 ± 28.2 pg/mL significantly different from mean concentration of 10.7 ± 6.3 pg/mL in 14 control individuals *1986*

Brain Natriuretic Peptide *Plasma* *Increase* In 26 patients with hypertrophic nonobstructive myopathy mean concentration of 211.9 ± 299.5 pg/mL significantly different from mean concentration of 6.3 ± 2.7 pg/mL in 14 control individuals *1986*

Endothelin-1 *Plasma* *Increase* In 26 patients with hypertrophic nonobstructive myopathy mean concentration of 2.31 ± 0.55 pg/mL significantly different from mean concentration of 1.47 ± 0.28 pg/mL in 14 control individuals *1986*

Epinephrine *Plasma* *No Effect* In 26 patients with hypertrophic nonobstructive myopathy mean concentration of 35.4 ± 48.1 pg/mL not significantly different from mean concentration of 37.3 ± 25.6 pg/mL in 14 control individuals *1986*

Norepinephrine *Plasma* *No Effect* In 26 patients with hypertrophic nonobstructive myopathy mean concentration of 337.6 ± 153.4 pg/mL not significantly different from mean concentration of 319.9 ± 71.7 pg/mL in 14 control individuals *1986*

359.80 Hypertrophic Obstructive Myopathy

Adrenomedullin *Plasma* *Increase* In 14 patients with hypertrophic obstructive myopathy mean concentration of 9.7 ± 5.6 pmol/L significantly different from mean concentration of 5.2 ± 0.4 pmol/L in 14 control individuals *1986*

Atrial Natriuretic Peptide *Plasma* *Increase* In 14 patients with hypertrophic obstructive myopathy mean concentration of 99.3 ± 74.7 pg/mL significantly different from mean concentration of 10.7 ± 6.3 pg/mL in 14 control individuals *1986*

Brain Natriuretic Peptide *Plasma* *Increase* In 14 patients with hypertrophic obstructive myopathy mean concentration of 430.6 ± 295.7 pg/mL significantly different from mean concentration of 6.3 ± 2.7 pg/mL in 14 control individuals *1986*

Endothelin-1 *Plasma* *Increase* In 14 patients with hypertrophic obstructive myopathy mean concentration of 2.68 ± 0.92 pg/mL significantly different from mean concentration of 1.47 ± 0.28 pg/mL in 14 control individuals *1986*

Epinephrine *Plasma* *No Effect* In 14 patients with hypertrophic obstructive myopathy mean concentration of 40.7 ± 34.7 pg/mL not significantly different from mean concentration of 37.3 ± 25.6 pg/mL in 14 control individuals *1986*

Norepinephrine *Plasma* *No Effect* In 14 patients with hypertrophic obstructive myopathy mean concentration of 297.4 ± 189.3 pg/mL not significantly different from mean concentration of 319.9 ± 71.7 pg/mL in 14 control individuals *1986*

359.90 Skeletal Muscle Disease

Alanine Aminotransferase *Serum* *Increase* May rarely cause increased ALT activity *4617*

360.11 Sympathetic Ophthalmitis

β_2-Microglobulin *Serum* *Increase* In patients with sympathetic ophthalmitis concentration increased in proportion to severity of disease with concentrations being high even at start of disease and decreased in remissions *316*

361.90 Retinal Detachment

Alkaline Phosphatase *Serum* *No Effect* No significant change observed in 10 patients following non-traumatic retinal detachment 72 to 96 hours after the event compared with matched controls *3732*

Calcium *Serum* *No Effect* No significant change observed in 10 patients with non-traumatic retinal detachment 72 to 96 hours after the event compared with matched controls *3732*

Creatinine *Serum* *No Effect* In 10 patients with non-trauatic retinal detachment no significant change observed 72 to 96 hours after the event compared with matched controls *3732*

γ-Glutamyltransferase *Serum* *No Effect* No significant effect observed in 10 patients with non-traumatic retinal detachment 72 to 96 hours after the event compared with matched controls *3732*

Osteocalcin *Serum* *No Effect* No significant change observed in 10 patients with non-traumatic detachment of retina after 72 to 96 hours of complete bed rest when mean concentration was 3.4 ± 1.1 ng/mL compared with 3.4 ± 1.2 ng/mL in healthy control population *3732*

Phosphate *Serum* *No Effect* In 10 patients with non-traumatic retinal detachment no significant change observed 72 to 96 hours after the event compared with matched controls *3732*

362.30 Retinal Artery Occlusion

Lipoprotein Lp(a) *Serum* *Increase* Mean concentration in 15 patients with central retinal artery occlusion of 20.4 ± 18.1 mg/dL significantly different from 10.0 ± 7.6 mg/dL in 20 healthy controls *3666*

362.30 Retinal Vein Occlusion

11-Dehydro-thromboxane B_2 *Urine* *No Effect* Mean excretion in 10 patients with retinal vein occlusion of 1,417 ± 549 pg/mg creatinine significantly different from 904 ± 292 pg/mg creatinine observed in 10 healthy controls *5781*

Lipoprotein Lp(a) *Serum* *Increase* Mean concentration in 20 patients with central retinal vein occlusion of 18.5 ± 21.7 mg/dL different from 10.0 ± 7.6 mg/dL in 20 healthy controls *3666*

363.20 Idiopathic Uveoretinitis

Anti-Endothelial Cell Antibodies *Serum* *Increase* Raised concentrations observed in 31% of 32 patients with isolated idiopathic uveoretinitis *5837*

Soluble Intercellular Adhesion Molecule-1 *Serum* *Increase* Mean concentration of 164 ng/mL in 32 patients with idiopathic uveoretinitis increased, with 295 ng/mL in 9 relapsed patients significantly increased compared with mean of 140 ng/mL in 22 normal controls *5837*
Serum *No Effect* Mean concentration of 23 ng/mL in 32 patients with idiopathic uveoretinitis (76 ng/mL in 9 relapsed patients) not significantly different from 37 ng/mL in 22 normal controls *5837*

von Willebrand Factor *Plasma* *Increase* In 32 patients with idiopathic uveoretinitis mean concentration of 90 units significantly higher than 65 units in 22 normal controls *5837*

363.20 Inflammation of Optic Nerve and Retina

Lymphocytes *Cerebrospinal Fluid* *Increase* CSF is normal or may show increased protein and up to 200 lymphocytes/µL *5544*

Protein *Cerebrospinal Fluid* *Increase* CSF is normal or may show increased protein and up to 200 lymphocytes/µL *5544*

364.04 Traumatic Uveitis

β_2-Microglobulin *Serum* *No Effect* No significant effect observed in patients with traumatic uveitis *316*

372.13 Vernal Keratoconjunctivitis

Substance P *Tears* *Increase* Mean concentration of 114.4 ± 35.1 pg/mL in 10 patients with vernal keratoconjunctivitis significantly higher than 70.9 ± 34.8 pg/mL observed in 65 healthy adults *1597*

372.14 Allergic Conjunctivitis

Substance P *Tears* *Increase* Mean concentration of 107. 7 ± 37.3 pg/mL in 10 patients with seasonal allergic conjunctivitis significantly higher than 70.9 ± 34.8 pg/mL observed in 65 healthy adults *1597*

377.30 Optic Neuritis

Anti-Neutrophil Cytoplasm Antibodies *Serum* *No Effect* In 0 of 2 patients (0%) with optic neuritis pANCA detected *3722*

Antinuclear Antibodies *Serum* *No Effect* In 0 of 2 patients (0%) with optic neuritis ANA detected *3722*

Glucose *Cerebrospinal Fluid* *No Effect* In 83 patients with acute optic neuritis glucose concentration normal *4412*

Leukocytes *Cerebrospinal Fluid* *Increase* In 83 patients with acute optic neuritis leukocyte concentration increased above 6 cells/µL in 36%, with highest count of 27 cells/µL *4412*

Oligoclonal Banding *Cerebrospinal Fluid* *Increase* In 76 patients with acute optic neuritis oligoclonal bands present in 28% of 39 patients with normal MRIs and in 73% of 37 patients with abnormal MRIs *4412*

Protein *Cerebrospinal Fluid* *Increase* In 83 patients with acute optic neuritis protein concentration increased above 50 mg/dL in 9.4% *4412*

380.10 Otitis Externa

Leukocytes *Blood* *Increase* When the infection is severe and there is mild fever, an elevated WBC will occur *900*

381.00 Otitis Media

Eosinophils *Blood* *Increase* In 48% of 70 patients hospitalized for this disorder *1576*

Leukocytes *Blood* *Increase* Acute exacerbations may produce elevated WBC *900* Usually accompanied by a mild leukocytosis with the appearance of less mature forms of neutrophils *900*

Lymphocytes *Blood* *Increase* In 66% of 70 patients hospitalized for this disorder *1576*

Neutrophils *Blood* *Decrease* In 53% of 70 patients hospitalized for this disorder *1576*
Blood *Increase* Usually accompanied by a mild leukocytosis with the appearance of less mature forms of neutrophils *900*

Transforming Growth Factor-β_1 *Serum* *Increase* In 125 children with bacterial acute otitis media median concentration of 11.5 pg/mL significantly different from value in 3.7 pg/mL in 59 children with nonbacterial acute otitis media compared with healthy controls in whom concentration was undetected *2096*

DISEASES OF THE CIRCULATORY SYSTEM

Acute Rheumatic Fever

390.00 Acute Rheumatic Fever

$CD3^+$ Lymphocytes *Blood* *No Effect* In 25 patients with acute rheumatic fever mean concentration of 3.44 ± 0.62 x 10^3 cells /μL not significantly different from 3.64 ± 0.58 x 10^3 cells /μL in 15 healthy controls *3737*

$CD4^+$:$CD8^+$ Lymphocyte Ratio *Blood* *Increase* In 25 patients with acute rheumatic fever mean ratio of 1.54 ± 0.26 significantly different from 1.10 ± 0.21 in 15 healthy controls *3737*

$CD4^+$ Lymphocytes *Blood* *Increase* In 25 patients with acute rheumatic fever mean concentration of 2.42 ± 0.24 x 10^3 cells/μL significantly different from 1.74 ± 0.32 x 10^3 cells/μL in 15 healthy controls *3737*

$CD8^+$ Lymphocytes *Blood* *No Effect* In 25 patients with acute rheumatic fever mean concentration of 1.52 ± 0.18 x 10^3 cells/μL significantly different from 1.60 ± 0.14 x 10^3 cells/μL in 15 healthy controls *3737*

$CD16^+$ Lymphocytes *Blood* *No Effect* In 25 patients with acute rheumatic fever mean concentration of 1.18 ± 0.21 x 10^3 cells/μL significantly different from 0.84 ± 0.166 x 10^3 cells/μL in 15 healthy controls *3737*

$CD19^+$ Lymphocytes *Blood* *No Effect* In 25 patients with acute rheumatic fever mean concentration of 1.02 ± 0.12 x 10^3 cells/μL not significantly different from 1.10 ± 0.09 x 10^3 cells/μL in 15 healthy controls *3737*

$CD25^+$ Lymphocytes *Blood* *Increase* In 25 patients with acute rheumatic fever mean concentration of 0.90 ± 0.22 x 10^3 cells/μL significantly different from 0.55 ± 0.14 x 10^3 cells/μL in 15 healthy controls *3737*

Interleukin-1α *Serum* *Increase* In 25 patients with acute rheumatic fever mean concentration of 5.4 ± 1.9 pg/mL significantly different from 3.1 ± 1.4 pg/mL in 15 healthy controls *3737*

Interleukin-2 *Serum* *Increase* In 25 patients with acute rheumatic fever mean concentration of 7.3 ± 5.9 pg/mL significantly different from 0.3 ± 0.47 pg/mL in 15 healthy controls *3737*

Neopterin *Serum* *Increase* In 9 patients with acute rheumatic fever mean concentration of 15.1 ± 10.7 nmol/L compared with 5.2 ± 2.1 nmol/L in healthy controls *4549*

Tumor Necrosis Factor-α *Serum* *No Effect* In 25 patients with acute rheumatic fever mean concentration of 6.9 ± 3.1 pg/mL not significantly different from 6.4 ± 4.6 pg/mL in 15 healthy controls *3737*

390.00 Rheumatic Disease

Amyloid A Protein *Serum* *Increase* In 42 patients with rheumatic disease mean concentration of 193 ± 239 mg/L significantly greater than 1.3 ± 0.6 mg/L in 30 normal individuals *2851*

Apolipoprotein A-I *Serum* *Decrease* In 42 patients with rheumatic disease mean concentration of 1.24 ± 0.20 g/L significantly less than 1.52 ± 0.17 g/L in 30 normal individuals *2851*

Apolipoprotein A-II *Serum* *Decrease* In 42 patients with rheumatic disease mean concentration of 0.22 ± 0.07 g/L significantly less than 0.29 ± 0.04 g/L in 30 normal individuals *2851*

Cholesterol *Serum* *Decrease* Mean concentration of 4.5 ± 1.2 mmol/L significantly less than 5.0 ± 0.6 mmol/L in 30 normal individuals *2851*

β-Endorphin *White Blood Cells* *Decrease* Concentration decreased in patients with rheumatic diseases *633*

Erythrocyte Sedimentation Rate *Blood* *Increase* In 138 of 1,480 ESRs in a hospital population rates were greater than 100 mm/h: in a further study of 90 patients with 163 final diagnoses 30 were attributable to rheumatologic diseases *3097*

HDL_2-Cholesterol *Serum* *Decrease* In 42 patients with rheumatic disease mean concentration of 0.4 ± 0.2 mmol/L significantly less than 0.8 ± 0.3 mmol/L in 30 healthy individuals *2851*

HDL_3-Cholesterol *Serum* *No Effect* In 42 patients with rheumatic disease mean concentration of 0.6 ± 0.2 mmol/L not significantly different from 0.6 ± 0.1 mmol/L in 30 healthy control individuals *2851*

HDL-Cholesterol *Serum* *Decrease* In 42 patients with rheumatic disease mean concentration of 1.0 ± 0.3 mmol/L significantly less than 1.3 ± 0.3 mmol/L in 30 healthy controls *2851*

LDL-Cholesterol *Serum* *No Effect* In 42 patients with rheumatic disease mean concentration of 2.9 ± 1.2 mmol/L not significantly different from 3.2 ± 0.6 mmol/L in 30 normal individuals *2851*

Nucleotide Pyrophosphohydrolase, Soluble *Serum* *No Effect* Mean activity in 41 patients with miscellaneous rheumatic disease of 1,199 ± 42 pmol nitrophenol/h/mL not significantly different from that in 85 healthy individuals of 1,141 ± 22 pmol nitrophenol/h/mL *691*

Triglycerides *Serum* *No Effect* In 42 patients with rheumatic disease mean concentration of 1.3 ± 0.5 mmol/L not significantly different from 1.2 ± 0.3 mmol/L in 30 normal individuals *2851*

390.00 Rheumatic Fever

Adenosine Deaminase *Serum* *Increase* Increased *3926 4956 1340*

Alanine Aminotransferase *Serum* *No Effect* Usually normal unless the patient has cardiac failure with liver damage *5544*

Albumin *Serum* *Decrease* Impaired hepatic synthesis. Decreased serum albumin with strikingly increased $alpha_2$- and γ- globulins *4707*
Urine *Increase* A high percentage of patients show some proteinuria *367* Slight febrile albuminuria. Indicates mild focal nephritis. Concomitant glomerulonephritis appears in up to 2.5% of cases *5544*

Anti-Streptolysin-O Titer *Serum* *Increase* Increased titers develop after 2nd week and peak in 4 - 6 weeks *1980* Increased titer is found in 80% of patients within the first 2 months. Magnitude of titer is not related to severity; rate of fall is not related to course of disease *5544* Antibodies appear in 7 days, peak 2 - 4 weeks later and may remain elevated for months. Rising titer suggests infections *5619* Titer of 250 Todd U in adults and 333 in children is considered diagnostic of preceding streptococcal infection *2304*

Antibody Titer *Serum* *Increase* Antifibrinolysin titer is increased in this disease and in recent hemolytic streptococcus infections. 1 of the 3 titers (ASO, antihyaluronidase, antifibrinolysin elevated in 95% of cases. If all are normal, a diagnosis is less likely. Antihyaluronidase titer of 1,000 - 1,500 follows recent streptococcus A disease and up to 4,000 with rheumatic fever. Average titer is higher in early rheumatic activity than in subsiding or inactive rheumatic fever. Increased as often as ASO and antifibrinolysin titers *5544*

Antinuclear Antibodies *Serum* *No Effect* No significant increase in frequency *4068*

Aspartate Aminotransferase *Serum* *Increase* May occur as a result of chronic passive congestion in congestive heart failure or as a result of hepatotoxicity following salicylate therapy *1980* Serum level related to severity in the early stages *1290* The incidence and mechanism of occurrence is not clear. Usual values < 50 U/L *1025*

Casts *Urine* *Increase* Often mild abnormality of Addis count (protein, casts, RBC WBC) indicates mild focal nephritis. Concomitant glomerulonephritis appears in up to 2.5% of cases *5544*

Catecholamines *Urine* *Increase* Epinephrine and norepinephrine increase in proportion to the severity of circulatory failure. Catecholamine excretion, especially norepinephrine, is significantly raised in grades 3 and 4 of hemodynamic disturbance *5735*

Complement C_1 *Serum* *No Effect* Mean concentration typically normal or slightly increased in patients with rheumatic fever *4682*

Complement C_1q *Serum* *No Effect* Mean concentration typically normal or slightly increased in patients with rheumatic fever *4682*

Complement C_2 *Serum* *No Effect* Mean concentration typically normal or slightly increased in patients with rheumatic fever *4682*

390.00 Rheumatic Fever *(continued)*

Complement C_3 *Serum Increase* Elevated during the acute stages of disease, coinciding with other indices of acute inflammation *4551*
Serum No Effect Mean concentration typically normal or slightly increased in patients with rheumatic fever *4682*

Complement C_4 *Serum No Effect* Mean concentration typically normal or slightly increased in patients with rheumatic fever *4682*

Complement C_5 *Serum No Effect* Mean concentration typically normal or slightly increased in patients with rheumatic fever *4682*

Complement CH50 *Serum No Effect* Mean concentration typically normal or slightly increased in patients with rheumatic fever *4682*

Complement, Total *Serum Decrease* In general, normal or elevated. A small number of patients have reduced levels during the acute phase without any clear relation to severity or particular clinical manifestation *1980*
Serum Increase During the acute stage *4551* Elevated during activity inflammation and subsides with remission *4683* In general, normal or elevated. A small number of patients have reduced levels during the acute phase without any clear relation to severity or particular clinical manifestation *1980*
Serum No Effect In general, normal or elevated. A small number of patients have reduced levels during the acute phase without any clear relation to severity or particular clinical manifestation *1980* Elevated during activity inflammation and subsides with remission *4683* During the acute stage *4551*
Synovial Fluid Decrease The early and late components of the complement system are decreased *5097*

Copper *Serum Increase* In acute disease *5544* Has been used as an index of disease activity *1290* Statistically significant *4871*

Coproporphyrin *Urine Increase* Reported effect *1290*

C-Reactive Protein *Serum Increase* Almost always positive in the early stages of untreated disease and the most sensitive indicator of activity. Remains positive in the presence of active carditis *1980* Test is frequently positive and is not influenced by anemia, but is frequently positive with congestive heart failure from any cause *2304*

Cryofibrinogen *Plasma Increase* Reported effect *3417*

Epinephrine *Urine Increase* Epinephrine and norepinephrine increase in proportion to the severity of circulatory failure. Catecholamine excretion, especially norepinephrine, is significantly raised in grades 3 and 4 of hemodynamic disturbance *5735*

Erythrocyte Sedimentation Rate *Blood Decrease* May be decreased in the presence of congestive heart failure *2304*
Blood Increase Typically seen in the myocarditis of rheumatic fever *1980* Almost always elevated early in the course of untreated cases. May be decreased in the presence of congestive heart failure but not usually to the normal range *2304* Sensitive test of rheumatic activity; returns to normal with adequate treatment with ACTH or salicylates. It may remain increased after WBC becomes normal. Becomes normal with onset of congestive heart failure even in the presence of rheumatic activity *5544*

Erythrocytes *Urine Increase* Often mild abnormality of Addis count (protein, casts, RBC, WBC) indicates mild focal nephritis. Concomitant glomerulonephritis appears in up to 2.5% of cases *5544* Moderate increase *367*

Fibrinogen *Plasma Increase* Reported effect *1980*

α_1-Globulin *Serum Increase* Moderate increase in the early stages *1290*

α_2-Globulin *Serum Increase* Increases occur in the acute phase (parallel with the serum C-reactive protein), and fall during quiescence or following steroid therapy *1290* Serum proteins are altered, with decreased serum albumin and increased α_2- and γ- globulins. Streptococcus A infections do not increase α_2- globulin *5544*

γ-Globulin *Serum Increase* Serum proteins are altered, with decreased serum albumin and increased alpha$_2$- and γ- globulins *5544*

Haptoglobin *Serum Increase* Conditions associated with increased ESR and α_2-globulin; increases in collagen disease *5544*

Hematocrit *Blood Decrease* Anemia is common, gradually improves as activity subsides; microcytic types. Anemia may be related to increased plasma volume that occurs in early phase *5544* Anemia correlates closely with the degree of inflammation; persistence of anemia suggests continued rheumatic activity *1980* Usually normochromic and normocytic and resolves without specific treatment *2304*

Hemoglobin *Blood Decrease* Anemia is common (hemoglobin usually 8 - 12 g/dL); gradually improves as activity subsides; microcytic type. May be related to increased plasma volume that occurs in early phase *5544* Usually normochromic and normocytic and resolves without specific treatment *2304* Anemia correlates closely with the degree of inflammation; persistence of anemia suggests continued rheumatic activity *1980*

Immunoglobulin A *Serum Increase* Increased immunoglobulins, particularly of IgG and IgA, and elevated immune responses to streptococcal cellular and extracellular products *4551* Increase in the globulin fraction of the serum proteins is frequent and mainly due to an increase in IgG and IgA *2304*

Immunoglobulin G *Serum Increase* Increased immunoglobulins, particularly of IgG and IgA, and elevated immune responses to streptococcal cellular and extracellular products *4551* Increase in the globulin fraction of the serum proteins is frequent and mainly due to an increase in IgG and IgA *2304*

Immunoglobulins *Serum Increase* Increased immunoglobulins, particularly of IgG and IgA, and elevated immune responses to streptococcal cellular and extracellular products *4551*

Lactate Dehydrogenase *Serum Increase* In some cases of acute rheumatic carditis *1290*

Leukocytes *Blood Increase* Common leukocytosis with counts of 12,000 - 24,000 /µL and increased percentage of polymorphonuclear cells *367* Increase may persist for weeks after fever subsides. Count may decrease with salicylate and ACTH therapy *5544* Frequently present early in disease *2304*
Synovial Fluid Increase Increased number of white cells in synovial fluid, ranging from 300 - 98,000 /µL *5544* 10,000 - 15,000 /µL *1980*
Urine Increase Indicates mild focal nephritis *5544* Moderate increase in RBCs and WBCs in urine *367*

Mucoprotein *Serum Increase* Observed effect *1980*

Neutrophils *Blood Increase* Reported effect *5677*
Synovial Fluid Increase Increased number neutrophils, ranging from 8 - 98 /µL *5544*

Norepinephrine *Urine Increase* Epinephrine and norepinephrine increase in proportion to the severity of circulatory failure. Catecholamine excretion, especially norepinephrine, is significantly raised in grades 3 and 4 of hemodynamic disturbance *5735*

Properdin Factor B *Plasma No Effect* Mean concentration typically normal or slightly increased in patients with rheumatic fever *4682*

Protein *Serum Increase* Increase in the globulin fraction of the serum proteins is frequent and mainly due to an increase in IgG and IgA *2304*
Urine Increase Proteinuria may occur *367* Slight febrile albuminuria. Indicates mild focal nephritis. Concomitant glomerulonephritis appears in up to 2.5% of cases *5544*

Rheumatoid Factor *Serum No Effect* Concentration may be normal *5544*

Vanillylmandelic Acid *Urine Increase* Increased VMA excretion was observed in cases of grade 4 hemodynamic disturbance *5735*

VDRL *Serum Positive* Not uncommon to encounter biologic false positive reactions *367*

Viscosity *Synovial Fluid Decrease* Reported effect *1980*

398.90 Rheumatic Heart Disease

Carnitine, Free *Plasma Decrease* Mean concentration in 11 patients with rheumatic heart disease of 80.9 ± 28.2 µmol/L significantly less than 89.5 ± 48.2 µmol/L in healthy controls *3736*
Tissue Decrease Mean concentration in myocardium of 11 patients with rheumatic heart disease of 0.72 ± 0.37 µmol/g dry weight significantly less than 1.44 ± 1.03 µmol/g dry weight in myocardium from healthy controls *3736*

CD3+ Lymphocytes *Blood* *No Effect* In 15 patients with chronic rheumatic heart disease mean concentration of 3.10 ± 0.90 x 10^3 cells/µL not significantly different from 3.64 ± 0.58 x 10^3 cells/µL in 15 healthy controls *3737*

CD4+:CD8+ Lymphocyte Ratio *Blood* *No Effect* In 15 patients with chronic rheumatic heart disease mean ratio of 1.01 ± 0.14 not significantly different from 1.10 ± 0.21 in 15 healthy controls *3737*

CD4+ Lymphocytes *Blood* *Increase* Three groups were included: 13 patients with active RHD, 12 with non-active RHD, and 14 control children. T helper (CD4+) cells did not differ significantly between groups *5849*
Blood *No Effect* In 15 patients with chronic rheumatic heart disease mean concentration of 1.74 ± 0.26 x 10^3 cells/µL not significantly different from 1.74 ± 0.32 x 10^3 cells/µL in 15 healthy controls *3737*

CD8+ Lymphocytes *Blood* *Increase* In 15 patients with chronic rheumatic heart disease mean concentration of 1.66 ± 0.26 x 10^3 cells/µL significantly different from 1.60 ± 0.14 x 10^3 cells/µL in 15 healthy controls *3737* Three groups were included: 13 patients with active RHD, 12 with non-active RHD, and 14 control children. A decrease in CD8+ cells may be related to rheumatic activity *5849*

CD16+ Lymphocytes *Blood* *No Effect* In 15 patients with acute chronic rheumatic heart disease mean concentration of 0.76 ± 0.16 x 10^3 cells/µL not significantly different from 0.84 ± 0.166 x 10^3 cells/µL in 15 healthy controls *3737*

CD19+ Lymphocytes *Blood* *No Effect* In 15 patients with chronic rheumatic heart disease mean concentration of 0.94 ± 0.18 x 10^3 cells/µL not significantly different from 1.10 ± 0.09 x 10^3 cells/µL in 15 healthy controls *3737*

CD25+ Lymphocytes *Blood* *No Effect* In 15 patients with chronic rheumatic heart disease mean concentration of 0.48 ± 0.16 x 10^3 cells/µL not significantly different from 0.55 ± 0.14 x 10^3 cells/µL in 15 healthy controls *3737*

Interleukin-1α *Serum* *No Effect* In 15 patients with chronic rheumatic heart disease mean concentration of 2.7 ± 2.3 pg/mL not significantly different from 3.1 ± 1.4 pg/mL in 15 healthy controls *3737*

Interleukin-2 *Serum* *Increase* Evaluated in children with rheumatic heart disease (RHD). Three groups were included: 13 patients with active RHD, 12 with non-active RHD, and 14 control children. Serum IL-2 was measured by radioimmunoassay and monoclonal antibodies respectively. Patients with active RHD showed a significant increase in IL-2 concentrations compared with controls with a mean (SEM) IL-2 of 3.48 (0.62) v 1.26 (0.16) U/mL *5849*
Serum *No Effect* In 15 patients with chronic rheumatic heart disease mean concentration of 0.4 ± 0.05 pg/mL not significantly different from 0.3 ± 0.47 pg/mL in 15 healthy controls *3737*

Tumor Necrosis Factor-α *Serum* *No Effect* In 15 patients with chronic rheumatic heart disease mean concentration of 6.6 ± 3.9 pg/mL not significantly different from 6.4 ± 4.6 pg/mL in 15 healthy controls *3737*

Hypertensive Diseases

401.00 Malignant Hypertension

Albumin *Urine* *Increase* May occur from leaking glomerular capillaries. significant proteinuria 500 mg/d or > 1+ by qualitative estimation) occurs very rarely in benign essential hypertension; their presence suggests the malignant phase or primary renal parenchymal disease *900*

Aldosterone *Plasma* *Increase* Most patients *2034*

Ammonia *Blood* *Decrease* Decreased arterial ammonia in azotemic patients, (mean of 34 ± 1.4 mmol/L) *4213*

Bicarbonate *Serum* *Increase* Metabolic alkalosis may occur with potassium loss *1980*

Carbon Dioxide Partial Pressure *Blood* *Increase* Metabolic alkalosis may occur with potassium loss *1980*

Catecholamines *Urine* *Increase* Slightly increased *5544*

Cholesterol *Serum* *Increase* Mean concentration was 199.7 ± 7.5 mg/dL in 24 male patients compared to 170.9 ± 6.3 in controls *795*

Cholesterol Esters *Serum* *Increase* Mean concentration was 118.0 ± 8.4 mg/dL in 24 male patients (normal 101.7 ± 6.3 mg/dL) *795*

Erythrocytes *Urine* *Increase* Malignant phase of hypertension. May occur from leaking glomerular capillaries. Hematuria occurs very rarely in benign essential hypertension; its presence suggests the malignant phase or primary renal parenchymal disease *900*

Hematocrit *Blood* *Decrease* Many patients show evidence of microangiopathic hemolytic anemia *2034*

Hemoglobin *Blood* *Decrease* Many patients show evidence of microangiopathic hemolytic anemia *2034*

17-Hydroxycorticosteroids *Urine* *Increase* Slightly increased *5544*

17-Ketogenic Steroids *Urine* *Increase* Slightly increased *5544*

pH *Blood* *Increase* Metabolic alkalosis may occur with potassium loss *1980*

Phospholipids *Serum* *Increase* In 24 male patients, mean concentration was 234.7 ± 13.5 mg/dL compared to 204.1 ± 3.5 mg/dL in normals *795*

Potassium *Serum* *Decrease* Many diseases including hyperaldosteronism are characterized by low serum concentration *2304*

Renin Activity *Plasma* *Increase* Most patients *2034* *2304*

Triglycerides *Serum* *Increase* In 24 male patients, mean concentration was 93.4 ± 6.3 mg/dL compared to 76.1 ± 3.7 in controls *795*

Vanillylmandelic Acid *Urine* *Increase* May occur *2034*

401.90 Essential Hypertension

Adrenomedullin *Plasma* *Increase* In 35 patients with essential hypertension mean concentration in those with WHO stage I disease of 2.9 ± 0.2 fmol/mL and of 3.4 ± 0.3 fmol/mL in those with stage II disease significantly higher than that in normal individuals, mean concentration of 2.3 ± 0.2 fmol/mL *2356* Mean concentration in 15 patients with essential hypertension of 3.4 fmol/mL significantly different from 2.7 fmol/mL in 10 normotensive controls *3802*

Albumin *Serum* *Decrease* Occasionally observed *5544*
Serum *No Effect* In 45 patients with essential hypertension concentration of 42 ± 3 g/L not significantly different from 42 ± 2 g/L in 20 healthy controls *1802*
Urine *Increase* In 165 patients with mild to moderate essential hypertension mean excretion of 20.6 ± 25.3 mg/d *2922* In 20 normotensives morning excretion of 12.65 ± 1.43 µg/min compared with 11.05 ± 1.18 µg/min at night and 43.21 ± 4.57 µg/min in 20 hypertensives in the morning compared with 20.77 ± 2.14 µg/min at night *5880* Median excretion of 13.2 mg/d in 26 patients with essential hypertension significantly different from 5.56 mg/d in 16 normotensive healthy controls *276* In hypertensive men and women significant positive slope observed with diastolic blood pressure with mean slope of 78.6 mm Hg *3768* In mild hypertensives with hypertension of < 5, 5 - 10, 10 -15 and > 15 years duration mean excretion in 12 h overnight urine specimens was 2.33, 2.4, 4.7 and 12.58 µg/min, respectively. In moderate hypertensives excretion was 4.2 and 14.0 µg/min in patients with history of < 5 years and 5 - 10 years respectively. Controls excreted a mean of 2.48 ± 2.4 µg/min *5087* In 29 patients with essential hypertension mean excretion of 29.21 ± 26.44 mg/d significantly greater than 9.08 ± 3.92 mg/d in 39 healthy controls *3087*

Aldolase *Serum* *Increase* There was a high correlation between systolic and diastolic BP and aldolase activity *310*

Aldosterone *Plasma* *Increase* Decreased metabolic clearance rate *3835* Mean peak of about 16 ng/dL in 10 hypertensives higher than peak of 13 ng/dL in 10 normotensives and trough of about 7 ng/dL higher than trough of 4 ng/dL in 10 normotensives *4180*
Urine *Decrease* Decreased metabolic clearance rate of aldosterone *3835*

Alkaline Phosphatase *Serum* *Increase* Mean activity as observed in a population of 6,000 adults increased significantly from 55.8 U/L in women with systolic blood pressure 150 - 159 mm Hg of 71.8 U/L significantly higher than 55.8 U/L in women with mean systolic blood pressure of 100 - 109 mm Hg: effect in men somewhat less marked but still highly significant *1823*

401.90 Essential Hypertension *(continued)*

Amino-terminal Propeptide of Type I I Procollagen *Serum Increase* In 15 patients with essential hypertension mean concentration of 11.20 ± 0.76 ng/mL significantly higher than 8.47 ± 0.77 ng/mL in 30 normotensive controls *2940*

Ammonia *Blood Decrease* Decreased arterial ammonia in azotemic patients, mean of 34 ± 1.4 mmol/L *4213*

Angiotensin-converting Enzyme *Serum Increase* Mean concentration in 55 patients with untreated essential hypertension 28 ± 1 U/mL compared with 28.5 ± 3 U/mL in 11 patients with untreated renovasular hypertension and 21 ± 1.5 U/mL in 23 normotensive individuals *3776*
Serum No Effect Normal levels for 14 patients with this disorder *4561* *1272* No difference was detected between men and woman and between normotensives and hypertensives *1272* Normal levels for 14 patients with this disorder *5427*

Antidiuretic Hormone *Plasma Decrease* Concentration significantly reduced in patients with low renin essential hypertension than in normal subjects *124*
Plasma Increase Concentration higher in patients with malignant hypertension than in normal controls *124*

α_2-Antiplasmin *Plasma No Effect* In 99 hypertensives (41 men, 58 women) mean concentration of 109 ± 11% normal not significantly different compared with 107 ± 11% normal in 286 normotensive controls (134 men, 152 women) *1760*

Antithrombin III *Plasma No Effect* In 54 hypertensives median thrombin-antithrombin III concentration of 2.9 µg/L not significantly different from 2.6 µg/L in 54 age-matched healthy controls *1208*

α_1-Antitrypsin *Urine Increase* In 29 patients with essential hypertension mean excretion of 0.48 ± 0.96 mg/d significantly greater than 0.12 ± 0.44 mg/d in 39 healthy controls *3087*

Apolipoprotein A *Serum Increase* In 38 female hypertensives mean concentration of 180.2 ± 6.7 mg/dL significantly different from 185.1 ± 12.3 mg/dL in 58 healthy female controls, and 155.8 ± 7.5 mg/dL in 27 hypertensive men not significantly different from 158.4 ± 7.5 mg/dL in 47 healthy normotensive women *1507*
Serum No Effect In 10 hypertensives with microalbuminuria mean concentration of 154 mg/dL not significantly different from 156 mg/dL in 15 hypertensives without microalbuminuria and 157 mg/dL in 20 normotensive controls *437*

Apolipoprotein A-I *Serum Decrease* In 8 patients with untreated essential hypertension mean concentration of 1.04 ± 0.18 g/L significantly different from 1.15 ± 0.18 g/L in 8 age-matched healthy controls *4424* Significantly reduced to 130 ± 28 mg/dL in 50 outpatients with essential hypertension compared with 145 ± 28 mg/dL in 50 age and sex matched normotensive controls *738*
Serum No Effect In 99 hypertensives (41 men, 58 women) mean concentration of 137 ± 28 mg/dL not significantly different compared with 137 ± 31 mg/dL in 286 normotensive controls (134 men, 152 women) *1760*

Apolipoprotein A-II *Serum Decrease* Significant reduction to 33 ± 10 mg/dL in 50 outpatients with essential hypertension compared with 40 ± 11 mg/dL in 50 age and sex matched normotensive controls *738*

Apolipoprotein B *Serum Increase* In 8 patients with untreated essential hypertension mean concentration of 1.11 ± 0.12 g/L significantly different from 0.86 ± 0.27 g/L in 8 age-matched healthy controls *4424* In 99 hypertensives (41 men, 58 women) mean concentration of 147 ± 40 mg/dL significantly different compared with 136 ± 41 mg/dL in 286 normotensive controls (134 men, 152 women) *1760* In 38 female hypertensives mean concentration of 113.9 ± 5.6 mg/dL significantly different from 89.2 ± 8.5 mg/dL in 58 healthy female controls, and 110.5 ± 5.8 mg/dL in 27 hypertensive men not significantly different from 88.8 ± 4.9 mg/dL in 47 healthy normotensive women *1507*
Serum No Effect No significant difference observed between concentrations of 50 outpatients with essential hypertension and 50 normotensive age and sex matched controls *738* In 10 hypertensives with microalbuminuria mean concentration of 110 mg/dL not significantly different from 109.5 mg/dL in 15 hypertensives without microalbuminuria and 104 mg/dL in 20 normotensive controls *437*

Apolipoprotein C-II *Serum Decrease* In 50 outpatients with essential hypertension significant reduction to 4.0 ± 2.6 mg/dL compared with 5.4 ± 2.9 mg/dL in 50 normotensive age and sex matched controls *738*

Apolipoprotein C-III *Serum No Effect* No significant difference observed between concentrations in 50 outpatients with essential hypertension and 50 normotensives age and sex matched *738*

Apolipoprotein E *Serum Decrease* Significant reduction to 5.0 ± 1.8 mg/dL in 50 outpatients with essential hypertension compared with 4.3 ± 1.8 mg/dL in 50 normotensive age and sex matched controls *738*

Ascorbic Acid *Serum Decrease* In 168 healthy individuals significant inverse relationship observed between plasma concentration and systolic blood pressure (r = -.0.18) and diastolic blood pressure (r = -0.20) *3594*

Aspartate Aminotransferase *Serum Increase* In 29% of 101 patients hospitalized for this disorder *1576*

Atrial Natriuretic Peptide *Plasma Increase* Concentration higher (16.34 ± 2.67 fmol/mL) in 8 low renin patients than in both 11 modulators (10.59 ± 4.29 fmol/mL) and 12 non-modulators (9.85 ± 2.64 fmol/mL) with essential hypertension and in 7 normotensive controls (9.88 ± 2.05 fmol/mL) *3169* In 21 hypertensives mean concentration of 45 ± 3 pg/mL versus 36 ± 3 pg/mL in sex, race and age matched controls *3580* Mean peak concentration in early morning of 105 pg/mL compared with 70 pg/mL in normotensives and mean nadir of 50 pg/mL occurred earlier than nadir of 25 pg/mL in evening in normotensives *4180* In patients with untreated essential hypertension significantly higher concentration observed, 92.9 ± 12.9 pg/mL, compared with 37.8 ± 6.0 pg/mL in age-matched controls *5071* In 21 hypertensive patients with low urinary kallikrein excretion mean ANP concentration of 42.2 ± 2.1 pg/mL significantly higher than 33.8 ± 2.5 pg/mL in normal urinary kallikrein excretion group (54 patients) *1131* In 10 patients with untreated uncomplicated mild to moderate essential hypertension mean concentration of 38.4 ± 6.9 pg/mL significantly higher than in 15 normotensive controls (18.3 ± 1.8 pg/mL) *5177* In 30 hypertensive patients concentration of 46.8 ± 3.3 pg/mL compared with 36.8 ± 3.3 pg/mL in 22 normotensive controls *3773* Significantly higher in hypertensives than in normotensives and borderline hypertensives. Highest concentrations occur in patients with left ventricular hypertrophy. Positive correlation observed between mean blood pressure and plasma ANP concentrations *2741* In many patients with essential hypertension mean concentration increased *4509* Mean concentration in patients with essential hypertension of 58.7 ± 6.7 pg/mL compared with 42.0 ± 4.1 pg/mL in normotensives *3774* Mean concentration in 15 patients with essential hypertension of 22 pg/mL significantly different from 11 pg/mL in 10 normotensive controls *3802*
Plasma No Effect No significant difference between concentrations in patients with essential hypertension (38.5 ± 2.8 pg/mL) and healthy normotensives (37.9 ± 1.4 pg/mL) *5774* Mean concentration in 44 patients with mild untreated essential hypertension of 13.2 (SEM 1.5) ng/L compared with 13.0 (1.3) ng/L in 48 normotensive controls *2924* In patients with essential hypertension concentrations not increased except in the severe form with diastolic pressure above 110 mm Hg *683* No significant difference observed between concentrations in 4 normotensive individuals (mean 24.3 to 27.9 pg/mL) compared with mean of 26.3 to 37.2 pg/mL in 4 hypertensives *1518*

Bicarbonate *Serum Increase* In 59% of 98 patients hospitalized for this disorder *1576*

Bradykinin *Urine Decrease* Compared with a healthy control group, a significantly lower mean kinin excretion was found in patients with essential hypertension *4975*

Brain Natriuretic Peptide *Plasma Increase* Mean concentration in 15 patients with essential hypertension of 13 pg/mL significantly different from 7 pg/mL in 10 normotensive controls *3802*

Cadmium *Serum Increase* No association between subclinical cadmium exposure and hypertension but confirmed relationship with cigarette smoking *368* There was a high correlation between systolic and diastolic BP and cadmium levels *310*

Calcium *Serum Decrease* Concentration reduced in 60 hypertensive individuals compared with that in 37 normotensive controls but to a lesser extent than that of ionized calcium *1646*

Serum *No Effect* No significant correlation observed between blood pressure and serum total calcium concentration *623* No significant difference observed between the concentrations in patients with essential arterial hypertension and of controls *5376*
Urine *Increase* Significantly increased excretion observed in 60 hypertensive individuals compared with 37 normotensive controls *1646*

Calcium, Complexed *Serum* *Decrease* In hypertensive individuals mean concentration reduced by 0.23 mg/dL compared with normotensive controls *1520*

Calcium, Protein-bound *Serum* *Increase* In hypertensive individuals mean concentration increased by 0.36 mg/dL compared with normotensive controls *1520*

Calcium, Ultrafiltrable *Serum* *Decrease* Mean concentration reduced in hypertensive individuals (by 0.32 mg/dL) compared with control individuals *1520*

Carcinoembryonic Antigen *Serum* *Increase* 28% of patients had values > 2.5 ng/mL *4891* In 156 patients with hypertension, 72% had concentrations less than 2.5 ng/mL, 26% had concentrations between 2.6 and 5.0 ng/mL, 2% had concentrations between 5.1 and 10.0 ng/mL and 0% had concentrations greater than 10.0 ng/mL *2010*

Catecholamines *Plasma* *Increase* Raised plasma catecholamines in some patients with primary hypertension *1073*
Urine *Increase* Up to 100 µg/d may be excreted *1290*

Cholesterol *Serum* *Increase* In 27 nondiabetic salt-sensitive normal and high renin hypertensive patients who were unable to modulate their adrenal and renal blood flow responses to a change in dietary sodium mean concentration of 209 ± 7 mg/dL and 238 ± 11 mg/dL in 19 modulators significantly different from normal range of 110 - 200 mg/dL *1616* Frequently elevated *2034* In 38 female hypertensives mean concentration of 260.6 ± 8.7 mg/dL not significantly different from 241.4 ± 23.8 mg/dL in 58 healthy female controls, and 235.1 ± 8.6 mg/dL in 27 hypertensive men not significantly different from 214.8 ± 8.2 mg/dL in 47 healthy normotensive women *1507* In 15 patients with mean age of 47.2 ± 1.6 years and essential hypertension mean concentration of 6.3 ± 0.1 mmol/L significantly greater than 5.6 ± 0.2 mmol/L in 15 normotensive men with mean age of 47.2 ± 1.6 years *2993* Hypertension often associated with increased serum cholesterol concentration *929* In 10 hypertensives with microalbuminuria mean concentration of 5.77 mmol/L not significantly higher than 4.99 mmol/L in 15 hypertensives without microalbuminuria and 5.02 mmol/L in 20 normotensive controls *437*
Serum *No Effect* In 23 hypertensive men with normal renin-sodium profiles, 9 with low renin-sodium profiles and 13 with high renin-sodium profiles mean concentrations of 224 ± 37 mg/dL, 211 ± 33 mg/dL and 234 ± 52 mg/dL respectively not significantly different from 224 ± 41 mg/dL in hypertensive population as a whole *4123* Mean concentration in patients with essential hypertension not significantly different from that in normotensives: 8 low renin patients 4.6 ± 0.1 mmol/L, 11 non-modulators 4.7 ± 0.1 mmol/L, 12 modulators 4.7 ± 0.1 mmol/L and 7 normotensives 4.3 ± 0.2 mmol/L *3169* In 8 patients with untreated essential hypertension mean concentration of 6.44 ± 1.28 mmol/L not significantly different from 6.20 ± 1.28 mmol/L in 8 age-matched healthy controls *4424* In 25 previously untreated patients with mild essential hypertension mean concentration of 205.5 ± 40.8 mg/dL not significantly different from 199.4 ± 35.8 mg/dL in 22 normotensive controls *4452* In 99 hypertensives (41 men, 58 women) mean concentration of 252 ± 65 mg/dL not significantly different compared with 241 ± 56 mg/dL in 286 normotensive controls (134 men, 152 women) *1760* In 8 non-insulin resistant nonobese patients with untreated essential hypertension mean concentration of 5.2 ± 0.7 mmol/L not significantly different from 5.6 ± 0.7 mmol/L in 8 healthy normotensive controls *232* In 60 women with moderate essential hypertension aged over 65 years mean concentration of 219.5 ± 48.9 mg/dL not significantly different from 207.6 ± 58.0 mg/dL in 46 normotensive women of similar age *131* No significant difference observed between 50 outpatients with essential hypertension and 50 age and sex matched normotensive controls *738* Median concentration of 6.3 mmol/L and lower and upper quartiles 5.4 and 7.1 mmol/L repectively compared with reference interval of 4.0 - 7.5 mmol/L *1208* Mean concentration of 222 ± 32 mg/dL observed in 15 hypertensive patients not significantly different from 206 ± 8 mg/dL in 23 normotensive controls *2887* In 45 patients with essential hypertension concentration of 5.3 ± 0.9 mmol/L not significantly different from 5.2 ± 0.7 mmol/L in 20 healthy controls *1802*

Cholesterol Ester Transfer Protein *Serum* *No Effect* In 8 patients with newly diagnosed essential hypertension mean concentration of about 57 ± 29 AU/L not significantly different from 67 ± 27 AU/L in 8 healthy controls *3057*

Cholesterol:HDL-Cholesterol Ratio *Serum* *Increase* In 38 female hypertensives mean ratio of 4.3 not significantly different from 4.1 in 58 healthy female controls, and 5.3 in 27 hypertensive men not significantly different from 4.4 in 47 healthy normotensive women *1507*

Cholesterol:Phospholipid Ratio *Red Blood Cells* *Decrease* In 8 patients with untreated essential hypertension mean ratio of 0.94 ± 0.09 significantly different from 1.03 ± 0.05 in 8 age-matched healthy controls *4424*

Cholinesterase *Serum* *Increase* There was a high correlation between systolic and diastolic BP and cholinesterase levels *310*

Chromogranin-A *Serum* *Increase* Mean concentration of 24.1 ± 12.9 U/L in 24 patients with renovascular hypertension higher than that in 21 healthy volunteers in heparin/glutathione plasma (16.3 - 21.5 U/L with upper limit of normal of 30.4 U/L) with 4 patients having concentrations greater than the upper limit of normal *524*

Copper *Serum* *No Effect* No significant difference observed between concentrations of patients with essential arterial hypertension and of healthy controls *5376*

Cortisol *Plasma* *Increase* In 10 hypertensives mean peak of about 18 µg/dL at 08:00 h not significantly different from mean peak of about 17 µg/dL in 10 normotensives and mean trough of about 7 µg/dL at 20:00 h not different from 7 µg/dL at 20:00 h in 10 normotensives *4180*
Plasma *No Effect* Mean concentration of 14.3 ± 3.9 mg/dL observed in 15 hypertensive patients not significantly different from 14.2 ± 0.9 mg/dL in 26 normotensive controls *2887*

Creatinine *Serum* *Increase* In 45 patients with essential hypertension concentration of 79 ± 19 µmol/L significantly different from 56 ± 12 µmol/L in 20 healthy controls *1802* In 49% of 106 patients hospitalized for this disorder *1576*
Serum *No Effect* In 165 patients with mild to moderate essential hypertension mean concentration of 94.7 ± 17.6 µmol/L *2922* Mean concentration of 79.5 ± 16.6 µmol/L in 8 low renin essential hypertensives not significantly different from 88.4 ± 8.8 µmol/L in 11 non-modulators, 88.5 ± 8.8 µmol/L in 12 modulators and 79.5 ± 8.7 µmol/L in 7 normotensive controls *3732* Concentrations nonsignificantly changed to 71.7 ± 9.2 µmol/L in 16 hypertensive patients with impaired glucose tolerance, cholesterol > 5.20 mmol/L and triglycerides > 1.8 mmol/L compared with 72.3 ± 9.3 µmol/L in 22 healthy control individuals *1469* Mean concentration in 15 patients with essential hypertension of 0.9 ± 0.1 mg/dL not significantly different from 0.8 ± 0.2 mg/dL in 10 normotensive controls *3802* Median concentration of 87.5 µmol/L in 26 patients with essential hypertension not significantly different from 93.5 µmol/L in 16 normotensive healthy controls *276* In 25 previously untreated patients with mild essential hypertension mean concentration of 1.01 ± 0.16 mg/dL not significantly different from 0.99 ± 0.13 mg/dL in 22 normotensive controls *4452* In 14 men with borderline hypertension mean concentration of 103 µmol/L not significantly higher than 101 µmol/L in 14 normotensive controls *4827*
Urine *No Effect* In 10 hypertensives receiving 100 mmol sodium and 80 mmol potassium per day diet mean excretion of 1.4 ± 0.3 mmol/d not significantly different from 1.2 ± 0.2 mmol/d in 10 healthy controls on same diet *4180* Mean excretion in 48 individuals aged 18 to 27 y with essential hypertension of 13.2 ± 0.9 mmol/d not significantly different from 14.1 ± 0.9 mmol/d in 25 age-matched controls *4517*

Creatinine Clearance *Urine* *Decrease* In 165 patients with mild to moderate essential hypertension mean clearance 20.6 ± 25.3 mL/s *2922*
Urine *No Effect* In 60 women with moderate essential hypertension aged over 65 years mean clearance of 89.8 ± 14.8 mL/min not significantly different from 92.2 ± 15.2 mL/min in 46 normotensive women of similar age *131*

D-Dimer *Plasma* *No Effect* In 99 hypertensives (41 men, 58 women) mean concentration of 0.10 ± 0.03 µg/mL not significantly different compared with 0.10 ± 0.03 µg/mL in 286 normotensive controls (134 men, 152 women) *1760*

3,4-Dihydroxyphenylalanine *Plasma* *No Effect* In 48 individuals aged 18 to 27 y with essential hypertension mean concentration of 13 ± 1 nmol/L not significantly different from 14 ± 1 nmol/L in 25 age-matched controls *4517*

401.90 Essential Hypertension *(continued)*

2,3-Dinor-6-Keto-Prostaglandin $F_{1\alpha}$ *Urine Decrease* In 46 patients with mild essential hypertension excretion ranged from less than 5 to more than 100 ng/g creatinine with significant negative correlation between excretion and blood pressure. Reduction of excretion of 100 ng/g creatinine was associated with increase of arterial pressure of 14 mm Hg (systolic) and 8 mm Hg (diastolic) *3507*
Urine No Effect In 15 patients with mean age of 47.2 ± 1.6 years and essential hypertension mean excretion of 99 ± 14 pg/mg creatinine not significantly different from 113 ± 9 pg/mg creatinine in 15 normotensive men with mean age of 47.2 ± 1.6 years *2993*

2,3-Dinor-Thromboxane B_2 *Urine No Effect* No significant correlation observed between excretion and blood pressure *3507* In 15 patients with mean age of 47.2 ± 1.6 years and essential hypertension mean excretion of 209 ± 27 pg/mg creatinine not significantly different from 242 ± 29 pg/mg creatinine in 15 normotensive men with mean age of 47.2 ± 1.6 years *2993*

Dopamine *Plasma Increase* Patients with essential hypertension had increased concentrations compared with those in controls *2955*
Urine Increase In 10 hypertensive individuals mean excretion of 266 ± 26 µg/d significantly higher than 186 ± 12 µg/d in 20 borderline hypertensives but not significantly different from 232 ± 19 µg/d in 20 normotensive controls *2603* In 48 patients aged 18 to 27 years with essential hypertension mean excretion of 1,920 ± 80 nmol/d significantly higher than 1,520 ± 130 nmol/d in 25 age-matched normotensive individuals *4517*

Dopamine β-Hydroxylase *Cerebrospinal Fluid No Effect* Mean concentration in 17 patients with essential hypertension of 30.9 ± 2.15 ng/mL compared with 31.7 ± 1.7 ng/mL in 15 healthy individuals *3855*
Serum Increase Mean concentration in 17 patients with essential hypertension of 9.50 ± 1.57 ng/mL compared with 8.78 ± 1.42 ng/mL in 15 healthy controls *3855*

Endothelin *Plasma Increase* In patients with essential hypertension and target organ damage mean concentration significantly increased *3739*
Urine Decrease Urinary excretion in individuals with essential hypertension of 68% from normal of 9- ± 16 ng/d to 29 ± 3 ng/d significantly higher than in healthy individuals *6*

Endothelin-1 *Plasma Increase* Concentrations significantly changed to approximately 1.6 pg/mL in 16 hypertensive patients with impaired glucose tolerance, cholesterol > 5.20 mmol/L and triglycerides > 1.8 mmol/L compared with 0.5 pg/mL in 22 healthy control individuals *1469* In several studies of patients with essential hypertension mean concentration increased typically 0.9 to 2.2-fold over appropriate normals regardless of stage of disease: in 8 patients with pregnancy induced hypertension mean concentration increased by 1.3-fold over reference range in nonpregnant women *328*
Plasma No Effect Under basal conditions mean concentration of 1.32 ± 0.63 pg/mL in 11 hypertensives not significantly different from 1.39 ± 0.57 pg/mL in 9 normotensive controls *3538* Essential hypertensive patients do not appear to have increased production of endothelin *4633* In 17 adult patients with essential hypertension mean concentration of 1.1 ± 0.3 pg/mL not significantly different from 1.3 ± 0.1 pg/mL in 19 healthy adult controls *2198* Essential hypertensive patients do not appear to have increased production of endothelin *4520* No significant difference observed between concentrations in 15 hypertensive non-pregnant women, 3.8 ng/L (range 2.4 - 5.8), compared with 3.6 ng/L (range 2.0 - 5.4), in 23 normotensive non-pregnant women *1512* Mean concentration of 0.40 ± 0.12 pmol/L in 8 pregnant women with chronic hypertension not significantly different from 0.25 ± 0.04 pmol/L in 11 normotensive pregnant women *5066*
Urine Decrease In 17 adult patients with essential hypertension mean excretion of 29 ± 3 ng/d versus 109 ± 21 ng/d in healthy adult controls *2198*

Epinephrine *Plasma Increase* In 30 hypertensives mean concentration of 70.8 ± 10.5 pg/mL compared with 54.8 ± 9.7 pg/mL in 22 normotensive controls *3773* May be observed *1552*
Urine No Effect In 10 hypertensives mean excretion of 8.1 ± 0.9 µg/d not significantly different from 6.9 ± 0.7 µg/d in 20 normotensive controls *2603*

Erythrocytes *Blood Increase* In 14 men with borderline hypertension mean concentration of 5.19 million/µL significantly higher than 4.83 million/µL in 14 normotensive controls *4827*

Erythropoietin *Serum No Effect* In 14 men with borderline hypertension mean concentration of 150 mIU/mL not significantly higher than 145 mIU/mL in 14 normotensive controls *4827*

Estradiol *Plasma Decrease* In 9 hypertensive men with low renin-sodium profile mean concentration of 22.6 ± 3.9 pg/mL different from 26.2 ± 5.3 pg/mL in 23 hypertensives with normal renin-sodium profiles *4123*
Plasma Increase In 13 hypertensive men with high renin-sodium profile mean concentration of 30.1 ± 6.5 pg/mL different from 26.2 ± 5.3 pg/mL in 23 hypertensives with normal renin-sodium profiles *4123*
Plasma No Effect In 23 hypertensive men with normal renin-sodium profile mean concentration of 26.2 ± 5.3 pg/mL not significantly different from 26.6 ± 3.9 pg/mL in hypertensive population as a whole *4123*

Factor VII *Plasma Increase* In men median concentration of 137% significantly higher than 100% in age-matched healthy controls but in hypertensive women median of 147% not significantly different from 139% in age-matched healthy controls *1208*

Factor VIII Coagulant *Plasma Increase* In 54 hypertensive patients median concentration of 116% significantly higher than median of 96% in 50 healthy aged matched controls *1208*

Fatty Acids (FFA), Free *Serum No Effect* In 8 patients with newly diagnosed essential hypertension mean concentration of about 420 µmol/L not significantly different from 430 µmol/L in 8 healthy controls *3057*

Fibrinogen *Plasma Increase* In 99 hypertensives (41 men, 58 women) mean concentration of 332 ± 61 mg/dL significantly increased compared with 311 ± 67 mg/dL in 286 normotensive controls (134 men, 152 women) *1760*
Plasma No Effect In 45 patients with essential hypertension concentration of 2.28 ± 0.68 g/L not significantly different from 2.47 ± 0.29 g/L in 20 healthy controls *1802* In 54 hypertensive patients no significant difference from reference interval of 1.7 - 4.0 g/L *1208*

Fibronectin *Plasma Increase* In 84 patients (50 men, 34 women) with newly diagnosed essential hypertension mean concentration of 99 ± 48% not significantly higher than 86 ± 30% in healthy controls *2708*

Filtration Rate *Red Blood Cells Increase* In 45 patients with essential hypertension red cell filtration rate significantly decreased by 22% to 66.2 ± 21.2 µL/s from 84.8 ± 15.0 µL/s in 20 healthy controls *1802*

Glucose *Serum Increase* In 45 patients with essential hypertension concentration of 5.6 ± 0.6 mmol/L significantly different from 5.2 ± 0.5 mmol/L in 20 healthy controls *1802* Significant increase in glucose and insulin response to a 75 g oral glucose challenge *4493*
Serum No Effect In 25 previously untreated patients with mild essential hypertension mean concentration of 88.3 ± 18.2 mg/dL not significantly different from 91.3 ± 12.8 mg/dL in 22 normotensive controls *4452* In 60 women with moderate essential hypertension aged over 65 years mean concentration of 117.0 ± 49.5 mg/dL not significantly different from 112.8 ± 34.4 mg/dL in 46 normotensive women of similar age *131* In 23 hypertensive men with normal renin-sodium profiles, 9 with low renin-sodium profiles and 13 with high renin-sodium profiles mean concentrations of 85.4 ± 16.5 mg/dL, 89.9 ± 7.8 mg/dL and 90.1 ± 14.1 mg/dL respectively not significantly different from 87.6 ± 14.4 mg/dL in hypertensive population as a whole *4123* In 27 nondiabetic salt-sensitive normal and high renin hypertensive patients who were unable to modulate their adrenal and renal blood flow responses to a change in dietary sodium mean concentration of 87 ± 3 mg/dL not significantly different from 82 ± 2 mg/dL in 19 modulators and normal range of 65 - 95 mg/dL *1616* Mean concentration in 8 patients with low renin essential hypertension, 4.3 ± 0.2 mmol/L, in 11 non-modulators 4.7 ± 0.2 mmol/L, and in 12 modulators 4.6 ± 0.3 mmol/L not significantly different from 4.1 ± 0.1 mmol/L in 7 normotensive controls *3732* In 8 patients with newly diagnosed essential hypertension mean concentration of 5.0 ± 0.5 mmol/L not significantly different from 4.8 ± 0.5 mmol/L in 8 healthy controls *3057*

β-Glucuronidase *Urine Increase* Moderately elevated (33.7 ± 23.4 U/L). Approximately half of the values were above normal *1805*

γ-Glutamyltransferase *Urine* *Increase* In 20 normotensives morning excretion of 23.48 ± 2.85 mU/min compared with 17.00 ± 2.20 mU/min at night and 48.19 ± 5.14 mU/min in 20 hypertensives in the morning compared with 21.84 ± 1.65 mU/min at night *5880*

HDL-Cholesterol *Serum* *Decrease* In 8 patients with untreated essential hypertension mean concentration of 0.98 ± 0.25 mmol/L significantly different from 1.36 ± 0.24 mmol/L in 8 age-matched healthy controls *4424* Concentrations significantly changed to 0.53 ± 0.9 mmol/L in 16 hypertensive patients with impaired glucose tolerance, cholesterol > 5.20 mmol/L and triglycerides > 1.8 mmol/L compared with 1.98 ± 0.16 mmol/L in 22 healthy control individuals *1469* In 45 patients with essential hypertension concentration of 1.3 ± 0.4 mmol/L significantly different from 1.6 ± 0.2 mmol/L in 20 healthy controls *1802* In 99 hypertensives (41 men, 58 women) mean concentration of 42 ± 15 mg/dL significantly decreased compared with 45 ± 15 mg/dL in 286 normotensive controls (134 men, 152 women) *1760*
Serum *Increase* Significant correlation with systolic blood pressure, but not diastolic, in men but not women *5654*
Serum *No Effect* In 10 hypertensives with microalbuminuria mean concentration of 1.29 mmol/L not significantly different from 1.46 mmol/L in 15 hypertensives without microalbuminuria and 1.42 mmol/L in 20 normotensive controls *437* In 54 hypertensives median concentration of 1.2 mmol/L and lower and upper quartiles 0.9 and 1.4 mmol/L respectively compared with reference interval of 0.9-1.7 mmol/L *1208* In 38 female hypertensives mean concentration of 67.1 ± 4.4 mg/dL not significantly different from 66.7 ± 5.0 mg/dL in 58 healthy female controls, and 47.6 ± 3.0 mg/dL in 27 hypertensive men not significantly different from 55.5 ± 3.8 mg/dL in 47 healthy normotensive women *1507* In 8 non-insulin resistant nonobese patients with untreated essential hypertension mean concentration of 1.3 ± 0.2 mmol/L not significantly different from 1.4 ± 0.2 mmol/L in 8 healthy controls *232* No significant difference observed between 50 outpatients with essential hypertension and 50 age and sex matched normotensive controls *738*

Hematocrit *Blood* *Increase* In 14 men with borderline hypertension mean of 0.462 significantly higher than 0.433 in 14 normotensive controls *4827*
Blood *No Effect* In 45 patients with essential hypertension value of 0.42 ± 0.04 not significantly different from 0.44 ± 0.08 in 20 healthy controls *1802* Mean of 46.8 ± 1.0% observed in 21 hypertensive patients not significantly different from 44.4 ± 0.9% in 29 normotensive controls *2887*

Hemoglobin *Blood* *Increase* In 14 men with borderline hypertension mean concentration of 159 g/L significantly higher than 147 g/L in 14 normotensive controls *4827*

Hemoglobin A_{1c} *Blood* *No Effect* In 8 nonobese non-insulin resistant patients with essential hypertension mean % of total 4.2% as in 8 healthy normotensive controls *232*

Hepatocyte Growth Factor *Serum* *No Effect* In 22 patients with peripheral arterial disease and hypertension mean concentration of 0.39 ± 0.02 ng/mL not significantly different from 0.42 ± 0.03 ng/mL in 15 normotensive patients with peripheral arterial disease *5817*

Homocysteine *Plasma* *Increase* Mean concentration in individuals being screened for cardiac risk factors showed mean concentration of 10.2 ± 1.2 µmol/L in 82 hypertensives significantly greater than mean of 8.9 ± 1.4 µmol/L in 126 normotensives *3251*

Homovanillic Acid *Urine* *Decrease* In 24 patients with established hypertension mean excretion of 17.6 ± 6.2 nmol/mL, in 14 patients with borderline hypertension of 16.1 ± 5.9 nmol/mL compared with 23.7 ± 8.9 nmol/mL in 18 normotensive controls *1327*

Hydrogen Peroxide *Plasma* *Increase* Mean concentration of 3.16 ± 0.14 µmol/L observed in 21 hypertensive patients significantly different from 2.50 ± 0.16 µmol/L in 29 normotensive controls *2887*

4-Hydroxy-3-Methoxy-Phenylglycol *Urine* *No Effect* No significant difference observed in excretions in 24 patients with established hypertension (7.8 ± 4.1 nmol/mL), 14 patients with borderline hypertension (7.0 ± 3.9 nmol/mL) and 18 normotensive controls (9.6 ± 3.9 nmol/mL) *1327*

25-Hydroxy Vitamin D *Serum* *Decrease* Of 290 medical patients, 103 had hypertension which had a correlation of p = 0.009 with hypovitaminosis *5212*

18-Hydroxycorticosterone *Urine* *No Effect* In 10 patients with essential hypertension mean excretion of 3.1 ± 0.6 µg/d not significantly different from 3.6 ± 0.5 µg/d in 11 normotensive controls *3535*

18-Hydroxycortisol *Urine* *No Effect* In 10 patients with essential hypertension mean excretion of 172 ± 15 µg/d not significantly different from 142 ± 35 µg/d in 11 normotensive controls *3535*

5-Hydroxyindoleacetic Acid *Cerebrospinal Fluid* *Increase* In 20 individuals with sustained hypertension concentration significantly higher than in 15 healthy controls *4759*

Immunoglobulin G *Serum* *No Effect* No significant difference observed between concentrations in 87 hypertensive and 87 normotensive controls *1051*
Urine *Increase* Median excretion of 4.52 mg/d in 26 patients with essential hypertension significantly different from 3.41 mg/d in 16 normotensive healthy controls *276*

Immunoglobulin M *Serum* *No Effect* No significant difference observed between concentrations in 87 hypertensive and 87 normotensive patients *1051*

Insulin *Plasma* *Decrease* In 9 hypertensive men with low renin-sodium profile mean concentration of 14.4 ± 5.5 µU/mL different from 21.1 ± 11.6 µU/mL in 23 hypertensives with normal renin-sodium profiles *4123*
Plasma *Increase* Concentration may be increased *4493* Significant increase in glucose and insulin response to a 75 g oral glucose *4746* Mean concentration of 87.0 ± 10.8 pmol/L in 11 patients with non-modulating essential hypertension significantly higher than mean concentrations in low renin patients (54.6 ± 16.4 pmol/L), modulators (68.4 ± 15.6 pmol/L) and normotensives (63.1 ± 21.6 pmol/L) *3169* In 13 hypertensive men with high renin-sodium profile mean concentration of 27.2 ± 17.5 µU/mL different from 21.1 ± 11.6 µU/mL in 23 hypertensives with normal renin-sodium profiles *4123* In 27 nondiabetic salt-sensitive normal and high renin hypertensive patients who were unable to modulate their adrenal and renal blood flow responses to a change in dietary sodium mean concentration of 17 ± 2 µU/mL significantly different from 10 ± 2 µU/mL in 19 modulators and normal range of 4 - 11 µU/mL *1616* Mean effect size of 0.28 between diastolic blood pressure and plasma insulin concentration as observed in several studies *1121*
Plasma *No Effect* In 8 patients with newly diagnosed essential hypertension mean concentration of 72 ± 34 pmol/L not significantly different from 55 ± 32 pmol/L in 8 healthy controls *3057* In 23 hypertensive men with normal renin-sodium profile mean concentration of 21.1 ± 11.6 µU/mL not significantly different from 21.4 ± 13.1 µU/mL in hypertensive population as a whole *4123* Mean concentration in 8 patients with low renin essential hypertension, 54.6 ± 16.4 pmol/L, and in 12 patients with modulating essential hypertension, 68.4 ± 15.6 pmol/L, not significantly different from 63.1 ± 21.6 pmol/L in 7 normotensive controls *3732*

Ionized Calcium *Serum* *Decrease* In 60 hypertensive patients concentration significantly lower than in 37 normotensive controls *1646* In hypertensive individuals mean concentration reduced by 0.07 mg/dL compared with normotensive controls *1520*
Serum *No Effect* No correlation observed in hypertensives between blood pressure and serum ionized calcium concentration *623*

Kallikrein *Urine* *No Effect* Excretion not significantly different from that in normotensives although in older hypertensives (over 40 years of age) excretion actually decreased *2763*

6-Keto-Prostaglandin $F_{1\alpha}$ *Plasma* *Decrease* In 26 hypertensive individuals significant decrease observed in comparison with concentration in 25 normotensive controls *802*
Urine *Decrease* In 46 patients with mild essential hypertension excretion rate ranged from 5 to 100 ng/g creatinine with significant negative correlation with blood pressure. A reduction of 100 ng/g creatinine was associated with an increased pressure of 19 mm Hg (systolic) and 12 mm Hg (diastolic) *3507*

LDL-Cholesterol *Serum* *Increase* Concentrations significantly changed to 5.57 ± 0.51 mmol/L in 16 hypertensive patients with impaired glucose tolerance, cholesterol > 5.20 mmol/L and triglycerides > 1.8 mmol/L compared with 2.51 ± 0.2 mmol/L in 22 healthy control individuals *1469* In 10 hypertensives with microalbuminuria mean concentration of 3.9 mmol/L not significantly different from 2.9 mmol/L in 15 hypertensives without microalbuminuria and 2.87 mmol/L in 20 normotensive

401.90 Essential Hypertension *(continued)*

LDL-Cholesterol *(continued)*
controls *437* In 38 female hypertensives mean concentration of 178.6 ± 9.4 mg/dL significantly different from 139.8 ± 10.3 mg/dL in 58 healthy female controls, and 164.9 ± 7.6 mg/dL in 27 hypertensive men significantly different from 138.0 ± 8.5 mg/dL in 47 healthy normotensive women *1507*
Serum *No Effect* In 99 hypertensives (41 men, 58 women) mean concentration of 149 ± 48 mg/dL not significantly different compared with 156 ± 45 mg/dL in 286 normotensive controls (134 men, 152 women) *1760* In 8 non-insulin resistant nonobese patients with untreated essential hyprtension mean concentration of 3.2 ± 0.7 mmol/L not significantly different from 3.5 ± 0.8 mmol/L in 8 healthy controls *232* In 54 hypertensives median concentration of 4.2 mmol/L and lower and upper quartile of 3.2 and 4.8 mmol/L respectively compared with reference interval of 3.0 - 5.0 mmol/L *1208* No significant difference observed between 50 outpatients with essential hypertension and 50 normotensive age and sex matched controls *738*

Lead *Blood* *Increase* A significant correlation between high blood lead levels and high blood pressure *368*

Lecithin:Cholesterol Acyltransferase *Serum* *No Effect* In 8 patients with newly diagnosed essential hypertension mean concentration of about 68 ± 25 AU/L not significantly different from 51 ± 17 AU/L in 8 healthy controls *3057*

Lecithin:Cholesterol Acyltransferase:Cholesterol Ester Transfer Protein Ratio *Serum* *Increase* In 8 patients with newly diagnosed essential hypertension mean ratio of 1.40 ± 0.64 significantly different from 0.79 ± 0.15 in 8 healthy controls *3057*

Lipoprotein A *Serum* *Increase* In 10 hypertensives with microalbuminuria mean concentration of 24.8 mg/dL significantly higher than 9.4 mg/dL in 15 hypertensives without microalbuminuria and 3.8 mg/dL in 20 normotensive controls *437*

Lipoprotein Lp(a) *Serum* *Increase* In 51 patients with untreated hypertension median concentration of 142 mg/L significantly different from 43 mg/L in 69 healthy volunteers, with 16.2% above 95th percentile of 361 mg/L *5417* In 38 female hypertensives median concentration of 200.5 mg/L significantly different from 94.0 mg/L in 58 healthy female controls, and 130.1 g/L in 27 hypertensive men not significantly different from 118 mg/L in 47 normotensive male controls *1507* Significant positive relationship observed in hypertensives between systolic blood pressure but not in other individuals. Borderline independent relationship observed between diastolic blood pressure and Lp(a) concentration in men *4892*
Serum *No Effect* In 54 hypertensives median concentration of 122 mg/L and lower and upper quartiles 57 and 338 mg/L respectively compared with reference interval of 0 - 300 mg/L *1208* In 99 hypertensives (41 men, 58 women) mean concentration of 30 ± 33 mg/dL not significantly different compared with 28 ± 32 mg/dL in 286 normotensive controls (134 men, 152 women) *1760* No significant correlation observed with either systolic or diastolic blood pressure in either men or women *4892*

Magnesium *Serum* *No Effect* No significant difference observed between concentrations in 60 hypertensive individuals and 37 normotensive controls *1646* No significant difference observed between the concentrations of patients with essential arterial hypertension and of controls *5376*
Urine *Increase* Significantly increased excretion observed in 60 hypertensive patients compared with excretion in 37 normotensive controls although serum concentrations similar *1646*

Metanephrine *Urine* *Increase* In 138 hypertensive men mean excretion of 0.3 to 2.0 μmol/d and in 185 hypertensive women mean excretion of 0.2 to 1.3 μmol/d *2529*
Urine *No Effect* In 977 patients with essential hypertension mean excretion of 1.7 ± 0.9 μmol/d not significantly different compared with 1.8 ± 1.3 μmol/d in 16 patients with cured pheochromocytoma *2131*

3-Methoxy-5-hydroxyphenylglycol
Cerebrospinal Fluid *Increase* In 20 hypertensives significantly increased concentration observed in comparison with 15 controls *4759*

Monoamine Oxidase *Platelets* *Decrease* Significantly lower MAO-B activities were observed in hypertensive patients, both men and women, when compared to normotensive controls *1905*

Na/K-ATPase *Red Blood Cells* *Decrease* Mean activity of 104.60 ± 29.37 nmol P/mg protein/h in 15 middle-aged hypertensives significantly reduced compared with 171.87 ± 34.42 nmol P/mg protein/h in 15 normotensive controls *5364*

N-Acetyl-Glucosaminidase *Urine* *Increase* In 20 normotensives morning excretion of 7.34 ± 0.51 mU/min compared with 6.55 ± 0.39 mU/min at night and 19.10 ± 1.81 mU/min in 20 hypertensives in the morning compared with 10.92 ± 0.87 mU/min at night *5880*

Norepinephrine *Plasma* *Increase* In 30 hypertensive patients mean concentration of 230.8 ± 52.3 pg/mL compared with 138.0 ± 19.6 pg/mL in 22 normotensive controls *3773* Patients with essential hypertension had increased concentrations compared with those in controls *2955*
Urine *Increase* In age matched individuals excretion slightly higher in hypertensives under age 40 years than in normotensive controls and significantly higher in individuals older than 40 years *2982* Mean excretion in 48 individuals aged 18 to 27 y with essential hypertension of 216 ± 11 nmol/d significantly greater than 179 ± 12 nmol/d in 25 normotensive controls *4517*
Urine *No Effect* In 10 hypertensives mean excretion of 40.3 ± 4.8 μg/d not significantly different from 37.4 ± 2.1 μg/d in 20 normotensive controls *1003*

Normetanephrine *Urine* *Increase* In 17 men aged 16 to 35 years mean excretion of 0.7 to 3.4 μmol/d and in 121 older than 35 years of 0.8 to 5.1 μmol/d: in 41 women aged 16 to 35 years mean excretion of 0.5 to 21 μmol/d and in 144 women older than 35 years 0.6 to 3.3 μmol/d *2529*

Parathyroid Hormone *Plasma* *Decrease* Significant negative association of intact PTH concentration with body mass in hypertensive individuals aged 20 to 39 years but not in those aged 40 to 69 years *1878*
Plasma *Increase* In 90 young individuals with mildly raised blood pressure significantly increased concentration (mean 2.3 pmol/L) compared with mean 1,5 pmol/L in 40 normotensive age-matched controls *5722*

Plasminogen *Plasma* *Increase* In 99 hypertensives (41 men, 58 women) mean concentration of 116 ± 19% normal significantly increased compared with 110 ± 17% normal in 286 normotensive controls (134 men, 152 women) *1760*

Plasminogen Activator Inhibitor *Plasma* *Increase* In 99 hypertensives (41 men, 58 women) mean concentration of 24 ± 27 U/mL significantly increased compared with 16 ± 15 U/mL in 286 normotensive controls (134 men, 152 women) *1760*

Plasminogen Activator Inhibitor Antigen *Plasma* *Increase* In 99 hypertensives (41 men, 58 women) mean concentration of 39 ± 35 ng/mL significantly increased compared with 30 ± 33 ng/mL in 286 normotensive controls (134 men, 152 women) *1760*

Platelet Aggregation *Blood* *Increase* Significant increase observed in 26 patients with essential hypertension compared with concentration in 25 normotensive controls *802*

Platelet-derived Growth Factor *Plasma* *Increase* In 25 previously untreated patients with mild essential hypertension mean concentration of 0.63 ± 0.23 ng/mL significantly different from 0.45 ± 0.14 ng/mL in 22 normotensive controls *4452*

Platelets *Blood* *No Effect* In 25 previously untreated patients with mild essential hypertension mean concentration of 236.5 ± 58.2 x 10^3/L not significantly different from 229.3 ± 39.4 x 10^3/L in 22 normotensive controls *4452*

Potassium *Red Blood Cells* *Decrease* Mean concentration of 86.79 ± 5.20 mmol/L in 15 middle-aged hypertensives significantly lower than 96.52 ± 4.66 mmol/L in 15 normotensive controls *5364*
Serum *Decrease* Untreated hypertensive patients frequently presented with low serum concentrations unassociated with acidosis or alkalosis *4527* Characterized by low serum concentration *2304*
Serum *No Effect* No significant difference observed in the concentrations of controls and of individuals with essential arterial hypertension *5376* Mean concentration of 4.81 ± 0.41 mmol/L in 15 middle-aged hypertensives not significantly different from 4.58 ± 0.45 mmol/L in 15 normotensive controls *5364* In 60 women with moderate essential hypertension aged over 65 years mean concentration of 4.08 ± 0.26 mmol/L not significantly different from 4.21 ± 0.27 mmol/L in 46 normotensive women of

similar age *131* In 27 nondiabetic salt-sensitive normal and high renin hypertensive patients who were unable to modulate their adrenal and renal blood flow responses to a change in dietary sodium mean concentration of 4.3 ± 0.1 mmol/L not significantly different from 4.2 ± 0.1 mmol/L in 19 modulators and normal range of 3.6 - 4.8 mmol/L *1616*
Urine No Effect In 10 hypertensives on 100 mmol sodium and 80 mmol potassium per day diet mean excretion of 40 ± 4 mmol/d not significantly different from 37 ± 5 mmol/d in 10 controls on same diet *4180*

Prorenin *Plasma No Effect* In 8 hypertensives mean concentration of 17 ± 2.4 ng angiotensin U/mL/h not significantly different from 21 ± 2.5 ng angiotensin U/mL/h in 8 healthy controls *5284*
Red Blood Cells No Effect In 8 individuals with hypertension mean activity of 58 ± 7 pg angiotensin U/mL/h not significantly different from 68 ± 10 pg angiotensin U/mL/h in 8 healthy controls *5284*

Prostaglandin E_2 *Urine Decrease* Excretion decreased to 403 ± 91 ng/d in 10 women with essential hypertension compared with 509 ± 80 ng/d in 7 normal women *2798*

Prostaglandins *Plasma Decrease* Reduced levels of A_2 in patients with essential hypertension as opposed to normal controls *2966*

Protein *Serum Decrease* Occasionally observed *5544*
Urine Increase May occur with accompanying renal functional impairment *2304*

Renin *Plasma Increase* In individuals with essential hypertension mean concentration of 136.5 ± 14.6 pg/mL compared with 1053 ± 8.6 pg/mL in normal controls *5073*

Renin Activity *Plasma Decrease* Mean activity of 0.99 ± 0.4 ng/mL/h in 21 hypertensives with low urinary kallikrein excretion significantly less than 1.35 ± 0.2 ng/mL/h in 54 hypertensive patients with normal urinary kallikrein excretion *1131* Suppressed plasma renin activity *780* Can be high, low or normal *2304* Decreased in 20% of patients at diagnosis *5544*
Plasma Increase Can be high, low or normal *2304* Mean level, measured after 1 h supine rest, was significantly higher in the hypertensive subjects, while the upright PRA was normal *2534* Greater in plasma of hypertensive patients and uremic patients than in plasma of normotensive control subjects *2791* In hypertensives mean peak activity of about 1.7 ng/mL/h and trough activity of about 1.0 ng/mL/h higher than peak of 1.3 ng/mL/h and trough of 0.6 ng/mL/h in normotensives *4180* In 11 hypertensives mean concentration of 1.83 ± 1.22 ng/mL/h not significantly higher than 1.40 ± 0.84 ng/mL/h in 9 normotensive controls *3538*
Plasma No Effect Can be high, low or normal *2304*

Retinol *Serum No Effect* No significant association observed between blood pressure and plasma retinol concentration in 168 healthy individuals *3594*

Retinol-binding Protein *Urine Increase* Median excretion of 0.15 mg/d in 26 patients with essential hypertension significantly different from 0.08 mg/d in 16 normotensive healthy controls *276*

Selenium *Serum No Effect* No significant association between blood pressure and selenium concentration in 168 healthy individuals *3594*

Sex-Hormone Binding Globulin *Serum Decrease* In 13 hypertensive men with high renin-sodium profile mean concentration of 23.2 ± 11.2 nmol/L different from 30.0 ± 12.7 nmol/L in 23 hypertensives with normal renin-sodium profiles *4123*
Serum Increase In 9 hypertensive men with low renin-sodium profile mean concentration of 38.8 ± 15.8 nmol/L different from 30.0 ± 12.7 nmol/L in 23 hypertensives with normal renin-sodium profiles *4123*
Serum No Effect In 23 hypertensive men with normal renin-sodium profile mean concentration of 30.0 ± 12.7 nmol/L not significantly different from 29.8 ± 13.8 nmol/L in hypertensive population as a whole *4123*

Sodium *Red Blood Cells Increase* Mean concentration of 22.34 ± 4.77 mmol/L in 15 middle-aged hypertensives significantly higher than 13.40 ± 3.32 mmol/L in 15 normotensive controls *5364*
Serum Decrease Slight but highly significant depression in circulating concentration. Mean in 130 hypertensives was 137.7 mmol/L and 140.4 mmol/L in 123 normotensives *4707*
Serum No Effect In 60 women with moderate essential hypertension aged over 65 years mean concentration of 139.7 ± 2.4 mmol/L not significantly different from 140.1 ± 2.6 mmol/L in 46 normotensive women of similar age *131* Mean concentration of 141.16 ± 2.12 mmol/L in 15 middle-aged hypertensives not significantly different from 142.13 ± 2.33 mmol/L in 15 normotensive controls *5364* In 14 men with borderline hypertension mean concentration of 142 mmol/L not significantly higher than 141 mmol/L in 14 normotensive controls *4827* Sodium homeostasis is usually maintained in gradual renal failure *4439* No significant differences observed between concentrations of control subjects and those with essential arterial hypertension *5376*
Urine Decrease In 60 women with moderate essential hypertension aged over 65 years mean concentration of 80.7 ± 24.8 mmol/d significantly different from 112.2 ± 45.1 mmol/d in 46 normotensive women of similar age *131*
Urine Increase Significantly higher excretion in subjects with diastolic blood pressure between 95 and 109 mm Hg than in the group with diastolic blood pressure below 90 mm Hg *1233*
Urine No Effect In 10 hypertensives mean excretion of 149 ± 11 mmol/d not significantly different from 145 ± 7 mmol/d in 20 normotensive controls *2603* Mean excretion in 48 individuals aged 18 to 27 y with essential hypertension of 183 ± 9 nmol/d not significantly different from 171 ± 8 nmol/d in 25 age-matched controls *4517* No significant difference in excretions in 10 hypertensive individuals on a fixed intake of 100 mmol sodium and 80 mmol potassium per day of 97 ± 4 mmol/d and in normotensives 102 ± 4 mmol/d *4180*

Soluble Fibrin Monomer *Plasma Increase* In 54 hypertensives median concentration of 13.5 nmol/L significantly higher than 10.6 nmol/L in 50 healthy age-matched controls *1208*

Soluble Intercellular Adhesion Molecule-1 *Serum Increase* In 45 patients with uncontrolled essential hypertension mean concentration of 68 ± 30 ng/mL significantly increased compared with 47 ± 17 ng/mL in 40 normotensive age- and sex-matched controls *478*

Taurine *Plasma No Effect* No significant association observed between blood pressure and plasma taurine concentration in 168 healthy individuals *3594*

Testosterone *Serum No Effect* In 23 hypertensive men with normal renin-sodium profile, 9 with low renin-sodium profile and 13 with high renin-sodium profiles mean concentrations of 4.86 ± 1.54 ng/mL, 5.60 ± 1.41 ng/mL and 5.58 ± 1.81 ng/mL respectively not significantly different from concentrations in hypertensive population as a whole *4123*

β-Thromboglobulin *Plasma Increase* In 25 previously untreated patients with mild essential hypertension mean concentration of 17.1 ± 6.3 U/mL significantly different from 12.7 ± 3.2 U/mL in 22 normotensive controls *4452*
Urine No Effect In 15 patients with mean age of 47.2 ± 1.6 years and essential hypertension mean excretion of 61 ± 6 pg/mg creatinine not significantly different from 62 ± 4 pg/mg creatinine in 15 normotensive men with mean age of 47.2 ± 1.6 years *2993*

Thrombomodulin *Plasma No Effect* In patients with essential hypertension concentration not significantly different from normal *3739*

Thromboxane A_2 *Plasma Increase* Observed effect *4902*

Thromboxane B_2 *Plasma Increase* Significant increase observed in 26 patients with essential hypertension compared with 25 normotensives *802*
Urine Decrease In 46 patients with mild essential hypertension no significant correlation between blood pressure and excretion *3507*

Tissue Plasminogen Activator *Plasma Decrease* In 99 hypertensives (41 men, 58 women) mean concentration of 0.63 ± 0.56 IU/mL significantly decreased compared with 0.76 ± 1.27 IU/mL in 286 normotensive controls (134 men, 152 women) *1760*
Urine No Effect Activity not detectable in the urine of two hypertensive patients *2139*

Tissue Plasminogen Activator Antigen *Plasma Increase* In 99 hypertensives (41 men, 58 women) mean concentration of 8.9 ± 2.9 ng/mL significantly increased compared with 7.9 ± 8.5 ng/mL in 286 normotensive controls (134 men, 152 women) *1760*

α-Tocopherol *Serum No Effect* No significant association between blood pressure and plasma α-tocopherol concentration in 168 healthy individuals *5364*

Transferrin *Urine Increase* Median excretion of 0.81 mg/d in 26 patients with essential hypertension significantly different from 0.33 mg/d in 16 normotensive healthy controls *276*

401.90 Essential Hypertension *(continued)*

Triglycerides *Serum* *Increase* In 38 female hypertensives mean concentration of 160.1 ± 21.1 mg/dL significantly different from 118.2 ± 14.0 mg/dL in 58 healthy female controls, and 180.7 ± 22.9 mg/dL in 27 hypertensive men not significantly different from 151.7 ± 38.1 mg/dL in 47 healthy normotensive women *1507* In 27 nondiabetic salt-sensitive normal and high renin hypertensive patients who were unable to modulate their adrenal and renal blood flow responses to a change in dietary sodium mean concentration of 182 ± 19 mg/dL and 210 ± 43 mg/dL in 19 modulators significantly different from normal range of 70 - 175 mg/dL *1616* Frequently elevated *2034* In 99 hypertensives (41 men, 58 women) mean concentration of 389 ± 600 mg/dL significantly increased compared with in 286 normotensive controls (134 men, 152 women) *1760* In 60 women with moderate essential hypertension aged over 65 years mean concentration of 141.7 ± 50.1 mg/dL significantly different from 118.9 ± 48.3 mg/dL in 46 normotensive women of similar age *131* Concentrations nonsignificantly changed to 2.01 ± 0.24 mmol/L in 16 hypertensive patients with impaired glucose tolerance, cholesterol > 5.20 mmol/L and triglycerides > 1.8 mmol/L compared with 1.02 ± 0.09 mmol/L in 22 healthy control individuals *1469* In 10 hypertensives with microalbuminuria mean concentration of 1.8 mmol/L significantly higher than 1.37 mmol/L in 15 hypertensives without microalbuminuria and 1.21 mmol/L in 20 normotensive controls *437* In 50 outpatients with essential hypertension significant increase to 135 ± 74 mg/dL compared with 90 ± 34 mg/dL in 50 age and sex matched normotensive controls *738* In 45 patients with essential hypertension concentration of 1.6 ± 1.4 mmol/L significantly different from 1.4 ± 0.6 mmol/L in 20 healthy controls *1802*
Serum *No Effect* In 54 hypertensives median concentration of 1.8 mmol/L and lower and upper quartiles of 1.3 and 2.2 mmol/L respectively compared with reference interval of 0.8 - 2.0 mmol/L *1208* Mean concentration of 186 ± 88 mg/dL observed in 15 hypertensive patients not significantly different from 154 ± 18 mg/dL in 23 normotensive controls *2887* In 8 non-insulin resistant nonobese patients with untreated essential hypertension mean concentration of 1.4 ± 0.3 mmol/L compared with 1.3 ± 0.3 mmol/L in 8 healthy controls *232* In 25 previously untreated patients with mild essential hypertension mean concentration of 106.5 ± 47.5 mg/dL not significantly different from 97.7 ± 35.5 mg/dL in 22 normotensive controls *4452* Mean concentration in patients with essential hypertension not significantly different from healthy controls: 1.7 mmol/L in 8 with low renin, 1.8 mmol/L in 11 non-modulators, 1.7 mmol/L in 12 modulators, compared with 1.6 mmol/L in 7 normotensives *3169* In 15 patients with mean age of 47.2 ± 1.6 years and essential hypertension mean concentration of 1.5 ± 0.1 mmol/L not significantly greater than 1.5 ± 0.2 mmol/L in 15 normotensive men with mean age of 47.2 ± 1.6 years *2993*

Urea Nitrogen *Serum* *Increase* Observed effect *4213* Concentrations increased nonsignificantly to 5.79 ± 0.69 mmol/L in 16 hypertensive patients with impaired glucose tolerance, cholesterol > 5.20 mmol/L and triglycerides > 1.8 mmol/L compared with 5.21 ± 0.81 mmol/L in 22 healthy control individuals *1469*
Serum *No Effect* Mean concentration of 10.5 ± 3.6 mmol/L in 8 low renin essential hypertensive patients not significantly different from 11.4 ± 2.5 mmol/L in 11 non-modulators, 9.8 ± 3.2 mmol/L in 12 modulators and 10.7 ± 2.9 mmol/L in 7 normotensives *3169*

Uric Acid *Serum* *Increase* Reported effect *1980* Significant correlation observed in women with both systolic and diastolic blood pressure *5654* Hyperuricemia probably indicates hypertensive vascular damage and is associated with a relatively diminished uric acid excretion rate in arterial hypertension *4236* In 54% of 102 patients hospitalized for this disorder *1576* In 15 patients with mean age of 47.2 ± 1.6 years and essential hypertension mean concentration of 396 ± 25 µmol/L significantly greater than 327 ± 16 µmol/L in 15 normotensive men with mean age of 47.2 ± 1.6 years *2993* Found in 58% of 470 patients (27% of 333 untreated patients). Degree or occurrence of hyperuricemia did not correlate with severity of hypertension *568*
Serum *No Effect* No significant correlation observed in men with either systolic or diastolic blood pressure *5654*

Vanillylmandelic Acid *Urine* *No Effect* No significant differences observed in mean excretions of 13.3 ± 5.9 nmol/mL in 24 patients with established hypertension, 14.0 ± 6.3 nmol/mL in 14 patients with borderline hypertension and in 18 normotensive controls (12.3 ± 5.5 nmol/mL) *1327* In 142 hypertensive men reference interval of 10 to 54 µmol/d and in 184 hypertensive women of 9 to 38 µmol/d *2529*

Viscosity *Blood* *Increase* In 45 patients with essential hypertension blood viscosity significantly increased over the shear range of 4.5 to 450 /s compared with that in 20 healthy controls *1802*

VLDL-Cholesterol *Serum* *Increase* In 38 female hypertensives mean concentration of 18.6 ± 3.4 mg/dL significantly different from 11.3 ± 1.4 mg/dL in 58 healthy female controls, and 3.2 ± 4.1 mg/dL in 27 hypertensive men significantly different from 13.8 ± 1.3 mg/dL in 47 healthy normotensive men *1507* Significant increase to 27 mg/dL from 18 mg/dL in 50 outpatients with essential hypertension compared with age and sex matched normotensive controls *738* Concentrations significantly changed to 0.41 ± 0.08 mmol/L in 16 hypertensive patients with impaired glucose tolerance, cholesterol > 5.20 mmol/L and triglycerides > 1.8 mmol/L compared with 0.21 ± 0.05 mmol/L in 22 healthy control individuals *1469* In 10 hypertensives with microalbuminuria mean concentration of 0.81 mmol/L not significantly different from 0.62 mmol/L in 15 hypertensives without microalbuminuria and 0.55 mmol/L in 20 normotensive controls *437*

Volume *Urine* *No Effect* In 10 hypertensives daily urinary volume of 947 ± 80 mL compared with 1,026 ± 72 mL in 20 age matched controls *2603*

von Willebrand Factor *Plasma* *Increase* In 45 patients with uncontrolled essential hypertension mean concentration of 1.31 ± 0.32 kU/L significantly increased compared with 1.00 ± 0.42 kU/L in 40 normotensive age- and sex-matched controls *478*
Plasma *No Effect* In 54 hypertensive patients median concentration of 85% not significantly different from median of 98% in 50 healthy age-matched controls *1208*

von Willebrand Factor Antigen *Plasma* *Increase* In 84 patients (50 men, 34 women) with newly diagnosed essential hypertension mean concentration of 149 ± 65% significantly higher than 98 ± 40% in healthy controls *2708*

Zinc *Serum* *Increase* There was a high correlation between systolic and diastolic BP and zinc levels *310*
Serum *No Effect* No significant difference observed between concentrations of patients with essential arterial hypertension and healthy controls *5376*
Urine *Increase* In patients with essential arterial hypertension excretion increased although reason not understood *5875*

401.90 Hypertension

Adenosine-N6-diethylthioether-N1-pyridinoximine 5'-phosphate *Serum* *No Effect* In 6 patients with hypertension concentrations ranged from 47.2 - 205.0 nmol/dL not significantly different from concentration in healthy individuals in whom the mean concentration was 162.2 nmol/dL *5294*

Aldosterone *Plasma* *No Effect* In 15 patients with primary hypertension mean basal concentration not significantly different from that in 15 normotensive controls *3876*

Angiotensin-II *Plasma* *No Effect* In 15 patients with primary hypertension mean basal concentration not significantly different from that in 15 normotensive controls *3876*

Angiotensinogen *Plasma* *No Effect* Mean angiotensinogen activity of 1,267 ± 265 ng/mL/h in 65 hypertensives aged 79 ± 6 y not significantly different from 1,354 ± 239 ng/mL/h in 26 normotensive controls aged 77 ± 8 years *5277*

α_1-Antichymotrypsin *Serum* *No Effect* Mean concentration within reference interval of 47.9 ± 8.1 mg/dL in two examined patients with hypertension *3044*

Apolipoprotein A-I *Serum* *No Effect* In 36 hypertensive men mean concentration of 1.3 g/L not significantly different from 1.4 g/L in 40 normotensive age-matched controls *3658*

Apolipoprotein B *Serum* *Increase* In 36 hypertensive men mean concentration of 1.4 g/L significantly different from 1.2 g/L in 40 normotensive age-matched controls *3658*

Cholesterol *Serum* *Increase* In 36 hypertensive men mean concentration of 6.2 mmol/L not significantly different from 5.6 mmol/L in 40 normotensive age-matched controls *3658*

Serum *No Effect* In 1,900 male patients with mild to moderate hypertension mean concentration of 5.72 ± 1.14 mmol/L not significantly different from that in healthy controls *70* Mean concentration of 229 ± 44 mg/dL in 65 hypertensives aged 79 ± 6 y not significantly different from 216 ± 56 mg/dL in 26 normotensive controls aged 77 ± 8 years *5277*

Creatinine *Serum* *Increase* Mean concentration of 0.87 ± 0.22 mg/dL in 65 hypertensives aged 79 ± 6 y significantly different from 0.73 ± 0.13 mg/dL in 26 normotensive controls aged 77 ± 8 years *5277*
Serum *No Effect* In 36 hypertensive men mean concentration of 83 μmol/L not significantly different from 81 μmol/L in 40 normotensive age-matched controls *3658*
Urine *Decrease* In 10 hypertensive black patients mean excretion of 13.0 ± 9.9 mmol/L significantly less than 17.4 ± 9.7 mmol/L in 10 normotensive blacks *4709*
Urine *No Effect* In 10 hypertensive Indians mean excretion of 10.5 ± 6.3 mmol/L not significantly different from 10.2 ± 6.1 mmol/L in 10 normotensive Indians *4709*

Endothelin-1 *Plasma* *Increase* In 8 patients with hypertension mean concentration in hepatic vein of 12.4 ± 2.4 pg/mL significantly different from 9.6 ± 1.6 pg/mL in hepatic vein of 10 normotensive controls: similar differences observed in femoral artery blood *3567*

Endothelin-3 *Plasma* *Increase* In 8 patients with hypertension mean concentration in hepatic vein of 14.2 ± 1.3 pg/mL significantly different from 10.0 ± 1.4 pg/mL in hepatic vein of 10 normotensive controls: similar differences observed in femoral artery blood *3567*

Fibrinogen *Plasma* *No Effect* In 36 hypertensive men mean concentration of 2.6 g/L not significantly different from 2.7 g/L in 40 normotensive age-matched controls *3658*

HDL-Cholesterol *Serum* *Decrease* In 36 hypertensive men mean concentration of 1.0 mmol/L significantly different from 1.2 mmol/L in 40 normotensive age-matched controls *3658*

High Molecular Weight β-Thromboglobulin *Urine* *Increase* In 36 hypertensive men mean nocturnal excretion of 2.5 ng/mmol creatinine and mean resting urinary excretion of 2.7 ng/mmol creatinine not significantly different from 1.9 ng/mmol creatinine and 2.3 ng/mmol creatinine in the nocturnal and resting urine of 36 and 34 normotensive controls respectively *3658*

Kallikrein *Urine* *Decrease* In 10 hypertensive black patients mean excretion of 2.3 ± 0.9 ng/μg protein less than 2.6 ± 1.9 ng/μg protein in 10 normotensive blacks and 1.2 ± 0.7 ng/μg protein in 10 hypertensive Indians significantly less than 2.6 ± 2.3 ng/μg protein in 10 normotensive Indians *4709*

LDL-Cholesterol *Serum* *Increase* In 36 hypertensive men mean concentration of 4.3 mmol/L not significantly different from 3.8 mmol/L in 40 normotensive age-matched controls *3658*

Lipoprotein Lp(a) *Serum* *No Effect* In 36 hypertensive men mean concentration of 3.8 mg/dL not significantly different from 4.2 mg/dL in 40 normotensive age-matched controls *3658*

Mean Platelet Volume *Blood* *No Effect* In 35 hypertensive men mean volume of 7.1 x 10^{-15}/L not significantly different from 7.1 x 10^{-15}/L in 40 normotensive controls *3658*

Nicotine *Serum* *No Effect* In 13 smoking hypertensive men mean concentration of 2.3 ng/mL not significantly different from 2.5 ng/mL in 19 normotensive age-matched smoking controls *3658*

Oubain-like Substance *Serum* *Increase* In 98 hypertensive NIDDM patients serum mean concentrations of 0.918 ± 0.212 nmol/L significantly higher than 0.589 ± 0.162 nmol/L in 60 normotensive NIDDM patients. Serum OLS concentration correlated positively with systolic blood pressure (r = 0.544) and with diastolic blood pressure (r = 0.488) *767*

Phosphate *Serum* *Decrease* Hypertension is less common cause of hypophosphatemia *969*

Platelets *Blood* *Increase* In 35 hypertensive men mean concentration of 219 x 10^9/L not significantly different from 214 x 10^9/L in 40 normotensive controls *3658*

Potassium *Serum* *No Effect* Mean concentration of 4.2 ± 0.4 mmol/L in 65 hypertensives aged 79 ± 6 y not significantly different from 4.2 ± 0.4 mmol/L in 26 normotensive controls aged 77 ± 8 years *5277*
Urine *Decrease* In 10 hypertensive blacks mean excretion of 61 ± 31 mmol/L different from 72 ± 24 mmol/L in 10 normotensive Indians *4709*
Urine *No Effect* In 10 hypertensive Indians mean excretion of 105 ± 44 mmol/L not significantly different from 115 ± 42 mmol/L in 10 normotensive Indians *4709* In 1,900 male patients with mild to moderate hypertension mean excretion of 60 mmol/d not significantly different from that in healthy controls *70*

Prekallikrein *Plasma* *No Effect* In 15 patients with primary hypertension mean basal concentration not significantly different from that in 15 normotensive controls *3876*

Prorenin *Plasma* *No Effect* Mean prorenin activity of 14.6 ± 8.6 ng/mL/h in 65 hypertensives aged 79 ± 6 y not significantly different from 15.1 ± 7.0 ng/mL/h in 26 normotensive controls aged 77 ± 8 years *5277*

Renin Activity *Plasma* *No Effect* Mean activity of 1.7 ± 1.6 ng/mL/h in 65 hypertensives aged 79 ± 6 y not significantly different from 1.5 ± 0.8 ng/mL/h in 26 normotensive controls aged 77 ± 8 years *5277* In 1,900 male patients with mild to moderate hypertension mean concentration of 0.53 ng/L/s not significantly different from that in healthy controls *70* In 15 patients with primary hypertension mean basal concentration not significantly different from that in 15 normotensive controls *3876*

Sodium *Urine* *Decrease* In 10 hypertensive black patients mean excretion of 105 ± 56 mmol/L significantly less than 210 ± 158 mmol/L in 10 normotensive blacks and 1.2 ± 0.7 mmol/L in 10 hypertensive Indians significantly less than 2.6 ± 2.3 mmol/L in 10 normotensive Indians *4709*
Urine *No Effect* In 1,900 male patients with mild to moderate hypertension mean excretion of 126 mmol/d not significantly different from that in healthy controls *70*

Thiocyanate *Serum* *No Effect* In 36 hypertensive men mean concentration of 70 μmol/L not significantly different from 70 μmol/L in 40 normotensive age-matched controls *3658*

β-Thromboglobulin *Plasma* *Increase* In 33 hypertensive men mean concentration of 2.5 ng/mL significantly different from 25 ng/mL in 40 normotensive controls *3658*

Tissue Kallikrein *Plasma* *No Effect* In 15 patients with primary hypertension mean basal concentration not significantly different from that in 15 normotensive controls *3876*

Triglycerides *Serum* *Increase* In 36 hypertensive men mean concentration of 1.6 mmol/L significantly different from 1.0 mmol/L in 40 normotensive age-matched controls *3658*

Urea Nitrogen *Serum* *No Effect* In 1,900 male patients with mild to moderate hypertension mean concentration of 5.68 ± 1.82 mmol/L not significantly different from that in healthy controls *70*

Uric Acid *Serum* *No Effect* Mean concentration of 5.7 ± 1.5 mg/dL in 65 hypertensives aged 79 ± 6 y not significantly different from 5.6 ± 1.3 mg/dL in 26 normotensive controls aged 77 ± 8 years *5277*
Urine *Decrease* May reduce renal excretion of urate *1357*

Volume *Urine* *No Effect* In 1,900 male patients with mild to moderate hypertension mean excretion of 1.32 L/d not significantly different from that in healthy controls *70*

401.90 Labile Hypertension

Dopamine *Plasma* *No Effect* Patients with labile hypertension had concentrations comparable to those in controls *2955*

5-Hydroxytryptamine *Plasma* *Decrease* Patients with labile hypertension had concentrations that correlated negatively with blood pressure and norepinephrine concentrations *2955*

Norepinephrine *Plasma* *Increase* Patients with labile hypertension had increased concentrations compared with those in controls *2955*

405.91 Renovascular Hypertension

Albumin *Urine* *Increase* In 8 patients with secondary hypertension: renovascular hypertension mean excretion of 57.12 ± 70.84 mg/d significantly greater than 9.08 ± 3.92 mg/d in 39 healthy controls *3087*

α_1-Antitrypsin *Urine* *Increase* In 8 patients with secondary hypertension: renovascular hypertension mean excretion of 8.14 ± 11.95 mg/d significantly greater than 0.12 ± 0.44 mg/d in 39 healthy controls *3087*

Atrial Natriuretic Peptide *Plasma* *Increase* Increased in hypertensive patients with mild to moderate chronic renal failure and may support the homeostasis of sodium balance *5064*

405.91 Renovascular Hypertension (continued)

Chloride *Serum* *Increase* Acidosis which is out of proportion to the degree of azotemia *1980*

Cholesterol *Serum* *Increase* Predisposes to development of arteriosclerosis *2033*

Creatinine *Urine* *Increase* Confirmatory evidence of greater water reabsorption as a cause of the decreased volume from the suspected kidney *2304*

Creatinine Clearance *Urine* *Decrease* Renal functional impairment *1980*

Glomerular Filtration Rate *Urine* *Decrease* Renal functional impairment *1980*

Glucose *Serum* *Increase* Associated with diabetes mellitus *2033*

Inulin Clearance *Urine* *Decrease* Renal functional impairment *1980*

Lipoproteins *Serum* *Increase* More than 50% of the patients showed obviously abnormal profiles of serum lipoproteins, which returned to normal or near-normal when the disease was ameliorated or corrected surgically *5515*

Osmolality *Urine* *Decrease* Renal functional impairment *1980*

pH *Blood* *Decrease* Acidosis which is out of proportion to the degree of azotemia *1980*
Urine *Decrease* Acidosis which is out of proportion to the degree of azotemia *1980*

Sodium *Urine* *Decrease* A 50% or greater decrease in volume excreted and a 15% or greater decrease in sodium concentration indicated renal artery obstruction and reversible renovascular hypertension *2304*

Specific Gravity *Urine* *Decrease* Renal functional impairment *1980*

Triglycerides *Serum* *Increase* Predisposes to development of arteriosclerosis *2033*

Uric Acid *Serum* *Increase* Increased incidence of hyperuricemia *2033*

Volume *Urine* *Increase* A 50% or greater decrease in volume excreted and a 15% or greater decrease in sodium concentration indicated renal artery obstruction and reversible renovascular hypertension *2304*

Diseases of the Heart

410.90 Acute Myocardial Infarction

α_1-Acid Glycoprotein *Serum* *Increase* During acute phase, from day 1 to 5, concentration may be increased *5869* One of the most reliable indicators of acute inflammation *4853* *4241* *2597* *4696* *3713* In 19 patients with acute myocardial infarction mean concentration on admission in those who developed complications of 0.91 g/L and 1.68 g/L 7 days later. In those who did not develop complications mean concentration on admission of 1.22 g/L and 1.97 g/L 7 days later *718* One of the most reliable indicators of acute inflammation *4373* In 40 patients with AMI peak concentration increased 8-fold above normal value 3 days after AMI *722*

Adrenomedullin *Plasma* *Increase* In 15 patients with AMI mean concentration on admission of 9.4 ± 1.3 fmol/mL significantly higher than 2.8 ± 0.2 fmol/mL in 15 age- and sex-matched healthy controls *2730* In patients with acute myocardial infarction mean concentration of 10.6 ± 1.9 pmol/L in right atrium significantly increased compared with 5.2 ± 0.3 pmol/L in controls *5818*
Serum *Increase* In 25 patients with acute myocardial infarction mean concentration was significantly different at 14.0 ± 9.0 pmol/L at 24 h from 5.1 ± 2.3 pmol/L in 46 healthy controls, with concentration declining to almost the reference range at 4 weeks *3536*

Alanine Aminotransferase *Serum* *Increase* Observed only when resulting cardiac tissue necrosis is great enough to cause a rise in AST equivalent to 150 spectrophotometric Units *5737* Normal or only minimally elevated *1025* In 49% of 18 patients hospitalized for this disorder *1576* Generally parallels AST but the increase is less marked *5544*
Serum *No Effect* Usually not increased unless there is liver damage due to congestive heart failure, drug therapy, etc *5544*

Albumin *Serum* *Decrease* In 22% of 111 patients hospitalized for this disorder *1576*
Serum *Increase* From day 5, concentration may show a rapid decrease and return to normal in the third week *5869*
Serum *No Effect* In 11 patients with AMI or unstable angina no significant change observed 24 to 48 hours after onset of pain *3732*
Urine *Increase* In 13 of 22 patients with acute myocardial infarction excretion increased above normal on admission: mean 0.82 µmol/L on day of admission, 0.30 µmol/L on day 1, 0.22 µmol/L on day 2 and 0.09 µmol/L on day 3 *1336*

Aldolase *Serum* *Increase* Rises after 3 h to a peak by 24 h (2 - 15 times normal), falling to normal by 4 - 7 days. There is a semiquantitative relation between the amount of necrosis and the peak level in the serum *1290* With cell destruction *5544* Activity increases in myocardial infarction in a time pattern similar to that of aspartate aminotransferase *2952*

Aldosterone *Plasma* *Increase* In 335 patients with acute myocardial infarction mean concentration of 22 ± 22 ng/dL (mean 12 days after infarction) significantly higher than 17 ± 7 ng/dL in 38 control individuals *4321*

Alkaline Phosphatase *Serum* *Increase* Increased in conjunction with normal levels of bilirubin indicate congestive heart failure or myocardial infarction - 28%, carcinoma - 25%, hepatobiliary - 16%, and other miscellaneous diseases *420* Some patients; usually during phase of organization *5544* Ten cases of acute transmural infarction were accompanied by a rise of 50 - 400% in serum concentration several h after onset of symptoms and lasted 3 - 5 d *4660* Significant increases evident within 2 - 3 h and persist 3 - 5 d in some cases *4707*
Serum *No Effect* In 11 patients with AMI or unstable angina no significant change observed 24 to 48 hours after onset of pain *3732*

Amino-terminal Propeptide of Type III Procollagen
Serum *Increase* In 38 patients with transmural myocardial infarction mean concentration increased significantly from baseline of 0.53 ± 0.20 U/mL at baseline to 0.75 ± 0.20 U/mL at 6 months and 0.76 ± 0.10 U/mL at 12 months *3541*

Amyloid A Protein *Serum* *Increase* In 29 patients with acute myocardial infarction on admission to hospital concentration increased above 0.3 mg/dL in 22 *3093* In 19 patients with acute myocardial infarction mean concentration in patients who developed complications was 420 mg/L on admission and 1090 mg/L after 7 days, and in those without complications it was 112 mg/L on admision and 526 mg/L after 7 days *718* In 40 patients with AMI, peak concentration increased 5,000-fold above normal value 3 days after AMI *722*

Anti-Heart Mitochondrial Antibodies *Serum* *Increase* In 15 of 35 patients (45.4%) with acute myocardial infarction anti-heart mitochondrial antibodies identified peaking between days 12 and 14 *4632*

α_1-Antichymotrypsin *Serum* *Increase* In 19 patients with AMI mean concentration on admission in those who developed complications 0.42 g/L and 0.96 g/L 7 days later. In those who did not develop complications mean concentration on admission 0.60 g/L and 1.07 g/L 7 days later *718* In 40 patients with AMI peak concentration increased 8-fold above normal value 3 days after AMI *722* During acute phase, from day 1 to 5, concentration may be increased *5869* Following myocardial infarction, a large rapid increase was noted to a maximum at day 5 *2457*

Antidiuretic Hormone *Plasma* *Increase* In 335 patients with acute myocardial infarction mean concentration of 1.6 ± 8.2 pg/mL (mean 12 days after infarction) significantly higher than 0.7 ± 0.3 pg/mL in 38 control individuals *4321*

Antithrombin III *Plasma* *Decrease* Significant decrease *3858* Found to be significantly diminished when measured by the Von Kaulla method; otherwise found to show a significant increase 3 months after an acute ischemic episode *3134*
Plasma *Increase* Found to be significantly diminished when measured by the Von Kaulla method; otherwise found to show a significant increase 3 months after an acute ischemic episode *3134*

α_1-Antitrypsin *Serum* *Increase* Showed a significant increase when compared to controls and remained elevated for 3 months after ischemic episode *3134* Significantly elevated in patients with AMI (n = 48) compared with controls (n = 19) *1735*

During acute phase, from day 1 to 5, concentration may be increased *5869*

Apolipoprotein A-I *Serum* *Decrease* In 49 male survivors of premature myocardial infarction mean concentration of 111.9 ± 2.5 mg/dL lower than 129.3 ± 3.4 mg/dL in 49 healthy controls *3523*

Apolipoprotein A-I:Apolipoprotein B Ratio
Serum *Decrease* In 18 patients with AMI and coronary artery disease mean ratio of 0.99 ± 0.23 and of 1.31 ± 0.32 in 20 patients with AMI but without coronary artery disease lower than 1.47 ± 0.43 in 24 age and sex matched controls *1851*

Apolipoprotein A-II *Serum* *Decrease* Mean concentration of 44.0 ± 1.2 mg/dL in 49 male survivors of premature myocardial infarction lower than 47.9 ± 1.1 mg/dL in 49 healthy controls *3523*

Apolipoprotein B *Serum* *Increase* In 49 male survivors of premature myocardial nfarction mean concentration of 129.7 ± 4.5 mg/dL higher than 118.2 ± 4.1 mg/dL in 49 healthy controls *3523*

Apolipoproteins *Serum* *Decrease* Apolipoprotein A-I and A-II were associated with decreased risk *4978*
Serum *Increase* Apolipoprotein B-100 was associated with increased risk *4978*

Aspartate Aminotransferase *Serum* *Increase* May cause increased AST activity *4617*

Atrial Natriuretic Peptide *Plasma* *Increase* On the second day in 30 patients with AMI mean concentration of 48 ± 34 pg/mL significantly increased compared with control values of 15 ± 7 pg/mL *3706* In 25 patients with acute myocardial infarction mean concentration was significantly different at 56.2 ± 63.5 pg/mL on admission from approximately 18 pg/mL in 46 healthy controls, with concentration declining but not to the reference range at 4 weeks *3536* In 145 patients on day 3 following infarct, median concentration of 30.3 pmol/L compared with upper limit of normal of 24 pmol/L, but with patients with higher concentrations having poorer prognosis *3911* In 335 patients with acute myocardial infarction mean concentration of 65 ± 64 pg/mL (mean 12 days after infarction) significantly higher than 21 ± 9 pg/mL in 38 control individuals *4321*
Plasma *No Effect* In 15 patients with uncomplicated myocardial infarction no remarkable variation in concentration observed and concentration not correlated with serum myoglobin, CK and CK-MB *5482*
Serum *Increase* Mean concentration in 14 patients with AMI, who died, of 60.2 ± 35 pmol/L significantly different from 29.5 ± 22 pmol/L in 61 patients who survived AMI *1014*

Basic Fibroblast Growth Factor *Serum* *No Effect* In 45 patients with acute myocardial infarction concentrations increased from 14.4 ± 5.7 pg/mL on day 1, to 7.4 ± 2.4 pg/mL on day 2, 7.3 ± 2.5 pg/mL on day 3, 11.7 ± 2.5 pg/mL on day 7, 7.8 ± 2.4 pg/mL on day 14, 6.6 ± 1.3 pg/mL on day 21 and 4.9 ± 1.3 pg/mL on day 28, not significantly different from controls *2599*

Basophils *Blood* *Decrease* In 29 post-myocardial infarction patients mean concentration of 0.04 ± 0.01 x 10^9/L significantly different from 0.06 ± 0.01 x 10^9/L in 20 apparently healthy controls *5543*

Bilirubin *Serum* *No Effect* Usual finding *5544*

Brain Natriuretic Peptide *Plasma* *Increase* On the second day in 30 patients with AMI mean concentration of 139 ± 104 pg/mL significantly increased compared with control values of 11 ± 8 pg/mL *3706* In 25 patients with acute myocardial infarction mean concentration was significantly different at 40.6 ± 37.5 pg/mL on admission (peaking at 155.4 ± 79.0 pg/mL at 24 h after admission) from approximately 12 pg/mL in 46 healthy controls, with concentration declining but not to the admision value at 4 weeks *3536* In patients with acute myocardial infarction plasma concentration of brain natriuretic peptide increased within hours of onset to more than 100 times normal concentration and highly correlated inversely with the cardiac index *3644* Mean concentration in 14 patients with AMI who died of 45.9 ± 18 pmol/L significantly different from 18.6 ± 10 pmol/L in 61 patients who survived AMI *1014*

C_1-Esterase Inhibitor *Serum* *Increase* Concentration not measurably reduced at the onset of acute coronary syndrome, but did increase to higher amounts during the the post-acute period *2201*
Serum *No Effect* Concentration not measurably reduced at the onset of acute coronary syndrome, but did increase to higher amounts during the the post-acute period *2201*

Calcium *Serum* *No Effect* In 11 patients with AMI or unstable angina no significant change observed 24 to 48 hours after pain onset *3732* Plasma concentration measured in 18 patients several days after admission showed a fall in 13 cases. Correction of values to a fixed albumin level removed the apparent tendency to hypocalcemia *5663*

Carbonic Anhydrase III *Serum* *No Effect* Not elevated in acute myocardial infarction *3554* No significant change observed in 26 patients after AMI (concentration remained within range of 18 to 25 µg/L during 5 days observation) *5377*

Catecholamines *Plasma* *Increase* The adrenal medulla can release circulating catecholamines as the result either of the generalized sympathetic stress reaction or of arterial hypoxia. Patients with higher plasma levels of catecholamines and free fatty acids may have a higher incidence of severe arrhythmias, shock, and death than patients with lower levels *2304*
Urine *Increase* Total urinary catecholamines were significantly elevated in the first 48 h *1091*

CD9 (p24) *Platelets* *No Effect* In 16 patients with AMI who responded to antithrombolytic therapy mean log amplification of fluorescence intensity of 48.4 ± 9.6 compared with 51.2 ± 10.3 in 5 patients who failed to respond to antithrombolytic treatment and 41.1 ± 11.4 in 10 healthy controls *1928*

Chlamydia pneumoniae Antibodies *Serum* *Increase* Seropositivity observed in 75% of patients with MI compared with 66% in control population without MI *117*

Cholesterol *Serum* *Increase* In 26 Greek-Caucasians who had had an AMI within the previous 6 - 17 months mean concentration of 6.1 ± 0.6 mmol/L significantly different from 5.5 ± 1.0 mmol/L in 26 age-matched healthy controls *5206* Very significantly elevated. Mean value was 212.2 ± 15.0 mg/dL in females and 209.1 ± 4.4 in males. Normal was 168.3 ± 4.2 and 170.9 ± 6.3 in females and males, respectively *795* Mean concentration of 5.57 ± 0.76 mmol/L in 20 patients with AMI without coronary artery disease and 6.08 ± 1.02 mmol/L in 18 patients with AMI and coronary artery disease higher than 5.38 ± 0.97 mmol/L in 24 age and sex matched controls *1851* Mean concentration of 6.2 ± 0.9 mmol/L in 116 patients who had survived an acute myocardial infarction significantly different from 5.8 ± 1.2 mmol/L in 116 matched controls *472* Tends to slowly decrease for a few weeks after infarction *2304*
Serum *No Effect* Mean concentration of 176 ± 11 mg/dL in 16 patients with AMI not significantly different from 172 ± 7 mg/dL in 13 control individuals *4805* In 49 male survivors of premature myocardial infarction (mean concentration of 220.3 ± 5.5 mg/dL) no significant change from normal observed (mean concentration of 211.9 ± 5.6 mg/dL) *3523*

Cholesterol Esters *Serum* *Increase* Mean concentration was 134.0 ± 13.6 mg/dL compared to 92.6 ± 6.7 mg/dL in women, and 129.2 ± 3.7 md/dL compared to 101.7 ± 5.6 mg/dL in men *795*

Cholinesterase *Serum* *Decrease* May occur with decrease in serum albumin *5544*

Copper *Red Blood Cells* *No Effect* In 21 patients with acute myocardial infarction mean concentration of 9.3 ± 3.0 µmol/L on day of infarction not significantly different from 9.0 ± 2.1 µmol/L 15 days later *181*
Serum *Decrease* In 21 patients with acute myocardial infarction mean concentration of 16.0 ± 6.5 µmol/L on day of infarction significantly different from 18.7 ± 5.3 µmol/L 15 days later although increased to 19.6 ± 5.8 µmol/L on day 4 *181*
Serum *Increase* Mean concentration of 123 µg/dL observed in 27 patients *5605* Increased concentrations reported immediately following acute myocardial infarction *3499* After infarction, a significant increase in serum copper and a decrease in zinc were observed *5462*

Cortisol *Plasma* *Increase* Observed reaction to stress *2304* In 69 patients with AMI mean concentration of 827 nmol/mL significantly higher than 414 nmol/mL in 315 patients without AMI *5222* In 22 of 25 patients studied within 24 hours of acute AMI mean morning concentration increased to 1421 nmol/L and evening concentration to 1134 nmol/L with loss of diurnal rhythmicity of cortisol but concentrations returned to normal within 4 days *67*

C-Reactive Protein *Serum* *Increase* In 29 patients with acute myocardial infarction on admission to hospital mean con-

410.90 Acute Myocardial Infarction *(continued)*

C-Reactive Protein *(continued)*
centration increased above 0.3 mg/dL in 22 *3093* Significant increase *3858* During acute phase, from day 1 to 5, concentration may be increased *5869* Mean concentration in 47 patients with MI 2.05 ± 0.36 mg/dL compared with 0.54 ± 0.08 mg/dL in 133 controls *117* In 19 patients with AMI mean concentration on admission in those who developed complications was 21 mg/L and 88 mg/L after 7 days. In those who did not develop complications mean concentration on admission of 12 mg/L and 60 mg/L after 7 days *718* Mean baseline concentration in 24 patients with acute myocardial infarction mean peak concentration of 69.2 ± 29.9 mg/L significantly different from normal of 1.2 ± 4.7 mg/L *4233* In 12 cases of AMI who had a cardiac rupture following AMI mean concentration of 28.1 mg/dL versus 9.7 mg/dL in 28 patients with AMI but without cardiac rupture (normal < 0.2 mg/dL) *5342* Appears within 24 - 48 h, begin to fall by the 3rd day and become negative after 1 - 2 weeks *5544* In 40 patients with AMI peak concentration increased 100-fold above normal value 3 days after AMI *722* In 11 patients with AMI mean concentration of 0.6 mg/dL on admission increased during admission to 12.4 ± 1.74 mg/dL after 48 h *633* Concentration increased 2 d after AMI. Mean values in patients who died within 3, 3 to 6, 6 to 12 and 12 to 24 mo were 166, 136, 85 and 74 mg/L, respectively, compared with 65 mg/L in those who survived *4131*

Creatine Kinase *Serum Increase* In 26 patients with AMI mean concentration was significantly increased to 600 U/L on day of admission, 1,000 U/L 1 day later, 400 U/L on day 2, 200 U/L on day 3 and had returned to normal on day 5 *5377* In 12 cases of AMI who had a cardiac rupture following AMI mean peak activity was no different from that in 28 individuals who had AMI but without cardiac rupture, but significantly different from that in healthy individuals *5342* Allows early diagnosis because increases appear within the appearance of CK-MB in the serum, the isoenzyme found only in the myocardium, is specific for myocardial damage *2039* Increased in > 90% of patients when blood is drawn at appropriate time *5544* In 69 patients with AMI mean activity of 172 U/L significantly higher than 84.5 U/L in 315 patients without AMI *5222* Mean activity in several men of 1669.2 ± 910.7 UL on second day post-infarction significantly greater than 394.4 ± 529.2 U/L on first day post-infarct and 761.4 ± 770.5 U/L on third day post-infarction *968* The incidence of elevation is approximately equal to AST and LD, but is more specific *1025* In 29 patients with AMI mean activity increased to 1,110 ± 850 U/L (upper limit of normal in men 80 U/L and 70 U/L in women) and to 295 ± 185 μg/L (upper limit of normal of 5 μg/L) *2957* In 64 patients with AMI serum concentrations peak at 7.5 ± 4.1 h after reperfusion *5158* Peak levels may be 50 - 100 times normal *1642* In 15 patients with acute myocardial infarction mean plasma activity increased to 1640 μg/L at about 16 hours after infarction *1752* Rises in 3 h reaching peak by 36 h (10 - 25 times normal), returning to normal by 4 days. Prolonged elevation indicates bad prognosis *1290* Mean peak activity in 14 patients with AMI who died of 2,684 ± 2,137 U/L significantly different from 1,681 ± 1,412 U/L in 61 patients who survived AMI *1014*
Serum No Effect In 29 patients with acute myocardial infarction on admission to hospital activity of 136.2 ± 77 U/L not different from reference range of 30 - 230 U/L *3093*

Creatine Kinase Isoenzymes *Serum Increase* For acute myocardial infarction sensitivities for CK-MB of 37% (0 - 5 h), 97% (6 - 11 h), 97% (12 - 23 h), 97% (24 - 47 h), 56% (48 - 95 h) and 88% (greater than 96 h) *5744*

Creatine Kinase MB-Isoenzyme *Serum Increase* In 69 patients with AMI mean concentration of 6.05 ng/mL significantly higher than 0.7 ng/mL in 315 patients without AMI *5222* Of serum CK-MB, cTnI and myoglobin, CK-MB had clinical sensitivity > 93% 6 - 24 h after onset of chest pain, remained highly sensitive for 48 h. Between 72 and 150 h after onset of chest pain had a sensitivity of only 18% *5740* Six percent of more implies acute infarction. Usual peak is 12 to 24 hours after onset *1626*

Creatinine *Serum Increase* In 59% of 98 patients at initial hospitalization for this disorder *1576* 9 of 22 patients showed elevations within 6 days of infarction. Initial and peak means were 0.101 ± 0.022 and 0.117 ± 0.025 μmol/L, respectively *5664*
Serum No Effect In 11 patients with AMI or unstable angina no significant change observed 24 to 48 hours after onset of acute chest pain *3732*

Cytomegalovirus Antibodies *Serum Increase* Seropositivity observed in 75% of patients with MI compared with 77% in control population without MI *117*

D-Dimer *Plasma Increase* In 60 patients with acute myocardial infarction median concentration of 376.0 ng/mL compared with 34.5 ng/mL in 30 healthy controls *2546*

Dehydroepiandrosterone Sulfate *Plasma Decrease* In 49 men following premature myocardial infarction mean concentration of 1473.59 ± 116.51 ng/mL significantly lower than 1867.92 ± 118 .85 ng/mL in 49 healthy controls *3523*

β-Endorphin *White Blood Cells Decrease* In 11 patients with AMI mean concentration of 30.2 ± 6.9 pg x 10^6 mononuclear cells on admission not significantly different from reference interval of 20 - 40 pg x 10^6 mononuclear cells but concentration decreased during admission to 6.9 ± 1.9 pg x 10^6 mononuclear cells after 48 h *633*
White Blood Cells No Effect In 11 patients with AMI mean concentration of 30.2 ± 6.9 pg x 10^6 mononuclear cells on admission not significantly different from reference interval of 20 - 40 pg x 10^6 mononuclear cells but concentration decreased during admission to 6.9 ± 1.9 pg x 10^6 mononuclear cells after 48 h *633*

Endothelial Cell Adhesion Molecule-1 *Platelets Increase* In 16 patients with AMI who responded to antithrombolytic therapy mean log amplification of fluorescence intensity of 50.2 ± 2.8 significantly different when compared with 57.1 ± 2.8 in 5 patients who failed to respond to antithrombolytic treatment: (44.5 ± 3.8 in 10 healthy controls) *1928*

Endothelin *Plasma Increase* Concentration significantly increased in patients with acute myocardial infarction, especially those associated with cardiogenic shock *3739* In 29 patients with AMI mean concentration increased to 9.4 ± 3.2 ng/L compared with 5.16 ± 0.7 ng/L in 22 healthy volunteers *2957*

Endothelin-1 *Plasma Increase* These results indicate that endothelin-1 is elevated in accordance with cardiac and pulmonary circulatory distress in patients with acute myocardial infarction, *5246* In 25 patients with infarcts but no cardiac failure mean concentration of 1.97 ± 0.69 pg/mL, in 16 with heart failure of 2.74 ± 1.02 pg/mL, in 13 with pulmonary edema of 4.54 ± 1.17 pg/mL and in 5 with cardiogenic shock of 8.91 ± 3.16 pg/mL compared with normal controls of 1.51 ± 0.39 pg/mL *5246* These results indicate that endothelin-1 is elevated in accordance with cardiac and pulmonary circulatory distress in patients with acute myocardial infarction, *5013* Mean concentration on admission in 6 patients with myocardial infarction of 0.746 ± 0.122 pg/mL compared with 0.428 ± 0.047 pg/mL in 27 healthy controls. Concentration increased to 0.868 ± 0.109 pg/mL after 6 h followed by a decrease to 0.597 ± 0.122 pg/mL after 72 h *4251* In 7 studies concentrations typically increased 1.9 to 3.7-fold, although in one 10.9-fold, above appropriate normal values *328*

Eosinophils *Blood No Effect* In 29 post-myocardial infarction patients mean concentration of 0.20 ± 0.02 x 10^9/L not significantly different from 0.20 ± 0.03 x 10^9/L in 20 apparently healthy controls *5543*

Epinephrine *Plasma Decrease* Significantly reduced in the first few days following infarction *2723* In 145 patients with AMI, on day 3 after infarct median concentration of 0.12 nmol/L not significantly different from upper limit of normal of 0.40 nmol/L, with patients having higher concentrations having poorer prognosis *3911*
Plasma Increase Mean concentration in 30 patients with acute MI of 0.65 ± 0.17 nmol/L and 0.41 ± 0.20 nmol/L on days 1 and 3 respectively compared with 0.20 ± 0.10 nmol/L and 0.08 ± 0.02 nmol/L respectively in 8 patients with chest pain but no MI *3912* Evidence for a sympathoadrenal response is found in the increased blood and urinary concentration of norepinephrine, epinephrine, or their metabolic products *2304* Correlates with fasting plasma free fatty acids, which are associated with increased incidence of serious arrhythmias after infarctions *1919*
Urine Increase Evidence for a sympathoadrenal response is found in the increased blood and urinary concentration of norepinephrine, epinephrine, or their metabolic products *2304*

In patients developing heart failure or cardiogenic shock, the urinary level of both free catecholamines rose notably in the 1st week after infarction. In uncomplicated cases, a moderate rise in the norepinephrine level in the 1st week was associated with only a transient rise in the epinephrine level *2444*

Erythrocyte Sedimentation Rate *Blood* *Increase* Rises slowly and may persist for weeks even though no complications are present *2039* Increased, usually by 2 - 3 days; peaks in 4 - 5 days; persists for 2 - 6 months. Sometimes more sensitive than WBC as it may occur before fever and persists after temperature and WBC have returned to normal. Degree of increase does not correlate with severity or prognosis *5544* May be a crude indication of the extent of myocardial damage. A normal ESR during the 2nd week suggests absence of or small myocardial infarction *1980*

Erythrocytes *Blood* *No Effect* In 29 post-myocardial infarction patients mean concentration of 4.65 ± 0.10 x 10^{12}/L not significantly different from 4.95 ± 0.10 x 10^{12}/L in 20 apparently healthy controls *5543*

Estradiol *Plasma* *No Effect* No significant effect observed in 49 male survivors of premature myocardial infarction (mean concentration of 33.2 ± 2.54 pg/mL) compared with 32.0 ± 2.53 pg/mL in 49 healthy controls *3523*

Estrogens *Plasma* *Increase* 34 of 35 male survivors of myocardial infarction, aged 24 - 48 y, had higher plasma concentration of estradiol than age matched controls. 29 of 35 had elevated concentration of estrone *1372*

Factor IV *Plasma* *Increase* A mean of 95 ng/mL was found in 21 patients, compared to normal 16 ± 4 in controls. Patients with chest pain but without evidence of infarction had a mean of 29 ng/mL. Elevation persisted for 1 week and returned to normal *1997*

Factor VII Coagulant *Plasma* *Increase* In 18 patients with AMI and coronary artery disease mean concentration of 105.7 ± 37.3% and of 107.1 ± 20.1% in 20 patients with AMI but without coronary artery disease higher than 95.5 ± 19.2% in 24 age and sex matched controls *1851*

Factor XIII *Plasma* *Decrease* Substantial depression developed with concomitant significant increases in the proportion and concentration of plasma high molecular weight fibrinogen complexes (HMWFC). An inverse correlation between factor XIII and percentage of HMWFC was demonstrated in the early stages of the illness *3253*

Fatty Acid-binding Protein *Serum* *Increase* In 15 patients with acute myocardial infarction mean plasma concentration increased to 144 µg/L at about 4 hours after infarction returning to reference interval within 24 h *1752*

Fatty Acid-binding Protein, Cytoplasmic Heart Type *Serum* *Increase* Mean concentration in 99 patients with acute myocardial infarction of 29.1 µg/L with a range of 13.4 - 87 µg/L significantly higher than that in 104 healthy volunteers, 4.1 µg/L with a range of 3.2 - 6.0 µg/L *2354*

Fatty Acids (FFA), Free *Serum* *Increase* High values (> 1,000 µmol/L) were associated with an increased incidence of serious cardiac arrhythmias after infarction *1919* May be partially related to pituitary-sympathoadrenal stimulation. Patients with higher plasma levels of catecholamines and free fatty acids may have a higher incidence of severe arrhythmias, shock, and death than patients with lower levels *2304* Tend to rise in the first 48 h *1091* Maximum values occurred within 8 h after infarction. Patients with values > 1,200 µmol/L had increased prevalence of serious arrhythmias and disorder of conductance *4867* Observed effect *3158*

Ferritin *Monocytes* *Increase* In 20 patients with AMI during their first 10 days of hospitalization a gradual increase of ferritin occurred on the 5th day (34.3 ± 6.8 ng/10^6 cells) compared with that on day zero (13.5 ± 1.3 ng/10^6 cells) *3613*
Serum *Increase* In 20 patients with AMI during their first 10 days of hospitalization a gradual increase of serum ferritin occurred starting on day 2 reaching a maximum of four times the initial level on the 6th day (470 ± 162 ng/mL) with a subsequent gradual decrease, although the concentration remained high at 286 ± 64 ng/mL *3613*

Fibrin Degradation Products *Plasma* *Increase* Clinical severity of infarction is related to the degree of elevation. Mortality rate was 22% among patients with values 20 µg/dL and 11% in those < 20 µg/dL *3898*

Fibrinogen *Plasma* *Increase* Substantial depression of factor XIII developed with concomitant significant increases in the proportion and concentration of plasma high molecular weight fibrinogen complexes (HMWFC). An inverse correlation between factor XIII and percentage of HMWFC was demonstrated in the early stages of the illness *3253* During acute phase, from day 1 to 5, concentration may be increased *5869* In 18 patients with AMI and coronary artery disease mean concentration of 2.82 ± 0.94 g/L and of 2.55 ± 0.61 g/L in 20 patients with AMI but without coronary artery disease higher than 2.27 ± 0.54 g/L in 24 age and sex matched controls *1851* Significant increase *3858*
Plasma *No Effect* Mean concentration of 3.4 ± 1.1 g/L in 116 patients who had survived an acute myocardial infarction not significantly different from 3.1 ± 0.5 g/L in 116 matched controls *472*

Fibrinopeptide A *Plasma* *Increase* Several studies have shown an increased concentration compared with those with stable angina indicating increased thrombin generation *2201* Mean concentration of 13.1 ± 3.1 ng/mL in 19 patients with AMI who died significantly different from 3.9 ± 1.2 ng/mL in 45 patients with AMI who survived *3031*

Glucose *Serum* *Increase* Mean concentration of 5.5 ± 1.3 mmol/L in 116 patients who had survived an acute myocardial infarction significantly different from 4.9 ± 1.0 mmol/L in 116 matched controls *472* May be partially related to pituitary-sympathoadrenal stimulation. May occur in patients who are not obviously diabetic; attributed to adrenal stimulation secondary to stress and shock *2304* In 70% of 119 patients hospitalized for this disorder *1576* Patients have higher fasting concentrations and dispose of an oral glucose load less efficiently than controls *4707* Glycosuria and hyperglycemia occur in up to 50% of patients *5544*
Urine *Increase* Glycosuria and hyperglycemia occur in up to 50% of patients *5544* May occur in patients who are not obviously diabetic; attributed to adrenal stimulation secondary to stress and shock *2304*

Glucose Tolerance *Serum* *Decrease* Some patients will have abnormal curves when checked months later *2304*

γ-Glutamyltransferase *Serum* *Increase* Activity reportedly increased in a variety of diseases including diseases of the pancreas, myocardium, kidney and lung as well as in diabetes *4617* Usually remains in the normal range for 3 - 4 days, then increases to reach a peak about the 8 - 11th day after infarction *1400* Activity is raised in association with anoxic damage to the liver, and also in association with recovery and repair *1290* Increased activity reported with myocardial infarction *3625* Observed in some patients with liver involvement *914* Increased in 50% of patients with shock or acute right heart failure, may have early peak within 48 h with rapid decline followed by later rise *5544*
Serum *No Effect* In 11 patients with AMI or unstable angina no significant change observed 24 to 48 hours after onset of chest pain *3732*

Glycogen Phosphorylase BB Isoenzyme *Serum* *Increase* Concentration increased typically between 1 and 4 h after chest pain onset *3235* In 32 patients with AMI all had concentrations increased above 7.0 µg/L in first 12 hours following infarction *4256*

GP Ib *Platelets* *No Effect* In 16 patients with AMI who responded to antithrombolytic therapy mean log amplification of fluorescence intensity of 121.9 ± 13.2 compared with 118.5 ± 17.1 in 5 patients who failed to respond to antithrombolytic treatment and 133.6 ± 8.0 in 10 healthy controls *1928*

GP IIb *Platelets* *No Effect* In 16 patients with AMI who responded to antithrombolytic therapy mean log amplification of fluorescence intensity of 34.4 ± 2.2 compared with 30.6 ± 2.6 in 5 patients who failed to respond to antithrombolytic treatment and 37.2 ± 1.7 in 10 healthy controls *1928*

GP IIb/GP IIIa *Platelets* *No Effect* In 16 patients with AMI who responded to antithrombolytic therapy mean log amplification of fluorescence intensity of 56.5 ± 8.0 compared with 57.2 ± 9.0 in 5 patients who failed to respond to antithrombolytic treatment and 53.0 ± 7.0 in 10 healthy controls *1928*

GP IIIa *Platelets* *No Effect* In 16 patients with AMI who responded to antithrombolytic therapy mean log amplification of fluorescence intensity of 334.1 ± 22.7 compared with 321.9 ± 43.5 in 5 patients who failed to respond to antithrombolytic treatment and 320.3 ± 25.2 in 10 healthy controls *1928*

410.90 Acute Myocardial Infarction *(continued)*

Granulocytes *Blood Increase* In 69 patients with AMI mean concentration of 7.6 x 10^9/L significantly higher than 4.5 x 10^9/L in 315 patients without AMI *5222*

Haptoglobin *Serum Increase* During acute phase, from day 1 to 5, concentration may be increased *5869* Significant increase *3858*

HDL-Cholesterol *Serum Decrease* In 26 Greek-Caucasians who had had an AMI within the previous 6 - 17 months mean concentration of 0.8 - 1.0 mmol/L significantly different from 0.9 - 1.2 mmol/L in 26 age-matched healthy controls *5206* In 18 patients with AMI and coronary artery disease mean concentration of 1.18 ± 0.25 mmol/L significantly lower than 1.38 ± 0.32 mmol/L in 24 age and sex matched controls *1851* Mean concentration of 1.2 ± 0.3 mmol/L in 116 patients who had survived an acute myocardial infarction significantly different from 1.6 ± 0.4 mmol/L in 116 matched controls *472* In 49 men who survived premature myocardial infarction mean concentration of 40.4 ± 1.5 mg/dL lower than 49.3 ± 2.0 mg/dL in 49 healthy controls *3523*
Serum No Effect In 20 patients with AMI but without coronary artery disease mean concentration of 1.39 ± 0.40 mmol/L not significantly different from 1.38 ± 0.32 mmol/L in 24 age and sex matched controls *1851*

Helicobacter pylori Antibodies *Serum Increase* Seropositivity observed in 54% of patients with MI compared with 50% in control population without MI *117*

Hemagglutination Inhibition *Serum Increase* Using the passive hemagglutination reaction, a 4-fold or greater rise in antibodies to saline extracts of human heart in 46% of 50 patients was found. Highest titers and highest frequency of elevated titers occurred 2 - 4 weeks after onset *2097*

Hematocrit *Blood Decrease* After an initial small increase, decreased 12% until day 9 and remained constant thereafter *4912* Significant increases in plasma volume, reflected by changes in hematocrit. Average change was 12%. For the patients with accompanying pulmonary edema, the change was 17% *5705*
Blood Increase Volume may be decreased, together with a slight increase in hematocrit *2304* After an initial small increase, decreased 12% until day 9 and remained constant thereafter *4912*

β-Hexosaminidase *Serum Increase* Increase in total concentration (hexosaminidase A and B) *3850*

High Molecular Weight Kininogen *Plasma Increase* Increased generation of bradykinin observed in association with AMI, as a result of kallikrein activation *2201*

Homocysteine *Plasma Increase* In addition, total homocysteine is an independent risk factor for premature cardiovascular diseases *5346* Levels of homocyst(e)ine were higher in cases than in controls (11.1 ± 4.0 [SD] vs 10.5 ± 2.8 nmol/mL; p = 0.03). The difference was attributable to an excess of high values among men who later had MIs. The relative risk for the highest 5% vs the bottom 90% of homocyst(e)ine levels was 3.1 (95% confidence interval, 1.4 to 6.9; p = 0.005). Moderately high levels of plasma homocyst(e)ine are associated with subsequent risk of MI independent of other coronary risk factors *4977* In 12 of 68 patients with AMI moderate hyperhomocysteinemia (> 17.3 µmol/L) observed with mean concentration increasing from 13.1 ± 4.6 µmol/L to 14.8 ± 4.8 µmol/L after 6 weeks *2907*
Plasma No Effect In 92 male cases mean concentration of 9.83 ± 3.00 µmol/L compared with 9.82 ± 3.17 µmol/L in 141 controls and 9.39 ± 2.42 µmol/L in 99 female cases mean concentration compared with 9.28 ± 2.59 µmol/L in 128 controls *76*

17-Hydroxycorticosteroids *Urine Increase* Reported effect *2304*

Hypoxanthine *Serum Increase* Myocardial ischemia in 18 patients resulted in an increase of coronary sinus hypoxanthine levels from 1.20 ± 0.52 mg/dL during pain *4322*

Immunoglobulin A *Serum Increase* In 145 individuals with previous myocardial infarction plasma IgA concentration (3.60 ± 1.68 g/L) higher than in healthy controls (2.73 ± 1.22 g/L), patients with angina pectoris and those with acute myocardial infarction (2.65 ± 1.46 g/L). 30% individuals had concentrations above 4.5 g/L compared with 3% in healthy controls *3684* Concentration in 135 men who had a MI or had sudden cardiac death of 274 mg/dL compared with 245 mg/dL in 135 control individuals matched for lipid concentrations *2797*

Immunoglobulin E *Serum Increase* Concentration in 135 men who had a MI or had sudden cardiac death of 1.2 mg/dL compared with 0.91 mg/dL in 135 control individuals matched for lipid concentrations *2797*

Immunoglobulin G *Serum Increase* Concentration in 135 men who had a MI or had sudden cardiac death of 1,230 mg/dL compared with 1,115 mg/dL in 135 control individuals matched for lipid concentrations *2797* From day 5, concentration may show a rapid decrease and return to normal in the third week *5869*
Serum No Effect No significant difference observed in patients who had a previous myocardial infarction and in healthy controls and patients with angina pectoris *3684*

Immunoglobulin M *Serum No Effect* Concentration in 135 men who had a MI or had sudden cardiac death of 132 mg/dL not significantly different when compared with 124 mg/dL in 135 control individuals matched for lipid concentrations *2797* In 145 patients with previous myocardial infarction no significant difference in concentration observed from that in healthy controls and patients with angina pectoris *3684*

Insulin-like Growth Factor-I *Serum Increase* In 34 patients with AMI mean concentration on admission of 280.8 ± 35.3 ng/mL not significantly different from 207.0 ± 29.5 ng/mL in 17 age-matched normal controls *2975*

Insulin-like Growth Factor-I, Free *Serum Increase* In 34 patients with AMI mean concentration on admission of 1.13 ± 0.2 ng/mL significantly different from 0.56 ± 0.28 ng/mL in 17 age-matched normal controls *2975*

Insulin-like Growth Factor Binding Protein-1
Serum Decrease In 34 patients with AMI mean concentration on admission of 39.9 ± 8.5 ng/mL significantly different from 69.5 ± 10.5 ng/mL in 17 age-matched normal controls *2975*

Insulin-like Growth Factor Binding Protein-3
Serum Increase In 34 patients with AMI mean concentration on admission of 2,919 ± 157 ng/mL significantly different from 2,397 ± 144 ng/mL in 17 age-matched normal controls *2975*

Interleukin-1 Receptor Antagonist *Serum Increase* In patients with severe acute myocardial infarction concentration greatly increased compared with concentration in patients with uncomplicated AMI *2933*

Interleukin-1β *Serum Increase* Mean baseline concentration in 24 patients with acute myocardial infarction mean peak concentration of 22.2 ± 8.6 pg/mL significantly different from normal of < 10 pg/mL *4233*
Serum No Effect IL-1β not detectable in any of 7 patients after severe acute myocardial infarction (Killip class 3 or 4) *2933*

Interleukin-6 *Serum Increase* Examined serum interleukin 6 (IL-6) levels in 12 patients with acute myocardial infarction (AMI). IL-6 levels became elevated in all patients, following the rise of serum creatine kinase (CK) activity *2324* In patients with AMI mean concentration of IL-6, which is synthesized in the myocardium, increases *633* Mean baseline concentration in 24 patients with acute myocardial infarction mean peak concentration of 184.9 ± 134.7 pg/mL significantly different from normal of 15.57 ± 2.9 pg/mL *4233*

Interleukin-8 *Serum Increase* Mean baseline concentration in 24 patients with acute myocardial infarction mean peak concentration of 103.0 ± 23.4 pg/mL significantly different from normal of < 30 pg/mL *4233* In 5 studied patients transient but significant rise in serum IL-8 concentration (13 - 1100 ng/L) observed within 22 hoursafter the onset of symptoms, whereas no increase observed in patients with angina pectoris or normal controls *13*
Serum No Effect Not detectable in the plasma of any of 7 patients after severe acute myocardial infarction (Killip class 3 or 4) *2933*

Iron *Serum Decrease* Observed response *5677 1998* Decrease in concentration observed following myocardial infarction *2952*

Isocitrate Dehydrogenase *Serum No Effect* Concentrations were within normal limits in assays performed within 24 h after onset of symptoms *5008*

Kallikrein-like Activity *Plasma Increase* Increased activity observed in association with AMI *2201*

Lactate *Blood* *Increase* Observed effect *1484* Patients may develop arterial and tissue hypoxia and metabolic acidosis with a decrease in arterial pH and pO_2, together with an increase in blood lactate concentration *2304*

Lactate Dehydrogenase *Serum* *Increase* Rises 2 - 10 fold after the first 12 h and reaches a peak by 24 - 48 h. The increase is roughly parallel to the degree of cardiac damage and also to the serum AST *1290* Increase begins several hours after onset of infarction *219* Moderate elevations in almost all patients (92-98%) with proven infarction. The complication by shock leads to higher values of AST and LD and to abnormal levels of enzymes that reflect hepatic injury (ALT, ICD) *1025* May remain elevated up to 10 - 14 days after onset; therefore is particularly useful when patient is first seen after sufficient time has elapsed for CK and AST to become normal *5544* Concentrations above 2,000 U/L suggest a poor prognosis *5544* In patients with acute myocardial infarction 8 hours after onset of pain activity increased in 83% patients *5838*

Lactate Dehydrogenase Isoenzyme-1 *Serum* *Increase* In 15 patients with acute myocardial infarction mean plasma activity increased to 530 µg/L at about 20 hours after infarction *1752*

Lactate Dehydrogenase Isoenzyme-5 *Serum* *Increase* Almost invariably increased, beginning 12 h after infarction and peaking after 48 h *3033* Parallels increase of fast moving LD with peak (3 - 4 times normal) in 48 h and persistent elevation for up to 2 weeks *5544*

Lactate Dehydrogenase Isoenzymes *Serum* *Increase* LD_1 is markedly increased *2226* Increased LD_1 and LD_2. May remain elevated after total LD is normalized. In small infarctions, LD_1 may be increased when total LD remains normal. In acute infarction with congestive heart failure, LD_1 and LD_5 are elevated. Distinguish infarction from other diseases which elevate total LD. Heat-stable, fast moving fractions increased in infarction *5544*

LDL-Cholesterol *Serum* *Increase* Mean concentration of 4.0 ± 0.9 mmol/L in 116 patients who had survived an acute myocardial infarction significantly different from 3.6 ± 1.1 mmol/L in 116 matched controls *472* In 26 Greek-Caucasians who had had an AMI within the previous 6 - 17 months mean concentration of 4.5 ± 0.5 mmol/L significantly different from 3.9 ± 0.9 mmol/L in 26 age-matched healthy controls *5206*

Leukocytes *Blood* *Increase* Mean count was significantly elevated in 464 patients, measured, on the average, 16.8 months before the infarction occurred. Total WBC was closely related to development of infarct and to cigarette smoking *1575* Almost invariable. 75 - 90% neutrophils with only a slight shift to the left. Leukocytosis is likely to develop before fever *5544* In 69 patients with AMI mean concentration of 10.4 x 10^9/L significantly higher than 7.2 x 10^9/L in 315 patients without AMI *5222* Patients with transmural infarcts had a significantly higher count than patients with nontransmural infarcts *2962* In 20 patients with AMI concentration of 10,740 ± 678 /µL on admission significantly greater than 6,536 ± 398 /µL in 14 healthy controls *3030*
Blood *No Effect* In 29 post-myocardial infarction patients with angina mean concentration of 7.66 ± 0.34 x 10^9/L not significantly different from 6.69 ± 0.30 x 10^9/L in 20 apparently healthy controls *5543*

Lipoprotein Lp(a) *Serum* *Decrease* In 97 male cases mean concentration of 73 mg/L compared with 108 mg/L in 148 controls *76*
Serum *Increase* In 18 patients with AMI and coronary artery disease mean concentration of 294 ± 308 mg/L and 270 ± 283 mg/L in 20 patients with AMI but no coronary artery disease markedly higher than 140 ± 154 mg/L in 24 age and sex matched controls *1851* In 97 female cases mean concentration of 113 mg/L compared with 91 mg/L in 121 controls *76* Reportedly increased concentrations of Lp(a) observed following acute myocardial infarction in association with acute phase reaction *2827*

α-Lipoproteins *Serum* *Increase* From day 5, concentration may show a rapid decrease and return to normal in the third week *5869*

Low Density Lipoprotein *Serum* *Decrease* In 26 Greek-Caucasians who had had an AMI within the previous 6 - 17 months mean concentration of 28 - 42 mg/dL significantly different from 45 - 76 mg/dL in 26 age-matched healthy controls *5206*

Low Density Lipoprotein-2 *Serum* *No Effect* In 26 Greek-Caucasians who had had an AMI within the previous 6 - 17 months mean concentration of 81 - 124 mg/dL not significantly different from 90 - 124 mg/dL in 26 age-matched healthy controls *5206*

Low Density Lipoprotein-3 *Serum* *Increase* In 26 Greek-Caucasians who had had an AMI within the previous 6 - 17 months mean concentration of 67 - 127 mg/dL not significantly different from 22 - 57 mg/dL in 26 age-matched healthy controls *5206*

Lymphocytes *Blood* *No Effect* In 29 post-myocardial infarction patients mean concentration of 1.91 ± 0.11 x 10^9/L not significantly different from 1.89 ± 0.13 x 10^9/L in 20 apparently healthy controls *5543* In 69 patients with AMI mean concentration of 1.9 x 10^9/L not significantly different from 2.1 x 10^9/L in 315 patients without AMI *5222*

Lysophosphatidylcholine *Serum* *Decrease* In patients with AMI significant reduction observed 24 - 48 h after onset of AMI *2916*
Serum *Increase* In patients following AMI increase observed 60 - 72 hours after onset of AMI *2916*

Magnesium *Serum* *Decrease* Hypomagnesemia is observed in about one quarter of patients with myocardial infarction *3195*

Malate Dehydrogenase *Serum* *Increase* Level rises after 6 - 24 h to a peak at 24 - 48 h (2 to 15 times normal), falling to normal by 5 days. The peak precedes AST and LD, and degree is similar to rise in AST *1290* Always elevated, sometimes strikingly *454* Elevated 2 to 10 times above normal in all cases of clinically proved infarction *5506*

Manganese Superoxide Dismutase *Serum* *Increase* An early small elevation was observed at approximately 16.2 hours and a high elevation at approximately 108 hours after the onset of symptoms *5093*

MCHC *Blood* *Increase* In 29 post-myocardial infarction patients MCHC significantly different from that in 20 apparently healthy controls *5543*

Monocytes *Blood* *No Effect* In 29 post-myocardial infarction patients mean concentration of 0.60 ± 0.04 x 10^9/L not significantly different from 0.54 ± 0.03 x 10^9/L in 20 apparently healthy controls *5543*

Myoglobin *Serum* *Increase* Most acute myocardial infarction patients have concentrations of 0.15 - 0.5 µg/mL compared with normal up to 0.09 µg/mL *2952* In 29 patients with AMI mean activity of 1320 ± 875 U/L observed (upper limit of normal 75 µg/L) *2957* In 30 patients with acute myocardial infarction mean time to first increased value 4.2 h, mean time to peak concentration 7 h, mean time to normalization more than 26 h with the increased concentration providing 55 multiples of the discriminant limit for acute myocardial infarction *702* In 9 patients with acute myocardial infarction serum myoglobin increased within 8 hours (before total CK or CK-MB) *3234* Very common; first appears in serum within a few h after infarction, reaching a peak before the peak of CK activity. Did not correlate with infarct size as estimated by CK *2525* Mean concentration in 26 patients with AMI on day of admission of 450 µg/L and of 200 µg/L on day 1 significantly increased compared with healthy individuals *5377* Mean concentration in 99 patients with acute myocardial infarction of 196 µg/L (range 95 - 472 µg/L) significantly higher than that in 104 healthy volunteers, 54 µg/L with a range of 41 - 70 µg/L *2354* In 22 of 25 patients studied within 24 h of a myocardial infarction concentration increased to a mean of 315.5 ng/mL but with return to normal within 4 days *67* Of serum CK-MB, cTnI and myoglobin, myoglobin had the highest clinical sensitivity (50%) when blood was collected between 0 and 6 h after onset of chest pain, and with clinical sensitivity > 93% 6 - 24 h after onset of chest pain. Between 72 and 150 h after onset of chest pain had a sensitivity of only 21% *5740* In 15 patients with acute myocardial infarction mean plasma concentration increased to 1,020 µg/L at about 4 hours after infarction returning to reference interval within 24 h *1752*
Urine *Increase* Sporadic; ischemic *5544*

Myoglobin:Fatty Acid-binding Protein Ratio
Serum *Increase* Serum ratio in patients with acute myocardial infarction approximately 5 *1752*

Myosin Light Chain I *Serum* *Increase* In 64 patients with AMI serum concentrations peak at 55 ± 28 h after reperfusion *5158*

410.90 Acute Myocardial Infarction (continued)

Neopterin *Urine* *Increase* In 13 patients with AMI mean excretion increased to 419 ± 202 µmol/mol creatinine compared with 121 ± 28 µmol/mol creatinine in 7 healthy controls *3446*

Neuropeptide Y *Plasma* *Increase* In 30 patients with MI mean concentration of 46.0 ± 6.4 pmol/L on day 1 and 60.8 ± 5.7 pmol/L on day 3 (peak concentration significantly increased) compared with 42.6 ± 12.3 pmol/L on day 1 and 34.4 ± 5.6 pmol/L on day 3 in 8 control patients with chest pain but no MI *3912*

Neutrophils *Blood* *Increase* Increase of polymorphonuclear leukocytes, with an increase in young forms *2304* In 58% of 100 patients hospitalized for this disorder *1576*
Blood *No Effect* In 29 post-myocardial infarction patients mean concentration of 4.86 ± 0.30 x 10^9/L not significantly different from 3.91 ± 0.24 x 10^9/L in 20 apparently healthy controls *5543*

Nickel *Serum* *Decrease* Decreases occur soon after infarction (within 24 h for Caucasian males and before the 3rd day in Caucasian females and Black males), followed by a sharp rise to > 2 times normal value *5605*
Serum *Increase* Decrease occurs soon after infarction (within 24 h for Caucasian males and before the 3rd day in Caucasian females and Black males), followed by a sharp rise to > 2 times normal value *5605* Mean concentration of 5.2 µg/L (n = 33) compared with mean in controls of 2.6 µg/L (n = 42) *3428*

Norepinephrine *Plasma* *Increase* Evidence for a sympathoadrenal response is found in the increased blood and urinary concentration or norepinephrine, epinephrine, or their metabolic products *2304* In 30 patients with acute MI mean concentrations on day 1 and 3 of 5.4 ± 0.6 nmol/L and 4.2 ± 1.6 nmol/L respectively compared with 2.8 ± 0.7 nmol/L and 1.5 ± 0.5 nmol/L in 8 control patients with chest pain but no MI *3912* Observed effect *2444* In 335 patients with acute myocardial infarction mean concentration of 278 ± 173 pg/mL (mean 12 days after infarction) significantly higher than 231 ± 87 pg/mL in 38 control individuals *4321*
Plasma *No Effect* In 145 patients with AMI, on day 3 following infarct median concentration of 2.29 nmol/L not significantly different from upper limit of normal of 2.40 nmol/L, but with poorer prognosis observed in patients with higher concentrations *3911*
Urine *Increase* In patients developing heart failure or cardiogenic shock, the urinary level of both free catecholamines rose notably in the 1st week after infarction. In uncomplicated cases, a moderate rise in the norepinephrine level in the 1st week was associated with only a transient rise in the epinephrine level *2444* Evidence for sympathoadrena response is found in the increased blood and urinary concentration or norepinephrine, epinephrine, or their metabolic products *2304*

Osteocalcin *Serum* *Decrease* Mean concentration of 2.0 ± 0.9 ng/mL in 11 patients with acute myocardial infarction or unstable angina 2.0 ± 0.9 ng/mL 24 to 48 hours after pain significantly less than 3.1 ± 1.1 ng/mL in healthy controls. Probable stress related effect *3732*

Oxidase *Plasma* *Increase* In 22 patients with AMI mean plasma oxidase activity of 233 ± 13 U/L significantly greater than 84 ± 5 U/L in 12 healthy controls *2931*

Oxygen Partial Pressure *Blood* *Decrease* Arterial pO_2 falls, but rarely below 70 mm Hg if there is reasonable cardiovascular function. In left ventricular failure with associated pulmonary edema, the arterial pO_2 may fall to 50 mm Hg *1290* Patients may develop arterial and tissue hypoxia and metabolic acidosis with a decrease in arterial pH and pO_2 *2304* Very frequent complication; occurs in 60% of uncomplicated cases. The intensity of hypoxemia is greatest after 2 - 3 days. The most intense and persisting hypoxemia was seen in patients with shock and/or acute left ventricular failure. Present even 6 months after onset in 25% *5662*

Oxygen Saturation *Blood* *Decrease* Arterial pO_2 falls, but rarely below 70 mm Hg if there is reasonable cardiovascular function. In left ventricular failure with associated pulmonary edema, the arterial pO_2 may fall to 50 mm Hg *1290* Patients may develop arterial and tissue hypoxia and metabolic acidosis with a decrease in arterial pH and pO_2 *2304* Very frequent complication; occurs in about 60% of uncomplicated cases. The intensity of hypoxemia is greatest after 2 - 3 days. The most intense and persisting hypoxemia was seen in patients with shock and/or acute left ventricular failure. Present even 6 months after onset in 25% *5662*

pH *Blood* *Decrease* Following cardiac arrest, acidosis rapidly develops, and, if not corrected, can result in the inability to defibrillate the heart in ventricular fibrillation *1980* Patients may develop arterial and tissue hypoxia and metabolic acidosis with an increase in blood lactate concentration *2304* Slight metabolic acidosis was observed on the first day of the disease in 37% of the cases, while severe metabolic acidosis was found in 50 - 60% of the cases during 1 year after myocardial infarction *5662*
Cerebrospinal Fluid *Decrease* In patients who developed severe anoxia after cardiac arrest, the normal cisternal-lumbar pH gradient was reversed, cisternal fluid was more acid (pH 6.815 vs 6.953), and cisternal potassium concentration was twice that of lumbar (6.7 vs 3.5 mmol/L). During anoxia, potassium and hydrogen ions flow from brain cells into the brain extracellular fluid. Acute changes are reflected more accurately by cisternal than by lumbar fluid *2536*

Phosphate *Serum* *No Effect* In 11 patients with AMI or unstable angina no significant change observed 24 to 48 hours after onset of acute pain *3732*

Phosphoglycerate Mutase *Plasma* *Increase* Peak activity occurred 5 hours after onset of acute myocardial infarction *5807*

Phospholipase A *Serum* *Increase* Increased activities in association with a wide variety of nonpancreatic disorders *2615*

Phospholipase A_2 *Serum* *Increase* In patients with AMI significant increase observed from 24 - 48 h of onset of infarction *2916*

Phospholipids *Serum* *Increase* Mean concentration was increased to 249.5 ± 7.6 mg/L in 69 male patients, compared to 204.1 ± 3.5 mg/L in normals *795*

α_2-Plasmin Inhibitor *Plasma* *No Effect* In 60 patients with acute myocardial infarction median concentration of 82% not significantly from that in 30 healthy controls *2546*

Plasminogen Activator Inhibitor-1 *Plasma* *No Effect* In 18 patients with AMI and coronary artery disease mean concentration of 29.5 ± 13.2 µg/L and in 20 patients with AMI but without coronary artery disease 24.3 ± 7.3 µg/L not significantly different from 23.2 ± 7.2 µg/L in 24 age and sex matched controls *1851*

Platelet Activating Factor *Serum* *No Effect* In 13 male patients with AMI mean concentration of 0.16 ± 0.04 ng/mL not significantly different from 0.25 ± 0.05 ng/mL in 10 normal males *1838*

Platelet Aggregation *Blood* *Decrease* Significantly reduced the first few days *2723*

Platelet-derived Growth Factor *Plasma* *Increase* In 29 post-myocardial infarction patients mean concentration of 58.4 ± 1.66 ng/L significantly different from 53.7 ± 2.01 ng/L in 20 apparently healthy controls *5543*

Platelets *Blood* *No Effect* In 29 post-myocardial infarction patients mean concentration of 270 ± 20 x 10^9/L not significantly different from 248 ± 12 x 10^9/L in 20 apparently healthy controls *5543*

Potassium *Cerebrospinal Fluid* *Increase* Of 41 patients with cardiac arrest studied, 20 regained consciousness and 21 did not. In those who did not, was a significant increase in the K^+ concentration found in samples obtained between 40 - 50 min and between 50 - 60 min after cardiac arrest. Potassium concentration of cisternal CSF obtained soon after cardiac arrest might give an indication of the degree of cerebral damage *4831* In patients who developed severe anoxia after a cardiac arrest, the cisternal K^+ concentration was twice that of lumbar (6.7 vs 3.5 mmol/L). During anoxia, K^+ and H^+ flow from brain cells into the brain extracellular fluid. Acute changes are reflected more accurately by cisternal than by lumbar fluid *2536*

Pro-Atrial Natriuretic Peptide (1-98) *Serum* *Increase* Significant negative correlation so that as left ventricular ejection fraction decreases concentration of pro-ANP increases *514*

Prostate-specific Antigen *Serum* *Decrease* Mean concentration in several men of 2.45 ± 2.58 µg/L on second day post-infarction significantly less than 2.81 ± 3.05 µg/L on first day post-infarct and 2.98 ± 3.21 µg/L on third day post-infarction *968*

Prothrombin Fragment 1.2 *Plasma* *Increase* Mean concentration of prothrombin fragment 1.2 in platelet-poor plasma from 15 patients with acute myocardial infarction of 5.3 ± 4.7 nmol/L significantly higher than 0.51 nmol/L (95% reference interval 0.21 - 2.78 nmol/L) in 268 healthy individuals less than 44 years of age *1860* Mean concentration of 6.7 ± 1.2 nmol/L in 19 patients with AMI who died significantly different from 3.7 ± 0.5 nmol/L in 45 patients with AMI who survived *3031*

P-Selectin *Serum* *Increase* Mean concentration of 83 ± 13 ng/mL in 16 patients with AMI on admission significantly different from 24 ± 5 ng/mL in 13 control individuals. Peak concentration reached 115 ± 17 ng/mL about 4 hours after admission *4805* In 16 patients with AMI who responded to antithrombolytic therapy mean log amplification of fluorescence intensity of 28.1 ± 1.9 significantly different when compared with 33.7 ± 1.2 in 5 patients who failed to respond to antithrombolytic treatment: (25.1 ± 2.6 in 10 healthy controls) *1928*

Pyridoxal Phosphate *Serum* *Decrease* Marked significant reduction in concentration of pyridoxal-5-phosphate concentration observed in patients with recent myocardial infarction *4965*

Renin Activity *Plasma* *Increase* In 335 patients with acute myocardial infarction mean activity 2.4 ± 2.9 ng/mL/h (mean 12 days after infarction) significantly higher than 1.2 ± 1.2 ng/mL/h in 38 control individuals *4321*

Retinol-binding Protein *Urine* *Increase* In 8 of 22 patients with acute myocardial infarction concentration increased above normal on day of admission: 1.43 mg/L on day 0, 0.27 mg/L on day 1, 0.20 mg/L on day 2 and 0.06 mg/L on day 3 *1336*

Rheumatoid Factor *Serum* *Increase* Found in 12% of patients *306* *874*

S-100ao Protein *Serum* *Increase* In 21 patients with AMI mean concentration increased to 4.74 ± 5.27 µg/L at admission and to peak at 8 h of 23.5 ± 27.7 µg/L compared with 0.12 ± 0.08 µg/L in healthy controls *5375*

Sex-Hormone Binding Globulin *Serum* *Increase* In 7 male patients with AMI mean concentration on admission 49.4 ± 8.8 nmol/L significantly greater than 28 ± 5.1 nmol/L in 7 control patients *3891*

Sodium *Serum* *Decrease* Frequent hyponatremia, degree of loss seems to correlate with severity of myocardial involvement *4707*

Soluble E-Selectin *Serum* *Increase* In 23 patients with acute myocardial infarction mean concentration of 26.4 ± 1.3 ng/mL on admission to hospital compared to 22.9 ± 1.1 ng/mL in 10 healthy controls. Concentrations increased to 28.8 ± 1.8 ng/mL after 3 hours, 25.6 ± 1.4 ng/mL after 6 hours, 25.7 ± 1.2 ng/mL after 12 hours and 24.6 ± 1.2 ng/mL after 24 hours *1927* In 24 patients with acute myocardial infarction mean peak concentration of 145.1 ± 74.5 ng/mL significantly different from normal of 29.1 - 63.4 ng/mL *4233* In 20 patients with AMI concentration of 37.2 ± 3.9 ng/mL on admission increased significantly to 46.1 ± 4.1 ng/mL after 6 h, 41.1 ± 3.8 ng/mL after 12 h, 41.6 ± 3.7 ng/mL after 24 h and 37.4 ± 3.3 ng/mL after 48 h compared with 32.5 ± 5.4 ng/mL in 14 healthy controls *3030*

Soluble Intercellular Adhesion Molecule-1 *Serum* *Increase* In 20 patients with AMI concentration of 250.7 ± 23.4 ng/mL on admission increased significantly to 271.2 ± 24.5 ng/mL after 6 h, 267.9 ± 18.8 ng/mL after 12 h, 265.1 ± 15.8 ng/mL after 24 h and 270.9 ± 20.4 ng/mL after 48 h compared with 204.0 ± 14.6 ng/mL in 14 healthy controls *3030* Mean baseline concentration in 24 patients with acute myocardial infarction mean peak concentration of 328.8 ± 168.5 ng/mL significantly different from normal of 189.1 - 42.3 ng/mL *4233*

Soluble P-Selectin *Serum* *Increase* Mean concentration of 272 ng/mL in 116 patients who had survived an acute myocardial infarction significantly different from 190 ng/mL in 116 matched controls *472*

Soluble Tumor Necrosis Factor Receptor-I *Serum* *Increase* Concentration significantly increased in patients with severe acute myocardial infarction compared with patients in whom AMI was uncomplicated *2933*

Soluble Vascular Cell Adhesion Molecule-1 *Serum* *Increase* In 23 patients with acute myocardial infarction mean concentration of 596 ± 28 ng/mL on admission to hospital compared to 349 ± 36 ng/mL in 10 healthy controls. Concentrations increased to 647 ± 29 ng/mL after 3 hours, 596 ± 32 ng/mL after 6 hours, 643 ± 34 ng/mL after 12 hours and 640 ± 38 ng/mL after 24 hours *1927*
Serum *No Effect* In 20 patients with AMI concentration of 734.5 ± 58.3 ng/mL on admission changed nonsignificantly to 753.4 ± 48.1 ng/mL after 6 h, 780.4 ± 40.7 ng/mL after 12 h, 782.8 ± 51.9 ng/mL after 24 h and 773.1 ± 54.9 ng/mL after 48 h compared with 766.1 ± 67.7 ng/mL in 14 healthy controls *3030*

Testosterone *Serum* *Decrease* In 49 men after premature myocardial infarction mean concentration of 423.0 ± 24.9 ng/dL less than 502.5 ng/dL in 49 healthy controls *3523*
Serum *No Effect* In 7 men with AMI at time of admission mean concentration of 13.0 ± 3.4 nmol/L not significantly different from 11.7 ± 1.4 nmol/L in 7 controls with no significant change with time *3891*

Testosterone, Free *Serum* *Decrease* In 49 men after premature myocardial infarction mean concentration of 12.13 ± 0.54 ng/dL compared with 13.77 ± 0.79 ng/dL in 49 healthy controls *3523*

Tetranectin *Serum* *Decrease* In 60 patients with acute myocardial infarction median concentration of 8.27 mg/L significantly less than 12.10 mg/L in 30 healthy controls *2546*

Thrombin/Antithrombin III Complex *Plasma* *Increase* Mean concentration of 27.3 ± 5.7 ng/mL in 19 patients with AMI who died significantly different from 11.2 ± 2.6 ng/mL in 45 patients with AMI who survived *3031*

β-Thromboglobulin *Plasma* *Increase* In 24 patients with AMI mean concentration on admission (3.5 ± 1.5 h after onset of symptoms) 105 ± 27 IU/mL compared with normal range of 35 ± 18 IU/mL *4542*

Thromboxane A_2 *Plasma* *Increase* Observed effect *4677*

Tissue Plasminogen Activator *Plasma* *No Effect* In 18 patients with AMI and coronary artery disease mean concentration of 7.1 ± 2.8 µg/L and 5.7 ± 3.3 µg/L in 20 with AMI but no coronary artery disease not significantly different from 6.2 ± 1.8 µg/L in 24 age and sex matched controls *1851*

Tissue Plasminogen Activator:Plasminogen Activator Inhibitor-1 Antigen Ratio *Plasma* *Increase* In 50 patients with acute myocardial infarction median ratio of 0.90 significantly different from 0.53 in healthy controls *127*

Transferrin *Serum* *Increase* From day 5, concentration may show a rapid decrease and return to normal in the third week *5869*

Tri-iodothyronine (T3) *Serum* *Decrease* Decreased to 66% at day 9 and then returned to normal within 2 months *4912*

Triglycerides *Serum* *Increase* Mean concentration of 2.0 mmol/L in 116 patients who had survived an acute myocardial infarction significantly different from 1.5 mmol/L in 116 matched controls *472* Tends to be moderately elevated for a few weeks following a brief decrease *2304* In 20 patients with AMI without coronary artery disease mean concentration of 1.55 ± 0.96 mmol/L and in 18 with AMI with coronary artery disease 2.09 ± 1.01 mmol/L higher than 1.15 ± 0.48 mmol/L in 24 age and sex matched controls *1851* In 26 Greek-Caucasians who had had an AMI within the previous 6 - 17 months mean concentration of 1.3 - 1.9 mmol/L significantly different from 1.0 - 1.5 mmol/L in 26 age-matched healthy controls *5206* Mean concentration was 92.5 ± 3.5 mg/dL in 69 male patients, compared to 76.1 ± 3.7 in controls *795* In 49 male survivors of premature myocardial infarction mean concentration of 173.7 ± 13.2 mg/dL higher than 135.2 ± 10.9 mg/dL in 49 healthy controls *3523* Rises to peak in 3 weeks; the increase may persist for 1 year *5544*
Serum *No Effect* Mean concentration of 147 ± 23 mg/dL in 16 patients with AMI not significantly different from 120 ± 22 mg/dL in 13 control individuals *4805*

Troponin I *Serum* *Increase* In 64 patients with AMI serum concentrations peak at 6.1 ± 3.5 h after reperfusion *5158* Concentrations increased in 98% patients with acute myocardial infarction as early as 30 min after infarction and remain increased for up to 10 days *2649* Of serum CK-MB, cTnI and myoglobin, cTnI had clinical sensitivity > 93% 6 - 24 h after onset of chest pain, remained highly sensitive for 48 h. Between 72 and 150 h after onset of chest pain had a sensitivity of 70%, much better than for myoglobin and CK-MB *5740*

Troponin T *Serum* *Increase* In 64 patients with AMI serum concentrations peak at 6.8 ± 4.0 h after reperfusion *5158* Significant correlation of cardiac troponin T concentration observed (r = 0.73) with myocardial infarct size *3236* In 90 patients with AMI admitted to CCU TnT concentrations at 24 h 1.00 - 55.76 ng/mL and 0.10 - 37.60 ng/mL significantly higher concentrations following CABG at 24 h (0.37 - 3.74 ng/mL) and at 96 h (0.09 -

410.90 Acute Myocardial Infarction *(continued)*

Troponin T *(continued)*
2.58 ng/mL) *5271* Concentrations increased in patients with acute myocardial infarction slightly later than troponin I and remains increased longer than troponin I *2649* Using a cutoff of 0.1 ng/mL sensitivities observed of 55% (0 - 5 h), 97% (6 - 11 h), 100% (12 - 23 h), 100% (24 - 47 h), 100% (48 - 95 h), and 100% (greater than 96 h) for acute myocardial infarction *5741* After 8 hours after onset of cardiac pain increased concentration observed in 93% of patients with acute myocardial infarction *5838* TnT concentration rose in parallel with both CK-MB and AST, but remained increased significantly longer: significant association of ratio of TnT to CK-MB with activity of ALT *3683*
Serum No Effect In 29 patients with acute myocardial infarction on admission to hospital concentration undetectable *3093*

Tumor Necrosis Factor-α *Serum Increase* TNF-α observed in the plasma of 6 of 7 patients following severe acute myocardial infarction (Killip class 3 or 4) *2933* Tumor necrosis factor-α was elevated *5093* In 24 patients with acute myocardial infarction mean peak concentration of 46.8 ± 21.3 pg/mL significantly different from normal of 4.35 ± 0.76 pg/mL *4233*
Serum No Effect In 11 patients with uncomplicated myocardial infarction (Killip class I) no TNF detected. Likewise no TNF detected in the plasma of control patients without AMI *2933*

Urea Nitrogen *Serum Increase* 18 of 22 patients showed elevations at some time during the study, usually within 3 days after admission *5664* In 36% of 119 patients hospitalized for this disorder *1576*

Uric Acid *Serum Increase* Frequently occurs *1235* In 60% of 110 patients hospitalized for this disorder *1576* In several studies, mean concentration ranged from 5.13 ± 1.10 to 7.32 mg/dL. Males were found to have a higher concentration (8.25 ± 1.21 mg/dL) than females (7.16 ± 1.17 mg/dL) compared to normal, 3.59 ± 0.80 mg/dL, 3.01 ± 0.32 mg/dL, respectively *4866*

Vascular Endothelial Growth Factor *Serum Increase* In 45 patients with acute myocardial infarction concentrations increased from 26.2 ± 5.4 pg/mL on day 1, to 30.1 ± 5.2 pg/mL on day 2, 56.6 ± 17.8 pg/mL on day 3, 256.3 ± 38.4 pg/mL on day 7, 205.7 ± 36.3 pg/mL on day 14, 165.7 ± 30.0 pg/mL on day 21 and 130.0 ± 23.8 pg/mL on day 28, significantly higher than controls on days 7, 14, 21 and 28 *2599*

Vasoactive Intestinal Polypeptide *Plasma Increase* In 9 patients with acute myocardial infarction mean concentration of 6.3 ± 0.7 pg/mL within 1 hour of admission significantly increased compared with 2.8 ± 0.9 pg/mL in 17 healthy controls *1939*

Viscosity *Serum Increase* Observed response *2414* Due to alterations in serum proteins during the acute phase of illness *2304*

Vitronectin Receptor *Platelets No Effect* In 16 patients with AMI who responded to antithrombolytic therapy mean log amplification of fluorescence intensity of 61.8 ± 6.3 compared with 60.9 ± 7.1 in 5 patients who failed to respond to antithrombolytic treatment and 59.8 ± 6.0 in 10 healthy controls *1928*

VLA-2 *Platelets No Effect* In 16 patients with AMI who responded to antithrombolytic therapy mean log amplification of fluorescence intensity of 40.4 ± 2.1 compared with 40.2 ± 3.5 in 5 patients who failed to respond to antithrombolytic treatment and 41.4 ± 2.1 in 10 healthy controls *1928*

Volume *Plasma Decrease* Probably the result of reflex adrenergic discharge and vasoconstriction, pooling or trapping of blood, sweating, or the development of pulmonary edema *2304*
Plasma Increase Significant increases in plasma volume, reflected by changes in hematocrit. Average change was 12%. For the patients with accompanying pulmonary edema, the change was 17% *5705*

von Willebrand Factor *Plasma Increase* Mean concentration of 128 ± 37 IU/dL in 116 patients who had survived an acute myocardial infarction significantly different from 100 ± 33 IU/dL in 116 matched controls *472*

Zinc *Red Blood Cells Increase* In 21 patients with acute myocardial infarction mean concentration of 168 ± 30 µmol/L on day of infarction significantly different from 155 ± 38 µmol/L 15 days later *181*
Serum Decrease Falls immediately to low levels following a myocardial infarction, rising to the orginal normal level over the next 10 - 14 days *1980* A significant decrease was observed *5462*

Zinc, Ultrafiltrable *Serum No Effect* In 16 patients with acute myocardial infarction mean concentration of 0.41 ± 0.14 µmol/L on day of infarction significantly different from 0.44 ± 0.10 µmol/L 15 days later although decreased to 0.38 ± 0.08 µmol/L on day 4 *181*

Zinc, Unexchangeable *Serum Increase* In 10 patients with acute myocardial infarction mean concentration of 1.9 ± 0.9 µmol/L on day of infarction significantly different from 3.0 ± 2.2 µmol/L 15 days later although decreased to 1.2 ± 0.7 µmol/L on day 5 *181*

410.90 Coronary Artery Thrombosis

Antiphospholipid Antibodies *Serum Increase* About 18% of patients with premature coronary artery thrombosis have antiphospholipid antibodies *441*

413.90 Angina Pectoris

Amyloid A Protein *Serum Increase* In 4 of 32 patients with stable angina mean concentration increased above 0.3 mg/dL and in 1 of 31 with unstable angina mean concentration increased above 0.3 mg/dL. In all other patients concentration normal *3093*

α_1-Antitrypsin *Serum No Effect* In patients with unstable angina mean concentration remained within normal range *3936*

Aspartate Aminotransferase *Serum No Effect* Usual finding *5544*

Basophils *Blood Increase* In 25 patients with angina pectoris mean concentration of 0.09 ± 0.01 x 10^9/L significantly different from 0.06 ± 0.01 x 10^9/L in 20 apparently healthy controls *5543*

Bilirubin *Serum No Effect* Typical observation *5544*

C_1-Esterase Inhibitor *Serum No Effect* In 35 patients with unstable angina pectoris on admission to hospital mean concentration of 105.6 ± 4.3% and in 25 patients with stable angina mean concentration of 106.3 ± 4.9% not significantly different from 112.5 ± 4.1% in 25 healthy controls *2202*

Cholesterol *Serum Increase* Mean concentration of 203 ± 9 mg/dL in 15 patients with angina significantly different from 172 ± 7 mg/dL in 13 control individuals *4805*
Serum No Effect In 19 patients with stable angina mean concentration of 202 ± 7 mg/dL not significantly different from 219 ± 9 mg/dL in 16 healthy controls *3860*

C-Reactive Protein *Serum Increase* In 4 of 32 patients with stable angina mean concentration increased above 0.3 mg/dL but in 20 of 31 with unstable angina mean concentration increased above 0.3 mg/dL *3093*
Serum No Effect In patients with unstable angina pectoris mean concentration fell within normal range *3936*

Creatine Kinase *Serum No Effect* In 31 with unstable angina mean activity 80 ± 53 U/L not significantly different from reference interval of 30 - 230 U/L *3093* Activity usually normal *5544*

Creatinine *Serum Increase* In 60% of 50 patients hospitalized for this disorder *1576*

D-Dimer *Plasma No Effect* In 25 patients with stable angina mean concentration of 358.1 ± 51.8 ng/mL not significantly different from 272.4 ± 71.2 ng/mL in 25 healthy controls *2202*

Endothelin *Plasma Increase* In patients with vasospastic angina pectoris concentration significantly increased even before coronary spasm, without further increase during spasm *3739*

Endothelin-1 *Plasma Increase* In 2 studies of patients with vasospastic angina pectoris mean concentrations increased 1.7 to 1.8-fold above appropriate normals and in 3 studies of patients with stable angina mean concentrations increased 0.8 to 1.6-fold above appropriate normals *328* Unstable angina is associated with an increase in endothelin-1 plasma levels during the acute phase, levels were similar in unstable angina, 0.635 ± 0.052 pg/mL [log(1 + x)], and myocardial infarction, 0.746 ± 0.122, and significantly higher than in controls, 0.428 ± 0.047, and stable angina patients, 0.449 ± 0.052 ($p < 0.01$) *4247* In 29 patients with unstable angina on admission to hospital mean concentration of 0.635 ± 0.052 pg/mL comparable to that in patients with myocardial infarction and significantly higher than in healthy control subjects (0.428 ± 0.047 pg/mL) and stable angina patients (0.449 ± 0.052 pg/mL) *4251*

Eosinophils *Blood* *No Effect* In 25 patients with angina pectoris mean concentration of 0.16 ± 0.02 x 10^9/L not significantly different from 0.20 ± 0.03 x 10^9/L in 20 apparently healthy controls *5543*

Erythrocyte Sedimentation Rate *Blood* *No Effect* May be helpful in distinguishing this entity from acute myocardial infarction *1980*

Erythrocytes *Blood* *No Effect* In 25 patients with angina mean concentration of 4.90 ± 0.08 x 10^{12}/L not significantly different from 4.95 ± 0.10 x 10^{12}/L in 20 apparently healthy controls *5543*

Factor IV *Plasma* *Increase* Patients with chest pain but without evidence of infarction had a mean of 29 ng/mL. Elevation persisted for 1 week and returned to normal *1997*

Factor XII *Plasma* *Decrease* In 35 patients with unstable angina pectoris on admission to hospital mean concentration of 95.8 ± 5.2% significantly different from 117.0 ± 4.5% in 25 healthy controls *2202*
Plasma *No Effect* In 25 patients with stable angina mean concentration of 107.7 ± 6.0% not significantly different from 117.0 ± 4.5% in 25 healthy controls *2202*

β-Factor XIIa Inhibition *Plasma* *No Effect* In 35 patients with unstable angina pectoris on admission to hospital mean concentration of 136.8 ± 7.8% and in 25 patients with stable angina mean concentration of 128.3 ± 6.6% not significantly different from 149.8 ± 8.3% in 25 healthy controls *2202*

Fatty Acid-binding Protein, Cytoplasmic Heart Type *Serum* *No Effect* Mean concentration in 99 patients with angina pectoris of 5.6 µg/L with a range of 3.8 - 8.7 µg/L not significantly higher than that in 104 healthy volunteers, 4.1 µg/L with a range of 3.2 - 6.0 µg/L *2354*

Fibrinogen *Plasma* *Increase* Concentration increased in patients with stable angina but not to the extent observed in patients with unstable angina *2201* In 35 patients with unstable angina pectoris on admission to hospital mean concentration of 370 ± 18 mg/dL and in 25 patients with stable angina mean concentration of 372 ± 23 mg/dL significantly different from 300 ± 12 mg/dL in 25 healthy controls *2202*

Glycogen Phosphorylase BB Isoenzyme *Serum* *Increase* In patients with stable angina concentration similar to that in healthy individuals or patients without angina *3235*
Serum *No Effect* In 14 patients with chronic stable angina pectoris concentrations less than 7 µg/L as in 116 healthy individuals upper limit of normal (97.5 percentile) was 7.0 µg/L *4256*

HDL-Cholesterol *Serum* *No Effect* In 19 patients with stable angina mean concentration of 36 ± 3 mg/dL not significantly different from 45 ± 3 mg/dL in 16 healthy controls *3860* In 21 patients with stable angina mean concentration of 41 ± 10 mg/dL not significantly different from 49 ± 14 mg/dL in 27 controls *3517*

High Molecular Weight Kininogen *Plasma* *No Effect* In 25 patients with stable angina mean concentration of 83.9 ± 4.9% not significantly different from 87.7 ± 3.9% in 25 healthy controls *2202*

immunoglobulin A *Serum* *Increase* In 26 patients with angina pectoris mean concentration of 2.87 ± 0.83 g/L not significantly higher than 2.73 ± 1.22 g/L in controls *3684*

Inhibitor-bound Urokinase Plasminogen Activator *Plasma* *No Effect* In 47 patients with stable angina pectoris with coronary occlusion mean concentration of 1.1 ± 0.06 ng/mL not significantly different from 0.9 ± 0.01 ng/mL in right atria of 13 patients with stable angina but without coronary occlusion *4003*

Intercellular Adhesion Molecule-1 *Serum* *Increase* In 33 patients with variant angina mean concentration of 271 ± 13 ng/mL and 213 ± 13 ng/mL in 22 patients with stable angina significantly different from 187 ± 16 ng/mL in 20 healthy volunteers *3531*
Serum *No Effect* In 19 patients with stable angina mean concentration of 126 ± 8 ng/mL not significantly different from 120 ± 10 ng/mL in 16 healthy controls *3860*

Interleukin-6 *Serum* *Increase* In 6 of 29 patients (21%) with stable angina concencentrations greater than < 3 pg/mL were detected in contrast to healthy controls in whom no IL-6 was detected *439*

Interleukin-8 *Serum* *No Effect* No change from normal observed in 2 patients with stable angina *13*

Kallikrein Inhibition *Plasma* *Increase* In 35 patients with unstable angina pectoris on admission to hospital mean concentration of 118.3 ± 3.5% and in 25 patients with stable angina mean concentration of 123.8 ± 4.1% significantly different from 106.4 ± 4.7% in 25 healthy controls *2202*

Kallikrein-like Activity *Plasma* *No Effect* In 25 patients with stable angina mean activity of 31.7 ± 3.8 U/L not significantly different from 27.4 ± 1.3 U/L in 25 healthy controls *2202*

Lactate Dehydrogenase *Serum* *No Effect* Typical observation *5544* In 89% of 75 patients hospitalized for this disorder *1576*

Lactate Dehydrogenase Isoenzyme-5 *Serum* *No Effect* Activity usually normal *5544*

LDL-Cholesterol *Serum* *No Effect* In 21 patients with stable angina mean concentration of 131 ± 37 mg/dL not significantly different from 109 ± 21 mg/dL in 27 controls *3517*

Leukocytes *Blood* *No Effect* In 25 patients with angina mean concentration of 7.38 ± 0.36 x 10^9/L not significantly different from 6.69 ± 0.30 x 10^9/L in 20 apparently healthy controls *5543*

Lipoprotein Lp(a) *Serum* *Increase* In 18 patients with unstable angina mean concentration of 319 ± 193 mg/L compared with 191 ± 141 mg/L in 18 patients with stable exertional angina *3936*
Serum *No Effect* In 29 individuals with angina pectoris mean and median concentrations of 165 and 112 mg/L not significantly different from 180 and 105 mg/L respectively in 1498 control individuals *4892*

Lymphocytes *Blood* *No Effect* In 25 patients with angina pectoris mean concentration of 2.13 ± 0.11 x 10^9/L not significantly different from 1.89 ± 0.13 x 10^9/L in 20 apparently healthy controls *5543*

Lysophosphatidylcholine *Serum* *No Effect* In patients with angina pectoris no significant increase observed *2916*

MCHC *Blood* *No Effect* In 25 patients with angina pectoris MCHC not significantly different from that in 20 apparently healthy controls *5543*

Monocytes *Blood* *No Effect* In 25 patients with angina pectoris mean concentration of 0.55 ± 0.05 x 10^9/L not significantly different from 0.54 ± 0.03 x 10^9/L in 20 apparently healthy controls *5543*

Myoglobin *Serum* *Increase* Mean concentration in 66 patients with acute myocardial infarction of 72 µg/L (range 51 - 104 µg/L) significantly higher than that in 104 healthy volunteers, 54 µg/L with a range of 41 - 70 µg/L *2354*

Neutrophils *Blood* *No Effect* In 25 patients with angina mean concentration of 4.45 ± 0.30 x 10^9/L not significantly different from 3.91 ± 0.24 x 10^9/L in 20 apparently healthy controls *5543*

Oxidase *Plasma* *Increase* In 28 patients with angina mean plasma oxidase activity of 127 ± 5 U/L significantly greater than 84 ± 5 U/L in 12 healthy controls *2931*

Phospholipase A_2 *Serum* *No Effect* No significant change observed in patients with angina pectoris *2916*

Plasmin-α_2-Plasmin Inhibitor Complex *Plasma* *Increase* In 18 patients with unstable angina mean concentration of 0.78 ± 0.42 µg/mL significantly higher than 0.41 ± 0.13 µg/mL in 18 patients with stable exertional angina *3936*

Plasmin-Antiplasmin Complex *Plasma* *No Effect* In 47 patients with stable angina pectoris with coronary occlusion mean concentration of 0.9 ± 0.1 µg/mL not significantly different from 1.1 ± 0.3 µg/mL in right atria of 13 patients with stable angina but without coronary occlusion *4003*

Plasminogen *Plasma* *No Effect* In 35 patients with unstable angina pectoris on admission to hospital mean concentration of 119.9 ± 4.4% and in 25 patients with stable angina mean concentration of 124.7 ± 6.3% not significantly different from 115.0 ± 7.5% in 25 healthy controls *2202*

413.90 Angina Pectoris *(continued)*

Plasminogen Activator Inhibitor-1 *Plasma* *No Effect* In 47 patients with stable angina pectoris with coronary occlusion mean concentration of 14.9 ± 1.0 U/mL not significantly different from 11.2 ± 1.9 U/mL in right atria of 13 patients with stable angina but without coronary occlusion *4003* In 25 patients with stable angina mean concentration of 6.5 ± 1.3 AU/mL not significantly different from 4.6 ± 1.6 AU/mL in 25 healthy controls *2202*

Platelet-derived Growth Factor *Plasma* *No Effect* In 25 patients with angina mean concentration of 59.2 ± 1.55 ng/L not significantly different from 53.7 ± 2.01 ng/L in 20 apparently healthy controls *5543*

Platelets *Blood* *No Effect* In 25 patients with angina mean concentration of 254 ± 10 x 10^9/L not significantly different from 248 ± 12 x 10^9/L in 20 apparently healthy controls *5543*

Prekallikrein *Plasma* *No Effect* In 35 patients with unstable angina pectoris mean concentration on hospital admission of 103.9 ± 5.1% and in 25 patients with stable angina mean concentration of 101.3 ± 3.8% not significantly different from 111.2 ± 6.8% in 25 healthy controls *2202*

Prothrombin Fragment 1.2 *Plasma* *No Effect* In 47 patients with stable angina pectoris with coronary occlusion mean concentration of 2.3 ± 0.2 nmol/L not significantly different from 2.7 ± 0.3 nmol/L in right atria of 13 patients with stable angina but without coronary occlusion *4003*

P-Selectin *Serum* *No Effect* Mean concentration of 28 ± 4 ng/mL in 15 patients with angina not significantly different from 24 ± 5 ng/mL in 13 control individuals *4805*

Soluble E-Selectin *Serum* *Increase* In 33 patients with variant angina mean concentration of 45 ± 2 ng/mL and 40 ± 3 ng/mL in 22 patients with stable angina significantly different from 38 ± 3 ng/mL in 20 healthy volunteers *3531*

Soluble Vascular Cell Adhesion Molecule-1
Serum *Increase* In 33 patients with variant angina mean concentration of 828 ± 56 ng/mL and 780 ± 39 ng/mL in 22 patients with stable angina not significantly different from 707 ± 39 ng/mL in 20 healthy volunteers *3531*

Thrombin/Antithrombin III Complex *Plasma* *Increase* In 18 patients with unstable angina pectoris mean concentration of 3.6 ± 1.3 ng/mL compared with 1.9 ± 0.5 ng/mL in 18 patients with stable exertional angina pectoris *3936*
Plasma *No Effect* In 35 patients with unstable angina pectoris on admission to hospital mean concentration of 7.9 ± 1.7 µg/L and in 25 patients with stable angina mean concentration of 4.9 ± 0.8 µg/L not significantly different from 4.5 ± 0.7 µg/L in 25 healthy controls *2202* In 47 patients with stable angina pectoris with coronary occlusion mean concentration of 9.9 ± 1.8 µg/L not significantly different from 8.9 ± 1.3 µg/L in right atria of 13 patients with stable angina but without coronary occlusion *4003*

β-Thrombomodulin *Urine* *Increase* Mean excretion in 21 patients with unstable angina over 12 hours of 4.94 ± 3.91 mg/mmol creatinine compared with 1.77 ± 1.48 mg/mmol creatinine in 6 patients with non-cardiac chest pain *1562*

Thromboxane A_2 *Plasma* *Increase* Observed effect *4677*

Tissue Factor *Plasma* *No Effect* n 21 patients with stable angina mean concentration of tissue factor antigen of 184 ± 46 pg/mL not significantly increased compared with 177 ± 37 pg/mL in 27 controls *3517*

Tissue Plasminogen Activator *Plasma* *Increase* In 47 patients with stable angina pectoris with coronary occlusion mean concentration of 10.5 ± 0.7 ng/mL significantly different from 7.5 ± 0.9 ng/mL in right atria of 13 patients with stable angina but without coronary occlusion *4003* In 35 patients with unstable angina pectoris on admission to hospital mean concentration of 15.9 ± 1.9 ng/mL and in 25 patients with stable angina mean concentration of 10.4 ± 1.0 ng/mL significantly different from 5.1 ± 0.4 ng/mL in 25 healthy controls *2202*

Tissue Plasminogen Activator Antigen *Plasma* *Increase* 1.44-fold higher mean concentration observed in patients exhibiting angina at rest than in patients exhibiting angina only after physical exercise *1699*

Triglycerides *Serum* *No Effect* Mean concentration of 143 ± 24 mg/dL in 15 patients with angina not significantly different from 120 ± 22 mg/dL in 13 control individuals *4805* In 21 patients with stable angina mean concentration of 125 ± 112 mg/dL not significantly different from 130 ± 56 mg/dL in 27 controls *3517* In 19 patients with stable angina mean concentration of 151 ± 15 mg/dL not significantly different from 165 ± 19 mg/dL in 16 healthy controls *3860*

Troponin I *Serum* *No Effect* Concentrations not increased in patients with stable angina pectoris *2649*

Troponin T *Serum* *Increase* In 38 of 142 patients with angina pectoris cocentration increased when cutoff of 0.2 µg/L used *892*
Serum *No Effect* In 28 of 38 patients (61%) with stable angina troponin T concencentrations were less than 0.1 mg/dL *439* Concentrations not increased in patients with stable angina pectoris *2649* In 31 with unstable angina mean concentration of 0.02 ± 0.04 µg/L not different from reference interval of 0 - 0.2 µg/L *3093*

Uric Acid *Serum* *Increase* In 55% of 72 patients hospitalized for this disorder *1576*

Urokinase Plasminogen Activator Activity
Plasma *No Effect* In 47 patients with stable angina pectoris with coronary occlusion mean concentration of 1.5 ± 0.03 ng/mL not significantly different from 1.8 ± 0.05 ng/mL in right atria of 13 patients with stable angina but without coronary occlusion *4003*

Urokinase Plasminogen Activator Activity:Plasminogen Activator Ratio *Plasma* *Decrease* In 47 patients with stable angina pectoris with coronary occlusion mean ratio of 59.0 ± 0.06% significantly different from 65.3 ± 2.9% in right atria of 13 patients with stable angina but without coronary occlusion *4003*

Urokinase Plasminogen Activator Antigen
Plasma *No Effect* In 47 patients with stable angina pectoris with coronary occlusion mean concentration of 2.7 ± 0.06 ng/mL not significantly different from 2.8 ± 0.05 ng/mL in right atria of 13 patients with stable angina but without coronary occlusion *4003*

413.90 Angina Pectoris, Unstable

Amyloid A *Serum* *Increase* Median concentration on admission in 26 patients with unstable angina and high C-reactive protein concentrations increased in the majority of patients and increased concentration in 21 of 26 patients 3 months after discharge. In those patients with lower or normal concentrations on admission many had abnormal concentrations on discharge *438*

Chlamydia pneumoniae Antibodies *Serum* *Increase* 21 of 26 patients with unstable angina and high C-reactive protein concentrations demonstrated antibodies to Chlamydia pneumoniae on admission to hospital with 13 positive at a dilution of 1:32 or more *438*

Cholesterol *Serum* *No Effect* In 20 patients with unstable angina mean concentration of 209 ± 8 mg/dL not significantly different from 219 ± 9 mg/dL in 16 healthy controls *3860* In 21 patients with unstable angina mean concentration of 203 ± 36 mg/dL not significantly different from 184 ± 23 mg/dL in 27 controls *3517* *3517*

C-Reactive Protein *Serum* *Increase* In 965 patients with unstable angina, tertiles of < 2 mg/L, 2 - 10 mg/L and > 10 mg/L with increased numbers of patients dying or having AMIs with increasing concentration *5263* Increase acute phase reactants, such as CRP, observed in patients with unstable angina *358* Median concentration on admission in 26 patients with unstable angina of 9.9 mg/L (increased in 24 patients) and increased concentration in 21 of 26 patients 3 months after discharge. In those patients with lower or normal concentrations on admission many had normal concentrations on discharge *438* In 35 of 48 patients with severe unstable angina without increased serum CK, troponin T and lactate dehydrogenase, had increased C-reactive protein on admission to hospital *3094* In 28 of 38 patients (61%) with unstable angina concencentrations greater than 3 mg/LL were observed with median concentration of 6.4 µg/L *439*

Creatine Kinase MB-Isoenzyme *Serum* *No Effect* Mean concentration increased above 3.1 ng/mL in 22 (24%) of 91 patients admitted to a CCU but with normal CK-MB concentration *1631*

D-Dimer *Plasma* *Increase* Constant observation in patients with unstable angina due to breakdown of fibrin *2201*

Factor XII Inhibition *Plasma* *Decrease* Inhibition capacity significantly reduced in patients with unstable angina as observed when they were admitted to hospital *2201*

Fibrinogen *Plasma* *Increase* In patients with an increased concentration above 300 mg/dL was associated with increased risk of death, AMI or spontaneous ischemia *358* Concentration increased in patients with unstable angina when they were admitted to hospital *2201* In 965 patients with unstable angina, tertiles of < 338 mg/dL, 338 - 399 mg/dL and > 399 mg/dL with increased numbers of patients dying or having AMIs with increasing concentration *5263*

Fibrinopeptide A *Plasma* *Increase* Several studies have shown that patients with unstable angina have shown increased thrombin activity *2201* Several studies have shown an increased concentration compared with those with stable angina indicating increased thrombin generation *2201*
Urine *Increase* Several studies have shown that patients with unstable angina have shown increased thrombin activity *2201*

Glycogen Phosphorylase BB Isoenzyme *Serum* *Increase* Concentration increased above upper reference limit in the majority of patients with unstable angina *3235*

HDL-Cholesterol *Serum* *No Effect* In 21 patients with unstable angina mean concentration of 44 ± 13 mg/dL not significantly different from 49 ± 14 mg/dL in 27 controls *3517* In 20 patients with unstable angina mean concentration of 45 ± 5 mg/dL not significantly different from 45 ± 3 mg/dL in 16 healthy controls *3860*

Helicobacter pylori Antibodies *Serum* *Increase* 21 of 26 patients with unstable angina and high C-reactive protein concentrations demonstrated antibodies to Helicobacter pylori on admission to hospital with median titers of 28.9 ± 55 U/L *438*

High Molecular Weight Kininogen *Plasma* *Decrease* Increased generation of bradykinin observed in patients with unstable angina, which may be partly explained by systemic heparinization *2201*

Homocysteine *Plasma* *Increase* In 587 patients with angiographically confirmed coronary artery disease mean concentration of 0.4 µmol/L higher in those with unstable angina than in those with stable symptoms *3844*

Intercellular Adhesion Molecule-1 *Serum* *Increase* In 20 patients with unstable angina mean concentration of 217 ± 14 ng/mL significantly different from 120 ± 10 ng/mL in 16 healthy controls *3860*

Interleukin-6 *Serum* *Increase* In 23 of 28 patients (61%) with unstable angina concencentrations greater than < 3 pg/mL were detected in contrast to healthy controls in whom no IL-6 was detected *439*

Kallikrein Inhibition *Plasma* *No Effect* Inhibition capacity not changed significantly in patients with unstable angina *2201*

LDL-Cholesterol *Serum* *No Effect* In 21 patients with unstable angina mean concentration of 129 ± 34 mg/dL not significantly different from 109 ± 21 mg/dL in 27 controls *3517*

Lipoprotein Lp(a) *Serum* *Increase* In 167 patients who were admitted to hospital with final diagnosis of unstable angina, 56 who had increased troponin T concentrations (> 0.2 ng/mL) also had increased Lp(a) concentrations with mean of 22.3 mg/dL compared with 6 mg/dL in others *5052*
Serum *No Effect* In 15 patients with unstable angina mean concentration on admission to hospital 15.5 mg/dL not significantly different from normal range of 14.4 ± 1.8 mg/dL *3896*

Plasminogen Activator Inhibitor *Plasma* *Increase* In 15 patients with unstable angina mean concentration on admission to hospital of 11.4 ± 1.4 IU/mL significantly different from normal range of 4.9 ± 1.0 IU/mL *3896* Constant observation in patients with unstable angina *2201*

Plasminogen Activator Inhibitor-1 *Plasma* *Increase* Concentration increased in patients with unstable angina when they were admitted to hospital and may stay increased for 10 days *2201*

Prekallikrein *Plasma* *No Effect* Concentration not changed significantly in patients with unstable angina *2201*

Prothrombin Fragment 1.2 *Plasma* *Increase* Mean concentration of prothrombin fragment 1.2 in platelet-poor plasma from 8 patients with unstable angina pectoris of 5.9 ± 4.1 nmol/L significantly higher than 0.51 nmol/L (95% reference interval 0.21 - 2.78 nmol/L) in 268 healthy individuals less than 44 years of age *1860*

Thrombin/Antithrombin III Complex *Plasma* *Increase* Several studies have shown that patients with unstable angina have shown increased thrombin activity: complexes persist for several days after clinical stabilization of the patients *2201*

Tissue Factor Antigen *Plasma* *Increase* In 21 patients with unstable angina mean concentration of tissue factor antigen of 240 ± 75 pg/mL significantly increased compared with 177 ± 37 pg/mL in 27 controls *3517*

Tissue Plasminogen Activator Activity *Plasma* *Decrease* Activity may be normal or reduced in patients with unstable angina *2201*
Plasma *No Effect* Activity may be normal or reduced in patients with unstable angina *2201*

Tissue Plasminogen Activator Antigen *Plasma* *Increase* In 15 patients with unstable angina mean concentration on admission to hospital of 8.7 ± 0.9 ng/mL significantly different from normal range of 4.9 ± 0.4 ng/mL *3896* Concentration increased in patients with unstable angina when they were admitted to hospital and may stay increased for 10 days *2201*

Triglycerides *Serum* *No Effect* In 20 patients with unstable angina mean concentration of 176 ± 21 mg/dL not significantly different from 165 ± 19 mg/dL in 16 healthy controls *3860*

Troponin I *Serum* *Increase* Concentrations increased in 30 - 45% patients with unstable angina pectoris with percentage increase of TnI higher than that of TnT *2649* Mean concentration increased above 3.1 ng/mL in 22 (24%) of 91 patients admitted to a CCU but with normal CK-MB concentration *1631* In 106 patients with unstable angina with chest discomfort at rest only 68% of patients with increased troponin I were free of cardiac events compared with 90% of those without increases *1631*

Troponin T *Serum* *Increase* Substantial increase in concentration observed in 20 patients who had unstable angina based on prolonged chest pain for less than 30 minotes at rest without hekp from nitrates *1305* Concentrations increased in 30 - 45% patients with unstable angina pectoris with percentage increase of TnI higher than that of TnT *2649* In 167 patients who were admitted to hospital with final diagnosis of unstable angina, 56 who had increased troponin T concentrations (> 0.2 ng/mL) also had increased Lp(a) concentrations with mean of 22.3 mg/dL compared with 6 mg/dL in others *5052*
Serum *No Effect* In 28 of 38 patients (61%) with unstable angina troponin T concencentrations were less than 0.1 mg/dL *439*

413.90 Syndrome X

Angiotensin-converting Enzyme *Serum* *No Effect* In 18 women with cardiological syndrome X mean activity 87.9 ± 22 U/L not significantly different from 88.7 ± 27 U/L in 18 healthy controls *4226*

Glucose Tolerance *Serum* *Increase* Mildly impaired glucose tolerance observed with disease, associated with insulin resistance and compensatory hyperinsulinemia *3395* In a group of hyperinsulinemic patients integrated plasma glucose response for 2 h was significantly higher at 13.4 ± 0.4 mmol/L compared with 11.0 ± 0.4 mmol/L in nonhyperinsulinemic patients *5846*

HDL-Cholesterol *Serum* *Decrease* In a group of hyperinsulinemic patients mean concentration was significantly lower at 1.06 ± 0.05 mmol/L compared with 1.32 ± 0.5 mmol/L in nonhyperinsulinemic patients *5846* Reduced concentration observed with disease *3395*

Triglycerides *Serum* *Increase* In a group of hyperinsulinemic patients mean concentration was significantly higher at 2.4 ± 0.2 mmol/L compared with 1.4 ± 0.1 mmol/L in nonhyperinsulinemic patients *5846* Increased concentration observed with disease *3395*

Uric Acid *Serum* *Increase* In a group of hyperinsulinemic patients mean concentration was significantly higher at 5.3 ± 0.2 mg/dL compared with 4.4 ± 0.2 mg/dL in nonhyperinsulinemic patients *5846*

414.00 Coronary Artery Disease

α_1-Acid Glycoprotein *Serum* *Increase* Significant progressive increase observed from mean control concentration (70 individuals) of 62.8 ± 1.0 mg/dL to 74.4 ± 1.0 mg/dL in 57 patients with Gensini's score of greater than 43 *3604*

Albumin *Serum* *Decrease* In 170 cases of early coronary artery disease mean concentration of 42.5 ± 3.3 g/L significantly less than 44.2 ± 3.4 g/L in 168 healthy controls *5746*

Alkaline Phosphatase *Serum* *Increase* Mean concentration of 11.7 μmol/L in 50 patients with CAD significantly greater than 9.9 μmol/L in 50 matched controls *3577*

Angiotensin-converting Enzyme *Serum* *Increase* Mean activity of 46 U/L in 100 patients with CHD significantly higher than 36 U/L in 57 age-matched controls: difference almost entirely due to differences in individuals less than 55 years of age *309*

Anti-Chlamydia pneumoniae Antibodies *Serum* *Increase* In 220 consecutive male survivors of myocardial infarction 59 had no detectable antibodies, 74 had intermediate titers of 1/8 to 1/32 dilution and 80 were seropositive at 1/64 dilution *1924*

Anticardiolipin Antibodies *Serum* *Increase* 232 patients enrolled in the European Concerted Action on Thrombosis Angina Pectoris Study were studied. aCL were not found to be a marker of either progressive cardiovascular disease or recurrent thrombotic events *5299*

Antiplasmin *Plasma* *Decrease* Reduction observed in large studies associated with the presence of coronary heart disease *2201*

Antithrombin III *Plasma* *Decrease* Reduction observed in large studies associated with the presence of coronary heart disease *2201*

α_1-Antitrypsin *Serum* *Decrease* Reduction observed in large studies associated with the presence of coronary heart disease *2201*
Serum *Increase* Significant progressive increase observed from mean control concentration (70 individuals) of 205.8 ± 4.6 mg/dL to 225.2 ± 4.9 mg/dL in 57 patients with Gensini's score of greater than 43 *3604*

Apolipoprotein A-I *Serum* *Decrease* In 145 men (mean age 51 y) with coronary artery disease mean concentration significantly less than in 135 healthy controls (mean age 49 y) *1691* In 321 men with angiographically proved premature CAD mean concentration of 114 ± 26 mg/dL significantly less than 136 ± 32 mg/dL in 901 control individuals *1692* In 20 patients with coronary artery disease mean concentration of 1117 ± 183 mg/L significantly different from 1455 ± 166 mg/L in 20 healthy controls *3483* In 18 patients with CAD mean concentration of 1.27 ± 0.22 g/L significantly less than 1.59 ± 0.26 g/L in 18 healthy controls *1850* In 731 men with coronary artery disease in those with 3 narrowed vessels mean concentration of 1.00 g/L significantly different from 1.08 g/L in those with 0 narrowed vessels. In 323 women with coronary artery cisease mean concentration in those with 3 narrowed vessels 1.11 g/L significantly different from 1.19 g/L in those with no narrowed vessels *2882* In 26 white male patients with premature vascular disease mean concentration of 81.4 ± 4.3 mg/dL not significantly different from 90.0 ± 3.3 mg/dL in 32 age-matched white male controls *5384* Mean concentration in 59 Chinese patients with coronary artery disease of 870 ± 120 mg/L significantly different from 1,080 ± 160 mg/L in 95 age-matched controls *5743* In 55 patients with more than 50% stenosis in at least one main coronary artery mean concentration of 1.39 ± 0.27 g/L significantly different from 1.65 ± 0.28 g/L in 100 healthy controls *2959*
Serum *No Effect* Mean concentration in 34 patients with coronary artery disease of 122 ± 23 mg/dL not significantly different from 140 ± 27 mg/dL in 11 healthy controls *1085*

Apolipoprotein A-II *Serum* *Decrease* In 20 patients with coronary artery disease mean concentration of 293 ± 62 mg/L significantly different from 344 ± 61 mg/L in 20 healthy controls *3483*

Apolipoprotein B *Serum* *Increase* Mean concentration in 59 Chinese patients with coronary artery disease of 860 ± 220 mg/L significantly different from 760 ± 200 mg/L in 95 age-matched controls *5743* In 171 patients with severe coronary disease mean concentration of 1,193 ± 347 mg/L greater than 1,078 ± 327 mg/L in 83 normal controls with concentration increasing with severity of CAD *3014* In 145 men (mean age 51 y) with CAD mean concentration significantly greater than in 135 healthy control men (mean age 49 y) *1691* In 18 patients with CAD mean concentration of 1.33 ± 0.32 g/L not significantly greater than 1.18 ± 0.33 g/L in 18 healthy controls *1850* In 731 men with coronary artery disease in those with 3 narrowed vessels mean concentration of 0.98 g/L significantly different from 0.87 g/L in those with 0 narrowed vessels. In 323 women with coronary artery disease mean concentration in those with 3 narrowed vessels of 1.00 g/L significantly different from 0.89 g/L in those with no narrowed vessels *2882* In 321 men with angiographically proved CAD mean concentration of 131 ± 37 mg/dL significantly higher than 108 ± 33 mg/dL in 901 control individuals *1692*
Serum *No Effect* In 55 patients with more than 50% stenosis in at least one main coronary artery mean concentration of 1.34 ± 0.34 g/L not significantly different from 1.36 ± 0.29 g/L in 100 healthy controls *2959* Mean concentration in 34 patients with coronary artery disease of 120 ± 29 mg/dL not significantly different from 109 ± 38 mg/dL in 11 healthy controls *1085*

Apolipoprotein B-100 *Serum* *Increase* In 26 white male patients with premature vascular disease mean concentration of 106.0 ± 5.3 mg/dL significantly different from 81.3 ± 5.5 mg/dL in 32 age-matched white male controls *5384*

Apolipoprotein C-II *Serum* *Increase* In 18 patients with CAD mean concentration of 51.6 ± 17.6 mg/L significantly higher than mean of 30.3 ± 8.1 mg/L in 18 healthy controls *1850*

Apolipoprotein C-III *Serum* *Decrease* In 145 men (mean age 51 y) with CAD mean concentration of 0.027 ± 0.008 g/L significantly less than 0.036 ± 0.020 g/L in 135 control men (mean age 49 y) *1691*
Serum *Increase* In 18 patients with CAD mean concentration of 98.6 ± 34.1 mg/L not significantly greater than 75.7 ± 30.5 mg/L in 18 healthy controls *1850*

Apolipoprotein E *Serum* *Decrease* In 145 men (mean age 51 y) mean concentration of 0.040 ± 0.015 g/L significantly less than 0.055 ± 0.029 g/L in 135 healthy men (mean age 49 y) *1691*
Serum *No Effect* In 55 patients with more than 50% stenosis in at least one main coronary artery mean concentration of 6.29 ± 1.99 mg/dL not significantly different from 6.69 ± 1.97 mg/dL in 100 healthy controls *2959*

Apolipoprotein Lp(a) *Urine* *Increase* In 116 patients with angiographically proved coronary artery disease 25th and 75th percentiles 3.25 and 10.35 μg/dL significantly higher than in 109 clinically healthy controls in whom 25th and 75th percentiles were 1.43 and 3.50 μg/dL *2788*

Bilirubin *Serum* *Decrease* In 171 patients with severe coronary disease mean concentration of 5.7 ± 2.1 mg/L less than 6.7 ± 3.2 mg/L in 83 normal controls with concentration decreasing with severity of CAD *3014*

C_4b-Binding Protein *Serum* *No Effect* Nonsignificant change observed from mean control concentration (70 individuals) of 21.1 ± 1.0 mg/dL to 22.0 ± 1.0 mg/dL in 57 patients with Gensini's score of greater than 43 *3604*

Ceruloplasmin *Serum* *Increase* Significant progressive increase observed from mean control concentration (70 individuals) of 32.2 ± 1.0 mg/dL to 35.2 ± 1.0 mg/dL in 57 patients with Gensini's score of greater than 43 *3604*

Cesium *Blood* *Increase* Mean concentration in a group of patients with coronary heart disease of 4.7 ± 1.4 μg/kg significantly different from 3.0 ± 0.52 μg/kg in healthy controls *2806*

Chlamydia pneumoniae Antibodies *Serum* *No Effect* Seropositivity observed in 68% patients with CAD, compared with 65% of controls without CAD *117*

Cholesterol *Serum* *Decrease* In 55 patients with more than 50% stenosis in at least one main coronary artery mean concentration of 5.89 ± 1.34 mmol/L significantly different from 6.25 ± 1.07 mmol/L in 100 healthy controls *2959*
Serum *Increase* In 171 patients with severe coronary disease mean concentration of 1,891 ± 400 mg/L greater than 1,780 ± 399 mg/L in 83 normal controls with concentration increasing with severity of CAD *3014* In 23 patients with coronary artery disease mean concentration of 226 ± 63 mg/dL significantly different from 178 ± 17 mg/dL in 25 age- and sex-matched controls *5067* In 587 patients with angiographically confirmed coronary artery disease mean concentration increased progressively with number of main coronary arteries with significant stenosis from 6.32 mmol/L with one, 6.69 mmol/L with two, 6.76 mmol/L with

three and 7.01 mmol/L with four *3844* Mean concentration in 30 male patients with coronary atherosclerosis of 5.62 ± 0.77 mmol/L significantly different from 5.02 ± 0.77 mmol/L in 20 healthy controls *1176* Mean concentration in 170 cases of early coronary artery disease 5.84 ± 1.02 mmol/L significantly higher than 5.53 ± 1.06 mmol/L in 168 healthy controls *5746* In 321 men with angiographically documented premature CAD mean concentration of 224 ± 53 mg/dL compared with 214 ± 36 mg/dL in 901 control individuals *1692* In 731 men with coronary artery disease in those with 3 narrowed vessels mean concentration of 2.34 g/L significantly different from 2.15 g/L in those with 0 narrowed vessels. In 323 women with coronary artery disease mean concentration in those with 3 narrowed vessels 2.49 g/L significantly different from 2.31 g/L in those with no narrowed vessels *2882* In patients with NIDDM, in the 9 with CAD mean concentration of 5.26 ± 1.03 mmol/L significantly higher than the mean baseline of 5.04 ± 1.00 mmol/L in the 131 who did not have CAD *3852* Mean concentration in patients with severe CAD higher than in controls and healthy adults *3795* In 116 patients with angiographically proved coronary artery disease mean concentration of 219.80 ± 47.6 mg/dL significantly higher than in 109 clinically healthy controls in whom mean was 189.8 ± 43.3 mg/dL *2788*
Serum *No Effect* In 26 white male patients with premature vascular disease mean concentration of 5.43 ± 0.19 mmol/L not significantly different from 5.19 ± 0.19 mmol/L in 32 age-matched white male controls *5384* In 30 individuals with single artery disease mean concentration of 6.95 ± 1.38 mmol/L, 6.90 ± 1.42 mmol/L in double vessel disease and 6.72 ± 1.50 mmol/L in triple vessel disease not significantly different from 6.97 ± 1.45 mmol/L in 30 control individuals without coronary artery disease *4926* In 43 patients with coronary atherosclerosis mean concentration of 2,070 ± 630 mg/L not significantly different from 1,900 ± 450 mgL in 31 healthy controls *4873* Mean concentration in 59 Chinese patients with coronary artery disease of 1,830 ± 450 mg/L not significantly different from 1,860 ± 370 mg/L in 95 age-matched controls *5743* In 20 patients with coronary artery disease mean concentration of 1,839 ± 242 mg/L not significantly different from 1,807 ± 291 mg/L in 20 healthy controls *3483* In 18 patients with coronary artery disease mean concentration of 5.54 ± 1.06 mmol/L not significantly different from 5.41 ± 1.07 mmol/L in matched controls *1850* Mean concentration in 34 patients with coronary artery disease of 202 ± 37 mg/dL not significantly different from 207 ± 51 mg/dL in 11 healthy controls *1085* In patients with coronary atherosclerosis patients, 40 with triple vessel disease had a mean concentration of 193 ± 6 mg/dL not significantly different from 188 ± 6 mg/dL in 22 patients with normal coronary arteries *3803*

Cholesterol, Esterified *Serum* *Decrease* In 30 individuals with single artery disease mean concentration of 5.11 ± 1.08 mmol/L, 4.60 ± 1.25 mmol/L in double vessel disease and 4.75 ± 1.42 mmol/L in triple vessel disease significantly different from 5.18 ± 1.50 mmol/L in 30 control individuals without coronary artery disease *4926*

Cholesterol, Nonesterified *Serum* *Increase* In 30 individuals with single artery disease mean concentration of 1.94 ± 0.85 mmol/L, 1.85 ± 0.71 mmol/L in double vessel disease and 1.97 ± 0.72 mmol/L in triple vessel disease significantly different from 1.79 ± 1.32 mmol/L in 30 control individuals without coronary artery disease *4926*

Citrate *Plasma* *No Effect* Mean concentration in 30 male patients with coronary atherosclerosis of 8.6 ± 1.4 µmol/L not significantly different from 9.4 ± 1.4 µmol/L in 20 healthy controls *1176*

C-Reactive Protein *Serum* *Increase* Significant progressive change observed from mean control concentration (70 individuals) of 145.5 ± 1.2 mg/dL to 314.2 ± 1.2 mg/dL in 57 patients with Gensini's score of greater than 43 *3604* Mean concentration in 219 patients with CAD of 1.32 ± 0.22 mg/dL compared with 0.58 ± 0.11 mg/dL in 109 without CAD *117*
Serum *No Effect* Median concentration in 34 patients with severe coronary artery disease of 1.3 mg/L not significantly different from 1.99 mg/L in 30 healthy controls *1068*

Creatinine *Serum* *Increase* Mean concentration of 92 ± 20 µmol/L in 170 cases of early coronary artery disease significantly greater than 85 ± 19 µmol/L in 168 healthy controls *5746*
Serum *No Effect* In patients with coronary atherosclerosis patients 40 with triple vessel disease had a mean concentration of 0.9 ± 0.06 mg/dL not significantly different from 0.9 ± 0.03 mg/dL in 22 patients with normal coronary arteries *3803*

Cytomegalovirus Antibodies *Serum* *No Effect* Seropositivity observed in 77% patients with CAD, compared with 74% of controls without CAD *117*

Factor VII *Plasma* *Increase* Mean concentration observed to be increased in survivors of myocardial infarction *3922*

Factor VIII Coagulant *Plasma* *Increase* Concentration observed to be higher in survivors of myocardial infarctions *3922*

Fatty Acids (FFA), Free *Serum* *No Effect* In 30 individuals with single artery disease mean concentration of 0.26 ± 0.02 mmol/L, 0.34 ± 0.07 mmol/L in double vessel disease and 0.33 ± 0.04 mmol/L in triple vessel disease not significantly different from 0.29 ± 0.08 mmol/L in 30 control individuals without coronary artery disease *4926*

Fibrinogen *Plasma* *Increase* In 23 patients with coronary artery disease mean concentration of 408 ± 118 mg/dL significantly different from normal values of 180 ± 300 mg/dL *5067* In survivors of myocardial infarction mean concentration increased *3922* Median concentration in 34 patients with severe coronary artery disease of 2.87 g/L significantly different from 2.09 g/L in 30 healthy controls *1068*
Plasma *No Effect* Nonsignificant change observed from mean control concentration (70 individuals) of 262.4 ± 1.0 mg/dL to 273.1 ± 1.0 mg/dL in 57 patients with Gensini's score of greater than 43 *3604*

Folate *Serum* *Decrease* In 500 elderly individuals in a long-term healthcare facility 219 patients had a history of AMI or angina pectoris. Mean concentration of 6.6 µg/L in 69 men with coronary artery disease compared with mean of 10.3 µg/L in 84 men without coronary artery disease, with 6.4 µg/L in 150 women with CAD versus 10.4 µg/L in 197 women without *182*
Serum *Increase* In 27 patients with coronary artery disease mean concentration increased to 30 ± 20 nmol/L *3099*

Glucose *Serum* *Increase* In 170 cases of early coronary artery disease mean concentration of 5.31 ± 2.15 mmol/L significantly greater than 4.71 ± 0.93 mmol/L in 168 controls *5746*
Serum *No Effect* In 55 patients with more than 50% stenosis in at least one main coronary artery mean concentration of 5.49 ± 1.73 mmol/L not significantly different from 5.30 ± 0.97 mmol/L in 100 healthy controls *2959*

Haptoglobin *Serum* *Decrease* Significant change observed from mean control concentration (70 individuals) of 159.2 ± 1.1 mg/dL to 130.3 ± 1.1 mg/dL in 57 patients with Gensini's score of greater than 43 *3604*

HDL_2-Cholesterol *Serum* *Decrease* In 30 individuals with single artery disease mean concentration of 0.76 ± 0.25 mmol/L, 0.48 ± 0.10 mmol/L in double vessel disease and 0.49 ± 0.15 mmol/L in triple vessel disease significantly different from 0.99 ± 0.21 mmol/L in 30 control individuals without coronary artery disease *4926*

HDL_{2a}-Apolipoprotein A-I *Serum* *Decrease* In 20 patients with coronary artery disease mean concentration of about 420 mg Apo A-I/L significantly different from about 560 mg Apo A-I/L in 20 healthy controls, but not significantly different as a proportion of total Apo A-I *3483*

HDL_{2b}-Apolipoprotein A-I *Serum* *Decrease* In 20 patients with coronary artery disease mean concentration of about 250 mg Apo A-I/L significantly different from about 350 mg Apo A-I/L in 20 healthy controls, but not significantly different as a proportion of total Apo A-I *3483*

HDL_3-Apolipoprotein A-I *Serum* *Decrease* In 20 patients with coronary artery disease mean concentration of about 310 mg Apo A-I/L significantly different from about 400 mg Apo A-I/L in 20 healthy controls, but not significantly different as a proportion of total Apo A-I *3483*

HDL_3-Cholesterol *Serum* *Decrease* In 30 individuals with single artery disease mean concentration of 0.13 ± 0.08 mmol/L, 0.15 ± 0.05 mmol/L in double vessel disease and 0.12 ± 0.09 mmol/L in triple vessel disease significantly different from 0.16 ± 0.09 mmol/L in 30 control individuals without coronary artery disease *4926*

HDL-Cholesterol *Serum* *Decrease* In 116 patients with angiographically proved coronary artery disease mean concentration of 34.7 ± 11.3 mg/dL significantly less than in 109 clinically healthy controls in whom mean was 46.6 ± 14.6 mg/dL *2788* In 587 patients with angiographically confirmed coronary artery disease mean concentration decreased progressively with number of main coronary arteries with significant stenosis from 1.20 mmol/L with one, 1.03 mmol/L with two, 1.04 mmol/L with

414.00 Coronary Artery Disease *(continued)*

HDL-Cholesterol *(continued)*
three and 1.04 mmol/L with four *3844* Mean concentration in 34 patients with coronary artery disease of 37 ± 9 mg/dL significantly different from 50 ± 16 mg/dL in 11 healthy controls *1085* Mean concentration of 1.01 ± 0.31 mmol/L in 170 individuals with early coronary artery disease significantly reduced compared with 1.17 ± 0.33 mmol/L in 168 healthy controls *5746* Mean concentration in 59 Chinese patients with coronary artery disease of 290 ± 80 mg/L significantly different from 430 ± 130 mg/L in 95 age-matched controls *5743* In 145 men (mean age 51 y) with CAD mean concentration significantly less than in 135 healthy men (mean age 49 y) *1691* In 321 men with angiographically proved premature CAD mean concentration of 36 ± 11 mg/dL significantly less than 45 ± 12 mg/dL in 901 control individuals *1692* In 18 patients with coronary artery disease mean concentration of 1.10 ± 0.26 mmol/L significantly reduced compared with mean concentration of 1.39 ± 0.37 mmol/L in matched controls *1850* In 323 women with coronary artery disease mean concentration in those with 3 narrowed vessels of 0.49 g/L significantly different from 0.54 g/L in those with no narrowed vessels *2882* Of patients with NIDDM, in the 70 with CAD mean concentration of 0.82 ± 0.19 mmol/L significantly less than mean concentration of 0.98 ± 0.32 mmol/L in the 114 who did not have CAD *3852* Mean concentration in 30 male patients with coronary atherosclerosis of 0.88 ± 0.26 mmol/L significantly different from 1.27 ± 0.23 mmol/L in 20 healthy controls *1176* In patients with coronary atherosclerosis patients, 40 with triple vessel disease had a mean concentration of 37 ± 1 mg/dL significantly different from 48 ± 2 mg/dL in 22 patients with normal coronary arteries *3803* In 23 patients with coronary artery disease mean concentration of 47 ± 11 mg/dL significantly different from 53 ± 3 mg/dL in 25 age- and sex-matched controls *5067* In 171 patients with severe coronary disease mean concentration of 372 ± 144 mg/L less than 412 ± 156 mg/L in 83 normal controls with concentration decreasing with severity of CAD *3014* In 30 individuals with single artery disease mean concentration of 0.89 ± 0.29 mmol/L, 0.63 ± 0.20 mmol/L in double vessel disease and 0.61 ± 0.15 mmol/L in triple vessel disease significantly different from 1.15 ± 0.36 mmol/L in 30 control individuals without coronary artery disease *4926* In 43 patients with coronary atherosclerosis mean concentration of 450 ± 120 mg/L significantly different from 570 ± 150 mgL in 31 healthy controls *4873* In patients with severe CAD mean concentration significantly less than in healthy 85-year olds and controls *3795* In 20 patients with coronary artery disease mean concentration of 377 ± 67 mg/L significantly different from 640 ± 102 mg/L in 20 healthy controls *3483*
Serum No Effect In 731 men with coronary artery disease in those with 3 narrowed vessels mean concentration of 0.40 g/L not significantly different from 0.42 g/L in those with 0 narrowed vessels *2882* In 26 white male patients with premature vascular disease mean concentration of 0.83 ± 0.05 mmol/L not significantly different from 0.92 ± 0.04 mmol/L in 32 age-matched white male controls *5384*

HDL-Cholesterol:Cholesterol Ratio *Serum Increase* In 30 individuals with single artery disease mean concentration of 0.13, 0.09 in double vessel disease and 0.09 in triple vessel disease significantly different from 0.16 in 30 control individuals without coronary artery disease *4926*

Helicobacter pylori Antibodies *Serum No Effect* Seropositivity observed in 58% patients with CAD, compared with 46% of controls without CAD *117*

Heparin-releasable Platelet Factor 4 *Plasma Increase* Significant increase to 100.1 ± 38.1 observed in patients with CAD 5 minutes after intravenous heparin compared with controls (61.0 ± 24.0) *4498*

Hexosamine *Serum Decrease* Considerably higher plasma levels of non-protein-bound hexosamine (500 nmol/mL) and lower levels of protein-bound hexosamines (3,770 nmol/mL) were observed in the ischemic heart disease group, compared with the plasma levels of non-protein-bound hexosamine (320 nmol/mL) and protein-bound hexosamine (4,260 nmol/mL) of the control group *3908*
Serum Increase Considerably higher plasma levels of non-protein-bound hexosamine (500 nmol/mL) and lower levels of protein-bound hexosamines (3,770 nmol/mL) were observed in the ischemic heart disease group, compared with the plasma levels of non-protein-bound hexosamine (320 nmol/mL) and protein-bound hexosamine (4,260 nmol/mL) of the control group *3908*

Homocysteine *Plasma Increase* In 587 patients with angiographically confirmed coronary artery disease mean concentration increased progressively with number of main coronary arteries with significant stenosis from 10.9 µmol/L with one, 10.9 µmol/L with two, 10.9 µmol/L with three and 11.4 µmol/L with four *3844* Patients with coronary artery disease had a higher homocyst(e)ine level than control subjects (13.66 ± 6.44 versus 10.93 ± 4.92 nmol/mL, p less than 0.001) *1693* In 27 patients with coronary artery disease mean concentration increased to 12 ± 6 µmol/L *3099* Mean concentration in 69 80-year old men with CAD of 18 ± 5 µmol/L significantly higher than 14 ± 3 µmol/L in 84 80-year old men without CAD. In 150 women aged 80 years with CAD mean concentration of 17 ± 3 µmol/L significantly higher than 11 ± 4 µmol/L in 197 80-year old women without CAD *182* Mean concentration in 170 cases of early coronary artery disease 13.4 ± 4.78 µmol/L significantly greater than 10.1 ± 3.09 µmol/L in 168 healthy controls *5746*

Homocystine *Plasma Increase* In patients with early CAD plasma concentration of 1.2 to 1.3 times that in healthy controls and in peripheral and cerebrovascular disease ratio increased to 1.5 to 1.8 times that in healthy controls *5346*

Interleukin-1β *Serum No Effect* Median concentration in 34 patients with severe coronary artery disease of 3.0 pg/mL not significantly different from 3.0 pg/mL in 30 healthy controls *1068*

Interleukin-6 *Serum No Effect* Median concentration in 34 patients with severe coronary artery disease of 3.0 pg/mL not significantly different from 3.0 pg/mL in 30 healthy controls *1068*

6-Keto-Prostaglandin $F_{1\alpha}$ *Plasma No Effect* In 30 patients with atherosclerosis mean concentration of 7.5 ± 6.5 pg/mL not significantly different from 10 ± 5 pg/mL in healthy controls *1067*

Lactate *Plasma Increase* In 30 individuals with single artery disease mean concentration of 0.75 ± 0.25 mmol/L, 1.38 ± 0.30 mmol/L in double vessel disease and 1.00 ± 0.28 mmol/L in triple vessel disease significantly different from 0.65 ± 0.18 mmol/L in 30 control individuals without coronary artery disease *4926*

LDL-Cholesterol *Serum Increase* In 321 men with angiographically proved premature CAD mean concentration of 156 ± 51 mg/dL significantly higher than 138 ± 33 mg/dL in 901 control individuals *1692* In 116 patients with angiographically proved coronary artery disease mean concentration of 148.5 ± 38.2 mg/dL significantly higher than in 109 clinically healthy controls in whom mean was 124.7 ± 33.4 mg/dL *2788* Of patients with NIDDM, in the 70 who had CAD mean concentration of 3.40 ± 0.87 mmol/L significantly higher than mean concentration of 3.13 ± 0.88 mmol/L in the 114 who did not have CAD *3852* In 30 individuals with single artery disease mean concentration of 5.22 ± 0.90 mmol/L, 5.17 ± 0.86 mmol/L in double vessel disease and 5.12 ± 0.87 mmol/L in triple vessel disease significantly different from 5.03 ± 1.15 mmol/L in 30 control individuals without coronary artery disease *4926* In 731 men with coronary artery disease in those with 3 narrowed vessels mean concentration of 1.67 g/L significantly different from 1.50 g/L in those with 0 narrowed vessels. In 323 women with coronary artery disease mean concentration in those with 3 narrowed vessels 1.73 g/L significantly different from 1.54 g/L in those with no narrowed vessels *2882* Mean concentration in 30 male patients with coronary atherosclerosis of 3.93 ± 0.95 mmol/L significantly different from 3.13 ± 0.67 mmol/L in 20 healthy controls *1176* In 23 patients with coronary artery disease mean concentration of 134 ± 38 mg/dL significantly different from 103 ± 19 mg/dL in 25 age- and sex-matched controls *5067*
Serum No Effect Mean concentration in 59 Chinese patients with coronary artery disease of 1,170 ± 420 mg/L not significantly different from 1,160 ± 390 mg/L in 95 age-matched controls *5743* In 26 white male patients with premature vascular disease mean concentration of 3.66 ± 0.19 mmol/L not significantly different from 3.31 ± 0.18 mmol/L in 32 age-matched white male controls *5384* In 43 patients with coronary atherosclerosis mean concentration of 1,240 ± 510 mg/L not significantly different from 1,110 ± 550 mgL in 31 healthy controls *4873* Mean concentration in 34 patients with coronary artery disease of 131 ± 36 mg/dL not significantly different from 123 ±

45 mg/dL in 11 healthy controls *1085* In 170 individuals with early coronary artery disease mean concentration of 3.85 ± 0.92 mmol/L not significantly increased compared with 3.67 ± 0.94 mmol/L in 168 healthy controls *5746*

Lecithin:Cholesterol Acyltransferase *Serum* *Decrease* In 30 individuals with single artery disease mean activity of 55.35 ± 15.40 nmol/mL/h, 31.60 ± 14.80 nmol/mL/h in double vessel disease and 16.37 ± 8.35 nmol/mL/h in triple vessel disease significantly different from 107.35 ± 27.30 nmol/mL/h in 30 control individuals without coronary artery disease *4926* In 20 patients with coronary artery disease mean LCAT activity of 56.5 ± 20.7 mmol/L/h significantly different from 83.3 ± 20.7 mmol/L/h in 20 healthy controls *3483*

Leukocytes *Blood* *Increase* In 55 patients with more than 50% stenosis in at least one main coronary artery mean concentration of 8,236 ± 2,443 x 10^9/L not significantly different from 7,140 ± 2,083 x 10^9/L in 100 healthy controls *2959*

Lipoprotein A-I *Serum* *Decrease* Mean concentration in 34 patients with coronary artery disease of 39 ± 14 mg/dL significantly different from 48 ± 10 mg/dL in 11 healthy controls *1085*

Lipoprotein A-I:Lipoprotein A-II Ratio *Serum* *No Effect* Mean ratio in 34 patients with coronary artery disease of 84 ± 19 not significantly different from 95 ± 20 in 11 healthy controls *1085*

Lipoprotein Lp(a) *Serum* *Increase* Significantly higher concentration observed in patients with angiographically diagnosed CHF *2827* In 587 patients with angiographically confirmed coronary artery disease mean concentration increased progressively with number of main coronary arteries with significant stenosis from 115 U/L with one, 206 U/L with two, 303 U/L with three and 305 U/L with four *3844* Mean concentration in 59 Chinese patients with coronary artery disease of 214 ± 159 mg/L significantly different from 115 ± 123 mg/L in 95 age-matched controls *5743* In 731 men with coronary artery disease in those with 3 narrowed vessels mean concentration of 123 mg/L significantly different from 67 mg/L in those with 0 narrowed vessels. In 323 women with coronary artery disease mean concentration in those with 3 narrowed vessels 92 mg/L significantly different from 79 mg/L in those with no narrowed vessels *2882* In 26 white male patients with premature vascular disease mean concentration of 28.1 ± 5.5 mg/dL not significantly different from 11.9 ± 5.0 mg/dL in 32 age-matched white male controls *5384* In 23 patients with coronary artery disease mean concentration of 90 ± 78 mg/dL significantly different from 30 ± 25 mg/dL in 25 age- and sex-matched controls *5067* In 321 men with angiographically proved premature CAD mean concentration of 19.9 ± 19 mg/dL significantly higher than 14.9 ± 17.5 mg/dL in 901 control individuals *1692* In 116 patients with angiographically proved coronary artery disease 25th and 75th percentiles of 10.00 and 49.50 mg/dL significantly higher than in 109 clinically healthy controls in whom 25th and 75th percentiles were 5.75 and 27.50 mg/dL *2788* Significant change observed from mean control concentration (70 individuals) of 8.9 ± 1.2 mg/dL to 16.4 ± 1.2 mg/dL in 57 patients with Gensini's score of greater than 43 *3604*
Serum *No Effect* Of patients with NIDDM, mean concentration of 18.65 ± 19.36 mg/dL in the 96 with CAD not significantly higher than mean concentration of 16.67 ± 19.40 mg/dL in 131 patients who did not have CAD *3852*

Lymphocytes *Blood* *Decrease* Concentration of 29% (compared with normal of 20.3 - 46.7%) in 211 patients with known or suspected CAD with 5-year survival significantly less in those with low counts *3913*

α_2-Macroglobulin *Serum* *Decrease* Reduction observed in large studies associated with the presence of coronary heart disease *2201*
Serum *Increase* Significant progressive increase observed from mean control concentration (70 individuals) of 194.4 ± 1.0 mg/dL to 221.4 ± 1.0 mg/dL in 57 patients with Gensini's score of greater than 43 *3604*

Phospholipids *Serum* *No Effect* In 30 individuals with single artery disease mean concentration of 2.78 ± 0.42 mmol/L, 3.15 ± 0.46 mmol/L in double vessel disease and 2.86 ± 0.40 mmol/L in triple vessel disease not significantly different from 2.90 ± 0.50 mmol/L in 30 control individuals without coronary artery disease *4926*

Preβ1-HDL-Apolipoprotein A-I *Serum* *Increase* In 20 patients with coronary artery disease mean concentration of about 90 mg Apo A-I/L significantly different from about 70 mg Apo A-I/L in 20 healthy controls and significantly different as a proportion of total plasma Apo A-I *3483*

Preβ2-HDL-Apolipoprotein A-I *Serum* *No Effect* In 20 patients with coronary artery disease mean concentration of about 50 mg Apo A-I/L not significantly different from about 55 mg Apo A-I/L in 20 healthy controls, and not significantly different as a proportion of total Apo A-I *3483*

Preβ3-HDL-Apolipoprotein A-I *Serum* *No Effect* In 20 patients with coronary artery disease mean concentration of about 10 mg Apo A-I/L not significantly different from about 15 mg Apo A-I/L in 20 healthy controls, and not significantly different as a proportion of total Apo A-I *3483*

Protein *Serum* *No Effect* Mean concentration in 170 cases of early coronary artery disease of 71.1 ± 4.4 g/L not significantly greater than 70.5 ± 4.8 g/L in 168 healthy controls *5746*

Protein C *Plasma* *Decrease* Reduction observed in large studies associated with the presence of coronary heart disease *2201*

Pyridoxal Phosphate *Serum* *Increase* In 27 patients with coronary artery disease mean concentration increased to 69 ± 49 nmol/L *3099*

Rubidium *Blood* *No Effect* Mean concentration in a group of patients with coronary heart disease of 2,540 ± 6,000 µg/kg not significantly different from 2,805 ± 408 µg/kg in healthy controls *2806* Mean concentration of 2,805 ± 408 µg/kg in healthy controls as determined by ICP-MS after microwave digestion *2806*

Superoxide Dismutase *Red Blood Cells* *No Effect* In 43 patients with coronary atherosclerosis mean concentration of CuZn superoxide dismutase of 3,475 ± 1,018 U/g hemoglobin not significantly different from 3,618 ± 1,042 U/g in 31 healthy controls *4873*

Thiobarbituric Acid-reacting Substances *Serum* *Increase* Mean concentration in 30 male patients with coronary atherosclerosis of 5.7 ± 0.7 µmol/L significantly different from 2.5 ± 0.6 µmol/L in 20 healthy controls *1176*

Tissue Plasminogen Activator Antigen *Plasma* *Increase* In 366 patients with coronary artery stenosis mean concentration increased significantly with number of stenosed major coronary arteries *1699*

Tissue Plasminogen Activator:Plasminogen Activator Inhibitor-1 Complex *Plasma* *Increase* In 23 patients with coronary artery disease mean concentration of 10.3 ± 5.7 ng/mL significantly different from 3.4 ± 1.3 ng/mL in 25 age- and sex-matched controls *5067*

Transferrin *Serum* *No Effect* Nonsignificant change observed from mean control concentration (70 individuals) of 269.4 ± 8.6 mg/dL to 266.9 ± 6.6 mg/dL in 57 patients with Gensini's score of greater than 43 *3604*

Triglycerides *Serum* *Increase* Mean concentration in 30 male patients with coronary atherosclerosis of 1.84 ± 0.43 mmol/L significantly different from 1.35 ± 0.23 mmol/L in 20 healthy controls *1176* In 23 patients with coronary artery disease mean concentration of 188 ± 115 mg/dL significantly different from 110 ± 27 mg/dL in 25 age- and sex-matched controls *5067* In 18 patients mean concentration of 2.03 ± 0.74 mmol/L not significantly increased compared with 1.17 ± 0.52 mmol/L in matched controls *1850* In patients with NIDDM, in the 95 who had CAD the mean concentration of 2.66 ± 1.88 mmol/L was significantly higher than 2.33 ± 1.78 mmol/L in the 130 who did not have CAD *3852* In 171 patients with severe coronary disease mean concentration of 1,755 ± 1,083 mg/L greater than 1,340 ± 682 mg/L in 83 normal controls with concentration increasing with severity of CAD *3014* In 731 men with coronary artery disease in those with 3 narrowed vessels mean concentration of 1.19 g/L significantly different from 1.12 g/L in those with 0 narrowed vessels. In 323 women with coronary artery disease mean concentration in those with 3 narrowed vessels of 1.31 g/L significantly different from 0.99 g/L in those with no narrowed vessels *2882* In 321 men with angiographically proved premature CAD mean concentration of 189 ± 95 mg/dL significantly higher than 141 ± 104 mg/dL in 901 control individuals *1692* Mean concentration significantly higher in 145 men (mean age 51 y) than in 135 healthy control men *1691* In 116 patients with angiographically proved coronary artery disease mean concentration of 192.2 ± 89.2 mg/dL significantly higher than in 109 clinically healthy controls in whom mean was 106.9

414.00 Coronary Artery Disease (continued)

Triglycerides *(continued)*
± 53.6 mg/dL *2788* Mean concentration in 170 individuals with early coronary artery disease of 2.2 ± 1.26 mmol/L significantly higher than 1.52 ± 1.04 mmol/L in 168 healthy controls *5746* In 43 patients with coronary atherosclerosis mean concentration of 2,050 ± 1,370 mg/L significantly different from 1,120 ± 550 mgL in 31 healthy controls *4873* In patients with severe CAD mean concentration significantly higher than in healthy elderly and controls *3795* In 30 individuals with single artery disease mean concentration of 1.86 ± 0.51 mmol/L, 2.43 ± 0.63 mmol/L in double vessel disease and 2.17 ± 0.72 mmol/L in triple vessel disease significantly different from 1.73 ± 0.45 mmol/L in 30 control individuals without coronary artery disease *4926* In 55 patients with more than 50% stenosis in at least one main coronary artery mean concentration of 1.87 ± 0.62 mmol/L significantly different from 1.44 ± 0.63 mmol/L in 100 healthy controls *2959* In 20 patients with coronary artery disease mean concentration of 1,148 ± 371 mg/L not significantly different from 978 ± 477 mg/L in 20 healthy controls *3483* Mean concentration in 34 patients with coronary artery disease of 168 ± 62 mg/dL significantly different from 124 ± 70 mg/dL in 11 healthy controls *1085*
Serum No Effect In 26 white male patients with premature vascular disease mean concentration of 2.3 ± 0.21 mmol/L not significantly different from 2.0 ± 0.52 mmol/L in 32 age-matched white male controls *5384* Mean concentration in 59 Chinese patients with coronary artery disease of 1,410 ± 640 mg/L not significantly different from 1,300 ± 1,040 mg/L in 95 age-matched controls *5743* In patients with coronary atherosclerosis patients, 40 with triple vessel disease had a mean concentration of 125 ± 16 mg/dL not significantly different from 112 ± 10 mg/dL in 22 patients with normal coronary arteries *3803*

Tumor Necrosis Factor-α *Serum No Effect* Median concentration in 34 patients with severe coronary artery disease of 8.7 pg/mL not significantly different from 8.8 pg/mL in 30 healthy controls *1068*

Uric Acid *Serum Increase* Mean concentration in 170 individuals with early coronary artery disease of 377 ± 84 µmol/L significantly greater than 305 ± 86 µmol/L in 168 healthy controls *5746*
Serum No Effect In patients with coronary atherosclerosis patients, 40 with triple vessel disease had a mean concentration of 5.5 ± 0.2 mg/dL not significantly different from 5.4 ± 0.2 mg/dL in 22 patients with normal coronary arteries *3803*

Vitamin B_{12} *Serum Decrease* In 500 elderly individuals in a long-term healthcare facility 219 patients had a history of AMI or angina pectoris. Mean concentration of 434 ng/mL in 69 men with coronary artery disease compared with mean of 593 ng/mL in 84 men without coronary artery disease, with 427 ng/mL in 150 women with CAD versus 594 ng/mL in 197 women without *182*
Serum Increase In 27 patients with coronary artery disease mean concentration increased to 295 ± 126 pmol/L *3099*

VLDL-Cholesterol *Serum Increase* In 23 patients with coronary artery disease mean concentration of 34 ± 13 mg/dL significantly different from 22 ± 5 mg/dL in 25 age- and sex-matched controls *5067* Mean concentration in 170 individuals with early coronary artery disease 1.00 ± 0.65 mmol/L significantly greater than 0.64 ± 0.49 mmol/L in 168 healthy controls *5746*
Serum No Effect In 26 white male patients with premature vascular disease mean concentration of 0.94 ± 0.11 mmol/L not significantly different from 0.99 ± 0.17 mmol/L in 32 age-matched white male controls *5384*

von Willebrand Factor Antigen *Plasma Increase* Mean concentration increased in survivors of myocardial infarction *3922*

414.80 Ischemic Heart Disease

Apolipoprotein A-I *Serum Decrease* In each major study group mean high density lipoproteins were lower in persons with coronary heart disease than in those without the disease. The average difference was small--typically 3 - 4 mg/dL -- but statistically significant *732*

Apolipoprotein B *Serum Increase* Patients with coronary artery disease had increased levels *3289*

Apolipoproteins *Serum Decrease* Significantly lower apolipoprotein A-I levels *1691* Apolipoprotein A-I was a strong negative risk factor *4835* Significantly lower apolipoprotein A-I levels *1692*
Serum Increase Significantly higher apolipoprotein B levels *1691* The results of multivariate analysis showed that apolipoprotein B was a significant independent risk factor but apolipoprotein A-I was a stronger negative risk factor. Apolipoprotein B was a highly significant risk factor in a univariate analysis but not in a multivariate analysis when serum cholesterol was included *4835* Significantly higher apolipoprotein B levels *1692*

Basic Fibroblast Growth Factor *Serum Increase* bFGF detected in 60% of patients with stable or unstable angina without significant CAD, 39% of patients with stable and unstable angina with significant coronary artery stenosis and 25% of post-infarction patients compared with undetectable amounts in 20 healthy controls *2041*

Bicarbonate *Serum Increase* In 62% of 434 patients hospitalized for this disorder *1576*

Carcinoembryonic Antigen *Serum Increase* 39% of patients had values > 2.5 ng/mL *4891*

Catecholamines *Plasma Increase* Epinephrine and norepinephrine increase in proportion to the severity of circulatory failure. Catecholamine excretion, especially norepinephrine, is significantly raised in grades 3 and 4 of hemodynamic disturbance *5735*
Urine Increase Epinephrine and norepinephrine increase in proportion to the severity of circulatory failure. Catecholamine excretion, especially norepinephrine, is significantly raised in grades 3 and 4 of hemodynamic disturbance *5735*

Cholesterol *Serum Increase* Mean concentration in hypercholesterolemic patients with IHD of 365 ± 87 mg/dL higher than in those without IHD 316 ± 42 mg/dL *5510* Studies of patients with coronary atherosclerotic heart disease and of their families have indicated a significantly higher incidence (16 - 44%) of elevated plasma cholesterol and/or triglyceride levels, usually classified as type II or type IV *2304* Increased risk of heart disease associated with Lp(a) concentrations above 30 mg/dL and 3rd tertile (> 236 mg/dL) of cholesterol concentrations *681* In 30 patients with ischemic heart disease free of an end-point after 49 months mean concentration of 6.1 ± 0.8 mmol/L and in 24 patients with an end-point mean concentration of 6.1 ± 1.9 mmol/L different from normal *471*

Copper *Serum Decrease* Epidemiologic and metabolic data are consistent with the hypothesis that a metabolic imbalance in regard to zinc and copper is a major factor in the etiology of coronary heart disease. A metabolic imbalance is either a relative or an absolute deficiency of copper characterized by a high ratio of zinc to copper. The imbalance results in hypercholesterolemia and an increased mortality due to coronary heart disease *2705*

Creatine Kinase *Serum Increase* In 30 patients with ischemic heart disease free of an end-point after 49 months mean activity of 796 U/L and in 24 patients with an end-point mean activity of 997 U/L different from normal *471*

Creatinine *Serum Increase* In 58% of 312 patients hospitalized for this disorder *1576*

Cryoglobulins *Serum Increase* Variable elevation of cryoglobulins *4707*

D-Dimer *Plasma No Effect* In hypercholesterolemic patients with IHD mean concentration of 124 ± 53 ng/mL not significantly different from 110 ± 62 ng/mL in patients without IHD *5510*

Endothelin-1 *Plasma Increase* In one study of 5 patients with myocardial ischemia mean concentration increased 1.4 times compared with healthy controls *328*

Epinephrine *Urine Increase* Increased in proportion to the severity of circulatory failure. Catecholamine excretion is significantly raised in grades 3 and 4 of hemodynamic disturbance *5735*

Fibrinogen *Plasma Increase* In 30 patients with ischemic heart disease free of an end-point after 49 months, mean concentration of 3.3 ± 0.9 g/L and in 24 patients with an end-point mean concentration of 3.4 ± 0.7 g/L different from normal *471*

Fibrinopeptide A *Plasma No Effect* In hypercholesterolemic patients with IHD mean concentration of 4.12 ± 2.83 ng/mL not significantly different from 5.29 ± 7.50 ng/mL in patients without IHD *5510*

α_2-Globulin *Serum* *Increase* Rapid increase occurs before the rise in the γ- fraction *1290*

Glucose Tolerance *Serum* *Decrease* Reported in as many as 50% of patients with coronary artery disease *1980*

HDL-Cholesterol *Serum* *Decrease* In 30 patients with ischemic heart disease free of an end-point after 49 months mean concentration of 1.23 ± 0.38 mmol/L and in 24 patients with an end-point mean concentration of 1.07 ± 0.31 mmol/L different from normal *471* In hypercholesterolemic patients with IHD mean concentration of 46.8 ± 11.3 mg/dL compared with 53.7 ± 14.8 mg/dL in those without *5510*

Homocysteine *Plasma* *Increase* Mean concentration of 13.1 µmol/L in 229 men with ischemic heart disease significantly higher than 11.8 µmol/L in controls *5527* The patients were compared to age- and sex-matched controls. Significantly more patients than controls had hyperhomocysteinemia, 16/58 vs. 4/65, defined as fasting total homocysteine above 18.6 µmol/L *399*

Hypoxanthine *Serum* *Increase* Myocardial ischemia in 18 patients resulted in an increase of coronary sinus hypoxanthine levels from 1.20 ± 0.52 mg/dL during pain *4322*

Lactate *Blood* *Increase* Early lactate production occurred frequently before angina was noted *4322*

LDL-Cholesterol *Serum* *Increase* In 30 patients with ischemic heart disease free of an end-point after 49 months mean concentration of 4.1 ± 0.8 mmol/L and in 24 patients with an end-point mean concentration of 4.2 ± 1.0 mmol/L different from normal *471* In hypercholesterolemic patients with IHD mean concentration of 281 ± 54 mg/dL compared with 237 ± 51 mg/dL in patients without IHD *5510* Increased risk of heart disease associated with Lp(a) concentrations above 30 mg/dL and 2nd and 3rd tertile (> 134 mg/dL) of cholesterol concentrations *681*

Lipids *Serum* *Increase* The severity of atherosclerosis was slightly positively correlated with triglyceride concentration, especially in the younger patients and (not significantly) with plasma cholesterol concentration. Hyperlipidemia was present in 58.8% of patients *1031* Studies of patients with coronary atherosclerotic heart disease and of their families have indicated a significantly higher incidence (16 - 44%) of elevated plasma cholesterol and/or triglyceride levels, usually classified as type II or type IV *2304*

Lipoprotein Lp(a) *Serum* *Increase* Increased risk of heart disease associated with Lp(a) concentrations above 30 mg/dL and 2nd and 3rd tertile of cholesterol concentrations *681* In hypercholesterolemic patients with IHD mean concentration of 31.5 ± 24.8 mg/dL significantly greater than 21.1 ± 13.6 mg/dL in patients without IHD *5510*

Lymphocytes *Blood* *Decrease* Proportion reduced below normal of 20.3 to 46.7% in association with stress of left ventricular dysfunction *3914*

Magnesium *Serum* *Decrease* May occur in the course of the disease *4711*

Norepinephrine *Urine* *Increase* Increased in proportion to the severity of circulatory failure. Catecholamine excretion especially norepinephrine, is significantly raised in grades 3 and 4 of hemodynamic disturbance *5735*

pH *Blood* *Increase* In 48% of 184 patients hospitalized for this disorder *1576*

Plasmin-α_2-Plasmin Inhibitor Complex *Plasma* *No Effect* In hypercholesterolemic patients with IHD mean concentration of 0.61 ± 0.37 µg/mL not significantly different from 0.51 ± 0.24 µg/mL in those without IHD *5510*

Plasminogen Activator Inhibitor-1 *Plasma* *No Effect* Mean concentration of 22.2 ± 13.0 ng/mL in 6 patients with IHD not significantly different from 22.78 ± 8.29 ng/mL in 15 healthy controls *4718* In hypercholesterolemic patients with IHD mean concentration of 83.2 ± 70.8 ng/mL not significantly different from 64.9 ± 67.6 ng/mL in those without IHD *5510*

Prostacyclin *Plasma* *No Effect* Mean concentration of 17.6 ± 8.8 pg/mL in 6 patients with IHD not significantly higher than 19.1 ± 5.3 pg/mL in 20 healthy controls *4718*

Semicarbazide-sensitive Amine Oxidase *Serum* *No Effect* In 21 patients with chronic ischemic heart disease mean activity of 14.7 ± 4.0 nmol benzylamine/mL plasma/h not significantly different from 15.9 ± 3.9 nmol benzylamine/mL in 24 healthy controls *1659*

Soluble E-Selectin *Serum* *Increase* In 30 patients with ischemic heart disease free of an end-point after 49 months mean concentration of 54 ± 23 ng/mL and in 24 patients with an end-point mean concentration of 60 ± 30 ng/mL different from normal *471*

Soluble Tumor Necrosis Factor Receptor-p55
Serum *No Effect* In 20 patients with post AMI ischemic heart disease mean concentration of 1.65 ± 0.58 ng/mL compared with 1.90 ± 0.63 ng/mL in 20 age and sex matched controls *474*

Soluble Tumor Necrosis Factor Receptor-p75
Serum *Increase* In 20 patients with peripheral vascular disease mean concentration of 3.39 ± 0.98 ng/mL compared with 2.41 ± 0.75 ng/mL in 20 age and sex matched controls *474*

Thrombin/Antithrombin III Complex *Plasma* *No Effect* In hypercholesterolemic patients with IHD mean concentration of 9.95 ± 6.11 ng/mL not significantly different from 7.92 ± 9.94 ng/mL in patients without IHD *5510*

Thrombomodulin *Plasma* *Increase* Mean concentration of 49.2 ± 15.4 ng/mL in 6 patients with IHD significantly higher than 35.9 ± 8.1 ng/mL in 21 healthy controls *4718* In hypercholesterolemic patients with IHD mean concentration of 4.64 ± 1.09 ng/dL significantly higher than 3.5 ± 0.43 mg/dL in those without IHD *5510* In 30 patients with ischemic heart disease free of an end-point after 49 months mean concentration of 49 ± 19 ng/mL and in 24 patients with an end-point mean concentration of 65 ± 24 ng/mL different from normal *471*

Tissue Plasminogen Activator *Plasma* *Increase* Mean concentration of 20.96 ± 14.2 ng/mL in 6 patients with IHD significantly higher than 7.88 ± 10.1 ng/mL in 21 healthy controls *4718*
Plasma *No Effect* Mean concentration of 12.7 ± 5.48 ng/mL in hypercholesterolemic patients with IHD not significantly different from 11.9 ± 8.42 ng/mL in those without IHD *5510*

Triglycerides *Serum* *Increase* In 30 patients with ischemic heart disease free of an end-point after 49 months mean concentration of 1.7 mmol/L and in 24 patients with an end-point mean concentration of 2.0 mmol/L different from normal *471* Studies of patients with coronary atherosclerotic heart disease and of their families have indicated a significantly higher incidence (16 - 44%) of elevated plasma cholesterol and/or triglyceride levels, usually classified as type II or type IV *2304* The severity of atherosclerosis was positively correlated with plasma concentration, especially in the younger patients ($r = 0.29$, $p < 0.05$), and (not significantly) with plasma cholesterol concentration *1031*
Serum *No Effect* In hypercholesterolemic patients with IHD mean concentration of 174 ± 75 mg/dL not significantly different from 204 ± 194 mg/dL in patients without IHD *5510*

Troponin T *Serum* *Increase* Insignificant differences observed in patients with AMI, unstable angina pectoris, or undergoing PTCA with results obtained with first generation and second generation BMC Enzymun Troponin T assay performed on BMC ES 300 or 700 analyzers *333*

Tumor Necrosis Factor *Serum* *Increase* In 20 patients with post-AMI ischemic heart disease mean concentration of 1.88 ± 0.48 pg/mL compared with 1.19 ± 0.46 pg/mL in 20 age and sex matched controls *474*

Uric Acid *Serum* *Increase* Occurs frequently. In 92 young adults with coronary heart disease, mean level was 5.13 - 0.12, ranging from 3.0 - 7.8 mg/dL *1235* In 59% of 475 patients hospitalized for this disorder *1576* Reported effect *4866*

Vanillylmandelic Acid *Urine* *Increase* Increased excretion was observed in cases of grade 4 hemodynamic disturbance *5735*

von Willebrand Factor *Plasma* *Increase* In 20 patients with post-AMI ischemic heart disease mean concentration of 131 ± 33 IU/dL compared with 101 ± 26 IU/dL in 20 age and sex matched controls *474*
Plasma *No Effect* In hypercholesterolemic patients with IHD mean concentration of 130 ± 32% not significantly different from 118 ± 39% in those without IHD *5510*

Zinc *Serum* *Increase* Epidemiologic and metabolic data are consistent with the hypothesis that a metabolic imbalance in regard to zinc and copper is a major factor in the etiology of coronary heart disease. A metabolic imbalance is either a relative or an absolute deficiency of copper characterized by a high ratio of zinc to copper. The imbalance results in hypercholesterolemia and an increased mortality due to coronary heart disease *2705*

415.00 Cor Pulmonale

Ammonia *Blood Increase* Due to hepatic congestion *5394*

Carbon Dioxide Partial Pressure *Blood Increase* Increased when cor pulmonale is secondary to chest deformities or pulmonary emphysema *5544* The degree of arterial pCO_2 elevation is in direct proportion to the inadequacy of alveolar ventilation in relation to metabolic production of CO_2 *2304*

Catecholamines *Plasma Increase* Epinephrine and norepinephrine increase in proportion to the severity of circulatory failure. Catecholamine excretion, especially norepinephrine, is significantly raised in grades 3 and 4 of hemodynamic disturbance *5735*
Urine Increase Epinephrine and norepinephrine increase in proportion to the severity of circulatory failure. Catecholamine excretion, especially norepinephrine, is significantly raised in grades 3 and 4 of hemodynamic disturbance *5735*

Epinephrine *Urine Increase* Increased in proportion to the severity of circulatory failure. Catecholamine excretion is significantly raised in grades 3 and 4 of hemodynamic disturbance *5735*

Erythrocytes *Blood Increase* Secondary polycythemia *5544* Erythrocytosis, secondary to chronic hypoxemia may be prominent, especially in bronchitic patients *2304*

Hematocrit *Blood Increase* Secondary polycythemia *4775*

Hemoglobin *Blood Increase* Secondary polycythemia *4775*

Norepinephrine *Urine Increase* Increased in proportion to the severity of circulatory failure. Catecholamine excretion, especially norepinephrine, is significantly raised in grades 3 and 4 of hemodynamic disturbance *5735*

Oxygen Partial Pressure *Blood Decrease* Acute hypoxia and hypermetabolism associated with fever and infection *2304*

Oxygen Saturation *Blood Decrease* Acute hypoxia and hypermetabolism associated with fever and infection *2304*

Theophylline *Serum Increase* Cor pulmonale reported to decrease elimination of theophylline *5034*

Vanillylmandelic Acid *Urine Increase* Increased excretion observed in cases of grade 4 hemodynamic disturbance *5735*

Viscosity *Serum Increase* An increase in blood viscosity, red blood cell mass, and blood volume is thought to further compromise the pressure-flow relationships of the constricted and restricted pulmonary vascular bed *2304*

Volume *Plasma Increase* An increase in blood viscosity, red blood cell mass, and blood volume is thought to further compromise the pressure-flow relationships of the constricted and restricted pulmonary vascular bed *2304*

415.10 Pulmonary Embolism

Alkaline Phosphatase *Serum Increase* Since lung is rich source of enzyme, activity may increase with diseases of lung such as pneumonia or pulmonary embolism *4617*

Anticardiolipin Antibodies *Serum Increase* A control was matched by age, smoking history, and length of follow-up to each of the 90 patients with deep venous thrombosis or pulmonary embolus. The anticardiolipin antibody titers were higher in case patients with pulmonary embolus than in their matched controls (P =0.01) *2891*

D-Dimer *Plasma Increase* Concentrations increasd above 500 µg/L in all but 5 of 73 patients with pulmonary embolism *3510* Diagnosis in outpatients excluded in outpatients with concentrations less than 500 µg/L *4086* Normal concentration could exclude pulmonary embolism in 28% of 101 outpatients *5387*
Plasma No Effect Normal concentrations occurred in 47 of 98 patients with pulmonary embolism *2869*

Fibrinopeptide A *Urine Increase* Mean excretion in 7 patients with pulmonary embolism 41.1 ± 2.6 ng/mg creatinine significantly higher than 4.8 ± 2.5 ng/mg creatinine in 22 patients without pulmonary embolism *5320*

Lipoprotein Lp(a) *Serum Increase* In 25 patients with pulmonary embolism mean concentration of 21.4 ± 23.0 mg/dL significantly higher than 6.7 ± 6.1 mg/dL in 25 control blood donors *977*

Troponin T *Serum Increase* Concentration increased in 9 patients with pulmonary embolism (4 with TNT > 0.1 ng/mL) *5838*

415.10 Pulmonary Embolism and Infarction

Alanine Aminotransferase *Serum Increase* Slight increase *1980*

Aldolase *Serum Increase* Moderate increase found, with no sharp peak as in myocardial infarction *1290*

Alkaline Phosphatase *Serum Increase* Elevation is temporary and found at maximum value within 1 - 3 weeks after embolism *1171* In 30% of 19 patients at initial hospitalization for this disorder *1576*

Amylase *Pleural Fluid Increase* Normal or low *4493* May occur *3482*
Pleural Fluid No Effect Usually less than or equal to serum level *4493*

Antithrombin Titer *Plasma Decrease* About 2% of venous thromboembolism is due to antithrombin III deficiency *2304*

Aspartate Aminotransferase *Serum Increase* Slight increase *1980* Rises later and slower than after cardiac infarction. Possibly related to associated congestive failure *1290* In a small proportion of patients with this disease slightly elevated values occur by 3 or 4 days after the bout of chest pain *1025* Characterized by increased LD and usually by normal AST values. Incidence of elevation has varied from 0 - 30% and the elevations are slight to moderate. The rise is delayed for 3 - 5 days after onset of pain *5544*

Bilirubin, Unconjugated *Serum Increase* Pulmonary embolism with infarction is associated with unconjugated hyperbilirubinemia *3625*

Carbon Dioxide Partial Pressure *Blood Decrease* In 62% of 19 patients at initial hospitalization for this disorder *1576* pO_2 and pCO_2 are both low *3848* Decreased pO_2 associated with normal or decreased pCO_2 *5544*
Blood No Effect Decreased pO_2 associated with normal or decreased pCO_2 *5544*

Cold Agglutinins *Serum Increase* Implicated as cause of intravascular thrombosis, but their role is neither clear nor constant *2304*

Creatine Kinase *Serum Increase* For reasons that are still unclear some cases may have high levels *1642*
Serum No Effect Enzyme activity usually normal *911* Activity usually unaffected *1980* The absence of elevated CK and the presence of increased LD in conjunction with other diagnostic techniques can be used to distinguish pulmonary from myocardial infarction *5544*

Cryofibrinogen *Plasma Increase* Implicated as a cause of intravascular thrombosis, but their role is neither clear nor constant *2304*

Cryoglobulins *Serum Increase* Implicated as a cause of intravascular thrombosis, but their role is neither clear nor constant *2304*

Cryomacroglobulins *Serum Increase* Implicated as a cause of intravascular thrombosis, but their role is neither clear nor constant *2304*

Erythrocyte Sedimentation Rate *Blood Increase* Elevated in most patients *2039*

Erythrocytes *Pleural Fluid Increase* 1000 - 100,000 /µL *4493* In about 10% of cases *1025* Pleural effusions in association with infarction often are bloody *2304*
Sputum Increase Blood-streaked or grossly bloody sputum *2304*

Factor IV *Plasma Increase* Markedly elevated in patients with embolic or cardiorespiratory failure *1997*

Fibrin Degradation Products *Plasma Increase* 42% of 24 patients suspected of acute thrombophlebitis and 50% of 14 patients with documented pulmonary emboli had positive fibrinogen tests *704*

Fibrinogen *Plasma Increase* Implicated as a cause of intravascular thrombosis, but their role is neither clear nor constant *2304*

Glucose *Pleural Fluid No Effect* Pleural fluid and serum concentrations are similar *4493*
Serum Increase In 44% of 21 patients at initial hospitalization for this disorder *1576*

Lactate Dehydrogenase *Pleural Fluid Increase* Exudate *126*
Serum Increase Characteristically a rise of activity and in about 50% of cases no rise of AST activity. Initially considered to be diagnostic, has been shown repeatedly to be not the case

2304 2 to 4 times normal values. Increased within 24 h of onset of pain 1025 Combination of increased LD and a normal AST present in 60 - 75% of patients 2039 Frequently elevated within 5 days after the embolic event. Too nonspecific to be diagnostic 1980
Serum No Effect Values may be normal in the presence of embolism 2304

Lactate Dehydrogenase Isoenzyme-5 *Serum Increase* Elevated to 8.4% of the total LD value of 736 U/L in 5 cases of pulmonary embolism 1756

Lactate Dehydrogenase Isoenzymes *Serum Increase* LD_3 without hemorrhage into lung. LD_1, LD_2, LD_3: with hemorrhage into lung. LD_3 and LD_5, embolus with acute cor pulmonale causing acute congestion of liver 5544 There is some disagreement about whether the LD is elevated in pulmonary infarction, but elevated levels of LD_3 are found 5544 1642

Leukocytes *Blood Increase* Characteristically rises to 10,000 - 15,000 /µL, and occasionally higher. Usually a modest preponderance of polymorphonuclear cells 2304 In 44% of 24 patients at initial hospitalization for this disorder 1576 Usually normal in pulmonary embolism. With pulmonary infarction there may be a relative increase in neutrophils and a leukocytosis 1980
Blood No Effect Count rarely exceeds 15,000 /µL and is usually < 10,000 /µL with little shift to left. This aids in the differential diagnosis of pulmonary embolism and pneumonia 4760 Usually normal with pulmonary embolism. With pulmonary infarction there may be a relative increase in neutrophils and a leukocytosis 1980

Neutrophils *Blood Increase* With pulmonary infarction there may be a relative increase in neutrophils and a leukocytosis 1980 In 40% of 22 patients at initial hospitalization for this disorder 1576
Pleural Fluid Increase Neutrophils predominate in pleural fluid 3052 Predominant cell type 4493

Oxygen Partial Pressure *Blood Decrease* Abnormal alveolar-arterial gradient for oxygen and resting hypoxemia. Arterial pO_2 fails to exceed 55 mm Hg following 100% oxygen breathing 1980 pO_2 and pCO_2 are both low 3848 pO_2 > 80 mm Hg excludes diagnosis of pulmonary embolism in almost all cases 4760 In 86% of 17 patients at initial hospitalization for this disorder 1576

Oxygen Saturation *Blood Decrease* pO_2 > 80 mm Hg excludes diagnosis of pulmonary embolism in almost all cases 4760 pO_2 and pCO_2 are both low 3848 Abnormal alveolar-arterial gradient for oxygen and resting hypoxemia. Arterial pO_2 fails to exceed 55 mm Hg following 100% oxygen breathing 1980

pH *Blood Increase* In 89% of 19 patients at initial hospitalization for this disorder 1576 May be alkaline in the acute stages 3848
Pleural Fluid Decrease Exudate (pH < 7.3) 126

Platelets *Blood Increase* In 19% of 15 patients at initial hospitalization for this disorder 1576 Implicated as a cause of intravascular thrombosis, but their role is neither clear nor constant 2304

Protein *Pleural Fluid Increase* Exudative effusion in about 50% of cases 1025

Specific Gravity *Pleural Fluid Increase* Exudate (> 1.016) 126

Urobilinogen *Urine Increase* Hemorrhage into tissues 5544

416.00 Primary Pulmonary Hypertension

Anti-Ku Antibodies *Serum Increase* Anti-Ku antibodies were found in 23% of patients with PPH and none of 24 normal controls (PPH versus controls, p = 0.01) 2351 5788

Endothelin-1 *Plasma Increase* Reported effect 751 In 3 studies mean concentrations increased to 1.52 ± 0.45 pg/mL, 3.5 ± 2.5 pg/mL and 20.7 ± 1.8 pg/mL increased 5.8-fold, 2.4-fold and 1.6-fold respectively above appropriate normal values 328

Fibrinogen *Plasma Increase* In 25 patients with primary pulmonary hypertension mean of 374.3 ± 12.8 mg/dL significantly greater than 324.1 ± 16.5 mg/dL in 25 healthy controls 2272

Glutathione *BAL Fluid Increase* In 8 patients with primary pulmonary hypertension mean airway concentration of 0.9 ± 0.1 µmol/L significantly different from 0.55 ± 0.04 µmol/L in 8 healthy controls 2551

Glutathione Peroxidase *BAL Fluid No Effect* In 8 patients with primary pulmonary hypertension mean airway concentration of 29 ± 4 mU/mL not significantly different from 29 ± 6 mU/mL in 8 healthy controls 2551

Hematocrit *Blood Increase* In 25 patients with primary pulmonary hypertension mean of 46.3 ± 1.2% not significantly greater than 45.0 ± 0.9% in 25 healthy controls 2272

5-Hydroxytryptamine *Plasma Increase* In 16 patients with primary pulmonary hypertension mean concentration increased to 30.1 ± 9.2 nmol/L compared with 0.6 ± 0.1 nmol/L in 16 age and sex matched controls 2134
Platelets Decrease In 16 patients with primary pulmonary hypertension mean concentration decreased to 1.8 ± 0.6 x 10^{-18} mol/platelet compared with 3.2 ± 0.2 x 10^{-18} mol/platelet in 16 age and sex matched controls 2134

Nitric Oxide *BAL Fluid Decrease* In 8 patients with primary pulmonary hypertension mean airway concentration of 0.69 ± 0.21 µmol/L significantly different from 3.3 ± 1.05 µmol/L in 8 healthy controls 2551
Breath Decrease In 8 patients with primary pulmonary hypertension mean airway gas concentration of 2.8 ± 0.9 ppb significantly different from 8 ± 1 ppb in 8 healthy controls 2551

Plasminogen Activator Inhibitor-1 *Plasma Increase* In 25 patients with primary pulmonary hypertension mean of 6.2 ± 0.8 U/mL significantly different from 4.7 ± 0.8 U/mL in 25 healthy controls 2272

Superoxide Dismutase *BAL Fluid No Effect* In 8 patients with primary pulmonary hypertension mean airway concentration of 1.1 ± 0.1 U/mL not significantly different from 1.0 ± 0.2 U/mL in 8 healthy controls 2551

Tissue Plasminogen Activator *Plasma Decrease* In 25 patients with primary pulmonary hypertension mean of 0.08 ± 0.05 IU/mL significantly different from 0.27 ± 0.13 IU/mL in 25 healthy controls 2272

Tissue Plasminogen Activator Antigen *Plasma No Effect* In 25 patients with primary pulmonary hypertension mean of 7.5 ± 0.8 ng/mL not significantly different from 7.6 ± 3.1 ng/mL in 25 healthy controls 2272

Uric Acid *Serum Increase* Mean concentration in 90 patients with primary pulmonary hypertension significantly increased to 7.5 mg/dL compared with 4.9 mg/dL in 30 controls, with the increase proportional to the severity of the disease 3707

416.90 Cardiopulmonary Disease

Carcinoembryonic Antigen *Serum Increase* In 106 patients with cardiopulmonary disease, 75.5% had concentrations of 0.0 - 3.0 ng/mL, 12.3% had concentrations from 3.1 - 5.0 ng/mL, 10.4% had concentrations from 5.1 - 10.0 ng/mL and 1.9% had concentrations greater than 10.0 ng/mL when measured by method on Bayer Technicon Immuno 1® system compared with 95.9%, 3.5%, 0.6% and 0.0% respectively in 173 healthy nonsmokers 339

420.90 Acute Pericarditis

Aspartate Aminotransferase *Serum Increase* 50% incidence of slightly elevated values reported. Usual values < 48.2 U/L 1025 Modest elevations occur. This is especially likely to happen when pericardial effusion produces venous hypertension and hepatic congestion 2304

Cells *Pericardial Fluid Increase* Few lymphocytes or RBCs typically observed 1539

Creatine Kinase *Serum No Effect* Activity usually within normal limits 5544

Glucose *Pericardial Fluid No Effect* Same as serum level 1539

Lactate Dehydrogenase *Pericardial Fluid Decrease* Less than 60% of serum levels 1539

Leukocytes *Blood Decrease* Normal or low in viral or tuberculous pericarditis 1539

420.90 Acute Pericarditis *(continued)*

Leukocytes *(continued)*
Blood Increase Often increased but may be within normal limits *2304* Usually increased in proportion to fever; normal or low in viral disease and tuberculous pericarditis; markedly increased in suppurative bacterial pericarditis *5544*
Blood No Effect Normal or low in viral or tuberculous pericarditis *1539*

Protein *Pericardial Fluid Decrease* Less than 50% of serum levels *1539*

421.00 Bacterial Endocarditis

Albumin *Serum Decrease* Mildly depressed, mean of 3.0 ± 0.1 g/dL. Lowest values found in pneumococcal infection 2.4 ± 0.4 g/dL *4067*
Urine Increase Almost invariably present, even when no renal lesions are found with bacterial endocarditis *5545*

Carbon Dioxide Partial Pressure *Blood Decrease* In 14 narcotic addicts with bacterial endocarditis the arterial CO_2 tension, at 27.8 ± 1.7 mm Hg, was significantly lower than a group of narcotics with other disorders, at 40.1 ± 3.7 mm Hg *3862*

Complement C_3 *Serum Decrease* Decreased total C_3 and C_4, with conversion products of both, in subacute endocarditis *5651* Decreased total hemolytic complement or C_3 in 8 of 17 or 47% of patients tested. 7 of the 8 had evidence of renal disease *4067*

Complement C_4 *Serum Decrease* Decreased total C_3 and C_4, with conversion products of both, in subacute endocarditis *5651*

Complement, Total *Serum Decrease* Decreased total hemolytic complement in 8 of 17 or 47% of patients tested. 7 of the 8 had evidence of renal disease *4067* Decreased total C_3 and C_4, with conversion products of both, in subacute endocarditis *5651*

Coombs' Test *Serum Positive* Rarely there is hemolytic anemia with a positive Coombs' test *5544*

Creatinine *Serum Increase* Increase parallels BUN elevation; higher concentration found in fatal cases than in survivors *4067* Elevated in patients with diffuse glomerulonephritis and chronic infective endocarditis *900*

Cryoglobulins *Serum Increase* Variable elevation of cryoglobulins *4707*

Erythrocyte Casts *Urine Increase* Casts are seen in the occasional patient with diffuse glomerulonephritis *900* Found in 12% of patients *4067*

Erythrocyte Sedimentation Rate *Blood Increase* Increased in 90% of cases. A normal ESR is useful in excluding this diagnosis *1980* Elevated in 90% of cases but is of no differential aid in the work-up of fever of unknown origin *2304* Increased in 90% of cases. A normal ESR is useful in excluding this diagnosis *5583* Usually elevated with a mean of 57.3 ± 3.6 mm/h. Mean ESR in survivors, 77.5 mm/h, was significantly higher than in fatalities, 40.7 mm/h *4067*

Erythrocytes *Urine Increase* Microscopic hematuria found in 55% of patients *4067* Hematuria even without renal involvement *5583* Hematuria (usually microscopic) occurs at some stage in many cases due to glomerulitis or renal infarct or focal embolic glomerulonephritis *5544*

γ-Globulin *Serum Increase* With renal parenchymal disease *5583* Mean = 3.7 ± 0.1 g/dL in 125 cases of various types of infection *4707* Seen in about 50% of patients *2039* Mean concentration of 3.7 ± 0.1 g/dL in 125 cases of various types of infection *4067*

Hematocrit *Blood Decrease* Rarely there is a hemolytic anemia with a positive Coombs' test *5544* Normocytic normochromic anemia commonly presents with mean hematocrit of 35.5 ± 0.6%. Lowest hematocrits found in gram-negative (29.8 ± 3.1%) and culture-negative cases (30.4 ± 1.6%). Degree of anemia is related to duration of illness, not virulence of organism *4067* Normochromic, normocytic anemia occurs in 60 - 70% of cases *2304* Anemia is more common in long-standing infection and has no specificity *900*

Hemoglobin *Blood Decrease* Rarely there is a hemolytic anemia with a positive Coombs' test *5544* Normocytic normochromic anemia commonly present with mean hematocrit of 35.5 ± 0.6%. Lowest hematocrits found in gram-negative (29.8 ± 3.1%) and culture- negative cases (30.4 ± 1.6%). Degree of anemia is related to duration of illness, not virulence of organism *4067* Anemia is more common in long-standing infection and has no specificity *900* Normochromic, normocytic anemia occurs in 60 - 70% of cases *2304*

Interleukin-6 *Serum No Effect* In the sera from 10 patients with subacute enterococcal or streptococcal endocarditis concentrations were normal. However, the levels were low or undetectable in patients with bacterial endocarditis *2644*

Iron *Serum Decrease* Observed effect *5544*

Leukocytes *Blood Decrease* Of little value in bacterial endocarditis, in which normal, high, and low counts may occur *1980* Occasional leukopenia *5544*
Blood Increase Typical observation *1980* Normal in about 50% of patients and elevated up to about 15,000 /µL in the rest, with 65 - 85% neutrophils. Higher count indicates presence of a complication. Occasionally there is leukopenia *5544* Counts ranged widely; mean = 12,700 ± 600 /µL. Highest in pneumococcal (17,300 ± 3,400 /µL), gram-negative (16,800 ± 4,300 /µL) and S. Aureus (13,900 ± 1,000 /µL) *4067* Only slight leukocytosis is expected in subacute cases, and even this is absent in about 50% of patients. Leukocytosis of 15,000 /µL is common with acute disease *2039*
Blood No Effect Excretion usually within normal limits *1223* Normal in about 50% of patients and elevated up to about 15,000 /µL in the rest *5544* *5583* May be normal, low, or elevated. Normal counts are just as prevalent as elevated counts *2304*
Cerebrospinal Fluid Increase May reach 100 /µL, mostly polymorphonuclears and lymphocytes in bacterial endocarditis with embolism *367*

Monocytes *Blood Increase* Found in 15 - 20% of patients but is not correlated with the presence or number of peripheral phagocytic reticuloendothelial cells *999* Elevated WBC up to about 15,000 /µL in 50%. Monocytosis may be pronounced *5544*

Neutrophils *Blood Increase* Usually increased numbers of immature granulocytes are found in the blood *2039* Normal or elevated to 15,000 /µL with 65 - 85% neutrophils *5583* Elevated WBC in 50% of patients with 65 - 85% neutrophils *5544*

pH *Blood Increase* In 14 narcotic addicts with bacterial endocarditis, the blood pH, at 7.47 ± 0.01 was significantly higher than in a group of narcotics with other disorders, at 7.36 ± 0.06 *3862*

Platelets *Blood Decrease* Usually normal but occasionally it is decreased; rarely purpura occurs *5544*
Blood No Effect Usually normal but occasionally it is decreased; rarely purpura occurs *5544*

Protein *Cerebrospinal Fluid Increase* Slightly elevated in infection with embolism *367*
Urine Increase Mild to moderate proteinuria is common as a result of joint and muscle inflammation *367*

Rheumatoid Factor *Serum Increase* Rheumatoid factor may be observed in certain patients with subacute bacterial endocarditis *2473* Positive in 17 of 36 patients but did not correlate with renal failure *4067* 13 (24%) of 55 patients were seropositive at some point in their courses. More severe cases were more likely to develop rheumatoid factor *4766* Elevated levels of IgG and IgM rheumatoid factor were found in patients with subacute infection *707* Mean concentration increased in patients with subacute bacterial endocarditis *2472* May be used to confirm the diagnosis. Following remission, titers fall to 0 *1980*

Tumor Necrosis Factor-α *Serum Increase* In the sera from 10 patients with subacute enterococcal or streptococcal endocarditis, however, the levels were low or undetectable *2644*

Urea Nitrogen *Serum Increase* Reported effect *4067* Increased -- usually 25 - 75 mg/dL *5545*

421.00 Infective Endocarditis

Blood *Urine Increase* In 143 cases, hematuria observed at start of treatment *3899*

C-Reactive Protein *Serum* *Increase* Mean concentration increased at the start of treatment in 96% of 179 patients with infective endocarditis *3899* In 147 of 197 cases mean CRP concentration of 110 mg/L at the start of treatment significantly higher than the upper reference limit of 10 mg/L *3899*

Creatinine *Serum* *No Effect* In 125 cases mean concentration of 108 µmol/L at the start of treatment but with concentrations increasing to 124 µmol/L after 4 weeks treatment *3899*

Creatinine Clearance *Urine* *Decrease* In 125 cases mean clearance of 1.17 mL/s at the start of treatment but with deterioration to 1.124 mL/s after 2 weeks of antibiotic treatment and 1.07 mL/s after 4 weeks treatment *3899*

Erythrocyte Sedimentation Rate *Blood* *Increase* In 147 (67% of 197) cases mean ESR of 50 mm/h at the start of treatment significantly higher than upper reference limit *3899*

Hemoglobin *Blood* *Decrease* In 125 cases mean concentration at the start of treatment 120 g/L declining every week during treatment *3899*

Immunoglobulin E *Serum* *Increase* In 125 cases mean concentration of 12.8 g/L at the start of treatment with concentrations greater than 14.9 g/L observed in 41 (33%) of the episodes *3899*

Leukocytes *Blood* *Increase* In 109 of 178 cases mean WBC concentration of 11.2 x 10^9/L at the start of treatment significantly higher than the upper reference limit of 10 x 10^9/L *3899*

Platelets *Blood* *Decrease* In 155 cases mean platelet concentration of 227 x 10^9/L at the start of treatment with 40 (26%) lower than the lower reference limit of 150 x 10^9/L *3899*
Blood *Increase* Mean concentration increased above 350,000 /µL at the start of treatment in 14% of 155 episodes in 178 patients with infective endocarditis *2956* Mean concentration decreased below 150,000 /µL at the start of treatment in 26% of 155 episodes in 178 patients with infective endocarditis *2956* In 155 cases mean platelet concentration of 227 x 10^9/L at the start of treatment with 21 (14%) higher than the upper reference limit of 350 x 10^9/L *3899*

Procollagen Type II Peptide *Serum* *Increase* .Observed effect *1054*

421.00 Löffler's Endocarditis

Eosinophils *Blood* *Increase* Marked eosinophilia of the blood associated with diffuse organ infiltration by eosinophils *2304* Eosinophilia up to 70%; may be absent at first but appears sooner or later *5544*

Immunoglobulin M *Serum* *Increase* Especially when particulate antigenic material is present in the blood stream *1290*

Leukocytes *Blood* *Increase* Frequently increased *5544*

422.00 Acute Myocarditis

Aspartate Aminotransferase *Serum* *Increase* Marked elevation signals a poor prognosis *2304*

Complement Fixation *Serum* *Increase* Positive in helminthic myocarditis *2304*

Creatine Kinase *Serum* *Increase* Elevated cardiac enzymes may be the earliest evidence of myocarditis *2304* Increase observed in only 8% of patients with myocarditis *2936*

Creatine Kinase MB-Isoenzyme *Serum* *Increase* Increase observed in only 2% of patients with myocarditis *2936*

Eosinophils *Blood* *Increase* Characteristic of helminthic myocarditis *2304*

Lactate Dehydrogenase *Serum* *Increase* Elevated cardiac enzymes may be the earliest evidence of myocarditis *2304*

Neutralizing Antibodies *Serum* *Increase* In viral myocarditis *2304*

Neutrophils *Blood* *Decrease* Crisis is characterized by acute neutropenia and respiratory alkalosis *2304*

pH *Blood* *Increase* Crisis is characterized by acute neutropenia and respiratory alkalosis *2304*

Troponin T *Serum* *Increase* Mean concentration of 0.59 ng/mL found in patients with biopsy-proven myocarditis, with increase overall in 53% of patients with myocarditis *2936*

423.20 Constrictive Pericarditis

Albumin *Serum* *Decrease* Decreased with normal total protein *5544*

Lactate Dehydrogenase *Pleural Fluid* *Decrease* Transudate *126*

pH *Pleural Fluid* *Increase* Transudate (pH > 7.3) *126*

Protein *Pleural Fluid* *Decrease* Transudate secondary to increased hydrostatic pressure. (< 3 g/dL) *126*
Serum *Decrease* Enteric loss of plasma protein *4891*

Specific Gravity *Pleural Fluid* *Decrease* Transudate (< 1.016) *126*

425.40 Cardiomyopathy

Anti-Mitochondrial M7 Antibody *Serum* *Increase* May be present in some patients with various cardiomyopathies *1778*

Aspartate Aminotransferase *Serum* *Increase* Increased, often to extremely high levels; these may rise even further after recovery from shock in cobalt beer cardiomyopathy *5544*

Atrial Natriuretic Peptide *Plasma* *Increase* In 15 patients with asymptomatic nonobstructive hypertrophic cardiomyopathy mean concentration of about 42 ± 4 fmol/L compared with about 13 ± 1 fmol/L in 10 healthy controls *5812*

Brain Natriuretic Peptide *Plasma* *Increase* In 15 patients with asymptomatic nonobstructive hypertrophic cardiomyopathy mean concentration of 98.6 ± 30.8 fmol/L compared with 1.9 ± 0.4 fmol/L in 10 age-matched controls *5812*

BSP Retention *Serum* *Increase* Disordered liver function in advanced cases of obliterative cardiomyopathy *2304*

Calcium *Serum* *No Effect* In 17 men with dilated cardiomyopathy mean concentration of 2.3 ± 0.2 mmol/L not significantly different from 2.4 ± 0.2 mmol/L in 50 healthy male controls *3942*

Copper *Serum* *Increase* Mean concentration in 17 men with dilated cardiomyopathy of 1,544 ± 280 µg/L significantly higher than 1,111 ± 340 µg/L in 17 healthy controls *3942*

Creatine Kinase *Serum* *Increase* Increased, often to extremely high levels; may rise even further after recovery from shock in cobalt beer cardiomyopathy *5544*

Eosinophils *Blood* *Increase* Observed effect *4933* Mild to moderate eosinophilia. Marked in Loeffler's eosinophilic cardiomyopathy *2304*

Erythrocyte Sedimentation Rate *Blood* *Increase* Often elevated in Loeffler's disease *2304*

Erythrocytes *Ascitic Fluid* *Increase* Ascitic fluid and pericardial fluid are usually blood-stained or serous and contain leukocytes in obliterative cardiomyopathies *2304*
Blood *Increase* Increased, often to extremely high levels; may rise even further after recovery from shock in cobalt beer cardiomyopathy *5544*
Pericardial Fluid *Increase* Ascitic fluid and pericardial fluid are usually blood-stained or serous and contain leukocytes in obliterative cardiomyopathies *2304*

γ-Globulin *Serum* *Increase* May be found and are probably the result of hepatic insufficiency due to heart failure *2304*

Hematocrit *Blood* *Decrease* A slight degree of anemia with obliterative cardiomyopathies *2304*

Hemoglobin *Blood* *Decrease* A slight degree of anemia in obliterative cardiomyopathies *2304*

Iron *Serum* *Decrease* Occasionally low *2304*
Serum *No Effect* In 17 men with dilated cardiomyopathy mean concentration of 1,050 ± 458 µg/L not significantly different from 985 ± 272 µg/L in 50 controls *3942*

Kynurenine *Serum* *Increase* In patients with dilated cardiomyopathy concentration significantly increased and correlated with severity of dilated cardiomyopathy *4474*

Lactate *Blood* *Increase* Lactic acidosis and shock in cobalt beer myopathies *5544*

Lactate Dehydrogenase *Serum* *Increase* Increased, often to extremely high levels; may rise even further after recovery from shock in cobalt beer cardiomyopathy *5544*

Leukocytes *Ascitic Fluid* *Increase* Ascitic fluid and pericardial fluid are usually blood-stained or serous and contain leukocytes in obliterative cardiomyopathies *2304*

425.40 Cardiomyopathy *(continued)*

Leukocytes *(continued)*
Pericardial Fluid *Increase* Ascitic fluid and pericardial fluid are usually blood-stained or serous and contain leukocytes in obliterative cardiomyopathies *2304*

Lymphocytes *Blood* *Decrease* Proportion reduced below normal of 20.3 to 46.7% in patients with dilated cardiomyopathy in association with stress of left ventricular dysfunction *3914*

Magnesium *Serum* *No Effect* In 17 men with dilated cardiomyopathy mean concentration of 0.82 ± 0.1 mmol/L not significantly different from 0.83 ± 0.1 mmol/L in 50 healthy controls *3942*

Neopterin *Serum* *Increase* In patients with dilated cardiomyopathy concentration increased and correlated with severity of cardiomyopathy *4474*

Potassium *Serum* *No Effect* In 17 men with dilated cardiomyopathy mean concentration of 4.1 ± 0.5 mmol/L not significantly different from 4.2 ± 0.4 mmol/L in 50 healthy controls *3942*

Selenium *Serum* *Decrease* Mean concentration in 17 men with dilated cardiomyopathy of 47.8 ± 16.2 µg/L significantly less than 75 ± 12 µg/L in 50 healthy controls *3942*

Sodium *Serum* *No Effect* In 17 men with dilated cardiomyopathy mean concentration of 137 ± 5 mmol/L not significantly different from 140 ± 3 mmol/L in 50 healthy control men *3942*

Troponin T *Serum* *Increase* 2 of 11 patients with end-stage cardiomyopathy had increased concentrations of 0.17 and 0.67 µg/L due to ischemia *1556*

Zinc *Serum* *Decrease* In 17 men with dilated cardiomyopathy mean concentration of 745 ± 195 µg/L significantly reduced compared with 931 ± 178 µg/L in 17 healthy controls *3942*

425.40 Cardiomyopathy, Hypertrophic

Atrial Natriuretic Peptide *Plasma* *Increase* Mean concentration of 155 ± 171 pg/mL in 23 patients significantly higher than 33 ± 15 pg/mL in 14 matched normotensive controls *3326*

Brain Natriuretic Peptide *Plasma* *Increase* Mean concentration of 71 ± 46 pg/mL in 23 patients significantly higher than 34 ± 20 pg/mL in 14 matched normotensive controls *3326*

Copper *Serum* *Increase* Increased concentrations reported in patients with dilated cardiomyopathy *3499*

Creatine Kinase Isoenzymes *Serum* *Increase* In 22 patients with hypertrophic cardiomyopathy mean MMa, MMb and MMc activities were 19.4 ± 4.1%, 26.7 ± 2.5% and 33.5 ± 7.0% of total CK-MM compared with 11.3 ± 3.0%, 21.5 ± 4.4% and 40.7 ± 7.0% respectively in 14 healthy controls *1985*

Creatine Kinase MB-Isoenzyme *Serum* *Increase* In 22 patients with hypertrophic cardiomyopathy mean activity of CK-MB 7.8 ± 3.8 U/L compared with 0.4 ± 0.8 U/L in 14 normal controls *1985*

Endothelin-1 *Plasma* *Increase* In 3 patients with level I idiopathic hypertrophic cardiomyopathy mean concentration of 2.5 ± 0.7 pg/mL, in 7 with level II disease of 6.0 ± 0.9 pg/mL and 6 with level II disease of 10.7 ± 3.9 pg/mL, 1.6-fold, 3.7-fold and 6.7-fold respectively above normal values *328*

427.31 Atrial Fibrillation

Albumin *Serum* *No Effect* Mean concentration in 25 patients with untreated chronic atrial fibrillation not significantly different from that in 31 age-matched controls *2947*

Alkaline Phosphatase *Serum* *No Effect* Mean activity in 25 patients with untreated chronic atrial fibrillation not significantly different from that in 31 age-matched controls *2947*

Atrial Natriuretic Peptide *Plasma* *Increase* In 25 patients with untreated chronic atrial fibrillation concentration of 23.9 ± 14.2 pmol/L significantly higher than 6.7 ± 3.0 pmol/L in 31 age-matched controls *2947* Median atrial natriuretic peptide concentration of 213 ng/L observed in 26 patients with mild to moderate stable congestive heart failure and chronic atrial fibrillation *5393*

Calcium *Serum* *No Effect* Mean concentration in 25 patients with untreated chronic atrial fibrillation not significantly different from that in 31 age-matched controls *2947*

Creatinine *Serum* *No Effect* Mean concentration in 25 patients with chronic untreated atrial fibrillation not significantly different from that in 31 age-matched controls *2947*

D-Dimer *Plasma* *Increase* In 37 patients with chronic atrial fibrillation median concentration of 158 ng/mL (interquartile range 81 - 292 ng/mL) significantly different from 76 ng/mL (interquartile range 53 - 103 ng/mL) in 158 controls with sinus rhythm *1740*

Fibrinogen *Plasma* *Increase* In 37 patients with chronic atrial fibrillation median concentration of 3.78 g/L (interquartile range 3.0 - 4.7 g/L) significantly different from 2.60 g/L (interquartile range 2.24 - 2.99 g/L) in 158 controls with sinus rhythm *1740*

Magnesium *Monocytes* *No Effect* Mean concentration of 0.118 ± 0.090 µmol/mg protein in 25 patients with untreated chronic atrial fibrillation not significantly different from 0.133 ± 0.093 µg/mg protein in 31 age-matched controls *2947*
Red Blood Cells *No Effect* Mean concentration of 2.42 ± 0.36 mmol/L in 25 untreated patients with chronic atrial fibrillation not significantly different from 2.41 ± 0.53 mmol/L in 31 age-matched controls *2947*
Serum *No Effect* Mean concentration of 0.81 ± 0.09 mmol/L in 25 patients with untreated chronic atrial fibrillation not significantly different from 0.81 ± 0.11 mmol/L in 31 age-matched controls *2947*

Phosphate *Serum* *No Effect* Mean concentration in 25 patients with untreated chronic atrial fibrillation not significantly different from that in 31 age-matched controls *2947*

Potassium *Serum* *No Effect* Mean concentration in 25 patients with untreated chronic atrial fibrillation not significantly different from that in 31 age-matched controls *2947*

Sodium *Serum* *No Effect* No significant differences observed in mean concentrations of 25 patients with untreated chronic atrial fibrillation and 31 age-matched controls *2947*

Urea Nitrogen *Serum* *No Effect* Mean concentration in 25 patients with untreated chronic atrial fibrillation not significantly different from that in 31 age-matched controls *2947*

von Willebrand Factor *Plasma* *Increase* In 37 patients with chronic atrial fibrillation median concentration of 152 IU/dL (interquartile range of 108 - 198 IU/dL) significantly different from 105 IU/dL (interquartile range of 80 - 147 IU/dL) in 158 controls with sinus rhythm *1740*

427.50 Cardiac Arrest

Creatine Kinase *Serum* *Increase* Increased activity occurred above 80 U/L in 49% of 107 adults admitted to hospital (91 of whom had suffered an out of hospital arrest), rising to 90% by 24 h *3656*

Creatine Kinase MB-Isoenzyme *Serum* *Increase* Increased activity occurred above 10 U/L in 71% of 107 adults admitted to hospital (91 of whom had suffered an out of hospital arrest), rising to 78% by 24 h *3656*

Neuron-specific Enolase *Serum* *Increase* Serum NSE concentration increased from day zero to day five in the persistently comatose patients (maximum 2,907 ng/mL) with concentrations greater than 33 ng/dL providing 100% specificity and 100% positive predictive value for predicting persistent coma *1517* In 43 patients who had had a cardiac arrest, concentrations greater than 33 ng/mL predicted persistent coma with a high specificity *1517*

428.00 Congestive Cardiac Failure

Adenosine Monophosphate *Plasma* *Increase* Concentration significantly increased with congestive cardiac failure and related to severity of the heart failure and plasma norepinephrine concentration and pulmonary artery pressure *3861*

Alanine Aminotransferase *Serum* *Increase* Increased in about 12% of patients *5544* Depending on the severity and chronicity of cardiac failure *900* 33% of 9 patients showed increases (range 6.3 - 76.3 U/L) *3161* Heart failure or shock with attendant hepatic necrosis may lead to elevated values *1025*

Albumin *Serum* *Decrease* In 63 patients with stable chronic congestive cardiac failure mean concentration of 43.8 ± 3.1 g/L significantly decreased compared with 45.4 ± 2.3 g/L in 20 con-

trols *136* Common with cardiac fibrosis of liver *5544* Increase in plasma volume without increase in total protein *1290*
Urine Increase Slight albuminuria (< 1 g/day) is common *5544* The urinalysis frequently demonstrates reversible proteinuria *900*

Aldosterone *Plasma Increase* In 53 patients with stable chronic congestive cardiac failure mean concentration of 699 ± 91 pmol/L significantly different from 279. ± 42 pmol/L in 16 healthy controls *135* In 17 patients with congestive cardiac failure median concentration of 411 pmol/L compared with 103 pmol/L in 17 healthy control individuals *4055* Enhanced ADH and aldosterone activity *4707* In far-advanced failure, or in moderate failure under vigorous therapy with diuretics, increases in production and excretion, ranging from detectable to very striking, have been noted *2304*
Plasma No Effect In 44 patients with congestive cardiac failure with atrial fibrillation median concentration of 116 pg/mL not significantly different from 100 pg/mL in 225 patients with congestive cardiac failure with sinus rhythm within normal range of 50 - 250 pg/mL *5319*
Urine Increase May be increased in edematous states of cardiac failure *1290* In far-advanced failure, or in moderate failure under vigorous therapy with diuretics, increases in production and excretion, ranging from detectable to very striking, have been noted *2304*

Alkaline Phosphatase *Serum Increase* Increase in conjunction with normal levels of bilirubin indicate congestive heart failure or myocardial infarction in 28% of cases *420* Usually elevated with cardiac cirrhosis *900* Mild to moderate increase (30 - 135 U/L) in 45% of cases *5544*

Alkaline Phosphatase Isoenzymes *Serum Increase* All 5 patients showed elevations of isoenzyme I *2557*

Amino Acids *Plasma Increase* Slight increase *1290*

Ammonia *Blood Increase* In patients with azotemia, arterial levels were elevated to 88 mmol/L *4213*

Amylase *Pleural Fluid Increase* May occur *3482*
Pleural Fluid No Effect Usually less than or equal to serum level *4493*
Serum Decrease Possibly decreased in some cases *1290*

Angiotensin-II *Plasma Increase* Concentration significantly higher in 17 patients with congestive cardiac failure (median 81 pmol/L) compared with median of 12 pmol/L in 17 control individuals *4055*

α_1-Antichymotrypsin *Serum Increase* Mean concentration increased above reference interval of 47.9 ± 8.1 mg/dL in 1 of 1 patient (100%) with congestive cardiac failure *3044*

Antidiuretic Hormone *Plasma Increase* In 8 patients with congestive cardiac failure mean concentration of 8.6 ± 3.3 pg/mL significantly different from 0 - 8 pg/mL in healthy individuals *5* Enhanced ADH and aldosterone activity *4707* In 17 patients with congestive cardiac failure median concentration of arginine vasopressin of 5.3 pmol/L compared with 2.0 pmol/L in 17 healthy controls *4055*

Antinuclear Antibodies *Pleural Fluid Increase* ANA antibodies observed in 2 of 15 pleural fluid specimens *2665*

Aspartate Aminotransferase *Serum Increase* Mild elevation occurred in 33% of 9 cases: levels ranged from 11 - 39 U/L, with the upper limit of normal at 24 U/L *3161* Usually < 100 U/L *1025* Depending on the severity and chronicity of cardiac failure *900* In 552 patients with symptomatic cardiac failure and evidence of cardiomegaly on X-ray, AST activity of 46 U/L was associated with 3-year survival rate of 34% compared with 60% in those with lower activities *326*

Aspartate Aminotransferase:Alanine Aminotransferase Ratio
Serum Increase Ratio greater than 3.0 with AST activity exceeding 500 U/L (normal < 40 U/L) is suggestive of circulatory disturbances, especially left ventricular failure, or malignant diseases involving the liver *4617*

Atrial Natriuretic Peptide *Plasma Increase* Mean concentration in 5 patients with class I CHF of 68.6 ± 36.7 pg/mL, 72.1 ± 18.2 pg/mL in 10 with class II and 187 ± 40.9 pg/mL in 16 with class III all significantly higher than the mean in 19 healthy controls of 251 ± 31.5 pg/mL *229* In patients with severe heart failure the sicker they were the higher the serum ANP concentration *3708* In 58 patients on hospital admission with chronic heart failure detectable ANP concentration higher in those patients with increased concentration of TnT *4744* In 15 patients with severe congestive heart failure mean concentration of 152.7 ± 96.9 pg/mL significantly different from 67.1 ± 48.3 pg/mL in 57 patients with mild congestive heart failure and 12.7 ± 6.4 pg/mL in 25 age-matched normal controls *3200* In 44 patients with congestive cardiac failure with atrial fibrillation median concentration of 380 pmol/L significantly different from 285 pmol/L in 225 patients with congestive cardiac failure with sinus rhythm above normal range of 15 - 35 pmol/L *5319* Concentrations increased in patients with congestive heart failure *2952* Median atrial natriuretic peptide concentration of 213 ng/L observed in 26 patients with mild to moderate stable congestive heart failure and chronic atrial fibrillation *5393* In 10 patients with congestive cardiac failure mean concentration more than 3 times higher than in control individuals *4102* In patients with acute myocardial infarction and congestive cardiac failure mean concentration in right atrium of 50 ± 12 pg/mL significantly increased compared with 30 ± 7 pg/mL in patients with AMI but without congesttive cardiac failure and 7 ± 1 pg/mL in healthy controls *5818* Although concentration low or undetectable in 8 healthy individuals and 9 control patients without cardiac disease it was increased in 17 patients with CCF *5232* Elevated cardiac filling pressure is associated with increased circulating concentrations *643* Levels were directly related to the severity of heart disease. It was well correlated with mean pulmonary arterial pressure *2170*

Bicarbonate *Serum Decrease* Acidosis occurs when renal insufficiency is associated or there is CO_2 retention due to pulmonary insufficiency *5544*
Serum Increase Alkalosis occurs in uncomplicated failure; hyperventilation, alveolar-capillary block due to associated pulmonary fibrosis; hypochloremic alkalosis due to K^+ depletion *5544*
Serum No Effect No significant change usually observed *5544*

Bilirubin *Serum Increase* Frequently increased (indirect more than direct); usually 1 - 5 mg/dL. It usually represents combined right- and left-sided failure with hepatic engorgement and pulmonary infarcts. May suddenly rise rapidly if superimposed myocardial infarction occurs *5544* In 552 patients with symptomatic cardiac failure and evidence of cardiomegaly on X-ray, bilirubin concentration of > 20 μmol/L (> 1.2 mg/dL) was associated with 3-year survival rate of 41% compared with 68% in those with lower concentrations *326* Depending on the severity and chronicity of cardiac failure *900*
Urine Increase With jaundice *5544*

Bilirubin, Indirect *Serum Increase* Unconjugated hyperbilirubinemia reflects reduced hepatic blood flow *367* Concentration may be increased in patients with hypoxia due to, for example, pulmonary fibrosis or heart failure. Condition arises because conjugation of bilirubin requires UDP-glucuronic acid which, in turn, requires oxygen *4617*

Brain Natriuretic Peptide *Plasma Increase* In patients with acute myocardial infarction and congestive cardiac failure mean concentration in right atrium of 177 ± 61 pg/mL significantly increased compared with 40 ± 1 pg/mL in patients with AMI but without congesttive cardiac failure and 5 ± 1 pg/mL in healthy controls *5818* In 15 patients with severe congestive heart failure mean concentration of 690.6 ± 491.1 pg/mL significantly different from 86.8 ± 82.6 pg/mL in 57 patients with mild congestive heart failure and 15.2 ± 11.2 pg/mL in 25 age-matched healthy controls *3200* In 7 patients with congestive cardiac failure mean concentration of 168.3 (SE 67.8) ng/L compared with normal determined in 5 individuals of 5.9 (SE 0.8) ng/L *5242*

BSP Retention *Serum Increase* Hepatic dysfunction, often with structural damage to the liver, may result in moderate BSP retention *2304* The most frequently abnormal test. It may indicate circulatory stasis as well as cellular damage *5544*

CA 125 *Serum Increase* In patients with severe heart failure the sicker they were the higher the serum CA 125 concentration *3708*

Carbon Dioxide Partial Pressure *Blood Decrease* Acidosis occurs when renal insufficiency is associated or there is CO_2 retention due to pulmonary insufficiency *5544*
Blood Increase Alkalosis occurs in uncomplicated failure; hyperventilation, alveolar-capillary block due to associated pulmonary fibrosis; hypochloremic alkalosis due to potassium depletion *5544*

Chloride *Serum Decrease* Tends to fall but may be normal before treatment *5544*

428.00 Congestive Cardiac Failure *(continued)*

Chloride *(continued)*
Serum *No Effect* Tends to fall but may be normal before treatment *5544*

Cholesterol *Serum* *Decrease* With severe hepatic congestion *1290*

Cholesterol Esters *Serum* *Decrease* Reported effect *5544*

Cholinesterase *Serum* *Decrease* Some patients *5544*

Copper *Serum* *Increase* Statistically significant *4871*

Cortisol *Plasma* *Increase* In 45 patients with congestive heart failure mean concentration of 462 ± 121 nmol/L significantly different from 326 ± 84 nmol/L in 14 control patients *3113*
Plasma *No Effect* In 63 patients with stable chronic congestive cardiac failure mean concentration of 413 ± 107 nmol/L not significantly increased compared with 370 ± 109 nmol/L in 20 controls *136* In 53 patients with stable chronic congestive cardiac failure mean concentration of 415 ± 15 nmol/L not significantly different from 372 ± 30 nmol/L in 16 healthy controls *135*

C-Peptide *Plasma* *Increase* In 45 patients with congestive heart failure mean concentration of 1.1 nmol/L significantly different from 0.72 nmol/L in 14 control patients *3113*

Creatine Kinase MB-Isoenzyme *Serum* *Increase* In 35 patients with congestive cardiac failure mean concentration of 4.8 ± 0.7 ng/mL different from that in 55 healthy blood donors in whom the mean concentration was 3.5 ± 0.5 ng/mL *3515* In 33 patients with stable congestive cardiac failure mean concentration of 2.97 ng/mL significantly higher than in a matched group of 47 healthy blood donors *3514*

Creatinine *Serum* *Increase* Causes reduced blood flow leading to prerenal azotemia *1290* Diminished renal excretion *1290* In 63 patients with stable chronic congestive cardiac failure mean concentration of 129 ± 53 μmol/L significantly increased compared with 91 ± 8 μmol/L in 20 controls *136* In 53 patients with stable chronic congestive cardiac failure mean concentration of 125 ± 6 μmol/L significantly different from 92. ± 2 μmol/L in 16 healthy controls *135* Causes reduced blood flow leading to prerenal azotemia *5544*

Creatinine Clearance *Urine* *Decrease* Diminished renal excretion with severe failure *1290* Significant reduction observed in patients with congestive cardiac failure *4055*

Dehydroepiandrosterone *Plasma* *Decrease* In 53 patients with stable chronic congestive cardiac failure mean concentration of 10.4 ± 1.0 nmol/L significantly different from 15.3 ± 2.4 nmol/L in 16 healthy controls *135* In 63 patients with stable chronic congestive cardiac failure mean concentration of 9.9 ± 6.9 nmol/L significantly decreased compared with 15.6 ± 8.3 nmol/L in 20 controls *136*

Dehydroepiandrosterone:Cortisol Ratio *Plasma* *Increase* In 63 patients with stable chronic congestive cardiac failure mean ratio of 69.6 ± 62.4 not significantly increased compared with 44.0 ± 77.0 in 20 controls *136*

Dopamine *Plasma* *No Effect* In 44 patients with congestive cardiac failure with atrial fibrillation median concentration of 17 pg/mL not significantly different from 20 pg/mL in 225 patients with congestive cardiac failure with sinus rhythm within normal range of 5 - 50 pg/mL *5319*

β-Endorphin *Plasma* *Increase* In patients with congestive cardiac failure, concentration increased with increasing NYHA functional class: class I 37.1 ± 3.1 fmol/mL, class II 52.4 ± 3.0 fmol/mL, class III 87.6 ± 2.9 fmol/mL, class IV 116.0 ± 18.0 fmol/mL *3329*

Endothelin *Plasma* *Increase* In 22 patients with severe but stable chronic heart failure mean concentration of 10.2 ± 34 pg/mL compared with 5.9 ± 1.8 pg/mL in healthy controls *5273* Significant increase to 12.4 ± 0.6 pmol/L observed in 47 patients with CHF compared with 6.4 ± 0.3 pmol/L in 16 healthy age and sex matched controls *3426* In 44 patients with congestive cardiac failure with atrial fibrillation median concentration of 7.0 pg/mL significantly different from 4.9 pg/mL in 225 patients with congestive cardiac failure with sinus rhythm and above normal range of 1 - 5 pg/mL *5319*

Endothelin-1 *Plasma* *Increase* In 15 patients with severe congestive heart failure mean concentration of 3.56 ± 1.67 pg/mL significantly different from 2.21 ± 0.67 pg/mL in 57 patients with mild congestive heart failure and 1.5 ± 0.9 pg/mL in 20 age-matched healthy controls *3200* In 3 studies mean concentrations typically increased 1.8 to 2.5-fold, although in one the increase was 5.0-fold above appropriate normal values *328* In 102 patients with CHF mean concentration of 2.1 ± 0.1 pg/mL in those with NYHA functional class II and 4.0 ± 0.4 pg/mL in those with functional classes III and IV compared with 1.5 ± 0.2 pg/mL in healthy individuals *5312* Plasma endothelin concentrations were evaluated in 53 chronic, congestive heart failure (CHF) patients with or without history of systemic hypertension. In patients with CHF, big endothelin-1 was significantly greater than in hypertensive patients with normal cardiac function and in control subjects (both $p < 0.0001$). Patients with severe CHF had significantly greater big endothelin-1 values than did those with moderate CHF *3967*

Endothelin-1, Big *Plasma* *Increase* Using a nonextractable ELISA procedure mean concentration in patients with NHYA class: I 0.7 ± 0.2 pmol/L, class II 1.1 ± 0.5 pmol/L, class III 1.2 ± 0.6 pmol/L, and 2.1 ± 0.7 pmol/L compared with 0.5 ± 0.1 pmol/L in healthy controls *2061*

Endothelin, Big *Plasma* *Increase* In 8 patients with congestive cardiac failure mean concentration of 13.0 ± 2.9 pmol/L significantly different from 5.02 - 6.54 pmol/L in healthy individuals *5*

Epinephrine *Plasma* *Increase* In 8 patients with congestive cardiac failure mean concentration of 90 ± 42 pg/mL significantly different from 0 - 82 pg/mL in healthy individuals *5* In 45 patients with congestive heart failure mean concentration of 0.31 nmol/L not significantly different from 0.23 nmol/L in 14 control patients *3113* In 53 patients with stable chronic congestive cardiac failure mean concentration of 1.29 ± 0.22 nmol/L significantly different from 0.51 ± 0.04 nmol/L in 16 healthy controls *135*
Plasma *No Effect* In 44 patients with congestive cardiac failure with atrial fibrillation median concentration of 47 pg/mL not significantly different from 36 pg/mL in 225 patients with congestive cardiac failure with sinus rhythm within normal range of 10 - 70 pg/mL *5319*

Erythrocyte Sedimentation Rate *Blood* *Decrease* May be decreased because of decreased serum fibrinogen *5544* As a result of decreased synthesis of fibrinogen by the liver which is passively congested *1980*
Blood *Increase* In 552 patients with symptomatic cardiac failure and evidence of cardiomegaly on X-ray, ESR > 11 mm/h was associated with 3-year survival rate of 62% compared with 56% in those with lower concentrations *326* In 47 patients with chronic heart failure mean rate of 21 ± 3 mm/h significantly higher than 4 ± 1 mm/h in 17 healthy controls *137*

Erythrocytes *Ascitic Fluid* *Increase* > 10,000 cells/μL seen in 10% of cases *233*
Pleural Fluid *Increase* May be present *126*
Urine *Increase* There are isolated RBC and WBC, hyaline and sometimes granular casts *5544*

Estradiol *Plasma* *Increase* In 53 patients with stable chronic congestive cardiac failure mean concentration of 69.2 ± 7.0 pmol/L significantly different from 45.4 ± 8.5 pmol/L in 16 healthy controls *135*
Plasma *No Effect* In 63 patients with stable chronic congestive cardiac failure mean concentration of 65.3 ± 48.8 pmol/L not significantly increased compared with 47.9 ± 32.0 pmol/L in 20 controls *136*

Fatty Acids (FFA), Free *Serum* *Increase* In 45 patients with congestive heart failure mean concentration of 603 ± 284 μmol/L significantly different from 469 ± 143 μmol/L in 14 control patients *3113*

Fibrinogen *Plasma* *Decrease* Decreased secondary to impaired liver function *2304*

Glomerular Filtration Rate *Urine* *Decrease* With a fall in effective cardiac output, a commensurate reduction in renal blood flow generally occurs *4707* *2304*

Glucagon *Plasma* *No Effect* In 45 patients with congestive heart failure mean concentration of 37.3 ± 5.7 pmol/L not significantly different from 34.5 ± 4.6 pmol/L in 14 control patients *3113*

Glucagon:Insulin Ratio *Plasma* *No Effect* In 45 patients with congestive heart failure mean ratio of 6.1 ± 3.2 pmol/munits not significantly different from 5.7 ± 2.7 pmol/munits in 14 control patients *3113*

Glucose *Peritoneal Fluid* *Increase* High concentrations *4165*

Pleural Fluid *No Effect* Pleural fluid and serum concentrations are similar *4493*
Serum *Decrease* May occur if cardiac output is severely curtailed and liver congestion is marked *367*
Serum *Increase* Abnormal increases in the fasting blood sugar are common *1980*
Serum *No Effect* In 45 patients with congestive heart failure mean concentration of 5.2 ± 0.7 mmol/L not significantly different from 5.5 ± 0.3 mmol/L in 14 control patients *3113*

γ-Glutamyltransferase *Serum* *Increase* Due to anoxic damage to the liver *1290* All 9 patients had elevated activity, secondary to hepatic damage. Mean activity of 180 U/L, range 58 - 568 U/L *3161*

Granular Casts *Urine* *Increase* There are isolated RBC and WBC, hyaline and sometimes granular casts *5544*

Growth Hormone *Plasma* *Increase* In 53 patients with stable chronic congestive cardiac failure mean concentration of 1.8 ± 0.5 ng/mL not significantly different from 1.1 ± 0.4 ng/mL in 16 healthy controls *135* In 45 patients with congestive heart failure mean concentration of 2.0 μg/L significantly different from 0.35 μg/L in 14 control patients *3113*

Guanosine Monophosphate *Plasma* *Increase* In ethanol-extracted specimens mean concentration of 8.012 ± 3.289 nmol/L compared with 3.439 ± 1.226 nmol/L in healthy blood donors and in unextracted specimens concentration of 9.983 ± 2.971 nmol/L compared with 5.301 ± 1.456 nmol/L in healthy blood donors *2405* Concentration significantly increased in patients with congestive cardiac failure with concentration increasing with severity of heart failure and pulmonary artery pressure and decreased sharply with treatment although still remaining at a high value *3861* Mean concentration significantly higher in NYHA stage IV (10.5 μmol/L) compared with 9.0 μmol/L in NYHA stage III and 5.0 μmol/L in NYHA stage II patients *2406* In 18 patients with congestive cardiac failure mean concentration of 16.7 ± 9.7 pmol/L significantly higher than 4.0 ± 1.0 pmol/mL in 15 controls *4818*
Urine *Increase* In 50 patients with heart failure mean concentration of 1.49 ± 1.43 μmol/g creatinine significantly higher than 0.39 ± 0.24 μmol/g in 76 healthy volunteers *2406*

Hematocrit *Blood* *Decrease* Slightly decreased but red cell mass may be increased *5544*

Hyaline Casts *Urine* *Increase* There are isolated RBC and WBC, hyaline and sometimes granular casts *5544*

Insulin *Plasma* *Increase* In 53 patients with stable chronic congestive cardiac failure mean concentration of 77.8 ± 7.5 pmol/L significantly different from 40.6 ± 6.9 pmol/L in 16 healthy controls *135* In 45 patients with congestive heart failure mean concentration of 6.1 mU/L not significantly different from 6.7 mU/L in 14 control patients *3113*

Insulin-like Growth Factor-I *Serum* *No Effect* In 53 patients with stable chronic congestive cardiac failure mean concentration of 146 ± 8 ng/mL not significantly different from 148 ± 11 ng/mL in 16 healthy controls *135*

Interferon-γ *Serum* *Decrease* In 47 patients with chronic heart failure mean concentration of 0.66 ± 0.03 IU/mL significantly lower than 0.79 ± 0.06 IU/mL in 17 healthy controls *137*

Interleukin-1 Receptor Antagonist *Serum* *Increase* Mean concentration in 80 patients with congestive cardiac failure due to coronary artery disease or hypertension increased above 95th percentile of 400 pg/mL in 19%, 25%, 45% and 65% of functional classes I, II, III and IV respectively *5200*

Interleukin-1β *Serum* *Increase* In 47 patients with chronic heart failure mean concentration of 0.35 ± 0.06 pg/mL not significantly higher than 0.23 ± 0.06 pg/mL in 17 healthy controls *137* Mean concentration in 80 patients with congestive cardiac failure due to coronary artery disease or hypertension increased above 95th percentile of 8 pg/mL in 25% and 37% of functional classes III and IV respectively *5200*

Interleukin-2 *Serum* *No Effect* Mean concentration in 80 patients with congestive cardiac failure due to coronary artery disease or hypertension increased above 95th percentile of < 312 pg/mL in 2 patients only *5200*

Interleukin-6 *Serum* *Increase* In 9 cases with CHF and no cachexia mean concentration of 12.0 ± 13.9 pg/mL and 9 with CHF and cachexia of 16.9 ± 18.2 pg/mL significantly higher than 0.3 - 8.3 pg/mL in 14 normal volunteers *3182* Mean concentration in 80 patients with congestive cardiac failure due to coronary artery disease or hypertension increased above 95th percentile of 10 pg/mL in 58% of functional class IV *5200* In 47 patients with chronic heart failure mean concentration of 3.62 ± 0.47 pg/mL significantly higher than 0.97 ± 0.17 pg/mL in 17 healthy controls *137* In 70 patients with CCF spread through NYHA classes I to IV mean concentrations of 4.1 ± 0.8 pg/mL, 4.0 ± 1.0 pg/mL, 10.0 ± 3.6 pg/mL and 53.9 ± 19.3 pg/mL, respectively, with the latter one significantly higher than 2.5 ± 0.2 pg/mL in 62 healthy controls *3801* In 45 patients with congestive heart failure mean concentration of 5.3 ng/L not significantly different from 2.7 ng/L in 14 control patients *3113*

Interleukin-10 *Serum* *Decrease* In 47 patients with chronic heart failure mean concentration of 1.87 pg/mL significantly lower than 5.31 pg/mL in 17 healthy controls *137*

8-iso-Prostaglandin $F_{2\alpha}$ *Pericardial Fluid* *Increase* Concentration of 27.0 ± 2.5 pg/mL significantly higher in symptomatic patients than in asymptomatic patients with concentration of 11.1 ± 1.6 pg/mL *3254*

Ketones *Serum* *Increase* In 45 patients with congestive heart failure mean blood concentration of 267 μmol/L significantly different from 150 μmol/L in 14 control patients *3113*

Lactate *Blood* *Increase* Increased formation from glucose due to hypoxia *367*
Blood *No Effect* In 45 patients with congestive heart failure mean concentration of 0.74 mmol/L not significantly different from 0.66 mmol/L in 14 control patients *3113*

Lactate Dehydrogenase *Serum* *Increase* Increased in about 40% of patients *5544*

Lactate Dehydrogenase Isoenzyme-5 *Serum* *Increase* Elevated to 14.5% of total LD in 12 patients with passive congestion *1756* LD_1 and $_5$ are elevated *4746* May occur *5544*

Lactate Dehydrogenase Isoenzymes *Serum* *Decrease* LD_2 was decreased in 12 patients with passive congestion. Mean value = 28.8% of total LD (normal = 36%) *1756*

Leucine Aminopeptidase *Serum* *Increase* Slight elevations were found in the sera of 9 patients. Mean for the group 33 U/L, range 15 - 62 U/L *3161*

Leukocytes *Ascitic Fluid* *Increase* Less than 1,000 /μL *233*
Blood *Increase* In 47 patients with chronic heart failure mean concentration of 7,100 ± 300 /μL significantly higher than 5,100 ± 300 /μL in 17 healthy controls *137*
Pleural Fluid *Increase* < 1000 /μL *4493*
Urine *Increase* There are isolated RBC and WBC, hyaline and sometimes granular casts *5544* Occasionally WBC may be seen with hyaline or granular casts *900*

Magnesium *Serum* *Decrease* In 3 of 81 patients with magnesium concentration of less than 0.72 mmol/L patients had congestive cardiac failure *3159*

Malondialdehyde *Serum* *Increase* Mean concentration of 2.65 ± 1.0 μmol/L in 30 patients with CCF significantly different from 1.45 ± 0.77 μmol/L in 16 healthy individuals *1159*

MCV *Blood* *Increase* Overall hypervolemia involving both plasma and red cell volume *3710*

Metanephrine *Plasma* *Increase* In 16 patients with heart failure false positive increase of plasma metanephrine or normetanephrine concentration observed *2994*

3-Methylxanthine *Serum* *Decrease* Patients with congestive cardiac failure receiving theophylline reported to be associated with significantly decreased elimination of 3-methylxanthine *5034*

Monocytes *Pleural Fluid* *Increase* Predominant cell type *4493*

Myoglobin *Serum* *Increase* In 35 patients with congestive cardiac failure mean concentration of 44.4 ± 19.0 ng/mL different from that in 55 healthy blood donors in whom the mean concentration was 10.7 ± 2.1 ng/mL *3515*

Neuropeptide Y *Plasma* *Increase* Concentration increased at rest in 17 patients with congestive cardiac failure (551 ± 48 pg/mL) versus 311 ± 22 pg/mL in 14 healthy controls *3237* In 8 patients with congestive cardiac failure mean concentration of 51.6 ± 4.6 pmol/L significantly different from 28 - 49.6 pmol/L in healthy individuals *5*

Norepinephrine *Plasma* *Increase* In 53 patients with stable chronic congestive cardiac failure mean concentration of 3.41 ± 0.32 nmol/L significantly different from 1.94 ± 0.17 nmol/L in 16 healthy controls *135* In 45 patients with congestive heart failure mean concentration of 1.9 nmol/L significantly different from 1.2 nmol/L in 14 control patients *3113* In patients with severe heart failure the sicker they were the higher the serum norepineh-

428.00 Congestive Cardiac Failure *(continued)*

Norepinephrine *(continued)*
phrine concentration *3708* In 15 patients with severe congestive heart failure mean concentration of 1032 ± 1042 pg/mL significantly different from 260 ± 218 pg/mL in 57 patients with mild congestive heart failure *3200* In 44 patients with congestive cardiac failure with atrial fibrillation median concentration of 506 pg/mL not significantly different from 519 pg/mL in 225 patients with congestive cardiac failure with sinus rhythm higher than upper limit of normal of 500 pg/mL *5319* Consistently elevated. Typically average concentration of 700 - 800 pg/mL *1547* In 8 patients with congestive cardiac failure mean concentration of 1,057 ± 384 pg/mL significantly different from 125 - 473 pg/mL in healthy individuals *5* In 102 patients with CHF mean concentration of 317 ± 23 pg/mL in those with NYHA functional class II and 614 ± 70 pg/mL in those with functional classes III and IV significantly increased compared with concentration in healthy individuals *5312* Concentration increased at rest in 17 patients with congestive cardiac failure of (306 ± 73 pg/mL) compared with 124 ± 22 pg/mL in 14 healthy controls *3237*

Normetanephrine *Plasma Increase* In 16 patients with heart failure false positive increase of plasma metanephrine or normetanephrine concentration observed *2994*

N-terminal Atrial Natriuretic Peptide *Plasma Increase* In 44 patients with congestive cardiac failure with atrial fibrillation median concentration of 1.46 nmol/L significantly different from 1.00 nmol/L in 225 patients with congestive cardiac failure with sinus rhythm above normal range of 0.15 - 0.50 nmol/L *5319*

N-terminal Pro-Atrial Natriuretic Peptide *Plasma Increase* Mean concentration in 25 individuals with heart failure of 1,030 ± 411 pmol/L significantly greater than that in 33 healthy individuals of 188 ± 71 pmol/L *3839*

Ornithine Carbamoyltransferase *Serum Increase* Liver cell damage *5544*

pH *Blood Decrease* Acidosis occurs when renal insufficiency is associated or there is CO_2 retention due to pulmonary insufficiency, low plasma sodium, or ammonium chloride toxicity *5544*
Blood Increase Occurs in uncomplicated heart failure *5544*
Urine No Effect Usually within normal limits *5544*

Potassium *Serum Decrease* Most often due to the kaliuretic action of diuretics without adequate potassium replacement *1980* Deficiency is common and excess is occasionally noted in patients under therapy. When failure is severe, an accelerated excretion rate may result from secondary hyperaldosteronism *2304*
Serum Increase Less common than hypokalemia. A common complication in patients on potassium supplements who are not responding to their diuretics *1980* Deficiency is common and excess is occasionally noted in patients under therapy *2304*
Serum No Effect Normal or slightly increased (because of shift from hypochloremic alkalosis due to some diuretics) *5544* In 53 patients with stable chronic congestive cardiac failure mean concentration of 4.0 ± 0.05 mmol/L not significantly different from 3.9. ± 0.05 mmol/L in 16 healthy controls *135*
Urine No Effect Concentration usually unaffected *5544*

Pro-Atrial Natriuretic Peptide *Serum Increase* In 45 patients with congestive heart failure mean concentration of 1.46 nmol/L significantly different from 0.44 nmol/L in 14 control patients *3113* In 8 patients with congestive cardiac failure mean concentration of 2,663 ± 421 pmol/L significantly different from < 1,200 pmol/L in healthy individuals *5*

Pro-Atrial Natriuretic Peptide (1-30) *Serum Increase* Mean concentration in 5 patients with class I CHF of 1,452 ± 580 pg/mL, 4,141 ± 1,640 pg/mL in 10 with class II and 6,648 ± 1,130 pg/mL in 16 with class III all significantly higher than the mean in 19 healthy controls of 251 ± 31.5 pg/mL *229*

Protein *Ascitic Fluid No Effect* Variable amounts between 1.5 - 5.0 g/dL *233*
Pleural Fluid Decrease Consistent with a transudate *413*
Serum Increase In 63 patients with stable chronic congestive cardiac failure mean concentration of 70.3 ± 4.4 g/L significantly increased compared with 67.1 ± 2.8 g/L in 20 controls *136*
Urine Increase Mild to moderate proteinuria varying from 0.5 - 4 g/d is not unusual; may be greater in severe failure with a marked decrease in GFR and renal blood flow *2304*

Prothrombin Time *Plasma Increase* May be slightly increased, with increased sensitivity to anticoagulant drugs *5544* Frequently elevated *900*

Renin *Plasma Increase* In 44 patients with congestive cardiac failure with atrial fibrillation median concentration of 100 µU/mL not significantly different from 74 µU/mL in 225 patients with congestive cardiac failure with sinus rhythm higher than normal range of 5 - 50 µU/mL *5319*

Renin Activity *Plasma Increase* In 53 patients with stable chronic congestive cardiac failure mean activity of 11.7 ± 2.0 ng/mL/h significantly different from 1.3 ± 0.2 ng/mL/h in 16 healthy controls *135*

Selenium *Serum Decrease* In 57 hospitalized patients with congestive cardiac failure mean plasma concentration of 77.8 ± 18.4 µg/L compared with 104.6 ± 18.0 µg/L in 45 healthy age-matched controls *2950*

Sodium *Serum Decrease* In 53 patients with stable chronic congestive cardiac failure mean concentration of 137.7 ± 0.4 mmol/L significantly different from 139.0 ± 0.5 mmol/L in 16 healthy controls *135* May be the result of over-vigorous use of diuretics in an already dehydrated patient who is on a sodium-restricted diet. A common hyponatremic syndrome is observed in patients who continue to have edema and clinical heart failure. Total body sodium in these patients is increased, but the amount of retained water is even greater. Is true dilutional hyponatremia *1980*
Serum Increase Sodium retention *4439* In 552 patients with symptomatic cardiac failure and evidence of cardiomegaly on X-ray sodium concentration < 135 mmol/L was associated with 3-year survival rate of 55% compared with 61% in those with lower concentrations *326*
Urine Decrease Sodium retention *4439* Patients may, when renal function is intact, reduce urinary sodium concentration virtually to zero. They may retain nearly 100% of the sodium offered them. Hypervolemia and edema result *2304* As the heart improves, urinary output increases but is low in sodium and has a high specific gravity *367*

Soluble CD14 Receptor *Serum Increase* In 47 patients with chronic heart failure mean concentration of 3,401 ± 134 ng/mL significantly higher than 2,714 ± 121 ng/mL in 17 healthy controls *137*

Soluble E-Selectin *Serum Increase* In 47 patients with chronic heart failure mean concentration of 49 ± 3 ng/mL significantly higher than 37 ± 3 ng/mL in 17 healthy controls *137*

Soluble Fas Antigen *Serum Increase* In 70 patients with CCF spread through NYHA classes I to IV mean concentrations of 2.2 ± 0.2 ng/mL, 3.1 ± 0.2 ng/mL, 3.9 ± 0.3 ng/mL and 5.1 ± 0.6 ng/mL, respectively, with the latter two significantly higher than 2.2 ± 0.1 ng/mL in 62 healthy controls *3801*

Soluble Fas Ligand Antigen *Serum Increase* In 70 patients with CCF spread through NYHA classes I to IV mean concentrations of 0.44 ± 0.01 ng/mL, 0.44 ± 0.01 ng/mL, 0.44 ± 0.02 ng/mL and 0.48 ± 0.02 ng/mL, respectively, not significantly different from 0.43 ± 0.01 ng/mL in 62 healthy controls *3801*

Soluble Intercellular Adhesion Molecule-1 *Serum Increase* In 102 patients with CHF mean concentration of 207 ± 9.4 ng/mL in those with NYHA functional class II and 293 ± 18 ng/mL in those with functional classes III and IV compared with 149 ± 10 ng/mL in healthy individuals *5312* In 47 patients with chronic heart failure mean concentration of 383 ± 13 ng/mL significantly higher than 277 ± 13 ng/mL in 17 healthy controls *137*

Soluble Interleukin-2 Receptor-α *Serum No Effect* Mean concentration in 80 patients with congestive cardiac failure due to coronary artery disease or hypertension increased above 95th percentile of 3.2 pg/mL in 7 patients only *5200*

Soluble Interleukin-6 Receptor *Serum Increase* Mean concentration in 80 patients with congestive cardiac failure due to coronary artery disease or hypertension increased above 95th percentile of 51 pg/mL in 15%, 25% and 34% of functional classes II, III and IV respectively *5200*

Soluble Tumor Necrosis Factor Receptor-I *Serum Increase* In 63 patients with stable chronic congestive cardiac failure significant positive correlation of r = 0.70 with serum creatinine concentration *136* In 63 patients with stable chronic congestive cardiac failure mean concentration of 128.9 ± 84.5 pg/mL significantly increased compared with 63.6 ± 23.3 pg/mL in 20 controls *136* In 47 patients with chronic heart failure mean concentration of 1,323 ± 112 pg/mL significantly higher than 629 ± 59 pg/mL in 17 healthy controls *137*

Soluble Tumor Necrosis Factor Receptor-II
Serum Increase Mean concentration in 80 patients with congestive cardiac failure due to coronary artery disease or hypertension increased above 95th percentile of 2.8 pg/mL in 55% and 95% of functional classes III and IV respectively *5200* In 63 patients with stable chronic congestive cardiac failure mean concentration of 250.1 ± 109.5 pg/mL significantly increased compared with 187.0 ± 92.3 pg/mL in 20 controls *136* In 63 patients with stable chronic congestive cardiac failure significant positive correlation of r = 0.52 with serum TNF-α concentration *136* In 45 patients with congestive heart failure mean concentration of 1,890 ng/L significantly different from 1,336 ng/L in 14 control patients *3113* In 47 patients with chronic heart failure mean concentration of 2,626 ± 163 pg/mL significantly higher than 1,972 ± 250 pg/mL in 17 healthy controls *137*

Specific Gravity *Urine Decrease* May be high during the phases of salt and water retention and low during periods of diuresis *2304*
Urine Increase May be high during the phases of salt and water retention and low during periods of diuresis *2304* Urine is concentrated, with specific gravity 1.020. Oliguria is a characteristic feature of right-sided failure *5544*

Testosterone *Serum No Effect* In 63 patients with stable chronic congestive cardiac failure mean concentration of 11.2 ± 5.9 nmol/L not significantly increased compared with 10.0 ± 3.0 nmol/L in 20 controls *136* In 53 patients with stable chronic congestive cardiac failure mean concentration of 11.2 ± 0.9 nmol/L not significantly different from 9.9 ± 0.5 nmol/L in 16 healthy controls *135*

Theophylline *Serum Increase* Congestive cardiac failure reported to decrease elimination of theophylline *5034*

Thyroid Stimulating Hormone *Serum No Effect* In 53 patients with stable chronic congestive cardiac failure mean concentration of 2.1 ± 0.2 µU/mL not significantly different from 1.5 ± 0.2 µU/mL in 16 healthy controls *135*

Tri-iodothyronine, Reverse (rT3) *Serum Increase* In 53 patients with stable chronic congestive cardiac failure mean concentration of 0.52 ± 0.04 nmol/L significantly different from 0.31 ± 0.01 nmol/L in 16 healthy controls *135*

Troponin I *Serum Increase* In 35 patients with congestive cardiac failure mean concentration of 72.1 ± 15.8 pg/mL significantly greater than that in 55 healthy blood donors in whom the mean concentration was 20.4 ± 3.2 pg/mL *3515*

Troponin T *Serum Increase* In 58 patients on hospital admission with chronic heart failure detectable TnT (> 0.2 ng/mL) observed in 30 (51.7%), with 91.7% in NYHA class IV patients, 68% of NYHA class III patients and 18.2% of NYHA class II patients due to leakage from cardiomyocytes *4744* In 33 patients with stable congestive cardiac failure mean concentration of 0.163 ng/mL significantly higher than in a matched group of 47 healthy blood donors *3514* In 110 patients with renal impairment serum cardiac troponin-T concentration detectable with concentrations ranging from 0 - 17.2 µg/L and in the 6 who also had CCF median concentration of 2.8 µg/mL *891*

Tumor Necrosis Factor-α *Serum Increase* In 70 patients with CCF spread through NYHA classes I to IV mean concentrations of 5.9 ± 2.0 pg/mL, 10.0 ± 3.3 pg/mL, 11.3 ± 5.5 pg/mL and 121.0 ± 26.3 pg/mL, respectively, with the latter one significantly higher than 4.2 ± 0.6 pg/mL in 62 healthy controls *3801* Mean concentration in 80 patients with congestive cardiac failure due to coronary artery disease or hypertension increased above 95th percentile of 3.8 pg/mL in 25% and 42% of functional classes III and IV respectively *5200* In 47 patients with chronic heart failure mean concentration of 10.7 ± 1.34 pg/mL not significantly different from 7.05 ± 0.67 pg/mL in 17 healthy controls *137* In 63 patients with stable chronic congestive cardiac failure significant positive correlation of r = 0.43 with serum creatinine concentration *136* Mean concentration in 33 patients with chronic heart failure of 115 ± 25 U/mL compared with 9 ± 3 U/mL in 33 age-matched healthy controls *3010* In 9 cases with CHF and no cachexia mean concentration of 3.3 ± 3.1 pg/mL and 9 with CHF and cachexia of 4.3 ± 2.8 pg/mL significantly higher than 0.5 - 1.2 pg/mL in 14 normal volunteers *3182*
Serum No Effect In 63 patients with stable chronic congestive cardiac failure mean concentration of 9.8 ± 8.6 pg/mL not significantly increased compared with 5.8 ± 2.7 pg/mL in 20 controls *136* In 53 patients with stable chronic congestive cardiac failure mean concentration of 9.5 ± 1.2 pg/mL not significantly different from 7.0 ± 0.7 pg/mL in 16 healthy controls *135* In 45 patients with congestive heart failure mean concentration of 19 ng/L not significantly different from 14 ng/L in 14 control patients *3113*

Urea *Serum Increase* In 63 patients with stable chronic congestive cardiac failure mean concentration of 9.7 ± 5.6 mmol/L significantly increased compared with 5.7 ± 1.2 mmol/L in 20 controls *136*

Urea Nitrogen *Serum Increase* Moderate azotemia (BUN usually < 60 mg/dL) is evident with severe oliguria; may increase with vigorous diuresis *5544* May be as high as 80 - 100 mg/dL as a result of prerenal azotemia *900* Observed with renal impairment *1642*

Uric Acid *Serum Increase* In 552 patients with symptomatic cardiac failure and evidence of cardiomegaly on X-ray, urate concentration of > 500 µmol/L (> 8.4 mg/dL) was associated with 3-year survival rate of 47% compared with 69% in those with lower concentrations *326* Frequently elevated from either prerenal azotemia or, more commonly, the use of diuretics *900* Significant inversee relationship observed between serum uric acid and maximum blood flow after exercise *138*

Urobilinogen *Urine Increase* With hepatic anoxia *1290*

Volume *Plasma Increase* Overall hypervolemia involving both plasma and red cell volume *3710* May be normal or increased *2304*
Red Blood Cells Increase Overall hypervolemia involving both plasma and red cell volume *3710*
Urine Decrease Volume significantly reduced in patients with congestive cardiac failure compared with healthy controls *4055* With edema *1290*

Water Clearance, Free *Urine Decrease* Clearance reduced in patients with congestive cardiac failure compared with that in controls *4055*

428.10 Acute Cardiogenic Lung Edema

Mucin-associated Antigen *Serum No Effect* Mean concentration of 9.0 ± 3.1 ng/mL observed in 5 patients with acute cardiogenic lung edema not significantly different from 9.9 ± 0.8 ng/mL observed in 59 healthy individuals *4797*

429.00 Myocarditis

Creatine Kinase MB-Isoenzyme *Serum Increase* Observed effect *248*

γ-Glutamyltransferase *Serum Increase* Activity reportedly increased in a variety of diseases including diseases of the pancreas, myocardium, kidney and lung as well as in diabetes *4617*

Soluble Intercellular Adhesion Molecule-1 *Serum Increase* Mean concentration of 343.5 ± 128.9 ng/mL in 8 patients with myocarditis significantly different from 161.6 ± 54.0 ng/mL in 14 age- and sex-matched healthy volunteer controls *5275*

Troponin I *Serum Increase* Patients with myocarditis and perimyocarditis may show increased TnI and TnT concentrations if myocardial tissue is involved in the inflammatory process *2649*

Troponin T *Serum Increase* Patients with myocarditis and perimyocarditis may show increased TnI and TnT concentrations if myocardial tissue is involved in the inflammatory process *2649*

429.20 Cardiovascular Disease

Anti-Platelet Factor 4-heparin Antibodies *Serum Increase* In 76 patients receiving emergency care for cardiovascular problems positive titer (more than 2 SD above mean in 140 healthy men or women) observed in 9 (11.8%) *5536*

Atrial Natriuretic Peptide *Plasma Increase* In 269 elderly individuals with clinically stable cardiovascular disease mean concentration of 29.0 ± 1.9 pmol/L significantly higher than that in 90 healthy elderly in whom the mean concentration was 11.4 ± 1.1 pmol/L which, in turn, was significantly higher than 3.0 ± 0.3 pmol/L in 24 healthy young individuals *1037*

CA 72-4 *Serum Increase* In 62 patients with cardiovascular disease 6 (10%) had a concentration greater than cut-off of 2.5 U/mL with median concentration of 1.5 U/mL *4505*

429.20 Cardiovascular Disease *(continued)*

Carcinoembryonic Antigen *Serum* *Increase* In 62 patients with cardiovascular disease 15 (24%) had a concentration greater than cut-off of 3 ng/mL with median concentration of 1.9 ng/mL *4505*

429.40 Postcardiotomy Syndrome

Antibody Titer *Serum* *Increase* Excellent correlation between the titer of circulating antiheart antibodies and the development of this syndrome in postoperative patients *2304*

429.90 Heart Disease

Carcinoembryonic Antigen *Serum* *Increase* In 289 patients with heart disease 61% had concentrations less than 2.5 ng/mL, 32% had concentrations between 2.6 and 5.0 ng/mL, 5% had concentrations between 5.1 and 10.0 ng/mL and 2% had concentrations greater than 10.0 ng/mL *2010*

Cerebrovascular Disease

430.00 Subarachnoid Hemorrhage

Cholesterol *Serum* *Decrease* In patients who had a stroke for whatever cause poor outcome was associated with low cholesterol concentration with relative hazard that was 9% lower for each 1.0 mmol/L (39 mg/dL) increase in cholesterol concentration *1276*

D-Dimer *Cerebrospinal Fluid* *Increase* Values greater than 500 µg/L are consistent with subarachnoid hemorrhage, recent CNS bleeding or other CNS pathology *2952*

Endothelin *Urine* *Increase* Urinary excretion in individuals with subarachnoid hemorrhage reported to be significantly higher than in healthy individuals *6*

Endothelin-1 *Cerebrospinal Fluid* *Increase* A considerable quantity of endothelin-like immunoreactivity was demonstrated as present in the CSF of patients with subarachnoid hemorrhage. The endothelin levels in the CSF raised from 0.4 ± 0.2 (mean ± SD) pmol/L at day 0 - 1 to 2.2 ± 0.6 pmol/L at day 6 and the levels decreased gradually *5092* In 11 patients with subarachnoid aneurysmal hemorrhage mean concentration increased to 2.2 ± 0.6 pg/mL, 5.5 times normal range *328*
Plasma *Increase* In 1 study of patients with subarachnoid aneurysmal hemorrhage mean concentration increased to 7.7 ± 3.3 pg/mL (n = 12), 5.1 times appropriate normal range *328*

Interleukin-6 *Cerebrospinal Fluid* *Increase* Samples from 12 patients were analyzed. Dramatically increased levels of IL-6 were detected in the CSF in 11 of the 12 patients; slightly elevated levels of soluble CD8 were observed in six patients IL-6 levels were higher on day 6 than on days 3 and 9 *3348*
Cerebrospinal Fluid *No Effect* Samples from 12 patients were analyzed. The increases were not paralleled by increased values in the serum samples *3348*

β_2-Microglobulin *Cerebrospinal Fluid* *Increase* In patients with subarachnoid hemorrhage mean concentration of 1.96 mg/L significantly higher than mean of 1.01 mg/L in 57 control patients *5421*

Soluble CD8$^+$ *Cerebrospinal Fluid* *Increase* Samples from 12 patients were analyzed. CD8 was observed in six patients *3348*
Cerebrospinal Fluid *No Effect* Samples from 12 patients were analyzed. The increases were not paralleled by increased values in the blood samples *3348*

Soluble Interleukin-2 Receptor *Cerebrospinal Fluid* *Increase* Samples from 12 patients were analyzed. Moderately increased levels of soluble IL-2R were detected in the CSF in 11 of the 12 patients *3348*
Cerebrospinal Fluid *No Effect* Samples from 12 patients were analyzed. The increases were not paralleled by increased values in the serum samples *3348*

431.00 Cerebral Hemorrhage

α_1-Antichymotrypsin *Cerebrospinal Fluid* *Increase* Increased in patients with meningitis or mild hemorrhage, but equal to normal in patients with encephalitis, epilepsy, degenerative disorders or diseases of the CNS *187*

Antidiuretic Hormone *Plasma* *Increase* Associated with excessive ADH production resulting in sodium loss *4707*

Carnosinase *Serum* *Decrease* In 48 patients with cerebral infarction or primary intracerebral hemorrhage median concentration of 113 nmol/mL/min significantly less than 223 nmol/mL/min in 39 age and gender matched controls *5589*

Cholesterol *Serum* *Decrease* In patients who had a stroke for whatever cause poor outcome was associated with low cholesterol concentration with relative hazard that was 9% lower for each 1.0 mmol/L (39 mg/dL) increase in cholesterol concentration *1276*

Eosinophils *Blood* *Increase* In 45% of 13 patients hospitalized for this disorder *1576*

Epinephrine *Plasma* *Increase* Plasma concentrations were 0.65 ± 0.11 ng/mL in subarachnoid hemorrhage patients *384*

Erythrocytes *Cerebrospinal Fluid* *Increase* All 17 patients with hemorrhagic vascular lesions had RBC counts > 5,000 /µL *5713* RBCs reach the CSF by seeping into the ventricle after hypertensive hemorrhage. CSF may remain clear if hemorrhage was small and wholly confined to the brain substance *2039* In 75% of the patients with intracerebral hemorrhage, the CSF was either grossly bloody or xanthochromic: in 25%, the CSF was clear *2969*

Fibrinogen *Plasma* *Increase* The greater the degree of initial neurological deficit the greater were plasma high molecular weight fibrinogen complex (HMWFC) values, which were associated with poor clinical outcome. Values were significantly higher in patients with intracerebral hemorrhage, subarachnoid hemorrhage and cerebral embolism *1508*

Glomerular Filtration Rate *Urine* *Increase* Associated excess ADH may tend to accelerate GFR *4707*

Glucose *Serum* *Increase* In 29% of 13 patients hospitalized for this disorder *1576*
Urine *Increase* Transient glucosuria *2033*

Hemoglobin F *Cerebrospinal Fluid* *Increase* Increased percentage in CSF indicates neonatal subarachnoid hemorrhage *783*

Lactate Dehydrogenase *Cerebrospinal Fluid* *Increase* In the acute stage of the disease. The increase seems to be the result of blood and plasma reaching the CSF in hemorrhage *5736* Elevated in all 27 determinations of CSF in 17 patients with hemorrhagic vascular lesions and in 13 of 30 patients with nonhemorrhagic lesions *5713*
Serum *Increase* In 40% of 10 patients hospitalized for this disorder *1576*

Leukocytes *Blood* *Increase* In 51% of 15 patients hospitalized for this disorder *1576* Increased (15,000 - 20,000 /µL) (higher than in cerebral occlusion, e.g., embolism, thrombosis) *5544*
Cerebrospinal Fluid *Increase* Count will be commensurate with the amount of bleeding, 1 WBC/1,000 RBC. Increase is caused by the inflammatory reaction in the meninges and may reach levels of 500 /µL *367*

α_1-Microglobulin *Cerebrospinal Fluid* *Increase* Of 4 patients with cerebral hemorrhage mean concentration in 3 greater than that in 15 healthy controls of 34.8 ± 16.0 µg/L *2370*

Monocytes *Cerebrospinal Fluid* *Increase* Mononuclear cells are increased *2039*

Neuron-specific Enolase *Serum* *Increase* 9 of 13 patients with intracerebral hemorrhage demonstrated NSE peaks above 20 ng/mL 24 to 72 h after initial hemorrhage *4611*

Neutrophils *Blood* *Increase* In 45% of 13 patients hospitalized for this disorder *1576*

Norepinephrine *Plasma* *Increase* Plasma concentrations were greatly increased compared to normals, cardiac catheterization patients, and patients with other illnesses. Mean for all the hemorrhagic patients was 0.94 ± 0.10 ng/mL. Patients with poor prognosis had initially higher and markedly higher follow-up concentrations than those with good prognosis *384*

Occult Blood *Cerebrospinal Fluid* *Increase* In early subarachnoid hemorrhage (< 8 h after onset of symptoms), test may be positive before xanthochromia develops in CSF *5544*

Plasminogen *Cerebrospinal Fluid* *Decrease* In 11 infants with intraventricular hemorrhage median concentration of 0.55% compared with value of 0.74% in reference population *5653*

Protein *Cerebrospinal Fluid* *Increase* Usually elevated to around 100 mg/dL with maximum levels 8 - 10 days after bleeding *367*

S-100 Protein *Serum* *Increase* In 13 patients with primary intra-cerebral hemorrhage mean concentration on admission to hospital of 0.43 ± 0,23 μg/L significantly different from concentration of 0.11 ± 0.03 μg/L in 51 healthy age, sex and race matched controls *19*

Sodium *Serum* *Decrease* Associated with excessive ADH production *4707* Serum sodium is usually less than 130 mEq/L *126*
Urine *Increase* Urine is almost always hypertonic to plasma *126*

Uric Acid *Cerebrospinal Fluid* *Increase* Markedly increased with decreased CSF:blood ratio, possibly due to cellular breakdown and nucleoprotein catabolism *5100*
Serum *Increase* Increased in both blood and CSF with a lowered CSF:blood ratio, possibly due to cellular breakdown and nucleoprotein catabolism *5100*
Urine *Increase* Increased excretion in neurological and psychiatric disorders; progressive rise in urinary level following slight rise in blood, due to disturbed purine metabolism *5100*

433.10 Carotid Artery Stenosis

Cholesterol *Serum* *Increase* In 592 patients with severe stenosis mean concentration of 5.92 mmol/L compared with mean concentration of 5.82 mmol/L in 826 patients with moderate stenosis and 5.65 mmol/L in 214 patients with mild stenosis *1664*

HDL-Cholesterol *Serum* *Increase* In 592 patients with severe stenosis mean concentration of 1.78 mmol/L compared with mean concentration of 1.68 mmol/L in 826 patients with moderate stenosis and 1.11 mmol/L in 214 patients with mild stenosis *1664*

LDL-Cholesterol *Serum* *Increase* In 592 patients with severe stenosis mean concentration of 4.08 mmol/L compared with mean concentration of 3.77 mmol/L in 826 patients with moderate stenosis and 3.70 mmol/L in 214 patients with mild stenosis *1664*

434.00 Cerebral Thrombosis

Antidiuretic Hormone *Plasma* *Increase* Associated with excessive ADH production resulting in sodium loss *4707*

Antiphospholipid Antibodies *Serum* *Increase* About 60% of patients with cerebrovascular thrombosis have antiphospholipid antibodies *441*

α_1-Antitrypsin *Serum* *Increase* Increased *4763 4371 4373 4241 83*

Aspartate Aminotransferase *Serum* *Increase* Increased the following week in 50% of cases *5544* Values may be up to 50 U/L *1025*

Creatine Kinase *Serum* *Increase* 15 of 21 patients with acute stroke had raised levels at some time during the 1st week after ictus. Values ranged from 28.3 - 710 U/L *1244* Increases in 50% of patients with extensive brain infarction. Maximum levels in 3 days; increase may not appear before 2 days; levels usually less than in acute myocardial infarction and remain increased for longer time; return to normal within 14 days; high mortality associated with levels > 300 U/L *5544*

Erythrocytes *Cerebrospinal Fluid* *No Effect* Never causes blood in the spinal fluid unless the infarct is especially congested, then a very faint xanthochromia may occur *2033*

Fibrin Degradation Products *Plasma* *Decrease* A decrease in fibrinolytic activity was noticed *281*

Fibrinogen *Plasma* *Increase* Significant increase was noted in cerebral thromboembolic stroke in young patients *4762*

Glomerular Filtration Rate *Urine* *Increase* Associated excess ADH may tend to accelerate GFR *4707*

Lactate Dehydrogenase *Cerebrospinal Fluid* *Increase* All of the 17 patients with hemorrhagic lesions showed elevations. 13 of 30 patients with nonhemorrhagic lesions showed similar but smaller elevations in the CSF. Serum elevations were less frequent and independent of those in the CSF *5713*
Serum *Increase* Serum elevations were less frequent and independent of those in the CSF *5713*

Leukocytes *Cerebrospinal Fluid* *Increase* A slight increase is common in the 1st few days. Rarely, and for unexplained reasons, a brisk transient pleocytosis (400 - 2,000 polymorphonuclears/μL) occurs on the 3rd day *2033*

Lipoproteins, Pre-β *Serum* *Increase* Significant rise was noticed in all patients *281*

Nickel *Serum* *Increase* Mean concentration of 5.2 μg/L (n = 33) compared with mean of 2.6 μg/L (n = 42) in controls *3428* Increased *4746*

Protein *Cerebrospinal Fluid* *Increase* The total amount may be normal, but frequently it is raised to 50 - 80 mg/dL. Rarely it is over 100 mg/dL, in which case some other diagnosis should be considered *2033*
Cerebrospinal Fluid *No Effect* The total amount may be normal, but frequently it is raised to 50 - 80 mg/dL. Rarely it is over 100 mg/dL, in which case some other diagnosis should be considered *2033*

Semicarbazide-sensitive Amine Oxidase *Serum* *No Effect* In 42 patients with cerebral thrombosis mean activity of 13.3 ± 5.2 nmol benzylamine/mL plasma/h not significantly different from 15.9 ± 3.9 nmol benzylamine/mL in 24 healthy controls *1659*

Sodium *Serum* *Decrease* Associated with excessive ADH production *4707* Serum sodium is usually less than 130 mEq/L *126*
Urine *Increase* Urine is almost always hypertonic to plasma *126*

Triglycerides *Serum* *Increase* Significant rise noticed in all patients *281*

Uric Acid *Cerebrospinal Fluid* *Increase* Markedly increased with decreased CSF:blood ratio, possibly due to cellular breakdown and nucleoprotein catabolism *5100*
Serum *Increase* In 24% of 12 patients hospitalized for this disorder *1576* Increased in both blood and CSF with a lowered CSF:blood ratio, possibly due to cellular breakdown and nucleoprotein catabolism *5100* Found in 25% of patients of both sexes with acute stroke *4050*
Urine *Increase* Increased excretion in neurological and psychiatric disorders; progressive rise in urinary level following slight rise in blood, due to disturbed purine metabolism *5100*

434.10 Cerebral Embolism

Antidiuretic Hormone *Plasma* *Increase* Associated with excessive ADH production resulting in sodium loss *4707*

Aspartate Aminotransferase *Serum* *Increase* Values may be up to 50 U/L *1025* Increased the following week in 50% of cases *1290*

Creatine Kinase *Serum* *Increase* Peak values occur at 48 h, falling in 3 - 4 days. Bad prognosis is indicated by an early rise, and by its magnitude. No increase is associated with brain stem infarction and angiomata *1290*

Erythrocytes *Cerebrospinal Fluid* *Increase* Usually findings are the same as in cerebral thrombosis. 33% of patients develop hemorrhagic infarction, usually producing slight xanthochromia several days later; some cases may have grossly bloody CSF (10,000 RBC/μL) *5544*

Fibrinogen *Plasma* *Increase* The greater the degree of initial neurological deficit the greater were plasma high molecular weight fibrinogen complexes values, which were associated with poor clinical outcome. Values were significantly higher in patients with intracerebral hemorrhage, subarachnoid hemorrhage and cerebral embolism *1508*

Glomerular Filtration Rate *Urine* *Increase* Associated excess ADH may tend to accelerate GFR *4707*

Glucose *Cerebrospinal Fluid* *No Effect* CSF concentration usualy unaffected *2033*
Serum *No Effect* Concentration typically unaffected by disease *5544*

434.10 Cerebral Embolism *(continued)*

Leukocytes *Cerebrospinal Fluid* *Increase* Septic embolism (e.g., bacterial endocarditis) may cause increased WBC, up to 200 /µL with variable lymphocytes and polymorphonuclear leukocytes *5544*

Neutrophils *Cerebrospinal Fluid* *Increase* In septic embolus, the proportion of lymphocytes and polymorphonuclears varies with the acuteness of the septic process *2033*

Protein *Cerebrospinal Fluid* *Increase* Elevated in septic emboli *2033*
Serum *Increase* In septic embolism *5544*

Semicarbazide-sensitive Amine Oxidase *Serum* *No Effect* In 26 patients with cerebral embolism mean activity of 14.6 ± 7.5 nmol benzylamine/mL plasma/h not significantly different from 15.9 ± 3.9 nmol benzylamine/mL in 24 healthy controls *1659*

Sodium *Serum* *Decrease* Serum sodium is usually less than 130 mEq/L *126* Associated with excessive ADH production *4707*
Urine *Increase* Urine is almost always hypertonic to plasma *126*

Uric Acid *Cerebrospinal Fluid* *Increase* Markedly increased with decreased CSF:blood ratio, possibly due to cellular breakdown and nucleoprotein catabolism *5100*
Serum *Increase* Increased in both blood and CSF with a lowered CSF:blood ratio, possibly due to cellular breakdown and nucleoprotein catabolism *5100* Found in 25% of patients of both sexes with acute stroke *4050*
Urine *Increase* Increased excretion in neurological and psychiatric disorders; progressive rise in urinary level following slight rise in blood, due to disturbed purine metabolism *5100*

434.91 Cerebral Infarction

Amyloid β-Protein *Cerebrospinal Fluid* *No Effect* In 8 patients with cerebral infarction concentrations ranged from 0.06 to 5.45 pmol/mL not significantly different from mean concentration of 4.00 ± 2.92 pmol/mL *3716*

Amyloid β-Protein Precursor *Cerebrospinal Fluid* *Decrease* In 8 patients with cerebral infarction concentrations ranged from 0.50 to 1.58 integrated OD units not significantly different in some from mean concentration of 1.35 ± 0.38 integrated OD units in 25 normal controls but decreased in others *3716*
Cerebrospinal Fluid *No Effect* In 8 patients with cerebral infarction concentrations ranged from 0.50 to 1.58 integrated OD units not significantly different in some from mean concentration of 1.35 ± 0.38 integrated OD units in 25 normal controls but decreased in others *3716*

α_1-Antichymotrypsin *Cerebrospinal Fluid* *Increase* In 8 patients with cerebral infarction concentrations ranged from 1.80 to 20.95 µg/mL significantly different from mean concentration of 2.27 ± 1.40 µg/mL in 25 normal controls *3716*

α_1-Antitrypsin *Serum* *Increase* High molecular weight fibrinogen complexes, native fibrinogen, alpha$_1$-antitrypsin and alpha$_2$-macroglobulin were significantly increased in cerebral infarction patients *1508*

Aspartate Aminotransferase *Cerebrospinal Fluid* *Increase* Increased for some days after infarction or cerebrovascular accident without a corresponding rise in CSF ALT *1290*
Serum *Increase* Increased the following week in 50% of cases *1290* Values may be up to 50 U/L *1025* May cause increased AST activity *4617*

Carbonic Anhydrase II *Cerebrospinal Fluid* *Increase* In 20 patients with brain infarction median concentration of 66.5 µg/L significantly higher than median of 7.9 µg/L in 97 controls *4012*

Cells *Cerebrospinal Fluid* *No Effect* In 8 patients with cerebral infarction concentrations ranged from 0.3 to 3.0 cells/µL not significantly different from normal *3716*

Cholesterol *Serum* *Decrease* In patients who had a stroke for whatever cause poor outcome was associated with low cholesterol concentration with relative hazard that was 9% lower for each 1.0 mmol/L (39 mg/dL) increase in cholesterol concentration *1276* In all patients a significant reduction in total lipids, cholesterol, triglyceride and all lipoproteins was demonstrated after the acute cerebrovascular accident presumably due to the stress situation *2493*

Copper *Cerebrospinal Fluid* *Increase* Patients with cerebral infarctions had abnormally high concentrations in plasma and CSF. The plasma Cu:Zn ratio was also significantly elevated *500*
Serum *Increase* Abnormally high concentrations in plasma and CSF. The plasma Cu:Zn ratio was also significantly elevated *500*

Creatine Kinase *Cerebrospinal Fluid* *Increase* Of 10 patients with cerebral infarction 2 had increases above upper limit of normal of 10 U/L *4780*
Serum *Increase* Peak values occur at 48 h, falling in 3 - 4 days. Bad prognosis is indicated by an early rise, and by its magnitude. No increase is associated with brain stem infarction or angiomata *1290*

Creatine Kinase BB-Isoenzyme *Serum* *Increase* Observed effect *248*

Erythrocytes *Cerebrospinal Fluid* *No Effect* In 20 patients with brain infarction median concentration of 2 x 10^6/L not significantly different from median of 1 x 10^6/L in 97 controls *4012*

Factor XIII *Plasma* *Decrease* Substantial depression developed together with concomitant significant increases in the proportion and concentration of plasma high molecular weight fibrinogen complexes (HMWFC). An inverse correlation between factor XIII and percentage of HMWFC was demonstrated in the early stages of the illness *3253*

Fibrinogen *Plasma* *Increase* High molecular weight fibrinogen complexes, native fibrinogen, alpha$_1$-antitrypsin and alpha$_2$-macroglobulin were significantly increased in cerebral infarction patients *1508* Substantial depression of factor XIII concentrations developed together with concomitant significant increases in the proportion and concentration of plasma high molecular weight fibrinogen complexes (HMWFC). An inverse correlation between factor XIII and percentage of HMWFC was demonstrated in the early stages of the illness *3253*

Leukocytes *Blood* *Increase* In patients with ischemic cerebral infarction 3 days after stroke mean concentration increased. Higher counts observed in patients with more severe neurological impairment and larger infarct size *4202*
Cerebrospinal Fluid *No Effect* In 20 patients with brain infarction median concentration of 1 x 10^6/L not significantly different from median of 1 x 10^6/L in 97 controls *4012*

Lipids *Serum* *Decrease* In all patients a significant reduction in total lipids, cholesterol, triglyceride and all lipoproteins was demonstrated after the acute cerebrovascular accident presumedly due to the stress situation *2493*

Lipoproteins *Serum* *Decrease* In all patients a significant reduction in total lipids, cholesterol, triglyceride and all lipoproteins was demonstrated after the acute cerebrovascular accident presumedly due to the stress situation *2493*

α_2-Macroglobulin *Serum* *Increase* High molecular weight fibrinogen complexes, native fibrinogen, alpha$_1$-antitrypsin, and alpha$_2$-macroglobulin were significantly increased in cerebral infarction patients *1508*

α_1-Microglobulin *Cerebrospinal Fluid* *Increase* Of 13 patients with cerebral infarction mean concentration in 4 greater than that in 15 healthy controls of 34.8 ± 16.0 µg/L *2370*

Monocytes *Cerebrospinal Fluid* *Increase* Mononuclear cells are increased in CSF early in the course of the disease *2039*

Neuron-specific Enolase *Serum* *Increase* Concentration in 10 of 11 patients with Glasgow outcome scale 1 (GOS 1) increased above upper limit of normal of normal range of 2 - 20 ng/mL, 7 of 12 with GOS3 increased above 30 ng/mL, 1 with GOS 4 and none of 6 with GOS 5 *4611*

Protein *Cerebrospinal Fluid* *Increase* In 8 patients with cerebral infarction concentrations ranged from 22 to 112 mg/dL significantly different in half the patients from normal mean of 29 mg/dL *3716* Slight elevations of 60 - 75 mg/dL are found in 20% of patients *367*
Cerebrospinal Fluid *No Effect* In 20 patients with brain infarction median concentration of 455 mg/L not significantly higher than median of 400 mg/L in 97 controls *4012*

Superoxide Dismutase *Cerebrospinal Fluid* *Increase* In 36 acute ischemic stroke patients activity on day 1 and day 4 after symptom onset the amount was increased. It was significantly correlated with the size of the infarction on computed tomography *5038*

Triglycerides *Serum* *Decrease* In all patients a significant reduction in total lipids, cholesterol, triglyceride and all lipoproteins was demonstrated after the acute cerebrovascular accident presumedly due to the stress situation *2493*

Uric Acid *Cerebrospinal Fluid* *Increase* Markedly increased with decreased CSF:blood ratio, possibly due to cellular breakdown and nucleoprotein catabolism *5100*
Serum *Increase* In 36% of 115 cases of acute infarction *4050* Increased in both blood and CSF with a lowered CSF:blood ratio, possibly due to cellular breakdown and nucleoprotein catabolism *5100*
Urine *Increase* Increased excretion in neurological and psychiatric disorders; progressive rise in urinary level following slight rise in blood, due to disturbed purine metabolism *5100*

435.90 Transient Cerebral Ischemia

Adenosine Monophosphate *Platelets* *Decrease* Mean concentration of cAMP of 4.06 ± 0.92 pmol x 10^9/L in 59 patients during acute stage of cerebral ischemia significantly different from 5.21 ± 1.71 pmol x 10^9/L in 57 patients 1 year following episode *154*

Antiphospholipid Antibodies *Serum* *Increase* About 37% of patients with TIAs have antiphospholipid antibodies *441* Observed effect in patients with transient cerebral ischemia *5282*

Bicarbonate *Serum* *Increase* In 70% of 31 patients hospitalized for this disorder *1576*

Carbonic Anhydrase II *Cerebrospinal Fluid* *No Effect* In 20 patients with brain infarction median concentration of 11.2 µg/L not significantly different from median of 7.9 µg/L in 97 controls *4012*

Cholesterol *Serum* *Increase* In 16 patients with TIA or minor stroke mean concentration of 231.7 ± 42.8 mg/dL during 12 - 48 h after the event significantly higher than 192.2 ± 36.0 mg/dL in specimens collected between 49 and 168 hours affter the event *215*
Serum *No Effect* Mean concentration of 5.94 ± 0.95 mmol/L in 59 patients during acute stage of cerebral ischemia not significantly different from 5.97 ± 1.04 mmol/L in 57 patients 1 year following episode *154*

Erythrocyte Sedimentation Rate *Blood* *No Effect* In 48 patients with TIA mean rate of 10 ± 9 mm/h *1344*

Erythrocytes *Cerebrospinal Fluid* *No Effect* In 20 patients with brain infarction median concentration of 2 x 10^6/L not significantly different from median of 1 x 10^6/L in 97 controls *4012*

Fibrinogen *Plasma* *No Effect* In 48 patients with TIA mean concentration of 3.9 ± 1.1 mg/L *1344*

Glucose *Serum* *No Effect* Median concentration of 5.4 mmol/L in 59 patients during acute stage of cerebral ischemia not significantly different from 5.6 mmol/L in 57 patients 1 year following episode *154*

Guanosine Monophosphate *Platelets* *No Effect* Mean concentration of cGMP of 0.76 ± 0.19 pmol x 10^9/L in 59 patients during acute stage of cerebral ischemia not significantly different from 0.75 ± 0.28 pmol x 10^9/L in 57 patients 1 year following episode *154*

HDL-Cholesterol *Serum* *No Effect* Mean concentration of 1.26 ± 0.32 mmol/L in 59 patients during acute stage of cerebral ischemia not significantly different from 1.30 ± 0.37 mmol/L in 57 patients 1 year following episode *154* In 16 patients with TIA or minor stroke mean concentration of 41.3 ± 8.7 mg/dL during 12 - 48 h after the event not significantly different from 37.6 ± 12.6 mg/dL in specimens collected between 49 and 168 hours affter the event *215*

Hematocrit *Blood* *Increase* In 29% of 48 patients hospitalized for this disorder *1576*

Hemoglobin *Blood* *Increase* In 25% of 48 patients hospitalized for this disorder *1576*

Hemoglobin A_{1c} *Blood* *No Effect* In 48 patients with TIA mean concentration of 4.9 ± 0.3% *1344*

LDL-Cholesterol *Serum* *Increase* In 16 patients with TIA or minor stroke mean concentration of 161.7 ± 42.3 mg/dL during 12 - 48 h after the event significantly higher than 129.3 ± 28.5 mg/dL in specimens collected between 49 and 168 hours affter the event *215*
Serum *No Effect* Mean concentration of 3.99 ± 0.90 mmol/L in 59 patients during acute stage of cerebral ischemia not significantly different from 3.92 ± 0.92 mmol/L in 57 patients 1 year following episode *154*

LDL-Cholesterol:HDL-Cholesterol Ratio *Serum* *No Effect* Mean ratio of 3.31 ± 1.03 in 59 patients during acute stage of cerebral ischemia not significantly different from 3.22 ± 1.13 in 57 patients 1 year following episode *154*

Leukocytes *Blood* *Increase* Mean concentration of 7.9 ± 2.0 x 10^9/L in 59 patients during acute stage of cerebral ischemia significantly different from 7.0 ± 1.8 x 10^9/L in 57 patients 1 year following episode *154*
Blood *No Effect* In 48 patients with TIA mean concentration of 6.8 ± 2.0 x 10^9 /L *1344*
Cerebrospinal Fluid *No Effect* In 20 patients with brain infarction median concentration of 2 x 10^6/L not significantly different from median of 1 x 10^6/L in 97 controls *4012*

Neutrophil Gelatinase-associated Lipocalcin
Plasma *Decrease* Mean concentration of 126 ± 48 µg/L in 59 patients during acute stage of cerebral ischemia significantly different from 157 ± 58 µg/L in 57 patients 1 year following episode *154*
Serum *Increase* In 48 patients with TIA median concentration of 110 µg/L significantly different from 97 µg/L in 36 healthy controls *1344*

Neutrophil Proteinase 4 *Serum* *Increase* In 48 patients with TIA median concentration of 31 µg/L significantly different from 24 µg/L in 36 healthy controls *1344*

Platelets *Plasma* *No Effect* Mean concentration in platelet-rich plasma of 387 ± 104 x 10^9/L in 59 patients during acute stage of cerebral ischemia not significantly different from 369 ± 102 x 10^9/L in 57 patients 1 year following episode *154*

Protein *Cerebrospinal Fluid* *No Effect* In 20 patients with brain infarction median concentration of 466 mg/L not significantly different from median of 400 mg/L in 97 controls *4012*

Soluble Tumor Necrosis Factor Receptor-I
Serum *Decrease* Mean concentration of 2.59 ± 1.3 µg/L in 59 patients during acute stage of cerebral ischemia significantly different from 3.50 ± 2.20 µg/L in 57 patients 1 year following episode *154*
Serum *No Effect* In 48 patients with TIA median concentration of 2.0 µg/L not significantly different from 2.1 µg/L in 36 healthy controls *1344*

Triglycerides *Serum* *No Effect* In 16 patients with TIA or minor stroke mean concentration of 130.7 ± 33.0 mg/dL during 12 - 48 h after the event not significantly different from 142.1 ± 67.0 mg/dL in specimens collected between 49 and 168 hours affter the event *215* Mean concentration of 1.70 ± 0.96 mmol/L in 59 patients during acute stage of cerebral ischemia not significantly different from 1.68 ± 0.90 mmol/L in 57 patients 1 year following episode *154*

Tumor Necrosis Factor-α *Serum* *No Effect* In 48 patients with TIA median concentration of 0 µg/L not significantly different from 0 µg/L in 36 healthy controls *1344*

Uric Acid *Serum* *Increase* In 46% of 50 patients hospitalized for this disorder *1576*

436.00 Apoplexy

Collagenase-like Peptidase *Serum* *No Effect* Mean activity of 0.54 ± 0.03 nmol/min/mL in 42 patients with apoplexy not significantly less than that in 55 healthy individuals in whom mean activity 0.60 ± 0.03 nmol/min/mL *2380*

Dipeptidyl Aminopeptidase *Serum* *No Effect* Mean activity of 75.9 ± 3.31 nmol/min/mL in 45 patients with apoplexy not significantly different from than that in 117 healthy individuals in whom mean activity 70.1 ± 0.37 nmol/min/mL *2380*

436.00 Cerebrovascular Accident

α_1-Antichymotrypsin *Serum* *Increase* Mean concentration increased above reference interval of 47.9 ± 8.1 mg/dL in 2 of 8 patients (25%) with cerebovascular accident *3044*

Carnosinase *Serum* *Decrease* In 53 patients with cerebrovascular accidents mean activity of 74.6 nmol/mL/min significantly different from 161 ± 7 nmol/mL/min in 16 healthy controls *5590*

436.00 Cerebrovascular Accident *(continued)*

Prothrombin Fragment 1.2 *Plasma Increase* Mean concentration of prothrombin fragment 1.2 in platelet-poor plasma from 8 patients with cerebrovascular accident of 4.6 ± 3.7 nmol/L significantly higher than 0.51 nmol/L (95% reference interval 0.21 - 2.78 nmol/L) in 268 healthy individuals less than 44 years of age *1860*

436.00 Stroke

α_1-Acid Glycoprotein *Serum Increase* In 41 patients with stroke mean concentration of 70 ± 22 mg/dL significantly greater than 34 ± 11 mg/dL in 20 healthy elderly controls *348*

Albumin:Globulin Ratio *Serum Decrease* In 41 patients with stroke mean ratio of 1.49 ± 0.29 significantly less than 1.71 ± 0.24 in 20 healthy elderly controls *348*

Anti-Interferon-γ Autoantibodies
Cerebrospinal Fluid No Effect Mean concentration of 0.0053 ± 0.005 ng/mL in 15 patients with stroke compared with 0.0044 ± 0.004 ng/mL in 15 healthy adults *1333*
Serum No Effect Mean concentration of 0.005 ± 0.004 ng/mL in 15 patients with stroke compared with 0.006 ± 0.005 ng/mL in 15 healthy adults *1333*

Anti-Interleukin-4 Autoantibodies
Cerebrospinal Fluid Increase Mean concentration of 0.034 ± 0.01 ng/mL in 15 patients with stroke compared with 0.005 ± 0.004 ng/mL in 15 healthy adults *1333*
Serum Increase Mean concentration of 0.0055 ± 0.005 ng/mL in 15 patients with stroke compared with 0.013 ± 0.007 ng/mL in 15 healthy adults *1333*

Anti-Interleukin-10 Autoantibodies
Cerebrospinal Fluid Increase Mean concentration of 0.019 ± 0.013 ng/mL in 15 patients with stroke compared with 0.0048 ± 0.004 ng/mL in 15 healthy adults *1333*
Serum No Effect Mean concentration of 0.01 ± 0.0069 ng/mL in 15 patients with stroke compared with 0.01 ± 0.006 ng/mL in 15 healthy adults *1333*

Anti-Tumor Necrosis Factor-α Autoantibodies
Cerebrospinal Fluid Increase Mean concentration of 0.0069 ± 0.006 ng/mL in 15 patients with stroke compared with 0.0046 ± 0.004 ng/mL in 15 healthy adults *1333*
Serum Increase Mean concentration of 0.008 ± 0.0069 ng/mL in 15 patients with stroke compared with 0.0042 ± 0.004 ng/mL in 15 healthy adults *1333*

Anticardiolipin Antibodies *Serum Increase* 232 patients enrolled in the European Concerted Action on Thrombosis Angina Pectoris Study were studied. aCL were not found to be a marker of either progressive cardiovascular disease or recurrent thrombotic events *5299*
Serum No Effect A control was matched by age, smoking history, and length of follow-up to each of the 100 patients with ischemic stroke. The anticardiolipin antibody titers in patients with ischemic stroke and controls were not significantly different ($p > 0.2$) *4537*

Antiphospholipid Antibodies *Serum Increase* Observed in some patients following stroke *5282*

Antithrombin III *Plasma Decrease* In 86 patients with acute ischemic stroke mean concentration of 95 ± 14% significantly different from 108 ± 10% in 60 healthy controls *96*
Plasma No Effect In acute phase (within 7 days of onset) in 23 patients with cardioembolic stroke mean concentration of 82 ± 14%, in 10 with atherothrombotic stroke of 88 ± 14% and 98 ± 17% in 12 with lacunar stroke no significant difference from 93 ± 15% in 27 healthy controls *5787*

α_1-Antitrypsin *Serum Increase* In 41 patients with stroke mean concentration of 184 ± 42 mg/dL significantly greater than 156 ± 32 mg/dL in 20 healthy elderly controls *348*

Apolipoprotein A *Serum No Effect* In patients with stroke no significant difference observed in concentrations compared with healthy controls *2539*

Apolipoprotein B *Serum No Effect* No significant difference observed between concentrations in healthy individuals and in those with stroke *2539*

C_4b-Binding Protein *Serum Increase* In 4 of 8 patients with stroke mean concentrations were above normal range of 68 - 140% *699*

Carnosinase *Serum Decrease* In 48 acute stroke patients median concentration of 135 nmol/mL/min significantly less than 223 nmol/mL/min in 39 age and gender matched controls *5589*

Cholesterol *Serum Decrease* In patients who had a stroke for whatever cause poor outcome was associated with low cholesterol concentration with relative hazard that was 9% lower for each 1.0 mmol/L (39 mg/dL) increase in cholesterol concentration *1276*
Serum No Effect No significant difference observed in concentrations of healthy individuals and of those with stroke *2539*

Cobalamin *Serum No Effect* In 162 consecutively studied patients with stroke mean concentration of 242 pmol/L (range 55 - 15,090) not significantly different from 246 pmol/L (range 68 - 13,900) in an age and sex matched control group *3067*

C-Reactive Protein *Serum No Effect* In 41 patients with stroke mean concentration of 0.6 ± 1.2 µg/mL not significantly greater than 0.5 ± 0.2 µg/mL in 20 healthy elderly controls *348*

Creatinine *Serum No Effect* In 162 consecutively studied patients with stroke mean concentration of 86 µg/L (range 40 - 197) not significantly different from 84 µg/L (range 55 - 230) in an age and sex matched control group *3067*

D-Dimer *Plasma Increase* In 86 patients with acute ischemic stroke mean concentration of 894 ± 1,436 µg/L significantly different from 220 ± 133 µg/L in 60 healthy controls *96* In acute phase (within 7 days of onset) in 23 patients with cardioembolic stroke mean concentration of 731 ± 959 ng/mL and in 10 patients with atherothrombotic stroke 221 ± 143 ng/mL significantly increased compared with 90 ± 71 ng/mL in 27 healthy controls *5787*
Plasma No Effect In acute phase (within 7 days of onset of stroke) mean concentration in 12 patients with lacunar stroke 125 ± 81 ng/mL not significantly different from 90 ± 71 ng/mL in 27 healthy controls *5787*

Endothelin-1 *Plasma Increase* There was a marked (four-fold) elevation in plasma endothelin-1 levels in the patients (median, 11.7 pg/mL; 25th and 75th centiles, 5.4 and 13.2 pg/mL) compared with those in a control group *5871*

Erythrocyte Sedimentation Rate *Blood Increase* In 208 patients with ischemic stroke poor outcome was associated with mean rate of 34.7 mm/h versus 17.1 mm/h in those with a good outcome *759* In 72 patients with stroke mean rate of 21 ± 19 mm/h *1344*

Fibrinogen *Plasma Increase* In 41 patients with stroke mean concentration of 418 ± 136 mg/dL significantly greater than 334 ± 39 mg/dL in 20 healthy elderly controls *348*
Plasma No Effect In 72 patients with stroke mean concentration of 4.6 ± 1.2 mg/L *1344*

Fibrinopeptide A *Plasma Increase* Mean concentrations in acute phase in 23 patients with cardioembolic stroke 14.1 ± 17.0 ng/mL and in 10 with atherothrombotic stroke 13.1 ± 15.3 ng/mL both significantly increased and in 12 patients with lacunar stroke of 5.2 ± 4.4 ng/mL nonsignificantly increased compared with 4.1 ± 3.3 ng/mL in 27 healthy controls *5787*

Folate *Blood No Effect* In 162 consecutively studied patients with stroke mean concentration of 330 nmol/L (range 50 - 1,275) not significantly different from 294 nmol/L (range 144 - 1,024) in an age and sex matched control group *3067*

Glial Fibrillary Acidic Protein *Cerebrospinal Fluid Increase* Transient increase observed during first week following ischemic stroke. Extent of increase correlated with size of infarct and clinical state *217*

Glucose *Serum Increase* Glucose concentrations above 144 mg/dL in 750 nondiabetics predicted increased mortality *5620*

HDL-Cholesterol *Serum Decrease* In patients with stroke concentration significantly less than in healthy control individuals *2539*

Hemoglobin A_{1c} *Blood No Effect* In 72 patients with stroke mean concentration of 4.8 ± 0.5% *1344*

Homocysteine *Plasma Increase* In 17 patients with stroke mean concentration at a median of 583 days following cerebral infarction of 14.5 µg/L significantly greater than 11.4 µg/L although not significantly different from 13.8 µg/L in an age and sex matched control group *3067* Hyperhomocysteinaemia was present in 57 of 142 survivors with stroke (40%) and in four of

66 controls (6%) *563* Plasma homocyst(e)ine levels in 41 patients with acute strokes, 27 patients with transient ischemic attacks, 31 patients with recognized risk factors for but no recent symptoms of cerebrovascular disease, and 31 normal volunteers (controls). Plasma homocyst(e)ine concentration was moderately but significantly higher in the patients than in the controls (p less than 0.0001). Approximately 30% of the patients had homocyst(e)ine levels higher than the controls *944*
Plasma No Effect In 241 consecutively studied patients with stroke mean concentration of 13.4 μg/L not significantly different from 13.8 μg/L in an age and sex matched control group *3067* In 42 male cases mean concentration of 10.4 ± 2.72 μmol/L compared with 9.82 ± 3.17 μmol/L in 141 controls and in 32 female cases mean concentration of 10.1 ± 3.23 μmol/L compared with 9.28 ± 2.59 μmol/L in 128 controls *76*

Interleukin-1 Receptor Antagonist *Serum Increase* In 41 patients with stroke mean concentration of 354 ± 270 pg/mL significantly greater than 139 ± 113 pg/mL in 20 healthy elderly controls *348*

Interleukin-6 *Serum Increase* In 41 patients with stroke mean concentration of 4.6 ± 4.2 pg/mL significantly greater than 1.0 ± 0.9 pg/mL in 20 healthy elderly controls *348*

LDL-Cholesterol *Serum No Effect* No significant difference observed between concentrations of patients with stroke and of healthy controls *2539*

Leukocytes *Blood No Effect* In 72 patients with stroke mean concentration of 8.0 ± 2.6 x 10^9 /L *1344*

Lipoprotein Lp(a) *Serum Decrease* In 42 male cases mean concentration of 79 mg/L compared with 108 in 148 controls *76*
Serum Increase In 28 female cases mean concentration of 158 mg/L compared with 91 mg/L in 121 controls *76* Several studies report higher concentrations in patients with stroke *2827* In patients with stroke mean concentration of 218.9 ± 21.6 mg/L compared with 157.8 ± 19.7 mg/L in healthy controls *2539*
Serum No Effect No significant difference observed in mean concentration of 0.12 g/L in 164 patients with cardiovascular disease at least 21 days after a stroke and concentration of 0.12 g/L in 91 spousal controls *3302*

Neutrophil Gelatinase-associated Lipocalcin
Serum Increase In 72 patients with stroke median concentration of 122 μg/L significantly different from 97 μg/L in 36 healthy controls *1344*

Neutrophil Proteinase 4 *Serum Increase* In 72 patients with stroke median concentration of 35 μg/L significantly different from 24 μg/L in 36 healthy controls *1344*

Oligoclonal Banding *Cerebrospinal Fluid Increase* Oligoclonal IgG bands detected in patients with stroke *3261*

Plasmin-α_2-Plasmin Inhibitor Complex *Plasma Increase* In 23 patients with cardioembolic stroke in acute phase (within 7 days of onset) mean concentration of 2.2 ± 3.5 μg/mL significantly greater than 0.8 ± 0.4 μg/mL in 27 healthy controls *5787*
Plasma No Effect In acute phase (within 7 days of onset) mean concentration of 0.8 ± 0.3 μg/mL in 10 patients with atherothrombotic stroke and in 12 patients with lacunar stroke mean concentration of 0.5 ± 0.2 μg/mL not significantly different from 0.8 ± 0.4 μg/mL in 27 healthy controls *5787*

Plasminogen *Plasma Decrease* In 86 patients with acute ischemic stroke mean concentration of 100 ± 17% significantly different from 110 ± 8% in 60 healthy controls *96*

Plasminogen Activator Inhibitor-1 *Plasma Increase* In 86 patients with acute ischemic stroke mean concentration of 38 ± 42 μg/L significantly different from 21 ± 12 μg/L in 60 healthy controls *96*

Platelet Activating Factor *Serum Increase* In 11 out of 17 patients with ischemic stroke PAF detected compared with only in 3 of 25 age-matched healthy controls *4592*

Platelet Activating Factor-like Lipids *Serum Increase* In 17 patients with ischemic stroke mean concentration of 294 ± 211 pg/mL compared with 140 ± 122 pg/mL in 25 age-matched controls *4592*

Protein C *Plasma Decrease* In acute phase (within 7 days of onset) in 23 patients with cardioembolic stroke mean concentration of 102 ± 25% significantly decreased but in 10 patients with atherothrombotic stroke 130 ± 26% and 143 ± 27% in 12 patients with lacunar stroke nonsignificant increase compared with 124 ± 21% in 27 healthy controls *5787*
Plasma No Effect In 86 patients with acute ischemic stroke mean concentration of 96 ± 17% not significantly different from 102 ± 14% in 60 healthy controls *96*

Protein C Antigen *Plasma Decrease* In acute phase (within 7 days of onset) in 23 patients with cardioembolic stroke mean concentration of 97 ± 24% significantly reduced, but in 10 with atherothrombotic stroke mean concentration of 134 ± 22% and in 12 patients with lacunar stroke 148 ± 25% not significantly different from 122 ± 20% in 27 healthy children *5787*

Protein S *Plasma Increase* In 86 patients with acute ischemic stroke mean concentration of 118 ± 22% significantly different from 102 ± 26% in 60 healthy controls *96*
Plasma No Effect In 8 stroke patients mean concentrations ranged from 57% to 112% (with only one result below lower limit of reference interval) compared with normal range of 70 - 140% *699*

Protein S, Free *Plasma Decrease* In 8 stroke patients although total protein S concentration within reference interval free protein S concentration reduced with results ranging from 10 to 50% compared with reference interval of 50 - 130% *699*
Plasma No Effect In 86 patients with acute ischemic stroke mean concentration of 100 ± 29% not significantly different from 93 ± 26% in 60 healthy controls *96*

S-100 Protein *Cerebrospinal Fluid Increase* In 28 patients who had ischemic stroke transient increase during first week after stroke. Extent of increase correlated with size of infarct and clinical state *217*
Serum Increase In 68 patients with ischemic stroke mean concentration of 0.27 ± 0.09 μg/L on admission to hospital significantly different from concentration of 0.11 ± 0.03 μg/L in 51 healthy age, sex and race matched controls *19*

Semicarbazide-sensitive Amine Oxidase *Serum No Effect* In 68 stroke patients mean activity of 13.8 ± 6.1 nmol benzylamine/mL plasma/h not significantly different from 15.9 ± 3.9 nmol benzylamine/mL in 24 healthy controls *1659*

Soluble E-Selectin *Serum No Effect* Mean concentration of 31 ± 19 ng/mL in 10 patients with acute stroke not significantly different from 30 ± 9 ng/mL in 12 healthy control individuals *3885*

Soluble Tumor Necrosis Factor Receptor-I *Serum Increase* In 72 patients with stroke median concentration of 3.1 μg/L significantly different from 2.1 μg/L in 36 healthy controls *1344*

Thrombin/Antithrombin III Complex *Plasma Increase* In patients within acute phase (7 days) of a stroke, in 23 with cardioembolic stroke mean concentration of 18.0 ± 17.2 ng/mL significantly increased, and in 10 with atherothrombotic stroke of 5.4 ± 3.9 ng/mL and in 12 with lacunar stroke of 3.1 ± 1.8 ng/mL nonsignificantly increased compared with 2.6 ± 1.4 ng/mL in 27 healthy controls *5787* In 86 patients with acute ischemic stroke mean concentration of 8 ± 14.8 μg/L significantly different from 1.3 ± 0.3 μg/L in 60 healthy controls *96*

Tissue Plasminogen Activator *Plasma Increase* In 86 patients with acute ischemic stroke mean concentration of 15 ± 14 μg/L significantly different from 5.1 ± 3 μg/L in 60 healthy controls *96*

Triglycerides *Serum No Effect* No significant difference observed between concentrations in ptients with ischemic strokes and healthy controls *2539*

Tumor Necrosis Factor-α *Serum No Effect* In 72 patients with stroke median concentration of 0 μg/L not significantly different from 0 μg/L in 36 healthy controls *1344*

Diseases of the Arteries and Veins

440.00 Atherosclerosis

Alkaline Phosphatase *Serum Increase* Mean concentration of 15.7 μmol/L in 25 patients with multivascular atherosclerosis significantly greater than 10.8 μmol/L in 25 matched controls *3577*

Apolipoprotein A-I *Serum Decrease* An excellent predictor of this condition *5167* Patients with angiographically documented coronary artery disease were found to have elevated levels of apolipoprotein B and decreased levels of A-I or A-II compared with individuals without the disease *4356 4967 4921*

Apolipoprotein A-II *Serum Decrease* Patients with angiographically documented coronary artery disease were found to have elevated levels of apolipoprotein B and decreased levels of A-I or A-II compared with individuals without the disease *4967 4356 4921*

440.00 Atherosclerosis *(continued)*

Apolipoprotein B *Serum* *Increase* Patients with angiographically documented coronary artery disease were found to have elevated levels of apolipoprotein B and decreased levels of A-I or A-II compared with individuals without the disease *4356* *4921* *4967*

Apolipoproteins *Serum* *No Effect* In middle-aged women the relationship to risk was weak and did not approach statistical significance *883*

Bicarbonate *Serum* *Increase* In 56% of 67 patients hospitalized for this disorder *1576*

Cadmium *Serum* *Increase* The highest blood cadmium level was observed in smokers with coronary heart disease plus hypertension *34*

Ceruloplasmin *Serum* *Increase* High concentrations of Zn, Cu and ceruloplasmin were found in 13 patients when compared with controls. The Zn:Cu ratio is much higher in arteriosclerotic patients than in healthy subjects *650*

Cholesterol *Serum* *Increase* Nonfasting levels are related to the development of coronary heart disease in both men and women aged 19 years and older *4746* Correlates highly with the risk of myocardial infarction *2033* Severity of disease correlated (not significantly) with plasma cholesterol concentration *1031* Reported effect *731* Elevated fasting plasma concentration was frequently found in 219 male and 63 female patients *270*

Copper *Serum* *Increase* High concentrations found in 13 patients when compared with controls. The Zn:Cu ratio is much higher in arteriosclerotic patients than in healthy subjects *650* Statistically significant *4871*

Cotinine *Serum* *No Effect* In middle-aged women the relationship to risk was weak and did not approach statistical significance *883*

Creatinine *Serum* *Increase* In 64% of 36 patients hospitalized for this disorder *1576* May occur with kidney involvement *1025*

Cryomacroglobulins *Serum* *Increase* Reported effect *1774*

Dehydroepiandrosterone Sulfate *Plasma* *No Effect* In middle-aged women the relationship to risk was weak and did not approach statistical significance *883*

Endothelin-1 *Plasma* *Increase* In 2 studies of patients with atherosclerosis mean concentrations increased by means of 2.3 and 2.4-fold above appropriate normal values *328*

Erythrocytes *Blood* *Increase* True polycythemia with a considerable increase of red cell volume may occur *3710*

Factor VIII *Plasma* *Increase* In atherosclerosis *932*

Glucose *Serum* *No Effect* In 26 NIDDM patients with symptomatic atherosclerotic vascular disease mean concentration of 8.3 ± 2.9 mmol/L not significantly different from 91 ± 2.8 mmol/L in 75 NIDDM patients without symptomatic atherosclerotic vascular disease *3948*

Glycated Hemoglobin A_{1c} *Blood* *Increase* In nondiabetics relative risk of significant atherosclerosis increases with increasing proportion of hemoglobin A_{1c} *5481*

HDL-Cholesterol *Serum* *Decrease* Non fasting HDL is inversely related to the development of coronary heart disease in both men and women aged 49 years and older *731*
Serum *No Effect* In 26 NIDDM patients with symptomatic atherosclerotic vascular disease mean concentration of 1.36 ± 0.42 mmol/L not significantly different from 1.40 ± 0.49 mmol/L in 75 NIDDM patients without symptomatic atherosclerotic vascular disease *3948*

Hemoglobin A_{1c} *Blood* *No Effect* In 26 NIDDM patients with symptomatic atherosclerotic vascular disease mean concentration of 7.2 ± 2.0% not significantly different from 7.6 ± 1.7% in 75 NIDDM patients without symptomatic atherosclerotic vascular disease *3948*

Homocysteine *Plasma* *Increase* Hyperhomocysteinemia has been shown to constitute an independent risk factor for premature occlusive arterial disease *796*

LDL-Cholesterol *Serum* *No Effect* In 26 NIDDM patients with symptomatic atherosclerotic vascular disease mean concentration of 3.00 ± 0.80 mmol/L not significantly different from 3.16 ± 0.85 mmol/L in 75 NIDDM patients without symptomatic atherosclerotic vascular disease *3948*

Lipids *Serum* *Increase* Reported effect *1031* Hyperlipidemia was present in 43.9% of patients with atherosclerosis of the legs. Hyperlipidemia was frequently found in 219 male and 63 female patients. No significant relationship was found between uric acid and cholesterol or triglyceride *270*

Lipoproteins *Serum* *Increase* Hyperuricemia and hyperlipidemia were frequently found in 219 male and 63 female patients. No significant relationship was found between uric acid and cholesterol or triglyceride, when the males were divided into lipoprotein types it was found that those who were normolipoproteinemic or who had type IV hyperlipoproteinemia had a significantly higher mean uric acid level *270*

α_2-Macroglobulin *Serum* *Increase* Reported effect *3134*

Osteocalcin *Serum* *No Effect* Mean concentration of 4.70 ± 0.28 ng/mL in 34 women with aortic atherosclerosis not significantly different from 4.70 ± 0.15 ng/mL in 79 women without aortic atherosclerosis *2445*

Osteocalcin, Bound *Serum* *Decrease* Mean concentration of 2.55 ± 0.17 ng/mL in 34 women with aortic atherosclerosis different from 2.77 ± 0.09 ng/mL in 79 women without aortic atherosclerosis *2445*

Osteocalcin, Free *Serum* *Increase* Mean concentration of 2.16 ± 0.15 ng/mL in 34 women with aortic atherosclerosis different from 1.93 ± 0.08 ng/mL in 79 women without atherosclerosis *2445*

Selenium *Serum* *Decrease* Low concentrations of selenium in plasma in coronary atherogenesis *3585*

Soluble Vascular Cell Adhesion Molecule-1
Serum *Increase* In 26 NIDDM patients with symptomatic atherosclerotic vascular disease mean concentration of 789 ± 187 ng/mL significantly different from 664 ± 175 ng/mL in 75 NIDDM patients without symptomatic atherosclerotic vascular disease *3948*

Tissue Plasminogen Activator:Plasminogen Activator Inhibitor-1 Antigen Ratio *Plasma* *Increase* In 7 atherosclerotic individuals median ratio of 0.66 not significantly different from 0.53 in healthy controls *127*

Triglycerides *Serum* *Increase* Frequently found in 219 male and 63 female patients. No significant relationship was found between uric acid and triglyceride *270* The severity of disease showed a slight positive correlation with plasma triglyceride concentrations, especially in the younger patients *1031*
Serum *No Effect* In 26 NIDDM patients with symptomatic atherosclerotic vascular disease mean concentration of 1.60 ± 0.86 mmol/L not significantly different from 2.01 ± 1.30 mmol/L in 75 NIDDM patients without symptomatic atherosclerotic vascular disease *3948*

Urea Nitrogen *Serum* *Increase* Several mechanisms are involved *1025* In 36% of 75 patients hospitalized for this disorder *1576*

Uric Acid *Serum* *Increase* In 59% of 71 patients hospitalized for this disorder *1576* Increased in 80% of patients with elevated serum triglycerides *5544* Frequently found in 219 male and 63 female patients. No significant relationship was found between uric acid and serum lipids *270*

Volume *Red Blood Cells* *Decrease* RBC volume is decreased in the hypertension resulting from renal artery stenosis *3710*
Red Blood Cells *Increase* True polycythemia with a considerable increase of red cell volume may occur *3710*

Zinc *Serum* *Increase* High serum concentrations were found in 13 patients when compared with controls. The Zn:Cu ratio is much higher in arteriosclerotic patients than in healthy subjects *650*

440.10 Renal Artery Stenosis

Creatinine *Serum* *Increase* Median concentration of 107 ± 61 µmol/L in 104 patients with renal artery stenosis significantly different from 91 ± 41 µmol/L in 251 patients with essential hypertension *449*

Creatinine Clearance *Urine* *Decrease* Median clearance of 78 ± 29 ml/min in 104 patients with renal artery stenosis significantly different from 95 ± 29 ml/min in 251 patients with essential hypertension *449*

Metanephrine *Plasma* *Increase* In 6 patients with renal artery stenosis false positive increase of plasma metanephrine or normetanephrine concentration observed *2994*

Normetanephrine *Plasma* *Increase* In 6 patients with renal artery stenosis false positive increase of plasma metanephrine or normetanephrine concentration observed *2994*

Potassium *Serum* *No Effect* Median concentration of 3.8 ± 0.4 mmol/L in 104 patients with renal artery stenosis not significantly different from 3.8 ± 0.4 mmol/L in 251 patients with essential hypertension *449*

Renin Activity *Plasma* *Increase* Median activity of 2.0 nmol/L/h in 104 patients with renal artery stenosis significantly different from 1.0 nmol/L/h in 251 patients with essential hypertension *449*

441.00 Dissecting Aortic Aneurysm

Alanine Aminotransferase *Serum* *No Effect* Unless complications occur *5544*

Amylase *Serum* *Increase* Hyperamylasemia has been reported, although mechanism is unclear *1338* *3410*

Aspartate Aminotransferase *Serum* *Increase* Not helpful since modest elevations may occur in both dissection and infarction *2304*

Serum *No Effect* Unless complications occur *5544*

Creatine Kinase *Serum* *Increase* Elevated levels were found in 14 of 22 patients (64%). The CK was 95% CK-MM *1026*

Serum *No Effect* Unless complications occur *5544*

Lactate Dehydrogenase *Serum* *No Effect* Unless complications occur *5544*

Lactate Dehydrogenase Isoenzyme-5 *Serum* *No Effect* Unless complications occur *5544*

Occult Blood *Feces* *Increase* Reported effect *4891*

441.50 Ruptured Aortic Aneurysm

Hematocrit *Pleural Fluid* *Increase* Values approaching those found in blood are more indicative of frank hemorrhage, and such levels would be found in traumatic hemothorax or bleeding associated with pneumothorax or ruptured aortic aneurysm *1980*

Hemoglobin *Pleural Fluid* *Increase* Values approaching those found in blood are more indicative of frank hemorrhage, and such levels would be found in traumatic hemothorax or bleeding associated with pneumothorax or ruptured aortic aneurysm *1980*

443.00 Raynaud's Disease

Angiotensin-converting Enzyme *Serum* *No Effect* In 13 patients with primary Raynaud's disease mean activity of 6.33 ± 1.29 U/mL not significantly different from 7.79 ± 0.76 U/mL in 50 healthy controls *4535*

Endothelin-1 *Plasma* *Increase* In 4 studies of patients with Raynaud's disease mean increases of 1.0 to 3.1 fold observed *328*

5-Hydroxytryptamine *Plasma* *No Effect* In 12 patients with primary Raynaud's phenomenon median concentration of 0.6 ng/mL (IQR 0.3 - 2.4 ng/mL) not significantly different from median of 0.9 ng/mL (IQR 0.7 - 1.8 ng/mL) in 19 normal controls *871*

IgG Antiendothelial Antibodies *Serum* *Increase* In 13 patients with primary Raynaud's disease antibodies detected in 3 *4535*

von Willebrand Factor Antigen *Plasma* *Increase* In 13 patients with primary Raynaud's disease mean concentration of 1.19 ± 0.58 IU/mL significantly different from 0.80 ± 0.52 IU/mL in 58 healthy controls *4535*

443.10 Buerger's Disease

Endothelin-1 *Plasma* *Increase* In !3 patients with Buerger's disease mean concentration increased to 4.8 ± 0.6 pg/mL, mean 3.0-fold above appropriate normals *328*

443.90 Intermittent Claudication

Cholesterol *Serum* *No Effect* In 113 men with intermittent claudication mean concentration of 194 ± 37 mg/dL not significantly different from 189 ± 36 mg/dL in 2,311 men without intermittent claudication *682*

Lipoprotein Lp(a) *Serum* *Increase* In 113 men with intermittent claudication mean concentration of 46 ± 45 mg/dL significantly different from 33 ± 35 mg/dL in 2311 men without intermittent claudication *682*

443.90 Peripheral Arterial Disease

Angiogenin *Serum* *Increase* Mean concentration in 38 patients with stage IV peripheral arterial occlusive disease of 467 ± 26 ng/mL significantly increased compared with 358 ± 16 ng/mL in healthy individuals *635*

Anti-Platelet Factor 4-heparin Antibodies *Serum* *Increase* In 80 patients with peripheral arterial disease positive titer (more than 2 SD above mean in 140 healthy men or women) observed in 6 (7.5%) *5536*

Apolipoprotein A-I *Serum* *Decrease* In 17 white male patients with premature vascular disease mean concentration of 85.4 ± 4.3 mg/dL not significantly different from 90.0 ± 3.3 mg/dL in 32 age-matched white male controls *5384*

Apolipoprotein B-100 *Serum* *Increase* In 17 white male patients with premature vascular disease mean concentration of 100.9 ± 5.9 mg/dL not significantly different from 81.3 ± 5.5 mg/dL in 32 age-matched white male controls *5384*

Cholesterol *Serum* *Increase* In 119 patients with hypercholesterolemia and symptomatic for peripheral artery disease mean concentration of 6.6 ± 1.4 mmol/L significantly different from 5.5 ± 1.0 mmol/L in 132 age and sex matched asymptomatic controls *477* In 121 patients with peripheral arterial disease mean concentration of 7.34 ± 0.14 mmol/L significantly greater than 6.82 ± 0.10 mmol/L in 126 healthy controls *4903*

Serum *No Effect* In 46 patients with peripheral arterial disease mean concentration of 202 - 243 mg/dL not significantly different from 188 - 247 mg/dL in 76 healthy controls *4121* Mean concentration of 5.91 ± 1.32 mmol/L in 52 male patients with peripheral artery disease and 6.21 ± 1.34 mmol/L in 30 women with peripheral artery disease not significantly different from 5.41 ± 0.92 mmol/L in 58 control men and 5.50 ± 0.89 mmol/L in 38 control women, respectively *2538* In 17 white male patients with premature vascular disease mean concentration of 5.25 ± 0.20 mmol/L not significantly different from 5.19 ± 0.19 mmol/L in 32 age-matched white male controls *5384*

Cholesterol:HDL-Cholesterol Ratio *Serum* *Increase* Mean ratio of 5.94 ± 1.67 in 52 male patients with peripheral artery disease and 5.32 ± 1.39 in 30 women with peripheral artery disease significantly different from 4.42 ± 1.32 in 58 control men and 4.12 ± 1.07 in 38 control women, respectively *2538*

C-Reactive Protein *Serum* *Increase* Significant increase to 1.99 mg/L in patients who developed peripheral artery disease compared with 1.34 mg/L in patients who did not, with probability of PAD rising with increasing concentration *4350*

D-Dimer *Plasma* *Increase* In 193 patients with stable peripheral arterial disease mean concentration of 797 ± 802 ng/mL compared with 163 ± 54 ng/mL in healthy volunteers *407*

Factor VII Coagulant *Plasma* *No Effect* In 46 patients with peripheral arterial disease nonsignificant difference in activity of 82 - 103% compared with 80 - 103% in 76 healthy controls *4121*

Fibrinogen *Plasma* *Increase* In 119 patients with hypercholesterolemia and symptomatic for peripheral artery disease mean concentration of 3.7 ± 0.8 g/L significantly different from 3.0 ± 0.5 g/L in 132 age and sex matched asymptomatic controls *477* In 46 patients with peripheral arterial disease mean concentration of 280 - 360 mg/dL significantly different from 240 - 305 mg/dL in 76 healthy controls *4121*

HDL_2-Cholesterol *Serum* *Decrease* Mean concentration of 0.24 ± 0.11 mmol/L in 52 male patients with peripheral artery disease and 0.29 ± 0.15 mmol/L in 30 women with peripheral artery disease significantly different from 0.39 ± 0.17 mmol/L in 58 control men and 0.48 ± 0.19 mmol/L in 38 control women, respectively *2538*

443.90 Peripheral Arterial Disease (continued)

HDL_2-Cholesterol:HDL_3-Cholesterol Ratio *Serum Decrease* Mean ratio of 0.42 ± 0.19 in 52 male patients with peripheral artery disease and 0.43 ± 0.20 in 30 women with peripheral artery disease significantly different in men but not significantly different in women from 0.57 ± 0.22 in 58 control men and 0.51 ± 0.22 in 38 control women, respectively *2538*

HDL_3-Cholesterol *Serum Decrease* Mean concentration of 0.63 ± 0.19 mmol/L in 52 male patients with peripheral artery disease and 0.74 ± 0.21 mmol/L in 30 women with peripheral artery disease significantly different from 0.75 ± 0.24 mmol/L in 58 control men and 0.98 ± 0.25 mmol/L in 38 control women, respectively *2538*

HDL-Cholesterol *Serum Decrease* In 121 patients with peripheral arterial disease mean concentration of 1.36 ± 0.04 mmol/L significantly less than 1.52 ± 0.04 mmol/L in 126 healthy controls *4903* Mean concentration of 1.06 ± 0.30 mmol/L in 52 male patients with peripheral artery disease and 1.15 ± 0.27 mmol/L in 30 women with peripheral artery disease significantly different from 1.22 ± 0.27 mmol/L in 58 control men and 1.39 ± 0.34 mmol/L in 38 control women, respectively *2538*
Serum Increase In 119 patients with hypercholesterolemia and symptomatic for peripheral artery disease mean concentration of 1.26 ± 0.33 mmol/L significantly different from 1.45 ± 0.34 mmol/L in 132 age and sex matched asymptomatic controls *477*
Serum No Effect In 17 white male patients with premature vascular disease mean concentration of 0.95 ± 0.06 mmol/L not significantly different from 0.92 ± 0.04 mmol/L in 32 age-matched white male controls *5384*

Hepatocyte Growth Factor *Serum Increase* In 37 patients with peripheral arterial disease mean concentration of 0.40 ± 0.02 ng/mL compared with 0.19 ± 0.01 ng/mL in 40 control individuals, with concentration tending to be higher in patients with collaterals *5817*

Homocysteine *Plasma Increase* 214 patients with symptomatic (claudication, rest pain, gangrene, amputation) lower extremity arterial occlusive disease and/or symptomatic (stroke, cerebral transient ischemic attacks) cerebral vascular disease and in 103 control persons. Mean plasma homocyst(e)ine was significantly higher in patients than in controls (14.37 ± 6.89 nmol/mL vs 10.10 ± 2.16 nmol/mL, p less than 0.05). Thirty-nine percent of patients (83 of 214) had plasma homocyst(e)ine values greater than control mean + 2 standard deviations *5176*

Laminin *Serum Increase* Mean concentration in 38 patients with stage IV peripheral arterial occlusive disease of 826 ± 97 ng/mL significantly increased compared with 379 ± 21 ng/mL in healthy individuals *635*

LDL-Cholesterol *Serum Increase* In 119 patients with hypercholesterolemia and symptomatic for peripheral artery disease mean concentration of 4.4 ± 1.3 mmol/L significantly different from 3.4 ± 0.9 mmol/L in 132 age and sex matched asymptomatic controls *477*
Serum No Effect In 17 white male patients with premature vascular disease mean concentration of 3.64 ± 0.19 mmol/L not significantly different from 3.31 ± 0.18 mmol/L in 32 age-matched white male controls *5384*

Lipoprotein Lp(a) *Serum Increase* In 89 patients with peripheral vascular disease mean concentration of 21 ± 2.2 mg/dL significantly higher than 13 ± 1.3 mg/dL in 129 healthy controls, but no significant difference observed between those patients with moderate and severe distal ischemia *4059* In 17 white male patients with premature vascular disease mean concentration of 44.8 ± 6.8 mg/dL significantly different from 11.9 ± 5.0 mg/dL in 32 age-matched white male controls *5384*

Plasminogen Activator Antigen-1 Activity *Plasma Increase* In 46 patients with peripheral arterial disease mean concentration of 12.1 - 26.8 U/mL significantly different from 4.4 - 14.9 U/mL in 76 healthy controls *4121*

Plasminogen Activator Inhibitor *Plasma Increase* In 121 patients with peripheral arterial disease mean concentration of 128.3% pool significantly greater than 108.2% pool in 126 healthy controls *4903*

Plasminogen Activator Inhibitor-1 *Plasma No Effect* Mean concentration of 21.64 ± 14.1 ng/mL in 14 patients with POAD not significantly different from 22.78 ± 8.29 ng/mL in 15 healthy controls *4718* In 16 patients mean concentration of 21.8 ± 7.2 ng/mL not significantly different from 22.78 ± 8.29 ng/mL in 15 healthy controls *4718*

Prostacyclin *Plasma Increase* Mean concentration of 27.5 ± 17.6 pg/mL in 15 patients significantly higher than 19.1 ± 5.3 pg/mL in 20 healthy controls *4718*
Plasma No Effect Mean concentration of 23.9 ± 12.7 pg/mL in 14 patients with POAD not significantly higher than 19.1 ± 5.3 pg/mL in 20 healthy controls *4718*

Protein C *Plasma Decrease* Mean percentage of normal 86 ± 26% in 193 patients with stable peripheral arterial disease compared with 100 ± 20% in normals *407*

Protein S *Plasma Decrease* In 193 patients with stable peripheral arterial disease mean percentage of normal 83 ± 24% compared with 100 ± 20% in normals *407*

Soluble Intercellular Adhesion Molecule-1 *Serum Increase* In 119 patients with hypercholesterolemia and symptomatic for peripheral artery disease, mean concentration of 359 ± 124 ng/mL significantly different from 298 ± 103 ng/mL in 132 age and sex matched asymptomatic controls *477*

Soluble Vascular Cell Adhesion Molecule-1
Serum Increase In 119 patients with hypercholesterolemia and symptomatic for peripheral artery disease mean concentration of 661 ± 216 ng/mL significantly different from 595 ± 159 ng/mL in 132 age and sex matched asymptomatic controls *477*

Thrombomodulin *Plasma Increase* Mean concentration in 16 patients of 49.6 ± 17.2 ng/mL significantly higher than 35.9 ± 8.1 ng/mL in 21 healthy controls *4718* Mean concentration of 51.3 ± 19.7 ng/mL in 15 patients with POAD significantly higher than 35.9 ± 8.1 ng/mL in 21 healthy controls *4718*

Tissue Plasminogen Activator *Plasma Increase* In 193 patients with peripheral arterial disease mean concentration of 7.1 ± 4.5 ng/mL compared with 2.3 ± 1.6 ng/mL in healthy volunteers *407* In 121 patients with peripheral arterial disease mean concentration of 7.54 ng/mL significantly greater than 6.23 ng/mL in 126 healthy controls *4903* Mean concentration of 12.4 ± 4.2 ng/mL in 16 patients significantly higher than 7.88 ± 10.1 ng/mL in 21 healthy controls *4718* Mean concentration of 15.38 ± 11.2 ng/mL in 14 patients with POAD significantly higher than 7.88 ± 10.1 ng/mL in 21 healthy controls *4718*

Triglycerides *Serum Increase* In 121 patients with peripheral arterial disease mean concentration of 1.68 mmol/L significantly greater than 1.28 mmol/L in 126 healthy controls *4903* In 119 patients with hypercholesterolemia and symptomatic for peripheral artery disease mean concentration of 1.8 mmol/L significantly different from 1.4 mmol/L in 132 age and sex matched asymptomatic controls *477* Mean concentration of 1.73 ± 0.52 mmol/L in 52 male patients with peripheral artery disease and 1.45 ± 0.39 mmol/L in 30 women with peripheral artery disease significantly different from 1.30 ± 0.38 mmol/L in 58 control men and 0.96 ± 0.31 mmol/L in 38 control women, respectively *2538*
Serum No Effect In 17 white male patients with premature vascular disease mean concentration of 1.8 ± 0.13 mmol/L not significantly different from 2.0 ± 0.52 mmol/L in 32 age-matched white male controls *5384*

VLDL-Cholesterol *Serum No Effect* In 17 white male patients with premature vascular disease mean concentration of 0.66 ± 0.08 mmol/L not significantly different from 0.99 ± 0.17 mmol/L in 32 age-matched white male controls *5384*

von Willebrand Factor *Plasma Decrease* In 46 patients with peripheral arterial disease significant difference in activity of 112 - 192% compared with 156 - 262% in 76 healthy controls *4121*

443.90 Peripheral Vascular Disease

α_1-Antichymotrypsin *Serum No Effect* Mean concentration within reference interval of 47.9 ± 8.1 mg/dL in one examined patient with peripheral vascular disease *3044*

Cholesterol *Serum Increase* Mean concentration of 6.4 ± 1.3 mmol/L in 170 patients with peripheral vascular disease significantly different from 5.6 ± 1.2 mmol/L in 119 healthy controls *475*

Fibrinogen *Plasma Increase* Mean concentration of 3.6 ± 0.7 g/L in 170 patients with peripheral vascular disease significantly different from 3.0 ± 0.5 g/L in 119 healthy controls *475*

Mean concentration in 55 patients with peripheral vascular disease of 4.1 ± 0.8 g/L significantly different from 3.1 ± 0.9 mmol/L in 55 matched controls *473*

Glucose *Serum* *Increase* Mean concentration of 5.5 ± 0.3 mmol/L in 170 patients with peripheral vascular disease not significantly different from 5.2 ± 0.4 mmol/L in 119 healthy controls *475*

HDL-Cholesterol *Serum* *Decrease* Mean concentration in 55 patients with peripheral vascular disease of 1.2 ± 0.4 mmol/L significantly different from 1.4 ± 0.3 mmol/L in 55 matched controls *473* Mean concentration of 1.3 ± 0.3 mmol/L in 170 patients with peripheral vascular disease significantly different from 1.4 ± 0.4 mmol/L in 119 healthy controls *475*

LDL-Cholesterol *Serum* *Increase* Mean concentration of 4.2 ± 1.1 mmol/L in 170 patients with peripheral vascular disease significantly different from 3.6 ± 1.0 mmol/L in 119 healthy controls *475* Mean concentration in 55 patients with peripheral vascular disease of 4.4 ± 1.0 mmol/L significantly different from 3.5 ± 1.0 mmol/L in 55 matched controls *473*

Platelets *Blood* *Decrease* Mean concentration of 187 ± 86 x 10^9 cells/mL in 84 patients with HIV-1 infection significantly different from 295 ± 56 x 10^9 cells/mL in 84 healthy controls *476*

Soluble P-Selectin *Plasma* *Increase* Median concentration of 222.5 ng/mL in 84 patients with HIV-1 infection significantly different from 200 ng/mL in 84 healthy controls *476*
Serum *Increase* Mean concentration in 55 patients with peripheral vascular disease of 6.5 ± 1.4 mmol/L significantly different from 5.6 ± 1.0 mmol/L in 55 matched controls *473* Median concentration of 287 ng/mL in 170 patients with peripheral vascular disease significantly different from normal range of 45 ± 700 ng/mL derived from 119 healthy controls *475*

Soluble Tumor Necrosis Factor Receptor-p55
Serum *No Effect* In 20 patients with peripheral vascular disease mean concentration of 2.22 ± 1.46 ng/mL compared with 1.90 ± 0.63 ng/mL in 20 age and sex matched controls *474*

Soluble Tumor Necrosis Factor Receptor-p75
Serum *Increase* In 20 patients with peripheral vascular disease mean concentration of 3.92 ± 1.43 ng/mL compared with 2.41 ± 0.75 ng/mL in 20 age and sex matched controls *474*

β-Thromboglobulin *Plasma* *Increase* Mean concentration in 55 patients with peripheral vascular disease of 46 ± 14 ng/mL significantly different from 37 ± 12 ng/mL in 55 matched controls *473*

Thrombomodulin *Plasma* *Increase* Mean concentration in 55 patients with peripheral vascular disease of 55 ± 15 ng/mL significantly different from 46 ± 14 ng/mL in 55 matched controls *473*

Triglycerides *Serum* *Increase* Median concentration of 1.8 mmol/L in 170 patients with peripheral vascular disease significantly different from 1.4 mmol/L in 119 healthy controls *475* Mean concentration in 55 patients with peripheral vascular disease of 2.0 mmol/L significantly different from 1.5 mmol/L in 55 matched controls *473*

Tumor Necrosis Factor *Serum* *Increase* In 20 patients with peripheral vascular disease mean concentration of 1.78 ± 0.59 pg/mL compared with 1.19 ± 0.46 pg/mL in 20 age and sex matched controls *474*

von Willebrand Factor *Plasma* *Increase* Mean concentration in 55 patients with peripheral vascular disease of 133 ± 34 IU/dL significantly different from 102 ± 30 IU/dL in 55 matched controls *473* Mean concentration of 168 ± 50 IU/dL in 84 patients with HIV-1 infection significantly different from 104 ± 35 IU/dL in 84 healthy controls *476* In 20 patients with peripheral vascular disease mean concentration of 129 ± 29 IU/dL compared with 101 ± 26 IU/dL in 20 age and sex matched controls *474*

444.90 Arterial Embolism and Thrombosis

Acid Phosphatase *Serum* *Increase* Acid hyperphenylphosphatasia which lasted from 3 - 6 days and reached a maximum of 4.1, 5.8, and 7 U/L, respectively, was noted after each of the 3 episodes of thromboembolism *4661* Peak activity is reached 2 - 3 days after onset of symptoms *4707*

Albumin *Urine* *Increase* Constant finding among 31 patients *2304*

Aspartate Aminotransferase *Serum* *Increase* In 38% of 37 patients hospitalized for this disorder *1576*

Creatinine *Serum* *Increase* In 50% of 21 patients hospitalized for this disorder *1576*

Lactate Dehydrogenase *Serum* *Increase* In 32% of 37 patients hospitalized for this disorder *1576*

Leukocytes *Blood* *Increase* In 47% of 46 patients hospitalized for this disorder *1576*

Myoglobin *Urine* *Increase* Sporadic; ischemia *5544* Sudden muscle damage due to ischemia, e.g., thrombosis of artery supplying a large muscle mass *1290*

Neutrophils *Blood* *Increase* In 50% of 40 patients hospitalized for this disorder *1576*

Urea Nitrogen *Serum* *Increase* In 34% of 42 patients hospitalized for this disorder *1576* Progressive azotemia *2304*

446.00 Microscopic Polyangitis

Anti-Myeloperoxidase Antibodies *Serum* *Increase* In 51 patients with microscopic polyangitis antibodies to myeloperoxidase present in 31 patients *1910*

Anti-Myeloperoxidase-Antineutrophil Cytoplasmic Autoantibodies *Serum* *Increase* In 22 patients with microscopic polyangitis 14 (64%) demonstrated anti-myeloperoxidase-ANCA positivity *2879*

Anti-Neutrophil Cytoplasm Antibodies *Serum* *Increase* Antibodies detected in 2.5% of 78 patients *162* In 51 patients with microscopic polyangitis ANCA present in 38 (74.5%) of which 33 had a perinuclear staining pattern and 5 had a cytoplasmic staining pattern *1910*

Anti-Proteinase 3--Antineutrophil Cytoplasmic Autoantibodies *Plasma* *Increase* In 22 patients with microscopic polyangitis 2 (9%) demonstrated anti-proteinase 3-ANCA positivity *2879*

Antibodies to Proteinase 3 *Serum* *Increase* In 51 patients with microscopic polyangitis antibodies to proteinase 3 present in 4 patients *1910*

Blood *Urine* *Increase* In 67 patients with microscopic polyangitis and renal signs hematuria present in 45 patients (67.2%) *1910*

c-Antineutrophil Cytoplasmic Autoantibodies
Plasma *Increase* In 22 patients with microscopic polyangitis 2 (9%) demonstrated c-ANCA positivity *2879*

Creatinine *Serum* *Increase* In 85 patients with microscopic polyangitis mean serum concentration of 2.59 ± 2.96 mg/dL with renal signs present in 67 patients (78.8%) *1910*

Elastase Antineutrophil Cytoplasmic Autoantibodies
Serum *Increase* Antibodies detected in 78.2% of 78 patients *162*

Leukocytes *Urine* *Increase* In 67 patients with microscopic polyangitis and renal signs leukocyturia present in 30 patients (44.8%) *1910*

Myeloperoxidase Antineutrophil Cytoplasmic Autoantibodies
Serum *Increase* Antibodies detected in 78.2% of 78 patients *162*

p-Antineutrophil Cytoplasmic Autoantibodies
Plasma *Increase* In 22 patients with microscopic polyangitis 20 (91%) demonstrated p-ANCA positivity *2879*

Perinuclear Antineutrophil Cytoplasmic Autoantibodies
Serum *Increase* Antibodies detected in 88.4% of 78 patients *162*

Protein *Urine* *Increase* In 85 patients with microscopic polyangitis and renal signs proteinuria (0.5 - 6 g/d) present in 54 patients (80.6%) *1910*

Proteinase 3-Antineutrophil Cytoplasmic Autoantibodies
Serum *Increase* Antibodies detected in 5.1% of 78 patients *162*

446.00 Periarteritis

Complement C_1 *Serum* *Increase* Mean concentration typically slightly increased or normal in patients with periarteritis *4682*

446.00 Periarteritis *(continued)*

Complement C_1q *Serum* *Increase* Mean concentration typically slightly increased or normal in patients with periarteritis *4682*

Complement C_2 *Serum* *Increase* Mean concentration typically slightly increased or normal in patients with periarteritis *4682*

Complement C_3 *Serum* *Increase* Mean concentration typically slightly increased or normal in patients with periarteritis *4682*

Complement C_4 *Serum* *Increase* Mean concentration typically slightly increased or normal in patients with periarteritis *4682*

Complement C_5 *Serum* *Increase* Mean concentration typically slightly increased or normal in patients with periarteritis *4682*

Complement CH50 *Serum* *Increase* Mean concentration typically slightly increased or normal in patients with periarteritis *4682*

Properdin Factor B *Plasma* *Increase* Mean concentration typically slightly increased or normal in patients with periarteritis *4682*

446.00 Polyarteritis

Anti-DNA Antibodies *Serum* *No Effect* In 10 patients with microscopic polyarteritis none were positive for anti-DNA antibodies *3029*

Anti-Endothelial Cell Antibodies *Serum* *Increase* 2% of patients with microscopic polyarteritis had anti-endothelial cell antibodies *5425* Observed effect *5798*

Anti-Myeloperoxidase Antibodies *Serum* *Increase* In 8 patients with microscopic polyarteritis all were positive for anti-myeloperoxidase antibodies *3029*

Anti-Neutrophil Cytoplasm Antibodies *Serum* *Increase* Circulating antibodies are found in about 80% of active cases of Wegener's granulomatosis and microscopic polyarteritis *4601* Particularly associated with various forms of vasculitis including Wegener's granulomatosis, Kawasaki disease and microscopic polyarteritis *1174* Observed effect *4953*

Antinuclear Factor *Serum* *Increase* In 10 patients with microscopic polyarteritis 3 were positive for ANCA *3029*

Soluble Intercellular Adhesion Molecule-1 *Serum* *Increase* In 2 patients with active vasculitis mean concentration of 498 ng/mL significantly higher than mean concentration of 270 ± 47 ng/mL in 10 healthy controls: no significant difference in concentrations between patients with active and inactive vasculitis *2461*

446.00 Polyarteritis Nodosa

Albumin *Serum* *Decrease* Hypoalbuminemia occurs only in those patients with the nephrotic syndrome *1980*
Urine *Increase* Abnormal urinalysis is far more frequent (70 - 80%) than azotemia (25 - 30%) *900*

Ammonium Ions *Urine* *Increase* May be associated with classic distal renal tubular acidosis which is associated with hyokalemia, hyperchloremic metabolic acidosis, urine pH > 5.5, increased urinary ammonium ion excretion, a negative urine anion gap, increased urinary osmol gap, decreased urinary citrate and increased urinary calcium in some patients *4071*

Anion Gap *Urine* *Decrease* May be associated with classic distal renal tubular acidosis which is associated with hyokalemia, hyperchloremic metabolic acidosis, urine pH > 5.5, increased urinary ammonium ion excretion, a negative urine anion gap, increased urinary osmol gap, decreased urinary citrate and increased urinary calcium in some patients *4071*

Anti-Neutrophil Cytoplasm Antibodies *Serum* *Increase* In 2 of 5 patients (40%) with polyarteritis nodosa pANCA detected *3722*
Serum *No Effect* Antibodies not detected in any of 18 patients *162*

Antinuclear Antibodies *Serum* *Increase* Infrequently seen and, when present, are in low titer *1980* In 2 of 5 patients (40%) with polyarteritis nodosa ANA detected *3722* Usually absent, and when present should suggest that the arteritis is part of another disorder *4551*

Calcium *Urine* *Increase* May be associated with classic distal renal tubular acidosis which is associated with hyokalemia, hyperchloremic metabolic acidosis, urine pH > 5.5, increased urinary ammonium ion excretion, a negative urine anion gap, increased urinary osmol gap, decreased urinary citrate and increased urinary calcium in some patients *4071*

Cellular Casts *Urine* *Increase* Found in patients with glomerular disease *2039*

Chloride *Serum* *Increase* May be associated with classic distal renal tubular acidosis which is associated with hyokalemia, hyperchloremic metabolic acidosis, urine pH > 5.5, increased urinary ammonium ion excretion, a negative urine anion gap, increased urinary osmol gap, decreased urinary citrate and increased urinary calcium in some patients *4071*

Cholesterol *Serum* *Increase* Leading to nephrosis *5544*

Citrate *Urine* *Decrease* May be associated with classic distal renal tubular acidosis which is associated with hyokalemia, hyperchloremic metabolic acidosis, urine pH > 5.5, increased urinary ammonium ion excretion, a negative urine anion gap, increased urinary osmol gap, decreased urinary citrate and increased urinary calcium in some patients *4071*

Cold Agglutinins *Serum* *Increase* Have been reported *1980*

Complement, Total *Serum* *Decrease* Depression of titers may be found in early, acute phases *1315* Subsides with remission *4683*
Serum *Increase* Elevated during active inflammation and subsides with remission *4683* Possibly the result of low utilization or a rapid rate of production *1980* In some patients *65*

Coombs' Test *Serum* *Negative* Usual observation *1315*

C-Reactive Protein *Serum* *Increase* Mean concentration of 78 mg/L in 15 patients significantly greater than in healthy controls *208*

Creatinine *Serum* *Increase* With renal involvement *2034*

Cryoglobulins *Serum* *Increase* Cryoglobulinemia is rarely reported, but this may reflect late collection or improper handling of specimens *4551* Variable elevation of cryoglobulins *4707*

Elastase Antineutrophil Cytoplasmic Autoantibodies *Serum* *No Effect* Antibodies not detected in any of 18 patients *162*

Eosinophils *Blood* *Increase* Hallmark of patients with allergic granulomatosis and angiitis is eosinophilia > 400 /µL, and usually > 1,500 /µL. This degree of eosinophilia is rarely seen in patients with polyarteritis in whom the lungs are spared *1315* Eosinophilia is almost exclusively related to the variants of necrotizing angiitis with pulmonary involvement, it is uncommonly seen in classical polyarteritis *1980*

Erythrocyte Sedimentation Rate *Blood* *Increase* Almost a prerequisite for diagnosis *900* Mean rate of 68 mm/h in 16 patients with active disease significantly greater than in healthy controls *208* Almost always elevated in active untreated polyarteritis *4551* Generally reflects the intensity of the disease activity *2039* Generally elevated (often exceeding 80 mm/h Westergren) *1980*

Erythrocytes *Urine* *Increase* Abnormal urinalysis is far more frequent (70 - 80%) than azotemia (25 - 30%) *900* Hematuria is likely to be intermittent *1980* Microscopic hematuria is found in patients with glomerular disease *2039*

Fibrinogen *Plasma* *Increase* Mean concentration of 5.8 g/L in 16 patients with active disease significantly greater than in healthy controls *208*

α_1-Globulin *Serum* *Increase* Moderate increase *1290*

α_2-Globulin *Serum* *Increase* Marked increase *1290*

β-Globulin *Serum* *Increase* Moderate increase in some cases *1290*

γ-Globulin *Serum* *Increase* Frequently found *1980*
Serum *No Effect* Concentration usually normal *5544*

Granular Casts *Urine* *Increase* Hyaline and granular casts indicate renal involvement *367* Abnormal urinalysis is far more frequent (70 - 80%) than azotemia (25 - 30%) *900*

Hematocrit *Blood* *Decrease* Anemia is found chiefly in cases complicated by renal insufficiency or blood loss *1980* Mild anemia is frequently present due either to blood loss or to chronic renal insufficiency *1315* Almost a prerequisite for diagnosis *900*

Hemoglobin *Blood* *Decrease* Almost a prerequisite for diagnosis *900* Anemia is found chiefly in cases complicated by renal insufficiency or blood loss *1980* Mild anemia is frequently present due either to blood loss or to chronic renal insufficiency *1315*

Hepatitis B Surface Antigen *Serum* *Increase* Found in approximately 25% of patients, independent of apparent liver involvement *1980* In cases associated with hepatitis B infection the hepatitis B surface antigen is persistently detectable, usually at high titers, throughout the illness *4551*

Hyaline Casts *Urine* *Increase* Hyaline and granular casts indicate renal involvement *367*

Immune Complexes *Serum* *Increase* Mean concentration of 317 µg/mL in 12 patients with active disease significantly greater than in healthy controls *208*

Immunoglobulin D *Serum* *Increase* Reported effect *1290*

Immunoglobulins *Serum* *No Effect* Usually within normal limits *4551*

Iron *Serum* *Increase* Anemia may be due to chronic blood loss *1980* *1315*

Iron-binding Capacity, Total *Serum* *Increase* Anemia may be due to chronic blood loss *1315* *1980*

Iron Saturation *Serum* *Decrease* Anemia may be due to chronic blood loss *1315* *1980*

Leukocytes *Blood* *Increase* Polymorphonuclear leukocytosis (the result of inflammatory and necrotic lesions) occurs in the majority of patients *1980* Usually associated with leukocytosis, often 15,000 /µL or more *2039* Almost a prerequisite for diagnosis *900* In about 80% of cases, there is mild leukocytosis with a shift to the left *4551*
Urine *Increase* Found in patients with glomerular disease *2039*

MCH *Blood* *Decrease* Microcytic hypochromic anemia may occur due to blood loss, increased demand or dietary inadequacy. MCH < 27 pg, MCV < 80 fL *1098* Mild anemia is frequently present due either to blood loss or to chronic renal failure *1315* Anemia is found chiefly in cases complicated by renal insufficiency or blood loss *1980*

MCHC *Blood* *Decrease* Anemia is found chiefly in cases complicated by renal insufficiency or blood loss *1980* Mild anemia is frequently present due either to blood loss or to chronic renal failure *1315*

MCV *Blood* *Decrease* Microcytic hypochromic anemia may occur due to blood loss, increased demand or dietary inadequacy. MCH < 27 pg, MCV < 80 fL *1098*

Monocytes *Blood* *Increase* Has been reported *3246*

Myeloperoxidase Antineutrophil Cytoplasmic Autoantibodies
Serum *No Effect* Antibodies not detected in any of 18 patients *162*

Net Acid Excretion *Urine* *Increase* May be associated with classic distal renal tubular acidosis which is associated with hyokalemia, hyperchloremic metabolic acidosis, urine pH > 5.5, increased urinary ammonium ion excretion, a negative urine anion gap, increased urinary osmol gap, decreased urinary citrate and increased urinary calcium in some patients *4071*

Neutrophil Proteinase 3 *Serum* *Increase* In 4 patients with active polyarteritis nodosa mean concentration of 236 ± 117 µg/mL and mean of 158 ± 51 µg/mL in 4 patients with inactive disease significantly higher than mean of 78 ± 30 µg/mL in 21 normal individuals *2120*

Neutrophils *Blood* *Increase* In about 80% of cases, there is mild leukocytosis with a shift to the left *4551*

Osmolal Gap *Urine* *Increase* May be associated with classic distal renal tubular acidosis which is associated with hyokalemia, hyperchloremic metabolic acidosis, urine pH > 5.5, increased urinary ammonium ion excretion, a negative urine anion gap, increased urinary osmol gap, decreased urinary citrate and increased urinary calcium in some patients *4071*

Perinuclear Antineutrophil Cytoplasmic Autoantibodies
Serum *No Effect* Antibodies not detected in any of 18 patients *162*

pH *Urine* *Increase* May be associated with classic distal renal tubular acidosis which is associated with hyokalemia, hyperchloremic metabolic acidosis, urine pH > 5.5, increased urinary ammonium ion excretion, a negative urine anion gap, increased urinary osmol gap, decreased urinary citrate and increased urinary calcium in some patients *4071*

Platelets *Blood* *Increase* Counts > 500,000 /µL frequently found *2039*

Potassium *Serum* *Decrease* May be associated with classic distal renal tubular acidosis which is associated with hyokalemia, hyperchloremic metabolic acidosis, urine pH > 5.5, increased urinary ammonium ion excretion, a negative urine anion gap, increased urinary osmol gap, decreased urinary citrate and increased urinary calcium in some patients *4071*

Protein *Urine* *Increase* With renal involvement *1980* Found in patients with glomerular disease *2039*

Proteinase 3-Antineutrophil Cytoplasmic Autoantibodies
Serum *No Effect* Antibodies not detected in any of 18 patients *162*

Rheumatoid Factor *Serum* *Increase* Present in some patients *2039*
Serum *No Effect* Usually absent, and when present should suggest that the arteritis is part of another disorder *4551*

Ristocetin Cofactor *Plasma* *Increase* Mean activity of 266 ± 90% of normal in 16 patients with active disease significantly greater than 103 ± 20% in 20 healthy controls *208*

Urea Nitrogen *Serum* *Increase* With renal involvement *2034*

von Willebrand Factor Antigen *Plasma* *Increase* Mean concentration of 237 ± 106% of normal in 16 patients with active disease significantly increased compared with 72 ± 21% in 20 healthy controls *208*

446.10 Bronchiolitis

Eosinophil Cationic Protein *Serum* *Increase* Mean concentration of > 16 µg/L observed in 14 of 92 children on admission to hospital for acute bronchiolitis *4315*

446.10 Kawasaki Disease

Alanine Aminotransferase *Serum* *Increase* In 40 patients with Kawasaki disease mean activity of > 40 U/L in 17 significantly different from none in 106 controls *2353*

Albumin *Serum* *Decrease* In 40 patients with Kawasaki disease mean concentration of < 35 g/L in 23 significantly different from none in 106 controls *2353*

Angiotensin-converting Enzyme *Serum* *Decrease* Mean activity of 2.8 ± 1.7 pmol/mol/min in 12 children with active Kawasaki disease significantly lower than 4.8 ± 2.7 pmol/mol/min in 12 healthy control children *1412*

Anti-Endothelial Cell Antibodies *Serum* *Increase* 3 of 18 patients with KD and 8 of 20 febrile control patients had AECA (p value not significant) *1938* AECA have been detected in systemic lupus erythematosus, scleroderma and dermatomyositis but are also found in systemic vasculitis, Kawasaki disease, hemolytic uremic syndrome, thrombotic thrombocytopenic purpura and renal allograft recipients at the time of rejection *1174*

Anti-Neutrophil Cytoplasm Antibodies *Serum* *Increase* We found that 7 of 18 patients with Kawasaki disease (KD) and 6 of 20 febrile control patients had ANCA (by immunofluorescence or ELISA, p value not significant) *1938* Particularly associated with various forms of vasculitis including Wegener's granulomatosis, Kawasaki disease and microscopic polyarteritis *1174*

Blood *Urine* *Increase* In 40 patients with Kawasaki disease blood present in 7, significantly different from none in 106 controls *2353*

Cholesterol *Serum* *Decrease* In 23 patients (16 boys) with Kawasaki disease mean concentration reduced to 3.32 ± 0.85 mmol/L within 30 days of disease *4534*

C-Reactive Protein *Serum* *Increase* Median concentration in acute stage of 8.3 mg/dL in 20 patients with Kawasaki disease significantly different from normal of 0.1 mg/dL *3203* In 40 patients with Kawasaki disease mean concentration of 103 ± 58 mg/L significantly different from < 5 mg/L in 106 controls *2353* Mean concentration of 23 ± 5 mg/dL in 12 children with active Kawasaki disease significantly higher than < 0.25 mg/dL in 12 healthy control children *1412*

Endothelin-1 *Plasma* *Increase* Plasma immunoreactive endothelin (iET) levels were investigated in patients with Kawasaki disease (KD). The iET level was 2.49 ± 0.13 pg/mL in KD patients and 1.32 ± 0.06 in age-matched control subjects, showing a significant increase with KD *3607*

446.10 Kawasaki Disease *(continued)*

Epstein Barr Virus Antibodies *Serum* *Increase* Forty-nine (86%) of 57 patients and 15 (68%) or 22 patients with recurrent disease had serological evidence of primary infection during the first month after the onset of their disease based on the results of a sensitive method of detecting antibody to viral capsid antigen *2677*

Erythrocyte Sedimentation Rate *Blood* *Increase* Mean rate of 80 ± 23 mm/h in 12 children with active Kawasaki disease significantly higher than 7 ± 6 mm/h in 12 healthy control children *1412*

HDL-Cholesterol *Serum* *Decrease* In 23 patients (16 boys) mean concentration reduced to 0.54 ± 0.25 mmol/L within 30 days of onset of disease *4534*

Hemoglobin *Blood* *Decrease* In 40 patients with Kawasaki disease mean concentration of < 100 g/L in 12 of 40 patients significantly different from none in 106 controls *2353* Mean concentration of 8.5 ± 1.1 g/dL in 12 children with active Kawasaki disease significantly lower than 11.5 ± 1.7 g/dL in 12 healthy control children *1412*

Interferon-γ *Serum* *Increase* In 15 patients with Kawasaki disease concentration during active phase of the disease 0.4 - 1.6 U/mL significantly higher than 0.2 - 1.2 U/mL in the convalescent phase and 0.3 - 0.7 U/mL in controls *2168*

Interleukin-4 *Serum* *Increase* In 15 patients with Kawasaki disease concentration during active phase of the disease of 7 - 108 pg/mL significantly higher than 0 - 24 pg/mL in the convalescent phase and 4 - 21 pg/mL in controls *2168*

Interleukin-6 *Serum* *Increase* Determined in 25 patients with Kawasaki disease (KD) and in healthy children. IL-6 activity in the sera of patients was seen to increase during the acute stage *3357* Serum IL-6 levels were increased in acute KD as well as in febrile controls *5366* In 24 patients with Kawasaki disease mean peak concentration of 78 ± 111 pg/mL in first week significantly different from < 8 pg/mL in 20 controls *2353*
Serum *No Effect* In 23 patients with Kawasaki disease mean peak concentration of < 8 pg/mL in first week not significantly different from < 8 pg/mL in 20 controls *2353*
Urine *Increase* Urinary IL-6 levels were consistently elevated in patients with acute KD, but much lower in febrile controls *5366*

Interleukin-10 *Serum* *Increase* Mean concentration in 23 patients with Kawasaki disease of 125.037 ± 111.161 pg/mL significantly higher than that in 13 individuals hospitalized for elective surgery, 16.042 ± 5.088 pg/mL *3819* In 15 patients with Kawasaki disease concentration during active phase of the disease 6 - 305 pg/mL significantly higher than 1 - 615 pg/mL in the convalescent phase and 3 - 19 pg/mL in controls *2168*

Interleukin-11 *Serum* *No Effect* In 20 patients with Kawasaki disease mean peak concentration of < 16 pg/mL in first week not significantly different from < 16 pg/mL in 20 controls *2353*

Leukemia Inhibitory Factor *Serum* *No Effect* In 20 patients with Kawasaki disease mean peak concentration of < 16 pg/mL in first week not significantly different from < 16 pg/mL in 20 controls *2353*

Leukocytes *Blood* *Increase* Mean concentration of 32,000 ± 16,000 /µL in 12 children with active Kawasaki disease significantly higher than 6,850 ± 1,900 /µL in 12 healthy control children *1412* Median concentration in acute stage of 14.9 x 10^3/µL in 20 patients with Kawasaki disease significantly higher than normal of 8.7 x 10^3 /µL *3203* In 40 patients with Kawasaki disease mean concentration of 13.2 ± 3.9 x 10^9/L significantly different from 8.5 ± 2.6 x 10^9/L in 106 controls *2353*
Blood *No Effect* Median concentration in acute stage of 36.5 x 10^4 /µL in 20 patients with Kawasaki disease not significantly different from normal of 32.3 x 10^4 /µL *3203*

β_2-Microglobulin *Urine* *Increase* Urinary levels of N-acetyl-β-D-glucosaminidase (NAG) and β_2-microglobulin (beta 2-m) were also elevated during the acute phase of this disease *5366*

N-Acetyl-Glucosaminidase *Urine* *Increase* Urinary levels of N-acetyl-β-D-glucosaminidase (NAG) and β_2-microglobulin (beta 2-m) were also elevated during the acute phase of this disease *5366*

Nerve Growth Factor *Serum* *Increase* Mean concentration in 12 children with active disease of 1,220 ± 1,600 pg/mL significantly different from 277 ± 246 pg/mL in inactive phase of disease and 6.5 ± 2.0 pg/mL in 12 healthy control children *1412*

Neutrophils *Blood* *Increase* In 40 patients with Kawasaki disease mean concentration of 8.5 ± 3.7 x 10^9/L significantly different from 3.3 ± 1.5 x 10^9/L in 106 controls *2353*

Platelets *Blood* *Decrease* In 12 patients with Kawasaki disease mean concentrations ranged from 47 to 457 x 10^9/L *3529*
Blood *Increase* Mean concentration of 620 ± 324 x 10^3 /µL in 12 children with active Kawasaki disease significantly higher than 380 ± 90 x 10^3 /µL in 12 healthy control children *1412*
Blood *No Effect* In 12 patients with Kawasaki disease mean concentrations ranged from 47 to 457 x 10^9/L *3529* In 40 patients with Kawasaki disease mean concentration of 318 ± 88 x 10^9/L not significantly different from 320 ± 68 x 10^9/L in 106 controls *2353*

Protein *Urine* *Increase* In 40 patients with Kawasaki disease blood present in 7, significantly different from none in 106 controls *2353*

Soluble Tumor Necrosis Factor Receptor-p60
Serum *Increase* In 48 pediatric patients with acute Kawasaki disease mean concentration of 6.3 ± 4.2 ng/mL significantly higher than 1.5 ± 0.5 ng/mL in 30 control children *1610*

Thrombopoietin *Plasma* *Increase* In 40 patients with Kawasaki disease mean peak concentration of 5.69 ± 2.66 fmol/mL in first week significantly different from 1.94 ± 0.69 fmol/mL in 106 controls *2353* In 11 patients with Kawasaki disease mean concentrations ranged from 107 to 294 pg/mL compared with undetectable levels in controls *3529*

Tumor Necrosis Factor-α *Serum* *Increase* Determined in 25 patients with Kawasaki disease (KD) and in healthy children. Levels in patients increased during the acute stage *3357*

Vascular Endothelial Growth Factor *Serum* *Increase* Median concentration in acute stage of Kawasaki disease in 3 patients with coronary artery lesions of 156.4 pg/mL and of 356.6 pg/mL in 17 patients with Kawasaki disease without coronary artery lesions significantly different from normal of 117.4 pg/mL *3203*

446.10 Mucocutaneous Lymph Node Syndrome

Amyloid A Protein *Serum* *Increase* In 8 patients mean concentration in acute phase of 2.71 ± 0.38 mg/L *3728*

C-Reactive Protein *Serum* *Increase* In 8 patients mean concentration in acute phase of 1.91 ± 0.33 mg/L *3728*

446.20 Churg-Strauss Syndrome

Anti-Neutrophil Cytoplasm Antibodies *Serum* *No Effect* Antibodies not detected in any of 6 patients *162* In 0 of 2 patients (0%) with Churg-Strauss syndrome pANCA detected *3722*

Antinuclear Antibodies *Serum* *No Effect* In 0 of 2 patients (0%) with Churg-Strauss syndrome ANA detected *3722*

Elastase Antineutrophil Cytoplasmic Autoantibodies
Serum *No Effect* Antibodies not detected in any of 6 patients *162*

Myeloperoxidase Antineutrophil Cytoplasmic Autoantibodies
Serum *Increase* Antibodies detected in 83.3% of 6 patients *162*

Perinuclear Antineutrophil Cytoplasmic Autoantibodies
Serum *Increase* Antibodies detected in 66.7% of 6 patients *162*

Proteinase 3-Antineutrophil Cytoplasmic Autoantibodies
Serum *No Effect* Antibodies not detected in any of 6 patients *162*

446.20 Collagen Vascular Disease

KL-6 Antigen *Serum* *Increase* In 11 patients with collagen vascular disease mean concentration of 1,051 ± 417 U/mL significantly different from 207 ± 6 U/mL in 237 healthy controls *5134*

446.21 Goodpasture's Syndrome

Anti-Myeloperoxidase Antibodies *Serum* *Increase* Weakly positive results may occur in patients with Goodpasture's syndrome *2952*

Antibody Titer *Serum* *Increase* Glomerular and alveolar basement membrane antibodies *3712* Circulating antibodies to glycopeptide antigen are found in over 90% of cases *126*

Complement C_1 *Serum* *No Effect* Mean concentration typically normal in patients with chronic glomerulonephritis or Goodpasture's syndrome *4682*

Complement C_1q *Serum* *No Effect* Mean concentration typically normal in patients with chronic glomerulonephritis or Goodpasture's syndrome *4682*

Complement C_2 *Serum* *No Effect* Mean concentration typically normal in patients with chronic glomerulonephritis or Goodpasture's syndrome *4682*

Complement C_3 *Serum* *No Effect* Mean concentration typically normal in patients with chronic glomerulonephritis or Goodpasture's syndrome *4682* Almost always normal *126*

Complement C_4 *Serum* *No Effect* Almost always normal *126*

Complement C_5 *Serum* *No Effect* Mean concentration typically normal in patients with chronic glomerulonephritis or Goodpasture's syndrome *4682*

Complement CH50 *Serum* *No Effect* Mean concentration typically normal in patients with chronic glomerulonephritis or Goodpasture's syndrome *4682*

Complement, Total *Serum* *No Effect* Almost always normal *126*

Creatinine *Serum* *Increase* Progressive renal failure *126*

Glomerular Basement Membrane Antibody *Serum* *Increase* Increased concentrations often above 250 units occur in patients with Goodpasture's syndrome (glomerulonephritis and pulmonary hemorrhage) *2952*

Hematocrit *Blood* *Decrease* Secondary to prolonged pulmonary bleeding *126*

Hemoglobin *Blood* *Decrease* Secondary to prolonged pulmonary bleeding *126*

HLA Antigens *Blood* *Present* HLA-DR2 is twenty five times more likely in patients with this disease and caries with it a worse prognosis *5428*

Iron *Serum* *Decrease* Secondary to prolonged pulmonary bleeding *126*

Iron-binding Capacity, Total *Serum* *Increase* Secondary to prolonged pulmonary bleeding *126*

Iron Saturation *Serum* *Decrease* Secondary to prolonged pulmonary bleeding *126*

MCHC *Blood* *Decrease* Secondary to prolonged pulmonary bleeding *126*

Oxygen Partial Pressure *Blood* *Decrease* Secondary to prolonged pulmonary bleeding *126*

Procollagen Type IV Peptide *Serum* *Increase* Sequential serum concentrations in one patient with active Goodpasture's syndrome were marginally elevated (less than 11 ng/mL) *2623*

Properdin Factor B *Plasma* *No Effect* Mean concentration typically normal in patients with chronic glomerulonephritis or Goodpasture's syndrome *4682*

Soluble Intercellular Adhesion Molecule-1 *Serum* *Increase* In 6 patients with active vasculitis mean concentration of 508 ± 126 ng/mL significantly higher than mean concentration of 270 ± 47 ng/mL in 10 healthy controls: no significant difference between concentrations in active and inactive vasculitis *2461*

Urea Nitrogen *Serum* *Increase* Progressive renal failure *126*

446.40 Granulomatous Angiitis

Oligoclonal Banding *Cerebrospinal Fluid* *Increase* Oligoclonal IgG bands detected with granulomatous angiitis *3261*

446.40 Wegener's Granulomatosis

Anti-Endothelial Cell Antibodies *Serum* *Increase* Only 19% of patients with Wegener's granulomatosis had anti-endothelial cell antibodies(AECA) *5425* IgG AECA were demonstrated in 59% and IgM AECA in 68% of patients *5400*

Anti-Myeloperoxidase-Antineutrophil Cytoplasmic Autoantibodies *Serum* *Increase* In 21 patients with Wegener's granulomatosis 4 (19%) demonstrated anti-myeloperoxidase-ANCA positivity *2879*

Anti-Neutrophil Cytoplasm Antibodies *Serum* *Increase* Antibodies detected in 84.2% of 108 patients *162* 84 - 100% have increased Cytoplasmic ANCA *4953* In 21 of 23 patients with generalized (92%) or localized (62%) Wegener's granulomatosis indirect immunofluorescent test was positive whereas all healthy control blood donors were negative *1676* In multiple studies sensitivities for disease of 34 - 92% and specificities of 88 - 100%, with sensitivities greater for active than inactive disease *4276* In 3 patients with active disease mean concentration of 46 SLI units significantly higher than < 22 SLI units in 4 patients with disease in remission *3872* Median concentration of 1:64 observed in 57 patients with Wegener's granulomatosis *5561* Circulating antibodies are found in about 80% of active cases of Wegener's granulomatosis and microscopic polyarteritis *4601* PR3-ANCA are serological markers for Wegener's granulomatosis (WG) *1886* Particularly associated with various forms of vasculitis including Wegener's granulomatosis, Kawasaki disease and microscopic polyarteritis *1174*

Anti-Proteinase 3--Antineutrophil Cytoplasmic Autoantibodies *Plasma* *Increase* In 21 patients with Wegener's granulomatosis 15 (71%) demonstrated anti-proteinase 3-ANCA positivity *2879*

Anticardiolipin Antibodies *Serum* *Increase* Reported effect *2126*

Antiproteinase 3 Antibodies *Serum* *Increase* In 2 patients with active disease mean concentration of 50 U/mL significantly higher than < 10.0 U/mL in 5 patients with disease in remission, although 2 patients with active disease also had concentrations less than 10.0 U/mL *3872* 19 patients with active disease had a mean concentration of 72 U/mL *3638*

c-Antineutrophil Cytoplasmic Autoantibodies *Plasma* *Increase* In 21 patients with Wegener's granulomatosis 17 (81%) demonstrated c-ANCA positivity *2879*

Complement, Total *Serum* *No Effect* Hypocomplementemia is not seen despite the presence of circulating immune complex *565*

C-Reactive Protein *Serum* *Increase* In 4 patients with active disease mean concentration of 760 ± 530 mg/L significantly higher than 30 ± 10 mg/L in 5 patients with inactive disease *3872* Mean concentration of 11 ± 3.0 mg/L observed in 57 patients *5561* In 13 patients with major disease activity mean concentration of 107 mg/L and 70 mg/L in 9 with minor disease activity *4992*

Creatinine *Serum* *Increase* With renal involvement *565*

Elastase Antineutrophil Cytoplasmic Autoantibodies *Serum* *Increase* Antibodies detected in 7.4% of 108 patients *162*

Erythrocyte Sedimentation Rate *Blood* *Increase* Markedly elevated *565* In 4 patients with active disease mean rate of 48.3 ± 5.9 mm/h significantly higher than 7.8 ± 4.6 mm/h in 5 patients with inactive disease *3872* Mean rate of 37.3 ± 4.3 mm/h observed in 57 patients *5561*

Hematocrit *Blood* *Decrease* Mild anemia *565*

Hemoglobin *Blood* *Decrease* Mild anemia *565*

immunoglobulin A *Serum* *Increase* Mild hypergammaglobulinemia, particularly of the IgA class *565*

Intercellular Adhesion Molecule-1 *Serum* *Increase* 19 patients with active disease had a mean concentration of 499 ng/mL significantly higher than 347 ng/mL in 6 patients in remission and 245 ng/mL in 10 healthy controls *3638*

Lactate Dehydrogenase *Serum* *Increase* In 4 patients with active disease mean activity of 412.8 ± 82.3 U/L not significantly higher than 354.8 ± 39.3 U/L in 5 patients with inactive disease *3872*

Leukocytes *Blood* *Increase* Mild elevation *565* In 4 patients with active disease mean concentration of 11,650 ± 1,836 /μL significantly higher than 4,720 ± 896 /μL in 5 patients with inactive disease *3872*

Monocyte Chemotactic Protein-1 *Serum* *Decrease* Mean concentration undetectable in 1 patient with Wegener's granulomatosis compared with 101 ± 24 pg/mL in 16 healthy women and men *4460*

446.40 Wegener's Granulomatosis *(continued)*

Monocyte Chemotactic Protein-1 *(continued)*
Urine *Increase* In 1 patient with Wegener's granulomatosis mean concentration of 425 pg/mg creatinine significantly different when compared with mean concentration of 130 ± 30 pg/mg creatinine in 30 healthy women and 32 healthy men *4460*

Myeloperoxidase Antineutrophil Cytoplasmic Autoantibodies
Serum *Increase* Antibodies detected in 7.4% of 108 patients *162*

Neutrophil Proteinase 3 *Serum* *Increase* In 4 patients with active Wegener's granulomatosis mean concentration of 416 ± 39 µg/mL significantly higher than mean of 154 ± 80 µg/mL in 8 patients with inactive disease and 78 ± 30 µg/mL in 21 normal controls *2120*

Oxygen Partial Pressure *Blood* *Decrease* May be seen with pulmonary involvement *565*

Oxygen Saturation *Blood* *Decrease* May be seen with pulmonary involvement *565*

p-Antineutrophil Cytoplasmic Autoantibodies
Plasma *Increase* In 21 patients with Wegener's granulomatosis 4 (19%) demonstrated p-ANCA positivity *2879*

Perinuclear Antineutrophil Cytoplasmic Autoantibodies
Serum *Increase* Antibodies detected in 4.6% of 108 patients *162*

Platelets *Blood* *Increase* In 4 patients with active disease mean concentration of 430,000 ± 77,000 /µL significantly higher than 191,000 ± 34,000 /µL in 5 patients with inactive disease *3872* Thombocytosis may be seen as an acute pase reactant *565*

Proteinase 3-Antineutrophil Cytoplasmic Autoantibodies
Serum *Increase* Antibodies detected in 78.7% of 108 patients *162*

Rheumatoid Factor *Serum* *Increase* Mild elevation *565*

Soluble CD30 *Serum* *Increase* Concentrations ranged from 2.5 ± 46.7 U/mL (mean 21.4 ± 1.4 U/mL) observed in 57 patients compared with 8.8 ± 0.9 U/mL in 21 healthy control individuals. Higher concentrations associated with increased disease activity *5561*

Soluble E-Selectin *Serum* *Increase* 19 patients with active disease and 6 with inactive disease had a mean concentration not significantly different from 48 ng/mL in 10 healthy controls *3638*

Soluble Intercellular Adhesion Molecule-1 *Serum* *Increase* In 6 patients with active vasculitis mean concentration of 594 ± 118 ng/mL significantly higher than mean concentration of 270 ± 47 ng/mL in 10 healthy controls: no significant difference between concentrations in active and inactive vasculitis *2461* In 13 patients with major disease activity and 9 with minor disease activity median concentration on diagnosis of 520 ng/mL (range 165 - 864 ng/mL) compared with mean of 328 ± 77.4 ng/mL in 57 healthy controls *4992*
Serum *No Effect* In 13 patients with major disease activity and 9 with minor disease activity median concentration on diagnosis of 44.9 ng/mL (range 37.7 - 81.3 ng/mL) not significantly different from mean of 42.7 ± 13.6 ng/mL in 57 healthy controls *4992*

Soluble Interleukin-2 Receptor *Serum* *Increase* Soluble IL-2R levels were higher in patients with generalized and active disease than in those with limited and inactive disease. In 25 patients with complete clinical remission, sIL-2R levels were significantly elevated, although levels of CRP and c-ANCA were normal *4652*

Soluble Vascular Cell Adhesion Molecule-1
Serum *Increase* 19 patients with active disease had a mean concentration of 1,130 ng/mL significantly greater than 582 ng/mL in 10 healthy donors *3638* In 13 patients with major disease activity and 9 with minor disease activity median concentration on diagnosis of 1,119 ng/mL (range 396 - 3,029 ng/mL) compared with mean of 588 ± 158.6 ng/mL in 57 healthy controls *4992*

Thrombomodulin *Plasma* *Increase* Mean concentration of 80 ng/mL observed in 8 patients with active disease significantly higher than 10 ng/mL in 10 healthy controls *3873* In 4 patients with active disease mean concentration of 85 ± 45 ng/mL significantly higher than 12 ng/mL in 5 patients with disease in remission and 10 ng/mL in 66 normal controls *3872*

Urea Nitrogen *Serum* *Increase* With renal involvement *565*

446.50 Cranial Arteritis and Related Conditions

Albumin *Serum* *Decrease* In 30% of 16 patients hospitalized for this disorder *1576*

Aldolase *Serum* *No Effect* Activity usually normal *413*

Alkaline Phosphatase *Serum* *Increase* Abnormal liver test results, have been found, but biopsies have shown only minor nonspecific changes *1160*

Antinuclear Antibodies *Serum* *No Effect* Characteristically absent *4551*

Aspartate Aminotransferase *Serum* *No Effect* Activity usually normal *413*

Complement, Total *Serum* *Increase* In 6 patients, 50% had increased values *4925*
Serum *No Effect* No significant change observed *4551*

Creatine Kinase *Serum* *No Effect* Activity usually normal *413*

Erythrocyte Sedimentation Rate *Blood* *Increase* The only laboratory abnormality of significance is a very rapid ESR, often reaching 100 mm/h (Westergren method) *4551* Elevated to > 80 mm/h (Westergren) in polymyalgia rheumatica *367* A striking elevation of ESR is characteristic *1988*

Fibrinogen *Plasma* *Increase* Parallels the rapid ESR *4551*

α_2-Globulin *Serum* *Increase* Parallels the rapid ESR *4551*

γ-Globulin *Serum* *Increase* May occur in temporal arteritis *5545*

Hematocrit *Blood* *Decrease* Mild anemia is common, especially in older patients, in polymyalgia rheumatica *367* Hypoproliferative anemia is common and may be significant, with hematocrits in the 25 - 30% range *2081* In 30% of 16 patients hospitalized for this disorder *1576*

Hemoglobin *Blood* *Decrease* Hypoproliferative anemia is common and may be significant *2081* Mild anemia is common, especially in older patients, in polymyalgia rheumatica *367* In 49% of 16 patients hospitalized for this disorder *1576*

HLA Antigens *Blood* *Present* Association noted with HLA-DR4 *5428*

Lactate Dehydrogenase *Serum* *No Effect* Activity usually normal *413*

LE Cells *Blood* *No Effect* Not usually observed in patients with cranial arteritis *5545*

Leukocytes *Blood* *Increase* Slightly increased with shift to the left in temporal arteritis *5545* In 36% of 16 patients hospitalized for this disorder *1576*

Monocytes *Blood* *Increase* Has been reported *3246*

Neutrophils *Blood* *Increase* In 42% of 14 patients hospitalized for this disorder *1576*

Protein *Cerebrospinal Fluid* *Increase* May occur due to intracerebral artery involvement *5545*

Rheumatoid Factor *Serum* *Increase* Present in serum in 7.5% of patients with polymyalgia rheumatica *5545*
Serum *No Effect* Characteristically absent *4551*

446.50 Giant Cell Arteritis

α_1-Acid Glycoprotein *Serum* *Increase* Mean concentration of 2.28 ± 0.13 mg/mL in 25 patients with giant cell arteritis significantly different from 0.4 - 1.2 mg/mL in 20 healthy volunteers *4390*

Alkaline Phosphatase *Serum* *Increase* Mean activity of 318 ± 39 U/L in 25 patients with giant cell arteritis significantly different from 53 - 120 U/L in 20 healthy volunteers *4390*

C-Reactive Protein *Serum* *Increase* Mean concentration of 91 ± 9.6 µg/mL in 25 patients with giant cell arteritis significantly different from < 2.3 µg/mL in 20 healthy volunteers *4390*

Creatinine *Serum* *Decrease* Mean concentration of 79 ± 7 nmol/mL in 25 patients with giant cell arteritis not significantly different from 40 - 120 nmol/mL in 20 healthy volunteers *4390*

Haptoglobin *Serum* *Increase* Mean concentration of 6.65 ± 0.29 mg/mL in 25 patients with giant cell arteritis significantly different from 0.5 - 3.2 mg/mL in 20 healthy volunteers *4390*

Interleukin-6 *Serum* *Increase* Mean concentration of 59.4 ± 18 pg/mL in 25 patients with giant cell arteritis significantly different from 3.3 ± 0.9 pg/mL in 20 healthy volunteers *4390*

Leukemia Inhibitory Factor *Serum* *Increase* Reportedly detected in serum of patients with giant cell arteritis but not in other vasculitis *1614*

Soluble CD23 *Serum* *Increase* Mean concentration of 1.6 ± 0.24 U/mL in 25 patients with giant cell arteritis significantly different from 0.82 ± 0.24 U/mL in 20 healthy volunteers *4390*

Soluble E-Selectin *Serum* *No Effect* In 45 patients with giant cell arteritis mean concentration of 44.5 ± 28.0 ng/mL not significantly different from 38.3 ± 31.1 ng/mL in 33 healthy controls *893*

Soluble Intercellular Adhesion Molecule-1 *Serum* *Increase* In 45 patients with giant cell arteritis mean concentration of 361 ± 130 ng/mL significantly different from 243 ± 47 ng/mL in 33 healthy controls *893*

Soluble Intercellular Adhesion Molecule-3 *Serum* *No Effect* In 45 patients with giant cell arteritis mean concentration of 38.4 ± 20.6 ng/mL not significantly different from 35.3 ± 24.7 ng/mL in 33 healthy controls *893*

Soluble L-Selectin *Serum* *No Effect* In 45 patients with giant cell arteritis mean concentration of 540 ± 321 ng/mL not significantly different from 467 ± 234 ng/mL in 33 healthy controls *893*

Soluble Vascular Cell Adhesion Molecule-1 *Serum* *No Effect* In 45 patients with giant cell arteritis mean concentration of 705 ± 279 ng/mL not significantly different from 661 ± 255 ng/mL in 33 healthy controls *893*

446.50 Polymyalgia Rheumatica

α_1-Acid Glycoprotein *Serum* *Increase* In 25 patients with myalgia rheumatica median concentration of 1.8 g/L significantly higher than upper limit of normal of 1.0 g/L *5549*

Cholesterol *Serum* *No Effect* In 25 patients with myalgia rheumatica median concentration of 4.6 mmol/L not different from upper limits of normal of 7.7 mmol/L in men and 8.2 mmol/L in women *5549*

C-Reactive Protein *Serum* *Increase* In 25 patients with myalgia rheumatica median concentration of 45.0 mg/L significantly higher than upper limit of normal of 5 mg/L *5549*

C-terminal Propeptide of Type I Procollagen *Serum* *Decrease* Mean concentration of 104 ± 34 µg/L in 40 patients significantly less than 116 ± 27 µg/L in 35 age-matched controls *3189*

Deoxypyridinoline *Urine* *Increase* Mean concentration of 14.3 ± 6.5 µg/L in 40 patients 90% higher than in age-matched controls *3189*

Erythrocyte Sedimentation Rate *Blood* *Increase* In 25 patients with myalgia rheumatica median rate of 74 mm/h significantly higher than upper limit of normal of 20 mm/h *5549*

γ-Globulin *Serum* *Increase* In 22 patients with polymyalgia rheumatica mean concentration of 1.53 ± 0.38 g/dL *3904*

Haptoglobin *Serum* *Increase* In 25 patients with myalgia rheumatica median concentration of 4.3 g/L significantly higher than upper limit of normal of 2.5 g/L *5549*

immunoglobulin A *Serum* *Increase* In 22 patients with polymyalgia rheumatica mean concentration of 463.6 ± 143.8 mg/dL *3904*

Immunoglobulin G *Serum* *Increase* In 22 patients with polymyalgia rheumatica mean concentration of 1,947.7 ± 719.2 mg/dL *3904*

Immunoglobulin M *Serum* *Increase* In 22 patients with polymyalgia rheumatica mean concentration of 196.7 ± 92.6 mg/dL *3904*

Lipoprotein Lp(a) *Serum* *No Effect* In 25 patients with myalgia rheumatica median concentration of 183 mg/mL not different from upper limit of normal of 480 mg/mL in healthy individuals *5549*

Pyridinoline *Urine* *Increase* Mean excretion of 74.9 ± 29 µg/L in 40 patients, 153% higher than in age-matched controls *3189*

Soluble CD4+ *Serum* *Decrease* In 19 patients mean concentration of 9.7 ± 12.8 U/mL significantly less than 19.0 ± 11.4 U/mL in 41 healthy controls *4538*

Soluble CD8+ *Serum* *Increase* In 19 patients mean concentration of 410 ± 142 U/mL significantly greater than 327 ± 132 U/mL in 41 healthy controls *4538*

Soluble Intercellular Adhesion Molecule-1 *Serum* *Increase* In 16 patients mean concentration of 666 ± 204 ng/mL significantly greater than 389 ± 140 ng/mL in 41 healthy controls *4538*

Soluble Interleukin-2 Receptor *Serum* *Increase* In 19 patients mean concentration of 815 ± 395 U/mL significantly greater than 262 ± 49 U/mL in 41 healthy controls *4538*

Triglycerides *Serum* *No Effect* In 25 patients with myalgia rheumatica median concentration of 1.2 mmol/L not different from upper limit of normal of 2.2 mmol/L in healthy individuals *5549*

446.50 Temporal Arteritis

Anticardiolipin Antibodies *Serum* *Increase* Reported effect *1532*

Immunoglobulin G *Serum* *Increase* Increased levels have been found *565*

Interleukin-6 *Serum* *Increase* 15 initially untreated patients with PMR/GCA. Interleukin-6 activity was significantly elevated in all untreated patients *1020*

446.60 Thrombotic Thrombocytopenic Purpura

Anti-Endothelial Cell Antibodies *Serum* *Increase* AECA have been detected in systemic lupus erythematosus, scleroderma and dermatomyositis but are also found in systemic vasculitis, Kawasaki disease, hemolytic uremic syndrome, thrombotic thrombocytopenic purpura and renal allograft recipients at the time of rejection *1174* *4248*

Bilirubin *Serum* *Increase* Elevated in 90% of patients *5677*

Bilirubin, Indirect *Serum* *Increase* In 90% of patients *5677*

Bleeding Time *Patient* *Increase* Varies depending upon the platelet count *4551*

Capillary Fragility *Blood* *Increase* Positive tourniquet test *5699*

Casts *Urine* *Increase* With kidney involvement *1980*

Cells *Bone Marrow* *Increase* Increased number of megakaryocytes but with marginal platelets *5545*

Clot Retraction *Blood* *Decrease* Varies depending upon the platelet count *4551* Absent or deficient due to thrombocytopenia *5699*

Clotting Time *Blood* *No Effect* Clotting time usually normal *4979* *112*

Coombs' Test *Serum* *Positive* Rarely *3828*

Creatinine *Serum* *Increase* Renal function may be impaired *1980* In 135 patients with thrombotic thrombocytopenic purpura mean concentration of 173.9 µmol/L on entry into study significantly different from 40 - 110 µmol/L in normal individuals *4395*

D-Dimer *Plasma* *No Effect* Mean concentration of 451 ± 436 ng/mL in 13 patients with TTP not significantly different from 621 ± 58 ng/mL in 50 healthy controls *5508*

Eosinophils *Blood* *Increase* WBC generally normal or slightly increased, often with a relative lymphocytosis and eosinophilia *4551*

Bone Marrow *Increase* Increased numbers of young megakaryocytes and often an increase in eosinophils *3172*

Erythrocytes *Urine* *Increase* Gross or microscopic hematuria *1980*

Factor V *Plasma* *Decrease* Slight decrease in 2 cases *2999*

Fibrinogen *Plasma* *No Effect* In 13 patients with TTP mean concentration of 261 ± 59 mg/dL not significantly different from normal *5508*

Glomerular Filtration Rate *Urine* *Decrease* Renal function may be impaired *1980*

Haptoglobin *Serum* *Decrease* May accompany elevated indirect bilirubin, indicating intravascular RBC destruction *5699*

446.60 Thrombotic Thrombocytopenic Purpura *(continued)*

Hematocrit *Blood Decrease* Anemia secondary to blood loss may be present *4551* In 135 patients with thrombotic thrombocytopenic purpura mean concentration of 0.26 on entry into study significantly different from 0.35 - 0.50 in normal individuals *4395*

Hemoglobin *Blood Decrease* In 135 patients with thrombotic thrombocytopenic purpura mean concentration of 8.96 g/dL on entry into study significantly different from 12.0 - 17.5 g/dL in normal individuals *4395* Anemia secondary to blood loss may be present *4551* 5.5 g/dL in 33% of patients *5677* *5699* *Plasma Increase* May accompany elevated indirect bilirubin, indicating intravascular RBC destruction *5699*

Iron-binding Capacity, Total *Serum Decrease* Anemia from blood loss may be present *5677*

Iron Saturation *Serum Increase* Anemia from blood loss may be present *5677*

Lactate Dehydrogenase *Serum Increase* In 135 patients with thrombotic thrombocytopenic purpura mean activity of 1,363 U/L on entry into study significantly different from 100 - 225 U/L in normal individuals *4395*

LE Cells *Blood Positive* Positive initially in 10 - 20% of patients *112*

Leukocytes *Blood Increase* Generally normal or slightly increased, often with a relative lymphocytosis, atypical lymphocytes (particularly in children), and eosinophilia *4551* *Urine Increase* With kidney involvement *1980*

Lymphocytes *Blood Increase* Often with a relative lymphocytosis, atypical lymphocytes (particularly in children), and eosinophilia *4551*

Neutrophils *Blood Increase* Leukocytosis in 50% with a shift to the left and appearance of immature granulocytes *5699*

Partial Thromboplastin Time *Plasma No Effect* PTT typically normal *4979*

Plasmin-α_2-Plasmin Inhibitor Complex *Plasma No Effect* Mean concentration of 1.1 ± 1.1 µg/mL in 13 patients with TTP not significantly different from 1.45 ± 0.36 µg/mL in 50 healthy controls *5508*

Plasminogen Activator Inhibitor-1 *Plasma No Effect* In 13 patients with TTP mean concentration of 30.5 ± 5.6 ng/mL not significantly different from 28.1 ± 7.2 ng/mL in 50 healthy controls *5508*

Plasminogen Activator Inhibitor-2 *Plasma No Effect* PAI-II not detected in 13 patients with TTP *5508*

Platelet Aggregating Factor *Serum Increase* In 88 patients with thrombotic thrombocytopenic purpura a platelet aggregating factor was observed in 52 on entry into study *4395*

Platelet-associated IgG *Blood Increase* In 135 patients with thrombotic thrombocytopenic purpura mean concentration of 28.1 fg/plt on entry into study significantly different from < 5.5 fg/plt in normal individuals *4395*

Platelet Survival *Blood Decrease* Increased platelet destruction results in thrombocytopenia or shortened platelet survival (i.e., compensated thrombocytolytic states) *2573*

Platelets *Blood Decrease* Decreased count- no bleeding until count less than 60,000 /µL *5545* In 135 patients with thrombotic thrombocytopenic purpura mean concentration of 25.3 ± 19.4 x 10^9/L on entry into study significantly different from 150 - 400 x 10^9/L in normal individuals *4395* Usually concentration is within range of 10,000 - 50,000 /µL *5677*

Protein *Urine Increase* With kidney involvement *1980* Proteinuria or hematuria in 90% of patients *5677*

Prothrombin Time *Plasma No Effect* PT usually normal *4979* *112*

Reticulocytes *Blood Increase* In most cases *5699* Averaged 20% *112* In 135 patients with thrombotic thrombocytopenic purpura mean concentration of 293 x 10^9/L on entry into study significantly different from 15 - 150 x 10^9/L in normal individuals *4395*

Soluble Fas Antigen *Serum Increase* In 24 patients with thrombotic thrombocytopenic purpura and 9 with hemolytic uremic syndrome mean concentration of 2.39 ± 1.62 ng/mL significantly higher than 1.01 ± 0.24 ng/mL in 25 healthy individuals *2229*

Soluble Fas Ligand Antigen *Serum Increase* In 24 patients with thrombotic thrombocytopenic purpura and 9 with hemolytic uremic syndrome mean serum concentration of 0.307 ± 0.230 ng/mL significantly higher than 0.057 ± 0.039 ng/mL in 25 healthy individuals *2229*

Thrombin Time *Blood No Effect* Time usually normal *4979*

Thrombin/Antithrombin III Complex *Plasma Increase* Mean concentration of 26.3 ± 16.7 ng/mL in 13 patients with TTP higher than 18.5 ± 9.0 ng/mL in 50 healthy controls *5508*

Thrombomodulin *Plasma Increase* In 24 patients with thrombotic thrombocytopenic purpura and in 9 with hemolytic uremic syndrome mean serum concentration of 46.6 ± 26.6 ng/mL significantly higher than 10.5 ± 1.9 ng/mL in 25 healthy individuals *2229* In 13 patients with TTP mean concentration of 10.0 ± 2.8 ng/mL significantly higher than 5.4 ± 1.4 ng/mL in 50 healthy controls *5508*

Tissue Plasminogen Activator *Plasma No Effect* In 13 patients with TTP mean concentration of 23.9 ± 10.8 ng/mL not significantly different from 19.3 ± 3.2 ng/mL in 50 healthy controls *5508*

Urea *Serum Increase* In 135 patients with thrombotic thrombocytopenic purpura mean concentration of 13.3 mmol/L on entry into study significantly different from 1.8 - 8.7 mmol/L in normal individuals *4395*

Urea Nitrogen *Serum Increase* Renal function may be impaired *1980* Elevated initially in 50% of patients and more terminally *5677*

VDRL *Serum Positive* In 10% of patients (biological false positive) *112*

von Willebrand Factor *Plasma Increase* In 135 patients with thrombotic thrombocytopenic purpura mean activity of 221%/mL on entry into study significantly different from 40 - 150%/mL in normal individuals *4395* *Plasma No Effect* In 13 patients with TTP mean concentration of 66.7 ± 41.5% not significantly different from normal *5508*

von Willebrand Factor Antigen *Plasma Decrease* In 13 patients with TTP mean concentration of 80.6 ± 40.7% reduced compared with concentration of 152 ± 14% in 50 healthy controls *5508*

446.70 Pulseless Disease (Aortic Arch Syndrome)

Erythrocyte Sedimentation Rate *Blood Increase* Consistently elevated to high levels *4551* May be present *4674*

γ-Globulin *Serum Increase* Serum proteins abnormal with increased γ-globulins, mostly composed of IgM *5544* May be present *4674*

HLA Antigens *Blood Present* Frequency of HLA-Bw52 greater in affected Asians *5428*

Immunoglobulin M *Serum Increase* May be present *4674* Serum proteins abnormal with increased γ-globulins, mostly composed of IgM *5544*

Leukocytes *Blood Increase* May be present *4674* Mild *4551* *Blood No Effect* Usually normal *5544*

446.70 Takayasu's Arteritis

Endothelin-1 *Plasma Increase* Mean concentration increased with disease activity *53* In 23 patients mean concentration increased to 5.3 ± 0.7 pg/mL, mean 3.3-fold above normal *328*

Erythrocyte Sedimentation Rate *Blood Increase* Mean rate increased with disease activity *53*

Fibrinogen *Plasma No Effect* Mean concentration of 341.8 ± 12.1 mg/dL in 59 patients with Takayasu's arteritis significantly different from 314.5 ± 36.5 ng/mL in 36 healthy control individuals *3818*

Soluble Intercellular Adhesion Molecule-1 *Serum Increase* Mean concentration of 191.1 ± 12.5 ng/mL in 73 patients with Takayasu's arteritis significantly different from 165.2 ± 11.5 ng/mL in 36 healthy control individuals *3818*

Soluble Vascular Cell Adhesion Molecule-1 *Serum* *Increase* Mean concentration of 871.4 ± 71.9 ng/mL in 73 patients with Takayasu's arteritis significantly different from 607.9 ± 31.7 ng/mL in 36 healthy control individuals *3818*

Thrombomodulin *Plasma* *No Effect* Mean concentration did not correlate with disease activity *53*

447.60 Systemic Vasculitis

Anti-Myeloperoxidase-Antineutrophil Cytoplasmic Autoantibodies *Serum* *Increase* In 43 patients with systemic vasculitis 18 demonstrated anti-myeloperoxidase-ANCA positivity *2879*

Anti-Proteinase 3--Antineutrophil Cytoplasmic Autoantibodies *Plasma* *Increase* In 43 patients with systemic vasculitis 17 demonstrated anti-proteinase 3-ANCA positivity *2879*

c-Antineutrophil Cytoplasmic Autoantibodies *Plasma* *Increase* In 43 patients with systemic vasculitis 19 demonstrated c-ANCA positivity *2879*

p-Antineutrophil Cytoplasmic Autoantibodies *Plasma* *Increase* In 43 patients with systemic vasculitis 24 demonstrated p-ANCA positivity *2879*

447.60 Vasculitis

Anti-Endothelial Cell Antibodies *Serum* *Increase* In patients with sytemic vasculitis AECA have been detected *1174*

Anti-Entactin Antibodies *Serum* *Increase* In 38 patients with systemic vasculitis IgG anti-entactin antibodies observed in 2 *4604*

Anti-Myeloperoxidase Antibodies *Serum* *Increase* Increased concentration observed in patients with vasculitis usually involving kidneys (necrotizing pauciimmune glomerulonephritis) *2952*

Anti-Neutrophil Cytoplasm Antibodies *Serum* *Increase* In 14 of 28 patients with vasculitis serum positive for ANCA with indirect immunofluorescent test *1676* Positive test observed in 43 patients with systemic vasculitis, with high positivity associated with relapses *2879*

Complement C_1 *Serum* *Decrease* Mean concentration typically slightly reduced in patients with cryoglobulinemia or vasculitis *4682*

Complement C_1q *Serum* *Decrease* Mean concentration typically slightly reduced in patients with cryoglobulinemia or vasculitis *4682*

Complement C_2 *Serum* *Decrease* Mean concentration typically slightly reduced or normal in patients with cryoglobulinemia or vasculitis *4682*

Complement C_3 *Serum* *Decrease* Mean concentration typically slightly reduced or normal in patients with cryoglobulinemia or vasculitis *4682*

Complement C_4 *Serum* *Decrease* Mean concentration typically slightly reduced in patients with cryoglobulinemia or vasculitis *4682*

Complement C_5 *Serum* *No Effect* Mean concentration typically normal in patients with cryoglobulinemia or vasculitis *4682*

Complement CH50 *Serum* *Decrease* Mean concentration typically slightly reduced in patients with cryoglobulinemia or vasculitis *4682*

Hyaluronan *Serum* *Increase* In 10 patients with systemic vasculitis and acute renal failure mean concentration of 674 ± 495 µg/L significantly higher than 90 ± 37 µg/L in 31 age and gender matched controls, although concentration in remission had concentrations within the reference interval *5591*

Properdin Factor B *Plasma* *No Effect* Mean concentration typically normal in patients with cryoglobulinemia or vasculitis *4682*

447.80 Carotid Arterial Disease

Folate *Serum* *Decrease* In 22 older men with 40 - 100% extracranial carotid arterial disease mean concentration of 6.3 ± 2.1 µg/L significantly different from 9.5 ± 3.2 µg/L in 99 older men with ECAD of 0 - 39%: 6.3 ± 1.4 µg/L and 9.5 ± 3.1 µg/L in corresponding groups of older women *183*

Homocysteine *Plasma* *Increase* In 22 older men with 40 - 100% extracranial carotid arterial disease mean concentration of 19 ± 6 µmol/L significantly different from 14 ± 4 µmol/L in 99 older men with ECAD of 0 - 39%: 17 ± 4 µmol/L and 13 ± 5 µmol/L in corresponding groups of older women *183*

Vitamin B_{12} *Serum* *Decrease* In 22 older men with 40 - 100% extracranial carotid arterial disease mean concentration of 454 ± 215 ng/L significantly different from 553 ± 154 ng/L in 99 older men with ECAD of 0 - 39%: 433 ± 126 ng/L and 533 ± 157 ng/L in corresponding groups of older women *183*

451.90 Phlebitis and Thrombophlebitis

Acid Phosphatase *Serum* *Increase* 8 of 9 female patients with thrombophlebitis of the lower extremities had elevations. Activities of 11 - 16.1 U/L during the acute phase of disease, a fall to borderline values of 9 U/L during convalescence, and a return to normal values of 1.6 - 6.5 U/L after recovery *4659*

Alkaline Phosphatase *Serum* *Increase* In 28% of 51 patients at initial hospitalization for this disorder *1576*

Antithrombin III *Plasma* *Decrease* Significant decrease *4522*

Antithrombin Titer *Plasma* *Decrease* About 2% of venous thromboembolism is due to antithrombin III deficiency *2304*

Aspartate Aminotransferase *Serum* *Increase* In 25% of 51 patients at initial hospitalization for this disorder *1576*

Eosinophils *Blood* *Increase* In 40% of 49 patients at initial hospitalization for this disorder *1576*

Fibrin Degradation Products *Plasma* *Increase* 42% of 24 patients suspected of acute thrombophlebitis had positive fibrinogen tests *704*

Leukocytes *Blood* *Increase* In 28% of 51 patients at initial hospitalization for this disorder *1576*

Neutrophils *Blood* *Increase* In 36% of 49 patients at initial hospitalization for this disorder *1576*

Platelet Adhesiveness *Blood* *Increase* Increased in 7 cases *4522*

β-Thromboglobulin *Plasma* *Increase* Increased in 7 cases *4522*

451.90 Thrombophlebitis

Fibrinopeptide A *Plasma* *Increase* In 40 puerperal patients mean concentration in those with septic pelvic thrombophlebitis of 23.8 ng/mL compared with 7 ng/mL in those with endometritis *5617*

453.00 Budd-Chiari Syndrome

Anticardiolipin-specific IgG Antibodies *Serum* *Increase* In 19 patients with Budd-Chiari syndrome mean concentration of 13.8 ± 13.3 GPL units significantly different from 6.3 ± 4.4 GPL units in 11 healthy controls *42*

453.30 Renal Vein Thrombosis

Ammonium Ions *Urine* *Increase* May lead to proximal renal tubular acidosis which is associated with hypokalemia, hyperchloremic metabolic acidosis, urine pH < 5.5, increased urinary ammonium ion excretion, a negative urine anion gap, increased urinary osmol gap, normal urinary citrate, normal urinary calcium excretion and Fanconi syndrome *4071*

Anion Gap *Urine* *Decrease* May lead to proximal renal tubular acidosis which is associated with hypokalemia, hyperchloremic metabolic acidosis, urine pH < 5.5, increased urinary ammonium ion excretion, a negative urine anion gap, increased urinary osmol gap, normal urinary citrate, normal urinary calcium excretion and Fanconi syndrome *4071*

453.30 Renal Vein Thrombosis *(continued)*

Bicarbonate *Serum* *Decrease* May lead to proximal renal tubular acidosis which is associated with hypokalemia, hyperchloremic metabolic acidosis, urine pH < 5.5, increased urinary ammonium ion excretion, a negative urine anion gap, increased urinary osmol gap, normal urinary citrate, normal urinary calcium excretion and Fanconi syndrome *4071*

Calcium *Urine* *No Effect* May lead to proximal renal tubular acidosis which is associated with hypokalemia, hyperchloremic metabolic acidosis, urine pH < 5.5, increased urinary ammonium ion excretion, a negative urine anion gap, increased urinary osmol gap, normal urinary citrate, normal urinary calcium excretion and Fanconi syndrome *4071*

Chloride *Serum* *Increase* May lead to proximal renal tubular acidosis which is associated with hypokalemia, hyperchloremic metabolic acidosis, urine pH < 5.5, increased urinary ammonium ion excretion, a negative urine anion gap, increased urinary osmol gap, normal urinary citrate, normal urinary calcium excretion and Fanconi syndrome *4071*

Citrate *Urine* *No Effect* May lead to proximal renal tubular acidosis which is associated with hypokalemia, hyperchloremic metabolic acidosis, urine pH < 5.5, increased urinary ammonium ion excretion, a negative urine anion gap, increased urinary osmol gap, normal urinary citrate, normal urinary calcium excretion and Fanconi syndrome *4071*

Glucose *Urine* *Increase* May lead to proximal renal tubular acidosis which is associated with hypokalemia, hyperchloremic metabolic acidosis, urine pH < 5.5, increased urinary ammonium ion excretion, a negative urine anion gap, increased urinary osmol gap, normal urinary citrate, normal urinary calcium excretion and Fanconi syndrome *4071*

Osmolal Gap *Urine* *Increase* May lead to proximal renal tubular acidosis which is associated with hypokalemia, hyperchloremic metabolic acidosis, urine pH < 5.5, increased urinary ammonium ion excretion, a negative urine anion gap, increased urinary osmol gap, normal urinary citrate, normal urinary calcium excretion and Fanconi syndrome *4071*

pH *Urine* *Decrease* May lead to proximal renal tubular acidosis which is associated with hypokalemia, hyperchloremic metabolic acidosis, urine pH < 5.5, increased urinary ammonium ion excretion, a negative urine anion gap, increased urinary osmol gap, normal urinary citrate, normal urinary calcium excretion and Fanconi syndrome *4071*

Phosphate *Serum* *Decrease* May lead to proximal renal tubular acidosis which is associated with hypokalemia, hyperchloremic metabolic acidosis, urine pH < 5.5, increased urinary ammonium ion excretion, a negative urine anion gap, increased urinary osmol gap, normal urinary citrate, normal urinary calcium excretion and Fanconi syndrome *4071*

Potassium *Serum* *Decrease* May lead to proximal renal tubular acidosis which is associated with hypokalemia, hyperchloremic metabolic acidosis, urine pH < 5.5, increased urinary ammonium ion excretion, a negative urine anion gap, increased urinary osmol gap, normal urinary citrate, normal urinary calcium excretion and Fanconi syndrome *4071*

Uric Acid *Serum* *Decrease* May lead to proximal renal tubular acidosis which is associated with hypokalemia, hyperchloremic metabolic acidosis, urine pH < 5.5, increased urinary ammonium ion excretion, a negative urine anion gap, increased urinary osmol gap, normal urinary citrate, normal urinary calcium excretion and Fanconi syndrome *4071*

453.80 Deep Vein Thrombosis

Anticardiolipin Antibodies *Serum* *Increase* A control was matched by age, smoking history, and length of follow-up to each of the 90 patients with deep venous thrombosis or pulmonary embolus. The anticardiolipin antibody titers were higher in case patients than in their matched controls (p = 0.01) *1736*

γ-Carboxyglutamic Acid, Free *Plasma* *Increase* In 14 hospitalized patients with deep venous thrombosis mean concentration of 372 ± 244 pmol/mL significantly higher than that in 19 healthy men and women aged between 35 and 65 years in whom mean concentration was 146 ± 34 pmol/mL *2014*

D-Dimer *Plasma* *Increase* In 16 patients with DVT mean concentration of 5,141 ng/mL significantly greater than 3,024 ng/mL in patients without *2805* In the blood of 107 patients with proved deep venous thrombosis concentrations increased in 88% as measured by enzyme immunoassay *784*

Eosinophils *Blood* *Increase* In 1 patient with venous thrombosis of the calf and asthma mean concentration of 966 x 10^6/L significantly different from upper limit of normal of 440 x 10^6/L in 29 normal individuals *607*

Histamine *Plasma* *No Effect* In 1 patient with venous thrombosis of calf and asthma mean concentration of < 1.8 nmol/L not significantly different from mean concentration of 4.0 nmol/L in 29 normal individuals *607*

Laminin *Serum* *Increase* Mean concentration in 23 patients with deep venous thrombosis of 534 ± 61 ng/mL increased compared with 379 ± 21 ng/mL in 15 healthy individuals *635*

Lipoprotein Lp(a) *Serum* *Increase* In 63 patients with deep venous thrombosis median concentration of 63 mg/L significantly different from 43 mg/L in 69 healthy volunteers, but with 3.2% above 95th percentile of 361 mg/L *5417*

Prothrombin Fragment 1.2 *Plasma* *Increase* Mean concentration of prothrombin fragment 1.2 in platelet-poor plasma from 7 patients with venous thrombosis of 4.6 ± 3.7 nmol/L significantly higher than 0.51 nmol/L (95% reference interval 0.21 - 2.78 nmol/L) in 268 healthy individuals less than 44 years of age *1860*

453.90 Venous Embolism and Thrombosis

Folate *Serum* *No Effect* In 220 patients with venous thromboembolism mean concentration of 4.38 ± 2.9 ng/mL was not significantly different from 4.95 ± 2.2 ng/mL in 220 healthy controls *1688*

Homocysteine *Plasma* *Increase* In 269 patients with deep-vein thrombosis 28 (10%) had plasma concentrations (median 12.9 μmol/L) above the 95th percentile for the controls as compared with 13 of 269 controls in whom the median concentration was 12.3 μmol/L *1116* In 220 patients with venous thromboembolism mean concentration of 11.7 ± 10.8 μmol/L was significantly greater than 9.1 ± 6.6 μmol/L in 220 healthy controls *1688*

Vitamin B_{12} *Serum* *No Effect* In 220 patients with venous thromboembolism mean concentration of 308 ± 150 pg/mL was not significantly different from 297 ± 93 pg/mL in 220 healthy controls *1688*

453.90 Venous Thrombosis

Antiphospholipid Antibodies *Serum* *Increase* About 25% of patients with unexplained venous thrombosis have antiphospholipid antibodies *441*

455.60 Hemorrhoids

Carcinoembryonic Antigen *Serum* *Increase* In 49 patients with hemorrhoids 67% had concentrations less than 2.5 ng/mL, 28% had concentrations between 2.6 and 5.0 ng/mL, 4% had concentrations between 5.1 and 10.0 ng/mL and 1% had concentrations greater than 10.0 ng/mL *2010*

Occult Blood *Feces* *Increase* In 124 patients who presented at an ER with gastrointestinal bleeding 6.4% had hemorrhoids or polyps *1383*

456.00 Esophageal Varices

Occult Blood *Feces* *Increase* In 93 patients who presented at an ER with upper gastrointestinal tract bleeding 12% had esophageal varices *1383*

Urea Nitrogen:Creatinine Ratio *Serum* *Increase* Ratio of more than 36 is strongly suggestive of upper gastrointestinal tract bleeding *1383*

456.40 Varicocele

β-Chorionic Gonadotropin *Urine* *Increase* In 7 patients with varicocele mean excretion of 1.84 ± 0.54 mIU/mL significantly increased compared with 1.13 ± 0.08 mIU/mL in 31 normal controls *1964*

457.10 Intestinal Lymphangiectasia

Immunoglobulin E *Serum* *Increase* In 10 patients with intestinal lymphangiectasia mean concentration of 112 ng/mL (range 18.6 - 676) significantly higher than mean of 96 ng/mL (range 24 - 386) in 74 healthy controls *2323*

458.00 Hypotension, Orthostatic

Atrial Natriuretic Peptide *Plasma* *Increase* Marked increase observed in overnight recumbent and upright plasma ANP in patients with orthostatic hypotension with overnight clearance being significantly lower than in normal individuals *5325*

459.90 Amyloid Angiopathy

Amyloid β-Protein *Cerebrospinal Fluid* *No Effect* In 1 patient concentration was 2.92 pmol/mL not significantly different from mean concentration of 4.00 ± 2.92 pmol/mL *3716*

Amyloid β-Protein Precursor *Cerebrospinal Fluid* *Decrease* In 1 patient concentration was 0.52 integrated OD units significantly different from mean concentration of 1.35 ± 0.38 integrated OD units in 25 normal controls *3716*

α_1-Antichymotrypsin *Cerebrospinal Fluid* *Increase* In 1 patient concentration was 20.05 µg/mL significantly different from mean concentration of 2.27 ± 1.40 µg/mL in 25 normal controls *3716*

Cells *Cerebrospinal Fluid* *No Effect* In 1 patient concentration of 0.3 cells/µL not significantly different from normal of 3 cells/µL *3716*

Protein *Cerebrospinal Fluid* *No Effect* In 1 patient concentration of 18 mg/dL not significantly different from normal of 28 mg/dL in 25 healthy controls *3716*

459.90 Hepatic Veno-occlusive Disease

Plasminogen Activator Inhibitor-1 *Plasma* *Increase* In 31 of 186 consecutive patients undergoing bone marrow transplantation who developed hyperbilirubinemia mean concentration increased to 322 ± 161 ng/mL in 7 patients with vascular occlusive disease compared with reference interval of 4 - 43 ng/mL *4529*

DISEASES OF THE RESPIRATORY SYSTEM

463.00 Acute Tonsillitis

Leukocytes *Blood* *Increase* Acute localized infections cause leukocytosis *5544*

465.90 Respiratory Syncitial Virus Infection

Amyloid A Protein *Serum* *Increase* In 70 patients mean concentration in acute phase of 1.49 ± 0.76 mg/L *3728*

C-Reactive Protein *Serum* *Increase* In 70 patients mean concentration in acute phase of 0.76 ± 0.58 mg/dL *3728*

Protein *BAL Fluid* *Increase* In 18 children (median age 3.1 mo) median concentration of 0.49 mg/mL with range of 0.13 - 2.46 mg/mL compared with median of 0.36 mg/mL and range of 0.07 - 1.65 mg/L in 16 ventilated surgical controls *2647*

Surfactant Protein A *BAL Fluid* *Decrease* In 18 children (median age 3.1 mo) median concentration of 5.6 µg/mL with range of 0.6 - 151.9 µg/mL compared with median of 9.0 µg/mL and range of 0.5 - 139.6 µg/L in 16 ventilated surgical controls *2647*

Surfactant Protein B *BAL Fluid* *Decrease* In 18 children (median age 3.1 mo) median concentration of 12.0 ng/mL with range of 0 - 60.8 ng/mL compared with median of 118.1 ng/mL and range of 0 - 778.2 ng/L in 16 ventilated surgical controls *2647*

Surfactant Protein D *BAL Fluid* *Decrease* In 18 children (median age 3.1 mo) median concentration of 130.3 ng/mL with range of 0 - 1,486.0 ng/mL compared with median of 600.4 ng/mL and range of 0 - 1,869.0 ng/L in 16 ventilated surgical controls *2647*

473.90 Chronic Sinusitis

Hematocrit *Blood* *Increase* In 54% of 11 patients at initial hospitalization for this disorder *1576*

Hemoglobin *Blood* *Increase* In 63% of 11 patients at initial hospitalization for this disorder *1576*

Sodium *Blood* *Increase* Urine is almost always hypertonic to plasma *126*

474.00 Chronic Tonsillitis

Macrophage Colony Stimulating Factor *Serum* *No Effect* In 12 patients with chronic tonsillitis mean concentration of 0.60 ± 0.36 ng/mL not significantly different from 0.63 ± 0.05 ng/mL in 5 healthy volunteers *3362*

477.90 Allergic Rhinitis

Cedar Pollen-specific IgE Antibodies *Serum* *Increase* In 47 patients with seasonal allergic rhinitis mean concentration of 23.9 ± 24.8 U/mL before pollen season increased by 32.1 ± 47.6% to 27.9 ± 25.7 U/mL during the pollen season *3871*

D. farinae-specific IgE Antibodies *Serum* *No Effect* In 49 patients with perennial allergic rhinitis mean concentration of approximately 84 ARU/mL significantly higher than that in 14 non-atopic adults *3870*

Interleukin-4 *Serum* *No Effect* In 49 patients with perennial allergic rhinitis mean concentration of 13.4 pg/mL significantly higher than that in 14 non-atopic adults, in whom mean concentration was 1.94 ± 1.83 pg/mL *3870*

Soluble Interleukin-2 Receptor *Serum* *Increase* In 47 patients with seasonal allergic rhinitis mean concentration of 411 ± 171 U/mL before pollen season increased by 30.5 ± 65.0% to 530 ± 374 U/mL during the pollen season *3871*

477.90 Hay Fever

Eosinophils *Blood* *Increase* May occur during the season, but its presence or absence has little diagnostic value, since it is variable *900* Characterized by a mild, persistent eosinophilia despite rather profound tissue involvement *5677*

Immunoglobulin E *Serum* *Increase* Increased in atopic diseases. Occurs in about 30% of patients *5544* During the pollen season *1290* Allergic persons usually have values 2 to 6 times normal *2039*

480.90 Viral Pneumonia

Alkaline Phosphatase *Serum* *Increase* In 70% of 10 patients at initial hospitalization for this disorder *1576*

Antidiuretic Hormone *Plasma* *Increase* Inappropriate increase *5679*

Aspartate Aminotransferase *Serum* *Increase* In 80% of 10 patients at initial hospitalization for this disorder *1576*

Carbon Dioxide Partial Pressure *Blood* *Increase* Low pO_2 with normal or high pCO_2 *5863*

Carcinoembryonic Antigen *Pleural Fluid* *Increase* Benign inflammatory effusions (tuberculosis, empyema, pneumonia) had mean activity of 6.2 ± 3.4 ng/mL, higher than effusions caused by congestive heart failure (2.9 ± 1.5 ng/mL) and other noninflammatory effusions *4369*

Cholesterol *Serum* *Decrease* In 40% of 10 patients at initial hospitalization for this disorder *1576*

Complement-fixing Antibodies *Serum* *Positive* Complement-fixing antibodies appear 8 - 9 days after onset *4314*

Eosinophils *Blood* *Increase* In 32% of 15 patients at initial hospitalization for this disorder *1576*

480.90 Viral Pneumonia *(continued)*

Eosinophils *(continued)*
Pleural Fluid *Increase* Eosinophilia greater than 10% may be present *126*

Erythrocytes *Sputum* *Increase* Sputum in acute pneumonia is rusty, blood-streaked and mucopurulent *2039*

Glucose *Pleural Fluid* *Decrease* Exudate *126*

Hematocrit *Blood* *Decrease* In 49% of 16 patients at initial hospitalization for this disorder *1576*

Hemoglobin *Blood* *Decrease* In 55% of 16 patients at initial hospitalization for this disorder *1576*

Isocitrate Dehydrogenase *Serum* *No Effect* No effect on activity *5008*

Lactate Dehydrogenase *Pleural Fluid* *Increase* Usually higher than in serum; commonly found in chronic pleural effusions and is not useful in differential diagnosis *5544*
Serum *Increase* In 60% of 10 patients at initial hospitalization for this disorder *1576* The increases that did occur were in cases of viral pneumonia *2350*

Lactate Dehydrogenase Isoenzyme-5 *Serum* *Increase* Abnormally elevated to 6.3% of the total LD value of 774 U/mL in 6 cases of lobar pneumonia *1756*

Leukocytes *Blood* *Decrease* Normal or low with a relative lymphocytosis *4314*
Blood *Increase* In 48% of 16 patients at initial hospitalization for this disorder *1576*
Blood *No Effect* Normal or low with a relative lymphocytosis *4314*

Lymphocyte T-Cells *Blood* *Decrease* Normal *1588*

Lymphocytes *Blood* *Decrease* In 52% of 15 patients at initial hospitalization for this disorder *1576*
Blood *Increase* Normal or low WBC with a relative lymphocytosis *4314* In 39% of 15 patients at initial hospitalization for this disorder *1576*

Neopterin *Urine* *Increase* Increased in viral infections *4772*

Neutrophils *Blood* *Decrease* In 52% of 15 patients at initial hospitalization for this disorder *1576*
Blood *Increase* In 39% of 15 patients at initial hospitalization for this disorder *1576*

Oxygen Partial Pressure *Blood* *Decrease* Low pO_2 with normal or high pCO_2 *5863*

pH *Pleural Fluid* *Decrease* Pleural fluid pH of < 7.20 or 0.15 below arterial pH frequently occurs in parapneumonic effusions *3052*

Protein *Pleural Fluid* *Increase* Exudate (> 3 g/dL) *126*

Specific Gravity *Pleural Fluid* *Increase* Exudate (> 1.016) *126*

Standard Bicarbonate *Serum* *Increase* Increased standard bicarbonate in blood *1290*

482.90 Bacterial Pneumonia

Albumin *Serum* *Decrease* In 50% of 17 patients at initial hospitalization for this disorder *1576*
Urine *Increase* Common *5252*

Amylase *Pleural Fluid* *No Effect* Usually less than or equal to serum level *4493*
Serum *Increase* Early reports emphasized that increased activity can occur, but no more recent documentation of this is available *4537* Early reports emphasized that it can occur, but no more recent documentation of this is available *4171*

Anti-Streptolysin-O Titer *Serum* *Increase* In group A streptococcal infections *1980*

Antidiuretic Hormone *Plasma* *Increase* Inappropriate increase *5679*

Aspartate Aminotransferase *Serum* *Increase* In 54% of 18 patients at initial hospitalization for this disorder *1576*
Serum *No Effect* Typical observation *5544*

Bilirubin *Serum* *Increase* Occasionally present *1980*
Serum *No Effect* Typical observation *5544*

Carbon Dioxide Partial Pressure *Blood* *Decrease* In 63% of 14 patients at initial hospitalization for this disorder *1576*

Carcinoembryonic Antigen *Pleural Fluid* *Increase* Benign inflammatory effusions (tuberculosis, empyema, pneumonia) had mean activity of 6.2 ± 3.4 ng/mL, higher than effusions caused by congestive heart failure (2.9 ± 1.5) and other noninflammatory effusions *4369*
Serum *Increase* 47% of patients had values > 2.5 ng/mL *4891*

Cells *Sputum* *Increase* Gram's stain of sputum reveals many polymorphonuclear leukocytes, and many gram-positive cocci in pairs and singly in pneumonoccal pneumonia *5545*

Chloride *Urine* *Decrease* Excretion of chlorides is decreased *5252*

Cholesterol *Serum* *Decrease* Infections associated with liver damage; possibly severe pneumonia *1290* In 45% of 17 patients at initial hospitalization for this disorder *1576*

Complement C_3 *Serum* *Decrease* Mean concentrations in acute infection was slightly decreased *926*

Copper *Serum* *Increase* Statistically significant *4871*

C-Reactive Protein *Serum* *Increase* Nonspecific indicator of acute infection *413*

Eosinophils *Pleural Fluid* *Increase* Eosinophilia greater than 10% may be present *126*

Erythrocyte Sedimentation Rate *Blood* *Increase* Nonspecific indicator of acute infection *413*

Erythrocytes *Sputum* *Increase* Sputum in acute pneumonia is rusty, blood-streaked and mucopurulent *2039*

Fibrin Degradation Products *Plasma* *Increase* Elevation is much more common in fatal cases than in survivors in acute respiratory infection *4881*

Glucose *Pleural Fluid* *Decrease* Levels less than 3.3 mmol/L (60 mg/dL) *396*
Serum *Increase* In 48% of 18 patients at initial hospitalization for this disorder *1576*

Granular Casts *Urine* *Increase* Protein, WBC, hyaline and granular casts in small amounts are common *5544*

Hematocrit *Blood* *Decrease* Anemia is common in pneumococcal but not in staphylococcal pneumonia *5252* In 40% of 19 patients at initial hospitalization for this disorder *1576*

Hemoglobin *Blood* *Decrease* In 38% of 18 patients at initial hospitalization for this disorder *1576* Anemia is common in pneumococcal but not in staphylococcal pneumonia *5252*

Hyaline Casts *Urine* *Increase* Protein, WBC, hyaline and granular casts in small amounts are common *5544*

Immunoglobulin E *Pleural Fluid* *Increase* Immunoglobulins are present in large amount *4327*

Immunoglobulin G *Pleural Fluid* *Increase* Predominant immunoglobulin found in effusions *4327*

Immunoglobulin M *Pleural Fluid* *Increase* Immunoglobulins are present in large amounts forming a series declining from the IgG (70% of serum concentration) to the IgM (50% of serum concentration) *4327*

Immunoglobulins *Pleural Fluid* *Increase* Immunoglobulins are present in large amounts forming a series declining from the IgG (70% of serum concentration) to the IgM (50% of serum concentration) *4327*

Interleukin-6 *Serum* *Increase* In a group of patients with bacterial pneumonia mean concentration of 10 ± 13 pg/mL compared with 3 ± 4 pg/mL in healthy controls *1079*

Ketones *Urine* *Increase* Ketones may occur with severe infection *5544*

Lactate Dehydrogenase *Pleural Fluid* *Increase* Usually higher than in serum; commonly found in chronic pleural effusions and is not useful in differential diagnosis *5544*
Serum *Increase* In some cases *5252* In 32% of 17 patients at initial hospitalization for this disorder *1576*
Serum *No Effect* Reported observation *1290* Normal in 45 of 50 cases of uncomplicated pneumonia. The increases that did occur were in cases of viral pneumonia. Unreliable screening methods were suggested to account for the increase in LD in pneumonia in a previous study *2350*

Leukocytes *Blood* *Decrease* Leukopenia with a shift to the left occurs in fulminating pneumococcal infections, particularly in the presence of bacteremia and in alcoholics *367* Normal or low WBC in aged, in overwhelming infection, or with other causative organisms such as Klebsiella pneumoniae *5545*
Blood *Increase* Already present at initial chill *5252* In 66% of 19 patients at initial hospitalization for this disorder *1576*

Total count ranges from 15,000 - 40,000 /µL or higher with a shift to the left in differential count *367*
Pleural Fluid *Increase* A markedly elevated leukocyte count 10,000 /µL), especially with a preponderance of neutrophils, is highly suggestive of a pyogenic infection *1980*
Sputum *Increase* Sputum contains very many leukocytes with intracellular gram-positive cocci in staphylococcal pneumonia *5545*
Urine *Increase* Protein, WBC, hyaline and granular casts in small amounts are common *5544*

Lipoproteins *Pleural Fluid* *Increase* Pleural effusions in patients with bacterial pleurisy contain low density lipoproteins (33% of the serum LDL concentration on average) but almost no very low density lipoproteins (about 1% of the serum VLDL concentration on average) *4327*

Low Density Lipoprotein *Pleural Fluid* *Present* Pleural effusions in patients with bacterial pleurisy contain low density lipoproteins (33% of the serum LDL concentration on average) but almost no very low density lipoproteins (about 1% of the serum VLDL concentration on average) *4327*

Neutrophils *Blood* *Increase* A polymorphonuclear leukocytosis of above 15,000 /µL. However, the count may be normal and in some instances of overwhelming infection a leukopenia may be present *900* In 55% of 18 patients at initial hospitalization for this disorder *1576*
Pleural Fluid *Increase* Predominant cell type *4493*

Nitrate plus Nitrite *Serum* *No Effect* In a group of patients with bacterial pneumonia mean concentration of 37 ± 28 µmol/L not significantly different compared with 30 ± 9 µmol/L in healthy controls *1079*

Nitroblue Tetrazolium Test *Blood* *Increase* Elevated in 29 of 33 lobar pneumonia patients, mean of 33.5% (control mean of 5.4%). Useful in differential diagnosis of pulmonary infection and thromboembolism (3 of 55 with abnormal scores) *2107*

Oxygen Partial Pressure *Blood* *Decrease* Low pO_2 with normal or high pCO_2 *5863* In 98% of 14 patients at initial hospitalization for this disorder *1576*

pH *Blood* *Increase* In 91% of 14 patients at initial hospitalization for this disorder *1576*
Pleural Fluid *Decrease* Exudate (pH < 7.3) *126*

Procalcitonin *Plasma* *Increase* In a group of patients with cardiogenic shock mean concentration of 2.4 ± 3.7 ng/mL on days 5 and 10 compared with < 0.1 ng/mL in healthy controls *1079*

Protein *Pleural Fluid* *Increase* High total protein concentrations *774*
Urine *Increase* Protein, WBC, hyaline and granular casts in small amounts are common *5544*

Rheumatoid Factor *Pleural Fluid* *Increase* May be present with rheumatoid disease, but may also be found in other types of pleural effusions (e.g., carcinoma, tuberculosis, bacterial pneumonia) *5544*
Serum *Increase* Positive latex fixation in 22% of 50 patients *927*

Soluble Tumor Necrosis Factor Receptor-p55
Serum *Increase* In a group of patients with bacterial pneumonia mean concentration of 5.5 ± 4.1 ng/mL compared with 1.1 ± 0.7 ng/mL in healthy controls *1079*

Soluble Tumor Necrosis Factor Receptor-p75
Serum *Increase* In a group of patients with bacterial pneumonia mean concentration of 9.5 ± 4.8 ng/mL compared with 2.4 ± 1.4 ng/mL in healthy controls *1079*

Specific Gravity *Pleural Fluid* *Increase* Exudate (> 1.016) *126*

Tissue Polypeptide Antigen *Serum* *No Effect* In 3 patients with bronchopneumonia mean concentration of 65.7 ± 21.1 U/L not significantly different from 72.7 ± 19.2 U/L in 19 healthy controls *5845*

Tumor Necrosis Factor-α *Serum* *Increase* In a group of patients with bacterial pneumonia mean concentrations of 32 ± 17 pg/mL compared with 6 ± 1.5 pg/mL in healthy controls *1079*

VeryLow Density Lipoprotein *Pleural Fluid* *Decrease* Pleural effusions in patients with bacterial pleurisy contain low density lipoproteins (33% of the serum LDL concentration on average) but almost no very low density lipoproteins (about 1% of the serum VLDL concentration on average) *4327*

Zinc *Serum* *Decrease* Statistically significant *4871*

482.90 Pneumonia

α_1-Acid Glycoprotein *Serum* *Increase* In 42 adults on admission to hospital mean concentration of 1.95 ± 0.48 g/L compared with less than 0.50 g/L in 30 healthy controls *721*

Alkaline Phosphatase *Serum* *Increase* Since lung is rich source of enzyme, activity may increase with diseases of lung such as pneumonia or pulmonary embolism *4617*

Amyloid A Protein *Serum* *Increase* In 42 adult patients on admission to hospital mean concentration of 696 ± 325 mg/L compared with less than 1.5 mg/L in 30 healthy controls *721*

Anti-Entactin Antibodies *Serum* *Increase* In 20 patients IgM anti-entactin antibodies observed in one *4604*

α_1-Antichymotrypsin *Serum* *Increase* Mean concentration in 42 adults on admission to hospital of 0.82 ± 0.10 g/L compared with less than 0.50 g/L in 30 healthy controls *721*

Carcinoembryonic Antigen *Serum* *Increase* In 28 patients with pneumonia 54% had concentrations less than 2.5 ng/mL, 42% had concentrations between 2.6 and 5.0 ng/mL, 4% had concentrations between 5.1 and 10.0 ng/mL and 1% had concentrations greater than 10.0 ng/mL *2010*

C-Reactive Protein *Serum* *Increase* In 42 adults on admission to hospital mean concentration of 44 ± 32 mg/L compared with concentration of less than 3 mg/L in 30 healthy controls *721* In 28 patients with community-acquired pneumonia 100% had CRP concentration > 50 mg/L on admission to hospital, with 75% with concentrations greater than 100 mg/L *4911*

Eosinophils *Blood* *Increase* In 38 trauma patients who developed pneumonia mean concentration of 816 ± 651 /µL significantly greater than 406 ± 582 /µL in 62 patients who did not develop pneumonia *1177*

Immunoglobulin E *Serum* *Increase* In 38 trauma patients who developed pneumonia mean concentration significantly greater than in 62 patients who did not develop pneumonia *1177*

Leukocytes *Blood* *Increase* In 28 patients with community-acquired pneumonia 62% had WBC > 10,000 /µL on admission to hospital *4911*

Neuron-specific Enolase *Serum* *Increase* In 8 of 60 patients (13.3%) with pneumonia with/without COPD, concentration increased above upper limit of normal. Median concentration of 6.0 µg/L (range 3.5 - 29 µg/L) compared with upper limit of normal of 10 µg/L *885*

Phospholipase A_2 Type II *Serum* *Increase* Increase in concentration observed of 26 µg/L in patients with pneumonia compared with 2 and 4 µg/L in healthy controls *3767*

Retinol *Urine* *Increase* In 18 patients with pneumonia mean excretion of 0.64 µmol/d compared with less than 0.01 µmol/d in 8 healthy controls *5007*

Retinol-binding Protein *Urine* *Increase* In 17 of 29 patients with pneumonia and sepsis detectable amounts of RBP detected: mean excretion of 2.8 µmol/d in the 17 patients compared with undetectable amounts in 8 healthy controls *5007*

Theophylline *Serum* *Increase* Pneumonia reported to decrease elimination of theophylline *5034*

Vitamin A *Urine* *Increase* In 18 patients with pneumonia or sepsis mean excretion of 0.78 µmol/d compared with 0.0016 µmol/d in 8 healthy controls *5007*

483.01 Mycoplasma Pneumoniae Infection

Amyloid A Protein *Serum* *Increase* In 53 patients mean concentration in acute phase of 2.00 ± 0.62 mg/L *3728*

Antibody Titer *Serum* *Increase* IgM antibodies present in 13 of 14 patients tested *3461*

Bilirubin, Indirect *Serum* *Increase* Occasional patients have been reported with hemolytic anemia *900*

Cold Agglutinins *Serum* *Increase* Elevated titers may persist for weeks or months *4551* 50% of patients, mostly severely ill, will develop reaction at the end of the 1st or the beginning of the 2nd week *367* In over 50% of patients and is related to the *4746* Significant titers in 50% of patients during the 2nd to 4th weeks, disappearing by the 6th to 8th weeks *5619* Fourfold or greater rise in titer during the illness is considered diagnostic *900* Elevated titers may persist for weeks or months *1448*

Complement Fixation *Serum* *Increase* Demonstration of CF antibodies of IgM type in week 2 provides early specific

483.01 Mycoplasma Pneumoniae Infection *(continued)*

Complement Fixation *(continued)* diagnosis *1358* A 4-fold or greater rise in titer of paired sera obtained during acute and convalescent phases is diagnostic of recent mycoplasma infection *5619* Proved to be inappropriate for the early etiological diagnosis of infections, since the high titers were distributed undifferentially among the various patient groups and many sera (38%) showed anticomplementary activity *712*

Coombs' Test *Serum Positive* Direct test may be positive in convalescence *5252* May occur *367*

C-Reactive Protein *Serum Increase* In 53 patients mean concentration in acute phase of 1.14 ± 0.47 mg/dL *3728*

Eosinophils *Blood Increase* May be observed *128*

Erythrocyte Sedimentation Rate *Blood Increase* Usually elevated *367*

Erythrocyte Survival *Red Blood Cells Decrease* Occasional patients have been reported with hemolytic anemia *900*

Haptoglobin *Serum Decrease* Usually normal but, in some cases, decreases rapidly with bacteremia *5252* Reported observation *1475*

Hemagglutination Inhibition *Serum Increase* Titer of at least 1:128 (preferably 1:512) points to the presence of a M. pneumoniae infection, especially if clinical, radiological, and laboratory data suggest a nonbacterial or mixed pneumonia *712*

Hematocrit *Blood Decrease* Sometimes seen in convalescence *1471* Occasional patients have been reported with hemolytic anemia *900*

Hemoglobin *Blood Decrease* Occasional patients have been reported with hemolytic anemia *900* Sometimes seen in convalescence *1471*
Plasma Increase Observed finding *1475* Reported observation *5677* Hemolysis has been reported in severe cases *5252* *3238*

Indirect Fluorescent Antibodies *Sputum Increase* Detects antibodies in the bronchial secretions of patients with mycoplasma infection; sensitive and specific test *440*

Lactate Dehydrogenase *Serum Increase* May be elevated *5252*

Leukocytes *Blood Increase* 27% of patients had counts > 10,000 /µL and 5% > 15,000 /µL *1542* Usually > 15,000 /µL, peaks in the first few days unless complications develop *5252* Usually below 10,000 /µL but up to 20,000 /µL in 10% of clinical cases *2039*
Blood No Effect Counts are usually < 10,000 /µL, but may go higher *900*

Lymphocytes *Blood Increase* May occur during the period of acute illness *367*

Neutrophils *Blood Increase* Slight neutrophilia occurs with counts of 60 - 85% neutrophils *367*

pH *Pleural Fluid Decrease* Exudate (pH < 7.3) *126*

Protein *Pleural Fluid Increase* Rare effusion which is usually small and an exudate (> 3g/dL) *126*

Reticulocytes *Blood Increase* Sometimes seen in convalescence *1471*

Specific Gravity *Pleural Fluid Increase* Exudate (> 1.016) *126*

VDRL *Serum Positive* False positive reactions in screening tests are common *5252*

486.00 Atypical Pneumonia

C-Reactive Protein *Serum Increase* In 9 patients with atypical pneumonia mean concentration of 122 ± 68 mg/L significantly greater than normal concentration of less than 10 mg/L *4038*

Granulocyte Colony Stimulating Factor *Serum Increase* In 8 patients with atypical pneumonia mean concentration of 60 ± 33 ng/L significantly greater than normal concentration of less than 39 ng/L *4038*

Interleukin-6 *Serum Increase* In 9 patients with atypical pneumonia mean concentration of 52 ± 25 ng/L significantly greater than normal concentration of less than 20 ng/L *4038*

Lactoferrin *Plasma No Effect* In 6 patients with atypical pneumonia mean concentration of 69 ± 17 µg/L not different from normal concentration of 40 - 215 µg/L *4038*

Leukocytes *Blood No Effect* In 9 patients with atypical pneumonia mean count of 7,500 ± 2,000 /µ/L not different from normal count of 4,000 - 9,000 /µL *4038*

Monocytes *Blood No Effect* In 9 patients with atypical pneumonia mean count of 1,900 ± 600 /µ/L not different from normal count of 2,000 - 3,000 /µL *4038*

Myeloperoxidase *Serum Increase* In 32 patients with atypical pneumonia mean concentration of 1,155 ± 752 µg/L significantly greater than normal concentration of 107 - 678 µmg/L *4038*

Neutrophils *Blood No Effect* In 9 patients with atypical pneumonia mean count of 5,600 ± 1,600 /µ/L not different from normal count of 2,000 - 6,000 /µL *4038*

Phosphate *Serum Decrease* Atypical pneumonia is less common cause of hypophosphatemia due to shift of phosphate into the cells and reduced absorption of phosphate from intestinal tract *969*

486.00 Parapneumonia

Carcinoembryonic Antigen *Pleural Fluid Increase* Mean concentration increased in 4 of 8 effusions in patients with complicated parapneumonia and 2 of 6 patients with border complicated paraneumonia and 1 of 23 in patients with typical parapneumonia *1649*

486.01 Resolving Pneumonia

Aspartate Aminotransferase *Serum Increase* In 40% of 65 patients at initial hospitalization for this disorder *1576*

Bicarbonate *Serum Decrease* Respiratory alkalosis may occur *1980*

Carbon Dioxide Partial Pressure *Blood Decrease* Moderate to severe hypoxia and respiratory alkalosis in pneumocystis pneumonitis *2283* Impaired gas diffusion and the accompanying hyperventilation results in a low pCO_2, unless the defect is severe and CO_2 retention occurs *4707* Respiratory alkalosis may occur *1980* In 40% of 43 patients at initial hospitalization for this disorder *1576*

Hematocrit *Blood Decrease* In 47% of 79 patients at initial hospitalization for this disorder *1576*

Hemoglobin *Blood Decrease* In 42% of 79 patients at initial hospitalization for this disorder *1576*

Lactate Dehydrogenase *Serum Increase* In 33% of 62 patients at initial hospitalization for this disorder *1576*
Serum No Effect Levels were normal in 45/50 cases of uncomplicated pneumonia. Increases that did occur were in cases of viral pneumonia. Unreliable screening methods were suggested to account for the increases in a previous study *2350*

Leukocytes *Blood Increase* In 51% of 79 patients at initial hospitalization for this disorder *1576*

Lymphocytes *Lung Tissue Increase* In 13 patients with lymphocytic interstitial pneumonitis, lung biopsies in all cases showed diffuse interstitial infiltrations consisting of mature lymphocytes and plasma cells *5050*

Neutrophils *Blood Increase* In 37% of 81 patients at initial hospitalization for this disorder *1576*
Pleural Fluid Increase Neutrophils predominate in pleural fluid *3052*

Oxygen Partial Pressure *Blood Decrease* Moderate to severe hypoxia and respiratory alkalosis in pneumocystis pneumonitis *2283* In 76% of 41 patients at initial hospitalization for this disorder *1576* Low pO_2 with normal or high pCO_2 *5863*

Oxygen Saturation *Blood Decrease* Moderate to severe hypoxia and respiratory alkalosis in pneumocystis pneumonitis *2283* Low pO_2 with normal or high pCO_2 *5863*

pH *Blood Increase* Moderate to severe hypoxia and respiratory alkalosis in pneumocystis pneumonitis *2283* Respiratory alkalosis may occur *1980* In 79% of 42 patients at initial hospitalization for this disorder *1576*

Plasma Cells *Lung Tissue* *Increase* In 13 patients with lymphocytic interstitial pneumonitis, lung biopsies in all cases showed diffuse interstitial infiltrations consisting of mature lymphocytes and plasma cells *5050*

487.00 Influenza

Albumin *Urine* *Increase* Febrile albuminuria may occur *5252* Mild albuminuria will be found in most febrile conditions *900*

Alkaline Phosphatase *Serum* *Increase* In some cases, even in the absence of discernible complications *5252*

Amyloid A Protein *Serum* *Increase* In 25 patients mean concentration in acute phase of 1.80 ± 0.50 mg/L *3728*

Aspartate Aminotransferase *Serum* *Increase* Usually elevated *1980*

Bilirubin *Serum* *Increase* Hemolytic anemia *5677* *4222*

Complement Fixation *Serum* *Increase* May become positive during the 2nd week of illness *1980* A very high titer is suggestive of recent infection. Recent immunization with inactivated influenza virus vaccine has little effect upon titer obtained when S antigen is used. A 4-fold or greater rise between paired sera is accepted as evidence of infection *900*

C-Reactive Protein *Serum* *Increase* In 25 patients mean concentration in acute phase 0.75 ± 0.63 mg/L *3728*

Creatine Kinase *Serum* *Increase* Higher in the acute stage than during the convalescence out of bed, while the controls showed higher activities when ambulant than during bed rest *1580*

Erythrocyte Survival *Red Blood Cells* *Decrease* Hemolytic anemia *5677* *4222*

Factor II *Plasma* *Decrease* May be associated with defibrination resulting in platelet and coagulation factor consumption *5677*

Factor IV *Plasma* *Decrease* May be associated with defibrination resulting in platelet and coagulation factor consumption *5677*

Fibrinogen *Plasma* *Decrease* May be associated with defibrination resulting in platelet and coagulation factor consumption *5677*

Hemagglutination Inhibition *Serum* *Increase* Appears to be more useful in detecting influenza A than complement-fixation tests (CF). 23% of cases verified by HI were missed by CF *4243* A 4-fold or greater rise in antibody level between paired sera is accepted as evidence of infection *900* May become positive during the second week of illness *1980*

Hematocrit *Blood* *Decrease* Hemolytic anemia *4222* *5677*

Hemoglobin *Plasma* *Increase* Hemolytic anemia *4222* *5677*

Leukocytes *Blood* *Decrease* Occurs in 50% of patients *5545* Leukopenia frequently associated with infectious diseases *2239* In many cases *5252* Often seen early in influenza but mild leukocytosis is more common. Brisk leukocytosis 15,000 /µL) suggests a secondary bacterial infection *2039*
Blood *Increase* Leukopenia is often seen early in influenza but mild leukocytosis is more common. Brisk leukocytosis (> 15,000 /µL) suggests a secondary bacterial infection. Moderate leukocytosis (10,000 - 20,000 /µL) may occur *2039* Usually elevated *1980*
Blood *No Effect* Total and differential counts are within normal limits in the majority of cases *5252*

Lymphocytes *Blood* *Decrease* Leukopenia and lymphopenia are often seen early in influenza but mild leukocytosis is more common *2039* The numbers of circulating lymphocytes are sharply and regularly reduced *5650*
Blood *Increase* The percentage of T-lymphocytes was decreased but a relative and absolute increase of non-T-lymphocytes occurred *2424*

Neutralizing Antibodies *Serum* *Increase* May become positive during the 2nd week of illness *1980* A 4-fold or greater rise in antibody level between paired sera is accepted as evidence of infection *900*

Neutrophils *Blood* *Decrease* Leukopenia frequently associated with infectious diseases *2239*
Blood *Increase* Secondary bacterial infection commonly leads to a polymorphonuclear leukocytosis in excess of 15,000 /µL *900*

Platelets *Blood* *Decrease* May be associated with defibrination resulting in platelet and coagulation factor consumption *5677*

Prothrombin Consumption *Blood* *Increase* May be associated with defibrination resulting in platelet and coagulation factor consumption *5677*

Rheumatoid Factor *Serum* *Increase* Rheumatoid factor may be observed in certain patients *2473* Concentration may be increased in influenza as in other diseases with chronic inflammation *2952* Mean concentration increased in patients with influenza *2472*

491.00 Chronic Bronchitis

α_1-Antichymotrypsin *Serum* *Increase* A study of patients with emphysema, bronchitis or asthma revealed there was no deficiency similar to that of alpha$_1$-antitrypsin. In fact, the levels were increased in all the disease states studied *953*

Bicarbonate *Serum* *Increase* In 59% of 18 patients at initial hospitalization for this disorder *1576*

Carbon Dioxide Partial Pressure *Blood* *Decrease* Can occur due to compensatory increase in ventilatory rate *4920*

Carcinoembryonic Antigen *Serum* *Increase* 33% of patients had values > 2.5 ng/mL *4891* In 61 patients with bronchitis 67% had concentrations less than 2.5 ng/mL, 25% had concentrations between 2.6 and 5.0 ng/mL, 7% had concentrations between 5.1 and 10.0 ng/mL and 1% had concentrations greater than 10.0 ng/mL *2010*

Cells *Sputum* *Increase* Observed effect *900*

Copper *Serum* *Increase* Statistically significant *4871*

Creatine Kinase BB-Isoenzyme *Serum* *No Effect* Virtually the same level as in normal subjects *3762*

Endothelin-1 *BAL Fluid* *Increase* In 5 patients with chronic bronchitis mean concentration of 0.08 ± 0.03 pg/mL (1.5 times appropriate normal) *328*
BAL Fluid *No Effect* In chronic bronchitics mean concentration of 4.2 ± 0.2 pg/mL not significantly different from 4.4 ± 0.2 pg/mL in healthy controls *328*

Eosinophils *Blood* *Increase* Increased if there is allergic basis or component *5544* In 36% of 24 patients at initial hospitalization for this disorder *1576*
Sputum *Increase* More than 3% eosinophils indicates an allergic state *900*

Erythrocyte Sedimentation Rate *Blood* *Increase* Present during the course of infection *900*

Leukocytes *Blood* *Increase* Normal or increased *5544*

Mucin-associated Antigen *Serum* *Increase* Mean concentration of 21.8 ± 1.9 ng/mL observed in 28 patients with chronic bronchitis and other pulmonary diseases significantly different from 9.9 ± 0.8 ng/mL observed in 59 healthy individuals *4797*

Neutrophils *Blood* *Increase* Neutrophilic cells are present only during the course of an infection *900*

Oxygen Partial Pressure *Blood* *Decrease* 66% of nonasthmatic chronic lung disease patients (bronchitis and emphysema) had a mean pO_2 of 72.7 mm Hg. Bronchitics but not emphysemics showed a positive correlation between pO_2 and ventilatory performance *5184* In 61% of 19 patients at initial hospitalization for this disorder *1576* Arterial O_2 tension in 54 patients with chronic nonspecific lung disease, indicated subnormal results to be more frequent among bronchitics (79% with hypoxemia) than among emphysematous patients (63% with hypoxemia *3272* Tendency to decrease witH the increase in dyspnea severity was apparent *3271*

Oxygen Saturation *Blood* *Decrease* Tendency to decrease with the increase in dyspnea severity was apparent *3271*

pH *Blood* *Decrease* In 60% of 20 patients at initial hospitalization for this disorder *1576*
Blood *Increase* Can occur due to compensatory increase in ventilatory rate *4920*

Rheumatoid Factor *Serum* *Increase* Found in 62% of patients *306* *874*

Tissue Polypeptide Antigen *Serum* *No Effect* In 11 patients mean concentration of 100.1 ± 68.5 U/L not significantly different from 72.7 ± 19.2 U/L in 19 healthy controls *5845*

Zinc *Serum* *Decrease* Statistically significant *4871*

491.20 Chronic Obstructive Airways Disease

Carbon Dioxide Partial Pressure *Urine Increase* In 20 patients with COAD mean of 6.72 ± 1.25 kPa significantly different from 5.12 ± 0.62 kPa in 10 healthy controls *1809*

Erythrocytes *Blood Increase* In 20 patients with COAD mean concentration of 5.36 ± 0.81 x 10^{12}/L significantly different from 4.72 ± 0.56 x 10^{12}/L in 10 healthy controls *1809*

Ferritin *Serum No Effect* In 20 patients with COAD mean concentration of 220 ± 124 µg/L not significantly different from 235 ± 103 µg/L in 10 healthy controls *1809*

Hematocrit *Blood Increase* In 20 patients with COAD mean of 0.47 ± 0.06 not significantly different from 0.43 ± 0.05 in 10 healthy controls *1809*

Hemoglobin *Blood Increase* In 20 patients with COAD mean concentration of 152.8 ± 17.9 g/L not significantly different from 149.3 ± 9.5 g/L in 10 healthy controls *1809*

Iron *Serum Decrease* In 20 patients with COAD mean concentration of 12.7 ± 3.7 µmol/L not significantly different from 13.9 ± 6.2 µmol/L in 10 healthy controls *1809*
Urine Increase In 20 patients with COAD mean excretion of 24.6 ± 20.8 µmol/d significantly different from 9.7 ± 7.6 µmol/d in 10 healthy controls *1809*

Iron-binding Capacity, Unsaturated *Serum No Effect* In 20 patients with COAD mean concentration of 32.5 ± 12.3 µmol/L not significantly different from 31.7 ± 15.2 µmol/L in 10 healthy controls *1809*

MCH *Blood Decrease* In 20 patients with COAD mean of 28.3 ± 3.3 pg not significantly different from 31.5 ± 2.1 pg in 10 healthy controls *1809*

MCHC *Blood Decrease* In 20 patients with COAD mean of 324.0 ± 19.3 g/L significantly different from 347.0 ± 11.6 g/L in 10 healthy controls *1809*

MCV *Blood Decrease* In 20 patients with COAD mean of 86.8 ± 6.9 fL not significantly different from 90.8 ± 4.5 fL in 10 healthy controls *1809*

Oxygen Partial Pressure *Urine Decrease* In 20 patients with COAD mean of 6.47 ± 0.71 kPa significantly different from 8.81 ± 0.71 kPa in 10 healthy controls *1809*

pH *Urine Decrease* In 20 patients with COAD mean of 7.41 ± 0.06 significantly different from 7.45 ± 0.04 µmol/d in 10 healthy controls *1809*

Phosphate *Serum Decrease* Chronic obstructive airways disease is less common cause of hypophosphatemia due to increased renal loss of phosphate *969*

Transferrin *Serum Decrease* In 20 patients with COAD mean concentration of 1.91 ± 0.56 g/L not significantly different from 2.23 ± 0.41 g/L in 10 healthy controls *1809*

492.80 Pulmonary Emphysema

Ammonia *Blood Increase* Found in high percentage of patients without evidence of congestive failure or liver disease *4707*

Angiotensin-converting Enzyme *Serum Increase* In 10 patients with emphysema mean concentration of 150 ± 18 U/L significantly higher than 108 ± 13 U/L in 85 healthy control individuals *5338*

α_1-Antitrypsin *Serum Decrease* α_1-Antitrypsin deficiency trait may account for up to 10% of emphysema cases *3525*

Carbon Dioxide Partial Pressure *Blood Decrease* In 10 patients with emphysema mean of 39 ± 11 mm Hg significantly different from 52 ± 9 mm Hg in 85 healthy control individuals *5338*
Blood Increase Respiratory acidosis may occur *1980* Arterial blood oxygen decreased and CO_2 increased *5544*

Carcinoembryonic Antigen *Serum Increase* In 49 patients with pulmonary emphysema 43% had concentrations less than 2.5 ng/mL, 37% had concentrations between 2.6 and 5.0 ng/mL, 16% had concentrations between 5.1 and 10.0 ng/mL and 4% had concentrations greater than 10.0 ng/mL *2010* 57% of patients had values > 2.5 ng/mL *4891*

Erythrocytes *Blood Increase* Secondary polycythemia *5544*

Hematocrit *Blood Increase* Rises in later stages *900*

Hemoglobin *Blood Increase* Rises in later stages *900*

Interleukin-8 *Serum Increase* Mean concentration in 15 patients with chronic pulmonary emphysema of 33 ± 11 pg/mL significantly different from < 13 pg/mL in 10 healthy controls *2548*

Leukocytes *Sputum Increase* Often infected on smear; increased WBC and epithelial debris *900*

Oxygen Partial Pressure *Blood Decrease* In 10 patients with emphysema mean of 48 ± 3 mm Hg significantly different from 69 ± 9 mm Hg in 85 healthy control individuals *5338*

Oxygen Saturation *Blood Decrease* 66% of nonasthmatic chronic lung disease patients (bronchitis and emphysema) had a mean pO_2 of 72.7 mm Hg. Bronchitics, but not emphysemics, showed a positive correlation between pO_2 and ventilatory performance *5184* Arterial tension in 54 patients with chronic nonspecific lung disease, indicated subnormal results to be more frequent among bronchitics (79% with hypoxemia) than among emphysematous patients (63% with hypoxemia) *3272*

pH *Blood Decrease* Respiratory acidosis may occur *1980*
Blood No Effect In 10 patients with emphysema mean of 7.37 ± 1.29 not significantly different from 7.40 ± 1.30 in 85 healthy control individuals *5338*

Potassium *Serum Increase* Rises in acidosis but total body potassium is usually depressed *900*
Serum No Effect Usually no significant effect *5544*
Urine No Effect Usually unaffected *5544*

Renin Activity *Plasma Increase* In 10 patients with emphysema mean activity of 3.78 ± 0.48 ng/mL/h significantly higher than 2.76 ± 0.64 ng/mL/h in 85 healthy control individuals *5338*

Sodium *Serum No Effect* Usual finding *5544*

Volume *Plasma Increase* Normal or increased *5544*
Plasma No Effect Normal or increased *5544*
Urine No Effect Usually normal *5544*

493.90 Asthma

Adrenomedullin *Plasma Increase* Mean concentration of 98 ± 32 pg/mL in 9 patients with acute asthma significantly different from 21 ± 3 pg/mL 7 stable asthmatic patients and 18 ± 2 pg/mL in 30 normal controls *2743*

Albumin *Sputum No Effect* Concentration in 14 asthmatic patients of 0.88 ± 0.14 mg/mL not significantly different from 0.93 ± 0.23 mg/mL in healthy controls *4816*

Amino-terminal Propeptide of Type I Procollagen
Serum No Effect In 14 prepubertal children with newly detected perennial asthma mean concentration of 13.8 nmol/L not significantly different from 14.9 nmol/L in 21 healthy children *4944*

Amino-terminal Propeptide of Type III Procollagen
Serum No Effect In 14 prepubertal children with newly detected perennial asthma mean concentration of 7.8 µg/L not significantly different from 17.8 µg/L in 21 healthy children *4944*

Angiotensin-converting Enzyme *Serum Increase* In 23 patients with extrinsic asthma mean concentration of 141 ± 25 U/L significantly higher than 108 ± 13 U/L in 85 healthy control individuals *5338*
Serum No Effect In 24 patients with intrinsic asthma mean concentration of 98 ± 15 U/L not significantly different from 108 ± 13 U/L in 85 healthy control individuals *5338*

Anti-Mitochondrial Antibodies *Serum Increase* In 20% of cases *456*

α_1-Antichymotrypsin *Serum Increase* Mean concentration in 136 asthmatic patients of 55.8 ± 16 mg/dL significantly different from 47.9 ± 8.1 mg/dL in 110 healthy controls *3044* A study of patients with emphysema, bronchitis or asthma revealed there was no deficiency similar to that of alpha$_1$-antitrypsin. In fact, the levels were increased in all the disease states studied *953*

Antidiuretic Hormone *Plasma Increase* In status asthmaticus *2569*

Aspartate Aminotransferase *Serum Increase* Possibly due to anoxic tissue damage in status asthmaticus *1290* Increased in 90% of acute untreated asthma patients *2569*

Bicarbonate *Serum Decrease* May be decreased in early stages and may be increased in later stages *5544*
Serum Increase In 40% of 95 patients at initial hospitalization for this disorder *1576* May be decreased in early stages and increased in later stages *5544*

Serum *No Effect* In a moderate to severe attack the partial pressure of CO_2 is reduced, while normal values are obtained for bicarbonate and pH. As the condition worsens the pCO_2 and bicarbonate will rise and pH fall *900*

CA 19-9 *Serum* *Increase* The percentage of patients with positive serum levels was 42.3% with pulmonary disease (14.5% in asbestosis, 27.3% in bronchial asthma, 59.4% in bronchiectasis, 81.3% in idiopathic pulmonary fibrosis and 61.5% in pulmonary tuberculosis) *2026*

Carbon Dioxide Partial Pressure *Blood* *Decrease* In 30% of 91 patients at initial hospitalization for this disorder *1576* pH, total plasma CO_2 and pCO_2 are decreased as a result of metabolic acidosis in status asthmaticus *4423* Reduced in a moderate to severe attack, while normal values are obtained for bicarbonate and pH. As the condition worsens the pCO_2 while the pH falls *900*
Blood *Increase* CO_2 retention, indicating alveolar hypoventilation, has a grave prognostic significance *2039* Reduction in arterial oxygen tension without concomitant elevation of arterial pCO_2 in moderately severe asthma. Elevation of pCO_2 is dependent upon total reduction in ventilation or will be seen when severe mucus plugging is present *900* Reduced in a moderate to severe attack, while normal values are obtained for bicarbonate and pH. As the condition worsens the pCO_2 will rise while the pH falls *900*
Blood *No Effect* The finding of a normal pCO_2 in a patient experiencing a severe asthmatic attack should alert the clinician to impending respiratory failure *900* In 23 patients with extrinsic asthma mean of 50 ± 10 mm Hg and 50 ± 10 mm Hg in 24 patients with intrinsic asthma not significantly different from 52 ± 9 mm Hg in 85 healthy control individuals *5338*

Cells *Sputum* *No Effect* In 12 untreated patients with asthma mean concentration of 0.64 x 10^6/mL not significantly different from 0.49 x 10^6/mL in normal individuals *238* In 43 patients with chronic bronchial asthma total cell count similar to that in 20 healthy individuals *4422*

Ceruloplasmin *Serum* *Increase* In 50 patients with bronchial asthma mean concentration of 618 ± 172 mg/L significantly greater than that in 250 healthy people, in whom the mean concentration was 315 ± 119 mg/L *1377*

Ceruloplasmin Ferroxidase *Serum* *Increase* In 50 patients with bronchial asthma mean activity of 1,057 ± 292 U/L significantly greater than that in 250 healthy people in whom the mean concentration was 537 ± 201 U/L *1377*

Chloride *Sweat* *Increase* High concentrations found in sweat of chronic asthmatics and their relatives *5043*

Ciliated Cells *Sputum* *No Effect* Concentration in 14 asthmatic patients of 1.1 ± 0.3% not significantly different from 0.8 ± 0.4% in healthy controls *4816*

Complement C_3 *Serum* *Increase* In patients with acute asthma significantly higher concentration observed than in normal controls *4486*

Complement C_3b *Serum* *No Effect* No significant difference observed between concentrations in patients with acute asthma and healthy controls *4486*

Complement C_3d *Serum* *No Effect* Concentration in asthmatic patients not significantly different from healthy controls *4486*

Complement C_4 *Serum* *Decrease* Decreased serum concentrations of C_4 and factor B were found in 3 of 15 skin-test positive asthmatic children. Confirming the involvement of complement in the pathogenesis of immediate type reaction *2256*
Serum *No Effect* Usually normal *2569*

Complement, Total *Serum* *No Effect* In the absence of any immunoglobulin deficiency, the levels of the immunoglobulins as well as complement are within normal limits *4551*

Copper *Serum* *Increase* Statistically significant *4871* In 50 patients with bronchial asthma mean concentration of 24.50 ± 9.64 µmol/L significantly greater than that in 250 healthy people, mean concentration of 15.82 ± 4.15 µmol/L *1377*

Cortisol *Plasma* *Decrease* In 36 asthmatic children 8:00 a.m. plasma concentrations were compared with changes in their total eosinophil count (TEC) from 8:00 a.m. to 9:30 a.m. All children with low cortisol levels had decreases in TEC of < 2%, whereas 78% of children with normal cortisol had decreases > 15%. All children with decreases 15% had normal cortisol levels *491* Concentrations of about 27 ng/dL in 57 symptomatic asthmatics significantly higher than 18 ng/dL in 72 asymptomatic patients and 10 ng/dL in normal individuals *2956*
Plasma *No Effect* In 36 asthmatic children 8:00 a.m. plasma concentrations were compared with changes in their total eosinophil count (TEC) from 8:00 a.m. to 9:30 a.m. All children with low cortisol levels had decreases in TEC of < 2%, whereas 78% of children with normal cortisol had decreases 15%. All children with decreases > 15% had normal cortisol levels *491*

Creatine Kinase *Serum* *Increase* Increases correlated with severity of symptoms (subjective) and objective measurement of airway obstruction *639* High in 38% of acute untreated asthma patients *2569*

C-terminal Propeptide of Type I Collagen *Serum* *No Effect* In 14 prepubertal children with newly detected perennial asthma mean concentration of 3.2 nmol/L not significantly different from 3.2 nmol/L in 21 healthy children *4944*

Cysteinyl-containing Leukotrienes *Serum* *Increase* In 31 asthmatic patients mean concentration of 500 ± 31 pmol/L significantly greater than 112.1± 8.27 pmol/L in 10 normal healthy donors *3283*

2,3-Diphosphoglycerate *Red Blood Cells* *Increase* In acute untreated attacks *2569*

Dipyridinoline *Urine* *No Effect* In 14 prepubertal children with newly detected perennial asthma mean excretion of 18.4 nmol/mmol creatinine not significantly different from 18.4 nmol/mmol creatinine in 21 healthy children *4944*

Dopamine *Plasma* *Increase* Concentrations of about 32 pmol/mL in 57 symptomatic asthmatics significantly higher than 20 pmol/mL in 72 asymptomatic patients and 13 pmol/mL in normal individuals *2956*

Endothelin-1 *BAL Fluid* *Increase* In 6 patients with asthma mean concentration of 0.25 ± 0.05 pg/mL (5.4 fold rise compared with normal) and in 1 with status asthmaticus concentration of 0.3 pg/mL (6.0 times appropriate normal value) *328*
BAL Fluid *No Effect* In stable asthmatics mean concentration slightly increased at 5.2 ± 0.2 pg/mL compared with 4.4 ± 0.2 pg/mL in healthy controls *328*

Eosinophil Cationic Protein *Serum* *Increase* In 33 asthmatic patients mean concentration of 12.6 µg/L significantly different from 4.6 µg/L in 6 healthy controls *3791* Mean concentration of 54.3 ± 23.0 µg/L in 10 patients with atopic asthma *1931* In 19 patients with severe asthma 7 patients had concentrations above 20 µg/L as measured by Pharmacia procedure during 21 exacerbations of the disease with fourfold increase above baseline in 12 exacerbations *1060* Concentration in 14 asthmatic patients of 9.3 ± 1.6 ng/mL significantly different from 1.5 ± 0.8 ng/mL in healthy controls *4816* Mean concentration in 60 patients with childhood asthma of approximately 15 µg/L *4627*
Serum *No Effect* In 12 untreated patients with asthma mean concentration of 6.8 µg/L not significantly different from 4 µg/L in normal individuals *238*
Sputum *Increase* Median concentration in 9 patients with asthma who smoked of 0.16 µg/L and of 0.22 µg/L in 10 who did not smoke *4667* Concentration in 14 asthmatic patients of 697.7 ± 141.3 ng/mL significantly different from 88.0 ± 31.5 ng/mL in healthy controls *4816* In 12 untreated patients with asthma mean concentration of 165 µg/L significantly different from 34 µg/L in normal individuals *238* Mean concentration of 984.5 ± 1245.5 µg/L/g in 10 patients with atopic asthma *1931*

Eosinophil Protein X *Serum* *Increase* In 12 children with atopic asthma mean concentration of 94.7 µg/L significantly different when compared with 30.8 µg/L in 9 control children *2825* Mean concentration in 60 patients with childhood asthma of approximately 45 µg/L *4627*
Serum *No Effect* In 12 untreated patients with asthma mean concentration of 20 µg/mL not significantly different from 11 µg/L in normal individuals *238*
Sputum *Increase* In 12 untreated patients with asthma mean concentration of 360 µg/L significantly different from 41 µg/L in normal individuals *238*
Urine *Increase* In 12 children with atopic asthma mean concentration of 116.4 µg/mmol creatinine compared with 43.0 µg/mmol creatinine in 9 control children *2825*

Eosinophils *BAL Fluid* *Increase* In 33 asthmatic patients mean concentration of 0.7% significantly different from 0.0% in 6 healthy controls *3791*
Blood *Increase* Mean concentration of 310 x 10^6/L in 10 patients with atopic asthma *1931* In 12 untreated patients with asthma mean proportion of 3.8% significantly different from 1.8% in normal individuals *238* Mean concentration in 9 patients with asthma who did not smoke of 391 ± 90.6 x 10^6/L and of 202 ±

493.90 Asthma *(continued)*

Eosinophils *(continued)*
45.7 x 10^6/L in 10 who smoked *4667* In 80 asthmatic children aged between 6 months and 15 years total eosinophil count ranged from 10 to 2,100 /µL with upper limit of normal of 400 cells/µL with mean cell count increasing with clinical severity, 220 /µL for intermittent disease, 441 /µL for mild persistent disease, 725 /µL for moderate persistent disease and 1,591 /µL for severe persistent disease *2543* Mean concentration of 246 x 10^6/L in 10 patients with chronic obstructive pulmonary disease *1931* In 33 asthmatic patients mean concentration of 350.0 x 10^6/L significantly different from 120.0 x 10^6/L in 6 healthy controls *3791* In 55% of 122 patients at initial hospitalization for this disorder *1576* In 3 patients with asthma (2 acute, 1 non-acute) mean concentrations of 525 x 10^6/L significantly different from upper limit of normal of 440 x 10^6/L in 29 normal individuals *607* In 52 patients with active bronchial asthma (not on steroid therapy), total eosinophil counts were > 350 /µL. Counts showed inverse correlation (r = -0.74) with specific airway conductance *2231* In 8 patients with bronchial asthma and eosinophilia mean concentration of 1,190 ± 600 /µL compared with less than 500 /µL in 100 normal individuals and 299 ± 91.3 /µL in 6 patients with bronchial asthma but without eosinophilia *5776* In more than 60% of patients tested *849* Tended to increase after bronchial provocation test but the increase did not correlate with the occurrence of the immediate type bronchial provocation test reaction *2256*
Sputum Increase In 43 patients with chronic bronchial asthma proportion of eosinophils of 14% compared with 0.6% in 20 healthy individuals, concentration correlating with severity of asthma *4422* Stained sputum is usually found to contain eosinophils; pointed elongated crystals derived from eosinophilic granules (Charcot-Leyden crystals) and spiral mucocellular bronchial casts (Curschmann's spirals) are also found *2039* Concentration in 14 asthmatic patients of 38.8 ± 8.2% significantly higher than 0.3 ± 0.2% in healthy controls *4816* In 12 untreated patients with asthma mean concentration of 14.8% significantly different from 0.0% in normal individuals *238* Often found; although suggestive of asthma in both allergic and infective types, they are not pathognomonic *4551*
Tissue Increase In 33 asthmatic patients mean concentration in bronchial tissue of 45.5 /mm² significantly different from 2.5 /mm² in 6 healthy controls *3791*

Epinephrine *Plasma Increase* Concentrations of about 138 pg/mL in 57 symptomatic asthmatics significantly higher than 98 pg/mL in 72 asymptomatic patients and 75 pg/mL in normal individuals *2956*

Epinephrine:Norepinephrine Ratio *Plasma Increase* Ratio significantly increased in 57 patients with asthma *2955*

Glucose *Serum Increase* May be due to epinephrine or corticosteroids *900* May be found in corticosteroid-treated patients *4551*

Granulocyte-Macrophage Colony Stimulating Factor
Serum No Effect Not detected in the serum of any of 8 patients with condition *2744*

Haptoglobin *Serum Increase* Mean concentration in acute exacerbations of 228.5 ± 80.8 mg/dL in 50 children with asthma significantly increased compared with152.3 ± 49.8 mg/dL in clinical remission *2739*

Hematocrit *Blood Increase* In 37% of 122 patients at initial hospitalization for this disorder *1576*

Hemoglobin *Blood Increase* In 37% of 121 patients at initial hospitalization for this disorder *1576*

Histamine *Plasma Increase* In 3 patients with asthma (2 acute, 1 non-acute) mean concentrations of 11.8 - 24.8 nmol/L significantly different from mean concentration of 4.0 nmol/L in 29 normal individuals *607*

5-Hydroxytryptamine *Platelets Decrease* Concentration significantly decreased in 57 patients with asthma *2955* Concentrations of about 100 ng/mL in 57 symptomatic asthmatics significantly lower than 150 ng/mL in 72 asymptomatic patients and 200 ng/mL in normal individuals *2956*

5-Hydroxytryptamine, Free *Plasma Increase* Concentrations of free serotonin of about 10 ng/mL in 57 symptomatic asthmatics significantly higher than 2 ng/mL in 72 asymptomatic patients and < 1.3 ng/mL in normal individuals *2956* Concentration significantly increased in 57 patients with asthma *2955*
Platelets Increase Concentration significantly increased in 57 patients with asthma *2955*

Immunoglobulin A, Secretory *Sputum Increase* Median concentration in 9 patients with asthma who smoked of 54 mg/L and of 8 mg/L in 10 who did not smoke *4667*

Immunoglobulin E *Serum Increase* In 6 atopic asthmatic children mean concentration of 605.7 IU/mL compared with 27 IU/mL in 12 age-matched controls *5161* In 6 asthmatic individuals mean concentration of 263 kU/L significantly greater than 24.9 kU/L in 6 healthy controls *4548*
Serum No Effect Usual effect observed is no change from normal *1315* Elevated in most patients with allergic asthma but not in most patients with intrinsic asthma. At this time, however, the IgE level should not be used by itself to differentiate intrinsic from extrinsic asthma. Elevated in 75-81% of the children with asthma, nasal allergy, and atopic dermatitis. Elevated serum IgE concentration or blood eosinophilia, or both, was noted in 85% of the patients *849* In 6 nonatopic asthmatic children mean concentration of 9.0 IU/mL compared with 27 IU/mL in 12 age-matched controls *5161* Usually found in patients with allergic asthma but not with other forms *2460*

Immunoglobulins *Serum No Effect* In the absence of any immunoglobulin deficiency, the levels of the immunoglobulins as well as complement are within normal limits *4551*

Interleukin-3 *Serum No Effect* Not detected in the serum of any of 8 patients with condition *2744*

Interleukin-4 Receptor *Serum Increase* The serum levels were examined in children with allergic diseases, and compared with those in non-allergic controls of the same age and sex. The serum concentration of IL-4 was elevated in all allergic groups, including cases of atopic eczema, bronchial asthma and anaphylaxis to food, compared with non-allergic controls *3369*

Interleukin-5 *Serum Increase* Detected in the serum of 1 of 8 patients with bronchial asthma *2744*
Sputum Increase Concentration in 14 asthmatic patients of 1.03 ± 7.1 pg/mL significantly different from not detectable amount in healthy controls *4816*

Interleukin-8 *Serum No Effect* Mean concentration in 19 patients with bronchial asthma of < 13 pg/mL not significantly different from < 13 pg/mL in 10 healthy controls *2548*
Sputum No Effect Concentration in 14 asthmatic patients of 1.31 ± 0.40 ng/mL not significantly different from 1.52 ± 0.44 ng/mL in healthy controls *4816*

Lactate *Blood Increase* Increased arterial blood lactate in acute untreated attacks *2569* Lactic acid, pyruvic acid and the lactic/pyruvic ratio are increased in some patients *4423*

Lactate Dehydrogenase Isoenzyme-5 *Serum Increase* Raised activities of LD_3 and LD_5 comprised the bulk of the increase in total activity. The increment in LD_3 activity arose from lung involvement whereas the major portion of the increment in LD_5 activity was derived from the liver *5374*

Lactate Dehydrogenase Isoenzymes *Serum Increase* Raised activities of LD_3 and LD_5 comprised the bulk of the increase in total activity. LD_1 and LD_2 were unaltered. The increment in LD_3 activity arose from lung involvement whereas the major portion of the increment in LD-5 activity was derived from the liver in patients with asthma *5374*

Lactoferrin *Sputum Increase* Median concentration in 9 patients with asthma who smoked of 63 mg/L and of 25 mg/L in 10 who did not smoke *4667*

Leukocytes *Blood Increase* In 53% of 122 patients at initial hospitalization for this disorder *1576*
Blood No Effect In 12 untreated patients with asthma mean concentration of 6.25 x 10^3/mL not significantly different from 6.3 x 10^3/mL in normal individuals *238*

Leukotriene B_4 *BAL Fluid Increase* In 2 children during asthmatic attacks mean concentrations of 315.0 and 57.1 pg/mg protein compared with undetectable amounts before extubation and in two healthy controls *5835*
Plasma Increase In 29 asthmatic patients mean concentration of 483 ± 75 pmol/L significantly greater than 140 ± 12.1 pmol/L in 10 normal healthy donors. Concentration in asthmatics during attacks of 432 ± 62 pmol/L significantly greater than 325 ± 109 pmol/L between attacks *3283*

Leukotriene C_4 *BAL Fluid Increase* In 2 children during asthmatic attacks mean concentrations of 303.0 and 102.8 pg/mg protein compared with undetectable amounts before extubation and in two healthy controls *5835*

Lymphocytes *Sputum No Effect* In 12 untreated patients with asthma mean concentration of 0.0% not significantly different from 3.7% in normal individuals *238*

Macrophages *Sputum Increase* Concentration in 14 asthmatic patients of 19.8 ± 4.8% significantly different from 36.0 ± 4.4% in healthy controls *4816*
Sputum No Effect In 12 untreated patients with asthma mean concentration of 37% not significantly different from 70% in normal individuals *238*

Myelin Basic Protein *Serum Increase* In 8 patients with bronchial asthma and eosinophilia mean concentration of 93.8 ± 34.1 ng/mL but in 6 patients with bronchial asthma but without eosinophilia mean concentration of 50.0 ± 13.5 ng/mL compared with mean of 41 ± 19 ng/mL in 100 normal individuals *5776*

Myeloperoxidase *Serum Increase* Mean concentration in 60 patients with childhood asthma of approximately 1,280 µg/L *4627*
Sputum Increase Median concentration in 9 patients with asthma who smoked of 8 mg/L and of 6 mg/L in 10 who did not smoke *4667*

Neutrophils *Blood Increase* In 38% of 122 patients at initial hospitalization for this disorder *1576* Modest changes in the peripheral WBC count occur along with an occasional increase in the percentage of polymorphonuclear WBC *900*
Sputum Decrease Concentration in 14 asthmatic patients of 38.3 ± 7.4% significantly different from 60.9 ± 4.2% in healthy controls *4816*
Sputum Increase In 43 patients withasthma proportion of neutrophils 14.4% compared with 8.8% in 20 healthy individuals *4422*
Sputum No Effect In 12 untreated patients with asthma mean concentration of 34.5% not significantly different from 27.3% in normal individuals *238* Concentration in 14 asthmatic patients of 2.1 ± 0.4% not significantly different from 1.9 ± 0.6% in healthy controls *4816*

Norepinephrine *Plasma Increase* Concentrations of about 360 pg/mL in 57 symptomatic asthmatics significantly higher than 290 pg/mL in 72 asymptomatic patients and 220 pg/mL in normal individuals *2956*

Osteocalcin *Serum Decrease* In 14 prepubertal children with newly detected perennial asthma mean concentration of 11.5 µg/L significantly different from 21 µg/L in 21 healthy children *4944*

Oxygen Partial Pressure *Blood Decrease* In 74% of 89 patients at initial hospitalization for this disorder *1576* In 23 patients with extrinsic asthma mean of 44 ± 7 mm Hg significantly different from 69 ± 9 mm Hg in 85 healthy control individuals *5338* In general, with moderate asthma of whatever type, and even sometimes when there is no obvious distress, a modest reduction of arterial oxygen pressure to 60 - 70 mm Hg may be found. As an attack becomes more severe, a further reduction may yield values as low as 50 - 60 mm Hg *3431*
Blood No Effect In 24 patients with intrinsic asthma mean of 61 ± 9 mm Hg not significantly different from 69 ± 9 mm Hg in 85 healthy control individuals *5338*

pH *Blood Decrease* pH, total plasma CO_2 and pCO_2 are decreased as a result of metabolic acidosis in status asthmaticus *4423* In a moderate to severe attack; bicarbonate and pH are lowered. As the condition worsens the pCO_2 will rise while bicarbonate and pH fall *900*
Blood Increase In 59% of 92 patients at initial hospitalization for this disorder *1576*
Blood No Effect Usually within normal limits in moderate to severe attack *900* In 23 patients with extrinsic asthma mean of 7.34 ± 0.99 and 7.39 ± 1.00 in 24 patients with extrinsic asthma not significantly different from 7.40 ± 1.30 in 85 healthy control individuals *5338*

Phosphate *Serum Decrease* In 40% of 107 patients at initial hospitalization for this disorder *1576*

Phospholipase A *Serum Increase* Status asthmaticus *2200*

Platelet Aggregation response to ADP *Blood Increase* Aggregation of 62.9 ± 13.8% in 57 symptomatic asthmatics significantly higher than 32.9 ± 14.7% in 72 asymptomatic patients and 22.9 ± 9.8% in normal individuals *2956*

Platelet Aggregation response to Collagen *Blood Increase* Aggregation of 66.9 ± 9.8% in 57 symptomatic asthmatics significantly higher than 34.6 ± 15.2% in 72 asymptomatic patients and 25.8 ± 11.2% in normal individuals *2956*

Potassium *Serum Decrease* Hypokalemia caused by therapy or gastrointestinal fluid losses in children may intensify or induce respiratory failure by producing muscle weakness *900* May be found in corticosteroid-treated patients *4551*

Procollagen Type III Peptide *Serum No Effect* Our results showed that the concentration of procollagen peptide in blood samples from patients with asthma was 5.8 ± 2.4, 4.9 ± 1.8 in patients with COPD and 11.1 ± 3.6 in healthy subjects. There was no significant difference between patients with asthma, COPD and healthy subjects ($p < 0.01$) *2752*

Protein 1 *BAL Fluid Positive* In patients with asthma protein 1 detectable *2371*

Pyridinoline *Urine No Effect* In 14 prepubertal children with newly detected perennial asthma mean excretion of 150 nmol/mmol creatinine not significantly different from 128 nmol/mmol creatinine in 21 healthy children *4944*

Pyridoxal Phosphate *Red Blood Cells Decrease* Mean concentration of 59 ± 35 nmol/L in 15 adult asthmatics significantly less than 111 ± 61 nmol/L in 16 healthy controls *4336*
Serum Decrease Mean concentration of 21 ± 15 nmol/L in 15 adult asthmatics significantly less than 73 ± 41 nmol/L in 16 healthy controls *4336*

Pyruvate *Blood Increase* Lactic acid, pyruvic acid, and the lactic/pyruvic ratio are increased in some patients *4423*

Renin Activity *Plasma No Effect* In 23 patients with extrinsic asthma mean activity of 2.75 ± 1.30 ng/mL/h and 2.90 ± 0.50 ng/mL/h in 24 patients with intrinsic asthma not significantly different from 2.76 ± 0.64 ng/mL/h in 85 healthy control individuals *5338*

Rheumatoid Factor *Serum Increase* Found in 17% of patients *874 306*

Soluble Intercellular Adhesion Molecule-1 *Serum Increase* In 20 patients with atopic bronchial asthma during asthma attacks mean concentration of 50.7 ± 20.6 U/mL significantly higher than those in stable condition (38.3 ± 9.3 U/mL) *2732* In 17 atopic asthmatic patients in stable condition mean concentration of 37.0 ± 13.3 U/mL compared with 29.1 ± 4.6 U/mL in 17 normal subjects. During asthmatic attacks mean concentration in 10 patients increased to 41.7 ± 7.9 U/mL from baseline of 33.6 ± 12.6 U/mL *2050* In 45 asthmatic children (15 mild, 15 moderate and 15 severe) mean concentration of 390.0 ± 108.3 ng/mL significantly higher than 193.2 ± 33.95 ng/mL in 20 healthy control children. Concentration increased progressively in asthmatics with severity of illness *1349*

Soluble Interleukin-2 Receptor *Serum Increase* Mean concentration in 44 acutely ill asthmatic patients of 42 pmol/L not significantly different from 41 pmol/L in 47 asthmatic patients in remission but significantly greater than 27 pmol/L in 50 healthy controls *3631*

Soluble Interleukin-6 Receptor *Serum Increase* In 20 patients with bronchial asthma mean concentration of 132 ± 31 ng/mL significantly higher than that in 111 normal control individuals in whom the mean concentration was 111 ± 16 ng/mL *5804*
Serum No Effect In 10 patients with stable bronchial asthma mean concentration of 113 ± 21 ng/mL was not significantly different from that in 10 normal control individuals in whom the mean concentration was 112 ± 22 ng/mL *5804*

Spasmogenic Cysteinyl Leukotrienes *Serum Increase* In 31 asthmatic patients mean concentration of 529 ± 40 pmol/L during attacks significantly greater than 413± 50.4 pmol/L between attacks *3283*

Thromboxane B_2 *BAL Fluid No Effect* In 2 children during asthmatic attacks mean concentrations undetectable compared with undetectable amounts before extubation and in two healthy controls *5835*

Tryptase *Serum No Effect* Mean concentration in 60 patients with childhood asthma not significantly different from that in healthy individuals *4627*
Sputum Increase Median concentration in 9 patients with asthma who smoked of 2.5 mg/L and of 8 mg/L in 10 who did not smoke *4667*

Tumor Necrosis Factor-α *Serum Increase* In 14 patients with atopic bronchial asthma during asthma attacks mean concentration of 71.0 ± 52.1 pg/mL significantly higher than those in stable condition (27.9 ± 16.3 pg/mL) *2732*
Serum No Effect In 13 children with bronchial asthma mean concentration not significantly different from that in 11 healthy controls *5079*

493.90 Asthma (continued)

Type I Collagen Cross-linked N-telopeptide *Urine Decrease* In 14 prepubertal children with newly detected perennial asthma mean excretion of 532 nmol/mmol creatinine not significantly different from 659 nmol/mmol creatinine in 21 healthy children *4944*

Type I Collagen Teleopeptide *Serum No Effect* In 14 prepubertal children with newly detected perennial asthma mean concentration of 1.22 nmol/L not significantly different from 1.24 nmol/L in 21 healthy children *4944*

Uric Acid *Serum Increase* Has been observed and is thought to be a consequence of the excessive use of sympathomimetic drugs *2036*

494.00 Bronchiectasis

α_1-Antichymotrypsin *Serum No Effect* Mean concentration within reference interval of 47.9 ± 8.1 mg/dL in all 2 patients with bronciectasis *3044*

Arylsulfatase *Serum Increase* 30 - 50% increase in activity *1279*

CA 19-9 *Serum Increase* The percentage of patients with positive serum levels was 42.3% with pulmonary disease (14.5% in asbestosis, 27.3% in bronchial asthma, 59.4% in bronchiectasis, 81.3% in idiopathic pulmonary fibrosis and 61.5% in pulmonary tuberculosis) *2026*

Cells *Sputum Increase* Polymorphonuclear and lymphocytic, as well as bronchial epithelial cells with varying degrees of metaplasia *900*

Cold Agglutinins *Serum Increase* Elevated titers may persist for weeks or months *4551*

Erythrocyte Sedimentation Rate *Blood Increase* Nonspecific elevation seen with acute infections *4920*

γ-Globulin *Serum Decrease* Seen when chronic uncontrolled infection persists *900* May be increased with chronic infection or decreased if congenital agammaglobulinemia is the underlying disease *2039*
Serum Increase Seen when chronic uncontrolled infection persists *900* May be increased with chronic infection or decreased if congenital agammaglobulinemia is the underlying disease *2039*

Hematocrit *Blood Decrease* When chronic uncontrolled infection persists, normochromic normocytic anemia is common *900*

Hemoglobin *Blood Decrease* Leukocytosis and anemia are common *2039* When chronic uncontrolled infection persists, normochromic normocytic anemia is common *900*

Leukocytes *Blood Increase* Leukocytosis and anemia are common *2039* During acute sepsis *900*
Blood No Effect Usually normal unless pneumonitis is present *5544*

Lymphocytes *Sputum Increase* Microscopic examination reveals polymorphonuclear and lymphocytic, as well as bronchial epithelial cells with varying degrees of metaplasia *900*

Neutrophils *Sputum Increase* Polymorphonuclear and lymphocytic, as well as bronchial epithelial cells with varying degrees of metaplasia *900*

Oxygen Partial Pressure *Blood Decrease* Mild to moderate hypoxemia secondary to venous mixture with arterial blood *4920*

495.00 Farmer's Lung Disease

KL-6 Antigen *Serum Increase* In 5 patients with Farmer's lung disease mean concentration of 1,305 ± 42 U/mL significantly different from 207 ± 6 U/mL in 237 healthy controls *5134*

495.80 Cryptogenic Fibrosing Alveolitis

Acid Phosphatase, Tartrate Resistant *Serum No Effect* No significant effect observed in patients with cryptogenic fibrosing alveolitis *2618*

495.90 Allergic Alveolitis

Carbon Dioxide Partial Pressure *Blood No Effect* Arterial blood gases show decreased pO_2 with either slight respiratory alkalosis or normal pH and pCO_2 *900*

Eosinophils *Blood Increase* Eosinophilia up to 45% *5544* Eosinophilia is exceptional *900*

γ-Globulin *Serum Increase* Elevation in the range of 2 - 3 g/dL *900*

Leukocytes *Blood Increase* Normal WBC; increased in presence of infection *5544*

Neutrophils *Blood Increase* During the acute febrile episodes there is a polymorphonuclear leukocytosis of 15,000 - 25,000 /µL *900*

Oxygen Partial Pressure *Blood Decrease* Arterial blood gases show decreased pO_2 with either slight respiratory alkalosis or normal pH and pCO_2 *900*

Oxygen Saturation *Blood Decrease* Arterial blood gases show decreased pO_2 with either slight respiratory alkalosis or normal pH and pCO_2 *900*

pH *Blood Increase* Arterial blood gases show decreased pO_2 with either slight respiratory alkalosis or normal pH and pCO_2 *900*

Precipitins *Serum Increase* Found in 17 - 18%, particularly against the thermophilic actinomycete M. faeni and also, against T. vulgaris and fungi such as the genus Aspergillus and Mucormycosis *4073*

495.90 Allergic Bronchopulmonary Disease

Aspergillus Antibody *Serum Increase* Antibodies are observed in]/- 70% of patients with allergic bronchopulmonary disease *2952*

495.90 Allergy

Eosinophil Cationic Protein *Serum Increase* In 75 children sensitized to mite allergens median concentration of 15 µg/L compared with 5 µg/L in 16 children without sensitization to 7 inhalant allergens *2843*

Eosinophils *Blood Increase* In 75 children sensitized to mite allergens median concentration of 350 /µL compared with 150 /µL in 16 children without sensitization to 7 inhalant allergens *2843*

495.90 Hypersensitivity Pneumonitis

$CD4^+:CD8^+$ Lymphocyte Ratio *BAL Fluid Decrease* Mean ratio in 10 patients with hypersensitivity pneumonitis of 1.1 ± 0.2 *1989*

Lymphocytes *BAL Fluid Increase* Mean proportion of total cells in 10 patients with hypersensitivity pneumonitis of 67 ± 4.1% significantly different from 12 ± 1% in 21 control individuals *1989*

Protein *BAL Fluid Increase* Mean concentration in 10 patients with hypersensitivity pneumonia of 401 ± 178 mg/mL significantly different from 82 ± 16 mg/mL in 21 control individuals *1989*

Surfactant Protein A *BAL Fluid Increase* Mean concentration in 10 patients with hypersensitivity pneumonia of 9.0 ± 1.7 µg/mL significantly different from 4.0 ± 0.3 µg/mL in 21 control individuals *1989*

496.00 Chronic Obstructive Pulmonary Disease

Alanine *Muscle No Effect* In 12 adults with stable chronic obstructive pulmonary disease mean concentration of 1,134 ± 66 µmol/kg wet weight not significantly different from 1,254 ± 113 µmol/kg wet weight in 8 healthy age matched controls *4196*
Plasma Decrease In 12 adults with stable chronic obstructive pulmonary disease mean concentration of 254 ± 10 µmol/L significantly different from 375 ± 25 µmol/L in 8 healthy age matched controls *4196*

Aldosterone *Plasma Increase* Plasma renin and aldosterone tended to have higher than normal baseline values, especially in hypercapnic patients *1420*

Ammonia *Blood Increase* Venous levels were significantly influenced by pH and pCO_2 *1110*

α_1-Antichymotrypsin *Serum Increase* Mean concentration increased above reference interval of 47.9 ± 8.1 mg/dL in 5 of 16 patients (31%) with COPD *3044*

α_1-Antitrypsin *Serum Decrease* Homozygotes for alpha$_1$-antitrypsin deficiency traits usually develop chronic obstructive lung disease by age 40. Heterozygotes have levels intermediate between normals and homozygotes, and frequently develop this disease *3525*

Arginine *Muscle Increase* In 12 adults with stable chronic obstructive pulmonary disease mean concentration of 341 ± 37 µmol/kg wet weight significantly different from 198 ± 27 µmol/kg wet weight in 8 healthy age matched controls *4196*
Plasma No Effect In 12 adults with stable chronic obstructive pulmonary disease mean concentration of 90 ± 4 µmol/L not significantly different from 90 ± 5 µmol/L in 8 healthy age matched controls *4196*

Asparagine *Muscle No Effect* In 12 adults with stable chronic obstructive pulmonary disease mean concentration of 142 ± 8 µmol/kg wet weight not significantly different from 143 ± 14 µmol/kg wet weight in 8 healthy age matched controls *4196*
Plasma Decrease In 12 adults with stable chronic obstructive pulmonary disease mean concentration of 48 ± 2 µmol/L significantly different from 58 ± 4 µmol/L in 8 healthy age matched controls *4196*

Bicarbonate *Serum Increase* Suggests chronic hypoventilation *1980* In 82% of 69 patients at initial hospitalization for this disorder *1576*

Cancer-associated Serum Antigen *Serum Increase* 3 of 53 patients with obstructive lung disease had concentrations above 9 U/mL *1135*

Carbon Dioxide Partial Pressure *Blood Increase* In 33% of 75 patients at initial hospitalization for this disorder *1576* Decreased pO_2 associated with increased pCO_2 *5544* In 10 patients with hypercapnia, mean renal net acid excretion was elevated and correlated with arterial pCO_2, blood pH and urinary pH *3223*

Cells *Sputum No Effect* In 18 patients with COPD total cell count similar to that in 20 healthy individuals *4422*

Chloride *Serum Decrease* Suggests chronic hypoventilation *1980* In 44% of 71 patients at initial hospitalization for this disorder *1576*

Cholesterol *Serum Decrease* Decreased in decompensated patients. Amount of decrease correlates with degree of hypoxemia *4571*

Citrulline *Muscle Increase* In 12 adults with stable chronic obstructive pulmonary disease mean concentration of 121 ± 15 µmol/kg wet weight significantly different from 62 ± 15 µmol/kg wet weight in 8 healthy age matched controls *4196*
Plasma No Effect In 12 adults with stable chronic obstructive pulmonary disease mean concentration of 54 ± 2 µmol/L not significantly different from 48 ± 2 µmol/L in 8 healthy age matched controls *4196*

CYFRA 21-1 *Serum Increase* Mean concentration in 33 patients with COPD of 2.3 ± 1.0 ng/mL compared with 1.1 ± 0.3 ng/mL in 29 healthy controls with a positivity rate of 12.1% *3665*

Desmosine *Urine Increase* In 22 patients with COPD mean excretion of 11.8 ± 5.1 µg/g creatinine higher than 7.5 ± 1.4 µg/g creatinine in 21 never smokers *5032*

2,3-Diphosphoglycerate *Red Blood Cells Increase* Synthesis is increased *380*

Elastin Peptide *Serum Increase* In 10 patients with chronic obstructive pulmonary disease mean concentration of 66.8 ± 5.8 ng/L compared with 23.4 ± 4.6 ng/mL in 12 nonsmokers *4675*
Urine Increase In 10 patients with chronic obstructive pulmonary disease mean concentration of 910.8 ± 105.6 ng/mL compared with 281.0 ± 67.8 ng/mL in 12 healthy smokers *4675*

Eosinophil Cationic Protein *Serum Increase* Mean concentration of 83.3 ± 79.2 µg/L in 10 patients with chronic obstructive pulmonary disease *1931*
Sputum Increase Median concentration in 9 patients with COPD of 0.15 mg/L *4667* Mean concentration of 417.5 ± 363.5 µg/L/g in 10 patients with chronic obstructive pulmonary disease *1931*

Eosinophils *Blood Increase* Mean concentration in 9 patients with COPD of 169 ± 31.1 x 10^6/L *4667* In 37% of 79 patients at initial hospitalization for this disorder *1576* In 21 patients treated with budesonide and 19 patients treated with budesonide plus prednisolone mean concentrations 125 and 84 /µL, respectively *4324*
Sputum No Effect In 18 patients with COPD proportion of eosinophils of 0.8% compared with 0.6% in 20 healthy individuals *4422*

Erythrocytes *Blood Increase* Erythrocytosis, secondary to chronic hypoxemia may be prominent, especially in bronchitic patients *2304*

Gastrin *BAL Fluid Increase* In 25 patients with COPD median values of 17.3 pg/100 U LDH *1231*
Serum Increase In 25 patients with COPD median values of 50.5 pg/100 U LDH *1231*

Glomerular Filtration Rate *Urine Decrease* Hypercapnic patients showed low effective renal plasma flow, impaired water and sodium excretion compared to normocapnic patients and normal controls *1420*

Glutamic Acid *Muscle Decrease* In 12 adults with stable chronic obstructive pulmonary disease mean concentration of 1,988 ± 107 µmol/kg wet weight significantly different from 2,610 ± 197 µmol/kg wet weight in 8 healthy age matched controls *4196*
Plasma Decrease In 12 adults with stable chronic obstructive pulmonary disease mean concentration of 91 ± 5 µmol/L significantly different from 130 ± 10 µmol/L in 8 healthy age matched controls *4196*
Red Blood Cells Increase Erythrocyte L-glutamate was significantly elevated only in hypercapnic patients *5394*

Glutamine *Muscle Increase* In 12 adults with stable chronic obstructive pulmonary disease mean concentration of 10,782 ± 770 µmol/kg wet weight significantly different from 7,844 ± 293 µmol/kg wet weight in 8 healthy age matched controls *4196*
Plasma Decrease In 12 adults with stable chronic obstructive pulmonary disease mean concentration of 580 ± 17 µmol/L significantly different from 641 ± 17 µmol/L in 8 healthy age matched controls *4196*

γ-Glutamyltransferase *Serum Increase* Increased activity reported with COPD *3625*

Glycine *Muscle No Effect* In 12 adults with stable chronic obstructive pulmonary disease mean concentration of 762 ± 49 µmol/kg wet weight not significantly different from 634 ± 33 µmol/kg wet weight in 8 healthy age matched controls *4196*
Plasma No Effect In 12 adults with stable chronic obstructive pulmonary disease mean concentration of 242 ± 11 µmol/L not significantly different from 253 ± 20 µmol/L in 8 healthy age matched controls *4196*

Hematocrit *Blood Decrease* Even minor degrees of anemia are poorly tolerated by patients. Because of the high incidence of peptic ulcer associated with this disease, an anemia may be due to occult or clinically evident gastrointestinal bleeding *1980*
Blood Increase In 42% of 80 patients at initial hospitalization for this disorder *1576* Polycythemia, suggesting a significant degree of chronic hypoxemia *1980*

Hemoglobin *Blood Decrease* Even minor degrees of anemia are poorly tolerated by patients. Because of the high incidence of peptic ulcer associated with this disease, an anemia may be due to occult or clinically evident gastrointestinal bleeding *1980*
Blood Increase In 39% of 80 patients at initial hospitalization for this disorder *1576* Polycythemia, suggesting a significant degree of chronic hypoxemia *1980* In 25 patients with severe disease, blood hemoglobin exhibited a significant increase indicating an improved oxygen transport. In most patients a leftward shifting of the oxygen dissociation curve occurred. Hemoglobin was significantly increased in all patients, regardless of degree of hypoxia *2274*

Histidine *Muscle No Effect* In 12 adults with stable chronic obstructive pulmonary disease mean concentration of 232 ± 16 µmol/kg wet weight not significantly different from 161 ± 8 µmol/kg wet weight in 8 healthy age matched controls *4196*
Plasma No Effect In 12 adults with stable chronic obstructive pulmonary disease mean concentration of 79 ± 2 µmol/L not significantly different from 88 ± 3 µmol/L in 8 healthy age matched controls *4196*

496.00 Chronic Obstructive Pulmonary Disease *(continued)*

Hydroxylysylpyridinoline *Urine* *Increase* In 12 patients with COPD mean excretion of 51.5 ± 24 9 nmol/mmol creatinine significantly higher than 24.9 ± 6.1 nmol/mmol creatinine in 19 never smoking controls *5032*

Immunoglobulin A, Secretory *Sputum* *Increase* Median concentration in 9 patients with COPD of 51 mg/L *4667*

Immunoglobulin E *Serum* *Increase* In 21 patients treated with budesonide and 19 patients treated with budesonide plus prednisolone mean concentrations 39 and 22 IU/mL, respectively *4324*

Isodesmosine *Urine* *Increase* In 12 patients wit COPD mean excretion of 11.3 ± 5.0 µg/g creatinine significantly higher than 6.9 ± 1.3 µg/g creatinine in 22 never smoking controls *5032*

Isoleucine *Muscle* *No Effect* In 12 adults with stable chronic obstructive pulmonary disease mean concentration of 51 ± 3 µmol/kg wet weight not significantly different from 50 ± 4 µmol/kg wet weight in 8 healthy age matched controls *4196*
Plasma *No Effect* In 12 adults with stable chronic obstructive pulmonary disease mean concentration of 63 ± 4 µmol/L not significantly different from 69 ± 4 µmol/L in 8 healthy age matched controls *4196*

Lactoferrin *Sputum* *Increase* Median concentration in 9 patients with COPD of 61 mg/L *4667*

Leptin *Serum* *Decrease* Mean concentration in 31 patients with COPD of 1.14 ± 1.17 ng/mL significantly different from 2.47 ± 2.01 ng/mL in 15 age-matched healthy controls *5122*

Leucine *Muscle* *No Effect* In 12 adults with stable chronic obstructive pulmonary disease mean concentration of 104 ± 5 µmol/kg wet weight not significantly different from 113 ± 7 µmol/kg wet weight in 8 healthy age matched controls *4196*
Plasma *No Effect* In 12 adults with stable chronic obstructive pulmonary disease mean concentration of 122 ± 6 µmol/L not significantly different from 136 ± 5 µmol/L in 8 healthy age matched controls *4196*

Leukocytes *Blood* *Increase* In 42% of 80 patients at initial hospitalization for this disorder *1576*

Lipids *Serum* *Decrease* Decreased in decompensated patients. Amount of decrease correlates with degree of hypoxemia *4571*

β-Lipoprotein *Serum* *Decrease* Decreased in decompensated patients. Amount of decrease correlates with degree of hypoxemia *4571*

Lysine *Muscle* *No Effect* In 12 adults with stable chronic obstructive pulmonary disease mean concentration of 536 ± 70 µmol/kg wet weight not significantly different from 350 ± 44 µmol/kg wet weight in 8 healthy age matched controls *4196*
Plasma *No Effect* In 12 adults with stable chronic obstructive pulmonary disease mean concentration of 179 ± 9 µmol/L not significantly different from 194 ± 14 µmol/L in 8 healthy age matched controls *4196*

Lysylpyridinoline *Urine* *Increase* In 12 patients with COPD mean excretion of 12.9 ± 5.9 nmol/mmol creatinine higher than 4.9 ± 2.0 nmol/mmol creatinine in 19 never smokers *5032*

α_2-Macroglobulin *Serum* *Decrease* Reported effect *642*

Methionine *Muscle* *No Effect* In 12 adults with stable chronic obstructive pulmonary disease mean concentration of 29 ± 3 µmol/kg wet weight not significantly different from 26 ± 3 µmol/kg wet weight in 8 healthy age matched controls *4196*
Plasma *No Effect* In 12 adults with stable chronic obstructive pulmonary disease mean concentration of 26 ± 1 µmol/L not significantly different from 28 ± 1 µmol/L in 8 healthy age matched controls *4196*

Myeloperoxidase *Sputum* *Increase* Median concentration in 9 patients with COPD of 12 mg/L *4667*

Neutrophils *Blood* *Increase* In 42% of 79 patients at initial hospitalization for this disorder *1576*
Sputum *Increase* In 18 patients with COPD proportion of neutrophils 47.5% compared with 8.8% in 20 healthy individuals *4422*

Nitrate plus Nitrite *Serum* *Increase* In 21 patients with COPD mean concentration of 14.48 ± 2.76 µmol/L compared with 3.48 ± 0.40 µmol/L in 11 healthy controls *212*

Ornithine *Muscle* *Increase* In 12 adults with stable chronic obstructive pulmonary disease mean concentration of 154 ± 23 µmol/kg wet weight significantly different from 86 ± 4 µmol/kg wet weight in 8 healthy age matched controls *4196*
Plasma *No Effect* In 12 adults with stable chronic obstructive pulmonary disease mean concentration of 74 ± 6 µmol/L not significantly different from 61 ± 2 µmol/L in 8 healthy age matched controls *4196*

Oxygen Partial Pressure *Blood* *Decrease* In 82% of 70 patients at initial hospitalization for this disorder *1576* Decreased pO_2 associated with increased pCO_2 *5544* Greatest declines in arterial oxygen saturation occurred during sleep, with intermittent decreases as great as 44% saturation (range of 12 - 44% saturation) *1509*

Oxygen Saturation *Blood* *Decrease* Decreased pO_2 associated with increased pCO_2 *5544* Greatest declines in arterial oxygen saturation occurred during sleep, with intermittent decreases as great as 44% saturation (range, 12 - 44% saturation) *1509*

pH *Blood* *Decrease* Blood pH was significantly lower in 10 patients with chronic obstructive lung disease than in normocapnic controls. Renal net acid excretion was elevated but urinary pH was not significantly raised *3223* In 48% of 74 patients at initial hospitalization for this disorder *1576*

Phenylalanine *Muscle* *No Effect* In 12 adults with stable chronic obstructive pulmonary disease mean concentration of 52 ± 3 µmol/kg wet weight not significantly different from 48 ± 3 µmol/kg wet weight in 8 healthy age matched controls *4196*
Plasma *No Effect* In 12 adults with stable chronic obstructive pulmonary disease mean concentration of 53 ± 1 µmol/L not significantly different from 53 ± 1 µmol/L in 8 healthy age matched controls *4196*

Potassium *Serum* *Decrease* Suggests a coexisting primary metabolic alkalosis *1980*
Serum *Increase* When acidemia is present, may be falsely high because of potassium ions moving from the extracellular space *1980*

Procollagen Type III Peptide *Serum* *No Effect* The concentration of procollagen peptide in blood samples from patients with asthma was 5.8 ± 2.4, 4.9 ± 1.8 in patients with COPD and 11.1 ± 3.6 in healthy subjects. There was no significant difference between patients with asthma, COPD and healthy subjects ($p < 0.01$) *2752*

Renin Activity *Plasma* *Increase* Plasma renin and aldosterone tended to have higher than normal baseline values, especially in hypercapnic patients *1420*

Serine *Muscle* *No Effect* In 12 adults with stable chronic obstructive pulmonary disease mean concentration of 352 ± 24 µmol/kg wet weight not significantly different from 281 ± 18 µmol/kg wet weight in 8 healthy age matched controls *4196*
Plasma *No Effect* In 12 adults with stable chronic obstructive pulmonary disease mean concentration of 120 ± 5 µmol/L not significantly different from 121 ± 5 µmol/L in 8 healthy age matched controls *4196*

Sodium *Urine* *Decrease* Hypercapnic patients showed low effective renal plasma flow, impaired water and sodium excretion compared to normocapnic patients and normal controls *1420*

Soluble Tumor Necrosis Factor Receptor-p55
Serum *Increase* Mean concentration in 31 patients with COPD of 1.16 ± 0.47 ng/mL significantly different from 0.67 ± 0.13 ng/mL in 15 age-matched healthy controls *5122*

Soluble Tumor Necrosis Factor Receptor-p75
Serum *Increase* Mean concentration in 31 patients with COPD of 3.65 ± 1.29 ng/mL significantly different from 2.25 ± 0.43 ng/mL in 15 age-matched healthy controls *5122*

Taurine *Muscle* *No Effect* In 12 adults with stable chronic obstructive pulmonary disease mean concentration of 14,830 ± 1,200 µmol/kg wet weight not significantly different from 15,235 ± 3,537 µmol/kg wet weight in 8 healthy age matched controls *4196*
Plasma *No Effect* In 12 adults with stable chronic obstructive pulmonary disease mean concentration of 57 ± 3 µmol/L not significantly different from 55 ± 5 µmol/L in 8 healthy age matched controls *4196*

Thiol Groups, Total *Serum* *Decrease* In 16 patients with COPD mean concentration of 248 ± 25 µmol/L compared with 520 ± 19 µmol/L in 7 healthy controls *212*

Threonine *Muscle No Effect* In 12 adults with stable chronic obstructive pulmonary disease mean concentration of 499 ± 34 µmol/kg wet weight not significantly different from 494 ± 21 µmol/kg wet weight in 8 healthy age matched controls *4196*
Plasma No Effect In 12 adults with stable chronic obstructive pulmonary disease mean concentration of 127 ± 8 µmol/L not significantly different from 134 ± 8 µmol/L in 8 healthy age matched controls *4196*

Triglycerides *Serum Decrease* Decreased in decompensated patients. Amount of decrease correlates with degree of hypoxemia *4571*

Tryptase *Sputum Increase* Median concentration in 9 patients with COPD of 3.5 mg/L *4667*

Tryptophan *Muscle No Effect* In 12 adults with stable chronic obstructive pulmonary disease mean concentration of 13 ± 1 µmol/kg wet weight not significantly different from 12 ± 1 µmol/kg wet weight in 8 healthy age matched controls *4196*
Plasma No Effect In 12 adults with stable chronic obstructive pulmonary disease mean concentration of 41 ± 1 µmol/L not significantly different from 43 ± 1 µmol/L in 8 healthy age matched controls *4196*

Tumor Necrosis Factor-α *Serum Increase* Mean concentration in 31 patients with COPD of 6.59 ± 1.92 pg/mL significantly different from 5.41 ± 1.60 pg/mL in 15 age-matched healthy controls *5122*

Tyrosine *Muscle No Effect* In 12 adults with stable chronic obstructive pulmonary disease mean concentration of 57 ± 3 µmol/kg wet weight not significantly different from 56 ± 3 µmol/kg wet weight in 8 healthy age matched controls *4196*

Valine *Muscle No Effect* In 12 adults with stable chronic obstructive pulmonary disease mean concentration of 179 ± 7 µmol/kg wet weight not significantly different from 179 ± 13 µmol/kg wet weight in 8 healthy age matched controls *4196*

Viscosity *Serum Increase* An increase in blood viscosity, red blood cell mass, and blood volume is thought to further compromise the pressure-flow relationships of the constricted and restricted pulmonary vascular bed *2304*

Volume *Plasma Increase* An increase in blood viscosity, red blood cell mass, and blood volume is thought to further compromise the pressure- flow relationships of the constricted and restricted pulmonary vascular bed *2304*

500.00 Anthracosis

Bicarbonate *Serum Increase* CO_2 retention may occur *900*

Carbon Dioxide Partial Pressure *Blood Increase* Impaired gas exchange in established cases *367*

Erythrocyte Sedimentation Rate *Blood Increase* Increased ESR generally indicates secondary infection *900*

Erythrocytes *Blood Increase* Secondary polycythemia *5544* May become progressively elevated *900*

Hematocrit *Blood Decrease* Secondary anemia *5544*
Blood Increase May become progressively elevated *900*

Hemoglobin *Blood Decrease* Secondary anemia *5544*
Blood Increase May become progressively elevated *900*

Leukocytes *Blood Increase* Increased with associated infection *5544*

Oxygen Partial Pressure *Blood Decrease* Impaired gas exchange in established cases *367* Arterial oxygen saturation may fall *900*

Oxygen Saturation *Blood Decrease* Arterial oxygen saturation may fall *900*

Rheumatoid Factor *Serum Increase* 42% of patients without associated arthritis had a positive sheep cell agglutination test, while 80% with associated rheumatoid arthritis were found to be seropositive *1980*

501.00 Asbestosis

Bicarbonate *Serum Increase* CO_2 retention may occur *900*

CA 19-9 *Serum Increase* The percentage of patients with positive serum levels was 42.3% with pulmonary disease (14.5% in asbestosis, 27.3% in bronchial asthma, 59.4% in bronchiectasis, 81.3% in idiopathic pulmonary fibrosis and 61.5% in pulmonary tuberculosis) *2026*

Carbon Dioxide Partial Pressure *Blood Decrease* Impaired gas diffusion and the accompanying hyperventilation results in a low pCO_2, unless the defect is severe and CO_2 retention occurs *4707*
Blood Increase Impaired gas exchange in established cases *367*

Erythrocyte Sedimentation Rate *Blood Increase* Increased ESR generally indicates secondary infection *900*

Erythrocytes *Blood Increase* Secondary polycythemia *5544* May become progressively elevated *900*
Pleural Fluid Increase Often blood pleural effusions *367*

Hematocrit *Blood Decrease* Secondary anemia *5544*
Blood Increase May become progressively elevated *900*

Hemoglobin *Blood Decrease* Secondary anemia *5544*
Blood Increase May become progressively elevated *900*

Leukocytes *Blood Increase* Increased with associated infection *5544*

Oxygen Partial Pressure *Blood Decrease* Arterial oxygen saturation may fall *900* Impaired gas exchange in established cases *367*

Oxygen Saturation *Blood Decrease* Arterial oxygen saturation may fall *900*

Rheumatoid Factor *Serum Increase* 21% positivity *874 306*

502.00 Silicosis

Angiotensin-converting Enzyme *Serum Increase* Elevated and associated with a progression of the disease *3183 3825*

Bicarbonate *Serum Increase* CO_2 retention may occur *900*

Carbon Dioxide Partial Pressure *Blood Increase* Impaired gas exchange in established cases *367*

1,25-Dihydroxy Vitamin D_3 *Serum Increase* Observed effect *126*

Erythrocyte Sedimentation Rate *Blood Increase* Increased ESR generally indicates secondary infection *900*

Erythrocytes *Blood Increase* May become progressively elevated *900*

Hematocrit *Blood Decrease* Secondary anemia *5544*
Blood Increase May become progressively elevated *900*

Hemoglobin *Blood Decrease* Secondary anemia *5544*
Blood Increase May become progressively elevated *900*

Leukocytes *Blood Increase* Increased with associated infection *5544*

Oxygen Partial Pressure *Blood Decrease* Arterial oxygen saturation may fall *900* Impaired gas exchange and movement of respiratory cage due to noncompliant lungs *367* Impaired gas exchange in established cases *367*

Oxygen Saturation *Blood Decrease* Impaired gas exchange and movement of respiratory cage due to noncompliant lungs *367* Arterial oxygen saturation may fall *900*

Procollagen Type III Peptide *Serum No Effect* In patients with silicosis normal serum concentrations of both parameters were found *4680*

Rheumatoid Factor *Serum Increase* Positive in 15% of patients *874 306*

Tissue Polypeptide Antigen *Serum No Effect* Mean concentration in one patient of 51.2 U/L not significantly different from 72.7 ± 19.2 U/L in 19 healthy controls *5845*

503.00 Berylliosis

Bicarbonate *Serum Increase* CO_2 retention may occur *900*

Calcium *Urine Increase* Hypercalciuria may occur *900*

Carbon Dioxide Partial Pressure *Blood Decrease* Impaired gas diffusion and the accompanying hyperventilation results in a low pCO_2, unless the defect is severe and CO_2 retention occurs *4707*
Blood Increase Impaired gas exchange in established cases *367*

Erythrocyte Sedimentation Rate *Blood Increase* Increased ESR generally indicates secondary infection *900*

Erythrocytes *Blood Increase* Secondary polycythemia *5544* May become progressively elevated *900*

503.00 Berylliosis *(continued)*

γ-Globulin *Serum* *Increase* Occasional transient hypergammaglobulinemia *5544*

Hematocrit *Blood* *Decrease* Secondary anemia *5544*
Blood *Increase* May become progressively elevated *900* Secondary polycythemia *5544*

Hemoglobin *Blood* *Decrease* Secondary anemia *5544*
Blood *Increase* Secondary polycythemia *5544* May become progressively elevated *900*

Leukocytes *Blood* *Increase* Increased with associated infection *5544*

Oxygen Partial Pressure *Blood* *Decrease* Arterial oxygen saturation may fall *900* Hypoxemia is frequent *5848* Impaired gas exchange in established cases *367*

Oxygen Saturation *Blood* *Decrease* Hypoxemia is frequent *5848* Arterial oxygen saturation may fall *900*

510.00 Empyema

α_1-Antichymotrypsin *Serum* *Increase* A study of patients with emphysema, bronchitis or asthma revealed there was no deficiency similar to that of alpha$_1$-antitrypsin. In fact, the levels were increased in all the disease states studied *953*

Carcinoembryonic Antigen *Pleural Fluid* *Increase* Benign inflammatory effusions (tuberculosis, empyema, pneumonia) had mean activity of 6.2 ± 3.4 ng/mL, higher than effusions caused by congestive heart failure (2.9 ± 1.5) and other noninflammatory effusions *4369* Mean concentration increased in all 5 effusions in patients with empyema *1649*

Glucose *Cerebrospinal Fluid* *No Effect* In subdural empyema *413*
Pleural Fluid *Decrease* 0-60 mg/dL *4493* Levels less than 3.3 mmol/L (60 mg/dL) *396*

Leukocytes *Blood* *Increase* Total counts may become extremely high *5677* In subdural empyema. (20,000 - 40,000 /μL) *413*
Cerebrospinal Fluid *Increase* In subdural empyema. (50 - 1,000 /μL, 20 - 80% neutrophils) *413*
Pleural Fluid *Increase* 25,000 - 100,000 /μL *4493*

Neutrophils *Pleural Fluid* *Increase* Very high counts occur; cells tend to degenerate, with blurred nuclei which do not stain in characteristic purple color *3052*

Oxygen Partial Pressure *Blood* *Decrease* Empyema or tuberculous effusion *1604*

Oxygen Saturation *Blood* *Decrease* Empyema or tuberculous effusion *1604*

pH *Pleural Fluid* *Decrease* May occur in non-neoplastic inflammatory pleural effusion (empyema, rheumatoid disease, tuberculosis) *1604* All 10 patients had a pleural fluid pH of < 7.30. Pleural fluid pH values < 7.30 are likely to result in loculation of the pleural space *4190*

Protein *Cerebrospinal Fluid* *Increase* In subdural empyema. (75 - 300 mg/dL) *413*
Pleural Fluid *Increase* Exudate *4493*

511.00 Pleurisy

Tissue Polypeptide Antigen *Serum* *No Effect* In 6 patients with nonspecific pleurisy mean concentration of 48.6 ± 37.1 U/L not significantly different from 72.7 ± 19.2 U/L in 19 healthy controls *5845*

513.00 Abscess of Lung

Albumin *Urine* *Increase* Frequent *5544*

Erythrocyte Sedimentation Rate *Blood* *Increase* Markedly elevated *900*

Hematocrit *Blood* *Decrease* Normochromic normocytic anemia in chronic stage *5544*

Hemoglobin *Blood* *Decrease* Characteristic leukocytosis and moderate or even severe anemia *2039* Normochromic normocytic anemia in chronic stage *5544*

Leukocytes *Blood* *Increase* In most patients there is a leukocytosis in the range of 20,000 - 30,000 /μL. The debilitated or elderly patients may fail to respond to the infection with a leukocytosis *900*

Neutrophils *Blood* *Increase* In most patients there is a leukocytosis in the range of 20,000 - 30,000 cells/μL. The debilitated or elderly patients may fail to respond to the infection with a leukocytosis *900*

Tissue Polypeptide Antigen *Serum* *No Effect* In 4 patients mean concentration of 78.3 ± 47.2 U/L not significantly different from 72.7 ± 19.2 U/L in 19 healthy controls *5845*

514.00 Pulmonary Congestion and Hypostasis

Bicarbonate *Serum* *Decrease* Respiratory alkalosis may occur *1980*

Carbon Dioxide Partial Pressure *Blood* *Decrease* Respiratory alkalosis may occur *1980*

pH *Blood* *Increase* Respiratory alkalosis may occur *1980*

Protein *Pleural Fluid* *Decrease* Transudate (< 3 g/dL) *1025*

515.00 Pulmonary Fibrosis

α_1-Antichymotrypsin *Serum* *Increase* Mean concentration increased above reference interval of 47.9 ± 8.1 mg/dL in 1 of 1 patient (100%) with pulmonary fibrosis *3044*

Bilirubin, Indirect *Serum* *Increase* Concentration may be increased in patients with hypoxia due to, for example, pulmonary fibrosis or heart failure. Condition arises because conjugation of bilirubin requires UDP-glucuronic acid which, in turn, requires oxygen *4617*

CYFRA 21-1 *Serum* *Increase* In 19 patients with pulmonary fibrosis concentrations were increased above the upper limit of normal of 1.9 ng/mL in 10 *4740*

Protein 1 *BAL Fluid* *Positive* In patients with pulmonary fibrosis protein 1 detected *2371*

515.00 Pulmonary Fibrosis with Cardiovascular Disease

Albumin *BAL Fluid* *Increase* In 19 patients mean concentration of 183.1 ± 72.0 μg/mL significantly different from 52.8 ± 7.8 μg/mL in 13 healthy control volunteers *1595*

$CD4^+$:$CD8^+$ Lymphocyte Ratio *BAL Fluid* *No Effect* In 19 patients mean ratio of 4.4 ± 2.5 not significantly different from 3.8 ± 0.9 in 13 healthy control volunteers *1595*

Cells *BAL Fluid* *No Effect* In 19 patients mean concentration of 328.2 ± 67.2 x 10^3/mL not significantly different from 147.5 ± 59.3 x 10^3/mL in 13 healthy control volunteers *1595*

Eosinophil Cationic Protein *BAL Fluid* *Increase* In 19 patients mean concentration of 63.5 ± 18.8 ng/L significantly different from 12.5 ± 1.7 ng/L in 13 healthy control volunteers *1595*

Eosinophils *BAL Fluid* *Increase* In 19 patients mean concentration of 5.73 ± 2.39 x 10^3/mL significantly different from 0.03 ± 0.01 x 10^3/mL in 13 healthy control volunteers *1595*

Lactate Dehydrogenase *BAL Fluid* *Increase* In 19 patients mean activity of 60.6 ± 14.9 U/L not significantly different from 22.8 ± 5.4 U/L in 13 healthy control volunteers *1595*

Lymphocytes *BAL Fluid* *Increase* In 19 patients mean concentration of 117.8 ± 50.9 x 10^3/mL significantly different from 7.0 ± 2.4 x 10^3/mL in 13 healthy control volunteers *1595*

Macrophages *BAL Fluid* *No Effect* In 19 patients mean concentration of 192.6 ± 43.9 x 10^3/mL not significantly different from 139.0 ± 56.6 x 10^3/mL in 13 healthy control volunteers *1595*

Neutrophils *BAL Fluid* *Increase* In 19 patients mean concentration of 12.0 ± 4.4 x 10^3/mL significantly different from 1.5 ± 0.5 x 10^3/mL in 13 healthy control volunteers *1595*

Protein *BAL Fluid* *Increase* In 19 patients mean concentration of 54.6 ± 17.9 mg/dL significantly different from 16.1 ± 1.4 mg/dL in 13 healthy control volunteers *1595*

Type III Procollagen Amino-terminal Peptide-related Antigen *BAL Fluid* *Increase* In 19 patients mean concentration of 63.1 ± 44.9 ng/L significantly different from 0.5 ± 0.1 ng/L in 13 healthy control volunteers *1595*

516.00 Pulmonary Alveolar Proteinosis

Albumin *BAL Fluid* *Increase* In 10 patients mean concentration of 564 mg/L versus less than 29.1 mg/L in 8 controls *1598*

Carbon Dioxide Partial Pressure *Blood* *Decrease* Impaired gas diffusion and the accompanying hyperventilation results in a low pCO_2, unless the defect is severe and CO_2 retention occurs *4707*

Carcinoembryonic Antigen *BAL Fluid* *Increase* In 10 patients mean concentration of 70 ng/mL versus less than 1.0 ng/mL in 8 controls *1598*
Serum *Increase* In 10 patients mean concentration of 5.7 ng/mL versus less than 1.0 ng/mL in 8 controls *1598*

KL-6 Antigen *Serum* *Increase* In 4 patients with pulmonary alveolar proteinosis mean concentration of 6,119 ± 895 U/mL significantly different from 207 ± 6 U/mL in 237 healthy controls *5134*

Lactate Dehydrogenase *Serum* *Increase* Values for all 12 patients were above the normal upper limit *3314* Increases when protein accumulates in lungs and drops to normal when infiltrate resolves *5544*

Oxygen Partial Pressure *Blood* *Decrease* In 4 patients with pulmonary alveolar proteinosis Pa_{O_2} less than 70 mm Hg *5134*

Oxygen Saturation *Blood* *Decrease* May be normal or reduced *367*

516.10 Idiopathic Pulmonary Hemosiderosis

Anisocytes *Blood* *Increase* Peripheral blood displays the classic changes of severe iron depletion: anisocytosis, poikilocytosis, microcytosis, and hypochromia *5677*

Bilirubin *Urine* *Increase* Excretion may be increased by the increased porphyrin catabolism *5677*

Bilirubin, Indirect *Serum* *Increase* Occasional findings of hemolytic type of anemia *5544*

Carbon Dioxide Partial Pressure *Blood* *Decrease* Impaired gas diffusion and the accompanying hyperventilation results in a low pCO_2, unless the defect is severe and CO_2 retention occurs in primary pulmonary hemosiderosis *4707*

Carcinoembryonic Antigen *Serum* *Increase* Increases reported *1601* *4551*

Eosinophils *Blood* *Increase* Eosinophilia of moderate degree occurs in about 12% of the cases *5677* In up to 20% of patients *5544*

Erythrocytes *Urine* *Increase* Microscopic hematuria in some cases. Gross hematuria occurs infrequently *5677*

Glomerular Basement Membrane Antibody *Serum* *Increase* Increased concentrations often above 250 units occur rarely in patients with idiopathic pulmonary hemosiderosis *2952*

Iron *Serum* *Decrease* Peripheral blood displays the classic changes of severe iron depletion: anisocytosis, poikilocytosis, microcytosis, and hypochromia *5677*
Serum *No Effect* Hypochromic microcytic anemia due to pulmonary hemorrhages with normal serum iron and iron-binding capacity *5544*

Iron-binding Capacity, Total *Serum* *Increase* Reported effect *5677*
Serum *No Effect* Hypochromic microcytic anemia due to pulmonary hemorrhages with normal serum iron and iron-binding capacity *5544*

MCV *Blood* *Decrease* Peripheral blood displays the classic changes of severe iron depletion: anisocytosis, poikilocytosis, microcytosis, and hypochromia *5677*

Occult Blood *Feces* *Increase* Stools may contain occult blood as a result of swallowed blood-laden sputum *5677*

Poikilocytes *Blood* *Increase* Peripheral blood displays the classic changes of severe iron depletion: anisocytosis, poikilocytosis, microcytosis, and hypochromia *5677*

Urobilinogen *Urine* *Increase* Occasional findings of hemolytic type of anemia *5544* Excretion may be increased by the increased porphyrin catabolism *5677*

516.30 Fibrosing Alveolitis

Ammonium Ions *Urine* *Increase* May be associated with classic distal renal tubular acidosis which is associated with hyokalemia, hyperchloremic metabolic acidosis, urine pH > 5.5, increased urinary ammonium ion excretion, a negative urine anion gap, increased urinary osmol gap, decreased urinary citrate and increased urinary calcium in some patients *4071*

Anion Gap *Urine* *Decrease* May be associated with classic distal renal tubular acidosis which is asociated with hyokalemia, hyperchloremic metabolic acidosis, urine pH > 5.5, increased urinary ammonium ion excretion, a negative urine anion gap, increased urinary osmol gap, decreased urinary citrate and increased urinary calcium in some patients *4071*

Calcium *Urine* *Increase* May be associated with classic distal renal tubular acidosis which is asociated with hyokalemia, hyperchloremic metabolic acidosis, urine pH > 5.5, increased urinary ammonium ion excretion, a negative urine anion gap, increased urinary osmol gap, decreased urinary citrate and increased urinary calcium in some patients *4071*

Chloride *Serum* *Increase* May be associated with classic distal renal tubular acidosis which is asociated with hyokalemia, hyperchloremic metabolic acidosis, urine pH > 5.5, increased urinary ammonium ion excretion, a negative urine anion gap, increased urinary osmol gap, decreased urinary citrate and increased urinary calcium in some patients *4071*

Citrate *Urine* *Decrease* May be associated with classic distal renal tubular acidosis which is asociated with hyokalemia, hyperchloremic metabolic acidosis, urine pH > 5.5, increased urinary ammonium ion excretion, a negative urine anion gap, increased urinary osmol gap, decreased urinary citrate and increased urinary calcium in some patients *4071*

Net Acid Excretion *Urine* *Increase* May be associated with classic distal renal tubular acidosis which is associated with hyokalemia, hyperchloremic metabolic acidosis, urine pH > 5.5, increased urinary ammonium ion excretion, a negative urine anion gap, increased urinary osmol gap, decreased urinary citrate and increased urinary calcium in some patients *4071*

Osmolal Gap *Urine* *Increase* May be associated with classic distal renal tubular acidosis which is associated with hyokalemia, hyperchloremic metabolic acidosis, urine pH > 5.5, increased urinary ammonium ion excretion, a negative urine anion gap, increased urinary osmol gap, decreased urinary citrate and increased urinary calcium in some patients *4071*

pH *Urine* *Increase* May be associated with classic distal renal tubular acidosis which is associated with hyokalemia, hyperchloremic metabolic acidosis, urine pH > 5.5, increased urinary ammonium ion excretion, a negative urine anion gap, increased urinary osmol gap, decreased urinary citrate and increased urinary calcium in some patients *4071*

Potassium *Serum* *Decrease* May be associated with classic distal renal tubular acidosis which is asociated with hyokalemia, hyperchloremic metabolic acidosis, urine pH > 5.5, increased urinary ammonium ion excretion, a negative urine anion gap, increased urinary osmol gap, decreased urinary citrate and increased urinary calcium in some patients *4071*

516.30 Idiopathic Fibrosing Alveolitis

Amino-terminal Propeptide of Type III Procollagen *BAL Fluid* *Increase* In 18 patients with fibrosing alveolitis mean concentration of 1.9 ± 6.1 µg/L significantly different from 0.1 ± 0.5 µg/L in 17 controls with minor respiratory symptoms *2902*
Serum *Increase* In 18 patients with fibrosing alveolitis mean concentration of 3.7 ± 1.1 µg/L significantly different from 2.7 ± 0.9 µg/L in 17 controls with minor respiratory symptoms *2902*

C-terminal Propeptide of Type III Procollagen *BAL Fluid* *Increase* In 18 patients with fibrosing alveolitis mean concentration of 13.6 ± 25.9 µg/L significantly different from 0.0 ± 0.0 µg/L in 17 controls with minor respiratory symptoms *2902*

516.30 Idiopathic Fibrosing Alveolitis *(continued)*

C-terminal Propeptide of Type III Procollagen *(continued)*
Serum No Effect In 18 patients with fibrosing alveolitis mean concentration of 111.3 ± 29.0 μg/L not significantly different from 107.0 ± 38.8 μg/L in 17 controls with minor respiratory symptoms *2902*

Tissue Polypeptide Antigen *Serum No Effect* In 12 patients with idiopathic fibrosing alveolitis mean concentration of 67.0 ± 65.1 U/L not significantly different from 72.7 ± 19.2 U/L in 19 healthy controls *5845*

516.30 Idiopathic Pulmonary Fibrosis

Albumin *BAL Fluid No Effect* In 27 patients mean concentration of 134.2 ± 50.3 μg/mL not significantly different from 52.8 ± 7.8 μg/mL in 13 healthy control volunteers *1595*

CA 19-9 *Serum Increase* The percentage of patients with positive serum levels was 42.3% with pulmonary disease (14.5% in asbestosis, 27.3% in bronchial asthma, 59.4% in bronchiectasis, 81.3% in idiopathic pulmonary fibrosis and 61.5% in pulmonary tuberculosis) *2026*

CD4⁺:CD8⁺ Lymphocyte Ratio *BAL Fluid Decrease* In 27 patients mean ratio of 2.1 ± 0.5 not significantly different from 3.8 ± 0.9 in 13 healthy control volunteers *1595*

Cells *BAL Fluid Increase* In 42 patients with IPF mean concentration of 16.1 ± 1.6 x 10^6/L significantly higher than 9.7 ± 1.3 x 10^6/L in 20 control individuals *5859*
BAL Fluid No Effect In 27 patients mean concentration of 260.3 ± 39.1 x 10^3/mL not significantly different from 147.5 ± 59.3 x 10^3/mL in 13 healthy control volunteers *1595*

C-Reactive Protein *Serum Increase* In 42 patients with IPF mean concentration of 1.6 ± 0.3 mg/dL significantly different from 0.3 ± 0.1 mg/dL in 20 control individuals *5859*

Endothelin-1 *Plasma Increase* Mean concentration of 10.14 ± 0.52 pg/mL in 37 patients with idiopathic pulmonary fibrosis significantly greater than 7.86 ± 0.65 pg/mL in 27 healthy controls *5353*

Eosinophil Cationic Protein *BAL Fluid Increase* In 27 patients mean concentration of 106.2 ± 35.8 ng/L significantly different from 12.5 ± 1.7 ng/L in 13 healthy control volunteers *1595*

Eosinophils *BAL Fluid Increase* In 27 patients mean concentration of 9.60 ± 3.27 x 10^3/mL significantly different from 0.03 ± 0.01 x 10^3/mL in 13 healthy control volunteers *1595* In 42 patients with IPF mean proportion of 1.8 ± 0.5% significantly different from 0.0 ± 0.0% in 20 control individuals *5859*

Interleukin-8 *Serum Increase* In 42 patients with IPF mean concentration of 54.7 ± 7.5 pg/mL significantly different from 5.2 ± 0.8 pg/mL in 20 control individuals *5859*

KL-6 Antigen *Serum Increase* In 16 patients with idiopathic pulmonary fibrosis mean concentration of 1,204 ± 264 U/mL significantly different from 207 ± 6 U/mL in 237 healthy controls *5134*

Lactate Dehydrogenase *BAL Fluid Increase* In 27 patients mean activity of 53.5 ± 11.6 U/L not significantly different from 22.8 ± 5.4 U/L in 13 healthy control volunteers *1595*
Serum Increase In one patient mean activity of 1,300 U/L significantly different from reference interval of 200 to 450 U/L *5407* In 42 patients with IPF mean activity of 216 ± 11 U/L significantly different from 160 ± 7 U/L in 20 control individuals *5859*

Leukocytes *BAL Fluid Increase* In 42 patients with IPF mean concentration of 716 ± 112 pg/mL significantly different from 67 ± 10 pg/mL in 20 control individuals *5859*
Blood Increase In 42 patients with IPF mean concentration of 8.9 ± 0.5 x 10^6/L significantly different from 6.5 ± 0.5 x 10^6/L in 20 control individuals *5859*

Lymphocytes *BAL Fluid Increase* In 27 patients mean concentration of 55.2 ± 15.9 x 10^3/mL significantly different from 7.0 ± 2.4 x 10^3/mL in 13 healthy control volunteers *1595* In 42 patients with IPF mean proportion of 10.1 ± 1.9% not significantly different from 5.6 ± 1.0% in 20 control individuals *5859*

Macrophages *BAL Fluid Decrease* In 42 patients with IPF mean proportion of 78.3 ± 2.9% significantly different from 93.9 ± 1.0% in 20 control individuals *5859*
BAL Fluid No Effect In 27 patients mean concentration of 179.2 ± 22.4 x 10^3/mL not significantly different from 139.0 ± 56.6 x 10^3/mL in 13 healthy control volunteers *1595*

Neutrophils *BAL Fluid Increase* In 42 patients with IPF mean proportion of 9.8 ± 2.4% significantly different from 0.3 ± 0.1% in 20 control individuals *5859* In 27 patients mean concentration of 14.9 ± 7.1 x 10^3/mL significantly different from 1.5 ± 0.5 x 10^3/mL in 13 healthy control volunteers *1595*

Protein *BAL Fluid Increase* In 27 patients mean concentration of 30.7 ± 8.6 mg/dL significantly different from 16.1 ± 1.4 mg/dL in 13 healthy control volunteers *1595*

Surfactant Protein A *BAL Fluid Decrease* One report described significantly reduced concentrations in 28 patients with idiopathic pulmonary fibrosis *1989*

Type III Procollagen Amino-terminal Peptide-related Antigen
BAL Fluid Increase In 27 patients mean concentration of 47.1 ± 25.0 ng/L significantly different from 0.5 ± 0.1 ng/L in 13 healthy control volunteers *1595*

Type IV Collagen 7S Domain *Serum Increase* In 11 patients with idiopathic pulmonary fibrosis mean concentration of 5.0 ± 1.5 ng/mL compared with 2.7 ± 0.9 ng/mL in 10 healthy controls *2601*

516.80 Interstitial Pneumonia

KL-6 Antigen *Serum Increase* In a patient with radiation pneumonia concentration increased. Serum KL-6 antigen concentration more sensitive as a measure of activity than lactate dehydrogenase and procollagen III N-terminal peptide *1984*

Mucin-associated Antigen *Serum Increase* Concentration reportedly increased in patients with interstitial pneumonia *4797*

518.00 Pulmonary Collapse

Bicarbonate *Serum Decrease* Respiratory alkalosis may occur *1980*

Carbon Dioxide Partial Pressure *Blood Decrease* Acute massive atelectasis produces a picture of an intrapulmonary right-to-left shunt with a drop in pCO_2 *900* Respiratory alkalosis may occur *1980*

Leukocytes *Blood Increase* May occur *900*

Oxygen Partial Pressure *Blood Decrease* Acute massive atelectasis produces a picture of an intrapulmonary right-to-left shunt with a drop in pO_2 *900*

Oxygen Saturation *Blood Decrease* Acute massive atelectasis produces a picture of an intrapulmonary right-to-left shunt with a drop in pO_2 *900*

pH *Blood Decrease* Active massive atelectasis produces a picture of intrapulmonary right-to-left shunt with a decrease in pH *900*
Blood Increase Respiratory alkalosis may occur *1980*

518.10 Pneumomediastinum

Leukocytes *Blood Increase* Variable and nonspecific leukocytosis *5544*

518.30 Chronic Eosinophilic Pneumonia

CD4⁺ Lymphocytes *BAL Fluid Increase* Mean concentration in 21 patients with chronic eosinophilic pneumonia of 5.4 ± 1.8% significantly different from 0.9 ± 0.6% in 19 controls *2858*

Cells *BAL Fluid Increase* Mean concentration in 21 patients with chronic eosinophilic pneumonia of 2.85 ± 0.34 x 10^5 /mL significantly greater than 1.54 ± 0.25 x 10^5 /mL in 19 controls *2858*

Eosinophils *BAL Fluid Increase* Mean concentration in 21 patients with chronic eosinophilic pneumonia of 31.2 ± 6.9% significantly different from 0.5 ± 0.1% in 19 controls *2858*
Blood Increase Mean concentration in 21 patients with chronic eosinophilic pneumonia of 22.6 ± 4.3% significantly greater than 1.1 ± 0.2% in 19 controls *2858*

Leukocytes *Blood Increase* Mean concentration in 21 patients with chronic eosinophilic pneumonia of 8.2 ± x 10^3 cells/μL significantly greater than 4.7 ± 0.8 x 10^3 cells/μL in 19 controls *2858*

Lymphocytes *BAL Fluid Increase* Mean concentration in 21 patients with chronic eosinophilic pneumonia of 21.7 ± 5.5% significantly different from 5.9 ± 1.3% in 19 controls *2858*

Macrophage Inflammatory Protein-1α *BAL Fluid No Effect* Mean concentration in 16 patients with chronic eosinophilic pneumonia of 125 pg/mg albumin not significantly different from 95 pg/mg albumin in 13 controls *2858*

Macrophages *BAL Fluid Decrease* Mean concentration in 21 patients with chronic eosinophilic pneumonia of 38.8 ± 5.8% significantly different from 91.0 ± 1.0% in 19 controls *2858*

Neutrophils *BAL Fluid Increase* Mean concentration in 21 patients with chronic eosinophilic pneumonia of 8.1 ± 2.6% significantly different from 2.4 ± 0.5% in 19 controls *2858*

RANTES *BAL Fluid Increase* Mean concentration in 16 patients with chronic eosinophilic pneumonia of 107 ± 27 pg/mg albumin significantly different from 1.4 pg/mg albumin in 13 controls *2858*

518.30 Pulmonary Infiltration with Eosinophilia

Granulocyte-Macrophage Colony Stimulating Factor *Serum No Effect* Not detected in the serum of any of 6 patients with condition *2744*

Interleukin-3 *Serum No Effect* Not detected in the serum of any of 6 patients with condition *2744*

Interleukin-5 *Serum Increase* Detected in the serum of 2 of 6 patients with pulmonary infiltration with eosinophilia *2744*

518.40 Pulmonary Edema

Carbon Dioxide Partial Pressure *Blood Decrease* Decreased pO_2 associated with normal or decreased pCO_2 *5544* *Blood No Effect* Decreased pO_2 associated with normal or decreased pCO_2 *5544*

Creatine Kinase *Serum Increase* For reasons that are still unclear some cases may have high levels *1025 1642*

Oxygen Partial Pressure *Blood Decrease* Decreased pO_2 associated with normal or decreased pCO_2 *5544* Mean arterial O_2 tension measured in 71 patients breathing room air was 59 mm Hg. The 14 acidemic patients had markedly lower pO_2, all under 60 mm Hg *1153*

Oxygen Saturation *Blood Decrease* Mean arterial O_2 tension measured in 71 patients breathing room air was 59 mm Hg. The 14 acidemic patients had markedly lower pO_2, all under 60 mm Hg *1153* Decreased pO_2 associated with normal or decreased pCO_2 *5544*

pH *Blood Decrease* Of 71 patients breathing room air, 14 were acidemic; 35 alkalemic and 33 had a pH in the normal range *1153*
Blood Increase Of 71 patients breathing room air, 14 were acidemic; 35 alkalemic and 33 had a pH in the normal range. The acidemic group had markedly lower pO_2, all under 60 mm Hg *1153*

Theophylline *Serum Increase* Acute pulmonary edema reported to decrease elimination of theophylline *5034*

518.89 Benign Lung Disease

Amino-terminal Propeptide of Type I Collagen *Serum No Effect* Mean concentration of 26.56 ± 8.41 μg/L observed in 12 patients with benign lung disease not significantly different from 30.01 ± 2.43 μg/L in 18 healthy matched control individuals *2731*

Cancer-associated Serum Antigen *Serum Increase* 10 of 157 patients (6%) with benign lung disease had concentrations above 9 U/mL *1135*

Carcinoembryonic Antigen *Serum No Effect* In 85 patients with benign lung disease median concentration of 1.1 ng/mL *3809*

Cells *BAL Fluid Increase* In 19 patients with benign lung diseases mean concentration of 2.5 ± 1.7 x 10^6/L not significantly different from 1.9 ± 1.0 x 10^6/L in 13 healthy controls *961*

C-terminal Telopeptide of Type I Collagen *Serum No Effect* Mean concentration of 3.26 ± 0.54 μg/L observed in 12 patients with benign lung disease not significantly different from 2.74 ± 0.15 μg/L in 18 healthy matched control individuals *2731*

CYFRA 21-1 *Serum No Effect* In 85 patients with benign lung disease median concentration of 0.8 ng/mL *3809*

Fibronectin *BAL Fluid Increase* In 19 patients with benign lung disease median concentration of 920 ng/mL significantly different from 363 ng/mL in 13 healthy controls *961*

γ-Glutamyltransferase *Serum Increase* Activity reportedly increased in a variety of diseases including diseases of the pancreas, myocardium, kidney and lung as well as in diabetes *4617*

Lymphocytes *BAL Fluid Increase* In 19 patients with benign lung diseases mean concentration of 6.2 ± 3.1% not significantly different from 5.4 ± 5.7% in 13 healthy controls *961*

Macrophages *BAL Fluid Increase* In 19 patients with benign lung diseases mean concentration of 41 ± 32% not significantly different from 81 ± 14% in 13 healthy controls *961*

Neutrophils *BAL Fluid Increase* In 19 patients with benign lung diseases mean concentration of 44 ± 32% significantly different from 10 ± 11% in 13 healthy controls *961*

pS2-Protein *Serum No Effect* In 17 patients with non-cancerous diseases of the lung median concentration of 127.0 pg/mL and mean concentration of 153.3 ± 121.5 pg/mL not significantly different compared with median of 148.8 pg/mL and mean of 167.7 ± 134.0 pg/mL in 91 healthy individuals *2152*

Tissue Polypeptide Antigen *Serum Increase* In 85 patients with benign lung disease median concentration of 49 U/L *3809*

518.89 Benign Pulmonary Disease

CA 549 *Serum No Effect* In 26 patients with benign disease of the lung one had a concentration greater than 30.0 kU/L with BRESMARQ assay *764*

CYFRA 21-1 *Serum Increase* In 48 patients with benign lung disease median concentration of 1.8 ng/mL significantly different from that in 50 healthy individuals with median concentration of 1.2 ng/mL and range of 0.5 - 2.4 ng/mL *3559* Mean concentration in 50 patients with benign pulmonary diseases of 2.9 ± 3.6 ng/mL compared with 1.1 ± 0.3 ng/mL in 29 healthy controls with a positivity rate of 16.0% *3665*

Glutathione S-Transferase-pi *Serum No Effect* Mean concentration in 25 patients with benign pulmonary disease of 24.8 ± 9.7 ng/mL not significantly different from 22.2 ± 9.7 ng/mL in 30 healthy volunteers *2150*

Sialic Acid *Serum Increase* In 106 patients with benign pulmonary disease mean concentration of 89.7 ± 0.12 mg/dL significantly higher than 64.3 ± 8.5 mg/dL in 84 healthy controls *2530*

Sialic Acid, Lipid-associated *Serum Increase* In 107 patients with primary lung cancer mean concentration of 21.5 ± 0.053 mg/dL significantly higher than 15.5 ± 3.4 mg/dL in 207 healthy controls *2530*

518.89 Pulmonary Disease

Erythropoietin *Serum Increase* In 37 patients with polycythemia associated with unspecified pulmonary diseases mean concentration of 22 ± 26 IU/L compared with 9 ± 4 IU/L in 79 reference controls *4320*

Hemoglobin *Blood Increase* In 37 patients with polycythemia associated with unspecified pulmonary diseases mean concentration of 18.1 ± 0.93 g/dL compared with 14.0 ± 1.1 g/dL in 79 reference controls *4320*

518.89 Pulmonary Infection

Neutrophil Proteinase 3 *Serum Increase* In 8 patients with severe pulmonary infections mean concentration of 225 ± 87 μg/mL significantly higher than mean of 78 ± 30 μg/mL in 21 normal individuals *2120*

519.80 Acute Respiratory Infection

Adenosine-N6-diethylthioether-N1-pyridinoximine 5'-phosphate *Serum No Effect* In 3 patients with acute respiratory infection concentrations ranged from 64.1 - 426.2 nmol/dL not significantly different from concentration in healthy individuals in whom the mean concentration was 162.2 nmol/dL *5294*

C-Reactive Protein *Serum Increase* In 10 children aged 5 months to 15 years mean concentration during febrile phase 6.1 ± 4.2 mg/dL significantly higher than 1.0 ± 2.0 mg/dL during convalescent phase *2046*

Interleukin-6 *Serum Increase* During febrile phase in 10 children aged 5 months to 15 years mean concentration of 25.1 ± 20.2 pg/mL significantly increased compared with 6.6 ± 11.3 pg/mL in convalescent phase *2046* In 59 outpatients with acute respiratory infection 22 had concentrations above 15 pg/mL *2046*

Thyroxine (T4) *Serum Decrease* In 10 children aged 5 months to 15 years mean concentration of 118 ± 4.5 nmol/L during febrile phase nonsignificantly lower than 135 ± 33 nmol/L in convalescent phase *2046*

Tri-iodothyronine (T3) *Serum Decrease* In 10 patients aged 5 months to 15 years during febrile phase mean concentration of 1.8 ± 0.6 nmol/L less than 2.3 ± 0.4 nmol/L during convalescent phase *2046*

519.80 Liddle's Syndrome

Aldosterone *Plasma Decrease* In one patient with Liddle's syndrome 2 years after renal transplant concentration of 7.3 ng/dL on normal sodium diet and 24.9 ng/dL on low sodium diet compared with 11.7 ± 6.1 ng/dL and 50.0 ± 17.6 ng/dL respectively in 10 azathioprine treated control renal transplant recipients. Prior to transplantation urine aldosterone negligible *537*
Urine Decrease In 18 individuals affected with Liddle's syndrome mean excretion of 369 ± 388 ng/12 h compared with 1,903 ± 425 ng/12 h in 15 unaffected members and 2,625 ± 520 ng/12 h in 10 not at risk members of the same family. Mean aldosterone:potassium ratio of 22 ± 23, 171 ± 26 and 148 ± 32 in the three groups respectively *537*

Bicarbonate *Serum No Effect* In 18 individuals with Liddle's syndrome mean concentration of 28 ± 1 mmol/L not significantly different when compared with 27 ± 1 mmol/L in 15 unaffected individuals and 26 ± 1 mmol/L in 10 not at risk individuals in the same family *537*

Creatinine Clearance *Urine No Effect* In 18 individuals with Liddle's syndrome 12 hour creatinine clearance of 90 ± 9 mL/min compared with 75 ± 11 mL/min in 15 unaffected individuals and 94 ± 13 mL/min in 10 not at risk members of the same family *537*

Potassium *Serum Decrease* In 18 individuals with Liddle's syndrome mean concentration of 3.6 ± 0.1 mmol/L compared with 4.2 ± 0.1 mmol/L in 15 unaffected individuals and 4.3 ± 0.1 mmol/L in 10 not at risk individuals in the same family *537*

Renin Activity *Plasma Decrease* In one patient 2 years after renal transplantation for Liddle's syndrome activity on normal sodium diet 0.7 ng/mL/h and 3.0 ng/mL/h on low sodium diet compared with 1.6 ± 0.6 ng/mL/h and 4.9 ± 1.3 ng/mL/h respectively in 10 azathioprine treated renal transplant recipient controls. Response to sodium restriction normal and similar to that in control transplant recipients *537*

519.80 Nonmalignant Disease

Epidermal Growth Factor *Serum Increase* In 15 patients with extra-pancreatic disease mean concentration of 26.9 ± 5.6 µg/L significantly different from 17.7 ± 3.8 µg/L in 22 healthy controls *3439*

Insulin-like Growth Factor-I *Serum Increase* In 23 patients with extrapancreatic disease mean concentration of 208.2 ± 43.4 µg/L significantly different from 103.3 ± 22.0 µg/L in 22 healthy controls *3439*

Somatostatin *Plasma No Effect* In 23 patients with extrapancreatic disease mean concentration of 34.1 ± 7.1 ng/L not significantly different from 29.7 ± 6 3 ng/L in 22 healthy controls *3439*

T23 Protein *Serum Increase* Protein detected in serum of 1 of 15 patients with various non-malignant diseases compared with none in controls *1781*

DISEASES OF THE DIGESTIVE SYSTEM

520.30 Fluorosis

Albumin *Serum Decrease* Mean concentration of 42.8 ± 5.0 g/L in 25 patients with skeletal fluorosis not significantly different from 47.8 ± 5.0 g/L in 13 healthy controls *5088*

C-Reactive Protein *Serum Increase* Mean concentration of 5.67 ± 6.95 mg/dL in 25 patients with skeletal fluorosis significantly different from 0.66 ± 0.52 mg/dL in 13 healthy controls *5088*

Erythrocyte Sedimentation Rate *Blood Increase* Mean rate of 20.1 ± 11.6 mm/h in 20 male patients with skeletal fluorosis and 42.4 ± 24.5 mm/h in 14 female patients with skeletal fluorosis significantly greater than 8.3 ± 5.4 mm/h in 15 healthy male controls and 15.3 ± 12.0 mm/h in 10 healthy female controls *5088*

Fluoride *Serum Increase* Mean concentration in 49 patients with fluorosis of 0.22 ± 0.12 mg/L significantly greater than 0.03 ± 0.02 mg/L in 36 healthy controls *5088*
Urine Increase Mean concentration in 24-hour urine of 49 patients with fluorosis of 3.52 ± 2.76 mg/L significantly greater than 0.38 ± 0.21 mg/L in 36 healthy controls *5088*

Haptoglobin *Serum Increase* Mean concentration of 1.88 ± 0.64 g/L in 25 patients with skeletal fluorosis significantly different from 1.39 ± 0.57 g/L in 13 healthy controls *5088*

523.10 Gingivitis

Cystatin *Saliva Increase* In 67 patients mean concentration of 0.12 mg/mL higher than 0.08 mg/mL in 19 healthy individuals *2121*

523.40 Periodontal Inflammation

Platelet Activating Factor *Saliva Increase* Significant positive correlation with severity of periodontal inflammation. In 69 patients mean concentration increased from 2,364 ± 900 fmol equivalents of 16:0-AGEPC/mL saliva at probe depth of greater than 4 mm (no sites) to above 10,000 fmol equivalents of 16:0-AGEPC/mL in patients with 37 - 75 sites at same probe depth *1657*

523.40 Periodontitis

Antioxidant Capacity *Saliva Decrease* Significant difference observed between mean concentration of 175 ± 53 mmol/L in 18 patients with periodontal disease and 254 ± 110 mmol/L in 16 individuals without periodontal disease *788*
Serum No Effect No significant difference observed between mean concentration of 480 ± 77 µmol/L in 18 patients with periodontal disease and 500 ± 95 µmol/L in 16 individuals without periodontal disease *788*

α_1-Antitrypsin *Saliva No Effect* Mean concentration of 69 ± 104 ng/mL in 8 patients with moderate to severe periodontitis not significantly different from 60 ± 101 ng/mL in 5 healthy individuals *4058*

Calcium *Saliva Decrease* Mean concentration reduced to 1,024 ± 410 µg/dL in 14 patients with periodontitis from mean of 1,446 ± 435 µg/dL in 10 healthy controls *2856*
Serum Increase Mean concentration increased to 10.5 ± 0.3 mg/dL in 14 patients with periodontitis compared with 9.9 ± 0.7 mg/dL in 10 healthy controls *2856*

C-Reactive Protein *Saliva No Effect* Mean concentration of 10.2 ± 5.3 pg/mL in 8 patients with moderate to severe periodontitis not significantly different from 67 ± 6.5 pg/mL in 5 healthy individuals *4058*

Cystatin *Saliva* *Increase* In 60 patients mean concentration of 0.18 mg/mL higher than 0.08 mg/mL in 19 healthy individuals *2121*

α_2-Macroglobulin *Saliva* *Increase* Mean concentration of 873 ± 1,665 ng/mL in 8 patients with moderate to severe periodontitis significantly different from 38.1 ± 32.3 ng/mL in 5 healthy individuals *4058*

Magnesium *Saliva* *No Effect* In 14 patients with periodontitis mean concentration of 100 ± 81 µg/dL compared with 72 ± 36 µg/dL in 10 healthy adult controls (nonsignificant increase) *2856*
Serum *No Effect* In 14 patients with periodontitis mean concentration of 2.38 ± 0.15 mg/dL compared with 2.35 ± 0.21 mg/dL in 10 healthy controls *2856*

Polymorphonuclear Elastase *Saliva* *No Effect* Mean concentration of 17.4 ± 16.9 ng/mL in 8 patients with moderate to severe periodontitis not significantly different from 22.3 ± 32.4 ng/mL in 5 healthy individuals *4058*

Testosterone *Saliva* *Increase* Significant increase to mean of 139 ± 17 pg/mL in 14 patients with periodontitis compared with 116 ± 14 pg/mL in 10 healthy controls *2856*
Serum *No Effect* In 14 patients with periodontitis mean concentration of 4,617 ± 387 pg/mL compared with 4,700 ± 431 pg/mL in 10 healthy controls *2856*

Zinc *Saliva* *No Effect* Nonsignificant increase from mean baseline of 11.2 ± 4.8 µg/dL in 10 healthy adult controls to 12.4 ± 6.2 µg/dL in 14 patients with periodontitis *2856*
Serum *Decrease* Significant reduction from mean baseline of 168 ± 26 µg/dL in 10 healthy adult controls to 135 ± 34 µg/dL in 14 patients with periodontitis *2856*

526.89 Cherubism

Calcium *Urine* *Increase* In 4 children aged 9 to 14 years concentration high for age *4947*

Deoxypyridinoline *Urine* *Increase* In 4 children aged 9 to 14 years concentration high for age *4947*

Hydroxyproline *Urine* *Increase* In 4 children aged 9 to 14 years concentration high for age *4947*

Osteocalcin *Serum* *No Effect* In 4 children aged 9 to 14 years concentration normal *4947*

Parathyroid Hormone *Plasma* *No Effect* In 4 children aged 9 to 14 years concentration normal *4947*

Pyridinoline *Urine* *Increase* In 4 children aged 9 to 14 years concentration high for age *4947*

527.90 Diseases of the Salivary Glands

Amylase *Serum* *Increase* Salivary gland disease: mumps, suppurative inflammation, duct obstruction due to calculus *5544*

528.20 Stomatitis, Aphthous

Prostaglandin E_2 *Saliva* *Decrease* In 6 patients with stage I recurrent aphthous stomatitis mean concentration of 220 ± 62 pg/mL (108 ± 25 pg/min), of 112 ± 19 pg/mL (63 ± 12 pg/min) (significant) in 15 with stage II disease and 468 ± 121 pg/mL (235 ± 69 pg/min) different from 447 ± 123 pg/mL (215 ± 30 pg/min) in 12 healthy controls *5750*

Protein *Saliva* *Decrease* In 6 patients with stage I recurrent aphthous stomatitis mean concentration of 1.69 ± 0.33 mg/mL, of 1.49 ± 0.13 mg/mL (significant) in 15 with stage II disease and 1.60 ± 0.22 mg/mL different from 2.34 ± 0.53 mg/mL in 12 healthy controls *5750*

Volume *Saliva* *No Effect* In 6 patients with stage I recurrent aphthous stomatitis mean flow rate of 0.53 ± 0.07 mL/min, of 0.55 ± 0.04 mL/min in 15 with stage II disease and 0.52 ± 0.07 mL/min not significantly different from 0.58 ± 0.07 mL/min in 12 healthy controls *5750*

Disease of the Gastrointestinal Tract

530.10 Esophagitis

Ferritin *Serum* *Decrease* In 725 patients with serum ferritin concentration of less than 50 ng/mL detected in 15 patients with esophagitis grades III or IV *2968*

Occult Blood *Feces* *Increase* In 93 patients who presented at an ER with upper gastrointestinal tract bleeding 5.6% had esophagitis *1383*

Urea Nitrogen:Creatinine Ratio *Serum* *Increase* Ratio of more than 36 is strongly suggestive of upper gastrointestinal tract bleeding *1383*

530.70 Mallory-Weiss Syndrome

Occult Blood *Feces* *Increase* In 93 patients who presented at an ER with upper gastrointestinal tract bleeding 4% had Mallory-Weiss syndrome *1383*

Urea Nitrogen:Creatinine Ratio *Serum* *Increase* Ratio of more than 36 is strongly suggestive of upper gastrointestinal tract bleeding *1383*

531.00 Gastric Ulcer

Carcinoembryonic Antigen *Serum* *Increase* In 94 patients with gastric ulcer 55% had concentrations less than 2.5 ng/mL, 29% had concentrations between 2.6 and 5.0 ng/mL, 15% had concentrations between 5.1 and 10.0 ng/mL and 1% had concentrations greater than 10.0 ng/mL *2010*

Ferritin *Serum* *Decrease* In 725 patients with serum ferritin concentration of less than 50 ng/mL detected in 31 patients with gastric or duodenal ulcer with erosions *2968*

Gastrin *Serum* *No Effect* Patients with gastric ulcer typically have moderately increased serum concentrations *2952*

Pepsinogen I *Serum* *Increase* Characteristic finding *68*
Serum *No Effect* In 46 patients with gastric ulcer mean concentration of 51.2 ± 24.8 µg/L not significantly different from 49.0 ± 30.8 µg/L in 116 healthy controls *2761* No significant difference, regardless of location of ulcer, when compared with age and sex-matched controls (99.6 ± 44.8 ng/mL) *776*

Pepsinogen II *Serum* *Increase* In 46 patients with gastric ulcer mean concentration of 23.9 ± 13.1 µg/L significantly different from 18.1 ± 13.3 µg/L in 116 healthy controls *2761*

532.00 Duodenal Ulcer

α_1-Antitrypsin *Serum* *Decrease* In 5 of 50 patients with duodenal ulcer concentration reduced and patients had SZ and S phenotype. Mean concentration in patients with DU of 2.12 ± 0.11 g/L compared with 2.47 ± 0.08 g/L *4752*

Carcinoembryonic Antigen *Serum* *Increase* In 166 patients with duodenal ulcer 70% had concentrations less than 2.5 ng/mL, 22% had concentrations between 2.6 and 5.0 ng/mL, 6% had concentrations between 5.1 and 10.0 ng/mL and 2% had concentrations greater than 10.0 ng/mL *2010*

Corticotropin *Plasma* *No Effect* Mean resting concentration in 13 patients with duodenal ulcer within normal range *2495*

Cortisol *Plasma* *Increase* Patients with duodenal ulcer had concentrations that were increased compared with those in controls *2955*
Plasma *No Effect* Mean resting concentration in 13 patients with duodenal ulcer within normal range *2495*

Dopamine *Plasma* *Increase* Patients with duodenal ulcer had concentrations that were increased compared with those in controls *2955*

Epinephrine *Plasma* *Increase* Patients with duodenal ulcer had concentrations that were increased compared with those in controls *2955*

Epinephrine:Norepinephrine Ratio *Plasma* *Increase* Patients with duodenal ulcer had ratios (> 0.5) that were increased compared with those in controls *2955*

Ferritin *Serum* *Decrease* In 725 patients with serum ferritin concentration of less than 50 ng/mL detected in 31 patients with gastric or duodenal ulcer with erosions *2968*

532.00 Duodenal Ulcer *(continued)*

Gastrin *Serum* *No Effect* Patients with duodenal ulcer typically have normal serum concentrations *2952*

5-Hydroxytryptamine, Free *Plasma* *Increase* Patients with duodenal ulcer had concentrations that were increased compared with those in controls *2955*

Lipase *Serum* *Increase* In patients with abdominal diseases such as duodenal ulcer may be increased enzyme activity *5231*

Norepinephrine *Plasma* *Increase* Mean resting concentration in 13 patients with duodenal ulcer of 0.26 ng/mL significantly higher than 0.18 ng/mL in 14 individuals with no history of abdominal pain *2495* Patients with duodenal ulcer had concentrations that were increased compared with those in controls *2955*

Pepsinogen I *Serum* *Increase* In 23 patients with duodenal ulcer mean concentration of 66.0 ± 22 6 µg/L significantly different from 49.0 ± 30.8 µg/L in 116 healthy controls *2761* Characteristic finding *5078*

Pepsinogen II *Serum* *No Effect* In 23 patients with duodenal ulcer mean concentration of 21.9 ± 9.5 µg/L not significantly different from 18.1 ± 13.3 µg/L in 116 healthy controls *2761*

Pepsinogen A *Serum* *Increase* In 19 men with duodenal ulcer mean concentration of 108.2 ± 58.3 µg/L compared with 51.5 ± 20.8 µg/L in 68 control men. In 15 women with duodenal ulcer mean concentration of 105.9 ± 56.3 µg/L compared with 52.0 ± 23.4 µg/L in 82 healthy women *1227*

Platelet Aggregation *Blood* *Increase* Patients with duodenal ulcer had platelet aggregability that was increased compared with that in controls *2955*

533.90 Peptic Ulcer

Amylase *Peritoneal Fluid* *Increase* With perforation *5544*
Serum *Increase* Extremely high values found in any condition in which the GI tract is perforated or loses viability *4707* Mild-moderate elevation with active ulcer and no associated pancreatitis. Rise is directly related to the size and duration of perforation, and amount of fluid accumulated in peritoneal cavity. Free perforations not in contact with pancreas may lead to hyperamylasemia also *4537*

Angiotensin-converting Enzyme *Serum* *Increase* Significant increase regardless of whether ulceration was gastric or duodenal *1213*

Bicarbonate *Duodenal Contents* *Decrease* Bicarbonate level has been shown to be 1/2 of controls *1936*
Serum *Increase* Pyloric obstruction with vomiting and loss of gastric secretion results in hypochloremia, hyponatremia, hypokalemia, elevated serum pH and carbon dioxide content, and azotemia *1980*

Bleeding Time *Patient* *Increase* In 56 patients with duodenal ulcer and 48 patients with gastric ulcer mean bleeding time normal (360 s) in three quarters and prolonged to 830 s in one quarter *2118*

Calcium *Serum* *Increase* Due to excessive alkali intake if the antacid contains calcium, or if milk is taken in excess *1290*

Carcinoembryonic Antigen *Serum* *Increase* 14% of patients had positive assay (values > 12.5 ng/mL) *528* About 10% patients have increased concentration *4891*

Chloride *Serum* *Decrease* May fall below 100 mmol/L in an ulcer complicated by obstruction. With persistent marked obstruction, may reach as low as 60 mmol/L *900* Pyloric obstruction with vomiting and loss of gastric secretion results in hypochloremia, hyponatremia, hypokalemia, elevated serum pH and carbon dioxide content, and azotemia *1980*

CYFRA 21-1 *Serum* *Increase* In 13 patients with peptic ulcer median concentration of 2.5 ng/mL significantly different from that in 50 healthy individuals with median concentration of 1.2 ng/mL and range of 0.5 - 2.4 ng/mL *3559*

Endothelin-1 *Plasma* *Increase* Mean concentrations in patients with active ulcer and healing ulcer of 5.26 ± 0.78 pg/mL and 3.47 ± 0.58 pg/mL significantly higher than 2.08 ± 0.24 pg/mL in patients with ulcers in scarring stage and 1.87 ± 0.27 pg/mL in healthy controls *3342*

Erythrocyte Sedimentation Rate *Blood* *Increase* Elevation of the WBC, increased ESR and related phenomena are, to be expected in the event of perforation, massive hemorrhage, and toxic or infectious complications *1980*
Blood *No Effect* Normal in peptic ulcer, but accelerated in carcinoma of the stomach *1980*

Gastrin *Serum* *Increase* May occur after meals *3413* Tends to be elevated in gastric ulcer and correlates with decreased acid secretion *367*
Serum *No Effect* Fasting serum concentrations are normal in patients with ordinary duodenal ulcer disease. Although the mean increase in concentration after a meal is higher in duodenal ulcer than in normal subjects, this test is not helpful diagnostically *4891* Fasting concentration is generally normal despite hypersecretion of gastric acid. May occur after meals *3413*

α_1-Globulin *Serum* *Increase* May be increased *5544*

α_2-Globulin *Serum* *Increase* May be increased *5544*

Glucose *Serum* *Decrease* A high frequency of spontaneous hypoglycemia occurs in these patients *4707*

Glucose Tolerance *Serum* *Decrease* Significantly greater rise in glucose concentration and higher output of insulin was observed in patients with duodenal ulcer *2297*

Hematocrit *Blood* *Decrease* In 56 patients with duodenal ulcer and 48 patients with gastric ulcer in those in whom bleeding time was normal median 33% and in those in whom it was prolonged median 29% *2118* An ulcer that bleeds chronically will cause a varying degree of iron deficiency anemia *1980* A few patients will have anemia because of chronic blood loss *900*
Blood *No Effect* Uncomplicated peptic ulcer is not associated with anemia *1980*

Hemoglobin *Blood* *Decrease* An ulcer that bleeds chronically will cause a varying degree of iron deficiency anemia *1980* In 56 patients with duodenal ulcer and 48 patients with gastric ulcer in those in whom bleeding time was normal median concentration of 111 g/L and in those in whom it was prolonged median concentration of 94 g/L *2118* A few patients will have anemia because of chronic blood loss *900*
Blood *No Effect* Uncomplicated peptic ulcer is not associated with anemia *1980*

5-Hydroxytryptamine *Plasma* *No Effect* Not increased in gastric and duodenal ulcer disease *4164*

Iron *Serum* *Decrease* An ulcer that bleeds chronically will cause a varying degree of iron deficiency anemia *1980*

Iron-binding Capacity, Total *Serum* *Increase* An ulcer that bleeds chronically will cause a varying degree of iron deficiency anemia *1980*

Iron Saturation *Serum* *Decrease* An ulcer that bleeds chronically will cause a varying degree of iron deficiency anemia *1980*

Lactate Dehydrogenase *Gastric Material* *Increase* Moderately increased activity *1290*

Leukocytes *Blood* *Increase* Elevation of the WBC, increased ESR and related phenomena are to be expected in the event of perforation, massive hemorrhage, and toxic or infectious complications *1980* Increased with shift to left *5544*

Lipase *Serum* *Increase* Perforated or penetrating peptic ulcer especially with involvement of the pancreas *5544*

Lysolecithin *Gastric Material* *Increase* Found to be high *2464*

MCH *Blood* *Decrease* A few patients will have anemia because of chronic blood loss *900* An ulcer that bleeds chronically will cause a varying degree of iron deficiency anemia *1980*

MCHC *Blood* *Decrease* An ulcer that bleeds chronically will cause a varying degree of iron deficiency anemia *1980* A few patients will have anemia because of chronic blood loss *900*

MCV *Blood* *Decrease* An ulcer that bleeds chronically will cause a varying degree of iron deficiency anemia *1980* A few patients will have anemia because of chronic blood loss *900*

Occult Blood *Feces* *Increase* In 93 patients who presented at an ER with upper gastrointestinal tract bleeding 12% had a peptic ulcer *1383*

Partial Thromboplastin Time *Plasma* *No Effect* In 56 patients with duodenal ulcer and 48 patients with gastric ulcer in those in whom bleeding time was normal median 30 s and in those in whom it was prolonged median 30 s, both within reference interval *2118*

Pepsinogen *Serum* *Increase* Serum acid protease activity at pH 1.8 (pepsin) shows slightly higher levels than normal *3511* An elevated serum concentration appears to be a subclinical marker of the ulcer diathesis in families with the autosomal dominant form of peptic ulcer disease. Elevated immunoreactive pepsinogen I (> 100 ng/mL) segregated as a dominant trait in the affected families *4458*

pH *Blood* *Increase* May exceed 7.45. Complicated by obstruction *900* Pyloric obstruction with vomiting and loss of gastric secretion results in hypochloremia, hyponatremia, hypokalemia, elevated serum pH and CO_2 content, and azotemia *1980*
Gastric Material *Decrease* True achlorhydria virtually excludes peptic ulcer disease. In gastric ulcer the average basal gastric secretion is decreased or normal *297*
Gastric Material *Increase* No single test of gastric secretion shows abnormal hypersecretion in more than 50% of duodenal ulcer patients *297* Characteristic finding with disease *1218*

Platelets *Blood* *No Effect* In 56 patients with duodenal ulcer and 48 patients with gastric ulcer in those in whom bleeding time was normal median concentration of 245 x 10^9/L and in those in whom it was prolonged median concentration of 216 x 10^9/L *2118*

Potassium *Serum* *Decrease* Pyloric obstruction with vomiting and loss of gastric secretion results in hypochloremia, hyponatremia, hypokalemia, elevated serum pH and carbon dioxide content, and azotemia *1980* May be < 3.5 mmol/L when complicated by obstruction *900*

Prothrombin Time *Plasma* *No Effect* In 56 patients with duodenal ulcer and 48 patients with gastric ulcer in those in whom bleeding time was normal median 80% and in those in whom it was prolonged median concentration of 85%, both within reference interval *2118*

Sodium *Serum* *Decrease* Pyloric obstruction with vomiting and loss of gastric secretion results in hypochloremia, hyponatremia, hypokalemia, elevated serum pH and carbon dioxide content, and azotemia *1980* May be < 135 mmol/L when complicated by obstruction *900*

Trypsin *Serum* *No Effect* Mean concentration of trypsin-like immunoreactivity in 14 patients with a peptic ulcer did not exceed concentration in 85 healthy control individuals (42.78 ± 10.26 ng/mL) *3330*

Urea Nitrogen *Serum* *Increase* Pyloric obstruction with vomiting and loss of gastric secretion results in hypochloremia, hyponatremia, hypokalemia, elevated serum pH and carbon dioxide content, and azotemia *1980*

Urea Nitrogen:Creatinine Ratio *Serum* *Increase* Ratio of more than 36 is strongly suggestive of upper gastrointestinal tract bleeding *1383*

von Willebrand Factor *Plasma* *Increase* In 56 patients with duodenal ulcer and 48 patients with gastric ulcer in those in whom bleeding time was normal, median concentration of 179% and in those in whom it was prolonged median concentration of 161%, both within reference interval *2118*

535.10 Atrophic Gastritis

Parietal Cell Antibodies *Serum* *Increase* Approximately 60% of patients with atrophic gastritis have antibodies to gastric parietal cells *2952*

535.10 Chronic Gastritis

Pepsinogen I *Serum* *No Effect* In 44 patients with chronic gastritis mean concentration of 56.3 ± 34.2 µg/L not significantly different from 49.0 ± 30.8 µg/L in 116 healthy controls *2761*

Pepsinogen II *Serum* *No Effect* In 44 patients with chronic gastritis mean concentration of 20.1 ± 13.0 µg/L not significantly different from 18.1 ± 13.3 µg/L in 116 healthy controls *2761*

535.50 Gastritis

Albumin *Serum* *Decrease* Secondary to protein-losing enteropathy in atrophic gastroenteritis *4707* May be low in patients with giant hypertrophic gastritis who exude protein into the lumen *900*

Antibody Titer *Serum* *Increase* Parietal cell antibody detected by CF tests using gastric mucosal homogenate or by direct immunofluorescence on sections of gastric mucosa is present in approximately 60% of patients with idiopathic atrophic gastritis *1210*

Antithyroglobulin Antibodies *Serum* *Increase* With atrophic gastritis *4891*

Aspartate Aminotransferase *Serum* *Increase* In 33% of 37 patients at initial hospitalization for this disorder *1576*

CA 72-4 *Serum* *Increase* In 30 patients with gastritis or gastric ulcer 2 (7%) had a concentration greater than cut-off of 2.5 U/mL with median value of 1.6 U/mL *4505*

Carcinoembryonic Antigen *Serum* *Increase* In 30 patients with gastritis or gastric ulcer 4 (13%) had a concentration greater than cut-off of 3 ng/mL with median value of 1.9 ng/mL *4505*

Eosinophils *Blood* *Increase* Peripheral eosinophilia in eosinophilic gastritis *4891*

Gastrin *Serum* *Increase* The combination of high serum gastrin and low pepsinogen is commonly found in patients with atrophic gastritis *4891* Increased in chronic atrophic gastritis *5049* The combination of high serum gastrin and low pepsinogen is commonly found in patients with atrophic gastritis *4545*

Hematocrit *Blood* *Decrease* May be low in patients with bleeding *900*

Hemoglobin *Blood* *Decrease* May be low in patients with bleeding *900* Hypochromic microcytic anemia due to blood loss *5544*

Hydrochloric Acid *Gastric Fluid* *Decrease* Transient hypochlorhydria or achlorhydria may be observed during episodes of acute gastritis *4891* Most patients with Menetrier's disease have achlorhydria. However, some patients may have hypersecretion *4960*

Iron-binding Capacity, Total *Serum* *Increase* Anemia may be due to chronic blood loss *1980* *1315*

Iron Saturation *Serum* *Decrease* Anemia may be due to chronic blood loss *1315* *1980*

Lactate Dehydrogenase *Gastric Material* *Increase* Moderately increased activity *1290*

Leukocytes *Blood* *Increase* May be present in cases of corrosive or phlegmonous gastritis *900*

MCH *Blood* *Decrease* May be low in patients with bleeding *900*

MCHC *Blood* *Decrease* May be low in patients with bleeding *900*

MCV *Blood* *Decrease* May be low in patients with bleeding *900*
Blood *Increase* Secondary to B_{12} deficiency with atrophic gastritis *4891*

Neutrophils *Blood* *Increase* In 40% of 36 patients at initial hospitalization for this disorder *1576*

Occult Blood *Feces* *Increase* Upper GI bleeding *4891* In 93 patients wł. presented at an ER with upper gastrointestinal tract bleeding 18.5% had gastritis *1383*

Pepsin *Gastric Material* *Decrease* In Menetrier's Disease hyposecretion is usual finding *851*

Pepsinogen *Serum* *Decrease* The combination of high serum gastrin and low pepsinogen is commonly found in patients with atrophic gastritis *4891*

pH *Gastric Material* *Decrease* Erosive hemorrhagic gastritis appears to be due to pathologic back diffusion of hydrogen ions caused by a breakdown of the gastric mucosal barrier *4957* In Menetrier's disease hyposecretion of gastric acid is usual finding *851* Most patients with Menetrier's disease have achlorhydria, but some may have hypersecretion *2320*
Gastric Material *Increase* Most patients with Menetrier's Disease have achlorhydria. However, some patients may have hypersecretion *4960* Transient hypochlorhydria or achlorhydria may be observed during episodes of acute gastritis *4891*

Protein *Feces* *Increase* An increased sensitivity of atrophic mucosa to exogenous irritants is suggested by the observation that patients with atrophic gastritis lost excessive amounts of plasma protein when they ingested ethanol *832*
Serum *Decrease* An increased sensitivity of atrophic mucosa to exogenous irritants is suggested by the observation that patients with atrophic gastritis lost excessive amounts of plasma

535.50 Gastritis *(continued)*

Protein *(continued)*
protein when they ingested ethanol *832* In Menetrier's disease hypoproteinemia is often seen *851*

Urea Nitrogen:Creatinine Ratio *Serum Increase* Ratio of more than 36 is strongly suggestive of upper gastrointestinal tract bleeding *1383*

Uropepsinogen *Urine Decrease* With atrophic gastritis *1218*

Vitamin B_{12} *Serum Decrease* With atrophic gastritis *4891*

537.00 Pyloric Stenosis, Acquired

Bicarbonate *Serum Increase* Metabolic alkalosis secondary to vomiting *1218*

Chloride *Serum Decrease* Metabolic alkalosis secondary to vomiting *1218*

Hydrochloric Acid *Gastric Fluid Increase* Due to excess circulating gastrin *1218*

pH *Gastric Material Decrease* Due to excess circulating gastrin *1218*

Potassium *Serum Decrease* Secondary to vomiting *1218*
Urine No Effect Concentration usually normal *5544*

Sodium *Serum Decrease* Secondary to vomiting *1218*

537.40 Fistula of Stomach and Duodenum

Alkaline Phosphatase *Serum Increase* Leading to secondary osteomalacia *1290*

Bicarbonate *Serum Decrease* Metabolic acidosis may occur *1980*

Carbon Dioxide Partial Pressure *Blood Decrease* Metabolic acidosis may occur *1980*

Carcinoembryonic Antigen *Serum Increase* Found in 15% (2.5 ng/mL) *1218*

Chloride *Serum Decrease* In gastric fistula, hypokalemic, hypochloremic alkalosis may result *4891*

Fat *Feces Increase* Excessively rapid passage of intestinal contents. Increased fat in feces with gastrocolic fistula *1290*

Hematocrit *Blood Decrease* Anemia and hypoproteinemia reflect malnutrition and chronic disease *4891*
Blood Increase Will reflect the degree of hemoconcentration *4891*

Hemoglobin *Blood Decrease* Anemia and hypoproteinemia reflect malnutrition and chronic disease *4891*

Leukocytes *Blood Increase* May be elevated with sepsis *4891*

Nitrogen *Feces Increase* Observed effect *1290*

Occult Blood *Feces Increase* The most common presentation. False negative and positives occur *5625*

pH *Blood Decrease* With high output proximal small bowel or pancreatic fistulas, the patients may be acidotic, because the lost pancreatic and biliary secretions are alkaline *4891* Metabolic acidosis may occur *1980*
Blood Increase In gastric fistula, hypokalemic, hypochloremic alkalosis may result *4891*

Potassium *Serum Decrease* In gastric fistula, hypokalemic, hypochloremic alkalosis may result *4891* Renal wasting leads to hypokalemic state *3735*

Protein *Serum Decrease* Anemia and hypoproteinemia reflect malnutrition and chronic disease *4891*

Sodium *Serum Decrease* Small intestinal aspiration or fistula. The loss of sodium/day (430 mmol) is > the loss of chloride (270 mmol) *1290*

537.90 Benign Gastric Disease

CA 549 *Serum No Effect* In 16 patients with benign disease of the stomach none had a concentration greater than 30.0 kU/L with BRESMARQ assay *764*

540.90 Acute Appendicitis

Amylase *Serum Increase* In a series of 149 cases, 57 had hyperamylasemia. The highest value was 800 Su/100 mL without an obstructed gangrenous appendix *4537* In a series of 149 cases, 57 had hyperamylasemia. The highest value was 800 SU/100 mL with no obstructed, gangrenous appendix *645* 57 of 149 cases had increased concentration. Highest value was 1,480 U/L in a patient with an obstructed gangrenous appendix *645*

C-Reactive Protein *Serum Increase* Most patients with complicated appendicitis had increased concentrations of CRP *1881* In 116 patients with edematous appendicitis mean concentration of 33 ± 3 mg/L and 109 ± 12 mg/L in 29 with perforated appendix or appendiceal abscess higher than 22 ± 4 mg/L in 31 patients without appendicitis or other manifest inflammatory disease *1880* Using an upper limit of the reference range of 5 mg/L 98 patients with acute appendicitis had a mean concentration of 50.9 ± 58.9 mg/L compared with 19.1± 33.1 mg/L in 159 with diseases other than acute appendicitis *1970* Using a CRP cutoff of 50 mg/L (10 times ULN) in children with appendicitis, this provided a sensitivity of 76%, specificity of 82%, positive predictive value of 91% and accuracy of 78% for perforation *847* In 8 of 11 patients with acute appendicitis concentration greater than 1.0 mg/dL *4886* In a meta-analysis of 22 articles with 3,436 patients sensitivity of serum C-reactive protein for diagnosing acute appendicitis sensitivity ranged from 0.40 to 0.99 and specificity ranged from 0.27 to 0.90 using cutoff values for a positive test from 5 to 25 mg/L *1969* While clinical factors provided a discriminant of 0.854 for acute appendicitis, leukocyte counts greater than 10,000 /µL improved discriminant to 0.901 and addition of C-reactive protein concentrations above 5 mg/L increased the discriminant further *1970* Preoperative mean concentration of 128.5 mg/L in 28 patients with perforated appendicitis higher than 33.8 mg/L in 62 patients with nonperforated appendicitis higher than 5 mg/L those with normal appendices *1930*
Serum No Effect In 14 patients with phlegmatous appendicitis, 39 with gangrenous appendicitis and 52 with perforated appendices mean concentrations on admission of 14, 39 and 52 mg/L respectively not significantly different from 55 g/L in 13 patients with normal appendices *1379* Most patients with uncomplicated appendicitis had normal concentrations of CRP *1881*

Erythrocyte Sedimentation Rate *Blood Increase* Using an upper limit of the reference range of 20 mm/h 98 patients with acute appendicitis had a mean rate of 17.2 ± 18.3 mm/h compared with 11.8 ± 12.5 in 159 with diseases other than acute appendicitis *1970* With abscess formation or peritonitis, the rate increases rapidly *1980*
Blood No Effect While clinical factors provided a discriminant of 0.854 for acute appendicitis, leukocyte counts greater than 10,000 /µL improved discriminant to 0.901 and addition of C-reactive protein concentrations above 5 mg/L increased the discriminant further, as did a neutrophil count above 75%, but an ESR greater than 20 mm/h provided no further enhancement to the discrimant *1970* In unruptured acute appendicitis, the ESR is normal during the first 24 h, even when the appendix is suppurative or gangrenous *1980*

Erythrocytes *Urine Increase* In 66 patients with acute appendicitis more than 4 rbc/hpf observed in 32 (48%) before appendectomy decreasing to 9 (14%) on the first postoperative day *4240* Small numbers are found in the urine in about 25% of patients *4891*

Glucose *Serum Increase* In 34% of 52 patients at initial hospitalization for this disorder *1576*

5-Hydroxytryptamine *Plasma Increase* Values for patients with subsequently confirmed appendicitis (median 70 nmol/L) significantly exceeded (p = 0.005) those for patients with abdominal pain in whom appendicitis was only a possible diagnosis (median 20 nmol/L) *4865*

Interleukin-6 *Serum Increase* In 11 patients with perforated appendices mean concentration on admission of 100 ng/L significantly different from 22 ng/L in 14 patients with normal appendices *1379*
Serum No Effect In 28 patients with phlegmatous appendicitis and 45 with gangrenous appendicitis mean concentrations on admission of 19 and 24 ng/L respectively not significantly different from 22 ng/L in 14 patients with normal appendices *1379*

Leukocyte Elastase *Serum Increase* In 12 patients with perforated appendices mean concentration on admission of 98 ± 21 µg/L significantly different from 74 ± 12 µg/L in 14 patients with normal appendices *1379*
Serum No Effect In 28 patients with phlegmatous appendicitis mean concentration on admission of 69 ± 8 µg/L and 74 ± 12 µg/L in 45 patients with gangrenous appendicitis not significantly different from 74 ± 12 µg/L in 14 patients with normal appendices *1379* In 165 patients with acute appendicitis mean concentration of 69 ± 8 µg/L in 28 patients with phlegmonous appendices, 74 ± 7 µg/L in 45 patients with gangrenous appendices and 98 ± 21 µg/L in 12 patients with perforated appendices compared with 74 ± 1 µg/L in 14 patients with normal appendices *1382*

Leukocytes *Blood Increase* Counts above 10,900 /µL observed in 1.710 of 1,919 proved cases of acute appendicitis *882* Using an upper limit of the reference range of 10 x 10^9 98 patients with acute appendicitis had a mean count of 14.6 ± 3.6 x 10^9 compared with 10.2 ± 4.6 x 10^9 in 159 with diseases other than acute appendicitis *1970* In 116 patients with edematous appendicitis mean concentration of 14,200 ± 300 /µL and 15,800 ± 900 /µL in 29 with perforated appendix or appendiceal abscess higher than 10,800 ± 800 /µL in 31 patients without appendicitis or other manifest inflammatory disease *1880* In 82% of 108 patients at initial hospitalization for this disorder *1576* Most women with uncomplicated appendicitis had counts greater than 9,000 /µL and most men greater than 10,000 /µL: also observed in patients with complicated acute appendicitis *1881* WBC count of 15,863 /µL in 56 patients with perforated appendix not significantly different from 15,582 /µL in 22 children with appendicitis but without perforation *847* In all 11 patients with acute appendicitis in one study concentrations greater than 11,000 /µL *4886* Raised total count in 42%, a raised neutrophil percentage in 93% and a raised absolute neutrophil count in 77% *1219* While clinical factors provided a discriminant of 0.854 for acute appendicitis, leukocyte counts greater than 10,000 /µL improved discriminant to 0.901 *1970* In 28 patients with phlegmatous appendicitis, 45 with gangrenous appendicitis and 12 with perforated appendices mean concentrations on admission of 11.8 ± 0.8, 12.4 ± 0.5 and 15.3 ± 0.7 x 10^9/L respectively significantly different from 9.9 ± 0.7 x 10^9/L in 14 patients with normal appendices *1379* In 165 patients with acute appendicitis mean concentration of 11.8 ± 0.8 x 10^9/L in 28 patients with phlegmonous appendices, 12.4 ± 0.5 x 10^9/L in 45 patients with gangrenous appendices and 15.3 ± 0.7 x 10^9/L in 12 patients with perforated appendices compared with 9.9 ± 0.7 x 10^9/L in 14 patients with normal appendices *1382* 96% of patients had either an abnormal total or differential count. Leukocytosis > 10,000 /µL or a differential in excess of 75% neutrophils supports this clinical diagnosis *4263*
Blood No Effect Normal count of 3,800 to 10,900 /µL observed in 209 of 1,919 proved cases of acute appendicitis *882*
Urine Increase In 66 patients with acute appendicitis more than 4 WBC/hpf observed in 32 (48%) before appendectomy decreasing to 9 patients (14%) on the first postoperative day *4240* Small numbers are found in the urine in about 25% of patients *4891*

Lymphocytes *Blood Decrease* In 80% of 105 patients at initial hospitalization for this disorder *1576*

Neutrophils *Blood Increase* 96% of patients had either an abnormal total or differential WBC count. Leukocytosis > 10,000 /µL or a differential in excess of 75% neutrophils supports this clinical diagnosis *4263* In 8 of 11 patients with acute appendicitis neutrophil count greater than 75% *4886* While clinical factors provided a discriminant of 0.854 for acute appendicitis, leukocyte counts greater than 10,000 /µL improved discriminant to 0.901 and addition of C-reactive protein concentrations above 5 mg/L increased the discriminant further, as did a neutrophil count above 75% *1970* Using an upper limit of the reference range of the neutrophil proportion of total leukocyte count of 75% 98 patients with acute appendicitis had a mean count of 82.2 ± 8.5% compared with 73.6 ± 11.8% in 159 with diseases other than acute appendicitis *1970* Raised total leukocyte count in 42%, a raised neutrophil percentage in 93% and a raised absolute neutrophil count in 77% *1219* In 71% of 106 patients at initial hospitalization for this disorder *1576*

Phospholipase A_2 *Serum Increase* In 116 patients with edematous appendicitis mean concentration of 38 ± 6 µg/L and 134 ± 25 µg/L in 29 with perforated appendix or appendiceal abscess higher than 15 ± 5 µg/L in 31 patients without appendicitis or other manifest inflammatory disease *1880*

Phospholipase A_2 Type II *Serum Increase* Increase in concentration observed of 134 µg/L in severe acute appendicitis compared with 2 and 4 µg/L in healthy controls *3767*

Protein *Urine Increase* In 66 patients with acute appendicitis excretion of more than 0.5 g/L observed in 32 (48%) before appendectomy decreasing to 9 (14%) on the first postoperative day *4240*

553.30 Hernia, Diaphragmatic

Carbon Dioxide Partial Pressure *Blood Increase* 11 out of 20 infants with congenital hernia survived. Of the 9 nonsurvivors, arterial pCO_2 levels were markedly higher (61.3 ± 15.4 mm Hg) and pO_2 levels lower (49.8 ± 14.2 mm Hg) than in survivors (44.3 ± 7.9 mm Hg, 307.9 ± 142.3 mm Hg respectively) *507* Severe hypercarbia may be present *900*

Hematocrit *Blood Decrease* Microcytic anemia (due to loss of blood) may be present *5544*

Hemoglobin *Blood Decrease* Microcytic anemia (due to loss of blood) may be present *5544*

MCH *Blood Decrease* Microcytic anemia (due to loss of blood) may be present *5544*

MCV *Blood Decrease* Microcytic anemia (due to loss of blood) may be present *5544*

Occult Blood *Feces Increase* May be positive *5544*

Oxygen Partial Pressure *Blood Decrease* Severe hypoxia may be present *900* 11 out of 20 infants with congenital hernia survived. Of the 9 nonsurvivors, arterial pCO_2 levels were markedly higher (61.3 ± 15.4 mm Hg) and pO_2 levels lower (49.8 ± 14.2 mm Hg) than in survivors (44.3 ± 7.9 mm Hg, 307.9 ± 142.3 mm Hg, respectively) *507*

Oxygen Saturation *Blood Decrease* Severe hypoxia may be present *900* 11 out of 20 infants with congenital hernia survived. Of the 9 nonsurvivors, arterial pCO_2 levels were markedly higher (61.3 ± 15.4 mm Hg) and pO_2 levels lower (49.8 ± 14.2 mm Hg) than in survivors (44.3 ± 7.9 mm Hg, 307.9 ± 142.3 mm Hg, respectively) *507*

pH *Blood Decrease* Severe acidosis may be present *900*

553.90 Hernia

Carcinoembryonic Antigen *Serum Increase* In 103 patients with hernias, 77% had concentrations less than 2.5 ng/mL, 22% had concentrations between 2.6 and 5.0 ng/mL, 1% had concentrations between 5.1 and 10.0 ng/mL and 0% had concentrations greater than 10.0 ng/mL *2010*

555.10 Granulomatous Colitis

Carcinoembryonic Antigen *Serum Increase* In 59 patients with granulomatous colitis 53% had concentrations less than 2.5 ng/mL, 27% had concentrations between 2.6 and 5.0 ng/mL, 15% had concentrations between 5.1 and 10.0 ng/mL and 5% had concentrations greater than 10.0 ng/mL *2010*

555.90 Crohn's Disease

α_1-Acid Glycoprotein *Serum Increase* Median concentration in 68 patients with Crohn's disease 27 µmol/L in 27 with index of activity of 0 - 5 and 37 µmol/L in 41 with index of activity > 5 *4120* Mean concentration in 256 patients with Crohn's disease about 0.84 g/L *1861* In 10 of 54 patients concentraton increased above upper limit of normal although 12 had active disease *2* Mean concentration of 197 mg/dL in 13 patients with acute Crohn's disease significantly greater than 127 mg/dL in 14 patients with 17 patients with Crohn's disease in remission and 119 mg/dL in 20 healthy controls *4344* Positive correlation of r = 0.209 with Crohn's disease activity index *4472*

Alanine Aminotransferase *Serum Increase* Activity in patients with Crohn's disease increased in 13 of 100 patients *5488*

Albumin *Serum No Effect* Median concentration in 68 patients with Crohn's disease of 41 g/L in 27 with index of activity of 0 - 5 and 37 g/L in 41 with index of activity > 5 *4120*

555.90 Crohn's Disease *(continued)*

Alkaline Phosphatase *Serum Increase* Activity in patients with Crohn's disease increased in 25 of 100 patients *5488* *Serum No Effect* In two studies mean alkaline phosphatase activity was unchanged *3697*

Alkaline Phosphatase, Bone Isoenzyme *Serum Increase* Activity in patients with Crohn's disease increased in 16 of 100 patients *5488*

Alkaline Phosphatase, Fast Liver Isoenzyme *Serum Increase* Activity in patients with Crohn's disease increased in 64 of 100 patients *5488*

Alkaline Phosphatase, Intestinal *Serum Increase* Activity in patients with Crohn's disease increased in 8 of 100 patients *5488*

Alkaline Phosphatase, Liver Isoenzyme *Serum Increase* Activity in patients with Crohn's disease increased in 84 of 100 patients *5488*

Amylase, Pancreatic Isoenzyme *Serum Increase* Median activity in 46 patients with Crohn's disease of 105 U/L *2094*

Angiotensin-converting Enzyme *Serum No Effect* No significant difference was noted between active Crohn's, inactive Crohn's, and normal controls. However, patients who had active disease and were receiving steroid therapy had significantly lower levels *3840*

Anti-Endomysial IgA Antibodies *Serum Increase* Antibodies observed in 11 of 19 specimens from patients with Crohn's disease *109*

Anti-Endothelial Cell Antibodies *Serum Increase* Levels were elevated in ulcerative colitis ($p < 0.0001$) and Crohn's disease ($p < 0.05$) compared with healthy controls *5012*

Anti-Neutrophil Cytoplasm Antibodies *Serum Increase* In 2 of 25 patients with Crohn's disease positive antibodies observed *2021* Observed effect in some patients with Crohn's disease *4923*

Anti-Saccharomyces cerevisiae Antibodies *Serum Increase* Detected in about 60 - 70% of patients with Crohn's disease *4485*

α_2-Antiplasmin *Plasma No Effect* In 28 patients with Crohn's disease mean concentration of 95 ± 1.3% compared with 93 ± 0.9% in 60 healthy blood donor controls *4948*

Antithrombin III *Plasma No Effect* In 36 patients with active Crohn's disease median concentration of 102% (25th and 75th quartiles 89 and 106 respectively) and in 45 patients with moderate Crohn's disease median 102 (25th and 75th quartiles 96 and 108 respectively) compared with upper limit of normal of > 70% *4725*

α_1-Antitrypsin *Feces Increase* Mean concentration in 15 patients with Crohn's disease 3482.4 µg/g (278.50 mg/d) not significantly different from 987.91 µg/g (47.43 mg/d) in 20 healthy controls *4521*

Ascorbic Acid *Serum Decrease* Mean concentration of 273 ± 125 µmol/L in 8 children with Crohn's disease significantly different from 420 ± 114 µmol/L in 12 healthy control children *2196*

Aspartate Aminotransferase *Serum Increase* Activity in patients with Crohn's disease increased in 17 of 100 patients *5488*

Basic Fibroblast Growth Factor *Serum No Effect* In 44 children with ulcerative colitis mean concentration of 8.64 ± 1.30 pg/mL not significantly different from 10.72 ± 1.38 pg/mL in 49 control children *546* In 64 children with Crohn's disease mean concentration of 12.72 ± 1.36 pg/mL not significantly different from 10.72 ± 1.38 pg/mL in 49 control children *546*

Bilirubin *Serum Increase* Concentration of greater than 10 x 10^9/L observed in 37% of 100 patients with Crohn's disease *5488* Concentration in patients with Crohn's disease increased in 8 of 100 patients *5488*

C_4b-Binding Protein *Serum Increase* In 54 patients with Crohn's disease mean concentration of 107.3% compared with 88.9% in 30 healthy controls *2*

CA 19-9 *Serum No Effect* In none of 11 patients with Crohn's disease was concentration increased *5406*

CA-M43 *Serum No Effect* In none of 11 patients with Crohn's disease was concentration increased *5406*

Carcinoembryonic Antigen *Serum Increase* In 29 patients with Crohn's disease, 86% had concentrations less than 2.5 ng/mL, 12% had concentrations between 2.6 and 5.0 ng/mL, 2% had concentrations between 5.1 and 10.0 ng/mL and 0% had concentrations greater than 10.0 ng/mL *2010* *Serum No Effect* In none of 11 patients with Crohn's disease was concentration increased *5406*

β-Carotene *Serum No Effect* In 22 to 24 children with Crohn's disease mean concentration of 0.4 ± 0.3 µmol/L not significantly different from 0.4 ± 0.3 µmol/L in 20 to 23 healthy control children *2196*

CD8+ Lymphocytes *Blood No Effect* In 28 patients with Crohn's disease mean proportion of T cells 22.7 ± 2.6% not significantly different from 21.2 ± 0.3% in 22 healthy controls *3753*

Cells *Synovial Fluid Increase* In 1 patient mean concentration of 15,000 /µL *4343*

Cholesterol *Serum Decrease* In 30 patients with Crohn's disease and partial ileal resection mean concentration of 160 mg/dL significantly less than 168 mg/dL in 21 patients with Crohn's disease without ileal resection which was significantly less than 198 mg/dL in 63 healthy controls *359*

Cortisol *Plasma Increase* In 256 patients with Crohn's disease mean concentration about 11.9 µg/dL compared with upper reference limit of 7.2 µg/dL *1861*

C-Reactive Protein *Serum Increase* Positive correlation of r = 0.134 observed with Crohn's disease activity index *4472* In 256 patients with Crohn's disease mean concentration about 5 mg/L *1861* Mean concentration of 5.9 mg/dL in 13 patients with acute Crohn's disease significantly different from 1.9 mg/dL in 17 patients with Crohn's disease in remission and 0.7 mg/dL in 20 healthy controls *4344* In 16 of 54 patients concentration incrased above upper limit of normal although only 12 were identified as having active disease *2* In 31 patients with Dutch activity index of more than 100 mean concentration of 7.0 mg/L compared with < 3 mg/L in 14 patients with Dutch activity index of less than 100 and < 3 mg/L in 20 healthy controls *5388*

D-Dimer *Plasma Increase* In 36 patients with active Crohn's disease median concentration of 331 µg/L (25th and 75th quartiles 248 and 581 respectively) and in 45 patients with moderate Crohn's disease median 204 µg/L (25th and 75th quartiles 169 and 364 respectively) compared with upper limit of normal of < 500 µg/L *4725* In 31 patients with Dutch activity index of more than 100 mean concentration of 500 ng FE/mL compared with < 500 ng FE/mL in 14 patients with Dutch activity index of less than 100 and < 500 ng FE/mL in 20 healthy controls *5388*

β-Endorphin *White Blood Cells Decrease* Concentration decreased in patients with Crohn's disease *633*

Erythrocyte Sedimentation Rate *Blood Increase* Median rate in 68 patients with Crohn's disease of 10 mm/h in 27 with index of activity 0 - 5 and 22 mm/h in 41 with index of activity > 5 *4120* In 22 of 54 patients rate increased above normal whereas only 12 were identified as having active disease *2* In 31 patients with Dutch activity index of more than 100 mean rate 20 mm/h compared with 12 mm/h in 14 patients with Dutch activity index of less than 100 and 7 mm/h in 20 healthy controls *5388* In 1 patient mean rate 32 mm/h *4343*

Factor XIII *Plasma No Effect* In 36 patients with active Crohn's disease median concentration of 97.5% (25th and 75th quartiles 76 and 116 respectively) and in 45 patients with moderate Crohn's disease median concentration of 111% (25th and 75th quartiles 98 and 139 respectively) compared with normal limits of 70 - 140% *4725*

Factor XIII Activity *Plasma Decrease* In 31 patients with Dutch activity index of more than 100 mean concentration of 92% compared with 119% in 14 patients with Dutch activity index of less than 100 and 112% in 20 healthy controls *5388*

Fibrin Degradation Products *Plasma Increase* In 31 patients with Dutch activity index of more than 100, mean concentration of 420 ng FE/mL compared with 320 ng FE/mL in 14 patients with Dutch activity index of less than 100 and 300 ng FE/mL in 20 healthy controls *5388*

Fibrinogen *Plasma Increase* In 36 patients with active Crohn's disease median concentration of 425 mg/dL (25th and 75th quartiles 317 and 603 respectively) and in 45 patients with moderate Crohn's disease median 333 mg/dL (25th and 75th quartiles 290 and 385 respectively) compared with upper limit of normal of < 400 mg/dL *4725* In 31 patients with Dutch activity index of more than 100 mean concentration of 8.2 g/L compared with 3.0 g/L in 14 patients with Dutch activity index of less than 100 and 2.9 g/L in 20 healthy controls *5388*

Fibrinogen Degradation Products *Plasma* *Increase* In 31 patients with Dutch activity index of more than 100 mean concentration of 275 ng FE/mL compared with 170 ng FE/mL in 14 patients with Dutch activity index of less than 100 and 175 ng FE/mL in 20 healthy controls *5388*

β-Galactosidase *Feces* *Decrease* In 8 patients with active Crohn's disease production during incubation significantly reduced compared with healthy individuals, increase unrelated to initial β-D-galactosidase *1436*

γ-Glutamyltransferase *Serum* *Increase* Activity in patients with Crohn's disease increased in 28 of 100 patients *5488*

Glutathione *Blood* *Increase* Mean concentration of 7.4 ± 1.1 µmol/g hemoglobin in 12 children with Crohn's disease significantly different from 6.4 ± 1.0 µmol/g hemoglobin in 12 healthy control children but not different from reference interval of 4.5 - 8.7 µmol/g hemoglobin *2196*

Glutathione Peroxidase *Serum* *Increase* Mean activity of 1,248 ± 499 U/L in 12 children with Crohn's disease significantly different from 763 ± 131 U/L in 20 - 23 healthy control children but not different from reference interval of 603 - 1288 U/L *2196*

HDL-Cholesterol *Serum* *Increase* In 30 patients with Crohn's disease and partial ileal resection mean concentration of 48 mg/dL significantly higher than 41 mg/dL in 63 healthy controls *359*

Hematocrit *Blood* *Decrease* Villous atrophy associated with Crohn's disease may cause absorptive failure leading to low iron concentrations and anemia *5174*

Hemoglobin *Blood* *Decrease* Villous atrophy associated with Crohn's disease may cause absorptive failure leading to low iron concentrations and anemia *5174* Mean concentration of 145 ± 28 g/L in 12 children with Crohn's disease significantly different from 161 ± 14 g/L in 12 healthy control children but not different from reference interval of 120 - 180 g/L *2196* Median concentration in 68 patients with Crohn's disease of 8.3 mmol/L in 27 with index of activity of 0 - 5 and 7.9 mmol/L in 41 with index of activity > 5 *4120* In 36 patients with active Crohn's disease median concentration of 134 g/L (25th and 75th quartiles 125 and 175 respectively) and in 45 patients with moderate Crohn's disease median of 146 g/L (25th and 75th quartiles 135 and 175 respectively) compared with upper limits of normal of 140 g/L in men and 120 g/L in women *4725*
Feces *Increase* Mean concentration in 15 patients with colorectal cancer of 27.0 µg/g (4.60 mg/d) significantly different from 1.5 µg/g (0.15 mg/d) in 20 healthy controls *4521*

IgA Anti-Neutrophil Cytoplasm Antibodies *Serum* *Increase* In 20 children with Crohn's disease 40% had detectable IgA ANCA compared with 11% in control children *2197*

IgA Anti-Saccharomyces cerevisiae Antibodies *Serum* *Increase* In 20 children with Crohn's disease 60% had detectable IgA ASCA compared with 11% in control children *2197*

IgG Anti-Saccharomyces cerevisiae Antibodies *Serum* *Increase* In 20 children with Crohn's disease 60% had detectable IgG ASCA compared with 11% in control children *2197*

Immunoglobulin A *Serum* *Increase* Median concentration in 68 patients with Crohn's disease of 2.32 g/L in 27 with index of activity of 0 - 5 and 2.49 g/L in 41 with index of activity > 5 significantly different from median of 1.71 g/L in healthy adults *4120*

Immunoglobulin G *Serum* *Increase* Median concentration in 68 patients with Crohn's disease of 11.5 g/L in 27 with index of activity of 0 - 5 and 11.5 g/L in 41 with index of activity > 5 significantly different from median of 9.94 g/L in healthy adults *4120*

Immunoglobulin G_1 *Serum* *Decrease* Median concentration in 68 patients with Crohn's disease of 7.4 g/L in 27 with index of activity of 0 - 5 and 6.7 g/L in 41 with index of activity > 5 significantly different from median of 8.01 g/L in healthy adults *4120*

Immunoglobulin G_2 *Serum* *Increase* Median concentration in 68 patients with Crohn's disease of 3.6 g/L in 27 with index of activity of 0 - 5 and 3.8 g/L in 41 with index of activity > 5 significantly different from median of 2.17 g/L in healthy adults *4120*

Immunoglobulin G_3 *Serum* *Decrease* Median concentration in 68 patients with Crohn's disease of 0.45 g/L in 27 with index of activity of 0 - 5 and 0.44 g/L in 41 with index of activity > 5 significantly different from median of 0.94 g/L in healthy adults *4120*

Immunoglobulin G_4 *Serum* *Increase* Median concentration in 68 patients with Crohn's disease of 0.34 g/L in 27 with index of activity of 0 - 5 and 0.29 g/L in 41 with index of activity > 5 significantly different from median of 0.08 g/L in healthy adults *4120*

Immunoglobulin M *Serum* *Decrease* Median concentration in 68 patients with Crohn's disease of 1.25 g/L in 27 with index of activity of 0 - 5 and 1.46 g/L in 41 with index of activity > 5 significantly different from median of 1.56 g/L in healthy adults *4120*

Insulin *Plasma* *No Effect* In 29 children with Crohn's disease in relapse mean concentration (and 95% CI) 9.3 (5.3 - 13.0) mU/L not significantly different from 12.0 (11.0 - 14.0) mU/L in age and sex matched controls *5209*

Insulin-like Growth Factor-I *Serum* *Decrease* Mean (and 95% CI) in 29 children with Crohn's disease in relapse of 0.54 (0.29 - 0.90) U/mL compared with 1.58 (1.11-2.00) U/mL in age and sex matched controls *5209*

Insulin-like Growth Factor Binding Protein-1 *Serum* *No Effect* In 29 children with Crohn's disease in relapse mean concentration (and 95% CI) of 55.0 (41.0-89.4) µg/L compared with 57.0 (42.0-80.0) µg/L in age and sex matched controls *5209*

Interferon-γ *Serum* *Increase* Concentration increased in patients with Crohn's disease especially in those with active or nonresected disease *4583*

Interleukin-1 Receptor Antagonist *Serum* *Increase* In a group of patients with moderate or severe Crohn's disease mean concentration of approximately 1,200 pg/mL significantly higher than 307 ± 27 pg/mL in 24 controls *2310*

Interleukin-1β *Serum* *Increase* Patients with concentrations > 75 pg/mL had shorter time to relapse than patients with lower concentrations *4669*

Interleukin-6 *Serum* *Increase* Detectable concentrations observed in 18 of 21 patients with Crohn's disease (median 47, range < 20 to 250 pg/L) but in only 2 patients with ulcerative colitis and in 2 control individuals *3231* The serum concentration of IL-6 was determined in 70 patients with Crohn's disease (CD). Serum IL-6 concentrations were significantly (p less than 0.005) increased in patients with CD (mean ± SEM, 6.8 ± 0.9 U/mL) compared with patients with UC (mean, less than 4 U/mL) and healthy controls. Of patients with CD, 68.5% had serum IL-6 concentrations of greater than or equal to 4 U/mL, compared with 0% of healthy controls *1885* Serum concentrations of IL-6 were measured in 10 patients with CD before, at day 10 and 2 years after resection of inflamed bowel segments. The corresponding IL-6 serum concentrations were 37 ± 6 U/mL in CD (controls: 11 ± 0.6 U/mL; p less than 0.0036). Serum IL-6, elevated in 7 patients with CD at day 10 postoperatively, had returned to normal in all patients by this time *4685*

Interleukin-8 *Serum* *Increase* Thirty-eight per cent (8/20) of patients with active Crohn's disease had high levels of IL-8 but there was no significant difference between active and inactive disease *2485*

Interleukin-10 *Serum* *Increase* In 18 patients with active disease mean concentration of 132 ± 32 pg/mL significantly higher than 52 ± 17 pg/mL in 22 patients with inactive disease and 44 ± 9.5 pg/mL in 30 healthy controls *2840*

Iron *Serum* *Decrease* Villous atrophy associated with Crohn's disease may cause absorptive failure leading to low iron concentrations and anemia *5174*

Lactate Dehydrogenase *Serum* *No Effect* Activity in patients with Crohn's disease increased in only 1 of 100 patients *5488*

555.90 Crohn's Disease *(continued)*

LDL-Cholesterol *Serum* *Decrease* In 30 patients with Crohn's disease and partial ileal resection mean concentration of 84 mg/dL significantly less than 114 mg/dL in 21 patients with Crohn's disease without ileal resection which was significantly less than 140 mg/dL in 63 healthy controls *359*

Leukocytes *Blood* *Increase* In 36 patients with active Crohn's disease median concentration of 8,100 /µL (25th and 75th quartiles 6,500 and 11,200 respectively) and in 45 patients with moderate Crohn's disease median of 6,900 /µL (25th and 75th quartiles 5,100 and 8,500 respectively) compared with upper limit of normal of 10,500 /µL *4725*

Lysozyme *Serum* *Increase* Activity may be increased in Crohn's disease *2952*
Urine *Increase* Activity may be increased in Crohn's disease *2952*

β_2-Microglobulin *Serum* *No Effect* Mean concentration of 2.70 ± 1.38 mg/dL in 13 patients with acute Crohn's disease not significantly greater than 1.74 ± 1.37 mg/dL in 17 patients with Crohn's disease in remission and 2.50 ± 1.28 mg/dL in 20 healthy controls *4344*

Neopterin *Urine* *Increase* Positive correlation of r = 0.429 observed between neopterin:creatinine ratio and Crohn's disease activity index *4472*

Neutrophil Elastase *Feces* *Increase* Mean concentration in 15 patients with colorectal cancer of 41.5 µg/g (10.24 mg/d) significantly different from 0.6 µg/g (0.11 mg/d) in 20 healthy controls *4521*

Partial Thromboplastin Time *Plasma* *No Effect* In 36 patients with active Crohn's disease median time of 40 s (25th and 75th quartiles of 36 and 43 s respectively) and in 45 patients with moderate Crohn's disease median 38 s (25th and 75th quartiles 34 and 41 s respectively) compared with upper limit of normal of 45 s *4725*

Perinuclear Antineutrophil Cytoplasmic Autoantibodies
Serum *Increase* Detected at a dilution of 1:100 in about 5 - 10% of patients with Crohn's disease *4485*

Phospholipase A_2 *Serum* *Increase* In chronic inflammatory diseases such as Crohn's disease and ulcerative colitis serum concentration of PLA2-II correlates with activity of the disease *3766*

Phospholipase A_2 Type II *Serum* *Increase* Considerable increase in concentration observed correlating well with the activity of the disease *3767*

Plasmin-α_2Antiplasmin Complex *Plasma* *Increase* In 36 patients with active Crohn's disease median concentration of 505 µg/L (25th and 75th quartiles of 334 and 660 respectively) and in 45 patients with moderate Crohn's disease median concentration of 373 µg/L (25th and 75th quartiles 284 and 579 respectively) compared with upper limit of normal of < 400 µg/L *4725*

Plasminogen *Plasma* *No Effect* In 28 patients with Crohn's disease mean concentration of 107 ± 4.9% compared with 109.9 ± 1.1% in 60 healthy blood donor controls *4948*

Plasminogen Activator Inhibitor-1 *Plasma* *Decrease* In 28 patients with Crohn's disease mean concentration significantly decreased to 8.5 ± 1.1 ng/mL compared with 17.8 ± 1.1 ng/mL in 60 healthy blood donor controls *4948*
Plasma *No Effect* In 36 patients with active Crohn's disease median concentration of 2.1 U/mL (25th and 75th quartiles 1.6 and 2.7 respectively) and in 45 patients with moderate Crohn's disease median 2.3 (25th and 75th quartiles 1.6 and 3.5 respectively) compared with upper limit of normal of < 3.5 U/mL *4725*

Platelets *Blood* *Increase* In 36 patients with active Crohn's disease median concentration of 353,000 /µL (25th and 75th quartiles of 292,000 and 420,000 respectively) and in 45 patients with moderate Crohn's disease median of 266,000 /µL (25th and 75th quartiles of 241,000 and 343,000 respectively) compared with upper limit of normal of 350,000 /µL *4725*

Protein C *Plasma* *No Effect* Mean concentration of 105.2% in 54 patients with Crohn's disease not significantly different from 101.7% in 30 healthy controls *2*

Protein S, Free *Plasma* *Decrease* In 31 of 54 patients with Crohn's disease mean concentration below normal lower limit of 70%: mean in all patients with Crohn's disease of 72.2% compared with 97.5% in 30 healthy controls *2*

Prothrombin Fragment 1.2 *Plasma* *Increase* In 36 patients with active Crohn's disease median concentration of 0.7 nmol/L (25th and 75th quartiles 0.5 and 1.2 respectively) and in 45 patients with moderate Crohn's disease median of 0.8 nmol/L (25th and 75th quartiles 0.6 and 1.0 respectively) compared with upper limit of normal of < 1.1 nmol/L *4725*

Pyridinoline *Synovial Fluid* *Increase* In 1 patient mean concentration of 13.8 pmol/mL *4343*

Retinol *Serum* *Increase* Mean concentration of 1.80 ± 0.67 µmol/L in 12 children with Crohn's disease significantly different from 1.60 ± 0.31 µmol/L in 12 healthy control children but not different from reference interval of 0.66 - 2.69 µmol/L *2196*
Serum *No Effect* In 22 to 24 children with Crohn's disease mean concentration of 1.55 ± 0.57 µmol/L not significantly different from 1.60 ± 0.31 µmol/L in 20 to 23 healthy control children *2196*

Retinol-binding Protein *Serum* *No Effect* Mean concentration of 39 ± 15 mg/L in 12 children with Crohn's disease not significantly different from 36 ± 10 mg/L in 12 healthy control children and reference interval of 30 - 60 mg/L *2196*

Selenium *Serum* *No Effect* Mean concentration of 1.7 ± 0.4 µmol/L in 12 children with Crohn's disease not significantly different from 1.5 ± 0.2 µmol/L in 12 healthy control children and reference interval of 1.28 - 2.35 µmol/L *2196*

Sialic Acid *Serum* *Increase* Mean concentration of 116.3 ± 34.2 mg/dL in 13 patients with acute Crohn's disease significantly greater than 55.7 ± 17.8 mg/dL in 17 patients with ulcerative colitis in remission and 64.7 ± 3.2 mg/dL in 20 healthy controls *4344*

Soluble CD44 Splice Variant 6 *Serum* *No Effect* Median concentration in 20 patients with Crohn's disease of 219 ng/mL not significantly different from that in 20 healthy donors of 221 ng/mL *4317*

Soluble Intercellular Adhesion Molecule-1 *Serum* *Increase* Median concentration of 365 ng/mL in 31 patients with active Crohn's disease significantly higher than 245 ng/mL in 29 healthy controls *3783*

Soluble Interleukin-2 Receptor *Serum* *Increase* Serum concentrations of the soluble IL-2 receptor (sIL-2R) measured in 10 patients with CD before, at day 10, and 2 years after resection of inflamed bowel segments. Preoperatively, mean sIL-2R concentration was 495 ± 62 U/mL (mean ± SEM; healthy controls; 210 ± 25 U/mL; p < 0.02) in CD. Two years postoperatively, sIL-2R was still elevated in 6 out of 9 patients in both disease groups. These patients did not differ from the remaining group with respect to disease activity *4685*

Thrombin/Antithrombin III Complex *Plasma* *No Effect* In 36 patients with active Crohn's disease median concentration of 2.5 µg/L (25th and 75th quartiles 2.0 and 3.5 respectively) and in 45 patients with moderate Crohn's disease median concentration of 2.3 µg/L (25th and 75th quartiles 2.0 and 2.5 respectively) compared with upper limit of normal of < 4.0 µg/L *4725*

Tissue Plasminogen Activator *Plasma* *No Effect* In 28 patients with Crohn's disease mean concentration of 4.95 ± 0.54 ng/mL compared with 5.13 ± 0.4 ng/mL in 60 healthy blood donor controls *4948*

Tissue Transglutaminase Antibodies *Serum* *Increase* Antibodies observed in most of specimens positive for endomysium antibodies from patients with Crohn's disease *109*

α-Tocopherol *Serum* *Increase* Mean concentration of 26 ± 4 µmol/L in 12 children with Crohn's disease significantly different from 20 ± 4 µmol/L in 12 healthy control children but not different from reference interval of 9 - 47 µmol/L *2196*

γ-Tocopherol *Serum* *No Effect* In 22 to 24 children with Crohn's disease mean concentration of 6 ± 3 µmol/L not significantly different from 5 ± 2 µmol/L in 20 to 23 healthy control children *2196* Mean concentration of 7 ± 3 µmol/L in 22 - 24 children with Crohn's disease not significantly different from 5 ± 2 µmol/L in 12 healthy control children *2196*

α-Tocopherol:Lipids Ratio *Serum* *Increase* Mean concentration of 418 ± 139 µmol/g in 12 children with Crohn's disease not significantly different from 325 ± 46 µmol/g in 12 healthy control children but not different from reference interval of > 186 µmol/g *2196* In 22 to 24 children with Crohn's disease mean concentration of 395 ± 163 µmol/g significantly different from 325 ± 46 µmol/g in 20 to 23 healthy control children *2196*

Triglycerides *Serum* *Increase* In 30 patients with Crohn's disease and partial ileal resection mean concentration of 138 mg/dL significantly higher than 98 mg/dL in 63 healthy controls *359*

Tumor Necrosis Factor-α *Serum* *Increase* Concentration increased in most patients *3180* Patients with concentrations > 70 pg/mL had considerable risk of relapsing *4669*

Urokinase Plasminogen Activator *Plasma* *Decrease* In 28 patients with Crohn's disease mean concentration of 0.38 ± 0.03 ng/mL significantly reduced compared with 0.47 ± 0.014 ng/mL in 60 healthy blood donor controls *4948*

Vitamin A *Serum* *Decrease* Concentration reduced in 54 patients in relation to activity of the disease *4656*

Zinc *Lymphocytes* *Decrease* In one study mean concentration was decreased *3697*
Lymphocytes *No Effect* In two studies mean concentration was unchanged *3697*
Monocytes *Decrease* In one study mean concentration was decreased *3697*
Neutrophils *No Effect* In three studies in polymophonuclear cells mean concentration was unchanged *3697*
Red Blood Cells *Decrease* In two studies mean concentration was decreased *3697*
Red Blood Cells *No Effect* In two studies mean concentration was unchanged *3697*
Serum *Decrease* In patients with Crohn's disease concentration is typically reduced *2952* Villous atrophy associated with Crohn's disease may cause absorptive failure leading to low zinc concentrations *5174* In 54 patients with Crohn's disease concentration reduced in relation to activity of disease *4656* In 20 studies mean concentration was reduced to about 80% of that in healthy controls *3697*
White Blood Cells *No Effect* In two studies mean concentration was unchanged *3697*

555.90 Regional Enteritis or Ileitis

α_1-Acid Glycoprotein *Serum* *Increase* One of the most reliable indicators of acute inflammation *4241* *3713* *4373* *4853* *2597* *4696*

Alanine Aminotransferase *Serum* *Increase* Liver abnormalities are common *2034*

Albumin *Serum* *Decrease* A reasonably accurate indication of the patient's overall condition *4891* Occurs frequently and is probably due largely to the leakage of protein from the diseased gut *5540* In 32 patients, 13 fell into a distinct group of low tryptophan serum concentrations. Patients in this group ate less, had lower albumin levels and greater intestinal protein loss than normal tryptophan patients *365*

Alkaline Phosphatase *Serum* *Increase* Indicates hepatic involvement *900* Frequently abnormal in patients who otherwise show no indication of liver disease *4891*
White Blood Cells *Increase* Markedly increased *2750*

Angiotensin-converting Enzyme *Serum* *Decrease* Significantly depressed compared with normal controls and those with inactive disease *1213*
Serum *No Effect* Wide variation observed *1213* No significant difference was noted between active Crohn's, inactive Crohn's, and normal controls. However, patients who had active disease and were receiving steroid therapy had significantly lower levels *3840*

Antibody Titer *Serum* *Increase* Antibodies to reticulin *3712*

α_1-Antichymotrypsin *Serum* *Increase* Serum concentrations were associated with increasing severity *5608*

Aspartate Aminotransferase *Serum* *Increase* Liver abnormalities are common *2034* Due to associated liver disease *465*

Bile Acids *Serum* *Decrease* In patients with Crohn's disease whether resected or not the postprandial level of bile acids is low *2137*

Bilirubin *Serum* *Increase* Due to associated liver disease *465*

Calcium *Urine* *Increase* High levels may be found *581*

Carcinoembryonic Antigen *Serum* *Increase* 14% of 58 patients had positive assay. There was no correlation between CEA concentration and extent or activity of disease, but those with elevated levels all had the disease for > 7 y, mean = 18.1 y duration *528* 40% of patients had values > 2.5 ng/mL *4891* In 97 patients with regional ileitis 60% had concentrations less than 2.5 ng/mL, 27% had concentrations between 2.6 and 5.0 ng/mL, 11% had concentrations between 5.1 and 10.0 ng/mL and 2% had concentrations greater than 10.0 ng/mL *2010*

Carotene *Serum* *Decrease* With malabsorption *4891*

Chenodeoxycholic Acid *Serum* *No Effect* Fasting values were in the normal range but postprandial increase was lower than in healthy controls *2137*

Cholic Acid *Serum* *No Effect* Fasting values were in the normal range but postprandial increase was lower than in healthy controls *2137*

Erythrocyte Sedimentation Rate *Blood* *Increase* Tend to suggest that the inflammatory process is active *4891* Elevation takes place during acute exacerbations *900*

Fat *Feces* *Increase* Deficient intraluminal bile acids *4891*

Folate *Serum* *Decrease* Decreased with extensive skin disease *5230* Deficiency may result in anemia *1098* Decreased with extensive skin disease *772* *602*

γ-Globulin *Serum* *Decrease* May be elevated in some patients but are normal or low in others *4891*
Serum *Increase* May be elevated in some patients but are normal or low in others *4891*
Serum *No Effect* May be elevated in some patients but are normal or low in others *4891*

γ-Glutamyltransferase *Serum* *Increase* Observed in some patients *1290* In the presence of pericholangitis *4891*

Haptoglobin *Serum* *Increase* Haptoglobin concentrations rise with increasing clinical activity of the disease, while the prealbumin fraction declines *3303* Reported effect *4551*

Hematocrit *Blood* *Decrease* Frequently moderate anemia, most often iron deficiency, but occasionally macrocytic caused by poor diet or failure to absorb vitamin B_{12} normally *4891* Anemia in approximately 70% of cases *4551* Iron deficiency is common *1980* Anemia when present can be a result of iron loss or of reduced absorption of vitamin B_{12} *900*

Hemoglobin *Blood* *Decrease* Frequently moderate anemia, most often iron deficiency, but occasionally macrocytic caused by poor diet or failure to absorb vitamin B_{12} normally *4891* Anemia when present can be a result of iron loss or of reduced absorption of vitamin B_{12} *900* Iron deficiency is common *1980* Anemia in approximately 70% of cases *4551*

HLA Antigens *Blood* *Present* If associated arthritis HLA-B_27 found more frequently than control group *5428*

immunoglobulin A *Serum* *Increase* Reported effect *1290*

Immunoglobulins *Serum* *No Effect* Conentrations of all commonly measured immunoglobulins usually normal *4551* Patterns vary widely within a given patient, and most workers report no consistent deviations in the mean levels of the major Ig classes (including IgE) in sera of patients compared with healthy controls *2807*

Iron *Bone Marrow* *Decrease* As a result of chronic blood loss *4891* Iron deficiency defined by the absence of marrow hemosiderin was found with anemia in 36% of 41 patients with ulcerative colitis, and 22% of 64 with Crohn's disease. An additional 32% and 2%, respectively, had iron deficiency with normal erythropoiesis *5218*
Serum *Decrease* As a result of chronic blood loss *4891* Iron deficiency is common *1980* Iron deficiency anemia was found in 36% of 41 patients with ulcerative colitis, and 22% of 64 patients with Crohn's disease. An additional 32% and 2%, respectively, had iron deficiency with normal erythropoiesis *5218*

Iron-binding Capacity, Total *Serum* *Increase* Frequent iron deficiency anemia. Severity depends upon rate and duration of bleeding *4891*

Iron Saturation *Serum* *Decrease* Frequent iron deficiency anemia. Severity depends upon rate and duration of bleeding *4891*

Lactate Dehydrogenase *Serum* *Increase* Liver abnormalities are common *2034*

Leukocytes *Blood* *Increase* Leukocytosis (usually mild) *4551* Tend to suggest that the inflammatory process is active *4891* Elevation takes place during acute exacerbations *900*
Feces *Increase* Large numbers *4891*

Lysozyme *Serum* *Increase* Particularly when the inflammatory process is active *1411* *4891*

555.90 Regional Enteritis or Ileitis (continued)

Magnesium *Serum* *Decrease* Common feature of severe colitis *4551*

MCH *Blood* *Decrease* Frequently moderate anemia, most often iron deficiency, but occasionally macrocytic caused by poor diet or failure to absorb vitamin B_{12} normally *4891*

MCHC *Blood* *Decrease* Frequently moderate anemia, most often iron deficiency, but occasionally macrocytic caused by poor diet or failure to absorb vitamin B_{12} normally *4891*

MCV *Blood* *Decrease* As a result of chronic blood loss *4891*
Blood *Increase* Macrocytic, megaloblastic anemia may indicate folic acid or vitamin B_{12} deficiency *4891* Macrocytic anemia may occur due to vitamin B_{12} or folate deficiency. MCV > 100 fL *1098*

Monocytes *Blood* *Increase* Relative lymphocytopenia may occur as a result of absolute increase in monocytes and polymorphonuclear cells *5205*

Neutrophils *Blood* *Increase* Relative lymphocytopenia may occur as a result of absolute increase in monocytes and polymorphonuclear cells *5205* Count increases with increasing disease activity *2550*

Occult Blood *Feces* *Increase* Stools are not grossly bloody, insidious blood loss with guaiac positive stools is the rule *1980* Observed in some patients *2039* Chronic blood loss *4891*

Oxalate *Urine* *Increase* Due to associated liver disease *465*

Platelets *Blood* *Increase* May be present *4891*

Potassium *Serum* *Decrease* Common feature of severe colitis *4551*

Prealbumin *Serum* *Decrease* Haptoglobin concentrations rise with increasing clinical activity of the disease, while the prealbumin fraction declines *3303*

Protein *Serum* *Decrease* Often present; due in some part to diminished intake, but mainly result from excessive enteric protein loss *4891*

Sodium *Serum* *Decrease* Common feature of severe colitis *4551*

Thyroxine Binding Globulin *Serum* *Increase* Mean levels were high in these patients, mainly due to the high levels in female patients *2420*

Tri-iodothyronine (T3) *Serum* *Increase* The concentration was lower in severely ill patients than in those who were mildly-moderately ill, while T4 and TBG were not affected by the severity of the disease *2420*

Tryptophan *Plasma* *Decrease* In 32 patients, 13 fell into a distinct group of low tryptophan serum concentrations. Patients in this group ate less, had low albumin levels and greater intestinal protein loss than normal tryptophan patients *365*

Uric Acid *Urine* *Increase* High levels may be found *581*

Vitamin B_{12} *Serum* *Decrease* Frequently moderate anemia, most often iron deficiency, but occasionally macrocytic caused by poor diet or failure to absorb vitamin B_{12} normally *4891* Tests may be abnormal *367*

Xylose Tolerance Test *Urine* *No Effect* Typical observation *5544*

Zinc *Serum* *Decrease* In patients with regional enteritis concentration is typically reduced *2952*

556.90 Ulcerative Colitis

α_1-Acid Glycoprotein *Serum* *Increase* Mean concentration of 302 mg/dL in 9 patients with acute ulcerative colitis significantly greater than 103 mg/dL in 14 patients with ulcerative colitis in remission and 119 mg/dL in 20 healthy controls *4344* Median concentration in 66 patients with ulcerative colitis 16 µmol/L in 24 with index of activity 0 - 1 and 29 µmol/L in 42 with index of activity 2 - 3 *4120*

Alanine Aminotransferase *Serum* *Increase* With liver involvement *900*

Albumin *Serum* *Decrease* Portends a worse prognosis, probably because the degree of abnormality parallels clinical severity *4891* Deficiency may result in anemia *1098* Occurs frequently and is probably due largely to the leakage of protein from the diseased gut *5540*
Serum *No Effect* Median concentration in 66 patients with ulcerative colitis 45 g/L in 24 with index of activity 0 - 1 and 41 g/L in 42 with index of activity 2 - 3 *4120*

Alkaline Phosphatase *Serum* *Increase* Often increased slightly *5544*
White Blood Cells *Increase* Markedly increased *2750*

Angiotensin-converting Enzyme *Serum* *No Effect* Similar levels as controls *1213*

Anti-Endothelial Cell Antibodies *Serum* *Increase* levels were elevated in ulcerative colitis ($p < 0.0001$) and Crohn's disease ($p < 0.05$) compared with healthy controls *5012*

Anti-Neutrophil Cytoplasm Antibodies *Serum* *Increase* ANCA were found in 26 IBD sera (25%) and in none of 51 controls. Twenty-two positive sera (85%) were from patients with ulcerative colitis (UC). The pattern of distribution of immunofluorescence was always perinuclear (P-ANCA) *4413* 16 of 21 patients (76%) with ulcerative colitis had positive results *2021* Observed in some patients with ulcerative colitis *4923*

Anti-Saccharomyces cerevisiae Antibodies *Serum* *Increase* Detected in about 10 - 15% of patients with ulcerative colitis *4485*

α_1-Antichymotrypsin *Serum* *Increase* Serum concentrations were associated with increasing severity *5608*

α_2-Antiplasmin *Plasma* *Increase* In 9 patients with severe disease mean concentration of 800 µg/L compared with 530 µg/L in 19 patients with mild disease, 995 µg/L in 15 in remission and 335 µg/L in 20 healthy controls *5388*
Plasma *No Effect* In 84 patients with ulcerative colitis mean concentration of 92 ± 1.05% compared with 93 ± 0.9% in 60 healthy blood donor controls *4948*

α_1-Antitrypsin *Feces* *Increase* Mean concentration in 27 patients with ulcerative colitis of 1,465.2 µg/g (278.50 mg/d) not significantly different from 327.4 µg/g (47.43 mg/d) in 20 healthy controls *4521*
Serum *Increase* Increased compared to control subjects. There was a correlation between the level and disease activity *446*

Ascorbic Acid *Serum* *Decrease* Mean concentration of 295 ± 136 µmol/L in 7 children with ulcerative colitis not significantly different from 420 ± 114 µmol/L in 12 healthy control children *2196*
Serum *No Effect* In 7 children with ulcerative colitis mean concentration of 295 ± 136 µmol/L not significantly different from 420 ± 114µmol/L in 12 healthy control children *2196*

Aspartate Aminotransferase *Serum* *Increase* With liver involvement *900*

CA 19-9 *Serum* *Increase* In 3 of 17 patients with ulcerative colitis concentrations increased (74.0, 41.0, and 43.0 U/mL) above cutoff limit *5406*

CA-M43 *Serum* *Increase* In one of 17 patients concentration increased to 7.6 U/mL just above cutoff of 7.5 U/mL *5406*

Calcium *Serum* *Decrease* Usually deficient *2034*
Urine *Increase* High levels may be found *581*

Carbon Dioxide *Feces* *No Effect* In 25 patients with ulcerative colitis mean production of carbon dioxide of 0.95 ± 0.27 mL/g dry weight after 1 hour and 17.29 ± 2.27 mL/g dry weight after 4 hours not significantly different from 0.32 ± 0.11 mL/g dry weight after 1 hour and 14.91 ± 1.38 mL/g dry weight in 17 controls *3011*

Carcinoembryonic Antigen *Serum* *Increase* Increase observed in almost 20% patients *1601* Elevated in as many as 27% of patients *4477* Serial measurements done of 57 patients yield significant correlations between peak CEA concentration and disease severity and extent of colonic involvement *1653* In 146 patients with ulcerative colitis 69% had concentrations less than 2.5 ng/mL, 18% had concentrations between 2.6 and 5.0 ng/mL, 8% had concentrations between 5.1 and 10.0 ng/mL and 5% had concentrations greater than 10.0 ng/mL *2010* In 46 patients with ulcerative colitis 84.8% had concentrations up to 3.0 ng/mL, 10.9% had concentrations between 3.1 - 5.0 ng/mL and 4.3% between 5.1 - 10.0 ng/mL in contrast to concentrations in 151 healthy nonsmokers in whom 95.4% had concentrations between 0 and 3.0 ng/mL and 4.6% between 4.1 and 10.0 ng/mL *11* Increase observed in almost 20% patients *4551* Increase occurs in about 20% patients *4891* 11% of 61 patients had positive assays. There was no correlation between CEA and length of history, degree of activity, or extent of colonic involvement *528*

Serum *No Effect* In none of 17 patients with ulcerative colitis was the concentration increased *5406*

β-Carotene *Serum* *No Effect* Mean concentration of 0.4 ± 0.4 μmol/L in 10 - 12 children with ulcerative colitis not significantly different from 0.4 ± 0.2 μmol/L in 20 - 23 healthy control children and reference interval of 0.1 - 1.6 μmol/L *2196* In 10 to 12 children with ulcerative colitis mean concentration of 0.4 ± 0.4 μmol/L not significantly different from 0.4 ± 0.2 μmol/L in 20 to 23 healthy control children *2196*

Catecholamines *Plasma* *Increase* Circulating levels *2034*
Urine *Increase* Circulating levels *2034*

CD4+ Lymphocytes *Blood* *No Effect* In 15 patients with ulcerative colitis mean proportion of T cells of 44.1 ± 4.2% not significantly different from 43.1 ± 2.6% in 22 healthy controls *3753*

CD8+ Lymphocytes *Blood* *No Effect* In 15 patients with ulcerative colitis mean proportion of T cells 21.2 ± 2.5% not significantly different from 21.2 ± 0.3% in 22 healthy controls *3753*

Cholesterol *Feces* *Increase* The fecal excretion of cholesterol, coprostanol, and cholestane-38 beta, 5 alpha, 6 β-triol was higher in these patients than in other control and patient groups *4299*

Complement, Total *Serum* *Increase* Mean titer increased in 16 patients *1516*

Coombs' Test *Serum* *Positive* Has been described *4891*

Copper *Serum* *Increase* In 8 patients with moderate clinical activity median concentration of 137 μg/dL not significantly different from 113 μg/dL in 10 healthy controls *5059*

C-Reactive Protein *Serum* *Increase* In 9 patients with severe disease mean concentration of 35 mg/L compared with 3 mg/L in 19 patients with mild disease, < 3 mg/L in 15 in remission and < 3 mg/L in 20 healthy controls *5388*
Serum *No Effect* Mean concentration of 0.7 mg/dL in 9 patients with acute ulcerative colitis and 0.6 mg/dL in 14 patients with ulcerative colitis in remission not significantly different from 0.7 mg/dL in 20 healthy controls *4344*

D-Dimer *Plasma* *Increase* In 9 patients with severe disease mean concentration of 1,000 ng FE/mL compared with 500 ng FE/mL in 19 patients with mild disease, < 500 ng FE/mL in 15 in remission and in 20 healthy controls *5388*

Erythrocyte Sedimentation Rate *Blood* *Increase* In 9 patients with severe disease mean rate of 26 mm/h compared with 12 mm/h in 19 patients with mild disease, 15 mm/h in 15 in remission and 7 mm/h in 20 healthy controls *5388* Often normal or only slightly increased *5544*
Blood *No Effect* Median concentration in 66 patients with ulcerative colitis 5 mm/h in 24 with index of activity 0 - 1 and 10 mm/h in 42 with index of activity 2 - 3 *4120*

Factor XIII Activity *Plasma* *Decrease* In 9 patients with severe disease mean concentration of 63% compared with 114% in 19 patients with mild disease, 105% in 15 in remission and 109% in 20 healthy controls *5388*

Fibrin Degradation Products *Plasma* *Increase* In 9 patients with severe disease mean concentration of 1,000 ng FE/mL compared with 460 ng FE/mL in 19 patients with mild disease, 532 ng FE/mL in 15 in remission and 300 ng FE/mL in 20 healthy controls *5388*

Fibrinogen *Plasma* *Increase* In 9 patients with severe disease mean concentration of 4.2 g/L compared with 3.3 g/L in 19 patients with mild disease, 3.1 g/L in 15 in remission and 2.9 g/L in 20 healthy controls *5388*

Fibrinogen Degradation Products *Plasma* *Increase* In 9 patients with severe disease mean concentration of 310 ng FE/mL compared with 230 ng FE/mL in 19 patients with mild disease, 225 ng FE/mL in 15 in remission and 175 ng FE/mL in 20 healthy controls *5388*

Folate *Serum* *Decrease* May be the cause of anemia *900*

α_1-Globulin *Serum* *Increase* Serum orosomucoid was well correlated with clinical activity, intestinal protein loss, serum albumin, fractional catabolic rates of albumin, and IgG synthesis rate *2439*

α_2-Globulin *Serum* *Increase* May be increased *5544*

γ-Glutamyltransferase *Serum* *Increase* Observed in some patients *900* Increased with associated liver damage and correlates with other liver enzymes *1290*

Glutathione *Blood* *No Effect* Mean concentration of 7.1 ± 1.4 μmol/g hemoglobin in 10 - 12 children with ulcerative colitis not significantly different from 6.4 ± 1.0 μmol/g hemoglobin in 20 - 23 healthy control children and reference interval of 4.5 - 8.7 μmol/g hemoglobin *2196*

Glutathione Peroxidase *Serum* *Decrease* In 8 patients with moderate clinical activity median activity of 339 U/L significantly different from 396 U/L in 10 healthy controls *5059*
Serum *No Effect* Mean activity of 973 ± 233 U/L in 10 - 12 children with ulcerative colitis not significantly different from 763 ± 131 U/L in 20 - 23 healthy control children and reference interval of 603 - 1,288 U/L *2196*

Haptoglobin *Serum* *Increase* Reported effect *4551* Haptoglobin concentrations rise with increasing clinical activity of the disease, while the prealbumin fraction declines *3303*

Hematocrit *Blood* *Decrease* Anemia secondary to colonic blood loss. Severity varies, depending on the rate and duration of bleeding *4891* Anemia may be due to blood loss, simple iron deficiency, deficiencies in folic acid, pyridoxine, or vitamin B_{12} *900* Anemia in approximately 70% of cases *4551*

Hemoglobin *Blood* *Decrease* Anemia secondary to colonic blood loss. Severity varies, depending on the rate and duration of bleeding *4891* Anemia in approximately 70% of cases *4551* Median concentration in 66 patients with ulcerative colitis of 8.2 mmol/L in 24 with index of activity 0 - 1 and 8.2 mmol/L in 42 with index of activity 2 - 3 *4120* Anemia may be due to blood loss, simple iron deficiency, deficiencies in folic acid, pyridoxine, or vitamin B_{12} (frequently 6 g/dL) *5544*
Blood *No Effect* Mean concentration of 147 ± 18 g/L in 10 - 12 children with ulcerative colitis not significantly different from 161 ± 14 g/L in 20 - 23 healthy control children and reference interval of 120 - 180 g/L *2196*
Feces *Increase* Mean concentration in 27 patients with colorectal cancer of 824.7 μg/g (206.19 mg/d) significantly different from 1.5 μg/g (0.15 mg/d) in 20 healthy controls *4521*

HLA Antigens *Blood* *Present* If associated arthritis HLA-B_27 found more frequently than control group *5428*

Hydrogen *Feces* *No Effect* In 25 patients with ulcerative colitis mean production of hydrogen of 0.0083 ± 0.0039 mL/g dry weight after 1 hour and 0.29 ± 0.067 mL/g dry weight after 4 hours not significantly different from 0.0092 ± 0.0023 mL/g dry weight after 1 hour and 0.20 ± 0.064 mL/g dry weight in 17 controls *3011*

Hydrogen Sulfide *Feces* *Increase* In 25 patients with ulcerative colitis mean production of hydrogen sulfide of 0.041 ± 0.025 mL/g dry weight after 1 hour and 0.27 ± 0.054 mL/g dry weight after 4 hours significantly different from 0.0069 ± 0.0013 mL/g dry weight after 1 hour and 0.095 ± 0.014 mL/g dry weight in 17 controls *3011*

IgA Anti-Neutrophil Cytoplasm Antibodies *Serum* *Increase* In 25 children with ulcerative colitis 80% had detectable IgA ANCA compared with 11% in control children *2197*

IgA Anti-Saccharomyces cerevisiae Antibodies *Serum* *Increase* In 25 children with ulcerative colitis 12% had detectable IgA ASCA compared with 4% in control children *2197*

IgG Anti-Saccharomyces cerevisiae Antibodies *Serum* *Increase* In 25 children with ulcerative colitis 12% had detectable IgG ASCA compared with 4% in control children *2197*

Immunoglobulin A *Serum* *Increase* Median concentration in patients with ulcerative colitis of 2.74 g/L in 24 with index of activity 0 - 1 and 2.03 g/L in 42 with index of activity 2 - 3 significantly different from median of 1.71 g/L in healthy adults *4120* In 19 men with ulcerative colitis mean concentration of 261 ± 105 mg/dL significantly different from 201 ± 89 mg/dL in 106 healthy control men *2278*
Serum *No Effect* In 11 women with ulcerative colitis mean concentration of 173 ± 97 mg/dL not significantly different from 174 ± 80 mg/dL in 150 healthy control women *2278*

Immunoglobulin G *Serum* *Increase* In 19 men with ulcerative colitis mean concentration of 1,285 ± 299 mg/dL significantly different from 1,148 ± 224 mg/dL in 106 healthy controls *2278* Median concentration in patients with ulcerative colitis of 12.8 g/L in 24 with index of activity 0 - 1 and 10.7 g/L in 42 with index of activity 2 - 3 significantly different from median of 9.94 g/L in healthy adults *4120*
Serum *No Effect* In 11 women with ulcerative colitis mean concentration of 1,299 ± 284 mg/dL not significantly different from 1,157 ± 271 mg/dL in 150 healthy control women *2278*

556.90 Ulcerative Colitis (continued)

Immunoglobulin G_1 *Serum No Effect* Median concentration in 66 patients with ulcerative colitis of 7.4 g/L in 24 with index of disease activity of 0 - 1 and 8.1 g/L in 42 with index of disease activity 2 - 3 not significantly different from median of 8.01 g/L in healthy adults *4120*

Immunoglobulin G_2 *Serum Increase* Median concentration in 66 patients with ulcerative colitis of 3.2 g/L in 24 with 0 - 1 index of disease activity and 3.1 g/L in 42 with index of activity 2 - 3 significantly different from median of 2.17 g/L in healthy adults *4120*

Immunoglobulin G_3 *Serum Decrease* Median concentration in patients with ulcerative colitis of 0.52 g/L in 24 with index of activity 0 - 1 and 0.47 g/L in 42 with index of activity 2 - 3 significantly different from median of 0.94 g/L in healthy adults *4120*

Immunoglobulin G_4 *Serum Increase* Median concentration in patients with ulcerative colitis of 0.38 g/L in 24 with index of activity 0 - 1 and 0.37 g/L in 42 with index of activity 2 - 3 significantly different from median of 0.08 g/L in healthy adults *4120*

Immunoglobulin M *Serum No Effect* Median concentration in patients with ulcerative colitis of 1.66 g/L in 24 with index of activity 0 - 1 and 1.40 g/L in 42 with index of activity 2 - 3 not significantly different from median of 1.56 g/L in healthy adults *4120* In 19 men with ulcerative colitis mean concentration of 54 ± 19 mg/dL not significantly different from 61 ± 36 mg/dL in 106 healthy controls and in 11 women with ulcerative colitis mean concentration of 64 ± 28 mg/dL not significantly different from 77 ± 39 mg/dL in 150 healthy control women *2278*

Immunoglobulins *Serum No Effect* Patterns vary widely within a given patient, and most workers report no consistent deviations in the mean levels of the major Ig classes (including IgE) in sera of patients compared with healthy controls *2807* Concentrations usually normal *4551*

Interleukin-1 Receptor Antagonist *Serum Increase* In a group of patients with moderate or severe ulcerative colitis mean concentration approximately 1,300 pg/mL significantly higher than 307 ± 27 pg/mL in 24 controls *2310*

Interleukin-6 *Serum Increase* Serum concentrations of IL-6 were measured in 10 patients with UC before, at day 10 and 2 years after resection of inflamed bowel segments. The IL-6 serum concentrations were 33 ± 6 U/mL in UC. Serum IL-6, elevated in 6 patients with UC at day 10 postoperatively, had returned to normal in all patients by this time *4685* The serum concentration of IL-6 was determined in 23 patients with ulcerative colitis (UC). Of patients with UC, 21.7% had serum IL-6 concentrations of greater than or equal to 4 U/mL, compared with 0% of healthy controls *1885*
Serum No Effect In only 2 of 20 patients with ulcerative colitis was interleukin-6 detectable in serum *3231*

Interleukin-10 *Serum Increase* In 20 patients with active disease mean concentration of 144 ± 34 pg/mL significantly higher than 73 ± 19 pg/mL in 24 patients with inactive disease and 44 ± 9.5 pg/mL in 30 healthy controls *2840*

Iron *Bone Marrow Decrease* Iron deficiency defined by the absence of marrow hemosiderin was found with anemia in 36% of 41 patients. An additional 32% had iron deficiency with normal erythropoiesis *5218*
Serum Decrease Commonly iron deficient *4891* In 8 patients with moderate clinical activity median concentration of 64 µg/dL significantly different from 118 µg/dL in 10 healthy controls *5059* Iron deficiency defined by the absence of marrow hemosiderin was found with anemia in 36% of 41 patients. An additional 32% had iron deficiency with normal erythropoiesis *5218*

Iron-binding Capacity, Total *Serum Increase* Frequent iron deficiency anemia. Severity depends upon rate and duration of bleeding *4891*

Iron Saturation *Serum Decrease* Frequent iron deficiency anemia. Severity depends upon rate and duration of bleeding *4891*

Isocitrate Dehydrogenase *Serum No Effect* Activity unaffected *5008*

Lactate Dehydrogenase *Serum Increase* With liver involvement *900*

Leukocytes *Blood Increase* Leukocytosis (usually mild) *4551* Commonly associated with the more severe varieties. May be marked, with total counts as high as 40,000 - 50,000 /µL *4891*
Blood No Effect Usually normal unless complication occurs (e.g., abscess) *5544*

Lysozyme *Serum Increase* Increased in severely affected cases *2750*

Magnesium *Serum Decrease* Common feature of severe colitis *4551*

MCH *Blood Decrease* Anemia in approximately 70% of cases *4551* Anemia secondary to colonic blood loss. Severity varies, depending on the rate and duration of bleeding *4891*

MCHC *Blood Decrease* Anemia secondary to colonic blood loss. Severity varies, depending on the rate and duration of bleeding *4891* Anemia in approximately 70% of cases *4551*

MCV *Blood Decrease* Anemia in approximately 70% of cases *4551* Anemia secondary to colonic blood loss. Severity varies, depending on the rate and duration of bleeding *4891*

Methane *Feces No Effect* In 25 patients with ulcerative colitis mean production of methane of 0.013 ± 0.0042 mL/g dry weight after 1 hour and 0.44 ± 0.17 mL/g dry weight after 4 hours not significantly different from 0.017 ± 0.0077 mL/g dry weight after 1 hour and 0.56 ± 0.26 mL/g dry weight in 17 controls *3011*

Methanethiol *Feces No Effect* In 25 patients with ulcerative colitis mean production of methanethiol of 0.013 ± 0.0065 mL/g dry weight after 1 hour and 0.12 ± 0.024 mL/g dry weight after 4 hours not significantly different from 0.0055 ± 0.0013 mL/g dry weight after 1 hour and 0.10 ± 0.016 mL/g dry weight in 17 controls *3011*

β_2-Microglobulin *Serum No Effect* Mean concentration of 2.48 ± 0.51 mg/dL in 9 patients with acute ulcerative colitis not significantly greater than 1.72 ± 0.49 mg/dL in 14 patients with ulcerative colitis in remission and 2.50 ± 1.28 mg/dL in 20 healthy controls *4344*

Monocytes *Blood Increase* Relative lymphocytopenia may occur as a result of absolute increase in monocytes and polymorphonuclear cells *5205*

Neutral Sterols *Feces Increase* The fecal excretion of cholesterol, coprostanol, and cholestane-38 beta, 5 alpha, 6 β-triol was higher in patients with ulcerative colitis than in other control and patient groups *4299*

Neutrophil Elastase *Feces Increase* Mean concentration in 27 patients with colorectal cancer of 54.8 µg/g (15.14 mg/d) significantly different from 0.6 µg/g (0.11 mg/d) in 20 healthy controls *4521*

Neutrophils *Blood Increase* Relative lymphocytopenia may occur as a result of absolute increase in monocytes and polymorphonuclear cells *5205* Count increases with increasing disease activity *2550*

Occult Blood *Feces Increase* Positive for blood (gross and/or occult) *5544* Lower GI bleeding *4891*

Perinuclear Antineutrophil Cytoplasmic Autoantibodies *Serum Increase* Detected at a dilution of 1:100 in about 60 - 70% of patients with ulcerative colitis *4485*

pH *Blood Increase* Increased progressively with increased severity of the colitis and as the lesions became more widespread. Significant differences were observed in values between the mild/moderate and severe forms and between the severe and complicated forms (toxic megacolon) *687*

Phospholipase A_2 *Serum Increase* In patients with chronic inflammatory diseases such as ulcerative colitis serum concentration of PLA2-II correlates with activity of the disease *3766*

Phospholipase A_2 Type II *Serum Increase* Considerable increase in concentration observed correlating well with the activity of the disease *3767*

Plasminogen *Plasma No Effect* In 84 patients with ulcerative colitis mean concentration of 107 ± 4.9% compared with 109.9 ± 1.1% in 60 healthy blood donor controls *4948*

Plasminogen Activator Inhibitor-1 *Plasma Decrease* In 84 patients with ulcerative colitis mean concentration significantly decreased to 8.9 ± 1.1 ng/mL compared with 17.8 ± 1.1 ng/mL in 60 healthy blood donor controls *4948*

Platelets *Blood Increase* Most commonly in those patients having marked leukocytosis. Not associated with coagulation defects *4891*

Potassium *Serum* *Decrease* Common feature of severe colitis *4551* Portends a worse prognosis, probably because the degree of abnormality parallels clinical severity *4891* Serum electrolytes may show losses due to diarrhea, especially hypokalemia, which may contribute to colonic atony and may portend acute toxic dilatation *900*

Prealbumin *Serum* *Decrease* Haptoglobin concentrations rise with increasing clinical activity of the disease, while the prealbumin fraction declines *3303*

Protein *Serum* *Decrease* Malnutrition with protein deficiency *900* Fever, hypovolemia, tachycardia and hypoproteinemia are major manifestations *2039*

Prothrombin Time *Plasma* *Increase* Hypoprothrombinemia (prolonged time) is a commonly found defect in moderate or severe disease *4891*

Pyridoxine *Serum* *Decrease* Anemia may be due to blood loss, simple iron deficiency, deficiencies in folic acid, pyridoxine, or vitamin B_{12} *900*

Retinol *Serum* *No Effect* Mean concentration of 1.30 ± 0.31 µmol/L in 10 - 12 children with ulcerative colitis not significantly different from 1.60 ± 0.31 µmol/L in 20 - 23 healthy control children and reference interval of 0.66 - 2.69 µmol/L *2196*

Retinol-binding Protein *Serum* *No Effect* Mean concentration of 32 ± 10 mg/L in 10 - 12 children with ulcerative colitis not significantly different from 36 ± 10 mg/L in 20 - 23 healthy control children and reference interval of 30 - 60 mg/L *2196*

Rheumatoid Factor *Serum* *No Effect* Usually negative even with associated arthritis *4891*

Selenium *Serum* *Decrease* In 8 patients with moderate clinical activity median concentration of 43 µg/dL significantly different from 60 µg/dL in 10 healthy controls *5059*
Serum *No Effect* Mean concentration of 1.6 ± 0.2 µmol/L in 10 - 12 children with ulcerative colitis not significantly different from 1.5 ± 0.2 µmol/L in 20 - 23 healthy control children and reference interval of 1.28 - 2.35 µmol/L *2196*

Sialic Acid *Serum* *Increase* Mean concentration of 92.4 ± 29.4 mg/dL in 9 patients with acute ulcerative colitis not significantly greater than 65.9 ± 12.3 mg/dL in 14 patients with ulcerative colitis in remission and 64.7 ± 3.2 mg/dL in 20 healthy controls *4344*

Sodium *Serum* *Decrease* Common feature of severe colitis *4551*

Soluble CD44 Splice Variant 6 *Serum* *Decrease* Median concentration in 15 patients with clinically active ulcerative colitis of 153 ng/mL significantly reduced compared with that in 20 healthy donors of 221 ng/mL *4317*

Soluble Intercellular Adhesion Molecule-1 *Serum* *Increase* Median concentration of 300 ng/mL in 10 patients with active ulcerative colitis significantly higher than 245 ng/mL in 29 healthy controls *3783*

Soluble Interleukin-2 Receptor *Serum* *Increase* Serum concentrations of the soluble IL-2 receptor (sIL-2R) measured in 10 patients with UC before, at day 10 and 2 years after resection of inflamed bowel segments. Preoperatively, mean sIL-2R concentration was 495 ± 62 U/mL (mean ± SEM; healthy controls; 210 ± 25 U/mL; $p < 0.02$) in CD and 705 ± 120 U/mL ($p < 0.00002$) in UC. Two years postoperatively, sIL-2R was still elevated in 6 out of 9 patients in both disease groups. These patients did not differ from the remaining group with respect to disease activity *4685*

Thyroxine Binding Globulin *Serum* *Increase* Mean serum values were high in these patients, mainly due to the high levels in female patients *2420*

Tissue Plasminogen Activator *Plasma* *No Effect* In 84 patients with ulcerative colitis mean concentration of 5.79 ± 0.37 ng/mL compared with 5.13 ± 0.4 ng/mL in 60 healthy blood donor controls *4948*

α-Tocopherol *Serum* *No Effect* Mean concentration of 24 ± 12 µmol/L in 10 - 12 children with ulcerative colitis not significantly different from 20 ± 4 µmol/L in 20 - 23 healthy control children and reference interval of 9 - 47 µmol/L *2196*

γ-Tocopherol *Serum* *No Effect* Mean concentration of 5 ± 4 µmol/L in 10 - 12 children with ulcerative colitis not significantly different from 5 ± 2 µmol/L in 20 - 23 healthy control children *2196* In 10 to 12 children with ulcerative colitis mean concentration of 5 ± 4 µmol/L not significantly different from 5 ± 2 µmol/L in 20 to 23 healthy control children *2196*

α-Tocopherol:Lipids Ratio *Serum* *No Effect* Mean concentration of 372 ± 186 µmol/g in 10 - 12 children with ulcerative colitis not significantly different from 325 ± 46 µmol/g in 20 - 23 healthy control children and reference interval of > 186 µmol/g *2196*

Tri-iodothyronine (T3) *Serum* *Decrease* The concentration was lower in the severely ill patients than in those who were mildly-moderately ill, while T4 and TBG were not affected by the severity of the disease *2420*

Tumor Necrosis Factor-α *Serum* *Increase* Concentration increased in the majority of patients *3180*

Uric Acid *Urine* *Increase* High levels may be found *581*

Urokinase Plasminogen Activator *Plasma* *Increase* In 84 patients with ulcerative colitis mean concentration of 0.52 ± 0.025 ng/mL significantly increased compared with 0.47 ± 0.014 ng/mL in 60 healthy blood donor controls *4948*

Vitamin B_{12} *Serum* *Decrease* Anemia may be due to blood loss, simple iron deficiency, deficiencies in folic acid, pyridoxine, or vitamin B_{12} *900*

Volume *Plasma* *Decrease* Fever, hypovolemia, tachycardia and hypoproteinemia are major manifestations *2039*

Xylose Tolerance Test *Urine* *No Effect* Typical observation *5544*

Zinc *Serum* *Decrease* In patients with ulcerative colitis concentration is typically reduced *2952*
Serum *No Effect* In 8 patients with moderate clinical activity median concentration of 83 µg/dL not significantly different from 87 µg/dL in 10 healthy controls *5059*

557.00 Intestinal Infarction

Creatine Kinase *Serum* *No Effect* In 8 individuals with intestinal infarction activity not significantly different from that in individuals with other intraabdominal catastrophes or that in healthy controls *1573*

Creatine Kinase BB-Isoenzyme *Serum* *Increase* Reported effect *248*

Creatine Kinase Isoenzymes *Serum* *Increase* In 8 patients with intestinal infarction mean concentration of CK-BB of 22.3 ± 5.3 ng/mL significantly greater than 11.0 ± 0.8 ng/mL in 22 individuals with other forms of intraabdominal catastrophe and 5.8 ± 0.7 ng/mL in 20 controls *1573*
Serum *No Effect* In 8 patients with intestinal infarction mean concentration of CK-MB not significantly different from that in individuals with other intraabdominal catastrophes or in healthy controls *1573*

Lipase *Serum* *Increase* Activity may be increased in patients with abdominal diseases such as intestinal infarction *5231*

557.00 Mesenteric Artery Embolism

Alkaline Phosphatase *Serum* *Increase* A selective elevation of the intestinal isoenzyme has been described in acute intestinal ischemia *900* Peak activity is reached 2 - 3 days after onset of symptoms *4707*

Alkaline Phosphatase Isoenzymes *Serum* *Increase* A selective elevation of the intestinal isoenzyme has been described in acute intestinal ischemia *900*

Amylase *Serum* *Increase* May occur with mesenteric infarction *645*

Aspartate Aminotransferase *Serum* *Increase* After intestinal infarction *1290*

Fat *Feces* *Increase* Excessive fecal fat loss from recurrent ischemic damage to the intestinal mucosal function resulting in malabsorption *2304*

Hematocrit *Blood* *Increase* Will reflect the hemoconcentration secondary to fluid loss into the bowel and peritoneal cavity following bowel infarction *900*

Lactate Dehydrogenase *Serum* *Increase* Reported effect *900*

Leukocytes *Blood* *Increase* Reflects hemoconcentration and documents the cellular response to the endotoxins released by the involved bowel *900* Marked increase (15,000 - 25,000 /µL or more) with shift to the left *5544*

Occult Blood *Feces* *Increase* Upper GI bleeding *4891*

557.00 Mesenteric Artery Embolism *(continued)*

pH *Blood Decrease* Serum electrolytes usually show a depressed CO_2-combining power from the induced severe metabolic acidosis *900*

Phosphate *Serum Increase* Of 7 patients with massive intestinal infarction, all had elevated concentrations *2413*

Urea Nitrogen *Serum Increase* Will reflect the hemoconcentration secondary to fluid loss into the bowel and peritoneal cavity following bowel infarction *900*

557.00 Necrotizing Enterocolitis

Acetylhydrolase *Serum Decrease* In newborns with necrotizing encephalitis mean activity of acetylhydrolase (platelet activating factor degrading enzyme) of 10.6 ± 0.7 nmol/mL/min significantly lower than 23 ± 1.4 nmol/mL/min in control premature infants *2263*

Epidermal Growth Factor *Saliva Decrease* Mean concentration of approximately 1,600 ± 300 pg/mg saliva in 15 patients with NEC compared with 6,700 ± 1,200 pg/mg saliva in 12 healthy gestational and postnatal age-matched control infants *2108*
Serum Decrease Mean concentration of approximately 15 ± 5 pg/mL in 8 patients with NEC compared with 270 ± 100 pg/mL in 5 healthy gestational and postnatal age-matched control infants *2108*

Platelet Activating Factor *Serum Increase* In newborns with necrotizing encephalitis mean concentration of 18.1 ± 3.6 ng/mL significantly higher than 3.1 ± 0.9 ng/mL in control premature infants *2263*

Tumor Necrosis Factor-α *Serum Increase* In newborns with necrotizing encephalitis mean concentration of 136 ± 75 U/mL significantly higher than 1.5 ± 0.8 U/mL in control premature infants *2263*

558.90 Acute Diarrhea

Retinol *Urine Increase* In 44 children with diarrhea excretion on day of admission to hospital of 1.44 ± 2.94 µmol/d significantly greater than 0.00 ± 0.001 µmol/d in 44 healthy controls *101*

558.90 Colitis

Amylase, Pancreatic Isoenzyme *Serum Increase* Median activity in 21 patients with indeterminate colitis of 73 U/L *2094*

Ferritin *Serum Decrease* In 725 patients with serum ferritin concentration of less than 50 ng/mL detected in 4 patients with colitis *2968*

558.90 Diarrhea

Ammonia *Urine Increase* In prolonged diarrhea *1290*

Bicarbonate *Serum Decrease* Reported effect *5544*

Bilirubin *Feces Increase* In severe diarrhea a little bilirubin may be present *1290*

Calcitonin *Plasma Increase* In 2 of 142 specimens (1.4%) from patients with chronic diarrhea of non-tumor origin concentration increased above upper limit of normal of 71 pg/mL *4635*

Chloride *Feces Increase* During moderate diarrhea the output may increase to 60 mmol/day. In very severe diarrhea the fecal composition approaches that of ileal fluid, and up to 500 mmol of chloride can be lost in 24 h *1290*
Serum Decrease Observed effect *5544*
Urine Decrease Excessive loss, due to severe diarrhea *1290*

Creatinine *Serum Increase* Leading to reduced renal blood flow (prerenal azotemia) *5544*

Cyclosporine *Blood Decrease* Secondary diarrhea causes reduced absorption from the gut with a large decrease in the area under the curve and trough blood concentrations *671*
Serum Decrease Secondary diarrhea causes reduced absorption from the gut with a large decrease in the area under the curve and trough blood concentrations *671*

Fat *Feces Increase* Excessively rapid passage of intestinal contents. With severe diarrhea *1290*

Gastrin-releasing Peptide *Serum Increase* In 9 of 162 specimens (5.6%) from patients with chronic diarrhea of non-tumor origin concentration increased above upper limit of normal of 542 pg/mL *4635*

Hematocrit *Blood Increase* When salt and water are lost in isotonic proportions, a contraction of the extracellular fluid compartment occurs and hemoconcentration develops *4891*

Hemoglobin *Blood Increase* When salt and water are lost in isotonic proportions, a contraction of the extracellular fluid compartment occurs and hemoconcentration develops *4891*

Motilin *Plasma Increase* In 23 of 70 specimens (32.9%) from patients with chronic diarrhea of non-tumor origin concentration increased above upper limit of normal of 125 pg/mL *4635*

Neurotensin *Plasma Increase* In 14 of 171 specimens (8.2%) from patients with chronic diarrhea of non-tumor origin concentration increased above upper limit of normal of 250 pg/mL *4635*

Nitrogen *Feces Increase* Increased total nitrogen observed *1290*

Pancreatic Polypeptide *Plasma Increase* In 31 of 175 specimens (17.7%) from patients with chronic diarrhea of non-tumor origin concentration increased above upper limit of normal of 465 pg/mL *4635*

pH *Blood Decrease* Tends to fall *1290*
Urine Decrease Observed effect *5544*

Potassium *Serum Decrease* Depletion may develop with any severe diarrhea *4891*
Urine Decrease Normal or decreased *5544*

Sodium *Serum Decrease* 60 mmol/day may be lost *1290* Hyponatremia commonly results *4891*
Serum Increase In osmotic diarrhea water loss is proportionately greater than that of sodium. Dehydration with hypernatremia may occur *4891*

Somatostatin *Plasma Increase* In 5 of 163 specimens (3.1%) from patients with chronic diarrhea of non-tumor origin concentration increased above upper limit of normal of 68 pg/mL *4635*

Substance P *Plasma Increase* In 11 of 171 specimens (6.4%) from patients with chronic diarrhea of non-tumor origin concentration increased above upper limit of normal of 240 pg/mL *4635*

Urea Nitrogen *Serum Increase* Observed in patients with diarrhea and severe dehydration, who were rapidly dehydrated with concomitant fall of BUN to normal or subnormal levels *1627*

Vasoactive Intestinal Polypeptide *Plasma Increase* In 6 of 190 specimens (3.2%) from patients with chronic diarrhea of non-tumor origin concentration increased above upper limit of normal of 84 pg/mL *4635*

Volume *Plasma Decrease* When salt and water are lost in isotonic proportions, a contraction of the extracellular fluid compartment occurs and hemoconcentration develops *4891*

558.90 Diarrheal Diseases

Soluble Interleukin-2 Receptor *Serum Increase* In 9 children diarrheal disease with no pathogens identified mean concentration of 2,061 U/mL not significantly different from 1,826 U/mL in age-matched controls. In 4 with pathogens identified mean 2,592 U/mL significantly different from 1,188 U/mL in age-matched controls *769*

558.90 Enterocolitis

α_1-Acid Glycoprotein *Serum Increase* Mean concentration in 13 adult patients with enterocolitis of 1.12 ± 0.54 g/L compared with less than 0.50 g/L in 30 healthy controls *721*

Amyloid A Protein *Serum Increase* In 8 patients mean concentration in acute phase of 2.19 ± 1.03 mg/L *3728* Mean concentration in 13 adults on admission to hospital of 394 ± 172 mg/L compared with less than 1.5 mg/L in 30 healthy controls *721*

α_1-Antichymotrypsin *Serum Increase* Mean concentration in 13 adult patients with enterocolitis of 0.64 ± 0.32 g/L compared with less than 0.50 g/L in 30 healthy controls *721*

C-Reactive Protein *Serum* *Increase* In 8 patients mean concentration in acute phase of 1.32 ± 0.75 mg/L *3728* In 13 adult patients with enterocolitis mean concentration of 40 ± 12 mg/L compared with less than 3 mg/L in 30 healthy controls *721*

558.90 Gastroenteritis

CA 72-4 *Serum* *Increase* In 9 patients with gastroenteritis 1 (11%) had a concentration greater than cut-off of 2.5 U/mL with median concentration of 1.3 U/mL *4505*

Carcinoembryonic Antigen *Serum* *Increase* In 11 patients with gastritis or gastric ulcer 2 (18%) had a concentration greater than cut-off of 3 ng/mL with median value of 1.9 ng/mL *4505*

Enteroglucagon *Plasma* *Increase* In 11 infants suffering from acute gastroenteritis mean concentration in acute state of 1,292 (SEM 312) pmol/L compared with 79 (SEM 27) pmol/L in healthy control infants *2946*

Glucagon, Pancreatic *Plasma* *Increase* In 11 infants with acute gastroenteritis mean concentration of 17.8 pmol/L compared with 6.3 pmol/L in healthy controls *2946*

Hemoglobin *Blood* *Decrease* Abnormal blood tests were found in 76 of 116 cases of acute gastroenteritis (67.2%) including 16.1% with abnormal hemoglobin concentrations *697*

Ketones *Urine* *Increase* Increased urinary ketones observed in 15 (12.9%) of 116 patients with acute gastroenteritis *697*

Leukocytes *Blood* *Increase* Abnormal blood tests were found in 76 of 116 cases of acute gastroenteritis (67.2%) including 47.8% with abnormal leukocyte counts *697*
Feces *Increase* Positive fecal tests for leukocytes observed in 14 of 26 patients (53.8%) with acute gastroenteritis *697*

Motilin *Plasma* *Increase* In 11 infants with acute gastroenteritis mean concentration of 217.6 pol/L significantly higher than 98.5 pmol/L in healthy controls *2946*

Neurotensin *Plasma* *No Effect* In 11 infants with acute gastroenteritis no significant difference observed compared with healthy controls *2946*

Nitrate *Serum* *Increase* Median concentration of 117.7 µmol/L in 20 patients with inflammatory bowel disease significantly different from 32.8 µmol/L in 20 healthy controls *1277*

Occult Blood *Feces* *Increase* Positive fecal occult blood tests observed in 8 of 26 patients (30.8%) with acute gastroenteritis *697*

Pancreatic Polypeptide *Plasma* *No Effect* In 11 infants with acute gastroenteritis no significant difference observed when concentration compared with that in healthy controls *2946*

Peptide Tyrosine Tyrosine *Plasma* *Increase* In 11 infants with acute gastroenteritis mean concentration increased to 114.6 pmol/L compared with 37.0 pmol/L in healthy controls *2946*

Potassium *Serum* *Decrease* Abnormal blood tests were found in 76 of 116 cases of acute gastroenteritis (67.2%) including 13.7% with abnormal potassium concentrations *697*
Serum *Increase* Abnormal blood tests were found in 76 of 116 cases of acute gastroenteritis (67.2%) including 13.7% with abnormal potassium concentrations *697*

Sodium *Serum* *Decrease* Abnormal blood tests were found in 76 of 116 cases of acute gastroenteritis (67.2%) including 16.5% with abnormal sodium concentrations *697*
Serum *Increase* Abnormal blood tests were found in 76 of 116 cases of acute gastroenteritis (67.2%) including 16.5% with abnormal sodium concentrations *697*

Urea Nitrogen *Serum* *Increase* Abnormal blood tests were found in 76 of 116 cases of acute gastroenteritis (67.2%) including 16.5% with abnormal urea nitrogen concentrations *697*

Vasoactive Intestinal Polypeptide *Plasma* *No Effect* In 11 infants with acute gastroenteritis no significant difference observed when compared with healthy controls *2946*

558.90 Gastroenteritis and Colitis

Albumin *Serum* *Decrease* Hypoalbuminemia and persistent diarrhea in cytomegalovirus enteritis *5359*

Bicarbonate *Serum* *Decrease* May be noted *900*

Chloride *Serum* *Decrease* Either increase or decrease may be noted *900*
Serum *Increase* Reflects the loss of greater volumes of fluid than salt. Either increase or decrease may be noted *900*

Glucose *Cerebrospinal Fluid* *Decrease* In children with severe dehydration *900*
Serum *Decrease* Of 868 infants with dehydration from gastroenteritis, 7.9% of cases had blood sugar levels of 0 - 50 mg/dL. A high mortality rate was found in patients with hypoglycemia *1765*
Serum *Increase* Of 868 infants with dehydration from gastroenteritis, blood sugar levels in 10.2% were > 200 mg/dL. High mortality rate was found in patients with hyperglycemia *1765*

Hematocrit *Blood* *Increase* Normal to elevated, depending on the amount of dehydration *900*

Hemoglobin *Blood* *Increase* Hemoglobin and hematocrit are normal to elevated, depending on the amount of dehydration *900*

Leukocytes *Blood* *No Effect* Usually within the normal limits of 5,000 - 10,000 /µL *900*

Lymphocytes *Blood* *Decrease* In viral gastroenteritis, during acute illness, a transient lymphopenia was noted which involved all lymphocyte subpopulations *1199*
Cerebrospinal Fluid *No Effect* Normal except when aseptic meningoencephalitis is part of the overall syndrome. Then lymphocytic pleocytosis is found *900*

Magnesium *Serum* *Decrease* Mean serum level of 2.06 ± 0.62 mg/dL in 54 patients with noncholeric gastroenteritis. 7 (13%) had values below the lower normal limit *1268*

pH *Blood* *Decrease* May be noted *900*
Blood *Increase* Increased progressively with increased severity. The lesions became more widespread. Statistically significant differences were observed in pH values between the mild/moderate and severe forms and between the severe and complicated forms *687*

Protein *Serum* *Decrease* Enteric loss of plasma protein *4891*

Sodium *Serum* *Decrease* Either increase or decrease may be noted *900*
Serum *Increase* Reflects the loss of greater volumes of fluid than salt. Either increase or decrease may be noted *900*

558.90 Indeterminate Colitis

Tumor Necrosis Factor-α *Serum* *Increase* Concentration increased in the majority of patients *3180*

560.90 Intestinal Obstruction

Albumin *Serum* *Decrease* In 35% of 42 patients at initial hospitalization for this disorder *1576* 6% mortality in cases with > 3 g/dL; 33% mortality with < 3 g/dL *1290*
Serum *No Effect* Concentration may be unaffected *1290*

Alkaline Phosphatase *Serum* *Increase* In 31% of 42 patients at initial hospitalization for this disorder *1576*

Amylase *Serum* *Increase* Moderate hyperamylasemia without evidence of associated pancreatitis. Values > 1,850 U/L may indicate strangulated or necrotic bowel *4537* Often marked elevation *4707*

Aspartate Aminotransferase *Serum* *Increase* In 33% of 42 patients at initial hospitalization for this disorder *1576*

Bicarbonate *Serum* *Increase* Metabolic alkalosis secondary to vomiting *5544* In 46% of 47 patients at initial hospitalization for this disorder *1576*

Carbon Dioxide Partial Pressure *Blood* *Decrease* Metabolic acidosis secondary to lactic acidosis *413*

Chloride *Serum* *Decrease* Metabolic alkalosis secondary to vomiting *5544*
Serum *Increase* With dehydration *4891*

Cholesterol *Serum* *Decrease* In 39% of 42 patients at initial hospitalization for this disorder *1576*

Creatinine *Serum* *Increase* With dehydration *4891*

Erythrocytes *Ascitic Fluid* *Increase* Bloody ascitic fluid *413*

Glucose *Serum* *Increase* In 42% of 46 patients at initial hospitalization for this disorder *1576*

560.90 Intestinal Obstruction *(continued)*

Hematocrit *Blood* *Increase* Normal early, but later increased, with dehydration *5544*

Hemoglobin *Blood* *Increase* Normal early, but later increased, with dehydration *5544*

Lactate Dehydrogenase *Serum* *Increase* In 32% of 42 patients at initial hospitalization for this disorder *1576* Increase may indicate strangulation (infarction) of small intestine *5544*

Leukocytes *Blood* *Decrease* Leukopenia with left shift suggest infarction with sepsis *413*
Blood *Increase* In 40% of 47 patients at initial hospitalization for this disorder *1576* May be normal in early cases of simple or strangulation obstruction. With advanced cases, may range from 12,000 - 15,000 /µL or more. Counts of 25,000 - 30,000 /µL or more strongly indicate vascular occlusion to the bowel as by mesenteric thrombosis *900*

Lipase *Serum* *Increase* Activity may be increased in patients with abdominal diseases such as bowel obstruction *5231*

Neutrophils *Blood* *Increase* In 39% of 44 patients at initial hospitalization for this disorder *1576*

Occult Blood *Feces* *Increase* Gross rectal blood suggests carcinoma of colon or intussusception *5544*
Gastric Material *Increase* Positive test suggests strangulation; there may be gross blood if strangulated segment is high in jejunum *5544*

pH *Blood* *Decrease* Metabolic acidosis secondary to lactic acidosis *413* Reflects the course of the patient and therapy *5544*

Potassium *Serum* *Decrease* Metabolic alkalosis secondary to vomiting *5544*

Sodium *Serum* *Increase* Secondary to dehydration *2034*
Urine *Increase* Specific gravity increases, with deficit of water and electrolytes unless pre-existing renal disease is present *5544*

Specific Gravity *Urine* *Increase* Increases with deficit of water and electrolytes unless pre-existing renal disease is present. Urinalysis helps rule out renal colic, diabetic acidosis, etc *5544* Urinalysis may be entirely normal in intestinal obstruction with the exception of relatively high specific gravity *900*

Urea Nitrogen *Serum* *Increase* Azotemia may be striking; also with massive hemorrhage *1025* Increase suggests blood in intestine or renal damage *5544*

Volume *Urine* *Decrease* Urinary output diminishes early in the disease *367*

562.10 Diverticulosis

α_1-Acid Glycoprotein *Serum* *No Effect* Mean concentration of 98 mg/dL in 11 patients with diverticulosis not significantly different from 119 mg/dL in 20 healthy controls *4344*

Carcinoembryonic Antigen *Serum* *Increase* In 58 patients with diverticulosis 59% had concentrations less than 2.5 ng/mL, 38% had concentrations between 2.6 and 5.0 ng/mL, 3% had concentrations between 5.1 and 10.0 ng/mL and 0% had concentrations greater than 10.0 ng/mL *2010* Increases reported in patients with diverticular disease *4891*

C-Reactive Protein *Serum* *Increase* Mean concentration of 2.1 mg/dL in 13 patients with diverticulosis not significantly different from 0.7 mg/dL in 20 healthy controls *4344*

Erythrocyte Sedimentation Rate *Blood* *Increase* May be mildly elevated in patients with diverticular disease *900*

Hematocrit *Blood* *Decrease* Blood loss is usually minimal but massive bleeding may occur in patients with diverticular disease *4891*

Hemoglobin *Blood* *Decrease* Blood loss is usually minimal but massive bleeding may occur in patients with diverticular disease *4891*

Iron *Serum* *Decrease* Some cases of diverticular disease mat show effect *4891*

Iron-binding Capacity, Total *Serum* *Increase* Some cases of diverticular disease may show effect *4891*

MCH *Blood* *Decrease* Some cases of diverticular disease may show effect *4891*

MCHC *Blood* *Decrease* Observed in some cases of diverticular disease *4891*

β_2-Microglobulin *Serum* *No Effect* Mean concentration of 2.85 ± 1.48 mg/dL in 13 patients with diverticulosis not significantly different from 2.50 ± 1.28 mg/dL in 20 healthy controls *4344*

Occult Blood *Feces* *Increase* May occur in patients with diverticular disease *4891*

Sialic Acid *Serum* *No Effect* Mean concentration of 66.2 ± 8.3 mg/dL in 13 patients with diverticulosis not significantly greater than 64.7 ± 3.2 mg/dL in 20 healthy controls *4344*

562.11 Diverticulitis

α_1-Acid Glycoprotein *Serum* *Increase* Mean concentration of 239 mg/dL in 7 patients with diverticulitis significantly different from 119 mg/dL in 20 healthy controls *4344*

CA 19-9 *Serum* *No Effect* In none of 7 patients with diverticulitis was concentration increased *5406*

CA-M43 *Serum* *No Effect* In none of 7 patients with diverticulitis was concentration increased *5406*

Carcinoembryonic Antigen *Serum* *Increase* Increased concentrations may be observed *4551* Increased concentrations reported *1601* In 84 patients with diverticulitis 73% had concentrations less than 2.5 ng/mL, 20% had concentrations between 2.6 and 5.0 ng/mL, 5% had concentrations between 5.1 and 10.0 ng/mL and 2% had concentrations greater than 10.0 ng/mL *2010*
Serum *No Effect* In none of 7 patients with diverticulitis was concentration increased *5406*

C-Reactive Protein *Serum* *Increase* Mean concentration of 5.2 mg/dL in 7 patients with diverticulitis significantly different from 0.7 mg/dL in 20 healthy controls *4344*

Erythrocytes *Urine* *Increase* Although urinalysis may be normal hematuria may signal involvement of the bladder or ureter *900*

Iron *Serum* *Decrease* Some cases *4891*

Iron-binding Capacity, Total *Serum* *Increase* Some cases *4891*

Leukocytes *Blood* *Increase* Symptoms are chronic constipation punctuated by episodes of acute abdominal pain, fever, and leukocytosis *2039* Usually elevated with the appearance of less mature forms of neutrophils, but this finding might be lacking in elderly or debilitated patients *900* In 51% of 35 patient at initial hospitalization for this disorder *1576*

MCH *Blood* *Decrease* Some cases *4891*

MCHC *Blood* *Decrease* Some cases *4891*

β_2-Microglobulin *Serum* *No Effect* Mean concentration of 2.90 ± 1.13 mg/dL in 7 patients with diverticulitis not significantly different from 2.50 ± 1.28 mg/dL in 20 healthy controls *4344*

Neutrophils *Blood* *Increase* Leukocytosis with an increase in polymorphonuclear forms *4891* In 51% of 36 patients at initial hospitalization for this disorder *1576*

Occult Blood *Feces* *Increase* In 124 patients who presented at an ER with gastrointestinal bleeding 6.4% had diverticulitis *1383* Observed effect in some patients *4891*

Sialic Acid *Serum* *No Effect* Mean concentration of 87.6 ± 28.6 mg/dL in 7 patients with diverticulitis not significantly greater than 64.7 ± 3.2 mg/dL in 20 healthy controls *4344*

564.10 Irritable Bowel Syndrome

Anti-Neutrophil Cytoplasm Antibodies *Serum* *Increase* Increased perinuclear ANCA *4606*

Cortisol *Plasma* *Increase* Patients with irritable bowel syndrome and diarrhea had concentrations significantly increased compared with those in controls and IBS patients with spastic colons *2955*

Dopamine *Plasma* *Increase* Patients with irritable bowel syndrome and diarrhea had concentrations significantly increased compared with those in controls and IBS spastic colon patients *2955*

Epinephrine *Plasma* *Increase* Patients with irritable bowel syndrome and diarrhea had concentrations significantly increased compared with those in controls and IBS patients with spastic colons *2955*

5-Hydroxytryptamine *Plasma* *Increase* Patients with irritable bowel syndrome and spastic colon had concentrations significantly decreased compared with those in controls and IBS patients with diarrhea *2955*
Platelets *Decrease* Concentrations higher in patients with IBS and spastic colon than in controls and patients with IBS and controls *2955*

5-Hydroxytryptamine, Free *Plasma* *Increase* Patients with irritable bowel syndrome and diarrhea had concentrations significantly increased compared with those in controls and IBS patients with spastic colons *2955*

Nitrate *Serum* *No Effect* Median concentration of 35.5 μmol/L in 12 patients with irritable bowel syndrome not significantly different from 32.8 μmol/L in 20 healthy controls *1277*

Norepinephrine *Plasma* *Increase* Patients with irritable bowel syndrome and diarrhea had concentrations significantly increased compared with those in controls and IBS patients with spastic colons *2955*

Platelet Aggregation *Blood* *Increase* Patients with irritable bowel syndrome and diarrhea had significantly increased aggregability compared with that in controls and IBS patients with spastic colons *2955*

564.20 Postgastrectomy Dumping Syndrome

Fat *Feces* *Increase* Malabsorption from poor mixing and rapid transit *2034*

Glucagon *Plasma* *Increase* Hypoglycemia following gastrectomy, gut glucagon levels in the plasma are raised *1290*

Glucose *Serum* *Decrease* Rapid absorption of carbohydrate by smaller intestine leads to release of insulin which continues to act after most of the carbohydrate has been absorbed and stored *1290*
Serum *Increase* Rapid and prolonged alimentary hyperglycemia with subsequent delayed absorption *2034*

Glucose Tolerance *Serum* *Decrease* Characteristically the curve consists of a rise in blood glucose to between 200 - 300 mg/dL, 30 min after oral administration of glucose. This is followed by a rapid fall in the next hour to hypoglycemic levels, at which point symptoms occur *1980*

Hematocrit *Blood* *Decrease* Iron deficiency and vitamin B_{12} deficiency are common following subtotal gastrectomy *1980*

Hemoglobin *Blood* *Decrease* Iron deficiency and vitamin B_{12} deficiency are common following subtotal gastrectomy *1980*

Iron *Serum* *Decrease* Iron deficiency and vitamin B_{12} deficiency are common following subtotal gastrectomy *1980*

MCH *Blood* *Decrease* Iron deficiency and vitamin B_{12} deficiency are common following subtotal gastrectomy *1980*

MCHC *Blood* *Decrease* Iron deficiency and vitamin B_{12} deficiency are common following subtotal gastrectomy *1980*

MCV *Blood* *Decrease* Iron deficiency and vitamin B_{12} deficiency are common following subtotal gastrectomy *1980*

Potassium *Serum* *Decrease* Jejunal hypersecretion of water and electrolytes, especially potassium *2034*

Vitamin B_{12} *Serum* *Decrease* Iron deficiency and vitamin B_{12} deficiency are common following subtotal gastrectomy *1980*

Volume *Plasma* *Decrease* Jejunal hypersecretion of water and electrolytes, with resultant reduced plasma volume *2034*

567.90 Peritonitis

Albumin *Serum* *Decrease* Increase in plasma volume without increase in total protein *1290*

Aldosterone *Plasma* *Increase* Increased adrenal production *2034*
Urine *Increase* Increased adrenal production *2034*

Amylase *Serum* *Increase* Hyperamylasemia up to 405 U/L without appreciable pancreatic disease *4261*

CA 125 *Serum* *Increase* False positive result *3909* High levels were mainly associated with spontaneous bacterial peritonitis *3560*

Catecholamines *Plasma* *Increase* Increased adrenal production *2034*
Urine *Increase* Increased adrenal production *2034*

Eosinophils *Ascitic Fluid* *Increase* Ascites associated with eosinophilic enteritis and peritonitis has a high eosinophil count *4891*

Erythrocytes *Ascitic Fluid* *Increase* < 10,000 cells/μL is unusual. Normally more seen *233* May be bloody *413*
Peritoneal Fluid *Increase* Bloody ascites may be seen with tuberculous peritonitis *4891*

Glucocorticoids *Plasma* *Increase* Increased adrenal production *2034*

Glucose *Ascitic Fluid* *Decrease* Seen with tuberculous peritonitis *413*

Hematocrit *Blood* *Increase* Secondary; may be increased owing to hemoconcentration from extracellular fluid loss into the peritoneal cavity *900*

Hemoglobin *Blood* *Increase* May be increased owing to hemoconcentration from extracellular fluid loss into the peritoneal cavity *900*

Interleukin-1β *Serum* *No Effect* Mean undetectable concentration in 4 patients with spontaneous bacterial peritonitis not significantly different from not detectable amount in 17 healthy controls *4228*

Interleukin-6 *Ascitic Fluid* *Increase* Mean concentration in 10 patients with spontaneous bacterial peritonitis of 103 ± 24 ng/mL *4228*
Serum *Increase* Mean concentration in 4 patients with spontaneous bacterial peritonitis of 1,736 ± 394 ng/mL significantly different from not detectable amount in 17 healthy controls *4228*

6-Keto-Prostaglandin $F_{1\alpha}$ *Ascitic Fluid* *Increase* Mean concentration in 10 patients with spontaneous bacterial peritonitis of 113 ± 38 pg/mL *4228*
Plasma *No Effect* Mean concentration of 6.7 ± 4.7 pg/mL in 4 patients with spontaneous bacterial peritonitis not significantly different from 8.8 ± 1.4 pg/mL in 16 healthy controls *4228*

Leukocytes *Ascitic Fluid* *Increase* > 1,000 /μL predominantly polymorphonuclear cells *233* Elevated counts (> 250 /μL) indicate peritoneal irritation *367* Mean total count of 5,500 /μL *2487*
Blood *Increase* Elevated (20,000 - 50,000 /μL) and consists predominantly of polymorphonuclear neutrophils. May not occur in the older age group and those on steroids *900*

Leukotriene B_4 *Ascitic Fluid* *No Effect* Mean concentration not detectable in 10 patients with spontaneous bacterial peritonitis of 10 ± 1.6 mg/mL *4228*
Plasma *Increase* Mean concentration of 54 ± 54.6 pg/mL in 4 patients with spontaneous bacterial peritonitis significantly different from not detectable amount in 17 healthy controls *4228*

Lymphocytes *Ascitic Fluid* *Increase* A high percentage suggests tuberculous peritonitis *367*

Monocytes *Ascitic Fluid* *Increase* Seen with tuberculous peritonitis *413*
Peritoneal Fluid *Increase* Most patients have > 80% mononuclear forms characterizing chronic inflammatory disease, especially tuberculosis *4891*

Neutrophils *Ascitic Fluid* *Increase* 10 of 11 patients with bacterial peritonitis had counts > 250/μL. Very few patients with other diseases had comparable granulocyte counts *2487*
Blood *Increase* Secondary; WBC is elevated with a major increase in polymorphonuclear granulocytes. May not be present in the older age group and those on steroids *900*
Pleural Fluid *Increase* Neutrophils predominate in pleural fluid *3052*

Phospholipase A_2 Type I *Serum* *Increase* Concentration reported as high as 440 μg/L in peritonitis compared with 2 and 4 μg/L in healthy controls *3767*

Potassium *Serum* *Decrease* Secondary to increased aldosterone production *2034*

Prostaglandin E_2 *Ascitic Fluid* *Increase* Mean concentration in 10 patients with spontaneous bacterial peritonitis of 79 ± 20.7 pg/mL *4228*
Plasma *No Effect* Mean concentration of 52 ± 48.0 pg/mL in 4 patients with spontaneous bacterial peritonitis not significantly different from 70 ± 13.0 pg/mL in 16 healthy controls *4228*

567.90 Peritonitis *(continued)*

Protein *Ascitic Fluid* *Increase* Mean concentration in 7 patients with spontaneous bacterial peritonitis of 10 ± 1.6 mg/mL *4228* Often > 2.5 g/dL in ascitic fluid *233*
Peritoneal Fluid *Increase* Exceeds 2.5 g/dL in 85 - 100% of patients with tuberculous peritonitis. Exudate with protein concentration > 3.0 g/dL usually found with tuberculous and bacterial peritonitis *4891*

Sodium *Serum* *Increase* Secondary to increased aldosterone production *2034*

Soluble Intercellular Adhesion Molecule-1
Ascitic Fluid *Increase* Mean concentration in 10 patients with spontaneous bacterial peritonitis of 215 ± 27 ng/mL *4228*
Serum *Increase* Mean concentration in 3 patients with spontaneous bacterial peritonitis of 1,204 ± 271 ng/mL significantly different from 228 ± 24 ng/mL in 17 healthy controls *4228*

Specific Gravity *Peritoneal Fluid* *Increase* Exudate with specific gravity > 1.016 usually found with tuberculous and bacterial peritonitis *4891*

Thromboxane B_2 *Ascitic Fluid* *Increase* Mean concentration in 10 patients with spontaneous bacterial peritonitis of 53 ± 3.2 pg/mL *4228*
Plasma *No Effect* Mean concentration of 127 ± 32 pg/mL in 2 patients with spontaneous bacterial peritonitis not significantly different from 153 ± 67 pg/mL in 16 healthy controls *4228*

Tumor Necrosis Factor-α *Serum* *No Effect* Mean undetectable concentration in 3 patients with spontaneous bacterial peritonitis not significantly different from not detectable amount in 17 healthy controls *4228*

Urea Nitrogen *Serum* *Increase* Secondary; may be increased owing to hemoconcentration from extracellular fluid loss into the peritoneal cavity *900*

Volume *Plasma* *Decrease* Exudation of fluid leads to reduction in effective circulating volume *2034*

569.84 Multiple Angiodysplasia

Ferritin *Serum* *Decrease* In 725 patients with serum ferritin concentration of less than 50 ng/mL detected in 9 patients with multiple angiodysplasia *2968*

569.89 Proctosigmoiditis

α_1-Acid Glycoprotein *Serum* *No Effect* Mean concentration of 111 mg/dL in 13 patients with nonulcerative proctosigmoiditis not significantly different from 119 mg/dL in 20 healthy controls *4344*

C-Reactive Protein *Serum* *Increase* Mean concentration of 1.4 mg/dL in 13 patients with acute nonulcerative proctosigmoiditis not significantly different from 0.7 mg/dL in 20 healthy controls *4344*

β_2-Microglobulin *Serum* *No Effect* Mean concentration of 2.16 ± 1.02 mg/dL in 13 patients with nonulcerative proctosigmoiditis not significantly different from 2.50 ± 1.28 mg/dL in 20 healthy controls *4344*

Sialic Acid *Serum* *No Effect* Mean concentration of 70.1 ± 17.9 mg/dL in 13 patients with nonulcerative proctosigmoiditis not significantly greater than 64.7 ± 3.2 mg/dL in 20 healthy controls *4344*

569.90 Benign Colon Disease

CA 549 *Serum* *No Effect* In 65 patients with benign disease of the colon none had a concentration greater than 30.0 kU/L with BRESMARQ assay *764*

569.90 Benign Gastrointestinal Disease

Carcinoembryonic Antigen *Serum* *Increase* Mean concentration increased in 37% of patients with benign gastrointestinal disease compared with 11% in healthy individuals *3191* In 78 patients with gastrointestinal disease, 74.4% had concentrations of 0.0 - 3.0 ng/mL, 17.9% had concentrations from 3.1 - 5.0 ng/mL, 7.7% had concentrations from 5.1 - 10.0 ng/mL and 0.0% had concentrations greater than 10.0 ng/mL when measured by method on Bayer Technicon Immuno 1® system compared with 95.9%, 3.5%, 0.6% and 0.0% respectively in 173 healthy nonsmokers *339*

Chymotrypsin *Feces* *Decrease* In 35 patients with gastrointestinal disease mean activity of 10 ± 1 U/g significantly reduced compared with 15 ± 1 U/g in 50 healthy controls *3133*

Colon Specific Antigen *Serum* *Increase* In patients with benign gastrointestinal disease 10 % had increased concentration compared with 8% in healthy controls *3191*

Elastase 1 *Feces* *No Effect* In 35 patients with gastrointestinal disease mean concentration of 546 ± 62 µg/g not significantly reduced compared with 602 ± 38 µg/g in 50 healthy controls *3133*

SP2 *Serum* *No Effect* 1 of 10 patients with benign gastrointestinal disease had a concentration of 14 U/mL when the upper limit of normal was 14 U/mL with 9 having lower concentrations *5260*

Tennessee Antigen *Serum* *Increase* In patients with benign gastrointestinal disease, 36% had increased concentration compared with 7% healthy controls who had increased concentrations *3191*

569.90 Inflammatory Bowel Disease

α_1-Acid Glycoprotein *Serum* *Increase* Median concentration of 32 µmol/L in patients with active inflamatory bowel disease and 29 µmol/L in inactive IBD significantly higher than 20 µmol/L in 29 healthy controls *3783*

α_2-Antiplasmin *Plasma* *Increase* In 9 patients with severe disease median concentration of 800 µg/L significantly greater than 335 µg/L in 20 healthy controls *5388*
Plasma *No Effect* In 112 patients with inflammatory bowel disease mean concentration of 93 ± 0.85% compared with 93 ± 0.9% in 60 healthy blood donor controls *4948*

Ascorbic Acid *Serum* *Decrease* Mean concentration of 284 ± 125 µmol/L in 15 children with IBD significantly different from 420 ± 114 µmol/L in 12 healthy control children *2196* In 15 children with Crohn's disease mean concentration of 284 ± 125 µmol/L significantly different from 420 ± 114 µmol/L in 12 healthy control children *2196*

CA 125 *Serum* *Increase* In 10 patients with inflammatory bowel disease median concentration of 14.3 U/L *2090* Median concentration of 14 µg/L in 10 patients with inflammatory bowel disease *5191*

β-Carotene *Serum* *No Effect* Mean concentration of 0.4 ± 0.3 µmol/L in 22 - 24 children with IBD not significantly different from 0.4 ± 0.2 µmol/L in 12 healthy control children and reference interval of 0.1 - 1.6 µmol/L *2196*

C-Reactive Protein *Serum* *Increase* Median concentration of 7 mg/L in patients with active inflammatory bowel disease and 5 mg/L in inactive IBD significantly higher than 1 mg/L in 29 healthy controls *3783*

CYFRA 21-1 *Serum* *No Effect* Median concentration of 2.1 µg/L in 10 patients with inflammatory bowel disease not different from 1.9 µg/L in 40 healthy controls *5191*

Glutathione *Blood* *Increase* Mean concentration of 7.3 ± 1.3 µmol/g hemoglobin in 22 - 24 children with IBD significantly different from 6.4 ± 1.0 µmol/g hemoglobin in 12 healthy control children but not different from reference interval of 4.5 - 8.7 µmol/g hemoglobin *2196*

Glutathione Peroxidase *Serum* *Increase* Mean activity of 1,117 ± 411 U/L in 22 - 24 children with IBD significantly different from 763 ± 131 U/L in 20 - 23 healthy control children but not different from reference interval of 603 - 1,288 U/L *2196*

Hemoglobin *Blood* *Decrease* Mean concentration of 146 ± 23 g/L in 22 - 24 children with IBD significantly different from 161 ± 14 g/L in 12 healthy control children but not different from reference interval of 120 - 180 g/L *2196*

M3/M21 *Serum* *No Effect* In 10 patients with inflammatory bowel disease median concentration of 49.6 U/L compared with that in 40 healthy blood donors in whom the median concentration was 25.2 U/L *2090*

Neopterin *Urine* *Increase* Concentrations increased with active disease and may be used to monitor progress of disease *121*

Nitrate *Serum* *No Effect* Median concentration of 35.1 µmol/L in 19 patients with inflammatory bowel disease not significantly different from 32.8 µmol/L in 20 healthy controls *1277*

Plasminogen *Plasma* *No Effect* In 112 patients with inflammatory bowel disease mean concentration of 106 ± 1.8% compared with 109.9 ± 1.1% in 60 healthy blood donor controls *4948*

Plasminogen Activator Inhibitor-1 *Plasma* *Decrease* In 112 patients with inflammatory bowel disease mean concentration significantly decreased to 8.8 ± 1.1 ng/mL compared with 17.8 ± 1.1 ng/mL in 60 healthy blood donor controls *4948*

Retinol *Serum* *No Effect* Mean concentration of 1.55 ± 0.57 µmol/L in 22 - 24 children with IBD not significantly different from 1.60 ± 0.31 µmol/L in 12 healthy control children but not different from reference interval of 0.66 - 2.69 µmol/L *2196*

Retinol-binding Protein *Serum* *No Effect* Mean concentration of 36 ± 13 mg/L in 22 - 24 children with IBD not significantly different from 36 ± 10 mg/L in 12 healthy control children and reference interval of 30 - 60 mg/L *2196*

Selenium *Serum* *No Effect* Mean concentration of 1.6 ± 0.3 µmol/L in 22 - 24 children with IBD not significantly different from 1.5 ± 0.2 µmol/L in 12 healthy control children and reference interval of 1.28 - 2.35 µmol/L *2196*

Soluble Intercellular Adhesion Molecule-1 *Serum* *Increase* Median concentration of 355 ng/mL in 58 patients with active inflammatory bowel disease significantly higher than 245 ng/mL in 29 healthy controls *3783*

Soluble Interleukin-2 Receptor *Serum* *Increase* Median concentration of 715 U/mL in patients with active inflammatory bowel disease and 645 U/mL in inactive IBD significantly higher than 500 U/mL in 29 healthy controls *3783*

Tissue Plasminogen Activator *Plasma* *No Effect* In 112 patients with inflammatory bowel disease mean concentration of 5.57 ± 0.31 ng/mL compared with 5.13 ± 0.4 ng/mL in 60 healthy blood donor controls *4948*

α-Tocopherol *Serum* *Increase* Mean concentration of 25 ± 9 µmol/L in 22 - 24 children with IBD significantly different from 20 ± 4 µmol/L in 12 healthy control children but not different from reference interval of 9 - 47 µmol/L *2196*

γ-Tocopherol *Serum* *No Effect* Mean concentration of 6 ± 3 µmol/L in 22 - 24 children with IBD not significantly different from 5 ± 2 µmol/L in 12 healthy control children *2196*

α-Tocopherol:Lipids Ratio *Serum* *Increase* Mean concentration of 395 ± 163 µmol/g in 22 - 24 children with IBD significantly different from 325 ± 46 µmol/g in 12 healthy control children but not different from reference interval of > 186 µmol/g *2196*

Trypsin *Serum* *No Effect* Mean concentration of trypsin-like immunoreactivity in 27 patients with inflammatory bowel disease either during active or symptom-free period did not exceed concentration in 85 healthy control individuals (42.78 ± 10.26 ng/mL) *3330*

Urokinase Plasminogen Activator *Plasma* *No Effect* In 112 patients with inflammatory bowel disease mean concentration of 0.49 ± 0.02 ng/mL compared with 0.47 ± 0.014 ng/mL in 60 healthy blood donor controls *4948*

569.90 Non-inflammatory Bowel Disease, Intestinal Inflammation

CD4+ Lymphocytes *Blood* *No Effect* In 11 patients with noninflammatory bowel disease intestinal inflammation mean proportion of T cells of 44.1 ± 3.9% not significantly different from 43.1 ± 2.6% in 22 healthy controls *3753*

CD8+ Lymphocytes *Blood* *No Effect* In 11 patients with noninflammatory bowel disease intestinal inflammation mean proportion of T cells 21.4 ± 3.1% not significantly different from 21.2 ± 0.3% in 22 healthy controls *3753*

Diseases of the Liver, Gallbladder, and Pancreas

570.00 Acute and Subacute Necrosis of the Liver

α_1-Acid Glycoprotein *Serum* *Increase* Sensitivity of 65% and a specificity of 80% with severe liver disease *1439*

Alanine Aminotransferase *Serum* *Increase* Observed effect *3141* Sometimes reaches levels of 2,000 U/L. Activity falls slowly reaching normal levels in about 2 - 3 months, unless complications occur *5544* Mean activity of 199 ± 78 U/L observed in 3 patients with acute liver necrosis compared with < 40 U/L in 27 healthy controls *3793* Levels are higher in acute hepatitis than in obstructive jaundice *1025* Peak values between 200 and 1,500 U/L are typical *2033* Sometimes reaches levels of 2,000 U/L. Activity falls slowly reaching normal levels in about 2 - 3 months, unless complications occur *1642* A marked increase occurs which is relatively higher than the rise in AST. The level is raised in nonicteric attacks. In liver disease results of ALT and sorbitol dehydrogenase run parallel with AST results *1290*

Albumin *Serum* *Decrease* Mean concentration of 29 ± 2 g/L observed in 3 patients with acute liver necrosis compared with 42 ± 1.0 g/L in 27 healthy controls *3793*
Serum *No Effect* Concentration usually normal *5544*

Aldolase *Serum* *Increase* Cell destruction. Normal or may be slightly increased *5544*
Serum *No Effect* Normal or may be slightly increased *5544*

Alkaline Phosphatase *Serum* *Increase* Higher in obstructive jaundice than in acute hepatitis. The basis for elevation in patients with hepatobiliary disease is obscure. Increased formation by hepatic parenchymal or ductal cells, perhaps supplemented by impaired excretion, is the apparent mechanism *1025* With jaundice *390* Up to 16 U/L *5544* Mean activity of 639 ± 177 U/L observed in 3 patients with acute liver necrosis compared with 151 ± 20 U/L in 27 healthy controls *3793* Up to 16 U/L *1642* Most commonly between 65 and 160 U/L *1290* With jaundice *2124* Incidence of elevation is 80 - 100%; usual range 25 - 80 U/L *1025*
White Blood Cells *Increase* Markedly increased; may remain increased for years after jaundice has disappeared *5544*

Amino Acids *Cerebrospinal Fluid* *Increase* In massive liver necrosis the amount present in CSF is proportional to the degree of liver damage *1290*
Plasma *Increase* In acute yellow atrophy, the plasma concentration is roughly proportional to the degree of liver damage. Methionine and tyrosine show the highest increase *1290*
Urine *Increase* In massive liver necrosis the amount present in urine is proportional to the degree of liver damage *4707*

Ammonia *Blood* *Increase* In acute hepatic necrosis and cirrhosis; may increase after portacaval anastomosis *5544*

Amylase *Serum* *Decrease* Decrease possible due to liver damage *1290*

Antithrombin III *Plasma* *Decrease* Decreased in parenchymatous liver disease *3472* *5220*

α_1-Antitrypsin *Serum* *No Effect* Concentration usually normal *5544*

Aspartate Aminotransferase *Serum* *Increase* In liver diseases, may be 10 - 100 times normal and remain elevated for long periods of time *1642* *1290* Higher in acute hepatitis than in obstructive jaundice *1025* Mean elevation in 17 cases of hepatitis was 36.5 times the normal upper limit (24 U/L). All patients showed elevation, mean of 766 U/L *3161*

Bilirubin *Serum* *Increase* Rarely exceeds 15 - 20 mg/dL *2039* May be > 30 mg/dL *5544* Mean activity of 156 ± 105 µmol/L observed in 3 patients with acute liver necrosis compared with 9.4 ± 0.8 µmol/L in 27 healthy controls *3793*
Urine *Increase* May precede the onset of jaundice by several days *2039*

Bilirubin, Direct *Serum* *Increase* Normal or slight increase (< 15% of total) *5544*

BSP Retention *Serum* *Increase* Commonly observed *2033*
Serum *No Effect* In patients with ascites, BSP dye may be lost into abdomen. Results may falsely appear normal *5544*

CA 19-9 *Serum* *Increase* Positive analyses have been encountered *3657* *2026*

570.00 Acute and Subacute Necrosis of the Liver *(continued)*

Carcinoembryonic Antigen *Serum* *Increase* Found in 50% of 16 patients with acute liver damage. Levels increased with increasing clinical severity. In acute damage, peak CEA occurs later than the time of maximum liver necrosis, suggesting that the rise is associated with regeneration. Higher levels occur in those patients with greater disturbance of liver function suggesting altered metabolism or excretion of CEA *628*

Cholesterol *Red Blood Cells* *Increase* An increase was detected in most patients with hepatocellular disease or cholestatic jaundice but the alteration in RBC lipid content did not correlate with RBC survival *4201* 25 - 50% increase in the membrane concentration, resulting in the characteristic target cell *5699*
Serum *Decrease* Due to severe liver damage *1290* Mean concentration of 2.4 ± 0.4 mmol/L observed in 3 patients with acute liver necrosis compared with 5.9 ± 0.2 mmol/L in 27 healthy controls *3793*
Serum *Increase* Greater elevations are more characteristic of hepatocanalicular jaundice (intrahepatic cholestasis) than of posthepatic jaundice *1025* In patients with obstructive jaundice or intrahepatic cholestasis concentration is usually elevated to 250 - 500 mg/dL; greater elevations occur occasionally *1025* *1290*

Cholinesterase *Serum* *Decrease* Depression of enzyme concentration tends to be more marked in patients ill with chronic liver disease, such as cirrhosis, than in those ill with acute conditions, such as viral hepatitis, ascending cholangitis, and acute anoxic hepatomegaly. Peaks and depressions in cholinesterase activity in acute liver disease are related to the extent of hepatic parenchymal damage *5498*

Coproporphyrin *Urine* *Increase* In liver disease, coproporphyrinuria may not indicate increased formation of the pigment, but rather its diversion from bile to urine *367*

Creatine Kinase *Serum* *No Effect* Activity usually within normal limits *5544*

Erythrocyte Survival *Red Blood Cells* *Decrease* Decreased survival; mild to moderate hemolysis *4199*

Erythrocytes *Urine* *Increase* In a few patients, slight hematuria *2033*

Estrogens *Urine* *Increase* Observed effect *5544*

Ferritin *Serum* *Increase* Increased in acute hepatitis. Exceeded the upper limit of the normal values in most cases *5883* Increased in acute hepatocellular damage due to acetaminophen overdosage *1287*

α-Fetoprotein *Serum* *Increase* 10 - 20% of nonmalignant liver diseases of all types have elevated serum levels, which tend to be fluctuating or transient. Steady or rising levels indicate malignancy *5759* Increased in hepatitis, especially in infants (when levels exceed 40 ng/mL) *1290* Up to 40% of patients with massive hepatic necrosis *4891* Reported effect *75*

Fibrin Degradation Products *Plasma* *Increase* Patients with severe acute hepatic necrosis may have findings compatible with intravascular coagulation, thrombocytopenia and increased levels of fibrinogen/fibrin degradation products *2161* Reported effect *5677*

Fibrinogen *Plasma* *Decrease* Formation is depressed in liver failure, resulting in decreased plasma levels *1290*
Plasma *Increase* Patients with severe acute hepatic necrosis may have findings compatible with intravascular coagulation, thrombocytopenia and increased levels of fibrinogen/fibrin degradation products *2161*

Folate *Serum* *Decrease* Decreased in some cases of liver disease due to inadequate intake *5544*

α_1-Globulin *Serum* *Decrease* Tend to be low in hepatocellular disease falling in parallel with serum albumin *5189*

α_2-Globulin *Serum* *Decrease* α- and β-globulins decrease when hepatocellular failure impairs their synthesis *367*
Serum *Increase* If the necrosis is not too extensive there may be a slight increase *1290*

β-Globulin *Serum* *Decrease* α- and β-globulins decrease when hepatocellular failure impairs their synthesis *367*

γ-Globulin *Serum* *Increase* Mildly elevated due to increased γ-globulin *2033*

Glucose *Serum* *Decrease* Observed effect *1290* Lowered levels result from massive hepatic necrosis or a deficiency of enzymes necessary for glycogenolysis *367* Diffuse severe disease - primary or metastatic tumor *5544*

Glucose Tolerance *Serum* *Decrease* Decreased tolerance:excessive peak-decreased formation of glycogen with low fasting levels and subsequent hypoglycemia *5544* Decreased because of inability to form glycogen from administered glucose *1290*

β-Glucuronidase *Serum* *Decrease* Decreased *1777* *1498*

γ-Glutamyltransferase *Serum* *Increase* Mean activity of 198 ± 2 U/L observed in 3 patients with acute liver necrosis compared with < 50 U/L in 27 healthy controls *3793* In acute hepatitis, elevation is less marked than that of other liver enzymes, but it is the last to return to normal *5544* The estimation may be useful in monitoring duration of the disease, since raised activity persists longer than do ALT or AST activities *1290* Observed effect *1025*

Haptoglobin *Serum* *Decrease* Mild to moderate hemolysis usually occurs *4199*

Hematocrit *Blood* *Decrease* Mild to moderate hemolysis usually occurs *4199*
Blood *No Effect* Anemia is not a feature *2033*

Hemoglobin *Blood* *Decrease* Mild to moderate hemolysis usually occurs *4199*
Blood *No Effect* Anemia is not a feature *2033*
Plasma *Increase* Mild to moderate hemolysis usually occurs *4199*

Hepatitis B Surface Antigen *Serum* *Increase* 31 of 59 patients with acute uncomplicated hepatitis had detectable hepatitis B antigen *790*

Heterophile Antibody *Serum* *Increase* May be positive but guinea pig kidney cell absorption removes the antibody *2033*

β-Hexosaminidase *Serum* *Increase* Increase in total concentration (hexosaminidase A and B) *3850*

5-Hydroxytryptamine *Plasma* *No Effect* Reported effect *492*

^{131}I Uptake *Serum* *Increase* In hepatic disease *4707*

immunoglobulin A *Serum* *Increase* Slightly increased or normal *2033*

Immunoglobulin M *Serum* *Increase* Reported effect *1290*

Iron *Serum* *Increase* High serum concentrations, more than can be explained by high ferritin levels are found in acute hepatitis *5883* In acute hepatitis the serum iron level is increased, presumably due to the liberation of stored iron from necrosing liver cells *1290* The degree of increase parallels the amount of hepatic necrosis *5544*

Iron-binding Capacity, Total *Serum* *Increase* May be increased with hepatitis *5544*

Lactate Dehydrogenase *Serum* *Increase* Total LD is increased in 50% of the cases. Relatively slight elevations or not at all *1025* *1642* Occasionally increased *2034* Characteristically observed *2257*

Lactate Dehydrogenase Isoenzyme-5 *Serum* *Increase* Most marked increase, which occurs during prodromal stage and is greatest at time of onset of jaundice *5544* Present in increased amounts *1290*

Lactate Dehydrogenase Isoenzymes *Serum* *Increase* Increase attributable to LD_4 and LD_5 *1642* Most marked increase is of LD_5, which occurs during prodromal stage and is greatest at time of onset of jaundice *5544*

Lecithin *Red Blood Cells* *Increase* 25 - 50% increase in the membrane concentration, resulting in the characteristic target cell *5699*

Leucine Aminopeptidase *Serum* *Increase* Moderately increased *1290*

Leukocytes *Blood* *Decrease* Mild leukopenia *2033* WBC is normal or low during acute hepatitis and leukopenia may be observed *2039*
Blood *Increase* Up to 50,000 /μL with massive necrosis *5544*

Lipase *Serum* *Decrease* Lack of bile salts results in the failure to activate pancreatic lipase in the intestinal lumen *4707*

Lipids *Serum* *Increase* Increased in acute hepatitis *1290*

Lymphocytes *Blood* *Decrease* Transient *2033*
Blood *Increase* Relative lymphocytosis *2033* Atypical lymphocytes varying between 2 - 20% are common during the acute phase *2033*

Magnesium *Serum* *Increase* Pathological increase in serum with liver disease *1290*

Neutrophils *Blood* *Decrease* Transient *2033*
Blood *Increase* May be associated with a moderate to severe neutrophilia *5677*

N-Formiminoglutamic Acid *Urine* *Increase* Reported effect *5544*

Nitrogen *Serum* *Decrease* Reduction of total nitogen observed *1290*

5'-Nucleotidase *Serum* *Increase* Increased (although low levels have been reported with very severe liver damage), especially if intrahepatic cholestasis present *1290*

Ornithine Carbamoyltransferase *Serum* *Increase* Liver cell damage *5544*

Phospholipids *Red Blood Cells* *Increase* An increase in RBC phospholipid was detected in most patients with hepatocellular disease or cholestatic jaundice but the alteration in RBC lipid content did not correlate with RBC survival *4201*

Plasminogen Antigen *Plasma* *Decrease* With massive necrosis *3141*

Platelets *Blood* *Decrease* Patients with severe acute hepatic necrosis may have findings compatible with intravascular coagulation, thrombocytopenia and increased levels of fibrinogen/fibrin degradation products *2161*

Protein *Urine* *Increase* In a few patients minimal proteinuria *2033*

Prothrombin Time *Plasma* *Increase* Increased time indicates degree of parenchymal damage; marked prolongation (> 20 sec) is an early reflection of massive necrosis *367* Due to poor fat absorption *5544*

Pyruvate *Blood* *Increase* Very advanced liver stage *1290*

Reticulocytes *Blood* *Increase* Mild *2033*

Somatomedin *Plasma* *Decrease* Observed effect *3141*

Sulfate *Urine* *Decrease* Patients with liver disease often have reduced urinary sulfate *4707*

Thromboplastin Time *Plasma* *Increase* Mean activity of 0.36 ± 0.08 observed in 3 patients with acute liver necrosis compared with 0.70 - 1.30 in 27 healthy controls *3793*

Triglycerides *Serum* *Decrease* Mean concentration of 0.8 ± 0.1 mmol/L observed in 3 patients with acute liver necrosis compared with 1.1 ± 0.1 mmol/L in 27 healthy controls *3793*

Tyrosine Crystals *Urine* *Increase* Acute yellow atrophy *5544*

Urea Nitrogen *Serum* *Decrease* Abnormally low levels have been attributed to liver failure. This is not a rare finding today and its significance should not be overlooked. Values of 5 mg/dL or less observed in 1% of 16,000 determinations *1627*

Urobilinogen *Urine* *Increase* Early hepatitis (usually the first 48 h, but it may persist for 1 - 2 days longer in some cases). Also in hepatic necrosis *1290* May precede the onset of jaundice by several days *2039*

Vitamin B_{12} *Serum* *Increase* The blood level may be 3 - 8 times the normal concentration. Predominantly the free form is increased *1290*

Xylose Tolerance Test *Urine* *Abnormal* In patients with ascites, the urine excretion is low *5544*

Zinc *Serum* *Decrease* Found to be low in patients with hepatitis *2038*

570.00 Acute Hepatitis

Alcohol Dehydrogenase *Serum* *Increase* In 40 Nigerians with hepatitis mean activity of 4.3 ± 1.0 U/L significantly different from 0.7 ± 0.1 U/L in 120 healthy controls *3866*

Alkaline Phosphatase *Serum* *Increase* In 12 patients with acute hepatitis 92% had activities above 112 U/L *1406*

Aspartate Aminotransferase *Serum* *Increase* In 12 patients with acute hepatitis 100% had activities above 40 U/L *1406*

Bilirubin *Serum* *Increase* In 12 patients with acute hepatitis 100% had concentrations above 26 µmol/mL *1406*

CA 19-9 *Serum* *Increase* In 12 patients with acute hepatitis 100% had concentrations above 35 U/mL *1406*

Cholinesterase *Serum* *Decrease* In 12 patients with acute hepatitis 64% had activities less than 4,000 U/L *1406*

C-Reactive Protein *Serum* *Increase* In 12 patients with acute hepatitis 67% had concentrations above 5 mg/L *1406*

α-Fetoprotein *Serum* *No Effect* In 12 patients with acute hepatitis none had concentrations above 30 µg/L *1406*

Gelsolin *Serum* *Decrease* In 14 patients with early acute hepatitis mean concentration of 80 ± 40 µg/mL compared with 226 ± 52 µg/mL in 43 healthy individuals but concentration returned to normal as the disease resolved *2362*

α_1-Globulin *Serum* *Decrease* Concentration may be decreased in patients with acute viral hepatitis *4617*

γ-Glutamyltransferase *Serum* *Increase* In 12 patients with acute hepatitis 100% had activities above 55 U/L *1406*

Multiubiquitin Chains *Serum* *Increase* In 30 specimens from 7 patients with acute viral hepatitis mean concentration of 9.62 ± 4.58 µg/cells in 1 L blood significantly different from that in 45 healthy men and 51 healthy women) in whom the mean concentration was 3.86 ± 1.56 µg/cells from 1 liter of blood) *5125*

Neopterin *Serum* *Increase* Highest concentrations in people with liver disease observed in those with acute liver hepatitis with good correlation with liver function tests *997*

Prothrombin Time *Plasma* *Increase* Prolongation of the prothrombin time usually indicates that the disease is a chronic one, such as advanced cirrhosis: if it increases in acute liver disease it usually indicates the disease is a fulminant one, as in acute viral hepatitis *4617*

Soluble E-Selectin *Serum* *Increase* In 12 patients with acute hepatitis 33% had concentrations above 86 µg/L *1406*

Soluble Intercellular Adhesion Molecule-1 *Serum* *Increase* In 12 patients with acute hepatitis, 100% had concentrations above 286 µg/L *1406*

Soluble Vascular Cell Adhesion Molecule-1 *Serum* *Increase* In 12 patients with acute hepatitis 100% had concentrations above 872 µg/L *1406*

Ubiquitin, Free *Blood* *No Effect* In 30 specimens from 7 patients with acute viral hepatitis mean concentration of 133 ± 57.2 µg/cells in 1 L blood not significantly different from that in 45 healthy men and 51 healthy women in whom the mean concentration was 126 ± 24.4 µg/cells from 1 liter of blood *5125*

Urea Nitrogen *Serum* *Increase* In 12 patients with acute hepatitis 25% had concentrations above 8.6 mmol/mL *1406*

Zinc *Urine* *Increase* Excretion enhanced as a consequence of rapid cellular turnover resulting in moderate zincuria *5174*

570.00 Chronic End-stage Liver Disease

Cholestanol *Serum* *Increase* Marked increase in liver and serum concentrationsn not seen for other sterols *3794*

Lipoic Acid *Liver* *Decrease* Concentration in the liver of 41 patients with end-stage liver disease of 97 ± 48 ng/mg protein significantly less than that in 11 healthy individuals of 198 ± 61 ng/mg protein *253*

570.00 Drug-induced Liver Disease

Albumin *Serum* *Decrease* In 6 patients mean concentration of 41 ± 6 g/L different from normal range of 42 - 52 g/L *1371*

Anti-Mitochondrial M6 Antibody *Serum* *Increase* May be present in some patients with drug-induced hepatitis *1778*

Aspartate Aminotransferase *Serum* *Increase* In 6 patients mean activity of 0.8 ± 0.5 µkat/L different from normal range of < 0.6 µkat/L *1371*

Bilirubin *Serum* *Increase* In 6 patients mean concentration of 59 ± 118 µmol/L different from normal range of 4 - 21 µmol/L *1371*

Galactose Tolerance *Patient* *No Effect* In 6 patients mean mean $T_{1/2}$ 14 ± 0 min not different from normal range of < 17 min *1371*

Hyaluronic Acid *Serum* *Increase* Twenty patients with acetaminophen-induced acute liver damage of varying severity were studied. HYA rose rapidly with clinical deterioration to reach a median value of 27,510 µg/L, 7 days post-ingestion, which was significantly higher ($p < 0.005$) than in patients ($n = 7$) who exhibited only marked derangement of liver function tests without evidence of encephalopathy, HYA median value of 3,240 µg/L *560*

571.00 Alcoholic Fatty Liver

Alanine Aminotransferase *Serum Increase* In 15 patients with alcoholic fatty liver mean activity of 69 ± 3 U/L increased compared with 20 ± 2 U/L in 30 healthy controls *2269*

Albumin *Serum No Effect* In 15 patients with alcoholic fatty liver mean concentration of 4.6 ± 0.2 g/dL not significantly different when compared with 4.9 ± 0.1 g/dL in 30 healthy controls *2269*

Aspartate Aminotransferase *Serum Increase* In 15 patients with alcoholic fatty liver mean activity of 66 ± 4 U/L increased compared with 23 ± 1 U/L in 30 healthy controls *2269*

Bilirubin *Serum Increase* In 15 patients with alcoholic fatty liver mean concentration of 1.3 ± 0.1 mg/dL increased compared with 0.6 ± 0.1 mg/dL in 30 healthy controls *2269*

Cholesterol *Liver No Effect* In 12 patients with alcoholic fatty liver mean concentration of 4.1 ± 1.6 μmol/g in specimens obtained at autopsy not significantly higher than 3.8 ± 1.3 μmol/g in 9 control specimens from nonalcoholics *194*

Globulin *Serum No Effect* In 15 patients with alcoholic fatty liver mean concentration of 2.9 ± 0.1 g/dL not significantly different when compared with 2.8 ± 0.1 g/dL in 30 healthy controls *2269*

7α-Hydroperoxycholest-5-en-3β-ol *Liver Increase* In 12 patients with alcoholic fatty liver mean concentration of 12.4 ± 7.1 nmol/g in specimens obtained at autopsy significantly higher than 1.2 ± 1.7 nmol/g in 9 control specimens from nonalcoholics *194*

7β-Hydroperoxycholest-5-en-3β-ol *Liver Increase* In 12 patients with alcoholic fatty liver mean concentration of 25.0 ± 14.0 nmol/g in specimens obtained at autopsy significantly higher than 2.0 ± 3.3 nmol/g in 9 control specimens from nonalcoholics *194*

7α-Hydroperoxycholest-5-en-3β-ol:Cholesterol Ratio *Liver Increase* In 12 patients with alcoholic fatty liver mean ratio of 0.33 ± 0.20 (nmol/g:μmol/g) in specimens obtained at autopsy significantly different from 0.027 ± 0.029 in 9 control specimens from nonalcoholics *194*

7β-Hydroperoxycholest-5-en-3β-ol:Cholesterol Ratio *Liver Increase* In 12 patients with alcoholic fatty liver mean ratio of 0.71 ± 0.43 (nmol/g:μmol/g) in specimens obtained at autopsy significantly different from 0.045 ± 0.054 in 9 control specimens from nonalcoholics *194*

571.10 Alcoholic Hepatitis

Alanine Aminotransferase *Serum Increase* Mean activity on admission to hospital of 62 ± 7 U/L in 20 patients with alcoholic hepatitis higher than 10 - 28 U/L in normal individuals *2156* In 32 patients with alcoholic hepatitis mean activity of 156 ± 6 U/L increased compared with 20 ± 2 U/L in 30 healthy controls *2269*

Albumin *Serum Decrease* In 32 patients with alcoholic hepatitis mean concentration of 4.2 ± 0.2 g/dL decreased compared with 4.8 ± 0.1 g/dL in 30 healthy controls *2269*

Aspartate Aminotransferase *Serum Increase* Diagnosis made on clinical grounds with AST activity less than 300 to 500 U/L *3625* In 32 patients with alcoholic hepatitis mean activity of 225 ± 8 U/L increased compared with 23 ± 1 U/L in 30 healthy controls *2269* Mean activity on admission to hospital of 146 ± 15 U/L in 20 patients with alcoholic hepatitis higher than 107 ± 15 U/L in normal individuals *2156*

Aspartate Aminotransferase:Alanine Aminotransferase Ratio *Serum Increase* Diagnosis made on clinical grounds with AST:ALT ratio usually greater than 2 *3625*

Bilirubin *Serum Increase* In 32 patients with alcoholic hepatitis mean concentration of 3.7 ± 0.1 mg/dL increased compared with 0.6 ± 0.2 mg/dL in 30 healthy controls *2269*

C-Reactive Protein *Serum Increase* Mean concentration of 48 mg/L observed in 59 survivors of acute alcoholic hepatitis and 49 mg/L in 13 nonsurvivors *1923*

Globulin *Serum Increase* In 32 patients with alcoholic hepatitis mean concentration of 3.1 ± 0.1 g/dL increased compared with 2.8 ± 0.1 g/dL in 30 healthy controls *2269*

Hyaluronan *Serum Increase* Mean concentration on admission to hospital of 542 ± 31 ng/mL in 20 patients with alcoholic hepatitis significantly higher than normal of 10 - 100 ng/mL *2156*

Interleukin-1α *Serum Increase* Mean cytokine concentrations were elevated in cirrhotic patients and alcoholic hepatitis patients compared with controls and alcoholic patients without liver disease. IL-1α concentrations remained elevated for up to 6 mo after diagnosis of alcoholic hepatitis *2667*

Interleukin-6 *Serum Increase* Plasma levels of interleukin-6 (IL-6) were assayed in 96 samples from 58 patients with severe alcoholic hepatitis, and 69 patients in control groups (21 normal, 10 alcoholic without liver disease, 10 inactive alcoholic cirrhosis, 18 chronic liver disease, 10 chronic renal failure). Plasma IL-6 levels were markedly elevated in patients with alcoholic hepatitis when compared with all control groups (p less than 0.001) *4779* Evaluated serial plasma interleukin-6 levels in 30 consecutive patients with moderate to severe alcoholic hepatitis. Mean admission plasma interleukin-6 activity was markedly increased (49.8 ± 8.5 U/mL, normal less than 5 U/mL) in patients with alcoholic hepatitis, and levels decreased with clinical improvement to 15.6 ± 6.1 U/mL at 6 months *2157* Mean cytokine concentrations were elevated in cirrhotic patients and alcoholic hepatitis patients compared with controls and alcoholic patients without liver disease. Interleukin-6 normalized in parallel with clinical recovery *2667*

Interleukin-8 *Serum Increase* Serial plasma interleukin-8 concentrations were measured in 40 consecutive patients with moderate-to-severe alcoholic hepatitis over a 6-mo period. Two control groups included 10 patients without clinically important liver disease admitted for treatment of alcohol dependence and 12 healthy male volunteers. The mean plasma interleukin-8 level on admission was markedly increased: 695 ± 146 pg/mL in the alcoholic hepatitis patients. The alcohol-dependent control group and the normal volunteer controls had mean interleukin-8 concentrations of 106 ± 28 pg/mL and 10 ± 5 pg/mL, respectively *2158*

International Normalized Ratio *Plasma Increase* In 32 patients with alcoholic hepatitis mean ratio of 1.6 ± 0.1 increased compared with reference range of < 1.2 *2269*

Leukocytes *Blood No Effect* Mean concentration on admission to hospital of 9.8 ± 0.9 x 10^3/μL in 20 patients with alcoholic hepatitis not significantly different from 4.8 - 10.8 x 10^3/μL in normal individuals *2156*

Neopterin *Serum Increase* Mean concentration of 8.35 nmol/L in chronic alcoholics with hepatitis significantly higher than in 12 healthy controls *1808*

Neutrophils *Blood Increase* In 30 patients with alcoholic cirrhosis mean concentration of 5.8 ± 0.3 x 10^3/μL different when compared with 3.7 ± 0.1 x 10^3/μL in 30 healthy controls *2269* In 32 patients with alcoholic hepatitis mean concentration of 7.1 ± 0.3 x 10^3/μL different when compared with 3.7 ± 0.1 x 10^3/μL in 30 healthy controls *2269*
Serum No Effect Mean concentration on admission to hospital of 6.8 ± 0.9 x 10^3/μL in 20 patients with alcoholic hepatitis not significantly different from 1.4 - 6.5 x 10^3/μL in normal individuals *2156*

Prothrombin Time *Plasma Increase* Prolongation of the prothrombin time usually indicates that the disease is a chronic one, such as advanced cirrhosis: if it increases in acute liver disease it usually indicates the disease is a fulminant one, as in severe alcoholic hepatitis *4617* Increased time suggests deteriorating liver function in patients with alcoholic hepatitis *5276*

Soluble Intercellular Adhesion Molecule-1 *Serum Increase* Mean concentration on admission to hospital of 488 ± 70 ng/mL in 20 patients with alcoholic hepatitis significantly higher than normal of 100 - 200 ng/mL *2156*

Tumor Necrosis Factor-α *Serum Increase* Mean cytokine concentrations were elevated in cirrhotic patients and alcoholic hepatitis patients compared with controls and alcoholic patients without liver disease. Tumor necrosis factor-α concentrations remained elevated for up to 6 mo after diagnosis of alcoholic hepatitis *2667*

571.20 Alcoholic Hepatic Fibrosis

Multiubiquitin Chains *Serum No Effect* In 11 patients with alcoholic hepatic fibrosis mean concentration of 3.0 ± 0.7 ng/mL not significantly different from 4.1 ± 1.7 ng/mL in 10 healthy controls *5126*

Ubiquitin, Free *Serum* *No Effect* In 11 patients with alcoholic hepatic fibrosis mean concentration of 34.8 ± 16.3 ng/mL not significantly different from 29.6 ± 6.6 ng/mL in 10 healthy controls *5126*

571.20 Alcoholic Liver Disease

Alanine Aminotransferase *Serum* *Increase* In 9 patients with alcoholic liver disease median activity of 59 U/L compared with 34 U/L in 13 patients with alcoholism and 26 U/L in 8 healthy controls *4146*

Albumin *Serum* *Decrease* In 9 patients with alcoholic liver disease median concentration of 3.1 g/dL compared with 4.1 g/dL in 13 patients with alcoholism and 4.7 g/dL in 8 healthy controls *4146*
Serum *No Effect* In 11 patients mean concentration of 46 ± 3 g/L not different from normal range of 42 - 52 g/L *1371*

Amylase *Serum* *Increase* In 12 patients with alcoholic liver disease mean activity of 55.6 ± 4.8 U/L significantly increased compared with 37.0 ± 3.0 U/L in 21 healthy controls *1086*

Amylase, Pancreatic Isoenzyme *Serum* *No Effect* Mean activity in 12 patients with alcoholic liver disease 21.7 ± 2.0 U/L not significantly different from 19.0 ± 1.7 U/L in 21 healthy controls *1086*

Amylase, Salivary Isoenzyme *Serum* *Increase* In 12 patients with alcoholic liver disease mean activity of 33.9 ± 4.4 U/L significantly greater than 17.9 ± 2.0 U/L in 21 healthy controls *1086* In patients with alcoholic liver disease significant increase observed but not observed in chronic alcohol misusers in relapse or remission *1086*

Apolipoprotein A-I *Serum* *Increase* Concentrations are increased with alcoholic steatosis to a greater extent than wirh established cirrhosis *1778*

Aspartate Aminotransferase *Serum* *Increase* In 9 patients with alcoholic liver disease median activity of 59 U/L compared with 29 U/L in 13 patients with alcoholism and 26 U/L in 8 healthy controls *4146* In 11 patients mean activity of 1.1 ± 1.0 µkat/L different from normal range of < 0.6 µkat/L *1371* Ratio greater than 2.0 with AST activity not exceeding 200 U/L (normal < 40 U/L) is suggestive of alcoholic liver disease *4617*

Aspartate Aminotransferase:Alanine Aminotransferase Ratio *Serum* *Increase* Ratio greater than 2.0 with AST activity not exceeding 200 U/L (normal < 40 U/L) is suggestive of alcoholic liver disease *4617* Ratio of > 2:1 characteristic of alcoholic liver disease *1778*

Bilirubin *Serum* *No Effect* In 11 patients mean concentration of 14 ± 5 µmol/L not different from normal range of 4 - 21 µmol/L *1371*

Cholesterol *Serum* *Decrease* Concentrations are usually normal but may fall as liver damage becomes so severe as to reduce the synthesis of lecithin cholesterol acyltransferase activity *1778* In 9 patients with alcoholic liver disease median concentration of 3.3 mmol/L compared with 4.9 mmol/L in 8 healthy controls *4146*
Serum *No Effect* Concentrations are usually normal but may fall as liver damage becomes so severe as to reduce the synthesis of lecithin cholesterol acyltransferase activity *1778*

β-Chorionic Gonadotropin *Plasma* *Increase* Mean concentration increased from 63 ng/mL in mild cases with fibrosis to 80 ng/mL in severe cases above upper limit of normal of about 78 ng/mL *5315*

Coproporphyrin *Urine* *Increase* Excretion of coproporphyrins increased *1778*

Erythrocyte Sedimentation Rate *Blood* *Increase* Rate increased *1778*

Erythrocytes *Blood* *Decrease* In 9 patients with alcoholic liver disease median concentration of 3.7 x 10^6/µL compared with 4.7 x 10^6/µL in 13 patients with alcoholism and 4.6 x 10^6/µL in 8 healthy controls *4146*

Ferritin *Serum* *Increase* Concentrations often increased with alcoholic liver disease, either as part of an acute phase response or release from damaged hepatocytes, but not to the same extent as with iron overload *1778* Plasma concentration may be increased but not to the same extent as in hemochromatosis *5276*

Folate *Serum* *Decrease* May be decreased alone or with Vitamin B_{12} *1778*

Galactose Tolerance *Patient* *No Effect* In 11 patients mean $T_{1/2}$ of 14 ± 2 min not different from normal range of < 17 min *1371*

γ-Glutamyltransferase *Serum* *Increase* Activity increased out of proportion to other hepatic enzymes *1778* In 9 patients with alcoholic liver disease median activity of 263 U/L compared with 66 U/L in 13 patients with alcoholism and 23 U/L in 8 healthy controls *4146*

HDL-Cholesterol *Serum* *Increase* Concentration increased *1778*

Hyaluronan *Serum* *No Effect* Concentration ranged from 14 - 78 µg/L in patients with alcoholic liver disease within reference range of 10 - 100 µg/L *3072*

Hyaluronic Acid *Serum* *Increase* 62 patients with alcoholic liver disease were evaluated. All but six patients had elevated serum levels *1725*

5-Hydroxytryptophol *Urine* *Increase* Excretion increased so that ratio of 5-hydroxytryptophol to 5-hydroxyindoleacetic acid in urine collected 12 hours after drinking in a dose dependent manner in both alcohol misusers and healthy volunteers *1778*

immunoglobulin A *Serum* *Increase* Concentration increased *1778*

Immunoglobulin G *Serum* *Increase* Concentration may be slightly increased *1778*

Immunoglobulin M *Serum* *No Effect* Concentration usually normal *1778*

6-Keto-Prostaglandin $F_{1\alpha}$ *Plasma* *No Effect* In 9 patients with alcoholic liver disease median concentration of 63.5 pg/mL compared with 71.2 pg/mL in 13 patients with alcoholism and 67.0 pg/mL in 8 healthy controls *4146*

Laminin *Serum* *Increase* Mean concentration increased to about 135 ng/mL in mild cases with fibrosis to 200 ng/mL in severe cases, greater than upper limit of 140 ng/mL *5315*

MCV *Blood* *Increase* In 9 patients with alcoholic liver disease median MCV of 98 fL compared with 92 fL in 13 patients with alcoholism and 91 fL in 8 healthy controls *4146* Volume increased *1778*

Neopterin *Serum* *Increase* In 30 patients with alcoholic liver disease mean concentration of 14.8 ± 5.1 nmol/L, with mean in 7 without cirrhosis of 11.4 ± 3.0 nmol/L and 15.5 ± 6.2 nmol/L in 23 with cirrhosis different from 6.0 ± 2.2 nmol/L in healthy controls *5682*

Platelets *Blood* *Decrease* In 9 patients with alcoholic liver disease median count of 137 x 10^3 /µL compared with 250 x 10^3 /µL in 13 patients with alcoholism and 255 x 10^3 /µL in 8 healthy controls *4146*

Procollagen Type III Peptide *Serum* *Increase* Increased concentration was useful in assessing extent of hepatic fibrosis *5276* Mean concentration increased to about 13 ng/mL in mild cases with fibrosis to 16 ng/mL in severe cases, greater than upper limit of 12 ng/mL *5315*

Triglycerides *Serum* *Increase* Median concentration of 1.7 mmol/L in 13 patients with alcoholism and 0.9 mmol/L in 8 healthy controls *4146* Increased in fasting state *1778*
Serum *No Effect* In 9 patients with alcoholic liver disease median concentration of 1.1 mmol/L compared with 0.9 mmol/L in 8 healthy controls *4146*

Type IV Collagen 7S Domain *Serum* *Increase* Mean concentration increased to about 4.6 ng/mL in mild cases with fibrosis to 8.2 ng/mL in severe cases, greater than upper limit of 4.4 ng/mL *5315*

Type IV Collagen, Triple-helix Domain *Serum* *Increase* Mean concentration increased to about 110 ng/mL in mild cases with fibrosis to 270 ng/mL in severe cases, greater than upper limit of 90 ng/mL *5315*

Vitamin B_{12} *Serum* *Decrease* May be decreased alone or with folate *1778*

571.20 Laennec's or Alcoholic Cirrhosis

Acid-soluble Carnitine, Total *Serum* *No Effect* In 15 patients with alcoholic cirrhosis mean concentration of 35.1 ± 27.5 µmol/L not significantly different from 28.0 ± 16.7 µmol/L in 28 healthy volunteer controls *2810*

Acylcarnitine *Serum* *No Effect* Unchanged plasma concentration observed in patients with alcohol-induced liver cirrhosis compared with healthy controls *2809*

571.20 Laennec's or Alcoholic Cirrhosis *(continued)*

Acylcarnitine, Long Chain *Serum Increase* Significantly increased plasma concentration observed in patients with alcohol-induced liver cirrhosis compared with healthy controls *2809*

Acylcarnitine, Short Chain *Serum Increase* In 15 patients with alcoholic liver cirrhosis mean concentration of 18.8 ± 14.1 µmol/L not significantly different from 12.7 ± 6.8 µmol/L in 28 healthy volunteer controls *2810* Significantly increased plasma concentration observed in patients with alcohol-induced liver cirrhosis compared with healthy controls *2809*

Alanine Aminotransferase *Serum Increase* Ranged from 20 - 258 U/L (maximum normal limit 35 U/L) *5738* In 30 patients with alcoholic cirrhosis mean activity of 73 ± 5 U/L increased compared with 20 ± 2 U/L in 30 healthy controls *2269* Usually much lower than the AST *2039*
Serum No Effect Normal in most cases of portal cirrhosis *5008*

Albumin *Serum Decrease* In 95 patients, there was a significant decrease in mean albumin concentration, increase in mean γ-globulins, while mean α- and β-globulins were normal. Characteristic electrophoresis pattern revealed a lack of demarcation between β and γ peaks (β-γ bridging) *5082* In 30 patients with alcoholic cirrhosis mean concentration of 3.5 ± 0.3 g/dL decreased compared with 4.8 ± 0.1 g/dL in 30 healthy controls *2269* Decreased concentration observed with decreased plasma concentration of carnitine in 14 of 36 patients with alcohol-induced liver cirrhosis *2809* In 36 postmenopausal women with alcoholic cirrhosis mean concentration of 30 ± 1 g/L significantly different from 47 ± 1 g/L in 27 alcohol abstaining postmenopausal women *1675*
Serum No Effect In 6 alcoholic patients with liver cirrhosis mean concentration of 36 ± 2 g/L and in 12 former alcoholic patients with liver cirrhosis mean concentration of 35 ± 2 g/L not significantly different from normal range of 35 - 50 g/L *2932*

Aldosterone *Plasma Increase* Increased secretion *4707*
Urine Increase May be increased in edematous states of hepatic cirrhosis *1290* High renal output is due to increased secretion and decreased catabolism. Renal clearance rate may be reduced *4707*

Alkaline Phosphatase *Serum Increase* Closely parallels serum bilirubin *4707* In 35 patients with alcoholic liver cirrhosis median activity of 239 U/L significantly different from 125 U/L in 90 healthy controls *2572* Incidence of elevation: 40%; usual range of values: 25 - 85 U/L; 5% incidence of values > 107 U/L. Jaundice may be absent or present. Usually normal or only mildly elevated *1025* Observed with liver damage *2803* Up to 16 U/L in Laennec's cirrhosis *1642* Associated with jaundice *5738*

Alkaline Phosphatase Isoenzymes *Serum Increase* Alkaline phosphatase-I was the major elevated isoenzyme in 12 of 14 cases. Isoenzyme-IV was raised in 5 of the 14 patients *2557*

Amino Acids *Plasma Increase* Increased amino acids (glycine, glutamine, serine, threonine, tyrosine, and alanine) in portal cirrhosis *4577*

Ammonia *Blood Increase* Increased in terminal portal cirrhosis *1290*

Angiotensin-converting Enzyme *Serum Increase* In patients with alcoholic liver disease mean activity of 30.8 U/mL compared with 22.8 in controls. 30% of patients had elevated levels *532*

Anti-Mitochondrial Antibodies *Serum Increase* Reported effect *4176* Low incidence of the autoimmune serological markers - ANA (13%) and SMA (13%) *1792* Reported effect *4551* *5658*
Serum No Effect Not a significantly increased frequency compared with healthy controls *4176*

Antinuclear Antibodies *Serum Increase* Low incidence of the autoimmune serological markers antinuclear antibody (13%) and smooth muscle antibody (13%) *1792* 7% of patients were positive (2% of controls) *4176* Increased frequency observed *4551*

Aspartate Aminotransferase *Serum Increase* 50 - 145 U/L *2039* Consistently elevated and higher than ALT activity *5738* In 6 alcoholic patients with liver cirrhosis mean activity of 66 ± 9 U/L and in 12 former alcoholic patients with liver cirrhosis mean activity of 50 ± 4 U/L significantly different from normal range of 10 - 40 U/L *2932* In 30 patients with alcoholic cirrhosis mean activity of 141 ± 7 U/L increased compared with 23 ± 1 U/L in 30 healthy controls *2269* In 36 postmenopausal women with alcoholic cirrhosis mean activity of 50.8 ± 14.3 U/L significantly different from 28.6 ± 2.3 U/L in 27 alcohol abstaining postmenopausal women *1675*

Bile Acids *Serum Increase* In 30 patients with alcoholic liver cirrhosis, portal hypertension and bleeding esophageal varices *2452* In 30 patients with alcoholic liver cirrhosis portal hypertension and bleeding esophageal varices *1873* Total bile acids were elevated in all patients with alcoholic liver cirrhosis. This test was found to discriminate most efficiently between acute alcohol intoxication and liver cirrhosis *2453*

Bilirubin *Serum Increase* Mean concentration of 1.4 ± 0.3 mg/dL in 6 patients with alcoholic liver cirrhosis significantly greater than 0.6 ± 0.3 mg/dL in 23 healthy controls *5493* Increased concentration observed with decreased plasma concentration of carnitine in 14 of 36 patients with alcohol-induced liver cirrhosis *2809* Elevated ranging from 2.4 - 9.5 mg/dL *5738* In 30 patients with alcoholic cirrhosis mean concentration of 2.5 ± 0.2 mg/dL increased compared with 0.6 ± 0.1 mg/dL in 30 healthy controls *2269* In 6 alcoholic patients with liver cirrhosis mean concentration of 2.0 ± 0.4 mg/dL and in 12 former alcoholic patients with liver cirrhosis mean concentration of 2.0 ± 0.1 mg/dL significantly different from normal range of 0.1 - 1.0 mg/dL *2932*

Bilirubin, Direct *Serum Increase* Occasionally acute alcoholic disease presents with a predominant elevation in the serum conjugated bilirubin suggesting extrahepatic obstruction of the biliary system *2039*

CA 19-9 *Serum Increase* In 49 patients with alcoholic cirrhosis median concentration of 70 kU/L significantly higher than upper limit of normal of 35 kU/L, with 73% of patients having abnormal values *3218*

CA 125 *Serum Increase* False positive result *3909* Abnormal in 60% of patients *3560*

Calcitonin *Plasma Increase* Immunoreactive calcitonin was increased in relation to raised alkaline phosphatase activity *2143*

Calcium *Serum Decrease* In 35 patients with alcoholic liver cirrhosis median concentration of 2.11 mmol/L not significantly different from 2.35 mmol/L in 90 healthy controls *2572* Low concentrations correlated well with high AST activity in 78 cirrhotic patients *3467*

Carcinoembryonic Antigen *Serum Increase* Positive assays were obtained in 40 of 88 patients with severe alcoholic liver disease but in none of 14 patients with nonalcoholic liver disease. Values usually were lower than in colonic or pancreatic cancer *3587* In 49 patients with alcoholic cirrhosis median concentration of 5 µg/L significantly higher than upper limit of normal of 14 µg/L, with 26% of patients having abnormal values *3218* Increase frequently observed *4891* About 50% of patients with severe alcoholic liver disease have elevated (> 2.5 ng/mL) values, usually < 5 and rarely 10 ng/mL *3588*

Carnitine *Serum Decrease* Decreased plasma concentration observed in 14 of 36 patients with alcohol-induced liver cirrhosis *2809*
Serum Increase Both free and acylcarnitine levels were significantly higher than normal. Chiefly due to increased free carnitine concentrations *87* High in alcoholic liver cirrhosis due to an increased amount of esterified carnitine *111* Increased plasma concentration observed in 8 of 11 patients with alcohol-induced liver cirrhosis *2809*
Urine Increase Not significantly increased urinary concentration observed in patients with alcohol-induced liver cirrhosis compared with healthy controls *2809*

Carnitine, Free *Serum Increase* Not significantly increased plasma concentration observed in patients with alcohol-induced liver cirrhosis compared with healthy controls *2809*
Serum No Effect In 15 patients with alcoholic cirrhosis mean concentration of 16.3 ± 17.4 µmol/L not significantly different from 15.3 ± 10.5 µmol/L in 28 healthy volunteer controls *2810*

Cells *Bone Marrow Increase* Normal or increased *2684*

Cholesterol *Liver No Effect* In 12 patients with alcoholic cirrhosis mean concentration of 3.9 ± 1.5 µmol/g in specimens obtained at autopsy not significantly higher than 3.8 ± 1.3 µmol/g in 9 control specimens from nonalcoholics *194*
Red Blood Cells Increase 25 - 50% increase in the membrane concentration, resulting in the characteristic target cell *5699*

Serum *Decrease* Mean concentration of 139 ± 16 mg/dL in 6 patients with alcoholic liver cirrhosis significantly less than 191 ± 33 mg/dL in 23 healthy controls *5493*
Serum *Increase* In fatty infiltration of the liver the serum concentration was significantly increased, as compared with the normal values and with the figures obtained in the cases of chronic inflammatory liver disease *1440*

β-Chorionic Gonadotropin *Plasma* *Increase* Mean concentration increased to about 125 ng/mL in alcoholic cirrhosis above upper limit of normal of 78 ng/mL *5315*

Cold Agglutinins *Serum* *Increase* Elevated titers may persist for weeks or months *4468* *4551*

Complement C_3 *Serum* *Decrease* Low levels of C_3, C_4 and factor B were common with cirrhosis and confined to those cases with severe reduction in serum albumin and/or prothrombin index *790*

Complement C_4 *Serum* *Decrease* Low levels of C_3, C_4 and factor B were common with cirrhosis and confined to those cases with severe reduction in serum albumin and/or prothrombin index *790*

Complement, Total *Serum* *Decrease* Low levels of C_3, C_4 and factor B were common with cirrhosis and confined to those cases with severe reduction in serum albumin and/or prothrombin index *790*

Creatinine *Serum* *Increase* Increased plasma concentration observed in 8 of 11 patients with alcohol-induced liver cirrhosis *2809*

Erythrocyte Sedimentation Rate *Blood* *Increase* Extreme elevation is found *5544*

Erythrocyte Survival *Red Blood Cells* *Decrease* Moderately shortened in 48 of 68 alcoholic liver disease patients *2684* *4769* Especially in patients with predominant indirect bilirubinemia *1457* Moderately shortened in 48 of 68 alcoholic liver disease patients *5699*

Estradiol *Plasma* *Increase* In 36 postmenopausal women with alcoholic cirrhosis mean concentration of 61.1 ± 16.9 pg/mL significantly higher than 27.5 ± 3.3 pg/mL in 27 alcohol abstaining postmenopausal women *1675*

Factor VIII *Plasma* *Increase* Increased activity in alcoholic liver disease *1855*

Fatty Acids (FFA), Free *Serum* *Increase* Significantly increased plasma concentration observed in patients with alcohol-induced liver cirrhosis compared with healthy controls *2809*

α-Fetoprotein *Serum* *Increase* Concentrations above 30 ng/mL were found in 14% of patients *75*

Fibrin Degradation Products *Plasma* *Increase* Fibrinolytic activity is significantly increased in advanced cirrhosis. Total fibrinogen concentration was normal *3082*

Fibrinogen *Plasma* *No Effect* Fibrinolytic activity is significantly increased in advanced cirrhosis. Total fibrinogen concentration was normal *3082*

Follicle Stimulating Hormone *Plasma* *Decrease* In 36 postmenopausal women with alcoholic cirrhosis mean concentration of 19.6 ± 4.2 mIU/mL significantly different from 63.3 ± 5.5 mIU/mL in 27 alcohol abstaining postmenopausal women *1675*

Globulin *Serum* *Increase* In 30 patients with alcoholic cirrhosis mean concentration of 4.1 ± 0.3 g/dL increased compared with 2.8 ± 0.1 g/dL in 30 healthy controls *2269*

α_1-Globulin *Serum* *No Effect* Concentration usually normal *5544*

α_2-Globulin *Serum* *Increase* Moderate increase *1290*
Serum *No Effect* Concentration usually normal *5544*

β-Globulin *Serum* *No Effect* Concentration usually within normal limits *5544*

γ-Globulin *Serum* *Increase* In 6 alcoholic patients with liver cirrhosis mean concentration of 21 ± 2 g/L and in 12 former alcoholic patients with liver cirrhosis mean concentration of 19 ± 5 g/L significantly different from normal range of 6 - 16 g/L *2932* In 95 patients, there was a significant increase in mean concentration, while mean α- and β-globulins were normal. Characteristic electrophoresis pattern reveals a lack of demarcation between β and γ peaks (β-γ bridging) *5082* Usually increased; it reflects inflammation and parallels the severity of the inflammation *5544* Mean total globulin values were found to be lowest in the healthy subjects followed by acute viral hepatitis, primary hepatocellular carcinoma and cirrhosis in that order *1459*

Glucagon *Plasma* *Increase* May occur *4781*

Glucose *Serum* *Decrease* Replacement or destruction of functioning hepatic tissue may evoke hypoglycemia *4707*

Glucose Tolerance *Serum* *Decrease* A diabetic curve may occur and is a reflection of endogenous insulin resistance *2033*

γ-Glutamyltransferase *Serum* *Increase* Increases with liver damage *1290* In 36 postmenopausal women with alcoholic cirrhosis mean activity of 113.4 ± 21.3 U/L significantly different from 25.7 ± 2.7 U/L in 27 alcohol abstaining postmenopausal women *1675*

Hematocrit *Blood* *Decrease* Approximately 75% of chronic liver disease patients have anemia, usually mild *2684* *4769*

Hemoglobin *Blood* *Decrease* Approximately 75% of chronic liver disease patients have anemia, usually mild *2684* *4769*
Blood *No Effect* In 6 alcoholic patients with liver cirrhosis mean concentration of 13 ± 1 g/dL and in 12 former alcoholic patients with liver cirrhosis mean concentration of 13 ± 0.9 g/dL significantly different from normal range of 13 - 17 g/dL *2932*

Hyaluronan *Serum* *Increase* Concentration ranged from 205-800 µg/L in patients with alcoholic liver cirrhosis and higher concentrations when combined with hepatitis *3072*

Hyaluronic Acid *Serum* *Increase* The median serum concentrations in alcoholic cirrhosis (467 µg/L) were significantly increased in comparison with controls *1371*

7α-Hydroperoxycholest-5-en-3β-ol *Liver* *No Effect* In 12 patients with alcoholic cirrhosis mean concentration of 2.3 ± 3.5 nmol/g in specimens obtained at autopsy not significantly higher than 1.2 ± 1.7 nmol/g in 9 control specimens from nonalcoholics *194*

7β-Hydroperoxycholest-5-en-3β-ol *Liver* *No Effect* In 12 patients with alcoholic cirrhosis mean concentration of 3.2 ± 5.8 nmol/g in specimens obtained at autopsy not significantly higher than 2.0 ± 3.3 nmol/g in 9 control specimens from nonalcoholics *194*

7α-Hydroperoxycholest-5-en-3β-ol:Cholesterol Ratio
Liver *No Effect* In 12 patients with alcoholic cirrhosis mean ratio of 0.079 ± 0.13 (nmol/g:µmol/g) in specimens obtained at autopsy not significantly different from 0.027 ± 0.029 in 9 control specimens from nonalcoholics *194*

7β-Hydroperoxycholest-5-en-3β-ol:Cholesterol Ratio
Liver *No Effect* In 12 patients with alcoholic cirrhosis mean ratio of 0.11 ± 0.22 (nmol/g:µmol/g) in specimens obtained at autopsy not significantly different from 0.045 ± 0.054 in 9 control specimens from nonalcoholics *194*

β-Hydroxybutyrate *Serum* *Increase* Significantly increased plasma concentration observed in patients with alcohol-induced liver cirrhosis compared with healthy controls *2809*

Immunoglobulin A *Serum* *Increase* Reported effect *4551* Moderate hypergammaglobulinemia, especially IgA *1792*

Immunoglobulin G *Serum* *Increase* Elevated in about 50% of the patients *4198*

Immunoglobulin M *Serum* *No Effect* Concentration usually normal *5544*

Insulin *Plasma* *Increase* The majority of cirrhotics demonstrated increased levels of circulating insulin due to decreased hormonal catabolism *2468*

Interleukin-1 *Serum* *Increase* Mean IL-1α concentrations were elevated in cirrhotic patients and alcoholic hepatitis patients compared with controls and alcoholic patients without liver disease *2667*

Interleukin-1β *Serum* *Increase* Mean concentration of 41.4 ± 16.0 pg/mL in 33 alcoholics significantly higher than 20.7 ± 17.5 pg/mL in 43 healthy controls *1169*

Interleukin-6 *Serum* *Increase* Mean concentration of 32.3 ± 13.9 pg/mL in 33 alcoholics significantly higher than 17.9 ± 11.0 pg/mL in 43 healthy controls *1169* Mean cytokine concentrations were elevated in cirrhotic patients and alcoholic hepatitis patients compared with controls and alcoholic patients without liver disease. Interleukin-6 normalized in parallel with clinical recovery *2667*

International Normalized Ratio *Plasma* *Increase* In 30 patients with alcoholic cirrhosis mean ratio of 1.7 ± 0.1 increased compared with reference range of < 1.2 *2269*

Iron *Liver* *Increase* Iron deposition in the liver is common *1980*
Serum *Increase* Presumably due to the liberation of stored iron from necrosing liver cells *1290*

571.20 Laennec's or Alcoholic Cirrhosis *(continued)*

Iron-binding Capacity, Total *Serum* *Decrease* Significantly reduced *3681* Observed effect *5863*

Iron Saturation *Serum* *Increase* Moderate to marked rise in percent saturation in hepatic cirrhosis *5863*

Isocitrate Dehydrogenase *Serum* *No Effect* Mean serum activity was normal with portal cirrhosis *5008*

Lactate Dehydrogenase *Serum* *Increase* Slight increase *1980* High in 6 of 20 patients with portal cirrhosis *5008*

Lactate Dehydrogenase Isoenzyme-5 *Serum* *Increase* LD 4 and 5 are elevated *1025*

Lactate Dehydrogenase Isoenzymes *Serum* *Increase* LD 4 and 5 are elevated *1025*

Laminin *Serum* *Increase* In patients with alcoholic cirrhosis mean concentration of 2.94 U/mL compared with a mean of 1.28 U/mL for healthy patients *5420* Mean concentration increased to about 225 ng/mL, greater than upper limit of 140 ng/mL *5315* In patients with alcoholic cirrhosis mean concentration of 2.94 U/mL compared to a mean of 1.28 U/mL for healthy patients *3786*

Lecithin *Red Blood Cells* *Increase* 25 - 50% increase in the membrane concentration, resulting in the characteristic target cell *5699*

Leptin *Serum* *Increase* In 10 cirrhotic women leptin concentration of 23.1 ± 4.4 ng/mL was significantly increased compared with 9.3 ± 1.6 ng/mL in 8 healthy controls *3401* In 18 cirrhotic men leptin concentration of 3.6 ± 0.7 pg/mL and of 3.1 ± 0.5 pg/mL in 10 cirrhotic women were significantly increased compared with 1.0 ± 0.2 pg/mL in 15 healthy control men and 8 control women *3401*
Serum *No Effect* In 18 cirrhotic men leptin concentration of 5.9 ± 0.9 ng/mL was not significantly increased compared with 5.6 ± 0.8 ng/mL in 15 healthy controls *3401*

Leukocytes *Ascitic Fluid* *Increase* In 58 culture-negative patients the ascitic fluid count range was 28 - 1,800 and 50% of counts were > 300 /µL. The percentage of polymorphonuclear leukocytes ranged from 2 - 98% *4263* In 57 uncomplicated alcoholic liver disease patients, total ascitic WBC counts were often markedly elevated. Mean 360 /µL *2487*
Blood *Decrease* May result from hypersplenism, a direct effect of alcohol or folate deficiency *2033*
Blood *Increase* Leukocytosis may be pronounced *2039*
Blood *No Effect* In 6 alcoholic patients with liver cirrhosis mean concentration of 7,167 ± 1,133 x 10^6/L and in 12 former alcoholic patients with liver cirrhosis mean concentration of 6,221 ± 995 x 10^6/L not significantly different from normal range of 4,500 - 10,000 x 10^6/L *2932*

Lipids *Serum* *Increase* In 28 patients, 13 showed hypercholesterolemia, 16 increased serum triglyceride and 8 increased serum phospholipid *2154* In fatty infiltration of the liver the serum cholesterol, triglyceride and total lipid concentrations were significantly increased, as compared with the normal values and with the figures obtained in the cases of chronic inflammatory liver disease *1440*

β-Lipoprotein *Serum* *Increase* In fatty infiltration of the liver the serum total lipid concentrations were significantly increased, as compared with the normal values and with the figures obtained in the cases of chronic inflammatory liver disease. Beta and prebeta lipoprotein were increased *1440*

Luteinizing Hormone *Plasma* *Decrease* In 36 postmenopausal women with alcoholic cirrhosis mean concentration of 5.3 ± 1.4 mIU/mL significantly different from 24.0 ± 2.8 mIU/mL in 27 alcohol abstaining postmenopausal women *1675*

Lymphocytes *Blood* *No Effect* In 6 alcoholic patients with liver cirrhosis mean concentration of 2,187 ± 356 x 10^6/L and in 12 former alcoholic patients with liver cirrhosis mean concentration of 2,089 ± 224 x 10^6/L not significantly different from normal range of 1,300 - 4,000 x 10^6/L *2932*

α_2-Macroglobulin *Serum* *Increase* Significantly increased *3681*

Magnesium *Red Blood Cells* *Decrease* The mean concentration (4.7 mmol/L packed cells) was significantly below normal values *5547*
Serum *Decrease* May occur *5507* 4 of 11 patients had abnormally low concentration. Mean concentration (1.85 mmol/L) was significantly lower than the normal mean *5547*

MCV *Blood* *Increase* Occasionally mild macrocytosis, but rarely > 115 fL in the absence of megaloblastic changes in marrow. Reported incidence varies from 33 - 65% *5699*

Metallothionein *Serum* *No Effect* Since not associated with increased copper in the liver no significant effect observed in patients with alcoholic cirrhosis *3646*

Multiubiquitin Chains *Serum* *Increase* In 10 patients with alcoholic liver cirrhosis mean concentration of 7.5 ± 4.6 ng/mL significantly higher than 4.1 ± 1.7 ng/mL in 10 healthy controls *5126*

5'-Nucleotidase *Serum* *Increase* Elevations ranging from 32.7 - 265 U/L (normal 2 - 11 U/L) were observed in 36 patients. In 20 cases of Laennec's cirrhosis with acute fatty infiltration the range was 18.8 - 56.9 *2803*

Ornithine Carbamoyltransferase *Serum* *Increase* Liver cell damage *5544*

Parathyroid Hormone, Intact *Plasma* *No Effect* In 35 patients with alcoholic liver cirrhosis median concentration of 39.5 µg/L not significantly different from 35.2 µg/L in 90 healthy controls *2572*

Phospholipids *Serum* *Increase* 45 patients suffering from steatosis of the liver have been examined with reference to serum lipid abnormalities. 28 of the patients were chronic alcoholics. 13 patients showed hypercholesterolemia, 16 increased serum triglyceride and 8 increased serum phospholipid *2154*
Serum *No Effect* In 6 patients with alcoholic liver cirrhosis mean concentration of 224 ± 13 mg/dL not significantly increased compared with 214 ± 13 mg/dL in 23 healthy controls *5493*

Platelets *Blood* *Decrease* May result from hypersplenism, a direct effect of alcohol or folate deficiency *2033* Mild; in about 50% of cases *4769*

Potassium *Serum* *Decrease* Often present in these patients and may represent gastrointestinal losses, decreased oral intake, or increased urinary excretion through acquired renal tubular acidosis *2039*

Procollagen Type III Peptide *Serum* *Increase* For the detection of cirrhosis the P-III-P concentration was 94% sensitive and 81% specific *5183* Mean concentration increased to about 25 ng/mL in patients with alcoholic cirrhosis greater than upper limit of 12 ng/mL *5315*

Prolactin *Plasma* *Increase* In 36 postmenopausal women with alcoholic cirrhosis mean concentration of 13.7 ± 2.3 ng/mL significantly different from 5.7 ± 0.4 ng/mL in 27 alcohol abstaining postmenopausal women *1675*

Protein *Ascitic Fluid* *Decrease* Ascitic fluid is usually a transudate with protein < 3.0 g/dL and specific gravity < 1.016. However, protein may exceed 2.5 g/dL in up to 30% of patients *4891*

Prothrombin Time *Plasma* *Increase* Increased time observed with decreased plasma concentration of carnitine in 14 of 36 patients with alcohol-induced liver cirrhosis *2809* Severe clotting factor deficiencies are common *2033*

Reticulocytes *Blood* *Decrease* Reticulocytosis can be suppressed by alcohol *5699* *2415*
Blood *Increase* Average proportion of 8.6%, ranging from 2.3 - 24.6% in 16 patients *2415*

Rheumatoid Factor *Serum* *Increase* Found in 36% of patients *306* *874*

Sodium *Serum* *Decrease* Frequent in patients with ascites or edema *2033*

Specific Gravity *Ascitic Fluid* *Decrease* Ascitic fluid is usually a transudate with protein < 3.0 g/dL and specific gravity < 1.016. However, protein may exceed 2.5 g/dL in up to 30% of patients *4891*

Substance P *Plasma* *Increase* In 9 patients with alcoholic cirrhosis mean concentration of 50.8 ± 6.4 pg/mL significantly higher than 32.9 ± 1.0 pg/mL in 53 healthy controls and directly correlated with severity of condition *2964*

Testosterone *Serum* *Decrease* In 36 postmenopausal women with alcoholic cirrhosis mean concentration of 0.47 ± 0.05 ng/mL significantly different from 0.74 ± 0.06 ng/mL in 27 alcohol abstaining postmenopausal women *1675*

Thyroid Stimulating Hormone *Serum* *Increase* The mean serum TSH level was 3.1 µU/mL in the normals and 7.1 µU/mL in the cirrhotic patients. 15% of the hepatic patients had serum TSH values above 10 µU/mL *3822*

Thyroxine (T4) *Serum* *Increase* The mean free T4 value was significantly higher (3.3 ng/dL) than in the normal subjects (2.1 ng/dL) *3822*

Tissue Inhibitor of Metalloproteinase *Serum* *No Effect* Mean concentration of about 220 ng/mL, less than upper limit of 250 ng/mL *5315*

Tri-iodothyronine (T3) *Serum* *Decrease* The mean serum T3 value, 85 ng/dL, was significantly reduced in the hepatic patients as compared to a mean serum T3 value of 126 ng/dL in the normal subjects, while the free T3 value was 0.28 ng/dL in both groups. The reduction of the serum total and free T3 values were closely correlated with the degree of liver damage *3822*

Triglycerides *Serum* *Increase* In 6 patients with alcoholic liver cirrhosis mean concentration of 117 ± 51 mg/dL higher than 87 ± 23 mg/dL in 23 healthy controls *5493* In 28 patients, 13 showed hypercholesterolemia, 16 increased serum triglyceride and 8 increased serum phospholipid *2154* In fatty infiltration of the liver the serum cholesterol, triglyceride and total lipid concentrations were significantly increased, as compared with the normal values and with the figures obtained in the cases of chronic inflammatory liver disease *1440*

Tumor Necrosis Factor-α *Serum* *Increase* Mean cytokine concentrations were elevated in cirrhotic patients and alcoholic hepatitis patients compared with controls and alcoholic patients without liver disease. Tumor necrosis factor-α concentrations remained elevated for up to 6 mo after diagnosis of alcoholic hepatitis *2667* Mean concentration of 18.9 ± 15.1 pg/mL in 33 alcoholics significantly higher than 4.64 ± 6.99 pg/mL in 43 healthy controls *1169*

Type IV Collagen 7S Domain *Serum* *Increase* Mean concentration increased to about 10.2 ng/mL, greater than upper limit of 4.4 ng/mL *5315*

Type IV Collagen, Triple-helix Domain *Serum* *Increase* Mean concentration increased to about 300 ng/mL, greater than upper limit of 90 ng/mL *5315*

Ubiquitin, Free *Serum* *Increase* In 10 patients with alcoholic liver cirrhosis mean concentration of 63.5 ± 33.7 ng/mL significantly higher than 29.6 ± 6.6 ng/mL in 10 healthy controls *5126*

Urea Nitrogen *Serum* *Decrease* With severe cirrhosis *2033*

Uric Acid *Serum* *Decrease* Serum concentration was 4.18 ± 0.25 mg/dL in 22 male patients, significantly lower than in age-matched controls, 6.44 ± 0.19. An inverse correlation (r = 0.70) was found with serum bilirubin *3476*
Serum *Increase* Hyperuricemia resulting from depressed urinary excretion of uric acid parallels lactic acidosis *367*

Urobilinogen *Urine* *No Effect* Normal or increased *5544*

Vitamin E *Serum* *No Effect* In 6 patients with alcoholic liver cirrhosis mean concentrations of 24.1 ± 3.8 µmol/L and 5.02 ± 0.43 µmol/g in 6 patients with alcoholic liver cirrhosis not significantly different from 26.0 ± 4.4 µmol/L and 5.28 µmol/g lipids respectively in 23 healthy controls *5493*

Volume *Plasma* *Increase* In 64% of patients *3710* Averages 15% above normal. Hemodilution exaggerates anemia *2684* With nutritional cirrhosis; usually moderate and occurs in approximately 33% of the patients *2799*
Urine *Decrease* With ascites and edema *1290*

Zinc *Serum* *Decrease* Found to be low in patients with alcoholic cirrhosis or hepatitis, and elevated in alcoholics with normal or fatty liver *2038*
Urine *Increase* Excretion enhanced as a consequence of rapid cellular turnover resulting in moderate zincuria *5174*

571.30 Alcoholic Foamy Degeneration of Liver

Alkaline Phosphatase *Serum* *Increase* Transient increased activity observed above 300 U/L with more prolonged increase in alkaline phosphatase activity *3625*

Aspartate Aminotransferase *Serum* *Increase* Transient increased activity observed above 300 U/L *3625*

Bilirubin *Serum* *Increase* Increased concentration observed in most cases *3625*

Cholesterol *Serum* *Increase* Increased concentration observed in most cases *3625*

Leukocytes *Blood* *No Effect* Concentration typically normal *3625*

571.41 Chronic Persistent Hepatitis

Alanine Aminotransferase *Serum* *Increase* Mean activity of 65 ± 39 U/L in 23 patients with chronic persistent hepatitis significantly different from 20 ± 7 U/L in 29 healthy controls *3668* In 12 chronic persistent hepatitis patients mean activity of 68 ± 18 U/L significantly different from 14 ± 8 U/L in 20 healthy volunteers *2372* In 30 patients with CPH mean activity of 142 ± 56 U/L not significantly different from normal *2381*

Albumin *Serum* *No Effect* Mean concentration of 4.1 ± 0.3 g/dL in 23 patients with chronic persistent hepatitis not significantly different from 4.5 ± 0.3 g/dL in 29 healthy controls *3668* In 8 patients mean concentration of 47 ± 5 g/L not different from normal range of 42 - 52 g/L *1371* In 30 patients with CPH mean concentration of 4.3 ± 0.2 g/dL not significantly different from normal *2381*

Alkaline Phosphatase *Serum* *No Effect* In 30 patients with CPH mean activity of 174 ± 53 U/L not significantly different from normal *2381*

Aspartate Aminotransferase *Serum* *Increase* Mean activity of 45 ± 25 U/L in 23 patients with chronic persistent hepatitis significantly different from 24 ± 5 U/L in 29 healthy controls *3668* In 8 patients mean activity of 0.8 ± 0.4 µkat/L different from normal range of < 0.6 µkat/L *1371*
Serum *No Effect* In 30 patients with CPH mean activity of 82 ± 26 U/L not significantly different from normal *2381*

Bilirubin *Serum* *No Effect* In 30 patients with CPH mean concentration of 1.0 ± 0.2 mg/dL not significantly different from normal *2381* In 8 patients mean concentration of 17 ± 11 µmol/L not different from normal range of 4 - 21 µmol/L *1371* Mean concentration of 0.7 ± 0.2 mg/dL in 23 patients with chronic persistent hepatitis not significantly different from 0.6 ± 0.1 mg/dL in 29 healthy controls *3668* In 12 chronic persistent hepatitis patients mean concentration of 0.4 ± 0.3 mg/dL not significantly different from 0.5 ± 0.3 mg/dL in 20 healthy volunteers *2372*

Ferritin *Serum* *No Effect* In 30 patients with CPH mean concentration of 276 ± 96 ng/mL not significantly different from normal *2381*

Galactose Tolerance *Patient* *No Effect* In 8 patients mean mean $T_{1/2}$ 15 ± 4 min not different from normal range of < 17 min *1371*

γ-Globulin *Serum* *No Effect* In 30 patients with CPH mean concentration of 1.5 ± 0.3 g/dL not significantly different from normal *2381* In 12 chronic persistent hepatitis patients mean concentration of 1.2 ± 0.3 g/dL not significantly different from 1.1 ± 0.3 g/dL in 20 healthy volunteers *2372*

γ-Glutamyltransferase *Serum* *Increase* In 12 chronic persistent hepatitis patients mean activity of 34 ± 12 U/L significantly different from 10 ± 3 U/L in 20 healthy volunteers *2372*
Serum *No Effect* In 30 patients with CPH mean activity of 43 ± 21 U/L not significantly different from normal *2381*

immunoglobulin A *Serum* *No Effect* In 30 patients with CPH mean concentration of 346 ± 92 mg/dL not significantly different from normal *2381*

Immunoglobulin G *Serum* *No Effect* In 30 patients with CPH mean concentration of 1,920 ± 180 mg/dL not significantly different from normal *2381*

Immunoglobulin M *Serum* *No Effect* In 30 patients with CPH mean concentration of 142 ± 24 mg/dL not significantly different from normal *2381*

Indocyanine Green Clearance *Serum* *No Effect* In 12 chronic persistent hepatitis patients mean retention ratio in 15 minutes 8 ± 4% *2372*

Interleukin-1 *Serum* *Increase* IL-1β and IL-2 values in serum from 28 patients with chronic hepatitis B diagnosed by liver biopsy and 23 healthy controls were measured by the radioimmunoassay (RIA) method. In general, high values of serum IL-1β and IL-2 were seen in patients with chronic persistent hepatitis. Serum IL-1β and IL-2 values of all patients with chronic hepatitis were higher than in healthy controls (p < 0.001) *3961*

571.41 Chronic Persistent Hepatitis (continued)

Interleukin-2 *Serum* *Increase* IL-1β and IL-2 values in serum from 28 patients with chronic hepatitis B diagnosed by liver biopsy and 23 healthy controls were measured by the radioimmunoassay (RIA) method. In general, high values of serum IL-1β and IL-2 were seen in patients with chronic persistent hepatitis. Serum IL-1β and IL-2 values of all patients with chronic hepatitis were higher than in healthy controls ($p < 0.001$) *3961*

Lymphocytes *Blood* *No Effect* In 30 patients with CPH mean concentration of 2,230 ± 654 /μL not significantly different from normal *2381*

Lysyl Oxidase *Serum* *Increase* In patients with chronic persistent hepatitis activity increased 1.6-fold compared with healthy controls *3670*

Macrophage Colony Stimulating Factor *Serum* *No Effect* In 12 patients with chronic persistent hepatitis mean concentration of about 2.2 ng/mL not significantly different from 1.95 ± 0.44 ng/mL in 20 healthy volunteers *2372*

Neuron-specific Enolase *Serum* *Increase* In 2 of 15 patients with CPH concentration exceeded upper limit of normal of 11 μg/L *887*

Pro-Matrix Metalloproteinase 1 *Serum* *No Effect* Mean concentration of 183 ± 34 ng/mL in 23 patients with chronic persistent hepatitis not significantly different from 155 ± 17 ng/mL in 29 healthy controls *3668*

Procollagen Type III Peptide *Serum* *No Effect* Measured in paired serum samples from 133 patients with various chronic liver diseases and from 50 healthy age-matched controls. In 24 (of the 133) patients with autoimmune chronic liver disease, follow-up determination was performed during therapeutic treatment with immunosuppressive drugs. Compared with controls P-III-NP concentrations (medians) were not significantly elevated in patients with chronic persistent hepatitis ($p = 0.06$) *4270*

Protein *Serum* *No Effect* In 30 patients with CPH mean concentration of 7.5 ± 0.5 g/dL not significantly different from normal *2381*

Prothrombin Time *Plasma* *No Effect* In 30 patients with CPH mean time of 80 ± 22% not significantly different from normal *2381*

Soluble Interleukin-2 Receptor *Serum* *Increase* Mean concentration in 10 patients with chronic persistent hepatitis of 724 ± 262 U/mL significantly higher than 389 ± 77 U/mL in 72 normal controls *3608* In 30 patients with chronic persistent hepatitis C mean concentration of 1,010 ± 451 U/mL significantly different from normal *2381*

Tissue Inhibitor of Metalloproteinase-1 *Serum* *Increase* In 37 patients with chronic persistent hepatitis (11 type B, 17 type C and 9 cryptogenic) mean concentration of 179.1 ± 30.6 ng/mL not significantly higher than 147.8 ± 22.0 ng/mL in 53 normal individuals *3690*
Serum *No Effect* Mean concentration of 74 ng/mL in one patient with chronic persistent hepatitis C not significantly different from 66 ng/mL in the platelet-poor plasma of one healthy individual *3667*

Tissue Inhibitor of Metalloproteinase-2 *Serum* *No Effect* Mean concentration of 61 ± 13 ng/mL in 23 patients with chronic persistent hepatitis not significantly different from 61 ± 13 ng/mL in 29 healthy controls *3668*

571.49 Autoimmune Hepatitis

Acetylcholine Receptor Binding Antibodies *Serum* *Increase* Unexplained positive results are observed frequently in patients with autoimmune liver disease *2952*

Alanine Aminotransferase *Serum* *Increase* Activity increased as part of hepatitic pattern of changes *1778*

Albumin *Serum* *No Effect* Concentrations usually normal *1778*

Alkaline Phosphatase *Serum* *No Effect* Activity normal as part of hepatitic pattern of changes *1778*

Anti-Actin *Serum* *Increase* Characteristically found with classic type of disease (type 1) *2817*

Anti-Asialoglycoprotein Receptor *Serum* *Increase* Characteristically found with classic type of disease (type 1) *2817* Occurs at high titers in almost all patients with active disease *1778*

Anti-Endomysial IgA Antibodies *Serum* *Increase* In 181 patients with autoimmune hepatitis anti-endomysial antibodies observed in eight *5492*

Anti-Gliadin Antibodies *Serum* *Increase* In 181 patients with autoimmune hepatitis anti-gliadin antibodies observed in six. All six were among the eight with anti-endomysial antibodies *5492*

Anti-Liver Cytosol 1 Antibodies *Serum* *Increase* Rarely found with classic type (type 1) of disease, but characteristic of type 2 (anti-LKM -1) *2817*

Anti-Liver Cytosolic Antigen *Serum* *Increase* Occurs at high titers in 20 - 50% patients with active disease *1778*

Anti-Liver-Pancreas Protein Antibodies *Serum* *Increase* Occasionally found with type 1 disease (classic type) *2817*

Anti-Mitochondrial Antibodies *Serum* *Increase* Occasionally found with type 1 disease (classic type) *2817* About 20% of patients with chronic autoimmune hepatitis had detectable antimitochondrial antibodies *2885*

Anti-Neutrophil Cytoplasm Antibodies *Serum* *Increase* In 10 of 20 patients (50%) with autoimmune hepatitis positive antibodies observed *2021*

Anti-Smooth Muscle Antibodies *Serum* *Increase* Type 1 autoimmune hepatitis is characterized by presence of antinuclear or smooth muscle antibodies at titers of at least 1:80 *3625* Characteristically found with classic type of disease (type 1) *2817* Concentration typically increased in about 80% patients *1778*

Anti-Soluble Liver Antigen *Serum* *Increase* Type 3 autoimmune hepatitis is characterized by presence of antibodies to soluble liver antigen *3625* Occasionally found with type 1 disease (classic disease) *2817* Occurs at high titers in 20 - 50% patients with active disease *1778*

Antibodies to Liver/Kidney Microsome Type I *Serum* *Increase* Characteristic of type 2 (anti-LKM -1) disease *2817* Concentration increased in about 3 - 4% patients usually without ANA and SMA *1778* Type 2 autoimmune hepatitis is characterized by presence of antibodies to liver/kidney microsome type 1 *3625*

Antinuclear Antibodies *Serum* *Increase* Concentration typically increased in about 80% patients *1778* Characteristically found with classic disease (type 1), and rarely with type 2 of disease (anti-LKM-1) *2817* Type 1 autoimmune hepatitis is characterized by presence of antinuclear or smooth muscle antibodies at titers of at least 1:80 *3625*

Aspartate Aminotransferase *Serum* *Increase* Activity increased as part of hepatitic pattern of changes *1778*

Bilirubin *Serum* *Increase* Concentration increased as part of hepatitic pattern of changes *1778*

CA 19-9 *Serum* *Increase* In 11 patients withautoimmune hepatitis median concentration of 31 kU/L not significantly different from upper limit of normal of 35 kU/L, but 36% of patients had abnormal values *3218*

Carcinoembryonic Antigen *Serum* *Increase* In 11 patients with autoimmune hepatitis median concentration of 7.5 μg/L not different from upper limit of normal of 14 μg/L, but 12% of patients had abnormal values *3218*

CD8+ Lymphocytes *Blood* *Increase* Significantly higher as compared with normal controls *3916*

Ferritin *Serum* *Increase* Plasma concentration may be increased but not to the same extent as in hemochromatosis *5276*

γ-Globulin *Serum* *Increase* Concentration may be increased up to 6 - 8 g/L in patients with autoimmune chronic active liver disease *4617*

γ-Glutamyltransferase *Serum* *Increase* Activity may be increased, sometimes markedly, but of uncertain significance *1778*

immunoglobulin A *Serum* *No Effect* Concentration typically normal *1778*

Immunoglobulin G *Serum* *Increase* Concentration typicaly markedly and selectively increased *1778*

Immunoglobulin M *Serum* *Increase* Concentration typically normal, but may be moderately increased in severe disease *1778*

Serum *No Effect* Concentration typically normal, but may be moderately increased in severe disease *1778*

Interleukin-1α-Autoantibody *Serum* *No Effect* In 20 patients with autoimmune hepatitis proportion with autoantibody 15% compared with 12.6% in 838 healthy controls *2374*

Neopterin *Serum* *Increase* In 15 patients with autoimmune hepatitis mean concentration of 11.1 ± 1.2 nmol/L, with mean in 6 without cirrhosis of 10.2 ± 2.4 nmol/L and 11.7 ± 1.4 nmol/L in 9 with cirrhosis different from 6.0 ± 2.2 nmol/L in healthy controls *5682*

Transforming Growth Factor-β_1 *Serum* *Increase* In 18 patients with active autoimmune hepatitis median concentration of 109 ng/mL significantly different from 34 ng/mL in remission *343*

571.49 Chronic Active Autoimunne Hepatitis

Alanine Aminotransferase *Serum* *Increase* In 8 patients mean activity 98 ± 34 U/L compared with less than 30 U/L in 838 healthy controls *2374*

Antibodies to Liver/Kidney Microsome Type I *Serum* *Increase* Increased concentration observed in patients with autoimmune chronic hepatitis (type 2) *2952*

γ-Glutamyltransferase *Serum* *Increase* In 8 patients mean concentration of 2.8 ± 0.3 U/L compared with undetectable amounts in 838 healthy controls *2374*

Interleukin-1α-Autoantibody *Serum* *No Effect* In 8 patients proportion with autoantibody 12.5% compared with 12.6% in 838 healthy controls *2374*

571.49 Chronic Active Hepatitis

Alanine Aminotransferase *Serum* *Increase* In patients with severe liver injury mean activity of 137.6 ± 20.1 U/L greater than 126.7 ± 19.2 U/L in those with moderate injury, greater than 69.8 ± 14.1 U/L in those with mild injury and 20.0 ± 1.9 U/L in healthy controls *1329* Mild elevation *1980* In 30 chronic active hepatitis patients mean activity of 308 ± 201 U/L significantly different from 14 ± 8 U/L in 20 healthy volunteers *2372* Continuing or phasic release of transaminase enzymes from damaged liver cells, depending upon the degree of hepatocellular necrosis: serum levels range from 300 - 1,000 U/L during exacerbations *4337* Mean activity of 104 ± 74 U/L in 33 patients with liver cirrhosis significantly different from 24 ± 5 U/L in 29 healthy controls *3668* Mean activity of 176 ± 164 U/L in 34 patients with chronic active hepatitis significantly different from 20 ± 7 U/L in 29 healthy controls *3668* Usually increased (up to 10 times normal range) *5544* In 90% of 15 patients at initial hospitalization for this disorder *1576*

Albumin *Serum* *Decrease* In 36% of 19 patients at initial hospitalization for this disorder *1576* Active phases with hepatocellular necrosis are marked by signs of hepatic dysfunction *4551* Mean concentration of 3.8 ± 0.4 g/dL in 34 patients with chronic active hepatitis significantly different from 4.5 ± 0.3 g/dL in 29 healthy controls *3668* In patients with severe liver injury mean concentration of 38.3 ± 1.2 g/L less than 40.4 ± 0.7 g/L in those with moderate injury, less than 42.4 ± 1.0 g/L in those with mild injury and 47.4 ± 1.1 g/L in healthy controls *1329*

Alkaline Phosphatase *Serum* *Increase* In patients with severe liver injury mean activity of 91.0 ± 11.4 U/L greater than 84.5 ± 6.2 U/L in those with moderate injury, greater than 88.0 ± 23.6 U/L in those with mild injury and 84.2 ± 10.3 U/L in healthy controls *1329* Only slight increases *4551* Approximately 90% of patients with toxic hepatocellular jaundice have elevated values. Almost always < 88 U/L and in most < 50 U/L. Approximately 5% of patients with hepatocellular jaundice may have levels of 88 - 135 U/L. In jaundiced patients with higher levels, posthepatic jaundice should be suspected *1025* In 60% of 19 patients at initial hospitalization for this disorder *1576* Occasionally *1980* Moderately elevated (times 2) or normal *2033*

Ammonium Ions *Urine* *Increase* May be associated with classic distal renal tubular acidosis which is asociated with hyokalemia, hyperchloremic metabolic acidosis, urine pH > 5.5, increased urinary ammonium ion excretion, a negative urine anion gap, increased urinary osmol gap, decreased urinary citrate and increased urinary calcium in some patients *4071*

Amylase *Serum* *Increase* Activity greater than 220 U/L observed in 19% patients with chronic active hepatitis *4110*

Anion Gap *Urine* *Decrease* May be associated with classic distal renal tubular acidosis which is associated with hyokalemia, hyperchloremic metabolic acidosis, urine pH > 5.5, increased urinary ammonium ion excretion, a negative urine anion gap, increased urinary osmol gap, decreased urinary citrate and increased urinary calcium in some patients *4071*

Anti-Mitochondrial Antibodies *Serum* *Increase* Present in 30% of patients *4778* Positive in 85% of cases *4176* Found in 10 - 20% of patients *2033* Reaction is highly positive (an incidence of 60 - 70%). True incidence could be even higher if tests were done only in phases of activity *4551* Found in 66% of patients compared to 2% of controls *4176* Found in about 50 - 66% of patients *1980* In a high percentage of cases. More frequent in HBsAg negative cases *2033* Positive in 85% of cases *4991*

Antibody Titer *Serum* *Increase* Increased incidence of high titers of serum autoantibodies *4778*

Antinuclear Antibodies *Serum* *Increase* Raised more often than LE cell phenomenon positive *1290* Recognized by immunofluorescence, with an incidence of positive tests of 60% *4893* Increased incidence of high titers of serum autoantibodies *4778* Common (20 - 60% of cases) *2033* Observed effect *4551* 57% of patients were positive compared to 2% of controls *4176*

Antithrombin III *Plasma* *Decrease* Decreased in parenchymatous liver disease *3472* *5220*

α_1-Antitrypsin *Serum* *Increase* Increased *4373* *83* *4371* *4241* *4763*
Serum *No Effect* No differences with controls noted *1422*

Apolipoprotein A-I *Serum* *Decrease* The levels of prebeta and alpha lipoprotein were decreased *1440*

Aspartate Aminotransferase *Serum* *Increase* Mild elevation *1980* Mean activity of 114 ± 119 U/L in 34 patients with chronic active hepatitis significantly different from 24 ± 5 U/L in 29 healthy controls *3668* In 97% of 18 patients at initial hospitalization for this disorder *1576* In patients with severe liver injury mean activity of 120.4 ± 16.0 U/L greater than 84.1 ± 12.1 U/L in those with moderate injury, greater than 42.9 ± 5.8 U/L in those with mild injury and 24.3 ± 2.2 U/L in healthy controls *1329* Usually increased (up to 10 times normal range) *5544* Continuing or phasic release of transaminase enzymes from damaged liver cells, depending upon the degree of hepatocellular necrosis: serum concentrations range from 145 - 500 U/L during exacerbations *4337*

Aspartate Aminotransferase:Alanine Aminotransferase Ratio *Serum* *Decrease* In patients with severe liver injury mean ratio of 0.91 ± 0.06 greater than 0.74 ± 0.08 in those with moderate injury, greater than 0.66 ± 0.06 in those with mild injury but less than 1.29 ± 0.11 in healthy controls *1329*

Bile Acids *Serum* *Increase* Postprandial levels were significantly higher *1873*

Bilirubin *Serum* *Increase* In 51% of 19 patients at initial hospitalization for this disorder *1576* In patients with severe liver injury mean concentration of 9.4 ± 1.1 mg/L greater than 8.4 ± 1.6 mg/L in those with moderate injury, greater than 5.3 ± 1.0 mg/L in those with mild injury and 5.7 ± 0.5 mg/L in healthy controls *1329* Active phases with hepatocellular necrosis are marked by signs of hepatic dysfunction *4551* Usually moderately increased (3 - 10 mg/dL) but rarely exceeds 20 mg/dL *2033*
Serum *No Effect* In 30 chronic active hepatitis patients mean concentration of 0.8 ± 0.3 mg/dL not significantly different from 0.5 ± 0.3 mg/dL in 20 healthy volunteers *2372* Mean concentration of 0.8 ± 0.3 mg/dL in 34 patients with chronic active hepatitis not significantly different from 0.6 ± 0.1 mg/dL in 29 healthy controls *3668*

Biotin *Serum* *Increase* Significantly high in autoimmune hepatitis *3703*

BSP Retention *Serum* *Increase* Noted even during inactive phase of disease *2033* Active phases with hepatocellular necrosis are marked by signs of hepatic dysfunction *4551*

CA 15-3 *Serum* *Increase* In 7 patients with chronic active hepatitis mean concentration of 25.4 ± 13 U/mL higher than cutoff of 22 U/mL, with 3 having concentrations greater than 25 U/mL, 2 with concentrations above 35 U/mL and 1 with a concentration above 40 U/mL *2076*

CA 125 *Serum* *Increase* Elevated in 4% of patients *3560*

571.49 Chronic Active Hepatitis *(continued)*

Calcium *Urine Increase* May be associated with classic distal renal tubular acidosis which is asociated with hyokalemia, hyperchloremic metabolic acidosis, urine pH > 5.5, increased urinary ammonium ion excretion, a negative urine anion gap, increased urinary osmol gap, decreased urinary citrate and increased urinary calcium in some patients *4071*

Carbohydrate-deficient Transferrin *Serum Increase* Reported to increase concentration *3090*

Carbon Dioxide Partial Pressure *Blood Decrease* Reduced in a high percentage of chronic as well as acute hepatitis patients *4707*

Carcinoembryonic Antigen *Serum Increase* 4 of 7 patients showed elevated values (> 12.5 ng/mL) *528*

CD4+ Lymphocytes *Blood No Effect* No significant increase *3916*

CD8+ Lymphocytes *Blood Increase* Significantly higher as compared with normal controls *3916*

Ceruloplasmin *Serum Increase* Alpha$_2$-glycoproteins, ceruloplasmin, and transferrin were elevated *3681*

Chenodeoxycholic Acid *Serum Increase* 3-β-Hydroxy-5-cholenoic acid was elevated in hepatobiliary disease. Normal 0.184 mmol/L, chronic active hepatitis 2.364 *5149* Degree of elevation is related to the severity of illness as judged by other biochemical and clinical parameters. Bile acids return to normal in patients who respond to therapy *2426*

Chloride *Serum Increase* May be associated with classic distal renal tubular acidosis which is asociated with hyokalemia, hyperchloremic metabolic acidosis, urine pH > 5.5, increased urinary ammonium ion excretion, a negative urine anion gap, increased urinary osmol gap, decreased urinary citrate and increased urinary calcium in some patients *4071*

Cholesterol *Serum Decrease* Significant decrease in concentration noted in 34 patients with chronic active hepatitis compared with that in 34 controls with unrelated diseases *853* Significantly reduced *1440*

Cholic Acid *Serum Increase* Mean fasting and 3 h total cholic acid conjugates were significantly higher *2480* Degree of elevation is related to the severity of illness as judged by other biochemical and clinical parameters. Bile acids return to normal in patients who respond to therapy *2426* Elevated in 80% of Patients *2137*

Cholinesterase *Serum Decrease* In 16 patients with chronic active hepatitis mean activity of 4,112 ± 1,177 U/L significantly less than 5,902 ± 1,233 U/L in 16 healthy individuals *2632*

Citrate *Urine Decrease* May be associated with classic distal renal tubular acidosis which is asociated with hyokalemia, hyperchloremic metabolic acidosis, urine pH > 5.5, increased urinary ammonium ion excretion, a negative urine anion gap, increased urinary osmol gap, decreased urinary citrate and increased urinary calcium in some patients *4071*

Complement Fixation *Serum Increase* Incidence of positivity to anticytoplasmic antibodies (titer > 8) was reported to be 27 - 30% in contrast to an incidence of 3 - 4% in controls and 7 - 12% in other types of liver disease *3186*

Complement, Total *Serum Decrease* Normal or mildly decreased *2033*
Serum No Effect Concentration unaffected by disease *4551* No characteristic alterations have been reported for levels of complement or complement components *4188*

Coombs' Test *Serum Positive* Sometimes present *5544*

Copper Zinc Superoxide Dismutase *Serum Decrease* Total activity was decreased in both active and inactive phases *809*

Factor IX *Plasma Decrease* In 16 patients with chronic active hepatitis mean concentration of 54 ± 11% significantly less than 100 ± 4% in 16 healthy individuals *2632*

Factor X *Plasma Decrease* In 16 patients with chronic active hepatitis mean concentration of 91 ± 23% not significantly less than 113 ± 22% in 16 healthy individuals *2632*

Fatty Acids (FFA), Free *Serum Decrease* In 11 cases a depression of the essential fatty acid concentration (linoleic and arachidonic) was noted with concomitant elevation of oleic, palmitic, and palmitoleic acids *1617*
Serum Increase The pattern in 11 cases of hepatitis accompanied by jaundice showed elevated levels of oleic, palmitic, and palmitoleic acids attributed to the decreased ability of the liver to desaturate the endogenous saturated and monounsaturated acids to polyunsaturated ones *1617*

α-Fetoprotein *Serum Increase* Observed effect *711* Concentrations above 30 ng/mL were found in 58% of patients *75* Elevated in 42% of cases *4728*

Fibrin Degradation Products *Plasma Increase* Significantly increased *3082*

Fibrinogen *Plasma No Effect* Fibrinolytic activity is increased but total fibrinogen is normal *3082*

γ-Globulin *Serum Increase* Hyperglobulinemia is usually found. Provides a good index of activity and remission; fluctuations are synchronous with those of transaminase enzymes *3184* Hyperglobulinemia is usually found Provide a good index of activity and remission; fluctuations are synchronous with those of transaminase enzymes *2039* Elevated and remain raised without normalizing late in convalescence *5189* Levels (> 2 g/dL) common, particularly with abundant plasma cell infiltration of liver *2033*
Serum No Effect In 30 chronic active hepatitis patients mean concentration of 1.5 ± 0.4 g/dL not significantly different from 1.1 ± 0.3 g/dL in 20 healthy volunteers *2372*

Glucose *Serum Decrease* Replacement or destruction of functioning hepatic tissue may evoke hypoglycemia *4707*

γ-Glutamyltransferase *Serum Increase* In 30 chronic active hepatitis patients mean activity of 148 ± 87 U/L significantly different from 10 ± 3 U/L in 20 healthy volunteers *2372* In 90% of 10 patients at initial hospitalization for this disorder *1576*

Glycated Protein *Serum Increase* Alpha$_2$-glycoproteins, ceruloplasmin, and transferrin were elevated *3681*

Haptoglobin *Serum Decrease* The only protein to be significantly reduced *3681*

HDL-Cholesterol *Serum Increase* Increased *325 5707 3327*

Hematocrit *Blood Decrease* Anemia, leukopenia and thrombocytopenia occur in 40 - 60% of patients *5544* Slight to moderate anemia with leukopenia and thrombocytopenia are seen, particularly in patients with splenomegaly *4551*

Hemoglobin *Blood Decrease* Anemia, leukopenia, and thrombocytopenia occur in 40 - 60% of patients *5544* Slight to moderate anemia with leukopenia and thrombocytopenia are seen, particularly in patients with splenomegaly *4551*

Hepatitis B Surface Antigen *Serum Increase* 25 - 30% of patients. Occurring more frequently in men than women *367*

HLA Antigens *Blood Present* HLA-DR3 present in 68% of patients versus 24% of controls *5678*

Hyaluronic Acid *Serum Increase* Measured in paired serum samples from 133 patients with various chronic liver diseases from 50 healthy age-matched controls. In 24 (of the 133) patients with autoimmune chronic liver disease, follow-up determination was performed during therapeutic treatment with immunosuppressive drugs. Serum concentrations (medians) of HA were increased (p = 0.0058) in 32% of patients with chronic active hepatitis. The difference was statistically significant *4270*
Serum No Effect The median level in chronic persistent hepatitis (42 µg/L) did not differ significantly from the corresponding value in the control group (36 µg/L) *1371*

immunoglobulin A *Serum Increase* Reported effect *4551* In 50 patients, mean levels of all three major classes of immunoglobulin, IgG, IgM and IgA, were increased but only IgG was markedly raised *3185* Mean concentration in 9 patients with chronic active hepatitis of about 900 mg/dL significantly higher than 288 ± 121 mg/dL in 18 healthy blood donors *54*

Immunoglobulin G *Serum Increase* Mean concentration in 9 patients with chronic active hepatitis of about 3,600 mg/dL significantly higher than 1,200 ± 319 mg/dL in 18 healthy blood donors *54* Elevated levels were present in about 50% of the patients *4198* In 50 patients, mean levels of all 3 major classes of immunoglobulin, IgG, IgM, and IgA, were increased but only IgG was markedly raised *3185*

Immunoglobulin M *Serum Increase* Reported effect *4551* Mean concentration in 9 patients with chronic active hepatitis of about 300 mg/dL significantly higher than 80 ± 29 mg/dL in 18 healthy blood donors *54* In 50 patients, mean levels of all 3 major classes of immunoglobulin, IgG, IgM and IgA, were increased but only IgG was markedly raised *3185*

Immunoglobulins *Serum* *Increase* Pronounced reflecting the immunological aberrations *4551*

Indocyanine Green Clearance *Serum* *No Effect* In 30 chronic active hepatitis patients mean retention ratio in 15 minutes 9 ± 4% *2372*

β1-Integrin *Serum* *Increase* In 21 patients with chronic active hepatitis mean concentration of 3.4 ± 0.1μg/mL significantly higher than 2.1 ± 0.1 μg/mL in 18 healthy adult controls *5785*

β3-Integrin *Serum* *Increase* In 21 patients with chronic active hepatitis mean concentration of 10.5 ± 1.2 μg/mL μg/mL significantly higher than 5.5 ± 0.5 μg/mL in 18 healthy adult controls *5785*

Interleukin-1 *Serum* *Increase* IL-1β and IL-2 values in serum from 28 patients with chronic hepatitis B diagnosed by liver biopsy and 23 healthy controls were measured by the radioimmunoassay (RIA) method. In general low values of serum IL-1β and IL-2 were seen in patients with chronic active hepatitis (severe). Serum IL-1β and IL-2 values of all patients with chronic hepatitis were higher than in healthy controls ($p < 0.001$) *3961*

Interleukin-2 *Serum* *Increase* IL-1β and IL-2 values in serum from 28 patients with chronic hepatitis B diagnosed by liver biopsy and 23 healthy controls were measured by the radioimmunoassay (RIA) method. In general low values of serum IL-1β and IL-2 were seen in patients with chronic active hepatitis (severe). Serum IL-1β and IL-2 values of all patients with chronic hepatitis were higher than in healthy controls ($p < 0.001$) *3961*

Iron-binding Capacity, Total *Serum* *Increase* Alpha$_2$-glycoproteins, ceruloplasmin and transferrin were elevated *3681*

Laminin P1 *Serum* *Increase* Mean concentration significantly increased compared with healthy controls *3670*

LE Cells *Blood* *Positive* Positive in 10 - 35% of cases *2033* Found in about 50 - 66% of patients *1980* Positivity differs from that obtained in SLE, in that preparations show fewer typical LE cells and positive tests are more transient or intermittent *3185*

Leukocytes *Blood* *Decrease* Anemia, leukopenia, and thrombocytopenia occur in 40 - 60% of patients *5544* Slight to moderate anemia with leukopenia and thrombocytopenia are seen, particularly in patients with splenomegaly *4551*

Lidocaine Index *Serum* *Decrease* After administration of 1 mg/kg of 20 g/L lidocaine mean index of 586.6 ± 52.9 μg/L/h in 14 patients with severe hepatitis less than 623.2 ± 32.3 μg/L/h in 21 patients with moderate hepatitis, 670.0 ± 39.3 μg/L/h in 5 patients with mild hepatitis compared with an index of 675.0 ± 66.4 μg/L/h in 12 apparently healthy volunteers *1329*

Lidocaine Index:Monoethylglycinexylidide Index Ratio *Serum* *Increase* After administration of 1 mg/kg of 20 g/L lidocaine mean ratio of 16.0 ± 3.2 in 14 patients with severe hepatitis greater than 12.3 ± 3.4 in 21 patients with moderate hepatitis, 9.2 ± 2.4 in 5 patients with mild hepatitis compared with an index of 10.6 ± 1.5 in 12 apparently healthy volunteers *1329*

Lipase *Serum* *Increase* Activity greater than 270 U/L observed in 4% patients with chronic active hepatitis *4110*

Lymphocyte T-Cells *Blood* *Decrease* Normal *1588*

Lysyl Oxidase *Serum* *Increase* Compared with healthy controls mean activity increased 4.4-fold *3670*

α$_2$-Macroglobulin *Serum* *Increase* Moderate elevation *3480* *2249* Significant increase *3681*

β$_2$-Macroglobulin *Serum* *Increase* An increased serum concentration is characteristic *2586*

Macrophage Colony Stimulating Factor *Serum* *Increase* In 30 patients with chronic active hepatitis mean concentration of about 3.4 ng/mL significantly different from 1.95 ± 0.44 ng/mL in 20 healthy volunteers *2372*

Magnesium *Red Blood Cells* *Decrease* Mean RBC concentration of 3.99 ± 0.61 compared to 5.08 ± 0.25 mmol/L *508* *Serum* *Decrease* Mean concentration of 1.28 ± 0.18 mmol/L. Normal concentration of 1.73 ± 0.13 mmol/L *508*

Manganese *Serum* *Increase* Significant $p < 0.001$ *5460*

Manganese Superoxide Dismutase *Serum* *Decrease* Total activity in blood was decreased in both active and inactive phases *809*

Metallothionein *Serum* *No Effect* Since condition not associated with accumulation of copper in the liver plasma concentration not increased *3646*

Monoethylglycinexylidide Index *Serum* *Decrease* After administration of 1 mg/kg of 20 g/L lidocaine mean index of 74.7 ± 10.0 μg/L/h in 14 patients with severe hepatitis less than 105.1 ± 8.7 μg/L/h in 21 patients with moderate hepatitis, 119.4 ± 18.2 μg/L/h in 5 patients with mild hepatitis compared with an index of 104.7 ± 10.1 μg/L/h in 12 apparently healthy volunteers *1329* *Serum* *No Effect* After administration of 1 mg/kg of 20 g/L lidocaine mean index of 74.7 ± 10.0 μg/L/h in 14 patients with severe hepatitis less than 105.1 ± 8.7 μg/L/h in 21 patients with moderate hepatitis, 119.4 ± 18.2 μg/L/h in 5 patients with mild hepatitis compared with an index of 104.7 ± 10.1 μg/L/h in 12 apparently healthy volunteers *1329*

Net Acid Excretion *Urine* *Increase* May be associated with classic distal renal tubular acidosis which is associated with hyokalemia, hyperchloremic metabolic acidosis, urine pH > 5.5, increased urinary ammonium ion excretion, a negative urine anion gap, increased urinary osmol gap, decreased urinary citrate and increased urinary calcium in some patients *4071*

Neuron-specific Enolase *Serum* *No Effect* In none of 15 patients with CAH was concentration increased above upper limit of normal of 11 μg/L *887*

5'-Nucleotidase *Serum* *Increase* In 6 patients mean activity of 31 U/L (range 13 - 43 U/L) compared with mean of 3.8 U/L in healthy controls. Isoform % for NTP1 40%, NTP2 13% and NTP3 46% compared with 12%, 30% and 58% respectively in healthy individuals *3993*

Osmolal Gap *Urine* *Increase* May be associated with classic distal renal tubular acidosis which is associated with hyokalemia, hyperchloremic metabolic acidosis, urine pH > 5.5, increased urinary ammonium ion excretion, a negative urine anion gap, increased urinary osmol gap, decreased urinary citrate and increased urinary calcium in some patients *4071*

pH *Urine* *Increase* May be associated with classic distal renal tubular acidosis which is associated with hyokalemia, hyperchloremic metabolic acidosis, urine pH > 5.5, increased urinary ammonium ion excretion, a negative urine anion gap, increased urinary osmol gap, decreased urinary citrate and increased urinary calcium in some patients *4071*

Plasma Cells *Blood* *Increase* Increased plasma cells in bone marrow and may appear in peripheral blood *5544* *Bone Marrow* *Increase* Plasmacytosis in the bone marrow is part of the abnormal immunological response *2423*

Platelets *Blood* *Decrease* Slight to moderate anemia with leukopenia and thrombocytopenia are seen, particularly in patients with splenomegaly *4551* Anemia, leukopenia, and thrombocytopenia occur in 40 - 60% of patients *5544*

Potassium *Serum* *Decrease* May be associated with classic distal renal tubular acidosis which is associated with hyokalemia, hyperchloremic metabolic acidosis, urine pH > 5.5, increased urinary ammonium ion excretion, a negative urine anion gap, increased urinary osmol gap, decreased urinary citrate and increased urinary calcium in some patients *4071*

Prealbumin *Serum* *Decrease* In 16 patients with chronic active hepatitis mean concentration of 19.0 ± 3.5 mg/dL significantly less than 29.0 ± 5.5 mg/dL in 16 healthy individuals *2632*

Pro-Matrix Metalloproteinase 1 *Serum* *No Effect* Mean concentration of 210 ± 48 ng/mL in 34 patients with chronic active hepatitis not significantly different from 155 ± 17 ng/mL in 29 healthy controls *3668*

Procollagen Type III Peptide *Serum* *Increase* Measured in paired serum samples from 133 patients with various chronic liver diseases and from 50 healthy age-matched controls. In 24 (of the 133) patients with autoimmune chronic liver disease, follow-up determination was performed during therapeutic treatment with immunosuppressive drugs. Compared with controls P-III-NP concentrations (medians) were significantly elevated in 65% of patients with chronic active hepatitis ($p = 0.00097$).The difference was not statistically significant *4270*

Procollagen Type IV Peptide *Serum* *Increase* The serum concentrations were 4.2 ± 0.9 ng/mL in controls, 6.5 ± 2.5 ng/mL in chronic inactive hepatitis, 9.5 ± 3.8 ng/mL in chronic active hepatitis *5765* The serum concentrations were 4.2 ± 0.9 ng/mL in controls, 14.4 ± 7.5 ng/mL in liver cirrhosis *5765*

Proline Hydroxylase *Serum* *Increase* Activity significantly increased compared with healthy controls *3670*

Protein C *Plasma* *Decrease* In 16 patients with chronic active hepatitis mean concentration of 66 ± 23% significantly less than 95 ± 12% in 16 healthy individuals *2632*

571.49 Chronic Active Hepatitis *(continued)*

Protein Z *Plasma* *Decrease* In 16 patients with CAH mean concentration of 2,051 ± 322 µg/L significantly less than 2,820 ± 336 µg/L in 16 healthy individuals *2632* Mean protein Z concentration in patients with chronic active (aggressive) hepatitis of 2,051 ± 322 µg/L significantly different from 2,820 ± 336 µg/L in healthy controls *2645*

Prothrombin Time *Plasma* *Increase* In patients with severe liver injury mean time of 12.6 ± 0.3 s greater than 12.1 ± 0.2 s in those with moderate injury, greater than 11.1 ± 0.3 s in those with mild injury and 11.7 ± 0.2 s in healthy controls *1329* Often prolonged *2033* Patients with marked prolongation, despite vitamin K replacement and a positive LE cell test, have the worst prognosis *1980*

Soluble Interleukin-2 Receptor *Serum* *Increase* Mean concentration in 27 patients with chronic active hepatitis of 838 ± 250 U/mL significantly higher than 389 ± 77 U/mL in 72 normal controls *3608*

Superoxide Dismutase *Blood* *Decrease* Total activity was decreased in both active and inactive phases of chronic persistent hepatitis but was did not fall significantly in chronic active hepatitis *809*

Tissue Inhibitor of Metalloproteinase-1 *Serum* *Increase* In 72 patients with chronic active hepatitis (33 type B, 31 type C, 2 type B and type C and 6 cryptogenic) mean concentration of 228.6 ± 98.5 ng/mL significantly higher than 147.8 ± 22.0 ng/mL in 53 normal individuals *3690*

Tissue Inhibitor of Metalloproteinase-2 *Serum* *No Effect* Mean concentration of 72 ± 15 ng/mL in 34 patients with chronic active hepatitis not significantly different from 61 ± 13 ng/mL in 29 healthy controls *3668*

Tissue Plasminogen Activator *Plasma* *Increase* Concentration increased above 8.3 ng/mL in 46.2% of 39 patients with chronic active hepatitis *3887*

VLDL-Cholesterol *Serum* *Increase* Marked elevation *126*

Zinc *Serum* *Decrease* Significant $p < 0.001$ *5460*

571.49 Chronic Active Hepatitis 2A Type B

N-terminal Peptide of Type III Procollagen *Serum* *Increase* Mean concentration in 19 patients with chronic active hepatitis 2A-B of 0.93 ± 0.23 U/mL compared with reference interval of 0.35 - 0.65 U/mL *3669*

Prolyl 4-Hydroxylase β-subunit *Serum* *No Effect* Mean concentration in 21 patients with chronic active hepatitis 2A type B of 65 ± 14 ng/mL compared with 38 - 74 ng/mL in 30 control individuals *3669*

571.49 Chronic Active Hepatitis 2A Type C

N-terminal Peptide of Type III Procollagen *Serum* *Increase* Mean concentration in 19 patients with chronic active hepatitis 2A-C of 0.98 ± 0.24 U/mL compared with reference interval of 0.35 - 0.65 U/mL *3669*

Prolyl 4-Hydroxylase β-subunit *Serum* *No Effect* Mean concentration in 21 patients with chronic active hepatitis 2A type C of 67 ± 15 ng/mL compared with 38 - 74 ng/mL in 30 control individuals *3669*

571.49 Chronic Active Hepatitis 2B Type B

N-terminal Peptide of Type III Procollagen *Serum* *Increase* Mean concentration in 19 patients with chronic active hepatitis 2B-B of 1.21 ± 0.37 U/mL compared with reference interval of 0.35 - 0.65 U/mL *3669*

Prolyl 4-Hydroxylase β-subunit *Serum* *No Effect* Mean concentration in 21 patients with chronic active hepatitis 2B type B of 73 ± 20 ng/mL compared with 38 - 74 ng/mL in 30 control individuals *3669*

571.49 Chronic Active Hepatitis 2B Type C

N-terminal Peptide of Type III Procollagen *Serum* *Increase* Mean concentration in 19 patients with chronic active hepatitis 2B-C of 1.24 ± 0.42 U/mL compared with reference interval of 0.35 - 0.65 U/mL *3669*

Prolyl 4-Hydroxylase β-subunit *Serum* *No Effect* Mean concentration in 21 patients with chronic active hepatitis 2B type C of 73 ± 18 ng/mL compared with 38 - 74 ng/mL in 30 control individuals *3669*

571.49 Chronic Active Hepatitis C

Alanine Aminotransferase *Serum* *No Effect* In 30 patients with mild CAH mean activity of 121 ± 62 U/L and in 21 with severe CAH mean activity of 162 ± 88 U/L not significantly different from normal *2381*

Albumin *Serum* *No Effect* In 30 patients with mild CAH mean concentration of 4.1 ± 0.7 g/dL and in 21 with severe CAH mean concentration of 3.9 ± 0.3 g/dL not significantly different from normal *2381*

Alkaline Phosphatase *Serum* *No Effect* In 30 patients with mild CAH mean activity of 190 ± 52 U/L and in 21 with severe CAH mean activity of 192 ± 45 U/L not significantly different from normal *2381*

Aspartate Aminotransferase *Serum* *No Effect* In 30 patients with mild CAH mean activity of 82 ± 46 U/L and in 21 with severe CAH mean activity of 88 ± 47 U/L not significantly different from normal *2381*

Bilirubin *Serum* *No Effect* In 30 patients with mild CAH mean concentration of 0.9 ± 0.3 mg/dL and in 21 with severe CAH mean concentration of 0.9 ± 0.1 mg/dL not significantly different from normal *2381*

Ferritin *Serum* *No Effect* In 30 patients with mild CAH mean concentration of 218 ± 146 ng/mL and in 21 with severe CAH mean concentration of 218 ± 56 ng/mL not significantly different from normal *2381*

γ-Globulin *Serum* *No Effect* In 30 patients with mild CAH mean concentration of 4.1 ± 0.7 g/dL and in 21 with severe CAH mean concentration of 3.9 ± 0.3 g/dL not significantly different from normal *2381*

γ-Glutamyltransferase *Serum* *No Effect* In 30 patients with mild CAH mean activity of 54 ± 36 U/L and in 21 with severe CAH mean activity of 48 ± 35 U/L not significantly different from normal *2381*

immunoglobulin A *Serum* *Increase* In 21 patients with severe CAH mean concentration of 135 ± 54 mg/dL significantly different from normal *2381*
Serum *No Effect* In 30 patients with mild CAH mean concentration of 321 ± 103 mg/dL not significantly different from normal *2381*

Immunoglobulin G *Serum* *No Effect* In 30 patients with mild CAH mean concentration of 1,923 ± 351 mg/dL and in 21 with severe CAH mean concentration of 2,102 ± 354 mg/dL not significantly different from normal *2381*

Immunoglobulin M *Serum* *No Effect* In 30 patients with mild CAH mean concentration of 184 ± 96 mg/dL and in 21 with severe CAH mean concentration of 154 ± 72 mg/dL not significantly different from normal *2381*

Interferon-γ *Serum* *Increase* In 89 patients with chronic active hepatitis C mean concentration of 0.52 ± 0.41 IU/mL compared with 0.2 ± 0.15 IU/mL in 40 matched healthy donor controls *2450*

Interleukin-6 *Serum* *No Effect* In 16 patients with chronic active hepatitis C concentration normal in both patients that did and did not respond to interferon-α *1804*

Lipopolysaccharides *Serum* *Increase* Sixteen of 89 (18%) of patients with chronic active hepatitis C showed circulating LPS (2.72 ± 2.85 pg/mL) whereas none was detected in 40 matched healthy donor controls *2450*

Lymphocytes *Blood* *No Effect* In 30 patients with mild CAH mean concentration of 1,986 ± 624 /µL and in 21 with severe CAH mean concentration of 2,124 ± 641 /µL not significantly different from normal *2381*

Protein *Serum* *No Effect* In 30 patients with mild CAH mean concentration of 7.5 ± 0.6 g/dL and in 21 with severe CAH mean concentration of 7.3 ± 0.3 g/dL not significantly different from normal *2381*

Prothrombin Time *Plasma* *No Effect* In 30 patients with mild CAH mean time of 95 ± 12% and in 21 with severe CAH mean activity of 80 ± 7% not significantly different from normal *2381*

Soluble CD14+ *Serum* *Increase* In 89 patients with chronic active hepatitis C mean concentration of 4.50 ± 1.15 ng/mL compared with 2.94 ± 1.55 ng/mL in 40 matched healthy donor controls *2450*

Thyroid Microsomal Antibodies *Serum* *Increase* Prevalence in male patients with chronic HCV was < 2%. Prevalence in women significantly higher at 22.1% versus 1.6% in HBV controls and not significantly higher than 13.5% in normal controls *2268*

Tissue Inhibitor of Metalloproteinase-1 *Serum* *Increase* Mean concentration of 143 ng/mL in one patient with chronic active hepatitis C significantly different from 66 ng/mL in the platelet-poor plasma of one healthy individual *3667*

Tumor Necrosis Factor-α *Serum* *Increase* Tendency for concentration to be increased with that in nonresponders tending to be higher than in responders *1804*

571.49 Chronic Hepatitis

Alanine Aminotransferase *Serum* *Increase* Mean activity of 106 ± 103 U/L in 30 patients with chronic hepatitis significantly different from 27 ± 5 U/L in 29 healthy controls *5316* In 80 patients mean activity of 123 ± 82 U/L compared with less than 30 U/L in 838 healthy controls *2374* In 28 patients with chronic hepatitis mean activity of 74.14 ± 32.27 U/L significantly higher than 28.50 ± 6.55 U/L in 69 healthy blood donor controls *3591*
Serum *No Effect* In 21 patients with chronic hepatitis mean activity of 30 U/L not different from reference interval of < 40 U/L *2071*

Albumin *Serum* *No Effect* In 21 patients with chronic hepatitis mean concentration of 4.4 ± 0.3 g/L not different from reference interval of 3.8 - 5.3 g/L *2071*

Aldolase *Serum* *No Effect* Activity typically normal or slightly increased in patients with chronic hepatitis *2952*

Alkaline Phosphatase *Serum* *No Effect* In 21 patients with chronic hepatitis mean activity of 137 U/L not different from reference interval of 90 - 250 U/L *2071*

Apolipoprotein A-I *Serum* *No Effect* Mean concentration of 1,418 ± 224 mg/L in 9 patients with chronic hepatitis not significantly different from 1,522 ± 212 mg/L in 21 healthy controls *5063*

Aspartate Aminotransferase *Serum* *Increase* In patients with chronic viral hepatitis aspartate aminotransferase activity correlated with increased plasma ferritin concentration. Iron probably released from hepatocellular stores associated with necrosis *1145* In 28 patients with chronic hepatitis mean activity of 72.35 ± 30.40 U/L significantly higher than 22.81 ± 7.95 U/L in 69 healthy blood donor controls *3591* Mean activity of 69 ± 54 U/L in 30 patients with chronic hepatitis significantly different from 27 ± 5 U/L in 29 healthy controls *5316*

Aspartate Aminotransferase:Alanine Aminotransferase Ratio
Serum *Decrease* Significantly higher prevalence of ratios less than 1.0 in patients with chronic hepatitis (170 of 177) compared with those with cirrhosis (41 of 130) *1723*

Basic Fibroblast Growth Factor *Serum* *Increase* Mean concentration of 3.8 pg/mL (range 2.2 - 10.4 pg/mL) in 22 patients not significantly different from 4.8 pg/mL (range 2.9 - 9.5 pg/mL) in 40 healthy individuals, but with 9.1% abnormal *2262*

Bilirubin *Serum* *No Effect* In 21 patients with chronic hepatitis mean concentration of 0.7 mg/dL not different from reference interval of 0.2 - 1.0 mg/dL *2071*

CA 19-9 *Serum* *Increase* In 180 patients with chronic hepatitis positive rate of 12% observed using cut-off from normals and 7% at 90% specificity *2594*

CA 242 *Serum* *Increase* In 180 patients with chronic hepatitis positive rate of 2% observed using cut-off from normals and 7% at 90% specificity *2594*

Carcinoembryonic Antigen *Serum* *Increase* In 59 patients with hepatitis 67.8% had concentrations up to 3.0 ng/mL, 16.9% had concentrations between 3.1 - 5.0 ng/mL, 8.5% between 5.1 - 10.0 ng/mL and 6.8% had concentrations above 10.1 ng/mL in contrast to concentrations in 151 healthy nonsmokers in whom 95.4% had concentrations between 0 and 3.0 ng/mL and 4.6% between 4.1 and 10.0 ng/mL *11*

Ceruloplasmin *Serum* *Decrease* Concentration typically reduced in patients with chronic hepatitis *3499*

Cholesterol *Serum* *No Effect* Mean concentration of 1,673 ± 466 mg/L in 9 patients with chronic hepatitis not significantly different from 1,892 ± 233 mg/L in 21 healthy controls *5063*

CYFRA 21-1 *Serum* *Increase* In 51 patients with chronic hepatitis concentrations ranged from 0.9 - 9.2 μg/L with a positive rate of 33% compared with upper limit of normal of 1.9 ng/mL *4740*

Descarboxyprothrombin *Serum* *Increase* Four of 57 patients (7%) had a mean concentration that exceeded 40 mAU/mL in 273 normal individuals *3897*

Endothelin-1 *Plasma* *Decrease* ET-1 levels (2.05 ± .37 pg/mL) were slightly lower than those in healthy controls (2.18 ± 0.37 pg/mL) *5340* ET-1 levels (2.05 ± 0.37 pg/mL) were slightly lower than those in healthy controls (2.18 ± 0.37 pg/mL) *5339*

Ferritin *Serum* *Increase* In 80 patients with chronic viral hepatitis increased concentrations observed in 30% men and 8% women *1145*

α-Fetoprotein *Serum* *Increase* Concentrations may be moderately increased in patients with chronic hepatitis and liver cirrhosis *5285* Occasionally may have concentrations up to 500 μg/L with or without hepatic cirrhosis *1778* In 55 patients with hepatitis 85.5% had concentrations up to 15.0 ng/mL, 0.0% had concentrations between 15.1 - 20.0 ng/mL, 7.3% between 20.1 - 100 ng/mL, 5.5% had concentrations between 100.1 - 350.0 ng/mL and 1.8% had concentrations above 350.0 ng/mL in contrast to concentrations in 400 healthy individuals in whom 99.2% had concentrations between 0 and 15.0 ng/mL, 0.2% between 15.1 and 20.0 ng/mL and 0.5%% between 20.1 and 100 ng/mL *11* Median concentration of 10.5 ng/mL in 30 patients with chronic hepatitis significantly different from 2.0 ng/mL in 29 healthy controls *5316*
Serum *No Effect* In 28 patients with chronic hepatitis mean concentration of 4.99 ± 9.71 U/mL lower than the normal upper limit of normal of 8.5 U/mL *3591*

Fibronectin *Plasma* *Increase* Increased concentration was useful in assessing extent of hepatic fibrosis *5276*

Follistatin, Free *Serum* *Increase* Mean concentration in 11 patients with chronic hepatitis of 4.4 ± 0.7 μg/L different from that in 60 normal adults of 3.5 ± 0.2 μg/L *4523*

γ-Glutamyltransferase *Serum* *Increase* In 80 patients mean concentration of 1.3 ± 0.4 U/L compared with undetectable amounts in 838 healthy controls *2374*

Granulocyte-Macrophage Colony Stimulating Factor
Serum *No Effect* In 66 patients with chronic viral liver disease mean concentration not significantly different from that in 99 healthy adults *5782*

HDL_2-Cholesterol *Serum* *No Effect* Mean concentration of 162 ± 81 mg/L in 9 patients with chronic hepatitis not significantly different from 231 ± 107 mg/L in 21 healthy controls *5063*

HDL_3-Cholesterol *Serum* *No Effect* Mean concentration of 255 ± 44 mg/L in 9 patients with chronic hepatitis not significantly different from 292 ± 52 mg/L in 21 healthy controls *5063*

HDL-Cholesterol *Serum* *Decrease* Mean concentration of 417 ± 99 mg/L in 9 patients with chronic hepatitis significantly different from 523 ± 117 mg/L in 21 healthy controls *5063*

Hepatitis B Surface Antigen *Serum* *Positive* In 21 patients with chronic hepatitis 3 were HbsAg-positive *2071*

Hepatitis C Virus Antibodies *Serum* *Positive* In 21 patients with chronic hepatitis 18 were HCV-antibody positive *2071*

Hepatocyte Growth Factor *Serum* *No Effect* In patients with chronic hepatitis mean concentration of 0.30 ng/mL compared with mean concentration in 10 normal individuals of 0.25 ± 0.06 ng/mL *3714*

Hyaluronic Acid *Serum* *Increase* Mean concentration in patients with chronic hepatitis of 66.3 ± 48.5 ng/mL compared with 24.9 ± 12.8 ng/mL in healthy controls *3365*

Interferon-γ *Serum* *Increase* In 66 patients with chronic viral liver disease mean concentration significantly different from that in 99 healthy adults *5782*

571.49 Chronic Hepatitis *(continued)*

Interleukin-1α-Autoantibody *Serum* *No Effect* In 80 patients proportion with autoantibody 15.3% compared with 12.6% in 838 healthy controls *2374*

Interleukin-1β *Serum* *No Effect* In 66 patients with chronic viral liver disease mean concentration not significantly different from that in 99 healthy adults *5782*

Interleukin-2 *Serum* *Increase* In 66 patients with chronic viral liver disease mean concentration significantly different from that in 99 healthy adults *5782*

Interleukin-6 *Serum* *No Effect* In 66 patients with chronic viral liver disease mean concentration of about 40 pg/mL similar to that in 99 healthy adults *5782*

Interleukin-8 *Serum* *Increase* In 66 patients with chronic viral liver disease mean concentration significantly different from that in 99 healthy adults *5782*

Iron *Serum* *Increase* Increase in concentration to above 150 µg/dL observed in chronic hepatitis *2952* In 80 patients with chronic viral hepatitis increased iron concentrations observed in 36% *1145*

Laminin *Serum* *Increase* Increased concentration was useful in assessing extent of hepatic fibrosis *5276*

Myeloperoxidase *Serum* *No Effect* In 20 patients with chronic hepatitis mean concentration of 222.6 ± 17.2 ng/mL compared with 219.5 ± 5.7 ng/mL in healthy controls *3718*

Neopterin *Serum* *Increase* In patients with chronic liver disease due to non-A, non-B viral hepatitis concentration significantly increased compared with those in B viral and alcoholic patients *997*
Urine *Increase* Excretion increased in patients with chronic viral hepatitis *121* In patient with chronic liver disease rate of abnormality than rate of abnormality of serum neopterin *997*

Phospholipids *Serum* *No Effect* Mean concentration of 1,883 ± 356 mg/L in 9 patients with chronic hepatitis not significantly different from 1,928 ± 193 mg/L in 21 healthy controls *5063*

Platelets *Blood* *Decrease* In 21 patients with chronic hepatitis mean concentration of 15.0 x 10^9/L less than reference interval of 17 - 39 x 10^9/L *2071*

Proapolipoprotein A-I *Serum* *Increase* Mean concentration of 93 ± 20 mg/L in 9 patients with chronic hepatitis significantly different from 69 ± 25 mg/L in 21 healthy controls *5063*

Procollagen Type III Peptide *Serum* *Increase* Increased concentration was useful in assessing extent of hepatic fibrosis *5276*

Prolyl Hydroxylase *Serum* *Increase* Increased activity was useful in assessing extent of hepatic fibrosis *5276* *5276*

Tissue Polypeptide Antigen *Serum* *Increase* Median concentration of 176.8 U/L in 30 patients with chronic hepatitis significantly different from 25.2 U/L in 29 healthy controls *5316* In 28 patients with chronic hepatitis mean concentration of 296.68 ± 221.94 U/L significantly greater than 37.73 ± 20.76 U/L in 69 healthy blood donor controls *3591*

Triglycerides *Serum* *Increase* Mean concentration of 1,347 ± 699 mg/L in 9 patients with chronic hepatitis not significantly different from 1,005 ± 397 mg/L in 21 healthy controls *5063*

Tumor Necrosis Factor-α *Serum* *No Effect* In 66 patients with chronic viral liver disease mean concentration not significantly different from that in 99 healthy adults *5782*

Type IV Collagen 7S Domain *Serum* *Increase* Increased concentration was useful in assessing extent of hepatic fibrosis *5276*

571.49 Chronic Liver Disease

Alkaline Phosphatase *Serum* *Increase* In 55 patients with mild chronic liver disease 25% had activities above 112 U/L *1406*

Aspartate Aminotransferase *Serum* *Increase* In 55 patients with mild chronic liver disease of 72% had activities above 40 U/L *1406*

Bilirubin *Serum* *Increase* In 55 patients with mild chronic liver disease 6% had concentrations above 26 µmol/L *1406*

CA 19-9 *Serum* *Increase* In 55 patients with mild chronic liver disease 26% had concentrations above 35 U/mL *1406*

γ-Carboxyglutamic Acid, Free *Plasma* *Decrease* In 12 patients with chronic liver disease mean concentration of 115 ± 55 pmol/mL significantly lower than that in 19 healthy men and women aged between 35 and 65 years in whom mean concentration was 146 ± 34 pmol/mL *2014*

Cholinesterase *Serum* *Decrease* In 55 patients with mild chronic liver disease 6% had activities less than 4,000 U/L *1406*

Collagen IV *Serum* *Increase* In 71 patients with chronic liver disease without cirrhosis who drink < 40 g alcohol/d mean concentration of 112 µg/L, and 151 µg/L in those drinking > 40 g/d mean concentration significantly higher than in healthy individuals *1405*

C-Reactive Protein *Serum* *Increase* In 55 patients with mild chronic liver disease 30% had concentrations above 5 mg/L *1406*

Cryoglobulins *Serum* *Increase* Cryoglobulinemia observed in 19 of 59 patients with chronic liver disease other than those caused by HBV or HCV infections *3165*

Estradiol *Plasma* *No Effect* In 40 women with amenorrhea who had chronic liver disease other than cirrhosis mean concentration of 0.07 ± 0.07 nmol/L not significantly different from reference interval of 0.08 - 0.11 nmol/L *375*

α-Fetoprotein *Serum* *Increase* In 55 patients with mild chronic liver disease 4% had activities above 30 µg/L *1406*

Follicle Stimulating Hormone *Plasma* *Increase* In 40 women with amenorrhea who had chronic liver disease other than cirrhosis mean concentration of 54 ± 22 IU/L significantly different from upper limit of reference interval of less than 12 IU/L *375*

Follistatin, Free *Serum* *Increase* Mean concentration in 20 patients with chronic liver disease of 8.1 ± 1.1 µg/L significantly different from that in 60 normal adults of 3.5 ± 0.2 µg/L *4523*

γ-Glutamyltransferase *Serum* *Increase* In 55 patients with mild chronic liver disease 58% had activities above 55 U/L *1406*

Intercellular Adhesion Molecule-1 *Serum* *Increase* Mean concentration in 58 patients with mild chronic liver disease of approximately 450 µg/L significantly increased compared with mean concentration in 28 healthy blood donors of 215.5 µg/L (95% confidence limits of mean 198.1 - 232.9 µg/L) *4143*

Luteinizing Hormone *Plasma* *Increase* In 40 women with amenorrhea who had chronic liver disease other than cirrhosis mean concentration of 27 ± 12 IU/L significantly different from upper limit of reference interval of less than 12 IU/L *375*

Macrocytes *Blood* *Increase* In 75 elderly patients with macrocytosis chronic liver disease was responsible in 2 *3232*

N-terminal Peptide of Type III Procollagen *Serum* *Increase* In 71 patients with chronic liver disease without cirrhosis who drink < 40 g alcohol/d mean concentration of 0.90 U/mL, and 1.08 U/mL in those drinking > 40 g/d mean concentration significantly higher than in healthy individuals *1405*

Procollagen 1 C-terminal Peptide *Serum* *Increase* In 71 patients with chronic liver disease without cirrhosis who drink < 40 g alcohol/d mean concentration of 899 µg/L, and 1,118 µg/L in those drinking > 40 g/d mean concentration significantly higher than in healthy individuals *1405*

Prolactin *Plasma* *No Effect* In 40 women with amenorrhea who had chronic liver disease other than cirrhosis mean concentration of 235 ± 139 mIU/L not significantly different from reference interval of 50 - 700 mIU/L *375*

Prolyl Hydroxylase *Serum* *Increase* In 71 with chronic liver disease without cirrhosis who drink < 40 g alcohol/d mean concentration of 78 µg/L, and 88 µg/L in those drinking > 40 g/d mean concentration significantly higher than in healthy individuals *1405*

Rheumatoid Factor *Serum* *Increase* Mean concentration increased in patients with chronic liver disease *2472* Rheumatoid factor may be observed in certain patients *2473*

Sex-Hormone Binding Globulin *Serum* *No Effect* In 40 women with amenorrhea who had chronic liver disease other than cirrhosis mean concentration of 66 ± 33 nmol/L not significantly different from reference interval of 30 - 90 nmol/L *375*

Soluble E-Selectin *Serum* *Increase* In 55 patients with mild chronic liver disease 38% had concentrations above 86 µg/L *1406*

Soluble Intercellular Adhesion Molecule-1 *Serum* *Increase* In 55 patients with mild chronic liver disease, 77% had concentrations above 286 µg/L *1406*

Soluble Vascular Cell Adhesion Molecule-1
Serum *Increase* In 55 patients with mild chronic liver disease, 70% had concentrations above 872 µg/L *1406*

Testosterone *Serum* *No Effect* In 40 women with amenorrhea who had chronic liver disease other than cirrhosis mean concentration of 1.1 ± 1.3 nmol/L not significantly different from reference interval of 0.3 - 2.8 nmol/L *375*

Urea Nitrogen *Serum* *Increase* In 55 patients with mild chronic liver disease 9% had concentrations above 8.6 mmol/L *1406*

571.50 Cirrhosis of Liver

Acetate *Serum* *Increase* In 6 cirrhotics mean concentration of 95 ± 25 µmol/L not significantly different from 79 ± 20 µmol/L in 6 healthy individuals *1460*

α_1-Acid Glycoprotein *Serum* *Decrease* Compared with mean and SD in healthy adults of 0.691 ± 0.165 g/L concentration in 12 cirrhotics with mild liver dysfunction 0.550 ± 0.280 g/L, in 22 with moderate dysfunction 0.478 ± 0.230 g/L and in 13 with severe dysfunction 0.525 ± 0.310 g/L *5464*
Serum *Increase* Sensitivity of 65% and a specificity of 80% with severe liver disease *1439*

Acid-soluble Carnitine, Total *Serum* *No Effect* In 57 patients with cirrhotic liver disease mean concentration of 32.8 ± 27.0 µmol/L not significantly different from 28.0 ± 16.7 µmol/L in 28 healthy volunteer controls *2810*

Acylcarnitine, Short Chain *Serum* *No Effect* In 57 patients with cirrhotic liver disease mean concentration of 15.3 ± 11.4 µmol/L not significantly different from 12.7 ± 6.8 µmol/L in 28 healthy volunteer controls *2810*

Adenosine Deaminase *Serum* *Increase* Increased *3926* *1340* *4956*

Adrenomedullin *Plasma* *Increase* In 28 patients with cirrhosis without ascites mean concentration of 8.2 ± 2.3 fmol/mL and in 12 with ascites mean concentration of 12.7 ± 4.5 fmol/mL significantly different from 5.8 ± 0.8 fmol/mL in 10 healthy controls *2745*

Alanine Aminotransferase *Serum* *Increase* In 24 patients with liver cirrhosis mean activity of 49 U/L higher than reference interval of < 40 U/L *2071* In 5 patients with Child-Pugh grade A disease mean activity of 105 ± 11 U/L, in 10 with Child-Pugh grade B disease of 66 ± 24 U/L and in 13 with Child-Pugh grade C disease of 75 ± 27 U/L, with the diseased patients significantly different from 30 ± 16 U/L in 19 healthy controls *4533* Mean activity of 104 ± 74 U/L in 33 patients with liver cirrhosis significantly different from 24 ± 5 U/L in 29 healthy controls *3668* Mean activity of 102 ± 114 U/L in 33 patients with liver cirrhosis significantly different from 20 ± 7 U/L in 29 healthy controls *3668* Mean activity in 32 patients with hepatic cirrhosis of 54 ± 26 U/L significantly different from < 30 U/L in 28 healthy controls *152* Values are modestly elevated (300 U/L). Much lower than the respective values for AST. In cirrhosis of the liver, even with jaundice, the moderate AST level and the lower ALT level are in contrast with the high levels of both transaminases observed in acute viral hepatitis *1025* In 20 patients with cirrhosis mean activity of 76 ± 25 U/L significantly different from 14 ± 8 U/L in 20 healthy volunteers *2372* In 52% of 48 patients at initial hospitalization for this disorder *1576* In 11 patients with cirrhosis mean activity of 138.55 ± 91.96 U/L significantly higher than 28.50 ± 6.55 U/L in 69 healthy blood donor controls *3591* In 48 patients mean activity 65 ± 21 U/L compared with less than 30 U/L in 838 healthy controls *2374* Slight elevation occurred in 33% of patients with cirrhosis. Values ranged from 11-77 U/L *3161*
Serum *No Effect* In 23 patients with chronic active hepatitis C with cirrhosis mean activity of 145 ± 102 U/L not significantly different from normal *2381*

Albumin *Ascitic Fluid* *Decrease* Concentrations less than 2.0 g/dL reliably differentiate hepatic cirrhosis from other causes of ascites *1921*
Serum *Decrease* In 11 patients with alcoholic cirrhosis mean concentration of 34 ± 6 g/L different from normal range of 42 - 52 g/L *1371* Parallels functional status of parenchymal cells and may be useful for following progress of liver disease; but it may be normal in the presence of considerable liver damage *5544* In 28 patients with cirrhosis without ascites mean concentration of 38 ± 5 g/L and in 12 with ascites mean concentration of 30 ± 7 g/L significantly lower than 43 ± 2 g/L in 10 healthy controls *2745* In 128 patients with liver cirrhosis mean concentration of 40.5 ± 4.2 g/L for Child-Pugh score A, 35 ± 4.9 g/L for Child-Pugh score B and 29.8 ± 5 g/L for Child-Pugh score C significantly decreased compared with 44 ± 8 g/L in healthy controls *1654* Mean concentration of 31.8 ± 5.9 g/L significantly less than 42.1 ± 4.3 g/L in 30 healthy controls *855* In 24 patients with cirrhosis mean concentration of 390 µmol/L (range 280 - 622 µmol/L) generally reduced below reference interval of 540 - 800 µmol/L *3566* Mean concentration of 3.3 ± 0.5 g/dL in 33 patients with liver cirrhosis significantly different from 4.5 ± 0.3 g/dL in 29 healthy controls *3668* In 5 patients with Child-Pugh grade A disease mean concentration of 2.96 ± 0.67 g/dL, in 10 with Child-Pugh grade B disease 2.16 ± 1.01 g/dL and in 13 with Child-Pugh grade C disease 2.44 ± 0.39 g/dL, with the diseased patients significantly different from 4.42 ± 0.62 g/dL in 19 healthy controls *4533* In 29 male patients with liver cirrhosis mean concentration of 3.75 ± 0.07 g/dL and 3.61 ± 0.10 g/dL in 39 female patients with liver cirrhosis mean concentration significantly different compared with normal range of 3.9 - 5.0 g/dL *4803* Mean concentration of 29 ± 6 g/L observed in 27 patients with cirrhosis *3315* In 9 patients with cirrhosis without ascites and 25 patients with cirrhosis and ascites mean concentration of 34 ± 2 g/L and 27 ± 1 g/L, respectively, significantly lower than 47 ± 1 g/L in 17 healthy controls *1904* Mean values were found to be highest in the healthy subjects followed by acute viral hepatitis, primary hepatocellular carcinoma and cirrhosis, in that order. Both the mean albumin and mean total globulin of each group, were significantly different from the respective means of the other 3 groups *1459* Mean concentration in 32 patients with hepatic cirrhosis of 3.2 ± 0.5 g/dL significantly different from > 40 g/dL in 28 healthy controls *152* In 33 patients with decompensated hepatic cirrhosis mean concentration of 29 ± 1 g/L significantly less than 38 ± 1 g/L in 31 compensated cirrhotic patients *2964* In 14 patients with alcoholic cirrhosis mean concentration of 33 ± 6 g/L different from normal range of 42 - 52 g/L *1371* In 51% of 69 patients at initial hospitalization for this disorder *1576* In 15 patients with Child's group A disease mean 38 ± 5 g/L, in 16 with Child's group B 31 ± 6 g/L and 10 with Child's group C 25 ± 5 g/L less than that in healthy adults *638* In 10 patients with liver cirrhosis without ascites mean concentration of 3.6 ± 0.4 g/dL and 2.8 ± 0.2 g/dL in 11 patients with cirrhosis and ascites significantly different from mean concentration of 4.9 ± 0.3 g/dL in 10 healthy controls *5349* In 21 patients with cirrhosis but without ascites mean concentration of 35 g/L and 29 g/L in 19 with cirrhosis and ascites compared with normal values of 35 - 50 g/L *5347*
Serum *No Effect* In 24 patients with liver cirrhosis mean concentration of 3.9 ± 0.4 g/L not different from reference interval of 3.8 - 5.3 g/L *2071* Usually parallels functional status of parenchymal cells, but may be normal in the presence of considerable liver cell damage *5544* In 23 patients with chronic active hepatitis C with cirrhosis mean concentration of 4.0 ± 0.4 g/dL not significantly different from normal *2381*

Alcohol Dehydrogenase *Serum* *Increase* In 60 Nigerians with cirrhosis of the liver mean activity of 2.7 ± 0.5 U/L significantly different from 0.7 ± 0.1 U/L in 120 healthy controls *3866*

Aldolase *Serum* *Increase* Normal or slightly increased *1980*
Serum *No Effect* Activity typically normal or slightly increased in patients with portal cirrhosis *2952* Normal or slightly increased *1980*

Aldosterone *Plasma* *Increase* Increased secretion *4707* Mean concentration in 10 non-azotemic cirrhotics of 241 ± 67 pg/mL significantly increased compared with normal *3877* In 10 patients with liver cirrhosis without ascites mean concentration of 108 ± 26 pg/mL (not significant) and 218 ± 194 pg/mL in 11 patients with cirrhosis and ascites significantly different from mean concentration of 75 ± 51 pg/mL in 10 healthy controls *5349* In 20 patients with hepatic cirrhosis mean plasma aldosterone concentration of 334 ± 79 pg/mL not significantly different from 125 ± 15 pg/mL in 19 healthy individuals *1464* Increased levels *4289* In 25 patients with cirrhosis with ascites mean concentration of 157 ± 48 ng/dL significantly higher than 12 ± 4 ng/dL in 9 patients with cirrhosis but without ascites and 27 ± 4 ng/dL in 17 healthy controls *1904* In 10 patients with liver cirrhosis and ascites mean concentration of 740 pg/mL significantly higher than 133 pg/mL in 7 patients with liver cirrhosis without ascites *1650*
Urine *Increase* May be increased in edematous states of hepatic cirrhosis *1290*

571.50 Cirrhosis of Liver (continued)

Alkaline Phosphatase *Serum Increase* In 21 patients with cirrhosis but without ascites mean activity of 338 U/L and 378 U/L in 19 with cirrhosis and ascites compared with normal values of 100 - 300 U/L *5347* In 24 patients with cirrhosis mean activity of 405 U/L (range 106 - 1139 U/L) generally higher than reference interval of 50 - 275 U/L *3566* In 47% of 67 patients at initial hospitalization for this disorder *1576* Average elevation in 6 cases 3.5 times normal upper limit *3161* In 5 patients with Child-Pugh grade A disease mean activity of 112 ± 38 U/L, in 10 with Child-Pugh grade B disease 110 ± 36 U/L and in 13 with Child-Pugh grade C disease 121 ± 38 U/L, with the latter two groups of diseased patients significantly different from 80 ± 35 U/L in 19 healthy controls *4533* Mean activity in 32 patients with hepatic cirrhosis of 205 ± 90 U/L significantly different from < 200 U/L in 28 healthy controls *152* In 33 patients with cirrhosis of the liver 61% had activities above 112 U/L *1406* Non-specifically elevated in cirrhosis but often reaches levels exceeding 160 U/L *900* 50% incidence of elevation usually in the range of 25 - 188 U/L in postnecrotic cirrhosis *1025*
Serum No Effect In 23 patients with chronic active hepatitis C with cirrhosis mean activity of 218 ± 7- U/L not significantly different from normal *2381* In 24 patients with liver cirrhosis mean activity of 180 U/L within reference interval of 90 - 250 U/L *2071*
White Blood Cells Increase Slightly increased in 30% of patients *5544*

Amino Acids *Cerebrospinal Fluid Increase* Increased in advanced cirrhosis in proportion to the degree of liver damage *1290*
Urine Increase Increased in advanced cirrhosis in proportion to the degree of liver damage *1290* Mean amino acid clearance (glycine, glutamine, serine, threonine, alanine, and tyrosine) were raised in Indian childhood cirrhosis patients *4577*

Ammonia *Blood Increase* In 6 cirrhotics mean concentration of 129 ± 35 mg/dL significantly different from 86 ± 19 mg/dL in 6 healthy individuals *1460* Increased in liver coma and cirrhosis and with portacaval shunting of blood *5544*

Amylase *Pleural Fluid No Effect* Usually less than or equal to serum level *4493*
Serum Increase Activity greater than 220 U/L observed in 42% patients with hepatic cirrhosis *4110* High incidence of pancreatic abnormality in patients with no clinical evidence of pancreatic acinar disease *5378*
Urine Increase High incidence of pancreatic abnormality in patients with no clinical evidence of pancreatic acinar disease *5378*

Amylase, Pancreatic Isoenzyme *Serum Increase* Activity increased in some patients with hepatic cirrhosis who had high total amylase activities *4110*

Angiotensin-converting Enzyme *Serum Increase* In 10 patients with non-azotemic cirrhosis mean activity increased to 25.8 ± 1.8 U/L *3877*

Anti-Mitochondrial Antibodies *Serum Increase* Positive in a majority of patients with postnecrotic cirrhosis, independent of the presence of HBsAg or LE cells *4160* Found in 5 - 30% of patients with postnecrotic cirrhosis depending upon the technique used *4160* Observed effect *4778*

Antibody Titer *Serum Increase* Increased incidence of high titers of serum autoantibodies *4778* Patients with cirrhosis appear to have antibodies to a larger number of enteric bacteria though not higher titers to individual strains *4160* Increased incidence of antithyroid antibodies *4960*

Anticardiolipin-specific IgG Antibodies *Serum Increase* In 18 patients with cirrhosis mean concentration of 15.1 ± 14.9 GPL units significantly different from 6.3 ± 4.4 GPL units in 11 healthy controls *42*

Antidiuretic Hormone *Plasma Decrease* In 10 patients with liver cirrhosis without ascites mean concentration of 1.0 ± 0.8 pg/mL and 1.3 ± 1.1 pg/mL in 11 patients with cirrhosis and ascites not significantly different from mean concentration of 0.8 ± 0.7 pg/mL in 10 healthy controls *5349*

Antinuclear Antibodies *Serum Increase* Increased incidence of high titers of serum autoantibodies *4778* With postnecrotic cirrhosis *367*

α_2-Antiplasmin *Plasma Decrease* Values of 4.24 and 2.56 mg/dL for compensated and decompensated liver cirrhosis compared to 6.2 mg/dL for controls *4543* Significant decrease in hepatic cirrhosis and in several other liver diseases. Mean value of 73 ± 15% compared to 100 ± 8% for controls *5187* Values of 4.24 and 2.56 mg/dL for compensated and decompensated liver cirrhosis compared to 6.2 mg/dL for controls *157*

Antithrombin III *Plasma Decrease* Decreased *3472 5220* In 18 patients mean concentration of 9.4 ± 4.9 U/mL significantly less than 11.8 ± 1.1 U/mL in 30 healthy controls *855*

Antithyroglobulin Antibodies *Serum Increase* Increased incidence of antithyroid antibodies *2320*

α_1-Antitrypsin *Serum Increase* Increased *4763 4371 4373 4241 83*

Apolipoprotein A-I *Serum Decrease* Prebeta and alpha lipoprotein were decreased *1440* Mean concentration of 913 ± 221 mg/L in 6 patients with decompensated liver cirrhosis and 1052 ± 217 mg/L in 17 patients with compensated liver cirrhosis significantly different from 1522 ± 212 mg/L in 21 healthy controls *5063*

Arginine *Plasma No Effect* Concentrations of 98.7 ± 41.7 µmol/L in 13 patients with Child-Turcotte subgroup C liver cirrhosis not significantly different from 110 ± 23.9 µmol/L in 66 healthy controls *3292*
Urine No Effect Excretions of 17.4 ± 35.3 µmol/g creatinine in 13 patients with Child-Turcotte subgroup C liver cirrhosis significantly different from 20.9 ± 15.9 µmol/g creatinine in 66 healthy controls *3292*

Argininic Acid *Serum No Effect* Concentrations of < 0.015 - 0.130 µmol/L in 13 patients with Child-Turcotte subgroup C liver cirrhosis significantly different from < 0.015 - 0.440 µmol/L in 66 healthy controls *3292*
Urine No Effect Excretions of 5.33 ± 2.76 µmol/g creatinine in 13 patients with Child-Turcotte subgroup C liver cirrhosis not significantly different from 6.73 ± 2.80 µmol/g creatinine in 66 healthy controls *3292*

Aspartate Aminotransferase *Serum Increase* In 33 patients with cirrhosis of the liver 85% had activities above 40 U/L *1406* In 89% of 69 patients at initial hospitalization for this disorder *1576* In 11 patients with nonalcoholic cirrhosis mean activity of 2.2 ± 2.6 µkat/L different from normal range of < 0.6 µkat/L *1371* In 14 patients with alcoholic cirrhosis mean activity of 2.0 ± 1.5 µkat/L different from normal range of < 0.6 µkat/L *1371* Mean activity in 32 patients with hepatic cirrhosis of 52 ± 24 U/L significantly different from < 20 U/L in 28 healthy controls *152* 60 - 70% incidence of elevated activities: up to 145 U/L in 65 - 75% of cases *5544* In 24 patients with cirrhosis mean activity 79 U/L (range 30 - 261 U/L) higher than reference interval of 10 - 40 U/L *3566* In 11 patients with cirrhosis mean activity of 142.91 ± 139.15 U/L significantly higher than 22.81 ± 7.95 U/L in 69 healthy blood donor controls *3591* Mild elevation occurred in 86% of 6 cases. Mean elevation was twice normal upper limit *3161*
Serum No Effect In 23 patients with chronic active hepatitis C with cirrhosis mean activity of 103 ± 88 U/L not significantly different from normal *2381*

Aspartate Aminotransferase:Alanine Aminotransferase Ratio *Serum Decrease* Ratios less than 1.0 in observed in 41 of 130 patients with hepatic cirrhosis who typically had low Child-Pugh scores *1723*

Atrial Natriuretic Peptide *Plasma Increase* In 20 patients with hepatic cirrhosis mean atrial natriuretic peptide concentration of 72 ± 9 pg/mL significantly different from 32 ± 5 pg/mL in 19 healthy individuals *1464* In 10 patients with cirrhosis and ascites mean concentration of 81.3 ± 8.5 pg/mL significantly higher than 29.8 ± 3.2 pg/mL in 6 healthy controls *2447* In 25 patients with cirrhosis with ascites mean concentration of 63 ± 7 fmol/mL and 45 ± 10 fmol/mL in 9 patients with cirrhosis but without ascites significantly higher than 18 ± 1 fmol/mL in 17 healthy controls *1904* In patients with cirrhosis increased plasma atrial natriuretic peptide concentrations were related to the degree of hemodilution, increased pulmonary arterial pressure and the degree of portal hypertension, but not by arterial oxygenation levels *3595*

Basic Fibroblast Growth Factor *Serum Increase* Mean concentration of 8.7 pg/mL (range 3.8 - 44.2 pg/mL) in 21 patients not significantly different from 4.8 pg/mL (range 2.9 - 9.5 pg/mL) in 40 healthy individuals, but with 42.9% abnormal *2262*

Bile Acids *Serum* *Increase* Significant increase of total and individual bile acids observed in 20 patients with moderate post-hepatic cirrhosis *1854*
Serum *No Effect* Serum bile acids did not discriminate between anicteric patients with fatty liver (n = 10) and liver cirrhosis (n = 9) and normal controls (n = 27), *1312*
Urine *Increase* Mean values for bile acids in urine: control 1.9 µg/mL, obstructive jaundice µg/mL and cirrhosis of 15.14 µg/mL (compensated) and 11.84 µg/mL (uncompensated) *5148*

Bile Acids, Conjugated *Serum* *Increase* Mean concentration of total conjugated bile acids of 4.171 ± 1.406 µg/mL in 20 patients with moderate post-hepatitis cirrhosis significantly higher than 0.432 ± 0.104 µg/mL in 20 healthy controls *1854*

Bilirubin *Serum* *Increase* Mean concentration of 56 µmol/L (5 - 265 U/L) generally higher than reference interval of 2 - 17 µg/L *3566* Most is indirect unless cirrhosis is of the cholangiolitic type. Higher and more stable in postnecrotic cirrhosis; lower and more fluctuating levels occur in Laennec's cirrhosis. Terminal icterus may be constant and severe *5544* Usually elevated except in well-compensated liver disease. A direct bilirubin > 0.3 mg/dL means liver disease unless severe hemolysis or the rare congenital syndromes of bilirubin metabolism are present *900* Values range from 7.8 - 8 mg/dL in postnecrotic cirrhosis *5738* In 11 patients with nonalcoholic cirrhosis mean concentration of 63 ± 115 µmol/L different from normal range of 4 - 21 µmol/L *1371* In 21 patients with cirrhosis but without ascites mean concentration of 21 µmol/L and 67 µmol/L in 19 with cirrhosis and ascites compared with normal values of 5 - 21 µmol/L *5347* In 14 patients with alcoholic cirrhosis mean concentration of 56 ± 70 µmol/L different from normal range of 4 - 21 µmol/L *1371* In 5 patients with Child-Pugh grade A disease mean concentration of 0.91 ± 0.53 mg/dL, in 10 with Child-Pugh grade B disease 1.53 ± 0.73 mg/dL and in 13 with Child-Pugh grade C disease 2.97 ± 1.18 mg/dL, with the diseased patients significantly different from 0.56 ± 0.36 mg/dL in 19 healthy controls *4533* In 29 male patients with liver cirrhosis mean concentration of 1.23 ± 0.09 mg/dL and 1.33 ± 0.08 mg/dL in 39 female patients with liver cirrhosis mean concentration significantly different compared with normal range of 0.3 - 1.2 mg/dL *4803* In 54% of 68 patients at initial hospitalization for this disorder *1576* In 33 patients with cirrhosis of the liver 52% had concentrations above 26 µmol/L *1406* Mean concentration of 167.6 ± 203.5 µmol/L observed in 27 patients with cirrhosis *3315* In 10 patients with liver cirrhosis without ascites mean concentration of 1.1 ± 0.3 mg/dL and 2.3 ± 1.8 mg/dL in 11 patients with cirrhosis and ascites significantly different from mean concentration of 0.7 ± 0.2 mg/dL in 10 healthy controls *5349* In 33 patients with decompensated hepatic cirrhosis mean concentration of 2.0 ± 0.4 mg/dL significantly higher than 1.2 ± 0.1 mg/dL in 31 compensated cirrhotic patients *2964* Mean concentration of 3.8 ± 2.5 mg/dL in 33 patients with liver cirrhosis significantly different from 0.6 ± 0.1 mg/dL in 29 healthy controls *3668* In 20 patients with cirrhosis mean concentration of 1.4 ± 0.5 mg/dL significantly different from 0.5 ± 0.3 mg/dL in 20 healthy volunteers *2372* In 9 patients with cirrhosis without ascites and 25 patients with cirrhosis and ascites mean concentration of 1.6 ± 0.2 mg/dL and 6.8 ± 2.0 mg/dL, respectively, significantly higher than 0.7 ± 0.1 mg/dL in 17 healthy controls *1904* In 15 patients with Child's group A disease mean 1.3 ± 0.5 mg/dL, in 16 with Child's group B 4.8 ± 4.1 mg/dL and 10 with Child's group C 9.3 ± 8.1 mg/dL greater than that in healthy adults *638* In 28 patients with cirrhosis without ascites mean concentration of 1.4 ± 1.1 mg/dL and in 12 with ascites mean concentration of 2.5 ± 1.4 mg/dL significantly higher than 0.6 ± 0.1 mg/dL in 10 healthy controls *2745* Mean concentration in 32 patients with hepatic cirrhosis of 3.2 ± 2.8 mg/dL significantly different from < 1.0 mg/dL in 28 healthy controls *152*
Serum *No Effect* In 23 patients with chronic active hepatitis C with cirrhosis mean concentration of 0.9 ± 0.3 mg/dL not significantly different from normal *2381* In 24 patients with liver cirrhosis mean concentration of 0.8 mg/dL within reference interval of 0.2 - 1.0 mg/dL *2071*

Bilirubin, Direct *Serum* *Increase* In 87% of 29 patients at initial hospitalization for this disorder *1576*

Bilirubin, Indirect *Serum* *Increase* In 71% of 27 patients at initial hospitalization for this disorder *1576*

Biotin *Serum* *Decrease* Significantly low in decompensated liver cirrhosis compared to healthy controls *3703*

Bleeding Time *Patient* *Increase* In 28 of 70 patients (40%) with cirrhosis following a variety of causes abnormal bleeding time of more than 10 minutes observed *5477*

BSP Retention *Serum* *Increase* Decreased removal of dye in advanced cirrhosis of liver *1290* Sensitive index of liver function and is most useful in the absence of jaundice to follow the course of disease when the other liver function tests are normal *5544*

c-erb-B_2 Oncoprotein *Serum* *Increase* Abnormal concentrations observed in 10 of 26 (38.5%) of patients *3564*

CA 15-3 *Serum* *Increase* In 26 patients with cirrhosis mean concentration of 26.8 ± 19 U/mL higher than cutoff of 22 U/mL, with 10 having concentrations greater than 25 U/mL and 6 having concentrations greater than 40 U/mL *2076* Elevated in 11.6% of 86 cirrhotic patients *886*

CA 19-9 *Serum* *Increase* CA 19-9 concentration increased in some patients with hepatic cirrhosis *1253* Positive analyses have been encountered *3657* *2026* In patients with hepatic cirrhosis false positive rate observed in 50 of 211 patients *1404* CA 19-9 concentration increased in 62% of 118 patients with liver cirrhosis *1253* CA 19-9 concentration increased above 37 U/mL in 23.7% patients with hepatic cirrhosis *1253* In 33 patients with cirrhosis of the liver 61% had concentrations above 35 U/mL *1406* Increased concentrations observed in 47% patients with cirrhosis and other benign liver diseases *5276* In one study 57% of patients had concentrations above cutoff of 60 U/mL *3120* In 162 patients with liver cirrhosis positive rate of 12% observed using cut-off from normals and 9% at 90% specificity *2594*

CA 27-29 *Serum* *Increase* In 21% of 19 women concentration above 36 U/mL *766*

CA 72-4 *Serum* *No Effect* In one study no patients had concentrations above cutoff value of 4.0 U/mL *3120*

CA 125 *Serum* *Increase* Median concentration of 293 µg/L in 20 patients with liver cirrhosis *5191* In 20 patients with hepatic cirrhosis median concentration of 293 U/L *2090* In one study 54% of patients had concentrations above cutoff of 35 U/mL *3120* In 40 patients with liver cirrhosis mean concentration of 191.6 ± 191.9 U/mL with 67.5% having concentrations above 35 U/mL *2636*

CA 195 *Serum* *Increase* False positive results occurred in 100% of patients *3228*

CA 242 *Serum* *Increase* In 162 patients with liver cirrhosis positive rate of 7% observed using cut-off from normals and 8% at 90% specificity *2594*

Calcium *Serum* *Decrease* In 38% of 68 patients at initial hospitalization for this disorder *1576* Low concentrations correlated well with high AST activity in 78 cirrhotic patients *3467*

Carcinoembryonic Antigen *Pleural Fluid* *Increase* Mean concentration increased in 1 of 11 effusions in patients with liver cirrhosis *1649*
Serum *Increase* Increase observed *4551* In 120 patients with alcoholic cirrhosis 30% had concentrations less than 2.5 ng/mL, 44% had concentrations between 2.6 and 5.0 ng/mL, 24% had concentrations between 5.1 and 10.0 ng/mL and 2% had concentrations greater than 10.0 ng/mL *2010* In 62 patients with cirrhosis of the liver 53.2% had concentrations up to 3.0 ng/mL, 19.4% had concentrations between 3.1 - 5.0 ng/mL, 22.6% between 5.1 - 10.0 ng/mL and 4.8% had concentrations greater than 10.1 ng/mL in contrast to concentrations in 151 healthy nonsmokers in whom 95.4% had concentrations between 0 and 3.0 ng/mL and 4.6% between 4.1 and 10.0 ng/mL *11* In one study 32% of patients had concentrations above cutoff value of 5.0 ng/mL *3120* Increase observed in some patients *1601* In 34 patients with cirrhosis 41.2% had concentrations of 0.0 - 3.0 ng/mL, 23.5% had concentrations from 3.1 - 5.0 ng/mL, 17.6% had concentrations from 5.1 - 10.0 ng/mL and 17.6% had concentrations greater than 10.0 ng/mL when measured by method on Bayer Technicon Immuno 1® system compared with 95.9%, 3.5%, 0.6% and 0.0% respectively in 173 healthy nonsmokers *339*
Serum *No Effect* Positive assays were obtained in 40 of 88 patients with severe alcoholic liver disease but in none of 14 patients with nonalcoholic liver disease. Values usually were lower than in colonic or pancreatic cancer *3587*

Cardiac Output *Patient* *Increase* In 20 patients with hepatic cirrhosis mean cardiac output of 5,917 ± 205 mL/min significantly different from 4,825 ± 174 mL/min in 19 healthy individuals *1464*

571.50 Cirrhosis of Liver *(continued)*

Carnitine *Serum* *Increase* Patients with liver disease had increased plasma concentrations of free (96 µmol/L) and total (144 µmol/L) compared with controls (free = 45 µmol/L) and total (58 µmol/L) *5638*

Carnitine, Free *Serum* *Increase* In 57 patients with cirrhotic liver disease mean concentration of 17.5 ± 18.4 µmol/L not significantly different from 15.3 ± 10.5 µmol/L in 28 healthy volunteer controls *2810*

Carvedilol *Serum* *Increase* In patients with cirrhotic liver disease concentration of carvedilol on average about 4 to 6 times higher than in healthy individuals *4915*

Cathepsin D *Serum* *Increase* Mean concentration in 92 patients with liver cirrhosis of 65.7 ± 3 9 nmol/L significantly increased compared with 10.0 ± 0.71 nmol/L in 98 healthy controls *3004* Concentration increased in 70-75% of patients *595*

CD4+ Lymphocytes *Blood* *No Effect* No significant rise *3916*

CD8+ Lymphocytes *Blood* *Increase* Significantly higher as compared with normal controls *3916*

Cells *Bone Marrow* *Increase* Normal or increased *2684*

Ceruloplasmin *Serum* *Increase* Elevated in various forms of acute and chronic liver disease *1898*

Chenodeoxycholic Acid *Serum* *Increase* 3-β-Hydroxy-5-cholenoic acid concentration was increased in hepatobiliary disease. Normal - 0.184 mmol/L. Cirrhosis: compensated 0.433 mmol/L and uncompensated 1.636 mmol/L *5149* Raised fasting levels were found in 29 of 49 patients *5239*

Cholesterol *Ascitic Fluid* *Decrease* Concentrations less than 55 mg/dL reliably differentiate hepatic cirrhosis from other causes of ascites *1921*
Ascitic Fluid *Increase* In 73 specimens from patients with cirrhosis or hepatocellular carcinoma mean concentration of 0.70 ± 0.05 mmol/L but significantly less than 3.14 ± 0.24 mmol/L in 21 specimens from patients with peritoneal neoplasia *728*
Serum *Decrease* Mean concentration of 1,300 ± 314 mg/L in 6 patients with decompensated liver cirrhosis and 1,435 ± 308 mg/L in 17 patients with compensated liver cirrhosis significantly different from 1,892 ± 233 mg/L in 21 healthy controls *5063* Mean concentration in 32 patients with hepatic cirrhosis of 140 ± 42 mg/dL significantly different from 150 - 230 mg/dL in 28 healthy controls *152* In 26 alcoholic cirrhotics mean concentration of 4.43 ± 1.24 mmol/L significantly less than 5.68 ± 1.39 mmol/L in 10 age and sex matched controls *3345* Significant decrease in concentration noted in 34 patients with hepatic cirrhosis compared with that in 34 patients with chronic active hepatitis and 34 controls with unrelated diseases, with decrease progressing with increased severity of disease *853* Significantly reduced. Prebeta and alpha lipoprotein were decreased also *1440* In 24% of 61 patients at initial hospitalization for this disorder *1576*
Serum *No Effect* In 37 individuals with hepatic cirrhosis mean concentration of 5.04 ± 1.70 mmol/L not significantly different from 5.47 ± 0.95 mmol/L in 98 healthy controls aged 24 to 55 years with method performed on ILab® 900 automated analyzer *4848*

Cholesterol, Esterified *Cerebrospinal Fluid* *No Effect* In 21 patients with Alzheimer's disease mean concentration of 0.25 ± 0.29 mg/dL not significantly different from 0.42 ± 0.34 mg/dL in 28 matched controls *3645*

Cholesterol Esters *Serum* *Decrease* Decreased esters reflect more severe parenchymal cell damage *5544*

Cholesterol, Free *Cerebrospinal Fluid* *No Effect* In 21 patients with Alzheimer's disease mean concentration of 0.13 ± 0.19 mg/dL not significantly different from 0.25 ± 0.19 mg/dL in 27 matched controls *3645*

Cholic Acid *Serum* *Increase* Raised fasting levels were found in 19 of 49 patients (39%) *5239* Elevated in 97% of patients *2137*

Cholinesterase *Serum* *Decrease* In 10 patients with liver cirrhosis without ascites mean activity of 0.48 ± 0.12 δ pH and 0.22 ± 0.07 δ pH in 11 patients with cirrhosis and ascites significantly different from mean activity of 0.84 ± 0.14 δ pH in 10 healthy controls *5349* In 33 patients with cirrhosis of the liver 45% had activities below 4,000 U/L *1406* In 128 patients with liver cirrhosis mean concentration of 5,976 ± 2,625 U/L for Child-Pugh score A, 3,649 ± 1,834 U/L for Child-Pugh score B and 2,106 ± 1,498 U/L for Child-Pugh score C significantly decreased compared with 9,500 ± 5,000 U/L in healthy controls *1654* In 18 patients with hepatic cirrhosis mean activity of 2302 ± 1072 U/L significantly less than 5902 ± 1233 U/L in 16 healthy individuals *2632* In 21 patients with cirrhosis but without ascites mean activity of 0.42 U/L and 0.23 U/L in 19 with cirrhosis and ascites compared with normal values of 0.6 - 1.2 U/L *5347* Tends to be more marked in chronic liver disease, such as cirrhosis than in acute disorders. Sixty patients with chronic liver disease showed a serum cholinesterase range of 0.73 - 0.008 *5498*
Serum *Increase* In active cirrhosis *1290*

β-Chorionic Gonadotropin *Ascitic Fluid* *No Effect* Concentration below 10 mIU/mL in all but 1 of 55 patients with hepatic cirrhosis *1702*

Chylomicrons *Peritoneal Fluid* *Increase* Present *3242*

Collagen IV *Serum* *Increase* In 100 patients with cirrhosis who drink < 40 g alcohol/d mean concentration of 283 µg/L, and 342 µg/L in those drinking > 40 g/d mean concentration significantly higher than in healthy individuals *1405*

Complement C_3 *Serum* *Decrease* Low levels of C_3, C_4, and factor B were common with cirrhosis and confined to those cases with severe reduction in serum albumin and/or prothrombin time *790*

Complement C_4 *Serum* *Decrease* Low levels of C_3, C_4, and factor B were common with cirrhosis and confined to those cases with severe reduction in serum albumin and/or prothrombin time *790* Decreased C_3 and C_4 occasionally occur *2332*

Complement, Total *Serum* *Decrease* Depressed in patients with chronic liver disease; does not correlate with immune phenomena, but appears to be related to impaired hepatic protein synthesis *367* Decreased C_3 and C_4 occasionally occurs *2332*

Copper *Serum* *Increase* Elevated in various forms of acute and chronic liver disease *1290* *1898*

Coproporphyrin *Urine* *Increase* In liver disease, coproporphyrinuria may not indicate increased formation of the pigment, but rather its diversion from bile to urine *367*

C-Reactive Protein *Serum* *Increase* In 33 patients with cirrhosis of the liver 67% had concentrations above 5 mg/L *1406*

Creatine *Serum* *No Effect* Concentrations of 16.5 ± 11.5 µmol/L in male patients and 56.6 ± 50.2 µmol/L in female patients with Child-Turcotte subgroup C liver cirrhosis not significantly different from 30.1 ± 12.3 µmol/L in male and 54.8 ± 21.0 µmol/L in female healthy controls respectively *3292*
Urine *No Effect* Excretions of 25 - 170 µmol/g creatinine in male patients and 30 ± 4,680 µmol/g creatinine in female patients with Child-Turcotte subgroup C liver cirrhosis not significantly different from 30 - 1,700 µmol/g creatinine in male and 30 - 3,200 µmol/g creatinine in female healthy controls respectively *3292*

Creatine Kinase *Serum* *No Effect* No significant effect observed *1980*

Creatine Kinase MB-Isoenzyme *Serum* *No Effect* In 32 patients with cirrhosis and normal ECG cardiac mass CK-MB concentration normal in all patients *4034*

Creatinine *Serum* *Decrease* Concentrations of 65.5 ± 18.3 µmol/L in male patients with Child-Turcotte subgroup C liver cirrhosis significantly different from 80.8 ± 17.7 µmol/L in male healthy controls *3292*
Serum *No Effect* In 9 patients with cirrhosis without ascites and 25 patients with cirrhosis and ascites mean concentration of 1.0 ± 0.1 mg/dL and 1.6 ± 0.3 mg/dL, respectively, not significantly different from 0.9 ± 0.04 mg/dL in 17 healthy controls *1904* In 10 patients with liver cirrhosis without ascites mean concentration of 1.1 ± 0.2 mg/dL and 1.3 ± 0.3 mg/dL in 11 patients with cirrhosis and ascites not significantly different from mean concentration of 1.1 ± 0.3 mg/dL in 10 healthy controls *5349* In 28 patients with cirrhosis without ascites mean concentration of 0.8 ± 0.3 mg/dL and in 12 with ascites mean concentration of 1.0 ± 0.4 mg/dL not significantly different from 1.1 ± 0.3 mg/dL in 10 healthy controls *2745* In 21 patients with cirrhosis but without ascites mean concentration of 71 µmol/L and 88 µmol/L in 19 with cirrhosis and ascites compared with normal values of 26 - 80 µmol/L *5347* Concentrations of 54.2 ± 19.8 µmol/L in female patients with Child-Turcotte subgroup C liver cirrhosis not significantly different from 65.3 ± 19.7 µmol/L in

male healthy controls *3292* In 24 patients with cirrhosis mean concentration of 88 µmol/L (range 45 - 142 µmol/L) generally not different from reference interval of 49 - 121 µmol/L *3566*

Creatinine Clearance *Urine Decrease* In 10 patients with liver cirrhosis without ascites mean clearance of 88 ± 15 mL/min and 62 ± 14 mL/min in 11 patients with cirrhosis and ascites significantly different from mean clearance of 113 ± 25 mL/min in 10 healthy controls *5349* In 21 patients with cirrhosis but without ascites mean clearance of 107 mL/min and 62 mL/min in 19 with cirrhosis and ascites compared with normal values of 90 - 170 mL/min *5347*
Urine No Effect In 20 patients with hepatic cirrhosis mean clearance of 96 ± 5 mL/min not significantly different from 110 ± 11 mL/min in 19 healthy individuals *1464*

CYFRA 21-1 *Serum Increase* In 34 patients with liver cirrhosis median concentration of 2.9 ng/mL significantly different from that in 50 healthy individuals with median concentration of 1.2 ng/mL and range of 0.5 - 2.4 ng/mL *3559* Median concentration of 4.7 µg/L in 20 patients with liver cirrhosis significantly different from 1.9 µg/L in 40 healthy controls *5191*

D-Dimer *Plasma Increase* In patients with either compensated or decompensated alcoholic liver cirrhosis concentration significantly compared with controls, but concentration higher in decompensated cirrhosis *1841*

Descarboxyprothrombin *Serum Increase* Five of 60 patients (8.3%) had a mean concentration that exceeded 40 mAU/mL in 273 normal individuals *3897*

Endothelin *Plasma Decrease* Early papers reported subnormal or normal concentrations *3568*
Plasma Increase Typically increased concentrations reported in patients with cirrhosis of the liver, with higher concentrations in patients with fluid retention and the highest concentrations in patients with functional renal failure. Concentrations very high when cirrhosis is complicated by hepatocellular carcinoma *3568* In 25 patients with cirrhosis with ascites mean concentration of 29 ± 4 pg/mL significantly higher than 13 ± 8 pg/mL in 9 patients with cirrhosis but without ascites and 5 ± 0.4 pg/mL in 17 healthy controls *1904* In 10 patients with liver cirrhosis and ascites mean concentration of 11.2 pg/mL significantly higher than 7.6 pg/mL in 7 patients with liver cirrhosis without ascites *1650*
Plasma No Effect Early papers reported subnormal or normal concentrations *3568*

Endothelin-1 *Plasma Decrease* Plasma levels of endothelin (ET) were determined by radioimmunoassay in 11 healthy volunteers and 34 patients with liver cirrhosis. The results revealed that the mean ET plasma level was significantly lower in 34 cirrhotic patients than in normal subjects (40.21 ± 4.38 ng/L vs 84.55 ± 7.88 ng/L, p < 0.01) *807*
Plasma Increase In 96 patients with cirrhosis mean concentration of 8.4 ± 0.3 pg/mL significantly different from 5.1 ± 0.3 pg/mL in 56 age- and sex-matched healthy controls *5297* ET-1 levels (3.71 ± 1.17 pg/mL) were significantly higher than those in healthy controls (2.18 ± 0.37 pg/mL) *5339* The plasma endothelin concentration was significantly higher in patients with cirrhosis with ascites than in normal controls (8.3 ± 2.3 pg/mL vs. 3.3 ± 1.4 pg/mL, mean ± S.D., p less than 0.001), *5340* In 24 patients with cirrhosis mean brachial venous concentration of 3.40 pg/mL (range of 1.25 - 7.84 pg/mL) significantly higher than 1.53 pg/mL (range of 0.78 - 2.12 pg/mL) in 11 controls *3566* Concentrations reported to be high in cirrhosis of various etiologies in children *3568* In 41 patients with cirrhosis mean concentration in hepatic vein of 21.2 ± 0.9 pg/mL significantly different from 9.6 ± 1.6 pg/mL in hepatic vein of 10 normotensive controls: similar differences observed in femoral artery blood *3567*

Endothelin-3 *Plasma Increase* In 41 patients with cirrhosis mean concentration in hepatic vein of 19.0 ± 1.4 pg/mL significantly different from 10.0 ± 1.4 pg/mL in hepatic vein of 10 normotensive controls: similar differences observed in femoral artery blood *3567* In 96 patients with cirrhosis mean concentration of 23.9 ± 1.7 pg/mL significantly different from 18.2 ± 2.3 pg/mL in 56 age- and sex-matched healthy controls *5297*

Erythrocyte Sedimentation Rate *Blood Increase* Extreme elevation is found *5544*

Erythrocyte Survival *Red Blood Cells Decrease* Moderately shortened in 48 of 68 alcoholic liver disease patients *4769* Mild to moderate hemolysis *4199* Especially in patients with predominant indirect bilirubinemia *1457* Moderately shortened in 48 of 68 alcoholic liver disease patients *2684 5699*

Erythrocytes *Ascitic Fluid Increase* > 10,000 cells/µL seen in 1% of cases *233*
Blood Decrease Anemia reflects increased plasma volume and some increased destruction of RBCs. If more severe, rule out hemorrhage in gastrointestinal tract, folic acid deficiency, excessive hemolysis, etc *5544*

Estradiol *Plasma Increase* Estradiol is the most active estrogen *457 91 1267* In 29 male patients with liver cirrhosis mean concentration of 66.24 ± 4.23 pg/mL and 59.38 ± 6.49 pg/mL in 39 female patients with liver cirrhosis mean concentration significantly different compared with normal range of 20 - 59 pg/mL *4803*
Plasma No Effect In 38 women with amenorrhea and alcoholic cirrhosis mean concentration of 0.10 ± 0.08 nmol/L and of 0.09 ± 0.04 nmol/L in 12 amenorrheic women with other cirrhoses not significantly different from reference interval of 0.08 - 0.11 nmol/L *375*

Estrogens *Plasma Increase* Inability to conjugate estrogens *4960*

Factor V *Plasma Decrease* Impaired hepatic synthesis *875*

Factor VII *Plasma Decrease* In 10 cirrhotics mean concentration in all below reference range of 0.54 - 1.23 U/mL *417*

Factor VIII *Plasma Increase* Increased activity in alcoholic liver disease *1855*

Factor IX *Plasma Decrease* In 18 patients with liver cirrhosis mean concentration of 54 ± 11% significantly less than 100 ± 4% in 16 healthy individuals *2632* In 10 cirrhotics mean concentration in 7 below reference range of 60 - 100% *417*

Factor X *Plasma Decrease* In 18 patients with hepatic cirrhosis mean concentration of 69 ± 19% significantly less than 113 ± 22% in 16 healthy individuals *2632* In 10 cirrhotics mean concentration in 5 below reference range of 60 - 100% *417*

Fat *Feces Increase* May be excessive amounts of fecal fat *4707*

Fatty Acids *Cerebrospinal Fluid Decrease* In 30 patients with Alzheimer's disease mean concentration of 4.5 ± 3.2 mg/dL significantly different from 28.0 ± 18.5 mg/dL in 31 matched controls *3645*

Fatty Acids (FFA), Free *Serum No Effect* In 6 cirrhotics mean concentration of 0.326 ± 0.380 mEq/L significantly different from 0.357 ± 0.202 mEq/L in 6 healthy individuals *1460*

Ferritin *Serum Increase* In one study 21% of patients had concentrations above cutoff value of 500 ng/mL *3120*
Serum No Effect In 23 patients with chronic active hepatitis C with cirrhosis mean concentration of 315 ± 165 ng/mL not significantly different from normal *2381*

α-Fetoprotein *Serum Increase* Occasionally may have concentrations up to 100 µg/L without evidence of hepatocellular carcinoma *1778* In 33 patients with cirrhosis of the liver 16% had concentrations above 30 µg/L *1406* False positive rate observed of 39 of 211 patients probably due to cellular proliferation and necrosis *1404* In 6% of patients in one study concentrations were above the cutoff value of 200 ng/mL *3120* In 11 patients with cirrhosis mean concentration of 60.93 ± 117.27 U/mL significantly higher than normal upper limit of normal of 8.5 U/mL *3591* 10 - 20% of nonmalignant liver diseases of all types have elevated serum concentrations, which tend to be fluctuating or transient. Steady or rising levels indicate malignancy *5759* In 87 patients with cirrhosis of the liver 89.7% had concentrations up to 15.0 ng/mL, 2.3% had concentrations between 15.1 - 20.0 ng/mL, 5.7% between 20.1 - 100 ng/mL, 1.1% had concentrations between 100.1 - 350.0 ng/mL and 1.1% had concentrations above 350.0 ng/mL in contrast to concentrations in 400 healthy individuals in whom 99.2% had concentrations between 0 and 15.0 ng/mL, 0.2% between 15.1 and 20.0 ng/mL and 0.5%% between 20.1 and 100 ng/mL *11* Elevated above 10 ng/mL in 34% of cases *4728* Concentrations may be moderately increased in patients with chronic hepatitis and liver cirrhosis *5285* Mean activity in 32 patients with hepatic cirrhosis of 24 ± 14 ng/mL significantly different from < 15 ng/mL in 28 healthy controls *152*

Fibrin Degradation Products *Plasma Increase* Reported effect *5677* Fibrinolytic activity is significantly increased in advanced cirrhosis and chronic aggressive hepatitis. Total fibrinogen concentration was normal *3082* Reported effect *2161*

Fibrinogen *Plasma Decrease* Impaired hepatic synthesis *875*

571.50 Cirrhosis of Liver *(continued)*

Fibrinogen *(continued)*
Plasma *No Effect* Fibrinolytic activity is significantly increased in advanced cirrhosis and chronic aggressive hepatitis. Total fibrinogen concentration was normal *3082*

Fibronectin *Plasma* *Decrease* Mean fasting concentration in 15 patients with hepatic cirrhosis of 20.8 ± 11.8 mg/dL significantly lower than that in 28 normal men, 32.5 ± 7.1 mg/dL, and 31.6 ± 5.7 mg/dL in 34 normal women, although values were normal in one half of patients and markedly reduced in others (mainly those with decompensated liver cirrhosis) *4811*

Follicle Stimulating Hormone *Plasma* *No Effect* In 38 women with amenorrhea and alcoholic cirrhosis mean concentration of 33 ± 30 IU/L and of 33 ± 21 IU/L in 12 amenorrheic women with other cirrhoses not significantly different from upper limit of reference interval of less than 12 IU/L *375*

Follistatin, Free *Serum* *Increase* Mean concentration in 9 patients with hepatic cirrhosis of 13.1 ± 1.2 µg/L significantly different from that in 60 normal adults of 3.5 ± 0.2 µg/L *4523*

Fractional Excretion of Sodium *Urine* *Decrease* In 21 patients with cirrhosis but without ascites mean fractional excretion of 0.88% and 0.35% in 19 with cirrhosis and ascites compared with normal values of 0.5 - 1.0% *5347*

Fucosidase *Serum* *Increase* In 36 patients with cirrhosis mean activity of α-L-fucosidase 71.3 ± 6 nkat/L compared with 51.4 ± 4.5 nkat/L in 30 healthy controls *1132*

Galactose Eliminating Capacity *Urine* *Decrease* In 128 patients with liver cirrhosis galactose eliminating capacity of 332 ± 106 mg/min for Child-Pugh score A, 278 ± 90 mg/min for Child-Pugh score B and 234 ± 80 mg/min for Child-Pugh score C significantly decreased compared with 508 ± 64 mg/min in healthy controls *1654*
Urine *No Effect* Galactose eliminating capacity of 508 ± 64 mg/min in healthy controls *1654* In 42 patients with cirrhosis mean clearance of 1.68 ± 0.09 mmol/min significantly reduced when compared with normal range of > 1.7 mmol/min in men and > 1.4 mmol/min in women *3567*

Galactose Tolerance *Patient* *Increase* In 11 patients with alcoholic cirrhosis mean $T_{1/2}$ of 28 ± 8 min different from normal range of < 17 min *1371* In 14 patients with alcoholic cirrhosis mean $T_{1/2}$ of 34 ± 15 min different from normal range of < 17 min *1371*

Gastrin *Serum* *Increase* Mean fasting concentration was elevated (41.6 ± 3.1 pmol/L) compared to normal (26.3 ± 3.4 pmol/L) in cirrhotic patients *2898*

γ-Globulin *Serum* *Increase* Usually increased; it reflects inflammation and parallels the severity of the inflammation *5544* Hypergammaglobulinemia exceeding 3 g/dL. Suggests chronic active hepatitis or primary biliary cirrhosis *900* Mean total values were found to be lowest in the healthy subjects followed by acute viral hepatitis primary hepatocellular carcinoma and cirrhosis in that order *1459* Mean concentration in 32 patients with hepatic cirrhosis of 2.5 ± 0.6 g/dL significantly different from < 1.5 g/dL in 28 healthy controls *152* Concentration may be increased up to 6 - 8 g/L in patients with autoimmune chronic active liver disease: in cirrhosis the increase is more modest *4617* The increase in γ- fraction is polyclonal in nature and is due first to increase in IgM fraction followed by an increase in IgG fraction *5189*
Serum *No Effect* In 23 patients with chronic active hepatitis C with cirrhosis mean concentration of 1.9 ± 0.4 g/dL not significantly different from normal *2381* In 20 patients with cirrhosis mean concentration of 1.7 ± 0.3 g/dL not significantly different from 1.1 ± 0.3 g/dL in 20 healthy volunteers *2372*

Glomerular Filtration Rate *Urine* *Decrease* In 25 patients with cirrhosis and ascites mean GFR of 54 ± 4 mL/min significantly different from 117 ± 16 mL/min in 9 cirrhotics without ascites *1904*

Glucagon *Plasma* *Increase* Concentration was raised 2 - 6 fold in patients with spontaneous portal systemic shunting or surgically induced portacaval shunting. Increased levels were due to hypersecretion rather than decreased catabolism *4782* In cirrhotic patients glucagon concentration increased in comparison with healthy controls, and has inverse relationship with liver function *2809*

Glucose *Peritoneal Fluid* *Increase* High concentrations *4165*
Pleural Fluid *No Effect* Pleural fluid and serum concentrations are similar *4493*
Serum *Decrease* Observed in advanced disease *4707* Can occur with various types of liver disease. Hepatic hypoglycemia is a fasting hypoglycemia and often only relieved by food *1980*
Serum *Increase* In 6 cirrhotics mean concentration of 6.3 ± 1.6 mmol/L significantly different from 5.1 ± 0.7 mmol/L in 6 healthy individuals *1460*

Glucose-6-Phosphatase *Serum* *Increase* Moderate rise *1290*

Glucose Tolerance *Serum* *Decrease* A diabetic-type curve may occur and is a reflection of endogenous insulin resistance *2033*

β-Glucuronidase *Serum* *Increase* Increased *1777* *1498*

γ-Glutamyltransferase *Saliva* *Increase* Significantly higher (8.3 U/L) versus normal controls (5.12 U/L) *2448*
Serum *Increase* In 48 patients mean activity of 1.8 ± 0.2 U/L compared with undetectable amounts in 838 healthy controls *2374* Mean activity in 32 patients with hepatic cirrhosis of 56 ± 24 U/L significantly different from < 28 U/L in 28 healthy controls *152* In 33 patients with cirrhosis of the liver 49% had activities above 55 U/L *1406* In 5 patients with cirrhosis of liver, the mean GGT elevation (132 U/L) was 4.4 times the normal upper limit *3161* In inactive cases, average values are lower than in chronic hepatitis. Increases > 10 - 20 times in cirrhotic patients suggest superimposed primary carcinoma of the liver *5544* In 23 patients with chronic active hepatitis C with cirrhosis mean activity of 132 ± 165 U/L significantly different from normal *2381* In 5 patients with Child-Pugh grade A disease mean activity of 35 ± 7 U/L, in 10 with Child-Pugh grade B disease of 70 ± 41 U/L and in 13 with Child-Pugh grade C disease of 86 ± 34 U/L, with the latter two groups of diseased patients significantly different from 24 ± 18 U/L in 19 healthy controls *4533* In 79% of 34 patients at initial hospitalization for this disorder *1576*

Glutathione *Plasma* *Decrease* Mean concentration in 80 patients with liver cirrhosis of 3.0 µmol/L significantly different from 10.2 µmol/L in 40 healthy individuals *3106*
Red Blood Cells *Decrease* Mean concentration in 80 patients with liver cirrhosis of 1.6 mmol/L significantly different from 2.6 mmol/L in 40 healthy individuals *3106*

Glutathione Peroxidase *Serum* *Increase* In 15 patients with Child's group A disease mean 115 ± 40 mU/mL, in 16 with Child's group B 160 ± 60 mU/mL greater and in 10 with Child's group C 200 ± 90 mU/mL significantly greater than 130 ± 10 mU/mL in 13 healthy adults *638*

Glyco-conjugated Bile Acids *Serum* *Increase* Mean concentration of 2.163 ± 0.619 µg/mL in 20 patients with moderate post-hepatitis ciirhosis significantly greater than 0.222 ± 0.96 µg/mL in 20 healthy controls *1854*

Glycocalicin *Plasma* *No Effect* In 8 patients with hepatic cirrhosis mean concentration of 1.90 ± 0.16 µg/mL not significantly different from 2.04 ± 0.14 µg/mL in 11 healthy controls *366*

Glycochenodeoxycholic Acid *Serum* *Increase* Mean concentration of 1.675 ± 0.466 µg/mL in 20 patients with moderate post-hepatitis cirrhosis significantly greater than 0.121 ± 0.074 µg/mL in 20 healthy controls *1854*

Glycocholic Acid *Serum* *Increase* Mean concentration of 0.352 ± 0.094 µg/mL in 20 patients with moderate post-hepatitis cirrhosis significantly higher than 0.075 ± 0.012 µg/mL in 20 healthy controls *1854*

Glycodeoxycholic Acid *Serum* *Increase* Mean concentration of 0.126 ± 0.055 µg/mL in 20 patients with moderate post-hepatitis cirrhosis significantly higher than 0.026 ± 0.010 µg/mL in 20 healthy controls *1854*

Glycolithocholic Acid *Serum* *Increase* Mean concentration of 0.010 ± 0.004 µg/L in 20 moderate post-hepatitis cirrhosis significantly greater than trace measurement in 20 healthy controls *1854*

GP Ib *Platelets* *Increase* In 8 patients with hepatic cirrhosis mean concentration of total GPIb of 46,000 ± 5,000 molecules/P not significantly different from 39,500 ± 2,000 molecules/P in 11 healthy controls *366*

GP IIIa *Platelets* *No Effect* In 8 patients with hepatic cirrhosis mean concentration of surface expressed GPIIIa of 40,000 ± 3,000 molecules/P not significantly different from 40,000 ± 4,000 molecules/P in 11 healthy controls *366*

Growth Hormone *Plasma* *Increase* In 47 patients with liver cirhosis, those with Child's score of 9 greater than upper limit of normal of 11.5 mU/L *2812* In patients with cirrhosis mean basal concentration of 3.9 µg/L significantly increased compared with 0.19 µg/L in healthy control subjects *2060*

Growth Hormone Binding Protein *Serum* *Decrease* In cirrhotic patients mean concentration of 14.6 ± 3.9% significantly reduced compared with normal individuals 20.4 ± 4.7% *2060* In healthy controls mean concentration of 11.3 ± 0.5%/ 50 µL serum higher than 9.7 ± 0.5%/50 µL in 31 Pugh's class A patients and 7.2 ± 0.5%/50 µL in 21 Pugh's class B and C patients *313*
Serum *Increase* In 47 patients with liver cirhosis, those with Child's scores of 5 through 8 greater than upper limit of normal of 6% *2812*

Guanidine *Serum* *No Effect* Concentrations of < 0.06 - 0.400 µmol/L in 13 patients with Child-Turcotte subgroup C liver cirrhosis not significantly different from < 0.06 - 0.210 µmol/L in 66 healthy controls *3292*
Urine *No Effect* Excretions of 10.8 ± 4.23 µmol/g creatinine in 13 patients with Child-Turcotte subgroup C liver cirrhosis significantly different from 9.75 ± 3.38 µmol/g creatinine in 66 healthy controls *3292*

Guanidinoacetic Acid *Serum* *Increase* Concentrations of 5.20 ± 2.95 µmol/L in male patients and 4.36 ± 2.64 µmol/L in female patients with Child-Turcotte subgroup C liver cirrhosis significantly different from 2.61 ± 0.517 µmol/L in male and 2.01 ± 0.572 µmol/L in female healthy controls respectively *3292*
Urine *No Effect* Excretions of 205 ± 152 µmol/g creatinine in 13 patients with Child-Turcotte subgroup C liver cirrhosis not significantly different from 223 ± 128 µmol/g creatinine in 66 healthy controls *3292*

γ-Guanidinobutyric Acid *Serum* *No Effect* Concentrations of < 0.013 µmol/L in 13 patients with Child-Turcotte subgroup C liver cirrhosis not significantly different from < 0.013 - 0.055 µmol/L in 66 healthy controls *3292*
Urine *Decrease* Excretions of 4.14 ± 2.43 µmol/g creatinine in 13 patients with Child-Turcotte subgroup C liver cirrhosis significantly different from 11.8 ± 9.29 µmol/g creatinine in 66 healthy controls *3292*

β-Guanidinopropionic Acid *Urine* *No Effect* Excretions of up to 0.620 µmol/g creatinine in 13 patients with Child-Turcotte subgroup C liver cirrhosis not significantly different from up to 1.00 µmol/g creatinine in 66 healthy controls *3292*

Guanidinosuccinic Acid *Serum* *Decrease* Concentrations of 0.097 ± 0.133 µmol/L in 13 patients with Child-Turcotte subgroup C liver cirrhosis significantly different from 0.259 ± 0.096 µmol/L in 66 healthy controls *3292*
Urine *Decrease* Excretions of 9.87 ± 14.5 µmol/g creatinine in 13 patients with Child-Turcotte subgroup C liver cirrhosis significantly different from 25.0 ± 9.03 µmol/g creatinine in 66 healthy controls *3292*

Guanosine Monophosphate *Plasma* *No Effect* In 9 patients all concentrations fell within normal range of 3.19 ± 1.98 nmol/L *2406*
Urine *Increase* In 9 patients with hepatic cirrhosis concentration significantly higher than 1.65 ± 1.56 µmol/g creatinine in healthy controls *2406* In 20 patients with hepatic cirrhosis mean urinary excretion cyclic guanosine phosphate of approximately 800 pg/mL/min significantly different from about 100 pg/mL/min in 19 healthy individuals *1464*

HDL_2-Cholesterol *Serum* *No Effect* Mean concentration of 241 ± 76 mg/L in 6 patients with decompensated liver cirrhosis and 259 ± 135 mg/L in 17 patients with compensated liver cirrhosis not significantly different from 231 ± 107 mg/L in 21 healthy controls *5063*

HDL_3-Cholesterol *Serum* *Decrease* Mean concentration of 153 ± 42 mg/L in 6 patients with decompensated liver cirrhosis and 176 ± 58 mg/L in 17 patients with compensated liver cirrhosis significantly different from 292 ± 52 mg/L in 21 healthy controls *5063*

HDL-Cholesterol *Serum* *Decrease* Decreased *5707* Significant decrease in concentration noted in 34 patients with hepatic cirrhosis compared with that in 34 patients with chronic active hepatitis and 34 controls with unrelated diseases, with decrease progressing with severity of disease *853* Mean concentration of 394 ± 102 mg/L in 6 patients with decompensated liver cirrhosis and 436 ± 146 mg/L in 17 patients with compensated liver cirrhosis significantly different from 523 ± 117 mg/L in 21 healthy controls *5063* In 26 alcoholic cirrhotics mean concentration of 1.25 ± 0.41 mmol/L not significantly reduced below mean concentration of 1.53 ± 0.48 mmol/L age and sex matched controls *3345* Decreased *325* In 37 individuals with hepatic cirrhosis mean concentration of 0.99 ± 0.36 mmol/L significantly different from 1.09 ± 0.27 mmol/L in 98 healthy controls aged 24 to 55 years with direct homogeneous method from Daiichi (Tokyo) performed on ILab® 900 automated analyzer *4848* Decreased *3327*

HDL-Triglycerides *Serum* *Increase* In 26 alcoholic cirrhotics mean concentration of 0.21 ± 0.11 mmol/L significantly higher than 0.08 ± 0.03 mmol/L in 10 healthy age and sex matched controls *3345*

Hematocrit *Blood* *Decrease* In 34% of 70 patients at initial hospitalization for this disorder *1576* Anemia reflects increased plasma volume and some increased destruction of RBCs *5544* Approximately 75% of chronic liver disease patients have anemia, usually mild *2684* *4769* In 15 patients with Child's group A disease mean 40 ± 8%, in 16 with Child's group B 36 ± 7% and 10 with Child's group C 36 ± 9% less than 43 ± 5% in 13 healthy controls *638*

Hemoglobin *Blood* *Decrease* Anemia reflects increased plasma volume and some increased destruction of RBCs *5544* Approximately 75% of chronic liver disease patients have anemia, usually mild *4769* In 36% of 69 patients at initial hospitalization for this disorder *1576* Approximately 75% of chronic liver disease patients have anemia, usually mild *2684*
Plasma *Increase* Mild to moderate hemolysis usually occurs *4199*

Hepatic Sorbitol Clearance *Urine* *Decrease* In 128 patients with liver cirrhosis hepatic sorbitol clearance of 595 ± 258 mL/min for Child-Pugh score A, 425 ± 225 mL/min for Child-Pugh score B and 343 ± 217 mL/min for Child-Pugh score C significantly decreased compared with 911 ± 137 mL/min in healthy controls *1654*

Hepatitis B Surface Antigen *Serum* *Positive* In 24 patients with liver cirrhosis 2 were HBsAg positive *2071*

Hepatitis C Virus Antibodies *Serum* *Positive* In 24 patients with cirrhosis of liver 22 were HCV-antibody positive *2071*

Hepatocyte Growth Factor *Serum* *Increase* In patients with hepatic cirrhosis mean concentration of 0.52 ng/mL compared with mean concentration in 10 normal individuals of 0.25 ± 0.06 ng/mL *3714*

β-Hexosaminidase *Serum* *Increase* Increase in total concentration (hexosaminidase A and B) *3850*

High Molecular Weight Multimers *Plasma* *Decrease* In 8 patients with hepatic cirrhosis mean proportion of 25.0 ± 1.1% of total significantly different from 31.7 ± 0.8% in 11 healthy controls *366*

Homoarginine *Plasma* *No Effect* Concentrations of 1.79 ± 0.670 µmol/L in male patients and 1.62 ± 1.03 µmol/L in female patients with Child-Turcotte subgroup C liver cirrhosis not significantly different from 1.98 ± 0.634 µmol/L in male and 1.51 ± 0.609 µmol/L in female healthy controls respectively *3292*
Urine *No Effect* Excretions of up to 15 µmol/g creatinine in 13 patients with Child-Turcotte subgroup C liver cirrhosis significantly different from up to 6 µmol/g creatinine in 66 healthy controls *3292*

Hyaluronic Acid *Serum* *Increase* The median serum concentrations in nonalcoholic cirrhosis (357 µg/L) were significantly increased in comparison with controls *1371* Mean concentration in patients with hepatic cirrhosis 214 ± 121 ng/mL compared with 14.9 ± 12.8 ng/mL in healthy controls *3365* Measured in paired serum samples from 133 patients with various chronic liver diseases and from 50 healthy age-matched controls. In 24 (of the 133) patients with autoimmune chronic liver disease, follow-up determination was performed during therapeutic treatment with immunosuppressive drugs. Serum concentrations (medians) of HA were increased ($p = 0.0058$) in 91% of patients with active cirrhosis ($p < 6 \times 10^{-7}$). The difference in active cirrhosis was statistically significant *4270* Mean concentration in 49 patients with cirrhosis of 371.6 ± 292.4 ng/mL significantly increased compared with 19.8 ± 16.9 ng/mL in 100 healthy controls *4570*

Hydrogen *Blood* *No Effect* In 6 cirrhotics mean concentration of 12 ± 7 ppm not significantly different from 13 ± 11 ppm in 6 healthy individuals *1460*

25-Hydroxy Vitamin D_3 *Serum* *Decrease* In patients with stable cirrhosis, values were slightly depressed, mean of 18.9 ± 8.9 ng/mL. Lower normal limit of 21 ng/mL *4657*

571.50 Cirrhosis of Liver *(continued)*

5-Hydroxyindoleacetic Acid *Plasma Decrease* In 30 patients with cirrhosis mean concentration of 1.5 ± 0.1 nmol/L significantly less than 2.3 ± 0.1 nmol/L in age-matched controls, but no correlation with severity of cirrhosis or hepatic venous pressure gradient *352*

5-Hydroxytryptamine *Blood Decrease* In 30 patients with cirrhosis mean concentration of 158 ± 28 nmol/L significantly less than 332 ± 19 nmol/L in age-matched controls, but no correlation with severity of cirrhosis *352*

5-Hydroxytryptamine, Conjugated *Plasma Increase* In 30 patients with cirrhosis mean concentration of 32.2 ± 8.1 nmol/L significantly higher than 16.4 ± 1.4 nmol/L in age-matched controls, with concentration in cirrhotics not significantly higher than concentrations in controls except in those with Pugh grade A in whom concentration also significantly higher than in grade C patients *352*

5-Hydroxytryptamine, Free *Plasma Increase* In 30 patients with cirrhosis mean concentration of unconjugated 5-hydroxytryptamine of 6.8 ± 1.7 nmol/L significantly higher than 3.4 ± 0.5 nmol/L in age-matched controls, with significantly higher concentrations in patients with Pugh grade A than grade C cirrhotic patients *352*

^{131}I Uptake *Serum Increase* In hepatic disease *4707*

IDL-Cholesterol *Serum No Effect* In 26 alcoholic cirrhotics mean concentration of 0.13 ± 0.08 mmol/L not significantly different from 0.12 ± 0.05 mmol/L in 10 age and sex matched controls *3345*

IDL-Triglycerides *Serum No Effect* In 26 alcoholic cirrhotics mean concentration of 0.12 ± 0.09 mmol/L not significantly different from 0.12 ± 0.06 mmol/L in 10 age and sex matched controls *3345*

Immunoglobulin A *Serum Increase* Reported effect *900* Mean concentration in 22 patients with alcoholic cirrhosis of 720 mg/dL significantly higher than 288 ± 121 mg/dL in 18 healthy blood donors *54* Hypergammaglobulinemia is common, involving all classes of immunoglobulins *367*
Serum No Effect In 23 patients with chronic active hepatitis C with cirrhosis mean concentration of 358 ± 96 mg/dL not significantly different from normal *2381*

Immunoglobulin G *Serum Increase* The increase in γ- fraction is polyclonal in nature and is due first to increase in IgM fraction followed by an increase in IgG fraction *5189* Mean concentration in 22 patients with alcoholic cirrhosis of 3,300 mg/dL significantly higher than 1,200 ± 319 mg/dL in 18 healthy blood donors *54* In about 50% of the patients with cryptogenic cirrhosis, alcoholic cirrhosis, and chronic active hepatitis *4198*
Serum No Effect In 23 patients with chronic active hepatitis C with cirrhosis mean concentration of 2,265 ± 407 mg/dL not significantly different from normal *2381*

Immunoglobulin M *Serum Increase* Mean concentration in 22 patients with alcoholic cirrhosis of 220 mg/dL significantly higher than 80 ± 29 mg/dL in 18 healthy blood donors *54* The increase in γ- fraction is polyclonal in nature and is due first to increase in IgM fraction followed by an increase in IgG fraction *5189* Reported effect *4160*
Serum No Effect In 23 patients with chronic active hepatitis C with cirrhosis mean concentration of 186 ± 124 mg/dL not significantly different from normal *2381*

Indocyanine Green Clearance *Serum Decrease* In 42 patients with cirrhosis mean clearance of 0.28 ± 0.04 L/min significantly reduced when compared with normal range of 0.30 ± 0.70 L/min *3567*
Serum Increase In 10 patients with liver cirrhosis without ascites mean retention at 15 minutes of 23.2 ± 10.1% and 48.4 ± 15.2% in 11 patients with cirrhosis and ascites significantly different from mean retention of 7.1 ± 2.1% in 10 healthy controls *5349* In 20 patients with cirrhosis mean retention ratio in 15 minutes of 25 ± 6% *2372*

Insulin *Plasma Increase* In 6 cirrhotics mean concentration of 265 ± 211 pmol/L significantly different from 94 ± 76 pmol/L in 6 healthy individuals *1460* The majority of cirrhotics demonstrated increased levels of circulating insulin due to decreased hormonal catabolism *2468*

Insulin-like Growth Factor-I *Serum Decrease* In patients with cirrhosis significant inverse correlation observed with Child scores: in Child class A mean concentration of 133 ± 48 ng/mL, class B 75 ± 29 ng/mL and class C mean 43 ± 20 ng/mL, compared with normal range of 190 ± 43 ng/mL in healthy 21 - 30 year olds *2813* Observed effect *2166* Basal mean concentration of 177 ± 116 ng/mL in 18 patients with active disease, 250 ± 135 ng/mL in 11 patients with inactive disease significantly reduced compared with 810 ± 297 ng/mL in 30 healthy controls *800*
Serum Increase In 47 patients with liver cirhosis, those with Child's scores of 5 and 6 greater than upper limit of normal of 56 µg/L *2812*

Insulin-like Growth Factor Binding Protein-1
Serum Increase In 47 patients with liver cirhosis, those with Child's scores of 7 through 10 greater than upper limit of normal of 38 µg/L *2812*

Insulin-like Growth Factor Binding Protein-2
Serum Increase In 47 patients with liver cirhosis, those with Child's scores of 9 greater than upper limit of normal of 0.72 mg/L *2812*

Insulin-like Growth Factor Binding Protein-3
Serum Decrease Basal mean concentration of 1.71 ± 1.29 µg/mL in 18 patients with active disease, 2.98 ± 0.96 µg/mL in 11 patients with inactive disease significantly reduced compared with 6.82 ± 1.31 µg/mL in 30 healthy controls *800*
Serum Increase In 47 patients with liver cirhosis, those with Child's scores of 5 greater had higher concentrations than upper limit of normal of 1.85 mg/L *2812*

β1-Integrin *Serum Increase* In 17 patients with hepatic cirrhosis mean concentration of 4.9 ± 0.3 µg/mL significantly higher than 2.1 ± 0.1 µg/mL in 18 healthy adult controls *5785*

β3-Integrin *Serum Increase* In 17 patients with hepatic cirrhosis mean concentration of 13.6 ± 1.5 µg/mL significantly higher than 5.5 ± 0.5 µg/mL in 18 healthy adult controls *5785*

Intercellular Adhesion Molecule-1 *Serum Increase* Mean concentration in 94 patients with liver cirrhosis of approximately 1,200 µg/L significantly increased compared with mean concentration in 28 healthy blood donors of 215.5 µg/L (95% confidence limits of mean 198.1 - 232.9 µg/L) *4143*

Interleukin-1α-Autoantibody *Serum No Effect* In 48 patients proportion with autoantibody 18.8% compared with 12.6% in 838 healthy controls *2374*

Interleukin-1β *Serum No Effect* Mean undetectable concentration in 17 patients with liver cirrhosis not different from undetectable amount in 17 healthy controls *4228*

Interleukin-6 *Ascitic Fluid Increase* Mean concentration in 53 patients with liver cirrhosis of 12 ± 1.8 ng/mL *4228*
Serum Increase In 5 patients with Child-Pugh grade A disease mean concentration of 12.67 ± 1.53 pg/mL, in 10 with Child-Pugh grade B disease 18.65 ± 7.38 pg/mL and in 13 with Child-Pugh grade C disease 23.43 ± 7.04 pg/mL, with the latter two significantly different from 14.16 ± 3.93 pg/mL in 19 healthy controls *4533* Mean concentration in 24 patients with liver cirrhosis of 1,191 ± 358 pg/mL significantly different from not detectable amount in 17 healthy controls *4228*

International Normalized Ratio *Plasma Increase* In 5 patients with Child-Pugh grade A disease mean ratio of 1.10 ± 0.05, in 10 with Child-Pugh grade B disease 1.27 ± 0.11 and in 13 with Child-Pugh grade C disease 1.68 ± 0.30, with the latter two groups ofdiseased patients significantly different from 1.01 ± 0.08 in 19 healthy controls *4533*

Iron *Serum Decrease* In 28% of 21 patients at initial hospitalization for this disorder *1576*

Iron-binding Capacity, Total *Serum Decrease* The only protein significantly reduced *3681* Reported effect *5863* In 51% of 21 patients at initial hospitalization for this disorder *1576*

Iron Saturation *Serum Increase* Moderate to marked rise in percent saturation in hepatic cirrhosis *5863*

Isocitrate Dehydrogenase *Serum Increase* Normal or slightly increased in 20% of patients. A large increase suggests a poorer prognosis *5544*

α-Keto-δ-Guanidinovaleric Acid *Serum No Effect* Concentrations of < 0.035 - 0.150 µmol/L in 13 patients with Child-Turcotte subgroup C liver cirrhosis not significantly different from < 0.035 - 0.200 µmol/L in 66 healthy controls *3292*

Urine *No Effect* Excretions of up to 35 µmol/g creatinine in 13 patients with Child-Turcotte subgroup C liver cirrhosis not significantly different from up to 35 µmol/g creatinine in 66 healthy controls *3292*

6-Keto-Prostaglandin $F_{1\alpha}$ *Ascitic Fluid* *Increase* Mean concentration in 47 patients with liver cirrhosis of 145 ± 62 pg/mL *4228*
Plasma *Increase* Mean concentration in 23 patients with liver cirrhosis of 104 ± 67.4 pg/mL significantly different from 8.8 ± 1.4 pg/mL in 16 healthy controls *4228*

Lactate Dehydrogenase *Ascitic Fluid* *Increase* In 73 specimens from patients with cirrhosis or hepatocellular carcinoma mean activity of 103 ± 6 U/L but significantly less than 823 ± 107 U/L in 21 specimens from patients with peritoneal neoplasia. Ascitic fluid:serum ratio of activity in 58 specimens from patients with cirrhosis or hepatocellular carcinoma of 0.41 ± 0.04 significantly less than 3.85 ± 0.96 in 9 specimens from patients with peritoneal neoplasia *728*
Pleural Fluid *Decrease* Transudate *126*
Serum *Increase* Slight increase *1980* In 32% of 69 patients at initial hospitalization for this disorder *1576*

Lactate Dehydrogenase Isoenzyme-5 *Serum* *Increase* LD 4 and 5 are moderately elevated *1025*

Lactate Dehydrogenase Isoenzymes *Serum* *Increase* LD 4 and 5 are moderately elevated *1025*

Laminin *Serum* *Increase* Increased concentration was useful in assessing extent of hepatic fibrosis *5276*

Laminin P1 *Serum* *Increase* Mean concentration significantly increased compared with healthy controls *3670*

Lathosterol *Serum* *Decrease* In patients with cirrhosis low concentrations observed in both plasma and liver reflecting decreased cholesterol synthesis *3794*

LDL-Cholesterol *Serum* *Decrease* Significant decrease in concentration noted in 34 patients with hepatic cirrhosis compared with that in 34 patients with chronic active hepatitis and 34 controls with unrelated diseases, with decrease progressing with severity of disease *853* In 26 alcoholic cirrhotics mean concentration of 2.90 ± 1.01 mmol/L significantly reduced compared with 3.76 ± 1.02 mmol/L in 10 age and sex matched controls *3345*

LDL-Triglycerides *Serum* *Increase* In 26 alcoholic cirrhotics mean concentration of 0.48 ± 0.28 mmol/L significantly increased compared with 0.21 ± 0.08 mmol/L in 10 age and sex matched controls *3345*

LE Cells *Blood* *Positive* Reported in about 33% of patients with postnecrotic cirrhosis at some time during their illness. Cells tended to be present during active disease and absent during remission *4160*

Leptin *Serum* *Increase* In 39 female patients with liver cirrhosis mean concentration significantly different compared with controls *4803*
Serum *No Effect* In 29 male patients with liver cirrhosis mean concentration not significantly different compared with controls *4803*

Leucine Aminopeptidase *Serum* *Increase* 92% of 25 patients had mean peak values which were moderate to highly elevated. Mean = 523 ± 204 and range = 189 - 900 U/L (normal = 322 U/L) *579*

Leukocytes *Ascitic Fluid* *Increase* A total WBC exceeding 300 /µL with predominantly polymorphonuclear leukocytes indicates associated peritonitis *900* Less than 250 cells/µL *4746*
Blood *Decrease* Decreased with hypersplenism *5544*
Blood *No Effect* Usually normal with active cirrhosis *5544*
Pleural Fluid *Increase* < 500 /µL *4493*

Leukotriene B_4 *Ascitic Fluid* *Increase* Mean concentration in 47 patients with liver cirrhosis of 21 ± 5.4 pg/mL *4228*
Plasma *Increase* Mean concentration in 23 patients with liver cirrhosis of 22 ± 16.3 pg/mL significantly different from undetectable amount in 17 healthy controls *4228*

Leukotriene E_4 *Urine* *Increase* In 9 patients with cirrhosis without ascites median concentration of 1.24 nmol/L or 82 nmol/mol creatinine and in 19 with ascites 1.17 nmol/L or 264 nmol/mol creatinine higher than median excretion of 0.52 nmol/L (range of 0.34 - 0.270 nmol/L) or 40 nmol/mol creatinine (range of 29 - 52 nmol/mol creatinine) in 10 healthy individuals *5347*

Lipase *Serum* *Increase* Activity greater than 270 U/L observed in 29% patients with hepatic cirrhosis *4110*

Lipids *Serum* *Increase* Gross elevation noted in acute alcoholic liver injury and primary biliary cirrhosis *900*

Lipoprotein Lp(a) *Serum* *Decrease* In 20 patients with hepatic cirrhosis median concentration of 11 mg/L significantly different from 43 mg/L in 69 healthy volunteers, with none having a concentration above 95th percentile of 361 mg/L *5417* Since Lp(a) is synthesized in the liver concentration may be reduced with impaired liver function *2827*

Luteinizing Hormone *Plasma* *No Effect* In 38 women with amenorrhea and alcoholic cirrhosis mean concentration of 16 ± 16 IU/L and of 14 ± 11 IU/L in 12 amenorrheic women with other cirrhoses not significantly different from upper limit of reference interval of less than 12 IU/L *375*

Lymphocytes *Blood* *No Effect* In 23 patients with chronic active hepatitis C with cirrhosis mean count of 1,740 ± 524 /µL not significantly different from normal *2381*

Lysyl Oxidase *Serum* *Increase* Compared with healthy controls mean activity increased 11.8-fold *3670*

M3/M21 *Serum* *Increase* In 20 patients with cirrhosis of the liver median concentration of 281.8 U/L compared with that in 40 healthy blood donors in whom the median concentration was 25.2 U/L *2090*

α_2-Macroglobulin *Serum* *Increase* High concentrations were found in decompensated hepatic cirrhosis, 2.8 ± 0.8 g/L compared to normal, 2.3 ± 0.6 g/L *4615* Significantly increased in patients with cryptogenic cirrhosis, alcoholic cirrhosis and chronic active hepatitis *3681* Moderate elevation *2249*

Macrophage Colony Stimulating Factor *Serum* *Increase* In 20 patients with liver cirrhosis mean concentration of about 3.2 ng/mL significantly different from 1.95 ± 0.44 ng/mL in 20 healthy volunteers *2372*

Magnesium *Red Blood Cells* *Decrease* The mean concentration in cirrhotic patients (4.7 mmol/L packed cells) was significantly below normal values *5547*
Serum *Decrease* In 35% of 14 patients at initial hospitalization for this disorder *1576* 4 of 11 patients had abnormally low concentrations. The mean concentration for the cirrhotic patients, 1.85 mmol/L, was significantly lower than the normal mean *5547*

Manganese *Serum* *Increase* Significant $p < 0.001$ *5460*

MCV *Blood* *Increase* Occasionally mild macrocytosis, but rarely > 115 fL in the absence of megaloblastic changes in marrow. Reported incidence varies from 33 - 65% *5699*

Metallopanstimulin *Serum* *No Effect* In none of 4 patients with cirrhosis of the liver mean concentration exceeded upper limit of normal of < 10 ng/mL in healthy individuals aged 19 - 88 years *1462*

Methylguanidine *Urine* *No Effect* Excretions of up to 10 µmol/g creatinine in 13 patients with Child-Turcotte subgroup C liver cirrhosis significantly different from 2.99 ± 1.24 µmol/g creatinine in 66 healthy controls *3292*

β_2-Microglobulin *Serum* *Increase* In one study 63% of patients had concentrations above cutoff of 2.0 mg/mL *3120*

Monocytes *Pleural Fluid* *Increase* Predominant cell type *4493*

Mucoprotein *Serum* *Decrease* Observed effect *1025*

Myeloperoxidase *Serum* *Increase* Mean concentration in 41 patients with cirrhosis 309.1 ± 17.2 ng/mL compared with 219.5 ± 5.7 ng/mL in healthy controls *3718*

Myoglobin *Serum* *No Effect* In 32 patients with cirrhosis and normal ECG cardiac concentration normal in all patients *4034*

α-N-Acetylarginine *Serum* *No Effect* Concentrations of < 0.015 - 0.600 µmol/L in 13 patients with Child-Turcotte subgroup C liver cirrhosis significantly different from < 0.015 - 0.620 µmol/L in 66 healthy controls *3292*
Urine *No Effect* Excretions of 21.7 ± 9.32 µmol/g creatinine in 13 patients with Child-Turcotte subgroup C liver cirrhosis not significantly different from 22.2 ± 9.63 µmol/g creatinine in 66 healthy controls *3292*

N-Acetyl-Leukotriene E_4 *Urine* *Increase* In 9 patients with cirrhosis without ascites median concentration of 0.35 nmol/L or 25 nmol/mol creatinine and in 19 with ascites 0.29 nmol/L or 64 nmol/mol creatinine higher than median excretion of 0.14 nmol/L (range of 0.08 - 0.23 nmol/L) or 13 nmol/mol creatinine (range of 7 - 20 nmol/mol creatinine) in 10 healthy individuals *5347*

571.50 **Cirrhosis of Liver** *(continued)*

Neopterin *Serum Increase* Mean concentration of 8.3 nmol/L in 68 cirrhotic alcoholics compared with 5.21 nmol/L in 37 alcoholic non-cirrhotics and 2.91 nmol/L in 12 healthy controls *1808*

Neuron-specific Enolase *Serum Increase* In 3 of 86 patients with cirrhosis concentration exceeded upper limit of normal of 11 µg/L *887*

Nickel *Serum Decrease* Mean concentration of 1.6 µg/L (n = 18) compared with mean concentration in controls of 2.6 µg/L (n = 42) *3428*

N-Methylnicotinamide *Serum Increase* In 29 adult patients with cirrhosis mean and median basal concentrations were 42 ng/mL and 35 ng/mL respectively in 19 Child type A patients and 50 ng/mL and 45 ng/mL in 10 Child type B patients compared with mean and median of 21 ng/mL in 16 healthy controls *985*
Urine Increase In 29 adult patients with cirrhosis mean basal excretion of 21mg/d compared with mean 9 mg/d in 7 healthy controls *985*

Norepinephrine *Plasma Increase* In 20 patients with hepatic cirrhosis mean plasma aldosterone concentration of 392 ± 66 pg/mL not significantly different from 243 ± 44 pg/mL in 19 healthy individuals *1464* In 10 patients with liver cirrhosis without ascites mean concentration of 363 ± 70 pg/mL and 425 ± 110 pg/mL in 11 patients with cirrhosis and ascites significantly different from mean concentration of 188 ± 79 pg/mL in 10 healthy controls *5349* In 25 patients with cirrhosis with ascites mean concentration of 626 ± 74 pg/mL significantly higher than 366 ± 70 pg/mL in 9 patients with cirrhosis but without ascites and 248 ± 36 pg/mL in 17 healthy controls *1904* Median activity in 19 patients with cirrhosis and ascites of 828 pg/mL significantly different from reference range of 50 - 400 pg/mL *5347* In 21 patients with cirrhosis but without ascites mean concentration of 212 pg/mL and 828 pg/mL in 19 with cirrhosis and ascites compared with normal values of 50 - 400 pg/mL *5347*
Plasma No Effect Median activity in 9 patients with cirrhosis but without ascites of 212 pg/mL not significantly different from reference range of 50 - 400 pg/mL *5347*

N-terminal Peptide of Type III Procollagen *Serum Increase* In 100 patients with cirrhosis who drink < 40 g alcohol/d mean concentration of 1.31 U/mL, and 1.7- U/mL in those drinking > 40 g/d mean concentration significantly higher than in healthy individuals *1405*

5'-Nucleotidase *Serum Increase* Increased in 50% of patients *5544* In 34 patients with liver cirrhosis mean activity 9 U/L (range 2 - 35 U/L) compared with mean of 3.8 U/L in healthy individuals, with mean % isoforms of 25%, 17% and 52% for NTP1, NTP2 and NTP3 whose mean activities are 12%, 30% and 58% respectively in healthy individuals *3993*

Ornithine Carbamoyltransferase *Serum Increase* Liver cell damage *5544*

Osmolality *Serum Decrease* Mean osmolality of 279 ± 51 mOsm/kg in 11 patients with cirrhosis and ascites significantly different from mean osmolality of 287 ± 3 mOsm/kg in 10 healthy controls *5349*
Serum No Effect In 10 patients with liver cirrhosis without ascites mean osmolality of 286 ± 3 mOsm/kg not significantly different from mean osmolality of 287 ± 3 mOsm/kg in 10 healthy controls *5349*

Partial Thromboplastin Time *Plasma Increase* Severe clotting factor deficiencies are common *2033*

pH *Pleural Fluid Increase* Transudate (pH > 7.3) *126*

Phosphate *Serum Decrease* In 40% of 68 patients at initial hospitalization for this disorder *1576* Pronounced hypophosphatemic response in cirrhotic patients after glucose administration *2719*

Phospholipids *Cerebrospinal Fluid Decrease* In 30 patients with Alzheimer's disease mean concentration of 0.2 ± 0.1 mg/dL significantly different from 3.5 ± 5.0 mg/dL in 31 matched controls *3645*
Serum Decrease Mean concentration of 1,468 ± 217 mg/L in 6 patients with decompensated liver cirrhosis and 1,684 ± 255 mg/L in 17 patients with compensated liver cirrhosis significantly different from 1,928 ± 193 mg/L in 21 healthy controls *5063*

Platelets *Blood Decrease* Platelet count below 88,000 /µL carried an odds ratio of 5.5 for large esophageal varices and of 4.5 for large or gastric varices *5836* In patients withhepatic cirrosis mean count 97, 000 /µL significantly reduced compared with normal, possibly related to decreased production of thrombopoietin by the liver *3917* Mean concentration of 8.0 ± 4.6 x 10^4/µL significantly different from 24.5 ± 7.3 x 10^4/µL observed in 30 healthy volunteer controls *2604* In 24 patients with liver cirrhosis mean concentration of 12.3 x 10^9/L significantly below reference interval of 17 - 39 x 10^9/L *2071* Mean concentration of 58 ± 24 x 10^9/L observed in 27 patients with cirrhosis *3315* Mild; in about 50% of cases *4769* Patients with severe acute hepatic necrosis may have findings compatible with intravascular coagulation, thrombocytopenia and increased levels of fibrinogen/fibrin degradation products *2161* In 38% of 48 patients at initial hospitalization for this disorder *1576*
Blood Increase In 20 of 70 patients (29%) with cirrhosis following a variety of causes mean platelet count less than 100,000 /µL *5477* Increased in miscellaneous disease states *5544*

Porphobilinogen *Urine Increase* Occasionally observed *367*

Potassium *Serum Decrease* Frequent in patients with ascites and edema *2033*

Prealbumin *Serum Decrease* In 18 patients with hepatic cirrhosis mean concentration of 10.6 ± 4.2 mg/dL significantly less than 29.0 ± 5.5 mg/dL in 16 healthy individuals *2632*

Prekallikrein *Plasma Decrease* Mean concentration of 69.8 ± 32.8% in 18 patients significantly less than 100.0 ± 23.1% in 30 healthy controls *855*

Pro-Matrix Metalloproteinase 1 *Serum Increase* Mean concentration of 253 ± 64 ng/mL in 33 patients with hepatic cirrhosis significantly different from 155 ± 17 ng/mL in 29 healthy controls *3668*

Proapolipoprotein A-I *Serum Increase* Mean concentration of 88 ± 25 mg/L in 6 patients with decompensated liver cirrhosis not significantly different and 105 ± 36 mg/L in 17 patients with compensated liver cirrhosis significantly different from 69 ± 25 mg/L in 21 healthy controls *5063*

Procollagen 1 C-terminal Peptide *Serum Increase* In 100 patients with cirrhosis who drink < 40 g alcohol/d mean concentration of 1,234 µg/L, and 1,488 µg/L in those drinking > 40 g/d mean concentration significantly higher than in healthy individuals *1405*

Procollagen Type III Peptide *Serum Increase* In patients in Egypt with hepatic cirrhosis mean concentration in systemic blood 3.2 ± 1.5 ng/mL compared with 1.8 ± 0.6 ng/mL in patients without abnormal liver function *4492*

Progesterone *Plasma Increase* Raised in 36 of 50 men with liver disease compared with 20 healthy male control subjects. Significantly higher in men with nonalcoholic cirrhosis with gynaecomastic than those without *1428*

Prolactin *Plasma Increase* Found in 14% of men with liver disease. Levels unrelated to presence of gynecomastia *1428*
Plasma No Effect In 38 women with amenorrhea and alcoholic cirrhosis mean concentration of 561 ± 473 mIU/L and of 688 ± 593 IU/L in 12 amenorrheic women with other cirrhoses not significantly different from reference interval of 50 - 700 mIU/L *375*

Proline Hydroxylase *Serum Increase* Mean activity significantly increased compared with healthy controls *3670*

Prolyl Hydroxylase *Serum Increase* In 100 patients with cirrhosis who drink < 40 g alcohol/d mean concentration of 94 µg/L, and 110 µg/L in those drinking > 40 g/d mean concentration significantly higher than in healthy individuals *1405*

Prostaglandin E_2 *Ascitic Fluid Increase* Mean concentration in 47 patients with liver cirrhosis of 27 ± 3.2 pg/mL *4228*
Plasma No Effect Mean concentration in 23 patients with liver cirrhosis of 67 ± 21.1 pg/mL not significantly different from 70 ± 30 pg/mL in 16 healthy controls *4228*

Prostate-specific Antigen *Serum Increase* In 58 men with cirrhosis of the liver 91.4% had concentrations between 0 and 4.0 ng/mL and 8.9% between 4.1 and 10.0 ng/mL compared with upper limit of normal of 4.0 ng/mL *11*

Protein *Ascitic Fluid Decrease* Concentrations less than 2.5 g/dL reliably differentiate hepatic cirrhosis from other causes of ascites *1921* Ascitic fluid is usually a transudate with protein < 3.0 g/dL and specific gravity < 1.016. However, protein may exceed 2.5 g/dL in up to 30% of patients *4891* < 2.5 g/dL in ascitic fluid *233*

Ascitic Fluid *Increase* Mean concentration in 46 patients with cirrhosis of the liver of 26 ± 2.4 mg/mL *4228* Mean concentration in 72 specimens from patients with cirrhosis or hepatocellular carcinoma of 19.19 ± 1.26 g/L. Mean ascitic fluid:serum concentration ratio of 0.29 ± 0.02. Note both concentration and ratio significantly less than in patients with peritoneal neoplasia *728*
Pleural Fluid *Decrease* Transudate (< 3 g/dL) *4493* May cause pleural effusion by several mechanisms; most important of these is transfer of fluid from the peritoneal cavity via either direct diaphragmatic defect or lymphatics *464*
Serum *Decrease* Total serum protein is usually normal or decreased *5544*
Serum *Increase* Increased serum globulin may cause increased total protein especially in posthepatic cirrhosis *5544*
Serum *No Effect* In 23 patients with chronic active hepatitis C with cirrhosis mean concentration of 7.5 ± 0.6 g/dL not significantly different from normal *2381*

Protein C *Plasma* *Decrease* In 18 patients with hepatic cirrhosis mean concentration of 38 ± 11% significantly less than 95 ± 12% in 16 healthy individuals *2632* In 10 cirrhotics mean concentration in all below reference range of 72 - 106% *417* In 50 patients with alcoholic or viral cirrhosis mean concentration of 62 ± 79% significantly less than 118 ± 14% in 40 healthy controls *652* Mean concentration in 18 patients of 49.3 ± 35.3% significantly less than 105.0 ± 35.0% in 30 healthy controls *855*

Protein S *Plasma* *No Effect* In 50 patients with alcoholic or viral cirrhosis mean concentration of 101± 30% not significantly different from 99 ± 18% in 40 healthy controls *652*

Protein S, Free *Plasma* *No Effect* In 50 patients with alcoholic or viral cirrhosis mean concentration of 130 ± 31% not significantly different from 113 ± 23% in 40 healthy controls *652*

Protein Z *Plasma* *Decrease* In 18 patients with liver cirrhosis mean concentration of 1,061 ± 345 μg/L significantly less than 2,820 ± 336 μg/L in 16 healthy individuals *2632* Mean protein Z concentration in patients with hepatic cirrhosis of 1,061 ± 345 μg/L significantly different from 2,820 ± 336 μg/L in healthy controls *2645*

Prothrombin *Plasma* *Decrease* In 10 cirrhotics mean concentration in 7 below reference range of 60 - 150% *417*

Prothrombin Time *Plasma* *Decrease* Mean time in 26 patients with chronic viral hepatitis and cirrhosis of 71 ± 13% significantly different from that observed in 30 healthy volunteer controls *2604* In 9 patients with cirrhosis without ascites and 25 patients with cirrhosis and ascites mean time of 71 ± 7% and 61 ± 18%, respectively, significantly lower than 98 ± 1% in 17 healthy controls *1904* Median time (as % of control) in 9 patients with cirrhosis and ascites of 43% different from reference range of 70 - 100% *5347* Mean activity in 32 patients with hepatic cirrhosis of 66 ± 26% significantly different from 80 - 100% in 28 healthy controls *152* In 128 patients with liver cirrhosis mean time of 80 ± 16% for Child-Pugh score A, 59 ± 13% for Child-Pugh score B and 45 ± 12% for Child-Pugh score C significantly decreased compared with 100 ± 30% in healthy controls *1654*
Plasma *Increase* Hypoprothrombinemia unresponsive to parenteral vitamin K is indicative of severe hepatocellular dysfunction *900* In 10 patients with liver cirrhosis without ascites mean time of 12.7 ± 0.9 s and 15.0 ± 1.4 s in 11 patients with cirrhosis and ascites significantly different from mean retention of 11.8 ± 0.8 s in 10 healthy controls *5349* Mean prothrombin time of 15.3 ± 4.3 s observed in 27 patients with cirrhosis *3315* In 18 patients mean INR of 1.44 ± 0.45 significantly higher than 1.05 ± 0.11 in 30 healthy controls *855* In 33 patients with decompensated hepatic cirrhosis mean PT of 16.8 ± 1.4 s significantly higher than 13.3 ± 0.2 s in 31 compensated cirrhotic patients *2964* In 15 patients with Child's group A disease mean 13.2 ± 0.8 s, in 16 with Child's group B 14.4 ± 1.3 s and 10 with Child's group C 18.1 ± 2.4 s greater than normal range of 1 - 13 s in healthy adults *638* Prolongation of the prothrombin time usually indicates that the disease is a chronic one, such as advanced cirrhosis *4617*
Plasma *No Effect* Median time in 9 patients with cirrhosis but without ascites of 72% (as % of control) not different from reference range of 70 -100% *5347* In 23 patients with chronic active hepatitis C with cirrhosis mean time of 85 ± 10% not significantly different from normal *2381*

Pseudouridine *Ascitic Fluid* *Increase* In 51 specimens from patients with cirrhosis or hepatocellular carcinoma mean concentration of 3.78 ± 0.27 μmol/L but significantly less than 7.48 ± 0.72 μmol/L in 10 specimens from patients with peritoneal neoplasia *728*

Putrescine *Urine* *Increase* Mean excretion in 32 patients with hepatic cirrhosis of 23.2 ± 9.1 nmol/mg creatinine significantly different from 11.2 ± 1.5 nmol/mg creatinine in 28 healthy controls *152*

Putrescine, Free *Urine* *Increase* Mean excretion in 32 patients with hepatic cirrhosis of 2.1 ± 1.7 nmol/mg creatinine significantly different from 0.9 ± 0.4 nmol/mg creatinine in 28 healthy controls *152*

Putrescine, N-monoacetylated *Urine* *Increase* Mean excretion in 32 patients with hepatic cirrhosis of 19.9 ± 8.4 nmol/mg creatinine significantly different from 11.2 ± 1.5 nmol/mg creatinine in 28 healthy controls *152*

Renal Plasma Flow *Patient* *Decrease* In 25 patients with cirrhosis and ascites mean plasma flow of 311 ± 40 mL/min significantly different from 601 ± 70 mL/min in 9 cirrhotics without ascites *1904*

Renin Activity *Plasma* *Increase* Increased levels *4289* In 21 patients with cirrhosis but without ascites mean activity of 0.51 ng/mL/h and 6.0 ng/mL/h in 19 with cirrhosis and ascites compared with normal values of 0.5 - 2.0 ng/mL/h *5347* In 25 patients with cirrhosis with ascites mean activity of 6.5 ± 2 ng/mL/h significantly higher than 0.4 ± 0.01 ng/mL/h in 9 patients with cirrhosis but without ascites and 1 ± 0.2 ng/mL/h in 17 healthy controls *1904* In 10 patients with liver cirrhosis without ascites mean activity of 1.9 ± 1.5 ng/mL/h (not significant) and 3.5 ± 3.4 ng/mL/h in 11 patients with cirrhosis and ascites significantly different from mean activity of 0.9 ± 0.8 ng/mL/h in 10 healthy controls *5349* In 10 patients with liver cirrhosis and ascites mean concentration of 14.6 ng/mL/h significantly higher than 1.8 ng/mL/h in 7 patients with liver cirrhosis without ascites *1650* In 20 patients with hepatic cirrhosis mean plasma renin activity of 2.8 ± 0.7 ng/mL/h not significantly different from 1.0 ± 0.2 ng/mL/h in 19 healthy individuals *1464*
Plasma *No Effect* Median activity in 9 patients with cirrhosis but without ascites of 0.51 ng/mL/h not significantly different from reference range of 0.5 - 2.0 ng/mL/h *5347*

Reticulocytes *Blood* *Decrease* Reticulocytosis can be suppressed by alcohol *5699* *2415*
Blood *Increase* Average of 8.6%, ranging from 2.3 to 24.6% in 16 patients *2415*

Rheumatoid Factor *Serum* *Increase* Dysproteinemias and paraproteinemias present significant seropositivity *1980*

Ristocetin Cofactor Activity *Plasma* *Increase* In 8 patients with hepatic cirrhosis mean concentration of 494 ± 82% of normal significantly different from 100% in 11 healthy controls *366*

Selenium *Serum* *Decrease* In 15 patients with Child's group A disease mean 10.8 ± 2.8 μg/dL, in 16 with Child's group B 10.0 ± 2.5 μg/dL significantly less and in 10 with Child's group C 8.6 ± 1.9 μg/dL also significantly less than 13.8 ± 1.6 μg/dL in 13 healthy adults *638*

Selenoprotein P *Serum* *Decrease* In 15 patients with Child's group A disease mean 0.80 ± 0.30 mU/mL, in 16 with Child's group B 0.65 ± 0.25 mU/mL significantly less and in 10 with Child's group C 0.45 ± 0.20 mU/mL also significantly less than 0.90 ± 0.20 mU/mL in 13 healthy adults *638*

Sex-Hormone Binding Globulin *Serum* *Increase* Increased concentrations reported in men with liver cirrhosis but changes in women not significant *1424*
Serum *No Effect* In 38 women with amenorrhea and alcoholic cirrhosis mean concentration of 59 ± 30 nmol/L and of 62 ± 37 nmol/L in 12 amenorrheic women with other cirrhoses not significantly different from reference interval of 30 - 90 nmol/L *375*

Sodium *Serum* *Decrease* In 25 patients with cirrhosis and ascites mean concentration of 127 ± 2 mmol/L significantly different from 137 ± 1 mmol/L in 17 healthy controls *1904* Especially in patients with ascites *4707* Characteristic *5674* Mean concentration of 135 ± 4 mmol/L in 11 patients with cirrhosis and ascites significantly different from mean concentration of 139 ± 2 mmol/L in 10 healthy controls *5349* In 28 patients with cirrhosis without ascites mean concentration of 137.4 ± 3.3 mmol/L and in 12 with ascites mean concentration of 133.0 ± 5.7 mmol/L significantly different from 140.9 ± 0.9 mmol/L in 10 healthy controls

571.50 **Cirrhosis of Liver** *(continued)*

Sodium *(continued)*
2745 In 24 patients with cirrhosis mean concentration of 133 mmol/L (range 112 - 143 mmol/L) slightly lower than reference interval of 136 - 146 mmol/L *3566*
Serum *No Effect* In 10 patients with liver cirrhosis without ascites mean concentration of 139 ± 2 mmol/L not significantly different from mean concentration of 139 ± 2 mmol/L in 10 healthy controls *5349* In 9 patients with cirrhosis without ascites mean concentration of 135 ± 2 mmol/L not significantly different from 137 ± 1 mmol/L in 17 healthy controls *1904*
Urine *Decrease* In 20 patients with hepatic cirrhosis mean excretion of 32 ± 5 mmol/24 h significantly different from 54 ± 5 mmol/24 h in 19 healthy individuals *1464* Mean excretion of 62 ± 25 mmol/d in 11 patients with cirrhosis and ascites significantly different from mean concentration of 110 ± 26 mmol/d in 10 healthy controls *5349* In 25 patients with cirrhosis and ascites mean excretion of 8 ± 2 mmol/d significantly different from 38 ± 5 mmol/d in 17 healthy controls *1904*
Urine *No Effect* Mean excretion of 91 ± 19 mmol/d in 10 patients with liver cirrhosis without cirrhosis not significantly different from mean concentration of 110 ± 26 mmol/d in 10 healthy controls *5349* In 24 patients with cirrhosis mean excretion of 65 mmol/d (range 15 - 156 mmol/d) towards lower limit of reference interval of 50 - 150 mmol/d *3566* In 9 patients with cirrhosis without ascites mean excretion of 37 ± 4 mmol/d not significantly different from 38 ± 5 mmol/d in 17 healthy controls *1904*

Soluble E-Selectin *Serum* *Increase* In 33 patients with cirrhosis of the liver 36% had concentrations above 86 µg/L *1406*

Soluble Intercellular Adhesion Molecule-1
Ascitic Fluid *Increase* Mean concentration in 53 patients with liver cirrhosis of 151 ± 16 ng/mL *4228*
Serum *Increase* In 33 patients with cirrhosis of the liver, 94% had concentrations above 286 µg/L *1406* Mean concentration in 24 patients with liver cirrhosis of 731 ± 141 ng/mL significantly different from 228 ± 24 ng/mL in 17 healthy controls *4228*

Soluble Interleukin-2 Receptor *Serum* *Increase* In 30 patients with mild chronic active hepatitis C mean concentration of 1,014 ± 335 U/mL and in 21 cases with severe disease mean concentration of 1,847 ± 451 U/mL significantly different from normal *2381*

Soluble Vascular Cell Adhesion Molecule-1
Serum *Increase* In 33 patients with cirrhosis of the liver 93% had concentrations above 872 µg/L *1406*

Somatomedin *Plasma* *Decrease* Observed effect *3141*

Specific Gravity *Ascitic Fluid* *Decrease* Ascitic fluid is usually a transudate with protein < 3.0 g/dL and specific gravity < 1.016. However, protein may exceed 2.5 g/dL in up to 30% of patients *4891*
Pleural Fluid *Decrease* Transudate (< 1.016) *126*

Spermidine *Urine* *Increase* Mean excretion in 32 patients with hepatic cirrhosis of 12.3 ± 3.5 nmol/mg creatinine significantly different from 5.9 ± 1.1 nmol/mg creatinine in 28 healthy controls *152*

Spermidine, Free *Urine* *Increase* Mean excretion in 32 patients with hepatic cirrhosis of 0.6 ± 0.7 nmol/mg creatinine significantly different from 0.2 ± 0.1 nmol/mg creatinine in 28 healthy controls *152*

Spermidine, N^1-acetylated *Urine* *Increase* Mean excretion in 32 patients with hepatic cirrhosis of 4.4 ± 1.1 nmol/mg creatinine significantly different from 2.5 ± 0.4 nmol/mg creatinine in 28 healthy controls *152*

Spermidine, N^8-acetylated *Urine* *Increase* Mean excretion ratio in 32 patients with hepatic cirrhosis of 1.7 ± 0.5 significantly different from 1.3 ± 0.2 in 28 healthy controls *152*

Spermine, Free *Urine* *Increase* Mean excretion in 32 patients with hepatic cirrhosis of 0.6 ± 0.5 nmol/mg creatinine significantly different from 0.3 ± 0.3 nmol/mg creatinine in 28 healthy controls *152*

Spermine, N-acetylated *Urine* *No Effect* Mean excretion in 32 patients with hepatic cirrhosis of not detectable not different from not detectable in 28 healthy controls *152*

Squamous Cell Carcinoma Antigen *Serum* *Increase* In 86 patients with hepatic cirrhosis mean concentration of 1.39 µg/L with 9 patients having a concentration higher than in 100 healthy individuals (64 men, 36 women with mean age 56.4 years) without hepatitis B in whom the upper limit of normal was 2.3 µg/L *888*

Substance P *Plasma* *Increase* In 33 patients with decompensated hepatic cirrhosis mean concentration of 52.2 ± 2.8 pg/mL significantly higher than 38.8 ± 2.3 pg/mL in 31 compensated cirrhotic patients *2964* In 64 patients with hepatic cirrhosis mean concentration of 45.7 ± 2.0 pg/mL significantly higher than 32.9 ± 1.0 pg/mL in 53 healthy controls and directly correlated with severity of condition *2964* In 10 patients with liver cirrhosis without ascites mean concentration of 151 ± 55 pg/mL and 323 ± 143 pg/mL in 11 patients with cirrhosis and ascites significantly different from mean concentration of 57 ± 19 pg/mL in 10 healthy controls *5349* In 20 patients with hepatic cirrhosis mean substance P concentration of 63 ± 5 pg/mL significantly different from 22.8 ± 5 pg/mL in 19 healthy individuals *1464*

Sulfate *Urine* *Decrease* Patients with liver disease often have reduced urinary sulfate *4707*

Tauro-conjugated Bile Acids *Serum* *Increase* Mean concentration in 20 patients with moderate post-hepatitis cirrhosis of 2.008 ± 0.787 µg/mL significantly greater than 0.210 ± 0.107 µg/mL in 20 healthy controls *1854*

Taurochendeoxycholic Acid *Serum* *Increase* Mean concentration of 1.308 ± 0.475 µg/mL in 20 patients with moderate post-hepatitis cirrhosis significantly higher than 0.103 ± 0.051 µg/mL in 20 healthy controls *1854*

Taurocholic Acid *Serum* *Increase* Mean concentration of 0.562 ± 0.242 µg/mL in 20 patients with moderate post-hepatitis cirrhosis significantly higher than 0.069 ± 0.038 µg/mL in 20 healthy controls *1854*

Taurodeoxycholic Acid *Serum* *Increase* Mean concentration of 0.105 ± 0.068 µg/mL in 20 patients with moderate post-hepatitis cirrhosis significantly higher than 0.038 ± 0.018 µg/mL in 20 healthy controls *1854*

Taurolithocholic Acid *Serum* *Increase* Mean concentration of 0.033 ± 0.017 µg/mL in 20 patients with moderate post-hepatitis cirrhosis significantly higher than trace measurement in 20 healthy controls *1854*

Testosterone *Serum* *No Effect* In 38 women with amenorrhea and alcoholic cirrhosis mean concentration of 1.0 ± 1.0 nmol/L and of 0.7 ± 0.2 nmol/L in 12 amenorrheic women with other cirrhoses not significantly different from reference interval of 0.3 - 2.8 nmol/L *375*

Thiobarbituric Acid-reacting Substances *Serum* *Increase* Mean concentration of thiobarbituric acid-reactive substances in serum of 13 patients with hepatic cirrhosis of 1.36 ± 0.33 µmol/L compared with 1.01 ± 0.21 µmol/L in 47 healthy individuals *5585*

Thrombin/Antithrombin III Complex *Plasma* *Increase* In patients with either compensated or decompensated alcoholic liver cirrhosis concentration significantly increased compared with healthy controls *1841*

Thromboplastin Generation *Blood* *Increase* Reflects various abnormalities *5544*

Thrombopoietin *Plasma* *Decrease* Concentration undetectable in 23 of 27 patients with cirrhosis *3315*
Plasma *No Effect* Mean concentration of 1.21 ± 0.55 fmol/mL not significantly different from 1.26 ± 0.74 fmol/mL observed in 30 healthy volunteer controls *2604*

Thromboxane B_2 *Ascitic Fluid* *Increase* Mean concentration in 46 patients with liver cirrhosis of 57 ± 8.1 pg/mL *4228*
Plasma *No Effect* Mean concentration in 17 patients with liver cirrhosis of 256 ± 126 pg/mL not significantly different from 153 ± 67 pg/mL in 14 healthy controls *4228*

Thyroid Stimulating Hormone *Serum* *Increase* The mean serum TSH level was 3.1 µU/mL in the normals and 7.1 µU/mL in the cirrhotic patients. 15% of the hepatic patients had serum TSH values above 10 µU/mL *3822*
Serum *No Effect* Patients with severe alcoholic hepatitis often are euthyroid sick with low T3, low T4 and elevated rT3 and normal TSH *673*

Thyroxine Binding Globulin *Serum* *Decrease* In chronic liver disease *126*
Serum *Increase* Increased *4289*

Thyroxine (T4) *Serum* *Decrease* Typically associated with decreased TBG concentration in hepatic cirrhosis *1965*

Serum *Increase* In 11 patients with decompensated cirrhosis, the free T4 index and free T4 by dialysis method and its absolute value were significantly raised, due to disturbance in the protein binding capacity *1687*

Thyroxine (T4) Index, Free *Serum* *Increase* In 11 patients with decompensated cirrhosis, the free T4 index and free T4 by dialysis method and its absolute value were significantly raised, due to disturbance in the protein binding capacity *1687*

Tissue Inhibitor of Metalloproteinase-1 *Serum* *Increase* In 75 patients with liver cirrhosis (5 primary biliary cirrhosis, 7 alcoholic, 14 type B, 45 type C, 1 type B and type C, and 3 cryptogenic) mean concentration of 256.1 ± 121.5 ng/mL significantly higher than 147.8 ± 22.0 ng/mL in 53 normal individuals *3690*

Tissue Inhibitor of Metalloproteinase-2 *Serum* *Increase* Mean concentration of 93 ± 21 ng/mL in 33 patients with liver cirrhosis significantly different from 61 ± 13 ng/mL in 29 healthy controls *3668*

Tissue Plasminogen Activator *Plasma* *Increase* In 50% of 78 patients with uncompensated liver cirrhosis and in 85.7% of 84 patients with decompensated liver cirrhosis mean concentration increased above 8.3 ng/mL *3887* Concentration significantly increased in patients with either compensated or decompensated alcoholic liver cirrhosis *1841*

Tissue Plasminogen Activator Antigen *Plasma* *Increase* Concentration increased in patients with either compensated or decompensated alcoholic cirrhosis *1841*

Tissue Polypeptide Antigen *Serum* *Increase* In 11 patients with cirrhosis mean concentration of 1,076.80 ± 878.66 U/L significantly greater than 37.73 ± 20.76 U/L in 69 healthy blood donor controls *3591*

Transforming Growth Factor-β_1 *Serum* *Increase* In 94 patients with hepatic cirrhosis, 13.9% had concentrations greater than the upper limit of normal of 20 ng/mL *5181*
Urine *Increase* Median concentration of 30.3 µg/g creatinine in 94 patients with hepatic cirrhosis significantly higher than 12.2 µg/g creatinine in 50 healthy adults *5181*

Tri-iodothyronine, Reverse (rT3) *Serum* *Increase* Mean serum reverse T3 and free reverse T3 (450 pg/dL) were increased in hepatic cirrhosis *827* Patients with severe alcoholic hepatitis often are euthyroid sick with low T3, low T4 and elevated rT3 and normal TSH *673*

Triglycerides *Serum* *Decrease* In 37 individuals with hepatic cirrhosis mean concentration of 1.22 ± 0.64 mmol/L significantly different from 1.70 ± 1.23 mmol/L in 98 healthy controls aged 24 to 55 years with method performed on ILab® 900 automated analyzer *4848*
Serum *No Effect* Mean concentration of 857 ± 457 mg/L in 6 patients with decompensated liver cirrhosis and 1,007 ± 347 mg/L in 17 patients with compensated liver cirrhosis significantly different from 1,005 ± 397 mg/L in 21 healthy controls *5063* In 26 alcoholic cirrhotics mean concentration of 1.25 ± 0.70 mmol/L not significantly different from 1.10 ± 0.44 mmol/L in 10 age and sex matched controls *3345*

Troponin I *Serum* *Increase* In 32 patients with cirrhosis and normal ECG cardiac troponin I concentration increased in 10 patients (range of 0.06 - 0.25 µg/L *4034*

Trypsin *Serum* *Increase* High incidence of pancreatic abnormality in patients with no clinical evidence of pancreatic acinar disease *5378*
Serum *No Effect* Mean concentration of trypsin-like immunoreactivity in 13 patients with liver cirrhosis did not exceed concentration in 85 healthy control individuals (42.78 ± 10.26 ng/mL) *3330*

Tryptophan *Cerebrospinal Fluid* *Increase* Increased concentrations due to decreased plasma branched chain amino acids *3918*

Tumor Necrosis Factor-α *Serum* *No Effect* Mean undetectable concentration in 17 patients with liver cirrhosis not different from undetectable amount in 17 healthy controls *4228*

Tyrosine *Plasma* *Increase* In 30 patients with alcoholic liver cirrhosis, portal hypertension and bleeding esophageal varices *2452*

Urea *Serum* *Decrease* Concentrations of 3.18 ± 2.06 µmol/L in 13 patients with Child-Turcotte subgroup C liver cirrhosis not significantly different from 4.42 ± 1.10 µmol/L in 66 healthy controls *3292*
Urine *No Effect* Excretions of 145 ± 71.8 µmol/g creatinine in 13 patients with Child-Turcotte subgroup C liver cirrhosis significantly different from 185 ± 48.6 µmol/g creatinine in 66 healthy controls *3292*

Urea Nitrogen *Serum* *Decrease* Often decreased (< 10 mg/dL) *5544*
Serum *Increase* In 25 patients with cirrhosis and ascites mean concentration of 39 ± 7 mg/dL significantly higher than 16 ± 1 mg/dL in 17 healthy controls *1904* In 33 patients with cirrhosis of the liver 18% had concentrations above 8.6 mmol/L *1406* In 10 patients with liver cirrhosis without ascites mean concentration of 15 ± 2 mg/dL and 17 ± 6 mg/dL in 11 patients with cirrhosis and ascites not significantly different from mean concentration of 11 ± 4 mg/dL in 10 healthy controls *5349* Increased with gastrointestinal hemorrhage *5544*
Serum *No Effect* In 9 patients with cirrhosis without ascites mean concentration of 14 ± 6 mg/dL not significantly different from 16 ± 1 mg/dL in 17 healthy controls *1904* In 28 patients with cirrhosis without ascites mean concentration of 14.9 ± 7.1 mg/dL and in 12 with ascites mean concentration of 15.3 ± 7.6 mg/dL not significantly different from 14.5 ± 4.1 mg/dL in 10 healthy controls *2745*

Uric Acid *Serum* *Increase* In 98 patients with cirrhosis mean concentration of 6.1 mg/dL was significantly higher than 5.5 mg/dL in age and sex-matched healthy controls. Concentration was unrelated to stage of disease or ERPF *2974* In 52% of 68 patients at initial hospitalization for this disorder *1576*
Serum *No Effect* No significant difference in concentration observed between cirrhotics without ascites and healthy matched controls *2974*

Urobilinogen *Urine* *Increase* In early and recovery stages *5544* In patients with advanced liver cirrhosis excretion may increase to 6 - 8 mg/d compared with upper limit of normal of 4 mg/d *2952*
Urine *No Effect* Normal or increased *5544*

Vitamin B_{12} *Serum* *Increase* May be 3 - 8 times the normal concentration. The increase is mainly in the α-globulin bound fraction *1290* Markedly increased; mean = 608 pg/mL in 33 patients *4448*

Vitamin B_{12} Binding Capacity *Serum* *Increase* Significant elevation; usually correlated with WBC in peripheral blood *4448*

Vitamin B_{12} Binding Capacity, Unsaturated
Serum *Decrease* Decreased concentrations observed during hepatic cirrhosis *2952*

VLDL-Cholesterol *Serum* *Decrease* In 26 alcoholic cirrhotics mean concentration of 0.19 ± 0.12 mmol/L significantly less than 0.37 ± 0.09 mmol/L in 10 age and sex matched controls *3345*

VLDL-Triglycerides *Serum* *Decrease* In 26 alcoholic cirrhotics mean concentration of 0.45 ± 0.30 mmol/L significaantly less than mean concentration of 0.66 ± 0.46 mmol/L in 10 age and sex matched controls *3345*

Volume *Blood* *Increase* In 20 patients with hepatic cirrhosis mean blood volume of 4,490 ± 168 mL significantly different from 3,312 ± 308 mL in 19 healthy individuals *1464*
Plasma *Increase* Averages 15% above normal. Hemodilution exaggerates anemia *2684* In 64% of patients *3710*
Red Blood Cells *Decrease* 25% of patients *3710*
Urine *Decrease* With ascites and edema *1290*
Urine *No Effect* Median excretion in 9 patients with cirrhosis but without ascites of 234 mL/4 h and in 19 with ascites of 256 mL/4 h not significantly different from 222 mL/4 h in 10 healthy controls *5347*

von Willebrand Factor Antigen *Plasma* *Increase* In 8 patients with hepatic cirrhosis mean concentration of 462 ± 103% of normal significantly different from 100% in 11 healthy controls *366*

Xylose Tolerance Test *Urine* *No Effect* Typical observation *5544*

Zinc *Cerebrospinal Fluid* *Decrease* Mean CSF concentration of 2.8 ± 1.8 µg/dL. Normal mean for control group was 4.0 ± 2.6 µg/dL *5725*
Serum *Decrease* Lower concentrations of total serum zinc (540 ± 111 mg/L), and of albumin-bound serum zinc (295 ± 113 mg/L) and a higher concentration of alpha$_2$-macroglobulin-bound zinc (245 ± 69 mg/L) were found in 28 healthy patients with decompensated hepatic cirrhosis, compared to 28 healthy subjects (835 ± 91; 679 ± 83; 156 ± 27 mg/1 respectively) *1622* Patients had serum levels < 70 µg/dL with a mean of 53.4 ± 11

571.50 Cirrhosis of Liver *(continued)*

Zinc *(continued)*
µg/dL (normal mean concentration of 85 µg/dL) *5725* In patients with hepatic cirrhosis concentration is typically reduced *2952* Significant p < 0.001 *5460* *4871*

571.50 Cryptogenic Cirrhosis

Metallothionein *Serum* *No Effect* Since cryptogenic cirrhosis not associated with increased liver copper plasma concentration unaffected *3646*

Substance P *Plasma* *Increase* In 7 patients with hepatic cirrhosis mean concentration significantly higher than 32.9 ± 1.0 pg/mL in 53 healthy controls and directly correlated with severity of condition *2964*

571.50 Hepatic Fibrosis

Neuron-specific Enolase *Serum* *Increase* In 2 of 15 patients with hepatic fibrosis concentration exceeded upper limit of normal of 11 µg/L *887*

Platelets *Blood* *Decrease* Mean concentration of 18.6 ± 3.9 x 10^4/µL in 14 patients with chronic viral hepatitis and stage 1 fibrosis and 16.0 ± 5.8 x 10^4/µL in five with stage 2 fibrosis markedly different from 24.5 ± 7.3 x 10^4/µL observed in 30 healthy volunteer controls *2604* In patients with severe fibrosis mean count 130, 000 /µL, 158,000 /µL in patients with mild fibrosis *3917*

Procollagen Type III Peptide *Serum* *Increase* In patients with hepatic fibrosis, in some of whom it may have been due to schistosomiasis, mean concentration in systemic blood of 4.1 ± 0.9 ng/mL compared with 1.8 ± 0.6 ng/mL in healthy controls *4492*

Prothrombin Time *Plasma* *Decrease* Mean time in 14 patients with chronic viral hepatitis and stage 1 fibrosis 94 ± 7% and in three with stage 3 fibrosis of 83 ± 6% markedly different from that observed in 30 healthy volunteer controls *2604*

Thrombopoietin *Plasma* *Increase* In 14 patients with chronic viral hepatitis and fibrosis stage 1 mean concentration of 2.50 ± 1.60 fmol/mL and in five with stage 2 disease mean concentration of 1.89 ± 0.65 fmol/mL significantly higher than 1.26 ± 0.74 fmol/mL in 30 healthy volunteer controls *2604*

571.50 Posthepatitic Cirrhosis

Acid-soluble Carnitine, Total *Serum* *Decrease* In 22 patients with alcoholic cirrhosis mean concentration of 21.8 ± 13.0 µmol/L significantly different from 28.0 ± 16.7 µmol/L in 28 healthy volunteer controls *2810*

Acylcarnitine, Free *Urine* *No Effect* In 22 HBsAg-positive, nonalcoholic cirrhotic patients free acylcarnitine excretion unchanged in comparison with healthy controls *2809*

Acylcarnitine, Long Chain *Serum* *Increase* In 22 HBsAg-positive, nonalcoholic cirrhotic patients long chain acylcarnitine concentration increased in comparison with healthy controls *2809*

Acylcarnitine, Short Chain *Serum* *No Effect* In 22 patients with post-hepatitic liver cirrhosis mean concentration of 10.8 ± 5.6 µmol/L not significantly different from 12.7 ± 6.8 µmol/L in 28 healthy volunteer controls *2810*
Urine *No Effect* In 22 HBsAg-positive, nonalcoholic cirrhotic patients short chain acylcarnitine excretion unchanged in comparison with healthy controls *2809*

Carnitine *Serum* *Increase* In 15 HBsAg-positive, nonalcoholic cirrhotic patients (Child B and C) carnitine concentration increased in comparison with healthy controls *2809*
Urine *No Effect* In 22 HBsAg-positive, nonalcoholic cirrhotic patients carnitine concentration unchanged in comparison with healthy controls *2809*

Carnitine, Free *Serum* *Decrease* In 15 patients with alcoholic cirrhosis mean concentration of 11.2 ± 9.1 µmol/L significantly different from 15.3 ± 10.5 µmol/L in 28 healthy volunteer controls *2810*

β-Chorionic Gonadotropin *Plasma* *Increase* Mean concentration increased to about 130 ng/mL in non-alcoholic cirrhosis above upper limit of normal of 78 ng/mL *5315*

Laminin *Serum* *Increase* Mean concentration increased to about 195 ng/mL, greater than upper limit of 140 ng/mL *5315*

Multiubiquitin Chains *Serum* *No Effect* In 6 patients with alcoholic hepatic fibrosis mean concentration of 4.2 ± 1.3 ng/mL not significantly different from 4.1 ± 1.7 ng/mL in 10 healthy controls *5126*

Procollagen Type III Peptide *Serum* *Increase* Mean concentration increased to about 22 ng/mL in patients with cirrhosis, greater than upper limit of 12 ng/mL *5315*

Tissue Inhibitor of Metalloproteinase *Serum* *No Effect* Mean concentration of about 195 ng/mL, less than upper limit of 250 ng/mL *5315*

Tissue Inhibitor of Metalloproteinase-1 *Serum* *Increase* Mean concentration of 222 ng/mL in one patient with posthepatitis C cirrhosis significantly different from 66 ng/mL in the platelet-poor plasma of one healthy individual *3667*

Type IV Collagen 7S Domain *Serum* *Increase* Mean concentration increased to 8.3 ng/mL, greater than upper limit of 4.4 ng/mL *5315*

Type IV Collagen, Triple-helix Domain *Serum* *Increase* Mean concentration increased to about 200 ng/mL, greater than upper limit of 90 ng/mL *5315*

Ubiquitin, Free *Serum* *No Effect* In 6 patients with alcoholic hepatic fibrosis mean concentration of 28.8 ± 7.5 ng/mL not significantly different from 29.6 ± 6.6 ng/mL in 10 healthy controls *5126*

571.60 Primary Biliary Cirrhosis

Acid-soluble Carnitine, Total *Serum* *Increase* In 15 patients with primary biliary cirrhosis mean concentration of 52.5 ± 40.0 µmol/L significantly different from 28.0 ± 16.7 µmol/L in 28 healthy volunteer controls *2810*

Acylcarnitine, Free *Urine* *Increase* In 15 patients with primary biliary cirrhosis carnitine urinary excretion, normalized for creatinine excretion, increased by a factor of two in comparison with healthy controls *2809*

Acylcarnitine, Short Chain *Serum* *Increase* In 15 patients with primary biliary cirrhosis mean concentration of 20.0 ± 14.0 µmol/L significantly different from 12.7 ± 6.8 µmol/L in 28 healthy volunteer controls *2810*
Urine *Increase* In 15 patients with primary biliary cirrhosis carnitine urinary excretion, normalized for creatinine excretion, increased by a factor of two in comparison with healthy controls *2809*

Adenosine Deaminase *Serum* *Increase* Activity was raised in all cases of infectious hepatitis, three-quarters of the cases of hepatic cirrhosis and approximately half the cases of biliary cirrhosis and drug jaundice *1784*

Alanine Aminotransferase *Serum* *Increase* In 12 patients with PBC mean activity of 58 ± 11 U/L compared with less than 30 U/L in 838 healthy controls *2374* Usually only mildly elevated *1980* Mean activity of 130 ± 24 U/L observed in 8 patients with PBC compared with < 40 U/L in 27 healthy controls *3793* Modestly elevated (300 U/L) in most of these patients. Values are as high or higher than those of AST *1025*
Serum *No Effect* In patients with PBC characteristically cholestatic pattern of abnormal liver tests observed *1778*

Albumin *Serum* *Decrease* Normal or slightly decreased early; later more markedly decreased *5544* Mean concentration of 26 ± 2 g/L observed in 8 patients with PBC compared with 42 ± 1.0 g/L in 27 healthy controls *3793* In 57 patients with PBC mean concentration of 38 ± 6 g/L different from normal range *1371* In patients with PBC characteristically cholestatic pattern of abnormal liver tests observed with hypoalbuminemia seen mainly in patients with long-standing and end-stage disease *1778*
Serum *No Effect* Mean concentration in 77 patients with PBC of 41 ± 0.6 g/L not significantly different from that observed in 255 healthy elderly controls *2802*

Alkaline Phosphatase *Serum* *Increase* Increased activity detected in patients with PBC *3625* Striking elevations. Incidence of elevation is 100%. Usual range of values of 270 - 375 U/L *4746* Mean activity in 77 patients with PBC of 553 ± 33 U/L different from that observed in 255 healthy elderly controls

2802 In patients with PBC characteristically cholestatic pattern of abnormal liver tests observed *1778* In 15 patients with primary biliary cirrhosis activity increased *2809* Mean activity of 1,168 ± 426 U/L observed in 8 patients with PBC compared with 151 ± 20 U/L in 27 healthy controls *3793* Increased activity observed in 90% patients *5276*

Amino Acids *Urine* *Increase* Aminoaciduria, especially cystine and threonine, may be found *5544*

Ammonium Ions *Urine* *Increase* May be associated with classic distal renal tubular acidosis which is associated with hyokalemia, hyperchloremic metabolic acidosis, urine pH > 5.5, increased urinary ammonium ion excretion, a negative urine anion gap, increased urinary osmol gap, decreased urinary citrate and increased urinary calcium in some patients *4071*

Anion Gap *Urine* *Decrease* May be associated with classic distal renal tubular acidosis which is asociated with hyokalemia, hyperchloremic metabolic acidosis, urine pH > 5.5, increased urinary ammonium ion excretion, a negative urine anion gap, increased urinary osmol gap, decreased urinary citrate and increased urinary calcium in some patients *4071*

Anti-Endomysial IgA Antibodies *Serum* *No Effect* In 62 patients with primary biliary cirrhosis anti-endomysial antibodies not observed in any *5492*

Anti-Gliadin IgA Antibodies *Serum* *No Effect* In 62 patients with primary biliary cirrhosis anti-gliadin IgA antibodies not observed in any *5492*

Anti-Gliadin IgG Antibodies *Serum* *Increase* In 62 patients with primary biliary cirrhosis anti-gliadin IgA antibodies observed in 11 (16%) *5492*

Anti-Mitochondrial Antibodies *Serum* *Increase* 40% positive *4991* Occurs in up to 50% of patients *4160* Found in almost 100% of cases, while incidence is only 10% in extrahepatic biliary obstruction *4160* Reported effect *1980* Present in > 90% of patients compared with 2 - 3% of obstructive bile duct patients *4778* In patients with PBC titer may be increased, with types M2, M4, M8 and M9 with M2 antibody most specific for PBC *1778* 40% positive *4176* Reported effect *4176* 79 - 94% of all cases give positive results *1290* Increase reported *4551* Reported incidence of 10 - 50%, depending on the titer selected for positivity *1211* Detected in patients with PBC *3625*
Serum *No Effect* 35 of 597 women (5.8%) with PBC had undetectable antibodies *2885*

Anti-Mitochondrial M2 Antibody *Serum* *Increase* In patients with PBC titer may be increased, with types M2, M4, M8 and M9 with M2 antibody most specific for PBC *1778*

Anti-Mitochondrial M4 Antibody *Serum* *Increase* In patients with PBC titer may be increased, with types M2, M4, M8 and M9 with M2 antibody most specific for PBC *1778*

Anti-Mitochondrial M8 Antibody *Serum* *Increase* In patients with PBC titer may be increased, with types M2, M4, M8 and M9 with M2 antibody most specific for PBC *1778*

Anti-Mitochondrial M9 Antibody *Serum* *Increase* In patients with PBC titer may be increased, with types M2, M4, M8 and M9 with M2 antibody most specific for PBC *1778*

Anti-Smooth Muscle Antibodies *Serum* *Increase* In patients with PBC titer may be > 1:40 in about 30% patients *1778* Patients with PBC and undetectable antimitochondrial antibodies had higher incidence of anti-smooth muscle antibodies (50% compared to 38% with antimitochondrial antibodies) *2885*

Antibody Titer *Serum* *Increase* Increased incidence of high titers of serum autoantibodies *4778*

Antinuclear Antibodies *Serum* *Increase* Increased frequency observed *4068* Increased incidence of high titers of serum autoantibodies *4778* Moderate incidence (24%), but the reaction is relatively weak *4551* In patients with PBC titer may be > 1:40 in about 30% patients *1778* Patients with PBC and undetectable antimitochondrial antibodies had higher incidence of antinuclear antibodies (79% compared to 36% with antimitochondrial antibodies) *2885* Found in 40% of patients and 2% of controls *4176*

Apolipoprotein A-I *Serum* *Decrease* In 4 female patients compared with 6 age and sex matched controls *314* Low in patients with cholestatic liver disease *1511*

Apolipoprotein A-II *Serum* *Decrease* Low in patients with cholestatic liver disease *1511* In 4 female patients compared with 6 age and sex matched controls *314*

Apolipoprotein E *Serum* *Decrease* Low in patients with cholestatic liver disease *1511*

Aspartate Aminotransferase *Serum* *Increase* Modest elevations (usually < 145 U/L) *1025* Usually only mildly elevated *1980* Hepatocellular necrosis is slight as judged by low serum transaminase levels, and hepatocellular function is well preserved *4551* In 57 patients with PBC mean activity of 1.5 ± 1.0 µkat/L different from normal range of < 0.6 µkat/L *1371*
Serum *No Effect* In patients with PBC characteristically cholestatic pattern of abnormal liver tests observed *1778*

Bile Acids *Serum* *Increase* In 15 patients with primary biliary cirrhosis concentration increased *2809*

Bilirubin *Serum* *Increase* In patients with PBC characteristically cholestatic pattern of abnormal liver tests observed *1778* Mean activity of 313 ± 42 µmol/L observed in 8 patients with PBC compared with 9.4 ± 0.8 µmol/L in 27 healthy controls *3793* Mean concentration in 77 patients with PBC of 1.5 ± 0.2 mg/dL different from that observed in 255 healthy elderly controls *2802* Concentrations vary with disease. Normal concentrations observed in early stages of the disease and increased concentration occurs with disease progression and a poor prognosis *3625* In 15 patients with primary biliary cirrhosis concentration increased *2809* In 57 patients with PBC mean concentration of 45 ± 72 µmol/L different from normal range of 4 - 21 µmol/L *1371* Usually conjugated, representing posthepatic cell obstruction. At times, a large proportion may be unconjugated reflecting impaired hepatic function *4960* Usually conjugated bilirubinemia and total concentration range from 3 - 20 mg/dL or higher. In the final stages, concentrations may exceed 50 mg/dL *2033*
Serum *No Effect* Concentrations vary with disease. Normal concentrations observed in early stages of the disease and increased concentration occurs with disease progression and a poor prognosis *3625*

Bilirubin, Conjugated *Serum* *Increase* In patients with PBC characteristically cholestatic pattern of abnormal liver tests observed, with conjugated and unconjugated fractions increased *1778*

Bilirubin, Direct *Serum* *Increase* Usually conjugated, representing posthepatic cell obstruction *4960* Usually conjugated bilirubinemia and total concentrations range from 3 - 20 mg/dL or higher. In the final stages, concentrations may exceed 50 mg/dL *2033* Increases in the serum bilirubin, mostly of the direct fraction *1980*

Bilirubin, Indirect *Serum* *Increase* Total concentration is usually 5 - 10 mg/dL but may vary between normal and 25 mg/dL. Usually conjugated and therefore represents posthepatic cell obstruction, but at times a large proportion of unconjugated bilirubin may be present in the serum as a reflection of impaired hepatic function *4960*

Bilirubin, Unconjugated *Serum* *Increase* In patients with PBC characteristically cholestatic pattern of abnormal liver tests observed, with conjugated and unconjugated fractions increased *1778*

CA 19-9 *Serum* *Increase* In 20 patients with primary biliary sclerosis median concentration of 74 kU/L significantly higher than upper limit of normal of 35 kU/L, with 60% of patients having abnormal values *3218*

Calcium *Urine* *Increase* May be associated with classic distal renal tubular acidosis which is asociated with hyokalemia, hyperchloremic metabolic acidosis, urine pH > 5.5, increased urinary ammonium ion excretion, a negative urine anion gap, increased urinary osmol gap, decreased urinary citrate and increased urinary calcium in some patients *4071*

Carbohydrate-deficient Transferrin *Serum* *Increase* Reported to increase concentration *3090*

Carcinoembryonic Antigen *Serum* *Increase* In 20 patients with primary biliary sclerosis median concentration of 5 µg/L not different from upper limit of normal of 14 µg/L, but 12% of patients had abnormal values *3218*

Carnitine *Serum* *No Effect* In 15 patients with primary biliary cirrhosis carnitine plasma pool unchanged in comparison with healthy controls *2809*

Carnitine, Free *Serum* *Increase* In 15 patients with primary biliary cirrhosis mean concentration of 32.5 ± 27.2 µmol/L significantly different from 15.3 ± 10.5 µmol/L in 28 healthy volunteer controls *2810*

571.60 Primary Biliary Cirrhosis *(continued)*

CD4+ Lymphocytes *Blood* *No Effect* No significant increase observed in patients with primary biliary cirrhosis *3916* No significant increase in patients with primary biliary cirrhosis when compared to controls *3916*

CD8+ Lymphocytes *Blood* *Increase* Significantly higher as compared with normal controls in patients with primary biliary cirrhosis *3916*

Ceruloplasmin *Serum* *Increase* Elevated in 46 of 46 cases *1087*

Chenodeoxycholic Acid *Serum* *Increase* In 15 patients with primary biliary cirrhosis, 13 had increased fasting levels *4552* Severe cholestasis *2426*

Chloride *Serum* *Increase* May be associated with classic distal renal tubular acidosis which is asociated with hyokalemia, hyperchloremic metabolic acidosis, urine pH > 5.5, increased urinary ammonium ion excretion, a negative urine anion gap, increased urinary osmol gap, decreased urinary citrate and increased urinary calcium in some patients *4071*

Cholesterol *Serum* *Increase* Moderate to marked elevations up to 1,800 mg/dL *1025* Characteristic observation in patients with PBC *4419* Marked increase in total cholesterol and phospholipids takes place, with normal triglycerides; serum is not lipemic. The increase is associated with xanthomas and xanthelasmas *5544* Hypercholesterolemia of an extreme degree (2,000 mg/dL) may be present *2039* Hypercholesterolemia occurs in about half the patients on presentation *3625*
Serum *No Effect* Mean concentration in 77 patients with PBC of 278 ± 13 mg/dL not significantly different from that observed in 255 healthy elderly controls *2802* Mean concentration of 5.9 ± 2.1 mmol/L observed in 8 patients with PBC compared with 5.9 ± 0.2 mmol/L in 27 healthy controls *3793*

Cholesterol, Free:Cholesterol Ratio *Serum* *Increase* In late stages of disease ratio shows a progressive increase *4419*
Serum *No Effect* In early stages of disease ratio is normal *4419*

Cholic Acid *Serum* *Increase* In 15 patients with primary biliary cirrhosis, 13 had increased fasting levels *4552* Severe cholestasis *2426*

Citrate *Urine* *Decrease* May be associated with classic distal renal tubular acidosis which is asociated with hyokalemia, hyperchloremic metabolic acidosis, urine pH > 5.5, increased urinary ammonium ion excretion, a negative urine anion gap, increased urinary osmol gap, decreased urinary citrate and increased urinary calcium in some patients *4071*

Copper *Liver* *Increase* Elevated in 43 of 45 patients, > 400 µg/g dry weight were found almost exclusively in patients with advanced histological disease *1087* 8 of 13 patients had liver copper content as high as seen in patients with hepatolenticular degeneration (250 µg/g dry wt) *4367*
Urine *Increase* Elevated in 42 of 46 patients. A correlation was found (r = 0.68) between urinary and hepatic copper *1087*

Cryoglobulins *Serum* *Increase* Found in high concentration in 90% of patients (undetectable in controls). Composed of IgM (60%), IgG-IgM (25%), and IgA-IgM (5%) *5557*

Enzyme Inhibitory Antibody to Pyruvate Dehydrogenase *Serum* *Increase* 80 - 90% positive cases observed in patients with primary biliary cirrhosis *2470*

Fibrinogen *Plasma* *Decrease* Formation is depressed in liver failure, resulting in decreased plasma levels *1290*

Fibronectin *Plasma* *Increase* No significant differences were found between the plasma fibronectin levels of patients with primary biliary cirrhosis and those of controls *4154*

Galactose Tolerance *Patient* *Increase* In 57 patients with PBC mean $T_{1/2}$ of 19 ± 8 min different from normal range of < 17 min *1371*

α_2-Globulin *Serum* *Increase* Moderate increases *1290*

β-Globulin *Serum* *Increase* Marked increase *1290*

γ-Globulin *Serum* *Increase* Usually elevated, particularly IgM *1980* Serum globulins (especially β and α_2) are increased *4960* Hypergammaglobulinemia is mainly due to an elevation of IgM *1447* Serum globulins (especially β and α_2) are increased *5544*

Glucose *Serum* *Decrease* Replacement or destruction of functioning hepatic tissue may evoke hypoglycemia *4707*

β-Glucuronidase *Serum* *Increase* Increased *1777* *1498*

γ-Glutamyltransferase *Serum* *Increase* Mean activity of 284 ± 136 U/L observed in 8 patients with PBC compared with < 50 U/L in 27 healthy controls *3793* In patients with PBC characteristically cholestatic pattern of abnormal liver tests observed *1778* Elevation is marked *5544* In 12 patients with PBC mean concentration of 2.1 ± 0.3 U/L compared with undetectable amounts in 838 healthy controls *2374*

Granulocyte-Macrophage Colony Stimulating Factor *Serum* *Decrease* In 25 patients with symptomatic PBC and 39 with asymptomatic PBC mean concentration significantly different from that in 99 healthy adults *5782*

HDL-Cholesterol *Serum* *Decrease* Significant decrease observed in advanced disease *4419* Mean concentration ranged from 0.25 to 1.02 mmol/L in 8 patients with PBC compared with 1.7 ± 0.1 mmol/L in 27 healthy controls *3793*
Serum *Increase* In 7 female patients compared to 6 normal age matched controls *325* *314* *5707* Marked increase characteristic observation in patients with early PBC *4419* In 7 female patients compared to 6 normal age matched controls *3327*

β-Hexosaminidase *Serum* *Increase* High specificity and sensitivity for primary biliary cirrhosis *3073*

Hyaluronan *Serum* *Increase* Concentration ranged from 21-800 µg/L. In patients with PBC and cirrhosis grade 4 had concentrations above the reference range. Optimal predicting value of 25 µg/L calculated *3072*

Hyaluronic Acid *Serum* *Increase* Determined in 76 patients with primary biliary cirrhosis (PBC). The HA and PIII NP concentrations were significantly increased compared with controls ($p < 0.001$) *3842* In patients with primary biliary cirrhosis significant increases were found in serum laminin, hyaluronate and P-III-P and, more important, a significant correlation was found between the histological stage of the disease and serum hyaluronate *4154* The median serum concentrations in primary biliary cirrhosis (150 µg/L) were significantly increased in comparison with controls *1371*

Hydroxyproline *Urine* *No Effect* Not different from age matched controls *2191*

immunoglobulin A *Serum* *Increase* Hypergammaglobulinemia is common, involving all classes of immunoglobulins (IgG, IgA, IgM), although IgM may be selectively increased *367* In patients with PBC concentration may be slightly increased but are usually normal *1778*
Serum *No Effect* In patients with PBC concentration may be slightly increased but are usually normal *1778*

Immunoglobulin G *Serum* *Increase* IgG is more likely to be elevated in chronic hepatitis and cryptogenic cirrhosis, whereas IgM is high in biliary cirrhosis *4160* Hypergammaglobulinemia is common, involving all classes of serum immunoglobulins (IgG, IgA, IgM), although IgM may be selectively increased *367*

Immunoglobulin M *Serum* *Increase* Elevated in about 80% of patients *2033* Reported effect *1980* Hypergammaglobulinemia is common, involving all classes of immunoglobulins, although IgM may be selectively increased *367* In patients with PBC characteristically increased concentration of IgM *1778* Increased concentration detected in patients with PBC *3625* Hypergammaglobulinemia is mainly due to an elevation of IgM *1447* Increased concentration observed in 90% patients *5276* Reported effect *4551*

Interferon-γ *Serum* *Increase* Significant increase reported in patients with primary biliary cirrhosis *394* In 25 patients with symptomatic PBC and 39 with asymptomatic PBC mean concentration significantly different from that in 99 healthy adults *5782*

Interleukin-1α-Autoantibody *Serum* *No Effect* In 12 patients with PBC proportion with autoantibody 16.7% compared with 12.6% in 838 healthy controls *2374*

Interleukin-1β *Serum* *Increase* Significant increase reported in patients with primary biliary cirrhosis *394*
Serum *No Effect* In 25 patients with symptomatic PBC and 39 with asymptomatic PBC mean concentration not significantly different from that in 99 healthy adults *5782*

Interleukin-2 *Serum* *Increase* In 28 patients with primary biliary cirrhosis mean concentration of 39 ± 13 U/mL compared with 0.8 ± 0.5 U/mL in healthy controls *3491* In 25 patients with symptomatic PBC and 39 with asymptomatic PBC mean concentration significantly different from that in 99 healthy adults

5782 Significant increase reported in patients with primary biliary cirrhosis *394*

Interleukin-6 *Monocytes Increase* Significant increase reported in patients with primary biliary cirrhosis *394*
Serum Decrease In 39 patients with asymptomatic PBC mean concentration significantly less than 34.1 pg/mL in 99 healthy adults *5782*
Serum Increase Significant increase reported in patients with primary biliary cirrhosis *394*
Serum No Effect In 25 patients with symptomatic PBC mean concentration not significantly different from 34.1 pg/mL in 99 healthy adults *5782*

Interleukin-8 *Serum Increase* In 25 patients with symptomatic PBC and 39 with asymptomatic PBC mean concentration significantly different from that in 99 healthy adults *5782*

International Normalized Ratio *Plasma No Effect* In patients with PBC characteristically normal INR *1778*

Iron-binding Capacity, Total *Serum Decrease* In hepatic cirrhosis *5863*

Iron Saturation *Serum Increase* Moderate to marked rise in percent saturation in hepatic cirrhosis *5863*

Laminin *Serum Increase* Increased concentration was useful in assessing extent of hepatic fibrosis *5276* In patients with this primary biliary cirrhosis the mean level (2.14 U/mL) was significantly higher than healthy controls (mean 1.28 U/mL) *5420* In patients with primary biliary cirrhosis significant increases were found in serum laminin, hyaluronate and P-III-P *4154*

LDL-Cholesterol *Serum Increase* Marked increase characteristic observation in patients with early PBC: also seen in advanced disease *4419*

Lipids *Serum Increase* Common *2033*

Lipoprotein X *Serum Increase* Characteristic observation in advanced disease together with marked increase of LDL-cholesterol concentration *4419*

Lipoprotein Lp(a) *Serum Decrease* In 42 patients with primary biliary cirrhosis mean concentration of 28.5 mg/L compared with 75.0 mg/L in healthy controls *1865*
Serum No Effect No significant difference observed between mean concentration of 2.55 mg/dL in 39 women with PBC and 5.2 mg/dL in healthy controls *4419*

Metallothionein *Serum Increase* In patients with primary biliary cirrhosis concentrations ranged from 1.8 to 52.2 ng/mL compared with 2.4 to 4.8 ng/mL in controls. Concentrations in stage I or II typically normal but increased in stage III and abnormal in all stage IV *3646*

Neopterin *Serum Increase* In 46 patients with primary biliary cirrhosis mean concentration of 11.0 ± 1.0 nmol/L, with mean in 35 without cirrhosis of 11.0 ± 1.1 nmol/L and 11.1 ± 2.9 nmol/L in 11 with cirrhosis different from 6.0 ± 2.2 nmol/L in healthy controls *5682*

Net Acid Excretion *Urine Increase* May be associated with classic distal renal tubular acidosis which is asociated with hyokalemia, hyperchloremic metabolic acidosis, urine pH > 5.5, increased urinary ammonium ion excretion, a negative urine anion gap, increased urinary osmol gap, decreased urinary citrate and increased urinary calcium in some patients *4071*

5'-Nucleotidase *Serum Increase* In 18 patients levels ranged from 32.7 - 265 U/L, mean activity of 127.8 ± 79.5 U/L *2803*

Osmolal Gap *Urine Increase* May be associated with classic distal renal tubular acidosis which is asociated with hyokalemia, hyperchloremic metabolic acidosis, urine pH > 5.5, increased urinary ammonium ion excretion, a negative urine anion gap, increased urinary osmol gap, decreased urinary citrate and increased urinary calcium in some patients *4071*

Osteocalcin *Serum Decrease* In 15 premenopausal females with this disorder *2191*

pH *Urine Increase* May be associated with classic distal renal tubular acidosis which is asociated with hyokalemia, hyperchloremic metabolic acidosis, urine pH > 5.5, increased urinary ammonium ion excretion, a negative urine anion gap, increased urinary osmol gap, decreased urinary citrate and increased urinary calcium in some patients *4071*

Phospholipids *Serum Decrease* In 4 female patients compared to 6 normal age matched controls *314*
Serum Increase Marked increase in total cholesterol and phospholipids takes place, with normal triglycerides; serum is not lipemic. The increase is associated with xanthomas and xantholasmas *5544*

Platelets *Blood Decrease* In patients with primary biliary cirrhosis platelet counts of less than 200 x 10^9/L strongly associated with variceal hemorrhages *4156*

Potassium *Serum Decrease* May be associated with classic distal renal tubular acidosis which is asociated with hyokalemia, hyperchloremic metabolic acidosis, urine pH > 5.5, increased urinary ammonium ion excretion, a negative urine anion gap, increased urinary osmol gap, decreased urinary citrate and increased urinary calcium in some patients *4071*

Procollagen Type III Peptide *Serum Increase* Increased concentration was useful in assessing extent of hepatic fibrosis *5276* Among patients with primary biliary cirrhosis, both PGA index and P-III-P concentration correlated well with the severity of the disease, determined by the Mayo score (r = 0.72 and 0.66 respectively) *5183* Significant increases were found in serum laminin, hyaluronate and P-III-P in patients with primary biliary cirrhosis *4154* Determined in 76 patients with primary biliary cirrhosis (PBC), the HA and PIIINP concentrations were significantly increased compared with controls (p less than 0.001) *3842*

Prothrombin Time *Plasma Increase* Laboratory findings of steatorrhea but prothrombin time is normal or restored to normal by parenteral vitamin K *5544* Increased time suggests deteriorating liver function in patients with end-stage primary biliary cirrhosis *5276*

Sodium *Serum Decrease* Frequently found, especially in patients with ascites *4707*

Superoxide Dismutase *Serum Increase* In patients with primary biliary cirrhosis mean concentration of manganese superoxide dismutase of 407 ± 35 ng/mL significantly increased in comparison with concentrations in patients with other liver diseases including hepatocellular carcinoma, liver cirrhosis, chronic hepatitis and obstructive jaundice *3919*

Thromboplastin Time *Plasma Increase* Mean activity of 0.48 ± 0.06 observed in 8 patients with PBC compared with 0.70 - 1.30 in 27 healthy controls *3793*

Thyroxine Binding Globulin *Serum Increase* Observed effect *126*

Triglycerides *Serum Increase* Mean concentration of 1.8 ± 0.5 mmol/L observed in 8 patients with PBC compared with 1.1 ± 0.1 mmol/L in 27 healthy controls *3793* With time, all lipids rise, including triglycerides *4960*
Serum No Effect Marked increase in total cholesterol and phospholipids takes place, with normal triglycerides; serum is not lipemic *5544*

Tumor Necrosis Factor-α *Serum Increase* In 28 patients with primary biliary cirrhosis mean concentration of 549 ± 162 pg/mL compared with undetectable concentrations in healthy controls *3491* Significant increase reported in patients with primary biliary cirrhosis *394*
Serum No Effect In 25 patients with symptomatic PBC and 39 with asymptomatic PBC mean concentration not significantly different from that in 99 healthy adults *5782*

Uric Acid *Serum Decrease* May occur *5544*

Urobilinogen *Urine Increase* Urine contains urobilinogen and bilirubin *5544*

Vitamin E *Serum Decrease* Deficiency might be expected in patients with defective fat absorption *4707*

Vitamin K *Serum Decrease* Median concentration of vitamin K_1 in 77 patients with PBC of 0.65 nmol/L significantly different from 0.95 nmol/L observed in 255 healthy elderly controls *2802*

571.80 Hepatic Steatosis

Alanine Aminotransferase *Serum Increase* Increased activity, but less than 3 times upper limit of normal, is the most common biochemical activity in patients with nonalcoholic steatohepatitis *3625*

Albumin *Serum No Effect* Normal concentration is characteristic in patients with nonalcoholic steatohepatitis *3625*

Alkaline Phosphatase *Serum Increase* Swelling of liver against the fibrous Glisson's capsule that occurs with steatosis hinders blood flow and causes increased enzyme activity *4617*

571.80 Hepatic Steatosis *(continued)*

Aspartate Aminotransferase *Serum Increase* Increased activity, but less than 3 times the upper limit of normal, is the most common biochemical activity in patients with nonalcoholic steatohepatitis *3625*

Aspartate Aminotransferase:Alanine Aminotransferase Ratio *Serum Decrease* Ratio of less than 1.0, in the absence of cirrhosis, is characteristic in patients with nonalcoholic steatohepatitis *3625*

Bilirubin *Serum Increase* Increased concentration is unusual in patients with nonalcoholic steatohepatitis *3625*

Cathepsin D *Serum Increase* Mean concentration in 16 patients with benign hepatic steatosis of 23.1 ± 3.5 nmol/L significantly increased compared with 10.0 ± 0.71 nmol/L in 98 healthy controls *3004*
Serum No Effect No significant change observed in patients with liver steatosis *595*

Desialylated Transferrin:Transferrin Ratio *Serum No Effect* A normal ratio differentiates patients with nonalcoholic steatohepatitis from those with excessive alcohol ingestion *3625*

Ferritin *Serum Increase* Increased concentration in patients with nonalcoholic steatohepatitis has been described but most likely arises from underlying hepatic necroinflammatory activity *3625*

Glucose *Serum Increase* Nonalcoholic steatohepatitis is associated with increased concentration *3625*

Neuron-specific Enolase *Serum Increase* In 1 of 6 patients with hepatic steatosis concentration exceeded upper limit of normal of 11 µg/L *887*

Transferrin Saturation *Serum Increase* Increased saturation in patients with nonalcoholic steatohepatitis has been described but most likely arises from underlying hepatic necroinflammatory activity *3625*

571.80 Hepatosplenomegaly

Acid Ribonuclease *Serum Increase* Median activity in 11 patients with hepatosplenomegaly of 54.4 U/L significantly different from 42.0 U/L in 32 healthy controls *2566*

Alanine Aminotransferase *Serum Increase* Median activity in 11 patients with hepatosplenomegaly of 90 U/L significantly different from 22 U/L in 32 healthy controls *2566*

Albumin *Serum No Effect* Median concentration in 11 patients with hepatosplenomegaly of 3.4 g/dL not significantly different from 3.7 g/dL in 32 healthy controls *2566*

Alkaline Phosphatase *Serum Increase* Median activity in 11 patients with hepatosplenomegaly of 116 U/L significantly different from 63 U/L in 32 healthy controls *2566*

Alkaline Ribonuclease *Serum Increase* Median activity in 11 patients with hepatosplenomegaly of 70.8 U/L significantly different from 67.4 U/L in 32 healthy controls *2566*

Bilirubin *Serum Increase* Median concentration in 11 patients with hepatosplenomegaly of 1.9 mg/dL significantly different from 0.7 mg/dL in 32 healthy controls *2566*

Creatinine *Serum Increase* Median concentration in 11 patients with hepatosplenomegaly of 1.0 mg/dL not significantly different from 0.7 mg/dL in 32 healthy controls *2566*

Urea *Serum Increase* Median concentration in 11 patients with hepatosplenomegaly of 40 mg/dL significantly different from 31 mg/dL in 32 healthy controls *2566*

571.80 Non-alcoholic Fatty Liver

Alanine Aminotransferase *Serum Increase* In 26 patients with non-alcoholic fatty liver mean activity of 61 ± 2 U/L increased compared with 20 ± 2 U/L in 30 healthy controls *2269*

Albumin *Serum No Effect* In 26 patients with non-alcoholic fatty liver mean concentration of 4.9 ± 0.1 g/dL not different when compared with 4.8 ± 0.1 g/dL in 30 healthy controls *2269*

Aspartate Aminotransferase *Serum Increase* In 26 patients with non-alcoholic fatty liver mean activity of 57 ± 4 U/L increased compared with 23 ± 1 U/L in 30 healthy controls *2269*

Bilirubin *Serum Increase* In 26 patients with non-alcoholic fatty liver mean concentration of 1.0 ± 0.1 mg/dL increased compared with 0.6 ± 0.1 mg/dL in 30 healthy controls *2269*

Globulin *Serum No Effect* In 26 patients with non-alcoholic fatty liver mean concentration of 2.9 ± 0.0 g/dL not different when compared with 2.8 ± 0.1 g/dL in 30 healthy controls *2269*

Neutrophils *Blood No Effect* In 15 patients with non-alcoholic fatty liver mean concentration of 4.2 ± 0.2 x 10^3/µL not different when compared with 3.7 ± 0.1 x 10^3/µL in 30 healthy controls *2269* In 26 patients with non-alcoholic fatty liver mean concentration of 3.8 ± 0.2 x 10^3/µL not different when compared with 3.7 ± 0.1 x 10^3/µL in 30 healthy controls *2269*

Tissue Inhibitor of Metalloproteinase-1 *Serum Increase* In 23 patients with non-alcoholic fatty liver mean concentration of 168.6 ± 39.1 ng/mL not significantly higher than 147.8 ± 22.0 ng/mL in 53 normal individuals *3690*

572.00 Liver Abscess (Pyogenic)

Alanine Aminotransferase *Serum Increase* Increases during preicteric phase to peaks 500 U/L) by the time jaundice appears; then rapid fall in several days; become normal 2 - 5 weeks after onset of jaundice *5544* Regardless of cause may be associated with increase in activity, usually near normal but may be increased 3 - 4-fold *3406*
Serum No Effect Transaminase levels are often normal in the absence of biliary tract infections in acute liver abscess *367*

Albumin *Serum Decrease* Levels below 3.0 g/dL are common *900* Decreased synthesis and increased catabolism of albumin cause hypoproteinemia in the majority of patients with acute liver abscess *367* Hypoalbuminemia is a frequent finding *3406*

Alkaline Phosphatase *Serum Increase* 25 - 80 U/L in over 80% of cases; 80 - 375 U/L in 100% of cases during obstructive phase *5544* In patients with space-occupying lesions such as liver abscess, the degree of elevation may be striking (270-535 U/L) with little or no rise in the serum bilirubin values. This pattern of hepatic dysfunction is useful in the recognition of these space-occupying lesions particularly in the recognition of metastasis to the liver in patients with carcinomatosis *1642* Elevated in 75% of cases *4891* In patients with space-occupying lesions such as liver abscess, the degree of elevation may be striking (270 - 535 U/L) with little or no rise in the serum bilirubin values. This pattern of hepatic dysfunction is useful in the recognition of these space-occupying lesions particularly in the recognition of metastasis to the liver in patients with carcinomatosis *1025* Observed with liver damage *900*

Amylase *Serum Decrease* Severe liver damage *5544*

Aspartate Aminotransferase *Serum Increase* Both rise during preicteric phase to peaks 240 U/L) by the time jaundice appears; then rapid fall in several days; become normal 2 - 5 weeks after onset of jaundice *5544* Regardless of cause may be associated with increase in activity, usually near normal but may be increased 3 - 4-fold *3406* May exhibit a mild to moderate elevation *900*
Serum No Effect Transaminase levels are often normal in the absence of biliary tract infections in acute liver abscess *367*

Bilirubin *Serum Increase* Regardless of cause may be associated with moderate increase in concentration *3406* Elevated in 50% of cases *4891* Moderate increase in about 33% of patients. Usually indicates pyogenic rather than amebic and suggests poorer prognosis because of more tissue destruction *5544*

BSP Retention *Serum No Effect* BSP dye may be lost into abdomen. Results may falsely appear normal *5544*

Cholinesterase *Serum Decrease* Liver diseases, especially hepatitis. Lowest level corresponds to peak of disease and becomes normal with recovery *5544*

Erythrocyte Sedimentation Rate *Blood Increase* Markedly raised rate is characteristic of condition *3406*

Erythrocyte Survival *Red Blood Cells Decrease* Decreased RBC survival; mild to moderate hemolysis *4199*

α-Fetoprotein *Serum Increase* 10 - 20% of nonmalignant liver diseases of all types have elevated serum AFP levels, which tend to be fluctuating or transient. Steady or rising levels indicate malignancy *5759*

γ-Globulin *Serum Increase* Hypergammaglobulinemia is a frequent finding *3406*

Glucose *Serum Decrease* Replacement or destruction of functioning hepatic tissue may evoke hypoglycemia *4707*

γ-Glutamyltransferase *Serum* *Increase* In 5 patients with liver granulomas, including miliary tuberculosis and sarcoidosis, serum GGT levels were all elevated, mean activity of 303 U/L, range 116 - 740 U/L *3161*

Hematocrit *Blood* *Decrease* A mild normochromic anemia is common *4891* Mild to moderate anemia *900* Anemia is characteristic of condition *3406*

Hemoglobin *Blood* *Decrease* A mild normochromic anemia is common *4891* Anemia is characteristic of condition *3406* Mild to moderate anemia *900*
Plasma *Increase* Mild to moderate hemolysis usually occurs *4199*

International Normalized Ratio *Plasma* *Increase* Prolonged INR may be observed in protracted illness *3406*

Isocitrate Dehydrogenase *Serum* *Increase* 500 - 2000 U/L in 1st week; < 800 U/L after 2 weeks; slightly elevated in 3rd week *5544*

Leucine Aminopeptidase *Serum* *Increase* In 12 patients with granulomatous hepatitis, all showed elevated LAP levels, varying from 380 - 1,000 U/L, with a mean of 622 (normal 322 U/L) *579*

Leukocytes *Blood* *Increase* Marked leukocytosis is characteristic of condition *3406* Increase in WBC due to increase in granulocytes *5544* Marked leukocytosis with WBC above 20,000 /μL *900*

Neutrophils *Blood* *Increase* Polymorphonuclear leukocytosis in > 90% of patients; usually over 20,000 /μL *5544*

Ornithine Carbamoyltransferase *Serum* *Increase* Liver cell damage *5544*

Partial Thromboplastin Time *Plasma* *Increase* Reported effect *900*

Platelets *Blood* *No Effect* No significant effect usually observed *900*

Prothrombin Time *Plasma* *Increase* Increased in cases of severe liver damage due to poisons, hepatitis, cirrhosis *5544*

Sulfate *Urine* *Decrease* Patients with liver disease often have reduced urinary sulfate *4707*

Vitamin B_{12} *Serum* *Increase* High concentrations of vitamin B_{12} often exceeding 1,000 ng/L *3406*

572.20 Hepatic Encephalopathy

Acid Ribonuclease *Serum* *Increase* Median activity in 9 patients with hepatic encephalopathy of 66.9 U/L significantly different from 42.0 U/L in 32 healthy controls *2566*

Alanine Aminotransferase *Serum* *Increase* Median activity in 9 patients with hepatic encephalopathy of 291 U/L significantly different from 22 U/L in 32 healthy controls *2566*

Albumin *Serum* *Decrease* Median concentration in 9 patients with hepatic encephalopathy of 3.3 g/dL significantly different from 3.7 g/dL in 32 healthy controls *2566* Marked decrease *3918*

Alkaline Phosphatase *Serum* *Increase* Median activity in 9 patients with hepatic encephalopathy of 193 U/L significantly different from 63 U/L in 32 healthy controls *2566*

Alkaline Ribonuclease *Serum* *Increase* Median activity in 9 patients with hepatic encephalopathy of 84.7 U/L significantly different from 67.4 U/L in 32 healthy controls *2566*

Ammonia *Blood* *Increase* Elevated in about 60% of patients. Poor correlation between the level of blood ammonia and the depth of the hepatic coma *1980* Elevated in most patients *3192*
Cerebrospinal Fluid *Increase* Elevated in most patients *3192*

Bicarbonate *Serum* *Decrease* Respiratory alkalosis may occur *1980*

Bilirubin *Serum* *Increase* Median concentration in 9 patients with hepatic encephalopathy of 4.0 mg/dL significantly different from 0.7 mg/dL in 32 healthy controls *2566*

Carbon Dioxide Partial Pressure *Blood* *Decrease* Respiratory alkalosis may occur *1980*

Creatinine *Serum* *Increase* Median concentration in 9 patients with hepatic encephalopathy of 1.4 mg/dL significantly different from 0.7 mg/dL in 32 healthy controls *2566*

Dopamine β-Hydroxylase *Serum* *Decrease* A decrease in H^3-dopamine uptake was demonstrated in the blood platelets of 22 hepatic encephalopathy patients when compared to that of patients with liver cirrhosis but without hepatic encephalopathy, and controls. There was a direct correlation between the stage of hepatic encephalopathy and the decrease in H^3-dopamine uptake *3596*

Factor VII *Plasma* *Decrease* All 7 patients with values < 8% of normal failed to regain consciousness from hepatic coma due to fulminant hepatic failure *1680*

Fatty Acids (FFA), Free *Cerebrospinal Fluid* *Increase* Short and medium chain fatty acids with lengths C_5- C_8 are often elevated in blood and CSF *3192*
Serum *Increase* Short and medium chain fatty acids with lengths C_5-C_8 are often elevated in blood and CSF *3192* Significant elevation *3918* Plasma free fatty acids are commonly elevated *367*

α-Fetoprotein *Serum* *Increase* In fulminant hepatic failure, 15 of the 64 patients (23%) had raised levels but in only 2 did they exceed 50 ng/mL. Of the 23 survivors, 11 (48%) had elevated levels. This rise was found early after the development of a grade IV coma and constitutes an encouraging prognostic sign at a time when the liver function tests and EEG are not helpful *3680*

Fibrinogen *Plasma* *Decrease* Low levels of clotting factors found in fulminant hepatic failure are due to decrease in liver synthesis aggravated by increased consumption *1680*

Gc-Globulin *Serum* *Decrease* In 79 patients with hepatic encephalopathy mean concentration of 122 ± 85 mg/L significantly lower than 365 ± 57 mg/L in healthy individuals with significant reductions observed in patients who subsequently developed cardiovascular failure, intracranial hypertension and infections *4637*

Gc-Globulin, Free *Serum* *Decrease* In 79 patients with hepatic encephalopathy mean concentration of 83 ± 74 mg/L significantly lower than 328 ± 77 mg/L in healthy individuals with significant reductions observed in patients who subsequently developed cardiovascular failure, intracranial hypertension and infections *4637*

β-Glucuronidase *Serum* *Decrease* Decreased *1777* *1498*

Glutamine *Cerebrospinal Fluid* *Increase* An end product in ammonia metabolism *3192*
Plasma *Increase* An end product in ammonia metabolism *3192*

Isoleucine *Plasma* *Decrease* Branched chain amino acids are generally reduced *3192*

Leucine *Plasma* *Decrease* Branched chain amino acids are generally reduced *3192*

Methionine *Plasma* *Increase* Frequently increased and is implicated in the pathogenesis of the disorder *3192*

Nickel *Serum* *Decrease* Thought to be caused by hypoalbuminemia *3428*

pH *Blood* *Increase* Respiratory alkalosis may occur *1980*

Phenylalanine *Plasma* *Increase* Consistently elevated *3192*

Potassium *Serum* *Increase* Decreased concentrations indirectly induce hepatic coma by its effect on ammonia metabolism. Renal production of ammonia increases in the presence of potassium deficiency *1620*

Prothrombin Time *Plasma* *Increase* Prolonged in liver disease *1980*

Sodium *Urine* *Decrease* Hyponatremia (< 130 mmol/L) occurred in 61% of patients with hepatic failure due to decompensated cirrhosis of liver *793*

Tryptophan *Cerebrospinal Fluid* *Increase* The only amino acid with increased CSF concentrations compared to normals and stable cirrhotics, probably attributable to increased plasma free tryptophan in hepatic coma patients *3918*
Plasma *Increase* The only amino acid with increased CSF concentrations compared to normals and stable cirrhotics, probably attributable to increased plasma free tryptophan in hepatic coma patients *3918*

Urea *Serum* *Increase* Median concentration in 9 patients with hepatic encephalopathy of 58 mg/dL significantly different from 31 mg/dL in 32 healthy controls *2566*

Valine *Plasma* *Decrease* Branched chain amino acids are generally reduced *3192*

572.20 Hepatic Encephalopathy (continued)

Vitamin B_{12} *Serum Increase* May increase to 30 - 40 times the normal level. The increase is mainly in the free form *1290*

572.30 Portal Hypertension

Laminin *Serum Increase* Increased concentration was useful in assessing extent of hepatic fibrosis *5276*

572.40 Gallstones

Alkaline Phosphatase *Serum Increase* Since enzyme is produced by the biliary tract at all levels from the canaliculi to to the mucosa of the gallbladder and the large bile ducts, enzyme, activity may increase with diseases that cause impedance of bile flow such as biliary calculi impacted in the common bile duct *4617*

Amylase *Serum Increase* In 15 cases of acute pancreatitis with gallstones median serum amylase activity of 870 U/L was higher than 194 U/L in 41 cases without gallstones *2689*

CA 19-9 *Serum Increase* Concentrations may be increased markedly with obstruction of bilary tract by gallstones *1778*

Cholesterol *Serum No Effect* In 30 hypertensive men with gallstone disease mean concentration of 5.6 mmol/L not significantly different from 5.8 mmol/L in 231 hypertensive men without gallstone disease and 5.1 mmol/L in 17 normotensive men with gallstone disease not significantly different from 5.8 mmol/L in 242 normotensive controls *3787*

Glucose *Serum Increase* In 30 hypertensive men with gallstone disease mean concentration of 5.9 mmol/L significantly different from 5.0 mmol/L in 231 hypertensive men without gallstone disease *3787*
Serum No Effect In 17 normotensive men with gallstone disease mean concentration of 5.0 mmol/L not significantly different from 4.5 mmol/L in 242 normotensive men without gallstone disease *3787*

HDL-Cholesterol *Serum No Effect* In 30 hypertensive men with gallstone disease mean concentration of 1.1 mmol/L not significantly different from 1.2 mmol/L in 231 hypertensive men without gallstone disease and 1.1 mmol/L in 17 normotensive men with gallstone disease not significantly different from 1.2 mmol/L in 242 normotensive controls *3787*

Insulin *Plasma Increase* In 30 hypertensive men with gallstone disease mean concentration of 24.3 mU/L significantly different from 17.1 mU/L in 231 hypertensive men without gallstone disease *3787*
Plasma No Effect In 17 normotensive men with gallstone disease mean concentration of 12.3 mU/L not significantly different from 13.3 mU/L in 242 normotensive men without gallstone disease *3787*

LDL-Cholesterol *Serum No Effect* In 30 hypertensive men with gallstone disease mean concentration of 3.4 mmol/L not significantly different from 3.6 mmol/L in 231 hypertensive men without gallstone disease and 3.2 mmol/L in 17 normotensive men with gallstone disease not significantly different from 3.8 mmol/L in 242 normotensive controls *3787*

Lipase *Serum Increase* In 15 cases of acute pancreatitis with gallstones median serum lipase activity of 10,082 U/L was higher than 1,218 U/L in 41 cases without gallstones *2689*

Triglycerides *Serum No Effect* In 30 hypertensive men with gallstone disease mean concentration of 2.4 mmol/L not significantly different from 1.9 mmol/L in 231 hypertensive men without gallstone disease and 1.6 mmol/L in 17 normotensive men with gallstone disease not significantly different from 1.6 mmol/L in 242 normotensive controls *3787*

572.40 Hepatic Failure

Alanine Aminotransferase *Serum Increase* May be increased or normal *1025* Observed effect *3141*

Alkaline Phosphatase *Serum Increase* May be normal or increased *1025*

Ammonia *Blood Increase* Characteristic of liver failure *4707*

Aspartate Aminotransferase *Serum Increase* May be normal or increased *1025* Mean activity of 1,640 U/L (range 48 - 8,490 U/L) in 46 patients with fulminant hepatic failure compared with 10 - 40 U/L in normal controls *2281*

Bicarbonate *Serum Increase* Persistent alkalosis in patients with hepatic failure *4016*

Biliprotein *Serum Increase* In 43 patients with fulminant hepatic failure on admission mean concentration of 13.2 mg/L (range of 6.3 - 100.7 mg/L) significantly increased compared to mean of 1.3 mg/L (range of 0 - 4.1 mg/L) in 7 healthy controls *2281*

Bilirubin *Serum Increase* Mean concentration in 46 patients with fulminant hepatic failure of 143 µmol/L (range 21 - 639 µmol/L) compared with 0 - 17 U/L in healthy controls *2281* May be increased or normal *1025*

Carbon Dioxide Partial Pressure *Blood Decrease* Characteristic of liver failure *4707*

Cholesterol *Serum Decrease* When the serum cholesterol decreases in a patient with a high serum cholesterol associated with liver disease, this may be indicative of hepatic failure *4617*

Creatinine *Serum Increase* Mean concentration in 46 patients with fulminant hepatic failure of 390 µmol/L (56 - 984 µmol/L) compared with normal range of 45 - 105 µmol/L *2281* High values (> 1.6 mg/dL) in 22 of 50 cases of hepatic failure due to decompensated cirrhosis or attacks of acute viral hepatitis *793*

Erythrocytes *Urine Increase* WBC, RBC, and hyaline casts were found in 26% of patients with hepatic failure due to decompensated cirrhosis or attacks of acute viral hepatitis *793*

Factor II *Plasma Decrease* Low levels of clotting factors found in fulminant hepatic failure are due to decrease in liver synthesis aggravated by increased consumption *1680*

Factor V *Plasma Decrease* Low levels of clotting factors found in fulminant hepatic failure are due to decrease in liver synthesis aggravated by increased consumption *1680*

Factor VII *Plasma Decrease* All 7 patients with values 8% of normal failed to regain consciousness from hepatic coma due to fulminant hepatic failure *1680*

α-Fetoprotein *Serum Increase* Concentrations above 500 µg/L are virtually diagnostic of HCC *1778* In fulminant hepatic failure, 15 of the 64 patients (23%) had raised levels but in only 2 did they exceed 50 ng/mL. Of the 23 survivors, 11 (48%) had elevated levels. This rise was found early after the development of a grade IV coma and constitutes an encouraging prognostic sign at a time when the liver function tests and EEG are unhelpful *3680* Reported effect *1025* Mean concentration of 28 ng/mL (range 1.4 - 403 ng/mL) in 46 patients with fulminant hepatic failure compared with normal range of 0 - 15 ng/mL *2281*

Fibrinogen *Plasma Decrease* Low levels of clotting factors found in fulminant hepatic failure are due to decrease in liver synthesis aggravated by increased consumption *1680*

Glomerular Filtration Rate *Urine Decrease* Reduced GFR was highly significant in 6 and mild-moderate in 14 of 50 cases of hepatic failure due to decompensated cirrhosis of liver *793* GFR varied from 1 - 24 mL/min in 25 of 43 hepatic failure patients. Only one of these survived *5673*

Glucose *Serum Decrease* Replacement or destruction of functioning hepatic tissue may evoke hypoglycemia *4707* The incidence is low *1025*

Glucose Tolerance *Serum Decrease* There is a rapid rise of the blood sugar to abnormal levels and a slow return to normal *1025*

β-Glucuronidase *Serum Decrease* Decreased *1777 1498*

Haptoglobin *Serum Decrease* Reported effect *1025*

HDL-Cholesterol *Serum Increase* Increased *3327 5707 325*

Hepatocyte Growth Factor *Serum Increase* In 23 patients with fulminant hepatic failure mean concentration of 8.06 ng/mL compared with mean concentration in 10 normal individuals of 0.25 ± 0.06 ng/mL *3714* Mean concentration in 34 patients with acetaminophen-induced hepatic failure of 7.4 ng/mL (range of of 0.45 - 48.4 ng/mL) and in 9 patients with fulminant hepatic failure from other causes of 3.8 ng/mL (range of 1.72 - 25.1 ng/mL) compared with mean of 0.24 ng/mL (range of 0 - 0.5 ng/mL) in 30 normal individuals *2281*

Hyaline Casts *Urine* *Increase* WBC, RBC, and hyaline casts were found in 26% of patients with hepatic failure due to decompensated cirrhosis or attacks of acute viral hepatitis *793*

Insulin-like Growth Factor-I *Serum* *Decrease* Observed effect *2166*

Lactate Dehydrogenase *Serum* *Increase* May be increased or normal *1025*

Leucine *Urine* *Increase* Observed effect *1025*

Leukocytes *Urine* *Increase* WBC, RBC, and hyaline casts were found in 26% of patients with hepatic failure due to decompensated cirrhosis or attacks of acute viral hepatitis *793*

Magnesium *Serum* *Decrease* Hypomagnesemia is common in hepatic failure *4016*

Nickel *Serum* *Decrease* Thought to be caused by hypoalbuminemia *3428*

pH *Blood* *Increase* Persistent alkalosis in patients with hepatic failure *4016*

Phosphate *Serum* *Decrease* Hypophosphatemia may occur in hepatic failure as a result of intravenous carbohydrate feeding, gram-negative septicemia, endotoxemia, and large dose steroid treatment *4016*

Platelets *Blood* *Decrease* As a result of hypersplenism *1025*

Prothrombin Time *Plasma* *Increase* Mean time in 46 individuals with fulminant hepatic failure 65 s (range 14 - 240 s) compared with normal range of 12 - 15 s *2281*

Sodium *Serum* *Decrease* Hyponatremia (< 130 mmol/L) occurred in 61% of patients with hepatic failure due to decompensated cirrhosis of liver *793* In hepatic failure patients, sodium loss in urine may be high if the GFR falls below 24 mL/min *5673* Frequently depressed in hepatic failure. Severe hyponatremic states are found in end-stage hepatic cirrhosis with uniformly poor prognosis *4016*
Serum *Increase* Marked sodium retention (9 mmol/24 h) may occur in fulminant hepatic failure when GFR exceeds 40 mL/min *5673*
Urine *Decrease* Hyponatremia (< 130 mmol/L) occurred in 61% of patients with hepatic failure due to decompensated cirrhosis of liver *793* Marked sodium retention (9 mmol/24 h) may occur in fulminant hepatic failure when GFR exceeds 40 mL/min *5673*
Urine *Increase* In hepatic failure patients, sodium loss in urine may be high if the GFR falls below 24 mL/min *5673*

Urea Nitrogen *Serum* *Decrease* Only if hepatic tissue is severely damaged *4707*
Serum *Increase* Blood levels of urea were raised in 20 cases (40%) of which in 9 cases it was > 60 mg/dL in patients with hepatic failure arising from decompensated cirrhosis or attacks of acute viral hepatitis *793*

572.80 Hepatic Granuloma

Alkaline Phosphatase *Serum* *Increase* Increased activity in the absence of other abnormal liver function tests is suggestive of hepatic infiltration by tumor, granuloma or fat *4617*

573.30 Ischemic Hepatitis

Alanine Aminotransferase *Serum* *Increase* Markedly increased activity observed in ischemic hepatitis with poor hepatic perfusion leading to centrizonal hepatocyte necrosis *3625*

Alanine Aminotransferase:Lactate Dehydrogenase Ratio *Serum* *Increase* Ratio of less than 1.5 has been used to differentiate ischemic hepatitis from acute viral hepatitis *3625*

Alkaline Phosphatase *Serum* *Increase* Mildly increased activity, rarely higher than 2 times normal, observed in ischemic hepatitis with poor hepatic perfusion leading to centrizonal hepatocyte necrosis *3625*

Aspartate Aminotransferase *Serum* *Increase* Markedly increased activity observed in ischemic hepatitis with poor hepatic perfusion leading to centrizonal hepatocyte necrosis *3625*

Bilirubin *Serum* *Increase* Mildly increased concentration, rarely higher than 4 times normal, observed in ischemic hepatitis with poor hepatic perfusion leading to centrizonal hepatocyte necrosis *3625*

Lactate Dehydrogenase *Serum* *Increase* Markedly increased activity observed in ischemic hepatitis with poor hepatic perfusion leading to centrizonal hepatocyte necrosis *3625*

Prothrombin Time *Plasma* *Increase* Time may or may not be prolonged in ischemic hepatitis with poor hepatic perfusion leading to centrizonal hepatocyte necrosis *3625*
Plasma *No Effect* Time may or may not be prolonged in ischemic hepatitis with poor hepatic perfusion leading to centrizonal hepatocyte necrosis *3625*

573.30 Toxic Hepatitis

α_1-Acid Glycoprotein *Serum* *Increase* Sensitivity of 65% and a specificity of 80% with severe liver disease *1439*

Alanine Aminotransferase *Serum* *Increase* Levels depend upon severity. In severe toxic hepatitis, serum enzymes may be 10 - 20 times higher than in acute hepatitis and show a different pattern, i.e., increase in LD > AST > ALT (acute icteric period) *5544* Observed effect *3141* Rises precipitously *900* Elevations in toxic hepatitis due to carbon tetrachloride occur within 24 h and may reach peaks of up to 27,000 U/L. Other toxins (chlorpromazine salicylates, azaserine and pyrazinamide) will cause smaller elevations *5737*

Aldolase *Serum* *Increase* Due to carbon tetrachloride and other poisons *1290*

Alkaline Phosphatase *Serum* *Increase* Elevated to > 3 times normal *900* Found in 6 patients with toxic drug hepatitis with values of 134 ± 19.8 U/L *2803* Striking increase *4707* Drugs particularly likely to produce this type of jaundice are chlorpromazine or organic arsenicals. Alkaline phosphatase values are at least as high as in posthepatic jaundice *1025*

Amylase *Serum* *Decrease* Severe liver damage *5544*

Anti-Mitochondrial Antibodies *Serum* *Increase* Especially in drug-induced hepatitis due to halothane or chlorpromazine *4160*

Antithrombin III *Plasma* *Increase* Elevated in the acute hepatitis following renal transplantation *3472* *5220*

α_1-Antitrypsin *Serum* *Increase* Increased *4371* *4763* *4241* *4373* *83*

Aspartate Aminotransferase *Serum* *Increase* Concentration depend upon severity. In severe cases, (especially carbon tetrachloride poisoning), serum enzymes may be 10 - 20 times higher than in acute hepatitis and show a different pattern (i.e., increase in LD > AST > ALT) *5544* Elevations of ALT reflects acute hepatic disease somewhat more specifically than is true of AST *1025* Elevations in toxic hepatitis due to carbon tetrachloride exposure occur within 24 h and may reach peaks of up to 13,000 U/L. Other toxins (chlorpromazine, salicylates, azaserine, and pyrazinamide) will cause smaller increases *4746* Usual values of 240 - 1,900 U/L. Values > 145 U/L are usual and > 240 U/L are frequent *1025*

Bilirubin, Direct *Serum* *Increase* Increased early *5544*

Bilirubin, Indirect *Serum* *Increase* Increased predominantly *5544*

Cholesterol *Serum* *Decrease* Normal or mildly depressed in hepatitis; but markedly depressed in severe hepatitis *1025* Liver damage due to cinchophen, chloroform, carbon tetrachloride, or phosphate *1290*

α-Fetoprotein *Serum* *No Effect* Curiously absent *4891*

Glucose *Serum* *Decrease* Can occur with various types of liver disease. Hepatic hypoglycemia is a fasting hypoglycemia and often only transiently relieved by food *1980* Due to organic arsenic, carbon tetrachloride, chloroform, cinchophen, phosphate, alcohol, acute paracetamol poisoning *1290*

Glucose-6-Phosphatase *Serum* *Increase* After liver damage with carbon tetrachloride the serum level reaches its peak values by 6 h *1290*

β-Glucuronidase *Serum* *Increase* Increased with extensive cell necrosis *1777* *1498*

γ-Glutamyltransferase *Serum* *Increase* Raised enzyme activity may be the only evidence of moderate liver damage due to drugs *1290*

Hyaluronic Acid *Serum* *No Effect* The median level in patients with drug induced liver reaction (33 μg/L) did not differ significantly from the corresponding value in the control group (36 μg/L) *1371*

573.30 Toxic Hepatitis *(continued)*

Isocitrate Dehydrogenase *Serum Increase* Hepatitis of liver poisons, normal in 2 - 3 weeks *5544*

Lactate Dehydrogenase *Serum Increase* LD 4 and 5 due to chemical poisoning *1642*

Lactate Dehydrogenase Isoenzyme-5 *Serum Increase* Due to chemical poisoning *5544*

Lactate Dehydrogenase Isoenzymes *Serum Increase* LD_4, LD_5 due to chemical poisoning *1642*

α_2-Macroglobulin *Serum Increase* Reported effect *3480*

β_2-Macroglobulin *Serum Increase* An increased serum concentration is characteristic *2586*

Manganese *Serum Increase* During acute phase increase up to four times that seen in normal subjects *5460*

Nickel *Serum Decrease* Thought to be caused by hypoalbuminemia *3428*

5'-Nucleotidase *Serum Increase* Six cases of toxic drug hepatitis showed activities ranging from 91.3 - 155.7 U/L (normal 2 - 11 U/L) *2803*

Protein *Serum Decrease* Enteric loss of plasma protein *4891*

Prothrombin Time *Plasma Increase* Prolongation of the prothrombin time usually indicates that the disease is a chronic one, such as advanced cirrhosis: if it increases in acute liver disease it usually indicates the disease is a fulminant one, as after ingestion of a toxic dose of chemicals, e.g., acetaminophen *4617* Increased in cases of severe liver damage due to poisons *5544*

Thyroxine Binding Globulin *Serum Increase* Increased levels *4289*

Urea Nitrogen *Serum Decrease* With severe damage due to hepatotoxic agents *4707*

Urobilinogen *Urine Increase* Normal or increased during preicteric phase *5544*
Urine No Effect Typical observation *5544*

VLDL-Cholesterol *Serum Increase* Marked elevation *126*

573.80 Hepatocellular Jaundice

CA 19-9 *Serum Increase* CA 19-9 concentration increased in some patients with hepatocellular jaundice *1253*

Cholesterol *Serum Decrease* Concentration of LCAT in the liver may be decreased in patients with acute hepatocellular disease which may lead to a decrease in the amount of circulating cholesterol *4617*

Cholesterol, Nonesterified *Serum Decrease* Concentration of LCAT in the liver may be decreased in patients with acute hepatocellular disease which may lead to a decrease in the amount of circulating cholesterol, but this is esterified and an increase in nonesterified cholesterol *4617*

573.90 Benign Liver Disease

CA 19-9 *Serum Increase* In 27 patients with benign liver disease 15% had a serum concentration greater than 37 U/mL *1957*

CA 242 *Serum Increase* In 27 patients with benign liver disease, 7% had a serum concentration greater than 20 U/mL *1957*

CA 549 *Serum Increase* In 27 patients with benign liver disease, 7 had a concentration of 11 U/mL, 6 with a concentration of 12 U/mL and 5 with a concentration of 13 U/mL with an upper limit of normal of 11 U/mL *5260*
Serum No Effect In 75 patients with benign disease of the liver none had a concentration greater than 30.0 kU/L with BRESMARQ assay *764*

Enzyme Inhibitory Antibody to Pyruvate Dehydrogenase *Serum Increase* 1% positive cases observed in patients with other liver diseases *2470*

Ferritin *Serum Increase* In 46 male patients with benign liver disease mean concentration of 735 ± 876 ng/mL significantly different from 165 ± 17 ng/mL in 35 healthy men, and 494 ± 657 ng/mL in 15 women with bengn liver disease significantly greater than 55 ± 37 ng/mL in 35 healthy women *3121*

SP2 *Serum No Effect* 12 of 27 patients with benign liver disease had a concentration of 14 U/mL and 11 had a concentration of 15 U/mL when the upper limit of normal was 14 U/mL *5260*

573.90 Hepatobiliary Disease

CA 19-9 *Serum Increase* In 11.7% of 60 patients with hepatobiliary disease concentration increased above cut-off of 37 U/mL *2854*

Carcinoembryonic Antigen *Serum Increase* In 11.7% of 60 patients with hepatobiliary disease concentration increased above cut-off of 37 U/mL *2854*

EL-1 *Serum Increase* In 11.7% of 60 patients with hepatobiliary disease concentration increased above cut-off of 37 U/mL *2854*

Leucine Aminopeptidase *Serum Increase* Although activity is found in many tissues, including pancreas, brain, heart, intestine and blood vessels, activity in serum only increases in in patients with hepatobiliary disease *4617*

Scan1 *Serum Increase* In 26.7% of 60 patients with hepatobiliary disease concentration increased above cut-off of 37 U/mL *2854*

573.90 Liver Disease

Acid-soluble Carnitine, Total *Serum No Effect* In 22 patients with non-cirrhotic liver disease mean concentration of 34.4 ± 21.7 µmol/L not significantly different from 28.0 ± 16.7 µmol/L in 28 healthy volunteer controls *2810*

Acylcarnitine, Short Chain *Serum No Effect* In 22 patients with non-cirrhotic liver disease mean concentration of 12.2 ± 5.3 µmol/L not significantly different from 12.7 ± 6.8 µmol/L in 28 healthy volunteer controls *2810*

Alkaline Phosphatase, Bone Isoenzyme *Serum Increase* In patients with chronic liver disease slight increase observed *4217*

Alpidem *Serum Decrease* Because of decreased synthesis of albumin and α_1-acid glycoprotein and possibly due to dilutional effect of peripheral edema and ascites the bound fraction of the drug may be decreased with an increase in the free fraction. Effect on bound fraction only is listed here *5869*

Amylobarbital *Serum Decrease* Because of decreased synthesis of albumin and α_1-acid glycoprotein and possibly due to dilutional effect of peripheral edema and ascites the bound fraction of the drug may be decreased with an increase in the free fraction. Effect on bound fraction only is listed here *5869*

Carcinoembryonic Antigen *Serum Increase* In 29 patients with unspecified liver disease 58.6% had concentrations of 0.0 - 3.0 ng/mL, 17.2% had concentrations from 3.1 - 5.0 ng/mL, 17.2% had concentrations from 5.1 - 10.0 ng/mL and 6.9% had concentrations greater than 10.0 ng/mL when measured by method on Bayer Technicon Immuno 1® system compared with 95.9%, 3.5%, 0.6% and 0.0% respectively in 173 healthy non-smokers *339*

Carnitine, Free *Serum Increase* In 22 patients with non-cirrhotic liver disease mean concentration of 22.2 ± 17.0 µmol/L not significantly different from 15.3 ± 10.5 µmol/L in 28 healthy volunteer controls *2810*

Clonazepam *Serum Decrease* Because of decreased synthesis of albumin and α_1-acid glycoprotein and possibly due to dilutional effect of peripheral edema and ascites the bound fraction of the drug may be decreased with an increase in the free fraction. Effect on bound fraction only is listed here *5869*

3,3'-Di-iodothyronine *Serum Increase* In 22 patients with liver disease mean concentration of 72.6 ± 56.7 pmol/L not significantly different from that in 22 healthy age and sex-matched controls in whom the mean plasma concentration was 45.5 ± 16.3 pmol/L *4138*

Diazepam *Serum Decrease* Because of decreased synthesis of albumin and α_1-acid glycoprotein and possibly due to dilutional effect of peripheral edema and ascites the bound fraction of the drug may be decreased with an increase in the free fraction. Effect on bound fraction only is listed here *5869*

Digitoxin *Serum* *No Effect* Because of decreased synthesis of albumin and α_1-acid glycoprotein and possibly due to dilutional effect of peripheral edema and ascites the bound fraction of the drug may be decreased with an increase in the free fraction. Effect on bound fraction only is listed here *5869*

Disopyramide *Serum* *Decrease* Because of decreased synthesis of albumin and α_1-acid glycoprotein and possibly due to dilutional effect of peripheral edema and ascites the bound fraction of the drug may be decreased with an increase in the free fraction. Effect on bound fraction only is listed here *5869*

Erythromycin *Serum* *Decrease* Because of decreased synthesis of albumin and α_1-acid glycoprotein and possibly due to dilutional effect of peripheral edema and ascites the bound fraction of the drug may be decreased with an increase in the free fraction. Effect on bound fraction only is listed here *5869*

Etomidate *Serum* *Decrease* Because of decreased synthesis of albumin and α_1-acid glycoprotein and possibly due to dilutional effect of peripheral edema and ascites the bound fraction of the drug may be decreased with an increase in the free fraction. Effect on bound fraction only is listed here *5869*

Ferritin *Serum* *Increase* Ferritin is an acute phase reactant and inflammation increases serum ferritin concentration 3- to 5-fold *4784*

α-Fetoprotein mRNA *Serum* *Increase* In rare cases AFP mRNA detectable in peripheral blood from patients with nonmalignant liver disease, especially after liver surgery *5285*

Furosemide *Serum* *Decrease* Because of decreased synthesis of albumin and α_1-acid glycoprotein and possibly due to dilutional effect of peripheral edema and ascites the bound fraction of the drug may be decreased with an increase in the free fraction. Effect on bound fraction only is listed here. Bound fraction may be decreased or unchanged *5869*

Serum *No Effect* Because of decreased synthesis of albumin and α_1-acid glycoprotein and possibly due to dilutional effect of peripheral edema and ascites the bound fraction of the drug may be decreased with an increase in the free fraction. Effect on bound fraction only is listed here. Bound fraction may be decreased or unchanged *5869*

β-Hexosaminidase *Serum* *Increase* Activity increased in patients with liver disorders *2291*

β-Hexosaminidase Isoenzyme P *Serum* *Increase* Activity substantially increased in patients with liver disorders *2291*

Interleukin-6 *Serum* *Increase* Mean concentration not detected in 22.2% of 9 patients with liver disease with or without disseminated intravascular coagulation compared with undetectable amounts in patients with hematologic malignancies or obstetric disorders *3890*

Kallistatin *Plasma* *Decrease* Mean concentration in 9 patients with liver disease of 7.2 ± 2.5 µg/mL significantly less compared with 21.2 ± 3.5 µg/mL in 30 healthy controls *781*

Lidocaine *Serum* *No Effect* Because of decreased synthesis of albumin and α_1-acid glycoprotein and possibly due to dilutional effect of peripheral edema and ascites the bound fraction of the drug may be decreased with an increase in the free fraction. Effect on bound fraction only is listed here *5869*

MCV *Blood* *Increase* In 100 patients with macrocytosis (MCV greater than 110 fL) 2 had liver disease *4924*

Naproxen *Serum* *Decrease* Because of decreased synthesis of albumin and α_1-acid glycoprotein and possibly due to dilutional effect of peripheral edema and ascites the bound fraction of the drug may be decreased with an increase in the free fraction. Effect on bound fraction only is listed here *5869*

Osteocalcin *Serum* *Increase* In patients with chronic liver disease slight increase observed *4217*

Oxprenolol *Serum* *Decrease* Because of decreased synthesis of albumin and α_1-acid glycoprotein and possibly due to dilutional effect of peripheral edema and ascites the bound fraction of the drug may be decreased with an increase in the free fraction. Effect on bound fraction only is listed here *5869*

Penbutolol *Serum* *Decrease* Because of decreased synthesis of albumin and α_1-acid glycoprotein and possibly due to dilutional effect of peripheral edema and ascites the bound fraction of the drug may be decreased with an increase in the free fraction. Effect on bound fraction only is listed here *5869*

Phenylbutazone *Serum* *Decrease* Because of decreased synthesis of albumin and α_1-acid glycoprotein and possibly due to dilutional effect of peripheral edema and ascites the bound fraction of the drug may be decreased with an increase in the free fraction. Effect on bound fraction only is listed here *5869*

Phenytoin *Serum* *Decrease* Because of decreased synthesis of albumin and α_1-acid glycoprotein and possibly due to dilutional effect of peripheral edema and ascites the bound fraction of the drug may be decreased with an increase in the free fraction. Effect on bound fraction only is listed here *5869*

Plasminogen Activator Inhibitor-1 *Plasma* *No Effect* In 31 of 186 consecutive patients undergoing bone marrow transplantation who developed hyperbilirubinemia mean concentration of 45 ± 33 ng/mL in 17 patients with hepatic injury compared with reference interval of 4 - 43 ng/mL *4529*

Propranolol *Serum* *Decrease* Because of decreased synthesis of albumin and α_1-acid glycoprotein and possibly due to dilutional effect of peripheral edema and ascites the bound fraction of the drug may be decreased with an increase in the free fraction. Effect on bound fraction only is listed here *5869*

Quinidine *Serum* *Decrease* Because of decreased synthesis of albumin and α_1-acid glycoprotein and possibly due to dilutional effect of peripheral edema and ascites the bound fraction of the drug may be decreased with an increase in the free fraction. Effect on bound fraction only is listed here *5869*

Salicylate *Serum* *Decrease* Because of decreased synthesis of albumin and α_1-acid glycoprotein and possibly due to dilutional effect of peripheral edema and ascites the bound fraction of the drug may be decreased with an increase in the free fraction. Effect on bound fraction only is listed here *5869*

Soluble E-Selectin *Serum* *No Effect* Mean concentration in 4 patients with liver disease and disseminated intravascular coagulation of 53.3 ± 18.3 ng/mL not significantly different from about 48 ng/mL in 5 patients without DIC *3890*

Sulfadiazine *Serum* *Decrease* Because of decreased synthesis of albumin and α_1-acid glycoprotein and possibly due to dilutional effect of peripheral edema and ascites the bound fraction of the drug may be decreased with an increase in the free fraction. Effect on bound fraction only is listed here *5869*

Sulfisoxazole *Serum* *Decrease* Because of decreased synthesis of albumin and α_1-acid glycoprotein and possibly due to dilutional effect of peripheral edema and ascites the bound fraction of the drug may be decreased with an increase in the free fraction. Effect on bound fraction only is listed here *5869*

Thiopental *Serum* *Decrease* Because of decreased synthesis of albumin and α_1-acid glycoprotein and possibly due to dilutional effect of peripheral edema and ascites the bound fraction of the drug may be decreased with an increase in the free fraction. Effect on bound fraction only is listed here *5869*

Tianeptine *Serum* *Decrease* Because of decreased synthesis of albumin and α_1-acid glycoprotein and possibly due to dilutional effect of peripheral edema and ascites the bound fraction of the drug may be decreased with an increase in the free fraction. Effect on bound fraction only is listed here *5869*

Tolbutamide *Serum* *Decrease* Because of decreased synthesis of albumin and α_1-acid glycoprotein and possibly due to dilutional effect of peripheral edema and ascites the bound fraction of the drug may be decreased with an increase in the free fraction. Effect on bound fraction only is listed here *5869*

Tolfenamic Acid *Serum* *Decrease* Because of decreased synthesis of albumin and α_1-acid glycoprotein and possibly due to dilutional effect of peripheral edema and ascites the bound fraction of the drug may be decreased with an increase in the free fraction. Effect on bound fraction only is listed here *5869*

Transglutaminase *Serum* *Decrease* In 12 patients with liver disease mean plasma concentration of 14.0 ± 5.1 pmol/100 µL/h significantly different from 19.7 ± 4.6 pmol/100 µL/h in 19 control patients without liver disease *1599*

Tumor Necrosis Factor-α *Serum* *No Effect* Mean concentration not detected in 9 patients with liver disease with or without disseminated intravascular coagulation compared with undetectable amounts in patients with hematologic malignancies or obstetric disorders *3890*

Valproic Acid *Serum* *Decrease* Because of decreased synthesis of albumin and α_1-acid glycoprotein and possibly due to dilutional effect of peripheral edema and ascites the bound fraction of the drug may be decreased with an increase in the free fraction. Effect on bound fraction only is listed here *5869*

573.90 Liver Disease *(continued)*

Verapamil *Serum* *Decrease* Because of decreased synthesis of albumin and α_1-acid glycoprotein and possibly due to dilutional effect of peripheral edema and ascites the bound fraction of the drug may be decreased with an increase in the free fraction. Effect on bound fraction only is listed here *5869*

573.90 Multifactorial Liver Disease

Neopterin *Serum* *Increase* In 28 patients with multifactorial liver disease mean concentration of 22.1 ± 7.8 nmol/L, with mean in 6 without cirrhosis of 8.8 ± 1.4 nmol/L and 25.1 ± 9.4 nmol/L in 22 with cirrhosis different from 6.0 ± 2.2 nmol/L in healthy controls *5682*

573.90 Non-malignant Disease of the Liver

5-Nucleotide Phosphodiesterase Isoenzyme V *Serum* *Increase* Mean activity was increased in the plasma of 59% of 161 patients with non-malignant disease of the liver, pancreas or biliary system *1781*

574.20 Cholelithiasis

Alanine Aminotransferase *Serum* *No Effect* In neither men nor women with gallstones were significant differences from controls observed *78*

Albumin *Serum* *Increase* Concentration significantly increased in women with gallstones compared with healthy controls but no such difference observed in men *78*

Alkaline Phosphatase *Serum* *Increase* In both men and women with gallstones activity significantly higher than in age and sex matched healthy controls *78*

Bilirubin *Serum* *Decrease* In women with gallstones concentration significantly reduced compared with control women but no such difference observed in men *78*

Carcinoembryonic Antigen *Bile* *Increase* Mean concentration in 5 patients with intrahepatic calculi of 57.4 ng/mL *3729* *Serum* *Increase* In 51 patients with cholelithiasis, 82% had concentrations less than 2.5 ng/mL, 17% had concentrations between 2.6 and 5.0 ng/mL, 1% had concentrations between 5.1 and 10.0 ng/mL and 0% had concentrations greater than 10.0 ng/mL *2010*

Cholesterol *Serum* *Decrease* Concentration significantly reduced in women with gallstones compared with controls but no such difference observed in men *78*

Glucose *Serum* *Increase* In both men and women patients with gallstones had significantly higher concentrations than in control individuals *78*

Protein *Serum* *Increase* Concentration significantly higher in women with gallstones than in control women but no such difference observed in men *78*

Triglycerides *Serum* *No Effect* In neither men nor women with gallstones were differences from normal observed *78*

Vitamin E *Serum* *Decrease* In 40 patients with gall stones and cholelithiasis with jaundice mean concentration of 8.5 ± 0.4 µg/mL and in 24 without jaundice 9.6 ± 0.6 µg/mL compared with 12.2 ± 0.5 µg/L in age matched controls *5296*

574.20 Cholestasis

Albumin *Serum* *Decrease* In 9 patients with intrahepatic cholestasis mean concentration of 36 g/L compared with normal values of 35 - 50 g/L *5347*

Alkaline Phosphatase *Serum* *Increase* In 9 patients with intrahepatic cholestasis mean activity of 1,011 U/L compared with normal values of 100 - 300 U/L *5347*

Aspartate Aminotransferase *Serum* *Increase* Median activity in 9 patients with intrahepatic cholestasis of 51 U/L significantly different from reference range of 5 - 28 U/L *5347*

Bilirubin *Serum* *Increase* Median concentration in 9 patients with intrahepatic cholestasis of 74 µmol/L significantly different from reference range of 5 - 21 µmol/L *5347*

Cholesterol *Serum* *Increase* Concentration may be increased in patients with prolonged cholestasis caused by a marked increase in serum cholesterol concentration *4617*

Cholinesterase *Serum* *Decrease* In 9 patients with intrahepatic cholestasis mean activity of 0.53 U/L compared with normal values of 0.6 - 1.2 U/L *5347*

Creatinine *Serum* *No Effect* In 9 patients with intrahepatic cholestasis mean concentration of 53 µmol/L compared with normal values of 26 - 80 µmol/L *5347*

Creatinine Clearance *Urine* *No Effect* In 9 patients with intrahepatic cholestasis mean clearance of 108 mL/min compared with normal values of 90 - 170 mL/min *5347*

Fractional Excretion of Sodium *Urine* *No Effect* In 9 patients with intrahepatic cholestasis mean fractional excretion of 0.81% compared with normal values of 0.5 - 1.0% *5347*

β-Globulin *Serum* *Increase* Concentration may be increased in patients with prolonged cholestasis caused by a marked increase in serum cholesterol concentration *4617*

Lecithin *Serum* *Increase* Concentration may be increased in patients with prolonged cholestasis caused by a marked increase in serum cholesterol concentration as a result of hyperlecithinemia *4617*

Leukotriene E_4 *Urine* *Increase* In 25 patients with extrahepatic cholestasis median excretion of 1078 pmol/L (range 853 - 1663 pmol/L) or 74 nmol/mol creatinine (range 52 - 93 nmol/mol creatinine) significantly greater than medians of 182 pmol/L and 14 nmol/mol creatinine in 25 age and sex matched controls *3386* In 9 patients with intrahepatic cholestasis median concentration of 1.03 nmol/L or 221 nmol/mol creatinine higher than median excretion of 0.52 nmol/L (range of 0.34 - 0.70 nmol/L) or 40 nmol/mol creatinine (range of 29 - 52 nmol/mol creatinine) in 10 healthy individuals *5347*

Lipoprotein X *Serum* *Increase* Presence of protein is specific for cholestasis but is not for a specific disease *4617*

N-Acetyl-Leukotriene E_4 *Urine* *Increase* In 9 patients with intrahepatic cholestasis median concentration of 0.25 nmol/L or 61 nmol/mol creatinine higher than median excretion of 0.14 nmol/L (range of 0.08 - 0.23 nmol/L) or 13 nmol/mol creatinine (range of 7 - 20 nmol/mol creatinine) in 10 healthy individuals *5347*

5'-Nucleotidase *Serum* *Increase* In 13 patients with extrahepatic cholestasis mean activity of 43 U/L (range 9 - 217 U/L) compared with mean of 3.8 U/L in healthy controls. Isoform % NTP1 50%, NTP2 15% and NTP3 35% compared with 12%, 30% and 58% respectively in healthy individuals *3993*

Prothrombin Time *Plasma* *No Effect* In 9 patients with intrahepatic cholestasis mean time of 86% compared with normal values of 70 - 100% *5347*

Volume *Urine* *No Effect* Median excretion in 9 patients with intrahepatic cholestasis of 278 mL/4 h not different from median of 222 mL/4 h in 10 healthy controls *5347*

574.20 Intrahepatic Cholestasis of Pregnancy

Alanine Aminotransferase *Serum* *Increase* Activity may vary from normal to values found in viral hepatitis *1778* *Serum* *No Effect* Activity may vary from normal to values found in viral hepatitis *1778*

Alkaline Phosphatase *Serum* *Increase* Activity may be increased up to 4 - 10 times the upper limit of the reference interval, with the hepatic isoenzyme predominating *1778*

Alkaline Phosphatase, Liver Isoenzyme *Serum* *Increase* Activity may be increased up to 4 - 10 times the upper limit of the reference interval, with the hepatic isoenzyme predominating *1778*

Aspartate Aminotransferase *Serum* *Increase* Activity may vary from normal to values found in viral hepatitis *1778* *Serum* *No Effect* Activity may vary from normal to values found in viral hepatitis *1778*

Bile Acids *Serum* *Increase* Concentration is increased 10 to 100-fold and occasionally may be the only abnormality *1778*

Bilirubin *Serum* *Increase* Concentrations may be increased up to 100 µmol/L *1778*

574.50 Cholecystolithiasis

CA 72-4 *Serum Increase* In 61 patients with cholecystolithiasis 5 (8%) had a concentration greater than cut-off of 2.5 U/mL with median concentration of 1.4 U/mL *4505*

Carcinoembryonic Antigen *Serum Increase* In 61 patients with cholecystolithiasis 13 (21%) had a concentration greater than cut-off of 3 ng/mL with median concentration of 1.9 ng/mL *4505*

575.00 Acute Cholecystitis

Alanine Aminotransferase *Serum Increase* May be mildly elevated even in the absence of intrahepatic infection or common bile duct obstruction *4891* 4 of 8 patients showed elevated levels. Mean value of 44 U/L, range of 8 - 154 U/L *3161* Occasionally increased *2034*

Alkaline Phosphatase *Serum Increase* Average elevation of 3 times the maximum normal limit in 75% of 8 cases studied *3161* May be mildly elevated even in the absence of intrahepatic infection or common bile duct obstruction *4891* Increased in some cases, even if serum bilirubin is normal *5544* In 30% of 16 patients at initial hospitalization for this disorder *1576*

Alkaline Phosphatase Isoenzymes *Serum Increase* All 11 patients with biliary tree disease, including 5 with cholecystitis and 6 with pericholangitis, showed elevated isoenzyme I. 7 of the 11 had raised isoenzyme-IV *2557*

Amylase *Serum Decrease* Decreased in some cases *1290*
Serum Increase May exceed 1,000 U/L. May or may not indicate concomitant acute pancreatitis, because elevations in this range may be seen in acute cholecystitis without any changes in the pancreas *4555 4891*

Aspartate Aminotransferase *Serum Increase* In 8 cases, 4 showed moderate elevation. The mean value for the group was 38 U/L, while the normal upper limit was 24 U/L *3161* May be mildly elevated even in the absence of intrahepatic infection or common bile duct obstruction *4891* May be increased in 75% of patients *5544* In 57% of 15 patients at initial hospitalization for this disorder *1576* Occasionally increased *2034*

Bilirubin *Serum Increase* Mild hyperbilirubinemia occasionally occurs *2039* Usually mild (< 4.0 mg/dL) *4891*
Serum No Effect Observed in some cases *5544*
Urine Increase Occasionally found *2039*

BSP Retention *Serum Increase* Increased BSP retention (some cases) even if serum bilirubin is normal *5544*

CA 19-9 *Serum Increase* Positive analyses have been encountered *2026 3657*

CA 125 *Serum Increase* Reported low incidence of positives in patients with cholecystitis *3797*

Carcinoembryonic Antigen *Serum Increase* In 39 patients with cholecystitis 77% had concentrations less than 2.5 ng/mL, 17% had concentrations between 2.6 and 5.0 ng/mL, 5% had concentrations between 5.1 and 10.0 ng/mL and 1% had concentrations greater than 10.0 ng/mL *2010* 23% of patients had values > 2.5 ng/mL *4891*

Cholesterol *Serum Decrease* Lower concentrations of total and low-density-lipoprotein (LDL) cholesterol in patients with cholecystitis than in control subjects *4808*

Erythrocyte Sedimentation Rate *Blood Increase* Increased ESR, WBC (up to 20,000 /μL) and other evidences of acute inflammatory process *5544*

γ-Globulin *Serum No Effect* Concentration usually normal *5544*

γ-Glutamyltransferase *Saliva Increase* Significantly higher (18.3 U/L) versus controls (5.12 U/L) *2448*
Serum Increase In 8 patients, the mean (210 U/L) was 7.0 times the normal upper limit *3161*

HDL-Cholesterol *Serum No Effect* There was no appreciable difference in high-density-lipoprotein (HDL) cholesterol and triglycerides between control subjects and men either with gallstones or after cholecystectomy *4808*

5-Hydroxytryptamine *Plasma No Effect* Reported effect *41*

LDL-Cholesterol *Serum Decrease* Lower concentrations of total and low-density-lipoprotein (LDL) cholesterol in patients with cholecystitis than in control subjects *4808*

Leucine Aminopeptidase *Serum Increase* 7 patients had raised concentrations varying from 385 - 450 U/L, while in those with chronic disease, only 4 of 8 cases showed mild elevation *579* Moderate increase *1290*

Leukocytes *Blood Increase* During an acute attack, the count averages 12,000 - 15,000 /μL with a neutrophilic leukocytosis and an increase in band forms *4891* Increased ESR, WBC (up to 20,000 /μL) and other evidences of acute inflammatory process *5544* In 655% of 15 patients at initial hospitalization for this disorder *1576*

Lipase *Serum Increase* In some cases *5544* Activity may be increased in patients with abdominal disease such as acute cholecystitis *5231* In 25% of cases *4960*

Neutrophils *Blood Increase* Neutrophilic leukocytosis *4891* In 60% of 15 patients at initial hospitalization for this disorder *1576*

5'-Nucleotidase *Serum Increase* Slight hepatic inflammation and partial biliary obstruction *413*

Ornithine Carbamoyltransferase *Serum Increase* Liver cell damage *5544*

Triglycerides *Serum No Effect* There was no appreciable difference in high-density-lipoprotein (HDL) cholesterol and triglycerides between control subjects and men either with gallstones or after cholecystectomy *4808*

Urobilinogen *Urine Increase* Usually disappears within 24 - 48 h after the attack subsides *4891*

575.90 Benign Biliary Disease

CA 19-9 *Serum Increase* In 43 patients with benign biliary disease 28% had a serum concentration greater than 37 U/mL *1957* CA 19-9 concentration increased in some patients with biliary disease *1253*

CA 195 *Serum Increase* Mean concentration of 45.9 ± 77.4 U/mL in 21 patients with benign biliary tract disease and obstructive disease significantly higher than cutoff of 12 U/mL: 12 patients with concentrations greater than 12 U/mL *122*
Serum No Effect Mean concentration of 9.7 ± 17.2 U/mL in 61 patients with benign biliary tract disease without obstructive disease not significantly higher than cutoff of 12 U/mL: however, 11 patients had concentrations greater than 12 U/mL *122*

CA 242 *Serum Increase* In 43 patients with benign biliary disease 15% had a serum concentration greater than 20 U/mL *1957*

575.90 Gallbladder Disease

Alanine Aminotransferase *Serum Increase* In 197 patients with gallstone hepatitis mean activity 255 ± 208 U/L *2360*

Amylase *Serum Increase* In 197 patients with gallstone hepatitis mean activity of 382 ± 733 Caraway units (normal < 135) *2360*

Aspartate Aminotransferase *Serum Increase* In 197 patients with gallstone hepatitis mean activity of 319 ± 375 U/L *2360*

Bilirubin *Serum Increase* In 197 patients with gallstone hepatitis jaundice was present in 49 (24.9%): mean concentration of 3.4 ± 2.5 mg/dL *2360*

Leukocytes *Blood Increase* In 197 patients with gallstone hepatitis mean concentration of 10,700 ± 5,100 /μL *2360*

576.00 Postcholecystectomy Syndrome

Amylase *Serum Increase* If tests are performed repeatedly, immediately after attacks, some abnormalities will appear if there is an organic cause of the syndrome *2034*

Leukocytes *Blood Increase* If tests are performed repeatedly, immediately after attacks, some abnormalities will appear if there is an organic cause of the syndrome *2034*

Lipase *Serum Increase* If tests are performed repeatedly, immediately after attacks, some abnormalities will appear if there is an organic cause of the syndrome *2034*

576.10 Autoimmune Cholangiopathy

Alanine Aminotransferase *Serum Increase* In largest series of patients cholestatic features predominate with mean ALT activity of 119 U/L *3625*

Alkaline Phosphatase *Serum Increase* In largest series of patients cholestatic features predominate with mean alkaline phosphatase activity of 631 U/L *3625*

Anti-Mitochondrial Antibodies *Serum Increase* In largest series of patients there are both AMA-positive and negative patients *3625*

Aspartate Aminotransferase *Serum Increase* In largest series of patients cholestatic features predominate with mean AST activity of 104 U/L *3625*

Bilirubin *Serum Increase* In largest series of patients cholestatic features predominate with mean bilirubin concentration of 2.7 mg/dL *3625*

Cholesterol *Serum Increase* In largest series of patients cholestatic features predominate with mean cholesterol concentration of 278 mg/dL *3625*

576.10 Autoimmune Cholangitis

Enzyme Inhibitory Antibody to Pyruvate Dehydrogenase *Serum Increase* 9% positive cases observed in patients with autoimmune cholangitis *2470*

576.10 Cholangitis

Alanine Aminotransferase *Serum Increase* 77% of 13 patients showed mild elevation with a mean of 46 and range of 11 - 96 U/L *3161* With parenchymal cell necrosis and malfunction *5544*

Alkaline Phosphatase *Serum Increase* Values indicate extrahepatic obstruction *367* Elevation (mean = 255 U/L) observed in 100% of 13 cases *3161*

Alkaline Phosphatase Isoenzymes *Serum Increase* All 11 patients with biliary tree disease, including 5 with cholecystitis and 6 with pericholangitis, showed elevated isoenzyme I. 7 of the 11 had raised isoenzyme-IV *2557*

Aspartate Aminotransferase *Serum Increase* Mean elevation of 48 U/L, twice the normal upper limit, was found in 13 cases. 77% of the patients had elevated levels *3161* Usually remaining < 100 U/L, but values of 240 are found, followed by a sharp drop within 48 h *367* In 70% of 10 patients at initial hospitalization for this disorder *1576* With parenchymal cell necrosis and malfunction *5544*

Bilirubin *Serum Increase* Values are usually in the range of 2 - 4 mg/dL and are uncommonly higher than 10 mg/dL *367*

CA 19-9 *Serum Increase* CA 19-9 concentration increased to above 1,000 U/mL in some patients with acute cholangitis, returning to normal with appropriate decompression of the common duct *1253* Marked elevation *4127* Concentrations of 10,000 to 50,000 U/L have been obtained in patients with acute cholangitis secondary to gallstones *5276* The possibility of benign biliary tract disease should be considered in patients showing an extraordinarily high serum value (60,000 U/mL) *3674* Positive analyses have been encountered *3657*

CA 50 *Serum Increase* Marked elevation *4127*

CA 195 *Serum Increase* Practically all patients with acute cholangitis had marked elevations *4127*

Creatinine *Serum Increase* In 37 of 225 patients with nonmalignant acute cholangitis (16.4%) serum creatinine concentration greater than, or equal to, 1.5 mg/dL with mortality higher in population with high serum creatinine group than in normal serum creatinine group *5121*

Glucose *Serum Decrease* Often accompanies mental changes *4891*

γ-Glutamyltransferase *Serum Increase* A mean elevation of 249 U/L (8.3 times normal maximum) was found in 13 patients *3161*

Leucine Aminopeptidase *Serum Increase* In 13 patients, 77% showed elevations. Mean = 46 U/L, 2.1 times the normal value *3161*

Leukocytes *Blood Increase* Usually exceeds 20,000 /µL in suppurative cholangitis. Marked increase, up to 30,000 /µL with increase in granulocytes *5544* In 36% of 11 patients at initial hospitalization for this disorder *1576*

Neutrophils *Blood Increase* In 36% of 11 patients at initial hospitalization for this disorder *1576* Marked increase, up to 30,000 /µL with increase in granulocytes in suppurative cholangitis *5544*

5'-Nucleotidase *Serum Increase* Elevated levels indicate extrahepatic obstruction *367*

Platelets *Blood Decrease* Characteristic of the acute phase *4891*

Trypsinogen-2 *Urine Increase* Urinary dipstick gave false positive result for acute pancreatitis in 3 patients with purulent cholangitis *2633*

Urobilinogen *Urine Increase* With infection of the biliary tract. In cholangitis very high concentrations are attained *1290* With parenchymal cell necrosis and malfunction *5544*

576.10 Primary Sclerosing Cholangitis

Alanine Aminotransferase *Serum Increase* Mild to moderate increases of less than 3 times the upper reference limit observed in most patients *1778*

Albumin *Serum Decrease* In 12 patients with mean concentration of 39 ± 8 g/L different from normal range of 4 - 21 µmol/L *1371*

Alkaline Phosphatase *Serum Increase* During early, asymptomatic, period increased alkaline phosphatase activity may be the only abnormality *3625* Characteristically increased activity observed, but not increased to the same extent as in PBC *1778* In 32 children with primary sclerosing cholangitis the majority had increased activities *5684* Increased activity observed invariably *5276*

Anti-Neutrophil Cytoplasm Antibodies *Serum Increase* Present in some patients with primary sclerosing cholangitis *4923* In 30 children with primary sclerosing cholangitis 9 had positive antibodies (6 perinuclear and 3 cytoplasmic) *5684* Increased titers may occur *5276* Antibodies observed in 6 of 8 patients with primary sclerosing cholangitis *2021*

Anti-Smooth Muscle Antibodies *Serum Increase* In 31 children with primary sclerosing cholangitis 19 had positive antibodies *5684*

Antinuclear Antibodies *Serum Increase* In 30 children with primary sclerosing cholangitis 14 had positive antibodies *5684*

Aspartate Aminotransferase *Serum Increase* Mild to moderate increases of less than 3 times the upper reference limit observed in most patients *1778* In 12 patients with mean activity of 1.8 ± 1.6 µkat/L different from normal range of < 0.6 µkat/L *1371*

Bilirubin *Serum Increase* Increased concentration observed inconsistently *5276* In 12 patients with mean concentration of 26 ± 21 µmol/L different from normal range of 4 - 21 µmol/L *1371* In early stages of disease concentration typically normal, but increases gradually as disease progresses *1778* In 32 children with primary sclerosing cholangitis 12 had increased concentrations *5684*
Serum No Effect In early stages of disease concentration typically normal, but increases gradually as disease progresses *1778*

CA 19-9 *Serum Increase* Concentrations increased in patients with PSC who develop cholangiocarcinoma *1778* In 31 patients with primary sclerosing cholangitis median concentration of 50 kU/L significantly higher than upper limit of normal of 35 kU/L, with 61% of patients having abnormal values *3218*

Carcinoembryonic Antigen *Bile Increase* Mean concentration in 6 patients with primary sclerosing cholangitis of 21.6 ng/mL *3729*
Serum Increase Concentrations increased in patients with PSC who develop cholangiocarcinoma *1778* In 31 patients with primary sclerosing cholangitis median concentration of 2 µg/L not different from upper limit of normal of 14 µg/L, but 16% of patients had abnormal values *3218*

Ceruloplasmin *Serum Increase* As in other chronic cholestatic liver diseases concentration may be increased *1778* Increased concentration may occur *5276*

Cholesterol *Serum* *Increase* In 22 patients with stage I or II primary sclerosing cholangitis mean concentration of 206 ± 62 mg/dL and in 34 patients with stage III or IV disease 248 ± 79 mg/dL: 30% of patients had concentrations exceeding the 95th percentile for age and sex *2496*

Copper *Urine* *Increase* Increased excretion may occur *5276* As in other chronic cholestatic liver diseases concentration may be increased *1778*

Galactose Tolerance *Patient* *Increase* In 12 patients mean T1/2 of 25 ± 6 min different from normal range of < 17 min *1371*

γ-Globulin *Serum* *Increase* Hyper-γ-globulinemia largely attributable to polyclonal increase of IgG *1778*

γ-Glutamyltransferase *Serum* *Increase* Characteristically increased activity observed *1778* Increased activity observed invariably *5276*

HDL-Cholesterol *Serum* *Increase* In 22 patients with stage I or II primary sclerosing cholangitis mean concentration of 61 ± 19 mg/dL and in 34 patients with stage III or IV disease of 58 ± 28 mg/dL: concentration increased in 20% patients *2496*

immunoglobulin A *Serum* *Increase* Hyper-γ-globulinemia largely attributable to polyclonal increase of IgG, but modest increases of IgA and IgM may be observed *1778*

Immunoglobulin G *Serum* *Increase* Hyper-γ-globulinemia largely attributable to polyclonal increase of IgG *1778* In 31 children with primary sclerosing cholangitis the majority had increased concentrations *5684*

Immunoglobulin M *Serum* *Increase* Hyper-γ-globulinemia largely attributable to polyclonal increase of IgG, but modest increases of IgA and IgM may be observed *1778*

Metallothionein *Serum* *Increase* In patients with primary sclerosing cholangitis concentrations ranged from 1.8 to 52.2 ng/mL compared with 2.4 to 4.8 ng/mL in healthy controls *3646*

Triglycerides *Serum* *Increase* In 22 patients with stage I or II primary sclerosing cholangitis mean concentration of 94 ± 34 mg/dL and in 34 patients with stage III or IV disease 99 ± 47 mg/dL: triglyceride concentration increased in 17% of patients *2496*

Vitamin A *Serum* *Decrease* In 22 patients with stage I or II primary sclerosing cholangitis mean concentration of 437 ± 174 µg/L and in 34 patients with stage III or IV disease 407 ± 179 µg/L: vitamin A concentration decreased below normal range in 82% of patients *2496*

Vitamin D *Serum* *Decrease* In 22 patients with stage I or II primary sclerosing cholangitis mean concentration of 38 ± 17 ng/mL and in 34 patients with stage III or IV disease 28 ± 13 ng/mL: vitamin A concentration decreased below normal range in 57% of patients *2496*

576.20 Biliary Atresia

1,25-Dihydroxy Vitamin D *Serum* *Increase* In 5 patients with biliary atresia mean concentration of 51.7 ± 17.6 ng/L significantly different from that in 50 healthy individuals in whom the mean concentration was 32.2 ± 8.5 ng/L as measured by RIA method of Hollis et al *2209*

Hyaluronic Acid *Serum* *Increase* Measured serum levels at presentation and 1 year follow-up in 37 infants who presented with hepatobiliary disease in the first 6 months of life. In patients at presentation, the hyaluronic acid concentration was raised in 11 of 15 with biliary atresia. One year later, the 9 patients who developed progressive liver disease showed 2 - 6-fold increases in hyaluronic acid concentration while no increase was observed in the 28 with undetectable or mild disease *5283*

576.20 Biliary Obstruction

Aldosterone *Plasma* *Increase* Mean concentration in 43 patients with biliary tract obstruction of 156 ± 72 pg/mL significantly different from 43 ± 20 pg/mL in 14 healthy control individuals *1628*

Alkaline Phosphatase *Serum* *Increase* Since enzyme is produced by the biliary tract at all levels from the canaliculi to to the mucosa of the gallbladder and the large bile ducts, enzyme, activity may increase with diseases that cause impedance of bile flow *4617*

Amylase *Serum* *No Effect* In 11 patients with biliary obstruction median concentration of 148 U/L (range 43 - 403) not higher than 180 U/L (range 60 - 300) in 120 healthy controls *2089*

Atrial Natriuretic Peptide *Plasma* *Increase* Mean concentration in 43 patients with biliary tract obstruction of 118 ± 46 pg/mL significantly different from 40 ± 16 pg/mL in 14 healthy control individuals *1628*

Bilirubin *Serum* *Increase* Concentration may increase with diseases that cause impedance of bile flow *4617*

CA 19-9 *Serum* *Increase* In one study of patients with biliary obstruction or liver diseases other than hepatitis, cirrhosis or hepatocellular carcinoma 60% had concentrations above cutoff value of 60 U/mL *3120* In 14 patients with benign obstructive jaundice positive rate of 79% observed using cut-off from normals and 65% at 90% specificity *2594*

CA 72-4 *Serum* *Increase* In one study 60% of patients with biliary obstruction or liver diseases other than hepatocellular carcinoma, hepatitis or cirrhosis had concentrations greater than cutoff of 4.0 U/mL *3120*

CA 125 *Serum* *Increase* In one study of patients with biliary obstruction and liver diseases other than cirrhosis, hepatitis or hepatocellular carcinoma 55% had concentrations above cutoff value of 35 U/mL *3120*

CA 242 *Serum* *Increase* In 14 patients with benign obstructive jaundice positive rate of 21% observed using cut-off from normals and 21% at 90% specificity *2594*

Carcinoembryonic Antigen *Serum* *Increase* In 25% of patients with biliary obstruction or liver diseases other than hepatocellular carcinoma, cirrhosis or hepatitis serum concentrations increased above cutoff value of 5.0 ng/mL *3120*

Ferritin *Serum* *Increase* In one study of patients with biliary obstruction and liver diseases other than cirrhosis, hepatitis or hepatocellular carcinoma 64% had concentrations above cutoff value of 500 ng/mL *3120*

α-Fetoprotein *Serum* *No Effect* In one study of patients with biliary obstruction and other liver diseases none had concentrations above cutoff of 200 ng/mL *3120*

β_2-Microglobulin *Serum* *Increase* In one study of patients with biliary obstruction or liver diseases other than hepatocellular carcinoma, hepatitis or cirrhosis 77% had concentrations greater than cutoff value of 2.0 ng/mL *3120*

Renin *Plasma* *Increase* Mean concentration in 43 patients with biliary tract obstruction of 24.5 ± 32.0 pg/mL not significantly different from 9.6 ± 5.4 pg/mL in 14 healthy control individuals *1628*

Trypsin-2-α_1-Antitrypsin *Serum* *Increase* In 11 patients with biliary obstruction median concentration of 6.0 µg/L (range 3.8 - 23) higher than 4.2 µg/L (range 2.1 - 14) in 120 healthy controls *2089*

Trypsinogen-2 *Serum* *No Effect* In 11 patients with biliary obstruction median concentration of 37 µg/L (range 9.6 - 347) not higher than 39 µg/L (range 11 - 233) in 120 healthy controls *2089*

Urobilinogen *Urine* *Decrease* In patients with early complete bile duct obstruction may decrease below 1 mg/d compared with upper limit of normal of 4 mg/d *2952*

576.20 Extrahepatic Biliary Obstruction

Alanine Aminotransferase *Serum* *Increase* 10 - 100 U/L; returns to normal within 1 week after obstruction is relieved *5544* Increased activity in all cases of biliary tract obstruction. Common duct obstruction due to stones, pancreatitis, tumor, duct carcinoma, and leukemia nodes showed values of 64 - 400 U/L. Calculous biliary obstruction was associated with ALT activity of 42 - 45 U/L *5738* In obstruction due to benign or malignant disease *5008*

Albumin *Serum* *No Effect* Median concentration in 9 patients with obstructive jaundice of 34 g/L not significantly different from reference range of 35 - 50 g/L *5347*

Aldolase *Serum* *Increase* Normal or slightly increased *1980* *Serum* *No Effect* Activity typically normal or slightly increased in patients with obstructive jaundice *2952*

Alkaline Phosphatase *Serum* *Increase* Median activity in 9 patients with obstructive jaundice of 880 U/L significantly different from reference range of 100 - 300 U/L *5347* Markedly increased, related to the completeness of obstruction. Up to 376

576.20 Extrahepatic Biliary Obstruction *(continued)*

Alkaline Phosphatase *(continued)*
U/L in complete biliary obstruction *5544* Closely parallels serum bilirubin *4707* 95% - 100% incidence of elevation usually ranging from 60 - 140 U/L. Incidence of values > 105 U/L = 40% *1025* Associated with increase of 53 - 240 U/L. Common duct obstruction due to stones had values of 53 - 110 U/L *5738* May become elevated in attack in the absence of hyperbilirubinemia *900*
White Blood Cells *Increase* Parallels alkaline phosphatase *5544*

Alkaline Phosphatase Isoenzymes *Serum* *Increase* 10 jaundiced patients with extrahepatic biliary obstruction had elevated isoenzyme-I and 8 of the 10 had raised isoenzyme-IV *2557* Two main isoenzymes are present: alpha$_2$-globulin, derived directly from the liver cells, which contributed the major fraction, and the 2nd, present in smaller proportions and represents the regurgitation of bile alkaline phosphatase as a result of obstruction to the normal flow of bile *4216* 15 of 17 patients with obstructive jaundice showed a couplet of liver isoenzymes in the alpha$_1$ and alpha$_2$ areas. Mean levels were 4.7 and 20.5 respectively *4341*

Amylase *Serum* *Increase* Occurs in calculus common duct obstruction without pancreatitis due to an increase in pancreatic isoenzyme *5580* Values > 1,000 U/L usually indicate choledocholithiasis *32* Marked elevations should point to the diagnosis of acute pancreatitis of primary nature or secondary to calculus biliary tract disease *900*
Urine *Increase* Increased excretion in obstruction due to stone in common bile duct *1290*

Anti-Mitochondrial Antibodies *Serum* *Increase* 11% of patients were positive and 6% of controls *4991* *4176*
Serum *No Effect* No significant increase in frequency *4176*

Antinuclear Antibodies *Serum* *Increase* Positive in 11% of patients (2% in controls) *4176*

Aspartate Aminotransferase *Serum* *Increase* Median activity in 9 patients with obstructive jaundice of 111 U/L significantly different from reference range of 5 - 28 U/L *5347* Up to 145 U/L; returns to normal within 1 week after obstruction is relieved *5544* Increased activity in all cases of biliary tract obstruction. Common duct obstruction due to stones, pancreatitis, tumor, duct carcinoma, and leukemia nodes showed values of 31 - 193 U/L *5738*

Bile Acids *Urine* *Increase* Mean values for bile acids in urine: control 1.9 µg/mL, obstructive jaundice µg/mL, cirrhosis of 15.14 µg/mL (compensated) and 11.84 (uncompensated) *5148*

Bilirubin *Feces* *Decrease* Marked decrease. Clay colored stools observed *5544*
Serum *Increase* During or soon after an attack of biliary colic. Increased in about 33% of patients *5544* Median concentration in 9 patients with obstructive jaundice of 102 µmol/L significantly different from reference range of 5 - 21 µmol/L *5347*
Serum *No Effect* Remains normal in the presence of serum alkaline phosphatase that is markedly increased with the obstruction of one hepatic bile duct *5544*
Urine *Increase* During or soon after an attack of biliary colic. Increased in about 33% of patients *5544* Values of 1 - 5 mg/dL are common in an episode of cholecystitis. Levels higher than 5 mg/dL are usually the result of common bile duct obstruction, particularly if there is a predominance of the direct-reacting fraction of bilirubin *900*

Bilirubin, Indirect *Serum* *Increase* Normal or slight increase *5544*

BSP Retention *Serum* *Increase* Normal or may later become only slightly increased *5544*

Carcinoembryonic Antigen *Serum* *Increase* Circulating levels are elevated in benign extrahepatic biliary tract obstruction and inflammation *5060* 43% of patients had values > 2.5 ng/mL *2010* Slight increases may be observed *4891*

Chenodeoxycholic Acid *Serum* *Increase* Serum bile acids elevate promptly during the acute episode and indicate biliary tract disease *2426* 3-β-Hydroxy-5-cholenoic acid was elevated in hepatobiliary disease. Normal concentration of 0.184 mmol/L, obstructive jaundice concentration of 6.783 mmol/L *5149*

Cholesterol *Red Blood Cells* *Increase* 25 - 50% increase in the membrane concentration, resulting in the characteristic target cell *5699* An increase in RBC cholesterol and phospholipid was detected in most patients with hepatocellular disease or cholestatic jaundice but the alteration in RBC lipid content did not correlate with RBC survival *4201*
Serum *Increase* In 15 patients, (aged 16 - 78 y), compared to controls, there was an increase in total cholesterol due to an increase in the unesterified fraction *3516* Continues to rise for some time after obstruction has been established, reaching extreme heights. Persists for a long period, falling when the obstruction is relieved *3263*

Cholesterol, Free *Serum* *Increase* In simple biliary obstruction the increase is greater in the free fraction *1290*

Cholic Acid *Serum* *Increase* Serum bile acids elevate promptly during the acute episode indicate biliary tract disease *2426*

Cholinesterase *Serum* *Decrease* In 9 patients with obstructive jaundice mean activity of 0.52 U/L compared with normal values of 0.6 - 1.2 U/L *5347*

Creatine Kinase *Serum* *No Effect* Activity usually within normal limits *1980*

Creatinine *Serum* *No Effect* Median concentration in 9 patients with obstructive jaundice of 71 µmol/L not significantly different from reference range of 26 - 80 µmol/L *5347*

Creatinine Clearance *Urine* *Decrease* Median clearance in 9 patients with obstructive jaundice of of 78 mL/min not significantly different from reference range of 90 - 170 mL/min *5347*

Fat *Feces* *Increase* May be excessive amounts of fecal fat *4707* Deficient intraluminal bile acids *4891*

Fractional Excretion of Sodium *Urine* *No Effect* In 9 patients with obstructive jaundice mean fractional excretion 0.91% compared with normal values of 0.5 - 1.0% *5347*

α_1-Globulin *Serum* *Increase* α- and β-Globulins increase in infection or obstructive jaundice *367*

α_2-Globulin *Serum* *Increase* In cholestasis, the increase in alpha$_2$- and β-globulin components correlates with the height of serum lipid values and is a useful point in distinguishing between biliary obstructive lesions and other nonobstructive types of jaundice *5189* α- and β-Globulins increase in infection or obstructive jaundice *367*

β-Globulin *Serum* *Increase* In cholestasis, the increase in alpha$_2$- and β-globulin components correlates with the height of serum lipid values and is a useful point in distinguishing between biliary obstructive lesions and other nonobstructive types of jaundice *5189*

γ-Glutamyltransferase *Serum* *Increase* Increase is faster and greater than that of serum alkaline phosphatase and LAP *5544* Increased with obstructive jaundice *1290*

Haptoglobin *Serum* *Increase* Can be variable or increased. Increased in 33% of patients with obstructive biliary disease *5544*

Isocitrate Dehydrogenase *Serum* *Increase* 100 - 500 U/L *5544*
Serum *No Effect* Within the normal range in patients with obstruction due to benign or malignant disease *5008*

Lactate Dehydrogenase *Serum* *Increase* Slight increase *1980* In obstruction due to benign or malignant disease *5008*

Lactate Dehydrogenase Isoenzyme-5 *Serum* *Increase* Was markedly elevated in 3 cases. Mean elevation = 11.0% of total LD value *1756*

Lactate Dehydrogenase Isoenzymes *Serum* *Increase* LD$_4$ was elevated to 9.3% of total LD value in 3 cases *1756*

Lecithin *Red Blood Cells* *Increase* 25 - 50% increase in the membrane concentration, resulting in the characteristic target cell *5699*

Leucine Aminopeptidase *Serum* *Increase* 9 patients with obstruction due to stones had highly elevated serum values, ranging from 48 - 990 U/L *579*
Urine *Increase* Moderate increase with simple obstruction *1290*

Leukocytes *Blood* *Increase* A moderate leukocytosis of 10,000 - 15,000 /µL found in the majority of patients with an attack. Higher elevations in the range of 20,000 - 25,000 /µL or the appearance of many less mature forms are indicative of complications such as suppuration or cholangitis *900* Normal or increased *2039*
Blood *No Effect* Normal WBC observed in most cases *5544*

Leukotriene E_4 *Urine* *Increase* In 9 patients with obstructive jaundice median concentration of 1.21 nmol/L or 142 nmol/mol creatinine higher than median excretion of 0.52 nmol/L (range of 0.34 - 0.70 nmol/L) or 40 nmol/mol creatinine (range of 29 - 52 nmol/mol creatinine) in 10 healthy individuals *5347*

Lipase *Serum* *Decrease* Lack of bile salts result in the failure to activate pancreatic lipase in the intestinal lumen *4707*
Serum *Increase* Marked elevations should point to the diagnosis of acute pancreatitis of primary nature or secondary to calculus biliary tract disease *900*

Lipids *Serum* *Increase* In cholestasis, the increase in alpha$_2$- and β-globulin components correlates with the height of serum lipid values and is a useful point in distinguishing between biliary obstructive lesions and other nonobstructive types of jaundice *5189*

Lipoproteins *Serum* *Increase* Alpha$_2$- and β-globulins contain lipoproteins which may be markedly increased in cholestatic lesions of the liver *5189*

Mucoprotein *Serum* *Increase* Observed effect *1025*

N-Acetyl-Leukotriene E_4 *Urine* *Increase* In 9 patients with obstructive jaundice median concentration of 0.26 nmol/L or 47 nmol/mol creatinine higher than median excretion of 0.14 nmol/L (range of 0.08 - 0.23 nmol/L) or 13 nmol/mol creatinine (range of 7 - 20 nmol/mol creatinine) in 10 healthy individuals *5347*

Norepinephrine *Plasma* *No Effect* In 9 patients with obstructive jaundice mean concentration of 282 pg/mL compared with normal values of 50 - 400 pg/mL *5347*

5'-Nucleotidase *Serum* *Increase* Increased in extra-hepatic biliary obstruction *1290*

Occult Blood *Feces* *Increase* May be positive or negative in patients with extrahepatic biliary obstruction *2039*

Ornithine Carbamoyltransferase *Serum* *Increase* Liver cell damage *5544*

Osmotic Fragility *Red Blood Cells* *Decrease* Thin, flat erythrocytes are more resistant than normal cells and have decreased osmotic fragility *1980*

Phospholipids *Red Blood Cells* *Increase* An increase in RBC phospholipid was detected in most patients with hepatocellular disease or cholestatic jaundice but the alteration in RBC lipid content did not correlate with RBC survival *4201*
Serum *Increase* In 15 patients (aged 16 - 78), compared to 23 controls (aged 18 - 63), there was an increased in cholesterol and phospholipids and increase in phospholipid to cholesterol ratio *3516*

Prothrombin Time *Plasma* *Increase* Prolonged, with response to parenteral vitamin K more frequent than in hepatic parenchymal cell disease *5544*
Plasma *No Effect* Median time as % of control in 9 patients with obstructive jaundice of 82% not significantly different from reference range of 70 - 100% *5347*

Renin Activity *Plasma* *Increase* Median activity in 9 patients with obstructive jaundice of 3.0 ng/mL/h higher than reference range of 0.5 - 2.0 ng/mL/h *5347*

Triglycerides *Serum* *Increase* A marked and persistent elevation. The increase is of similar magnitude to that for cholesterol and phospholipid. Following relief of obstruction the triglycerides returned to normal. Associated with a clear serum and negative cold aggregation test in contrast to the changes in cases of endogenous (type IV) hypertriglyceridemia *3516*

Urobilinogen *Feces* *Decrease* When very high serum bilirubin levels are attained, a little bilirubin may diffuse into the bowel, resulting in the appearance of small quantities of urobilinogen in the stools. Otherwise none is detected *1290* Marked decrease. Clay colored stools *5544*
Urine *Increase* With infection of the biliary tract. In cholangitis very high concentrations of urine urobilinogen are attained. Probably bacteria act in the proximal parts of the bile-ducts, on the bile-pigments *1290*

Vitamin K *Serum* *Decrease* Due to fat malabsorption *4707*

Volume *Urine* *Increase* Median excretion in 9 patients with obstructive jaundice of 288 mL/4 h not significantly different from 222 mL/4 h in 10 healthy controls *5347*

576.50 Spasm of Sphincter of Oddi

Amylase *Serum* *Increase* Obstruction of the pancreatic duct by drug-induced spasm of sphincter (e.g., opiates, codeine, methyl choline, chlorothiazide) *5544*

Lipase *Serum* *Increase* Obstruction of the pancreatic duct by drug-induced spasm of the sphincter (e.g.,by opiates, codeine, methyl choline) *5544*

576.80 Byler's Disease

Alanine Aminotransferase *Serum* *Increase* Usually becomes apparent in first year of life with intermittent jaundice initially, later persistent. Activity may be markedly increased, indicating hepatic necrosis *3406*

Aspartate Aminotransferase *Serum* *Increase* Usually becomes apparent in first year of life with intermittent jaundice initially, later persistent. Activity may be markedly increased, indicating hepatic necrosis *3406*

Bilirubin *Serum* *Increase* Usually becomes apparent in first year of life with intermittent jaundice initially, later persistent *3406*

576.80 Choledochal Cysts

Carcinoembryonic Antigen *Bile* *Increase* Mean concentration in 5 patients with choledochal cysts of 20.0 ng/mL *3729*

576.90 Biliary Tract Disease

Carcinoembryonic Antigen *Bile* *No Effect* Mean concentration in 34 patients with benign biliary strictures of 10.1 ng/mL *3729*

Epidermal Growth Factor *Serum* *Increase* In 15 patients with biliary tract disease mean concentration of 27.2 ± 7.0 µg/L significantly different from 17.7 ± 3.8 µg/L in 22 healthy controls *3439*

Insulin-like Growth Factor-I *Serum* *Increase* In 15 patients with biliary tract disease mean concentration of 145.1 ± 37.2 µg/L not significantly different from 103.3 ± 22.0 µg/L in 22 healthy controls *3439*

Somatostatin *Plasma* *Increase* In 15 patients with biliary tract disease mean concentration of 50.1 ± 12.8 ng/L significantly different from 29.7 ± 6.3 ng/L in 22 healthy controls *3439*

Trypsin *Serum* *No Effect* Mean concentration of trypsin-like immunoreactivity in 13 patients with either gall-bladder or common bile duct stones did not exceed concentration in 85 healthy control individuals (42.78 ± 10.26 ng/mL) *3330*

576.90 Non-malignant Disease of the Biliary Tract

Epinephrine *Plasma* *Increase* Biliary dyskinesia associated with increased concentration *2955*

5-Hydroxytryptamine *Plasma* *Increase* Biliary dyskinesia associated with increased concentration *2955*

Norepinephrine *Plasma* *Increase* Biliary dyskinesia associated with increased concentration *2955*

5-Nucleotide Phosphodiesterase Isoenzyme V
Serum *Increase* Mean activity was increased in the plasma of 59% of 161 patients with non-malignant disease of the liver, pancreas or biliary system *1781*

577.00 Acute Pancreatitis

Adrenomedullin *Plasma* *Increase* In 6 patients with acute pancreatitis mean concentration of 13.8 ± 3.8 fmol/mL significantly different from 5.1 ± 0.2 fmol/mL in healthy controls *5343*

Alanine Aminotransferase *Serum* *Increase* In 163 patients with necrotizing pancreatitis mean activity of 113.5 U/L and 120.0 U/L in 376 patients with edematous pancreatitis *5151* 4 of 10 patients showed elevations. Values ranged from 10 - 50 U/L mean concentration of 26.5 U/L (upper limit of normal of 24 U/L) *3161*

577.00 Acute Pancreatitis *(continued)*

Albumin *Ascitic Fluid* *Increase* Elevated level (> 2.9 g/dL) is characteristic *4891*
Serum *Decrease* In 163 patients with necrotizing pancreatitis mean concentration of 32.0 g/L and 38.0 g/L in 376 patients with edematous pancreatitis *5151* In 66% of 21 patients at initial hospitalization for this disorder *1576*

Aldolase *Serum* *Increase* Other nonspecific serum enzymes may also be increased *5544*

Alkaline Phosphatase *Ascitic Fluid* *Increase* Ranged from 0.3 to 11.2 mmol p-nitrophenol/h/mL *1695*
Serum *Increase* In 45% of 21 patients at initial hospitalization for this disorder *1576* Anicteric cases had normal levels. Cases with some degree of common bile duct obstruction were all elevated *2803* Parallels serum bilirubin *5544* In 163 patients with necrotizing pancreatitis mean activity of 206.5 U/L and 196.0 U/L in 376 patients with edematous pancreatitis *5151*

Amino Acids *Plasma* *Decrease* In patients with acute hemorrhagic necrotizing pancreatitis *4455*
Urine *Increase* In some patients with familial pancreatitis the urine may contain an excess amount of amino acids, especially cystine and lysine *900*

Amylase *Ascitic Fluid* *Increase* Ascites may develop, 0.5-2 liters in volume, containing increased amylase with a level higher than that of serum *5544* Concentration in ascitic fluid is usually 1,000 U/L *192* Varied from 1,060 - 48,000 U/L in ascites *1695*
Pleural Fluid *Increase* With pancreatic pseudocyst *4493* Pleural effusions occur in about 10% of patients, with amylase commonly elevated *3052* Elevated in primary or metastatic lung cancer, pancreatitis, or esophageal perforation *4537* Pleural effusion has been reported in about 6% of patients with acute pancreatitis. These effusions contain pleural fluid amylase. May occur in other conditions including metastatic carcinoma *1025* May contain very high concentration, even with normal serum level. If the concentrations are lower than the serum, pancreatitis is virtually excluded as the cause *4891* With pancreatic pseudocyst *3054*
Saliva *Increase* Increased α-amylase in parotid saliva *1875*
Serum *Decrease* Extensive marked destruction of pancreas. Decreased levels are clinically significant only in occasional cases of fulminant pancreatitis *5544*
Serum *Increase* Increase begins in 3 - 6 h, rises to over 250 U/L within 8 h in 75% of patients, reaches maximum in 20 - 30 h, and may persist for 48 - 72 h. May be up to 40 times normal, but the height of the increase does not correlate with the severity of the disease. More than 10% of patients may have normal values even in terminal stage *5544* Rises within 24 - 48 h of acute onset, normalizing within 3 - 5 days *4537* Amylase isoenzyme, P3, is elevated in acute pancreatitis but not in other conditions *1584* In 14 patients with acute pancreatitis and sepsis and in 36 without early sepsis mean activity greater than 3 SD of mean in healthy individuals *536* In 56 cases of acute pancreatitis median serum amylase activity of 277 U/L was higher in 31 nonalcoholic cases than 209 U/L in 25 cases with other causes *2689* In 29 patients with acute pancreatiitis median concentration of 969 U/L (range 151 - 7,020) higher than 180 U/L (range 60 - 300) in 120 healthy controls *2089* In 163 patients with necrotizing pancreatitis mean activity of 1,689 U/L and 1,490 U/L in 376 patients with edematous pancreatitis *5151* Mean activity increased above 220 U/L in 153 of 158 patients *1*
Serum *No Effect* Occasionally seen; probably following a transient rise and fall, extensive necrosis or acute exacerbation of chronic pancreatitis in which the pancreas cannot produce amylase *4537*
Urine *Increase* Tends to reflect serum changes by a time lag of 6 - 10 h, but sometimes increased urine levels are higher and of longer duration than serum levels *5544* Often elevated and persists up to the 3rd day after the onset of the disease *900* Increased renal clearance *402* Elevation has been used to diagnose acute pancreatitis in the absence of renal failure. Levels higher than 6,000 U/24 h or 300 U/h are usually seen in patients with acute attacks *367* In 14 patients with acute pancreatitis and sepsis and in 36 without early sepsis mean activity greater than 3 SD of mean in healthy individuals *586*

Anionic Trypsinogen *Serum* *Increase* In 30 patients with acute pancreatitis mean anionic trypsinogen concentration of 47 (6 to 180) fold higher than mean of 11.5 µg/L (normal range 4.2 - 31.5) with return to normal within 2 to 3 weeks *2831*

Antithrombin III *Plasma* *Decrease* In both survivors (n = 10) and fatal cases (n = 4) a high frequency of reduced values were found during the first week after admission. Values were significantly more reduced in the fatal cases *4*

α_1-Antitrypsin *Ascitic Fluid* *Decrease* Ranged from 15 - 170 mg/dL in ascites (normal serum value of 200 - 400 mg/dL) *1695*
Serum *Decrease* Decreased *4241* *83* *4373* *4763* *4371*

Arylsulfatase *Ascitic Fluid* *Increase* Varied from 89 - 5,170 pmol/min/mL *1695*

Ascorbic Acid *Serum* *Decrease* In 29 patients with acute pancreatiitis median concentration of vitamin C and ascorbic acid were respectively 2.8 (0.3 - 10) µg/mL and < 0.5 (< 0.5 - 6.0) µg/mL compared with 15 (6.3 - 19) µg/mL and 12 (4.5 - 18) µg/mL in 30 healthy volunteers *4701*

Aspartate Aminotransferase *Serum* *Increase* Both normal and elevated levels have been reported. Usual values of 20 - 700 U/L *5544* No apparent correlation with damage to pancreas, serum lipase, amylase, or calcium, but there is direct correlation with the serum bilirubin level suggesting increase due to biliary obstruction *1290* In 163 patients with necrotizing pancreatitis mean activity of 110.0 U/L and 105.0 U/L in 376 patients with edematous pancreatitis *5151* In 87% of 21 patients at initial hospitalization for this disorder *1576* Mild elevation (mean = 36.2 U/L) in 80% of 10 cases (normal maximum = 24 U/L) *3161* Both normal and elevated levels have been reported. Usual values of 20-700 U/L *1025*

Bilirubin *Serum* *Increase* In 32% of 21 patients at initial hospitalization for this disorder *1576* Seen in about 20% of patients *2039* May be moderately elevated as a consequence of edema of the head of the pancreas with resultant obstruction of the common bile duct *1980* In 163 patients with necrotizing pancreatitis mean concentration of 22.2 µmol/L and 29.1 µmol/L in 376 patients with edematous pancreatitis *5151*
Serum *No Effect* May be increased when pancreatitis of biliary tract origin but is usually normal in alcoholic pancreatitis *5544*
Urine *Increase* Seen in about 20% of patients *2039*

Bilirubin, Direct *Serum* *Increase* In 80% of 10 patients at initial hospitalization for this disorder *1576*

Bilirubin, Indirect *Serum* *Increase* In 40% of 10 patients at initial hospitalization for this disorder *1576*

CA 19-9 *Serum* *Increase* Positive analyses have been encountered *2026* The serum concentration was above the normal value of 37 U/mL in 21% of patients *4507* CA 19-9 concentration increased above 37 U/mL in 4 of 15 (26.6%) patients with acute pancreatitis and in 11% of 37 patients in another study *1253* Positive analyses have been encountered *3657*

CA 50 *Serum* *Increase* Marked elevation *4127*

CA 125 *Serum* *Increase* False positive result *3909*

CA 195 *Serum* *Increase* Large number of false positives (60%) *4127*

Calcium *Serum* *Decrease* In 163 patients with necrotizing pancreatitis mean concentration of 2.14 mmol/L and 2.25 mmol/L in 376 patients with edematous pancreatitis *5151* Total and ionized calcium were low or in the low normal range in 11 clearly documented cases *5621* Mean = 7.3 ± 1.5 mg/dL in the 12 patients (range = 4.6 - 9.9). The 5 patients who did not recover had the lowest concentrations *1695* Often found with a low serum albumin; when correction of serum calcium is made for hypoalbuminemia, most patients are found to be normocalcemic *79* Decreased concentrations are seen in acute pancreatitis *2952* Decreased in severe cases 1 - 9 days after onset. Usually occurs after amylase and lipase levels have become normal. Values < 7.0 mg/dL indicates poor prognosis *367*
Serum *Increase* Occasionally, in patients whose pancreatitis is related to hyperparathyroidism, it may be elevated even during the acute attack *900*
Serum *No Effect* In 20 patients with acute pancreatitis mean concentration on admission to hospital of 2.59 ± 0.25 mmol/L not significantly different from 2.51 ± 0.28 mmol/L in healthy blood donor controls *2834*

Carcinoembryonic Antigen *Pleural Fluid* *Increase* Mean concentration increased in 1 of 1 effusion in a patient with acute pancreatitis *1649*
Serum *Increase* May be found *1109* Increases may occur *4891* Slight increases may be observed *4551* Increases may be observed *1601*

Catecholamines *Urine Increase* May be marked; increased due to severe stress *5544*

Cationic Trypsinogen *Serum Increase* Mean concentration in 30 patients with acute pancreatitis shows a 9-fold increase (range 1 - 35 fold) compared with normal concentration with mean of 20.9 µg/L (normal range 11.4 - 38.0 µg/L) returning to normal range within 2 to 3 weeks *2831*

Cholesterol *Serum Decrease* In 42% of 21 patients at initial hospitalization for this disorder *1576*
Serum Increase In 163 patients with necrotizing pancreatitis mean concentration of 4.40 mmol/L and 4.45 mmol/L in 376 patients with edematous pancreatitis *5151*

Chylomicrons *Serum Increase* Increased *4358 3017 4372*

C-Peptide *Plasma Increase* In 15 patients with acute pancreatitis mean concentration on admission of 1.90 ± 1.12 nmol/L significantly different from 1.11 ± 0.46 nmol/L 10 days later when measured by Byk-Mallinckrodt kit *2577*
Plasma No Effect In 15 patients with acute pancreatitis mean concentration on admission of 0.48 ± 0.50 nmol/L not significantly different from 0.52 ± 0.25 nmol/L 10 days later when measured by Novo procedure using M-1221 antibodies *2577*

C-Reactive Protein *Serum Increase* Sensitivity, specificity and diagnostic accuracy for establishing the severity of acute pancreatitis (using cutoff of 11 mg/L) was 8%, 95% and 64% respectively *4114* In 24 patients with mild acute pancreatitis mean concentration of 27.2 ± 6 µg/mL and 41.9 ± 14 µg/mL in 19 patients with severe acute pancreatitis at the time of admission to hospital *414* Concentration increased in 12 of 15 patients with severe acute pancreatitis and 13 of 25 who had mild acute pancreatitis, but with no significant differences between mean concentrations *4115* In 20 patients with acute pancreatitis median concentrations ranged from 125 to 212 mg/L in patients with severe disease and 36 to 75 mg/L in those with mild disease *3589* Median plasma concentrations of C-reactive protein were significantly higher in patients with 'severe' illness ($p < 0.001$) than those with 'mild' illness. A particularly marked increase of interleukin-6 was found in two patients with necrotising pancreatitis and fatal outcome *5467*

Creatine Kinase *Serum Increase* Was found to indicate a more severe or prolonged course than in cases with normal levels, but to have little diagnostic value *4363*

Creatinine *Serum Increase* In 163 patients with necrotizing pancreatitis mean concentration of 97.2 mmol/L and 79.6 mmol/L in 376 patients with edematous pancreatitis *5151* In 42% of 14 patients at initial hospitalization for this disorder *1576*
Serum No Effect In 6 patients with acute pancreatitis mean concentration of 0.68 ± 0.10 mg/dL not significantly different from that in healthy controls *5343*

Elastase *Neutrophils Increase* Activity correlated with severity of pancreatitis. Sensitivity and specificity of test greater than 90% with a positive severity predictive value of almost 80% at the time of admission and 97% after 24 h and a negative predictive value of approximately 98% *1201*

Eosinophils *Pleural Fluid Increase* Eosinophilia greater than 10% may be present *126*

Epinephrine *Plasma Increase* Increased circulating epinephrine *1290*

Erythrocytes *Ascitic Fluid Increase* In hemorrhagic pancreatitis *413*
Ascitic Fluid No Effect Variable amount noted *233*
Pleural Fluid Increase 1,000 - 10,000 /µL *4493*

Fibronectin *Plasma Decrease* Studied in 32 patients with pancreatitis. Patients were subdivided by clinical and biochemical criteria: severe acute pancreatitis (n = 10), moderate acute pancreatitis (n = 17), and acute attack of chronic pancreatitis (n = 5). Serum and plasma samples were collected on days 1 - 7, 10, 14, and 21 *36*

Fibronectin Fragment *Urine Increase* Maximum levels were seen on the first day of admission *5140*

Glucagon *Plasma Increase* Increased concentrations lead to the release of calcitonin and resultant depression of serum calcium *2039*

Glucose *Serum Increase* Seen in about 25% of patients *2039* In 45% of 21 patients at initial hospitalization for this disorder *1576* Often found and signifies involvement of pancreatic islet cells *900* Transient hyperglycemia is not rare *4891* In 163 patients with necrotizing pancreatitis mean concentration of 8.83 mmol/L and 6.61 mmol/L in 376 patients with edematous pancreatitis *5151*
Urine Increase Routine urinalysis is usually normal but there may be glucose in the urine *900* Appears in 25% of the patients *5544*

α-Glucosidase *Serum Increase* Patients with pancreatitis associated with trauma or complicated by severe necrosis, hemorrhage, or abscess also displayed greater increases *4182*

β-Glucuronidase *Ascitic Fluid Increase* Ranged from 850 to 16,500 µg phenolphthalein/h/dL *1695*

γ-Glutamyltransferase *Saliva Increase* Significantly higher (15.1 U/L) versus controls (5.12 U/L) *2448*
Serum Increase Was elevated to a mean level of 300 U/L (10 times normal) in all 10 cases *3161* Always elevated *5544* Observed in some patients *4484*

Hematocrit *Blood Decrease* In 163 patients with necrotizing pancreatitis mean value of 43.5% and 41.2% in 376 patients with edematous pancreatitis *5151*
Blood Increase Probably reflects intravascular volume contraction *1980* Occasionally because of hemoconcentration *900*

Hemoglobin *Blood Increase* Usually normal but may be high occasionally due to hemoconcentration *900* In 163 patients with necrotizing pancreatitis mean concentration of 148 g/L and 138 g/L in 376 patients with edematous pancreatitis *5151*

Hyaluronic Acid *Serum Increase* A total of 52 patients with pancreatitis were studied (acute pancreatitis =17; chronic pancreatitis = 35) and compared to 194 controls. Patients with pancreatitis displayed elevated levels in all groups, when compared with the controls *3107* Studied in 32 patients with pancreatitis. Patients were subdivided by clinical and biochemical criteria: severe acute pancreatitis (n = 10), moderate acute pancreatitis (n = 17), and acute attack of chronic pancreatitis (n = 5). Serum and plasma samples were collected on days 1 - 7, 10, 14, and 21. In moderate acute pancreatitis concentrations fluctuated around the upper reference limit, but declined to mid-normal levels at day 21. In severe acute pancreatitis all three parameters increased. In patients who died as a consequence of sepsis and multi-organ failure the increase was much more pronounced *36*

17-Hydroxycorticosteroids *Urine Increase* May be marked; increased due to severe stress *5544*

Hydroxyproline *Urine Increase* High levels were observed on the second to fifth day *5140*

Insulin *Plasma Increase* In 13 patients with acute pancreatitis mean concentration on admission of 0.17 ± 0.17 nmol/L not significantly different from 0.11 ± 0.15 nmol/L 10 days later *2577*

Interleukin-1 Receptor Antagonist *Serum Increase* In 14 patients with acute pancreatitis and sepsis mean concentration of 10,339 ± 63,412 pg/mL and in 36 without early sepsis mean concentration of 578 ± 1,934 pg/mL greater than upper limit of normal of < 200 pg/mL *586*

Interleukin-1β *Serum No Effect* In 14 patients with acute pancreatitis and sepsis mean concentration of 8.3 ± 5.7 pg/mL and in 36 without early sepsis mean concentration of 5.8 ± 1.9 pg/mL. Only 6% had abnormally high concentration *586*

Interleukin-6 *Serum Increase* Sensitivity, specificity and diagnostic accuracy for establishing the severity of acute pancreatitis (using cutoff of 2.7 pg/mL) was 100%, 86% and 91% respectively *4114* Concentration increased in 40 patients with acute pancreatitis compared with 40 healthy controls, with significant difference between concentrations in 15 patients with severe acute pancreatitis (25 µg/L) and 25 who had mild acute pancreatitis (2 µg/L *4115* In 50 patients with acute pancreatitis, 46 (92%) had increased concentrations of IL-6 in their plasma, 1,512 ± 635 pg/mL compared with reference upper limit of less than 10 pg/mL *586* In 24 patients with mild acute pancreatitis mean concentration of 861 ± 20 pg/mL and 33,600 ± 17,600 pg/mL in 19 patients with severe acute pancreatitis at the time of admission to hospital *414* Median plasma concentrations of interleukin-6, were significantly higher in patients with 'severe' illness ($p < 0.001$) than those with 'mild' illness. A particularly marked increase in interleukin-6 was found in two patients with

577.00 Acute Pancreatitis *(continued)*

Interleukin-6 *(continued)*
necrotising pancreatitis and fatal outcome *5467* In 50 patients with acute pancreatitis, the serum concentration of interleukin-6 was determined daily during the first week of hospitalization. Patients were divided into three groups according to clinical criteria: mild pancreatitis (less than or equal to 1 complication; n = 25), severe pancreatitis (greater than or equal to 2 complications; n = 15), and lethal outcome (n = 10). Patients with mild disease showed initially slightly elevated levels of interleukin-6 (22.0 ± 9.8 U/mL) that decreased to low levels within 4 days (5.0 ± 1.0 U/mL). In patients with severe pancreatitis, serum concentrations of interleukin-6 were initially clearly elevated (35.0 ± 7.5 U/mL) and remained slightly elevated until day 7 (13.0 ± 2.0 U/mL). Patients with lethal outcome had markedly elevated initial interleukin-6 concentrations (61.0 ± 15.0 U/mL) that decreased but were still elevated at day 7 (26.0 ± 2.5 U/mL) *3001*

Interleukin-8 *Serum Increase* Sensitivity, specificity and diagnostic accuracy for establishing the severity of acute pancreatitis (using cutoff of 30 pg/mL) was 100%, 81% and 88% respectively *4114* In 24 patients with mild acute pancreatitis mean concentration of 2.3 ± 0.7 pg/mL and 9.8 ± 3.7 pg/mL in 19 patients with severe acute pancreatitis at the time of admission to hospital *414* Patients with complicated pancreatitis had statistically significant (p less than 0.05) higher mean values of IL-8 (121 ± 41 pg/mL vs. 13 ± 6 pg/mL, mean ± SEM) than patients with uncomplicated disease *1884*

Interleukin-10 *Serum Increase* In 14 patients with acute pancreatitis and sepsis mean concentration of 107.4 ± 24.7 pg/mL and in 36 without early sepsis mean concentration of 85.0 ± 18.2 pg/mL greater than upper limit of normal of < 10 pg/mL *586* In 24 patients with mild acute pancreatitis mean concentration of 33 ± 5 pg/mL and 25.8 ± 2.7 pg/mL in 19 patients with severe acute pancreatitis at the time of admission to hospital *414* On the first day of acute pancreatitis in 17 patients with mild disease mean concentration of 424 ± 389 pg/mL significantly higher than 15 ± 6 pg/mL in 21 patients with severe disease and undetectable IL-10 observed in 12 healthy individuals *4113*

Ionized Calcium *Serum Decrease* Elevated PTH concentration and inversely correlated with serum ionized calcium *5621*

17-Ketogenic Steroids *Urine Increase* May be marked; increased due to severe stress *5544*

Lactate Dehydrogenase *Pleural Fluid Increase* Exudate *126*
Serum Increase In 163 patients with necrotizing pancreatitis mean activity of 510 U/L and 320 U/L in 376 patients with edematous pancreatitis *5151* Nonspecific serum enzymes may also be increased *5544* In 45% of 21 patients at initial hospitalization for this disorder *1576* In some cases *1290*

Lactate Dehydrogenase Isoenzyme-5 *Serum Increase* Elevated to 8.3% of the total value of 861 U/L in 3 cases. Increases occurred in LD isoenzymes 4 and 5 *1756*

Lactate Dehydrogenase Isoenzymes *Serum Increase* LD_4 was elevated above the normal value in 3 cases. LD_4 comprised 8.4% of total LD of 861 U/L (= 4%) *1756*

Laminin *Serum Increase* Studied in 32 patients with pancreatitis. Patients were subdivided by clinical and biochemical criteria: severe acute pancreatitis (n = 10), moderate acute pancreatitis (n = 17), and acute attack of chronic pancreatitis (n = 5). Serum and plasma samples were collected on days 1 - 7, 10, 14, and 21. In moderate acute pancreatitis concentrations fluctuated around the upper reference limit, but declined to mid-normal levels at day 21. In severe acute pancreatitis all three parameters increased *36* A total of 52 patients with pancreatitis were studied (acute pancreatitis =17; chronic pancreatitis = 35) and compared to 194 controls. Patients with pancreatitis displayed elevated levels in all groups, when compared with the controls *3107*

Leucine Aminopeptidase *Serum Increase* Transient moderate rise in acute but no increase in chronic pancreatitis *1290* Of 6 patients, 67% had abnormally high values, ranging from 195 - 455 U/L (322 U/L upper limit of normal) *579*

Leukocytes *Ascitic Fluid No Effect* Variable *233*
Blood Increase WBC is slightly to moderately increased (10,000 - 20,000 /µL) *5544* In 163 patients with necrotizing pancreatitis mean concentration of 16,440 /µL and 11,000 /µL in 376 patients with edematous pancreatitis *5151* In 60% of 21 patients at initial hospitalization for this disorder *1576* Usually elevated *900*
Pleural Fluid Increase 5,000 - 20,000 /µL *4493*

Lipase *Ascitic Fluid Increase* May be elevated *192*
Pleural Fluid Increase May contain very high concentration, even with normal serum level. If the concentration is lower than the serum, pancreatitis is virtually excluded as the cause *4891*
Serum Increase Lipase activity increases within 4 to 8 hours of onset of acute pancreatitis, peaking at 24 hours and decreasing within 8 to 14 days. Sensitivity in diagnosis of acute pancreatitis between 56% and 100% and specificity between 42 and 100% *5231* Activity increased in 40 patients with acute pancreatitis compared with 40 healthy controls, but no significant difference between activities in 15 patients with severe acute pancreatitis and 25 who had mild acute pancreatitis *4115* In 14 patients with acute pancreatitis and sepsis and in 36 without early sepsis mean activity greater than 3 SD of mean in healthy individuals *586* Elevated in 90% of cases *4935* Mean activity increased above 270 U/L in all of 158 patients *1* Usually rises in parallel with the amylase activity, reaching its peak in 72 or 96 h with a gradual fall; values > 2.0 mL of N/100 NaOH are significant *367* Increases in 50% of patients and may remain elevated as long as 14 days after amylase returns to normal *5544* Elevated in 63%, amylase in 70%, and 83% had parallel elevation of both enzymes *192* In 56 cases of acute pancreatitis median serum lipase activity of 2,454 U/L was not significantly different in 31 nonalcoholic cases from 2,223 U/L in 25 cases with other causes *2689*

Lipase:Amylase Ratio *Serum Increase* Mean ratio of 2.2 was best for differentiating alcoholic from nonalcoholic pancreatitis *1*

Lipids *Serum Increase* Transient; subsides shortly after the onset of the disease and reappears with recurrences. These features differentiate the hyperlipidemia of acute pancreatitis from pancreatitis secondarily associated with primary abnormalities of lipid metabolism *900* Patients with disease caused by alcohol may exhibit milky serum as a result of marked elevation of lipids *4891*

Lipoproteins *Serum Increase* May be present *4891*

α_2-Macroglobulin *Ascitic Fluid Increase* Ascites had concentrations from 44 - 400 mg/dL. Normal serum level is 200 - 400 mg/dL *1695*
Serum Increase Reported effect *3480*

Magnesium *Red Blood Cells Decrease* In 20 patients with acute pancreatitis mean concentration on admission to hospital 2.38 ± 0.50 mmol/L significantly different from 2.85 ± 0.42 mmol/L in healthy blood donor controls *2834*
Serum Decrease Concentration is reduced in association with malabsorption of acute pancreatitis *2952* Observed in a few patients and could partly account for the failure of hypocalcemia to respond to exogenous calcium *4891* In 20 patients with acute pancreatitis mean concentration on admission to hospital 0.89 ± 0.18 mmol/L significantly different from 0.95 ± 0.17 mmol/L in healthy blood donor controls *2834* Low or in the low normal range *5621*

Malate Dehydrogenase *Serum Increase* Slight increase *1290* Nonspecific serum enzymes may be increased *5544*

Methemalbumin *Ascitic Fluid Increase* Ranged from 2.6 - 35 g/dL in the patients with hemorrhagic pancreatitis *1695*
Serum Increase May be present in serum in acute hemorrhagic pancreatitis and not in nonhemorrhagic pancreatitis *4891* Appears after 12 h, reaching peak values by 4 - 5 days. There is a much higher mortality in acute hemorrhagic pancreatitis than in edematous acute pancreatitis *1290* Consistent methemalbuminemia in patients with hemorrhagic pancreatitis, whereas in patients with acute edematous pancreatitis, none could be detected in serum or ascites *1694*

β_2-Microglobulin *Serum Increase* Sensitivity, specificity and diagnostic accuracy for establishing the severity of acute pancreatitis (using cutoff of 2.1 mg/L) was 58%, 81% and 73% respectively *4114* In 20 patients with acute pancreatitis median concentrations ranged from 1.55 to 2.12 mg/L in patients with severe disease and 1.25 to 1.52 mg/L in those with mild disease *3589*

Neutrophil Elastase *Plasma Increase* Patients with complicated pancreatitis had statistically significant (p less than 0.05) higher mean values of neutrophil elastase (547 ± 35 ng/mL vs. 250 ± 20 ng/mL) than patients with uncomplicated disease *1884*

Neutrophils *Blood* *Increase* In 75% of 20 patients at initial hospitalization for this disorder *1576* Usually elevated *900*
Pleural Fluid *Increase* Predominant cell type *4493*

5'-Nucleotidase *Serum* *Increase* Six patients showed elevations ranging from 16.1 - 67.1 U/L (normal 2 - 11 U/L) *2803*

Occult Blood *Feces* *Increase* Reported effect *4891*

Oxygen Partial Pressure *Blood* *Decrease* Blood gases often reveal a moderate lowering of pO_2 *4891*

Oxygen Saturation *Blood* *Decrease* Blood gases often reveal a moderate lowering of pO_2 *4891*

Pancreatic Secretory Trypsin Inhibitor *Serum* *Increase* In all cases of acute pancreatitis concentration increased to 35.0 - 4,500 ng/mL compared with normal mean of 9.4 ng/mL *3949* In 15 of 15 cases concentration of PSTI increased to mean of 317.7 ± 155.6 ng/mL *3719*

Parathyroid Hormone *Plasma* *Increase* Elevated and inversely correlated with serum ionized calcium *5621*

pH *Pleural Fluid* *Decrease* Exudate (pH < 7.3) *126*

Phosphate *Serum* *Decrease* In 41% of 21 patients at initial hospitalization for this disorder *1576* In 78 patients with acute pancreatitis 47 (60%) developed significant hypophosphatemia (less than 0.8 mmol/L) within 4 days of hospitalization but returned to normal within 14 days *4496* Low or in the low normal range *5621*

Phospholipase A *Serum* *Increase* Within 48 hours after start of acute pancreatitis an up to tenfold increase was demonstrable *620* Maximal diagnostic accuracy obtained for the initial activities of amylase, lipase and phospholipase A were 0.83, 0.83, and 0.76 at cutoff values of 650, 650, and 41 U/L respectively *2615* Median plasma concentrations of phospholipase A activity were significantly higher in patients with 'severe' illness (p < 0.001) than those with 'mild' illness. A particularly marked increase in interleukin-6 was found in two patients with necrotising pancreatitis and fatal outcome *5467*

Phospholipase A_2 *Serum* *Increase* Increased concentrations reported *46* Increase in acute pancreatitis is correlated with severity of the disease but probably arising from outside the pancreas. Both PLA2-I and PLA2-II affected in early stages of acute pancreatitis. Activity of PLA2 greater in sera of patients with severe necrotizing acute pancreatitis but no correlation between activity of PLA2-I and severity so activity in acute pancreatitis largely due to PLA2-II *3766*

Phospholipase A_2 Type I *Serum* *Increase* Considerable increase in concentration observed in patients with acute pancreatitis, but is not helpful in assessing the severity of the disease. Concentration reported as high as 563 µg/L in severe acute pancreatitis and 177 µg/L in moderate acute pancreatitis compared with 2 and 4 µg/L in healthy controls *3767*

Polymorphonuclear Elastase *Serum* *Increase* In 20 patients with acute pancreatitis median concentrations ranged from 120 to 2.74 µg/L in patients with severe disease and 71 to 116 µg/L in those with mild disease *3589* In 24 patients with mild acute pancreatitis mean concentration of 113.1 ± 17.5 ng/mL and 239.8 ± 54 ng/mL in 19 patients with severe acute pancreatitis at the time of admission to hospital *414*

Potassium *Serum* *Decrease* Usually normal or only slightly depressed *4891*

Procollagen Type III Peptide *Serum* *Increase* A total of 52 patients with pancreatitis were studied (acute pancreatitis = 17; chronic pancreatitis = 35) and compared to 194 controls. Patients with pancreatitis displayed elevated levels in all groups, when compared with the controls *3107* Studied in 32 patients with pancreatitis. Patients were subdivided by clinical and biochemical criteria: severe acute pancreatitis (n = 10), moderate acute pancreatitis (n = 17), and acute attack of chronic pancreatitis (n = 5). Serum and plasma samples were collected on days 1 - 7, 10, 14, and 21. In moderate acute pancreatitis concentrations fluctuated around the upper reference limit, but declined to mid-normal levels at day 21. In severe acute pancreatitis all three parameters increased. In patients who died as a consequence of sepsis and multi-organ failure the increase was much more pronounced *36*

Proinsulin *Plasma* *Increase* In 15 patients with acute pancreatitis mean concentration on admission of 11.1 ± 12.6 pmol/L not significantly different from 7.5 ± 10.8 pmol/L 10 days later *2577*

Protein *Ascitic Fluid* *Increase* Variable but often > 2.5 g/dL in ascitic fluid *233* Total protein varied from 1.2 - 6.6 g/dL *1695*
Peritoneal Fluid *Increase* Greater than 30 g/L in 70% of cases of pancreatic ascites *1216*
Pleural Fluid *Increase* Exudate (> 3 g/dL) *126*

Soluble $CD4^+$ *Serum* *Decrease* In 22 patients with biliary pancreatitis mean concentration of 21 ± 3 U/mL and in 13 patients with nonbiliary pancreatitis of 14 ± 2 U/mL on day of admission and for next 3 days mean concentration significantly reduced compared with 10 - 40 U/mL in 40 healthy controls of mean age 65 years *4112*
Serum *No Effect* In 22 patients with biliary pancreatitis mean concentration of 23 ± 6 U/mL and in 13 patients with nonbiliary pancreatitis of 11 ± 3 U/mL on day of admission not significantly different from 10 - 40 U/mL in 40 healthy controls of mean age 65 years *4112*

Soluble $CD8^+$ *Serum* *Increase* In 35 patients with acute pancreatitis mean concentration on admission of 674 ± 62 U/mL in those with biliary pancreatitis and 553 ± 83 U/mL in those with nonbiliary pancreatitis significantly higher than 140 - 530 U/mL in 40 healthy controls with mean age of 65 years *4112*

Soluble Interleukin-2 Receptor *Serum* *Increase* In 35 patients with acute pancreatitis mean concentration on admission of 1,084 ± 213 U/mL in those with biliary pancreatitis and 685 ± 115 U/mL in those with nonbiliary pancreatitis significantly higher than 170 - 388 U/mL in 40 healthy controls with mean age of 65 years *4112*

Specific Gravity *Pleural Fluid* *Increase* Exudate (> 1.016) *126*

Triglycerides *Serum* *Increase* In 163 patients with necrotizing pancreatitis mean concentration of 1.31 mmol/L and 1.35 mmol/L in 376 patients with edematous pancreatitis *5151* Often imparts a lactescence to the serum. Elevated because of a transient inhibition to chylomicron removal from the circulation *1980* May reach 1,000 mg/dL or higher *4891*

Trypsin *Serum* *Increase* In 28 patients with acute pancreatitis mean concentration increased to 309.7 ± 197.8 ng/mL compared with 42.78 ± 10.26 ng/mL in 85 healthy controls *3330* 10 - 40 times higher than normal *4891*

Trypsin-2-α_1-Antitrypsin *Serum* *Increase* In 29 patients with acute pancreatiitis median concentration of 249 µg/L (range 52 - 2,170) higher than 4.2 µg/L (range 2.1 - 14) in 120 healthy controls *2089*

Trypsinogen-2 *Serum* *Increase* In 29 patients with acute pancreatiitis median concentration of 750 µg/L (range 75 - 4,750) higher than 39 µg/L (range 11 - 233) in 120 healthy controls *2089*
Urine *Increase* Urinary dipstick successfully detected acute pancreatitis in 50 out of 53 proven cases *2633*

Tumor Necrosis Factor-α *Serum* *Increase* In 14 patients with acute pancreatitis and sepsis mean concentration of 22.8 ± 7.5 pg/mL and in 36 without early sepsis mean concentration of 28.8 ± 10.6 pg/mL. 36% had abnormally high concentration *586*

Urea *Serum* *Increase* In 163 patients with necrotizing pancreatitis mean concentration of 16.78 mmol/L and 12.50 mmol/L in 376 patients with edematous pancreatitis *5151*

Urea Nitrogen *Serum* *Increase* Rarely exceeds 4 mg/dL *4891* Not uncommon with more severe cases, especially when shock and oliguria are present *367*

577.00 Pancreatitis

Alanine Aminotransferase *Serum* *Increase* Overall activity higher in patients with biliary pancreatitis than those with alcoholic pancreatitis *5022*

Alkaline Phosphatase *Serum* *Increase* Overall activity higher in patients with biliary pancreatitis than those with alcoholic pancreatitis *5022*

Amylase *Serum* *Increase* Mean activity in 25 patients with nonalcoholic pancreatitis of 1,320 U/L higher than 439 U/L in 11 patients with alcoholic pancreatitis and reference interval of 25 - 115 U/L *145* Overall activity higher in patients with biliary pancreatitis than those with alcoholic pancreatitis *5022* Activity of 3,503 U/L higher in patients with pancreatic necrosis than in those without necrosis *2359*
Urine *Increase* Overall activity higher in patients with biliary pancreatitis than those with alcoholic pancreatitis *5022*

Aspartate Aminotransferase *Serum* *Increase* Activity high but significantly higher in patients with pancreatic necrosis than

577.00 Pancreatitis *(continued)*

Aspartate Aminotransferase *(continued)* in those without necrosis *2359* Overall activity higher in patients with biliary pancreatitis than those with alcoholic pancreatitis *5022*

Bilirubin *Serum Increase* Concentration high but significantly higher in patients with pancreatic necrosis than in those without necrosis *2359*

CA 72-4 *Serum Increase* In 52 patients with pancreatitis 4 (8%) had a concentration greater than cut-off of 2.5 U/mL with median concentration of 1.3 U/mL *4505*

Carcinoembryonic Antigen *Serum Increase* In 52 patients with pancreatitis 15 (29%) had a concentration greater than cut-off of 3 ng/mL with median concentration of 1.9 ng/mL *4505* In 95 patients with pancreatitis 47% had concentrations less than 2.5 ng/mL, 31% had concentrations between 2.6 and 5.0 ng/mL, 18% had concentrations between 5.1 and 10.0 ng/mL and 1% had a concentration greater than 10.0 ng/mL *2010*

α-Fetoprotein *Serum No Effect* In 38 patients with pancreatitis 100.0% had concentrations up to 15.0 ng/mL in comparison with concentrations in 400 healthy individuals in whom 99.2% had concentrations between 0 and 15.0 ng/mL, 0.2% between 15.1 and 20.0 ng/mL and 0.5%% between 20.1 and 100 ng/mL *11*

Lactate Dehydrogenase *Serum Increase* Activity high but significantly higher in patients with pancreatic necrosis than in those without necrosis *2359*

Lactate Dehydrogenase:Aspartate Aminotransferase Ratio *Serum Decrease* Ratio low (less than 6) on postadmission days 1 and 2 *2359*
Serum Increase Ratio low (less than 6) on postadmission days 1 and 2 but then peaked at 19.2 to 97.5 on day 7 for 5 patients with pancreatic necrosis: ratio reached about 12 in 17 patients without necrosis and in 50 healthy controls *2359*

Lipase *Serum Increase* Mean activity in 25 patients with nonalcoholic pancreatitis of 226 U/L higher than 154 U/L in 11 patients with alcoholic pancreatitis and reference interval of 4 - 24 U/L *145*

Lipase:Amylase Ratio *Serum Increase* Ratio higher in patients with alcoholic pancreatitis than those with biliary pancreatitis *5022*

α_2-Macroglobulin *Serum Decrease* Concentration reduced in proteolytic diseases such as pancreatitis *2952*

MCV *Blood Increase* MCV higher in patients with alcoholic pancreatitis than those with biliary pancreatitis *5022*

Multiubiquitin Chains *Serum No Effect* In 5 patients with pancreatitis mean concentration of 5.7 ± 4.8 ng/mL not significantly different from 4.1 ± 1.7 ng/mL in 10 healthy controls *5126*

Triglycerides *Serum Increase* In patients with hyperlipidemic pancreatitis triglyceride concentration above 500 mg/dL (in one study they ranged from 600 to 17,770 mg/dL) *1533*

Ubiquitin, Free *Serum No Effect* In 5 patients with pancreatitis mean concentration of 33.6 ± 11.5 ng/mL not significantly different from 29.6 ± 6.6 ng/mL in 10 healthy controls *5126*

577.10 Chronic Pancreatitis

Albumin *Ascitic Fluid Increase* Elevation (> 2.9 g/dL) is characteristic *4891*
Serum Decrease In 27% of 11 patients at initial hospitalization for this disorder *1576* Mild depression may occur *4891*

Alkaline Phosphatase *Serum Increase* In 40% of 12 patients at initial hospitalization for this disorder *1576* In each of 6 male alcoholic patients with calcific disease, a marked elevation was associated with minimal elevation in serum bilirubin or BSP excretion *4918* Jaundice may occur not only during acute attacks but also during the silent stage. Usually due to extrahepatic cholestasis an elevated alkaline phosphatase and normal AST at the early stages tend to support this *900*

Amylase *Ascitic Fluid Increase* Greatly increased in pancreatic ascites *4891*
Pleural Fluid Increase With pancreatic pseudocyst *4746* Pleural effusions occur in about 10% of pancreatitis patients, with amylase commonly elevated *3052* Pleural fluid pH of < 7.20 or 0.15 below arterial pH frequently occurs in parapneumonic effusion *3052* Elevated in primary or metastatic lung cancer, pancreatitis, or esophageal perforation *4537*
Saliva Decrease Salivary output, amylase, and HCO_3 concentration decreased in 88% of patients *2531*
Serum Increase Hyperamylasemia in acute exacerbation sometimes accompanied by a transient elevation in salivary type isoamylase (S-amylase) *5526* Mean activity in 8 patients with chronic pancreatitis and diabetes mellitus of 98 ± 28 U/L significantly different from 56 ± 15 U/L in 3 patients with chronic pancreatitis but with normal OGTT *2175* Usually normal during quiescent phase. Rises as chronic damage progresses, but tends to become less pronounced. May actually be normal during relapse *4537* May be found, especially if the blood is drawn early in the attack. With each succeeding episode, however, pancreatic exocrine function decreases and the likelihood of finding an elevated amylase diminishes *2039*
Serum No Effect Usually normal during quiescent phase. Rises as chronic damage progresses but tends to become less pronounced. May actually be normal during relapse *4537* As disease progresses and more of the gland is destroyed, acute pancreatitis may occur without elevation *4891*

Androstanediol Glucuronide *Plasma No Effect* Mean concentration in 12 male patients with chronic pancreatitis of 21.6 ± 15.1 nmol/L not significantly different from 9.8 - 43.3 nmol/L in 40 healthy men *2416*

Androstenedione *Plasma No Effect* Mean concentration in 12 male patients with chronic pancreatitis of 5.7 ± 3.8 nmol/L not significantly different from 2.8 - 7.5 nmol/L in 40 healthy men *2416*

Aspartate Aminotransferase *Serum Increase* In 48% of 12 patients at initial hospitalization for this disorder *1576*

Bicarbonate *Saliva Decrease* Salivary output, amylase, and (HCO_3) concentration decreased in 88% of patients *2531*

CA 19-9 *Serum Increase* Majority of concentrations in 12 male patients with chronic pancreatitis less than 37 U/L *2416* In 105 patients with chronic pancreatitis positive rate of 24% observed using cut-off from normals and 20% at 90% specificity *2594* In 7.1% of 70 patients with cancer other than pancreatic cancer concentration increased above cut-off of 37 U/mL *2854* Positive analyses have been encountered *3657* CA 19-9 concentration increased above 37 U/mL in 2 of 30 (6.7%) patients with chronic pancreatitis in one study and 27% of 66 patients in another study *1253* Positive analyses have been encountered *2026* Concentration increased in 5 of 7 patients with chronic pancreatitis *411*

CA 242 *Serum Increase* In 105 patients with chronic pancreatitis positive rate of 14% observed using cut-off from normals and 21% at 90% specificity *2594*

Calcium *Serum Decrease* Malnutrition is the result of the malabsorption of fat, proteins, and fat-soluble vitamins which results in low concentrations *900*

Carcinoembryonic Antigen *Serum Increase* Concentration increased in 2 of 8 patients with chronic pancreatitis *411* In 14.3% of 70 patients with chronic pancreatitis concentration increased above cut-off of 37 U/mL *2854*

Carnitine *Serum Decrease* In 12 patients with chronic pancreatitis fasting mean serum concentration significantly less than in age and sex matched controls *2435*

Carnitine, Free *Serum Decrease* In 12 patients with chronic pancreatitis mean concentration significantly less than in age and sex matched healthy controls *2435*

Carotene *Serum Decrease* With malabsorption *4960*

Cholesterol *Serum Increase* Some cases *1290*

Chymotrypsin *Feces Decrease* In 8 patients with mild chronic pancreatic insufficiency mean excretion of 9.3 ± 3.6 U/g and 5 ± 1 U/g in 14 patients with moderate pancreatitis and 2 ± 1 U/g in 22 patients with severe chronic pancreatic insufficiency significantly reduced compared with 15 ± U/g in 50 healthy controls *3133* Found to be a more reliable measure of pancreatic function than trypsin activity. False positives have been noted in 10% of controls, and normal values may occur in patients *110*

C-Peptide *Plasma No Effect* Mean baseline concentration in 8 patients with chronic pancreatitis and diabetes mellitus of approximately 0.4 nmol/L not significantly different from approximately 0.5 nmol/L in 3 patients with chronic pancreatitis but with normal OGTT *2175*

Dehydroepiandrosterone Sulfate *Plasma* *No Effect* Mean concentration in 12 male patients with chronic pancreatitis of 5.0 ± 2.7 μmol/L not significantly different from 2.1 - 11.3 μmol/L in 40 healthy men *2416*

Dihydrotestosterone *Serum* *Increase* Mean concentration in 12 male patients with chronic pancreatitis of 4.1 ± 1.7 nmol/L significantly different from 0.9 - 5.8 nmol/L in 40 healthy men *2416*

EL-1 *Serum* *Increase* In 25.7% of 70 patients with chronic pancreatitis concentration increased above cut-off of 37 U/mL *2854*

Elastase 1 *Feces* *Decrease* In 8 patients with mild chronic pancreatic insufficiency mean excretion of 208 ± 88 μg/g and 28 ± 8 μg/g in 14 patients with moderate pancreatitis and 12.5 ± 5.6 μg/g in 22 patients with severe chronic pancreatic insufficiency significantly reduced compared with 602 ± 38 μg/g in 50 healthy controls *3133*

Eosinophils *Blood* *Increase* In 21 of 122 patients (17.2%) with chronic pancreatitis marked eosinophilia above 500 /μL observed *5243*
Pleural Fluid *Increase* Eosinophilia greater than 10% may be present *126*

Epidermal Growth Factor *Serum* *Increase* In 15 patients with chronic pancreatitis mean concentration of 24.2 ± 6.2 μg/L significantly different from 17.7 ± 3.8 μg/L in 22 healthy controls *3439*

Erythrocytes *Ascitic Fluid* *No Effect* Variable amount noted *233*
Pleural Fluid *Increase* 1,000 - 10,000 /μL *4493*

Fat *Feces* *Increase* Deficiency intraluminal pancreatic enzymes *4891* The number and size of fecal fat globules correlate with the degree of steatorrhea *1240*

Fibronectin *Plasma* *No Effect* Studied in 32 patients with pancreatitis. Patients were subdivided by clinical and biochemical criteria: severe acute pancreatitis (n = 10), moderate acute pancreatitis (n = 17), and acute attack of chronic pancreatitis (n = 5). During an acute attack all parameters were within the reference range *36*

Fibronectin Fragment *Urine* *Increase* Maximum levels were seen on the first day of admission for an acute exacerbation *5140*

Glucagon *Plasma* *Decrease* Decreased *618 1038 1290*
Plasma *No Effect* Mean baseline concentration in 8 patients with chronic pancreatitis and diabetes mellitus of approximately 24 pmol/L not significantly different from approximately 33 pmol/L in 3 patients with chronic pancreatitis but with normal OGTT *2175*

Glucagon-like Peptide-1 *Serum* *No Effect* Mean baseline concentration in 8 patients with chronic pancreatitis and diabetes mellitus of approximately 37 pmol/L not significantly different from approximately 28 pmol/L in 3 patients with chronic pancreatitis but with normal OGTT *2175*

Glucose *Pleural Fluid* *Decrease* Usually decreased in an exudate *126*
Serum *Increase* Mean concentration in 8 patients with chronic pancreatitis and diabetes mellitus of 8.7 ± 1.6 mmol/L significantly different from 4.6 ± 0.1 mmol/L in 3 patients with chronic pancreatitis but with normal OGTT *2175* In 27% of 11 patients at initial hospitalization for this disorder *1576* Increased circulating epinephrine *1290* Some cases *5544*

Glucose Tolerance *Serum* *Decrease* There will be a diabetic oral test in 65% of patients and frank diabetes in > 10% of patients *5544* Of 50 patients with chronic relapsing pancreatitis, 66% had evidence of glucose intolerance *1980*

γ-Glutamyltransferase *Serum* *Increase* Observed in some patients *4484* Increased when there is involvement of the biliary tract or active inflammation *5544*

Hemoglobin A_{1c} *Blood* *Increase* Mean concentration in 8 patients with chronic pancreatitis and diabetes mellitus of 8.0 ± 1.2% significantly different from 4.5 ± 0.8% in 3 patients with chronic pancreatitis but with normal OGTT *2175*

Hyaluronic Acid *Serum* *Increase* A total of 52 patients with pancreatitis were studied (acute pancreatitis = 17; chronic pancreatitis = 35) and compared to 194 controls. Patients with pancreatitis displayed elevated levels in all groups, when compared with the controls *3107*
Serum *No Effect* Studied in 32 patients with pancreatitis. Patients were subdivided by clinical and biochemical criteria: severe acute pancreatitis (n = 10), moderate acute pancreatitis (n = 17), and acute attack of chronic pancreatitis (n = 5). Serum and plasma samples were collected on days 1 - 7, 10, 14, and 21. During an acute attack all parameters were within the reference range *36*

Hydroxyproline *Urine* *Increase* High levels were observed on the second to fifth day after an acute exacerbation *5140*

Insulin *Plasma* *No Effect* Mean baseline concentration in 8 patients with chronic pancreatitis and diabetes mellitus of approximately 20 pmol/L not significantly different from approximately 30 pmol/L in 3 patients with chronic pancreatitis but with normal OGTT *2175*

Insulin-like Growth Factor-I *Serum* *Increase* In 15 patients with chronic pancreatitis mean concentration of 180.9 ± 46.4 μg/L not significantly different from 103.3 ± 22.0 μg/L in 22 healthy controls *3439*

Isocitrate Dehydrogenase *Serum* *No Effect* No effect observed on activity *5008*

Lactate Dehydrogenase *Pleural Fluid* *Increase* Exudate *126*

Laminin *Serum* *Increase* A total of 52 patients with pancreatitis were studied (acute pancreatitis = 17; chronic pancreatitis = 35) and compared to 194 controls. Patients with pancreatitis displayed elevated levels in all groups, when compared with the controls *3107*
Serum *No Effect* Studied in 32 patients with pancreatitis. Patients were subdivided by clinical and biochemical criteria: severe acute pancreatitis (n = 10), moderate acute pancreatitis (n = 17), and acute attack of chronic pancreatitis (n = 5). During an acute attack all parameters were within the reference range *36*

Leukocytes *Ascitic Fluid* *No Effect* Variable *233*
Blood *Increase* In 27% of 11 patients at initial hospitalization for this disorder *1576*
Pleural Fluid *Increase* 5,000 - 20,000 /μL *4493*

Lipase *Serum* *Increase* As functioning tissue is destroyed, it is not uncommon to find only normal levels *4960* Activity may be increased in chronic pancreatitis *5231*
Serum *No Effect* As functioning tissue is destroyed, it is not uncommon to find only normal levels *4960*

Lipids *Feces* *Increase* Reduced intraluminal pancreatic enzyme activity with maldigestion of lipid and protein *1980*
Serum *Increase* Reported effect *1290*

α_2-Macroglobulin *Serum* *Increase* Reported effect *3480*

Magnesium *Serum* *Decrease* Concentration is reduced in association with malabsorption of chronic pancreatitis *2952* May occur *5507*

β_2-Microglobulin *Serum* *Increase* In 34 patitients with chronic pancreatitis median concentration of 1.5 mg/L (range 1.0 - 4.5 mg/L) significantly higher than concentration in 40 healthy individuals (median 1.2 mg/L with central 95th percentile range of 0.9 - 1.6 mg/L) *4111*

Neutrophils *Blood* *Increase* In 36% of 11 patients at initial hospitalization for this disorder *1576*
Pleural Fluid *Increase* Predominant cell type *4493* Neutrophils predominate in pleural fluid *3052*

Nitrogen *Feces* *Increase* Increase of total nitrogen observed *1290* Excretion of > 2.5 g total nitrogen/d usually found in cases of chronic progressive pancreatitis compared with normal range of 1 - 2 g/d *2952*

Occult Blood *Feces* *Increase* Reported effect *4891*

pH *Pleural Fluid* *Decrease* Exudate (pH < 7.3) *126*

Phospholipids *Serum* *Increase* Increase in cholesterol, phospholipids and neutral fats *1290*

Procollagen Type III Peptide *Serum* *Increase* A total of 52 patients with pancreatitis were studied (acute pancreatitis = 17; chronic pancreatitis = 35) and compared to 194 controls. Patients with pancreatitis displayed elevated levels in all groups, when compared with the controls *3107*
Serum *No Effect* Studied in 32 patients with pancreatitis. Patients were subdivided by clinical and biochemical criteria: severe acute pancreatitis (n = 10), moderate acute pancreatitis (n = 17), and acute attack of chronic pancreatitis (n = 5). During an acute attack all parameters were within the reference range *36*

577.10 Chronic Pancreatitis *(continued)*

Protein *Ascitic Fluid* *Increase* Variable but often > 2.5 g/dL in ascitic fluid *233*
Feces *Increase* Reduced intraluminal pancreatic enzyme activity with maldigestion of lipid and protein *1980*
Peritoneal Fluid *Increase* Greater than 30 g/L in 70% of cases of pancreatic ascites *1216*
Pleural Fluid *Increase* Exudate (> 3 g/dL) *126*

Scan1 *Serum* *Increase* In 18.6% of 70 patients with chronic pancreatitis concentration increased above cut-off of 37 U/mL *2854*

Sodium *Sweat* *Increase* Concentrations exceeded 90 mmol/L in 26% and 120 mmol/L in 6% of noncalcific pancreatitis patients *278*

Soluble Interleukin-2 Receptor *Serum* *Increase* In 34 patients with chronic pancreatitis median concentration of 479 U/mL (range 125 - 1,268 U/mL) significantly higher than concentration in 40 healthy individuals (median 260 U/mL with central 95th percentile range of 170 - 388 U/mL) *4111*

Somatostatin *Plasma* *Increase* In 15 patients with chronic pancreatitis mean concentration of 89.1 ± 22.8 ng/L significantly different from 29.7 ± 6.3 ng/L in 22 healthy controls *3439*

Specific Gravity *Pleural Fluid* *Increase* Exudate (> 1.016) *126*

Testosterone *Serum* *Increase* Mean concentration in 12 male patients with chronic pancreatitis of 19.2 ± 5.8 nmol/L significantly different from 7.4 - 37 nmol/L in 40 healthy men *2416*

Thiobarbituric Acid-reacting Substances *Serum* *Increase* In 11 patients with chronic pancreatitis mean concentration of thiobarbituric acid-reactive substances of 1.45 ± 0.18 μmol/L compared with 1.01 ± 0.21 μmol/L in 47 healthy individuals *5585*

Triglycerides *Serum* *Increase* Increase in cholesterol, phospholipids, and neutral fats *1290*

Triolein ^{131}I Test *Feces* *Positive* Abnormal in 33% of patients *5544*

Trypsin *Serum* *Increase* Mean circulatory concentration in 16 cases was 433 U/L. Normal < 100 U/L *3734*

Trypsin-like Immunoreactivity *Serum* *Decrease* In 9 of 12 patients with severe pancreatic exocrine sufficiency (enzyme output below 25% of the normal minimum) had very low trypsin-like immunoreactivity *1911*
Serum *Increase* In 8 of 8 patients with mild or moderate pancreatic exocrine sufficiency (enzyme output above 25% of the normal minimum) mean concentration above normal range of 8 - 44 ng/mL in healthy adults *1911*

Trypsinogen-2 *Urine* *Increase* Urinary dipstick gave false positive result for acute pancreatitis in 2 patients with chronic pancreatitis *2633*

Vitamin A *Serum* *Decrease* Some cases *1290*

Xylose Tolerance Test *Urine* *Abnormal* With malabsorption *4960*

577.20 Pancreatic Cyst and Pseudocyst

Alkaline Phosphatase *Serum* *Increase* Increased in 10% of patients *5544*

Amylase *Ascitic Fluid* *Increase* Greatly increased in pancreatic ascites *4891*
Serum *Increase* Laboratory findings preceding acute pancreatitis are present (mild and unrecognized in 33% of cases). Persistent increase after an acute episode may indicate formation of a pseudocyst *5544* Persistent increase 4 - 6 weeks following onset of pancreatitis suggests pseudocyst. 77% of 78 patients had hyperamylasemia at diagnosis *4537*
Urine *Increase* Persistent increase 4 - 6 weeks after onset of pancreatitis suggests pseudocyst. Hyperamylasuria is usual but not invariable *4537*

Bicarbonate *Duodenal Contents* *Decrease* Duodenal contents after secretin-pancreozymin stimulation usually show decreased bicarbonate content (< 70 mmol/L) but normal volume and normal content of amylase, lipase, and trypsin *5544*

Bilirubin *Serum* *Increase* Serum direct bilirubin is increased (> 2 mg/dL) in 10% of patients *5544* Occasionally elevated *900*

Bilirubin, Direct *Serum* *Increase* Increased (> 2 mg/dL) in 10% of patients *5544*

Glucose *Pleural Fluid* *No Effect* Pleural fluid and serum concentrations are similar *4493*
Serum *Increase* Occasionally there is an associated elevation of the fasting blood sugar level *900*

Leukocytes *Pleural Fluid* *Increase* 5,000 - 20,000 /μL *4493*

Lipase *Duodenal Contents* *No Effect* Duodenal contents after secretin-pancreozymin stimulation usually show decreased bicarbonate content (< 80 mmol/L) but normal volume and normal content of amylase, lipase, and trypsin *5544*
Serum *Increase* Laboratory findings preceding acute pancreatitis are present (this is mild and unrecognized in 33% of the cases). Persistent increase of serum amylase and lipase after an acute episode may indicate formation of a pseudocyst *5544* May be elevated after recent attack of pancreatitis in pseudocyst *900*

pH *Pleural Fluid* *Decrease* Exudate (pH < 7.3) *126*

Protein *Pleural Fluid* *Increase* Exudate *4493*

Specific Gravity *Pleural Fluid* *Increase* Exudate (> 1.016) *126*

Trypsin *Duodenal Contents* *No Effect* Duodenal contents after secretin-pancreozymin stimulation usually show decreased bicarbonate content (< 80 mmol/L) but normal volume and normal content of amylase, lipase, and trypsin *5544*

Volume *Duodenal Contents* *No Effect* Duodenal contents after secretin-pancreozymin stimulation usually show decreased bicarbonate content (< 80 mmol/L) but normal volume and normal content of amylase, lipase, and trypsin *5544*

577.80 Obstruction of Pancreatic Duct

Lipase *Serum* *Increase* Activity mey be increased in patients with obstruction of the pancreatic duct *5231*

577.90 Benign Pancreatic Disease

CA 19-9 *Serum* *Increase* In 42 patients with benign pancreatic disease 12% had a serum concentration greater than 37 U/mL *1957*

CA 242 *Serum* *Increase* In 42 patients with benign pancreatic disease, 7% had a serum concentration greater than 20 U/mL *1957*

577.90 Non-malignant Disease of the Pancreas

γ-Glutamyltransferase *Serum* *Increase* Activity reportedly increased in a variety of diseases including diseases of the pancreas, myocardium, kidney and lung as well as in diabetes *4617* Increased activity reported with pancreatic disorders *3625*

5-Nucleotide Phosphodiesterase Isoenzyme V
Serum *Increase* Mean activity was increased in the plasma of 59% of 161 patients with non-malignant disease of the liver, pancreas or biliary system *1781*

578.90 Gastrointestinal Bleeding

Urea:Creatinine Ratio *Serum* *Increase* Mean ratio of 22.5 with upper gastrointestinal bleeding and 15.8 with lower gastrointestinal bleeding *756*

579.00 Celiac Disease

Acylcarnitine *Serum* *No Effect* In 12 children with active celiac disease mean concentration of 6.4 ± 4.2 μmol/L not significantly different from 9.1 ± 5.3 μmol/L in 7 with inactive disease and 9.9 ± 6.5 μmol/L in 17 control symptomatic children with gastrointestinal disorders. Normal range of 10.0 ± 7.4 μmol/L *2998*

Alanine Aminotransferase *Serum* *Increase* In 158 adults with celiac disease hypertransaminasemia was identified in 67 (42%) *293* In 158 adult patients with celiac disease mean activity increased in 67 (42%) to 61 U/L (range 25 to 470 U/L) *293*

Albumin *Serum* *Decrease* Reflects possible malabsorption of protein or protein-losing enteropathy *1980* May be diminished owing to excessive leakage of serum protein into the gut lumen *4891*

Alkaline Phosphatase *Serum* *Decrease* Reported effect *3160*
Serum *Increase* In 42 symptomatic adult patients mean activity of 27.6 ± 4.3 King-Armstrong units significantly different from reference range of 5 - 15 King-Armstrong units *3388* Leading to secondary osteomalacia *1290* Suggestive of secondary hyperparathyroidism *900*
Serum *No Effect* Mean activity in 9 children with celiac disease of 217 U/L not significantly different from 155 U/L in 28 healthy controls *757*

Amino Acids *Plasma* *Increase* Found in celiac disease and idiopathic steatorrhea if liver damage is also present *1290*

Anti-Endomysial IgA Antibodies *Serum* *Increase* Observed in 87% of 97 patients with celiac disease and in 1% of nonceliac controls *1442* In 55 patients with celiac disease in children < 5 y up to and including adults sensitivity for disease 98.2% and specificity 100% *196* In 100 patients with celiac disease 100 had detectable antibodies compared with 0 of 52 healthy controls *4588* In 21 of 27 children with coeliac disease (78%) IgA-antiendomysium antibodies at presentation *1879*

Anti-Gliadin Antibodies *Serum* *Increase* 24 of 27 children with coeliac disease (89%) had IgA-antigliadin antibodies at presentation *1879*

Anti-Gliadin IgA Antibodies *Feces* *Increase* In 19 patients with untreated celiac disease mean concentration of 24 AU significantly higher than 4.5 AU in 12 control individuals *1944*
Serum *Increase* Mean concentration in 19 patients with untreated celiac disease 44 AU compared with 2 AU in controls *1944* In 55 patients with celiac disease in children < 5 y up to and including adults sensitivity for disease 90.9% and specificity 98.5% *196* Observed in 69% of 97 patients with celiac disease and in 29% of nonceliac controls *1442* In 100 patients with celiac disease 55 had detectable antibodies compared with 0 of 52 healthy controls *4588*

Anti-Gliadin IgG Antibodies *Serum* *Increase* In 55 patients with celiac disease in children < 5 y up to and including adults sensitivity for disease 96.4% and specificity 69.2% *196* In 100 patients with celiac disease, 78 had detectable antibodies compared with 7 of 52 healthy controls *4588*

Anti-Jejunum Antibodies (Human) *Serum* *Increase* In 100 patients with celiac disease 100 had detectable antibodies compared with 0 of 52 healthy controls *4588* In 55 patients with celiac disease in children < 5 y up to and including adults sensitivity for disease 100% and specificity 72.3% *196*

Anti-Jejunum Antibodies (Rat) *Serum* *Increase* In 55 patients with celiac disease in children < 5 y up to and including adults sensitivity for disease 100% and specificity 83.1% *196*

Anti-Reticulin IgA Antibodies *Serum* *Increase* In 55 patients with celiac disease in children < 5 y up to and including adults sensitivity for disease 88.9% and specificity 72.3% *196*

Antibody Titer *Serum* *Increase* Antibodies to reticulin found in 78% of cases *3712*

Apolipoprotein A-I *Serum* *Decrease* In 17 Algerian patients with untreated celiac disease mean concentration of 1.04 ± 0.19 g/L significantly different from 1.22 ± 0.14 g/L in 34 healthy controls *3436*

Apolipoprotein A-II *Serum* *No Effect* In 17 Algerian patients with untreated celiac disease mean concentration of 0.27 ± 0.07 g/L not significantly different from 0.27 ± 0.08 g/L in 34 healthy controls *3436*

Apolipoprotein A-IV *Serum* *No Effect* In 17 Algerian patients with untreated celiac disease mean concentration of 0.16 ± 0.07 g/L not significantly different from 0.16 ± 0.05 g/L in 34 healthy controls *3436*

Apolipoprotein B *Serum* *No Effect* In 17 Algerian patients with untreated celiac disease mean concentration of 0.74 ± 0.15 g/L not significantly different from 0.83 ± 0.19 g/L in 34 healthy controls *3436*

Apolipoprotein C-II *Serum* *No Effect* In 17 Algerian patients with untreated celiac disease mean concentration of 0.010 ± 0.004 g/L not significantly different from 0.01 ± 0.00 g/L in 34 healthy controls *3436*

Apolipoprotein C-III *Serum* *No Effect* In 17 Algerian patients with untreated celiac disease mean concentration of 0.02 ± 0.01 g/L not significantly different from 0.02 ± 0.01 g/L in 34 healthy controls *3436*

Apolipoprotein E *Serum* *No Effect* In 17 Algerian patients with untreated celiac disease mean concentration of 0.06 ± 0.04 g/L not significantly different from 0.05 ± 0.02 g/L in 34 healthy controls *3436*

Ascorbic Acid *Serum* *No Effect* Concentration usually unaffected by disease *4960*

Aspartate Aminotransferase *Serum* *Increase* In 158 adult patients with celiac disease mean activity increased in 67 (42%) to 47 U/L (range 30 to 190 U/L) *293* In 158 adults with celiac disease hypertransaminasemia was identified in 67 (42%) *293*

Bicarbonate *Feces* *Increase* In occasional patients, significant metabolic acidosis can develop in association with bicarbonate loss in the stool *4891*
Serum *Decrease* If diarrhea is severe, marked electrolyte depletion *4891*

Calcium *Feces* *Increase* In steatorrhea *1290*
Serum *Decrease* In 50% of untreated patients, concentration may be less than 9 mg/dL *4960* Often decreased in patients with diarrhea and steatorrhea *4891* An indication of vitamin D and calcium malabsorption *1980*
Serum *No Effect* In 42 symptomatic adult patients mean concentration of 9.0 ± 0.2 mg/dL not different from reference range of 8.5 - 10.5 mg/dL *3388* Mean concentration in 9 children with celiac disease of 9.4 mg/dL not significantly different from 9.5 mg/dL in 28 healthy controls *757*

Carcinoembryonic Antigen *Serum* *Increase* In adult celiac disease, 2 of 9 patients had concentrations > 12.5 ng/mL (normal < 12.5 ng/mL) *528*

Carnitine *Serum* *Decrease* In 12 children with active celiac disease mean concentration of 39.7 ± 3.8 μmol/L significantly less than 50.1 ± 3.3 μmol/L in 7 with nonactive disease and 53.2 ± 5.1 μmol/L 17 symptomatic controls. Normal range of 51.5 ± 6.5 μmol/L *2998*

Carnitine, Free *Serum* *No Effect* In 12 patients with active celiac disease mean concentration of 33.7 ± 4.2 μmol/L not significantly different from 41.1 ± 9.2 μmol/L in 7 with nonactive disease and 43.4 ± 11.3 μmol/L in 17 symptomatic controls with other gastrointestinal diseases. Normal range of 38.5 ± 12.6 μmol/L *2998*

Carotene *Serum* *Decrease* Usually depressed in patients with sufficient intestinal involvement to produce steatorrhea *4891* At the time of the initial diagnosis, most patients have steatorrhea, low serum carotene levels, abnormal D-xylose absorption, and an abnormal small bowel X-ray pattern *2039* A useful indication of fat malabsorption low levels are found in as many as 80% of patients with steatorrhea *1980*

Ceruloplasmin *Serum* *Decrease* Moderate transient deficiencies in patients with nephrosis *5544*

Chloride *Serum* *Decrease* If diarrhea is severe, marked electrolyte depletion *4891*

Cholesterol *Serum* *Decrease* In 17 Algerian patients with untreated celiac disease mean concentration of 3.38 ± 0.64 mmol/L significantly different from 4.18 ± 0.59 mmol/L in 34 healthy controls *3436* Malnutrition due to malabsorption *1290* Usually depressed in patients with sufficient intestinal involvement to produce steatorrhea *4891* In 6 patients with celiac disease mean concentration of 3.66 mmol/L reduced below normal *5501*

Cholinesterase *Serum* *Decrease* May be decreased in some cases of malnutrition in which albumin is decreased *5544*

Complement C_3 *Serum* *Decrease* Found in 28% of patients *3550*

Copper *Serum* *Decrease* Decreased in sprue and celiac disease in infants as a result of the inability to synthesize the apoprotein *1290* Plasma zinc and copper depression was found in 10 adult patients. These findings further indicate that trace metal deficiency is another common nutritional complication *4929*

1,25-Dihydroxy Vitamin D *Serum* *Increase* Mean concentration in 9 children with celiac disease of 69.1 pg/mL significantly different from 24.1 pg/mL in 28 healthy controls *757*

24,25-Dihydroxy Vitamin D *Serum* *Decrease* Mean concentration in 9 children with celiac disease of 0.7 ng/mL significantly different from 2.0 ng/mL in 28 healthy controls *757*

579.00 Celiac Disease *(continued)*

Fat *Feces Increase* In small intestinal disease *4891* If the coefficient of fat absorption is < 93%, steatorrhea is present *4891* Due to allergy to gluten (wheat protein) *1290*

Ferritin *Serum Decrease* The most discriminating test to distinguish between untreated celiac disease and other gastrointestinal disorders in the pediatric age group *4945*

Folate *Serum Decrease* Folic acid deficiency occurring in idiopathic steatorrhea (up to 80 mg/h) *5544* Observed effect *367* Patients may show a megaloblastic anemia and leukopenia secondary to folic acid or vitamin B_{12} deficiency. In these instances low serum folate and B_{12} levels will be found *900*

γ-Globulin *Serum Decrease* May be diminished owing to excessive leakage of serum protein into the gut lumen *4891*

Glucose Tolerance *Serum Increase* Flat curve in celiac disease and diseases of intestinal wall and in monosaccharide malabsorption *367*

Growth Hormone *Plasma Decrease* Insulin-induced growth hormone secretion is inadequate in most cases during the active phase, but returns to normal on recovery provided the diet is gluten-free *5422*

HDL-Cholesterol *Serum Decrease* In 6 patients with celiac disease mean concentration of 0.89 ± 0.06 mmol/L reduced below normal *5501* In 17 Algerian patients with untreated celiac disease mean concentration of 0.98 ± 0.26 mmol/L significantly different from 1.34 ± 0.26 mmol/L in 34 healthy controls *3436*

HDL-Phospholipids *Serum Decrease* In 17 Algerian patients with untreated celiac disease mean concentration of 1.28 ± 0.19 mmol/L significantly different from 1.55 ± 0.20 mmol/L in 34 healthy controls *3436*

HDL-Triglycerides *Serum No Effect* In 17 Algerian patients with untreated celiac disease mean concentration of 0.45 ± 0.17 mmol/L not significantly different from 0.39 ± 0.09 mmol/L in 34 healthy controls *3436*

Hematocrit *Blood Decrease* Characteristic iron-deficiency anemia. The peripheral blood smear may show hypochromia. In some cases iron-deficiency anemia may be the predominant abnormality indicative of malabsorption *900*

Hemoglobin *Blood Decrease* Characteristic iron-deficiency anemia. The peripheral blood smear may show hypochromia. In some cases iron-deficiency anemia may be the predominant abnormality indicative of malabsorption *900*

HLA Antigens *Blood Present* HLA-DR3 found in 96% of patients versus 27% of controls *5678* HLA-B_8 and DRw3 are found *1588*

25-Hydroxy Vitamin D_3 *Serum Decrease* Reported effect *4960*
Serum No Effect In 42 symptomatic adult patients mean concentration of 22.7 ± 3.5 ng/dL not different from reference range of 8 - 40 ng/dL *3388*

25-Hydroxy Vitamin D *Serum No Effect* Mean concentration in 9 children with celiac disease of 29.2 ng/mL not significantly different from 31.5 ng/mL in 28 healthy controls *757*

17-Hydroxycorticosteroids *Urine Decrease* In patients with sufficient malabsorption to cause pituitary or adrenal insufficiency *5679*

5-Hydroxyindoleacetic Acid *Urine Increase* Excretion may be increased in patients with celiac disease due to overproduction of serotonin in the cells of the small intestine *1778* Abnormal tryptophan metabolism may result in elevated urinary excretion in patients with malabsorption *4891* In a 23-year old man celiac disease urinary excretion of 53 μmol/d observed compared with less than 42 μmol/d in 47 normal male volunteers *1168* Modest increases observed in patients with celiac disease *2952* Slightly increased level (12-16 mg/24 h) *2034*

5-Hydroxytryptamine *Blood Increase* In a 23-year old man celiac disease first presented with two fasting 5-HT concentrations of 542 and 798 μg/L compared with 85 ± 36 μg/L in 47 normal male volunteers *1168*
Plasma Increase In untreated disease. The values declined with treatment *4880*

IDL-Cholesterol *Serum Decrease* In 6 patients with celiac disease mean concentration of 0.07 ± 0.01 mmol/L reduced below normal *5501*

IgA Anti-Tissue Transglutaminase Antibodies
Serum Increase 99.1% patients had increased titers against tTG whereas 94.7% of the control sera were negative *1166*

immunoglobulin A *Serum Increase* May be increased *4960*

Immunoglobulin M *Serum Decrease* Reported low in 37% of patients *4960*

Insulin-like Growth Factor-I *Serum Decrease* Mean concentration in 9 children with celiac disease of 108 ng/mL significantly different from 240 ng/mL in 28 healthy controls *757*

Interleukin-1 Receptor Antagonist *Serum No Effect* In 1 of 14 patients with celiac disease mean concentration greater than upper limit of normal of 410 pg/mL (difference not significant) *1529*

Interleukin-1β *Serum No Effect* In 13 of 14 patients with celiac disease mean concentration greater than upper limit of normal of 3.9 pg/mL (difference not significant) *1529*

Interleukin-6 *Serum No Effect* In 12 of 16 patients with celiac disease mean concentration greater than upper limit of normal of 2.8 pg/mL *1529*

Iron *Serum Decrease* Very common, because the duodenal lesion usually impairs iron absorption in the untreated patient *4891* Characteristic iron-deficiency anemia. In some cases, may be the predominant abnormality indicative of malabsorption *900*

Iron-binding Capacity, Total *Serum Increase* Characteristic iron deficiency anemia *900*

Iron Saturation *Serum Decrease* Characteristic iron deficiency anemia *900*

17-Ketosteroids *Urine Decrease* In patients with sufficient malabsorption to cause pituitary or adrenal insufficiency *5679*

LDL-Apolipoprotein B *Serum No Effect* In 6 patients with celiac disease mean concentration of 58.2 ± 3.3 mg/dL not significantly different from 56.0 ± 3.5 mg/dL in healthy controls *5501*

LDL-Cholesterol *Serum Decrease* In 17 Algerian patients with untreated celiac disease mean concentration of 1.96 ± 0.51 mmol/L significantly different from 2.42 ± 0.54 mmol/L in 34 healthy controls *3436* In 6 patients with celiac disease mean concentration of 2.61 ± 0.19 mmol/L reduced below normal *5501*

LDL-Phospholipids *Serum Decrease* In 17 Algerian patients with untreated celiac disease mean concentration of 0.57 ± 0.21 mmol/L significantly different from 0.79 ± 0.22 mmol/L in 34 healthy controls *3436*

LDL-Triglycerides *Serum No Effect* In 17 Algerian patients with untreated celiac disease mean concentration of 0.43 ± 0.41 mmol/L not significantly different from 0.31 ± 0.15 mmol/L in 34 healthy controls *3436*

Leukocytes *Blood Decrease* Uncommon but may occur if severe folate or vitamin B_{12} deficiency is present *4891* Patients may show a megaloblastic anemia and leukopenia secondary to folic acid or vitamin B_{12} deficiency. In these instances low serum folate and B_{12} levels will be found *900*

Lipoprotein A *Serum Decrease* In 17 Algerian patients with untreated celiac disease mean concentration of 0.31 ± 0.09 g/L significantly different from 0.37 ± 0.05 g/L in 34 healthy controls *3436*

Lipoprotein Lp(a) *Serum No Effect* In 17 Algerian patients with untreated celiac disease mean concentration of 0.15 ± 0.20 g/L significantly different from 0.19 ± 0.14 g/L in 34 healthy controls *3436*

Lymphocytes *Blood Decrease* Uncommon but may occur if severe folate or vitamin B_{12} deficiency is present *4891* Often an absolute lymphopenia due to loss of lymphocytes into the small intestine *1980*

Magnesium *Serum Decrease* Often low. 10% of untreated patients may have levels < 1 mmol/L and may have symptoms from the deficiency *4960* May occur *5507*

MCH *Blood Decrease* Characteristic iron deficiency anemia. The peripheral blood smear may show hypochromia. In some cases iron deficiency anemia may be the predominant abnormality indicative of malabsorption *900*

MCHC *Blood Decrease* Characteristic iron deficiency anemia. The peripheral blood smear may show hypochromia. In some cases iron deficiency anemia may be the predominant abnormality indicative of malabsorption *900*

MCV *Blood Decrease* Characteristic of iron-deficiency anemia the peripheral blood smear may show microcytosis. In some cases iron-deficiency anemia may be the predominant abnormality indicative of malabsorption *900*
Blood Increase Macrocytic anemia may occur due to vitamin B_{12} or folate deficiency. MCV > 100 fL *1098*

Nitrogen *Feces Increase* Observed effect *1290*

Osteocalcin *Serum No Effect* Mean concentration in 9 children with celiac disease of 6.0 ng/mL not significantly different from 8.4 ng/mL in 28 healthy controls *757*

Oxalate *Urine Increase* 6 of 9 children with untreated disease had hyperoxaluria *3863*

Pancreatitis-associated Protein *Serum Increase* In 54 patients with celiac disease on a free diet mean concentration of 127.3 ± 56.8 ng/mL significantly different from 27.6 ± 9.0 ng/mL in 17 healthy controls. Mean concentration of 47.2 ± 20.5 ng/mL in 47 patients with celiac disease on a gluten free diet also higher than in the controls *706*

Parathyroid Hormone *Plasma Increase* Mean concentration in 9 children with celiac disease of 43 pg/mL not significantly different from 32 pg/mL in 28 healthy controls *757* Malabsorption of calcium results in increased parathyroid hormone production and renal tubular reabsorption of phosphate decreases, leading to mild hypophosphatemia *2719*
Plasma No Effect In 42 symptomatic adult patients mean concentration of 90.3 ± 18.0 pg/dL not different from reference range of 20 - 100 pg/dL *3388*

Phosphate *Serum Decrease* Malabsorption of calcium results in increased parathyroid hormone production and renal tubular reabsorption of phosphate decreases, leading to mild hypophosphatemia *2719* Low vitamin D absorption from small bowel *1290*
Serum No Effect Mean concentration in 9 children with celiac disease of 4.0 mg/dL not significantly different from 4.6 mg/dL in 28 healthy controls *757*
Urine Increase Malabsorption of calcium results in increased parathyroid hormone production and renal tubular reabsorption of phosphate decreases, leading to mild hypophosphatemia *2719*

Phospholipids *Serum Decrease* In 17 Algerian patients with untreated celiac disease mean concentration of 2.06 ± 0.31 mmol/L significantly different from 2.46 ± 0.29 mmol/L in 34 healthy controls *3436*

Platelets *Blood Increase* May be present and may reflect splenic atrophy *4891*

Potassium *Serum Decrease* If diarrhea is severe, marked electrolyte depletion *4891*

Protein *Serum Decrease* Defective amino acid absorption might contribute to the observed reduction in serum protein levels *4891* Enteric loss of plasma protein *4891*

Prothrombin Time *Plasma Increase* May be prolonged in celiac sprue owing to malabsorption of vitamin K *4891* An indication of vitamin K malabsorption *1980*

Pyridoxine *Serum Decrease* Lack of B_6 results in failure to metabolize tryptophan and high concentrations of tryptophan metabolites *4707*

Sodium *Serum Decrease* If diarrhea is severe, marked electrolyte depletion *4891*

Soluble Interleukin-2 Receptor *Serum Increase* In 8 children receiving gluten-containing diet mean concentration of 1,188 U/mL not significantly different from 688 U/mL in age-matched controls. In 3 on gluten-free diet mean concentration of 652 U/mL not significantly different from 602 U/mL in age-matched controls *769*

Thyroxine Binding Globulin *Serum Decrease* Decreased in hypoproteinemia *5544*

Thyroxine (T4) *Serum Decrease* Decreased in hypoproteinemia *5544*

Triglycerides *Serum Decrease* In 6 patients with celiac disease mean concentration of 0.75 ± 0.11 mmol/L reduced below normal *5501*
Serum No Effect In 17 Algerian patients with untreated celiac disease mean concentration of 0.94 ± 0.41 mmol/L not significantly different from 0.92 ± 0.31 mmol/L in 34 healthy controls *3436*

Triolein ^{131}I Test *Feces Positive* Positive test for lipid droplets in the stool, but results are inconsistent *1980*

Tryptophan *Plasma Decrease* In 15 children with untreated celiac disease concentration significantly reduced to 13 ± 4 µmol/L compared with 31 ± 13 µmol/L in 12 treated children and 81 ± 22 µmol/L in 12 control children *2254*

Urea Nitrogen *Serum Decrease* Impaired protein absorption *5544*

Uric Acid *Serum Decrease* Slight *5544*

Vitamin A *Serum Decrease* Due to faulty fat absorption *1290*

Vitamin B_{12} *Serum Decrease* If severe ileal disease is present, vitamin B_{12} absorption is abnormally low both with and without added intrinsic factor *4891* Patients may show a megaloblastic anemia and leukopenia secondary to folic acid or vitamin B_{12} deficiency. Malabsorption *5544*

Vitamin E *Serum Decrease* Decreased *4596*

Vitamin K *Serum Decrease* Due to malabsorption *5677*

VLDL-Cholesterol *Serum Decrease* In 6 patients with celiac disease mean concentration of 0.19 ± 0.04 mmol/L reduced below normal *5501*
Serum No Effect In 17 Algerian patients with untreated celiac disease mean concentration of 0.44 ± 0.31 mmol/L significantly different from 0.39 ± 0.13 mmol/L in 34 healthy controls *3436*

VLDL-Phospholipids *Serum No Effect* In 17 Algerian patients with untreated celiac disease mean concentration of 0.23 ± 0.17 mmol/L not significantly different from 0.21 ± 0.08 mmol/L in 34 healthy controls *3436*

VLDL-Triglycerides *Serum No Effect* In 17 Algerian patients with untreated celiac disease mean concentration of 0.36 ± 0.38 mmol/L not significantly different from 0.27 ± 0.16 mmol/L in 34 healthy controls *3436*

Xylose Tolerance Test *Blood Abnormal* The 1 h value was found to be more reliable than was fecal fat analysis in screening children for celiac disease *653* One h after 5 g xylose, the blood xylose concentration is 20 mg/dL or more in treated disease or in cases other than celiac disease. In untreated disease, the 1 h blood-xylose is < 20 mg/dL *1290* Usually found at the time of initial diagnosis *2039*
Urine Abnormal Abnormal absorption observed *4891*

Zinc *Serum Decrease* Depression of plasma zinc and lowered taste discrimination were observed in untreated patients. With confirmation of plasma copper depression indicates that trace metal deficiency is a common nutritional complication of adult celiac disease *4929*

579.00 Gluten-sensitive Enteropathy

Alanine Aminotransferase *Serum Increase* High prevalence of increased activity reported in patients with gluten-sensitive enteropathy, usually receding on treatment with gluten-free diet *3625*

Aspartate Aminotransferase *Serum Increase* High prevalence of increased activity reported in patients with gluten-sensitive enteropathy, usually receding on treatment with gluten-free diet *3625*

579.10 Sprue

Zinc *Serum Decrease* In patients with sprue concentration is typically reduced *2952*

579.10 Tropical Sprue

5-Hydroxyindoleacetic Acid *Urine Increase* Modest increases observed in patients with tropical sprue *2952*

579.80 Food Intolerance

Histidine *Urine Decrease* In 20 patients with food intolerance median excretion of 383.5 µmol/d significantly different from 371 - 1,771 µmol/d in 25 nonallergic volunteers *1292*

Immunoglobulin E *Serum Increase* In 20 patients with food intolerance median concentration of 60 significantly different from normal range *1292*

579.80 Protein-losing Enteropathy

Albumin *Serum* *Decrease* Excessive enteric loss usually leads to the development of edema *4707* Responsible for excessive loss from circulation with subsequent decreased serum concentration *4617*

α_1-Antitrypsin *Feces* *Increase* In 32 patients with protein-losing enteropathy mean concentration of 1.31 ± 0.71 mg/g, fecal loss of 450 ± 255 mg/d and intestinal clearance of 124 ± 86 mL/d all significantly higher than 0.21 ± 0.17 mg/g, 23.9 ± 20.3 mg/d and 8.47 ± 7.56 mL/d respectively in 30 people without gastrointestinal disorders *3749*

Complement C_2 *Serum* *Decrease* Found in 50% of patients *3910*

Eosinophils *Blood* *Increase* Occasional eosinophilia *5544*

Factor B *Plasma* *Decrease* Found in 50% of patients *4431* *5229*

α_1-Globulin *Serum* *Increase* In protein-losing enteropathy *5544*

α_2-Globulin *Serum* *Increase* In protein-losing enteropathy *5544*

γ-Globulin *Serum* *Decrease* In protein-losing enteropathies *5544*

Hematocrit *Blood* *Decrease* There may be a moderate anemia *900*

Hemoglobin *Blood* *Decrease* There may be a moderate anemia *900*

Thyroxine Binding Globulin *Serum* *Decrease* Decreased in nephrosis and other causes of marked hypoproteinemia *5544*

Thyroxine (T4) *Serum* *Decrease* Decreased T4 with hypoproteinemia *5544*

579.80 Steatorrhea

Calcium *Serum* *Decrease* Decreased concentrations are seen in steatorrhea *2952*

579.90 Malabsorption

Albumin *Serum* *Decrease* Marked hypoproteinemia *900* Decreased in malabsorption syndrome *367*

Alkaline Phosphatase *Serum* *Increase* An indication of vitamin D and calcium malabsorption *1980*

Amylase *Serum* *Increase* Increased in chronic malabsorption with intestinal villous atrophy *1290*

α_1-Antichymotrypsin *Duodenal Contents* *Increase* Concentration in duodenal juice from children with malabsorption disease is elevated relative to children with pancreatic insufficiency *2628*

α_1-Antitrypsin *Serum* *Decrease* These conditions reduce activity *2091*

Ascorbic Acid *Serum* *Decrease* In steatorrhea *456*

Bicarbonate *Serum* *Decrease* Normal or decreased *5544*

CA 19-9 *Serum* *No Effect* In 7 patients with nonpancreatic malabsorption mean concentration below cutoff of 37 U/mL *4998*

Calcium *Feces* *Increase* In diarrheas of all sorts, but especially steatorrheas, large fecal calcium losses occur. One patient with steatorrhea (nontropical sprue) was observed to excrete all ingested calcium plus the amount calculated to have been derived from 8 liters of intestinal juices which are normally excreted into the tract, a deficit amounting to 500 mg of calcium daily *2252*
Serum *Decrease* Decreased in hypoproteinemia *1025* An indication of vitamin D and calcium malabsorption *1980* Particularly in small bowel disease *367*

Carotene *Serum* *Decrease* Decreased in malabsorption syndrome *367* A useful indication of fat malabsorption low levels are found in as many as 80% of patients with steatorrhea *1980*

Chloride *Serum* *No Effect* Concentration usually unchanged *5544*

Cholesterol *Serum* *Decrease* Decreased in malabsorption syndrome *367*

Cholinesterase *Serum* *Decrease* May be decreased in some cases of malnutrition in which albumin is decreased *5544*

Chymotrypsin *Feces* *Decrease* Found to be a more reliable measure of pancreatic function than trypsin activity. False positives have been noted in 10% of controls, and normal values may occur in patients *110*

Complement C_2 *Serum* *Decrease* Observed effect *4746*

Factor II *Plasma* *Decrease* Malabsorption of fat-soluble vitamin K results in hypoprothrombinemia *367*

Fat *Feces* *Increase* In malabsorption syndrome *367* The number and size of fecal fat globules correlates with the degree of steatorrhea *1240*

Folate *Serum* *Decrease* Particularly in small bowel disease *367* Macrocytic anemia may occur due to vitamin B_{12} or folate deficiency. MCV > 100 fL *1098*

Glucose Tolerance *Serum* *Increase* Flat curve in celiac disease and diseases of intestinal wall and in monosaccharide malabsorption *367*

Hematocrit *Blood* *Decrease* There may be moderate anemia in idiopathic hypoproteinemia *900*

Hemoglobin *Blood* *Decrease* Mild anemia *900*

25-Hydroxy Vitamin D_3 *Serum* *Decrease* 66% of patients with malabsorption had low (< 21 ng/mL) serum concentrations. Only 1 of 31 patients had a value > 21 ng/mL and 20 had assays < 12 ng/mL *4657*

Indican *Urine* *Increase* Found in several malabsorptive states as well as bacterial overgrowth *2034*

Iron-binding Capacity, Total *Serum* *Increase* Observed effect *367*

Magnesium *Serum* *Decrease* Hypomagnesemia may occur *5507*

MCH *Blood* *Decrease* Microcytic hypochromic anemia may occur due to blood loss, increased demand or dietary inadequacy. MCH < 27 pg, MCV < 80 fL *1098*

MCV *Blood* *Decrease* Microcytic hypochromic anemia may occur due to blood loss, increased demand or dietary inadequacy. MCH < 27 pg, MCV < 80 fL *1098*
Blood *Increase* Macrocytic anemia may occur due to vitamin B_{12} or folate deficiency. MCV > 100 fL *1098*

Parathyroid Hormone *Plasma* *Increase* Malabsorption of calcium results in increased parathyroid hormone production and renal tubular reabsorption of phosphate decreases, leading to mild hypophosphatemia *2719*

pH *Urine* *Decrease* Normal or decreased *5544*

Phosphate *Serum* *Decrease* An indication of vitamin D and calcium malabsorption *1980* Malabsorption of calcium results in increased parathyroid hormone production and renal tubular reabsorption of phosphate decreases, leading to mild hypophosphatemia *2719*
Urine *Increase* Malabsorption of calcium results in increased parathyroid hormone production and renal tubular reabsorption of phosphate decreases, leading to mild hypophosphatemia *2719*

Prothrombin Time *Plasma* *Increase* An indication of vitamin K malabsorption *1980*

Thyroxine Binding Globulin *Serum* *Decrease* Decreased with hypoproteinemia *5544*

Thyroxine (T4) *Serum* *Decrease* Decreased with hypoproteinemia *5544*

Triolein ^{131}I Test *Feces* *Positive* Positive test for lipid droplets in the stool, results are inconsistent *1980*

Vitamin B_{12} *Serum* *Decrease* Particularly in tropical sprue and bacterial overgrowth *367*

Vitamin K *Serum* *Decrease* Deficiency and resulting bleeding tendency is to be expected with fat malabsorption *4707*

Volume *Feces* *Increase* Unabsorbed fats and fatty acids cause stools to be bulky and voluminous *367*
Urine *No Effect* Usually unaffected *5544*

Xylose Tolerance Test *Urine* *Abnormal* Abnormal absorption observed *2034*

Zinc *Serum* *Decrease* Decreased *5083*

DISEASES OF THE GENITOURINARY SYSTEM

580.00 Acute Postinfectious Glomerulonephritis

Complement C_1 *Serum Decrease* Mean concentration typically slightly decreasedin patients with early acute postinfectious glomerulonephritis *4682*
Serum No Effect Mean concentration typically normal in patients with late acute postinfectious glomerulonephritis *4682*

Complement C_1q *Serum Decrease* Mean concentration typically decreased in patients with early acute postinfectious glomerulonephritis *4682*
Serum No Effect Mean concentration typically normal in patients with late acute postinfectious glomerulonephritis *4682*

Complement C_2 *Serum Decrease* Mean concentration typically slightly decreased in patients with early acute postinfectious glomerulonephritis *4682*
Serum No Effect Mean concentration typically normal in patients with late acute postinfectious glomerulonephritis *4682*

Complement C_3 *Serum Decrease* Mean concentration typically slightly decreased in patients with either early or late acute postinfectious glomerulonephritis *4682*

Complement C_4 *Serum Decrease* Mean concentration typically slightly decreased in patients with early acute postinfectious glomerulonephritis *4682* Mean concentration typically normal in patients with late acute postinfectious glomerulonephritis *4682*

Complement C_5 *Serum No Effect* Mean concentration typically normal in patients with acute postinfectious glomerulonephritis although concentration may be slightly decreased in the early phase *4682*

Complement CH50 *Serum Decrease* Mean concentration typically slightly decreased in patients with early or late acute postinfectious glomerulonephritis *4682*

Properdin Factor B *Plasma No Effect* Mean concentration typically normal in patients with acute postinfectious glomerulonephritis although may be slightly reduced in early phase *4682*

580.00 Acute Poststreptococcal Glomerulonephritis

Alanine Aminotransferase *Urine Increase* Increased *2508 5671 4096*

Albumin *Serum Decrease* May be low as a result of urinary loss and excessive catabolism of protein *2034*
Urine Increase Common although it rarely exceeds 3 g/d *900* Usually occurs, with size of proteins indicating degree of glomerular damage. Albumin is nearly always present *5686*

Aldosterone *Plasma Increase* The decreased GFR and increased aldosterone secretion lead to retention of sodium and water with resultant hypervolemia *2304*
Urine Decrease Occurs in the presence of edema in children *5545*
Urine Increase The decreased GFR and increased aldosterone secretion lead to retention of sodium and water with resultant hypervolemia *2304*

Ammonia *Urine Decrease* Decreased in nephritis with damage to the distal renal tubules *1290*

Anti-Streptolysin-O Titer *Serum Increase* Usually raised indicating recent streptococcal infection but may fall rapidly with the use of antimicrobials *367* In 75 patients hospitalized for poststreptococcal glomerulonephritis ASO titers were highest in those with an increased plasma concentration of IgG *5642* Titer usually exhibits a rise some time during the course of the disease and may be the only evidence of antecedent β-hemolytic streptococcal infection *2039*

α_1-Antitrypsin *Serum No Effect* Concentration usually normal *5544*

Arylsulfatase *Serum Increase* 30 - 50% increase in activity *1279*

Bicarbonate *Serum Decrease* Metabolic acidosis *126*

Calcium *Urine Decrease* Decreased excretion in acute nephritis, partly due to decreased intestinal absorption *1290*

Cells *Urine Increase* 36% renal epithelial cells were found in tubular nephrosis (necrosis) and in glomerulonephritis *3071*

Ceruloplasmin *Serum Increase* Found regularly with hypoproteinemia *2210*

Chloride *Serum Decrease* Seen in azotemic or oliguric patients *126*

Cholesterol *Serum Increase* Sometimes elevated even when serum albumin is not greatly decreased *2034*

Complement C_1q *Serum Decrease* Particularly during diuretic phase *126*

Complement C_3 *Serum Decrease* Persistently low with C_3 conversion products and normal C_4 *5651*
Serum Increase Particularly during diuretic phase *126*

Complement C_4 *Serum Decrease* Usually less than that of C_3 *572*
Serum No Effect C_3 was persistently low with C_3 conversion products and normal C_4 *5651*

Complement, Total *Serum Decrease* Marked reduction coincident with development of nephritis *367*

Copper *Serum Increase* Found regularly with hypoproteinemia *2210*

Creatinine *Serum Increase* Mild renal failure with plasma values of 1.5 - 4.0 mg/dL is very common in the initial stages *367*

Eosinophils *Blood Increase* Occasionally *5677*

Erythrocyte Casts *Urine Increase* Microscopic examination reveals numerous red blood cells and variable numbers of casts. Indicate bleeding from the glomerulus *367*

Erythrocyte Sedimentation Rate *Blood Increase* Usually moderately raised *367*

Erythrocytes *Urine Increase* Hematuria, gross or only microscopic. May occur during the initial febrile upper respiratory infection then reappear with nephritis in 1 - 2 weeks. It lasts 2 to 12 weeks; usual duration is 2 months *5545* Hematuria usually occurs in conjunction with proteinuria, but may occur alone in some cases *5686*

Factor VIII *Plasma Increase* Patients who made a complete recovery upon 4 year follow-up had normal initial values, while those who developed persistent renal damage had high factor VIII values. Other coagulation factors are of no prognostic significance *1315*

Fatty Casts *Urine Increase* May appear within the first few weeks *2034*

Fibrin Degradation Products *Plasma Increase* Increased (> 10 μg/mL) in 28% of acute cases. Mean value was 8.4 ± 5.6 μg/mL (normal: 3.2 ± 1.2 μg/mL) *2863* Raised serum or urine levels are common without other evidence of enhanced fibrinolysis *2646*
Urine Increase Raised serum or urine levels are common without other evidence of enhanced fibrinolysis *2646*

α_1-Globulin *Serum Increase* Moderate increase *1290*

α_2-Globulin *Serum Increase* There is a moderate increase appearing in the early stages *1290*

Glomerular Filtration Rate *Urine Decrease* The decreased GFR and increased aldosterone secretion lead to retention of sodium and water with resultant hypervolemia *2304*

Glucose *Urine Increase* Occasional glycosuria occurs *367*

β-Glucuronidase *Urine Increase* 31 of 38 patients with active disease had elevated activities, with a mean value of 70.0 ± 50.4. Of the 38 patients with inactive glomerulonephritis, 17 had elevated activities *3373*

Granular Casts *Urine Increase* Granular and epithelial cell casts are found *5545* Usually present *367*

Haptoglobin *Serum No Effect* Concentration usually normal *5544*

Hematocrit *Blood Decrease* Dilutional anemia *2304* Normocytic, normochromic anemia occurs as a result of hemodilution *900*

Hemoglobin *Blood Decrease* Slightly reduced to 11-12 g/dL as a result of dilution *367* Anemia is usually present, its severity varying directly with the severity of the azotemia *2039*

Hemoglobin Casts *Urine Increase* Indicate bleeding from the glomerulus *367*

β-Hexosaminidase *Urine Decrease* Decreased levels in urine *5229*

580.00 Acute Poststreptococcal Glomerulonephritis *(continued)*

^{131}I Uptake *Serum* *Decrease* In renal disease *4707*

Immunoglobulin A *Serum* *Increase* In 39 patients hospitalized for poststreptococcal glomerulonephritis 11 (28%) had an increased concentration of IgA *5642*

Immunoglobulin G *Serum* *Increase* In 75 patients hospitalized for poststreptococcal glomerulonephritis 33 (44%) had an increased concentration of IgG *5642*

Leukocytes *Blood* *Increase* Increased neutrophils in children *5545*
Urine *Increase* Large numbers of red and white cells are found *367*

Lipids *Urine* *Increase* Lipid droplets may appear within the first few weeks *2034*

Lipoproteins *Serum* *Increase* More than 50% of the patients with glomerulonephritis, nephrotic syndrome and renovascular hypertension showed obviously abnormal lipoprotein profiles, which returned to normal or near-normal when the disease was ameliorated or corrected surgically *5515*

Magnesium *Serum* *Decrease* Majority of cases showed a fall in both serum and urinary levels, associated with hypoproteinemia and hypoalbuminemia *4013* Hypomagnesemia may occur in some cases *5507*
Urine *Decrease* Majority of cases showed a fall in both serum and urinary levels, associated with hypoproteinemia and hypoalbuminemia *4013*

Neutrophils *Urine* *Increase* In interstitial nephritis and nephrosclerosis patients, the percentage of polymorphonuclear granulocytes was 76 - 85% *3071*

pH *Urine* *Decrease* May occur early in the course of the illness *2034*

Protein *Pleural Fluid* *Decrease* Pleural effusions are usually transudates (< 3 g/dL) *126*
Serum *Decrease* Occasionally lowered with reversed A/G ratio *2039*
Urine *Increase* Usually occurs, with size of proteins indicating degree of glomerular damage. Albumin is nearly always present *5686* May reach over 6 - 8 g/d, but is more often below 2 g/d *5545*

Sodium *Serum* *Decrease* The decreased GFR and increased aldosterone secretion lead to retention of sodium and water with resultant hypervolemia *2304*
Urine *Decrease* Reflects avid salt reabsorption in the distal nephron *126* Very low (< 15 mmol/L) *2034*

Specific Gravity *Urine* *Increase* May occur early in the course of the illness *2034*

Tryptophan *Plasma* *Increase* Tyrosine and tryptophan usually rise in acute and chronic glomerulonephritis *4707*

Tyrosine *Plasma* *Increase* Tyrosine and tryptophan usually rise in acute and chronic glomerulonephritis *4707*

Urea Nitrogen *Serum* *Increase* Elevated in 50% of patients *2034* All fractions of nonprotein nitrogen increase *1642*

Volume *Plasma* *Increase* The decreased GFR and increased aldosterone secretion lead to retention of sodium and water with resultant hypervolemia *2304* Plasma volume may be as much as 50% above normal during edematous phase *3710*
Urine *Decrease* The disease is sometimes ushered in by oliguria which may progress to complete anuria *2034*

580.90 Glomerulonephritis

Albumin *Urine* *Increase* In a group of patients with IgAGN and normal renal function mean excretion 269.7 ± 420.2 mg/d, 154.4 ± 209.5 mg/d in IgAGN with chronic renal failure, and 158.6 ± 182.3 mg/d in membranous glomerulonephritis compared with 5.4 ± 3.2 mg/d in healthy controls *4391*

Anti-Neutrophil Cytoplasm Antibodies *Serum* *Increase* Anti-neutrophil cytoplasmic antibodies (ANCA) are associated with different forms of both primary and secondary vasculitis and glomerulonephritis *1955*

Atrial Natriuretic Peptide *Plasma* *No Effect* In a group of patients with IgAGN and normal renal function mean concentration of 112 ± 81 pg/mL, 159 ± 111 pg/mL in IgAGN with chronic renal failure, and 145 ± 139 pg/mL in membranous glomerulonephritis compared with 25 ± 111 pg/mL in healthy controls *4391*

Blood *Urine* *Increase* In 26 of 31 patients (84%) with IgA glomerulonephritis mean excretion greater than 500,000 /mL *220*

Creatinine *Serum* *Increase* In 6 of 21 patients (19%) with IgA glomerulonephritis mean concentration greater than 0.11 mmol/L *220*

Endothelin-1 *Plasma* *Increase* In a group of patients with IgAGN and normal renal function mean concentration of 9.2 ± 7.0 pg/mL, 5.1 ± 3.2 pg/mL in IgAGN with chronic renal failure, and 6.9 ± 4.7 pg/mL in membranous glomerulonephritis compared with 3.5 ± 4.1 pg/mL in healthy controls *4391*
Urine *Increase* In a group of patients with IgAGN and normal renal function mean excretion of 0.035 ± 0.017 ng/min, 0.032 ± 0.011 ng/min in IgAGN with chronic renal failure, and 0.028 ± 0.013 ng/min in membranous glomerulonephritis compared with 0.019 ± 0.005 ng/min in healthy controls *4391*
Urine *No Effect* In 10 children with glomerulonephritis mean excretion of 12.2 pmol/sq m/d not significantly different from 12.9 (lower and upper quartiles 10.0 - 15.2 pmol/sq m/d) in 60 healthy children *5733*

Glomerular Basement Membrane Antibody *Serum* *Increase* Increased concentrations often above 250 units occur in patients with glomerulonephritis without pulmonary hemorrhage *2952*

Guanosine Monophosphate *Urine* *Decrease* In a group of patients with IgAGN with chronic renal failure of 0.186 ± 0.117 nmol/min in membranous glomerulonephritis compared with 0.330 ± 0.050 nmol/min in healthy controls *4391*
Urine *No Effect* In a group of patients with IgAGN and normal renal function mean excretion of 0.378 ± 0.110 nmol/min and 0.338 ± 0.064 nmol/min in membranous glomerulonephritis compared with 0.330 ± 0.050 nmol/min in healthy controls *4391*

Magnesium *Urine* *Increase* Excretion is increased in association with chronic glomerulonephritis *2952*

β_2-Microglobulin *Urine* *Increase* In a group of patients with IgAGN and normal renal function mean excretion of 104.6 ± 100.1 µg/d, 5,650.2 ± 620.7 µg/d in IgAGN with chronic renal failure, and 1,92.2 ± 365.0 µg/d in membranous glomerulonephritis compared with 83.8 ± 87.1 µg/d in healthy controls *4391*

N-Acetyl-Glucosaminidase *Urine* *Increase* In a group of patients with IgAGN and normal renal function mean excretion of 3.97 ± 5.85 U/d, 14.82 ± 10.83 U/d in IgAGN with chronic renal failure, and 4.81 ± 2.46 U/d in membranous glomerulonephritis compared with 1.58 ± 1.31 U/d in healthy controls *4391*

Protein *Urine* *Increase* In 25 of 31 patients (81%) with IgA glomerulonephritis mean excretion greater than 0.2 g/d *220*

Type IV Collagen Peptide *Serum* *Increase* In 15 patients with active glomerulonephritis mean concentration of 14 ± 8.2 ng/mL compared with 7.8 ± 3.0 ng/mL in 32 patients with chronic interstitial nephritis and 8.1 ± 2.4 ng/mL in 17 patients with various chronic kidney diseases and 9.1 ± 1.7 ng/mL in 23 ambulatory kidney transplant patients *2623*

581.30 Glomerulonephritis, Minimal Change

Alanine Aminotransferase *Urine* *Increase* Increased *4096* *5671* *2508*

Albumin *Serum* *Decrease* Occurs as a result of heavy protein loss, especially low molecular weight plasma proteins such as albumin and transferrin in the urine *367*
Urine *Increase* Characterized by heavy proteinuria, consisting almost entirely of low molecular weight plasma proteins, especially albumin and transferrin. Values are > 5 g/d *367*

Anti-Streptolysin-O Titer *Serum* *Increase* Above normal titers may occur *3953*

Ceruloplasmin *Serum* *Increase* Found regularly with hypoproteinemia *2210*

Cholesterol *Serum* *Increase* Usually occurs *367*

Complement C_3 *Serum* *No Effect* No significant effect observed *3021*

Complement C_4 *Serum* *No Effect* No significant effect observed *3021*

Copper *Serum* *Increase* Found regularly with hypoproteinemia *2210*

Erythrocytes *Urine* *Increase* Microscopic hematuria is seen in a minority of patients *5685*

Fatty Casts *Urine* *Increase* Hyaline, granular, and fatty casts are found *367*

Granular Casts *Urine* *Increase* Hyaline, granular, and fatty casts are found *367*

β-Hexosaminidase *Urine* *Decrease* Decreased levels in urine *5229*

Hyaline Casts *Urine* *Increase* Hyaline, granular, and fatty casts are found *367*

immunoglobulin A *Serum* *Decrease* Usually normal or modestly decreased *872*

Immunoglobulin E *Serum* *Increase* May be increased *872*

Immunoglobulin G *Serum* *Decrease* May be profoundly depressed during relapse *872*

Immunoglobulin M *Serum* *Increase* May be increased *872*

Interleukin-6 *Serum* *No Effect* Mean concentration in 8 patients with minimal change glomerulonephritis of 0.3 ± 0.5 pg/mL not significantly different from 0.3 ± 0.6. pg/mL in 48 healthy controls *4566*
Urine *No Effect* Mean concentration in 8 patients with minimal change glomerulonephritis of 1.6 ± 2.9 pg/mL not significantly different from 0.3 ± 0.5. pg/mL in 48 healthy controls *4566*

Iron-binding Capacity, Total *Serum* *Decrease* Decreased as a result of heavy protein loss in the urine, especially low molecular weight proteins, such as albumin and transferrin *367*

α_2-Macroglobulin *Serum* *Increase* Reported effect *2088*

Plasma Cells *Blood* *Increase* Elevated *5230* *1399* *1343*

Procollagen Type IV Peptide *Urine* *Increase* The highest urinary concentrations were found in seven patients with minimal change glomerulonephritis (7.5 ± 3.2 ng/mL) *2623*

Protein *Pleural Fluid* *Decrease* Pleural effusions are usually transudates (< 3 g/dL) *126*
Urine *Increase* Characterized by heavy proteinuria consisting almost entirely of low molecular weight plasma proteins, especially albumin and transferrin. Values are > 5 g/d *367* Marked proteinuria - usually > 4.5 g/d; usually exclusively albuminuria in children with lipoid nephrosis, but in glomerulonephritis high- and low-molecular weight proteins are present with nephrotic syndrome *5545*

Soluble Fas Antigen *Serum* *No Effect* Mean concentration in 8 patients with minimal change glomerulonephritis of 2.3 ± 0.6 ng/mL not significantly different from 2.1 ± 0.5 ng/mL in 48 healthy controls *4566*
Urine *No Effect* Mean concentration in 8 patients with minimal change glomerulonephritis of 0.0 ± 0.9 ng/mL not significantly different from 0.0 ± 0.0 ng/mL in 48 healthy controls *4566*

Soluble Fas Ligand Antigen *Serum* *No Effect* Mean concentration in 8 patients with minimal change glomerulonephritis of 0.47 ± 0.4 ng/mL not significantly different from 0.55 ± 0.13 ng/mL in 48 healthy controls *4566*

Tryptophan *Plasma* *Increase* Tyrosine and tryptophan usually rise in acute and chronic glomerulonephritis *4707*

Tumor Necrosis Factor-α *Serum* *No Effect* Mean concentration in 8 patients with minimal change glomerulonephritis of 4.2 ± 5.6 pg/mL not significantly different from 4.1 ± 6.0 pg/mL in 48 healthy controls *4566*
Urine *No Effect* Mean concentration in 8 patients with minimal change glomerulonephritis of 0.0 ± 0.0 pg/mL not significantly different from 0.0 ± 0.0 pg/mL in 48 healthy controls *4566*

Tyrosine *Plasma* *Increase* Tyrosine and tryptophan usually rise in acute and chronic glomerulonephritis *4707*

581.90 Nephropathy

Antithrombin III *Plasma* *No Effect* In 17 patients with nondiabetic nephropathy mean concentration of 97 U/dL compared with reference interval of 80 - 120 U/dL *4640*

Fibrinogen *Plasma* *Increase* In 17 patients with nondiabetic nephropathy mean concentration of 5.82 g/L compared with reference interval of 1.50 - 3.85 g/L *4640*

Lipoprotein Lp(a) *Serum* *Increase* In 17 patients with nondiabetic nephropathy mean concentration of 39 mg/dL compared with reference interval of < 25 mg/dL *4640*

Plasminogen Activator Inhibitor-1 *Plasma* *No Effect* In 17 patients with nondiabetic nephropathy mean concentration of 16.9 U/mL compared with reference interval of 0 - 24 U/mL *4640*

Protein C *Plasma* *No Effect* In 17 patients with nondiabetic nephropathy mean concentration of 127 U/dL compared with reference interval of 65 - 140 U/dL *4640*

581.90 Nephrotic Syndrome

α_1-Acid Glycoprotein *Serum* *Decrease* In patients with nephrotic syndrome much of α_1-AG is lost in the urine and rate of synthesis in the liver cannot keep pace *2613* In 31 patients with nephrotic syndrome mean concentration of 0.59 ± 0.04 g/L significantly reduced compared with 0.71 ± 0.05 g/L in 10 healthy individuals *5004* In 22 patients with nephrotic syndrome mean plasma concentration of 0.62 ± 0.32 g/L significantly reduced compared with 0.98 ± 0.28 g/L in 22 healthy matched controls *2498*
Urine *Increase* Excretion significantly increased in patients with nephrotic syndrome *2613*

Aggregation Index *Red Blood Cells* *Increase* In 29 children with nephrotic syndrome mean aggregation index of 23.8 ± 5.3 significantly different from reference range of 17.3 ± 5.0 *125*

Albumin *Saliva* *Decrease* In 10 children with steroid-sensitive nephrotic syndrome in remission mean concencentration of 49 mg/L significantly different from 94 mg/L in 11 healthy controls *3764*
Serum *Decrease* Responsible for excessive loss from circulation with subsequent decreased serum concentration *4617* In 10 children with steroid-sensitive nephrotic syndrome in remission mean concencentration of 17.1 g/L significantly different from 18.9 g/L in 11 healthy controls *3764* Median concentration of 1.74 ± 0.68 g/dL in 16 children with nephrosis significantly different from 3.83 ± 0.54 g/dL in 16 normotensive healthy controls *458* In 31 patients with nephrotic syndrome mean concentration of 19 ± 1 g/L significantly less than 38 ± g/L in 10 healthy controls *5004* In 62 patients with nephrotic syndrome mean concenration of 18 ± 1 g/L significantly different from 38 ± 1 g/L in 12 healthy controls *5003* In 39 patients with nephrotic syndrome mean concentration of 22 ± 16 g/L significantly different from concentration in 32 normal volunteers *5436* In patients with nephrotic syndrome plasma concentration reduced due to loss in the urine *2613* Massive loss in urine results in low serum concentration despite increased synthesis *4707* In 7 patients with nephrotic syndrome albumin concentration as measured by bromcresol green method on Kodak Ektachem® 700XR from 20 to 200% higher (up to 16 g/L higher) than as measured by protein electrophoresis *1826* Contributes to hypercoagulable state in nephrotic syndrome and associated with an excessive risk of thromboembolic complications: albumin concentration often less than 25 g/L *3931* Invariably reduced to < 3 g/dL, usually between 1 - 3 g/dL, with occasional values of < 0.5 g/dL in hypovolemia *367* Plasma albumin concentration may decrease to 25% of the normal value. Most albumin filtered at glomerulus is excreted into urine. Hypoalbuminemia is largely due to the inability of liver to increase albumin synthesis sufficiently to replace urinary losses *2613* In 22 patients with nephrotic syndrome mean plasma concentration of 19.04 ± 6.28 g/L significantly less than 41.80 ± 2.68 g/L in 22 healthy matched controls *2498*
Urine *Increase* Massive loss in urine *4707* In patients with nephrotic syndrome increased loss in urine observed *2613* In 22 patients with nephrotic syndrome mean excretion of 7.7 ± 4.1 g/d significantly greater than in 22 healthy matched controls *2498* Albumin comprises about 70% of urinary protein in nephrotic syndrome. Albumin synthesis is increased (typically 3- to 4- fold) and catabolism is reduced in nephrotic syndrome. Absolute rate of albumin catabolism is reduced in nephrotic patients *2613* The principal protein found in the urine. Despite the fact that its concentration may be greatly reduced in the plasma *2039*

Aldosterone *Plasma* *Increase* Excess contributes to the development of edema *4707* Secretion is augmented in response to decreased plasma values *2034*

Alkaline Phosphatase *Serum* *Increase* In 40% of 25 patients at initial hospitalization for this disorder *1576*
White Blood Cells *Decrease* Untreated disease *5544*

Antiplasmin *Plasma* *Decrease* In 39 patients with nephrotic syndrome mean concentration of 81 ± 6.0% significantly different from 100 ± 2.0% in 32 normal volunteers *5436*

α_2-Antiplasmin *Plasma* *Decrease* In 39 patients with nephrotic syndrome mean concentration of 56 ± 2.2 µg/mL significantly different from 66 ± 1.9 µg/mL in 32 normal volunteers

581.90 Nephrotic Syndrome *(continued)*

α_2-Antiplasmin *(continued)*
5436 A slight decrease in patients with nephrotic syndrome, but a normal level in patients with chronic latent glomerulonephritis *5117*
Plasma Increase Contributes to hypercoagulable state in nephrotic syndrome and associated with an excessive risk of thromboembolic complications *3931*
Urine Increase In 39 patients with nephrotic syndrome mean excretion of 169.0 ± 71.0 mg/g creatinine significantly different from undetectable amount in 32 normal volunteers *5436*

Antithrombin III *Plasma Decrease* Greatly reduced concentration and activity *5438* In 22 patients with nephrotic syndrome mean plasma concentration of 0.27 ± 0.07 g/L significantly reduced compared with 0.32 ± 0.04 g/L in 22 healthy matched controls *2498* Contributes to hypercoagulable state in nephrotic syndrome and associated with an excessive risk of thromboembolic complications: concentration often less than 75% of normal *3931* In infants this has been suggested to explain hypercoagulability *3132 5220* Mean concentration decreased in patients with nephrotic syndrome due to small size and increased glomerular selectivity *2613* In infants this has been suggested to explain hypercoagulability *3472* In 29 children with nephrotic syndrome mean concentration of 81 ± 21% significantly reduced compared with reference values of 100 ± 10% *125*
Urine Increase Excretion increased in patients with nephrotic syndrome due to small molecular size and increased permselectivity *2613*

α_1-Antitrypsin *Serum Decrease* In 29 children with nephrotic syndrome mean concentration of 1.7 ± 0.9 g/L significantly less than reference range of 2.7 ± 0.4 g/L *125* In 39 patients with nephrotic syndrome mean concentration of 209 ± 13 mg/dL not significantly different from 233 ± 12 mg/dL in 32 normal volunteers *5436* These conditions reduce activity *2091* In 22 patients with nephrotic syndrome mean plasma concentration of 0.90 ± 0.21 g/L significantly reduced compared with 1.69 ± 0.41 g/L in 22 healthy matched controls *2498*
Serum Increase Increased *83 4373 4241 4763 4371*
Urine Increase In 39 patients with nephrotic syndrome mean excretion of 88.5 ± 24.0 mg/g creatinine significantly different from undetectable amount in 32 normal volunteers *5436*

α_1-Antitrypsin Activity *Serum Decrease* In 39 patients with nephrotic syndrome mean activity of 9[illegible] ± 3.9% significantly different from 117 ± 2.0% in 32 normal volunteers *5436*

Apolipoprotein A *Serum No Effect* Concentration typically normal *3526*

Apolipoprotein A-I *Serum Decrease* In 10 children with congenital nephrotic syndrome mean concentration of 47.4 ± 11.6 mg/dL significantly decreased compared with 105.4 ± 18.0 mg/dL in comparable controls *149* In severe, fully developed cases, increase in low density lipoproteins with normal or decreased alpha lipoproteins has been described *1980* Median concentration of 75.8 ± 16.3 mg/dL in 16 children with nephrosis significantly different from 99.3 ± 12.1 mg/dL in 16 normotensive healthy controls *458* Untreated uncomplicated nephrotic syndrome is characterized by increased low (beta) and very low (prebeta) density lipoproteins and a diminution of high density (alpha) lipoprotein. Changes correlated strictly with albumin concentration were more pronounced with albumin concentration < 20 g/L *1717*
Serum Increase In 22 patients with nephrotic syndrome mean plasma concentration of 1.57 ± 0.20 g/L not significantly different from 1.44 ± 0.30 g/L in 22 healthy matched controls *2498* In 62 patients with nephrotic syndrome mean concentration of 1.67 ± 0.06 g/L significantly different from 1.30 ± 0.07 g/L in 12 healthy controls *5003* Mean concentration of 1.64 ± 0.08 g/L significantly higher than 1.26 ± 0.06 g/L in 10 healthy controls *5004*
Serum No Effect No significant change observed in patients with the nephrotic syndrome *2613* In 10 patients with primary renal disease and nephrotic syndrome mean concentration of 181 ± 10 mg/dL and in 8 with diabetic nephropathy with nephrotic syndrome mean concentration of 168 ± 15 mg/dL not significantly different from normal *5569*

Apolipoprotein A-II *Serum Decrease* In 22 patients with nephrotic syndrome mean plasma concentration of 0.29 ± 0.11 g/L significantly reduced compared with 0.38 ± 0.13 g/L in 22 healthy matched controls *2498* In 10 children with congenital nephrotic syndrome mean concentration of 8.6 ± 1.9 mg/dL significantly decreased compared with 28.7 ± 2.4 mg/dL in comparable controls *149*
Serum No Effect Concentration remained unchanged in patients with nephrotic syndrome *2613*

Apolipoprotein A:Apolipoprotein B Ratio *Serum Decrease* Since concentration of apolipoprotein B is usually increased and that of apolipoprotein A is typically normal, ratio is reduced *3526*

Apolipoprotein B *Serum Increase* In 31 patients with nephrotic syndrome mean concentration of 2.40 ± 0.15 g/L significantly higher than 0.91 ± 0.06 g/L in 10 healthy controls *5004* In 10 children with congenital nephrotic syndrome mean concentration of 91.5 ± 10.1 mg/dL significantly increased compared with 77.1 ± 14.1 mg/dL in comparable controls *149* In 22 patients with nephrotic syndrome mean plasma concentration of 1.81 ± 0.78 g/L significantly greater than 1.23 ± 0.31 g/L in 22 healthy matched controls *2498* In 62 patients with nephrotic syndrome mean concentration of 2.43 ± 0.11 g/L significantly different from 0.90 ± 0.05 g/L in 12 healthy controls *5003* In 10 patients with primary renal disease and nephrotic syndrome mean concentration of 182 ± 13 mg/dL and in 8 with diabetic nephropathy with nephrotic syndrome mean concentration of 172 ± 13 mg/dL significantly higher than normal *5569* Concentration increased in patients with nephrotic syndrome *2613* Concentration typically increased *3526*

Apolipoprotein B-I *Serum Increase* Median concentration of 85.6 ± 19.9 mg/dL in 16 children with nephrosis significantly different from 53.8 ± 13.6 mg/dL in 16 normotensive healthy controls *458*

Apolipoprotein B:Apolipoprotein A-I Ratio *Serum Increase* In 62 patients with nephrotic syndrome mean ratio of 1.6 ± 0.1 significantly different from 0.7 ± 0.1 in 12 healthy controls *5003*

Apolipoprotein C-II *Serum Increase* In 22 patients with nephrotic syndrome mean plasma concentration of 68.4 ± 36.1 mg/L not significantly increased compared with 52.3 ± 27.6 mg/L in 22 healthy matched controls *2498*
Serum No Effect Concentration remains unchanged in patients with nephrotic syndrome *2613*

Apolipoprotein C-III *Serum Increase* In 22 patients with nephrotic syndrome mean plasma concentration of 161.8 ± 60.7 mg/L significantly increased compared with 101.7 ± 36.2 mg/L in 22 healthy matched controls *2498* Concentration increased in patients with nephrotic syndrome *2613*

Apolipoprotein E *Serum Increase* In 22 patients with nephrotic syndrome mean plasma concentration of 76.8 ± 24.3 mg/L significantly increased compared with 37.6 ± 9.2 mg/L in 22 healthy matched controls *2498*

Apolipoprotein Lp(a) *Serum Increase* Hyperlipidemia constitutes a risk factor for vascular disease in nephrotic syndrome: Apolipoprotein Lp(a) concentration increased irrespective of the apolipoprotein A isoform class *3931*

Atrial Natriuretic Peptide *Plasma Increase* In 9 patients with nephrotic syndrome mean concentration of 19 ± 4 pmol/L higher than 11 ± 2 pmol/L in 10 healthy controls *5004*
Plasma No Effect Mean concentration in 11 patients with nephrotic syndrome of 19.3 ± 23.6 fmol/mL not significantly different from that in 37 healthy volunteers, 18.6 ± 11.4 fmol/mL although considerable variability observed with concentration in one patient markedly increased *3325*
Urine No Effect Mean concentration in 11 patients with nephrotic syndrome of 23.0 ± 21.1 fmol/mL not significantly different from that in 37 healthy volunteers, 16.1 ± 6.1 fmol/mL *3325*

Basophils *Blood Increase* Some cases *5544*

Calcium *Feces Increase* May be high indicating malintestinal absorption *3338*
Serum Decrease In 76% of 25 patients at initial hospitalization for this disorder *1576* Reduced proportionately to the fall in albumin concentration in the early stages with true hypocalcemia evident later in the disease *3338*
Urine Decrease Low urinary excretion is common *3338*

Calcium, Ultrafiltrable *Serum Decrease* In 12 patients with nephrotic syndrome and 14 nephrotic patients during clinical remission, mean ionized calcium of 1.08 ± 0.10 and 1.21 ± 0.10 mmol/L ultrafiltrate respectively, significantly lower than the normal mean (1.28 ± 0.06 mmol/L) *3060*

Carnitine *Serum* *Decrease* Median concentration of 31.3 ± 10.9 mg/dL in 16 children with nephrosis significantly different from 41.9 ± 12.2 mg/dL in 16 normotensive healthy controls *458*

Casts *Urine* *Increase* Sediment may be abnormal early in the disease before clinical signs of the syndrome become manifest, characterized by hyaline, granular, and waxy casts and plain casts with inclusions of RBC, WBC, tubular cells, and refractile fat bodies *1980*

Ceruloplasmin *Serum* *Decrease* Concentration typically reduced in patients with nephrotic syndrome *3499* Found regularly with hypoproteinemia *710* Moderate transient deficiencies *5544*
Serum *Increase* In 22 patients with nephrotic syndrome mean plasma concentration of 0.55 ± 0.25 g/L significantly increased compared with 0.27 ± 0.15 g/L in 22 healthy matched controls *2498*

Cholesterol *Serum* *Decrease* Normal or low cholesterol suggests poor nutrition and suggests a poor prognosis *413*
Serum *Increase* In 10 patients with primary renal disease and nephrotic syndrome mean concentration of 395 ± 20 mg/dL and in 8 with diabetic nephropathy with nephrotic syndrome mean concentration of 381 ± 26 mg/dL significantly higher than normal *5569* In patients with nephrotic syndrome and chronic renal failure 90% had cholesterol concentrations exceeding 240 mg/dL *2575* In 22 patients with nephrotic syndrome mean plasma concentration of 10.83 ± 4.96 mmol/L significantly greater than 5.98 ± 1.02 mmol/L in 22 healthy matched controls *2498* In 62 patients with nephrotic syndrome mean concentration of 9.9 ± 0.3 mmol/L significantly different from 4.9 ± 0.2 mmol/L in 12 healthy controls *5003* Hyperlipidemia constitutes a risk factor for vascular disease in nephrotic syndrome: VLDL-, IDL-, and LDL-cholesterol all contribute to increased plasma cholesterol concentration: increased concentration due to overproduction and impaired catabolism of apolipoprotein B-containing lipoproteins *3931* In 39 patients with nephrotic syndrome mean concentration of 403 ± 81 mg/dL significantly different from that in 32 normal volunteers *5436* In 31 patients with nephrotic syndrome mean concentration of 10.1 ± 0.5 mmol/L significantly higher than 4.9 ± 0.2 mmol/L in 10 healthy controls *5004* In 50% of 14 patients at initial hospitalization for this disorder *1576* Median concentration of 414 ± 86 mg/dL in 16 children with nephrosis significantly different from 122 ± 11 mg/dL in 16 normotensive healthy controls *458* Commonly increased in patients with nephrotic syndrome *3746* Characteristic finding *3526* In 10 children with congenital nephrotic syndrome mean concentration of 6.95 ± 1.59 mmol/L significantly increased compared with 4.04 ± 0.92 mmol/L in comparable controls *149* Typically elevated *1980* In 9 hypertriglyceridemic patients mean concentration of 11.06 ± 5.31 mmol/L compared with 6.42 ± 1.10 mmol/L in the same patients in remission and 7.99 ± 4.17 mmol/L in 10 normotriglyceridemic patients compared with 5.69 ± 1.12 mmol/L in the same patients in remission compared with 5.54 ± 0.97 mmol/L in 38 healthy controls *2499* In 25 individuals with nephrotic syndrome mean concentration of 8.43 ± 3.49 mmol/L significantly different from 5.47 ± 0.95 mmol/L in 98 healthy controls aged 24 to 55 years with method performed on ILab® 900 automated analyzer *4848*

Cholesterol:HDL-Cholesterol Ratio *Serum* *Increase* Since HDL-cholesterol concentration may be normal the cholesterol:HDL-cholesterol risk ratio is high *3526*

Cholinesterase *Serum* *Increase* 18 of 19 patients had values elevated above 12.5 U/mL *5498*

Chylomicrons *Serum* *Increase* Increased *4358* *3017* *4372*

Colloid Osmotic Pressure *Serum* *Decrease* In 22 patients with nephrotic syndrome mean plasma value of 15.1 ± 3.2 mm Hg significantly less than 27.2 ± 3.5 mm Hg in 22 healthy matched controls *2498*

Complement C_1 *Serum* *No Effect* Mean concentration typically normal in patients with nephrotic syndrome *4682*

Complement C_1q *Serum* *No Effect* Mean concentration typically normal or slightly decreased in patients with nephrotic syndrome *4682*

Complement C_2 *Serum* *No Effect* Mean concentration typically normal in patients with nephrotic syndrome *4682*

Complement C_3 *Serum* *Decrease* In 22 patients with nephrotic syndrome mean plasma concentration of 0.89 ± 0.28 g/L significantly reduced compared with 1.16 ± 0.22 g/L in 22 healthy matched controls *2498*
Serum *No Effect* Mean concentration typically normal in patients with nephrotic syndrome *4682*

Complement C_4 *Serum* *Increase* In 22 patients with nephrotic syndrome mean plasma concentration of 0.38 ± 0.16 g/L significantly increased compared with 0.23 ± 0.10 g/L in 22 healthy matched controls *2498*
Serum *No Effect* Mean concentration typically normal in patients with nephrotic syndrome *4682*

Complement C_5 *Serum* *No Effect* Mean concentration typically normal in patients with nephrotic syndrome *4682*

Complement CH50 *Serum* *No Effect* Mean concentration typically normal or slightly decreased in patients with nephrotic syndrome *4682*

Copper *Serum* *Decrease* In patients with nephrotic syndrome binding protein is lost in the urine with a resulting decrease in serum concentration *3931* Found regularly with hypoproteinemia *710*

Corticosteroids *Plasma* *Decrease* In patients with nephrotic syndrome binding protein is lost in the urine with a resulting decrease in serum concentration *3931*

Cortisol *Plasma* *Decrease* In patients with nephrotic syndrome binding protein is lost in the urine with a resulting decrease in serum concentration *3931*

C-Reactive Protein *Serum* *No Effect* In 22 patients with nephrotic syndrome mean plasma concentration of 3.5 ± 3.2 mg/L not significantly increased compared with 3.3 ± 2.1 mg/L in 22 healthy matched controls *2498*

Creatinine *Serum* *Increase* In 48% of 24 patients at initial hospitalization for this disorder *1576* In 39 patients with nephrotic syndrome mean concentration of 1.9 ± 0.2 mg/dL (range of 0.7 - 3.3 mg/dL) not significantly different from in 32 normal volunteers *5436*

D-Dimer *Plasma* *Increase* In 39 patients with nephrotic syndrome mean concentration of 437 ± 69 ng/mL significantly different from 116 ± 6 ng/mL in 32 normal volunteers *5436*
Urine *Increase* In 25 patients with nephrotic syndrome median concentration of 1.78 ng/mL significantly different from that in normal controls in whom the mean concentration was 0.69 ± 0.60 ng/mL *4789*

Disopyramide *Serum* *No Effect* Normal binding of protein observed resulting in no modifications to plasma concentration of drug *5869*

Endothelin-1 *Urine* *No Effect* In 6 children with nephrotic syndrome mean excretion of 10.0 pmol/sq m/d not significantly different from 12.9 (lower and upper quartiles 10.0 - 15.2 pmol/sq m/d) in 60 normal children *5733*

Eosinophils *Blood* *Increase* In 42% of 26 patients at initial hospitalization for this disorder *1576*

Erythrocyte Sedimentation Rate *Blood* *Increase* Due to increased fibrinogen *413*

Erythrocytes *Ascitic Fluid* *Increase* > 10,000 cells/μL is unusual *233*
Urine *Increase* Microscopic hematuria is present in 33% of cases but casts are rare and there is no evidence of prior streptococcal infection *2039*

Erythropoietin *Serum* *No Effect* In 26 patients with nephrotic syndrome mean concentration of 6.2 ± 4.5 mIU/mL not significantly different from 6.7 ± 2.4 mIU/mL in 12 normal control individuals *5437*
Urine *Increase* Increased excretion observed in 26 patients with nephrotic syndrome compared with that in 12 normal controls *5437*

Factor IV *Plasma* *Increase* Thrombocytosis contributes to hypercoagulable state in nephrotic syndrome and associated with an excessive risk of thromboembolic complications *3931*

Factor V *Plasma* *Decrease* Contributes to hypercoagulable state in nephrotic syndrome and associated with an excessive risk of thromboembolic complications *3931*
Plasma *Increase* May occur *5144*

Factor VII *Plasma* *Increase* May occur *5144*

Factor VIII *Plasma* *Decrease* Contributes to hypercoagulable state in nephrotic syndrome and associated with an excessive risk of thromboembolic complications *3931*
Plasma *Increase* May occur *5144*

581.90 Nephrotic Syndrome *(continued)*

Factor VIII Antigen *Plasma* *Increase* In 29 children with nephrotic syndrome mean concentration of 231 ± 68% significantly increased compared with reference values of 100 ± 20% *125*

Factor VIII Coagulant *Plasma* *Increase* In 29 children with nephrotic syndrome mean concentration of 267 ± 77% significantly increased compared with reference values of 100 ± 20% *125*

Factor IX *Plasma* *Decrease* Contributes to hypercoagulable state in nephrotic syndrome and associated with an excessive risk of thromboembolic complications *3931*

Factor X *Plasma* *Increase* May occur *5144*

Factor XI *Plasma* *Decrease* Contributes to hypercoagulable state in nephrotic syndrome and associated with an excessive risk of thromboembolic complications *3931* In part due to excessive urinary loss *5219*

Factor XII *Plasma* *Decrease* In part due to excessive urinary loss *5219* In 29 children with nephrotic syndrome mean concentration of 45 ± 20% significantly reduced compared with reference values of 100 ± 15% *125*

Ferritin *Serum* *No Effect* In 22 patients with nephrotic syndrome mean plasma concentration of 148 ± 130 μg/L not significantly increased compared with 118 ± 69 μg/L in 22 healthy matched controls *2498*

α-Fetoprotein *Serum* *Increase* Markedly raised maternal serum and amniotic fluid AFP levels were found in 2 cases of congenital nephrotic syndrome of the fetus *4735*

Fibrin Degradation Products *Urine* *Increase* The greater the degree of proteinuria the greater the level of fibrinogen degradation product in the urine *771*

Fibrin/Fibrinogen Degradation Product E *Urine* *Increase* In 15 patients with nephrotic syndrome mean excretion of 105.5 ± 150.1 ng/mL significantly different from 1.68 ± 1.05 ng/mL in 30 controls *4790*

Fibrinogen *Plasma* *Increase* Plasma clotting factors, especially fibrinogen, have been elevated in many patients and returned to normal when remission was induced by adrenal corticosteroids *2304* Contributes to hypercoagulable state in nephrotic syndrome and associated with an excessive risk of thromboembolic complications *3931* In 29 children with nephrotic syndrome mean concentration of 5.9 ± 1.8 g/L significantly increased compared with reference values of 3.0 ± 0.5 g/L *125* Mean concentration may be increased in the plasma of patients with nephrotic syndrome and contribute to hypercoagulable state *2613* In 22 patients with nephrotic syndrome mean plasma concentration of 6.78 ± 3.99 g/L significantly greater than 2.82 ± 0.59 g/L in 22 healthy matched controls *2498*

Fibrinopeptide A *Plasma* *Increase* Marked increase *2035*

Filtration Index *Blood* *No Effect* In 29 children with nephrotic syndrome mean index of 12.0 ± 7.2 not significantly different when compared with reference values of 12.5 ± 5.4 *125*

α_1-Globulin *Serum* *Decrease* Normal or decreased *4671*
Urine *Increase* Significant quantities are found *2034*

α_2-Globulin *Serum* *Increase* There is an increase with poor separation from the β-globulin band *1290* Hypoproteinemia is primarily due to a decrease in the albumin fraction and an increase in the alpha$_2$-globulin fraction *1980*

β-Globulin *Serum* *Increase* There is a marked increase with incomplete separation from the alpha$_2$ fraction *1290*
Urine *Increase* Significant quantities are found *2034*

γ-Globulin *Urine* *Increase* Significant quantities are found *2034*

Glomerular Filtration Rate *Urine* *Decrease* Increased total body sodium and water occurs as a result of reduced GFR and causes the characteristic edema *367* In 31 patients with nephrotic syndrome mean GFR of 67 ± 6 mL/min *5004* In 62 patients with nephrotic syndrome mean rate of 77 ± 4 mL/min significantly different from 106 ± 5 mL/min in 12 healthy controls *5003*

β-Glucuronidase *Urine* *Increase* 8 of 13 patients had activities > 30 U/L: mean for the entire group was 44.3 ± 25.3 U/L *3373*

Haptoglobin *Serum* *Increase* Conditions associated with increased ESR and alpha$_2$-globulin *5544* In 22 patients with nephrotic syndrome mean plasma concentration of 2.34 ± 1.08 g/L significantly greater than 1.13 ± 0.37 g/L in 22 healthy matched controls *2498*

HDL$_2$-Cholesterol *Serum* *Decrease* Marked reduction observed in patients with nephrotic syndrome *2613*
Serum *No Effect* In 10 patients with primary renal disease and nephrotic syndrome mean concentration of 12 ± 2 mg/dL and in 8 with diabetic nephropathy with nephrotic syndrome mean concentration of 11 ± 2 mg/dL not significantly different from normal *5569*

HDL$_3$-Cholesterol *Serum* *Increase* Modest increase observed in patients with nephrotic syndrome *2613*
Serum *No Effect* In 10 patients with primary renal disease and nephrotic syndrome mean concentration of 42 ± 4 mg/dL and in 8 with diabetic nephropathy with nephrotic syndrome mean concentration of 42 ± 5 mg/dL not significantly different from normal *5569*

HDL-Cholesterol *Serum* *Decrease* In patients with nephrotic syndrome concentration unchanged or decreased *2613* In 10 children with congenital nephrotic syndrome mean concentration of 0.55 ± 0.23 mmol/L not significantly different from 1.38 ± 0.33 mmol/L in comparable controls *149* Decreased *325* *3327* *5707* Characteristically normal or decreased *3526* In patients with nephrotic syndrome and chronic renal failure 50% had HDL-cholesterol concentrations less than 35 mg/dL *2575*
Serum *Increase* In 25 individuals with nephrotic syndrome mean concentration of 1.26 ± 0.30 mmol/L significantly different from 1.09 ± 0.27 mmol/L in 98 healthy controls aged 24 to 55 years with direct homogeneous method from Daiichi (Tokyo) performed on ILab® 900 automated analyzer *4848* In 31 patients with nephrotic syndrome mean concentration of 1.5 ± 0.1 mmol/L significantly higher than 1.3 ± 0.05 mmol/L in 10 healthy controls *5004* In patients with nephrotic syndrome reported to be low, normal or increased *3746*
Serum *No Effect* In 62 patients with nephrotic syndrome mean concentration of 1.4 ± 0.1 mmol/L not significantly different from 1.3 ± 0.1 mmol/L in 12 healthy controls *5003* In 9 hypertriglyceridemic patients mean concentration of 1.32 ± 1.01 mmol/L compared with 1.44 ± 0.38 mmol/L in the same patients in remission and 1.42 ± 1.21 mmol/L in 10 normotriglyceridemic patients compared with 1.54 ± 0.52 mmol/L in the same patients in remission compared with 1.29 ± 0.27 mmol/L in 38 healthy controls *2499* Characteristically normal or decreased *3526* In patients with nephrotic syndrome reported to be low, normal or increased *3746* In 10 patients with primary renal disease and nephrotic syndrome mean concentration of 53 ± 5 mg/dL and in 8 with diabetic nephropathy with nephrotic syndrome mean concentration of 55 ± 6 mg/dL not significantly different from normal *5569*
Serum *Normal* Hyperlipidemia constitutes a risk factor for vascular disease in nephrotic syndrome: VLDL-, IDL-, and LDL-cholesterol all contribute to increased plasma cholesterol concentration but HDL-cholesterol concentration usually remains normal *3931*

HDL-Phospholipids *Serum* *No Effect* In 10 patients with primary renal disease and nephrotic syndrome mean concentration of 108 ± 10 mg/dL and in 8 with diabetic nephropathy with nephrotic syndrome mean concentration of 108 ± 11 mg/dL not significantly different from normal *5569*

HDL-Triglycerides *Serum* *No Effect* In 10 patients with primary renal disease and nephrotic syndrome mean concentration of 21 ± 3 mg/dL not significantly different from normal but in 8 with diabetic nephropathy with nephrotic syndrome mean concentration of 40 ± 6 mg/dL significantly higher than normal *5569* In 9 hypertriglyceridemic patients mean concentration of 0.24 ± 0.10 mmol/L compared with 0.22 ± 0.05 mmol/L in the same patients in remission and 0.21 ± 0.08 mmol/L in 10 normotriglyceridemic patients compared with 0.20 ± 0.04 mmol/L in the same patients in remission compared with 0.18 ± 0.02 mmol/L in 38 healthy controls *2499*

Hemoglobin *Blood* *Decrease* In 26 patients with nephrotic syndrome mean concentration of 125 ± 25 g/L compared with 148 ± 11 g/L in 12 normal control individuals *5437*

Hemopexin *Serum* *Decrease* In 22 patients with nephrotic syndrome mean plasma concentration of 0.35 ± 0.12 g/L significantly reduced compared with 0.83 ± 0.25 g/L in 22 healthy matched controls *2498*

25-Hydroxy Vitamin D_3 *Serum Decrease* Range in 26 patients was 1 - 18.6 ng/mL, mean concentration of 8.6 ± 1 ng/mL. Normal values of 21.8 ± 2.3 ng/mL. Values were inversely correlated with degree of proteinuria and directly related to serum albumin *1795*

25-Hydroxy Vitamin D *Serum Decrease* Nephrotic syndrome significantly correlated with hypovitaminosis D (p = 0.04) *5212*

^{131}I Uptake *Serum Increase* Urinary loss of TBG results in lowering of most blood thyroid hormones and increased T3 uptake *1980*

IDL-Cholesterol *Serum Increase* Mean concentration increased due to increased synthesis and decreased catabolism *2613* Hyperlipidemia constitutes a risk factor for vascular disease in nephrotic syndrome *3931* In 9 hypertriglyceridemic patients mean concentration of 1.39 ± 0.47 mmol/L compared with 0.59 ± 0.19 mmol/L in the same patients in remission and 0.78 ± 0.19 mmol/L in 10 normotriglyceridemic patients compared with 0.17 ± 0.13 mmol/L in the same patients in remission compared with 0.11 ± 0.09 mmol/L in 38 healthy controls *2499* In 22 patients with nephrotic syndrome mean plasma concentration of 0.91 ± 0.61 mmol/L significantly greater than 0.23 ± 0.10 mmol/L in 22 healthy matched controls *2498*

IDL-Cholesterol, Esterified *Serum Increase* Hyperlipidemia constitutes a risk factor for vascular disease in nephrotic syndrome: Lipoprotein IDL- and LDL classes tend to be enriched in cholesterol ester *3931*

IDL-Triglycerides *Serum Increase* In 22 patients with nephrotic syndrome mean plasma concentration of 1.10 ± 0.61 mmol/L significantly greater than 0.24 ± 0.08 mmol/L in 22 healthy matched controls *2498* In 9 hypertriglyceridemic patients mean concentration of 1.14 ± 0.60 mmol/L compared with 0.17 ± 0.11 mmol/L in the same patients in remission and 0.45 ± 0.27 mmol/L in 10 normotriglyceridemic patients compared with 0.14 ± 0.09 mmol/L in the same patients in remission compared with 0.11 ± 0.06 mmol/L in 38 healthy controls *2499*

immunoglobulin A *Serum Decrease* Observed effect *5544*
Serum Increase In 22 patients with nephrotic syndrome mean plasma concentration of 3.80 ± 1.22 g/L significantly greater than 2.84 ± 1.04 g/L in 22 healthy matched controls *2498* Usually normal or elevated *872*

Immunoglobulin E *Serum Increase* Samples of serum and PBMC were collected at the same time from 42 pediatric patients with idiopathic nephrotic syndrome (INS) and 28 age-matched healthy individuals. The level of IgE in healthy individuals was 50 - 100 U/mL, and that in the INS patients was on the average 380 - 1,000 U/mL *5789* Usually normal or elevated *872*

Immunoglobulin G *Serum Decrease* Higher IgM and lower IgG serum concentrations were found in nephrotic patients than in normal controls (929 ± 537 mg/dL) *5798* In 22 patients with nephrotic syndrome mean plasma concentration of 6.51 ± 2.99 g/L significantly less than 11.04 ± 1.95 g/L in 22 healthy matched controls *2498* In patients with nephrotic syndrome concentration in plasma reduced to greatest extent of immunoglobulins due, in part, to loss in the urine due to increased glomerular permselectivity. As permselectivity is lost clearance approaches that of albumin. Fractional rate of IgG catabolism is inappropriately increased *2613* May be significantly reduced *872* In patients with nephrotic syndrome significant reduction observed due to loss in the urine *2613*
Urine Increase In patients with nephrotic syndrome significant increase observed in urine due to renal damage *2613* Excretion reduced due to normal or inappropriately increased synthesis but also increased excretion *2613*

Immunoglobulin G_1 *Saliva Decrease* In 10 children with steroid-sensitive nephrotic syndrome in remission mean concencentration of 8.7 mg/L not significantly different from 12.8 mg/L in 11 healthy controls *3764*
Serum Decrease In 10 children with steroid-sensitive nephrotic syndrome in remission mean concencentration of 2.3 g/L significantly different from 3.9 g/L in 11 healthy controls *3764*

Immunoglobulin G_4 *Saliva Decrease* In 10 children with steroid-sensitive nephrotic syndrome in remission mean concencentration of 0.43 mg/L not significantly different from 0.48 mg/L in 11 healthy controls *3764*
Serum Decrease In 10 children with steroid-sensitive nephrotic syndrome in remission mean concencentration of 90 mg/L significantly different from 280 mg/L in 11 healthy controls *3764*

Immunoglobulin M *Serum Decrease* Concentration may be decreased in the plasma of patients with nephrotic syndrome even though very little of the protein is lost in the urine because of its large molecular size *2613*
Serum Increase Higher IgM and lower IgG serum concentrations were found in nephrotic patients than in normal controls (157 ± 108 mg/dL vs 127 ± 38 mg/dL) *5798* Observed effect *872* Concentration may be increased in nephrotic syndrome. Little excretion occurs in urine even in nephrotic syndrome because of size of molecule *2613*
Serum No Effect Concentration usually normal *5544* In 22 patients with nephrotic syndrome mean plasma concentration of 1.77 ± 1.17 g/L not significantly different from 1.81 ± 0.88 g/L in 22 healthy matched controls *2498*

Immunoglobulins *Serum Decrease* Usually more pronounced in children, averaging about 0.2 g/dL, which explains the high susceptibility to infection *4707*
Urine Increase Severe urinary loss *4707*

Interleukin-4 *Serum Increase* Samples collected at the same time from 42 pediatric patients with idiopathic nephrotic syndrome (INS) and 28 age-matched healthy individuals. The level of IL4 in the healthy controls was 400 - 500 pg/mL and that in the INS patients was on the average 1,080 - 4,000 pg/mL *5789*

ionized Calcium *Serum Decrease* In 12 patients with nephrotic syndrome and 14 nephrotic patients during clinical remission, mean ionized calcium of 1.08 ± 0.10 and 1.21 ± 0.10 mmol/L ultrafiltrate respectively, significantly lower than the normal mean (1.28 ± 0.06 mmol/L) *3060*

Iron *Serum Decrease* In patients with nephrotic syndrome binding protein is lost in the urine with a resulting decrease in serum concentration *3931* Probably related to loss of specific iron binding serum globulin in the urine *1290*

Iron-binding Capacity, Total *Serum Decrease* Excessive loss of protein-bound iron with low total IBC *1290* Observed effect *2034*

17-Ketosteroids *Urine Decrease* Marked decrease *1025* Excretion may be decreased in patients with nephrosis *2952*

Lactate Dehydrogenase *Pleural Fluid Decrease* Transudate *126*
Serum Increase In 44% of 25 patients at initial hospitalization for this disorder *1576*

Lactate Dehydrogenase Isoenzyme-5 *Serum Increase* May be slightly increased *5544*

LDL-Cholesterol *Serum Increase* In 10 patients with primary renal disease and nephrotic syndrome mean concentration of 278 ± 21 mg/dL and in 8 with diabetic nephropathy with nephrotic syndrome mean concentration of 253 ± 30 mg/dL significantly higher than normal *5569* Hyperlipidemia constitutes a risk factor for vascular disease in nephrotic syndrome *3931* In patients with nephrotic syndrome and chronic renal failure 85% had LDL-cholesterol concentrations exceeding 130 mg/dL *2575* Marked elevation secondary to direct secretion by liver and decrease catabolism *126* In 10 children with congenital nephrotic syndrome mean concentration of 3.51 ± 1.09 mmol/L significantly increased compared with 2.43 ± 0.61 mmol/L in comparable controls *149* Hyperlipidemia occurs as a result of increased synthesis and decreased catabolism of lipoproteins *2613* In 9 patients with nephrotic syndrome mean concentration of 7.1 ± 1.1 mmol/L significantly different from 3.7 ± 0.1 mmol/L in 41 healthy controls *5003* Commonly increased in patients with nephrotic syndrome *3746* In 9 hypertriglyceridemic patients mean concentration of 6.75 ± 4.21 mmol/L compared with 3.97 ± 1.17 mmol/L in the same patients in remission and 5.27 ± 2.50 mmol/L in 10 normotriglyceridemic patients compared with 3.72 ± 1.18 mmol/L in the same patients in remission compared with 3.87 ± 0.77 mmol/L in 38 healthy controls *2499* In 22 patients with nephrotic syndrome mean plasma concentration of 7.30 ± 2.41 mmol/L significantly greater than 3.87 ± 0.69 mmol/L in 22 healthy matched controls *2498*

LDL-Cholesterol, Esterified *Serum Increase* Hyperlipidemia constitutes a risk factor for vascular disease in nephrotic syndrome: Lipoprotein IDL- and LDL classes tend to be enriched in cholesterol ester *3931*

LDL-Cholesterol:HDL-Cholesterol Ratio *Serum Increase* Mean ratio in 31 patients with nephrotic syndrome of 5.6 ± 0.5 significantly higher than 2.6 ± 0.2 in 10 healthy controls *5004*

581.90 Nephrotic Syndrome *(continued)*

LDL-Cholesterol:HDL-Cholesterol Ratio *(continued)*
Ratio increased in patients with nephrotic syndrome due to increased LDL- and unchanged or reduced HDL-cholesterol concentration *2613*

LDL-Phospholipids *Serum* *Increase* In 10 patients with primary renal disease and nephrotic syndrome mean concentration of 188 ± 14 mg/dL and in 8 with diabetic nephropathy with nephrotic syndrome mean concentration of 177 ± 15 mg/dL significantly higher than normal *5569*

LDL-Triglycerides *Serum* *Increase* In 9 hypertriglyceridemic patients mean concentration of 0.66 ± 0.43 mmol/L compared with 0.29 ± 0.12 mmol/L in the same patients in remission and 0.35 ± 0.07 mmol/L in 10 normotriglyceridemic patients compared with 0.22 ± 0.12 mmol/L in the same patients in remission compared with 0.21 ± 0.11 mmol/L in 38 healthy controls *2499* In 10 patients with primary renal disease and nephrotic syndrome mean concentration of 76 ± 9 mg/dL and in 8 with diabetic nephropathy with nephrotic syndrome mean concentration of 76 ± 10 mg/dL significantly higher than normal *5569* In 22 patients with nephrotic syndrome mean plasma concentration of 0.56 ± 0.36 mmol/L significantly greater than 0.25 ± 0.10 mmol/L in 22 healthy matched controls *2498*

Leukocytes *Ascitic Fluid* *Increase* Less than 250 cells/µL *233*
Blood *Increase* In 56% of 24 patients at initial hospitalization for this disorder *1576*

Lipids *Serum* *Increase* Characterized by a great increase of all lipid constituents with both quantitative and qualitative alterations in lipoproteins *1980* Characteristic hyperlipidemia occurs with elevations in cholesterol, phospholipids, and triglycerides *367*
Urine *Increase* Lipiduria is a regular feature of the nephrotic syndrome. It is recognized in the fatty casts present in great numbers as well as in the cells which appear to be shed by the kidney *2039* All fractions increased *5544*

β-Lipoprotein *Serum* *Increase* In severe, fully developed cases, increase in low density lipoproteins with normal or decreased alpha lipoproteins has been described *1980* Untreated uncomplicated nephrotic syndrome is characterized by increased low (beta) and very low (prebeta) density lipoproteins and a diminution of high density (alpha) lipoprotein. Changes correlated strictly with albumin concentration were more pronounced with albumin concentration < 20 g/L *1717*

Lipoprotein Lp(a) *Serum* *Increase* In 22 patients with nephrotic syndrome mean plasma concentration of 0.98 g/L significantly greater than 0.17 g/L in 22 healthy matched controls *2498* Concentration increased in many renal diseases including nephrotic syndrome but mechanism for this in nephrotic disease unknown *2613* In 62 patients with nephrotic syndrome mean concentration of 46 (range 2 - 414) mg/dL significantly different from 7 (range 1 - 15) mg/dL in 12 healthy controls *5003* In patients with nephrotic syndrome with chronic renal failure 60% had Lp(a) concentrations greater than 30 mg/dL *2575* In 31 patients with nephrotic syndrome mean concentration of 49.0 mg/dL (range 19.4 - 79.0 mg/dL) significantly greater than 7.0 mg/dL in 10 healthy controls *5004* Characteristic finding *3526* In 62 patients with nephrotic syndrome mean concentration of 69 ± 10 mg/dL (median 46 mg/dL) significantly higher than mean of 18 ± 2 mg/dL (median 9 mg/dL) in 91 healthy controls *5570* In 9 hypertriglyceridemic patients mean concentration of 1,429 ± 914 mg/L compared with 185 ± 204 mg/L in the same patients in remission and 1,152 ± 604 mg/L in 10 normotriglyceridemic patients compared with 282 ± 101 mg/L in the same patients in remission compared with 173 ± 202 mg/L in 38 healthy controls *2499* Lp(a) concentration increased *2827*
Serum *No Effect* In 10 patients with primary renal disease and nephrotic syndrome mean concentration of 57 ± 21 mg/dL and in 8 with diabetic nephropathy with nephrotic syndrome mean concentration of 50 ± 14 mg/dL not significantly significantly different from normal *5569*

Lipoproteins *Serum* *Increase* More than 50% of the patients with glomerulonephritis, nephrotic syndrome and renovascular hypertension showed obviously abnormal lipoprotein profiles, returning to normal or near-normal when the disease was ameliorated or corrected surgically *5515*

Lipoproteins, Pre-β *Serum* *Increase* Untreated uncomplicated nephrotic syndrome is characterized by increased low (beta) and very low (prebeta) density lipoproteins and a diminution of high density (alpha) lipoprotein. Changes correlated strictly with albumin concentration and were more pronounced with albumin concentration < 20 g/L *1717*

Lymphocytes *Blood* *Decrease* In 41% of 26 patients at initial hospitalization for this disorder *1576*

α_2-Macroglobulin *Serum* *Decrease* In 39 patients with nephrotic syndrome mean concentration of 436 ± 31 mg/dL significantly different from 198 ± 14 mg/dL in 32 normal volunteers *5436*
Serum *Increase* Marked elevations *91* Primarily due to decreased plasma values and selective retention of the high molecular weight protein. Increased synthesis may also be a factor *2710* In 22 patients with nephrotic syndrome mean plasma concentration of 4.25 ± 1.72 g/L significantly greater than 1.43 ± 0.56 g/L in 22 healthy matched controls *2498* In 29 children with nephrotic syndrome mean concentration of 9.6 ± 3.4 g/L significantly increased compared with reference values of 2.85 ± 0.65 g/L *125* Concentration increased in proportion to the severity of protein loss in nephrotic syndrome *2952* Marked elevations *3778* Elevations as high as 1.0 g/dL have been noted *2937* In 39 patients with nephrotic syndrome mean activity of 197 ± 26% significantly different from 128 ± 8% in 32 normal volunteers *5436*
Urine *Increase* In 39 patients with nephrotic syndrome mean excretion of 27.8 ± 6.2 mg/g creatinine significantly different from undetectable amount in 32 normal volunteers *5436*

β_2-Macroglobulin *Serum* *Decrease* An increase in urine and a decrease in serum levels is seen *2586*
Urine *Increase* An increase in urine and a decrease in serum levels is seen *2586*

Magnesium *Serum* *Decrease* In a majority of cases, serum levels were low with concomitant increase in urinary concentration due to massive albuminuria, as 35% of Mg is bound to albumin *4013*
Urine *Increase* In a majority of cases, serum levels were low with concomitant increase in urinary concentration due to massive albuminuria, as 35% of Mg is bound to albumin *4013*

α_1-Microglobulin *Serum* *Decrease* In 22 patients with nephrotic syndrome mean plasma concentration of 56.7 ± 54.0 mg/L slightly reduced compared with 82.7 ± 27.2 mg/L in 22 healthy matched controls *2498*

N-Acetyl-Glucosaminidase B *Urine* *Increase* In 15 patients with nephrotic syndrome mean concentration of 9.0 ± 8.4 µg/L or 13.5 ± 11.9 µg/g creatinine significantly different from concentrations in 40 healthy adults in whom mean excretion was 3.1 ± 3.0 µg/L or 2.9 ± 2.0 µg/g creatinine *3838*

Neutrophils *Blood* *Increase* In 49% of 26 patients at initial hospitalization for this disorder *1576*

Nickel *Serum* *Decrease* Thought to be caused by hypoalbuminemia *3428*

Oncotic Pressure *Serum* *Decrease* Observed in conjunction with hypoalbuminemia in patients with nephrotic syndrome *3931*

Oval Fat Bodies *Urine* *Increase* The lipoid material is usually degenerative fatty vacuoles, neutral fat droplets, oval fat bodies, and doubly refractile fat bodies *1980*

pH *Pleural Fluid* *Increase* Transudate (pH > 7.3) *126*

Phosphate *Serum* *Increase* In 60% of 25 patients at initial hospitalization for this disorder *1576*

Phospholipids *Serum* *Increase* Typically elevated *1980* In 10 patients with primary renal disease and nephrotic syndrome mean concentration of 366 ± 13 mg/dL and in 8 with diabetic nephropathy with nephrotic syndrome mean concentration of 369 ± 20 mg/dL significantly higher than normal *5569* Elevated cholesterol with lipiduria can be demonstrated; however, phospholipids and triglycerides are even more consistently and strikingly elevated *1025*

Plasminogen *Plasma* *Decrease* Contributes to hypercoagulable state in nephrotic syndrome and associated with an excessive risk of thromboembolic complications *3931*
Plasma *Increase* In 39 patients with nephrotic syndrome mean concentration of 13.9 ± 0.7 mg/dL significantly different from 10.6 ± 0.3 mg/dL in 32 normal volunteers *5436*
Urine *Increase* In 39 patients with nephrotic syndrome mean excretion of 12.3 ± 2.5 mg/g creatinine significantly different from undetectable amount in 32 normal volunteers *5436*

Plasminogen Activator Inhibitor *Plasma* *Decrease* In 39 patients with nephrotic syndrome mean concentration of 7.5 ± 1.5 AU/mL not significantly different from 11.3 ± 1.6 AU/mL in 32 normal volunteers *5436*

Platelets *Blood* *Increase* In 43% of 18 patients at initial hospitalization for this disorder *1576* In 29 children with nephrotic syndrome mean concentration of 524 ± 172 10^9/L significantly increased compared with reference values of 250 ± 50 10^9/L *125* Mildly increased *5144* Thrombocytosis contributes to hypercoagulable state in nephrotic syndrome and associated with an excessive risk of thromboembolic complications *3931*

Prealbumin *Serum* *No Effect* In 22 patients with nephrotic syndrome mean plasma concentration of 0.27 ± 0.13 g/L not significantly reduced compared with 0.28 ± 0.25 g/L in 22 healthy matched controls *2498*

Prednisolone *Serum* *Decrease* Renal loss of cortisol binding globulin which also binds prednisolone probably responsible for reduced concentration of the drug *5869*

Prednisolone, Free *Serum* *Increase* In patients with nephrotic syndrome hypoalbuminemia increases the proportion of free drug producing toxicity *3931*

Properdin Factor B *Plasma* *No Effect* Mean concentration typically normal in patients with nephrotic syndrome *4682*

Protein *Ascitic Fluid* *Decrease* < 2.5 g/dL in ascitic fluid *233*
Pleural Fluid *Decrease* Transudate secondary to decreased albumin. (< 3 g/dL) *126*
Serum *Decrease* In 22 patients with nephrotic syndrome mean plasma concentration of 53.39 ± 5.07 g/L significantly less than 73.40 ± 5.21 g/L in 22 healthy matched controls *2498* Median concentration of 3.97 ± 0.74 g/dL in 16 children with nephrosis significantly different from 7.3 ± 0.74 g/dL in 16 normotensive healthy controls *458* In 29 children with nephrotic syndrome mean concentration of 43.9 ± 4.7 g/L significantly reduced compared with reference values of 65 ± 2.5 g/L *125*
Urine *Increase* High concentrations were observed in 19 patients, including adults and children *5498* In 22 patients with nephrotic syndrome mean excretion of 9.4 ± 6.2 g/d significantly greater than < 0.1 g/d in 22 healthy matched controls *2498* Contributes to hypercoagulable state in nephrotic syndrome and associated with an excessive risk of thromboembolic complications: protein excretion often more than 10 g/d *3931* In 39 patients with nephrotic syndrome mean excretion of 9.2 ± 1.3 g/d significantly different from excretion in 32 normal volunteers *5436* In 31 patients with nephrotic syndrome mean excretion significantly increased to 8.8 ± 0.7 g/d *5004* Heavy proteinuria must be present for this diagnosis *2039* In 62 patients with nephrotic syndrome mean excretion of 8.5 ± 0.5 g/d significantly different from dipstick negative amount in 12 healthy controls *5003* Median excretion of 89.9 ± 45.7 mg/m²/h in 16 children with nephrosis significantly different from 3.8 ± 45.7 mg/m²/h in 16 normotensive healthy controls *458*

Protein C *Plasma* *Decrease* Because of small size protein is lost in the urine as a result of increased permselectivity of the glomeruli *2613*
Plasma *Increase* In 29 children with nephrotic syndrome mean concentration of 153 ± 46% significantly increased compared with reference values of 95 ± 12.5% *125* Contributes to hypercoagulable state in nephrotic syndrome and associated with an excessive risk of thromboembolic complications *3931*
Urine *Increase* Excretion increased in urine because of increased glomerular permselectivity *2613*

Protein S *Plasma* *Decrease* Concentration reduced in patients with nephrotic syndrome because of its small molecular size and increased glomerular permselectivity *2613*
Plasma *Increase* Contributes to hypercoagulable state in nephrotic syndrome and associated with an excessive risk of thromboembolic complications *3931* In 29 children with nephrotic syndrome mean concentration of 117 ± 29% significantly increased compared with reference values of 95 ± 12.5% *125*
Urine *Increase* Excretion increased in urine due to small size and increased glomerular permselectivity *2613*

Protein S, Free *Plasma* *No Effect* In 29 children with nephrotic syndrome mean concentration of 91 ± 33% not significantly different when compared with reference values of 95 ± 12.5% *125*

Relative Viscosity *Blood* *Increase* In 29 children with nephrotic syndrome mean relative viscosity of 7.9 ± 0.9 mPa/s at shear rate 3.2 s^{-1} significantly increased versus 7.1 ± 0.6 mPa/s in controls and 4.7 ± 0.3 mPa/s versus 4.6 ± 0.2 mPa/s at shear rate 20.4 s^{-1} and 3.3 ± 0.2 mPa/s versus 3.0 ± 0.2 mPa/s at shear rate 128 s^{-1} after treatment for 3 weeks with steroids *125*

Sodium *Urine* *Decrease* Results from increased aldosterone secretion and reduced GFR *367* Mean excretion of 7.9 ± 2.5 mmol/h in 9 patients with nephrotic syndrome lower than 13.1 ± 1.5 mmol/h in 10 healthy controls *5004*

Specific Gravity *Pleural Fluid* *Decrease* Transudate (< 1.016) *126*

T3-Uptake *Serum* *Increase* Low T4 and raised resin uptake due to reduced TBG concentration occurs with protein loss *5863* Urinary loss of TBG results in lowering of most blood thyroid hormones and increased T3 uptake *1980*

β-Thromboglobulin *Plasma* *Increase* Thrombocytosis contributes to hypercoagulable state in nephrotic syndrome and associated with an excessive risk of thromboembolic complications *3931*

Thromboplastin Generation *Blood* *Increase* Has been noted *2634*

Thyroxine Binding Globulin *Serum* *Decrease* Concentration reduced due to loss in urine *1965* Decreased concentrations observed in patients with nephrotic syndrome *2952* Low T4 and raised resin uptake due to reduced TBG concentration occurs with protein loss *5863* Urinary loss of TBG results in lowering of most blood thyroid hormones and increased T3 uptake *1980* Decreased concentration observed due to renal loss *206*

Thyroxine (T4) *Serum* *Decrease* Low T4 and raised resin uptake due to reduced TBG concentration occurs with protein loss *5863* Urinary loss of TBG results in lowering of most blood thyroid hormones and increased T3 uptake *1980* Decreased concentration observed due to renal loss of TBG *206* In patients with nephrotic syndrome binding protein is lost in the urine with a resulting decrease in serum concentration *3931*

Tissue Plasminogen Activator Antigen *Plasma* *Increase* In 39 patients with nephrotic syndrome mean concentration of 5.2 ± 0.8 ng/mL significantly different from 3.6 ± 0.3 ng/mL in 32 normal volunteers *5436*

Transferrin *Saliva* *No Effect* In 10 children with steroid-sensitive nephrotic syndrome in remission mean concencentration of 4.1 mg/L significantly different from 5.8 mg/L in 11 healthy controls *3764*
Serum *Decrease* Concentrations as low as 40 mg/dL observed in patients with nephrotic syndrome *2952* In 22 patients with nephrotic syndrome mean plasma concentration of 1.26 ± 0.49 g/L significantly reduced compared with 2.86 ± 0.32 g/L in 22 healthy matched controls *2498* In patients with nephrotic syndrome due to loss in the urine *2613* In 10 children with steroid-sensitive nephrotic syndrome in remission mean concencentration of 1.7 g/L significantly different from 2.0 g/L in 11 healthy controls *3764*
Urine *Increase* In patients with nephrotic syndrome significant loss in the urine observed *2613*

Tri-iodothyronine (T3) *Serum* *Decrease* Typically associated with loss of TBG in urine *1965* Urinary loss of TBG results in lowering of most blood thyroid hormones and increased T3 uptake *1980*

Triglycerides *Serum* *Increase* Typically elevated *1980* In 31 patients with nephrotic syndrome mean concentration of 2.8 ± 0.3 mmol/L significantly greater than 1.0 ± 0.05 mmol/L in 10 healthy controls *5004* Elevated cholesterol with lipiduria can be demonstrated; however, phospholipids and triglycerides are even more consistently and strikingly elevated *1025* Hyperlipidemia constitutes a risk factor for vascular disease in nephrotic syndrome: VLDL-, IDL-, and LDL-triglycerides all contribute to increased plasma triglyceride concentration: overproduction and impaired catabolism of apolipoprotein B-containing lipoproteins observed *3931* In 9 hypertriglyceridemic patients mean concentration of 4.13 ± 1.38 mmol/L compared with 1.49 ± 0.69 mmol/L in the same patients in remission and 1.90 ± 0.91 mmol/L in 10 normotriglyceridemic patients compared with 1.24 ± 0.27 mmol/L in the same patients in remission compared with 1.10 ± 0.24 mmol/L in 38 healthy controls *2499* In 10 children with congenital nephrotic syndrome mean concentration of 8.40 ± 4.34 mmol/L significantly increased compared with 0.96 ± 0.34

581.90 Nephrotic Syndrome *(continued)*

Triglycerides *(continued)*
mmol/L in comparable controls *149* In patients with nephrotic syndrome and chronic renal failure 60% had triglyceride concentrations greater than 200 mg/dL *2575* Characteristic finding *3526* In 62 patients with nephrotic syndrome mean concentration of 3.0 ± 0.3 mmol/L significantly different from 1.0 ± 0.1 mmol/L in 12 healthy controls *5003* Commonly increased in patients with nephrotic syndrome *3746* In 25 individuals with nephrotic syndrome mean concentration of 2.27 ± 1.50 mmol/L significantly different from 1.70 ± 1.23 mmol/L in 98 healthy controls aged 24 to 55 years with method performed on ILab® 900 automated analyzer *4848* In 10 patients with primary renal disease and nephrotic syndrome mean concentration of 286 ± 60 mg/dL and in 8 with diabetic nephropathy with nephrotic syndrome mean concentration of 414 ± 58 mg/dL significantly higher than normal *5569* In 22 patients with nephrotic syndrome mean plasma concentration of 3.98 ± 1.12 mmol/L significantly greater than 1.25 ± 0.30 mmol/L in 22 healthy matched controls *2498*

Urea Nitrogen *Serum Decrease* Some patients *5544*
Serum Increase In 51% of 26 patients at initial hospitalization for this disorder *1576*

Uric Acid *Serum Increase* In 52% of 25 patients at initial hospitalization for this disorder *1576*

Viscosity *Blood Increase* In 29 children with nephrotic syndrome mean viscosity of 10.7 ± 1.6 mPa/s at shear rate of 3.2 /s, 6.2 ± 0.7 mPa/s at shear rate of 20.4 /s and 4.4 ± 0.5 mPa/s at shear rate of 128 /s significantly increased compared with reference values at corresponding shear rates of 9.0 ± 1.0 mPa/s, 5.5 ± 0.4 mPa/s and 3.9 ± 0.3 mPa/s respectively with no significant differences at shear rates of 0.20 mPa/s and 0.51 mPa/s *125*
Blood No Effect In 29 children with nephrotic syndrome mean viscosity of 21.1 ± 3.8 mPa/s not significantly different from reference range of 27.5 ± 5.2 mPa/s at shear rate 0.20 s^{-1}, and 19.3 ± 2.6 mPa/s versus 19.3 ± 2.8 mPa/s at shear rate 0.51 s *125*
Plasma Decrease In 22 patients with nephrotic syndrome mean plasma viscosity of 1.02 ± 0.10 mPa/s significantly less than 1.11 ± 0.09 mPa/s in 22 healthy matched controls *2498*
Plasma Increase With loss of low and intermediate molecular weight proteins in urine the amount of higher molecular weight proteins is increased and plasma viscosity is ncreased *2613* In 29 children with nephrotic syndrome mean viscosity of 1.35 ± 0.15 mPa/s significantly increased compared with reference values of 1.27 ± 0.04 mPa/s *125*

Vitamin D Binding Protein *Serum Decrease* Mean concentration of 371 ± 46 µg/mL significantly less than 436 ± 33 µg/mL in normal controls *2738*

VLDL-Cholesterol *Serum Increase* In 9 patients with nephrotic syndrome mean concentration of 3.7 ± 1.4 mmol/L significantly different from 0.3 ± 0.1 mmol/L in 41 healthy controls *5003* In patients with nephrotic syndrome increased synthesis and decreased catabolism observed *2613* In 9 hypertriglyceridemic patients mean concentration of 1.60 ± 0.59 mmol/L compared with 0.42 ± 0.22 mmol/L in the same patients in remission and 0.52 ± 0.23 mmol/L in 10 normotriglyceridemic patients compared with 0.26 ± 0.18 mmol/L in the same patients in remission compared with 0.27 ± 0.20 mmol/L in 38 healthy controls *2499* Commonly increased in patients with nephrotic syndrome *3746* Hyperlipidemia constitutes a risk factor for vascular disease in nephrotic syndrome *3931* Marked elevation with uremia *126* In 22 patients with nephrotic syndrome mean plasma concentration of 1.19 ± 0.66 mmol/L significantly greater than 0.38 ± 0.16 mmol/L in 22 healthy matched controls *2498* In 10 patients with primary renal disease and nephrotic syndrome mean concentration of 64 ± 16 mg/dL and in 8 with diabetic nephropathy with nephrotic syndrome mean concentration of 74 ± 18 mg/dL significantly higher than normal *5569* In 10 children with congenital nephrotic syndrome mean concentration of 1.80 ± 0.78 mmol/L significantly increased compared with 0.16 ± 0.10 mmol/L in comparable controls *149*

VLDL-Phospholipids *Serum Increase* In 10 patients with primary renal disease and nephrotic syndrome mean concentration of 70 ± 15 mg/dL and in 8 with diabetic nephropathy with nephrotic syndrome mean concentration of 84 ± 10 mg/dL significantly higher than normal *5569*

VLDL-Triglycerides *Serum Increase* In 9 hypertriglyceridemic patients mean concentration of 2.09 ± 3.07 mmol/L compared with 0.81 ± 0.22 mmol/L in the same patients in remission and 0.89 ± 0.52 mmol/L in 10 normotriglyceridemic patients compared with 0.68 ± 0.18 mmol/L in the same patients in remission compared with 0.60 ± 0.20 mmol/L in 38 healthy controls *2499* In 10 children with congenital nephrotic syndrome mean concentration of 4.52 ± 2.26 mmol/L significantly increased compared with 0.44 ± 0.29 mmol/L in comparable controls *149* In 10 patients with primary renal disease and nephrotic syndrome mean concentration of 187 ± 56 mg/dL and in 8 with diabetic nephropathy with nephrotic syndrome mean concentration of 315 ± 63 mg/dL significantly higher than normal *5569* In 22 patients with nephrotic syndrome mean plasma concentration of 2.11± 1.12 mmol/L significantly greater than 0.61 ± 0.20 mmol/L in 22 healthy matched controls *2498* In 9 patients with nephrotic syndrome mean concentration of 4.0 ± 1.0 mmol/L significantly different from 0.7 ± 0.1 mmol/L in 41 healthy controls *5003*

Volume *Blood Decrease* Contributes to hypercoagulable state in nephrotic syndrome and associated with an excessive risk of thromboembolic complications *3931*
Plasma Decrease Contributes to hypercoagulable state in nephrotic syndrome and associated with an excessive risk of thromboembolic complications *3931* In nephrotic syndrome, even with edema, blood volume is normal or decreased *3710*

Warfarin, Free *Plasma Increase* In patients with nephrotic syndrome hypoalbuminemia increases the proportion of free drug possibly producing toxicity *3931*

Zinc *Serum Decrease* In patients with nephrotic syndrome binding protein is lost in the urine with a resulting decrease in serum concentration *3931* Associated protein loss *4296* Decreased *5083*

582.10 Focal Glomerulosclerosis

Endothelin *Urine Increase* Urinary excretion in individuals with focal glomerulosclerosis reported to be significantly higher than in healthy individuals and correlated significantly with excretion of NAG, β-microglobulin and albumin *6*

582.90 Chronic Renal Disease

Albumin *Serum Decrease* Mean concentration in 42 patients with chronic renal disease of 37 ± 7 g/L significantly different from 44 ± 2 g/L in 75 healthy controls *4510*

Bicarbonate *Serum Decrease* Mean concentration of total carbon dioxide in 9 patients with chronic renal disease of 17 ± 3.9 mmol/L significantly different from 24 ± 2.1 mmol/L in 9 age and sex-matched controls *5801*

Chloride *Serum No Effect* Mean concentration in 9 patients with chronic renal disease of 101 ± 6.9 mmol/L not significantly different from 102 ± 4.4 mmol/L in 9 age and sex-matched controls *5801*

Cholesterol *Serum Increase* Mean concentration of 242 ± 113 mg/dL in 368 patients with impaired renal function significantly different from 180 ± 83 mg/d L in 163 healthy controls *2787*

Creatinine *Serum Increase* Mean concentration in 22 diabetics with chronic renal disease (creatinine < 2.0 mg/dL) of 0.92 ± 0.06 mg/dL significantly different from 0.77 ± 0.03 mg/dL in 20 healthy controls *1592*

Fractional Excretion of Sodium *Urine Increase* Mean concentration in 9 patients with chronic renal disease of 11.11 ± 2.54% significantly different from 1.49 ± 0.31% in 9 age and sex-matched controls *5801*

Glomerular Filtration Rate *Urine Decrease* Mean concentration in 9 patients with chronic renal disease of 9.2 ± 2.4 mL/min significantly different from 105.2 ± 3.9 mL/min in 9 age and sex-matched controls *5801*

γ-Glutamyltransferase *Serum Increase* Activity reportedly increased in a variety of diseases including diseases of the pancreas, myocardium, kidney and lung as well as in diabetes *4617*

Growth Hormone *Plasma Increase* Mean concentration in 22 diabetics with chronic renal disease (creatinine < 2.0 mg/dL) of 2.3 ± 1.0 ng/mL not significantly different from 1.8 ± 1.0 ng/mL in 20 healthy controls *1592*

HDL-Cholesterol *Serum* *Decrease* Mean concentration of 43 ± 19 mg/dL in 368 patients with impaired renal function significantly different from 49 ± 23 mg/dL in 163 healthy controls *2787*

Insulin-like Growth Factor-I *Serum* *No Effect* Mean concentration in 22 diabetics with chronic renal diease (creatinine < 2.0 mg/dL) of 254 ± 51 ng/mL not significantly different from 230 ± 14 g/mL in 20 healthy controls *1592*

Ionized Magnesium *Serum* *No Effect* Mean concentration in 42 patients with chronic renal disease of 0.57 ± 0.05 mmol/L not significantly different from 0.56 ± 0.05 mmol/L in 75 healthy controls *4510*

Ionized Magnesium:Total Magnesium Ratio *Serum* *Increase* Mean ratio in 42 patients with chronic renal disease of 0.73 ± 0.08 significantly different from 0.69 ± 0.04 in 75 healthy controls *4510*

LDL-Cholesterol *Serum* *Increase* Mean concentration of 162 ± 91 mg/dL in 368 patients with impaired renal function significantly different from 132 ± 61 mg/d L in 163 healthy controls *2787*

Lipoprotein Lp(a) *Serum* *Increase* Median concentration of 14.9 mg/dL in 368 patients with impaired renal function significantly different from 12.0 mg/dL in 163 healthy controls *2787*
Urine *Increase* Median concentration of 14.8 mg/dL in 368 patients with impaired renal function significantly different from 31.0 mg/dL in 163 healthy controls *2787*

Magnesium *Serum* *No Effect* Mean concentration in 42 patients with chronic renal disease of 0.80 ± 0.11 mmol/L not significantly different from 0.81 ± 0.07 mmol/L in 75 healthy controls *4510*

Potassium *Serum* *No Effect* Mean concentration in 9 patients with chronic renal disease of 4.3 ± 0.7 mmol/L not significantly different from 4.4 ± 0.4 mmol/L in 9 age and sex-matched controls *5801*

Renin Activity *Plasma* *Decrease* Mean concentration in 9 patients with chronic renal disease of 1.63 ± 0.17 ng/mL/h significantly different from 3.24 ± 0.62 ng/mL/h in 9 age and sex-matched controls *5801*

Sodium *Serum* *No Effect* Mean concentration in 9 patients with chronic renal disease of 131 ± 5.5 mmol/L not significantly different from 136 ± 0.7 mmol/L in 9 age and sex-matched controls *5801*
Urine *Decrease* Mean concentration in 9 patients with chronic renal disease of 143 ± 28 mmol/d significantly different from 293 ± 54 mmol/d in 9 age and sex-matched controls *5801*

Triglycerides *Serum* *Increase* Mean concentration of 227 ± 270 mg/dL in 368 patients with impaired renal function significantly different from 108 ± 139 mg/dL in 163 healthy controls *2787*

Urea Nitrogen *Serum* *Increase* Mean concentration in 22 diabetics with chronic renal disease (creatinine < 2.0 mg/dL) of 17 ± 1 mg/dL not significantly different from 15 ± 1 mg/dL in 20 healthy controls *1592*

582.90 Glomerulonephritis, Chronic

Aluminum *Bone* *Increase* In 10 patients with chronic glomerulonephritis receiving regular hemodialysis mean concentration of 13.0 ± 4.7 µg/g wet weight *1167*

Arginine *Plasma* *No Effect* In 22 patients with chronic glomerulonephritis without dialysis concentrations of 93 - 182 ng/mL not different from 63 - 508 ng/mL in 10 normal controls *2331*

Complement C_1 *Serum* *No Effect* Mean concentration typically normal in patients with chronic glomerulonephritis or Goodpasture's syndrome *4682*

Complement C_1q *Serum* *No Effect* Mean concentration typically normal in patients with chronic glomerulonephritis or Goodpasture's syndrome *4682*

Complement C_2 *Serum* *No Effect* Mean concentration typically normal in patients with chronic glomerulonephritis or Goodpasture's syndrome *4682*

Complement C_3 *Serum* *No Effect* Mean concentration typically normal in patients with chronic glomerulonephritis or Goodpasture's syndrome *4682*

Complement C_4 *Serum* *No Effect* Mean concentration typically normal in patients with chronic glomerulonephritis or Goodpasture's syndrome *4682*

Complement C_5 *Serum* *No Effect* Mean concentration typically normal in patients with chronic glomerulonephritis or Goodpasture's syndrome *4682*

Complement CH50 *Serum* *No Effect* Mean concentration typically normal in patients with chronic glomerulonephritis or Goodpasture's syndrome *4682*

Creatine *Serum* *Increase* In 22 patients with chronic glomerulonephritis concentrations of 20 - 607 ng/mL higher than 7 - 128 ng/mL in 10 normal controls *2331*

Creatinine *Serum* *Increase* In 22 patients with chronic glomerulonephritis concentrations of 952 - 2,595 ng/mL higher than 17 - 103 ng/mL in 10 normal controls *2331*

D-Dimer *Urine* *No Effect* In 45 patients with chronic glomerulonephritis median concentration of 0.44 ng/mL not significantly different from that in normal controls in whom the mean concentration was 0.69 ± 0.60 ng/mL *4789*

Fibrin/Fibrinogen Degradation Product E *Urine* *Increase* In 30 patients with chronic glomerulonephritis mean excretion of 8.89 ± 8.98 ng/mL significantly different from 1.68 ± 1.05 ng/mL in 30 controls *4790*

Guanidine *Serum* *Increase* In 22 patients with chronic glomerulonephritis concentrations of 0.13 - 0.44 ng/mL higher than undetectable amounts in 10 normal controls *2331*

Guanidinoacetic Acid *Serum* *Increase* In 22 patients with chronic glomerulonephritis concentrations of 1.13 - 3.15 ng/mL higher than 0.58 - 2.03 ng/mL in 10 normal controls *2331*

γ-Guanidinobutyric Acid *Serum* *Increase* In 22 patients with chronic glomerulonephritis concentrations of 0 - 3.02 ng/mL not different from undetectable amounts in 10 normal controls *2331*

β-Guanidinopropionic Acid *Serum* *Increase* In 22 patients with chronic glomerulonephritis concentrations of 0 - 3.62 ng/mL higher than undetectable amounts in 10 normal controls *2331*

Guanidinosuccinic Acid *Serum* *Increase* In 22 patients with chronic glomerulonephritis concentrations of 4.86 - 39.51 ng/mL higher than undetectable amounts in 10 normal controls *2331*

Intercellular Adhesion Molecule-1 *Serum* *No Effect* In 10 patients with active disease mean concentration of 347 ng/mL not significantly different from 245 ng/mL in 10 healthy controls *3638*

Methylguanidine *Serum* *Increase* In 6 patients with diabetic nephropathy concentrations of 1.47 - 7.28 ng/mL higher than undetectable amounts in 10 normal controls *2331*

Monocyte Chemotactic Protein-1 *Serum* *Decrease* Mean concentration of 46 ± 46 pg/mL in 3 patients with chronic glomerulonephritis compared with 101 ± 24 pg/mL in 16 healthy women and men *4460*
Urine *Increase* In 3 patients with chronic glomerulonephritis mean concentration of 4,069 ± 1,929 pg/mg creatinine significantly different when compared with mean concentration of 130 ± 30 pg/mg creatinine in 30 healthy women and 32 healthy men *4460*

Properdin Factor B *Plasma* *No Effect* Mean concentration typically normal in patients with chronic glomerulonephritis or Goodpasture's syndrome *4682*

Soluble E-Selectin *Serum* *Increase* 10 patients with active disease had a mean concentration not significantly different from 48 ng/mL in 10 healthy controls *3638*

Soluble Vascular Cell Adhesion Molecule-1 *Serum* *Increase* 10 patients with active disease had a mean concentration of 1,259 ng/mL significantly greater than 582 ng/mL in 10 healthy donors *3638*

Taurocyamine *Serum* *Increase* In 22 patients with chronic glomerulonephritis concentrations of 0 - 1.37 ng/mL different from undetectable amounts in 10 normal controls *2331*

583.00 Glomerulonephritis-1, Membranoproliferative

CD45 Leukocytes *Tissue* *Increase* In 1 patient with membranoproliferative glomerulonephritis-1 number of positive cells 673 cells/mm² in renal tissue *3026*

583.00 Glomerulonephritis-1, Membranoproliferative *(continued)*

Complement, Total Hemolytic *Serum* *Decrease* Concentration decreased below 30 U/mL in 13 of 26 patients *4931*

Creatinine *Serum* *Increase* In 1 patient with membranoproliferative glomerulonephropathy-1 concentration of 1.05 mg/dL different from 0.88 ± 0.17 mg/dL in 20 healthy controls *3026*

Intercellular Adhesion Molecule-1 *Tissue* *Increase* In 1 patient with membranoproliferative glomerulonephritis-1 percentage of ICAM-1 positive renal tubuli 14.0% *3026*

Protein *Urine* *Increase* Concentration increased to 2.9 ± 0.9 g/d in 13 patients with hypocomplementemia *4931* In 1 patient with membranoproliferative glomerulonephritis-1 excretion of 2.33 mg/mg creatinine *3026*

Soluble Intercellular Adhesion Molecule-1 *Serum* *Increase* In 1 patient with membranoproliferative glomerulonephritis-1 concentration of soluble ICAM-1 of 540 ng/mL compared with 306 ± 52 ng/mL in 20 healthy controls *3026*
Urine *Increase* In 1 patient with membranoproliferative glomerulonephritis-1 excretion of soluble ICAM-1 of 35.0 ng/mL or 31.8 ng/mg creatinine compared with 2.6 ± 1.7 ng/mL or 2.5 ± 3.0 ng/mg creatinine in 20 healthy controls *3026*

583.10 Glomerulonephritis, Membranous

Alanine Aminotransferase *Urine* *Increase* Increased *4096 2508 5671*

Albumin *Urine* *Increase* Usually occurs, with size of proteins indicating degree of glomerular damage *5686* In excess of 3 g/d is characteristic *900*

Amino Acids *Plasma* *Decrease* Mean concentration of essential amino acids and tyrosine were significantly lower, resulting in a low essential/total ratio *3409*

Anti-Streptolysin-O Titer *Serum* *Increase* Above normal titers may occur *3953*

Ceruloplasmin *Serum* *Increase* Found regularly with hypoproteinemia *2210*

Cholesterol *Serum* *Increase* Occurs, but is less frequent than in minimal change glomerulonephritis *367*

Complement C_3 *Serum* *No Effect* Nearly always *872*

Complement C_4 *Serum* *No Effect* Nearly always *872*

Complement, Total *Serum* *No Effect* Nearly always *872*

Copper *Serum* *Increase* Found regularly with hypoproteinemia *2210*

Creatinine Clearance *Urine* *Decrease* Progression of the disease is characterized by declining creatinine clearance *900*

Erythrocytes *Urine* *Increase* Hematuria usually occurs in conjunction with proteinuria, but may occur alone in some cases *5686* Microscopic hematuria is common *669* Gross hematuria is uncommon even though microscopic hematuria is observed in 40% of the patients *900*

Factor B *Plasma* *Increase* Elevated in 38% of 26 females with acne between ages of 27 and 42 y *4431 5229*

Glucose *Serum* *Increase* Chemical or overt diabetes appears more common than might be expected by chance *850*

Granular Casts *Urine* *Increase* Usually present *900*

β-Hexosaminidase *Urine* *Decrease* Decreased levels in urine *5229*

Hyaline Casts *Urine* *Increase* Usually present *900*

Interleukin-1β *Urine* *Increase* In 21 patients mean excretion of 403 ± 48 pg/mg creatinine significantly increased compared with 172 ± 27 pg/mg creatinine in 13 healthy controls *2985*

Protein *Pleural Fluid* *Decrease* Pleural effusions are usually transudates (< 3 g/dL) *126*
Serum *Decrease* Usually occurs, with size of proteins indicating degree of glomerular damage. Albumin is nearly always present *5686* Onset of disease was marked by proteinuria without nephrotic syndrome in 24.2% of patients *3817* Proteinuria is nonselective, distinguishing it from minimal change glomerulonephritis *367*
Urine *Increase* Proteinuria is nonselective, distinguishing it from minimal change glomerulonephritis *367* Usually occurs, with size of proteins indicating degree of glomerular damage. Albumin is nearly always present *5686* Onset of disease was marked by proteinuria without nephrotic syndrome in 24.2% of patients *3817*

Tryptophan *Plasma* *Increase* Tyrosine and tryptophan usually rise in acute and chronic glomerulonephritis *4707*

Tumor Necrosis Factor-α *Urine* *Increase* In 21 patients mean excretion of 37.2 ± 2.6 pg/mg creatinine significantly increased compared with 13.5 ± 1.5 pg/mg creatinine in 13 healthy controls *2985*

Tyrosine *Plasma* *Decrease* Mean concentration of essential amino acids and tyrosine were significantly lower, resulting in a low essential/total ratio *3409*
Plasma *Increase* Tyrosine and tryptophan usually rise in acute and chronic glomerulonephritis *4707*

Urea Nitrogen *Serum* *Increase* Occurs late in course *872*

583.20 Glomerulonephritis, Membranoproliferative

Alanine Aminotransferase *Urine* *Increase* Increased *2508 5671 4096*

Albumin *Serum* *Decrease* Mean concentration in 7 patients with membranoproliferative glomerulonephritis of 38 ± 5 g/L different from 43 ± 3 g/L in 8 patients with minimal change glomerulonephritis *4566*

Anti-Streptolysin-O Titer *Serum* *Increase* In about 40% of patients *668*

α_2-Antiplasmin *Plasma* *No Effect* A slight decrease in patients with nephrotic syndrome, but a normal level in patients with chronic latent glomerulonephritis *5117*

Ceruloplasmin *Serum* *Increase* Found regularly with hypoproteinemia *2210*

Chloride *Serum* *Increase* 16 patients with membranoproliferative glomerulonephritis had a mean value significantly higher than that in normal subjects or patients with nephrotic syndrome *1234*

Complement C_1 *Serum* *No Effect* Mean concentration typically normal in patients with membranoproliferative glomerulonephritis *4682*

Complement C_1q *Serum* *No Effect* Mean concentration typically normal in patients with membranoproliferative glomerulonephritis *4682*

Complement C_2 *Serum* *No Effect* Mean concentration typically normal in patients with membranoproliferative glomerulonephritis *4682*

Complement C_3 *Serum* *Decrease* Permanent depression of C_3 is found in 60 - 80% of patients *5545* Profound prolonged depression ascribed to anticomplementary factors *2034* In 70% of cases *668* Mean concentration typically slightly reduced in patients with membranoproliferative glomerulonephritis *4682*

Complement C_4 *Serum* *No Effect* Mean concentration typically normal in patients with membranoproliferative glomerulonephritis *4682* Concentration usually normal *572*

Complement C_5 *Serum* *Decrease* Mean concentration typically slightly reduced in patients with membranoproliferative glomerulonephritis *4682*

Complement CH50 *Serum* *Decrease* Mean concentration typically slightly decreased in patients with membranoproliferative glomerulonephritis *4682*

Complement, Total *Serum* *Decrease* Characteristic of membranoproliferative glomerulonephritis *5686*

Copper *Serum* *Increase* Found regularly with hypoproteinemia *2210*

C-Reactive Protein *Serum* *Increase* Mean concentration in 7 patients with membranoproliferative glomerulonephritis of 0.14 ± 0.13 mg/dL different from 0.06 ± 0.03 mg/dL in 8 patients with minimal change glomerulonephritis *4566*

Creatinine *Serum* *Increase* Mean concentration in 7 patients with membranoproliferative glomerulonephritis of 106.1 ± 17.7 µmol/L different from 70.7 ± 26.5 µmol/L in 8 patients with minimal change glomerulonephritis *4566* BUN and creatinine rise as GFR decreases *1980*

Creatinine Clearance *Urine* *Decrease* Mean excretion in 7 patients with membranoproliferative glomerulonephritis of 60.8 ± 15.5 mL/min different from 103.9 ± 25.5 mL/min in 8 patients with minimal change glomerulonephritis *4566*

Endothelin *Urine* *Increase* Urinary excretion in individuals with membranous proliferative glomerulonephritis reported to be significantly higher than in healthy individuals and correlated significantly with excretion of NAG, β-microglobulin and albumin *6*

Erythrocyte Sedimentation Rate *Blood* *Decrease* Normal or low *2093*

Glomerular Filtration Rate *Urine* *Decrease* BUN and creatinine rise as GFR decreases *1980* In 50% of cases *668*

Hematocrit *Blood* *Decrease* In over 50% of the cases *668* Mild anemia which is normocytic and normochromic develops as azotemia occurs *1980*

Hemoglobin *Blood* *Decrease* In over 50% of the cases *668* Mild anemia which is normocytic and normochromic develops as azotemia occurs *1980* Mean concentration in 7 patients with membranoproliferative glomerulonephritis of 12.4 ± 1.2 g/dL different from 13.8 ± 1.4 g/dL in 8 patients with minimal change glomerulonephritis *4566*

β-Hexosaminidase *Urine* *Decrease* Decreased levels in urine *5229*

Interleukin-6 *Serum* *Increase* Mean concentration in 7 patients with membranoproliferative glomerulitis of 1.8 ± 3.1 pg/mL not significantly different from 0.4 ± 0.6 pg/mL in 42 healthy controls *4566*
Urine *Increase* Mean concentration in 7 patients with membranoproliferative glomerulitis of 7.4 ± 7.3 pg/mL significantly different from 0.4 ± 0.7 pg/mL in 42 healthy controls *4566*

Leukocytes *Blood* *Decrease* Mean concentration in 7 patients with membranoproliferative glomerulonephritis of 7.1 ± 2.0 x 10^3 /µL different from 6.4 ± 1.9 x 10^3 /µL in 8 patients with minimal change glomerulonephritis *4566*

α_2-Macroglobulin *Serum* *Increase* Reported effect *2088*

Monocyte Chemotactic Protein-1 *Serum* *Increase* Mean concentration of 222 ± 22 pg/mL in 3 patients with MPGN compared with 101 ± 24 pg/mL in 16 healthy women and men *4460*
Urine *Increase* In 3 patients with membroproliferative glomerulonephritis mean concentration of 1,181 ± 481 pg/mg creatinine significantly different when compared with mean concentration of 130 ± 30 pg/mg creatinine in 30 healthy women and 32 healthy men *4460*

Phosphate *Serum* *Increase* As functional loss becomes severe (GFR 50% of normal or less), there is usually a rise in serum phosphate and uric acid *1980*

Procollagen Type IV Peptide *Serum* *Increase* The highest serum concentrations were found in nine patients with membranoproliferative glomerulonephritis (16 ± 9.4 ng/mL) *2623*

Properdin Factor B *Plasma* *Decrease* Mean concentration typically slightly reduced in patients with membranoproliferative glomerulonephritis *4682*

Protein *Pleural Fluid* *Decrease* Pleural effusions are usually transudates (< 3 g/dL) *126*
Serum *Decrease* Mean concentration in 7 patients with membranoproliferative glomerulonephritis of 68 ± 11 g/L different from 73 ± 7 g/L in 8 patients with minimal change glomerulonephritis *4566* *4566*
Urine *No Effect* Mean excretion in 7 patients with membranoproliferative glomerulonephritis of 1.03 ± 0.79 g/d not different from 0.97 ± 1.24 g/d in 8 patients with minimal change glomerulonephritis *4566*

Soluble Fas Antigen *Serum* *Increase* Mean concentration in 7 patients with membranoproliferative glomerulitis of 3.9 ± 1.5 ng/mL significantly different from 2.2 ± 0.6 ng/mL in 42 healthy controls *4566*
Urine *No Effect* Mean concentration in 7 patients with membranoproliferative glomerulitis of 0.0 ± 0.0 ng/mL not significantly different from 0.0 ± 0.0 ng/mL in 42 healthy controls *4566*

Soluble Fas Ligand Antigen *Serum* *No Effect* Mean concentration in 7 patients with membranoproliferative glomerulitis of 0.69 ± 0.09 ng/mL not significantly different from 0.56 ± 0.14 ng/mL in 42 healthy controls *4566*
Urine *Increase* Mean concentration in 7 patients with membranoproliferative glomerulitis of 1.0 ± 1.7 pg/mL not significantly different from 0.0 ± 0.0 pg/mL in 42 healthy controls *4566*

Tyrosine *Plasma* *Increase* Tyrosine and tryptophan usually rise in acute and chronic glomerulonephritis *4707*

Urea Nitrogen *Serum* *Increase* BUN and creatinine rise as GFR decreases *1980* Mean concentration in 7 patients with membranoproliferative glomerulonephritis of 3.0 ± 0.9 mmol/L different from 2.1 ± 0.8 mmol/L in 8 patients with minimal change glomerulonephritis *4566*

Tryptophan *Plasma* *Increase* Tyrosine and tryptophan usually rise in acute and chronic glomerulonephritis *4707*

Tumor Necrosis Factor *Urine* *Increase* In 8 patients with MPGN mean concentration of 126.7 ± 63.2 pg/mL significantly higher than in healthy controls *3962*

Tumor Necrosis Factor-α *Serum* *Increase* Mean concentration in 7 patients with membranoproliferative glomerulitis of 12.1 ± 17.1 pg/mL not significantly different from 4.4 ± 6.4 pg/mL in 42 healthy controls *4566*

583.20 Glomerulonephritis, Mesangioproliferative

α_1-Acid Glycoprotein *Serum* *Increase* In 97 patients with MPGN median concentration of 0.86 ± 0.21 g/L significantly greater than 0.72 ± 0.07 g/L in 45 healthy controls with concentration higher in those with moderate to severe albuminuria than in those with heavy range albuminuria *5193*

α_1-Antitrypsin *Serum* *Increase* In 31 patients with MPGN median concentration of 1.54 ± 0.28 g/L significantly greater than 1.22 ± 0.08 g/L in 45 healthy controls with concentration higher in those with mild to moderate albuminuria than in those with heavy range albuminuria *5193*

CD45 Leukocytes *Tissue* *Increase* In 1 patient with mesangioproliferative glomerulonephritis number of positive cells 590 cells/mm² renal tisue *3026*

C-Reactive Protein *Serum* *No Effect* In 97 patients with MPGN median concentration of 5 ± 0 mg/L not significantly different from 5.0 ± 0 mg/L in 45 healthy controls *5193*

Creatinine *Serum* *Increase* In 1 patient with mesangioproliferative glomerulonephritis concentration of 1.48 mg/dL different from 0.88 ± 0.17 mg/dL in 20 healthy controls *3026*

Haptoglobin *Serum* *Increase* In 97 patients with MPGN median concentration of 2.21 ± 0.67 g/L significantly greater than 1.53 ± 0.42 g/L in 45 healthy controls with concentration higher in those with heavy range albuminuria than in those with mild to moderate albuminuria *5193*

Intercellular Adhesion Molecule-1 *Tissue* *Increase* In 1 patient with mesangioproliferative glomerulonephritis percentage of ICAM-1 positive renal tubuli 1.0% *3026*

Interleukin-6 *Serum* *Increase* A prospective study of plasma interleukin-6 (IL-6) levels was performed in 54 patients. Interleukin-6 was found in plasma of nine patients *2235*
Urine *Increase* Interleukin-6 was not detected in the urine of 10 patients with rheumatoid arthritis with raised plasma IL-6 *2235* A prospective study of plasma and urinary interleukin-6 (IL-6) levels was performed in 54 patients. Interleukin-6 was found in the urine of twenty-two patients. Interleukin-6 was not detected in the urine of 10 healthy controls or the urine of 10 patients with rheumatoid arthritis with raised plasma IL-6. Interleukin-6 was found in the urine of only one out of an additional seven patients with lupus nephritis *2235*

N-Acetyl-Glucosaminidase B *Urine* *Increase* In 12 patients with mesangeal glomerulonephritis mean concentration of 10.1 ± 7.6 µg/L or 10.6 ± 10.1 µg/g creatinine significantly different from concentrations in 40 healthy adults in whom mean excretion was 3.1 ± 3.0 µg/L or 2.9 ± 2.0 µg/g creatinine *3838*

Protein *Urine* *Increase* In 1 patient with mesangioproliferative glomerulonephritis excretion of 1.31 mg/mg creatinine *3026*

Soluble Intercellular Adhesion Molecule-1 *Serum* *Increase* In 1 patient with mesangioproliferative glomerulonephritis concentration of soluble ICAM-1 of 440 ng/mL compared with 306 ± 52 ng/mL in 20 healthy controls *3026*
Urine *Increase* In 1 patient with mesangioproliferative glomerulonephritis excretion of soluble ICAM-1 of 5.3 ng/mL or 7.6 ng/mg creatinine compared with 2.6 ± 1.7 ng/mL or 2.5 ± 3.0 ng/mg creatinine in 20 healthy controls *3026*

583.20 Mesangial Proliferative Glomerulonephritis

Albumin *Serum* *No Effect* Mean concentration in 10 patients with mesangial proliferative glomerulonephritis of 42 ± 4 g/L not different from 43 ± 3 g/L in 8 patients with minimal change glomerulonephritis *4566*

583.20 Mesangial Proliferative Glomerulonephritis *(continued)*

C-Reactive Protein *Serum* *Increase* Mean concentration in 10 patients with mesangial proliferative glomerulonephritis of 0.19 ± 0.20 mg/dL different from 0.06 ± 0.03 mg/dL in 8 patients with minimal change glomerulonephritis *4566*

Creatinine *Serum* *Increase* Mean concentration in 10 patients with mesangial proliferative glomerulonephritis of 106.1 ± 26.5 μmol/L different from 70.7 ± 26.5 μmol/L in 8 patients with minimal change glomerulonephritis *4566*

Creatinine Clearance *Urine* *Decrease* Mean clearance in 10 patients with mesangial proliferative glomerulonephritis of 74.4 ± 23.9 mL/min different from 103.9 ± 25.5 mL/min in 8 patients with minimal change glomerulonephritis *4566*

Hemoglobin *Blood* *No Effect* Mean concentration in 10 patients with mesangial proliferative glomerulonephritis of 14.1 ± 1.9 g/dL not different from 13.8 ± 1.4 g/dL in 8 patients with minimal change glomerulonephritis *4566*

Interleukin-6 *Serum* *Increase* Mean concentration in 10 patients with mesangial proliferative glomerulonephritis of 2.0 ± 3.4 pg/mL not significantly different from 0.4 ± 0.7 pg/mL in 60 healthy controls *4566*
Urine *Increase* Mean concentration in 10 patients with mesangial proliferative glomerulonephritis of 5.2 ± 6.1 pg/mL not significantly different from 0.3 ± 0.6 pg/mL in 60 healthy controls *4566*

Leukocytes *Blood* *No Effect* Mean concentration in 10 patients with mesangial proliferative glomerulonephritis of 6.8 ± 1.8 x 10^3 /μL not different from 6.4 ± 1.9 x 10^3 /μL in 8 patients with minimal change glomerulonephritis *4566*

Protein *Serum* *No Effect* Mean concentration in 10 patients with mesangial proliferative glomerulonephritis of 74 ± 5 g/L not different from 73 ± 7 g/L in 8 patients with minimal change glomerulonephritis *4566*
Urine *Increase* Mean excretion in 10 patients with mesangial proliferative glomerulonephritis of 1.26 ± 1.28 g/d different from 0.97 ± 1.24 g/d in 8 patients with minimal change glomerulonephritis *4566*

Soluble Fas Antigen *Serum* *Increase* Mean concentration in 10 patients with mesangial proliferative glomerulonephritis of 3.4 ± 0.9 ng/mL significantly different from 2.1 ± 0.4 ng/mL in 60 healthy controls *4566*
Urine *No Effect* Mean concentration in 10 patients with mesangial proliferative glomerulonephritis of 0.0 ± 0.0 ng/mL not significantly different from 0.0 ± 0.0 ng/mL in 60 healthy controls *4566*

Soluble Fas Ligand Antigen *Serum* *No Effect* Mean concentration in 10 patients with mesangial proliferative glomerulonephritis of 0.53 ± 0.09 ng/mL not significantly different from 0.55 ± 0.13 ng/mL in 60 healthy controls *4566*

Tumor Necrosis Factor-α *Serum* *Increase* Mean concentration in 10 patients with mesangial proliferative glomerulonephritis of 12.8 ± 17.9 pg/mL not significantly different from 4.2 ± 6.1 pg/mL in 60 healthy controls *4566*
Urine *Increase* Mean concentration in 10 patients with mesangial proliferative glomerulonephritis of 0.5 ± 1.2 pg/mL not significantly different from 0.0 ± 0.0 pg/mL in 60 healthy controls *4566*

Urea Nitrogen *Serum* *Increase* Mean concentration in 10 patients with mesangial proliferative glomerulonephritis of 2.7 ± 0.6 mmol/L different from 2.1 ± 0.8 mmol/L in 8 patients with minimal change glomerulonephritis *4566*

583.40 Glomerulonephritis, Rapidly Progressive

Alanine Aminotransferase *Urine* *Increase* Increased *2508* *4096* *5671*

Albumin *Urine* *Increase* Usually occurs; with size of proteins indicating degree of glomerular damage *5686*

Anti-Myeloperoxidase III Antibodies *Serum* *Increase* All p-ANCA-positive patients had titers of anti-MPO antibodies *4503*

Anti-Streptolysin-O Titer *Serum* *Increase* May be found in 30% of patients without other evidence of streptococcal etiology *5685*

Calcium *Serum* *Decrease* Decreases renal failure develops *1980*

Casts *Urine* *Increase* Observed effect *5686*

Ceruloplasmin *Serum* *Increase* Found regularly with hypoproteinemia *2210*

Complement C_3 *Serum* *No Effect* No significant effect observed *3021*

Complement C_4 *Serum* *No Effect* No significant effect observed *3021*

Complement, Total *Serum* *No Effect* Concentration usually normal *3021* *1980*

Copper *Serum* *Increase* Found regularly with hypoproteinemia *2210*

Creatinine *Serum* *Increase* Over 2.5 mg/dL at time of biopsy in all cases *3614* BUN and creatinine rise as GFR decreases *1980*

Erythrocytes *Urine* *Increase* Hematuria is usually microscopic, and it is a rather constant feature indicating activity *1980* Microscopic hematuria in 15 of 29 patients *3614* Hematuria usually occurs in conjunction with proteinuria, but may occur alone in some cases *5686*

Glomerular Filtration Rate *Urine* *Decrease* BUN and creatinine rise as GFR decreases *1980*

Hematocrit *Blood* *Decrease* Anemia which is normocytic and normochromic develops as azotemia occurs *1980*

Hemoglobin *Blood* *Decrease* Anemia which is normocytic and normochromic develops as azotemia occurs *1980*

β-Hexosaminidase *Urine* *Decrease* Decreased levels in urine *5229*

Myeloperoxidase *Serum* *Increase* All p-ANCA-positive patients had measurable myeloperoxidase activity, not demonstrated in normal individuals *4503*

Phosphate *Serum* *Increase* As functional loss becomes severe (GFR 50% of normal or less), there is usually a rise in serum phosphate and uric acid *1980*

Platelets *Blood* *Decrease* Observed occasionally *572*

Protein *Urine* *Increase* Exceeds 2.5 g/d in 8 of 29 cases *3614* Proteinuria is always present *1980* Usually occurs; with size of proteins indicating degree of glomerular damage. Albumin is nearly always present *5686*

Specific Gravity *Urine* *Decrease* Concentrating capacity is impaired, with urine specific gravity around 1.010 *1980*

Tryptophan *Plasma* *Increase* Tyrosine and tryptophan usually rise in acute and chronic glomerulonephritis *4707*

Tyrosine *Plasma* *Increase* Tyrosine and tryptophan usually rise in acute and chronic glomerulonephritis *4707*

Urea Nitrogen *Serum* *Increase* Usually > 80 mg/dL *5545* BUN and creatinine rise as GFR decreases *1980*

Uric Acid *Serum* *Increase* As functional loss becomes severe (GFR 50% of normal or less), there is usually a rise in serum phosphate and uric acid *1980*

Volume *Urine* *Decrease* Oliguria < 500 mL/24 h was present in 20 of 29 cases and dialysis was required in 22 *3614*

583.60 Renal Cortical Necrosis

Aspartate Aminotransferase *Serum* *Increase* May cause increased AST activity *4617*

583.81 Lupus Nephritis

Ammonium Ions *Urine* *Decrease* May cause distal renal tubular acidosis (type IV) is associated with hyperkalemia, hyperchloremic metabolic acidosis, urine pH < 5.5, decreased urinary ammonium ion excretion, a positive urine anion gap, normal urinary citrate and urinary calcium excretion *4071*

Anion Gap *Urine* *Increase* May cause distal renal tubular acidosis (type IV) is associated with hyperkalemia, hyperchloremic metabolic acidosis, urine pH < 5.5, decreased urinary ammonium ion excretion, a positive urine anion gap, normal urinary citrate and urinary calcium excretion *4071*

Anti-DNA Antibodies *Serum Increase* In 7 patients with WHO class II disease mean concentration of 9 U/mL (25% to 75% range 7 - 33): in 10 patients with class IV disease mean of 112 U/mL (range 61 - 758) and in 9 with class V disease mean of 25 U/mL (9.5 - 60) *2377*

Calcium *Urine No Effect* May cause distal renal tubular acidosis (type IV) is associated with hyperkalemia, hyperchloremic metabolic acidosis, urine pH < 5.5, decreased urinary ammonium ion excretion, a positive urine anion gap, normal urinary citrate and urinary calcium excretion *4071*

CD45 Leukocytes *Tissue Increase* In 6 patients with lupus nephritis mean number of positive cells 563 ± 329 cells/mm^2 in renal tissue *3026*

Chloride *Serum Increase* May cause distal renal tubular acidosis (type IV) is associated with hyperkalemia, hyperchloremic metabolic acidosis, urine pH < 5.5, decreased urinary ammonium ion excretion, a positive urine anion gap, normal urinary citrate and urinary calcium excretion *4071*

Citrate *Urine No Effect* May cause distal renal tubular acidosis (type IV) is associated with hyperkalemia, hyperchloremic metabolic acidosis, urine pH < 5.5, decreased urinary ammonium ion excretion, a positive urine anion gap, normal urinary citrate and urinary calcium excretion *4071*

Complement CH50 *Serum No Effect* In 7 patients with WHO class II disease mean concentration of 25 mg/dL (25% to 75% range 12 - 32) compared with normal range of 32 - 41 U/mL): in 10 with class IV disease mean 9.5 U/mL (range 9 - 18) and in 9 with class V disease mean 35 U/mL (range 26 - 38) *2377*

Creatinine *Serum Increase* In 6 patients with lupus nephritis mean concentration of 1.21 ± 0.51 mg/dL higher than 0.88 ± 0.17 mg/dL in 20 healthy controls *3026*
Serum No Effect In 7 patients with WHO class II disease mean concentration of 0.6 mg/dL (25% to 75% range of 0.5 - 0.7): in 10 with class IV disease mean 1.1 mg/dL (range of 0.8 - 1.7) and in 9 with class V disease mean 0.6 mg/dL (range of 0.5 - 0.8) *2377*

Endothelin *Urine Increase* Urinary excretion in individuals with lupus nephritis reported to be significantly higher than in healthy individuals and correlated significantly with excretion of NAG, β-microglobulin and albumin *6*

Intercellular Adhesion Molecule-1 *Tissue Increase* In 6 patients with lupus nephritis mean percentage of ICAM-1 positive renal tubuli 5.2 ± 7.8% *3026*

Interleukin-6 *Serum Increase* In 7 patients with WHO class II disease mean concentration of 60 pg/mL (25 to 75% range 53 - 71): in 10 patients with class IV disease mean of 55 pg/mL (46 - 91) and in 9 with class V disease mean of 52 pg/mL (48 - 54) *2377*
Urine Increase In 7 individuals with WHO class II disease mean excretion of 7.8 ng/d with 25% - 75% range 5 - 17 ng/d: in 10 patients wth class IV disease 91.0 ng/d (45 - 115) and in 9 with class V disease 10.8 ng/d (5 - 18) *2377*

pH *Urine Decrease* May cause distal renal tubular acidosis (type IV) is associated with hyperkalemia, hyperchloremic metabolic acidosis, urine pH < 5.5, decreased urinary ammonium ion excretion, a positive urine anion gap, normal urinary citrate and urinary calcium excretion *4071*

Potassium *Serum Increase* May cause distal renal tubular acidosis (type IV) which is associated with hyperkalemia, hyperchloremic metabolic acidosis, urine pH < 5.5, decreased urinary ammonium ion excretion, a positive urine anion gap, normal urinary citrate and urinary calcium excretion *4071*

Protein *Urine Increase* In 6 patients with lupus nephritis mean excretion of 1.65 ± 0.85 mg/mg creatinine *3026* In 7 patients with WHO class II disease mean excretion of 0.3 g/d with 25% to 75% range of 0.2 - 0.5: in 10 patients with class IV disease mean excretion of 1.6 g/d (0.6 - 6.0), and in 9 with class V disease 3.3 g/d (1.2 - 3.5) *2377*

Soluble Intercellular Adhesion Molecule-1 *Serum Increase* In 6 patients with lupus nephritis mean concentration of soluble ICAM-1 of 373 ± 144 ng/mL compared with 306 ± 52 ng/mL in 20 healthy controls *3026*
Urine Increase In 6 patients with lupus nephritis mean excretion of soluble ICAM-1 of 22.4 ± 21.6 ng/mL or 12.0 ± 9.8 ng/mg creatinine compared with 2.6 ± 1.7 ng/mL or 2.5 ± 3.0 ng/mg creatinine in 20 healthy controls *3026*

583.89 Basement Membrane Thickening

Blood *Urine Increase* In 30 of 71 patients (42%) with basement membrane disease mean excretion greater than 500,000 /mL *220*

Creatinine *Serum Increase* In 5 of 71 patients (7%) with basement membrane disease mean concentration greater than 0.11 mmol/L *220*

N-Acetyl-Glucosaminidase B *Urine No Effect* In 22 patients with basement membrane thickening mean concentration of 2.6 ± 1.7 µg/L or 4.9 ± 3.5 µg/g creatinine not significantly different from concentrations in 40 healthy adults in whom mean excretion was 3.1 ± 3.0 µg/L or 2.9 ± 2.0 µg/g creatinine *3838*

Protein *Urine Increase* In 30 of 71 patients (42%) with basement membrane disease mean excretion greater than 0.2 g/d *220*

583.89 Crescentric Glomerulonephritis

Anti-Neutrophil Cytoplasm Antibodies *Serum Increase* Observed effect *4953*

583.89 Glomerulonephritis, Transplant-associated

Monocyte Chemotactic Protein-1 *Serum Increase* Mean concentration of 178 pg/mL in one patient with transplant-associated glomerulonephritis compared with 101 ± 24 pg/mL in 16 healthy women and men *4460*
Urine Increase In 1 patient with tranplant-associated glomerulonephritis mean concentration of 4,300 pg/mg creatinine significantly different when compared with mean concentration of 130 ± 30 pg/mg creatinine in 30 healthy women and 32 healthy men *4460*

583.89 IgA Nephropathy

α_1-Acid Glycoprotein *Serum Increase* In 38 patients with IgA nephropathy median concentration of 1.0 ± 0.18 g/L significantly greater than 0.72 ± 0.07 g/L in 45 healthy controls *5193*

Albumin *Serum No Effect* In 24 patients with IgA nephropathy mean concentration of 37 ± 1 g/L *5004* Normal; at least early in the disease *565*

Anti-Endothelial Cell Antibodies *Serum Increase* Detected in IgA subtype ($p < 0.001$) *5563*

Anti-Streptococcal Polysaccharide Antibody *Serum Increase* Measured using an enzyme-linked immunosorbent assay in 41 children with IgA nephropathy. The titers of ASP of the IgA and IgG classes, were significantly increased *3727*

Anti-Streptolysin-O Antibody *Serum Increase* Measured using an enzyme-linked immunosorbent assay in 41 children with IgA nephropathy. The titers of ASO of the IgA and IgM classes, were significantly increased *3727*

α_1-Antitrypsin *Serum Increase* In 38 patients with IgA nephropathy median concentration of 1.47 ± 0.21 g/L significantly greater than 1.22 ± 0.08 g/L in 45 healthy controls *5193*

Apolipoprotein A-I *Serum Increase* In 24 patients with IgA nephropathy mean concentration of 1.46 ± 0.05 g/L significantly higher than 1.26 ± 0.06 g/L in 10 healthy controls *5004*

Apolipoprotein B *Serum Increase* In 24 patients with IgA nephropathy mean concentration of 1.45 ± 0.08 g/L significantly higher than 0.91 ± 0.06 g/L in 10 healthy controls *5004*

CD45 Leukocytes *Tissue Increase* In 12 patients with IgA nephropathy mean number of positive cells 549 ± 398 cells/mm^2 in renal tissue *3026*

Cholesterol *Serum Increase* In 24 patients with IgA nephropathy mean concentration of 6.9 ± 0.3 mmol/L significantly increased compared with 4.9 ± 0.2 mmol/L in 10 healthy controls *5004*

Complement, Total *Serum No Effect* Normal; at least early in the disease *565*

C-Reactive Protein *Serum No Effect* In 38 patients with IgA nephropathy median concentration of 5 ± 0 g/L not significantly different from 5.0 ± 0 g/L in 45 healthy controls *5193*

583.89 IgA Nephropathy *(continued)*

Creatinine *Serum* *Increase* In 20 patients with mild IgA nephropathy mean concentration of 0.77 ± 0.04 mg/dL and 0.97 ± 0.07 mg/dL in 20 patients with advanced stage IgA nephropathy *4819* Normal; at least early in the disease *565* In 12 patients with IgA nephropathy mean concentration of 2.06 ± 1.32 mg/dL higher than 0.88 ± 0.17 mg/dL in 20 healthy controls *3026*

Creatinine Clearance *Urine* *Decrease* In 18 patients with IgA nephropathy mean clearance of 73.0 ± 10.2 mL/min significantly different from 104.0 ± 10.3 mL/min in 12 patients with chronic tonsillitis *3362*

Endothelin *Urine* *Increase* Urinary excretion in individuals with IgA nephropathy reported to be significantly higher than in healthy individuals and correlated significantly with excretion of NAG, β-microglobulin and albumin *6*

Erythrocytes *Urine* *Increase* Macroscopic hematuria apparently heralds the onset of the disease in some patients *2505*

Glomerular Filtration Rate *Urine* *Decrease* In 24 patients with IgA nephropathy mean GFR of 67 ± 5 mL/min *5004*

Haptoglobin *Serum* *Increase* In 38 patients with IgA nephropathy median concentration of 2.23 ± 0.6 g/L significantly greater than 1.53 ± 0.42 g/L in 45 healthy controls *5193*

HDL-Cholesterol *Serum* *Decrease* In 24 patients with IgA nephropathy mean concentration of 1.0 ± 0.06 mmol/L significantly less than 1.3 ± 0.05 mmol/L in 10 healthy controls *5004*

Immunoglobulin A *Serum* *Increase* In 18 patients with IgA nephropathy mean concentration of 427 ± 28 mg/dL significantly different from 288 ± 39 mg/dL in 12 patients with chronic tonsillitis *3362* Increased in 30 - 50% of patients *1004*

Immunoglobulin E *Serum* *Increase* Mean concentration in 99 cases of primary IgA nephropathy of 122.0 IU/mL significantly higher than 43.7 IU/mL in 33 healthy controls *4821*

Intercellular Adhesion Molecule-1 *Tissue* *Increase* In 12 patients with IgA nephropathy mean percentage of ICAM-1 positive renal tubuli 10.6 ± 16.3% *3026*

Interleukin-1β *Serum* *No Effect* In 16 patients with IgA nephropathy and Schonlein-Henoch purpura IL-β not detected in any as in none of 16 patients with other nephropathies or who were normal *5747*
Urine *Increase* In 16 patients with IgA nephropathy and Schonlein-Henoch purpura IL-1β detected in 10 at a mean concentration of 144.10 ± 45.14 pg/mL compared with 2 of 16 patients with other nephropathies or who were normal in whom the concentration was 8.67 ± 2.39 pg/mL *5747*

Interleukin-2 *Serum* *No Effect* In 16 patients with IgA nephropathy and Schonlein-Henoch purpura IL-2 not detected in any as in none of 16 patients with other nephropathies or who were normal *5747*
Urine *No Effect* In 16 patients with IgA nephropathy and Schonlein-Henoch purpura IL-2 detected in 3 at a mean concentration of 64.77 ± 8.74 pg/mL compared with 5 of 16 patients with other nephropathies or who were normal in whom the concentration was 47.60 ± 19.26 pg/mL *5747*

Interleukin-4 *Serum* *No Effect* In 16 patients with IgA nephropathy and Schonlein-Henoch purpura IL-4 not detected in any as in none of 16 patients with other nephropathies or who were normal *5747*
Urine *No Effect* In 16 patients with IgA nephropathy and Schonlein-Henoch purpura IL-4 detected in 10 at a mean concentration of 22.49 ± 6.63 pg/mL compared with 13 of 16 patients with other nephropathies or who were normal in whom the concentration was 24.01 ± 5.59 pg/mL *5747*

Interleukin-6 *Urine* *Increase* The levels of urinary IL-6 in patients with the advanced stage were significantly higher than those in patients with the mild stage of the disease or in healthy adults *5245*
Urine *No Effect* In 16 patients with IgA nephropathy and Schonlein-Henoch purpura IL-6 detected in 5 at a mean concentration of 87.47 ± 94.83 pg/mL compared with 6 of 16 patients with other nephropathies or who were normal in whom the concentration was 104.00 ± 90.88 pg/mL *5747*

Interleukin-12 *Serum* *No Effect* In 16 patients with IgA nephropathy and Schonlein-Henoch purpura IL-12 not detected in any as in none of 16 patients with other nephropathies or who were normal *5747*
Urine *No Effect* In 16 patients with IgA nephropathy and Schonlein-Henoch purpura IL-12 not detected in any compared with none of 16 patients with other nephropathies or who were normal *5747*

LDL-Cholesterol:HDL-Cholesterol Ratio *Serum* *Increase* In 24 patients with IgA nephropathy mean ratio of 5.6 ± 0.5 significantly higher than 2.6 ± 0.2 in 10 healthy controls *5004*

Lipoprotein Lp(a) *Serum* *Increase* In 24 patients with IgA nephropathy mean concentration of 9.7 mg/dL (range 4.8 - 17.0 mg/dL) significantly higher than 7.0 mg/dL in 10 healthy controls *5004*

Macrophage Colony Stimulating Factor *Serum* *Increase* In 18 patients with severe IgA nephropathy mean concentration of 0.80 ± 0.44 ng/mL not significantly higher than 0.63 ± 0.05 ng/mL in 5 healthy volunteers *3362*
Urine *Increase* In 12 patients with chronic tonsillitis mean excretion of 3.10 ± 0.43 μg/g creatinine significantly higher than 1.88 ± 0.21 μg/g creatinine in 5 healthy volunteers *3362* In 18 patients with severe IgA nephropathy mean excretion of 4.83 ± 0.54 μg/g creatinine significantly higher than 1.88 ± 0.21 μg/g creatinine in 5 healthy volunteers *3362*

Monocyte Chemotactic Protein-1 *Serum* *Decrease* Mean concentration of 57 pg/mL in 2 patients with IgA nephropathy compared with 101 ± 24 pg/mL in 16 healthy women and men *4460*
Urine *Increase* In 5 patients with IgA nephropathy mean concentration of 902 ± 314 pg/mg creatinine significantly different when compared with mean concentration of 130 ± 30 pg/mg creatinine in 30 healthy women and 32 healthy men *4460*

Protein *Serum* *No Effect* In 18 patients with IgA nephropathy mean concentration of 69 ± 1 g/L not significantly different from 71 ± 1 g/L in 12 patients with chronic tonsillitis *3362*
Urine *Increase* Urine Protein excretion rates are usually less than 3.5 g/day; not uncommonly it is normal or only mildly increased *565* In 24 patients with IgA nephropathy mean excretion of 1.3 ± 0.1 g/d *5004* In 20 patients with mild IgA nephropathy mean excretion of 1,032 ± 152 mg/g creatinine and 2,760 ± 479 mg/g creatinine in 20 patients with advanced stage IgA nephropathy *4819* In 12 patients with IgA nephropathy mean excretion of 2.51 ± 2.77 mg/mg creatinine *3026* In 18 patients with IgA nephropathy mean excretion of 0.7 ± 0.3 g/d significantly different from < 0.1 g/d in 12 patients with chronic tonsillitis *3362*
Urine *No Effect* Urine protein excretion rate is usually less than 3.5 g/d; not uncommonly it is normal or only mildly increased *565*

Soluble Fas Antigen *Serum* *Increase* In 20 patients with mild IgA nephropathy mean concentration of 1.79 ± 0.19 ng/mL and 2.62 ± 0.18 ng/mL in 20 patients with advanced stage IgA nephropathy *4819*

Soluble Intercellular Adhesion Molecule-1 *Serum* *No Effect* In 12 patients with IgA nephropathy mean concentration of soluble ICAM-1 of 325 ± 94 ng/mL compared with 306 ± 52 ng/mL in 20 healthy controls *3026*
Urine *Increase* In 12 patients with IgA nephropathy mean excretion of soluble ICAM-1 of 11.2 ± 9.7 ng/mL or 13.4 ± 18.4 ng/mg creatinine compared with 2.6 ± 1.7 ng/mL or 2.5 ± 3.0 ng/mg creatinine in 20 healthy controls *3026*

Triglycerides *Serum* *Increase* In 24 patients with IgA nephropathy mean concentration of 2.0 ± 0.2 mmol/L significantly increased compared with 1.0 ± 0.05 mmol/L in healthy controls *5004*

Tumor Necrosis Factor-α *Urine* *Increase* In 16 patients with IgA nephropathy and Schonlein-Henoch purpura TNF-α detected in 11 at a mean concentration of 84.76 ± 46.63 pg/mL compared with 1 of 16 patients with other nephropathies or who were normal in whom the concentration was 30.37 pg/mL *5747*

Urea Nitrogen *Serum* *Increase* Normal; at least early in the disease *565* In 20 patients with mild IgA nephropathy mean concentration of 13.6 ± 0.7 mg/dL and 16.5 ± 0.9 mg/dL in 20 patients with advanced stage IgA nephropathy *4819*

583.89 Interstitial Nephritis

CD45 Leukocytes *Tissue* *Increase* In 5 patients with interstitial nephritis mean number of positive cells 1165 ± 726 cells/mm^2 in renal tissue *3026*

Creatinine *Serum* *Increase* In 5 patients with minimal change disease mean concentration of 6.10 ± 6.15 mg/dL significantly different from 0.88 ± 0.17 mg/dL in 20 healthy controls *3026*

Intercellular Adhesion Molecule-1 *Tissue* *Increase* In 5 patients with interstitial nephritis mean percentage of ICAM-1 positive renal tubuli 29.0 ± 26.4% *3026*

Protein *Urine* *Increase* In 5 patients with interstitial nephritis mean excretion of 1.46 ± 0.90 mg/mg creatinine *3026*

Soluble Intercellular Adhesion Molecule-1 *Serum* *Increase* In 5 patients with interstitial nephritis mean concentration of soluble ICAM-1 of 461 ± 198 ng/mL compared with 306 ± 52 ng/mL in 20 healthy controls *3026*
Urine *No Effect* In 5 patients with interstitial nephritis mean excretion of soluble ICAM-1 of 4.6 ± 4.7 ng/mL or 6.2 ± 5.7 ng/mg creatinine compared with 2.6 ± 1.7 ng/mL or 2.5 ± 3.0 ng/mg creatinine in 20 healthy controls *3026*

583.89 Minimal Change Disease

Albumin *Serum* *Decrease* In 10 patients with minimal change disease who responded to prednisone mean concentration of 22.4 ± 4.0 g/L and of 17.3 ± 4.1 g/L in 4 who failed to respond to prednisone significantly different from normal *4005*

CD45 Leukocytes *Tissue* *Increase* In 5 patients with minimal change disease mean number of positive cells 157 ± 60 cells/mm^2 in renal tissue *3026*

Creatinine *Serum* *No Effect* In 10 patients with minimal change disease who responded to prednisone mean concentration of 1.10 ± 0.16 mg/dL and of 1.12 ± 0.10 mg/dL in 4 who failed to respond to prednisone not significantly different from normal *4005* In 5 patients with minimal change disease mean concentration of 0.85 ± 0.29 mg/dL not significantly different from 0.88 ± 0.17 mg/dL in 20 healthy controls *3026*

Intercellular Adhesion Molecule-1 *Tissue* *No Effect* In 5 patients with minimal change disease mean percentage of ICAM-1 positive renal tubuli 0.4 ± 0.5% *3026*

Protein *Urine* *Increase* In 10 patients with minimal change disease who responded to prednisone, mean excretion of 6.06 ± 3.09 g/d and of 12.0 ± 11.4 g/d in 4 who failed to respond to prednisone significantly different from normal *4005* In 5 patients with lupus nephritis mean excretion of 7.05 ± 1.77 mg/mg creatinine *3026*

Soluble HLA-I *Serum* *Increase* In 10 patients with minimal change disease, who responded to prednisone mean concentration of 1,040 ± 1,066 ng/mL and of 668 ± 315 ng/mL in 4 who failed to respond to prednisone significantly higher than 415 ± 256 ng/mL in 45 healthy volunteer controls *4005*
Urine *Increase* In 4 patients with minimal change disease who failed to respond to prednisone, mean excretion of 541 ± 239 ng/mg creatinine and 100 ± 42 ng/mg creatinine in 10 patients who responded to prednisone significantly higher than undetectable amounts in 45 healthy volunteer controls *4005*

Soluble Intercellular Adhesion Molecule-1 *Serum* *No Effect* In 5 patients with minimal change disease mean concentration of soluble ICAM-1 of 290 ± 140 ng/mL compared with 306 ± 52 ng/mL in 20 healthy controls *3026*
Urine *Increase* In 5 patients with minimal change disease mean excretion of soluble ICAM-1 of 40.9 ± 25.0 ng/mL or 26.3 ± 3.9 ng/mg creatinine compared with 2.6 ± 1.7 ng/mL or 2.5 ± 3.0 ng/mg creatinine in 20 healthy controls *3026*

583.90 Balkan Nephropathy

Ammonium Ions *Urine* *Increase* May be associated with classic distal renal tubular acidosis which is associated with hyokalemia, hyperchloremic metabolic acidosis, urine pH > 5.5, increased urinary ammonium ion excretion, a negative urine anion gap, increased urinary osmol gap, decreased urinary citrate and increased urinary calcium in some patients *4071*

Anion Gap *Urine* *Decrease* May be associated with classic distal renal tubular acidosis which is associated with hyokalemia, hyperchloremic metabolic acidosis, urine pH > 5.5, increased urinary ammonium ion excretion, a negative urine anion gap, increased urinary osmol gap, decreased urinary citrate and increased urinary calcium in some patients *4071*

Calcium *Urine* *Increase* May be associated with classic distal renal tubular acidosis which is associated with hyokalemia, hyperchloremic metabolic acidosis, urine pH > 5.5, increased urinary ammonium ion excretion, a negative urine anion gap, increased urinary osmol gap, decreased urinary citrate and increased urinary calcium in some patients *4071*

Chloride *Serum* *Increase* May be associated with classic distal renal tubular acidosis which is associated with hyokalemia, hyperchloremic metabolic acidosis, urine pH > 5.5, increased urinary ammonium ion excretion, a negative urine anion gap, increased urinary osmol gap, decreased urinary citrate and increased urinary calcium in some patients *4071*

Citrate *Urine* *Decrease* May be associated with classic distal renal tubular acidosis which is associated with hyokalemia, hyperchloremic metabolic acidosis, urine pH > 5.5, increased urinary ammonium ion excretion, a negative urine anion gap, increased urinary osmol gap, decreased urinary citrate and increased urinary calcium in some patients *4071*

β_2-Microglobulin *Urine* *Increase* In 23 individuals with Balkan nephropathy 87% demonstrated increased excretion of β_2-microglobulin *2254*

Net Acid Excretion *Urine* *Increase* May be associated with classic distal renal tubular acidosis which is associated with hyokalemia, hyperchloremic metabolic acidosis, urine pH > 5.5, increased urinary ammonium ion excretion, a negative urine anion gap, increased urinary osmol gap, decreased urinary citrate and increased urinary calcium in some patients *4071*

Osmolal Gap *Urine* *Increase* May be associated with classic distal renal tubular acidosis which is associated with hyokalemia, hyperchloremic metabolic acidosis, urine pH > 5.5, increased urinary ammonium ion excretion, a negative urine anion gap, increased urinary osmol gap, decreased urinary citrate and increased urinary calcium in some patients *4071*

pH *Urine* *Increase* May be associated with classic distal renal tubular acidosis which is associated with hyokalemia, hyperchloremic metabolic acidosis, urine pH > 5.5, increased urinary ammonium ion excretion, a negative urine anion gap, increased urinary osmol gap, decreased urinary citrate and increased urinary calcium in some patients *4071*

Potassium *Serum* *Decrease* May be associated with classic distal renal tubular acidosis which is associated with hyokalemia, hyperchloremic metabolic acidosis, urine pH > 5.5, increased urinary ammonium ion excretion, a negative urine anion gap, increased urinary osmol gap, decreased urinary citrate and increased urinary calcium in some patients *4071*

583.90 Glomerular Disease

Brain Natriuretic Peptide *Urine* *Increase* In 12 patients with primary glomerular disease mean excretion of 5.72 ± 0.44 pmol/d significantly different from that in 11 healthy individuals in whom the mean excretion was 3.82 ± 0.62 pmol/d *5265*

Creatinine *Serum* *Increase* Mean concentration in 20 patients with chronic glomerular disease of 1.3 ± 0.2 mg/dL compared with 0.9 ± 0.3 mg/dL in 9 healthy controls *5153*
Serum *No Effect* In 20 patients with chronic glomerular disease mean concentration of 1.3 ± 0.3 mg/dL not significantly greater than 0.9 ± 0.3 mg/dL in 9 healthy controls *5153*

Creatinine Clearance *Urine* *Decrease* In 11 patients with primary glomerular disease mean clearance of 68.6 ± 10.2 mL/min significantly different from that in 11 healthy individuals *5265*

Hepatocyte Growth Factor *Urine* *No Effect* Mean concentration in 20 patients with chronic glomerular disease not significantly different from 1.5 ± 0.2 ng/g creatinine in 9 healthy controls *5153* In 20 patients with chronic glomerular disease mean excretion not significantly different from that in 9 healthy controls in whom the mean excretion was 1.5 ± 0.2 ng/g creatinine *5153*

Tissue Plasminogen Activator *Urine* *Increase* In 28 of 43 patients with glomerular disease urinary t-PA detectable *2139*

583.90 Glomerulonephritis, Focal

Alanine Aminotransferase *Urine* *Increase* Increased *4096* *5671* *2508*

Albumin *Urine* *Increase* Noted to have slight but persistent proteinuria *900*

583.90 Glomerulonephritis, Focal (continued)

Amino Acids *Plasma Decrease* Mean concentration of essential amino acids and tyrosine were significantly lower, resulting in a low essential/total ratio *3409*
Urine Increase May be found *1947*

Anti-Streptolysin-O Titer *Serum Increase* Above normal titers may occur *3953*

Calcium *Serum Decrease* Decreases as metabolic acidosis develops *1980*

Ceruloplasmin *Serum Increase* Found regularly with hypoproteinemia *2210*

Complement C_3 *Serum No Effect* No significant effect observed *872*

Copper *Serum Increase* Found regularly with hypoproteinemia *2210*

Erythrocyte Sedimentation Rate *Blood Increase* High ESR may be found in patients with abnormal plasma protein levels *1980*

Erythrocytes *Urine Increase* Noted to have slight persistent proteinuria accompanied by microscopic hematuria *900* Microscopic or massive hematuria *1980*

Glucose *Urine Increase* May be found *1947*

β-Hexosaminidase *Urine Decrease* Decreased levels in urine *5229*

Immunoglobulin G *Serum Decrease* May be significantly reduced *872*

Lymphocytes *Urine Increase* May be found *1947*

α_2-Macroglobulin *Serum Increase* Reported effect *2088*

Osmolality *Urine Decrease* Concentrating capacity is impaired, with urine specific gravity around 1.010 *1980*

Protein *Pleural Fluid Decrease* Pleural effusions are usually transudates (< 3 g/dL) *126*
Urine Increase May persist for years, even after other manifestations cease *1980*

Specific Gravity *Urine Decrease* Concentrating capacity is impaired, with urine specific gravity around 1.010 *1980*

Tryptophan *Plasma Increase* Tyrosine and tryptophan usually rise in acute and chronic glomerulonephritis *4707*

Tyrosine *Plasma Decrease* Mean concentration of essential amino acids and tyrosine were significantly lower, resulting in a low essential/total ratio *3409*
Plasma Increase Tyrosine and tryptophan usually rise in acute and chronic glomerulonephritis *4707*

Uric Acid *Serum Increase* As functional loss becomes severe (GFR 50% of normal or less), there is usually a rise in serum phosphate and uric acid *1980*

583.90 Glomerulonephritis, Postinfectious

CD45 Leukocytes *Tissue Increase* In 1 patient with postinfectious glomerulonephritis number of positive cells 297 cells/mm^2 in renal tissue *3026*

Creatinine *Serum Increase* In 1 patient with postinfectious glomerulonephropathy concentration of 1.21 mg/dL different from 0.88 ± 0.17 mg/dL in 20 healthy controls *3026*

Intercellular Adhesion Molecule-1 *Tissue No Effect* In 1 patient with postinfectious glomerulonephritis percentage of ICAM-1 positive renal tubuli 0.0% *3026*

Monocyte Chemotactic Protein-1 *Serum Increase* Mean concentration of 238 ± 94 pg/mL in 4 patients with infection-associated glomerulonephritis compared with 101 ± 24 pg/mL in 16 healthy women and men *4460*
Urine Increase In 3 patients with infection-associated glomerulonephritis mean concentration of 12,199 ± 5,956 pg/mg creatinine significantly different when compared with mean concentration of 130 ± 30 pg/mg creatinine in 30 healthy women and 32 healthy men *4460*

Protein *Urine Increase* In 1 patient with postinfectious glomerulonephritis excretion of 0.70 mg/mg creatinine *3026*

Soluble Intercellular Adhesion Molecule-1 *Serum No Effect* In 1 patient with postinfectious glomerulonephritis concentration of soluble ICAM-1 of 270 ng/mL compared with 306 ± 52 ng/mL in 20 healthy controls *3026*
Urine Increase In 1 patient with postinfectious glomerulonephritis excretion of soluble ICAM-1 of 7.2 ng/mL or 6.2 ng/mg creatinine compared with 2.6 ± 1.7 ng/mL or 2.5 ± 3.0 ng/mg creatinine in 20 healthy controls *3026*

583.90 Nephritis

S Protein-membrane Attack Complex (SC_5b-9)
Urine Increase In 18 of 38 patients with glomerulopathies, excretions ranged from 200 to 20,000 ng/mg creatinine but concentrations did not differentiate between patients with membranous nephropathy and those with other causes of glomerulopathy *3865*

583.90 Nephropathy, Membranous

α_1-Acid Glycoprotein *Serum No Effect* In 31 patients with membranous nephropathy median concentration of 0.8 ± 0.16 g/L not significantly greater than 0.72 ± 0.07 g/L in 45 healthy controls *5193*

Albumin *Serum No Effect* In 11 patients with membranous nephropathy mean concentration of 36.7 ± 9.0 g/L not significantly different from normal *4005* Mean concentration in 7 patients with membranous nephropathy of 41 ± 3 g/L not different from 43 ± 3 g/L in 8 patients with minimal change glomerulonephritis *4566*

α_1-Antitrypsin *Serum Increase* In 31 patients with membranous nephropathy median concentration of 1.49 ± 0.45 g/L significantly greater than 1.22 ± 0.08 g/L in 45 healthy controls *5193*

CD45 Leukocytes *Tissue Increase* In 9 patients with membranous nephropathy mean number of positive cells 652 ± 459 cells/mm^2 in renal tissue *3026*

C-Reactive Protein *Serum No Effect* Mean concentration in 7 patients with membranous nephropathy of 0.06 ± 0.05 mg/dL not different from 0.06 ± 0.05 mg/dL in 8 patients with minimal change glomerulonephritis *4566* In 31 patients with membranous nephropathy median concentration of 5 ± 2.5 mg/L not significantly different from 5.0 ± 0 mg/L in 45 healthy controls but with concentration higher in those with heavy range albuminuria than in those with mild to moderate albuminuria *5193*

Creatinine *Serum Decrease* Mean concentration in 7 patients with membranous nephropathy of 61.9 ± 8.8 μmol/L different from 70.7 ± 26.5 μmol/L in 8 patients with minimal change glomerulonephritis *4566*
Serum Increase In 9 patients with membranous nephropathy mean concentration of 1.83 ± 1.74 mg/dL higher than 0.88 ± 0.17 mg/dL in 20 healthy controls *3026*
Serum No Effect In 10 patients with membranous nephropathy mean concentration of 1.20 ± 0.18 mg/dL not significantly different from normal *4005*

Creatinine Clearance *Urine No Effect* Mean clearance in 7 patients with membranous nephropathy of 75.5 ± 14.8 mL/min different from 103.9 ± 25.5 mL/min in 8 patients with minimal change glomerulonephritis *4566*

Haptoglobin *Serum Increase* In 31 patients with membranous nephropathy median concentration of 3.14 ± 1.13 g/L significantly greater than 1.53 ± 0.42 g/L in 45 healthy controls with concentration higher in those with heavy range albuminuria than in those with mild to moderate albuminuria *5193*

Hemoglobin *Blood No Effect* Mean concentration in 7 patients with membranous nephropathy of 13.5 ± 0.9 g/dL not different from 13.8 ± 1.4 g/dL in 8 patients with minimal change glomerulonephritis *4566*

Intercellular Adhesion Molecule-1 *Tissue Increase* In 9 patients with membranous nephropathy mean percentage of ICAM-1 positive renal tubuli 14.1 ± 19.2% *3026*

Interleukin-6 *Serum No Effect* Mean concentration in 7 patients with membranous nephropathy of 0.6 ± 0.9 pg/mL not significantly different from 0.4 ± 0.8 pg/mL in 48 healthy controls *4566*
Urine No Effect Mean concentration in 7 patients with membranous nephropathy of 2.3 ± 3.2 pg/mL not significantly different from 0.4 ± 0.6 pg/mL in 48 healthy controls *4566*

Leukocytes *Blood No Effect* Mean concentration in 7 patients with membranous nephropathy of 5.8 ± 2.2 x 10^3/μL not different from 6.4 ± 1.9 x 10 /μL in 8 patients with minimal change glomerulonephritis *4566*

Monocyte Chemotactic Protein-1 *Serum Decrease* Mean concentration of 73 ± 73 pg/mL in 2 patients with membranous nephropathy compared with 101 ± 24 pg/mL in 16 healthy women and men *4460*
Urine Increase In 3 patients with membranous nephropathy mean concentration of 425 ± 61 pg/mg creatinine significantly different when compared with mean concentration of 130 ± 30 pg/mg creatinine in 30 healthy women and 32 healthy men *4460*

Protein *Serum No Effect* Mean concentration in 7 patients with membranous nephropathy of 74 ± 4 g/L not different from 73 ± 7 g/L in 8 patients with minimal change glomerulonephritis *4566*
Urine Increase In 9 patients with membranous nephropathy mean excretion of 3.09 ± 1.03 mg/mg creatinine *3026* In 10 patients with membranous nephropathy mean excretion of 7.72 ± 5.43 g/d significantly different from normal *4005*
Urine No Effect Mean excretion in 7 patients with membranous nephropathy of 1.01 ± 0.40 g/d not different from 0.97 ± 1.24 g/d in 8 patients with minimal change glomerulonephritis *4566*

Soluble Fas Antigen *Serum No Effect* Mean concentration in 7 patients with membranous nephropathy of 2.2 ± 0.7 ng/mL not significantly different from 2.2 ± 0.6 ng/mL in 48 healthy controls *4566*
Urine No Effect Mean concentration in 7 patients with membranous nephropathy of 0.0 ± 0.0 ng/mL not significantly different from 0.0 ± 0.0 ng/mL in 48 healthy controls *4566*

Soluble Fas Ligand Antigen *Serum No Effect* Mean concentration in 7 patients with membranous nephropathy of 0.47 ± 0.04 ng/mL not significantly different from 0.55 ± 0.13 ng/mL in 48 healthy controls *4566*

Soluble HLA-I *Serum No Effect* In 10 patients with membranous nephropathy, mean concentration of 445 ± 86 ng/mL not significantly different from 415 ± 256 ng/mL in 45 healthy volunteer controls *4005*
Urine Increase In 10 patients with membranous nephropathy, mean excretion of 125 ± 28 ng/mg creatinine significantly higher than undetectable amount in 45 healthy volunteer controls *4005*

Soluble Intercellular Adhesion Molecule-1 *Serum No Effect* In 9 patients with membranous nephropathy mean concentration of soluble ICAM-1 of 353 ± 159 ng/mL compared with 306 ± 52 ng/mL in 20 healthy controls *3026*
Urine Increase In 9 patients with membranous nephropathy mean excretion of soluble ICAM-1 of 20.2 ± 19.4 ng/mL or 21.0 ± 21.5 ng/mg creatinine compared with 2.6 ± 1.7 ng/mL or 2.5 ± 3.0 ng/mg creatinine in 20 healthy controls *3026*

Tumor Necrosis Factor-α *Serum No Effect* Mean concentration in 7 patients with membranous nephropathy of 4.1 ± 5.1 pg/mL not significantly different from 4.3 ± 5.8 pg/mL in 48 healthy controls *4566*
Urine No Effect Mean concentration in 7 patients with membranous nephropathy of 0.0 ± 0.0 pg/mL not significantly different from 0.0 ± 0.0 pg/mL in 48 healthy controls *4566*

Urea Nitrogen *Serum Increase* Mean concentration in 7 patients with membranous nephropathy of 2.4 ± 0.5 mmol/L different from 2.1 ± 0.8 mmol/L in 8 patients with minimal change glomerulonephritis *4566*

583.90 Tubulointerstitial Disease

Ammonium Ions *Urine Decrease* May cause distal renal tubular acidosis (type IV) is associated with hyperkalemia, hyperchloremic metabolic acidosis, urine pH < 5.5, decreased urinary ammonium ion excretion, a positive urine anion gap, normal urinary citrate and urinary calcium excretion *4071*

Calcium *Urine No Effect* May cause distal renal tubular acidosis (type IV) is associated with hyperkalemia, hyperchloremic metabolic acidosis, urine pH < 5.5, decreased urinary ammonium ion excretion, a positive urine anion gap, normal urinary citrate and urinary calcium excretion *4071*

Chloride *Serum Increase* May cause distal renal tubular acidosis (type IV) is associated with hyperkalemia, hyperchloremic metabolic acidosis, urine pH < 5.5, decreased urinary ammonium ion excretion, a positive urine anion gap, normal urinary citrate and urinary calcium excretion *4071*

Citrate *Urine No Effect* May cause distal renal tubular acidosis (type IV) is associated with hyperkalemia, hyperchloremic metabolic acidosis, urine pH < 5.5, decreased urinary ammonium ion excretion, a positive urine anion gap, normal urinary citrate and urinary calcium excretion *4071*

pH *Urine Decrease* May cause distal renal tubular acidosis (type IV) is associated with hyperkalemia, hyperchloremic metabolic acidosis, urine pH < 5.5, decreased urinary ammonium ion excretion, a positive urine anion gap, normal urinary citrate and urinary calcium excretion *4071*

Potassium *Serum Increase* May cause distal renal tubular acidosis (type IV) which is associated with hyperkalemia, hyperchloremic metabolic acidosis, urine pH < 5.5, decreased urinary ammonium ion excretion, a positive urine anion gap, normal urinary citrate and urinary calcium excretion *4071*

583.99 Renal Disease

Carcinoembryonic Antigen *Serum Increase* In 11 patients with kidney disease 54.5% had concentrations of 0.0 - 3.0 ng/mL, 27.3% had concentrations from 3.1 - 5.0 ng/mL, 9.1% had concentrations from 5.1 - 10.0 ng/mL and 9.1% had concentrations greater than 10.0 ng/mL when measured by method on Bayer Technicon Immuno 1® system compared with 95.9%, 3.5%, 0.6% and 0.0% respectively in 173 healthy nonsmokers *339*

Carvedilol *Serum Increase* Although carvedilol is mainly metabolized by the liver in patients with hypertension and renal insufficiency mean AUC of carvedilol increased and plasma concentrations approximately 40 to 50% higher than in hypertensives with normal renal function. Mean peak plasma concentrations only approximately 12 to 26% higher *4915*

Cysteine *Plasma No Effect* Mean concentration in 12 patients with renal disease of 248 ± 53 µmol/L not significantly different from 231 ± 30 µmol/L in 10 healthy controls *2395*

Dopamine β-Hydroxylase *Cerebrospinal Fluid No Effect* Mean concentration of 34.7 ± 5.1 ng/mL in 11 patients with renal disease not significantly different from 31.3 ± 1.4 ng/mL in 32 healthy individuals *3855*
Serum Increase Mean concentration of 22.2 ± 3.9 ng/mL in 11 patients with renal disease significantly higher than 9.24 ± 1.11 ng/mL in 32 healthy controls *3855*

Epidermal Growth Factor *Urine Decrease* In 11 children with renal disease but wih normal renal function mean excretion of 13.6 ± 5.1 ng/mg creatinine (11.3 ± 3.6 µg/d) not significantly less than that in 180 healthy children aged 7 - 15 y in whom mean excretion was 15.2 ± 6.5 ng/mg creatinine (10.6 ± 4.8 µg/d) *5300*

Erythrocyte Sedimentation Rate *Blood Increase* In 138 of 1,480 ESRs in a hospital population rates were greater than 100 mm/h: in a further study of 90 patients with 163 final diagnoses 25 were attributable to renal diseases *3097*

γ-Glutamyltransferase *Serum Increase* Activity reportedly increased in a variety of diseases including diseases of the pancreas, myocardium, kidney and lung as well as in diabetes *4617*

Glutathione *Plasma Increase* Mean concentration in 12 patients with renal disease mean concentration of 23.5 ± 13.1 µmol/L significantly different from 10.4 ± 8.8 µmol/L in 10 healthy controls *2395*

Lipoic Acid *Plasma Increase* Concentration in plasma of 22 patients with renal disease of 4.6 ± 1.1 ng/mg protein significantly greater than that in 92 healthy individuals of 3.1 ± 0.9 ng/mg protein *253*

Lipoprotein Lp(a) *Serum Increase* In 5 men with predialysis renal disease mean concentration of 519 U/L different from 385 U/L in 23 healthy controls and 890 U/L in 15 women different from mean of 367 U/L in 33 control women *1673*

Magnesium *Lymphocytes Increase* In 12 patients prior to renal transplant mean concentration of 0.88 ± 0.27 µg/mg protein significantly different from 0.72 ± 0.1 µg/mg protein in 11 healthy controls *4377*
Serum Increase In 12 patients prior to renal transplant mean concentration of 1.07 ± 0.14 mmol/L compared with 0.86 ± 0.09 mmol/L in controls *4377*

583.99 Renal Disease *(continued)*

Prostate-specific Antigen *Serum Increase* In 102 men with nonmalignant renal disease, 87.3% had concentrations between 0 and 4.0 ng/mL, 10.9% between 4.1 and 10.0 ng/mL and 2.0% between 10.1 and 30.0 ng/mL compared with upper limit of normal of 4.0 ng/mL *11*

Soluble HLA-I *Urine Increase* Known to be present in urine of people with chronic renal disease *216*

584.00 Acute Renal Failure

Adenosine Monophosphate *Plasma Increase* Elevated in uremia *1987*

Albumin *Serum Decrease* In 8 patients with acute renal failure mean concentration of 26.2 ± 1.5 g/L *1239*

Alkaline Phosphatase *Serum Increase* Not related to degree of azotemia *5544*

Amino Acids *Plasma Increase* Increased total concentration due to rise in nonessential amino acids. Proline, hydroxyproline, glycine, citrulline, ornithine, were increased. Valine and tryptophan were decreased *1100*

Ammonia *Blood Decrease* Decreased arterial ammonia in azotemic patients mean of 34 ± 1.4 mmol/L *4213*
Urine Decrease With severe renal damage. May be < 1% of the urea nitrogen *4707*

Amylase *Serum Increase* May be increased without evidence of pancreatitis in early stage *5545* Mild elevation may occur with renal insufficiency but rarely more than above twice the normal upper limit *4537*

Angiotensin-converting Enzyme *Serum Decrease* Level increased with normalization of renal function *4417*

Aspartate Aminotransferase *Serum Increase* In 63% of 11 patients at initial hospitalization for this disorder *1576*

Bicarbonate *Serum Decrease* Observed with acidosis *1980* Metabolic acidosis *1583* In 74% of 12 patients at initial hospitalization for this disorder *1576* Falls 1 - 2 mmol/L each day during oliguric phase *572*

Calcium *Serum Decrease* Hypocalcemia in acute (anuria) and chronic renal failure *1025* May occur in early stage *5545* In the range of 6.3 - 8.3 mg/dL *3339* In 72% of 11 patients at initial hospitalization for this disorder *1576* In 8 patients with acute renal failure mean concentration of 1.06 ± 0.05 mmol/L significantly different from reference interval of 1.17 - 1.37 mmol/L in 28 healthy controls *1239*
Serum Increase In one study of 40 patients with 40 patients with hypercalcemia and low intact PTH concentrations, 2 were attributable to acute renal failure *3280*

Carbon Dioxide Partial Pressure *Blood Decrease* Metabolic acidosis may occur *1980*

Carcinoembryonic Antigen *Serum Increase* Increased in about 50% of the patients *5544*

Carnitine *Serum Increase* Total carnitine, free carnitine, short-chain and long chain acylcarnitine values of patients with acute renal failure were markedly elevated compared with healthy controls *5571*

Cholesterol *Serum No Effect* In 8 patients with acute renal failure mean concentration of 128 ± 7 mg/dL significantly different from 211 ± 8 mg/dL in 28 healthy controls *1239*

Cortisol *Plasma Increase* Normal or slightly elevated *1369*

Creatine *Cerebrospinal Fluid Increase* High concentrations in blood and CSF have been associated with azotemia *4707*
Serum Increase High concentrations in blood and CSF have been associated with azotemia *4707*

Creatinine *Serum Increase* Characteristic *3521* In 99% of 12 patients at initial hospitalization for this disorder *1576* In 8 patients with acute renal failure mean concentration of 5.4 ± 0.6 mg/dL *1239* In 24 patients with acute renal failure mean concentration of 862 ± 361 mmol/L significantly greater than 93 ± 14 mmol/L in 20 healthy controls *3383*
Urine Decrease Excretion during initial phase was 1.49 ± 2.20 mmol significantly less than 2.94 ± 3.37 mmol in recovery phase *5301*

1,25-Dihydroxy Vitamin D_3 *Serum Decrease* In 8 patients with acute renal failure mean concentration of 4 ± 2 pg/mL significantly different from 32 ± 3 pg/mL in 28 healthy controls *1239*

Endothelin *Urine Increase* Excretion increased in patients with acute renal failure *6*

Endothelin-1 *Plasma Increase* In 7 patients with acute renal failure mean concentration increased to 10.4 ± 5.1 pg/mL, 6.9 times normal values *328* Reported effect *1489*

Eosinophils *Blood Increase* In 32% of 12 patients at initial hospitalization for this disorder *1576*

Epidermal Growth Factor *Serum No Effect* Excretions of 566 ± 132, 554 ± 129 and 569 ± 134 pmol/L noted during initial, recovery and normal phases, respectively *5301*
Urine Decrease Low urinary excretions noted during initial and recovery phases whereas higher concentrations were found during the normal stage *5301*

Erythrocyte Casts *Urine Increase* Associated with active glomerulonephritis *900*

Erythrocytes *Urine Increase* In the early stage *5545*

Fatty Acids (FFA), Free *Serum Increase* Elevated in acute renal failure, but normal or low in chronic failure *3135*

Ferritin *Serum Increase* In 24 patients with acute renal failure mean concentration of 1000 ± 752 ng/mL significantly greater than 105.0 ± 43 ng/mL in 20 healthy controls *3383* In 24 patients with acute renal failure mean concentration of 1,000 ng/dL *3383*

Fetal Antigen 1 *Serum Increase* Significant effect of acute renal failure observed on concentration in 20 patients receiving dialysis with median about 350 ng/mL compared with reference interval of 12.3 - 46.6 ng/mL *2436*

Fibrin Degradation Products *Plasma Increase* In 25 patients with acute failure due to falciparum malaria, marked increase in plasma fibrinogen fibrin degradation products were observed. The other coagulation parameters were within the normal limits *4878*

Gastrin *Serum Increase* In both acute and chronic failure *1122*

Glomerular Filtration Rate *Urine Decrease* Decreased cortical renal blood flow was noted in acute failure due to falciparum malaria *4878* Decreased due to reduced number of functioning glomeruli *1290*

Glucagon *Plasma Increase* Elevated 2 to 10 times above normal and remains essentially unchanged by dialysis *452*

Glucose *Serum Increase* Hyperglycemia and impaired glucose tolerance are common. Elevated ratio of insulin/glucose during glucose tolerance testing is found consistently *1583*

Glucose Tolerance *Serum Decrease* Hyperglycemia and impaired glucose tolerance are common in renal failure. Elevated ratio of insulin/glucose during glucose tolerance testing is found consistently *1583*

β-Glucuronidase *Urine Increase* All 8 patients revealed high values of urinary activity above the normal limit of 30 with a mean value of 148.1 ± 158.3 U/L *1805*

Growth Hormone *Plasma Increase* Consistently occurring hypersecretion may be induced by severe uremia *1583*
Urine Increase Marked elevation *3144*

HDL-Cholesterol *Serum Decrease* In 8 patients with acute renal failure mean concentration of 34 ± 7 mg/dL significantly different from 64 ± 4 mg/dL in 28 healthy controls *1239*

Hematocrit *Blood Decrease* In 24 patients with acute renal failure mean value of 31.8 ± 4.4% significantly different from 42.9 ± 3.1% in 20 healthy controls *3383* May fall to the low 20's *572*

Hemoglobin *Blood Decrease* In 24 patients with acute renal failure mean concentration of 10.5 ± 1.7 g/dL significantly different from 14.8 ± 1.1 g/dL in 20 healthy controls *3383*
Urine Increase May appear in the urine of a patient with intravascular hemolysis or myoglobin in trauma *900*

β-Hexosaminidase *Urine Increase* Extremely high values observed in acute renal failure following hypotensive episodes *3373*

25-Hydroxy Vitamin D_2 *Serum Decrease* In 8 patients with acute renal failure mean concentration of 17 ± 7 nmol/mL significantly different from 81 ± 9 nmol/mL in 28 healthy controls *1239*

17-Hydroxycorticosteroids *Urine Increase* Both free and glucuronide fraction of 17 OHCS are elevated in acute but not chronic failure *467*

^{131}I Uptake *Serum Decrease* In renal disease *4707*

Iron *Serum* *Decrease* In 24 patients with acute renal failure mean concentration of 82.8 ± 67.3 µg/dL significantly less than 144.0 ± 43 µg/dL in 20 healthy controls *3383*

17-Ketogenic Steroids *Urine* *Increase* Both free and glucuronide fraction of 17 OHCS are elevated in acute but not chronic failure *467*

Lactate Dehydrogenase *Serum* *Increase* In 72% of 11 patients at initial hospitalization for this disorder *1576*
Urine *Increase* In acute tubular necrosis *5544*

LDL-Cholesterol *Serum* *Decrease* In 8 patients with acute renal failure mean concentration of 80 ± 4 mg/dL significantly different from 134 ± 8 mg/dL in 28 healthy controls *1239*

Leukocytes *Blood* *Increase* In 65% of 12 patients at initial hospitalization for this disorder *1576* Often 10,000 /µL *572* Increased even without infection in the early stage *5545*

Lipase *Serum* *Increase* May be increased without evidence of pancreatitis in early stage *5545*

β_2-Macroglobulin *Serum* *Decrease* An increase in urine and a decrease in serum levels is seen in disorders of renal tubular function *2586*
Urine *Increase* An increase in urine and a decrease in serum levels is seen in disorders of renal tubular function *2586*

Magnesium *Serum* *Increase* Pathological increase with renal failure *1290*

Neutrophils *Blood* *Increase* In 74% of 12 patients at initial hospitalization for this disorder *1576*

Osmolality *Urine* *Decrease* < 350 mOsm/kg in intrarenal acute renal failure *3494* Manifested by oliguria, increasing serum creatinine, a urine osmolality of < 400 mOsm/kg and a urine/plasma osmolality ratio of < 1 - 5 *3521*
Urine *Increase* > 500 mOsm/kg in prerenal acute renal failure *3494*

Osteocalcin *Serum* *Decrease* In 8 patients with acute renal failure mean concentration of 18.5 ± 5.0 ng/mL significantly different from 22.9 ± 1.2 ng/mL in 28 healthy controls *1239*

Osteocalcin, Carboxylated *Serum* *No Effect* In 8 patients with acute renal failure mean concentration of 1.15 ± 0.3 ng/mL not significantly different from 1.1 ± 0.1 ng/mL in 28 healthy controls *1239*

Osteocalcin, Total *Serum* *Decrease* In 8 patients with acute renal failure mean concentration of 17.3 ± 5.0 ng/mL significantly different from 21.8 ± 1.1 ng/mL in 28 healthy controls *1239*

Parathyroid Hormone *Plasma* *Decrease* In one study of 40 patients with nonmalignant causes of low intact PTH concentration and hypercalcemia 2 cases were attributed to acute renal failure *3280*
Plasma *Increase* In 8 patients with acute renal failure mean concentration of 120 ± 31 pg/mL significantly different from 17 ± 3 pg/mL in 28 healthy controls *1239*

pH *Blood* *Decrease* Mild acidosis is common *1583* Metabolic acidosis increases within 2nd week *5545*
Urine *Increase* Normal or increased *5544*

Phosphate *Serum* *Increase* Reduction in GFR leads to increased serum concentration *969* In 72% of 11 patients at initial hospitalization for this disorder *1576* Hyperphosphatemia may occur depending on the duration and severity of disease *367* Serum phosphate concentration may be increased in patients with acute renal failure *5204*

Platelets *Blood* *Decrease* As a consequence of peripheral destruction *2024*

Potassium *Serum* *Decrease* Large urinary potassium excretion may cause decreased serum concentration in diuretic stage *5545* May occur early in renal failure due to diarrhea, vomiting, or spontaneous potassium loss in urine *367*
Serum *Increase* Liberated during body cell breakdown, and is not excreted completely in the urine *1290* During oliguric phase *572* May occur depending on the duration and severity of the disease *367*
Urine *Decrease* In acute tubular necrosis the kidney loses it ability to reabsorb sodium, and an increased concentration of urine sodium with a relative decrease in urine potassium will be noted *900*

Protein *Serum* *Decrease* In 8 patients with acute renal failure mean concentration of 55.5 ± 3.3 g/L *1239*
Urine *Increase* In the early stage *5545*

Renin Activity *Plasma* *Increase* Increased in failure due to falciparum malaria *4878*

Sodium *Serum* *Decrease* Often decreased, in the 2nd week *5545*
Urine *Increase* In acute tubular necrosis the kidney loses its ability to reabsorb sodium, and an increased concentration of urine sodium with a relative decrease in urine potassium will be noted *900*

Specific Gravity *Urine* *Decrease* A low, fixed specific gravity indicates tubular damage *900*
Urine *Increase* May be high in the early stage *5545*

Sulfate *Serum* *Increase* In metabolic acidosis accompanying renal failure. Serves as a reliable index of insufficiency *4707*

Triglycerides *Serum* *Increase* In 8 patients with acute renal failure mean concentration of 168 ± 19 mg/dL significantly different from 110 ± 10 mg/dL in 28 healthy controls *1239*

Troponin I *Serum* *Increase* One patient with acute renal failure had a troponin-I concentration greater than 1 µg/L *890*

Troponin T *Serum* *Increase* One patient with acute renal failure had a troponin-T concentration greater than 0.2 µg/L by both ELISA and Enzymun procedures *890* Mean concentration increased above 0.2 µg/L in 75% patients with acute renal failure *334*

Urea Nitrogen *Saliva* *Increase* A near perfect correlation (r = 0.97) was found for saliva, plasma urea nitrogen ratios in 56 pairs of samples from patients with renal failure. The mean serum concentration before dialysis was 81.2 ± 30.9 mg/dL. In unstimulated saliva, the urea nitrogen saliva: plasma ratio remained constant at 1.3 *4756*
Serum *Increase* Rises < 20 mg/dL/day in transfusion reaction. Rises > 50 mg/dL/day in overwhelming infection or severe crushing injuries in early stage. Continues to rise for several days after onset of diuresis in the 2nd week *5545* Excessive tubular reabsorption of urea and several other nonprotein nitrogen constituents may play a role in diseases producing this state *1025* In 99% of 12 patients at initial hospitalization for this disorder *1576* In 8 patients with acute renal failure mean concentration of 70.9 ± 8.0 mg/dL *1239* In 24 patients with acute renal failure mean concentration of 47.5 ± 20.5 mmol/L significantly greater than 6.3 ± 1.03 mmol/L in 20 healthy controls *3383*

Uric Acid *Serum* *Increase* In 99% of 11 patients at initial hospitalization for this disorder *1576*

Viscosity *Serum* *Increase* Significantly increased in 15 patients with acute failure due to falciparum malaria *4878*

Vitamin A *Serum* *Decrease* In 8 patients with acute renal failure mean concentration of 213 ± 24 ng/mL significantly less than 520 ± 41 ng/mL in 28 healthy controls *1239*
Serum *No Effect* In 8 patients with acute renal failure mean concentration of 53 ± 8 mg/L not significantly different from 47 ± 3 mg/L in 28 healthy controls *1239*

Vitamin E *Serum* *Decrease* In 8 patients with acute renal failure mean concentration of 6 ± 2 µg/mL significantly different from 15 ± 1 µg/mL in 28 healthy controls *1239*

Vitamin K *Serum* *No Effect* In 8 patients with acute renal failure mean concentration of 1,360 ± 687 pg/mL not significantly different from 301 ± 21 pg/mL in 28 healthy controls *1239*

VLDL-Cholesterol *Serum* *No Effect* In 8 patients with acute renal failure mean concentration of 9 ± 1 mg/dL not significantly different from 12 ± 2 mg/dL in 28 healthy controls *1239*

VLDL-Triglycerides *Serum* *No Effect* In 8 patients with acute renal failure mean concentration of 38 ± 7 mg/dL not significantly different from 34 ± 6 mg/dL in 28 healthy controls *1239*

Volume *Plasma* *Decrease* Initial hypovolemia followed by hyper- or normovolemia in acute renal failure due to falciparum malaria *4878*
Plasma *Increase* Initial hypovolemia followed by hyper- or normovolemia in acute renal failure due to falciparum malaria *4878*
Urine *Decrease* Manifested by oliguria, urine osmolality of < 400 mOsm/kg and a urine/plasma osmolality ratio of < 1 - 5 *3521* Urine is scant in volume (often < 50 mL/day) for 2 weeks, in the early stage. Daily volume of 400 mL indicates onset of tubular recovery. Daily volume of 1,000 mL occurs in several days or < 2 weeks *5545*

584.50 Acute Tubular Necrosis

CD45 Leukocytes *Tissue Increase* In 1 patient with acute tubular necrosis number of positive cells 235 cells/mm^2 in renal tissue *3026*

Creatinine *Serum Increase* In 25 patients with acute tubular necrosis mean concentration of 4.0 ± 1.6 mg/dL significantly greater than 0.9 ± 0.3 mg/dL in 9 healthy controls *5153* Mean concentration in 25 patients with ATN 4.0 ± 1.6 mg/dL compared with 0.9 ± 0.3 mg/dL in 9 healthy controls *5153* In 1 patient with acute tubular necrosis concentration of 4.25 mg/dL significantly different from 0.88 ± 0.17 mg/dL in 20 healthy controls *3026*

Endothelin-1 *Plasma Increase* In one patient 0.9-fold increase observed *328*

Erythropoietin *Serum Decrease* In 10 patients with ATN mean concentration significantly less for degree of anemia and remained low after restoration of excretory function as measured by GFR due to defective synthesis of erythropoietin *3785*

Hepatocyte Growth Factor *Urine Increase* Mean concentration in 25 patients with ATN of 11.8 ± 2.1 ng/g creatinine compared with 1.5 ± 0.2 ng/g creatinine in 9 healthy controls *5153* In 25 patients with acute tubular necrosis mean excretion of 11.8 ± 2.1 ng/g creatinine significantly different from that in 9 healthy controls in whom the mean excretion was 1.5 ± 0.2 ng/g creatinine *5153*

Intercellular Adhesion Molecule-1 *Tissue Increase* In 1 patient with acute tubular necrosis percentage of ICAM-1 positive renal tubuli 5.0% *3026*

Monocyte Chemotactic Protein-1 *Serum Decrease* Mean concentration undetectable in 1 patient with mesangial/proliferative ATN compared with 101 ± 24 pg/mL in 16 healthy women and men *4460*
Urine Increase In 1 patient with mesangial/proliferative ATN mean concentration of 266 pg/mg creatinine significantly different when compared with mean concentration of 130 ± 30 pg/mg creatinine in 30 healthy women and 32 healthy men *4460*

Protein *Urine Increase* In 1 patient with acute tubular necrosis excretion of 2.16 mg/mg creatinine *3026*

Soluble Intercellular Adhesion Molecule-1 *Serum No Effect* In 1 patient with acute tubular necrosis concentration of soluble ICAM-1 of 320 ng/mL compared with 306 ± 52 ng/mL in 20 healthy controls *3026*
Urine Increase In 1 patient with acute tubular necrosis excretion of soluble ICAM-1 of 9.0 ng/mL or 7.1 ng/mg creatinine compared with 2.6 ± 1.7 ng/mL or 2.5 ± 3.0 ng/mg creatinine in 20 healthy controls *3026*

584.50 Renal Tubular Disease

N-Acetyl-Glucosaminidase B *Urine Increase* In 15 patients with tubular lesions mean concentration of 9.5 ± 10.4 µg/L or 18.5 ± 26.6 µg/g creatinine significantly different from concentrations in 40 healthy adults in whom mean excretion was 3.1 ± 3.0 µg/L or 2.9 ± 2.0 µg/g creatinine *3838*

585.00 Chronic Renal Failure

Acetaminophen *Serum No Effect* No interference observed at creatinine concentrations up to 17 mg/dL (1,500 µmol/L) with method on Du Pont aca *1241*

α_1-Acid Glycoprotein *Serum Increase* Mean concentration in 18 non-dialyzed uremic patients of 1.27 ± 0.47 g/L compared with 0.79 ± 0.09 g/L in 20 healthy controls *5431* Concentration increased significantly with increase in serum creatinine concentration *1192* In 25 uremic patients mean activity of 1.20 ± 0.40 g/L compared with 0.83 ± 0.17 g/L in 17 control individuals *5432*
Urine Increase In 25 uremic individuals mean excretion of 126 ± 160 mg/d compared with 3 ± 1 mg/d in 17 control individuals *5432*

Acid Phosphatase *Red Blood Cells Increase* Activity in urine, erythrocytes, and serum was increased. Marked increase occurred in all 3 specimens in the terminal stage *2728* A 2-fold increase was found in uremic patients compared to normal controls. After hemodialysis both the serum phosphate and acid phosphatase activity were reduced *3450*
Serum Increase Activity in urine, erythrocytes, and serum was increased. Marked increase occurred in all 3 specimens in the terminal stage *2728*
Urine Increase Activity in urine, erythrocytes, and serum was increased in patients with renal failure. Marked increases occur in all 3 specimens in the terminal stage *2728*

Acid Phosphatase, Tartrate Resistant *Serum Increase* In 30 patients with chronic renal failure without hepatopathy mean activity of 9.2 ± 7.6 U/L significantly greater than 6.8 ± 0.9 U/L in 16 healthy controls *1677* In 10 patients with CRF mean concentration of 311 (range 230 - 375) µg/L, 12.0 (5.8 - 20.1) U/L significantly greater than mean concentration and range of 178 (41 - 288) µg/L, 5.6 (1.8 - 10.3) U/L in 29 healthy premenopausal women, 302 (range 129 - 348) µg/L, 7.5 (range 4.2 - 12.9) U/L in 12 healthy postmenopausal women and 197 (range 61 - 301) U/L, 6.5 (range 2.1 - 11) U/L in 25 healthy men *812*

Acylcarnitine *Serum Increase* In 34 uremic nondialyzed patients mean concentration of 28.7 µmol/L compared with 6.2 µmol/L in 49 apparently healthy adult controls *4401*

Adenosine Monophosphate *Plasma Increase* Elevated in uremia *1987*

Adenosine Triphosphate *Red Blood Cells Increase* In 7 patients with uremia mean concentration before hemodialysis of 2,029 ± 467 nmol/L significantly greater than that in healthy individuals in whom the reported concentration is 1,200 - 1,400 nmol/mL *626*

Adrenomedullin *Plasma Increase* In patients with renal impairment and essential hypertension mean concentration in those with creatinine concentration of 1.5 - 3 mg/dL 4.1 ± 0.5 fmol/mL, in those with creatinine of 3 - 6 mg/dL 5.3 ± 0.6 fmol/mL, and in those with creatinine > 6 mg/dL of 7.3 ± 1.3 fmol/mL compared with mean concentration of 2.3 ± 0.2 fmol/mL in 17 normal individuals *2356*

Alanine *Plasma Decrease* Decreased *237 555 4798*
Plasma Increase In 10 patients with chronic renal failure undergoing regular hemodialysis mean concentration of 278 ± 24 µmol/L significantly greater than 221 ± 9 µmol/L in 31 healthy age and sex matched controls *1656*
Urine Increase Increases up to 4 times normal value *424*

Alanine Aminotransferase *Serum Increase* In 38% of 142 patients at initial hospitalization for this disorder *1576*

Albumin *Serum Decrease* Mean concentration significantly reduced in patients with chronic renal failure *3050* Concentrations are normal or low in chronic uremia *2136* Tend to be diminished as a result of urinary protein loss *4746* In 20 patients with uremia mean concentration of 37.7 g/L significantly reduced compared with 42.1 g/L in 67 healthy controls *3392* In 43% of 141 patients at initial hospitalization for this disorder *1576* In 68 patients with chronic renal disease mean concentration of 4.15 ± 0.47 g/dL significantly different from 4.5 ± 0.32 g/dL in 73 healthy normal volunteers *3487*
Urine Increase Proteinuria and granular casts suggest chronic parenchymal renal disease *900*

Aldosterone *Plasma Increase* Observed in some patients *2034*
Urine Increase Observed in some patients *2034*

Alkaline Phosphatase *Serum Increase* In 30 patients with chronic renal failure without hepatopathy mean activity of 81 ± 64 U/L significantly greater than 66 ± 14 U/L in 16 healthy controls *1677* In 15 patients with severe renal insufficiency mean activity of 144 ± 15 U/L significantly different from 97 ± 6 U/L in 14 with moderate insufficiency and 88 ± 6 U/L in 13 with mild insufficiency *1410* Not significant increase to mean of 87.2 ± 35.6 U/L in 19 patients with predialytic chronic renal failure compared with 81.0 ± 22.5 U/L in 38 healthy controls *870* In 29% of 139 patients at initial hospitalization for this disorder *1576*
Serum No Effect In 19 children with end-stage renal disease mean activity of 190 ± 69 U/L compared with reference interval of 80 - 225 U/L *527* In 26 patients with chronic renal failure without secondary hyperparathyroidism median activity of 145 U/L not significantly different from 125 U/L in 90 healthy controls *2572*
Urine Increase 69% of cases showed elevation *1670*

Alkaline Phosphatase, Bone Isoenzyme *Serum Increase* In patients with chronic renal failure with hemodialysis moderate increase observed *4217*

Aluminum *Serum Increase* Accumulates in all patients with renal failure *5461*

Amino Acids *Plasma Increase* Increased total concentration due to rise in nonessential amino acids. Proline, hydroxyproline, glycine, citrulline, ornithine were increased. Valine, and tryptophan were decreased *1100*
Urine Increase As GFR decreases, amino acid clearance and excretion increases. Increased levels of alanine (4 times normal), threonine, cystine, valine, and leucine (2 - 3 times normal), and proline are found in urine *424*

Ammonia *Blood Decrease* Decreased arterial ammonia in azotemic patients, (mean of 34 ± 1.4 mmol/L) *4213*
Blood Increase Despite reduced excretion, renal failure does not usually lead to arterial excess, unless hepatic failure occurs *4707*
Urine Decrease With severe renal damage may be < 1% of the urea nitrogen *4707*

Amphotericin B *Serum Decrease* Uremia is associated with decreased binding of acidic drugs to plasma proteins. Effect on bound fraction only is listed here *5869*

Amylase *Serum Increase* Mean activity in 42 patients with chronic renal failure 531 ± 392 U/L significantly different from 183 ± 54 U/L in 47 healthy controls *1015* In 63 patients with chronic renal failure mean activity of 280 ± 128 U/L significantly different from 148 ± 64 U/L in 34 healthy volunteer controls *3331* In 87 patients with renal failure but without abdominal pain 74% had increased serum amylase activity but not to above 5 times the upper limit of normal *3063* Mean activity of 166 ± 111 U/L in 25 patients with chronic renal failure significantly greater than 91 ± 20 U/L in 10 healthy individuals *2687* Patients with severe failure may have significant hyperamylasemia in the absence of clinical symptoms or signs of acute pancreatitis *5185* Mild elevation may occur with renal insufficiency but rarely more than above twice the normal upper limit *4537*
Urine Decrease Mean activity in 42 patients with chronic renal failure of 102 ± 82 U/L significantly different from 220 ± 296 U/L in 47 healthy controls *1015*
Urine Increase In patients with severe renal insufficiency, the amylase to creatinine ratios were significantly raised. Clearance ratios of pancreatic and salivary isoamylase to creatinine changed in parallel to that of total amylase. The results suggest that in severe renal failure the loss of nephrons results in decreased fractional reabsorption of amylase in the tubules *4024*

Amylase, Pancreatic Isoenzyme *Serum Increase* In 78% of 87 patients with renal failure but without abdominal pain increased enzyme activity observed *3063* Mean activity in 42 patients with chronic renal failure of 392 ± 268 U/L significantly different from 84 ± 30 U/L in 47 healthy controls *1015* In 63 patients with chronic renal failure mean activity of 138 ± 70 U/L significantly different from 80 ± 46 U/L in 34 healthy volunteer controls *3331*
Urine Decrease Mean activity in 42 patients with chronic renal failure of 61 ± 72 U/L significantly different from 132 ± 186 U/L in 47 healthy controls *1015*

Amylase, Salivary Isoenzyme *Serum Increase* Mean activity in 42 patients with chronic renal failure of 171 ± 164 U/L significantly different from 98 ± 55 U/L in 47 healthy controls *1015*
Urine Decrease Mean activity in 42 patients with chronic renal failure of 38 ± 28 U/L significantly different from 92 ± 152 U/L in 47 healthy controls *1015*

Amylin *Plasma Increase* In patients whose creatinine clearance was less than 20 mL/min mean concentration of 17.9 ± 1.7 pg/mL compared with 8.8 ± 1.2 pg/mL in patients whose clearance exceeded 80 mL/min *5595*

Androstenedione *Plasma Decrease* Significant reduction observed in 14 male patients with nondiabetic end stage renal disease compared with 28 age-matched healthy controls *695*

Angiotensin-converting Enzyme *Serum Increase* Elevated regardless of severity of disease *4843* Significantly higher than in an age - matched control group *3528* It is thought that an enlarged pulmonary vascular bed and accelerated cellular breakdown were the cause *1272*

1,5-Anhydroglucitol *Serum Decrease* In 20 uremic undialyzed individuals mean concentration as measured by LC/MS 85.4 ± 15.2 µmol/L and 106 ± 21.3 µmol/L by enzymatic method significantly reduced compared with 151.8 ± 11.6 µmol/L and 159.8 ± 9.8 µmol/L respectively in 20 normal controls *3812* In 13 non-diabetic patients with end stage renal disease not on dialysis mean concentration of 6.22 ± 2.10 µg/mL significantly less than 24.20 ± 7.50 µg/mL in healthy controls *1359*

Anti-Interleukin-1 Antibodies *Serum Positive* Anti-IL-1α antibodies observed in 8.9% of patients with chronic renal failure *5084*

Antinuclear Antibodies *Serum Increase* Increased in 11 of 86 patients who had never been dialyzed and 52 of 243 chronic dialysis patients. Significantly lower hematocrits and WBC counts were noted with the presence of these antibodies *3820*

Antioxidant Capacity *Serum Decrease* Activity reduced in patients with chronic renal failure with lowest levels observed in those requiring regular hemodialysis *2861*
Serum Increase In 22 patients with chronic renal failure mean concentration predialysis 571 ± 31 µmol/L Trolox eq. significantly higher than 427 ± 34 µmol/L Trolox eq. in healthy controls *2385*

Antithrombin III *Plasma Decrease* Concentration significantly lower in 14 hemodialysis patients compared with 14 age and sex matched controls *2722*

Antithrombin III Activity *Plasma Decrease* In 14 hemodialysis patients mean activity significantly lower than in 14 age and sex matched controls *2722*

Antithyroglobulin Antibodies *Serum No Effect* Serum thyroglobulin was elevated in 92% of 38 patients in the early stage of this disorder. After two months of corticosteroid treatment the levels were significantly decreased in 25 patients who could be rechecked *3582*

Apolipoprotein A *Serum Decrease* Significant reduction observed in patients with chronic renal failure *1590*

Apolipoprotein A-I *Serum Decrease* In 68 patients with chronic renal disease mean concentration of 129 ± 40 mg/dL significantly different from 152 ± 31 mg/dL in 73 healthy normal volunteers *3487* Mean concentration in 117 patients with uremia of 1.16 ± 0.28 g/L different from 1.85 ± 0.27 g/L in 110 healthy controls *4002* Mean concentration reduced in patients with chronic renal failure compared with that in healthy controls *211*
Serum Increase Significant increase observed in uremic patients to 0.27 ± 0.07 g/L in patients on hemodialysis and 0.22 ± 0.08 g/L in those with end stage renal failure *1270*
Serum No Effect In 39 patients with chronic renal failure and normal nutrition mean concentration of 1.41 ± 0.07 g/L not significantly different from 1.40 ± 0.07 g/L in 44 patients with chronic renal failure but with malnutrition *5005* In 13 patients with chronic renal failure, but dialysis independent, mean concentration of 1.26 ± 0.29 g/L not significantly different from 1.56 ± 0.59 g/L in 27 healthy controls *935*

Apolipoprotein A-I:Apolipoprotein B Ratio
Serum Decrease Ratio is typically in the low-normal range *3526*

Apolipoprotein A-II *Serum Decrease* Mean concentration reduced in patients with chronic renal failure compared with that in healthy controls *211*

Apolipoprotein A-IV *Serum Increase* In patients with end-stage renal disease mean concentration of 59 ± 19 mg/dL observed in those treated by hemodialysis, 51 ± 12 mg/dL in those treated by peritoneal dialysis compared with 18 ± 6 mg/dL in healthy controls *1164*

Apolipoprotein B *Serum Increase* Mean concentration in 117 patients with uremia of 1.38 ± 0.65 g/L different from 1.11 ± 0.31 g/L in 110 healthy controls *4002*
Serum No Effect In 68 patients with chronic renal disease mean concentration of 140 ± 38 mg/dL not significantly different from 135 ± 31 mg/dL in 73 healthy normal volunteers *3487* In 13 patients with chronic renal failure, but dialysis independent, mean concentration of 0.97 ± 0.31 g/L not significantly different from 0.87 ± 0.20 g/L in 27 healthy controls *935* In patients with chronic renal failure no significant difference observed from concentration in healthy individuals *211*

Apolipoprotein C-I *Serum No Effect* No significant difference from normal observed in 56 patients with chronic renal failure *211*

Apolipoprotein C-II *Serum Increase* Significant increase in mean concentration observed in 56 patients with chronic renal failure *211*

Apolipoprotein C-III *Serum Increase* In 56 patients with chronic renal failure mean concentration markedly increased *211*

Apolipoprotein E *Serum Decrease* Marked reduction, especially in men, in 56 patients with chronic renal failure *211*

585.00 **Chronic Renal Failure** *(continued)*

Apolipoprotein Lp(a) *Serum* *Increase* Mean concentration of 23.5 mg/dL in 24 uremics before initiation of dialysis compared with mean of 4.7 mg/dL in 18 healthy controls *2549*

Aprindine *Serum* *Increase* Uremia is associated with changed binding of basic or neutral drugs to plasma proteins. Effect on bound fraction only is listed here *5869*

Arginine *Plasma* *Decrease* Children with mild renal insufficiency showed a significant decrease in tyrosine and arginine *424*
Plasma *No Effect* In 10 patients with chronic renal failure undergoing regular hemodialysis mean concentration of 73 ± 7 μmol/L not significantly different from 66 ± 2 μmol/L in 31 healthy age and sex matched controls *1656*

Arsenic *Serum* *Increase* In 19 uremic patients not receiving dialysis mean concentration of 5.12 ± 5.58 μg/L significantly different from reference interval of 0.96 ± 1.52 μg/L *5855*

Arsenobetaine *Serum* *Increase* In 19 uremic patients not receiving dialysis mean concentration of 3.55 ± 4.59 μg/L significantly different from reference interval for total arsenic of 0.96 ± 1.52 μg/L in 23 healthy adults *5855*

Ascorbic Acid *Serum* *Decrease* In 22 patients with chronic renal failure mean concentration predialysis 10.5 ± 1.7 μmol/L significantly lower than 41.6 ± 8.3 μmol/L in healthy controls *2385*

Aspartic Acid *Plasma* *Decrease* In 10 patients with chronic renal failure undergoing regular hemodialysis mean concentration of 38 ± 3 μmol/L significantly less than 130 ± 7 μmol/L in 31 healthy age and sex matched controls *1656*

Atrial Natriuretic Peptide *Plasma* *Increase* Mean concentration in 10 patients with chronic renal failure of 104.7 ± 11.4 pmol/L significantly higher than 5.6 ± 1.7 pmol/L in 11 healthy male subjects aged 20 - 23 years *2911* In 17 patients on long-term continuous ambulatory peritoneal dialysis concentration significantly higher than in healthy individuals *2894* Mean concentration in 10 patients with chronic renal failure of 28.9 ± 21.3 fmol/mL higher than that in 37 healthy volunteers, 18.6 ± 11.4 fmol/mL *3325* In 11 patients with chronic renal failure before dialysis median concentration of 23 pg/mL, in 13 patients on chronic dialysis 34 pg/mL compared with concentration in 28 control individuals (19 pg/mL) *2442* In 30 patients with mean age 57 years with chronic renal failure mean predialysis concentration of 240.2 ± 28.7 pg/mL significantly higher than 50.7 ± 4.1 pg/mL in 20 control individuals of mean age 55 years *2062* In patients with chronic renal failure mean concentration of 60.6 ± 9.1 pmol/L higher than 13.6 ± 1.9 pmol/L in healthy controls *3469* Significantly higher in children with end-stage renal disease than in healthy children and children with advanced renal failure without evidence of volume expansion *4281* In 57 patients with chronic renal failure the mean level (173 pg/mL) was significantly higher than in normal subjects (37.6 pg/mL) *2042* In patients with chronic renal failure mean concentration of 173 ± 17.0 pg/mL compared with 37.6 ± 1.9 pg/mL in healthy normal controls *2042*
Urine *No Effect* Mean concentration in 10 patients with chronic renal failure of 18.0 ± 12.6 fmol/mL not significantly different from that in 37 healthy volunteers, 16.1 ± 6.1 fmol/mL *3325*

Azapropazone *Serum* *Decrease* Uremia is associated with decreased binding of acidic drugs to plasma proteins. Effect on bound fraction only is listed here *5869*

Azlocillin *Serum* *Decrease* Uremia is associated with decreased binding of acidic drugs to plasma proteins. Effect on bound fraction only is listed here *5869*

$7B_2$ *Serum* *Increase* Significant increase of immunoreactive $7B_2$ (novel pituitary polypeptide) in patients with chronic renal failure undergoing hemodialysis to 502 ± 36 pg/mL compared with 52.9 ± 1.7 pg/mL in male controls and 55.8 ± 1.3 pg/mL in women *2317*

Bactericidal Permeability-increasing Protein (BPI)
Serum *Increase* In 28 undialyzed patients with chronic renal failure mean concentration of 3,785 ± 2,842 pg/mL significantly higher than that in 15 healthy volunteers in whom the mean concentration was 2,582 ± 921 pg/mL *4077*

Bicarbonate *Serum* *Decrease* Metabolic acidosis may occur *1980* In 59% of 146 patients at initial hospitalization for this disorder *1576*

Bilirubin *Serum* *Decrease* Uremia is associated with decreased binding of acidic drugs to plasma proteins. Effect on bound bilirubin fraction only is listed here *5869*
Serum *Increase* In 22 patients with chronic renal failure mean concentration predialysis 9.9 ± 0.5 μmol/L not significantly higher than 7.8 ± 0.4 μmol/L in healthy controls *2385*
Serum *No Effect* Within normal limits in all 26 cases *3104*

Bone Sialoprotein *Serum* *Increase* In 26 patients with chronic renal failure without secondary hyperparathyroidism mean concentration of 23.0 ± 14.7 μg/L significantly higher than that in 90 healthy controls in whom the mean concentration was 12.1 ± 5.0 μg/L *2572*

Brain Natriuretic Peptide *Plasma* *Increase* In 30 patients with mean age 57 years with chronic renal failure mean predialysis concentration of 192.1 ± 24.9 pg/mL significantly higher than 8.6 ± 1.0 pg/mL in 20 control individuals of mean age 55 years *2062* In 10 patients with chronic renal failure mean concentration of 21.0 ± 3.8 pmol/L compared with 1.3 ± 0.2 pmol/L in healthy control individuals *2911*
Urine *Increase* In 9 patients with chronic renal failure mean excretion of 11.07 ± 1.73 pmol/d significantly different from that in 11 healthy individuals in whom the mean excretion was 3.82 ± 0.62 pmol/d *5265*

CA 19-9 *Serum* *No Effect* In 10 patients with chronic renal failure on either peritoneal dialysis or hemodialysis mean concentration below upper limit of normal of 37 U/mL *4998*

CA 125 *Serum* *Increase* In 50 patients with renal failure mean concentration of 46.9 ± 103.6 U/mL with 44.2% with concentrations above 35 U/mL *2636* False positive result *3909*

CA 549 *Serum* *Increase* In 14 patients with chronic renal failure 2 had a concentration of 11 U/mL, 2 with a concentration of 12 U/mL and 2 with a concentration of 13 U/mL with an upper limit of normal of 11 U/mL *5260*

Cadmium *Blood* *Increase* In 11 smoking patients with chronic renal failure mean concentration of 5.05 μg/dL compared with 2.38 μg/dL in 17 smoking controls: in 5 nonsmoking patients with chronic renal failure mean concentration of 3.86 μg/dL compared with 2.02 μg/dL in nonsmoker controls *5667*
Serum *Decrease* Probably due to proteinuria and a loss of cadmethionein in urine *34*

Calcitonin *Plasma* *Increase* Basal plasma concentrations were increased to a mean of 185.88 ± 16.36 pg/mL *2967*

Calcium *Serum* *Decrease* In 15 patients with severe renal insufficiency mean concentration of 8.6 ± 0.2 mg/dL significantly different from 9.1 ± 0.2 mg/dL in 14 with moderate insufficiency and 9.3 ± 0.2 mg/dL in 13 with mild insufficiency *1410* In 19 patients with predialytic chronic renal failure mean concentration of 9.09 ± 0.51 mg/dL significantly less than 9.65 ± 0.42 mg/dL in 38 healthy controls *870* In 47% of 142 patients at initial hospitalization for this disorder *1576* Falls late in renal failure, often reaching 6 mg/dL and occasionally 4 mg/dL *367* In a study of 28 patients with hypocalcemia and low intact parathyroid hormone concentration, 2 had chronic renal failure *3280* Hypocalcemia in acute (anuria) and chronic renal failure *1025* Usually reduced primarily as a result of diminished synthesis of active metabolites of vitamin D, particularly in the setting of high levels of intracellular phosphate *2304*
Serum *Increase* In 26 patients with chronic renal failure without secondary hyperparathyroidism median concentration of 2.65 mmol/L not significantly different from 2.35 mmol/L in 90 healthy controls *2572* In 40 patients with nonmalignant causes of low intact PTH concentrations and hypercalcemia 20 were due to excess 1α-hydroxycholecalciferol in chronic renal failure *3280*
Serum *No Effect* In one study of 59 patients with normocalcemia and low intact PTH concentration, 10 had chronic renal failure *3280*
Sweat *Increase* Concentrations of Ca, Mg and phosphate in sweat were significantly elevated due to an increase in the secretion of these electrolytes in the secretory portion of the sweat gland, while that in the reabsorptive duct is normal *4225*
Urine *Decrease* Falls early, to < 100 mg/24 h, before there is any drop in serum levels, reflecting the fall of GFR *367*

Calmodulin *Red Blood Cells* *Increase* In 25 uremic patients on regular hemodialysis mean concentration of 11.45 ± 0.66 fg/cell compared with 8.62 ± 0.37 fg/cell in controls *3583*
White Blood Cells *Increase* In 25 uremic patients on regular hemodialysis mean concentration of 590.5 fg/cell significantly higher than in healthy controls, 130 ± 30 fg/cell *3583*

Carbamazepine *Serum* *No Effect* Uremia is associated with changed binding of basic or neutral drugs to plasma proteins. Effect on bound fraction only is listed here *5869*

Carbamylated Hemoglobin *Blood* *Increase* In 30 patients with chronic renal failure mean concentration of 164 ± 87.7 µg carbamylated valine/g hemoglobin compared with 41 ± 11.5 µg carbamylated valine/g hemoglobin in 25 controls *2875* In 167 individuals with a wide variety of renal diseases markedly increased concentrations (mean greater than 80 ng isopropyl hydantoin/mg globin) observed in chronic renal failure, dialysis patients and transplant patients with renal failure *4914*

Carbamylated Protein *Serum* *Increase* In 24 uremic patients before dialysis mean concentration of 0.289 ± 0.11 absorbance U/mg protein significantly higher than 0.088 ± 0.04 absorbance U/mg protein in 14 normal individuals *262*

Carbon Dioxide Partial Pressure *Blood* *Decrease* Metabolic acidosis may occur *1980* In 63% of 31 patients at initial hospitalization for this disorder *1576*

Carnitine *Serum* *Increase* Mean concentration in undialysed uremics of 92.5 ± 37.5 µmol/L compared with mean of 53.3 ± 8.4 µmol/L in healthy controls *4401*

Carnitine, Free *Serum* *Increase* In 34 uremic undialyzed patients mean concentration of 63.8 µmol/L compared with 47.1 µmol/L in 49 apparently healthy controls *4401*

Carnosinase *Serum* *Decrease* Significant reduction observed in patients with chronic renal failure *263*

Carvedilol *Serum* *Increase* Although carvedilol is mainly metabolized by the liver in patients with hypertension and renal insufficiency mean AUC of carvedilol increased and plasma concentrations approximately 40 to 50% higher than in hypertensives with normal renal function. Mean peak plasma concentrations only approximately 12 to 26% higher *4915*

Casts *Urine* *Increase* With renal parenchymal disease *1727*

Catalase *Red Blood Cells* *Increase* In 12 patients with chronic renal failure mean activity of 0.117 ± 0.03 K/s.g hemoglobin significantly different from 0.086 ± 0.025 K/s.g hemoglobin in 11 controls *3323*

Catecholamines *Plasma* *Increase* Moderate increase *1326* With fluorescence methods due to interfering substances *3269*

Cefazolin *Serum* *Decrease* Uremia is associated with decreased binding of acidic drugs to plasma proteins. Effect on bound fraction only is listed here *5869*

Cefoxitin *Serum* *Decrease* Uremia is associated with decreased binding of acidic drugs to plasma proteins. Effect on bound fraction only is listed here *5869*

Ceftriaxone *Serum* *Decrease* Uremia is associated with decreased binding of acidic drugs to plasma proteins. Effect on bound fraction only is listed here *5869*

Cells *Bone Marrow* *Increase* Tends to be moderately hypercellular *5699* *662*
Urine *Increase* Renal epithelial cells were increased to 49% of total cells in benign endemic nephropathy *3071*

Chemiluminescence *Blood* *Increase* Mean value of 260 ± 250 counts/10 s in 104 patients with chronic renal failure receiving chronic hemodialysis significantly different from 119 ± 98 counts/10 s in 98 healthy controls *803*
Neutrophils *Increase* Mean value of 419 ± 141 counts/10^6 cells/10 s in 104 patients with chronic renal failure receiving chronic hemodialysis significantly different from 141 ± 103 counts/10^6 cells/10 s in 98 healthy controls *803*

Chloramphenicol *Serum* *Decrease* Uremia is associated with decreased binding of acidic drugs to plasma proteins. Effect on bound fraction only is listed here *5869*

Chloride *Serum* *Decrease* Decreased or normal *5544*
Serum *No Effect* Decreased or normal *5544*

Chlorpromazine *Serum* *No Effect* Uremia is associated with changed binding of basic or neutral drugs to plasma proteins. Effect on bound fraction only is listed here *5869*

Cholesterol *Platelets* *No Effect* In 14 patients with uremia mean concentration of 97.8 ± 17.0 µg/10^9 cells not significantly different from 91.7 ± 26.0 µg/10^9 cells in 14 healthy volunteer controls *5440*
Serum *Decrease* In 104 patients with end-stage renal disease receiving hemodialysis mean concentration of 181.5 ± 4.9 mg/dL significantly different from 212.2 ± 3.4 mg/dL in healthy controls *1488*
Serum *Increase* Characteristic finding *3526* Mean concentration in 12 patients with chronic renal failure and uremia of 5.14 ± 1.46 mmol/L compared with 4.82 ± 1.08 mmol/L in 9 healthy controls *2230* Most studies show only a modest increase *2304* Characteristic finding *3526* May be elevated *2136* In patients with chronic renal failure without nephrotic syndrome 30% had cholesterol concentrations exceeding 240 mg/dL *2575*
Serum *No Effect* Mean concentration in 117 patients with uremia of 5.54 ± 1.53 mmol/L not significantly different from 4.71 ± 0.89 mmol/L in 110 healthy controls *4002* In 68 patients with chronic renal disease mean concentration of 205 ± 46 mg/dL not significantly different from 201 ± 32 mg/dL in 73 healthy normal volunteers *3487* Nonsignificant decrease to 193 mg/dL in uremic patients compared with 201 mg/dL in controls *726* In 39 patients with chronic renal failure and normal nutrition mean concentration of 6.0 ± 0.2 mmol/L not significantly different from 6.1 ± 0.3 mmol/L in 44 patients with chronic renal failure but with malnutrition *5005* In 13 patients with chronic renal failure, but dialysis independent, mean concentration of 6.06 ± 1.68 mmol/L not significantly different from 6.34 ± 0.78 mmol/L in 27 healthy controls *935*

Cholesterol, Free *Serum* *No Effect* In 13 patients with chronic renal failure, but dialysis independent, mean concentration of 1.42 ± 0.43 mmol/L not significantly different from 1.54 ± 0.21 mmol/L in 27 healthy controls *935*

Cholesterol:HDL-Cholesterol Ratio *Serum* *Increase* Ratio is typically abnormally high *3526* In 68 patients with chronic renal disease mean ratio of 5.2 ± 1.7 significantly different from 4.1 ± 1.2 in 73 healthy normal volunteers *3487*

Choline *Plasma* *Increase* Concentration in uremic patients immediately before renal transplantation 29.8 ± 1.86 µmol/L *22*

Chromogranin-A *Serum* *Increase* Concentration very high in uremics *5860*

Cimetidine *Serum* *Increase* Uremia is associated with changed binding of basic or neutral drugs to plasma proteins. Effect on bound fraction only is listed here *5869*

Citrulline *Plasma* *Increase* Compared with healthy controls significant increase observed with mild renal failure and increased progressively with progression of renal failure *746* In 10 patients with chronic renal failure undergoing regular hemodialysis mean concentration of 85 ± 4 µmol/L significantly greater than 32 ± 1 µmol/L in 31 healthy age and sex matched controls *1656*

Clofibrate *Serum* *Decrease* Uremia is associated with decreased binding of acidic drugs to plasma proteins. Effect on bound fraction only is listed here *5869*

Clonazepam *Serum* *No Effect* Uremia is associated with changed binding of basic or neutral drugs to plasma proteins. Effect on bound fraction only is listed here *5869*

Clonidine *Serum* *Increase* Uremia is associated with changed binding of basic or neutral drugs to plasma proteins. Effect on bound fraction only is listed here *5869*

Complement C_3d *Serum* *Increase* Observed in patients with serum creatinine concentrations above 200 µmol/L regardless of type of kidney disease *2818*

Copper Zinc Superoxide Dismutase
Red Blood Cells *Increase* In patients with chronic renal failure mean activity of 2,243 ± 205 U/g hemoglobin in 12 with creatinine clearance of 51 - 90 mL/min, 2,434 ± 163 U/g hemoglobin in 12 with clearance 21 - 50 mL/min and in 12 with clearance < 20 mL/min activity of 2,709 ± 203 U/g hemoglobin significantly different when compared with 1,920 ± 140 U/g hemoglobin in 13 healthy controls with clearance > 90 mL/min *3502*
Serum *Increase* Mean value of 331.3 ± 107.7 ng/mL in 104 patients with chronic renal failure receiving chronic hemodialysis significantly different from 33.4 ± 26.0 ng/mL in 98 healthy controls *803*

Corticotropin *Saliva* *No Effect* Mean concentration in 10 patients with chronic renal failure of 9.9 ± 5.8 pmol/L not significantly different from range in 50 healthy Caucasian volunteers 9.3 - 4.0 pmol/L *3605*

Cortisol *Plasma* *Increase* In 14 patients with nondiabetic end stage renal disease concentration significantly higher than in 28 healthy age-matched controls *695* Normal or slightly elevated *1369*

585.00 Chronic Renal Failure *(continued)*

Cortisol *(continued)*
Plasma No Effect Concentration normal or may be increased *876* Mean concentration of 387 ± 98 nmol/L in 10 patients with chronic renal failure not significantly different from that in 50 healthy Caucasian volunteers, 344 ± 81 nmol/L *3605*
Saliva No Effect Mean concentration in 10 patients with chronic renal failure of 25.1 ± 10.4 nmol/L not significantly different from range in 50 healthy Caucasian volunteers of 17.9 - 7.6 nmol/L *3605*

Cortisone *Plasma Decrease* Mean concentration of 18.4 ± 3.6 nmol/L in 10 patients with chronic renal failure significantly different from that in 50 healthy Caucasian volunteers, 51.4 ± 16.7 nmol/L *3605*
Saliva Increase Mean concentration in 10 patients with chronic renal failure of 0.38 ± 0.11 nmol/L not significantly different from range in 50 healthy Caucasian volunteers 0.50 - 0.19 nmol/L *3605*

CPC-precipitable Uronic Acid *Serum Increase* In patients with chronic renal failure mean concentration of 13.7 mg/L (range 7.1 - 23.6 mg/L) significantly higher than 9.6 mg/L (range 5.1 - 13.9 mg/L) in healthy controls due to increased concentrations of low sulfated chondroitin sulfate *548*
Urine Increase Excretion increased in patients with chronic renal failure compared with healthy controls *548*

C-Peptide *Plasma Increase* In 71 patients with end stage renal disease mean concentration of 5.0 ± 1.8 ng/mL significantly higher than 3.3 ± 1.5 ng/mL in 30 healthy volunteers *2221*

C-Reactive Protein *Serum Increase* In 39 patients with chronic renal failure and normal nutrition mean concentration of 25 ± 4 mg/L significantly different from 13 ± 3 mg/L in 44 patients with chronic renal failure but with malnutrition *5005*
Serum No Effect No significant change observed in 99 patients with uncomplicated terminal uremia on conservative therapy *1191*

Creatine *Cerebrospinal Fluid Increase* High concentrations in blood and CSF have been associated with azotemia *4707*
Serum Increase High concentrations in blood and CSF have been associated with azotemia *4707*

Creatine Kinase *Serum Increase* Two of 12 patients with chronic renal failure receiving medical treatment had activity above upper limit of normal *3686*

Creatine Kinase Isoenzymes *Serum Increase* In 88 patients with chronic renal failure receiving maintenance hemodialysis mean activity increased for CK-MB, 5.9 U/L versus 4.8 U/L, and for CK-BB, 5.5 ng/mL versus 3.2 ng/mL *2398*

Creatine Kinase MB-Isoenzyme *Serum Increase* Four of 12 patients with chronic renal failure receiving medical treatment had concentration above upper limit of normal *3686* May be due to accompanying myopathy *768*

Creatinine *Serum Increase* Mean concentration of 10.8 ± 2.5 mg/dL in 104 patients with chronic renal failure receiving chronic hemodialysis significantly different from 1.0 ± 0.2 mg/dL in 98 healthy controls *803* In 23 patients with chronic renal failure mean concentration of 862 ± 150 mmol/L significantly greater than 93 ± 14 mmol/L in 20 healthy controls *3383* Appears to rise more slowly in the presence of renal disease than the BUN. It is less useful than the BUN to assess effectiveness of hemodialysis in the treatment of renal failure, since it does not decrease as rapidly as BUN *1025* Mean concentration in 9 patients with chronic renal failure not requiring dialysis 5.0 ± 0.4 mg/dL compared with 0.9 ± 0.3 mg/dL in 9 healthy controls *5153* In 10 patients with chronic renal failure not requiring dialysis mean concentration of 5.0 ± 0.4 mg/dL significantly greater than 0.9 ± 0.3 mg/dL in 9 healthy controls *5153* In 97% of 144 patients at initial hospitalization for this disorder *1576* In 19 predialytic patients with chronic renal failure mean concentration of 4.06 ± 1.15 mg/dL significantly increased compared with 0.85 ± 0.12 mg/dL in controls *870* In 12 children with chronic renal failure median concentration of 160 µmol/L significantly different from 52 µmol/L in 8 healthy pediatric controls *2346* In 11 children with chronic renal failure median concentration of 160 mmol/L not significantly different from 52 mmol/L in 10 healthy children *2347* Mean concentration in 26 diabetics with chronic renal failure (creatinine > 2.0 mg/dL) of 5.67 ± 0.59 mg/dL significantly different from 0.77 ± 0.03 mg/dL in 20 healthy controls *1592* Mean concentration in 17 uremic patients pre-dialysis of 1.0 ± 0.3 mmol/L significantly greater than upper limit of < 0.1 mmol/L in 10 healthy controls *3811* Higher concentration of Jaffe chromogens *3489* In late failure *367*

Creatinine Clearance *Urine Decrease* Mean clearance in 22 patients with glomerular disease of 66 ± 7 mL/min and in 22 patients with tubulointestitial disease of 70 ± 7 mL/min *3398* Less than 20 mL/min *2991* In 19 patients with predialytic chronic renal failure mean 23.2 ± 12.4 mL/min significantly less than 115 ± 12.5 mL/min in 38 normal controls *870* In 15 patients with severe renal insufficiency mean concentration of 10 ± 1 mL/min significantly different from 44 ± 3 mL/min in 14 with moderate insufficiency and 81 ± 5 mL/min in 13 with mild insufficiency *1410* In 9 patients with chronic renal failure mean clearance of 22.2 ± 6.9 mL/min significantly different from that in 11 healthy individuals *5265*
Urine No Effect In 19 children with end-stage renal disease mean clearance of 35 ± 15 mL/min/1.73 sq m compared with reference interval of 25 ± 18 mL/min/1.73 sq m *527*

C-terminal Propeptide of Type I Procollagen
Serum Increase Concentration of 165.1 ± 33.5 µg/L in 15 patients with chronic renal failure significantly higher than 132.1 ± 41.3 µg/L in 8 healthy controls *2839* In 30 patients with chronic renal failure without hepatopathy mean concentration of 217 ± 154 µg/mL significantly greater than 129 ± 33 µg/mL in 16 healthy controls *1677*
Serum No Effect In 19 children with end-stage renal disease mean concentration of 413 ± 190 µg/L compared with reference interval of 77 - 626 µg/L *527*

C-terminal Telopeptide of Type I Collagen *Serum Increase* In 19 children with end-stage renal disease mean concentration of 52 ± 35 µg/L compared with reference interval of 6 - 19 µg/L *527*

CYFRA 21-1 *Serum Increase* In 24 patients with chronic renal failure median concentration of 2.9 ng/mL significantly different from that in 50 healthy individuals with median concentration of 1.2 ng/mL and range of 0.5 - 2.4 ng/mL *3559*

Cysteine *Plasma Increase* Mean concentration in 14 patients on maintenance hemodialysis before hemodialysis of 556 ± 258 µmol/L significantly higher than 231 ± 30 µmol/L in 10 healthy controls *2395* In 10 patients with chronic renal failure undergoing regular hemodialysis mean concentration of 110 ± 12 µmol/L significantly greater than 50 ± 2 µmol/L in 31 healthy age and sex matched controls *1656*

Cystine *Plasma Increase* Children with renal failure showed a decrease in most amino acids but an increase in cystine and glycine. 14 of 31 children (45%) had cystine concentrations above the normal upper limit *424* Significant increase observed in patients with mild renal failure and increased progressively with progression of renal failure *746*

Dapsone *Serum No Effect* Uremia is associated with changed binding of basic or neutral drugs to plasma proteins. Effect on bound fraction only is listed here *5869*

D-Dimer *Urine Increase* In 24 patients with chronic renal failure median concentration of 12.2 ng/mL significantly different from that in normal controls in whom the mean concentration was 0.69 ± 0.60 ng/mL *4789*

Dehydroepiandrosterone *Plasma Decrease* Significant reduction observed in 14 patients with nondiabetic end stage renal disease than in 28 healthy age-matched controls *695*

3-Deoxyglucosone *Serum Increase* In 17 uremic nondiabetics mean concentration before dialysis 6.96 ± 1.02 µmol/L compared with mean concentration in 18 healthy individuals of 1.94 ± 0.17 µmol/L *3814*

Dexamethasone Suppression *Patient Abnormal* In patients with chronic renal failure hemodialysis enhances the clearance of dexamethasone and may also be associated with diminished dexamethasone absorption from the gi-tract and diminished cortisol clearance from the circulation leading to false positive results with dexamethasone suppression test *5723*

Diazepam *Serum Decrease* Uremia is associated with changed binding of basic or neutral drugs to plasma proteins. Effect on bound fraction only is listed here *5869*

Diazoxide *Serum Decrease* Uremia is associated with decreased binding of acidic drugs to plasma proteins. Effect on bound fraction only is listed here *5869*

Dicloxacillin *Serum Decrease* Uremia is associated with decreased binding of acidic drugs to plasma proteins. Effect on bound fraction only is listed here *5869*

Diflunisal *Serum* *Decrease* Uremia is associated with decreased binding of acidic drugs to plasma proteins. Effect on bound fraction only is listed here *5869*

Digitoxin *Serum* *Decrease* Uremia is associated with changed binding of basic or neutral drugs to plasma proteins. Effect on bound fraction only is listed here *5869*

Digoxin *Serum* *Increase* May be affected if beta counting method used *749*

1,25-Dihydroxy Vitamin D *Serum* *Decrease* Significant correlation observed between reduction in total 1,25 (OH)2D and worsening renal function (r = 0.974) *2738* In 11 patients with CRF mean concentration of 9.3 ± 3.4 ng/L significantly different from that in 50 healthy individuals in whom the mean concentration was 32.2 ± 8.5 ng/L as measured by RIA method of Hollis et al *2209* Decreased concentrations observed in patients with chronic renal failure *2952*
Serum *No Effect* In 19 children with end-stage renal disease mean concentration of 89 ± 54 pmol/L compared with reference interval of 39 - 102 pmol/L *527*

1,25-Dihydroxy Vitamin D_2 *Serum* *Decrease* In 15 patients with severe renal insufficiency mean concentration of 11 ± 4 pg/mL significantly different from 29 ± 5 pg/mL in 14 with moderate insufficiency and 38 ± 9 pg/mL in 13 with mild insufficiency *1410*

1,25-Dihydroxy Vitamin D_3 *Serum* *Decrease* Decreased concentration observed with end-stage renal failure *519* Observed effect *126* In 31 patients with chronic renal failure with mild renal impairment (GFR 45-90 mL/min) mean concentration of 28.9 ± 2.7 pg/mL compared with 39.5 ± 1.9 pg/mL in 16 normal individuals *3147*

1,25-Dihydroxy Vitamin D, Free *Serum* *Decrease* Significant correlation observed between reduction in concentration and worsening renal function (r = 0.974) *2738*

Dimethylarsinic Acid *Serum* *Increase* In 19 uremic patients not receiving dialysis mean concentration of 0.82 ± 1.05 µg/L (16.0% of total arsenic concentration) significantly different from reference interval *5855*

2,3-Diphosphoglycerate *Red Blood Cells* *Increase* Intracellular concentration is appropriately increased in response to anemia *817* *5677* In patients with uremia mean concentration significantly increased *626*

Dipyridinoline *Serum* *Increase* In 29 patients with chronic renal failure mean concentration of 82.9 ± 93.7 nmol/L significantly greater than undetectable amount in 19 healthy controls *2313*
Urine *Increase* In 29 patients with chronic renal failure mean excretion of 66.5 ± 116.8 µmol/mol creatinine significantly greater than 9.1 ± 3.6 µmol/mol in 19 healthy controls *2313*

Disopyramide *Serum* *Increase* Uremia is associated with changed binding of basic or neutral drugs to plasma proteins. Effect on bound fraction only is listed here *5869*

Dopamine *Urine* *Increase* Mean excretion in 22 patients with glomerular disease of 1,195 ± 119 nmol/d and in 22 patients with tubulointestitial disease 1,141 ± 120 nmol/d *3398*

Dopamine β-Hydroxylase *Serum* *Decrease* Concentration of dopamine-β-hydroxylase decreased in uremia but doubled following hemodialysis *5860*

Doxycycline *Serum* *Decrease* Uremia is associated with decreased binding of acidic drugs to plasma proteins. Effect on bound fraction only is listed here *5869*

D-Tubocurarine *Serum* *No Effect* Uremia is associated with changed binding of basic or neutral drugs to plasma proteins. Effect on bound fraction only is listed here *5869*

Endothelin *Plasma* *Increase* Significantly increased to 57.5 ± 5 pg/mL in chronically uremic patients compared with 20.8 ± 0.8 pg/mL in healthy controls *1125* In 38 undialyzed patients with chronic renal failure mean concentration of 0.82 ± 0.13 pmol/L, in 20 patients with chronic renal failure on CAPD mean of 2.81 ± 0.63 pmol/L and in 14 patients on hemodialysis mean of 4.52 ± 1.21 pmol/L *5578* Significant increase observed in 33 patients with chronic end stage renal disease with or without hemodialysis *4668* Mean concentration in 4.59 ± 2.09 pg/mL compared with 1.88 ± 0.6 pg/mL in healthy controls *5024* In 17 patients on long-term continuous ambulatory peritoneal dialysis significantly higher than in healthy individuals *2894*
Plasma *No Effect* Normal concentrations observed in uremia and in renal failure *4093*
Urine *Increase* Urinary excretion in individuals with end stage renal disease reported to be significantly higher than in healthy individuals *6*

Endothelin-1 *Plasma* *Increase* In 2 studies mean concentrations increased 2.4-fold and 1.4-fold above normal values respectively *328* In 2 studies mean concentrations increased by 3.3-fold (n = 12) and 1.8-fold (n = 24) above respective normal values *328* Both in hemolyzed and nonhemolyzed patients with chronic renal failure concentration significantly increased *4519*
Urine *Decrease* In patients with chronic renal failure, both dialyzed and undialyzed, mean concentration and excretion significantly reduced *4519*
Urine *Increase* In 16 children with chronic renal failure mean excretion of 30.3 pmol/sq m/d significantly different from 12.9 (lower and upper quartiles 10.0 - 15.2 pmol/sq m/d) in 60 normal children *5733*

Epidermal Growth Factor *Urine* *Decrease* In 19 children with chronic renal failure mean excretion of 6.9 ± 3.0 ng/mg creatinine (3.1 ± 1.6 µg/d) significantly less than that in 180 healthy children aged 7 - 15 y in whom mean excretion was 15.2 ± 6.5 ng/mg creatinine (10.6 ± 4.8 µg/d) *5300*

Epinephrine *Plasma* *Increase* Moderate increase *1326*

Erythrocyte Sedimentation Rate *Blood* *Increase* Characteristic increase as a result of increased plasma fibrinogen *367*

Erythrocyte Survival *Red Blood Cells* *Decrease* Shortened RBC life span and inhibitor of heme synthesis cause anemia in renal insufficiency *1495* Shortened to about half normal when the blood urea exceeds 200 mg/dL *367* Slightly to moderately reduced *5699*

Erythrocytes *Blood* *Decrease* In chronic renal insufficiency, anemia is commonly caused by a relative or absolute deficiency of red cell production *3710*
Urine *Increase* With renal parenchymal disease *1727*

Erythropoietin *Serum* *Decrease* Decreased secretion of erythropoietin of renal origin *3710* Reduced in chronic failure causing relative hypoplasia of the marrow *367*
Serum *Increase* May be elevated to varying degrees in patients with anemia associated with end-stage renal disease. The increase in erythropoietin titer was apparently not sufficient to meet the increase in demand for new RBCs created by their shortened life span and the inhibitors of heme synthesis *1495* Mean concentration of 17.9 ± 18.2 mIU/mL in 104 patients with chronic renal failure receiving chronic hemodialysis not significantly different from 13.2 ± 16.2 mIU/mL in 98 healthy controls *803*

Estrone *Plasma* *Increase* Concentration significantly higher in 14 patients with end stage renal disease than in 28 healthy age-matched controls *695*

Etomidate *Serum* *Decrease* Uremia is associated with changed binding of basic or neutral drugs to plasma proteins. Effect on bound fraction only is listed here *5869*

Euglobulin Fibrinolytic Activity *Plasma* *Decrease* In 71 patients with end stage renal disease mean activity of 91.2 ± 20.9 BAU correlated reversely with plasma insulin concentration *2221*

Factor V *Plasma* *Decrease* Occasionally observed *367*

Factor VII *Plasma* *Decrease* Occasionally observed *367*

Factor VIII *Plasma* *Increase* Dramatic increase in both factor VIII/von Willebrand antigen and activity (315 ± 30% vs. 104 ± 9% in control, and 402 ± 48% activity in patients vs. 111 ± 5% controls) *5577* Increased activity has been reported *1307*

Fatty Acids (FFA), Free *Serum* *Decrease* Elevated in acute renal failure, but normal or low in chronic failure *3135*
Serum *No Effect* No significant effect observed in patients with chronic renal failure *3050*

Fentanyl *Serum* *Increase* Uremia is associated with changed binding of basic or neutral drugs to plasma proteins. Effect on bound fraction only is listed here *5869*

Ferritin *Serum* *No Effect* In 23 patients with chronic renal failure mean concentration of 90 ± 56 ng/mL not significantly different from 105.0 ± 43 ng/mL in 20 healthy controls *3383* In 23 patients with chronic renal failure mean concentration of 90 ng/dL *3383*

Fibrin Degradation Products *Plasma* *Increase* Elevated levels (> 10 µg/mL) occurred in 73% of chronic nephritic patients. Mean value was 16.0 ± 5.9 µg/mL *2863*

585.00 Chronic Renal Failure *(continued)*

Fibrin/Fibrinogen Degradation Product E *Urine Increase* In 29 patients with chronic renal failure mean excretion of 156.5 ± 204.5 ng/mL significantly different from 1.68 ± 1.05 ng/mL in 30 controls *4790*

Fibrinogen *Plasma Increase* Usually raised about 30%, resulting in characteristic rise of ESR *367*

Fibronectin *Plasma Decrease* Significantly reduced concentration observed in patients with uremia before and after hemodialysis *4625*

Fluoxetine *Serum No Effect* Uremia is associated with changed binding of basic or neutral drugs to plasma proteins. Effect on bound fraction only is listed here *5869*

Follicle Stimulating Hormone *Plasma Increase* In 7 patients with chronic renal failure prior to dialysis mean concentration significantly increased *5596* In 25 uremic patients mean concentrations of 10.3 ± 6.5 IU/L (by RIA) and 8.5 ± 4.4 IU/L (by IRMA) significantly greater than 4.7 ± 2.5 IU/L (by RIA) and 4.2 ± 2.2 IU/L (by IRMA) in 57 healthy normal controls *3438*

Follistatin, Free *Serum Increase* Mean concentration in 42 patients with chronic renal disease of 6.7 ± 0.9 µg/L significantly different from that in 60 normal adults of 3.5 ± 0.2 µg/L *4523*

Fructosamine *Serum Increase* Mean concentration in 20 patients with uremia of 2.35 ± 0.36 mmol/L significantly greater than 2.16 ± 0.29 mmol/L in 67 healthy controls *3392*
Serum No Effect In 20 uremic undialyzed patients mean concentration of 282 ± 13 µmol/L not significantly different from 261 ± 5 µmol/L in 20 healthy controls *3812*

Furosemide *Serum Decrease* Uremia is associated with decreased binding of acidic drugs to plasma proteins. Effect on bound fraction only is listed here *5869*

Gastric Inhibitory Polypeptide *Plasma Increase* Markedly increased in uremic patients prior to dialysis compared with healthy controls *4875*
Plasma No Effect No significant change observed in patients with uremia *1953*

Gastrin *Serum Increase* Mean concentration of 689 pg/mL observed in 12 uremic patients with linear correlation between serum concentrations of creatinine and gastrin: mean concentration in controls 118 pg/mL *1320* In both acute and chronic failure *2771* Concentration significantly increased in uremic patients *1953* Minimal increase observed in uremic patients prior to hemodialysis *4875* Elevated; no apparent correlation with calcitonin levels *2967*

Gastrin-releasing Peptide *Serum Increase* Concentration of 7.1 ± 2.1 pmol/L observed in group of individuals with chronic renal failure on hemodialysis compared with mean of 2.1 pmol/L in healthy controls *2019*

α_1-Globulin *Serum Increase* Moderate increases *1290*

α_2-Globulin *Serum Increase* Biochemical abnormalities are those seen in the nephrotic syndrome *1980* There is a moderate increase *1290*

β-Globulin *Serum No Effect* Concentration usually normal *5544*

γ-Globulin *Serum No Effect* Concentration usually normal *5544*

Glomerular Filtration Rate *Urine Decrease* BUN and creatinine rise as GFR decreases *1980*

Glucagon *Plasma Increase* Fasting immunoreactive glucagon was elevated to 534 ± 2 pg/mL in chronic failure. Normal value was 113 ± 9 pg/mL *2846* Concentration significantly increased in patients with uremia *1953* Glucagon is elevated 2 to 10 times above normal and remains essentially unchanged by dialysis *452*

Glucose *Serum Decrease* Depressed glucose concentration observed with whole blood measurement by Boehringer Mannheim AccuChek II and Lifescan One-touch reflectance systems *5379*
Serum Increase Mean concentration of 5.71 ± 0.93 mmol/L in 20 uremic patients significantly greater than 5.02 ± 0.96 mmol/L in 67 controls *3392* Increased mean plasma concentration in chronic failure *2607* Hyperglycemia and impaired glucose tolerance are common in renal failure. Elevated ratio of insulin/glucose during glucose tolerance testing is found consistently *1583* In 71 patients with end stage renal disease mean concentration of 100.6 ± 12.1 mg/dL significantly higher than 90.6 ± 1.2 mg/dL in 30 healthy volunteers *2221*
Serum No Effect No effect of uremia observed with whole blood measurements using Nova Stat Profile 5 whereas reflectance systems show reduced concentrations *5379*
Urine Increase With renal parenchymal disease *1727*

Glucose-6-Phosphatase *Serum Increase* Slight rise with renal disease *1290*

Glucose Tolerance *Serum Decrease* More than 50% of patients in late renal failure have glucose intolerance as severe as in mild diabetes but with normal fasting blood dextrose and often without glycosuria *367*

Glutamic Acid *Plasma Decrease* Mean concentration of serine, threonine, and glutamic acid decreased with deteriorating renal function in children with renal failure *424*

γ-Glutamyltransferase *Serum Increase* Increased activity reported with uremia *3625*

Glutathione *Plasma Increase* In 19 patients with chronic renal failure mean concentration of 5.4 ± 1.9 µmol/L significantly different from 14.39 ± 4.10 µmol/L in 14 controls *3323*
Plasma No Effect Mean concentration in 14 patients on maintenance hemodialysis before hemodialysis of 9.1 ± 7.5 µmol/L not significantly different from 10.4 ± 8.8 µmol/L in 10 healthy controls *2395*

Glutathione, Oxidized *Plasma Decrease* In 19 patients with chronic renal failure mean concentration of 9.36 ± 2.40 mg/dL significantly different from 12.2 ± 2.0 mg/dL in 14 controls *3323*

Glutathione Peroxidase *Red Blood Cells Decrease* In 14 patients with chronic renal failure mean activity of 15.88 ± 3.5 U/g hemoglobin significantly different from 20.04 ± 2.0 U/g hemoglobin in 14 controls *3323*
Red Blood Cells Increase In patients with chronic renal failure mean activity of 59.8 ± 5.2 U/g hemoglobin in 12 with creatinine clearance of 51 - 90 mL/min, 61.7 ± 5.6 U/g hemoglobin in 12 with clearance of 21 - 50 mL/min and in 12 with clearance < 20 mL/min activity of 75.8 ± 6.9 U/g hemoglobin significantly different when compared with 41.8 ± 3.9 U/g hemoglobin in 13 healthy controls with clearance > 90 mL/min *3502* Mean activity of 41.8 ± 3.9 U/g hemoglobin in 13 healthy controls with renal clearance > 90 mL/min *3502* In 14 patients with chronic renal failure mean activity of 15.88 ± 3.5 U/g hemoglobin significantly different from 20.04 ± 2.0 U/g hemoglobin in 11 controls *3323*
Serum Decrease In 87 patients with chronic renal failure mean activity of 106 ± 2.7 U/L significantly less than 281 ± 3.6 U/L in controls *4461*
Serum No Effect In 87 patients with chronic renal failure mean immunoreactive concentration changed insignificantly from 14.1 ± 1.26 µg/mL compared with 15.2 ± 1.6 µg/mL in controls *4461* Mean value of 7,554 ± 6,317 ng/mL in 104 patients with chronic renal failure receiving chronic hemodialysis not significantly different from 7,297 ± 3,795 ng/mL in 98 healthy controls *803*

Glutathione, Reduced *Plasma Decrease* In 19 patients with chronic renal failure mean activity of 37.65 ± 17.0 mg/dL significantly different from 119.98 ± 36.0 mg/dL in 14 controls *3323*
Plasma Increase In 14 patients with chronic renal failure mean concentration of 5.34 ± 1.90 µmol/L significantly different from 14.39 ± 4.10 µmol/L in 11 controls *3323*

Glutathione Reductase *Red Blood Cells Increase* In 13 patients with chronic renal failure mean activity of 2.99 ± 0.6 U/g hemoglobin significantly different from 4.39 ± 0.7 U/g hemoglobin in 13 controls *3323*

Glutathione Transferase *Red Blood Cells Increase* In 12 patients with chronic renal failure mean activity of 4.32 ± 1.50 U/g hemoglobin significantly different from 2.87 ± 0.57 U/g hemoglobin in 15 controls *3323*

Glycerol *Serum Increase* Increased mean plasma concentration in chronic failure *2607*

Glycine *Plasma Increase* A significant rise in mean concentration occurred in children whose GFR was < 15 mL/min/1.73 m^3. 34% had values above normal upper limit *424* In 10 patients with chronic renal failure undergoing regular hemodialysis mean concentration of 281 ± 14 µmol/L significantly greater than 249 ± 8 µmol/L in 31 healthy age and sex matched controls *1656*

Granular Casts *Urine Increase* Proteinuria and granular casts suggest chronic parenchymal renal disease *900*

Growth Hormone *Plasma Increase* Consistently occurring hypersecretion may be induced by severe uremia *1583* Mean concentration in 26 diabetics with chronic renal failure (creatinine > 2.0 mg/dL) of 3.0 ± 0.8 ng/mL significantly different from 1.8 ±

1.0 ng/mL in 20 healthy controls *1592* Basal concentration increased with hyperresponsiveness to insulin hypoglycemia observed but paradoxical increase during glucose tolerance tests and with TRH infusions *876* Mean concentration in 27 uremic patients of 3.6 ± 0.6 µg/L significantly higher than 2.5 ± 0.5 µg/L in normal controls *741* Reported effect *2304* Increased mean plasma concentration in chronic failure *2607*
Urine Increase Marked elevation *3144*

Growth Hormone Binding Protein *Serum Decrease* In 9 patients undergoing hemodialysis binding reduced to 24.6 ± 6%, in 8 patients undergoing CAPD binding reduced to 25.7 ± 7.6%, in 9 patients 3 months after renal transplantation reduced to 25.1 ± 8.6% and in 11 patients with renal disease who were off dialysis reduced to 16.8 ± 5.6% compared with 39.3 ± 8.0% in 26 normal individuals *3230*

Guanosine Monophosphate *Plasma Increase* In patients with renal failure mean concentration in ethanol-extracted specimens of 10.52 ± 2.444 nmol/L compared with 3.439 ± 1.226 nmol/L in healthy blood donors and in nonextracted specimens of 12.602 ± 1.895 nmol/L compared with 5.301 ± 1.456 nmol/L in healthy blood donors *2405* Mean concentration in chronic renal failure of 14.3 ± 2.9 pmol/mL significantly greater than 6.5 ± 1.1 pmol/mL in healthy controls *3469*
Urine Decrease In 29 patients with chronic renal failure mean concentration of about 0.2 µmol/g creatinine significantly less than 0.39 ± 0.5 µmol/g creatinine in healthy controls *2406*

Guanosine Triphosphate *Red Blood Cells Increase* In patients with uremia mean concentration significantly increased *626*

HDL_2-Cholesterol *Serum No Effect* In 13 patients with chronic renal failure, but dialysis independent, mean concentration of 0.54 ± 0.30 mmol/L not significantly different from 0.73 ± 0.31 mmol/L in 27 healthy controls *935*

HDL_3-Cholesterol *Serum No Effect* In 13 patients with chronic renal failure, but dialysis independent, mean concentration of 0.72 ± 0.22 mmol/L not significantly different from 0.80 ± 0.12 mmol/L in 27 healthy controls *935*

HDL-Cholesterol *Serum Decrease* Mean concentration in 117 patients with uremia of 1.08 ± 0.31 mmol/L different from 1.43 ± 0.31 mmol/L in 110 healthy controls *4002* In patients with chronic renal failure without nephrotic syndrome 35% had HDL-cholesterol concentrations less than 35 mg/dL *2575* Mean concentration reduced to 40 mg/dL in uremics from 50 mg/dL in healthy controls *726* In 68 patients with chronic renal disease mean concentration of 42 ± 11 mg/dL significantly different from 54 ± 11 mg/dL in 73 healthy normal volunteers *3487* In 104 patients with end-stage renal disease receiving hemodialysis mean concentration of 35.9 ± 1.2 mg/dL significantly different from 48.8 ± 1.1 mg/dL in healthy controls *1488* Mean concentration in 12 patients with chronic renal failure and uremia of 1.19 ± 0.34 mmol/L compared with 1.44 ± 0.28 mmol/L in 9 healthy controls *2230* Significant decrease observed in patients with chronic renal failure *1590*
Serum No Effect In 39 patients with chronic renal failure and normal nutrition mean concentration of 1.2 ± 0.1 mmol/L not significantly different from 1.3 ± 0.1 mmol/L in 44 patients with chronic renal failure but with malnutrition *5005* In 13 patients with chronic renal failure, but dialysis independent, mean concentration of 1.26 ± 0.42 mmol/L not significantly different from 1.53 ± 0.39 mmol/L in 27 healthy controls *935*

HDL-Triglycerides *Serum Increase* Mean concentration in 12 patients with chronic renal failure and uremia of 0.21 ± 0.07 mmol/L compared with 0.15 ± 0.06 mmol/L in 9 healthy controls *2230*

Hematocrit *Blood Decrease* Anemia occurs in almost all chronic patients. Uremia without anemia suggests acute renal failure. RBCs are normochromic or have slightly reduced MCHC, about 30 - 31 *367* Mean value of 26.6 ± 5.7% in 104 patients with chronic renal failure receiving chronic hemodialysis significantly different from 45.3 ± 10.2% in 98 healthy controls *803* In 89% of 146 patients at initial hospitalization for this disorder *1576* Hydremia and dehydration are common. Changes will exaggerate or minimize the degree of anemia *5699* In 34 patients with chronic renal failure mean value of 25.3 ± 4.1% significantly different from 42.9 ± 3.1% in 20 healthy controls *3383* Characteristically normocytic and normochromic, and is associated with a normal or slightly decreased number of reticulocytes *5677*

Hemoglobin *Blood Decrease* In patients with chronic renal failure mean concentration of 115 ± 24.7 g/L in 12 with creatinine clearance of 51 - 90 mL/min, 114 ± 27.3 g/L in 12 with clearance 21 - 50 mL/min and in 12 with clearance < 20 mL/min concentration of 108 ± 17.3 g/L significantly different when compared with 124 ± 18.7 g/L in 13 healthy controls with clearance > 90 mL/min *3502* In 23 patients with chronic renal failure mean concentration of 8.1 ± 1.4 g/dL significantly different from 14.8 ± 1.1 g/dL in 20 healthy controls *3383* In 89% of 146 patients at initial hospitalization for this disorder *1576* Anemia is characteristic of chronic failure, normal hemoglobin suggests acute failure *367* Hydremia and dehydration are common. Changes will exaggerate or minimize the degree of anemia *5699* Normocytic and normochromic, and associated with a normal or slightly decreased number of reticulocytes *5677* Mean concentration of 9.0 ± 1.9 g/dL in 104 patients with chronic renal failure receiving chronic hemodialysis significantly different from 14.4 ± 2.5 g/dL in 98 healthy controls *803*
Plasma Increase Mild hemolysis may occur *3710*

Hemoglobin A_{1c} *Blood Increase* In 20 patients with uremia mean concentration of 8.43% significantly greater than 6.41% in 67 healthy controls *3392*

Heparan Sulfate *Urine Decrease* Excretion not detected in patients with chronic renal failure compared with normals in whom it is a major glycosaminoglycan *548*

Hepatocyte Growth Factor *Urine No Effect* Mean concentration in 10 patients with chronic renal failure not significantly different from 1.5 ± 0.2 ng/g creatinine in 9 healthy controls *5153*

β-Hexosaminidase *Urine Increase* Urinary levels often increased in chronic renal disease and are very sensitive to degree of renal damage *3373*

Hippuric Acid *Serum Increase* In patients with acute or chronic renal failure concentration ranged from 0.11-16.2 mg/dL with moderately close correlation with serum creatinine concentration *2315*

Histamine *Plasma Increase* In 6 hemodialysis patients with pruritus mean concentration of 368 ± 103 pg/mL compared with 146 ± 22 pg/mL in 5 uremic patients without pruritus and 142 ± 16 pg/mL in 5 normal controls *1554*

Histidine *Plasma Increase* In 7 elderly individuals with renal failure concentration significantly increased compared with controls *701* In 10 patients with chronic renal failure undergoing regular hemodialysis mean concentration of 87 ± 3 µmol/L significantly greater than 68 ± 2 µmol/L in 31 healthy age and sex matched controls *1656*

Homocysteine *Plasma Increase* Mean concentration of 31.7 pmol/L observed in 167 patients with end stage renal disease, with highest concentrations observed in individuals who had cardiac events *3635* We conclude that hyperhomocysteinemia is present from the early stage of chronic renal failure and may constitute a risk factor for premature arteriosclerosis in uremic patients *4334* In patients with chronic renal failure mean concentration of 18.2 ± 1.7 µmol/L in those with serum creatinine less than 300 µmol/L, 27.3 ± 3.2 µmol/L in those with serum creatinine over 300 µmol/L compared with 8.0 ± 0.3 µmol/L in 45 controls *4942*

Hyaluronic Acid *Serum Increase* In 22 patients with renal insufficiency and 40 with end stage renal failure concentrations significantly increased compared with age and sex-matched healthy controls: significant correlation observed between concentration and degree of renal failure *1974* In 176 adult patients and 15 children receiving hemodialysis for chronic renal failure hyaluronic acid concentration increased to more than 80 µg/L in more than 90% with median value 182 µg/L. ?Concentration did not correlate with serum creatinine *5333* Serum levels were measured in 105 renal patients and 22 normal controls. Median HA concentrations were 23 µg/L in controls, 47 µg/L in patients with chronic renal failure (CRF, not on dialysis; p less than 0.001), 75 µg/L on CAPD (p less than 0.001) vs. controls, p = 0.045 vs. CRF), and 167 µg/L on hemodialysis (p less than 0.001 vs. controls, CRF, and CAPD), respectively *2222*

Hydrocortisone *Serum Decrease* Uremia is associated with changed binding of basic or neutral drugs to plasma proteins. Effect on bound fraction only is listed here *5869*

585.00 Chronic Renal Failure *(continued)*

Hydroxylysylpyridinoline *Serum* *No Effect* Mean concentration in 34 uremic patients pre-hemodialysis of 78.3 ± 7.0 nmol/L significantly higher than that in 10 healthy individuals, 3.2 ± 0.2 nmol/L *3813*

5-Hydroxytryptamine *Blood* *Decrease* Mean concentration in 39 patients with chronic renal failure on conservative treatment of 779 ± 66 nmol/L significantly different from that in 35 healthy controls of 1,039 ± 69 nmolL *5016*

^{131}I Uptake *Serum* *Decrease* In renal disease *4707*

IDL-Apolipoprotein B *Serum* *Increase* Mean concentration in 12 patients with chronic renal failure and uremia of 7 ± 4 mmol/L compared with 4 ± 1 mmol/L in 4 healthy controls *2230*

IDL-Cholesterol *Serum* *Increase* Mean concentration in 12 patients with chronic renal failure and uremia of 0.43 ± 0.24 mmol/L compared with 0.15 ± 0.07 mmol/L in 9 healthy controls *2230*

IDL-Triglycerides *Serum* *Increase* Mean concentration in 12 patients with chronic renal failure and uremia of 0.10 ± 0.07 mmol/L compared with 0.07 ± 0.03 mmol/L in 9 healthy controls *2230*

Indapamide *Serum* *Decrease* Uremia is associated with decreased binding of acidic drugs to plasma proteins. Effect on bound fraction only is listed here *5869*

Indican *Serum* *Increase* In 20 uremic patients undergoing regular hemodialysis mean concentration prior to hemodialysis of 238.8 ± 33.6 nmol/mL significantly greater than that in 12 healthy controls in whom mean concentration was 2.6 ± 0.4 nmol/mL *2149*

Indole *Feces* *Increase* In 20 patients with chronic renal failure undergoing regular hemodialysis concentration ranged from 210 ± 75 nmol/mg feces compared with that in 12 healthy controls in whom mean concentration was 120 ± 28 nmol/mg feces *2149*

Indomethacin *Serum* *Decrease* Uremia is associated with decreased binding of acidic drugs to plasma proteins. Effect on bound fraction only is listed here *5869*

Inosine Triphosphate *Red Blood Cells* *Increase* In patients with uremia mean concentration significantly increased *626*

Insulin *Plasma* *Increase* In 71 patients with end stage renal disease mean concentration of 8.3 ± 4.9 µU/mL significantly higher than 5.2 ± 2.9 µU/mL in 30 healthy volunteers *2221* Usual observation in chronic renal failure *2304* Increased basal immunoreactive insulin levels in chronic uremia may be due to prolonged half-life *245*
Urine *Increase* Markedly elevated *3144*

Insulin-like Growth Factor-I *Serum* *Increase* Mean concentration of 331 ± 88 ng/mL in 19 patients with predialytic chronic renal failure significantly greater than 220 ± 71 ng/mL in 20 healthy controls *870*
Serum *No Effect* In 27 uremic patients mean concentration of 305 ± 24 µg/L not significantly different from 262 ± 16 µg/L in normal controls *741* Concentration normal in children with end stage renal failure compared with healthy controls *490* In 19 children with end-stage renal disease mean concentration of 23 ± 15 nmol/L *527* Mean concentration in 26 diabetics with chronic renal failure (creatinine > 2.0 mg/dL) of 234 ± 25 ng/mL not significantly different from 230 ± 14 g/mL in 20 healthy controls *1592*

Insulin-like Growth Factor-II *Serum* *No Effect* In children with end stage renal failure mean concentration unchanged from that in healthy children *490*

Insulin-like Growth Factor Binding Protein-1
Serum *Increase* Markedly increased concentration observed in children with end stage renal failure compared with healthy children *490*

Insulin-like Growth Factor Binding Protein-2
Serum *Increase* Significant increase observed in children with end stage renal disease compared with healthy control children *490*

Insulin-like Growth Factor Binding Protein-3
Serum *Increase* Marked increase observed in children with end stage renal disease compared with healthy children *490*
Serum *No Effect* In 19 children with end-stage renal disease mean concentration of 3.7 ± 1.40 mg/L *527*

Intercellular Adhesion Molecule-1 *Serum* *Increase* In 10 patients with chronic renal failure receiving hemodialysis mean concentration of 405 ng/mL significantly higher than 245 ng/mL in 10 healthy controls *3638*

Interleukin-1β *Serum* *Increase* In 1 of 11 children with chronic renal failure was IL-1β at a concentration of 8,570 pg/mL detected in serum *2347*
Serum *No Effect* In 8 children with chronic renal failure mean concentration of 0.08 ± 0.05 ng/mL compared with 0.07 ± 0.02 ng/mL in 8 controls *5391*
Urine *No Effect* In 1 of 11 children with chronic renal failure was IL-1β detected in urine *2347* In none of 11 children with chronic renal failure was IL-6 detected in urine *2347*

Interleukin-2 *Serum* *Increase* In 76 patients with chronic renal failure mean concentration increased to 24.2 ng/L before hemodialysis *3977*

Interleukin-6 *Serum* *Increase* In only 1 of 11 children with chronic renal failure was IL-6 detected in serum, at a concentration of 660 pg/mL *2347* In 5 out of 9 uremic patients detectable concentrations observed with range from 20 - 64 pg/mL compared with only 2 of 5 healthy control individuals having detectable concentrations *744* Forty-eight patients with end-stage renal failure, including 32 long-term HD patients and 16 chronic uremic patients undergoing their first dialysis session, were tested for plasma IL-6 using both biological and immunoreactive assays. Plasma IL-6 activity was significantly increased in patients with chronic renal failure ($p < 0.001$) compared to its level in normal individuals *2123* Increased concentration observed in chronic renal failure *4093*
Serum *No Effect* In 8 children with chronic renal failure concentration of < 20 ng/L compared with < 20 ng/L in 8 controls *5391*

Interleukin-8 *Serum* *Increase* In 2 of 11 children with chronic renal failure was IL-8 at concentrations of 860 and 6,700 pg/mL detected in serum *2347*

Iron *Serum* *Decrease* Normal in mild cases, but with severe failure, both hypo- and hyperferremia have been observed *1316 1485 5699* In 23 patients with chronic renal failure mean concentration of 59.8 ± 27.3 µg/dL significantly less than 144.0 ± 43 µg/dL in 20 healthy controls *3383*
Serum *Increase* Normal in mild cases, but with severe failure, both hypo- and hyperferremia have been observed *5699 1485 1316*

Iron-binding Capacity, Total *Serum* *Decrease* In 64% of 17 patients at initial hospitalization for this disorder *1576* Low in both mild and severe renal failure, with the lowest levels found in patients with poor nutritional state *3921*

Isoleucine *Plasma* *Decrease* Significant but moderate decrease observed in patients with marked chronic renal failure *746* In 10 patients with chronic renal failure undergoing regular hemodialysis mean concentration of 41 ± 2 µmol/L significantly less than 50 ± 2 µmol/L in 31 healthy age and sex matched controls *1656*

Kallikrein *Urine* *Decrease* In 22 patients with chronic renal failure excretion reduced in both normotensive and hypertensive individuals *981*

Lactate Dehydrogenase *Pleural Fluid* *Decrease* Transudate *126*
Serum *Increase* Occasional increase but to no clinically useful degree *5544* Patients with chronic renal disease, especially those with nephrotic syndrome or hemolytic anemia, also have increased values *1025*
Serum *No Effect* Within normal limits *3449*
Urine *Increase* 38% of cases showed elevation *1670*

Lactoferrin *Plasma* *Increase* Mean value of 288.6 ± 226.5 ng/mL in 104 patients with chronic renal failure receiving chronic hemodialysis not significantly different from 225.9 ± 101.8 ng/mL in 98 healthy controls *803*

LDL-Apolipoprotein B *Serum* *No Effect* Mean concentration in 12 patients with chronic renal failure and uremia of 72 ± 30 mmol/L compared with 66 ± 24 mmol/L in 9 healthy controls *2230*

LDL-Cholesterol *Serum* *Decrease* In 104 patients with end-stage renal disease receiving hemodialysis mean concentration of 109.3 ± 4.1 mg/dL significantly different from 137.0 ± 3.0 mg/dL in healthy controls *1488* Mean concentration reduced to 100 mg/dL in uremics compared with 118 mg/dL in controls *726*
Serum *Increase* In patients with chronic renal failure without nephrotic syndrome 10% had LDL-cholesterol concentrations

exceeding 130 mg/dL *2575* Mean concentration in 117 patients with uremia of 3.42 ± 1.14 mmol/L different from 2.6 ± 0.6 mmol/L in 110 healthy controls *4002*
Serum No Effect Mean concentration in 12 patients with chronic renal failure and uremia of 2.51 ± 0.79 mmol/L compared with 2.66 ± 0.81 mmol/L in 9 healthy controls *2230* In 13 patients with chronic renal failure, but dialysis independent, mean concentration of 4.09 ± 1.45 mmol/L not significantly different from 4.32 ± 0.74 mmol/L in 27 healthy controls *935* In 39 patients with chronic renal failure and normal nutrition mean concentration of 3.7 ± 0.2 mmol/L not significantly different from 3,5 ± 0.2 mmol/L in 44 patients with chronic renal failure but with malnutrition *5005* In 68 patients with chronic renal disease mean concentration of 128 ± 43 mg/dL not significantly different from 127 ± 29 mg/dL in 73 healthy normal volunteers *3487*

LDL-Triglycerides *Serum Increase* Mean concentration in 12 patients with chronic renal failure and uremia of 0.34 ± 0.21 mmol/L compared with 0.27 ± 0.13 mmol/L in 9 healthy controls *2230*

Leptin *Serum Increase* Mean concentration in 141 patients with end-stage renal disease of 26.8 ± 5.7 μg/L in men and 38.4 ± 5.6 μg/L in women significantly greater than 11.9 ± 3.1 μg/L in normal men and 21.2 ± 3.0 μg/L in normal women *3344* Significant increase in concentration may be observed, probably as a result of decreased renal clearance *5542*

Leu-Enkephalin *Plasma Decrease* In 28 patients with chronic renal failure mean concentration suppressed *5873*

Leucine *Plasma Decrease* In 10 patients with chronic renal failure undergoing regular hemodialysis mean concentration of 76 ± 4 μmol/L significantly less than 97 ± 3 μmol/L in 31 healthy age and sex matched controls *1656* Significant but moderate decrease in patients with marked renal failure *746*

Leukocytes *Blood Decrease* Mean concentration of 4.9 ± 1.5 x 10^3/μL in 104 patients with chronic renal failure receiving chronic hemodialysis significantly different from 6.1 ± 2.1 x 10^3/μL in 98 healthy controls *803*
Blood Increase Slight neutrophilic leukocytosis may be observed *662* *5699* In 26% of 146 patients at initial hospitalization for this disorder *1576*
Blood No Effect In 12 children with chronic renal failure median concentration of 7.1 x 10^9/L not significantly different from 8.9 x 10^9/L in 8 healthy pediatric controls *2346* In 11 children with chronic renal failure median concentration of 7.1 x 10^{-9}/L not significantly different from 8.9 x 10^9/L in 10 healthy children *2347*
Urine Increase With renal parenchymal disease *1727*

Lidocaine *Serum Increase* Uremia is associated with changed binding of basic or neutral drugs to plasma proteins. Effect on bound fraction only is listed here *5869*

Lipase *Serum Increase* In 80% of 87 patients with renal failure but without abdominal pain hyperlipasemia observed with 2.3% having activity more than 10 times the upper limit of normal *3063* Mean activity of 270 ± 182 U/L in 25 patients with chronic renal failure significantly greater than 84 ± 20 U/L in 10 healthy individuals *2687* In 63 patients with chronic renal failure mean activity of 292 ± 211 U/L significantly different from 122 ± 62 U/L in 34 healthy volunteer controls *3331* Activity increased in inverse relationship to renal clearance *5231*

Lipids *Serum Increase* Raised in late renal failure, mainly due to a rise in triglycerides; phospholipids and cholesterol are normal or slightly elevated *367*

Lipopolysaccharide-binding Protein *Serum Increase* In 28 undialyzed patients with chronic renal failure mean concentration of 8,513 ± 797 ng/mL significantly higher than that in 15 healthy volunteers in whom the mean concentration was 5,424 ± 749 ng/mL *4077*

β-Lipoprotein *Serum Increase* Increased mean plasma concentration in chronic failure *2607*

Lipoprotein Lp(a) *Serum Increase* In 39 patients with chronic renal failure and normal nutrition median concentration of 11.7 mg/dL significantly different from 19.5 mg/dL in 44 patients with chronic renal failure but with malnutrition compared with median of 6.9 mg/dL in 259 healthy controls *5005* In 104 patients with end-stage renal disease receiving hemodialysis mean concentration of 30.1 ± 2.9 mg/dL significantly different from 17.1 ± 1.5 mg/dL in healthy controls *1488* In patients with chronic renal failure without nephrotic syndrome 45% had Lp(a) concentrations greater than 30 mg/dL *2575* In 68 patients with chronic renal disease receiving CAPD mean concentration of 23.13 ± 22.12 mg/dL (median 15.1 mg/dL) significantly different from 16.38 ± 20.32 mg/dL (median 6.1 mg/dL) in 73 healthy normal volunteers *3487* In 84 patients with chronic renal failure receiving regular hemodialysis median concentration of 34.3 mg/dL significantly higher than 19.7 mg/dL in 104 healthy controls *230*

Lipoproteins *Serum Increase* 42 of 100 patients had type IV hyperlipoproteinemia, which did not correlate with degree of disease, or age, sex, weight or diet of patient *5709* Characteristically increased. Type IV hyperlipoproteinemia occurs commonly secondary to renal failure *2136*

Lipoproteins, Pre-β *Serum Increase* Consistent rise in late renal failure *367* Increased mean plasma concentration in chronic failure *2607*

Luteinizing Hormone *Plasma Increase* In 25 patients with chronic uremia mean concentration as measured by RIA of 48.9 ± 16.5 U/L (18.8 ± 8.6 U/L by IRMA) significantly greater than 14.0 ± 5.2 U/L as measured by RIA and 7.0 ± 4.3 U/L as measured by IRMA in 57 healthy normal controls *3438* Concentration significantly higher in 14 patients with nondiabetic end stage renal disease compared with 28 healthy age-matched controls *695*

Lymphocytes *Blood Decrease* In 66% of 141 patients at initial hospitalization for this disorder *1576*

Lysine *Plasma No Effect* In 10 patients with chronic renal failure undergoing regular hemodialysis mean concentration of 148 ± 10 μmol/L not significantly different from 144 ± 4 μmol/L in 31 healthy age and sex matched controls *1656*

Lysozyme *Urine Increase* Marked increase *4224*

Lysylpyridinoline *Serum No Effect* Mean concentration in 34 uremic patients pre-hemodialysis of 16.4 ± 2.9 nmol/L significantly higher than that in 10 healthy individuals, 0.3 ± 0.07 nmol/L *3813*

$β_2$-Macroglobulin *Serum Decrease* An increase in urine and a decrease in serum levels is seen in disorders of renal tubular function *2586*
Urine Increase An increase in urine and a decrease in serum levels is seen in disorders of renal tubular function *2586*

Magnesium *Red Blood Cells Increase* Of 15 patients with a variety of renal lesions and a wide range of BUN, 9 had elevated erythrocyte magnesium levels. Mean concentration for the whole group was significantly raised, 6.7 mmol/L packed cells *5547*
Serum Decrease Depletion occurs in rare instances *3457*
Serum Increase In 43% of 60 patients at initial hospitalization for this disorder *1576* Increases when GFR falls to < 30 mL/min *5545*
Sweat Increase Concentrations of Ca, Mg and phosphate in sweat were significantly elevated due to an increase in the secretion of these electrolytes in the secretory portion of the sweat gland, while that in the reabsorptive duct is normal *4225*

Malondialdehyde *Serum Increase* Increase observed in patients with chronic renal failure with highest concentrations observed in those with lowest serum antioxidant activity *2861* In 10 patients with chronic renal failure mean blood concentration of 133.0 ± 20.5 nmol/g significantly different from 101.5 ± 17.0 nmol/g in 12 controls *3323* In 22 patients with chronic renal failure mean concentration predialysis of 2.94 ± 0.28 μmol/L significantly higher than 1.45 ± 0.15 μmol/L in healthy controls *2385*

Maprotiline *Serum No Effect* Uremia is associated with changed binding of basic or neutral drugs to plasma proteins. Effect on bound fraction only is listed here *5869*

MCHC *Blood Decrease* Slightly reduced, to about 30 - 31% *367*

MCV *Blood Increase* Slight macrocytosis has been observed *3104*

Met-Enkephalin *Plasma Increase* In 28 patients with chronic renal failure mean concentration markedly increased and significantly correlated with plasma creatinine concentration (r = 0.60) and to plasma urea (r = 0.36) *5873*

Metanephrines, Total *Urine No Effect* Normal urinary excretion *1326*

Methotrexate *Serum Decrease* Uremia is associated with decreased binding of acidic drugs to plasma proteins. Effect on bound fraction only is listed here *5869*

585.00 Chronic Renal Failure *(continued)*

3-Methylhistidine *Plasma Increase* Significant increase observed in patients with mild renal failure which increased progressively with progression of renal failure *746*

Methylmalonate *Serum Increase* Concentration above upper limit of normal in 36 of 37 patients with end stage renal disease on chronic hemodialysis. Mean at 0 mo 0.60 µmol/L, 0.55 µmol/L after 1 mo, 0.70 µmol/L after 2 mo, 0.76 µmol/L after 3 mo compared with normal of 0.52 - 0.66 µmol/L *3543*

Metoclopramide *Serum No Effect* Uremia is associated with changed binding of basic or neutral drugs to plasma proteins. Effect on bound fraction only is listed here *5869*

β_2-Microglobulin *Serum Increase* In 28 patients without increased urinary protein but with marginally increased serum urea and/or creatinine mean concentration of 5.9 ± 1.7 mg/L and in 42 patients with increased serum urea and/or creatinine together with increased urinary protein mean concentration of 11 ± 10 mg/L significantly greater than 1.6 ± 0.5 mg/L in 30 healthy controls *4863* In 26 patients with chronic renal failure receiving hemodialysis mean concentration of 57.9 ± 3.0 mg/L compared with 1.51 ± 0.03 mg/L in 17 healthy controls *3547* Impaired renal function inhibits clearance and increases serum concentration *228*

Midazolam *Serum No Effect* Uremia is associated with changed binding of basic or neutral drugs to plasma proteins. Effect on bound fraction only is listed here *5869*

Monocytes *Urine Increase* 29 - 33% mononuclear cells found in lupus nephritis and endemic benign nephropathy *3071*

Morphine *Serum Increase* Uremia is associated with changed binding of basic or neutral drugs to plasma proteins. Effect on bound fraction only is listed here *5869*

Moxaprindine *Serum Increase* Uremia is associated with changed binding of basic or neutral drugs to plasma proteins. Effect on bound fraction only is listed here *5869*

Myeloperoxidase *Serum Increase* Mean value of 50.8 ± 49.3 ng/mL in 104 patients with chronic renal failure receiving chronic hemodialysis significantly different from 7.6 ± 6.0 ng/mL in 98 healthy controls *803*

Myoglobin *Serum Increase* All 12 of 12 patients with chronic renal failure receiving medical treatment had concentration above upper limit of normal *3686*

N-Acetyl-Glucosaminidase *Serum Decrease* In 12 patients with chronic renal failure mean activity of 184 ± 44 U/L significantly less than 390 ± 65 U/L in 23 healthy blood donors *3111*
Urine Increase In random urine specimens activity 20 times higher in specimens from uremic patients than from healthy individuals *3076*

N-Acetylcysteine *Serum Increase* In 11 patients with chronic renal failure mean plasma concentration prior to administration of N-acetylcysteine and hemodialysis of 4.0 ± 2.1 µmol/L compared with reported concentrations of 0.31, 0.08 and 0.26 µmol/L in healthy individuals *1493*

Naproxen *Serum Decrease* Uremia is associated with decreased binding of acidic drugs to plasma proteins. Effect on bound fraction only is listed here *5869*

Neuropeptide Y *Plasma Increase* Concentrations ranged from 5.3 to 5.9 pmol/L significantly different from reference interval of 1.8 - 2.4 pmol/L *3847*

Neutrophils *Blood Increase* Slight neutrophilic leukocytosis may be observed *662* In 67% of 141 patients at initial hospitalization for this disorder *1576* Slight neutrophilic leukocytosis may be observed *5699*
Blood No Effect In 11 children with chronic renal failure median concentration of 2.3 x 10^{-9}/L not significantly different from 4.3 x 10^9/L in 10 healthy children *2347* In 12 children with chronic renal failure median concentration of 2.3 x 10^9/L not significantly different from 4.3 x 10^9/L in 8 healthy pediatric controls *2346*

Norepinephrine *Plasma Increase* In patients with mild renal failure norepinephrine clearance reduced by 20% and in patients on hemodialysis reduced by 40% *5860* Moderate increase *1326*

Ornithine *Plasma Increase* Increased significantly with mild renal failure but did not increase with progression of renal failure *746*
Plasma No Effect In 10 patients with chronic renal failure undergoing regular hemodialysis mean concentration of 68 ± 4 µmol/L not significantly different from 76 ± 3 µmol/L in 31 healthy age and sex matched controls *1656*

Osmolality *Urine Decrease* With renal parenchymal disease *1727*
Urine No Effect 250 - 400 mOsm/kg; becomes fixed close to plasma level of 280 - 295 mOsm/kg *413*

Osmotic Fragility *Red Blood Cells No Effect* Usually no significant effect *3104*

Osteocalcin *Serum Increase* In 20 patients with chronic renal failure mean concentration of 36.2 ± 26 µg/L (range 7 to 100) compared with 12.2 ± 4.5 µg/L in 30 normal women as measured by CIA *2556* Significant increase observed in 35 patients with chronic renal failure (10.2 ± 14.6 nmol/L) occurring when creatinine clearance decreased below 20 mL/min *2454* In 14 patients with secondary hyperparathyroidism mean concentrations by sandwich EIA and RIA of 17.6 ± 27.4 µg/L and 46.5 ± 60.0 µg/L compared with mean concentrations 4.2 ± 1.2 µg/L and 6.6 ± 1.4 µg/L by sandwich EIA and RIA methods respectively in 20 healthy individuals *2246* In 19 patients with predialytic chronic renal failure mean concentration of 23 ± 19 ng/mL significantly greater than 7 ± 3 ng/mL in 38 healthy controls *870* In 30 patients with chronic renal failure without hepatopathy mean concentration of 14 ± 8.7 ng/mL significantly greater than 3.2 ± 0.9 ng/mL in 16 healthy controls *1677* Inverse relationship between calculated creatinine clearance and serum osteocalcin concentration *1574* Markedly elevated *1375* In 96 patients with predialysis chronic renal failure mean concentration of 69 ± 63 µg/L (11.9 nmol/L) significantly different from that in healthy adults (men 25 ± 5 µg/L, women 20 ± 6 µg/L) *541* Using the Diagnostic Systems Laboratories' method mean concentration of 49 ± 33 µg/L in 10 patients with chronic renal failure significantly higher than that in 68 healthy adults (4 ± 3.6 µg/L) *1149* In patients with chronic renal failure with hemodialysis moderate increase observed *4217* In 19 children with end-stage renal disease mean concentration of 32 ± 10 µg/L compared with reference interval of 4 - 20 µg/L *527*

Oxalate *Serum Increase* In 15 patients with chronic renal failure mean concentration of 74.8 ± 18.5 µmol/L and 129.9 ± 47.7 µmol/L in 31 patients on chronic hemodialysis compared with normal range of 16.8 ± 6.0 µmol/L *259* In end stage renal disease accumulation of oxalate is a common finding. In 14 patients receiving CAPD mean concentration of 30.2 ± 11.2 µmol/L as high as in patients receiving peritoneal hemodialysis preceding dialysis (31.9 ± 11.1 µmol/L) *5784*

Oxazepam *Serum Increase* Uremia is associated with changed binding of basic or neutral drugs to plasma proteins. Effect on bound fraction only is listed here *5869*

p-Cresol *Feces Increase* In 20 patients with chronic renal failure undergoing regular hemodialysis concentration ranged from 850 ± 150 nmol/mg feces compared with that in 12 healthy controls in whom mean concentration was 423 ± 80 nmol/mg feces *2149*
Serum Increase Mean concentration in 17 uremic patients pre-dialysis of 50 ± 29 µmol/L significantly greater than 4.5 ± 5.1 µmol/L in 10 healthy controls *3811* In 20 uremic patients undergoing regular hemodialysis mean concentration prior to hemodialysis of 116.0 ± 30.6 nmol/mL significantly greater than that in 12 healthy controls in whom mean concentration was 5.8 ± 2.7 nmol/g feces *2149*

Pancreatic Polypeptide *Plasma Increase* Concentration significantly increased in uremic patients *1953* Markedly increased concentration observed in uremic patients prior to hemodialysis compared with healthy controls *4875*

Pancreatic Secretory Trypsin Inhibitor *Serum Increase* Concentration increased in 6 of 6 patients to 412.8 ± 98.2 ng/mL *3719*

Papaverine *Serum Decrease* Uremia is associated with changed binding of basic or neutral drugs to plasma proteins. Effect on bound fraction only is listed here *5869*

Paraoxonase *Serum Decrease* Mean concentration in 117 patients with uremia of 100 U/mL different from about 190 U/mL in 110 healthy controls *4002*
Serum No Effect Mean activity of 0.19 ± 0.16 U/mL in 47 patients with end-stage renal disease not significantly different from 0.20 ± 0.14 U/mL in 156 healthy controls when paraoxon used as substrate but significantly reduced when 4-nitrophenyl acetate used as substrate *1011*

Parathyroid Hormone *Plasma Decrease* In a study involving 28 patients with hypocalcemia and low intact PTH concentration, 2 had chronic renal failure *3280* In one study 20 of 40 patients with low intact PTH and hypercalcemia not due to malignant disease 20 had excess 1α-hydroxycholecalciferol in chronic renal failure *3280* In a study of 59 patients with low intact PTH concentrations and normocalcemia 10 had chronic renal failure *3280*
Plasma Increase In 12 of 17 patients on long-term continuous ambulatory peritoneal dialysis concentration significantly increased *2894* In 68 patients with chronic renal disease mean concentration of 129 ± 142 pg/mL significantly different from 34 ± 16 pg/mL in 73 healthy normal volunteers *3487* In 10 patients mean concentration of 491 ± 359 ng/L compared with 29.8 ± 13.8 ng/L in 57 healthy adults *1150* In 30 patients with chronic renal failure without hepatopathy mean concentration of 353 ± 343 pg/mL significantly greater than 30 ± 15 pg/mL in 16 healthy controls *1677* Increased nearly in all patients. be extremely high. Rough inverse correlation with renal function *4318* Elevated in chronic uremia *2136* Mean concentration of 236 ± 225 pg/mL in 104 patients with chronic renal failure receiving chronic hemodialysis significantly different from 35 ± 33 pg/mL in 98 healthy controls *803* Reaches 10 times normal late in renal failure *367* In 19 patients with predialytic chronic renal failure mean concentration of C-terminal PTH of 1.57 ± 1.47 ng/mL compared with 0.34 ± 0.19 ng/mL in 38 healthy controls: in patients intact PTH of 140 ± 149 pg/mL compared with 21 ± 7 pg/mL in controls *870*
Plasma No Effect In 19 children with end-stage renal disease mean concentration of 45 ng/L compared with reference interval of 10 - 55 ng/L *527*

Parathyroid Hormone 1-84 *Plasma Increase* Mean concentration in 30 patients with chronic renal failure of 30.3 pmol/L (range 2.0 - 190 pmol/L) significantly different from mean 2.21 pmol/L (range 1.0 - 5.0 pmol/L) in 57 healthy laboratory staff *3105*

Parathyroid Hormone, Intact *Plasma Increase* In 15 patients with severe renal insufficiency mean concentration of 271 ± 43 pg/mL significantly different from 95 ± 29 pg/mL in 14 with moderate insufficiency and 37 ± 5 pg/mL in 13 with mild insufficiency *1410*
Plasma No Effect In 26 patients with chronic renal failure without secondary hyperparathyroidism median concentration of 45.5 μg/L not significantly different from 35.2 μg/L in 90 healthy controls *2572*

PDN-21 *Serum Increase* In 16 patients with chronic renal failure concentrations in most patients marginally exceeded the upper limit of normal of 67 pg/mL in 98 healthy controls *5137*

Penicillin G *Serum Decrease* Uremia is associated with decreased binding of acidic drugs to plasma proteins. Effect on bound fraction only is listed here *5869*

Pentosidine *Serum Increase* In 24 uremic individuals mean concentration of 2,620 ± 1,310 μmol/L significantly higher than 151 ± 55 μmol/L in 19 healthy individuals *5160* Mean concentration in serum from patients with end-stage renal disease requiring hemodialysis of 1,267 ± 695 nmol/L compare with 77 ± 40 nmol/L in 33 healthy individuals *5130*

pH *Blood Decrease* In 31% of 31 patients at initial hospitalization for this disorder *1576* Metabolic acidosis is an invariable concomitant of chronic failure *2304* Mild acidosis is common in renal failure *1583*
Pleural Fluid Increase Transudate (pH > 7.3) *126*

Phenol *Feces Increase* In 20 patients with chronic renal failure undergoing regular hemodialysis concentration ranged from 65 ± 25 nmol/mg feces compared with that in 12 healthy controls in whom mean concentration was 46 ± 6 nmol/mg feces *2149*
Serum Increase Mean concentration in 17 uremic patients pre-dialysis 14 ± 15 μmol/L significantly greater than 2.0 ± 1.8 μmol/L in 10 healthy controls *3811* In 20 uremic patients undergoing regular hemodialysis mean concentration prior to hemodialysis of 29.2 ± 13.7 nmol/mL significantly greater than that in 12 healthy controls in whom mean concentration was 6.9 ± 0.7 nmol/mL *2149*

Phentolamine Test *Patient Increase* Probably related to impaired excretion of drug *1618*

Phenylalanine *Plasma Increase* In 10 patients with chronic renal failure undergoing regular hemodialysis mean concentration of 43 ± 1 μmol/L significantly greater than 38 ± 1 μmol/L in 31 healthy age and sex matched controls *1656*

Phenylbutazone *Serum Decrease* Uremia is associated with decreased binding of acidic drugs to plasma proteins. Effect on bound fraction only is listed here *5869*

Phenytoin *Serum Decrease* Uremia is associated with decreased binding of acidic drugs to plasma proteins. Effect on bound fraction only is listed here *5869*

Phosphate *Serum Increase* In 15 patients with severe renal insufficiency mean concentration of 5.3 ± 0.4 mg/dL significantly different from 3.7 ± 0.2 mg/dL in 14 with moderate insufficiency and 3.5 ± 0.1 mg/dL in 13 with mild insufficiency *1410* Increases when creatinine clearance falls to approximately 25 mL/min *5545* Hyperphosphatemia may occur in association with secondary hyperparathyroidism *5204* In 19 patients with predialytic chronic renal failure mean concentration of 4.08 ± 0.85 mg/dL not significantly increased compared with 3.75 ± 0.37 mg/dL in 38 healthy controls *870* Plasma levels rise late in renal failure and are unrelated to the serum calcium levels *367* Serum phosphate concentration may be increased in patients with chronic renal failure *5204* Reduction in GFR leads to increased serum concentration *969* In 75% of 141 patients at initial hospitalization for this disorder *1576*
Sweat Increase Concentrations of Ca, Mg and phosphate in sweat were significantly elevated due to an increase in the secretion of these electrolytes in the secretory portion of the sweat gland, while that in the reabsorptive duct is normal *4225*

Phospholipase A_2 *Serum Increase* Activity generally eight fold higher in uremic plasma than in normal plasma *942*

Phospholipase A_2 Type I *Serum Increase* In 10 patients with chronic renal failure mean concentration of 38.1 μg/L (range 11.1 μg/L to 69.2 μg/L) significantly higher than 4.0 μg/L (range 1.7 μg/L to 5.6 μg/L) in 20 reference individuals *4108*

Phospholipase A_2 Type II *Serum Increase* In 11 uremic patients median concentration of 1025 μg/L (range 52 - 3,320) significantly greater than 9.2 μg/L (range 4.6 - 17.5) in 13 controls and activities median 6.5 μmol/min/L and 0.49 μmol/min/L respectively *1224*
Serum No Effect In 10 patients with chronic renal failure mean concentration of 7.6 μg/L (range 3.3 μg/L to 20.4 μg/L) not significantly different from 5.0 μg/L (range 2.1 μg/L to 25.3 μg/L) in 20 reference individuals *4108*

Phospholipids *Platelets Decrease* In 14 patients with uremia mean concentration of 338.0 ± 79 nmol/10^9 cells significantly different from 511.6 ± 125 nmol/10^9 cells in 14 healthy volunteer controls *5440*

Pindolol *Serum No Effect* Uremia is associated with changed binding of basic or neutral drugs to plasma proteins. Effect on bound fraction only is listed here *5869*

Plasminogen Activator Inhibitor-1 *Plasma Increase* In 71 patients with end stage renal disease mean activity of 6.2 ± 2.6 ng/mL with reverse correlation with euglobulin fibrinolytic activity *2221*

Platelet Aggregation response to ADP *Blood Decrease* In 14 patients with uremia main increase in the percentage of light transmittance recorded for 5 min of 55.0 ± 17% significantly different from 73.3 ± 11.6% in 14 healthy volunteer controls *5440*

Platelet Aggregation response to Arachidonic Acid *Blood Decrease* In 14 patients with uremia main increase in the percentage of light transmittance recorded for 5 min of 66.1 ± 13% significantly different from 82.1 ± 6.3% in 14 healthy volunteer controls *5440*

Platelet Aggregation response to Collagen *Blood Decrease* In 14 patients with uremia main increase in the percentage of light transmittance recorded for 5 min of 28.0 ± 29% significantly different from 73.1 ± 10.8% in 14 healthy volunteer controls *5440*

Platelet Aggregation response to Epinephrine *Blood Decrease* In 14 patients with uremia main increase in the percentage of light transmittance recorded for 5 min of 58.6 ± 23% significantly different from 77.7 ± 5.4% in 14 healthy volunteer controls *5440*

Platelets *Blood Decrease* In 14 hemodialysis patients platelet count significantly lower than in 14 age and sex matched controls *2722*
Blood Increase Normal or slightly increased. However, platelet function may be severely impaired *5699* *662*

Potassium *Feces Increase* May represent an important adaptive response *2075*

585.00 Chronic Renal Failure *(continued)*

Potassium *(continued)*
Red Blood Cells *Increase* In 36 patients, a normal or high erythrocyte potassium was found *2443*
Serum *Decrease* May occur *572*
Serum *Increase* Liberated during body cell breakdown, and is not excreted completely in the urine *1290*

Prazosin *Serum* *No Effect* Uremia is associated with changed binding of basic or neutral drugs to plasma proteins. Effect on bound fraction only is listed here *5869*

Prealbumin *Serum* *Increase* In 68 patients with chronic renal disease mean concentration of 36 ± 9 mg/dL significantly different from 29.5 ± 6 mg/dL in 73 healthy normal volunteers *3487* In patients requiring dialysis concentration higher in those receiving hemodialysis (7.96 ± 1.68 μmol/L) than in those receiving CAPD 7.33 ± 2.40 μmol/L) and in controls (5.81 ± 0.50 μmol/L) *4832*

Prednisolone *Serum* *Decrease* Uremia is associated with changed binding of basic or neutral drugs to plasma proteins. Effect on bound fraction only is listed here *5869*

Prolactin *Plasma* *Increase* Basal concentrations are increased in uremia but suppression with levodopa is impaired *876* Concentration significantly higher in 14 patients with end stage renal disease than in 28 healthy age-matched controls *695* Increased levels *3394* Significantly decreased in patients with impaired renal function, both in patients on drug therapy and in those not taking any drugs affecting plasma prolactin. No relation was found with age, sex, underlying diagnosis, or duration of uremia *950* Significant increase to 270 mU/L observed in 62 patients with moderate chronic renal failure and to 562 mU/L in 13 patients with severe chronic renal failure compared with 168 mU/L in 100 healthy hospital personnel *951*

Prolactin response to TRH *Plasma* *Decrease* In 7 patients with end stage renal disease prior to treatment with erythropoietin response to TRH blunted *5596*

Proline *Plasma* *Increase* In 10 patients with chronic renal failure undergoing regular hemodialysis mean concentration of 346 ± 49 μmol/L significantly greater than 134 ± 5 μmol/L in 31 healthy age and sex matched controls *1656*

Propafenone *Serum* *Increase* Uremia is associated with changed binding of basic or neutral drugs to plasma proteins. Effect on bound fraction only is listed here *5869*

Propoxyphene *Serum* *No Effect* Uremia is associated with changed binding of basic or neutral drugs to plasma proteins. Effect on bound fraction only is listed here *5869*

Propranolol *Serum* *Increase* Uremia is associated with changed binding of basic or neutral drugs to plasma proteins. Effect on bound fraction only is listed here *5869*
Serum *No Effect* Uremia is associated with changed binding of basic or neutral drugs to plasma proteins. Effect on bound fraction only is listed here *5869*

Prostate-specific Antigen *Serum* *No Effect* No significant difference observed in 39 patients aged 40 - 49 years with end-stage renal disease (mean 1.256 ± 0.1 ng/dL) compared with 1.138 ± 0.09 ng/dL in 40 healthy screened men aged 40 - 49 years, 1.026 ± 0.11 ng/dL in 22 patients aged 50 - 59 years with end-stage renal disease compared with 1.146 ± 0.11 ng/dL in 56 screenees aged 50 - 59 years and 3.602 ± 0.20 ng/dL in 21 patients aged over 60 years compared with 3.530 ± 0.22 ng/dL in 73 screenees aged over 60 years *3622*

Protein *Pleural Fluid* *Decrease* Transudate secondary to decreased albumin. (< 3 g/dL) *126*
Serum *Decrease* Total protein is decreased with chronic renal insufficiency *5545* In 20 patients with uremia mean concentration of 67.5 ± 7.1 g/L significantly less than 72.3 ± 4.7 g/L in 67 healthy controls *3392*
Urine *Increase* Mean excretion in 22 patients with glomerular disease 2.9 ± 0.8 g/d significantly greater than that in 22 patients with tubulointestitial disease in whom the excretion was 0.3 ± 0.1 g/d *3398* With renal parenchymal disease *1727*

Protein 1 *Serum* *Increase* Mean concentration significantly increased in 25 patients with renal failure with good correlation (r = 0.77) with serum creatinine concentration *2375*

Protein C *Plasma* *Decrease* In patients with renal insufficiency and terminal uremia protein C activity was significantly decreased: probable correlation between decreasing protein C concentration and progressive renal failure *4940*

Protoporphyrin *Red Blood Cells* *Increase* May be moderately increased *5699* *3104*

Pseudouridine *Serum* *Increase* Concentration increased in patients both on and not on hemodialysis and correlated best with inverse of creatinine clearance *1278*

Pyridinoline *Serum* *Increase* In 29 patients with chronic renal failure mean concentration of 268.5 ± 334.4 nmol/L significantly greater than 5.9 ± 1.5 μmol/mol in 19 healthy controls *2313*
Urine *Increase* In 29 patients with chronic renal failure mean excretion of 244.6 ± 436.5 μmol/mol creatinine significantly greater than 28.9 ± 6.3 μmol/mol creatinine in 19 healthy controls *2313*

Pyridinoline Cross-linked Telopeptide of Type I Collagen
Serum *Increase* Concentration of 23.4 ± 10.9 μg/L significantly higher in 15 patients with renal disease than 3.2 ± 0.48 μg/L in 8 healthy controls *2839* In patients with impaired renal function concentration increase becomes significant when GFR falls below 50 mL/min per 1.73 sq m *4366*

Quinidine *Serum* *Increase* Uremia is associated with changed binding of basic or neutral drugs to plasma proteins. Effect on bound fraction only is listed here *5869*
Serum *No Effect* Uremia is associated with changed binding of basic or neutral drugs to plasma proteins. Effect on bound fraction only is listed here *5869*

Renin Activity *Plasma* *Increase* Activity significantly higher in 10 uremic patients at both pH 7.4 and 5.7 than in 10 normal individuals *2792* In 17 patients on long-term continuous ambulatory peritoneal dialysis concentration significantly higher than in healthy individuals *2894*

Reticulocytes *Blood* *Decrease* In patients with chronic renal failure mean concentration of 32.7 ± 15.4 x 10^9/L in 12 with creatinine clearance of 51 - 90 mL/min, 31.5 ± 17.3 x 10^9/L in 12 with clearance 21 - 50 mL/min and in 12 with clearance < 20 mL/min concentration of 28.6 ± 18.1 x 10^9/L significantly different when compared with 46.8 ± 19.5 x 10^9/L in 13 healthy controls with clearance > 90 mL/min *3502* Anemia is characteristically normocytic and normochromic, and is associated with a normal or slightly decreased number of reticulocytes *5677*
Blood *Increase* Highest values (6%) observed when the BUN was 300 - 350 mg/dL *4764* May be moderately increased *3104* *5699* 1- 4 times normal after correction for reduced RBC *367*

Retinol *Serum* *Increase* In 22 patients with chronic renal failure mean concentration predialysis 2.51 ± 0.30 μmol/L significantly higher than 1.89 ± 0.14 μmol/L in healthy controls *2385*

Retinol-binding Protein *Serum* *Increase* In uremic patients requiring dialysis concentration higher in those receiving hemodialysis (8.84 ± 1.59 μmol/L) than in those receiving CAPD (6.28 ± 2.82 μmol/L) and in controls (2.34 ± 0.32 μmol/L) *4832*

Ristocetin Cofactor *Plasma* *Increase* In 12 patients with chronic renal failure mean von Willebrand factor activity increased to 1.88 μg/mL from 1.07 μg/mL in normals *1840*

Salicylate *Serum* *Decrease* Uremia is associated with decreased binding of acidic drugs to plasma proteins. Effect on bound fraction only is listed here *5869*

Selenium *Serum* *Decrease* Mean concentration in 11 nondialyzed uremic patients of 11.9 ± 1.9 μg/dL compared with 11.3 ± 1.0 μg/dL in 27 dialyzed uremic patients, both significantly less than the mean of 13.6 ± 0.8 μg/dL in 40 healthy individuals *2537*

Serine *Plasma* *Decrease* Significant decrease observed in patients with mild renal failure *746* In 10 patients with chronic renal failure undergoing regular hemodialysis mean concentration of 66 ± 2 μmol/L significantly less than 113 ± 3 μmol/L in 31 healthy age and sex matched controls *1656*

Sialic Acid *Serum* *Increase* Concentration significantly increased in plasma of patients with chronic glomerulonephritis and those with chronic renal failure maintained on hemodialysis *3958*

Sialic Acid, Lipid-associated *Serum* *Increase* In patients with chronic glomerulonephritis and those with chronic renal failure maintained on chronic hemodialysis mean concentration significantly increased *3958*

Sodium *Red Blood Cells* *Decrease* Erythrocyte sodium values showed a wide range, from very high to very low, and the rate constant for Na^+ efflux was found to be higher than normal *2443*
Red Blood Cells *Increase* Erythrocyte sodium values showed a wide range, from very high to very low, and the rate constant

for Na efflux was found to be higher than normal *2443* In 25% of uremic patients *5628*
Serum Decrease Decreased because of tubular damage with loss in urine, vomiting, diarrhea, diet restriction, etc *5545*
Serum Increase Much less common *572*
Serum No Effect Usually normal *572*
Urine Decrease Excretion slightly lower in patients with CRF compared with controls *3469*

Soluble E-Selectin *Serum No Effect* In 12 children with chronic renal failure median concentration of 55 ng/mL not significantly different from 55 ng/mL in 8 healthy pediatric controls *2346*

Soluble HLA-I *Sweat Increase* Known to be present in small amounts in sweat of people with chronic renal disease *216*

Soluble Interleukin-2 Receptor *Serum Increase* Soluble interleukin-2 receptor concentration increases in patients with chronic renal failure *4094* In 76 patients with chronic renal failure mean concentration increased to 9.9 ng/L prior to hemodialysis *3977* Concentration increases in patients with chronic renal failure *4095*

Soluble Tumor Necrosis Factor Receptor *Serum Increase* Mean concentration in 26 patients with chronic renal failure without dialysis of 16.7 ± 7.2 ng/mL significantly higher than 3.5 ± 0.7 ng/mL in 34 healthy blood donors *1982*

Soluble Tumor Necrosis Factor Receptor-p55
Serum Increase Mean concentration of 22 ± 1 ng/mL in 14 patients with chronic renal failure undergoing regular hemodialysis significantly greater than 1.2 ± 0.3 ng/mL in healthy controls *2020* In 4 patients with end-stage renal disease prior to any dialysis mean concentration of 27.0 ± 7.7 ng/mL significantly different from 2.68 ± 0.94 ng/mL in 5 normal controls *588* In 8 children with chronic renal failure mean concentration ranged from 17 ± 6 ng/mL compared with 1.4 ± 1 ng/mL in 8 controls *5391*

Soluble Tumor Necrosis Factor Receptor-p75
Serum Increase In 8 children with chronic renal failure mean concentrations ranged from 27 ± 7 ng/mL compared with 4.2 ± 1 ng/mL in 8 controls *5391* Mean concentration of 25 ± 2 ng/mL in 14 patients with chronic renal failure significantly greater than 2.0 ± 0.3 ng/mL in healthy controls *2020* In 4 patients with end-stage renal disease prior to any dialysis mean concentration of 19.57 ± 7.5 ng/mL significantly different from 2.36 ± 0.8 ng/mL in 5 normal controls *588*

Soluble Vascular Cell Adhesion Molecule-1
Serum No Effect In 12 children with chronic renal failure median concentration of 1,250 ng/mL not significantly different from 1,200 ng/mL in 8 healthy pediatric controls *2346*

Somatostatin *Plasma Increase* In 24 non-diabetic uremic patients mean concentration of somatostatin-like immunoreactivity of 43.5 ± 7.2 pg/mL compared with 5.0 ± 0.7 pg/mL in 60 healthy individuals *5582* Concentration significantly increased in both pre- and post-dialysis specimens in uremic patients in comparison with age and sex matched healthy controls *1866*
Plasma No Effect No significant effect observed in patients with uremia *1953*

SP2 *Serum No Effect* 4 of 14 patients with chronic renal failure had a concentration of 14 U/mL and 4 had a concentration of 15 U/mL when the upper limit of normal was 14 U/mL *5260*

Specific Gravity *Pleural Fluid Decrease* Transudate (< 1.016) *126*
Urine Decrease With decreased renal function, specific gravity is 1.020, as renal impairment is more severe, specific gravity approaches 1.010. The test is sensitive for early loss of renal function, but a normal finding does not necessarily rule out active kidney disease *5544*

Squamous Cell Carcinoma Antigen *Serum Increase* In 61 patients with uremia mean concentration of 4.0 ± 4.2 µg/L compared with upper limit of normal of 2.5 µg/L *3561*

α-Subunit of Glycoprotein Hormones *Plasma Increase* In 25 patients with chronic uremia mean concentration of 5.5 ± 3.0 µg/L significantly greater than 0.4 ± 0.2 µg/L in 57 normal controls *3438*

Sulfadiazine *Serum Decrease* Uremia is associated with decreased binding of acidic drugs to plasma proteins. Effect on bound fraction only is listed here *5869*

Sulfamethoxazole *Serum Decrease* Uremia is associated with decreased binding of acidic drugs to plasma proteins. Effect on bound fraction only is listed here *5869*

Sulfate *Serum Increase* In metabolic acidosis accompanying renal failure. Serves as a reliable index of insufficiency *4707*

Sulfonamides *Serum Decrease* Uremia is associated with decreased binding of acidic drugs to plasma proteins. Effect on bound fraction only is listed here *5869*

Superoxide Dismutase *Serum Increase* In 11 patients with chronic renal failure mean activity of 7.37 ± 4.20 U/mL not significantly different from 5.50 ± 1.47 U/mL in 14 controls *3323*

Taurine *Plasma Increase* Significant increase observed in mild renal failure but did not increase in parallel with progression of renal failure *746*

Tertatolol *Serum No Effect* Uremia is associated with changed binding of basic or neutral drugs to plasma proteins. Effect on bound fraction only is listed here *5869*

Theophylline *Serum Decrease* Uremia is associated with changed binding of basic or neutral drugs to plasma proteins. Effect on bound fraction only is listed here *5869* Uremia is associated with decreased binding of acidic drugs to plasma proteins. Effect on bound fraction only is listed here *5869*
Serum Increase Concentration may be increased by 3 to 5 µg/mL in therapeutic range due to 3-methylxanthine as measured by method on Kodak Ektachem® systems *2078*

Thiobarbituric Acid-reacting Substances *Serum Increase* Mean concentration of thiobarbituric acid-reactive substances of 2.25 ± 0.33 µmol/L in 20 patients with renal insufficiency and chronic dialysis compared with 1.01 ± 0.21 µmol/L in 47 healthy individuals *5585*

Thiol Groups, Total *Serum Increase* In 22 patients with chronic renal failure mean concentration predialysis of 328 ± 16 µmol/L not significantly higher than 297 ± 13 µmol/L in healthy controls *2385*

Thiopental *Serum Decrease* Uremia is associated with decreased binding of acidic drugs to plasma proteins. Effect on bound fraction only is listed here *5869*

Threonine *Plasma Decrease* Mean concentration decreased with deteriorating renal function in children *424* In 10 patients with chronic renal failure undergoing regular hemodialysis mean concentration of 86 ± 6 µmol/L significantly less than 107 ± 4 µmol/L in 31 healthy age and sex matched controls *1656*

β-Thromboglobulin *Plasma Increase* Mean concentration in 14 hemodialysis patients significantly higher than in 14 age and sex matched controls *2722*

Thyroid Stimulating Hormone *Serum No Effect* Serum thyroglobulin was elevated in 92% of 38 patients in the early stage of this disorder. After two months of corticosteroid treatment the levels were significantly decreased in 25 patients who could be rechecked *3582* Concentration normal in uremia *876* In 25 patients with chronic uremia mean concentration of 1.5 ± 0.8 mU/L not significantly different from 1.4 ± 0.6 mU/L in 57 age and sex matched controls *3438*

Thyroxine Binding Globulin *Serum Decrease* Mean concentration significantly reduced in patients with chronic renal failure *3050*

Thyroxine Binding Prealbumin *Serum Increase* Mean concentration significantly increased in patients with chronic renal failure *3050*

Thyroxine (T4) *Serum Decrease* Normal or decreased *3582* Uremia is associated with decreased binding of acidic drugs to plasma proteins. Effect on bound fraction only is listed here *5869* In 56% of 26 patients at initial hospitalization for this disorder *1576* Significant decrease in total and free T4; total T4 mean concentration of 5.3 ± 1.9 µg/dL. Levels were even further depleted in terminal failure *2751* Mean concentration reduced in patients with chronic renal failure *3050*

Thyroxine (T4), Free *Serum Decrease* Mean concentration in patients with chronic renal failure decreased when determined by direct equilibrium dialysis *3050* In 25 individuals with uremia mean concentration of 9.21 ± 1.2 pmol/L significantly less than 11.3 ± 1.8 pmol/L in 57 normal controls *3438*

Tienilic Acid *Serum Decrease* Uremia is associated with decreased binding of acidic drugs to plasma proteins. Effect on bound fraction only is listed here *5869*

Tissue Plasminogen Activator *Plasma No Effect* In 71 patients with end stage renal disease mean activity of 1.7 ± 0.9 ng/mL *2221*

585.00 Chronic Renal Failure *(continued)*

α-Tocopherol *Serum* *Decrease* In 22 patients with chronic renal failure mean concentration predialysis 23.2 ± 3.0 µmol/L not significantly lower than 28.2 ± 2.7 µmol/L in healthy controls *2385*

Tolfenamic Acid *Serum* *Decrease* Uremia is associated with decreased binding of acidic drugs to plasma proteins. Effect on bound fraction only is listed here *5869*

Tolmetin *Serum* *Decrease* Uremia is associated with decreased binding of acidic drugs to plasma proteins. Effect on bound fraction only is listed here *5869*

Tri-iodothyronine, Free (fT3) *Serum* *Decrease* In 25 patients with chronic uremia mean concentration of 4.5 ± 1.2 pmol/L significantly less than 6.8 ± 1.3 pmol/L in 57 normal controls *3438* Mean concentration as determined by equilibrium dialysis reduced in patients with chronic renal failure *3050*

Tri-iodothyronine, Reverse (rT3) *Serum* *No Effect* Reverse T3 is normal but free reverse T3 is usually elevated *3582* Mean concentration unchanged in patients with chronic renal failure *3050*

Tri-iodothyronine (T3) *Serum* *Decrease* Decreased *3582* Although mean serum total T3 concentration was normal, 43% had low serum T3 and 54% had low serum free T3 concentrations *4954* Mean concentration reduced in patients with chronic renal failure *3050* Reduced total and free T3, mean total T3 concentration of 65.4 ± 17.4 ng/dL *2751*
Urine *Decrease* Reduced excretion, 27 ± 44 ng/24h *2751*

Triamterene *Serum* *Decrease* Uremia is associated with changed binding of basic or neutral drugs to plasma proteins. Effect on bound fraction only is listed here *5869*

Triglycerides *Serum* *Increase* Characteristically increased. Type IV hyperlipoproteinemia occurs commonly secondary to renal failure *2136* In 68 patients with chronic renal disease mean concentration of 178 ± 82 mg/dL significantly different from 116 ± 60 mg/dL in 73 healthy normal volunteers *3487* Mean concentration in 12 patients with chronic renal failure and uremia of 1.64 ± 0.60 mmol/L compared with 0.99 ± 0.30 mmol/L in 9 healthy controls *2230* Present in most patients whether or not they are dialyzed *2304* Characteristically increased with impaired renal function *367* Increased mean plasma concentration in chronic failure *2607* Significant increase observed in patients with chronic renal failure *1590* Hypertriglyceridemia was found in 43% of patients. 20 men had values > 200 mg/dL and 23 women had 150 mg/dL or greater *5709* In 104 patients with end-stage renal disease receiving hemodialysis mean concentration of 190.5 ± 12.9 mg/dL significantly different from 119.4 ± 5.4 mg/dL in healthy controls *1488* Mean concentration increased to 200 mg/dL in uremic patients compared with 111 mg/dL in controls *726* Endogenous VLDL triglyceride production rate was significantly raised in 13 patients who were not on dialysis treatment *957* Characteristic finding *3526* Mean concentration in 117 patients with uremia of 2.34 ± 1.48 mmol/L different from 1.06 ± 0.52 mmol/L in 110 healthy controls *4002* In patients with chronic renal failure without nephrotic syndrome 40% had triglyceride concentrations greater than 200 mg/dL *2575*
Serum *No Effect* In 39 patients with chronic renal failure and normal nutrition mean concentration of 2.5 ± 0.2 mmol/L not significantly different from 2.3 ± 0.2 mmol/L in 44 patients with chronic renal failure but with malnutrition *5005* In 13 patients with chronic renal failure, but dialysis independent, mean concentration of 1.69 ± 0.63 mmol/L not significantly different from 1.77 ± 0.77 mmol/L in 27 healthy controls *935*

Trimethoprim *Serum* *No Effect* Uremia is associated with changed binding of basic or neutral drugs to plasma proteins. Effect on bound fraction only is listed here *5869*

Troponin I *Serum* *Increase* In 37 patients with chronic renal failure 36 had troponin-I concentrations of less than 1 µg/L and 1 had a concentration greater than 1 µg/L *890* One of 12 patients with chronic renal failure receiving medical treatment had concentration above upper limit of normal *3686*

Troponin T *Serum* *Increase* In 8 of 18 patients receiving hemodialysis concentrations ranged from 0.03 - 1.73 µg/L greater than diagnostic cutoff of 0.2 µg/L *5272* Mean concentration increased above 0.2 µg/L in 40% patients with chronic renal failure *334* In 67 uremic patients with chronic renal failure mean concentration of 0.24 µg/L (range of 0.01 - 3.7 µg/L) with 31 (46.3%) in the pathological range having a concentration greater than 0.1 µg/L *1954* Concentrations of cardiac troponin-T increased above 0.2 µg/L in 15 of 51 patients (29%) undergoing chronic hemodialysis *2585* Seven of 12 patients with chronic renal failure receiving medical treatment had concentration above upper limit of normal *3686* In 37 patients with chronic renal failure 32 had troponin-T concentrations of less than 0.2 µg/L and 5 with concentrations greater than 0.2 µg/L by ELISA method and 36 had concencentrations less than 0.2 µg/L and 1 greater than 0.2 µg/L as measured by Enzymun procedure *890* In 10 patients with CRF not receiving dialysis mean concentration of 0.17 ± 0.29 µg/L and median concentration of 0.03 µg/L. Concentration increased in 3 patients (30%) *1556* In 110 patients with renal impairment serum cardiac troponin-T concentration detectable with concentrations ranging from 0 - 17.2 µg/L *891* Increased steady-state plasma concentration of ≥0.2 µg/L 39% of a population of hemodialysis patients with first generation cTnT ELISA and 29% with second generation with a cutoff of ≥0.15 µg/L *1973* Increased concentrations observed in 6 of 30 patients with chronic renal failure *333* In 82 patient specimens with creatinine concentrations greater than 2 mg/dL, 52 (63.4%) had increased concentrations of cardiac troponin T, most of which were less than 1.0 ng/mL (upper limit of normal 0.1 ng/mL) *3028*

Trypsin *Serum* *No Effect* Mean concentration of trypsin-like immunoreactivity in 30 patients with severe chronic renal failure receiving hemodialysis did not exceed concentration in 85 healthy control individuals (42.78 ± 10.26 ng/mL) *3330*

Trypsinogen *Serum* *Increase* Mean concentration of 215 ± 193 ng/mL in 25 patients with chronic renal failure significantly greater than 24 ± 4 ng/mL in 10 healthy individuals *2687*

Tryptophan *Plasma* *Decrease* In 7 elderly patients with renal failure significant decrease observed *701* Uremia is associated with decreased binding of acidic drugs to plasma proteins. Effect on bound fraction only is listed here *5869*

TSH response to TRH *Serum* *Decrease* Response blunted in 7 individuals with chronic renal failure prior to treatment with erythropoietin *5596* Slight diminution observed in both nondialyzed and dialyzed patients *876*

Tumor Necrosis Factor *Urine* *No Effect* Mean concentration of 24.3 ± 10.2 pg/mL in 4 patients with chronic renal failure not significantly different from that in healthy controls *3962*

Tumor Necrosis Factor-α *Serum* *Increase* Mean concentration in 9 patients with chronic renal failure of 45 ± 25 U/mL compared with 9 ± 3 U/mL in 33 control individuals *3010* Prior to hemodialysis mean concentration in 76 patients increased to 21.3 ng/L *3977* In 1 of 11 children with chronic renal failure median TNF-α detected in serum *2347*
Serum *No Effect* Mean concentration of 0.9 ± 0.2 ng/mL in 14 patients with chronic renal failure undergoing regular hemodialysis not significantly different from 0.7 ± 0.2 ng/mL in healthy controls *2020*
Urine *Increase* In none of 11 children with chronic renal failure was TNF-α detected in serum *2347*

Tumor Necrosis Factor-binding Protein-1 *Serum* *Increase* Increase observed in patients with renal insufficiency as a result of decrease in the glomerular filtration rate *2917*

Tyrosine *Plasma* *Decrease* In 7 elderly patients with renal failure significant decrease observed *701* Children with mild renal insufficiency showed a significant decrease in tyrosine and arginine and an increase in cystine. Tyrosine showed a linear correlation between decreasing plasma concentration and GFR (r = 0.4) *424*
Plasma *No Effect* In 10 patients with chronic renal failure undergoing regular hemodialysis mean concentration of 39 ± 2 µmol/L not significantly different from 43 ± 1 µmol/L in 31 healthy age and sex matched controls *1656*

Ubiquitin *Serum* *Increase* In 19 patients with chronic renal failure who had not undergone dialysis mean concentration of 38.0 ± 22.2 ng/mL significantly higher than 11.2 ± 4.4 ng/mL in 10 control individuals *3888*

Urea *Serum* *Increase* Mean concentration in 17 uremic patients pre-dialysis of 28.9 ± 3.5 mmol/L significantly greater than upper limit of < 7.1 mmol/L in 10 healthy controls *3811*

Urea Nitrogen *Saliva* *Increase* A near perfect correlation (r = 0.97) was found for saliva: plasma urea nitrogen ratios in 56 pairs of samples from patients with renal failure. The mean serum urea nitrogen level for renal failure patients before dialysis was 81.2 ± 30.9 mg/dL. In unstimulated saliva, the urea nitrogen saliva: plasma ratio remained constant at 1.3 *4756*

Serum Increase In 23 patients with chronic renal failure mean concentration of 45.5 ± 11.0 mmol/L significantly greater than 6.3 ± 1.03 mmol/L in 20 healthy controls *3383* Mean concentration in 26 diabetics with chronic renal failure (creatinine > 2.0 mg/dL) of 55 ± 4 mg/dL significantly different from 15 ± 1 mg/dL in 20 healthy controls *1592* In 98% of 148 patients at initial hospitalization for this disorder *1576* Damage to the nephrons leads to faulty urine formation and excretion. The blood urea begins to rise when the equivalent of one kidney is lost, or when the GFR falls below 10 mL/min *1290*

Uric Acid *Serum Increase* In 91% of 140 patients at initial hospitalization for this disorder *1576* Increase is usually < 10 mg/dL *5545* Rise begins very early, but is so slight that the level becomes consistently abnormal only when the GFR falls to about 15 mL/min. In late renal failure there is a further increase in fractional urate clearance so that plasma urate rises less steeply than plasma urea or creatinine *367* In 22 patients with chronic renal failure mean concentration predialysis of 398 ± 15 µmol/L significantly higher than 300 ± 21 µmol/L in healthy controls *2385*

Uric Acid Clearance *Urine Increase* Increases slightly early in renal failure and again in the late stages, causing plasma urate to rise less steeply than urea or creatinine *367*

Uronic Acid *Serum Increase* Mean concentration of cetylpyridinium chloride precipitable uronic acid in 34 patients with renal failure of 13.7 mg/L (range 7.1 - 23.6 mg/L) significantly higher than mean of 9.6 mg/L in healthy controls *548*
Urine Increase Mean excretion of cetylpyridinium chloride precipitable uronic acid in 34 patients with chronic renal failure of 4.74 mg/d (range 2.46 to 8.40 mg/d) increased compared with mean 2.55 mg/d (range 1.73 to 3.27 mg/d) *548*

Uroporphyrin *Serum Increase* In 7 patients with end stage renal disease on continuous ambulatory peritoneal dialysis mean concentration of 25.4 ± 26.0 nmol/L and in 7 receiving hemodialysis of 36.7 ± 11.7 nmol/L compared with 2.0 ± 0.7 nmol/L in 7 healthy controls *3262*

Valine *Plasma Decrease* In 7 elderly patients with renal failure significantly decreased concentration observed *701* In 10 patients with chronic renal failure undergoing regular hemodialysis mean concentration of 137 ± 9 µmol/L significantly less than 177 ± 6 µmol/L in 31 healthy age and sex matched controls *1656* Significant but moderate decrease observed in patients with marked renal failure *746*

Valproic Acid *Serum Decrease* Uremia is associated with decreased binding of acidic drugs to plasma proteins. Effect on bound fraction only is listed here *5869*

Vancomycin *Serum No Effect* In specimens with creatinine concentrations up to 17 mg/dL interference of less than 10% observed with fluorescence polarization immunoassay used with Roche Cobas Fara II analyzer *2441*

Vanillylmandelic Acid *Urine Decrease* Probably due to toxicity and impaired excretion *3572*
Urine No Effect Normal urinary excretion *1326*

Verapamil *Serum No Effect* Uremia is associated with changed binding of basic or neutral drugs to plasma proteins. Effect on bound fraction only is listed here *5869*

Vitamin A *Serum Increase* Concentration increased in patients receiving dialysis with concentration higher in patients receiving hemodialysis (5.18 ± 1.75 µg/L) than in those receiving CAPD (4.77 ± 2.11 µmol/L) and in control group (2.27 ± 0.49 µmol/L) *4832*

Vitamin D Binding Protein *Serum Increase* Mean concentration in 9 children with chronic renal failure not receiving CAPD of 569.9 ± 35.7 µg/mL significantly higher than 437.4 ± 21.5 µg/mL in 18 healthy control children *805*
Serum No Effect In patients with moderate renal failure and in those on chronic hemodialysis concentration not significantly different from that in normal individuals *2738*

VLDL-Apolipoprotein B *Serum Increase* Mean concentration in 12 patients with chronic renal failure and uremia of 9 ± 6 mmol/L compared with 6 ± 2 mmol/L in 4 healthy controls *2230*

VLDL-Cholesterol *Serum Increase* Mean concentration increased to 52 mg/dL in uremics compared with 32 mg/dL in controls *726* Mean concentration in 12 patients with chronic renal failure and uremia of 0.73 ± 0.49 mmol/L compared with 0.41 ± 0.24 mmol/L in 9 healthy controls *2230* Significant increase observed in patients with chronic renal failure *1590* Marked elevation with uremia *126*
Serum No Effect In 13 patients with chronic renal failure, but dialysis independent, mean concentration of 0.68 ± 0.39 mmol/L not significantly different from 0.61 ± 0.51 mmol/L in 27 healthy controls *935*

VLDL-Cholesterol Esters *Serum No Effect* In 13 patients with chronic renal failure, but dialysis independent, mean concentration of 0.42 ± 0.25 mmol/L not significantly different from 0.38 ± 0.32 mmol/L in 27 healthy controls *935*

VLDL-Cholesterol, Free *Serum No Effect* In 13 patients with chronic renal failure, but dialysis independent, mean concentration of 0.26 ± 0.16 mmol/L not significantly different from 0.23 ± 0.18 mmol/L in 27 healthy controls *935*

VLDL-Triglycerides *Serum Increase* Mean concentration increased to 133 mg/dL compared with 69 mg/dL in controls *726* Mean concentration in 12 patients with chronic renal failure and uremia of 0.77 ± 0.42 mmol/L compared with 0.45 ± 0.19 mmol/L in 9 healthy controls *2230*
Serum No Effect In 13 patients with chronic renal failure, but dialysis independent, mean concentration of 1.01 ± 0.51 mmol/L not significantly different from 0.91 ± 0.59 mmol/L in 27 healthy controls *935*

Volume *Plasma Decrease* Hydremia and dehydration are common. Changes will exaggerate or minimize the degree of anemia *5699*
Plasma Increase Hydremia and dehydration are common. Changes will exaggerate or minimize the degree of anemia *5699*
Urine Decrease With renal parenchymal disease *1727* Terminal chronic nephritis *1290*

von Willebrand Factor *Plasma Increase* In 12 children with chronic renal failure median concentration of 1.03 U/mL significantly different from 0.55 U/mL in 8 healthy pediatric controls *2346*

von Willebrand Factor Antigen *Plasma Increase* Mean concentration increased to 2.77 µg/mL from normal of 1.01 µg/mL in 11 patients with chronic renal failure *1840*

Warfarin *Plasma Decrease* Uremia is associated with decreased binding of acidic drugs to plasma proteins. Effect on bound fraction only is listed here *5869*

Zidovudine *Serum Increase* In 4 patients with end stage renal disease the four hour trough concentration was 0.43 ± 0.12 µg/mL compared with 0.16 µg/mL in controls *3997*

Zidovudine Glucuronide *Serum Increase* In 4 patients with end stage renal disease mean 4-hour trough concentration of 23 to 440 times the concentration in normal individuals and decreases by half with each hemodialysis *3997*

Zinc *Serum Decrease* Hypozincemia is regularly observed in patients with chronic renal failure *5174*

Zolpidem *Serum Increase* Uremia is associated with changed binding of basic or neutral drugs to plasma proteins. Effect on bound fraction only is listed here *5869*

Zomepirac *Serum Decrease* Uremia is associated with decreased binding of acidic drugs to plasma proteins. Effect on bound fraction only is listed here *5869*

586.00 Multiple Organ Failure

Endotoxin *Serum Increase* In 15 patients with sepsis and multiple organ failure mean concentration of 6.5 ± 5.1 pg/mL compared with 4.0 ± 1.5 pg/mL in 8 patients with multiple organ failure without sepsis *1363*

Soluble E-Selectin *Serum Increase* In 15 patients with sepsis and multiple organ failure mean concentration of 345 ± 103 ng/mL compared with 122 ± 81 ng/mL in 8 patients with multiple organ failure without sepsis *1363*

Soluble Fas Antigen *Serum Increase* In 10 patients with multiple organ failure without disseminated intravascular coagulation mean concentration of 4.45 ± 2.57 ng/mL significantly higher than 1.01 ± 0.24 ng/mL in 25 healthy individuals *2229*

Soluble Fas Ligand Antigen *Serum Increase* In 10 patients with multiple organ failure mean serum concentration of 0.229 ± 0.150 ng/mL significantly higher than 0.057 ± 0.039 ng/mL in 25 healthy individuals *2229*

Soluble Intercellular Adhesion Molecule-1 *Serum Increase* In 15 patients with sepsis and multiple organ failure mean concentration of 1,103 ± 342 ng/mL compared with 356 ± 138 ng/mL in 8 patients with multiple organ failure without sepsis *1363*

586.00 Multiple Organ Failure *(continued)*

Soluble Vascular Cell Adhesion Molecule-1
Serum *Increase* In 15 patients with sepsis and multiple organ failure mean concentration of 2,655 ± 1,784 ng/mL compared with 945 ± 512 ng/mL in 8 patients with multiple organ failure without sepsis *1363*

Thrombomodulin *Plasma* *Increase* In 10 patients with mean serum concentration of 39.3 ± 15.8 ng/mL significantly higher than 10.5 ± 1.9 ng/mL in 25 healthy individuals *2229*

586.00 Renal Failure

Aldosterone *Plasma* *Increase* Without dichloromethane extraction, concentrations significantly higher with 3 radioimmunoassays in renal failure than when extraction used although assays on normal plasma showed no difference between extracted and nonextracted specimens *2782*

Amylin *Plasma* *Increase* Significant increase of plasma amylin when kidney function, expressed by creatinine clearance fell below 20 mL/min (17.9 ± 1.7) versus 8.8 ± 1.2 pg/mL (p = 0.0005) when clearance exceeded 80 mL/min *5595*

Carvedilol *Serum* *Increase* Although carvedilol is mainly metabolized by the liver in patients with hypertension and renal insufficiency mean AUC of carvedilol increased and plasma concentrations approximately 40 to 50% higher than in hypertensives with normal renal function. Mean peak plasma concentrations only approximately 12 to 26% higher *4915*

Homocysteine *Plasma* *Increase* Plasma homocysteine in three different groups of patients with chronic renal failure (one group without dialysis, one with CAPD and one with hemodialysis) was increased compared to controls *2286*
Plasma *No Effect* In 13 patients with renal failure aged 2 months to 10 years median concentration of 5.7 µmol/L, and in 1 child aged 11 - 15 y of 7.0 µmol/L, compared with 5.8 µmol/L, and 6.6 µmol/L in healthy children in the same age groups *5471*

Homocystine *Plasma* *Increase* Moderate to marked increase (up to 50 µmol/L) observed in patients with renal failure and is positively correlated with the serum creatinine concentration *5346*

Laminin *Serum* *Increase* Observed effect *2056*

β_2-Microglobulin *Serum* *Increase* In 42 patients with renal failure mean concentration of 20.52 ± 13.2 mg/L (median 17.56 mg/L) significantly different from mean of 1.71 ± 0.46 mg/L (median 1.55 mg/L) in 81 healthy controls *4166*

Osteocalcin *Serum* *Increase* Plasma levels up to 200 fold higher than control values have been reported in patients with renal osteodystrophy and end stage renal disease *1106*

Phenytoin *Serum* *Increase* In a small number of patients over recovery of values may occur with method on Bayer Technicon Immuno 1® system *340*

Progesterone *Plasma* *Decrease* In patients with renal failure may be over or under recovery of progesterone when measured by method on Bayer Technicon Immuno 1® system *341*
Plasma *Increase* In patients with renal failure may be over or under recovery of progesterone when measured by method on Bayer Technicon Immuno 1® system *341*

586.00 Renal Insufficiency

Albumin *Urine* *Increase* In 10 children with serum creatinine concentrations greater than 120 µmol/L mean overnight excretion of 155 mg (4.7 - 591) compared with 58.7 mg (0.48 - 8100) in 10 with serum creatinine concentrations less than 120 µmol/L and 0.4 mg (0 - 18) in 10 healthy controls *5332*

Carvedilol *Serum* *Increase* Although carvedilol is mainly metabolized by the liver in patients with hypertension and renal insufficiency mean AUC of carvedilol increased and plasma concentrations approximately 40 to 50% higher than in hypertensives with normal renal function. Mean peak plasma concentrations only approximately 12 to 26% higher *4915*

Growth Hormone *Urine* *Increase* In 10 children with serum creatinines greater than 120 µmol/L mean overnight excretion of 2,649 /µU (804 - 8,556) significantly greater than 7.5 /µU (1.0 - 85 /µU) in 10 with serum creatinines less than 120 µmol/L and 4.0 /µU (2.6 - 7.3 /µU) in 10 healthy controls *5332*

β_2-Microglobulin *Urine* *Increase* In 10 children with serum creatinines greater than 120 µmol/L mean overnight excretion of 11,637 µg (875 - 15,400) compared with 32 µg (1 - 104) in 10 children with serum creatinines less than 120 µmol/L and 8 µg (3 - 18.7) in 10 healthy controls *5332*

Troponin I *Serum* *No Effect* In 9 patients with renal impairment all had troponin-I concentrations of less than 1 µg/L *890*

Troponin T *Serum* *No Effect* In 9 patients with renal impairment all had troponin-T concentrations of less than 0.2 µg/L by ELISA and Enzymun procedures *890* Only small differences observed in patients with renal failure with results obtained with first generation and second generation BMC Enzymun Troponin T assay performed on BMC ES 300 or 700 analyzers *333*

587.00 Focal Segmental Glomerular Sclerosis

Albumin *Serum* *No Effect* In 11 patients with focal segmental glomerular sclerosis mean concentration of 38.8 ± 11.7 g/L not significantly different from normal *4005*

CD45 Leukocytes *Tissue* *Increase* In 6 patients with FSGS mean number of positive cells 597 ± 401 cells/mm^2 in renal tissue *3026*

Creatinine *Serum* *Increase* In 6 patients with FSGS mean concentration of 1.30 ± 0.34 mg/dL higher than 0.88 ± 0.17 mg/dL in 20 healthy controls *3026*
Serum *No Effect* In 11 patients with focal segmental glomerular sclerosis mean concentration of 1.07 ± 0.21 mg/dL not significantly different from normal *4005*

Intercellular Adhesion Molecule-1 *Tissue* *Increase* In 6 patients with FSGS mean percentage of ICAM-1 positive renal tubuli 10.7 ± 16.7% *3026*

Monocyte Chemotactic Protein-1 *Serum* *Decrease* Mean concentration of 51 ± 33 pg/mL in 6 patients with FSGS compared with 101 ± 24 pg/mL in 16 healthy women and men *4460*
Urine *Increase* In 6 patients with FSGS mean concentration of 537 ± 221 pg/mg creatinine significantly different when compared with mean concentration of 130 ± 30 pg/mg creatinine in 30 healthy women and 32 healthy men *4460*

Protein *Urine* *Increase* In 6 patients with FSGS mean excretion of 3.33 ± 6.15 mg/mg creatinine *3026* In 11 patients with focal segmental glomerulosclerosis mean excretion of 7.72 ± 5.43 g/d significantly different from normal *4005*

Soluble HLA-I *Serum* *Increase* In 11 patients with focal segmental glomerular sclerosis, mean concentration of 713 ± 790 ng/mL significantly higher than 415 ± 256 ng/mL in 45 healthy volunteer controls *4005*
Urine *Increase* In 11 patients with focal segmental glomerular sclerosis, mean excretion of 457 ± 247 ng/mg creatinine significantly higher than undetectable amount in 45 healthy volunteer controls *4005*

Soluble Intercellular Adhesion Molecule-1 *Serum* *No Effect* In 6 patients with FSGS mean concentration of soluble ICAM-1 of 347 ± 72 ng/mL compared with 306 ± 52 ng/mL in 20 healthy controls *3026*
Urine *Increase* In 6 patients with FSGS mean excretion of soluble ICAM-1 of 13.6 ± 17.4 ng/mL or 10.1 ± 13.3 ng/mg creatinine compared with 2.6 ± 1.7 ng/mL or 2.5 ± 3.0 ng/mg creatinine in 20 healthy controls *3026*

587.00 Renal Sclerosis

Arginine *Plasma* *Increase* In 14 patients with renal sclerosis concentrations of 63 - 1,043 ng/mL higher than 63 - 508 ng/mL in 10 normal controls *2331*

Creatine *Serum* *Increase* In 14 patients with renal sclerosis concentrations of 20 - 273 ng/mL higher than 7 - 128 ng/mL in 10 normal controls *2331*

Creatinine *Serum* *Increase* In 14 patients with renal sclerosis concentrations of 6.9 - 32.2 mg/L higher than 1.7 - 10 3 mg/L in 10 normal controls *2331*

Guanidine *Serum* *Increase* In 14 patients with renal sclerosis concentrations of 0 - 0.56 ng/mL higher than undetectable amounts in 10 normal controls *2331*

Guanidinoacetic Acid *Serum* *Increase* In 14 patients with renal sclerosis concentrations of 1.11 - 5.22 ng/mL higher than 0.58 - 2.03 ng/mL in 10 normal controls *2331*

γ-Guanidinobutyric Acid *Serum* *No Effect* In 14 patients with renal sclerosis concentrations of 0 ng/mL not different from undetectable amounts in 10 normal controls *2331*

β-Guanidinopropionic Acid *Serum* *Increase* In 14 patients with renal sclerosis concentrations of 0 - 0.31 ng/mL higher than undetectable amounts in 10 normal controls *2331*

Guanidinosuccinic Acid *Serum* *Increase* In 14 patients with renal sclerosis concentrations of 2.24 - 10.42 ng/mL higher than undetectable amounts in 10 normal controls *2331*

Methylguanidine *Serum* *Increase* In 14 patients with renal sclerosis concentrations of 0 - 0.46 ng/mL higher than undetectable amounts in 10 normal controls *2331*

Taurocyamine *Serum* *Increase* In 14 patients with renal sclerosis concentrations of 0 - 0.46 ng/mL different from undetectable amounts in 10 normal controls *2331*

588.00 Renal Dwarfism

Alkaline Phosphatase *Serum* *Increase* Usually elevated *367*

Calcium *Serum* *Decrease* May be quite low but is more commonly in the low-normal range *367* May lead to hypocalcemia or low normal serum calcium levels. In time there will be significant parathyroid hyperplasia, and the serum calcium may become inappropriately elevated *2039*
Serum *Increase* May be normal or elevated. When both phosphate and calcium are high, metastatic calcifications in subcutaneous tissues and conjunctiva may develop *2039*
Serum *No Effect* May be normal or elevated. When both phosphate and calcium are high, metastatic calcifications in subcutaneous tissues and conjunctiva may develop *2039*

Phosphate *Serum* *Increase* May be normal or elevated. When both phosphate and calcium are high, metastatic calcifications in subcutaneous tissues and conjunctiva may develop *2039*
Serum *No Effect* May be normal or elevated. When both phosphate and calcium are high, metastatic calcifications in subcutaneous tissues and conjunctiva may develop *2039*

588.00 Renal Osteodystrophy

Alkaline Phosphatase *Serum* *Decrease* Reported effect with end-stage osteopenia and chronic renal osteodystrophy *3160*

Alkaline Phosphatase, Bone Isoenzyme *Serum* *Increase* Median activity of 20.9 U/L observed in 86 patients with renal osteodystrophy significantly different from median of 15.5 U/L in 30 control individuals *3576*

C-terminal Telopeptide of Type I Collagen *Serum* *Increase* Median concentration of 38.8 µg/L observed in 86 patients with renal osteodystrophy significantly different from median of 2.5 µg/L in 30 control individuals *3576*

Hydroxyproline, Free *Plasma* *Increase* Serum free levels were significantly elevated in the patient group with conservatively treated end-stage renal failure (n = 14) and in the patient group on chronic hemodialysis (n = 107), with the latter group showing the highest value *5345*

Interleukin-6 *Serum* *Increase* Median concentration of 16.5 pg/mL observed in 86 patients with renal osteodystrophy significantly different from median of 1.0 pg/mL in 30 control individuals *3576*

Osteocalcin *Serum* *Increase* In 42 patients with renal osteodystrophy undergoing chronic hemodialysis mean concentration of 64.0 ± 74.8 ng/mL significantly greater than 6.2 ± 2.2 ng/mL in healthy controls *789* Median concentration of 143.8 ng/mL observed in 86 patients with renal osteodystrophy significantly different from median of 14.2 ng/mL in 30 control individuals *3576*

Parathyroid Hormone *Plasma* *Increase* Median concentration of 279.8 pg/mL observed in 86 patients with renal osteodystrophy significantly different from median of 27.8 pg/mL in 30 control individuals *3576*

588.10 Diabetes Insipidus, Nephrogenic

Creatinine *Serum* *Increase* Mean concentration of 1.4 ± 0.2 mg/dL in 7 patients with nephrogenic diabetes insipidus significantly different from 0.7 ± 0.2 mg/dL in 27 healthy controls *1084*

Creatinine Clearance *Urine* *Decrease* Mean clearance of 81 ± 35 mL/min in 7 patients with nephrogenic diabetes insipidus significantly different from 108 ± 10 mL/min in 27 healthy controls *1084*

Fractional Excretion of Sodium *Urine* *No Effect* Mean excretion of 0.7 ± 0.2% in 7 patients with nephrogenic diabetes insipidus not significantly different from 0.5 ± 0.2% in 27 healthy controls *1084*

Fractional Excretion of Urea *Urine* *Increase* Mean excretion of 62 ± 19% in 7 patients with nephrogenic diabetes insipidus significantly different from 45 ± 7.5% in 27 healthy controls *1084*

Fractional Excretion of Uric Acid *Urine* *No Effect* Mean excretion of 9.0 ± 3.0% in 7 patients with nephrogenic diabetes insipidus not significantly different from 8.2 ± 2.0% in 27 healthy controls *1084*

Osmolality *Urine* *No Effect* Mean excretion of 132 ± 19 mOsm/kg in 7 patients with nephrogenic diabetes insipidus not significantly different from 50 - 1,000 mOsm/kg in 27 healthy controls *1084*

Protein *Serum* *No Effect* Mean concentration of 7.5 ± 0.6 g/dL in 7 patients with nephrogenic diabetes insipidus not significantly different from 7.2 ± 0.7 g/dL in 27 healthy controls *1084*

Renin Activity *Plasma* *Increase* Mean activity of 17.0 ± 6.0 ng/mL/h in 6 patients with nephrogenic diabetes insipidus significantly different from 1.5 ± 0.6 ng/mL/h in 27 healthy controls *1084*

Sodium *Serum* *Increase* Mean concentration of 152 ± 4 mmol/L in 7 patients with nephrogenic diabetes insipidus significantly different from 140 ± 2.5 mmol/L in 27 healthy controls *1084*

Urea *Serum* *No Effect* Mean concentration of 36 ± 10 mg/dL in 7 patients with nephrogenic diabetes insipidus not significantly different from 32 ± 7 mg/dL in 27 healthy controls *1084*

Uric Acid *Serum* *Increase* Mean concentration of 5.7 ± 0.8 mg/dL in 7 patients with nephrogenic diabetes insipidus significantly different from 4.3 ± 0.9 mg/dL in 27 healthy controls *1084*
Urine *No Effect* Mean excretion of 598 ± 80 mg/d in 7 patients with nephrogenic diabetes insipidus not significantly different from 548 ± 100 mg/d in 27 healthy controls *1084*

588.80 Secondary Hyperparathyroidism

Alkaline Phosphatase *Serum* *No Effect* In 25 patients with renal secondary hyperparathyroidism median activity of 133 U/L not significantly different from 125 U/L in 90 healthy controls *2572*

Bone Sialoprotein *Serum* *Increase* In 25 patients with chronic renal failure and secondary hyperparathyroidism mean concentration of 30.6 ± 18.9 µg/L significantly higher than that in 90 healthy controls in whom the mean concentration was 12.1 ± 5.0 µg/L *2572*

Calcium *Serum* *Decrease* In 25 patients with renal secondary hyperparathyroidism median concentration of 2.09 mmol/L not significantly different from 2.35 mmol/L in 90 healthy controls *2572*

Deoxypyridinoline *Urine* *Increase* In 18 patients with secondary hyperparathyroidism mean excretion of 8.59 ± 5.87 nmol/mmol creatinine compared with 5.71 ± 1.59 nmol/mmol creatinine in 79 healthy controls as measured by assay on Ciba Corning ACS:180 system *804*

Deoxypyridinoline, Free *Urine* *Increase* Mean excretion in 18 patients aged 32 - 66 years of approximately 6.5 nmol/mol creatinine significantly different from approximately 4.0 nmol/mol creatinine in healthy controls, although still within normal range *4383* In 14 patients with secondary hyperparathyroidism mean excretion of 9.2 ± 5.1 µmol/mol creatinine significantly different from 1.7 - 5.9 µmol/mol creatinine in healthy men and 3.1 - 8.1 µmol/mol creatinine in healthy women wnen measure by CLIA technique *4427*

588.80 Secondary Hyperparathyroidism *(continued)*

Osteocalcin *Serum* *Increase* In 14 patients with secondary hyperparathyroidism mean concentrations by sandwich EIA and RIA of 10.2 ± 7.1 μg/L and 11.4 ± 4.1 μg/L compared with mean concentrations 4.2 ± 1.2 μg/L and 6.6 ± 1.4 μg/L by sandwich EIA and RIA methods respectively in 20 healthy individuals *2246*

Parathyroid Hormone, Intact *Plasma* *Increase* In 25 patients with renal secondary hyperparathyroidism median concentration of 145.2 μg/L significantly different from 35.2 μg/L in 90 healthy controls *2572*

588.81 Proximal Renal Tubular Acidosis (Type II)

Alkaline Phosphatase *Serum* *Increase* Increased in Albricht-type renal tubular acidosis, as in Fanconi Syndrome, but no aminoaciduria *1290* Observed in some patients *1025*

Amino Acids *Urine* *Increase* Found in children *900*

Bicarbonate *Serum* *Decrease* Low bicarbonate level *4979* Low levels in the presence of alkaline urine; very low levels with acid urine *413* Hereditary or sporadic proximal renal tubular acidosis is associated with hypokalemia, hyperchloremic metabolic acidosis, urine pH < 5.5, increased urinary ammonium ion excretion, a negative urine anion gap, increased urinary osmol gap, normal urinary citrate and normal urinary calcium excretion *4071*

Calcium *Serum* *Decrease* Renal tubular acidosis or Fanconi Syndrome must be considered in patients with osteomalacia. Normal to decreased values observed *1025*
Serum *Increase* Hypercalcemia in 5 of 17 patients with transient primary renal tubular acidosis *3954*
Serum *No Effect* Renal tubular acidosis or Fanconi Syndrome must be considered in patients with osteomalacia. Normal to decreased values observed *1025*
Urine *Increase* The hypercalciuria results in nephrocalcinosis or nephrolithiasis which,in the absence of generalized aminoaciduria, aids in the differentiation of this disease from the more common De Toni-Debre-Fanconi Syndrome *900*

Chloride *Serum* *Increase* Hereditary or sporadic proximal renal tubular acidosis is associated with hypokalemia, hyperchloremic metabolic acidosis, urine pH < 5.5, increased urinary ammonium ion excretion, a negative urine anion gap, increased urinary osmol gap, normal urinary citrate and normal urinary calcium excretion *4071*

Glomerular Filtration Rate *Urine* *Decrease* Usually reduced *4979*

Glucose *Serum* *Decrease* Hereditary or sporadic proximal renal tubular acidosis is associated with hypokalemia, hyperchloremic metabolic acidosis, urine pH < 5.5, increased urinary ammonium ion excretion, a negative urine anion gap, increased urinary osmol gap, normal urinary citrate and normal urinary calcium excretion, glycosuria in the absence of hyperglycemia, hypouricemia and hypophosphatemia *4071*
Urine *Increase* Found in children *900*

Parathyroid Hormone *Plasma* *Increase* Secondary to hypocalcemia *572*

pH *Blood* *Decrease* Tends to fall *1290*
Urine *Increase* Always relatively high with the gradient defect, no matter how severe the systemic acidosis *4979*

Phosphate *Serum* *Decrease* Low in the early stages and increasing to normal values with increasing azotemia *900* Hereditary or sporadic proximal renal tubular acidosis is associated with hypokalemia, hyperchloremic metabolic acidosis, urine pH < 5.5, increased urinary ammonium ion excretion, a negative urine anion gap, increased urinary osmol gap, normal urinary citrate and normal urinary calcium excretion *4071* Low in the early stages and increasing to normal values with increasing azotemia *1025*
Urine *Increase* Excessive loss in urine *5544*

Potassium *Serum* *Decrease* Normal or decreased *5023* *5515* May be a life-threatening complication *900* Hydrogen ion and ammonium ion production by the renal tubule cells is diminished, with excessive loss of potassium in the urine. In any case of severe renal damage, potassium conservation may be impaired *1290* Renal wasting leads to hypokalemic state *3735*
Serum *No Effect* Normal or decreased *413*
Urine *Increase* Renal wasting of potassium *3735* May result in severe hypokalemic paralysis *4979*

Sodium *Serum* *Decrease* Hyponatremia may develop *4979* Normal or decreased *413*
Serum *No Effect* Normal or decreased *413*

Uric Acid *Serum* *Decrease* Hereditary or sporadic proximal renal tubular acidosis is associated with hypokalemia, hyperchloremic metabolic acidosis, urine pH < 5.5, increased urinary ammonium ion excretion, a negative urine anion gap, increased urinary osmol gap, normal urinary citrate and normal urinary calcium excretion *4071* Hypouricemia, secondary to increased renal clearance of uric acid, is present in some patients (children) *900*
Urine *Increase* Hypouricemia, secondary to increased renal clearance of uric acid, is present in some patients (children) *900*

Uric Acid Clearance *Urine* *Increase* Hypouricemia, secondary to increased renal clearance of uric acid, is present in some patients (children) *900*

Volume *Urine* *Increase* Characterized by polyuria *4979*

588.82 Classic Distal Renal Tubular Acidosis (Type I)

Ammonium Ions *Urine* *Increase* Classic dRTA may be hereditary or sporadic and is asociated with hyokalemia, hyperchloremic metabolic acidosis, urine pH > 5.5, increased urinary ammonium ion excretion, a negative urine anion gap, increased urinary osmol gap, decreased urinary citrate and increased urinary calcium in some patients *4071*

Anion Gap *Urine* *Decrease* Classic dRTA may be hereditary or sporadic and is asociated with hyokalemia, hyperchloremic metabolic acidosis, urine pH > 5.5, increased urinary ammonium ion excretion, a negative urine anion gap, increased urinary osmol gap, decreased urinary citrate and increased urinary calcium in some patients *4071*

Calcium *Urine* *Decrease* Classic dRTA may be hereditary or sporadic and is asociated with hyokalemia, hyperchloremic metabolic acidosis, urine pH > 5.5, increased urinary ammonium ion excretion, a negative urine anion gap, increased urinary osmol gap, decreased urinary citrate and increased urinary calcium in some patients *4071*

Chloride *Serum* *Decrease* Classic dRTA may be hereditary or sporadic and is asociated with hyokalemia, hyperchloremic metabolic acidosis, urine pH > 5.5, increased urinary ammonium ion excretion, a negative urine anion gap, increased urinary osmol gap, decreased urinary citrate and increased urinary calcium in some patients *4071*

Citrate *Urine* *Decrease* Classic dRTA may be hereditary or sporadic and is asociated with hyokalemia, hyperchloremic metabolic acidosis, urine pH > 5.5, increased urinary ammonium ion excretion, a negative urine anion gap, increased urinary osmol gap, decreased urinary citrate and increased urinary calcium in some patients *4071*

Net Acid Excretion *Urine* *Increase* Classic dRTA may be hereditary or sporadic and is asociated with hyokalemia, hyperchloremic metabolic acidosis, urine pH > 5.5, increased urinary ammonium ion excretion, a negative urine anion gap, increased urinary osmol gap, decreased urinary citrate and increased urinary calcium in some patients *4071*

Osmolal Gap *Urine* *Increase* Classic dRTA may be hereditary or sporadic and is asociated with hyokalemia, hyperchloremic metabolic acidosis, urine pH > 5.5, increased urinary ammonium ion excretion, a negative urine anion gap, increased urinary osmol gap, decreased urinary citrate and increased urinary calcium in some patients *4071*

Potassium *Serum* *Decrease* Classic dRTA may be hereditary or sporadic and is asociated with hyokalemia, hyperchloremic metabolic acidosis, urine pH > 5.5, increased urinary ammonium ion excretion, a negative urine anion gap, increased urinary osmol gap, decreased urinary citrate and increased urinary calcium in some patients *4071*

588.82 Distal Renal Tubular Acidosis

Bicarbonate *Serum* *Decrease* Alkaline urine regardless of bicarbonate level *413*

Urine *Increase* Alkaline urine regardless of bicarbonate level in blood *413*

Calcium *Urine* *Increase* An almost constant feature and frequently results in the formation of renal calculi *367*

Chloride *Serum* *Increase* Normal anion gap *413*

β_2-Macroglobulin *Serum* *Decrease* An increase in urine and a decrease in serum levels is seen *2586*
Urine *Increase* An increase in urine and a decrease in serum levels is seen *2586*

Parathyroid Hormone *Plasma* *Increase* Secondary to reduced calcium *868*

pH *Urine* *Increase* Inappropriately high *1283* Cardinal clinical finding is a urine pH which is never lower than 6.0, even with severe metabolic acidosis *367*

Phosphate *Serum* *Decrease* Typical feature of Type I *367*

Potassium *Serum* *Decrease* Commonly occurs in Type I *367*
Serum *Increase* Some cases *413*
Urine *Increase* Commonly occurs in Type I *367*

Sodium *Urine* *Increase* Characteristic complication of metabolic acidosis *4581*

588.82 Distal Renal Tubular Acidosis (Type IV)

Anion Gap *Urine* *Increase* Distal renal tubular acidosis (type IV) is associated with hyperkalemia, hyperchloremic metabolic acidosis, urine pH < 5.5, decreased urinary ammonium ion excretion, a positive urine anion gap, normal urinary citrate and urinary calcium excretion *4071*

Calcium *Urine* *No Effect* Distal renal tubular acidosis (type IV) is associated with hyperkalemia, hyperchloremic metabolic acidosis, urine pH < 5.5, decreased urinary ammonium ion excretion, a positive urine anion gap, normal urinary citrate and urinary calcium excretion *4071*

Chloride *Serum* *Increase* Distal renal tubular acidosis (type IV) is associated with hyperkalemia, hyperchloremic metabolic acidosis, urine pH < 5.5, decreased urinary ammonium ion excretion, a positive urine anion gap, normal urinary citrate and urinary calcium excretion *4071*

Citrate *Urine* *No Effect* Distal renal tubular acidosis (type IV) is associated with hyperkalemia, hyperchloremic metabolic acidosis, urine pH < 5.5, decreased urinary ammonium ion excretion, a positive urine anion gap, normal urinary citrate and urinary calcium excretion *4071*

pH *Urine* *Decrease* Distal renal tubular acidosis (type IV) is associated with hyperkalemia, hyperchloremic metabolic acidosis, urine pH < 5.5, decreased urinary ammonium ion excretion, a positive urine anion gap, normal urinary citrate and urinary calcium excretion *4071*

Potassium *Serum* *Increase* Distal renal tubular acidosis (type IV) is associated with hyperkalemia, hyperchloremic metabolic acidosis, urine pH < 5.5, decreased urinary ammonium ion excretion, a positive urine anion gap, normal urinary citrate and urinary calcium excretion *4071*

588.82 Voltage-dependent Distal Renal Tubular Acidosis Type I)

Ammonium Ions *Urine* *Increase* May be associated with hyerkalemia, hyperchloremic metabolic acidosis, urine pH > 5.5, increased urinary ammonium ion excretion, a positive urine anion gap, increased urinary osmol gap, low urinary citrate and high or normal urinary calcium excretion *4071*

Anion Gap *Urine* *Decrease* May be associated with hyerkalemia, hyperchloremic metabolic acidosis, urine pH > 5.5, increased urinary ammonium ion excretion, a positive urine anion gap, increased urinary osmol gap, low urinary citrate and high or normal urinary calcium excretion *4071*

Calcium *Urine* *Increase* May be associated with hyerkalemia, hyperchloremic metabolic acidosis, urine pH > 5.5, increased urinary ammonium ion excretion, a positive urine anion gap, increased urinary osmol gap, low urinary citrate and high or normal urinary calcium excretion *4071*

Chloride *Serum* *Increase* May be associated with hyerkalemia, hyperchloremic metabolic acidosis, urine pH > 5.5, increased urinary ammonium ion excretion, a positive urine anion gap, increased urinary osmol gap, low urinary citrate and high or normal urinary calcium excretion *4071*

Citrate *Urine* *Decrease* May be associated with hyerkalemia, hyperchloremic metabolic acidosis, urine pH > 5.5, increased urinary ammonium ion excretion, a positive urine anion gap, increased urinary osmol gap, low urinary citrate and high or normal urinary calcium excretion *4071*

Net Acid Excretion *Urine* *Increase* May be associated with hyerkalemia, hyperchloremic metabolic acidosis, urine pH > 5.5, increased urinary ammonium ion excretion, a positive urine anion gap, increased urinary osmol gap, low urinary citrate and high or normal urinary calcium excretion *4071*

Osmolal Gap *Urine* *Decrease* May be associated with hyerkalemia, hyperchloremic metabolic acidosis, urine pH > 5.5, increased urinary ammonium ion excretion, a positive urine anion gap, increased urinary osmol gap, low urinary citrate and high or normal urinary calcium excretion *4071*

pH *Urine* *Increase* May be associated with hyerkalemia, hyperchloremic metabolic acidosis, urine pH > 5.5, increased urinary ammonium ion excretion, a positiv urine anion gap, increased urinary osmol gap, low urinary citrate and high or normal urinary calcium excretion *4071*

Potassium *Serum* *Increase* May be associated with hyerkalemia, hyperchloremic metabolic acidosis, urine pH > 5.5, increased urinary ammonium ion excretion, a positive urine anion gap, increased urinary osmol gap, low urinary citrate and high or normal urinary calcium excretion *4071*

590.00 Chronic Pyelonephritis

Alanine Aminotransferase *Urine* *Increase* Increased *5671* *2508* *4096*

Albumin *Urine* *Increase* Qualitative proteinuria may be absent but if present is mild *900*

Alkaline Phosphatase *Urine* *Increase* Almost invariably elevated in a group of 10 patients *1670*

Ammonium Ions *Urine* *Increase* May be associated with classic distal renal tubular acidosis which is associated with hyokalemia, hyperchloremic metabolic acidosis, urine pH > 5.5, increased urinary ammonium ion excretion, a negative urine anion gap, increased urinary osmol gap, decreased urinary citrate and increased urinary calcium in some patients *4071*

Anion Gap *Urine* *Decrease* May be associated with classic distal renal tubular acidosis which is associated with hyokalemia, hyperchloremic metabolic acidosis, urine pH > 5.5, increased urinary ammonium ion excretion, a negative urine anion gap, increased urinary osmol gap, decreased urinary citrate and increased urinary calcium in some patients *4071*

Calcium *Urine* *Increase* May be associated with classic distal renal tubular acidosis which is associated with hyokalemia, hyperchloremic metabolic acidosis, urine pH > 5.5, increased urinary ammonium ion excretion, a negative urine anion gap, increased urinary osmol gap, decreased urinary citrate and increased urinary calcium in some patients *4071*

Casts *Urine* *Increase* As in acute pyelonephritis, the leukocyte cast in the absence of other cellular casts is a most helpful finding and strongly supports the diagnosis. The urine sediment may be normal but repeated examination will usually reveal pyuria and cylindruria *900* With renal parenchymal disease *1727*

Ceruloplasmin *Serum* *Increase* Found in 84 patients with exacerbated disease. Raised levels indicate the amount of activity of the pathologic process and distinguishes it from glomerulonephritis *5238*

Chloride *Serum* *Increase* Hyperchloremia frequently accompanies chronic pyelonephritis *1980* May be associated with classic distal renal tubular acidosis which is associated with hyokalemia, hyperchloremic metabolic acidosis, urine pH > 5.5, increased urinary ammonium ion excretion, a negative urine anion gap, increased urinary osmol gap, decreased urinary citrate and increased urinary calcium in some patients *4071*

590.00 Chronic Pyelonephritis *(continued)*

Citrate *Urine* *Decrease* May be associated with classic distal renal tubular acidosis which is associated with hyokalemia, hyperchloremic metabolic acidosis, urine pH > 5.5, increased urinary ammonium ion excretion, a negative urine anion gap, increased urinary osmol gap, decreased urinary citrate and increased urinary calcium in some patients *4071*

Creatinine Clearance *Urine* *Decrease* Decreased 24 h clearance *5545*

Erythrocytes *Urine* *Increase* With renal parenchymal disease *1727* Microscopic hematuria may be present *900*

α_1-Globulin *Serum* *Increase* Moderate increases *1290*

α_2-Globulin *Serum* *Increase* Moderate increase *1290*

Glomerular Filtration Rate *Urine* *Decrease* Decreased due to reduced filtration surface (fewer functioning glomeruli) *1290* A decrease proportional to progress of renal disease *5545*

Glucose *Urine* *Increase* With renal parenchymal disease *1727*

β-Glucuronidase *Urine* *Increase* All 15 patients showed elevated activity (mean 61.9 ± 39.1), whereas 11 of 13 patients with inactive disease showed normal values (mean 24.0 ± 7.8 U) *1805*

Haptoglobin *Serum* *Increase* Increased serum levels found in 84 chronic patients correlated with activity of pathologic process and distinguished it from glomerulonephritis *5238*

Hematocrit *Blood* *Decrease* A normocytic, normochromic anemia may be present as in other forms of renal insufficiency. May be more severe, since chronic infection will act synergistically with renal insufficiency to depress bone marrow function *900*

Hemoglobin *Blood* *Decrease* A normocytic, normochromic anemia may be present as in other forms of renal insufficiency. May be more severe, since chronic infection will act synergistically with renal insufficiency to depress bone marrow function *900*

β-Hexosaminidase *Urine* *Decrease* Decreased levels in urine *5229*

Lactate Dehydrogenase *Urine* *Increase* Urinary activity was almost invariably elevated *1670*

Leukocytes *Urine* *Increase* WBCs, bacteria, and little protein are common urinary findings *367*

Magnesium *Serum* *Decrease* Hypomagnesemia may occur *5507*

Net Acid Excretion *Urine* *Increase* May be associated with classic distal renal tubular acidosis which is associated with hyokalemia, hyperchloremic metabolic acidosis, urine pH > 5.5, increased urinary ammonium ion excretion, a negative urine anion gap, increased urinary osmol gap, decreased urinary citrate and increased urinary calcium in some patients *4071*

Osmolal Gap *Urine* *Increase* May be associated with classic distal renal tubular acidosis which is associated with hyokalemia, hyperchloremic metabolic acidosis, urine pH > 5.5, increased urinary ammonium ion excretion, a negative urine anion gap, increased urinary osmol gap, decreased urinary citrate and increased urinary calcium in some patients *4071*

Osmolality *Urine* *Decrease* With renal parenchymal disease *1727*

pH *Urine* *Increase* May be associated with classic distal renal tubular acidosis which is associated with hyokalemia, hyperchloremic metabolic acidosis, urine pH > 5.5, increased urinary ammonium ion excretion, a negative urine anion gap, increased urinary osmol gap, decreased urinary citrate and increased urinary calcium in some patients *4071*

Potassium *Serum* *Decrease* May be associated with classic distal renal tubular acidosis which is associated with hyokalemia, hyperchloremic metabolic acidosis, urine pH > 5.5, increased urinary ammonium ion excretion, a negative urine anion gap, increased urinary osmol gap, decreased urinary citrate and increased urinary calcium in some patients *4071*

Protein *Urine* *Increase* With renal parenchymal disease *1727* Slight, usually < 3 g/d *367*

Sialic Acid *Serum* *Increase* Increased in 84 chronic patients, correlated with activity of pathologic process and distinguished it from glomerulonephritis *5238*

Specific Gravity *Urine* *Decrease* The urine is usually of low specific gravity or at least no more than isosmotic plasma *900*

Thyroxine (T4) *Urine* *Increase* Urinary loss exceeds the normal mean 10-fold *1487*

Urea Nitrogen *Serum* *Increase* May be elevated *367*

Volume *Urine* *Decrease* With renal parenchymal disease *1727*

590.10 Acute Pyelonephritis

Albumin *Urine* *Increase* Often present but minimal in degree *900*

Alkaline Phosphatase *Serum* *Increase* In 29% of 13 patients at initial hospitalization for this disorder *1576* Significant elevation can be found in some patients. This occurs in cases with clinical or histological evidence of severe disease, occasionally associated with papillary necrosis and gram-negative septicemia. Widespread renal inflammatory destruction results in release of enzyme from the tubular cells into the blood stream *1535*

Aspartate Aminotransferase *Serum* *Increase* In 28% of 14 patients at initial hospitalization for this disorder *1576*

Casts *Urine* *Increase* With renal parenchymal disease *1727* Essentially diagnostic *1980* Generally interpreted as indicative of renal parenchymal inflammation and which in the absence of other types of cellular casts provides strong support for a diagnosis of pyelonephritis *900*

C-Reactive Protein *Serum* *Increase* In 43 women with acute pyelonephritis mean concentration on admission to hospital of 72.7 mg/L significantly higher than in controls *2394* Marked increase indicates an acute infection *413*

Creatinine *Serum* *Increase* In 48% of 16 patients at initial hospitalization for this disorder *1576*

Creatinine Clearance *Urine* *Decrease* Decreased 24 h clearance *5545*

Erythrocyte Sedimentation Rate *Blood* *Increase* In 43 women with acute pyelonephritis mean rate on admission to hospital of 35 ± 3 mm/h significantly higher than in controls *2394*

Erythrocytes *Urine* *Increase* With renal parenchymal disease *4746* The finding of gross or microscopic hematuria is variable but not uncommon *900*

Fibrin Degradation Products (D-Dimer) *Urine* *Increase* FDP-D detected in the urine of 60% patients with acute pyelonephritis *4557*

α_1-Globulin *Serum* *Increase* Moderate increases *1290*

α_2-Globulin *Serum* *Increase* Moderate increase *1290*

Glomerular Filtration Rate *Urine* *Decrease* Decreased due to reduced filtration surface (fewer functioning glomeruli) *1290*

Glucose *Urine* *Increase* With renal parenchymal disease *1727*

β-Glucuronidase *Urine* *Increase* All 15 patients with active disease showed elevated activity (mean 61.9 ± 39.1 U/L), whereas 11 of 13 patients with inactive disease showed normal values (mean 24.0 ± 7.8 U/L) *1805*

Interleukin-1 Receptor Antagonist *Urine* *Decrease* In 40 children with first time acute pyelonephritis IL-1ra detectable in 98% specmens with median concentration of 239 pg/μmol creatinine and in 7 children with recurrent acute pyelonephritis IL-1ra detected in 86% and median concentration of 17 pg/μmol creatinine compared with 100% detection rate and median concentration of 1,019 pg/μmol creatinine in 10 healthy children *5322*

Interleukin-1α *Urine* *No Effect* In 40 children with first time acute pyelonephritis, IL-1α detectable in 68% specmens with median concentration of 3.6 pg/μmol creatinine and in 7 children with recurrent acute pyelonephritis IL-1α detected in 29% and nondetectable median concentration compared with detection rate of 50% and median concentration of 1.4 pg/μmol creatinine in 10 healthy children *5322*

Interleukin-6 *Serum* *Increase* In 43 women with acute pyelonephritis mean concentration on admission to hospital of 75 ± 12 pg/mL (median 55 pg/mL) significantly higher than not detectable concentration in controls *2394*
Urine *Increase* In 43 women with acute pyelonephritis mean concentration on admission to hospital of 80 ± 16 pg/mL (median 44 pg/mL) significantly higher than not detectable concentration in controls *2394*

Interleukin-8 *Serum* *Increase* In 43 women with acute pyelonephritis mean concentration on admission to hospital 245 pg/mL (median 73 pg/mL) significantly higher than not detectable concentration in controls *2394*
Urine *Increase* In 43 women with acute pyelonephritis mean concentration on admission to hospital of 1,499 ± 240 pg/mL (median 870 pg/mL) significantly higher than not detectable concentration in controls *2394*

Isocitrate Dehydrogenase *Serum* *No Effect* No effect on activity observed *5008*

Lactate Dehydrogenase *Urine* *Increase* Increased in 25% of patients *5544*

Leukocytes *Blood* *Increase* In 68% of 16 patients at initial hospitalization for this disorder *1576* Most patients exhibit a leukocytosis of 15,000 - 20,000 /µL with an increase of immature neutrophils in the differential count *900* In 43 women with acute pyelonephritis mean concentration on admission to hospital 11.7 ± 0.6 10^9/L significantly higher than in controls *2394*
Urine *Increase* With renal parenchymal disease *1727*
Urine *No Effect* Typical observation *572* Acute pyelonephritis may exist in the absence of pyuria and bacteriuria. This may occur in the patient with hematogenous dissemination of infection to the renal parenchyma without communication to urinary drainage, as in renal carbuncle or perinephric abscess *900*

Magnesium *Serum* *Decrease* May occur *5507*

α_1-Microglobulin *Urine* *Increase* Concentration significantly increased compared with that in acute cystitis and asymptomatic bacteriuria *4557*

β_2-Microglobulin *Urine* *Increase* Concentration significantly increased compared with that in acute cystitis and in those with asymptomatic bacteriuria *4557*

N-Acetyl-Glucosaminidase *Urine* *Increase* Concentration in urine significantly increased compared with that in acute cystitis and asymptomatic bacteriuria *4557*

Neutrophils *Blood* *Increase* In 63% of 14 patients at initial hospitalization for this disorder *1576* Most patients exhibit a leukocytosis of 15,000 - 20,000 /µL with an increase of immature neutrophils in the differential count *900*

Protein *Urine* *Increase* Proteinuria is usually mild, rarely exceeding 1.5 - 2.0 g/d *1980* Usually < 2 g/d *1025* With renal parenchymal disease *1727*

Retinol-binding Protein *Urine* *Increase* Concentration significantly increased compared with that in acute cystitis and asymptomatic bacteriuria *4557*

Specific Gravity *Urine* *Decrease* Urine concentrating ability is impaired relatively early *1980*

Urea Nitrogen *Serum* *Increase* In 24% of 16 patients at initial hospitalization for this disorder *1576* Uncomplicated disease does not characteristically exhibit evidence of renal insufficiency; however, a nonspecific elevation of BUN may be a reflection of volume contraction and dehydration *900*

Volume *Urine* *Decrease* With renal parenchymal disease *1727* *1290*

590.10 Pyonephrosis

C-Reactive Protein *Serum* *Increase* In 16 patients with pyonephrosis mean C-reactive protein concentration of 11.7 ± 5.2 mg/dL significantly higher than 1.2 ± 1.1 mg/dL in 9 patients with uncomplicated hydronephrosis *5748*

Erythrocyte Sedimentation Rate *Blood* *Increase* In 16 patients with pyonephrosis mean ESR of 88.8 ± 34.8 mm/h significantly higher than 42.9 ± 34.6 mm/h in 9 individuals with uncomplicated hydronephrosis *5748*

590.80 Pyelonephritis

N-Acetyl-Glucosaminidase B *Urine* *Increase* In 14 patients with pyelonephritis mean concentration of 29.0 ± 39.8 µg/L or 13.5 ± 11.9 µg/g creatinine significantly different from concentrations in 40 healthy adults in whom mean excretion was 3.1 ± 3.0 µg/L or 2.9 ± 2.0 µg/g creatinine *3838*

Phospholipase A *Serum* *Increase* Reported effect *2200*

591.00 Hydronephrosis

Alanine Aminotransferase *Urine* *Increase* Increased *4096* *5671* *2508*

Albumin *Urine* *No Effect* In uninfected hydronephrosis the urine is negative. If infection supervenes, WBC and albumin are noted *900*

C-Reactive Protein *Serum* *Increase* In 9 patients with uncomplicated hydronephrosis mean C-reactive protein of 1.2 ± 1.1 mg/dL *5748*

Creatinine *Serum* *Increase* In 70% of 10 patients at initial hospitalization for this disorder *1576*

Erythrocyte Sedimentation Rate *Blood* *Increase* In 9 patients with uncomplicated hydronephrosis mean ESR of 42.9 ± 34.6 mm/h *5748*

Erythrocytes *Blood* *Increase* True polycythemia with a considerable increase of red cell volume may occur *3710*

Hematocrit *Blood* *Decrease* In cases of advanced renal damage elevation of the BUN and secondary anemia may be noted secondary to uremia *900*

Hemoglobin *Blood* *Decrease* In cases of advanced renal damage elevation of the BUN and secondary anemia may be noted secondary to uremia *900*

Leukocytes *Blood* *Increase* In 27% of 11 patients at initial hospitalization for this disorder *1576*
Urine *No Effect* In uninfected cases the urine is negative. If infection supervenes, WBC and albumin are noted *900*

Magnesium *Serum* *Decrease* Hypomagnesemia may occur *5507*

Urea Nitrogen *Serum* *Increase* In 20% of 10 patients at initial hospitalization for this disorder *1576* In cases of advanced renal damage elevation of the BUN and secondary anemia may be noted secondary to uremia *900*

Volume *Red Blood Cells* *Increase* True polycythemia with a considerable increase of red cell volume may occur *3710*

591.00 Infected Hydronephrosis

C-Reactive Protein *Serum* *Increase* In 13 patients with infected hydronephrosis mean C-reactive protein concentration of 7.5 ± 4.7 mg/dL significantly higher than 1.2 ± 1.1 mg/dL in 9 patients with uncomplicated hydronephrosis *5748*

Erythrocyte Sedimentation Rate *Blood* *Increase* In 13 patients with infected hydronephrosis mean ESR of 84.6 ± 44.4 mm/h significantly higher than 42.9 ± 34.6 mm/h in 9 individuals with uncomplicated hydronephrosis *5748*

592.00 Nephrolithiasis

Angiotensin-converting Enzyme *Urine* *Increase* Activity was found to be significantly elevated *534*

Calcium *Serum* *Decrease* May represent presenting manifestations *1025*
Serum *No Effect* Mean concentration of 4.7 ± 0.2 mg/dL observed in 26 patients with calcium nephrolithiasis compared with 4.7 ± 0.2 mg/dL in 14 healthy controls *2363* In a study of 59 patients with normocalcemia and low intact PTH concentrations 3 had renal calculi without hypercalciuria *3280*
Urine *Increase* Increased in the majority of patients with calcareous calculi, but will be normal in patients whose primary problem is infection *367* In 64 patients with low renal phosphate threshold in 18 with renal calculi mean concentration of 6.0 ± 0.6 mmoL/d significantly different from 3.5 ± 0.4 mmoL/d in 46 without renal lithiasis *4215* 35% of patients have increased urinary concentration (> 250 mg/24 h in females and > 300 mg/24 h in males) *5545*
Urine *No Effect* Mean excretion of 157.7 ± 56.7 mg/g creatinine observed in 26 patients with calcium nephrolithiasis compared with 153.0 ± 135.5 mg/g creatinine in 14 healthy controls *2363*

Citrate *Urine* *No Effect* Mean excretion of 372.9 ± 249.8 mg/g creatinine observed in 26 patients with calcium nephrolithiasis compared with 425.4 ± 268.9 mg/g creatinine in 14 healthy controls *2363*

592.00 Nephrolithiasis *(continued)*

1,25-Dihydroxy Vitamin D *Serum* *Increase* In 64 patients with low renal phosphate threshold in 18 with renal calculi mean concentration of 49.3 ± 2.8 pg/mL significantly different from 37.6 ± 1.9 pg/mL in 46 without renal lithiasis *4215*

Erythrocytes *Urine* *Increase* Microscopic hematuria is found *367*

Glomerular Filtration Rate *Urine* *No Effect* In 64 patients with low renal phosphate threshold in 18 with renal calculi mean clearance of 85 ± 3 mL/min/sq m not significantly different from 89 ± 2 mL/min/sq m in 46 without renal lithiasis *4215*

25-Hydroxy Vitamin D_3 *Serum* *Decrease* Significantly lower in 29 untreated patients with recurrent calcium containing kidney stones (15.8 ± 9.8 ng/mL) than in controls (23.6 ± 9.8 ng/mL). Deficiency is possible due to low milk diet followed by recurrent stone patients *5449*

ionized Calcium *Serum* *No Effect* In 64 patients with low renal phosphate threshold in 18 with renal calculi mean concentration of 1.20 ± 0.01 mmol/L not significantly different from 1.21 ± 0.02 mmol/L in 46 without renal lithiasis *4215*

Lactate Dehydrogenase *Urine* *No Effect* Usually within normal limits *5544*

Leukocytes *Urine* *Increase* Few to many WBCs and microscopic hematuria are found *367*

β-Lipoprotein *Serum* *Increase* With corresponding increase in beta:alpha ratio *5426*

Oxalate *Urine* *Increase* Mean excretion of 30.1 ± 10.8 mg/g creatinine observed in 26 patients with calcium nephrolithiasis significantly different when compared with 17.6 ± 8.3 mg/g creatinine in 14 healthy controls *2363*

Parathyroid Hormone *Plasma* *Decrease* In a study of 59 patients with normocalcemia and low intact PTH concentration, 3 had renal calciuria without hypercalciuria *3280*
Plasma *No Effect* In 64 patients with low renal phosphate threshold in 18 with renal calculi mean concentration of 33 ± 2 pg/mL not significantly different from 38 ± 2 pg/mL in 46 without renal lithiasis *4215*

Phosphate *Serum* *No Effect* In 64 patients with low renal phosphate threshold in 18 with renal calculi mean concentration of 0.79 ± 0.02 mmol/L not significantly different from 0.77 ± 0.02 mmol/L in 46 without renal lithiasis *4215*

Pyridoxine *Serum* *Decrease* A relationship may exist between deficient B_6 and endogenous oxalic acid production and stone formation *4707*

Thyroxine (T4) *Urine* *Decrease* In male renal calcium stone patients aged 20 - 40 years, urinary T4 is lower than in age-matched controls *4697*

Tubular Maximum for Phosphate *Urine* *No Effect* In 64 patients with low renal phosphate threshold in 18 with renal calculi mean $TmPO_4$ of 0.60 ± 0.02 mmol/L not significantly different from 0.58 ± 0.01 mmol/L in 46 without renal lithiasis *4215*

Uric Acid *Serum* *Decrease* Mean concentration of 5.6 ± 1.2 mg/dL observed in 26 patients with calcium nephrolithiasis compared with 6.7 ± 0.9 mg/dL in 14 healthy controls *2363*
Urine *No Effect* Mean excretion of 485.0 ± 184.3 mg/g creatinine observed in 26 patients with calcium nephrolithiasis compared with 447.8 ± 101.6 mg/g creatinine in 14 healthy controls *2363*

592.10 Ureter Calculus

Albumin *Urine* *Increase* The urinalysis often shows no significant alteration from normal but may progress through the stages of mild pyuria to moderate pyuria with albuminuria and onto frank infection or passage of renal casts *900*

Erythrocyte Casts *Urine* *Increase* The urinalysis often shows no significant alteration from normal but may progress through the stages of mild pyuria to moderate pyuria with albuminuria and onto frank infection or passage of renal casts *900*
Urine *No Effect* The urinalysis often shows no significant alteration from normal *900*

Leukocytes *Urine* *Increase* The urinalysis often shows no significant alteration from normal but may progress through the stages of mild pyuria to moderate pyuria with albuminuria and onto frank infection or passage of renal casts *900*
Urine *No Effect* Children usually have no WBC in their unspun microscopic urine examination. WBC are not always present in these lower tract obstructions even with moderate symptoms unless infection is present *900* Urinalysis often shows no significant alteration from normal *900*

593.20 Renal Cyst

Erythropoietin *Serum* *Increase* In 15 patients with polycythemia associated with renal cysts mean concentration of 19 ± 12 IU/L compared with 9 ± 4 IU/L in 79 reference controls *4320*

Hemoglobin *Blood* *Increase* In 15 patients with polycythemia associated with renal cysts mean concentration of 18.8 ± 1.46 g/dL compared with 14.0 ± 1.1 g/dL in 79 reference controls *4320*

593.70 Vesicoureteric Reflux

N-Acetyl-Glucosaminidase *Urine* *Increase* In 43 grade III patients mean activity of 6.024 U/g creatinine, in 28 grade IV patients 0.059 U/g creatinine and in 13 with grade V disease 17.290 IU/g creatinine compared with 4.98 ± 0.756 U/g creatinine in non-refluxing age and sex-matched controls *3534*

593.81 Renal Artery Embolism

Alanine Aminopeptidase *Urine* *Increase* In a patient with renal artery embolism mean concentration increased to 30 U/g creatinine 15 days after onset of symptoms, 19 U/g creatinine 24 days and 9 U/g creatinine 33 days after onset of symptoms (normal range of 0.9 - 6.9 U/g creatinine) *1205*

Amylase *Serum* *Increase* In a patient with renal artery embolism mean concentration increased from 326 U/L on admission to 537 U/L 7 days after onset of symptoms *1205*

Creatinine *Serum* *Increase* In a patient with renal artery embolism mean concentration increased from normal concentration to 19 mg/L 7 days after onset of symptoms *1205*

Creatinine Clearance *Urine* *Decrease* In a patient with renal artery embolism mean clearance decreased to 52 mL/min 7 days after onset of symptoms *1205*

Leukocytes *Blood* *Increase* In a patient with renal artery embolism mean concentration increased from 10,400 /μL on admission to 21,400 /μL 7 days after onset of symptoms *1205*

Lysozyme *Urine* *Increase* In a patient with renal artery embolism mean concentration increased to 1.9 mg/L 15 days after onset of symptoms (normal range of 0 - 0.3 mg/L) *1205*

N-Acetyl-Glucosaminidase *Urine* *Increase* In a patient with renal artery embolism mean concentration increased to 587 μmol/h/g creatinine 15 days after onset of symptoms, 524 μmol/h/g 24 days and 69 μmol/h/g creatinine 33 days after onset of symptoms *1205*

593.81 Renal Infarction

Alanine Aminotransferase *Serum* *Increase* Increased if area of infarction is large; peak by 2nd day; return to normal by 5th day with arterial infarction of kidney *5545*

Aspartate Aminotransferase *Serum* *Increase* Increased if area of infarction is large; peaks by 2nd day; returns to normal by 5th day with arterial infarction of kidney *5545* In unilateral renal arterial infarction. Reaches a peak within several days then gradually falls *4707*

C-Reactive Protein *Serum* *Increase* With large infarction *413*

Creatine Kinase *Serum* *No Effect* Activity usually normal *413*

Erythrocytes *Urine* *Increase* Common *413*

Lactate Dehydrogenase *Serum* *Increase* Occasional increase but to no clinically useful degree. May be increased markedly with arterial infarction of kidneys. Peak on 3rd day; return to normal by 10th day *5545* Observed in some patients *1025*
Urine *Increase* May be increased markedly with arterial infarction of kidney. LD peaks on 3rd day; returns to normal by 10th day *5545*

Leukocytes *Blood* *Increase* Increased if area of infarction is large; peaks by 2nd day; returns to normal by 5th day with arterial infarction of kidney *5545*

Protein *Urine* *Increase* Common *413*

593.89 Nephropathy, Obstructive

Ammonium Ions *Urine* *Decrease* May cause distal renal tubular acidosis (type IV) is associated with hyperkalemia, hyperchloremic metabolic acidosis, urine pH < 5.5, decreased urinary ammonium ion excretion, a positive urine anion gap, normal urinary citrate and urinary calcium excretion *4071*

Anion Gap *Urine* *Increase* May cause distal renal tubular acidosis (type IV) is associated with hyperkalemia, hyperchloremic metabolic acidosis, urine pH < 5.5, decreased urinary ammonium ion excretion, a positive urine anion gap, normal urinary citrate and urinary calcium excretion *4071*

Calcium *Urine* *No Effect* May cause distal renal tubular acidosis (type IV) is associated with hyperkalemia, hyperchloremic metabolic acidosis, urine pH < 5.5, decreased urinary ammonium ion excretion, a positive urine anion gap, normal urinary citrate and urinary calcium excretion *4071*

Chloride *Serum* *Increase* May cause distal renal tubular acidosis (type IV) is associated with hyperkalemia, hyperchloremic metabolic acidosis, urine pH < 5.5, decreased urinary ammonium ion excretion, a positive urine anion gap, normal urinary citrate and urinary calcium excretion *4071*

Citrate *Urine* *No Effect* May cause distal renal tubular acidosis (type IV) is associated with hyperkalemia, hyperchloremic metabolic acidosis, urine pH < 5.5, decreased urinary ammonium ion excretion, a positive urine anion gap, normal urinary citrate and urinary calcium excretion *4071*

pH *Urine* *Decrease* May cause distal renal tubular acidosis (type IV) is associated with hyperkalemia, hyperchloremic metabolic acidosis, urine pH < 5.5, decreased urinary ammonium ion excretion, a positive urine anion gap, normal urinary citrate and urinary calcium excretion *4071*

Potassium *Serum* *Increase* May cause distal renal tubular acidosis (type IV) which is associated with hyperkalemia, hyperchloremic metabolic acidosis, urine pH < 5.5, decreased urinary ammonium ion excretion, a positive urine anion gap, normal urinary citrate and urinary calcium excretion *4071*

593.90 Renal Dysfunction

Deoxypyridinoline *Urine* *Increase* In 22 patients with renal dysfunction mean excretion of 8.75 ± 7.23 nmol/mmol creatinine compared with 5.71 ± 1.59 nmol/mmol creatinine in 79 healthy controls as measured by assay on Ciba Corning ACS:180 system *804*

Deoxypyridinoline, Free *Urine* *No Effect* Mean excretion in 26 patients aged 28 - 76 years of approximately 4.5 nmol/mol creatinine not significantly different from approximately 4.0 nmol/mol creatinine in healthy controls *4383*

Immunoglobulin E *Serum* *Increase* In 10 trauma patients with renal dysfunction mean concentration significantly greater than in 90 patients who did not develop renal dysfunction *1177*

593.90 Salt-wasting Nephritis

Ammonium Ions *Urine* *Decrease* May cause distal renal tubular acidosis (type IV) is associated with hyperkalemia, hyperchloremic metabolic acidosis, urine pH < 5.5, decreased urinary ammonium ion excretion, a positive urine anion gap, normal urinary citrate and urinary calcium excretion *4071*

Anion Gap *Urine* *Increase* May cause distal renal tubular acidosis (type IV) is associated with hyperkalemia, hyperchloremic metabolic acidosis, urine pH < 5.5, decreased urinary ammonium ion excretion, a positive urine anion gap, normal urinary citrate and urinary calcium excretion *4071*

Calcium *Urine* *No Effect* May cause distal renal tubular acidosis (type IV) is associated with hyperkalemia, hyperchloremic metabolic acidosis, urine pH < 5.5, decreased urinary ammonium ion excretion, a positive urine anion gap, normal urinary citrate and urinary calcium excretion *4071*

Chloride *Serum* *Increase* May cause distal renal tubular acidosis (type IV) is associated with hyperkalemia, hyperchloremic metabolic acidosis, urine pH < 5.5, decreased urinary ammonium ion excretion, a positive urine anion gap, normal urinary citrate and urinary calcium excretion *4071*

Citrate *Urine* *No Effect* May cause distal renal tubular acidosis (type IV) is associated with hyperkalemia, hyperchloremic metabolic acidosis, urine pH < 5.5, decreased urinary ammonium ion excretion, a positive urine anion gap, normal urinary citrate and urinary calcium excretion *4071*

pH *Urine* *Decrease* May cause distal renal tubular acidosis (type IV) is associated with hyperkalemia, hyperchloremic metabolic acidosis, urine pH < 5.5, decreased urinary ammonium ion excretion, a positive urine anion gap, normal urinary citrate and urinary calcium excretion *4071*

Potassium *Serum* *Increase* May cause distal renal tubular acidosis (type IV) which is associated with hyperkalemia, hyperchloremic metabolic acidosis, urine pH < 5.5, decreased urinary ammonium ion excretion, a positive urine anion gap, normal urinary citrate and urinary calcium excretion *4071*

594.10 Bladder Calculus

β-Chorionic Gonadotropin *Urine* *Increase* In 7 patients with bladder calculus mean excretion of 1.21 ± 0.37 mIU/mL not significantly increased compared with 1.13 ± 0.08 mIU/mL in 31 normal controls *1964*

595.00 Acute Cystitis

Fibrin Degradation Products (D-Dimer) *Urine* *Increase* FDP-D detected in the urine of one third of patients with acute pyelonephritis *4557*

597.80 Urethritis

Bicarbonate *Serum* *Decrease* Reveals the degree of renal impairment *900*

Calcium *Serum* *Decrease* Reveals the degree of renal impairment *900*

Chloride *Serum* *Increase* Reveals the degree of renal impairment *900*

Creatinine *Serum* *Increase* Reveals the degree of renal impairment *900*

Leukocytes *Urine* *Increase* Renal impairment *900*

Phosphate *Serum* *Increase* Reveals the degree of renal impairment *900*

Potassium *Serum* *Increase* Reveals the degree of renal impairment *900*

Sodium *Serum* *Decrease* Reveals the degree of renal impairment *900*

Urea Nitrogen *Serum* *Increase* Reveals the degree of renal impairment *900*

599.00 Urinary Tract Infection

α_1-Acid Glycoprotein *Serum* *Increase* In 22 hospitalized children aged 1 to 14 years mean concentration at time of admission of 1.96 g/L compared with less than 0.50 g/L in normals *717* In 28 adult patients with urinary tract infection mean concentration on admission to hospital of 2.05 ± 0.45 g/L compared with less than 0.50 g/L in 30 healthy controls *721*

Amyloid A Protein *Serum* *Increase* In 10 patients mean concentration in acute phase of 2.16 ± 0.73 mg/L *3728* In 22 hospitalized children aged 1 to 14 years at time of admission mean concentration of 1,084 mg/L compared with normal of less than 1 mg/L *717* In 28 adults with urinary tract infection mean concentration on admission to hospital of 829 ± 73 mg/L compared with normal of less than 1.5 mg/L *721*

Angiotensin-converting Enzyme *Urine* *Increase* Activity was found to be significantly elevated *534*

α_1-Antichymotrypsin *Serum* *Increase* In 28 adult patients with urinary tract infection mean concentration on admission to hospital of 1.26 ± 0.30 g/L compared with less than 0.50 g/L in

599.00 Urinary Tract Infection *(continued)*

α_1-Antichymotrypsin *(continued)*
30 healthy controls *721* In 22 hospitalized children aged 1 to 14 years mean concentration at time of admission of 1.11 g/L compared with normal of less than 0.50 g/L *717*

Casts *Urine* *Increase* In uncomplicated acute symptomatic infections, urine sediment usually contains numbers of pus cells and WBC casts *1980*

C-Reactive Protein *Serum* *Increase* In 22 hospitalized children aged 1 to 14 years mean concentration at time of admission of 122 mg/L compared with normal of less than 3 mg/L *717* In 28 adult patients with urinary tract infection mean concentration on admission to hospital 190 ± 52 mg/L compared with normal of less than 3 mg/L *721* In 10 patients mean concentration in acute phase of 1.39 ± 0.78 mg/L *3728*
Urine *Increase* In 20 patients with urinary tract infection mean concentration of 6 - 460 µg/L significantly different from < 6 µg/L in 34 patients with normal courses *4994*
Urine *No Effect* In 20 patients with urinary tract infection mean concentration of < 6 µg/L not significantly different from < 6 µg/L in 34 patients with normal courses *4994*

Erythrocyte Casts *Urine* *No Effect* A variable number of RBCs may be present, but there are no RBC casts *1980*

Erythrocytes *Urine* *Increase* A variable number of RBCs may be present, but there are no RBC casts *1980*

Fibrin Degradation Products *Plasma* *Increase* Elevation is much more common in fatal cases than in survivors *4881*

β-Glucuronidase *Urine* *Increase* Of the 13 patients with positive bladder and negative ureteral cultures, 6 showed elevated activity. The mean value was 29.5 ± 15.7 U. Of 25 ureteral specimens (right or left) with negative cultures, 7 showed elevated activity (mean 25.5 ± 10.8 U) *1805*

Immunoglobulin A *Urine* *Increase* Mean concentration of 3.3 mg/24 h. Secretory IgA locally produced in the bladder *2587*

Interleukin-1 *Urine* *No Effect* A concomitant study revealed increases in urine IL-6, but not IL-1β, and tumor necrosis factor-α levels in patients with UTI *2727*

Interleukin-6 *Urine* *Increase* A concomitant study revealed increases in urine IL-6, but not IL-1β, and tumor necrosis factor-α levels in patients with UTI *2727*

Interleukin-8 *Urine* *Increase* Of 113 patients, 112 had elevated levels of IL-8 in their urine (1,078.0 ± 181.5 pg/mL), regardless of whether they had an upper or lower UTI; this was in contrast to undetectable levels (less than 16 pg/mL) in the urine of all of the 20 normal individuals and 74 control patients without UTI *2727*

Leukocytes *Urine* *Increase* In uncomplicated acute symptomatic infections, urine sediment usually contains numbers of pus cells and WBC casts *1980*

α_2-Macroglobulin *Urine* *Increase* In 29 patients with urinary tract infection mean concentrations of 220 - 9,000 µg/L significantly different from < 180 µg/L in 34 patients with normal courses *4994*
Urine *No Effect* In 11 patients with urinary tract infection mean concentration of < 180 µg/L not significantly different from < 180 µg/L in 34 patients with normal courses *4994*

Myeloperoxidase *Urine* *Increase* In 40 patients with urinary tract infection mean concentration of 730 µg/L significantly different from < 200 µg/L in 34 renal transplant patients with normal courses *4994*

Neutrophils *Urine* *Increase* The median values for polymorphonuclear granulocytes were > 90% in bacterial renal or urinary tract disease and in polycystic kidney disease *3071*

Protein *Urine* *Increase* Proteinuria to the extent of +2 (usually < 2 g/d) occurs *1980*

Tumor Necrosis Factor-α *Urine* *No Effect* A concomitant study revealed no increase in patients with UTI *2727*

599.60 Urinary Tract Obstruction

Ammonium Ions *Urine* *Increase* May be associated with voltage-dependent distal renal tubular acidosis which is associated with hyerkalemia, hyperchloremic metabolic acidosis, urine pH > 5.5, increased urinary ammonium ion excretion, a positive urine anion gap, increased urinary osmol gap, low urinary citrate and high or normal urinary calcium excretion *4071*

Anion Gap *Urine* *Decrease* May be associated with voltage-dependent distal renal tubular acidosis which is associated with hyerkalemia, hyperchloremic metabolic acidosis, urine pH > 5.5, increased urinary ammonium ion excretion, a positive urine anion gap, increased urinary osmol gap, low urinary citrate and high or normal urinary calcium excretion *4071*

Calcium *Urine* *Increase* May be associated with voltage-dependent distal renal tubular acidosis which is associated with hyerkalemia, hyperchloremic metabolic acidosis, urine pH > 5.5, increased urinary ammonium ion excretion, a positive urine anion gap, increased urinary osmol gap, low urinary citrate and high or normal urinary calcium excretion *4071*

Chloride *Serum* *Increase* May be associated with voltage-dependent distal renal tubular acidosis which is associated with hyerkalemia, hyperchloremic metabolic acidosis, urine pH > 5.5, increased urinary ammonium ion excretion, a positive urine anion gap, increased urinary osmol gap, low urinary citrate and high or normal urinary calcium excretion *4071*

Citrate *Urine* *Decrease* May be associated with voltage-dependent distal renal tubular acidosis which is associated with hyerkalemia, hyperchloremic metabolic acidosis, urine pH > 5.5, increased urinary ammonium ion excretion, a positive urine anion gap, increased urinary osmol gap, low urinary citrate and high or normal urinary calcium excretion *4071*

Net Acid Excretion *Urine* *Increase* May be associated with voltage-dependent distal renal tubular acidosis which is associated with hyerkalemia, hyperchloremic metabolic acidosis, urine pH > 5.5, increased urinary ammonium ion excretion, a positive urine anion gap, increased urinary osmol gap, low urinary citrate and high or normal urinary calcium excretion *4071*

Osmolal Gap *Urine* *Decrease* May be associated with voltage-dependent distal renal tubular acidosis which is associated with hyerkalemia, hyperchloremic metabolic acidosis, urine pH > 5.5, increased urinary ammonium ion excretion, a positive urine anion gap, increased urinary osmol gap, low urinary citrate and high or normal urinary calcium excretion *4071*

pH *Urine* *Increase* May be associated with voltage-dependent distal renal tubular acidosis which is associated with hyerkalemia, hyperchloremic metabolic acidosis, urine pH > 5.5, increased urinary ammonium ion excretion, a positive urine anion gap, increased urinary osmol gap, low urinary citrate and high or normal urinary calcium excretion *4071*

Potassium *Serum* *Increase* May be associated with voltage-dependent distal renal tubular acidosis which is associated with hyerkalemia, hyperchloremic metabolic acidosis, urine pH > 5.5, increased urinary ammonium ion excretion, a positive urine anion gap, increased urinary osmol gap, low urinary citrate and high or normal urinary calcium excretion *4071*

Prostate-specific Antigen *Serum* *Increase* Large increases observed in patients with obstructive uropathy in the absence of malignant disease *3407*

599.90 Benign Urinary Tract Disorders

BTA TRAK *Urine* *Increase* Mean concentration of 32.6 U/mL in patients with benign genitourinary tract disease significantly greater than 4.1 U/mL in healthy blood donors *539*

β-Chorionic Gonadotropin *Urine* *Increase* In 64 patients with benign urinary tract disorders mean excretion of 1.49 ± 0.15 mIU/mL significantly increased compared with 1.13 ± 0.08 mIU/mL in 31 normal controls *1964*

Nuclear Matrix Protein 22 *Urine* *Increase* Median concentration of 4.4 U/mL significantly different from 2.9 U/mL in healthy blood donors *539*

599.90 Genitourinary Tract Disease

α-Fetoprotein *Serum* *No Effect* In 42 patients with nonmalignant genitourinary tract disease 100.0% had concentrations up to 15.0 ng/mL in comparison with concentrations in 400 healthy individuals in whom 99.2% had concentrations between 0 and 15.0 ng/mL, 0.2% between 15.1 and 20.0 ng/mL and 0.5%% between 20.1 and 100 ng/mL *11*

Nuclear Matrix Protein 22 *Urine* *No Effect* Mean concentration of 3.3 U/mL in 117 patients with benign genitourinary tract disease not significantly different from 2.9 U/mL in 175 volunteers *1534*

Prostate-specific Antigen *Serum Increase* In 101 men with nonmalignant genitourinary tract disease 86.1% had concentrations between 0 and 4.0 ng/mL, 8.9% between 4.1 and 10.0 ng/mL and 5.0% between 10.1 and 30.0 ng/mL compared with upper limit of normal of 4.0 ng/mL *11*

599.90 Nonmalignant Urogenital Disease

Prostate-specific Antigen *Serum Increase* Of 102 patients with nonmalignant urogenital disease 69.4% had values below upper limit of normal of 4.0 ng/mL as measured by method on Bayer Technicon Immuno 1®, 21.6% had values between 4.0 and 10.0 ng/mL and 8.8% had values between 10.0 and 40.0 ng/mL *342*

600.00 Benign Prostatic Hypertrophy

Acid Phosphatase *Serum Increase* Ordinary digital rectal palpation of the prostate produced significantly raised activities in 3 of 24 patients *1008* May have slight elevations after vigorous prostatic massage *1025* Elevated in 7% of 141 cases *3677*

Acid Phosphatase, Prostatic *Serum Increase* Approximately 10% of patients with benign prostatic disease have increased prostatic acid phosphatase activity *228*

Acid Phosphatase, Tartrate Inhibitable *Serum Increase* In 59 specimens from patients with BPH mean activity of 2.64 ± 0.55 U/L significantly higher than 1.95 ± 0.89 U/L in 300 specimens from healthy men. Ratio of serum tartrate-inhibitable acid phosphatase to total protein in 59 specimens from patients with BPH 46.64 ± 7.82 nU/g compared with 19.14 ± 8.44 nU/g in 300 specimens from healthy control men *4101*

Adenosine-N6-diethylthioether-N1-pyridinoximine 5'-phosphate *Serum No Effect* In 3 patients with BPH, concentrations ranged from 61.2 - 205.4 nmol/dL not significantly different from concentration in healthy individuals in whom the mean concentration was 162.2 nmol/dL *5294*

Albumin *Urine Increase* The urinalysis may be completely normal or may reveal albuminuria, pyuria, and hematuria as a result of obstruction with infection or stone formation *900*

Amylase *Serum Increase* Reported in 95% of patients with benign disease and 70% of carcinomas. Similar results have not been reported elsewhere *1996*

Androgens *Plasma Increase* Increased testosterone; especially in older patients *1993*

Cholesterol *Serum Increase* In patients with residual urine, nonesterified cholesterol was elevated in 42.1% and total levels in 61.4%. Patients with no residual urine had normal cholesterol *2503*

β-Chorionic Gonadotropin *Urine Increase* In 8 patients with prostatic hyperplasia mean excretion of 1.37 ± 0.17 mIU/mL significantly increased compared with 1.13 ± 0.08 mIU/mL in 31 normal controls *1964*

Creatinine *Serum Increase* In 246 patients with BPH mean creatinine concentration was 1.12 mg/dL with 11% having increased concentrations which occurred twice as often in the men with a history of diabetes or hypertension *1701* In 53% of 58 patients at initial hospitalization for this disorder *1576*

Erythrocytes *Urine Increase* The urinalysis may be completely normal or may reveal albuminuria, pyuria, and hematuria as a result of obstruction with infection or stone formation *900*
Urine No Effect The urinalysis may be completely normal or may reveal albuminuria, pyuria, and hematuria as a result of obstruction with infection or stone formation *900*

Estradiol *Urine No Effect* No significant difference observed between excretions in healthy middle-aged men and those with BPH *4275*

Estriol *Urine No Effect* No significant difference in excretion between middle-aged normal men and those with BPH *4275*

Estrone *Urine No Effect* No significant difference observed in excretions between healthy middle-aged men and those with BPH *4275*

Free Prostate-specific Antigen:Total Prostate-specific Antigen Ratio *Serum Decrease* Median of 0.2 (range of 0.041 - 0.485) in 99 patients with benign prostatic hyperpasia. At PSA concentration of < 4 ng/mL median ratio of 0.2, in range of 4 - 10 ng/mL median of 0.22 and over 10 ng/mL 0.15 *3006*
Serum Increase In 156 patients with BPH mean ratio of 0.195 ± 0.09 significantly higher than cutoff of 0.13 *1481*
Serum No Effect In 53 men with benign prostatic hypertrophy mean ratio of 21.7 ± 10.3 not significantly different from that in 35 healthy individuals *5451*

Gonadotropin, Pituitary *Plasma Decrease* Patients with both malignant and benign prostatic disease showed lower concentrations of luteinizing hormone when compared with age-matched controls *1992*

Hematocrit *Blood Decrease* Anemia may be present secondary to uremia *900*

Hemoglobin *Blood Decrease* Anemia may be present secondary to uremia *900*

Insulin-like Growth Factor *Serum Increase* Median concentration in 12 patients with cancer of the prostate of 482 ± 39 µg/L significantly different from 358 ± 50 µg/L in 7 patients with no known prostate abnormality *2181*

Insulin-like Growth Factor-I *Serum No Effect* Median concentration in 12 patients with cancer of the prostate of 124 ± 18 µg/L not significantly different from 117 ± 17 µg/L in 7 patients with no known prostate abnormality *2181*

Insulin-like Growth Factor-II *Serum Increase* Median concentration in 12 patients with cancer of the prostate of 359 ± 26 µg/L significantly different from 241 ± 37 µg/L in 7 patients with no known prostate abnormality *2181*

Insulin-like Growth Factor Binding Protein-2
Serum No Effect Median concentration in 12 patients with cancer of the prostate of 364 ± 61 µg/L not significantly different from 367 ± 44 µg/L in 7 patients with no known prostate abnormality *2181*

Insulin-like Growth Factor Binding Protein-3
Serum Increase Median concentration in 12 patients with cancer of the prostate of 2,871 ± 386 µg/L significantly different from 1,909 ± 364 µg/L in 7 patients with no known prostate abnormality *2181*

Interleukin-8 *Serum No Effect* In 53 men with benign prostatic hypertrophy mean concentration of 6.5 pg/mL not significantly different from that in 35 healthy individuals in whom the mean concentration was 6.8 ± 3.6 pg/mL *5451*

Leukocytes *Urine Increase* The urinalysis may be completely normal or may reveal albuminuria, pyuria, and hematuria as a result of obstruction with infection or stone formation *900*
Urine No Effect The urinalysis may be completely normal or may reveal albuminuria, pyuria, and hematuria as a result of obstruction with infection or stone formation *900*

Luteinizing Hormone *Plasma Decrease* Patients with both malignant and benign prostatic disease showed lower concentrations when compared with age-matched controls *1992*

Matrix Metalloproteinase-2 *Serum No Effect* Mean concentration of 580.8 ± 162.2 ng/mL in 76 patients with benign prostatic hypertrophy not significantly different from 538.0 ± 91.2 ng/mL in 70 healthy controls *1772*

Metallopanstimulin *Serum Increase* In 54% of 37 patients with benign prostatic hypertrophy mean concentration exceeded upper limit of normal of < 10 ng/mL in healthy individuals aged 19 - 88 years *1462*

Monocytes *Blood Increase* In 63% of 73 patients at initial hospitalization for this disorder *1576*

Neutrophils *Blood Increase* In 44% of 73 patients at initial hospitalization for this disorder *1576*

Pro-Kallikrein 2 *Serum Increase* In 63 patients with benign prostatic hypertrophy mean concentration of 0.09 µg/L (range of 0.0 - 0.78 µg/L) significantly higher than 0.02 µg/L (range of 0.0 - 0.08 µg/L) in 20 healthy men *4500*

Progesterone *Plasma Increase* Increased; especially in older patients *1993*

Prostate Secretory Protein *Serum Increase* Concentration increased in 20 of 49 patients with BPH, with a range in all patients of 0.6 - 27.6 µg/L compared with mean of 5.8 µg/L (SD 3.8) in men of 50 years of age or older *2266*

Prostate-specific Antigen *Serum Decrease* Patients with BPH typically had low basal concentrations with small increases following digital rectal examination *5221*
Serum Increase In 48 patients, biopsy proved negative for cancer, mean concentration as determined by Delphia assay of 8.9 µg/L (range 2.7 - 39.1) *4211* Median of 6.7 ng/mL (range 1 - 24 ng/mL) in 99 patients with benign prostatic hyperplasia

600.00 Benign Prostatic Hypertrophy *(continued)*

Prostate-specific Antigen *(continued)*
3006 In 7 patients with consistently high PSA concentrations above 20 ng/mL for 34 months 4 of 15 biopsies showed benign prostatic hypertrophy *2670* In 26 patients with prostatic hyperplasia and chronic inflammation mean concentration of 5.6 ng/mL compared with 2.1 ng/mL in 81 men undergoing prostatic resection for bladder outlet obstruction *4181* In men with BPH concentration increases by about 0.3 ng/mL per gram of tissue *4370* In 63 patients with benign prostatic hypertrophy mean concentration of 5.17 µg/L (range of 0.24 -22.9 µg/L) compared with mean of 0.43 µg/L (range of 0.03 - 1.73 µg/L) in healthy men *4500* In 476 men with benign prostatic hypertrophy, 45.8% of values less than 2.5 ng/mL, 11.1% between 2.6 and 4.0 ng/mL, 29.2% between 4.0 and 10.0 ng/mL, 13.5% between 10 and 40 ng/mL and 0.4% over 40 ng/mL: similar values with BPH with prostatitis *489* Elevated in 21% to 68% of cases *4267* In 156 patients with BPH mean concentration of 4.77 ± 4.42 µg/L higher than upper limit of normal of 4.0 µg/L *1481* In 121 patients who had transurethral prostatectomy performed for BPH mean concentration of 4.5 ng/mL, median 2.6 ng/mL and 1 SD 7.2 ng/mL *877* 25 - 30% of patients with BPH have concentrations of PSA above 4 ng/mL *1254* Median concentration in 12 patients with cancer of the prostate of 2.0 µg/L significantly different from 0.6 µg/L in 7 patients with no known prostate abnormality *2181* In 43 patients with BPH mean concentration as determined by Hybritech enzyme immunoassay 7.6 ng/mL (range 1.0 to 45.7) *5031* In 209 men with BPH 78.5% had concentrations between 0 and 4.0 ng/mL, 16.3% between 4.1 and 10.0 ng/mL, 4.3% between 10.1 and 30.0 ng/mL and 1.0% between 30.1 - 60.0 ng/mLcompared with upper limit of normal of 4.0 ng/mL *11* Of 303 men with benign prostatic hypertrophy 60.1% had values below upper limit of normal of 4.0 ng/mL as measured by method on Bayer Technicon Immuno 1®, 28.4% had values between 4.0 and 10.0 ng/mL and 11.6% had values between 10.0 and 40.0 ng/mL *342* More than 15% of patients with benign prostatic hypertrophy have increased activity *228* Elevated in 21% to 68% of cases *2273*
Serum No Effect In 53 men with benign prostatic hypertrophy mean concentration of 7.1 ± 4.0 ng/mL not significantly different from that in 35 healthy individuals *5451*

Prostate-specific Antigen, Free *Serum Increase* In 63 patients with benign prostatic hypertrophy mean concentration of 0.86 µg/L (range of 0.0 - 5.12 µg/L) *4500* In 48 patients, biopsy proved negative for cancer, mean concentration as determined by Delphia assay of 8.9 µg/L (range 2.7 - 39.1) with free percentage of 17.1 ± 6.2% (median 16.5%) *4211*

Prostatic Inhibin-like Peptide *Plasma Increase* Concentration significantly increased to mean of 107.8 ± 19 ng/mL from 10.2 ± 1 ng/mL in control men and 88.7 ± 9 ng/mL in men with prostatic cancer *5194*
Urine Increase In patients with benign prostatic hyperplasia mean concentration of 294 ± 49 µg/d compared with very low excretion of 23.6 ± 5 µg/d in prostatic cancer and 137.6 ± 10 µg/d in healthy control men *5194*

Protein *Serum Decrease* In 59 specimens from patients with BPH, mean concentration of 65.81 ± 9.56 g/L compared with 72.88 ± 8.03 g/L in 300 normal specimens *4101*
Urine Increase Normal or increased *413*
Urine No Effect Normal or increased *413*

Soluble CD44 Splice Variant 5 *Serum Decrease* Mean concentration in 30 patients with benign prostatic hypertrophy of 34 ± 15 µg/L significantly different from 54 ± 23 µg/L in 30 control men *2988*
Serum No Effect Mean concentration in 30 patients with BPH not significantly different from that in healthy men of 54.1 ± 22.7 µg/L *2507*

Soluble CD44 Splice Variant 6 *Serum Decrease* Mean concentration in 30 patients with BPH, of 159 ± 38 µg/L not significantly different from 179 ± 64 µg/L in 30 control men *2988*
Serum No Effect Mean concentration in 30 patients with BPH not significantly different from that in healthy men of 179 ± 64 µg/L *2507*

Soluble CD44 Standard *Serum No Effect* Mean concentration in 30 patients with BPH, of 499 ± 130 µg/L not significantly different from 501 ± 87 µg/L in 30 control men *2988* Mean concentration in 30 patients with BPH not significantly different from that in healthy men of 501 ± 87 µg/L *2507*

Testosterone *Serum Decrease* In 11 patients with BPH, mean concentration as measured by DPC radioimmunoassay was 336 ng/dL (range 250 to 597) *5031*
Serum Increase Increased; especially in older patients *1993*

Transforming Growth Factor-β_1 *Serum No Effect* In 10 patients with BPH median concentration of 26.9 ng/mL significantly different from value in matched healthy controls *5711*

Urea Nitrogen *Serum Increase* In 29% of 80 patients at initial hospitalization for this disorder *1576*

Uric Acid *Serum Increase* In 48% of 80 patients at initial hospitalization for this disorder *1576*

601.00 Acute Prostatitis

Prostate-specific Antigen *Serum Increase* In 16 patients with acute prostatitis mean concentration of 5.6 ng/mL compared with 2.1 ng/mL in 81 men undergoing prostatic resection for bladder outlet obstruction *4181* In 7 patients with consistently high PSA concentrations above 20 ng/mL for 34 months 5 of 15 biopsies showed acute prostatitis *2670* In 24 patients with acute bacterial prostatitis mean concentration of 23.4 µg/L (range 8.9 to 63.2) compared with < 4 µg/L in 12 healthy volunteers *1261*

Prostate-specific Membrane Antigen Reverse Transcriptase Assay *Plasma Increase* In 24 patients with acute bacterial prostatitis 10 (41.6%) had a positive assay compared with none of 12 healthy volunteers *1261*

601.10 Chronic Prostatitis

Prostate-specific Antigen *Serum Increase* In 7 patients with consistently high PSA concentrations above 20 ng/mL for 34 months 7 of 15 biopsies showed chronic prostatitis *2670*

601.90 Prostatitis

Amylase *Serum Increase* Moderate increase in total concentration *5580*

Aspartate Aminotransferase *Serum Increase* In 26% of 15 patients at initial hospitalization for this disorder *1576*

Eosinophils *Blood Increase* In 45% of 13 patients at initial hospitalization for this disorder *1576*

Isocitrate Dehydrogenase *Serum No Effect* No significant effect on activity observed *5008*

Leukocytes *Prostatic Fluid Increase* In the chronic form, prostatic fluid usually shows 10 - 15 WBCs (pus cells) with prostatitis *5545* Since the presence of increased number of leukocytes and oval fat bodies are seen equally in cases of chronic bacterial prostatitis and nonbacterial prostatitis, the microscopic appearance of the expressed prostatic secretions is not specifically diagnostic *900*
Urine Increase Following prostatic massage the last portion of voided urine shows an increased WBC compared with the first portion *413*

Neutrophils *Blood Increase* In 30% of 13 patients at initial hospitalization for this disorder *1576*

Oval Fat Bodies *Prostatic Fluid Increase* Since the presence of increased number of leukocytes and oval fat bodies are seen equally in cases of chronic bacterial prostatitis and nonbacterial prostatitis, the microscopic appearance of the expressed prostatic secretions is not specifically diagnostic *900*

pH *Prostatic Fluid Increase* The pH of prostatic secretions of males with chronic bacterial prostatitis reached a mean value of 8.1 during inflammation. Values for males without inflammatory prostatic disease was 6.7 *4116*

Prostate-specific Antigen *Serum Increase* In 80 men with prostatitis 81.2% had concentrations between 0 and 4.0 ng/mL, 12.5% between 4.1 and 10.0 ng/mL and 6.2% between 10.1 and 30.0 ng/mL compared with upper limit of normal of 4.0 ng/mL *11* In 72 men with mean age of 39 y PSA concentration was increased above 4 ng/mL in 5 of 7 patients with acute bacterial prostatitis, 2 of 13 patients with chronic bacterial prostatitis and 2 of 32 patients with abacterial prostatitis and none of 20 patients with prostatodynia *3992* Elevated due to acute bacterial prostatitis in 2 patients *4267* *1002* Prostatitis can cause up to a fivefold increase in PSA independent of any associated cancer of the prostate *1543*

Protein *Prostatic Fluid* *Decrease* Average amount of protein and protein-like substance was low at 28.0 g/L, range 15.0 - 37.7, compared to normal 42.6, range 37.5-64 *207*

602.80 Prostatic Infarction

Acid Phosphatase *Serum* *Increase* Sometimes to high levels *5544*

Prostate-specific Antigen *Serum* *Increase* Reported effect *4267*

602.90 Benign Prostatic Disease

CA 549 *Serum* *No Effect* In 81 patients with benign disease of the prostate none had a concentration greater than 30.0 kU/L with BRESMARQ assay *764*

Carcinoembryonic Antigen *Serum* *Increase* In 24 men with benign prostate disease 87.5% had concentrations of 0.0 - 3.0 ng/mL, 12.5% had concentrations from 3.1 - 5.0 ng/mL, 0.0% had concentrations from 5.1 - 10.0 ng/mL and 0.0% had concentrations greater than 10.0 ng/mL when measured by method on Bayer Technicon Immuno 1® system compared with 95.9%, 3.5%, 0.6% and 0.0% respectively in 173 healthy nonsmokers *339*

Prostate-specific Antigen *Serum* *No Effect* In 103 patients with benign prostate disease mean concentration of 4.46 ± 5.90 μg/L *80*

Prostate-specific Antigen, Complexed *Serum* *No Effect* In 103 patients with benign prostate disease mean concentration of 3.89 ± 5.48 μg/L *80*

Prostate-specific Antigen, Free *Serum* *No Effect* In 103 patients with benign prostate disease mean concentration of 0.85 ± 1.01 μg/L *80*

606.90 Infertility in Males

Cadmium *Serum* *No Effect* No significant difference from fertile male controls *4981*

Copper *Serum* *Increase* Infertile men (n = 8) had higher mean concentrations than those of proven fertility (n = 38). The difference was statistically significant. (P < 0.01) but was of small magnitude (about 1.5 μmol/L) *4981*

5-Hydroxytryptamine *Plasma* *Increase* Concentration increased in psychogenic infertile men *2955*

immunoglobulin A *Semen* *Increase* 20 Patients tested and 50% were positive for sperm-bound IgA *859*

Immunoglobulin G *Semen* *Positive* 20 Patients tested and 100% were positive for sperm-bound IgG *859*

Immunoglobulin M *Semen* *No Effect* 20 patients tested and 0% positive for sperm-bound IgM *859*

Inhibin-A *Plasma* *No Effect* Concentration undetectable in 29 men with primary testicular disease of varying causes with increased plasma FSH, as in 16 healthy men aged 19 - 45 y *113*

Inhibin-B *Plasma* *Decrease* Mean concentration of 37 ± 6 pg/mL in 29 men with infertility of varying causes with increased plasma FSH concentration significantly less than 187 ± 28 pg/mL in 16 healthy men aged 19 - 45 y *113*

Interleukin-2 *Semen* *Increase* In the seminal plasma of 23 infertile men the mean concentration was 443.3 ± 40.5 fmol/mL significantly greater than 251.3 ± 42.7 fmol/mL in the seminal plasma of 20 fertile men *4000*

Lead *Blood* *No Effect* No significant difference from fertile male controls *4981*
Red Blood Cells *No Effect* No significant difference between fertile and infertile males *4981*

Leukocytes *Semen* *Increase* In the seminal plasma of 23 infertile men the mean count was 1 - 20 x 10^5/mL significantly different from < 2 x 10^5/mL in the seminal plasma of 20 fertile men *4000*

Pro-α-C-related Peptide *Plasma* *Decrease* Mean concentration of approximately 700 pg/mL in 29 men with infertility of varying causes with increased plasma FSH concentration not significantly different from 880 pg/mL in 16 healthy men aged 19 - 45 y *113*

Prolactin *Plasma* *Increase* Four patients with oligospermia were found to have slightly to moderately elevated levels *5718* Hyperprolactinemia observed in psychogenic infertile men in association with hyperserotoninemia *2955*

Sperm Count *Semen* *Decrease* In the seminal plasma of 23 infertile men the mean sperm count was 0 - 18 x 10^6/mL significantly different from > 20 x 10^6/mL in the seminal plasma of 20 fertile men *4000* Count decreased in psychogenic infertile men in association with hyperserotoninemia *2955*

Sperm Morphology *Semen* *Decrease* In the seminal plasma of 23 infertile men the mean sperm normal morphology was 10 - 60% significantly different from > 50% in the seminal plasma of 20 fertile men *4000*

Sperm Motility *Semen* *Decrease* In the seminal plasma of 23 infertile men the mean sperm motility was 0 - 60% significantly different from > 50% in the seminal plasma of 20 fertile men *4000* Motility decreased in psychogenic infertile men in association with hyperserotoninemia *2955*

Volume *Semen* *No Effect* In the seminal plasma of 23 infertile men the mean ejaculate volume was 1.4 - 6.0 mL not significantly different from 1.8 - 6.5 mL in the seminal plasma of 20 fertile men *4000*

Zinc *Red Blood Cells* *No Effect* No significant difference between fertile and infertile males *4981*
Serum *No Effect* No significant difference from fertile male controls *4981*

607.89 Peyronie's Disease

Anti-α-Elastin Antibodies *Serum* *Increase* In 8 patients with Peyronie's disease mean optical density of 1.377 ± 0.078 significantly higher than 0.979 ± 0.051 in 8 healthy controls *5015*

Anti-Tropoelastin Antibodies *Serum* *Increase* In 8 patients with Peyronie's disease mean optical density of 1.053 ± 0.142 significantly higher than 0.811 ± 0.144 in 8 healthy controls *5015*

Type 1 Anti-Collagen Antibodies *Serum* *No Effect* In 8 patients with Peyronie's disease mean optical density of 0.638 ± 0.066 not significantly higher than 0.537 ± 0.055 in 8 healthy controls *5015*

Type 2 Anti-Collagen Antibodies *Serum* *No Effect* In 8 patients with Peyronie's disease mean optical density of 1.166 ± 0.099 not significantly higher than 1.049 ± 0.099 in 8 healthy controls *5015*

610.10 Fibrocystic Disease of Breast

Apolipoprotein A-I *Serum* *No Effect* In 23 women with fibrocystic disease of the breast mean concentration of 157.2 ± 8.9 mg/dL not significantly different from 167.5 ± 11.0 mg/dL in 13 women with benign breast masses *2910*

Apolipoprotein A-I:Apolipoprotein B Ratio
Serum *Decrease* In 23 women with fibrocystic disease of the breast mean concentration of 1.8 ± 0.1 significantly different from 2.4 ± 0.3 in 13 women with benign breast masses *2910*

Apolipoprotein A-II *Serum* *Increase* In 23 women with fibrocystic disease of the breast mean concentration of 80.5 ± 4.4 mg/dL significantly different from 69.9 ± 5.6 mg/dL in 13 women with benign breast masses *2910*

Apolipoprotein B *Serum* *Increase* In 23 women with fibrocystic disease of the breast mean concentration of 99.1 ± 5.4 mg/dL significantly different from 76.6 ± 4.8 mg/dL in 13 women with benign breast masses *2910*

Apolipoprotein C-III *Serum* *No Effect* In 23 women with fibrocystic disease of the breast mean concentration of 12.4 ± 0.9 mg/dL not significantly different from 11 ± 0.8 mg/dL in 13 women with benign breast masses *2910*

Apolipoprotein D *Serum* *Increase* In 23 women with fibrocystic disease of the breast mean concentration of 16.3 ± 1.1 mg/dL significantly different from 13.3 ± 1.7 mg/dL in 13 women with benign breast masses *2910*

610.10 Fibrocystic Disease of Breast *(continued)*

Apolipoprotein E *Serum* *No Effect* In 23 women with fibrocystic disease of the breast mean concentration of 15.6 ± 0.9 mg/dL not significantly different from 15.1 ± 1.2 mg/dL in 13 women with benign breast masses *2910*

c-erb-B_2 Oncoprotein *Serum* *No Effect* In 28 women with fibrocystic disease of the breast none had concentrations exceeding 15 U/mL *3562*

CA 15-3 *Serum* *No Effect* In 28 women with fibrocystic disease of the breast none had concentrations exceeding 35 U/mL *3562*

Carcinoembryonic Antigen *Serum* *No Effect* In 28 women with fibrocystic disease of the breast none had concentrations exceeding 5 ng/mL *3562*

Cholesterol *Serum* *No Effect* In 23 women with fibrocystic disease of the breast mean concentration of 204.5 ± 8.5 mg/dL not significantly different from 191.0 ± 8.8 mg/dL in 13 women with benign breast masses *2910*

Dehydroepiandrosterone Sulfate *Breast Cyst Fluid* *No Effect* In 30 patients with cyst fluid K/Na < 3 mean concentration was 29.6 ± 24.5 mol/L and in 30 with cyst fluid K/Na > 3 mean concentration was 230.5 ± 127.1 mol/L significantly different from plasma concentration of 5.2 ± 3.1 mol/L in 50 controls *3317*
Plasma *No Effect* In 30 patients with cyst fluid K/Na < 3 mean concentration was 4.0 ± 1.9 mol/L and in 30 with cyst fluid K/Na > 3 mean concentration was 4.8 ± 2.0 mol/L not significantly different from 5.2 ± 3.1 mol/L in 50 controls *3317*

Estradiol *Breast Cyst Fluid* *Increase* In 30 patients with cyst fluid K/Na < 3 mean concentration was 2,390 ± 1,413 pmol/L and in 30 with cyst fluid K/Na > 3 mean concentration was 10,973 ± 2,724 pmol/L significantly different from plasma concentration of 444 ± 236 pmol/L in 50 controls *3317*
Plasma *No Effect* In 30 patients with cyst fluid K/Na < 3 mean concentration was 371 ± 290 pmol/L and in 30 with cyst fluid K/Na > 3 mean concentration was 389 ± 191 pmol/L not significantly different from 444 ± 236 pmol/L in 50 controls *3317*

HDL-Cholesterol *Serum* *No Effect* In 23 women with fibrocystic disease of the breast mean concentration of 59.6 ± 4.0 mg/dL not significantly different from 59.9 ± 7.1 mg/dL in 13 women with benign breast masses *2910*

17-Hydroxyprogesterone *Breast Cyst Fluid* *Increase* In 30 patients with cyst fluid K/Na < 3 mean concentration was 47.8 ± 39.3 nmol/L and in 30 with cyst fluid K/Na > 3 mean concentration was 156.1 ± 81.1 nmol/L significantly different from plasma concentration of 2.4 ± 0.9 nmol/L in 50 controls *3317*
Plasma *No Effect* In 30 patients with cyst fluid K/Na < 3 mean concentration was 1.8 ± 1.2 nmol/L and in 30 with cyst fluid K/Na > 3 mean concentration was 2.1 ± 1.2 nmol/L not significantly different from 2.4 ± 0.9 nmol/L in 50 controls *3317*

LDL-Cholesterol *Serum* *Increase* In 23 women with fibrocystic disease of the breast mean concentration of 121.9 ± 7.5 mg/dL significantly different from 103.9 ± 7.5 mg/dL in 13 women with benign breast masses *2910*

Lipoprotein Lp(a) *Serum* *No Effect* In 23 women with fibrocystic disease of the breast mean concentration of 27.6 ± 9.2 mg/dL not significantly different from 26.7 ± 12.5 mg/dL in 13 women with benign breast masses *2910*

Platelet Factor 4 *Breast Cyst Fluid* *Increase* Concentrations in cyst fluids from 50 patients ranged from 8 - 225 ng/mL (median 25 ng/mL). Concentration within normal plasma range of 6.5 - 25 ng/mL in 34 (68%) patients *3495*

Progesterone *Breast Cyst Fluid* *Increase* In 30 patients with cyst fluid K/Na < 3 mean concentration was 135.1 ± 63.6 nmol/L and in 30 with cyst fluid K/Na > 3 mean concentration was 167.6 ± 79.2 nmol/L significantly different from plasma concentration of 18.8 ± 13.7 nmol/L in 50 controls *3317*
Plasma *No Effect* In 30 patients with cyst fluid K/Na < 3 mean concentration was 17.2 ± 11.1 nmol/L and in 30 with cyst fluid K/Na > 3 mean concentration was 14.9 ± 11.1 nmol/L not significantly different from 18.8 ± 13.7 nmol/L in 50 controls *3317*

Testosterone *Breast Cyst Fluid* *Increase* In 30 patients with cyst fluid K/Na < 3 mean concentration was 3.2 ± 1.4 nmol/L and in 30 with cyst fluid K/Na > 3 mean concentration was 9.6 ± 2.8 nmol/L significantly different from plasma concentration of 1.7 ± 1.0 nmol/L in 50 controls *3317*
Serum *No Effect* In 30 patients with cyst fluid K/Na < 3 mean concentration was 1.7 ± 0.7 nmol/L and in 30 with cyst fluid K/Na > 3 mean concentration was 1.7 ± 0.7 nmol/L not significantly different from 1.7 ± 1.0 nmol/L in 50 controls *3317*

β-Thromboglobulin *Breast Cyst Fluid* *Increase* Concentrations in cyst fluids from 50 patients ranged from < 4 - 330 ng/mL. Concentration within normal plasma range of 14 - 80 ng/mL in 24 (48%) patients *3495*

Thrombospondin *Breast Cyst Fluid* *Increase* Median concentration in cyst fluids from 50 patients of 2,500 ng/mL significantly higher than concentrations in plasma (57 - 216 ng/mL) *3495* Mean concentration of 15,277 ng/mL, with mean concentration for type II (Na^+) cysts 35,289 ng/mL and 4,355 ng/mL for type I (K^+) cysts *2074*

Thyroid Stimulating Hormone *Breast Cyst Fluid* *Decrease* In 30 patients with cyst fluid K/Na < 3 mean concentration was 0.2 ± 0.2 mU/L and in 30 with cyst fluid K/Na > 3 mean concentration was 0.2 ± 0.2 mU/L significantly different from serum concentration of 1.8 ± 0.9 mU/L in 50 controls *3317*
Serum *No Effect* In 30 patients with cyst fluid K/Na < 3 mean concentration was 1.97 ± 0.7 mU/L and in 30 with cyst fluid K/Na > 3 mean concentration was 1.8 ± 1.0 mU/L not significantly different from 1.8 ± 0.9 mU/L in 50 controls *3317*

Thyroxine (T4) *Breast Cyst Fluid* *Decrease* In 30 patients with cyst fluid K/Na < 3 mean concentration was 52.7 ± 9.0 nmol/L and in 30 with cyst fluid K/Na > 3 mean concentration was 51.5 ± 6.4 nmol/L significantly different from serum concentration of 117.1 ± 16.7 nmol/L in 50 controls *3317*
Serum *No Effect* In 30 patients with cyst fluid K/Na < 3 mean concentration was 114.5 ± 18.0 nmol/L and in 30 with cyst fluid K/Na > 3 mean concentration was 115.8 ± 14.1 nmol/L not significantly different from 117.1 ± 16.7 nmol/L in 50 controls *3317*

Thyroxine (T4), Free *Breast Cyst Fluid* *Decrease* In 30 patients with cyst fluid K/Na < 3 mean concentration was 5.1 ± 3.8 pmol/L and in 30 with cyst fluid K/Na > 3 mean concentration was 5.1 ± 3.8 pmol/L significantly different from serum concentration of 19.3 ± 3.8 pmol/L in 50 controls *3317*
Serum *No Effect* In 30 patients with cyst fluid K/Na < 3 mean concentration was 20.6 ± 2.6 pmol/L and in 30 with cyst fluid K/Na > 3 mean concentration was 19.3 ± 2.6 pmol/L not significantly different from 19.3 ± 3.8 pmol/L in 50 controls *3317*

Tri-iodothyronine, Free (fT3) *Breast Cyst Fluid* *Increase* In 30 patients with cyst fluid K/Na < 3 mean concentration was 15.8 ± 14.6 pmol/L and in 30 with cyst fluid K/Na > 3 mean concentration was 69.4 ± 30.9 pmol/L significantly different from serum concentration of 5.2 ± 1.4 pmol/L in 50 controls *3317*
Serum *No Effect* In 30 patients with cyst fluid K/Na < 3 mean concentration was 5.1 ± 0.9 pmol/L and in 30 with cyst fluid K/Na > 3 mean concentration was 4.6 ± 1.4 pmol/L not significantly different from 5.2 ± 1.4 pmol/L in 50 controls *3317*

Triglycerides *Serum* *No Effect* In 23 women with fibrocystic disease of the breast mean concentration of 107.7 ± 9.5 mg/dL not significantly different from 93.5 ± 15.2 mg/dL in 13 women with benign breast masses *2910*

VLDL-Cholesterol *Serum* *No Effect* In 23 women with fibrocystic disease of the breast mean concentration of 21.9 ± 2.0 mg/dL not significantly different from 18.9 ± 3.3 mg/dL in 13 women with benign breast masses *2910*

611.10 Gynecomastia

Estradiol *Plasma* *No Effect* In 44 men with previous testicular disorders mean concentration of 41.1 ± 19 ng/L and 38.1 ± 13 ng/L in 444 men without antecedent testicular disorders not significantly different from 39.5 ± 10 ng/L in 41 healthy controls *330*

Follicle Stimulating Hormone *Plasma* *Increase* In 44 men with previous testicular disorders mean concentration of 5.5 ± 3.3 IU/L significantly different from mean concentration of 4.0 ± 3.8 IU/L in 444 men without antecedent testicular disorders and 4.2 ± 1.9 IU/L in 41 healthy controls *330*

Luteinizing Hormone *Plasma* *Increase* In 44 men with previous testicular disorders mean concentration of 6.1 ± 3.0 IU/L significantly different from 4.9 ± 5.0 IU/L in 444 men without antecedent testicular disorders and 4.3 ± 1.9 IU/L in 41 healthy controls *330*

Prolactin *Plasma No Effect* In 34 men with previous testicular disorders mean concentration of 11.3 ± 5.8 µg/L and 11.9 ± 7.2 µg/L in 369 men without antecedent testicular disorders not significantly different from 13.3 ± 9.2 µg/L in 41 healthy controls *330*

Sex-Hormone Binding Globulin *Serum No Effect* No apparent effect on concentration *4234*

Testosterone *Serum Decrease* In 44 men with previous testicular disorders mean concentration of 6.02 ± 2.8 µg/L and 7.2 ± 2.1 µg/L in 444 men without antecedent testicular disorders significantly different from 8.2 ± 1.4 µg/L in 41 healthy controls *330*

614.00 Acute Adnexitis

C-Reactive Protein *Serum Increase* In 115 women with acute adnexitis correlated well with acute inflammatory pelvic disease *4651*

614.20 Salpingitis

CA 125 *Serum Increase* In patients with salpingitis (grades 1 - 3) positive predictive value of concentrations above 16 U/mL was 97% *1260*

614.20 Tubo-ovarian Abscess

C-Reactive Protein *Serum Increase* Mean concentration on admission in 51 women with PID 149.2 mg/L versus 76.9 mg/L in others *4319* Concentration increased to mean of 149.2 ± 65.2 mg/L in patients with tubo-ovarian abscess compared with cut-off of less than 6 mg/L *3451*

Erythrocyte Sedimentation Rate *Blood Increase* Mean rate on admission in 51 women with PID of 90.0 mm/h versus 42.0 mm/h in others *4319*

Leukocytes *Blood Increase* Concentration increased to mean of 16,200 ± 5,399 /µL in patients with tubo-ovarian abscess compared with cut-off of less than 10,000 /µL *3451* Mean concentration on admission in 51 women with PID 16,200 /µL versus 11,830 /µL in others *4319*

614.40 Pelvic Inflammatory Disease

CA 15-3 *Serum No Effect* In 20 women with proved PID mean concentration of 17.1 ± 6.1 U/mL not significantly different from 19.4 ± 5.9 U/mL in 20 women in whom PID was ruled out and 17.3 ± 4.9 U/mL in 50 controls *3636*

CA 19-9 *Serum No Effect* In 20 women with proved PID mean concentration of 19.2 ± 19.8 U/mL not significantly different from 13.3 ± 6.9 U/mL in 20 women in whom PID was ruled out and 13.9 ± 11.1 U/mL in 50 controls *3636*

CA 125 *Serum Increase* False positive result *3909* Median concentration of 19 µg/L in 38 patients with pelvic inflammatory disease *5191* In 36 women with PID mean concentration greater than 30 U/mL compared with reference interval of < 17 U/mL. Highest mean concentrations of 427 U/mL in patients with advanced disease with pelvic mass *3557* In 50 patients with provisional diagnosis of pelvic inflammatory disease 66% on admission had concentrations in excess of cutoff of 16 U/mL (range 20 to 1,300 U/mL). Concentration correlated with extent of inflammatory peritoneal involvement (eta = 0.74) *1260* False positive result *1963* In 38 patients with PID median concentration of 18.8 U/L *2090* In 20 women with proved PID mean concentration of 78.8 ± 42.0 U/mL significantly higher than 28.0 ± 23.1 U/mL in 20 women in whom PID was ruled out and 24.1 ± 13.1 U/mL in 50 controls *3636*

Carcinoembryonic Antigen *Serum No Effect* In 20 women with proved PID mean concentration of 3.8 ± 0.3 ng/mL not significantly different from 3.8 ± 0.3 ng/mL in 20 women in whom PID was ruled out and 3.9 ± 0.3 ng/mL in 50 controls *3636*

C-Reactive Protein *Serum Increase* Mean concentration on admission in 51 women with PID increased above 5 mg/L in 96.1% *4319* Concentration increased to mean of 76.9 ± 79.8 mg/L in patients with PID without tubo-ovarian abscess compared with cut-off of less than 6 mg/L *3451*

CYFRA 21-1 *Serum No Effect* Median concentration of 1.3 µg/L in 38 patients with pelvic inflammatory disease not different from 1.9 µg/L in 40 healthy controls *5191*

Erythrocyte Sedimentation Rate *Blood Increase* Rate increased to mean of 60.8 ± 36.6 mm/h in patients with PID without tubo-ovarian abscess compared with cut-off of less than 15 mm/h *3451* Rate increased to mean of 89.9 ± 33.1 mm/h in patients with tubo-ovarian abscess compared with cut-off of less than 15 mm/h *3451* Mean rate on admission in 51 women with PID increased above 15 mm/h in 92.1% *4319*

α-Fetoprotein *Serum No Effect* In 70 patients with acute pelvic inflammatory disease median concentration of 1.2 kIU/L (range of 0.5 - 5.9 kIU/L) within the normal range for non-pregnant women *840*

Insulin-like Growth Factor-I *Serum No Effect* In 20 women with proved PID mean concentration of 1.0 ± 0.5 U/mL not significantly different from 1.1 ± 0.4 U/mL in 20 women in whom PID was ruled out and 0.8 ± 0.3 U/mL in 50 controls *3636*

Leukocytes *Blood Increase* Mean concentration on admission in 51 women with PID increased above 10,000 /µL in 70.6% *4319* Concentration increased to mean of 11,830 ± 4,210 /µL in patients with PID without tubo-ovarian abscess compared with cut-off of less than 10,000 /µL *3451* In 36 women with PID mean concentration greater than 10,000 cells/µL in moderate cases of PID increasing to counts > 15,000 cells/µL in patients with severe disease *3557*

M3/M21 *Serum No Effect* In 38 patients with PID median concentration of 12.4 U/L compared with that in 40 healthy blood donors in whom the median concentration was 25.2 U/L *2090*

614.90 Benign Disease of Female Genital Tract

CA 125 *Serum No Effect* In 20 women with benign disease of the genital tract (5 with endometriosis, 5 with fibromas, 7 with cervicitis and 3 with vaginitis) median concentration of 13.5 U/mL (range 3.0 - 103 U/mL) not significantly different from median of 8.3 U/mL (range 3.0 - 23.5 U/mL) in 15 healthy controls *4575*
Vaginal Fluid Increase In 20 women with benign disease of the genital tract (5 with endometriosis, 5 with fibromas, 7 with cervicitis and 3 with vaginitis) median concentration of 1,780 U/mL (range 140 - 65,100 U/mL) not significantly different from median of 358 U/mL (range 104 - 4,232 U/mL) in 15 healthy controls *4575*

Carcinoembryonic Antigen *Serum No Effect* In 20 women with benign disease of the genital tract (5 with endometriosis, 5 with fibromas, 7 with cervicitis and 3 with vaginitis) median concentration of 0.9 ng/mL (range of 0.9 - 2.9 ng/mL) not significantly different from median of 1.0 ng/mL (range of 0.5 - 2.5 ng/mL) in 15 healthy controls *4575*
Vaginal Fluid Increase In 20 women with benign disease of the genital tract (5 with endometriosis, 5 with fibromas, 7 with cervicitis and 3 with vaginitis) median concentration of 395 ng/mL (range 75 - 5,420 ng/mL) significantly different from median of 171 ng/mL (range 13 - 672 ng/mL) in 15 healthy controls *4575*

Squamous Cell Carcinoma Antigen *Serum No Effect* In 20 women with benign disease of the genital tract (5 with endometriosis, 5 with fibromas, 7 with cervicitis and 3 with vaginitis) median concentration of 1.1 ng/mL (range of 0.4 - 3.5 ng/mL) not significantly different from median of 0.8 ng/mL (range of 0.3 - 2.7 ng/mL) in 15 healthy controls *4575*
Vaginal Fluid Increase In 20 women with benign disease of the genital tract (5 with endometriosis, 5 with fibomas, 7 with cervicitis and 3 with vaginitis) median concentration of 3,375 ng/mL (range 85 - 13,000 ng/mL) significantly different from median of 1,340 ng/mL (range 27 - 5,430 ng/mL) in 15 healthy controls *4575*

614.90 Upper Female Genital Tract Infection

C-Reactive Protein *Serum Increase* In 120 women with acute upper genital tract infection odds ratio for an increased C-reactive protein concentration of 4.6 *4060*

614.90 Upper Female Genital Tract Infection *(continued)*

Erythrocyte Sedimentation Rate *Blood* *Increase* In 120 women with acute upper genital tract infection odds ratio for an increased ESR 2.5 *4060*

Leukocytes *Blood* *Increase* In 120 women with acute upper genital tract infection leukocyte counts > 3 per hpf had specificity of 88% and positive predictive value, also of 88%: odds ratio for an increased WBC count 10.0 *4060* In 120 women with acute upper genital tract infection leukocyte counts > 3 per hpf had specificity of 88% *4060*
Vaginal Fluid *Increase* In 120 women with acute upper genital tract infection leukocyte counts > 3 per hpf observed had sensitivity of 78% *4060*

615.90 Endometritis

Fibrinopeptide A *Plasma* *Increase* In patients with puerperal endometritis mean concentration of 7 ng/mL, higher than in healthy individuals *5617*

617.90 Endometrioma

CA 19-9 *Serum* *Increase* In 38 patients with endometometrioma cysts mean concentration of 32.2 ± 44.9 U/mL compared with mean of 12.8 ± 19.7 U/mL in those with nonendometriotic cysts *1903* *1903*

CA 125 *Serum* *Increase* In 38 patients with endometometrioma cysts mean concentration increased in parallel with serum CA 19-9 concentration *1903* In one woman with a ruptured endometrioma concentration increased to 9,300 IU/mL, with return to markedly lower level with elimination of endometriosis *2459*

617.90 Endometriosis

Anticardiolipin Antibodies *Serum* *Increase* Incidence of 9.4% in 64 patients significantly higher than 3.1% in 97 healthy controls *156*

Antiphosphatidic Acid Antibodies *Serum* *Increase* Incidence of 1.6% in 64 patients not significantly higher than 0.0% in 97 healthy controls *156*

Antiphosphatidylethanolamine Antibodies *Serum* *No Effect* Incidence of 6.3% in 64 patients not significantly different from 0.0% in 97 healthy controls *156*

Antiphosphatidylglycerol Antibodies *Serum* *No Effect* Incidence of 3.1% in 64 patients not significantly different from 0.0% in 97 healthy controls *156*

Antiphosphatidylinositol Antibodies *Serum* *Increase* Incidence of 6.3% in 64 patients not significantly higher than 2.1% in 97 healthy controls *156*

Antiphosphatidylserine Antibodies *Serum* *Increase* Incidence of 12.5% in 64 patients significantly higher than 5.2% in 97 healthy controls *156*

CA 19-9 *Serum* *Increase* In one patient with probable pelvic endometriosis concentration increased above 150 U/mL during menses but not after menses: in luteal and premenstrual phases the concentration returned to normal *2328*

CA 27-29 *Serum* *No Effect* In none of 30 women with endometriosis was concentration increased above 36 U/mL *766*

CA 72 *Serum* *No Effect* In 7 patients with stage I disease mean concentration of 1.4 ± 1.1 U/mL, in 3 with stage II of 2.0 ± 1.0 U/mL, in 6 with stage III disease of 1.5 ± 1.9 U/mL and in 3 with stage IV disease of 2.3 ± 2.0 U/mL not significantly different from 2.7 ± 2.1 U/mL in 16 patient controls with normal pelvis *3571*

CA 72-4 *Serum* *Increase* In one patient with probable pelvic endometriosis concentration increased above 10 U/mL during menses but not after menses: in luteal and premenstrual phases the concentration returned to the normal range *2328*

CA 125 *Serum* *Increase* Commonly associated with increased concentration *1350* Median concentration of 63 µg/L in 10 patients with endometriosis *5191* In one patient with probable pelvic endometriosis concentration increased above 1,000 U/mL during menses but not after menses: in luteal and premenstrual phases the concentration returned to within the normal range *2328* In 4 patients with endometriosis median concentration of 62.9 U/L *2090* In 18 women with endometriosis mean concentration of 22.2 ± 35.5 U/mL with 11.1% with concentrations above 35 U/mL *2636* The mean value was significantly higher than that observed in normal women (28.6 U/mL versus 11.1 U/mL) *291* In women with endometriosis concentration increased and correlated with the presence and volume of endometriomas and of deeply infiltrating endometriosis. Diagnostic sensitivity and speciicity of CA-125 for endometriosis 25% and 87% respectively and for endometriomas and deeply infiltrating endometriosis 36% and 87% for a cutoff concentration of 25 U/mL *2757* False positive result *3909*
Serum *No Effect* In 7 patients with stage I disease mean concentration of 11.9 ± 11.6 U/mL, in 3 with stage II 16.7 ± 7.6 U/mL, in 6 with stage III disease 13.3 ± 8.2 U/mL and in 3 with stage IV disease 15.0 ± 7.6 U/mL not significantly different from 16.3 ± 11.8 U/mL in 16 patient controls with normal pelvis *3571*

Carbonic Anhydrase Antibodies *Serum* *Increase* In 16 of 23 (69.6%) of patients with endometriosis antibodies to bovine carbonic anhydrase detected in contrast to 2 of 17 controls *2671*

CYFRA 21-1 *Serum* *No Effect* Median concentration of 1.0 µg/L in 10 patients with endometriosis not different from 1.9 µg/L in 40 healthy controls *5191*

Endometrial Antibodies *Peritoneal Fluid* *Increase* Concentration significantly higher than in patients without endometriosis *242*
Serum *Increase* Concentration significantly higher in patients with endometriosis than in control patients, but unrelated to severity of disease *242*

Estradiol *Plasma* *Increase* Mean concentration in 29 patients in follicular phase of cycle of 365 ± 45 pmol/L in luteal phase significantly higher than 239 ± 32 pmol/L in 23 controls, and of 383 ± 45 pmol/L in luteal phase not significantly higher than 367 ± 55 pmol/L in healthy controls *62* In 10 infertile patients with endometriosis mean concentration of 126.1 ± 11.1 pg/mL not significantly greater than 111.1 ± 5.0 pg/mL in 10 controls studied in follicular phase *3990*

17β-Estradiol *Peritoneal Fluid* *No Effect* The peritoneal fluid levels of 17 β-estradiol in women with minimal stage endometriosis were not significantly altered *302*

Follicle Stimulating Hormone *Plasma* *Decrease* In 10 infertile patients with endometriosis mean concentration of 6.3 ± 0.9 mIU/mL not significantly less than 7.1 ± 1.5 mIU/mL in 10 controls studied in follicular phase *3990*
Plasma *Increase* In 10 infertile patients with endometriosis mean concentration of 6.9 ± 1.2 mIU/mL not significantly greater than 5.1 ± 0.4 mIU/mL in 10 controls studied in follicular phase *3990*

β_2-Glycoprotein I-dependent Anticardiolipin Antibodies
Serum *Increase* Incidence of 6.3% in 64 patients significantly higher than 0.0% in 97 healthy controls *156*

Interleukin-4 *Serum* *Increase* Significant increase observed in patients with endometriosis *2258*

Interleukin-4 mRNA *Serum* *Increase* Significant increase observed in patients with endometriosis, with highest concentrations associated with most severe disease *2258*

6-Keto-Prostaglandin $F_{1\alpha}$ *Peritoneal Fluid* *No Effect* No difference observed between concentrations in women with endometriosis and healthy normal women *3639*

M3/M21 *Serum* *No Effect* In 10 patients with endometriosis median concentration of 4.05 U/L compared with that in 40 healthy blood donors in whom the median concentration was 25.2 U/L *2090*

Monocyte Chemotactic Protein-1 *Peritoneal Fluid* *Increase* In 13 patients with minimal endometriosis median concentration of 70 pg/mL, in 15 women with mild endometriosis 135 pg/mL, in 24 with moderate endometriosis 205 pg/mL and in 8 with severe endometriosis 1,165 pg/mL, with the latter two groups significantly different from 137 pg/mL in 18 reference women without endometriosis *175*
Serum *Increase* Median concentration in 27 patients with stage I disease of 163 pg/mL, in 20 patients with stage II disease of 180 pg/mL and in 10 with stage III or IV disease of 195 pg/mL significantly different from undetectable amount in 44 healthy controls *62*

Placental Protein 14 *Serum* *Increase* In women with endometriosis concentration increased and correlated with the presence and volume of endometriomas and of deeply infiltrating endometriosis *2757*

Progesterone *Peritoneal Fluid* *Decrease* In the peritoneal fluid there was a significant reduction in progesterone and its ratio with 17 β-estradiol in women with minimal stage endometriosis ($p < 0.03$, $p < 0.04$, respectively) *302*
Plasma *Decrease* Mean concentration in 30 patients in follicular phase of cycle of 1.5 ± 0.3 pmol/L in luteal phase not significantly lower than 2.4 ± 1.1 pmol/L in 23 controls *62*
Plasma *Increase* Mean concentration of 25.8 ± 4.6 pmol/L in 20 patients in luteal phase not significantly higher than 19.7 ± 3.2 pmol/L in 18 healthy controls *62*

Prolactin *Plasma* *No Effect* No significant difference in mean concentration observed in patients with endometriosis compared with normal women *3991* Serum prolactin levels were studied in 43 infertile patients. The mean prolactin level in the endometriotic group was 372 mIU/L (range 187 - 752) while that in the controls was 333 mIU/L (range 124 - 767). There was no statistical difference ($t = 1.12$) *190*

Prolactin response to Insulin *Plasma* *No Effect* No significant difference observed in patients with endometriosis compared with healthy controls *3991*

Prolactin response to TRH *Plasma* *No Effect* No significant difference observed between patients with endometriosis and healthy controls *3991*

620.20 Ovarian Cyst

CA 125 *Serum* *Increase* In 90 patients with benign ovarian cysts median concentration of 17.3 U/L *2090* Median concentration of 17 µg/L in 90 patients with benign ovarian cysts *5191*

CYFRA 21-1 *Serum* *No Effect* Median concentration of 1.3 µg/L in 90 patients with benign ovarian cysts not different from 1.9 µg/L in 40 healthy controls *5191*

M3/M21 *Serum* *Decrease* In 90 patients with benign ovarian cysts median concentration of 6.3 U/L compared with that in 40 healthy blood donors in whom the median concentration was 26.3 U/L *2090*

Pregnanediol *Urine* *Increase* Increased in luteal cysts of ovary *5545*

Progesterone *Plasma* *Increase* Increased in luteal cysts of ovary *5545*

620.90 Benign Ovarian Disease

CA 125 *Serum* *Increase* In 106 women with benign ovarian disease 16 (15.1%) had concentrations above 65 U/mL *1896* Using a cutoff of > 35 U/L sensitivity for ovarian cancer 82% *1134*

CA 549 *Serum* *No Effect* In 52 patients with benign disease of the ovary none had a concentration greater than 30.0 kU/L with BRESMARQ assay *764*

Cancer-associated Serum Antigen *Serum* *Increase* Using a cutoff of > 4 U/L sensitivity for ovarian cancer 87% *1134*

Tissue Polypeptide Antigen *Serum* *Increase* Using a cutoff of > 80 U/L sensitivity for ovarian cancer 92% *1134*

621.80 Endometrial Cysts

Macrophage Colony Stimulating Factor *Serum* *No Effect* In 71 patients with endometrial cysts mean concentration of 763.8 ± 183.9 U/mL not significantly lower than baseline normal of 1,056 U/mL *5094*

621.90 Benign Endometrial Disease

CA 549 *Serum* *No Effect* In 87 patients with benign disease of the endometrium none had a concentration greater than 30.0 kU/L with BRESMARQ assay *764*

621.90 Benign Uterine Diseases

CA 72-4 *Serum* *No Effect* In 48 women with benign uterine diseases 0 (0%) had concentrations above 6 U/mL *1896*

CA 125 *Serum* *No Effect* In 48 women with benign uterine diseases 0 (0%) had concentrations above 65 U/mL *1896*

622.10 Cervical Dysplasia

CA 125 *Serum* *No Effect* In 5 women with severe dysplasia of the genital tract median concentration of 9.4 U/mL (range 6.0 - 17.5 U/mL) not significantly different from median of 8.3 U/mL (range 3.0 - 1,590 U/mL) in 15 healthy controls *4575*
Vaginal Fluid *No Effect* In 5 women with severe dysplasia of the genital tract median concentration of 552 U/mL (range 101 - 3,067 U/mL) not significantly different from median of 358 U/mL (range 104 - 4,232 U/mL) in 15 healthy controls *4575*

Carcinoembryonic Antigen *Serum* *No Effect* In 5 women with severe dysplasia of the genital tract median concentration of 0.7 ng/mL (range of 0.5 - 2.5 ng/mL) not significantly different from median of 1.0 ng/mL (range of 0.5 - 2.5 ng/mL) in 15 healthy controls *4575*
Vaginal Fluid *No Effect* In 5 women with severe dysplasia of the genital tract median concentration of 116 ng/mL (range 31 - 275 ng/mL) not significantly different from median of 171 ng/mL (range 13 - 672 ng/mL) in 15 healthy controls *4575*

Squamous Cell Carcinoma Antigen *Serum* *No Effect* In 5 women with severe dysplasia of the genital tract median concentration of 0.7 ng/mL (range of 0.5 - 1.2 ng/mL) not significantly different from median of 0.8 ng/mL (range of 0.3 - 2.7 ng/mL) in 15 healthy controls *4575*
Vaginal Fluid *No Effect* In 5 women with severe dysplasia of the genital tract median concentration of 440 ng/mL (range 220 - 2,110 ng/mL) not significantly different from median of 1,340 ng/mL (range 27 - 5,430 ng/mL) in 15 healthy controls *4575*

625.80 Benign Gynecological Disease

Lysophosphatidic Acid *Serum* *No Effect* In 17 patients with benign gynecologic diseases median concentration of 0.5 µmol/L not significantly different from 0.1 µmol/L in 48 healthy controls *5758*

627.20 Menopausal and Postmenopausal Symptoms

Estrogens *Urine* *Decrease* The urinary excretion of total estrogens will be below 10 µg/d. Values above 20 µg/d are suggestive of a pathologic process such as a granulosa cell tumor *900*

Follicle Stimulating Hormone *Plasma* *Increase* Observed effect *900*

Luteinizing Hormone *Plasma* *Increase* Observed effect *900*

627.20 Postmenopause

Acid Phosphatase, Tartrate Resistant *Serum* *Increase* Mean activity of 7.31 ± 0.58 U/L in 41 healthy postmenopausal women significantly different from 4.66 ± 0.37 U/L in 31 healthy premenopausal women *4715*

Adenosine Monophosphate *Urine* *No Effect* Mean concentration of 0.057 ± 0.003 mg/mg creatinine in 41 healthy postmenopausal women significantly different from 0.058 ± 0.006 mg/mg creatinine in 31 healthy premenopausal women *4715*

Aldosterone *Plasma* *Decrease* Decreased despite increases in systolic blood pressure *4179*

Alkaline Phosphatase *Serum* *Increase* Mean activity of 61.1 ± 2.7 U/L in 41 healthy postmenopausal women significantly different from 38.3 ± 3.3 U/L in 31 healthy premenopausal women *4715* These changes in bone-related variables did not generally occur until the level of follicle-stimulating hormone exceeded approximately 50 IU/L *3824*

Amyloid P *Serum* *Increase* Observed effect *2051*

Antithrombin *Plasma* *Increase* Significant increase compared with men of the same age *3432*

627.20 Postmenopause *(continued)*

Antithrombin III *Plasma* *No Effect* No significant effect observed with menopause *2051*

α_1-Antitrypsin *Serum* *Decrease* Decreased after menoopause and increased by estrogen therapy *2051*
Serum *Increase* Observed effect *2051*

α_2-AP-Glycoprotein *Serum* *Decrease* Decreased after menoopause and increased by estrogen therapy *2051*

Apolipoprotein A-I *Serum* *No Effect* Concentration in healthy postmenopausal women of 1.56 - 0.28 g/L not significantly different from 1.52 ± 0.28 g/L when concentrations adjusted for age differences *908*

Apolipoprotein B *Serum* *Increase* Concentration in healthy postmenopausal women of 1.05 - 0.25 g/L significantly different from 0.88 ± 0.24 g/L in healthy premenopausal women *909*

Atrial Natriuretic Peptide *Plasma* *Increase* Suggests that the increase in plasma levels found in postmenopusal women is related with age and that ANP does not play a direct role in the physiologic hormonal changes of menopause *4179*

Bicarbonate *Serum* *Increase* These changes in bone-related variables did not generally occur until the level of follicle-stimulating hormone exceeded approximately 50 IU/L *3824*

CA 125 *Serum* *No Effect* 258 postmenopausal volunteers who were not seeking gynecologic care had CA 125 meausred. Only one subject had a level greater than 35 U/mL. The mean value was 5.6 ± 3.5 U/mL *5646*

Calcium *Serum* *Increase* These changes in bone-related variables did not generally occur until the level of follicle-stimulating hormone exceeded approximately 50 IU/L *3824*
Serum *No Effect* Mean concentration of 9.49 ± 0.08 mg/dL in 41 healthy postmenopausal women not significantly different from 9.25 ± 0.09 mg/dL in 31 healthy premenopausal women *4715*
Urine *Increase* These changes in bone-related variables did not generally occur until the level of follicle-stimulating hormone exceeded approximately 50 IU/L *3824*
Urine *No Effect* Mean concentration of 0.12 ± 0.01 mg/mg creatinine in 41 healthy postmenopausal women significantly different from 0.12 ± 0.01 mg/mg creatinine in 31 healthy premenopausal women *4715*

Ceruloplasmin *Serum* *No Effect* No significant change observed with menopause *2051*

Cholesterol *Serum* *Increase* Increased significantly as a consequence of menopause and all increases occurred within 6 months of the cessation of menstrual periods *2438*

1,25-Dihydroxy Vitamin D_3 *Serum* *No Effect* Mean concentration of 25.7 ± 1.2 pg/mL in 41 healthy postmenopausal women not significantly different from 27.8 ± 1.5 pg/mL in 31 healthy premenopausal women *4715*

Dipyridinoline *Urine* *Increase* Mean concentration of 19.1 ± 1.9 nmol/mmol creatinine in 41 healthy postmenopausal women significantly different from 12.1 ± 0.8 nmol/mmol creatinine in 31 healthy premenopausal women *4715*

Estradiol *Plasma* *Decrease* Abrupt decrease *808*

Estrogens *Plasma* *Decrease* Deficiency of rapid onset *141*

Factor VII *Plasma* *Increase* Large increase in activity compared to men of the same age. Greater levels found in those women experiencing a natural compared to a surgical menopause *3432*

Fibrinogen *Plasma* *Increase* Large increase in activity compared to men of the same age. Greater levels found in those women experiencing a natural compared to a surgical menopause *3432*

Follicle Stimulating Hormone *Plasma* *Increase* Observed effect *808*
Plasma *No Effect* In 42 postmenopausal women with biopsy diagnosed breast cancer mean concentration of 47.55 ± 3.18 IU/L not significantly different from reference range of 19 - 130 IU/L *2789*

β_2-Glycoprotein I *Serum* *No Effect* No significant change observed with menopause *2051*

β_2-Glycoprotein III *Serum* *Decrease* Decreased after menoopause and increased by estrogen therapy *2051*

Haptoglobin *Serum* *Increase* Observed effect *2051*

HDL-Cholesterol *Serum* *Decrease* Decreased significantly (p less than 0.05) as a consequence of menopause, but the decline occured gradually over the 2 years preceding cessation of menses *2438*
Serum *No Effect* Concentration in healthy postmenopausal women of 0.55 - 0.15 g/L not significantly different from 0.56 ± 0.14 g/L when concentrations adjusted for age differences *908*

Hemopexin *Serum* *No Effect* No significant effect observed with menopause *2051*

α_2-HS Glycoprotein *Serum* *Decrease* Decreased after menoopause and increased by estrogen therapy *2051*

25-Hydroxy Vitamin D_3 *Serum* *Increase* Mean concentration of 22.6 ± 1.2 ng/mL in 41 healthy postmenopausal women significantly different from 18.8 ± 1.1 ng/mL in 31 healthy premenopausal women *4715*

Hydroxyproline *Urine* *Increase* These changes in bone-related variables did not generally occur until the level of follicle-stimulating hormone exceeded approximately 50 IU/L *3824* Mean concentration of 0.040 ± 0.003 mg/mg creatinine in 41 healthy postmenopausal women significantly different from 0.029 ± 0.002 mg/mg creatinine in 31 healthy premenopausal women *4715*

Immunoglobulin G *Serum* *No Effect* No significant effect of menopause noted *2051*

Immunoglobulin M *Serum* *No Effect* No significant effect of menopause noted *2051*

Insulin-like Growth Factor-I *Serum* *Decrease* Mean concentration of 75.9 ± 5.1 ng/mL in 41 healthy postmenopausal women significantly different from 105.3 ± 9.2 ng/mL in 31 healthy premenopausal women *4715*

Ionized Calcium *Serum* *No Effect* Mean concentration of 1.22 ± 0.009 mmol/L in 41 healthy postmenopausal women not significantly different from 1.20 ± 0.008 mmol/L in 31 healthy premenopausal women *4715*

LDL-Cholesterol *Serum* *Increase* Increased significantly as a consequence of menopause and all increases occurred within 6 months of the cessation of menstrual periods *2438*

Lipoprotein A-I *Serum* *Decrease* Decreased after menoopause and increased by estrogen therapy *2051*

β-Lipoprotein *Serum* *Increase* Observed effect *2051*

Luteinizing Hormone *Plasma* *Increase* Observed effect *808*
Plasma *No Effect* In 42 postmenopausal women with biopsy diagnosed breast cancer mean concentration of 20.27 ± 1.83 IU/L not significantly different from reference range of 12 - 58 IU/L *2789*

Methylmalonate *Serum* *Increase* Mean concentration in women older than 60 years had on average 0.037 µmol/L higher than younger women *4284*

Osteocalcin *Serum* *Increase* Mean concentration of 4.51 ± 0.26 ng/mL in 41 healthy postmenopausal women significantly different from 3.41 ± 0.25 ng/mL in 31 healthy premenopausal women *4715* Significant increase in women more thn 2 years into menopause *1095*

Parathyroid Hormone *Plasma* *No Effect* Mean concentration of 31.5 ± 1.7 pg/mL in 41 healthy postmenopausal women not significantly different from 28.3 ± 2.2 pg/mL in 31 healthy premenopausal women *4715*

Phosphate *Serum* *Decrease* Concentration reported to both increase and decrease after the menopause, or to be unaffected by it *969*
Serum *Increase* Serum phosphate concentration may be increased with postmenopausal state *5204* These changes in bone-related variables did not generally occur until the level of follicle-stimulating hormone exceeded approximately 50 IU/L *3824* Concentration reported to both increase and decrease after the menopause, or to be unaffected by it *969*
Serum *No Effect* Concentration reported to both increase and decrease after the menopause, or to be unaffected by it *969*

Prealbumin *Serum* *No Effect* No significant effect of menopause noted *2051*

Prolactin *Plasma* *Increase* Slight increase *808*

Pyridinoline *Urine* *Increase* Mean concentration of 59.5 ± 5.5 nmol/mmol creatinine in 41 healthy postmenopausal women significantly different from 39.0 ± 2.0 nmol/mmol creatinine in 31 healthy premenopausal women *4715*

Pyridinoline:Dipyridinoline Ratio *Urine No Effect* Mean ratio of 3.3 ± 0.11 in 41 healthy postmenopausal women not significantly different from 3.3 ± 0.11 in 31 healthy premenopausal women *4715*

Renin Activity *Plasma Decrease* Plasma renin activity was decreased despite increases in systolic blood pressure in 103 postmenopausal women *4179*

Retinol-binding Protein *Serum No Effect* No significant effect of menopause noted *2051*

Testosterone *Serum No Effect* No change *808*

Triglycerides *Serum Increase* Increased significantly as a consequence of menopause and all increases occurred within 6 months of the cessation of menstrual periods *2438*

628.00 Normogonadotropic Anovulation

Androgen Index, Free (FAI) *Plasma No Effect* Mean index in 13 patients of 2.6 ± 1.3 not significantly different from 3.1 ± 1.0 in 8 healthy women during during the early follicular phase of their menstrual cycle *4638*

Androstenedione *Plasma No Effect* Mean concentration in 13 patients of 7.9 ± 2.8 nmol/L not significantly different from 10.5 ± 3.2 nmol/L in 8 healthy women during during the early follicular phase of their menstrual cycle *4638*

Follicle Stimulating Hormone *Plasma No Effect* Mean concentration in 13 patients of 4.3 ± 1.2 IU/L not significantly different from 5.4 ± 1.2 IU/L in 8 healthy women during during the early follicular phase of their menstrual cycle *4638*

Luteinizing Hormone *Plasma No Effect* Mean concentration in 13 patients of 4.0 ± 1.9 IU/L not significantly different from 3.5 ± 1.3 IU/L in 8 healthy women during during the early follicular phase of their menstrual cycle *4638*

Testosterone *Serum No Effect* Mean concentration in 13 patients of 1.3 ± 0.5 nmol/L not significantly different from 1.8 ± 0.5 nmol/L in 8 healthy women during during the early follicular phase of their menstrual cycle *4638*

628.90 Infertility, Unexplained

Anticardiolipin Antibodies *Serum Increase* Incidence of 12.3% in 65 patients not significantly higher than 3.1% in 97 healthy controls *156*

Antiphosphatidic Acid Antibodies *Serum Increase* Incidence of 3.1% in 65 patients not significantly higher than 0.0% in 97 healthy controls *156*

Antiphosphatidylethanolamine Antibodies *Serum No Effect* Incidence of 9.2% in 65 patients not significantly different from 0.0% in 97 healthy controls *156*

Antiphosphatidylglycerol Antibodies *Serum No Effect* Incidence of 4.6% in 65 patients not significantly different from 0.0% in 97 healthy controls *156*

Antiphosphatidylinositol Antibodies *Serum Increase* Incidence of 6.2% in 65 patients not significantly higher than 2.1% in 97 healthy controls *156*

Antiphosphatidylserine Antibodies *Serum Increase* Incidence of 10.8% in 65 patients not significantly higher than 5.2% in 97 healthy controls *156*

β_2-Glycoprotein I-dependent Anticardiolipin Antibodies *Serum Increase* Incidence of 1.5% in 65 patients not significantly higher than 0.0% in 97 healthy controls *156*

629.90 Benign Pelvic Diseases

CA 125 *Serum Increase* In 156 women with benign pelvic diseases 31% had values greater than 35 U/mL compared with 5% in apparently healthy women overall when measured by Centocor second generation assay *2637*

PREGNANCY, COMPLICATIONS OF PREGNANCY AND THE PUERPERIUM

630.00 Hydatidiform Mole

Carcinoembryonic Antigen *Serum No Effect* Only 1 of 17 patients had a value > 2.5 ng/mL in serum. In all cases, the hydatid fluid had values > 2.5 and the range was 3 - 40 ng/mL *1179*

β-Chorionic Gonadotropin *Plasma Increase* Human chorionic somatomammotropin was > normal in 8 of 13 patients with intact mole, ranging from 10 - 910 ng/mL *3533* In 30 patients with molar pregnancy in remission mean concentration of 435 ± 89 IU/mL significantly higher than 100 ± 8 IU/mL in 23 healthy pregnant women during the first trimester *4747* High concentrations of chorionic gonadotropin and reduced pregnanediol indicate diagnosis *4707* 0.5 - 2,830 IU/mL and less than 200 IU/mL in 36% of the patients *3705* Median concentration of 101,300 mIU/mL in 4 patients with partial mole, 174,800 mIU/mL in 21 with complete mole and 833 mIU/mL in 27 with persistent mole different from 3 mIU/mL in 58 nonpregnant controls *1929*
Urine Increase A rising titer at the end of the first trimester is significant. Titers can rise to 1,000 IU/L or more *1290*

Estrogens *Plasma Increase* Plasma unconjugated estradiol was greater than normal in 6 of 13 patients with intact mole, ranging from 1.82 - 8.10 ng/mL at 15 - 19 weeks gestation *3533*

Factor II *Plasma Decrease* May be associated with defibrination resulting in platelet and coagulation factor consumption *5677*

Factor IV *Plasma Decrease* May be associated with defibrination resulting in platelet and coagulation factor consumption *5677*

α-Fetoprotein *Serum No Effect* Undetectable in 100% of patients with intact mole, but > 10 ng/mL in 18 of 23 normal pregnancies *3533*

Fibrin Degradation Products *Plasma Increase* Increased circulating amounts with associated prolonged thrombin time indicate hypercoagulability *3124*

Fibrinogen *Plasma Decrease* Decreased as a result of excess utilization due to release of tissue thromboplastin *1290* May be associated with defibrination resulting in platelet and coagulation factor consumption *5677*

Hemoglobin F *Blood Increase* Observed effect *5544*

Inhibin *Plasma Increase* In 5 women with hydatidiform moles mean concentration of 4,200 ± 850 U/L significantly higher than 1,550 ± 1,020 U/L in 26 women at same stage of pregnancy *244*

Interleukin-1β *Serum Decrease* In 30 patients with molar pregnancy in remission mean concentration of 16.45 ± 0.57 pg/mL significantly lower than 26.2 ± 1.71 pg/mL in 23 healthy pregnant women during the first trimester *4747*
Serum Increase In 12 patients with progressive molar pregnancy mean concentration of 798 ± 177 pg/mL significantly higher than 26.2 ± 1.71 pg/mL in 23 healthy pregnant women during the first trimester *4747*

Interleukin-6 *Serum Increase* In 30 patients with molar pregnancy in remission and in 12 with progressive disease mean concentrations of 55.9 ± 9.38 pg/mL and 6,625 ± 1,031 pg/mL, respectively, significantly higher than 30.5 ± 1.31 pg/mL in 23 healthy pregnant women during the first trimester *4747*

Leptin *Serum Increase* Since leptin is produced by trophoblastic tissue as well as in adipocytes, concentrations increase with disease progression *5542*

Major Basic Protein *Serum Increase* Median concentration of 1,826 ng/mL in 4 patients with partial mole, 921 ng/mL in 21 with complete mole and 235 ng/mL in 27 with persistent mole different from 129 ng/mL in 58 nonpregnant controls *1929*

Partial Thromboplastin Time *Plasma Decrease* Mean time was 32.9/37.1 s in patients compared to 33.6/35.9 in normal pregnancy. Associated with prolonged thrombin time and indicates hypercoagulability *3124*

Platelets *Blood Decrease* May be associated with defibrination resulting in platelet and coagulation factor consumption *5677*

630.00 Hydatidiform Mole *(continued)*

Pregnanediol *Urine Decrease* High concentrations of chorionic gonadotropin and reduced pregnanediol suggests diagnosis *4707*

Progesterone *Plasma Decrease* High concentrations of chorionic gonadotropin and reduced pregnanediol indicate diagnosis *4707*
Plasma Increase Higher progesterone concentration than found in normal pregnant women in 8 of 13 patients with intact mole, ranging from 17.5 - 79.2 ng/mL *3533*

Prothrombin Consumption *Blood Increase* May be associated with defibrination resulting in platelet and coagulation factor consumption *5677*

Thrombin Time *Blood Increase* Mean time was 21.1/16.6 s in patients compared to 17.6/15.9 in normal pregnancy. Prolonged time and associated reduction of partial thromboplastin time indicates hypercoagulability and high fibrinogen turnover rate *3124*

Thyroid Stimulating Hormone *Serum Increase* 9 of 14 patients were hyperthyroid. Found in high concentrations in 13 preoperative patients. Close correlation with human chorionic gonadotropins suggests that the hCG molecule, when present in large amounts, stimulates thyroid function *2153*

Thyroxine (T4) *Serum Increase* 9 of 14 patients were hyperthyroid. T4 varied from 18 - 34 mg/dL *2153* In patients with gestational trophoblastic disease without signs of hyperthyroidism, the mean serum total and free T4 concentrations were 43% and 92% higher than those in normal pregnancy *3933*

Tri-iodothyronine (T3) *Serum Increase* 9 of 14 patients were hyperthyroid. Serum T3 ranged from 300 - 800 ng/dL. Correlated closely with chorionic gonadotropins *2153* High in 13 of 15 patients with molar pregnancy, paralleling the concentration of T4 *5581*

Tumor Necrosis Factor-β *Serum Increase* In 12 patients with progressive molar pregnancy in remission mean concentration of 724 ± 197 pg/mL significantly different from upper limit of normal in first trimester of 32.6 pg/mL in 23 healthy pregnant women *4747*
Serum No Effect In 30 patients with molar pregnancy in remission mean concentration of 13.55 ± 1.05 pg/mL not significantly different from upper limit of normal in first trimester of 32.6 pg/mL in 23 healthy pregnant women *4747*

630.00 Placental-site Trophoblastic Tumor

β-Chorionic Gonadotropin *Plasma Increase* Median concentration of 76 mIU/mL in 5 patients with PSTT different from 3 mIU/mL in 58 nonpregnant controls *1929*

Major Basic Protein *Serum Increase* Median concentration of 199 ng/mL in 5 patients with PSTT different from 129 ng/mL in 58 nonpregnant controls *1929*

632.00 Missed Abortion

β-Chorionic Gonadotropin *Plasma Decrease* In 30 women with missed abortions mean concentration of 8,835 ± 13,132 mIU/mL significantly different from 37,553 ± 30,133 mIU/mL in 30 women with ongoing pregnancies *1013*

Creatine Kinase *Serum No Effect* In 30 women with missed abortions mean activity of 84.8 ± 49.3 U/L not significantly different from 81.5 ± 40.3 U/L in 30 women with ongoing pregnancies *1013*

Progesterone *Plasma Decrease* In 30 women with missed abortions mean concentration of 17.7 ± 14.4 ng/mL significantly different from 63.2 ± 27.2 ng/mL in 30 women with ongoing pregnancies *1013*

633.00 Ectopic Pregnancy

Amylase *Serum Increase* Associated with ruptured ectopic pregnancy *2626* Elevated levels *5618* Values of 2,000 U/L have been reported *1504*

CA 125 *Serum Increase* Concentration in women with ectopic pregnancies likely to be higher than in those with intrauterine pregnancies *4499*

β-Chorionic Gonadotropin *Plasma Decrease* Decreased *3777* 82.6% of 23 women with proven ectopic pregnancies had abnormally low first trimester hCG levels *564* Decreased *455* *4736* In 30 women with ectopic pregnancy mean concentration of 15,190 ± 26,903 mIU/mL significantly different from 37,553 ± 30,133 mIU/mL in 30 women with ongoing pregnancies *1013* Decreased *552*
Urine Decrease Low values for the stage of pregnancy *1290*

Creatine Kinase *Serum Increase* In 21 patients with proved ectopic pregnancy mean activity of 53.4 U/L significantly higher than in all other pregnancies studied *1263*
Serum No Effect In 11 patients with symptomatic tubal pregnancy mean activity of 59 ± 10.1 U/L and 58.5 ± 12.4 U/L not significantly different from 58.5 ± 7.2 U/L in 20 women with normal pregnancies *5483* In 30 women with ectopic pregnancy mean activity of 81.4 ± 66.2 U/L not significantly different from 81.5 ± 40.3 U/L in 30 women with ongoing pregnancies *1013*

Erythrocyte Sedimentation Rate *Blood Increase* Rises in the first 24 h *1980*

Glucose *Serum Increase* In 45% of 11 patients at initial hospitalization for this disorder *1576*

Hematocrit *Blood No Effect* May be normal, even in view of acute rupture of an ectopic pregnancy, as the patient has not had time for fluid stabilization *900*

Lactate Dehydrogenase *Serum Increase* In 4 of 10 patients at initial hospitalization for this disorder *1576*

Leukocytes *Blood Increase* May increase but rarely to significantly high levels *900*
Blood No Effect No significant change in count usually observed *900*

Lipase *Serum No Effect* Normal levels *4289*

Progesterone *Plasma Decrease* In 30 women with ectopic pregnancy mean concentration of 33.7 ± 26.5 ng/mL significantly different from 63.2 ± 27.2 ng/mL in 30 women with ongoing pregnancies *1013*

Relaxin *Plasma Decrease* On days 39 - 70 of pregnancy mean serum relaxin concentration significantly lower in 10 resorbing ectopic gestations than in a normal control group of 13 intrauterine pregnancies *1644*

633.00 Ectopic Tubal Pregnancy

Creatine Kinase *Serum Increase* Mean activity in 20 women who had an ectopic tubal pregnancy of 34.2 U/L compared with 18.7 U/L in women matched for age and duration of pregnancy *4512*

Creatine Kinase MB-Isoenzyme *Serum No Effect* Mean activity in 20 women who had an ectopic tubal pregnancy not significantly different compared with that in women matched for age and duration of pregnancy *4512*

634.90 Recurrent Abortions

Anticardiolipin Antibodies *Serum Increase* Incidence of 7.7% in 130 patients not significantly higher than 3.1% in 97 healthy controls *156*

Antiphosphatidic Acid Antibodies *Serum Increase* Incidence of 3.1% in 130 patients not significantly higher than 0.0% in 97 healthy controls *156*

Antiphosphatidylethanolamine Antibodies *Serum No Effect* Incidence of 4.6% in 130 patients not significantly different from 9.3% in 97 healthy controls *156*

Antiphosphatidylglycerol Antibodies *Serum No Effect* Incidence of 0.0% in 130 patients not significantly different from 0.0% in 97 healthy controls *156*

Antiphosphatidylinositol Antibodies *Serum Increase* Incidence of 3.8% in 130 patients not significantly higher than 2.1% in 97 healthy controls *156*

Antiphosphatidylserine Antibodies *Serum Increase* Incidence of 13.1% in 130 patients not significantly higher than 5.2% in 97 healthy controls *156*

Antiphospholipid Antibodies *Serum Increase* About 60% of patients with recurrent fetal loss (recurrent miscarriage syndrome) have antiphospholipid antibodies *441*

β_2-Glycoprotein I-dependent Anticardiolipin Antibodies *Serum* *Increase* Incidence of 5.4% in 130 patients not significantly higher than 4.1% in 97 healthy controls *156*

637.90 Abortion

Anticardiolipin Antibodies *Serum* *Increase* An elevated IgG anticardiolipin antibody level at the first prenatal visit was the only aPL measurement that was significantly associated with fetal loss (relative risk, 3.5; CI, 1.56 to 8.07) *3176*

CA 125 *Serum* *Increase* Although marker is routinely present in amniotic fluid highest maternal serum concentrations occurred in first trimester: 6 of 10 women with CA 125 concentrations above 150 U/mL aborted compared with 4 of 92 with concentrations less than 150 U/mL *797*

Ceruloplasmin *Serum* *Decrease* Significant decrease in 20 patients observed 3 hours after induced abortion *3964*

Copper *Serum* *Decrease* In 20 patients 3 hours after induced abortion significant reduction in concentration observed *3964*

Creatine Kinase *Serum* *No Effect* Mean activity in 30 patients with spontaneous abortions of 84.8 ± 49.3 not significantly different from 81.5 ± 40.3 U/L in 30 patients with on-going normal pregnancies *1013*

Gravidin *Plasma* *Decrease* In 28 women in first trimester administration of RU-486 caused mean decrease from 100% to 94% after 2 days *5692*

Homocysteine *Plasma* *Increase* Hyperhomocysteinemia was diagnosed in 21 women of the study group (21%). In the parous women of the study group, the prevalence of hyperhomocysteinemia was more than two times greater compared with the nulliparous subjects (33% and 14%, respectively). Hyperhomocysteinemia is a risk factor in women with unexplained recurrent early pregnancy loss *5734*

Interleukin-2 *Serum* *Decrease* In women with recurrent miscarriage a decrease in IL-2 serum levels ($p < 0.05$) were compared to women with normal pregnancies. These results support the concept that disturbances of immune tolerance of the fetus may account for some cases of recurrent miscarriage *3257*

Malondialdehyde *Serum* *Decrease* Mean concentrations before abortion by suction curettage of 2.67 nmol/mL, emcredil-induced 3.22 nmol/L and spontaneous 3.49 nmol/mL compared with 1.91, 1.97 and 1.95 nmol/mL respectively after abortion *4564*

Thyroxine Binding Globulin *Serum* *Decrease* Significantly lower concentrations observed in spontaneously aborting women in early pregnancy *4885*

Thyroxine (T4) *Serum* *Decrease* Slightly lower concentration observed in spontaneously aborting women at same stage of pregnancy *4885*

Tissue Polypeptide Antigen *Serum* *No Effect* No significant change observed during abortion *570*

Tri-iodothyronine (T3) *Serum* *Decrease* Slightly lower concentration observed at same stage of pregnancy in spontaneously aborting women *4885*

Tumor Necrosis Factor-α *Serum* *Increase* In women with recurrent miscarriage an increase in TNF-α (p less than 0.05) were compared to women with normal pregnancies. These results support the concept that disturbances of immune tolerance of the fetus may account for some cases of recurrent miscarriage *3257*

Zinc *Serum* *No Effect* No significant change observed in 20 patients 3 hours after induced abortion *3964*

640.00 Threatened Abortion

β-Chorionic Gonadotropin *Plasma* *Decrease* Decreased *552 455 602 3777*
Urine *Decrease* Low values for stage of pregnancy. Low values in early pregnancy are found in habitual abortion *1290*

Creatine Kinase *Serum* *No Effect* In 15 patients with theatened abortion mean activity of 73 ± 11.4 U/L not significantly different from 58.5 ± 7.2 U/L in 20 women with normal pregnancies *5483*

α-Fetoprotein *Serum* *No Effect* In patients with premature labor, the majority of concentrations were significantly below the normal range, and the peak levels were achieved approximately 1 month earlier than normal. In patients whose pregnancies were terminated by abortion, the levels exhibited a significant rise within a few h after induction because of resorption of fetal elements into the maternal circulation *2069*

Leucine Aminopeptidase *Serum* *Increase* High prior to abortion *1290*

Pregnanediol *Urine* *Decrease* Sometimes *5544*

Progesterone *Plasma* *Decrease* Has been reported to be low, but is often normal prior to spontaneous abortion *4707*

641.20 Abruptio Placentae

CA 125 *Serum* *Increase* Sensitivity and specificity for abruptio placentae were 70% and 94% respectively. The data supports a decidual source for CA 125 and may indicate a utility as a marker of this condition *5704*

642.40 Pre-eclampsia

Alanine Aminotransferase *Serum* *Increase* Degree of abnormality closely parallels the severity *964* In 12 preeclamptic patients activity of 26 ± 12 U/L not significantly different when compared with 23 ± 6 U/L in 12 normotensive controls *4482* In 79 pregnant women with preeclampsia median activity of 15 U/L significantly greater than that in 87 normotensive pregnant women in whom the median activity was 4 U/L *2712* In about 20 women with preeclampsia at weeks 24 - 29 and 30 - 35 mean activities of 0.91 ± 0.48 and 0.82 ± 0.32 µkat/L significantly higher than 0.33 ± 0.02 and 0.30 ± 0.02 µkat/L in healthy pregnant women at the corresponding times and < 0.60 µkat/L in healthy control women *2080* Degree of abnormality closely parallels the severity *3617 5115* In about 20% of patients with mild cases *811*
Serum *No Effect* Usually activity not elevated. When transaminases are found to be elevated, either pronounced hepatic or marked myocardial alterations have occurred *900* In about 20 women with preeclampsia mean activity at weeks 36 - 40 of 0.27 ± 0.03 µkat/L not significantly different from < 0.60 µkat/L in healthy nonpregnant control women *2080* In 67 women with preeclampsia mean activity of 15 U/L not significantly different from 7 U/L in 41 women with normotensive pregnancies *2714*

Albumin *Serum* *Decrease* Significantly reduced below the levels for normal pregnancy *900* In 20 pregnant women in third trimester with severe pre-eclampsia mean concentration of 34 ± 3 g/L significantly less than 36 ± 2 g/L in 17 hypertensive pregnant women *600*
Urine *Increase* Characteristic but may appear late in the course of the disease. Fluctuates from day to day *811* Mean albumin/creatinine excretion of 1.4 (0.6 - 3.6) mg/mmol in 20 pregnant women in third trimester with severe pre-eclampsia significantly higher than 0.7 (0.4 - 1.2) mg/mmol in 38 women with mild pre-eclampsia, 0.7 (0.4 - 1.4) mg/mmol in 17 women with essential hypertension, 0.7 (0.6 - 0.9) mg/mmol in 40 normal pregnant women and 0.6 (0.5 - 0.9) mg/mmol in 26 nonpregnant women. Albumin excretion rate of 13 (7 - 32) mg/d in the women with severe pre-eclampsia significantly higher than 7 (5 - 8) mg/d in 9 normal pregnant women *600*

Aldosterone *Plasma* *Decrease* In pregnant women with preeclampsia one week before delivery mean activity in 16 who had a Cesarean section of 26.9 ± 5.8 ng/dL significantly different from 44.4 ± 21.1 ng/dL in 11 pregnant women without preeclampsia and 24.0 ± 5.2 ng/dL in 14 with preeclampsia who had a vaginal delivery significantly different from 37.9 ± 7.3 ng/dL in 8 who had a vaginal delivery *1608* In pre-eclamptic women mean concentration significantly less than in pregnant healthy controls *4745* The secretory rate is somewhat depressed, but often falls within the lower range of normal for pregnancy. In severe cases, concentration was found to be within the range for nonpregnant women (10% of that of normal pregnancy) *5592* Concentration depressed in the plasma of 21 preeclamptic women compared with that in 15 healthy normotensive pregnant controls *3881* Significantly suppressed during the last trimester despite levels of renin substrate and progesterone that were not significantly different from those observed in normotensive preg-

642.40 **Pre-eclampsia** *(continued)*

Aldosterone *(continued)*
nancy *5616* In 8 preeclamptic women in their third trimester mean concentration of 871 ± 156 pmol/L significantly less than that in 7 normotensive pregnant women in their third trimester in whom the mean concentration was 1,495 ± 241 pmol/L *2914*
Plasma Increase In 13 pre-eclamptic women mean concentration increased in parallel with severity of pre-eclampsia *2177* At term, hypertensive, toxemic pregnant women had elevated aldosterone and plasma renin activity, which remained elevated > 1 week after delivery *139* Mean concentration of 1395 ± 261 pmol/L significantly increased compared with concentration in nonpregnant control women (652 ± 78 pmol/L) but less than in normal pregnant women (2665 ± 350 pmol/L) *856*
Plasma No Effect During normal pregnancy, plasma levels of renin, angiotensin II, and aldosterone are increased. Paradoxically with pregnancy-induced hypertension they commonly decrease towards the normal *4223* In hypertensive groups, plasma renin activity and aldosterone concentration were significantly suppressed during the last trimester despite levels of renin substrate and progesterone that were not significantly different from those observed in normotensive pregnancy *5616*
Urine Decrease Significantly suppressed during the last trimester despite levels of renin substrate and progesterone that were not significantly different from those observed in normotensive pregnancy *5616* The secretory rate is somewhat depressed, but often falls within the lower range of normal for pregnancy. In severe cases, concentration was found to be within the range for nonpregnant women (10% of that of normal pregnancy) *5592*
Urine Increase At term, hypertensive, toxemic pregnant women had elevated aldosterone and plasma renin activity, which remained elevated > 1 week after delivery *139*
Urine No Effect In hypertensive groups, plasma renin activity and aldosterone concentration were significantly suppressed during the first trimester despite levels of renin substrate and progesterone that were not significantly different from those observed in normotensive pregnancy *5616* During normal pregnancy, plasma levels of renin, angiotensin II, and aldosterone are increased. Paradoxically with pregnancy-induced hypertension, they commonly decrease towards the normal *4223*

Alkaline Phosphatase *Serum Increase* Exaggerated increases may occur and could indicate placental as well as hepatic damage *811* May be elevated above the normal increase found in pregnancy. This is due to a rise in the heat-stable (placental) isoenzyme *4546*
Serum No Effect Usually not elevated. When elevated, either pronounced hepatic or marked myocardial alterations have occurred *900* Activity usually normal *4546*

Alkaline Phosphatase Isoenzymes *Serum Increase* May be elevated above the normal increase found in pregnancy, due to a rise in the heat-stable (placental) isoenzyme *4546*

Alkaline Phosphatase, Tissue Unspecific *Urine Increase* Mean excretion of 2.77 ± 0.22 U/g creatinine in 26 mildly pre-eclamptic women (6 of 26 abnormal) and of 3.75 ± 0.14 U/g creatinine in 26 severely pre-eclamptic women (20 of 26 abnormal) significantly greater than 2.02 ± 0.13 U/g creatinine in 20 normotensive control pregnant women *4748*

Aminopeptidase A *Serum Increase* Activity increased in preeclampsia but not to the same extent as in normal pregnancy *3539*

Amylase *Serum Increase* In 13 patients with severe pre-eclampsia mean concentration of 1.6 µmol/L compared with 1.1 µmol/L in 30 normal pregnancies *2066*

Angiotensin-I *Plasma Decrease* In 8 preeclamptic pregnant women mean concentration of 12.6 ± 1.5 fmol/mL significantly different from 28.0 ± 3.7 fmol/mL in seven normotensive pregnant women in their third trimester *2914*

Angiotensin-converting Enzyme *Serum No Effect* In 8 preeclamptic women mean activity of 17.5 ± 1.1 nmol hippuric acid/min/mL not significantly different from that in 7 normotensive pregnant women in their third trimester in whom the mean concentration was 16.6 ± 0.8 nmol/min/mL *2914*

Antidiuretic Hormone *Plasma Increase* Positive correlation between severity of toxemia and circulating ADH *4707*

Antithrombin III *Plasma Decrease* Noted in one patient with severe pre-eclampsia toxemia *629* Concentration in preeclamptic women significantly lower than in healthy pregnant women in both second and third trimesters *2179* Concentration decreased but only in severe preeclampsia *4064* In 19 women with preeclampsia mean concentration of 73% significantly different from 93% in 18 normal pregnant women *4033*

Ascorbic Acid *Serum Decrease* Mean concentration of 11.0 nmol/mL in 14 patients at 35.1 ± 2.9 weeks with preeclampsia significantly different from 21.1 nmol/mL in 17 healthy women at 39.9 ± 0.8 weeks *2271*
Serum No Effect In 12 patients with severe preeclampsia mean values of 0.5 ± 0.5 mg/dL and of 0.7 ± 0.6 mg/dL in 14 patients with mild preeclampsia not significantly different from 0.7 ± 0.4 mg/dL in 20 healthy controls *3955*

Aspartate Aminotransferase *Serum Increase* Degree of abnormality closely parallels the severity *3617* In about 20 women with preeclampsia at weeks 24 - 29 and 30 - 35 mean activities of 0.74 ± 0.27 and 0.82 ± 0.17 µkat/L significantly higher than 0.45 ± 0.02 and 0.43 ± 0.02 µkat/L in healthy pregnant women at the corresponding times and < 0.60 µkat/L in healthy control women *2080* In 26 women with mild pre-eclampsia mean concentration of 19.1 ± 17.5 U/L and in 8 with severe pre-eclampsia 33.0 ± 26.7 U/L compared with 12.0 ± 7.5 U/L in 39 healthy controls *3353* Degree of abnormality closely parallels the severity *964* In about 20% of patients with mild cases *811* Degree of abnormality closely parallels the severity *5115* In 23 women with pregnancies complicated by preeclampsia or HELLP syndrome median activity of 125 U/L *2713* In 12 preeclamptic patients activity of 35 ± 16 U/L not significantly different when compared with 28 ± 18 U/L in 12 normotensive controls *4482*
Serum No Effect In about 20 women with preeclampsia mean activity at weeks 36 - 40 of 0.45 ± 0.04 µkat/L not significantly different from < 0.60 µkat/L in healthy nonpregnant control women *2080* In 25 patients with preeclampsia concentration of 43.4 ± 47 U/L not significantly different from 24.5 ± 11.9 U/L in 11 control pregnant women *3059* Usually activity not elevated. When elevated, either pronounced hepatic or marked myocardial alterations have occurred *900* In 67 women with preeclampsia mean activity of 17 U/L not significantly different from 9 U/L in 41 women with normotensive pregnancies *2714*

Atrial Natriuretic Peptide *Plasma Increase* Concentration higher at same stage of pregnancy than in non-preeclamptic control pregnant women: mean of 12.9 pg/mL in first trimester, 18.5 pg/mL in second trimester and 31.1 pg/mL in third trimester *3247* Nonsignificant increase to 93 ± 36 pmol/L in preeclamptic women compared with 55 ± 8 pmol/L in normal pregnancy and 53 ± 3 in nonpregnant controls *856* In 21 preeclamptic women median concentration of 11.9 pmol/L significantly different from 7.5 pmol/L in 12 healthy pregnant women *4195* Mean concentration in 9 mild preeclamptics 127 ± 60 ng/L and in 6 individuals with severe preeclampsia 392 ± 225 ng/L compared with 37 ± 19 ng/L in 25 young nonpregnant control women *5217* In pre-eclamptic women mean concentration significantly higher than in healthy pregnant controls *4745* In 49 patients with gestational hypertension median concentration of 13.6 pmol/L significantly different from 7.5 pmol/L in 49 matched pregnant controls, with concentrations in severe preeclampsia (19.2 pmol/L) higher than in mild preeclampsia (12.3 pmol/L) *4194*

Bicarbonate *Serum Decrease* Changes in electrolytes are usually insignificant. In severe cases, the bicarbonate may be lowered *811*

Bleeding Time *Patient Increase* In 9 of 26 patients with pre-eclampsia prolonged bleeding time observed in comparison with none in a control pregnant population *2629*

BSP Retention *Serum Increase* A larger proportion of hypertensive women have increased retention than normal pregnant women, (> 5% in 45 min), but many are in the range of normal *811*

γ-Butyric Acid *Plasma Increase* In pre-eclamptic patients during third trimester concentration similar to that in normal pregnant women in third trimester (158 ± 9 pmol/mL in pre-eclamptics versus 176 ± 6 pmol/mL in normal women) but 13 ± 3% lower during labor *949*

Calcitonin *Plasma No Effect* No significant difference observed in third trimester in pre-eclampsia or in normal pregnancy compared with nonpregnant controls *4056*

Calcitonin Gene-related Peptide *Serum No Effect* In 21 patients with severely eclamptic pregnancies mean concentration of 29.8 ± 4.2 pmol/L not significantly different from 28.5 ± 5.4 pmol/L in 21 non-pregnant women *4631*

Calcium *Serum Decrease* Significantly lower with preeclampsia (but not significantly different from concentration in normal pregnancy) than 3 and 6 months after pregnancy *4056*
Serum No Effect In 12 preeclamptic women mean concentration of 1.17 ± 0.04 mmol/L not significantly different from 1.22 ± 0.01 mmol/L in 33 normal pregnant women and 1.22 ± 0.01 mmol/L in 42 nonpregnant women *2000* In 9 patients with preeclampsia mean concentrations of 2.65 ± 0.13 mmol/L, 2.34 ± 0.09 mmol/L and 2.26 ± 0.7 mmol/L in the first, second and third trimesters not significantly different from 2.44 ± 0.06 mmol/L, 2.40 ± 0.07 mmol/L and 2.28 ± 0.05 mmol/L in the first, second and third trimesters of 22 healthy control women *4980*
Urine Decrease In 12 preeclamptic women in their third trimester mean concentration of 2.9 ± 0.7 mmol/d significantly different from 6.5 ± 0.2 mmol/d in 24 normotensive women in their third trimester *4712* Mean excretion of 42 ± 29 mg/d in preeclamptic women in third trimester significantly less than in normal pregnant women, 313 ± 140 mg/d *5173*

Cationic Trypsinogen *Serum Increase* In 13 patients with severe preeclampsia mean concentration of 64 ng/mL compared with 22 ng/mL in 30 women with normal pregnancies *2066*

Cholesterol *Serum Decrease* In 5 preeclamptic women median concentration of 6.88 mmol/L not significantly different from 7.35 mmol/L in 8 healthy control individuals *4594*

β-Chorionic Gonadotropin *Plasma Increase* Mean of MoM in 34 pregnant women with preeclampsia of 1.67 compared with 1 in 5,776 control pregnant women at 15 to 18 weeks of pregnancy *3650* In 41 primigravids who developed preeclampsia concentration significantly higher than in 41 age and gestation matched pregnant control women *4515* Severe cases often are associated with high urinary and serum concentrations, and mild cases are not *3126*
Plasma No Effect Average serum and urinary concentrations were the same in pre-eclamptic as in normal pregnant women *5175*
Urine Increase Severe cases often are associated with high urinary and serum concentrations, and mild cases are not *3126*
Urine No Effect Average concentrations in urine and sera were the same in pre-eclamptic as in normal pregnant women *5175*

Colloid Osmotic Pressure *Serum Decrease* Significant reduction observed in patients with preeclampsia related to severity of preeclampsia and degree of proteinuria but best correlation with plasma fibronectin concentration suggesting that endothelial injury rather than proteinuria is cause *434*

Complement, Total *Serum Increase* Significantly higher than in late normal pregnancy *5056 860*

Copper *Serum Decrease* Concentration in maternal serum reduced in women with pre-eclampsia in comparison with control pregnant women *2672*

Creatinine *Serum Decrease* Low BUN (9 ± 2 mg/dL) and low creatinine (0.75 ± 0.2 mg/dL) in late pregnancy are indicative of toxemia *367*
Serum Increase Concentration higher in severe pre-eclamptics than in mild pre-eclamptics and in healthy pregnant women controls *2591* In 16 preeclamptic women mean concentration of 1.0 ± 0.03 mg/dL significantly higher than in 11 normal pregnant women (0.74 ± 0.03 mg/dL) *856* If the hypertension has reached relatively severe levels, may be elevated, indicating renal damage *900* Mean concentration of 70 ± 19.9 μmol/L in 26 mildly pre-eclamptic women (nonsignificant increase) and of 131 ± 10.2 μmol/L in 26 severely pre-eclamptic women significantly greater than 62 ± 12 μmol/L in 20 normotensive control pregnant women *4748*
Serum No Effect In 20 pregnant women in third trimester with severe pre-eclampsia mean concentration of 0.08 ± 0.01 mmol/L not significantly different from 0.07 ± 0.01 mmol/L in 38 with mild pre-eclampsia and 0.07 ± 0.01 mmol/L in 17 pregnant women with essential hypertension *600* In 20 preeclamptic pregnant women mean concentration of 0.86 ± 0.08 mg/dL not significantly different from that in 25 healthy nonpregnant women in whom the mean concentration was 0.82 ± 0.07 mg/dL *2697* In 23 women with pregnancies complicated by preeclampsia or HELLP syndrome median concentration of 82 μmol/L *2713* In 20 pregnant women with pre-eclampsia mean concentration of 0.86 ± 0.08 mmol/L not significantly different from 0.80 ± 0.04 mmol/L in 25 healthy nonpregnant control women *2698* In 20 preeclamptic pregnant women mean concentration of 0.86 ± 0.08 mmol/L not different from 0.80 ± 0.04 mmol/L in 25 healthy nonpregnant women *2699*
Urine Decrease Mean excretion in 30 patients with preeclampsia 69.9 ± 8.6 mg/dL significantly less than 114.2 ± 8.1 mg/dL in 30 matched controls *2259* In 20 pregnant women in third trimester with severe pre-eclampsia mean excretion of 9.7 ± 2.7 mmol/d not significantly less than 10.1 ± 2.5 mmol/d in 38 patients with mild pre-eclampsia, 10.1 ± 2.9 mmol/d in 17 pregnant women with essential hypertension, 11.1 ± 2.7 mmol/d in 40 normal women compared with 11.3 ± 2.3 mmol/d in 26 nonpregnant women *600*

Creatinine Clearance *Urine Decrease* In comparison with clearance in normal pregnant women mean clearance reduced in third trimester (102 mL/min) versus 118 mL/min in normal third trimester and 5 days after delivery, 106 mL/min versus 119 mL/min *4056* In 16 preeclamptic women mean clearance of 103 ± 5 mL/min significantly less than in 11 normal pregnant women (126 ± 6 mL/min) *856* In 12 preeclamptic women in their third trimester mean concentration of 1.88 ± 0.18 mL/s not significantly different from 2.12 ± 0.17 mL/s in 24 normotensive women in their third trimester *4712* Mean clearance of 176 ± 37.7 mL/min in 26 mildly pre-eclamptic women (nonsignificant decrease) and of 86 ± 14.8 mL/min in 26 severely pre-eclamptic women significantly less than 195 ± 40 mL/min in 20 normotensive control pregnant women *4748* In 20 pregnant women in third trimester with severe pre-eclampsia mean clearance of 1.5 ± 0.5 mL/s and 1.7 ± 0.4 mL/s in 36 women with mild pre-eclampsia, 1.8 ± 0.6 mL/s in 17 pregnant women with essential hypertension significantly less than 2.2 ± 0.4 mL/s in 9 normal pregnant women *600*

Cryofibrinogen *Plasma Increase* Suggest that slow, chronic, intravascular clotting is taking place *5677*

Cytidine Deaminase *Serum Increase* Increased activity observed in 42.9% of patients with severe pre-eclampsia, 9.1% of patients with mild pre-eclampsia and in 8.6% normal pregnancies *252*

D-Dimer *Plasma No Effect* In 19 women with preeclampsia mean concentration not significantly different from that in 18 normal pregnant women *4033*

Dehydroepiandrosterone *Plasma Increase* Concentration significantly increased at 32 and 36 weeks in preeclamptic pregnancies compared with normal pregnancies *4444*

Dehydroepiandrosterone Sulfate *Plasma No Effect* No significant difference observed in concentrations at 32 and 36 weeks between preeclamptic and normal pregnancies *4444*

Deoxycorticosterone *Plasma Decrease* Plasma concentrations averaged 10.2 ± 2.7 ng/dL, which is about half the value found in normal pregnant women *5622*

1,25-Dihydroxy Vitamin D *Serum Decrease* In 12 preeclamptic women in their third trimester mean concentration of 1,72.1 ± 18.5 pmol/L significantly different from 2,19.6 ± 12.7 pmol/L in 24 normotensive women in their third trimester *4712*
Serum No Effect No significant difference observed between concentrations in third trimester in normal pregnant, hypertensive and preeclamptic women *5173*

Dopamine *Plasma Increase* In pre-eclamptic women mean arterial concentration significantly higher than in normotensive pregnant controls. Venous plasma concentration also significantly higher *3882*

Dopamine, Free *Plasma Increase* In 21 preeclamptic women mean concentration of free dopamine of 137 ± 35 pg/mL compared with 55 ± 6 pg/mL in 15 normotensive pregnant women *3881*

α_1-Easily Precipitable Glycoprotein *Serum Increase* Concentration of alpha$_1$-easily precipitable glycoprotein increased greatly despite large urinary losses, indicating augmented synthesis *5055* Concentration of alpha$_1$ easily precipitable glycoprotein increased greatly despite large urinary losses, indicating augmented synthesis *5056*
Urine Increase Large urinary losses of alpha$_1$ easily precipitable glycoprotein *5056 5055*

Eicosapentaenoic Acid *Serum Decrease* Significant reduction observed in pre-eclamptic women at term compared with nonpregnant controls *5565*

Endothelin *Plasma Increase* In pregnant women with preeclampsia one week before delivery mean concentration in 16 who had a Cesarean section of 1.52 ± 0.1 pg/mL significantly higher than 1.04 ± 0.04 pg/mL in 11 pregnant women without preeclampsia but 1.21 ± 0.1 pg/mL in 14 with preeclampsia who had a vaginal delivery not significantly different from 1.00 ± 0.07 pg/mL in 8 who had a vaginal delivery *1608* Increased concen-

642.40 **Pre-eclampsia** *(continued)*

Endothelin *(continued)*
trations observed with pre-eclampsia *4093* Significant increase observed in women with pre-eclampsia compared with normal pregnant women *5178* Mean concentration significantly increased in women with preeclampsia during the third trimester but normalized with postpartum decrease of blood pressure *5310* In 16 pregnant women with preeclampsia mean concentration of 22.6 ± 2.0 pmol/L significantly higher than mean 12.0 ± 1.0 pmol/L in 11 gestation-matched pregnant women and 10.4 ± 1.3 pmol/L in nonpregnant controls *856* In preeclampsia mean concentration of 22.6 ± 2.0 pmol/L significantly higher than 12.0 ± 1.0 pmol/L in normal pregnant women and 10.4 pmol/L in nonpregnant control women *856*

Endothelin-1 *Amniotic Fluid Decrease* Concentrations not significantly decreased to 16.0 ± 2.3 pmol/L in 35 women with severe pre-eclampsia compared with 19.4 ± 4.2 pmol/L in 31 women with normal pregnancies *5712*
Plasma Increase Mean concentration of 5.0 (2.1 - 12.4) ng/L significantly increased compared with mean of 3.6 ng/L in normotensive nonpregnant women and 2.1 ng/L in pregnant women *1512* In patients with mild and severe pre-eclampsia mean concentrations of 14.3 ± 2.2 pg/mL and 27.2 ± 8.6 pg/mL significantly higher than in nonpregnant state of 10.7 ± 2.5 pg/mL *2319* In 2 studies of women with pre-eclampsia but without hemolysis mean concentrations increased 1.4- and 1.9-fold compared with pregnant women at the same stage of pregnancy *328* Concentrations increased to 2.8 ± 0.6 pmol/L in 35 women with severe pre-eclampsia in retroplacental (and other blood) compared with 2.3 ± 0.3 pmol/L in 31 women with normal pregnancies *5712* In 4 women with pre-eclampsia and hemolysis mean concentration of 2.2 times appropriate normals and 33 women in two other studies means were 1.4 and 1.9 times normal values *328* The mean level among the women with preeclampsia (29.9 ± 13.2 fmol/mL) was significantly higher than those of the chronically hypertensive women (16.1 ± 7.3 fmol/mL, p = 0.002) and of the control pregnant women (19.7 ± 9.2 fmol/mL, p = 0.011) *4630* Mean concentration in 12 patients with severe preeclampsia of 11.0 ± 6.6 pg/mL significantly different from 8.4 - 6.7 pg/mL in normotensive patients *4482* Mean concentration in 11 women with preeclampsia of 0.75 ± 0.28 pmol/L significantly higher than 0.25 ± 0.04 pmol/L in 11 normotensive pregnant women *5066* In 21 preeclamptic women median concentration of 6.2 pmol/L significantly higher than 4.8 pmol/L in 32 healthy pregnant women *4195*
Plasma No Effect In toxemic pregnancies no significant differences observed in comparison with normal pregnancies *3946*

Endothelin-1, Big *Amniotic Fluid Decrease* Concentrations not significantly decreased to 15.1 ± 2.2 pmol/L in 35 women with severe pre-eclampsia compared with 16.8 ± 1.6 pmol/L in 31 women with normal pregnancies *5712*
Plasma Increase Concentrations significantly increased to 5.1 ± 0.4 pmol/L in 35 women with severe pre-eclampsia in retroplacental (and other blood) compared with 3.9 ± 0.3 pmol/L in 31 women with normal pregnancies *5712* Mean concentration of 1.87 ± 0.62 pmol/L in 11 preeclamptic women significantly greater than 0.99 ± 0.21 pmol/L in 11 normotensive pregnant women and 1.49 ± 0.15 pmol/L in 16 nonpregnant women *5066*

Epinephrine *Plasma Increase* In 21 preeclamptic women plasma free epinephrine concentration was 45 ± 5 pg/mL versus 27 ± 2 pg/mL in 15 healthy control normotensive pregnant women *3881* In arterial plasma concentration significantly higher (on average 3 times) in preeclamptics than in normotensive pregnant women. In venous plasma concentration also higher in preeclamptics than in normotensives *3882*

Epinephrine, Free *Plasma Increase* In 21 preeclamptic women plasma free epinephrine concentration was 45 ± 5 pg/mL versus 27 ± 2 pg/mL in 15 healthy control normotensive pregnant women *3881*

Erythrocyte Volume *Blood No Effect* Increase observed in pre-eclamptic pregnancies similar to that in normal pregnancies *3064*

Erythropoietin *Serum Increase* In 19 pre-eclamptic patients mean concentration of 26.9 ± 31.2 mIU/mL compared with mean of 6.5 mIU/mL in nonpregnant female controls: higher but not significantly so than in pregnant women. Concentrations highest in most severe pre-ecamptic women *2591*
Urine Increase Erythropoietin detected in the urine of 9 of 19 pre-eclamptic women *2591*

Estradiol *Plasma Decrease* Concentration of total estradiol significantly reduced in preeclamptic patients at 32 and 36 weeks compared with normal pregnancies *4444*
Urine Decrease In preeclamptic pregnancies significant reduction observed at 32 and 36 weeks compared with normal pregnancies *4444*

Estradiol, Unconjugated *Plasma No Effect* No significant difference in concentration observed between preeclamptic and normal pregnancies at 32 and 36 weeks *4444*

Estrogens *Plasma Decrease* Average serum and urinary estrogens were reduced in pre-eclampsia compared to normal pregnancy, but there was considerable overlap in values *5175*
Urine Decrease Average serum and urinary estrogens were reduced in pre-eclampsia compared to normal pregnancy, but there was considerable overlap in values *5175* In 99 pre-eclamptic patients, the incidence of subnormal concentrations was 76% *5683* Low values were found in 36% (23 of 64) patients *5036* In a series of 794 patients, hypoglycemia had a significant association with low estriol excretion, fetal growth retardation, and perinatal mortality *3115*

Estrone *Plasma Decrease* Concentration of total estrone significantly reduced in pre-eclamptic pregnancies compared with normal pregnancies at 32 and 36 weeks *4444*

Estrone, Unconjugated *Plasma No Effect* No difference observed at 32 and 36 weeks between concentrations in pre-eclamptic and normal pregnancies *4444*

Factor VIII *Plasma Decrease* In the ratio between factor VIII-related antigen and factor VIII activity a highly significant increase was observed during the 3rd trimester. The highest ratios were associated with either a perinatal death or with the delivery of a severely growth retarded infant *5226*

Factor X *Plasma Decrease* Factor XII was significantly higher in 12 patients than in the normal group, while factors XI and X were slightly lower *899*

Factor XI *Plasma Decrease* Factor XII was significantly higher in 12 patients than in the normal group, while factors XI and X were slightly lower *899*

Factor XII *Plasma Increase* Factor XII was significantly higher in 12 patients than in the normal group, while factors XI and X were slightly lower *899*

Fatty Acids (FFA), Free *Serum Increase* In 16 women with overt pre-eclampsia mean concentration of 0.74 ± 0.25 mmol/L significantly higher than 0.42 ± 0.14 mmol/L in 16 healthy pregnant women and 0.50 ± 0.15 mmol/L in 19 women who eventually developed pre-eclampsia concentration significantly higher than 0.34 ± 0.11 mmol/L in 19 women with uneventful pregnancies *3130*

Fatty Acids, Polyunsaturated *Serum Decrease* Significantly reduced in pre-eclamptic women at term compared with nonpregnant women *5565*

Fibrin Degradation Products *Plasma Decrease* Plasma fibrinolytic activity may be more depressed than in normal pregnancy *517* Reported effect *5677*
Plasma Increase In second trimester significant increase observed in preeclamptic pregnant women compared with normal pregnant women *2179* Elevated levels (> 10 µg/mL) occurred in all patients. Mean level was 35 µg/mL *2863* Suggest that slow, chronic, intravascular clotting is taking place *5677*

Fibrinogen *Liver Increase* Fibrin outlining the hepatic sinusoids was found in all 12 cases; in 2 of them there were also large nodular deposits of fibrin and to a lesser extent of IgG, IgM, and C_3 in areas of necrosis *174*
Plasma Increase Significant increase observed in second trimester in pre-eclamptic pregnant women compared with healthy pregnant women *2179* Increased by about 70% and 145% in pre-eclampsia and eclampsia, respectively *794*
Plasma No Effect Concentration typically the same as in normal pregnancy *5677* Levels of fibrinogen and of other clotting factors do not differ from those found in normal late pregnancy *1630* In essential hypertension, the level remains more or less the same as in normal pregnancy *794* In 19 women with preeclampsia mean concentration not significantly different from that in 18 normal pregnant women *4033*

Fibronectin *Plasma Decrease* Significant reduction observed in patients with preeclampsia *5053*

Plasma Increase In preeclamptic women at 38-41 weeks of pregnancy concentration significantly higher than in women with normal pregnancy at same stage of gestation *1380* In 18 preeclamptic peripartum women concentration significantly higher than in 19 normal control women. Magnitude of increase is not a predictor of severity of pre-eclampsia *665* Concentrations increased in pregnant women who subsequently develop preeclampsia *1778* Mean concentration of 243 ± 9 mg/L in 26 preeclamptic pregnant women in first trimester, 241 ± 8 mg/L in second trimester and 333 ± 18 mg/L in third trimester significantly higher than in normotensive pregnant women at same stage of pregnancy *3966* In 19 women with preeclampsia mean concentration of 410 mg/L significantly different from 262 mg/L in 18 normal pregnant women *4033*

Fractional Excretion of Calcium *Urine Decrease* In 12 preeclamptic women in their third trimester mean concentration of 1.42 ± 0.01% significantly different from 2.68 ± 0.01% in 24 normotensive women in their third trimester *4712*

α_1-Globulin *Serum Increase* Significantly elevated *900*

α_2-Globulin *Serum Increase* Significantly elevated *900*

γ-Globulin *Serum Decrease* Significantly reduced below the levels for normal pregnancy *900*

Glomerular Filtration Rate *Urine Decrease* Reduced 25 - 30% below the rate in normal pregnancy *4707*

Glucose *Serum Decrease* The patients with severe pre-eclampsia had significantly lower fasting plasma glucose levels than those with mild pre-eclampsia and normal pregnancies *4864* In the total series of 794 patients, hypoglycemia had a significant association with low estriol excretion, fetal growth retardation, and perinatal mortality *3115*

Glutathione *Blood Decrease* In 8 women with pregnancies complicated by preeclampsia median concentration of 624 μmol/L compared with 750 μmol/L in 22 normotensive pregnant women *2713*

Glutathione S-Transferase Alpha 1-1 *Serum Increase* In 79 pregnant women with preeclampsia median concentration of 4.1 μg/L significantly greater than that in 87 normotensive pregnant women in whom the median concentration was 1.0 μg/L *2712*

Glutathione S-Transferase-pi 1-1 *Serum Increase* In 67 women with preeclampsia median concentration of 15.7 μg/L significantly different from 7.9 μg/L in 81 healthy nonpregnant female volunteers *2714*

Glutathione:Hemoglobin Ratio *Blood Decrease* In 8 women with pregnancies complicated by preeclampsia median ratio of 0.076 compared with 0.101 in 22 normotensive pregnant women *2713*

Glycated Protein *Urine Increase* Increased urinary loss observed with pre-eclampsia *811*

Haptoglobin *Serum Decrease* In 67 women with preeclampsia median concentration of 0.5 g/L significantly different from 0.92 g/L in 81 healthy nonpregnant female volunteers *2714*

HDL-Cholesterol *Serum Decrease* In 5 preeclamptic women median concentration of 1.43 mmol/L significantly different from 1.70 mmol/L in 8 healthy control individuals *4594*

Hematocrit *Blood Increase* Hemoconcentration is an index of severity; with grave prognosis if it increases or persists *811* Usually thrombocytopenia and high hematocrit values *1812*
Blood No Effect Mean of 35.5 ± 2.3% in 14 patients at 35.1 ± 2.9 weeks with preeclampsia not significantly different from 35.5 ± 2.3% in 17 healthy women at 39.9 ± 0.8 weeks *2271* In 19 patients with gestational hypertension mean value of 35 ± 4% not significantly different from 34 ± 3% in 70 healthy pregnant women *4194* In 21 preeclamptic women mean of 35 ± 4% not significantly different from 36 ± 2% in 32 healthy pregnant women *4195* In 12 patients with severe preeclampsia mean values of 40.7 ± 6.4% and of 35.4 ± 5.9% in 14 patients with mild preeclampsia not significantly different from 35.5 ± 2.6% in 20 healthy controls *3955* No significant difference observed between preeclamptic and normal pregnant women *856* No difference observed from concentration in normal pregnant women *2591*

Hemoglobin *Blood No Effect* In 12 patients with severe preeclampsia mean values of 14.1 ± 2.6 g/dL and of 12.1 ± 2.2 g/dL in 14 patients with mild preeclampsia not significantly different from 11.8 ± 1.2 g/dL in 20 healthy controls *3955* No significant difference observed from concentration in normal pregnant women *2591* In 23 women with pregnancies complicated by preeclampsia or HELLP syndrome median concentration of 7.9 mmol/L not different from 7.45 mmol/L in 22 women wih normal pregnancies *2713*

Hemopexin *Serum Decrease* Found to be significantly lower than in normal pregnancy *5056*
Serum No Effect No change was found compared to normal late pregnancy *860*

25-Hydroxy Vitamin D *Serum No Effect* In 12 preeclamptic women in their third trimester mean concentration of 73.9 ± 7.5 nmol/L not significantly different from 89.8 ± 11.7 nmol/L in 24 normotensive women in their third trimester *4712*

IDL-Protein *Serum Decrease* In 5 preeclamptic women median concentration of 93 mg/dL not significantly different from 123 mg/dL in 8 healthy control individuals *4594*

Immunoglobulin D *Serum Decrease* Significantly lower than in normal late pregnancy *5054*

Immunoglobulin E *Serum Increase* Concentration significantly higher in 20 primigravid women preeclampsia than in 17 women with normal pregnancy *64*

Immunoglobulin G *Serum Decrease* Significantly lower than in normal late pregnancy *391 2232 5054* Mean concentration not significantly less than in nonpregnant state and no different from that in normal pregnancy *634*

Immunoglobulin M *Serum No Effect* Mean concentration in 36 women did not differ significantly from that in 12 women with normal pregnancies and in healthy nonpregnant controls *634*

Immunoglobulins *Serum Decrease* Decreased; may predispose to infection, especially urinary tract infections *5056 5055*

Insulin *Plasma Decrease* Both the fasting plasma insulin and insulin response following glucose injection were lower in patients with severe pre-eclampsia than in those with mild pre-eclampsia or a normal pregnancy. The differences however were not statistically significant *4864*

Interleukin-2 *Serum Increase* Increase observed in pre-eclampsia *4095* Concentration increased in patients with pre-eclampsia *4094* Increased in the plasma of patients with pre-eclampsia *4093*

Interleukin-12 (p40 Subunit) *Serum Increase* Concentrations increased in women with severe pre-eclampsia *1250*

Interleukin-12 p75 Dimer *Serum Increase* Concentrations increased in women with severe pre-eclampsia *1250*

Ionized Calcium *Red Blood Cells Increase* In 20 preeclamptic pregnant women mean membrane concentration of 1.21 ± 0.35 μmol/g membrane protein significantly different from 0.83 ± 0.16 μmol/g membrane protein in 25 healthy nonpregnant women *2699*
Serum Decrease In 20 preeclamptic pregnant women mean concentration of 1.98 ± 0.16 mmol/L significantly different from 2.43 ± 0.14 mmol/L in 25 healthy nonpregnant women *2699*
Serum No Effect No significant difference in concentrations in third trimester observed in preeclamptic, hypertensive and normal pregnant women *5173* In 9 patients with preeclampsia mean concentrations of 1.4 ± 0.02 mmol/L, 1.14 ± 0.02 mmol/L and 1.17 ± 0.03 mmol/L in the first, second and third trimesters not significantly different from 1.17 ± 0.01 mmol/L, 1.15 ± 0.01 mmol/L and 1.13 ± 0.01 mmol/L in the first, second and third trimesters of 22 healthy control women *4980* In 12 preeclamptic women in their third trimester mean concentration of 1.20 ± 0.01 mmol/L not significantly different from 1.26 ± 0.01 mmol/L in 24 normotensive women in their third trimester *4712*

Ionized Magnesium *Red Blood Cells Decrease* In 20 preeclamptic pregnant women mean membrane concentration of 0.28 ± 0.09 mmol/g membrane protein significantly less than that in 25 healthy nonpregnant women in whom the mean membrane concentration was 0.55 ± 0.13 mmol/g membrane protein *2697*
Serum Decrease In 20 preeclamptic pregnant women mean concentration of 0.70 ± 0.12 mmol/L significantly less than that in 25 healthy nonpregnant women in whom the mean concentration was 0.93 ± 0.06 mmol/L *2697* In 12 preeclamptic women mean concentration of 0.48 ± 0.01 mmol/L similar to 0.48 ± 0.01 mmol/L in 33 normal pregnant women but significantly less than 0.60 ± 0.005 mmol/L in 42 nonpregnant women *2000*

642.40 Pre-eclampsia *(continued)*

Ionized Magnesium *(continued)*
Serum *No Effect* In 9 patients with preeclampsia mean concentrations of 1.16 ± 0.03 mg/dL, 1.10 ± 0.05 mg/dL and 1.07 ± 0.04 mg/dL in the first, second and third trimesters not significantly different from 1.17 ± 0.03 mg/dL, 1.10 ± 0.03 mg/dL and 1.04 ± 0.03 mg/dL in the first, second and third trimesters of 22 healthy control women *4980*

Iron Saturation *Serum* *Decrease* Found to be significantly lower than in normal pregnant women *5056*
Serum *No Effect* No change was found compared to normal late pregnancy *860*

Isocitrate Dehydrogenase *Serum* *Increase* Frequently increased indicating placental degeneration within previous 48 h *1290*

6-Keto-Prostaglandin $F_{1\alpha}$ *Plasma* *Increase* In 18 pre-eclamptic patients peripartum concentration significantly greater than in 19 normal pregnant controls *665*
Urine *Decrease* In pre-eclamptic women mean excretion of 105.3 ± 28.2 pg/mg creatinine compared with 211.1 ± 33.8 pg/mg creatinine in controls *5772*

Lactate *Blood* *Decrease* Lower in pre-eclamptic women in the 3rd trimester than in normal pregnant women *1408*

Lactate Dehydrogenase *Serum* *Increase* In 67 women with preeclampsia median activity of 289 U/L significantly different from 147 U/L in 81 healthy nonpregnant female volunteers *2714* In 23 women with pregnancies complicated by preeclampsia or HELLP syndrome median activity of 807 U/L *2713* In 12 preeclamptic patients peak activity of 809 ± 232 U/L significantly different when compared with 554 ± 267 U/L in 12 normotensive controls *4482* In about 20 preeclamptic women activities at weeks 24 - 29, 30 - 35 and 36 - 40 of 15.16 ± 3.10, 11.45 ± 1.05 and 9.42 ± 0.72 µkat/L significantly higher than that in healthy pregnant women in whom mean activities were 6.38 ± 0.19 µkat/L at weeks 24 - 29 and 6.80 ± 0.21 µkat/L at weeks 30 - 35 and normal range of 3.9 - 8.0 µkat/L *2080* Rose to a mean value of 384.1 ± 31.8 U/L in severe pre-eclampsia, over the normal value in pregnancy of 154.5 - 12.2 U/L *4546* Usually not elevated. When transaminases are found to be elevated, either pronounced hepatic or marked myocardial alterations have occurred *900*

Laminin *Serum* *Increase* In 21 women with pre-eclampsia in the third trimester of their pregnancy mean concentration of 299.9 ± 16.0 ng/mL significantly higher than 127.8 ± 8.0 ng/mL in 22 healthy nonpregnant controls *1609*

LDL-Protein *Serum* *Decrease* In 5 preeclamptic women median concentration of 279 mg/dL not significantly different from 345 mg/dL in 8 healthy control individuals *4594*

Leucine Aminopeptidase, Placental *Serum* *Increase* In normal pregnancies and in mild preeclamptic pregnancies up to week 33 no significant difference in activities observed but thereafter activities significantly higher in preeclamptics. In severe preeclamptics maximum activity occurred at week 31 *3537*

Leukocytes *Blood* *No Effect* In 12 patients with severe preeclampsia mean values of 9.9 ± 3.7 x 10^9/L and of 11.2 ± 3.9 x 10^9/L in 14 patients with mild preeclampsia not significantly different from 10.3 ± 1.9 x 10^9/L in 20 healthy controls *3955* Mean concentration in 6 preeclamptic patients in their 30th week of pregnancy of 8,233 ± 1,089 /µL not significantly different from that in 8 healthy individuals, 8,438 ± 1,089 /µL *2073*

Lipase, Hepatic *Serum* *Increase* In 5 preeclamptic women median activity of 28.5 µmol fatty acd/mL/h significantly different from 18 µmol fatty acid/mL/h in 8 healthy control individuals *4594*

Lipolytic Activity *Serum* *Increase* In 16 women with overt pre-eclampsia mean activity of 0.88 ± 0.28 mmol/L/24 h significantly higher than 0.35 ± 0.17 mmol/L/24 h in 16 women with uneventful pregnancies but mean activity of 0.36 ± 0.15 mmol/L/24 h in 19 women who eventually developed pre-eclampsia mean activity not significantly higher than 0.34 ± 0.14 mmol/L/24 h in 19 healthy pregnant women *3130*

β-Lipoprotein *Serum* *Increase* Higher than in normal late pregnancy *2232* *860* *5056* Significantly elevated *900*

Low Density Lipoprotein-I *Serum* *Decrease* In 5 preeclamptic women median concentration of 22 mg/dL significantly different from 62 mg/dL in 8 healthy control individuals *4594*

Low Density Lipoprotein-2 *Serum* *Decrease* In 5 preeclamptic women median concentration of 55 mg/dL significantly different from 211 mg/dL in 8 healthy control individuals *4594*

Low Density Lipoprotein-3 *Serum* *Increase* In 5 preeclamptic women median concentration of 170 mg/dL significantly different from 55 mg/dL in 8 healthy control individuals *4594*

Lymphocytes *Blood* *Increase* Mean concentration in 6 preeclamptic patients in their 30th week of pregnancy of 2,313 ± 574 /µL significantly different from that in 8 healthy individuals, 1,569 ± 449 /µL *2073*

α_2-Macroglobulin *Serum* *Decrease* Mild *2233*
Serum *Increase* Low concentration of albumin and other small proteins may stimulate almost indiscriminate synthesis of many proteins. Larger molecules cannot leak through the glomeruli and accumulate in the blood *5056* *5055*

Macrophage Colony Stimulating Factor *Serum* *Increase* Mean concentration in 6 preeclamptic patients in their 30th week of pregnancy of 1,807 ± 450 U/mL significantly different from that in 8 healthy individuals, 1,099 ± 323 U/mL *2073*

Magnesium *Red Blood Cells* *Decrease* In 20 pregnant women with preeclampsia mean concentration of 1.02 ± 0.16 mmol/L significantly different from 1.79 ± 0.10 mmol/L in 25 healthy nonpregnant control women *2698*
Serum *No Effect* In 20 pregnant women with preeclampsia mean concentration of 0.70 ± 0.12 mmol/L significantly different from 0.93 ± 0.06 mmol/L in 25 healthy nonpregnant control women *2698* In 9 patients with preeclampsia mean concentrations of 1.73 ± 0.06 mg/dL, 1.53 ± 0.04 mg/dL and 1.55 ± 0.04 mg/dL in the first, second and third trimesters not significantly different from 1.77 ± 0.03 mg/dL, 1.75 ± 0.04 mg/dL and 1.58 ± 0.05 mg/dL in the first, second and third trimesters of 22 healthy control women *4980* In 12 preeclamptic women mean concentration of 0.76 ± 0.02 mmol/L similar to 0.77 ± 0.01 mmol/L in 33 normal pregnant women but less than 0.83 ± 0.06 mmol/L in 42 nonpregnant women *2000*

Matrix Metalloproteinase-8 *Serum* *No Effect* Mean concentration of 106 ± 159 ng/mL 21 preeclamptic women not significantly different from 57 ± 118 ng/mL in 21 healthy pregnant controls *2749*

Matrix Metalloproteinase-9 *Serum* *No Effect* Mean concentration of 425 ± 323 ng/mL 21 preeclamptic women not significantly different from 542 ± 318 ng/mL in 21 healthy pregnant controls *2749*

β_2-Microglobulin *Serum* *Increase* Significant increase observed in 15 patients with severe preeclampsia compared with normal pregnant women *3883*
Urine *Decrease* Significant decrease observed in patients with severe preeclampsia compared with normal pregnant women *3883*

Monocytes *Blood* *Decrease* Mean concentration in 6 preeclamptic patients in their 30th week of pregnancy of 344 ± 219 /µL lower but not significantly different from that in 8 healthy individuals, 503 ± 210 /µL *2073*

N-Acetyl-Glucosaminidase *Urine* *Increase* Excretion in preeclampsia increased above the normal increase observed during third trimester of normal pregnancy *2290*

Neutrophils *Blood* *Decrease* Mean concentration in 6 preeclamptic patients in their 30th week of pregnancy of 5,385 ± 540 /µL lower but not significantly different from that in 8 healthy individuals, 6,273 ± 1,463 /µL *2073*

Nitrogen *Urine* *Increase* Urinary amines are increased in hypertension resulting from pregnancy *5882*

Norepinephrine *Plasma* *Increase* In preeclamptics mean arterial concentration higher than in normotensive pregnant women *3882*

N-terminal Pro-Atrial Natriuretic Peptide *Plasma* *Increase* In 49 patients with gestational hypertension median concentration of 571 pmol/L significantly different from 266 pmol/L in 49 matched pregnant controls, with concentrations in severe preeclampsia (766 pmol/L) higher than in mild preeclampsia (492 pmol/L) *4194*

Oxygen Partial Pressure *Blood* *Decrease* In 9 patients with severe pre-eclampsia, there was a significant increase in alveolar-to-arterial pO_2 difference and physiological shunt, indicating a degree of pulmonary ventilation/perfusion imbalance *5192*

Oxygen Saturation *Blood Decrease* In 9 patients with severe pre-eclampsia, there was a significant increase in alveolar-to-arterial pO_2 difference and physiological shunt, indicating a degree of pulmonary ventilation/perfusion imbalance *5192*

Parathyroid Hormone *Plasma Decrease* During third trimester mean concentration lower than in nonpregnant control women *4056*
Plasma Increase In 12 preeclamptic women in their third trimester mean concentration of 29.9 ± 4.3 ng/L significantly different from 15.4 ± 1.3 ng/L in 24 normotensive women in their third trimester *4712*
Plasma No Effect Tendency for concentration to be higher but not significantly so after delivery *4056*

Partial Thromboplastin Time *Plasma No Effect* In 19 women with preeclampsia mean time not significantly different from that in 18 normal pregnant women *4033*

Phosphate *Serum Increase* Concentration higher 3 months after delivery in pre-eclamptic women than in nonpregnant controls but concentration not different from that in normal pregnant women *4056*
Serum No Effect No significant difference observed in concentrations during third trimester of pregnancy in normal, hypertensive and preeclamptic women *5173*

Phospholipase A_2 Type II *Serum Increase* Increase in concentration observed: 23 µg/L in mild preeclampsia and 54 µg/L in severe preeclampsia compared with 2 and 4 µg/L in healthy controls *3767* In 25 patients with preeclampsia concentration increased: in 6 with mild preeclampsia mean concentration of 6.1 ± 3.0 ng/mL (not significantly different from 6.0 ± 3.2 ng/mL in 23 controls), but in severe preeclampsia in 19 women mean concentration was 19.9 ± 12.3 ng/mL *3059*

Placental Isoferritin *Serum Decrease* In 85 pregnant women at risk of developing preeclampsia of 14.8 ± 3.9 U/mL significantly different from 19.0 ± 2.6 U/mL in 146 low risk controls *284*

Placental Lactogen *Plasma Increase* In primigravid women with preeclampsia during 36 - 40 weeks significant increase observed whereas no significant effect observed in multigravid women with preeclampsia *3849*

Placental Protein 5 *Serum Increase* In normal pre-eclamptic or eclamptic pregnancy PP5 concentration increased compared with normal pregnancy *2709*

Placental-type Plasminogen Activator Inhibitor
Plasma Decrease In pre-eclampsia significantly reduced concentration of placental-type plasminogen activator inhibitor observed although total concentration increased *1048*

Plasmin-Plasmin Inhibitor Complex *Plasma Increase* Mean concentration in 6 preeclamptic patients in their 30th week of pregnancy of 0.70 ± 0.41 µg/mL higher but not significantly different from that in 8 healthy individuals, 0.59 ± 0.34 µg/mL *2073*

Plasminogen Activator Inhibitor-1 *Plasma Increase* Mean concentration of 303 ± 159 ng/mL 21 preeclamptic women significantly different from 182 ± 126 ng/mL in 21 healthy pregnant controls *2749* In pre-eclampsia significantly increased concentrations of total plasminogen activator inhibitor observed but significantly reduced concentrations of placental-type activator inhibitor *1048* In 14 preeclamptic pregnant women concentration significantly higher in second trimester than in healthy pregnant women *2179*

Platelet-activating Factor Acetylhydrolase *Serum Decrease* In severe preeclampsia concentration of 12.5 ± 3.9 nmol/min/mL was significantly lower than in normal pregnancy *3355*
Serum Increase In mild preeclampsia activity at 28 - 41 weeks gestation of 28.0 ± 1.0 nmol/min/mL sinificantly higher than in age-matched healthy pregnant women of 21.3 ± 0.8 nmol/min/mL. In severe preeclampsia concentration of 12.5 ± 3.9 nmol/min/mL was significantly lower than in normal pregnancy *3355*

Platelets *Blood Decrease* In 20 pregnant women in third trimester with severe pre-eclampsia mean concentration of 231,000 ± 80,000 /µL not significantly less than 263,000 ± 71,000 /µL in 38 patients with mild pre-eclampsia and 278,000 ± 83,000 /µL in 17 pregnant women with essential hypertension *600* In 23 women with pregnancies complicated by preeclampsia or HELLP syndrome median concentration of 88 x 10^9/L low *2713* Evidence of intravascular coagulation, as shown by elevated levels of fibrin degradation products and reduced platelet counts, has been found in many women *518* Nine of 26 patients (34%) showed thrombocytopenia *2629* Usually thrombocytopenia and high hematocrit values *1812* In 16 preeclamptic women mean concentration of 184,000 ± 17,000 /µL not significantly lower than 201,000 ± 15,000 /µL in 11 normal pregnant women *856* In 12 preeclamptic patients lowest concentration of 180,000 ± 66,000 /µL significantly different when compared with 248,000 ± 80,000 /µL in 12 normotensive controls *4482* In about 20 pregnant women with preeclampsia mean concentrations at weeks 24 - 29, 30 - 35 and 36 - 40 of 213 ± 20.9, 198 ± 10.0 and 212 ± 17.0 x 10 ^{9}/L significantly less than those in 20 healthy pregnant women in whom mean concentrations of 255 ± 9.1 x 10^9/L at weeks 24 - 29 and 245 ± 11.0 x 10 ^{9}/L at weeks 30 - 35 not significantly different from normal range of 150 - 400 x 10^9/L *2080* An occasional patient is mildly to moderately thrombocytopenic *517*
Blood Increase In 21 preeclamptic women 5 weeks postpartum mean concentration of 285 ± 13.8 x 10^9/L significantly higher than 234 ± 15.6 x 10^9/L in healthy women at same time but within normal range of 150 - 400 x 10^9/L *2080*
Blood No Effect In 21 preeclamptic women mean count of 237,000 ± 93,000 /µL not significantly different from 287,000 ± 77,000 /µL in 12 healthy pregnant women *4195* Usually within the normal range *4776* In 19 women with preeclampsia mean concentration not significantly different from that in 18 normal pregnant women *4033* Even in severe preeclampsia count unaffected *4064* In 12 patients with severe preeclampsia mean values of 189 ± 101 x 10^9/L and of 215 ± 88 x 10^9/L in 14 patients with mild preeclampsia not significantly different from 227 ± 47 x 10^9/L in 20 healthy controls *3955* In 19 patients with gestational hypertension mean value of 252,000 ± 78,100 /µL not significantly different from 275,000 ± 87,100 /µL in 70 healthy pregnant women *4194* In 25 patients with preeclampsia concentration of 180,000 ± 65,000 /µL not significantly different from 216,000 ± 11,900 /µL in 11 control pregnant women *3059*

Potassium *Serum Increase* In 12 preeclamptic women mean concentration of 4.85 ± 0.11 mmol/L significantly greater than 4.06 ± 0.05 mmol/L in 33 normal pregnant women and 4.37 ± 0.04 mmol/L in 42 nonpregnant women *2000* Concentration increased in the plasma of 21 preeclamptic women compared with that in 15 normotensive pregnant controls *3881*
Serum No Effect In 9 patients with preeclampsia mean concentrations of 4.21 ± 0.09 mmol/L, 4.27 ± 0.20 mmol/L and 4.10 ± 0.02 mmol/L in the first, second and third trimesters not significantly different from 4.28 ± 0.06 mmol/L, 4.09 ± 0.08 mmol/L and 4.14 ± 0.07 mmol/L in the first, second and third trimesters of 22 healthy control women *4980* In 20 preeclamptic pregnant women mean concentration of 4.1 ± 0.4 mmol/L not different from 4.4 ± 0.2 mmol/L in 25 healthy nonpregnant women *2699* In 20 preeclamptic pregnant women mean concentration of 4.1 ± 0.4 mmol/L not significantly different from that in 25 healthy nonpregnant women in whom the mean concentration was 4.3 ± 0.2 mmol/L *2697* In 20 pregnant women with pre-eclampsia mean concentration of 4.1 ± 0.4 mmol/L not significantly different from 4.4 ± 0.2 mmol/L in 25 healthy nonpregnant control women *2698*

Pregnancy-associated Protein A *Serum Increase* Preeclamptic toxemia causes significant increase compared with concentration in normal pregnancy: concentration higher in severe preeclampsia with albuminuria and when preeclampsia occurred relatively early in pregnancy *2709*

Pregnanediol *Urine Decrease* Reduced compared to normal pregnant women, but there was considerable overlap in values *5175* In 58 women with mild pre-eclampsia, mean of 29.5 mg/24 h, ranging from 6 - 63.8. The average decrease of 40% was not found significant because of the wide range of values in both normo- and hypertensive patients *2552*

Progesterone *Plasma Decrease* Reduced compared to normal pregnant women, but there was considerable overlap in values *5175* In 58 women with mild pre-eclampsia, mean of 29.5 mg/24 h, ranging from 6 - 63.8 mg/24 h. The average decrease of 40% was not found significant because of the wide range of values in both normo- and hypertensive patients *2552*
Plasma No Effect No significant difference observed at 32 and 36 weeks in concentrations in pre-eclamptic and normal pregnancies *4444*

Protein *Serum Decrease* Significantly reduced below the levels for normal pregnancy *900* In 26 women with mild pre-eclampsia mean concentration of 59.8 ± 5.6 g/L and in 8 with severe pre-eclampsia 58.3 ± 5.6 g/L compared with 63.4 ± 4.1 g/L in 39 healthy controls *3353*
Urine Increase In 21 preeclamptic women mean daily excretion of 2,778 ± 2,958 mg significantly higher than < 300 mg in 32

642.40 Pre-eclampsia *(continued)*

Protein *(continued)*
healthy pregnant women *4195* Mean excretion in 30 patients with preeclampsia 2.6 g/L significantly higher than < 0.3 g/L in 30 matched controls *2259* In 12 patients with severe preeclampsia mean values of 3.0 ± 2.0 g/d and of 1.9 ± 1.4 g/d in 14 patients with mild preeclampsia not significantly different from 0 g/d in 20 healthy controls *3955* In 8 women with mild pre-eclampsia mean excretion of 2.4 ± 2.6 g/L and in 8 with severe pre-eclampsia 5.7 ± 3.9 g/L compared with 0 in 39 healthy controls *3353* Hypertension, edema, and proteinuria characterize toxemia of pregnancy *367* This diagnosis is questionable without the presence of proteinuria. Renal leakage of small molecular weight proteins is characteristic *811* In 49 patients with preeclampsia mean excretion of less than 2,354 ± 2,790 mg/d significantly different from < 300 mg/d in 70 healthy pregnant women *4194* In 8 women with preeclampsia mean excretion of 4.21 ± 1,15 g/d significantly higher than < 0.1 g/d in 7 normotensive pregnant women in their third trimester *2914* In 9 of 13 preeclamptic patients protein detected by dipstick compared with 1 in 12 normotensive controls *4482* In 16 preeclamptic women mean excretion of 1.67 ± 0.57 g/d significantly increased compared with 0.20 ± 0.05 g/d in 11 healthy normal pregnant women *856* In 23 women with pregnancies complicated by preeclampsia or HELLP syndrome median excretion of 1 g/L *2713* In normal pregnant women ratio of protein to creatinine did not exceed 200 mg/g in random or 24-hour specimens although in pre-eclamptic women this ratio often exceeded *2425* In 20 preeclamptic pregnant women mean excretion of 1.39 ± 0.75 g/d significantly greater than 0.12 ± 0.05 g/d in 22 healthy pregnant women *2699* 1 to 4+ proteinuria observed in all 19 pre-eclamptic women studied *2591* In 20 pregnant women with preeclampsia mean excretion of 1.39 ± 0.75 g/d significantly greater than that in 22 healthy pregnant women in whom the mean excretion was 0.12 ± 0.05 g/d which was not significantly different from normal *2698* In 20 preeclamptic pregnant women mean excretion of 1.39 ± 0.75 g/d significantly greater than that in 25 healthy nonpregnant women in whom the mean excretion was 0.12 ± 0.05 g/d *2697* In 25 patients with preeclampsia concentration increased to 30 - 100 ng/dL compared with < 30 ng/dL in 23 control pregnant women *3059*

Protein C *Plasma No Effect* In 19 women with preeclampsia mean concentration not significantly different from that in 18 normal pregnant women *4033*

Protein S *Plasma No Effect* In 19 women with preeclampsia mean concentration not significantly different from that in 18 normal pregnant women *4033*

Prothrombin Time *Plasma No Effect* In 19 women with preeclampsia mean time not significantly different from that in 18 normal pregnant women *4033*

Renin *Plasma Decrease* In pre-eclamptic women concentration significantly less than in pregnant healthy controls *4745*
Plasma No Effect In 26 women with mild pre-eclampsia mean concentration of 498.3 ± 246.1 ng/L and in 8 with severe pre-eclampsia of 579.0 ± 278.2 ng/L compared with 506.6 ± 253.2 ng/L in 39 healthy controls *3353*

Renin, Active *Plasma Decrease* In 8 preeclamptic women in their third trimester mean concentration of 11.3 ± 2.9 ng/L not significantly less than that in 7 normotensive pregnant women in their third trimester in whom the mean concentration was 17.3 ± 5.4 ng/L *2914*

Renin Activity *Plasma Decrease* In 13 pre-eclamptic women activity significantly less than in 13 healthy control pregnant women *2177* During normal pregnancy, plasma levels of renin, angiotensin II, and aldosterone are increased. Paradoxically with pregnancy-induced hypertension they commonly decrease towards the normal *4223* In hypertensive groups, plasma renin activity and aldosterone concentration were significantly suppressed during the last trimester despite levels of renin substrate and progesterone that were not significantly different from those observed in normotensive pregnancy *5616* Activity depressed in the plasma of 21 preeclamptic women compared with that in 15 normotensive pregnant controls *3881* In pregnant women with preeclampsia one week before delivery mean activity in 16 who had a Cesarean section of 73.3 ± 22.2 ng/mL/24 h not significantly different from 59.9 ± 17.3 ng/mL/24 h in 11 pregnant women without preeclampsia but 61.1 ± 21.3 ng/mL/24 h in 14 with preeclampsia who had a vaginal delivery significantly different from 124.3 ± 39.6 ng/mL/24 h in 8 who had a vaginal delivery *1608*
Plasma Increase Greater increase in pre-eclamptic than in normal pregnant women *5110* In preeclamptic women mean activity of 3.4 ± 1.1 ng/L/s nonsignificantly increased compared with concentration in pregnant women (2.8 ± 0.6 ng/L/s) and significantly increased compared with nonpregnant controls (0.7 ± 0.1 pmol/L) *856* At term, hypertensive, toxemic pregnant women had elevated aldosterone and plasma renin activity, which remained elevated > 1 week after delivery *139*
Plasma No Effect Renin activity was found to be about the same, or less, than in normotensive pregnant women *5441* No significant effect usually observed *811*

Sodium *Serum Decrease* Serum concentrations tend to decline as severity increases *4707* In 12 preeclamptic women mean concentration of 139.1 ± 0.9 mmol/L significantly less than 140.2 ± 0.5 mmol/L in 33 normal pregnant women and 142.4 ± 0.16 mmol/L in 42 nonpregnant women *2000* Rarely *811*
Serum No Effect In 20 preeclamptic pregnant women mean concentration of 140 ± 5 mmol/L not significantly different from that in 25 healthy nonpregnant women in whom the mean concentration was 142 ± 4 mmol/L *2697* In 20 preeclamptic pregnant women mean concentration of 140 ± 5 mmol/L not different from 142 ± 5 mmol/L in 25 healthy nonpregnant women *2699* In 20 pregnant women with preeclampsia mean concentration of 140 ± 5 mmol/L not significantly different from 142 ± 5 mmol/L in 25 healthy nonpregnant control women *2698* In 9 patients with preeclampsia mean concentrations of 137.8 ± 2.0 mmol/L, 141.3 ± 1.6 mmol/L and 142.1 ± 3.9 mmol/L in the first, second and third trimesters not significantly different from 139.5 ± 1.2 mmol/L, 139.0 ± 1.1 mmol/L and 140.1 ± 0.9 mmol/L in the first, second and third trimesters of 22 healthy control women *4980*
Urine Decrease Reduced to a greater extent than that in normal pregnancy *4707*
Urine Increase In 12 preeclamptic women in their third trimester mean concentration of 124 ± 13 mmol/d not significantly different from 100 ± 8 mmol/d in 24 normotensive women in their third trimester *4712*

Soluble Intercellular Adhesion Molecule-1 *Serum Increase* In 106 patients with mild preeclampsia mean concentration of 246 ± 107 ng/mL, 249 ± 81 ng/mL in 31 patients with severe preeclampsia and 268 ± 113 ng/mL in 20 patients with preeclampsia and fetal growth retardation not significantly different from 224.9 ± 4.0 µg/L in 76 healthy pregnant controls *1186*

Soluble Vascular Cell Adhesion Molecule-1
Serum Increase In 106 patients with mild preeclampsia mean concentration of 835 ± 197 ng/mL, 855 ± 203 ng/mL in 31 patients with severe preeclampsia, not significantly different from controls, and 855 ± 203 ng/mL in 20 patients with preeclampsia and fetal growth retardation significantly different from 668 ± 145 ng/mL in 76 healthy pregnant controls *1186*

Thiol Groups, Total *Serum Increase* Mean concentration of 646 nmol/mL in 14 patients at 35.1 ± 2.9 weeks with preeclampsia not significantly different from 516 nmol/mL in 17 healthy women at 39.9 ± 0.8 weeks *2271*

Thrombin/Antithrombin III Complex *Plasma Increase* Mean concentration in 6 preeclamptic patients in their 30th week of pregnancy of 14.18 ± 8.75 ng/mL higher but not significantly different from that in 8 healthy individuals, 10.26 ± 1.77 ng/mL *2073*

β-Thromboglobulin *Plasma Increase* In 8 primiparous preeclamptics mean concentration of 186.6 ± 29.9 ng/mL compared with 45.4 ± 31.8 ng/mL in a control group of 8 normal primiparous women *3046* In severe preeclampsia only concentration increased *4064*

Thrombomodulin *Plasma Increase* In 30 women with mild pre-eclampsia mean concentration of 43.0 ± 15.9 ng/mL significantly increased compared with 13.3 ± 8.6 ng/mL in 30 healthy normotensive pregnant women and 12.1 ± 8.0 ng/mL in 30 healthy normotensive nonpregnant control women *522*
Urine No Effect Mean excretion in 30 patients with preeclampsia of 138.6 ± 31.9 ng/mL not significantly higher than 130.4 ± 12.7 ng/mL in 30 matched controls, although thrombomodulin:creatinine ratio significantly increased to 1.67 ± 0.16 compared with 1.15 ± 0.09 in 30 matched controls *2259*

Thromboxane B_2 *Plasma No Effect* Concentration unchanged even in severe preeclampsia *4064*
Urine No Effect No significant difference observed between amounts excreted in normal pregnancy and in pre-eclamptics *5772*

Thyroid Stimulating Hormone *Serum Increase* Significantly increased concentration observed in preeclamptic women compared with healthy pregnant controls *2918* Significantly higher in third trimester in pre-eclamptic women than in normotensive pregnant women *2919*

Thyroxine Binding Globulin *Serum Decrease* Significantly reduced concentration in pre-eclamptic women compared with pregnant control women *2918*

Thyroxine (T4) *Serum Decrease* Concentration significantly reduced in preeclamptic patients compared with healthy pregnant women *2918*
Serum Increase The mean serum T4 and free T4 concentrations were significantly higher than those in normal pregnant women *3933*

Thyroxine (T4), Free *Serum Decrease* Significantly reduced in pre-eclamptic women in third trimester compared with normotensive women at same time *2919* Significantly reduced concentration observed in preeclamptic women compared with non-preeclamptic controls *2918*

Tissue Inhibitor of Metalloproteinase-1 *Serum No Effect* Mean concentration of 181 ± 124 ng/mL 21 preeclamptic women not significantly different from 161 ± 56 ng/mL in 21 healthy pregnant controls *2749*

Tissue Plasminogen Activator *Plasma Increase* In second and third trimester significantly higher than in healthy normally pregnant women: progressive and significant increase observed throughout preeclamptic pregnancy *2179*
Plasma No Effect Mean concentration of 8.9 ± 6.5 ng/mL 21 preeclamptic women not significantly different from 6.6 ± 3.8 ng/mL in 21 healthy pregnant controls *2749*

Triglycerides *Serum Increase* In 5 preeclamptic women median concentration of 3.65 mmol/L significantly greater than 1.93 mmol/L in 8 healthy control individuals *4594* In 12 patients with severe preeclampsia mean values of 337 ± 215 mg/dL and of 317 ± 147 mg/dL in 14 patients with mild preeclampsia not significantly different from 213 ± 88 mg/dL in 20 healthy controls *3955* In 16 women with overt pre-eclampsia mean concentration of 4.2 ± 1.4 mmol/L significantly higher than 2.4 ± 0.8 mmol/L in 16 healthy pregnant women and 1.3 ± 0.5 mmol/L in 19 women who eventually developed preclampsia significantly higher than 0.9 ± 0.3 mmol/L in 19 healthy pregnant women *3130*

Urea Nitrogen *Serum Decrease* Low (9 ± 2 mg/dL) and low creatinine (0.75 ± 0.2 mg/dL) in late pregnancy are indicative of toxemia *367*
Serum Increase If the hypertension has reached relatively severe levels, may be elevated, indicating renal damage *900* Mean concentration of 1.62 ± 0.2 mmol/L in 26 mildly pre-eclamptic women (nonsignificant increase) and of 2.0 ± 0.23 mmol/L in 26 severely pre-eclamptic women significantly greater than 1.5 ± 2.7 mmol/L in 20 normotensive control pregnant women *4748*

Uric Acid *Serum Increase* In 16 twin pregnancies with preeclampsia mean concentration of 7.7 mg/dL significantly higher than 5.4 mg/dL in 67 twin pregnancies without pre-eclampsia: mean concentration of 5.9 mg/dL in 10 pre-eclamptic singleton pregnancies significantly higher than mean of 4.7 mg/dL in 83 singleton pregnancies without pre-eclampsia *1492* Elevations of plasma urate is an early feature of pre-eclampsia *4305* In 30 women with mild pre-eclampsia mean concentration of 5.3 ± 1.3 mg/dL significantly increased compared with 4.2 ± 0.7 mg/dL in 30 healthy normotensive pregnant women and 4.4 ± 1.2 mg/dL in 30 healthy normotensive nonpregnant control women *522* In 16 preeclamptic women mean concentration of 7.1 ± 0.3 mg/dL significantly higher than in 11 normal pregnant women (3.8 ± 0.2 mg/dL) *856* Mean concentration of 0.33 ± 0.05 mmol/L in 26 mildly pre-eclamptic women (nonsignificant increase) and of 0.44 ± 0.025 mmol/L in 26 severely pre-eclamptic women significantly greater than 0.21 ± 0.045 mmol/L in 20 normotensive control pregnant women *4748* Concentration in severe pre-eclamptics of 7.5 ± 2.9 mg/dL compared with 5.8 ± 2.0 mg/dL and 4.9 ± 0.4 in healthy pregnant control women *2591* In 25 patients with preeclampsia concentration increased to 6.9 - 1.3 mg/dL compared with 3.9 ± 0.5 mg/dL in 23 control pregnant women *3059* In 34 women with pre-eclampsia mean concentration of 6.3 ± 0.2 mg/dL significantly higher than 4.9 ± 0.2 mg/dL in 6 pregnant control women *1609* Mean concentration of 6.4 ± 1.4 mg/dL in 14 patients at 35.1 ± 2.9 weeks with preeclampsia significantly different from 4.5 ± 1.2 mg/dL in 17 healthy women at 39.9 ± 0.8 weeks *2271* In 8 women with preeclampsia mean concentration of 392 ± 36 µmol/L significantly higher than 285 ± 22 µmol/L in 7 normotensive pregnant women in their third trimester *2914* Perinatal mortality was markedly increased when maternal plasma urate concentrations were raised, generally in associated with severe pre-eclampsia of early onset. Maternal hypertension, even severe, without hyperuricemia, was associated with an excellent prognosis for the fetus. When maternal hypertension was mild and hyperuricemia was severe, the prognosis for the fetus was poor *4306* Associated with cellular destruction *2707* Mean concentration of 0.40 ± 0.08 mmol/L in 20 pregnant women in third trimester with severe pre-eclampsia significantly higher than 0.31 ± 0.04 mmol/L in 17 pregnant women with essential hypertension *600* In 26 women with mild pre-eclampsia mean concentration of 354.9 ± 72.2 µmol/L and in 8 with severe pre-eclampsia of 407.4 ± 79.5 µmol/L compared with 276.1 ± 57.5 µmol/L in 39 healthy controls *3353* In 9 of 13 preeclamptic patients peak concentration of 6.7 ± 0.9 mg/dL significantly different when compared with 4.4 ± 1.0 mg/dL in 12 normotensive controls *4482*
Serum No Effect In 23 women with pregnancies complicated by preeclampsia or HELLP syndrome median concentration of 0.42 mmol/L *2713* Values may or may not be elevated in severe cases. When elevated, may represent liver or kidney dysfunction *900*

Urokinase Plasminogen Activator Receptor
Plasma No Effect Mean concentration of 1.1 ± 0.6 ng/mL in 21 preeclamptic women not significantly different from 1.1 ± 0.9 ng/mL in 21 healthy pregnant controls *2749*

Vasoactive Intestinal Polypeptide *Plasma Increase* Mean concentration of 13.9 pmol/L observed in 18 women with untreated gestational proteinuric hypertension at 32 to 40 weeks gestation compared with mean of 4.4 pmol/L in 8 women with normal pregnancies *2213*

Viscosity *Serum Increase* Apparent blood viscosity rises sharply as the hematocrit increases due to hemoconcentration *811*

Vitamin E *Serum Increase* Mean concentration of 25.7 nmol/mL in 14 patients at 35.1 ± 2.9 weeks with preeclampsia not significantly different from 21.3 nmol/mL in 17 healthy women at 39.9 ± 0.8 weeks *2271*

Vitamin E: Lipd Ratio *Serum Increase* Mean concentration of 2.8 nmol/µmoL lipid in 14 patients at 35.1 ± 2.9 weeks with preeclampsia not significantly different from 2.4 nmol/µmoL in 17 healthy women at 39.9 ± 0.8 weeks *2271*

VLD $Lipoprotein_1$ *Serum Increase* In 5 preeclamptic women median concentration of 184 mg/dL significantly different from 68 mg/dL in 8 healthy control individuals *4594*

VLD $Lipoprotein_2$ *Serum Increase* In 5 preeclamptic women median concentration of 146 mg/dL significantly different from 76 mg/dL in 8 healthy control individuals *4594*

Volume *Plasma Decrease* Hemoconcentration is an index of severity and prognosis *811* Increase that normally occurs with pregnancy less in pre-eclamptic women *3064*
Red Blood Cells No Effect In 14 cases in the late stages, mean red cell volume was identical with that of normal pregnant women in the same gestational period *481*

Zinc *Serum Decrease* Concentration significantly reduced in pre-eclamptic women compared with control pregnant women *2672*

642.60 Eclampsia

Alanine Aminotransferase *Serum Increase* Degree of abnormality closely parallels the severity *3617* Presumably due to ischemic damage to liver cells *647* All 14 patients had normal activities on the day of convulsion. On the 2nd day, the test became progressively abnormal and peaked on the 5 - 7th day postpartum *1021*

Albumin *Serum Decrease* Significantly reduced below the levels for normal pregnancy *900*
Urine Increase Characteristic finding. Reflects severity of disease *811*

642.60 **Eclampsia** *(continued)*

Aldosterone *Plasma Increase* At term, hypertensive, toxemic pregnant women had elevated aldosterone and plasma renin activity, which remained elevated > 1 week after delivery *139*
Urine Decrease Less than concentrations usually found in normal pregnancy *1290*

Alkaline Phosphatase, Tissue Unspecific *Urine Increase* Mean excretion of 13.8 ± 4.4 U/g creatinine observed in 20 eclamptic patients compared with 2.02 ± 0.13 U/g creatinine in 20 healthy normotensive control pregnant women (abnormal excretions observed in 18 of 20 patients) *4748*

Amylase *Serum Decrease* Severe liver damage *5544*

Antidiuretic Hormone *Plasma Increase* Positive correlation between severity of toxemia and circulating ADH *4707*

Antithrombin III *Plasma Decrease* Decreased as the gestosis index increased *2070*

Ascorbic Acid *Serum No Effect* In 13 patients with eclampsia mean values of 0.6 ± 0.5 mg/dL not significantly different from 0.7 ± 0.4 mg/dL in 20 healthy controls *3955*

Aspartate Aminotransferase *Serum Increase* Degree of abnormality closely parallels the severity *964 3617* Presumably due to ischemic damage to liver cells *647*

Bicarbonate *Serum Decrease* Usually reduced. Not uncommon to see values < 13.5 mmol/L *1291*

Bilirubin *Serum Increase* Elevated in only 3 of 134 patients, and those cases were only minimally elevated *897* Uncommon. In 134 women, including 45 with eclampsia, only 3 had levels > 1.2 mg/dL, with 2.3 mg/dL as the highest value *4223*
Serum No Effect Seldom elevated, even in severe eclampsia *811*

Bradykinin *Plasma Increase* Reported effect *2070*

Calcium *Serum No Effect* Concentration not usually affected *1291*

Catecholamines *Urine Increase* Increased due to severe stress *5544*

Chloride *Serum Decrease* With marked edema *1291*

β-Chorionic Gonadotropin *Plasma Increase* Not demonstrable in all cases *4906*
Urine Increase Not demonstrable in all cases *4906*

Clotting Time *Blood Decrease* Markedly reduced *2079*

Complement, Total *Serum No Effect* No significant effect observed *3979*

Creatinine *Serum Decrease* Low BUN (9 ± 2 mg/dL) and low creatinine (0.75 ± 0.2 mg/dL) in late pregnancy are indicative of toxemia *367*
Serum Increase Mean concentration of 145 ± 8.5 µmol/L in 20 eclamptic women significantly greater than 62 ± 12 µmol/L in 20 normotensive control pregnant women *4748* If the hypertension has reached relatively severe levels, may be elevated, indicating renal damage *900*

Creatinine Clearance *Urine Decrease* Mean clearance of 75 ± 13.8 mL/min in 20 eclamptic women significantly less than 195 ± 40 mL/min in 20 normotensive control pregnant women *4748*

Dopamine *Plasma No Effect* Mean concentration of 32.3 ± 7.3 pg/mL in 21 eclamptic women not significantly higher than 27.9 ± 6.5 pg/mL in 15 normotensive pregnant women *2666*

Epinephrine *Plasma Increase* Mean concentration of 150.2 ± 35.6 pg/mL in 21 eclamptic women significantly higher than 42.3 ± 13.9 pg/mL in 15 normotensive pregnant women *2666*

Estrogens *Plasma Decrease* Typical response *4907*

Fibrinogen *Plasma Decrease* A serious complication *2079*
Plasma Increase Increased by about 70% and 145% in pre-eclampsia and eclampsia, respectively *794*

α_1-Globulin *Serum Increase* Significantly elevated *900*

α_2-Globulin *Serum Increase* Significantly elevated *900*

γ-Globulin *Serum Decrease* Significantly reduced below the levels for normal pregnancy *900*

Glomerular Filtration Rate *Urine Decrease* Reduced 25 - 30% below the rate in normal pregnancy *4707*

Glucose *Serum Increase* Occasionally following eclamptic fit *1291*

Glucose Tolerance *Serum Decrease* Due to either hepatic dysfunction or relative insulin resistance *647*

Glutathione *Plasma No Effect* Concentration not usually affected *1291*

Hematocrit *Blood Increase* Hemoconcentration is an index of severity; with grave prognosis if it increases or persists *811*
Blood No Effect In 13 patients with eclampsia mean values of 37.2 ± 5.4% not significantly different from 35.5 ± 2.6% in 20 healthy controls *3955*

Hemoglobin *Blood No Effect* In 13 patients with eclampsia mean values of 12.8 ± 1.9 g/dL not significantly different from 11.8 ± 1.2 g/dL in 20 healthy controls *3955*

17-Hydroxycorticosteroids *Urine Increase* Increased due to severe stress *5544*

Immunoglobulins *Serum Decrease* Predisposes patients to infections, especially urinary tract infections *5056 5055*

17-Ketogenic Steroids *Urine Increase* Increased due to severe stress *5544*

Lactate *Blood Increase* Only after convulsions *1291*

Leukocytes *Blood Increase* In 13 patients with eclampsia mean values of 16.4 ± 4.4 x 10^9/L significantly different from 10.3 ± 1.9 x 10^9/L in 20 healthy controls *3955* Intoxications due to metabolic causes can cause leukocytosis *5544*

Lipids *Urine Increase* Lipids in the urine include all fractions. Double refractile (cholesterol) bodies can be seen. There is a high protein content *5544*

β-Lipoprotein *Serum Increase* Significantly elevated *900*

Magnesium *Cerebrospinal Fluid Decrease* Both serum and CSF concentrations were found to be low *234*
Serum Decrease Both serum and CSF concentrations were found to be low *234*

Neutrophils *Blood Increase* May be associated with a moderate to severe neutrophilia *5677*

Nitrogen *Serum Increase* Blood urea tends to decrease, but amino acids and unknown substances are increased *1290*
Urine Increase Urinary amines are increased in hypertension resulting from pregnancy *5882*

Norepinephrine *Plasma Increase* Mean concentration of 537.7 ± 215.7 pg/mL in 21 eclamptic women significantly higher than 269.9 ± 118.5 pg/mL in 15 normotensive pregnant women *2666*

Phosphate *Serum Increase* Slight increase *1291*

Plasminogen *Plasma Decrease* Decreased as the gestosis index increased *2070*

Platelets *Blood Decrease* Marked reduction in some patients with severe toxemia *2079*
Blood No Effect In 13 patients with eclampsia mean values of 175 ± 90 x 10^9/L not significantly different from 227 ± 47 x 10^9/L in 20 healthy controls *3955*

Progesterone *Plasma Decrease* Appears to be unrelated to the severity of the condition *4707*

Protein *Serum Decrease* Significantly reduced below the levels for normal pregnancy *900*
Serum Increase Secondary to hemoconcentration *2079*
Urine Increase As a result of hemoconcentration *1291* In 13 patients with eclampsia mean values of 2.6 ± 1.6 g/d significantly different from 0 g/d in 20 healthy controls *3955* Hypertension, edema, and proteinuria characterize toxemia of pregnancy *367* Constant finding *811*

Prothrombin Time *Plasma Increase* Higher than normal in pregnant patients *2079*

Renin Activity *Plasma Decrease* During normal pregnancy, plasma levels of renin, angiotensin II, and aldosterone are increased. Paradoxically with pregnancy-induced hypertension, they commonly decrease towards the normal *4223* In hypertensive groups, plasma renin activity and aldosterone concentration were significantly suppressed during the last trimester despite levels of renin substrate and progesterone that were not significantly different from those observed in normotensive pregnancy *5616*
Plasma Increase At term, hypertensive, toxemic pregnant women had elevated aldosterone and plasma renin activity, which remained elevated > 1 week after delivery *139*
Plasma No Effect Activity usually normal *5441* Average concentration and activity are slightly less than in normotensive pregnancies, but nearly all values in each group are in the same range *811*

Sodium *Serum* *Decrease* Reduced concentrations as a result of hemodilution. Averages 4 - 8 mmol/L lower than in normal nonpregnant women *4707* Rarely *811*
Urine *Decrease* Reduced to a greater extent than that in normal pregnancy *4707*

Triglycerides *Serum* *Increase* In 13 patients with eclampsia mean values of 296 ± 127 mg/dL not significantly different from 213 ± 88 mg/dL in 20 healthy controls *3955*

Urea Nitrogen *Serum* *Decrease* Low (9 ± 2 mg/dL) and low creatinine (0.75 ± 0.2 mg/dL) in late pregnancy are indicative of toxemia *367* Tends to decrease *1290*
Serum *Increase* Mean concentration of 2.1 ± 0.31 mmol/L in 20 eclamptic women significantly greater than 1.5 ± 2.7 mmol/L in 20 normotensive control pregnant women *4748*
Serum *No Effect* No significant increase *1291*

Uric Acid *Serum* *Increase* Serial determinations to follow therapeutic response and estimate prognosis *5544* Consistently observed *1291* Hyperuricemia usually precedes the development of azotemia due to reduced urate clearance *367* Mean concentration of 0.5 ± 0.036 mmol/L in 20 eclamptic women significantly greater than 0.21 ± 0.045 mmol/L in 20 normotensive control pregnant women *4748*

Viscosity *Serum* *Increase* Apparent blood viscosity rises sharply as the hematocrit increases due to hemoconcentration *811*

Volume *Plasma* *Decrease* In severe cases *1291* Hemoconcentration is an index of severity and prognosis *811*
Red Blood Cells *No Effect* In 14 cases in the late stages of eclampsia and pre-eclampsia, mean red cell volume was identical with that of normal pregnant women in the same gestational period *481*

642.90 Hypertension complicating Pregnancy

Alanine Aminotransferase *Serum* *Increase* In 48 pregnant women with hypertension complicating pregnancy median activity of 7 U/L significantly greater than that in 87 normotensive pregnant women in whom the median activity was 4 U/L *2712*
Serum *No Effect* In 35 women with pregnancy induced hypertension mean activity of 7 U/L not significantly different from 7 U/L in 41 women with normotensive pregnancies *2714*

Antithrombin III *Plasma* *No Effect* In 13 women with chronic pregnancy-related hypertension mean concentration of 86% not significantly different from 93% in 18 normal pregnant women *4033*

Apolipoprotein A-I *Serum* *No Effect* In 35 women with hypertension complicating pregnancy median concentration of 183.5 mg/dL not significantly different from median of 184.0 mg/dL in 35 women with uncomplicated pregnancies *3007*

Apolipoprotein B *Serum* *No Effect* In 35 women with hypertension complicating pregnancy median concentration of 126.0 mg/dL not significantly different from median of 134.0 mg/dL in 35 women with uncomplicated pregnancies *3007*

Aspartate Aminotransferase *Serum* *No Effect* In 35 women with pregnancy induced hypertension mean activity of 10 U/L not significantly different from 9 U/L in 41 women with normotensive pregnancies *2714*

Atrial Natriuretic Peptide *Plasma* *Increase* In 11 women with gestational hypertension median concentration of 10.7 pmol/L significantly different from 7.5 pmol/L in 12 healthy pregnant women *4195* In 19 patients with gestational hypertension median concentration of 10.7 pmol/L significantly different from 9.1 pmol/L in 19 matched pregnant controls *4194*

Cholesterol *Serum* *Decrease* In 35 women with hypertension complicating pregnancy median concentration of 6.0 mmol/L not significantly different from median of 6.4 mmol/L in 35 women with uncomplicated pregnancies *3007*

β-Chorionic Gonadotropin *Plasma* *Increase* Mean of MoM in 234 pregnant women with pregnancy-induced hypertension of 1.15 compared with 1 in 5,776 control pregnant women at 15 to 18 weeks of pregnancy *3650*

D-Dimer *Plasma* *No Effect* In 13 women with chronic pregnancy-related hypertension mean concentration not significantly different from that in 18 normal pregnant women *4033*

Endothelin-1 *Plasma* *Increase* In 11 women with gestational hypertension median concentration of 5.6 pmol/L not significantly higher than 4.8 pmol/L in 32 healthy pregnant women *4195*

Fibrinogen *Plasma* *No Effect* In 13 women with chronic pregnancy-related hypertension mean concentration not significantly different from that in 18 normal pregnant women *4033*

Fibronectin *Plasma* *Increase* Mean concentration of 240 ± 5 mg/L in 119 hypertensive pregnant women in first trimester, 236 ± 4 mg/L in second trimester and 294 ± 7 mg/L in third trimester significantly higher than in normotensive pregnant women at same stage of pregnancy *3966*
Plasma *No Effect* In 13 women with chronic pregnancy-related hypertension mean concentration of 296 mg/L not significantly different from 262 mg/L in 18 normal pregnant women *4033*

Glutathione S-Transferase Alpha 1-1 *Serum* *Increase* In 48 pregnant women with hypertension complicating pregnancy median concentration of 1.5 µg/L significantly greater than that in 87 normotensive pregnant women in whom the median concentration was 1.0 µg/L *2712*

Glutathione S-Transferase-pi 1-1 *Serum* *Increase* In 35 women with pregnancy-induced hypertension median concentration of 14.2 µg/L significantly different from 7.9 µg/L in 81 healthy nonpregnant female volunteers *2714*

Haptoglobin *Serum* *No Effect* In 35 women with pregnancy-induced hypertension median concentration of 0.92 g/L not significantly different from 0.92 g/L in 81 healthy nonpregnant female volunteers *2714*

HDL-Cholesterol *Serum* *No Effect* In 35 women with hypertension complicating pregnancy median concentration of 1.8 mmol/L not significantly different from median of 1.9 mmol/L in 35 women with uncomplicated pregnancies *3007*

Hematocrit *Blood* *Increase* In 19 patients with gestational hypertension mean value of 37 ± 3% significantly different from 34 ± 3% in 70 healthy pregnant women *4194*
Blood *No Effect* In 11 women with gestational hypertension mean of 38 ± 3% not significantly different from 36 ± 2% in 32 healthy pregnant women *4195*

Lactate Dehydrogenase *Serum* *Increase* In 35 women with hypertensive pregnancies median activity of 229 U/L significantly different from 147 U/L in 81 healthy nonpregnant female volunteers *2714*

LDL-Cholesterol *Serum* *Decrease* In 35 women with hypertension complicating pregnancy median concentration of 3.0 mmol/L not significantly different from median of 3.5 mmol/L in 35 women with uncomplicated pregnancies *3007*

Lipoprotein Lp(a) *Serum* *Decrease* In 35 women with hypertension complicating pregnancy median concentration of 14.8 mg/dL not significantly different from median of 21.2 mg/dL in 35 women with uncomplicated pregnancies *3007*

N-terminal Pro-Atrial Natriuretic Peptide *Plasma* *Increase* In 19 patients with gestational hypertension median concentration of 407 pmol/L significantly different from 230 pmol/L in 19 matched pregnant controls *4194*

Partial Thromboplastin Time *Plasma* *No Effect* In 13 women with chronic pregnancy-related hypertension mean time not significantly different from that in 18 normal pregnant women *4033*

Phospholipase A_2 Type II *Serum* *Increase* Increase in concentration observed in pregnancy-induced hypertension *3767*

Platelets *Blood* *No Effect* In 11 women with gestational hypertension mean count of 234,000 ± 63,000 /µL not significantly different from 287,000 ± 77,000 /µL in 12 healthy pregnant women *4195* In 13 women with chronic pregnancy-related hypertension mean concentration not significantly different from that in 18 normal pregnant women *4033* In 19 patients with gestational hypertension mean value of 239,000 ± 63,500 /µL not significantly different from 275,000 ± 87,100 /µL in 70 healthy pregnant women *4194*

Protein *Urine* *Increase* In 11 women with gestational hypertension mean daily excretion of < 300 mg not significantly different from < 300 mg in 32 healthy pregnant women *4195*
Urine *No Effect* In 19 patients with gestational hypertension mean excretion of less than 300 mg/d not significantly different from < 300 mg/d in 70 healthy pregnant women *4194*

642.90 Hypertension complicating Pregnancy *(continued)*

Protein C *Plasma No Effect* In 13 women with chronic pregnancy-related hypertension mean concentration not significantly different from that in 18 normal pregnant women *4033*

Protein S *Plasma No Effect* In 13 women with chronic pregnancy-related hypertension mean concentration not significantly different from that in 18 normal pregnant women *4033*

Prothrombin Time *Plasma No Effect* In 13 women with chronic pregnancy-related hypertension mean time not significantly different from that in 18 normal pregnant women *4033*

Triglycerides *Serum Increase* In 35 women with hypertension complicating pregnancy median concentration of 2.9 mmol/L significantly different from median of 2.3 mmol/L in 35 women with uncomplicated pregnancies *3007*

643.10 Emesis Gravidarum

β-Chorionic Gonadotropin *Plasma Decrease* Significantly lower concentration observed in late pregnancy in women with emesis gravidarum compared with concentration in pregnant women without emesis *2421*
Plasma Increase Significantly higher concentration observed in early pregnancy compared with pregnant women without emesis *2421*

643.10 Hyperemesis Gravidarum

Alanine Aminotransferase *Serum Increase* In one patient with hyperemesis for one week ALT activity of 550 U/L observed but mechanism of jaundice in hyperemesis gravidarum not understood *3924* Activity may be increased up to 200 U/L *1778*

Alkaline Phosphatase *Serum Increase* Two to four-fold increase may be observed indicating cholestasis *1778*
Serum No Effect In one patient with hyperemesis for one week normal activity observed but mechanism of jaundice in hyperemesis gravidarum not understood *3924*

Aspartate Aminotransferase *Serum Increase* Activity may be increased up to 200 U/L *1778*

Bilirubin *Serum Increase* Jaundice may be mild with plasma bilirubin concentrations rarely exceeding 75 µmol/L: both conjugated and unconjugated fractions are affected, related to impaired excretion of bilirubin *1778*

Bilirubin, Conjugated *Serum Increase* In one patient with hyperemesis for one week concentration of 106 µmol/L observed but mechanism of jaundice in hyperemesis gravidarum not understood *3924* Jaundice may be mild with plasma bilirubin concentrations rarely exceeding 75 µmol/L: both conjugated and unconjugated fractions are affected *1778*

Bilirubin, Unconjugated *Serum Increase* Jaundice may be mild with plasma bilirubin concentrations rarely exceeding 75 µmol/L: both conjugated and unconjugated fractions are affected *1778*

BSP Retention *Serum Increase* In patients with hyperemesis increased retention observed unlike those pregnant women with mild or no vomiting *3924*

γ-Glutamyltransferase *Serum Increase* Two to four-fold increase may be observed indicating cholestasis *1778*

Prothrombin Time *Plasma No Effect* In one patient with hyperemesis for one week normal time observed but mechanism of jaundice in hyperemesis gravidarum not understood *3924*

Thyroxine (T4) *Serum Increase* In about one third of hyperemesis women have a raised T4 compared with normal pregnant women *1965*

Thyroxine (T4), Free *Serum Increase* In about one third women with hyperemesis concentration higher than that in normal pregnant women. Plasma concentration correlates with hCG concentration in women with hyperemesis but not in normal pregnant women *1965*

Tri-iodothyronine, Free (fT3) *Serum Increase* In about 20% pregnant women with hyperemesis concentration higher than in normal pregnant women *1965*

Tri-iodothyronine (T3) *Serum Increase* In about 20% pregnant women with hyperemesis concentration higher thn in normal pregnant women *1965*

646.70 Acute Fatty Liver of Pregnancy

Alanine Aminotransferase *Serum Increase* Activity markedly increased in many cases *1778*

Alkaline Phosphatase *Serum Increase* Activity markedly increased in many cases *1778*

Ammonia *Plasma Increase* Concentration increased with hepatic encephalopathy *1778*

Aspartate Aminotransferase *Serum Increase* Activity markedly increased in many cases *1778*

Bilirubin *Serum Increase* Hyperbilirubinemia is invariable and is usually severe with a rise primarily of conjugated bilirubin *1778*

Bilirubin, Conjugated *Serum Increase* Hyperbilirubinemia is invariable and is usually severe with a rise primarily of conjugated bilirubin *1778*

Glucose *Serum Decrease* Hypoglycemia is often present *1778*

Leukocytes *Blood Increase* Increased leukocyte count above 15 x 10^9/L often observed in condition *1778*

Uric Acid *Serum Increase* Hyperuricemia may be present *1778*

646.80 Pregnancy complicated by Intrauterine Growth Retardation

Apolipoprotein B *Serum Decrease* In 20 pregnant women with intrauterine growth retardation median concentration of 171.0 mg/dL not significantly different from median of 184.0 mg/dL in 35 women with uncomplicated pregnancies *3007* In 20 pregnant women with intrauterine growth retardation median concentration of 120.0 mg/dL not significantly different from median of 134.0 mg/dL in 35 women with uncomplicated pregnancies *3007*

Cholesterol *Serum Decrease* In 20 pregnant women with intrauterine growth retardation median concentration of 5.9 mmol/L not significantly different from median of 6.4 mmol/L in 35 women with uncomplicated pregnancies *3007*

HDL-Cholesterol *Serum No Effect* In 20 pregnant women with intrauterine growth retardation median concentration of 1.8 mmol/L not significantly different from median of 1.9 mmol/L in 35 women with uncomplicated pregnancies *3007*

LDL-Cholesterol *Serum Decrease* In 20 pregnant women with intrauterine growth retardation median concentration of 3.2 mmol/L not significantly different from median of 3.5 mmol/L in 35 women with uncomplicated pregnancies *3007*

Lipoprotein Lp(a) *Serum Decrease* In 20 pregnant women with intrauterine growth retardation median concentration of 16.3 mg/dL not significantly different from median of 21.2 mg/dL in 35 women with uncomplicated pregnancies *3007*

Triglycerides *Serum No Effect* In 20 pregnant women with intrauterine growth retardation median concentration of 2.1 mmol/L not significantly different from median of 2.3 mmol/L in 35 women with uncomplicated pregnancies *3007*

648.80 Gestational Diabetes Mellitus

Intercellular Adhesion Molecule-1 *Serum No Effect* In patients with gestational diabetes mean serum concentration not significantly different from that in controls *5519*

Soluble E-Selectin *Serum Increase* In patients with gestational diabetes mean serum concentration significantly different from that in controls with concentration remaining increased post-partum *5519*

Soluble Vascular Cell Adhesion Molecule-1
Serum Increase In patients with gestational diabetes mean serum concentration significantly different from that in controls with concentration remaining increased post-partum *5519*

656.40 Pregnancy Complicated by Intrauterine Death

β-Chorionic Gonadotropin *Urine No Effect* Concentration usually normal *5544*

Estrogens *Urine Decrease* Observed effect *1290*

Pregnanediol *Urine* *Decrease* Fetal death. If < 5 mg/24 h then abortion is inevitable *1290*

Progesterone *Plasma* *Decrease* Fetal death. If < 5 mg/24 h then abortion is inevitable *1290*

Uric Acid *Serum* *Increase* Perinatal mortality was markedly increased when maternal plasma-urate concentrations were raised, generally in association with severe pre-eclampsia of early onset. Maternal hypertension, even severe, without hyperuricemia, was associated with an excellent prognosis for the fetus. When maternal hypertension was mild and hyperuricemia was severe, the prognosis for the fetus was poor *4306*

658.40 Chorioamnionitis

C-Reactive Protein *Serum* *Increase* In pregnant women with premature rupture of the membranes and chorioamnionitis mean concentration of 0.8 mg/dL compared with 0.2 mg/dL in those with negative amniotic fluid cultures *5811*

Leukocytes *Amniotic Fluid* *Increase* In pregnant women with premature rupture of the membranes and chorioamnionitis mean concentration of 268 /μL compared with 2 /μL in those with negative amniotic fluid cultures *5811*
Blood *Increase* In pregnant women with premature rupture of the membranes and chorioamnionitis mean concentration of 11,300 /μL compared with 9,400 /μL in those with negative amniotic fluid cultures *5811*

Macrophage Inflammatory Protein-1α
Amniotic Fluid *Increase* Mean concentration in 8 women with chorioamnionitis of about 1,000 pg/mL significantly different from that in 29 women not in labor in whom the mean concentration was about 2 pg/mL *1251*

674.90 Obstetric Disorder

Interleukin-6 *Serum* *Increase* Mean concentration detected in 12.5% of 13 patients with obstetric disorders with or without disseminated intravascular coagulation *3890*

Soluble E-Selectin *Serum* *No Effect* Mean concentration in 2 patients with obstetric disorders and disseminated intravascular coagulation of 32.1 ± 16.8 ng/mL not significantly different from about 40 ng/mL in 5 patients without DIC *3890*

Tumor Necrosis Factor-α *Serum* *No Effect* Mean concentration not detected in 13 patients with obstetric disorders with or without disseminated intravascular coagulation compared with undetectable amounts in patients with liver disease or hematologic malignancies *3890*

DISEASES OF THE SKIN AND SUBCUTANEOUS TISSUE

682.90 Cellulitis

α_1-Antichymotrypsin *Serum* *Increase* Mean concentration increased above reference interval of 47.9 ± 8.1 mg/dL in 1 of 1 patient (100%) with cellulitis *3044*

691.80 Atopic Dermatitis

Eosinophil Cationic Protein *Serum* *Increase* In 19 patients with atopic dermatitis significantly increased and concentration correlated with degree of activity. Concentration declined with response to treatment *988* In 43 patients with atopic dermatitis mean concentration of 25.9 ± 24.4 ng/mL significantly different from 12.2 ± 9.8 ng/mL in 55 healthy controls *1607*

Eosinophils *Blood* *Increase* In 20 patients with atopic dermatitis and eosinophilia mean concentration of 1,200 ± 1,180 /μL but in 18 patients with atopic dermatitis but without eosinophilia mean concentration of 229 ± 159 /μL compared with less than 500 /μL in 100 normal individuals *5776* In 43 patients with atopic dermatitis mean concentration of 507 ± 432 /μL significantly different from 127 ± 92 /μL in 55 healthy controls *1607*

Immunoglobulin E *Serum* *Increase* In 19 patients with atopic dermatitis significantly increased concentration observed which was not affected by treatment *988* In 43 patients with atopic dermatitis mean concentration of 2,714 ± 3,218 U/mL significantly different from 75 ± 72 U/mL in 55 healthy controls *1607*

Interleukin-4 *Serum* *Increase* The IL-4 levels in patients with atopic dermatitis were significantly higher than those in normal controls *4085*
Serum *No Effect* IL-4 detected in 23 of 43 patients with atopic dermatitis with a mean concentration in those in whom it was detected of 1.83 ± 2.75 pg/mL not significantly different from 2.18 ± 2.86 pg/mL in the 20 of 45 healthy controls in whom it was detected *1607*

Myelin Basic Protein *Serum* *Increase* In 20 patients with atopic dermatitis and eosinophilia mean concentration of 97.2 ± 91.3 ng/mL (not significantly increased) but in 18 patients with atopic dermatitis but without eosinophilia mean concentration of 40.0 ± 24.0 ng/mL (not significantly different) compared with mean of 41 ± 19 ng/mL in 100 normal individuals *5776*

Soluble CD14+ *Serum* *No Effect* In 43 patients with atopic dermatitis mean concentration of 2.87 ± 0.77 μg/mL not significantly different from 2.89 ± 0.85 μg/mL in 55 healthy controls *1607*

Soluble CD30 *Serum* *Increase* Mean concentration of 74.75 U/mL in 16 patients with atopic dermatitis significantly higher than that in 15 healthy controls of 6.60 U/mL *1262*

Soluble E-Cadherin *Serum* *Increase* Mean concentration in serum from 17 patients with atopic dermatitis or drug eruptions of 5.5 ng/mL significantly higher than that in 31 healthy volunteers of 3.6 ± 1.1 ng/mL *3371*

Soluble E-Selectin *Serum* *Increase* In 43 patients with atopic dermatitis mean concentration of 51.0 ± 42.5 ng/mL significantly different from 30.6 ± 10.6 ng/mL in 55 healthy controls *1607* Mean concentration of 81 ± 7 ng/mL in 24 patients significantly different from 44 ± 4 ng/mL in 16 healthy volunteer controls *989*

Soluble Interleukin-2 Receptor *Serum* *Increase* In 19 patients with atopic dermatitis mean concentration significantly increased and correlated with degree of disease activity. Concentration did not change with treatment *988*

Substance P *Tears* *No Effect* Mean concentration of 65.0 ± 34.2 pg/mL in 10 patients with atopic dermatitis not significantly different from 70.9 ± 34.8 pg/mL observed in 65 healthy adults *1597*

Tumor Necrosis Factor-α *Serum* *Increase* In 15 children with atopic dermatitis mean concentration increased compared with concentrations in 11 healthy controls *5079*

691.80 Atopic Eczema

Adenosine Monophosphate *Lymphocytes* *Decrease* Individuals in the severe eczema group were shown to have a significant diminution in their unstimulated lymphocyte cAMP concentrations and absolute responses *4009*

Eosinophils *Blood* *Increase* Observed effect *5677*

Immunoglobulin E *Serum* *Increase* Total serum concentration was elevated in 75 - 81% of the children with asthma, nasal allergy and atopic dermatitis and an elevated serum concentration or blood eosinophilia, or both, was noted in 85% of the patients *849* Atopic subjects tend to have moderate increases *1290* Some patients *4551*

Interleukin-4 *Serum* *Increase* The serum level of IL-4 was examined in children with allergic diseases, and compared with those in non-allergic controls of the same age and sex. The serum concentration of IL-4 was elevated in all allergic groups, including cases of atopic eczema, bronchial asthma and anaphylaxis to food, compared with non-allergic controls *3369*

Soluble Intercellular Adhesion Molecule-1 *Serum* *Increase* In 18 patients with severe atopic eczema mean concentration of 565 ± 99 ng/mL significantly higher than 296 ± 46 ng/mL in 22 healthy controls *2801* In 18 patients with severe atopic eczema mean concentration of 89.7 ± 29.9 ng/mL significantly higher than 48.8 ± 22.7 ng/mL in 22 healthy controls *2801*

Soluble Interleukin-2 Receptor *Serum* *Increase* Significant elevation of sIL-2R was observed in sera from children with atopic eczema or history of an anaphylactic reaction to food, as compared with that in non-allergic controls *3369*

691.80 Chronic Eczema

Eosinophils *Blood* *Increase* In 3 patients with chronic eczema and eosinophilia mean concentration of 858 ± 388 /µL compared with less than 500 /µL in 100 normal individuals and in one patient with chronic eczema but without eosinophilia *5776*

Growth Hormone *Plasma* *Increase* Mean concentration of 2.7 ± 1.7 mU/L in 5 patients with eczema compared with 1.2 ± 0.6 mU/L in 6 normal controls but higher mean largely attributable to increased concentration in one individual *4220*

Myelin Basic Protein *Serum* *Increase* In 3 patients with chronic eczema and eosinophilia mean concentration of 120 ± 76.4 ng/mL and in 1 patient with chronic eczema but without eosinophilia mean concentration of 108 ng/mL compared with mean of 41 ± 19 ng/mL in 100 normal individuals *5776*

692.90 Contact Dermatitis

Soluble CD30 *Serum* *No Effect* Mean concentration of 6.90 U/mL in 10 patients with allergic contact dermatitis not significantly different from that in 15 healthy controls of 6.60 U/mL *1262*

692.90 Nonatopic Eczema

Eosinophil Cationic Protein *Serum* *No Effect* In 24 patients with nonatopic eczema mean concentration of 14.4 ± 11.9 ng/mL not significantly different from 12.2 ± 9.8 ng/mL in 55 healthy controls *1607*

Eosinophils *Blood* *Increase* In 24 patients with nonatopic eczema mean concentration of 242 ± 154 /µL not significantly different from 127 ± 92 µL in 55 healthy controls *1607*

Immunoglobulin E *Serum* *Increase* In 24 patients with nonatopic eczema mean concentration of 273 ± 525 U/mL significantly different from 75 ± 72 U/mL in 55 healthy controls *1607*

Interleukin-4 *Serum* *No Effect* IL-4 detected in 12 of 24 patients with atopic dermatitis with a mean concentration in those in whom it was detected of 2.71 ± 3.3 pg/mL not significantly different from 2.18 ± 2.86 pg/mL in the 20 of 45 healthy controls in whom it was detected *1607*

Soluble CD14+ *Serum* *No Effect* In 24 patients with nonatopic eczema mean concentration of 2.93 ± 1.08 µg/mL not significantly different from 2.89 ± 0.85 µg/mL in 55 healthy controls *1607*

Soluble E-Selectin *Serum* *Increase* In 24 patients with nonatopic eczema mean concentration of 42.9 ± 21.0 ng/mL significantly different from 30.6 ± 10.6 ng/mL in 55 healthy controls *1607*

694.00 Dermatitis Herpetiformis

Antibody Titer *Serum* *Increase* Reticulin antibodies *3712*

Eosinophils *Blood* *Increase* In 36% of 11 patients at initial hospitalization for this disorder *1576* Occurs in some skin diseases *5544*

Fat *Feces* *Increase* In small intestinal disease *4891*

HLA Antigens *Blood* *Present* HLA-B_8 and HLA-Bw15 associated with this disease *4879* HLA-DR3 found in 77% of patients versus 20% of controls *5678* HLA antigen DR2 found in 97% of patients with this disease compared to 25% of controls *4584*

Lactate Dehydrogenase *Serum* *Increase* In 25% of 12 patients at initial hospitalization for this disorder *1576*

Monocytes *Blood* *Increase* In 63% of 11 patients at initial hospitalization for this disorder *1576*

Neutrophils *Blood* *Increase* In 45% of 11 patients at initial hospitalization for this disorder *1576*

694.40 Pemphigus

Albumin *Serum* *Decrease* In untreated patients in the advanced stage of disease. Often drops to 25% of normal *1499*

Antibody Titer *Serum* *Increase* Numerous studies have confirmed the presence of autoantibodies specific for an intercellular substance of skin and mucosa in serum from patients with active pemphigus *1315*

Complement Fixation *Serum* *Increase* 50 - 75% of bullous pemphigoid patients have serum antibodies capable of fixing complement to the basement membrane *4551*

Complement, Total *Serum* *Decrease* Cryoproteins observed in patients with pemphigus have been shown to contain IgG, complement components, and other serum proteins *3532*

Cryoglobulins *Serum* *Increase* When observed in patients with pemphigus have been shown to contain IgG, complement components, and other serum proteins. Appeared in the clinically active stage and disappeared subsequent to clinical improvement *3532*

Eosinophils *Blood* *Decrease* In severely ill patients the percentage, even if previously high, drops off - often to 0% *1499* *Blood* *Increase* Moderately increased percentage in pemphigus vulgaris *1499* Slight or absent eosinophilia in pemphigus foliaceous *1499*

Erythrocyte Sedimentation Rate *Blood* *Increase* Increased globulin, especially fibrinogen, probably accounts for the increased ESR *367*

Hematocrit *Blood* *Decrease* Anemia is common and may be due to inanition, serum loss and infection *367*

Hemoglobin *Blood* *Decrease* Anemia is common and may be due to inanition, serum loss and infection *367*

Immunoglobulin E *Serum* *Increase* Significant increase in 70% of bullous pemphigoid patients *4551*

Immunoglobulin M *Serum* *Increase* About 70% of patients with this condition have elevated levels *5280*

Indirect Fluorescent Antibodies *Serum* *Increase* Numerous studies have confirmed the presence of autoantibodies specific for an intercellular substance of skin and mucosa in serum from patients with active pemphigus *1315*

Leukocytes *Blood* *Increase* Usually elevated with an increase of immature forms *367*

Protein *Serum* *Decrease* May fall to 50% of normal in untreated patients with advanced disease *1499* Total serum protein may fall as low as 3.6 g/dL with a correspondingly low level of albumin *367*

694.40 Pemphigus Vulgaris

Intercellular Adhesion Molecule-1 *Serum* *No Effect* In 9 patients with pemphigus vulgaris median concentration of 194 ng/mL (range 101 - 406) not significantly different compared with median of 203 ng/mL and range of 90 - 343 ng/mL in 20 healthy individuals *1022*

Soluble E-Cadherin *Serum* *Increase* Mean concentration in serum from 17 patients with pemphigus vulgaris of 5.0 ng/mL significantly higher than that in 31 healthy volunteers of 3.6 ± 1.1 ng/mL *3371*

Soluble E-Selectin *Serum* *Increase* In 9 patients with pemphigus vulgaris median concentration of 45 ng/mL (range 33 - 110) significantly increased compared with median of 28.5 ng/mL and range of 6.4 - 48 ng/mL in 20 healthy individuals *1022*

694.50 Bullous Pemphigoid

Eosinophils *Blood* *Increase* In 3 patients with bullous pemphigoid and eosinophilia mean concentration of 4,410 ± 1,820 /µL compared with less than 500 /µL in 100 normal individuals and in 1 patient with bullous pemphigoid but without eosinophilia *5776*

Intercellular Adhesion Molecule-1 *Serum* *No Effect* In 15 patients with bullous pemphigoid median concentration of 211 ng/mL (range 159 - 386) not significantly different compared with median of 203 ng/mL and range of 90 - 343 ng/mL in 20 healthy individuals *1022*

Myelin Basic Protein *Serum* *Increase* In 3 patients with bullous pemphigoid and eosinophilia mean concentration of 615 ± 74.5 ng/mL and in 1 patient with bullous pemphigoid but without eosinophilia concentration of 25 ng/mL (not significantly different) compared with mean of 41 ± 19 ng/mL in 100 normal individuals *5776*

Soluble E-Cadherin *Blister Fluid* *Increase* Mean concentration in blister fluid from 31 patients with bullous pemphigoid of 14 ng/mL significantly higher than that in blister fluid from 31 healthy volunteers of 6.9 ± 1.5 ng/mL *3371*
Serum *Increase* Mean concentration in serum from 31 patients with bullous pemphigoid of 6.9 ng/mL significantly higher than that in 31 healthy volunteers of 3.6 ± 1.1 ng/mL *3371*

Soluble E-Selectin *Serum* *Increase* In 15 patients with bullous pemphigoid median concentration of 47 ng/mL (range 30 - 94) significantly increased compared with median of 28.5 ng/mL and range of 6.4 - 48 ng/mL in 20 healthy individuals *1022*

695.10 Erythema Multiforme

Eosinophils *Blood* *Increase* Occurs in some infectious diseases *5544*

695.10 Scalded Skin Syndrome

Albumin *Serum* *Decrease* Responsible for excessive loss from circulation in some patients with subsequent decreased serum concentration *4617*

695.10 Stevens-Johnson Syndrome

5-Oxoproline *Red Blood Cells* *Decrease* Value of 1.66 mmol/L observed in one patient with Stevens-Johnson syndrome significantly decreased compared with 2.36 ± 0.37 mmol/L in 100 healthy controls *3384*
Urine *Increase* Value of 320 mmol/mol creatinine observed in one patient with Stevens-Johnson syndrome significantly increased compared with < 50 mmol/mol creatinine in 100 healthy controls *3384*

695.89 Exfoliative Dermatitis

Albumin *Serum* *Decrease* Responsible for excessive loss from circulation in some patients with subsequent decreased serum concentration *4617*

696.00 Psoriatic Arthritis

Anti-Endothelial Cell Antibodies *Serum* *No Effect* In patients with undefined connective tissue disease (n = 57), ankylosing spondylitis (n = 109), and psoriatic arthritis (n = 58), the frequency of AECA corresponded to that of the random population sample *3845*

Melanoma Inhibitory Factor *Serum* *No Effect* In 29 patients mean concentration of 4.8 ± 3.2 ng/mL showed no significant difference from 3.6 ± 2.8 ng/mL in 120 healthy controls *3655*

696.10 Psoriasis

α_1-Acid Glycoprotein *Serum* *Increase* Elevated levels in states associated with cell proliferation *4853* *2597* *4241* *3713* *4373* *4696*

Angiotensin-converting Enzyme *Serum* *No Effect* Not significantly different in psoriatic arthritis (n = 12) from normal controls *3141* Normal in cutaneous psoriasis *5207* Levels remained normal *5207*

Dehydroepiandrosterone *Plasma* *Decrease* Observed effect *5229* *602* *5679*

Endothelin *Plasma* *Increase* Mean concentration of 5.4 ± 1.7 pg/mL in 65 treated patients with psoriasis significantly greater than 2.8 ± 0.6 pg/mL in 40 healthy controls *5833*

Endothelin-1 *Plasma* *Increase* In 15 patients with psoriasis median concentration of endothelin-1 of 0.9 pg/mL significantly increased compared with median concentration of 0.6 pg/mL in 15 healthy controls *516*

Fat *Feces* *Increase* Steatorrhea has been reported in association with psoriasis; degree correlated with extent of involvement *4824* *1499*

Folate *Serum* *Decrease* Decreased with extensive skin disease *5230* *772* *602*

Glycosaminoglycans *Urine* *Increase* Points towards increased dermal metabolism *4941*

Growth Hormone *Plasma* *Increase* In 12 fasting patients with psoriasis mean concentration of 4.4 ± 1.4 mU/L compared with 1.2 ± 0.3 mU/L in 6 normal individuals *4220*

HLA Antigens *Blood* *Present* HLA-Cw6 present in 50% of caucasian patients versus 23% of controls *5678* HLA-$B_2$7 associated with psoriatic spondylitis *4879*

Homocystine *Plasma* *Increase* Moderate increase observed in patients with psoriasis *5346*

Hyaluronic Acid *Serum* *Increase* Significantly elevated levels were found compared with healthy controls and atopic dermatitis *3164*

Interferon-γ *Serum* *Increase* In a study population 21 patients with psoriasis vulgaris, together with 21 healthy controls, the mean serum levels of interferon-γ were significantly elevated *1803*

Interleukin-1 *Serum* *No Effect* In a study population patients with psoriasis vulgaris, together with 21 healthy controls, the mean serum levels were not significantly different from those in controls *1803*

Interleukin-2 *Serum* *Increase* In 24 patients with acute phase psoriasis mean concentration of 0.91 ± 0.92 U/mL significantly different from 0.47 ± 0.35 U/mL in 20 healthy controls *1072*

β_2-Microglobulin *Serum* *Increase* In 24 patients with acute phase psoriasis mean concentration of 2.5 ± 1.3 ng/mL significantly different from 1.3 ± 0.3 ng/mL in 20 healthy controls *1072*

Procollagen Type III Peptide *Serum* *Increase* In patients with psoriatic arthritis an increased aminoterminal propeptide of type III procollagen may be related to the joint disease. 38% of patients with psoriatic arthritis had an increased aminoterminal propeptide of type III procollagen in the absence of detectable liver fibrosis *5832*

Soluble CD4+ *Serum* *Increase* In 24 patients with acute phase psoriasis mean concentration of 69 ± 24 U/mL significantly different from 29 ± 10 U/mL in 20 healthy controls *1072*

Soluble CD8+ *Serum* *Increase* In 24 patients with acute phase psoriasis mean concentration of 372 ± 146 U/mL significantly different from 276 ± 69 U/mL in 20 healthy controls *1072*

Soluble Cytokeratin 19 Fragment *Serum* *No Effect* In 24 patients with acute phase psoriasis mean concentration of about 0.66 ng/mL not significantly different from about 0.4 ng/mL in 20 healthy controls *1072*

Soluble E-Selectin *Serum* *Increase* Mean concentration of 99 ± 13 ng/mL in 16 patients significantly different from 44 ± 4 ng/mL in 16 healthy volunteer controls *989*

Soluble Intercellular Adhesion Molecule-1 *Serum* *Increase* In 24 patients with acute phase psoriasis mean concentration of 509 ± 154 ng/mL significantly different from 215 ± 92 ng/mL in 20 healthy controls *1072* Mean concentration of approximately 490 ng/mL in 32 patients with psoriasis significantly different from 400 ng/mL in 112 healthy controls *1871*

Soluble Intercellular Adhesion Molecule-3 *Serum* *Increase* Mean concentration of approximately 200 ng/mL in 32 patients with psoriasis significantly different from 120 ng/mL in 112 healthy controls *1871*

Soluble Interleukin-2 Receptor *Serum* *Increase* In 24 patients with acute phase psoriasis mean concentration of 906 ± 569 U/mL significantly different from 627 ± 174 U/mL in 20 healthy controls *1072*

Soluble p55 *Serum* *Increase* Mean concentration in 6 patients of 0.43 ± 0.04 ng/mL compared with 0.07 ng/mL in 3 healthy controls *1394*

Soluble Tumor Necrosis Factor Receptor-I *Serum* *Increase* Mean concentration of approximately 2.8 ng/mL in 32 patients with psoriasis significantly different from 1.4 ng/mL in 112 healthy controls *1871*

696.10 Psoriasis *(continued)*

Squamous Cell Carcinoma Antigen *Serum* *Increase* In 24 patients with acute phase psoriasis mean concentration of about 6.4 ng/mL significantly different from about 1.2 ng/mL in 20 healthy controls *1072*

Tumor Necrosis Factor-α *Serum* *No Effect* In a study population of 21 patients with psoriasis vulgaris, together with 21 healthy controls, the mean serum levels of tumor necrosis factor-α were not significantly different from those in controls *1803*

Uric Acid *Serum* *Increase* Increased with increased extent and severity of cutaneous lesions *1499* Increased nucleic acid turnover *5863* Slight elevation may occur, especially in male patients *2900* Found in 30 - 40% of patients *4707*

Zinc *Serum* *Decrease* Decreased *5083* *1852*

696.10 Psoriasis Vulgaris

Soluble E-Cadherin *Serum* *Increase* Mean concentration in serum from 17 patients with psoriasis vulgaris of 5.1 ng/mL significantly higher than that in 31 healthy volunteers of 3.6 ± 1.1 ng/mL *3371*

701.00 Morphea

C-terminal Propeptide of Type I Procollagen
Serum *Increase* In 9 patients with morphea mean concentration of 162 ± 70 ng/mL not significantly higher than 139 ± 83 ng/mL in 30 healthy control volunteers *2675*

704.01 Alopecia

3α-Androstanediol *Plasma* *Increase* In 20 premenopausal women with androgenic alopecia mean concentration of 0.69 ± 0.06 nmol/L significantly higher than 0.41 ± 0.03 nmol/L in 10 female controls *2981*

3α-Androstanediol Glucuronide *Plasma* *Increase* In 20 premenopausal women with androgenic alopecia mean concentration of 11.1 ± 2.3 nmol/L significantly higher than 6.2 ± 0.47 nmol/L in 10 female controls *2981*

3α-Androstanediol Sulfate *Plasma* *Increase* In 20 premenopausal women with androgenic alopecia mean concentration of 197.6 ± 27.3 nmol/L significantly higher than 67.2 ± 4.2 nmol/L in 10 female controls *2981*

Androsterone Glucuronide *Plasma* *Increase* In 20 premenopausal women with androgenic alopecia mean concentration of 158.7 ± 27.8 nmol/L significantly higher than 73 ± 4.6 nmol/L in 10 female controls *2981*

Androsterone Sulfate *Plasma* *Increase* In 20 premenopausal women with androgenic alopecia mean concentration of 3,618 ± 686 nmol/L significantly higher than 2,038 ± 200 nmol/L in 10 female controls *2981*

Soluble Interleukin-2 Receptor *Serum* *Increase* In patients with alopecia areata in active phase concentrations significantly higher than in patients with stable disease and healthy controls *5386*

704.10 Hirsutism

Androgen Index, Free (FAI) *Plasma* *Increase* In 37 hirsute women mean index of 11.3 ± 2.8 in obese patients significantly higher than 6.2 ± 0.8 in lean patients *1387*

5α-Androstane-3α-17β-Diol-Glucuronide *Plasma* *Increase* In 25 hyperandrogenic hirsute women mean concentration of 5.7 ± 1.3 ng/mL compared with 3.2 ± 0.7 ng/mL in 15 normoandrogenic hirsute women and 1.8 ± 0.6 ng/mL in 15 healthy age-matched women *4155*

Androstanediol *Plasma* *No Effect* After adjustment for the effects of age and BMI there was no significant association between the degree of hirsutism and the level of androstanediol *3628*

Androstanediol Glucuronide *Plasma* *No Effect* No correlation observed in 23 women with facial hirsutism and plasma concentration of 5α-androstane-3α,17β-diol glucuronide *4532* No significant difference observed between mean concentration of 2.2 ± 0.8 nmol/L in 15 women with polycystic ovary disease and hirsutism and 7 with polycystic ovary disease and no hirsutism and 2.2 ± 0.8 nmol/L in 20 healthy control women *4609*

3α-Androstanediol Glucuronide *Plasma* *Increase* Mean concentration in 8 hirsute women with oligomenorrhea of 510 ng/dL significantly different from 270 ng/dL in 12 hirsute women with regular ovulatory cycles and 230 ng/dL in 20 non-obese healthy women controls *2669* Serum 3AG levels in each group of HF were significantly higher (p less than 0.01 - 0.001) than those in normal females [normal: 2.9 ± 0.94 nmol/L (n = 28)]. However, normal 3AG levels (less than 5.2 nmol/L) were present in 50 - 67% of HF in each group *3989* In 23 hirsute women mean concentration of 5.8 ± 2.0 ng/mL compared with 2.5 ± 1.3 ng/mL in 30 premenopausal women *1148* In 22 hirsute women aged 17 - 45 y median and mean concentrations of 5.5 ng/mL and 5.8 ± 2.4 ng/mL significantly different from median of 3.0 ng/mL and mean of 3.1 ± 1.4 ng/mL in 16 healthy control women *3445*

3α-17β-Androstanediol Glucuronide *Urine* *Increase* Increased excretion is associated with increased dihydrotestosterone production *2952*

Androstenedione *Plasma* *Increase* 27 patients with hirsutism, compared with the hormone levels of 27 female patients without endocrine disorders. Of the androgens, only androstenedione showed a slightly significant elevation in hirsutism *4647* In 25 hyperandrogenic women mean concentration of 14.1 ± 4.5 nmol/L compared with 6.7 ± 2.1 nmol/L in 15 normoandrogenic hirsute women and 5.7 ± 1.9 nmol/L in healthy women of similar age *4155* Concentration often increased in hirsutism *2952*
Plasma *No Effect* Insignificant change to mean of 8.6 nmol/L in 50 hirsute women compared with mean and SD of 8.7 ± 3.7 nmol/L in 19 healthy controls of same age group (17 - 39 years) *3938*

Androsterone Sulfate *Plasma* *No Effect* The mean Andros-S level in idiopathic hirsutism (3.5 ± 0.5) was not significantly different from levels in normal women (3.0 ± 0.5) *5885*

Cortisol *Plasma* *Increase* 27 patients with hirsutism, compared with the hormone levels of 27 female patients without endocrine disorders. Of the androgens, only androstenedione showed a slightly significant elevation in hirsutism *4647*

Dehydroepiandrosterone Sulfate *Plasma* *Increase* In 25 hyperandrogenic hirsute women mean concentration of 7.3 ± 3.9 µmol/L compared with 5.1 ± 1.2 µmol/L in 15 normoandrogenic women and 4.3 ± 1.0 µmol/L in 15 age matched control women *4155* Mean concentration in 8 hirsute women with oligomenorrhea of 227.9 µg/mL different from 221.6 µg/mL in 12 hirsute women with regular ovulatory cycles *2669* Increased concentrations may be associated with hirsutism in women *2952* In 50 hirsute women aged 17 - 44 years mean concentration of 8.7 µmol/L compared with mean and SD of 5.5 ± 1.7 µmol/L in 19 healthy women aged 17 - 39 years *3938*

Dihydrotestosterone *Serum* *Increase* Hirsute women presented significantly higher levels of dihydrotestosterone (0.54 ± 0.07 nmol/L vs 0.32 ± 0.03 nmol/L; $p < 0.02$) *4072*

Estrogens *Plasma* *No Effect* No differences were observed between serum estrogen concentrations in patients with hirsutism and controls *4072*

Follicle Stimulating Hormone *Plasma* *Decrease* Mean concentration in 8 hirsute women with oligomenorrhea of 5.30 IU/L different from 6.31 IU/L in 12 hirsute women with regular ovulatory cycles *2669*

HDL-Cholesterol *Serum* *Decrease* p less than 0.01 *5666*

Luteinizing Hormone *Plasma* *Increase* Mean concentration in 8 hirsute women with oligomenorrhea of 11.55 IU/L different from 3.69 IU/L in 12 hirsute women with regular ovulatory cycles *2669*

Luteinizing Hormone:Follicle Stimulating Hormone Ratio
Plasma *Increase* Mean ratio in 8 hirsute women with oligomenorrhea of 2.15 significantly different from 0.63 in 12 hirsute women with regular ovulatory cycles *2669*

Prolactin *Plasma* *Increase* Both baseline and stimulated levels were highly significantly elevated in hirsutism *4647*

Prostate-specific Antigen *Serum* *Increase* In 22 hirsute women aged 17 - 45 y median and mean concentrations of 4 pg/mL and 43 ± 127 pg/mL significantly different from median of 2 pg/mL and mean of 4 ± 4.8 pg/mL in 16 healthy control women *3445* In 37 hirsute women mean concentration of 12.8 ± 5.4 pg/mL in obese patients significantly higher than 6.2 ± 1.5 pg/mL in lean patients *1387* In 37 hirsute women PSA was detected in 32 compared with 0 pg/mL in all 11 healthy controls *1387*

Sex-Hormone Binding Globulin *Serum* *Decrease* In 50 hirsute women mean concentration of 30.9 nmol/L (range 10 - 66 nmol/L) compared with 67.2 nmol/L (30 - 99 nmol/L) in 5 healthy nonpregnant women *5657* Variable reduction observed *4234* Reduced concentration observed in women with clinical manifestations of hyperandrogenism *1424* In 14 hirsute women mean concentration of 37 ± 21 nmol/L significantly less than in 10 normal women 65 ± 39 nmol/L as measured by a time-resolved immunofluorometric assay *3788* In 37 hirsute women mean concentration of 266 ± 36 µg/dL in obese patients significantly lower than 451 ± 41 µg/dL in lean patients *1387*
Serum *No Effect* Mean concentration in 50 hirsute women aged 17 - 44 years 43 nmol/L compared with mean and SD in healthy women of the same age of 43 ± 16 nmol/L *3938*

Testosterone *Saliva* *Increase* In 50 hirsute women aged 17 - 44 years mean concentration of 105 pmol/L compared with mean and SD in women of same age of 52 ± 18 pmol/L *3938*
Serum *Increase* In 50 hirsute women mean concentration of 2.6 nmol/L compared with mean and SD of 1.75 ± 0.7 nmol/L in 19 healthy control women aged 17 - 39 years *3938* Hirsute women presented significantly higher levels of testosterone than controls (1.49 ± 0.38 vs 0.59 ± 0.05 nmol/L, mean ± SEM; $p < 0.05$) *4072* In 25 hyperandrogenic women mean concentration of 2.4 ± 0.4 nmol/L compared with 1.3 ± 0.1 nmol/L in 15 normoandrogenic women and 0.8 ± 0.4 nmol/L in 15 healthy women of similar age *4155* Mean concentration in 8 hirsute women with oligomenorrhea of 130 ng/dL significantly different from 86 ng/dL in 12 hirsute women with regular ovulatory cycles and 73 ng/dL in 20 non-obese healthy women controls *2669*
Serum *No Effect* In 37 hirsute women mean concentration of 71 ± 11 ng/dL in obese patients not significantly different from 71 ± 4 ng/dL in lean patients *1387*

Testosterone, Free *Serum* *Increase* Mean concentration in 8 hirsute women with oligomenorrhea of 4.7 pg/mL significantly different from 1.8 pg/mL in 12 hirsute women with regular ovulatory cycles and reference interval of 0.2 - 3.2 pg/mL in healthy women *2669* In 25 hyperandrogenic hirsute women mean concentration of 10.8 ± 6.1 pmol/L significantly higher than 6.7 ± 2.1 pmol/L in 15 normoandrogenic hirsute women and 3.8 ± 2.0 pmol/L in 15 healthy women of similar age *4155*

Thyroid Stimulating Hormone *Serum* *Increase* In 27 women with hirsutism, and the results were compared with those recorded in 45 female control persons. Baseline concentrations of TSH prior to stimulation were significantly elevated in hirsutism *4647*

Thyroxine (T4) *Serum* *Decrease* Hypothyroidism is a significant finding *4647*

Triglycerides *Serum* *Increase* p less than 0.01 *5666*

VLDL-Cholesterol *Serum* *Increase* p less than 0.01 *5666*

704.10 Idiopathic Hirsutism

Androgen Index, Free (FAI) *Plasma* *No Effect* In 24 women with idiopathic hirsutism mean index of 4.33 ± 2.62 not significantly greater than 3.67 ± 1.96 in 12 normal women *1389* In 17 women with idiopathic hirsutism mean index of 4.0 ± 2.2 not significantly different from 2.4 ± 1.8 in 17 healthy control women *1388*

3α-Androstanediol Glucuronide *Plasma* *Increase* Concentration increased in women with idiopathic hirsutism *1148*

Androstenedione *Plasma* *No Effect* In 17 women with idiopathic hirsutism mean concentration of 2.9 ± 0.8 ng/mL not significantly different from 2.5 ± 0.8 ng/mL in 17 healthy control women *1388* In 12 young women with idiopathic hirsutism mean concentration of 10.9 ± 1.1 nmol/L not different from normal range of 1.4 - 15.0 nmol/L *3546* Mean concentration in 57 women with idiopathic hirsutism and acne of 4.50 ± 1.25 nmol/L not significantly different from 20 healthy premenopausal women in follicular phase 4.18 ± 1.46 nmol/L *1479*

δ⁴-Androstenedione *Plasma* *No Effect* In 24 women with idiopathic hirsutism mean baseline concentration of 2.8 ± 0.8 ng/mL not significantly different from 2.6 ± 0.8 ng/mL in 12 normal women *1389*

Cortisol *Plasma* *No Effect* In 17 women with idiopathic hirsutism mean concentration of 15.7 ± 7.4 µg/dL not significantly different from 15.3 ± 4.6 µg/dL in 17 healthy control women *1388* In 24 women with idiopathic hirsutism mean baseline concentration of 17 ± 7 µg/dL not significantly different from 16 ± 6 µg/dL in 12 normal women *1389*

Dehydroepiandrosterone *Plasma* *No Effect* In 24 women with idiopathic hirsutism mean baseline concentration of 9.4 ± 4.9 ng/mL not significantly different from 8.1 ± 4.1 ng/mL in 12 normal women *1389* Mean concentration in 57 women with idiopathic hirsutism and acne of 19.72 ± 7.95 nmol/L not significantly different from that in 20 healthy premenopausal women in follicular phase 18.60 ± 8.10 nmol/L *1479*

Dehydroepiandrosterone Sulfate *Plasma* *Increase* In 17 women with idiopathic hirsutism mean concentration of 2,654 ± 1,157 ng/mL not significantly different from 1,902 ± 705 ng/mL in 17 healthy control women *1388*
Plasma *No Effect* In 12 young women with idiopathic hirsutism mean concentration of 6.6 ± 0.2 µmol/L not different from normal range of 3.1 - 9.4 µmol/L *3546* In 24 women with idiopathic hirsutism mean baseline concentration of 2,598 ± 820 ng/mL not significantly different from 1,994 ± 756 ng/mL in 12 normal women *1389*

11-Deoxycortisol *Plasma* *No Effect* Mean concentration in 57 women with idiopathic hirsutism and acne of 1.35 + 1.04 nmol/L not significantly different from 20 healthy premenopausal women in follicular phase 1.81 ± 0.56 nmol/L *1479* In 24 women with idiopathic hirsutism mean baseline concentration of 3.5 ± 2.0 ng/mL not significantly different from 3.8 ± 2.2 ng/mL in 12 normal women *1389* In 17 women with idiopathic hirsutism mean concentration of 2.6 ± 1.1 ng/mL not significantly different from 3.2 ± 2.1 ng/mL in 17 healthy control women *1388*

21-Deoxycortisol *Plasma* *No Effect* Mean concentration in 57 women with idiopathic hirsutism and acne of 0.34 + 0.28 nmol/L not significantly different from 20 healthy premenopausal women in follicular phase 0.20 ± 0.14 nmol/L *1479*

Estradiol *Plasma* *No Effect* In 12 young women with idiopathic hirsutism mean concentration of 90 ± 10 pmol/L not different from normal range of 70 - 150 pmol/L *3546*

Follicle Stimulating Hormone *Plasma* *No Effect* In 12 young women with idiopathic hirsutism mean concentration of 4.7 ± 0.4 IU/L not different from normal range of 1.5 - 11.0 IU/L *3546*

Growth Hormone *Plasma* *No Effect* Mean concentration of 3.3 ± 4.1 ng/mL in 17 women with idiopathic hirsutism not significantly different from that in healthy control women *1388*

11β-Hydroxyandrostenedione *Plasma* *No Effect* Mean concentration in 57 women with idiopathic hirsutism and acne of 6.86 + 3.00 nmol/L not significantly different from that in 20 healthy premenopausal women in follicular phase 5.74 ± 2.61 nmol/L *1479*

17-Hydroxypregnenolone *Plasma* *No Effect* Mean concentration in 57 women with idiopathic hirsutism and acne of 7.47 + 3.51 nmol/L not significantly different from 20 healthy premenopausal women in follicular phase 5.16 ± 3.15 nmol/L *1479*

17-Hydroxyprogesterone *Plasma* *Increase* In 24 women with idiopathic hirsutism mean baseline concentration of 1.3 ± 0.7 ng/mL significantly different from 0.8 ± 0.3 ng/mL in 12 normal women *1389*
Plasma *No Effect* In 17 women with idiopathic hirsutism mean concentration of 1.2 ± 0.7 ng/mL not significantly different from 0.8 ± 0.3 ng/mL in 17 healthy control women *1388* In 12 young women with idiopathic hirsutism mean concentration of 2.2 ± 0.2 nmol/L not different from normal range of 1.0 - 3.0 nmol/L *3546* Mean concentration in 57 women with idiopathic hirsutism and acne of 2.26 + 1.81 nmol/L not significantly different from 20 healthy premenopausal women in follicular phase 1.40 ± 0.69 nmol/L *1479*

Insulin-like Growth Factor-I *Serum* *No Effect* Mean concentration of 197 ± 79 ng/mL in 17 women with idiopathic hirsutism not significantly different from that in healthy control women *1388*

Insulin-like Growth Factor Binding Protein-3
Serum *No Effect* Mean concentration in 15 women of 2.9 ± 0.7 µg/mL in 17 women with idiopathic hirsutism not significantly different from that in healthy control women *1388*

Luteinizing Hormone *Plasma* *No Effect* In 12 young women with idiopathic hirsutism mean concentration of 3.6 ± 0.6 IU/L not different from normal range of 1.0 - 25.0 IU/L *3546*

704.10 Idiopathic Hirsutism *(continued)*

Progesterone *Plasma* *No Effect* In 17 women with idiopathic hirsutism mean concentration of 0.8 ± 0.3 ng/mL not significantly different from 0.7 ± 0.2 ng/mL in 17 healthy control women *1388*

Prostate-specific Antigen *Serum* *Increase* In 15 women with idiopathic hirsutism median concentration of 4 pg/mL compared with 0 pg/mL in 11 healthy controls *1387*

Sex-Hormone Binding Globulin *Serum* *Decrease* In 17 women with idiopathic hirsutism mean concentration of 226 ± 89 µg/dL significantly different from 351 ± 138 µg/dL in 17 healthy control women *1388*

Testosterone *Serum* *Increase* In 24 women with idiopathic hirsutism mean concentration of 45 ± 14 ng/dL greater than 39 ± 14 ng/dL in 12 normal women *1389*
Serum *No Effect* In 17 women with idiopathic hirsutism mean concentration of 46 ± 15 ng/dL not significantly different from 40 ± 14 ng/dL in 17 healthy control women *1388* In 12 young women with idiopathic hirsutism mean concentration of 1.7 ± 0.1 nmol/L not different from normal range of < 3.0 nmol/L *3546* Mean concentration in 57 women with idiopathic hirsutism and acne of 1.28 + 0.40 nmol/L not significantly different from 20 healthy premenopausal women in follicular phase 1.00 ± 0.52 nmol/L *1479*

Testosterone, Free *Serum* *No Effect* In 12 young women with idiopathic hirsutism mean concentration of 8.2 ± 0.6 pmol/L not different from normal range of 2.4 - 12.5 pmol/L *3546*

706.10 Acne

Androgens *Plasma* *Increase* In a group of 34 women with this condition 80% had an androgen excess *4664* Elevated in 38% of 26 females with acne between ages of 27 and 42 y *4648*

Androstenedione *Plasma* *Increase* Elevated in 38% of 26 females with acne between ages of 27 and 42 y *4648*

Dehydroepiandrosterone Sulfate *Plasma* *Increase* Elevated in 38% of 26 females with acne between ages of 27 and 42 y *4648* Women with acne and hirsutism had increased levels compared to a group with acne only *2100* In about 100 prepubertal, premenarchal girls with comedonal acne mean concentration of about 2,200 nmol/L significantly different from about 1,800 nmol/L in 52 like girls without acne *3149*

Estradiol *Plasma* *No Effect* In about 100 prepubertal, premenarchal girls with comedonal acne mean concentration of about 30 pmol/L not significantly different from about 26 pmol/L in 52 like girls without acne *3149*

Ferritin *Serum* *Increase* 19 of 24 males had increased levels *4746*

Hematocrit *Blood* *Decrease* 25% of patients with severe nodulocystic disease had mild anemia *4746*

Hemoglobin *Blood* *Decrease* 25% of patients with severe nodulocystic disease had mild anemia *4746* Reported effect *3025*

Immunoglobulin G *Serum* *Increase* Significant increase observed in patients with very low grade or severe acne *2208*

Iron *Serum* *Decrease* Found in 75% of patients with severe nodulocystic disease *4746*

Iron-binding Capacity, Total *Serum* *No Effect* Normal concentration usually observed *3025* Normal levels in 29 patients with severe nodulocystic disease *4746*

Iron Saturation *Serum* *Decrease* 11 of 24 patients with severe nodulocystic disease had decreased levels *4746*

Progesterone *Plasma* *No Effect* In about 100 prepubertal, premenarchal girls with comedonal acne mean concentration of about 850 pmol/L not significantly different from about 650 pmol/L in 52 like girls without acne *3149*

Sex-Hormone Binding Globulin *Serum* *Decrease* In women with clinical manifestations of hyperandrogenism such as hirsutism and severe acne plasma concentration of SHBG may be reduced *1424*
Serum *No Effect* In about 100 prepubertal, premenarchal girls with comedonal acne mean concentration of about 44 nmol/L not significantly different from about 46 nmol/L in 52 like girls without acne *3149*

Testosterone *Serum* *Increase* Elevated in 38% of 26 females with acne between ages of 27 and 42 y *4648*
Serum *No Effect* In about 100 prepubertal, premenarchal girls with comedonal acne mean concentration of about 650 pmol/L not significantly different from about 700 pmol/L in 52 like girls without acne *3149* Free and total testosterone were measured in 34 men and 14 women suffering from acne but otherwise healthy *5077* No significant difference observed in either men or women with acne when compared against age matched controls *5077*

Testosterone, Free *Serum* *No Effect* In about 100 prepubertal, premenarchal girls with comedonal acne mean concentration of about 10 pmol/L not significantly different from about 11 pmol/L in 52 like girls without acne *3149* No significant difference observed in either men or women when matched against healthy age-matched controls without acne *5077*

708.80 Muckle-Wells Syndrome

Alanine Aminotransferase *Serum* *No Effect* In one patient with Muckle-Wells syndrome activity remained within normal limits *1704*

Alkaline Phosphatase *Serum* *No Effect* In one patient with Muckle-Wells syndrome activity remained within normal limits *1704*

Aspartate Aminotransferase *Serum* *No Effect* In one patient with Muckle-Wells syndrome activity remained within normal limits *1704*

Bilirubin *Serum* *No Effect* In one patient with Muckle-Wells syndrome concentration remained within normal limits *1704*

Cholesterol *Serum* *No Effect* In one patient with Muckle-Wells syndrome concentration remained within normal limits *1704*

Complement C_1q *Serum* *No Effect* In one patient with Muckle-Wells syndrome concentration remained within normal limits *1704*

Complement C_3 *Serum* *No Effect* In one patient with Muckle-Wells syndrome concentration remained within normal limits *1704*

Complement C_3dg *Serum* *No Effect* In one patient with Muckle-Wells syndrome concentration remained within normal limits *1704*

Complement C_4 *Serum* *No Effect* In one patient with Muckle-Wells syndrome concentration remained within normal limits *1704*

Complement CH50 *Serum* *Increase* In one patient with Muckle-Wells syndrome concentration increased to 464 E/mL *1704*

Corticotropin *Plasma* *Decrease* In one patient with Muckle-Wells syndrome increased concentration observed with nadir of < 1.0 ng/L associated with peak of cortisol of 700 nmol/L coincident with the climax of the urticaria *1704*

Cortisol *Plasma* *Increase* In one patient with Muckle-Wells syndrome increased concentration observed with peak of 700 nmol/L coincident with the climax of the urticaria *1704*

C-Reactive Protein *Serum* *Increase* In one patient with Muckle-Wells syndrome concentration increased to 58 mg/L *1704*

Creatinine *Serum* *No Effect* In one patient with Muckle-Wells syndrome concentration remained within normal limits *1704*

Creatinine Clearance *Urine* *No Effect* In one patient with Muckle-Wells syndrome clearance remained within normal limits (74 mL/min) *1704*

Erythrocyte Sedimentation Rate *Blood* *Increase* In one patient with Muckle-Wells syndrome rate increased to 45 mm/h *1704*

Ferritin *Serum* *Decrease* In one patient with Muckle-Wells syndrome low to normal concentration observed *1704*

Fibrinogen *Plasma* *Increase* In one patient with Muckle-Wells syndrome in the presence of urticaria increased concentration observed *1704*

α_2-Globulin *Serum* *Increase* In one patient with Muckle-Wells syndrome increased concentration observed *1704*

Hematocrit *Blood* *Decrease* In one patient with Muckle-Wells syndrome mild normo- to hypochromic anemia observed *1704*

Hemoglobin *Blood* *Decrease* In one patient with Muckle-Wells syndrome mild normo- to hypochromic anemia observed *1704*

Interleukin-6 *Serum* *Increase* In one patient with Muckle-Wells syndrome concentration increased to 91 pg/mL in the evening but not in samples taken in the morning or at noon *1704*

Iron *Serum* *Decrease* In one patient with Muckle-Wells syndrome low to normal concentration observed *1704*

Leukocytes *Blood* *Increase* In one patient with Muckle-Wells syndrome leukocytosis of up to 11.7 x 10^9/L with normal differential observed *1704*

Partial Thromboplastin Time *Plasma* *No Effect* In one patient with Muckle-Wells syndrome in the presence of urticaria normal time observed *1704*

Platelets *Blood* *Increase* In one patient with Muckle-Wells syndrome thrombocytosis of up to 453 x 10^9/L with normal differential observed *1704*

Potassium *Serum* *No Effect* In one patient with Muckle-Wells syndrome concentration remained within normal limits *1704*

Protein *Serum* *Increase* In one patient with Muckle-Wells syndrome increased concentration of 82.4 g/L observed *1704*

Reptilase® Time *Blood* *Increase* In one patient with Muckle-Wells syndrome in the presence of urticaria slightly prolonged time observed *1704*

Thrombin Time *Blood* *Decrease* In one patient with Muckle-Wells syndrome in the presence of urticaria shortened time observed *1704*

Thromboplastin Time *Plasma* *No Effect* In one patient with Muckle-Wells syndrome in the presence of urticaria normal time observed *1704*

Triglycerides *Serum* *No Effect* In one patient with Muckle-Wells syndrome concentration remained within normal limits *1704*

Urea Nitrogen *Serum* *No Effect* In one patient with Muckle-Wells syndrome concentration remained within normal limits *1704*

708.90 Urticaria

Calcium *Serum* *No Effect* In acute and chronic urticaria, mean serum values did not differ significantly from control groups. Only 7 cases had abnormal values. Abnormal calcium metabolism is not associated with urticaria and calcium treatment is not indicated *2458*

Complement C_3 *Serum* *No Effect* Patients with hereditary angioedema have decreased levels of C_1 esterase inhibitor and C_4 in the presence of normal amounts of C_3 and C_1q. Normal values for these complement components are found in persons with allergic angioedema *562*

Complement C_4 *Serum* *Decrease* Low C_4 or C_1 esterase confirms clinical diagnosis of hereditary angioedema *1555* Patients with hereditary angioedema have decreased levels of C_1 esterase inhibitor and C_4 in the presence of normal amounts of C_3 and C_1q. Normal values for these complement components are found in persons with allergic angioedema *562*

Complement, Total *Serum* *Decrease* Patients with hereditary angioedema have decreased levels of C_1 esterase inhibitor and C_4 in the presence of normal amounts of C_3 and C_1q. Normal values for these complement components are found in persons with allergic angioedema *562* 10 of 72 patients were found to have decreased total complement hemolytic activity *3352* Reported effect *1499*

Eosinophil Cationic Protein *Serum* *No Effect* In 13 patients with urticaria mean concentration of 10.0 ± 7.1 ng/mL not significantly different from 12.2 ± 9.8 ng/mL in 55 healthy controls *1607*

Eosinophils *Blood* *Increase* Characterized by a mild, persistent eosinophilia despite rather profound tissue involvement *5677* In 1 patient with non-parasitic giant urticaria and asthma mean concentration of > 440 x 10^6/L significantly different from upper limit of normal of 440 x 10^6/L in 29 normal individuals *607* In 13 patients with urticaria mean concentration of 200 ± 124 /µL not significantly different from 127 ± 92 µL in 55 healthy controls *1607* In 34% of 28 patients at initial hospitalization for this disorder *1576*

Histamine *Plasma* *Increase* In 1 patient with nonparasitic giant urticaria and asthma mean concentration of 48.2 nmol/L significantly different from mean concentration of 4.0 nmol/L in 29 normal individuals *607*
Urine *Increase* Increased excretion observed in patients with urticaria *2952*

Immunoglobulin E *Serum* *Increase* In 13 patients with urticaria mean concentration of 152 ± 126 U/mL significantly different from 75 ± 72 U/mL in 55 healthy controls *1607*

Interleukin-4 *Serum* *No Effect* IL-4 detected in 4 of 13 patients with atopic dermatitis with a mean concentration in those in whom it was detected of 1.02 ± 1.3 pg/mL not significantly different from 2.18 ± 2.86 pg/mL in the 20 of 45 healthy controls in whom it was detected *1607*

Monocytes *Blood* *Increase* In 50% of 28 patients at initial hospitalization for this disorder *1576*

Neutrophils *Blood* *Increase* In 28% of 28 patients at initial hospitalization for this disorder *1576*

Soluble CD14+ *Serum* *No Effect* In 13 patients with urticaria mean concentration of 2.98 ± 0.55 µg/mL not significantly different from 2.89 ± 0.85 µg/mL in 55 healthy controls *1607*

Soluble E-Selectin *Serum* *No Effect* In 13 patients with urticaria mean concentration of 36.3 ± 14.5 ng/mL not significantly different from 30.6 ± 10.6 ng/mL in 55 healthy controls *1607*

DISEASES OF THE MUSCULOSKELETAL SYSTEM AND CONNECTIVE TISSUE

710.00 Systemic Lupus Erythematosus

α_1-Acid Glycoprotein *Serum* *Increase* One of the most reliable indicators of acute inflammation *3713 4853 2597 4241 4696 4373*

Alanine Aminotransferase *Serum* *Increase* May be found in patients with myositis *900* In 16 patients with SLE in whom anti-PL 4 detected abnormal liver function tests observed in 4 (25%) *3295*

Albumin *Serum* *Decrease* Indicates the severity of excessive protein loss; tends to rise in the improving patient *1578* Low serum concentration (2.5 g/dL) were found in 8% of 39 patients *4662* Found in 50 - 66% of patients *1393*
Serum *No Effect* In 39 patients serum concentrations were stable throughout the course of SLE *4662* In patients with low grade activity and those in remission the serum concentrations remain within the normal range *724*
Urine *Increase* The most common abnormality ranging from mild to intermittent to nephrotic levels (> 3.56 g/d) *900*

Aldolase *Serum* *Increase* May be found in patients with myositis *900*

Alkaline Phosphatase *Serum* *Increase* In 16 patients with SLE in whom anti-PL 4 detected abnormal liver function tests observed in 4 (25%) *3295* In 39 adult patients with SLE mean activity of 110.7 ± 12.4 U/L significantly different from 57.4 ± 1.5 U/L in 122 healthy control adults *2006*

Alkaline Phosphatase Band-10 Isoenzyme *Serum* *Increase* In 39 adult patients with SLE mean activity of 12.62 ± 2.57 U/L significantly different from 10.0 ± 0.69 U/L in 122 healthy control adults *2006*

Amylase *Pleural Fluid* *Increase* Elevation in pleural fluid may occur *3482*

Amyloid A *Serum* *Increase* In patients with active systemic lupus erythematosus concentrations typically 2.4 times higher than reference interval determined by Behring Nephelometer II of < 0.17 - 10.1 mg/L *2961*

Angiotensin-converting Enzyme *Serum* *Increase* Observed effect *4488 3041*

Anti-β_2-Glycoprotein I Antibodies *Serum* *Increase* In 24 patients with SLE 100% had antibodies before an episode of thrombosis, 88% during thrombosis and 100% following thrombosis, compared with 17% of 102 SLE patients without thrombosis *1801*

Anti-DNA Antibodies *Serum* *Increase* Relation noted between flares of activity in SLE patients and high antibody concentration *5874* In 65 of 85 consecutive patients anti-DNA

710.00 Systemic Lupus Erythematosus *(continued)*

Anti-DNA Antibodies *(continued)*
antibodies observed *4237* In 13 patients with SLE 5 were positive for anti-DNA antibodies *3029*

Anti-ds DNA Antibodies *Serum Increase* Found in 49% of cases *4897* Positivity observed in 100% of 9 specimens in patients with SLE during relapses compared with 50% in 6 specimens from patients in remission *4380* Concentration significantly higher in patients with active disease than in those with inactive disease *601* Positive results with IgG antibodies to ds-DNA occur in about 60% patients with SLE *2952* ds-DNA antibodies detected in 97% of 33 Arabs with SLE *66* In 16 patients with SLE antibodies detected in 10 (63%) *3295* In 12 of 21 patients with active SLE serum ds-DNA activity greater than 36% *1937*

Anti-Endothelial Cell Antibodies *Serum Increase* IgG anti-endothelial antibodies (AEA), as measured by ELISA or immunoblotting technique could be detected in serum samples of 56 out of 64 patients with SLE (88%) *5400* AECAs of the IgA and IgG subtype were detected in lupus nephritis LN ($p < 0.001$) *5563* AECA have been detected *1174*

Anti-Entactin Antibodies *Serum Increase* In 79 patients IgM antientactin antibodies observed in 7, anti-entactin antibodies in 19 and both in 5 *4604*

Anti-Histone Antibodies *Serum Increase* Found in 100% of patients with drug induced SLE *126* Found in 50% of patients *5428* Found in 46% of cases *4897*

Anti-Ku Antibodies *Serum Increase* 9 of 9 patients with SLE had anti-Ku antibodies *921* 15 - 50% of patients with this disease *5788* In 16 patients with SLE antibodies detected in 1 (6%) *3295*

Anti-La Antibodies *Serum Increase* RNP antibodies detected in 7.5% of 33 Arabs with SLE *66* In 16 patients with SLE antibodies detected in 1 (6%) *3295*

Anti-Mitochondrial Antibodies *Serum Increase* Positive in 12% of patients and 6% of controls *4991* *4176* Found in 18% of patients and 2% of controls *4176* 8% of patients were positive *1290*
Serum No Effect Rarely observed *4551* Uniformly absent *5658*

Anti-Myeloperoxidase Antibodies *Serum Increase* In 13 patients with SLE 7 were positive for anti-myeloperoxidase antibodies *3029* Weakly positive results may occur in patients with SLE *2952*

Anti-Neutrophil Cytoplasm Antibodies *Serum Increase* In 1 of 2 patients (50%) with SLE pANCA detected *3722* ANCA observed in 40 of 157 sera (25%) from patients with SLE. Only pANCA not a cANCA pattern seen *4653*
Serum No Effect Antibodies not detected in any of 64 patients *162*

Anti-PL 4 *Serum Increase* In 16 patients with SLE antibody detected and associated with severe renal disease and haematological disease *3295*

Anti-Ribonuclear Protein Antibodies *Serum Increase* Increased concentration observed in 35 - 40% patients with SLE *2952* Found in 34% of cases *4897*

Anti-Ro Antibodies *Serum Increase* RNP antibodies detected in 18.5% of 33 Arabs with SLE *66* In 16 patients with SLE antibodies detected in 1 (6%) *3295*

Anti-Sjögren's Syndrome A Antibodies (SSA[Ro])
Serum Increase Found in 35% of cases *4897* Found in 100% of neonatal SLE cases *126*

Anti-Sjögren's Syndrome B Antibodies (SSB[La])
Serum Increase 15% of cases *3712* Increased concentration observed in patients with SLE *2952* Found in 5% of cases *4897*

Anti-Smith Antibodies *Serum Increase* Increased concentration observed in patients with SLE but lacks sensitivity *2952* Present in 30% of cases. Highly diagnostic *3712* In 16 patients with SLE antibodies detected in 2 (13%) *3295* Anti-Sm antibodies detected in 3 of 14 patients with renal disease and 6 of 13 patients without renal disease in 33 Arabs with SLE *66* Found in 23% of cases *4897*

Anti-ss DNA Antibodies *Serum Increase* Found in 42% of cases *4897*

Anti-U1RNP Antibodies *Serum Increase* In 16 patients with SLE antiphospholipid IgG antibodies detected in 2 (25%) *3295*

Antibodies to Human Leukocyte Interferon *Serum Increase* Antibodies to human leukocyte interferon occuring spontaneously without prior treatment observed in certain clinical conditions although their significance is unknown *4392*

Anticardiolipin Antibodies *Plasma Increase* Anticardiolipin antibodies observed in 184 of 390 outpatients with SLE (47%) *21*
Serum Increase None of the patients with syphilis or healthy controls was positive for any GPI-dependent aPL. By contrast, 40% were detected in patients with SLE *3360* In 22 of 83 consecutive patients anticardiolipin antibodies observed *4237* Increased concentrations of IgG aCL in 54 (51.4%), IgM aCL in 27 (25.7%) and both IgG aCL and IgM aCL in 21 (25.7%) observed in 105 patients *1719* RNP antibodies detected in 2.5% of 33 Arabs with SLE *66* Studied 75 outpatients with documented SLE who were attending their hospital clinics: 57 were aCL positive and 18 were aCL negative *2891* In 30 children with SLE 26 (87%) initially positive for either IgG or IgM anticardiolipin antibodies (24 had IgG ACLs and 15 had IgM ACLs) *4290* In 16 of 50 patients with SLE anticardiolipin antibody detected *3359*

Anticardiolipin-specific IgG Antibodies *Serum Increase* 24 patients with SLE 13% had antibodies before an episode of thrombosis, 38% during thrombosis and 33% following thrombosis *1801*

Anticardiolipin-specific IgM Antibodies *Serum Increase* In 24 patients with SLE 13% had antibodies before an episode of thrombosis, 29% during thrombosis and 33% following thrombosis *1801*

α_1-Antichymotrypsin *Serum Increase* Collagen vascular diseases *2628* Reported effect *2457*

Antinuclear Antibodies *Pleural Fluid Increase* Indicates SLE *1980* ANA antibodies observed in 6 of 8 pleural fluid specimens *2665*
Serum Increase Titers were higher in patients with nephritis than in a control group of SLE patients without nephritis but were no higher than in scleroderma *4011* Appearance of antibody to DNA frequently (40% of the time) heralds an approaching clinical flare within several months *1578* Found in 100% of cases *4897* Increased concentration observed in almost all patients with SLE *2952* Nearly all patients with active SLE are positive. Titers vary according to the intensity of disease activity *2039* 9 of 9 patients with SLE had anti-nuclear antibodies *921* Present in 97.7% of patients (44 of 45) tested using immunofluorescent technique *646* In 2 of 2 patients (100%) with SLE ANA detected *3722* In 89 of 90 consecutive patients antinuclear antibodies observed *4237* 95 - 100% positivity *4068* Present in high titer but only low titers were found in other rheumatoid diseases *3834* Observed effect *1444*
Serum No Effect Of 165 patients with SLE a subgroup of 8 patients with active SLE yet with persistently negative tests for antinuclear factor and LE cells was identified *1747* 10 patients with clinical signs of disease had persistently negative ANA tests. Raynaud's phenomenon, excessive hair fall and oral ulcers were frequent in this subgroup *1472*
Synovial Fluid Increase Increased frequency observed *1980*

Antinuclear Antibodies, (HEp-2 cells) *Serum Increase* In 16 patients with SLE antibody detected in all (100%) *3295*

Antinuclear Factor *Serum Increase* Antinuclear factor detected in 89.5% of 33 Arabs with SLE *66* In 13 patients with SLE all were positive for ANCA *3029*

Antioxidative Enzyme Activity *Serum Increase* In 10 children with SLE mean activity of 34.36 ± 17.54 µmol H_2O_2/mL/min higher than 11.06 ± 0.23 µmol H_2O_2/mL/min in 20 healthy control children *3268*

Antiphosphatidic Acid Antibodies *Serum Increase* In 13 of 50 patients with SLE antiphosphatidyl antibody detected *3359* In 7 of 50 patients with SLE antiphosphatidic acid antibody detected *3359* None of the patients with syphilis or healthy controls was positive for any GPI-dependent aPL. By contrast, 12% were detected in patients with SLE *3360*

Antiphosphatidylethanolamine Antibodies *Serum Increase* None of the patients with syphilis or healthy controls was positive for any GPI-dependent aPL. By contrast, 8% were detected in patients with SLE *3360*

Antiphosphatidylinositol Antibodies *Serum Increase* In 6 of 50 patients with SLE antiphosphatidyl inositol antibody detected *3359* None of the patients with syphilis or healthy controls was positive for any GPI-dependent aPL. By contrast, 18% were detected in patients with SLE *3360*

Antiphosphatidylserine Antibodies *Serum* *Increase* None of the patients with syphilis or healthy controls was positive for any GPI-dependent aPL. By contrast, 20% were detected in patients with SLE *3360*

Antiphospholipid Antibodies *Serum* *Increase* In 16 patients with SLE antiphospholipid IgG antibodies detected in 3 (19%) *3295* Increased concentrations of antiphospholipid antibodies observed in 60 of 105 patients (57.1%) *1719* IgG anticardiolipin antibodies (IgG ACL) were looked for using an ELISA technique in 92 consecutive SLE patients seen over a one-year period. Twenty-four SLE patients presented with neurological manifestations (40 episodes): 15/24 (62.5%) were found positive for APL antibodies versus 22/68 patients (32%) without neurological symptoms ($p < 0.01$). APL antibodies antedated neurological symptoms in 13/16 cases *1797*

α_1-Antitrypsin *Serum* *Increase* Increased *4763* *5544* *83* *4241* *4373* *4371*

Aspartate Aminotransferase *Serum* *Increase* May be found in patients with myositis *900* In 16 patients with SLE in whom anti-PL 4 detected abnormal liver function tests observed in 4 (25%) *3295*

bcl-2 Protein *Lymphocytes* *Increase* In SLE patients a significant proportion of T cell lymphocytes expressed increased amounts of bcl-2 protein *176*

Bilirubin *Serum* *Increase* In 16 patients with SLE in whom anti-PL 4 detected abnormal liver function tests observed in 4 (25%) *3295*

Biological False-positive Serologic Test for Syphilis *Serum* *Increase* Detected in 7.0% of 256 patients with SLE *5314*

Biopterin *Serum* *No Effect* In 23 patients with SLE mean concentration of 9.71 ± 3.47 nmol/L not significantly less than 11.32 ± 3.00 nmol/L in 21 healthy controls *1956*

C_4b-Binding Protein *Serum* *No Effect* No significant difference observed between patients with SLE and lupus anticoagulant who were antiphospholipid negative (202.8 ± 30.7 µg/mL), LA-positive (198.2 ± 52.8 µg/mL), aPL-positive (182.5 ± 50.8 µg/mL), and LA/aPL-positive (185.5 ± 32.5 µg/mL) and healthy controls (200.4 ± 27.3 µg/mL) *3359*

CA 125 *Serum* *Increase* Among patients with active disease, values higher than the generally accepted upper limit of 35 U/mL were found in 10 of 28 cases *3573*

Carbon Dioxide Partial Pressure *Blood* *Decrease* Impaired gas diffusion and the accompanying hyperventilation results in a low pCO_2, unless the defect is severe and CO_2 retention occurs *4707*

Cholesterol *Serum* *Increase* Leading to nephrosis *5544*

Chylomicrons *Synovial Fluid* *Increase* Chylous effusions have been reported *3770* *4487*

Clotting Time *Blood* *Increase* Circulating anticoagulants are not rare but do not usually cause bleeding *1980*

Cold Agglutinins *Serum* *Increase* Have been detected *1980*

Complement C_1 *Serum* *Decrease* Mean concentration typically slightly reduced in patients with active SLE *4682*

Complement C_1q *Serum* *Decrease* Observed effect *4683* Mean concentration typically slightly reduced in patients with active SLE *4682*

Complement C_1r *Serum* *Decrease* Observed effect *4683*

Complement C_1s *Serum* *Decrease* Observed effect *4683*

Complement C_2 *Serum* *Decrease* Mean concentration typically slightly reduced or normal in patients with active SLE *4682* Found in 50% of patients *4683*

Complement C_3 *Pericardial Fluid* *Decrease* Low or absent *1550* *1789*
Pleural Fluid *Decrease* Observed effect *126*
Serum *Decrease* In 16 patients with SLE in whom anti-PL 4 detected low concentration observed in 13 (81%) *3295* Reduced levels arise from increased catabolism and reduced synthesis which always occurs at some stage of active SLE *4890* 21 children had 52 episodes of C_3 depression (mean duration 25 weeks); only 11 had active nephritis when concentrations were depressed *4869* In patients with active SLE concentration significantly lower than in those with inactive disease *601* Concentration of 63 ± 8 mg/dL in patients with subendothelial deposits, compared to 142 ± 27 mg/dL in controls *389* In 10 of 21 patients with active SLE serum C_3 concentration less than 80 mg/dL *1937* Relation noted between flares of activity in SLE patients and low concentration *5874* Reduced levels arise from increased catabolism and reduced synthesis which always occurs at some stage of active SLE *3416* Especially low in patients with active nephritis. C_5 is usually normal *4683* Reduced concentration observed in 55% of 9 specimens in patients with SLE during relapses with abnormal excretion of sIL-2R compared with 17.6% in those with normal sIL-2R excretion *4380* Caused by hypercatabolism *785* Mean concentration typically slightly reduced in patients with active SLE *4682* Caused by hypercatabolism *2694* *1033* Low concentration is consistent with active SLE whereas undetectable amounts suggest congenital C_3 deficiency *2952*
Serum *Increase* C_3 hypocomplementemia observed in 12 of 31 (38.5%) Arabs with SLE, 10 of 16 with renal disease and 2 of 15 without renal disease *66* Early in active disease the acute inflammatory response may cause increased C_3 and C_4 production *3416*
Synovial Fluid *Decrease* Complement levels are very low *900*

Complement C_3d *Serum* *Increase* Concentration significantly higher in patients with active disease than in those with inactive disease *601*

Complement C_4 *Cerebrospinal Fluid* *Decrease* Abnormally low C_4 levels *144* Low CSF levels of C_4 occur in patients with CNS involvement, due to in vivo immune reaction *4683*
Pericardial Fluid *Decrease* Low or absent *1550* *1789*
Pleural Fluid *Decrease* Observed effect *126*
Serum *Decrease* In 9 of 18 patients with active SLE serum C_4 concentration less than 18.5 mg/dL *1937* Mean concentration typically slightly decreased in patients with active SLE *4682* Relation noted between flares of activity in SLE patients and low concentration *5874* Reduced levels arise from increased catabolism synthesis which always occurs at some stage of active disease *3416* Concentration significantly lower in patients with active SLE than in those with inactive disease *601* Reduced levels arise from increased catabolism synthesis which always occurs at some stage of active disease *4890* Especially low in patients with active nephritis. C_5 is usually normal *4683* Serum C_4 levels was 8 ± 2 mg/dL in patients with subendothelial deposits, compared to 27 ± 6 mg/dL in patients with deposits *389* C_4 occasionally remained depressed longer than C_3, perhaps reflecting continuing subclinical disease activity *4869* In 16 patients with SLE in whom anti-PL 4 detected low concentration observed in 13 (81%) *3295*
Serum *Increase* Early in active disease the acute inflammatory response may cause increased C_3 and C_4 production *3416*
Synovial Fluid *Decrease* Complement levels are very low *900*
Urine *Increase* In 19 patients with SLE mean excretion of 124 ± 178 µg/d significantly different from 8.3 ± 4.0 µg/d in 4 normal individuals *5344*

Complement C_5 *Serum* *Decrease* Mean concentration typically slightly reduced or normal in patients with active SLE *4682*

Complement CH50 *Serum* *Decrease* In 16 patients with SLE in whom anti-PL 4 detected low concentration observed in 13 (81%) *3295* Mean concentration typically slightly reduced in patients with active SLE *4682*

Complement, Total *Pericardial Fluid* *Decrease* Low or absent *1550* *1789*
Pleural Fluid *Decrease* Low complement (< 10 U/mL) in 11 of 12 patients with SLE or rheumatoid pleuritis *3052* 5 of 7 cases showed reduced levels of CH50, C_1, C_1 inhibitor and C_2 in pleural fluid *1759*
Serum *Decrease* Reduced levels arise from increased catabolism and reduced synthesis which always occurs at some stage of active SLE *4890* Low C_1 (C_1q and C_1s), C_2, C_3, and C_4 occur in active SLE. Especially low in patients with active nephritis. C_5 is usually normal *4683* Found in 80 (57%) patients *1444* Reduced in about 75% of patients with active disease. Reduction may be correlated with the activity of the illness and varies inversely with ANA titers *4684* Reduced levels arise from increased catabolism and reduced synthesis which always occurs at some stage of active SLE *3416* In 35 patients, 77% had decreased values. In discoid lupus, 57% had elevated levels *4925*
Serum *Increase* Normal or elevated *367* Early in active SLE the acute inflammatory response may cause increased C_3 and

710.00 Systemic Lupus Erythematosus *(continued)*

Complement, Total *(continued)*
C_4 production *3416* In discoid lupus, 57% had elevated levels *4925*
Synovial Fluid Decrease Compared to total protein, levels are low in 60 - 70% of joint effusions *631* May be markedly reduced below the complement level of serum *144* Low levels may occur in some patients *4683* Marked decrease in synovial fluids *4063*

Coombs' Test *Serum Positive* Coomb's test positive in 7 of 29 (24%) Arabs with SLE *66* A positive test is frequently associated with active hemolysis but may be seen in individuals without markedly shortened RBC survival *2039* About 5% of patients may develop hemolytic anemia. Direct Coombs' test is almost always positive in these cases *1980* Positive in 18 - 65% of patients in different studies, but only 10% of these manifest significant hemolysis *624*

Coombs' Test, Direct *Serum Positive* Positive test significantly associated with the presence of anticardiolipin antibodies observed in 147 of 390 outpatients (47%) *21* In 22 of 88 consecutive patients positive direct Coombs' test observed *4237*

Coombs' Test, Indirect *Serum Positive* Positive test significantly associated with the presence of anticardiolipin antibodies observed in 147 of 390 outpatients (47%) *21*

Copper *Serum Increase* Increase in collagen diseases *5544* Increased *4586* Increase in collagen diseases *1290* Increased *3900*

C-Reactive Protein *Serum Increase* In patients with active systemic lupus erythematosus concentrations typically 5.8 times higher than reference interval determined by Behring Nephelometer II of < 0.17 - 10.1 mg/L *2961* C-reactive proteins and other acute phase reactants are elevated and remain elevated to some degree during periods of apparent remission *2039* In 20 patients with SLE median concentration of 5.4 mg/L significantly different from upper limit of normal of 2.6 mg/L *1612*
Serum No Effect Mean concentration of 8 mg/L in 8 patients with active SLE not significantly greater than in healthy controls *208* In 20 patients with SLE median concentration of 5.4 mg/L not significantly greater than median of 3 mg/L in 20 healthy blood donors *1614*

Creatine *Serum Increase* Correlates well with severity of morphologic lesions *2159*
Urine Increase Increased breakdown *5544*

Creatine Kinase *Serum Increase* May be found in patients with myositis *900*

Creatinine *Serum Increase* Most reliable variable for estimation of renal involvement *1578* Serum creatinine and BUN were increased, indicating uremia *2685*
Serum No Effect In 37 patients with systemic lupus erythematosus mean concentration of 81.3 ± 19.4 µmol/L not significantly different from 77.8 ± 13.3 µmol/L in 57 heathy volunteers *4399*

Creatinine Clearance *Urine Decrease* Mean decrease in clearance of 18% was accompanied by a 14% inulin clearance fall, and correlated with the prostaglandin E levels *2685*

Cryoglobulins *Serum Increase* Increased cryoglobulins were found in patients with severe lesions and in no instance did it occur simultaneously with rheumatoid factor which was found in milder lesions *2159* Variable elevations of cryoglobulins *4707* Found in 7 - 90% of patients in various studies; associated with disease activity especially nephritis *837*

Dehydroepiandrosterone Sulfate *Plasma Decrease* Mean concentration in 11 male patients of 1.29 ± 0.32 µg/mL compared with 3.04 ± 0.33 µg/mL in 13 male controls and 0.75 ± 0.12 µg/mL in 24 female patients compared with 2.16 ± 0.18 µg/mL in 28 female controls *5042*

Elastase Antineutrophil Cytoplasmic Autoantibodies
Serum No Effect Antibodies not detected in any of 64 patients *162*

Endothelial Cell Protein C Receptor *Plasma Increase* In 16 patients with SLE mean concentration of 272.9 ± 167.7 ng/mL significantly different from 133.4 ± 53.4 ng/mL in 18 controls *2862*

Endothelin *Plasma Increase* In 15 SLE patients without Raynaud's phenomenon mean concentration of 6.6 ± 1.7 pg/mL and in 15 with Raynaud's phenomenon 7.4 ± 2.2 pg/mL significantly higher than 3.9 ± 2.5 pg/mL in 10 normal controls *3361*

Endothelin-1 *Plasma Increase* In one study of 23 patients mean concentration increased to 12.4 ± 3.8 pg/mL (4.3-fold increase) *328* In 2 studies mean increases of 4.3-fold observed, with 60% attributable to primary and 40% attributable to secondary symptoms *328*
Plasma No Effect In one study of 7 patients mean concentration of 1.2 ± 0.2 pg/mL (0.9-fold normal value) *328*

Erythrocyte Casts *Urine Increase* In lupus glomerulonephritis it is not unusual to find a sediment in which all the formed elements and casts seen in various stages *1980* Red cells or casts observed in 44.4% of 9 specimens in patients with SLE during relapses compared with 0% in 6 specimens from patients in remission *4380*

Erythrocyte Sedimentation Rate *Blood Increase* In 16 patients with SLE in whom anti-PL 4 detected raised ESR observed in 16 (100%) *3295* Mean rate of 33 mm/h in 9 patients with active disease significantly greater than in healthy controls *208* Frequently and markedly elevated, even in the presence of apparently mild disease activity due to the presence of abnormal globulins *1980* Significantly higher in patients with active disease than in those with inactive disease *601* In 12 of 17 patients with active SLE mean rate greater than 30 mm/h and corrected ESR over 30 mm/h in 8 of 17 *1937*
Blood No Effect No relationship noted between flares of activity in SLE patients and ESR *5874*

Erythrocytes *Urine Increase* Red cells or casts observed in 44.4% of 9 specimens in patients with SLE during relapses compared with 0% in 6 specimens from patients in remission *4380* Proteinuria and other urine abnormalities including RBCs > 5 /hpf observed in 54% of Arabs with SLE *66* Levels of hematuria and proteinuria correlate well with severity of morphologic lesions *2159*

Factor B *Plasma Decrease* Found in 50% of patients *4431* *5229*

Fibrin Degradation Products *Plasma Increase* Elevated levels (> 10 µgl/mL) occurred in 100% of lupus nephritis patients. Mean value was 21.4 ± 7.6 µg/mL *2863*

Fibrinogen *Plasma Increase* Frequently elevated *1980*
Plasma No Effect Mean concentration of 2.8 g/L in 8 patients with active SLE not significantly greater than in healthy controls *208*

Fibronectin *Plasma No Effect* Mean fasting concentration in 15 patients with SLE of 36.1 ± 10.2 mg/dL not significantly different from that in 28 normal men, 32.5 ± 7.1 mg/dL, and 31.6 ± 5.7 mg/dL in 34 normal women *4811*

Fructosamine *Serum Increase* In 37 patients with SLE mean concentration of 278 ± 47 µmol/L different from 258 ± 23 µmol/L in 57 heathy volunteers *4399*

β-Galactosidase *Serum Decrease* Mean serum concentration was 0.139 ± 0.019 mmol/min/L, compared with 0.243 ± 0.038 in controls *2288*

Gelatinase *Serum Increase* In 17 patients with SLE mean concentration of 685.9 ± 97.7 ng/mL significantly higher than 408.9 ± 28.0 ng/mL in 53 healthy controls *5878*

α_1-Globulin *Serum Increase* Moderate increase *1290*

α_2-Globulin *Serum Increase* Marked increase *1290* A less specific but frequent abnormality *900* May be elevated in lupus nephritis *1980*

γ-Globulin *Serum Increase* Increase in about 70% of patients *1393* Serum globulin concentrations in excess of 4.0 g/dL are seen in over 50% of cases *2039* A less specific but frequent abnormality *900* Marked increase occur in patient with proteinuria *4308*

Glucose *Pleural Fluid No Effect* Concentration same as in plasma *1980*
Serum No Effect In 37 patients with systemic lupus erythematosus mean concentration of 4.8 ± 0.7 mmol/L not significantly different from 5.2 ± 0.5 mmol/L in 57 heathy volunteers *4399*
Synovial Fluid Decrease Less than 25 mg/dL, lower than blood *1367*

Glycated Protein *Serum Increase* Have been found to be elevated but are nonspecific *1980*

β_2-Glycoprotein IgG Antibodies *Serum* *Increase* Antibodies detected in 10.1% of 308 patients with SLE *5314*

β_2-Glycoprotein IgM Antibodies *Serum* *Increase* Antibodies detected in 5.8% of 308 patients with SLE *5314*

Granular Casts *Urine* *Increase* In lupus glomerulonephritis it is not unusual to find a sediment in which all the formed elements and casts seen in various stages *1980*

Haptoglobin *Serum* *Decrease* Decreased if associated with hemolytic anemia *5544*

HDL-Cholesterol *Serum* *No Effect* Total lipid concentration was found to be low but HDL fraction was normal *3129*

Hematocrit *Blood* *Decrease* In 14 of 21 patients with active SLE mean value of less than 40% *1937* Reflects disease activity in patients both with and without renal disease *1578* Hemolytic anemia observed in 21% of Arabs with SLE *66* Less than 30% in 53% of patients *1445* The most common hematologic abnormality occurring in 57 - 78% of patients. May be caused by hypersplenism, iron deficiency, renal disease, drugs, antierythrocyte antibody and complement *624* Significant anemia, usually normocytic, normochromic, found in 58% (81) of cases *1444*
Blood *No Effect* No relationship noted between flares of activity in SLE patients and hematocrit *5874*

Hemoglobin *Blood* *Decrease* Hemolytic anemia observed in 21% of Arabs with SLE *66* Anemia, usually normocytic, is present in the majority of cases and is frankly hemolytic with a positive Coombs' test in < 10% of the cases *900* In 14 of 21 patients with active SLE mean concentration less than 13 g/dL *1937* Significant anemia, usually normocytic, normochromic, found in 58% (81) of cases *1444* The most common hematologic abnormality occurring in 57 - 78% of patients. May be caused by hypersplenism, iron deficiency, renal disease, drugs, antierythrocyte antibody and complement *624* In 16 patients with SLE in whom anti-PL 4 detected anemia with hemoglobin of less than 11 g/dL observed in 9 (56%) *3295*

Hexosamine *Serum* *Increase* Hexosamine and other acute-phase reactants are elevated and remain so to some degree during period of apparent remission *2039* Have been found to be elevated but are nonspecific *1980*

HLA Antigens *Blood* *Present* HLA-A17, HLA-B_8, HLA-DR2 and HLA-DR3 associated with this disease *4879* HLA-DR3 present in 70% of patients versus 28% of controls *5678* HLA-DR2 and HLA-DR3 frequently associated with whites with this disease *5428*

IgG Antiendothelial Antibodies *Serum* *Increase* Antibodies detected in 38 of 41 patients with SLE *5399*

Immune Complexes *Serum* *Increase* Mean concentration of 190 µg/mL in 4 patients with active disease not significantly greater than in healthy controls *208*

Immunoglobulin A *Cerebrospinal Fluid* *Increase* Elevation of IgG index was noted in 70% of patients, IgA index in 77% and IgM index in 100% of 13 patients when compared with 20 controls with other neurological disorders *4289*
Serum *Increase* Level decreased progressively after the first trimester *1055* Slightly elevated except in the presence of protein-losing nephropathy *1980* Mean concentrations were within the normal range at diagnosis (271 ± 171 mg/dL) but increased significantly to 349 ± 210 mg/dL during follow-up ($p < 0.05$) in 39 patients *4662*

Immunoglobulin D *Serum* *Increase* Reported effect *1290*

Immunoglobulin G *Cerebrospinal Fluid* *Increase* In 8 patients with neuropsychiatric SLE mean concentration of 8.84 ± 1.80 mg/dL significantly higher than 2.11 ± 1.03 mg/dL in 20 patients with CNS non-inflammation controls *5295* Elevation of IgG index was noted in 70% of patients, IgA index in 77% and IgM index in 100% of 13 patients when compared with 20 controls with other neurological disorders *4289*
Serum *Increase* Slightly elevated except in the presence of protein-losing nephropathy *1980* The IgG dynamics differed from those of IgA and IgM by high mean IgG concentrations at diagnosis (1,492 ± 835 mg/dL) and a significant decrease to 1,195 ± 748 mg/dL during follow-up. The pattern was characterized by an inverse relation of IgA and IgG; while IgA concentrations increased significantly during follow-up, a parallel decrease in IgG occurred *4662* Marked increase in untreated patients of 18.7 ± 5.1 g/L, with only a moderate correlation with disease activity *2159*

Immunoglobulin M *Cerebrospinal Fluid* *Increase* Elevation of IgG index was noted in 70% of patients, IgA index in 77% and IgM index in 100% of 13 patients when compared with 20 controls with other neurological disorders *4289*
Serum *Increase* Slightly elevated except in the presence of protein-losing nephropathy *1980* Increased from a mean value of 88 ± 52 mg/dL at diagnosis to 113 ± 181 mg/dL during follow-up *4662* Reported effect *724*

Immunoglobulins *Serum* *Increase* In 16 patients with SLE in whom anti-PL 4 detected increased concentration observed in 11 (67%) *3295*

Intercellular Adhesion Molecule-1 *Serum* *No Effect* In 30 patients with active disease mean concentration of 267 ng/mL and 319 ng/mL in 20 patients with inactive disease not significantly different from 245 ng/mL in 10 healthy controls *3638*

Interferon-α *Cerebrospinal Fluid* *No Effect* In 8 patients with neuropsychiatric SLE INF-α not detectable *5295*

Interleukin-1 Receptor Antagonist *Serum* *Increase* Median concentration in 20 patients with SLE of 0.63 ng/mL not significantly higher than 0.27 ng/mL in 20 healthy controls *1612* Mean concentration in 35 patients with SLE of 592.5 ± 114.5 pg/mL significantly different from 243.4 ± 12.9 pg/mL in 41 healthy controls *5042*

Interleukin-1β *Cerebrospinal Fluid* *No Effect* In 8 patients with neuropsychiatric SLE IL-1β not detectable *5295*
Serum *No Effect* In 52 patients with SLE median concentration undetectable not different from normal *1612*

Interleukin-2 *Serum* *Increase* Mean concentration in 35 patients with SLE of 27.6 ± 4.2 pg/mL significantly different from 4.2 ± 0.9 pg/mL in 41 healthy controls *5042*

Interleukin-3 *Serum* *Increase* The serum level of IL-3 determined by ELISA was found to be higher in a cohort of 16 patients with SLE in comparison to healthy controls *1496*

Interleukin-6 *Cerebrospinal Fluid* *Increase* Paired serum and cerebrospinal fluid (CSF) specimens from 14 patients with systemic lupus erythematosus (SLE) and central nervous system (CNS) involvement were studied for interleukin-6 (IL-6). 23 patients with noninflammatory neurologic diseases, and 9 SLE patients without CNS involvement were also studied. CSF IL-6 activity was elevated only in SLE patients with CNS involvement *2173* In all 8 patients with neuropsychiatric SLE concentration increased to mean of 71.40 ± 5.89 pg/mL whereas it was only detected in 2 of 20 controls *5295*
Serum *Increase* Mean concentration in 35 patients with SLE of 7.1 ± 1.2 pg/mL significantly different from undetectable amount in 41 healthy controls *5042* Increased concentrations characteristic of active disease but normal in inactive disease *3999* In 52 patients with SLE median concentration of 293 pg/mL significantly different from upper limit of normal *1612* Increased IL-6 is characteristic of SLE and higher in active SLE than in inactive SLE but concentration in inactive SLE higher than in controls *3074* Sixteen consecutive patients who developed an exacerbation were analysed in this study. Blood samples were drawn in EDTA monthly. At the time of maximal disease activity during exacerbation, IL-6 plasma concentrations were increased (greater than or equal to 6 pg/mL) in 12 out of the 16 cases *4964* Measured urinary levels of interleukin 6 (IL-6) in 29 patients with active lupus nephritis, detected IL-6 activity in the urine of 24 (83%) of 29 patients before the initiation of therapy. The median value of urinary IL-6 levels in patients with a histologic diagnosis of WHO class IV on renal biopsy was significantly higher than that in patients with other classes ($p < 0.01$) *5099* Mean concentration of 56.9 ± 14.8 pg/mL in 20 patients with SLE significantly different from 11.4 ± 1.9 pg/mL in healthy blood donors *1130*
Serum *No Effect* Paired serum and cerebrospinal fluid (CSF) specimens from 14 patients with systemic lupus erythematosus (SLE) and central nervous system (CNS) involvement were studied for interleukin-6 (IL-6). 23 patients with noninflammatory neurologic diseases, and 9 SLE patients without CNS involvement were also studied. There was no significant difference in serum IL-6 activity among the 3 groups *2173*
Urine *No Effect* Interleukin-6 was found in the urine of only one out of an additional seven patients with lupus nephritis *2235*

Inulin Clearance *Urine* *Decrease* A mean decrease of 14% was observed in 7 female patients *2685*

Lactate Dehydrogenase *Serum* *Increase* Significantly higher in patients with diffuse proliferative lupus nephritis *2338*
Urine *Increase* With nephritis *5544*

710.00 Systemic Lupus Erythematosus *(continued)*

Lactate Dehydrogenase Isoenzymes *Serum Increase* Significantly higher in patients with diffuse proliferative lupus nephritis. Serum levels of total LD, LD_1 and LD_2 *2338* LD_3 and LD_4 *5544*

LE Cells *Blood Positive* Of 165 patients, 8 patients with active disease yet with persistently negative tests for ANA and LE cells were identified *1747* Most patients will develop positive tests during their illnesses but SLE is not excluded without a positive test *2039* Lupus cells detected in 10 of 31 (32%) Arabs with SLE *66* The LE test was concluded to be insensitive, nonspecific, and did not correspond to clinical activity of the patient *1679* Found in 76% (107) of 140 patients *1444* 28 of 45 (63.5%) patients had positive results *646*
Synovial Fluid Positive May be present in synovial fluid *5545*

Leukocytes *Blood Decrease* Leukopenia (< 4,000 /µL) is common, and frequently is important in implicating SLE rather than infection or other inflammatory diseases which may cause similar clinical manifestations *900* Mild leukopenia in 68 patients (49%) with counts between 2,000 - 4,000 /µL *1444* Reduction in total count in almost 50% of all patients *624* A moderate leukopenia (1,800 - 4,000 /µL) is seen in 70% of patients at some point in their courses and is often associated with a lymphopenia *2039* Leukopenia observed in 30% of Arabs with SLE *66* In 4 of 21 patients with active SLE mean concentration less than 4,000 /µL *1937*
Synovial Fluid Increase 5,000 /µL *1980* Usually low (< 5,000 /µL) with a low percentage of neutrophils *900* Usually does not not exceed 3,000 /µL *144*
Urine Increase Leukocytes > 10 /hpf observed in 33.3% of 9 specimens in patients with SLE during relapses compared with 0% in 6 specimens from patients in remission *4380*

Lipids *Serum Decrease* Total lipid concentration was found to be low but HDL fraction was normal *3129*

Lipoprotein Lp(a) *Serum Increase* In 34 patients with SLE mean concentration of 42 ± 35 mg/dL higher than 26 ± 25 mg/dL in 66 healthy controls *529*

Lupus Anticoagulant *Plasma Increase* Detected in 8.2% of 184 patients with SLE *5314* An analysis of 29 published series (comprising over 1,000 patients with SLE) yielded an average frequency of 34% for the lupus anticoagulant and 44% for anticardiolipin *3139* Increased concentrations of lupus anticoagulant observed in 9 of 105 patients (8.6%) all of whom were associated with anticardiolipin antibodies *1719* In 15 of 50 patients with SLE lupus anticoagulant detected *3359*

Lymphoblasts *Urine Increase* Lymphoblasts/plasma cells observed in 77.8% of 9 specimens in patients with SLE during relapses compared with 0% in 6 specimens from patients in remission *4380*

Lymphocyte T-Cells *Blood Decrease* Normal *1588*

Lymphocytes *Blood Decrease* In 16 patients with SLE in whom anti-PL 4 detected lymphopenia observed in all *3295* Overall depression of peripheral blood leukocytes frequently with a lymphopenia and a slight shift to the left in the granulocytic series *900* In 10 of 21 patients with active SLE mean concentration less than 1,100 /µL *1937* In 158 patients with active, untreated disease, lymphopenia was present in 75%, and another 18% of those patients developed lymphopenia subsequent to disease reactivation. Lymphopenia of < 1,500 occurred more frequently than any of the preliminary criteria and it was the most prevalent initial laboratory abnormality *4374*

Mannose-binding Protein *Serum Increase* In patients with active systemic lupus erythematosus concentrations typically 2.1 times higher than reference interval determined by Behring Nephelometer II of < 0.17 - 10.1 mg/L *2961*

Melanoma Inhibitory Factor *Serum No Effect* In 39 patients mean concentration of 4.4 ± 2.3 ng/mL showed no significant difference from 3.6 ± 2.8 ng/mL in 120 healthy controls *3655*

α_1-Microglobulin *Cerebrospinal Fluid No Effect* Of 4 patients with SLE mean concentration in none greater than that in 15 healthy controls of 34.8 ± 16.0 µg/L *2370*

Monocyte Chemotactic Protein-1 *Serum Increase* Mean concentrations of 353, 528 and 195 pg/mL in one patients with each of types III, IV and V SLE compared with 101 ± 24 pg/mL in 16 healthy women and men *4460*
Urine Increase In 3 patients with SLE mean concentrations of 376, 6,400 and 120 pg/mg creatinine for one patient in each of types III, IV and V significantly different when compared with mean concentration of 130 ± 30 pg/mg creatinine in 30 healthy women and 32 healthy men *4460*

Monocytes *Blood Increase* Was reported *3246*
Urine Increase 29 - 33% mononuclear cells were found in lupus nephritis and endemic benign nephropathy *3071* Monocytes observed in 66.7% of 9 specimens in patients with SLE during relapses compared with 0% in 6 specimens from patients in remission *4380*

Mucopolysaccharides *Urine Increase* Have been found to be elevated but are nonspecific *1980*

Mucoprotein *Serum Increase* Mucoproteins and other acute-phase reactants are elevated and persist to some degree during periods of apparent remission *2039*

Multiubiquitin Chains *Serum No Effect* In 38 patients with SLE mean concentration of 3.88 ± 1.32 µg/cells in 1 L blood not significantly different from that in 45 healthy men and 51 healthy women in whom the mean concentration was 3.86 ± 1.55 µg/cells from 1 liter of blood *5125*

Myeloperoxidase Antineutrophil Cytoplasmic Autoantibodies *Serum Increase* Antibodies detected in 15.6% of 64 patients *162*

Neopterin *Serum Increase* Mean concentration of 12.2 ± 5.1 nmol/L in 5 patients with SLE significantly greater than that in 18 healthy control individuals, 6.4 ± 1.8 nmol/L *3864* In 23 patients with SLE mean concentration of 43.08 ± 13.9 nmol/L significantly greater than 26.13 ± 9.72 nmol/L in 21 healthy controls *1956*
Urine Increase Concentrations increased with active disease and may be used to monitor progress of disease *121* Concentration in 28 patients with active disease of 290 (138 - 704) µmol/mol creatinine compared with 208 (90 - 433) µmol/mol creatinine in 18 patients with inactive disease and 163 (62 - 270) µmol/mol creatinine in 37 controls *601*

Neutrophil Proteinase 3 *Serum Increase* In 8 patients with active SLE mean concentration of 216 ± 41 µg/mL and mean of 131 ± 59 µg/mL in 8 patients with inactive disease significantly higher than mean of 78 ± 30 µg/mL in 21 normal individuals *2120*

Neutrophils *Blood Decrease* There is usually an overall depression of peripheral blood leukocytes, frequently with a lymphopenia and a slight shift to the left in the granulocytic series *900* In 16 patients with SLE in whom anti-PL 4 detected neutropenia with neutrophil count of less than 2 x 10^9/L observed in 6 (38%), and severe neutropenia (count of less than 1 x 10^9/L) in 4 (25%) *3295* Reduced counts in 7 of 21 cases. 62% had a subnormal response to etiocholanolone challenge, indicating reduced marrow reserves *2683* Present in well over 50% of patients *933*
Bone Marrow Decrease Reduced counts in 7 of 21 cases. 62% had a subnormal response to etiocholanolone challenge, indicating reduced marrow reserves *2683*
Synovial Fluid Decrease WBC are usually low (< 5,000 /µL) with a low percentage of neutrophils *900*

5'-Nucleotidase *Serum Increase* In 2 cases elevated to 13 and 26 U/L *2803*

Oligoclonal Banding *Cerebrospinal Fluid Increase* Oligoclonal IgG bands detected with neurolupus *3261*

Partial Thromboplastin Time *Plasma Increase* Prolonged time significantly associated with the presence of anticardiolipin antibodies observed in 147 of 390 outpatients (47%) *21* Reported effect *1980*

Pentosidine *Serum No Effect* In 37 patients with SLE mean concentration of 63.2 ± 59.6 nmol/L not significantly different from 48.3 ± 11.5 nmol/L in 57 heathy volunteers *4399*

Perinuclear Antineutrophil Cytoplasmic Autoantibodies *Serum Increase* Antibodies detected in 75% of 64 patients *162*

pH *Pleural Fluid Decrease* Exudate (pH < 7.3) *126*

Phospholipase A_2 *Serum Increase* Considerable increase in activity observed in patients with SLE correlating well with the activity of the disease *3767*

Phospholipase A_2 Type II *Serum Increase* Considerable increase in concentration observed in patients with SLE correlating well with the activity of the disease *3767*

Plasma Cells *Urine* *Increase* Lymphoblasts/plasma cells observed in 77.8% of 9 specimens in patients with SLE during relapses compared with 0% in 6 specimens from patients in remission *4380*

Platelet Activating Factor *Serum* *Increase* In 8 of 10 patients with active systemic lupus erythematosus detectable amounts of PAF observed (5.4 ± 2.9 ng/mL) during the most active phase of the disease but not detectable during inactive phases of the disease or in healthy individuals *5202*

Platelet-activating Factor Acetylhydrolase *Serum* *Decrease* Marked reduction observed in patients with active SLE compared with patients with inactive SLE and in healthy controls *5202*

Platelets *Blood* *Decrease* Thrombocytopenia significantly associated with the presence of anticardiolipin antibodies observed in 147 of 390 outpatients (47%) *21* In 16 patients with SLE in whom anti-PL 4 detected thrombocytopenia with platelet count of less than 100 x 10^9/L observed in 7 (44%) *3295* Thrombocytopenia (< 100,000 /µL) is common and is most frequently mild without purpura. Severe thrombocytopenia may occur, but purpura is rarely the presenting manifestation *900* May occur, due to increased destruction *624* Thrombocytopenia observed in 21% of Arabs with SLE *66* Mild thrombocytopenia in 32 patients (23%). Purpura or bleeding noted in 5 cases *1444*
Blood *No Effect* Most patients have increased production and increased peripheral destruction, with a normal circulating platelet count *624*

Potassium *Serum* *Increase* Two patients with long standing disease had persistent hyperkalemia apparently due to defect in renal tubular secretion *1088*

Precipitins *Serum* *Increase* Found in 15% of patients and 3% of controls *700*

Procollagen Type II Peptide *Serum* *Increase* Raised serum IgG anti-type II collagen antibody levels were present in 11% of patients with RA, 30% with SLE, 44% with PSS and 42% with OL *1600* *1532*

Progesterone *Plasma* *Decrease* In 26 women with inactive or quiescent SLE lower peak and day-7 postovulation concentration during menstrual cycle significantly lower than in 21 normally menstruating control women *179*

Properdin Factor B *Plasma* *Decrease* Mean concentration typically slightly reduced or normal in patients with active SLE *4682*

Prostaglandin E *Urine* *Increase* The mean pretreatment excretion of urinary immunoreactive prostaglandin E, 42.7 ± 6.4 ng/h, was significantly higher than the value of 29.0 ± 1.9 ng/h for normal subjects *2685*

Prostaglandin E_2 *Cerebrospinal Fluid* *Increase* Mean concentration of 0.97 ± 0.50 pg/mL in 8 patients with neuropsychiatric SLE slightly higher than 0.20 ± 0.07 pg/mL in 20 patients with CNS non-inflammation (controls) *5295*

Protein *Cerebrospinal Fluid* *Increase* In patients with neurologic symptoms *144*
Serum *No Effect* In 39 patients serum total protein and albumin concentrations were stable throughout the course of disease *4662* In 37 patients with systemic lupus erythematosus mean concentration of 44 ± 6 g/L not significantly different from 42 ± 8 g/L in 57 heathy volunteers *4399* In 37 patients with systemic lupus erythematosus mean concentration of 72 ± 9 g/L not significantly different from 72 ± 4 g/L in 57 heathy volunteers *4399*
Synovial Fluid *Decrease* Synovial fluid may be a transudate with low protein content (< 3 g/dL), especially in patients with asymptomatic joint effusions associated with nephritis and edema. In other patients with inflammatory joint signs, the fluid is an exudate with increased protein content (3 - 5 g/dL) *900*
Synovial Fluid *Increase* Synovial fluid may be a transudate with low protein content (< 3 g/dL), especially in patients with asymptomatic joint effusions associated with nephritis and edema. In other patients with inflammatory joint signs, the fluid is an exudate with increased protein content (3 - 5 g/dL) *900*
Urine *Increase* Proteinuria and other urine abnormalities observed in 54% of Arabs with SLE *66* Levels of hematuria and proteinuria correlate well with severity of morphologic lesions *2159* Changes in the amount of proteinuria do not reflect histologic changes in the kidneys *1980* Generally precedes hematuria and red cell casts, although small degrees of renal involvement may occur without proteinuria *1578* Protein > 2^+ observed in 88.9% of 9 specimens in patients with SLE during relapses compared with 100% in 6 specimens from patients in remission *4380*

Protein S *Plasma* *No Effect* No significant difference observed between patients with SLE and lupus anticoagulant who were antiphospholipid negative (81.9 ± 2.3%), LA-positive (79.0 ± 3.8%), aPL-positive (75.2 ± 9.2%), and LA/aPL-positive (77.5 ± 5.0%) and healthy controls (77.5 ± 4.0%) *3359*

Protein S, Free *Plasma* *No Effect* No significant difference observed between patients with SLE and lupus anticoagulant who were antiphospholipid negative (86.5 ± 11.6%), LA-positive (86.5 ± 11.2%), aPL-positive (77.3 ± 13.3%), and LA/aPL-positive (82.5 ± 8.5%) and healthy controls (82.0 ± 4.0%) *3359*

Protein S, Functional *Plasma* *No Effect* No significant difference observed between patients with SLE and lupus anticoagulant who were antiphospholipid negative (74.2 ± 9.3%), LA-positive (74.3 ± 7.4%), aPL-positive (71.5 ± 9.7%), and LA/aPL-positive (73.0 ± 5.7%) and healthy controls (79.9 ± 5.5%) *3359*

Proteinase 3-Antineutrophil Cytoplasmic Autoantibodies *Serum* *No Effect* Antibodies not detected in any of 64 patients *162*

Prothrombin Fragment 1.2 *Plasma* *Increase* Mean concentration of prothrombin fragment 1.2 in platelet-poor plasma from 11 patients with SLE of 4.2 ± 2.4 nmol/L significantly higher than 0.51 nmol/L (95% reference interval 0.21 - 2.78 nmol/L) in 268 healthy individuals less than 44 years of age *1860*

Prothrombin Time *Plasma* *Increase* A prolonged time may suggest the possibility of a circulating anticoagulant, which is particularly likely to be found in patients with a chronic false positive serologic test for syphilis *900*

Rheumatoid Factor *Serum* *Increase* Rheumatoid factor detected in 5 of 31 (16%) Arabs with SLE *66* Rheumatoid factor may be observed in certain patients *2473* In 15% of cases *144* Concentration may be increased as in other diseases with chronic inflammation *2952* Positive tests (titer of 1:80 or more) were found in 50% (61) of patients *1444* Rheumatoid factors are present in almost 50% of patients at some time during their course, but intermittently and at low titer *2039* Mean concentration increased in patients with SLE *2472*

Ristocetin Cofactor *Plasma* *Increase* Mean activity of 311 ± 134% of normal in 9 patients with active SLE significantly greater than 103 ± 20% in 20 healthy controls *208*

RNP Antibodies *Serum* *Increase* RNP antibodies detected in 11% of 33 Arabs with SLE *66*

Soluble E-Selectin *Serum* *Increase* 30 patients with active disease and 20 with inactive disease had a mean concentration not significantly different from 48 ng/mL in 10 healthy controls *3638*

Soluble Endothelial Leukocyte Adhesion Molecule *Serum* *Increase* Mean concentration in 35 patients with SLE of 50.0 ± 3.9 ng/mL significantly different from 36.3 ± 2.3 ng/mL in 41 healthy controls *5042*

Soluble HLA-I *Serum* *Increase* In 27 patients with SLE, mean concentration of 1.85 ± 1.15 µg/mL significantly increased compared with 0.41 ± 0.20 µg/mL in 30 normal controls *5306* Mean concentration of 4,120 ± 2,400 cpm/mL observed in 58 patients with SLE significantly different from 2,900 ± 1,540 cpm/mL in 82 controls, with concentration of 6,180 ± 2,100 cpm/mL significantly higher in 22 patients with active disease than 2,860 ± 1,600 cpm/mL in 36 patients with inactive disease *576*

Soluble HLA-FHC *Serum* *Increase* Mean concentration of 800 ± 550 cpm/mL observed in 58 patients with SLE significantly different from 160 ± 100 cpm/mL in 82 controls, with concentration of 810 ± 600 cpm/mL significantly higher in 22 patients with active disease than 590 ± 324 cpm/mL in 36 patients with inactive disease *576*

Soluble Intercellular Adhesion Molecule-1 *Serum* *Increase* In 18 children with systemic lupus erythmatosus mean concentration of 513 ± 139 ng/mL significantly greater than 210 ± 95 ng/mL in 25 healthy control children *2935* Mean concentration in 35 patients with SLE of 389.2 ± 19.6 ng/mL significantly different from 249.4 ± 10.0 ng/mL in 41 healthy controls *5042* In 9 patients with active vasculitis mean concentration of 509 ± 71 ng/mL significantly higher than mean concentration of 270 ± 47 ng/mL in 10 healthy controls: no significant difference between concentrations in active and inactive vasculitis *2461*

710.00 Systemic Lupus Erythematosus *(continued)*

Soluble Interleukin-2 Receptor *Serum* *Increase* Mean concentration in 35 patients with SLE of 893.4 ± 75.4 U/mL significantly different from 560.9 ± 20.4 U/mL in 41 healthy controls *5042* Higher in inactive SLE than in controls and significantly increased in active disease but with decrease when disease became inactive *5716* Concentration significantly higher in patients with active disease than in those with inactive disease *601*
Urine *Increase* Concentrations > 1,100 U/mL observed in 66.7% of 9 specimens in patients with SLE during relapses compared with 0% in 6 specimens from patients in remission *4380*

Soluble Interleukin-6 Receptor *Serum* *Increase* Mean concentration in 35 patients with SLE of 37.5 ± 2.3 ng/mL significantly different from 27.4 ± 1.0 ng/mL in 41 healthy controls *5042*

Soluble Tumor Necrosis Factor Receptor-p55 *Serum* *Increase* In 52 patients with SLE median concentration of 3 ng/mL significantly different from median concentration of 1 ng/mL in 22 patients with rheumatoid arthritis and that in normal individuals. In a second study median concentration in 20 patients with SLE of 3.8 ng/mL higher than median of 2.7 ng/mL in 20 patients with rheumatoid arthritis and 2.6 ng/mL in 18 patients with spondyloarthropathy and 2.1 ng/mL in 20 healthy controls *1612*

Soluble Tumor Necrosis Factor Receptor-p75 *Serum* *Increase* In 52 patients with SLE median concentration of 7.15 ng/mL significantly different from median concentration of 4.3 ng/mL in 22 patients with rheumatoid arthritis and that in normal individuals *1612* Median concentration in 20 patients with SLE of 18 ng/mL higher than 6.9 ng/mL in 20 healthy controls *1612*

Soluble Vascular Cell Adhesion Molecule-1 *Serum* *Increase* Mean concentration in 35 patients with SLE of 1,030.9 ± 57.2 ng/mL significantly different from 657.6 ± 27.6 ng/mL in 41 healthy controls *5042* 30 patients with active disease had a mean concentration of 893 ng/mL significantly greater than 582 ng/mL in 10 healthy donors *3638*

Specific Gravity *Pleural Fluid* *Increase* Exudate (> 1.016) *126*

Stromelysin *Plasma* *Increase* In 17 patients with SLE mean concentration of 258.4 ± 34.6 ng/mL significantly higher than 50.0 ± 4.4 ng/mL in 53 healthy controls *5878*

Thrombomodulin *Plasma* *Increase* In 15 patients with SLE and Raynaud's phenomenon mean concentration of 42.4 ± 11.0 ng/mL and in 15 without Raynaud's phenomenon of 35.0 ± 7.6 ng/mL significantly greater than 3.8 ± 2.4 ng/mL in 10 normal controls *3361* In 16 patients with active disease mean concentration of approximately 78 ng/mL compared with about 20 ng/mL in 8 patients wth inactive disease and 10 ng/mL in healthy controls *3873* In 42 patients with SLE mean concentration of 20.9 ± 18.3 ng/mL significantly different from 10.7 ± 11.0 ng/mL in 18 controls *2862*

Thromboplastin Generation *Blood* *Increase* The type of anticoagulant most commonly found inhibits the conversion of prothrombin to thrombin and exhibits prolonged thromboplastin and prothrombin times *1980*

Thromboxane A_2 *Plasma* *Increase* With kidney involvement *4036*

Tissue Inhibitor of Metalloproteinase *Serum* *Increase* Mean concentration of 48.29 ± 23.86 units in 75 patients with SLE significantly higher than than 42.77 ± 16.71 units in 70 healthy blood donor controls with concentrations higher in patients with active disease than those with inactive disease *1524*

Tissue Plasminogen Activator *Urine* *Increase* Urinary t-PA detectable in 6 of 8 patients *2139*

Tumor Necrosis Factor-α *Cerebrospinal Fluid* *No Effect* In 8 patients with neuropsychiatric SLE TNF-α not detectable *5295*
Serum *Increase* In 52 patients with SLE median concentration of 40.1 pg/mL significantly different from upper limit of normal *1612*

Ubiquitin, Free *Blood* *Decrease* In 38 patients with SLE mean concentration of 63.9 ± 24.7 µg/cells in 1 L blood less than that in 45 healthy men and 51 healthy women in whom the mean concentration was 126 ± 24.4 µg/cells from 1 liter of blood *5125*

Urea Nitrogen *Serum* *Increase* Elevated, usually > 100 mg/dL. Indicates uremia *2685* Correlates well with severity of morphologic lesions *2159*
Serum *No Effect* In 37 patients with systemic lupus erythematosus mean concentration of 6.5 ± 3.3 mmol/L not significantly different from 6.1 ± 1.5 mmol/L in 57 heathy volunteers *4399*

Vascular Endothelial Growth Factor *Serum* *No Effect* Mean concentration in 17 patients with SLE of 242 ± 109 pg/mL not significantly different from 184 ± 62 pg/mL in 20 healthy individuals *2674*

VDRL *Serum* *Positive* Biologic false positive results in 14% of patients *1444* A persistent biologic false positive serologic test for syphilis may precede overt manifestations by many months or years *2039* VDRL test positive in 2 of 22 (9%) Arabs with SLE *66* Incidence of false positive reactions is 15% *2304*

Viscosity *Serum* *Increase* Modest increases may be seen, but no hyperviscosity syndromes have been reported *4768*
Synovial Fluid *Decrease* Slightly decreased *1980*

Vitamin B_{12} Binding Capacity *Serum* *Increase* Significant elevation; usually correlated with WBC in peripheral blood *4448*

von Willebrand Factor *Plasma* *Increase* In 15 SLE patients with Raynaud's phenomenon mean concentration of 140 ± 30 % and in 15 without Raynaud's phenomenon of 158 ± 33 % compared with 78 ± 22 % in 10 healthy controls *3361*

von Willebrand Factor Antigen *Plasma* *Increase* Mean concentration of 243 ± 157% of normal in 9 patients with active SLE significantly higher than 72 ± 21% in 20 healthy controls *208*

710.10 CREST Syndrome

Anti-Topoisomerase-I Antigen *Serum* *Increase* Antibodies detected in 2 of 22 patients (9%) *4815*

Anticentromere Antibody *Serum* *Increase* Concentration increased in patients with CREST syndrome *2952*

Occult Blood *Feces* *Increase* 22 of 144 patients with SSC/CREST syndrome had at least one episode of gastrointestinal hemorrhage *1249*

710.10 Progressive Systemic Sclerosis

Albumin *Urine* *Increase* Appears during renal failure *900*

Anti-ds DNA Antibodies *Serum* *No Effect* Found in 0% of cases *4897*

Anti-Ribonuclear Protein Antibodies *Serum* *Increase* Found in 5% of cases *4897*

Anti-Scl-70 Antibodies *Serum* *Increase* Found in 23% of cases (10% with CREST syndrome) *4897*

Anti-Sjögren's Syndrome A Antibodies (SSA[Ro]) *Serum* *Increase* Found in 33% of cases *4897*

Anti-Sjögren's Syndrome B Antibodies (SSB[La]) *Serum* *Increase* Found in 6% of cases *4897*

Anti-Smith Antibodies *Serum* *No Effect* Found in 0% of cases *4897*

Anti-ss DNA Antibodies *Serum* *Increase* Found in 14% of cases *4897*

Antibody Titer *Serum* *Increase* The anticentromere antibody is thought to be closely associated with the CREST variant of scleroderma. It may be a useful prognostic indicator *4197*

Anticentromere Antibody *Serum* *Increase* Found in 10% of cases (77% with CREST syndrome) *4897*

α_1-Antichymotrypsin *Serum* *Increase* Reported effect *2457* Collagen vascular diseases *2628*

Antinuclear Antibodies *Serum* *Increase* Reported effect *4011* Found in 58% of cases *4897* Found in the sera of 40-90% of patients. In most cases the titers are relatively low, as compared to those found in SLE *4551* Present in 60% of 47 serum samples in titers of 1:16 or greater *4456* Detected in low titer in 50 - 60% of cases and usually related to the nucleolar and ill-defined glycoprotein antigens *2039* 75 - 80% positivity *4068*

Aspartate Aminotransferase *Serum Increase* Moderate to marked increase with associated myositis *1025*

Ceruloplasmin *Serum Increase* Believed to occur as a non-specific response (acute phase reactant) *4551* Mean level of ceruloplasmin, but not copper were raised in these patients, although both were raised in the 2 patients with the most aggressive disease *2428*

Chylomicrons *Serum Increase* Moderate increase secondary to presence of IgG or IgM that binds heparin and thereby decreases the activity of lipoprotein lipase *126*

Cold Agglutinins *Serum Increase* Increased titer *413*

Complement, Total *Serum Decrease* In 27 patients, 44% had decreased values *4925* Occasionally *4683*
Serum Increase In 27 patients, 19% had increased values *4925*
Serum No Effect Normal in all but a few patients *5274* Concentration usually unaffected by disease *4551*

Copper *Serum Increase* Increased *4586 3900 4871*

Creatine Kinase *Serum Increase* Moderate to marked increase with associated myositis *1025*

Creatinine *Serum Increase* Renal function may be impaired *1980*

Cryofibrinogen *Plasma Increase* Small amounts *2308*

Eosinophils *Blood Increase* Eosinophilia has been observed but is uncommon *1980* Early in the disease, the blood count is normal save for rare eosinophilia *144*

Erythrocyte Casts *Urine Increase* Appears during renal failure *900*

Erythrocyte Sedimentation Rate *Blood Decrease* Decreased in 33% of patients *5545*
Blood Increase Increased in 33% of patients *5545*
Blood No Effect Normal in 33%, decreased in 33%, and increased in 33% of patients *5545*

Erythrocytes *Urine Increase* Appears during renal failure *900*

Fat *Feces Increase* Defects of multiple stages of digestion-absorption *4891*

γ-Globulin *Serum Increase* Occurs in about 50% of patients; usually only moderate (1.4 - 2.0 g/dL), values of 3.5 g/dL and higher have been observed *4551* Frequently found but is nonspecific *900*

Glomerular Filtration Rate *Urine Decrease* The earliest demonstrable change in renal scleroderma *1980* Renal function may be impaired *1980*

Glycosaminoglycans *Urine Increase* Possibly reflecting the severity of the disease *2022*

Hematocrit *Blood Decrease* A mild hypochromic microcytic anemia may be present *900* Found in up to 25% of patients *1980*

Hemoglobin *Blood Decrease* Found in up to 25% of patients *1980* A mild hypochromic microcytic anemia may be present *900*

Hyaluronic Acid *Serum Increase* Serum levels were measured using an affinoimmunoenzymatic assay in patients with distal (n = 16) and proximal (n = 15) progressive systemic sclerosis (PSS) and in 31 controls. The mean sHA was significantly higher in the patients with PSS than in controls (mean ± SD:80 ± 43.4 μg/L vs. 42.3 ± 19.1 μg/L, p less than 0.001). sHA was significantly higher in patients with proximal PSS than in patients with distal PSS (106.4 ± 44.6 μg/L vs. 55.4 ± 23.8 μg/L, p less than 0.001) *948* The circulating levels of hyaluronate were determined in 36 patients with scleroderma and in 36 control subjects matched for age and sex. The mean serum concentration in patients with the disorder (n = 25) was 131 μg/L and significantly greater ($p < 0.001$) than that of the controls (mean 49 μg/L) *1370*

Hydroxyproline *Urine Increase* Increased in some patients, especially those with active disease *367*

Immunoglobulin A *Serum Increase* Reported effect *4456* Usually slightly elevated *1980*

Immunoglobulin G *Serum Increase* In most cases and in greatest measure, the increase involves IgG; less often the levels of IgA and IgM are elevated *4551* Usually slightly elevated *1980*

Immunoglobulin M *Serum Increase* Reported effect *4456* Usually slightly elevated *1980*

Lactate Dehydrogenase *Serum Increase* Moderate to marked increase with associated myositis *1025*

LE Cells *Blood Positive* Occasionally positive *2039*

Leukocytes *Blood No Effect* WBC and differential are usually normal *1980*

MCH *Blood Decrease* A mild hypochromic microcytic anemia may be present *900* Found in up to 25% of patients *1980*

MCHC *Blood Decrease* Found in up to 25% of patients *1980* A mild hypochromic microcytic anemia may be present *900*

MCV *Blood Decrease* Found in up to 25% of patients *1980* A mild hypochromic microcytic anemia may be present *900*

Platelets *Blood Decrease* Has been reported *1980*

Procollagen Type II Peptide *Serum Increase* Raised serum IgG anti-type II collagen antibody levels were present in 11% of patients with RA, 30% with SLE, 44% with PSS and 42% with OL *1600*

Procollagen Type III Peptide *Serum Increase* Serum P-III-P levels were elevated in patients with PSS and MCTD/overlap syndrome, suggesting a high rate of collagen biosynthesis by fibroblasts. Patients with RA showed no significant elevation of serum P-III-P compared with normal control group *155*

Protein *Urine Increase* In urinalysis proteinuria may be the only manifestation *1980* May be present for extended periods without clinical evidence of progressive renal dysfunction *1980* Renal involvement *144*

Renin Activity *Plasma Increase* Extremely elevated levels are a frequent accompaniment of renal scleroderma *1980*

Rheumatoid Factor *Serum Increase* Present in 33% of sera from 47 patients with scleroderma *4456* 25 - 33% of patients have positive tests. In most cases the titers have been 1:320 or less *4551* Almost 50% of patients have factor present in serum but it does not correlate with the existence of joint disease *2039*

Urea Nitrogen *Serum Increase* Renal function may be impaired *1980*

VDRL *Serum Positive* Occasionally there are biologic false positive tests *144*

Vitamin B_{12} *Serum Decrease* A selective vitamin B_{12} deficiency only or a decrease in iron stores may be present without other obvious signs of the malabsorption syndrome *1980*

710.10 Scleroderma

Anti-Endothelial Cell Antibodies *Serum Increase* AECA have been detected in systemic lupus erythematosus, scleroderma and dermatomyositis but are also found in systemic vasculitis, Kawasaki disease, hemolytic uremic syndrome, thrombotic thrombocytopenic purpura and renal allograft recipients at the time of rejection *4248 1174 5780*

Anti-Entactin Antibodies *Serum Increase* In 20 patients IgM anti-entactin antibodies observed in one *4604*

Anti-Ku Antibodies *Serum Increase* Isolation and characterization of cDNA encoding the 80-kDa subunit protein of the human autoantigen Ku (p70/p80) recognized by autoantibodies from patients with scleroderma-polymyositis overlap syndrome *5788 3503* 4 of 4 patients with scleroderma had anti-Ku antibodies *921*

Anti-Neutrophil Cytoplasm Antibodies *Serum No Effect* Antibodies not detected in any of 10 patients *162*

Antinuclear Antibodies *Serum Increase* 4 of 4 patients with scleroderma had anti-nuclear antibodies *921*

Autoantibodies to Scl 70 Antigen *Serum Increase* Concentration increased in 20 - 60% of patients with scleroderma: more prevalent in the diffuse form of scleroderma *2952*

Complement C_1 *Serum No Effect* Mean concentration typically normal or slightly increased in patients with scleroderma *4682*

Complement C_1q *Serum No Effect* Mean concentration typically normal or slightly increased in patients with scleroderma *4682*

Complement C_2 *Serum No Effect* Mean concentration typically normal or slightly increased in patients with scleroderma *4682*

Complement C_3 *Serum No Effect* Mean concentration typically normal or slightly increased in patients with scleroderma *4682*

710.10 Scleroderma *(continued)*

Complement C_4 *Serum* *No Effect* Mean concentration typically normal or slightly increased in patients with scleroderma *4682*

Complement C_5 *Serum* *No Effect* Mean concentration typically normal or slightly increased in patients with scleroderma *4682*

Complement CH50 *Serum* *No Effect* Mean concentration typically normal or slightly increased in patients with scleroderma *4682*

C-terminal Propeptide of Type I Procollagen *Serum* *Increase* In 39 patients with localized scleroderma mean concentration of 300 ± 252 ng/mL and of 478 ± 296 ng/mL in 15 patents with generalized scleroderma significantly higher than 139 ± 83 ng/mL in 30 healthy control volunteers *2675*

CYFRA 21-1 *Serum* *Increase* In 14 patients with scleroderma median concentration of 1.9 ng/mL significantly different from that in 50 healthy individuals with median concentration of 1.2 ng/mL and range of 0.5 - 2.4 ng/mL *3559*

Elastase Antineutrophil Cytoplasmic Autoantibodies *Serum* *Increase* Antibodies detected in 20% of 10 patients *162*

Endothelin-1 *Plasma* *Increase* In 19 patients concentrations increased to 10.7 ± 7.3 pg/mL, mean 2.9-fold above appropriate normals *328* Radioimmunoassay demonstrated a mean ± SD plasma level of 10.7 ± 7.3 pg/mL in the patients (n = 19) and 3.7 ± 2 pg/mL in the control subjects (n = 16) (p less than 0.005) *2526*

Gelatinase *Serum* *Increase* In 9 patients with scleroderma mean concentration of 632.8 ± 129.8 ng/mL significantly higher than 408.9 ± 28.0 ng/mL in 53 healthy controls *5878*

5-Hydroxytryptamine *Plasma* *No Effect* Median concentration of 0.7 ng/mL (IQR 0.5 - 1.5 ng/mL) in 11 patients with scleroderma not significantly different from 0.9 ng/mL (IQR 0.7 - 1.8 ng/mL) in 19 normal individuals *871*

Interferon-γ *Serum* *No Effect* Serum concentrations measured in 78 scleroderma patients and 73 controls, using enzyme-linked immunosorbent assay, radioimmunoassay, and bioassay techniques. IFN-γ was not detected in any sera *3750*

Interleukin-1 *Serum* *No Effect* Serum concentrations measured in 78 scleroderma patients and 73 controls, using enzyme-linked immunosorbent assay, radioimmunoassay, and bioassay techniques. IL-1α was found with equal frequency in patient and control sera *3750*

Interleukin-2 *Serum* *Increase* Serum concentrations measured in 78 scleroderma patients and 73 controls, using enzyme-linked immunosorbent assay, radioimmunoassay, and bioassay techniques. IL-2 was detected more frequently in sera from scleroderma patients than in sera from controls *3750*

Interleukin-4 *Serum* *Increase* Serum concentrations measured in 78 scleroderma patients and 73 controls, using enzyme-linked immunosorbent assay, radioimmunoassay, and bioassay techniques. IL-4 was detected more frequently in sera from scleroderma patients than in sera from controls *3750*

Interleukin-6 *Serum* *Increase* Serum concentrations measured in 78 scleroderma patients and 73 controls, using enzyme-linked immunosorbent assay, radioimmunoassay, and bioassay techniques. IL-6 was detected more frequently in sera from scleroderma patients than in sera from controls *3750*

Myeloperoxidase Antineutrophil Cytoplasmic Autoantibodies *Serum* *Increase* Antibodies detected in 10% of 10 patients *162*

Nucleotide Pyrophosphohydrolase, Soluble *Serum* *Increase* Mean activity in 28 patients with scleroderma of 1,565 ± 65 pmol nitrophenol/h/mL significantly different from that in 85 healthy individuals 1,141 ± 22 pmol nitrophenol/h/mL *691*

Occult Blood *Feces* *Increase* One of 6 patients with scleroderma had at least one episode of gastrointestinal hemorrhage *1249*

Perinuclear Antineutrophil Cytoplasmic Autoantibodies *Serum* *Increase* Antibodies detected in 20% of 10 patients *162*

Properdin Factor B *Plasma* *No Effect* Mean concentration typically normal or slightly reduced in patients with scleroderma *4682*

Proteinase 3-Antineutrophil Cytoplasmic Autoantibodies *Serum* *No Effect* Antibodies not detected in any of 10 patients *162*

Soluble Interleukin-2 Receptor *Serum* *Increase* In 48 patients with localized scleroderma mean concentration of 105 ± 124 pmol/L significantly different from 54 ± 29 pmol/L in 20 healthy controls *2322*

Stromelysin *Plasma* *Increase* In 9 patients with scleroderma mean concentration of 109.1 ± 18.8 ng/mL significantly higher than 50.0 ± 4.4 ng/mL in 53 healthy controls *5878*

Tumor Necrosis Factor-α *Serum* *No Effect* Serum concentrations measured in 78 scleroderma patients and 73 controls, using enzyme-linked immunosorbent assay, radioimmunoassay, and bioassay techniques. TNF-α was found with equal frequency in patient and control sera *3750*

710.10 Systemic Sclerosis

α_1-Acid Glycoprotein *Serum* *Increase* In 8 patients with limited systemic sclerosis mean 0.93 g/L (range of 0.65 - 1.19) and 1.17 g/L (range of 0.58 - 1.70) in 16 with diffuse sclerosis mean compared with normal individuals *4619*

Adenosine Deaminase *Serum* *Increase* In 48 patients with progressive systemic sclerosis mean plasma activity of 18.65 ± 6.58 U/L significantly greater than 9.53 ± 3.0 U/L in 48 reference plasmas *3464*

Amino-terminal Propeptide of Type III Procollagen *Serum* *Increase* Concentration increased in comparison with that in healthy age and sex-matched controls *4618*

Angiotensin-converting Enzyme *Serum* *No Effect* In 31 patients with limited systemic sclerosis mean activity of 5.85 ± 1.21 U/mL and 6.49 ± 1.30 U/mL in 25 patients with diffuse systemic sclerosis not significantly different from 7.79 ± 0.76 U/mL in 58 healthy controls *4535*

Anti-DNA Topomerase I *Serum* *Increase* In 265 patients with systemic sclerosis antibodies detected in 68 and not in 197 *2871*

Anti-Ku Antibodies *Serum* *Increase* In 274 patients with systemic sclerosis antibodies detected in 7 and not in 267 *2871*

Anti-RNAP Antibodies *Serum* *Increase* In 275 patients with systemic sclerosis antibodies detected in 14 and not in 261 *2871*

Anti-Scl-70 Antibodies *Serum* *Increase* Antibodies observed in 12 of 31 sera from patients with systemic sclerosis with all but one patient having sclerodermatous skin involvement above the MCP level *2151*

Anti-Th RNP Antibodies *Serum* *Increase* In 273 patients with systemic sclerosis antibodies detected in 5 and not in 268 *2871*

Anti-Topoisomerase-I Antigen *Serum* *Increase* Antibodies detected in 72 of 191 patients (37%) *4815*

Anti-U1RNP Antibodies *Serum* *Increase* In 246 patients with systemic sclerosis antibodies detected in 67 and not in 179 *2871* Antibodies observed in 6 of 31 sera from patients with systemic sclerosis *2151*

Anti-U3 RNP *Serum* *Increase* In 275 patients with systemic sclerosis antibodies detected in 10 and not in 267 *2871*

Anticardiolipin Antibodies *Serum* *Increase* Antibodies observed in 9 of 31 sera from patients with systemic sclerosis *2151*

Anticentromere Antibody *Serum* *Increase* In 274 patients with systemic sclerosis antibodies detected in 44 and not in 230 *2871*

Antinuclear Antibodies *Serum* *Increase* Antibodies observed in 27 of 31 sera from patients with systemic sclerosis *2151*

Autoantibodies to Scl 70 Antigen *Serum* *Increase* In 46 specimens observed in 26% of 397 patients in one study with positivity of 8 - 36% in this study *4815*

Cholesterol *Serum* *No Effect* Mean concentration in 20 patients with systemic sclerosis of 4.3 ± 0.2 mmol/L not significantly different from 4.8 ± 0.2 mmol/L in 18 healthy controls *3597*

Creatinine *Serum* *No Effect* Mean concentration in 20 patients with systemic sclerosis of 95.5 ± 5.8 μmol/L not significantly different from 89.7 ± 3.2 μmol/L in 18 healthy controls *3597*

Creatinine Clearance *Urine* *No Effect* Mean clearance in 20 patients with systemic sclerosis of 98.1 ± 9.1 mL/min not significantly different from 103.5 ± 5.9 mL/min in 18 healthy controls *3597*

EDTA Clearance *Urine* *Decrease* In 8 patients with limited systemic sclerosis mean clearance 97% and 84% in 16 with diffuse sclerosis mean compared with 100% in normal individuals *4619*

Endothelin-1 *Plasma* *Increase* In one study of 7 patients mean concentration increased to 1.8 ± 0.3 pg/mL (1.5 times appropriate normal) and in the other of 7 patients mean concentration increased to 4.5 ± 1.3 pg/mL (1.1 times normal) *328* Mean concentration in 20 patients with systemic sclerosis of 1.72 ± 0.8 pg/mL significantly different from 0.63 ± 0.06 pg/mL in 18 healthy controls *3597*

Erythrocyte Sedimentation Rate *Blood* *Increase* In 8 patients with limited systemic sclerosis mean rate of 11 mm/h (range 6 - 56) and 25 mm/h (range 6 - 52) in 16 with diffuse sclerosis mean compared with normal individuals *4619*

Fab-PIINP *Serum* *Increase* In patients with systemic sclerosis concentration increased compared to healthy controls matched for age and sex *4618*

Glucose *Serum* *No Effect* Mean concentration in 20 patients with systemic sclerosis of 5.0 ± 0.6 mmol/L not significantly different from 5.1 ± 0.1 mmol/L in 18 healthy controls *3597*

Hepatocyte Growth Factor *Serum* *Increase* In 30 patients with systemic sclerosis median concentration of approximately 270 pg/mL (310 pg/mL in 20 patients with diffuse sclerosis and 240 pg/mL in 10 patients with limited sclerosis) significantly different from approximately 200 pg/mL in 60 healthy controls *2595*

Hyaluronan *Serum* *Increase* In patients with systemic sclerosis concentration increased compared with that in age and sex matched controls *4618*

IgG Anti-Calpastatin Antibodies *Serum* *Increase* In 63 patients with systemic sclerosis antibodies detected in 15 (24%) *4590*

IgG Antiendothelial Antibodies *Serum* *Increase* In 36 patients with limited systemic sclerosis and 31 with diffuse sclerosis antibodies detected in 16 and 31, respectively *4535*

IgM Anti-Calpastatin Antibodies *Serum* *Increase* In 63 patients with systemic sclerosis antibodies detected in 14 (22%) *4590*

Intercellular Adhesion Molecule-1 *Serum* *Decrease* In 7 patients with sclerotic systemic sclerosis mean concentration of 124 ± 17 ng/mL not significantly different from 150 ± 18 ng/mL in 36 healthy controls *1893*
Serum *Increase* In 5 patients with early edematous systemic sclerosis mean concentration of 229 ± 39 ng/mL significantly different from 150 ± 18 ng/mL in 36 healthy controls *1893*

Interleukin-1β *Serum* *Increase* In 18 patients with mean concentration of 36.3 ± 18.5 pg/mL significantly different from 4.2 ± 1.2 pg/mL in 25 healthy controls *5113*

Interleukin-2 *Serum* *Increase* In 18 patients with mean concentration of 348.8 ± 20.2 pg/mL significantly different from 100.0 ± 20 pg/mL in 25 healthy controls *5113* In a study of 48 patients with systemic sclerosis (SSc). elevated serum levels of soluble interleukin 2 (IL-2) were noted in 44% of early untreated patients with SSc *862*

Interleukin-4 *Serum* *Increase* Median concentration of 2.6 pg/mL in 55 patients with systemic sclerosis significantly increased compared with < 1.8 pg/mL in 20 healthy controls *2043* In 18 patients with mean concentration of 1.2 ± 1.25 ng/mL significantly different from 0.75 ± 0.1 ng/mL in 25 healthy controls *5113*

Interleukin-6 *Serum* *Increase* In 9 patients with early diffuse cutaneous systemic sclerosis median concentration of 4.6 pg/mL significantly greater than < 0.7 pg/mL in 20 healthy controls *2044* In 18 patients with mean concentration of 159.6 ± 120.5 pg/mL significantly different from 14.3 ± 7.9 pg/mL in 25 healthy controls *5113*
Serum *No Effect* In 12 patients with early limited cutaneous systemic sclerosis, 22 with late limited cutaneous systemic sclerosis, and 12 with late diffuse cutaneous systemic sclerosis median concentration of < 0.7 pg/mL as in 20 healthy controls *2044*

Interleukin-8 *Serum* *Increase* In 18 patients with mean concentration of 321.0 ± 204.1 pg/mL significantly different from 3.5 ± 0.9 pg/mL in 25 healthy controls *5113*

Interleukin-10 *Serum* *Increase* Median concentration of 76 pg/mL in 52 patients with systemic sclerosis significantly increased compared with 34 pg/mL in 20 healthy controls *2043*

Interleukin-13 *Serum* *Increase* Median concentration of 3.7 pg/mL in 73 patients with systemic sclerosis significantly increased compared with 2.2 pg/mL in 20 healthy controls *2043*

Melanoma Inhibitory Factor *Serum* *No Effect* In 10 patients mean concentration of 3.5 ± 2.8 ng/mL showed no significant difference from 3.6 ± 2.8 ng/mL in 120 healthy controls *3655*

Neopterin *Serum* *Increase* In a study of 48 patients with systemic sclerosis (SSc). elevated serum levels of neopterin (indicators of lymphocyte/monocyte activation) were noted in 40% of early untreated patients with SSc *862*

Occult Blood *Feces* *Increase* 22 of 144 patients with SSC/CREST syndrome had at least one episode of gastrointestinal hemorrhage *1249*

Oncostatin M *Serum* *Increase* In one 70-year old patient with diffuse cutaneous systemic sclerosis of 11 years duration with pulmonary fibrosis and a leg ulcer had a very high concentration of oncostatin M, typically not detectable in 20 healthy controls *2044*
Serum *No Effect* In 55 patients with systemic sclerosis median concentration, typically not detectable, not significantly different from that in 20 healthy controls *2044*

Phospholipase A_2 *Serum* *Decrease* In sera of patients with systemic sclerosis persistent subnormal amounts of PLA2 catalytic activity and of pancreatic PLA2-I concentration observed possibly related to abnormal arachidonic metabolism *3766*

Procollagen Type I Peptide *Serum* *Increase* In 61 patients with systemic sclerosis (SSc) and in 21 control subjects the mean P1CP level in the SSc patients was significantly higher than in the normal controls (mean ± SD, 326 ± 319 vs 128 ± 87 ng/mL; $p < 0.005$). In 36% of the SSc patients, the serum P1CP level was significantly elevated more than two standard deviations above the mean control value *2673* *4620*

Procollagen Type III Peptide *Serum* *Increase* In 82 patients with SSc, serum concentrations of aminoterminal type III procollagen peptide (PIII NP), smaller PIII NP-related antigens (Fab PIII NP) and hyaluronan (HA) were increased as compared to healthy controls matched for age and sex *4618*

P-Selectin *Serum* *Decrease* In 7 patients with sclerotic systemic sclerosis mean concentration of 185 ± 64 ng/mL not significantly different from 262 ± 85 ng/mL in 36 healthy controls *1893*
Serum *Increase* In 5 patients with early edematous systemic sclerosis mean concentration of 360 ± 106 ng/mL not significantly different from 262 ± 85 ng/mL in 36 healthy controls *1893*

Soluble E-Selectin *Serum* *Decrease* In 7 patients with sclerotic systemic sclerosis mean concentration of 37 ± 9 ng/mL not significantly different from 48 ± 19 ng/mL in 36 healthy controls *1893*
Serum *Increase* In 80 patients mean concentration of 83.7 ± 30.7 ng/mL significantly higher than 53.5 ± 14.6 ng/mL in 20 healthy controls *2321* In 5 patients with early edematous systemic sclerosis mean concentration of 59 ± 11 ng/mL not significantly different from 48 ± 19 ng/mL in 36 healthy controls *1893*

Soluble gp130 *Serum* *No Effect* In 55 patients with systemic sclerosis median concentration of 311 pg/mL (range 180 - 800 pg/mL) not significantly different from median of 316 pg/mL (range 232 - 520 pg/mL) in 20 healthy controls *2044*

Soluble Intercellular Adhesion Molecule-1 *Serum* *Increase* In 80 patients significant positive correlation with sVCAM-1 concentration *2321* Mean concentration in 12 patients with systemic sclerosis ranged from 15 to 81 ng/mL compared with 25 ± 12 ng/mL (range 13 - 42) in 30 healthy controls *2086*

Soluble Interleukin-2 Receptor *Serum* *Increase* In 20 patients with systemic sclerosis mean concentration of 154 ± 185 pmol/L significantly different from 54 ± 29 pmol/L in 20 healthy controls *2322* In 18 patients with mean concentration of 6,026 ± 4,300 pg/mL significantly different from 4,704 ± 1,400 pg/mL in 25 healthy controls *5113* In a study of 48 patients with systemic sclerosis (SSc). elevated serum levels of soluble interleukin 2 receptor (IL-2R), were noted in 100% of early untreated patients with SSc *862*

Soluble Interleukin-6 Receptor *Serum* *Increase* In 55 patients with systemic sclerosis median concentration of 820 pg/mL (range 390 - 1,400 pg/mL) significantly greater than median of 650 pg/mL (range 430 - 1,000 pg/mL) in 20 healthy controls *2044*

710.10 Systemic Sclerosis *(continued)*

Soluble Interleukin-6 Receptor *(continued)*
Serum No Effect In 22 patients with early diffuse cutaneous systemic sclerosis median concentration of 640 pg/mL (range 520 - 1,220 pg/mL) and in 12 patients with late diffuse cutaneous systemic sclerosis median concentration of 770 pg/mL (range 440 - 1,170 pg/mL not significantly greater than median of 650 pg/mL (range 430 - 1,000 pg/mL) in 20 healthy controls *2044*

Soluble Vascular Cell Adhesion Molecule-1
Serum Decrease In 7 patients with sclerotic systemic sclerosis mean concentration of 437 ± 179 ng/mL not significantly different from 497 ± 43 ng/mL in 36 healthy controls *1893*
Serum Increase In 80 patients mean concentration of 786.6 ± 297.6 ng/mL significantly higher than 506.8 ± 127.3 ng/mL in 20 healthy controls *2321* In 5 patients with early edematous systemic sclerosis mean concentration of 952 ± 177 ng/mL significantly different from 497 ± 43 ng/mL in 36 healthy controls *1893*

Thrombomodulin *Plasma Increase* Mean concentration of 65 ng/mL in 6 patients significantly higher than 10 ng/mL in 66 healthy controls *3873*
Plasma No Effect In 30 patients with limited systemic sclerosis mean concentration of 41.33 ± 14.25 ng/mL and 50.07 ± 14.57 ng/mL in 27 patients with diffuse systemic sclerosis significantly different from 23.32 ± 8.53 ng/mL in 40 healthy controls *4535*

Triglycerides *Serum No Effect* Mean concentration in 20 patients with systemic sclerosis of 1.0 ± 0.2 mmol/L not significantly different from 1.3 ± 0.1 mmol/L in 18 healthy controls *3597*

Tumor Necrosis Factor-α *Serum Increase* In 18 patients with mean concentration of 11.0 ± 6.0 pg/mL significantly different from 5.8 ± 2.3 pg/mL in 25 healthy controls *5113*

Vascular Endothelial Growth Factor *Serum Increase* Mean concentration in 40 patients with systemic sclerosis of 360 ± 233 pg/mL significantly different from 184 ± 62 pg/mL in 20 healthy individuals *2674*

von Willebrand Factor *Plasma Increase* In 8 patients with limited systemic sclerosis mean concentration of 240% and 262% in 16 with diffuse sclerosis mean compared with 100% in normal individuals *4619*

710.20 Sjögren's Syndrome

Acid *Urine Increase* In 18 of 27 patients with Sjögren's syndrome renal tubular acidosis observed *1381*

Albumin *Serum Decrease* Common *900*

Amino Acids *Urine No Effect* In none of 27 patients with Sjögren's syndrome was abnormal excretion of amino acids observed *1381*

Ammonium Ions *Urine Increase* May be associated with classic distal renal tubular acidosis which is asociated with hyokalemia, hyperchloremic metabolic acidosis, urine pH > 5.5, increased urinary ammonium ion excretion, a negative urine anion gap, increased urinary osmol gap, decreased urinary citrate and increased urinary calcium in some patients *4071* May lead to proximal renal tubular acidosis which is associated with hypokalemia, hyperchloremic metabolic acidosis, urine pH < 5.5, increased urinary ammonium ion excretion, a negative urine anion gap, increased urinary osmol gap, normal urinary citrate, normal urinary calcium excretion and Fanconi syndrome *4071*

Angiotensin-converting Enzyme *Serum Increase* A study of 21 cases of this syndrome revealed that only 2 cases had elevated levels and these were only modest increases *3183 3041 4488*
Serum No Effect Raised activity isn't usually associated with this syndrome *3183*

Anion Gap *Urine Decrease* May be associated with classic distal renal tubular acidosis which is asociated with hyokalemia, hyperchloremic metabolic acidosis, urine pH > 5.5, increased urinary ammonium ion excretion, a negative urine anion gap, increased urinary osmol gap, decreased urinary citrate and increased urinary calcium in some patients *4071* May lead to proximal renal tubular acidosis which is associated with hypokalemia, hyperchloremic metabolic acidosis, urine pH < 5.5, increased urinary ammonium ion excretion, a negative urine anion gap, increased urinary osmol gap, normal urinary citrate, normal urinary calcium excretion and Fanconi syndrome *4071*

Anti-ds DNA Antibodies *Serum No Effect* Found in 0% of cases *4897*

Anti-Mitochondrial Antibodies *Serum Increase* May occur *4767* Found in 18% of patients and 2% of controls *4176*

Anti-Neutrophil Cytoplasm Antibodies *Serum No Effect* Antibodies not detected in any of 10 patients *162*

Anti-Ribonuclear Protein Antibodies *Serum Increase* Found in 5% of cases *4897*

Anti-Sjögren's Syndrome A Antibodies (SSA[Ro])
Serum Increase Found in 70% of cases *4897* Increased concentration observed in 40 - 50% patients with Sjogren's syndrome *2952* In 25 patients with Sjogren's syndrome mean concentration increased above normal in 61% of patients on initial examination *275*

Anti-Sjögren's Syndrome B Antibodies (SSB[La])
Serum Increase In 25 patients with Sjogren's syndrome mean concentration increased above normal in 36% of patients on initial examination *275* Increased concentration observed in 40 - 50% patients with Sjogren's syndrome *2952* Found in 60% of cases *4897*

Anti-Smith Antibodies *Serum No Effect* Found in 0% of cases *4897*

Anti-ss DNA Antibodies *Serum No Effect* Found in 0% of cases *4897*

Antibody Titer *Serum Increase* Antibodies to reticulin. 75% of patients exhibit antibodies to salivary duct epithelium *3712*

α_1-Antichymotrypsin *Serum Increase* Reported effect *2457* Collagen vascular diseases *2628*

Antinuclear Antibodies *Serum Increase* Present in about 60% (fluorescent technique) *2039* In 9 of 35 tested patients with postpartum thyroiditis titers of greater than 1:40 observed *1899* Demonstrable in close to 70% of patients *484* 40 - 75% positivity *4068* Observed increased positivity *4551*

Antithyroglobulin Antibodies *Serum Increase* Rare *123*

Bicarbonate *Serum Decrease* May lead to proximal renal tubular acidosis which is associated with hypokalemia, hyperchloremic metabolic acidosis, urine pH < 5.5, increased urinary ammonium ion excretion, a negative urine anion gap, increased urinary osmol gap, normal urinary citrate, normal urinary calcium excretion and Fanconi syndrome *4071*

Calcium *Urine Increase* May be associated with classic distal renal tubular acidosis which is associated with hyokalemia, hyperchloremic metabolic acidosis, urine pH > 5.5, increased urinary ammonium ion excretion, a negative urine anion gap, increased urinary osmol gap, decreased urinary citrate and increased urinary calcium in some patients *4071*
Urine No Effect May lead to proximal renal tubular acidosis which is associated with hypokalemia, hyperchloremic metabolic acidosis, urine pH < 5.5, increased urinary ammonium ion excretion, a negative urine anion gap, increased urinary osmol gap, normal urinary citrate, normal urinary calcium excretion and Fanconi syndrome *4071*

Chloride *Serum Increase* May lead to proximal renal tubular acidosis which is associated with hypokalemia, hyperchloremic metabolic acidosis, urine pH < 5.5, increased urinary ammonium ion excretion, a negative urine anion gap, increased urinary osmol gap, normal urinary citrate, normal urinary calcium excretion and Fanconi syndrome *4071* May be associated with classic distal renal tubular acidosis which is associated with hyokalemia, hyperchloremic metabolic acidosis, urine pH > 5.5, increased urinary ammonium ion excretion, a negative urine anion gap, increased urinary osmol gap, decreased urinary citrate and increased urinary calcium in some patients *4071*

Citrate *Urine Decrease* May be associated with classic distal renal tubular acidosis which is associated with hyokalemia, hyperchloremic metabolic acidosis, urine pH > 5.5, increased urinary ammonium ion excretion, a negative urine anion gap, increased urinary osmol gap, decreased urinary citrate and increased urinary calcium in some patients *4071* In 20 of 27 patients with Sjögren's syndrome excretion less than > 2.50 mmol/d in healthy women *1381*

Urine *No Effect* May lead to proximal renal tubular acidosis which is associated with hypokalemia, hyperchloremic metabolic acidosis, urine pH < 5.5, increased urinary ammonium ion excretion, a negative urine anion gap, increased urinary osmol gap, normal urinary citrate, normal urinary calcium excretion and Fanconi syndrome *4071*

Complement C_3 *Serum* *Decrease* Caused by hypercatabolism *785* *2694* *1588* *1033*

Complement C_3d *Serum* *Increase* In 25 patients with Sjogren's syndrome mean concentration increased above normal in 5% of patients on initial examination *275*

Complement, Total *Serum* *Decrease* Occasionally decreased, especially with cryoglobulinemia *4683*

Coombs' Test *Serum* *Positive* May occur *4767*

Copper *Serum* *Increase* Increased *4871* *3900* *4586*

C-Reactive Protein *Serum* *Increase* In 25 patients with Sjogren's syndrome mean concentration increased above normal in 7% of patients on initial examination *275*

Cryoglobulins *Serum* *Increase* Variable elevation of cryoglobulins *4707*

1,25-Dihydroxy Vitamin D *Serum* *Increase* In 25 patients with Sjogren's syndrome mean concentration of 60 ± 12 pg/mL on initial examination and 26 ± 9 pg/mL at two years's follow-up examination compared with normal of 33 ± 9 pg/mL *275*

Elastase Antineutrophil Cytoplasmic Autoantibodies
Serum *No Effect* Antibodies not detected in any of 10 patients *162*

Eosinophils *Blood* *Increase* Occurs in about 25% of the patients *4767*

Epstein Barr Virus Antibodies *Serum* *Increase* The average IgG antibody titers to domains of the five EBV nuclear antigens (EBNA-1,2,3,4, and 6), especially the amino-terminal domain of EBNA-2 in sera of patients with this syndrome were slightly higher than those in normal sera *2337*

Erythrocyte Sedimentation Rate *Blood* *Increase* In approximately 66% of patients *4767*

Fractional Excretion of Sodium *Urine* *No Effect* In none of 27 patients with Sjögren's syndrome was abnormal fractional excretion of sodium observed *1381*

γ-Globulin *Serum* *Increase* Electrophoresis shows increase globulins largely due to 7S γ-globulin *5545* Hypergammaglobulinemia characterized by a diffuse increase in IgG, IgA, and IgM is found especially in those patients with the sicca complex not accompanied by a connective tissue disease *1913* Present in most cases *2039*

Glucose *Urine* *Increase* May lead to proximal renal tubular acidosis which is associated with hypokalemia, hyperchloremic metabolic acidosis, urine pH < 5.5, increased urinary ammonium ion excretion, a negative urine anion gap, increased urinary osmol gap, normal urinary citrate, normal urinary calcium excretion and Fanconi syndrome *4071*
Urine *No Effect* In none of 27 patients with Sjögren's syndrome was abnormal excretion of glucose observed *1381*

γ-Glutamyltransferase *Saliva* *Increase* Significantly higher (19.6 U/L) versus controls (5.12 U/L) *2448*

Hematocrit *Blood* *Decrease* Mild normochromic, normocytic anemia occurs in about 25% of patients *900* Anemia is seen in 33% of patients *4767*

Hemoglobin *Blood* *Decrease* Anemia is seen in 33% of patients *4767* Mild normochromic, normocytic anemia occurs in about 25% of patients *900*

HLA Antigens *Blood* *Present* HLA-DR3 present in 75% of patients versus 21% of controls *5678* Increased frequency of HLA-DR2 and HLA-DR3 and decrease. HLA-DR4 in primary disease and increased DR4 with normal freq. DR2 and DR3 in secondary *5428* HLA-DR3 found found in 84% of patients with this disease compared to 24% of controls *4584*

25-Hydroxy Vitamin D *Serum* *Decrease* In 25 patients with Sjogren's syndrome mean concentration of 21 ± 7 ng/mL on initial examination and 20 ± 10 ng/mL at two years's follow-up examination compared with normal of 28 ± 12 ng/mL *275*

immunoglobulin A *Serum* *Increase* Reported effect *4551* In 25 patients with Sjogren's syndrome mean concentration increased above normal in 63% of patients on initial examination *275* Hypergammaglobulinemia characterized by a diffuse increase in IgG, IgA, and IgM is found especially in those patients with the sicca complex not accompanied by a connective tissue disease *1913*

Immunoglobulin G *Serum* *Increase* The elevated globulin is usually 7S γ-globulin IgG and is not monoclonal *900* In 25 patients with Sjogren's syndrome mean concentration increased above normal in 66% of patients on initial examination *275* Hypergammaglobulinemia characterized by a diffuse increase in IgG, IgA, and IgM is found especially in those patients with the sicca complex not accompanied by a connective tissue disease *1913*

Immunoglobulin M *Serum* *Increase* Reported effect *4551* Hypergammaglobulinemia characterized by a diffuse increase in IgG, IgA, and IgM is found especially in those patients with the sicca complex not accompanied by a connective tissue disease *1913* In 25 patients with Sjogren's syndrome mean concentration increased above normal in 22% of patients on initial examination *275*

LE Cells *Blood* *Positive* Found in 15 - 20% of patients *4767*

Leukocytes *Blood* *Decrease* Occurs in 25% of patients *4767* Occurs in about 25% of the patients *900*

β_2-Macroglobulin *Saliva* *Increase* Normal *1588*
Serum *Increase* Often elevated and correlates well with the degree of lymphocytic infiltration seen on biopsy *4767*

α_1-Microglobulin *Urine* *Increase* In 11 of 27 patients with Sjögren's syndrome increased excretion above 10 mg/L in heathy individuals observed *1381*

β_2-Microglobulin *Serum* *Increase* In 25 patients with Sjogren's syndrome mean concentration increased above normal in 41% of patients on initial examination *275*

Myeloperoxidase Antineutrophil Cytoplasmic Autoantibodies
Serum *No Effect* Antibodies not detected in any of 10 patients *162*

N-Acetyl-Glucosaminidase *Urine* *Increase* In 7 of 27 patients with Sjögren's syndrome increased excretion above 8μkat/mol creatinine observed in healthy individuals *1381*

Net Acid Excretion *Urine* *Increase* May be associated with classic distal renal tubular acidosis which is associated with hyokalemia, hyperchloremic metabolic acidosis, urine pH > 5.5, increased urinary ammonium ion excretion, a negative urine anion gap, increased urinary osmol gap, decreased urinary citrate and increased urinary calcium in some patients *4071*

Osmolal Gap *Urine* *Increase* May be associated with classic distal renal tubular acidosis which is asociated with hyokalemia, hyperchloremic metabolic acidosis, urine pH > 5.5, increased urinary ammonium ion excretion, a negative urine anion gap, increased urinary osmol gap, decreased urinary citrate and increased urinary calcium in some patients *4071* May lead to proximal renal tubular acidosis which is associated with hypokalemia, hyperchloremic metabolic acidosis, urine pH < 5.5, increased urinary ammonium ion excretion, a negative urine anion gap, increased urinary osmol gap, normal urinary citrate, normal urinary calcium excretion and Fanconi syndrome *4071*

Perinuclear Antineutrophil Cytoplasmic Autoantibodies
Serum *Increase* Antibodies detected in 30% of 10 patients *162*

pH *Urine* *Decrease* May lead to proximal renal tubular acidosis which is associated with hypokalemia, hyperchloremic metabolic acidosis, urine pH < 5.5, increased urinary ammonium ion excretion, a negative urine anion gap, increased urinary osmol gap, normal urinary citrate, normal urinary calcium excretion and Fanconi syndrome *4071*
Urine *Increase* May be associated with classic distal renal tubular acidosis which is associated with hyokalemia, hyperchloremic metabolic acidosis, urine pH > 5.5, increased urinary ammonium ion excretion, a negative urine anion gap, increased urinary osmol gap, decreased urinary citrate and increased urinary calcium in some patients *4071*

Phosphate *Serum* *Decrease* May lead to proximal renal tubular acidosis which is associated with hypokalemia, hyperchloremic metabolic acidosis, urine pH < 5.5, increased urinary ammonium ion excretion, a negative urine anion gap, increased urinary osmol gap, normal urinary citrate, normal urinary calcium excretion and Fanconi syndrome *4071*

Potassium *Serum* *Decrease* In 1 of 27 patients with Sjögren's syndrome hypokalemia observed in association with

710.20 Sjögren's Syndrome *(continued)*

Potassium *(continued)*
incomplete renal tubular acidosis *1381* May be associated with classic distal renal tubular acidosis which is asociated with hyokalemia, hyperchloremic metabolic acidosis, urine pH > 5.5, increased urinary ammonium ion excretion, a negative urine anion gap, increased urinary osmol gap, decreased urinary citrate and increased urinary calcium in some patients *4071* May lead to proximal renal tubular acidosis which is associated with hypokalemia, hyperchloremic metabolic acidosis, urine pH < 5.5, increased urinary ammonium ion excretion, a negative urine anion gap, increased urinary osmol gap, normal urinary citrate, normal urinary calcium excretion and Fanconi syndrome *4071*

Proteinase 3-Antineutrophil Cytoplasmic Autoantibodies
Serum *No Effect* Antibodies not detected in any of 10 patients *162*

Rheumatoid Factor *Serum* *Increase* Detected in > 70% of cases, regardless of the presence or absence of rheumatoid arthritis *4767* Rheumatoid factor may be observed in certain patients *2473* 96% positivity *874* High incidence even when not associated with a connective disease; the incidence of seropositivity is greatest in definite RA *1980* Mean concentration increased in patients with Sjogren's disease *2472*

Rheumatoid Factor (IgA) *Serum* *Increase* In 25 patients with Sjogren's syndrome mean concentration increased above normal in 80% of patients on initial examination *275*

Rheumatoid Factor (IgM) *Serum* *Increase* In 25 patients with Sjogren's syndrome mean concentration increased above normal in 83% of patients on initial examination *275*

Soluble Intercellular Adhesion Molecule-1 *Serum* *No Effect* Mean concentration in 12 patients with Sjogren's syndrome ranged from 13 to 44 ng/mL compared with 25 ± 12 ng/mL (range 13 - 42) in 30 healthy controls *2086*

SSA Antibodies *Serum* *Positive* 17 of 35 patients with postpartum thyroiditis were anti-SSA positive after the postpartum period and all except 3 were positive at follow-up *1899*

SSB Antibodies *Serum* *Positive* In 13 of 35 patients with postpartum thyroiditis induced Sjogren's syndrome SSB antibodies observed *1899*

Thrombomodulin *Plasma* *No Effect* In 35 patients with Sjogren's syndrome mean concentration of 16 ng/mL not significantly different from 10 ng/mL in 66 healthy controls *3873*

Tubular Maximum for Phosphate *Urine* *Decrease* In 18 of 27 patients with Sjögren's syndrome tubular reabsorption less than > 79% in normal adults *1381*

Uric Acid *Serum* *Decrease* May lead to proximal renal tubular acidosis which is associated with hypokalemia, hyperchloremic metabolic acidosis, urine pH < 5.5, increased urinary ammonium ion excretion, a negative urine anion gap, increased urinary osmol gap, normal urinary citrate, normal urinary calcium excretion and Fanconi syndrome *4071*
Urine *No Effect* In none of 27 patients with Sjögren's syndrome was abnormal excretion of uric acid observed *1381*

710.40 Dermatomyositis

Aldolase *Serum* *Increase* Increased activities observed in patients with dermatomyositis *2952*

Anti-Endothelial Cell Antibodies *Serum* *Increase* AECA have been detected in systemic lupus erythematosus, scleroderma and dermatomyositis but are also found in systemic vasculitis, Kawasaki disease, hemolytic uremic syndrome, thrombotic thrombocytopenic purpura and renal allograft recipients at the time of rejection *1174*

Autoantibodies to Jo1 Antigen *Serum* *Increase* Concentration increased in 10% of patients with dermatomyositis *2952*

Creatine *Urine* *Increase* Urinary creatine may be significantly increased in patients with dermatomyositis *2952*

Neopterin *Serum* *Increase* In 15 patients with primary dermatositis mean concentration of 20.6 ± 11.3 nmol/L significantly greater than 5.2 ± 1.8 nmol/L in healthy controls, with 92% having values greater than the 95th percentile in healthy controls *4550*

Soluble Interleukin-2 Receptor *Serum* *Increase* In 15 patients with primary dermatomyositis mean concentration of 883 ± 553 U/mL significantly greater than 509 ± 207 U/mL in healthy controls, with 38% having a value greater than the 95th percentile in the healthy controls *4550*

Soluble Tumor Necrosis Factor Receptor-p55
Serum *Increase* In 15 patients with primary dermatositis mean concentration of 4.33 ± 2.61 ngmL significantly greater than 2.55 ± 0.7 ng/mL in healthy controls, with 46% having values greater than the 95th percentile in the healthy controls *4550*

Vascular Endothelial Growth Factor *Serum* *Increase* Mean concentration in 49 patients with polymyositis/dermatositis of 352 ± 273 pg/mL significantly different from 184 ± 62 pg/mL in 20 healthy individuals *2674*

710.40 Dermatomyositis/Polymyositis

Alanine Aminotransferase *Serum* *Increase* In general, serum enzymes correlate well with the disease activity and are useful therapeutic and prognostic indicators *900* Elevated at some time in nearly every patient *505*

Aldolase *Serum* *Increase* Released as a result of destructive myopathy. Almost invariably elevated in the acute or subacute stages *4051* Elevated at some time in nearly every patient *505*

Angiotensin-converting Enzyme *Serum* *Increase* Observed effect *3041* Reported effect *4488*

Anti-ds DNA Antibodies *Serum* *Increase* Found in 25% of cases of dermatomyositis *4897*

Anti-Ribonuclear Protein Antibodies *Serum* *No Effect* Found in 0% of cases *4897*

Anti-Smith Antibodies *Serum* *No Effect* Found in 0% of cases of dermatomyositis *4897*

Antibody Titer *Serum* *Increase* Occasionally patients with dermatomyositis display antibodies to striated muscle *3712*

Antinuclear Antibodies *Serum* *Increase* 40% of patients were ANA positive and LE cell negative *646* *646* Reported to be positive in 25%, positive only in a few cases of uncomplicated disease; positive titer in 2%, contrary to other reports. Higher titers were found in patients with other complications *505* Positive in 35% of patients tested, although only 2% of patients with pure disease had detectable levels *4051* Reported effect *4068* Found in 82% of cases of polymyositis *4897* Reported effect *4551*

Aspartate Aminotransferase *Serum* *Increase* Released as a result of destructive myopathy. Almost invariably elevated in the acute or subacute stages *4051* Observed effect *1980* May be increased in the absence of clinical evidence of muscle wasting. Steroid therapy causes the level to fall towards normal *1290* Moderate to marked increase. Usual values < 145 U/L *1025* Elevated at some time in nearly every patient *505*

Cholinesterase *Serum* *Decrease* With serum albumin *5544*

Complement, Total *Serum* *Decrease* In 15 patients, 20% had decreased values *4925*
Serum *Increase* Elevated during active inflammation and subsides with remission *4683* In 15 patients, 13% had increased values *4925*

Copper *Serum* *Increase* Increased *4586* *4871* *3900*

Creatine *Urine* *Increase* Urine shows a moderate increase in creatine and a decrease in creatinine *5544*

Creatine Kinase *Serum* *Increase* Released as a result of destructive myopathy *4051* Elevated at some time in nearly every patient. Most consistent of the serum enzymes and correlated best with clinical course and parameters of activity *505* Almost invariably elevated in the acute stages, whereas in the clinically inactive cases or in those in remission they are often normal *4551*

Creatine Kinase MB-Isoenzyme *Serum* *Increase* Reported effect *248*

Creatinine *Urine* *Decrease* Active disease. As the urine creatine increases, so the urine creatinine falls *1290*

Eosinophils *Blood* *Increase* Frequently increased *5544*

Erythrocyte Sedimentation Rate *Blood* *Increase* Moderately to markedly increased; may be normal *5544*
Blood *No Effect* Moderately to markedly increased; may be normal *5544*

α_2-Globulin *Serum* *Increase* Commonly elevated *367*

γ-Globulin *Serum* *Increase* Commonly elevated *367*

Haptoglobin *Serum* *Increase* Conditions associated with increased ESR and α_2-globulin; increases in collagen diseases *5544*

Hematocrit *Blood* *Decrease* Mild anemia may be expected *900*

Hemoglobin *Blood* *Decrease* Mild anemia may be expected *900*

Immunoglobulin D *Serum* *Increase* Reported effect *1290*

Lactate Dehydrogenase *Serum* *Increase* Elevated at some time in nearly every patient *505* Elevation in both acute and chronic polymyositis *2226* Moderate to marked increase *1025* Increased but less sensitive indicator of muscle injury *1980*

Lactate Dehydrogenase Isoenzyme-5 *Serum* *Increase* In cases of chronic polymyositis, a relative but mild rise was noted *2226* May be increased, paralleling the increased LD *5544*

Lactate Dehydrogenase Isoenzymes *Serum* *Increase* In cases of chronic polymyositis, a relative but mild rise was noted *2226*

LE Cells *Blood* *Positive* 40% of patients were ANA positive and LE cell negative *646* About 5% of patients have positive test *367*

Leukocytes *Blood* *Increase* Mild leukocytosis occurs, especially in acute cases *367* May be expected *900*

Malate Dehydrogenase *Serum* *Increase* May be increased but offers no additional diagnostic value *5544*

Myoglobin *Urine* *Increase* In severe cases *5544*

Rheumatoid Factor *Serum* *Increase* Positive (> 1:40) in 18 of 82 recorded (20%): including 5 patients (6%) with pure polymyositis (Type I), 4 (5%) with pure dermatomyositis (Type II), and 9 (10%) with the overlap type (Type V) *4551* Reported to be positive in 40%. Positive only in a few cases of uncomplicated disease. Positive titer in 10% contrary to other reports. Higher titers were found in patients with other complications *505* Positive in 10 - 50% of patients *367*

710.40 Myositis

Aspartate Aminotransferase *Serum* *Increase* May cause increased AST activity *4617*

Complement C_1 *Serum* *No Effect* Mean concentration typically normal or slightly increased in patients with myositis *4682*

Complement C_1q *Serum* *No Effect* Mean concentration typically normal or slightly increased in patients with myositis *4682*

Complement C_2 *Serum* *No Effect* Mean concentration typically normal or slightly increased in patients with myositis *4682*

Complement C_3 *Serum* *No Effect* Mean concentration typically normal or slightly increased in patients with myositis *4682*

Complement C_4 *Serum* *No Effect* Mean concentration typically normal or slightly increased in patients with myositis *4682*

Complement C_5 *Serum* *No Effect* Mean concentration typically normal or slightly increased in patients with myositis *4682*

Complement CH50 *Serum* *No Effect* Mean concentration typically normal or slightly increased in patients with myositis *4682*

Properdin Factor B *Plasma* *No Effect* Mean concentration typically normal or slightly increased in patients with myositis *4682*

710.40 Polymyositis

Aldolase *Serum* *Increase* Increased activities observed in patients with poliomyositis *2952*

Anti-Ku Antibodies *Serum* *Increase* Isolation and characterization of cDNA encoding the 80-kDa subunit protein of the human autoantigen Ku (p70/p80) recognized by autoantibodies from patients with scleroderma-polymyositis overlap syndrome *3503* *5788*

Autoantibodies to Jo1 Antigen *Serum* *Increase* Concentration increased in 30% of patients with polymyositis *2952*

C-Reactive Protein *Serum* *No Effect* In 15 patients with polymyositis/dermatomyositis mean concentration of 0.48 ± 0.26 mg/dL not significantly different from normal *1613*

Erythrocyte Sedimentation Rate *Serum* *Increase* In 15 patients with polymyositis/dermatomyositis mean rate of 21 ± 24.5 mm/h significantly different from normal *1613*

Interleukin-1 Receptor Antagonist *Serum* *Increase* In 15 patients with polymyositis/dermatomyositis mean concentration of 755 ± 4,374 pg/mL significantly different from normal *1613*

Interleukin-1β *Serum* *No Effect* In 15 patients with polymyositis/dermatomyositis mean concentration of 15 ± 0 pg/mL not significantly different from normal *1613*

Interleukin-6 *Serum* *Increase* In 15 patients with polymyositis/dermatomyositis mean concentration of 21 ± 21 pg/mL significantly different from normal *1613* Significant elevations of IL-6 levels were observed in the sera of patients with polymyositis (119 ± 72 pg/mL), when compared to those of controls ($p < 0.05$) *4800*

Manganese Superoxide Dismutase *Serum* *Increase* Markedly higher in the serum of patients with untreated form of this disease *5761*

Neopterin *Serum* *Increase* In 15 patients with primary polymyositis mean concentration of 11.3 ± 4.6 nmol/L significantly greater than 5.2 ± 1.8 nmol/L in healthy controls, with 60% having a value greater than the 95th percentile in the healthy controls *4550*

Rheumatoid Factor *Serum* *Increase* Concentration may be increased as in other diseases with chronic inflammation *2952*

Soluble Interleukin-2 Receptor *Serum* *Increase* In 15 patients with primary polymyositis mean concentration of 685 ± 409 U/mL significantly greater than 509 ± 207 U/mL in healthy controls, with 20% having a value greater than the 95th percentile in the healthy controls *4550*

Soluble Tumor Necrosis Factor Receptor-p55 *Serum* *Increase* In 15 patients with primary polymyositis mean concentration of 3.26 ± 1.45 ngmL significantly greater than 2.55 ± 0.7 ng/mL in healthy controls, with 13% having values greater than the 95th percentile in the healthy controls *4550* In 15 patients with polymyositis/dermatomyositis mean concentration of 3.5 ± 2.02 ng/mL significantly different from normal *1613*

Soluble Tumor Necrosis Factor Receptor-p75 *Serum* *Increase* In 15 patients with polymyositis/dermatomyositis mean concentration of 8.9 ± 5.05 ng/mL significantly different from normal *1613*

Thrombomodulin *Plasma* *Increase* Mean concentration in 7 patients with myositis or dermatomyositis of 75 ng/mL significantly higher than 10 ng/mL in 66 healthy controls *3873*

Tumor Necrosis Factor-α *Serum* *No Effect* In 15 patients with polymyositis/dermatomyositis mean concentration of 30 ± 9 pg/mL not significantly different from normal *1613*

Vascular Endothelial Growth Factor *Serum* *Increase* Mean concentration in 49 patients with polymyositis/dermatositis of 352 ± 273 pg/mL significantly different from 184 ± 62 pg/mL in 20 healthy individuals *2674*

710.50 Eosinophilia-Myalgia Syndrome

Antinuclear Antibodies *Serum* *Increase* Antinuclear antibodies detected in 61.5% of 39 patients with L-tryptophan-associated eosinophilia-myalgia syndrome *2589*

710.90 Connective Tissue Disease

Brain Natriuretic Peptide *Urine* *Increase* In 8 patients with connective tissue disease mean excretion of 6.28 ± 0.98 pmol/d significantly different from that in 11 healthy individuals in whom the mean excretion was 3.82 ± 0.62 pmol/d *5265*

Creatinine Clearance *Urine* *Decrease* In 7 patients with connective tissue disease mean clearance of 59.7 ± 14.0 mL/min significantly different from that in 11 healthy individuals *5265*

Soluble HLA-I *Cerebrospinal Fluid* *No Effect* In 2 patients with connective tissue disease mean concentration undetectable *216*

Soluble HLA-II *Cerebrospinal Fluid* *Increase* In 2 patients with connective tissue disease, mean concentration of 230 U/mL *216*

710.90 Mixed Connective Tissue Disease

Angiotensin-converting Enzyme *Serum* *Increase* Mean concentration of 26.4 ± 14.0 mU/mL in 6 patients with MCTD and pulmonary hypertension compared with 16.5 ± 3.9 mU/mL in 18 controls *3957*
Serum *No Effect* Mean activity of 16.8 ± 4.1 mU/mL in 18 patients with MCTD but without pulmonary hypertension compared with 16.5 ± 3.9 mU/mL in 18 controls *3957*

Anti-ds DNA Antibodies *Serum* *Increase* Found in 25% of cases *4897*

Anti-Ku Antibodies *Serum* *Increase* 5 - 15% of patients with this disease *5788*

Anti-Neutrophil Cytoplasm Antibodies *Serum* *No Effect* In 0 of 2 patients (0%) with mixed connective tissue disease pANCA detected *3722*

Anti-Ribonuclear Protein Antibodies *Serum* *Increase* Found in 100% of cases *4897*

Anti-Smith Antibodies *Serum* *Increase* Found in 8% of cases *4897*

Antinuclear Antibodies *Serum* *Increase* In 2 of 2 patients (100%) with mixed connective tissue disease ANA detected *3722* Usually high titers (> 1:1000), speckled pattern *126*

Complement, Total *Serum* *Decrease* In 30% of cases *126*

Creatine Kinase MB-Isoenzyme *Serum* *Increase* Observed effect *248*

γ-Globulin *Serum* *Increase* Diffuse hypergammaglobulinemia *126* *126*

Hematocrit *Blood* *Decrease* Anemia *126*

Hemoglobin *Blood* *Decrease* Anemia *126*

Hyaluronic Acid *Serum* *Increase* The greatest increases were in patients with overlap syndrome. Mean value of 202 µg/L compared to 49 µg/L in controls *1370*

Leukocytes *Blood* *Decrease* Leukopenia *126*

Platelets *Blood* *Decrease* Thrombocytopenia *126*

Procollagen Type III Peptide *Serum* *Increase* Serum P-III-P levels were elevated in patients with PSS and MCTD/overlap syndrome, suggesting a high rate of collagen biosynthesis by fibroblasts. Patients with RA showed no significant elevation of serum P-III-P compared with normal control group *155*

Rheumatoid Factor *Serum* *Increase* Found in over 50% of cases. Titer is usually very high *126* Rheumatoid factor may be observed in certain patients *2473* Mean concentration increased in patients with mixed connective tissue disease *2472*

710.90 Overlap Syndrome

Procollagen Type II Peptide *Serum* *Increase* Raised serum IgG anti-type II collagen antibody levels were present in 11% of patients with RA, 30% with SLE, 44% with PSS and 42% with OL *1600*

710.90 Undifferentiated Connective Tissue Disease

Angiotensin-converting Enzyme *Serum* *No Effect* Mean activity of 16.8 ± 4.1 mU/mL in 14 patients with MCTD but without pulmonary hypertension compared with 16.5 ± 3.9 mU/mL in 18 controls *3957*

Anti-Ku Antibodies *Serum* *Increase* 7 of 7 patients with undifferentiated connective tissue disease had anti-Ku antibodies *921*

Antinuclear Antibodies *Serum* *Increase* 7 of 7 patients with undifferentiated connective tissue disease had anti-nuclear antibodies *921*

711.00 Acute Arthritis (Pyogenic)

Complement, Total *Synovial Fluid* *Decrease* Compared to total protein, levels are low in 60 - 70% of joint effusions *631*

C-Reactive Protein *Serum* *Increase* In 12 positive culture patients, 4 of whom had positive gram stains, mean concentration of 145 mg/L and in 12 culture-negative patients, one of whom was gram-stain positive, mean concentration of 120 mg/L *2778*

Glucose *Serum* *Decrease* Low in most cases *2039*

Lactate *Synovial Fluid* *Increase* Reported effect *413*

Leukocytes *Blood* *Increase* Counts frequently exceed 50,000 /µL, higher than in other types of arthritis *2039* Routine blood studies should reflect the presence of a closed space infection with a polymorphonuclear leukocytosis *900* Elevated total WBC count *1328*
Synovial Fluid *Increase* May vary from 10,000 - 300,000 /µL, depending upon the stage of infection and inflammatory response. The cells are predominantly polymorphonuclear *900* In 12 positive culture patients, 4 of whom had positive gram stains, mean leukocyte count 94,000 /µL and in 12 culture-negative patients, one of whom was gram-stain positive, mean count 49,000 cells/µL *2778* Infected fluid is characteristically turbid or purulent, with a count of 100,000 /µL or more, with a differential of 90% polymorphonuclears *5573*

L-Lactate *Synovial Fluid* *Increase* In 12 positive culture patients, 4 of whom had positive gram stains, mean concentration of 13.5 mmol/L and in 12 culture-negative patients, one of whom was gram-stain positive, mean concentration of 7.1 mmol/L *2778*

Neutrophils *Blood* *Increase* An elevated absolute neutrophil count *1328*
Synovial Fluid *Increase* Increase in number, ranging from 75 - 100 /µL *5544*

Nitroblue Tetrazolium Test *Blood* *Increase* NBT positive cells were found in synovial fluid of 7 of 8 patients, while only 4 showed positive peripheral blood tests *1922*
Synovial Fluid *Increase* NBT positive cells were found in synovial fluid of 7 of 8 patients, while only 4 showed positive peripheral blood tests *1922*

pH *Synovial Fluid* *Decrease* Close correlation (r = -0.092) was found between decreasing pH and increasing WBC in synovial fluid. The high WBC usually found in acute and chronic arthritis results in low pH which may contribute to the poor response to treatment with aminoglycoside antibiotics *5574*

Protein *Synovial Fluid* *Decrease* 30 - 40% of the plasma concentration *4398*

711.00 Purulent Arthritis

Phospholipase A_2 Type II *Synovial Fluid* *Increase* Considerable increase in catalytic activity observed in patients with purulent arthritis *3767*

711.00 Septic Arthritis

Prostaglandin E_2 *Synovial Fluid* *Increase* Mean concentration in 3 patients of 11.9 nmol/L *3366*

711.90 Infectious Arthritis

Interleukin-10 *Serum* *No Effect* In 8 patients with infectious arthritis mean concentration of 6.4 ± 4.5 U/mL not significantly different from 8.8 ± 1.9 U/mL in 22 healthy controls *986*
Synovial Fluid *No Effect* In 3 patients with inflammatory arthritis mean concentration of 3.0 ± 1.9 U/mL not significantly different from 8.8 ± 1.9 U/mL in serum of 22 healthy controls *986*

711.90 Inflammatory Arthritis

Amino-terminal Propeptide of Type III Collagen
Saliva *No Effect* In 20 patients with inflammatory joint disease median concentration of < 0.1 µg/L (range < 0.1 - 8.3 µg/L) not significantly different from < 0.1 µg/L (range < 0.1 - 2.7 µg/L) in 13 fit healthy volunteers *4773*

C-terminal Propeptide of Type I Procollagen
Saliva *Increase* In 20 patients with inflammatory joint disease median concentration of 10.5 µg/L (range < 0.1 - 219 µg/L) significantly higher than < 0.1 µg/L (range < 0.1 - 6.2 µg/L) in 13 fit healthy volunteers *4773*

Hyaluronic Acid *Serum* *Increase* In 20 patients with inflammatory joint disease median concentration of 91 µg/L (range 29 - 438 µg/L) higher than 61.5 µg/L (range 15 - 130 µg/L) in 13 fit healthy volunteers *4773*

Interleukin-10 *Serum* *No Effect* In 3 patients with inflammatory arthritis mean concentration of 0 U/mL not significantly different from 8.8 ± 1.9 U/mL in 22 healthy controls *986*
Synovial Fluid *No Effect* In 3 patients with inflammatory arthritis mean concentration of 4.9 ± 1.4 U/mL not significantly different from 8.8 ± 1.9 U/mL in serum of 22 healthy controls *986*

714.00 Rheumatoid Arthritis

α_1-Acid Glycoprotein *Serum* *Increase* One of the most reliable indicators of acute inflammation *4696* *4373* In 51 patients with rheumatoid arthritis median concentration of 1.7 and 1.3 g/L on two occasions significantly higher than upper limit of normal of 1.0 g/L in healthy individuals *5549* One of the most reliable indicators of acute inflammation *3713* Mean value for orosomucoid was elevated compared with that in control subjects *4174* One of the most reliable indicators of acute inflammation *4853* *2597* *4241*

Acid Phosphatase *Synovial Fluid* *Increase* Of 155 patients with different joint disorders, patients with rheumatoid arthritis showed significantly higher levels than those with bacterial arthritis, osteoarthritis and noninflammatory joint effusions. About 70% of the patients with RA had higher concentrations than those found among the patients with nonrheumatoid diseases *362*

Alanine Aminotransferase *Serum* *Increase* In 117 patients with rheumatoid arthritis mean value of 18.0 U/L compared with reference range of 10 - 41 U/L with 5.1% outside reference range *428*
Serum *No Effect* Generally normal *1980*

Albumin *Serum* *Decrease* Frequent finding attributed to generalized hypermetabolism. Corticosteroid administration accentuates hypoalbuminemia *4707* In 50 patients with rheumatoid arthritis with amyloidosis mean concentration of 3.4 ± 0.4 g/dL compared with 3.3 ± 0.5 g/dL in 45 patients with rheumatoid arthritis without amyloidosis less than 4.1 ± 0.2 g/dL in 41 healthy controls *5767* In 117 patients with rheumatoid arthritis mean value of 31.6 g/L compared with reference range of 32 - 52 g/L with 41.6% outside reference range *428*
Serum *No Effect* In 60 patients with rheumatoid arthritis mean concentration of 44 ± 5 g/L not significantly different from 42 ± 8 g/L in 57 heathy volunteers *4399*
Urine *Increase* No abnormalities are found in the urinalysis except for proteinuria *900*

Aldolase *Serum* *No Effect* In 40 patients with classic or definite rheumatoid arthritis mean activity normal *4565*

Alkaline Phosphatase *Serum* *Decrease* In 57 patients with rheumatoid arthritis median activity of 8.1 KA U/dL significantly different from 13 KA U/dL in healthy controls: increased activity found in 5.3% of rheumatoid arthritis *430*
Serum *Increase* In 117 patients with rheumatoid arthritis mean value of 98.3 U/L compared with reference range of 36 - 120 U/L with 17.9% outside reference range *428* In 57 adult patients with rheumatoid arthritis mean activity of 118.9 ± 12.6 U/L significantly different from 57.4 ± 1.5 U/L in 122 healthy control adults *2006* Characteristically abnormal when the arthritis is active *900*
Serum *No Effect* Generally normal *1980*

Alkaline Phosphatase Band-10 Isoenzyme *Serum* *Increase* In 57 adult patients with rheumatoid arthritis mean activity of 15.72 ± 2.33 U/L significantly different from 10.0 ± 0.69 U/L in 122 healthy control adults *2006*

Alkaline Phosphatase, Bone Isoenzyme *Serum* *No Effect* In 57 patients with rheumatoid arthritis median activity of 10.8 ng/mL not significantly different from normal *430*
Synovial Fluid *Increase* In 37 patients mean concentration of 10.4 ± 15.3 µg/L significantly higher than 2.6 ± 1.6 µg/L in 29 patients with osteoarthritis *1044*

Amino Acids *Plasma* *Decrease* Frequent hypoaminoacidemia. Arginine, glutamine, tyrosine, and histidine are low *4707*

Amino-terminal Propeptide of Type I Procollagen *Serum* *Increase* In 57 patients with rheumatoid arthritis mean concentration of 48.1 ± 21.8 µg/L significantly different from 36.8 ± 15.6 µg/L in 90 controls *1961*
Synovial Fluid *Increase* In 59 patients median concentration was 782 µg/L *1961*

Amino-terminal Propeptide of Type III Procollagen *Serum* *Increase* In 57 patients with rheumatoid arthritis mean concentration of 5.3 ± 2.7 µg/L significantly different from 3.5 ± 0.8 µg/L in 90 controls *1961*
Synovial Fluid *Increase* In 59 patients median concentration was 1,478 µg/L *1961*

Amylase *Pleural Fluid* *No Effect* Usually less than or equal to serum level *4493*

Amyloid A *Serum* *Increase* In patients with active rheumatoid arthritis concentrations typically 4.2 times higher than reference interval determined by Behring Nephelometer II of < 0.17 - 10.1 mg/L *2961* In 200 patients with acute phase reaction concentrations increased up to 2,200 mg/L compared with median of 3.0 mg/L in healthy individuals *5668*

Amyloid A Protein *Serum* *Increase* In 51 patients with early rheumatoid arthritis mean concentration of 36 mg/L *5408*

Angiotensin-converting Enzyme *Serum* *Increase* Observed effect *3041* *4488*
Serum *No Effect* Not significantly different (n = 48) from normal controls (n = 26) *3141*

Anti-ds DNA Antibodies *Serum* *Increase* Found in 2% of cases *4897* *413*

Anti-Entactin Antibodies *Serum* *Increase* In 25 patients IgM anti-entactin antibodies observed in 6 *4604*

Anti-Histone Antibodies *Serum* *Increase* Found in 15 - 20% of cases *126* Found in 10% of cases *4897*

Anti-Ku Antibodies *Serum* *Increase* 3 of 3 patients with rheumatoid arthritis had anti-Ku antibodies *921*

Anti-Mitochondrial Antibodies *Serum* *Increase* Reported effect *4551* Positive in 10% of patients *5658* Occasionally positive in low titer *4160*

Anti-Neutrophil Cytoplasm Antibodies *Serum* *No Effect* ANCA not observed in the sera of patients with rheumatoid arthritis *2502* In 0 of 2 patients (0%) with rheumatic arthritis pANCA detected *3722*

Anti-Ribonuclear Protein Antibodies *Serum* *Increase* Found in 1% of cases *4897*

Anti-Scl-70 Antibodies *Serum* *No Effect* Found in 0% of cases *4897*

Anti-Sjögren's Syndrome A Antibodies (SSA[Ro]) *Serum* *Increase* Found in 4% of cases *4897*

Anti-Sjögren's Syndrome B Antibodies (SSB[La]) *Serum* *Increase* Found in 1% of cases *4897*

Anti-Smith Antibodies *Serum* *Increase* Found in 5% of cases *4897*

Anti-ss DNA Antibodies *Serum* *Increase* Found in 4% of cases *4897*

Anti-Streptolysin-O Titer *Serum* *Increase* Above normal titers may occur *3953*

Antibody Titer *Serum* *Increase* Antibodies to reticulin *3712*

Anticentromere Antibody *Serum* *No Effect* Found in 0% of cases *4897*

α_1-Antichymotrypsin *Serum* *Increase* Significant rise *554* *2780*
Synovial Fluid *Increase* Significant rise *554* *2780*

Antinuclear Antibodies *Serum* *Increase* Of 119 patients with rheumatoid arthritis 44.4% of those with abnormal thyroid function had positive ANA compared with 43.8% in those without thyroid disease *4812* Found in 56% of cases *4897* 25-60% positivity *4068* 3 of 3 patients with rheumatoid arthritis had anti-nuclear antibodies *921* In 37% of patients increased titers observed *2502* Present in serum of 10 - 50% of patients (depending on the technique used) but is also usually in low titer compared to that in SLE *2039* 30 of 42 (73%) severely affected patients were antinuclear factor positive and 19 were LE cell negative *646* 30 of 42 (73.2%) severely affected patients were antinuclear factor positive and 19 of them were LE cell negative *646* In 2 of 2 patients (100%) with rheumatic arthritis ANA detected *3722* Highly sensitive tests will detect them in 60% of patients. Titers are generally lower than in SLE; predominantly IgM *1980*
Synovial Fluid *Increase* Occasionally positive *1980*

α_2-Antiplasmin/Plasmin Complex *Plasma* *Increase* In 20 patients with active disease mean concentration of 1.58 ± 3.08 µg/mL significantly higher than 0.53 ± 0.23 µg/mL in 9 patients with inactive disease and normal range of < 0.8 µg/mL *1615*

714.00 **Rheumatoid Arthritis** *(continued)*

Antithrombin III *Plasma Decrease* No significant correlation between low levels and thromboembolic disease *499*

α_1-Antitrypsin *Serum Increase* In patients with RA complicated by Amyloidosis *3378*
Synovial Fluid Increase Elevated in 36 patients with involvement of the knee joint *4384*

Apolipoprotein A-I *Serum No Effect* In 50 patients with rheumatoid arthritis with amyloidosis mean concentration of 116 ± 26 mg/dL compared with 124 ± 29 mg/dL in 45 patients with rheumatoid arthritis without amyloidosis less than 133 ± 29 mg/dL in 41 healthy controls *5767* In 54 female patients found to be in normal range *3129*

Apolipoprotein A-I:Apolipoprotein A-II Ratio
Serum Increase In 50 patients with rheumatoid arthritis with amyloidosis mean ratio of 4.55 compared with 5.88 in 45 patients with rheumatoid arthritis without amyloidosis more than 3.70 in 41 healthy controls *5767*

Apolipoprotein A-II *Serum Decrease* In 50 patients with rheumatoid arthritis with amyloidosis mean concentration of 25 ± 6 mg/dL compared with 21 ± 7 mg/dL in 45 patients with rheumatoid arthritis without amyloidosis less than 35 ± 6 mg/dL in 41 healthy controls *5767*

Apotranscobalamin II *Serum Increase* Concentration significantly increased in 30 patients with active rheumatoid arthritis compared with concentration in 27 patients in clinical remission *180*

Arginine *Plasma Decrease* Frequently low *4707*

Aspartate Aminotransferase *Serum Increase* In 117 patients with rheumatoid arthritis mean value of 15.5 U/L compared with reference range of 11 - 36 U/L with 0.8% outside reference range *428* Characteristically abnormal when the arthritis is active *900*
Serum No Effect Generally normal *1980*

Bile Acids *Serum Increase* In a series of 20 patients with RA and without prior causes of hepatic damage. Elevated in 80% of patients *97* In 117 patients with rheumatoid arthritis mean value of of 2.3 µmol/L compared with reference range of 0 - 6 µmol/L with 3.4% outside reference range *428*

Bilirubin *Serum No Effect* In 117 patients with rheumatoid arthritis mean value of 7.6 µmol/L compared with reference range of 3 - 26 µmol/L with 0.0% outside reference range *428*

Biopterin *Serum No Effect* In 21 patients with rheumatoid arthritis mean concentration of 10.02 ± 1.68 nmol/L not significantly less than 11.32 ± 3.00 nmol/L in 21 healthy controls *1956*
Synovial Fluid Increase In 21 patients with RA mean concentration of 22.11 nmol/L significantly greater than 16.61 ± 7.47 nmol/L in 21 patients with osteoarthritis *1956*

BSP Retention *Serum Increase* In a series of 20 patients with RA and without prior causes of hepatic damage. Elevated in 60% of patients *97* At times increased *900*

Calcitonin Gene-related Peptide *Serum Increase* In patients with rheumatoid arthritis mean concentration higher than in controls *2928*

Calcium *Serum Increase* After correction for hypoalbuminemia, 113/229 female and 65/135 male patients had hypercalcemia *2638* In 13 patients with rheumatoid arthritis and high ESR mean concentration of 2.42 ± 0.09 mmol/L significantly higher than 2.34 ± 0.07 mmol/L in 15 healthy controls *2455*
Serum No Effect Generally normal *1980*
Urine Increase Patients with active disease (ESR > 28 mm/h and Ritchie articular index > 8) had a significant higher excretion (42% higher) than in patients with inactive disease *1311*

Carbon Dioxide Partial Pressure *Blood Decrease* Impaired gas diffusion and the accompanying hyperventilation results in a low pCO_2, unless the defect is severe and CO_2 retention occurs *4707*
Pleural Fluid Increase 60 - 70 mm Hg *1604*

Carcinoembryonic Antigen *Serum Increase* In seropositive cases *1290*

β-Carotene *Serum Decrease* Mean concentration of 92.9 ± 52.1 µg/L in 14 patients with rheumatoid arthritis nonsignificantly reduced compared with 150.4 ± 144.5 µg/L in 27 healthy controls *2101*

Catecholamines *Urine Decrease* The more severe the stage and class of the arthritis, the lower the epinephrine, and the closer to normal norepinephrine values. Norepinephrine seems to reflect a compensation in catecholamine metabolism rather than adrenal cortex system influence *2316*

CD25+ Lymphocytes *Blood Decrease* In 5 patients with active rheumatoid arthritis concentrations ranged from 24 to 100 cells/µL compared with normal concentration range of 135 - 315 /µL *941*

Cells *Synovial Fluid Increase* In 5 patients mean concentration of 10,400 ± 3,972 /µL *4343*

Ceruloplasmin *Serum Increase* Significantly raised in rheumatoid disease in both sexes *4703* In 33 patients with rheumatoid arthritis mean concentration of 286.2 ± 86.38 U/L significantly higher than 149.4 ± 32.7 U/L in 34 controls *3963* May cause green color of plasma *5544*
Synovial Fluid Increase Characteristic of rheumatoid effusions *4704*

Cholesterol *Pericardial Fluid Increase* High levels (2.6 - 5.2 mmol/L; 100 to 200 mg/dL) *566*
Serum Decrease Median concentration in 17 patients with rheumatoid arthritis of 5.7 mmol/L significantly different from 7.25 mmol/L in 16 healthy controls *5548* Reduced; appears to be related to the severity and activity of the disease; not affected by therapy *1980*
Serum No Effect Mean concentration of 192 ± 42 mg/dL in 131 patients with rheumatoid arthritis not significantly higher than 185 ± 42 mg/dL in 200 healthy controls *195* In 51 patients with rheumatoid arthritis median concentrations of 5.6 mmol/L on two occasions significantly higher than upper limit of normal of 7.7 mmol/L in healthy men and 8.2 mmol/L in healthy women *5549*

Chondrex *Serum Increase* Mean concentration of 156.9 ± 122.1 µg/L in 56 patients with active rheumatoid arthritis significantly different from 50.7 ± 38.6 µg/L in 329 apparently healthy controls *2040*
Serum No Effect Mean concentration of 51.4 ± 30.9 µg/L in 9 patients with inactive rheumatoid arthritis not significantly different from 50.7 ± 38.6 µg/L in 329 apparently healthy controls *2040*

Chylomicrons *Synovial Fluid Increase* Chylous effusions have been reported *4487 3770*

Collagenase-like Peptidase *Serum Decrease* Mean activity of 0.36 ± 0.01 nmol/min/mL in 107 patients with rheumatoid arthritis significantly less than that in 55 healthy individuals in whom mean activity was 0.60 ± 0.03 nmol/min/mL *2380*

Complement C_1 *Serum Increase* Mean concentration typically slightly increased or normal in patients with moderate rheumatoid arthritis *4682*
Serum No Effect Mean concentration typically normal or slightly reduced in patients with severe rheumatoid arthritis *4682*

Complement C_1q *Serum Increase* Mean concentration typically slightly increased or normal in patients with moderate rheumatoid arthritis *4682* Observed effect *4683*
Serum No Effect Mean concentration typically normal or slightly reduced in patients with severe rheumatoid arthritis *4682*

Complement C_1r *Serum Decrease* Observed effect *4746*

Complement C_2 *Serum Increase* Mean concentration typically slightly increased or normal in patients with moderate rheumatoid arthritis *4682* Found in 50% of patients *4683*
Serum No Effect Mean concentration typically normal in patients with severe rheumatoid arthritis *4682*

Complement C_3 *Pericardial Fluid Decrease* Low or absent *1550 1789*
Pleural Fluid Decrease In about 5% of cases *126*
Serum Decrease Caused by hypercatabolism *1588 785 1033 2694*
Serum Increase The mean plasma C_3e level in these samples (3.0 ± 1.3 mg/dL) was significantly increased as compared to that in patients with degenerative joint disease (0.9± 0.4 mg/dL) and healthy blood donors (0.8 ± 0.5 mg/dL). C_3d levels were increased by more than 2 SD in 79% of RA samples. In most RA patients, the C_3d levels were higher in synovial fluid than in plasma *3843* Mean concentration typically slightly increased or normal in patients with moderate rheumatoid arthritis *4682*
Serum No Effect Mean concentration typically normal or slightly reduced in patients with severe rheumatoid arthritis *4682*

Synovial Fluid *Decrease* Marked reduction of C_1, C_2, C_3 and C_4 in seropositive patients. Only C_4 was significantly decreased in seronegative patients *4683*
Synovial Fluid *Increase* The mean plasma C_3e level in these samples (3.0 ± 1.3 mg/dL) was significantly increased as compared to that in patients with degenerative joint disease (0.9 ± 0.4 mg/dL). C_3d levels were increased by more than 2 SD in 79% of RA samples. In most patients, the C_3d levels were higher in synovial fluid than in plasma *3843*

Complement C_4 *Pericardial Fluid* *Decrease* Low or absent *1789* *1550*
Pleural Fluid *Decrease* In about 5% of cases *126*
Serum *Increase* Mean concentration typically slightly increased or normal in patients with moderate rheumatoid arthritis *4682*
Serum *No Effect* Mean concentration typically normal or slightly reduced in patients with severe rheumatoid arthritis *4682*
Synovial Fluid *Decrease* Marked reduction of C_1, C_2, C_3, and C_4 in seropositive patients. Only C_4 was significantly decreased in seronegative patients *4683*

Complement C_5 *Serum* *Increase* Mean concentration typically slightly increased or normal in patients with moderate rheumatoid arthritis *4682*
Serum *No Effect* Mean concentration typically normal in patients with severe rheumatoid arthritis *4682*

Complement CH50 *Serum* *Increase* Mean concentration typically slightly increased or normal in patients with moderate rheumatoid arthritis *4682*
Serum *No Effect* Mean concentration typically normal or slightly reduced in patients with severe rheumatoid arthritis *4682*

Complement, Total *Pericardial Fluid* *Decrease* Low or absent *1550* *1789*
Pleural Fluid *Decrease* Low complement (< 10 U/mL) in 11 of 12 patients with SLE or rheumatoid pleuritis *3052* Seropositive patients had decreased CH50, C_1, C_2, and C_1 inhibitor in pleural and pericardial fluids *1759*
Serum *Decrease* In 64 patients, 19% had decreased values *4925* In rare instances and with a highly acute onset, may be low *1980*
Serum *Increase* Activity tends to be elevated in patients with mild disease, lower levels were found in seropositive than seronegative patients *4683* In 64 patients, 16% had increased values *4925*
Serum *No Effect* No significant effect observed *413*
Synovial Fluid *Decrease* Intra-articular depletion of whole complement activity in the presence of normal or elevated serum levels is in proportion to the titer of rheumatoid factor in serum or synovial fluid *4683* Low compared to that in other types of inflammatory joint effusions, especially in relation to the total protein concentration *2039* Low values associated with more severe disease and poorer prognosis *630* Compared to total protein, levels are low in 60 - 70% of joint effusions *631* Whole complement activity is reduced *2087* Marked reduction of C_1, C_2, C_3, and C_4 in seropositive patients. Only C_4 was significantly decreased in seronegative patients *4683*

Connective Tissue Activating Protein-III *Serum* *Increase* Increased amounts detected in plasma of patients with rheumatoid arthritis *5114*

Copper *Serum* *Increase* Elevated in excess of the binding capacity of ceruloplasmin, resulting in raised free copper levels *3127* Both serum Cu and ceruloplasmin were measured in 189 RA patients and were found to be significantly elevated. An inverse relation was found between serum iron and copper and a strong direct correlation between serum antioxidant activity and ceruloplasmin *4703*
Synovial Fluid *Increase* Characteristic of rheumatoid effusions *4704*
Urine *Increase* Patients show an abnormal copper excretion pattern compared with nonrheumatoid subjects *3427*

Copper Zinc Superoxide Dismutase
Red Blood Cells *Decrease* Significantly decreased values compared with age and sex matched controls before but not after copper supplementation *1182*

Cortisol *Plasma* *No Effect* Mean concentration of approximately 190 nmol/L in 29 patients with rheumatoid arthritis not significantly different from approximately 170 nmol/L in 23 control patients with osteoarthritis *1064*

C-Reactive Protein *Serum* *Increase* Severe disease is characterized by increased concentration *3999* In 51 patients with early rheumatoid arthritis mean concentration of 34 mg/L *5408* Nearly always abnormal and generally reflects the degree of disease activity *4551* In 51 patients with rheumatoid arthritis median concentration of 19.0 mg/L on one occasion significantly higher than upper limit of normal of 5 mg/L in healthy individuals *5549* In 99 adult patients with rheumatoid arthritis of less than 1 year's duration mean concentration of 33.8 mg/L (median 27.0 mg/L) significantly higher than upper limit of reference interval *2790* In 31 patients median concentration of 30 µg/mL *5287* In patients with active rheumatoid arthritis concentrations typically 10 times higher than reference interval determined by Behring Nephelometer II of < 0.17 - 10.1 mg/L *2961* In 114 patients with active rheumatoid arthritis mean concentration in 38 with IgA rheumatoid factor of 1.80 ± 1.51 (on a scale from 1 - 12) significantly different from 0.66 ± 1.20 in 76 without IgA rheumatoid factor and significantly higher than in healthy controls *3973* Mean concentration of 30 ± 21 mg/dL in 20 men, 35 ± 30 mg/dL in 14 premenopausal women and 36 ± 30 mg/dL in 28 postmenopausal women significantly higher than in healthy controls *1833* In 143 patients with rheumatoid arthritis significant positive correlation with serum IL-6 concentraton of r = 0.50 *879* Increased inconsistently *5544* In 20 patients with rheumatoid arthritis median concentration of 38.4 mg/L significantly different from upper limit of normal of 2.6 mg/L *1612* In 20 patients with rheumatoid arthritis median concentration of 38.5 mg/L significantly greater than median of 3 mg/L in 20 healthy blood donors *1614* Mean concentration of 22 ± 10.0 mg/L observed in 25 patients *5561* In 13 patients with rheumatoid arthritis mean concentration of 3.90 ± 0.89 mg/dL higher than in controls *5439*

Creatine Kinase *Serum* *Decrease* In 40 patients with classic or definite rheumatoid arthritis mean activity of 37.6 U/L significantly less than 77.7 U/L in 40 control patients *4565*

Creatine Kinase MB-Isoenzyme *Serum* *Increase* Observed effect *248*

Creatinine *Serum* *No Effect* In 60 patients with rheumatoid arthritis mean concentration of 74.3 ± 16.8 µmol/L not significantly different from 77.8 ± 13.3 µmol/L in 57 heathy volunteers *4399*

Cross-linked C-terminal Telopeptide of Type I Collagen
Serum *Increase* In 59 patients with rheumatoid arthritis mean concentration of 6.4 ± 4.1 µg/L significantly different from 3.1 ± 0.8 µg/L in 90 controls *1961*
Synovial Fluid *Increase* In 59 patients median concentration was 16.7 µg/L *1961* *1961*

Cryoglobulins *Serum* *Increase* Demonstrated occasionally but do not appear to have diagnostic significance *1980* Variable elevation of cryoglobulins *4707*

C-terminal Propeptide of Type I Procollagen
Serum *Decrease* In 119 women with rheumatoid arthritis mean concentration of 105 ± 32 µg/L compared with 117 ± 38 µg/L in 47 healthy female controls *2826*

C-terminal Telopeptide of Type I Collagen *Urine* *No Effect* In 18 postmenopausal women aged 51 - 69 y with rheumatoid arthritis mean excretion of 367 ± 442 µg/mmol creatinine in 2-hour not significantly different from than that in 30 healthy premenopausal women aged 24 - 50 y with regular menstrual cycle in whom the mean excretion was 263 ± 117 µg/mmol creatinine in 2-hour morning collection. In 20 postmenopausal women with rheumatoid arthritis mean excretion of 421 ± 183 µg/mmol creatinine also not significantly different from 546 ± 257 µg/mmol creatinine in 22 matched post-menopausal controls *5131*

Cytidine Deaminase *Serum* *No Effect* In 16 patients with rheumatoid arthritis median activity of 8.97 U/L not significantly different from median activity of 5.73 U/L in 12 patients with seronegative polyarthritis *5290*
Synovial Fluid *Increase* In 16 patients with rheumatoid arthritis median activity in knee synovial fluid of 55.8 U/mL significantly higher than median activity of 8.11 U/mL in synovial fluid from knees of 12 patients with seronegative polyarthritis *5290*

Cytomegalovirus Antibodies *Serum* *Increase* The titers of antibody were found to increase with the disease duration *1468*

D-Dimer *Plasma* *Increase* In 20 patients with active disease mean concentration of 462.7 ± 360.4 ng/mL significantly higher than 112.8 ± 33.4 ng/mL in 9 patients with inactive disease and normal range of < 150 ng/mL *1615*
Plasma *No Effect* Mean concentration in 29 patients of 354.1 ± 340.8 ng/mL significantly greater than 51.1 ± 20.9 ng/mL in 40 healthy adults *1615*

714.00 **Rheumatoid Arthritis** *(continued)*

Dehydroepiandrosterone Sulfate *Plasma Decrease* Mean concentration in 29 patients with rheumatoid arthritis 540 nmol/L significantly reduced compared with 2100 nmol/L in control population of 23 patients with osteoarthritis *1064*

Deoxypyridinoline *Urine Increase* Mean excretion of 64 ± 35 nmol/8 h in 62 patients with rheumatoid arthritis significantly greater than 34 ± 19 nmol/8 h in 56 healthy controls although difference in premenopausal women not significant *1833* Increased excretion observed in conjunction with increased disease activity *1833*

Dipeptidyl Aminopeptidase *Serum Decrease* Mean activity of 45.0 ± 1.37 nmol/min/mL in 101 patients with rheumatoid arthritis significantly less than that in 117 healthy individuals in whom mean activity was 70.1 ± 0.37 nmol/min/mL *2380*

Dipyridinoline *Urine Increase* In 18 postmenopausal women aged 51 - 69 y with rheumatoid arthritis mean excretion of total dipyridinoline of 13.2 ± 5.6 nmol/mmol creatinine in 2-hour not significantly different from than that in 30 healthy premenopausal women aged 24 - 50 y with regular menstrual cycle in whom the mean excretion was 9.1 ± 4.0 nmol/mmol creatinine in 2-hour morning collection *5131*

Dipyridinoline, Free *Urine Increase* In 18 postmenopausal women aged 51 - 69 y with rheumatoid arthritis mean excretion of 4.9 ± 3.1 nmol/mmol creatinine in 2-hour significantly greater than that in 30 healthy premenopausal women aged 24 - 50 y with regular menstrual cycle in whom the mean excretion was 2.4 ± 1.7 nmol/mmol creatinine in 2-hour morning collection *5131*

Dipyridinoline, Peptide-bound *Urine No Effect* In 18 postmenopausal women aged 51 - 69 y with rheumatoid arthritis mean excretion of 8.4 ± 4.5 nmol/mmol creatinine in 2-hour not significantly different from than that in 30 healthy premenopausal women aged 24 - 50 y with regular menstrual cycle in whom the mean excretion was 6.7 ± 3.3 nmol/mmol creatinine in 2-hour morning collection. In 20 postmenopausal women with rheumatoid arthritis mean excretion of 14.5 ± 7.0 nmol/mmol creatinine also significantly different from 11.4 ± 10.2 nmol/mmol creatinine in 22 matched post-menopausal controls *5131*

Eosinophils *Blood Increase* Eosinophilia has been reported in patients with pleural or pulmonary manifestations *1980*

Epithelial-neutrophil Activating Protein-78
Synovial Fluid Increase Detected in synovial fluid of patients with rheumatoid arthritis, and to a greater extent than in patients with osteoarthritis *5114*

Epstein Barr Virus Antibodies *Serum No Effect* Few heightened serologic responses were noted in the average IgG antibody titers to domains of the five EBV nuclear antigens (EBNA-1,2,3,4, and 6), especially the amino-terminal domain of EBNA-2 in sera of patients with this disorder *2337*

Erythrocyte Sedimentation Rate *Blood Increase* In 114 patients with active rheumatoid arthritis mean ESR in 38 with IgA rheumatoid factor of 32.4 mm/h not significantly different from 26.2 ± 15.9 mm/h in 76 without IgA rheumatoid factor but significantly higher than in healthy controls *3973* In a study of 137 patients with rheumatoid arthritis mean rate of 47 ± 32 mm/h significantly greater than in healthy controls *3460* In 143 of patients with rheumatoid arthritis significant positive correlation with serum IL-6 of r = 0.41 observed *879* At times, although joint inflammation has subsided, ESR will remain accelerated because of the continued elevation of serum globulins *1980* Mean of 31 ± 24 mm/h in 20 men, 39 ± 26 mm/h in 14 premenopausal women, and 42 ± 32 mm/h in 28 postmenopausal women with rheumatoid arthritis significantly higher than in healthy controls *1833* In 100 patients, correlated with disease activity and stage of disease *3615* In 31 patients median rate of 62 mm/h *5287* In 99 adult patients with rheumatoid arthritis of less than 1 year's duration mean rate of 46.4 mm/h (median 44.0 mm/h) significantly higher than upper limit of reference interval *2790* In 51 patients with early rheumatoid arthritis mean rate 50 mm/h *5408* In 5 patients mean rate of 54 ± 27 mm/h *4343* Severe disease is characterized by increased ESR *3999* In 51 patients with rheumatoid arthritis median rate of 46 and 40 mm/h on two occasions significantly higher than upper limit of normal of 20 mm/h in healthy individuals *5549* Nearly always abnormal and generally reflects the degree of disease activity *4551* Mean rate of 37.0 ± 7.1 mm/h observed in 25 patients *5561*
Blood No Effect Elevated when the classic case is active, normal when the disease is quiet because of its natural course or as a result of therapy *900* The majority of patients who are in complete remission will have a normal ESR *1980*

Factor B *Synovial Fluid Decrease* Found in 50% of patients *3141*

Ferritin *Serum Increase* In 20 patients with rheumatoid arthritis mean concentration of 310 ± 580 ng/mL *3945*
Serum No Effect Mean concentration in 19 of 35 patients with iron deficiency of 51.6 µg/L compared with 257.4 µg/L in 10 with adequate iron stores (normal 10 - 120 µg/L in women and 15 - 300 µg/L in men) *3784*
Synovial Fluid Increase In 41 patients with rheumatoid arthritis mean concentration of 1,068 ± 1,104 ng/mL *3945*

Fibrin Degradation Products *Plasma No Effect* Mean concentration of 6.82 ± 3.60 µg/mL in 20 patients with active disease significantly higher than 4.23 ± 1.13 µg/mL in 9 patients with inactive disease but within normal range of < 10 µg/mL *1615*

Fibrinogen *Plasma Increase* In 20 patients with active disease mean concentration of 477.8 ± 126.4 mg/dL higher than normal range of 200 - 400 mg/dL *1615* Can be used to assess disease activity *1290*
Plasma No Effect In 9 patients with inactive disease mean concentration of 395.8 ± 64.9 mg/dL not significantly different from normal range of 200 - 400 mg/dL *1615*

Follicle Stimulating Hormone *Plasma Increase* In 12 male patients with rheumatoid arthritis mean concentration of 343 ± 212 µg/L significantly different from 177 ± 98 µg/L in 70 healthy male controls *3309*

Fructosamine *Serum Increase* In 60 patients with rheumatoid arthritis mean concentration of 278 ± 43 µmol/L different from 258 ± 23 µmol/L in 57 heathy volunteers *4399*

β-Galactosidase *Serum Decrease* Mean serum concentration was 0.139 ± 0.019 mmol/min/L, compared with 0.243 ± 0.038 in controls *2288*

Gastrin *Serum Increase* Patients tend to have higher than normal serum concentration. There appears to be poor correlation with acid secretion *4425*

Gelatinase *Serum No Effect* In 73 patients with rheumatoid arthritis mean concentration of 484.9 ± 31.5 ng/mL not significantly higher than 408.9 ± 28.0 ng/mL in 53 healthy controls *5878*

α_1-Globulin *Serum Increase* Moderate increase *1290*
Serum No Effect Generally not significantly changed *1980*

α_2-Globulin *Serum Increase* Elevation occurs in some 50% of all patients and in the majority with progressive chronic disease *2039* Elevated and does not fall with steroid therapy *1290* α_2- and β-globulin fractions are often elevated in the acute active phase, whereas during the chronic active phase, γ-globulin fractions are elevated *900*

β-Globulin *Serum Increase* α_2- and β-globulin fractions are often elevated in the acute phase, whereas during the chronic active phase, γ-globulin fractions are elevated *900*
Serum No Effect Generally not significantly changed *1980*

γ-Globulin *Pericardial Fluid Increase* γ-Globulin complexes found to be present in rheumatoid pericarditis *266*
Serum Increase α_2- and β-globulin fractions are often elevated in the acute active phase, whereas during the chronic active phase, γ-globulin fractions are elevated *900* Elevation occurs in some 50% of all patients and in the majority with progressive chronic disease *2039* In 21 patients with elderly onset of rheumatoid arthritis mean concentration of 1.22 ± 0.28 g/dL *3904* Severe disease is characterized by hyper-γ-globulinemia *3999*

Glucose *Pericardial Fluid Decrease* With rheumatoid pericarditis a low concentration, often < 1.7 mmol/L (30 mg/dL) is seen *1550*
Pleural Fluid Decrease Concentrations are invariably < 30 mg/dL *3052* Markedly reduced, 20 mg/dL or less, is very suggestive and virtually diagnostic of rheumatoid disease. A low level in the range of 40 mg/dL can be found in infectious processes and in malignant pleural effusions *1980*
Serum No Effect In 60 patients with rheumatoid arthritis mean concentration of 5.4 ± 1.0 mmol/L not significantly different from 5.2 ± 0.5 mmol/L in 57 heathy volunteers *4399*

Synovial Fluid *Decrease* Slightly reduced glucose content *2039* In 16 patients with rheumatoid arthritis median concentration in knee synovial fluid of 57.9 mg/dL significantly lower than median concentration of 84.5 mg/dL in synovial fluid from knees of 12 patients with seronegative polyarthritis *5290* Normal or low *413*
Synovial Fluid *No Effect* Normal or low *413*

Glucose Tolerance *Serum* *Decrease* Moderate intolerance in most patients. More severe in patients with associated infection and inflammation *4707* Characteristically depressed with active disease; easy to produce hypoglycemia if this abnormality is treated with oral hypoglycemic agents *900*

Glutamic Acid *Plasma* *Increase* Usually the only elevated serum amino acid *4707*
Urine *Decrease* Reported effect *4707*

Glutamine *Plasma* *Decrease* Frequently low *4707*

γ-Glutamyltransferase *Serum* *Increase* Increased activity reported with rheumatoid arthritis *3625* In a series of 20 patients with RA and without prior causes of hepatic damage. Elevated in 55% of patients *97* In 117 patients with rheumatoid arthritis mean value of 50.8 U/L compared with reference range of 8 - 45 U/L with 33.0% outside reference range *428*
Serum *No Effect* In 57 patients with rheumatoid arthritis median activity of 20 U/L not significantly different from normal: 59.7% of RA patients had increased activities *430*

Glycated Protein *Serum* *Decrease* Significant lowering of β-2 glycoprotein concentrations found *2779*

Glycosaminoglycans *Serum* *Increase* A corresponding increase has been reported in synovial fluid, serum and urine of patients with rheumatic diseases *2651*
Synovial Fluid *Increase* A corresponding increase has been reported in synovial fluid, serum and urine of patients with rheumatic diseases *2651*
Urine *Increase* Significant difference (median 33; n = 63) in comparison with unaffected individuals (median 20.2; n = 38) *2651*

Glycosylated Ferritin *Serum* *Increase* In 20 patients with rheumatoid arthritis mean proportion of 65.9 ± 15.0% *3945*
Synovial Fluid *Increase* In 41 patients with rheumatoid arthritis mean proportion of 11.9 ± 10.7% *3945*

Granulocyte Colony Stimulating Factor
Bone Marrow *Increase* In 25 patients with rheumatoid arthritis concentration in bone marrow serum increased in 8 with median concentration of 161 pg/mL. Median and mean concentrations of 113.5 pg/mL and 654.4 pg/mL respectively significantly higher than in 10 controls in whom concentration was undetectable in all *5157*

Granulocyte-Macrophage Colony Stimulating Factor
Bone Marrow *No Effect* In 25 patients with rheumatoid arthritis concentration in bone marrow serum close to or below the assay detection limit *5157*

Haptoglobin *Serum* *Increase* Usually parallels the activity of the ESR *1980* In 51 patients with rheumatoid arthritis median concentration of 3.6 and 3.2 g/L on two occasions significantly higher than upper limit of normal of 2.5 g/L in healthy individuals *5549*

HDL-Cholesterol *Serum* *Decrease* Median concentration in 17 patients with rheumatoid arthritis of 1.64 mmol/L significantly different from 1.88 mmol/L in 16 healthy controls *5548* In 54 female patients 36% reduction was noted *3129*
Serum *No Effect* Mean concentration of 50 ± 16 mg/dL in 131 patients with rheumatoid arthritis not significantly different from 50 ± 13 mg/dL in 200 healthy controls *195*

Hematocrit *Blood* *Decrease* Mild anemia occurs in approximately 40% of cases *2039* Normocytic, normochromic, or perhaps hypochromic anemia which may be severe when the disease is very active *900* Anemia may occur *1098*

Hemoglobin *Blood* *Decrease* In 13 patients with rheumatoid arthritis mean concentration of 12.5 ± 0.2 g/dL lower than in controls *5439* Mean concentration in 35 patients with rheumatoid arthritis of 105.5 ± 11.1 g/L significantly reduced compared with normal ranges of 110 - 160 g/L in women and 130 - 175 g/L in men *3784* In 51 patients with early rheumatoid arthritis mean concentration of 124 g/L *5408* Mild anemia occurs in approximately 40% of cases *2039* Normocytic, normochromic, or perhaps hypochromic anemia which may be severe when the disease is very active *900* Anemia may occur, hemoglobin < 13 g/dL *1098*

Blood *No Effect* In 16 patients with rheumatoid arthritis median concentration of 12.0 g/dL not significantly different from median concentration of 11.7 g/dL in 12 patients with seronegative polyarthritis *5290*
Urine *No Effect* In 810 women and 208 men with RA isolated hematuria observed in 10 and 5% respectively compared with 9 and 4% respectively in 352 healthy control women and 105 men controls *2772*

Heterophile Antibody *Serum* *Increase* One case *1025*

Hexosamine *Serum* *Increase* Usually parallels the activity of the ESR *1980*

β-Hexosaminidase *Urine* *Decrease* Decreased levels in urine *5229*

Histidine *Plasma* *Decrease* Frequently low *4707*

HLA Antigens *Blood* *Present* HLA-B_27 present in 35% of patients versus 11% of controls HLA-DR4 present in 56% of patients versus 15% of controls *5678* HLA antigen DR4 found in 54% of patients with this disease compared to 16% of controls *4584*

Hyaluronic Acid *Serum* *Increase* Concentration increases in rheumatoid arthritis in proportion to severity of disease *3365* Compared with the controls, the mean level of plasma HA was sevenfold higher in the RA group *1786* In early disease serum concentration indicates ongoing joint damage and is predictive of disease activity *3145* Immunoassays were used to measure levels in the serum of 35 patients with RA and a group of age- and sex-matched control subjects. Serum levels were significantly higher in the RA population than in the control group *5223* The increase in serum levels in subjects getting out of bed in the morning ranges from 10 to 63 μg/L in healthy persons and from 54 μg/L in patients with this disorder *3073* Serum levels were significantly higher in the RA population than in the control group *3273* Patients displayed highly elevated levels of hyaluronic acid (HA), while others exhibited normal levels *4174* Increased serum levels of hyaluronate (HA) have been found in patients with rheumatoid arthritis (RA) *3975*

Hydroxyproline *Urine* *Increase* Patients with active disease (ESR > 28 mm/h and Ritchie articular index > 8) had a significant higher excretion (42% higher) than in patients with inactive disease *1311*

Hydroxypyridinoline *Synovial Fluid* *No Effect* In 20 patients with rheumatoid arthritis mean concentration high at 25.3 ± 13.5 pmol/mL *4872*
Urine *Increase* In 20 patients with rheumatoid arthritis mean concentration of about 140 pmol/μmol creatinine significantly greater than mean of 90 pmol/μmol creatinine in 20 patients with osteoarthritis *4872*

immunoglobulin A *Saliva* *Increase* Significantly elevated in 24% of patients. 80% of the patients with elevated IgA concentrations had keratoconjunctivitis sicca as well *382*
Serum *Increase* Reported effect *5544* In 21 patients with elderly onset of rheumatoid arthritis mean concentration of 325.1 ± 138.9 mg/dL *3904* In 114 patients with active rheumatoid arthritis mean concentration in 38 with IgA rheumatoid factor of 4.12 ± 2.26 g/L not significantly different from 3.14 ± 2.21 g/L in 76 without IgA rheumatoid factor but significantly higher than in healthy controls *3973*

Immunoglobulin A, Secretory *Serum* *Increase* In 30 patients with active disease mean concentration of 0.091 ± 0.079 mg/mL significantly increased and in 33 patients with inactive disease 0.013 ± 0.026 mg/mL not significantly different from 0.002 ± 0.004 mg/mL in 30 healthy controls *2491*

Immunoglobulin D *Serum* *Increase* Reported effect *1290*

Immunoglobulin G *Serum* *Increase* In 21 patients with elderly onset of rheumatoid arthritis mean concentration of 1,427.7 ± 297.6 mg/dL *3904* In 114 patients with active rheumatoid arthritis mean concentration in 38 with IgA rheumatoid factor of 15.02 ± 4.93 g/L not significantly different from 13.95 ± 3.08 g/L in 76 without IgA rheumatoid factor but significantly higher than in healthy controls *3973*

Immunoglobulin M *Serum* *Increase* Reported effect *5544* In 21 patients with elderly onset of rheumatoid arthritis mean concentration of 133.1 ± 68.0 mg/dL *3904* In 114 patients with active rheumatoid arthritis mean concentration in 38 with IgA rheumatoid factor of 2.29 ± 1.02 g/L not significantly different from 1.89 ± 1.11 g/L in 76 without IgA rheumatoid factor but significantly higher than in healthy controls *3973*
Synovial Fluid *Increase* Very suggestive of this disease *345*

714.00 Rheumatoid Arthritis *(continued)*

Insulin-like Growth Factor-I *Serum* *Decrease* Mean concentration in 13 patients with untreated rheumatoid arthritis of 132 ± 62 μg/L significantly less than 179 ± 54 μg/L in 15 healthy controls *2455*

Insulin-like Growth Factor-II *Serum* *Decrease* Mean concentration in 13 untreated patients of 553 ± 199 μg/L significantly reduced compared with 714 ± 200 μg/L in 15 healthy controls *2455*

Insulin-like Growth Factor Binding Protein-3 *Serum* *No Effect* Mean concentration of about 4,000 μg/L in 13 patients with active rheumatoid arthritis not significantly different from about 4,500 μg/L in 15 healthy controls *2455*

Interferon-γ-inducible Protein-10 *Serum* *Increase* Very little amounts detected in plasma of patients with rheumatoid arthritis *5114*

Interleukin-1 *Serum* *Increase* Before treatment, activation of the monocyte-macrophage system had been signified by elevated serum levels as well as a marked in vitro production of IL-1 *2235*
Serum *No Effect* Plasma levels were compared with conventional measures of disease activity. The mean levels in the two groups were not significantly different and, within the patient group (n = 53), its measurement in plasma seems to offer little of clinical value *1286*

Interleukin-1 Receptor Antagonist *Serum* *No Effect* Median concentration in 20 patients with rheumatoid arthritis of 0.46 ng/mL not significantly higher than 0.27 ng/mL in 20 healthy controls *1612*

Interleukin-1α *Bone Marrow* *No Effect* In 25 patients with rheumatoid arthritis concentration in bone marrow serum close to or below the assay detection limit in 22 with generally mild increases in the other three *5157*

Interleukin-1β *Bone Marrow* *No Effect* In 25 patients with rheumatoid arthritis concentration in bone marrow serum close to or below the assay detection limit *5157*
Serum *No Effect* In 22 patients with rheumatoid arthritis median concentration undetectable not different from normal *1612* Median concentration in 17 patients with rheumatoid arthritis of 6.2 pg/mL not significantly different from 15 pg/mL or less in 16 healthy controls *5548*

Interleukin-2 *Bone Marrow* *No Effect* In 25 patients with rheumatoid arthritis concentration in bone marrow serum close to or below the assay detection limit *5157*
Serum *Increase* Measured the concentrations of TNF-α and IL-2 in plasma from 2 groups of patients suffering from rheumatoid arthritis (RA). One group had high and one had low disease activity. In addition, in connection with steroid treatment in the high disease activity group, TNF-α was significantly increased in plasma from RA patients with high disease activity compared with those of low disease activity (p = 0.0009) *1391*
Serum *No Effect* Not detectable in all except one of 47 patients with uncomplicate rheumatoid arthritis: also not detectable in 45 healthy controls *941*

Interleukin-3 *Bone Marrow* *No Effect* In 25 patients with rheumatoid arthritis concentration in bone marrow serum close to or below the assay detection limit *5157*

Interleukin-4 *Bone Marrow* *No Effect* In 25 patients with rheumatoid arthritis concentration in bone marrow serum close to or below the assay detection limit *5157*

Interleukin-6 *Bone Marrow* *Increase* In 25 patients with rheumatoid arthritis concentration in bone marrow serum concentration increased in 8. Median concentration of 46.5 pg/mL. In peripheral blood serum median and mean concentrations of 28.5 pg/mL and 34.6 pg/mL respectively significantly higher than 23 pg/mL in 10 healthy controls *5157*
Bone Marrow *No Effect* In 25 patients with rheumatoid arthritis concentration in bone marrow serum concentration increased in 8. Median concentration of 46.5 pg/mL. In peripheral blood serum median and mean concentrations of 28.5 pg/mL and 34.6 pg/mL respectively significantly higher than 23 pg/mL in 10 healthy controls *5157*
Serum *Increase* Serum levels were significantly higher in the RA population than in the control group *3273* Immunoassays were used to measure levels of 35 patients with RA and a group of age-and sex-matched control subjects. Serum levels of IL-6 were significantly higher in the RA population than in the control group *5223* Concentrations increased and correlated strongly with ESR and RF titers and to a lesser degree with platelets counts *1019* In 80% of 143 patients with rheumatoid arthritis mean concentration greater than 10 pg/mL with median 36 pg/mL (range 4 to 403 pg/mL) *879* Mean concentration of 82.7 ± 71.0 pg/mL in 22 patients with rheumatoid arthritis significantly different from 11.4 ± 1.9 pg/mL in healthy blood donors *1130* In 51 patients with early rheumatoid arthritis mean concentration of 51 ng/mL *5408* In 22 patients with rheumatoid arthritis median concentration of 288 pg/mL significantly different from upper limit of normal *1612* Median concentration in 17 patients with rheumatoid arthritis of 91.5 pg/mL significantly different from < 8.5 pg/mL or less in 16 healthy controls *5548* Concentration highly correlated with severity of disease *3999* In 25 patients with rheumatoid arthritis concentration in bone marrow serum concentration increased in 8. Median concentration of 46.5 pg/mL. In peripheral blood serum median and mean concentrations of 28.5 pg/mL and 34.6 pg/mL respectively significantly higher than 23 pg/mL in 10 healthy controls *5157* Before treatment, activation of the monocyte-macrophage system had been signified by elevated serum levels of IL-1, IL-6, CRP and neopterin as well as a marked in vitro production of IL-1, tumour necrosis factor-α (TNF-α) and IL-6 *2235*
Synovial Fluid *Increase* Mean concentration of 24.9 ± 49.7 ng/L in 22 patients with rheumatoid arthritis *1130* Highest concentrations in patients with arthritides observed in those with RA especially in those with very active general symptoms and severe joint pain *605* All of a population of patients with rheumatoid arthritis all had increased synovial fluid IL-6 concentrations *2250* Concentration highly correlated with severity of disease *3999*

Interleukin-7 *Bone Marrow* *No Effect* In 25 patients with rheumatoid arthritis concentration in bone marrow serum close to or below the assay detection limit *5157*

Interleukin-8 *Bone Marrow* *Increase* In 25 patients with rheumatoid arthritis concentration in bone marrow serum concentration increased in 23 and median 200 pg/mL. Median and mean concentrations of 270 and 458.2 pg/mL significantly higher than 42 pg/mL in 10 healthy controls *5157*
Serum *Increase* Detected in serum of patients with rheumatoid arthritis *5114*
Synovial Fluid *Increase* Detected in synovial fluid of patients with rheumatoid arthritis *5114* In 16 patients with rheumatoid arthritis mean concentration in knee synovial fluid of 2.35 ng/mL significantly higher than mean concentration of 0.22 ng/mL in synovial fluid from knees of 12 patients with seronegative polyarthritis *5290*

Interleukin-10 *Serum* *Increase* In 42 patients with rheumatoid arthritis mean concentration of 161.3 ± 25.4 U/mL significantly higher than 8.8 ± 1.9 U/mL in 22 healthy controls *986*
Synovial Fluid *Increase* In 42 patients with rheumatoid arthritis mean concentration of 84.6 ± 17.6 U/mL significantly different from 8.8 ± 1.9 U/mL in serum of 22 healthy controls *986*

Interleukin-11 *Serum* *No Effect* In 31 untreated patients median concentration of 79 pg/mL *5287*
Synovial Fluid *Increase* In 31 untreated patients median concentration of 120.5 pg/mL *5287*

Ionized Calcium *Serum* *No Effect* Mean concentration in 13 patients with rheumatoid arthritis and high ESR mean concentration of 1.20 ± 0.04 mmol/L not significantly different from 1.18 ± 0.02 mmol/L in 15 healthy controls *2455*

Iron *Serum* *Decrease* Serum iron < 50 μg/dL *1098* Mean concentration of 8.3 ± 3.7 μmol/L in 35 patients significantly less than normal range of 9.0 - 35.0 μmol/L *3784* Decrease in concentration observed in chronic diseases such as rheumatoid arthritis *2952* Seen frequently, often as a result of gastrointestinal blood loss *2039*

Iron-binding Capacity, Total *Serum* *Decrease* Total IBC < 200 - 300 μg/dL *1098* Low; rises with successful steroid therapy *1290*

Iron Saturation *Serum* *Decrease* Transferrin saturation < 20% *1098*

Isocitrate Dehydrogenase *Serum* *No Effect* No effect on activity observed *5008*

Keratan Sulfate *Serum* *Decrease* Single analyses of peripheral blood of rheumatoid arthritis (RA) patients showed a significant reduction in the mean value for keratan sulfate (KS) compared with that in control subjects *4174*

Lactate *Pleural Fluid* *Increase* High concentrations may be seen *1438*

Synovial Fluid *Increase* In 16 patients with rheumatoid arthritis median concentration in knee synovial fluid of 29.6 mg/dL significantly higher than median concentration of 16.6 mg/dL in synovial fluid from knees of 12 patients with seronegative polyarthritis *5290*

Lactate Dehydrogenase *Pericardial Fluid* *Increase* With rheumatoid pericarditis markedly elevated *1550*
Serum *Increase* Characteristically abnormal when the arthritis is active *900* Reported effect *2257*

LDL-Cholesterol *Serum* *Decrease* In 54 female patients 26% reduction was noted *3129* Median concentration in 17 patients with rheumatoid arthritis of 3.4 mmol/L significantly different from 4.95 mmol/L in 16 healthy controls *5548*
Serum *No Effect* Mean concentration of 119 ± 33 mg/dL in 131 patients with rheumatoid arthritis not significantly higher than 117 ± 31 mg/dL in 200 healthy controls *195*

LDL-Cholesterol:HDL-Cholesterol Ratio *Serum* *Decrease* Median ratio in 17 patients with rheumatoid arthritis of 2.05 not significantly different from 2.73 in 16 healthy controls *5548*

LE Cells *Blood* *Positive* Positive in up to 25% of patients. The number of cells seen in a preparation is less than in SLE *2039* Usually weakly reactive *5544* 30 of 42 (73%) severely affected patients were antinuclear factor positive and 19 were LE cell negative *646*

Leukemia Inhibitory Factor *Serum* *No Effect* Not detected in serum of patients with rheumatoid arthritis *1614*
Synovial Fluid *Increase* High concentrations observed in synovial fluid in approximately 25% of patients with rheumatoid arthritis *1614*

Leukocytes *Blood* *Decrease* Occasionally low; characteristically so in Felty's Syndrome in which granulocytes are depleted *2039*
Blood *Increase* About 25% of patients develop neutrophilic leukocytosis. These patients usually have arthritis of short duration with a high degree of activity and fever *4817* There may be a slight increase early in the active disease *5544* Usually normal but may be elevated or depressed. In children may be very high (70,000 /µL) *900*
Blood *No Effect* The majority of patients have normal counts *4817* In 31 patients median concentration of 8.8 x 10^3/L *5287* Usually normal but may be elevated or depressed *900*
Pleural Fluid *Increase* 1,000 - 20,000 /µL *4493*
Synovial Fluid *Increase* Elevated (3,000 to 60,000 /µL, with an average of around 10,000 /µL), with predominantly polymorphonuclear response at times of active disease *2039* Mean concentration of 7,500 ± 3,200 /µL in 33 patients *1161* Mean concentration in 6 patients with rheumatoid arthritis 18,000 ± 8,324 /µL compared with 300 /µL in 3 normal individuals *3344* Less than 15,000 /µL *1980* In 31 patients median concentration of 8.6 x 10^3/L *5287*

Leukotriene B_4 *Synovial Fluid* *Increase* Concentration significantly increased compared with that in osteoarthritis *45*

Leukotriene C_4 *Synovial Fluid* *Increase* Detected at concentrations of 51 - 214 pmol/L in 5 of 14 patients with rheumatoid arthritis *3366*

Lipids *Serum* *Decrease* In 54 female patients plasma lipid levels were low *3129*

Lipoprotein Lipase *Serum* *Decrease* Median activity without heparin in 17 patients with rheumatoid arthritis of 1.05 mU/mL significantly different from 1.32 mU/mL in 16 healthy controls. Post-heparin respective activities of 204 mU/mL and 279 mU/mL *5548*

Lipoprotein Lp(a) *Serum* *Increase* Median concentration of 19 mg/dL in 131 patients with rheumatoid arthritis significantly higher than 9 mg/dL in 200 healthy controls *195*
Serum *No Effect* In 51 patients with rheumatoid arthritis median concentrations of 172 and 165 mg/mL on two occasions not increased above upper limit of normal of 480 mg/mL in healthy individuals *5549*

Luteinizing Hormone *Plasma* *Increase* In 12 male patients with rheumatoid arthritis mean concentration of 53 ± 34 µg/L significantly different from 30 ± 12 µg/L in 70 healthy male controls *3309*

Lymphocyte T-Cells *Blood* *No Effect* Increased T4/T8 ratio *126*

Lysylpyridinoline *Synovial Fluid* *No Effect* In 20 patients with rheumatoid arthritis mean concentration undetectable *4872*
Urine *Increase* In 20 patients with rheumatoid arthritis mean concentration of about 25 pmol/µmol creatinine significantly greater than mean of 17 pmol/µmol creatinine in 20 patients with osteoarthritis *4872*

β_2-Macroglobulin *Synovial Fluid* *Increase* Increased concentration *5103* *5150*

Macrophage Inflammatory Protein-1α
Synovial Fluid *Increase* Concentration increased compared with that in patients with osteoarthritis *5114*

Macrophage Inflammatory Protein-1β
Synovial Fluid *Increase* Detectable but concentration decreased compared with that in patients with osteoarthritis *5114*

Malondialdehyde *Serum* *Increase* In 33 patients with rheumatoid arthritis mean concentration of 3.42 ± 0.8 µmol/L significantly higher than 2.62 ± 0.42 µmol/L in 34 controls *3963*

Mannose-binding Protein *Serum* *Increase* In patients with active rheumatoid arthritis concentrations typically 1.6 times higher than reference interval determined by Behring Nephelometer II of < 0.17 - 10.1 mg/L *2961*

MCH *Blood* *Decrease* Microcytic hypochromic anemia may occur due to blood loss, increased demand or dietary inadequacy. MCH < 27 pg, MCV < 80 fL *1098*

MCV *Blood* *Decrease* Microcytic hypochromic anemia may occur due to blood loss, increased demand or dietary inadequacy. MCH < 27 pg, MCV < 80 fL *1098*
Blood *Increase* Macrocytic anemia may occur due to vitamin B_{12} or folate deficiency. MCV > 100 fL *1098*

Melanoma Inhibitory Factor *Serum* *Increase* In 46 patients mean concentration of 10.3 ± 10.2 ng/mL significantly greater than 3.6 ± 2.8 ng/mL in 120 healthy controls *3655*

α_1-Microglobulin *Cerebrospinal Fluid* *No Effect* Of 2 patients with rheumatoid arthritis mean concentration in neither greater than that in 15 healthy controls of 34.8 ± 16.0 µg/L *2370*

Monocyte Chemotactic Protein-1 *Synovial Fluid* *Increase* Concentration increased compared with that in patients with osteoarthritis *5114*

Monocytes *Blood* *Increase* Has been reported *3246* In 41% of 91 patients at initial hospitalization for this disorder *1576*
Pleural Fluid *Increase* Predominant cell type *4493*

Multiubiquitin Chains *Serum* *Increase* In 38 patients with rheumatoid arthritis mean concentration of 5.47 ± 2.12 µg/cells in 1 L blood significantly different from that in 45 healthy men and 51 healthy womenin whom the mean concentration was 3.86 ± 1.55 µg/cells from 1 liter of blood *5125*

Myosin *Serum* *No Effect* In 40 patients with classic or definite rheumatoid arthritis mean concentration normal *4565*

Neopterin *Serum* *Increase* Before treatment, activation of the monocyte-macrophage system had been signified by elevated serum levels of neopterin *2235*
Serum *No Effect* In 21 patients with rheumatoid arthritis mean concentration of 21.63 ± 3.32 nmol/L not significantly different from 26.13 ± 9.72 nmol/L in 21 healthy controls *1956*
Synovial Fluid *Increase* In 21 patients with RA mean concentration of 74.96 ± 35.88 nmol/L 3 times the concentration in 21 patients with osteoarthritis *1956* Exacerbations of disease associated with increased concentrations, which are higher in inflammatory joints than in non-inflammatory joints *121*
Urine *Increase* Urinary excretion shows good correlation with disease stage and clinical activity *121*

Nerve Growth Factor *Serum* *Increase* Mean concentration of 36.9 ± 86 pg/mL in 33 patients *1161*
Synovial Fluid *Increase* Mean concentration of 12.5 ± 19.2 pg/mL in 26 patients *1161*

Nerve Growth Factor Autoantibodies *Serum* *Increase* Mean value of 0.74 ± 0.18 in 33 patients significantly different from 0.42 ± 0.13 in 30 healthy controls *1161*
Synovial Fluid *Increase* Mean value of 0.76 ± 0.39 in 33 patients *1161*

Neurokinin A *Synovial Fluid* *Decrease* In patients with rheumatoid arthritis mean concentration reduced compared with controls *2928*

Neuropeptide Y *Synovial Fluid* *Increase* Mean concentration significantly higher in patients with rheumatoid arthritis than in controls *2928*

Neutrophil-activating Protein-2 *Serum* *No Effect* Normal amounts detected in plasma of patients with rheumatoid arthritis *5114*

714.00 **Rheumatoid Arthritis** *(continued)*

Neutrophils *Blood Increase* About 25% of patients develop a significant neutrophilic leukocytosis. These patients usually have arthritis of short duration with a high degree of activity and fever *4817* In 60% of 92 patients at initial hospitalization for this disorder *1576*
Pleural Fluid Increase Predominant cells neutrophils or monocytes *4493*
Synovial Fluid Increase Increased number, ranging from 5 - 96 /µL *5544*

Nitrate *Urine Increase* In 10 patients with rheumatoid arthritis with mean age of 63 ± 12 y and duration of disease of 4.4 ± 5.8 y mean excretion of 223 ± 126 µmol/mmol creatinine compared with 83 ± 63 µmol/mmol creatinine in 18 age and sex comparable controls *5019*

5'-Nucleotidase *Lymphocytes Decrease* In 36 patients with rheumatoid arthritis median concentrations of 7.6, 5.1 and 5.5 nmol/10^6 lymphocytes/h in patients with good response, insufficient response and adverse reactions respectively significantly less than 9.0 nmol/10^6 lymphocytes/h in 14 healthy controls *2648*
Serum Increase May be found in up to 33% of patients with a greater increase in enzyme activity in the synovial fluid *1290*
Synovial Fluid Increase Slightly increased in cases showing more advanced X-ray changes *5136* In 58% with reduction to normal following corticosteroid therapy *1290*

Nucleotide Pyrophosphohydrolase, Sedimentable
Synovial Fluid Decrease Mean activity in 6 patients with rheumatoid arthritis 38 ± 11 pmol/h/mL compared with 172 ± 68 pmol/h/mL in 3 normal individuals *3344*

Nucleotide Pyrophosphohydrolase, Soluble
Serum No Effect Mean activity in 46 patients with seropositive rheumatoid arthritis of 1,166 ± 37 pmol nitrophenol/h/mL not significantly different from that in 85 healthy individuals 1,141 ± 22 pmol nitrophenol/h/mL *691*
Synovial Fluid Decrease Mean activity in 6 patients with rheumatoid arthritis 430 ± 74 pmol/h/mL compared with 606 ± 174 pmol/h/mL in 3 normal individuals *3344*

Osteocalcin *Serum Decrease* Mean concentration of 7.2 ± 2.3 µg/L in 119 women with rheumatoid arthritis compared with 8.7 ± 2.1 µg/L in 47 healthy female controls *2826* In 2 patients with rheumatoid arthritis mean concentration significantly less than in 40 healthy age and sex matched controls *907*
Serum Increase In 15 patients with definite rheumatoid arthritis concentration significantly increased in late onset rheumatoid arthritis compared with healthy controls and patients with early or advanced rheumatoid arthritis *3296*
Serum No Effect In 105 ambulant non-steroid treated patients there was no relationship to parameters of disease activity *1311*

Parathyroid Hormone *Plasma Decrease* In 13 patients with rheumatoid arthritis and high erythrocyte sedimentation rates mean concentration of 22.2 ± 5.0 ng/L significantly less than 29.6 ± 6.3 ng/L in 15 healthy controls *2455*

Partial Thromboplastin Time *Plasma No Effect* Mean time in 20 patients with active disease of 37.4 ± 4.6 s and 36.4 ± 2.9 s in 9 with inactive disease not statistically different from each other and within normal range of 29 - 42 s *1615*

Pentosidine *Serum Increase* In 60 patients with rheumatoid arthritis mean concentration of 108.4 ± 146.5 nmol/L significantly different from 48.3 ± 11.5 nmol/L in 57 heathy volunteers *4399*

pH *Pleural Fluid Decrease* 7.0-7.2 pH *1604*
Synovial Fluid Decrease Low pH correlates with increasing WBC count (r = 0.92) in synovial fluid of acute and chronic arthritis *5574*

Phosphate *Serum No Effect* Generally normal *1980*

Phospholipase A *Serum Increase* Reported effect *4229*

Phospholipase A_2 *Serum Increase* Increased concentrations reported *46* Catalytic activity of phospholipase A2 and concentration of PLA2-II increased in serum of patients with rheumatoid arthritis and other arthritides *3766* Considerable increase in catalytic activity observed in patients with rheumatoid arthritis correlating well with the activity of the disease *3767*
Serum No Effect In 15 untreated patients mean concentration of 35.87 ± 9.6 kU/L compared with range of 15.1 - 47.8 kU/L in 20 healthy individuals *1926*
Synovial Fluid Increase Considerable increase of PLA2-II observed in disease with activity correlating with severity of disease *3766* In 15 untreated patients mean concentration of 79.59 ± 19.96 kU/L significantly increased compared with range of 28.38 - 4.46 kU/L in 15 patients with osteoarthritis *1926*

Phospholipase A_2 Type II *Serum Increase* Considerable increase in concentration observed in patients with rheumatoid arthritis correlating well with the activity of the disease *3767* In patients with rheumatoid arthritis mean concentration higher than in osteoarthritis and in healthy controls. Highest concentrations observed in patients with active rheumatoid arthritis *4905*
Synovial Fluid Increase Considerable increase in catalytic activity observed in patients with rheumatoid arthritis *3767*

α_2-Plasmin Inhibitor *Plasma No Effect* Mean concentration in 20 patients with active disease of 186.5 ± 242.1% and 119.8 ± 15.9% in 9 with inactive disease not significantly different from each other and normal range of 70 - 130% *1615*

Plasminogen Activator Inhibitor *Plasma Increase* Mean concentration of 16.1 U/mL without vasculitis in 38 patients with rheumatoid arthritis without vasculitis significantly higher than 11.1 U/mL in 64 normal individuals *2934*

Platelets *Blood Increase* Severe disease is characterized by thrombocytosis *3999* Counts exceeding 400,000 /µL are common and correlate best with leukocytosis and highly active disease *1980* In 46% of 40 patients at initial hospitalization for this disorder *1576*
Blood No Effect In 13 patients with rheumatoid arthritis mean concentration of 372 ± 28 x 10^6/L not significantly different from normal *5439* In 51 patients with early rheumatoid arthritis mean concentration of 307 x 10^9/L within the normal range *5408*

Polyamine Oxidase *Synovial Fluid Increase* In patients with rheumatoid arthritis polyamine oxidases present in synovial fluid *1466*

Procollagen Type II Peptide *Serum Increase* Detected in the sera of a group of patients with rheumatoid arthritis by ELISA and by immunoblotting *622* Raised serum IgG anti-type II collagen antibody levels were present in 11% of patients with RA, 30% with SLE, 44% with PSS and 42% with OL *1600* Type II collagen were detected in 22.7% of sera from 480 patients with rheumatoid arthritis (RA) *1593*

Procollagen Type III Peptide *Serum Increase* Significant correlation observed between concentration and AIMS score: increased concentrations mainly reflect extent of synovial inflammation of major joints *1465* Serum P-III-P levels were elevated in patients with PSS and MCTD/overlap syndrome, suggesting a high rate of collagen biosynthesis by fibroblasts. Patients with RA showed no significant elevation of serum P-III-P compared with normal control group *155* Mean concentration in 29 patients of 0.53 ± 0.14 U/mL significantly higher than 0.44 ± 0.09 U/mL in 40 healthy adults *1615*
Serum No Effect Patients with RA showed no significant elevation of serum P-III-P compared with normal control group. But the group of RA patients with elevated ESR and/or serum CRP values showed high levels of serum P-III-P *155*
Synovial Fluid Increase The levels were one to three hundred times higher than serum levels, and they showed the positive correlation with serum levels, suggesting that serum P-III-P might be originated from synovial P-III-P *155*

Prolactin *Plasma Decrease* In men with RA mean concentration significantly reduced whereas only bioactive prolactin significantly reduced in women *3709*

Properdin Factor B *Plasma Increase* Mean concentration typically slightly increased or normal in patients with moderate rheumatoid arthritis *4682*
Plasma No Effect Mean concentration typically normal in patients with severe rheumatoid arthritis *4682*

Prostaglandin E_2 *Synovial Fluid Increase* Mean concentration in 6 untreated patients of about 3.6 nmol/L with concentration incresasing with stage of the disease *3366*

Prostaglandins *Synovial Fluid Increase* Prostaglandin E_2 usually predominates. Concentration does not seem to correlate with clinical course of disease *521*

Protein *Pericardial Fluid Increase* With rheumatoid pericarditis a high total protein is common *1550*
Pleural Fluid Increase Tends to produce high total protein concentration *774*
Serum No Effect In 60 patients with rheumatoid arthritis mean concentration of 71 ± 6 g/L not significantly different from 72 ± 4 g/L in 57 heathy volunteers *4399*
Synovial Fluid Increase Characteristically turbid with increased protein content *2039*

Prothrombin Time *Plasma* *No Effect* Mean time in 20 patients with active disease of 11.1 ± 0.4 s and 10.8 ± 0.2 s in 9 with inactive disease not significantly different and within normal range *1615*

Purine Nucleoside Phosphorylase *Lymphocytes* *Increase* In 36 patients with rheumatoid arthritis median concentrations of 102.5 ± 19.4, 83.8 ± 21.6 and 82.7 ± 22.9 nmol/10^6 lymphocytes/h in patients with good response, insufficient response and adverse reactions respectively significantly higher than 84 nmol/10^6 lymphocytes/h in 14 healthy controls *2648*

Pyridinoline *Synovial Fluid* *Increase* In 5 patients mean concentration of 32.4 ± 14.6 pmol/mL *4343*
Urine *Increase* In 62 patients with rheumatoid arthritis mean 8 h excretion of 254 ± 116 nmol/8 h significantly greater than 153 ± 84 nmol/8 h in 56 healthy controls although differences in postmenopausal women not significant *1833* Excretion increased significantly increased in patients with rheumatoid arthritis compared with controls *1833* In 18 postmenopausal women aged 51 - 69 y with rheumatoid arthritis mean excretion of total pyridinoline of 83.9 ± 26.7 nmol/mmol creatinine in 2-hour significantly greater than that in 30 healthy premenopausal women aged 24 - 50 y with regular menstrual cycle in whom the mean excretion was 44.8 ± 17.3 nmol/mmol creatinine in 2-hour morning collection. In 20 postmenopausal women with rheumatoid arthritis mean excretion of 115.4 ± 59.8 nmol/mmol creatinine also significantly different from 69.0 ± 45.8 nmol/mmol creatinine in 22 matched post-menopausal controls *5131*

Pyridinoline Cross-linked Telopeptide of Type I Collagen *Serum* *Increase* In 99 adult patients with rheumatoid arthritis of less than 1 year's duration mean concentration of 5.9 ± 2.2 μg/L (median 5.3 μg/L) compared with upper limit of reference interval of 4.6 μg/L with mean concentration of 6.6 ± 2.3 μg/L higher in those with general joint disease than 4.6 ± 1.3 μg/L in those with peripheral joint disease *2790*

Pyridinoline, Free *Urine* *Increase* In 18 postmenopausal women aged 51 - 69 y with rheumatoid arthritis mean excretion of immunologically measured free dipyridinoline of 6.8 ± 1.7 nmol/mmol creatinine in 2-hour not significantly different from than that in 30 healthy premenopausal women aged 24 - 50 y with regular menstrual cycle in whom the mean excretion was 4.9 ± 1.3 nmol/mmol creatinine in 2-hour morning collection. In 20 postmenopausal women with rheumatoid arthritis mean excretion of 9.2 ± 4.4 nmol/mmol creatinine also significantly different from 6.4 ± 1.7 nmol/mmol creatinine in 22 matched post-menopausal controls *5131*
Urine *No Effect* In 20 postmenopausal women with rheumatoid arthritis mean excretion of 34.2 ± 30.8 nmol/mmol creatinine not significantly different from 29.1 ± 20.4 nmol/mmol creatinine in 22 matched post-menopausal controls *5131*

Pyridinoline, Peptide-bound *Urine* *Increase* In 18 postmenopausal women aged 51 - 69 y with rheumatoid arthritis mean excretion of 50.5 ± 16.4 nmol/mmol creatinine in 2-hour significantly greater than that in 30 healthy premenopausal women aged 24 - 50 y with regular menstrual cycle in whom the mean excretion was 34.9 ± 15.2 nmol/mmol creatinine in 2-hour morning collection. In 20 postmenopausal women with rheumatoid arthritis mean excretion of 81.1 ± 42.9 nmol/mmol creatinine also significantly different from 39.8 ± 25.8 nmol/mmol creatinine in 22 matched post-menopausal controls *5131*

Pyridoxine *Urine* *Decrease* Patients with active disease excrete abnormally low B_6 and related metabolites *4707*

Pyrophosphate *Synovial Fluid* *No Effect* Near normal levels *2386*

Retinol *Serum* *No Effect* Mean concentration of 685 ± 135 μg/L in 14 patients with rheumatoid arthritis not different from 685 ± 111 μg/L in 27 healthy controls *2101*

Rheumatoid Factor *Serum* *Increase* Low values associated with more severe disease and poorer prognosis *630* Of 119 patients with rheumatoid arthritis 44.4% of those with thyroid disease had positive rheumatoid factor compared with 50.0% in those without thyroid disease *4812* The majority of rheumatoid sera give positive reactions; the incidence varies with different techniques, but at least 70%. A high degree of correlation of rheumatoid factors and subcutaneous nodules, symmetrical deforming arthritis of the hands and wrists, and various visceral manifestations of rheumatoid arthritis *4551* Correlated with anatomical stage, class and course of disease and ESR *1141* In 31 patients rheumatoid factor present in 19 and absent in 12 *5287* Mean concentration increased in patients with rheumatoid arthritis *2472* Mean concentration of 199.6 ± 84.3 U/L observed in 25 patients *5561* Significant increase to 347 ± 502 ng/mL observed in patients with rheumatoid arthritis *3365* Most patients with rheumatoid arthritis have a positive titer, although 25% have a nonreactive titer *2952* As few 28% of patients with rheumatoid arthritis may have positive RF measurements *5211* Rheumatoid factor may be observed in certain patients *2473*
Synovial Fluid *Increase* Low values associated with more severe disease and poorer prognosis *630*

Rheumatoid Factor (IgA) *Serum* *Increase* In 114 patients with active rheumatoid arthritis mean OD of 0.183 ± 0.170 significantly different from 0.028 ± 0.013 in 24 healthy controls. 38 of the 114 patients had demonstrable IgA rheumatoid factor *3973*

Rheumatoid Factor (IgM) *Serum* *Increase* In 114 patients with active rheumatoid arthritis mean titer in 38 with IgA rheumatoid factor of 1:256 significantly different from 1:128 in 76 without IgA rheumatoid factor significantly higher than in healthy controls *3973*

Selenium *Serum* *Decrease* Mean plasma concentration of 107.5 ± 23.8 μg/L in 60 patients with chronic rheumatoid arthritis significantly less than 168.5 ± 46.4 μg/L in 60 healthy controls *2781*
Serum *No Effect* Mean concentration of 60.0 ± 12.8 μg/L in 27 patients with rheumatoid arthritis not significantly different from 61.2 ± 12.2 μg/L in 51 healthy controls *2101*

Sodium *Saliva* *Increase* The concentrations of salivary sodium and IgA were significantly elevated in 24% of patients. 80% of the patients with elevated sodium and IgA concentrations had keratoconjunctivitis sicca as well *382*

Soluble CD4⁺ *Serum* *No Effect* In 26 patients with rheumatoid arthritis mean concentration of surface CD4 of 41 ± 60 not significantly different from 25 ± 20 in controls and most concentrations remained within normal range regardless of clinical response *1217*

Soluble CD8⁺ *Blood* *No Effect* Mean concentration of surface CD8 in 26 patients with rheumatoid arthritis of 510 ± 353 U/mL not significantly different from 405 ± 245 U/mL in healthy controls *1217*
Serum *Increase* Concentration increased compared with age-matched healthy controls *5111*
Synovial Fluid *Increase* Concentration increased compared with patients with osteoarthritis and age-matched healthy controls *5111*

Soluble CD30 *Serum* *Increase* Concentrations of 15.2 ± 2.1 U/mL observed in 25 patients compared with 8.8 ± 0.9 U/mL in 21 healthy control individuals *5561*

Soluble E-Selectin *Serum* *No Effect* In 13 patients with rheumatoid arthritis mean concentration of 49.3 ± 4.6 ng/mL not significantly different from 48.2 ± 3.9 ng/mL in controls *5439*

Soluble HLA-I *Serum* *Increase* In 8 blacks with active rheumatoid arthritis mean concentration of 556 ng/mL significantly higher than 357 ng/mL in normal blacks *25* In 16 patients with rheumatoid arthritis, mean concentration of 0.61 ± 0.34 μg/mL significantly increased compared with 0.41 ± 0.20 μg/mL in 30 normal controls *5306*

Soluble HLA-II *Synovial Fluid* *Increase* Known to be present in the synovial fluid of patients with rheumatoid arthritis *216*

Soluble Intercellular Adhesion Molecule-1 *Serum* *Increase* In 13 patients with rheumatoid arthritis mean concentration of 345.0 ± 29.8 ng/mL significantly higher than 238.0 ± 26.0 ng/mL in controls *5439*

Soluble Intercellular Adhesion Molecule-3 *Synovial Fluid* *Increase* Mean concentration of 40.5 ± 3.0 ng/mL in specimens from 39 patients *2244*

Soluble Interleukin-2 Receptor *Serum* *Increase* In 26 patients with rheumatoid arthritis mean concentration of 851 ± 313 U/mL significantly higher than 462 ± 151 U/mL. Mean concentration of 1,040 ± 283 U/mL higher in those who responded to NSAIDs than 751 ± 288 U/mL in those who did not *1217* Mean concentration of 81 pmol/L (range 40 - 350 pmol/L) significantly higher in 65 patients than in healthy controls *3367* Mean concentration of 1,288 ± 421 U/mL in 19 patients with active disease significantly higher than 686 ± 205 U/mL in 18 patients with inactive disease or 842 ± 414 U/mL in 5 with active disease undergoing treatment with cyclosporine *941* In 26 patients with rheumatoid arthritis median concentration of 81 pmol/L (range 40 - 350 pmol/L) significantly higher than median of 45 pmol/L (range 13 - 100 pmol/L) in 25 control patients with osteoarhtritis *3367* In a study of 137 patients with rheumatoid arthritis mean concentration of 980 ± 589 U/mL compared with mean of 446

714.00 Rheumatoid Arthritis *(continued)*

Soluble Interleukin-2 Receptor *(continued)*
U/mL in 47 healthy controls *3460* In 41 patients with rheumatoid arthritis with average duration of disease of 168 ± 110 months mean concentration increased to 910 ± 422 units *4167*
Synovial Fluid *Increase* Mean concentration of 125 pmol/L (range 52 - 460 pmol/L) in 10 healthy volunteers *3367* In 27 specimens from patients with rheumatoid arthritis median concentration of 125 pmol/L (range of 52 - 460 pmol/L) significantly higher than median of 37 pmol/L (range of 15 - 140 pmol/L) in 28 control specimens from patients with osteoarthritis and 2.5 pmol/L (range of 0 - 10 pmol/L) in 10 healthy control individuals *3367*

Soluble Interleukin-6 Receptor-α *Synovial Fluid* *Increase* Mean concentration of 24.7 ± 7.5 ng/mL in 22 patients with rheumatoid arthritis *1130*

Soluble P-Selectin *Serum* *Increase* In 13 patients with rheumatoid arthritis mean concentration of 332.8 ± 48.2 ng/mL significantly higher than 113.9 ± 10.2 ng/mL in controls *5439*
Synovial Fluid *Increase* Mean concentration of 72.4 ± 12.9 ng/mL in specimens from 39 patients *2244*

Soluble Transferrin Receptor *Serum* *No Effect* Mean concentration in 35 patients of 2.8 ± 1.4 mg/L not significantly different from normal range of 0.85 - 3.05 mg/L *3784*

Soluble Tumor Necrosis Factor Receptor-p55
Serum *Increase* Median concentration in 20 patients with rheumatoid arthritis of 2.7 ng/mL higher than 2.1 ng/mL in 20 healthy controls *1612*

Soluble Tumor Necrosis Factor Receptor-p55:Tumor Necrosis Factor-α Ratio *Serum* *Decrease* In 66 patients with rheumatoid arthritis mean ratio of 426 ± 178 significantly different from 1,042 ± 644 in 14 healthy controls *4378*

Soluble Tumor Necrosis Factor Receptor-p75
Serum *Increase* In 66 patients with rheumatoid arthritis mean concentration of 2,116 ± 857 pg/mL significantly higher than 738 ± 139 pg/mL in 14 healthy controls *4378* Median concentration in 20 patients with rheumatoid arthritis of 9 ng/mL higher than 6.9 ng/mL in 20 healthy controls *1612* In 66 patients with rheumatoid arthritis mean concentration of 4,545 ± 1,287 pg/mL significantly higher than 1,025 ± 219 pg/mL in 14 healthy controls *4378*

Soluble Tumor Necrosis Factor Receptor-p75:Tumor Necrosis Factor-α *Serum* *Decrease* In 66 patients with rheumatoid arthritis mean ratio of 921 ± 278 significantly different from 1,453 ± 930 in 14 healthy controls *4378*

Soluble Vascular Cell Adhesion Molecule-1
Serum *Increase* In 13 patients with rheumatoid arthritis mean concentration of 815.8 ± 42.5 ng/mL significantly higher than 592.5 ± 114.2 ng/mL in controls *5439*

Stromelysin *Plasma* *Increase* In 73 patients with rheumatoid arthritis mean concentration of 187.9 ± 13.8 ng/mL significantly higher than 50.0 ± 4.4 ng/mL in 53 healthy controls *5878*

Substance P *Synovial Fluid* *Decrease* No substance P detectable in synovial fluid of patients with rheumatoid arthritis *2928*

Testosterone *Serum* *No Effect* In 12 male patients with rheumatoid arthritis mean concentration of 4.09 ± 1.56 ng/mL not significantly different from 4.32 ± 1.07 ng/mL in 70 healthy male controls *3309*

Thrombin/Antithrombin III Complex *Plasma* *Increase* Mean concentration in 29 patients of 9.19 ± 11.93 ng/mL significantly greater than 1.23 ± 0.42 ng/mL in 40 healthy adults *1615*

β-Thromboglobulin *Plasma* *No Effect* Normal amounts detected in plasma of patients with rheumatoid arthritis *5114*

Thrombomodulin *Plasma* *Increase* In 12 patients with active disease mean concentration of 50 ng/mL compared with 15 ng/mL in 30 patients with inactive disease and 10 ng/mL in healthy controls *3873*

Thyroxine (T4) *Serum* *Decrease* In 119 patients with rheumatoid arthritis 18 had hypothyroidism *4812*

Tissue Plasminogen Activator Antigen *Plasma* *No Effect* In 38 patients with rheumatoid arthritis without vasculitis mean concentration without venous occlusion of 126% not significantly different from 139% in 64 normal individuals *2934*

α-Tocopherol *Serum* *Decrease* In 14 patients with rheumatoid arthritis mean concentration of 9.02 ± 2.30 mg/L not significantly reduced compared with 9.93 ± 2.55 mg/L in 27 healthy controls *2101*

Transferrin *Serum* *No Effect* Mean concentration in 19 patients with adequate iron stores of 23.3 ± 3.8 µmol/L significantly less compared with 26.9 ± 5.3 µmol/L in 10 patients with iron deficiency but still within normal range of 21 - 36 µmol/L *3784*

Triglycerides *Serum* *No Effect* In 51 patients with rheumatoid arthritis median concentrations of 1.3 and 1.4 mmol/L on two occasions not increased above upper limit of normal of 2.2 mmol/L in healthy individuals *5549* Median concentration in 17 patients with rheumatoid arthritis of 1.21 mmol/L not significantly different from 1.4 mmol/L in 16 healthy controls *5548* Mean concentration of 112 ± 69 mg/dL in 131 patients with rheumatoid arthritis not significantly higher than 125 ± 83 mg/dL in 200 healthy controls *195*

Trypsin Inhibitor *Synovial Fluid* *Increase* Elevated in 36 patients with involvement of the knee joint *4384*

Tumor Necrosis Factor-α *Bone Marrow* *No Effect* In 25 patients with rheumatoid arthritis concentration in bone marrow serum close to or below the assay detection limit *5157*
Serum *Increase* In 22 patients with rheumatoid arthritis median concentration of 25.6 pg/mL significantly different from upper limit of normal *1612* Immunoassays were used to measure levels of TNF-α in the serum of 35 patients with RA and a group of age-and sex-matched control subjects. Serum levels were significantly higher in the RA population than in the control group *5223* In 66 patients with rheumatoid arthritis mean concentration of 5.6 ± 4.7 pg/mL significantly higher than 0.9 ± 0.4 pg/mL in 14 healthy controls *4378* Serum levels of TNF-α were significantly higher in the RA population than in the control group *3273*
Serum *No Effect* Median concentration in 17 patients with rheumatoid arthritis of 19.3 pg/mL not significantly different from 20 pg/mL or less in 16 healthy controls *5548*
Synovial Fluid *Increase* Observed in joint fluid in some patients *4605*

Tumor Necrosis Factor-β *Bone Marrow* *No Effect* In 25 patients with rheumatoid arthritis concentration in bone marrow serum close to or below the assay detection limit *5157*
Serum *Increase* In 66 patients with rheumatoid arthritis mean concentration of 4.2 ± 9.1 pg/mL significantly higher than 0.0 ± 0.0 pg/mL in 14 healthy controls *4378*
Synovial Fluid *No Effect* Reported effect *4605*

Type IV Collagen 7S Domain *Serum* *Increase* In 29 patients mean concentration of 4.49 ± 0.58 ng/mL significantly greater than 3.82 ± 0.87 ng/mL in 40 healthy adults *1615*

Tyrosine *Plasma* *Decrease* Frequently low *4707*

Ubiquitin, Free *Blood* *Decrease* In 23 patients with rheumatoid arthritis mean concentration of 88.3 ± 43.5 µg/cells in 1 L blood less than that in 45 healthy men and 51 healthy women in whom the mean concentration was 126 ± 24.4 µg/cells from 1 liter of blood *5125*

Urea Nitrogen *Serum* *Increase* At times increased. Somewhat elevated (30 - 40 mg/dL) during active phase *900*
Serum *No Effect* In 60 patients with rheumatoid arthritis mean concentration of 6.7 ± 2.0 mmol/L not significantly different from 6.1 ± 1.5 mmol/L in 57 heathy volunteers *4399*

Uric Acid *Serum* *Increase* Slight elevation may occur, especially in male patients *2900*
Serum *No Effect* Generally normal *1980*

Varicella Zoster Antibodies *Serum* *Increase* The titers were not found to increase with the disease duration *1468*

Vascular Endothelial Growth Factor *Serum* *Increase* Mean concentration in 11 patients with rheumatoid arthritis of 563 ± 375 pg/mL significantly different from 184 ± 62 pg/mL in 20 healthy individuals *2674*

Vasoactive Intestinal Polypeptide *Synovial Fluid* *No Effect* No consistent increase or decrease observed with rheumatoid arthritis compared with controls *2928*

VDRL *Serum* *Positive* Biologic false positive tests reported in 5 - 10% of patients. Those patients are more likely to have positive LE cell tests *1980*

Viscosity *Plasma* *Increase* In 16 patients with rheumatoid arthritis median vicosity of 1.80 cP significantly different from median viscosity of 1.74 cP in 12 patients with seronegative polyarthritis *5290* In 58 patients with rheumatoid arthritis median of 1.83 ± 0.14 mPa significantly different from 1.72 mPa in healthy controls *430*

Vitamin B_{12} *Serum* *No Effect* Mean concentration of holo-transcobalamin I and II not significantly different between 30 patients with active rheumatoid arthritis and 27 in clinical remission *180*

von Willebrand Factor *Plasma* *No Effect* In 38 patients with rheumatoid arthritis without vasculitis mean concentration of 850 IU/L without venous occlusion not significantly different from 786 IU/L in 64 normal individuals *2934*

714.10 Felty's Syndrome

Anti-ds DNA Antibodies *Serum* *No Effect* Found in 0% of cases *4897*

Anti-Neutrophil Cytoplasm Antibodies *Serum* *Increase* In 33% of patients with Felty's syndrome increased titers observed *2502*

Anti-ss DNA Antibodies *Serum* *Increase* Found in 100% of cases *4897*

Antinuclear Antibodies *Serum* *Increase* Positive in 100% of cases *4068* Found in 75% of cases *4897* In 69% of patients increased titers observed *2502*

Complement, Total *Serum* *Decrease* Hypocomplementemia usually occurs *3513*

LE Cells *Blood* *Positive* Positive LE test is more frequent than in rheumatoid arthritis *5544*

Leukocytes *Blood* *Decrease* Leukopenia (usually due to neutropenia) occurs predisposing patients to infection *4962*

Neutrophils *Blood* *Decrease* Most patients appear to have increased cell margination probably with splenic sequestration. About 33% have impaired production *865* Leukopenia (usually due to neutropenia) occurs predisposing patients to infection *4962*

Rheumatoid Factor *Serum* *Increase* Serologic tests are positive; may be present in high titers *5544*

714.30 Juvenile Chronic Arthritis

Antioxidative Enzyme Activity *Serum* *Increase* In 72 children with juvenile chronic arthritis mean activity of 34.36 ± 17.54 µmol H_2O_2/mL/min significantly higher than 11.06 ± 0.23 µmol H_2O_2/mL/min in 20 healthy control children *3268*

Nerve Growth Factor *Serum* *Increase* Mean concentration of 254 ± 256 pg/mL in 17 children with systemic disease, 165 ± 301 pg/mL in 39 with polyarticular disease and 107 ± 112 pg/mL in 24 with pauciarticular disease significantly different from 6.0 ± 4.5 pg/mL in healthy controls *1413*

Soluble Intercellular Adhesion Molecule-1 *Serum* *Increase* In 37 children with juvenile chronic arthritis mean concentration of 609 ± 184 ng/mL significantly greater than 210 ± 95 ng/mL in 25 healthy control children *2935*

714.30 Juvenile Rheumatoid Arthritis

Alanine Aminotransferase *Serum* *Increase* Mild elevation is common in untreated and aspirin-treated children but increases are sporadic *4258*

Albumin *Serum* *Decrease* In acute systemic form *335*

Anti-ds DNA Antibodies *Serum* *Increase* Found in 5% of cases *4897*

Anti-Ribonuclear Protein Antibodies *Serum* *Increase* Found in 3% of cases *4897*

Anti-Sjögren's Syndrome A Antibodies (SSA[Ro]) *Serum* *No Effect* Found in 0% of cases *4897*

Anti-Sjögren's Syndrome B Antibodies (SSB[La]) *Serum* *No Effect* Found in 0% of cases *4897*

Anti-ss DNA Antibodies *Serum* *Increase* Found in 3% of cases *4897*

Anti-Streptolysin-O Titer *Serum* *Increase* Increased in 50% of cases *1588*

Antinuclear Antibodies *Serum* *Increase* Found in 57% of cases *4897* Frequently found in sera from patients with pauciarticular disease and children with mild disease activity *4451* Found in 13% of cases *4746*
Serum *No Effect* In acute systemic form *335*

Aspartate Aminotransferase *Serum* *Increase* Transiently but only moderately elevated in many children receiving high dosages of aspirin; decreases to normal as the dosage of salicylates is lowered *900* Mild elevation is common in untreated and aspirin-treated children but increases are sporadic *4258*

Complement C_3 *Serum* *Increase* Serum C_2, C_4, and C_9 were elevated, but only C_9 correlated well with ESR *4683*
Synovial Fluid *Decrease* Synovial fluid levels C_1q, C_3, C_4 and C_9 were consistently depressed in all seropositive patients, and in 5 of 14 seronegative patients *4683*

Complement C_4 *Serum* *Increase* Serum C_2, C_3, C_4, and C_9 were elevated, but only C_9 correlated well with ESR *4683*
Synovial Fluid *Decrease* Synovial fluid levels of C_1q, C_3, C_4, and C_9 were consistently depressed in all seropositive patients and in 5 of 14 seronegative patients *4683*

Complement, Total *Serum* *Decrease* In 22 patients, 32% had decreased values *4925*
Serum *Increase* Normal or increased *335* Serum C_2, C_3, C_4, and C_9 were elevated, but only C_9 correlated well with ESR. RF positive patients tend to have lower CH50 than do RF negative patients, but both groups show increased titers during active disease *4683* In 22 patients, 13% had increased values *4925*
Serum *No Effect* Normal or increased *335*
Synovial Fluid *Decrease* Synovial fluid levels of C_1q, C_3, C_4, and C_9 were consistently depressed in all seropositive patients and in 5 of 14 negative patients *4683*

C-Reactive Protein *Serum* *Increase* In acute systemic form *335*

Erythrocyte Sedimentation Rate *Blood* *Increase* Moderately increased; mean of 68 mm/h, and range of 38 - 104 mm/h in 6 children with chronic polyarthritis *956* ESR is usually elevated moderately when inflammatory disease is severe, but is often normal in the presence of reduced disease activity and is not a constant laboratory parameter *900*
Blood *No Effect* Usually elevated moderately when inflammatory disease is severe, but is often normal in the presence of reduced disease activity and is not a consistent laboratory parameter *900*

Ferritin *Serum* *Increase* Markedly increased, ranging from 120 - 2,000 µg/dL (mean = 822 µg/dL) compared to normals, 35 - 155 µg/dL. Fluctuations correlated closely with disease activity ($r = 0.954$, $p < 0.05$) *956*

Glucose *Synovial Fluid* *Decrease* Normal or low *335*

Hematocrit *Blood* *Decrease* Moderate anemia is common with hematocrit values of 30 - 34% *900*

Hemoglobin *Blood* *Decrease* Moderate anemia is common with hemoglobin concentrations of 9 - 11 g/dL *900*

25-Hydroxy Vitamin D *Serum* *Decrease* In children with polyarticular and systemic juvenile rheumatoid arthritis significant decrease of 25(OH)D observed compared with control children and in those with pauciarticular disease *436*

Immunoglobulin G *Serum* *Increase* Polyclonal increase *1588*

Interleukin-1α *Serum* *Increase* In 22 patients with pauciarticular JRA mean concentration of 262 pg/mL and 275 pg/mL in 26 patients with polyarticular JRA significantly higher than 77 pg/mL in controls *3197*

Interleukin-1β *Serum* *No Effect* In 22 patients with pauciarticular JRA mean concentration of 0.91 pg/mL and 0.92 pg/mL in 26 patients with polyarticular JRA not significantly different from 1.62 pg/mL in 29 controls and 2.75 pg/mL in 12 patients with systemic onset JRA *3197*

Interleukin-2 *Serum* *Increase* In 22 patients with pauciarticular JRA mean concentration of 37,864 pg/mL and 39,496 pg/mL in 26 patients with polyarticular JRA significantly higher than 372 pg/mL in 29 controls and 0 pg/mL in 14 patients with systemic onset JRA *3197*

714.30 Juvenile Rheumatoid Arthritis (continued)

Interleukin-6 *Serum* *Increase* Measured interleukin-6 (IL-6) levels in 70 serum samples obtained from 25 patients with systemic-onset juvenile rheumatoid arthritis (JRA), using the hybridoma cell line B_9. Patients with systemic-onset JRA had significantly elevated serum IL-6 levels during active disease ($p < 0.00001$ versus healthy age-matched controls), but not during remission. Serum IL-6 levels correlated with the extent and severity of joint involvement ($p < 0.001$) and with platelet counts ($p < 0.05$) *1046* In 22 patients with pauciarticular JRA mean concentration of 540 pg/mL and 955 pg/mL in 26 patients with polyarticular JRA significantly higher than 116.6 pg/mL in 29 controls and 0 pg/mL in 14 patients with systemic onset JRA *3197* Plasma IL-6 levels were higher in patients with polyarticular JRA than controls *3859*
Synovial Fluid *Increase* High concentrations observed in patients with juvenile RA with polyarticular onset of disease *605*

Iron *Serum* *Decrease* Normal or low *335*

Iron-binding Capacity, Total *Serum* *Decrease* Normal or low *335*

Leukocytes *Blood* *Increase* Leukocytosis in the range of 15,000 - 25,000 /µL is common and distinguishes it from the adult rheumatoid arthritis *367* Usually normal but may be slightly elevated and rarely leukemoid *900* There may be a high peripheral WBC (up to 50,000 /µL) *144*
Blood *No Effect* Usually normal but may be slightly elevated and rarely even leukemoid *900*

Leukotriene E_4 *Urine* *Increase* In 10 children and adolescents with juvenile rheumatoid arthritis mean excretion 26.9 nmol/mol creatinine compared with 8.1 nmol/mol creatinine in 10 age and sex matched controls *1432*

Lymphocytes *Synovial Fluid* *Increase* Abundant lymphocytes (sometimes > 50%) and immature lymphocytes and monocytes present in the synovial fluid *5544*

α_2-Macroglobulin *Serum* *Decrease* In acute systemic form *335*

Rheumatoid Factor *Serum* *Increase* No more than 10% of patients have a positive rheumatoid factor in sera *367* Found in only 10 - 20% of children *144*
Serum *No Effect* No more than 10% of patients have a positive rheumatoid factor in sera *367* In acute systemic form *335* Found in only 10 - 20% of children *144*
Synovial Fluid *No Effect* Absent in synovial fluid *5545*

Soluble Interleukin-2 Receptor *Serum* *Increase* In 12 patients with systemic onset juvenile rheumatoid arthritis mean concentration of 2,363 U/mL significantly higher than in patients with pauciarticular (1,326 U/mL) and polyarticular (1,131 U/mL) JRA and controls (1,285 U/mL) *3197*

Thrombomodulin *Plasma* *Increase* In 2 patients with juvenile rheumatoid arthritis mean concentration of 115 ng/mL compared with 10 ng/mL in 66 healthy controls *3873*

Tumor Necrosis Factor-α *Serum* *No Effect* In 13 patients with systemic onset JRA mean concentration of 24.6 pg/mL not significantly different from undetectable amounts in 20 patients with pauciarticular JRA, 18 patients with polyarticular JRA and in 29 controls *3197*

714.30 Still's Disease

Ferritin *Serum* *Increase* In 2 patients with adult Still's disease concentrations greater than 10,000 µg/L observed: concentrations decreased in response to treatment *4694*

Soluble Interleukin-2 Receptor *Serum* *Increase* Increased concentrations observed in the plasma of 2 patients with adult Still's disease *4694*

715.90 Osteoarthritis

Alkaline Phosphatase, Bone Isoenzyme
Synovial Fluid *Increase* In 29 patients mean concentration of 2.6 ± 1.6 µg/L *1044*

Angiotensin-converting Enzyme *Serum* *No Effect* Not significantly different (n = 11) from normal controls (n = 26) *3141*

Aspartate Aminotransferase *Serum* *Increase* In 23% of 120 patients at initial hospitalization for this disorder *1576*

Biopterin *Synovial Fluid* *Increase* In 21 patients with osteoarthritis mean concentration of 16.61 ± 7.47 nmol/L *1956*

Bone Sialoprotein *Serum* *Increase* In 38 patients with osteoarthritis mean concentration of 102 ng/mL in those with scintigraphic abnormalities significantly different from 82 ng/mL in those without scintigraphic changes *4099* Mean concentration of 143.3 ± 27.3 ng/dL in 48 patients with osteoarthritis of the hip *903*

Carcinoembryonic Antigen *Serum* *Increase* In 112 patients with osteoarthritis 70% had concentrations less than 2.5 ng/mL, 24% had concentrations between 2.6 and 5.0 ng/mL, 5% had concentrations between 5.1 and 10.0 ng/mL and 1% had concentrations greater than 10.0 ng/mL *2010* 30% of patients had values > 2.5 ng/mL *4891*

Cartilage Oligomeric Matrix Protein *Serum* *Increase* Mean concentration of 7.7 ± 1.2 µg/mL in 48 patients with osteoarthritis of the hip *903* In 38 patients with osteoarthritis mean concentration of 13 µg/mL in those with scintigraphic abnormalities significantly different from 11 µg/mL in those without scintigraphic changes *4099*

Cells *Synovial Fluid* *Increase* In 4 patients mean concentration of 500 ± 82 /µL *4343*

Cholesterol *Serum* *No Effect* In 809 patients with osteoarthritis mean concentration of 5.8 ± 1.1 mmol/L not significantly different from that in normal individuals, with no differences observed between individuals with hip and knee problems *5058*

Chondrex *Serum* *Increase* Mean concentration of 142.8 ± 131.9 µg/L in 27 patients with osteoarthritis significantly different from 50.7 ± 38.6 µg/L in 329 apparently healthy controls *2040*

Chondroitin Sulfate Epitope ($3B_3$) *Synovial Fluid* *Increase* In 35 patients mean concentration of 1.29 ± 0.78 µg/mL *4758*

C-Reactive Protein *Serum* *Increase* Mean concentration of 7.5 ± 14.6 mg/L in 48 patients with osteoarthritis of the hip *903*
Serum *No Effect* In 14 patients median concentration of 0.0 µg/mL not different from normal *5287*

C-terminal Telopeptide of Type I Collagen *Urine* *Decrease* In 62 postmenopausal women with osteoarthritis mean excretion of 286 ± 160 µg/mmol creatinine significantly different from 546 ± 257 µg/mmol creatinine in 22 matched post-menopausal controls *5131*

Dipyridinoline *Urine* *No Effect* In 62 postmenopausal women with osteoarthritis mean excretion of immunologically measured dipyridinoline of 7.2 ± 2.4 nmol/mmol creatinine not significantly different from 6.4 ± 1.7 nmol/mmol creatinine in 22 matched post-menopausal controls *5131*

Dipyridinoline, Free *Urine* *Decrease* In 62 postmenopausal women with osteoarthritis mean excretion of 3.8 ± 2.1 nmol/mmol creatinine significantly different from 6.5 ± 5.9 nmol/mmol creatinine in 22 matched post-menopausal controls *5131*

Dopamine β-Hydroxylase *Serum* *Increase* 2 times normal value *4553*
Synovial Fluid *Increase* 3 times normal value *4553*

Epithelial-neutrophil Activating Protein-78
Synovial Fluid *Increase* Detected in synovial fluid of patients with osteoarthritis but to a lesser extent than in rheumatoid arthritis *5114*

Erythrocyte Sedimentation Rate *Blood* *Increase* Occurs only during rare episodes of acute inflammation of the joints *1980*
Blood *No Effect* In 14 patients median rate 10 mm/h, not different from normal *5287* Usually normal *1980* In 4 patients mean rate of 5 ± 3 mm/h *4343*

Ferritin *Synovial Fluid* *Increase* In 11 patients with osteoarthritis mean concentration of 393 ± 210 ng/mL *3945*

Gelatinase *Serum* *No Effect* In 9 patients with osteoarthritis mean concentration of 460.8 ± 65.1 ng/mL not significantly higher than 408.9 ± 28.0 ng/mL in 53 healthy controls *5878*

Glucose *Synovial Fluid* *No Effect* Nearly equal to blood concentration *1367*

Glycosaminoglycans *Serum* *Increase* A corresponding increase has been reported in synovial fluid, serum and urine of patients with rheumatic diseases *2651*
Synovial Fluid *Increase* In 35 patients mean concentration of 71.5 ± 30.8 µg/mL *4758* A corresponding increase has been reported in synovial fluid, serum and urine of patients with rheumatic diseases *2651*

Urine *Increase* Significant difference (median 25.4; n = 24) in comparison with unaffected individuals (median 20.2; n = 38) *2651*

Glycosylated Ferritin *Synovial Fluid* *Increase* In 10 patients with osteoarthritis mean proportion of 6.9 ± 11.0% *3945*

β-Hexosaminidase *Urine* *Decrease* Observed effect *3141*

Hyaluronic Acid *Serum* *Increase* Compared with the controls, the mean level of plasma HA was twofold higher in the OA group *1786* Assayed using a radiometric method (Pharmacia) in 73 osteoarthritis patients and 39 controls. SH levels were significantly higher in patients with osteoarthritis than in controls (92 ± 66 μg/L and 39 ± 21 μg/L, respectively, p = 0.0001) *257*

25-Hydroxy Vitamin D_3 *Serum* *Increase* In 91 women mean concentration of 187 ± 13 nmol/L significantly different from 155 ± 15 nmol/L in 56 matched controls: in 52 postmenopausal women mean concentration of 189 ± 15 nmol/L not significantly different from 158 ± 26 nmol/L in 26 age and sex matched controls *5749*

Hydroxypyridinoline *Synovial Fluid* *Increase* In 20 patients with osteoarthritis mean concentration high at 23.2 ± 8.4 pmol/mL *4872*
Synovial Fluid *No Effect* In 20 patients with osteoarthritis mean concentration undetectable *4872*

Insulin *Plasma* *Increase* In 25 overweight patients with osteoarthritis mean concentration of 17.50 ± 8.63 μU/mL significantly higher than mean concentration of 11.73 ± 6.0 μU/mL in 23 overweight patients without osteoarthritis although no significant difference between normal weight individuals with and without osteoarthritis *4839*

Insulin-like Growth Factor-I *Serum* *No Effect* In 91 women mean concentration of 142 ± 5.1 ng/mL not significantly different from 142 ± 5.8 ng/mL in 56 matched controls *5749* In 52 postmenopausal women mean concentration of 145 ± 7.1 ng/mL not significantly different from 136 ± 10 ng/mL in 56 matched controls *5749*

Insulin-like Growth Factor-II *Serum* *Increase* In 91 women mean concentration of 470 ± 18 ng/mL significantly greater than 449 ± 14 ng/mL in 56 matched controls: in 52 postmenopausal women mean concentration of 462 ± 22 ng/mL significantly higher than 444 ± 25 ng/mL in 26 age and sex matched controls *5749*

Insulin-like Growth Factor Binding Protein-3
Serum *Increase* In 91 women mean concentration of 4.2 ± 0.1 mg/L significantly higher than 3.8 ± 0.1 mg/L in 56 matched controls: 4.1 ± 0.2 mg/L in 52 postmenopausal women significantly higher than 3.7 ± 0.1 mg/L in 26 postmenopausal controls *5749*

Interleukin-6 *Serum* *No Effect* Mean concentration of 12.4 ± 3 pg/mL in 5 patients with osteoarthritis not significantly different from 11.4 ± 1.9 pg/mL in healthy blood donors *1130*
Synovial Fluid *Increase* Mean concentration of 0.92 ± 1.2 ng/L in 5 patients with osteoarthritis *1130*

Interleukin-10 *Serum* *No Effect* In 11 patients with osteoarthritis mean concentration of 11.5 ± 4.0 U/mL not significantly different from 8.8 ± 1.9 U/mL in 22 healthy controls *986*
Synovial Fluid *No Effect* In 11 patients with rheumatoid arthritis mean concentration of 7.9 ± 6.9 U/mL not significantly different from 8.8 ± 1.9 U/mL in serum of 22 healthy controls *986*

Interleukin-11 *Serum* *No Effect* In 20 patients median concentration of 81 pg/mL *5287*
Synovial Fluid *Increase* In 20 patients median concentration of 268 pg/mL *5287*

Keratan Sulfate Epitope ($5D_4$) *Synovial Fluid* *Increase* In 35 patients mean concentration of 10.44 ± 5.84 μg/mL *4758*

Leukocytes *Blood* *No Effect* In 14 patients median concentration of 7.3 x 10^3/L *5287*
Synovial Fluid *Increase* Counts range from 200 - 2000 /μL *367* Mean concentration of 250 ± 160 /μL in 9 patients *1161* Synovial fluid is viscid and has few white cells in degenerative joint disease *2039*
Synovial Fluid *No Effect* Mean concentration in 7 patients with osteoarthritis 183 ± 36 /μL compared with 300 /μL in 3 normal individuals *3344* In 14 patients median concentration of 0.22 x 10^3/L *5287*

Leukotriene C_4 *Synovial Fluid* *Increase* Detected at concentrations of 46 - 144 pmol/L in 9 of 21 patients with osteoarthritis *3366*

Macrophage Inflammatory Protein-1α
Synovial Fluid *Increase* Detectable but concentration decreased compared with that in patients with rheumatoid arthritis *5114*

Macrophage Inflammatory Protein-1β
Synovial Fluid *Increase* Concentration increased compared with that in patients with rheumatoid arthritis *5114*

Melanoma Inhibitory Factor *Serum* *No Effect* In 12 patients mean concentration of 5.2 ± 1.4 ng/mL showed no significant difference from 3.6 ± 2.8 ng/mL in 120 healthy controls *3655*

Monocyte Chemotactic Protein-1 *Synovial Fluid* *Increase* Detectable but concentration decreased compared with that in patients with rheumatoid arthritis *5114*

Monocytes *Blood* *Increase* In 51% of 125 patients at initial hospitalization for this disorder *1576*

Neopterin *Synovial Fluid* *Increase* In 21 patients with osteoarthritis mean concentration of 25.64 ± 9.99 nmol/L *1956*
Urine *Increase* Concentrations not as high in osteoarthritis as in rheumatoid arthritis *121*

Nerve Growth Factor *Serum* *Increase* Mean concentration of 3.7 ± 10 pg/mL in 27 patients *1161*
Synovial Fluid *Increase* Mean concentration of 6.5 ± 19.7 pg/mL in 20 patients *1161*

Nerve Growth Factor Autoantibodies *Serum* *No Effect* Mean value of 0.50 ± 0.17 in 27 patients not significantly different from 0.42 ± 0.13 in 30 healthy controls *1161*
Synovial Fluid *Increase* Mean value of 0.36 ± 0.31 in 20 patients *1161*

Nucleotide Pyrophosphohydrolase, Sedimentable
Synovial Fluid *Increase* Mean activity in 7 patients with osteoarthritis 251 ± 76 pmol/h/mL compared with 172 ± 68 pmol/h/mL in 3 normal individuals *3344*

Nucleotide Pyrophosphohydrolase, Soluble
Serum *Increase* Mean activity in 43 patients with osteoarthritis of 1,412 ± 63 pmol nitrophenol/h/mL significantly different from that in 85 healthy individuals 1141 ± 22 pmol nitrophenol/h/mL *691*
Synovial Fluid *Increase* Mean activity in 7 patients with osteoarthritis 1,017 ± 200 pmol/h/mL compared with 606 ± 174 pmol/h/mL in 3 normal individuals *3344*

Osteocalcin *Serum* *Increase* In 18 patients with osteoarthritis mean concentration of 27 ± 6 μg/L (4.6 nmol/L) not significantly different from 29 ± 2 μg/L (5.0 nmol/L) in healthy postmenopausal women but significantly different from that in healthy young adults (men 25 ± 5 μg/L, women 20 ± 6 μg/L) *541*
Synovial Fluid *Increase* In 35 patients mean concentration of 5.8 ± 2.6 ng/mL with mean concentrations of 3.0 ± 0.6 ng/mL, 4.9 ± 1.9 ng/mL and 7.8 ± 3.0 ng/mL in patients with normal, abnormal and severely abnormal scans respectively *4758*

Parathyroid Hormone *Plasma* *No Effect* In 91 women mean concentration of 32 ± 1.6 ng/mL not significantly different from 30 ± 2.8 ng/mL in 56 matched controls: in 52 postmenopausal women mean concentration of 38 ± 2.7 ng/mL not significantly different from 31 ± 1.9 ng/mL in 26 age and sex matched controls *5749*

Phospholipase A *Serum* *Increase* Reported effect *4229*

Phospholipase A_2 *Serum* *No Effect* In 15 untreated patients mean activity of 31.63 ± 7.5 kU/L compared with range of 15.1 - 47.8 kU/L in 20 healthy individuals *1926*
Synovial Fluid *Increase* Synovial fluid concentration of PLA2-II considerably increased in patients with osteoarthritis, rheumatoid arthritis and crystal-associated arthritis *3766*

Phospholipase A_2 Type II *Synovial Fluid* *Increase* Considerable increase in catalytic activity observed in patients with osteoarthritis *3767*

Procollagen Type III Peptide *Synovial Fluid* *Increase* The levels were one to three hundred times higher than serum levels, and they showed the positive correlation with serum levels, suggesting that serum P-III-P might be originated from synovial P-III-P *155*

Prostaglandin E_2 *Synovial Fluid* *Increase* Mean concentration in 5 untreated patients of about 0.8 nmol/L *3366*

Pyridinoline *Synovial Fluid* *Increase* In 4 patients mean concentration of 19.3 ± 5.8 pmol/mL *4343*

715.90 Osteoarthritis *(continued)*

Pyridinoline *(continued)*
Urine *No Effect* In 62 postmenopausal women with osteoarthritis mean excretion of total pyridinoline of 61.0 ± 50.6 nmol/mmol creatinine not significantly different from 69.0 ± 45.8 nmol/mmol creatinine in 22 matched post-menopausal controls *5131*

Pyridinoline, Free *Urine* *No Effect* In 62 postmenopausal women with osteoarthritis mean excretion of 18.8 ± 8.5 nmol/mmol creatinine not significantly different from 29.1 ± 20.4 nmol/mmol creatinine in 22 matched post-menopausal controls *5131*

Pyridinoline, Peptide-bound *Urine* *No Effect* In 62 postmenopausal women with osteoarthritis mean excretion of 42.2 ± 49.5 nmol/mmol creatinine not significantly different from 39.8 ± 25.8 nmol/mmol creatinine in 22 matched post-menopausal controls *5131*

Pyrophosphate *Synovial Fluid* *Increase* Moderately elevated levels *2386* In 135 patients with osteoarthritis median concentration of 10.5 µmol/L *1198*

Rheumatoid Factor *Serum* *Increase* In 20 patients rheumatoid factor present in 1 and absent in 19 patients with gout *5287*
Serum *No Effect* Typical observation *5544*

Soluble Intercellular Adhesion Molecule-3
Synovial Fluid *Increase* Mean concentration of 24.3 ± 3.4 ng/mL in specimens from 9 patients *2244*

Soluble Interleukin-2 Receptor *Serum* *Increase* Slight increase to mean of 45 pmol/mL (range 13 - 100 pmol/L) in 25 patients with osteoarthritis *3367*
Synovial Fluid *Increase* Mean concentration of 37 pmol/L (range of 15 - 140 pmol/L) in 28 specimens from patients with osteoarthritis higher than median of 2.5 pmol/L (range of 0 - 10 pmol/L) in 10 specimens from healthy control individuals *3367*

Soluble Interleukin-6 Receptor-α *Synovial Fluid* *Increase* Mean concentration of 10.1 ± 5.0 ng/mL in 5 patients with osteoarthritis *1130*

Soluble P-Selectin *Synovial Fluid* *Increase* Mean concentration of 10.9 ± 2.5 ng/mL in specimens from 9 patients *2244*

Stromelysin *Plasma* *Increase* In 9 patients with osteoarthritis mean concentration of 115.4 ± 21.6 ng/mL significantly higher than 50.0 ± 4.4 ng/mL in 53 healthy controls *5878*

Viscosity *Synovial Fluid* *No Effect* Viscosity normal *1367*

716.00 Kashin-Beck Disease

Glutathione Peroxidase *Serum* *Decrease* In 207 Tibetan villagers with Kashin-Beck disease mean concentration of 210 U/L but greater than 153 U/L in 147 villagers without disease and significantly less than 294 U/L in 63 individuals in control village. Number of individuals with concentrations less than 100 U/L 23%, 29% and 0% respectively *3599*

Iodine *Urine* *Decrease* In 273 Tibetan villagers with Kashin-Beck disease mean concentration of 1.2 µg/dL less than 1.6 µg/dL in 212 villagers without disease and significantly less than 1.8 µg/dL in 72 individuals in control village. Number of individuals with concentrations less than 1 µg/dL 36%, 35% and 14% respectively *3599*

Selenium *Serum* *Decrease* In 265 Tibetan villagers with Kashin-Beck disease mean concentration of 10.3 ng/mL greater than 8.8 ng/mL in 201 villagers without disease and significantly less than 11.5 ng/mL in 55 individuals in control village. Number of individuals with concentrations less than 5 ng/mL 35%, 43% and 31% respectively *3599*

Thyroid Stimulating Hormone *Serum* *Increase* In 262 Tibetan villagers with Kashin-Beck disease mean concentration of 6.3 U/L greater than 5.9 mU/L in 202 villagers without disease and significantly greater than 3.9 mU/L in 72 individuals in control village. Number of individuals with concentrations greater than 10 mU/L, 23%, 22% and 4% respectively *3599*

Thyroxine Binding Globulin *Serum* *Decrease* In 268 Tibetan villagers with Kashin-Beck disease mean concentration of 18.6 ± 3.5 mg/L less than 20.2 ± 3.7 mg/L in 204 villagers without disease and significantly less than 20.3 ± 3.3 mg/L in 72 individuals in control village. Number of individuals with concentrations less than 18 mg/L, 45%, 25% and 19% respectively *3599*

Thyroxine (T4) *Serum* *Decrease* In 259 Tibetan villagers with Kashin-Beck disease mean concentration of 7.1 ± 2.6 µg/dL less than 7.5 ± 2.8 µg/dL in 201 villagers without disease and significantly less than 8.6 ± 2.3 µg/dL in 72 individuals in control village. Number of individuals with concentrations less than 6 µg/dL 31%, 27% and 11% respectively *3599*

Tri-iodothyronine (T3) *Serum* *Decrease* In 257 Tibetan villagers with Kashin-Beck disease mean concentration of 163 ± 33 ng/dL less than 167 ± 32 ng/dL in 201 villagers without disease and less than 170 ± 26 ng/dL in 72 individuals in control village. Number of individuals with concentrations less than 150 ng/dL 38%, 29% and 19% respectively *3599*

716.10 Posttraumatic Arthritis

Pyridinoline *Synovial Fluid* *Increase* In 2 patients mean concentration of 28.5 ± 14.1 pmol/mL *4343*

716.10 Traumatic Arthritis

Phospholipase A_2 Type II *Synovial Fluid* *Increase* Considerable increase in catalytic activity observed in patients with traumatic arthritis *3767*

Prostaglandin E_2 *Synovial Fluid* *Increase* Mean concentration in 3 patients of 0.71 nmol/L *3366*

716.59 Polyarthritis

C-Reactive Protein *Serum* *No Effect* Median concentration of 1.54 mg/dL in 12 patients with seronegative polyarthritis *5290*

Cytidine Deaminase *Serum* *No Effect* Median activity of 5.73 U/L in 12 patients with seronegative polyarthritis *5290*
Synovial Fluid *Increase* Median activity of 8.11 U/mL in synovial fluid from knees of 12 patients with seronegative polyarthritis *5290*

Glucose *Synovial Fluid* *Decrease* Median concentration of 84.5 mg/dL in synovial fluid from knees of 12 patients with seronegative polyarthritis *5290*

Hemoglobin *Blood* *No Effect* Median concentration of 11.7 g/dL in 12 patients with seronegative polyarthritis *5290*

Interleukin-8 *Synovial Fluid* *Increase* Mean concentration of 0.22 ng/mL in synovial fluid from knees of 12 patients with seronegative polyarthritis *5290*

Lactate *Synovial Fluid* *Increase* Median concentration of 16.6 mg/dL in synovial fluid from knees of 12 patients with seronegative polyarthritis *5290*

Nucleotide Pyrophosphohydrolase, Soluble
Serum *No Effect* Mean activity in 25 patients with seronegative polyarthritis of 1,235 ± 56 pmol nitrophenol/h/mL not significantly different from that in 85 healthy individuals 1,141 ± 22 pmol nitrophenol/h/mL *691*

Viscosity *Plasma* *No Effect* Median viscosity of 1.74 cP in 12 patients with seronegative polyarthritis *5290*

716.80 Chronic Rheumatic Disease

Soluble CD44+ *Serum* *No Effect* In 15 patients with chronic rheumatic diseases mean concentration of 2.2 ± 1.6 nmol/L not significantly different from 2.7 ± 1.1 nmol/L in 43 age and sex matched controls *1918*

716.80 HLA B27-associated Oligoarthritis

Melanoma Inhibitory Factor *Serum* *No Effect* In 12 patients mean concentration of 6.6 ± 3.0 ng/mL showed no significant difference from 3.6 ± 2.8 ng/mL in 120 healthy controls *3655*

716.80 Reactive Arthritis

C-Reactive Protein *Serum* *Increase* In 10 patients, 1 of whom had positive blood culture, mean concentration of 119 mg/L *2778*

Leukocytes *Synovial Fluid* *Increase* In 11 patients, none of whom had positive blood culture, mean concentration of 36,000 /µL *2778*

L-Lactate *Synovial Fluid* *Increase* In 11 patients, none of whom had positive blood culture, mean concentration of 5.0 mmol/L *2778*

716.90 Chronic Arthritis

Antinuclear Antibodies *Serum* *Increase* In 33 of 69 patients with juvenile chronic arthritis antinuclear antibodies observed (48%) *5415*

C-Reactive Protein *Serum* *Increase* Mean concentration of 10 mg/L in 34 patients with juvenile chronic arthritis *5415*

Erythrocyte Sedimentation Rate *Blood* *Increase* Mean rate of 28 mm/h in 34 patients with juvenile chronic arthritis *5415*

Rheumatoid Factor (IgM) *Serum* *Increase* In 9 of 69 patients with juvenile chronic arthritis IgM rheumatoid factor observed (13%) *5415*

Soluble Intercellular Adhesion Molecule-3 *Synovial Fluid* *Increase* Mean concentration of 43.3 ± 10.6 ng/mL in specimens from 13 patients with arthritdes other than rheumatoid arthritis and osteoarthritis *2244*

Soluble Interleukin-2 Receptor *Serum* *Increase* In 81 patients with pauciarticular-, polyarticular-, and systemic-onset juvenile chronic arthritis concentration significantly higher (both in inactive and active disease) than in healthy controls. Concentration may be increased despite the absence of clinical symptoms *1430*

Soluble P-Selectin *Synovial Fluid* *Increase* Mean concentration of 28.2 ± 7.9 ng/mL in specimens from 13 patients with arthritdes other than rheumatoid arthritis and osteoarthritis *2244*

720.00 Ankylosing Spondylitis

Alkaline Phosphatase *Serum* *Decrease* In 14 patients with ankylosing spondylitis median activity of 8.0 KA U/dL significantly different from upper limit of normal in healthy controls *430*
Serum *Increase* In 38 patients with ankylosing spondylitis mean activity of 135 ± 44 U/L slightly but significantly higher than 114 ± 35 U/L in healthy controls *1549*
Serum *No Effect* In 33 patients with ankylosing spondylitis mean activity of 63.1 ± 23.7 U/L not significantly different from 64.0 ± 37.4 U/L in 23 healthy controls *5269*

Alkaline Phosphatase, Bone Isoenzyme *Serum* *No Effect* In 14 patients with ankylosing spondylitis median concentration of 12.7 ng/mL not significantly different from upper limit of normal in healthy controls *430*

Androstenedione *Plasma* *No Effect* In 50 male patients with ankylosing spondylitis mean concentration of 4.2 ± 1.8 nmol/L not significantly different from 3.8 ± 1.7 nmol/L in 50 healthy controls: change also not significantly different in women *1734*

Anti-Endothelial Cell Antibodies *Serum* *No Effect* In patients with undefined connective tissue disease (n = 57), ankylosing spondylitis (n = 109), and psoriatic arthritis (n = 58), the frequency of AECA corresponded to that of the random population sample *3845*

Calcium *Serum* *No Effect* Mean concentration in 38 adults with ankylosing spondylitis not significantly different from that in healthy controls *1549* In 33 patients with ankylosing spondylitis mean concentration of 93.9 ± 3.7 mg/L not significantly different from 94.4 ± 3.6 mg/L in 23 healthy controls *5269* In 32 patients with ankylosing spondylitis mean concentration of 94.2 ± 3.8 mg/L not significantly different from 94.4 ± 3.7 mg/L in 25 healthy volunteer controls *5270*

C-Reactive Protein *Serum* *Increase* In 18 Japanese patients with ankylosing spondylitis mean CRP concentration was 28.1 ± 6.0 mg/L compared with < 3 mg/L in 30 healthy adults *5162*

Creatinine *Serum* *No Effect* In 38 adult patients with ankylosing spondylitis mean concentration not significantly different from that in healthy adult controls *1549*

Dehydroepiandrosterone Sulfate *Plasma* *No Effect* In 50 male patients with ankylosing spondylitis mean concentration of 7.9 ± 4.1 µmol/L not significantly different from 5.8 ± 2.5 µmol/L in 50 healthy controls: difference also not significant in women *1734*

1,25-Dihydroxy Vitamin D_3 *Serum* *Increase* Mean concentration in 38 adults with ankylosing spondylitis of 64.0 ± 34.5 pg/mL higher than 52.4 ± 6.7 pg/mL in normal healthy control adults *1549*

24,25-Dihydroxy Vitamin D *Serum* *No Effect* In 38 patients with ankylosing spondylitis mean concentration of 2.3 ± 1.7 ng/mL not significantly different from 2.5 ± 0.6 ng/mL in healthy control adults *1549*

Dipyridinoline, Free *Urine* *No Effect* In 32 patients with ankylosing spondylitis mean excretion of 7.47 ± 6.39 nmol/mmoL creatinine not significantly different from 6.32 ± 2.52 nmol/mmoL creatinine in 25 healthy volunteer controls *5270*

Erythrocyte Sedimentation Rate *Blood* *Increase* In 18 Japanese patients with ankylosing spondylitis mean ESR was 25.0 ± 6.0 mm/h compared with < 20 mm/h in 30 healthy adults *5162*
Blood *No Effect* Rate similar in patients with ankylosing spondylitis and healthy controls except in patients who were taking NSAIDs in whom rate increased *1549*

17β-Estradiol *Plasma* *No Effect* In 50 male patients with ankylosing spondylitis mean concentration of 61 ± 19 pmol/L not significantly different from 63 ± 16 pmol/L in 50 healthy controls: diierence also not significant in women *1734*

Glucose *Serum* *Increase* In 33 patients with ankylosing spondylitis mean concentration of 5.13 ± 0.1 mmol/L significantly different from 4.76 ± 0.5 mmol/L in 23 healthy controls *5269*

γ-Glutamyltransferase *Serum* *Decrease* In 14 patients with ankylosing spondylitis median activity of 23 U/L significantly different from upper limit of normal in healthy controls: increased activity observed in 50% of patients *430*
Serum *No Effect* In 14 patients with ankylosing spondylitis median activity of 19 U/L not significantly different from upper limit of normal in healthy controls: increased activity observed in 64.3% of patients *430* In patients with ankylosing spondylitis with raised alkaline phosphatase activity GGT activity normal *1549*

Growth Hormone *Plasma* *No Effect* In 33 patients with ankylosing spondylitis mean concentration of 0.51 ± 0.8 ng/mL not significantly different from 0.29 ± 0.4 ng/mL in 23 healthy controls *5269*

HLA-B27 *Serum* *Increase* Of 18 Japanese patients with ankylosing spondylitis 16 were HLA-B27 positive *5162*

25-Hydroxy Vitamin D_3 *Serum* *No Effect* In 32 patients with ankylosing spondylitis mean concentration of 24.1 ± 17.6 ng/mL not significantly different from 20.1 ± 11.6 ng/mL in 25 healthy volunteer controls *5270*

25-Hydroxy Vitamin D *Serum* *No Effect* In 38 patients with ankylosing spondylitis mean concentration of 21.6 ± 13.5 ng/mL not significantly different from 20.1 ± 3.2 ng/mL in healthy control adults *1549* In 33 patients with ankylosing spondylitis mean concentration of 25.4 ± 17.2 ng/mL not significantly different from 19.5 ± 11.7 ng/mL in 23 healthy controls *5269*

IgA Antibodies against Collagen *Serum* *Increase* In 18 Japanese patients with ankylosing spondylitis mean concentration was 433.6 ± 27.6 mg/L significantly higher than that in 30 healthy adults *5162*

IgA1 Antibodies against Collagen Type I *Serum* *Increase* In 18 Japanese adults with ankylosing spondylitis mean OD_{492} value was 0.082 ± 0.038 not significantly different from 0.037 ± 0.005 in 30 healthy controls *5162*

IgA1 Antibodies against Collagen Type II *Serum* *Increase* In 18 Japanese adults with ankylosing spondylitis mean OD_{492} value was 0.026 ± 0.006 significantly different from 0.012 ± 0.001 in 30 healthy controls *5162*

IgA1 Antibodies against Collagen Type III *Serum* *Increase* In 18 Japanese adults with ankylosing spondylitis mean OD_{492} value was 0.055 ± 0.016 not significantly different from 0.034 ± 0.005 in 30 healthy controls *5162*

IgA1 Antibodies against Collagen Type IV *Serum* *Increase* In 18 Japanese adults with ankylosing spondylitis mean OD_{492} value was 0.028 ± 0.004 significantly different from 0.018 ± 0.001 in 30 healthy controls *5162*

720.00 Ankylosing Spondylitis *(continued)*

IgA1 Antibodies against Collagen Type IV *(continued)*
Serum *No Effect* In 18 Japanese adults with ankylosing spondylitis mean OD_{492} value was 0.011 ± 0.002 not significantly different from 0.009 ± 0.001 in 30 healthy controls *5162*

IgA2 Antibodies against Collagen Type I *Serum* *Increase* In 18 Japanese adults with ankylosing spondylitis mean OD_{492} value was 0.107 ± 0.015 significantly different from 0.057 ± 0.004 in 30 healthy controls *5162*

IgA2 Antibodies against Collagen Type II *Serum* *No Effect* In 18 Japanese adults with ankylosing spondylitis mean OD_{492} value was 0.025 ± 0.005 not significantly different from 0.016 ± 0.002 in 30 healthy controls *5162*

IgA2 Antibodies against Collagen Type III *Serum* *Increase* In 18 Japanese adults with ankylosing spondylitis mean OD_{492} value was 0.089 ± 0.011 significantly different from 0.049 ± 0.004 in 30 healthy controls *5162*

Insulin *Plasma* *Decrease* In 33 patients with ankylosing spondylitis mean concentration of 75.85 ± 44.5 pmol/L significantly different from 98.84 ± 44.5 pmol/L in 23 healthy controls *5269*

Insulin-like Growth Factor-I *Serum* *No Effect* In 33 patients with ankylosing spondylitis mean concentration of 218.3 ± 72.4 ng/mL not significantly different from 212.1 ± 71.1 ng/mL in 23 healthy controls *5269*

Insulin-like Growth Factor Binding Protein-3
Serum *Decrease* In 33 patients with ankylosing spondylitis mean concentration of 3.29 ± 0.6 µg/mL significantly different from 3.63 ± 0.6 µg/mL in 23 healthy controls *5269*

β-isomerized Fragments of C-telopeptide of Type I Collagen
Urine *No Effect* In 32 patients with ankylosing spondylitis mean excretion of 247.1 ± 141.3 nmol/mmoL creatinine not significantly different from 236.4 ± 107.5 nmol/mmoL creatinine in 25 healthy volunteer controls *5270*

Luteinizing Hormone *Plasma* *No Effect* In 50 male patients with ankylosing spondylitis mean concentration of 2.8 ± 1.5 IU/L not significantly different from 2.7 ± 1.4 IU/L in 50 healthy controls: change also not significantly different in women *1734*

Osteocalcin *Serum* *Decrease* In 25 men with ankylosing spondylitis mean concentration of 1.7 ± 1.1 ng/mL compared with 3.2 ± 1.3 ng/mL in healthy controls: in women with ankylosing spondylitis mean concentration of 1.2 ± 1.1 ng/mL compared with 4.1 ± 1.7 ng/mL in healthy control women *1549*
Serum *No Effect* In 33 patients with ankylosing spondylitis mean concentration of 7.1 ± 3.2 ng/mL not significantly different from 6.9 ± 2.8 ng/mL in 23 healthy controls *5269* In 32 patients with ankylosing spondylitis mean concentration of 7.2 ± 3.2 ng/mL not significantly different from 7.2 ± 2.8 ng/mL in 25 healthy volunteer controls *5270*

Parathyroid Hormone *Plasma* *Increase* In 38 patients with ankylosing spondylitis mean concentration of 3.1 ± 0.7 mEq/mL not significantly greater than 2.7 ± 0.6 mEq/mL in healthy controls *1549*
Plasma *No Effect* In 33 patients with ankylosing spondylitis mean concentration of 24.2 ± 12.3 pg/mL not significantly different from 25.3 ± 11.6 pg/mL in 23 healthy controls *5269* In 32 patients with ankylosing spondylitis mean concentration of 23.7 ± 12.3 pg/mL not significantly different from 24.6 ± 11.6 pg/mL in 25 healthy volunteer controls *5270*

Phosphate *Serum* *No Effect* Concentration reported to be normal in patients with ankylosing spondylitis *5269* Mean concentration in 38 patients with ankylosing spondylitis not significantly different from that in healthy control adults *1549*

Procollagen Type II Peptide *Serum* *Increase* Reported effect *824*

Pyridinium Crosslinks *Urine* *Increase* Excretion reported to be increased in some patients with ankylosing spondylitis *5269*

Pyridinoline, Free *Urine* *No Effect* In 32 patients with ankylosing spondylitis mean excretion of 22.16 ± 7.63 nmol/mmoL creatinine not significantly different from 22.88 ± 7.73 nmol/mmoL creatinine in 25 healthy volunteer controls *5270*

Sex-Hormone Binding Globulin *Serum* *No Effect* In 50 male patients with ankylosing spondylitis mean concentration of 35 ± 14 IU/L not significantly different from 35 ± 13 IU/L in 50 healthy controls: change also not significantly different in women *1734*

Testosterone *Serum* *No Effect* In 50 male patients with ankylosing spondylitis mean concentration of 16 ± 4 nmol/L not significantly different from 15 ± 5 nmol/L in 50 healthy controls: difference also not significant in women *1734*

Viscosity *Plasma* *No Effect* In 14 patients with ankylosing spondylitis median of 1.78 ± 0.18 mPa not significantly different from 1.72 mPa in healthy controls *430*

720.00 Rheumatoid (Ankylosing) Spondylitis

Alkaline Phosphatase *Serum* *Increase* Elevation in 47.5% of 40 patients and in most cases was derived from bone *2635*

Angiotensin-converting Enzyme *Serum* *No Effect* Not significantly different (n = 24) from normal controls (n = 26) *3141*

Carbon Dioxide Partial Pressure *Blood* *Increase* Impaired movement of the respiratory cage *5863*

Ceruloplasmin *Serum* *Increase* Raised significantly, with the greatest increases in the worst cases *2428*

Complement C_4 *Serum* *Increase* Raised concentration of C_4 and complement inactivation products *4814* Mean levels of C_4 and IgA were significantly elevated in patients with sporadic disease *2691*

Complement, Total *Synovial Fluid* *Increase* Frequently occurs *4683*

Copper *Serum* *Increase* Raised significantly, with the greatest increases in the worst cases *2428*

C-Reactive Protein *Serum* *Increase* 90% of cases *413*

Cryoglobulins *Serum* *Increase* Variable elevation of cryoglobulins *4707*

Erythrocyte Sedimentation Rate *Blood* *Increase* Occurs in about 80% of patients but other acute phase reactants tend to be absent *1367* Elevated in most but not in all patients with active disease. May be normal in patients who are symptomatic *900*
Blood *No Effect* Elevated in most but not in all patients with active disease. May be normal in patients who are symptomatic *900*

γ-Globulin *Serum* *Increase* Electrophoresis may show an elevation of the globulin fractions without any specific pattern *900* 25% of 40 patients showed elevated and abnormal globulins, alkaline phosphatase and hemogloblin *2635*

Glucose *Synovial Fluid* *Decrease* Lower than blood *1367*

Glycosaminoglycans *Serum* *Increase* A corresponding increase has been reported in synovial fluid, serum and urine of patients with rheumatic diseases *2651*
Synovial Fluid *Increase* A corresponding increase has been reported in synovial fluid, serum and urine of patients with rheumatic diseases *2651*
Urine *Increase* Observed effect *5808*

HDL-Cholesterol *Serum* *No Effect* Total lipid concentration was found to be low but HDL fraction was normal *3129*

Hematocrit *Blood* *Decrease* Anemia occurs in < 33% of cases *1367* Anemia is occasionally present in more severe cases and is usually normocytic *900*

Hemoglobin *Blood* *Decrease* Anemia occurs in < 33% of cases *1367* Anemia is occasionally present in more severe cases and is usually normocytic *900*

HLA Antigens *Blood* *Present* HLA antigen B_27 found in 90% of caucasian patients with this disease compared to 8% of controls *4584* HLA-B_27 present in 90% of patients versus 8% of controls *5678*

immunoglobulin A *Serum* *Increase* Mean levels of C_4 and IgA were significantly elevated in patients with sporadic disease *2691*

Lipids *Serum* *Decrease* Total lipid concentration was found to be low *3129*

Oxygen Partial Pressure *Blood* *Decrease* Impaired movement of the respiratory cage *5863*

Protein *Cerebrospinal Fluid* *Increase* Observed in 33% of patients, most often those with severe back pain *1367*

Rheumatoid Factor *Serum* *Increase* Serologic tests are positive in 15% of patients with arthritis of the vertebral region in ankylosing spondylitis *5545*
Serum *No Effect* Occurs no more frequently than in the general population *1367*

Viscosity *Synovial Fluid* *Decrease* Lower than blood *1367*

720.00 Spondylitis

Complement C_1 *Serum* *No Effect* Mean concentration typically normal or slightly increased in patients with spondylitis *4682*

Complement C_1q *Serum* *No Effect* Mean concentration typically normal or slightly increased in patients with spondylitis *4682*

Complement C_2 *Serum* *No Effect* Mean concentration typically normal or slightly increased in patients with spondylitis *4682*

Complement C_3 *Serum* *No Effect* Mean concentration typically normal or slightly increased in patients with spondylitis *4682*

Complement C_4 *Serum* *No Effect* Mean concentration typically normal or slightly increased in patients with spondylitis *4682*

Complement C_5 *Serum* *No Effect* Mean concentration typically normal or slightly increased in patients with spondylitis *4682*

Complement CH50 *Serum* *No Effect* Mean concentration typically normal or slightly increased in patients with spondylitis *4682*

Properdin Factor B *Plasma* *No Effect* Mean concentration typically normal or slightly increased in patients with spondylitis *4682*

721.00 Cervical Spondylosis

Acetylcholinesterase G4 Isoenzyme *Serum* *No Effect* No significant deviation from normal observed in a small number of patients *5778*

α_1-Microglobulin *Cerebrospinal Fluid* *Increase* Of 5 patients with Guillain-Barre syndrome mean concentration in two exceeded that in 15 healthy controls of 34.8 ± 16.0 µg/L *2370*

721.90 Spondylarthritis

C-Reactive Protein *Serum* *Increase* In 23 patients median concentration of 13.0 µg/mL *5287*

Erythrocyte Sedimentation Rate *Blood* *Increase* In 23 patients median rate of 26 mm/h *5287*

Interleukin-11 *Serum* *No Effect* In 23 patients median concentration of 89 pg/mL *5287*
Synovial Fluid *Increase* In 23 patients median concentration of 124 pg/mL *5287*

Leukocytes *Blood* *No Effect* In 23 patients median concentration of 7.9 x 10^3/L *5287*
Synovial Fluid *Increase* In 23 patients median concentration of 6.4 x 10^3/L *5287*

Rheumatoid Factor *Serum* *Increase* In 23 patients rheumatoid factor present in 19 and absent in 4 patients with seronegative spondyloarthritis *5287*

721.90 Spondylarthropathy

C-Reactive Protein *Serum* *Increase* In 18 patients with spondylarthropathy median concentration of 31.7 mg/L significantly greater than median of 3 mg/L in 20 healthy blood donors *1614* In 14 patients with spondylarthropathies median concentration of 0.48 mg/dL significantly different from normal *1613* In 18 patients with spondylarthropathy median concentration of 31.7 mg/L significantly different from upper limit of normal of 2.6 mg/L *1612*

Interleukin-1 Receptor Antagonist *Serum* *No Effect* Median concentration in 18 patients with spondyloarthropathy of 0.35 ng/mL not significantly higher than 0.27 ng/mL in 20 healthy controls *1612*

Interleukin-6 *Serum* *Increase* In 14 patients with spondylarthropathies mean concentration of 15 - 292 pg/mL significantly different from normal (range 15 - 22 pg/mL) *1613*

Interleukin-10 *Serum* *Increase* In 13 patients with spondylarthropathy mean concentration of 243.1 ± 87.8 U/mL significantly higher than 8.8 ± 1.9 U/mL in 22 healthy controls *986*
Synovial Fluid *No Effect* In 13 patients with spondylarthropathy mean concentration of 4.5 ± 3.2 U/mL not significantly different from 8.8 ± 1.9 U/mL in serum of 22 healthy controls *986*

Leukocytes *Synovial Fluid* *Increase* Mean value of 8,700 ± 4,300 /µL in 10 patients *1161*

Nerve Growth Factor *Serum* *Increase* Mean concentration of 8 ± 16 pg/mL in 10 patients *1161*
Synovial Fluid *Increase* Mean concentration of 121.4 ± 251.8 pg/mL in 10 patients *1161*

Nerve Growth Factor Autoantibodies *Serum* *Increase* Mean value of 0.68 ± 0.36 in 10 patients significantly different from 0.42 ± 0.13 in 30 healthy controls *1161*
Synovial Fluid *Increase* Mean value of 1.23 ± 0.54 in 10 patients *1161*

Soluble Tumor Necrosis Factor Receptor-p55
Serum *Increase* Median concentration in 18 patients with spondyloarthropathy of 2.6 ng/mL higher than 2.1 ng/mL in 20 healthy controls *1612*
Serum *No Effect* In 14 patients with spondylarthropathy median concentration of 1.45 ng/mL not significantly different from normal *1613*

Soluble Tumor Necrosis Factor Receptor-p75
Serum *No Effect* Median concentration in 18 patients with spondyloarthropathy of 5.6 ng/mL not significantly different from 6.9 ng/mL in 20 healthy controls *1612* In 14 patients with spondylarthropathy median concentration of 3.75 ng/mL not significantly different from normal (median 4.65 pg/mL) *1613*

722.10 Lumbar Invertebral Disc Herniation

CD19+ Lymphocytes *Blood* *No Effect* In 33 medication-free patients with generalized social phobia 95% confidence interval of 140 - 242 /µL not significantly different from 124 - 195 /µL in 32 healthy volunteers *4278*

Soluble CD95 *Cerebrospinal Fluid* *No Effect* Mean concentration undetectable in 20 patients, not significantly different from healthy controls *5044*
Serum *No Effect* Mean concentration in 20 patients of 112 ± 18 U/mL, not significantly different from healthy controls *5044*

722.20 Vertebral Disc Herniation

β_2-Microglobulin *Cerebrospinal Fluid* *Increase* Nonsignificant increase to mean of 1.57 mg/L observed in patients with vertebral disk herniation compared with 1.01 mg/L in control patients *5421*

722.60 Disc Disease

Creatine Kinase *Cerebrospinal Fluid* *Increase* Of 17 patients with disk disease, 7 had increases above upper limit of normal of 10 U/L *4780*

724.09 Spinal Canal Stenosis

Albumin Index *Cerebrospinal Fluid* *Increase* Range in 13 patients with spinal canal stenosis of 8.8 - 79.9 significantly different from mean of 4.0 in 33 normal controls *3019*

Soluble Intercellular Adhesion Molecule-1
Cerebrospinal Fluid *Increase* Range in 13 patients with spinal canal stenosis of 2.2 - 19.4 ng/mL significantly different from mean of 1.51 ng/mL in 33 normal controls *3019*
Serum *No Effect* Range in 13 patients with spinal canal stenosis of 214.9 - 590.2 ng/mL not significantly different from mean of 285.1 ng/mL in 33 normal controls *3019*

β-Trace Protein *Cerebrospinal Fluid* *Increase* In 12 patients with spinal canal stenosis mean concentration of 29.2 ± 10.3 mg/L significantly different from 16.6 ± 3.6 mg/L in 27 normal controls *5323*

724.80 Ossification of Posterior Longitudinal Ligaments

Osteocalcin, Intact *Serum Increase* Median concentration of 38 ± 12 ng/mL in 40 patients with OPLL significantly higher than 17 ± 8 ng/mL in 36 healthy controls *3363*

Procollagen Type I Peptide *Serum Increase* Median concentration of 980 ± 350 ng/mL in 40 patients with OPLL significantly higher than 360 ± 130 ng/mL in 36 healthy controls *3363*

727.82 Calcium Pyrophosphate Dihydrate Deposition Disease

Cells *Synovial Fluid Increase* In 1 patient mean concentration of 10,000 /μL *4343*

Erythrocyte Sedimentation Rate *Blood Increase* In 1 patient mean rate 50 mm/h *4343*

Leukocytes *Synovial Fluid Increase* Mean concentration in 10 patients with CPPD 1,175 ± 824 /μL compared with 300 /μL in 3 normal individuals *3344*

Nucleotide Pyrophosphohydrolase, Sedimentable *Synovial Fluid Increase* Mean activity in 10 patients with CPPD 294 ± 113 pmol/h/mL compared with 172 ± 68 pmol/h/mL in 3 normal individuals *3344*

Nucleotide Pyrophosphohydrolase, Soluble *Synovial Fluid Increase* Mean activity in 10 patients with CPPD of 1,206 ± 305 pmol/h/mL compared with 606 ± 174 pmol/h/mL in 3 normal individuals *3344*

Pyridinoline *Synovial Fluid Increase* In 1 patient mean concentration of 84.6 pmol/mL *4343*

728.11 Fibrodysplasia

Basic Fibroblast Growth Factor *Urine Increase* In 39 patients with active fibrodysplasia ossificans progressiva median excretion of 8,739 μg/g creatinine significantly different from 2,705 μg/g creatinine in 54 healthy control volunteers *2558*
Urine No Effect In 39 patients with inactive fibrodysplasia ossificans progressiva median excretion of 5,058 μg/g creatinine not significantly different from 2,705 μg/g creatinine in 54 healthy control volunteers *2558*

Creatine Kinase *Serum No Effect* In 3 patients with fibrodysplasia (myositis) ossificans progressiva mean activities of 25, 64 and 60 U/L compared with upper limit of normal of 195 U/L *5659*

Creatine Kinase BB-Isoenzyme *Serum Increase* In 2 patients with fibrodysplasia (myositis) ossificans progressiva mean activities of < 3 and < 5 U/L (not detected %) compared with normal of 0 - 1% *5659* In 21patient with fibrodysplasia (myositis) ossificans progressiva mean activity of 8 U/L (14 %) compared with normal of 0 - 1% *5659*

728.89 Eosinophilic Fasciitis

Eosinophils *Blood Increase* In one patient with eosinophilic fasciitis mean concentration of 4,061/μL (31%) *3807* In 3 patients with eosinophilic fasciitis and eosinophilia mean concentration of 3,470 ± 2,060 /μL compared with less than 500 /μL in 100 normal individuals *5776*
Blood No Effect In one patient with eosinophilic fasciitis mean concentration of 451/μL not significantly different from normal *3807*

Hemoglobin *Blood No Effect* In one patient with eosinophilic fasciitis mean concentration of 13.1 g/dL not significantly different from normal *3807*

Interleukin-5 *Serum No Effect* In one patient with eosinophilic fasciitis mean concentration undetectable *3807*
Synovial Fluid No Effect In one patient with eosinophilic fasciitis mean concentration of 32 pg/mL *3807*

Leukocytes *Blood Increase* In one patient with eosinophilic fasciitis mean concentration of 13,100/μL *3807*

Myelin Basic Protein *Serum Increase* In 3 patients with eosinophilc fasciitis and eosinophilia mean concentration of 190 ± 49.5 ng/mL compared with mean of 41 ± 19 ng/mL in 100 normal individuals *5776*

728.89 Rhabdomyolysis

Carbonic Anhydrase III *Serum Increase* In 16 patients with rhabdomyolysis mean concentration of 2.51 ± 3.59 mg/L compared to 0.015 ± 0.011 mg/L in 74 healthy controls *5112*

Creatine Kinase *Serum Increase* In 20 patients with rhabdomyolysis peak concentrations ranged from 7,300 to 303,250 U/L *3103* In one patient activity increased to 69500 U/L after acute episode with peak of 1.2 million U/L on second hospital day *1486*

Creatine Kinase Isoenzymes *Serum Increase* Rhabdomyolysis was associated with increase of CK-MM activity (100%) *1486*

Creatine Kinase MB-Isoenzyme *Serum Increase* Increased with rhabdomyolysis *248*

Glutathione S-Transferase *Serum No Effect* In one patient with rhabdomyolysis concentration remained below upper limit of reference range *4309*

Hemoglobin *Urine Increase* In one patient with episode of acute rhabdomyolysis urine hemoglobin 4+ *1486*

Lactate Dehydrogenase *Serum Increase* In one patient with acute episode peak activity of 26,000 U/L observed on hospital day 2 with 85 - 95% LD_5 *1486*

Myoglobin *Serum Increase* In one individual after acute episode concentration increased to 34,000 μg/L on the first hospital day *1486*

Myosin Heavy-chain Fragments *Serum Increase* In 20 patients with severe rhabdomyolysis concentration greater than reference limits in all patients with peak value 70 times the upper reference value *3103*

Phosphate *Serum Increase* Breakdown of muscle tissue may lead to release of phosphate into the ECF and renal failure *969* Hyperphosphatemia may occur with rhabdomyolysis *5204*

Troponin I *Serum Increase* In 9 of 84 specimens from 20 patients with rhabdomyolysis concentrations were greater than the detection limit of 0.1 μg/L: for myocardial infarction; the peak value (average 0.17 μg/L) was increased in 6 of 20 patients (30%) *3103*
Serum No Effect In 3 patients with rhabdomyolysis cardiac troponin I could not be detected *2995*

Troponin T *Serum Increase* In 81 of 100 specimens from 20 patients with rhabdomyolysis concentrations were greater than the discriminator value of 2 μg/L: the peak value (average 5.21 μg/L) was increased in 19 of 20 patients *3103*

728.90 Inflammatory Disease

Carcinoembryonic Antigen *Serum Increase* In 49 patients with inflammatory disease 81.6% had concentrations of 0.0 - 3.0 ng/mL, 12.2% had concentrations from 3.1 - 5.0 ng/mL, 6.1% had concentrations from 5.1 - 10.0 ng/mL and 0.0% had concentrations greater than 10.0 ng/mL when measured by method on Bayer Technicon Immuno 1® system compared with 95.9%, 3.5%, 0.6% and 0.0% respectively in 173 healthy nonsmokers *339*

Erythrocyte Sedimentation Rate *Blood Increase* In 138 of 1,480 ESRs in a hospital population rates were greater than 100 mm/h: in a further study of 90 patients with 163 final diagnoses 7 were attributable to inflammatory diseases *3097*

Iron *Serum Decrease* In patients with chronic inflammatory disease serum iron concentration may be low especially with coexisting severe iron deficiency *4784*

Iron-binding Capacity, Total *Serum Decrease* May decrease TIBC to below typical reference range of 50 - 70 μmol/L *4784*

Plasminogen Activator Inhibitor-1 *Plasma Increase* Mean concentration appears to be increased in inflammatory conditions *5693*

Platelets *Blood Increase* In 732 patients with platelet counts greater than 500,000 /μL, 8.9% had chronic inflammatory disorders *1869*

Transferrin Saturation *Serum Decrease* May decrease TIBC to below typical reference range of 50 - 70 μmol/L *4784*

Tumor Necrosis Factor-α *Feces Increase* Concentration of 100 - 500 times greater than corrsponding serum values. Concentration in patients with inactive disease similar to that in controls, as in patients who underwent corrective surgery *556*

729.10 Fibromyalgia Syndrome

Insulin-like Growth Factor-I *Serum* *No Effect* In 27 patients with fibromyalgia mean concentration of 204 ± 70 ng/mL not significantly different from 204 ± 70 ng/mL in 30 healthy controls *621*

Insulin-like Growth Factor Binding Protein-3
Serum *No Effect* In 27 patients with fibromyalgia mean concentration of 3.3 ± 0.7 mg/L not significantly different from 3.2 ± 0.8 mg/L in 30 healthy controls *621*

Nucleotide Pyrophosphohydrolase, Soluble
Serum *Increase* Mean activity in 66 patients with fibromyalgia of 1,272 ± 31 pmol nitrophenol/h/mL significantly different from that in 85 healthy individuals 1,141 ± 22 pmol nitrophenol/h/mL *691*

Substance P *Cerebrospinal Fluid* *Increase* In 32 patients with fibromyalgia syndrome mean concentration of 42.8 ± 14.9 fmol/mL about 3 times higher than 16.3 ± 6.0 fmol/mL in 30 normal controls *4481*

730.00 Acute Hematogenous Osteomyelitis

C-Reactive Protein *Serum* *Increase* Concentration increased above 19 mg/L initially in 98% of 44 children with acute hematogenous osteomyelitis with mean value of 71 mg/L *5361* Rate increased in 43 of 45 cases in children on admission to hospital (mean of 74 ± 56 mg/L) *5362* In 36 children with osteomyelitis mean concentration on admission to hospital of 65 ± 42 mg/L declining to less than 20 mg/L on 7th day and subsequently. Concentrations somewhat higher when osteomyelitis involved adjacent joint *5363*

Erythrocyte Sedimentation Rate *Blood* *Increase* Rate increased above 20 mm/h initially in 92% of 44 children with acute hematogenous osteomyelitis with mean value of 45 mm/h *5361* In 36 children with osteomyelitis mean rate on admission to hospital 45 ± 22 mm/h declining to 29 ± 17 mm/h on 10th day and 14 ± 10 mm/h on 29th day. Rate somewhat higher when osteomyelitis involved adjacent joint *5363* In 37 of 40 cases in children rate increased (mean 44 ± 22 mm/h) *5362*

Leukocytes *Blood* *Increase* Concentration increased above 12 x 10^9 /L initially in 35% of 44 children with acute hematogenous osteomyelitis *5361* In 36 children with osteomyelitis mean concentration on admission to hospital 9.2 ± 3.3 x 10^9/L declining to 5.6 ± 2.0 x 10^9/L on 5th, 19th and 29th days. Concentrations somewhat higher when osteomyelitis involved adjacent joint *5363*
Blood *No Effect* Leukocyte count normal (less than 12,000 /µL) in 31 of 46 children on admission to hospital *5362*

730.00 Osteomyelitis

Alkaline Phosphatase *Serum* *Increase* In 36% of 24 patients at initial hospitalization for this disorder *1576*
Serum *No Effect* Normal in all 39 cases *5535*

Aspartate Aminotransferase *Serum* *Increase* In 36% of 25 patients at initial hospitalization for this disorder *1576*

Calcium *Serum* *No Effect* Normal in all 39 cases *5535*

Cholesterol *Serum* *Decrease* In 32% of 24 patients at initial hospitalization for this disorder *1576*

C-Reactive Protein *Serum* *Increase* In 44 children with acute hematogenous osteomyelitis, C-reactive protein was increased above 19 mg/L at the time of admission in 98% cases with mean concentration of 71 mg/L. Peak mean concentration of 83 mg/L reached on day 2 with rapid decrease to normal within one week *5361* Indicates active disease *413*

Erythrocyte Sedimentation Rate *Blood* *Increase* May be elevated or normal *5535* In 44 children with acute hematogenous osteomyelitis, ESR increased above 20 mm/h initially in 92% cases with mean value of 45 mm/h and mean peak value of 58 mm/h on days 3 - 5 after admission with value returning to normal in approximately 3 weeks *5361*

Hematocrit *Blood* *Decrease* Patients with initial episodes tended to be more anemic and have a more marked leukocytosis than patients with recurrent disease *5535*

Hemoglobin *Blood* *Decrease* Patients with initial episodes tended to be more anemic and have a more marked leukocytosis than patients with recurrent disease *5535*

Leukocytes *Blood* *Increase* May be increased, especially in acute cases *5544* In 44 children with acute hematogenous osteomyelitis, 35% of children had concentrations above 12,000 /µL at the time of hospitalization *5361* Total counts may become extremely high *5677* Patients with initial episodes tended to be more anemic and have a more marked leukocytosis than patients with recurrent disease *5535*
Blood *No Effect* Usually normal; especially in recurrent disease. Rarely > 16,000 /µL *5535*

Monocytes *Blood* *Increase* In 55% of 26 patients at initial hospitalization for this disorder *1576*

Neutrophils *Blood* *Increase* In 44% of 26 patients at initial hospitalization for this disorder *1576*

Phosphate *Serum* *Decrease* In 24% of 25 patients at initial hospitalization for this disorder *1576*
Serum *No Effect* Normal in all 39 cases *5535*

Phospholipase A *Serum* *Increase* Reported effect *2200*

731.00 Osteitis Deformans

Acid Phosphatase *Serum* *Increase* Elevated in very advanced cases and rare in early to moderate cases *1935* Seen occasionally in advanced disease *4707*
Serum *No Effect* Normal in a high percentage of patients *4707*

Alkaline Phosphatase *Serum* *Increase* Characteristic observation *4440* 20 cases were reported in which all patients showed elevated serum concentration *2803* Marked increase directly related to severity and extent of disease *5544* Gradually rises with the extension of the disease, rising rapidly if osteogenic sarcoma develops. ACTH or cortisone causes a transitory fall, often followed by a sharp rebound increase *1290*

Alkaline Phosphatase Isoenzymes *Serum* *Increase* All 7 patients had elevations of isoenzyme II *2557*

Calcium *Serum* *Increase* Usually normal but immobilization of affected individuals produces a high risk of hypercalcemia *2039*
Urine *Increase* Common *2039* Excretion is frequently increased and may lead to stone formation *367*

Eosinophils *Blood* *Increase* In 1 patient with osteitis deformans and asthma mean concentration of 735 x 10^6/L significantly different from upper limit of normal of 440 x 10^6/L in 29 normal individuals *607*

Histamine *Plasma* *Increase* In 1 patient with osteitis deformans and asthma mean concentration of 14.5 nmol/L significantly different from mean concentration of 4.0 nmol/L in 29 normal individuals *607*

Hydroxyproline *Urine* *Increase* Increase as evidence of enhanced remodeling activity *2039*

Leucine Aminopeptidase *Serum* *Increase* Slightly elevated in 14% of patients. Values ranged from 8 - 26 U/L (22 U/L normal upper limit) *3161*

Osteocalcin *Serum* *Increase* Elevated in 53% of patients *5672*

Phosphate *Serum* *Increase* Usually normal or slightly elevated *2039*
Serum *No Effect* Normal or slightly increased *5544*

731.00 Paget's Disease

Acid Phosphatase, Tartrate Resistant *Serum* *Increase* Activity increased as were other measures of bone turnover *2618* Mean activity of 4.3 ± 0.2 ng/mL in 27 patients with polyostotic disease significantly greater than 2.9 ± 0.1 U/L in 59 healthy controls *102* In patients with Paget's disease moderate increase observed *4217*
Serum *No Effect* Mean activity of 3.3 ± 0.3 U/L in 16 patients with monostotic disease not significantly greater than 2.9 ± 0.1 U/L in 59 healthy controls *102*

Alkaline Phosphatase *Serum* *Increase* Mean activity of 312 ± 49 U/L in 16 patients with monostotic disease and of 759 ± 121 U/L in 27 patients with polyostotic disease significantly greater than 147 ± 5 U/L in 59 healthy controls *102* Activity may be substantially increased in patients with active Paget's disease due to increased bone formation *4560* In 24 patients with Paget's disease of bone median activity of 267 U/L signifi-

731.00 **Paget's Disease** *(continued)*

Alkaline Phosphatase *(continued)*
cantly different from 125 U/L in 90 healthy controls *2572* In 13 patients with active Paget's disease mean highest activity of total alkaline phosphatase exceeded upper reference limit 15.3-fold mainly due to bone alkaline phosphatase *2518* In 14 patients with Paget's disease median activity of 406 U/L significantly higher than that in 75 healthy men in whom the median activity was 101 U/L and in 20 premenopausal women, 88 U/L, and in 38 postmenopausal women, 115 U/L *4716* About 85% of patients with Paget's disease have increased serum alkaline phosphatase activity. Activity is particularly high when certain bones, especially the skull, are affected *1284* In 26 patients with primary hyperparathyroidism median activity of 167 U/L significantly higher than that in 75 healthy men in whom the median activity was 101 U/L and in 20 premenopausal women, 88 U/L, and in 38 postmenopausal women, 115 U/L *4716*
Serum No Effect About 15% of patients with Paget's disease have normal serum alkaline phosphatase activity. This is particularly common in patients with monostotic disease *1284*

Alkaline Phosphatase, Bone Isoenzyme *Serum Increase* In 90 patients with Paget's disease median concentration of 51.6 μg/L (25th to 75th percentiles: 46.9 - 95.0 μg/L) significantly increased compared with mean of 13.2 μg/L in 200 healthy controls *604* Mean activity of 199.6 U/L in 114 patients with primary hyperparathyroidism significantly different from reference intervals of 15.0 - 41.3 U/L in men and 11.6 - 30.6 U/L in premenopausal women *1799* Mean activity of 42 ± 7 U/L in 16 patients with monostotic disease and of 98 ± 16 U/L in 27 patients with polyostotic disease significantly greater than 12.1 ± 0.5 U/L in 59 healthy controls *102* In 13 patients with active Paget's disease mean highest concentration exceeded upper reference limit 34.1-fold *2518* In patients with Paget's disease marked increase observed *4217*

Amino-terminal Propeptide of Type I Procollagen
Serum Increase Mean concentration of 90 ± 14 ng/mL in 16 patients with monostotic disease and of 293 ± 56 ng/mL in 27 patients with polyostotic disease significantly greater than 33 ± 2 ng/mL in 59 healthy controls *102*

Bone Sialoprotein *Serum Increase* In 24 patients with Paget's disease of bone mean concentration of 32.3 ± 17.3 μg/L significantly higher than that in 90 healthy controls in whom the mean concentration was 12.1 ± 5.0 μg/L *2572* In 14 patients with Paget's disease median concentration of 24.9 ng/mL significantly higher than that in 75 healthy men in whom the median concentration was 9.8 ng/mL and in 20 premenopausal women, 8.7 ng/mL, and in 38 postmenopausal women, 11.9 ng/mL *4716*

Calcium *Serum Increase* In one study of 40 patients with nonmalignant causes of hypercalcemia and low intact PTH concentrations 1 was attributable to Paget's disease *3280*
Serum No Effect In 14 patients with Paget's disease median concentration of 2.35 mmol/L not significantly higher than that in 75 healthy men in whom the median concentration was 2.38 mmol/L and in 20 premenopausal women, 2.39 mmol/L, and in 38 postmenopausal women, 2.41 mmol/L *4716* In 24 patients with Paget's disease of bone median concentration of 2.32 mmol/L not significantly different from 2.35 mmol/L in 90 healthy controls *2572* In a study of 59 patients with normocalcemia and low intact PTH concentration, 3 had Paget's diease *3280*

Creatine Kinase *Serum No Effect* In 1 patient with juvenile Paget's disease mean activity of 89 U/L compared with upper limit of normal of 195 U/L *5659*

Creatine Kinase BB-Isoenzyme *Serum No Effect* In 1 patient with juvenile Paget's disease mean activity of < 10 U/L (not detected %) compared with normal of 0 - 1% *5659*

C-terminal Propeptide of Type I Collagen *Serum Increase* Mean concentration of 145 ± 11 ng/mL in 16 patients with monostotic disease and of 191 ± 12 ng/mL in 27 patients with polyostotic disease significantly greater than 107 ± 4 ng/mL in 59 healthy controls *102*

C-terminal Telopeptide of Type I Collagen *Urine Increase* Mean excretion of 711 ± 63 μg/mmol creatinine in 27 patients with polyostotic disease significantly greater than 228 ± 30 μg/mmol creatinine in 59 healthy controls *102*
Urine No Effect Mean excretion of 267 ± 55 μg/mmol creatinine in 16 patients with monostotic not significantly greater than 228 ± 30 μg/mmol creatinine in 59 healthy controls *102*

Deoxypyridinoline *Urine Increase* In 13 patients with Paget's disease mean excretion of 10.12 ± 3.12 nmol/mmol creatinine compared with 5.71 ± 1.59 nmol/mmol creatinine in 79 healthy controls as measured by assay on Ciba Corning ACS:180 system *804* Mean excretion of 6.92 ± 0.66 nmol/mmol creatinine in 16 patients with monostotic disease and of 16.4 ± 2.1 nmol/mmol creatinine in 27 patients with polyostotic disease significantly greater than 5.06 ± 0.28 nmol/mmol creatinine in 59 healthy controls *102* In 74 patients with untreated Paget's disease 51% had excretions greater than reference interval of 0.4 - 6.4 nmol/mmol creatinine. Mean excretion was 7.8 (range of 0.5 - 41.5) nmol/mmol creatinine *4388* Mean excretion in 12 patients with Paget's disease of about 35 nmol/mmol creatinine significantly greater than 8 nmol/mmol creatinine in 11 premenopausal women and 11 men *423* In 14 patients with Paget's disease median excretion of 18.0 nmol/mmol creatinine significantly higher than that in 75 healthy men in whom the median excretion was 5.0 nmol/mmol creatinine and in 20 premenopausal women, 5.1 nmol/mmol creatinine, and in 38 postmenopausal women, 7.2 nmol/mmol creatinine *4716*

Deoxypyridinoline, Free *Urine Increase* Mean excretion in 28 patients aged 42 - 72 years of approximately 8.5 nmol/mol creatinine significantly different from upper limit of normal of up to 7.3 nmol/mol creatinine in healthy controls *4383* In 54 patients with untreated Paget's disease of the bone mean excretion of 12.7 ± 8.0 μmol/mol creatinine significantly different from 1.7 - 5.9 μmol/mol creatinine in healthy men and 3.1 - 8.1 μmol/mol creatinine in healthy women when measured by CLIA technique *4427*

24,25-Dihydroxy Vitamin D *Serum Decrease* Mean concentration in 24 untreated patients of 3.93 ± 0.5 nmol/L reduced below mean of reference interval of 1.3 - 16.4 nmol/L *1138*

Galactosyl-Hydroxylysine *Urine Increase* The average excretion rate was higher only in patients with more active disease *2622* Mean excretion in 12 patients with Paget's disease of about 1.7 μmol/mmol creatinine significantly greater than 0.8 μmol/mmol creatinine in 11 premenopausal women and 11 men *423*

Glucogalactyosyl-Hydroxylysine *Urine No Effect* The excretion rate was normal *2622*

Hydroxyproline *Urine Increase* The excretion rate was increased above normal in all patients with this disease *2622* Excretion may be substantially increased in patients with active Paget's disease due to breakdown of collagen-containing bone matrix *4560* Mean excretion in 12 patients with Paget's disease of about 70 μmol/mmol creatinine significantly greater than 10 μmol/mmol creatinine in 11 premenopausal women and 11 men *423* Mean excretion of 124 ± 13 nmol/mg creatinine in 16 patients with monostotic disease and of 292 ± 37 nmol/mg creatinine in 27 patients with polyostotic disease significantly greater than 75 ± 4.2 nmol/mg creatinine in 59 healthy controls *102*

N-terminal Telopeptide of Type I Collagen
Bone Marrow Increase Concentrations of 645, 360 and 184 nmol BCE/L in 3 patients with Paget's disease of the bone significantly higher than 61, 71 and 127 nmol/L BCE respectively in peripheral blood *861*
Serum Increase Mean concentration of 21.5 ± 15.8 nmol BCE/L in 7 patients with Paget's disease of the bone significantly higher than 4.7 ± 3.2 nmol BCE/L in 32 premenopausal women *861*
Urine Increase Mean excretion of 238 ± 44 nmol BCE/mmol creatinine in 16 patients with monostotic disease and of 1,022 ± 188 nmol BCE/mmol creatinine in 27 patients with polyostotic disease significantly greater than 33 ± 5.1 nmol BCE /mmol creatinine in 59 healthy controls *102* Mean excretion of 214.0 ± 90.2 nmol BCE/mmol creatinine in 7 patients with Paget's disease of the bone significantly higher than 36.2 ± 17.4 nmol BCE/mmol creatinine in 32 premenopausal women *861*

Osteocalcin *Serum Increase* Mean concentration of 26 ± 1.9 ng/mL in 16 patients with monostotic disease and of 41 ± 3.2 ng/mL in 27 patients with polyostotic disease significantly greater than 17 ± 0.9 ng/mL in 59 healthy controls *102* In 8 patients with Paget's disease mean concentration of 36 ± 9 μg/L (6.2 nmol/L) significantly different from that in healthy adults (men 25 ± 5 μg/L, women 20 ± 6 μg/L) *541* In 13 patients with active Paget's disease mean highest concentration exceeded upper reference limit 3.2-fold *2518* In patients with Paget's disease moderate increase observed *4217* The extent of the increases over control values varies from about 60% to 600%

depending on the assay used *1104* *3998* In 24 patients with Paget's disease mean pretreatment concentration of 22.3 ± 2.98 µg/L significantly higher than normal *1138* Using the Diagnostic Systems Laboratories' method mean concentration of 16 ± 7.8 µg/L in 10 patients with Paget's disease significantly higher than that in 68 healthy adults (4 ± 3.6 µg/L) *1149*
Serum *No Effect* Concentration tends not to be increased in Paget's disease *1284*

Parathyroid Hormone *Plasma* *Decrease* In one study of 40 patients with low intact PTH concentration and hypercalcemia not due to malignant disease 1 was attributable to Paget's disease *3280* In a study of 59 patients with low intact PTH concentration and normocalcemia 3 had Paget's disease *3280*
Plasma *Increase* In 10 patients mean concentration of 64.5 ± 58 ng/L compared with 29.8 ± 13.8 ng/L in 57 healthy adults *1150*

Parathyroid Hormone, Intact *Plasma* *No Effect* In 24 patients with Paget's disease of bone median concentration of 37.6 µg/L not significantly different from 35.2 µg/L in 90 healthy controls *2572*

Procollagen Type I Peptide *Serum* *Increase* Elevated serum levels of PICP in patients with Paget's disease, compared with normal subjects and correlated with serum alkaline phosphatase, have been previously described *1545*

Pyridinoline *Urine* *Increase* Mean excretion in 12 patients with Paget's disease of about 105 nmol/mmol creatinine significantly greater than 25 nmol/mmol creatinine in 11 premenopausal women and 11 men *423* In 74 patients with untreated Paget's disease 66% had excretions greater than reference interval of 5.0 - 21.8 nmol/mmol creatinine. Mean excretion of 29.7 (range 10.9 - 105.5) nmol/mmol creatinine *4388* Mean excretion of 50.3 ± 5.6 nmol/mmol creatinine (men) and 77.3 ± 12.8 nmol/mmol creatinine (women) in 16 patients with monostotic disease and of 108 ± 14 nmol/mmol creatinine (men) and 147 ± 34 nmol/mmol creatinine (women) in 27 patients with polyostotic disease significantly greater than 27 ± 2.5 nmol/mmol creatinine (men) and 45 ± 2.6 nmol/mmol creatinine (womem)in 59 healthy controls *102* In 30 patients with Paget's disease mean excretion of 61.8 ± 45.8 nmol/mmol creatinine significantly greater than 25.7 ± 10.4 and 33.1 ± 14.7 nmol/mol creatinine in healthy men and women respectively *167* In 14 patients with Paget's disease median excretion of 57.7 nmol/mmol creatinine significantly higher than that in 75 healthy men in whom the median excretion was 20.8 nmol/mmol creatinine and in 20 premenopausal women, 19.6 nmol/mmol creatinine, and in 38 postmenopausal women, 28.2 nmol/mmol creatinine *4716*

Type I Collagen Cross-linked C-telopeptide
Serum *Increase* In 15 patients with Paget's disease mean concentration of 339 ± 36% of premenopausal concentration *4054*
Urine *Increase* In 6 patients with Paget's disease mean concentration of 670 ± 314% of premenopausal concentration *4054*

Type I Collagen Teleopeptide *Serum* *Increase* Mean concentration of 3.87 ± 0.35 ng/mL in 16 patients with monostotic disease and of 6.23 ± 0.76 ng/mL in 27 patients with polyostotic disease significantly greater than 3.07 ± 0.08 ng/mL in 59 healthy controls *102*

732.10 Perthes' Disease

Insulin-like Growth Factor-I *Serum* *Decrease* In boys with early Perthes' disease normal physiologic increase with age was absent or diminished *3752*

732.90 Hungry Bone Syndrome

Phosphate *Serum* *Decrease* Hungry bone syndrome is less common cause of severe hypophosphatemia due to shift of phosphate into cells *969*

733.00 Kevin-Coffey Syndrome

Creatine Kinase *Serum* *Increase* In 1 patient with Kevin-Coffey syndrome mean activity of 227 U/L compared with upper limit of normal of 195 U/L *5659*

Creatine Kinase BB-Isoenzyme *Serum* *No Effect* In 1 patient with Kevin-Coffey syndrome mean activity of < 10 U/L (not detected %) compared with upper limit of normal of 0 - 1% *5659*

733.00 Osteoporosis

Acid Phosphatase, Tartrate Resistant *Serum* *Increase* In patients with osteoporosis slight increase observed *4217*
Serum *No Effect* Mean activity of 7.59 ± 0.39 U/L in 43 untreated postmenopausal osteoporotic women significantly different from 7.31 ± 0.58 U/L in 41 healthy postmenopausal women *4715*

Adenosine Monophosphate *Urine* *No Effect* Mean excretion of 0.060 ± 0.004 mg/mg creatinine in 43 untreated osteoporotic postmenopausal women not significantly different from 0.057 ± 0.003 mg/mg creatinine in 41 healthy postmenopausal women *4715*

Albumin *Serum* *No Effect* No significant difference observed between mean daytime concentration of 40.2 g/L in 15 healthy postmenopausal women and 39.7 g/L in 15 postmenopausal women with osteoporosis *1285*

Alkaline Phosphatase *Serum* *Increase* In 42 osteoporotic postmenopausal women mean activity of 90 ± 57 U/L significantly higher than 72 ± 14 U/L in 14 healthy age matched postmenopausal women *1162* In hypermetabolic osteopenia *2039*
Serum *No Effect* In postmenopausal osteoporosis no significant difference between 26 subjects and 24 controls *4133* Usual effect observed *900* *5544* In 35 postmenopausal women with osteoporosis median activity of 79.7 ± 4.0 U/L before treatment not different from reference range of 30 - 100 U/L *2876* Mean activity of 64.2 ± 4.0 U/L in 43 untreated postmenopausal osteoporotic women not significantly different from 61.1 ± 2.7 U/L in 41 healthy postmenopausal women *4715*

Alkaline Phosphatase, Bone Isoenzyme *Serum* *Increase* In 40 women with untreated postmenopausal (type I) osteoporosis mean activity of 30.4 ± 1.9 U/L significantly different from 20.3 ± 1.0 U/L in 40 normal postmenopausal women *2668* In patients with osteoporosis slight increase observed *4217* In 25 osteoporotic postmenopausal women mean activity of 17.6 ± 8.1 U/L significantly higher than 15 ± 1.8 U/L in 14 healthy age matched postmenopausal women *1162*
Serum *No Effect* In 35 postmenopausal women with osteoporosis median concentration of 11.0 ± 0.8 µg/L (activity of 21.2 ± 1.4 U/L) before treatment not different from reference ranges of 4.3 - 22.4 µg/L (14.8 - 43.4 U/L) *2876* Mean activity of 29.8 U/L in 32 patients with osteoporosis not significantly different from reference intervals of 15.0 - 41.3 U/L in men and 11.6 - 30.6 U/L in premenopausal women *1799*

Calcitonin *Plasma* *No Effect* In postmenopausal osteoporosis no significant difference between 26 subjects and 24 controls *4133*

Calcium *Serum* *Decrease* Hypocalcemia may be present in severe cases *2039*
Serum *No Effect* No significant difference observed between daytime concentrations of 2.39 mmol/L in 15 postmenopausal women with osteoporosis and 2.35 mmol/L in 15 healthy postmenopausal women *1285* In a study of 59 patients with normocalcemia and low intact PTH concentration, 26 had osteoporosis *3280* Usual effect observed *900* Mean concentration of 9.45 ± 0.08 mg/dL in 43 untreated postmenopausal osteoporotic not women significantly different from 9.49 ± 0.08 mg/dL in 41 healthy postmenopausal women *4715* Process is usually so gradual that homeostatic forces control the serum calcium *2252*
Urine *Decrease* May be increased, normal, or decreased but is not influenced by intake; calcium restriction does not produce the normal fall *5544*
Urine *Increase* May be increased, normal, or decreased but is not influenced by intake; calcium restriction does not produce the normal fall *5544* Characteristic observation *2039*
Urine *No Effect* Mean excretion of 0.19 ± 0.01 mg/mg creatinine in 43 untreated osteoporotic postmenopausal women significantly different from 0.12 ± 0.01 mg/mg creatinine in 41 healthy postmenopausal women *4715* In 15 healthy postmenopausal women mean daytime excretion of 1.47 mmol/8 h not significantly different from 1.59 mmol/8 h in 15 postmenopausal women with osteoporosis *1285*

733.00 **Osteoporosis** *(continued)*

Cells *Bone Marrow Increase* The iliac bone marrow specimens showed infiltrates consisting of elongated mast cells, eosinophils, plasma cells, and varying numbers of lymphocytes *5448*

C-Reactive Protein *Serum Increase* In 18 men with senile osteoporosis mean concentration of 4.9 ± 2.6 mg/dL and in 18 women with senile osteoporosis mean concentration of 10.0 ± 6.0 mg/dL significantly higher than upper limit of normal of 3.0 mg/dL *3376*

Creatinine Clearance *Urine No Effect* In 40 women with untreated postmenopausal (type I) osteoporosis mean clearance 70.1 ± 2.4 mL/min not significantly different from 72.5 ± 3.2 mL/min in 40 normal postmenopausal women *2668*

C-terminal Osteocalcin *Serum No Effect* In 42 osteoporotic postmenopausal women mean concentration of 1.8 ± 2.7 ng/mL not significantly different from 2.1 ± 0.8 ng/mL in 14 healthy age matched postmenopausal women *1162*

Deoxypyridinoline *Urine Increase* In 13 patients with osteoporosis mean excretion of 8.40 ± 3.86 nmol/mmol creatinine compared with 5.71 ± 1.59 nmol/mmol creatinine in 79 healthy controls as measured by assay on Ciba Corning ACS:180 system *804* In 40 women with untreated postmenopausal (type I) osteoporosis mean excretion of 18.8 ± 0.9 nmol/mmol creatinine significantly different from 13.0 ± 0.6 nmol/mmol creatinine in 40 normal postmenopausal women *2668* In 7 patients with osteoporosis mean concentration of deoxypyridinoline crosslinks of 9.48 ± 3.91 nmol/mmol creatinine *4019* In 108 patients with untreated Paget's disease 6% had excretions greater than reference interval of 0.4 - 6.4 nmol/mmol creatinine. Mean excretion was 4.2 (range 2.0 - 7.7) nmol/mmol creatinine *4388* Mean excretion in 13 women aged about 65 years of about 15 nmol/mmol creatinine significantly greater than 9 nmol/mmol creatinine in 11 healthy premenopausal women aged about 36 years *423*

Deoxypyridinoline, Free *Urine Increase* Mean excretion in 31 patients aged 40 - 80 years of approximately 7.0 nmol/mol creatinine compared with approximately 4.0 nmol/mol creatinine in healthy controls *4383* In 255 patients with untreated osteoporosis mean excretion of 7.5 ± 4.1 µmol/mol creatinine significantly different from 1.7 - 5.9 µmol/mol creatinine in healthy men and 3.1 - 8.1 µmol/mol creatinine in healthy women when measured by CLIA technique *4427*

1,25-Dihydroxy Vitamin D_3 *Serum No Effect* Mean concentration of 25.3 ± 1.5 pg/mL in 43 untreated postmenopausal osteoporotic not women significantly different from 25.7 ± 1.2 pg/mL in 41 healthy postmenopausal women *4715*

Dipyridinoline *Urine Increase* Mean excretion of 23.6 ± 1.8 nmol/mmol creatinine in 43 untreated osteoporotic postmenopausal women not significantly different from 19.1 ± 1.9 nmol/mmol creatinine in 41 healthy postmenopausal women *4715*

Eosinophils *Bone Marrow Increase* The iliac bone marrow specimens showed infiltrates consisting of elongated mast cells, eosinophils, plasma cells, and varying numbers of lymphocytes *5448*

Galactosyl-Hydroxylysine *Urine Increase* Mean excretion in 13 women aged about 65 years of about 1.3 µmol/mmol creatinine significantly greater than 0.8 µmol/mmol creatinine in 11 healthy premenopausal women aged about 36 years *423*

25-Hydroxy Vitamin D_3 *Serum Increase* In 29 women mean concentration of 221 ± 19 nmol/L significantly different from 155 ± 15 nmol/L in 56 matched controls: in 53 postmenopausal women mean concentration of 209 ± 21 nmol/L not significantly different from 158 ± 26 nmol/L in 26 age and sex matched controls *5749*
Serum No Effect Mean concentration of 22.3 ± 1.5 ng/mL in 43 untreated postmenopausal osteoporotic women not significantly different from 22.6 ± 1.2 ng/mL in 41 healthy postmenopausal women *4715*

Hydroxyproline *Urine Increase* In hypermetabolic osteopenia *2039* In 7 patients with osteoporosis mean concentration of 36.2 ± 15.0 mmol/mmol creatinine *4019* Mean excretion of 0.48 ± 0.005 mg/mg creatinine in 43 untreated osteoporotic postmenopausal women not significantly different from 0.040 ± 0.003 mg/mg creatinine in 41 healthy postmenopausal women *4715* By assuming the value of 12 µmol/g creatinine as the threshold value, the sensitivity of the test is 87% and the specificity 60% *3612*
Urine No Effect Mean excretion in 13 women aged about 65 years of about 15 µmol/mmol creatinine not significantly greater than 8 µmol/mmol creatinine in 11 healthy premenopausal women aged about 36 years *423* In postmenopausal osteoporosis no significant difference between 26 subjects and 24 controls *4133*

Insulin-like Growth Factor-I *Serum Decrease* In 98 women mean concentration of 121 ± 5.5 ng/mL significantly less than 142 ± 5.8 ng/mL in 56 matched controls *5749*
Serum No Effect In 53 postmenopausal women mean concentration of 132 ± 7.4 ng/mL not significantly different from 136 ± 10 ng/mL in 26 matched controls: in 43 men mean concentration of 121 ± 8.7 ng/mL not significantly different from controls *5749* Mean concentration of 83.6 ± 8.5 ng/mL in 43 untreated postmenopausal osteoporotic women not significantly different from 75.9 ± 5.1 ng/mL in 41 healthy postmenopausal women *4715*

Insulin-like Growth Factor-II *Serum Decrease* In 98 women mean concentration of 441 ± 23 ng/mL significantly less than 449 ± 14 ng/mL in 56 matched controls *5749*
Serum No Effect In 53 postmenopausal women mean concentration of 445 ± 33 ng/mL not significantly different from 444 ± 25 ng/mL in 26 matched controls: in 43 men mean concentration of 410 ± 17 ng/mL not significantly different from controls *5749*

Insulin-like Growth Factor Binding Protein-3
Serum Decrease In 98 women mean concentration of 3.3 ± 0.1 mg/L significantly less than 3.8 ± 0.1 mg/L in 56 matched controls: 3.0 ± 0.2 mg/L in 53 postmenopausal women significantly less than 3.7 ± 0.1 mg/L in 26 postmenopausal controls *5749*
Serum No Effect In 43 men mean concentration of 3.2 ± 0.2 mg/L not significantly different from 3.1 ± 0.3 mg/L in 5 matched controls *5749* In 17 men mean concentration of 3.7 ± 0.3 mg/L not significantly different from 3.1 ± 0.3 mg/L in 5 matched controls *5749*

Interleukin-1 Receptor Antagonist *Serum Decrease* In 40 women with untreated postmenopausal (type I) osteoporosis mean concentration of 143 ± 21 pg/mL significantly different from 189 ± 22 pg/mL in 40 normal postmenopausal women *2668*

Interleukin-1α *Serum No Effect* In 40 women with untreated postmenopausal (type I) osteoporosis mean concentration of 658 ± 68 pg/mL not significantly different from 577 ± 28 pg/mL in 40 normal postmenopausal women *2668*

Interleukin-1β *Serum No Effect* In 40 women with untreated postmenopausal (type I) osteoporosis mean concentration of 637 ± 120 pg/mL not significantly different from 671 ± 163 pg/mL in 40 normal postmenopausal women *2668*

Interleukin-6 *Serum Increase* In 18 men with senile osteoporosis mean concentration of 164 ± 129 pg/mL and in 18 women with senile osteoporosis mean concentration of 477 ± 265 pg/mL significantly higher than normal range of 60 ± 20 pg/mL *3376*
Serum No Effect In 40 women with untreated postmenopausal (type I) osteoporosis mean concentration of 2.8 ± 0.4 pg/mL not significantly different from 2.6 ± 0.4 pg/mL in 40 normal postmenopausal women *2668*

ionized Calcium *Serum No Effect* Mean concentration of 1.23 ± 0.009 mmol/L in 43 untreated postmenopausal osteoporotic not women significantly different from 1.22 ± 0.009 mmol/L in 41 healthy postmenopausal women *4715* In 15 healthy postmenopausal women mean concentrations 1.248 and 1.253 mmol/L (day and night) compared with 1.263 during day and night in 15 women with postmenopausal oseoporosis *1285*

Lymphocytes *Bone Marrow Increase* The iliac bone marrow specimens showed infiltrates consisting of elongated mast cells, eosinophils, plasma cells, and varying numbers of lymphocytes *5448*

Magnesium *Serum Decrease* In severe cases *2039*

Osteocalcin *Serum Decrease* Significantly lower in 26 patients with postmenopausal osteoporosis than in 24 control subjects ($p < 0.002$) *4133* Relative to values in controls, it has been reported that plasma concentrations in postmenopausal osteoporosis are increased, unchanged or decreased *5261*
Serum Increase In postmenopausal osteoporotic women mean concentration of 17.4 ± 8.6 ng/mL compared with means of 7.8 ng/mL in premenopausal and 10.1 ng/mL in healthy postmenopausal women *5790* In patients with osteoporosis

slight increase observed *4217* Relative to values in controls, it has been reported that plasma concentrations in postmenopausal osteoporosis are increased, unchanged or decreased *5261* In 15 postmenopausal women with osteoporosis mean concentrations during daytime of 9.70 ng/L and at night 10.19 ng/L not significantly higher than 8.91 ng/L during day and 9.31 ng/L at night in 15 healthy postmenopausal women *1285* In 41 patients with postmenopausal osteoporosis mean concentration of 25.7 ± 7 µg/L (4.3 nmol/L) not significantly different from 29 ± 2 µg/L (5.0 nmol/L) in healthy postmenopausal women but significantly different from that in healthy young adults (men 25 ± 5 µg/L, women 20 ± 6 µg/L) *541* In 40 women with untreated postmenopausal (type I) osteoporosis mean concentration of 10.2 ± 0.4 ng/mL significantly different from 9.0 ± 0.3 ng/mL in 40 normal postmenopausal women *2668*
Serum No Effect In 42 osteoporotic postmenopausal women mean concentration of 8.3 ± 6.0 ng/mL not significantly different from 10.5 ± 6.0 ng/mL in 14 healthy age matched postmenopausal women *1162* Mean concentration of 4.18 ± 0.27 ng/mL in 43 untreated postmenopausal osteoporotic women not significantly different from 4.51 ± 0.26 ng/mL in 41 healthy postmenopausal women *4715* Relative to values in controls, it has been reported that plasma concentrations in postmenopausal osteoporosis are increased, unchanged or decreased *5261* In 36 osteoporotic women mean concentration of 12.5 ± 6.2 µg/L compared with 12.2 ± 4.5 µg/L in 30 normal women as measured by CIA *2556*

Parathyroid Hormone *Plasma Decrease* In a study of 59 patients with low intact PTH concentration and normocalcemia 26 had osteoprosis *3280*
Plasma No Effect In 29 women mean concentration of 29 ± 1.6 ng/mL not significantly different from 30 ± 2.8 ng/mL in 56 matched controls: in 53 postmenopausal women mean concentration of 30 ± 2.4 ng/mL not significantly different from 31 ± 1.9 ng/mL in 26 age and sex matched controls *5749* In postmenopausal osteoporosis no significant difference between 26 subjects and 24 controls *4133* No significant difference observed between mean daytime concentration of 41 ng/L in 15 healthy postmenopausal women and 39 ng/L in 15 with osteoporosis *1285* Mean concentration of 29.9 ± 1.9 pg/mL in 43 untreated postmenopausal osteoporotic not women significantly different from 31.5 ± 1.7 pg/mL in 41 healthy postmenopausal women *4715*

Phosphate *Serum No Effect* Usually no effect on concentration *5544*

Plasma Cells *Bone Marrow Increase* The iliac bone marrow specimens showed infiltrates consisting of elongated mast cells, eosinophils, plasma cells, and varying numbers of lymphocytes *5448*

Pyridinoline *Urine Increase* In 108 patients with untreated osteoporosis 32% had excretions greater than reference interval of 5.0 - 21.8 nmol/mmol creatinine. Mean excretion of 19.3 (range 9.3 - 30.6) nmol/mmol creatinine *4388* In 7 patients with osteoporosis mean concentration of 47.6 ± 39.3 nmol/mmol creatinine *4019* In 40 women with untreated postmenopausal (type I) osteoporosis mean excretion of 55.5 ± 2.5 nmol/mmol creatinine significantly different from 42.7 ± 2.1 nmol/mmol creatinine in 40 normal postmenopausal women *2668* Mean excretion of 79.8 ± 6.3 nmol/mmol creatinine in 43 untreated osteoporotic postmenopausal women significantly different from 59.5 ± 5.5 nmol/mmol creatinine in 41 healthy postmenopausal women *4715* Mean excretion in 13 women aged about 65 years of about 40 nmol/mmol creatinine significantly greater than 25 nmol/mmol creatinine in 11 healthy premenopausal women aged about 36 years *423*

Pyridinoline Cross-linked Telopeptide of Type I Collagen *Serum Increase* In 40 women with untreated postmenopausal (type I) osteoporosis mean concentration of 4.8 ± 0.3 U/L significantly different from 3.3 ± 0.2 U/L in 40 normal postmenopausal women *2668*

Pyridinoline, Free *Urine Increase* Mean excretion in women with osteoporosis significantly greater than 16 - 32 nmol/mmol creatinine in healthy premenopausal women *1798*

Pyridinoline:Dipyridinoline Ratio *Urine No Effect* Mean ratio of 3.5 ± 0.16 in 43 untreated osteoporotic postmenopausal women not significantly different from 3.3 ± 0.11 in 41 healthy postmenopausal women *4715*

Tumor Necrosis Factor-α *Serum Increase* In 18 men with senile osteoporosis mean concentration of 21.3 ± 9.4 pg/mL and in 18 women with senile osteoporosis mean concentration of 26.3 ± 12.0 pg/mL significantly higher than normal range of 10 ± 4 pg/mL *3376*

Type I Collagen Cross-linked N-telopeptide *Urine Increase* In 7 patients with osteoporosis mean concentration of deoxypyridinoline crosslinks of 109.7 ± 60.8 BCE/mmol creatinine *4019*

733.99 Melorheostosis

Creatine Kinase *Serum No Effect* In 1 patient with melorheostosis mean activity of 30 U/L compared with upper limit of normal of 195 U/L *5659*

Creatine Kinase BB-Isoenzyme *Serum No Effect* In 1 patient with melorheostosis mean activity of < 3 U/L compared with normal of 0 - 1% *5659*

733.99 Relapsing Polychondritis

Melanoma Inhibitory Factor *Serum No Effect* In 10 patients mean concentration of 3.4 ± 2.7 ng/mL showed no significant difference from 3.6 ± 2.8 ng/mL in 120 healthy controls *3655*

737.30 Idiopathic Scoliosis

Calcium *Serum Increase* In 29 Saudi Arabian volunteer girls aged 12 to 16 years in generally good health mean concentration of 2.96 ± 0.14 mmol/L significantly different from 2.18 ± 0.18 mmol/L in 48 normal controls *99*

Carbon Dioxide Partial Pressure *Blood Increase* Thoracic bellows defects; decreased pO_2 associated with increased pCO_2 *5544* Mean pCO_2 increased and pO_2 decreased with age in idiopathic scoliosis *2521*

Cortisol *Plasma No Effect* In 29 Saudi Arabian volunteer girls aged 12 to 16 years in generally good health mean concentration of 379.2 ± 69.3 nmol/L not significantly different from 404.7 ± 83.7 nmol/L in 48 normal controls *99*

Growth Hormone *Plasma No Effect* In 29 Saudi Arabian volunteer girls aged 12 to 16 years in generally good health mean concentration of 16.14 ± 10.18 µg/L not significantly different from 14.29 ± 8.92 µg/L in 48 normal controls *99*

Oxygen Partial Pressure *Blood Decrease* Thoracic bellows defects (patients with kyphoscoliosis); decreased pO_2 associated with increased pCO_2 *5544* Mean pCO_2 increased and pO_2 decreased with age in idiopathic scoliosis *2521*

Oxygen Saturation *Blood Decrease* Thoracic bellows defects; decreased pO_2 associated with increased pCO_2 *5544* Mean pCO_2 increased and pO_2 decreased with age in idiopathic scoliosis *2521*

Parathyroid Hormone *Plasma Increase* In 29 Saudi Arabian volunteer girls aged 12 to 16 years in generally good health mean concentration of 41.23 ± 7.87 pmol/L significantly different from 23.97 ± 5.75 pmol/L in 48 normal controls *99*

Phosphate *Serum Increase* In 29 Saudi Arabian volunteer girls aged 12 to 16 years in generally good health mean concentration of 1.81 mmol/L significantly different from 1.42 ± 0.21 mmol/L in 48 normal controls *99*

Testosterone *Serum Increase* In 29 Saudi Arabian volunteer girls aged 12 to 16 years in generally good health mean concentration of 0.73 ± 0.09 nmol/L significantly different from 0.36 ± 0.05 nmol/L in 48 normal controls *99*

Thyroid Stimulating Hormone *Serum No Effect* In 29 Saudi Arabian volunteer girls aged 12 to 16 years in generally good health mean concentration of 1.66 ± 0.77 mU/L not significantly different from 1.84 ± 0.87 mU/L in 48 normal controls *99*

Thyroxine (T4) *Serum Increase* In 29 Saudi Arabian volunteer girls aged 12 to 16 years in generally good health mean concentration of 7.48 ± 1.29 nmol/L not significantly different from 5.55 ± 1.07 nmol/L in 48 normal controls *99*

Tri-iodothyronine (T3) *Serum No Effect* In 29 Saudi Arabian volunteer girls aged 12 to 16 years in generally good health mean concentration of 0.82 ± 0.17 nmol/L not significantly different from 0.85 ± 0.23 nmol/L in 48 normal controls *99*

737.30 Idiopathic Scoliosis *(continued)*

Tri-iodothyronine (T3) *(continued)*

CONGENITAL ANOMALIES

741.90 Spina Bifida

Growth Hormone *Plasma* *Decrease* In 6 prepubertal children with spinal bifida and shunted hydrocephalus mean concentration of 1.0 µg/L significantly less than 2.1 µg/L in 32 control prepubertal children and in 11 postpubertal affected children mean concentration of 2.7 µg/L less than 8.5 µg/L in 41 postpubertal children *3125*

Insulin-like Growth Factor-I *Serum* *Decrease* In 6 prepubertal children with spinal bifida and shunted hydrocephalus mean concentration of 5.2 nmol/L significantly less than 12.4 nmol/L in 32 control prepubertal children and in 11 postpubertal affected children mean concentration of 15.9 nmol/L less than 21.3 nmol/L in 41 postpubertal children *3125*

Insulin-like Growth Factor Binding Protein-3 *Serum* *Decrease* In 6 prepubertal children with spinal bifida and shunted hydrocephalus mean concentration of 1.9 mg/L significantly less than 3.7 mg/L in 32 control prepubertal children and in 11 postpubertal affected children mean concentration of 4.1 mg/L not significantly less than 4.3 mg/L in 41 postpubertal children *3125*

742.20 Lissencephaly

Amyloid β-Protein *Cerebrospinal Fluid* *No Effect* In 1 patient with lissencephaly concentration was 1.38 pmol/mL not significantly different from mean concentration of 4.00 ± 2.92 pmol/mL *3716*

Amyloid β-Protein Precursor *Cerebrospinal Fluid* *Decrease* In 1 patient with lissencephaly concentration was 0.66 integrated OD units significantly different from mean concentration of 1.35 ± 0.38 integrated OD units in 25 normal controls *3716*

α_1-Antichymotrypsin *Cerebrospinal Fluid* *No Effect* In 1 patient with lissencephaly concentration was 2.30 µg/mL not significantly different from mean concentration of 2.27 ± 1.40 µg/mL in 25 normal controls *3716*

Cells *Cerebrospinal Fluid* *No Effect* In 1 patient with lissencephaly concentration of 1.0 cells/µL not significantly different from normal of 3 cells/µL *3716*

Protein *Cerebrospinal Fluid* *No Effect* In 1 patient with lissencephaly concentration of 23 mgL not significantly different from normal of 28 mg/dL in 25 healthy controls *3716*

747.29 Congenital Heart Disease

Erythropoietin *Serum* *Increase* In 24 patients with congenital heart disease mean concentration of 122 ± 232 U/L compared with 9 ± 4 U/L in 79 reference controls *4320*

Hemoglobin *Blood* *Increase* In 24 patients with congenital heart disease mean concentration of 18.2 ± 1.5 g/dL compared with 14 ± 1.1 g/dL in 79 reference controls *4320*

750.50 Pyloric Stenosis, Infantile

Bicarbonate *Serum* *Increase* In 75 patients with pyloric stenosis mean concentration of 27.2 mmol/L significantly higher than 22.3 mmol/L in 75 patients with gastrointestinal reflux *4904*

Chloride *Serum* *Decrease* In 75 patients with pyloric stenosis mean concentration of 95.7 mmol/L significantly lower than 103.6 mmol/L in 75 patients with gastrointestinal reflux *4904*

Urea Nitrogen *Serum* *Increase* In 75 patients with pyloric stenosis mean concentration of 13.5 mg/dL significantly higher than 7.5 mg/dL in 75 patients with gastrointestinal reflux *4904*

751.69 Intrahepatic Biliary Hypoplasia

Alanine Aminotransferase *Serum* *Increase* Most cases present in early childhood with a conjugated hyperbilirubinemia and plasma hepatic enzyme activity increased up to 30 times the reference interval *3406*

Alkaline Phosphatase *Serum* *Increase* Most cases present in early childhood with a conjugated hyperbilirubinemia and plasma hepatic enzyme activity increased up to 30 times the reference interval *3406*

Aspartate Aminotransferase *Serum* *Increase* Most cases present in early childhood with a conjugated hyperbilirubinemia and plasma hepatic enzyme activity increased up to 30 times the reference interval *3406*

Bilirubin *Serum* *Increase* Most cases present in early childhood with a conjugated hyperbilirubinemia *3406*

Bilirubin, Conjugated *Serum* *Increase* Most cases present in early childhood with a conjugated hyperbilirubinemia *3406*

Cholesterol *Serum* *Increase* Most cases present in early childhood with a conjugated hyperbilirubinemia and plasma hepatic enzyme activity increased up to 30 times the reference interval: plasma cholesterol raised up to 3 times the reference interval in 80% of cases *3406*

γ-Glutamyltransferase *Serum* *Increase* Most cases present in early childhood with a conjugated hyperbilirubinemia and plasma hepatic enzyme activity increased up to 30 times the reference interval *3406*

Lactate Dehydrogenase *Serum* *Increase* Most cases present in early childhood with a conjugated hyperbilirubinemia and plasma hepatic enzyme activity increased up to 30 times the reference interval *3406*

Triglycerides *Serum* *Increase* Most cases present in early childhood with a conjugated hyperbilirubinemia and plasma hepatic enzyme activity increased up to 30 times the reference interval: plasma triglycerides raised up to 3 times the reference interval in 80% of cases *3406*

752.50 Cryptorchidism

Mullerian Inhibiting Substance *Serum* *No Effect* In 34 boys with normal testes and girls of mean age 1.2 y but with cryptorchidism, or male pseudohermaphroditism concentrations ranged from about 8.0 ng/mL to approximately 150 ng/mL compared with mean of 63.8 ng/mL and lowest value of 7.0 ng/mL in healthy boys of the same age *2970*

752.70 Hermaphroditism

Mullerian Inhibiting Substance *Serum* *Decrease* In 14 boys with abnormal testes and girls with mean age of 1.2 y with mixed gonadal dysgenesis, true hermaphroditism, Leydig-call hyperplasia or testicular regression, concentrations ranged from lower limit of sensitivity of 0.5 ng/mL to approximately 60 ng/mL compared with mean of 84.0 ng/mL and lowest value of 6.4 ng/mL in healthy boys of the same age *2970*

752.80 Anorchia

Mullerian Inhibiting Substance *Serum* *Decrease* In 12 boys with mean age of 4.1 y concentrations ranged from lower limit of sensitivity of 0.5 ng/mL to approximately 3.0 ng/mL compared with mean of 63.8 ng/mL and lowest value of 7.0 ng/mL in healthy boys of the same age *2970*

753.10 Polycystic Kidney Disease

Albumin *Urine* *Increase* Progressive albuminuria *367*

Amino Acids *Plasma* *Decrease* Mean concentration of essential amino acids and tyrosine were significantly lower, resulting in a low essential/total ratio *3409*

Ammonia *Blood* *Decrease* Decreased arterial ammonia in azotemic patients, (mean of 34 ± 1.4 mmol/L) due to reduced synthesis by diseased kidney *4213*

Calcium *Urine* *Increase* Found in nonuremic medullary cystic disease *367*

Creatinine *Serum* *Increase* Common *413* Mean concentration in 9 patients with polycystic kidney disease of 1.9 ± 0.4 mg/dL compared with 0.9 ± 0.3 mg/dL in 9 healthy controls *5153*
Serum *No Effect* In 9 patients with polycystic kidney disease mean concentration of 1.9 ± 0.4 mg/dL not significantly greater than 0.9 ± 0.3 mg/dL in 9 healthy controls *5153*

Creatinine Clearance *Urine* *Decrease* Diminished clearance with acidosis *900*

Erythrocytes *Urine* *Increase* Progressive hematuria *367* Intermittent hematuria is common, and gross hematuria may be seen occasionally *1980*

Erythropoietin *Cyst Fluid* *Increase* Increased values were found in 49 plasma samples and 14 cyst fluids of 92 patients with renal cell carcinoma or renal cyst. Highest values were found in patients developing metastases after removal of renal carcinoma *3525*
Serum *Increase* Increased values were found in 49 plasma samples and 14 cyst fluids of 92 patients with renal cell carcinoma or renal cyst. Highest values were found in patients developing metastases after removal of renal carcinoma *3525*

Hematocrit *Blood* *Decrease* Most of the patients show some degree of anemia *900* Characteristic *572*

Hemoglobin *Blood* *Decrease* Characteristic anemia *572* Most of the patients show some degree of anemia *900*

Hepatocyte Growth Factor *Urine* *No Effect* In 10 patients with chronic renal failure not requiring dialysis mean excretion not significantly different from that in 9 healthy controls in whom the mean excretion was 1.5 ± 0.2 ng/g creatinine *5153* In 9 patients with polycystic kidney disease mean excretion not significantly different from that in 9 healthy controls in whom the mean excretion was 1.5 ± 0.2 ng/g creatinine *5153* Mean concentration in 9 patients with polycystic kidney disease not significantly different from 1.5 ± 0.2 ng/g creatinine in 9 healthy controls *5153*

Lactate Dehydrogenase *Urine* *No Effect* Excretion usually within normal limits *5544*

Neutrophils *Urine* *Increase* The median values were higher than 90% in bacterial, renal, or urinary tract disease and in polycystic kidney disease *3071*

Protein *Urine* *Increase* Usually minimal or mild *1980*

Sodium *Serum* *Decrease* Renal salt wasting *572*

Tyrosine *Plasma* *Decrease* Mean concentration of essential amino acids and tyrosine were significantly lower, resulting in a low essential/total ratio *3409*

Urea Nitrogen *Serum* *Increase* Azotemia *4213*

Volume *Red Blood Cells* *Increase* True polycythemia with a considerable increase of red cell volume may occur *3710*
Urine *Increase* Common *413*

753.16 Medullary Cystic Disease

Ammonium Ions *Urine* *Increase* May lead to proximal renal tubular acidosis which is associated with hypokalemia, hyperchloremic metabolic acidosis, urine pH < 5.5, increased urinary ammonium ion excretion, a negative urine anion gap, increased urinary osmol gap, normal urinary citrate, normal urinary calcium excretion and Fanconi syndrome *4071*

Anion Gap *Urine* *Decrease* May lead to proximal renal tubular acidosis which is associated with hypokalemia, hyperchloremic metabolic acidosis, urine pH < 5.5, increased urinary ammonium ion excretion, a negative urine anion gap, increased urinary osmol gap, normal urinary citrate, normal urinary calcium excretion and Fanconi syndrome *4071*

Bicarbonate *Serum* *Decrease* May lead to proximal renal tubular acidosis which is associated with hypokalemia, hyperchloremic metabolic acidosis, urine pH < 5.5, increased urinary ammonium ion excretion, a negative urine anion gap, increased urinary osmol gap, normal urinary citrate, normal urinary calcium excretion and Fanconi syndrome *4071*

Calcium *Serum* *Decrease* Frequent, but not invariable *572*
Urine *Increase* Found in nonuremic medullary cystic disease *367*
Urine *No Effect* May lead to proximal renal tubular acidosis which is associated with hypokalemia, hyperchloremic metabolic acidosis, urine pH < 5.5, increased urinary ammonium ion excretion, a negative urine anion gap, increased urinary osmol gap, normal urinary citrate, normal urinary calcium excretion and Fanconi syndrome *4071*

Casts *Urine* *No Effect* Normal urinary sediment *572*

Chloride *Serum* *Increase* May lead to proximal renal tubular acidosis which is associated with hypokalemia, hyperchloremic metabolic acidosis, urine pH < 5.5, increased urinary ammonium ion excretion, a negative urine anion gap, increased urinary osmol gap, normal urinary citrate, normal urinary calcium excretion and Fanconi syndrome *4071*

Citrate *Urine* *No Effect* May lead to proximal renal tubular acidosis which is associated with hypokalemia, hyperchloremic metabolic acidosis, urine pH < 5.5, increased urinary ammonium ion excretion, a negative urine anion gap, increased urinary osmol gap, normal urinary citrate, normal urinary calcium excretion and Fanconi syndrome *4071*

Creatinine Clearance *Urine* *Decrease* Diminished with acidosis *900*

Glucose *Urine* *Increase* May lead to proximal renal tubular acidosis which is associated with hypokalemia, hyperchloremic metabolic acidosis, urine pH < 5.5, increased urinary ammonium ion excretion, a negative urine anion gap, increased urinary osmol gap, normal urinary citrate, normal urinary calcium excretion and Fanconi syndrome *4071*

Hematocrit *Blood* *Decrease* Most of the patients show some degree of anemia *900* Characteristic anemia *572*

Hemoglobin *Blood* *Decrease* Most of the patients show some degree of anemia *900* Characteristic anemia *572*

Osmolal Gap *Urine* *Increase* May lead to proximal renal tubular acidosis which is associated with hypokalemia, hyperchloremic metabolic acidosis, urine pH < 5.5, increased urinary ammonium ion excretion, a negative urine anion gap, increased urinary osmol gap, normal urinary citrate, normal urinary calcium excretion and Fanconi syndrome *4071*

pH *Blood* *Decrease* Characteristic acidosis *572*
Urine *Decrease* May lead to proximal renal tubular acidosis which is associated with hypokalemia, hyperchloremic metabolic acidosis, urine pH < 5.5, increased urinary ammonium ion excretion, a negative urine anion gap, increased urinary osmol gap, normal urinary citrate, normal urinary calcium excretion and Fanconi syndrome *4071*

Phosphate *Serum* *Decrease* May lead to proximal renal tubular acidosis which is associated with hypokalemia, hyperchloremic metabolic acidosis, urine pH < 5.5, increased urinary ammonium ion excretion, a negative urine anion gap, increased urinary osmol gap, normal urinary citrate, normal urinary calcium excretion and Fanconi syndrome *4071*

Potassium *Serum* *Decrease* May lead to proximal renal tubular acidosis which is associated with hypokalemia, hyperchloremic metabolic acidosis, urine pH < 5.5, increased urinary ammonium ion excretion, a negative urine anion gap, increased urinary osmol gap, normal urinary citrate, normal urinary calcium excretion and Fanconi syndrome *4071*

Sodium *Serum* *Decrease* Renal salt wasting *572*
Urine *Increase* Characteristic renal salt wasting *572*

Specific Gravity *Urine* *Decrease* Characteristic hyposthenuria *572*

Urea Nitrogen *Serum* *Increase* Characteristic azotemia *572*

Uric Acid *Serum* *Decrease* May lead to proximal renal tubular acidosis which is associated with hypokalemia, hyperchloremic metabolic acidosis, urine pH < 5.5, increased urinary ammonium ion excretion, a negative urine anion gap, increased urinary osmol gap, normal urinary citrate, normal urinary calcium excretion and Fanconi syndrome *4071*

Volume *Urine* *Increase* Polyuria *2034*

753.16 Nephronophthisis

CD45 Leukocytes *Tissue* *Increase* In 1 patient with nephronophthiasis number of positive cells 335 cells/mm^2 in renal tissue *3026*

Creatinine *Serum* *Increase* In 1 patient with nephronophthiasis concentration of 1.40 mg/dL different from 0.88 ± 0.17 mg/dL in 20 healthy controls *3026*

753.16 Nephronophthisis *(continued)*

Intercellular Adhesion Molecule-1 *Tissue* *No Effect* In 1 patient with nephronophthisis percentage of ICAM-1 positive renal tubuli 0.0% *3026*

Protein *Urine* *Increase* In 1 patient with nephronophthiasis excretion of 5.90 mg/mg creatinine *3026*

Soluble Intercellular Adhesion Molecule-1 *Serum* *Increase* In 1 patient with nephronophthisis concentration of soluble ICAM-1 of 400 ng/mL compared with 306 ± 52 ng/mL in 20 healthy controls *3026*
Urine *Increase* In 1 patient with nephronophthisis excretion of soluble ICAM-1 of 7.4 ng/mL or 12.3 ng/mg creatinine compared with 2.6 ± 1.7 ng/mL or 2.5 ± 3.0 ng/mg creatinine in 20 healthy controls *3026*

753.17 Medullary Sponge Kidney

Calcium *Urine* *Increase* Hypercalciuria in 19 of 36 patients tested *1317*

pH *Urine* *Increase* Impaired ability to concentrate or acidify the urine maximally has been reported *572* *1843*

Specific Gravity *Urine* *Decrease* Impaired ability to concentrate or acidify the urine maximally has been reported *1843* *572*

756.40 Chondrodystrophy

Alkaline Phosphatase *Serum* *Decrease* Following arrest of growth in childhood, falls rapidly to adult levels *1290* Reported effect with achondroplasia and cretinism in children *3160*

756.40 Osteopathia Striata

Creatine Kinase *Serum* *No Effect* In 1 patient with osteopathia striata and one with osteopathia striata/cranial sclerosis mean activities of 90 U/L and 49 U/L compared with upper limit of normal of 195 U/L *5659*

Creatine Kinase BB-Isoenzyme *Serum* *No Effect* In 1 patient with osteopathia striata and one with osteopathia striata/cranial sclerosis mean activities of < 10 U/L and < 5 U/L (not detected %) compared with normal of 0 - 1% *5659*

756.51 Osteogenesis Imperfecta

Acid Phosphatase *Serum* *Increase* Much higher than normal in all 8 patients (37 - 77 U/L) studied *1682*
Serum *No Effect* The levels in patients did not differ significantly from those in controls of the same age *2391*

Alkaline Phosphatase *Serum* *Increase* Increase observed in 2 cases *2803*
Serum *No Effect* In 78 patients with osteogenesis imperfecta mean activity generally normal compared with healthy controls *3162*

Amino-terminal Propeptide of Type I Procollagen
Serum *Decrease* In 78 patients with osteogenesis imperfecta mean concentration reduced compared with healthy controls *3162*

Amino-terminal Propeptide of Type III Procollagen
Serum *No Effect* In 78 patients with osteogenesis imperfecta mean concentration normal compared with healthy controls *3162*

Cross-linked C-terminal Telopeptide of Type I Collagen
Serum *Decrease* In 78 patients with osteogenesis imperfecta mean concentration reduced in children but normal in adults compared with healthy controls *3162*

C-terminal Propeptide of Type I Procollagen
Serum *Decrease* In 78 patients with osteogenesis imperfecta mean concentration reduced in children but normal in adults compared with healthy controls *3162*

Osteocalcin *Serum* *Increase* Reported effect *733*
Serum *No Effect* In 78 patients with osteogenesis imperfecta mean concentration normal compared with healthy controls *3162*

Procollagen Type I Peptide *Serum* *Increase* Serum concentrations of procollagen I C-terminal propeptide (PICP) were studied in 74 patients with various forms of non-lethal osteogenesis imperfecta and 27 unaffected family members. Using the standard deviation (SD) score, PICP concentrations were found to be > or = -1 SD in 16%, between -1 and -2 SD in 26% and < or = -2 SD in 58% of the patients with osteogenesis imperfecta compared to healthy controls *573*

Pyridinoline *Serum* *Decrease* In 78 patients with osteogenesis imperfecta mean concentration reduced in children but increased in adults compared with healthy controls *3162*

756.52 Osteopetrosis

Acid Phosphatase *Serum* *Increase* Sometimes increased *5544*

Alkaline Phosphatase *Serum* *No Effect* Activity usually unaffected *5544*

Calcium *Serum* *Decrease* Moderate hypocalcemia occasionally in children *2034*
Serum *No Effect* Often no effect on concentration *5544*

Creatine Kinase BB-Isoenzyme *Serum* *Increase* Elevated level in three patients with adult osteopetrosis *5810*

Erythrocytes *Blood* *Decrease* Anemia and pancytopenia *5545*

Hematocrit *Blood* *Decrease* Anemia and pancytopenia *5545*

Hemoglobin *Blood* *Decrease* Anemia and pancytopenia *5545*

Leukocytes *Blood* *Decrease* Anemia and pancytopenia *5545*

Lymphocytes *Blood* *Decrease* Relative lymphocytosis or lymphocytopenia may occur *5545*
Blood *Increase* Relative lymphocytosis or lymphocytopenia may occur *5545*

Phosphate *Serum* *Decrease* Occasionally in children *2034*
Serum *No Effect* Often concentration unaffected *5544*

Platelets *Blood* *Decrease* Anemia and pancytopenia *5545*

756.52 Osteopetrosis, Adult Type I

Creatine Kinase *Serum* *No Effect* In 2 patients mean activities of 84 U/L and 71 U/L, compared with upper limit of normal of 195 U/L *5659*

Creatine Kinase BB-Isoenzyme *Serum* *No Effect* In 2 patients mean activities of < 5 U/L and < 5 U/L (not detected as % of total CK) *5659*

756.52 Osteopetrosis, Adult Type II

Creatine Kinase *Serum* *Increase* In 5 patients mean activities of 336 U/L, 284 U/L, 172 U/L, 81 U/L and 100 U/L compared with upper limit of normal of 195 U/L *5659*

Creatine Kinase BB-Isoenzyme *Serum* *Increase* In 5 patients mean activities of 219 U/L, 227 U/L, 84 U/L, 36 U/L and 66 U/L (65%, 80%, 49%, 44% and 66%, respectively, of total CK) compared with normal of 0 - 1% *5659*

756.52 Osteopetrosis, Infantile Form

Creatine Kinase *Serum* *Increase* In 2 patients mean activities 330 U/L and 554 U/L compared with upper limit of normal of 195 U/L *5659*

Creatine Kinase BB-Isoenzyme *Serum* *Increase* In 2 patients mean activities of 23 U/L and 443 U/L (7% and 79%, respectively of total CK) compared with normal of 0 -1% in normals *5659*

756.52 Osteopetrosis, Intermediate Form

Creatine Kinase *Serum* *No Effect* In 3 patients mean activities of 76 U/L, 83 U/L and 60 U/L compared with upper limit of normal of 195 U/L *5659*

Creatine Kinase BB-Isoenzyme *Serum* *Increase* In 3 patients mean activities of 20 U/L, 15 U/L and 10 U/L (27%, 18% and 17%, respectively, of total CK), compared with normal of 0 - 1% *5659*

756.54 Polyostotic Fibrous Dysplasia

Alkaline Phosphatase *Serum* *Increase* Characteristically increased *2433* In some cases *1290* Characteristic observation *5544*

Calcium *Serum* *No Effect* In a study of 59 patients with normocalcemia and low intact PTH concentration, 1 had polyostotic fibrous dysplasia *3280*

Parathyroid Hormone *Plasma* *Decrease* In a study of 59 patients with low intact PTH concentration and normocalcemia 1 had polyostotic fibrous dysplasia *3280*

756.55 Infantile Cortical Hyperostosis

Erythrocyte Sedimentation Rate *Blood* *Increase* Increased (Caffey's disease) *5544*

Leukocytes *Blood* *Increase* Increased (Caffey's disease) *5544*

756.59 Chondrodysplasia Punctata

Chitotriosidase *Serum* *No Effect* Normal activity observed in both of two patients with chondrodysplasia punctata *1917*

756.83 Ehlers-Danlos Syndrome

Ammonium Ions *Urine* *Increase* May be associated with classic distal renal tubular acidosis which is asociated with hyokalemia, hyperchloremic metabolic acidosis, urine pH > 5.5, increased urinary ammonium ion excretion, a negative urine anion gap, increased urinary osmol gap, decreased urinary citrate and increased urinary calcium in some patients *4071*

Anion Gap *Urine* *Decrease* May be associated with classic distal renal tubular acidosis which is associated with hyokalemia, hyperchloremic metabolic acidosis, urine pH > 5.5, increased urinary ammonium ion excretion, a negative urine anion gap, increased urinary osmol gap, decreased urinary citrate and increased urinary calcium in some patients *4071*

Calcium *Urine* *Increase* May be associated with classic distal renal tubular acidosis which is asociated with hyokalemia, hyperchloremic metabolic acidosis, urine pH > 5.5, increased urinary ammonium ion excretion, a negative urine anion gap, increased urinary osmol gap, decreased urinary citrate and increased urinary calcium in some patients *4071*

Chloride *Serum* *Increase* May be associated with classic distal renal tubular acidosis which is associated with hyokalemia, hyperchloremic metabolic acidosis, urine pH > 5.5, increased urinary ammonium ion excretion, a negative urine anion gap, increased urinary osmol gap, decreased urinary citrate and increased urinary calcium in some patients *4071*

Citrate *Urine* *Decrease* May be associated with classic distal renal tubular acidosis which is associated with hyokalemia, hyperchloremic metabolic acidosis, urine pH > 5.5, increased urinary ammonium ion excretion, a negative urine anion gap, increased urinary osmol gap, decreased urinary citrate and increased urinary calcium in some patients *4071*

Net Acid Excretion *Urine* *Increase* May be associated with classic distal renal tubular acidosis which is associated with hyokalemia, hyperchloremic metabolic acidosis, urine pH > 5.5, increased urinary ammonium ion excretion, a negative urine anion gap, increased urinary osmol gap, decreased urinary citrate and increased urinary calcium in some patients *4071*

Osmolal Gap *Urine* *Increase* May be associated with classic distal renal tubular acidosis which is associated with hyokalemia, hyperchloremic metabolic acidosis, urine pH > 5.5, increased urinary ammonium ion excretion, a negative urine anion gap, increased urinary osmol gap, decreased urinary citrate and increased urinary calcium in some patients *4071*

Potassium *Serum* *Decrease* May be associated with classic distal renal tubular acidosis which is associated with hyokalemia, hyperchloremic metabolic acidosis, urine pH > 5.5, increased urinary ammonium ion excretion, a negative urine anion gap, increased urinary osmol gap, decreased urinary citrate and increased urinary calcium in some patients *4071*

756.83 Ehlers-Danlos Syndrome Type VI

Deoxypyridinoline *Urine* *Increase* In 3 affected children mean excretion ranged from 557 ± 53 to 633 ± 56 µmol/mol creatinine compared with 53 ± 22 µmol/mol in 26 normal children and 152 ± 4 µmol/mol creatinine in one affected adult compared with 8 ± 3 µmol/mol creatinine in 45 adults *4022*

Pyridinoline *Urine* *Decrease* In 3 children mean excretions ranged from 89 to 96 µmol/mol creatinine compared with 251 ± 114 µmol/mol creatinine in 26 healthy children under 10 years of age, and 31 ± 2 µmol/mol creatinine in one adult compared with excretion of 31 ± 11 µmol/mol creatinine in 45 normal adults *4022*

756.89 Craniometaphyseal Dysplasia

Creatine Kinase *Serum* *No Effect* In 1 patient with central osteosclerosis with ectodermal dysplasia mean activity of 92 U/L compared with upper limit of normal of 195 U/L *5659*

Creatine Kinase BB-Isoenzyme *Serum* *No Effect* In 1 patient with central osteosclerosis with ectodermal dysplasia mean activity of < 5 U/L (not detected %) compared with normal of 0 - 1% *5659*

757.10 Ichthyosis, X-linked

Chitotriosidase *Serum* *Increase* Normal activity observed in five of six patients with condition, but activity of 211 nmol/h/mL in the other *1917*

757.31 Ectodermal Dysplasia

Creatine Kinase *Serum* *No Effect* In 1 patient with central osteosclerosis with ectodermal dysplasia mean activity of 42 U/L compared with upper limit of normal of 195 U/L *5659*

Creatine Kinase BB-Isoenzyme *Serum* *No Effect* In 1 patient with central osteosclerosis with ectodermal dysplasia mean activity of < 5 U/L (not detected %) compared with normal of 0 - 1% *5659*

757.33 Urticaria Pigmentosa

Alkaline Phosphatase *White Blood Cells* *Decrease* Of 30 patients with urticaria pigmentosa, 2 had alkaline leukocyte phosphatase indices less than 20 *5253*
White Blood Cells *Increase* Of 30 patients with urticaria pigmentosa, 11 had alkaline leukocyte phosphatase indices greater than 80 *5253*

Antinuclear Antibodies *Serum* *Increase* Of 30 patients with urticaria pigmentosa, 3 had positive antibody titers *5253*

Eosinophils *Blood* *Increase* Of 30 patients with urticaria pigmentosa, 3 had proportions greater than 7% *5253*

Erythrocytes *Blood* *No Effect* Of 30 patients with urticaria pigmentosa, 0 had counts less than 3.8 million /µL *5253*

Folate *Serum* *Decrease* Of 30 patients with urticaria pigmentosa, 3 had serum concentrations less than 3 ng/mL (7 pmol/L) *5253*

Granulocyte-Macrophage Colony Stimulating Factor *Serum* *Increase* Of 30 patients with urticaria pigmentosa, 8 had concentrations greater than 20 pg/mL *5253*

Interleukin-3 *Serum* *No Effect* Of 30 patients with urticaria pigmentosa all had normal concentrations *5253*

Interleukin-6 *Serum* *Increase* Of 30 patients with urticaria pigmentosa, 10 had concentrations greater than 3 pg/mL *5253*

Leukocytes *Blood* *Increase* Of 30 patients with urticaria pigmentosa, 4 had counts greater than 10,000 /µL *5253*

757.33 Urticaria Pigmentosa *(continued)*

Methylimidazoleacetic Acid *Urine Increase* In 12 adult patients with urticaria pigmentosa median concentration of 3.0 mmol/mol creatinine compared with 0.4 - 2.4 mmol/mol creatinine in healthy individuals *1845*

β_2-Microglobulin *Serum Increase* Of 30 patients with urticaria pigmentosa, 3 had serum concentrations greater than 1.9 mg/dL *5253*

Neopterin *Serum Increase* Of 30 patients with urticaria pigmentosa, 6 had serum concentrations greater than 10 nmol/L *5253*

Platelets *Blood Increase* Of 30 patients with urticaria pigmentosa, 3 had counts greater than 400,000 /μL *5253*

Stem Cell Factor *Serum Decrease* Of 30 patients with urticaria pigmentosa, 9 had concentrations less than 1,184 pg/mL *5253*
Serum Increase Of 30 patients with urticaria pigmentosa, 1 had a concentration greater than 1,812 pg/mL *5253*

Tryptase *Serum Increase* In 12 adult patients with urticaria pigmentosa median concentration measured with B12 mAb-based fluoroimmunoassay of 56 μg/L compared with 2.2 - 8.8 μg/L in healthy individuals *1845*

Tumor Necrosis Factor-α *Serum Increase* Of 30 patients with urticaria pigmentosa, 6 had concentrations greater than 20 pg/mL *5253*

Vitamin B_{12} *Serum Decrease* Of 30 patients with urticaria pigmentosa, 1 had a serum concentration less than 200 pg/mL (150 pmol/L) *5253*

758.00 Down's Syndrome

Acid Phosphatase *Serum Decrease* May be low *5545*

α_1-Antichymotrypsin *Serum No Effect* In 48 patients with Down's syndrome mean concentration of 42 ± 33 mg/dL not significantly different from 44 ± 18 mg/dL in 48 controls *98* In 11 adult Down's syndrome patients mean concentration of 513.3 ± 80.3 mg/L not significantly different from 476.1 ± 70.4 mg/L in 11 age and sex matched controls *2165*

CA 125 *Serum Increase* In the first and second trimesters, maternal serum levels were found to be elevated compared with controls *2204*

Carnitine *Serum Decrease* Deficiency was not observed in a large percentage of children. Below average levels were noted in 39.1% of cases with severe deficiency noted in 4 cases *894*

Cholesterol *Serum No Effect* Plasma lipid levels were measured in 20 mongoloid and 16 nonmongoloid mentally retarded subjects. Significant elevations of plasma triglyceride levels were found in patients with Down's syndrome compared with mentally retarded controls. However, no significant difference was found in plasma cholesterol, phospholipid and free fatty acid levels between the mongoloids and control subjects *3800*

β-Chorionic Gonadotropin *Plasma Increase* In 4,412 pregnant women 48 were demonstrated to have Down's syndrome using serum screening tests before 14 weeks of gestation. Abnormality of total β-chorionic gonadotropin detected 29% of these. When used in conjunction with the serum concentration of pregnancy-associated protein A an maternal age the detection rate with hCG was 63% *1950*

β-Chorionic Gonadotropin, Free *Plasma Increase* In 4,412 pregnant women 48 were demonstrated to have Down's syndrome using serum screening tests before 14 weeks of gestation. Abnormality of free β-chorionic gonadotropin detected 25% of these. When used in conjunction with the serum concentration of pregnancy-associated protein A and maternal age the detection rate was 60% *1950*

Copper *Serum Increase* In 16 patients with Down's syndrome aged 4 - 23 y mean values of 1.34 ± 0.05 mg/L significantly different from 1.10 ± 0.05 mg/L in 16 age and sex-matched controls *2520*

Copper Zinc Superoxide Dismutase
Red Blood Cells Increase Significantly elevated in patients with Down's syndrome without Alzheimer's disease *4076*

Copper:Zinc Ratio *Serum Increase* In 16 patients with Down's syndrome aged 4 - 23 y mean values of 1.64 ± 0.08 significantly different from 1.16 ± 0.06 in 16 age and sex-matched controls *2520*

Dopamine β-Hydroxylase *Serum Decrease* Present in abnormally low plasma concentrations although norepinephrine is not reduced *2765*

Estriol, Unconjugated *Plasma Increase* In 4,412 pregnant women 48 were demonstrated to have fetuses with Down's syndrome using serum screening tests before 14 weeks of gestation. Abnormality of unconjugated estriol detected 4% of these *1950*

Fatty Acids (FFA), Free *Serum No Effect* Plasma lipid levels were measured in 20 mongoloid and 16 nonmongoloid mentally retarded subjects. Significant elevations of plasma triglyceride levels were found in patients with Down's syndrome compared with mentally retarded controls. However, no significant difference was found in plasma cholesterol, phospholipid and free fatty acid concentrations between the mongoloids and control subjects *3800*

α-Fetoprotein *Serum Increase* In 4,412 pregnant women 48 were demonstrated to have Down's syndrome using serum screening tests before 14 weeks of gestation. Abnormality of α-fetoprotein detected 17% of these *1950*

Folate *Red Blood Cells Decrease* Red cell values were very low *1708*
Red Blood Cells No Effect No significant difference observed between means in 18 children with Down's syndrome and 18 age and gender matched controls *4411*
Serum Decrease Mean serum folate was normal in this group, these individuals displayed decreasing concentrations with age *1708*
Serum No Effect In 18 children with Down's syndrome mean concentration not significantly different from that in 18 age and gender matched controls *4411*

Growth Hormone *Plasma No Effect* Concentrations may be normal in patients with Down's syndrome *5034*

Hematocrit *Blood Increase* In 18 children with Down's syndrome aged 2 - 6 y mean of 39.1% (range 35.8 - 41.8%) significantly greater than 36.9% (range 33.7 - 41.5%) in 18 age and gender matched controls *4411*

Hemoglobin F *Blood Increase* Patients with an extra G chromosome *5544*

Homocystine *Plasma Decrease* Concentration reduced in some patients with Down's syndrome *5346*

Immunoglobulin G_1 *Serum Increase* In children with Down's syndrome aged 1 - 2.5, 4 - 8 and 9 - 12 years concentration significantly increased compared with healthy children of same ages *140*

Immunoglobulin G_2 *Serum Decrease* In children with Down's syndrome aged 9 - 12 years mean concentration significantly reduced compared with healthy controls of same age *140*
Serum No Effect In children with Down's syndrome aged 1 - 2.5 and 4 - 8 years concentration unchanged compared with healthy children of the same ages *140*

Immunoglobulin G_3 *Serum Increase* In children with Down's syndrome aged 1 - 2.5, 4 - 8 and 9 - 12 years concentration significantly increased compared ith concentration in healthy children of same ages *140*

Immunoglobulin G_4 *Serum Decrease* In children with Down's syndrome aged 1 - 2.5, 4 - 8 and 9 - 12 years mean concentration significantly reduced compared with healthy controls of same age. In those aged 4 - 12 years 68% had concentrations below 2 SDs of the geometrical mean of the controls *140*

Inhibin *Plasma Increase* During 15 - 17 weeks gestation in pregnant women with Down syndrome median of MoM of 1.53 compared with 1.0 in women with normal pregnancies *1012*

Insulin-like Growth Factor-I *Serum Decrease* Production may be deficient in patients with Down's syndrome *5034*

Iron *Serum Increase* Patients with anicteric hepatitis whose serum contained hepatitis-B surface antigen, had lower levels than controls *369*

Iron-binding Capacity, Total *Serum Decrease* Patients with anicteric hepatitis whose serum contained HBsAg, had lower levels than controls *369*

Leukocytes *Blood Decrease* In 14 children aged 2 - 6 y with Down's syndrome mean of 6,600 /µL not significantly less than 8,200 /µL in age and gender matched controls *4411*

Magnesium *Serum No Effect* In 16 patients with Down's syndrome aged 4 - 23 y mean values of 21.7 ± 0.4 mg/L not significantly different from 21.0 ± 0.4 mg/L in 16 age and sex-matched controls *2520*

MCV *Blood Increase* As a whole, the group showed an increase. Macrocytosis increased with age *1708* In 18 children aged 2 - 6 y with Down's syndrome mean volume of 86.9 fL (range 81.8 - 97.80 fL) significantly greater than 80.6 fL (range 70.9 - 91.9 fL) in 18 age and gender matched controls *4411*

Phospholipids *Serum No Effect* Plasma lipid levels were measured in 20 mongoloid and 16 nonmongoloid mentally retarded subjects. Significant elevations of plasma triglyceride levels were found in patients with Down's syndrome compared with mentally retarded controls. However, no significant difference was found in plasma cholesterol, phospholipid and free fatty acid levels between the mongoloids and control subjects *3800*

Pregnancy-associated Protein A *Serum Decrease* Concentration reduced during first trimester to 0.60 multiples of the normal median but increased to 1.00 of the multiples of the normal median during the second trimester *50*
Serum Increase In 4,412 pregnant women 48 were demonstrated to have Down's syndrome using serum screening tests before 14 weeks of gestation. Abnormality of pregnancy-associated protein A detected 42% of these *1950*

Pregnancy-specific Glycoprotein *Serum Decrease* Reduction to 0.73 multiple of the normal median observed during first trimester but increased to 1.17 multiple of the normal median during the second trimester *50*

Pro-aC Inhibin *Serum Increase* During 15 - 17 weeks gestation in pregnant women with Down syndrome median of MoM 1.34 compared with 1.0 in women with normal pregnancies *1012*

Propranolol *Serum Increase* High plasma concentrations have been observed in patients with Down's syndrome suggesting that the drug's bioavailability may be increased *5751*

Prostate-specific Antigen *Amniotic Fluid No Effect* Median maternal serum PSA MoM of 0.80 not significantly different from that in controls in whom 10th and 90th centiles were 0.49 and 1.68 respectively *4955*
Serum No Effect Median maternal serum PSA MoM of 0.89 not significantly different from that in controls in whom 10th and 90th centiles were 0.22 and 4.56 respectively *4955*

Schwangerschaftsprotein 1 *Serum Increase* In maternal serum in weeks 5 - 9 MoM was 0.27 in 25 women with Down's syndrome and 1.28 in weeks 14 - 20 in 117 women with Down's syndrome significantly different from controls *4246*
Serum No Effect In maternal serum in weeks 10 - 12 MoM was 0.89 in 14 women with Down's syndrome not significantly different from controls *4246*

Selenium *Serum Decrease* In 16 patients with Down's syndrome aged 4 - 23 y mean values of 43.2 ± 1.7 µg/L significantly different from 50.1 ± 1.6 µg/L in 16 age and sex-matched controls *2520*

Soluble β-Amyloid Peptide 40 *Serum Increase* In 43 patients with Down's syndrome median concentration of 116 pg/mL significantly different from 53 pg/mL in 43 age-matched normal controls *3441*

Soluble β-Amyloid Peptide 42 *Serum Increase* In 43 patients with Down's syndrome median concentration of 186 pg/mL significantly different from 25 pg/mL in 43 age-matched normal controls *3441*

Theophylline *Serum Increase* Clearance prolonged in most of 6 infants aged 2 - 19 months *5034*

Thyroid Stimulating Hormone *Serum No Effect* In 17 children aged 2 - 6 y with Down's syndrome no significant difference observed from control age and gender-matched controls *4411*

Triglycerides *Serum Increase* Plasma lipid levels were measured in 20 mongoloid and 16 nonmongoloid mentally retarded subjects. Significant elevations of plasma triglyceride levels were found in patients with Down's syndrome compared with mentally retarded controls. However, no significant difference was found in plasma cholesterol, phospholipid and free fatty acid levels between the mongoloids and control subjects *3800*

Uric Acid *Serum Increase* Some cases *1290*

Zinc *Serum Decrease* In 16 patients with Down's syndrome aged 4 - 23 y mean values of 0.83 ± 0.02 mg/L significantly different from 0.96 ± 0.03 mg/L in 16 age and sex-matched controls *2520* Decreased *5083*

758.10 Trisomy 13

Hemoglobin F *Blood Increase* Patients with an extra D chromosome *5544*
Blood No Effect Translocation - normal mosaicism in D_1 trisomy *5689*

758.60 Turner's Syndrome

Antimicrosomal Antibodies *Serum Increase* In 92 of 478 girls with Turner's syndrome antimicrosomal or antiperoxidase antibodies detected *4259*

Antiperoxidase Antibodies *Serum Increase* In 92 of 478 girls with Turner's syndrome antimicrosomal or antiperoxidase antibodies detected *4259*

Antithyroglobulin Antibodies *Serum Increase* In 106 of 478 girls with Turner's syndrome TGA antibodies detected *4259*

Growth Hormone *Plasma Decrease* In children with Turner's syndrome mean 12 h concentration of 1.8 µg/L (1 SD range 1.0 - 3.2 µg/L) in 96 females significantly lower than 2.7 µg/L (1 SD range 1.4 - 5.1 µg/L) in 35 female controls *694*
Urine Decrease In 7 children aged 6 to 14 years mean excretion 2.3 ± 1.8 ng/d compared with 13.4 ± 3.2 ng/d in 16 healthy children of same age range *2742*

Growth Hormone Binding Protein *Serum Decrease* In children with Turner's syndrome mean concentration of 208 pmol/L (1 SD range 115 - 378 pmol/L) in 96 females not significantly lower than 228 pmol/L (1 SD range 115 - 378 pmol/L) in 228 female controls *694*

Insulin-like Growth Factor-I *Serum Decrease* In children with Turner's syndrome mean concentration of 141 µg/L (1 SD range 80 - 248 µg/L) in 96 females significantly lower than 308 µg/L (1 SD range 178 - 531 µg/L) in 35 female controls *694*

758.70 Klinefelter's Syndrome (XXY)

Androgens *Plasma Decrease* Testosterone reported to be low in most studies, although there is considerable overlap between normal males and Klinefelter males. Generally higher in mosaics than in pure Klinefelter patients *2264* Quite variable but often tends to be midway between the normal male and female *1980*

Cholesterol *Serum Increase* Hyperlipidemia found in 8 of 24 patients; in 6, only cholesterol was elevated *3171*

Estradiol *Plasma Increase* Total and free plasma concentrations of estradiol are normal or increased. Does not correlate with clinical findings such as gynecomastia or hypoandrogenicity *2264*
Plasma No Effect Total and free plasma concentrations of estradiol are normal or increased. Does not correlate with clinical findings such as gynecomastia or hypoandrogenicity *2264*

Estradiol, Free *Plasma Increase* Total and free plasma concentrations of estradiol are normal or increased. Does not correlate with clinical findings such as gynecomastia or hypoandrogenicity *2264*
Plasma No Effect Total and free plasma concentrations of estradiol are normal or increased. Does not correlate with clinical findings such as gynecomastia or hypoandrogenicity *2264*

Estrogens *Plasma Increase* Total and free plasma concentrations of estradiol are normal or increased. Does not correlate with clinical findings such as gynecomastia or hypoandrogenicity *2264*
Plasma No Effect Total and free plasma concentrations of estradiol are normal or increased. Does not correlate with clinical findings such as gynecomastia or hypoandrogenicity *2264*

Follicle Stimulating Hormone *Plasma Increase* Commonly elevated; a result of deficient testicular function *2264* Always increased as a result of the extensive tubular disease *367*

758.70 Klinefelter's Syndrome (XXY) *(continued)*

Follicle Stimulating Hormone *(continued)*
Urine *Increase* Observed effect *1290*

Glucose *Serum* *Increase* Mild diabetes is found in 10% *1980*

Glucose Tolerance *Serum* *Decrease* Decreased 25% *1980*

Gonadotropin, Pituitary *Urine* *Increase* Almost invariably increased *367* Commonly elevated; a result of deficient testicular function *2264*

Growth Hormone *Plasma* *No Effect* Usually normal *2264*

17-Hydroxycorticosteroids *Urine* *No Effect* Usually normal *2264*

Inhibin-A *Plasma* *No Effect* Concentration undetectable in 9 men with Klinefelter's syndrome, as in 16 healthy men aged 19 - 45 y *113*

Inhibin-B *Plasma* *Decrease* Mean concentration of 11 ± 3 pg/mL in 9 men with Klinefelter's syndrome significantly less than 187 ± 28 pg/mL in 16 healthy men aged 19 - 45 y *113*

17-Ketogenic Steroids *Urine* *No Effect* Usually normal *2264*

17-Ketosteroids *Urine* *Decrease* May be normal or decreased *1980*

Lipids *Serum* *Increase* Hyperlipidemia found in 8 of 24 patients; in 6, only cholesterol was elevated *3171*

Luteinizing Hormone *Plasma* *Increase* Commonly elevated; result of deficient testicular function *2264* May either be high or normal *367*
Urine *Increase* Observed effect *413*

Pro-α-C-related Peptide *Plasma* *Increase* Mean concentration of approximately 1,200 pg/mL in 9 men with Klinefelter's syndrome not significantly different from 880 pg/mL in 16 healthy men aged 19 - 45 y *113*

Prolactin *Plasma* *No Effect* Usually normal *2264*

Sex-Hormone Binding Globulin *Serum* *Increase* Increased concentration usually observed *4234*

Testosterone *Serum* *Decrease* Reported to be low in most studies, although there is considerable overlap between normal males and Klinefelter males. Generally higher in mosaics than in pure Klinefelter patients *2264* Quite variable but often tends to be midway between the normal male and female *1980*

Thyroid Stimulating Hormone *Serum* *Decrease* Administration of TRH revealed a decreased TSH reserve in the Klinefelter patients *4895*
Serum *No Effect* Usually normal *2264*

758.80 Syndromes due to Sex Chromosome Abnormalities

Androgens *Plasma* *Increase* High plasma testosterone in XYY males *1290*

Estradiol *Plasma* *Decrease* In Turner's Syndrome *91* *457* *1267*

Estrogens *Plasma* *Decrease* In Turner's syndrome *1025*
Urine *Decrease* Doesn't increase with administration of hCG *413*

Follicle Stimulating Hormone *Plasma* *Increase* In Turner's syndrome *5544* Observed effect *5545*
Urine *Increase* In Turner's syndrome *1290*

Gonadotropin, Pituitary *Plasma* *Increase* In Turner's syndrome *5545*
Urine *Increase* In Turner's syndrome *1290*

Luteinizing Hormone *Plasma* *Increase* Usually doesn't increase until puberty *413*

Testosterone *Serum* *Increase* In XYY males *1290*

759.60 von Hippel-Lindau Disease

Epinephrine *Plasma* *No Effect* In 26 patients with VHL disease and pheochromocytoma mean concentration of 22 pg/mL not significantly different from 18 pg/mL in 178 reference individuals *1313*
Urine *No Effect* In 26 patients with VHL disease and pheochromocytoma mean excretion of 5 µg/d not significantly different from 9 µg/d in 178 reference individuals *1313*

Metanephrine *Plasma* *No Effect* In 26 patients with VHL disease and pheochromocytoma mean concentration of 30 pg/mL not significantly different from 27 pg/mL in 178 reference individuals *1313*
Urine *Increase* In 26 patients with VHL disease and pheochromocytoma mean excretion of 163 µg/d significantly different from 38 µg/d in 178 reference individuals *1313* In 26 patients with VHL disease and pheochromocytoma mean excretion of 1.3 µg/d not significantly different from 0 - 1.2 µg/d in 178 reference individuals *1313*

Norepinephrine *Plasma* *Increase* In 26 patients with VHL disease and pheochromocytoma mean concentration of 938 pg/mL significantly different from 200 pg/mL in 178 reference individuals *1313*

Normetanephrine *Plasma* *Increase* In 26 patients with VHL disease and pheochromocytoma mean concentration of 401 pg/mL significantly different from 45 pg/mL in 178 reference individuals *1313*

Vanillylmandelic Acid *Urine* *No Effect* In 26 patients with VHL disease and pheochromocytoma mean excretion of 6.8 µg/d not significantly different from 0 - 7.9 µg/d in 178 reference individuals *1313*

759.80 Cornelia de Lange's Syndrome

Pregnancy-associated Protein A *Serum* *Decrease* In 15 pregnancies in which blood was collected between the 16th and 19th weeks after which women delivered infants with CdL syndrome multiple of gestational median was 0.20, a highly significant reduction compared with normal pregnancies *49*

759.82 Marfan's Syndrome

Ammonium Ions *Urine* *Increase* May be associated with classic distal renal tubular acidosis which is associated with hyokalemia, hyperchloremic metabolic acidosis, urine pH > 5.5, increased urinary ammonium ion excretion, a negative urine anion gap, increased urinary osmol gap, decreased urinary citrate and increased urinary calcium in some patients *4071*

Anion Gap *Urine* *Decrease* May be associated with classic distal renal tubular acidosis which is asociated with hyokalemia, hyperchloremic metabolic acidosis, urine pH > 5.5, increased urinary ammonium ion excretion, a negative urine anion gap, increased urinary osmol gap, decreased urinary citrate and increased urinary calcium in some patients *4071*

Calcium *Urine* *Increase* May be associated with classic distal renal tubular acidosis which is associated with hyokalemia, hyperchloremic metabolic acidosis, urine pH > 5.5, increased urinary ammonium ion excretion, a negative urine anion gap, increased urinary osmol gap, decreased urinary citrate and increased urinary calcium in some patients *4071*

Chloride *Serum* *Increase* May be associated with classic distal renal tubular acidosis which is associated with hyokalemia, hyperchloremic metabolic acidosis, urine pH > 5.5, increased urinary ammonium ion excretion, a negative urine anion gap, increased urinary osmol gap, decreased urinary citrate and increased urinary calcium in some patients *4071*

Citrate *Urine* *Decrease* May be associated with classic distal renal tubular acidosis which is associated with hyokalemia, hyperchloremic metabolic acidosis, urine pH > 5.5, increased urinary ammonium ion excretion, a negative urine anion gap, increased urinary osmol gap, decreased urinary citrate and increased urinary calcium in some patients *4071*

Net Acid Excretion *Urine* *Increase* May be associated with classic distal renal tubular acidosis which is associated with hyokalemia, hyperchloremic metabolic acidosis, urine pH > 5.5, increased urinary ammonium ion excretion, a negative urine anion gap, increased urinary osmol gap, decreased urinary citrate and increased urinary calcium in some patients *4071*

Osmolal Gap *Urine* *Increase* May be associated with classic distal renal tubular acidosis which is associated with hyokalemia, hyperchloremic metabolic acidosis, urine pH > 5.5, increased urinary ammonium ion excretion, a negative urine anion gap, increased urinary osmol gap, decreased urinary citrate and increased urinary calcium in some patients *4071*

pH *Urine* *Increase* May be associated with classic distal renal tubular acidosis which is associated with hyokalemia, hyperchloremic metabolic acidosis, urine pH > 5.5, increased urinary ammonium ion excretion, a negative urine anion gap, increased urinary osmol gap, decreased urinary citrate and increased urinary calcium in some patients *4071*

Potassium *Serum* *Decrease* May be associated with classic distal renal tubular acidosis which is associated with hyokalemia, hyperchloremic metabolic acidosis, urine pH > 5.5, increased urinary ammonium ion excretion, a negative urine anion gap, increased urinary osmol gap, decreased urinary citrate and increased urinary calcium in some patients *4071*

759.89 Alport's Syndrome

CD45 Leukocytes *Tissue* *Increase* In 1 patient with Alport's syndrome number of positive cells 420 cells/mm^2 in renal tissue *3026*

Creatinine *Serum* *Increase* In 1 patient with Alport's syndrome concentration of 1.40 mg/dL different from 0.88 ± 0.17 mg/dL in 20 healthy controls *3026*

Intercellular Adhesion Molecule-1 *Tissue* *Increase* In 1 patient with Alport's syndrome percentage of ICAM-1 positive renal tubuli 2.0% *3026*

Protein *Urine* *Increase* In 1 patient with Alport's syndrome excretion of 3.66 mg/mg creatinine *3026*

Soluble Intercellular Adhesion Molecule-1 *Serum* *Decrease* In 1 patient with Alport's syndrome concentration of soluble ICAM-1 of 235 ng/mL compared with 306 ± 52 ng/mL in 20 healthy controls *3026*

Urine *No Effect* In 1 patient with Alport's syndrome excretion of soluble ICAM-1 of 2.3 ng/mL or 2.2 ng/mg creatinine compared with 2.6 ± 1.7 ng/mL or 2.5 ± 3.0 ng/mg creatinine in 20 healthy controls *3026*

759.89 Fish Odor Syndrome

Trimethylamine *Urine* *Increase* In 10 adults with fish odor syndrome mean 24 h excretion of 220 - 620 μmol increasing to 1,895 - 4,500 μmol over 8 hours after ingestion of 600 mg trimethylamine *224*

Trimethylamine-N-Oxide *Urine* *Increase* In 10 adults with fish odor syndrome excretion ranged from 45 - 255 μmol/d and increased to 140 - 1240 μmol/8 h after ingestion of 600 mg trimethylamine (with N-oxide comprising 11 - 54% of total in basal state and 5 - 23% after trimethylamine compared with means of 88% under normal conditions and 89% after 600 mg trimethylamine in control individuals) *224*

759.89 Menkes' Syndrome

Ceruloplasmin *Serum* *Decrease* Concentration typically reduced in patients with Menkes' syndrome *3499*

Cytochrome c Oxidase *White Blood Cells* *Decrease* In children and young infants with Menkes' syndrome marked reduction of activity observed *3499*

759.89 Smith-Lemli-Opitz Syndrome

Cholesterol *Serum* *Decrease* In 5 children with the Smith-Lemil-Opitz syndrome plasma concentrations ranged from 8 to 101 mg/dL (0.20 to 2.60 mmol/L) which is below the 5th percentile for age and sex matched controls *5234*

7-Dehydrocholesterol *Serum* *Increase* In 5 children with Smith-Lemil-Opitz syndrome concentration increased to 11 to 31 mg/dL, more than 2000 times above normal *5234*

PERINATAL DISORDERS

760.79 Vitamin D Intoxication

Ammonium Ions *Urine* *Increase* May be associated with classic distal renal tubular acidosis which is associated with hyokalemia, hyperchloremic metabolic acidosis, urine pH > 5.5, increased urinary ammonium ion excretion, a negative urine anion gap, increased urinary osmol gap, decreased urinary citrate and increased urinary calcium in some patients *4071*

Anion Gap *Urine* *Decrease* May be associated with classic distal renal tubular acidosis which is associated with hyokalemia, hyperchloremic metabolic acidosis, urine pH > 5.5, increased urinary ammonium ion excretion, a negative urine anion gap, increased urinary osmol gap, decreased urinary citrate and increased urinary calcium in some patients *4071*

Calcium *Urine* *Increase* May be associated with classic distal renal tubular acidosis which is associated with hyokalemia, hyperchloremic metabolic acidosis, urine pH > 5.5, increased urinary ammonium ion excretion, a negative urine anion gap, increased urinary osmol gap, decreased urinary citrate and increased urinary calcium in some patients *4071*

Chloride *Serum* *Increase* May be associated with classic distal renal tubular acidosis which is associated with hyokalemia, hyperchloremic metabolic acidosis, urine pH > 5.5, increased urinary ammonium ion excretion, a negative urine anion gap, increased urinary osmol gap, decreased urinary citrate and increased urinary calcium in some patients *4071*

Citrate *Urine* *Decrease* May be associated with classic distal renal tubular acidosis which is associated with hyokalemia, hyperchloremic metabolic acidosis, urine pH > 5.5, increased urinary ammonium ion excretion, a negative urine anion gap, increased urinary osmol gap, decreased urinary citrate and increased urinary calcium in some patients *4071*

Net Acid Excretion *Urine* *Increase* May be associated with classic distal renal tubular acidosis which is associated with hyokalemia, hyperchloremic metabolic acidosis, urine pH > 5.5, increased urinary ammonium ion excretion, a negative urine anion gap, increased urinary osmol gap, decreased urinary citrate and increased urinary calcium in some patients *4071*

Osmolal Gap *Urine* *Increase* May be associated with classic distal renal tubular acidosis which is associated with hyokalemia, hyperchloremic metabolic acidosis, urine pH > 5.5, increased urinary ammonium ion excretion, a negative urine anion gap, increased urinary osmol gap, decreased urinary citrate and increased urinary calcium in some patients *4071*

pH *Urine* *Increase* May be associated with classic distal renal tubular acidosis which is associated with hyokalemia, hyperchloremic metabolic acidosis, urine pH > 5.5, increased urinary ammonium ion excretion, a negative urine anion gap, increased urinary osmol gap, decreased urinary citrate and increased urinary calcium in some patients *4071*

Phosphate *Serum* *Increase* Vitamin D intoxication may increase the serum phosphate concentration *969*

Potassium *Serum* *Decrease* May be associated with classic distal renal tubular acidosis which is associated with hyokalemia, hyperchloremic metabolic acidosis, urine pH > 5.5, increased urinary ammonium ion excretion, a negative urine anion gap, increased urinary osmol gap, decreased urinary citrate and increased urinary calcium in some patients *4071*

765.39 Camurati-Engelmann Disease

Creatine Kinase *Serum* *No Effect* In 2 patients mean activities of 23 U/L and 33 U/L compared with upper limit of normal of 195 U/L *5659*

Creatine Kinase BB-Isoenzyme *Serum* *No Effect* In 2 patients mean activities of < 3 U/L and < 3 U/L (not detected %) compared with normal of 0 - 1% *5659*

768.90 Asphyxia, Newborn

Erythrocytes, Nucleated *Blood* *Increase* Nucleated red cell count in umbilical blood of 46 asphyxiated infants averaged 34.5 (range of 1 to 451) with only 7 (15%) showing 5 or less significantly different from 3.4 (range of 0 - 12) with 5 or less in 62

768.90 Asphyxia, Newborn *(continued)*

Erythrocytes, Nucleated *(continued)*
(75%) in 83 normal infants *4118* In 153 neurologically impaired infants mean count of 30.3 per 100 cells compared with 3.4 in controls *2776*

770.70 Bronchopulmonary Dysplasia

Interleukin-1β *Amniotic Fluid* *Increase* Median concentration in mother's amniotic fluid of 359 pg/mL when infants had bronchopulmonary dysplasia (13 infants) significantly higher than 12.2 pg/mL when infants did not have bronchopulmonary dysplasia (56 infants) *5497*

Interleukin-6 *Amniotic Fluid* *Increase* Median concentration in mother's amniotic fluid of 50.6 ng/mL when infants had bronchopulmonary dysplasia (13 infants) significantly higher than 2.2 ng/mL when infants did not have bronchopulmonary dysplasia (56 infants) *5497*

Interleukin-8 *Amniotic Fluid* *Increase* Median concentration in mother's amniotic fluid of 67.5 pg/mL when infants had bronchopulmonary dysplasia (13 infants) significantly higher than 3.5 pg/mL when infants did not have bronchopulmonary dysplasia (56 infants) *5497*

Tumor Necrosis Factor-α *Amniotic Fluid* *Increase* Median concentration in mother's amniotic fluid of 113.9 pg/mL when infants had bronchopulmonary dysplasia (13 infants) significantly higher than 6.5 pg/mL when infants did not have bronchopulmonary dysplasia (56 infants) *5497*

770.80 Acute Lung Failure

Endothelin-1 *Plasma* *Increase* In 14 patients with acute lung failure with increased cardiac output and depressed total vascular resistance and simultaneous pulmonary hypertension mean concentration in venous plasma of 9.8 ± 1.2 pmol/L versus 2.1 ± 0.2 pmol/L in healthy controls *5520*

770.80 Acute Respiratory Distress Syndrome

Angiotensin-converting Enzyme *Serum* *Increase* Increased activities observed in acute respiratory distress syndrome in premature infants *2952*

α_1-Antitrypsin *Serum* *Decrease* Decreased *4241* *4371* *4373* *83* *4763*

Bicarbonate *Serum* *Decrease* Metabolic acidosis *1185*

Bilirubin *Serum* *Increase* Reported effect *1426*

Carbon Dioxide Partial Pressure *Blood* *Increase* Impaired ventilation *5544*

Complement C_3 *Serum* *Decrease* Neonatal ARDS associated with decreased concentration. Caused by hypercatabolism *785* Neonatal ARDS associated with decreased C_3 concentration. Caused by hypercatabolism *1588* Neonatal ARDS associated with decreased serum concentration. Caused by hypercatabolism *1033* Neonatal ARDS associated with decreased serum C_3 concentration. Caused by hypercatabolism *2694*

Cortisol *Plasma* *Decrease* 18 newborn infants of < 37 weeks gestation who developed moderate to severe disease had a significantly lower mean cord plasma cortisol concentration at birth than that observed in 67 unaffected infants of similar gestational age; mean values were 3.36 ± 0.42 and 5.58 ± 0.43 µgl/dL, respectively *5108*

C-Reactive Protein *Serum* *Increase* In 8 polytraumatized patients who developed ARDS mean concentration of 95.0 ± 67.4 mg/L significantly greater than 40.8 ± 26.5 mg/L in 47 polytraumatized patients who did not develop ARDS and 1.7 ± 1.3 mg/L in 34 healthy controls *1156*

2,3-Diphosphoglycerate *Red Blood Cells* *Decrease* Concentrations in newborns typically reduced *496*

Elastase *Neutrophils* *Increase* In 8 polytraumatized patients who developed ARDS mean concentration of 407.1 ± 194.5 µg/L significantly greater than 115.6 ± 99.3 µg/L in 47 polytraumatized patients who did not develop ARDS and 32.3 ± 10.9 µg/L in 34 healthy controls *1156*

Endothelin-1 *Plasma* *Increase* Plasma endothelin-1 levels were elevated (4.6 ± 0.6 SEM and 4.9 ± 0.6 pg/mL respectively) as compared with control subjects (0.9 ± 0.1 and 0.6 ± 0.1 pg/mL) *2915*

Eosinophils *Blood* *Increase* In 8 trauma patients with ARDS mean concentration of 986 ± 836 /µL significantly greater than 543 ± 612 /µL in 92 patients who did not develop ARDS *1177*

Epithelial Cell-derived Neutrophil Activator-78
BAL Fluid *Increase* In 36 adult patients with ARDS mean of about 1.0 ng/mL on day 3 in those who lived and 0.2 ng/mL in those who died compared with about 0.01 ng/mL in 8 controls *1814*

Estrogens *Plasma* *Decrease* The average concentrations of estradiol in umbilical cord plasma from newborns with the syndrome with or without hyaline membrane disease were lower by 25% than in controls *5109*

Ferritin *Serum* *Increase* Using serum ferritin of more than 270 ng/mL in women and 680 ng/mL in men increased concentration predicted in ARDS with a sensitivity of 83% in women and 60% in men and specificity of 71% in women and 90% in men *901*

Hyaluronic Acid *Serum* *Increase* The time-dependent concentrations of were determined in sera of 16 patients during treatment with an extracorporeal CO_2 removal device. At the beginning of treatment strongly elevated serum concentrations of all studied extracellular matrix components were found *2830* Accumulates in the lung in adult respiratory distress syndrome *1975*

Immunoglobulin E *Serum* *Increase* In 8 trauma patients with ARDS mean concentration significantly greater than in 92 patients who did not develop ARDS *1177*

Interleukin-1 Receptor Antagonist Protein
BAL Fluid *Increase* In 36 adult patients with ARDS mean of about 1 ng/mL on day 3 in those who lived and 3 ng/mL in those who died compared with about 0.1 ng/mL in 8 controls *1814*

Interleukin-1β *BAL Fluid* *Increase* In 36 adult patients with ARDS mean of about 30 ng/mL on day 3 in those who lived and 35 ng/mL in those who died compared with about 0.25 ng/mL in 8 controls *1814*

Interleukin-1β:Interleukin-1 Receptor Antagonist Protein Ratio
BAL Fluid *Increase* In 36 adult patients with ARDS mean ratio of about 30 on day 3 in those who lived and 10 in those who died compared with about 0.3 in 8 controls *1814*

Interleukin-8 *BAL Fluid* *Increase* In 36 adult patients with ARDS mean of about 0.5 ng/mL on day 3 in those who lived and 0.6 ng/mL in those who died compared with about 0.01 ng/mL in 8 controls *1814*
Pulmonary Edema Fluid *Increase* In 11 patients with acute respiratory distress syndrome without sepsis mean concentration of 14.8 ng/mL significantly different from 6.7 ng/mL in 11 patients with hydrostatic pulmonary edema *3490*
Serum *Increase* In 11 patients with acute respiratory distress syndrome without sepsis mean concentration of 3.0 ± 0.4 ng/mL not significantly different from 2.0 ± 3.8 ng/mL in 11 patients with hydrostatic pulmonary edema *3490*

Laminin *Serum* *Increase* The time-dependent concentrations were determined in sera of 16 patients during treatment with an extracorporeal CO_2 removal device. At the beginning of treatment strongly elevated serum concentrations of all studied extracellular matrix components were found *2830*

Lipids *Serum* *Increase* Plasma lipids, particularly triglycerides complexed with fibrins, were elevated several-fold in patients with adult respiratory distress. Plasma triglycerides complexed with fibrins were significantly higher in patients who died than in those who survived *2855*

Macrophage Inflammatory Protein-1α *BAL Fluid* *Increase* In 36 adult patients with ARDS mean of about 1 ng/mL on day 3 in those who lived and 0.95 ng/mL in those who died compared with about 0.06 ng/mL in 8 controls *1814*

Monocyte Chemotactic Protein-1 *BAL Fluid* *Increase* In 36 adult patients with ARDS mean concentration of about 0.8 ng/mL on day 3 in those who lived and 0.9 ng/mL in those who died compared with about 0.05 ng/mL in 8 controls *1814*

Mucin-associated Antigen *Serum* *Increase* Mean concentration of 53.8 ± 6.6 ng/mL observed in 13 patients with acute respiratory distress syndrome significantly different from 9.9 ± 0.8 ng/mL observed in 59 healthy individuals *4797*

Neutrophils *BAL Fluid* *Increase* In 85 adult patients with ARDS mean of 372 cells/µL on third day after onset, 180 cells/µL on day 7, 80 cells/µL on day 14 and 98 cells/µL on day 21 *1814*

Oxygen Partial Pressure *Blood* *Decrease* Impaired ventilation *5544*

Oxygen Saturation *Blood* *Decrease* Impaired ventilation *5544*

pH *Blood* *Decrease* Decreased typically to pH 7.3 or lower *1426* Acidosis is first respiratory, later also metabolic *4613* Decreased to 7.3 or less *5544*

Phosphate *Serum* *Decrease* Respiratory distress syndrome is less common cause of hypophosphatemia due to shift of phosphate into the cells and increased renal loss of phosphate *969*

Phospholipase A *Serum* *Increase* In a clinical study in 48 patients at risk for this disease, the level was elevated in sepsis *2625*

Phospholipids *Serum* *Decrease* Reported effect *4613*

Potassium *Serum* *Increase* Reported effect *1426* Increased catabolism *5544*

Procollagen Type III Peptide *Serum* *Increase* The time-dependent concentrations were determined in sera of 16 patients during treatment with an extracorporeal CO_2 removal device. At the beginning of treatment strongly elevated serum concentrations of all studied extracellular matrix components were found *2830*

Prostaglandins *Plasma* *Increase* During the acute phase, plasma concentrations of the primary prostaglandins E and F were significantly elevated. The ratio of prostaglandin E to F was reversed *1577*

Protein *BAL Fluid* *Increase* In 36 adult patients with ARDS concentration increased compared with that in 8 controls *1814*
Pulmonary Edema Fluid *Increase* In 11 patients with acute respiratory distress syndrome without sepsis mean concentration of 4.6 ± 1.2 g/dL *3490*
Serum *Increase* Reported effect *1426* In 11 patients acute respiratory distress syndrome without sepsis mean concentration of 5.0 ± 1.1 g/dL *3490*

Thromboxane A_2 *Plasma* *Increase* Observed effect *1476*

Tri-iodothyronine (T3) *Serum* *Decrease* In preterm infants with this disorder, cord blood T3 concentration was significantly lower than that in cord blood of babies without this disease (22 ± 2.6 vs 36 ± 5 ng/dL). There was no significant rise at 24 h of age (22 ± 2.6 vs 34.0 ± 8 ng/dL) and remained low for 3 weeks *9*

Triglycerides *Serum* *Increase* Plasma lipids, particularly triglycerides complexed with fibrins were elevated several-fold in patients with adult disease. Triglycerides complexed with fibrins were significantly higher in patients who died than in those who survived *2855*

Type IV Collagen 7S Domain *Serum* *Increase* Mean concentration in 13 patients with ARDS of 14.8 ± 9.7 ng/mL compared with 2.7 ± 0.9 ng/mL in 10 healthy controls *2601*

Urea Nitrogen *Serum* *Increase* Increased catabolism *5544*

Uric Acid *Serum* *Increase* Higher serum concentrations during the first 3 days of life, and the urinary excretion over the period of 12 - 36 h of age is also higher than in the normal infants. Neonatal hyperuricemia is not due to renal retention but to increased production of uric acid *4268*
Urine *Increase* Higher serum concentrations during the first 3 days of life, and the urinary excretion over the period of 12 - 36 h of age was also higher than in the normal infants. Neonatal hyperuricemia is not due to renal retention but to increased production of uric acid *4268*

770.80 Acute Respiratory Failure

Endothelin-1 *Plasma* *Increase* Mean concentration in 13 patients at the time of hospital admission with acute respiratory failure of 10.7 ± 5.0 pg/mL significantly higher than 1.5 ± 0.5 pg/mL in 16 healthy controls *3519*

771.00 Congenital Rubella

Hemagglutination Inhibition *Serum* *Increase* The finding of antibody after 6 - 8 months of age may be taken as evidence of congenital rubella *900* Persistently elevated titers during 1st y of life *5619*

Immunoglobulin M *Serum* *Increase* Presence in cord blood indicates congenital rubella infection *5619* Frequently increased levels in the first 4 months of life (immunoglobulin > 20 mg/dL). Detection of rubella-specific IgM indicates congenital disease *900*

773.00 Hemolytic Disease of Newborn (Erythroblastosis Fetalis)

Ammonia *Blood* *Increase* There is some evidence associating hyperammonemia with the pathogenesis of kernicterus *4707*

Bilirubin *Serum* *Increase* In the severely affected group, cord blood concentration may be 10 mg/dL (of which 33 - 66% is direct-acting bilirubin). Peak levels may climb despite treatment, into the 30 mg/dL range (of which 66% is direct- acting bilirubin) *900* Characteristic of disease *4613* After birth, the rate of rise is a reflection of both the severity of the hemolytic process and the degree of hepatic maturity *5677* After birth, the rate of rise is a reflection of both severity of the hemolytic process and the degree of hepatic maturity *5677*

Bilirubin, Direct *Serum* *Increase* Severely affected group *900*

Bilirubin, Indirect *Serum* *Increase* In mild cases on the 2nd - 5th day of life, depending upon the rapidity of increase in the degree of jaundice *900* Concentration > 4 mg/dL in cord blood suggest severe disease. Levels of > 50 mg/dL may be seen by the 3rd day of life in untreated, severely affected infants *5677*
Serum *No Effect* Intermediate moderately affected group: rarely a baby in this group will develop jaundice *900*

Coombs' Test *Serum* *Negative* Usually negative when due to anti-A antibodies. It becomes negative within a few days of effective exchange transfusion *5545* Infant RBCs show a negative direct Coombs' test (by standard methods) with ABO erythroblastosis *5545* Negative or only weakly positive in cases of hemolytic disease due to ABO incompatibility *5677*
Serum *Positive* Direct test is strongly positive on cord blood RBC when due to Rh, Kel, Kidd, Duffy antibodies *5545* Strongly positive in infants sensitized by Rh(D) red cells and by red cells with most of the rarely involved blood group antigens. Negative or only weakly positive in cases of hemolytic disease due to ABO incompatibility *5677*

Erythrocyte Sedimentation Rate *Blood* *Increase* Of 70 infants showing accelerated rate, 49 had signs of hemolytic disease. The test was found to be very sensitive, detecting ABO incompatibilities even in absence of marked bilirubinemia *4799*

Erythrocytes *Blood* *Decrease* Generally parallels the fall of hemoglobin *4613*

Glucose *Serum* *Decrease* In the more severely affected infants *5677*

Hematocrit *Blood* *Decrease* Intermediate moderately affected group will become severely anemic in the first 7 - 10 days of life (anemia neonatorum) *4891* Mild cases may develop mild anemia in the first 4 - 6 weeks of life from which they recover spontaneously *900*

Hemoglobin *Blood* *Decrease* Adult hemoglobin is increased with hemolytic disease of the newborn *5545* In mild cases, mild anemia may develop in the first 4 - 6 weeks of life with spontaneous recovery. Intermediate group will become severely anemic in the first 7 - 10 days of life (anemia neonatorum). Hemoglobin may drop below 2 g/dL and the child may die unless given a transfusion. Because hydrops fetalis is due to hepatic dysfunction, not anemia, some fetuses become hydropic with hemoglobin levels of 7 - 8 g/dL. Others are not hydropic with levels of 3 - 4 g/dL *900*

Hemoglobin F *Blood* *Decrease* Observed effect *5545*

Immunoglobulin D *Serum* *Increase* Reported effect *1290*

Lactate Dehydrogenase *Serum* *Increase* Derived from red blood cells *1290*

Leukocytes *Blood* *Increase* Moderate with high polymorphonuclear percentage *4613* Increased (usually 15,000 - 30,000 /µL) with hemolytic disease *5545*

773.00 Hemolytic Disease of Newborn (Erythroblastosis Fetalis) *(continued)*

MCHC *Blood* *No Effect* Usually unaffected by disease *5545*

Osmotic Fragility *Red Blood Cells* *Increase* Increased with ABO erythroblastosis *5545*

Platelets *Blood* *Decrease* Frequently present in the severely affected group. Although partially a result of exchange transfusion, it is predominantly caused by a reduction of marrow megakaryocytes as a result of excess erythropoiesis. Counts < 40,000/µL are not uncommon *900* May occur secondary to isoimmune or exchange transfusion *5677*

Reticulocytes *Blood* *Increase* Counts normally 5 - 10% may be markedly elevated in the erythroblastic infant (up to 25 - 50% in severe cases) *900* Correlates roughly with the level of hemoglobin in the cord blood, although well-compensated hemolysis may occur *5677* Percentage is a rough indicator of prognosis *4613*

Urobilinogen *Feces* *Increase* Parallels serum levels of indirect bilirubin *5545*
Urine *Increase* Excess consistent with exaggerated hemolysis *4613* Parallels serum levels *5545*

773.00 Rh Incompatibility

Glutathione Peroxidase *Serum* *Decrease* In 8 newborns with jaundice due to Rh incompatibility mean activity of 0.357 ± 0.093 U/mL not significantly different from 0.429 ± 0.084 U/mL in 12 healthy control babies *222*

Selenium *Serum* *Decrease* In 8 newborns with jaundice due to Rh incompatibility mean concentration of 27.3 ± 11.5 ng/mL not significantly different from 40.1 ± 15.6 ng/mL in 12 healthy control babies *222*

773.10 ABO Incompatibility

Glutathione Peroxidase *Serum* *Decrease* In 11 newborns with jaundice due to ABO incompatibility mean activity of 0.338 ± 0.066 U/mL not significantly different from 0.429 ± 0.084 U/mL in 12 healthy control babies *222*

Selenium *Serum* *No Effect* In 11 newborns with jaundice due to ABO incompatibility mean concentration of 40.3 ± 8.2 ng/mL not significantly different from 40.1 ± 15.6 ng/mL in 12 healthy control babies *222*

774.40 Jaundice Due to Hepatocellular Damage (Newborn)

Bilirubin *Feces* *Decrease* Normal or decreased *5544*
Feces *No Effect* Normal or decreased *5544*
Urine *No Effect* Typical observation *5544*

Bilirubin, Direct *Serum* *Increase* Normal or slight increase *5544*

α-Fetoprotein *Serum* *Increase* Elevations occur in many cases of neonatal hepatitis and may be helpful in differentiating this condition from biliary atresia *5851*

Leucine Aminopeptidase *Serum* *Increase* In 12 patients with obstructive jaundice, all showed elevations, ranging from 430 - 990 U/L *579*

Partial Thromboplastin Time *Plasma* *Increase* Markedly prolonged *900*

Prothrombin Time *Plasma* *Increase* Markedly prolonged *900*

Urobilinogen *Feces* *Decrease* Normal or decreased *5544*
Urine *No Effect* Typical observation *5544*

774.40 Neonatal Hepatitis

α-Fetoprotein *Serum* *Increase* Neonatal hepatitis of any cause is associated with an increased concentration *1778*

Soluble HLA-I *Cerebrospinal Fluid* *No Effect* In 2 patients with neonatal hepatitis, mean concentration undetectable *216*

Soluble HLA-II *Cerebrospinal Fluid* *Increase* In 2 patients with neonatal hepatitis, mean concentration undetectable in one and 248 U/mL in the other *216*

774.60 Neonatal Jaundice

Bilirubin, Unconjugated *Serum* *Increase* Neonatal jandice is associated with unconjugated hyperbilirubinemia *3625*

774.60 Physiological Jaundice

Glutathione Peroxidase *Serum* *Decrease* In 9 newborns with physiological jaundice mean activity of 0.350 ± 0.049 U/mL not significantly different from 0.429 ± 0.084 U/mL in 12 healthy control babies *222*

Selenium *Serum* *No Effect* In 9 newborns with physiological jaundice mean concentration of 40.3 ± 8.7 ng/mL not significantly different from 40.1 ± 15.6 ng/mL in 12 healthy control babies *222*

777.80 Congenital Hepatic Fibrosis

Alkaline Phosphatase *Serum* *Increase* Mild to moderately increased activity may be the only plasma biochemical abnormality detected *3406*

γ-Glutamyltransferase *Serum* *Increase* Activity may be increased in addition to that of alkaline phosphatase *3406*

SIGNS AND SYMPTOMS

780.30 Convulsions

Cholinesterase *Cerebrospinal Fluid* *Decrease* In 18 patients with convulsive disorders mean concentration of 0.13 ± 0.01 µmol substrate hydrolyzed (0.09 ± 0.01 mg protein/30 min) significantly different from 0.48 ± 0.01 µmol substrate hydrolyzed (0.18 ± 0.01 mg protein/30 min) in 10 age and sex matched control patients with nonspecific headaches *321*

Creatine Kinase *Serum* *Increase* Raised levels have been reported following convulsive seizures *1980*

Estrogens *Plasma* *Increase* The incidence of epileptic seizures was higher in women during the high estrogen period of the menstrual cycle. Number of seizures correlated positively to estrogen/progesterone ratio and negatively to progesterone levels *241*

Lactate *Blood* *Increase* May occur with febrile convulsions in children *4860* In 10 patients with idiopathic seizures studied < 3 h after the seizure, arterial and CSF lactate were elevated in association with a mild arterial metabolic acidosis *593*
Cerebrospinal Fluid *Increase* May occur with febrile convulsions in children *4860* In 10 patients with idiopathic seizures studied 3 h after the seizure, arterial and CSF lactate were elevated in association with a mild arterial metabolic acidosis. The elevated CSF lactate persisted despite a return to normal of the arterial concentration in 7 patients studied between 3 - 6 h after the seizure *593*

Myoglobin *Urine* *Increase* Sporadic; exertional *5544*

Neutrophils *Blood* *Increase* Reported effect *5677*

pH *Blood* *Decrease* In 10 patients with idiopathic seizures studied 3 h after the seizure, arterial and CSF lactate were elevated in association with a mild arterial metabolic acidosis *593*

Pregnanediol *Urine* *Decrease* The incidence of epileptic seizures was higher in women during the high estrogen period of the menstrual cycle. Number of seizures correlated positively to estrogen:progesterone ratio and negatively to progesterone levels *241*

Progesterone *Plasma* *Decrease* The incidence of epileptic seizures was higher in women during the high estrogen period of the menstrual cycle. Number of seizures correlated positively to estrogen:progesterone ratio and negatively to progesterone levels *241*

Pyruvate *Blood* *Increase* May occur with febrile convulsions in children *4860*

Cerebrospinal Fluid *Increase* May occur with febrile convulsions in children *4860*

Uric Acid *Serum* *Increase* Significant increases were found in 17 patients with 2 or more grand mal seizures within 24 h. In 6 cases, concentrations were reached at which hyperuricemic renal failure may develop *3153* Observed effect *4041*

780.30 Febrile Seizures

Interleukin-1β *Cerebrospinal Fluid* *No Effect* Median concentration in 20 children with prolonged febrile seizures of < 4 pg/mL not significantly different from < 4 pg/mL in 23 healthy controls *2314*

Interleukin-6 *Cerebrospinal Fluid* *No Effect* Median concentration in 20 children with prolonged febrile seizures of < 31.2 pg/mL not significantly different from < 31.2 pg/mL in 23 healthy controls *2314*

Tumor Necrosis Factor-α *Cerebrospinal Fluid* *No Effect* Median concentration in 20 children with prolonged febrile seizures of < 15 pg/mL not significantly different from < 15 pg/mL in 23 healthy controls *2314*

780.30 Seizures

Creatine Kinase *Serum* *No Effect* No significant change observed in children with seizures *2492*

Interleukin-1β *Cerebrospinal Fluid* *No Effect* In 20 children with prolonged febrile seizures mean concentration of < 4 pg/mL not different from normal concentration of < 4 pg/mL *2314*

Interleukin-6 *Cerebrospinal Fluid* *No Effect* In 20 children with prolonged febrile seizures mean concentration of < 31.2 pg/mL not different from normal concentration of < 31.2 pg/mL *2314*

Prolactin *Plasma* *Increase* In 6 neonates with seizures mean concentration of 170 ± 23 ng/mL significantly higher than 114 ± 12 ng/mL in 22 neonates without seizures *2979* In 11 infants aged less than 2 months old mean concentration of 368 ± 402 ng/mL following seizures compared with 150 ± 105 ng/mL in recovery period *3592* Marked increase (to above 3 times baseline) observed at 15 - 30 minutes after 20 - 25 generalized tonic-clonic seizures *5752* Following single epileptic seizure concentration frequently increased *5249*

Soluble HLA-I *Cerebrospinal Fluid* *Increase* In 6 patients with seizures, mean concentration undetectable in all *216*

Soluble HLA-II *Cerebrospinal Fluid* *Increase* In 6 patients with seizures, mean concentration of 350 U/mL *216*

Tumor Necrosis Factor-α *Cerebrospinal Fluid* *No Effect* In 20 children with prolonged febrile seizures mean concentration of < 15 pg/mL not different from normal concentration of < 15 pg/mL *2314*

780.53 Sleep Apnea

Albumin *Urine* *Increase* In 9 patients with obturative sleep apnea syndrome mean excretion of 30.05 ± 15.74 mg/d significantly greater than 9.08 ± 3.92 mg/d in 39 healthy controls *3087*

α_1-Antitrypsin *Urine* *Increase* In 9 patients with obturative sleep apnea syndrome mean excretion of 0.38 ± 0.53 mg/d significantly greater than 0.12 ± 0.44 mg/d in 39 healthy controls *3087*

Catecholamines *Plasma* *Increase* Concentration significantly increased in sleep apnea patients both during waking and sleep periods *2955*
Urine *Increase* Concentration significantly increased in sleep apnea patients both during waking and sleep periods *2955*

Erythropoietin *Serum* *Increase* Mean concentration of 45 ± 33 mIU/mL significantly higher than 17 ± 8 mIU/mL in control individuals *660*

Interleukin-1β *Serum* *Decrease* Mean concentration of 0.39 ± 0.14 pg/mL (detected in 66.7% patients) in 12 patients with sleep apnea not significantly different from 0.60 ± 0.29 pg/mL (detected in 50.0% individuals) in 10 healthy controls *5463*

Interleukin-6 *Serum* *Increase* Mean concentration of 3.25 ± 0.76 pg/mL in 12 patients with sleep apnea significantly different from 1.02 ± 0.42 pg/mL in 10 healthy controls *5463*

Tumor Necrosis Factor-α *Serum* *Increase* Mean concentration of 2.51 ± 0.13 pg/mL in 12 patients with sleep apnea significantly different from 1.17 ± 0.10 pg/mL in 10 healthy controls *5463*

780.54 Hypersomnia, Idiopathic

Interleukin-1β *Serum* *Decrease* Mean concentration of 0.11 ± 0.23 pg/mL (detected in 14.3% patients) in 8 patients with idiopathic hypersomnia not significantly different from 0.60 ± 0.29 pg/mL (detected in 50.0% individuals) in 10 healthy controls *5463*

Interleukin-6 *Serum* *Increase* Mean concentration of 1.40 ± 0.34 pg/mL in 8 patients with idiopathic hypersomnia not significantly different from 1.02 ± 0.42 pg/mL in 10 healthy controls *5463*

Tumor Necrosis Factor-α *Serum* *Increase* Mean concentration of 1.57 ± 0.12 pg/mL in 8 patients with idiopathic hypersomnia not significantly different from 1.17 ± 0.10 pg/mL in 10 healthy controls *5463*

780.57 Obstructive Sleep Apnea Syndrome

Soluble Intercellular Adhesion Molecule-1 *Serum* *Increase* In 7 men with OSAS mean concentration before sleep of 392.9 ± 48.5 ng/mL significantly different from 201.2 ± 55.0 ng/mL in 6 healthy male controls *3874*

Soluble L-Selectin *Serum* *Increase* In 7 men with OSAS mean concentration before sleep of 1,386.6 ± 77.9 ng/mL significantly different from 1,038.8 ± 78.6 ng/mL in 6 healthy male controls *3874*

Soluble Vascular Cell Adhesion Molecule-1 *Serum* *Increase* In 7 men with OSAS mean concentration before sleep of 811.0 ± 87.8 ng/mL significantly different from 574.2 ± 42.7 ng/mL in 6 healthy male controls *3874*

780.70 Chronic Fatigue Syndrome

ACTH response to CRH *Plasma* *Decrease* In 30 patients with chronic fatigue syndrome attenuated net integrated response to CRH observed (128.0 ± 26.4 pmol/L/min versus 225.4 ± 34.5 pmol/L/min) in 72 normal volunteers *1112*

Acylcarnitine *Serum* *Decrease* In 19 men with chronic fatigue syndrome mean concentration of 8.7 ± 3.3 µmol/L and in 19 women with chronic fatigue syndrome 8.4 ± 4.4 µmol/L markedly lower than 13.4 ± 4.6 µmol/L in 177 men and 15.5 ± 4.4 µmol/L in 131 women *2859* In 19 female patients with chronic fatigue syndrome mean concentration of 8.9 ± 7.0 µmol/L significantly lower than 15.5 ± 4.4 µmol/L in reference population. In 8 men with CFS mean of 9.3 ± 3.7 µmol/L significantly less than 13.4 ± 4.6 µmol/L in controls *4157*

Alanine Aminotransferase *Serum* *No Effect* In 541 patients with CFS mean activity of 23.5 ± 0.81 U/L not significantly different from 22.2 ± 2.0 U/L in 95 control patients *324*

Alkaline Phosphatase *Serum* *Increase* Age- and sex-adjusted odds ratios of abnormal results, comparing cases with control subjects: 4.2 (95% CI, 1.6-11) *324* In 418 patients with CFS mean activity of 70.9 ± 1.2 U/L significantly higher than 63.6 ± 2.6 U/L in 96 control patients *324*

Angiotensin-converting Enzyme *Serum* *Increase* In 2 studies mean concentration in 20 patients with CFS of 49.1 ± 10.2 U/mL compared with 30.9 ± 9.7 U/mL in one study and 39.6 ± 8.5 U/mL compared with 34.8 ± 8.9 U/mL in controls in the other study *3042*

Anti-Smooth Muscle Antibodies *Serum* *Increase* Reported effect *5364*

Antibodies *Serum* *Increase* Antibodies to Ebstein Barr Virus, Cytomegalovirus, Herpes Simplex Virus, Coxsackie B virus and Measles Virus have all been reported *5364*

Antimicrosomal Antibodies *Serum* *Increase* In 235 patients with CFS mean proportion of specimens with abnormalities 6% not significantly different from 2% in 50 control patients *324*

780.70 Chronic Fatigue Syndrome (continued)

Antinuclear Antibodies *Serum* *Increase* In 522 patients with CFS mean proportion of specimens with abnormalities 15% significantly different from 0% in 50 control patients *324* Detected in 15% of cases vs 0% in the control subjects *324*

Aspartate Aminotransferase *Serum* *No Effect* In 424 patients with CFS mean activity of 24.5 ± 0.83 U/L not significantly different from 23.1 ± 1.8 U/L in 95 control patients *324*

Atypical Lymphocytes *Blood* *Increase* In 207 patients with CFS mean proportion of 0.72 ± 0.067% significantly higher than 0.18 ± 0.11% in 85 control patients *324*

Bicarbonate *Serum* *Increase* In 330 patients with CFS mean concentration of 25.3 ± 0.14 mmol/L significantly higher than 24.5 ± 0.27 mmol/L in 96 control patients *324*

Carnitine *Serum* *Decrease* In 27 female patients with chronic fatigue syndrome mean concentration of 41.2 ± 9.5 μmol/L significantly lower than 51.5 ± 11.6 μmol/L in reference population. In 8 men with CFS mean of 49.9 ± 9.1 μmol/L significantly less than 59.3 ± 11.9 μmol/L in controls *4157*

Carnitine, Free *Serum* *Decrease* In 19 men with chronic fatigue syndrome mean concentration of free L-carnitine of 53.6 ± 8.5 μmol/L lower than 56.1 ± 10.7 μmol/L in 177 healthy control men *2859* In 38 female patients with chronic fatigue syndrome mean concentration of 32.1 ± 6.9 μmol/L significantly lower than 40.1 ± 9.5 μmol/L in reference population. In 8 males with CFS mean of 40.6 ± 8.9 μmol/L significantly less than 46.8 ± 10.0 μmol/L in reference population *4157*
Serum *Increase* In 19 women with chronic fatgue syndrome mean concentration of free L-carnitine of 46.8 ± 8.2 μmol/L nonsignificantly higher than 43.6 ± 10.0 μmol/L in 131 healthy women *2859*

$CD3^+$ Lymphocytes *Blood* *No Effect* In 28 patients with chronic fatigue syndrome mean absolute number of 1,446.6 ± 544.3 /μL compared with normal range of 976 - 2,486 /μL with 5 patients having values below and 2 above normal range *4100*

$CD4^+$-29^+ Lymphocytes *Blood* *No Effect* In 28 patients with chronic fatigue syndrome mean absolute number of 392.3 ± 156.3 compared with normal range of 222-688 with 4 patients having concentrations below lower limit of normal *4100*

$CD4^+$-45^+RA Lymphocytes *Blood* *No Effect* In 28 patents with chronic fatigue syndrome mean absolute number of 378.9 ± 261.7 /μL compared with normal range of 190 - 760 /μL with 4 patients having concentrations below and one above normal range *4100*

$CD4^+$ Lymphocytes *Blood* *Increase* Reported effect *5364*
Blood *No Effect* Reported effect *5364* In 28 patients with chronic fatigue syndrome mean absolute number of 932.7 ± 320.4 compared with normal range of 656 - 1,476 with 5 patients having values below and 2 above reference range *4100*

$CD8^+$ Lymphocytes *Blood* *Increase* Reported effect *5364*
Blood *No Effect* In 28 patients with chronic fatigue syndrome mean absolute number of 484.6 ± 273 /μL compared with normal range of 230 - 790 /μL with 3 patients having concentrations below and 3 having concentrations above reference interval *4100* Reported effect *5364*

$CD19^+$ Lymphocytes *Blood* *No Effect* In 28 patients with chronic fatigue syndrome mean absolute number of 178.4 ± 81.3 compared with normal range of 56 - 328 with 2 patients having concentrations above upper limit of normal *4100*

$CD56^+$ Lymphocytes *Blood* *No Effect* In 28 patients with chronic fatigue syndrome mean absolute number of 249.1 ± 162.7 /μL compared with normal range of 86 - 612 /μL with 3 patients having concentrations and 1 above reference range *4100*

Cholesterol *Serum* *Increase* Age- and sex-adjusted odds ratios of abnormal results, comparing cases with control subjects: total cholesterol, 2.1 (95% CI, 1.2 - 3.4) *324* In 351 patients with CFS mean concentration of 5.39 ± 0.05 U/L significantly higher than 5.00 ± 0.10 U/L in 96 control patients *324*

Corticotropin-releasing Hormone
Cerebrospinal Fluid *No Effect* In 30 patients with chronic fatigue syndrome mean concentration of 8.4 ± 0.6 pmol/L not significantly different from 7.7 ± 0.5 pmol/L in 72 normal volunteers *1112*

Cortisol *Saliva* *Decrease* Mean evening and morning concentrations in 14 female patients with chronic fatigue syndrome of 1.0 ± 0 nmol/L and 5.8 ± 4.4 nmol/L, respectively, significantly reduced in comparison with 1.5 ± 1.5 nmol/L and 7.0 ± 3.5 nmol/L in 131 matched controls *5048*

Cortisol, Free *Urine* *Decrease* In 21 patients with chronic fatigue syndrome mean excretion of 116.1 ± 10.7 nmol/d significantly different from 181.3 ± 42.9 nmol/d in 15 healthy control individuals *4700* In 30 patients with chronic fatigue syndrome mean 24-hour excretion of 122.7 ± 8.9 nmol/d compared with 203.1 ± 10.7 nmol/d in 72 healthy controls *1112*

Epstein Barr Virus Antibodies *Serum* *Increase* The antibody profiles were studied in 136 patients presenting with this syndrome. These profiles were compared with a panel of sera from blood donors. The patients exhibited higher titers in a combined assay for antibodies to the Restricted and Diffuse components of the early antigen complex than the controls (p less than 0.001) but titers against these antigens were not useful on an individual basis *5728*
Serum *No Effect* There were no group differences in antibody titers between 14 patients with this disorder compared with 12 healthy controls *5728*

Erythrocyte Sedimentation Rate *Blood* *No Effect* In 501 patients with CFS mean rate of 10.6 ± 0.42 mm/h not significantly higher than 9.3 ± 0.99 mm/h in 94 control patients *324*

Folate *Serum* *Increase* Assayed serum folate levels of 60 patients with chronic fatigue syndrome (CFS) and found that 50% had values below 3.0 micrograms/L *2396*

Glucocorticoids *Plasma* *Decrease* In 30 patients with chronic fatigue syndrome mean basal evening concentration of 89.0 ± 8.7 nmol/L significantly less than 148.4 ± 20.3 nmol/L in 72 normal volunteers *1112*

4-Hydroxy-3-Methoxy-Phenylglycol *Plasma* *Decrease* Determined in 19 patients meeting CDC research case criteria for chronic fatigue syndrome and in 17 normal individuals. Patients showed a significant reduction in basal plasma levels of MHPG *1113*

5-Hydroxyindoleacetic Acid *Plasma* *Increase* Determined in 19 patients meeting CDC research case criteria for chronic fatigue syndrome and in 17 normal individuals. Patients showed a significant increase in basal plasma levels of 5-HIAA *1113*

Immune Complexes *Serum* *Increase* In 87 of 178 cases (48%) of chronic fatigue syndrome mean concentration increased: sex and age adjusted odds ratio for increased immune complexes 26.5 *324* In 296 patients with CFS mean concentration of 0.81 ± 1.66 g/L significantly higher than 0.11 ± 0.68 g/L in 50 control patients *324*

Immunoglobulin A *Serum* *Increase* Reported effect *5364*
Serum *No Effect* In 496 patients with CFS mean concentration of 2.07 ± 0.86 g/L not significantly different from 1.86 ± 0.86 g/L in 50 control patients *324* In 28 patients with chronic fatigue syndrome mean concentration of 162.1 ± 100.7 mg/dL compared with 90 - 450 mg/dL in normal controls with 6 patients below and 1 patient above normal range *4100*

Immunoglobulin D *Serum* *Increase* Reported effect *5364*

Immunoglobulin E *Serum* *No Effect* Mean concentration in 28 patients with chronic fatigue syndrome of 68.2 ± 130 mg/dL compared with normal range of 10 - 150 mg/dL with 8 patients with values below and 3 patients with values above normal range *4100*

Immunoglobulin G *Serum* *Increase* In 87 of 178 cases (48%) of chronic fatigue syndrome mean concentration increased. Sex and age adjusted odds ratio for increased IgG 8.5 *324* In 497 patients with CFS mean concentration of 11.24 ± 2.88 g/L significantly higher than 9.54 ± 2.11 g/L in 50 control patients *324*
Serum *No Effect* In 28 patients with chronic fatigue syndrome mean concentration of 892.3 ± 156.1 mg/dL compared with normal range of 600 - 1,800 mg/dL with 11 having concentrations below lower limit of normal *4100*

Immunoglobulin G_1 *Serum* *No Effect* In 28 patients with chronic fatigue syndrome mean concentration of 474.8 ± 142.5 mg/dL compared with normal range of 422 - 1,292 mg/dL with 12 patients having concentrations below lower limit of normal *4100*

Immunoglobulin G_2 *Serum* *No Effect* In 28 patients with chronic fatigue syndrome mean concentration of 207.5 ± 110 mg/dL compared with normal range of 117-747 mg/dL with 8 patients having concentrations below the lower limit of normal *4100*

Immunoglobulin G_3 *Serum* *No Effect* In 28 patients with chronic fatigue syndrome mean concentration of 39.6 ± 25.4 mg/dL compared with normal concentration of 41 - 129 mg/dL with 18 patients having concentrations below the lower limit of normal *4100*

Immunoglobulin G_4 *Serum* *No Effect* In 28 patients with chronic fatigue syndrome mean concentration of 23.9 ± 26.3 mg/dL compared with normal range of 1 - 291 mg/dL with no patients having values outside reference interval *4100*

Immunoglobulin M *Serum* *Decrease* In 496 patients with CFS mean concentration of 1.55 ± 0.85 g/L significantly lower than 1.92 ± 2.98 g/L in 50 control patients *324*
Serum *Increase* Reported effect *5364*
Serum *No Effect* In 28 patients with chronic fatigue syndrome mean concentration of 181.9 ± 90.1 mg/dL compared with normal range of 60 - 250 mg/dL with 1 patient having a concentration below, and 7 having concentrations above, normal range *4100*

Insulin-like Growth Factor-I *Serum* *Increase* In 15 patients with chronic fatigue syndrome mean concentration of 223 ± 60 ng/mL and in 15 patients with chronic fatigue syndrome and fibromyalgia mean concentration of 232 ± 59 ng/mL not significantly different from 204 ± 70 ng/mL in 30 healthy controls *621*

Insulin-like Growth Factor Binding Protein-3
Serum *No Effect* In 15 patients with chronic fatigue syndrome mean concentration of 3.1 ± 0.3 mg/L and in 15 patients with chronic fatigue syndrome and fibromyalgia mean concentration of 3.3 ± 0.5 mg/L not significantly different from 3.2 ± 0.8 mg/L in 30 healthy controls *621*

Interleukin-2 *Serum* *Increase* Reported effect *5364*

Lactate Dehydrogenase *Serum* *Decrease* In 319 patients with CFS mean concentration of 160 ± 1.9 U/L significantly lower than 181 ± 3.6 U/L in 96 control patients *324*
Serum *Increase* Age- and sex-adjusted odds ratios of abnormal results, comparing cases with control subjects: 0.30 (95% CI, 0.16 - 0.56) *324*

Leukocytes *Blood* *Increase* In 563 patients with CFS mean concentration of 7.26 ± 0.079 /µL significantly higher than 6.57 ± 0.20 /µL in 96 control patients *324*

Lymphocytes *Blood* *Increase* Age- and sex-adjusted odds ratios of abnormal results, comparing cases with control subjects: atypical lymphocytosis 11.4 (95% CI, 1.4 - 94) *324* In 473 patients with CFS mean proportion of 30.5 ± 0.37% significantly higher than 28.1 ± 0.89% in 85 control patients *324*

Magnesium *Red Blood Cells* *Decrease* In the case-control study, 20 patients with CFS had lower red cell magnesium concentrations than did 20 healthy control subjects matched for age, sex, and social class (difference 0.1 mmol/L, 95% confidence interval [CI] 0.05 to 0.15) *954*
Red Blood Cells *No Effect* In 89 patients with CFS mean concentration of 1.93 ± 0.38 mmol/L not significantly different from 1.91 ± 0.28 mmol/L in age and sex-matched controls *2164*
Serum *No Effect* In 89 patients with CFS mean concentration of 0.74 ± 0.06 mmol/L not significantly different from 0.73 ± 0.08 mmol/L in age and sex-matched controls *2164*

Monocytes *Blood* *Increase* In 473 patients with CFS mean proportion of 5.47 ± 0.10% significantly higher than 4.58 ± 0.25% in 85 control patients *324*

Thyroid Stimulating Hormone *Serum* *No Effect* In 520 patients with CFS mean concentration of 1.99 ± 0.091 U/L not significantly different from 2.16 ± 0.29 U/L in 50 control patients *324*

780.80 Hyperhidrosis

Bicarbonate *Serum* *No Effect* Usually no abnormality observed *5544*

Chloride *Serum* *Decrease* Reported effect *5544*

Creatinine *Serum* *Increase* Leading to reduced renal blood flow (prerenal azotemia) *5544*

pH *Urine* *No Effect* Usually within normal limits *5544*

Potassium *Serum* *No Effect* Usual observation *5544*
Urine *No Effect* Usually unaffected *5544*

Urea Nitrogen *Serum* *Increase* Dehydration *1025* *1642* Salt and water depletion causes reduced renal blood flow leading to prerenal azotemia *5544*

Volume *Plasma* *No Effect* Usually unchanged *5544*
Urine *No Effect* Usually unaffected *5544*

780.90 Proteus Syndrome

Alanine Aminotransferase *Serum* *No Effect* In a child with Proteus syndrome followed from age 15 to 35 months mean concentration remained within reference limits *4473*

α_1-Antitrypsin *Serum* *No Effect* In a child with Proteus syndrome followed from age 15 to 35 months mean concentration remained within reference limits *4473*

Aspartate Aminotransferase *Serum* *No Effect* In a child with Proteus syndrome followed from age 15 to 35 months mean concentration remained within reference limits *4473*

Bilirubin *Serum* *No Effect* In a child with Proteus syndrome followed from age 15 to 35 months mean concentration remained within reference limits *4473*

Calcium *Serum* *No Effect* In a child with Proteus syndrome followed from age 15 to 35 months mean concentration remained within reference limits *4473*

Creatine Kinase *Serum* *No Effect* In a child with Proteus syndrome followed from age 15 to 35 months mean concentration remained within reference limits *4473*

Creatinine *Serum* *No Effect* In a child with Proteus syndrome followed from age 15 to 35 months mean concentration remained within reference limits *4473*

Erythrocyte Sedimentation Rate *Blood* *No Effect* In a child with Proteus syndrome followed from age 15 to 35 months mean concentration remained within reference limits *4473*

Erythrocytes *Blood* *No Effect* In a child with Proteus syndrome followed from age 15 to 35 months mean concentration remained within reference limits *4473*

γ-Glutamyltransferase *Serum* *No Effect* In a child with Proteus syndrome followed from age 15 to 35 months mean concentration remained within reference limits *4473*

Growth Hormone *Plasma* *Decrease* In a child with Proteus syndrome followed from age 15 to 35 months mean concentration of 13.2 ng/mL at 15 months, 3.4 ng/mL at 20 months and 8.9 ng/mL at 35 months lower than reference limits *4473*

Immunoglobulin A *Serum* *No Effect* In a child with Proteus syndrome followed from age 15 to 35 months mean concentration remained within reference limits *4473*

Immunoglobulin G *Serum* *Decrease* In a child with Proteus syndrome followed from age 15 to 35 months mean concentration of 5.3 - 4.6 g/L below reference limits of 10.5 - 21 g/L *4473*

Immunoglobulin M *Serum* *No Effect* In a child with Proteus syndrome followed from age 15 to 35 months mean concentration remained within reference limits *4473*

Insulin-like Growth Factor-I *Serum* *No Effect* In a child with Proteus syndrome mean concentrations of 38, 16 and 28 µg/L at 15, 20 and 35 months not significantly different from normal range of 25 - 146 µg/L *4473*

Insulin-like Growth Factor-II *Serum* *Decrease* In a child with Proteus syndrome mean concentrations of 117, 180 and 148 µg/L at 15, 20 and 35 months significantly less than normal range of 320 - 772 µg/L *4473*

Insulin-like Growth Factor Binding Protein-3
Serum *Decrease* In a child with Proteus syndrome mean concentrations of 0.77, 0.41 and < 0.10 mg/L at 15, 20 and 35 months significantly less than normal range of 1.41 - 2.97 mg/L *4473*

Lactate Dehydrogenase *Serum* *No Effect* In a child with Proteus syndrome followed from age 15 to 35 months mean concentration remained within reference limits *4473*

Leukocytes *Blood* *No Effect* In a child with Proteus syndrome followed from age 15 to 35 months mean concentration remained within reference limits *4473*

Phosphate *Serum* *No Effect* In a child with Proteus syndrome followed from age 15 to 35 months mean concentration remained within reference limits *4473*

780.90 Proteus Syndrome *(continued)*

Platelets *Blood* *No Effect* In a child with Proteus syndrome followed from age 15 to 35 months mean concentration remained within reference limits *4473*

Potassium *Serum* *No Effect* In a child with Proteus syndrome followed from age 15 to 35 months mean concentration remained within reference limits *4473*

Protein *Serum* *No Effect* In a child with Proteus syndrome followed from age 15 to 35 months mean concentration remained within reference limits *4473*

Sodium *Serum* *No Effect* In a child with Proteus syndrome followed from age 15 to 35 months mean concentration remained within reference limits *4473*

Urea Nitrogen *Serum* *No Effect* In a child with Proteus syndrome followed from age 15 to 35 months mean concentration remained within reference limits *4473*

781.00 Postencephalitic Spasm

Nerve Growth Factor *Cerebrospinal Fluid* *Increase* In 5 children with postencephalitic spasms mean concentration of 379 ± 118 pg/mL compared with 6.29 ± 1.14 pg/mL in controls *4360*

781.70 Tetany

Calcium *Serum* *No Effect* In two patients with tetany and reduced ionized calcium concentration total calcium concentration reduced to lower limit of normal range *4494*

Ionized Calcium *Serum* *Decrease* In two patients with tetany concentrations reduced by 30% and 27% respectively *4494*

Ionized Magnesium *Serum* *Decrease* In two patients with tetany concentration reduced by 29% and 44% respectively *4494*

Magnesium *Serum* *No Effect* In two patients with reduced ionized magnesium concentration of total magnesium reduced to lower limit of normal *4494*

781.90 Catatonia

Homovanillic Acid *Plasma* *Increase* In 37 catatonic patients mean concentration on admission of 140.9 ± 53.6 pmol/mL significantly higher than 80.1 ± 40.1 pmol/mL in 17 healthy control children *3831*

781.90 Neurological Disorders

Tau Protein *Cerebrospinal Fluid* *Increase* Mean concentration of 125.8 ± 103.6 ng/L in 39 patients with various neurological disorders (11 with multinfarct dementia, 18 with multiple sclerosis, 6 with neurodegenerative diseases and 4 with viral encephalitis) significantly higher than that in healthy controls, 51.1 ± 7.3 ng/L *1546*

782.40 Shunt Hyperbilirubinemia

Bilirubin, Unconjugated *Serum* *Increase* Shunt hyperbilirubinemia is associated with unconjugated hyperbilirubinemia *3625*

783.40 Idiopathic Short Stature

Growth Hormone *Plasma* *No Effect* In children with idiopathic short stature mean 12 h concentration of 2.2 μg/L (1 SD range 1.4 - 3.4 μg/L) in 446 males and 2.2 μg/L (1 SD range 1.3 - 3.5 μg/L) in 122 females significantly lower than 2.1 μg/L (1 SD range 1.2 - 3.5 μg/L) in 47 male and 2.7 μg/L (1 SD range 1.4 - 5.1 μg/L) in 35 female controls *694*
Urine *Increase* In 66 patients with idiopathic short stature mean excretion of 17.3 ± 8.71 ng/L (2.23 ± 1.16 ng/mmol creatinine) markedly different from those in healthy individuals *1698*

Growth Hormone Binding Protein *Serum* *Decrease* In children with idiopathic short stature mean concentration of 103 pmol/L (1 SD range 63 - 166 pmol/L) in 448 males and 131 pmol/L (1 SD range 81 - 213 pmol/L) in 124 females significantly lower than 183 pmol/L (1 SD range 103 -326 pmol/L) in 407 male and 228 pmol/L (1 SD range 133 - 394 pmol/L) in 366 female controls *694*

Insulin-like Growth Factor-I *Serum* *Decrease* In children with idiopathic short stature mean concentration of 108 μg/L (1 SD range 51 - 231 μg/L) in males and 120 μg/L (1 SD range 56 - 257 μg/L) in females significantly lower than 217 μg/L (1 SD range 130 - 363 μg/L) in 47 male and 308 μg/L (1 SD range 178 - 531 μg/L) in 35 female controls *694*
Serum *No Effect* In 16 children with short stature mean concentration of about 90 μg/L not significantly different from normal concentration of 90 - 360 μg/L *3332*

Insulin-like Growth Factor-II *Serum* *Decrease* In 16 children with short stature mean concentration of about 510 μg/L not significantly different from normal concentration of 490 - 1,056 μg/L *3332*
Urine *Decrease* In 24 children with idiopathic short stature mean excretion of 1.0 ± 0.1 pmol/kg (15.2 ± 2.0 nmol/mol creatinine) compared with 2.4 ± 0.2 pmol/kg body weight (33.2 ± 3.8 nmol/mol creatinine) in 40 healthy controls *4250*

Insulin-like Growth Factor Binding Protein-3
Serum *No Effect* In 10 children with short stature mean concentration of about 1.9 μg/mL not significantly different from normal range of 1.7 - 4.0 μg/mL *3332*

783.50 Polydipsia, Primary

Creatinine *Serum* *No Effect* Mean concentration of 0.8 ± 0.1 mg/dL in 7 patients with primary polydipsia not significantly different from 0.7 ± 0.2 mg/dL in 27 healthy controls *1084*

Creatinine Clearance *Urine* *No Effect* Mean clearance of 90 ± 30 mL/min in 3 patients with primary polydipsia not significantly different from 108 ± 10 mL/min in 27 healthy controls *1084*

Fractional Excretion of Sodium *Urine* *No Effect* Mean fractional excretion of 0.7 ± 0.2% in 3 patients with primary polydipsia not significantly different from 0.5 ± 0.2% in 27 healthy controls *1084*

Fractional Excretion of Urea *Urine* *Increase* Mean fractional excretion of 78 ± 9% in 3 patients with primary polydipsia not significantly different from 45 ± 7.5% in 27 healthy controls *1084*

Fractional Excretion of Uric Acid *Urine* *No Effect* Mean fractional excretion of 9.5 ± 3.5% in 3 patients with primary polydipsia not significantly different from 8.2 ± 2.0% in 27 healthy controls *1084*

Osmolality *Urine* *No Effect* Mean excretion of 130 ± 47 mOsm/kg in 7 patients with primary polydipsia not significantly different from 50 - 1,000 mOsm/kg in 27 healthy controls *1084*

Protein *Serum* *No Effect* Mean concentration of 7.1 ± 0.6 g/dL in 7 patients with primary polydipsia not significantly different from 7.0 ± 0.5 g/dL in 27 healthy controls *1084*

Renin Activity *Plasma* *No Effect* Mean concentration of 0.9 ± 0.5 ng/mL/h in 5 patients with primary polydipsia not significantly different from 1.5 ± 0.6 ng/mL/h in 27 healthy controls *1084*

Sodium *Serum* *No Effect* Mean concentration of 138 ± 3 mmol/L in 7 patients with primary polydipsia not significantly different from 140 ± 2.5 mmol/L in 27 healthy controls *1084*

Urea *Serum* *Decrease* Mean concentration of 22 ± 6 mg/dL in 7 patients with primary polydipsia significantly different from 32 ± 7 mg/dL in 27 healthy controls *1084*

Uric Acid *Serum* *Decrease* Mean concentration of 3.0 ± 0.75 mg/dL in 7 patients with primary polydipsia significantly different from 4.3 ± 0.9 mg/dL in 27 healthy controls *1084*
Urine *No Effect* Mean excretion of 390 ± 150 mg/d in 3 patients with primary polydipsia not significantly different from 548 ± 100 mg/d in 27 healthy controls *1084*

783.60 Bulimia

α_1-Acid Glycoprotein *Serum* *Increase* In 18 subjects compared with age and sex matched controls *2082*

Aldolase *Serum* *Increase* Effect observed in extreme cases *2148*

Amylase *Serum* *Increase* In 33 female patients with bulimia nervosa for an average of 4.4 years mean activity of 4.60 ± 2.3 μkat/L not higher than upper limit of normal of 5.0 μkat/L but with activity of 5.61 μkat/L observed in 10 patients with very poor outcomes *2829* Measured in 34 patients (average age 28.5 (18 - 64) years) with anorexia nervosa (9 patients) and bulimia (25 patients) hyperamylasaemia was demonstrated in 13 of the 34 patients (38%) *2110*

Amylase, Salivary Isoenzyme *Serum* *Increase* In 33 female patients with bulimia nervosa for an average of 4.4 years mean activity of 3.06 ± 1.9 μkat/L higher than upper limit of normal of 2.7 μkat/L with the highest activity of 3.95 μkat/L observed in 10 patients with very poor outcomes *2829*

Bicarbonate *Serum* *Decrease* Effect observed in extreme cases *2148*

Chloride *Serum* *Decrease* Effect observed in extreme cases *2148*

Cholecystokinin *Cerebrospinal Fluid* *Decrease* CSF concentrations of CCK-8 were measured in 11 drug-free female patients with DSM-III-R-defined bulimia nervosa and in 16 normal subjects. The bulimic patients had significantly lower levels of CCK-8 than the comparison subjects *3175*
Plasma *Increase* Baseline values were significantly increased in the anorectic group (1.8 ± 0.4 pmol/L compared with 0.6 ± 0.2 pmol/L in controls) *2608*
Plasma *No Effect* Baseline CCK values were similar in controls (0.6 ± 0.2 pmol/L) and bulimics (0.6 ± 0.1 pmol/L) *4122*

Cortisol *Plasma* *Increase* In comparison with healthy controls, women with bulimia had an exaggerated secretion of either the amount and/or the duration of insulin, cortisol and prolactin. Significantly increased baseline level *2610* Malnourished patients with bulimia had higher concentrations than in age- and sex-matched controls *2955* In 22 bulimic women mean 6-h mean concentration of 100 ± 30 nmol/L compared with 80 ± 20 nmol/L in 21 healthy control women *4695* In 16 female outpatients with bulimia with reversed neurovegatitive symptoms of depression mean concentration of 147.5 ± 58.1 nmol/L not significantly different from 162.1 ± 42 nmol/L in 14 matched healthy controls *3015*
Plasma *No Effect* No significant difference observed in overall circadian pattern in bulimic women but associated with moderate increase in concentration *5629*

Creatine Kinase *Serum* *Increase* Effect observed in extreme cases *2148*

Dynorphin *Cerebrospinal Fluid* *No Effect* No significant difference observed between mean concentration of 21.3 ± 7.8 pg/mL in women with bulimia and 22.7 ± 8.3 pg/mL in control women *582*

β-Endorphin *Cerebrospinal Fluid* *Decrease* In 11 women with bulimia mean concentration of 71.9 ± 23.0 pg/mL significantly lower than 98.0 ± 17.7 pg/mL in control women *582*

Epinephrine *Plasma* *Increase* Malnourished patients with bulimia had higher concentrations than in age- and sex-matched controls *2955*

Epinephrine:Norepinephrine Ratio *Plasma* *Increase* Binge-abstinent bulimic patients had significantly higher ratios than in age- and sex-matched controls *2955*

Estradiol *Plasma* *Decrease* In 22 bulimic women mean concentration in follicular phase of 150 ± 80 pmol/L not significantly less than 170 ± 100 pmol/L in 21 controls but in luteal phase mean concentration of 140 ± 60 pmol/L significantly less than 310 ± 170 pmol/L in controls *4695*

Estrogens *Plasma* *No Effect* Reported effect *819*

Fatty Acids (FFA), Free *Serum* *Increase* In the majority of a group of patients with bulimia concentration increased *4145*

Glucose *Serum* *Decrease* Mean concentration in 13 patients with bulimia significantly less than in 15 healthy controls *4670* In 22 women of normal body weight mean concentration of 4.0 ± 0.6 mmol/L compared with 4.6 ± 0.6 mmol/L in 19 age and weight matched controls *1137*

Growth Hormone *Plasma* *No Effect* No overall effect observed on circadian pattern in bulimic women but modest reduction in growth hormone secretion observed *5629*

Hematocrit *Blood* *Increase* Effect observed in extreme cases *2148*

Hemoglobin *Blood* *Increase* Effect observed in extreme cases *2148*

Homovanillic Acid *Cerebrospinal Fluid* *Decrease* Significantly lower concentrations in hospitalized bulimic patients with a history of binge eating more frequently than twice daily (n = 11) compared with controls (n = 17) *2449*
Cerebrospinal Fluid *No Effect* In 27 normal weight bulimic patients compared to 14 normal volunteers *2608*
Plasma *Increase* In 11 women with bulimia mean concentration of 20.8 ± 12.2 ng/mL compared with 13.4 ± 3.7 ng/mL in 29 healthy controls *549*

4-Hydroxy-3-Methoxy-Phenylglycol *Plasma* *No Effect* In 11 women with bulimia mean concentration 3.7 ± 1.1 ng/mL not significantly increased compared with 3.0 ± 0.5 ng/mL in 29 healthy controls *549*

β-Hydroxybutyrate *Serum* *Increase* Increased concentration observed in 13 patients with bulimia nervosa compared with 15 healthy controls *4670* In majority of a group of bulimic patients concentration of β-hydroxybutyric acid increased *4145* In 22 bulimic women mean morning fasting concentration β-hydroxybutyric acid of 110 ± 160 μmol/L not significantly different from 60 ± 120 μmol/L in 21 healthy control women *4695*

5-Hydroxyindoleacetic Acid *Cerebrospinal Fluid* *Decrease* Significantly lower concentrations in hospitalized bulimic patients with a history of binge eating more frequently than twice daily (n = 11) compared with controls (n = 17) *2449*
Cerebrospinal Fluid *No Effect* In 27 normal weight bulimic patients compared to 14 normal volunteers *2608* In 22 bulimics on admission to hospital mean concentration of 134.5 ± 35.7 nmol/L not significantly different from 146.3 ± 30.2 nmol/L in 8 healthy normals *1114*

5-Hydroxytryptamine *Blood* *Increase* Malnourished patients with bulimia had higher concentrations than in age- and sex-matched controls *2955*

Insulin *Plasma* *Decrease* Mean concentration significantly less in 13 patients with bulimia than in 15 healthy controls *4670* In 22 bulimic women mean 6-hour mean concentration of 90 ± 30 pmol/L significantly less than 120 ± 30 pmol/L in 21 control women *4695*

Kynurenic Acid *Cerebrospinal Fluid* *No Effect* In 22 bulimics on admission to hospital mean concentration of 2.2 ± 0.6 nmol/L not significantly different from 2.8 ± 1.2 nmol/L in 8 healthy normals *1114*

Kynurenine *Cerebrospinal Fluid* *No Effect* In 22 bulimics on admission to hospital mean concentration of 29.6 ± 6.4 nmol/L not significantly different from 34.4 ± 12.3 nmol/L in 8 healthy normals *1114*

Leptin *Serum* *Decrease* In 16 female patients with bulimia best predictor for serum leptin concentration is percentage body fat *3347*

Lipase *Serum* *Increase* Measured in 34 patients (average age 28.5 (18 - 64) years) anorexia nervosa (9 patients) and bulimia (25 patients). In only two of them was there an elevated concentration of lipase and human pancreatic lipase *2110*

Lipase, Pancreatic *Serum* *Increase* Measured in 34 patients (average age 28.5 (18 - 64) years) anorexia nervosa (9 patients) and bulimia (25 patients). In only two of them was there an elevated concentration of lipase and human pancreatic lipase *2110*

Lipoprotein Lipase *Serum* *No Effect* No significant difference observed between activities in 22 women with bulimia nervosa and 19 age and weight matched controls *1137*

Luteinizing Hormone *Plasma* *Decrease* In 22 bulimic women mean 12 h mean concentration of 2.4 ± 1.8 IU/L compared with 3.0 ± 1.6 IU/L in 21 control women *4695*

Melatonin *Plasma* *Decrease* Low levels of melatonin also occur *1976*
Plasma *No Effect* In 8 women with bulimia nervosa mean peak daily concentration of 310 ± 33 pmol/L not significantly different from 334 ± 30 pmol/L in 21 healthy normal cycling women *3621*

Monoamine Oxidase *Platelets* *Increase* Platelet levels were found to be lower in 16 consecutive female in-patients fulfilling the DSM-III criteria for bulimia nervosa than in 12 female controls *1976*

783.60 Bulimia *(continued)*

Neopterin *Cerebrospinal Fluid* *No Effect* In 22 bulimics on admission to hospital mean concentration of 11.8 ± 4.1 nmol/L not significantly different from 13.7 ± 4.5 nmol/L in 8 healthy normals *1114*

Norepinephrine *Cerebrospinal Fluid* *Decrease* In 27 normal weight bulimic patients compared to 14 normal volunteers. The levels were significantly lower *2608*

Oxytocin *Cerebrospinal Fluid* *No Effect* Normal in 12 underweight bulimic anorexic women and 35 normal weight women with bulimia nervosa when compared to 11 controls *1115*

Peptide YY *Cerebrospinal Fluid* *Increase* In normal-weight bulimic patients absent from pathological eating behavior for a month concentrations significantly increased *2609*

pH *Blood* *Decrease* Effect observed in extreme cases *2148*
Blood *Increase* Metabolic alkalosis secondary to vomiting and laxative use *565*

Phospholipase A *Serum* *No Effect* Measured in 34 patients (average age 28.5 years), anorexia nervosa (9 patients) and bulimia (25 patients). Normal in all patients *2110*

Potassium *Serum* *Decrease* Secondary to vomiting and laxative use *565* Effect observed in extreme cases *2148*

Progesterone *Plasma* *Decrease* In 22 bulimic women mean concentration in luteal phase of 9 ± 10 pmol/L significantly less than 24 ± 15 pmol/L in 21 control women in luteal phase *4695*

Prolactin *Plasma* *Decrease* In comparison with healthy controls, women with bulimia had an exaggerated secretion of either the amount and/or the duration of insulin, cortisol and prolactin. Significantly reduced baseline level *2610*
Plasma *No Effect* Modest increase observed in association with bingeing and vomiting and daytime circadian pattern of prolactin similar in bulimics and controls. However blunted nocturnal pattern observed in bulimic women *5629*

Quinolinic Acid *Cerebrospinal Fluid* *No Effect* In 22 bulimics on admission to hospital mean concentration of 12.5 ± 2.9 nmol/L not significantly different from 13.8 ± 4.3 nmol/L in 8 healthy normals *1114*

Sodium *Serum* *Decrease* Effect observed in extreme cases *2148*

Somatostatin *Plasma* *Increase* Measured before and after a standardized fat and protein-rich fluid test meal. Significantly elevated after the test meals *4144*

Testosterone *Serum* *Increase* Women with normal-weight bulimia nervosa (n = 11) displayed significantly higher serum levels of free testosterone than age-matched controls (6.0 ± 0.7 vs 3.9 ± 0.8 pmol/L; p = 0.03) *5081*

Thyroid Stimulating Hormone *Serum* *Decrease* Mean concentration significantly lower in 22 female patients with bulimia than in 19 age and weight matched controls *1137*

Tri-iodothyronine (T3) *Serum* *No Effect* In 22 bulimic women mean concentration of 1.7 ± 0.3 nmol/L not significantly different from 1.8 ± 0.2 nmol/L in 21 control women *4695*

Triglycerides *Serum* *Increase* Concentration higher in patients who binge *4554*

Tryptophan *Cerebrospinal Fluid* *No Effect* In 22 bulimics on admission to hospital mean concentration of 2.0 ± 0.4 nmol/L not significantly different from 2.1 ± 0.3 nmol/L in 8 healthy normals *1114*

Urea Nitrogen *Serum* *Increase* Effect observed in extreme cases *2148*

Vasopressin *Plasma* *No Effect* Reported effect *2610*

783.90 Mixed-Sclerosing-Bone Dystrophy

Creatine Kinase *Serum* *No Effect* In 3 patients mean activities of 75 U/L, 92 U/L and 78 U/L compared with upper limit of normal of 195 U/L *5659*

Creatine Kinase BB-Isoenzyme *Serum* *No Effect* In 3 patients mean activities of < 10 U/L, < 10 U/L and < 5 U/L (not detected %) compared with normal of 0 - 1% *5659*

784.00 Headache

Cortisol *Cerebrospinal Fluid* *Decrease* Significant reduction observed in all 73 patients with headaches studied *1351*
Plasma *Decrease* Significant decrease observed in men with headaches: claimed to be due to altered circadian rhythm *1351*

Follicle Stimulating Hormone *Cerebrospinal Fluid* *Increase* Significant amounts detected in all patients with headaches compared with undetectable amounts in healthy controls *1351*
Plasma *Increase* Significant increase observed in all 73 male and female patients studied *1351*

Luteinizing Hormone *Cerebrospinal Fluid* *Increase* In all 73 patients with headaches studied significant amounts detected compared with undetectable amounts in controls *1351*
Plasma *Increase* Significant increase observed in women with headaches but no significant effect observed in men *1351*
Plasma *No Effect* No significant effect observed in male patients with headaches *1351*

Prolactin *Cerebrospinal Fluid* *Increase* In all 73 patients with headaches studied significant amounts detected compared with undetectable amounts in controls *1351*
Plasma *No Effect* Concentration remained within normal limits in 73 patients with headaches *1351*

785.40 Gangrene

Aldolase *Serum* *Increase* Activity may be slightly increased in patients with gangrene *2952*

Alkaline Phosphatase *Serum* *Increase* In 45% of 32 patients hospitalized for this disorder *1576*

Aspartate Aminotransferase *Serum* *Increase* May produce slight elevations. Usual values of 50 U/L *1025* In 27% of 32 patients hospitalized for this disorder *1576* Found with extensive necrosis *413*

Bicarbonate *Serum* *Increase* In 37% of 28 patients hospitalized for this disorder *1576*

Carbon Dioxide Partial Pressure *Blood* *Decrease* In 22% of 13 patients hospitalized for this disorder *1576*

Chloride *Serum* *Decrease* In 39% of 28 patients hospitalized for this disorder *1576*

C-Reactive Protein *Serum* *Increase* Precedes the rise in ESR; with recovery disappearance precedes the return to normal of the ESR. Also disappears when inflammatory process is suppressed by steroids or salicylates *5544*

Creatine Kinase *Serum* *Increase* Found with extensive necrosis. Predominantly CK-MM *413*

Cryoglobulins *Serum* *Increase* Marked elevation of cryoglobulins *4707*

Lactate Dehydrogenase *Serum* *Increase* Slight elevation *2033* In 24% of 32 patients hospitalized for this disorder *1576*

Leukocytes *Blood* *Increase* Due to tissue necrosis *5544* In 66% of 34 patients hospitalized for this disorder *1576*

Neutrophils *Blood* *Increase* In 63% of 33 patients hospitalized for this disorder *1576*

Oxygen Partial Pressure *Blood* *Decrease* In 63% of 11 patients hospitalized for this disorder *1576*

pH *Blood* *Increase* In 74% of 13 patients hospitalized for this disorder *1576*

Sodium *Serum* *Decrease* In 47% of 27 patients hospitalized for this disorder *1576*

785.50 Shock

Alanine Aminotransferase *Serum* *Increase* Heart failure or shock with attendant hepatic necrosis may lead to elevated values *1025*

Amino Acids *Plasma* *Increase* In severe shock *1290*

Amylase *Serum* *Increase* May be associated with hyperamylasemia *3024*

Aspartate Aminotransferase *Serum* *Increase* Usual values of 20 - 900 U/L *1025*

Bicarbonate *Serum* *Decrease* Respiratory alkalosis may occur *1980*

Carbon Dioxide Partial Pressure *Blood* *Decrease* Respiratory alkalosis may occur *1980*

Creatine Kinase BB-Isoenzyme *Serum* *Increase* Observed effect *248*

Creatinine *Serum* *Increase* Causes reduced renal blood flow leading to prerenal azotemia *5544*

2,3-Diphosphoglycerate *Red Blood Cells* *Increase* Disturbed RBC 2,3-DPG metabolism results in reduced oxygen affinity and delivery to tissues *367*

Epinephrine *Plasma* *Increase* In patients with septicemic, traumatic or hemorrhagic shock. Plasma epinephrine and noradrenaline concentrations were increased above the normal range *385*

Erythrocytes *Blood* *Decrease* Disturbed RBC 2,3-DPG metabolism results in reduced oxygen affinity and delivery to tissues *367* Hemoconcentration (dehydration, burns) or hemodilution (hemorrhage, crush injuries, and skeletal trauma) takes place *5544*
Blood *Increase* Hemoconcentration (e.g., dehydration, burns) or hemodilution (e.g., hemorrhage, crush injuries, and skeletal trauma) takes place *5544*

Euglobulin Lysis Time *Blood* *Increase* Increased in circulatory collapse *5220* *597*

Fibrin Degradation Products *Plasma* *Increase* Raised serum or urine levels are common without other evidence of enhanced fibrinolysis *2646*
Urine *Increase* Raised serum or urine levels are common without other evidence of enhanced fibrinolysis *2646*

Fibrinogen *Plasma* *Decrease* Decreased after severe shock during operation or after trauma, as a result of excessive utilization due to release of tissue thromboplastin *1290*
Plasma *No Effect* In 26 patients with shock without meningitis mean concentration of 1,183 mg/L not significantly different from that in healthy individuals *5401*

Fibronectin *Plasma* *Decrease* Decrease rapidly with shock but concentration rebounds rapidly with recovery *1959*

Glomerular Filtration Rate *Urine* *Decrease* Decreased after shock due to decreased renal blood flow *1290*

Glucose *Serum* *Increase* Increased circulating epinephrine *1290* Hyperglycemia occurs early *5544*

Interleukin-1 Receptor Antagonist
Cerebrospinal Fluid *Increase* In 26 patients with shock without meningitis mean concentration of 1,800 pg/mL significantly different from that in healthy individuals *5401*
Serum *Increase* In 26 patients with shock without meningitis mean concentration of 145,000 pg/mL significantly different from that in healthy individuals *5401*

Interleukin-1 Receptor Antagonist Type II
Cerebrospinal Fluid *Increase* In 26 patients with shock without meningitis mean concentration of 3.1 ng/mL not significantly different from that in healthy individuals, < 2.5 ng/mL *5401*
Serum *Increase* In 26 patients with shock without meningitis mean concentration of 22.7 ng/mL significantly different from that in healthy individuals, 16.5 ± 2.8 ng/mL *5401*

Interleukin-1β *Cerebrospinal Fluid* *Increase* In 26 patients with shock without meningitis mean concentration of 67.5 pg/mL significantly different from that in healthy individuals *5401*
Serum *Increase* In 26 patients with shock without meningitis mean concentration of 1,401 pg/mL significantly different from that in healthy individuals *5401*

Lactate *Blood* *Increase* May increase following shock *1290* May be of some prognostic value *5544*
Plasma *Increase* In 26 patients with shock without meningitis mean concentration of 5,108 µmol/L significantly different from that in healthy individuals *5401*

Lactate Dehydrogenase *Serum* *Increase* 2 to 40 times normal values *1025*

Leukocytes *Blood* *Decrease* There may be leukopenia when shock is severe as in gram-negative bacteremia *5544*
Blood *Increase* Common, especially with hemorrhage *5544*
Blood *No Effect* In 26 patients with shock without meningitis mean concentration of 3.8 x 10^9/L not significantly different from that in healthy individuals *5401*
Cerebrospinal Fluid *No Effect* In 26 patients with shock without meningitis mean concentration of 15 x 10^6/L not significantly different from that in healthy individuals *5401*

Norepinephrine *Plasma* *Increase* In patients with septicemic, traumatic or hemorrhagic shock, epinephrine and norepinephrine concentrations were increased above the normal range. In patients who died, plasma norepinephrine concentrations remained persistently elevated above normal while in those who survived, there was a rapid decline towards the normal range *385*

Oxygen Saturation *Blood* *Decrease* Disturbed RBC 2,3-DPG metabolism results in reduced oxygen affinity and delivery to tissues *367*

pH *Blood* *Increase* Respiratory alkalosis may occur *1980*

Phosphate *Serum* *Increase* Hyperphosphatemia may occur with shock, partially from lactic acidosis *5204*

Platelets *Blood* *Decrease* In 26 patients with shock without meningitis mean concentration of 47 x 10^9/L lower than in healthy individuals *5401*

Urea Nitrogen *Serum* *Increase* A decrease in plasma volume secondary to dehydration, blood loss, hypotension or shock is often referred to as prerenal azotemia *1025* *1642*

785.51 Cardiogenic Shock

Endothelin-1 *Plasma* *Increase* Increase of 5 to 14 times observed in cardiogenic shock *328* Reported effect *751*

Interleukin-6 *Serum* *Increase* In a group of patients with cardiogenic shock mean concentrations 78 ± 74 pg/mL compared with 3 ± 4 pg/mL in healthy controls *1079*

Nitrate plus Nitrite *Serum* *No Effect* In a group of patients with cardiogenic shock mean concentration of 26 ± 13 µmol/L not significantly different compared with 30 ± 9 µmol/L in healthy controls *1079*

Procalcitonin *Plasma* *Increase* In a group of patients with cardiogenic shock mean concentration of 1.4 ± 1.9 ng/mL on days 5 and 10 compared with < 0.1 ng/mL in healthy controls *1079*

Soluble Tumor Necrosis Factor Receptor-p55
Serum *Increase* In a group of patients with cardiogenic shock mean concentration of 3.1 ± 2.9 ng/mL compared with 1.1 ± 0.7 ng/mL in healthy controls *1079*

Soluble Tumor Necrosis Factor Receptor-p75
Serum *Increase* In a group of patients with cardiogenic shock mean concentration of 4.0 ± 1.4 ng/mL compared with 2.4 ± 1.4 ng/mL in healthy controls *1079*

Tumor Necrosis Factor-α *Serum* *Increase* In a group of patients with cardiogenic shock mean concentrations of 11 ± 13 pg/mL compared with 6 ± 1.5 pg/mL in healthy controls *1079*

785.59 Hemorrhagic Shock

Interleukin-1β *Serum* *No Effect* IL-1β not detected, as in controls, in any of 29 patients with hemorrhagic shock on admission to hospital *1364*

Interleukin-2 *Serum* *No Effect* IL-2 not detected, as in controls, in any of 29 patients with hemorrhagic shock on admission to hospital *1364*

Interleukin-6 *Serum* *Increase* IL-6 was detected in 12 of 29 patients with hemorrhagic shock on admission to hospital with IL-6 concentration being significantly higher than in controls *1364*

Interleukin-8 *Serum* *Increase* IL-8 was detected in 12 of 29 patients with hemorrhagic shock on admission to hospital with IL-8 concentration being significantly higher than in controls *1364*

Tumor Necrosis Factor-α *Serum* *Increase* TNF-α was detected in 28 of 29 patients with hemorrhagic shock on admission to hospital with TNF-α concentration being significantly higher than in controls *1364*

785.59 Septic Shock

Adrenomedullin *Plasma* *Increase* In 30 patients with severe sepsis mean concentration of 193.5 ± 30.1 fmol/mL significantly different from 5.1 ± 0.2 fmol/mL in healthy controls *5343*

785.59 Septic Shock *(continued)*

Albumin *Serum Decrease* In 20 patients with septic shock on admission to hospital mean concentration of 24 ± 3 g/L significantly lower than in healthy adults *5364*

Antithrombin III *Plasma Decrease* Significant reduction observed in all patients with septic shock *2135* Significant reduction observed especially in fatal cases *3320*

Arginase *Serum Increase* In patients with septic shock mean concentration ranged from several hundred ng/mL to 7000 ng/mL *5564*

Atrial Natriuretic Peptide *Plasma Increase* In 14 patients with septic shock mean concentration of 162.2 ± 117.3 pg/mL fivefold higher than in 10 healthy individuals (31.7 ± 12 pg/mL) with improvement in shock state associated with decline from 162.7 ± 80 pg/mL to 103.7 ± 28.8 pg/mL *3518*

C_4b-Binding Protein *Serum No Effect* No significant increase observed in 13 patients with septic shock (118 ± 40%) compared with normals possibly due to increased consumption *2135*

Calcitonin Gene-related Peptide *Serum Increase* In 20 patients with septic shock at onset of hypotension mean concentration of 207 ± 41 pmol/L significantly higher than 16 ± 1 pmol/L in healthy adults *5364*

Corticotropin *Plasma Increase* Mean concentration of 11.5 ± 6.6 pg/mL 25 patients with septic shock higher than normal range of 6 - 11 pg/mL *2978*

Cortisol *Plasma Increase* Mean concentration of 37.2 ± 15.6 µg/dL 12 patients with septic shock significantly different from normal range of 5 - 25 µg/dL *2978*

Creatinine *Serum Increase* In 30 patients with septic shock mean concentration of 2.23 ± 0.33 mg/dL significantly different from that in healthy controls *5343* In 20 patients with septic shock on admission to hospital mean concentration of 208 ± 45 µmol/L significantly higher than in healthy adults *5364*

β-Endorphin *Plasma Increase* Mean concentration of 40.6 ± 30.3 pg/mL 25 patients with septic shock higher than normal range of < 30 pg/mL *2978*

Endothelin-1 *Plasma Increase* In 14 patients with septic shock mean concentration of 10.7 ± 6.0 pg/mL sevenfold greater than 1.5 ± 0.5 pg/mL in healthy individuals with improvement in septic shock state associated with decline from 10.1 ± 6.8 pg/mL to 4.3 ± 1.8 pg/mL *3518*

Erythropoietin *Serum Increase* In 16 patients with sepsis or septic shock mean concentration of 120 ± 26 mIU/mL significantly higher than 10 ± 2 mIU/mL in 10 healthy controls *2808*

Estrone *Plasma Increase* In men serum estrogen concentrations, especially estrone, increased with onset of septic shock with mean of 3,515 ± 884 pmol/L on day 1, 2,450 ± 292 pmol/L on day 2 and 1,043 ± 255 pmol/L on day 3 *833*

Factor XII *Plasma Decrease* Significant reduction observed especially in fatal cases *3320*

Hematocrit *Blood Decrease* In 20 patients with septic shock on admission to hospital mean value of 36.1 ± 2.7% significantly lower than in healthy adults *5364*

Hemoglobin *Blood Decrease* In 20 patients with septic shock on admission to hospital mean concentration of 109 ± 9 g/L significantly lower than in healthy adults *5364*

Hep 3B Erythropoietin *Plasma Increase* In 16 patients with sepsis or septic shock mean concentration of 216 ± 23 mIU/mL significantly higher than 152 ± 11 mIU/mL in 10 healthy controls *2808*

High Molecular Weight Kininogen *Plasma Decrease* Significant reduction observed especially in fatal cases *3320*

Interleukin-1β *Serum Increase* In 10 neutropenic patients mean concentration of 348.8 ± 956.8 pg/mL before chemotherapy significantly higher than 19.0 ± 1.8 pg/mL in 5 normal volunteers. No significant differences in patients with septic shock between those with and without neutropenia *2132* In septic shock increase of 3 to 4 fold observed where increase greatest in surviving patients *4095*

Interleukin-6 *Serum Increase* In 10 neutropenic patients mean concentration of 34.7 ± 32.8 pg/mL before chemotherapy significantly higher than 13.0 ± 1.9 pg/mL in 5 normal volunteers. No significant differences between neutropenic and non-neutropenic patients with septic shock *2132* In a group of patients with septic shock mean concentrations on days 0 and 1 385 ± 251 pg/mL, 262 ± 238 pg/mL on days 2 and 4, 85 ± 88 pg/mL on days 5 and 10 compared with 3 ± 4 pg/mL in healthy controls *1079* In 16 patients with sepsis or septic shock mean concentration of 12,405 ± 6,662 pg/mL significantly higher than 7 ± 1 pg/mL in 10 healthy controls *2808* In 30 patients with severe septic shock mean concentration of 27,256 ± 7,895 pg/mL significantly different from < 10 pg/mL in healthy controls *5343* In 25 patients with septic shock significant increase of concentration to 15,627 ± 4,336 pg/mL in nonsurvivors compared with mean concentration of 20 ± 6 pg/mL in healthy controls. Concentration of 3,947 ± 1,410 pg/mL in survivors also increased *3310*

Interleukin-8 *Serum Increase* In 29 patients with septic shock mean concentration of 6.28 ± 9.00 ng/mL significantly higher than less than 0.01 ng/mL in 20 normal volunteers *1362* In 30 patients with severe septic shock mean concentration of 2,492 ± 673 pg/mL significantly different from < 10 pg/mL in healthy controls *5343*

Interleukin-10 *Serum Increase* Median concentration in 21 patients with septic shock 58 pg/mL significantly higher than 11 pg/mL in patients with septicemia without shock *3287*

Lactate *Blood Increase* Circulatory shock associated with concentration above 2.0 mmol/L. Concentration in patients who died 6.6 mmol/L versus 4.7 mmol/L who did not *255*
Plasma Increase In 20 patients with septic shock on admission to hospital mean concentration of 3.1 ± 0.3 mmol/L significantly higher than in healthy adults *5364* In 22 patients with sepsis on admission to hospital mean concentration of 1.4 ± 0.2 mmol/L significantly higher than in healthy adults *5364*

Leukemia Inhibitory Factor *Serum Increase* Detected in serum in only a few patients with septic shock *1614*

Leukocytes *Blood Increase* In 6 patients with septic shock mean concentration of 18.8 ± 12.4 x 10^3/µL *3868* In 20 patients with septic shock on admission to hospital mean concentration of 15.3 ± 3.1 10^9/L significantly higher than in healthy adults *5364*

α_2-Macroglobulin *Serum Decrease* Significant reduction observed especially in fatal cases *3320*

Methemoglobin *Blood Increase* In 6 patients with septic shock mean concentration of 1.0% higher than 0.6 - 0.7% in patients without infections *3868*

Neuropeptide Y *Plasma Increase* In 20 patients with septic shock at onset of hypotension mean concentration of 26 ± 10 pmol/L significantly higher than 9 ± 2 pmol/L in healthy adults *5364*

Neutrophil Elastase *Plasma Increase* In 29 patients with septic shock mean concentration of 694.3 ± 434.6 ng/mL significantly higher than 72.3 ± 35.3 ng/mL in 20 normal volunteers *1362*

Nitrate plus Nitrite *Serum Increase* In a group of patients with septic shock mean concentrations on days 0 and 1 of 72 ± 60 µmol/L, 190 ± 252 µmol/L on days 2 and 4, 11 ± 99 µmol/L on days 5 and 10 compared with 30 ± 9 µmol/L in healthy controls *1079*

Phospholipase A_2 *Serum Increase* Increased catalytic activity observed in patients with septic shock, sepsis and Gram-negative infections. Activity correlated with concentration of immunoreactive synovial-type PLA2-II *3766* Increased concentrations reported *46*

Plasminogen Activator Inhibitor-1 *Plasma Increase* Significant increase of plasminogen activator inhibitor type I in 52 patients with septic shock compared with a control group with concentrations highest in those individuals dying within one week *4203*

Prekallikrein *Plasma Decrease* Significant reduction observed especially in fatal cases *3320*

Procalcitonin *Plasma Increase* In a group of patients with septic shock mean concentrations on days 0 and 1 of 96 ± 181 ng/mL, 135 ± 174 ng/mL on days 2 and 4, 72 ± 47 ng/mL on days 5 and 10 compared with < 0.1 ng/mL in healthy controls *1079*

Protein C *Plasma Decrease* Significantly reduced to 47 ± 20% in 13 patients with septic shock *2135*

Protein S *Plasma No Effect* No significant change observed in 13 patients with septic shock with concentration of 88 ± 20.0% compared with 96 ± 15% in normals *2135*

Protein S, Free *Plasma No Effect* In 13 patients with septic shock mean concentration of 30 ± 8.7% compared with 29 ± 9% in normals *2135*

Soluble Tumor Necrosis Factor Receptor-p55 *Serum Increase* In a group of patients with septic shock mean concentrations on days 0 and 1 16.1 ± 11.2 ng/mL, 20.3 ± 16.2 ng/mL on days 2 and 4, 10.2 ± 8.1 ng/mL on days 5 and 10 compared with 1.1 ± 0.7 ng/mL in healthy controls *1079*

Soluble Tumor Necrosis Factor Receptor-p75 *Serum Increase* In a group of patients with septic shock mean concentrations on days 0 and 1 30.2 ± 36.9 ng/mL, 39.8 ± 44.4 ng/mL on days 2 and 4, 18.5 ± 15.3 ng/mL on days 5 and 10 compared with 2.4 ± 1.4 ng/mL in healthy controls *1079*

Substance P *Plasma Decrease* In 20 patients with septic shock at onset of hypotension mean concentration of 58 ± 11 pmol/L significantly lower than 117 ± 7 pmol/L in healthy adults *5364*

Testosterone *Serum Decrease* In men with septic shock mean concentration decreased *833*

Thrombin/Antithrombin III Complex *Plasma Increase* High concentrations observed in 12 of 13 patients with septic shock *2135*

Thrombomodulin *Plasma Increase* In 30 patients with severe septic shock mean concentration of 8.2 ± 0.9 functional U/mL significantly different from < 4.5 functional U/mL in healthy controls *5343*

Tumor Necrosis Factor-α *Serum Increase* Concentration increased in 3 of 14 patients with septic shock and in 10 normal individuals whose blood samples were stimulated by lipopolysaccharide but in none of 96 unstimulated normal donor samples *3758* Mean concentration of 242.5 pg/mL observed in 18 newborns with sepsis significantly different from 61.5 pg/mL in 20 preterm and 20 full-term healthy control neonates *209* In a group of patients with septic shock mean concentrations on days 0 and 1 108 ± 132 pg/mL, 131 ± 92 pg/mL on days 2 and 4, 53 ± 27 pg/mL on days 5 and 10 compared with 6 ± 1.5 pg/mL in healthy controls *1079* In 30 patients with severe septic shock mean concentration of 138.6 ± 22.0 pg/mL significantly different from < 5 pg/mL in healthy controls *5343* In 25 patients with septic shock significant increase of concentration to 42 ± 7 pg/mL in nonsurvivors compared with mean concentration of 10 ± 5 pg/mL in healthy controls *3310* In 10 neutropenic patients mean concentration of 18.8 ± 8.4 pg/mL before chemotherapy significantly higher than 11.0 ± 2.2 pg/mL in 5 normal volunteers. Mean concentration in septic shock patients with neutropenia higher than in those without *2132*

Urea *Serum Increase* In 20 patients with septic shock on admission to hospital mean concentration of 21.5 ± 5.2 μmol/L significantly higher than in healthy adults *5364*

786.09 Apnea

Calcium *Serum Increase* In 7 infants aged 2 days to 3 months with apnea severe hypercalcemia observed in all, 6 of whom were otherwise healthy *2762*

786.09 Chronic Respiratory Insufficiency

Nitrate plus Nitrite *Serum Increase* In 19 patients with CRI mean concentration of 8.27 ± 0.95 μmol/L compared with 3.48 ± 0.40 μmol/L in 11 healthy controls *212*

Thiol Groups, Total *Serum Decrease* In 13 patients with CRI mean concentration of 281 ± 29 μmol/L compared with 520 ± 19 μmol/L in 7 healthy controls *212*

787.00 Vomiting

Ammonia *Urine Increase* Increase in urine ammonia in prolonged vomiting with associated achlorhydria and ketosis *1290*

Bicarbonate *Serum Increase* Metabolic alkalosis *1290*

Chloride *Urine Decrease* Excessive chloride loss, due to vomiting *1290*

Creatinine *Serum Increase* Leading to reduced renal blood flow (prerenal azotemia) *5544*

Ketones *Urine Increase* Children are more liable to develop ketosis than adults with persistent vomiting *1290*

pH *Blood Increase* Metabolic alkalosis *1290*

Phosphate *Serum Decrease* Of 100 patients with hypophosphatemia, 12% was due to vomiting, 40% to intravenous glucose feeding, and miscellaneous or unexplained in the rest *421*

Potassium *Serum Decrease* Deficiency results from decreased intake of potassium, loss in the vomitus, and most important, from renal potassium wasting *4891*

Sodium *Serum Increase* Resulting in relative depletion of chloride and hydrogen ions (developing metabolic alkalosis), can lead to an increase in plasma sodium concentration in the presence of gross dehydration *1290*

Urea Nitrogen *Serum Increase* Dehydration *1025* Salt and water depletion causes reduced renal blood flow leading to prerenal azotemia *5544* Dehydration *1642*

788.20 Urinary Retention

Prostate-specific Antigen *Serum Increase* Urinary retention can cause up to a fivefold increase in PSA independent of any associated cancer of the prostate *1543*

789.00 Abdominal Pain

Basic Fibroblast Growth Factor *Serum No Effect* In 20 children with functional abdominal pain mean concentration of 10.53 ± 1.88 pg/mL not significantly different from 10.72 ± 1.38 pg/mL in 49 control children *546*

789.00 Acute Abdomen

Amylase *Serum No Effect* In 34 patients with acute abdominal disorders median concentration of 178 U/L (range 78 - 711) not higher than 180 U/L (range 60 - 300) in 120 healthy controls *2089*

Ascorbic Acid *Serum Decrease* In 27 patients with acute abdominal crisis median concentrations of vitamin C and ascorbic acid were respectively 3.7 (0.6 - 15) μg/mL and 2.3 (< 0.5 - 15) μg/mL compared with 15 (6.3 - 19) μg/mL and 12 (4.5 - 18) μg/mL in 30 healthy volunteers *4701*

Trypsin-2-α_1-Antitrypsin *Serum Increase* In 34 patients with acute abdominal disorders median concentration of 7.6 μg/L (range 2.4 - 36) higher than 4.2 μg/L (range 2.1 - 14) in 120 healthy controls *2089*

Trypsinogen-2 *Serum No Effect* In 34 patients with acute abdominal disorders median concentration of 27 μg/L (range 7.6 - 145) higher than 39 μg/L (range 11 - 233) in 120 healthy controls *2089*

789.00 Infantile Colic

5-Hydroxyindoleacetic Acid *Urine Increase* In 16 patients with infantile colic mean concentration of 4.19 ± 0.95 μg/mL in random specimens significantly different from 1.35 ± 0.35 μg/mL in 10 healthy controls *2864*

790.99 Hyperthyroxine-binding Globulinemia

Thyroxine Binding Globulin *Serum Decrease* Observed as consequence of natural excess of thyroxine binding globulin *206*

Thyroxine (T4) *Serum Decrease* Observed as consequence of natural excess of thyroxine binding globulin *206*

791.00 Bence-Jones Myeloma

Albumin *Serum Decrease* Mean concentration in 4 patients with Bence-Jones myeloma of 4.1 ± 0.1 g/dL compared with 4.5 ± 0.1 g/dL in 11 healthy controls *4582*

Albumin:Globulin Ratio *Serum Increase* Mean ratio in 4 patients with Bence-Jones myeloma of 1.9 ± 0.1 *4582*

Erythrocytes *Blood Decrease* Mean concentration in 4 patients with Bence-Jones myeloma of 266 ± 25 x 10^4/μL *4582*

791.00 Bence-Jones Myeloma *(continued)*

immunoglobulin A *Serum* *No Effect* Mean concentration in 4 patients with Bence-Jones myeloma of 42 ± 32 mg/dL *4582*

Immunoglobulin G *Serum* *Increase* Mean concentration in 4 patients with Bence-Jones myeloma of 3,599 ± 1,234 mg/dL *4582*

Immunoglobulin M *Serum* *No Effect* Mean concentration in 4 patients with Bence-Jones myeloma of 16 ± 11 mg/dL *4582*

Leukocytes *Blood* *No Effect* Mean concentration in 4 patients with Bence-Jones myeloma of 4,563 ± 516 /µL *4582*

Platelets *Blood* *No Effect* Mean concentration in 4 patients with Bence-Jones myeloma of 22.1 ± 1.4 x 10^4 /µL *4582*

Protein *Serum* *No Effect* Mean concentration in 4 patients with Bence-Jones myeloma of 6.3 ± 0.2 g/dL *4582*

791.30 Myoglobinuria

Aldolase *Serum* *Increase* Found in paroxysmal myoglobinuria due to muscle destruction *1290*

Aspartate Aminotransferase *Serum* *Increase* Observed effect *1290*

Creatine *Serum* *Increase* Muscle destruction after crush injury *1290*

Creatine Kinase *Serum* *Increase* Increases in necrosis or acute atrophy of striated muscle *5544*

11-Hydroxycorticosteroids *Urine* *No Effect* Endocrine studies are normal *5544*

17-Hydroxycorticosteroids *Urine* *No Effect* No significant abnormality observed *5544*

17-Ketogenic Steroids *Urine* *No Effect* Usually no effect on excretion of 17-KS *5544*

799.90 Disease, Unspecified

Lipoprotein Lp(a) *Serum* *Increase* In 10 patients with unspecified diseases mean concentration of 0.274 ± 0.431 g/L significantly greater than 0.118 ± 0.193 g/L in 100 healthy controls *3505*

INJURY AND POISONING

820.80 Hip Fracture

Albumin *Serum* *Decrease* In 12 patients living in nursing homes prior to surgery mean concentration of 2.98 g/dL significantly less than 3.44 g/dL and had poorer outcome. 10 patients who died had a mean concentration of 2.94 g/dL lower than 3.42 g/dL in those who survived. 30% mortality in patients with concentrations < 3.0 g/dL compared with 21% in those with concentrations greater than 3.0 g/dL *641*
Serum *No Effect* In 58 elderly women mean initial concentration of 39 ± 4 g/L not significantly different from 40 ± 3 g/L in 58 age-matched controls *59*

Alkaline Phosphatase *Serum* *Increase* In 57 women with hip fractures mean activity of 3.6 ± 1.6 µkat/L significantly different from 3.1 ± 1.0 µkat/L in 93 postmenopausal women *5129*
Serum *No Effect* In 58 elderly women mean initial activity of 2.9 ± 1.0 µkat/L not significantly different from 3.3 ± 1.2 µkat/L in 58 age-matched controls *59*

Alkaline Phosphatase, Bone Isoenzyme *Serum* *Increase* In 57 women with hip fractures mean activity of 29.1 ± 16.2 U/L significantly different from 25.1 ± 9.3 U/L in 93 postmenopausal women *5129*

Bilirubin *Serum* *Increase* Concentration may be increased in patients with hematomas, such as after a fracture of the neck of the femur, due to enhanced bilirubin production induced by increased activity of heme oxygenase *4617*

Calcium *Serum* *No Effect* In 58 elderly women mean initial concentration of 2.40 ± 0.12 mmol/L not significantly different from 2.40 ± 0.16 mmol/L in 58 age-matched controls *59*

Creatinine *Serum* *No Effect* In 58 elderly women mean initial concentration of 88 ± 22 µmol/L not significantly different from 92 ± 18 µmol/L in 58 age-matched controls *59*

Osteocalcin *Serum* *Decrease* In 58 elderly women mean initial concentration of 7.2 ± 2.9 ng/mL significantly less than 10.3 ± 4.8 ng/mL in 58 age-matched controls *59*

829.00 Bone Fracture

Albumin *Serum* *No Effect* In 12 patients with traumatic bone fracture no significant change observed 24 to 48 hours after trauma *3732*

Alkaline Phosphatase *Serum* *Increase* In 54 postmenopausal women with vertebral fractures mean activity of 3.6 ± 1.3 µkat/L significantly different from 3.1 ± 1.0 µkat/L in 93 postmenopausal women *5129* Rises in proportion to the formation of new bone cells *1025* In 20 patients following isolated tibial shaft fracture activity increased significantly in first 14 days following injury *1032* In 20 individuals following fracture of a tibia activity rose to a significantly increased extent by day 14 but in only 3 specimens did activity exceed normal range *550* Rises in proportion to the formation of new bone cells *1642*
Serum *No Effect* In 195 elderly women who subsequently developed hip fractures mean activity of 82 ± 22 U/L not different from 80 ± 35 U/L in women who did not *1105* In 19 men with a hip fracture mean activity not significantly different from that in age-matched controls *5213* In 26 elderly patients with femoral neck fracture mean concentration of 221 U/L within 24 h, but significantly increased to 281 U/L 1 week later, in comparison with reference range in elderly of 98 - 280 U/L *5216* In 12 men aged 22 to 64 years mean activty of 150 ± 24 U/L 24 to 48 hours after trauma and 160 ± 30 U/L 1 week after trauma compared with 160 ± 29 U/L in healthy controls *3732*

Alkaline Phosphatase, Bone Isoenzyme *Serum* *Decrease* In 20 patients following isolated tibial shaft fracture activity started to decrease by the fourth day following injury *1032* In 20 individuals following fracture of a tibia concentration decreased to a significant extent by day 4 reaching a nadir by day 8 at which time it started to increase reaching a concentration higher than day 1 by week 10 *550*
Serum *Increase* In 20 individuals following fracture of a tibia concentration decreased to a significant extent by day 4 reaching a nadir by day 8 at which time it started to increase reaching a concentration higher than day 1 by week 10 *550* In 54 postmenopausal women with vertebral fractures mean activity of 30.0 ± 15.3 U/L significantly different from 25.1 ± 9.3 U/L in 93 postmenopausal women *5129* In 20 patients following isolated tibial shaft fracture activity started to increase after 14 days following injury and by week 10 was significantly higher than on day 1. Rise continued to increase to week 20 and mirrored total activity *1032*

Androgen Index, Free (FAI) *Plasma* *Decrease* Mean index of 14.1 in 19 men with a fractured hip signficantly less than 31.5 in age-matched controls *5213*

Calcium *Serum* *Decrease* Commonly observed in elderly individuals with hip fractures, more so than in age matched controls *2023*
Serum *No Effect* In 12 patients with traumatic bone fracture no significant change observed 24 to 48 hours after trauma *3732* Mean concentration in 19 men with hip fractures not significantly different from that in healthy age-matched controls *5213* In 26 elderly patients with femoral neck fracture mean concentration within 24 h of 2.26 mmol/L, 1 week later 2.28 mmol/L compared with reference range in elderly of 2.2 - 2.6 mmol/L *5216*

Carbon Dioxide Partial Pressure *Blood* *Decrease* Decreased arterial pO_2 associated with normal or decreased pCO_2 with associated fat embolism *5545*
Blood *Normal* Decreased arterial pO_2 associated with normal or decreased pCO_2 with associated fat embolism *5545*

Creatine *Urine* *Increase* Increased breakdown *5544*

Creatinine *Serum* *No Effect* In 195 elderly women mean concentration in those who subsequently developed hip fractures mean concentration of 9.2 ± mg/L not significantly different from 7.9 ± 2.3 mg/L in those who did not *1105* In 26 elderly patients with femoral neck fractures mean concentration of 98.0 µmol/L within 24 h of admission, 101 µmol/L 1 week after surgery in comparison with reference range in elderly of 60 - 120 µmol/L *5216* In 12 patients with traumatic bone fracture no significant change observed 24 to 48 hours after trauma *3732*

1,25-Dihydroxy Vitamin D *Serum* *No Effect* In 26 elderly patients with femoral neck fractures mean concentration prior to surgery 39.6 pmol/L compared with 43.7 pmol/L 1 week after surgery and reference range in elderly of 26.5-72.3 pmol/L *5216*

1,25-Dihydroxy Vitamin D_3 *Serum* *Decrease* In 18 elderly women with bone fractures mean concentration of 26.0 ± 17.0 ng/L compared with 38.0 ± 13.0 ng/L in age and sex matched controls *4435*

24,25-Dihydroxy Vitamin D_3 *Serum* *Decrease* Relative decrease observed in all 7 patients studied during long bone fracture repair, with absolute decrease observed in three to nondetectable concentrations *5171*

Fat *Serum* *Increase* Fat globules observed in 42 - 67% of cases *5545*
Sputum *Increase* Fat globules found in sputum of some patients *5545*
Urine *Increase* In 60% of cases *5545*

Fatty Acids (FFA), Free *Serum* *Increase* Reported effect *5545*

Fibrin Degradation Products *Plasma* *Increase* In 37 adults with a fracture of the lower extremity mean concentration of 7.8 ± 14 mg/L on day of admission and 1.8 ± 2.5 mg/L on next day significantly higher than < 0.3 mg/L in 10 healthy controls *4939*

Fibrinogen Degradation Products *Plasma* *Increase* In 37 adults with a fracture of the lower extremity mean concentration of 1.2 ± 2.2 mg/L on day of admission and 0.48 ± 0.34 mg/L on next day significantly higher than < 0.25 mg/L in 10 healthy controls *4939*

γ-Glutamyltransferase *Serum* *No Effect* In 12 patients with traumatic bone fracture no significant change observed 24 to 48 hours after trauma *3732*

Hemoglobin *Blood* *Decrease* Unexplained fall after traumatic fracture *5545*

25-Hydroxy Vitamin D_3 *Serum* *Decrease* Low concentrations commonly observed in patients with hip fracture who were old, incapable of independent daily life, had poor dietary habits, reduced nutritional status and spent insufficient time in sunlight. Osteoporosis commonly observed *2023*
Serum *No Effect* Concentration within normal range in 7 patients during large bone fracture repair *5171*

25-Hydroxy Vitamin D *Serum* *Decrease* In 26 elderly patients with fracture of femoral neck mean concentration prior to surgery 11.6 nmol/L, 8.9 nmol/L 1 week after surgery, in comparison with reference range in elderly of 15.1-53.5 nmol/L *5216* Mean concentration in 19 men with hip fracture 9.7 ng/mL significantly less than 21.5 ng/mL in age-matched controls *5213*
Serum *No Effect* In 195 elderly women in those who subsequently developed hip fractures mean concentration of 14 ± 8 ng/mL not significantly different from 17 ± 12 ng/mL in those who did not *1105*

Hydroxyproline *Urine* *No Effect* In 12 men 24 to 48 hours after trumatic bone fracture mean excretion of 0.010 ± 0.005 mol/mol creatinine and 0.015 ± 0.003 mol/mol creatinine 1 week after fracture not significantly different from 0.010 ± 0.005 mol/mol creatinine in control individuals *3732*

Insulin-like Growth Factor-I *Serum* *No Effect* No significant difference observed between concentrations in old women with (251 ± 34 μg/L) and without bone fractures (262 ± 48 μg/L) *4435*

Lipase *Serum* *Increase* In 30 - 50% of cases *5545*

Magnesium *Serum* *Decrease* Mean concentration of 0.77 mmol/L in 19 men with hip fractures significantly less than 0.85 mmol/L in age-matched controls *5213*

Osteocalcin *Serum* *Decrease* In 12 men aged 22 to 64 years mean concentration reduced to 1.7 ± 0.9 ng/mL 24 to 48 hours and 2.8 ± 1.1 ng/mL 1 week following traumatic bone fracture compared with 3.3 ± 1.3 ng/mL in healthy controls. Effect probably stress related *3732*
Serum *Increase* Mean concentrations of carboxylated (6.4 ± 3.2 ng/mL) and noncarboxylated (1.62 ± 1.16 ng/mL) osteocalcin in elderly institutionalized women who subseuently developed hip fractures higher than 5.4 ± 2.8 ng/mL and 0.94 ± 0.93 ng/mL in those who did not develop hip fractures *1105* In 20 individuals following fracture of a tibia concentration increased to a significant extent by day 4 but then declined to a nadir by week 5 when the concentration was not significantly different from that on day 1, but thereafter it rose progressively so that by week 20 it was significantly higher than at the time of the injury *550*
Serum *No Effect* In 26 elderly patients with femoral neck fracture mean concentration on admission 3.12 ng/mL significantly increased to 3.73 ng/mL 1 week after surgery but still within reference range in elderly, 3.2 - 8.1 ng/mL *5216* In 20 individuals following fracture of a tibia concentration increased to a significant extent by day 4 but then declined to a nadir by week 5 when the concentration was not significantly different from that on day 1, but thereafter it rose progressively so that by week 20 it was significantly higher than at the time of the injury *550*

Oxygen Partial Pressure *Blood* *Decrease* Decreased arterial pO_2 associated with normal or decreased pCO_2 with associated fat embolism *5545*

Oxygen Saturation *Blood* *Decrease* Decreased arterial pO_2 associated with normal or decreased pCO_2 with associated fat embolism *5545*

Parathyroid Hormone *Plasma* *Increase* In 20 of 39 elderly patients with hip fractures significant increases in intact parathyroid hormone concentration observed *5722* In 18 elderly women with bone fractures mean concentration of 58.5 ± 8.2 ng/L compared with 13.5 ± 2.7 ng/L in 18 elderly women without bone fractures *4435*
Plasma *No Effect* In 195 elderly women mean concentration in those who subsequently developed hip fractures of 62 ± 27 pg/mL compared with 50 ± 30 pg/mL in those who did not *1105* Mean concentration in 19 men with a hip fracture not significantly different from that in age-matched controls *5213*

Phosphate *Serum* *Increase* Observed in some patients *1290* Observed effect *5544*
Serum *No Effect* In 26 elderly patients with femoral neck fractures mean concentration of 1.15 mmol/L within 24 h of admission, 1.11 mmol/L 1 week later in comparison with reference range of 0.8-1.4 mmol/L in elderly *5216* In 12 patients with traumatic bone fracture no significant change observed 24 to 48 hours after trauma *3732* Mean concentration in 19 men with hip fractures not significantly different from that in healthy age-matched controls *5213*

Platelets *Blood* *Decrease* Observed effect in some patients *5545*

Prothrombin Fragment 1.2 *Plasma* *Increase* In 37 adults with a fracture of the lower extremity mean concentration of 2.1 ± 1.4 nmol/L on day of admission and 1.4 ± 1.0 nmol/L on next day significantly higher than median of 0.7 (range of 0.3 - 1.8) nmol/L in 10 healthy controls *4939*

Pyridoxal Phosphate *Serum* *Decrease* In 10 of 20 patients with femoral bone fractures mean concentration less than 13 nmol/L *4338*

Soluble Fibrin Monomer *Plasma* *Increase* In 37 adults with a fracture of the lower extremity mean concentration of 29 ± 30 nmol/L on day of admission and 17 ± 20 nmol/L on next day significantly higher than median of 4 (range < 3 - 19) nmol/L in 10 healthy controls *4939*

Testosterone *Serum* *Decrease* In 19 men with a fractured hip mean concentration of 6.7 mmol/L significantly less than mean of 12.5 nmol/L in age-matched controls *5213*

Thrombin/Antithrombin III Complex *Plasma* *Increase* In 37 adults with a fracture of the lower extremity mean concentration of 47 ± 34 ng/mL on day of admission and 25 ± 14 ng/mL on next day significantly higher than median of 1.7 (range 1.2 - 2.6) ng/mL in 10 healthy controls *4939*

Triglycerides *Serum* *Increase* After traumatic fracture *5545*

Vitamin D Binding Protein *Serum* *No Effect* In 26 elderly patients with femoral neck fractures mean concentration presurgery of 299 mg/L but significantly increased to 354 mg/L 1 week after surgery, in comparison with reference range in elderly of 284 - 373 mg/L *5216*

854.00 **Brain Trauma**

3,3'-Di-iodothyronine *Serum* *Decrease* In 15 patients with brain injury mean concentration of 36.2 ± 19.4 pmol/L not significantly different from that in 15 healthy age and sex-matched controls in whom the mean plasma concentration was 54.1 ± 19.3 pmol/L *4138*

Interleukin-6 *Cerebrospinal Fluid* *Increase* In 15 children ventricular CSF concentrations were 3,158 ± 622 pg/mL, 1,112 ± 337 pg/mL and 827 ± 194 pg/mL on days 1, 2 and 3 respectively following traumatic brain injury significantly increased in comparison with 21 ± 6 pg/mL in 20 control children *377*

854.00 Brain Trauma *(continued)*

Interleukin-10 *Cerebrospinal Fluid* *Increase* In 15 children ventricular CSF concentrations were 47.2 ± 12.9 pg/mL, 21.0 ±6.7 pg/mL and 15.5 ± 5.9 pg/mL on days 1, 2 and 3 respectively following traumatic brain injury significantly increased in comparison with 21 ± 6 pg/mL in 20 control children *377*

854.00 Head Injury

α_1-Antichymotrypsin *Serum* *Increase* Mean concentration increased above reference interval of 47.9 ± 8.1 mg/dL in 2 of 2 patients (100%) with head-injury dementia *3044*

Creatine Kinase BB-Isoenzyme *Cerebrospinal Fluid* *Increase* Increased activity and CK-B mass concentration observed in first 24 hours following brain injury, higher than in the next 48 hours in 80% patients *3629*

Interleukin-6 *Serum* *Increase* Thirty patients with Glasgow Coma Scale (GCS) scores of 3 through 10 were observed for 15 days after head injury. Peak elevation of plasma IL-6 occurred on admission (85 ± 12 U/mL; normal level is less than 2 U/mL) and then decreased during the hospital course to a level of 29 ± 4 U/mL on day 15 *3396*

Leu-Enkephalin *Cerebrospinal Fluid* *Increase* In 15 severe head trauma patients who survived mean concentrations of 1.7 ± 0.2 pmol/mL on day 1, 1.9 ± 0.2 pmol/mL on day 4 and 1.5 ± 0.4 pmol/mL on day 7 significantly different from 0.9 ± 0.5 pmol/mL in 16 controls with herniated lumbar discs *4972*
Cerebrospinal Fluid *No Effect* In 15 severe head trauma patients who died mean concentration of 1.3 ± 0.3 pmol/mL on day 1, 1.0 ± 0.2 pmol/mL at day 4 and 0.8 ± 0.2 pmol/mL on day 7 not significantly different from 0.9 ± 0.5 pmol/mL in 16 controls with herniated lumbar discs *4972*

Met-Enkephalin *Cerebrospinal Fluid* *Increase* In 15 severe head trauma patients who died mean concentration of 4.1 ± 0.4 pmol/mL on day 1, 4.2 ± 0.2 pmol/mL on day 4 and 4.4 ± 0.5 pmol/mL on day 7 and 4.1 ± 0.5 pmol/mL on day 1, 3.8 ± 0.4 pmol/mL on day 4 and 2.8 ± 0.3 pmol/mL on day 7 in 16 who survivedsignificantly different from 1.9 ± 0.2 pmol/mL in 16 controls with herniated lumbar discs *4972*

Neuron-specific Enolase *Cerebrospinal Fluid* *Increase* In 19 patients with severe brain injury mean concentration of 183.6 ng/mL in the first 24 hours following injury rising to 356.2 ng/mL in the next 48 hours *3629*

Neuropeptide Y *Cerebrospinal Fluid* *Increase* In 16 severe head trauma patients mean concentration of 54.9 ± 15.5 pg/mL in 3 who died significantly different from 25.9 ± 12.3 pg/mL in 5 healthy controls *4973*
Cerebrospinal Fluid *No Effect* In 16 severe head trauma patients mean concentration of 20.5 ± 4.7 pg/mL in 13 who survived not significantly different from 25.9 ± 12.3 pg/mL in 5 healthy controls *4973*

Prothrombin Fragment 1.2 *Plasma* *Increase* In 14 patients with isolated head injury mean concentration on admission to hospital of 5.7 ± 4.1 nmol/L significantly different from median of 0.7 nmol/L in control population *4938*

Thrombin/Antithrombin III Complex *Plasma* *Increase* In 15 patients with multiple trauma and head injury mean concentration on admission to hospital of 79 ± 129 ng/mL significantly different from median of 1.7 ng/mL in control population *4938*

861.01 Cardiac Contusion

Creatine Kinase MB-Isoenzyme *Serum* *Increase* All of six patients with cardiac contusion had increased concentration *31* *31*

Creatine Kinase MB-Isoenzyme:Creatine Kinase Ratio *Serum* *Increase* Three of six patients with cardiac contusion had increased ratio (greater than 5%) *31*

Troponin I *Serum* *Increase* All of six patients with cardiac contusion had increased concentration *31*

929.90 Crush Injury

α_1-Acid Glycoprotein *Serum* *Increase* One of the most reliable indicators of acute inflammation *4373* *3713* *4696* *2597* *4241* *4853*

Alanine Aminotransferase *Serum* *Increase* In 3 of 4 patients with crush syndrome following an earthquake mean activity increased *3530*

Amylase *Serum* *Increase* Crush injury to abdomen resulting in contusion, rupture or hemorrhage provokes hyperamylasemia *4707*

Aspartate Aminotransferase *Serum* *Increase* Observed effect *1290* *1980* Slightly to moderate increase *1025* In 3 of 4 patients with crush syndrome following an earthquake mean activity increased *3530*

Catecholamines *Urine* *Increase* Due to severe stress *2034*

Creatine *Urine* *Increase* Increased formation myopathy *5544*

Creatine Kinase *Serum* *Increase* Increases in necrosis or acute atrophy of striated muscle *5544* Most reliable measure of skeletal muscle damage *1025* In 4 of 4 patients with crush syndrome following an earthquake mean activity increased *3530* Raised for approximately 15 days, especially if associated arterial obstruction *1290*

Creatine Kinase Isoenzymes *Serum* *Increase* Increased release of non-myocardial CK. In most cases increase in total CK not increased percentage of CK-MB *4750*

17-Hydroxycorticosteroids *Urine* *Increase* Due to severe stress *2034*

17-Ketogenic Steroids *Urine* *Increase* Due to severe stress *2034*

Lactate Dehydrogenase *Serum* *Increase* In 3 of 4 patients with crush syndrome following an earthquake mean activity increased *3530*

Lipase *Serum* *Increase* Activity increases in some patients sustaining severe injury to adipose tissue *4707*

Myoglobin *Urine* *Increase* Sudden muscle damage *1290*

Platelets *Blood* *Increase* Count rises slowly, lasting for 3 weeks in trauma *5545*

949.00 Burns

α_1-Acid Glycoprotein *Serum* *Increase* Generally the plasma concentration is dramatically increased *5869* One of the most reliable indicators of acute inflammation *2597* *3713* Increase observed with maximum about 6 - 8 days after injury *3581* The serum concentrations reached their maximal values after day 5 and remained at a high level throughout the total period studied (7 weeks) *4184* One of the most reliable indicators of acute inflammation *4241* *4373* *4696* *4853*

Adrenomedullin *Plasma* *Increase* In 10 patients with major burns mean concentration of 20.5 ± 3.2 fmol/L significantly different from 5.1 ± 0.2 fmol/mL in healthy controls *5343*

Alanine Aminotransferase *Serum* *Increase* Mean activity increased 67.4% in burned patients during recovery and a 25.6% increase after discharge *813* Rises soon after burn *4707*

Albumin *Serum* *Decrease* In one patient with severe burn injuries to 60% of her body surface area on admission to a referral hospital 55 days after injury, concentration reduced to 22 g/L *4547* Superficial burns reduce capillary membrane semipermeability and cause a disproportionate loss of albumin *4707* Responsible for excessive loss from circulation with subsequent decreased serum concentration *4617* In burn patients concentration decreased rapidly by as much as 50% after severe injury but low concentrations persisted for many weeks *3581*

Aldolase *Serum* *Increase* Cell destruction *5544*

Amino Acids *Plasma* *Increase* In severe burns the peptides derived from the burnt tissues appear in the plasma *1290* Considerable muscle catabolism may occur with increased plasma concentrations of amino acids, zinc and other cellular products *5174*
Urine *Increase* Amino acids and peptides from burnt tissues are excreted in urine *1290*

Amylase *Serum* *Decrease* Decreased in severe burns *1290*
Serum *Increase* May be associated with hyperamylasemia *3024*

Amyloid A *Serum* *Increase* Increased concentration, especially shortly after accident, associated with unfavorable prognosis *720*

Amyloid A Protein *Serum* *Increase* In 45 adult patients with burns covering 20 to 95% of their body surface area on admission mean concentration in those who survived of 33 ± 32 mg/L compared with 122 ± 43 mg/L in those with fatal outcome and less than 1 mg/L in healthy controls *716*

Androstenediol *Plasma* *Decrease* In men following burn injury nonsignificant decrease observed 10 - 23 days post-burn *2996*

Androstenediol Sulfate *Plasma* *Decrease* Nonsignificant decrease observed in men 10 - 23 days following thermal injury *2996*

Androstenedione *Plasma* *Decrease* Significant decrease observed in men during first four weeks following thermal injury *2996*

Angiotensin-II *Plasma* *Increase* Concentration increased on admission in burn patients with 30 - 66% burn injury *975*

Angiotensin-converting Enzyme *Serum* *Decrease* Mean concentration in 17 patients with burned lungs reached nadir of 16 μmol/min/L on seventh day compared with normal range of 65 - 135 μmol/min/L *4152*

α_1-Antichymotrypsin *Serum* *Increase* Acutely burned children exhibited a rapid rise to a maximum on day 10 postburn, which remained elevated after 60 days *2457* Increased after burn injury with peak about 6 - 8 days *3581*

Antidiuretic Hormone *Plasma* *Increase* In patients with 30 - 66% burn injury mean concentration increased 50 times normal on day of admission but returned to normal by day 4 to 5 *975*

α_1-Antitrypsin *Serum* *Decrease* Decreased during acute phase of thermal burn *4373* *4763* *83* *4371* *4241* Measured acute-phase reactants including fibrinogen, α_1-antitrypsin, C_1 inhibitor, and α_2-plasmin inhibitor. After initial declines, these four proteins increased rapidly in survivors. The levels of acute phase proteins in nonsurvivors remained low *5351*
Serum *Increase* Increased *4373* *83* *4371* *4763* *4241* Measured acute-phase reactants including fibrinogen, α_1-antitrypsin, C_1 inhibitor, and α_2-plasmin inhibitor. After initial declines, these four proteins increased rapidly in survivors. The levels of acute phase proteins in nonsurvivors remained low *5351* Increased after burn injury with maximum about 6 - 8 days *3581*

Aspartate Aminotransferase *Serum* *Increase* Mean increase of 67.4% during recovery and 25.6% increase observed after discharge from hospital *813* Rises soon after burn *4707*

Atrial Natriuretic Peptide *Plasma* *Increase* In patients with 30 - 66% burn injury, concentration normal on first admission to hospital but significant increase observed on days 3 to 5 *975*

C_1-Inhibitor *Serum* *Decrease* Measured acute-phase reactants including fibrinogen, α_1-antitrypsin, C_1 inhibitor, and α_2-plasmin inhibitor. After initial declines, these four proteins increased rapidly in survivors. The levels of acute phase proteins in nonsurvivors remained low *5351* Sensitivity of 60% and specificity of 87% *1187*
Serum *Increase* Measured acute-phase reactants including fibrinogen, α_1-antitrypsin, C_1 inhibitor, and α_2-plasmin inhibitor. After initial declines, these four proteins increased rapidly in survivors. The levels of acute phase proteins in nonsurvivors remained low *5351*

Calcium *Serum* *No Effect* On average, free or ionized calcium were in the normal range. However they were weakly correlated with the severity of burn injury *1458*

Catecholamines *Urine* *Increase* With physical or emotional stress *4690* Increased due to severe stress *5544*

Ceruloplasmin *Serum* *Decrease* In one patient with severe burn injuries to 60% of her body surface area on admission to a referral hospital 55 days after injury, concentration reduced to 0.02 g/L (reference interval 0.2 - 0.4 g/L) *4547* Marked depression observed in patients with burn injury *526*

Complement C_1s *Serum* *Decrease* Observed effect *4746*

Complement C_3 *Serum* *Decrease* Caused by hypercatabolism *2694* *1588* *1033* *785*
Serum *Increase* Mean concentration in 17 patients with burned lungs reached significant increase of 1.2 g/L on tenth day compared with normal range of 0.55 - 1.20 g/L *4152*

Copper *Serum* *Decrease* Significant depression of concentration observed in patients with thermal injury with lowest concentrations observed in patients with more than 40% total body surface burns *526* In one patient with severe burn injuries to 60% of her body surface area on admission to a referral hospital 55 days after injury, concentration reduced to < 1 μmol/L (reference interval 12 - 20 μmol/L) *4547* In 31 patients with burn injuries mean concentration of 0.70 (0.1 - 1.6) mg/L compared with 0.7 - 1.6 mg/L in healthy controls: serum copper concentration inversely related to burn surface area (r = -0.611) *1828*
Urine *Increase* In patients with burns mean excretion increased reaching 2.5 times the upper limit of normal 2 weeks postburn *526*

Corticosteroid-Binding Globulin *Serum* *Decrease* In 12 severely burned adult patients mean concentration on day of hospitalization significantly reduced to 18 mg/L from reference interval of 35 to 45 mg/L *416*

Cortisol *Plasma* *Increase* Significant increase observed in men soon after thermal injury *2996*
Urine *Increase* In 12 severely burned adult patients mean excretion on day of hospitalization significantly increased to mean of 480 μg/d, above upper limit of reference interval of 145 μg/d *416*

Cortisol, Free *Plasma* *Increase* In 12 severely burned adult patients mean concentration on day of hospitalization significantly increased to 12.4 μg/dL, above reference interval *416*

C-Reactive Protein *Serum* *Increase* In 45 adult patients with burns covering 20 to 95% of their surface area mean concentration on admission in those who survived was 18 ± 17 mg/L compared with 22 ± 21 mg/L in those who had a fatal outcome and less than 3 mg/L in healthy controls *716* Increased following burn injury with peak increase after about 6 - 8 days *3581*

Creatine *Urine* *Increase* Increased breakdown *5544*

Creatine Kinase *Serum* *Increase* In 8 thermal burn patients there was a significant increase ($p < 0.01$) *1902*

Creatine Kinase Isoenzymes *Serum* *Increase* Increased release of non-myocardial CK. Can be greater than 10% of CK *768* *4750*

Creatinine *Serum* *No Effect* In 10 patients with major burns mean concentration of 0.68 ± 0.10 mg/dL not significantly different from that in healthy controls *5343*

Creatinine Clearance *Urine* *Increase* Mean clearance in 20 burned patients, measured between the 4 - 35 postburn day, was 172.1 ± 48.4 mL/min/1.73 m^2. 13 patients had values > 2 S.D. above the normal *3108*

Dehydroepiandrosterone *Plasma* *Decrease* Significant decrease observed in men during first four weeks following thermal injury *2996*

Diazepam, Free *Serum* *Increase* In 7 burned patients the free fraction of diazepam was higher at 3,5% than the 1.7% typically observed in healthy individuals *5869*

Endothelin-1 *Plasma* *Increase* In 14 patients with burns mean concentration of 6 ± 3 fmol/L significantly higher than < 0.5 fmol/L in healthy controls *2301*

Epinephrine *Plasma* *Increase* A drop in eosinophils with increased corticoid and epinephrine production are manifestations of stress *4730* In patients with 30 - 66% burn injury significant increase observed when patients admitted to hospital *975*
Urine *Increase* Urinary excretion of epinephrine and its metabolites are rough indicators of degree of stress *4730* With physical or emotional stress *4690*

Factor V *Plasma* *Increase* Factor V and VIII may be 4 - 8 times normal for up to 3 months *5545*

Factor VIII *Plasma* *Increase* Factor V and VIII may be 4 - 8 times normal for up to 3 months *5545*

Factor B *Plasma* *Decrease* Found in 50% of patients *4431* *5229*

Fibrinogen *Plasma* *Decrease* Measured acute-phase reactants including fibrinogen, α_1-antitrypsin, C_1 inhibitor, and α_2-plasmin inhibitor. After initial declines, these four proteins increased rapidly in survivors. The levels of acute phase proteins in nonsurvivors remained low *5351* Falls during first 36 h, then rises steeply for up to 3 months *5545*
Plasma *Increase* Falls during the first 36 h and then rises steeply for up to 3 months *5545* Measured acute-phase reactants including fibrinogen, α_1-antitrypsin, C_1 inhibitor, and α_2-plasmin inhibitor. After initial declines, these four proteins increased rapidly in survivors. The levels of acute phase proteins in nonsurvivors remained low *5351*

949.00 **Burns** *(continued)*

Fibronectin *Plasma Decrease* Decreases rapidly in response to insult but responds rapidly with recovery *1959* Significantly reduced concentrations observed in patients with burn injuries *980* Mean concentration in 17 patients with burned lungs reached nadir of 130 mg/L on second day compared with normal range of 200 - 350 mg/L *4152*

Glomerular Filtration Rate *Urine Increase* May rise to very high values *3108*

Glucagon *Plasma Increase* Increased *1290 1038 618*

Glucose *Serum Increase* A syndrome of glycosuria, dehydration, coma, and severe glycosuria without ketosis has been recognized in patients recovering from major burns. This syndrome is distinct from the transient hyperglycemia that occurs immediately after burns or acute trauma *4707*
Urine Increase A syndrome of glycosuria, dehydration, coma, and severe glycosuria without ketosis has been recognized in patients recovering from major burns. This syndrome is distinct from the transient hyperglycemia that occurs immediately after burns or acute trauma *4707*

Glutathione Peroxidase *Serum Decrease* Mean activity decreased in patients with burn injury reverting to baseline only after 20 days *397*

Haptoglobin *Serum Increase* In burn injury patients peak concentration reached about 10 - 12 days after injury *3581*

Hematocrit *Blood Decrease* In 60 patients with burns studied 5 day after injury, when burns < 20% of surface area hematocrit of 0.356 ± 0.15, in those with 20 - 40% 0.343 ± 0.14 and in those > 40% 0.291 ± 0.14 *2800*

Hemoglobin *Blood Decrease* In 60 patients 5 days after injury, in those with < 20% of surface area burned mean concentration of 122 ± 5 g/L, in those 20 - 40% burned of 118 ± 5 g/L and in those > 40% 100 ± 5 g/L *2800* In one patient with severe burn injuries to 60% of her body surface area on admission to a referral hospital 55 days after injury, concentration reduced to 8.1 g/dL *4547*
Plasma Increase Intravascular hemolysis due to thermal burns; injuring RBCs *5544*
Urine Increase Intravascular hemolysis due to thermal burns; injuring RBCs *5544*

β-Hexosaminidase *Urine Decrease* Decreased levels in urine *5229*

Hyaluronan *Serum Increase* In 10 severely burned patients (burn size 28 ± 5% of body surface area) serum concentration was 206 ± 71 μg/L at 24 hours after injury and remained moderately increased for the first week post-injury *3915*

17-Hydroxycorticosteroids *Urine Increase* Increased due to severe stress *5544* Significant increase observed in men following thermal injury *2996*

Imipramine, Free *Serum Decrease* In 7 burned patients a 3-fold increase in the α_1-glycoprotein concentration was associated with a a decrease in the free fraction of imipramine from about 15 to 6.5% *5869*

immunoglobulin A *Serum Decrease* Concentration decreased following burn injury but did not fall below lower limit of normal range and usually returned to normal by about the fourth day after injury *3581*

Immunoglobulin G *Serum Decrease* Lowest concentration observed at 4 - 5 days after injury but gradual return towards normal concentration thereafter which was reached by 8 - 9 days. In some severe cases concentration continued to increase above normal range *3581*

Immunoglobulin M *Serum Decrease* Concentration decreased following burn injury but usually remained within reference range and rise after decrease not so marked *3581*

Interleukin-1 *Serum Increase* 27 burned patients were serially screened by ELISA and compared with cytokine levels in 16 healthy laboratory employees. Plasma samples with detectable amounts of IL-1β were significantly more frequent in burned patients than in controls *1238* Thirty-one patients with second- or third-degree burns, covering 10% to 95% of body surface area. Initial concentrations of IL-1β were increased (mean 188 ± 31 pg/mL) *680*

Interleukin-2 *Serum Increase* IL-2 concentrations significantly increased to 651 ± 137 pg/mL at 36 h after injury in individuals burned less than 20% of their surface area, 1,176 ± 253 pg/mL in those burned 20 - 40% of surface area compared with 474 ± 84 pg/mL in those with burns affecting more than 40% of surface area and less than 390 pg/mL in healthy controls: concentrations continued to increase at day 5 after injury with greatest increases in most severely burned patiens *2800* Concentration increased in plasma of patients with severe burns *3832*

Interleukin-6 *Serum Increase* At 36 hours after injury mean concentration of 141 ± 18 pg/mL in patients with burns affecting less than 20% of surface area, 172 ± 20 pg/mL in those with 20 - 40% affected and 675 ± 266 pg/mL in those with more than 40% of surface area affected compared with 90 ± 5 pg/mL in healthy controls; declines observed in all burned groups observed at 5 days but still above control concentrations *2800* The level of IL-6 was already increased at the first day following injury, and after a dip at day 2 or 3 rapidly reached a second maximal value at day 4 or 5 *4184* 27 burned patients were serially screened by ELISA and compared with cytokine levels in 16 healthy laboratory employees. Plasma samples with detectable amounts of IL-6 were significantly more frequent in burned patients than in controls *1238* Measured levels of interleukin-6 in plasma samples from 18 consecutive burn patients, including three lethal cases, during the early postburn period. In survivors burn injury caused initial increases in interleukin-6 levels that peaked at 6 hours after burn; this was significantly higher than interleukin-6 levels in normal controls (718 ± 216 vs 70 ± 4 pg/mL; $p < 0.01$) *5351* Concentration increased on postburn day 1, peaked on day 6 and remained increased on day 21. Correlation between increases in IL-6 and acute phase reactants response, and also a correlation between % total body surface area burn *448* In 12 severely burned adult patients mean concentration on day of hospitalization significantly increased to 300 U/mL, above reference interval *416*

Interleukin-8 *Serum Increase* On admission 24 of 25 burned patients had a detectable concentration with median of 1,027 pg/mL compared with undetectable amounts in 9 of 10 controls: higher concentrations observed in patients with largest burns *5474*

17-Ketogenic Steroids *Urine Increase* Excretion may be increased in patients with the stress of burns *2952* Increased due to severe stress *5544*

17-Ketosteroids *Urine Decrease* Concentration reduced or unchanged in men in first four weeks following thermal injury *2996*

Leukocytes *Blood Increase* Due to tissue necrosis *5544* On admission 25 burned patients had a mean concentration of 13.9 x 10^9/L *5474* In 7 patients with burns mean concentration of 18.5 ± 9.8 x 10^3/μL *3868*
Blood No Effect In 60 patients with burns studied 5 days after injury, in those with < 20% surface area burned WBC of 10,300 ± 900 /μL, in those with 20 - 40% burned 8,300 ± 1,300 /μL and in those with more than 40% 9,200 ± 1,700 /μL *2800*

Leukotriene E_4 *Urine Increase* Peak excretion in individuals with severe burns approximately 20-fold higher than in healthy volunteers *5643*

Lidocaine, Free *Serum Decrease* In 7 burned patients one week after the burn injury the free fraction of the drug was decreased to 17% compared with 35% in controls *5869*

Lipoprotein A-I *Serum Decrease* Concentration fell markedly in severely burned patients with lowest concentrations from 4 - 9 days after injury with weak negative correlation between concentration and severity of injury *3581*

Luteinizing Hormone *Plasma Decrease* Concentration in burned men below normal during the first 4 days following the injury and remaining in the low or mid normal range thereafter *5487*
Plasma No Effect No significant change observed in men in first four weeks following thermal injury *2996*

α_2-Macroglobulin *Serum No Effect* Little change in concentration observed following burn injury with perhaps a very slight decrease observed in severe burns *3581*

Magnesium *Red Blood Cells Decrease* Moderate and short-lived decrease in serum and erythrocytes occurs immediately after burn *2880*
Serum Decrease Moderate and short-lived decrease in serum and erythrocytes occurs immediately after burn *2880*

Meperidine, Free *Serum* *Decrease* In 7 burned patients one week after the burn injury the free fraction of the drug was decreased to 37% compared with 48% in controls *5869*

Methemoglobin *Blood* *No Effect* In 7 patients with burns mean concentration of 0.7% *3868*

Myoglobin *Serum* *Increase* In 8 thermal burn patients there was a significant increase ($p < 0.01$) *1902*

Neuropeptide Y *Plasma* *Increase* Mean concentration significantly increased on admission of patients with 30 - 66% burn injury *975*

Nickel *Serum* *Increase* Mean concentration of 7.2 μg/L (n = 3) compared with mean in controls of 2.6 μg/L (n = 42) *3428*

Nitrogen Balance *Patient* *Negative* Rapidly becomes negative with massive protein catabolism *1959*

Norepinephrine *Plasma* *Increase* Significant increase observed in patients with 30 - 66% burn injury on first admission to hospital *975*

Osmotic Fragility *Red Blood Cells* *Increase* Increased after thermal injury *5544*

Phenytoin, Free *Serum* *Increase* In 7 burned patients one week after the burn injury the free fraction of the drug was increased to 5.5% compared with 1.7% in controls *5869*

Phosphate *Serum* *Decrease* Patients recovering from burns may remain hypophosphatemic and hypouricemic for months after the initial injury *2719* Severe burns are common cause of severe hypophosphatemia due to shift of phosphate into the cells and increased renal loss of phosphate *969*
Serum *Increase* White phosphorus burns may increase the serum phosphate concentration *969*

α_2-Plasmin Inhibitor *Plasma* *Decrease* Measured acute-phase reactants including fibrinogen, α_1-antitrypsin, C_1 inhibitor, and α_2-plasmin inhibitor. After initial declines, these four proteins increased rapidly in survivors. The levels of acute phase proteins in nonsurvivors remained low *5351*
Plasma *Increase* Measured acute-phase reactants including fibrinogen, α_1-antitrypsin, C_1 inhibitor, and α_2-plasmin inhibitor. After initial declines, these four proteins increased rapidly in survivors. The levels of acute phase proteins in nonsurvivors remained low *5351*

Platelets *Blood* *Decrease* Moderate thrombocytopenia is frequently present for 2 - 4 days following severe thermal injury to more than 10% of the body. Reduction is most pronounced in patients with sepsis. The degree of thrombocytopenia does not correlate closely with prognosis, but rising platelet levels are associated with clinical improvement *2127*
Blood *Increase* Count rises slowly, lasting for 3 weeks in burns and other types of trauma *5545*
Blood *No Effect* In 60 patients studied 5 days after injury, in those with burns over < 20% of surface area mean count of 273,000 ± 26,000 /μL, in those with 20 - 40% 207,000 ± 18,000 /μL and in those with > 40% 16,6000 ± 26,000 /μL *2800*

Propranolol, Free *Serum* *Decrease* In 7 burned patients one week after the burn injury the free fraction of the drug was decreased to 4.5% compared with 10.7% in controls *5869*

Prostaglandin E_2 *Plasma* *Increase* In 14 patients with burns mean concentration of 450 ± 580 pg/mL significantly higher than < 25 pg/mL in healthy controls *2301*

α_1-Protease Inhibitor *Serum* *Increase* The serum concentrations of alpha 1-protease inhibitor (PI) reached their maximal values after day 5 and remained at a high level throughout the total period studied (7 weeks) *4184* In burned patients concentration significantly increased with concentration remaining high even after 10 days post-burn *2989*

Retinol-binding Protein *Serum* *Decrease* Significant decrease observed in patients with serious burn injury with return to normal in 9 days in those in whom less than 20% body surface area damaged and in 13 days in whom more damage is present *987*

Salicylate, Free *Serum* *Increase* In 7 burned patients one week after the burn injury the free fraction of the drug was increased to 69% compared with 32% in controls *5869*

Selenium *Serum* *Decrease* Mean concentration decreased in patients with burn injury for up to 20 days *397* In one patient with severe burn injuries to 60% of her body surface area on admission to a referral hospital 55 days after injury, concentration reduced to 0.35 μmol/L (reference interval 0.75 - 1.80 μmol/L) *4547*

Sex-Hormone Binding Globulin *Serum* *No Effect* In burned men concentration normal or slightly low *5487*

Silver *Serum* *Increase* Normal concentration less than 2.3 μg/L but when patients treated with silver sulfadiazine concentration may rise to 50 μg/L within 6 h of treatment and can reach a maximum of 310 μg/L *5556*
Urine *Increase* Normal concentration less than 2 μg/d but after 1 day of treatment with silver sulfadiazine increased excretion detected and may reach a maximum of 400 μg/d *5556*

Sodium *Red Blood Cells* *Increase* Reduced concentration in plasma, but an increase in RBC concentration occurs even in minor burns *4707*
Serum *Decrease* Reduced concentration in plasma, but an increase in RBC concentration occurs even in minor burns *4707*

Testosterone *Serum* *Decrease* Mean concentration significantly reduced below normal in 37 of 41 burned male patients: concentration declined rapidly after injury and remained low for weeks, with the concentration being lowest with the most severe burns *5487* Significant decrease observed in men in first four weeks following thermal injury *2996*

Transferrin *Serum* *Decrease* In patients with severe burn injury concentrations fell to well below reference range after only 24 hours with lowest concentrations occurring about day 6 with gradual return to normal values which began about 2 weeks after injury *3581*

Tumor Necrosis Factor-α *Serum* *Increase* In 11 of 35 severely burned adult patients mean concentration detectable on day of hospitalization *416*

Uric Acid *Serum* *Decrease* Patients recovering from burns may remain hypophosphatemic and hypouricemic for months after the initial injury *2719*

Uric Acid Clearance *Urine* *Increase* Significantly increased renal clearance is found *5615*

Viscosity *Serum* *Increase* Rises acutely and remains elevated for 4 - 5 days although hematocrit has returned to normal *5545*

Vitamin A *Serum* *Decrease* Concentration significantly reduced by fourth day with return to normal by 9 days in patients in whom less than 20% of surface area burned with much longer recovery required in those with greater damage *987*

VLDL-Cholesterol *Serum* *Increase* Moderate increase secondary to increased secretion and decreased catabolism *126*

Volume *Plasma* *Decrease* Decreased plasma volume and blood volume follows marked drop in cardiac output. Greatest decrease occurs in first 12 h and continues at a slower rate for 6 - 12 h longer. In a 40% burn, plasma volume falls 25% *5545*

Zinc *Serum* *Decrease* In one patient with severe burn injuries to 60% of her body surface area on admission to a referral hospital 55 days after injury, concentration reduced to 9.5 μmol/L (reference interval 11 - 18 μmol/L) *4547* Mean concentration reduced to 0.55 (0.2 - 1.5) mg/L compared with 0.7 - 1.6 mg/L in healthy controls *1828*
Serum *Increase* Considerable muscle catabolism may cccur with increased plasma concentrations of amino acids, zinc and other cellular products *5174*
Urine *Increase* Considerable muscle catabolism may cccur with increased plasma concentrations of amino acids, zinc and other cellular products: zinc and amino acids form complexes in plasma and filtered at glomerulus. If not all zinc reabsorbed leads to hyperzincuria *5174*

952.90 Spinal Cord Injury

Follicle Stimulating Hormone *Plasma* *Increase* In 20 patients with spinal cord injury mean concentration of 7.7 ± 1.6 IU/L not significantly different from 4.8 ± 0.4 IU/L in 16 healthy controls *5305*

GH response to Arginine *Plasma* *Decrease* In 20 patients with spinal cord injury mean peak concentration of 5.9 ± 1.0 ng/mL significantly different from 14.1 ± 2.8 ng/mL in 16 healthy controls *5305*

HDL-Cholesterol *Serum* *No Effect* Mean concentration of 37 ± 1 mg/dL in 78 hyperinsulinemic patients with spinal cord injury not significantly different from 39 ± 1 mg/dL in 119 normal patients with spinal cord injury *5856*

952.90 Spinal Cord Injury *(continued)*

Insulin-like Growth Factor-I *Serum Decrease* In 20 patients with spinal cord injury mean concentration of 198 ± 18 ng/mL significantly different from 267 ± 27 ng/mL in 16 healthy controls *5305*

LDL-Cholesterol *Serum No Effect* Mean concentration of 126 ± 4 mg/dL in 78 hyperinsulinemic patients with spinal cord injury not significantly different from 123 ± 3 mg/dL in 119 normal patients with spinal cord injury *5856*

Luteinizing Hormone *Plasma Increase* In 20 patients with spinal cord injury mean concentration of 4.0 ± 0.5 IU/L not significantly different from 3.2 ± 0.2 IU/L in 16 healthy controls *5305*

Testosterone *Serum Decrease* In 20 patients with spinal cord injury mean concentration of 3.12 ± 0.29 ng/mL significantly different from 4.68 ± 0.28 ng/mL in 16 healthy controls *5305*

Testosterone, Free *Serum Decrease* In 20 patients with spinal cord injury mean concentration of 1.89 ± 0.18 ng/mL significantly different from 2.46 ± 0.22 ng/mL in 16 healthy controls *5305*

Triglycerides *Serum Increase* Mean concentration of 143 ± 9 mg/dL in 78 hyperinsulinemic patients with spinal cord injury significantly different from 109 ± 8 mg/dL in 119 normal patients with spinal cord injury *5856*

Uric Acid *Serum Increase* Mean concentration of 6.3 ± 0.2 mg/dL in 78 hyperinsulinemic patients with spinal cord injury significantly different from 5.1 ± 0.1 mg/dL in 119 normal patients with spinal cord injury *5856*

958.00 Gas Embolism

Creatine Kinase *Serum Increase* In all of 27 patients with arterial gas embolism activity increased above 175 U/L. 14 of 22 had activities above 900 U/L with maximum 15 ± 2 h after diving accident and fell rapidly thereafter compared with mean activity of 177 ± 23 U/L in diving control group *4910*

Creatine Kinase Isoenzymes *Serum Increase* In 20 patients with arterial gas embolism CK-MB observed in amounts from 1 to 18% of total activity (greater than 4% of total activity in 6 patients) with mean activity of CK-MB being 268 U/L *4910*

958.10 Fat Embolism

Calcium *Serum Decrease* Decreased calcium correlated with leukocytosis and low hemoglobin *3755*

Carbon Dioxide Partial Pressure *Blood Decrease* Decreased arterial pO_2 with normal or decreased pCO_2 *5544*
Blood No Effect Decreased arterial pO_2 with normal or decreased pCO_2 *5544*

Fat *Sputum Increase* Fat globules found in sputum of some patients *5545*
Urine Increase In 60% of cases *5545*

Fatty Acids (FFA), Free *Serum Increase* Not of diagnostic value *5544*

Hemoglobin *Blood Decrease* Decreased hemoglobin correlates with leukocytosis and hypocalcemia *3755*

Leukocytes *Blood Increase* Decreased hemoglobin correlates with leukocytosis and hypocalcemia *3755*

Lipase *Serum Increase* Increased in 30 - 50% of cases *5544*

Macrophages *BAL Fluid Increase* 4 patients with fat embolism syndrome had more than 70% fat cells compared with none of 11 patients with no evidence of fat embolism but with hypoxemia *3504*

Neutrophils *BAL Fluid Increase* 4 patients with fat embolism syndrome had more than 70% fat cells compared with none of 11 patients with no evidence of fat embolism but with hypoxemia *3504*

Oxygen Partial Pressure *Blood Decrease* Decreased arterial pO_2 with normal or decreased pCO_2 *5544*

Oxygen Saturation *Blood Decrease* Decreased arterial pO_2 with normal or decreased pCO_2 *5544*

Platelets *Blood Decrease* Sometimes quite severe *5677*

958.40 Traumatic Shock

Adrenomedullin *Plasma Increase* In 16 patients with traumatic shock mean concentration of 41.1 ± 7.8 fmol/mL significantly different from 5.1 ± 0.2 fmol/mL in healthy controls *5343*

Creatinine *Serum No Effect* In 16 patients with traumatic shock mean concentration of 1.01 ± 0.11 mg/dL not significantly different from that in healthy controls *5343*

Interleukin-6 *Serum Increase* In 16 patients with traumatic shock mean concentration of 870.1 ± 297.5 pg/mL significantly different from < 10 pg/mL in healthy controls *5343*

Interleukin-8 *Serum Increase* In 16 patients with traumatic shock mean concentration of 107.5 ± 26.4 pg/mL significantly different from < 10 pg/mL in healthy controls *5343*

Thrombomodulin *Plasma No Effect* In 16 patients with traumatic shock mean concentration of 4.5 ± 0.5 functional U/mL not significantly different from < 4.5 functional U/mL in healthy controls *5343*

Tumor Necrosis Factor-α *Serum Increase* In 16 patients with traumatic shock mean concentration of 28.7 ± 8.2 pg/mL significantly different from < 5 pg/mL in healthy controls *5343*

959.80 Multiple Injury

Phospholipase A_2 *Serum Increase* Increased concentrations reported *46*

959.90 Trauma

α_1-Acid Glycoprotein *Serum Increase* Increases 2 - 4 fold in response to inflammation and trauma *4093*

Adrenomedullin *Plasma Increase* In 11 patients following trauma mean concentration of 14.9 ± 2.5 fmol/L significantly different from 5.1 ± 0.2 fmol/mL in healthy controls *5343*

Alanine Aminotransferase *Serum Increase* In children with blunt abdominal liver trauma in all cases in whom enzyme activity was greater than 250 U/L liver injury was present *2115*

Albumin *Serum Decrease* In 8 trauma patients on admission to hospital mean concentration of 37 g/L decreased to 35 g/L within 4 days, and 32 g/L within 10 days *3626*
Urine Increase Excretion increased in first 24 h following trauma with tubular and glomerular proteinuria which subsided by second post-trauma day. Excretion positively correlated with injury severity *1829*

Alkaline Phosphatase *Serum Decrease* In 8 trauma patients mean activity on admission of 39 U/L remained constant at 38 U/L by 4 days but then increased to 59 U/L by 7 days and 78 U/L by 10 days: normal range 25 - 80 U/L *3626*

Alkaline Ribonuclease *Serum Increase* Significant increase observed in patients with severe injury following trauma *2431*
Urine Increase In patients with multiple injury following trauma urinary clearance of free alkaline ribonuclease increased by 220% although creatinine clearance not affected *2431*

Amino Acids *Plasma Increase* Considerable muscle catabolism may cccur with increased plasma concentrations of amino acids, zinc and other cellular products *5174*

Amino-terminal Propeptide of Type III Procollagen
Serum Increase In 9 patients following major abdominal surgery mean concentraton of aminoterminal compound increased from preoperative baseline of 2.6 ± 0.6 µg/L to 5.3 ± 1.0 µg/L on postoperative day 10. Lowest mean of 2.1 ± 0.5 µg/L occurred on postoperative day 1 *2065*

Amyloid A *Serum Increase* Increases several hundred fold in response to trauma and inflammation *4093*

Antiphospholipid Antibodies *Serum No Effect* In 45 acutely injured patients mean concentration of 4.1 ± 3.0 µg/mL obtained within 24 hours of injury not significantly different from 3.8 ± 1.6 µg/mL in controls *1421*

α_1-Antitrypsin *Serum Increase* Increases 2 - 4 fold in response to trauma and and inflammation *4093*

Arginine *Plasma Decrease* Significant decrease observed with trauma in geriatric patients *2432*

Aspartate Aminotransferase *Serum Increase* In children with blunt abdominal trauma activity over 450 U/L always indicated hepatic injury *2115*

Atrial Natriuretic Peptide *Plasma* *Increase* In 12 patients with multiple trauma on admission to hospital mean concentration of 337.5 ± 125.6 ng/L significantly higher than 40.1 ± 14.3 ng/L in 15 matched hospital control individuals with acute illness *5458*

Bradykinin *Plasma* *Increase* In all of a group of patients with cumulative trauma disorder concentration increased to mean of 1,642.8 ± 270.9 pg/mL compared with healthy controls of 246.0 ± 37.8 pg/mL *2227*

Calcitonin Gene-related Peptide *Serum* *Increase* In all of a group of patients with cumulative trauma disorder concentration increased to a mean of 44.5 ± 10.8 pg/mL compared with healthy controls of 20.7 ± 3.7 pg/mL *2227*

Ceruloplasmin *Serum* *Increase* Increases 50% or more in response to injury and inflammation *4093*

Cholesterol *Serum* *Decrease* In trauma patients the concentration of plasma cholesterol falls dramatically *693*

Citrulline *Plasma* *Increase* Significant increase observed in geriatric patients with trauma *2432*

Complement C_3 *Serum* *Increase* Increases 50% or more in response to trauma and inflammation *4093*

Complement C_3a *Serum* *Increase* Strong correlation between concentration and degree of severity of injury *4663*

Complement C_4 *Serum* *Increase* Increases 50% or more in response to trauma and inflammation *4093*

Copper *Serum* *Decrease* In 32 patients with major trauma mean concentration of 0.96 (0.6 - 1.6) mg/L compared with 0.7 - 1.6 mg/L in healthy controls *1828*

Corticotropin *Plasma* *Increase* In 12 patients with multiple trauma on admission to hospital mean concentration of 123.7 ± 41.3 pmol/L significantly higher than 15.6 ± 5.8 pmol/L in 15 matched hospital control individuals with acute illness *5458*

Cortisol *Plasma* *Increase* Increased concentration observed in all 59 military casualties with cortisol concentration directly related to glucose concentration *4599* Occurs as part of general stress response *1638* During severe illness plasma cortisol concentrations tend to be higher than in other conditions, e.g. with multiple trauma concentrations tend to rise from about 46 µg/dL when patients first hospitalized rising to about 48 µg/dL after 4 days then decreasing to about 30 µg/dL after 8 days *2901* In 12 patients with multiple trauma on admission to hospital mean concentration of 1.23 ± 0.28 µmol/L significantly higher than 0.37 ± 0.08 µmol/L in 15 matched hospital control individuals with acute illness *5458* Mean concentration of 23.7 ± 3.3 µg/dL in 11 nonobese young individuals, 29.7 ± 7.4 µg/dL in 5 obese individuals and 23.3 ± 3.2 µg/dL in 6 traumatized elderly patients compared with 17.4 ± 1.8 µg/dL, 14.5 ± 1.4 µg/dL and 13.0 ± 1.7 µg/dL respectively in control populations *2429*

C-Peptide *Plasma* *Increase* In 29 hypermetabolic and catabolic multiply injured trauma patients twofold increase in plasma concentration observed although urinary excretion further increased *2430* Mean concentration of 4.1 ± 0.5 ng/mL in 11 nonobese young individuals, 5.7 ± 1.2 ng/mL in 5 obese individuals and 4.0 ± 0.9 ngmL in 6 traumatized elderly patients compared with 1.8 ± 0.2 ng/mL, 3.2 ± 0.5 ng/mL and 2.9 ± 0.3 ng/mL respectively in control populations *2429*
Urine *Increase* In 29 severely injured hypermetabolic and catabolic multiple trauma patients excretion was increased to 3 times normal both absolutely and when referenced to creatinine excretion *2430*

C-Reactive Protein *Serum* *Increase* Increases several hundred fold in response to trauma and inflammation *4093* In 47 polytraumatized patients who did not develop ARDS mean concentration of 40.8 ± 26.5 mg/L significantly greater than 1.7 ± 1.3 mg/L in 34 healthy controls *1156* Mean concentration in 13 patients following severe trauma reached peak of about 160 mg/L 3 days after injury with upper limit of normal of 4.0 mg/L *1829* Tissue injury stimulates C-reactive protein production *1834* In 78 patients hospitalized following trauma increased concentration observed with higher concentrations observed in nonsurvivors than survivors. On third day using value of less than 200 mg/L 83% survived and above 200 mg/L predictive value for death of 63% *1827*

Creatine *Urine* *Increase* Urinary creatine may be significantly increased in patients with skeletal muscle necrosis of trauma *2952*

Creatine Kinase *Serum* *Increase* In 17 young previously healthy patients following severe trauma mean peak activity of 3,200 U/L compared with normal of < 200 U/L without evidence of cardiac injury *1299* In 11 patients with blunt trauma mean activity 249 ± 63 U/L compared with 177 ± 23 U/L in a diving control group *4910*

Creatine Kinase MB-Isoenzyme *Serum* *Increase* In 17 young previously healthy patients following severe trauma mean peak mass concentration of 20.4 µg/L compared with normal of < 7 µg/L without evidence of cardiac injury *1299*

Creatine Kinase MB-Isoenzyme:Creatine Kinase Ratio *Serum* *Increase* In 17 young previously healthy patients following severe trauma mean CK-MB:CK ratio was of no help in detecting cardiac disease *1299*

Creatinine *Serum* *No Effect* In 11 patients following trauma mean concentration of 0.73 ± 0.07 mg/dL not significantly different from that in healthy controls *5343*

Dopamine *Plasma* *Increase* In 7 patients with polytrauma mean concentration of 35.1 pmol/mL compared with 24.4 pmol/mL in 14 healthy controls *5731*

Dopamine, Free *Plasma* *No Effect* In 7 patients with polytrauma mean concentration of 0.93 pmol/mL compared with 0.90 pmol/mL in 14 healthy controls (3.9% of total in trauma patients compared with 4.3% in healthy controls) *5731*

Elastase *Neutrophils* *Increase* In 47 polytraumatized patients who did not develop ARDS mean concentration of 115.6 ± 99.3 µg/L significantly greater than 32.3 ± 10.9 µg/L in 34 healthy controls *1156*

Elastase-α_1-Proteinase Inhibitor Complex *Serum* *Increase* Trauma associated with increased plasma concentration and correlated with severity of injury *4663*

β-Endorphin *Plasma* *No Effect* No significant difference observed between mean concentrations of 12.1 ± 7.5 pg/mL in 47 patients with multiple trauma and 10.5 ± 5.2 pg/mL in 35 control individuals *1907*

Endothelin *Plasma* *Increase* In 11 patients after severe injury concentration increased (0.9 to 2.3 fmol/mL) on admission but increased further after 6 - 12 hours to 1.2 to 4.8 fmol/mL with highest concentrations in most severely injured. Concentrations began to decrease after 6 - 12 h *2753*

Endothelin-1 *Plasma* *Increase* In 12 patients with multiple trauma on admission to hospital mean concentration of 19.1 ± 7.6 ng/L significantly higher than 4.2 ± 1.2 ng/L in 15 matched hospital control individuals with acute illness *5458* In 11 patients with major trauma injuries mean concentration increased to 5.1 pg/mL, 1.5-fold above appropriate normal values *328*

Endothelin-1, Big *Plasma* *Increase* In 11 patients with major trauma injuries mean concentration increased to 24.3 pg/mL, 1.6-fold above normal values for study *328*

Endothelin, Big *Plasma* *Increase* In 11 severely injured patients concentration increased on admission (mean about 7 fmol/mL) and further increased to 6 - 12 hours (mean about 10 fmol/mL) after which it began to decline: possibly caused by leakage from injured vascular endothelial cells *2753*

Eosinophils *Blood* *Decrease* Concentration falls in response to increased cortisol secretion occurring as part of general response to trauma *1638*

Epinephrine *Plasma* *Increase* In 7 patients with polytrauma mean concentration of 7.5 pmol/mL compared with 1.59 pmol/mL in 14 healthy controls *5731*

Epinephrine, Free *Plasma* *Increase* In 7 patients with polytrauma mean concentration of 1.75 pmol/mL compared with 0.23 pmol/mL in 14 healthy controls (18.7% of total in trauma patients compared with 16.2% in healthy controls) *5731*

Fatty Acids (FFA), Free *Serum* *Increase* In patients following trauma concentration increases in proportion to degree of injury *693*

Fibrin Degradation Products *Plasma* *Increase* In 45 acutely injured patients mean concentration increased to 4,536 ± 3,959 ng/mL within 24 h of injury compared with 232 ± 24 ng/mL in controls *1421*

Fibrinogen *Plasma* *Increase* Increases 2 - 4 fold in response to trauma and inflammation *4093*

Fibrinogen Degradation Products *Plasma* *Increase* In 73 patients following traumatic injuries mean concentration significantly greater at 4,700 - 4,800 ng/mL than in healthy individuals in whom upper limit of normal was 232 ± 24 ng/mL *1236*

959.90 **Trauma** *(continued)*

Fibrinopeptide A *Plasma Increase* Correlation observed between degree of tissue injury and plasma concentration *4663*

Fibronectin *Plasma Decrease* Significantly lower concentrations observed in patients with multiple trauma *980* Rapid decrease with onset of trauma but recovers rapidly with treatment *1959*

Glucose *Serum Increase* Mean concentration of 118 ± 5 mg/dL in 11 nonobese young individuals, 122 ± 13 mg/dL in 5 obese individuals and 125 ± 9 mgdL in 6 traumatized elderly patients compared with 85 ± 3 mg/dL, 103 ± 7 mg/dL and 98 ± 3 mg/dL respectively in control populations *2429* Increased concentration observed in all 59 military casualties, with glucose concentration directly related to injury severity score *4599*

γ-Glutamyltransferase *Urine Increase* In 13 patients excretion significantly increased during first 24 h following trauma with glomerular and tubular proteinuria. Subsided during second 24 h *1829*

Growth Hormone *Plasma Decrease* Mean concentration of 0.92 ± 0.26 ng/mL in 11 nonobese young individuals, 0.39 ± 0.07 ng/mL in 5 obese individuals and 0.54 ± 0.13 ng/mL in 6 elderly traumatized patients compared with 2.92 ± 0.63 ng/mL, 1.14 ± 0.56 ng/mL and 0.42 ± 0.11 ng/mL respectively in control populations *2429*
Plasma Increase Observed as part of general response to injury *1638* In individuals with injury endogenous growth hormone concentration increased *2686*

Haptoglobin *Serum Decrease* In patients following major abdominal surgery decrease observed presumably due to removal of hemoglobin-haptoglobin complex *4974*
Serum Increase Increases 2 - 4 fold in response to trauma and inflammation *4093*

Insulin *Plasma Decrease* Secretion of insulin is suppressed following trauma causing a relative hypoinsulinemia compared with circulating glucose concentration *1638*
Plasma Increase Increased concentration observed in all 59 military casualties, with glucose concentration but not insulin concentration directly related to injury severity score *4599*
Plasma No Effect Mean concentration of 9.3 ± 1.2 μIU/mL in 11 nonobese young individuals, 18.3 ± 3.6 μIU/mL in 5 obese individuals and 12.9 ± 4.5 μIU/mL in 6 traumatized elderly patients compared with 6.3 ± 0.6 μIU/mL, 19.2 ± 2.4 μIU/mL and 11.4 ± 2.0 μIU/mL respectively in control populations *2429*

Insulin-like Growth Factor-I *Serum Decrease* In injured patients concentration decreased in spite of increased growth hormone concentration *2686* Mean concentration of 113 ± 14 ng/mL in 11 nonobese young individuals, 79 ± 7 ng/mL in 5 obese individuals and 80 ± 10 ng/mL in 6 traumatized elderly patients compared with 228 ± 21 ng/mL, 136 ± 16 ng/mL and 133 ± 16 ng/mL respectively in control populations *2429* Plasma concentration may fall to very low level following a severe injury, especially during the early part of the catabolic phase but begins to rise during later stages *5182*

Insulin-like Growth Factor Binding Protein-3 Protease *Serum Increase* Reportedly increased activity in the plasma following trauma *2103*

Interleukin-6 *Serum Increase* Concentration increased in response to trauma as in response to elective surgery, preceding response by acute phase reactants. Concentration rises in proportion to the degree of tissue injury *448* In 60 patients with multiple trauma significant increase of concentration to 317 ± 124 pg/mL in nonsurvivors compared with mean concentration of 20 ± 6 pg/mL in healthy controls. Concentration in survivors of 247 ± 41 pg/mL also increased *3310*
Serum No Effect In 12 critically patients after trauma no significant increase in concentration observed although concentration significantly increased in patients with sepsis *5459*

6-Keto-Prostaglandin $F_{1\alpha}$ *Plasma Increase* Concentration significantly increased in arterial and mixed venous blood in patients who had undergone recent trauma *5429*

Ketones *Serum Increase* Mean concentration of 607 ± 172 μmol/L in 11 obese young individuals, 245 ± 56 μmol/L in 5 obese individuals and 345 ± 107 μmol/dL in 6 traumatized elderly patients compared with 74 ± 18 μmol/L, 44 ± 5 μmol/L and 58 ± 8 μmol/L respectively in control populations *2429*

Leukocytes *Blood Increase* In 7 patients with multiple trauma mean concentration of 17.0 ± 5.6 x 10^3/μL *3868*

Leukotriene E_4 *Urine Increase* In 7 patients with multiple trauma but without adult respiratory distress syndrome excretion of 76.8 nmol/mol creatinine/d during first 10 days after trauma compared with 10 ±3 nmol/mol creatinine/d in healthy controls but 10-fold higher if ARDS also *1433*

Lymphocytes *Blood Decrease* Occurs in response to increased secretion of cortisol following general stress reaction *1638* In 1,042 hospitalized patients with lymphocytopenia 90 had had trauma or a hemorrhage *730*

Methemoglobin *Blood No Effect* In 7 patients with multiple trauma mean concentration of 0.6% *3868*

Methionine *Plasma Decrease* Significant decrease observed in geriatric patients with trauma *2432*

3-Methylhistidine *Urine Increase* Increased with muscle catabolism *1959*

Myoglobin *Urine Increase* Mechanical trauma producing acute muscle necrosis may cause myoglobinuria *5065*

Neurokinin A *Plasma No Effect* No significant difference observed between concentrations in a group of patients with cumulative trauma disorder and healthy controls *2227*

Neurokinin B *Plasma No Effect* No significant difference observed between concentrations in a group of patients with cumulative trauma disorder and healthy controls *2227*

Neuropeptide Y *Plasma Increase* Half of a group of patients with cumulative trauma disorder had an increased concentration compared with healthy controls *2227*

Nitrogen Balance *Patient Negative* Rapidly becomes negative with massive protein catabolism *1959*

Norepinephrine *Plasma Increase* Increased concentration observed in all 59 military casualties with norepinephrine concentration directly related to glucose concentration *4599* In 7 patients with polytrauma mean concentration of 13.47 pmol/mL compared with 4.45 pmol/mL in 14 healthy controls *5731*

Norepinephrine, Free *Plasma Increase* In 7 patients with polytrauma mean concentration of 7.7 pmol/mL compared with 1.79 pmol/mL in 14 healthy controls (44.7% of total in trauma patients compared with 43.0% in healthy controls) *5731*

Ornithine *Plasma Increase* Significant increase observed in geriatric patients with trauma *2432*

Pancreatic Secretory Trypsin Inhibitor *Serum Increase* Marked increase observed in 84% of 31 seriously injured patients with increase apparent on second or third post-traumatic day with maximum at day 5.8 on average. In uneventful cases concentration returned to admission concentration within 2 weeks *4791*

Phosphate *Serum Decrease* In trauma patients during first 24 hours post-injury significant decrease from 1.00 ± 0.30 mmol/L to 0.75 ± 0.23 mmol/L in the absence of phosphate supplementation *996*
Urine Increase In trauma patients during the first 24 hours following injury significantly increased excretion observed in the absence of phosphate supplementation which account for the decreased serum phosphate concentration *996*

Phospholipase A_2 *Serum Increase* Increased activity observed in sera of patients with multiple injuries especially after abdominal trauma or other pancreatic irritation *3766*

Phospholipase A_2 Type I *Serum Increase* Patients with multiple injuries often have increased group I PLA_2, and lipase and amylase activities when there is abdominal trauma or other pancreatic irritation *3767*

Phospholipase A_2 Type II *Serum Increase* Patients with multiple injuries often have endotoxemia and bacteriemia and increased group II PLA_2, and concentration effectively predicts lethal multiorgan failure in patients with multiple injuries *3767*

Plasminogen Activator Inhibitor *Plasma Increase* In 45 acutely injured patients concentration increased to 93.2 ± 56.0 ng/mL within 24 h of injury compared with 20.9 ± 9.2 ng/mL in controls *1421*

Plasminogen Activator Inhibitor-1 *Plasma Increase* In 73 patients following traumatic injuries mean concentration significantly greater at 84 ng/mL than in healthy individuals in whom upper limit of normal was < 48 ng/mL *1236*

Potassium *Serum* *Decrease* Hypokalemia occurs in 50 to 68% of trauma patients, with concentration usually decreasing within one hour of trauma and returning to normal within 24 hours without significant potassium replacement. Mean concentration in trauma patients of 3.55 mmol/L significantly less than than 3.95 mmol/L in 59 consecutive outpatient hernia controls *5424*

Propeptide of Type I Procollagen *Serum* *Increase* In 9 patients following major abdominal surgery mean concentration of carboxy-terminal concentration increased from mean baseline of 77 ± 34 µg/L to 128 ± 67 µg/L 2 months later. Secondary peak occurred on day 7 with a minimum on first postoperative day *2065*

Protein *Serum* *Decrease* Mean concentration reduced to 58 g/L in 8 trauma patients within 24 hours of admission compared with normal range of 60 - 80 g/L: concentration increased to 62 g/L within 10 days of admission *3626*
Urine *Increase* In 13 patients following trauma, tubular and glomerular proteinuria occurred during the first 24 h which subsided by the second post-trauma day. Excretion positively correlated with injury severity *1829*

Prothrombin Fragment 1.2 *Plasma* *Increase* In 15 patients with multiple trauma and head injury mean concentration on admission to hospital of 8.1 ± 7.8 nmol/L significantly different from median of 0.7 nmol/L in control population *4938*

Substance P *Plasma* *No Effect* No significant difference observed between concentrations in a group of patients with cumulative trauma disorder and healthy controls *2227*

Thrombin/Antithrombin III Complex *Plasma* *Increase* In 15 patients with multiple trauma and head injury mean concentration on admission to hospital of 88 ± 104 ng/mL significantly different from median of 1.7 ng/mL in control population *4938* In 45 acutely injured patients mean concentration of 32.8 ± 19.0 ng/mL observed within 24 h of injury compared with 2.1 ± 1.7 ng/mL in controls *1421* In 37 patients following traumatic injuries mean concentration significantly greater at 34 - 44 ng/mL than in healthy individuals in whom upper limit of normal was 2.5 ± 1.5 ng/mL *1236*

Thromboxane B_2 *Plasma* *Increase* Concentration significantly increased in arterial and mixed venous plasma in patients who had suffered recent trauma *5429*

Thyroid Stimulating Hormone *Serum* *No Effect* Secretion unaffected by injury or surgery *1638*

Tissue Factor Antigen *Plasma* *No Effect* In 45 acutely injured patients concentration within 24 h of injury not significantly different from controls *1421*

Tissue Factor Pathway Inhibitor *Plasma* *Increase* In 73 patients following traumatic injuries mean concentration significantly greater at 125 ng/mL than in healthy individuals in whom upper limit of normal was < 100 ng/mL *1236*
Plasma *No Effect* In 45 acutely injured patients mean concentration not significantly different from controls within 24 h of injury *1421*

Tissue Plasminogen Activator *Plasma* *Increase* In 45 acutely injured patients mean concentration increased to 19.5 ± 12.3 ng/mL compared with 3.1 ± 1.3 ng/mL in controls *1421* In 73 patients following traumatic injuries mean concentration significantly greater at 22 ng/mL than in healthy individuals in whom upper limit of normal was 3.1 ± 1.3 ng/mL *1236*

Transferrin *Serum* *Decrease* Following major abdominal surgery mean concentration severely depressed *4974*

Troponin I *Serum* *Increase* In 17 young previously healthy patients following severe trauma mean peak concentrations greater than 0.6 µg/L occurred in 6, who showed greater incidence of hypertension, greater early volume loading and more frequent multiple organ dysfunction syndrome *1299*

Tumor Necrosis Factor-α *Serum* *Increase* In 73 patients following traumatic injuries mean concentration significantly greater than in healthy individuals, but concentration decreased in acute post-traumatic phase but rose again at day 22 *1236*
Serum *No Effect* In 60 patients with multiple trauma non-significant increase of concentration to 13 ± 2 pg/mL in non-survivors compared with mean concentration of 10 ± 5 pg/mL in healthy controls *3310*

Urea Nitrogen *Serum* *No Effect* No deviation outside reference range of 5 - 26 mg/dL in 8 trauma patients but mean concentration of 14.1 mg/dL on admission, 16.5 mg/dL within 4 days, 20.5 mg/dL within 7 days and 18.3 mg/dL within 10 days *3626*

Vasoactive Inhibitory Peptide *Plasma* *Increase* Half of a group of patients with cumulative trauma disorder had an increased concentration compared with healthy controls *2227*

Zinc *Serum* *Decrease* In 8 male patients mean concentration within 24 hours of admission to hospital of 41 µg/dL in comparison with 87 µg/dL in healthy controls to which concentration that in the trauma patients rose within 10 days *3626* Mean concentration in 32 patients with major trauma 0.64 (0.3 - 1.1) mg/L compared with 0.7 - 1.6 mg/L in healthy controls *1828*
Serum *Increase* Considerable muscle catabolism may cccur with increased plasma concentrations of amino acids, zinc and other cellular products: zinc and amino acids form complexes in plasma and filtered at glomerulus. If not all zinc reabsorbed leads to hyperzincuria *5174*
Urine *Increase* Considerable muscle catabolism may cccur with increased plasma concentrations of amino acids, zinc and other cellular products: zinc and amino acids form complexes in plasma and filtered at glomerulus. If not all zinc reabsorbed leads to hyperzincuria *5174*

984.90 Toxic Effects of Lead and Its Compounds (including Fumes)

Alanine *Urine* *Increase* With lead intoxication *1813*

Amino Acids *Urine* *Increase* Results from changes in the epithelium of the proximal convoluted tubules in lead poisoning *367* Transient finding *596*

α-Amino-Nitrogen *Urine* *Increase* With lead intoxication *1813*

β-Aminoisobutyric Acid *Urine* *Increase* A result of the nephrotoxic effect of lead *1290*

δ-Aminolevulinic Acid *Serum* *Increase* In 50 cases, brain levels increased 4-fold, urine 8-fold and plasma only 2-fold compared to controls *994*
Urine *Increase* In lead poisoning *1813* In 50 cases, brain levels increased 4-fold, urine 8-fold and plasma only 2-fold compared to controls *994* δ-aminolevulinic acid is increased *5545*

δ-Aminolevulinic Acid Dehydratase
Red Blood Cells *Decrease* RBC concentration correlates negatively with serum lead concentration *596*

Basophilic Stippling *Blood* *Increase* Coarse basophilic stippling occurs to an extreme degree, with involvement of up to 1 - 2% of cells *5677* Occurs in 60% of childhood cases *596*

Bilirubin *Serum* *Increase* Hemolytic anemia may occur *993*

Citrate *Urine* *Increase* Citraturia results from changes in the proximal convoluted tubules *367*

Copper *Red Blood Cells* *Increase* RBC concentration may increase with poisoning *1290*

Coproporphyrin *Red Blood Cells* *Increase* Free erythrocyte coproporphyrin ranges from 1 - 20 µg/dL in lead poisoning (normal 0 - 2 µg/dL) *367*
Urine *Increase* Increase in urine coproporphyrin III is associated with an increase in urine uroporphyrin and red cell protoporphyrin *1290* A reliable sign of intoxication and is often demonstrable before basophilic stippling *5545*

Eosinophils *Blood* *Increase* Increases in poisoning *5544*

Erythrocyte Sedimentation Rate *Blood* *Increase* With arsenic and lead intoxication *5544*

Erythrocyte Survival *Red Blood Cells* *Decrease* Hemolysis *1290* Red cell life span and osmotic fragility are decreased *367*

Erythrocytes *Blood* *Decrease* Hemolytic anemia *993*
Urine *Increase* Renal damage may occur *1813*

Fructose *Urine* *Increase* Occurs as a result of changes in the epithelium of the proximal convoluted tubules *367*

Glucose *Urine* *Increase* Nephrotoxic effect of lead *1290*

Hematocrit *Blood* *Decrease* Acute hemolytic anemia with hemoglobinemia and hemoglobinuria occasionally occur in acute lead poisoning *367*

Hemoglobin *Blood* *Decrease* Acute hemolytic anemia with hemoglobinemia and hemoglobinuria occasionally occur in acute lead poisoning *367*
Plasma *Increase* With acute hemolytic crisis *367*
Urine *Increase* With acute hemolytic crisis *1753*

Iron *Serum* *Increase* With hemolysis *1290*

Lead *Blood* *Increase* Diagnosis of lead poisoning is confirmed by blood concentrations of 25 - 40 µg/dL *367* *5545*

984.90 Toxic Effects of Lead and Its Compounds (including Fumes) *(continued)*

Lead *(continued)*
Feces *Increase* Lead concentrations of > 1.1 mg/specimen constitutes lead poisoning in adults *367*
Urine *Increase* Urine lead > 80 µg/L for children and > 150 µg/L in adults indicated lead poisoning *5545* The urine output of lead may increase to more than 100 mg/24 h. This may be associated with an increased output of urine coproporphyrin III *1290*

Leukocytes *Blood* *Decrease* Pancytopenia may occur *3471*

Levulinic Acid *Urine* *Increase* In children, at least, measurement of ALA in urine more sensitive than measurement of blood lead for evaluation of lead poisoning *2952*

MCH *Blood* *Decrease* Microcytic hypochromic anemia may occur due to blood loss, increased demand or dietary inadequacy. MCH < 27 pg, MCV < 80 fL *1098*

MCHC *Blood* *Decrease* Hemolytic anemia *993*

MCV *Blood* *Decrease* Microcytic hypochromic anemia may occur due to blood loss, increased demand or dietary inadequacy. MCH < 27 pg, MCV < 80 fL *1098* Hemolytic anemia *993*
Blood *Increase* Rare increase with poisoning *1290*

Occult Blood *Feces* *Increase* Bloody diarrhea may occur *1753*

Osmotic Fragility *Red Blood Cells* *Decrease* Osmotic fragility is decreased and mechanic fragility is increased *367*

Phosphate *Urine* *Increase* Results from changes in the epithelium in the proximal convoluted tubules *367*

Platelets *Blood* *Decrease* Pancytopenia may occur *3471*

Protein *Cerebrospinal Fluid* *Increase* Increased, with normal cell count in encephalopathy *5545*
Urine *Increase* Renal damage may occur *1813*

Protoporphyrin *Red Blood Cells* *Increase* Log of RBC protoporphyrin level closely correlated to blood level (r = 0.72) in lead-exposed workers. Especially useful in the detection of mild increases in blood lead concentrations under conditions of occupational exposure *5247* Accumulates in the erythrocytes as a result of the blocks in the synthetic process *367* Free erythrocyte protoporphyrin ranges from 300 - 3,000 mg/dL (normal concentration of 15 - 60 mg/dL) *367*

Reticulocytes *Blood* *Increase* Hemolytic anemia *1813*

Urea Nitrogen *Serum* *Increase* May cause renal damage *4672*

Uric Acid *Serum* *Increase* Moonshine whiskey causing 'saturnine gout' *1290* Increased in serum due to reduced renal clearance *267*
Urine *Decrease* Reduced renal clearance *267*

Urobilinogen *Urine* *Increase* Possibly in some cases as evidence of increased red cell destruction *1290*

985.00 Mercury Poisoning

Levulinic Acid *Urine* *Increase* Heavy metals poison ALA dehydratase so that ALA accumulates and urinary excretion is increased *2952*

985.90 Toxic Effects of Non-medicinal Metals

Alanine Aminotransferase *Serum* *Increase* Hepatotoxicity may occur with arsenicals *3146*

Albumin *Urine* *Increase* Common in mercury intoxication *367*

Alkaline Phosphatase *Serum* *Increase* Hepatotoxicity may occur with arsenicals *3146*

Arsenic *Urine* *Increase* Patients with chronic arsenic poisoning excrete 0.1 mg/day of arsenic. Normal values average 0.015 mg/day *367*

Aspartate Aminotransferase *Serum* *Increase* Hepatotoxicity may occur with arsenicals *3146*

Bicarbonate *Serum* *Decrease* May be depressed in chronic mercury poisoning *1290*

Bilirubin *Serum* *Increase* Hepatotoxicity may occur with arsenicals *3146*

BSP Retention *Serum* *Increase* Hepatotoxicity may occur with arsenicals *3146*

Calcium *Serum* *Increase* Highly significant hypercalciuria and decreased serum inorganic phosphate was found in a group of workers with cadmium intoxication *4702*

Casts *Urine* *Increase* Nephrotoxicity may occur with therapeutic doses of arsenicals *1813 1335 3311*

Cholesterol *Serum* *Increase* Hepatotoxic effects of arsenicals may be marked *3146*

Coproporphyrin *Urine* *Increase* Increased markedly in chronic arsenic poisoning *367*

Creatinine *Serum* *Increase* Nephrotoxicity is common with therapeutic doses of arsenicals *1641*

Eosinophils *Blood* *Increase* Observed effect *1641* Usually 10 - 20% in arsenic poisoning *2001*

Erythrocyte Sedimentation Rate *Blood* *Increase* With arsenic and lead intoxication *5544*

Erythrocytes *Blood* *Decrease* Pancytopenia may occur in arsenic intoxication *993*
Urine *Increase* Marked hematuria may occur in arsenic intoxication *3311 1813 1753 1335* Common in mercury poisoning *367*

Glucose *Serum* *Decrease* Hepatotoxicity may occur with arsenicals *3146*

Guanase *Serum* *Increase* Hepatotoxicity may occur with arsenicals *3146*

Hematocrit *Blood* *Decrease* Pancytopenia may occur *993* Mild to moderate anemia occurs in chronic arsenic poisoning *367*

Hemoglobin *Blood* *Decrease* Mild to moderate anemia occurs in chronic arsenic poisoning *367*

Isocitrate Dehydrogenase *Serum* *Increase* Hepatotoxicity may occur with arsenicals *3146*

Leukocytes *Blood* *Decrease* Pancytopenia may occur *993* In chronic arsenic poisoning *367*
Blood *Increase* May be caused by poisoning by chemicals, drugs, venoms, etc. (e.g., mercury, epinephrine, black widow spider) *5544* Occurs with industrial nickel exposure *3404*

Occult Blood *Feces* *Increase* Bloody diarrhea occurs with arsenic and mercury poisoning *1813*

Phosphate *Urine* *Decrease* Highly significant hypercalciuria and decreased serum inorganic phosphate was found in a group of workers with cadmium intoxication *4702*

Platelets *Blood* *Decrease* Pancytopenia may occur in arsenic poisoning *993*

Protein *Urine* *Increase* Nephrotoxicity may occur in mercury poisoning *1813* With renal damage in arsenic poisoning *1641* Nephrotoxicity may occur in mercury poisoning *1335 3311*

Pyruvate *Blood* *Increase* Arsenic, antimony, gold, and mercury inhibit pyruvate oxidation *1290*

Reticulocytes *Blood* *Increase* Values up to 18% have been observed following toxicity with arsenicals *2001*

Sodium *Serum* *Decrease* May occur with established mercury poisoning *1290*

Urea Nitrogen *Serum* *Increase* Nephrotoxicity is common with therapeutic doses of arsenicals *1641*

986.00 Toxic Effects of Carbon Monoxide

Aldolase *Serum* *Increase* Often elevated *544*

Aspartate Aminotransferase *Serum* *Increase* From skeletal muscle, heart muscle, and brain *1290*

Creatine Kinase *Serum* *Increase* 11 of 13 cases of carbon monoxide poisoning showed elevation, often accompanied by aldolase and transaminase elevation as well *544*

Erythrocytes *Urine* *Increase* Occurs in severe cases *367*

Glomerular Filtration Rate *Urine* *Increase* Occurs 12 - 24 h after exposure *4999*

Leukocytes *Blood* *Increase* Occurs in severe cases *367*

Lipids *Urine* *Increase* Lipids in the urine include all fractions. Double refractile (cholesterol) bodies can be seen. There is a high protein content *5544*

Myoglobin *Urine* *Increase* Sporadic; metabolic myoglobinuria *5544*

pH *Blood* *Decrease* Markedly decreased (metabolic acidosis due to tissue hypoxia) *5545*

Phosphoglucomutase *Serum* *Increase* One case with serum level increased 250 times normal reported *1290*

Protein *Urine* *Increase* Nephrotoxicity *4672* Occurs in severe cases *367*

Urea Nitrogen *Serum* *Increase* Nephrotoxicity *4672* Occurs in severe cases *367*

989.50 Toxic Effects of Venom

Alanine Aminotransferase *Serum* *Increase* Found in 6 of 14 patients admitted for bee stings *4137*

Aspartate Aminotransferase *Serum* *Increase* Elevated in 9 of 17 patients admitted for wasp/bee stings *4137*

Clotting Time *Blood* *Increase* Increased clotting time indicates severe envenomation from snake bite *367*

Creatine Kinase *Serum* *Increase* 14 of 17 patients admitted for wasp/bee stings showed elevated activities, indicating presence of damage to muscle fibers *4137*

Eosinophils *Blood* *Increase* Increases in poisoning (e.g., phosphate, black widow spider bite) *5544*

Hematocrit *Blood* *Decrease* A drop indicates severe envenomization following snake bite *367*

Hemoglobin *Blood* *Decrease* A drop indicates severe envenomization following snake bite *367*

Lactate Dehydrogenase *Serum* *Increase* Analysis of 17 patients admitted for wasp stings showed elevated LD in 8/14 cases, elevated AST and CK in 9/17 and 14/17, respectively *4137*

Leukocytes *Blood* *Increase* May be caused by poisoning by chemicals, drugs, or venoms *5544* Polymorphonuclear leukocytosis of 20,000 - 30,000 /μL *2034*

Myoglobin *Urine* *Increase* Common after bites *1290* Sporadic elevation; metabolic myoglobinuria *5544*

Neutrophils *Blood* *Increase* May be caused by poisoning by chemicals, drugs, or venoms *5544* Polymorphonuclear leukocytosis of 20,000 - 30,000 /μL *2034*

Protein *Urine* *Increase* May cause nephrotoxicity *4672*

Prothrombin Time *Plasma* *Increase* May be greatly prolonged in severe cases of snake bite *367*

Urea Nitrogen *Serum* *Increase* May cause nephrotoxicity *4672*

990.00 Effects of X-ray Irradiation

Alanine Aminotransferase *Serum* *Increase* May be increased in cases of radiation injury, indicating major cell and tissue damage *367*

β-Aminoisobutyric Acid *Plasma* *Increase* Due to tissue destruction *3424*

Amylase *Serum* *Increase* Sharp rise following salivary gland irradiation. Peak values range from 9 - 18 times preirradiation values. Steady decline to normal within 2 - 3 days *801*

Aspartate Aminotransferase *Serum* *Increase* May be increased in cases of radiation injury, indicating major cell and tissue damage *367*

Bilirubin *Serum* *Increase* Transient hyperbilirubinemia may be observed in cases of radiation injury *367*

Creatine *Urine* *Increase* Due to tissue destruction *3424*

Deoxycytidine *Urine* *Increase* Due to tissue destruction *3424*

Eosinophils *Blood* *Increase* After repeated irradiation *332*

Erythrocytes *Blood* *Decrease* Predominant only after large doses *2034*

Factor VIII *Plasma* *Increase* Increased activity after total body irradiation *4876*

Ferritin *Serum* *Increase* Occurs within 2 h of deep X-ray therapy *1290*

Fibrinogen *Plasma* *Increase* Indicates tissue damage *142*

γ-Globulin *Serum* *Increase* Some cases *1290*

Hematocrit *Blood* *Decrease* After large doses *2034*

Hemoglobin *Blood* *Decrease* After large doses *2034*

Lactate Dehydrogenase *Serum* *Increase* May be increased in cases of radiation injury, indicating major cell and tissue damage *367*

Leucine Aminopeptidase *Urine* *Increase* Toxic damage due to released metabolites *4254*

Leukocytes *Blood* *Decrease* Within a few h after irradiation a neutrophilic leukocytosis appears. Following this, an oscillation in the neutrophil count occurs, the rate at which it falls to the minimum being a function of the dose of radiation *2034*
Blood *Increase* Within a few h after irradiation a neutrophilic leukocytosis appears. Following this, an oscillation in the neutrophilic count occurs, the rate at which it falls to the minimum being a function of the dose of radiation *2034*

Lymphocytes *Blood* *Decrease* Lymphopenia commences immediately becoming maximal within 24 - 36 h *2034* The earliest laboratory finding is lymphopenia, reaching absolute lymphocyte levels below 1,000 /μL within the first 48 postexposure h in cases of radiation injury *367*

Lysozyme *Urine* *Increase* Often seen for over 45 days following therapy *5236*

Neutrophils *Blood* *Decrease* A gradual fall begins during the first 2 weeks after exposure, reaches a plateau, and may even rise slightly, followed by a steep fall to a low point at 30 days postexposure in cases of radiation injury *367* Within a few h after irradiation a neutrophilic leukocytosis appears. Following this, an oscillation in the neutrophilic count occurs, the rate at which it falls to the minimum being a function of the dose of radiation *2034*
Blood *Increase* Increased in electric shock *5677* Within a few h after irradiation a neutrophilic leukocytosis appears. Following this, an oscillation in the neutrophilic count occurs, the rate at which it falls to the minimum being a function of the dose of radiation *2034*

Ornithine Carbamoyltransferase *Serum* *Increase* Reflects breakdown of tissue proteins *590*

Platelets *Blood* *Decrease* A gradual fall in the first 2 weeks postexposure and reaches a low point after 30 days in cases of radiation injury *367*

Properdin *Plasma* *Increase* Reflects breakdown of tissue proteins *1290*

Protein *Urine* *Increase* May cause renal damage *1290*

Reticulocytes *Blood* *Decrease* May decrease or disappear in the first 48 postexposure h in cases of radiation injury *367*

Taurine *Urine* *Increase* Tissue destruction *3424*

Urea Nitrogen *Serum* *Increase* May cause renal damage *4672*

Uric Acid *Serum* *Increase* Reflects cellular breakdown *1776*
Urine *Increase* Reflects cellular breakdown *1776*

992.00 Heat Stroke

α_1-Acid Glycoprotein *Serum* *Increase* One of the most reliable indicators of acute inflammation *4241* *4373* *2597* *4696* *3713* *4853*

Alanine Aminotransferase *Serum* *Increase* In 27 patients (9 men, 18 women) on admission to hospital with heat stroke mean activity of 32.2 ± 50.8 U/L significantly higher than normal of 6.3 ± 29 U/L *104* Increases (mean activity of 10 times normal) to a peak on the 3rd day and returns to normal by the 2nd week. Very high levels are associated with lethal outcome *5545*

Albumin *Serum* *Increase* By approximately 11.6% after heat exposure for 2 - 11 h *4731*

Aldosterone *Plasma* *Increase* Increases by 76% after 1 week of thermal stress *247*

Aspartate Aminotransferase *Serum* *Increase* In 27 patients (9 men, 18 women) on admission to hospital with heat stroke mean activity of 138.6 ± 166.5 U/L significantly higher than normal of 20.1 ± 9.2 U/L *104* In a case of malignant hyperpyrexia, the initial elevation (after 3 h) of 110 U/L was due to muscle damage. Later elevations (12 - 24 h) was 1,600 and

992.00 Heat Stroke *(continued)*

Aspartate Aminotransferase *(continued)* 3,440 U/L reflected damage of the liver *1118* Increased (mean 20 times normal) peaks on 3rd day and returns to normal in 2 weeks. Very high levels are often associated with lethal outcome *5545* Following severe heat stroke *1290*
Serum *No Effect* Normal in children *1129*

Bicarbonate *Serum* *No Effect* In 27 patients (9 men, 18 women) on admission to hospital with heat stroke mean concentration of 19.1 ± 6.3 mmol/L not significantly different from normal *104*

Bilirubin *Serum* *Increase* Clinically apparent jaundice appears 24 - 36 h after admission *2034*

Bleeding Time *Patient* *Increase* Observed effect *2034*

BSP Retention *Serum* *Increase* In almost 50% of patients with induced fever *479* Without liver disease *5544*

Calcium *Serum* *Decrease* Initially and consistently high phosphate levels resulted in the fall of serum calcium to 5 mg/dL after 24 h in a case of malignant hyperpyrexia *1118*

Chloride *Serum* *Increase* Normal to high in severe cases *367*
Serum *No Effect* In 27 patients (9 men, 18 women) on admission to hospital with heat stroke mean concentration of 104.4 ± 4.9 mmol/L not significantly different from normal *104*

Clotting Time *Blood* *Increase* Typical finding observed *2034*

Creatine Kinase *Serum* *Increase* Biochemical estimations in a fatal case of malignant hyperpyrexia showed very high serum CK, phosphate, and potassium *1118* In 27 patients (9 men, 18 women) on admission to hospital with heat stroke mean activity of 494.3 ± 654 U/L significantly higher than normal of 261 ± 385 U/L *104*

Creatinine *Serum* *Increase* Renal failure is a common complication *2034* In 27 patients (9 men, 18 women) on admission to hospital with heat stroke mean concentration of 142 ± 55 µmol/L slightly higher than normal *104*

Factor VIII *Plasma* *Increase* Increased activity as a result of fever *1310*

Fibrinogen *Plasma* *Decrease* Formation is moderately depressed in severe heat stroke *1290*

Glucose *Serum* *Decrease* Has been observed *143*

Hematocrit *Blood* *No Effect* In 27 patients (9 men, 18 women) on admission to hospital with heat stroke mean concentration of 0.39 ± 0.05 not significantly different from normal *104*

Hemoglobin *Blood* *Increase* In children *1129*

Ketones *Serum* *Increase* Increased ketones in blood. Carbohydrate requirement increased with fever *1290*
Urine *Increase* Children are more liable to develop ketosis than adults with fever *5544* *1290*

Lactate Dehydrogenase *Serum* *Increase* In 27 patients (9 men, 18 women) on admission to hospital with heat stroke mean activity of 165 ± 74 U/L slightly higher than normal of 157.7 ± 43 U/L *104* Increases to a mean value 5 times normal by the 3rd day and returns to normal in 2 weeks. Very high levels are often associated with lethal outcome *5545*
Serum *No Effect* Normal in children *1129*

Lactate Dehydrogenase Isoenzyme-1 *Serum* *Increase* In 27 patients (9 men, 18 women) on admission to hospital with heat stroke mean % activity of 31.8 ± 10.0% not significantly higher than normal of 25.8 ± 9.6% *104*

Lactate Dehydrogenase Isoenzyme-2 *Serum* *Increase* In 27 patients (9 men, 18 women) on admission to hospital with heat stroke mean % activity of 21.3 ± 7.7% not significantly higher than normal of 18.7 ± 6.7% *104*

Lactate Dehydrogenase Isoenzyme-3 *Serum* *No Effect* In 27 patients (9 men, 18 women) on admission to hospital with heat stroke mean % activity of 20.6 ± 3.9% not significantly different from normal of 22.9 ± 5.6% *104*

Lactate Dehydrogenase Isoenzyme-4 *Serum* *Decrease* In 27 patients (9 men, 18 women) on admission to hospital with heat stroke mean % activity of 15.7 ± 6.9% not significantly different from normal of 20.3 ± 7.1% *104*

Lactate Dehydrogenase Isoenzyme-5 *Serum* *No Effect* In 27 patients (9 men, 18 women) on admission to hospital with heat stroke mean % activity of 10.6 ± 5.4% not significantly different from normal of 11.0 ± 3.6% *104*

Lead *Blood* *Increase* Increased temperature may result in mobilization of fixed lead *596*

Myoglobin *Urine* *Increase* Sudden muscle damage *1290* Sporadic; metabolic myoglobinuria *5544*

Phosphate *Serum* *Decrease* Neuroleptic malignant syndrome is less common cause of hypophosphatemia due to increased renal loss of phosphate *969*
Serum *Increase* Concentrations were very high (9.5 - 15 mg/dL) throughout and later resulted in a fall in serum calcium in one case of malignant hyperpyrexia *1118* In children *1129*

Platelets *Blood* *Decrease* Low in severe cases *367*

Potassium *Serum* *Decrease* Serum K is low and Cl is high in severe cases *367*
Serum *Increase* In malignant hyperpyrexia, raised to 9.0 mmol/L (normal concentration of 3.5 - 5.4 mmol/L) 2 h after the anesthetic was started *1118*
Serum *No Effect* In 27 patients (9 men, 18 women) on admission to hospital with heat stroke mean concentration of 3.57 ± 0.71 mmol/L not significantly different from normal *104*

Protein *Serum* *Decrease* Reduced by 15.7% after 2 - 11 h heat exposure *4731*

Prothrombin Time *Plasma* *Increase* May occur with prolonged hot weather *2277*

Renin Activity *Plasma* *Increase* Plasma activity increased by 174% after 1 week of thermal stress *247*

Sodium *Serum* *No Effect* In 27 patients (9 men, 18 women) on admission to hospital with heat stroke mean concentration of 135.9 ± 5.7 mmol/L not significantly different from normal *104*

Urea *Serum* *No Effect* In 27 patients (9 men, 18 women) on admission to hospital with heat stroke mean concentration of 7.25 ± 2.7 mmol/L not significantly different from normal *104*

Urea Nitrogen *Serum* *Increase* Elevated in severe cases *367*

Uric Acid *Serum* *Increase* In children *1129*

Volume *Plasma* *Decrease* Reduced 13.6% after 2 - 11 h heat exposure *4731*
Urine *Decrease* Urine volume is low in severe cases *367*

994.60 Motion Sickness

Aldosterone *Plasma* *Increase* In 5 healthy men moderately prone to motion sickness after 25 stimuli mean concentration changed from 0.073 ± 0.022 ng/mL to 0.100 ± 0.015 ng/mL compared with normal concentration of 0.037 ± 0.010 ng/mL *4976*

Androstenedione *Plasma* *Increase* In 5 healthy men moderately prone to motion sickness after 25 stimuli mean concentration changed significantly from 1.540 ± 0.260 ng/mL to 2.490 ± 0.250 ng/mL compared with normal concentration of > 1.200 ng/mL *4976*

Corticosterone *Plasma* *Increase* In 5 healthy men moderately prone to motion sickness after 25 stimuli mean concentration changed significantly from 2.720 ± 1.560 ng/mL to 16.950 ± 1.770 ng/mL compared with normal concentration of 3.980 ± 2.100 ng/L *4976*

Cortisol *Plasma* *Increase* In 5 healthy men moderately prone to motion sickness after 25 stimuli mean concentration changed significantly from 67.900 ± 7.780 ng/mL to 119.900 ± 14.420 ng/mL compared with normal concentration of 104.000 ± 3.400 ng/mL *4976*

Cortisone *Plasma* *Decrease* In 5 healthy men moderately prone to motion sickness after 25 stimuli mean concentration changed from 15.500 ± 2.830 ng/mL to 14.100 ± 3.600 ng/mL compared with normal concentration of 20.600 ± 9.300 ng/mL *4976*

Dehydroepiandrosterone Sulfate *Plasma* *Increase* In 5 healthy men moderately prone to motion sickness after 25 stimuli mean concentration changed nonsignificantly from 2,933 ± 200 ng/mL to 2,880 ± 170 ng/mL compared with normal concentration of 2,000 ± 355 ng/mL *4976*

11-Deoxycorticosterone *Plasma* *Increase* In 5 healthy men moderately prone to motion sickness after 25 stimuli mean concentration changed from 0.027 ± 0.013 ng/mL to 0.277 ± 0.235 ng/mL compared with normal concentration of 0.045 ± 0.016 ng/mL *4976*

11-Deoxycortisol *Plasma* *Increase* In 5 healthy men moderately prone to motion sickness after 25 stimuli mean concentration changed significantly from 0.350 ± 280 ng/mL to 1.420 ± 0.520 ng/mL compared with normal concentration of 0.470 ± 0.210 ng/mL *4976*

17-Hydroxyprogesterone *Plasma* *Increase* In 5 healthy men moderately prone to motion sickness after 25 stimuli mean concentration changed significantly from 1.050 ± 0.010 ng/mL to 7.190 ± 0.940 ng/mL compared with normal concentration of 1.190 ± 0.370 ng/mL *4976*

Progesterone *Plasma* *Increase* In 5 healthy men moderately prone to motion sickness after 25 stimuli mean concentration changed from 0.098 ± 0.024 ng/mL to 0.446 ± 0.350 ng/mL compared with normal concentration of 0.160 ± 0.070 ng/mL *4976*

Testosterone *Serum* *No Effect* In 5 healthy men moderately prone to motion sickness after 25 stimuli mean concentration changed insignificantly from 5.800 ± 1.000 ng/mL to 5.900 ± 0.620 ng/mL compared with normal concentration of > 2.800 ng/mL *4976*

994.80 Effects of Electric Current

Adenosine Monophosphate *Urine* *Increase* Mean change from 4.2 µmol/24 h to 14.2 µmol/24 h *5648*

Albumin *Urine* *Increase* Albuminuria and hemoglobinuria occurs in presence of severe burns *5545* Characteristic *2034*

Aspartate Aminotransferase *Serum* *Increase* Indicates severe tissue damage *5545* Trauma following direct current countershock to convert arrhythmia to normal rhythm (from intercostal muscle damage *1290*

Creatine Kinase *Serum* *Increase* Rose to abnormal levels in 5 of 8 patients, while the AST values showed no rise in patients undergoing D.C. countershock *2299* Electrical cardiac defibrillation or countershock in 50% of patients; returns to normal in 48 - 72 h *5544* Electrocautery used within the preceding days to the test may also produce elevated levels *1642*

Creatine Kinase MB-Isoenzyme *Serum* *Increase* Increased release of non-myocardial CK following electrical injury. In most cases increase in total CK without increased percentage of CK-MB *768* Increased release of non-myocardial CK following electrical injury. In most cases increase in total CK not increased percentage of CK-MB *4750*

Dopamine β-Hydroxylase *Serum* *No Effect* No effect observed *5648*

Erythrocytes *Cerebrospinal Fluid* *Increase* Bloody spinal fluid as a result of widespread vascular injury *2034*

Hematocrit *Blood* *Increase* Immediately following major injury *2034*

Hemoglobin *Urine* *Increase* In many cases, probably secondary to severe burns *2034*

Leukocytes *Blood* *Increase* Leukocytosis with many large immature granulocytes is common after severe shock *2034*

Myoglobin *Urine* *Increase* Sporadic; exertional *5544* Sudden muscle damage due to high-voltage electric shock *1290*

Neutrophils *Blood* *Increase* Leukocytosis with many large immature granulocytes is common after severe shock *2034*

pH *Blood* *Decrease* Profound metabolic acidosis *2034*

Potassium *Serum* *Decrease* Unexplained acute hypokalemia leading to respiratory arrest and cardiac arrhythmias has developed in some patients between the 2nd and 4th weeks following injury *2034*

Protein *Urine* *Increase* May cause renal damage *4672*

Urea Nitrogen *Serum* *Increase* May cause renal damage *4672*

Volume *Plasma* *Decrease* Immediately following major injury *2034*

995.00 Anaphylaxis

Histamine *Urine* *Increase* Increased excretion observed in patients with anaphylaxis *2952*

Tryptase *Serum* *Increase* In one patient 4 and 5 days after onset of anaphylactic symptoms concentrations of 7.2 ng/mL and 5.1 ng/mL significantly increased compared with < 1.0 ng/mL in normal individuals *5476*

995.10 Angioedema

Complement C_3 *Serum* *No Effect* Patients with hereditary angioedema have decreased levels of C_1 esterase inhibitor and C_4 in the presence of normal amounts of C_3 and C_1q. Normal values for these complement components are found in persons with allergic angioedema *562*

Complement C_4 *Serum* *No Effect* Patients with hereditary angioedema have decreased levels of C_1 esterase inhibitor and C_4 in the presence of normal amounts of C_3 and C_1q. Normal values for these complement components are found in persons with allergic angioedema *562*

Complement, Total *Serum* *No Effect* Patients with hereditary angioedema have decreased levels of C_1 esterase inhibitor and C_4 in the presence of normal amounts of C_3 and C_1q. Normal values for these complement components are found in persons with allergic angioedema *562*

Eosinophils *Blood* *Increase* In 3 patients with angioedema and eosinophilia mean concentration of 8,950 ± 1,070 /µL compared with less than 500 /µL in 100 normal individuals *5776*

Granulocyte-Macrophage Colony Stimulating Factor *Serum* *No Effect* Not detected in the serum of any of 13 patients with condition *2744*

Interleukin-3 *Serum* *No Effect* Not detected in the serum of any of 13 patients with condition *2744*

Interleukin-5 *Serum* *Increase* Detected in the serum of 10 of 13 patients with angioedema *2744*

Myelin Basic Protein *Serum* *Increase* In 1 patient with angioedema and eosinophilia mean concentration of 300 ± 301 ng/mL compared with mean of 41 ± 19 ng/mL in 100 normal individuals *5776*

995.30 Allergy, Classical

Histidine *Urine* *Decrease* In 14 patients with atopic allergy median excretion of 402.5 µmol/d significantly different from 371 - 1,771 µmol/d in 25 nonallergic volunteers *1292*

Immunoglobulin E *Serum* *Increase* In 14 patients with atopic allergy median concentration of 78 significantly different from normal range *1292*

995.89 Malignant Hyperpyrexia

Phosphate *Serum* *Increase* Release of phosphate is characteristic of malignant hyperpyrexia following exposure to anesthetic agents in susceptible individuals *969*

995.89 Malignant Hyperthermia

Creatine Kinase MB-Isoenzyme *Serum* *Increase* Observed effect *248*

Phosphate *Serum* *Increase* Hyperphosphatemia may occur partially due to rhabdomyolysis *5204*

996.81 Renal Transplant Rejection

Albumin *Serum* *Decrease* Hypoalbuminemia post-transplantation predicted significantly greater chronic graft rejection *5098*

Ammonium Ions *Urine* *Increase* May lead to proximal renal tubular acidosis which is associated with hypokalemia, hyperchloremic metabolic acidosis, urine pH < 5.5, increased urinary ammonium ion excretion, a negative urine anion gap, increased urinary osmol gap, normal urinary citrate, normal urinary calcium excretion and Fanconi syndrome *4071* May be associated with classic distal renal tubular acidosis which is asociated with hyokalemia, hyperchloremic metabolic acidosis, urine pH > 5.5, increased urinary ammonium ion excretion, a negative urine anion gap, increased urinary osmol gap, decreased urinary citrate and increased urinary calcium in some patients *4071*

996.81 Renal Transplant Rejection *(continued)*

Anion Gap *Urine Decrease* May be associated with classic distal renal tubular acidosis which is asociated with hyokalemia, hyperchloremic metabolic acidosis, urine pH > 5.5, increased urinary ammonium ion excretion, a negative urine anion gap, increased urinary osmol gap, decreased urinary citrate and increased urinary calcium in some patients *4071* May lead to proximal renal tubular acidosis which is associated with hypokalemia, hyperchloremic metabolic acidosis, urine pH < 5.5, increased urinary ammonium ion excretion, a negative urine anion gap, increased urinary osmol gap, normal urinary citrate, normal urinary calcium excretion and Fanconi syndrome *4071*

Anti-Endothelial Cell Antibodies *Serum Increase* Antibodies detected in 27% cases at time of rejection or thrombosis *5061*

Anti-Epithelial Antibodies *Serum Increase* Antibodies detected in 24% cases at time of rejection or thrombosis *5061*

Bicarbonate *Serum Decrease* May lead to proximal renal tubular acidosis which is associated with hypokalemia, hyperchloremic metabolic acidosis, urine pH < 5.5, increased urinary ammonium ion excretion, a negative urine anion gap, increased urinary osmol gap, normal urinary citrate, normal urinary calcium excretion and Fanconi syndrome *4071*

Calcium *Urine Increase* May be associated with classic distal renal tubular acidosis which is asociated with hyokalemia, hyperchloremic metabolic acidosis, urine pH > 5.5, increased urinary ammonium ion excretion, a negative urine anion gap, increased urinary osmol gap, decreased urinary citrate and increased urinary calcium in some patients *4071*
Urine No Effect May lead to proximal renal tubular acidosis which is associated with hypokalemia, hyperchloremic metabolic acidosis, urine pH < 5.5, increased urinary ammonium ion excretion, a negative urine anion gap, increased urinary osmol gap, normal urinary citrate, normal urinary calcium excretion and Fanconi syndrome *4071*

Chloride *Serum Increase* May lead to proximal renal tubular acidosis which is associated with hypokalemia, hyperchloremic metabolic acidosis, urine pH < 5.5, increased urinary ammonium ion excretion, a negative urine anion gap, increased urinary osmol gap, normal urinary citrate, normal urinary calcium excretion and Fanconi syndrome *4071* May be associated with classic distal renal tubular acidosis which is asociated with hyokalemia, hyperchloremic metabolic acidosis, urine pH > 5.5, increased urinary ammonium ion excretion, a negative urine anion gap, increased urinary osmol gap, decreased urinary citrate and increased urinary calcium in some patients *4071*

Cholesterol *Serum Increase* Hypercholesterolemia post-transplantation predicted significantly greater chronic graft rejection *5098*

Citrate *Urine Decrease* May be associated with classic distal renal tubular acidosis which is asociated with hyokalemia, hyperchloremic metabolic acidosis, urine pH > 5.5, increased urinary ammonium ion excretion, a negative urine anion gap, increased urinary osmol gap, decreased urinary citrate and increased urinary calcium in some patients *4071*
Urine No Effect May lead to proximal renal tubular acidosis which is associated with hypokalemia, hyperchloremic metabolic acidosis, urine pH < 5.5, increased urinary ammonium ion excretion, a negative urine anion gap, increased urinary osmol gap, normal urinary citrate, normal urinary calcium excretion and Fanconi syndrome *4071*

C-Reactive Protein *Urine Increase* In 15 patients with interstitial rejection mean concentration of 120 µg/L and 8,459 µg/L in 6 patients with vascular rejection significantly different from < 6 µg/L in 34 patients with normal courses *4994*

Fractional Excretion of Sodium *Urine Increase* Episodes of rejection observed in 12 of 13 patients following renal transplantation with a rise identified. In 1 increase preceded and in 8 followed diagnosis of rejection *5655*

Glucose *Urine Increase* May lead to proximal renal tubular acidosis which is associated with hypokalemia, hyperchloremic metabolic acidosis, urine pH < 5.5, increased urinary ammonium ion excretion, a negative urine anion gap, increased urinary osmol gap, normal urinary citrate, normal urinary calcium excretion and Fanconi syndrome *4071*

HDL-Cholesterol *Serum Decrease* Hypo-LDL-cholesterolemia post-transplantation predicted significantly greater chronic graft rejection *5098*

Interleukin-1 Receptor Antagonist *Serum Increase* In patients with an uncomplicated postoperative course the highest plasma concentration during the first 2 weeks post-transplant was a mean of 1,135 pg/mL, decreasing to a mean of 542 pg/mL in weeks 3 and 4. With rejection concentration increased 1 - 3 days before symptoms of rejection were observed or infection *1009*

LDL-Cholesterol *Serum Increase* Hyper-LDL-cholesterolemia post-transplantation predicted significantly greater chronic graft rejection *5098*

α_2-Macroglobulin *Urine Increase* In 15 patients with interstitial rejection mean concentration of 1,500 µg/L and 22,000 µg/L in 6 patients with vascular rejection significantly different from < 180 µg/L in 34 patients with normal courses *4994*

Myeloperoxidase *Urine No Effect* In 15 patients with interstitial rejection mean concentration of < 200 µg/L and < 200 µg/L in 5 of 6 with vascular rejection not significantly different from < 200 µg/L in 34 patients with normal courses *4994*

N-Acetyl-Glucosaminidase *Urine Increase* Episodes of rejection observed in 12 of 13 patients following renal transplantation with a rise in activity identified in 11 cases, in 7 increase preceded, in 3 occurred simultaneously and in 1 followed diagnosis of rejection *5655*

Neopterin *Serum Increase* Increasing neopterin concentrations observed after kidney transplant rejection *121*

Net Acid Excretion *Urine Increase* May be associated with classic distal renal tubular acidosis which is associated with hyokalemia, hyperchloremic metabolic acidosis, urine pH > 5.5, increased urinary ammonium ion excretion, a negative urine anion gap, increased urinary osmol gap, decreased urinary citrate and increased urinary calcium in some patients *4071*

Osmolal Gap *Urine Increase* May lead to proximal renal tubular acidosis which is associated with hypokalemia, hyperchloremic metabolic acidosis, urine pH < 5.5, increased urinary ammonium ion excretion, a negative urine anion gap, increased urinary osmol gap, normal urinary citrate, normal urinary calcium excretion and Fanconi syndrome *4071* May be associated with classic distal renal tubular acidosis which is asociated with hyokalemia, hyperchloremic metabolic acidosis, urine pH > 5.5, increased urinary ammonium ion excretion, a negative urine anion gap, increased urinary osmol gap, decreased urinary citrate and increased urinary calcium in some patients *4071*

pH *Urine Decrease* May lead to proximal renal tubular acidosis which is associated with hypokalemia, hyperchloremic metabolic acidosis, urine pH < 5.5, increased urinary ammonium ion excretion, a negative urine anion gap, increased urinary osmol gap, normal urinary citrate, normal urinary calcium excretion and Fanconi syndrome *4071*
Urine Increase May be associated with classic distal renal tubular acidosis which is asociated with hyokalemia, hyperchloremic metabolic acidosis, urine pH > 5.5, increased urinary ammonium ion excretion, a negative urine anion gap, increased urinary osmol gap, decreased urinary citrate and increased urinary calcium in some patients *4071*

Phosphate *Serum Decrease* Postrenal transplantation is common cause of severe hypophosphatemia due to shift of phosphate into the cells, reduced absorption of phosphate from the intestinal tract and increased renal loss of phosphate *969* May lead to proximal renal tubular acidosis which is associated with hypokalemia, hyperchloremic metabolic acidosis, urine pH < 5.5, increased urinary ammonium ion excretion, a negative urine anion gap, increased urinary osmol gap, normal urinary citrate, normal urinary calcium excretion and Fanconi syndrome *4071*

Potassium *Serum Decrease* May lead to proximal renal tubular acidosis which is associated with hypokalemia, hyperchloremic metabolic acidosis, urine pH < 5.5, increased urinary ammonium ion excretion, a negative urine anion gap, increased urinary osmol gap, normal urinary citrate, normal urinary calcium excretion and Fanconi syndrome *4071* May be associated with classic distal renal tubular acidosis which is asociated with hyokalemia, hyperchloremic metabolic acidosis, urine pH > 5.5, increased urinary ammonium ion excretion, a negative urine anion gap, increased urinary osmol gap, decreased urinary citrate and increased urinary calcium in some patients *4071*

Protein *Urine Increase* Proteinuria post-transplantation predicted significantly greater chronic graft rejection *5098*

Soluble HLA-I *Serum* *Increase* Mean concentration increased in graft versus host disease *576* Concentration reportedly increased with episodes of rejection *5306*

Soluble HLA-FHC *Serum* *Increase* Mean concentration increased in allograft rejection *576*

Triglycerides *Serum* *Increase* Hypertriglyceridemia pre- and 3 weeks post-transplant predicted significantly worse graft function at one year *5098*

Uric Acid *Serum* *Decrease* May lead to proximal renal tubular acidosis which is associated with hypokalemia, hyperchloremic metabolic acidosis, urine pH < 5.5, increased urinary ammonium ion excretion, a negative urine anion gap, increased urinary osmol gap, normal urinary citrate, normal urinary calcium excretion and Fanconi syndrome *4071*

996.81 Renal Transplantation

Albumin *Serum* *Decrease* In 19 patients mean concentration changed from baseline of 32 ± 6 g/L to 27 ± 5 g/L one week after transplantation (significant), to 28 ± 4 g/L at discharge from hospital, median 16 days (significantly different from baseline) *4511* Mean concentration in 27 patients with renal transplants receiving cyclosporine of 40 ± 4 g/L significantly different from 44 ± 2 g/L in 75 healthy controls *4510*
Serum *Increase* In 19 patients mean concentration changed from baseline of 32 ± 6 g/L prior to transplantation to 36 ± 4 g/L after 6 months (significant) and 35 ± 3 g/L one year after transplantation (significant) *4511*
Urine *Increase* Peak observed with renal graft rejection *5000*

Aldosterone *Plasma* *Increase* In 8 patients following renal transplantation mean concentration significantly higher than in controls with loss of circadian variation, possibly due to immunosuppressive therapy *979*

Alkaline Phosphatase *Serum* *No Effect* In 10 patients with chronic glomerulonephritis who received a renal transplant mean activity of 148 U/L within the normal range *1167* In 17 patients with chronic renal failure renal transplantation caused serum alkaline phosphatase activity to rise but not above reference range *2483*

Alkaline Phosphatase, Bone Isoenzyme *Serum* *Increase* In 52 patients mean concentration increased from 7.9 ± 1.2 μg/L pretransplantation to 14.6 ± 1.8 μg/L 3 months following renal transplantation *5702* In 17 patients with chronic renal failure bone alkaline phosphatase activity at the lower end of reference range but rose sequentially increasing by 4 to 10 fold in the 4 months following transplantation *2483*

Aluminum *Bone* *Decrease* In 10 patients with chronic glomerulonephritis who received a renal transplant mean concentration of 7.2 ± 5.6 μg/g wet weight significantly reduced compared with the time when they were receiving regular hemodialysis when the mean concentration was 13.0 ± 4.7 μg/g wet weight *1167*

Ammonium Ions *Urine* *Decrease* May cause distal renal tubular acidosis (type IV) is associated with hyperkalemia, hyperchloremic metabolic acidosis, urine pH < 5.5, decreased urinary ammonium ion excretion, a positive urine anion gap, normal urinary citrate and urinary calcium excretion *4071*

Amylase *Serum* *Increase* In 23 patients who had undergone renal transplantation at least 6 months previously mean activity of 209 ± 93 U/L significantly different from 148 ± 64 U/L in 34 healthy volunteer controls *3331* Mean activity in 25 patients following renal transplantation of 333 ± 106 U/L significantly different from 183 ± 54 U/L in 47 healthy controls *1015*
Urine *Decrease* Mean activity in 25 patients following renal transplantation of 186 ± 162 U/L not significantly different from 220 ± 296 U/L in 47 healthy controls *1015*

Amylase, Pancreatic Isoenzyme *Serum* *Increase* Mean activity in 25 patients following renal transplantation of 208 ± 55 U/L significantly different from 84 ± 30 U/L in 47 healthy controls *1015* In 23 patients who had undergone renal transplantation at least 6 months previously mean activity of 114 ± 53 U/L significantly different from 80 ± 46 U/L in 34 healthy volunteer controls *3331*
Urine *No Effect* Mean activity in 25 patients following renal transplantation of 134 ± 147 U/L not significantly different from 132 ± 186 U/L in 47 healthy controls *1015*

Amylase, Salivary Isoenzyme *Serum* *Increase* Mean activity in 25 patients following renal transplantation of 125 ± 69 U/L not significantly different from 98 ± 55 U/L in 47 healthy controls *1015*
Urine *Decrease* Mean activity in 25 patients following renal transplantation of 53 ± 37 U/L not significantly different from 92 ± 152 U/L in 47 healthy controls *1015*

Amyloid A *Serum* *Increase* Significant increase observed in patients during all phases of renal allograft rejections: mean peak concentration of 446 mg/L compared with 1 mg/L in controls *3380* Significant increase associated with renal transplant rejection more useful than either β_2-microglobulin or C-reactive protein *3379*

Amyloid A Protein *Serum* *Increase* In 19 episodes of rejection mean concentration increased to 705 ± 170 mg/L with rejection occurring on day 1 to 4 post-surgery from 306 ± 78 mg/L on day 2 post-uncomplicated surgery and to 460 ± 192 mg/L with rejection on day 5 or later *715*

Anion Gap *Urine* *Increase* May cause distal renal tubular acidosis (type IV) is associated with hyperkalemia, hyperchloremic metabolic acidosis, urine pH < 5.5, decreased urinary ammonium ion excretion, a positive urine anion gap, normal urinary citrate and urinary calcium excretion *4071*

Anti-Endothelial Cell Antibodies *Serum* *Increase* Antibodies detected in 20 of 79 (25%) patients with renal transplants: antibodies detected in 27% cases at time of rejection or thrombosis *5061*

Anti-Epithelial Antibodies *Serum* *Increase* Antibodies detected in 21 of 79 (26%) patients with renal transplants: antibodies detected in 24% cases at time of rejection or thrombosis *5061*

Anti-Interleukin-1 Antibodies *Serum* *Positive* In 159 renal graft recipients anti-IL-1α antibodies observed in 5.6% *5084*

Anticardiolipin Antibodies *Serum* *Increase* In 11 of 20 patients with renal transplants anticardiolipin antibodies detected *1844*

Antithrombin III *Plasma* *Increase* In 39 patients with renal transplants concentration significantly higher than in 20 healthy individuals and 20 patient controls. Concentration higher in patients with rejection and higher in individuals with transplant for less than one year than longer *5721*

Apolipoprotein A *Serum* *Increase* Mean concentration of 3.61 ± 0.82 g/L in 57 renal transplantation patients (41 men, 16 women of mean age 40.5 ± 13.8 years, with mean of 28.6 ± 12.9 months after transplantation) significantly different from 2.32 ± 0.62 g/L in 29 healthy controls (13 men, 16 women of mean age 30.0 ± 6.8 years) *5188*

Apolipoprotein A-I *Serum* *Decrease* Significant reduction observed in renal transplant recipients between 3 and 24 months post-transplant *726*
Serum *Increase* In 10 children with congenital nephrotic syndrome renal transplantation caused mean concentration to increase from baseline of 47.4 ± 11.6 mg/dL to 118.7 ± 13.9 mg/dL *149* In 20 consecutive patients significant increase in concentration observed months after transplantation *463*
Serum *No Effect* Mean concentration of 2.48 ± 0.66 g/L in 57 renal transplantation patients (41 men, 16 women of mean age 40.5 ± 13.8 years, with mean of 28.6 ± 12.9 months after transplantation) not significantly different from 2.26 ± 0.57 g/L in 29 healthy controls (13 men, 16 women of mean age 30.0 ± 6.8 years) *5188* In 17 patients with chronic renal failure following renal transplantation mean concentration of 1.38 ± 0.3 g/L not significantly different from 1.56 ± 0.59 g/L in 27 healthy controls *935*

Apolipoprotein A-I:Apolipoprotein B Ratio
Serum *Decrease* Mean ratio of 1.53 ± 0.55 in 57 renal transplantation patients (41 men, 16 women of mean age 40.5 ± 13.8 years, with mean of 28.6 ± 12.9 months after transplantation) significantly different from 1.84 ± 0.72 in 29 healthy controls (13 men, 16 women of mean age 30.0 ± 6.8 years) *5188*

Apolipoprotein A-II *Serum* *Increase* In 10 children with congenital nephrotic syndrome renal transplantation caused mean concentration to increase from baseline of 8.6 ± 1.9 mg/dL to 32.7 ± 6.0 mg/dL *149*

996.81 Renal Transplantation *(continued)*

Apolipoprotein A:Apolipoprotein B Ratio *Serum Increase* Mean ratio of 2.21 ± 0.64 in 57 renal transplantation patients (41 men, 16 women of mean age 40.5 ± 13.8 years, with mean of 28.6 ± 12.9 months after transplantation) significantly different from 1.76 ± 0.55 in 29 healthy controls (13 men, 16 women of mean age 30.0 ± 6.8 years) *5188*

Apolipoprotein B *Serum Increase* In 20 consecutive patients 6 months following renal transplantation significant increase in concentration observed *463* Mean concentration of 1.71 ± 0.45 g/L in 57 renal transplantation patients (41 men, 16 women of mean age 40.5 ± 13.8 years, with mean of 28.6 ± 12.9 months after transplantation) significantly different from 1.32 ± 0.31 g/L in 29 healthy controls (13 men, 16 women of mean age 30.0 ± 6.8 years) *5188* Concentration significantly increased at 3 and 24 months in patients after renal transplantation *726*
Serum No Effect In 17 patients with chronic renal failure following renal transplantation mean concentration of 0.99 ± 0.30 g/L not significantly different from 0.87 ± 0.20 g/L in 27 healthy controls *935* In 10 children with congenital nephrotic syndrome renal transplantation caused mean concentration to change from baseline of 91.5 ± 10.1 mg/dL to 91.9 ± 12.5 mg/dL *149*

Apolipoprotein C *Serum Decrease* Significant reduction observed between 3rd and 24th month post-transplant in patients with renal transplantation *726*

Apolipoprotein C-II *Serum Increase* Mean concentration of 0.06 ± 0.02 g/L in 57 renal transplantation patients (41 men, 16 women of mean age 40.5 ± 13.8 years, with mean of 28.6 ± 12.9 months after transplantation) significantly different from 0.04 ± 0.01 g/L in 29 healthy controls (13 men, 16 women of mean age 30.0 ± 6.8 years) *5188*

Apolipoprotein C-II:Apolipoprotein C-III Ratio
Serum Decrease Mean ratio of 0.27 ± 0.07 in 57 renal transplantation patients (41 men, 16 women of mean age 40.5 ± 13.8 years, with mean of 28.6 ± 12.9 months after transplantation) significantly different from 0.39 ± 0.08 in 29 healthy controls (13 men, 16 women of mean age 30.0 ± 6.8 years) *5188*

Apolipoprotein C-III *Serum Increase* Mean concentration of 0.23 ± 0.09 g/L in 57 renal transplantation patients (41 men, 16 women of mean age 40.5 ± 13.8 years, with mean of 28.6 ± 12.9 months after transplantation) significantly different from 0.11 ± 0.03 g/L in 29 healthy controls (13 men, 16 women of mean age 30.0 ± 6.8 years) *5188*

Apolipoprotein E *Serum Increase* Mean concentration of 0.07 ± 0.03 g/L in 57 renal transplantation patients (41 men, 16 women of mean age 40.5 ± 13.8 years, with mean of 28.6 ± 12.9 months after transplantation) significantly different from 0.04 ± 0.02 g/L in 29 healthy controls (13 men, 16 women of mean age 30.0 ± 6.8 years) *5188*

Apolipoprotein Lp(a) *Serum Decrease* In 20 consecutive patients aged 46 ± 11 years concentration decreased from median of 403 U/L before transplantation to 184 U/L at one week and 170 U/L at 6 months after transplantation: decrease significantly correlated with the increase in creatinine clearance (r = -0.48) *463*

Atrial Natriuretic Peptide *Plasma Decrease* In patients whose graft functioned plasma concentration declined in parallel with serum creatinine concentration (mean change from 658 to 210 µmol/L) whereas concentration increased with creatinine in individuals whose graft did not function *4266*
Plasma Increase In patients whose graft functioned, plasma concentration declined in parallel with serum creatinine concentration (mean change from 658 to 210 µmol/L) whereas concentration increased with creatinine in individuals whose graft did not function *4266*

CA 15-3 *Serum Increase* In 30 patients with chronic renal failure on regular hemodialysis concentration significantly higher than in 23 patients with chronic renal failure on regular hemodialysis *5850*

CA 19-9 *Serum No Effect* No significant difference observed between concentrations in 30 individuals with successful renal transplants and 50 healthy volunteers *5850*

CA 125 *Serum No Effect* No significant difference observed between mean concentrations of 30 patients with successful renal transplants and 50 healthy volunteers *5850*

Calcium *Serum Decrease* In 19 patients mean concentration changed from baseline of 2.48 ± 0.28 mmol/L to 0.98 ± 0.40 mmol/L one week after transplantation (significant), to 2.23 ± 0.25 mmol/L at discharge from hospital, median 16 days (significantly different from baseline), to 2.42 ± 0.15 mmol/L after 6 months (not significantly different from baseline) and 2.40 ± 0.14 mmol/L one year after transplantation (not significantly different from baseline) *4511*
Serum Increase In 4 of 92 patients with renal transplants (mean time since surgery 63 months) adjusted calcium concentration increased above 2.60 mmol/L *5035*
Serum No Effect In 83 of 92 patients with renal transplants (mean 63 months since surgery) mean adjusted concentration of calcium fell within normal range *5035*
Urine No Effect May cause distal renal tubular acidosis (type IV) is associated with hyperkalemia, hyperchloremic metabolic acidosis, urine pH < 5.5, decreased urinary ammonium ion excretion, a positive urine anion gap, normal urinary citrate and urinary calcium excretion *4071*

Carbamylated Hemoglobin *Blood Increase* In patients with renal transplants and renal failure mean concentration above 80 ng isopropyl hydantoin/mg globin compared with 15 - 39 ng isopropyl hydantoin/mg globin in healthy individuals *4914*

Carcinoembryonic Antigen *Serum Decrease* Concentration significantly less in 30 patients with successful renal transplants than in 23 patients with chronic renal failure on regular hemodialysis *5850*
Serum Increase In 45 patients with renal transplants 44% had concentrations less than 2.5 ng/mL, 39% had concentrations between 2.6 and 5.0 ng/mL, 12% had concentrations between 5.1 and 10.0 ng/mL and 5% had concentrations greater than 10.0 ng/mL *2010*

Chloride *Serum Increase* May cause distal renal tubular acidosis (type IV) is associated with hyperkalemia, hyperchloremic metabolic acidosis, urine pH < 5.5, decreased urinary ammonium ion excretion, a positive urine anion gap, normal urinary citrate and urinary calcium excretion *4071*

Cholesterol *Serum Decrease* In 10 children with congenital nephrotic syndrome renal transplantation caused mean concentration to decrease from baseline of 6.95 ± 1.59 mmol/L to 5.27 ± 0.98 mmol/L *149*
Serum Increase In patients with renal transplants 60% had cholesterol concentrations exceeding 240 mg/dL *2575* In 84 patients with chronic renal failure 6 months to one year after renal transplantation mean concentration rose to 249 ± 6 mg/dL compared with 189 ± 9 mg/dL before surgery *230* In 16 hyperlipidemic renal transplant patients mean concentration of 8.24 ± 1.86 mmol/L significantly greater than 4.2 ± 0.85 mmol/L in 10 healthy control individuals *1126* Mean concentration of 2.32 ± 0.49 g/L in 57 renal transplantation patients (41 men, 16 women of mean age 40.5 ± 13.8 years, with mean of 28.6 ± 12.9 months after transplantation) significantly different from 1.76 ± 0.29 g/L in 29 healthy controls (13 men, 16 women of mean age 30.0 ± 6.8 years) *5188* Characteristic observation *3526* Mean concentration increased to 226 mg/dL 3 months after renal transplantation and 218 mg/dL 24 months after renal transplantation compared with 201 mg/dL in controls *726*
Serum No Effect In 17 patients with chronic renal failure following renal transplantation mean concentration of 6.62 ± 1.36 mmol/L not significantly different from 6.34 ± 0.78 mmol/L in 27 healthy controls *935* In 12 normolipidemic renal transplant patients mean concentration of 5.57 ± 1.19 mmol/L not significantly greater than 4.2 ± 0.85 mmol/L in 10 healthy control individuals *1126*

Cholesterol, Free *Serum No Effect* In 17 patients with chronic renal failure following renal transplantation mean concentration of 1.58 ± 0.44 mmol/L not significantly different from 1.54 ± 0.21 mmol/L in 27 healthy controls *935*

Choline *Plasma Decrease* In patients receiving a kidney, concentration decreased from 29.8 ± 1.86 µmol/L before transplantation to 15.7 ± 2.32 µmol/L one day after at which level was maintained for several months *22*

Citrate *Urine No Effect* May cause distal renal tubular acidosis (type IV) is associated with hyperkalemia, hyperchloremic metabolic acidosis, urine pH < 5.5, decreased urinary ammonium ion excretion, a positive urine anion gap, normal urinary citrate and urinary calcium excretion *4071*

C-Reactive Protein *Serum Increase* Concentration increased with rejection but C-reactive protein not as good as serum amyloid A protein as a marker of rejection *3379*

Creatine Kinase *Serum Increase* One of 17 patients with renal transplants with chronic renal failure receiving hemodialysis had concentration above upper limit of normal *3686*

Creatine Kinase MB-Isoenzyme *Serum Increase* Three of 17 patients with renal transplants with chronic renal failure receiving hemodialysis had concentration above upper limit of normal *3686*

Creatinine *Serum Decrease* In 19 patients mean concentration changed from baseline of 757 ± 196 µmol/L to 329 ± 291 µmol/L one week after transplantation (significant), to 148 ± 72 µmol/L at discharge from hospital, median 16 days (significantly different from baseline), to 127 ± 37 µmol/L after 6 months (significant) and 147 ± 72 µmol/L one year after transplantation (significant) *4511* In 8 men with renal transplantation serum creatinine concentration decreased from 1406 ± 88 µmol/L presurgery to 398 ± 97 µmol/L one day after surgery and 194 ± 27 µmol/L 5 days after surgery *5732*

CrossLaps™ *Urine Increase* Median excretion of CrossLaps™ during median 9 days of transplant of 161 ± 41 µmol/mol creatinine increased to 306 ± 91 µmol/mol creatinine after median of 34 days post-transplant *5703*

C-terminal Propeptide of Type I Procollagen *Serum Increase* In 52 patients mean concentration increased from 119 ± 19 µg/L pretransplantation to 179 ± 27 µg/L 3 months following renal transplantation *5702*

1,25-Dihydroxy Vitamin D *Serum Decrease* In 92 post transplant patients (mean 63 months since transplantation) 18 had a concentration below the lower limit of normal *5035* *Serum Increase* In 15 of 92 patients with renal transplants (mean 63 months since surgery) concentration increased above upper limit of normal *5035* *Serum No Effect* In 59 of 92 patients following renal transplantation (mean 63 months since surgery) concentration within normal range *5035*

1,25-Dihydroxy Vitamin D_3 *Serum Decrease* In 31 adult patients 3 - 30 months after renal transplantation with mild renal impairment (GFR 45 - 90 mL/min) mean concentration reduced and positively correlated with serum 25-hydroxy-vitamin D_3 *3147* *Serum Increase* Concentration restored to normal from low concentration associated with end-stage renal disease *519* In 19 patients mean concentration changed from baseline of 27 ± 18 pmol/L to 48 ± 43 pmol/L one week after transplantation (not significant), to 52 ± 34 pmol/L at discharge from hospital, median 16 days (significantly different from baseline), to 100 ± 32 pmol/L after 6 months (significant) and 89 ± 33 pmol/L one year after transplantation (significant) *4511*

24,25-Dihydroxy Vitamin D_3 *Serum Increase* In 19 patients mean concentration changed from baseline of 1.4 ± 0.8 nmol/L to 1.4 ± 0.7 nmol/L one week after transplantation (not significant), to 1.9 ± 0.8 nmol/L at discharge from hospital, median 16 days (not significantly different from baseline), to 3.2 ± 1.6 nmol/L after 6 months (significant) and 3.3 ± 1.2 nmol/L one year after transplantation (significant) *4511*

Endothelin-1 *Plasma Increase* In 3 patients after renal transplantation mean concentration increased 3.0-fold above appropriate normal range *328* *Urine Increase* In 12 children following renal transplantation mean excretion of 31.2 pmol/sq m/d significantly different from 12.9 (lower and upper quartiles 10.0 - 15.2 pmol/sq m/d) in 60 healthy children *5733*

Erythropoietin *Serum Increase* In 17 patients with polycythemia following renal transplantation mean concentration of 65 ± 61 IU/L compared with 9 ± 4 IU/L in 79 reference controls *4320* In post-transplant patients with erythrocytosis mean concentration of 35.6 ± 5.7 mIU/mL significantly higher than 18.8 ± 2.6 mIU/mL in nonerythocytotic patients and 22.5 ± 0.95 mIU/mL in normal individuals *770*

α-Fetoprotein *Serum Decrease* Concentration significantly less in 30 patients with successful renal transplants than in 23 patients with chronic renal failure on regular hemodialysis *5850*

Fibrinogen *Plasma Decrease* In 16 patients median concentration decreased from 5.1 g/L preoperatively to 3.6 g/L, 3.6 g/L and 3.8 g/L on postoperative days 1, 3 and 5 respectively *609*

Fibronectin *Plasma Decrease* Significant reduction observed in patients during acute and chronic graft rejection *4625* *Plasma No Effect* Mean concentration of 0.33 ± 0.09 g/L in 57 renal transplantation patients (41 men, 16 women of mean age 40.5 ± 13.8 years, with mean of 28.6 ± 12.9 months after transplantation) not significantly different from 0.35 ± 0.08 g/L in 29 healthy controls (13 men, 16 women of mean age 30.0 ± 6.8 years) *5188*

Follicle Stimulating Hormone *Plasma Decrease* In post-transplant patients mean concentration of 6.8 ± 2.9 IU/L significantly less than 13.7 ± 14 IU/L in male controls *770* *Plasma No Effect* In patients following renal or cardiac transplantation regardless of immunosuppressant therapy and low plasma concentration of testosterone concentration not affected *4272*

Gastric Inhibitory Polypeptide *Plasma Decrease* Concentration decreased from high of uremia to median of 9.5 pmol/L following renal transplantation *1953*

Gastrin *Serum Decrease* Significant reduction from high concentration of uremia to median of 5 pmol/L following transplantation *1953* *Serum Increase* Mean concentration of 281 pg/mL in 8 patients with renal transplants compared with mean of 118 pg/mL in 20 control patients *1320*

Glucagon *Plasma Decrease* Significant reduction from high observed with uremia to median of 92 pg/L following renal transplantation *1953*

γ-Glutamyltransferase *Serum Increase* In 41 of renal transplant patients increased activity observed, most often without increased urinary glucaric acid suggesting that it is a manifestation of hepatobiliary dysfunction and not due to hepatic enzyme induction *2509*

HDL_2-Cholesterol *Serum No Effect* In 17 patients with chronic renal failure following renal transplantation mean concentration of 0.63 ± 0.36 mmol/L not significantly different from 0.73 ± 0.31 mmol/L in 27 healthy controls *935*

HDL_3-Cholesterol *Serum Increase* In 17 patients with chronic renal failure following renal transplantation mean concentration of 0.90 ± 0.18 mmol/L significantly different from 0.80 ± 0.12 mmol/L in 27 healthy controls *935*

HDL-Cholesterol *Serum Decrease* Concentration variable *3526* In patients with end-stage renal disease treated by renal transplantation 15% had HDL-cholesterol concentrations less than 35 mg/dL *2575* *Serum Increase* In renal transplantation patients mean concentration increased to 63 mg/dL at 3 months after transplantation and 58 mg/dL after 24 months compared with 50 mg/dL in controls *726* In 10 children with congenital nephrotic syndrome renal transplantation caused mean concentration to increase from baseline of 0.55 ± 0.23 mmol/L to 1.33 ± 0.22 mmol/L *149* Concentration variable *3526* In 84 patients with chronic renal failure 6 months to one year after renal transplantation mean concentration rose to 56 ± 4 mg/dL compared with 36 ± 2 mg/dL before surgery *230* In 20 consecutive patients 6 months following renal transplantation significant increase in concentration observed *463* *Serum No Effect* Mean concentration of 0.45 ± 0.11 g/L in 57 renal transplantation patients (41 men, 16 women of mean age 40.5 ± 13.8 years, with mean of 28.6 ± 12.9 months after transplantation) not significantly different from 0.47 ± 0.12 g/L in 29 healthy controls (13 men, 16 women of mean age 30.0 ± 6.8 years) *5188* Concentration variable *3526* In 17 patients with chronic renal failure following renal transplantation mean concentration of 1.53 ± 0.48 mmol/L not significantly different from 1.53 ± 0.39 mmol/L in 27 healthy controls *935*

Hemoglobin *Blood Increase* In 17 patients with polycythemia following renal transplantation mean concentration of 18.0 ± 0.82 g/dL compared with 14.0 ± 1.1 g/dL in 79 reference controls *4320*

Hepatic Triglyceride Lipase *Plasma Decrease* After 100 IU/kg body weight after 20 min HTGL activity at 10 and 20 min in 12 normolipidemic renal transplant patients was 40/41% less than in 10 healthy controls and in 16 hyperlipidemic renal transplant patients was 29/32% less than in the controls *1126*

Homocysteine *Plasma Decrease* In 55 patients who had received a renal transplant mean concentration of 27.7 ± 14.8 µmol/L significantly reduced compared with 36.9 ± 21.3 µmol/L in pretransplant patients *178*

Hyaluronic Acid *Serum Decrease* In 13 patients pretransplantation median concentration of 150 (range 60 - 898) µg/L decreased to 30 (11 - > 500) µg/L after transplantation *5333*

996.81 Renal Transplantation *(continued)*

25-Hydroxy Vitamin D_3 *Serum Decrease* In 19 patients mean concentration changed from baseline of 41.9 ± 21.8 nmol/L to 29.3 ± 15.5 nmol/L one week after transplantation (significant), to 29.5 ± 11.9 nmol/L at discharge from hospital, median 16 days (significantly different from baseline) *4511*
Serum No Effect In 19 patients mean concentration changed from baseline of 41.9 ± 21.8 nmol/L to 56.6 ± 27.8 nmol/L after 6 months (significant) and 45.0 ± 24.6 nmol/L one year after transplantation (not significant) *4511*

5-Hydroxytryptamine *Blood Decrease* Mean concentration in 39 patients with chronic renal failure after renal transplantation of 648 ± 60 nmol/L significantly different from that in 35 healthy controls of 1,039 ± 69 nmolL *5016*

Immunoglobulin G *Urine Increase* Peak excretion observed with graft rejection *5000*

Interleukin-1 Receptor Antagonist *Serum Increase* In patients with an uncomplicated postoperative course the highest plasma concentration during the first 2 weeks post-transplant was a mean of 1,135 pg/mL, decreasing to a mean of 542 pg/mL in weeks 3 and 4 *1009*

Interleukin-2 *Serum Increase* Great increase observed during renal transplant rejection *4095* Concentration greatly increased in patients in whom kidney is being rejected *4094* Increased concentration observed with rejection *4093*
Urine Increase Concentration greatly increased with renal transplant rejection *4095* Increase observed with renal allograft rejection *4093* Concentration greatly increased in patients in whom kidney is being rejected *4094*

ionized Calcium *Serum No Effect* In 19 patients mean concentration changed from baseline of 1.26 ± 0.14 mmol/L to 1.20 ± 0.22 mmol/L one week after transplantation (not significant), to 1.26 ± 0.13 mmol/L at discharge from hospital, median 16 days (not significantly different from baseline), to 1.25 ± 0.07 mmol/L after 6 months (not significant) and 1.25 ± 0.06 mmol/L one year after transplantation (not significant) *4511* In 10 patients with chronic glomerulonephritis who received a renal transplant mean concentration of 2.4 mmol/L within the normal range *1167*

Ionized Magnesium *Serum Decrease* Mean concentration in 27 patients with renal transplants receiving cyclosporine of 0.53 ± 0.05 mmol/L significantly different from 0.56 ± 0.05 mmol/L in 75 healthy controls *4510*

Ionized Magnesium:Total Magnesium Ratio
Serum Increase Mean ratio in 27 patients with renal transplants receiving cyclosporine of 0.73 ± 0.07 significantly different from 0.69 ± 0.04 in 75 healthy controls *4510*

LDL-Cholesterol *Serum Decrease* In 10 children with congenital nephrotic syndrome renal transplantation caused mean concentration to decrease from baseline of 3.51± 1.09 mmol/L to 3.00 ± 0.66 mmol/L *149*
Serum Increase Mean concentration increased to 134 mg/dL in patients 3 months after renal transplantation, and 139 mg/dL after 24 months compared with 118 mg/dL in controls *726* Characteristic observation *3526* In 84 patients with chronic renal failure 6 months to one year after renal transplantation mean concentration rose to 142 ± 7 mg/dL compared with 111 ± 6 mg/dL before surgery *230* In patients with end stage renal disease treated by renal transplantation 60% had LDL-cholesterol concentrations exceeding 130 mg/dL *2575*
Serum No Effect In 17 patients with chronic renal failure following renal transplantation mean concentration of 4.42 ± 1.15 mmol/L not significantly different from 4.32 ± 0.74 mmol/L in 27 healthy controls *935*

Lipase *Serum Increase* In 23 patients who had undergone renal transplantation at least 6 months previously mean activity of 175 ± 77 U/L significantly different from 122 ± 62 U/L in 34 healthy volunteer controls *3331*

Lipoprotein Lipase *Serum Decrease* In 10 healthy controls total postheparin lipolytic activity 20 min after 100 IU/kg body weight 354% higher than in 16 hyperlipidemic renal transplant patients and 206% higher than in 12 normolipidemic renal transplant patients *1126*

Lipoprotein Lp(a) *Serum Decrease* Concentration normalizes *3526* Renal transplantation was associated with a highly significant reduction of Lp(a) concentration in 20 patients *2827*
Serum Increase In patients with end-stage renal disease treated by renal transplantation 25% had Lp(a) concentrations greater than 30 mg/dL *2575*

Serum No Effect In 67 men who had received a renal transplant mean concentration of 347 U/L not different from 385 U/L in 23 healthy controls and 356 U/L in 27 women not different from mean of 367 U/L in 33 control women *1673*

Luteinizing Hormone *Plasma Decrease* In post-transplant patients with erythrocytosis mean concentration of 8.0 ± 3.3 IU/L compared with 13.9 ± 11.7 IU/mL in control men *770*
Plasma No Effect In spite of low plasma testosterone concentration in patients with either heart or kidney transplants and regardless of immunosuppressant therapy concentration not affected *4272*

Magnesium *Serum Decrease* Mean concentration in 27 patients with renal transplants receiving cyclosporine of 0.71 ± 0.10 mmol/L significantly different from 0.81 ± 0.07 mmol/L in 75 healthy controls *4510*
Urine Increase In 12 patients prior to renal transplant mean clearance of 52 ± 29 mL/min significantly different from 142 ± 15 mL in post-transplant patients *4377*

MCV *Blood Increase* In 100 patients with macrocytosis (MCV greater than 110 fL) 2 had had renal transplants *4924*

β_2-Microglobulin *Serum Increase* Increase observed but not as good a marker of rejection as serum amyloid A protein *3379*

Muscle-specific Actin *Urine Increase* Mean excretion of 0.018 ± 0.027 µg/mL observed in 49 patients after organ transplantation without nephrotoxicity compared with 0.003 ± 0.007 µg/mL observed in 5 healthy individuals *1945*

Myoglobin *Serum Increase* Six of 17 patients with renal transplants with chronic renal failure receiving hemodialysis had concentration above upper limit of normal *3686*

N-Acetyl-Glucosaminidase *Serum Increase* In 43 post-renal transplant patients (some as long as several years after operation) mean activity of 526 ± 233 U/L significantly greater than 390 ± 65 U/L in 23 control blood donors *3111*
Urine Increase In renal transplant patients mean excretion decreased from median of 3.7 U/mmol creatinine on 3rd day to 1.2 U/mmol creatinine on 15th day post-transplant. Normal excretion in healthy individuals 0.26 U/mmol creatinine *2292*

N-Acetyl-Glucosaminidase B *Urine No Effect* Percentage of N-acetylglucosaminidase B did not change from normal in renal transplant patients *2292*

Neopterin *Urine No Effect* In 21 allograft recipients excretion remained normal or increased at a constant level even though this did not affect prognosis *2756*

Nucleotide Pyrophosphohydrolase, Soluble
Serum Increase Mean activity in 28 patients with renal transplant with cyclosporine of 1,725 ± 72 pmol nitrophenol/h/mL significantly different from that in 85 healthy individuals of 1,141 ± 22 pmol nitrophenol/h/mL *691*
Serum No Effect Mean activity in 9 patients with renal transplant without cyclosporine of 1,123 ± 95 pmol nitrophenol/h/mL not significantly different from that in 85 healthy individuals of 1,141 ± 22 pmol nitrophenol/h/mL *691*

Osteocalcin *Serum Decrease* In patients following renal transplantation concentration decreased to near normal at 60 - 90 days after surgery. Effect probably due to immunosuppressive corticosteroid therapy *506* In 19 patients mean concentration changed from baseline of 20.2 ± 15.2 µg/L to 2.0 ± 1.7 µg/L one week after transplantation (significant), to 3.2 ± 0.4 µg/L at discharge from hospital, median 16 days (significantly different from baseline), to 6.7 ± 3.3 µg/L after 6 months (significant) and 8.7 ± 6.0 µg/L one year after transplantation (significant) *4511*
Serum Increase In 67 patients following renal transplantation (mean 63 months since surgery) about 30 had increased concentration above upper limit of normal *5035* In 30 patients with functioning kidney grafts concentration markedly increased compared with 30 age- and sex-matched controls *4134*

Oxalate *Serum Decrease* In 8 men with renal transplantation serum creatinine concentration decreased from 97 ± 15 µmol/L presurgery to 21 ± 3 µmol/L one day after surgery and 15 ± 6 µmol/L 5 days after surgery *5732*
Urine Decrease In 8 men with renal transplantation serum creatinine concentration decreased from 1,244 ± 150 µmol/d presurgery to 476 ± 60 µmol/d one day after surgery and 430 ± 100 µmol/d 5 days after surgery *5732*

Pancreatic Polypeptide *Plasma Decrease* Significant reduction from high concentration of uremia to median of 145 pmol/L following renal transplantation *1953*

Paraoxonase *Serum* *No Effect* Mean activity of 0.20 ± 0.12 U/mL in 132 patients with end-stage renal disease treated by renal transplantation not significantly different from 0.22 ± 0.17 U/mL in 185 healthy controls when paraoxon used as substrate *1011*

Parathyroid Hormone *Plasma* *Decrease* Significant reduction observed in patients following kidney transplantation over 240 days following surgery but still remained above normal concentration *506*
Plasma *Increase* In 10 patients with chronic glomerulonephritis who received a renal transplant mean concentration of 12.7 pmol/L slightly increased compared with normal *1167* Mean concentration in 30 individuals with well-functioning kidney grafts significantly higher than in 30 age- and sex-matched controls *4134* In 51 of 92 patients after renal transplantation (mean 63 months after surgery) concentration increased above upper limit of normal, 55 pg/mL *5035*
Plasma *No Effect* In 19 patients mean concentration changed from baseline of 11.8 ± 10.7 pmol/L to 15.9 ± 9.4 pmol/L one week after transplantation (not significant), to 15.8 ± 13.9 pmol/L at discharge from hospital, median 16 days (not significantly different from baseline), to 9.0 ± 10.9 pmol/L after 6 months (not significant) and 9.9 ± 12.4 pmol/L one year after transplantation (not significant) *4511* In 37 of 92 patients with renal transplants (mean 63 months after surgery) concentration within normal range *5035*

pH *Urine* *Decrease* May cause distal renal tubular acidosis (type IV) is associated with hyperkalemia, hyperchloremic metabolic acidosis, urine pH < 5.5, decreased urinary ammonium ion excretion, a positive urine anion gap, normal urinary citrate and urinary calcium excretion *4071*

Phosphate *Serum* *Decrease* In 19 patients mean concentration changed from baseline of 1.53 ± 0.45 µmol/L to 0.98 ± 0.40 µmol/L one week after transplantation (significant), to 0.97 ± 0.31 µmol/L at discharge from hospital, median 16 days (significantly different from baseline), to 1.02 ± 0.27 µmol/L after 6 months (significant) and 1.12 ± 0.25 µmol/L one year after transplantation (significant) *4511*

Plasminogen Activator Inhibitor *Plasma* *No Effect* In 16 patients median concentration changed nonsignificantly from 14.0 IU/mL preoperatively to 11.0 IU/mL, 8.4 IU/mL and 9.7 IU/mL on postoperative days 1, 3 and 5 respectively *609*

Platelets *Blood* *Decrease* In 20 patients with renal transplants in whom anticardiolipin antibodies detected greater frequency of thrombocytopenia detected than in patients without antibodies *1844*

Postheparin Lipolytic Activity *Plasma* *Decrease* After 100 IU/kg body weight after 20 min PHLA at 10 and 20 min in 12 normolipidemic renal transplant patients was 36.6/30.5% less than in 10 healthy controls and in 16 hyperlipidemic renal transplant patients was 85 to 105% less than in the controls *1126*

Postheparin Lipoprotein Lipase *Plasma* *Increase* In 10 children with congenital nephrotic syndrome renal transplantation caused mean activity to increase from 20.4 ± 7.3 µmol FFA/mL/h to 25.0 ± 9.1 µmol FFA/mL/h and mass to increase from 200.0 ± 56.9 ng/mL to 227.2 ± 88.4 ng/mL *149*

Potassium *Serum* *Increase* May cause distal renal tubular acidosis (type IV) which is associated with hyperkalemia, hyperchloremic metabolic acidosis, urine pH < 5.5, decreased urinary ammonium ion excretion, a positive urine anion gap, normal urinary citrate and urinary calcium excretion *4071*

Prostate-specific Antigen *Serum* *No Effect* In 12 patients who underwent renal transplantation mean concentration changed nonsignificantly from 1.0 ng/dL to 0.092 ng/dL a mean of 13.6 months following transplantation *3622*

Protein C *Plasma* *Decrease* In 16 patients median concentration changed significantly from 127 units preoperatively to 95 units, 100 units and 121 units on postoperative days 1, 3 and 5 respectively *609*

Pyridinium Crosslinks *Urine* *Increase* Median excretion during median 9 days of transplant of 54 ± 9 nmol/mmol creatinine increased to 108 ± 14 nmol/mmol creatinine after median of 34 days post-transplant *5703*

Renin Activity *Plasma* *Increase* In 8 patients following renal transplantation mean concentration higher than in healthy controls with loss of circadian variation, poosibly due to immunosuppressive therapy *979*

Rheumatoid Factor (IgM) *Serum* *No Effect* Concentrations in patients having had renal transplants similar to those in other individuals *1940*

Soluble E-Selectin *Serum* *No Effect* 10 patients following renal transplantation had a mean concentration not significantly different from 48 ng/mL in 10 healthy controls *3638*

Soluble Interleukin-2 Receptor *Serum* *Increase* Concentration greatly increased in renal transplant rejection *4095* Concentration greatly increased in patients in whom kidney is being rejected *4094* In candidates for renal transplantation mean concentration of 1,943 ± 878 kU/L compared with 350 ± 101 kU/L in controls. After transplantation increased concentration returned to normal except in those patients who developed ATN *5877* Increased concentrations in patients undergoing renal allograft rejection *4093*

Soluble Tumor Necrosis Factor Receptor *Serum* *No Effect* Mean concentration in 11 patients following uncomplicated renal transplantation of 4.8 ± 1.3 ng/mL significantly higher than 3.5 ± 0.7 ng/mL in 34 healthy blood donors *1982*

Soluble Vascular Cell Adhesion Molecule-1 *Serum* *Increase* 10 patients following renal grafts had a mean concentration of 1,311 ng/mL significantly greater than 582 ng/mL in 10 healthy donors *3638*

Somatostatin *Plasma* *No Effect* No significant change observed in concentration in uremic patients when renal transplantation performed *1953*

Testosterone *Serum* *Decrease* In both renal and cardiac transplant patients concentration low regardless of immunosuppressant therapy *4272*
Serum *No Effect* In post-transplant patients mean concentration of 13.2 ± 6.2 nmol/L not significantly different from 13.1 ± 6.0 nmol/L in control patients *770*

Tissue Plasminogen Activator Antigen *Plasma* *Increase* In 16 patients median concentration increased from 1.9 ng/mL preoperatively to 2.8 ng/mL, 2.1 ng/mL and 1.9 ng/mL on postoperative days 1, 3 and 5 respectively *609*

Transferrin *Urine* *Increase* Peak observed with renal graft rejection *5000*

Triglycerides *Serum* *Decrease* In 10 children with congenital nephrotic syndrome renal transplantation caused mean concentration to decrease from baseline of 8.40 ± 4.34 mmol/L to 1.73 ± 0.70 mmol/L *149*
Serum *Increase* In 84 patients with chronic renal failure 6 months to one year after renal transplantation mean concentration rose nonsignificantly to 183 ± 21 mg/dL compared with 210 ± 24 mg/dL before surgery *230* In patients with end-stage renal disease treated by renal transplantation 35% had triglyceride concentrations greater than 200 mg/dL *2575* Mean concentration 3 months after transplantation of 118 mg/dL, and at 24 months after transplantation 135 mg/dL compared with 111 mg/dL in controls *726* Characteristic observation *3526* In 16 hyperlipidemic renal transplant patients mean concentration of 6.02 ± 3.33 mmol/L significantly greater than 1.15 ± 0.45 mmol/L in 10 healthy control individuals *1126* Mean concentration of 1.76 ± 0.89 g/L in 57 renal transplantation patients (41 men, 16 women of mean age 40.5 ± 13.8 years, with mean of 28.6 ± 12.9 months after transplantation) significantly different from 0.92 ± 0.33 g/L in 29 healthy controls (13 men, 16 women of mean age 30.0 ± 6.8 years) *5188*
Serum *No Effect* In 12 normolipidemic renal transplant patients mean concentration of 1.84 ± 0.39 mmol/L significantly greater than 1.15 ± 0.45 mmol/L in 10 healthy control individuals, although still within reference range *1126* In 17 patients with chronic renal failure following renal transplantation mean concentration of 1.72 ± 0.81 mmol/L not significantly different from 1.77 ± 0.77 mmol/L in 27 healthy controls *935*

Troponin I *Serum* *Increase* One of 17 patients with renal transplants with chronic renal failure receiving hemodialysis had concentration above upper limit of normal *3686*

Troponin T *Serum* *Increase* Three of 17 patients with renal transplants with chronic renal failure receiving hemodialysis had concentration above upper limit of normal *3686*

Tumor Necrosis Factor-α *Serum* *Increase* In patients with renal allografts acute rejection was associated with significantly higher TNF concentration with respect to acute tubular necrosis, cyclosporine A nephrotoxicity, uncomplicated transplants and healthy subjects *4714*

996.81 Renal Transplantation *(continued)*

Type I Collagen Cross-linked N-telopeptide *Urine Increase* Median excretion of N-telopeptides during median 9 days of transplant of 119 ± 26 µmol/mol creatinine increased to 154 ± 33 µmol/mol creatinine after median of 34 days post-transplant *5703*

Uric Acid *Serum Decrease* Significant effect over first 3 mo *4649*
Serum Increase 105 of 131 transplant patients (80%) treated with cyclosporine with prednisone had serum uric acid above 8.0 mg/dL and 13 (10%) had uric acid above 14 mg/dL. In 63 of 115 (55%) treated with azathioprine, prednisone and ALG had uric acid above 8 mg/dL *1825*

VLDL-Cholesterol *Serum Decrease* Mean concentration reduced to 26 mg/dL in patients 3 months after renal transplantation and 22 mg/dL 24 months after renal transplantation compared with 32 mg/dL in controls *726*
Serum Increase In 84 patients with chronic renal failure 6 months to one year after renal transplantation mean concentration rose to 63 ± 5 mg/dL compared with 41 ± 4 mg/dL before surgery *230*
Serum No Effect In 17 patients with chronic renal failure following renal transplantation mean concentration of 0.61 ± 0.51 mmol/L not significantly different from 0.61 ± 0.51 mmol/L in 27 healthy controls *935*

VLDL-Cholesterol Esters *Serum No Effect* In 17 patients with chronic renal failure following renal transplantation mean concentration of 0.34 ± 0.28 mmol/L not significantly different from 0.38 ± 0.32 mmol/L in 27 healthy controls *935*

VLDL-Cholesterol, Free *Serum No Effect* In 17 patients with chronic renal failure following renal transplantation mean concentration of 0.28 ± 0.23 mmol/L not significantly different from 0.23 ± 0.18 mmol/L in 27 healthy controls *935*

VLDL-Triglycerides *Serum Decrease* In 10 children with congenital nephrotic syndrome renal transplantation caused mean concentration to decrease from baseline of 4.52 ± 2.26 mmol/L to 0.96 ± 0.53 mmol/L *149* Mean concentration reduced to 64 mg/dL in patients 3 months after transplantation but increased to 81 mg/dL 24 months after transplantation compared with 69 mg/dL in controls *726*
Serum No Effect In 17 patients with chronic renal failure following renal transplantation mean concentration of 1.09 ± 0.70 mmol/L not significantly different from 0.91 ± 0.59 mmol/L in 27 healthy controls *935*

996.82 Liver Transplant Rejection

Amyloid A Protein *Serum Increase* In 12 patients who had rejections of their liver transplants the mean concentration was 16.94 ± 8.82 mg/dL significantly different from 9.75 ± 6.60 mg/dL following transplantation *1474*

C-Reactive Protein *Serum Increase* In 12 patients who had received liver transplants the mean concentration was 4.41 ± 2.38 mg/dL significantly different from normal range of up to 0.9 mg/dL in controls *1474*

Neopterin *Serum Increase* Increasing neopterin concentrations observed after liver transplant rejection *121*

Soluble HLA-I *Serum Increase* Mean concentration increased in graft versus host disease *576* Concentration reportedly increased with episodes of rejection *5306*

Soluble HLA-FHC *Serum Increase* Mean concentration increased in allograft rejection *576*

Soluble Interleukin-2 Receptor *Bile Increase* Increased concentrations found in the bile in liver transplant patients before and during liver rejection *4095*

996.82 Liver Transplantation

Alanine Aminotransferase *Serum Decrease* Mean baseline activity of 130 ± 24 U/L in 8 patients with PBC increased to 254 ± 73 U/L on post-op day 1 and 209 ± 42 U/L on post-op days 5 - 7 and then decreased to 105 ± 49 U/L on post-op days 28 - 35 *3793*
Serum Increase Mean baseline activity of 130 ± 24 U/L in 8 patients with PBC increased to 254 ± 73 U/L on post-op day 1 and 209 ± 42 U/L on post-op days 5 - 7 and then decreased to 105 ± 49 U/L on post-op days 28 - 35 *3793*

Albumin *Serum Decrease* Mean concentration of 25 ± 4 g/L observed in 17 patients with liver transplantation *3315*
Serum Increase Mean baseline concentration of 26 ± 2 g/L in 8 patients with PBC increased to 28 ± 1 g/L on post-op day 1, to 29 ± 1 g/L on post-op days 5 - 7 and to 30 ± 2 g/L on post-op days 28 - 35 *3793*

Alkaline Phosphatase *Serum Decrease* Reported effect with posthepatic resection and transplantation *3160* Mean baseline activity of 1,168 ± 426 U/L in 8 patients with PBC decreased to 366 ± 135 U/L on post-op day 1, to 413 ± 92 U/L on post-op days 5 - 7 and to 551 ± 153 U/L on post-op days 28 - 35 *3793*

Amyloid A Protein *Serum Increase* Before surgery in 37 liver transplant patients mean concentration increased slightly to 0.9 ± 1.8 mg/dL (compared to normal 0.1 ± 0.1 mg/dL) but on days 1 to 2 after transplant concentration reached highest of 15.8 ± 10.2 mg/dL with concentration persisting in some patients above 2.6 mg/dL for several months after surgery. Mean value increased to 3.7 ± 7.1 mg/dL 12 months after surgery *3259* In 12 patients who had received liver transplants the mean concentration was 9.75 ± 6.60 mg/dL significantly different from 0.98 ± 0.42 mg/dL in controls *1474*

Apolipoprotein A-I *Serum Decrease* Following liver transplantation in 37 individuals concentration decreased in first few postoperative days reaching a trough in 8 days in patients with uncomplicated clinical outcome and in 12 days in those with complicated outcome so that concentrations in uncomplicated group significantly higher *2147* In 37 liver transplant patients mean concentration decreased by about 50% from about 106 mg/dL on day 1 to about 50 mg/dL on day 5 or 6 after surgery. Concentration then stabilized at lowest between days 15 to 30 or 60 before rising to a concentration still 20% below normal. Concentration reverted to normal within one year of surgery *3259*

Apolipoprotein A-II *Serum Decrease* In 37 liver transplant patients decrease of about 50% observed from about 17 mg/dL on day 1 to about 8 mg/dL on day 5 or 6 after surgery. Concentration then stabilized at lowest between days 15 and 30 or 60 before rising to a concentration still 20% below normal. Concentration reverted to normal within one year *3259*

Apolipoprotein B *Serum Increase* In 37 liver transplant patients mean concentration increased from about 40 mg/dL on day 1 post-transplant to about 77 mg/dL on day 15 and continued to increase to day 17. After day 20 concentration returned to about normal. Concentration reverted to normal within one year *3259*

Apolipoprotein C-II *Serum Increase* In 37 liver transplantation patients mean concentration increased from about 2 mg/dL on day 1 post-surgery to about 4 mg/dL on days 5, 10 and 20 mg/dL with slight decline thereafter to normal concentration. After one year concentration normal *3259*

Apolipoprotein C-III *Serum Increase* In 37 liver transplant patients mean concentration increased from about 5 mg/dL on day 1 to 9 mg/dL on days 3 and 18 although concentration dipped to about 7 mg/dL between these peaks. After day 20 concentration returned to about normal. Concentration reverted to normal within one year *3259*

Bilirubin *Serum Decrease* Mean baseline concentration of 313 ± 42 µmol/L in 8 patients with PBC decreased to 124 ± 18 µmol/L on post-op day 1, to 67 ± 10 µmol/L on post-op days 5 - 7 and to 105 ± 68 µmol/L on post-op days 28 - 35 *3793*
Serum Increase Mean concentration of 220.6 ± 235.0 µmol/L observed in 17 patients following liver transplantation *3315*

CA 19-9 *Serum Increase* In liver transplant patients mean concentration increased but increased further during rejection (increase observed in 85%) *4544*

Cholesterol *Serum Decrease* Mean baseline concentration of 5.9 ± 2.1 mmol/L in 8 patients with PBC decreased to 4.0 ± 1.0 mmol/L on post-op day 1, 3.7 ± 0.5 mmol/L on post-op days 5 - 7 and increased to 6.3 ± 0.6 mmol/L on post-op days 28 - 35 *3793*
Serum Increase Mean baseline concentration of 5.9 ± 2.1 mmol/L in 8 patients with PBC decreased to 4.0 ± 1.0 mmol/L on post-op day 1, 3.7 ± 0.5 mmol/L on post-op days 5 - 7 and increased to 6.3 ± 0.6 mmol/L on post-op days 28 - 35 *3793*

C-Reactive Protein *Serum Increase* In 52 patients without histological evidence of liver transplants the mean concentration was 4.65 ± 2.90 mg/dL significantly different from normal range of up to 0.9 mg/dL in controls *1474*

Endothelin-1 *Plasma Increase* In 12 patients who underwent orthoptic liver transplantation mean concentration increased to 4.2 ± 0.7 pg/mL, mean 2.6-fold above appropriate normal values *328*

Eosinophil Cationic Protein *Serum Increase* In patients with liver transplant rejection concentration rose by at least 50% from the last nadir prior to rejection a median of 9 days prior to the diagnosis of rejection in 11 of 14 (79%) rejection episodes but the rise occurred significantly earlier than rises in ALT or GST *2282*

γ-Glutamyltransferase *Serum Decrease* Mean baseline activity of 284 ± 136 U/L in 8 patients with PBC decreased to 103 ± 70 U/L on post-op day 1 and then increased to 180 ± 49 U/L on post-op days 5 - 7 and to 247 ± 87 U/L on post-op days 28 - 35 *3793*
Serum Increase Mean baseline activity of 284 ± 136 U/L in 8 patients with PBC decreased to 103 ± 70 U/L on post-op day 1 and then increased to 180 ± 49 U/L on post-op days 5 - 7 and to 247 ± 87 U/L on post-op days 28 - 35 *3793*

Glutathione Peroxidase *Serum No Effect* In 5 patients 6 weeks following liver transplantation mean concentration changed nonsignificantly from 208 ± 66 mU/mL to 195 ± 89 mU/mL pretransplant *638*

HDL-Cholesterol *Serum Decrease* In 37 liver transplant patients from day 1 to 5 or 6 after surgery mean concentration decreased by about 50% (from about 32 mg/dL to 15 mg/dL). Concentration then remained stable at lowest values from day 6 to 15, but from day 15 to 30 or 60 progressive rise to concentration still 20% below normal. Concentration reverted to normal within one year *3259*

Hyaluronan *Serum Increase* Concentration rises with acute liver rejection prior to an increase in the serum bilirubin concentration *3072*

Hyaluronic Acid *Serum Increase* In patients with liver transplant rejection concentration rose significantly a median of 3 days prior to the diagnosis of rejection - at least 2 days earlier than all other liver function tests, including glutathione S-transferase, although the difference was not statistically significant *5292*

Interleukin-8 *Serum Increase* Marked increase observed in patients with acute graft rejection: In 4 of 6 rejection episodes IL-8 concentration rose to 75 ± 38 pg/mL 2 days before clinical diagnosis with increase to 109 ± 51 pg/mL on day 4 after rejection *5233*
Serum No Effect In patients with uneventful recovery after liver transplantation concentration undetectable *5233*

β_2-Microglobulin *Bile Increase* Concentration significantly increased during acute liver transplant rejection *28*
Serum Increase Concentration significantly increased in liver transplant patients with or without rejection *28*

Platelets *Blood Decrease* Mean concentration of 50 ± 19 x 10^9/L observed in 17 patients following liver transplantation *3315*

Prothrombin Time *Plasma Increase* Mean prothrombin time of 18 ± 2.9 s observed in 17 patients following liver transplantation *3315*

Selenium *Serum Increase* In 5 patients 6 weeks following liver transplantation mean concentration increased significantly from 9.3 ± 1.6 µg/dL to 12.9 ± 2.1 µg/dL pretransplant *638*

Selenoprotein P *Serum Increase* In 5 patients 6 weeks following liver transplantation mean concentration increased significantly from 0.43 ± 0.1 mU/mL to 0.83 ± 0.1 mU/mL pretransplant *638*

Soluble Interleukin-2 Receptor *Bile Increase* Increased concentrations found in the bile in liver transplant patients before and during liver rejection *4095*
Serum Decrease In liver transplant patients reduced concentrations observed before and during rejection of liver *4095*

Thromboplastin Time *Plasma Increase* Mean baseline concentration of 0.48 ± 0.06 in 8 patients with PBC increased to 0.53 ± 0.04 on post-operative day 1, to 0.85 ± 0.05 on post-operative days 5 - 7 and to 1.0 ± 0.08 on post-operative days 28 - 35 *3793*

Thrombopoietin *Plasma Decrease* Concentration undetectable in 16 of 17 patients following liver transplantation *3315*

Triglycerides *Serum Decrease* Mean baseline concentration of 1.8 ± 0.5 mmol/L in 8 patients with PBC decreased to 0.7 ± 0.1 mmol/L on post-op day 1, but then increased to 1.9 ± 0.3 mmol/L on post-op days 5 - 7 and to 2.5 ± 0.4 mmol/L on post-op days 28 - 35 *3793*
Serum Increase In 37 patients who underwent liver transplantation mean concentration increased from about 50 mg/dL on day 1 post surgery to about 210 mg/dL on day 5 but did not change from day 6 to 20 despite huge infusions of plasma. After day 20 to 60 concentration returned to normal. Concentration reverted to normal within one year *3259* Mean baseline concentration of 1.8 ± 0.5 mmol/L in 8 patients with PBC decreased to 0.7 ± 0.1 mmol/L on post-op day 1, but then increased to 1.9 ± 0.3 mmol/L on post-op days 5 - 7 and to 2.5 ± 0.4 mmol/L on post-op days 28 - 35 *3793*

Troponin T *Serum Increase* Mean concentration increased above 0.2 µg/L in 78% patients following renal transplantation *334*

Tumor Necrosis Factor-α *Serum Increase* In patients undergoing rejection mean concentration of 8.0 pg/mL, 4.0 pg/mL with infection, 7.0 pg/mL with cyclosporine A toxicity, and 10.4 pg/L with OKT3 therapy *2815*
Serum No Effect Concentrations not increased in patients with stable liver transplants, but in those undergoing a rejection episode concentration increased which preceded clinical diagnosis by 1 - 2 days. Concentration returned to baseline upon treatment of the rejection episode *2326*

996.83 Heart Transplant Rejection

Amino-terminal Propeptide of Type III Procollagen
Serum Increase One to 2 weeks following histologic diagnosis of severe rejection concentration increased 220 - 660% in 4 late incidents, 80% in one early incident and decreased in 60% in one other early incident, but at the time of relection concentrations were not increased in comparison with previous values *2248*

Amyloid A *Serum Increase* Median concentration in patients in rejection phase of 13 mg/dL significantly higher than approximately 5.75 mg/dL in transplant patients in stable phase *3653*

Neopterin *Serum Increase* Increasing neopterin concentrations observed after heart transplant rejection *121* Median concentration in patients with transplant rejection of approximately 37 nmol/L significantly different from approximately 12 nmol/L in transplant patients in stable phase *3653*

Soluble HLA-I *Serum Increase* Mean concentration increased in graft versus host disease *576* Concentration reportedly increased with episodes of rejection *5306*

Soluble HLA-FHC *Serum Increase* Mean concentration increased in allograft rejection *576*

996.83 Heart Transplantation

Acylcarnitine, Long Chain *Serum No Effect* Mean concentration of 4.1 ± 2.7 µmol/L in 19 heart transplanted patients not significantly different from 4.75 ± 4.0 µmol/L in 3 healthy controls *3901*

Acylcarnitine, Short Chain *Serum No Effect* Mean concentration of 7.3 ± 5.2 µmol/L in 19 heart transplanted patients not significantly different from normal *3901*

Alkaline Phosphatase Band-10 Isoenzyme *Serum No Effect* In 22 episodes of rejection mean activity (% of total) was 9.4% compared with 7.7% in 22 patients with stable graft function and 5.1% in 16 apparently healthy adults. Differences not significant *2247*

Amino-terminal Propeptide of Type III Procollagen
Serum Increase Median concentration increased from about 5 µg/L preoperatively to about 12 µg/L on postoperative day 1, 32 µg/L on postoperative day 2, 60 µg/L on postoperative day 3, peaking at about 62 µg/L on postoperative day 4, thereafter declining slowly *2248*

Amyloid A *Serum Increase* Concentration increased about 40-fold 1 - 2 days post-transplant and stayed elevated for about one week *4643* Median concentration in 13 patients in postoperative phase of 25 mg/dL significantly higher than approximately 5.75 mg/dL in transplant patients in stable phase *3653*

996.83 Heart Transplantation *(continued)*

Antithrombin III *Plasma* *No Effect* No significant difference observed between concentrations in 91 post-transplant patients and 94 untransplanted patients with coronary artery disease *1066*

Atrial Natriuretic Peptide *Plasma* *Decrease* In 10 patients with congestive cardiac failure heart transplantation caused a decrease from 5 times above normal to 2 times above normal over the next 12 weeks *1530* In patients with severe heart failure the high presurgical concentration tended to normalize *3708*
Plasma *No Effect* In 14 patients initial high concentration decreased to normal range of healthy adults 5 to 12 days following transplantation in 11 of the recipients *5647*

CA 125 *Serum* *Decrease* In patients with severe heart failure the high presurgical concentration tended to normalize *3708*

Carnitine *Serum* *No Effect* Mean concentration of total carnitine of 44.0 ± 9.7 µmol/L in 19 heart transplanted patients not significantly different from normal *3901*

Carnitine, Free *Serum* *No Effect* Mean concentration of 32.6 ± 6.6 µmol/L in 19 heart transplanted patients not significantly different from normal *3901*

Cholesterol *Serum* *Increase* In 100 patients 3 months after heart transplant mean concentration increased to 234 ± 7 mg/dL from 168 ± 7 mg/dL pretransplant *269*

C-Reactive Protein *Serum* *Increase* Mean and median concentrations of 49.0 and 38.0 mg/L respectively during 19 rejection episodes significantly higher than mean and median of 7.0 and 3.0 mg/L respectively in 130 controls *5489* In 19 patients undergoing rejection median concentration of 3.8 ± 3.1 mg/dL and in 95 patients with rejection median of 7.3 ± 9.0 mg/dL compared with 0.3 ± 0.7 mg/dL in 130 individuals with uncomplicated course following surgery *120*

Fibrinogen *Plasma* *No Effect* No significant difference observed between concentrations in 91 post-transplant patients and 94 nontransplanted patients with coronary artery disease *1066*

HDL-Cholesterol *Serum* *Increase* In 100 heart transplant patients mean concentration increased to 47 ± 1 mg/dL 3 months after surgery from 34 ± 1 mg/dL presurgery *269*
Serum *No Effect* In 47 patients with heart transplants for dilated cardiomyopathy of 48 ± 2.7 mg/dL and 5.4 ± 2.5 mg/dL in 60 heart transplant patients because of coronary artery disease not significantly different from 49 ± 1.9 mg/dL in 65 healthy controls *2215*

Homocysteine *Plasma* *Increase* Hyperhomocysteinemia observed in 50 - 100% patients shortly after transplantation *2390*

Immunoglobulin A *Serum* *No Effect* In immunosuppressed cardiac transplant patients no marked changes in concentration observed *5495*

Immunoglobulin E *Serum* *Decrease* In 19 immunosuppressed cardiac transplant patients average duration for 50% reduction in concentration of 16 ± 37 d *5495*

Immunoglobulin G *Serum* *No Effect* In immunosuppressed cardiac transplant patients no marked changes in concentration observed *5495*

Immunoglobulin M *Serum* *No Effect* In immunosuppressed cardiac transplant patients no marked changes in concentration observed *5495*

Insulin *Plasma* *Increase* In 91 heart transplant recipients mean concentration of 8.5 ± 0.5 mIU/L significantly higher than 6.2 ± 0.3 mIU/L nontransplanted patients with coronary artery disease *1066*

Intercellular Adhesion Molecule-1 *Serum* *Increase* In 15 patients who had had heart transplants and subsequently developed rejection mean concentrations increased to 523 ± 97 µg/L versus baseline of 369 ± 81 µg/L *1868*

Interleukin-1β *Serum* *No Effect* No correlation observed in 11 post transplant patients with presence or absence of biopsy evidence of rejection *5537*

LDL-Cholesterol *Serum* *Increase* In 100 patients mean concentration increased to 148 ± 6 mg/dL from 111 ± 6 mg/dL 3 months after heart transplantation *269*
Serum *No Effect* In 47 patients with heart transplants for dilated cardiomyopathy of 100 ± 4.4 mg/dL and 110 ± 3.3 mg/dL in 60 heart transplant patients because of coronary artery disease not significantly different from 105 ± 5.4 mg/dL in 65 healthy controls *2215*

LDL-Cholesterol, Oxidized *Serum* *Increase* In 47 patients with heart transplants for dilated cardiomyopathy mean concentration of 1.27 ± 0.14 mg/dL and 1.73 ± 0.13 mg/dL in 60 heart transplant patients because of coronary artery disease significantly different from 0.68 ± 0.039 mg/dL in 65 healthy controls *2215*

Lipoprotein Lp(a) *Serum* *No Effect* Has no effect on Lp(a) concentration *2827* In 91 post-transplant patients concentrations not significantly different from those in 94 nontransplanted patients with coronary artery disease *1066*

β_2-Microglobulin *Serum* *Increase* In 15 patients who had had heart transplants and subsequently developed rejection mean concentrations increased to 38 ± 19 mg/L versus baseline of 33 ± 18 mg/L *1868*

Neopterin *Serum* *Increase* Mean and median concentrations of 47.4 and 37.6 nmol/L respectively during 19 rejection episodes significantly higher than mean and median of 14.7 and 11.0 nmol/L respectively in 130 controls *5489* In 19 patients with identified rejection median concentration of 37.6 ± 31.0 nmol/L and 70.0 ± 76.5 nmol/L in 95 patients with infection compared with 11.0 ± 10.8 nmol/L in 130 patients with uncomplicated course after surgery *120*
Serum *No Effect* Median concentration in 13 patients in postoperative phase of approximately 23 nmol/L not significantly different from approximately 12 nmol/L in transplant patients in stable phase *3653*

Norepinephrine *Plasma* *Decrease* In patients with severe heart failure the high presurgical concentration tended to normalize *3708*

Plasminogen Activator Inhibitor-1 *Plasma* *No Effect* No significant difference observed between concentrations in 91 post-heart transplant patients and 94 nontransplanted patients with coronary artery disease *1066*

Platelet Activating Factor *Serum* *No Effect* No correlation observed with presence or absence of biopsy signs of rejection in 11 post heart transplant patients *5537*

Platelet Aggregation *Blood* *Increase* In first wave of ADP-induced aggregation in 91 heart transplant recipients mean of 29.1 ± 0.9% of maximal aggregation versus 25.1 ± 1.0% in 94 nontransplanted patients with coronary artery disease: in second wave 21.4 ± 1.4% versus 15.9 ± 1.1% *1066*

Renin Activity *Plasma* *Increase* In 10 patients following heart transplantation mean concentration significantly higher than in controls with loss of circadian variation, possibly due to immunosuppressive therapy *979*

Soluble Interleukin-2 Receptor *Serum* *Increase* In 6 post-transplant recipients concentration increased about 40-fold with peak on day 1 or 2, typically one day before peak of SAA, with values returning to baseline about 2 weeks later *4643* Mean concentration in pretransplant patients (592 ± 209 kU/L) significantly higher than in controls (350 ± 101 kU/L) but after transplant slowly decreased to baseline in successfully treated patients but rose to 1129 ± 215 kU/L with acute rejection *5877* In 52 patients who had an orthoptic heart transplant, concentration increased early after transplant to 1,197 ± 330 kU/L versus 596 ± 265 kU/L *2348*

Thromboxane B_2 *Plasma* *No Effect* No correlation observed with presence or absence of biopsy signs of rejection in 11 post heart transplant patients *5537*

Tissue Polypeptide Antigen *Serum* *Increase* In 19 patients undergoing rejection median concentration of 73.5 ± 16.2 U/L and in 95 with infection mean of 158.2 ± 144.6 U/L compared with 43.1 ± 25.7 U/L in 130 patients with uncomplicated surgery *120* Mean and median concentrations of 75.6 and 73.5 U/L respectively during 19 rejection episodes significantly higher than mean and median of 44.9 and 43.1 U/L respectively in 130 controls *5489*

Triglycerides *Serum* *Increase* In 100 heart transplantation patients mean concentration increased to 195 ± 10 mg/dL 3 months after surgery from 107 ± 6 mg/dL presurgery *269*

Serum *No Effect* In 47 patients with heart transplants for dilated cardiomyopathy mean concentration of 130 ± 8.3 mg/dL and 140 ± 7.0 mg/dL in 60 heart transplant patients because of coronary artery disease not significantly different from 130 ± 7.5 mg/dL in 65 healthy controls *2215*

Troponin T *Serum* *Increase* In 19 heart transplant patients mean concentration increased to a maximum of 3.6 ± 1.8 µg/L at 7.1 ± 4.2 days after operation and remained higher than 0.5 µg/L in all patients for at least 43 days (mean 59 ± 20 days). Pattern of serum troponin T was unchanged by acute or chronic rejection episodes *5868*

Tumor Necrosis Factor *Serum* *Increase* In 9 of 11 patients following heart transplantation TNF concentration was increased before biopsy results showed evidence of rejection and in 15 of 31 rejecting patients (47%) positive biopsy results could be predicted from TNF concentrations. In 21 of 31 patients (68%) true positive predictions observed. In 10% of patients true negative prediction observed with normal TNF concentrations. In 3 patients increased TNF observed with negative biopsy (19% false positive rate) *5537*

Vitamin E *Serum* *Decrease* In 91 heart transplant recipients mean concentration of 14.8 ± 0.4 mg/L compared with 16.9 ± 0.7 mg/L in 94 nontransplanted coronary artery disease patients *1066*

996.84 Lung Transplant Rejection

Neopterin *Serum* *Increase* Increasing neopterin concentrations observed after lung transplant rejection *121*

Soluble HLA-I *Serum* *Increase* Mean concentration increased in graft versus host disease *576*

Soluble HLA-FHC *Serum* *Increase* Mean concentration increased in allograft rejection *576*

996.84 Lung Transplantation

Lipoprotein Lp(a) *Serum* *No Effect* Has no effect on Lp(a) concentration *2827*

Mucin-associated Antigen *Serum* *Increase* Concentration reportedly increased in patients who have had lung transplants *4797*

996.85 Bone Marrow Rejection

Soluble Intercellular Adhesion Molecule-1 *Serum* *Increase* Patients with β-thalassemia who rejected early their bone marrow engraftment had significantly higher mean pretransplant concentration of 531 ng/mL than those with sustained bone marrow engraftment (400 ng/mL) *748*

996.85 Bone Marrow Transplantation

Alanine Aminotransferase *Serum* *Increase* In 32 patients receiving allogeneic bone marrow transplants enzyme activity increased in all except one patient but returned to nomal within 2 days, remaining so for several days before rising again immediately before the end of aplasia, culminating at 3.7 ± 3.8 times the upper limit of normal *227*

Alkaline Phosphatase *Serum* *Increase* In 32 patients receiving allogeneic bone marrow transplants enzyme activity increased in 88% of all recipients *227*

Anticardiolipin-specific IgG Antibodies *Serum* *Increase* In one 4 month-old child who developed a major cerebrovascular accident and acute pulmonary hypertension in association with persistently increased anticardiolipin titers rising from 2.2 pretransplant to 15.7 at 60 days, 16.4 at 80 days, 22.2 at 140 days and 2.2 at 190 days (normal range < 7.0) *4244*

Anticardiolipin-specific IgM Antibodies *Serum* *No Effect* In one 4 month-old child who developed a major cerebrovascular accident and acute pulmonary hypertension in association with persistently increased anticardiolipin titers rising from < 2.5 pretransplant to 2.7 at 60 days, < 2.5 at 80 days, < 2.5 at 140 days and < 2.5 at 190 days (normal range < 2.5) *4244*

α_2-Antiplasmin Inhibitor/Plasmin Complex *Plasma* *Increase* In 8 children who developed veno-occlusive disease following bone marrow transplantation mean concentration changed from baseline of 1.12 ± 0.602 µg/mL to 0.67 ± 0.089 µg/mL after 7 days and 0.96 ± 0.364 µg/mL after 21 days compared with baseline of 0.52 ± 0.032 µg/mL and 0.655 ± 0.091 µg/mL after 7 days and 0.426 ± 0.081 µg/mL after 21 days in 19 who did not develop veno-occlusive disease *4006*

Antithrombin III *Plasma* *Decrease* In 8 children who developed veno-occlusive disease following bone marrow transplantation mean concentration changed from baseline of 81.0 ± 12.1% to 71.8 ± 6.56% after 7 days and 66.8 ± 11.2% after 21 days compared with baseline of 101 ± 7.16% and 90.6 ± 3.36% after 7 days and 90.3 ± 6.60% after 21 days in 19 who did not develop veno-occlusive disease *4006*

Bilirubin *Serum* *Increase* In 180 patients who underwnt autologous bone marrow transplantation for hematological malignancies 92 (51%) developed hyperbilirubinemia during the initial 40 days posttherapy. Jaundice with bilirubin > 4.0 mg/dL developed in 46 (26%) patients *5586* In 32 patients receiving allogeneic bone marrow transplants serum concentration increased in 96% of all recipients *227*

CD3+ Lymphocytes *Blood* *Increase* In one 4 month-old child who developed a major cerebrovascular accident and acute pulmonary hypertension in association with persistently increased anticardiolipin titers concentration on admission 80% different from normal range of 66 ± 8% *4244*

CD4+ Lymphocytes *Blood* *Decrease* In one 4 month-old child who developed a major cerebrovascular accident and acute pulmonary hypertension in association with persistently increased anticardiolipin titers concentration on admission 15% different from normal range of 52 ± 3% *4244*

CD8+ Lymphocytes *Blood* *No Effect* In one 4 month-old child who developed a major cerebrovascular accident and acute pulmonary hypertension in association with persistently increased anticardiolipin titers concentration on admission 16% not different from normal range of 19 ± 6% *4244*

CD16+ Lymphocytes *Blood* *No Effect* In one 4 month-old child who developed a major cerebrovascular accident and acute pulmonary hypertension in association with persistently increased anticardiolipin titers concentration on admission 13% not different from normal range of 15 ± 9% *4244*

CD19+ Lymphocytes *Blood* *Decrease* In one 4 month-old child who developed a major cerebrovascular accident and acute pulmonary hypertension in association with persistently increased anticardiolipin titers concentration on admission < 0.5% different from normal range of 21 ± 9% *4244*

CD25+ Lymphocytes *Blood* *Increase* In one 4 month-old child who developed a major cerebrovascular accident and acute pulmonary hypertension in association with persistently increased anticardiolipin titers concentration on admission 66% different from normal range of < 10% *4244*

C-Peptide *Plasma* *Increase* External irradiation prior to bone marrow transplantation was associated with high basal and glucagon-stimulated concentrations *4754*

D-Dimer *Plasma* *Increase* In 8 children who developed veno-occlusive disease following bone marrow transplantation mean concentration changed from baseline of 0.715 ± 0.179 mg/dL to 0.812 ± 0.202 mg/dL after 7 days and 2.49 ± 0.912 mg/dL after 21 days compared with baseline of 0.817 ± 0.206 mg/dL and 1.50 ± 0.518 mg/dL after 7 days and 1.00 ± 0.337 mg/dL after 21 days in 19 who did not develop veno-occlusive disease *4006*

Eosinophils *Blood* *No Effect* In one 4 month-old child who developed a major cerebrovascular accident and acute pulmonary hypertension in association with persistently increased anticardiolipin titers concentration on admission of 1.78 x 10^9/L not different from normal range of 0 - 0.8 x 10^9/L *4244*

Estradiol *Plasma* *Decrease* In 144 women after external irradiation prior to bone marrow transplantation decreased concentrations were observed for 3 years although 9 showed evidence of recovery of ovarian function later *4754*

Factor VII *Plasma* *No Effect* In 8 children who developed veno-occlusive disease following bone marrow transplantation mean concentration changed from baseline of 93.5 ± 17.1% to 80.2 ± 12.0% after 7 days and 104 ± 22.9% after 21 days compared with baseline of 94.5 ± 12.4% and 81.8 ± 12.3% after 7 days and 94.6 ± 14.5% after 21 days in 19 who did not develop veno-occlusive disease *4006*

996.85 Bone Marrow Transplantation *(continued)*

Fibrin Degradation Products *Plasma* *Increase* In 8 children who developed veno-occlusive disease following bone marrow transplantation mean concentration changed from baseline of 3.88 ± 0.368 µg/mL to 4.16 ± 0.584 µg/mL after 7 days and 9.44 ± 3.42 µg/mL after 21 days compared with baseline of 5.95 ± 1.58 µg/mL and 7.46 ± 2.14 µg/mL after 7 days and 4.99 ± 0.452 µg/mL after 21 days in 19 who did not develop veno-occlusive disease *4006*

Fibrinogen *Plasma* *Increase* In 8 children who developed veno-occlusive disease following bone marrow transplantation mean concentration changed from baseline of 250 ± 23.8 mg/dL to 352 ± 53.4 mg/dL after 7 days and 164 ± 11.9 mg/dL after 21 days compared with baseline of 319 ± 32.1 mg/dL and 331 ± 25.4 mg/dL after 7 days and 252 ± 29.3 mg/dL after 21 days in 19 who did not develop veno-occlusive disease *4006*

Follicle Stimulating Hormone *Plasma* *Increase* In men after external irradiation prior to bone marrow transplantation increased concentrations were observed although return to normal may occur with time *4754*

Glucose Tolerance *Serum* *No Effect* External irradiation prior to bone marrow transplantation was not associated with abnormal IGTTs *4754*

Gonadotropins *Plasma* *Increase* In 144 women after external irradiation prior to bone marrow transplantation increased concentrations were observed for 3 years although 9 showed evidence of recovery of ovarian function later *4754*

Growth Hormone *Plasma* *No Effect* In majority of adults who received a bone marrow transplant following total body irradiation mean peak response to challnges normal *4754*

Hemoglobin *Blood* *Decrease* In one 4 month-old child who developed a major cerebrovascular accident and acute pulmonary hypertension in association with persistently increased anticardiolipin titers concentration on admission 9.5 g/dL different from normal range of 10.5 - 13.5 g/dL *4244*

Hemoglobin A_{1c} *Blood* *No Effect* External irradiation prior to bone marrow transplantation was not associated with abnormal hemoglobin A_{1c} concentrations *4754*

Immunoglobulin A *Serum* *Decrease* In one 4 month-old child who developed a major cerebrovascular accident and acute pulmonary hypertension in association with persistently increased anticardiolipin titers concentration on admission < 0.03 g/L different from normal range of 0.05 - 0.4 g/L *4244*

Immunoglobulin E *Serum* *Decrease* In one 4 month-old child who developed a major cerebrovascular accident and acute pulmonary hypertension in association with persistently increased anticardiolipin titers concentration on admission 683 kU/L different from normal range of < 4.0 kU/L *4244*

Immunoglobulin G *Serum* *Decrease* In one 4 month-old child who developed a major cerebrovascular accident and acute pulmonary hypertension in association with persistently increased anticardiolipin titers concentration on admission 0.51 g/L different from normal range of 2.1 - 7.7 g/L *4244*

Immunoglobulin M *Serum* *Decrease* In one 4 month-old child who developed a major cerebrovascular accident and acute pulmonary hypertension in association with persistently increased anticardiolipin titers concentration on admission < 0.05 g/L different from normal range of 0.15 - 0.7 g/L *4244*

Insulin *Plasma* *Increase* External irradiation prior to bone marrow transplantation was associated with high concentrations and the first phase insulin response was significantly higher than in controls *4754*

Leukocytes *Blood* *No Effect* In one 4 month-old child who developed a major cerebrovascular accident and acute pulmonary hypertension in association with persistently increased anticardiolipin titers concentration on admission of 8.1 x 10^9/L not different from normal range of 5 - 15 x 10^9/L *4244*

Lymphocytes *Blood* *Increase* In one 4 month-old child who developed a major cerebrovascular accident and acute pulmonary hypertension in association with persistently increased anticardiolipin titers concentration on admission of 4.37 x 10^9/L different from normal range of 1.5 - 4.0 x 10^9/L *4244*

Neutrophils *Blood* *Decrease* In one 4 month-old child who developed a major cerebrovascular accident and acute pulmonary hypertension in association with persistently increased anticardiolipin titers concentration on admission of 0.24 x 10^9/L different from normal range of 2 - 8.5 x 10^9/L *4244*

N-terminal Propeptide of Type III Procollagen *Serum* *No Effect* In 8 children who developed veno-occlusive disease following bone marrow transplantation mean concentration changed from baseline of 1.50 ± 0.00 U/mL to 1.34 ± 0.198 U/mL after 7 days and 2.64 ± 0.878 U/mL after 21 days compared with baseline of 1.39 ± 0.241 U/mL and 1.973 ± 0.428 U/mL after 7 days and 2.09 ± 0.376 U/mL after 21 days in 19 who did not develop veno-occlusive disease *4006*

Plasminogen *Plasma* *Decrease* In 8 children who developed veno-occlusive disease following bone marrow transplantation mean concentration changed from baseline of 87.8 ± 11.3% to 84.6 ± 4.70% after 7 days and 63.2 ± 16.8% after 21 days compared with baseline of 92.0 ± 4.37% and 95.8 ± 4.39% after 7 days and 89.9 ± 5.80% after 21 days in 19 who did not develop veno-occlusive disease *4006*

Plasminogen Activator Inhibitor-1 *Plasma* *Decrease* In 8 children who developed veno-occlusive disease following bone marrow transplantation mean concentration changed from baseline of 96.5 ± 35.8 ng/mL to 23.9 ± 4.61 ng/mL after 7 days and 51.8 ± 9.82 ng/mL after 21 days compared with baseline of 28.8 ± 3.99 ng/mL and 25.4 ± 3.78 ng/mL after 7 days and 29.1 ± 4.13 ng/mL after 21 days in 19 who did not develop veno-occlusive disease *4006*

Platelets *Blood* *Increase* In one 4 month-old child who developed a major cerebrovascular accident and acute pulmonary hypertension in association with persistently increased anticardiolipin titers concentration on admission of 511 x 10^9/L different from normal range of 150 - 450 x 10^9/L *4244*

Protein C *Plasma* *No Effect* In 8 children who developed veno-occlusive disease following bone marrow transplantation mean concentration changed from baseline of 89.8 ± 18.7% to 57.8 ± 10.5% after 7 days and 105 ± 30.8% after 21 days compared with baseline of 73.3 ± 12.6% and 70.2 ± 10.0% after 7 days and 92.3 ± 12.2% after 21 days in 19 who did not develop veno-occlusive disease *4006*

Soluble Intercellular Adhesion Molecule-1 *Serum* *Increase* In 10 patients with AML mean concentrations ranged from 188 ± 56 ng/mL to 567 ± 77 ng/mL before bone marrow transplantation rising steadily after transplantation with means ranging from 202 to 571 ng/mL on 10th day, to 201 to 581 ng/mL on 20th day, 228 to 899 ng/mL on 39th day, 242 to 1,010 ng/mL on 40th day and 255 to 1,256 ng/mL on 50th day, with all values that were markedly increased being associated with graft versus host disease *3202*

Testosterone *Serum* *No Effect* In men after external irradiation prior to bone marrow transplantation basal concentration usually remains within reference limits although in patients receiving BMT for lymphoma concentrations tend to be reduced *4754*

Thrombin/Antithrombin III Complex *Plasma* *Increase* In 8 children who developed veno-occlusive disease following bone marrow transplantation mean concentration changed from baseline of 1.88 ± 0.250 ng/mL to 2.74 ± 0.566 ng/mL after 7 days and 8.68 ± 3.42 ng/mL after 21 days compared with baseline of 2.00 ± 0.489 ng/mL and 2.15 ± 0.588 ng/mL after 7 days and 2.67 ± 0.840 ng/mL after 21 days in 19 who did not develop veno-occlusive disease *4006*

Thrombomodulin *Plasma* *Increase* In 8 children who developed veno-occlusive disease following bone marrow transplantation mean concentration changed from baseline of 6.08 ± 1.79 U/mL to 5.57 ± 1.45 U/mL after 7 days and 15.9 ± 6.22 U/mL after 21 days compared with baseline of 9.76 ± 1.15 U/mL and 7.03 ± 0.78 U/mL after 7 days and 11.6 ± 1.23 U/mL after 21 days in 19 who did not develop veno-occlusive disease *4006*

Thyroid Stimulating Hormone *Serum* *Increase* External irradiation to the neck prior to bone marrow transplantation may lead to mildly increased basal TSH concentration *4754*

Thyroxine (T4) *Serum* *No Effect* External irradiation to the neck prior to bone marrow transplantation may lead to mildly increased basal TSH concentration, but normal thyroxine concentration *4754*

Tissue Plasminogen Activator *Plasma* *Increase* In 8 children who developed veno-occlusive disease following bone marrow transplantation mean concentration increased from baseline of 4.13 ± 0.86 ng/mL to 7.93 ± 2.24 ng/mL after 7 days and 15.8 ± 2.32 ng/mL after 21 days compared with baseline of 5.84 ± 1.04 ng/mL and 8.97 ± 1.72 ng/mL after 7 days and 9.25 ± 1.70 ng/mL after 21 days in 19 who did not develop veno-occlusive disease *4006*

von Willebrand Factor *Plasma* *Increase* In 8 children who developed veno-occlusive disease following bone marrow transplantation mean concentration changed from baseline of 79.5 ± 26.3% to 108 ± 29.6% after 7 days and 86.6 ± 25.3% after 21 days compared with baseline of 60.7 ± 2.67% and 60.2 ± 2.57% after 7 days and 64.4 ± 2.70% after 21 days in 19 who did not develop veno-occlusive disease *4006*

996.85 Graft versus Host Disease

Granulocyte Colony Stimulating Factor *Serum* *No Effect* In 21 patients after bone marrow transplantation no significant correlation observed between acute GVHD and G-CSF concentration *1874*

Intercellular Adhesion Molecule-1 *Serum* *No Effect* In 21 patients after bone marrow transplantation no significant correlation observed between acute GVHD and ICAM-1 concentration *1874*

Interleukin-6 *Serum* *No Effect* In 21 patients after bone marrow transplantation no significant correlation observed between acute GVHD and IL-6 concentration *1874*

Interleukin-8 *Serum* *No Effect* In 21 patients after bone marrow transplantation no significant correlation observed between acute GVHD and IL-8 concentration *1874*

Neopterin *Serum* *Increase* Increasing neopterin concentrations observed with graft versus host disease *121*
Urine *Increase* 6 patients with persistent GVHD had persistently increased urinary excretion *1781*

Plasminogen Activator Inhibitor-1 *Plasma* *No Effect* In 31 of 186 consecutive patients undergoing bone marrow transplantation who developed hyperbilirubinemia mean concentration of 41 ± 21 ng/mL in 7 patients with graft versus host disease compared with reference interval of 4 - 43 ng/mL *4529*

Soluble HLA-I *Serum* *Increase* Concentration reportedly increased with condition *5306* Mean concentration increased in graft versus host disease *576*

Soluble HLA-FHC *Serum* *Increase* Mean concentration increased in graft versus host disease *576*

Soluble Interleukin-2 Receptor *Serum* *Increase* In 21 patients after bone marrow transplantation the maximum concentration of sIL-2R correlated significantly with the severity of acute GVHD *1874*

Soluble Tumor Necrosis Factor Receptor *Serum* *No Effect* In 21 patients after bone marrow transplantation no significant correlation observed between acute GVHD and sTNF-R concentration *1874*

Stem Cell Factor *Serum* *No Effect* In 21 patients after bone marrow transplantation no significant correlation observed between acute GVHD and stem cell factor concentration *1874*

996.86 Pancreas Transplant Rejection

Neopterin *Pancreatic Fluid* *Increase* Increasing neopterin concentrations observed after pancreas transplant rejection *121*
Serum *Increase* Increasing neopterin concentrations observed after pancreas transplant rejection *121*

Soluble HLA-I *Serum* *Increase* Mean concentration increased in graft versus host disease *576*

Soluble HLA-FHC *Serum* *Increase* Mean concentration increased in allograft rejection *576*

996.86 Pancreas Transplantation

Pancreatic Elastase 1 *Serum* *Increase* Activity rose to a peak within 6 days of transplantation, thereafter declining to stabilize after 4 - 6 weeks at an increased level (10 ng/mL) for approximately one year and from 2 - 8 years activity was increased (1 - 6 ng/mL) in 14 of 20 patients *3065*

Sialic Acid *Serum* *Decrease* In 9 IDDM patients who underwent pancreatic transplantation concentration decreased to 0.21 ± 0.07 mmol/L compared with 0.83 ± 0.19 mmol/L in 8 IDDM patients who underwent kidney transplants and 1.12 ± 0.42 mmol/L in 8 patients with end-stage renal disease *213*

Soluble Intercellular Adhesion Molecule-1 *Serum* *Increase* In 10 patients with stable stable graft function mean concentration of 375.5 ± 42.0 ng/L and in 7 with episodes of rejection mean concentration of 573.3 ± 90.3 ng/L significantly increased compared with 235.6 ± 13.2 ng/L in 7 healthy control individuals *5609*

996.89 Heart-lung Transplantation

5-Hydroxytryptamine *Plasma* *No Effect* In 6 patients with primary pulmonary hypertension mean concentration after transplantation of 36.7 ± 10.1 nmol/L not significantly different from 32.3 ± 13.0 nmol/L prior to transplantation *2134*
Platelets *No Effect* In 6 patients with primary pulmonary hypertension mean concentration after transplantation of 1.9 ± 0.7 x 10^{-18} mol/platelet not significantly different from 1.5 ± 0.6 x 10^{-18} mol/platelet prior to transplantation *2134*

996.89 Ureteric Transplant into Colon

Calcium *Serum* *No Effect* In a study of 59 patients with normocalcemia and low intact PTH concentration, 1 had had a transplant of ureters into the colon *3280*

Parathyroid Hormone *Plasma* *Decrease* In a study of 59 patients with normocalcemia and low intact PTH concentration, 1 had had a ureteric transplant into the colon *3280*

999.90 Milk-Alkali Syndrome

Alkaline Phosphatase *Serum* *Decrease* Reported effect *3160*

Calcium *Serum* *Increase* An unusual complication of intensive peptic ulcer therapy is the evolution of hypercalcemia from excessive intake of milk and absorbable alkali *2039*

Phosphate *Serum* *Increase* Normal or elevated *1025*

4 REFERENCES

1 Missing Reference

2 Aadland E, Odegaard OR, Roseth A et al. Free protein S deficiency in patients with Crohn's disease. *Scand J Gastroenterol*, 29, 333-335 (1994)

3 Aarli A J et al. Antibodies against nicotinic acetylcholine receptor and skeletal muscle in human and experimental myasthenia gravis. *Scand J Immunol*, 4, 849 (1975)

4 Aasen AO, Kierulf P, Ruud TE, Godal HC. Studies on pathological plasma proteolysis in patients with acute pancreatitis. a preliminary report. *Acta Chir Scand*, Suppl 509, 83-87 (1982)

5 Aaser E, Gullestad L, Tollofsrud S, et al. Effect of bolus injection versus continuous infusion of furosemide on diuresis and neurohormonal activation in patients with severe congestive heart failure. *Scand J Clin Lab Invest*, 57, 361-368 (1997)

6 Abassi ZA, Klein H, Golomb E et al. Urinary endothelin: a possible biological marker of renal damage. *Am J Hypertens*, 6, 1046-1054 (1993)

7 Abbascino V, Graziano L, Guerra S et al. Coagulation disorders and tumor markers in the diagnosis of pancreatic cancer. *Oncology*, 48, 377-382 (1991)

8 Abbasse AA et al. Gonadal function abnormalities in sickle cell anemia. *Ann Intern Med*, 85, 601-605 (1976)

9 Abbassi V et al. Postnatal triiodothyronine concentrations in healthy preterm infants and in infants with respiratory distress syndrome. *Pediatr Res*, 11, 802-804 (1977)

10 Abbott CA, Mackness MI, Kumar S, et al. Serum paraoxonase activity, concentration, and phenotype distribution in diabetes mellitus and its relationship to serum lipids and lipoproteins. *Arterioscler Thromb Vasc Biol*, 15, 1812-1818 (1995)

11 Abbott Diagnostics. Manufacturer's Literature on AxSYM Immunoassay Analyzer. Abbott Park, IL 60064 (1995)

12 Abdel Aziz MT, Abdel Aziz WM, Kamel M et al. Clinical evaluation of serum aminoterminal propeptide of type III procollagen as tumor marker in gynecologic malignancies. *Tumori*, 79, 219-223 (1993)

13 Abe Y, Kawakami M, Kuroki M et al. Transient rise in serum interleukin-8 concentration during acute myocardial infarction. *Br Heart J*, 70, 132-134 (1993)

14 Abeleu GI. α-Fetoprotein in ontogenesis and its association with malignant tumors. *Adv Cancer Res*, 14, 295-358 (1971)

15 Abelson JL, Glitz D, Cameron OG et al. Endocrine, cardiovascular, and behavioral response to clonidine in patients with panic disorder. *Biol Psychiat*, 32, 8-25 (1992)

16 Ablin RJ. Serum proteins in prostatic cancer. *Urology*, 7, 39-47 (1976)

17 Abou-Hatah K, Nixon LS, O'Mahony MS, et al. Plasma esterases in cystic fibrosis: the impact of a respiratory exacerbation and its treatment. *Eur J Clin Pharmacol*, 54, 937-941 (1999)

18 Aboulghar MA, Mansour RT, Serour GI, et al. Elevated concentrations of angiogenin in serum and ascitic fluid from patients with severe ovarian hyperstimulation syndrome. *Hum Reprod*, 13, 2068-2071 (1998)

19 Abraha HD, Butterworth RJ, Bath PMW, et al. Serum S-100 protein, relationship to clinical outcomes in acute stroke. *Ann Clin Biochem*, 34, 546-550 (1997)

20 Abraham J P et al. Hemorrhagic complications of polycythemia vera. *Henry Ford Hosp Bull*, 9, 11 (1961)

21 Abu-Shakra M, Gladman DD, Urowitz MB, et al. Anticardiolipin antibodies in systemic lupus erythematosus: clinical and laboratory correlations. *Am J Med*, 99, 624-628 (1995)

22 Acara M, Rennick B, LaGraff S et al. Effect of renal transplantation on the levels of choline in the plasma of uremic humans. *Nephron*, 35, 241-243 (1983)

23 Acevedo HF, Campbell EA, Frich JC Jr et al. Urinary cholesterol. VII. The significance of the excretion of nonesterified cholesterol in patients with uterine carcinomas. *Cancer*, 36, 1459-1469 (1975)

24 Acevedo HF et al. Urinary cholesterol. VIII. its excretion in women with ovarian neoplasms. *Cancer*, 37, 2847-57 (1976)

25 Adamashvili IM, McDonald JC, Fraser PA et al. Soluble class I HLA antigens in patients with rheumatoid arthritis and their families. *J Rheumatol*, 22, 1025-1031 (1995)

26 Adami H O et al. Thyroid disease and function in breast cancer patients and non-hospitalized controls evaluated by determination of TSH, T3, rT3, and T4 levels in serum. *Acta Chir Scand*, 144, 89-97 (1978)

27 Adami S, Braga V, Squarantl R, et al. Bone measurements in asymptomatic primary hyperparathyroidism. *Bone*, 22, 565-570 (1998)

28 Adams DH, Burnett D, Stockley RA et al. Biliary β_2-microglobulin in liver allograft rejection. *Hepatology*, 8, 1565-1570 (1988)

29 Adams EB, Macleod J N. Amebic liver abscess and its complications. *Medicine*, 56, 325-333 (1977)

30 Adams EC. Differentiation of myoglobin and hemoglobin in biological fluids. *Ann Clin Lab Sci*, 1, 208 (1971)

31 Adams JE, Davila-Roman VG, Bessey PO, et al. Improved detection of cardiac contusion with cardiac troponin I. *Am Heart J*, 131, 308-312 (1996)

32 Adams JT, et al. Significance of an elevated serum amylase. *Surgery*, 63, 877-884 (1968)

33 Adams PC, Bradley C, Henderson AR. Evaluation of the hepatic iron index as a diagnostic criterion for genetic hemochromatosis. *J Lab Clin Med*, 130, 509-514 (1997)

34 Adamska-Dyniewska H, Bala T, Florczak H, et al. Blood cadmium in healthy subjects and in patients with cardiovascular diseases. *Reference not available*

35 Addiss DG, Lengerich EJ. Hypokalemic myopathy induced by giardia lamblia. *N Engl J Med*, 330, 66 (1994)

36 Adler G, Kropf J, Grobe E, Gressner AM. Follow-up of the serum levels of extracellular matrix components in acute and chronic pancreatitis. *Eur J Clin Invest*, 20, 494-501 (1990)

37 Adler RA. Clinically important effects of alcohol on endocrine function. *J Clin Endocrinol Metab*, 74, 957-960 (1992)

38 Adlersberg D et al. Uric acid partition in gout and hepatic disease. *Arch Intern Med*, 70, 101 (1942)

39 Agardh CD, Agardh E, Isaksson A et al. Association between urinary N-acetyl-β-glucosaminidase and its isoenzyme patterns and microangiopathy in type 1 diabetes mellitus. *Clin Chem*, 37, 1696-1699 (1991)

40 Agarwal A, Soni A, Aehanowsky M et al. Hyponatremia in patients with acquired immune deficiency. *Nephron*, 53, 317-321 (1989)

41 Agayev BA, Kuliyev BG. Clinical importance of determination of blood serotonin level during surgical treatment of cholecystitis. *Klin Khir*, 10, 7-10 (1975)

42 Aggarwal R, Ravishankar B, Misra R, et al. Significance of elevated IgG anticardiolipin antibody levels in patients with Budd-Chiari syndrome. *Am J Gastroenterol*, 93, 954-957 (1998)

43 Agren H, Lundqvist G. Low levels of somatostatin in human CSF mark depressive episodes. *Psychoneuroendocrinology*, 9, 233-248 (1984)

44 Aguirre JC, del Arbo JL, Raya J et al. Plasma β-endorphin levels in chronic alcoholics. *Alcohol*, 7, 409-412 (1990)

45 Ahmadzadeh N, Shingu M, Nobuaga M et al. Relationship between leukotriene B_4 and immunological parameters in rheumatoid synovial fluids. *Inflammation*, 15, 497-503 (1991)

46 Aho HJ, Grenman R, Sipila J, et al. Group II phospholipase A_2 in nasal fluid, mucosa and paranasal sinuses. *Acta Otolaryngol*, 117, 860-863 (1997)

47 Aimaretti G, Corneli G, Razzore P, et al. Usefulness of IGF-I assay for the diagnosis of GH deficiency. *J Endocrinol Invest*, 21, 506-511 (1998)

48 Aisenberg A C et al. Serum alkaline phosphatase at the onset of Hodgkin's disease. *Cancer*, 26, 318 (1970)

49 Aitken DA, Ireland M, Berry E et al. Pregnancy associated plasma protein-A (PAPP-A) in maternal serum from pregnancies with Cornelia de Lange syndrome. *Proc Natl Meet ACB*, 84-85 (1995)

50 Aitken DA, McKinnon D, Crossley JA et al. Changes in the maternal serum concentrations of PAPP-A and SP-1 in Down's syndrome pregnancies between the first and second trimester. *Proc ACB Natl Meet*, 72 (1993)

51 Aiyathurai JE et al. The probable significance of hypertriglyceridemia in viral hepatitis. *Aust NZ J Med*, 6, 529-532 (1976)

52 Aizenberg D, Hermesh H, Gil-ad I et al. TRH stimulation test in obsessive compulsive patients. *Psychiat Res*, 38, 21-26 (1991)

53 Akazawa H, Ikeda U, Kuroda T, Shimada K. Plasma endothelin-1 levels in Takayasu's arteritis. *Cardiology*, 87, 303-305 (1996)

54 Akdamar K, Epps AC, Maumus LT et al. Immunoglobulin changes in liver disease. *Ann NY Acad Sci*, 101-107 (1971)

55 Akenami FOT, Koskiniemi M, Farkkila M, Vaheri A. Cerebrospinal fluid plasminogen, plasmin and protease inhibitors in multiple sclerosis. *Fibrinolysis Proteolysis*, 13, 99-103 (1999)

56 Akenami FOT, Koskiniemi M, Frkkil M, Vaheri A. Cerebrospinal fluid plasminogen activator inhibitor-1 in patients with neurological disease. *J Clin Pathol*, 50, 157-160 (1997)

57 Akenami FOT, Koskiniemi M, Mustjoki S, et al. Plasma and cerebrospinal fluid activities of tissue plasminogen activator, urokinase and plasminogen activator inhibitor-1 in multiple sclerosis. *Fibrinolysis Proteolysis*, 11, 109-113 (1997)

58 Akerfeldt S. Oxidation of N, N-dimethyl-p-phenylenediamine by serum from patients with mental disease. *Science*, 125, 117-119 (1957)

59 Akesson K, Vergnaud Ph, Delmas PD et al. Serum osteocalcin increases during fracture healing in elderly women with hip fracture. *Bone*, 16, 427-430 (1995)

60 Akinyanju P A. Plasma and red cell lipids in sickle cell disease. *Ann Clin Lab Sci*, 6, 521-524 (1976)

61 Akiyami K. Serum levels of soluble IL-2 receptor α, IL-6, and IL-1 receptor antagonist in schizophrenia before and after neuroleptic administration. *Schiz Res*, 37, 97-106 (1999)

62 Akoum A, Lemay A, McColl SR, et al. Increased monocyte chemotactic protein-1 level and activity in the peripheral blood of women with endometriosis. *Am J Obstet Gynecol*, 175, 1620-1625 (1996)

63 Al Muhaseb N, Al Yousuf AR, Bajaj JS. Apolipoprotein A-I, A-II, B, C-II and C-III in children with insulin-dependent diabetes mellitus. *Pediatrics*, 89, 936-941 (1992)

64 Alanen A. Serum IgE and smooth muscle antibodies in pre-eclampsia. *Acta Obstet Gynecol Scand*, 63, 581-582 (1984)

65 Alarcon-Segovia D. The necrotizing vasculitides. *Med Clin North Am*, 61, 241-260 (1975)

66 Al-Attia HM. Clinicolaboratory profile of 33 Arabs with systemic lupus erythematosus. *Postgrad Med J*, 72, 677-679 (1996)

67 Al-Bassam M, Al-Rawi RM, Aubais KH. Cortisol and myoglobin: biochemical markers of myocardial infarction. *Clin Biochem Rev*, 14, 233 (1993)

68 Albillos A, Alvarez-Mon M, Rossi I et al. Different HCl and pepsinogen I secretion patterns in anatomically defined gastric ulcer subsets. *Am J Gastroenterol*, 85, 535-538 (1990)

69 Alcabes P, Selwyn PA, Davenny K et al. Laboratory markers and the risk of developing HIV-1 disease among injecting drug users. *AIDS*, 8, 107-115 (1994)

70 Alderman M, Sealey J, Cohen H, et al. Urinary sodium excretion and myocardial infarction in hypertensive patients: a prospective cohort study. *Am J Clin Nutr*, 65 Suppl, 682S-686S (1997)

71 Aldinger KA et al. Thyroid-stimulating hormone and prolactin levels in breast cancer. *Arch Intern Med*, 138, 1638-1641 (1978)

72 Aleem FA et al. Plasma estrogen in patients with endometrial hyperplasia and carcinoma. *Cancer*, 38, 2101-2104 (1976)

73 Alertsen AR, Aukrust A, Skaug OE et al. Selenium concentrations in blood and serum from patients with mental diseases. *Acta Psychiat Scand*, 74, 217-219 (1986)

74 Alexander B et al. Congenital SPCA deficiency: a hitherto unrecognized coagulation defect with hemorrhage rectified by serum and serum factors. *J Clin Invest*, 30, 596 (1951)

75 Alexander MG et al. α-Fetoprotein in liver disease. *S Afr Med J*, 53, 433-436 (1978)

76 Alfthan G, Pekkanen J, Jauhiainen M et al. Relation of serum homocysteine and lipoprotein(a) concentrations to atherosclerotic disease in a prospective Finnish population based study. *Atherosclerosis*, 106, 9-19 (1994)

77 Ali S, Sun T, Narukar L. Oligoclonal banding in cerebrospinal fluids of Lyme disease patients. *Am J Clin Pathol*, 100, 335 (1993)

78 Al-Kassab AS, Malatani TMS. The pattern of serum biochemical abnormalities in patients with gallstones. *Eur J Clin Chem Clin Biochem*, 30, 21-25 (1992)

79 Allam B F et al. Serum ionized calcium in acute pancreatitis. *Br J Surg*, 64, 665-668 (1977)

80 Allard WJ , Zhou Z, Yeung KK. Novel immunoassay for the measurement of prostate-specific antigen in serum. *Clin Chem*, 44, 1216-1223 (1998)

81 Allen KR, Rushworth PA, Degg TJ, Barth JH. Measurement of urinary porphobilinogen and porphyrins: preliminary data from a pilot QA scheme. *Ann Clin Biochem*, 34, 553-555 (1997)

82 Allen UD, King SM, Gomez MP, et al. Serum immunoreactive erythropoietin levels and associated factors amongst HIV-infected children. *AIDS*, 12, 1785-1791 (1998)

83 Allison AC. *Structure and Function of Plasma Proteins.* New York, Plenum Press, 1 (1974)

84 Allison AC, Rees W. The binding of haemoglobin by plasma proteins (haptoglobins). *Br Med J*, 2, 1137 (1957)

85 Allott EN, Mcardle B. Further observations on familial periodic paralysis. *Clin Sci*, 3, 229 (1938)

86 Al-Muhtaseb N, Al-Yusef AR, Bajaj JS. Lipoprotein lipids and apolipoproteins (AI, AII, B, CII, CIII) in type 1 and type 2 diabetes mellitus in young Kuwaiti women. *Diabetic Med*, 8, 732-737 (1991)

87 Alonso de la Pena C, Rozas I et al. Free carnitine and acylcarnitine levels in sera of alcoholics. *Biochem Med Metab Biol*, 44, 77-83 (1990)

88 Al-Refaie FN, De Silva CE, Wonke B et al. Changes in transferrin saturation after treatment with the oral iron chelator deferiprone in patients with iron overload. *J Clin Pathol*, 48, 110-114 (1995)

89 Alsabti EA. Serum α-fetoprotein in bladder carcinoma. *Oncology*, 34, 78-79 (1977)

90 Al-Sarraf et al. Primary liver cancer - a review. *Cancer*, 33, 574-582 (1974)

91 Alsever RN, Gotlin RW. *Handbook of Endocrine Tests In Adults and Children*, Chigago IL, Year Book Medical Publishers (1978)

92 Al-Shoumer KAS, Anyaoku V, Richmond W, Johnston DG. Elevated leptin concentrations in growth hormone-deficient hypopituitary adults. *Clin Endocrinol*, 47, 153-159 (1997)

93 Al-Shoumer KAS, Cox KH, Hughes CL, et al. Fasting and postprandial lipid abnormalities in hypopituitary women receiving conventional replacement therapy. *J Clin Endocrinol Metab*, 82, 2653-2659 (1997)

94 Altemus M, Jacobson KR, Debellis M, et al. Normal CSF oxytocin and NPY levels in OCD. *Biol Psychiat*, 45, 931-933 (1999)

95 Altemus M, Pigott T, Kalogeras KT et al. Abnormalities in the regulation of vasopressin and corticotropin releasing factor secretion in obsessive-compulsive disorder. *Arch Gen Psychiat*, 49, 9-20 (1992)

96 Altes A, Abellan MT, Mateo J, et al. Hemostatic disturbances in acute ischemic stroke: a study of 86 patients. *Acta Haematol*, 94, 10-15 (1995)

97 Altomonte L et al. Serum concentration of bile acids in the diagnosis of liver lesions in rheumatoid arthritis. *Minerva Med*, 73, 1695-1698 (1982)

98 Altstiel LD, Lawlor B, Mohs R et al. Elevated α_1-antichymotrypsin serum levels in a subset of nondemented first-degree relatives of Alzheimer's disease patients. *Dementia*, 6, 17-20 (1995)

99 Al-Turaiki MH, Akbar AM, Al-Shammari FJ et al. Plasma mineral and hormone levels in girls with idiopathic scoliosis. *Med Sci Res*, 22, 415-416 (1994)

100 Alvarez C, Ramos A. Lipids, lipoproteins and apoproteins in serum during infection. *Clin Chem*, 32, 142-145 (1986)

101 Alvarez JO, Salazar-Lindo E, Kohatsu J et al. Urinary excretion of retinol in children with acute diarrhea. *Am J Clin Nutr*, 61, 1273-1276 (1995)

102 Alvarez L, Peris P, Pons F, et al. Relationship between biochemical markers of bone turnover and bone scintigraphic indices in assessment of Paget's disease activity. *Arth Rheum*, 40, 461-468 (1997)

103 Alvsaker JO. Genetic studies in primary gout: investigations on the plasma levels of the urate-binding alpha 1 - alpha 2 globulin in individuals from two gouty kindred. *J Clin Invest*, 47, 1254 (1968)

104 Alzeer AH, El-Hazmi MAF, Warsy AS, et al. Serum enzymes in heat stroke: prognostic implication. *Clin Chem*, 43, 1182-1187 (1997)

105 Amador Garcia JM, Mendoza Montero J, Exposito Hernandez J et al. The clinical usefulness of the serological study of IgG antibodies and IgA against the antigens associated with the Epstein-Barr virus in patients with nasopharnyngeal carcinoma. *Acta Otorinolaringol Esp*, 43, 31-36 (1991)

106 Ambrosi B, Peverelli S, Passini E et al. Abnormalities of endocrine function in patients with clinically "silent" adrenal masses. *Eur J Endocrinol*, 132, 422-428 (1995)

107 Ambrus CM, Ambrus JL, Courey N et al. Inhibitors of fibrinolysis in diabetic children, mothers, and their newborn. *Am J Hematol*, 7, 245-254 (1979)

108 Amemiya N, Yatomi Y, Endo T, et al. A case of hepatocellular carcinoma with marked hyperfibrinogenemia. *Acta Haematol*, 97, 236-238 (1997)

109 Amin M, Eckhardt T, Kapitza S, et al. Correlation between tissue transglutaminase antibodies and endomysium antibodies as diagnostic markers of coeliac disease. *Clin Chim Acta*, 282, 219-225 (1999)

110 Amman RW et al. Diagnostic value of fecal chymotrypsin and trypsin assessment for detection of pancreatic disease. *Am J Dig Dis*, 13, 123-146 (1968)

111 Amodio P, Angeli P, Merkel C et al. Plasma carnitine levels in liver cirrhosis: relationship with nutritional status and liver damage. *J Clin Chem Clin Biochem*, 28, 619-626 (1990)

112 Amorosi EC, Ultmann JE. Thrombotic thrombocytopenic purpura: report of 16 patients and review of the literature. *Medicine*, 45, 136 (1969)

113 Anawalt BD, Bebb RA, Matsumoto AM, et al. Serum inhibin B levels reflect Sertoli cell function in normal men and men with testicular dysfunction. *J Clin Endocrinol Metab*, 81, 341-3345 (1996)

114 Andersen OO et al. Glucose tolerance and insulin secretion in hyperthyroidism. *Acta Endocrinol*, 84, 578-587 (1977)

115 Anderson B, Vermeulen A, Marin P et al. Testosterone concentrations in women and men with NIDDM. *Diabetes Care*, 17, 405-411 (1994)

116 Anderson JA et al. Diagnostic value of thyroid antibodies. *J Clin Endocrinol Metab*, 27, 937 (1967)

117 Anderson JL, Carlquist JF, Muhlestein JB, et al. Evaluation of C-reactive protein, an inflammatory marker, and infectious serology as risk factors for coronary artery disease and myocardial infarction. *J Am Coll Cardiol*, 32, 35-41 (1998)

118 Anderssen N. The activity of lactic dehydrogenase in megaloblastic anemia. *Scand J Haematol*, 1, 212 (1964)

119 Andersson L-M, Fredman P, Lekman A, et al. Increased cerebrospinal fluid ganglioside GD3 concentrations as a marker of microglial activation in HIV type I infection. *AIDS Res Hum Retrovir*, 14, 1065-1069 (1998)

120 Andert S, Vogl MK, Muller MM. Tissue polypeptide specific antigen, neopterin and CRP in monitoring patients after heart transplantation. *Clin Biochem Rev*, 14, 201 (1993)

121 Andert SE, Muller MM. Neopterin: biochemistry and clinical usefulness. *J Int Fed Clin Chem*, 7, 70-76 (1995)

122 Andicoechea A, Vizoso F, Alexandre E, et al. Carbohydrate antigen 195 (CA 195) in the sera of patients with esophageal, hepatic and biliary tract carcinomas. *Int J Biol Mark*, 13, 102-104 (1998)

123 Ando K, Saito K, Takai T et al. Anti-T3 autoantibodies in a case of chronic thyroiditis associated with Sjögren syndrome and systemic lupus erythematosus. *J Jpn Soc Int Med*, 72, 1680-1685 (1984)

124 Ando T, Shimamoto K, Nakahashi Y et al. Plasma antidiuretic hormone levels in patients with normal and low renin essential hypertension, and secondary hypertension. *Endocrinol Jpn*, 30, 567-570 (1983)

125 Andre E, Voisin P, Andre JL, et al. Hemorheological and hemostatic parameters in children with nephrotic syndrome undergoing steroid therapy. *Nephron*, 68, 184-191 (1994)

126 Andreoli TE, Carpenter CT, Plum F, Smith LH. In. *Essentials of Internal Medicine*, Philadelphia PA, WB Saunders (1986)

127 Andreotti F, Kluft C, Hamilton J et al. Effect of age, time of day and arterial disease on the relation between tissue-type plasminogen activator and plasminogen activator inhibitor-1 in plasma. *Fibrinolysis*, 6, 52-54 (1992)

128 Andrews C et al. An epidemic respiratory infection due to mycoplasma pneumoniae in a civilian population. *Am Rev Resp Dis*, 95, 972 (1967)

129 Angel C, Leach BE, Martens S, Cohen M. Serum oxidation tests in schizophrenic and normal subjects. *Arch Neurol*, 78, 500-504 (1957)

130 Angeli P, Gatta A, Caregaro L et al. Hypophosphatemia and renal tubular dysfunction in alcoholics. *Gastroenterology*, 100, 502-512 (1991)

131 Angelo S, Mauro C, Rosanna BC et al. Plasma triglycerides and 24 hour urinary sodium excretion in elderly hypertensives: a pathogenetic connection? *Clin Exp Hypertens*, 15, 833-848 (1993)

132 Angeloupoulou K, Diamandis EP, Kellen J et al. Prevelance of antibodies against p53 protein in various cancers. *Clin Chem*, 39, 1192 (1993)

133 Angelsen A, Syversen U, Stridsberg M, et al. Use of neuroendocrine serum markers in the follow-up of patients with cancer of the prostate. *Prostate*, 31, 110-117 (1997)

134 Angelucci E, Brittenham GM, McLaren CE, et al. Hepatic iron concentration and total body iron stores in thalassemia major. *N Engl J Med*, 343, 327-331 (2000)

135 Anker SD, Chua TP, Ponikowski P, et al. Hormonal changes and catabolic/anabolic imbalance in chronic heart failure and their importance for cardiac cachexia. *Circulation*, 96, 526-534 (1997)

136 Anker SD, Clark AL, Kemp M, et al. Tumor necrosis factor and steroid metabolism in chronic heart failure: possible relation to muscle wasting. *J Am Coll Cardiol*, 30, 997-1001 (1997)

137 Anker SD, Egerer KR, Volk H-D, et al. Elevated soluble CD14 receptors and altered cytokines in chronic heart failure. *Am J Cardiol*, 79, 1426-1430 (1997)

138 Anker SD, Leyva F, Poole-Wilson PA, et al. Relation between serum uric acid and lower limb blood flow in patients with chronic heart failure. *Heart*, 78, 39-43 (1997)

139 Annat G et al. Maternal and fetal plasma renin and dopamine-β-hydroxylase activities in toxemic pregnancy. *Obstet Gynecol*, 52, 219-224 (1978)

140 Anneren G, Magnusson CGM, Lilja G et al. Abnormal serum IgG subclass pattern in children with Down's syndrome. *Arch Dis Child*, 67, 628-631 (1992)

141 Annesley TM, McKenna BJ. Ectopic creatine kinase MB production in metastatic cancer. *Am J Clin Pathol*, 79, 255-259 (1983)

142 Annuzzi G, Jansso E, Kaijser L et al. Increased removal rate of exogenous triglycerides after prolonged exercise in man: time course and effect of exercise duration. *Metabolism*, 36, 438-443 (1987)

143 Anonymous. 52 factors that can affect blood glucose levels. *Clin Toxicol*, 4, 297 (1971)

144 Anonymous. *Primer on the Rheumatic Diseases*. The Arthritis Foundation, 7

145 Ansari E, Talenti DA, Scopelliti JA, et al. Serum lipase and amylase ratio in acute alcoholic and nonalcoholic pancreatitis by using Dupont aca discrete clinical analyzer. *Dig Dis Sci*, 41, 1823-1827 (1996)

146 Ansari K A et al. Circulating IgE, allergy and multiple sclerosis. *Acta Neurol Scand*, 53, 39-50 (1976)

147 Anstey L et al. Leucocyte alkaline phosphatase activity in polycythemia rubra vera. *Br J Haematol*, 9, 91 (1963)

148 Antaraki A, Rangou D, Chlouverakis C. The renin-aldosterone axis in patients with diabetes insipidus. *Clin Endocrinol*, 40, 505-510 (1994)

149 Antikainen M, Holmberg C, Taskinen M-R. Short-term effects of renal transplantation on plasma lipids and lipoprotein lipase in children with congenital nephrosis. *Clin Nephrol*, 41, 284-289 (1994)

150 Anton RF, Moak DH, Crow H. Comparison of carbohydrate deficient transferrin (CDT) and γ-glutamyltransferase (GGT) as markers of heavy alcohol consumption. *Clin Chem*, 39, 1149 (1993)

151 Antoniazzi F, Radetti G, Zamboni G et al. Effects of 1,25-dihydroxyvitamin D_3 and growth hormone therapy on serum osteocalcin levels in children with growth hormone deficiency. *Bone Miner*, 21, 151-156 (1993)

152 Antoniello S, Auletta M, Magri P, Pardo F. Urinary excretion of free and acetylated polyamines in hepatocellular carcinoma. *Int J Biol Mark*, 13, 92-97 (1998)

153 Antuno PG, Ravanelli-Meyer J, Nicholson K et al. Leukocyte hexokinase activity in aging and Alzheimer's disease. *Dementia*, 6, 200-204 (1995)

154 Anwaar I, Gottsater A, Ohlsson K, et al. Increasing levels of leukocyte-derived inflammatory mediators in plasma and cAMP in platelets during follow-up after acute cerebral ischemia. *Cerebrovasc Dis*, 8, 310-317 (1998)

155 Aoki A, Hagiwara E, Atsumi Y et al. Serum type III procollagen N-terminal peptide in patients with collagen diseases. *Ryumachi*, 30, 81-84 (1990)

156 Aoki K, Dudkiewicz AB, Matsuura E et al. Clinical significance of β_2-glycoprotein I-dependent anticardiolipin antibodies in the reproductive autoimmune failure syndrome: correlation with conventional antiphospholipid antibody detection systems. *J Obstet Gynecol*, 172, 926-931 (1995)

157 Aoki N, Yamanaka T. The alpha 2 plasmin inhibitor levels in liver diseases. *Clin Chim Acta*, 84, 99-105 (1978)

158 Aoki Y, Yanagisawa Y, Ohfusa H et al. Elevation of serum CA 19-9 in parallel with HbA_{1C} in a diabetic female with the Lewis (A+B-) blood group. *Diab Res Clin Pract*, 13, 77-81 (1991)

159 Aoyagi K, Miyake Y, Urakami K et al. Enzyme immunoassay of immunoreactive progastrin-releasing peptide(31-98) as tumor marker for small-cell lung carcinoma: development and evaluation. *Clin Chem*, 41, 537-543 (1995)

160 Aoyagi T, Wada T, Kojima F et al. Enzymatic changes in cerebrospinal fluid of patients with Alzheimer-type dementia. *J Clin Biochem Nutr*, 14, 133-139 (1993)

161 Apel RL, Fernandes BJ. Malignant lymphoma presenting with an elevated serum CA-125 level. *Arch Pathol Lab Med*, 119, 373-376 (1995)

162 Apenberg S, Andrassy K, Worner I, et al. Antibodies to neutrophil elastase: a study in patients with vasculitis. *Am J Kid Dis*, 28, 178-185 (1996)

163 Appleyard JG, Stanley DA. The evaluation of the vitamin B_6 status in children with convulsions. *Med Lab Technol*, 29, 160 (1972)

164 Araga S, Kishimoto M, Adachi A et al. The $CD5^+$ B cells and myasthenia gravis. *Autoimmunity*, 20, 129-134 (1995)

165 Araki A, Sako Y, Ito H. Plasma homocysteine concentrations in methylcobalamin treatment. *Atherosclerosis*, 103, 149-157 (1993)

166 Aramendi M, Bonilla I, Orellana MA et al. Urine excretion of myoglobin: a new marker of incipient nephropathy? *Clin Biochem Rev*, 14, 205 (1993)

167 Arbault P, Grimaux M, Pradet V et al. Assessment of urinary pyridinoline excretion with a specific enzyme-linked immunosorbent assay in normal adults and in metabolic bone diseases. *Bone*, 16, 461-467 (1995)

168 Arcasoy A, Cavdar AO. Changes of trace minerals (serum iron, zinc, copper and magnesium) in thalassemia. *Acta Haematol*, 53, 341-346 (1975)

169 Ardiles LG, Olavarria F, Elgueta M, et al. Anticardiolipin antibodies in classic pediatric hemolytic-uremic syndrome: a possible pathogenic role. *Nephron*, 78, 278-283 (1998)

170 Ardizzoni A, Bonavia M, Viale M et al. Biologic and clinical effects of continuous infusion of interleukin-2 in patients with non-small cell lung cancer. *Cancer*, 73, 1353-1360 (1994)

171 Arends T et al. Serum proteins in Hodgkin's disease and malignant lymphoma. *Am J Med*, 16, 833 (1954)

172 Arendt J, Bhanji S, Franey C et al. Plasma melatonin levels in anorexia nervosa. *Br J Psychiat*, 161, 361-364 (1992)

173 Argiris A, Mathur-Wagh U, Wilets I, et al. Abnormalities of serum amylase in HIV-positive patients. *Am J Gastroenterol*, 94, 1248-1252 (1999)

174 Arias F et al. Hepatic fibrinogen deposits in pre-eclampsia. immunofluorescent evidence. *N Engl J Med*, 295, 578-582 (1976)

175 Arici A, Tazuke SI, Oral E, et al. Monocyte chemotactic protein-1 concentration in peritoneal fluid of women with endometriosis and its modulation of expression in mesothelial cells. *Fertil Steril*, 67, 1065-1072 (1997)

176 Aringer M, Wintersberger W, Steiner CW et al. High levels of bcl-2 protein in circulating lymphocytes, but not B lymphocytes, of patients with systemic lupus erythematosus. *Clin Exp Rheumatol*, 10, 1423-1430 (1994)

177 Armata J et al. Thrombocytosis in acute leukemia. *Pol Med Sci Hist Bull*, 14, 55 (1971)

178 Arnadottir M, Hultberg B, Wahlberg J, et al. serum total homocysteine concentration before and after renal transplantation. *Kid Int*, 54, 1380-1384 (1998)

179 Arnalich F, Benito-Urbina S, Gonzalez-Gancedo P et al. Inadequate production of progesterone in women with systemic lupus erythematosus. *Br J Rheumatol*, 31, 247-251 (1992)

180 Arnalich F, Zamorano AF, Benito-Urbina S et al. Increased apotranscobalamin II levels in rheumatoid arthritis. *Br J Rheumatol*, 29, 171-173 (1990)

181 Arnaud J, Faure H, Bourland P et al. Longitudinal changes in serum zinc concentration and distribution after acute myocardial infarction. *Clin Chim Acta*, 230, 147-156 (1994)

182 Aronow WS, Ahn C. Association between plasma homocysteine and coronary artery disease in older persons. *Am J Cardiol*, 80, 1216-1218 (1997)

183 Aronow WS, Ahn C, Schoenfeld MR. Association between plasma homocysteine and extracranial carotid arterial disease in older persons, 1432-1433 (1997)

184 Aronson SM et al. Cerebrospinal fluid enzymes in central nervous system lipidosis. *Proc Soc Exp Biol Med*, 111, 664 (1962)

185 Aronson SM et al. Progression of amaurotic family idiocy as reflected by serum and cerebrospinal fluid changes. *Am J Med*, 24, 390 (1958)

186 Aronsson B, Blomback M, Eriksson S et al. Low levels of coagulation inhibitors in patients with Clostridium difficile infection. *Infection*, 20, 58-60 (1992)

187 Aroor AR, Venkatesh A, Pattabiraman TN. Antitryptic and antichymotryptic activities in cerebrospinal fluid in health and disease. *Ind J Med Res*, 70, 268-274 (1979)

188 Arruda VR, Saad STO, Costa FF. Hairy-cell leukemia and glucose-6-phosphate dehydrogenase (1994)

189 Artiss JD, Yang W-C, Harake B, et al. Application of a sensitive and specific reagent for the determination of serum iron to the Bayer DAX48. *Am J Clin Path*, 108, 269-274 (1997)

190 Arumugam K. Serum prolactin levels in infertile patients with endometriosis. *Malay J Pathol*, 13, 43-45 (1991)

191 Arumugam R, LeBlanc A, Seilheimer DK, et al. Serum leptin and IGF-I levels in cystic fibrosis. *Endocrine Res*, 24, 247-257 (1998)

192 Arvanitakes C et al. Diagnostic tests of exocrine pancreatic function and disease. *Gastroenterology*, 74, 932-948 (1978)

193 Asakura H, Jokaji H, Saito M et al. Plasma levels of soluble thrombomodulin increase in cases of disseminated intravascular coagulation with organ failure. *Am J Hematol*, 38, 281-287 (1991)

194 Asano M, Adachi J, Ueno Y. Cholesterol-derived hydroperoxides in alcoholic liver disease. *Lipids*, 34, 557-561 (1999)

195 Asanuma Y, Kawai S, Aoshima H, et al. Serum lipoprotein(a) and apolipoprotein(a) phenotypes in patients with rheumatoid arthritis. *Arth Rheum*, 42, 443-447 (1999)

196 Ascger H, Hahn-Zoric M, Hanson LA, et al. Value of serologic markers for clinical diagnosis and population studies of coeliac disease. *Scand J Gastroenterol*, 31, 61-67 (1996)

197 Ashby CR Jr, Carr LA, Cook CL et al. Alteration of platelet serotonergic mechanisms and monoamine oxidase activity in premenstrual syndrome. *Biol Psychiat*, 24, 225-233 (1988)

198 Askenazy F, Candito M, Caci H, et al. Whole blood serotonin content, tryptophan concentrations, and impulsivity in anorexia nervosa. *Biol Psychiat*, 43, 188-195 (1998)

199 Aso Y, Inukai T, Takemura Y. Mechanisms of elevation of serum and urinary concentrations of soluble thrombomodulin in diabetic patients: possible application as a marker for vascular endothelial injury. *Metabolism*, 47, 362-365 (1998)

200 Asseo PP, Panidis DK. Creatine kinase activity and isoenzyme analysis in thyroid disorders. *Clin Chem*, 30, 1107-1108 (1984)

201 Assicot M, Carsin H, Guilbaud J et al. Calcitonin precursors as new markers of sepsis. *Ann Clin Biol*, 50, 441 (1992)

202 Assicot M, Garin D, Flechaire A et al. Dramatic increase in circulating procalcitonin in acute malaria. *Clin Biochem Rev*, 14, 208 (1993)

203 Assicot M, Gendrel D, Carsin H et al. High serum procalcitonin concentrations in patients with sepsis and infection. *Lancet*, 341, 515-518 (1993)

204 Aster RH. Pooling of platelets in the spleen: role in the pathogenesis of thrombocytopenia. *J Clin Invest*, 45, 645 (1966)

205 Astles R, Petros WP, Peters WP et al. Artifactual hypoglycemia with hematopoietic cytokines. *Clin Chem*, 41, S202 (1995)

206 Astra USA, Inc. Manufacturer's literature on Levothyroxine. Westborough, MA 01581 (1995)

207 Atanssov N et al. Disc electrophoresis of prostatic fluid relative mobility and molecular weight of some enzymes and proteins. *Clin Chim Acta*, 36, 213-221 (1972)

208 Ates E, Bakkaloglu A, Saatci U et al. von Willebrand factor antigen compared with other factors in vasculitic syndromes. *Arch Dis Child*, 70, 40-43 (1994)

209 Atici A, Satar M, Cetiner S, Yaman A. Serum necrosis factor-α in neonatal sepsis. *Am J Perinatol*, 14, 401-404 (1997)

210 Attal-Khemis S, Dalmeyda V, Michot J-L, et al. Increased total 7α-hydroxy-dehydroepiandrosterone in serum of patients with Alzheimer's disease. *J Gerontol Biol Sci*, 53A, B125-B132 (1998)

211 Attman P-O, Alaupovic P, Gustafson A. Serum apolipoprotein profile of patients with chronic renal failure. *Kidney Int*, 32, 368-375 (1987)

212 Atzori L, Cannas E, Dettori T, et al. Plasma nitrite/nitrate and total thiols as markers of nitric oxide production and oxidative stress in patients with chronic obstructive pulmonary disease and chronic respiratory insufficiency. *Med Sci Res*, 26, 375-376 (1998)

213 Auersvald LA, Perez RV, Lorber MI, et al. Serum sialic acid, a risk factor for cardiovascular disease, improves following pancreas transplantation. *Transplant Proc*, 27 (1995)

214 Aukrust P, Muller F, Froland SS. Elevated serum levels of interleukin-4 and interleukin-6 in patients with common variable immunodeficiency (CVI) are associated with chronic immune activation and low numbers of CD4+ lymphocytes. *Clin Immunol Immunopathol*, 70, 217-224 (1994)

215 Aull S, Lalouschek W, Schneider P, et al. Dynamic changes of plasma lipids and lipoproteins in patients after transient ischemic attack or minor stroke. *Am J Med*, 101, 291-298 (1996)

216 Aultman D, Adamashvili I, Yaturu K, et al. Soluble HLA in human body fluids. *Hum Immunol*, 60, 239-244 (1999)

217 Aurell A, Rosengren LE, Karlsson B et al. Determination of S-100 and glial fibrillary acidic protein concentrations in cerebrospinal fluid after brain infarction. *Stroke*, 22, 1254-1258 (1991)

218 Austin RF, Desforges JE. Hereditary elliptocytosis: an unusual presentation of hemolysis in the newborn associated with transient morphological abnormalities. *Pediatrics*, 44, 196 (1969)

219 Auvinen. Evaluation of serum enzyme tests in the diagnosis of acute myocardial infarction. *Acta Med Scand*, Suppl 539, 7-70 (1972)

220 Auwardt R, Savige J, Wilson D. A comparison of the clinical and laboratory features of thin basement membrane disease (TBMD) and IgA glomerulonephritis (IgA GN). *Clin Nephrol*, 52, 1-4 (1999)

221 Awais G M. Serum lactic dehydrogenase levels in the diagnosis and treatment of carcinoma of the ovary. *Am J Obstet Gynecol*, 116, 1053-1057 (1973)

222 Aydin A, Sayal A, Isimer A. Plasma glutathione peroxidase activity and selenium levels of newborns with jaundice. *Biol Trace Elem Res*, 58, 85-90 (1997)

223 Aydiner A, Topuz E, Disci R et al. Serum tumor markers for detection of bone metastasis in breast cancer patients. *Acta Oncol*, 33, 181-186 (1994)

224 Ayesh R, Mitchell SC, Zhang A et al. The fish odour syndrome: biochemical, familial, and clinical aspects. *Br Med J*, 307, 655-657 (1993)

225 Ayvazain JH, Ayvazain LF. Changes in serum and urinary uric acid with the development of symptomatic gout. *J Clin Invest*, 42, 1835 (1963)

226 Azar HA et al. Malignant lymphoma and lymphatic leukemia associated with myeloma-type serum proteins. *Am J Med*, 23, 239 (1957)

227 Azar N, Valla D, Abdel-Samad I, et al. Liver dysfunction in allogeneic bone marrow transplantation recipients: influence of pre- and posttransplantation hepatic lesions. *Transplantation*, 62, 56-61 (1996)

228 Aziz DC, Rittenhouse HJ, Ranken R. Use and interpretation of tests in oncology. *Specialty Laboratories, Santa Monica CA,* (1991)

229 Azizi C, Maistre G, Kalotka H, et al. Plasma levels and molecular forms of proatrial natriuretic peptides in healthy subjects and in patients with congestive heart failure. *J Endocrinol*, 148, 51-57 (1996)

230 Azrolan N, Brown CD, Thomas L et al. Cyclosporin A has divergent effects on plasma LDL cholesterol (LDL-C) and lipoprotein (a) [Lp(a)] levels in renal transplant recipients. *Arterioscler Thromb*, 14, 1393-1398 (1994)

231 Baast RC Jr, Siegal FP, Runowicz C et al. Elevation of serum CA 125 prior to diagnosis of an epithelial ovarian carcinoma. *Gynecol Oncol*, 22, 115-120 (1985)

232 Baba T, Kodama T, Ishizaki T. Effect of chronic treatment with enalapril on glucose tolerance and serum insulin in non-insulin-resistant Japanese patients with essential hypertension. *Eur J Clin Pharmacol*, 45, 23-27 (1993)

233 Babb RR. Ascites: differential diagnosis and treatment. *Hosp Med*, April, 129-155 (1988)

234 Babel CS et al. Serum and cerebrospinal fluid magnesium in epilepsy. *J Ass Physicians India*, 21, 481-487 (1973)

235 Babu CS, Kannan KB, Bharadwaj VP et al. Lymphocyte arginase activity in leprosy - a preliminary report. *Ind J Med Res*, 91, 193-196 (1990)

236 Baccala AA, Zhong H, Clift SM, et al. Serum vascular endothelial growth factor is a candidate biomarker of metastatic tumor response to ex vivo gene therapy of renal cell cancer. *Urology*, 51, 327-332 (1998)

237 Bacchus H. *Essentials of Metabolic Diseases and Endocrinology*. Baltimore MD, University Park Press (1976)

238 Bacci E, Cianchetti S, Ruocco L, et al. Comparison between eosinophilic markers in induced sputum and blood in asthmatic patients. *Clin Exp Allergy*, 28, 1237-1243 (1999)

239 Bach C et al. L'absences congenitale de B-lipoproteines: une nouvelle observation. *Arch Fr Pediat*, 24, 1093 (1967)

240 Bach F, Bach FW, Pedersen AG et al. Creatine kinase-BB in the cerebrospinal fluid as a marker of CNS metastases and leptomeningeal carcinomatosis in patients with breast cancer. *Eur J Cancer Clin Oncol*, 25, 1703-1709 (1989)

241 Backstrom T. Epileptic seizures in women related to plasma estrogen and progesterone during the menstrual cycle. *Acta Neurol Scand*, 54, 321-347 (1976)

242 Badawy SZA, Cuenca V, Freliech H et al. Endometrial antibodies in serum and peritoneal fluid of infertile patients with and without endometriosis. *Fertil Steril*, 53, 930-932 (1990)

243 Badcock NR, Szep DA, Zoanetti GD et al. Fecal coproporphyrin isomers in sporadic and familial porphyria cutanea tarda. *Clin Chem*, 41, 1315-1317 (1995)

244 Badonnel Y, Barbe F, Legagneur H et al. Inhbin as a marker for hydatidiform mole: a comparative study with the determinations of intact human chorionic gonadotropin and its free β-subunit. *Clin Endocrinol*, 41, 155-162 (1994)

245 Bagdade JD. Disorders of carbohydrate and lipid metabolism in uremia. *Nephron*, 14, 153 (1975)

246 Bagni B, Cavallini AR, Indelli M, Malacarne P. Evaluation of CA 549 in malignant neoplasms of the human breast. *J Nuc Med Allied Sci*, 34, 13-16 (1990)

247 Bailey RE, Bartos D, Bartos F, Castro A. Activation of aldosterone and renin secretion by thermal stress. *Experientia*, 28, 159 (1972)

248 Baillie EE. CK isoenzymes: Part I clinical aspects. *Lab Med*, 10, 269 (1979)

249 Bailly D, Vignau J, Racadot N et al. Platelet serotonin levels in alcoholic patients: changes related to physiological and pathological factors, 57-68 (1993)

250 Baines M. Detection and incidence of B and C vitamin deficiency in alcohol-related illness. *Ann Clin Biochem*, 15, 307-312 (1978)

251 Baines M, Lee M, Higgins G. Age and disease related changes in erythrocyte superoxide dismutase activity from control and diabetic populations. *Proc ACB Natl Meet*, 50 (1995)

252 Baines TJ, Clark A. Cytidine deaminase -- a marker for pre-eclampsia? *Ann Clin Biochem*, 22, 420-422 (1985)

253 Baker H, Deangelis B, Baker ER, et al. A practical assay of lipoate in biologic fluids and liver in health and disease. *Free Radic Biol Med*, 25, 473-479 (1998)

254 Bakiri F, Benmiloud M, Vallotton MB. The renin-angiotensin system in panhypopituitarism: dynamic studies and therapeutic effects in Sheehan's syndrome. *J Clin Endocrinol Metab*, 56, 1042-1047 (1983)

255 Bakker J, Gris P, Coffernils M, et al. Serial blood lactate levels can predict the development of multiple organ failure following septic shock. *Am J Surg*, 171, 221-226 (1996)

256 Balasch J, Jimenez W, Arroyo V et al. Immunoreactive endothelin plasma levels in severe ovarian hyperstimulation syndrome. *Fertil Steril*, 64, 65-68 (1995)

257 Balblanc JC, Hartmann D, Noyer D et al. Serum hyaluronic acid in osteoarthritise du rhumatisme. *Rev Rhum Ed Fr*, 60, 194-202 (1993)

258 Balcerzak SP et al. Effect of iron deficiency and red cell age on human erythrocyte catalase activity. *J Lab Clin Med*, 67, 742 (1966)

259 Balcke P. Oxalic acid in chronic renal insufficiency. *Wien Klin Wschr*, 97, 1-15 (1985)

260 Baldini M, pappalettera M, Lecchi L, et al. Human lymphocyte antigens in Graves' disease: correlation with persistent course of disease. *Am J Med Sci*, 309, 43-48 (1995)

261 Balfe JW, Cole C, Welt LG. Red cell transport in patients with cystic fibrosis and in their parents. *Science*, 162, 689 (1968)

262 Balion CM, Caines PS, Draisey TF et al. Carbamylated proteins as indices of chronic renal failure. *Clin Chem*, 39, 1136 (1993)

263 Balion CM, Mantha CV, Laxdal VA et al. Serum carnosine activity in disease states. *Clin Chem*, 37, 916 (1991)

264 Balis ME, Dalser JS, Brown GB. Amino acid levels in malignancy. *Cancer Chemother Rep*, 16, 487-489 (1962)

265 Balks HJ, Conlon JM, Creutzfeldt W et al. Circulating bradykinin-like immunoreactivity and the pentagastrin-induced carcinoid flush. *Clin Endocrinol*, 29, 141-151 (1988)

266 Ball GV, Schrohenloher R, Hester R. γ globulin complexes in rheumatoid pericardial fluid. *Am J Med*, 58, 123 (1975)

267 Ball GV, Sorensen LB. Pathogenesis of hyperuricemia in saturnine gout. *N Engl J Med*, 280, 1199 (1969)

268 Ball SG. The chemical pathology of AIDS. *Ann Clin Biochem*, 31, 401-409 (1994)

269 Ballantyne CM, Radovancevic B, Farmer JA et al. Hyperlipidemia after heart transplantation: report of a 6-year experience. with treatment recommendations. *J Am Coll Cardiol*, 19, 1315-1321 (1992)

270 Ballantyne D et al. Relationship of plasma uric acid to plasma lipids and lipoproteins in subjects with peripheral vascular disease. *Clin Chim Acta*, 70, 323-328 (1976)

271 Ballard HS, Marcus AJ. Hypercalcemia in chronic myelogenous leukemia. *N Engl J Med*, 282, 663 (1970)

272 Balleari E, Bason C, Visani G, et al. Serum levels of granulocyte-macrophage colony-stimulating factor and granulocyte colony stimulating factor in treated patients with chronic myelogenous leukemia in chronic phase. *Haematologica*, 79, 7-12 (1994)

273 Ballmaier M, Schulze H, Strauss G, et al. Thrombopoietin in patients with congenital thrombocytopenia and absent radii: elevated serum levels, normal receptor expression, but defective reactivity to thrombopoietin. *Blood*, 90, 612-619 (1997)

274 Bando Y, Ushiogi Y, Toya D, et al. Antibodies to glutamic acid decarboxylase (GAD) in non-obese Japanese diabetics without insulin therapy: a comparison of two commercial RIA kits based on recombinant and pig brain GAD. *Diabetes Res Clin Pract*, 41, 25-33 (1998)

275 Bang B, Asmussen K, Sorensen GH, Oxholm P. Reduced 25-hydroxyvitamin D levels in primary Sjogren's syndrome. *Scand J Rheumatol*, 28, 180-183 (1999)

276 Bang LE, Holm J, Svendsen TL. Retinol-binding protein and transferrin in urine: new markers of renal function in essential hypertension and white coat hypertension? *Am J Hypertens*, 9, 1024-1028 (1996)

277 Bangert SK, O"Connor J. Lp(a) and hypothyroidism. *Proc ACB Natl Meet*, 114 (1992)

278 Bank S et al. Sweat electrolytes in chronic pancreatitis. *Am J Dig Dis*, 23, 178-181 (1978)

279 Banki CM, Karmasci L, Bissette G. Cerebrospinal fluid neuropeptides in dementia. *Biol Psychiat*, 32, 452-456 (1992)

280 Bansal AS, Bruce J, Wilson PB, Anyiwo CE. Serum sCD23 in patients with lepromatous and tuberculoid leprosy. *Scand J Infect Dis*, 30, 133-135 (1998)

281 Bansal BC et al. Serum lipids, platelets, and fibrinolytic activity in cerebrovascular disease. *Stroke*, 9, 137-139 (1978)

282 Bansil S, Troiano R, Cook SD et al. Serum soluble interleukin-2 receptor levels in chronic, progressive, stable and steroid-treated multiple sclerosis. *Acta Neurol Scand*, 84, 282-285 (1991)

283 Banu N, Hara H, Okamura M et al. Urinary excretion of type IV collagen and laminin in the evaluation of nephropathy in NIDDM: comparison with urinary albumin and markers of tubular dysfunction and/or damage. *Diabetes Res Clin Pract*, 29, 57-67 (1995)

284 Bar J, Maymon R, Hod M, et al. Low serum placental isoferritin in pregnant women at risk of developing preeclampsia. *Hypertens Pregnancy*, 17, 315-321 (1998)

285 Barabas J, Nagy E, Degrell I. Ascorbic acid in cerebrospinal fluid - a possible protection against free radicals in the brain. *Arch Gerontol Geriat*, 21, 43-48 (1995)

286 Barak M, Doweck I, Greenberg E et al. CYFRA 21-1: a new potential tumor marker for squamous cell carcinoma of head and neck. *Clin Biochem Rev*, 14, 262 (1993)

287 Baranowska B, Wasilewska-Dziubinska E, Radzikowska M, et al. Neuropeptide Y, galanin, and leptin release in obese women and in women with anorexia nervosa. *Metabolism*, 46, 1384-1389 (1997)

288 Barbaro G, Di Lorenzo G, Ribersani M, et al. Serum ferritin and hepatic glutathione concentrations in chronic hepatitis C patients related to the hepatitis C virus genotype. *J Hepatol*, 30, 774-782 (1999)

289 Barbe P, Bennet A, Stebenet M et al. Sex-hormone-binding globulin and protein-energy malnutrition indexes as indicators of nutritional status in women with anorexia nervosa. *Am J Clin Nutr*, 57, 319-322 (1993)

290 Barbera GJ et al. Stool trypsin and chymotrypsin in the diagnosis of pancreatic insufficiency in cystic fibrosis. *Am J Dis Child*, 112, 536-540 (1966)

291 Barbieri RL, Niloff JM, Bast RC et al. Elevated serum concentrations of CA125 in patients with advanced endometriosis. *Fertil Steril*, 45, 630-634 (1986)

292 Barbosa J et al. Plasma insulin in patients with myotonic dystrophy and their relatives. *Medicine*, 53, 307-323 (1974)

293 Bardella MT, Fraquelli M, Quatrini M, et al. Prevalence of hypertransaminasemia in adult celiac patients and effect of gluten-free diet. *Hepatology*, 22, 833-836 (1995)

294 Barillari P, Bolognese A, Chirletti P et al. Role of CEA, TPA, and CA 19-9 in the early detection of localized and diffuse recurrent rectal cancer. *Dis Colon Rectum*, 35, 471-476 (1992)

295 Barlow KA. Hyperlipidemia in primary gout. *Metabolism*, 17, 289 (1968)

296 Barnton DF, Finch CH. The diagnosis of iron deficiency anemia. *Am J Med*, 37, 62 (1964)

297 Baron JH. An assessment of the augmented histamine test in the diagnosis of peptic ulcer. *Gut*, 4, 243-253 (1963)

298 Barrett-Connor E et al. An epidemic of trichinosis following ingestion of wild pig in Hawaii. *J Infect Dis*, 133, 473 (1976)

299 Barros F et al. Etudes sur la paramyloidose Portugaise a forme polyneuritique III alterations des proteines plasmatiques. *Acta Neuropathol*, 2, Suppl, 101-110 (1963)

300 Barrow EM et al. A study of the carrier state for plasma thromboplastin component (PTC, Christmas factor) deficiency, utilizing a new assay procedure. *J Lab Clin Med*, 55, 936 (1960)

301 Barry M, Russi M, Armstrong L et al. Treatment of a laboratory-acquired Sabia virus infection. *N Engl J Med*, 333, 294-296 (1995)

302 Barry-Kinsella C, Sharma SC, Cottrell E et al. Mid to late luteal phase steroids in minimal stage endometriosis and unexplained infertility. *Eur J Obstet Gynecol Reprod Biol*, 54, 113-118 (1994)

303 Bartalena L, Grasso L, Brogioni S et al. Serum interleukin-6 in amiodarone-induced thyrotoxicosis. *J Clin Endocrinol Metab*, 78, 423-427 (1994)

304 Bartalena L, Marcocci C, Bogazzi F, et al. Relation between therapy for hyperthyroidism and the course of Graves' ophthalmology. *N Engl J Med*, 338, 73-78 (1998)

305 Bartelloni RT et al. Changes in individual plasma amino acid metabolism in the regulation of gluconeogenesis. *Metabolism*, 21, 67 (1972)

306 Bartfeld H. Rheumatoid factors and their biological significance. Introduction. *Ann NY Acad Sci*, 168, 30 (1969)

307 Barth WF et al. Primary amyloidosis. *Ann Intern Med*, 69, 787-805 (1968)

308 Barth WF et al. Primary amyloidosis. Clinical, immunochemical and immunoglobulin metabolism studies in fifteen patients. *Am J Med*, 47, 259-273 (1969)

309 Bartlett WA, Payne MN, Said BT et al. Serum angiotensin-converting enzyme activity in coronary heart disease: a marker for premature disease. *Proc ACB Natl Meet*, 40 (1994)

310 Bartolin R, Bouvenot G, Delboy C, Joubert M. Cadmium, zinc, pseudo-cholinesterase and aldolase blood levels in hypertensive and alcoholic patients. preliminary statistical computerized study on 124 cases. *Sem Hop Paris*, 56, 1718-1719 (1980)

311 Barton DPJ, Blanchard DK, Michelini-Norris B et al. Serum soluble interleukin-2 receptor-α levels in patients with gynecologic cancers: early effect of surgery. *Am J Reprod Immunol*, 30, 202-206 (1993)

312 Barton JC, Patton MA, Edwards CQ et al. Blood lead concentrations in hereditary hemochromatosis. *J Lab Clin Med*, 124, 193-198 (1994)

313 Baruch Y, Amit T, Hertz P et al. Decreased serum growth hormone-binding protein in patients with liver cirrhosis. *J Clin Endocrinol Metab*, 73, 777-780 (1991)

314 Baruch Y, Brook JG, Eidelman S, Aviram M. Increased concentration of high density lipoprotein in plasma and decreased platelet aggregation in primary biliary cirrhosis. *Arteriosclerosis*, 53, 151-162 (1984)

315 Barzel US et al. Renal ammonium excretion and urinary pH in idiopathic uric acid lithiasis. *J Urol*, 91, 1 (1964)

316 Bascoul J, Goze C, Domergue N et al. Serum level of 7α-hydroxycholesterol in hypercholesterolemic patients treated with cholestyramine. *Biochim Biophys Acta Lipids Lipid Metab*, 1044, 357-360 (1990)

317 Bases. Elevation of serum acid phosphatase in certain myeloproliferative diseases. *N Engl J Med*, 266, 538-540 (1962)

318 Bashar H, Urano T, Fukuta K et al. Plasminogen activators and plasminogen activator inhibitor 1 in urinary tract cancer. *Urol Int*, 52, 4-8 (1994)

319 Bassen F A, Kornzwieg A L. Malformation of the erythrocyte in a case of atypical retinitis pigmentosa. *Blood*, 5, 381 (1950)

320 Bastard J-P, Bruckert E, Robert J-J et al. Are free fatty acids related to plasma plasminogen activator inhibitor 1 in android obesity? *Int J Obesity*, 18, 836-838 (1995)

321 Basu PS, Batabyal SK, Bhattacharya A et al. Cholinesterase activities in cerebrospinal fluid of patients with idiopathic convulsive disorders. *Clin Chim Acta*, 235, 107-112 (1995)

322 Basun H, Fratiglioni L, Winblad B. Cobalamin levels are not reduced in Alzheimer's disease. *J Am Geriatr Soc*, 42, 132-136 (1994)

323 Bates AS, Evans AL, Jones P, Clayton RN. Assessment of GH status in adults with GH deficiency using serum growth hormone, serum insulin-like growth factor -I and urinary growth hormone excretion. *Clin Endocrinol*, 42, 425-430 (1995)

324 Bates DW, Buchwald D, Lee J et al. Clinical laboratory test findings in patients with chronic fatigue syndrome. *Arch Intern Med*, 155, 97-103 (1995)

325 Bates HM. The laboratory in prevention: HDL cholesterol and coronary heart disease. *Lab Manage*, 18, 17-22 (1980)

326 Batin P, Wickens M, McEntergart D, et al. The importance of abnormalities of liver function tests in predicting mortality in chronic heart failure. *Eur Heart J*, 16, 1613-1618 (1995)

327 Battisti C, Formichi P, Federico A. Vitamin E serum levels are normal in ataxia telangectasia (Louis-Bar disease). *J Neurol Sci*, 141, 114-116 (1996)

328 Battistini B, D'Orleans-Juste P, Sirois P. Endothelins: circulating plasma levels and presence in other biologic fluids. *Lab Invest*, 68, 600-628 (1993)

329 Baudin E, Gigliotti A, Ducrieux M, et al. Neuron-specific enolase and chromogranin A as markers of neuroendocrine tumours. *Br J Cancer*, 78, 1102-1107 (1998)

330 Bauduceau B, Reboul P, Le Guyadec T et al. Profil hormonal des gynecomasties idiopathiques de l'adulte jeune. *Ann Endocrinol*, 54, 163-167 (1993)

331 Bauer J, Landgraf S, Schrell U et al. Rise in serum prolactin concentration, a possibly helpful test in the differential diagnosis of frontal lobe epilepsy. *Dtsch Med Wschr*, 116, 1824-1827 (1991)

332 Bauer JD, Ackermann PG, Toro G. *Bray's Clinical Laboratory Methods.* 7th edition. St Louis, MO, CV Mosby (1968)

333 Baum H, Braun S, Gerhardt W, et al. Multicenter evaluation of a second-generation assay for cardiac troponin T. *Clin Chem*, 43, 1877-1884 (1997)

334 Baum H, et al. Cardiac troponin T in patients with high creatinine concentration but normal creatine kinase activity in serum. *Clin Chem*, 42, 474-475 (1996)

335 Baum J. Juvenile arthritis. *Am J Dis Child*, 135, 557-560 (1981)

336 Baumgartner A, Graf K-J, Kurten I. Prolactin in patients with major depressive disorder and in healthy subjects. I. Cross-sectional study of basal and post-TRH and post-dexamethasone prolactin levels. *Biol Psychiat*, 24, 249-267 (1988)

337 Bayati N, Silverman AL, Gordon SC. Serum α-fetoprotein levels and liver histology in patients with chronic hepatitis C. *Am J Gastroenterol*, 93, 2452-2456 (1998)

338 Bayer AS, et al. Candida meningitis. *Medicine*, 55, 477-486 (1976)

339 Bayer Corporation, Business Group Diagnostics. Manufacturer's literature on Technicon Immuno 1® System Carcinoembryonic antigen. Tarrytown, NY 10591, November (1996)

340 Bayer Corporation, Business Group Diagnostics. Manufacturer's literature on Technicon Immuno 1® System Phenytoin. Tarrytown, NY 10591, September (1995)

341 Bayer Corporation, Business Group Diagnostics. Manufacturer's literature on Technicon Immuno 1® System Progesterone. Tarrytown, NY 10591, April (1996)

342 Bayer Corporation, Business Group Diagnostics. Manufacturer's literature on Technicon Immuno 1® System Prostate Specific Antigen. Tarrytown, NY 10591, November (1996)

343 Bayer EM, Herr W, Kanzler S, et al. Transforming growth factor-β_1 in autoimmune hepatitis: correlation of liver tissue expression and serum levels with disease activity. *J Hepatol*, 28, 803-811 (1998)

344 Bayerdorffer E, Mannes GA, Ochsenkuhn T et al. Variation of serum bile acids in patients with colorectal adenomas during a one-year follow-up. *Digestion*, 55, 121-129 (1994)

345 Bayliss CE et al. Laboratory diagnosis of rheumatoid arthritis. prospective study of 85 patients. *Ann Rheum Dis*, 34, 395-402 (1975)

346 Baysal A, Johnson BA, Linkswiler H. Vitamin B_6 depletion in man: blood vitamin B_6, plasma pyridoxal-phosphate, serum cholesterol, serum transaminase. *J Nutr*, 89, 19 (1966)

347 Bazzano. Effects of folic acid metabolism on serum cholesterol levels. *Arch Intern Med*, 124, 710-713 (1969)

348 Beamer NB, Coull BM, Clark WM et al. Interleukin-6 and interleukin-1 receptor antagonist in acute stroke. *Ann Neurol*, 37, 800-804 (1995)

349 Beamish MR et al. Transferrin iron, chelatable iron and ferritin in idiopathic hemochromatosis. *Br J Haematol*, 27, 219 (1974)

350 Beard MF et al. Serum concentrations of vitamin B_{12} in acute leukemia. *Ann Intern Med*, 41, 323 (1954)

351 Bearn AG et al. Renal function in Wilson's disease. *J Clin Invest*, 36, 1107 (1957)

352 Beaudry P, Hadengue A, Callebert J et al. Blood and plasma 5-hydroxytryptamine levels in patients with cirrhosis. *Hepatology*, 20, 800-803 (1994)

353 Bech K, Damsbo P, Eldrup E, et al. β-Cell function and glucose and lipid oxidation in Graves' disease. *Clin Endocrinol*, 44, 59-66 (1996)

354 Beck et al. Biochemical studies on leucocytes II. phosphatase activity in chronic lymphatic leucemia, acute leucemia and miscellaneous hematologic conditions. *J Lab Clin Med*, 38, 245-253 (1951)

355 Becker DJ. The endocrine responses to protein calorie malnutrition. *Ann Rev Nutr*, 3, 187-212 (1983)

356 Becker DM, Kramer S. The neurological manifestations of porphyria: a review. *Medicine*, 56, 411-423 (1977)

357 Becker KL et al. Calcitonin heterogeneity in lung cancer and medullary thyroid cancer. *Acta Endocrinol*, 89, 89-99 (1978)

358 Becker RC, Cannon CP, Bovill EG, et al. Prognostic value of plasma fibrinogen concentrations in patients with unstable angina and non-Q-wave myocardial infarction (TIM1 IIIB trial). *Am J Cardiol*, 78, 142-147 (1996)

359 Becker SA, McClave SA. Lipid profiles in Crohn's disease patients with and without ileal resection. *Am J Gastroenterol*, 91, 2452 (1996)

360 Becker U, Gluud C, Farholt S et al. Menopausal age and sex hormones in postmenopausal women with alcoholic and non-alcoholic liver disease. *J Hepatol*, 13, 25-32 (1991)

361 Beckett GJ, Kellett HA, Gow SM et al. Raised plasma glutathione-S-transferase values in hyperthyroidism and in hypothyroid patients receiving thyroxine replacement: evidence for hepatic damage. *Br Med J*, 291, 427-431 (1985)

362 Beckman G et al. Acid phosphatase activity in the synovial fluid of patients with rheumatoid arthritis and other joint disorders. *Acta Rheum Scand*, 17, 47-56 (1971)

363 Beckmann H, Saavedra JM, Gattaz WF. Low angiotensin-converting enzyme activity (kininase II) in cerebrospinal fluid of schizophrenics. *Biol Psychiat*, 19, 679-684 (1984)

364 Bede HK et al. Fibrinogen content and fibrinolytic activity of blood in diabetics, before and after antidiabetic drugs. *J Ass Physicians India*, 25, 181-185 (1977)

365 Beeken WL. Serum tryptophan in Crohn's disease. *Scand J Gastroenterol*, 11, 735-740 (1976)

366 Beer JH, Clerici N, Baillod P et al. Quantitative and qualitative analysis of platelet GPIb and von Willebrand factor in liver cirrhosis. *Thromb Haemostas*, 73, 601-609 (1995)

367 Beeson-McDermott. *Textbook of Medicine*. 14th edition. Philadelphia PA, WB Saunders (1975)

368 Beevers DG, Cruickshank JK, Yeoman WB et al. Blood-lead and cadmium in human hypertension. *J Environ Pathol Toxicol Oncol*, 4, 251-60 (1980)

369 Beisel WR. Trace elements in infectious processes. *Med Clin North Am*, 60, 831 (1976)

370 Beitz A, Muller G, Beitz J et al. Von Willebrand's disease and hemophilia are associated with diminished thromboxane A2 (TXA2) formation in clotting whole blood. *Prostaglandins Leukot Essent Fatty Acids*, 50, 49-52 (1994)

371 Belfiore F et al. Serum acid phosphatase activity in diabetes mellitus. *Am J Med Sci*, 266, 139-143 (1973)

372 Belfiore F et al. Serum enzymes in diabetes mellitus. *Clin Chem*, 19, 447 (1973)

373 Belgorosky A, Chahin S, Rivarola MA. Elevation of serum luteinizing hormone levels during hydrocortisone treatment in infant girls with 21-hydroxylase deficiency. *Acta Paediat*, 85, 1172-1175 (1996)

374 Bell A, Hippel T, Goodman H. Use of cytochemistry and FAB classification in leukemia and other pathological states. *Am J Med Technol*, 47, 437-471 (1981)

375 Bell H, Raknerud N, Falch JA et al. Inappropriately low levels of gonadotropins in amenorrhoeic women with alcoholic and non-alcoholic cirrhosis. *Eur J Endocrinol*, 132, 444-449 (1995)

376 Bell IR, Edman JS, Selhub J et al. Plasma homocysteine in vascular disease and in nonvascular dementia of depressed elderly people. *Acta Psychiat Scand*, 86, 386-390 (1992)

377 Bell MJ, Kochanek PM, Doughty LA, et al. Interleukin-6 and interleukin-10 in cerebrospinal fluid after severe traumatic brain injury in children. *J Neurotrauma*, 14, 451-457 (1997)

378 Bellabarba G, Davila DF, Torres A et al. Plasma renin activity in chagasic patients with and without congestive heart failure. *Int J Cardiol*, 47, 5-11 (1995)

379 Bellingham AJ, Detter JC, Lenfant C. Regulatory mechanisms of hemoglobin oxygen affinity in acidosis and alkalosis. *J Clin Invest*, 50, 700-706 (1971)

380 Bellingham AJ, Detter JC, Lenfant C. The red cell in adaptation to anaemic hypoxia. *Clin Haematol*, 3, 577-594 (1974)

381 Belliveau et al. Liver enzymes and pathology in Hodgkin's disease. *Cancer*, 34, 300-305 (1974)

382 Ben-Aryeh H et al. Sialochemistry of patients with rheumatoid arthritis. electrolytes, protein, and salivary IgA. *Oral Surg*, 45, 63-70 (1978)

383 Benassayag C, Christeff N, Auclair MC et al. Early released lipid-soluble cardiodepressant factor and elevated oestrogenic substances in human septic shock. *Eur J Clin Invest*, 14, 288-294 (1984)

384 Benedict CR et al. Clinical significance of plasma adrenaline and noradrenaline concentrations in patients with subarachnoid haemorrhage. *J Neurol Neurosurg Psychiatry*, 41, 113-117 (1978)

385 Benedict CR et al. Plasma noradrenaline and adrenaline concentrations and dopamine β-hydroxylase activity in patients with shock due to septicemia, trauma and hemorrhage. *Q J Med*, 185, 1-20 (1978)

386 Benigni A, Boccardo P, Noris M et al. Urinary excretion of platelet-activating factor in haemolytic uraemic syndrome. *Lancet*, 339, 835-836 (1992)

387 Bennett JM et al. Significance of leukocyte alkaline phosphatase in Hodgkin's disease. *Arch Intern Med*, 121, 338 (1966)

388 Bennett RM, Mohla C. A solid-phase radioimmunoassay for the measurement of lactoferrin in human plasma: variations with age, sex and disease. *J Lab Clin Med*, 88, 156-166 (1976)

389 Bennett WM et al. Silent renal involvement in systemic lupus erythematosus. *Int Arch Allergy Appl Immunol*, 55, 420-8 (1977)

390 Bensley et al. Estimation of serum acid phosphatase in the diagnosis of metastasizing carcinoma. *Can Med Ass J*, 58, 261-264 (1948)

391 Benster B et al. Immunoglobulin levels in normal pregnancy and pregnancy complicated by hypertension. *Br J Obstet Gynaecol*, 77, 518-522 (1970)

392 Bercroft DMO et al. Abetalipoproteinemia (Bassen-Kornzweig syndrome). *Arch Dis Child*, 40, 40 (1965)

393 Berg B et al. Urinary excretion of histamine and histamine metabolites in leukemia. *Scand J Haematol*, 8, 63 (1971)

394 Berg PA, Klein R, Rocken M. Cytokines in primary biliary cirrhosis. *Sem Liver Dis*, 17, 115-123 (1997)

395 Berg S, Brodin B, Hesselvik F et al. Elevated levels of plasma hyaluron in septicaemia. *Scand J Clin Lab Invest*, 48, 727-732 (1988)

396 Berger HW, Maher G. Decreased glucose concentration in malignant pleural effusions. *Am Rev Resp Dis*, 103, 427-429 (1971)

397 Berger MM, Cavadini C, Bart A et al. Selenium losses in 10 burned patients. *Clin Nutr*, 11, 75-82 (1992)

398 Bergeron C, Bansard JY, Le Moine P, et al. Erythrocyte spermine levels: a prognostic parameter in childhood common acute lymphoblastic leukemia. *Leukemia*, 11, 31-36 (1997)

399 Bergmark C, Mansoor MA, Swedenborg J et al. Hyperhomocysteinemia in patients operated for lower extremity ischaemia below the age of 50--effect of smoking and extent of disease. *Eur J Vasc Surg*, 7, 391-396 (1993)

400 Bergsagel DE et al. The treatment of plasma cell myeloma. *Adv Cancer Res*, 10, 311 (1967)

401 Bergstromm J et al. Lactic acid accumulation in connection with fructose administration. *Acta Med Scand*, 184, 359 (1968)

402 Berk JE. New dimensions in the laboratory diagnosis of pancreatic disease. *Am J Gastroenterol*, 69, 417-427 (1978)

403 Berk PD et al. Defective BSP clearance in patients with constitutional hepatic dysfunction (Gilbert's syndrome). *Gastroenterology*, 63, 472 (1972)

404 Berk PD et al. Inborn errors of bilirubin metabolism. *Med Clin North Am*, 59, 817-821 (1975)

405 Berlin NJ. Diagnosis and classification of polycythemia. *Semin Hematol*, 12, 339 (1975)

406 Berman PH et al. Congenital hyperuricemia, an inborn error of purine metabolism associated with psychomotor retardation, athetosis and self-mutilation. *Arch Neurol*, 20, 44 (1969)

407 Bermes EW Jr, Strano A, Walega JM et al. Molecular markers of coagulation/fibrinolysis in peripheral arterial disease. *Clin Biochem Rev*, 14, 359 (1993)

408 Bernard A, Lauwerys R, Noel A et al. Determination by latex immunoassay of protein 1 in normal and pathological urine. *Clin Chim Acta*, 201, 231-246 (1991)

409 Bernard GR, Wheeler AP, Russell JA, et al. The effects of ibuprofen on the physiology and survival of patients with sepsis. *N Engl J Med*, 336, 912-918 (1997)

410 Bernard JF et al. Human erythrocytic calcium concentration in hemolytic anemia. *Biomed Exp*, 23, 431-433 (1975)

411 Berndt C, Haubold K, Wenger F, et al. K-ras mutations in stools and tissue samples from patients with malignant and nonmalignant pancreatic diseases. *Clin Chem*, 44, 2103-2107 (1998)

412 Bernengo MG et al. Relationship between T and B lymphocyte values and prognosis in malignant melanoma. *Br J Dermatol*, 98, 655-62 (1978)

413 Berner JJ. *Effects of Diseases on Laboratory Tests*. New York NY, JB Lippincott (1983)

414 Berney T, Gasche Y, Robert J, et al. Serum profiles of interleukin-6, interleukin-8, and interleukin-10 in patients with severe and mild acute pancreatitis. *Pancreas*, 18, 371-377 (1999)

415 Berni L, Costantini A, Di Vano M. Monoclonal gammopathies in Alzheimer's disease. *Clin Chem*, 39, 166 (1995)

416 Bernier J, Jobin N, Emptoz-Bonneton A, et al. Decreased corticosteroid-binding globulin in burn patients: relationship with interleukin-6 and fat in nutritional support. *Crit Care Med*, 26, 452-460 (1998)

417 Bernstein DE, Jeffers L, Erhardtsen E, et al. Recombinant factor VIIa corrects prothrombin time in cirrhotic patients: a preliminary study. *Gastroenterology*, 113, 1930-1937 (1997)

418 Bertello P, Molino P, Veglio F et al. Plasma endothelin in NIDDM patients with and without complications. *Diabetes Care*, 17, 574-577 (1994)

419 Bessis M et al. Etude comparee du plasmocytome et du syndrome de Waldenström. *Nouv Rev Fr Hematol*, 3, 159 (1963)

420 Betro MG. Significance of increased alkaline phosphatase and lactate dehydrogenase activities coincident with normal serum bilirubin. *Clin Chem*, 18, 1427-1429 (1972)

421 Betro MG et al. Hypophosphatasemia and hyperphosphatasemia in a hospital population. *Br Med J*, 1, 273-276 (1972)

422 Betteridge DJ, Cooper MB, Saggerson ED et al. Platelet function in patients with hypercholesterolaemia. *Eur J Clin Invest*, 24, 30-33 (1994)

423 Bettica P, Moro L, Robins SP et al. Bone-resorption markers galactosyl hydroxylysine, pyridinium crosslinks, and hydroxyproline compared. *Clin Chem*, 38, 2313-2318 (1992)

424 Betts, Green. Plasma and urine amino acid concentrations in children with chronic renal insufficiency. *Nephron*, 18, 132-139 (1977)

425 Beutler E. The red cell indices in the diagnosis of iron deficiency anemia. *Ann Intern Med*, 50, 313 (1959)

426 Beutler E, Gelbart T. Plasma glutathione in health and in patients with malignant disease. *J Lab Clin Med*, 105, 581-584 (1985)

427 Beveridge BR et al. Hypochromic anemia. *Q J Med*, 34, 135 (1965)

428 Beyeler C, Reichen J, Thomann SR, et al. Quantitative liver function in patients with rheumatoid arthritis treated with low-dose methotrexate: a longitudinal study. *Br J Rheumatol*, 36, 338-344 (1997)

429 Beyne P, Lisovoski F, Got L, et al. La β_2-microglobuline du liquide cephalorachidien en neurologie. *Presse Med*, 24, 1071-1075 (1995)

430 Beywler C, Banks RE, Thompson D et al. Bone alkaline phosphatase in rheumatic diseases. *Ann Clin Biochem*, 32, 379-384 (1995)

431 Bezwoda W, Derman D, Bothwell T et al. Significance of serum concentrations of carcinoembryonic antigen, ferritin, and calcitonin in breast cancer. *Cancer*, 48, 1623-1628 (1981)

432 Bezwoda WR et al. An investigation into gonadal dysfunction in patients with idiopathic hemochromatosis. *Clin Endocrinol*, 6, 377-385 (1977)

433 Bhargava DK, Gupta M, Nijhawan S et al. Adenosine deaminase (ADA) in peritoneal tuberculosis: diagnostic value in ascitic fluid and serum. *Tubercle*, 71, 121-126 (1990)

434 Bhatia RK, Bottoms SF, Saleh AA et al. Mechanisms for reduced colloid osmotic pressure in preeclampsia. *Am J Obstet Gynecol*, 157, 106-108 (1987)

435 Bhutta ZA, Mansoorali N, Hussain R. Plasma cytokines in paedriatric typhoidal salmonellosis: correlation with clinical course and outcomes. *J Infect*, 35, 253-256 (1997)

436 Bianchi ML, Bardare M, Caraceni MP et al. Bone metabolism in juvenile rheumatoid arthritis. *Bone Miner*, 9, 153-162 (1990)

437 Bianchi S, Bigazzi R, Valtriani C et al. Elevated serum insulin levels in patients with essential hypertension and microalbuminuria. *Hypertension*, 23, 681-687 (1994)

438 Biasucci LM, Liuzzo G, Grillo RL, et al. Elevated levels of C-reactive protein at discharge in patients with unstable angina predict recurrent instability. *Circulation*, 99, 855-860 (1999)

439 Biasucci LM, Vitelli A, Liuzzo G, et al. Elevated levels of interleukin-6 in unstable angina. *Circulation*, 94, 874-877 (1996)

440 Biberfield G, Sterner G. Antibodies in bronchial secretions following natural infection with mycoplasma pneumoniae. *Acta Pathol Microbiol Immunol Scand*, 79B, 599-605 (1971)

441 Bick RL. Antiphospholipid-thrombosis syndromes. *Biomed Prog*, 13, 41-45 (2000)

442 Bick RL, Bick MD, Fekete LF. Antithrombin III patterns in disseminated intravascular coagulation. *Am J Clin Pathol*, 73, 577-583 (1980)

443 Bick RL, Laughlin WR. Myeloproliferative syndromes. *Lab Med*, 24, 770-776 (1993)

444 Bickel H. Proximal tubular defects. In:. *Renal Disease, DAK Black (ed)* (1964)

445 Biederman J, Herzog DB, Rivinus TM. Urinary MHPG in anorexia nervosa patients with and without a concomitant major depressive disorder. *J Psychiat Res*, 18, 149-160 (1984)

446 Biemond I, Selby WS, Jewell DP, Klasen EC. α_1-Antitrypsin serum concentration and phenotypes in ulcerative colitis. *Digestion*, 29, 124-128 (1984)

447 Bierman et al. Correlation of serum lactic dehydrogenase activity with the clinical status of patients with cancer, lymphomas, and the leukemias. *Cancer Res*, 16, 660-667 (1957)

448 Biffl WL, Moore EE, Moore FA, Peterson VM. Interleukin-6 in the injured patient: marker of injury or mediator of inflammation? *Ann Surg*, 224, 647-664 (1996)

449 Bijlstra PJ, Postma CT, de Boo T, Thien T. Clinical and biochemical criteria in the detection of renal artery stenosis. *J Hypertens*, 14, 1033-1040 (1996)

450 Bikle DD, Gennant HK, Cann C et al. Bone disease in alcohol abuse. *Ann Intern Med*, 103, 42-48 (1990)

451 Bikle DD, Stesin A, Halloran B et al. Alcohol-induced bone disease: relationship to age and parathyroid hormone levels. *Alcohol Clin Exp Res*, 17, 690-695 (1993)

452 Bilbrey GL et al. Hyperglucagonemia of renal failure. *J Clin Invest*, 53, 841 (1974)

453 Binder R, Gilbert S. Muramidase in polycythemia vera. *Blood*, 36, 228 (1970)

454 Bing RJ. Diagnostic value of activity of malic dehydrogenase and phosphohexose isomerase. *J Am Med Ass*, 164, 647 (1957)

455 Bio-Science Laboratories. Bio-Science Handbook. *12th edition*, Van Nuys, CA (1979)

456 Bio-Science Laboratories. *Bio-Science Handbook: Specialized Diagnostic Laboratory Tests.* 11th Edition, Van Nuys, CA (1977)

457 Bio-Science Laboratories. Bio-Science Reports. Van Nuys, CA (1980)

458 Bircan Z, Kaplan A, Soker M, et al. Serum levels of carnitine, apolipoprotein A I, and apolipoprotein B in children with nephrotic proteinuria (1980)

459 Bishop CR et al. Leukokinetic studies. XIV. Blood neutrophil kinetics in chronic steady state neutropenia. *J Clin Invest*, 50, 1678 (1971)

460 Bjorneboe G-EA, Bjorneboe A, Johnsen J et al. Calcium status and calcium-regulating hormones in alcoholics. *Alcohol Clin Exp Res*, 12, 229-232 (1988)

461 Blaakaer J, Micic S, Morris ID et al. Immunoreactive inhibin-production in post-menopausal women with malignant epithelial ovarian tumors. *Eur J Obstet Gynecol Reprod Biol*, 52, 105-110 (1993)

462 Blaaker J, Hogdall CK, Micic S et al. Ovarian carcinoma serum markers and ovarian steroid activity - is there a link in ovarian cancer? A correlation of inhibin, tetranectin and CA-125 to ovarian activity and the gonadotropin levels. *Eur J Obstet Gynecol Reprod Biol*, 59, 53-56 (1995)

463 Black IW, Wilcken DCL. Decreases in apolipoprotein(a) after renal transplantation: implications for lipoprotein(a) metabolism. *Clin Chem*, 38, 353-357 (1992)

464 Black LF. The pleural space and pleural fluid. *Mayo Clin Proc*, 47, 493 (1972)

465 Blacklow NR, Cukor G. Viral gastroenteritis. *N Engl J Med*, 304, 397-406 (1981)

466 Blade J, Fernandez-Llama P, Bosch F, et al. Renal failure in multiple myeloma: presenting features and predictors of outcome in 94 patients from a single institution. *Arch Intern Med*, 158, 1889-1893 (1998)

467 Blair AJ et al. The plasma 17-hydroxycorticosteroid levels in acute and chronic renal failure. *Can J Biochem*, 39, 1617 (1961)

468 Blair SL, Heerdt P, Sachar S, et al. Glutathione metabolism in patients with non-small cell lung cancers. *Cancer Res*, 57, 152-155 (1997)

469 Blanchaer et al. Plasma lactic dehydrogenase and phosphohexose isomerase in leukemia. *Blood*, 13, 245-257 (1958)

470 Blanchard P, Anton B, Larousse C et al. Plasma vitamin E, non-high-density lipoprotein cholesterol, and apolipoprotein B in diabetic patients. *Clin Chem*, 38, 2339-2340 (1992)

471 Blann AD, Amiral J, McCollum CN. Prognostic value of increased soluble thrombomodulin and increased soluble E-selectin in ischaemic heart disease. *Eur J Haematol*, 59, 115-120 (1997)

472 Blann AD, Faragher EB, McCollum CN. Increased soluble P-selectin following myocardial infarction: a new marker for the progression of atherosclerosis. *Blood Coag Fibrinolysis*, 8, 383-390 (1997)

473 Blann AD, Lip GYH, Beevers DG, et al. Soluble P-selectin in atherosclerosis: a comparison with endothelial cell and platelet markers. *Thromb Haemost*, 77, 1077-180 (1997)

474 Blann AD, McCollum CN. Increased levels of soluble tumor necrosis factor receptors in atherosclerosis. *Inflammation*, 22, 483-491 (1998)

475 Blann AD, Seigneur M, Boisseau MR, et al. soluble P selectin in peripheral vascular disease: relationship to the location and extent of atherosclerotic disease and its risk factors. *Blood Coag Fibrinolysis*, 7, 789-793 (1996)

476 Blann AD, Seigneur M, Constans J, et al. Soluble P-selectin, thrombocytopenia and von Willebrand factor in HIV infected patients. *Thromb Haemostas*, 77, 1221-1222 (1997)

477 Blann AD, Seigneur M, Steiner M, et al. Circulating ICAM-1 and VCAM-1 in peripheral artery disease and hypercholesterolaemia: relationship to the location of atherosclerotic disease, smoking and in the prediction of adverse events. *Thromb Haemost*, 79, 1080-1085 (1998)

478 Blann AD, Tse W, Maxwell SJR et al. Increased levels of the soluble adhesion molecule E-selectin in essential hypertension. *J Hypertens*, 12, 925-928 (1994)

479 Blaschke TF et al. Effects of induced fever on sulfobromophthalein kinetics in man. *Ann Intern Med*, 78, 221 (1973)

480 Blay J-Y, Farcet J-P, Lavaud A et al. Serum concentrations of cytokines in patients with Hodgkin's disease. *Eur J Cancer*, 30A, 321-324 (1994)

481 Blekta M et al. Volume of whole blood and absolute amount of serum proteins in the early stage of late toxemia of pregnancy. *Am J Obstet Gynecol*, 106, 10-13 (1970)

482 Blennow K, Davidsson P, Wallin A et al. Gangliosides in cerebrospinal fluid in "probable Alzheimer's disease". *Arch Neurol*, 48, 1032-1035 (1991)

483 Blind E, Raue F, Meinel T et al. Diagnostiche Bedeutung von Parathormone-related-Protein bei Tumorpatienten mit Hypercalcaemie. *Dtsch Med Wschr*, 118, 330-335 (1993)

484 Bloch KJ et al. Sjögren's syndrome: a clinical, pathological, and serological study of sixty-two cases. *Medicine*, 44, 187 (1965)

485 Bloom A et al. Factor VIII and its inherited disorders. *Br Med Bull*, 33, 219-24 (1977)

486 Bloom AL. The von Willebrand syndrome. *Semin Hematol*, 17, 215-227 (1980)

487 Bloom EJ, Abrams DI, Rodgers G. Lupus anticoagulant in the acquired immunodeficiency syndrome. *J Am Med Ass*, 256, 491 (1986)

488 Bloomer JR et al. Blood volume and bilirubin production in acute intermittent porphyria. *N Engl J Med*, 284, 17 (1971)

489 Bluestein B, Zhou A, Tewari P et al. Multi-site clinical evaluation of an automated chemiluminescent immunoassay for prostate specific antigen (ACS PSA). *Ciba Corning Diagnostics Cancer Care Diagnostics*, Ciba Corning Diagnostics, Medford MA (1992)

490 Blum WF. Insulin-like growth factors (IGFs) and IGF binding proteins in chronic renal failure: evidence for reduced secretion of IGFs. *Acta Paediat Scand*, 80, 24-31 (1991)

491 Blumberg MZ et al. The total eosinophil count and adrenal function in asthmatic children. *Ann Allergy*, 35, 377-81 (1975)

492 Blyuger AF, Raitsis AB. Blood serotonin content in acute and chronic liver diseases. *Klin Med (Mosk)*, 50, 95-101 (1972)

493 Boag F, Weerakoon J, Ginsburg J et al. Diminished creatinine clearance in anorexia nervosa: reversal with weight gain. *J Clin Pathol*, 38, 60-63 (1985)

494 Bock E, Rafaelsen OJ. Schizophrenia: proteins in blood and cerebrospinal fluid. *Dan Med Bull*, 21, 93-105 (1974)

495 Bock E, Weeke B, Rafaelson OJ. Serum proteins in acutely psychotic patients. *J Psychiat Res*, 9, 1-9 (1971)

496 Boda D et al. In vitro effects of inosine-pyruvate-phosphate on p50 values and DPG contents of fresh and stored blood from healthy neonates, symptom-free premature infants and premature infants with respiratory disease. *Biol Neonate*, 33, 25-30 (1978)

497 Boehme MWJ, Werle E, Kommerell B et al. Serum levels of adhesion molecules and thrombomodulin as indicators of vascular injury in severe Plasmodium falciparum malaria. *Clin Investig*, 72, 598-603 (1994)

498 Boelen A, Plavoet-Ter Schiphorst MC, Wiersinga WM. Association between serum interleukin-6 and serum 3,5,3'-triodothyronine in nonthyroidal illness. *J Clin Endocrinol Metab*, 77, 1695-1699 (1993)

499 Boey ML, Loizou S, Colaco CB et al. Antithrombin III in systemic lupus erythematosus. *Clin Exp Rheumatol*, 2, 53-56 (1984)

500 Bogden JD et al. Copper, zinc, magnesium, and calcium in plasma and cerebrospinal fluid of patients with neurological diseases. *Clin Chem*, 23, 485-489 (1977)

501 Bogden JD et al. Effect of pulmonary tuberculosis on blood concentrations of copper and zinc. *Am J Clin Pathol*, 67, 251-256 (1977)

502 Boggs DR et al. An unusual pattern of neutrophil kinetics in sickle cell anemia. *Blood*, 41, 59 (1973)

503 Boggs DR et al. Factors influencing the duration of survival of patients with chronic lymphocytic leukemia. *Am J Med*, 40, 243 (1966)

504 Boggs DR, Fahey JL. Serum protein changes in malignant disease. *J Natl Cancer Inst*, 25, 1381 (1960)

505 Bohan A et al. A computer-assisted analysis of 153 patients with polymyositis and dermatomyositis. *Medicine*, 56, 255-285 (1977)

506 Boiskin I, Epstein S, Ismail F et al. Serum osteocalcin and bone mineral metabolism following successful renal transplantation. *Clin Nephrol*, 31, 316-322 (1989)

507 Boix-Ochoa J et al. The important influence of arterial blood gases on the prognosis of congenital diaphragmatic hernia. *World J Surg*, 1, 783-87 (1977)

508 Bojanowicz K et al. Disturbances of fat, carbohydrate, magnesium and protein balance in liver disease. *Acta Hepatogastroenterol*, 24, 155-161 (1977)

509 Bokesch VA. The potential role of complement in dengue hemorrhagic shock syndrome. *N Engl J Med*, 289, 996-1006 (1973)

510 Bolbach R, Becker M, Rotthauwe HW. Serum immunoreactive trypsin and pancreatic lipase in cystic fibrosis. *Eur J Pediatr*, 144, 161-170 (1985)

511 Bolufer P, Lluch A, Molina R, et al. Epidermal growth factor in human breast cancer, endometrial carcinoma and lung cancer. Its relationship to epidermal growth factor receptor, estradiol receptor. *Clin Chim Acta*, 33215, 51-61 (1993)

512 Boman K, Backstrom T, Gerdes U et al. Progesterone, androstenedione, testosterone and clinical characteristics in endometrial carcinoma. *Anticancer Res*, 11, 2163-2166 (1991)

513 Bon GG, von Mensdorff-Pouilly S, Kenemans P, et al. Clinical and technical evaluation of ACS™ BR serum assay of MUCI gene-derived glycoprotein in breast cancer, and comparison with CA 15-3 assays. *Clin Chem*, 43, 585-593 (1997)

514 Bonarjee VVS, Omland T, Nilsen DWT, et al. Plasma proatrial natriuretic factor (1-98) concentration after myocardial infarction: relation to indices of cardiac and renal function. *Br Heart J*, 73, 511-516 (1995)

515 Bonfrer JMG, Gaarenstroom KN, Korse CM, et al. CYFRA 21-1 in monitoring cervical cancer: a comparison with tissue polypeptide antigen and squamous cell carcinoma antigen. *Anticancer Res*, 17, 2329-2334 (1997)

516 Bonifati C, Mussi A, Carducci M, et al. Endothelin-1 levels are increased in sera and lesional skin extracts of psoriatic patients and correlate with disease severity. *Acta Derm Venereol*, 78, 22-26 (1998)

517 Bonnar J et al. Coagulation and fibrinolytic systems in pre-eclampsia and eclampsia. *Br Med J*, 2, 12 (1971)

518 Bonnar J et al. The role of coagulation and fibrinolysis in preeclampsia. *Perspect Nephrol Hypertens*, 5, 85-93 (1976)

519 Bonnin MR, Gonzalez MT, Huguet J et al. 1,25-Dihydroxycholecalciferol as measured by a radioreceptor assay in normal subjects and patients after kidney transplantation. *Clin Chem*, 36, 389-390 (1990)

520 Bonnin R, Villabona C, Rivera A et al. Is salivary cortisol a better index than free cortisol in serum or urine for diagnosis of Cushing syndrome? *Clin Chem*, 39, 1353-1354 (1993)

521 Bonta IL et al. Prostaglandins and chronic inflammation. *Biochem Pharmacol*, 27, 1611-1624 (1978)

522 Bontis J, Vavilis D, Agorastos T et al. Maternal plasma level of thrombomodulin is increased in mild preeclampsia. *Eur J Obstet Gynecol*, 60, 139-141 (1995)

523 Bonuccelli U, Piccini P, Del Dotto P et al. Platelet monoamine oxidase B activity in Parkinsonian patients. *J Neurol Neurosurg Psych*, 53, 854-855 (1990)

524 Boomsma F, Bhaggoe UM, Man in t Veld AJ, et al. Sensitivity and specificity of a new ELISA method for determination of chromogranin A in the diagnosis of pheochromocytoma and neuroblastoma. *Clin Chim Acta*, 239, 57-83 (1995)

525 Boomsma F, Derkx HM, van den Meiracker AH et al. Plasma semicarbazide-sensitive amine oxidase activity is elevated in diabetes mellitus and correlates with glycosylated hemoglobin. *Clin Sci*, 88, 675-679 (1995)

526 Boosalis MG, McCall JT, Solem LD et al. Serum copper and ceruloplasmin levels and urinary copper excretion in thermal injury. *Am J Clin Nutr*, 44, 899-906 (1986)

527 Boot AM, Nauta J, de Jong MCJW, et al. Bone mineral density, bone metabolism and body composition of children with chronic renal failure, with and without growth hormone treatment. *Clin Endocrinol*, 49, 665-672 (1998)

528 Booth SN et al. Serum carcinoembryonic antigen in clinical disorders. *Gut*, 14, 794-99 (1973)

529 Borba EF, Santos RD, Bonfa E et al. Lipoprotein(a) levels in systemic lupus erythematosus. *J Rheumatol*, 21, 220-223 (1994)

530 Borg H, Fernlund P, Sundkvist G. Protein tyrosine phosphatase-like protein IA2-antibodies plus glutamic acid decarboxylase 65 antibodies (GADA) indicates autoimmunity as frequently as islet cell antibodies assay in children with recently diagnosed diabetes mellitus. *Clin Chem*, 43, 2358-2363 (1997)

531 Borg S, Helander A, Beck O et al. Biochemical markers of alcohol abuse. *Proc ACB Natl Meet*, 16 (1994)

532 Borowsky SA, Lieberman J, Strome S, Sastre A. Elevation of serum angiotensin-converting enzyme level: occurrence in alcoholic liver disease. *Arch Intern Med*, 142, 893-895 (1982)

533 Borre M, Nerstrom B, Overgaard J. Erythrocyte sedimentation rate - a predictor of malignant potential in early prostate cancer. *Acta Oncol*, 36, 689-694 (1997)

534 Borsatti A. Increased urine angiotensin I converting enzyme activity in patients with upper urinary tract infection. *Clin Chim Acta*, 109, 211-218 (1981)

535 Bosch X, Bernadich O. Increased serum prostate-specific antigen in a man and a woman with hepatitis A. *N Engl J Med*, 337, 1849-1850 (1997)

536 Bosi A, Borsotti M, Ghelli P et al. Serum angiotensin-I-converting enzyme and lysozyme levels in untreated and unsplenectomized patients with Hodgkin's disease. *Acta Haematol*, 71, 329-333 (1984)

537 Botero-Velez M, Curtis JJ, Warnock DG. Liddle's syndrome revisited - a disorder of sodium reabsorption in the distal tubule. *N Engl J Med*, 330, 178-181 (1994)

538 Bottger D. Prognostic significance of lymphopenia in pulmonary sarcoidosis. *Z Erkrank Atm-Org*, 149, 197-201 (1977)

539 Botti C, Seregni E, Mattioli S, et al. Bladder cancer monitoring using two novel urinary markers. *Int J Biol Markers*, 12, 174-180 (1997)

540 Bottinger LE et al. Serum lipids in alcoholics. *Acta Med Scand*, 199, 357-361 (1976)

541 Bouillon R, Vanderschueren D, Van Herck E et al. Homologous radioimmunoassay of human osteocalcin. *Clin Chem*, 38, 2055-2060 (1992)

542 Boulat O, Janin B, Francioli P et al. Plasma carnitines: reference values in an ambulatory population. *Eur J Clin Chem Clin Biochem*, 31, 585-589 (1993)

543 Boulenger J-P, Jerabeck I, Jolicouer FB, et al. Elevated plasma levels of neuropeptide Y in patients with panic disorder. *Am J Psychiatr*, 153, 114-116 (1996)

544 Bour H et al. Les enzymes du muscle au cours du coma oxycarbone. *Sem Hop Paris*, 38, 3152-3157 (1962)

545 Bourantas KL, Hatzmichael EC, Makis AC, et al. Serum β-2-microglobulin, TNF-α and interleukins in myeloproliferative disorders. *Br J Haematol*, 63, 19-25 (1999)

546 Bousvaros A, Zurakowski D, Fishman SJ, et al. Serum basic fibroblast growth factor in pediatric Crohn's disease: implications for wound healing. *Dig Dis Sci*, 42, 378-386 (1997)

547 Bower BR, Gordon GS. Hormonal effects on non-endocrine tumors. *Annu Rev Med*, 16, 83 (1965)

548 Bower L, Warren C, Manley G. Human serum and urine glycosaminoglycans in health and in patients with chronic renal failure. *Ann Clin Biochem*, 29, 190-195 (1992)

549 Bowers MB Jr, Mazure CM, Greenfield DG. Elevated plasma monoamine metabolites in eating disorders. *Psychiat Res*, 52, 11-15 (1994)

550 Bowles SA, Kurdy N, Davis AM, et al. Serum osteocalcin, total and bone-specific alkaline phosphatase following isolated tibial shaft fracture. *Ann Clin Biochem*, 33, 196-200 (1996)

551 Boyano MD, Garcia-Vazquez MD, Gardeazabal J, et al. Serum soluble IL-2 receptor and IL-6 levels in patients with melanoma. *Oncology*, 54, 400-416 (1997)

552 Boyko WL, Barret B. Detection and quantitation of the β-subunit of human chorionic gonadotropin in serum by RIA. *Fertil Steril*, 33, 141-150 (1980)

553 Braasch JW, Camer SJ. Periampullary carcinoma. *Med Clin North Am*, 59, 309-314 (1975)

554 Brackertz D, Hagmann J, Kueppers F. Proteinase inhibitors in rheumatoid arthritis. *Ann Rheum Dis*, 34, 225-230 (1975)

555 Brady RO. Sphingolipidoses. *Annu Rev Biochem*, 47, 687-713 (1978)

556 Braegger CP et al. *Lancet*, 339, 89- (1992)

557 Brakman P et al. Blood coagulation and fibrinolysis in acute leukemia. *Br J Haematol*, 18, 135 (1970)

558 Brambilla F, Belloi L, Perna G et al. Plasma interleukin-1 beta concentrations in panic disorder. *Psychiat Res*, 54, 135-142 (1994)

559 Brambilla F, Facchinetti F, Petraglia F et al. Secretion pattern of endogenous opioids in chronic schizophrenia. *Am J Psychiat*, 141, 1183-1189 (1984)

560 Bramley PN, Rathbone BJ, Forbes MA et al. Serum hyaluronate as a marker of hepatic derangement in acute liver damage. *J Hepatol*, 13, 8-13 (1991)

561 Brandtzaeg P, Oktedalen O, Kierulf P et al. Elevated VIP and endotoxin plasma levels in human gram-negative septic shock. *Regul Peptide*, 24, 37-44 (1989)

562 Brasher GW et al. Complement component analysis in angioedema. Diagnostic value. *Arch Dermatol*, 111, 1140-1142 (1975)

563 Brattstrom L, Lindgren A, Israelsson B et al. Hyperhomocysteinaemia in stroke: prevalence, cause, and relationships to type of stroke and stroke risk factors. *Eur J Clin Invest.*, 22, 214-221 (1992)

564 Braunstein GD et al. First trimester chorionic gonadotropin measurements as an aid in the diagnosis of early pregnancy disorders. *Am J Obstet Gynecol*, 131, 25-32 (1978)

565 Braunwald E, Isselbacher K, Petersdorf RG et al. *Principles of Internal Medicine*. 11th edition, New York NY, McGraw-Hill (1987)

566 Brawley RK, Vasco JS, Morrow AG. Cholesterol pericarditis. *Am J Med*, 41, 235-248 (1966)

567 Brayne C, Calloway P. Serum creatine kinase BB isoenzyme levels. *Acta Psychiat Scand*, 81, 6-8 (1990)

568 Breckinridge A. Hypertension in hyperuricemia. *Proc Roy Soc Med*, 59, 316-318 (1966)

569 Breiter DN et al. Serum copper and zinc measurements in patients with osteogenic sarcoma. *Cancer*, 42, 598-602 (1978)

570 Bremme K, Eneroth P, Nilsson B et al. Maternal and cord serum levels of tissue polypeptide antigen (TPA) in normal pregnancies. *Gynecol Obstet Invest*, 19, 118-123 (1985)

571 Bremner JD, Licinio J, Darnell A, et al. Elevated CSF corticotropin-releasing factor concentrations in posttraumatic stress disorder. *Am J Psychiat*, 154, 624-629 (1997)

572 Brenner BM, Rector FC (eds). *The Kidney*. Philadelphia PA, WB Saunders, II (1976)

573 Brenner RE, Schiller B, Vetter U et al. Serum concentrations of procollagen I C-terminal propeptide, osteocalcin and insulin-like growth factor-I in patients with non-lethal osteogenesis imperfecta. *Acta Paediat*, 82, 764-767 (1993)

574 Brent GA, Hershman JM, Reed AW et al. Serum angiotensin-converting enzyme in severe nonthyroidal illnesses associated with low serum thyroxine concentration. *Ann Intern Med*, 100, 680-683 (1984)

575 Brereton HD et al. Pretreatment serum lactate dehydrogenase predicting metastatic spread in Ewing's sarcoma. *Ann Intern Med*, 83, 352-354 (1975)

576 Bresciani A, Pirozzi G, Spera M, et al. Increased level of serum HLA class I antigens in patients with systemic lupus erythematosus. Correlation with disease activity. *Tissue Antigens*, 52, 44-50 (1998)

577 Breslau NA, McGuire JL, Zerwekh JE. Hypercalcemia associated with increased serum calcitriol levels in three patients with lymphoma. *Ann Intern Med*, 100, 1-7 (1984)

578 Breslin NA, Suddath RL, Bissette G et al. CSF concentrations of neurotensin in schizophrenia: an investigation of clinical and biochemical correlates. *Schiz Res*, 12, 35-41 (1994)

579 Bressler R et al. Serum leucine aminopeptidase activity in hepatobiliary and pancreatic disease. *J Lab Clin Med*, 56, 417-430 (1960)

580 Breuer B, Smith S, Thor A, et al. ErbB-2 protein in sera and tumors of breast cancer patients. *Breast Cancer Res Treat*, 49, 261-270 (1998)

581 Breuer RI et al. Urinary crystalloid excretion in patients with inflammatory bowel disease. *Gut*, 11, 314 (1970)

582 Brewerton TD, Lydiard RB, Laraia MT et al. CSF β-endorphin and dynorphin in bulimia nervosa. *Am J Psychiat*, 149, 1096-1090 (1992)

583 Briars GL, Dean TP, Murphy JL et al. Faecal interleukin-8 and tumour necrosis factor-α concentrations in cystic fibrosis. *Arch Dis Child*, 73, 74-76 (1995)

584 Briheim G, Fryden A, Tobiasson P. Serum bile acids in Gilbert's syndrome before and after reduced caloric intake. *Scand J Gastroenterol*, 17, 877-80 (1982)

585 Brissenden JE, Cox DW. α_2-Macroglobulin in patients with obstructive lung disease, with and without α_1-antitrypsin deficiency. *Clin Chim Acta*, 128, 241-8 (1983)

586 Brivet FG, Emillie D, Galanaud P. Pro- and anti-inflammatory cytokines during acute severe pancreatitis: an early and sustained response, although unpredictable of death. *Crit Care Med*, 27, 749-755 (1999)

587 Brock DJ et al. Serum α-fetoprotein in cystic fibrosis of the pancreas. *Clin Chim Acta*, 81, 101-103 (1978)

588 Brockhaus M, Bar-Khayim Y, Gurwicz S, et al. Plasma tumor necrosis factor soluble receptors in chronic renal failure. *Kidney Int*, 42, 663-667 (1992)

589 Broder G. Quantitation and clinical significance of urinary fat. *Lancet*, 2, 188 (1969)

590 Brohult A, Brohult J, Brohult S. Effects of alkoxyglycerols on the serum ornithine carbamoyl transferase in connection with radiation treatment. *Experientia*, 28, 146 (1972)

591 Bronson WR. Pseudohyperkalemia due to release of potassium from white blood cells during clotting. *N Engl J Med*, 274, 369 (1966)

592 Brook J et al. Leukocyte alkaline phosphatase levels in multiple myeloma. *J Lab Clin Med*, 90, 114-117 (1977)

593 Brooks BR et al. Cerebrospinal fluid acid-base and lactate changes after seizures in unanesthetized man. i. idiopathic seizures. *Neurology*, 25, 935-942 (1975)

594 Brooks JE, Herbert M, Walder CP et al. Prolactin and stress: some endocrine correlates of pre-operative anxiety. *Clin Endocrinol*, 24, 635-656 (1986)

595 Brouillet JP, Hanslick B, Maudelonde T et al. Increased plasma cathepsin D concentration in hepatic carcinoma and cirrhosis but not in breast cancer. *Clin Biochem*, 24, 491-496 (1991)

596 Browder AA et al. The problem of lead poisoning. *Medicine*, 52, 121 (1973)

597 Brown B. Hematology: *Principles and Procedures*. 3rd edition, Philadelphia PA, Lea and Febiger (1980)

598 Brown J et al. Autoimmune thyroid diseases -- Graves' and Hashimoto's. *Ann Intern Med*, 88, 379-391 (1978)

599 Brown JD, Dac AN. Tuberculous peritonitis. low ascitic fluid glucose concentration as a diagnostic aid. *Am J Gastroenterol*, 66, 277-282 (1976)

600 Brown MA, Wang M-X, Buddle ML et al. Albumin excretion rate in normal and hypertensive pregnancy. *Clin Sci*, 86, 251-255 (1994)

601 Brown NS, Hughes J, Lim KL et al. Urine neopterin is the best predictor of disease activity in systemic lupus erythematosus. *Proc ACB Natl Meet*, 96 (1993)

602 Brown SS, Mitchell FL, Young DS (eds). *Chemical Diagnosis of Disease*. Amsterdam, Elsevier North-Holland Biomedical Press (1979)

603 Brownstein M H, Billard H S. Hepatoma associated with erythrocytosis. *Am J Med*, 40, 206 (1966)

604 Broyles DL, Nielsen RG, Bussett EM, et al. Analytical and clinical performance characteristics of Tandem-MP Ostase, a new immunoassay for serum bone alkaline phosphatase. *Clin Chem*, 44, 2139-2147 (1998)

605 Brozik M, Rosztoczy I, Meretey K et al. Interleukin 6 levels in synovial fluids of patients with different arthritides: Correlation with local IgM rheumatoid factor and systemic acute phase protein production. *J Rheumatol*, 19, 63-68 (1992)

606 Brozmanova E et al. Serum alkaline phosphatase in malignant bone tumors (osteosarcoma, chondrosarcoma, fibrosarcoma, Ewing's sarcoma). *Neoplasma*, 20, 419-425 (1973)

607 Bruce C, Taylor WH. Plasma histamine in patients with tropical disorders and acute asthma who exhibit eosinophilia. *Ann Clin Biochem*, 33, 249-252 (1996)

608 Brunell P et al. Zoster in children. *Am J Dis Child*, 115, 432 (1968)

609 Brunkwall J, Bergqvist D, Almer L-O et al. Tissue plasminogen activator, its fast acting plasma inhibitor and protein C after renal transplantation. *Thromb Res*, 77, 105-111 (1995)

610 Bruno G, Cavallo-Perin P, Bargero G, et al. Association of fibrinogen with glycemic control and albumin excretion rate in patients with non-insulin-dependent diabetes mellitus. *Ann Intern Med*, 125, 653-657 (1997)

611 Bruserud O, Akselen PE, Bergheim J, Nesthus I. Serum concentrations of E-selectin, P-selectin, ICAM-1 and interleukin-6 in acute leukemia patients with chemotherapy-induced leukopenia and bacterial infections. *Br J Haematol*, 91, 394-402 (1995)

612 Bruserud O, Bergheim J, Shammas FV et al. Serum concentrations of tumour necrosis factor-α during chemotherapy-induced leukopenia in patients with acute leukemia and bacterial infections. *Leuk Res*, 18, 415-421 (1994)

613 Bruserud O, Halstensen A, Peen E, Solberg CO. Serum levels of adhesion molecules and cytokines in patients with acute leukaemia. *Leukemia Lymphoma*, 23, 423-430 (1996)

614 Brutigam C, Wevers RA, Jansen RJT, et al. Biochemical hallmarks of tyrosine hydroxylase deficiency. *Clin Chem*, 44, 1897-1904 (1998)

615 Bruyn G W, Lequin R M. Huntington's chorea. *Lancet*, 2, 1300 (1964)

616 Buamah PK, Skillen AW. Lactate dehydrogenase isoenzyme 1 activity in sera of patients with ovarian cancer. *Clin Chem*, 36, 707-708 (1993)

617 Buccheri G, et al. Haemostatic abnormalities in lung cancer: prognostic implications. *Eur J Cancer*, 33, 50-55 (1997)

618 Buchanan KD. The gastrointestinal hormones: general concepts. *Clin Endocrinol Metab*, 8, 249-263 (1979)

619 Buchanan TM et al. Brucellosis in the United States, 1960-72, part II. Diagnostic aspects. *Medicine*, 53, 415-426 (1974)

620 Buchler M, Malfertheiner P, Schadlich H et al. Prognostic value of serum phospholipase A in acute pancreatitis. *Klin Wschr*, 67, 186-189 (1989)

621 Buchwald D, Umali J, Stene M. Insulin-like growth factor-I (somatomedin C) levels in chronic fatigue syndrome and fibromyalgia. *J Rheumatol*, 23, 739-742 (1996)

622 Buckee C, Morgan K, Ayad S et al. Diversity of antibodies to type II collagen in patients with rheumatoid arthritis: detection by binding to α-chains and to cyanogen bromide peptides. *Br J Rheumatol*, 29, 254-258 (1990)

623 Buckley BM, Smith SC, Beevers M et al. Lack of evidence of low ionized calcium levels in systemic hypertension. *Am J Cardiol*, 59, 878-880 (1987)

624 Budman DR, Steinberg A. Hematologic aspects of systemic lupus erythematosus. *Ann Intern Med*, 86, 220-229 (1977)

625 Buer J, Probst M, Franzke A, et al. Elevated serum levels of S100 and survival in metastatic malignant melanoma. *J Cancer*, 75, 1373-1376 (1997)

626 Buffo B, Marlewski M, Smolenski RT, et al. Erythrocyte nucleotides and blood hypoxanthine in patients with uremia evaluated immediately and 24 hours after hemodialysis. *Renal Fail*, 18, 247-252 (1996)

627 Bulaj ZJ, Griffen LM, Jorde LB, et al. Clinical and biochemical abnormalities in people heterozygous for hemochromatosis. *N Engl J Med*, 335, 1799-1805 (1996)

628 Bullen AW et al. Diagnostic usefulness of plasma carcinoembryonic antigen levels in acute and chronic liver disease. *Gastroenterology*, 73, 673-678 (1977)

629 Buller HR, Weenink AH, Treffers PE et al. Severe antithrombin III deficiency in a patient with pre-eclampsia. Observation on the effect of human AT III concentrate transfusion. *Scand J Haematol*, 25, 81-86 (1980)

630 Bunch TW et al. Synovial fluid complement: usefulness in diagnosis and classification of rheumatoid arthritis. *Ann Intern Med*, 81, 32-35 (1974)

631 Bunch TW, Hunder GG, Mcduffie FC, O'Brien PC. Synovial fluid complement determination as a diagnostic aid in inflammatory joint disease. *Mayo Clin Proc*, 49, 715-720 (1974)

632 Bundred RJ, Ratcliffe WA, Walker RA et al. Parathyroid hormone related protein and hypercalcemia in breast cancer. *Br Med J*, 303, 1506-1509 (1991)

633 Buratti T, Schratzberger P, Dunzendorfer S, et al. Decreased levels of β-endorphin in circulating mononuclear leukocytes from patients with acute myocardial infarction. *Cardiology*, 90, 43-47 (1998)

634 Burdash NM, Blake JM Jr, Hester LL Jr. Immunoglobulin levels and liver function tests in normal and toxemic pregnancies. *Am J Obstet Gynecol*, 116, 827-830 (1973)

635 Burgmann H, Hollenstein U, Maca T, et al. Increased serum laminin and angiogenin concentrations in patients with peripheral arterial occlusive disease. *J Clin Pathol*, 49, 508-510 (1996)

636 Burgmann H, Hollenstein U, Wenisch C et al. Serum concentrations of MIP-1α and interleukin-8 in patients suffering from acute Plasmodium falciparum malaria. *Clin Immunol immunopathol*, 76, 32-36 (1995)

637 Burgmann H, Looareesuwan S, Viravan C, et al. Serum laminin and basic fibroblast growth factor concentrations in patients with complicated Plasmodium falciparum malaria. *J Clin Immunol*, 16, 278-282 (1996)

638 Burk RF, Early DS, Hill KE, et al. Plasma selenium in patients with cirrhosis. *Hepatology*, 27, 794-798 (1998)

639 Burki NK et al. Serum creatine phosphokinase activity in asthma. *Am Rev Resp Dis*, 116, 327-330 (1977)

640 Burman KD et al. Ionized and total serum calcium and parathyroid hormone in hyperthyroidism. *Ann Intern Med*, 84, 668-671 (1976)

641 Burness R, Horne G, Purdie G. Albumin levels and mortality in patients with hip fractures. *NZ Med J*, 109, 56-57 (1996)

642 Burnett D, Stockley RA. Serum and sputum α-2 macroglobulin in patients with chronic obstructive airways disease. *Thorax*, 36, 512-516 (1981)

643 Burnett JC, Kao PC, Hu DC et al. Atrial natriuretic peptide elevation in congestive heart failure in the human. *Science*, 231, 1145-1147 (1986)

644 Burnett MA, Morris ER, Bown EG et al. Plasma N-acetylglucosaminidase in type II diabetes measurement by MNP release on Cobas MIRA. *Proc ACB Natl Meet*, 90 (1992)

645 Burnett W, Ness TD. Serum amylase and acute abdominal disease. *Br Med J*, 2, 770 (1955)

646 Burnham TK. The immunofluorescent tumor imprint technique II. the frequency of antinuclear factors in connective tissue diseases and dermatoses. *Ann Intern Med*, 65, 9-19 (1966)

647 Burt RL. Combined and free plasma α-amino nitrogen in normal pregnancy and toxemia. *Am J Obstet Gynecol*, 65, 304 (1953)

648 Burt RW, Ratcliffe JG, Stack BHR et al. Serum biochemical markers in lung cancer. *Br J Cancer*, 37, 714-717 (1978)

649 Burton ME, Morris ER, Asti T et al. ELISA measurement of von Willebrand factor antigen in type II diabetic patients. *Proc ACB Natl Meet*, 91 (1992)

650 Bustamante JB et al. Zinc, copper and ceruloplasmin in arteriosclerosis. *Biomed Pharmacother*, 25, 244-245 (1976)

651 But I, Gorisek B. Preoperative value of CA 125 as a reflection of tumour grade in epithelial ovarian cancer. *Gynecol Oncol*, 63, 166-172 (1996)

652 Butler M, Santos M, Collier D et al. Protein C, protein S, and free protein S levels in patients with liver disease measured by ELISA. *Clin Chem*, 41, S170-S171 (1995)

653 Buts JP et al. One-hour blood xylose test: a reliable index of small bowel function. *J Pediatr*, 92, 729-33. (1978)

654 Bux J, Hofmann C, Welte K. Serum G-CSF levels are not increased in patients with antibody-induced neutropenia unless they are suffering from infectious diseases. *Br J Haematol*, 105, 616-617 (1999)

655 Buyalos RP, Bergman RN, Geffner ME et al. The influence of luteinizing hormone and insulin on sex steroids and sex hormone-binding globulin in the polycystic ovarian syndrome. *Fertil Steril*, 60, 626-633 (1993)

656 Buzaid AC, Sandler AB, Hayden CL et al. Correlation between lipid-associated sialic acid and tumor burden in melanoma. *Int J Biol Mark*, 9, 247-250 (1994)

657 Cacabelos R, Alvarex XA, Franco-Maside A et al. Serum tumor necrosis factor (TNF) in Alzheimer's disease and multi-infarct dementia. *Meth Find Exp Clin Pharmacol*, 16, 29-35 (1994)

658 Cadeau BJ et al. Increased incidence of placenta-like alkaline phosphatase activity in breast and genitourinary cancer. *Cancer Res*, 34, 729-732 (1974)

659 Caen J P et al. Congenital bleeding disorders with long bleeding times and normal platelet counts. *Am J Med*, 41, 4 (1966)

660 Cahan C, Decker MJ, Arnold JL et al. Diurnal variations in serum erythropoietin levels in healthy subjects and sleep apnea patients. *J Appl Physiol*, 72, 2112-2117 (1992)

661 Caillol N, Pasqualini E, Mas E, et al. Pancreatic bile-salt-dependent lipase activity in serum of diabetic patients: is there a relationship with glycation? *Clin Sci*, 94, 181-188 (1998)

662 Callen IR, Limarz LR. Blood and bone marrow studies in renal disease. *Am J Clin Pathol*, 20, 3 (1950)

663 Calo L, D'Angelo A, Cantaro S, et al. Increased urinary $NO_2^-/NO_3^-/NO_3^-$ and cyclic guanosine monophosphate in patients with Bartter.s syndrome: relationship to vascular reactivity. *Am J Kid Dis*, 27, 784-789 (1996)

664 Calogero AE, Minacapilli G, Nicolosi AMG et al. Limited clinical usefulness of plasma corticotropin-releasing hormone, adrenocorticotropin and β-endorphin measurements as markers of lung cancer. *J Endocrinol Invest*, 15, 581-586 (1992)

665 Calvin S, Weinstein L, Witte MH et al. Plasma levels of fibronectin and prostacyclin metabolite in peripartum preeclamptic women. *Am J Perinatol*, 7, 125-129 (1990)

666 Calvo R et al. Acute hemolytic anemia due to anti-i: frequent cold agglutinins in infectious mononucleosis. *J Clin Invest*, 44, 1033 (1965)

667 Camacho J, Arnalich F, Zamorano AF et al. Serum erythropoietin levels in the anaemia of chronic disorders. *J Intern Med*, 229, 49-54 (1991)

668 Cameron JS et al. Membranoproliferative glomerulonephritis and persistent hypocomplementemia. *Br Med J*, 4, 7 (1970)

669 Cameron JS et al. Membranous nephropathy. In: Glomerulonephritis Morphology, Natural History and Treatment. pt i. *Kincaid-Smith P et al (eds)*, New York NY, John Wiley, 473 (1973)

670 Cameron OG, Lee MA, Curtis GC et al. Endocrine and physiological changes during 'spontaneous' panic attacks. *Psychoneuroendocrinology*, 12, 321-331 (1987)

671 Campana C, Regazzi MB, Buggia I, Molinaro M. Clinically significant drug interactions with cyclosporin. *Clin Pharmacokinet*, 30, 141-179 (1996)

672 Campbell IM et al. Abnormal fatty acid composition and impaired oxygen supply in cystic fibrosis patients. *Pediatrics*, 57, 480-486 (1976)

673 Campra JL, Reynolds TB. Alcoholic liver disease: clue to acute and chronic changes. *Consultant*, 67, 69 (1985)

674 Camu W, Billiard M, Baldy-Moulinier M. Fasting plasma and CSF amino acid levels in amyotrophic lateral sclerosis: a subtype analysis. *Acta Neurol Scand*, 88, 51-55 (1993)

675 Candel S et al. Serum amylase and serum lipase in mumps. *Ann Intern Med*, 25, 88-96 (1946)

676 Candito M, Askenazy F, Myquel M, et al. Tryptophanemia and tyrosinemia in adolescents with impulsive behavior. *Int Clin Psychopharmacol*, 8, 129-132 (1993)

677 Candito M, Pringuey D, Iordache A et al. Circadian variation in total plasma tryptophan. Antidepressant treatment: drugs and phase advance. *Life Sci*, 50, PL71-PL74 (1992)

678 Canellos GP. Chronic granulocytic leukemia. *Med Clin North Am*, 60, 1001-1018 (1976)

679 Canivet E, Lavaud S, Wong T et al. Cuprophane but not synthetic membrane induces increases in serum tumor necrosis factor-α levels during hemodialysis. *Am J Kid Dis*, 23, 41-46 (1994)

680 Cannon JG, Friedberg JS, Gelfand JA et al. Circulating interleukin-1 beta and tumor necrosis factor-α concentrations after burn injury in humans. *Crit Care Med*, 20, 1414-1419 (1992)

681 Cantin B, Gagnon F, Moorjani S, et al. Lipoprotein(a) as an independent risk factor for ischemic heart disease in men. *J Am Coll Cardiol*, 31, 519-525 (1998)

682 Cantin B, Moorjani S, Dagenais GR et al. Lipoprotein(a) distribution in a French Canadian population and its relation to intermittent claudication (The Quebec cardiovascular study). *Am J Cardiol*, 75, 1224-1228 (1995)

683 Cantin M, Garcia R, Thibault G et al. Atrial natriuretic factor in experimental and human hypertension. *Eur Heart J*, 9, 21-27 (1988)

684 Cantini F, Arcangeli A, Bellandi F et al. Serum osteocalcin and diabetes mellitus. *Minerva Med*, 83, 129-133 (1992)

685 Caplan A, Gross S. Hematologic and serologic studies in cystic fibrosis. *J Pediatr*, 73, 540 (1968)

686 Capocaccia L et al. Octopamine and ammonia plasma levels in hepatic encephalopathy. *Clin Chim Acta*, 75, 99-105 (1977)

687 Caprilli R et al. Blood pH: a test for assessment of severity in proctocolitis. *Gut*, 17, 763-769 (1976)

688 Caramona MM, Cotrim MD, Ribeiro CF, Macedo T. Monoamine oxidase activity in blood platelets of migraine patients. *J Neural Trans*, 32, Suppl, 161-164 (1990)

689 Caraway W T. Chemical and diagnostic specificity of laboratory tests. *Am J Clin Pathol*, 37, 445-459 (1962)

690 Carballo-Dieguez A, Sahs J, Goetz R. The effect of methadone on immunological parameters among HIV-positive and HIV-negative drug users. *Am J Drug Alcohol Abuse*, 20, 317-329 (1994)

691 Cardenal A, Masuda I, Ono W, et al. Serum nucleotide pyrophosphohydrolase activity; elevated levels in osteoarthritis, calcium pyrophosphate crystal deposition disease, scleroderma and fibromyalgia. *J Rheumatol*, 25, 2175-2180 (1998)

692 Carlson K, Ljunghall S, Simonsson B et al. Serum osteocalcin concentrations in patients with multiple myeloma - correlation with disease stage and survival. *J Intern Med*, 231, 133-137 (1992)

693 Carlson LA, Holmquist L, Lindholm M. Plasma lipid metabolism at trauma: Appearance of characteristic apolipoproteins in high density lipoproteins. *Acta Chir Scand*, 150, 87-106 (1984)

694 Carlsson LMS, Attie KM, Compton PG et al. Reduced concentration of serum growth hormone-binding protein in children with idiopathic short stature. *J Clin Endocrinol Metab*, 78, 1325-1330 (1994)

695 Carlstrom K, Pousette A, Stege R et al. Serum hormone levels in men with end stage renal disease. *Scand J Urol Nephrol*, 24, 75-78 (1990)

696 Carmel R.. Pepsinogens and other serum markers in pernicious anemia. *Am J Pathol*, 90, 442-445 (1988)

697 Carmelly Y, Samore M, Shoshany O, et al. Utility of clinical symptoms versus laboratory tests for evaluation of acute gastroenteritis. *Digest Dis Sci*, 41, 1749-1753 (1996)

698 Carpelan-Holmstrom M, Haglund C, Lundin J, et al. Preoperative serum levels of CA 242 and CEA predict outcome in colorectal cancer. *Eur J Cancer*, 32A, 1156-1161 (1996)

699 Carr ME Jr, Zekert SL. Protein S and C_4b-binding protein levels in patients with stroke: implications for protein S regulation. *Haemostasis*, 23, 159-167 (1993)

700 Carr RI et al. Antibodies to bovine γ globulin (BGG) and the occurrence of a BGG-like substance in systemic lupus erythematosus sera. *J Allerg Clin Immunol*, 50, 18-30 (1972)

701 Carr S, Layward E, Bevington A et al. Plasma amino acid profile in the elderly with increasing uraemia. *Nephron*, 66, 228-230 (1994)

702 Carraro P, Piebani M, Varagnolo MC et al. A new immunoassay for the measurement of myoglobin in serum. *J Clin Lab Anal*, 8, 70-75 (1994)

703 Carrella M et al. An evaluation of urinary D-glucaric acid excretion during acute hepatitis in man. *Am J Dig Dis*, 23, 18-22 (1978)

704 Carretta RF et al. Early diagnosis of venous thrombosis using ^{125}I-fibrinogen. *J Nucl Med*, 18, 5-10 (1977)

705 Carroccio A, Fontana M, Spagnuolo MI, et al. serum pancreatic enzymes in human immunodeficiency virus-infected children. *Scand J Gastroenterol*, 33, 998-1001 (1998)

706 Carroccio A, Iovanna JL, Iacono G, et al. Pancreatitis-associated protein in patients with celiac disease: serum levels and immunocytochemical localization in small intestine. *Digestion*, 58, 98-103 (1997)

707 Carson DA et al. IgG rheumatoid factor in subacute bacterial endocarditis: relationship to IgM rheumatoid factor and circulating immune complexes. *Clin Exp Immunol*, 31, 100-103 (1978)

708 Carter ND, Heath R, Jeffery S. Serum carbonic anhydrase-III in Duchenne dystrophy. *Lancet*, 2, 542 (1980)

709 Cartwright GE et al. Studies on free erythrocyte protoporphyrin plasma iron and plasma copper in normal and anemic subjects. *Blood*, 5, 501 (1948)

710 Cartwright GE, Gubler CJ, Bush JA, Wintrobe M. Studies on copper metabolism. XI Copper and iron metabolism in the nephrotic syndrome. *J Clin Invest*, 33, 685-698 (1954)

711 Carulli N et al. α-fetoprotein in chronic hepatitis. In: *Chronic Hepatitis.* Gentilini P et al (eds), Basel, Karger, 60-64 (1976)

712 Caruntu F et al. Passive hemagglutination and complement fixation reactions in the early diagnosis of mycoplasma pneumoniae infections. *Virologie*, 27, 229-235 (1976)

713 Casanueva FF, Dieguez C. Neuroendocrine regulation and actions of leptin. *Frontiers Neuroendocrinology*, 20, 317-363 (1999)

714 Casey LC, Balk RA, Bone RC. Plasma cytokine and endotoxin levels correlate with survival in patients with the sepsis syndrome. *Ann Intern Med*, 119, 771-778 (1993)

715 Casi MT, Bulatovic G, Orlic P et al. Serum amyloid A protein monitoring for early diagnosis of kidney allograft rejection. *Clin Biochem Rev*, 14, 211 (1993)

716 Casi MT, Coen D. Serum amyloid A and C-reactive protein in predicting postburn complications and fatal outcome in patients with severe burns. *Clin Biochem Rev*, 14, 211 (1993)

717 Casi MT, Dunovic S, Maric S. Acute phase proteins in children with urinary tract infections. *Clin Biochem Rev*, 14, 210 (1993)

718 Casi MT, Giojnaric-Spasic I, Surina B et al. Acute phase proteins in patients who developed acute myocardial infarction. *Clin Biochem Rev*, 14, 233 (1993)

719 Casi MT, Glojnaric-Spasic I, Roguljic A. Acute phase proteins as possible tumor markers. *Clin Biochem Rev*, 14, 211 (1993)

720 Casi MT, Husnjak-Coen D, Bolijkovac D et al. Serum amyloid A protein in patients with severe burns in predicting possible outcomes. *Diag Lab*, 27, 156 (1991)

721 Casi MT, Pauro M. Acute phase proteins in bacterial infections. *Clin Biochem Rev*, 14, 211 (1993)

722 Casl MT, Surina B, Glojnaric-Spasic I et al. Serum amyloid A protein in patients with acute myocardial infarction. *Ann Clin Biochem*, 32, 196-200 (1995)

723 Casper RC, Schoeller DA, Kushner R et al. Total daily energy expenditure and activity level in anorexia nervosa. *Am J Clin Nutr*, 53, 1143-1150 (1991)

724 Cass RM et al. Immunoglobulins G, A, and M in systemic lupus erythematosus. relationship to serum complement titer, latex titer, antinuclear antibody and manifestations of clinical disease. *Ann Intern Med*, 69, 749 (1968)

725 Cassader M, Ruiu G, Gambino R, et al. Apolipoprotein H levels in diabetic subjects: correlation with cholesterol levels. *Metabolism*, 46, 522-525 (1997)

726 Cassader M, Ruiu G, Gambino R et al. Lipoprotein-apolipoprotein changes in renal transplant recipients: a 2-year follow-up. *Metabolism*, 40, 922-925 (1991)

727 Casslen B, Bossmar T, Lecander I et al. Plasminogen activators and plasminogen activator inhibitors in blood and tumour fluids of patients with ovarian cancer. *Eur J Cancer*, 30A, 1302-1309 (1994)

728 Castaldo G, Oriani G, Cimino L et al. Total discrimination of peritoneal malignant ascites from cirrhosis- and hepatocarcinoma-associated ascites by assays of ascitic cholesterol and lactate dehydrogenase. *Clin Chem*, 40, 478-483 (1994)

729 Castaneda MR, Guerrero G. Studies on the leucocytic picture in brucellosis. *J Infect Dis*, 78, 43 (1946)

730 Castelino DJ, McNair P, Kay TWH. Lymphocytopenia in a hospital population - what does it signify. *Aust NZ J Med*, 27, 170-174 (1997)

731 Castelli W, Garrison RJ, Wilson PWF. Incidence of coronary heart disease and lipoprotein cholesterol levels. *J Am Med Ass*, 256, 2835 (1986)

732 Castelli WP et al. HDL cholesterol and other lipids in coronary heart disease: the cooperative lipoprotein phenotyping study. *Circulation*, 55, 767-772 (1977)

733 Castells S, Yasamura S, Fusi MA. Plasma osteocalcin levels in osteogenesis imperfecta. *J Pediatr*, 109, 88-91 (1986)

734 Castro-Bello F et al. High serum glutamic acid levels in patients with carcinoma of the pancreas. *Digestion*, 14, 360-363 (1976)

735 Castro-Gago M, Eiris-Punal J, Novo-Rodriguez MI, et al. Serum carnitine levels in epileptic children before and during treatment with valproic acid, carbamazepine, and phenobarbital. *J Child Neurol*, 13, 546-549 (1998)

736 Catalan R, Sahuquillo J, Poca MA et al. Neuropeptide Y cerebrospinal fluid levels in patients with normal pressure hydrocephalus syndrome. *Biol Psychiat*, 36, 61-63 (1994)

737 Catalano C, Torffvit O. Urinary excretion of Tamm-Horsfall protein in normotensive, normo-albuminuric type 1 diabetic patients. *Nephron*, 72, 436-441 (1996)

738 Catalano M, Aronica A, Carzaniga G et al. Serum lipids and apolipoproteins in patients with essential hypertension. *Atherosclerosis*, 87, 17-22 (1991)

739 Catalona WJ, Partin AW, Slawin KM, et al. Use of the percentage of free prostate-specific antigen to enhance differentiation of prostate cancer from benign prostatic disease: a prospective multicenter clinical trial. *J Am Med Ass*, 279, 1542-1547 (1998)

740 Cattaneo R et al. Peripheral T-lymphocytes in juvenile-onset diabetics (JOD) and in maturity-onset diabetics (MOD). *Diabetes*, 25, 223-226 (1976)

741 Caufriez A, Abramowicz D, Vanherweghem et al. *J Endocrinol Invest*, 16, 691-696 (1993)

742 Caughney J E, Myrianthopoulos N C. *Dystrophia Myotonica and related Disorders*. Springfield IL, CC Thomas (1973)

743 Cauley JA, Gutai JP, Kuller LH et al. The epidemiology of serum sex hormones in postmenopausal women. *Am J Epidemiol*, 129, 1120-1131 (1989)

744 Cavaillon J-M, Poignet J-L, Fitting C et al. Serum interleukin-6 in long term hemodialyzed patients. *Nephron*, 60, 307-313 (1992)

745 Cavill I, Jacobs A, Worwood M. Diagnostic method for iron status. *Ann Clin Biochem*, 23, 168-171 (1986)

746 Ceballos I, Chauveau P, Guerrin V et al. Early alterations of plasma free amino acids in chronic renal failure. *Clin Chim Acta*, 188, 101-108 (1990)

747 Celik I, Akalin S, Erbas T. Serum levels of interleukin 6 and tumor necrosis factor-α in hyperthyroid patients before and after propylthiouracil treatment. *Eur J Endocrinol*, 132, 668-672 (1995)

748 Centis F, Delfini C, Annibali M, et al. Increased serum levels of circulating intercellular adhesion molecule 1 predict the risk of graft rejection after bone marrow transplantation for thalassemia. *Bone Marrow Transplant*, 20, 125-128 (1997)

749 Cerceo E, Elloso CA. Factors affecting the radioimmunoassay of digoxin. *Clin Chem*, 18, 539 (1972)

750 Ceriello A, Taboga C, Giacomello R et al. Fibrinogen plasma levels as a marker of thrombin activation in diabetes. *Diabetes*, 43, 430-432 (1994)

751 Cernacek P, Stewart DJ. Immunoreactive endothelin in human plasma: marked elevations in patients in cardiogenic shock. *Biochem Biophys Res Commun*, 161, 562-567 (1989)

752 Cerny A, Katzenstein-Sutro E. Die paroxysmale lahmung. *Arch Neurol*, 70, 259 (1952)

753 Cetkovsky P, Koza V, Cepelak V et al. Haemostasis in patients with acute myeloid leukemia treated with intermediate dose of cytosine arabinoside and mitoxantrone: the influence of chemotherapy, infection and remission status on haemostasis. *Fibrinolysis*, 9, 165-169 (1995)

754 Chadwick SJD, Mowbray JF, Dudley HAF. Plasma fibronectin and complement in surgical patients. *Br J Surg*, 71, 718-720 (1984)

755 Chakrabarty S, Huang S, Moskal TL et al. Elevated serum levels of transforming growth factor-α in breast cancer patients. *Cancer Lett*, 79, 157-160 (1994)

756 Chalasani N, Clark WS, Wison CM. Blood urea nitrogen to creatinine concentration in gastrointestinal bleeding: a reappraisal. *Am J Gastroenterol*, 92, 1796-1799 (1997)

757 Challa A, Moulas A, Cholevas V, et al. Vitamin D metabolites in patients with coeliac disease. *Eur J Pediatr*, 157, 262-263 (1998)

758 Chambers JP et al. Determination of serum acid phosphatase in Gaucher's disease using 4-methylumbelliferyl phosphate. *Clin Chim Acta*, 80, 67-77 (1977)

759 Chamorro A, Vila N, Ascaso C, et al. Early prediction of stroke severity: role of the erythrocyte sedimentation rate. *Stroke*, 26, 573-576 (1995)

760 Champeyroux J, Moinade S. α-2 Macroglobulinemie chez les diabetiques ayant une retinopathie. *Nouv Presse Med*, 8, 135 (1979)

761 Chan A, Wong F, Arumanayagam M. Serum ultrafiltrable copper, total copper and caeruloplasmin concentrations in gynaecological carcinomas. *Ann Clin Biochem*, 30, 545-549 (1993)

762 Chan CH. Primary carcinoma of the liver. *Med Clin North Am*, 59, 989-994 (1975)

763 Chan CHS, Chan TYK, Shek ACC et al. Severe hypercalcemia associated with miliary tuberculosis. *J Trop Med Hyg*, 97, 180-182 (1994)

764 Chan DW, Beveridge RA, Bhargava A et al. Breast cancer marker CA549: a multicenter study. *Am J Clin Pathol*, 101, 465-470 (1994)

765 Chan DW, Beveridge RA, Bruzek DJ et al. Monitoring breast cancer with CA 549. *Clin Chem*, 34, 2000-2004 (1988)

766 Chan DW, Miksch D, Bruzek D et al. Truquant BR - a marker for breast cancer. *Clin Chem*, 39, 1194 (1993)

767 Chan JCN, Butt A, Ho CS, et al. Relation between blood pressure and serum concentration of oubain-like substance in non-insulin dependent diabetes mellitus. *Lancet*, 351, 266 (1998)

768 Chan KM, Ladenson JH. Increased creatine kinase MB in the absence of acute myocardial infarction. *Clin Chem*, 32, 2044-2051 (1986)

769 Chan KN, Phillips AD, Walker-Smith JA et al. Serum interleukin-2 receptor in infants and young children. *Acta Paediat*, 84, 151-156 (1995)

770 Chan PCK, Wei DCC, Tam SCF et al. Post-transplant erythrocytosis: Role of erythropoietin and male sex hormones. *Nephrol Dial Transplant*, 7, 137-142 (1992)

771 Chan V, Yeung CK, Chan TK. Antithrombin III and fibrinogen degradation product (fragment E) in diabetic nephropathy. *J Clin Pathol*, 35, 661-666 (1982)

772 Chanarin I. *The Megaloblastic Anemias*. Oxford, Blackwell (1979)

773 Chanarin I. *The Megaloblastic Anemias*. Philadelphia PA, FA Davis (1969)

774 Chandrasekhar AJ, Palatao A, Dubin A et al. Pleural fluid lactic acid dehydrogenase activity and protein content. *Arch Intern Med*, 123, 48-50 (1969)

775 Chang C-C, Huang C-N, Chuang L-M. Autoantibodies to thyroid peroxidase in patients with type I diabetes in Taiwan. *Eur J Endocrinol*, 139, 44-48 (1998)

776 Chang F-Y, Lai K-H, Wang T-F et al. Serum pepsinogen I levels of gastric ulcer patients are determined by the location of the ulcer crater. *Gastroenterol Jpn*, 27, 9-14 (1992)

777 Chang KD, Keck Jr PE, Stanton SP, et al. Differences in thyroid function between bipolar manic and mixed states. *Biol Psychiat*, 43, 730-733 (1998)

778 Chang S. Measurement of complement of patient with bone sarcoma. *Jpn J*, 37, 97-106 (1967)

779 Chang S-C, Hsu Y-T, Chen Y-C et al. Usefulness of soluble interleukin-2 receptor in differentiating tuberculous and carcinomatous pleural effusions. *Arch Intern Med*, 154, 1097-1101 (1994)

780 Channick BJ et al. Suppressed plasma renin activity in hypertension. *Arch Intern Med*, 123, 131 (1969)

781 Chao J, Schmaier A, Chen L-M, et al. Kallistatin, a novel human tissue kallikrein inhibitor: levels in body fluids, blood cells, and tissues in health and disease. *J Lab Clin Med*, 127, 612-620 (1996)

782 Chapel HM, Esiri MM, Wilcock GK. Immunoglobulin and other proteins in the cerebrospinal fluid of patients with Alzheimer's disease. *J Clin Pathol*, 37, 697-699 (1984)

783 Chaplin ER. Fetal hemoglobin in the diagnosis of neonatal subarachnoid hemorrhage. *Pediatrics*, 58, 751-54 (1976)

784 Chapman CS, Akhtar N, Campbell S et al. The use of D-dimer assay by enzyme immunoassay and latex agglutination techniques in the diagnosis of deep venous thrombosis. *Clin Lab Haematol*, 12, 37-42 (1990)

785 Chapman JC. Reference values (normal range) of seven proteins in serum and EDTA plasma: a comparison. *Can J Med Technol*, 42, 29-30 (1980)

786 Chapman MK, Prabhudesai M, Erdman JW Jr. Vitamin A status of alcoholics upon admission and after two weeks of hospitalization. *J Am Coll Nutr*, 12, 77-83 (1993)

787 Chappell P, Leckman J, Goodman W, et al. Elevated cerebrospinal fluid corticotropin-releasing factor in Tourette's syndrome: comparison to obsessive compulsive disorder and normal controls. *Biol Psychiatr*, 39, 776-783 (1996)

788 Chapple ILC, Mason GI, Garner I, et al. Enhanced chemiluminescent assay for measuring the total antioxidant capacity of serum, saliva and cervicular fluid. *Ann Clin Biochem*, 34, 412-421 (1997)

789 Charhon SA, Delmas PD, Malaval L et al. Serum bone Gla-protein in renal osteodystrophy: comparison with bone histomorphometry. *J Clin Endocrinol Metab*, 63, 892-897 (1986)

790 Charlesworth JA et al. Acute hepatitis: significance of changes in complement components. *Clin Exp Immunol*, 28, 496-501 (1977)

791 Chase HP et al. Increased prostaglandin synthesis in childhood diabetes mellitus. *J Pediatr*, 94, 185-189 (1979)

792 Chase HP et al. Juvenile diabetes mellitus and serum lipids and lipoprotein levels. *Am J Dis Child*, 130, 1113-1117 (1976)

793 Chattehee A et al. Renal functional status and serum electrolyte changes in hepatic failure. *J Ass Physicians India*, 25, 475-482 (1977)

794 Chatterjee T et al. Studies on plasma fibrinogen level in pre-eclampsia and eclampsia. *Experientia*, 34, 562-563 (1978)

795 Chaudhuri S et al. Study of serum lipids and enzymes in myocardial infarction and hypertension. *Thromb Res*, 11, 163-170 (1977)

796 Chauveau P, Chadefaux B, Coude M et al. Hyperhomocysteinemia, a risk factor for atherosclerosis in chronic uremic patients. *Kidney Int*, 41, Suppl, S72-S77 (1993)

797 Check JH, Nowroozi K, Winkel CA et al. Serum CA 125 levels in early pregnancy and subsequent spontaneous abortion. *Obstet Gynecol*, 75, 742-744 (1990)

798 Chen C-J, Sikes CR, Dziewanowska ZE et al. The influence of blood chemistry on T4 and FT4I in major depression. *J Affect Disord*, 20, 159-163 (1990)

799 Chen DS et al. Serum α-fetoprotein in hepatocellular carcinoma. *Cancer*, 40, 779-783 (1977)

800 Chen HS, Lin HD. Serum IGF-I and IGFBP-3 levels for the assessment of disease activity of acromegaly. *J Endocrinol Invest*, 22, 98-103 (1999)

801 Chen JW et al. Radiation-induced change in serum and urinary amylase levels in man. *Radiat Res*, 54, 141 (1973)

802 Chen LS, Ito T, Ogawa K et al. Plasma concentrations of 6-keto-prostaglandin F(1α), thromboxane B_2 and platelet aggregation in patients with essential hypertension. *Jpn Heart J*, 25, 1001-1009 (1984)

803 Chen M-F, Chang C-L, Liou S-Y. Increase in resting levels of superoxide anion in the whole blood of uremic patients on chronic hemodialysis. *Blood Purif*, 16, 290-300 (1998)

804 Chen S-Y, Sickel M, Kline S et al. An automated chemiluminescent immunoassay for deoxypyridinoline: a specific urinary marker for bone reabsorption. *Clin Chem*, 41, S40 (1995)

805 Chen WC, Yamaoka K, Nakajima S et al. Evaluation of vitamin D-binding protein and vitamin D metabolite loss in children on continuous ambulatory peritoneal dialysis. *Bone Miner*, 17, 389-398 (1992)

806 Chen YDI, Varasteh BB, Reaven GM. Plasma lactate concentration in obesity and type 2 diabetes. *Diabete Metab*, 19, 348-354 (1993)

807 Chen YX, Wang SC, Zhao GN et al. Plasma endothelin levels in cirrhotic patients and their correlation with atrial natriuretic peptide. *Chin Med J (Engl)*, 106, 643-646 (1993)

808 Cheng GJ. Effect of menopause and sex hormones on plasma lipids. *Chun Hua Fu Chan Ko Tsa Chih*, 25, 202-204 (1990)

809 Cheng J, Chen JM. Plasma superoxide dismutase measurement in children with viral hepatitis. *Free Rad Res Comm*, 12-13, 669-673 (1991)

810 Chernoff AI. The clinical, hematologic and genetic characteristics of the hemoglobin E syndromes. *J Lab Clin Med*, 47, 455 (1956)

811 Chesley LC. *Hypertensive Disorders in Pregnancy*. New York NY, Appleton-Century-Crofts (1978)

812 Cheung CK, Pansear NS, Haines C et al. Immunoassay of a tartrate-resistant acid phosphatase in serum. *Clin Chem*, 41, 679-686 (1995)

813 Chiarelli A, Casadei A, Pornaro E et al. Alanine and aspartate aminotransferase serum levels in burned patients: a long-term study. *J Trauma*, 27, 790-794 (1987)

814 Chiba S, Sugiyama T, Matsumoto H, et al. Antibodies against Helicobacter pylori were detected in the cerebrospinal fluid obtained from patients with Guillain-Barre syndrome. *Ann Neurol*, 44, 686-688 (1998)

815 Child JA, Spati B, Illingworth S. Serum β_2-microglobulin and C-reactive protein in the monitoring of lymphomas: findings in a multicenter study and experience in selected patients. *Cancer*, 45, 318-326 (1980)

816 Childs PA, Rodin I, Martin NJ , et al. Effect of fluoxetine on melatonin in patients with seasonal affective disorder and matched controls. *Br J Psychiat*, 166, 196-198 (1995)

817 Chillar RK, Desforges JF. Red cell organic phosphates in patients with chronic renal failure on maintenance haemodialysis. *Br J Haematol*, 26, 549 (1974)

818 Chinayon S, Harnkanitwatana C, Pasatrat S et al. Serum magnesium level in female diabetic patients. *Clin Biochem Rev*, 14, 219 (1993)

819 Chiodera P, Volpi R, Capretti L et al. Effect of estrogen and insulin-induced hypoglycemia on plasma oxytocin levels in bulimia and anorexia nervosa. *Metabolism*, 40, 1226-1230 (1991)

820 Chiricu TAI et al. Urinary 17-ketosteroid fractions in young patients with breast cancer. *Endocrinologie*, 16, 135-137 (1978)

821 Chitab MS et al. Nitroblue tetrazolium test in tuberculous and pyogenic meningitis. *Ind J Pediatr*, 13, 447-450 (1976)

822 Chittar HS, Nihalani KD, Varthakavi PK et al. Lipid peroxide levels in diabetics with micro- and macro-angiopathies. *J Nutr Biochem*, 5, 442-445 (1994)

823 Chodos DDF, Ely RS, Kelly VC. Paper electrophoresis of duodenal fluid from patients with cystic fibrosis. *Proc Soc Exp Biol Med*, 99, 775 (1952)

824 Choi EKK, Gatenby PA, McGill NW et al. Autoantibodies to type II collagen: occurence in rheumatoid arthritis, other arthritides, autoimmune connective tissue diseases, and chronic inflammatory syndromes. *Ann Rheum Dis*, 47, 313-322 (1988)

825 Choi J-H, Oh JY, Ryu SK, et al. Detection of epidermal growth factor receptor in the serum of gastric carcinoma patients. *Cancer*, 79, 1879-1883 (1997)

826 Chopia D, Clerken EP. Hypercalcemia and malignant disease. *Med Clin North Am*, 59, 229-239 (1977)

827 Chopra TJ et al. Reciprocal changes in serum concentrations of 3,3',5-triiodothyronine (T3) in systemic illnesses. *J Clin Endocrinol Metab*, 41, 1043-1049 (1975)

828 Choremis C, et al. Amino-acid tolerance curves and amino-aciduria in Cooley's and sickle cell anemias. *J Clin Pathol*, 12, 245 (1959)

829 Chow CC, Mak TWL, Chan CHS et al. Euthyroid sick syndrome in pulmonary tuberculosis before and after treatment. *Ann Clin Biochem*, 32, 385-391 (1995)

830 Chow N-H, Chang C-J, Cheng P-E et al. Clinical significance of urinary ferritin excretion in patients with transitional cell carcinoma. *Clin Sci*, 88, 701-706 (1995)

831 Chow N-H, Liu H-S, Chang C-J, et al. Urinary excretion of transforming growth factor-α in patients with transitional cell carcinoma. *Anticancer Res*, 18, 2053-2058 (1998)

832 Chowdhury AR et al. Gastrointestinal protein loss during ethanol ingestion. *Gastroenterology*, 72, 37 (1977)

833 Christeff N, Carli A, Benassayag C et al. Relationship between changes in serum estrone levels and outcome in human males with septic shock. *Circ Shock*, 36, 249-255 (1992)

834 Christensen L, Hagen C, Henriksen JE, Haug E. Elevated levels of sex hormones and sex hormone binding globulin in male patients with insulin dependent diabetes mellitus. *Dan Med Bull*, 44, 547-50 (1997)

835 Christensen NJ. Plasma catecholamines in long-term diabetics with and without neuropathy and in hypophysectomized subjects. *J Clin Invest*, 51, 779 (1972)

836 Christensson T et al. Serum lipids before and after parathyroidectomy in patients with primary hyperparathyroidism. *Clin Chim Acta*, 78, 411-415 (1977)

837 Christian CL et al. Systemic lupus erythematosus. cryoprecipitation of sera. *J Clin Invest*, 42, 823-829 (1963)

838 Christiansen I, Gidlof C, Kalkner K-M, et al. Elevated serum levels of soluble ICAM-1 in non-Hodgkin's lymphomas correlate with tumour burden, disease activity and other prognostic markers. *Br J Haematol*, 92, 639-646 (1996)

839 Christiansen M, Andersen JR, Torning J et al. Serum α-fetoprotein and alcohol consumption. *Scand J Clin Lab Invest*, 54, 215-220 (1994)

840 Christiansen M, Hogdall CK, Brihmer C. α-Fetoprotein and the acute phase response. A study using acute pelvic inflammatory disease as a model system. *Clin Chim Acta*, 225, 71-79 (1995)

841 Chu C-M, Sheen I-S, Yeh C-T, et al. Serum levels of interferon-α and -γ in acute and chronic hepatitis B virus infection. *Dig Dis Sci*, 40, 2107-2112 (1995)

842 Chu et al. Comparative evaluation of serum acid phosphatase, urinary cholesterol, and androgens in diagnosis of prostatic cancer. *Urology*, 6, 291-294 (1975)

843 Chua, et al. Acid phosphatase levels in bone marrow: value in detecting early bone metastases from carcinoma of the prostate. *J Urol*, 103, 462-466 (1970)

844 Chuang L-Y, Hung W-C, Yang M-L et al. Urinary epidermal growth factor receptor-binding growth factors in patients with cancers of the digestive tract. *Clin Biochem*, 27, 485-489 (1994)

845 Chuang Y, Lin ATL, Chen K, et al. Paraneoplastic elevation of serum alkaline phosphatase in renal cell carcinoma: incidence and prognosis. *J Urol*, 158, 1684-1687 (1997)

846 Chung HC, Rha SY, Park JO, et al. Physiological and pathological changes of plasma urokinase-type plasminogen activator, plasminogen activator inhibitor-1, and urokinase-type plasminogen activator receptor levels in healthy females and breast cancer patients. *Breast Cancer Res Treat*, 49, 41-50 (1998)

847 Chung J, Kung M, Lin S, et al. Diagnostic value of C-reactive protein in children with perforated appendicitis. *Eur J Pediatr*, 155, 529-531 (1996)

848 Chung U-I, Tanaka Y, Fujita T. Association of interleukin-6 and hypoaldosteronism in patients with cancer. *New Engl J Med*, 334, 473 (1996)

849 Church JA et al. Routine laboratory determinations in pediatric allergic disease. *Ann Allergy*, 41, 136-139 (1978)

850 Churg J, Ehrenreich T. Membranous nephropathy. In: *Glomerulonephritis Morphology, Natural History and Treatment*. pt. i. Kincaid-Smith P et al (eds), New York NY, John Wiley, 443 (1973)

851 Chusid EL, Hirsch RL, Colcher H. Spectrum of hypertrophic gastropathy. *Arch Intern Med*, 114, 621-628 (1964)

852 Ciccarelli E, Grottoli S, Razzore P, et al. Hexarelin, a synthetic growth hormone releasing peptide, stimulates prolactin secretion in acromegalic but not in hyperprolactinaemic patients. *Clin Endocrinol*, 44, 67-71 (1996)

853 Cicognani C, Malavolti M, Morselli-Labate AM, et al. Serum lipid and lipoprotein patterns in patients with liver cirrhosis and chronic active hepatitis. *Arch Intern Med*, 157, 792-796 (1997)

854 Cid J, Lozano M. Hemoglobin levels and platelet counts after iron therapy in iron deficiency anemia. *Haematologica*, 83, 749 (1998)

855 Ciechanowicz A, Kawiak J, Miks B et al. Plasma prekallikrein levels in patients with hepatocellular carcinoma and liver cirrhosis: a pilot study. *Ann Clin Biochem*, 30, 445-448 (1993)

856 Clark BA, Halvorson L, Sachs B, et al. Plasma endothelin levels in preeclampsia: elevation and correlation with uric acid levels and renal impairment. *Am J Obstet Gynecol*, 166, 962-968 (1992)

857 Clark GWB, Ireland AP, Hagen JA, et al. Carcinoembryonic antigen measurements in the management of esophageal cancer: an indicator of subclinical recurrence. *Am J Surg*, 170, 597-601 (1995)

858 Clark PMS, Conway GS, Wong D. Hyperinsulinaemia in the polycystic ovary syndrome confirmed by immunometric assay for insulin. *Proc ACB Natl Meet*, 42 (1992)

859 Clarke GN, Stojanoff A, Cauchi MN et al. The immunoglobulin class of antispermatozoal antibodies in serum. *Am J Reprod Immunol*, 7, 143-147 (1985)

860 Clarke HGM et al. Serum proteins in normal pregnancy and mild pre-eclampsia. *Br J Obstet Gynaecol*, 78, 105-109 (1971)

861 Clemens JD, Herrick MV, Singer FR, Eyre DR. Evidence that serum NTx (collagen-type I N-telopeptides) can act as an immunochemical marker of bone resorption. *Clin Chem*, 43, 2058-2063 (1997)

862 Clements PJ, Peter JB, Agopian MS et al. Elevated serum levels of soluble interleukin 2 receptor, interleukin 2 and neopterin in diffuse and limited scleroderma: effects of chlorambucil. *J Rheumatol*, 17, 908-910 (1991)

863 Cline MJ. Anemia in macroglobulinemia. *Am J Med*, 34, 213 (1963)

864 Cline MJ, Berlin NJ. Anemia in Hodgkin's disease. *Cancer*, 16, 526 (1963)

865 Cline MJ, Golde D. Immune suppression of hematopoiesis. *Am J Med*, 64, 301-309 (1978)

866 Clodi M, Oberbauer R, Bondlaj G, et al. Urinary excretion of apolipoprotein(a) fragments in type I diabetes mellitus patients. *Metabolism*, 48, 369-372 (1999)

867 Cobert BL. Reye's syndrome. *Hosp Med*, 89 (1986)

868 Coe FL, Fupo JJ. Evidence for mild reversible hyperparathyroidism in distal renal tubular acidosis. *Arch Intern Med*, 135, 1485 (1975)

869 Coe JE, Aikawa JK. Cholesterol pleural effusion. *Arch Intern Med*, 108, 763-774 (1961)

870 Coen G, Mazzaferro S, Ballanti P et al. Plasma insulin-like growth factor-I and bone formation parameters in predialysis chronic renal failure. *Miner Elect Metab*, 17, 153-159 (1991)

871 Coffman JD, Cohen RA. Plasma levels of 5-hydroxytryptamine during sympathetic stimulation and in Raynaud's phenomenon. *Clin Sci*, 86, 269-273 (1994)

872 Coggins CL et al. Unpublished observations. *US Coop Study of Adult Idiopathic Nephrotic Syndrome* (1975)

873 Cohen AJ, Philips TM, Kessler CM. Circulating coagulation inhibitors in the acquired immunodeficiency syndrome. *Ann Intern Med*, 104, 175-180 (1986)

874 Cohen AS (ed). *Laboratory Diagnostic Procedures in Rheumatic Diseases.* Boston MA, Little, Brown Co (1967)

875 Cohen JA, Kaplan MM. The SGOT/SGPT ratio - an indicator of alcoholic liver disease. *Dig Dis Sci*, 24, 835-838 (1979)

876 Cohen KL. Metabolic, endocrine, and drug-induced interference with pituitary function tests: a review. *Metabolism*, 26, 1165-1177 (1977)

877 Cohen MK, Riggs MW, Brawn PN et al. Serum prostate-specific antigen levels in stage A1 prostatic cancer. *Am J Clin Pathol*, 100, 127-129 (1993)

878 Cohen S, Butcher GA. Comments on immunization. *Milit Med*, 134, 1191 (1969)

879 Cohick CB, Furst DE, Quagliata S et al. Analysis of elevated serum interleukin-6 levels in rheumatoid arthritis: correlation with erythrocyte sedimentation rate or C-reactive protein. *J Lab Clin Med*, 123, 721-727 (1994)

880 Colao A, Ferone D, Di Carno A, et al. Vasopressin levels in Cushing's disease: inferior petrosal sinus assay, response to corticotrophin-releasing hormone and comparison with patients without Cushing's disease. *Clin Endocrinol*, 45, 157-166 (1996)

881 Cole DEC, Landry DA, Boucher MJ et al. Sweat sulfate concentrations are decreased in cystic fibrosis. *Clin Chim Acta*, 135, 237-244 (1986)

882 Coleman C, Thompson JE, Bennion RS, et al. White blood cell count is a poor predictor of severity of disease in the diagnosis of appendicitis. *Am Surg*, 64, 983-985 (1998)

883 Coleman MP, Key TJ, Wang DY et al. A prospective study of obesity, lipids, apolipoproteins and ischemic heart disease in women. *Atherosclerosis*, 92, 177-185 (1992)

884 Coleman R, Mashiter G, Fogelman I et al. Osteocalcin: a potential marker of metastatic bone disease and respone to treatment. *Eur J Cancer Clin Oncol*, 24, 1211-1217 (1988)

885 Collazos J, Esteban C, Fernandez A. Neuron-specific enolase concentrations in serum in nonneoplastic patients with pneumonia. *Clin Chem*, 40, 266-267 (1994)

886 Collazos J, Genolla J, Ruibal A. CA 15.3 in nonmalignant liver diseases. *Int J Biol Mark*, 6, 188-192 (1991)

887 Collazos J, Genolla J, Ruibal A. Neuron-specific enolase concentrations in serum in benign liver diseases. *Clin Chem*, 37, 579-581 (1991)

888 Collazos J, Rodriguez J. Squamous cell carcinoma antigen in patients with cirrhosis. *Clin Chem*, 39, 548 (1993)

889 Collins GB, Brosnihan KB, Zuti RA et al. Neuroendocrine, fluid balance, and thirst responses to alcohol in alcoholics. *Alcohol Clin Exp Res*, 16, 228-233 (1992)

890 Collinson PO, Hadcocks L, Foo Y, et al. Cardiac troponins in patients with renal dysfunction. *Ann Clin Biochem*, 35, 380-386 (1998)

891 Collinson PO, Kuan HL, Siu L et al. Troponin T as a marker of cardiac damage in patients with renal dysfunction. *Proc ACB Natl Meet*, 115 (1995)

892 Collinson PO, Stubbs PJ, Moseley D, et al. Troponin T for the differential diagnosis of skeletal and cardiac muscle damage. *Proc ACB Natl Meet*, 33 (1993)

893 Coll-Vincent B, Vilardell C, Font C, et al. Circulating soluble adhesion molecules in patients with giant cell arteritis: correlation between soluble intercellular adhesion molecule-1 (sICAM-1) concentrations and disease activity. *Ann Rheum Dis*, 58, 189-192 (1999)

894 Colombo ML, Girardo E, Gallo M et al. Carnitine and Down's syndrome. *Minerva Pediatr*, 41, 173-176 (1989)

895 Colomer R, Sole LA, Navarro M et al. CA 15-3: early results of a new breast cancer marker. *Anticancer Res*, 6, 683-684 (1986)

896 Colussi G, Macaluso M, Brunati C et al. Calcium metabolism and calciotropic hormone levels in Gitelman's syndrome. *Miner Elect Metab*, 20, 294-301 (1994)

897 Combes B et al. Disorders of the liver in pregnancy. In:. *Pathophysiology of Gestation.* Assali NS, Brinkman CR III (eds), New York NY, New Academic Press, I, 479-522 (1972)

898 Concanon JP et al. The CEA assays in bronchogenic carcinoma. *Am J Proctol*, 34, 184 (1974)

899 Condie R G. A serial study of coagulation factors XII, XI and X in plasma in normal pregnancy and in pregnancy complicated by pre-eclampsia. *Br J Obstet Gynaecol*, 83, 636-39 (1976)

900 Conn JW, *Conn. Current Diagnosis. 4th edition*, Philadelphia PA, WB Saunders (1974)

901 Connelly KG, Moss M, Parsons PE, et al. Serum ferritin as a predictor of the acute respiratory distress syndrome. *J Respir Crit Care Med*, 155, 21-25 (1997)

902 Connors MH, Jefferson I, Dunger DB, et al. Diminished thyroxine-binding globulin in pubertal diabetic children. *Diabetes Care*, 19, 246-248 (1996)

903 Conrozier T, Saxne T, Fan CSS, et al. Serum concentrations of cartilage oligomeric matrix protein and bone sialoprotein in hip osteoarthritis: a one year prospective study. *Ann Rheum Dis*, 57, 527-532 (1998)

904 Consensus Conference. Office for Medical Applications of Research, National Institutes of Health: diagnosis and treatment of Reye's syndrome. *J Am Med Ass*, 246, 2441-2444 (1981)

905 Constantinescu CS, Goodman DBP, Grossman RI, et al. Serum angiotensin-converting enzyme in multiple sclerosis. *Arch Neurol*, 54, 1012-1015 (1997)

906 Contacos C, Barter PJ, Vrga L, Sullivan DR. Cholesteryl ester transfer in hypercholesterolaemia: fasting and postprandial studies with and without pravastatin. *Atherosclerosis*, 141, 87-98 (1998)

907 Conti A, Sartorio A, Ferrero S, et al. Modifications of biochemical markers of bone and collagen turnover during corticosteroid therapy. *J Endocrinol Invest*, 19, 127-130 (1996)

908 Contois JH, McNamara JR, Lammi-Keefe CL, et al. Reference intervals for plasma apolipoprotein A-I determined with a standardized commercial immunoturbidimetric assay: results from the Framingham offspring study. *Clin Chem*, 42, 507-514 (1996)

909 Contois JH, McNamara JR, Lammi-Keefe CL, et al. Reference intervals for plasma apolipoprotein B determined with a standardized commercial immunoturbidimetric assay: results from the Framingham offspring study. *Clin Chem*, 42, 515-523 (1996)

910 Controne G et al. Cerebrospinal fluid lactic acid levels in meningitis. *J Pediatr*, 91, 379-384 (1977)

911 Coodley EL. Enzyme profiles in the evaluation of pulmonary infarction. *J Am Med Ass*, 207, 1307-1309 (1969)

912 Coodley GO, Loveless MO, Nelson HD et al. Endocrine function in the HIV wasting syndrome. *J Acq Immune Defic Syndromes*, 7, 46-51 (1994)

913 Cook CD et al. Studies of respiratory physiology in children. *Pediatrics*, 24, 181 (1959)

914 Cook et al. Nonutility of measurement of serum γ-glutamyl transpeptidase activities in diagnosis of myocardial disease. *Clin Chem*, 19, 774-776 (1973)

915 Cook GC et al. Effect of systemic infection and raised serum IgG concentration on the D-xylose test. *Am J Gastroenterol*, 67, 570-573 (1977)

916 Cooke WT et al. Rickets, growth, and alkaline phosphatase in urban adolescents. *Br Med J*, 2, 293-297 (1974)

917 Cookson GH, Rimington C. Porphobilinogen. *Biochem J*, 57, 476 (1954)

918 Cookson JC, Silverstone T, Williams S et al. Plasma cortisol levels in mania: associated clinical ratings and changes during treatment with haloperidol. *Br J Psychiat*, 146, 498-502 (1985)

919 Coolen RB, Pragay DA, Nosanchuk JS et al. Elevation of brain-type creatine kinase in serum from patients with carcinoma. *Cancer*, 44, 1414-1418 (1979)

920 Cooley et al. Plasma acid phosphatase in idiopathic and secondary thrombocytopenias. *Arch Intern Med*, 119, 345-354 (1967)

921 Cooley HM, Melny BJ, Gleeson R, et al. Clinical and serological associations of anti-Ku antibody. *J Rheumatol*, 26, 563-567 (1999)

922 Coombes RC et al. Plasma immunoreactive calcitonin in patients with non-thyroid tumors. *Lancet*, 1, 1080 (1974)

923 Coombes RC, Powles TJ, Gazet J-C et al. Assessment of biochemical tests to screen for metastases in patients with breast cancer. *Lancet*, 1, 296-298 (1980)

924 Coombes RC, Powles TJ, Neville AM. Evaluation of biochemical markers in breast cancer. *Proc Roy Soc Med*, 70, 843-845 (1977)

925 Coombs FS et al. Renal function in patients with gout. *J Clin Invest*, 19, 525 (1940)

926 Coonrod JD et al. Complement levels in pneumococcal pneumonia. *Infect Immunol*, 18, 14-22 (1977)

927 Coonrod JD et al. Latex agglutination in the diagnosis of pneumococcal infection. *J Clin Microbiol*, 4, 168 (1976)

928 Cooper EH, Turner R, Geekie A et al. α-Globulins in the surveillance of colorectal cancer. *Biomedicine*, 24, 171-178 (1976)

929 Cooper GR, Myers GL, Smith J et al. Blood lipid measurements: variations and practical utility. *J Am Med Ass*, 267, 1652-1660 (1992)

930 Cooper LZ et al. Neonatal thrombocytopenic purpura and other manifestations of rubella contracted in utero. *Am J Dis Child*, 110, 416 (1965)

931 Cooper N. Personal communication. *Dept Molecular Immunol, Scripps Clinic and Research Foundation*, San Diego, CA (1981)

932 Cooperberg AA, Teitelbaum JI. The concentration of antihemophilic globulin (AHG) in patients with coronary artery disease. *Ann Intern Med*, 54, 899 (1961)

933 Copeland GD et al. Systemic lupus erythematosus: a clinical report of 47 cases with pathologic findings in 18. *Am J Med Sci*, 236, 318 (1958)

934 Corash L, Shafer B, Blaese RM. Platelet-associated immunoglobulin, platelet size and the effect of splenectomy in the Wiskott-Aldrich syndrome. *Blood*, 65, 1439 (1985)

935 Corboy J, Sutherland WH, Walker RJ et al. Cholesteryl ester transfer in patients with renal failure or renal transplants. *Kidney Int*, 46, 1147-1153 (1994)

936 Corder MP et al. Familial occurrence of von Willebrand's disease, thrombocytopenia, and severe gastrointestinal bleeding. *Am J Med Sci*, 265, 219 (1973)

937 Corica F, Allegra A, Buemi M, et al. Altered platelet magnesium and plasma and urinary soluble form of intercellular adhesion molecule I (sICAM-1) concentrations in insulin dependent diabetes mellitus (IDDM) patients with microalbuminuria. *Magnesium Res*, 9, 307-312 (1997)

938 Corlette MB et al. Amylase elevation attributable to an ovarian neoplasm. *Gastroenterology*, 74, 907-909 (1978)

939 Corral J, Miralles JM, Garcia-Pascual IJ et al. Increased serum N-acetyl-β-D-glucosaminidase and α-D-mannosidase activities in obese subjects. *Clin Investig*, 70, 880-884 (1992)

940 Corrigan DF et al. Parameters of thyroid function in patients with active acromegaly. *Metabolism*, 27, 209-216 (1978)

941 Corvetta A, Luchetti MM, Pomponio G et al. Interleukin-2, soluble interleukin-2 receptor and tumor necrosis factor in sera from patients with rheumatoid arthritis. *Res Clin Lab*, 20, 275-281 (1990)

942 Costello J, Franson RC, Landwehr K et al. Activity of phospholipase A_2 in plasma increases in uremia. *Clin Chem*, 36, 198-200 (1990)

943 Couchman S, Crook M, Tutt P et al. Plasma, platelet, erythrocyte and plasma ultrafiltrable magnesium in diabetes mellitus. *Proc ACB Natl Meet*, 101 (1994)

944 Coull BM, Malinow MR, Beamer N et al. Elevated plasma homocyst(e)ine concentration as a possible independent risk factor for stroke. *Stroke*, 21, 572-576 (1990)

945 Coulon-Brunet MP, Thenault D, Khalfon D et al. Immunofluorimetric determination of serum neuron-specific enolase and lung cancers. *Immuno-Anal Biol Spec*, 67-71 (1991)

946 Counts DR, Swirtsman H, Carlsson LM et al. The effect of anorexia nervosa and refeeding on growth hormone-binding protein, the insulin-like growth factors and the IGF-binding proteins. *J Clin Endocrinol Metab*, 75, 762-767 (1992)

947 Couper JJ, Bates DJ, Cocciolone R et al. Association of lipoprotein(a) with puberty in IDDM. *Diabetes Care*, 16, 869-880 (1993)

948 Courtois H, Levesque H, Baudot N et al. Clinical correlations and prognosis based on hyaluronic acid serum levels in patients with progressive systemic sclerosis. *Br J Dermatol*, 124, 423-428 (1991)

949 Couvaras JL, Gant NF, Kramer J et al. Plasma concentrations of γ-butyric acid throughout human gestation. *Hypertens Pregnancy*, 12, 153-162 (1993)

950 Cowden EA et al. Hyperprolactinemia in renal disease. *Clin Endocrinol*, 9, 241-248 (1978)

951 Cowden EA, Ratcliffe WA, Beastall GH et al. Laboratory assessment of prolactin status. *Ann Clin Biochem*, 16, 113-121 (1979)

952 Cowen PJ, Parry-Billings M, Newsholme EA. Decreased plasma tryptophan levels in major depression. *J Affect Disord*, 16, 27-31 (1989)

953 Cox DW, Hoeppner VH, Levison H. Protease inhibitors in patients with chronic obstructive pulmonary disease: the α_1-antitrypsin heterozygote controversy. *Am Rev Resp Dis*, 113, 601-606 (1976)

954 Cox IM, Campbell MJ, Dowson D. Red blood cell magnesium and chronic fatigue syndrome. *Lancet.*, 337, 757-760 (1991)

955 Cox R, Gyde OH, Leyland MJ. Serum ferritin levels in small cell lung cancer. *Eur J Clin Oncol*, 22, 831-835 (1986)

956 Craft AW et al. Serum ferritin in juvenile chronic polyarthritis. *Ann Rheum Dis*, 36, 271-273 (1977)

957 Cramp DG et al. Plasma triglyceride secretion and metabolism in chronic renal failure. *Clin Chim Acta*, 76, 237-241 (1977)

958 Crane GG et al. The role of plasma proteins in chronic expansion of plasma volume in tropical splenomegaly syndrome. III. the interrelationships of albumin, immunoglobulins and plasma volume. *Trans Roy Soc Trop Med Hyg*, 69, 212-220 (1975)

959 Crawhall JC et al. Elevation of serum creatine kinase in severe hypokalemic hyperaldosteronism. *Clin Biochem*, 9, 237-240 (1976)

960 Creage A, Belec L, Clair B, et al. Circulating transforming growth factor beta 1 (TGF-β) in Guillain-Barre syndrome: decreased concentrations in the early course and increase with motor function. *J Neurol Neurosurg Psychiat*, 64, 162-165 (1998)

961 Cremades MJ, Menendez R, Rubio V, Sanchis J. Fibronectin in bronchoalveolar lavage fluid in lung cancer: tumor or inflammatory marker? *Respiration*, 65, 178-182 (1998)

962 Crigler JF, Najjar VA. Congenital familial non-hemolytic jaundice with kernicterus. *Pediatrics*, 10, 169 (1952)

963 Crilly RG, Anderson C, Hogan D et al. Bone histomorphometry, bone mass, and related parameters in alcoholic males. *Calcif Tissue Int*, 43, 269-273 (1988)

964 Crisp WE et al. Serum glutamic oxaloacetic transminase levels in the toxemias of pregnancy. *Obstet Gynecol*, 13, 487-497 (1959)

965 Crocker AC et al. Niemann-Pick disease: a review of 18 patients. *Medicine*, 37, 1-95 (1951)

966 Crocker AC, Landing. Phosphatase studies in Gaucher's disease. *Metabolism*, 9, 341-362 (1960)

967 Croizat H. Circulating cytokines in sickle cell patients during steady state. *Br J Haematol*, 87, 592-597 (1994)

968 Crook M, Preston K, Lancaster I. Serum prostatic specific-antigen concentrations in acute myocardial infarction. *Clin Chem*, 43, 1670 (1997)

969 Crook M, Swaminathan R. Disorders of plasma phosphate and indications for its measurement. *Ann Clin Biochem*, 33, 376-396 (1996)

970 Crook MA, Tutt P, Pickup JC. Elevated serum sialic acid concentration in NIDDM and its relationship to blood pressure and retinopathy. *Diabetes Care*, 16, 57-60 (1993)

971 Crook MA, Yip J, Earle KE et al. Serum sialic acid, a risk factor for cardiovascular disease, is increased in IDDM patients with microalbuminuria and clinical proteinuria. *Diabetes Care*, 17, 305-310 (1994)

972 Crosby WH. Paroxysmal nocturnal hemoglobinuria. *Blood*, 15, 505 (1960)

973 Crosby WH. The metabolism of hemoglobin and bile pigment in hemolytic disease. *Am J Med*, 18, 112 (1955)

974 Crout et al. Sporotrichosis arthritis. *Ann Intern Med*, 86, 294 (1977)

975 Crum RL, Dominic W, Hansbrough JF et al. Cardiovascular and neurohumoral responses following burn injury. *Arch Surg*, 125, 1065-1069 (1990)

976 Crystal HA, Ortof E, Fishman WH et al. Serum vitamin B_{12} levels and incidence of dementia in a healthy elderly population: a report from the Bronx Longitudinal Aging Study. *J Am Geriatr Soc*, 42, 933-936 (1994)

977 Csazar A, Karadi I, Juhasz E et al. High lipoprotein (a) levels with predominance of high molecular weight apo (a) isoforms in patients with pulmonary embolism. *Eur J Clin Invest*, 25, 368-370 (1995)

978 Cucuianu M et al. Increased serum γ-glutamyltransferase in hypertriglyceridemia: comparison with serum pseudocholinesterase. *Clin Chim Acta*, 71, 419-427 (1976)

979 Cugini P, Battisi P, Di Palma L et al. Secondary aldosteronism documented by plasma renin and aldosterone circadian rhythm in subjects with kidney or heart transplantation. *Renal Fail*, 14, 69-76 (1992)

980 Cuigniez PH, Biesbrouck M, Van Hooren J. A simple and rapid nephelometric procedure for fibronectin. *Ann Clin Biochem*, 22, 514-518 (1985)

981 Cumming AD, Lambie AT. Urinary kallikrein excretion in chronic renal failure: Relationship to blood pressure and the acute effect of captopril. *Renal Fail*, 10, 161-167 (1987)

982 Cunningham JJ, Mearkle PL, Brown RG. Vitamin C: an aldolase reductase inhibitor that normalizes erythrocyte sorbitol in insulin-dependent diabetes mellitus. *J Am Coll Nutr*, 13, 344-350 (1994)

983 Cunningham RT, Morrow JI, Johnston CF et al. Serum neuron-specific enolase concentrations in patients with neurological disorders. *Clin Chim Acta*, 230, 117-124 (1994)

984 Cunningham SK, McKenna TJ. Adrenal androgen and glucocorticoid production in conditions of corticotropin excess. *Proc ACB Natl Meet*, 68 (1992)

985 Cuomo R, Dattilo M, Pumpo R et al. Nicotinamide methylation in patients with cirrhosis. *J Hepatol*, 20, 138-142 (1994)

986 Cush JJ, Splawski JB, Thomas R et al. Elevated interleukin-10 levels in patients with rheumatoid arthritis. *Arth Rheum*, 38, 96-104 (1994)

987 Cynober L, Desmoulins D, Lioret N et al. Significance of vitamin A and retinol binding protein serum levels after burn injury. *Clin Chim Acta*, 148, 247-253 (1985)

988 Czech W, Krutmann J, Schopf E et al. Serum eosinophil cationic protein (ECP) is a sensitive measure for disease activity in atopic dermatitis. *Br J Dermatol*, 126, 351-355 (1992)

989 Czech W, Schope E, Kapp A. Soluble E-selectin in sera of patients with atopic dermatitis and psoriasis - correlation with disease activity. *Br J Derm*, 134, 17-21 (1996)

990 Czekalski S, Widecka K, Gozdzik J et al. Atrial natriuretic peptide and cyclic guanosine monophosphate plasma concentrations in patients with thyrotoxicosis and atrial fibrillation. Effect of short-term methimazole therapy. *J Endocrinol Invest*, 17, 341-346 (1994)

991 Dacie JV. Autoimmune hemolytic anemia. *Arch Intern Med*, 135, 1293 (1975)

992 Dacie JV. Secondary or symptomatic hemolytic anemias. In: *The Haemolytic Anemias*. New York NY, Grune and Stratton, 908 (1967)

993 Dacie JV. *The Haemolytic Anaemias,* part IV. New York NY, Grune and Stratton (1967)

994 Dagg JH et al. The relationship of lead poisoning to acute intermittent porphyria. *Q J Med*, 34, 163 (1964)

995 Dahl-Jorgensen K. Biochemical markers of diabetic microangiography: past, present and future. *Horm Res*, 50 Suppl 1, 12-16 (1998)

996 Daily WH, Tonnesen AS, Allen SJ. Hypophosphatemia - Incidence, etiology, and prevention in the trauma patient. *Crit Care Med*, 18, 1210-1214 (1990)

997 Daito K, Suou T, Kawasaki H. Clinical significance of serum and urinary neopterin levels in patients with various liver diseases. *Am J Gastroenterol*, 87, 471-476 (1992)

998 Dajas F, Lista A, Barbeito L. High urinary norepinephrine excretion in major depressive disorders: effects of a new type of MAO inhibitor (Moclobemide, Ro 11-1163). *Acta Psychiat Scand*, 70, 432-437 (1984)

999 Daland GA et al. Hematologic observations in bacterial endocarditis. *J Lab Clin Med*, 48, 827 (1956)

1000 Dally S, Danan M, Buisine A et al. Increase of blood level in chronic alcoholism. Relationship to blood pressure. *Presse Med*, 15, 492-493 (1986)

1001 Dalovisia JR et al. Subacute thyroiditis with increased serum alkaline phosphatase. *Ann Intern Med*, 88, 505-507 (1978)

1002 Dalton DL. Elevated serum prostate-specific antigen due to acute bacterial prostatitis. *Urology*, 35, 373 (1990)

1003 Damas P, Ledoux D, Nys M et al. Cytokine serum level during sepsis in human: IL-6 as a marker of severity. *Ann Surg*, 215, 356-362 (1992)

1004 D'Amico G.. Clinical features and natural history in adults with IgA nephropathy. *Am J Kid Dis*, 12, 353 (1988)

1005 Damle SR et al. Studies on glycolytic enzymes in relation to cancer. *Ind J Cancer*, 11, 280-284 (1974)

1006 D'Amore PA, Brown RH Jr, Ku P-T et al. Elevated basic fibroblast growth factor in the serum of patients with Duchenne Muscular Dystrophy. *Ann Neurol*, 35, 362-365 (1994)

1007 Daneman D, Crompton CH, Balfe JW et al. Plasma prorenin as an early marker of nephropathy in diabetic (IDDM) adolescents. *Kidney Int*, 46, 1154-1159 (1994)

1008 Daniel et al. Rise of serum-acid phosphatase level following palpation of the prostate. *Lancet*, 262, 998-999 (1952)

1009 Daniel V, Pasker S, Weimer R, et al. Clinical relevance of interleukin-1 receptor antagonist plasma levels in renal transplant recipients. *Infusionsther Transfusionmed*, 25, 35-38 (1998)

1010 Daniel WL et al. Biochemical and genetic investigations of the de Lange syndrome. *Am J Dis Child*, 121, 401-405 (1971)

1011 Dantoine TF, Debord J, Charmes J-P, et al. Decrease of serum paraoxonase activity in chronic renal failure. *J Am Soc Nephrol*, 9, 2082-2088 (1998)

1012 D'Antona D, Wallace EM, Shearing C, et al. Inhibin A and pro-aC inhibin in Down syndrome and normal pregnancies. *Prenatal Diag*, 18, 1122-1126 (1998)

1013 Darai E, Vlastos G, Benifla JL, et al. Is maternal serum creatine kinase actually a marker for early diagnosis of ectopic pregnancy? *Eur J Obstet Gynaecol Reprod Biol*, 68, 25-27 (1996)

1014 Darbar D, Davidson NC, Gillespie N, et al. Diagnostic value of B-type natriuretic peptide concentrations in patients with acute myocardial infarction. *Am J Cardiol*, 78, 284-287 (1996)

1015 Dardamanis MA, Elisaf MS, Vasakos SA, et al. α-Amylase and isoamylase levels in renal transplant recipients compared to uremic patients. *Renal Fail*, 17, 715-719 (1995)

1016 Das BS, Mohanty S, Mishra K et al. Increased cerebrospinal fluid protein and lipid peroxidation products in patients with cerebral malaria. *Trans Roy Soc Trop Med Hyg*, 85, 733-734 (1991)

1017 Das BS, Thurnham DI, Das DB. Plasma α-tocopherol, retinol, and carotenoids in children with falciparum malaria. *Am J Clin Nutr*, 64, 94-100 (1996)

1018 Das I, Essali MA, de Belleroche J et al. Elevated platelet phosphatidylinositol biphosphate in medicated schizophrenics. *Schiz Res*, 12, 265-268 (1994)

1019 Dasgupta B, Corkill M, Kirkham B et al. Serial estimation of interleukin 6 as a measure of systemic disease in rheumatoid arthritis. *J Rheumatol*, 19, 22-25 (1992)

1020 Dasgupta B, Panayi GS. Interleukin-6 in serum of patients with polymyalgia rheumatica and giant cell arteritis. *Br J Rheumatol*, 29, 456-458 (1990)

1021 Dass A et al. Serum transaminases in toxaemia of pregnancy. *Br J Obstet Gynaecol*, 71, 727-734 (1964)

1022 D'Auria L, Cordiali Fei P, Pietravalle M, et al. The serum levels of sE-selectin are increased in patients with bullous pemphigoid or pemphigus vulgaris. Correlation with the number of skin lesions and recovery after corticosteroid therapy. *Br J Dermatol*, 137, 59-64 (1997)

1023 Davi G, Catalano I, Belevedre M et al. Effects of defibrotide on fibrinolytic activity in diabetic patients with stable angina pectoris. *Thromb Res*, 65, 211-220 (1992)

1024 Davidsohn E, Lee CL. The laboratory in the diagnosis of infectious mononucleosis (with additional notes on epidemiology, etiology, and pathogenesis). *Med Clin North Am*, 46, 225 (1962)

1025 Davidsohn I. *Clinical Diagnosis by Laboratory Methods.* Henry JB (ed), 16th edition, Philadelphia PA, WB Saunders (1979)

1026 Davidson E, Weinberger I, Rotenberg Z et al. Elevated serum creatine kinase levels: an early diagnostic sign of acute dissection of the aorta. *Arch Intern Med*, 148, 2184-2186 (1988)

1027 Davidson GP, Corey M, Morad-Hassel F et al. Immunoassay of serum conjugates of cholic acid in cystic fibrosis. *J Clin Pathol*, 33, 390-394 (1980)

1028 Davidson M, Davis KL. A comparison of homovanillic acid concentrations in schizophrenic patients and normal controls. *Arch Gen Psychiat*, 45, 561-563 (1988)

1029 Davies SF, Rohrbach MS, Thelen V et al. Elevated serum angiotensin-converting enzyme (SACE) activity in acute pulmonary histoplasmosis. *Chest*, 85, 307-310 (1984)

1030 Davies-Jones. Lactate dehydrogenase and glutamic oxalacetic transaminase of the cerebrospinal fluid in tumours of the central nervous system. *J Neurol Neurosurg Psychiatry*, 32, 324-327 (1969)

1031 Davignon J et al. Plasma lipids and lipoprotein patterns in angiographically graded atherosclerosis of the legs and in coronary heart disease. *Can Med Ass J*, 116, 1245-1250 (1977)

1032 Davis A, Kurdy N, Bowles SA et al. Changes in serum levels of total alkaline phosphatase and the bone isoenzyme following isolated tibial shaft fracture. *Proc ACB Natl Meet*, 64-65 (1995)

1033 Davis CA, Vallota EH, Forristal J. Serum complement levels in infancy: age related changes. *Pediatr Res*, 13, 1043-1046 (1979)

1034 Davis HL Jr, Brown RR, Leklem J. Tryptophan metabolism in breast cancer. Correlation with urinary steroid excretion. *Cancer*, 31, 1061-1064 (1973)

1035 Davis JW, Grandineti A, Waslien CI, et al. Observations on serum uric acid levels and the risk of idiopathic Parkinson's disease. *Am J Epidemiol*, 144, 480-484 (1996)

1036 Davis KL, Davidson M, Mohs RC et al. Plasma homovanillic acid concentration and the severity of schizophrenic illness. *Science*, 227, 1601-1602 (1985)

1037 Davis KM, Fish LC, Minaker KL, Elahi D. Atrial natriuretic peptide levels in the elderly: differentiating normal aging changes from disease. *J Gerontol*, 51A, M95-M101 (1996)

1038 Davis PJ. Ageing and endocrine function. *Clin Endocrinol Metab*, 8, 153-174 (1979)

1039 Davis PJ, Davis FB. Hyperthyroidism in patients over the age of 60. *Medicine*, 53, 161-181 (1974)

1040 Davis RE et al. Serum pyridoxal, folate, and vitamin B_{12} levels in institutionalized epileptics. *Epilepsia*, 16, 463-468 (1975)

1041 Davis TME, Li G-Q, Guo X-B et al. Serum ionized calcium, serum and intracellular phosphate, and serum parathormone concentrations in acute malaria. *Trans Roy Soc Trop Med Hyg*, 87, 49-53 (1993)

1042 Dawood MY, Khan-Dawood FS. Plasma insulin-like growth factor-I, CA-125, estrogen, and progesterone in women with leiomyomas. *Fertil Steril*, 61, 617-621 (1994)

1043 Day AP, Bellavia S, Jones OTG, Stansbie D. Effect of simvastatin therapy on cell membrane cholesterol content and membrane function as assessed by polymorphonuclear cell NADPH oxidase activity. *Ann Clin Biochem*, 34, 269-275 (1997)

1044 Day AP, Hillman S, Dieppe PA et al. Synovial fluid bone alkaline phosphatase levels in rheumatoid arthritis and osteoarthritis. *Proc ACB Natl Meet*, 65 (1995)

1045 De Bellis MD, Geracioti TD Jr, Altemus M et al. Cerebrospinal fluid monoamine metabolites in fluoxetine-treated patients with major depression and in healthy volunteers. *Biol Psychiat*, 33, 636-641 (1993)

1046 de Benedetti F, Massa M, Robbioni P et al. Correlation of serum interleukin-6 levels with joint involvement and thrombocytosis in systemic juvenile rheumatoid arthritis. *Arth Rheum*, 34, 1158-1163 (1991)

1047 de Boer H, Blok GJ, Voerman HJ et al. Serum lipid levels in growth hormone-deficient men. *Metabolism*, 43, 199-203 (1994)

1048 de Boer K, Lecander I, Ten Cate JW et al. Placental-type plasminogen activator inhibitor in preeclampsia. *Am J Obstet Gynecol*, 158, 518-522 (1988)

1049 de Bont ESJM, De Leu LHFM, Okken A et al. Increased plasma concentrations of interleukin-1 receptor antagonist in neonatal sepsis. *Pediatr Res*, 37, 626-629 (1995)

1050 de Bont ESJM, Martens A, van Raan J et al. Diagnostic value of plasma levels of tumor necrosis factor alpha (TNF-α) and interleukin-6 (IL-6) in newborns with sepsis. *Acta Paediat*, 83, 696-699 (1994)

1051 De Bruijn AM, Geers FCA, Hylkema RSAJ et al. Blood pressure and immunoglobulins. *Clin Sci*, 65, 665-667 (1983)

1052 de Bruijn HWA, ten Hoor KA, van der Zee AGJ. Serum and cystic fluid levels of soluble interleukin-2 receptor-α in patients with epithelial ovarian tumors are correlated. *Tumor Biol*, 19, 160-166 (1998)

1053 de Bruin TWA, van Barlingen H, van Linde-Sibenius Trip M et al. Lipoprotein(a) and apolipoprotein B plasma concentrations in hypothyroid, euthyroid, and hyperthyroid subjects. *J Clin Endocrinol Metab*, 76, 121-126 (1993)

1054 De Buyzere ML, De Scheerder IK, Delanghe JR et al. Measurement of autoimmune response against collagen types I, III, and IV by enzyme-linked innunosorbent assay, and its application in infective endocarditis. *Clin Chem*, 35, 246-250 (1989)

1055 De Flamingh JP, Van Der Merwe JV. A serum biochemical profile of normal pregnancy. *S Afr Med J*, 65, 552-555 (1984)

1056 De Fronzo RA et al. Renal function in patients with multiple myeloma. *Medicine*, 57, 151-166 (1978)

1057 de Groen PC, Gores J, LaRusso N et al, et al. Biliary tract cancers. *N Engl J Med*, 341, 1368-1378 (1999)

1058 de Jong J, van den Berg C, Wiijburg H et al. α-N-acetyl-galactsaminidase deficiency with mild clinical manifestations and difficult biochemical diagnosis. *J Pediatr*, 125, 385-391 (1994)

1059 De Jorge FB et al. Biochemical studies on serum copper, copper oxidase, magnesium, sulfur calcium and phosphorus in cancer of the breast. *Clin Chim Acta*, 12, 403-406 (1965)

1060 de Keijzer MH, Vermes J, van Gendt JWG et al. Levels of various inflammation markers during exacerbation in patients with severe asthma. *Clin Chem*, 41, S87 (1995)

1061 de la Monte SM, Ghanbari K, Frey WH, et al. Characterization of the AD7C-NTP cDNA expression in Alzheimer's disease and measurement of a 41-kD protein in cerebrospinal fluid. *J Clin Invest*, 100, 3093-3104 (1997)

1062 de la Piedra C, Carbo C, Laranaga J et al. Correlation among plasma osteocalcin, growth hormone, and somatomedin C in acromegaly. *Calcif Tissue Int*, 43, 44-45 (1988)

1063 de la Piedra C, Diaz Martin MA, Diaz Diego EM et al. Serum concentrations of carboxyterminal cross-linked teleopeptide of type I collagen (ICTP), serum tartrate resistant acid phosphatase, and serum levels of intact parathyroid hormone in parathyroid hyperfunction. *Scand J Clin Lab Invest*, 54, 11-15 (1994)

1064 de La Torre B, Hedman M, Nilsson E et al. Relationship between blood and joint tissue DHEAS levels in rheumatoid arthritis and osteoarthritis. *Clin Exp Rheumatol*, 11, 597-601 (1993)

1065 De Leacy EA, McLeay CD, Eadie MJ et al. Effects of subjects' sex, and intake of tobacco, alcohol and oral contraceptives on plasma phenytoin levels. *Br J Clin Pharmacol*, 8, 33-36 (1979)

1066 De Lorgeril M, Dureau G, Boissonnat P et al. Platelet function and composition in heart transplant recipients compared with nontransplanted coronary patients. *Arterioscler Thromb*, 12, 222-230 (1992)

1067 De Lorgeril M, Reber G, Righetti A et al. Endogenic prostacycline and coronary artery disease. Plasma 6-keto-PGF(1alpha) measurement. *Arch Mal Coeur*, 78, 1150-1153 (1985)

1068 de Maat MPM, Pietersma A, Kofflard M, et al. Association of plasma fibrinogen levels with coronary artery diseas, smoking and inflammatory markers. *Atherosclerosis*, 121, 185-191 (1996)

1069 De Moor et al. Results obtained from 75 patients operated upon for hyperparathyroidism: low cholesterol levels in overt primary hyperparathyroidism. *Ann Endocrinol*, 616-620 (1973)

1070 De Pablo F, Eastman RC, Roth J, Gorden P. Plasma prolactin in acromegaly before and after treatment. *J Clin Endocrinol Metab*, 53, 344-52 (1981)

1071 de Paterna LR, Arnaiz F, Estenoz J et al. Study of serum markers CEA, CA 15.3 and CA 27.29 as diagnostic parameters in patients with breast carcinoma. *Int J Biol Mark*, 10, 24-29 (1995)

1072 de Pita O, Frezzolini A, Cianetti A, et al. Squamous cell carcinoma-related antigen (SCCr-Ag), sICAM-1 and β2-microglobulin are useful markers of disease activity in psoriasis. *Acta Derm Venereol*, 79, 132-135 (1999)

1073 De Quattro V et al. Raised plasma-catecholamines in some patients with primary hypertension. *Lancet*, 1, 806-809 (1972)

1074 De Rosa G, Corsello SM, De Rosa E et al. Endocrine study of anorexia nervosa. *Exp Clin Endocrinol*, 82, 160-172 (1983)

1075 De Rosa G, Della Casa S, Corsello SM et al. Thyroid function in altered nutritional state. *Exp Clin Endocrinol*, 82, 173-177 (1983)

1076 De Simone C, Tzantzoglou S, Jirillo E et al. L-carnitine deficiency in AIDS patients. *AIDS*, 6, 203-205 (1992)

1077 De Torok D et al. Quantitative and qualitative plasma protein studies on alcoholics vs nonalcoholics. *Ann NY Acad Sci*, 273, 167 (1977)

1078 De Vos N, Song C, Lin A-h, et al. Lower serum zinc in relation to serum albumin and proinflammatory cytokines in detoxified alcohol-dependent patients without apparent liver disease. *Neuropsychobiology*, 39, 144-150 (1999)

1079 de Werra I, Jaccard C, Corradin SB, et al. Cytokines, nitrite/nitrate, soluble tumor necrosis factor receptors, and procalcitonin concentrations: comparisons in patients with septic shock, cardiogenic shock, and bacterial pneumonia. *Crit Care Med*, 25, 607-613 (1997)

1080 De Wit R, Raasveld MHM, Ten Berghe RJM et al. Interleukin-6 concentrations in the serum of patients with AIDS-associated Kaposi's sarcoma during treatment with interferon-α. *J Intern Med*, 229, 539-542 (1991)

1081 De Wit R, Sylvester R, Tsitsa C, et al. Tumour marker concentrations at the start of chemotherapy is a stronger predictor of treatment failure than marker half-life: a study in patients with disseminated non-seminomatous testicular cancer. *Br J Cancer*, 75, 432-435 (1997)

1082 Dean G, Barnes HD. Porphyria in Sweden and South Africa. *S Afr Med J*, 33, 274 (1959)

1083 Dean JD, Owens DR, Matthews SB. Apolipoprotein and lipid ratios in treated non-insulin dependent diabetics. *Diabetes Res*, 15, 21-25 (1990)

1084 Decaux G, Prospert F, Namias B, Soupart A. Hyperuricemia as a clue for central diabetes insipidus (lack of V_1 effect) in the differential diagnosis of polydipsia. *Am J Med*, 103, 376-382 (1997)

1085 Decossin C, Castro G, Derudas B, et al. Subclasses of LpA-I in coronary artery disease: distribution and cholesterol efflux ability. *Eur J Clin Invest*, 27, 299-307 (1997)

1086 Deenmamode JMJM, Sherwood RA, Sherman DIN et al. Total pancreatic and salivary iso-amylase activities in alcohol misusers in relapse and remission and in alcoholic liver disease. *Clin Chim Acta*, 223, 169-172 (1993)

1087 Deering TB et al. Effect of D-penicillamine on copper retention in patients with primary biliary cirrhosis. *Gastroenterology*, 72, 1208-1212 (1977)

1088 Defronzo RA et al. Impaired renal tubular potassium secretion in systemic lupus erythematosus. *Ann Intern Med*, 86, 2268-2271 (1977)

1089 Deftos LJ. Bone protein and peptide assays in the diagnosis and management of skeletal disease. *Clin Chem*, 37, 1143-1148 (1991)

1090 Deger O, Orem A, Akyol N, et al. Polymorphonuclear leukocyte elastase levels in patients with Behcet's disease. *Clin Chim Acta*, 236, 129-134 (1995)

1091 Degroot L et al. Serum antigens and antibodies in the diagnosis of thyroid cancer. *J Clin Endocrinol Metab*, 45, 1220-1223 (1977)

1092 Deiss A et al. Hemolytic anemia in Wilson's disease. *Ann Intern Med*, 73, 413 (1970)

1093 DeJaco P, Asselain B, Orlandi C et al. Evaluation of circulating tumor necrosis factor-α in patients and gynecological malignancies. *Int J Cancer*, 48, 375-378 (1991)

1094 Del Nero A, Esposito N, Curro A, et al. Evaluation of urinary level of NMP22 a diagnostic marker for stage pTa-pT1 bladder cancer: comparison with urinary cytology and BTA test. *Eur Urol*, 35, 93-97 (1999)

1095 del Pino J, Martin-Gomez, Martin-Rodriquez M. Influence of sex, age and menopause on serum osteocalcin levels. *Klin Wschr*, 69, 1135-1138 (1990)

1096 Del Santo P, Moneti G, Salvadori M et al. Levels of the adducts of 4-aminobiphenyl to hemoglobin in control subjects and bladder carcinoma patients. *Cancer Lett*, 60, 245-251 (1991)

1097 Delafosse B et al. Variation des acides amines plasmatiques au cours des hepatites graves avec encephalopathy. *Nouv Presse Med*, 6, 1207-12 (1977)

1098 Delamore JW et al. Haematological clues in systemic disease. *Practitioner*, 216, 27-36 (1976)

1099 Delana C, Carru C, Pes GM. Lipid profile in multiple symmetric lipomatosis. *Clin Biochem Rev*, 14, 225 (1993)

1100 Delaporte C et al. Free plasma and muscle amino acids in uremic children. *Am J Clin Nutr*, 31, 1647-1651 (1978)

1101 Delbruck A, Oepen H. Mucopolysaccharidstoffwechsel bei Huntingtonscher chorea. *Hum Genet*, 1, 105 (1964)

1102 Delmas P, Chatelain P, Malaval L et al. Serum bone Gla-protein in growth hormone deficient children. *J Bone Miner Res*, 1, 333-338 (1986)

1103 Delmas P, Damiaux B, Malaval L et al. Serum bone γ-carboxyglutamic acid-containing protein in primary hyperparathyroidism and in malignant hypercalcaemia. *Calcif Tissue Int*, 77, 985-991 (1986)

1104 Delmas P, Demiaux B, Malaval L et al. Serum bone GLA-protein is not a sensitive marker of bone turnover in Paget's disease of bone. *Calcif Tissue Int*, 38, 60-66 (1986)

1105 Delmas PD. Biochemical markers of bone turnover I: theoretical considerations and clinical use in osteoporosis. *Am J Med*, 95, 11S-16S (1993)

1106 Delmas PD, Wilson DM, Mann KG et al. Effect of renal function on plasma levels of bone Gla-protein. *J Clin Endocrinol Metab*, 57, 1028 (1983)

1107 Delpech B, Chevallier B, Reinhardt N et al. Serum hyaluronan (hyaluronic acid) in breast cancer patients. *Int J Cancer*, 46, 388-390 (1990)

1108 Delregato J A, Spjut H. *Cancer.* 5th edition, St Louis MO, CV Mosby (1977)

1109 Delwiche R et al. CEA in pancreatitis. *Cancer*, 31, 328 (1973)

1110 Demedts M et al. Respiratory failure: correlation between encephalopathy, blood gases and blood ammonia. *Respiration*, 33, 199-210 (1976)

1111 Demericin G, Oner A, Unver Y, et al. Erythrocyte superoxide dismutase activity and plasma malonidialdehyde levels in children with Henoch Schonlein purpura. *Acta Paediatr*, 87, 848-852 (1998)

1112 Demitrack MA, Dale JK, Straus SE et al. Evidence for impaired activation of the hypothalamic-pituitary-adrenal axis in patients with chronic fatigue syndrome. *J Clin Endocrinol Metab*, 73, 1224-1234 (1991)

1113 Demitrack MA, Gold PW, Dale JK et al. Plasma and cerebrospinal fluid monoamine metabolism in patients with chronic fatigue syndrome: preliminary findings. *Biol Psychiat*, 32, 65-77 (1992)

1114 Demitrack MA, Heyes MP, Altemus M et al. Cerebrospinal fluid levels of kynurenine pathway metabolites in patients with eating disorders: relation to clinical and biochemical variable. *Biol Psychiat*, 37, 512-520 (1995)

1115 Demitrack MA, Lesem MD, Listwak SJ et al. CSF oxytocin in anorexia nervosa and bulimia nervosa: clinicial and pathophysiological considerations. *Am J Psychiat*, 147, 882-886 (1990)

1116 den Heijer M, Koster T, Blom HJ, et al. Hyperhomocysteinemia as a risk factor for deep-vein thrombosis. *N Engl J Med*, 334, 759-762 (1996)

1117 den Ouden M, Ubachs JMH, Stoot JEGM, van Werscht JWJ. Thrombin-antithrombin III and D-dimer plasma levels in patients with benign or malignant ovarian tumors. *Scand J Clin Lab Invest*, 58, 555-560 (1998)

1118 Denborough et al. Biochemical changes in malignant hyperpyrexia. *J Clin Endocrinol*, 1, 1137-1138 (1970)

1119 Denis LJ et al. Lactic dehydrogenase in prostatic cancer. *Invest Urol*, 1, 101-111 (1963)

1120 Denizot Y, Fixe P, Liozon E, Praloran V. Serum interleukin-8 (IL-8) and IL-6 concentrations in patients with hematologic malignancies. *Blood*, 87, 4016-4017 (1996)

1121 Denker PS, Pollock VE. Fasting serum insulin levels in essential hypertension: a meta analysis. *Arch Intern Med*, 152, 1649-1651 (1992)

1122 Dent RI et al. Hypergastrinemia in patients with acute renal failure. *Surg Forum*, 23, 312 (1972)

1123 Dent RI et al. Hyperparathyroidism: gastric acid secretion and gastrin. *Ann Surg*, 176, 360 (1972)

1124 Deodhar SD, Singh B, Pathak CM, et al. Thyroid functions in lithium-treated psychiatric patients: a cross-sectional study. *Biol Trace Element Res*, 67, 151-163 (1999)

1125 Deray G, Carayon A, Maistre G et al. Endothelin in chronic renal failure. *Nephrol Dial Transplant*, 7, 300-305 (1992)

1126 Derfler K, Hayde M, Heinz G, et al. Decreased postheparin lipolytic activity in renal transplant recipients with cyclosporin A. *Kidney Int*, 40, 720-727 (1991)

1127 d'Eril GM, Trotti R, Brustia R et al. Anticardiolipin antibodies in HIV infection. *Clin Chem*, 41, S100 (1995)

1128 Desai M et al. Lipids and lipoproteins in thalassemia major. *Ind J Pediatr*, 13, 663 (1976)

1129 Deschamps J P, Lahrichi M. Biological values in the child and adolescent. In:. *Reference Values in Human Chemistry,* G. Siest (ed), 1973, 109

1130 Desgeorges A, Gabay C, Silacci P, et al. Concentrations and origins of soluble interleukin 6 receptor-α in serum and synovial fluid. *J Rheumatol*, 24, 1510-1516 (1997)

1131 Dessi-Fulgheri P, Espinosa E, Zingaretti O et al. Urinary kallikrein excretion and blood pressure response to angiotensin converting enzyme inhibitors and calcium antagonists in hypertensive patients. *J Hypertens*, 11, 725-730 (1993)

1132 Deugnier Y, David V, Brissot P et al. Serum α-L-fucosidase: a new marker for the diagnosis of primary hepatic carcinoma? *Hepatology*, 4, 889-892 (1984)

1133 Devine PL, McGuckin MA, Quin RJ et al. Serum markers CASA and CA 15-3 in ovarian cancer: all MUC_1 assays are not the same. *Tumor Biol*, 15, 337-344 (1994)

1134 Devine PL, McGuckin MA, Quin RJ, Ward BG. Predictive value of the combination of serum markers, CA125, CASA and TPS in ovarian cancer. *Int J Gynecol Cancer*, 5, 170-178 (1995)

1135 Devine PL, Siebert WJ, Morton SL, et al. Serum mucin antigen (CASA) as a marker of amiodarone-induced pulmonary toxicity. *Dis Mark*, 14, 169-173 (1998)

1136 Devinsky O, Emoto S, Nadi NS, Theodore WH. Cerebrospinal fluid levels of neuropeptides, cortisol, and aminoacids in patients with epilepsy. *Epilepsia*, 34, 255-261 (1993)

1137 Devlin MJ, Walsh T, Kral JG et al. Metabolic abnormalities in bulimia nervosa. *Arch Gen Psychiat*, 47, 144-148 (1990)

1138 Devlin RD, Retallack RW, Fenton AJ et al. Long-term elevation of 1,25-dihydroxyvitamin D after short-term intravenous administration of pamidronate (aminohydroxypropylidene biphosphonate, APD) in Paget's disease of bone. *J Bone Miner Res*, 9, 81-85 (1994)

1139 Devuyst O, Lambert M, Rodhain J et al. Haematological changes and infectious complications in anorexia nervosa: a case-controlled study. *Q J Med*, 86, 791-799 (1993)

1140 Deyase SK et al. Placental alkaline phosphatase (Regan isoenzyme) in cancerous patients sera. *Ind J Cancer*, 13, 257-61 (1976)

1141 Dezelic G et al. The photometric latex test for rheumatoid factors in patients with rheumatoid arthritis. III. clinical evaluation. *Z Rheumatol*, 37, 112-22 (1978)

1142 D'Hallewin M, Baert L. Initial evaluation of the bladder tumor antigen test in superficial bladded cancer. *J Urol*, 155, 475-476 (1996)

1143 Dhansay MA, Benade AJS, Donald PR. Plasma lecithin-cholesterol acyltransferase activity and plasma lipoprotein composition and concentrations in kwashiorkor. *Am J Clin Nutr*, 53, 512-519 (1991)

1144 Dharnidharka VR, Dabbagh S, Atiyeh B, et al. prevalence of microalbuminuria in children with sickle cell disease. *Pediatr Nephrol*, 12, 475-478 (1998)

1145 Di Bisceglie AM, Axiotis CA, Hoofnagle JH et al. Measurements of iron status in patients with chronic hepatitis. *Gastroenterology*, 102, 2108-2113 (1992)

1146 Di Minno G, Mancini M. Drugs affecting plasma fibrinogen levels. *Cardiovasc Drug Ther*, 6, 25-27 (1992)

1147 Di Sant-Agnese PA. Cystic fibrosis of the pancreas. *J Am Med Ass*, 172, 135 (1960)

1148 Diagnostic Systems. Product Insert: Active androstanediol glucuronide. Diagnostic Systems, Webster TX

1149 Diamandi A, Khosravi J, Muthukumaran N et al. A two-site immunoenzymometric assay for human osteocalcin in serum. *Clin Chem*, 41, S51 (1995)

1150 Diamandi A, Khosravi J, Muthukumaran N et al. Immunoenzymometric assay of intact human parathyroid hormone in serum. *Clin Chem*, 41, S33-S34 (1995)

1151 Diamandis EP, Nadkarni S, Bhaumik B, et al. Immunofluorometric assay of pepsinogen C and preliminary clinical applications. *Clin Chem*, 43, 1365-1371 (1997)

1152 Diamond HS et al. Hyperuricosuria and increased tubular secretion of urate in sickle cell anemia. *Am J Med*, 59, 796-802 (1975)

1153 Diamond NJ et al. Arterial blood gases in acute pulmonary edema. *J Am Coll Emer Phys*, 5, 497-500 (1976)

1154 Diamond T, Vine J, Smart R et al. Thyrotoxic bone disease in women: a potentially reversible disorder. *Ann Intern Med*, 120, 8-11 (1994)

1155 Diani G, Poma G, Novazzi F, et al. Increased serum lipase with associated normoamylasemia in cancer patients. *Clin Chem*, 44, 1043-1045 (1998)

1156 Diaz J, Tornel PL, Jara P et al. The value of polymorphonuclear elastase in adult respiratory distress syndrome. *Clin Chim Acta*, 236, 119-127 (1995)

1157 Diaz R et al. Rose bengal plate agglutination and counterimmunoelectrophoresis tests on spinal fluid in the diagnosis of brucella meningitis. *J Clin Microbiol*, 7, 236-237 (1978)

1158 Diaz-Martin MA, Traba ML, De La Piedra C, et al. Aminoterminal propeptide of type I collagen and bone alkaline phosphatase in the study of bone metatases associated with prostatic carcinoma. *Scand J Clin Lab Invest*, 59, 125-132 (1999)

1159 Diaz-Velez CR, Garcia-Castineiras S, Mendoza-Ramos E, Hernandez-Lopez E. Increased malondialdehyde in peripheral blood of patients with congestive heart failure. *Am Heart J*, 131, 146-152 (1996)

1160 Dickson ER et al. Systemic giant cell arteritis with polymyalgia rheumatica. reversible abnormalities of liver function. *J Am Med Ass*, 224, 1496 (1973)

1161 Dicou E, Perrot S, Menkes CJ, et al. Nerve growth factor (NGF) autoantibodies and NGF in the synovial fluid: implications in spondylarthropathies. *Autoimmunity*, 24, 1-9 (1996)

1162 Diego EMD, Martin MAD, de la Piedra C, Rapado A. Lack of correlation between levels of osteocalcin and bone alkaline phosphatase in healthy control and postmenopausal osteoporotic women. *Horm Metab Res*, 27, 151-154 (1995)

1163 Diekman T, Lansberg PJ, Kastelein JJP, et al. Prevalence and correction of hypothyroidism in a large cohort of patients referred for dyslipidemia. *Arch Intern Med*, 155, 1490-1495 (1995)

1164 Dieplinger H, Lobentanz E-M, Konig P et al. Plasma apolipoprotein A-IV metabolism in patients with chronic renal disease. *Eur J Clin Invest*, 22, 166-174 (1992)

1165 Dietemann-Molard A, Pelletier A, Pauli G et al. Practical value of the assay of serum angiotensin converting enzyme activity in sarcoidosis. *Rev Pneμmol Clin*, 40, 121-125 (1984)

1166 Dieterich W, Laag E, Schopper H, et al. Autoantibodies to tissue transglutaminase as predictors of celiac disease. *Gastroenterology*, 115, 1317-1321 (1998)

1167 Dietl KH, Winterberg B, Bertram HP, et al. Aluminum bone disease improved after kidney transplantation - determination by atomic absorption spectroscopy. *Trace Elem Elect*, 14, 113-115 (1997)

1168 Dietzen DJ, Wilhite TR, Kenagy DN, et al. Extraction of glyceric and glycolic acids from urine with tetrahydrofuran: utility in detection of primary hyperoxaluria. *Clin Chem*, 43, 1315-1320 (1997)

1169 Diez Ruiz A, Santos Perez JI, Lopez Martinez G, et al. Tumor necrosis factor, interleukin-1 and interleukin-6 in alcoholic cirrhosis. *Alcohol Alcoholism*, 28, 319-323 (1993)

1170 Diez-Ewald M et al. Mechanisms of hemolysis in iron-deficiency anemia. *Blood*, 32, 884 (1968)

1171 Dijkman JH et al. Increased serum alkaline phosphatase activity in pulmonary infarction. *Acta Med Scand*, 180, 273-281 (1966)

1172 Diliberti JH, McMurry MP, Connor WE et al. Hypercholesterolemia associated with α-antitrypsin deficiency and hepatitis: lipoprotein and apoprotein determinations, sterol balance and treatment. *Am J Med Sci*, 288, 81-85 (1984)

1173 DiLisi LE, Murphy DL, Karoum F et al. Phenylethylamine excretion in depression. *Psychiat Res*, 13, 193-201 (1984)

1174 Dillon MJ, Tizard EJ. Anti-neutrophil cytoplasmic antibodies and anti-endothelial cell antibodies. *Pediat Nephrol*, 5, 256-259 (1991)

1175 Dimopoulos MA, Barlogie B, Smith TL et al. High serum lactate dehydrogenase level as a marker for drug resistance and short survival in multiple myeloma. *Ann Intern Med*, 115, 931-935 (1991)

1176 Dincer Y, Konukoglu D, Akcay T, Hatemi H. Plasma levels of citrate and lipid peroxides in men with coronary atherosclerosis. *Med Sci Res*, 27, 197-199 (1999)

1177 DiPiro JT, Howdieshell TR, Hamilton RG, Mansberger AR Jr. Immunoglobulin E and eosinophil counts are increased after sepsis in trauma patients. *Crit Care Med*, 26, 465-469 (1998)

1178 Dirix LY, Vermeulen PB, Pawinski A, et al. Elevated levels of the angiogenic cytokines basic fibroblast growth factor and vascular endothelial growth factor in sera of cancer patients. *Br J Cancer*, 76, 238-243 (1997)

1179 Disaia P et al. Carcinoembryonic antigen in cancer of the female reproductive system. *Cancer*, 39, 2365-2370 (1977)

1180 Discala V A, Kinney M J. Effects of myxedema on the renal diluting and concentrating mechanism. *Am J Med*, 50, 325 (1971)

1181 Dische MR, Porro RS. The cardiac lesions in Bassen-Kornzweig syndrome. *Am J Med*, 49, 568 (1970)

1182 DiSilvestro RA, Marten J, Skehan M. Effects of copper supplementation on ceruloplasmin and copper-zinc superoxide dismutase in free-living rheumatoid arthritis patients. *J Am Coll Nutr*, 11, 177-180 (1992)

1183 Ditzel J. Oxygen transport impairment in diabetes. *Diabetes*, 25, 832-838 (1976)

1184 Ditzel J et al. Hyperlipoproteinemia, diabetes, and oxygen affinity of hemoglobin. *Metabolism*, 26, 141-150 (1977)

1185 Divertie MB. The adult respiratory distress syndrome. *Mayo Clin Proc*, 57, 371-378 (1982)

1186 Djurovic S, Schjetlein R, Wisloff F, et al. Increased levels of intercellular adhesion molecules and vascular cell adhesion molecules in pre-eclampsia. *Br J Obstet Gynaecol*, 104, 466-470 (1997)

1187 Dnistrian AM, Schwartz MK, Greenberg EJ et al. Evaluation of CA M26, CA M29, CA 15-3, and CEA as circulating tumor markers in breast cancer patients. *Tumor Biol*, 12, 82-90 (1991)

1188 Dnistrian DN, Schwartz MK, Schwartz DC et al. An evaluation of breast antigen BR 27.29 in serum of patients with breast cancer. *Clin Chem*, 39, 1192 (1993)

1189 Doan CA et al. Idiopathic and secondary thrombocytopenic purpura. *Ann Intern Med*, 53, 861 (1960)

1190 Dobs AS, Dempsy MA, Ladenson PW et al. Endocrine disorders in men infected with AIDS. *Am J Med*, 84, 611-616 (1988)

1191 Docci D, Bilancioni R, Buscaroli A et al. Elevated serum levels of C-reactive protein in hemodialysis patients. *Nephron*, 56, 364-367 (1990)

1192 Docci D, Bilancioni R, Pistocchi E et al. Serum α_1-acid glycoprotein in chronic renal failure. *Nephron*, 39, 160-163 (1985)

1193 Docherty I, Harrop JS, Hine KR, Hopton MR. Myoglobin concentration, creatine kinase activity, and creatine kinase B subunit concentrations in serum during thyroid disease. *Clin Chem*, 30, 42-45 (1984)

1194 Dodd R, Winkler CF, Williams ME, Bunn PA. Calcitriol levels in hypercalcemic patients with adult T-cell lymphoma. *Arch Intern Med*, 146, 1971 (1986)

1195 Dodson L, Sachan DS, Krauss S et al. Alterations of serum and urinary carnitine profiles in cancer patients: hypothesis of possible significance. *J Am Coll Nutr*, 2, 133-142 (1989)

1196 Dogan P, Dogan M, Klockenkamper R. Determination of trace elements in blood serum of patients with Behcet's disease by total reflection X-ray fluorescence analysis. *Clin Chem*, 39, 1037-1041 (1993)

1197 Dohan PH et al. Evaluation of urinary cyclic 3',5'-adenosine monophosphate in the differential diagnosis of hypercalcemia. *J Clin Endocrinol Metab*, 35, 775 (1972)

1198 Doherty M, Belcher C, Regan M, et al. Association between synovial fluid levels of inorganic pyrophosphate and short term radiographic outcome of kee osteoarthritis. *Ann Rheum Dis*, 55, 432-436 (1996)

1199 Dolin R et al. Lymphocyte populations in acute viral gastroenteritis. *Infect Immunol*, 14, 422-428 (1976)

1200 Dominguez AS, Olivie MAA, Sousa TR, et al. Plasma parathyroid hormone related-protein levels in patients with cancer, normocalcemic and hypercalcemic. *Clin Chim Acta*, 244, 163-172 (1996)

1201 Dominguez-Munoz JE, Carballo F, Garcia MJ et al. Clinical usefulness of polymorphonuclear elastase in predicting the severity of acute pancreatitis: results of a multicentre study. *Br J Surg*, 78, 1230-1234 (1991)

1202 Dominick JC, et al. Isoenzymes of alkaline phosphatase in the serum of patients with cystic fibrosis. *Z Kinderheilk*, 119, 261-267 (1975)

1203 Dominiczak AF, Semple PF, Fraser R et al. Hypokalaemia in alcoholics. *Scott Med J*, 34, 489-494 (1989)

1204 Domula M, Bykowska K, Wegrzynowicz Z et al. Plasma fibronectin concentrations in healthy and septic infants. *Eur J Pediatr*, 144, 49-52 (1985)

1205 Donadio C, Auner I, Giordani R et al. Serum and urinary activities in renal artery embolism. *Clin Chim Acta*, 160, 143-149 (1986)

1206 Donaldson EM et al. Erythropoietic protoporphyria: a family study. *Br Med J*, 1, 659 (1967)

1207 Donaldson ES, Van Nagell JR Jr, Pursell S et al. Multiple biochemical markers in patients with gynecologic malignancies. *Cancer*, 45, 948-953 (1980)

1208 Donders SHJ, Lustermans FATh, van Wersch JWJ. Coagulation factors and lipid composition of the blood in treated and untreated hypertensive patients. *Scand J Clin Lab Invest*, 53, 179-186 (1993)

1209 Dong Q, Hawker F, McWilliam D et al. Circulating immunoreactive inhibin and testosterone levels in men with critical illness. *Clin Endocrinol*, 36, 399-404 (1992)

1210 Doniach D et al. Autoimmune phenomena in pernicious anemia. *Br Med J*, 1, 1374 (1963)

1211 Doniach D et al. Tissue antibodies in primary biliary cirrhosis, active chronic (lupoid) hepatitis, cryptogenic cirrhosis and other liver diseases and their clinical implications. *Clin Exp Immunol*, 1, 237 (1966)

1212 Donnelly S, Shah BR. Erythropoietin deficiency in hyporeninemia. *Am J Kidney Dis*, 33, 947-953 (1999)

1213 D'Onofrio GM, Levitt S, Ilett KF. Serum angiotensin converting enzyme in Crohn's disease, ulcerative colitis and peptic ulceration. *Aust NZ J Med*, 14, 27-30 (1984)

1214 Donohugh DL. Tropical eosinophilia: an etiologic inquiry. *N Engl J Med*, 269, 1357 (1963)

1215 Donovan DS Jr, Papadopoulos A, Staron RB, et al. Bone mass and vitamin D deficiency in adults with advanced cystic fibrosis lung disease. *Am J Respir Crit Care Med*, 158, 1892-1899 (1998)

1216 Donowitz M, Kerstein MD, Spliro HM. Pancreatic ascites. *Medicine*, 53, 183-195 (1974)

1217 Dooley MA, Cush JJ, Lipsky PE et al. The effects of nonsteroidal antiinflammatory drug therapy in early rheumatoid arthritis on serum levels of soluble interleukin-2 receptor, CD4, and CD8. *J Rheumatol*, 20, 1857- 1862 (1993)

1218 Doos WG et al. CEA levels in patients with colorectal polyps. *Cancer*, 36, 1996-2003 (1975)

1219 Doraiswamy NV. The neutrophil count in childhood acute appendicitis. *Br J Surg*, 64, 342-344 (1977)

1220 Dore F, Bonfigli S, Gaviano E et al. Serum erythropietin levels in thalassemia intermedia. *Ann Hematol*, 67, 183-186 (1993)

1221 Dore F, Bonfigli S, Pardini S, Longinotti M. Serum interleukin-8 levels in thalassemia intermedia. *Haematologica*, 80, 431-433 (1995)

1222 Dore-Duffy P, Newman W, Balabanov R et al. Circulating, soluble adhesion proteins in cerebrospinal fluid and serum of patients with multiple sclerosis: correlation with clinical activity. *Ann Neurol*, 37, 55-62 (1995)

1223 Dormer A. Bacterial endocarditis: survey of patients treated between 1945 and 1956. *Br Med J*, 1, 63 (1958)

1224 Dorsam G, Harris L, Payne M et al. Development and use of ELISA to quantify type II phospholipase A_2 in normal and uremic syndrome. *Clin Chem*, 41, 862-866 (1995)

1225 Dosquet C, Schaetz A, Faucher C et al. Tumour necrosis factor-α, interleukin-1β and interleukin-6 in patients with renal cell carcinoma. *Eur J Cancer*, 30A, 162-167 (1994)

1226 Dotevall L, Rosengren LE, Hagberg L. Increased cerebrospinal fluid levels of glial fibrillary acidic protein (GFAp) in Lyme Neuroborreliosis. *Infection*, 24, 125-129 (1996)

1227 Dotto P, Vianello F, del Bianco T et al. Blood pepsinogen as a subclinical marker for duodenal ulcer. *Curr Ther Res*, 54, 172-176 (1993)

1228 Douglas DM, Claireaux AE. Hodgkin's disease in childhood. *Arch Dis Child*, 28, 222 (1953)

1229 Dover S, McAllister J, Moore MR et al. Normal serum α-fetoprotein in acute hepatic porphyria. *Ann Clin Biochem*, 31, 289-290 (1994)

1230 Doweck I, Barak M, Greenberg E et al. CYFRA 21-1: a new potential tumor marker for squamous cell carcinoma of head and neck. *Arch Otolaryngol Head Neck Surg*, 121, 177-181 (1995)

1231 Dowlati A, Bury T, Corhay J-L, et al. Gastrin levels in serum and bronchoalveolar lavage fluid of patients with lung cancer: comparison with patients with lung cancer. *Thorax*, 51, 1270-1272 (1996)

1232 Dowling P et al. Cytomegalovirus complement fixation antibody in Guillain-Barre syndrome. *Neurology*, 27, 1153-1156 (1977)

1233 Doyle AE et al. Urinary sodium, potassium and creatinine excretion in hypertensive and normotensive Australians. *Med J Aust*, 2, 898-900 (1976)

1234 Dreher WH et al. Hyperchloremia associated with membranoproliferative glomerulonephritis. *Nephron*, 18, 321-325 (1977)

1235 Dreyfuss F. The role of hyperuricemia in coronary heart disease. *Dis Chest*, 38, 332-334 (1960)

1236 Dries DJ, Walenga JM, Hoppensteadt D, Fareed J. Molecular markers of hemostatic activation and inflammation following major injury: effect of therapy with IFN-γ. *J Interferon Cytokine Res*, 18, 327-335 (1998)

1237 Drivsholm L, Osterlind K, Cooper EH et al. Neuron-specific enolase (NSE) in serum. Comparison of monoclonal versus polyclonal assay based on 392 blood samples. *Int J Biol Mark*, 10, 1-4 (1995)

1238 Drost AC, Burleson DG, Cioffi WG Jr et al. Plasma cytokines following thermal injury and their relationship with patient mortality, burn size, and time postburn. *J Trauma*, 35, 335-339 (1993)

1239 Druml W, Schwarzenhofer M, Apsner R, Horl WH. Fat-soluble vitamins in patients with acute renal failure. *Miner Electrolyte Metab*, 24, 220-226 (1998)

1240 Drummey GO et al. Microscopical examination of the stool for steatorrhea. *N Engl J Med*, 264, 85-87 (1961)

1241 Du Pont aca package insert for acetaminophen. Du Pont, Wilmington DE (10/84)

1242 Dubin A et al. Hyperuricemia in hypoparathyroidism. *Metals*, 5, 703-709 (1956)

1243 Dubin IN. Chronic idiopathic jaundice. *Am J Med*, 24, 268 (1958)

1244 Dubo H et al. Serum creatine kinase in cases of stroke, head injury, and meningitis. *J Clin Endocrinol*, 2, 743-748 (1967)

1245 Duboscq C, Quintana I, Bassilotta E, et al. Plasminogen: an important hemostatic parameter in septic patients. *Thromb Haemostas*, 77, 1090-1095 (1997)

1246 Dubrey SW, Reaveley DA, Leslie DG et al. Effect of insulin-dependent diabetes mellitus on lipids and lipoproteins: a study of identical twins. *Clin Sci*, 84, 537-542 (1993)

1247 Dubrow R, Chi Suk K, Eldred AK. Fecal lysozyme: an unreliable marker for colorectal cancer. *Am J Gastroenterol*, 87, 617-621 (1992)

1248 Duchin JS, Koster FT, Peters CJ et al. Hantavirus pulmonary syndrome: a clinical description of 17 patients with a newly recognized disease. *N Engl J Med*, 330, 949-955 (1994)

1249 Duchini A, Sessoms SL. Gastrointestinal heorrhage in patients with systemic sclerosis and CREST syndrome. *Am J Gastroenterol*, 93, 1453-1456 (1998)

1250 Dudley DJ, Hunter C, Mitchell MD, et al. Elevations of serum interleukin-12 concentrations in women with severe preeclampsia and HELLP syndrome. *J Reprod Immunol*, 31, 97-107 (1996)

1251 Dudley DJ, Hunter C, Mitchell MD, Varner MW. Elevations of amniotic fluid macrophage inflammatory protein-1α concentrations in women during term and preterm labor. *Obstet Gynecol*, 87, 94-98 (1996)

1252 Duffy M. Proteases as prognostic markers in cancer. *Clin Cancer Res*, 2, 613-618 (1996)

1253 Duffy MJ. CA 19-9 as a marker for gastrointestinal cancers: a review. *Ann Clin Biochem*, 35, 364-370 (1998)

1254 Duffy MJ. PSA as a marker for prostate cancer: a critical review. *Ann Clin Biochem*, 33, 511-519 (1996)

1255 Duffy MJ, Maguire TM, McDermott EW, O'Higgins N. Urokinase plasminogen activator: a prognostic marker in multiple types of cancer. *J Surg Oncol*, 71, 130-135 (1999)

1256 Duffy MJ, McDermott E, Fennelly J et al. Prognostic value of c-erb-B_2 oncoprotein in breast cancer as determined by ELISA. *Proc ACB Natl Meet*, 35 (1993)

1257 Duggan C, Colin AC, Agil A , et al. Vitamin A status in acute exacerbations of cystic fibrosis. *Am J Clin Nutr*, 64, 635-639 (1996)

1258 Duggan C, Maguire T, McDermott E, et al. Urokinase plasminogen activator and urokinase plasminogen activator receptor in breast cancer. *Int J Cancer*, 61, 597-600 (1995)

1259 Duits AJ, Schnog JB, Lard LR, et al. Elevated IL-8 levels during sickle cell crisis. *Eur J Haematol*, 61, 302-305 (1998)

1260 Duk JM, Kauer FM, Fleuren GJ et al. Serum CA 125 levels in patients with a provisional diagnosis of pelvic inflammatory disease. Clinical and theoretical implications. *Acta Obstet Gynecol Scand*, 68, 637-641 (1989)

1261 Dumas F, Eschwge P, Loric S. Acute bacterial prostatitis induces hematogenous dissemination of prostate epithelial cells. *Clin Chem*, 43, 2007-2008 (1997)

1262 Dummer W, Brocker E-B, Bastian BC. Elevated serum levels of soluble CD30 are associated with atopic dermatitis, but not with respiratory atopic disorders and allergic contact dermatitis. *Br J Dermatol*, 137, 183-187 (1997)

1263 Duncan WC, Sweeting VM, Cawood P et al. Measurement of creatine kinase activity and diagnosis of ectopic pregnancy. *Br J Obstet Gynaecol*, 102, 233-237 (1995)

1264 Dunlop O, Bruun JN, Myrvang B et al. Calprotectin in cerebrospinal fluid of the HIV infected: a diagnostic marker of opportunistic central nervous system infection? *Scand J Infect Dis*, 23, 717-721 (1991)

1265 Duquesnoy B, Noel C, Hubaud P et al. Metabolisme phosphocalcique et histomorphometrie osseuse dans i'ethylisme chronique. *Rev Rhum Mal Osteo-Artic*, 51, 75-80 (1984)

1266 Duren M, Siperstein AE, Shen W, et al. Value of stimulated serum thyroglobulin levels for detecting persistent or recurrent differentiated thyroid cancer in high- and low-risk patients. *Surgery*, 126, 13-19 (1999)

1267 Dussault JH, Morissette J, Laberge C. Blood thyroxine concentrations in lower birth-weight infants. *Clin Chem*, 25, 2047-2049 (1979)

1268 Dutta JK et al. Serum magnesium study in cholera and non-choleric gastroenteritis. *Trans Roy Soc Trop Med Hyg*, 71, 263-264 (1977)

1269 Dutta TK. Clinical evaluation of serum protein-bound fucose as a diagnostic and prognostic index in malignant tumors. *Ind J Cancer*, 13, 262-266 (1976)

1270 Duval F, Frommherz K, Atger V et al. Influence of end-stage renal failure on concentrations of free apolipoprotein A-I in serum. *Clin Chem*, 35, 963-966 (1989)

1271 DuVillard L, Guiguet M, Casanovas R-O et al. Diagnostic value of serum IL-6 level in monoclonal gammopathies. *Br J Haematol*, 89, 243-249 (1995)

1272 Dux S, Aron N, Boner G, Carmel A. Serum angiotensin converting enzyme activity in normal adults and patients with different types of hypertension. *Isr J Med Sci*, 20, 1138-1142 (1984)

1273 Dwivedi C, Dixit M, Hardy RE. Plasma lipid-bound sialic acid alterations in neoplastic diseases. *Experientia*, 46, 91-94 (1990)

1274 Dworkin B, Rosenthal WS, Jankowski RH et al. Low blood selenium levels in alcoholics with and without advanced liver disease: correlations with clinical and nutritional status. *Dig Dis Sci*, 30, 838-840 (1985)

1275 Dworkin BM, Rosenthal WS, Gordon GG et al. Diminished blood selenium levels in alcoholics. *Alcohol Clin Exp Res*, 8, 535-538 (1984)

1276 Dyker AC, Weir CJ, Lees KR. Influence of cholesterol on survival after stroke: retrospective study. *Br Med J*, 314, 1584-1588 (1997)

1277 Dykhuizen RS, Masson J, McKnight G, et al. Plasma nitrate concentration in infective gastroenteritis and inflammatory bowel disease. *Gut*, 39, 393-395 (1996)

1278 Dzarik R, Lajdovova I, Spustova V et al. Pseudouridine excretion in healthy subjects and its accumulation in renal failure. *Nephron*, 61, 64-67 (1992)

1279 Dzialoszynski LM et al. Some clinical aspects of arylsulfatase activity. *Clin Chim Acta*, 15, 381-386 (1967)

1280 Eales L et al. Sodium and potassium balance in relation to periodic paralysis and in a case of pyelonephritis with malignant hypertension. *S Afr Med J*, 32, 251 (1958)

1281 Eales L et al. The clinical biochemistry of the human hepatocutaneous porphyrias in the light of recent studies of newly identified intermediates and porphyrin derivatives. *Ann NY Acad Sci*, 244, 441 (1975)

1282 Eales L, Saunders S J. The diagnostic importance of faecal porphyrins in the differentiation of the porphyrias. *S Afr J Lab Clin Med*, 40, 63 (1966)

1283 Earley LE, Gollschalk (eds). *Diseases of the Kidney*. 3rd edition, Boston MA, Little Brown Co (1974)

1284 Eastell R. Biochemical markers of bone turnover in Paget's disease of bone. *Bone*, 24, 49S-50S (1999)

1285 Eastell R, Calvo MS, Burritt MF et al. Abnormalities in circadian patterns of bone resorption and renal calcium conservation in type I osteoporosis. *J Clin Endocrinol Metab*, 74, 487-494 (1992)

1286 Eastgate JA, Symons JA, Wood NC et al. Plasma levels of interleukin-1-α in rheumatoid arthritis. *Br J Rheumatol*, 30, 295-297 (1991)

1287 Eastham EJ et al. Serum ferritin levels in acute hepatocellular damage from paracetamol overdosage. *Br Med J*, 1, 750-751 (1976)

1288 Eastham et al. Serum cholesterol in mental retardation. *Br J Psychiat*, 115, 1013-1017 (1969)

1289 Eastham JM, Reilly JT, MacNeil S. Raised urinary calmodulin levels in idiopathic myelofibrosis: possible implications for the aetilogy of fibrosis. *Br J Haematol*, 86, 668-670 (1994)

1290 Eastham RD. *Biochemical Values in Clinical Medicine*. 5th edition, Baltimore MD, Williams and Wilkins (1975)

1291 Eastman, Hellman. *Obstetrics*. 13th edition (Williams), New York NY, Appleton-Century-Crofts (1966)

1292 Eaton KK, Howard M, Hunnisett A. Urinary histidine excretion in patients with classical allergy (type A allergy), food intolerance (type B allergy), and fungal-type dysbiosis. *J Nutr Biochem*, 9, 586-590 (1998)

1293 Ebert W, Muley T, Drings P. Does the assessment of serum markers in patients with lung cancer aid in the clinical decision making process? *Anticancer Res*, 16, 2161-2168 (1996)

1294 Ebihara I, Nakamura T, Shimada N, Koide H. Increased plasma metalloproteinase-9 concentrations precede development of microalbuminuria in non-insulin-dependent diabetes mellitus. *Am J Kid Dis*, 32, 544-550 (1998)

1295 Eborowicz D et al. The correlation of routine cytology with the contents of carcinoembryonic antigen and α-fetoprotein in pleural and peritoneal effusions. *Arch Geschwulstforsch*, 47, 231-235 (1977)

1296 Eckert ED, Pomeroy C, Raymond N, et al. Leptin in anorexia nervosa. *J Clin Endocrinol Metab*, 83, 791-795 (1998)

1297 Economidow J et al. Carcinoembryonic antigen in thyroid disease. *J Clin Pathol*, 30, 878-880 (1977)

1298 Edmondson JW et al. The relationship of serum ionized and total calcium in primary hyperparathyroidism. *J Lab Clin Med*, 87, 624-629 (1976)

1299 Edouard AR, Mimoz O, Sami K, et al. Circulating cardiac troponin I in trauma patients without cardiac contusion. *Intensive Care Med*, 24, 569-573 (1998)

1300 Edwards AJ, Lee M, Harcourt G. Serum immunoglobulins and C_3 complement concentrations in malignancy. *Clin Oncol*, 3, 65-73 (1977)

1301 Edwards CQ, Kushner JP. Current concepts: screening for hemochromatosis. *N Engl J Med*, 328, 1616-1620 (1993)

1302 Efran ML et al. Hydroxyprolinemia II. a rare metabolic disease due to a deficiency of hydroxyproline oxidase. *N Engl J Med*, 272, 1299 (1965)

1303 Efrati P, Yaari A, Resnitzky P. Micro-densitometric evaluation of human neutrophil granulocyte enzymes in normals and in different pathological states. *Haematologica*, 71, 293-298 (1986)

1304 Efron ML. Aminoaciduria. *N Engl J Med*, 272, 1058 (1965)

1305 Efthymiadis A, Lefkos N, Liatsis I et al. The diagnostic value of the determination of troponin T in unstable angina. *Acta Cardiol*, 5, 419-424 (1994)

1306 Egberg N et al. Fasting (acute energy deprivation) in man: effect on blood coagulation and fibrinolysis. *Am J Clin Nutr*, 30, 1963-1967 (1977)

1307 Egeberg O. Blood coagulation in renal failure. *Scand J Clin Lab Invest*, 14, 163 (1962)

1308 Egeberg O. Influence of thyroid function in the blood clotting activity. *Scand J Clin Lab Invest*, 15, 1 (1963)

1309 Egeberg O. The blood coagulability in diabetic patients. *Scand J Clin Lab Invest*, 15, 533 (1963)

1310 Egeberg O. The effect of unspecific fever induction on the blood clotting system. *Scand J Clin Lab Invest*, 14, 471 (1962)

1311 Eggelmeijer F, Papapoulos SE, Westedt MI et al. Bone metabolism in rheumatoid arthritis; relation to disease activity. *Br J Rheumatol*, 32, 387-391 (1993)

1312 Einarsson K, Angelin B, Bjorkem I, Glaumann H. The diagnostic value of fasting individual serum bile acids in anicteric alcoholic liver disease: relation to liver morphology. *Hepatology*, 5, 108-111 (1985)

1313 Eisenhofer G, Lenders JWM, Linehan WM, et al. Plasma normetanephrine and metanephrine for detecting pheochromocytoma in von Hippel-Lindau disease and multiple endocrine neoplasia type 2. *N Engl J Med*, 340, 1872-1879 (1999)

1314 Eisner E et al. Coomb's-positive hemolytic anemia in Hodgkin's disease. *Ann Intern Med*, 66, 258 (1967)

1315 Ekberg MR et al. Significance of increased factor VIII in early glomerulonephritis. *Ann Intern Med*, 83, 337-341 (1975)

1316 Eklund SG et al. Anemia in uremia. *Acta Med Scand*, 190, 435 (1971)

1317 Ekstrom T et al. Medullary sponge kidney. *Proc Third Int Congr Nephrol*, 2, 54 (1966)

1318 El-Ahmady O, Mansour M, Zoeir H, Mansour O. Elevated concentrations of interleukins and leukotriene in response to mycobacterium tuberculosis infection. *Ann Clin Biochem*, 34, 160-164 (1997)

1319 El-Bashir B, Rostom A, Wright J. Nutrition and IGF-I in patients with cancer cachexia. *Proc ACB Natl Meet*, 50 (1993)

1320 El-Ghonaimy E, Barsoum R, Soliman M et al. Serum gastrin in chronic renal failure: morphological and physiological correlations. *Nephron*, 39, 86-94 (1985)

1321 El-Haddad S et al. Value of serum copper measurement in acute leukaemia of childhood. *Gaz Egypt Paediatr Ass*, 26, 67-72 (1977)

1322 El-Hazmi M, Warsy A, Al-Fawaz I et al. Fetal hemoglobin level - effect of gender, age and hemoglobin disorders. *Clin Chem*, 39, 1131 (1993)

1323 El-Hazmi MAF, Warsy AS, Bahakim H. Blood proteins C and S in sickle cell disease. *Acta Haematol*, 90, 114-119 (1993)

1324 Eli Lilly and Company. Manufacturer's literature on Humatrope® . Indianapolis, IN 46285 (1996)

1325 Elias AN, Pandian MR, Naqvi F et al. Relationship between prorenin, IGF-binding proteins in diabetic patients using a novel renin assay. *Clin Chem*, 41, S35 (1995)

1326 Elias AN, Vaziri ND, Maksy M. Plasma norepinephrine, epinephrine, and dopamine levels in end-stage renal disease. *Arch Intern Med*, 145, 1013 (1985)

1327 Eliasson K, Sjoquist B. Urinary catecholamine metabolites in borderline and established hypertension. Relationship to body composition. *Acta Med Scand*, 216, 369-375 (1984)

1328 Elin RJ et al. Lack of specificity of the limulus lysate test in the diagnosis of pyogenic arthritis. *J Infect Dis*, 137, 507-513 (1978)

1329 Elin RJ, Fried MW, Sampson M, et al. Assesment of monoethylglycinexylidide as measure of liver function for patients with chronic viral hepatitis. *Clin Chem*, 43, 1952-1957 (1997)

1330 Elisaf M, Bairaktari E, Kalaitzidis R, Siamopoulos KC. Hypomagnesemia in alcoholic patients. *Alcohol Clin Exp Res*, 22, 134 (1998)

1331 Elisaf M, Bairaktari H, Siamopoulos KC. Lp(a) levels in Greek patients with heterozygous familial hypercholesterolemia. *Int J Cardiol*, 53, 314-316 (1996)

1332 Elisaf M, Panteli K, Theodorou J, Siamopoulos KC. Fractional excretion of magnesium in normal subjects and in patients with hypomagnesemia. *Magnesium Res*, 10, 315-320 (1997)

1333 Elkarim RA, Mustafa M, Kivisakk P, et al. Cytokine autoantibodies in multiple sclerosis, aseptic meningitis and stroke. *Eur J Clin Invest*, 28, 295-299 (1998)

1334 El-Khawad C, Jamart J, Donckier J et al. Hemostasis variables in type I diabetic patients without demonstrable vascular complications. *Diabetes Care*, 16, 1137-1145 (1993)

1335 Elking MP et al. Drug induced modifications of laboratory test values. *Am J Hosp Pharm*, 25, 485 (1968)

1336 Ellekilde G, von Eyben FE, Holm J et al. Above-normal urinary excretion of albumin and retinol-binding protein in patients with acute myocardial infarction. *Clin Chem*, 39, 2350-2351 (1993)

1337 Elliot BA, Fleming AF. Source of elevated serum enzyme activities in patients with megaloblastic erythropoiesis secondary to folic acid deficiency. *Br Med J*, 1, 626 (1965)

1338 Elliott DW et al. A reevaluation of serum amylase determinations. *Arch Surg*, 83, 130 (1961)

1339 Ellis D, Forrest KY-Z, Erbey J, Orchard TJ. Urinary measurement of transforming growth factor-β and type IV collagen as new markers of renal injury: application of diabetic neuropathy. *Clin Chem*, 44, 991-1001 (1998)

1340 Ellis G, Goldberg DM. A reduced nictotinamide adenine dinucleotide linked kinetic assay for adenosine dreaminase activity. *J Lab Clin Med*, 76, 507-517 (1970)

1341 Ellis LD et al. Marrow iron: an evaluation of depleted stores in a series of 1,322 needle biopsies. *Ann Intern Med*, 61, 44 (1964)

1342 Ellis LD et al. The effect of iron stores on ferrokinetics in polycythemia. *Br J Haematol*, 13, 892 (1967)

1343 Ellman GL, Courtney KD, Andres V Jr et al. A new and rapid colorimetric determination of acetylcholinesterase activity. *Biochem Pharmacol*, 7, 88-95 (1961)

1344 Elneihoum AM, Falke P, Axelsson L, et al. Leukocyte activation detected by increased plasma levels of inflammatory mediators in patients with ischemic cerebrovascular diseases. *Stroke*, 27, 1734-1738 (1996)

1345 Elpeleg ON, Saada AB, Shaag A, et al. Lipoamide dehydrogenase deficiency: a new cause for recurrent myoglobinuria. *Muscle Nerve*, 20, 238-240 (1997)

1346 El-Reshaid KAM, Hakim AA, Hourani HA et al. Endocrine abnormalities in patients with amyloidosis. *Renal Fail*, 16, 725-730 (1994)

1347 Elrod R, Peskind ER, DiGiacomo L, et al. Effects of Alzheimer's disease severity on cerebrospinal fluid norepinephrine concentration. *Am J Psychiat*, 154, 25-30 (1997)

1348 El-Sadr W et al. Acquired immune deficiency syndrome. *Diag Clin Immunol*, 2, 73-85 (1984)

1349 El-Sawy IH, Badr-El-Din OM, El-Azzouni OE, Motawae HA. Soluble intercellular adhesion molecule-1 in sera of children with bronchial asthma exacerbation. *Int Arch Allergy Immunol*, 119, 126-132 (1999)

1350 Eltabbakh GH, Belinson JL, Kennedy AW, et al. Serum CA-125 measurements > 65 U/mL. *J Reprod Med*, 42, 617-624 (1997)

1351 Elwan O, Abdella M, El Bayad AB et al. Hormonal changes in headache patients. *J Neurol Sci*, 106, 75-81 (1991)

1352 El-Yazigi A, Al-Saleh I, Al-Mefty O. Concentrations of Ag, Al, Au, Bi, Cd, Pb, Sb, and Se in cerebrospinal fluid of patients with cerebral neoplasms. *Clin Chem*, 30, 1358-1360 (1984)

1353 El-Yazigi A, Al-Saleh I, Al-Mefty O. Concentrations of zinc, iron, molybdenum, arsenic, and lithium in cerebrospinal fluid of patients with brain tumors. *Clin Chem*, 32, 2187-2190 (1986)

1354 Emad A, Rezalan GR. Lactate dehydrogenase in bronchoalveolar fluid of patients with active pulmonary tuberculosis. *Respiration*, 66, 41-45 (1999)

1355 Emerson PM, Wilkinson JH. Lactate dehydrogenase in the diagnosis and assessment of response to treatment of megaloblastic anemia. *Br J Haematol*, 12, 678 (1966)

1356 Emmanuel NP, Lydiard RB, Reynolds RD et al. Plasma pyridoxal phosphate in anxiety disorders. *Biol Psychiat*, 36, 606-608 (1994)

1357 Emmerson BT. The management of gout. *New Engl J Med*, 334, 445-451 (1996)

1358 Emmons J et al. An aid to the rapid diagnosis of mycoplasma pneumoniae infections. *J Infect Dis*, 179, 650 (1969)

1359 Emoto M, Tabata T, Inoue T et al. Plasma 1,5-anhydroglucitol concentration in patients with end-stage renal disease with and without diabetes mellitus. *Nephron*, 61, 181-186 (1992)

1360 Ende N. Studies of amylase in pleural effusions and ascites. *Cancer*, 13, 283-287 (1960)

1361 Endo K, Maehara Y, Baba H, et al. Elevated levels of serum and plasma metalloproteinases in patients with gastric cancer. *Anticancer Res*, 17, 2253-2258 (1997)

1362 Endo S, Inada K, Ceska M et al. Plasma interleukin 8 and polymorphonuclear leukocyte elastase concentrations in patients with septic shock. *J Inflamm*, 45, 136-142 (1995)

1363 Endo S, Inada K, Kasai T, et al. Levels of soluble adhesion molecules and cytokines in patients with septic multiple organ failure. *J Inflamm*, 46, 212-219 (1996)

1364 Endo S, Inada K, Yamada Y et al. Plasma endotoxin and cytokine concentrations in patients with hemorrhagic shock. *Crit Care Med*, 22, 949-955 (1994)

1365 Engfeldt B, Zellerstrom R. Osteodysmetamorphosis fetalis. *J Pediatr*, 45, 125 (1954)

1366 Engle WK et al. Metabolic studies and therapeutic trials. In:. *Motor Neuron Disease*, New York NY, Grune and Stratton (1969)

1367 Engleman EG, Engleman EP. Ankylosing spondylitis: recent advances in diagnosis and treatment. *Med Clin North Am*, 61, 347-367 (1977)

1368 Engler H, Riesen WF. Effect of thyroid function on concentration of Lp(a). *Clin Chem*, 39, 2466-2469 (1993)

1369 Englert E et al. Metabolism of free and conjugated 17-hydroxy-corticosteroids in subjects with uremia. *J Clin Endocrinol Metab*, 18, 36 (1958)

1370 Engstrom-Laurent A, Feltelius N, Hallgren R et al. Raised serum hyaluronate levels in scleroderma: an effect of growth factor induced activation of connective tissue cells. *Ann Rheum Dis*, 44, 614-620 (1985)

1371 Engstrom-Laurent A, Loof L, Nyberg A et al. Increased serum levels of hyaluronate in liver disease. *Hepatology*, 5, 638-642 (1985)

1372 Entrican JH. Raised plasma estradiol and estrone levels in young survivors of myocardial infarction. *Lancet*, 2, 487-489 (1978)

1373 Epstein DM, Kline LR, Albelda SM et al. Tuberculous pleural effusions. *Chest*, 91, 106-109 (1987)

1374 Epstein JH, Redeker AG. Porphyria cutanea tarda - a study of the effect of phlebotomy. *N Engl J Med*, 279, 1301 (1968)

1375 Epstein S, Traberg H, Raja R, Poser J. Serum and dialysate osteocalcin levels in hemodialysis and peritoneal dialysis patients and after renal transplantation. *J Clin Endocrinol Metab*, 60, 1253-1256 (1985)

1376 Erbil MK, Karayilanoglu T, Kutluay T. The role of ATP-citrate lyase (ACL) in chronic alcoholics and its effect on lipid metabolism. *Clin Chem*, 37, 929 (1991)

1377 Erel O. Automated measurement of serum ferroxidase activity. *Clin Chem*, 44, 2313-2319 (1998)

1378 Erickson AR, Enzenauer RJ, Nordstrom DM et al. The prevalence of hypothyroidism in gout. *Am J Med*, 97, 231-234 (1994)

1379 Erikkson S. Acute appendicitis: a study on diagnostic accuracy and conservative treatment with antibiotics. *Thesis*, Stockholm (1994)

1380 Eriksen HO, Kern Hansen P, Brooks V et al. Plasma fibronectin concentration in normal pregnancy and preeclampsia. *Acta Obstet Gynecol Scand*, 66, 25-28 (1987)

1381 Eriksson P, Denneberg T, Larsson L, Lindstrom F. Biochemical markers of renal disease in primary Sjogren's syndrome. *Scand J Urol Nephrol*, 29, 383-392 (1995)

1382 Eriksson S, Granstrom L, Olander B, Pira U. Leukocyte elastase as a marker in the diagnosis of acute appendicitis. *Eur J Surg*, 161, 901-905 (1995)

1383 Ernst AA, Haynes ML, Nick TG, et al. Usefulness of the blood urea nitrogen/creatinine ratio in gastrointestinal bleeding. *Am J Emerg Med*, 17, 70-72 (1999)

1384 Ersler AJ et al. Plasma erythropoietin in polycythemia. *Am J Med*, 66, 243-247 (1978)

1385 Erslev AJ, Atwater J. Effect of mean corpuscular hemoglobin concentration on viscosity. *J Lab Clin Med*, 62, 401 (1963)

1386 Erzegovesi S, Bellodi L, Smeraldi E. Serum cholinesterase in obsessive-compulsive disorder. *Psych Res*, 58, 265-268 (1995)

1387 Escobar-Morreale HF, Serrano-Gotarredona J, Avila S, et al. The increased circulating prostate-specific antigen concentrations in women with hirsutism do not respond to acute changes in adrenal or ovarian function. *J Clin Endocrinol Metab*, 83, 2580-2584 (1998)

1388 Escobar-Morreale HF, Serrano-Gotarredona J, Garcia-Robles R, et al. Abnormalities in the serum insulin-like growth factor-1 axis in women with hyperandrogenism. *Fertil Steril*, 70, 1090-1100 (1998)

1389 Escobar-Morreale HF, Serrano-Gotarredona J, Garcia-Robles R, et al. Mild adrenal and ovarian steroidogenic abnormalities in hirsute women without hyperandrogenemia: does idiopathic hirsutism exist? *Metabolism*, 46, 902-907 (1997)

1390 Eskelinen M, Tikanoja S, Brown J. Clinical evaluation of new serum tumor markers CA M26 and CA M29 in patients with primary breast cancer. *Anticancer Res*, 10, 959-962 (1990)

1391 Espersen GT, Vestergaard M, Ernst E, Grunnet N. Tumour necrosis factor alpha and interleukin-2 in plasma from rheumatoid arthritis patients in relation to disease activity. *Clin Rheumatol*, 10, 374-376 (1991)

1392 Espinoza LR et al. Joint manifestations of sickle cell disease. *Medicine*, 53, 295-306 (1974)

1393 Estes D et al. The natural history of systemic lupus erythematosus by prospective analysis. *Medicine*, 39, 85 (1960)

1394 Ettehadi P, Greaves MW, Wallach D et al. Elevated tumour necrosis factor-α (TNF-α) biological activity in psoriatic skin lesions. *Clin Exp Immunol*, 96, 146-151 (1994)

1395 Evans AS et al. Specificity, sensitivity, and persistence of heterophil and EB-virus specific IgM antibodies in clinical and subclinical infectious mononucleosis. *J Infect Dis*, 132, 546 (1975)

1396 Evans RS, Duane RT. Acquired hemolytic anemia. I. the relation of erythrocyte antibody production to activity of the disease III. the significance of thrombocytopenia and leukopenia. *Blood*, 4, 1196 (1949)

1397 Evans RS et al. Primary thrombocytopenic purpura and acquired hemolytic anemia. *Arch Intern Med*, 122, 353 (1968)

1398 Evans RS et al. Primary thrombocytopenic purpura and acquired hemolytic anemia: evidence for a common etiology. *Arch Intern Med*, 87, 48 (1951)

1399 Evans RT, Wroe J. Is serum cholinesterase activity a predictor of succinyl choline sensitivity? an assessment of four methods. *Clin Chem*, 24, 1762-1766 (1978)

1400 Ewen LM, Griffiths J. γ-Glutamyl transpeptidase: elevated activities in certain neurologic diseases. *Am J Clin Pathol*, 59, 2-9 (1973)

1401 Faber J, Horslev-Peterson K, Perrild H et al. Different levels of thyroid disease on serum levels of procollagen III N-peptide and hyaluronic acid. *J Clin Endocrinol Metab*, 71, 1016-1021 (1990)

1402 Faber J, Horslev-Peterson, Perrild H et al. Different levels of thyroid disease on serum levels of procollagen III N-peptide and hyaluronic acid. *J Clin Endocrinol Metab*, 67, 1244-1249 (1988)

1403 Faber J, Siersbaek-Nielsen K. Serum free 3,5,3'-triiodothyronine (T3) in non-thyroidal somatic illness, as measured by ultrafiltration and immunoextraction. *Clin Chim Acta*, 256, 115-123 (1996)

1404 Fabris C, Basso DA, Leandro G et al. Serum CA 19-9 and α-fetoprotein in primary hepatocellular carcinoma and liver cirrhosis. *Cancer*, 68, 1795-1798 (1991)

1405 Fabris C, Falleti E, Federico E, et al. A comparison of four serum markers of fibrosis in the diagnosis of cirrhosis. *Ann Clin Biochem*, 34, 151-155 (1997)

1406 Fabris C, Falleti E, Pirisi M, et al. Non-specific increase of serum carbohydrate antigen 19-9 in patients with liver disease associated with increased circulating levels of adhesion molecules. *Clin Chim Acta*, 243, 29-33 (1995)

1407 Facer CA, Agiostratidou G. High levels of anti-phospholipid antibodies in uncomplicated and severe Plasmodium falciparum and in P. vivax malaria. *Clin Exp Immunol*, 95, 304-309 (1994)

1408 Fadel HE et al. Hyperuricemia in pre-eclampsia: a reappraisal. *Am J Obstet Gynecol*, 125, 640-647 (1976)

1409 Fahey JL, Boggs DR. Serum protein changes in malignant disease, the acute leukemias. *Blood*, 16, 1479 (1960)

1410 Fajtova VT, Sayegh MH, Hickey N, et al. Intact parathyroid hormone levels in renal insufficiency. *Calcif Tissue Int*, 57, 329-335 (1995)

1411 Falchuk KR et al. Serum lysozyme in Crohn's disease, a useful index of disease activity. *Gastroenterology*, 69, 893 (1975)

1412 Falcini F, Cerinic MM, Ermini M, et al. Nerve growth factor circulating levels are increased in Kawasaki disease: correlation with disease activity and reduced angiotensin converting enzyme levels. *J Rheumatol*, 23, 1798-1802 (1996)

1413 Falcini F, Cerinic MM, Lombardi A, et al. Increased circulating nerve growth factor is directly correlated with disease activity in juvenile chronic arthritis. *Ann Rheum Dis*, 55, 745-748 (1996)

1414 Famodu AA, Adedeji MO, Reid HL. Serial plasma fibrinogen changes accompanying sickle cell pain crisis. *Clin Lab Haematol*, 12, 43-47 (1990)

1415 Fanconi G. Die familiare panmyelopathie. *Semin Hematol*, 4, 233 (1967)

1416 Fanget F, Terra JL, Dalery J et al. Melatonin circannual rhythm in manic depressive patients. *Encephale*, 16, 197-202 (1990)

1417 Faraj BA, Camp VM, Murray DR et al. Plasma L-dopa in the diagnosis of malignant melanoma. *Clin Chem*, 32, 159-161 (1986)

1418 Faraj BA, Davis DC, Camp VM et al. Platelet monoamine oxidase activity in alcoholics, alcoholics with drug dependence, and cocaine addicts. *Alcohol Clin Exp Res*, 18, 1114-1120 (1994)

1419 Faraj BA, Davis DC, Camp VM et al. The effect of cocaine abuse on plasma levels of sulfated dopamine and salsolinol in alcoholics. *Alcohol*, 11, 337-342 (1994)

1420 Farber MO et al. Studies of plasma vasopressin and renin-angiotensin-aldosterone system in chronic obstructive lung disease. *J Lab Clin Med*, 90, 373-380 (1977)

1421 Fareed J, Talle A, Dries D et al. Molecular markers of coagulation, fibrinolytic and vascular activation in trauma patients. *Clin Biochem Rev*, 14, 267 (1993)

1422 Fargion S, Klasen EC, Lalattta F et al. Alpha 1-antitrypsin in patients with hepatocellular carcinoma and chronic active hepatitis. *Clin Genet*, 19, 134-139 (1981)

1423 Farkkila M, Palo J, Saijonmaa O et al. Raised plasma endothelin during acute migraine attack. *Cephalalgia*, 12, 383-384, discussion 340 (1992)

1424 Farmos Diagnostica Product Insert. SHBG IRMA: Immunoradiometric assay for sex hormone binding globulin. Farmos Diagnostica, Orion Corporation, Oulunsalo, Finland (1991)

1425 Farr M et al. Lysozymurian diabetes. *Br Med J*, 1, 624-265 (1976)

1426 Farrell P, Avery M E. Hyaline membrane disease. *Am Rev Resp Dis*, 111, 657 (1975)

1427 Farrow LJ et al. Autoantibodies and the hepatitis-associated antigen in acute infective hepatitis. *Br Med J*, 2, 693 (1970)

1428 Farthing MJ, Green JR, Edwards CR, Dawson AM. Progesterone, prolactin, and gynaecomastia in men with liver disease. *Gut*, 23, 276-279 (1982)

1429 Fasching P, Veitl M, Rohac M, et al. Elevated concentrations of circulating adhesion molecules and their association with microvascular complications in insulin-dependent diabetes mellitus. *J Clin Endocrinol Metab*, 81, 4313-4317 (1996)

1430 Fassbender K, Michels H, Vogt P et al. Soluble interleukin-2 receptors in children with juvenile chronic arthritis. *Scand J Rheumatol*, 21, 120-123 (1992)

1431 Fatemi S, Ryzen E, Flores J et al. Effect of experimental human magnesium depletion of parathyroid hormone secretion and 1,25-dihydroxyvitamin D metabolism. *J Clin Endocrinol Metab*, 73, 1067-1072 (1991)

1432 Fauler J, Thon A, Tsikas D et al. Enhanced synthesis of cysteinyl leukotrienes in juvenile rheumatoid arthritis. *Arth Rheum*, 37, 93-97 (1994)

1433 Fauler J, Tsikas D, Holch M et al. Enhanced urinary excretion of leukotriene E_4 by patients with multiple trauma with or without adult respiratory distress syndrome. *Clin Sci*, 80, 497-504 (1991)

1434 Faure P, Corticelli P, Richard MJ et al. Lipid peroxidation and trace element status in diabetic ketotic patients: influence of insulin therapy. *Clin Chem*, 39, 789-793 (1993)

1435 Faustman WO, Bardgett M, Faull KF, et al. Cerebrospinal fluid glutamate inversely correlates with positive symptom severity in unmedicated male schizophrenic/schizoaffective patients. *Biol Psychiatr*, 45, 68-75 (1999)

1436 Favier C, Neut C, Mizon C, et al. Fecal β-D-galactosidase production and Bifidobacteria are decreased in Crohn's disease. *Dig Dis Sci*, 42, 817-822 (1997)

1437 Fayol V, Hassanein HI, El-Badrawy N et al. Aminoterminal propeptide of type III procollagen: a marker of disease activity in schistosomal patients. *Eur J Clin Chem Clin Biochem.*, 29, 731-741 (1991)

1438 Feagler JR, Sorenson GD, Rosenfeld MG et al. Rheumatoid pleural effusion. *Arch Pathol Lab Med*, 92, 257-266 (1971)

1439 Feger J. Measurement of serum α_1-acid glycoprotein and α_1-antitrypsin desialylation in liver disease. *Hepatology*, 3, 356-359 (1983)

1440 Feher J et al. Serum lipids and lipoproteins in chronic liver disease. *Acta Med Acad Sci Hung*, 33, 217-223 (1976)

1441 Feig SA et al. Increased erythrocyte calcium content in hereditary spherocytosis. *Pediatr Res*, 9, 928 (1975)

1442 Feighery C, et al. The diagnosis of gluten-sensitive enteropathy: is exclusive reliance on histology appropriate? *Eur J Gastroenterol Hepatol*, 10, 919-925 (1998)

1443 Feigin RD et al. Inappropriate secretion of antidiuretic hormone in children with bacterial meningitis. *Am J Clin Nutr*, 30, 1482-1484 (1977)

1444 Feinglass EJ et al. Neuropsychiatric manifestations of systemic lupus erythematosus: diagnosis, clinical spectrum and relationship to other features of the disease. *Medicine*, 55, 323-339 (1976)

1445 Feinstein DI, Rapaport SI. Acquired inhibitors of blood coagulation. *Prog Haemostas Thromb*, 1, 75 (1972)

1446 Feitelberg S, Epstein S, Ismail F et al. Deranged bone mineral metabolism in chronic alcoholism. *Metabolism*, 36, 211-218 (1987)

1447 Feizi T. Immunoglobulins in chronic liver disease. *Gut*, 9, 193 (1968)

1448 Feizi T. Monotypic cold agglutinins in infection by nature. *Nature*, 215, 540 (1967)

1449 Fekete M, Laszlo A. Serum serotonin level in infantile autistic children. *Clin Chem*, 41, S97 (1995)

1450 Fekkes D, Pepplinkhuizen L, Verheij R et al. Abnormal plasma levels of serine, methionine, and taurine in transient acute polymorphic psychosis. *Psychiat Res*, 51, 11-18 (1994)

1451 Feldman EB, Wallace SL. Hypertriglyceridemia in gout. *Circulation*, 29, 508 (1964)

1452 Feldman JM. Plasma amino acids in patients with the carcinoid syndrome. *Cancer*, 38, 2127-2131 (1976)

1453 Feldman JM. Urinary serotonin in the diagnosis of carcinoid tumors. *Clin Chem*, 32, 840-844 (1986)

1454 Feldman S, Billaud L, Thalabard J-C et al. Fertility in women with late-onset adrenal hyperplasia due to 21-hydroxylase deficiency. *J Clin Endocrinol Metab*, 74, 635-639 (1992)

1455 Feldman WE et al. Cerebrospinal fluid lactic acid dehydrogenase activity. *Am J Dis Child*, 129, 77-80 (1975)

1456 Felice KJ, North WA. Creatine kinase values in amyotrophic lateral sclerosis. *J Neurol Sci*, 160 Suppl 1, S30-S32 (1998)

1457 Felsher BF et al. Indirect reacting bilirubinemia in cirrhosis: its relation to red cell survival. *Am J Dig Dis*, 13, 598 (1968)

1458 Fenton JJ, Jones M, Hartford CE. Calcium fractions in serum of patients with thermal burns. *J Trauma*, 23, 863-866 (1983)

1459 Fenuku RI et al. Serum albumin and total globulin levels in common liver diseases in Accra (Ghana). *Trop Geog Med*, 30, 87-90 (1978)

1460 Fernandes J, Morali G, Wolever TMS et al. Effect of acute lactulose administration on serum acetate lvels in cirrhosis. *Clin invest Med*, 17, 218-225 (1994)

1461 Fernandez-Calle P, Jimenez-Jimenez FJ, Molina JA, et al. Serum levels of ascorbic acid (vitamin C) in patients with Parkinson's disease. *J Neurol Sci*, 118, 25-28 (1993)

1462 Fernandez-Pol JA. Metallopanstimulin as a novel tumor marker in sera of patients with various types of common cancers: implications for prevention and therapy. *Anticancer Res*, 16, 2177-2186 (1996)

1463 Fernandez-Rodriguez CM, Perez-Arguelles BS, Ledo L et al. Ascites adenosine deaminase activity in tuberculous ascites with low protein content. *Am J Gastroenterol*, 86, 1500-1503 (1991)

1464 Fernandez-Rodriguez CM, Quiroga PJ, Zozaya JM, et al. Enhanced urinary excretion of cGMP in liver cirrhosis: relationship to hemodynamic changes, neurohormonal activation, and urinary sodium excretion. *Dig Dis Sci*, 42, 1416-1420 (1997)

1465 Ferraccioli GF, Cavalieri F, Triose Rioda W et al. Relationship between procollagen III peptide serum levels, synovitis of weight bearing joints and disability in rheumatoid arthritis. *Scand J Rheumatol*, 20, 314-318 (1991)

1466 Ferrante A, Storer RJ, Cleland LJ. Polyamine oxidase activity in rheumatoid arthritis synovial fluid. *Clin Exp Immunol*, 80, 373-375 (1990)

1467 Ferrara F, Mirto S. Serum LDH value as a predictor of clinical outcome in acute myelogenous leukemia of the elderly. *Br J Haematol*, 62, 627-630 (1996)

1468 Ferraro AS, Newkirk MM. Correlative studies of rheumatoid factors and anti-viral antibodies in patients with rheumatoid arthritis. *Clin Exp Immunol*, 92, 425-431 (1993)

1469 Ferri C, Bellini C, Desideri G, et al. Elevated plasma endothelin-1 levels as an additional risk factor in non-obese essential hypertensive patients with metabolic abnormalities. *Diabetologia*, 40, 100-102 (1997)

1470 Ferriss JB et al. Low-renin (primary) hyperaldosteronism. differential diagnosis and distinction of sub-groups within the syndrome. *Am Heart J*, 95, 641-658 (1978)

1471 Ferzi T et al. The role of mycoplasma in human disease. *Proc Roy Soc Med*, 59, 1109 (1966)

1472 Fessel WJ. ANA-negative systemic lupus erythematosus. *Am J Med*, 64, 80-6 (1978)

1473 Feussner G, Feussner V, Ziegler R. Apolipoprotein (a) phenotypes and lipoprotein (a) concentrations in patients with type III hyperlipoproteinemia. *J Intern Med*, 235, 425-430 (1994)

1474 Feussner G, Stech C, Dobmeyer J, et al. Serum amyloid A protein (SAA): a marker for liver allograft rejection in humans. *Clin Investig*, 72, 1007-1011 (1994)

1475 Fiala M et al. Pathogenesis of anemia associated with Mycoplasma pneumoniae. *Acta Haematol*, 51, 297 (1974)

1476 Fiddler GI, Lumley P. Preliminary clinical studies with thromboxane synthase inhibitors and thromboxane receptor blockers. A review. *Circulation*, 81, Suppl 1, 169-178 (1990)

1477 Field JB, Williams HE. Artifactual hypoglycemia associated with leukemia. *N Engl J Med*, 265, 946 (1961)

1478 Fierro MT, Lisa F, Novelli M et al. Soluble interleukin-2 receptor, CD4 and CD8 levels in melanoma: a longitudinal study. *Dermatology*, 184, 182-189 (1992)

1479 Fiet J, Gosling JP, Soliman H et al. Hirsutism and acne in women: coordinated radioimmunoassays for eight relevant steroids. *Clin Chem*, 40, 2296-2305 (1994)

1480 Fiet J, Villette J-M, Galons H et al. The application of a new highly-sensitive radioimmunoassay for plasma 21-deoxycortisol to the detection of steroid-21-hydroxylase deficiency. *Ann Clin Biochem*, 31, 56-64 (1994)

1481 Filella X, Alcover J, Molina R, et al. Clinical evaluation of free PSA/total PSA (prostate-specific antigen ratio) in the diagnosis of prostate cancer. *Eur J Cancer*, 33, 1226-1229 (1997)

1482 Fillela X, Fuster J, Molina R, et al. TAG-72, CA 19-9 and CEA as tumor markers in gastric cancer. *Acta Oncol*, 33, 747-751 (1994)

1483 Fillit H, Wanhong D, Luc B. Elevated circulating tumor necrosis factor levels in Alzheimer's disease. *Neurosci Lett*, 129, 318-320 (1991)

1484 Fillmore SJ et al. Blood-gas changes and pulmonary hemodynamics following acute myocardial infarction. *Circulation*, 45, 583 (1972)

1485 Finch CA et al. Ferrokinetics in man. *Medicine*, 49, 17 (1970)

1486 Fink R, Pappas A, Drew MJ et al. Rhabdomyolysis: i) a case of survival after 1.2 million U/L serum creatine kinase elevation: III) retrospective study of rhabdomyolysis based on elevated total serum creatine kinase. *Am J Clin Pathol*, 100, 332-333 (1993)

1487 Finucane JF et al. Effects of chronic renal disease on thyroid hormone metabolism. *Acta Endocrinol*, 84, 750-758 (1977)

1488 Fiorini F, Masturzo P, Mij M et al. Lipoprotein(a) levels in hemodialysis patients: relation to glucose intolerance and hemodialysis duration. *Nephron*, 70, 500-501 (1995)

1489 Firth JD, Ratcliffe PJ, Raine AEG et al. Endothelin: an important factor in acute renal failure? *Lancet*, 2, 1179-1182 (1988)

1490 Fischer P, Gotz ME, Danielczyk W, et al. Blood transferrin and ferritin in Alzheimer's disease. *Life Sci*, 60, 2273-2278 (1997)

1491 Fischer P, Gotz ME, Ellinger B et al. Platelet monoamine oxidase B activity and vitamin B_{12} in dementia. *Biol Psychiat*, 35, 772-774 (1994)

1492 Fischer RL, Bianculli KW, Hediger ML et al. Maternal serum uric acid levels in twin gestations. *Obstet Gynecol*, 85, 60-64 (1995)

1493 Fisher DH, Bostom AG. Total N-acetylcysteine levels are elevated in the plasma of patients with chronic renal failure. *Anal Lett*, 30, 1823-1831 (1997)

1494 Fisher GL et al. Copper and zinc levels in serum from human patients with sarcomas. *Cancer*, 37, 356-363 (1976)

1495 Fisher JW et al. Studies on the mechanism of the anemia of renal insufficiency. *Rev Interam Radiol*, 6, 19-22, 42-49 (1976)

1496 Fishman P, Kamashta M, Ehrenfeld M et al. Interleukin-3 immunoassay in systemic lupus erythematosus patients: preliminary data. *Int Arch Allergy Immunol*, 100, 215-218 (1993)

1497 Fishman WH et al. Markers for ovarian cancer: Regan isoenzyme and other glycoproteins. *Semin Oncol*, 3, 211-216 (1975)

1498 Fishman WH, Kato K, Antiss CL, Green S. Human serum β-glucuronidase: its measurement and some of its properties. *Clin Chim Acta*, 15, 435-447 (1967)

1499 Fitzpatrick TB et al (eds). *Dermatology in General Medicine*. New York NY, McGraw-Hill (1971)

1500 Fizazi K, Cojean I, Pignon J-P, et al. Normal serum neuron specific enolase (NSE) value after the first cycle of chemotherapy. *Cancer*, 82, 1049-1055 (1998)

1501 Fizazi K, Farhat F, Theodore C, et al. Ca125 and neuron-specific enolase (NSE) as tumor markers for intra-abdominal desmoplastic small round-cell tumours. *Br J Cancer*, 75, 76-78 (1997)

1502 Flecchia D, Mazza E, Carlini M et al. Reduced serum levels of dehydroepiandrosterone sulphate in adrenal incidentalomas: a marker of adrenocortical tumour. *Clin Endocrinol*, 42, 129-134 (1995)

1503 Flegar-Mestric Z, Tadej D, Subic-Albert N. Validity of 5-aminolevulinate dehydratase activity (5-ALAD) for the discrimination of alcoholics and nonalcoholics with chronic liver disease. *Clin Biochem*, 20, 81-84 (1987)

1504 Flege JB. Ruptured tubal pregnancy with elevated serum amylase levels. *Arch Surg*, 92, 397 (1966)

1505 Fleming LW et al. Plasma and erythrocyte magnesium in Huntington's chorea. *J Neurol Neurosurg Psychiatry*, 30, 374 (1967)

1506 Fleming SC, Smith S, Saunders P et al. Comparison of prognostic markers in myeloma and MGUS. *Proc ACB Natl Meet*, 168-169 (1995)

1507 Flesch M, Sachinidis A, Ko YD et al. Plasma lipids and lipoproteins and essential hypertension. *Clin Investig*, 72, 944-950 (1994)

1508 Fletcher AP et al. Blood coagulation and plasma fibrinolytic enzyme system pathophysiology in stroke. *Stroke*, 7, 337-348 (1976)

1509 Flick MR et al. Continuous in-vivo monitoring of arterial oxygenation in chronic obstructive lung disease. *Ann Intern Med*, 86, 725-730 (1977)

1510 Flink EB. Magnesium deficiency in alcoholism. *Alcohol Clin Exp Res*, 10, 590-594 (1986)

1511 Flore CH, Gustafson A. Apolipoproteins A-I, A-II and E in cholestatic liver disease. *Scand J Clin Lab Invest*, 45, 103-108 (1985)

1512 Florijn KW, Derkx FHM, Visser W et al. Plasma immunoreactive endothelin-1 in pregnant women with and without pre-eclampsia. *J Cardiovasc Pharmacol*, 17, Suppl 7, S446-S448 (1991)

1513 Foberg U, Fryd'EN A, K'Agedal B, Tobiasson P. Serum bile acids in Gilbert's syndrome after oral load of chenodeoxycholic acid. *Scand J Gastroenterol*, 20, 325-329 (1985)

1514 Foekens JA, Schmitt M, Wim LJ et al. Plasminogen activator inhibitor-1 and prognosis in primary breast cancer. *J Clin Oncol*, 12, 1648-1658 (1994)

1515 Fogar P, Basso D, Paozzo MP et al. C-peptide pattern in patients with pancreatic cancer. *Anticancer Res*, 13, 2577-2580 (1993)

1516 Fogel BJ et al. A note on serum complement activity with particular reference to ulcerative colitis. *Milit Med*, 132, 282 (1967)

1517 Fogel W, Krieger D, Veith M, et al. Serum neuron-specific enolase as early predictor of outcome after cardiac arrest. *Crit Care Med*, 25, 1133-1138 (1997)

1518 Follenius M, Brandenberger G, Simon C. Nocturnal fluctuations of plasma atrial natriuretic peptide in normotensive and hypertensive men. *Life Sci*, 42, 1635-1639 (1988)

1519 Folsom AR, Qamhieh HT, Flack JM et al. Plasma fibrinogen: levels and correlates in young adults. *Am J Epidemiol*, 138, 1023-1036 (1993)

1520 Folsom AR, Smith CL, Prineas RJ et al. Serum calcium fractions in essential hypertensive and matched normotensive subjects. *Hypertension*, 8, 11-15 (1986)

1521 Fonda M, Da Col PG, La Verde R et al. Lipoprotein(a) serum concentration in familial combined hyperlipidemia. *Clin Chim Acta*, 223, 121-127 (1993)

1522 Fonseca V, Ball S, Marks V et al. Hypoglycemia associated with anorexia nervosa. *Postgrad Med J*, 67, 460-461 (1991)

1523 Fonseca VA, D'Souza V, Houlder S et al. Vitamin D deficiency and low osteocalcin concentrations in anorexia nervosa. *J Clin Pathol*, 41, 195-197 (1988)

1524 Font J, pallares L, Martorell J, et al. Elevated soluble CD27 levels in serum of patients with systemic lupus erythematosus. *Clin Immunol Immunopathol*, 81, 239-243 (1996)

1525 Foo Y, Konecny P. Hyperamylasaemia in asymptomatic HIV patients. *Ann Clin Biochem*, 34, 259-262 (1997)

1526 Ford C, Wells FE, Rogers JN. Assessment of iron status in association with excess alcohol consumption. *Ann Clin Biochem*, 32, 527-531 (1995)

1527 Ford ES, Will JC, Bowman BA, Narayan KMV. Diabetes mellitus and serum carotenoids: findings from the third National Health and Nutrition Examination survey. *Am J Epidemiol*, 149, 168-76 (1999)

1528 Forman SD, Bissette G, Yao J et al. Cerebrospinal fluid corticotropin-releasing factor increases following haloperidol withdrawal in chronic schizophrenia. *Schiz Res*, 12, 43-51 (1994)

1529 Fornari MC, Pedreira S, Niveloni S, et al. Pre- and post-treatment serum levels of cytolines IL-1β, IL-6, and IL-1 receptor antagonist in celiac disease. Are they related to the associated osteopenia? *Am J Gastroenterol*, 93, 413-418 (1998)

1530 Forslund T, Fyhrquist F, Tikkanen I et al. Plasma atrial natriuretic peptide in cardiac transplant recipients: a prospective study. *Acta Med Scand*, 224, 3-7 (1988)

1531 Forsyth J, Grunewald RA, Lennard MS, et al. Alltered caffeine metabolism in patients with Parkinson's disease. *Br J Clin Pharmacol*, 47, 579P (1999)

1532 Fort JG, Cowchock FS, Abruzzo JL et al. Anticardiolipin antibodies in patients with rheumatic diseases. *Arth Rheum*, 30, 752-760 (1987)

1533 Fortson MR, Freedman SN, Webster PD. Clinical assessment of hyperlipidemic pancreatitis. *Am J Gastroenterol*, 90, 2134-2139 (1995)

1534 Fossey MD, Lydiard RB, Ballenger JC, et al. Cerebrospinal fluid corticotropin-releasing factor concentrations in patients with anxiety disorders and normal comparison subjects. *Biol Psychiatr*, 39, 703-707 (1996)

1535 Fotino. Elevation of serum alkaline phosphatase in severe pyelonephritis and obstructive nephropathy. *Nephron*, 12, 197-210 (1974)

1536 Foulk et al. Constitutional hepatic dysfunction (Gilbert's disease) its natural history and related syndromes. *Medicine*, 38, 25 (1969)

1537 Fowler D et al. Aminoaciduria and megaloblastic anemia. *J Clin Pathol*, 13, 230 (1960)

1538 Fowler JE Jr, Taylor G, Blom J, Stutzman RE. Experience with serum α-fetoprotein and human chorionic gonadotropin in non-seminomatous testicular tumors. *J Urol*, 124, 365-368 (1980)

1539 Fowler NO. Differential diagnosis of cardiomyopathies. *Prog Cardiovasc Dis*, 14, 113-128 (1971)

1540 Fowler W. The erythrocyte sedimentation rate in syphilis. *Br J Vener Dis*, 52, 309-312 (1976)

1541 Fowler WM, Pearson CM. Diagnostic and prognostic significance of serum enzymes. III. neurologic diseases other than muscular dystrophy. *Arch Phys Med Rehabil*, 45, 125 (1963)

1542 Foy HM et al. Mycoplasma pneumoniae in an urban area. *J Am Med Ass*, 214, 1666 (1970)

1543 France MW, Seneviratne CJ. Screening for prostatic carcinoma: case finding is not a problem. *Ann Clin Biochem*, 34, 333-338 (1997)

1544 Franceschini G, Werba JP, D'Acquarica AL et al. Microsomal enzyme inducers raise plasma high-density lipoprotein cholesterol levels in healthy control subjects but not in patients with primary hypoalphalipoproteinemia. *Clin Pharmacol Ther*, 57, 434-440 (1995)

1545 Francini G, Gonnelli S, Petrioloi R et al. Procollagen type I carboxy-terminal propeptide as a marker of osteoblastic bone metastases. *Cancer Epidemiol Biomarkers Prev*, 2, 125-129 (1993)

1546 Franciotta D, Di Paolo E, Tinelli C, Melzi d'Eril G. Protein ˆ in cerebrospinal fluid of patients with Alzheimer's disease. *Clin Chem*, 44, 357-358 (1998)

1547 Francis. Catecholamine levels in CHF. *Cardiovasc Rep Rev*, 6, 445

1548 Francis RB Jr, Haywood LJ. Elevated immunoreactive tumor necrosis factor and interleukin-1 in sickle cell disease. *J Natl Med Ass*, 84, 611-615 (1992)

1549 Franck H, Keck E. Serum osteocalcin and vitamin D metabolites in patients with ankylosing spondylitis. *Ann Rheum Dis*, 52, 343-346 (1993)

1550 Franco AE, Levine HD, Hall AP. Rheumatoid pericarditis. Report of 17 cases diagnosed clinically. *Ann Intern Med*, 77, 837-844 (1972)

1551 Francois B, Trimoreau F, Vignon P, et al. Thrombocytopenia in the sepsis syndrome: role of hemophagocytosis and macrophage colony-stimulating factor. *Am J Med*, 103, 114-120 (1997)

1552 Franco-Morselli R et al. Increased plasma adrenaline concentrations in benign essential hypertension. *Br Med J*, 2, 1251-1254 (1977)

1553 Franconi F, Bennardini F, Mattana A et al. Plasma and platelet taurine are reduced in subjects with insulin-dependent diabetes mellitus: effects of taurine supplementation. *Am J Clin Nutr*, 61, 1115-1119 (1995)

1554 Francos GC, Kauh YC, Gittlen SD et al. Elevated plasma histamine in chronic uremia: effects of ketotifen on pruritus. *Int J Dermatol*, 30, 884-889 (1991)

1555 Frank MM et al. Hereditary angioedema: the clinical syndrome and its management. *Ann Intern Med*, 84, 580-593 (1976)

1556 Frankel WL, Herold DA, Ziegler TW, Fitzgerald RL. Cardiac troponin-T is elevated in asymptomatic patients with chronic renal failure. *Am J Clin Pathol*, 106, 118-123 (1996)

1557 Franklin AJ. Cytomegalovirus infection presenting as acute haemolytic anaemia in an infant. *Arch Dis Child*, 47, 474 (1972)

1558 Franzke A, Probst-Kepper M, Buer J, et al. Elevated pretreatment serum levels of soluble vascular cell adhesion molecule 1 and lactate dehydrogenase as predictors of survival in cutaneous metastatic malignant melanoma. *Br J Cancer*, 78, 40-45 (1998)

1559 Fraser. Hypophosphatasia. *Am J Med*, 22, 730-746 (1957)

1560 Fraser WD, Robinson J, Lawton R et al. Elevated parathyroid hormone related peptide is associated with increased metastatic spread in hypercalcaemia of malignancy. *Proc ACB Natl Meet*, 20 (1994)

1561 Fredenrich A, Giroux L-M, Tremblay M, et al. Plasma lipoprotein distribution of apoC-III in normolipidemic and hypertriglyceridemic subjects: comparison of the apoC-III to apoE ratio in different lipoprotein fractions. *J Lipid Res*, 38, 1421-1432 (1997)

1562 Fredericks S, Leatham E, Redwood S et al. Urinary β-thromboglobulin is increased in unstable angina. *Proc ACB Natl Meet*, 37 (1994)

1563 Fredman P, Wallin A, Blennow K et al. Sulfatide as a biochemical marker in cerebrospinal fluid of patients with vascular dementia. *Acta Neurol Scand*, 85, 103-106 (1992)

1564 Fredrickson DS, Levy RI, Lees. Fat transport in lipoproteins - an integrated approach to mechanisms and disorders (concluded). *N Engl J Med*, 276, 273-281 (1967)

1565 Fredrickson DS, Levy RI, Lees. Fat transport in lipoproteins - an integrated approach to mechanisms and disorders (continued). *N Engl J Med*, 276, 148-156 (1967)

1566 Fredrickson DS, Levy RI, Lees. Fat transport in lipoproteins - an integrated approach to mechanisms and disorders (continued). *N Engl J Med*, 276, 215-225 (1967)

1567 Frei K, Fredrikson S, Fontana A, Link H. Interleukin-6 is elevated in plasma in multiple sclerosis. *J Neuroimmunol*, 31, 147-153 (1991)

1568 Frenette PS, Thirlwell, Trudeau M et al. The diagnostic value of CA 27-29, CA 15-3, mucin-like carcinoma antigen, carcinoembryonic antigen and CA 19-9 in breast and gastrointestinal malignancies. *Tumor Biol*, 15, 247-254 (1994)

1569 Frenkel EP et al. Elevated serum acid phosphatase associated with multiple myeloma. *Arch Intern Med*, 110, 345-349 (1962)

1570 Frenkel JK. Toxoplasmosis: mechanisms of infection, laboratory diagnosis and management. *Curr Top Pathol*, 54, 28 (1971)

1571 Frezza M, di Padova C, Pozzato G et al. High blood alcohol levels in women; the role of decreased gastric alcohol dehydrogenase activity and first-pass metabolism. *N Engl J Med*, 322, 95-99 (1990)

1572 Fricker J, Fumeron F, Chabchoub S et al. Lack of association between dietary alcohol and HDL-concentrations in obese women. *Atherosclerosis*, 81, 119-125 (1990)

1573 Fried MW, Murthy UK, Hassig SR et al. Creatine kinase isoenzymes in the diagnosis of intestinal infarction. *Dig Dis Sci*, 36, 1589-1593 (1991)

1574 Friedman AL, Helliczer JD, Gundberg CM et al. Serum osteocalcin concentrations in children with chronic renal insufficiency who are not undergoing dialysis. *J Pediatr*, 116, S55-S59 (1990)

1575 Friedman GD et al. The leukocyte count as a predictor of myocardial infarction. *N Engl J Med*, 290, 1275-1278 (1974)

1576 Friedman RB. Author's own data gathered from patients hospitalized at the University of Wisconsin hospitals. Data were collected on a minimum of ten patients for each reported disease-test association. *Unpublished Observations* (1974-1979)

1577 Friedman Z et al. Essential fatty acids, prostaglandins, and respiratory distress syndrome of the newborn. *Pediatrics*, 61, 341-347 (1978)

1578 Fries JF. The clinical aspects of systemic lupus erythematosus. *Med Clin North Am*, 61, 229-239 (1977)

1579 Fries JF, Holman HR. Systemic lupus erythematosus: a clinical analysis. In:. *Major Problems In Internal Medicine,* Smith LH (ed), Philadelphia PA, WB Saunders, 5, 123 (1975)

1580 Friman G. Serum creatine phosphokinase in epidemic influenza. *Scand J Infect Dis*, 8, 13-20 (1976)

1581 Frimpter GW. Cystathioninuria in a patient with cystinuria. *Am J Med*, 46, 832 (1969)

1582 Frithz G, Ronquist G, Ericsson P. Serum sialyltransferase and fucosyltransferase activities in patients with multiple myeloma. *Eur J Cancer Clin Oncol*, 21, 913-917 (1985)

1583 Frohlich J et al. Carbohydrate metabolism in renal failure. *Am J Clin Nutr*, 31, 1541-1546 (1978)

1584 Frost SJ. A simple quantitative index of the P3 amylase isoenzyme in the diagnosis of acute pancreatitis. *Clin Chim Acta*, 87, 23-28 (1976)

1585 Fryden A et al. Demonstration of cerebrospinal fluid lymphocytes sensitized against virus antigens in mumps meningitis. *Acta Neurol Scand*, 57, 396-404 (1978)

1586 Fuchs D, Hausen A, Kofler M et al. Neopterin as an index of immune response in patients with tuberculosis. *Lung*, 162, 337-346 (1984)

1587 Fuchs F, Klopper A. *Endocrinology of Pregnancy.* New York NY, Harper and Row (1971)

1588 Fudenberg HH, Stites DP, Caldwell JJ, Wells JV. *Basal and Clinical Immunology.* 3rd edition, Los Altos CA, Lange Medical Publications (1980)

1589 Fuh MM, Shieh SM, Wu DA et al. Abnormalities of carbohydrate and lipid metabolism in patients with hypertension. *Arch Intern Med*, 147, 1035-1038 (1987)

1590 Fuh MMT, Lee C-M, Jeng C-Y, et al. Effect of chronic renal failure on high-density lipoprotein kinetics. *Kidney Int*, 37, 1295-1300 (1990)

1591 Fuji S, Konishi I, Suzuki A et al. Analysis of serum lactate dehydrogenase levels and its isoenzymes in ovarian dysgerminoma. *Gynecol Oncol*, 22, 65-72 (1985)

1592 Fujihara M, Uemasu J, Kawasaki H. Serum and urinary levels of insulin-like growth factor I in patients with chronic renal disease and diabetes mellitus. *Clin Nephrol*, 45, 372-378 (1996)

1593 Fujii K, Tsuji M, Kitamura A et al. The diagnostic significance of anti-type II collagen antibody assay in rheumatoid arthritis. *Int Orthop*, 16, 272-276 (1992)

1594 Fujimoto K, Ichimori Y, Kakizoe T et al. Increased serum levels of basic fibroblast growth factor in patients with renal cell carcinoma. *Biochem Biophys Res Commun*, 180, 386-392 (1991)

1595 Fujimoto K, Kubo K, Yamaguchi S et al. Eosinophil activation in patients with pulmonary fibrosis. *Chest*, 108, 48-54 (1995)

1596 Fujimoto S, Kubo T, Tanaka H et al. Urinary pyridinoline and deoxypyridinoline in healthy children and in children with growth hormone deficiency. *J Clin Endocrinol Metab*, 80, 1922-1928 (1995)

1597 Fujishima H, Takeyama M, Takeuchi T, et al. Elevated levels of substance P in tears of patients with allergic conjunctivitis and vernal keratoconjunctivitis. *Clin Exp Allergy*, 27, 372-378 (1997)

1598 Fujishima T, Honda Y, Shijubo N, et al. Increased carcinoembryonic antigen concentrations in sera and bronchoalveolar lavage fluids of patients with pulmonary alveolar proteinosis. *Respiration*, 62, 317-321 (1995)

1599 Fujita K, Honda M, Hayashi R, et al. Transglutaminase activity in serum and cerebrospinal fluid in sporadic amyotrophic lateral sclerosis: a possible use as an indicator of extent of the motor neuron loss. *J Neurol Sci*, 158, 53-57 (1998)

1600 Fukasawa Y, Kano S. Anti-type II collagen antibodies in collagen disease. *Rinsho Byori*, 41, 876-881 (1993)

1601 Fulks A et al. Carcinoembryonic antigen (CEA): molecular biology and clinical significance. *Biochem Biophys Res Commun*, 417, 123 (1975)

1602 Fuller RK, Hoppel CL. Plasma carnitine in alcoholism. *Alcohol Clin Exp Res*, 12, 639-642 (1988)

1603 Fulop M et al. Lactic acidosis in diabetic patients. *Arch Intern Med*, 136, 987-990 (1976)

1604 Funahashi A, Sarkar TK, Kory RC. pO_2, pCO_2, and pH in pleural effusion. *J Lab Clin Med*, 78, 1006 (1971)

1605 Fung YK, Meade AG, Rack EP et al. Determination of blood mercury concentrations in Alzheimer's patients. *Clin Toxicol*, 33, 243-247 (1995)

1606 Furkem FC. Serum muramidase in haematological disorders. *NZ Med J*, 1, 28 (1972)

1607 Furue M, Koga T, Yamashita N. Soluble E-selectin and eosinophil cationic protein are distinct serum markers that differentially represent clinical features of atopic dermatitis. *Br J Derm*, 140, 67-72 (1999)

1608 Furuhashi N, Kimura H, Nagae H et al. Maternal plasma endothelin levels and fetal status in normal and preeclamptic pregnancies. *Gynecol Obstet Invest*, 39, 88-92 (1995)

1609 Furuhashi N, Kimura H, Nagae H et al. Serum laminin levels in normal pregnancy and preeclampsia. *Gynecol Obstet Invest*, 36, 172-175 (1993)

1610 Furukawa S, Matsubara T, Umezawa Y et al. Serum levels of p60 soluble tumor necrosis factor receptor during acute Kawasaki disease. *J Pediatr*, 124, 721-725 (1994)

1611 Fusco FD, Rosen SW. Gonadotropin-producing anaplastic large cell carcinomas of the lung. *N Engl J Med*, 275, 507 (1966)

1612 Gabay C, Cakir N, Moral F, et al. Circulating levels of tumor necrosis factor soluble receptors in systemic lupus erythemaosus are significantly higher than in other rheumatic diseases and correlate with disease activity. *J Rheumatol*, 24, 303-308 (1997)

1613 Gabay C, Gay-Croisier F, Roux-Lombard P, et al. Elevated serum levels of interleukin-1 receptor antagonist in polymyositis/dermatomyositis. *Arth Rheum*, 37, 1744-1751 (1994)

1614 Gabay C, Singwe M, Genin B, et al. Circulating levels of IL-11 and leukemia inhibitory factor (LIF) do not significantly participate in the production of acute-phase proteins in the liver. *Clin Exp Imunol*, 105, 260-265 (1996)

1615 Gabazza EC, Osamu T, Yamakami T et al. Correlation between clotting and collagen metabolism markers in rheumatoid arthritis. *Thromb Haemostas*, 71, 199-202 (1994)

1616 Gaboury CL, Hollenberg NK, Hopkins PN et al. Metabolic derangements in nonmodulating hypertension. *Am J Hypertens*, 8, 870-875 (1995)

1617 Gabr Y et al. Fatty acid composition of serum lipids in bilharzial hepatic fibrosis and chronic active hepatitis. *Acta Biol Med Ger*, 34, 45-51 (1975)

1618 Gabriel R. Ethambutol and a false-positive screening test for phaeochromocytoma. *Br Med J*, 3, 332 (1972)

1619 Gabrijelic D, Svetic B, Spaic D et al. Cathepsins B, H and L in human breast cancer. *Eur J Clin Chem Clin Biochem*, 30, 69-74 (1992)

1620 Gabuzda GJ. Ammonia metabolism and hepatic coma. *Gastroenterology*, 53, 806-810 (1967)

1621 Gadducci A, Baicchi U, Marral R, et al. Pre-operative evaluation of D-dimer and CA 125 levels in differentiating benign from malignant ovarian masses. *Gynecol Oncol*, 60, 197-202 (1996)

1622 Gadler H et al. Increased serum α-fetoprotein levels in cytomegalovirus infections. *Scand J Infect Dis*, 10, 101-105 (1978)

1623 Gaillard O, Meillet D, Diemert MC et al. Time-resolved immunofluorometric assay of complement C_3: application to cerebrospinal fluid. *Clin Chem*, 39, 309-312 (1993)

1624 Gaillard O, Meillet D, Gervais A et al. Lipoprotein(a) in cerebrospinal fluid measured by highly sensitive time-resolved immunofluorometric assay. *Clin Chem*, 40, 1975-1976 (1994)

1625 Galea P, Vermot-Desroches C, Le Contel C, et al. Circulating cell adhesion molecules in HIV-1 infected patients as indicator markers for AIDS progression. *Res Immunol*, 148, 109-117 (1997)

1626 Galen RS. The enzyme diagnosis of myocardial infarction. *Hum Pathol*, 6, 141-155 (1975)

1627 Gallagher, Seligson D. Significance of abnormally low blood urea levels. *N Engl J Med*, 266, 492-495 (1962)

1628 Gallardo JM, Padillo J, Martin-Malo A, et al. Increased plasma levels of atrial natriuretic peptide and endocrine markers of volume depletion in patients with obstructive jaundice. *Br J Surg*, 85, 28-31 (1998)

1629 Gallou G, Guilhem I, Poirier J-Y et al. Increased serum ferritin in insulin-dependent diabetes mellitus: relation to glycemic control. *Clin Chem*, 40, 947-948 (1994)

1630 Galton M et al. Coagulation studies on the peripheral circulation of patients with toxemia of pregnancy: a study for the evaluation of. *J Reprod Med*, 6, 89 (1971)

1631 Galvani M, Ottani F, Ferrini D, et al. Prognostic influence of elevated values of cardiac troponin I in patients with unstable angina. *Circulation*, 95, 2053-2059 (1997)

1632 Galvez S, Farcas A, Monari M. The concentration of α-1-antitrypsin in cerebrospinal fluid and serum in a series of 40 intracranial tumors. *Clin Chim Acta*, 91, 191-196 (1979)

1633 Gama R, Norris F, Wright J, et al. The entero-insular axis in polycystic ovarian syndrome. *Ann Clin Biochem*, 33, 190-195 (1996)

1634 Gamba G, Fornasari P, Montani N, Biancardi M et al. Plasma levels of protease inhibitors in acute myeloid leukemia at the onset of the disease and during antiblastic therapy. *Thromb Res*, 17, 41-53 (1980)

1635 Gamklou R, Schersten T. Activity of α1,4-glucosidase in serum from patients with malignant tumor. *Cancer*, 32, 298-301 (1973)

1636 Gando S, Nanzaki S, Sasaki S, Kemmotsu O. Significant correlations between tissue factor and thrombin markers in trauma and septic patients with disseminated intravascular coagulation. *Thromb Haemost*, 79, 1111-1115 (1998)

1637 Ganguli R, Yang Z, Shurin G et al. Serum interleukin-6 concentration in schizophrenia: elevation associated with duration of illness. *Psychiat Res*, 51, 1-10 (1994)

1638 Gann DS, Lilly MP. The endocrine response to injury. *Prog Crit Care Med*, 1, 15-47 (1984)

1639 Ganrot, Narlin, Karin. Relative concentrations of albumin and IgG in cerebrospinal fluid in health and in acute meningitis. *Scand J Infect Dis*, 10, 57-60 (1978)

1640 Gansslen M et al. Die hamolytische konstitution. *Dtsch Arch Klin Med*, 146, 1 (1925)

1641 Garb S. *Clinical Guide to Undesirable Drug Interactions and Drug Interferences*. New York NY, Springer Publishing Co (1971)

1642 Garb S. *Laboratory Tests in Common Use*. 6th edition, New York NY, Springer Publishing Co, 46-121 (1976)

1643 Garcia A, Galinowski A, Guicheney P et al. Free and conjugated plasma homovanillic acid in schizophrenic patients. *Biol Psychiat*, 26, 87-96 (1989)

1644 Garcia A, Skurnick JH, Goldsmith LT et al. Human chorionic gonadotropin and relaxin concentrations in early ectopic and normal pregnancies. *Obstet Gynecol*, 75, 779-783 (1990)

1645 Garcia Monco JC, Wheeler CM, Benach JL et al. Reactivity of neuroborreliosis patients (Lyme disease) to cardiolipin and gangliosides. *J Neurol Sci*, 117, 206-214 (1993)

1646 Garcia Zozaya JL, Viloria MP, Castro A. Changes in calcium and magnesium metabolism in essential arterial hypertension. *South Med J*, 81, 350-353 (1988)

1647 Garcia-Alix A, Martin-Ancel A, Ramos MT et al. Cerebrospinal fluid β_2-microglobulin in neonates with central nervous system infections. *Eur J Pediatr*, 154, 309-313 (1995)

1648 Garcia-Borreguero D, Jacobsen FM, Nurphy DL et al. Hormonal responses to the administration of m-chlorophenylpiperazine in patients with seasonal affective disorder and controls. *Biol Psychiat*, 37, 740-749 (1995)

1649 Garcia-Pachon E, Padilla-Navas I, Dosda D, et al. Elevated levels of carcinoembryonic antigen in nonmalignant pleural effusions. *Chest*, 111, 643-647 (1997)

1650 Garcia-Sepulcre MF, Carnicer F, Mauri M, et al. Increased plasma endothelin in liver cirrhosis and response to plasma volume expansion. *Am J Gastroenterol*, 91, 2452-2453 (1996)

1651 Garcia-Unzueta MT, Berrazueta JR, Montalban C, et al. Plasma adrenomedullin levels in type 1 diabetes. *Diabetes Care*, 21, 999-1003 (1998)

1652 Gardner FH, Murphy S. Granulocyte and platelet functions in PNH. *Series Haematol*, 5, 78 (1972)

1653 Gardner RC et al. Serial carcinoembryonic antigen (CEA) levels in patients with ulcerative colitis. *Am J Dig Dis*, 23, 129-133 (1978)

1654 Garello E, Battista S, Bar F, et al. Evaluation of hepatic function in liver cirrhosis: clinical utility of galactose elimination capacity, hepatic clearance of D-sorbitol, and laboratory investigations. *Dig Dis Sci*, 44, 782-788 (1999)

1655 Garibaldi LR, Aceto T Jr, Weber C. The pattern of gonadotropin and estradiol secretion in exaggerated thelarche. *Acta Endocrinol*, 128, 345-350 (1993)

1656 Garibotto G, Gurreri G, Robaudo C et al. Erythropoietin treatment and amino acid metabolism in hemodialysis patients. *Nephron*, 65, 533-536 (1993)

1657 Garito ML, Prihoda TJ, McManus LM. Salivary PAF levels correlate with the severity of periodontal inflamation. *J Dent Res*, 74, 1048-1056 (1995)

1658 Garnero P, Vassy V, Bertholin A et al. Markers of bone turnover in hyperthyroidism and the effects of treatment. *J Clin Endocrinol Metab*, 78, 955-959 (1994)

1659 Garpenstrand H, Ekblom J, von Arbin M, et al. Plasma semicarbazide-sensitive amine oxidase in stroke. *Eur Neurol*, 41, 20-23 (1999)

1660 Garrel DR, Delmas PD, Malaval L et al. Serum bone Gla protein: a marker of bone turnover in hyperthyroidism. *J Clin Endocrinol Metab*, 62, 1052-1055 (1986)

1661 Garst JB et al. Urinary sodium, potassium and aldosterone in Duchenne muscular dystrophy. *J Clin Endocrinol Metab*, 44, 185-188 (1977)

1662 Gartner LA, Pfeifer MC, Albani C et al. Soluble interleukin 2 receptor levels in children with type I insulin-dependent diabetes mellitus. *Ann Clin Lab Sci*, 25, 44-51 (1995)

1663 Garvey MJ, Tuason VB. Urinary levels of 3-methoxy-4-hydroxyphenylglycol predict symptom severity in selected patients with unipolar depression. *Psychiatr Res*, 62, 171-176 (1996)

1664 Gaseecki AP, Eliasziw M, Fox AJ, et al. Serum cholesterol level is associated with the severity of carotid stenosis in symptomatic patients: results from NASCET. *Cerebrovasc Dis*, 4, 417-420 (1994)

1665 Gasim S, El-Hassan AM, Khalil EAG, et al. High levels of plasma IL-10 and expression of IL-10 by keratinocytes during visceral leishmaniasis predict subsequent development of post-kala-azar dermal leishmaniasis. *Clin Exp Immunol*, 111, 64-69 (1998)

1666 Gattaz WF, Dalgalarrondo P, Schroeder HC. Abnormalities in serum concentrations of interleukin-2, interferon-α and interferon-γ in schizophrenia not detected. *Schiz Res*, 6, 237-241 (1992)

1667 Gattaz WF, Schmitt A, Maras A. Increased platelet phospholipase A_2 activity in schizophrenia. *Schiz Res*, 16, 1-6 (1995)

1668 Gaudagni F, Roselli M, Amato T et al. Clinical evaluation of serum tumor-associated glycoprotein-72 as a novel tumor marker for colorectal cancer patients. *J Surg Oncol*, 48, 16-20 (1991)

1669 Gaughran F, O'Neill E, Cole M, et al. Increased soluble interleukin 2 receptor levels in schizophrenia. *Schiz Res*, 29, 263-267 (1998)

1670 Gault MH et al. Clinical significance of urinary LDH, alkaline phosphatase and other enzymes. *Can Med Ass J*, 101, 208-215 (1962)

1671 Gault MH et al. Serum enzymes in patients with carcinoma of lung: lactic-acid dehydrogenase, phosphohexose isomerase, alkaline phosphatase and glutamic oxaloacetic transaminase. *Can Med Ass J*, 96, 87-94 (1967)

1672 Gault MH et al. Urinary enzymes in benign and malignant urinary tract disorders: alkaline phosphatase and lactic acid dehydrogenase. *Br J Urol*, 39, 296-306 (1967)

1673 Gault MH, Longerich LI, Purchase L, et al. Comparison of Lp(a) concentrations and some potential effects in hemodialysis, CAPD, transplantation, and control groups, and review of the literature. *Nephron*, 70, 155-170 (1995)

1674 Gause A, Keymis S, Scholz R et al. Increased levels of circulating cytokines in patients with untreated Hodgkin's disease. *Lymphokine Cytokine Res*, 11, 109-113 (1992)

1675 Gavaler JS, Deal SR, Van Thiel DH et al. Alcohol and estrogen levels in postmenopausal women: the spectrum of effect. *Alcohol Clin Exp Res*, 17, 786-790 (1993)

1676 Gavaud C, Ninet J, Monier JC et al. Anti-neutrophil cytoplasm antibodies in Wegener's granulomatosis and systemic vasculitis. *Presse Med*, 22, 1679-1686 (1993)

1677 Gavilanes EL, Parra EG, de la Piedra C et al. Clinical usefulness of serum carboxyterminal propeptide of procollagen I and tartrate-resistant acid phosphatase determinations to evaluate bone turnover in patients with chronic renal failure. *Miner Elect Metab*, 20, 259-264 (1994)

1678 Gavish D, Kleinman Y, Morag A et al. Hepatitis and jaundice associated with measles in young adults. *Arch Intern Med*, 143, 674-677 (1983)

1679 Gay L et al. Laboratory procedures used in the diagnosis of systemic lupus erythematosus: a review. *Am J Med Technol*, 43, 856-863 (1977)

1680 Gazzard BG et al. Factor VII levels as guide to prognosis in fulminant hepatic failure. *Gut*, 17, 489-491 (1976)

1681 Gdansky E, Diamant YZ, Laron Z, et al. Increased number of IGF-1 receptors on erythrocytes of women with polycystic ovarian syndrome. *Clin Endocrinol*, 47, 185-190 (1997)

1682 Gebala A. Acid hyperphosphatasia in three families with osteogenesis imperfecta. *Lancet*, 2, 1084 (1956)

1683 Gebauer G, Muller-Ruchholtz W. Tumor marker concentrations in normal and malignant tissues of colorectal cancer patients and their prognostic relevance. *Anticancer Res*, 17, 2731-2734 (1997)

1684 Geisler LP, Miller GA, Lee H, et al. Relationship of preoperative serum CA 125 to survival in epithelial ovarian carcinoma. *J Reprod Med*, 41, 140-142 (1996)

1685 Geiss HC, Ritter MM, Richter WO, et al. Low lipoprotein (a) levels during acute viral hepatitis. *Hepatology*, 24, 1334-1337 (1996)

1686 Gelato MC, Rutherford C, San-Roman G et al. The insulin-like growth factor-II/mannose-6-phosphate receptor in normal and diabetic pregnancy. *Metabolism*, 42, 1031-1038 (1993)

1687 Gembicki M et al. Total and free thyroxine in patients with liver cirrhosis. *Pol Med Sci Hist Bull*, 15, 213-216 (1976)

1688 Gemmati D, Previati M, Serino ML, et al. Low folate levels and thermolabile methylenetetrahydrofolate reductase as primary determinant of mild hyperhomocystinemia in normal and thromboembolic subjects. *Arterioscler Thromb Vasc Biol*, 19, 1761-1767 (1999)

1689 Genazzani AR, Nappi G, Facchinetti F et al. Progressive impairment of CSF β-Ep levels in migraine sufferers. *Pain*, 18, 127-133 (1984)

1690 Gendrel D, Raymond J, Assicot M, et al. Procalcitonine, proteine C-reactive et interleukine 6 dans les meningites bacteriennes et virales de l'enfant. *Presse Med*, 27, 1135-1139 (1998)

1691 Genest JJ Jr, Bard JM, Fruchart J-C et al. Plasma apolipoprotein A-I, A-II, B, E, and C-III containing particles in men with premature coronary artery disease. *Atherosclerosis*, 90, 149-157 (1991)

1692 Genest JJ Jr, McNamara JR, Ordovas JM et al. Lipoprotein cholesterol, apolipoprotein A-I and B and lipoprotein (a) abnormalities in men with premature coronary artery disease. *J Am Coll Cardiol*, 19, 792-802 (1992)

1693 Genest JJ Jr, McNamara JR, Salem DN et al. Plasma homocyst(e)ine levels in men with premature coronary artery disease. *J Am Coll Cardiol*, 16, 1114-1119 (1990)

1694 Geokas MC et al. Methemalbumin in the diagnosis of acute hemorrhagic pancreatitis. *Ann Intern Med*, 81, 483-6 (1974)

1695 Geokas MC et al. Studies of the ascites fluid of acute pancreatitis in man. *Am J Dig Dis*, 23, 182-188 (1978)

1696 George MS, Rosenstein D, Rubinow DR et al. CSF magnesium in affective disorder: lack of correlation with clinical course of treatment. *Psychiat Res*, 51, 139-146 (1994)

1697 George PM, Conaghan C, Angus HB, et al. Comparison of histological and biochemical hepatic iron indexes in the diagnosis of genetic hemochromatosis. *J Clin Pathol*, 49, 159-163 (1996)

1698 Georges P, Liefooghe J, Ponchaux D, et al. Urinary growth hormone excretion: results of a multicenter study in France. *Horm Res*, 47, 30-37 (1997)

1699 Geppert A, Graf S, Beckmann R, et al. Concentrations of endogenous tPA antigen in coronary artery disease: relation to thrombotic events, aspirin treatment, hyperlipidemia, and multivessel disease. *Arterioscler Thromb Vasc Biol*, 18, 1634-1642 (1998)

1700 Geracioti TD Jr, Loosen PT, Ebert MH et al. Concentrations of corticotropin-releasing hormone, norepinephrine, MHPG, 5-hydroxyindoleacetic acid, and tryptophan in the cerebrospinal fluid of alcoholic patients: serial sampling studies. *Neuroendocrinology*, 60, 635-642 (1994)

1701 Gerber GS, Goldfischer ER, Karrison TG, et al. Serum creatinine measurements in men with lower urinary tract symptoms secondary to benign prostatic hypertrophy. *Urology*, 49, 697-702 (1997)

1702 Gerbes AL, Hoermann R, Mann K, et al. Human chorionic gonadotropin-β in the differentiation of malignancy-related and nonmalignant ascites. *Digestion*, 57, 113-117 (1996)

1703 Gerbes AL, Jungst D, Xie Y et al. Ascitic fluid analysis for the differentiation of malignancy-related and nonmalignant ascites: proposal of a diagnostic sequence. *Cancer*, 68, 1808-1814 (1991)

1704 Gerbig AW, Dahinden CA, Mullis P, Hunziker T. Circadian elevation of IL-6 levels in Muckle-Wells syndrome: a disorder of the neuro-immune axis? *Q J Med*, 91, 489-492 (1998)

1705 Gerbitz K-D, Summer J, Schumacher I et al. Enolase isoenzymes as tumour markers. *J Clin Chem Clin Biochem*, 24, 1009-1016 (1986)

1706 Gerdes JS, Polin RA. Sepsis screen in neonates with evaluation of plasma fibronectin. *Pediatr Infect Dis J*, 6, 443-446 (1987)

1707 Gerding H, Cremer-Bartels G, Krause K et al. Neopterin in patients with choroidal melanoma. *Eur J Clin Chem Clin Biochem*, 31, 221-224 (1993)

1708 Gericke GS et al. Leucocyte ultrastructure and folate metabolism in Down's syndrome. *S Afr Med J*, 51, 369-374 (1977)

1709 Gerli G, Locatelli GF, Mongiat R et al. Erythrocyte antioxidant activity, serum ceruloplasmin, trace element levels in subjects with alcoholic liver disease. *Am J Clin Pathol*, 97, 614-618 (1992)

1710 Gerlo EAM, Sevens C. Urinary and plasma catecholamines and urinary catecholamine metabolites in pheochromocytoma: diagnostic value in 19 cases. *Clin Chem*, 40, 250-256 (1994)

1711 Gerner RH, Cohen DJ, Fairbanks L et al. CSF neurochemistry of women with anorexia nervosa and normal women. *Am J Psychiat*, 141, 1441-1444 (1984)

1712 Gervais A, Schiller E. Fibronectin in plasma and CSF: evidence for its intrathecal synthesis. *J Neurol Sci*, 105, 200-205 (1991)

1713 Geuse A, Scholz R, Klein S et al. Increased levels of circulating interleukin-6 in patients with Hodgkin's disease. *Hematol Oncol*, 9, 307-313 (1991)

1714 Geynoso G et al. CEA assay in cancer of the colon and pancreas and other digestive tract disorders. *Am J Dig Dis*, 16, 1 (1971)

1715 Ghadimi H et al. A familial disturbance of histidine metabolism. *N Engl J Med*, 265, 221 (1965)

1716 Gharib H et al. Serum levels of thyroid hormones in Hashimoto's thyroiditis. *Mayo Clin Proc*, 47, 175-179 (1972)

1717 Gherardi E et al. Relationship among the concentrations of serum lipoproteins and changes in their chemical composition in patients with untreated nephrotic syndrome. *Eur J Clin Invest*, 7, 563-570 (1977)

1718 Ghigo E, Nicolosi M, Arvat E et al. Growth hormone secretion in Alzheimer's disease: studies with growth hormone-releasing hormone alone and combined with pyridostigmine or arginine. *Dementia*, 4, 315-320 (1993)

1719 Ghirardello A, Doria A, Ruffatti A et al. Antiphospholipid antibodies (aPL) in systemic lupus erythematosus. Are they specific tools for the diagnosis of aPL syndrome? *Ann Rheum Dis*, 53, 140-142 (1994)

1720 Ghose AC et al. Immunoglobulin studies in malaria and kala-azar infections. *Ind J Med Res*, 66, 566-569 (1977)

1721 Ghoshi K. Lactate dehydrogenase in CML. *Am J Clin Path*, 99, 113 (1993)

1722 Gianella RA. Pathogenesis of acute bacterial diarrheal disorders. *Annu Rev Med*, 32, 341-357 (1981)

1723 Giannini E, Botta F, Fasoli A, et al. Progressive liver functional impairment is associated with an decreased AST/ALT ratio. *Digest Dis Sci*, 44, 1249-1253 (1999)

1724 Gibbons RP et al. Manifestations of renal cell carcinoma. *Urology*, 8, 201-206 (1976)

1725 Gibson PR, Fraser JR, Brown TJ et al. Hemodynamic and liver function predictors of serum hyaluronan in alcoholic liver disease. *Hepatology*, 15, 1054-1059 (1992)

1726 Gibson T et al. The effect of acid loading on renal excretion of uric acid and ammonium in gout. *Adv Exp Med Biol*, 76(B), 46-55 (1977)

1727 Gifford R. Is the renin-sodium profile helpful in evaluating hypertension? *J Am Med Ass*, 244, 35-37 (1980)

1728 Gilbert HS et al. A study of histamine in myeloproliferative disease. *Blood*, 28, 795 (1966)

1729 Gilbert HS et al. Plasma and urinary urate findings in myeloproliferative disorders. *J Mt Sinai Hosp*, 30, 185 (1963)

1730 Gilbert HS et al. Serum vitamin B_{12} content and unsaturated vitamin B_{12} binding capacity (UBBC) in myeloproliferative disease: value in differential diagnosis and as parameters of disease. *Ann Intern Med*, 71, 719 (1969)

1731 Gilbert MG. Cushing's syndrome in infancy. *Pediatrics*, 46, 217 (1970)

1732 Gil-del-Alamo P, Saccomanno K, Lania A, et al. Serum levels of β-subunit of chorionic gonadotropin in patients with pituitary tumors. *Eur J Endocrinol*, 133, 33-37 (1995)

1733 Gillespie G, Elder JB, Smith IS, Kennedy F. An analysis of spontaneous gastric acid secretion in normal and duodenal ulcer subjects: new criterion for the insulin test. *Gastroenterology*, 62, 903-911 (1972)

1734 Giltay EJ, Popp-Snijders C, van Schaardenburg D, et al. Serum testosterone levels are not elevated in patients with ankylosing spondylitis. *J Rheumatol*, 25, 2389-2394 (1998)

1735 Gilutz H, Siegel Y, Paran E, Cristal N. Alpha 1-antitrypsin in acute myocardial infarction. *Br Heart J*, 49, 26-29 (1983)

1736 Ginsburg KS, Liang MH, Newcomer L et al. Anticardiolipin antibodies and the risk for ischemic stroke and venous thrombosis. *Ann Intern Med*, 117, 997-1002 (1992)

1737 Gion M, Plebani M, Mione R et al. Serum CA549 in primary breast cancer: comparison with CA15.3 and MCA. *Br J Cancer*, 69, 721-725 (1994)

1738 Giordano C et al. γ-Globulins patterns in CSF of inflammatory neurological diseases in tropical Africa. *Eur Neurol*, 17, 160-165 (1978)

1739 Giovannoni G, Lai M, Kidd D, et al. Daily urinary neopterin excretion as an immunological marker of disease activity in multiple sclerosis. *Brain*, 120, 1-13 (1997)

1740 Gip GYH, Lowe GDO, Rumley A et al. Increased markers of thrombogenesis in chronic atrial fibrillation: effects of warfarin treatment. *Br Heart J*, 73, 527-533 (1995)

1741 Girre C, Hispard E, Therond P et al. Effect of abstinence from alcohol on the depression of glutathione peroxidase activity and selenium and vitamin E levels in chronic alcoholic patients. *Alcohol Clin Exp Res*, 14, 909-912 (1990)

1742 Gisslen M, Larsson M, Norkrans G et al. Tryptophan concentrations increase in cerebrospinal fluid and blood after zidovudine treatment in patients with HIV type 1 infection. *AIDS*, 10, 947-951 (1994)

1743 Giuer S, Schelp C, Madry N, et al. Serum polysialylated neural cell adhesion molecule in childhood neuroblastoma. *Br J Cancer*, 78, 106-110 (1998)

1744 Gjerris A, Hammer M, Vendsborg P et al. Cerebrospinal fluid vasopressin: Changes in depression. *Br J Psychiat*, 147, 696-701 (1985)

1745 Gjerris A, Sorensen AS, Rafaelsen O et al. 5-HT and 5-HIAA in cerebrospinal fluid in depression. *J Affect Disord*, 12, 13-22 (1987)

1746 Gjerris A, Werdelin L, Rafaelson OJ et al. CSF dopamine increased in depression: CSF dopamine, noradrenaline and their metabolites in depressed patients and in controls. *J Affect Disord*, 13, 279-286 (1987)

1747 Gladman DD et al. Systemic lupus erythematosus with negative LE cells and antinuclear factor. *J Rheumatol*, 5, 142-147 (1978)

1748 Glaser NS, Shirali AC, Styne DM, Jones KL. Acid-base homeostasis in children with growth hormone deficiency. *Pediatrics*, 102, 1407-1414 (1998)

1749 Glass AR, Kikendall JW, Sobin LH et al. Serum 25-hydroxyvitamin D concentrations in colonic neoplasia. *Horm Metab Res*, 25, 397-398 (1993)

1750 Glass AR, Kikendall JW, Sobin LH et al. Serum concentrations of insulin-like growth factor I in colonic neoplasia (1994)

1751 Glass IB, Chalmers R, Bartlett S et al. Increased plasma carnitine in severe alcohol dependence. *Br J Addict*, 84, 689-693 (1989)

1752 Glatz JFC, van der Vusse GJ, Maessen JG, et al. Fatty acid-binding protein as marker of muscle injury: experimental findings and clinical application. *Acta Anaesthesiol Scand*, 41 Suppl 111), 292-294 (1997)

1753 Gleason MN, Gosslein RE, Hodge HC. *Clinical Toxicology of Commercial Products*. Baltimore, MD, Williams and Wilkins (1957)

1754 Gleave ME, Coupland D, Drachenberg D, et al. Ability of serum prostate-specific antigen levels to predict normal bone scans in patients with newly diagnosed prostate cancer. *Urology*, 47, 708-712 (1996)

1755 Glendenning P, Stuckey BGA, Gutteridge DH, et al. High prevalence of normal total calcium and intact PTH in 60 patients with proven primary hyperthyroidism: a challenge to current diagnosic criteria. *Aust NZ J Med*, 28, 173-178 (1998)

1756 Glick JH. Serum lactate dehydrogenase isoenzyme and total lactate dehydrogenase values in health and disease, and clinical evaluation of these tests by means of discriminant analysis. *Am J Clin Pathol*, 52, 320-328 (1969)

1757 Glorieux F, Scriver CR. Loss of a parathyroid-hormone-sensitive component of phosphate transport in X-linked hypophosphatemic rickets. *Science*, 173, 997 (1972)

1758 Glovinsky D, Kalogeras KT, Kirch DG et al. Cerebrospinal fluid oxytocin concentration in schizophrenic patients does not differ from control subjects and is not changed by neuroleptic medication. *Schiz Res*, 11, 273-276 (1994)

1759 Glovsky MM et al. Reduction of pleural fluid complement activity in patients with systemic lupus erythematosus and rheumatoid arthritis. *Clin Immunol Immunopathol*, 6, 31-41 (1976)

1760 Glueck CJ, Glueck HI, Hamer T et al. Beta blockers, Lp(a), hypertension, and reduced basal fibrinolytic actity. *Am J Med Sci*, 307, 317-324 (1994)

1761 Glueck CJ, Levy RI, Fredrickson DS. Immunoreactive insulin, glucose tolerance and carbohydrate inducibility in type II, III, IV, and V hyperlipoproteinemia. *Diabetes*, 18, 739 (1969)

1762 Glueck CJ, Tieger M, Kunkel R et al. Hypocholesterolemia and affective disorders. *Am J Med Sci*, 308, 218-225 (1994)

1763 Glueck HI et al. Cold precipitable fibrinogen, cryofibrinogen. *Arch Intern Med*, 113, 748 (1964)

1764 Gluud CH. Serum testosterone concentrations in men with alcoholic cirrhosis: background for variation. *Metabolism*, 36, 373-378 (1987)

1765 Glyn-Jones R. Blood sugar in infantile gastro-enteritis. *S Afr Med J*, 49, 1474-6 (1975)

1766 Gnudi A et al. Variation of blood glucose and serum growth hormone, prolactin and insulin in subjects with insulin-dependent diabetes. *Acta Diabetol Lat*, 14, 119-128 (1977)

1767 Go VLW. Carcinoembryonic antigen. *Cancer*, 37, 562-566 (1976)

1768 Gocze PM, Szabo DG, Than GN et al. Placental protein 4 as a possible tumor marker in ovarian tumors. *Gynecol Obstet Invest*, 32, 107-111 (1991)

1769 Goddard AW, Narayan M, Woods SW, et al. Plasma levels of γ-aminobutyric acid and panic disorder. *Psychiat Res*, 63, 23-225 (1996)

1770 Goedert JJ, Biggar RJ, Melbye M et al. Effect of T4 count and cofactors on the incidence of AIDS in homosexual men infected with human immunodeficiency virus. *J Am Med Ass*, 257, 331 (1987)

1771 Goerz G, Bunselmeyer S, Bolsen K, Schurer NY. Ferrochelatase activities in patients with erythropoietic protoporphyria and their families. *Br J Dermatol*, 134, 880-885 (1996)

1772 Gohji K, Fujimoto N, Hara I, et al. Serum matrix metalloproteinase-2 and its density in men with prostate cancer as a new predictor of disease extension. *Int J Cancer (Pred Oncol)*, 79, 96-101 (1998)

1773 Goka AKJ, Rolston DDK, Mathan VI, Farthing MG. Diagnosis of giardiasis by specific IgM antibody enzyme-linked immunosorbent assay. *J Clin Endocrinol*, 11, 184 (1986)

1774 Gokcen M. Cryoglobulins behaving as cold agglutinins. *Postgrad Med*, 39, A68 (1966)

1775 Golay A, Swislocki ALM, Chen YDL et al. Effect of obesity on ambient plasma glucose, free fatty acid, insulin, growth hormone, and glucagon concentrations. *J Clin Endocrinol Metab*, 63, 481 (1986)

1776 Gold GL et al. Hyperuricemia associated with the treatment of acute leukemia. *Ann Intern Med*, 47, 428 (1957)

1777 Goldbarg JA, Pineda EP, Blanks BM, Rutenberg AM. A method for the colorimetric determination of β-glucuronidase in urine, serum and tissue: assay of enzymatic activity in health and disease. *Gastroenterology*, 36, 193-201 (1959)

1778 Goldberg A. Porphyrins and porphyrias In:. *Recent Advances in Haematology,* A Goldberg, McBrain, (eds), New York NY, Churchill-Livingstone (1971)

1779 Goldberg A, Rimington C. *Diseases of porphyrin metabolism*. Springfield IL, CC Thomas (1962)

1780 Goldberg A, Rimington C. Hereditary coproporphyria. *Lancet*, 1, 632 (1967)

1781 Goldberg DM, Brown D. Biochemical tests in the diagnosis, classification, and management of patients with malignant lymphoma and leukemia. *Clin Chim Acta*, 169, 1-76 (1987)

1782 Goldberg DM et al. Elevation of serum alkaline phosphatase activity and related enzymes in diabetes mellitus. *Clin Biochem*, 10, 8-11 (1977)

1783 Goldberg DM et al. Serum amylase and related enzymes in diabetic ketoacidosis. *J Clin Pathol*, 26, 985 (1974)

1784 Goldberg DM, Fletcher MJ, Watts C. Serum adenosine deaminase activity in hepatic disease. *Clin Chim Acta*, 14, 720-728 (1966)

1785 Goldberg MF. Retinal vaso-occlusion in sickling hemoglobinopathies. *Birth Defects*, 12, 475-515 (1976)

1786 Goldberg RL, Huff JP, Lenz ME et al. Elevated plasma levels of hyaluronate in patients with osteoarthritis and rheumatoid arthritis. *Arth Rheum*, 34, 799-807 (1991)

1787 Goldborg et al. A method for the determination of γ-glutamyl transpeptidase in human serum; enzymatic activity in health and disease. *Gastroenterology*, 44, 127-133 (1963)

1788 Golden NH, Pepper GM, Sacker I et al. The effects of a dopamine antagonist on luteinizing hormone and prolactin release in women with anorexia nervosa and in normal controls. *J Adolesc Health*, 13, 155-160 (1992)

1789 Goldenberg DL, Leff G, Grayzel AI. Pericardial tamponade in systemic lupus erythematosus; with absent hemolytic complement activity in pericardial fluid. *NY State Med*, 75, 910-912 (1975)

1790 Goldenshon ES, Appel SH. *Scientific Approach to Clinical Neurology*. Philadelphia PA, Lea and Febiger (1977)

1791 Goldfarb AF et al. Polycystic ovarian disease: clinical considerations. *J Reprod Med*, 18, 135-138 (1977)

1792 Golding PL et al. Multisystem involvement in chronic liver disease: studies on the incidence and pathogenesis. *Am J Med*, 55, 772 (1973)

1793 Goldman AS et al. Dysgammaglobulinemic antibody deficiency syndrome. *J Pediatr*, 70, 16 (1967)

1794 Goldman J, Matz R, Mortimer R et al. High elevations of creatine phosphokinase in hypothyroidism. An isoenzyme analysis. *J Am Med Ass*, 238, 325-326 (1977)

1795 Goldstein DA et al. Blood levels of 25-hydroxyvitamin D in nephrotic syndrome. *Ann Intern Med*, 87, 664-667 (1977)

1796 Goldstein NS, Blue DE, Hankin R, et al. Serum α-fetoprotein levels in patients with chronic hepatitis C. *Am J Clin Pathol*, 111, 811-816 (1999)

1797 Golstein M, Meyer O, Bourgeois P et al. Neurological manifestations of systemic lupus erythematosus: role of antiphospholipid antibodies. *Clin Exp Rheumatol*, 11, 373-379 (1993)

1798 Gomez B, Ardakani S, Evans B et al. Bone reabsorption assessed with a new monoclonal antibody-based enzyme immunoassay for free pyridinium crosslinks. *Clin Chem*, 41, S34 (1995)

1799 Gomez B Jr, Ardakani S, Ju J et al. Monoclonal antibody assay for measuring bone-specific alkaline phosphatase activity in serum. *Clin Chem*, 41, 1560-1566 (1995)

1800 Gomez Saez JM, Fernandez Real JM, Fernandez Castaner M et al. Study on growth hormone and insulin secretion in myotonic dystrophy. *Clin Investig*, 72, 508-511 (1994)

1801 Gomez-Pacheo L, Villa AR, Drenkard C, et al. Serum anti-β_2-glycoprotein-I and anticardiolipin antibodies during thrombosis in systemic lupus erythematosus patients. *Am J Med*, 106, 417-423 (1999)

1802 Gomi T, Ikeda T, Ikegami F. Beneficial effect of α-blocker on hemorheology in patients with essential hypertension. *Am J Hypertens*, 10, 886-892 (1997)

1803 Gomi T, Shiohara T, Munakata T et al. Interleukin-1-α, tumor necrosis factor alpha, and interferon γ in psoriasis. *Arch Dermatol*, 127, 827-830 (1991)

1804 Gonano F, Pirisi M, Soardo G et al. Changes in lipid metabolism by treatment with interferon alpha in patients with chronic viral liver disease. *Clin Biochem Rev*, 14, 225 (1993)

1805 Gonick HC et al. Urinary β-glucuronidase activity in renal disease. *Arch Intern Med*, 132, 63-69 (1973)

1806 Gonzalez A, Vizoso F, Vazquez J, et al. Clinical significance of preoperative serum levels of CA 125 and TAG-72 in ovarian carcinoma. *Int J Biol Markers*, 12, 112-117 (1997)

1807 Gonzalez C, Martin T, Cacho J, et al. Serum zinc, copper, insulin and lipids in Alzheimer's disease epsilon 4 apolipoprotein E allele carriers. *Eur J Clin Invest*, 29, 637-642 (1999)

1808 Gonzalez-Reimers E, Santolaria-Fernandez F, Rodriguez-Rodriguez E et al. Serum neopterin levels in alcoholic liver disease. *Drug Alcohol Dep*, 33, 151-156 (1993)

1809 Gonzalez-Villaron L, Perez-Arellano J, de Castro S. Urinary iron excretion in patients with chronic obstructive airways disease (COAD). *Ann Clin Biochem*, 32, 417-418 (1995)

1810 Goode HF, Kelleher J, Walker BE. The effects of acute infection on indices of zinc status. *Clin Nutr*, 10, 550-559 (1991)

1811 Goodkin DE, Jacobsen DW, Galvez N et al. Serum cobalamin deficiency is uncommon in multiple sclerosis. *Arch Neurol*, 51, 1110-1114 (1994)

1812 Goodlin RC. Severe pre-eclampsia: another great imitator. *Am J Obstet Gynecol*, 125, 747-753 (1976)

1813 Goodman LS et al. *The Pharmacological Basis of Therapeutics.* 4th edition, New York NY, MacMillan and Co (1970)

1814 Goodman RB, Strieter RM, Martin DP, et al. Inflammatory cytokines in patients with persistence of the acute respiratory distress syndrome. *Am J Respir Crit Care Med*, 154, 602-611 (1996)

1815 Goodnight SH Jr. Bleeding and intravascular clotting in malignancy: a review. *Ann NY Acad Sci*, 230, 271 (1974)

1816 Goodpasture HC et al. Colorado tick fever: clinical, epidemiologic and laboratory aspects of 228 cases in Colorado in 1973-1974. *Ann Intern Med*, 88, 303-310 (1978)

1817 Goodwin RA et al. Chronic pulmonary histoplasmosis. *Medicine*, 55, 413-450 (1976)

1818 Goos G, Declercq P, Proesmans W. Serum proteins in the haemolytic uraemic syndrome. *Pediatr Nephrol*, 9, 292-294 (1995)

1819 Gorden P et al. Hyperuricemia, a concomitant of the congenital vasopressin-resistant diabetes insipidus in the adult: studies of uric acid metabolism and plasma vasopressin. *N Engl J Med*, 284, 1057 (1971)

1820 Gordon DA. The extrarenal manifestations of hypernephroma. *Can Med Ass J*, 88, 61-67 (1963)

1821 Gordon HH, Nitowsky HM. Some studies of tocopherol in infants and children. *Am J Clin Nutr*, 4, 391 (1956)

1822 Gordon MS, Nemunaitis J, Hoffman R et al. A phase I trial of recombinant human interleukin-6 in patients with myelodysplastic syndromes and thrombocytopenia. *Blood*, 85, 3066-3076 (1995)

1823 Gordon T. Factors associated with serum alkaline phosphatase level. *Arch Pathol Lab Med*, 117, 187-190 (1993)

1824 Goren R, Simons LA. Plasma cholesterol esterification in hypertriglyceridaemia. *Clin Chim Acta*, 74, 289-296 (1977)

1825 Gores PF, Fryd DS, Sutherland DER et al. Hyperuricemia after renal transplantation. *Am J Surg*, 156, 397-400 (1988)

1826 Gorus FK, Van Blerk M. Ektachem slides overestimate serum albumin in patients with nephrotic syndrome. *Eur J Clin Chem Clin Biochem*, 31, 159-163 (1993)

1827 Gosling P, Dickson G. Serum C-reactive protein in patients with serious trauma. *Proc ACB Natl Meet*, 56 (1991)

1828 Gosling P, Sheehan TMT, Rothe HM. Serum zinc and copper concentrations in patients following burn injury and trauma. *Proc ACB Natl Meet*, 74 (1992)

1829 Gosling P, Sutcliffe AJ. Proteinuria following trauma. *Ann Clin Biochem*, 23, 681-685 (1986)

1830 Goswitz F et al. Erythrocyte reduced glutathione, glucose-6-phosphate dehydrogenase, and 6-phosphogluconic dehydrogenase in patients with myelofibrosis. *J Lab Clin Med*, 67, 615 (1966)

1831 Gotoh M, Mizuno K, Matsui J, Kunii N. Serum angiotensin i converting enzyme activity in patients with hyperthyroidism and hypothyroidism: relation to renin and aldosterone. *Nippon Naibunpi Gakkai Zasshi*, 60, 835-845 (1984)

1832 Gotz ME, Fischer P, Gsell W, et al. Platelet monoamine oxidase B activity in dementia. *Dement Geriatr Cogn Disord*, 9, 74-77 (1998)

1833 Gough AKS, Peel NFA, Eastell R et al. Excretion of pyridinium crosslinks correlates with disease activity and appendicular bone loss in early rheumatoid arthritis. *Ann Rheum Dis*, 53, 14-17 (1994)

1834 Gozzard DI, Liu Yin JA, Delamore IW. The clinical usefulness of C-reactive protein measurements. *Br J Haematol*, 63, 411-414 (1986)

1835 Graeff JDE, Lameijer LD. Periodic paralysis. *Am J Med*, 39, 70 (1965)

1836 Graham EA, Felgenhauer J, Detter JC, Labbe RF. Elevated zinc protoporphyrin associated with thalassemia trait and hemoglobin E. *J Pediatr*, 129, 105-110 (1996)

1837 Graham RC, Bernier GM. The bone marrow in multiple myeloma: correlation of plasma cell ultrastructure and clinical state. *Medicine*, 54, 225-244 (1975)

1838 Graham RM, Strahan ME, Norman KW et al. Platelet and plasma platelet activating factor in sepsis and myocardial infarction. *J Lipid Mediat Cell Signal*, 9, 167-182 (1994)

1839 Graig FA et al. Serum creatine-phosphokinase in thyroid disease. *Metabolism*, 12, 57-59 (1963)

1840 Gralnick HR, McKeown LP, Williams SB et al. Plasma and platelet von Willebrand factor defects in uremia. *Am J Med*, 85, 806-810 (1988)

1841 Gram J, Duscha H, Zurborn KH et al. Increased levels of fibrinolysis reaction products (D-dimer) in patients with decompensated alcoholic cirrhosis. *Scand J Gastroenterol*, 26, 1173-1178 (1991)

1842 Granado F, Olmedilla B, Gil-Martinez E, et al. Carotenoids, retinol and tocopherols in patients with insulin-dependent diabetes mellitus and their immediate relatives. *Clin Sci*, 94, 189-195 (1998)

1843 Granberg PO et al. Renal function studies in medullary sponge kidney. *Scand J Urol Nephrol*, 5, 177 (1971)

1844 Grandtnerova B, Gregova H, Mocikova H, et al. Anticardiolipin antibodies after kidney transplantation in patients without connective tissue disease. *Transplant Proc*, 31, 1-00 (1999)

1845 Granerus G, Lonnqvist B, Nystrand J, Roupe G. Serum tryptase measured with B12 and G5 antibody-based immunoassays in mastocytosis patients and its relation to histamine turnover. *Br J Derm*, 139, 858-861 (1998)

1846 Grange JM, Mitchell DN, Kemp M, Kardjito T. Serum angiotensin-converting enzyme and delayed hypersensitivity in pulmonary tuberculosis. *Tubercle*, 65, 117-121 (1984)

1847 Granter SR, Doolittle MH, Renshaw AA. Predominance of neutrophils in the cerebrospinal fluid of AIDS patients with cytomrgalovirus radiculopathy. *Am J Clin Pathol*, 105, 364-366 (1996)

1848 Grau GE, Taylor TE, Molyneux ME et al. Tumor necrosis factor and disease severity in children with Falciparum Malaria. *N Engl J Med*, 320, 1586-1591 (1989)

1849 Gray CH. Acute porphyria. *Arch Intern Med*, 85, 459 (1950)

1850 Graziani MS, Zanolla L, Righetti G et al. Distribution of CII and CIII peptides in lipoprotein classes: methods and clinical significance. *Clin Chem*, 40, 240-244 (1994)

1851 Graziani MS, Zanolla L, Righetti G et al. Lipoprotein(a) concentrations are increased in patients with myocardial infarction and angiographically normal coronary arteries. *Eur J Clin Chem Clin Biochem*, 31, 135-137 (1993)

1852 Greaves M, Boyde TRC. Plasma zinc concentrations in patients with psoriasis, other dermatoses and venous leg ulcerations. *Lancet*, 2, 1019-1020 (1967)

1853 Grebourg T, Lerebours G, Delpech B et al. Serum hyaluronate in malignant pleural mesothelioma. *Cancer*, 59, 2104-2107 (1988)

1854 Greco AV, Mingrone G. Serum bile acid concentrations in mild liver cirrhosis. *Clin Chim Acta*, 221, 183-189 (1993)

1855 Green AJ, Ratnoff OD. Elevated antihemophilic factor (AHF, factor VIII) procoagulant activity and AHF like antigen in alcoholic cirrhosis of the liver. *J Lab Clin Med*, 83, 189 (1974)

1856 Green AJE, Giovannoni G, Miller RF, et al. Cerebrospinal fluid S-100b concentration in patients with HIV infection. *AIDS*, 13, 13 (1999)

1857 Green JB et al. The cholesterol and cholesterol ester content in cerebrospinal fluid in patients with multiple sclerosis and other neurological diseases. *J Neurol Neurosurg Psychiatry*, 22, 117 (1959)

1858 Green OC, Fefferman R, Nair S. Plasma growth hormone levels in children with cystic fibrosis and short stature. *J Clin Endocrinol Metab*, 27, 1059 (1967)

1859 Greenberg BH et al. Primary type V hyperlipoproteinemia. *Ann Intern Med*, 87, 526-534 (1977)

1860 Greenberg CS, Hursting MJ, Macik BG et al. Evaluation of preanalytical variables associated with measurement of prothrombin fragment 1.2. *Clin Chem*, 40, 1962-1969 (1994)

1861 Greenberg GR, Feagan BG, Martin F et al. Oral budesonide for active Crohn's disease. *N Engl J Med*, 331, 836-841 (1994)

1862 Greendyke RM, Sharma K, Gifford FR. Serum levels of erythropoietin and selected other cytokines in patients with anemia of chronic disease. *Am J Clin Pathol*, 101, 338-341 (1994)

1863 Greenwood BM et al. Lymphocyte changes in acute malaria. *Trans Roy Soc Trop Med Hyg*, 71, 408-10 (1977)

1864 Greenwood BM et al. Speckled antinuclear factor in African sera. *Clin Exp Immunol*, 7, 75 (1970)

1865 Gregory WL, Game FL, Farrer M et al. Reduced serum lipoprotein(a) levels in patients with primary biliary cirrhosis. *Atherosclerosis*, 105, 43-50 (1994)

1866 Grekas DM, Raptis S, Tourkantonis AA. Plasma secretin, pancreozymin, and somatostatin-like hormone in chronic renal failure patients. *Uremia Invest*, 85, 117-120 (1984)

1867 Griesmacher A, Kindhauser M, Andert SE, et al. Enhanced levels of thiobarbituric acid-reactive substances. *Am J Med*, 98, 469-474 (1995)

1868 Griesmacher A, Weigel G, Kindhauser M et al. Heart transplantation and adhesion molecules. *Eur J Clin Chem Clin Biochem*, 33, A84-A85 (1995)

1869 Griesshammer M, Bangerter M, Sauer T, et al. Aetiology and clinical significance of thrombocytosis: analysis of 732 patients with an elevated platelet count. *J Intern Med*, 245, 295-300 (1999)

1870 Griffin G, Vartukartis JL. Hormone secreting tumors. In:. *Cancer Markers*, Clifton NJ, Humana Press (1982)

1871 Griffiths CEM, Boffa MJ, Gallatin WM, Martin S. Elevated levels of circulating intercellular adhesion molecule-3 (cICAM-3) in psoriasis. *Acta Derm Venereol*, 76, 2-5 (1996)

1872 Griffiths KD, Lock S, Jones AP. Urinary glycosaminoglycan excretion in type I and type II diabetes. *Clin Biochem Rev*, 14, 355 (1993)

1873 Grigorescu M, Tapalaga D, Dumitra, Scu D. Diagnostic value of serum bile acid determination in chronic hepatitis and liver cirrhosis. *Med Interne*, 18, 401-406 (1980)

1874 Grimm J, Zeller W, Zander AR. Soluble interleukin-2 receptor serum levels after allogeneic bone marrow transplantation as a marker for GVHD. *Bone Marrow Transplant*, 21, 29-32 (1998)

1875 Grimmel K et al. Amylase activity of parotid saliva in acute and chronic pancreatitis. *Acta Hepatogastroenterol*, 23, 334-444 (1976)

1876 Grinspoon S, Gulick T, Askari H, et al. Serum leptin levels in women with anorexia nervosa. *J Clin Endocrinol Metab*, 81, 3861-3863 (1996)

1877 Grob U, Honcamp M, Daume E, et al. Hormonal oral contraceptives, urinary porphyrin excretion and porphyrias. *Horm Metab Res*, 27, 379-383 (1995)

1878 Grobbee DE, Hackeng WHL, Birkenhager JC et al. Intact parathyroid hormone (1-84) in primary hypertension. *Clin Exp Hypertens Theory Pract*, 8, 299-308 (1986)

1879 Grodzinsky E, Jansson G, Skogh T et al. Anti-endomysium and anti-gliadin antibodies as serological markers for coeliac disease in childhood: a clinical study to develop a practical routine. *Acta Paediat*, 84, 294-298 (1995)

1880 Gronroos JM, Forsstrom JJ, Irjala K et al. Phospholipase A2, C-reactive protein, and white blood cell count in the diagnosis of acute appendicitis. *Clin Chem*, 40, 1757-1760 (1994)

1881 Gronroos JM, Gronroos P. Leukocyte count and C-reactive protein in the diagnosis of acute appendicitis. *Br J Surg*, 86, 501-504 (1999)

1882 Gropp C et al. Carcinoembryonic antigen, alpha 1-fetoprotein (AFP), ferritin, and alpha 2-pregnancy associated glycoprotein in the serum of lung cancer patients and its demonstration in lung tumor tissues. *Oncology*, 34, 267-72 (1977)

1883 Gross S et al. The platelets in iron-deficiency anemia. i the response to oral and parenteral iron. *Pediatrics*, 34, 315 (1964)

1884 Gross V, Andreesen R, Leser HG et al. Interleukin-8 and neutrophil activation in acute pancreatitis. *Eur J Clin Invest*, 22, 200-203 (1992)

1885 Gross V, Andus T, Caesar I et al. Evidence for continuous stimulation of interleukin-6 production in Crohn's disease. *Gastroenterology*, 102, 514-519 (1992)

1886 Gross WL, Schmitt WH, Csernok E. ANCA and associated diseases: immunodiagnostic and pathogenetic aspects. *Clin Exp Immunol*, 91, 1-12 (1993)

1887 Grossen Y, Eales L. Patterns of faecal porphyrin excretion in the hepatocutaneous porphyrias. *S Afr Med J*, 47, 2162 (1973)

1888 Gruden G, Cavallo-Perin P, Bazzan M et al. PAI-1 and factor VII activity are higher in IDDM patients with microalbuminuria. *Diabetes*, 43, 426-429 (1994)

1889 Gruden G, Veglio M, Cavallo-Perin P, et al. Lipoprotein(a) in non-insulin-dependent diabetic patients with normo- and microalbuminuria. *Horm Metab Res*, 26, 489-490 (1994)

1890 Grunfeld C, Kolter DP, Hamadeh R et al. Hypertriglyceridemia in AIDS. *Am J Med*, 86, 27-31 (1989)

1891 Grunfeld C, Pang M, Doerrler W et al. Lipids, lipoproteins and triglyceride clearance and cytokines in human immunodeficiency virus infection and acquired immune syndrome. *J Clin Endocrinol Metab*, 74, 1403-1408 (1992)

1892 Grunfeld C, Pang M, Shigenaga JK, et al. Serum leptin levels in the acquired immunodeficiency syndrome. *J Clin Endocrinol Metab*, 81, 4342-4346 (1996)

1893 Gruschwitz MS, Hornstein OP, von den Driesch P. Correlation of soluble adhesion molecules in the peripheral blood of scleroderma patients with their in situ expression and with disease activity. *Arth Rheum*, 38, 184-189 (1995)

1894 Guadagni F, Roselli M, Amato T et al. Tumor-associated glycoprotein-72 serum levels complement carcinoembryonic antigen levels in monitoring patients with gastrointestinal carcinoma: a longitudinal study. *Cancer*, 68, 2443-2450 (1991)

1895 Guadagni F, Roselli M, Cosimelli M et al. Biologic evaluation of tumor-associated glycoprotein-72 and carcinoembryonic antigen expression in colorectal cancer. *Dis Colon Rectum*, 37, S16-S23 (1994)

1896 Guadagni F, Roselli M, Cosimelli M et al. CA 72-4 serum marker - a new tool in the management of carcinoma patients. *Cancer Invest*, 13, 227-238 (1995)

1897 Guadagni F, Roselli M, Cosimelli M et al. Correlation between positive CA 72-4 serum levels and lymph node involvement in patients with gastric carcinoma. *Anticancer Res*, 13, 2409-2414 (1993)

1898 Gubler CJ, Brown H, Markowitz H et al. Studies on copper metabolism XXIII. portal (Laennec's) cirrhosis of the liver. *J Clin Invest*, 36, 1208-1216 (1957)

1899 Gudbjornsson B, Karlsson-Parra A, Karlsson E et al. Clinical and laboratory features of Sjögren's syndrome in young women with previous postpartum thyroiditis. *J Rheumatol*, 21, 215-219 (1994)

1900 Gudjonsson B et al. Cancer of the pancreas: diagnostic accuracy and survival statistics. *Cancer*, 42, 2494-2506 (1978)

1901 Guechot J, Laudat A, Loria A, et al. Diagnostic accuracy of hyaluron and type III procollagen amino-terminal peptide serum assays as markers of liver fibrosis in chronic viral hepatitis C evaluated by ROC curve analysis. *Clin Chem*, 42, 558-563 (1996)

1902 Guechot J, Lioret N, Cynober L et al. Myoglobinemia after burn injury: relationship to creatine kinase activity in serum. *Clin Chem*, 32, 857-859 (1986)

1903 Guerriero S, Ajossa S, Paoletti AM, et al. Tumor markers and transvaginal ultrasonography in the diagnosis of endometrioma. *Obstet Gynecol*, 88, 403-407 (1996)

1904 Guevara M, Gines P, Jimenez W, et al. Increased adrenomedullin levels in cirrhosis: relationship with hemodynamic abnormalities and vasoconstrictor systems. *Gastroenterology*, 114, 336-343 (1996)

1905 Guicheney P, Soliman H, Launay JM et al. Circulating monamine oxidase B and phenolsulfotransferase activities in essential hypertensive patients. *Clin Exp Hypertens*, 10, Part A, 533-544 (1988)

1906 Guidet B, Piot O, Masliah J, et al. Secretory non-pancreatic phospholipase AS in severe sepsis: relation to endotoxin, cytokines and thromboxane B2. *Infection*, 24, 103-108 (1996)

1907 Guieu R, Devaux C, Albanese J et al. β-Endorphin in multiple trauma victims. *Can J Neurol Sci*, 22, 160-163 (1995)

1908 Guieu R, Sampieri F, Bechis G et al. Use of HPLC to measure circulating adenosine levels in migrainous patients. *Clin Chim Acta*, 227, 185-194 (1994)

1909 Guillausseau PJ, Charles MA, Paolaggi F et al. Comparison of HbA1 and fructosamine in diagnosis of glucose-tolerance abnormalities. *Diabetes Care*, 13, 898-900 (1990)

1910 Guillevin L, Durand-Gasselin B, Cevallos R, et al. Microscopic polyangitis: clinical and laboratory findings in eighty-five patients. *Arth Rheum*, 42, 421-430 (1999)

1911 Gullo L, Ventrucci M, Bonora G et al. Comparative study of serum trypsin levels and pancreatic exocrine function in chronic pancreatitis. *Scand J Gastroenterol*, 15, 27-28 (1980)

1912 Gumaste VV, Sereny G, Dave P et al. Serum lipase levels in chronic alcoholics. *J Clin Gastroenterol*, 13, 407-410 (1991)

1913 Gumpel JM, Hobbs JR. Serum immune globulins in Sjögren's syndrome. *Ann Rheum Dis*, 29, 681 (1970)

1914 Gunmaste VV, Sereny G, Dave P et al. Serum lipase activity in chronic alcoholism. *J Clin Gastroenterol*, 13, 407-410 (1991)

1915 Gunther H. Handbuch der krankheiten des blutes und der blutbildenden organe. *Handbuch Der Organe*, 2 (1925)

1916 Gunz F, Baikie AG. *Leukemia*. New York NY, Grune and Stratton, 403 (1973)

1917 Guo Y, He W, Boer AM, et al. Elevated plasma chittriosidase activity in various lysosomal storage disorders. *J Inher Metab Dis*, 18, 717-722 (1995)

1918 Guo Y-J, Liu G, Wang X et al. Potential use of soluble CD44 in serum as indicator of tumor burden and metasis in patients with gastric or colon cancer. *Cancer Res*, 54, 422-426 (1994)

1919 Gupta DK et al. Increased plasma free-fatty-acid concentrations and their significance in patients with acute myocardial infarction. *Lancet*, 2, 1209 (1969)

1920 Gupta JK et al. Multiple sclerosis and malabsorption. *Am J Gastroenterol*, 68, 560-565 (1977)

1921 Gupta R, Misra SP, Dwivedi M, et al. Diagnosing ascites: value of ascitic fluid total protein, albumin, cholesterol, their ratios, serum ascites albumin and cholesterol gradient. *J Gastroenterol Hepatol*, 10, 295-299 (1995)

1922 Gupta RC et al. Nitroblue tetrazolium test in the diagnosis of pyogenic arthritis. *Ann Intern Med*, 80, 723-726 (1974)

1923 Gupta S, et al. Serial measurement of serum C-reactive protein facilitates evaluation in alcoholic hepatitis. *Hepato-Gastroenterology*, 42, 516-521 (1995)

1924 Gupta S, Leatham EW, Carrington D, et al. Elevated Chlamydia pneumoniae antibodies, cardiovascular events, and azithromycin in male survivors of myocardial infarction. *Circulation*, 96, 404-407 (1997)

1925 Gupta SK, Shukla VK, Gupta V et al. Serum trace elements and Cu/Zn ratio in malignant lymphomas in children. *J Trop Pediatr*, 40, 185-187 (1994)

1926 Gurakar-Osborne A, Prete PE. Rapid assay of phospholipase A_2 in plasma and synovial fluid. *Clin Chem*, 41, 118-119 (1995)

1927 Gurbel PA, Serebruany VL. Soluble vascular cell adhesion molecule-1 and E-selectin in patients with acute myocardial infarction treated with thrombolytic agents. *Am J Cardiol*, 81, 772-775 (1998)

1928 Gurbel PA, Serebruany VL, Shustov AR, et al. Increased baseline levels of P-selectin, and platelet endothelial cell adhesion molecule-1 in patients with acute myocardial infarction as predictors of unsuccessful thrombolysis. *Coron Art Dis*, 9, 451-458 (1998)

1929 Gurian KV, Podratz KC, Eig SA, et al. Major basic protein as a marker of malignant potential in trophoblastic neoplasia. *Am J Obstet Gynecol*, 175, 632-637 (1996)

1930 Gurleyik E, Gurleyik G, Unalmiser S, et al. Accuracy of C-reactive protein measurements in diagnosis of acute appendicitis compared with surgeon's clinical impression. *Colon Rectum*, 38, 1270-1274 (1995)

1931 Gursel G, Turktas H, Gokcora N, Tekin IO. Comparison of sputum and serum eosinophil cationic protein (ECP) levels in nonatopic asthma and chronic obstructive pulmonary disease. *J Asthma*, 34, 313-319 (1997)

1932 Gustin M, Radermecker M. Significance of elevated serum ACE in pneumonology. *Poumon Coeur*, 38, 339-345 (1982)

1933 Gutman AB et al. An 'acid' phosphatase occurring in the serum of patients with metastasizing carcinoma of the prostate gland. *J Clin Invest*, 17, 473-478 (1938)

1934 Gutman AB, Yu TF. Renal function in gout. *Am J Med*, 23, 600 (1957)

1935 Gutman, Tyson , Gutman. Serum calcium, inorganic phosphorus and phosphatase activity in hyperparathyroidism, Paget's disease, multiple myeloma and neoplastic disease of the bones. *Arch Intern Med*, 57, 379-413 (1936)

1936 Guttierrez LV, Baron JH. A comparison of basal and stimulated gastric acid and duodenal bicarbonate secretion in patients with and without duodenal ulcer disease. *Am J Gastroenterol*, 66, 270-276 (1976)

1937 Guzman J, Cardiel MH, Arce-Salinas A et al. The contribution of resting heart rate and routine blood tests to the clinical assessment of disease activity in systemic lupus erythematosus. *J Rheumatol*, 21, 1845-1848 (1994)

1938 Guzman J, Fung M, Petty RE. Diagnostic value of anti-neutrophil cytoplasmic and anti-endothelial cell antibodies in early Kawasaki disease. *J Pediatr*, 124, 917-920 (1994)

1939 Gyongyosi M, Nemeth J, Varkonyi T. Elevated levels of plasma vasoactive intestinal peptide in human acute myocardial infarction. *Int J Cardiol*, 56, 159-161 (1996)

1940 Ha R, Jindal RM, Milgrom MM, et al. Prostate-specific antigen values and their clinical significance in renal transplant recipients. *S Med J*, 91, 847-850 (1998)

1941 Haak T, Jungmann E, Felber A et al. Increased plasma levels of endothelin in diabetic patients with hypertension. *Am J Hypertens*, 5, 161-166 (1992)

1942 Haak T, Marz W, Jungmann E et al. Elevated endothelin levels in patients with hyperlipoproteinemia. *Clin Investig*, 72, 580-584 (1994)

1943 Haanpaa M, Dastidar P, Weinberg A, et al. CSF and MRI findings in patients with acute herpes zoster. *Neurology*, 51, 1405-1411 (1998)

1944 Haas L, Meillet D, Kapel N et al. Increased concentrations of fecal anti-gliadin IgA antibodies in untreated celiac disease. *Clin Chem*, 39, 696-697 (1993)

1945 Haas M, Meehan SM, Josephson MA, et al. Smooth muscle-specific actin levels in the urine of renal transplant recipients: correlation with cyclosporine or tacrolimus nephrotoxicity. *Am J Kid Dis*, 34, 69-84 (1999)

1946 Haas RH, Nasirian F, Nakano K, et al. Low platelet mitochondrial complex I and complex II/III activity in early untreated Parkinson's disease. *Ann Neurol*, 37, 714-722 (1995)

1947 Habib R et al. The nephrotic syndrome. In:. *Pediatric Nephrology*. P Royer et al (eds), Philadelphia PA, WB Saunders, 262 (1974)

1948 Haboubi NA, Thurnham DI. Effect of ethanol on erythrocyte acetylcholinesterase activity. *Ann Clin Biochem*, 23, 458-462 (1986)

1949 Hack CE, Hart M, van Schijndel RJ et al. Interleukin-8 in sepsis: relation to shock and inflammatory mediators. *Infect Immunol*, 60, 2835-2842 (1992)

1950 Haddow JE, Palomaki GE, Knight GJ, et al. Screening of maternal serum for fetal Down's syndrome in the first trimester. *N Engl J Med*, 338, 955-961 (1998)

1951 Hafez M et al. Antibody production and complement system in protein energy malnutrition. *J Trop Med Hyg*, 80, 36-39 (1977)

1952 Hafez M et al. Calcium and phosphorus metabolic changes in children with hepatic bilharziasis. *Gaz Egypt Paediatr Ass*, 23, 243-252 (1975)

1953 Haffner JA, Linnestad P, Schrumpf E et al. The immediate effect of renal transplantation on basal and meal-stimulated levels of gastrointestinal hormones. *Scand J Gastroenterol*, 22, 42-46 (1987)

1954 Hafner G, Thome-Kromer B, Schaube J et al. Cardiac troponins in serum in chronic renal failure. *Clin Chem*, 40, 1790-1791 (1994)

1955 Hagen EC, Ballieux BE, Daha MR et al. Fundamental and clinical aspects of anti neutrophil cytoplasmic antibodies. *Autoimmunity*, 11, 199-207 (1992)

1956 Hagihara M, Nagatsu T, Ohhashi M et al. Concentrations of neopterin and biopterin in serum from patients with rheumatoid arthritis or systemic lupus erythematosus and in synovial fluid from patients with rheumatoid or osteoarthritis. *Clin Chem*, 39, 705-706 (1993)

1957 Haglund C, Lundin J, Kuusela P et al. CA 242, a new tumour marker for pancreatic cancer: a comparison with CA 19-9, CA 50 and CEA. *Br J Cancer*, 70, 487-492 (1994)

1958 Hahn TJ et al. Reduced serum 25-hydroxyvitamin D concentration and disordered mineral metabolism in patients with cystic fibrosis. *J Pediatr*, 94, 38-42 (1979)

1959 Haider M, Haider SQ. Assessment of protein-calorie malnutrition. *Clin Chem*, 30, 1286-1299 (1984)

1960 Haire WD, Pirruccelo SJ, Carson SD. Monocyte tissue factor in treated Hodgkin's disease. *Leukemia Lymphoma*, 12, 259-263 (1994)

1961 Hakala M, Aman S, Luukkainen R, et al. Application of markers of collagen metabolism in serum and ynovial fluid for assessment of disease process in patients with rheumatoid arthritis. *Ann Rheum Dis*, 54, 886-890 (1995)

1962 Halbreich U, Asnis GM, Zumoff B et al. Effect of age and sex on cortisol secretion in depressives and normals. *Psychiat Res*, 13, 221-229 (1984)

1963 Halila H, Stenman UG, Seppala M. Ovarian cancer antigen CA 125 levels in pelvic inflammatory disease and pregnancy. *Cancer*, 57, 1327-1329 (1986)

1964 Halim AB, Narakat M, El-Zayat AM et al. Urinary β-hCG in benign and malignant urinary tract diseases. *Dis Mark*, 12, 109-115 (1994)

1965 Hall R. The clinical and technical background to the use of free hormone measurements in thyroid disease. Amersham UK, Kodak Clinical Diagnostics (1992)

1966 Hall R et al. Radioimmunoassay of human serum thyrotropin. *Br Med J*, 1, 582 (1972)

1967 Hall SK, Robinson P, Green A. Could salivary phenylalanine concentrations replace blood concentrations? *Ann Clin Biochem*, 37, 222-223 (2000)

1968 Hall SM, Preston IW. The effect of the patient's acid-base balance on Azostix® strips estimation of blood urea. *Ann Clin Biochem*, 9, 208 (1972)

1969 Hallan S, Asberg A. The accuracy of C-reactive protein in diagnosing acute appendicitis. *Scand J Clin Lab Invest*, 57, 373-380 (1997)

1970 Hallan S, Asberg A, Edna T-H. Additional value of biochemical tests in suspected acute appendicitis. *Eur J Surg*, 163, 533-538 (1997)

1971 Hallee TJ et al. Infectious mononucleosis at the United States Military Academy: a prospective study of a single class over four years. *Yale J Biol Med*, 47, 182 (1974)

1972 Hallek M, Wanders L, Ostwald M, et al. Serum β_2-microglobulin and serum thymidine kinase are independent predictors of progression-free survival in chronic lymphocytic leukemia and immunocytoma. *Leukemia Lymphoma*, 22, 439-447 (1996)

1973 Haller C, Zehelein J, Remppis A, et al. Cardiac troponin T in patients with end-stage renal disease: absence of expression in truncal skeletal muscle. *Clin Chem*, 44, 930-938 (1998)

1974 Hallgren R, Engstrom-Laurent A, Nisbeth U. Circulating hyaluronate. A potential marker of altered metabolism of the connective tissue in uremia. *Nephron*, 46, 150-154 (1987)

1975 Hallgren R, Samuelsson T, Laurent TC et al. Accumulation of hyaluronan (hyaluronic acid) in the lung in adult respiratory distress syndrome. *Am Rev Resp Dis*, 139, 682-687 (1989)

1976 Hallman J, Sakurai E, Oreland L. Blood platelet monoamine oxidase. *Acta Psychiat Scand*, 81, 73-77 (1990)

1977 Hallman J, von Knorring L, Edman G, Oreland L. Personality traints and platelet monoamine oxidase activity in alcoholic women. *Addict Behavior*, 16, 533-541 (1991)

1978 Halmesmaki E, Autti I, Granstrom ML et al. Estradiol, estriol, progesterone, prolactin and human chorionic gonadotropin in pregnant women with alcohol abuse. *J Clin Endocrinol Metab*, 64, 153-156 (1987)

1979 Halmesmaki E, Teramo KA, Widness J et al. Maternal alcohol abuse is associated with elevated fetal erythropoietin levels. *Obstet Gynecol*, 76, 219-222 (1990)

1980 Halsted JA. *The Laboratory in Clinical Medicine*. Philadelphia PA, WB Saunders (1976)

1981 Halton JM, Nazir DJ, McQueen MJ, Barr RD. Blood lipid profiles in children with acute lymphoblastic leukemia. *Cancer*, 83, 379-384 (1998)

1982 Halwachs G, Tiran A, Reisinger EC et al. Serum levels of the soluble receptor for tumor necrosis factor in patients with renal disease. *Clin Investig*, 72, 473-476 (1994)

1983 Ham TH. Hemoglobinuria. *Am J Med*, 18, 990 (1955)

1984 Hamada H, Kohno N, Akiyama M et al. Monitoring of serum KL-6 antigen in a patient with radiation pneumonia. *Chest*, 101, 858-860 (1992)

1985 Hamada M, Ohtani T, Sekiya M et al. Serum creatine kinase MM isoforms in hypertrophic cardiomyopathy. *Clin Sci*, 81, 723-726 (1991)

1986 Hamada M, Shigematsu Y, Kawakami H, et al. Increased plasma levels of adrenomedullin in patients with hypertrophic cardiomyopathy: its relation to endothelin-I, natriuretic peptides and noradrenaline. *Clin Sci*, 94, 21-28 (1998)

1987 Hamet P et al. Studies of the elevated extracellular concentration of cyclic AMP in uremic man. *J Clin Invest*, 56, 339 (1975)

1988 Hamilton CR Jr, Tumulty PA. Giant cell arteritis including temporal arteritis and polymyalgia rheumatica. *Medicine*, 50, 1 (1971)

1989 Hamm H, Luhrs J, Guzman y Rotaeche J, et al. Elevated surfactant protein A in bronchoalveolar lavage fluids from sarcoidosis and hypersensitivity pneumonitis patients. *Chest*, 106, 1766-1770 (1994)

1990 Hammerle AF, Krafft P, Wagner OA et al. Evaluation of serum TNF-α measurements in septic patients. *Anaesthetist*, 39, 547-551 (1990)

1991 Hammett JF et al. McArdle's disease: three cases in an Australian family. *Proc Aust Assoc Neurol*, 4, 21-25 (1966)

1992 Hammond GL. Serum FSH, LH and prolactin in normal males and patients with prostatic diseases. *Clin Endocrinol*, 7, 129-135 (1977)

1993 Hammond GL et al. Serum steroids in normal males and patients with prostatic diseases. *Clin Endocrinol*, 9, 113-121 (1978)

1994 Hampel H, Schoen D, Schwarz MJ, et al. Interleukin-6 is not altered in cerebrospinal fluid of first-degree relatives and patients with Alzheimer's disease. *Neurosci Lett*, 228, 143-146 (1997)

1995 Hampel H, Sunderland T, Kotter HU, et al. Decreased soluble interleukin-6 receptor in cerebrospinal fluid of patients with Alzheimer's disease. *Brain Res*, 780, 356-359 (1998)

1996 Hanafy HM et al. Increased serum amylase levels in prostatic diseases. *Urology*, 1, 372 (1973)

1997 Handin RI et al. Elevation of platelet factor four in acute myocardial infarction: measurement by radioimmunoassay. *J Lab Clin Med*, 91, 340-349 (1978)

1998 Handjani AM et al. Serum iron in acute myocardial infarction. *Blut*, 23, 363 (1971)

1999 Handweger S et al. Glucose tolerance in cystic fibrosis. *N Engl J Med*, 281, 451 (1969)

2000 Handwerker SM, Altura BT, Altura BM. Ionized serum magnesium and potassium levels in pregnant women with preeclampsia and eclampsia. *J Reprod Med*, 40, 201-208 (1995)

2001 Hanger FM, Gutman AB. Postarsphenamine jaundice. *J Am Med Ass*, 115, 263 (1940)

2002 Hankin ME et al. An evaluation of laboratory tests for the detection and differential diagnosis of Cushing's syndrome. *Clin Endocrinol*, 6, 185-196 (1977)

2003 Hankinson SE, Willett WC, Colditz GA, et al. Circulating concentrations of insulin-like growth factor-I and risk of breast cancer. *Lancet*, 351, 1393-1396 (1998)

2004 Hanks GE, D'Amico A, Epstein BE et al. Prostatic-specific antigen doubling times in patients with prostate cancer: a potentially useful reflection of tumour doubling time. *Int J Radiation Oncol Biol Phys*, 27, 125-127 (1993)

2005 Hanks GE, Hanlon AL, Lee WR, et al. Pretreatment prostate-specific antigen doubling times: clinical utility of this predictor of prostate cancer behavior. *Int J Rad Oncol*, 34, 549-553 (1996)

2006 Hanna AN, Waldman WJ, Lott JA, et al. Increased alkaline phosphatase isoforms in autoimmune diseases. *Clin Chem*, 43, 1357-1364 (1997)

2007 Hanna GL, Ornitz EM, Hariharan M. Urinary catecholamine excretion and behavioral differences in ADHD and normal boys. *J Child Adolesc Psychopharmacol*, 6, 63-73 (1996)

2008 Hannuksela M, Kesaniemi YA, Savolainen MJ. Evaluation of plasma cholesteryl ester transfer protein (CETP) activity as a marker of alcoholism. *Alcohol Alcoholism*, 27, 557-562 (1992)

2009 Hansen C, Irmscher AK, Kuhlemann K, et al. Insulin-dependent diabetes mellitus and glycosaminoglycans. *Horm Metab Res*, 27, 555-558 (1995)

2010 Hansen HJ, Snyder BS, Miller E et al. Carcinoembryonic antigen (CEA) assay: a laboratory adjunct in the diagnosis and management of cancer. *Hum Pathol*, 5, 139-147 (1974)

2011 Hansen M et al. Small cell carcinoma of the lung: serum calcitonin and serum histaminase at basal levels and stimulated by pentagastrin. *Acta Med Scand*, 204, 257-261 (1978)

2012 Hansen NE. Plasma lysozyme- a measure of neutrophil turnover. *Series Haematol*, 7, 1 (1974)

2013 Hansen PB, Kjeldsen L, Dalhoff K et al. Cerebrospinal fluid β_2-microglobulin in adult patients with acute leukemia or lymphoma: a useful marker in early diagnosis and monitoring of CNS-involvement. *Acta Neurol Scand*, 85, 224-227 (1992)

2014 Hanss M, Coppere B, Gineyts E et al. Increased plasma free γ-carboxyglutamic acid levels during deep vein thrombosis and intravascular disseminated coagulation. *Thromb Res*, 73, 185-192 (1994)

2015 Hanss M, Ville D, Dechavanne M. Increased plasma tissue-type plasminogen activator levels in patients with chronic cytopenia. *Haemostasis*, 20, 341-346 (1990)

2016 Hanssen KF et al. Increased serum prolactin in diabetic ketoacidosis: correlation between serum sodium and serum prolactin concentration. *Acta Endocrinol*, 85, 372-378 (1977)

2017 Hantouche E, Piketty ML, Poirier MF et al. Thyroid function in obsessive-compulsive disorder. *Encephale*, 17, 493-496 (1991)

2018 Hara H, Ban Y. Plasma polymorphonuclear elastase in patients with hyperthyroidism. *Endocrine J*, 40, 711-714 (1993)

2019 Haraguchi Y, Sakamoto A, Yoshida T et al. Plasma CRP-like immunoreactivity in healthy and diseased subjects. *Gastroenterol Jpn*, 23, 247-250 (1988)

2020 Haran N, Gurwicz S, Gallati H et al. Effect of 1α-hydroxyvitamin D_3 treatment on production of tumor necrosis factor-α by peripheral blood mononuclear cells and on serum concentrations of soluble tumor necrosis factor receptors in hemodialysis patients. *Nephron*, 66, 262-266 (1994)

2021 Hardarson S, LaBrecque DR, Mitros FA et al. Antineutrophil cytoplasmic antibody in inflammatory bowel and hepatobiliary diseases: high prevalence in ulcerative colitis, primary sclerosing cholangitis, and autoimmune hepatitis. *Am J Clin Pathol*, 99, 277-281 (1993)

2022 Hardy KH, Rosevear JW, Sams WM et al. Scleroderma and urinary excretion of acidic glycosaminoglycans. *Mayo Clin Proc*, 46, 119-127 (1971)

2023 Harju E, Sotaniemi E, Puranen J et al. High incidence of low serum vitamin D concentration in patients with hip fracture. *Arch Orthop Traum Surg*, 103, 408-416 (1985)

2024 Harker LA. *Hemostasis Manual.* Philadelphia PA, FA Davis (1974)

2025 Harlozinska A, Sedlaczek P, van Dalen A, et al. TPS and CA 125 levels in serum, cyst fluid and ascites of patients with epithelial ovarian neoplasms. *Anticancer Res*, 17, 4473-4478 (1997)

2026 Harmenberg U, Wahren B, Wiechel KL. Tumor markers carbohydrate antigens CA 19-9 and CA-50 and carcinoembryonic antigen in pancreatic cancer and benign diseases of the pancreatobiliary tract. *Cancer Res*, 48, 1985-1988 (1988)

2027 Harris CC et al. Serum α_1-antitrypsin in patients with lung cancer or abnormal sputum cytology. *Cancer*, 38, 1655-1657 (1976)

2028 Harris H. Erythropoietic protoporphyria. *Arch Dermatol*, 91, 85 (1968)

2029 Harris-Jones J N. Hyperuricemia and essential hypercholesterolemia. *Lancet*, 1, 857 (1957)

2030 Harrison AA, Dunbar PR, Neale TJ. Immunoassay of platelet-derived growth factor in the blood of patients with diabetes mellitus. *Diabetologia*, 37, 1142-1146 (1994)

2031 Harrison HE. The Fanconi syndrome. *J Chron Dis*, 7, 346 (1958)

2032 Harrison HE et al. Growth disturbance in hereditary hypophosphatemia. *Am J Dis Child*, 112, 290 (1966)

2033 Harrison TR. *Principles of Internal Medicine.* 5th edition, New York NY, McGraw-Hill (1966)

2034 Harrison TR. *Principles of Internal Medicine.* 8th edition, New York NY, McGraw-Hill (1977)

2035 Harrison TR. *Principles of Internal Medicine.* 10th edition, New York NY, McGraw-Hill (1983)

2036 Harter JG. Serum uric acid levels in patients with bronchial asthma. *J Allerg Clin Immunol*, 42, 88 (1968)

2037 Harthoorn-Lasthuizen E, Lindemans J, Langenhuijsen MMAC. Combined use of erythrocyte zinc protoporphyrin and mean corpuscular volume in differentiation of thalassemia from iron deficiency anemia. *Eur J Haematol*, 60, 245-251 (1998)

2038 Hartoma TR et al. Serum zinc and serum copper and indices of drug metabolism in alcoholics. *Eur J Clin Pharmacol*, 12, 147-151 (1977)

2039 Harvey AM et al. *The Principles and Practice of Medicine.* 19th edition, New York NY, Appleton-Century-Crofts (1976)

2040 Harvey S, Weisman M, O'Dell J, et al. Chondrex: a new marker of joint disease. *Clin Chem*, 44, 509-516 (1998)

2041 Hasdai D, Barak V, Leibovitz E, et al. Serum basic fibroblast growth factor levels in patients with ischemic heart disease. *Int J Cardiol*, 59, 133-138 (1997)

2042 Hasegawa K, Matsushita Y, Inoue T et al. Plasma levels of atrial natriuretic peptide in patients with chronic renal failure. *J Clin Endocrinol Metab*, 63, 819-822 (1986)

2043 Hasegawa M, Fujimoto M, Kikuchi K, Takehara K. Elevated serum levels of interleukin-4 (IL-4), IL-10, and IL-13 in patients with systemic sclerosis. *J Rheumatol*, 24, 328-332 (1997)

2044 Hasegawa M, Sato S, Fujimoto M, et al. Serum levels of interleukin 6 (IL-6), oncostatin M, soluble IL-6 receptor, and soluble gp 130 in patients with systemic sclerosis. *J Rheumatol*, 25, 308-313 (1998)

2045 Hashim JA, Walsh A, Hart CA et al. Cerebrospinal fluid interleukin-6 and its diagnostic value in the investigation of meningitis. *Ann Clin Biochem*, 32, 289-296 (1995)

2046 Hashimoto H, Igarashi N, Yachie A et al. The relationship between serum levels of interleukin-6 and thyroid hormone in children with acute respiratory infection. *J Clin Endocrinol Metab*, 78, 288-291 (1994)

2047 Hashimoto K, Nishioka T, Takao T et al. Low plasma corticotropin-releasing hormone (CRH) levels in patients with non-insulin dependent diabetes mellitus. *Endocrine J*, 40, 705-709 (1993)

2048 Hashimoto R, Mizutani M, Ohta T et al. Changes in plasma tetrahydrobiopterin levels of depressives in depressive and remission phases: reconfirmed by meaurement with an internal standard. *Neuropsychobiology*, 29, 57-60 (1994)

2049 Hashimoto R, Ozaki N, Ohta T et al. Total biopterin levels of plasma in patients with depression. *Neuropsychobiology*, 17, 176-177 (1987)

2050 Hashimoto S, Imai K, Kobayashi T et al. Elevated levels of soluble ICAM-1 in sera from patients with bronchial asthma. *Allergy*, 48, 370-372 (1993)

2051 Hashimoto S, Miwa M, Akasofu K, Nishida E. Changes in 40 serum proteins of post-menopausal women. *Maturitas*, 13, 23-33 (1991)

2052 Hashimoto T, Aihara R, Tayama M et al. Reduced thyroid-stimulating hormone response to thyrotropin-releasing hormone in autistic boys. *Dev Med Child Neurol*, 33, 313-319 (1991)

2053 Hasholzner U, Baumgartner L, Stieber P, et al. Clinical significance of the tumour markers CA 125 II and CA 72-4 in ovarian carcinoma. *Int J Cancer (Pred Oncol)*, 69, 329-334 (1996)

2054 Hasim IA, Hart CA, Shenkin A. Cerebrospinal fluid IL-6 as a diagnostic discriminator between viral and bacterial meningitis. *Proc ACB Natl Meet*, 70 (1992)

2055 Hasselbalch H, Junker P, Lisse I et al. Circulating hyaluronan in the myelofibrosis/osteomyelosclerosis syndrome and other myeloproliferative disorders. *Am J Hematol*, 36, 1-8 (1991)

2056 Hasslacher CH, Brocks DG. Serum concentration of laminin in type I diabetic patients with and without microangiopathy. *Transplant Proc*, 8, 534 (1986)

2057 Hastka J, Lasserre J-J, Schwarzbeck A et al. Central role of zinc protoporphyrin in staging iron deficiency. *Clin Chem*, 40, 768-773 (1994)

2058 Hastrup B et al. Acid phosphatase in Niemann-Pick's disease and a therapeutic experiment with cortisone. *Acta Med Scand*, 149, 287-290 (1954)

2059 Hatch FE et al. Nature of the renal concentrating defect in sickle cell disease. *J Clin Invest*, 46, 336 (1967)

2060 Hattori N, Kurahachi H, Ikeubo K et al. Serum growth hormone-binding protein, insulin-like growth factor-I, and growth hormone in patients with liver cirrhosis. *Metabolism*, 41, 377-381 (1992)

2061 Haug C, Koenig W, Hoeher M, et al. Direct enzyme immunometric measurement of plasma big endothelin-1 concentrations and correlation with indicators of left ventricular function. *Clin Chem*, 44, 239-243 (1998)

2062 Haug C, Metzele A, Steffgen J et al. Changes in brain natriuretic peptide and atrial natriuretic peptide plasma concentrations during hemodialysis in patients with chronic renal failure. *Horm Metab Res*, 26, 246-249 (1994)

2063 Haug CJ, Aukrust P, Haug E, et al. Severe deficiency of 1,25-dihydroxyvitamin D_3 in human immunodeficiency virus infection: association with immunological hyperactivity and only minor changes in calcium homeostasis. *J Clin Endicrinol Metab*, 83, 3832-3838 (1998)

2064 Haugen HN. Glucose and acetone as sources of error in plasma creatinine determinations. *Scand J Clin Lab Invest*, 6, 17-21 (1954)

2065 Haukipuro K, Melkko J, Risteli L et al. Connective tissue response to major surgery and postoperative infection. *Eur J Clin Invest*, 22, 333-340 (1992)

2066 Haukland HH, Florholmen J, Oian P et al. The effect of severe pre-eclampsia on the pancreas: changes in the serum cationic trypsinogen and pancreatic amylase. *Br J Obstet Gynaecol*, 94, 765-767 (1987)

2067 Hauner H, Bender M, Haastert B, Hube F. Plasma concentrations of soluble TNF-α receptors in obese subjects. *Int J Obesity*, 22, 1239-1243 (1998)

2068 Hautman R et al. Diagnosis of renal tumor by γ-glutamyltranspeptidase. *Urology*, 7, 12-16 (1976)

2069 Hay DM et al. Maternal serum α-fetoprotein in abnormal pregnancies and during induced abortion. *J Reprod Med*, 19, 75-78 (1977)

2070 Hayakawa M, Maki M. Coagulation-fibrinolytic and kinin-forming systems in toxemia of pregnancy. *Gynecol Obstet Invest*, 26, 181-190 (1988)

2071 Hayasaka H, Suzuki N, Fujimoto N, et al. Elevated plasma levels of matrix metalloproteinase-9 (92-kd type IV collagenase/gelatinase B) in hepatocellular carcinoma. *Hepatology*, 24, 1058-1062 (1996)

2072 Hayashi H, Mizishuma N, Yashinaga H, et al. The relationship between lipoprotein(a) and low density lipoprotein receptors during treatment of hyperthyroidism. *Horm Metab Res*, 28, 384-387 (1996)

2073 Hayashi M, Numaguchi M, Watabe H, Yaoi Y. High blood levels of macrophage-colony stimulating factor in preeclampsia. *Blood*, 88, 4426-4428 (1996)

2074 Hayden K, Tetlow L, Byrne G, Bundred N. Radioimmunoassay for the measurement of thrombospondin in plasma and breast cyst fluid: validation and clinical application. *Ann Clin Biochem*, 37, 319-325 (2000)

2075 Hayes CP, Robinson RR. Fecal potassium excretion in patients on chronic intermittent hemodialysis. *Trans Am Soc Artif Intern Organ*, 11, 242 (1965)

2076 Hayes DF, Zurawaski VR Jr, Kufe DW. Comparison of circulating CA15-3 and carcinoembryonic antigen levels in patients with breast cancer. *J Clin Oncol*, 4, 1542-1550 (1986)

2077 Hayhoe FGJ et al. *The Cytology and Cytochemistry of Acute Leukemias*, London, HMO Stationery Office (1964)

2078 Haynes DC. Summary of interference testing data for Kodak Ektachem Clinical Chemistry systems, Personal Communication (1994)

2079 Haynes DM. *Medical Complications during Pregnancy.* New York NY, McGraw-Hill Blakiston Division (1969)

2080 He S, Bremme K, Kallner A et al. Increased concentrations of lactate dehydrogenase in pregnancy with preeclampsia: a predictor for the birth of small-for-gestational-age infants. *Gynecol Obstet Invest*, 39, 234-238 (1995)

2081 Healey LA, Wilske KR. Anemia as a presenting manifestation of giant cell arteritis. *Arth Rheum*, 14, 27 (1971)

2082 Healy D, Calvin J, Whitehouse AM et al. α-1-Acid glycoprotein in major depressive and eating disorders. *J Affect Disord*, 22, 13-20 (1991)

2083 Healy DL, Burger HG, Mamers P et al. Elevated serum inhibin concentrations in postmenopausal women with ovarian tumors. *N Engl J Med*, 329, 1539-1542 (1993)

2084 Heath R, Jeffrey S, Carter N. Radioimmunoassay of human muscle carbonic anhydrase III in dystrophic states. *Clin Chim Acta*, 11, 299-305 (1982)

2085 Heath R, Schwartz MS, Brown IRF et al. Carbonic anhydrase III in neuromuscular disorders. *J Neurol Sci*, 59, 383-388 (1983)

2086 Hebbar M, Lassalle P, Janin A et al. E-selectin expression in salivary endothelial cells and sera from patients with systemic sclerosis. *Arth Rheum*, 38, 406-412 (1995)

2087 Hedberg H. Studies on the depressed hemolytic complement activity of synovial fluid in adult rheumatoid arthritis. *Acta Rheum Scand*, 9, 165 (1963)

2088 Hedfors E, Kisner S. Serum level and urinary excretion of α-2 macroglobulin in patients with renal disease. *Acta Med Scand*, 190, 347-351 (1971)

2089 Hedstrom J, Leinonen J, Sainio V et al. Time-resolved immunofluorometric assay of trypsin-2 complexed with α_1-antitrypsin in serum. *Clin Chem*, 40, 1761-1765 (1994)

2090 Hefler L, Tempfer C, Heinzl H, et al. M3/M21 serum levels in women with adnexal masses and inflammatory diseases. *Int J Cancer (Pred Oncol)*, 79, 434-438 (1998)

2091 Heidelberger KP. α_1-Antitrypsin deficiency: a review. *Ann Clin Lab Sci*, 6, 1963-1975 (1976)

2092 Heidenreich F, Arendt G, Jander S et al. Serum and cerebrospinal fluid levels of soluble intercellular adhesion molecule-1 (sICAM-1) in patients with HIV-1 associated neurological diseases. *J Neuroimmunol*, 52, 117-126 (1994)

2093 Heidman RC et al. Chronic glomerulonephritis associated with low serum complement activity (chronic hypocomplementemic glomerulonephritis). *Medicine*, 49, 207 (1970)

2094 Heikius B, Niermela S, Lehtola J, et al. Elevated pancreatic enzymes in inflammatory disease are associated with extensive disease. *Am J Gastroenterol*, 94, 1062-1069 (1999)

2095 Heikkila R, Aho K, Heliovaara M, et al. Serum testosterone and sex hormone-binding globulin concentrations and the risk of prostate carcinoma. *Cancer*, 86, 312-315 (1999)

2096 Heikkinen T, Ghaffar F, Okorodudu AO, Chonmaitree T. Serum interleukin-6 in bacterial and nonbacterial acute otitis media. *Pediatrics*, 102, 296-299 (1998)

2097 Heine WI et al. Antibodies to cardiac tissue in acute ischemic heart disease. *Am J Cardiol*, 17, 798 (1966)

2098 Heiskala H. CSF ACTH and β-endorphin in infants with West syndrome and ACTH therapy. *Brain Develop*, 19, 339-342 (1997)

2099 Heits F, Katschinski DM, Wilmsen U, et al. Serum thrombopoietin and interleukin-6 concentrations in tumour patients and response to chemotherapy-induced thrombocytopenia. *Eur J Haematol*, 59, 53-58 (1997)

2100 Held BL, Nader S, Rodriguez-Rigau LJ et al. Acne and hyperandrogenism. *J Am Acad Dermatol*, 10, 223

2101 Heliovaara M, Knekt P, Aho K et al. Serum antioxidants and risk of rheumatoid arthritis. *Ann Rheum Dis*, 53, 51-53 (1994)

2102 Helle KB et al. Circulating dopamine-β-hydroxylase (DBH) and catecholamines in a pediatric phaeochromocytoma. *Clin Exp Pharmacol Physiol*, 3, 487-491 (1976)

2103 Helle SI, Lonning PE. Insulin-like growth factors in breast cancer. *Acta Oncol*, 35 Suppl 5, 19-22 (1996)

2104 Heller FR, Galanti L, Jamart J et al. Serum lipoprotein(a) in patients with diabetes mellitus. *Diabetes Care*, 16, 819-823 (1993)

2105 Heller P et al. Enzymes in anemia: a study of abnormalities of several enzymes of carbohydrate metabolism in the plasma and erythrocytes in patients with anemia, with preliminary observations of bone marrow enzymes. *Ann Intern Med*, 53, 898-913 (1963)

2106 Heller P et al. Glycolytic, citric acid cycle, and hexosemonophosphate shunt enzymes of plasma and erythrocytes in megaloblastic anemia. *J Lab Clin Med*, 55, 425 (1960)

2107 Hellum KB. Nitroblue tetrazolium test in pulmonary thromboembolism and pneumonia. *Scand J Infect Dis*, 9, 131-134 (1977)

2108 Helmrath MA, Shin CE, Fox JW, et al. Epidermal growth factor in saliva and serum of infants with necrotizing enterocolitis. *Lancet*, 351, 266-267 (1998)

2109 Hemmingsen L et al. Urinary excretion of the ten plasma proteins in patients with extrarenal epithelial carcinoma. *Acta Chir Scand*, 143, 177-183 (1977)

2110 Hempen I, Lehnert P, Fichter M, Teufel J. Hyperamylasemia in anorexia nervosa and bulimia nervosa. Indications of a pancreatic disease. *Deutsch Med Wschr*, 114, 1913-1916 (1989)

2111 Henderson M, Kessel D. Alterations in plasma sialyltransferase levels in patients with neoplastic disease. *Cancer*, 39, 1129-1134 (1977)

2112 Hendrick AM, Mitchell MD, Harris AL. Plasma prostaglandins in lung cancer. *Eur J Cancer Clin Oncol*, 24, 1069-1071 (1988)

2113 Hendrick JC, Franchimont P. Radio-immunoassay of casein in the serum of normal subjects and of patients with various malignancies. *Eur J Cancer*, 10, 725-730 (1974)

2114 Henle W et al. Epstein-Barr specific diagnostic tests in infectious mononucleosis. *Hum Pathol*, 5, 552 (1974)

2115 Hennes HM, Smith DS, Schneider K et al. Elevated liver transaminase levels in children with blunt abdominal trauma: a predictor of liver injury. *Pediatrics*, 86, 87-90 (1990)

2116 Henricks WH, England BG, Giacherio DA, et al. Serum percent-free PSA does not predict extraprostatic spread of prostate cancer. *Am J Clin Path*, 109, 533-539 (1998)

2117 Henriksen OA et al. Evaluation of the endocrine functions in dystrophia myotonica. *Acta Neurol Scand*, 58, 178-189 (1978)

2118 Henrikson AE, Nilsson TK, Bergqvist D. Bleeding time and concentrations of von Willebrand factor in patients with acute upper gastrointestinal bleeding. *Eur S Surg*, 162, 627-631 (1996)

2119 Henry RR, Gumbiner B, Ditzler T et al. Intensive conventional insulin therapy for type II diabetes: metabolic effects during a 6-mo outpatient trial. *Diabetes Care*, 16, 21-31 (1993)

2120 Henshaw TJ, Malone CC, Gabay JE et al. Elevations of neutrophil proteinase 3 in serum of patients with Wegener's granulomatosis and polyarteritis nodosa. *Arth Rheum*, 37, 104-112 (1994)

2121 Henskens YMC, van der Velden U, Veerman ECI et al. Cystatin C levels of whole saliva are increased in periodontal patients. *Ann NY Acad Sci*, 694, 280-282 (1993)

2122 Heptner G, Dkomschke S, Domschke W. Comparison of CA 72-4 with CA 19-9 and carcinoembryonic antigen in the serodiagnostics of gastrointestinal malignancies. *Scand J Gastroenterol*, 24, 745-750 (1989)

2123 Herbelin A, Urena P, Nguyen AT et al. Elevated circulating levels of interleukin-6 in patients with chronic renal failure. *Kidney Int*, 39, 954-960 (1991)

2124 Herbert FK. The estimation of prostatic phosphatase in serum and its use in the diagnosis of prostatic carcinoma. *Q J Med*, 15, 221-241 (1946)

2125 Herbert V, Jayatilleke E, Shaw S, et al. Serum ferritin iron, a new test, measures human body iron stores unconfounded by inflammation. *Stem Cells*, 15, 291-296 (1997)

2126 Hergesell O, Egbring R, Andrassy K. Presence of anticardiolipin antibodies discriminates between Wegener's granulomatosis and microscopic polyarteritis. *Adv Exp Med Biol*, 336, .393-396 (1993)

2127 Hergt K. Blood levels of thrombocytes in burned patients: observations on their behavior in relation to the clinical condition of the patient. *J Trauma*, 12, 599 (1972)

2128 Herishanu Y et al. The CSF lipid content in brain atrophy. *J Neurol Sci*, 26, 583-586 (1975)

2129 Herlyn M et al. Monoclonal antibody detection of a circulating tumor associated antigen. *J Clin Immunol*, 2, 135-140 (1982)

2130 Hernandez A, Sepulveda P, Fernandez-Cuartero B et al. Urinary porphyrinogens in normal subjects and in patients with porphyria cutanea tarda and acute intermittent porphyria. *Horm Metab Res*, 25, 454-455 (1993)

2131 Heron E, Chatellier G, Billaud E, et al. The urinary metanephrine-to-creatinine ratio for the diagnosis of pheochromocytoma. *Ann Intern Med*, 125, 300-303 (1996)

2132 Herrmann JL, Blanchard H, Brunengo P et al. TNF-α, IL-1β and IL-6 plasma levels in neutropenic patients after onset of fever and correlation with the C-reactive protein (CRP) kinetic values. *Infection*, 22, 309-315 (1994)

2133 Herve C, Beyne P, Letteron P, Delacoux E. Comparison of erythrocyte transketolase activity with thiamine and thiamine phosphate ester levels in chronic alcoholic patients. *Clin Chim Acta*, 234, 91-100 (1995)

2134 Herve P, Launay J-M, Scrobohaci M-L et al. Increased plasma serotonin in primary pulmonary hypertension. *Am J Med*, 99, 249-254 (1995)

2135 Hesselvik JF, Malm J, Dahlback B et al. Protein C, protein S, and C_4b-binding protein in severe infection and septic shock. *Thromb Haemostas*, 65, 126-129 (1991)

2136 Heuck CC et al. Serum lipids in renal insufficiency. *Am J Clin Nutr*, 31, 1547-1553 (1978)

2137 Heuman R, Sjodahl R, Tobiasson P, Tagesson C. Postprandial serum bile acids in resected and non-resected patients with Crohn's disease. *Scand J Gastroenterol*, 17, 137-140 (1982)

2138 Heuser I, Deuschle M, Luppa P, et al. Increased diurnal plasma concentrations of dhydroepiandrosterone in depressed patients. *J Clin Endocrinol Metab*, 83, 3130-3133 (1998)

2139 Heussen-Schemmer C, Barron JR, Swanepoel CR et al. Urinary tissue plasminogen activator in renal disease. *Nephron* (1992)

2140 Heyes MP, Brew BJ, Martin A et al. Quinolinic acid in cerebrospinal fluid and serum in HIV-1 infections: relationship to clinical and neurological status. *Ann Neurol*, 29, 202-209 (1991)

2141 Heyes MP, Rubinow D, Lane C, Markey SP. Cerebrospinal fluid quinolinic acid concentrations are increased in acquired immune deficiency syndrome. *Ann Neurol*, 26, 275-277 (1989)

2142 Heyes MP, Swartz KJ, Markey SP, Beal MF. Regional brain and cerebrospinal fluid quinolinic acid concentrations in Huntington's disease. *Neurosci Lett*, 122, 265-269 (1991)

2143 Heynen C. Le calcitonine serique dans la cirrhose ethylique. *Cr Soc Biol*, 171, 690 (1977)

2144 Heynen C, Franchimont. Human calcitonin radioimmunoassay in normal and pathological conditions. *Eur J Clin Invest*, 4, 213 (1974)

2145 Hibi S, Ikushima S, Fujiwara F et al. Serum and urine β-2-microglobulin in hemophagocytic syndrome. *Cancer*, 75, 1700-1705 (1995)

2146 Hickling RA. Leukaemia and related conditions in the blood - uric acid. *Lancet*, 1, 175 (1958)

2147 Hickman PE, Campbell B, Tate J et al. Plasma protein changes and liver transplantation. *Clin Biochem Rev*, 14, 200 (1993)

2148 Hicks JM, D'Angelo L. The laboratory's role in serving adolescent patients. *Lab Med*, 29, 581-586 (1997)

2149 Hida M, Aiba Y, Sawamura S, et al. Inhibition of the accumulation of uremic toxins in the blood and their precursors in the feces after oral administration of Lebenin® , a lactic acid bacteria preparation, to uremic patients undergoing hemodialysis. *Nephron*, 74, 349-355 (1996)

2150 Hida T, Kuwabara M, Ariyoshi Y et al. Serum glutathione S-transferase-pi level as a tumor marker for non-small cell lung cancer. *Cancer*, 73, 1377-1382 (1994)

2151 Hietarinta M, Lassila O, Hietaharju A. Association of anti-U1RNP- and anti-Scl-70-antibodies with neurological manifestations in systemic sclerosis (scleroderma). *Scand J Rheumatol*, 23, 64-67 (1994)

2152 Higashiyama M, Doi I, Kodama K, et al. Estimation of serum level of pS2 protein in patients with lung adenocarcinoma. *Anticancer Res*, 16, 2351-2356 (1996)

2153 Higgins PJ. The thyrotoxicosis of hydatidiform mole. *Ann Intern Med*, 83, 307-311 (1975)

2154 Hilden M et al. Studies on the serum lipid and lipoproteins in steatosis of the liver. *Acta Med Scand*, 198, 207-212 (1975)

2155 Hilgenfeldt U, Kienapfel G, Kellermann W et al. Renin-angiotensin system in sepsis. *Clin Exp Hypertens Theory Pract*, 9, 1493-1504 (1987)

2156 Hill DB, Deaciuc IV, McClain CJ. Hyperhyaluronanemia in alcoholic hepatitis is associated with increased levels of circulating soluble intercellular adhesion molecule-1. *Alcohol Clin Exp Res*, 22, 1324-1327 (1998)

2157 Hill DB, Marsano L, Cohen D et al. Increased plasma interleukin-6 concentrations in alcoholic hepatitis. *J Lab Clin Med*, 119, 547-552 (1992)

2158 Hill DB, Marsano LS, McClain CJ. Increased plasma interleukin-8 concentrations in alcoholic hepatitis. *Hepatology*, 18, 576-580 (1993)

2159 Hill GS et al. Systemic lupus erythematosus morphologic correlations with immunologic and clinical data at the time of biopsy. *Am J Med*, 64, 61-79 (1978)

2160 Hill KK, Hill DB, McClain MP et al. Serum insulin-like growth factor-I concentrations in the recovery of patients with anorexia nervosa. *J Am Coll Nutr*, 12, 475-478 (1993)

2161 Hillenbrand P et al. Significance of intravascular coagulation and fibrinolysis in acute hepatic failure. *Gut*, 15, 83 (1974)

2162 Hillman RS, Finch CA. Erythropoiesis: normal and abnormal. *Semin Hematol*, 4, 327 (1967)

2163 Hillmen P, Lewis SM, Bessler M et al. Natural history of paroxysmal nocturnal hemoglobinuria. *N Engl J Med*, 333, 1253-1258 (1995)

2164 Hinds G, Bell NP, McMaster D et al. Normal red cell magnesium concentrations and magnesium loading tests in patients with chronic fatigue syndrome. *Ann Clin Biochem*, 31, 459-461 (1994)

2165 Hinds TR, Kukull WA, van Belle G et al. Relationship between serum α_1-antichymotrypsin and Alzheimer's disease. *Neurobiol Aging*, 15, 21-27 (1994)

2166 Hintz. Human somatomedin plasma binding proteins. In:. *Somatomedin and Related Peptides,* G Giordano (ed), Amsterdam, Excerpta Med, 143 (1979)

2167 Hirai K, Nomura M, Nakajima Y et al. Serum levels of retinol, inorganic phosphate and polyunsaturated fatty acid and their relationship in diabetic patients with early nephropathy. *Nutr Res*, 14, 1135-1142 (1994)

2168 Hirao J, Hibi S, Andoh T, Ichimura T. High levels of circulating interleukin-4 and interleukin-10 in Kawasaki disease. *Int Arch Allergy Immunol*, 112, 152-156 (1997)

2169 Hirase Y, Makatsuka H, Kawai T et al. Stable blood cell counts after one-week storage at room temperature. *Bull Environ Contam Toxicol*, 49, 504-508 (1992)

2170 Hirata Y, Ishii M, Matsuoka H et al. Plasma concentrations of a human atrial natriuretic polypeptide and cyclic GMP in patients with heart disease. *Am Heart J*, 113, 1463-1469 (1987)

2171 Hirata Y, Mitaka C, Sato K, et al. Increased circulating adrenomedullin, a novel vasodilatory peptide, in sepsis. *J Clin Endocrinol Metab*, 81, 1449-1453 (1996)

2172 Hirayama C et al. Serum cholesterol and bile acid in primary hepatoma. *Clin Chim Acta*, 71, 21-25 (1976)

2173 Hirohata S, Miyamoto T. Elevated levels of interleukin-6 in cerebrospinal fluid from patients with systemic lupus erythematosus and central nervous system involvement. *Arth Rheum*, 33, 644-649 (1990)

2174 Hiroshige K, Nawata H. High plasma concentrations of endothelin-like immunoreactivities in patients with hepatocellular carcinoma. *Am J Gastroenterol*, 88, 248-252 (1993)

2175 Hiroyoshi M, Tateishi K, Yasunami Y, et al. Elevated glucagon-like peptide-1 after oral glucose ingestion in patients with pancreatic diabetes. *Am J Gastroenterol*, 94, 976-981 (1999)

2176 Hirschl MH, Derfler K, Bieglmayer C, et al. Hormonal derangements in patients with severe alcohol intoxication. *Alcohol Clin Exp Res*, 18, 761-766 (1994)

2177 Hjertberg R, Belfrage P, Bremme K et al. The renin-angiotensin-aldosterone system in pregnancy. Response to terbutaline provocation in preeclampsia. *Clin Exp Hypertens Preg*, 10, 385-389 (1991)

2178 Hjorth-Hansen H, Seidel C, Lamvik J, et al. Elevated serum concentrations of hepatocyte growth factor in acute myelocytic leukaemia. *Eur J Haematol*, 62, 129-134 (1999)

2179 Ho C-H, Yang Z-L. The predictive value of the hemostasis parameters in the development of preeclampsia. *Thromb Haemostas*, 67, 214-218 (1992)

2180 Ho et al. Serum acid phosphatase levels in untreated carcinoma patients. *Miss Med*, 289-290 (1975)

2181 Ho PJ, Baxter RC. Insulin-like growth factor-binding protein-2 in patients with prostate carcinoma and benign prostatic hyperplasia. *Clin Endocrinol*, 46, 333-342 (1997)

2182 Ho WKK et al. Comparison of plasma hormonal levels between heroin-addicted and normal subjects. *Clin Chim Acta*, 75, 415-419 (1977)

2183 Hoad K, Mallon D, French M et al. Parathyroid hormone secretion in patients with HIV infection. *Clin Biochem Rev*, 14, 250 (1993)

2184 Hoag GN, Franks CR, de Coteau WE. Creatine kinase isoenzymes in serum of patients with cancer of various organs. *Clin Chem*, 24, 1654-1660 (1978)

2185 Hober D, Benyoucef S, Bocket L, et al. Soluble tumor necrosis factor receptor type II (sTNFRII) in HIV-infected patients: relationship with the plasma level of HIV-1 RNA. *Immunol Lett*, 67, 91-94 (1999)

2186 Hober D, Benyoucef S, Delannoy A-S, et al. High plasma level of soluble tumor necrosis factor receptor type II (sTNFRII) in symptomatic HIV-1-infected patients. *Infection*, 24, 213-217 (1996)

2187 Hober D, Benyoucef S, Delannoy A-S, et al. Plasma levels of sTNFR p75 and IL-8 in patients with HIV-1 infection. *Immunol Lett*, 52, 57-60 (1996)

2188 Hober D, Delannoy A-S, Benyoucef S, et al. High levels of sTNFR p75 and TNFα in Dengue-infected patients. *Microbiol Immunol*, 40, 569-573 (1996)

2189 Hochman HI et al. Chloride-losing diarrhea and metabolic alkalosis in an infant with cystic fibrosis. *Arch Dis Child*, 51, 390 (1976)

2190 Hock C, Golombowski S, Muller-Spahn F, et al. Cerebrospinal fluid levels of amyloid precursor protein and amyloid β-peptide in Alzheimer's disease and major depression - inverse correlation with dementia severity. *Eur Neurol*, 39, 111-118 (1998)

2191 Hodgson SF, Dickson ER, Wahner HW et al. Bone loss and reduced osteoblast function in primary biliary cirrhosis. *Ann Intern Med*, 103, 855-860 (1985)

2192 Hoeprich PD. *Infectious Diseases,* 2nd edition, Baltimore MD, Harper and Row (1977)

2193 Hoffbrand AV et al. Megaloblastic anaemia in myelosclerosis. *Q J Med*, 37, 493 (1968)

2194 Hoffbrand BI. Haemolytic anemia in Hodgkin's disease associated with high immunoglobulin deficiency. *Br J Cancer*, 18, 98 (1964)

2195 Hoffbrand BI. Hodgkin's disease and hypogammaglobulinemia: a rare association. *Br Med J*, 1, 1156 (1964)

2196 Hoffenberg EJ, Deutsch J, Smith S, Sokol RJ. Circulating antioxidant concentrations in children with inflammatory bowel disease. *Am J Clin Nutr*, 65, 1482-1488 (1997)

2197 Hoffenberg EJ, Fidanza S, Sauaia A. Serologic testing for inflammatory bowel disease. *J Pediatr*, 134, 447-452 (1999)

2198 Hoffman A, Grossman E, Goldstein DS et al. Urinary excretion rate of endothelin-1 in patients with essential hypertension and salt sensitivity. *Kidney Int*, 45, 556-560 (1994)

2199 Hoffman IF, Jere CS, Taylor TE, et al. The effect of Plasmodium falciparum malaria on HIV-1 RNA blood plasma concentration. *AIDS*, 13, 487-494 (1999)

2200 Hoffmann GE, Hiefinger R, Steinbrueckner B. Serum phospholipase A in hospitalized patients. *Clin Chim Acta*, 183, 59-64 (1989)

2201 Hoffmeister HM, Heller W, Seipel L. Molecular markers of hemostasis and fibrinolysis and inhibitor levels in unstable angina pectoris. *Fibrinolysis Proteolysis*, 11 Suppl 1, 61-65 (1997)

2202 Hoffmeister HM, Jur M, Wendel HP et al. Alterations of coagulation and fibrinolytic and kallikrein-kinin systems in the acute and postacute phases in patients with unstable angina pectoris. *Circulation*, 91, 2520-2527 (1995)

2203 Hogdall CK, Mogensen O, Tabor A et al. The role of serum tetranectin, CA 125, and a combined index as tumor markers in women with pelvic tumors. *Gynecol Oncol*, 56, 22-28 (1995)

2204 Hogdall CP, Hogdall EV, Arends J et al. CA-125 as a maternal serum marker for Down's syndrome in the first and second trimesters. *Prenat Diag*, 12, 223-227 (1992)

2205 Hoheisel G, Izbicki G, Roth M, et al. Proinflammatory cytokine levels in patients with lung cancer and carcinomatous pleurisy. *Respiration*, 65, 183-186 (1998)

2206 Hohnoki K, Inoue A, Koh C-S. Elevated serum levels of IFN-γ, IL-4 and TNF-α/unelevated serum levels of IL-10 in patients with demyelinating diseases during the acute stage. *J Neuroimmunol*, 87, 27-32 (1998)

2207 Holborow EJ et al. Smooth muscle auto-antibodies in infectious mononucleosis. *Br Med J*, 3, 323 (1973)

2208 Holland DB, Chao SW, Hitchcock ER et al. IgG subclasses in acne vulgaris. *Br J Dermatol*, 114, 349-351 (1986)

2209 Hollis BW, Kamerud JQ, Kurkowski A, et al. Quantification of circulating 1,25-dihydroxyvitamin D by radioimmunoassay with an ^{125}I-labeled tracer. *Clin Chem*, 42, 586-592 (1996)

2210 Holmberg CG, Laurell CB. Oxidase reactions in human plasma caused by ceruloplasmin. *Scand J Clin Lab Invest*, 3, 107 (1951)

2211 Holmgren J, Linholm J, Persson B et al. Detection by monoclonal antibody of carbohydrate antigen CA 50 in serum of patients with carcinoma. *Br Med J*, i, 1479-1482 (1984)

2212 Holst FGE, Hemmer CJ, Foth C, et al. Low levels of fibrin stabilizing factor (Factor XIII) in human plasmodium falciparum malaria: correlations with clinical severity. *Am J Trop Med Hyg*, 60, 99-104 (1999)

2213 Holst N, Oian P, Aune B et al. Increased plasma levels of vasoactive intestinal polypeptide in pre-eclampsia. *Br J Obstet Gynaecol*, 98, 803-806 (1991)

2214 Holton JB et al. Biochemical investigation of histidinaemia. *J Clin Pathol*, 17, 671 (1974)

2215 Holvoet P, Stassen J-M, van Clemput J, et al. Oxidized low density lipoproteins in patients with transplant-associated coronary disease. *Arterioscler Thromb Vasc Biol*, 18, 100-107 (1998)

2216 Holzel A et al. Aminoaciduria in galactosemia. *Br Med J*, 1, 194 (1952)

2217 Holzel A et al. Galactosemia. *Am J Med*, 22, 703 (1957)

2218 Hombs KS et al. Serum prolactin levels in untreated primary hypoparathyroidism. *Am J Med*, 64, 782-787 (1978)

2219 Homma Y, Kobayashi T, Yamaguchi H et al. Decrease of plasma large, light LDL (LDL1), HDL_2 and HDL_3 levels with concomitant increase of cholesterylester transfer protein (CETP) activity by probucol in type II hyperlipoproteinemia. *Artery*, 20, 1-18 (1993)

2220 Hong R, Good RA. Limited heterogeneity of γ globulin in hypogammaglobulinemia. *Science*, 156, 1102 (1967)

2221 Hong SY, Yang DH. Insulin levels and fibrinolytic activity in patients with end-stage renal disease. *Nephron*, 68, 329-333 (1994)

2222 Honkanen E, Froseth B, Gronhagen-Riska C. Serum hyaluronic acid and procollagen III amino terminal propeptide in chronic renal failure. *Am J Nephrol*, 11, 201-216 (1991)

2223 Honza A, Jork R, Muller D. Determination of fucokinase activity in the blood of schizophrenic patients. *Psych Neurol Med Psych*, 41, 531-538 (1989)

2224 Hoogenberg K, Sluiter WJ, Dullaart RPF. Effect of growth hormone and insulin like growth factor-I on urinary albumin excretion: studies in acromegaly and growth hormone deficiency. *Acta Endocrinol*, 129, 151-157 (1993)

2225 Hooshmand H. Serum lactate dehydrogenase isoenzymes in neuromuscular diseases. *Dis Nerv Syst*, 36, 607-611 (1975)

2226 Hooshmand H et al. The use of serum lactate dehydrogenase isoenzymes in the diagnosis of muscle diseases. *Neurology*, 19, 26-31 (1969)

2227 Hoppensteadt D, Chinthagada M, Chejfec G et al. Studies on the role of neuropeptides in the pathogenesis of cumulative trauma disorders. *Clin Chem*, 41, S66 (1995)

2228 Hoppichler F, Sandholzer C, Moncayo R et al. Thyroid hormone (fT4) reduces lipoprotein(a) plasma levels. *Atherosclerosis*, 115, 65-71 (1995)

2229 Hori Y, Wada H, Mori Y, et al. Plasma sFas and sFas ligand levels in patients with thrombocytopenic purpura and in those with disseminated intravascular coagulation. *Am J Hematol*, 61, 21-25 (1999)

2230 Horkko S, Huttunen K, Korhonen T et al. Decreased clearance of low-density lipoprotein in patients with chronic renal failure. *Kidney Int*, 45, 561-570 (1994)

2231 Horn BR et al. Total eosinophil counts in the management of bronchial asthma. *N Engl J Med*, 292, 1152-1255 (1975)

2232 Horne CHW et al. Serum α_2-macroglobulin, transferrin, albumin, and IgG levels in pre-eclampsia. *J Clin Pathol*, 23, 514-516 (1970)

2233 Horne CHW, Howie PW, Weir RJ, Goudie RB. Effect of combined oestrogen-progestogen oral contraceptives on serum-levels of α_2-macroglobulin, transferrin, albumin and IgG. *Lancet*, 1, 49-51 (1970)

2234 Hornef S, Lux J, Rassner G. Neuron-specific enolase (NSE) - a suitable tumor marker for malignant melanoma? *Hautarzt*, 43, 77-80 (1992)

2235 Horneff G, Sack U, Kalden JR et al. Reduction of monocyte-macrophage activation markers upon anti-CD4 treatment. Decreased levels of IL-1, IL-6, neopterin and soluble CD14 in patients with rheumatoid arthritis. *Clin Exp Immunol*, 91, 207-213 (1993)

2236 Horng CJ, Hsiao KJ, Chen CH et al. Urinary neopterin and biopterin levels in patients with depression. *Abstracts*, 5th APCCB, Kobe (1991)

2237 Horobin JM, Browning MC, McFarlane NP et al. Potential use of tumor marker CA 15-3 in the staging and prognosis of patients with breast cancer. *J Roy Coll Surg Edin*, 36, 219-221 (1991)

2238 Horrobin DF. The roles of prostaglandins and prolactin in depression, mania and schizophrenia. *Postgrad Med J*, 53, 198-201 (1977)

2239 Horsfall FL, Tamm I (eds). *Viral and Rickettsial Infections of Man*, 4th edition, Philadelphia PA, Lippincott (1965)

2240 Hortin GL, Landt M, Powderly WG. Changes in plasma amino acid concentrations in response to HIV-1 infection. *Clin Chem*, 40, 785-789 (1994)

2241 Horton L et al. The haematology of hypothyroidism. *Q J Med*, 45, 101-23 (1976)

2242 Horton MA et al. Reversible C_3 hypocomplementaemia in megaloblastic anemia due to vitamin B_{12} deficiency. *Br J Haematol*, 36, 23-27 (1977)

2243 Horwitz DL et al. Proinsulin and C-peptide in diabetes. *Med Clin North Am*, 62, 723-733 (1978)

2244 Hosaka S, Shah MR, Pope RM, Koch AE. Soluble forms of P-selectin and intercellular adhesion molecule-3 in synovial fluids. *Clin Immunol Immunopathol*, 78, 276-282 (1996)

2245 Hoshino T, Yamada K, Masuoka K et al. Elevated adenosine deaminase activity in the serum of patients with diabetes mellitus. *Diabet Res Clin Pract*, 25, 97-102 (1994)

2246 Hosoda K, Eguchi H, Nakamoto T et al. Sandwich immunoassay for intact human osteocalcin. *Clin Chem*, 38, 2233-2238 (1992)

2247 Hossein-Nia M, Sainsbury CG, Reilly ME et al. The separation of alkaline phosphatase isoenzymes and isoforms in the detection of heart graft rejection. *Clin Chem*, 39, 1155 (1993)

2248 Host NB, Aldershvile J, Horslov-Petersen K, et al. Serum aminoterminal propeptide of type III procollagen after cardiac transplantation and the effect of rejection. *Am J Cardiol*, 78, 1406-1410 (1996)

2249 Housley J. Alpha$_2$-macroglobulin levels in disease in man. *J Clin Pathol*, 21, 27-31 (1968)

2250 Hovdenes J, Kvien TK, Hovdenes AB. IL-6 in synovial fluids, plasma and supernatants from cultured cells of patients with rheumatoid arthritis and other inflammatory arthritides. *Scand J Rheumatol*, 19, 177-182 (1990)

2251 Howard RL, Buddington B, Alfrey AC. Urinary albumin, transferrin and iron excretion in diabetic patients. *Kidney Int*, 40, 923-926 (1991)

2252 Howard, Thomas. Clinical disorders of calcium homeostasis. *Medicine*, 42, 25-45 (1963)

2253 Howell RR et al. Glucose-6-phosphatase deficiency glycogen storage disease. studies on the interrelationship of carbohydrate, lipids, and purine abnormalities. *Pediatrics*, 29, 553-565 (1967)

2254 Hrabar A, Aleraj B, Ceovic S et al. β_2-Microglobulin studies in endemic Balkan nephropathy. *Kidney Int*, 40, S38-S40 (1991)

2255 Hrgovcic M et al. Serum copper levels in lymphoma and leukemia: special reference to Hodgkin's disease. *Am J Med*, 50, 56 (1971)

2256 Hsieh KH. Changes of serum complement and eosinophil count in antigen induced bronchospasm. *Ann Allergy*, 41, 182-185 (1978)

2257 Hsieh KM, et al. Serum lactic dehydrogenase levels in various disease states. *Proc Soc Exp Biol Med*, 91, 626-630 (1956)

2258 Hsu C-C, Yang B-C, Wu M-H, Huang K-E. Enhanced interleukin-4 expression in patients with endometriosis. *Fertil Steril*, 67, 1059-1064 (1997)

2259 Hsu C-D, Lucas RB, Johnson TBR et al. Elevated urine thrombomodulin/creatinine ratio in severely preeclamptic pregnancies. *Am J Obstet Gynecol*, 171, 854-856 (1994)

2260 Hsu COD, Meaddough E, Aversa K, et al. Elevated amniotic fluid levels of leukemia inhibitory factor, interleukin 6, and interleukin 8 in intra-amniotic infection. *Am J Obstet Gynecol*, 179, 1257-1270 (1998)

2261 Hsu C-T, Yu M-H, Lee C-YG et al. Ectopic production of prolactin in uterine cervical carcinoma. *Gynecol Oncol*, 44, 166-171 (1992)

2262 Hsu P-I, Chow N-H, Lai K-H, et al. Implications of serum basic fibroblast growth factor levels in chronic liver diseases and hepatocellular carcinoma. *Anticancer Res*, 17, 2803-2810 (1997)

2263 Hsueh W, Caplan MS, Sun X et al. Platelet-activating factor, tumor necrosis factor, hypoxia and necrotizing enterocolitis. *Acta Paediat*, 396, Suppl, 11-17 (1994)

2264 Hsueh WA et al. Endocrine features of Klinefelter's syndrome. *Medicine*, 57, 447-462 (1978)

2265 Hua CT, Hopwood JJ, Carlsson SR, et al. Evaluation of the lysosomal-associated membrane protein LAMP-2 as a marker for lysosomal storage disorders. *Clin Chem*, 44, 2094-2102 (1998)

2266 Huang C-L, Liang HM, Brassil D et al. Two-site monoclonal antibody-based immunoradiometric assay for measuring prostate secretory protein in serum. *Clin Chem*, 38, 817-823 (1992)

2267 Huang CM, Ruddel M, Elin RJ. Enzyme abnormalities of patients with acquired immunodeficiency syndrome. *Clin Chem*, 34, 2574-2576 (1988)

2268 Huang M-J, Tsai T-L, Huang B-Y, et al. Prevalence and significance of thyroid autoantibodies in patients with chronic hepatitis C virus infection: a prospective controlled study. *Clin Endocrinol*, 50, 503-509 (1999)

2269 Huang Y-S, Chan C-Y, Wu J-C, et al. Serum levels of interleukin-8 in alcoholic liver disease: relationship with disease stage, biochemical parameters and survival. *J Hepatol*, 24, 377-384 (1996)

2270 Huang YS et al. Plasma lipids and lipoproteins in Friedreich's ataxia and familial spastic ataxia - evidence for an abnormal composition of high density lipoproteins. *Can J Neurol Sci*, 5, 149-156 (1978)

2271 Hubel CA, Kagan VE, Kisin ER, et al. Increased ascorbate radical formation and ascorbate depletion in plasma from women with preeclampsia: implications for oxidative stress. *Free Radical Biol Med*, 23, 597-609 (1997)

2272 Huber K, Beckmann R, Frank H et al. Fibrinogen, t-PA, and PAI-1 plasma levels in patients with pulmonary hypertension. *Am J Resp Crit Care Med*, 150, 929-933 (1994)

2273 Huber PR, Schnell Y, Hering F et al. Prostate specific antigen: experimental and clinical observations. *Scand J Urol Nephrol*, 104, Suppl, 33-39 (1987)

2274 Huckauf H et al. Oxygen affinity of haemoglobin and red cell acid-base status in patients with severe chronic obstructive lung disease. *Br J Cancer*, 12, 129-142 (1976)

2275 Hudson RW, Edwards AL. Testicular function in hyperthyroidism. *J Androl*, 13, 117-124 (1992)

2276 Huengsberg M, Waring R, Moffitt D, et al. Serum cysteine levels in HIV infection. *AIDS*, 12, 1245 (1998)

2277 Huff B et al. *Physicians' Desk Reference. Supplement B.* Oradell NJ, Medical Economics (1972)

2278 Hughes NR. Serum concentrations of γ-G, γ-A, and γ-M immunoglobulins in patients with carcinoma, melanoma, and sarcoma. *J Natl Cancer Inst*, 46, 1015-1028 (1971)

2279 Hughes NR. Serum group-specific (Gc) protein concentrations in patient with carcinoma, melanoma, sarcoma, and cancers of hematopoietic tissues as determined by radial immunodiffusion. *J Natl Cancer Inst*, 46, 665-675 (1971)

2280 Hughes NR. Serum transferrin and ceruloplasmin concentrations in patients with carcinoma, melanoma, sarcoma and cancers of haematopoietic tissues. *Aust J Exp Biol Med Sci*, 50, 97-107 (1972)

2281 Hughes RD, Zhang L, Tsubouchi H et al. Plasma hepatocyte growth factor and biliprotein levels and outcome in fulminant hepatic failure. *J Hepatol*, 20, 106-111 (1994)

2282 Hughes VF, Trull AK, Joshi O. Evaluation of eosinophilic cationic protein as a marker of immune activation leading to acute liver allograft rejection. *Proc ACB Natl Meet*, 151-152 (1995)

2283 Hughes WT et al. Signs, symptoms, and pathophysiology of pneumocystis carinii pneumonitis. *NCI Monogr*, 43, 77-88 (1976)

2284 Huizenga JR, Tangerman A, Gips CH. Determination of ammonia in biological fluids. *Ann Clin Biochem*, 31, 529-543 (1994)

2285 Hullin RP et al. Renin and aldosterone relationships in manic depressive psychosis. *Br J Psychiat*, 131, 575-581 (1977)

2286 Hultberg B, Andersson A, Sterner G. Plasma homocysteine in renal failure. *Clin Nephrol*, 40, 230-235 (1993)

2287 Hultberg B, Berglund M, Andersson A, Frank A. Elevated plasma homocysteine in alcoholics. *Alcohol Clin Exp Res*, 17, 687-689 (1993)

2288 Hultberg B et al. Diagnostic value of determinations of lysosomal hydrolases in CSF of patients with neurological disease. *Acta Neurol Scand*, 57, 201-415 (1978)

2289 Hultberg B, Isaksson A, Berglund M et al. Serum β-hexosaminidase isoenzyme: a sensitive marker for alcohol abuse. *Alcohol Clin Exp Res*, 15, 549-552 (1991)

2290 Hultberg B, Isaksson A, Krutzen E et al. Urinary excretion of N-acetyl-β-D-glucosaminidase in normal and complicated pregnancy. *J Clin Chem Clin Biochem*, 27, 487-489 (1989)

2291 Hultberg B, Isaksson A, Lindgren A, et al. β-Hexosaminidase isoenzymes A and B in middle-aged and elderly subjects: determinants of plasma levels and relation to vascular disease. *Ann Clin Biochem*, 33, 432-437 (1996)

2292 Hultberg B, Isaksson A, Sterner G et al. Enzyme immunoassay of urinary β-hexosaminidase isoenzymes in patients with renal transplants. *Clin Chim Acta*, 192, 107-114 (1990)

2293 Hulyalkar AR, Nora R, Manowitz P. Arylsulfatase A variants in patients with alcoholism. *Alcohol Clin Exp Res*, 8, 337-341 (1984)

2294 Humaloja K, Roine RP, Salmela K et al. Serum dolichols in different clinical conditions. *Scand J Clin Lab Invest*, 51, 705-709 (1991)

2295 Human JA, Ubbink JB, Jerling JJ, et al. The effect of simvastatin on the plasma antioxidant concentrations in patients with hypercholesterolemia. *Clin Chim Acta*, 263, 67-77 (1997)

2296 Hume R, Goldberg A. Actual and predicted normal red-cell and plasma volumes in primary and secondary polycythemia. *Clin Sci*, 26, 499 (1964)

2297 Humphrey CS. Glucose tolerance and insulin secretion in patients with chronic duodenal ulcer. *Br Med J*, 4, 393 (1972)

2298 Humphries JE, Siragy H. Significant hyponatremia following DDAVP administration in a healthy adult. *Am J Hematol*, 44, 12-15 (1993)

2299 Hunt et al. Enzyme changes following direct current countershock. *Am Heart J*, 76, 340-344 (1968)

2300 Hunter G et al. *Tropical Medicine,* 5th edition, Philadelphia PA, WB Saunders (1976)

2301 Huribal M, Cunningham ME, D'Ainto ML et al. Endothelin-1 and prostaglandin E_2 levels increase in patients with burns. *J Am Coll Surg*, 180, 318-322 (1995)

2302 Hurley JR. Thyroiditis. *DM*, 24, 13-15, 35-38 (1977)

2303 Hurst DW, Meyer OO. Giant follicular lymphoblastoma. *Cancer*, 14, 753 (1961)

2304 Hurst J, Willis (eds). *The Heart,* 4th edition, New York NY, McGraw-Hill (1978)

2305 Hurt RD, Briones ER, Offord KP et al. Plasma lipids and apolipoprotein A-I and A-II levels in alcoholic patients. *Am J Clin Nutr*, 43, 521-529 (1986)

2306 Hussa RO. Clinical utility of human chorionic gonadotropin and α-subunit measurements. *Obstet Gynecol*, 60, 1-12 (1982)

2307 Hussain MJ, Peakman M, Gallati H, et al. Elevated serum levels of macrophage-derived cytokines precede and accompany the onset of IDDM. *Diabetologia*, 39, 60-69 (1996)

2308 Hussan JM et al. Systemic sclerosis and cryoglobulinemia. *Clin Immunol Immunopathol*, 6, 77 (1976)

2309 Hutchesson ACJ, Murdoch-Davis C, Green A, et al. Biochemical monitoring of treatment for galactosaemia: biological variability in metabolite concentrations. *J Inher Metab Dis*, 22, 139-148 (1999)

2310 Hyams JS, Fitzgerald JE, Wyzga N et al. Characterization of circulating interleukin-1 receptor antagonist expression in children with inflammatory bowel disease. *Dig Dis Sci*, 39, 1893-1899 (1994)

2311 Ibe BO, Kurantsin-Mills J, Usha Raj J et al. Plasma and urinary leukotrienes in sickle cell cell disease: possible role in the inflammatory process. *Eur J Clin Invest*, 24, 57-64 (1994)

2312 Ibrahim KS, Marrs TC, Husain OAN. LDH in gastric juice and its limitation in the diagnosis of gastric cancer. *Ann Clin Biochem*, 18, 364-367 (1981)

2313 Ibrahim S, Mojiminiyi S, Barron JL. High-performance liquid chromatographic determination of pyridinium crosslinks in serum, urine and dialysate of patients in chronic renal failure. *Ann Clin Biochem*, 33, 31-35 (1996)

2314 Ichiyama T, Nishikawa M, Yoshitomi T, et al. Tumor necrosis factor-α, interleukin-1β, and interleukin-6 in cerebrospinal fluid from children with prolonged febrile seizures. *Neurology*, 50, 407-411 (1998)

2315 Igarashi P, Gulyassy P, Stanfel L et al. Plasma hippurate in renal failure: high performance liquid chromatography method and clinical application. *Nephron*, 47, 290-294 (1987)

2316 Igari T et al. Catecholamine metabolism in the patients with rheumatoid arthritis. *Tohoku J Exp Med*, 122, 9-20 (1977)

2317 Iguchi H, Natori S, Ou Y et al. Plasma levels of $7B_2$ (a novel pituitary polypeptide) and its molecular forms in plasma and urine in patients with chronic renal failure: possible degradation by the kidney. *Regul Peptide*, 21, 263-270 (1988)

2318 Iguchi H, Yasuda D, Yamada Y et al. $7B_2$, a possible marker for nonfunctioning pancreatic islet cell tumor. *Horm Metab Res*, 23, 486-489 (1991)

2319 Ihara Y, Sagawa N, Hasegawa M et al. Concentrations of endothelin-1 in maternal and umbilical cord blood at various stages of pregnancy. *J Cardiovasc Pharmacol*, 17, S443-S445 (1991)

2320 Ihde DC et al. Clinical manifestations of hepatoma. *Am J Med*, 56, 83-91 (1974)

2321 Ihn H, Sato S, Fujimoto M, er al. Increased serum levels of soluble vascular cell adhesion molecule-1 and E-selectin in patients with systemic sclerosis. *Br J Rheum*, 37, 1188-1192 (1998)

2322 Ihn H, Sato S, Fujimoto M, et al. Clinical significance of serum levels of soluble interleukin-2 receptor in patients with localized scleroderma. *Br J Derm*, 134, 843-847 (1996)

2323 Iio A, Strober W, Broder S et al. The metabolism of IgE in patients with immunodeficiency states and neoplastic conditions. *J Clin Invest*, 59, 743-755 (1977)

2324 Ikeda U, Ohkawa F, Seino Y et al. Serum interleukin 6 levels become elevated in acute myocardial infarction. *J Mol Cell Cardiol*, 24, 579-584 (1992)

2325 Ilio CD, Arduini A, Del Boccio G et al. Glutathione redox cycle enzyme activities in erythrocytes of multiple sclerosis patients. *Clin Physiol Biochem*, 4, 120-124 (1986)

2326 Imagawa DK, Millis JM, Olthoff KM et al. The role of tumor necrosis factor in allograft rejection. *Transplantation*, 50, 219-225 (1990)

2327 Imagawa K, Matsumoto Y, Numata Y, et al. Development of a sensitive ELISA for human leptin, using monoclonal antibodies. *Clin Chem*, 44, 2165-2171 (1998)

2328 Imai A, Horibe S, Takagi A, et al. Drastic elevation of serum CA125, CA72-4 and CA19-9 levels during menses in a patient with probable endometriosis. *Eur J Obstet Gynecol*, 78, 79-81 (1998)

2329 Imai Y, Odajima R, Shimizu T, Shishiba Y. Serum hyaluronan concentration determined by radiometric assay in patients with pretibial myxedema and Graves' ophthalmopathy. *Endocrinol Jpn*, 37, 749-752 (1990)

2330 Imperatore G, Rivellese A, Galasso R, et al. Lipoprotein(a) concentrations in non-insulin-dependent diabetes mellitus and borderline hyperglycemia: a population-based study. *Metabolism*, 44, 1293-1297 (1995)

2331 Inamoto Y, Inamoto S, Hanai T, et al. Chemical characterization of guanidino compounds in serum. *Am Clin Lab*, June, 12-14 (2000)

2332 Inar S et al. Serum level of the fourth component of complement in various diseases. *Biken J*, 10, 65-87 (1967)

2333 Ince E, Karagol U, Deda G. Excitatory amino acid levels in cerebrospinal fluid of patients with infantile spasms. *Acta Paediatr*, 86, 1333-1336 (1997)

2334 Ingenbleek Y et al. T3 resin uptake in protein-calorie malnutrition. *Acta Endocrinol*, 81, 283-287 (1976)

2335 Ingenbleek Y et al. Triiodothyronine and thyroid-stimulating hormone in protein calorie malnutrition. *Lancet*, 2, 845-848 (1975)

2336 Inoue K, Nago N, Matsuo H, et al. Serum insulin and lipoprotein(a) concentrations. *Diabetes Care*, 20, 1242-1247 (1997)

2337 Inoue N, Harada S, Miyasaka N et al. Analysis of antibody titers to Epstein-Barr virus nuclear antigens in sera of patients with Sjögren's syndrome and with rheumatoid arthritis. *J Infect Dis*, 164, 22-28 (1991)

2338 Inoue T, Okamura M, Amatsu K et al. Serum lactate dehydrogenase and its isozymes in lupus nephritis. *Arch Intern Med*, 146, 548 (1986)

2339 Inui T, Ochi Y, Chen W et al. Increased serum concentration of type IV collagen peptide and type III collagen peptide in hyperthyroidism. *Clin Chim Acta*, 205, 181-186 (1992)

2340 Inui Y, Kuwajima M, Kawata S et al. Impaired ketogenesis in patients with adult-type citrullinemia. *Gastroenterology*, 107, 1154-1161 (1994)

2341 Inutsuka SI. Plasma copper and zinc levels in patients with malignant tumors of digestive organs. *Cancer*, 42, 626-631 (1978)

2342 Invitti C, Brunani A, Pasqualinotto L et al. Plasma galanin concentrations in obese, normal weight and anorectic women. *Int J Obesity*, 19, 347-349 (1995)

2343 Invitti C, De Martin I, Bolla GB et al. Effect of octreotide on catecholamine plasma levels in patients with chromaffn cell tumors. *Horm Res*, 40, 156-160 (1993)

2344 Invitti C, Fatti L, Camboni MG, et al. Effect of chronic treatment with octreotide nasal powder on serum levels of growth hormone, insulin-like growth factor I, insulin-like growth factor binding proteins 1 and 3 in acromegalic patients. *J Endocrinol Invest*, 19, 548-555 (1996)

2345 Invitti C, Giraldi FP, Dubini A, et al. Galanin is released by adrenocorticotropin-secreting pituitary adenomas in vivo and in vitro. *J Clin Endocrinol Metab*, 84, 1351-1356 (1999)

2346 Inward CD, Pall AA, Adu D, et al. Soluble circulating cell adhesion molecules in haemolytic uraemic syndrome. *Pediatr Nephrol*, 9, 574-578 (1995)

2347 Inward CD, Varagunam M, Adu D, et al. Cytokines in haemolytic uraemic syndrome with serocytotoxin-producing Escherichia coli infection. *Arch Dis Child*, 77, 145-147 (1997)

2348 Ippoliti G, Vinante F, Rovati B et al. Serum levels of soluble interleukin-2 receptor (sIL-2R) fail to correlate with the occurrence and degree of rejection in heart transplant patients. *Clin Transplant*, 4, 1-4 (1990)

2349 Iqbal SJ, Brain A, Holland S et al. Raised serum pyridoxal-5-phosphate levels in hypophosphatasia. *Proc ACB Natl Meet*, 69 (1995)

2350 Irani FA et al. Serum lactic dehydrogenase in pneumonia. *South Med J*, 65, 858, 874 (1972)

2351 Isern RA, Yaneva M, Weiner E et al. Autoantibodies in patients with primary pulmonary hypertension: association with anti-Ku. *Am J Med*, 93, 307-312 (1992)

2352 Ishigami-Miyake TT, Nagao AT, Arslanian C, et al. Evaluation of serum levels of IgG subclasses and anti-ribosyl-ribitolphosphate IgG and IgG2 in children with Haemophilus influenzae B in memingitis. *J Trop Pediat*, 45, 130-134 (1999)

2353 Ishiguro A, Ishikita T, Shimbo T, et al. Elevation of serum thrombopoietin precedes thrombocytosis in Kawasaki disease. *Thromb Haemost*, 79, 1096-1100 (1998)

2354 Ishii J, Wang J-H, Naruse H, et al. Serum concentrations of myoglobin vs human heart-type cytoplasmic fatty acid-binding protein in early detection of acute myocardial infarction. *Clin Chem*, 43, 1372-1378 (1997)

2355 Ishikawa M, Hayashi H, Saitoh S et al. Clinical significance of manganese superoxide dismutase in ovarian carcinoma. *Acta Obstet Gynecol Jpn*, 43, 509-515 (1991)

2356 Ishimitsu T, Nishikimi T, Saito Y et al. Plasma levels of adrenomedullin, a newly identified hypotensive peptide, in patients with hypertension and renal failure. *J Clin Invest*, 94, 2158-2161 (1994)

2357 Ishimura E, Nishizawa Y, Shoji S, Morii H. Serum type III, IV collagens and TIMP in patients with type II diabetes mellitus. *Life Sci*, 58, 1331-1337 (1996)

2358 Isobe T, Osserman E. Patterns of amyloidosis and their association with plasma cell dyscrasias, monoclonal immunoglobulins and Bence-Jones proteins. *N Engl J Med*, 290, 473 (1974)

2359 Isogai M, Yamaguchi A, Hori A, et al. LDH to AST ratio in biliary pancreatitis - a possible indicator of pancreatic necrosis: preliminary results. *Am J Gastroenterol*, 93, 363-367 (1998)

2360 Isogal M, Hachisuka K, Yamaguchi A, Hori A. Biochemical prediction of acute cholangitis and symptomatic bile duct stones by gallstone hepatitis. *HPB Surgery*, 8, 267-273 (1995)

2361 Isojrvi JIT, Repo M, Pakarinen AJ, et al. Carbamazepine, phenytoin, sex hormones, and sexual function in men with epilepsy. *Epilepsia*, 36, 366-370 (1995)

2362 Ito H, Kambe H, Kimura Y et al. Depression of plasma gelsolin level during acute liver injury. *Gastroenterology*, 102, 1686-1692 (1992)

2363 Ito H, Kotake T, Nomura K, Masai M. Clinical and biochemical features of uric acid nephrolithiasis. *Eur Urol*, 27, 324-328 (1995)

2364 Ito H, Takagi Y, Ando Y, Kubo A. Serum ferritin levels in patients with cervical cancer. *Obstet Gynecol*, 55, 358-362 (1980)

2365 Ito N, Kawata S, Tamura S et al. Positive correlation of plasma transforming growth factor-β_1 levels with tumor vascularity in hepatocellular carcinoma. *Cancer Lett*, 89, 45-48 (1995)

2366 Ito S, Yamazaki M, Usami A et al. Urinary excretion rate and clearance of IgG_4 and α_2-macroglobulin in type 2 diabetic patients. *Horm Metab Res*, 27, 303-304 (1995)

2367 Ito T, Kimura T, Nawata H. Serum elastase I appears specific for cancer of the pancreatic head. *Am J Gastroenterol*, 86, 1778-1783 (1991)

2368 Itoh K, Aida S, Ishiwata S et al. Immunochemical detection of urinary 5-methyl-2'-deoxycytidine as a potential biologic marker for leukemia. *Clin Chim Acta*, 234, 37-45 (1995)

2369 Itoh T et al. Studies on serum gastrin of the patients with gastric cancer. *Am J Gastroenterol*, 68, 56-63 (1977)

2370 Itoh Y, Enomoto H, Takagi K, et al. Human alpha$_1$-microglobulin levels in neurological disorders. *Eur Neurol*, 22, 1-6 (1983)

2371 Itoh Y, Ishii S, Tamano O et al. Distribution of protein 1 in body fluids. *Clin Biochem*, 14, 207 (1993)

2372 Itoh Y, Okanoue T, Enjyo F et al. Serum levels of macrophage colony stimulating factor (M-CSF) in liver disease. *J Hepatol*, 21, 527-535 (1994)

2373 Itoh Y, Okanoue T, Ohnishi N, et al. Serum levels of soluble tumor necrosis factor receptors and effects of interferon therapy in patients with chronic hepatitis C virus infection. *Am J Gastroenterol*, 94, 1332-1340 (1999)

2374 Itoh Y, Okanoue T, Sakamoto S et al. Serum autoantibody against interleukin-1α is unrelated to the etiology or activity of liver disease but can be raised by interferon treatment. *Am J Gastroenterol*, 90, 777-782 (1995)

2375 Itoh Y, Okutani R, Ishii S et al. Protein 1 values in serum and urine. *Clin Chem*, 38, 961 (1992)

2376 Iversen N, Lindahl A-K, Abildgaard U. Elevated TFPI in malignant disease: relation to cancer type and hypercoagulation. *Br J Haematol*, 102, 889-895 (1998)

2377 Iwano M, Dohi K, Hirata E et al. Urinary levels of IL-6 in patients with active lupus nephritis. *Clin Nephrol*, 40, 16-21 (1993)

2378 Iwasaki Y, Ikeda K, Kinoshita M. Plasma amino acid levels in patients with amyotrophic lateral sclerosis. *J Neurol Sci*, 107, 219-222 (1992)

2379 Iwase H, Kobayashi S, Itoh Y et al. Evaluation of serum tumor markers in patients with advanced or recurrent breast cancer. *Breast Cancer Res Treat*, 33, 83-88 (1994)

2380 Iwase-Okada K, Kojima K, Kato T et al. Collagenase-like peptidase activity in serum from patients with rheumatoid arthritis. *Experientia*, 41, 487-488 (1985)

2381 Izzo F, Curley S, Maio P, et al. Correlation of soluble interleukin-2 receptor levels with severity of chronic hepatitis C virus liver injury and dvelopment of hepatocellular cancer. *Surgery*, 120, 100-105 (1996)

2382 Jaatinen T-A, Koskinen P, Matinlauri I et al. Serum total renin is elevated in women with polycystic ovarian syndrome. *Fertil Steril*, 63, 1000-1004 (1995)

2383 Jackle-Meyer I, Szukics B, Neubauer K et al. Extracellular matrix proteins as early markers in diabetic neuropathy. *Eur J Clin Chem Clin Biochem*, 33, 211-219 (1995)

2384 Jackson AM, Alexandroff AB, Kelly RW et al. Changes in urinary cytokines and soluble intercellular adhesion molecule-1 (ICAM-1) in bladder cancer patients after Bacillus Calmette-Guerin (BCG) immunotherapy. *Clin Exp Immunol*, 99, 369-375 (1995)

2385 Jackson P, Loughrey CM, Lightbody JH et al. Effect of hemodialysis on total antioxidant capacity and serum antioxidants in patients with chronic renal failure. *Clin Chem*, 41, 1135-1138 (1995)

2386 Jacobelli S, McCarty, Silcox DC, Mall JC. Calcium pyrophosphate dihydrate crystal deposition in neuropathic joints. four cases of polyarticular involvement. *Ann Intern Med*, 79, 340-347 (1973)

2387 Jacobs A, Jones D, Ricketts C et al. Serum ferritin concentration in early breast cancer. *Br J Cancer*, 34, 286-290 (1976)

2388 Jacobs ML, Nathoe HMW, Blankestijn PJ, et al. Growth hormone responses to growth hormone-releasing hormone and clonidine in patients with type I diabetes and in normal controls: effect of age, body mass index and sex. *Clin Endocrinol*, 44, 547-553 (1996)

2389 Jacobs SC, Mason J, Kosten TR et al. Urinary free cortisol and separation and anxiety early in the course of bereavement and threatened loss. *Biol Psychiat*, 22, 148-152 (1987)

2390 Jacobsen DW. Acquired hyperhomocysteinemia in heart transplant recipients. *Clin Chem*, 44, 2238-2239 (1998)

2391 Jacobsen JG et al. Serum acid phosphatase in osteogenesis imperfecta. *Metabolism*, 10, 483-488 (1961)

2392 Jacobsen LK, Frazier JA, Malhotra AK, et al. Cerebrospinal fluid monoamine metabolites in childhood-onset schizophrenia. *Am J Psychiat*, 154, 69-74 (1997)

2393 Jacobson JM, Greenspan JS, Spritzler J, et al. Thalidomide for the treatment of oral aphthous ulcers in patients with human immunodeficiency virus infection. *N Engl J Med*, 336, 1487-1493 (1997)

2394 Jacobson SH, Hylander B, Wretlind B et al. Interleukin-6 and interleukin-8 in serum and urine in patients with acute pyelonephritis in relation to bacterial-virulence-associated traits and renal function. *Nephron*, 67, 172-179 (1994)

2395 Jacobson SH, Moldeus P. Whole blood-, plasma- and red blood cell glutathione and cysteine in patients with kidney disease and during hemodialysis. *Clin Nephrol*, 42, 189-192 (1994)

2396 Jacobson W, Saich T, Borysiewicz LK et al. Serum folate and chronic fatigue syndrome. *Neurology*, 43, 2645-2647 (1993)

2397 Jaeger P, Otto S, Speck RF et al. Altered parathyroid gland function in severely immunocompromised patients infected with human immunodeficiency virus. *J Clin Endocrinol Metab*, 79, 1701-1705 (1994)

2398 Jaffe AS, Ritter C, Meltzer V et al. Unmasking artifactual increases in creatine kinase isoenzymes in patients with renal failure. *J Lab Clin Med*, 104, 193-202 (1984)

2399 Jager W, Kissing A, Cilaci S et al. Is an increase in CA 125 in breast cancer patients an indicator of pleural metastases? *Br J Cancer*, 70, 493-495 (1994)

2400 Jager W, Kramer S, Palapelas V, Norbert L. Breast cancer and clinical utility of CA- 15.3 and CEA. *Scand J Clin Lab Invest*, 55 Suppl 221, 87-92 (1995)

2401 Jagwe JG et al. A study of serum uric acid in adult patients with tropical splenomegaly syndrome. *East Afr Med J*, 54, 74-76 (1977)

2402 Jain SK, Palmer M. Effect of glucose-6-phosphate dehydrogenase deficiency on reduced and oxidized glutathione and lipid peroxide levels in the blood of African-Americans. *Clin Chim Acta*, 253, 181-183 (1996)

2403 Jain VK et al. Estimation of copper in serum, erythrocyte and urine in protein calorie malnutrition. *Ind J Pediatr*, 13, 767-770 (1976)

2404 Jais P, Bouizar Z, Vissuzaine C, et al. Parathyroid hormone-related protein in an esophageal squamous cell carcinoma with tumor-induced hypercalcemia. *Am J Gastroenterol*, 92, 343-346 (1997)

2405 Jakob G, Mair J, Puschendorf B. Direct determination of cyclic guanosine monophosphate in plasma. *Clin Chem*, 39, 2530-2531 (1993)

2406 Jakob G, Mair J, Vorderwinkler K-P et al. Clinical significance of urinary cyclic guanosine monophosphate in diagnosis of heart failure. *Clin Chem*, 40, 96-100 (1994)

2407 Jakobsen PH, Morris-Jones S, Theander TG et al. Increased plasma levels of soluble IL-2R are associated with severe plasmodium falciparum malaria. *Clin Exp Immunol*, 96, 98-103 (1994)

2408 Jakobsson B, Berg U. Effect of hydrochlorothiazide and indomethacin treatment on renal function in nephrogenic diabetes insipidus. *Acta Paediat*, 83, 522-525 (1994)

2409 Jakovljevic M, Muck-Seler D, Pivac N, et al. Seasonal influence on platelet 5-HT levels in patients with recurrent major depression and schizophrenia. *Biol Psychiat*, 41, 1028-1034 (1997)

2410 Jakubowicz DJ, Nestler JE. 17α-hydroxyprogesterone responses to leuprolide and serum androgens in obese women with and without polycystic ovary syndrome after dietary weight loss. *J Clin Endocrinol Metab*, 82, 556-560 (1997)

2411 James K. A study of the α-2-macroglobulin homologues of various species. *Immunology*, 8, 55-61 (1965)

2412 James K, Merriman J, Gray RS, Duncan LJP. Serum α_2-macroglobulin levels in diabetes. *J Clin Pathol*, 33, 163-166 (1980)

2413 Jamieson et al. Changes in serum phosphate levels associated with intestinal infarction and necrosis. *Surg Gynecol Obstet*, 140, 19-21 (1975)

2414 Jan KM et al. Observations on blood viscosity changes after acute myocardial infarction. *Circulation*, 51, 1079 (1975)

2415 Jandl J et al. The anemia of liver disease. *J Clin Invest*, 34, 390 (1955)

2416 Jansa R, Prezelj J, Kocijancic A, et al. Androstanediol glucuronide in patients with pancreatic cancer and in those with chronic pancreatitis. *Horm Metab Res*, 28, 381-383 (1996)

2417 Jaouhari J, Schiele F, Dragacci S et al. Avidin-biotin enzyme immunoassay of osteocalcin in serum or plasma. *Clin Chem*, 38, 1968-1974 (1992)

2418 Jaques G, Bepler G, Holle R et al. Prognostic value of pretreatment carcinoembryonic antigen, neuron-specific enolase, and creatine kinase-BB levels in sera of patients with small cell lung cancer. *Cancer*, 62, 125-134 (1988)

2419 Jaquhari J, Schiele F, Tarallo P et al. Development of a new enzyme immunoassay for human serum osteocalcin: application to the determination of osteocalcin level in alcoholic men. *Ann Clin Biol*, 50, 487 (1992)

2420 Jarnerot G et al. The thyroid in ulcerative colitis and Crohn's disease. *Acta Med Scand*, 199, 229-232 (1976)

2421 Jarnfelt-Samsioe A, Bremme K, Eneroth P. Non-steroid hormones and tissue polypeptide (TPA) in emetic and non-emetic pregnancy. *Acta Obstet Gynecol Scand*, 65, 745-751 (1986)

2422 Jarrett RF. Hodgkin's disease. *Clin Haematol*, 5, 57-79 (1992)

2423 Jarrold R, Vilter RW. Hematologic observations in patients with chronic hepatic insufficiency. *J Clin Invest*, 28, 286 (1949)

2424 Jarstrand C et al. Peripheral blood lymphocyte populations in influenza patients. *Scand J Infect Dis*, 9, 1-3 (1977)

2425 Jaschevatzky OE, Rosenberg RP, Shalit A et al. Protein/creatinine ratio in random urine specimens for quantitation of proteinuria in preeclampsia. *Obstet Gynecol*, 75, 604-606 (1990)

2426 Javitt NB. Cholestatic jaundice. *Med Clin North Am*, 59, 817-821 (1975)

2427 Jaynes PM, Feld RD. Creatine kinase isoenzymes in serum of a patient with gallbladder cancer. *Clin Chem*, 27, 1316-1317 (1981)

2428 Jayson MI et al. Serum copper and caeruloplasmin in ankylosing spondylitis, systemic sclerosis, and morphea. *Ann Rheum Dis*, 35, 443-445 (1975)

2429 Jeevanandam M, Holaday NJ, Shamos RF et al. Acute IGF-1 deficiency in multiple trauma victims. *Clin Nutr*, 11, 352-357 (1992)

2430 Jeevanandam M, Ramias L, Schiller WR. Elevated urinary C-peptide excretion in multiple trauma patients. *J Trauma*, 31, 334-341 (1991)

2431 Jeevanandam M, Ramias L, Schiller WR. Nutritional influence on the plasma and urine free alkaline ribonuclease levels in severe trauma victims. *J Parenter Enter Nutr*, 15, 241-246 (1991)

2432 Jeevanandam M, Young DH, Ramias L et al. Effect of major trauma on plasma free amino acid concentrations in geriatric patients. *Am J Clin Nutr*, 51, 1040-1045 (1990)

2433 Jeffree GM. Enzymes in fibroblastic lesions. *J Bone Joint Surg*, 54, 535-546 (1972)

2434 Jegatheesan et al. Correlation of serum glycolytic enzymes and acid phosphatases with sites of metastases in mammary carcinomatosis. *Br Med J*, 1, 831-834 (1962)

2435 Jenq SF, Jap TS, Chiang H. Determination of carnitine levels in patients with chronic pancreatitis. *Clin Biochem Rev*, 14, 349 (1993)

2436 Jensen CH, Krogh TN, Stoving RK, et al. Fetal antigen 1 (FA1), a circulating member of the epidermal growth factor (EGF) superfamily: ELISA development, physiology and metabolism in relation to renal function. *Clin Chim Acta*, 268, 1-20 (1997)

2437 Jensen H et al. The turnover of IgG and IgM in myotonic dystrophy. *Neurology*, 21, 68 (1971)

2438 Jensen J, Nilas L, Christiansen C. Influence of menopoause on serum lipids and lipoproteins. *Maturitas*, 12, 321-331 (1990)

2439 Jensen KB et al. Serum orosomucoid in ulcerative colitis: its relation to clinical activity, protein loss, and turnover of albumin and IgG. *Scand J Gastroenterol*, 11, 177-183 (1976)

2440 Jensen M, Schroder J, Blomberg M, et al. Cerebrospinal fluid Aβ42 is increased early in sporadic Alzheimer's disease and declines with disease progression. *Ann Neurol*, 45, 504-511 (1999)

2441 Jerome H, Farrenkopf B, Vitone S et al. Fluorescence polarization immunoassay for vancomycin on the Cobas Fara II analyzer. *Clin Chem*, 36, 1045 (1990)

2442 Jespersen B, Pedersen EB. Increased plasma level of atrial natriuretic peptide in patients with chronic renal failure: effect of noradrenaline infusion. *Nephrol Dial Transplant*, 3, 762-767 (1988)

2443 Jessop S et al. Erythrocyte electrolyte content and sodium efflux in chronic renal failure. *Nephron*, 18, 82-87 (1977)

2444 Jewitt DE et al. Free noradrenaline and adrenaline excretion in relation to the development of cardiac arrhythmias and heart failure in patients with acute myocardial infarction. *J Clin Endocrinol*, 1, 635-641 (1969)

2445 Jie K-SG, Bots ML, Vermeer C et al. Vitamin K intake and osteocalcin levels in women with and without aortic atherosclerosis: a population-based study. *Atherosclerosis*, 116, 117-123 (1995)

2446 Jilma B, Fasching P, Ruthner C, et al. Elevated circulating P-selectin in insulin dependent diabetes mellitus. *Thromb Hemostas*, 76, 328-332 (1996)

2447 Jimenez W, Gutkowsk J, Gines P et al. Molecular forms and biological activity of atrial natriuretic factor in patients with cirrhosis and ascites. *Hepatology*, 14, 601-607 (1991)

2448 Jimenez-Alonso J, Jaimez L, Barrios L et al. Salivary γ-glutamyltransferase activity internal diseases. *Arch Intern Med*, 144, 1804 (1984)

2449 Jimerson DC, Lesem MD, Kaye WH, Brewerton TD. Low serotonin and dopamine metabolite concentrations in cerebrospinal fluid. *Arch Gen Psychiat*, 49, 132-138 (1992)

2450 Jirillo E, Amati L, Caradonna L, et al. Soluble (s) CD14 and plasmatic lipopolysaccharides (LPS) in patients with chronic hepatitis C before and after treatment with interferon (IFN)-α. *Immunopharmacol Immunotoxicol*, 20, 1-14 (1998)

2451 Joborn C, Hetta J, Niklasson J et al. Cerebrospinal fluid calcium, parathyroid hormone, and monoamine and purine metabolites and the blood-brain barrier function in primary hyperparathyroidism. *Psychoneuroendocrinology*, 16, 311-322 (1991)

2452 Joelsson B, Hultberg B, Alwmark A et al. Total serum bile acids, γ-glutamyltransferase, prealbumin, and tyrosine: sensitive serum markers of hepatic dysfunction in alcoholic liver cirrhosis. *Scand J Gastroenterol*, 18, 497-501 (1983)

2453 Joelsson B, Hultberg B, Isaksson A et al. Total fasting serum bile acids and β-hexosaminidase in alcoholic liver disease. *Clin Chim Acta*, 31, 203-209 (1984)

2454 Johansen JS, Thomsen K, Christiansen C. Plasma bone Gla protein concentrations in healthy adults. Dependence on sex, age, and glomerular filtration. *Scand J Clin Lab Invest*, 47, 345-350 (1987)

2455 Johansson AG, Baylink DJ, Ekenstam E et al. Circulating levels of insulin-like growth factor-I and -II, and IGF-binding protein-3 in inflammation and after parathyroid hormone infusion. *Bone Miner*, 24, 25-31 (1994)

2456 Johansson B, Roos B. 5-HIAA and HVA in spinal fluid and herpes zoster oticus. *N Engl J Med*, 285, 637 (1971)

2457 Johansson BG, Kindmark CO, Trell EY et al. Sequential changes of plasma proteins after myocardial infarction. *Scand J Clin Lab Invest*, 29, Suppl 124, 117-126 (1972)

2458 Johansson EA et al. Free serum calcium in urticaria. *Acta Allergologica*, 29, 25-29 (1975)

2459 Johansson J, Santala M, Kauppila A. Explosive rise of serum CA 125 following the rupture of ovarian endometrioma. *Hum Reprod*, 13, 3503-3504 (1998)

2460 Johansson SGO. Raised levels of a new immunoglobulin class (IgD) in asthma. *Lancet*, 2, 951 (1967)

2461 John S, Neumayer H-H, Weber M. Serum circulating ICAM-1 levels are not useful to indicate active vasculitis or early renal allograft rejection. *Clin Nephrol*, 42, 369-373 (1994)

2462 John WG. Glycosylated haemoglobin levels in patients referred for oral glucose tolerance tests. *Diabetic Med*, 3, 46-48 (1986)

2463 Johnsen T. Effect upon serum insulin, glucose and potassium concentrations of acetazolamide during attacks of familial periodic hypokalemic paralysis. *Acta Neurol Scand*, 56, 533-541 (1977)

2464 Johnson AG, Mcdermott SG. Lysolecithin: a factor in the pathogenesis of gastric ulceration? *Gut*, 15, 710-713 (1974)

2465 Johnson et al. Clinical significance of serum acid phosphatase levels in advanced prostatic carcinoma. *Urology*, 8, 123-126 (1976)

2466 Johnson RD, Bahnisch J, Stewart B et al. Optimized spectrophotometric determination of aldehyde dehydrogenase activity in erythrocytes. *Clin Chem*, 38, 584-588 (1992)

2467 Johnston CS, Solomon E, Corte C. Vitamin C depletion is associated with alterations in blood histamine and plasma free carnitine in adults. *J Am Coll Nutr*, 15, 586-591 (1996)

2468 Johnston DG et al. Hyperinsulinism of hepatic cirrhosis: diminished degradation or hypersecretion. *Lancet*, 1, 10-13 (1977)

2469 Johnston J, McLelland A, O'Reilly DStJ. The relationship between serum cholesterol and serum thyroid hormones in male patients with suspected hypothyroidism. *Ann Clin Biochem*, 30, 256-259 (1993)

2470 Jois J, Omagari K, Rowley MJ, et al. Enzyme inhibitory antibody to pyruvate dehydrogenase: diagnostic utility in primary biliary cirrhosis. *Ann Clin Biochem*, 37, 67-73 (2000)

2471 Jokl R, Lyons TJ, Laimins M et al. Platelet plasminogen activator inhibitor 1 in patients with type II diabetes. *Diabetes Care*, 17, 818-823 (1994)

2472 Joliff C. Rheumatoid arthritis: two procedures to monitor the disease process. *Advance/Laboratory*, Oct, 1-4 (1994)

2473 Jolliff C, Weaver AL. Current concepts in the laboratory assessment of rheumatoid arthritis. *Spec Chem Today*, 7, 1-4 (1994)

2474 Joly JP, Sesboue R, Hillemand B et al. Serum trypsin-like activity in chronic alcoholized men: possible relationship with lipids, apoA-I and apoB lipoproteins. *Alcohol Alcoholism*, 27, 563-569 (1992)

2475 Jones AP, Lock S, Griffiths KD. Urinary N-acetyl-β-glucosaminidase activity in type I diabetes mellitus. *Ann Clin Biochem*, 32, 58-62 (1995)

2476 Jones B, Mitchell D, Horn DB et al. Cerebrospinal fluid angiotensin converting enzyme levels in the diagnosis of neurosarcoidosis. *Scott Med J*, 36, 144-145 (1991)

2477 Jones EMM, Wilson DC. Clinical features of yellow fever cases at Vom Christian hospital during the 1969 epidemic on the Jos plateau, Nigeria. *Bull WHO*, 46, 653-657 (1977)

2478 Jones JW, Ways P. Abnormalities of high density lipoproteins in abetalipoproteinemia. *J Clin Invest*, 46, 1151 (1967)

2479 Jones M, Mellirsh V. A comparison of the exercise response in various groups of neurotic patients, and a method of rapid determination of oxygen in expired air using a catharometer. *Psychosom Med*, 1, 192 (1946)

2480 Jones MB, Weinstock S, Koretz RL et al. Clinical value of serum bile acid levels in chronic hepatitis. *Dig Dis Sci*, 26, 978-983 (1981)

2481 Jones NF et al. Hypoproteinemia in anaphylactoid purpura. *Br Med J*, 2, 1166 (1966)

2482 Jones PAE et al. Ferritinemia in leukemia and Hodgkin's disease. *Br J Cancer*, 27, 212 (1973)

2483 Jones RG, Dyson EH, Fletcher S et al. The use of a two-site immunoradiometric assay to assess bone disease following renal transplantation and parathyroidectomy. *Clin Biochem Rev*, 14, 246 (1993)

2484 Jones RL. Fibrinopeptide A in diabetes mellitus. Relation to levels of glucose, fibrinogen disappearance, and hemodynamic changes. *Diabetes*, 34, 836-843 (1985)

2485 Jones SC, Evans SW, Lobo AJ et al. Serum interleukin-8 in inflammatory bowel disease. *J Gastroenterol Hepatol*, 8, 508-512 (1993)

2486 Jones SE. Autoimmune disorders and malignant lymphoma. *Cancer*, 31, 1092 (1973)

2487 Jones SR. The absolute granulocyte count in ascites fluid. *West J Med*, 126, 344 (1977)

2488 Jordan RM, Kendall JW, Seaich JL et al. Cerebrospinal fluid hormone concentration in the evaluation of pituitary tumors. *Ann Intern Med*, 85, 49-55 (1976)

2489 Jordan TW et al. Enzymic detection of metachromatic leukodystrophy patients and heterozygotes. *NZ Med J*, 85, 369-372 (1977)

2490 Jorge JA, Reimers S, Santolaria F et al. Comportamiento del calcio, fosforo y magnesio en la cirrhosis hepatica alcoholica. *Ann Med Intern (Madrid)*, 4, 275-280

2491 Jorgensen C, Bologna C, Gutierrez M et al. Serum levels of secretory IgA and in vitro production of IgA in rheumatoid arthritis. *Clin Exp Rheumatol*, 11, 541-544 (1993)

2492 Jorgensen FB, Badskjer J, Pedersen BS et al. Creatine kinase isoenzymes in serum from children - especially focusing on CK-BB. *Scand J Clin Lab Invest*, 44, 453-455 (1984)

2493 Jorgensen FS et al. Plasma lipids and lipoproteins in young patients with brain infarction. *Acta Neurol Scand*, 57, 432-437 (1978)

2494 Jorgensen LGM, Osterlind K, Hansen HH et al. Serum neuron-specific enolase (S-NSE) in progressive small-cell lung cancer (SCLC). *Br J Cancer*, 70, 759-761 (1994)

2495 Jorgensen LS, Christiansen P, Raundahl U et al. Autonomic nervous system function in patients with functional abdominal pain. *Scand J Gastroenterol*, 28, 63-68 (1993)

2496 Jorgensen RA, Lindor KD, Sartin JS et al. Serum lipid and fat-soluble vitamin levels in primary sclerosing cholangitis. *J Clin Gastroenterol*, 20, 215-219 (1995)

2497 Jossa F, Trevisan M, Krogh V et al. Correlates of high-density lipoprotein cholesterol in a sample of healthy workers. *Prev Med*, 20, 700-712 (1991)

2498 Joven J, Cliville X, Camps J, et al. Plasma protein abnormalities in nephrotic syndrome: effect on plasma colloid osmotic pressure and viscosity. *Clin Chem*, 43, 1223-1231 (1997)

2499 Joven J, Simo JM, Vilella E et al. Accumulation of atherogenic remnants and lipoprotein(a) in the nephrotic syndrome: relation to remission of proteinuria. *Clin Chem*, 41, 908-913 (1995)

2500 Joyce CD, Fiscus RR, Wang X et al. Calcitonin gene-related peptide levels are elevated in patients with sepsis. *Surgery*, 108, 1097-1101 (1990)

2501 Joypaul B, Browning M, Newman E et al. Comparison of serum CA 72-4 and CA 19-9 levels in gastric cancer patients and correlation with recurrence. *Am J Surg*, 169, 595-599 (1995)

2502 Juby A, Johnston C, Davis P et al. Antinuclear and antineutrophil cytoplasmic antibodies (ANCA) in the sera of patients with Felty's syndrome. *Br J Rheumatol*, 31, 185-188 (1992)

2503 Juengst D et al. Urinary cholesterol excretion in men with benign prostatic hyperplasia and carcinoma of the prostate. *Cancer*, 43, 353-359 (1979)

2504 Julander I, Jarstrand C. Serum triglyceride elevations in patients with septicemia. *Scand J Infect Dis*, 17, 129-130 (1985)

2505 Julian BA, Cannon VR, Waldo FB et al. Macroscopic hematuria and proteinuria preceding renal IgA deposition in patients with IgA nephropathy. *Am J Kid Dis*, 17, 472-479 (1991)

2506 Juma FD, Gitau W, Bwibo NO, Gachoka C. Haemoglobin A_{1C} in children with sickle cell disease. *East Afr Med J*, 61, 32-34 (1984)

2507 Jung K, Lein M, Weiss S, et al. Soluble CD44 molecules in serum of patients with prostate cancer and benign prostatic hyperplasia. *Eur J Cancer*, 32A, 627-630 (1996)

2508 Jung K, Scholz D. An optimized assay of alanine aminopeptidase activity in urine. *Clin Chem*, 26, 1251-1254 (1980)

2509 Jung K, Scholz D. Increased serum γ-glutamyltransferase activity in renal transplant recipients: liver damage or microsomal enzyme induction. *Clin Chim Acta*, 141, 1-5 (1984)

2510 Jung K, von Linggrff P, Brux B, et al. Preanalytical determinants of total and free prostate-specific antigen and their ratio: blood collection and storage conditions. *Clin Chem*, 44, 685-688 (1998)

2511 Jung LC, Cavalieri RP. T3 thyrotoxicosis due to metastatic thyroid carcinoma. *J Clin Endocrinol Metab*, 36, 215 (1973)

2512 Jungmann E, Felber A, Graeber S et al. Human atrial natriuretic peptide in patients with type 1 diabetes mellitus: is it related to the development of diabetic neuropathy? *Clin Investig*, 71, 604-609 (1993)

2513 Jurga L et al. Importance of determinations of serum hexokinase, aldolase, and lactate dehydrogenase activities, and of the lactate/pyruvate quotient in the diagnosis of malignant tumors. *Neoplasma*, 25, 95-106 (1978)

2514 Juul A, Pedersen SA, Sorensen S et al. Growth hormone (GH) treatment increases serum insulin-like growth factor binding protein-3, bone isoenzyme alkaline phosphatase and forearm bone mineral content in young adults with GH deficiency of childhood onset. *Eur J Endocrinol*, 131, 41-49 (1994)

2515 Kabadi UM. Serum T3 and reverse T3 concentrations: indices of metabolic control in diabetes mellitus. *Diabetes Res*, 3, 417-421 (1986)

2516 Kabakow B et al. Hypercalcemia in Hodgkin's disease. *N Engl J Med*, 256, 59 (1967)

2517 Kabat GC, Chang CJ, Sparano JA, et al. Urinary estrogen metabolites and breast cancer: a case-control study. *Cancer Epidemiol Biomark Prevent*, 6, 505-509 (1997)

2518 Kaddam IMS, Iqbal SJ, Holland S et al. Comparison of serum osteocalcin with total and bone specific alkaline phosphatase and urinary hydroxyproline:creatinine ratio in patients with Paget's disease of bone. *Ann Clin Biochem*, 31, 327-330 (1994)

2519 Kadmon D, Thompson TC, Lynch GR et al. Elevated plasma chromogranin-A concentrations in prostatic carcinoma. *J Urol*, 146, 358-361 (1991)

2520 Kadrabova J, Madaric A, Sustrova M, Ginter E. Changed serum trace element profile in Down's syndrome. *Biol Trace Elem Res*, 54, 201-206 (1996)

2521 Kafer ER. Idiopathic scoliosis. *J Clin Invest*, 58, 825-833 (1976)

2522 Kagan BL, Leskin G, Haas B, Wilkins J. Elevated lipid levels in Vietnam veterans with chronic posttraumatic stress disorder. *Biol Psychiat*, 45, 374-377 (1999)

2523 Kagan IG. Trichinosis: a review of biologic, serologic and immunologic aspects. *J Infect Dis*, 107, 65 (1960)

2524 Kagaya A, Uchitomi Y, Takezaki E, et al. Plasma levels of cyclic GMP, immune parameters and depressive status during interferon therapy. *Neuropsychobiology*, 35, 128-131 (1997)

2525 Kager L et al. Serum myoglobin in myocardial infarction: the staccato phenomenon. *Am J Med*, 62, 86-91 (1977)

2526 Kahaleh MB. Endothelin, an endothelial-dependent vasoconstrictor in scleroderma. Enhanced production and profibrotic action. *Arth Rheum*, 34, 978-983 (1991)

2527 Kahn RS, Davidson M, Hirschowitz J et al. Nocturnal growth hormone secretion in schizophrenic patients and healthy subjects. *Psychiat Res*, 41, 155-161 (1992)

2528 Kahri J, Groop P-H, Viberti G et al. Regulation of apolipoprotein A-I-containing lipoproteins in IDDM. *Diabetes*, 42, 1281-1288 (1993)

2529 Kairisto V, Koskinen P, Mattila K et al. Reference intervals for 24-h urinary normetanephrine, metanephrine, and 3-methoxy-4-hydroxymandelic acid in hypertensive patients. *Clin Chem*, 38, 416-420 (1992)

2530 Kakari S, Stringou E, Toumbis M et al. Five tumor markers in lung cancer: significance of total and lipid-bound sialic acid. *Anticancer Res*, 11, 2107-2110 (1991)

2531 Kakizaki G et al. A new diagnostic test for pancreatic disorders by examination of parotid saliva. *Am J Gastroenterol*, 65, 437-446 (1976)

2532 Kakumu S, Shinagawa T, Ishikawa T et al. Serum interleukin 6 levels in patients with chronic hepatitis B. *Am J Gastroenterol*, 86, 1804-1808 (1991)

2533 Kalabay L, Cseh K, Benedek S et al. Serum α_2-HS glycoprotein concentrations in patients with hematological malignancies. *Ann Hematol*, 63, 264-269 (1991)

2534 Kalberg BE et al. Age, blood pressure, renin and urinary electrolytes in primary hypertension and in the normotensive state. *Scand J Clin Lab Invest*, 38, 319-327 (1978)

2535 Kalbfleisch JM, Lindemann RD, Ginn HE et al. Effects of ethanol administration on urinary excretion of magnesium and other electrolytes in alcoholic and normal subjects. *J Clin Invest*, 42, 1471-1475 (1963)

2536 Kalin EM. Cerebrospinal fluid acid base and electrolyte changes resulting from cerebral anoxia in man. *N Engl J Med*, 293, 1013-1016 (1975)

2537 Kallistratos G, Evangelou A, Seferiadis K et al. Selenium and hemodialysis: serum selenium levels in healthy persons, non-cancer and cancer patients with chronic renal failure. *Nephron*, 41, 217-222 (1985)

2538 Kalofoutis A, Papapanagiotou A, Tzivras M. Clinical significance of plasma HDL subfractions (HDL_2, HDL_3) in patients with peripheral arterial disease (PAD) in the Greek population. *Clin Biochem*, 32, 149-152 (1999)

2539 Kalra J, Prasad M, Mantha SV et al. Status of various lipoproteins in ischemic stroke. *Clin Chem*, 39, 1149 (1993)

2540 Kalra J, Rajput AH, Mantha SV, Prasad K. Serum antioxidant enzyme activity in Parkinson's disease. *Mol Cell Biochem*, 110, 165-168 (1992)

2541 Kamel S, Brazier M, Picard C et al. Urinary excretion of pyridinolines crosslinks measured by immunoassay and HPLC techniques in normal subjects and in elderly patients with vitamin D deficiency. *Bone Miner*, 26, 197-208 (1994)

2542 Kamemoto H. Significance of plasma interleukin-6 in the diagnosis of renal cell carcinoma. *Hinyokika Kiyo*, 39, 301-316 (1993)

2543 Kamfar HZ, Koshak EE, Milaat WA. Is there a role for automated eosinophil count in asthma severity assessment? *J Asthma*, 36, 153-158 (1999)

2544 Kam-Hansen S et al. B and T lymphocytes in cerebrospinal fluid and blood in multiple sclerosis, optic neuritis and mumps meningitis. *Acta Neurol Scand*, 58, 95-103 (1978)

2545 Kamoi K, Tamura T, Tanaka K, et al. Hyponatremia and osmoregulation of thirst and vasopressin secretion in patients with adrenal insufficiency. *J Clin Endocrinol Metab*, 77, 1584-1588 (1993)

2546 Kamper EF, Kopeikina L, Mantas A, et al. Tetranectin levels in patients with acute myocardial infarction and their alterations during thrombolytic treatment. *Ann Clin Biochem*, 35, 400-407 (1998)

2547 Kanai M, Ray A, Goodman DS. Radioimmunoassay of human plasma retinol-binding protein. *J Clin Invest*, 47, 2025 (1968)

2548 Kanazawa H, Kurihara N, Otsuka T, et al. Clinical significance of serum concentration of interleukin-8 in patients with bronchial asthma or chronic pulmonary emphysema. *Respiration*, 63, 236-240 (1996)

2549 Kandoussi A, Cachera C, Pagniez D et al. Plasma level of lipoprotein Lp(a) is high in predialysis or hemodialysis, but not in CAPD. *Kidney Int*, 42, 424-425 (1992)

2550 Kane S et al. Indices of granulocyte activity in inflammatory bowel disease. *Gut*, 15, 953-959 (1974)

2551 Kaneko FT, Arroliga AC, Dweik RA, et al. Biochemical reaction products of nitric oxide as quantitative markers of primary pulmonary hypertension. *Am J Respir Crit Care Med*, 158, 917-923 (1998)

2552 Kankaanrinta T. On the pregnanediol excretion in the urine during the last trimester of normal and toxemic pregnancy. *Scand J Clin Lab Invest*, 15, Suppl, 74 (1963)

2553 Kanno K, Hirata Y, Shichiri M et al. Plasma endothelin-1in patients with diabetes mellitus with or without vascular complications. *J Cardiovasc Pharmacol*, 17, S475-S476 (1991)

2554 Kanno K, Sasaki S, Hirata Y et al. Urinary excretion of aquaporin-2 in patients with diabetes insipidus. *N Engl J Med*, 332, 1540-1545 (1995)

2555 Kano K, Ichimura T. Increased α-hydroxybutyrate dehydrogenase in serum from children with measles. *Clin Chem*, 38, 624-627 (1992)

2556 Kao PC, Riggs BL, Schryver PG. Development and evaluation of an osteocalcin chemiluminoimmunoassay. *Clin Chem*, 39, 1369-1374 (1993)

2557 Kaplan A et al. Separation of human serum-alkaline-phosphatase isoenzymes by polyacrylamide gel electrophoresis. *J Clin Endocrinol*, 2, 1029-1031 (1969)

2558 Kaplan F, Sawyer J, Connors S, et al. Urinary basic fibroblast growth factor. *Clin Orthop Related Res*, 346, 59-65 (1998)

2559 Kaplan NM et al. Single-voided urine metanephrine assays in screening for pheochromocytoma. *Arch Intern Med*, 137, 190 (1977)

2560 Kaplanski G, Farnarier C, Payan M-J, et al. Increased levels of soluble adhesion molecules in the serum of patients with hepatitis C: correlation with cytokine concentrations and liver inflammation and fibrosis. *Dig Dis Sci*, 42, 2277-2284 (1997)

2561 Kaplowitz N et al. Isolation of erythrocytes with normal protoporphyrin levels in erythropoietic porphyria. *N Engl J Med*, 278, 1077 (1968)

2562 Kappeler R et al. Klinik der makroglobulinamie waldenström: beschreibung van 21 fallen-ubersicht der literatur. *Clinics In Gastroenterology.* W Sircus (ed), Philadelphia PA, WB Saunders, 25, 54 (1958)

2563 Kaptein et al. Thyroid hormone indexes. *Arch Intern Med*, 144, 314 (1984)

2564 Kapur A, Wild G, Milford-Ward A et al. Carbohydrate deficient transferrin: a marker for alcohol abuse. *Br Med J*, 299, 427-431 (1989)

2565 Karasik A, Menczer J, Pariente C et al. Insulin-like growth factor-I (IGF-I) and IGF-binding protein-2 are increased in cyst fluids of epithelial ovarian cancer. *J Clin Endocrinol Metab*, 78, 271-276 (1994)

2566 Karawya EM, Al-Wabel A-HA. Elevated levels of ribonucleases in serum of patients with liver disease. *Saudi Med J*, 17, 42-46 (1996)

2567 Karege F, Bovier P, Hilleret H et al. Lack of effect of anxiety on total plasma MHPG in depressed patients. *J Affect Disord*, 28, 211-217 (1993)

2568 Karege F, Widmer J, Bovier P et al. Platelet serotonin and plasma tryptophan in depressed patients: effect of drug treatment and clinical outcome. *Neuropsychopharmacology*, 10, 207-214 (1994)

2569 Karetzky MS. Blood studies in untreated patients with acute asthma. *Am Rev Resp Dis*, 112, 607 (1975)

2570 Karkkainen P. Serum and urinary β-hexosaminidase as markers of heavy drinking. *Alcohol Alcoholism*, 25, 365-369 (1990)

2571 Karkkainen P, Poikolainen K, Salaspuro M. Serum β-hexosaminidase as a marker of heavy drinking. *Alcohol Clin Exp Res*, 14, 187-190 (1990)

2572 Karmatschek M, Maier I, Seibel MJ, et al. Improved purification of human bone sialoprotein and development of a homologous radioimmunoassay. *Clin Chem*, 43, 2076-2082 (1997)

2573 Karpatkin S et al. Autoimmune thrombocytopenic purpura and the compensated thrombocytolytic state. *Am J Med*, 51, 1 (1971)

2574 Karvountzis GG et al. Relation of α-fetoprotein in acute hepatitis to severity and prognosis. *Ann Intern Med*, 80, 156-160 (1974)

2575 Kasiske BL. Hyperlipidemia in patients with chronic renal damage. *Am J Kid Dis*, 5 Suppl 3, S142-S156 (1998)

2576 Kasper CK et al. Clinical aspects of iron deficiency. *J Am Med Ass*, 191, 359 (1965)

2577 Kasperska-Czyzyk T, Heding LG, Tronier B. The serum concentrations of insulin, C-peptide, and proinsulin in patients with acute pancreatitis. *Int J Pancreatol*, 19, 167-171 (1995)

2578 Katila H, Appelberg B, Hurme M et al. Plasma levels of interleukin-1β and interleukin-6 in schizophrenia, other psychoses, and affective disorders. *Schiz Res*, 12, 29-34 (1994)

2579 Kato H, Kinoshita T, Suzuki S, et al. Production and effects of interleukin-6 and other cytokines in patients with non-Hodgkin's lymphoma. *Leukemia Lymphoma*, 29, 71-79 (1998)

2580 Kato H, Morioka H, Aramaki S et al. Radioimmunoassay for tumor antigen of human cervical squamous cell carcinoma. *Cell Mol Biol*, 25, 51-56 (1979)

2581 Katsuki A, Sumida Y, Murashima S, et al. Acute and chronic regulation of serum sex hormone-binding globulin levels by plasma insulin concentrations in male noninsulin-dependent diabetes mellitus patients. *J Clin Endocrinol Metab*, 81, 2515-2519 (1996)

2582 Katsuki A, Sumida Y, Murashima S, et al. Serum levels of tumor necrosis factor-α are increased in obese patients with noninsulin-dependen diabetes mellitus. *J Clin Endocrinol Metab*, 83, 859-862 (1998)

2583 Katsura Y, Nishigori H, Okano T, et al. Hepatocyte growth factor in vitreous fluid of patients with proliferative diabetic retinopathy and other retinal disorders. *Diabetes Care*, 21, 1759-1763 (1998)

2584 Kattwinkel J et al. The effects of age on alkaline phosphatase and other serologic liver function tests in normal subjects and patients with cystic fibrosis. *J Pediatr*, 82, 234 (1973)

2585 Katus HA, Haller C, Muller-Bardorff M et al. Cardiac troponin T in end-stage renal disease patients undergoing chronic maintenance hemodialysis. *Clin Chem*, 41, 1201-1202 (1995)

2586 Katzmann JA, Greipp PR, O'Fallon WM et al. Serum β_2-microglobulin. *Mayo Clin Proc*, 61, 752-753 (1986)

2587 Kaufman DB et al. Secretory IgA in urinary tract infections. *Br Med J*, 4, 463-465 (1970)

2588 Kaufman DM et al. Subdural empyema: analysis of 17 recent cases and review of the literature. *Medicine*, 54, 485-498 (1975)

2589 Kaufman LD, Varga J, Gomez-Reino JJ et al. Autoantibodies in sera from patients with L-tryptophan-associated eosinophilia-myalgia syndrome. *Clin Immunol Immunopathol*, 76, 115-119 (1995)

2590 Kaulsay KK, Ng EH, Ji CY, et all. Serum IGF-binding protein-6 and prostate specific antigen in breast cancer. *Eur J Endocrinol*, 140, 164-168 (1999)

2591 Kaupke CJ, Vaziri ND, Powers DR et al. Erythropoietin in preeclampsia. *Obstet Gynecol*, 78, 795-799 (1991)

2592 Kauppinen R, Timonen K, Mustajoki P. Treatment of the porphyrias. *Ann Med*, 26, 31-38 (1994)

2593 Kawa S, Oguchi H, Kobayashi T et al. Elevated serum levels of Dupan-2 in pancreatic cancer patients negative for Lewis blood group phenotype. *Br J Cancer*, 64, 899-902 (1991)

2594 Kawa S, Tokoo M, Hasebe O et al. Comparative study of CA242 and CA 19-9 for the diagnosis of pancreatic cancer. *Br J Cancer*, 70, 481-486 (1994)

2595 Kawaguchi Y, Harigai M, Fukasawa C, Hara M. Increased levels of hepatocyte growth factor in sera of patients with systemic scerosis. *J Rheumatol*, 26, 1012-1013 (1999)

2596 Kawai N, Kanzaki S, Takano-Watou S, et al. Serum free insulin-like growth factor I (IGF-I), total IGF-I, and IGF-binding protein-3 concentrations in normal children and children with growth hormone deficiency. *J Clin Endocrinol Metam*, 84, 82-89 (1999)

2597 Kawai T. *Clinical Aspects of the Plasma Proteins*, Philadelphia PA, JB Lippincott (1973)

2598 Kawakita M, Yonemura Y, Miyake H, et al. Soluble c-kit molecule in serum from healthy individuals and patients with haemopoietic disorders. *Br J Haematol*, 91, 23-29 (1995)

2599 Kawamoto A, Kawata H, Akai Y, et al. Serum levels of VEGF and basic FGF in the subacute phase of myocardial infarction. *Int J Cardiol*, 67, 47-54 (1998)

2600 Kawamura M, Sueshige N, Imayoshi K, et al. Enzyme immunoassay to detect antituberculous glycolipid antigen (Anti-TBGL antigen) antibodies in serum for diagnosis of tuberculosis. *J Clin Lab Analysis*, 11, 140-145 (1997)

2601 Kawamura M, Yamassawa F, Ishizaka A et al. Serum concentration of 7S collagen and prognosis in patients with the adult respiratory distress syndrome. *Thorax*, 49, 144-146 (1994)

2602 Kawamura N, Ookawara T, Suzuki K et al. Increased glycated Cu, Zn-superoxide dismutase levels in erythrocytes of patients with insulin-dependent diabetes mellitus. *J Clin Endocrinol Metab*, 74, 1352-1354 (1992)

2603 Kawano Y, Kawasaki T, Kawazoe N et al. Circadian variations of urinary dopamine, norepinephrine, epinephrine and sodium in normotensive and hypertensive subjects. *Nephron*, 55, 277-282 (1990)

2604 Kawasaki T, Takeshita A, Souda K, et al. Serum thrombopoietin levels in patients with chronic hepatitis and liver cirrhosis. *Am J Gastroenterol*, 94, 1918-1922 (1999)

2605 Kay NH et al. Hypouricemia in Hodgkin's disease. *Cancer*, 32, 1508 (1973)

2606 Kayal S, Jais J-P, Aguini N, et al. Elevated circulating E-selctin, intercellular adhesion molecule-1, and von Willebrand factor in patients with severe infection. *Am J Respir Crit Care Med*, 157, 776-784 (1998)

2607 Kaye JP et al. Plasma lipids in patients with chronic renal failure. *Clin Chim Acta*, 44, 301-305 (1973)

2608 Kaye WH, Ballenger JC, Lydiard RB et al. CSF monoamine levels in normal-weight bulimia: evidence for abnormal noradrenergic activity. *Am J Psychiat*, 147, 225-229 (1990)

2609 Kaye WH, Berrettini W, Gwirtsman H et al. Altered cerebrospinal fluid neuropeptide Y and peptide YY immunoreactivity in anorexia and bulimia nervosa. *Arch Gen Psychiat*, 47, 548-556 (1990)

2610 Kaye WH, Gwirrtsman HE, George DT. The effect of bingeing and vomiting on hormonal secretion. *Biol Psychiat*, 25, 768-780 (1989)

2611 Kaye WH, Gwirtsman HE, George DT et al. Elevated cerebrospinal fluid levels of immunoreactive corticotropin-releasing hormone in anorexia nervosa: relation to state of nutrition, adrenal function, and intensity of depression. *J Clin Endocrinol Metab*, 64, 203-208 (1987)

2612 Kaysar N, Kronenberg J, Polliack M et al. Severe hypophosphataemia during binge eating in anorexia nervosa. *Arch Dis Child*, 66, 138-139 (1991)

2613 Kaysen GA. Plasma composition in the nephrotic syndrome. *Am J Nephrol*, 13, 347-359 (1993)

2614 Kazi S, Ali SS, Furrukh F, et al. Comparison of metal ions in biological samples of schizophrenic patients and control subjects. *Am Clin Lab*, 19, 8 (2000)

2615 Kazmierczak SC, Van Lente F, Hodges ED. Diagnostic and prognostic utility of phospholipase A activity in patients with acute pancreatitis: comparison with amylase and lipase. *Clin Chem*, 37, 356-360 (1991)

2616 Kazumi T, vaAbo K, Yoshido R, et al. Prevalence of high serum lipoprotein (a) levels in Japanese patients with NIDDM. *Horm Metab Res*, 28, 607-609 (1996)

2617 Kean BH et al. The complement-fixation test in the diagnosis of congenital toxoplasmosis. *Am J Dis Child*, 131, 21-28 (1977)

2618 Kehely A, Moss DW. Circulating levels of tartrate-resistant acid phosphatase in macrophage-activated lung disease. *Ann Clin Biochem*, 29, 172-175 (1992)

2619 Keinanen-Kiukaanniemi S, Kaapa P et al. Decreased thromboxane production in migraine patients during headache-free period. *Headache*, 24, 339-341 (1984)

2620 Kelder W, McArthur JC, Nance-Sproson T, et al. β-chemokines MCP-1 and RANTES are selectively increased in cerebrospinal fluid of patients with human immunodeficiency virus-associated dementia. *Ann Neurol*, 44, 831-835 (1998)

2621 Kelestimur F, Utas C, Ozbakir O, et al. The effects of octreotide in a patient with Nelson's syndrome. *Postgrad Med J*, 72, 53-54 (1996)

2622 Kelleher PC. Urinary excretion of hydroxyproline, hydroxylysine and hydroxylysine glycosides by patients with Paget's disease of bone and carcinoma with metastases in bone. *Clin Chim Acta*, 92, 373-379 (1979)

2623 Keller F, Lyteal Ser Y, Schuppan D. Raised concentrations of the carboxy terminal propeptide of type IV (basement membrane) procollagen (NCI) in serum and urine of patients with glomerulonephritis. *Eur J Clin Invest*, 22, 175-181 (1992)

2624 Keller RT et al. Hypercalcemia secondary to a primary hepatoma. *J Am Med Ass*, 193, 782 (1965)

2625 Kellermann W, Frentzel-Beyme R, Welte M et al. Phospholipase A in acute lung injury after trauma and sepsis: Its relation to the inflammatory mediators PMN-Elastase, C_3a, and neopterin. *Klin Wschr*, 67, 190-195 (1989)

2626 Kelley ML. Elevated serum amylase associated with ruptured ectopic pregnancy. *J Am Med Ass*, 164, 406-407 (1957)

2627 Kelly CB, Cooper SJ. Differences and variability in plasma noradrenaline between depressive and anxiety disorders. *J Psychopharmacol*, 12, 161-167 (1998)

2628 Kelly UL, Cooper EH, Alexander C, Stone J. The assessment of antichymotrypsin in cancer monitoring. *Biomed Pharmacother*, 28, 209-215 (1978)

2629 Kelton KG, Hunter DJS, Neame PB. A platelet function defect in preeclampsia. *Obstet Gynecol*, 65, 107-109 (1985)

2630 Kema IP, de Vries EGE, Schellings AMJ et al. Improved diagnosis of carcinoid tumors by measurement of platelet serotonin. *Clin Chem*, 38, 534-540 (1992)

2631 Kemali D, Maj M, Iorio G et al. Relationship between CSF noradrenaline levels, C-EEG indicators of activation and psychosis ratings in drug-free schizophrenic patients. *Acta Psychiat Scand*, 71, 19-24 (1985)

2632 Kemkes-Matthes B, Matthes KJ. Protein Z, a new haemostatic factor, in liver diseases. *Haemostasis*, 25, 312-316 (1995)

2633 Kemppainen EA, Hedstrom JI, Puolakkainen PA, et al. Rapid measurement of urinary trypsinogen-2 as a screening test. *N Engl J Med*, 336, 1788-1793 (1997)

2634 Kendall AG et al. Nephrotic syndrome: a hypercoagulable state. *Arch Intern Med*, 127, 1021 (1971)

2635 Kendall et al. Haematology and biochemistry of ankylosing spondylitis. *Br Med J*, 2, 235-237 (1973)

2636 Kenemans P, Bon GG, Kessler AC et al. Multicenter technical and clinical evaluation of a fully automated enyme immunoassay for CA 125. *Clin Chem*, 38, 1466-1471 (1992)

2637 Kenemans P, van Kamp GJ, Oehr P et al. Heterologous double-determinant immunoradiometric assay CA 125 II: reliable second-generation immunoassay for determining CA 125 in serum. *Clin Chem*, 39, 2509-2513 (1993)

2638 Kennedy AC et al. Abnormalities of mineral metabolism suggestive of parathyroid overactivity in rheumatoid arthritis. *Curr Med Res Opin*, 3, 345-58 (1975)

2639 Kennedy SH, Brown GM, McVey G et al. Pineal and adrenal function before and after refeeding in anorexia nervosa. *Biol Psychiat*, 30, 216-224 (1991)

2640 Kennedy SH, Kutcher SP, Ralevski E, Brown GM. Nocturnal melatonin and 24-hour 6-sulphatoxymelatonin levels in various phases of bipolar affective disorder. *Psychiat Res*, 63, 219-222 (1996)

2641 Kenyon FE, Hardy SM. A biochemical study of Huntington's chorea. *J Neurol Neurosurg Psychiat*, 26, 123 (1963)

2642 Kergoat M-J, Leclerc BS, PetitClerc C et al. Discriminant biochemical markers for evaluating the nutritional status of elderly patients in long-term care. *Am J Clin Nutr*, 46, 849-861 (1987)

2643 Kern P, Hemmer CJ, van Damme J et al. Elevated tumor necrosis factor alpha and interleukin-6 serum levels as markers for complicated Plasmodium falciparum malaria. *Am J Med*, 87, 139-143 (1989)

2644 Kern WV, Engel A, Schieffer S et al. Circulating tumor necrosis factor alpha (TNF), soluble TNF receptors, and interleukin-6 in human subacute bacterial endocarditis. *Infect Immunol*, 61, 5413-5416 (1993)

2645 Kernkes-Matthes B, Matthes KJ. Protein Z. *Biomed Prog*, 13, 51-54 (2000)

2646 Kernoff PA et al. Normal and abnormal fibrinolysis. *Br Med Bull*, 33, 239-244 (1977)

2647 Kerr MH, Paton JY. Surfactant protein levels in severe respiratory syncytial virus infection. *Am J Respir Crit Care Med*, 159, 1115-1118 (1999)

2648 Kerstens PJSM, Stolk JN, Boerbooms AMT et al. Purine enzymes in rheumatoid arthritis: possible association with response to azathioprine. A pilot study. *Ann Rheum Dis*, 53, 608-611 (1994)

2649 Kerth P. Troponin I: biochemical background and clinical utility. *Acta Anaes Scand*, 41 Suppl, 295-296 (1997)

2650 Kervinen K, Savolainen MJ, Kesaniemi YA. Multiple changes in apoprotein B containing lipoproteins after ethanol withdrawal in alcoholic men. *Ann Med*, 23, 407-413 (1991)

2651 Kery V, Orlovska M, Stancikova M et al. Urinary glycosaminoglycan excretion in rheumatic diseases. *Clin Chem*, 38, 841-846 (1992)

2652 Kes P, Reiner Z. Symptomatic hypomagnesemia associated with gentamicin therapy. *Magnesium Trace Elem*, 9, 54-60 (1990)

2653 Keshgegian AA (ed). Serum creatine kinase MB isoenzyme in chronic muscle disease (Lankenau Hospital Case Conference). *Clin Chem*, 30, 575-578 (1984)

2654 Kettelhack C, Schoter D, Matthias D et al. Serum erythropoietin levels in patients with solid tumours. *Eur J Cancer*, 30A, 1289-1291 (1994)

2655 Kew MC et al. Serum α-fetoprotein levels in acute viral hepatitis. *Gut*, 14, 939 (1973)

2656 Key Pharmaceuticals, Inc. Manufacturer's literature on Theo-dur® . Kenilworth, NJ 07033 (1995)

2657 Keye WR et al. Amenorrhea, hyperprolactinemia and pituitary enlargement secondary to primary hypothyroidism. successful treatment with thyroid replacement. *Obstet Gynecol*, 48, 697-702 (1976)

2658 Khafagy EZ et al. Significance of abnormalities in urinary neutral mucopolysaccharides in bilharziasis. *Egypt J Bilharz*, 2, 111-116 (1975)

2659 Khalifa AS et al. Immunoglobulins in idiopathic thrombocytopenic purpura in childhood. *Acta Haematol*, 56, 205 (1976)

2660 Khalil M et al. Red cell membrane lipids in thalassemia. *Gaz Egypt Paediatr Ass*, 23, 273-280 (1975)

2661 Khan AA, Qureshi MN, Bauer S. Levels of cholesterol, total protein, and LDH in body fluids as indicators of malignancy. *Am J Clin Pathol*, 100, 332 (1993)

2662 Khan R et al. Bone marrow acid phosphatase: another look. *J Urol*, 117, 79-80 (1977)

2663 Khan SN, Rahman MA, Samad A. Trace elements in serum from Pakistani patients with acute and chronic ischemic heart disease and hypertension. *Clin Chem*, 30/5, 644-648 (1984)

2664 Khanna SK et al. Value of lactic dehydrogenase in cerebrospinal fluid of tuberculous meningitis patients. *J Ind Med Ass*, 68, 4-6 (1977)

2665 Khare V, Baethge B, Lang S et al. Antinuclear antibodies in pleural fluid. *Chest*, 106, 866-871 (1994)

2666 Khatun S, Kanayama N, Hossain B, et al. increased concentrations of plasma epinephrine and norepinephrine in patients with eclampsia. *Eur J Obstet Gynecol*, 69, 61-67 (1996)

2667 Khoruts A, Stahnke L, McClain CJ et al. Circulating tumor necrosis factor, interleukin-1 and interleukin-6 concentrations in chronic alcoholic patients. *Hepatology*, 13, 267-276 (1991)

2668 Khosla S, Peterson JM, Egan K et al. Circulating cytokine levels in osteoporotic and normal women. *J Clin Endocrinol Metab*, 79, 707-711 (1994)

2669 Khoury MY, Vieira JGH, Baracat EC, et al. Serum levels of androstanediol glucuronide, total testosterone, and free testosterone in hirsute women. *Fertil Steril*, 62, 76-80 (1994)

2670 Kibel AS, Krithivas K, Shamel LB, et al. Constitutive expression of high levels of prostate-specific antigen in the absence of prostate carcinoma. *Urology*, 48, 741-746 (1996)

2671 Kiechle FL, Quattrociocchi-Longe TM, Brinton DA. Carbonic anhydrase antibody in sera from patients with endometriosis. *Am J Clin Pathol*, 101, 611-615 (1994)

2672 Kiilholma P, Paul P, Pakarinen P et al. Copper and zinc in pre-eclampsia. *Acta Obstet Gynecol Scand*, 63, 629-631 (1984)

2673 Kikuchi K, Ihn H, Sato S et al. Serum concentration of procollagen type I carboxyterminal propeptide in systemic sclerosis. *Arch Dermatol Res*, 286, 77-80 (1994)

2674 Kikuchi K, Kubo M, Kadono T, et al. Serum concentrations of vascular endothelial growth factor in collagen diseases. *Br J Derm*, 139, 1049-1051 (1998)

2675 Kikuchi K, Sato S, Kadano T et al. Serum concentration of procollagen type I carboxyterminal propeptide in localized scleroderma. *Arch Dermatol*, 130, 1269-1272 (1994)

2676 Kikuchi M, Inagaki T. Atrial natriuretic peptide in aged patients with iron deficiency anemia. *Arch Gerontol Geriat*, 28, 105-115 (1999)

2677 Kikuta H, Matsumoto S, Osato T. Kawasaki disease and Epstein-Barr virus. *Acta Paediat Jpn*, 33, 765-770 (1991)

2678 Kim DS, Paik SH, Lim CM, et al. Value of ICAM-1 expression and soluble ICAM-1 level as a marker of activity in sarcoidosis. *Chest*, 115, 1059-1065 (1999)

2679 Kim H et al. Plasma insulin disturbances in primary hyperparathyroidism. *J Clin Invest*, 50, 2596-2605 (1971)

2680 Kim TJ, Anasti JN, Flack MR, et al. Routine endocrine screening for patients with karyotypically normal spontaneous premature ovarian failure. *Obstet Gynecol*, 89, 777-779 (1997)

2681 Kim YK, Lee MS, Suh KY. Decreased interleukin-2 production in Korean schizophrenic patients. *Biol Psychiat*, 43, 701-704 (1998)

2682 Kim YS, Plaut A. β-Glucuronidase studies in gastric secretions from patients with gastric cancer. *Gastroenterology*, 49, 50 (1965)

2683 Kimbal HR et al. Marrow granulocyte reserves in rheumatic diseases. *Arth Rheum*, 16, 345-352 (1973)

2684 Kimber C et al. The mechanism of anemia in chronic liver disease. *Q J Med*, 34, 33 (1965)

2685 Kimberly RP et al. Elevated urinary prostaglandins and the effects of aspirin on renal function in lupus erythematosus. *Ann Intern Med*, 89, 336-41 (1978)

2686 Kimbrough TD, Shernan S, Ziegler TR et al. Insulin-like growth factor-I response is comparable following intravenous and subcutaneous administration of growth hormone. *J Surg Res*, 51, 472-476 (1991)

2687 Kimmel PL, Tenner S, Habwe VQ et al. Trypsinogen and other pancreatic enzymes in patients with renal disease: a comparison of high-efficiency hemodialysis and continuous ambulatory peritoneal dialysis. *Pancreas*, 10, 325-330 (1995)

2688 King JS, Warner A. Cystinuria with hyperuricemia and methioninuria: biochemical study of a case. *Am J Med*, 43, 125 (1967)

2689 King LG, Seelig CB, Ramney JE. The lipase to amylase ratio in acute pancreatitis. *Am J Gastroenterol*, 90, 67-69 (1995)

2690 Kinghorn GR. Value of erythrocyte sedimentation rate in primary genital herpes. *Br J Clin Pract*, 32, 49-51 (1978)

2691 Kinsella TD et al. Serum complement and immunoglobulin levels in sporadic and familial ankylosing spondylitis. *J Rheumatol*, 2, 308-313 (1975)

2692 Kirilov G, Dakovska L, Borisova SM et al. Increased plasma endothelin levels in patients with insulin-dependent diabetes mellitus and end-stage vascular complications. *Horm Metab Res*, 26, 119-120 (1994)

2693 Kirkali Z, Esen AA, Kirkali G et al. Ferritin: a tumor marker expressed by renal cell carcinoma. *Eur Urol*, 28, 131-134 (1995)

2694 Kirkpatrick A. Complement. Immunochemistry System (ICS-9). Beckman Instruments, Fullerton CA

2695 Kishida T, Sato J, Fujimori S, et al. Clinical significance of serum iron and ferritin in patients with colorectal cancer. *J Gastroenterol*, 29, 19-23 (1994)

2696 Kishida T, Shinozawa I, Tanaka S, et al. Significance of serum iron and ferritin in patients with colorectal adenomas. *Scand J Gastroenterol*, 32, 233-237 (1997)

2697 Kisters K, Korner J, Louwen F, et al. Plasma and membrane Mg^{++} concentrations in normal pregnancy and in preeclampsia as compared to healthy female subjects - a plasmalemmal membrane model. *Trace Elem Elect*, 14, 109-112 (1997)

2698 Kisters K, Korner J, Louwen F, et al. Plasma, intracellular, and membrane Mg^{2+} concentrations in normal pregnancy and in preeclampsia. *Hypertens Preg*, 17, 169-178 (1998)

2699 Kisters K, Korner J, Louwen R, et al. Plasma and membrane Ca^{++} concentrations in normal pregnancy and in preeclampsia. *Trace Elem Elect*, 15, 1-4 (1998)

2700 Kivitie-Kallio S, Rajantie J, Juvonen E, Norio R. Granulocytopenia in Cohen syndrome. *Br J Haematol*, 98, 308-311 (1997)

2701 Klatka J. Concentration of total and protein-bound hydroxyproline in serum and urine in patients with laryngeal neoplasms. *Otolaryngol Pol*, 45, 195-200 (1991)

2702 Klein B, Klein T, Figer A et al. Soluble HLA class I in colon cancer. *Cancer*, 4, 322-325 (1991)

2703 Kleinman JE, Weinberger DR, Rogol AD et al. Plasma prolactin concentrations and psychopathology in chronic schizophrenia. *Arch Gen Psychiat*, 39, 655-657 (1982)

2704 Klemow D, Einsphar D, Brown TA et al. Serum transferrin receptor measurements in hematologic malignancies. *Am J Hematol*, 34, 193-198 (1990)

2705 Klevay LM. Coronary heart disease: the zinc/copper hypothesis. *Am J Clin Nutr*, 28, 764-774 (1975)

2706 Klimik JJ et al. Mycoplasma pneumoniae meningoencephalitis and transverse myelitis in pediatrics. *Pediatrics*, 58, 133-135 (1976)

2707 Klinenberg JR. Hyperuricemia and gout. *Med Clin North Am*, 61, 299-312 (1977)

2708 Kloczko J, Wojtukiewicz MZ, Bielawiec M et al. Von Willebrand factor antigen and fibronectin in essential hypertension. *Thromb Res*, 79, 331-336 (1995)

2709 Klopper A. Specific pregnancy proteins. *Curr Topics Exp Endocrinol*, 4, 128-165 (1983)

2710 Kluthe R, Hagemann U. The turnover of α-$_2$ macroglobulin in nephrotic syndrome. *Vox Sang*, 12, 308-311 (1967)

2711 Knapen MECM, van Altena A, Peters WHM, et al. Liver function following pregnancy complicated by naecolthe HELLP syndrome. *Br J Obstet Gynaecol*, 105, 1208-1210 (1998)

2712 Knapen MFCM, Mulder TPJ, Bisseling JGA, et al. Plasma glutathione S-transferase alpha 1-1: a more sensitive marker for hepatocellular damage than serum alanine aminotransferase in hypertensive disorders of pregnancy. *Am J Obstet Gynecol*, 178, 161-165 (1998)

2713 Knapen MFCM, Mulder TPJ, van Rooij IALM, et al. Low whole blood glutathione levels in pregnancies complicated by preelampsia or the hemolysis, elevated liver enzymes, low platelets syndrome. *Obstet Gynecol*, 92, 1012-1015 (1998)

2714 Knapen MFCM, Peters WHM, Mulder TPJ, et al. Plasma glutathione S-transferase Pi 1-1 measurements in the study of hemolysis in hypertensive disorders of pregnancy. *Hypertens Pregnancy*, 18, 147-156 (1999)

2715 Knapp S, Irwin M. Plasma levels of tetrahydrobiopterin and folate in major depression. *Biol Psychiat*, 26, 156-162 (1989)

2716 Knebl J, DeFazio P, Clearfield MB et al. Plasma lipids and cholesterol esterification in Alzheimer's disease. *Mech Age Dev*, 73, 69-77 (1994)

2717 Knekt P, Aromaa A, Maatela J et al. Serum selenium and subsequent risk of cancer among Finnish men and women. *J Natl Cancer Inst*, 82, 864-868 (1990)

2718 Knight AH et al. Significance of hyperamylasemia and abdominal pain in diabetic ketoacidosis. *Br Med J*, 3, 128-131 (1973)

2719 Knochel JP. The pathophysiology and clinical characteristics of severe hypophosphatemia. *Arch Intern Med*, 137, 203-220 (1977)

2720 Knochel JP, Moore GE. Rhabdomyolysis in malaria. *N Engl J Med*, 329, 1206-1207 (1993)

2721 Knopfle G et al. Serum α_1-fetoprotein in cystic fibrosis. *Eur J Pediatr*, 122, 241-248 (1976)

2722 Knudsen F, Dyerberg J. Platelets and antithrombin III in uremia: the acute effect of hemodialysis. *Scand J Clin Lab Invest*, 45, 341-347 (1985)

2723 Knudsen JB, Gormsen J, Skagen K, Amtorp O. Changes in platelet functions, coagulation and fibrinolysis in uncomplicated cases of acute myocardial infarction. *Thromb Haemostas*, 42, 1513-1522 (1980)

2724 Ko CW, Koo JH. Recombinant human growth hormone in Gitelman's syndrome. *Am J Kid Dis*, 33, 778-781 (1999)

2725 Ko GTC, Chan JCN, Yeung VTF, et al. Antibodies to glutamic acid decarboxylase in young Chinese diabetic patients. *Ann Clin Biochem*, 35, 761-767 (1998)

2726 Ko GTC, Yeung YTF, Chow C-C, et al. Pseudohyponatremia secondary to hypercholesterolaemia. *Ann Clin Biochem*, 34, 324-325 (1997)

2727 Ko YC, Mukaida N, Ishiyama S et al. Elevated interleukin-8 levels in the urine of patients with urinary tract infections. *Infect Immunol*, 61, 1307-1314 (1993)

2728 Kobayashi K et al. Clinical and experimental studies of acid phosphatase in renal failure. *Clin Chim Acta*, 1971, 173-182

2729 Kobayashi K et al. Rapid turnover of serum proteins in fulminant hepatitis. *Gastroenterology*, 12, 455 (1977)

2730 Kobayashi K, Kitamura K, Hirayama N, et al. Increased plasma adrenomedullin in acute myocardial infarction. *Am Heart J*, 131, 676-680 (1996)

2731 Kobayashi T, Gabazza EC, Taguchi O, et al. Type I collagen metabolites as tumor markers in patients with lung carcinoma. *Cancer*, 85, 1951-1957 (1999)

2732 Kobayashi T, Hashimoto S, Imai K et al. Elevation of serum soluble intercellular adhesion molecule-1 (sICAM-1) and sE-selectin levels in bronchial asthma. *Clin Exp Immunol*, 96, 110-115 (1994)

2733 Kocen RS et al. Familial alpha lipoprotein deficiency with neurologic abnormalities. *Lancet*, 1, 1341 (1967)

2734 Kochanska-Dziurowicz A, Starzewski JJ, Dunal W. Estimation of the value of serum β_2-microglobulin concentration in the diagnosis of Hashimoto's disease. *Clin Chim Acta*, 233, 101-104 (1995)

2735 Kodera Y, Yamamura Y, Torii A, et al. The prognostic value of preoperative serum levels of CEA and CA 19-9 in patients with gastric cancer. *Am J Gastroenterol*, 91, 49-53 (1996)

2736 Koduri PR, Carandang G, DeMarais P et al. Hyperferritinemia in reactive hemopagocytic syndrome: Report of four adult cases. *Am J Hematol*, 49, 247-249 (1995)

2737 Koehler LH, Benz EJ. Serum adenosine deaminase: methodology and clinical applications. *Clin Chem*, 8, 133-140 (1962)

2738 Koenig KG, Linberg JS, Zerwekh JE et al. Free and total 1,25-dihydroxyvitamin D levels in subjects with renal disease. *Kidney Int*, 41, 161-165 (1992)

2739 Koh YY, Kim YW, Park JD, Oh JW. A comparison of serum haptoglobin levels between acute exacerbation and clinical remission in asthma. *Clin Exp Allergy*, 26, 1202-1209 (1996)

2740 Kohan J, Raghaven D. Tumor markers in malignant germ cell tumors. In:. *The Management of Testicular Tumors.* MJ Peckham (ed), New York NY, Arnold, 50-69 (1981)

2741 Kohni M, Yasunari K, Matsuura T et al. Circulating atrial natriuretic polypeptide in essential hypertension. *Am Heart J*, 113, 1160-1163 (1987)

2742 Kohno H, Honda S. Low urinary growth hormone values in patients with Turner's syndrome. *J Clin Endocrinol Metab*, 74, 619-622 (1992)

2743 Kohno M, Hanehira T, Hirata K, et al. An accelerated increase of plasma adrenomedullin in acute asthma. *Metabolism*, 45, 1323-1325 (1996)

2744 Koike T, Enokihara H, Arimura H, et al. Serum concentrations of IL-5, GM-CSF, and IL-3 and the production by lymphocytes in various eosinophilia. *Am J Haematol*, 50, 98-102 (1995)

2745 Kojima H, Tsujimoto T, Uemura M, et al. Significance of increased plasma adrenomedullin concentration in patients with cirrhosis. *J Hepatol*, 28, 840-846 (1998)

2746 Kokoglu E, Karaarslan I, Mehmet H et al. Elevated serum Lp(a) levels in the early and advanced stages of breast cancer. *Cancer Biochem Biophys*, 14, 133-136 (1994)

2747 Kolar OJ et al. Serum and cerebrospinal fluid immunoglobulins in multiple sclerosis. *Neurology*, 20, 1058-1061 (1970)

2748 Kolaric K et al. Serum copper levels in patients with solid tumors. *Tumori*, 61, 173-177 (1975)

2749 Kolben M, Lopens A, Blaser J, et al. Proteases and their inhibitors are indicative in gestational disease. *Eur J Obstet Gynecol*, 68, 59-65 (1996)

2750 Koldjaer O et al. Indices of granulocyte activity in ulcerative colitis and Crohn's disease. *Dan Med Bull*, 24, 72-76 (1977)

2751 Kolendorf K et al. The influence of chronic renal failure on serum and urinary thyroid hormone levels. *Acta Endocrinol*, 89, 80-88 (1978)

2752 Kolevska T, Jagic V, Cvoriscec B et al. Procollagen type 1 peptide levels in patients with bronchial asthma and COPD. *Plucne Bolesti*, 43, 59-61 (1991)

2753 Koller J, Mair P, Wieser C et al. Endothelin and big endothelin concentrations in injured patients. *N Engl J Med*, 325, 1518 (1991)

2754 Komaki G, Tamai H, Mukuta T et al. Alterations in endothelium-associated proteins and serum thyroid hormone concentrations in anorexia nervosa. *Br J Nutr*, 68, 67-75 (1992)

2755 Komorowski J. Increased interleukin-2 level in patients with primary hypothyroidism. *Clin Immunol Immunopathol*, 63, 200-202 (1992)

2756 Konig P, Margreiter R, Huber CH et al. Neopterin levels in long-term renal allograft recipients. *Immunobiology*, 169, 208-212 (1985)

2757 Koninckx PR, Riittinen L, Seppala M et al. CA-125 and placental protein 14 concentrations in plasma and peritoneal fluid of women with deeply infiltrating pelvic endometriosis. *Fertil Steril*, 57, 523-530 (1992)

2758 Konings CH, Kuiper MA, Bergmans PLM et al. Increased angiotensin-converting enzyme activity in cerebrospinal fluid of treated patients with Parkinson's disease. *Clin Chim Acta*, 231, 101-106 (1994)

2759 Konings CH, Kuiper MA, Mulder C, et al. CSF acetylcholinesterase in Parkinson disease: decreased enzyme activity and immunoreactivity in demented patients. *Clin Chim Acta*, 235, 101-105 (1995)

2760 Konings CH, Kuiper MA, Scheltens Ph et al. Re-evaluation of cerebrospinal fluid angiotensin-converting enzyme activity in patients with "probable" Alzheimer's disease. *Eur J Clin Chem Clin Biochem*, 31, 495-497 (1993)

2761 Konishi N, Matsumoto K, Hiasa Y et al. Tissue and serum pepsinogen I and II in gastric cancer identified using immunochemistry and rapid ELISA. *J Clin Pathol*, 48, 364-367 (1995)

2762 Kooh S-W, Binet A. Hypercalcemia in infants presenting with apnea. *Can Med Ass J*, 143, 509-512 (1990)

2763 Koolen MI, Daha MR, Frolich M et al. Direct and indirect measurement of urinary kallikrein excretion in patients with essential hypertension and normotensives: relation to age and plasma renin and aldosterone levels. *Eur J Clin Invest*, 14, 171-174 (1984)

2764 Koper NP, Massuger LFAG, Thomas CMG, et al. Serum CA 125 measurements to identify patients with endometrial cancer who require lymphadenectomy. *Anticancer Res*, 18, 1897-1902 (1998)

2765 Kopin IJ et al. Plasma levels of norepinephrine. *Ann Intern Med*, 88, 671-680 (1978)

2766 Koponen H, Riekknien PJ. Cerebrospinal fluid acetylcholinesterase in patients with dementia associated with schizophrenia or chronic alcoholism. *Acta Psychiat Scand*, 83, 441-443 (1991)

2767 Kopp A, Jonat W, Schmahl M, Knabbe C. Transforming growth factor β2 (TGF-β2) levels in plasma of patients with metastatic breast cancer treated with tamoxifen. *Cancer Res*, 55, 4512-4515 (1995)

2768 Kopp H-P, Hopmeier P, Schernthaner G. Concentrations of circulating P-selectin are increased in patients with newly diagnosed insulin-dependent diabetes mellitus. *Exp Clin Endocrinol Diabetes*, 106, 41-44 (1998)

2769 Kopp WL et al. Blood volume and hematocrit value in macroglobulinemia and myeloma. *Arch Intern Med*, 123, 394 (1969)

2770 Koprowski HZ et al. Colorectal carcinoma antigens detected by hybridoma antibodies. *Somatic Cell Genet*, 5, 957 (1979)

2771 Korman MG et al. Hypergastrinemia in chronic renal failure. *Br Med J*, I, 209 (1972)

2772 Korpela M, Mustonen J, Heikkinen A et al. Isolated microscopic hematuria in patients with rheumatoid arthritis compared with age and sex matched controls. A population based study. *J Rheumatol*, 22, 427-431 (1995)

2773 Korppi M, Kroger L. C-reactive protein in viral and bacterial respiratory infection in children. *Scand J Infect Dis*, 25, 207-213 (1992)

2774 Korrapati MR, Vestal RE, Loi C-M. Theophylline metabolism in healthy nonsmokers and in patients with insulin-dependent diabetes mellitus. *Clin Pharmacol Ther*, 57, 413-418 (1995)

2775 Korri U-M, Nuutinen H, Salaspuro M. Increased blood acetate: a new laboratory marker of alcoholism and heavy drinking. *Alcohol Clin Exp Res*, 9, 468-471 (1985)

2776 Korst LM, et al. Nucleated red blood cells: an update on the marker for fetal asphyxia. *Obstet Gynecol*, 175, 843-846 (1996)

2777 Korsten CB, et al. Carcinoembryonic antigen activity in urine of patients with bladder carcinoma. *J Clin Chem Clin Biochem*, 14, 389-393 (1976)

2778 Kortekangas P, Peltola O, Toivanen A, Aro HT. Synovial fluid L-lactic acid in acute arthritis of the adult knee joint. *Scand J Rheumatol*, 24, 98-101 (1995)

2779 Kosaka S. β-2 Glycoprotein I in rheumatoid arthritis. *Tohoku J Exp Med*, 122, 223 (1977)

2780 Kosaka S, Tazawa M. α_1- Antichymotrypsin in rheumatoid arthritis. *Tohoku J Exp Med*, 119, 369-375 (1976)

2781 Kose K, Dogan P, Kardas Y, Saraymen R. Plasma selenium levels in rheumatoid arthritis. *Biol Trace Elem Res*, 53, 51-56 (1996)

2782 Koshida H, Miyamori I, Miyazaki R et al. Falsely elevated plasma aldosterone concentrations by direct radioimmunoassay in chronic renal failure. *J Lab Clin Med*, 114, 294-300 (1989)

2783 Koshida K, Nishino A, Yamamoto H et al. The role of alkaline phosphatase isoenzymes as tumor markers for testicular germ cell tumors. *J Urol*, 146, 57-60 (1991)

2784 Koski CL, Khurana R, Mayer RF. Guillain-Barre syndrome. *Am Fam Physician*, 34, 202 (1986)

2785 Koskinen P, Irjala K, Viikari J et al. Serum fructosamine in the assessment of glycaemic control in diabetes mellitus. *Scand J Clin Lab Invest*, 47, 285-292 (1987)

2786 Kostina S I. Some particularities in diagnostic, clinical picture, and therapy of pulmonary sarcoidosis. *Z Erkrank Atm-Org*, 149, 280-282 (1977)

2787 Kostner KM, Clodi M, Bodlaj G, et al. Decreased urinary apolipoprotein (a) excretion in patients with impaired renal function. *Eur J Clin Invest*, 28, 447-452 (1998)

2788 Kostner KM, Huber K, Stefenelli T, Rinner H. Urinary apo(a) discriminates coronary artery disease patients from controls. *Atherosclerosis*, 129, 103-110 (1997)

2789 Kostoglou-Athanassiou I, Ntalles K, Gogas J, et al. Sex hormones in postmenopausal women with breast cancer on tamoxifen. *Horm Res*, 47, 116-120 (1997)

2790 Kotaniemi A, Isomaki H, Hakala M et al. Increased type I collagen degradation in early rheumatoid arthritis. *J Rheumatol*, 21, 1593-1596 (1994)

2791 Kotchen TA et al. Modification of renin reactivity by lipids extracted from normal, hypertensive, and uremic plasma. *J Clin Endocrinol Metab*, 43, 971-981 (1976)

2792 Kotchen TA, Guyenne TT, Corvol P et al. Enzymatic activity of renin in plasma of normal and uraemic subjects. *Clin Sci*, 67, 365-368 (1984)

2793 Kottel RH, Hoch SO, Parsons RG et al. Serum ribonuclease activity in cancer patients. *Br J Cancer*, 38, 280-286 (1978)

2794 Koukkou E, Panayiotidis P, Alevizou-Terzaki V et al. High levels of serum soluble interleukin-2 receptors in hyperthyroid patients: correlation with serum thyroid hormones and independence from the etiology of the hyperthyroidism. *J Clin Endocrinol Metab*, 73, 771-776 (1991)

2795 Kovace GL, Bezzegh A, Nyuli N. Stress hormone secretion during ethanol withdrawal. *Diag Lab*, 27, 91 (1991)

2796 Kovacs GL, Marko E, Toldy E et al. Regulatory hormones of fluid and electrolyte homeostasis in alcohol withdrawal. *Clin Biochem Rev*, 14, 199 (1993)

2797 Kovanen PT, Manttari M, Palosuo T, et al. Prediction of myocardial infarction in dyslipidemic men by elevated levels of immunoglobulin A, E and G, but not M. *Arch Intern Med*, 158, 1434-1439 (1998)

2798 Kovatz S, Arber I, Korzets Z et al. Urinary kallikrein in normal pregnancy, pregnancy with hypertension, and toxemia. *Nephron*, 40, 48-51 (1985)

2799 Kowalski HJ, Abelmann WH. The cardiac output at rest in Laennec's cirrhosis. *J Clin Invest*, 32, 1025 (1953)

2800 Kowal-Vern A, Walenga JM, Hoppensteadt D et al. Interleukin-2 and interleukin-6 in relation to burn size in the acute phase of thermal injury. *J Am Coll Surg*, 178, 357-362 (1994)

2801 Kowalzick L, Kleinheinz A, Neuber K et al. Elevated serum levels of soluble adhesion molecules ICAM-1 and ELAM-1 in patients with severe atopic eczema and influence of UVA1 treatment. *Dermatology*, 190, 14-18 (1995)

2802 Kowdley KV, Emond MJ, Sadowski JA, Kaplan MM. Plasma vitamin K_1 level is decreased in primary biliary cirrhosis. *Am J Gadtroenterol*, 92, 2059-2061 (1997)

2803 Kowlessar OD et al. Comparative study of serum leucine aminopeptidase, 5-nucleotidase and nonspecific alkaline phosphatase in diseases affecting the pancreas, hepatobiliary tree and bone. *Am J Med*, 31, 231-237 (1961)

2804 Kozakowska E, Korta T, Jablonska-Skwiecinska E. Observations on the red cell ATP of surgical patients during the premortal period. *Biomed Biochim Acta*, 43, S103-S104 (1984)

2805 Kozman H, Flemmer MC, Rahnama M. Deep venous thrombosis: prediction by D-dimer? *South Med J*, 90, 907-910 (1997)

2806 Krachler M, Scharfetter H, Wirnsberger GH. Evaluation of concentrations of cesium and rubidium in whole blood, plasma and serum in different diseases. *Trace Elem Elect*, 15, 22-27 (1998)

2807 Kraft SC, Kirsner JB. The immunology of ulcerative colitis and Crohn's disease: clinical and humoral aspects. In:. *Inflammatory Bowel Disease*, Philadelphia PA, Lea and Febiger, 60 (1975)

2808 Krafte-Jacobs B, Bock GH. Circulating erythropoietin and interleukin-6 concentrations increase in critically ill children with sepsis and septic shock. *Crit Care Med*, 24, 1455-1459 (1996)

2809 Krahenbuhl S. Carnitine metabolism in chronic liver disease. *Life Sci*, 59, 1579-1599 (1996)

2810 Krahenbuhl S, Reichen J. Carnitine metabolism in patients with chronic liver disease. *Hepatology*, 25, 148-153 (1996)

2811 Krantz SB. Erythropoietin. *Blood*, 77, 419 (1991)

2812 Kratzsch J, Blum WF, Schenker E, Keller E. Regulation of growth hormone (GH), insulin-like growth factor (IGF) I, IGF binding proteins -1, -2, -3 and GH binding protein during progression of liver cirrhosis. *Exp Clin Endocrinol*, 103, 285-291 (1995)

2813 Kratzsch J, Blum WF, Schenker E et al. Measurement of insulin-like growth factor I (IGF-I) in normal adults, patients with liver cirrhosis and acromegaly: experience with a new competitive enzyme immunoassay. *Exp Clin Endocrinol*, 101, 144-149 (1993)

2814 Kratzsch J, Blum WF, Ventz M et al. Growth hormone-binding protein-related immunoreactivity in the serum of patients with acromegaly is regulated inversely by growth hormone concentration. *Eur J Endocrinol*, 132, 306-312 (1995)

2815 Kraus T, Noronha IL, Manner M. Clinical value for cytokine determination for screening, differetiation and therapy monitoring of infections and noninfectious complications after orthoptic liver transplantation. *Transplant Proc*, 23, 1509-1512 (1991)

2816 Kravitz SC et al. Uremia complicating leukemia chemotherapy. *J Am Med Ass*, 146, 1595 (1951)

2817 Krawitt EL. Autoimmune hepatitis. *N Engl J Med*, 334, 897-903 (1996)

2818 Krediet RT, Asghar SS, Koomen GCM et al. Effects of renal failure on complement C_3d levels. *Nephron*, 59, 41-45 (1991)

2819 Kreisberg R A. Diabetic ketoacidosis: new concepts and trends in pathogenesis and treatment. *Ann Intern Med*, 88, 681-695 (1978)

2820 Kreisman SH, Hennessey JV. Consistent reversible elevations of serum creatinine levels in severe hypothyroidism. *Arch Intern Med*, 159, 79-82 (1999)

2821 Kreiss JK, Lawrence DN, Kasper CK et al. Antibody to human T-cell leukemia virus membrane antigens, β_2-microglobulin levels, and thymosin-α_1 levels in hemophiliacs and their spouses. *Ann Intern Med*, 100, 178-182 (1984)

2822 Krentz AJ, Clark PMS, Cox L et al. Insulin and proinsulin-like molecules in motor neurone disease. *Ann Clin Biochem*, 30, 195-197 (1993)

2823 Krieger C, Perry TL, Ziltener HJ. Amyotrophic lateral sclerosis: interleukin-6 levels in cerebrospinal fluid. *Can J Neurol Sci*, 19, 357-359 (1992)

2824 Kristensson-Aas A, Wallerstedt S, Alling C et al. Haematological findings in chronic alcoholics after heavy drinking with special reference to haemolysis. *Eur J Clin Invest*, 16, 178-183 (1986)

2825 Kristjansson S, Strannegard I-L, Strannegard O, et al. Urinary eosinophil protein X in children with atopic asthma: a useful marker of antiinflammatory treatment. *J Allerg Clin Immunol*, 97, 1179-1187 (1996)

2826 Kroger H, Risteli J, Risteli L et al. Serum osteocalcin and carboxyterminal propeptide of type I procollagen in rheumatoid arthritis. *Ann Rheum Dis*, 52, 338-342 (1993)

2827 Kronenberg F, Utermann G, Dieplinger H. Lipoprotein(a) in renal disease. *Am J Kid Dis*, 27, 1-25 (1996)

2828 Kroning H, Tager M, Thiel U, et al. Overproduction of IL-7, IL-10 and TGF-β1 in multiple myeloma. *Acta Haematol*, 98, 116-118 (1997)

2829 Kronvall P, Fahy TA, Isaksson A et al. The clinical relevance of salivary amylase monitoring in bulimia nervosa. *Biol Psychiat*, 32, 156-163 (1992)

2830 Kropf J, Grobe E, Knoch M et al. The prognostic value of extracellular matrix component concentrations in extracorporeal CO_2 removal. *Eur J Clin Chem Clin Biochem*, 29, 805-812 (1991)

2831 Kruger B, Emmrich J, Tessenow W et al. Anionic and cationic trypsin(ogen)-like immunoreactivity in the diagnosis of acute pancreatitis. *Clin Biochem Rev*, 14, 207 (1993)

2832 Krugman, Ward (eds). *Infectious Diseases*, 5th edition, St Louis MO, CV Mosby (1973)

2833 Kruskemper HL et al. Serum enzyme activities in disorders of thyroid function. *Germ Med*, 14, 55-58 (1969)

2834 Krzewicki J. Clinical study on magnesium and calcium level in the blood during acute pancreatitis. *Mag Res*, 11, 19-23 (1998)

2835 Ktiouet J, Susini de Luca H, Zouaghi H et al. Decrease of binding activity of transcortin (CBG) in major depression: a preliminary study. *Encephale*, 10, 215-216 (1984)

2836 Kubonishi I, Bandobashi K, Murata N, et al. High serum levels of CA125 and interleukin-6 in a patient with Ki-1 lymphoma. *Br J Haematol*, 98, 450-452 (1997)

2837 Kubota K, Tamura J, Kurabayashi H, et al. Evaluation of increased serum ferritin levels in patients with hyperthyroidism. *Clin Investig*, 72, 26-29 (1993)

2838 Kubota M, Teukamoto R, Krokawa K, et al. Elevated serum γ-interferon and interleukin-6 in patients with necrotizing lymphadeitis (Kikuvhi's disease). *Br J Haematol*, 95, 613-615 (1996)

2839 Kucharewicz B, Kilpatrick WS, Kilpatrick ES et al. Serum concentration of collagen fragments in patients with diabetes and renal failure. *Proc ACB Natl Meet*, 157 (1995)

2840 Kucharzik T, Stoll R, Lugering N et al. Circulating antiinflammatory cytokine IL-10 in patients with inflammatory bowel disease (IBD). *Clin Exp Immunol*, 100, 452-456 (1995)

2841 Kudo T, Iqbal K, Ravid R et al. Alzheimer's disease: correlation of cerebro-spinal fluid and brain ubiquitin levels. *Brain Res*, 639, 1-7 (1994)

2842 Kudolo GB, DeFronzo RA. Urinary platelet-activating factor excretion is elevated in non-insulin dependent diabetes mellitus. *Prostagland Lipid Mediators*, 57, 87-98 (1999)

2843 Kuehr J, Frischer T, Barth R et al. Eosinophils and eosinophilic cationic protein in children with and without sensitization to inhalant allergens. *Eur J Pediatr*, 153, 739-744 (1994)

2844 Kuhnel A, Gross U, Jacob K, Doss MO. Studies on coproporhyrin isomers in urine and feces. *Clin Chim Acta*, 282, 45-58 (1999)

2845 Kuiper MA, van Kamp GJ, Bergmans PL et al. Serum α_1-antichymotrypsin is not a useful marker for Alzheimer's disease or dementia in Parkinson's disease. *J Neur Transmiss*, 6, 145-149 (1993)

2846 Kuku SF et al. Heterogeneity of plasma glucagon. *J Clin Invest*, 58, 742-750 (1976)

2847 Kumano H, Kuboki T, Tawara R et al. Interrelationship between serum muscle enzymes and a low T3 in anorexia nervosa. *Endocrinol Jpn*, 37, 583-589 (1990)

2848 Kumar A et al. Hypercalcemia in leukemia. *Ind J Cancer*, 13, 277-79 (1976)

2849 Kumar BJ, Khurana ML, Ammini AC et al. Reproductive endocrine functions in men with primary hypothyroidism: effect of thyroxine replacement. *Horm Res*, 34, 215-218 (1990)

2850 Kumar MS et al. The relationship of thyroid-stimulating hormone (TSH), thyroxine (T4), and triiodothyronine (T3) in primary thyroid failure. *Am J Clin Pathol*, 68, 747-751 (1977)

2851 Kumon Y, Suehiro T, Ikeda Y et al. Influence of serum amyloid A protein on high-density lipoprotein in chronic inflammatory disease. *Clin Biochem*, 26, 505-511 (1993)

2852 Kung AWC, Pang RWC, Lauder I et al. Changes in serum lipoprotein(a) and lipids during treatment of hyperthyroidism. *Clin Chem*, 41, 226-231 (1995)

2853 Kunishima S, Tahara T, Kato T, et al. Serum thrombopoietin and plasma glycocalcin concentrations as useful diagnostic markers in thrombocytopenic disorders. *Eur J Haematol*, 57, 68-71 (1996)

2854 Kuno N, Kurimoto K, Fukushima M et al. Effectiveness of multivariate analysis of tumor markers in diagnosis of pancreatic carcinoma: a prospective study in multiinstitutions. *Pancreas*, 9, 725-730 (1994)

2855 Kunz F et al. Plasma lipids, coagulation factors, and fibrin formation after severe multiple trauma, and in adult respiratory distress syndrome. *J Trauma*, 18, 115-120 (1978)

2856 Kuraner T, Beksac MS, Kayakirilmaz K et al. Serum and parotid saliva testosterone, calcium, magnesium, and zinc levels in males, with and without periodontitis. *Biol Trace Elem Res*, 31, 43-49 (1991)

2857 Kurantsin-Mills J, Ibe BO, Natta CL et al. Elevated urinary levels of thromboxane and prostacyclin metabolites in sickle cell disease reflects activated platelets in the circulation. *Br J Haematol*, 87, 580-585 (1994)

2858 Kurashima K, Mukaida N, Fujimura M, et al. A specific elevation of RANTES in bronchoalveolar lavage fluids of patients with chronic eosinophilic pneumonia. *Lab Invest*, 76, 67-75 (1997)

2859 Kuratsune H, Yamaguti K, Takahashi M et al. Acylcarnitine deficiency in chronic fatigue syndrome. *Clin Infect Dis*, 18, S62-S67 (1994)

2860 Kurobe M, Kato A, Takei Y et al. Fluorometric enzyme immunoassay of basic fibroblast growth factor with monoclonal antibodies. *Clin Chem*, 38, 2121-2123 (1992)

2861 Kuroda M, Asaka S, Tofuku Y et al. Serum antioxidant activity in uremic patients. *Nephron*, 41, 293-298 (1985)

2862 Kurosawa S, Stearns-Kurosawa DJ, Carson CW, et al. Plasma levels of endothelial cell protein C receptor are elevated in patients with sepsis and systemic lupus erythematosus: lack of correlation with thrombomodulin suggests involvement of different pathological processes, 725 - 727 (1997)

2863 Kuroyanagi T et al. Fibrin degradation products in renal diseases. *Tohoku J Exp Med*, 119, 237-244 (1976)

2864 Kurtoglu S, Uzum K, Hallac JK, Coskun A. 5-Hydroxy-3-indole acetic levels in infantile colic: is serotoninergic tonus responsible for this problem? *Acta Paediatr*, 86, 764-765 (1997)

2865 Kuruvilla A, Peedicayil J, Srikrishna G et al. A study of serum prolactin levels in schizophrenia: a comparison of males and females. *Clin Exp Pharmacol Physiol*, 19, 603-606 (1992)

2866 Kuruvilla A, Srikrishna G, Peedicayil J et al. A study on serum prolactin levels in schizophrenia: correlation with positive and negative symptoms. *Int Clin Pychopharmacol*, 8, 177-179 (1993)

2867 Kurzrock R, Redman J, Cabanillas F et al. Serum interleukin 6 levels are elevated in lymphoma patients and correlate with survival in advanced Hodgkin's disease. *Cancer Res*, 53, 2118-2122 (1993)

2868 Kuschner JP et al. Idiopathic refractory sideroblastic anemia: clinical and laboratory investigation of 17 patients and review of the literature. *Medicine*, 50, 139 (1971)

2869 Kutinsky I, Blakley S, Roche V. Normal D-dimer levels in patients with pulmonary embolism. *Arch Intern Med*, 159, 1569-1572 (1999)

2870 Kuusela P, Haglund C, Roberts PJ. Comparison of a new tumor marker CA 242 with CA 19-9, CA 50 and carcinoembryonic antigen (CEA) in digestive tract diseases. *Br J Cancer*, 63, 636-640 (1991)

2871 Kuwana M, Kaburaki J, Okano Y, et al. Clinical and prognostic associations based on serum antinuclear antibodies in Japanese patients with systemic sclerosis. *Arth Rheum*, 37, 75-83 (1994)

2872 Kuwert E et al. Demonstration of complement in spinal fluid in multiple sclerosis. *Ann NY Acad Sci*, 122, 429 (1965)

2873 Kuylenstierna J, Karlberg B. Prostaglandin E_2 and the renin-angiotensin system in primary aldosteronism and Cushing's syndrome. *ProstaglandIns Leukot Med*, 17, 387-395 (1985)

2874 Kwa HG, de Jong-Bakker M, Engelman E et al. Plasma prolactin in human breast cancer. *Lancet*, 1, 433-434 (1974)

2875 Kwan JTC, Carr EC, Bending MR et al. Determination of carbamylated hemoglobin by high-performance liquid chromatography. *Clin Chem*, 36, 606-610 (1993)

2876 Kyd PA, De Vooght K, Kerkhoff F, et al. Clinical usefulness of bone alkaline phosphatase in osteoporosis. *Ann Clin Biochem*, 35, 717-725 (1998)

2877 Kyle RA. Multiple myeloma: review of 869 cases. *Mayo Clin Proc*, 50, 29 (1975)

2878 Kyle RA, Bayrd EO. Amyloidosis: review of 236 cases. *Medicine*, 54, 271-300 (1975)

2879 Kyndt X, Reumaux D, Bridoux F, et al. Serial measurement of antineutrophil cytoplasmic autoantibodies in patients with systemic vasculitis. *Am J Med*, 106, 527-533 (1999)

2880 La Fargue P et al. Evolution du magnesium serique et erythrocytaire chez les brules. *Clin Chim Acta*, 80, 17-21 (1977)

2881 Laaksonen R, Riihimaki A, Laitila J et al. Serum and muscle tissue ubiquinone levels in healthy subjects. *J Lab Clin Med*, 125, 517-521 (1995)

2882 Labeur C, De Bacquer D, De Backer G et al. Plasma lipoprotein(a) values and severity of coronary artery disease in a large population of patients undergoing coronary angiography. *Clin Chem*, 38, 2261-2266 (1992)

2883 Labib M, Ranganath L, Southgate J et al. Acute effect of ethanol intake on plasma osteocalcin concentration. *Ann Clin Biochem*, 26, 563-564 (1989)

2884 Labrune P, Benattar C, Ammoury N et al. Serum concentrations of albumin, C-reactive protein, α_2-macroglobulin, prealbumin, fibronectin, fibrinogen, transferrin, and retinol binding protein in 55 patients with hepatic glycogen storage diseases. *J Pediatr Gastroenterol Nutr*, 18, 41-44 (1994)

2885 Lacerda MA, Ludwig J, Dickson ER, et al. Antimitochondrial antibody-negative primary biliary cirrhosis. *Am J Gastroenterol*, 90, 247-249 (1995)

2886 Lacko AG et al. Serum cholesterol esterification in hyperthyroidism and hypothyroidism. *Horm Metab Res*, 10, 147-151 (1978)

2887 Lacy F, O'Connor DT, Schmid-Schonbein GW. Plasma hydrogen peroxide production in hypertensives and normotensive subjects at genetic risk of hypertension. *J Hypertens*, 16, 291-303 (1998)

2888 Laessle RG, Fischer M, Fichter MM et al. Cortisol levels and vigilance in eating disorder patients. *Psychoneuroendocrinology*, 17, 475-484 (1992)

2889 Lafferty FW. Primary hyperparathyroidism. *Arch Intern Med*, 141, 1761-1766 (1981)

2890 Lagrost L, Athias A, Lemort N, et al. Plasma lipoprotein distribution and lipid transfer activities in patients with type IIb hyperlipidemia treated with simvastatin. *Atherosclerosis*, 143, 415-425 (1999)

2891 Lahita RG, Rivkin E, Cavanagh I et al. Low levels of total cholesterol, high-density lipoprotein, and apolipoprotein A1 in association with anticardiolipin antibodies in patients with systemic lupus erythematosus. *Arth Rheum*, 36, 1566-1574 (1993)

2892 Lahoda F et al. Typing of uric acid level in CSF in neurological and psychiatric diseases. *Adv Exp Med Biol*, 76, 256-258 (1977)

2893 Lahteenmaki PM, Toppari J, Ruokenen A, et al. Low serum inhibin B concentrations in male survivors of childhood malignancy. *Eur J Cancer*, 35, 612-619 (1999)

2894 Lai KN, Li PKT, Woo KS et al. Vasoactive hormones in uremic patients on continuous ambulatory peritoneal dialysis. *Clin Nephrol*, 35, 218-223 (1991)

2895 Laidler P, Kowalski D, Siberring J. Arylsulfatase A in serum from patients with cancer of various organs. *Clin Chim Acta*, 204, 69-78 (1991)

2896 Laing I, Tames FJ, Owen DC et al. Serum lipid fractions in insulin resistant and non-insulin resistant patients with polycystic ovary syndrome. *Proc ACB Natl Meet*, 40 (1993)

2897 Laitinen K, Karkkainen M, Lalla M et al. Is alcohol an osteoporosis-inducing agent for young and middle-aged women? *Metabolism*, 42, 875-881 (1994)

2898 Lam SK. Hypergastrinemia in cirrhosis of liver. *Gut*, 17, 700-708 (1976)

2899 Lambana S. Clinical value of protein-bound fucose in patients with carcinoma and other diseases. *Gann*, 69, 379-388 (1976)

2900 Lambert JR et al. Serum uric acid levels in psoriatic arthritis. *Ann Rheum Dis*, 36, 264-267 (1977)

2901 Lamberts SWJ, Swanson J, Bruining HA, De Jong FH. Corticosteroid therapy in severe illness. *N Engl J Med*, 337, 1285-1292 (1997)

2902 Lammi L, Ryhanen L, Lakari E, et al. type III and type I procollagen markers in fibrosing alveolitis. *Am J Resir Crit Care Med*, 159, 818-823 (1999)

2903 Lamont NM et al. Porphyria in the African. *Q J Med*, 30, 373 (1961)

2904 Lamrs CBH et al. Serum albumin levels in patients with the Zollinger-Ellison syndrome. *Gastroenterology*, 73, 975-979 (1977)

2905 Landau H et al. Gonadotropin, thyrotropin and prolactin reserve in beta thalassemia. *Clin Endocrinol*, 9, 163-173 (1978)

2906 Landfield PW, Applegate MD, Schmitzer-Osborne SE et al. Phosphate/calcium alterations in the first stages of Alzheimer's disease: implications for etiology and pathogenesis. *J Neurol Sci*, 106, 221-229 (1991)

2907 Landgren F, Israelsson B, Lindgren A et al. Plasma homocysteine in acute myocardial infarction: homocysteine-lowering effect of folic acid. *J Intern Med*, 237, 381-388 (1995)

2908 Landin K, Blennow K, Wallin A et al. Low blood pressure and blood glucose levels in Alzheimer's disease: evidence for a hypometabolic disorder? *J Intern Med*, 233, 357-363 (1993)

2909 Landman D, Sarai A, Sathe SS. Use of pentoxifylline therapy for patients with AIDS-related wasting. *Clin Infect Dis*, 18, 97-99 (1994)

2910 Lane DM, Boatman KK, McConathy WJ. Serum lipids and apolipoproteins in women with breast masses. *Breast Cancer Res Treat*, 34, 161-169 (1995)

2911 Lang CC, Choy AMJ, Coutie WJ et al. Effect of haemodialysis on plasma levels of brain natriuretic peptide in patients with chronic renal failure. *Clin Sci*, 82, 127-131 (1992)

2912 Lang H. *Creatine Kinase Isoenzymes: Pathophysiology and Clinical Application*. Berlin, Springer-Verlag (1981)

2913 Lange PH. Testicular cancer markers. In:. *Cancer Markers*, Clifton NJ, Humana Press, II, 262 (1982)

2914 Langer B, Grima M, Coquard C, et al. Plasma active renin, angiotensin I, and angiotensin II during pregnancy and in preeclampsia. *Obstet Gynecol*, 91, 196-202 (1998)

2915 Langleben D, DeMarchie M, Laporta D et al. Endothelin-1 in acute lung injury and the adult respiratory distress syndrome. *Am Rev Resp Dis*, 148, 1646-1650 (1993)

2916 Langton SR, Jarnicki A. Phospholipase A2 activity elevation and lysophopholipid decreases following myocardil infarction or surgically-induced ischaemia. *Proc ACB Natl Meet*, 34 (1993)

2917 Lantz M, Thysell H, Nilsson E et al. On the binding of tumor necrosis factor (TNF) to heparin and the release in vivo of the TNF-binding protein I by heparin. *J Clin Invest*, 88, 2026-2031 (1991)

2918 Lao TT, Chin RKH, Swaminathan R. Thyroid function in pre-eclampsia. *Br J Obstet Gynaecol*, 95, 880-883 (1988)

2919 Lao TT, Chin RKH, Swaminathan R et al. Maternal thyroid hormones and outcome of pre-eclamptic pregnancies. *Br J Obstet Gynaecol*, 97, 71-74 (1990)

2920 Lapatsanis P et al. Phosphaturia in thalassemia. *Pediatrics*, 58, 885-892 (1976)

2921 Lappalainen R, Lindholm D, Riikonen R. Low levels of nerve growth factor in cerebrospinal fluid of children with Rett syndrome. *J Child Neurol*, 11, 296-300 (1996)

2922 Larochelle P. Effect of quinapril on the albumin excretion rate in patients with mild to moderate hypertension. *Am J Hypertens*, 9, 551-559 (1996)

2923 Larochelle P, Cusson JR, du Souich P et al. Renal effects of a nonhypotensive I.V. dose of felodipine. *J Clin Pharmacol*, 33, 732-737 (1993)

2924 Larochelle P, Cusson JR, Gutkowska J et al. Plasma atrial natriuretic factor concentrations in essential and renovascular hypertension. *Br Med J*, 294, 1249-1252 (1987)

2925 Laron Z, Wang XL, Klinger B, et al. Insulin-like growth factor-I decreases serum lipoprotein (a) during long-term treatment of patients with Laron syndrome. *Am J Hematol*, 53, 165-169 (1996)

2926 Larrain C, Ampeuero R, Pumarino H. Hematological changes in anorexia nervosa. *Rev Med Chile*, 117, 534-543 (1989)

2927 Larsson A, Flodin M, Kolberg H. Increased serum concentrations of carbohydrate-deficient transferrin (CDT) in patients with cystic fibrosis. *Upsala Med J*, 103, 231-236 (1998)

2928 Larsson J, Ekblom A, Henriksson K et al. Concentration of substance P, neurokinin A, calcitonin gene-related peptide, neuropeptide Y and vasoactive intestinal peptide in synovial fluid from knee joints in patients suffering from rheumatoid arthritis. *Scand J Rheumatol*, 20, 326-335 (1991)

2929 Larsson SD. Anemia and iron metabolism in hypothyroidism. *Acta Med Scand*, 157, 349 (1967)

2930 Larussa FM, Larocca LM, Rusciani L et al. OKT4/OKT8 ratio and serum beta 2-microglobulin in mycosis fungoides and chronic benign dermatitis. *Eur J Cancer Clin Oncol*, 22, 663-669 (1986)

2931 Lasala GP, Wright T, Osman K et al. Plasma oxidase assay for screening of myocardial infarction. *Am J Med Sci*, 308, 157-161 (1994)

2932 Laso FJ, Iglesias MC, Lopez A, et al. increased interleukin-12 serum levels in chronic alcoholism. *J Hepatol*, 28, 771-777 (1998)

2933 Latini R, Bianchi M, Correale E et al. Cytokines in acute myocardial infarction: selective increase in circulating tumor necrosis factor, its soluble receptor, and interleukin-1 receptor antagonist. *J Cardiovasc Pharmacol*, 23, 1-6 (1994)

2934 Lau CS, McLaren M, Hanslip J et al. Abnormal fibrinolysis in patients with rheumatoid arthritis and impaired endothelial fibrinolytic response in those complicated by vasculitis. *Ann Rheum Dis*, 52, 643-649 (1993)

2935 Laucella SA, Gaddi E, Balbaryski J, et al. Soluble intercellular adhesion molecule-1 in paediatric connective tissue diseases. *Acta Paediatr*, 88, 399-403 (1999)

2936 Lauer B, Niederau C, Kuhl U, et al. Cardiac troponin T in patients with clinically suspected myocarditis. *J Am Coll Cardiol*, 30, 1354-1359 (1997)

2937 Laurell C-B, Jeppson JO. Protease inhibitors in plasma. In:. *The Plasma Proteins, Structure, Function, and Genetic Control*. FW Putnam (ed), New York NY, Academic Press, 1, 229-264 (1975)

2938 Laurencet FM, Martinez T, Beris P. Spurious extreme reticulocytosis with an automated reticulocyte analyzer. *N Engl J Med*, 337, 1922-1923 (1997)

2939 Laursen EM, Lanng S, Rasmussen MH, et al. Normal spontaneous and stimulated GH levels despite decreased IGF-I concentrations in cystic fibrosis patients. *Eur J Endocrinol*, 140, 315-321 (1999)

2940 Laviades C, Mayor G, Diez J et al. Treatment with lisinopril normalizes serum concentrations of procollagen type III amino-terminal peptide in patients with essential hypertension. *Am J Hypertens*, 7, 52-58 (1994)

2941 Lawrence DM et al. Plasma testosterone and androstenedione levels during monitored induction of ovulation in infertile women with 'simple' amenorrhea and with the polycystic ovary syndrome. *Clin Endocrinol*, 5, 609-18 (1976)

2942 Lawrence JH, Rosenthal RL. Multiple myeloma associated with polycythemia: report of four cases. *Am J Med Sci*, 218, 149 (1949)

2943 Lawrence JR, Campbell GR, Barrington H, et al. Clinical and biochemical determinants of plasma lipid peroxide levels in type 2 diabetes. *Ann Clin Biochem*, 35, 387-392 (1998)

2944 Lawson D, Westcombe P, Saggar B. Pilot trial of an infant screening programme for cystic fibrosis: measurement of parotid salivary sodium at four months. *Arch Dis Child*, 44, 715-718 (1969)

2945 Lawson DH et al. Early mortality in the megaloblastic anemias. *Q J Med*, 41, 1 (1972)

2946 Lawson GR, Nelon R, Lakr MF et al. Gut regulatory peptides and intestinal permeability in acute infantile gastroenteritis. *Arch Dis Child*, 67, 272-276 (1992)

2947 Lawson N, Haidar S, Morris K et al. Plasma α-atrial natriuretic peptide and cellular magnesium concentrations in patients with atrial fibrillation. *Proc ACB Natl Meet*, 37-38 (1994)

2948 Lawson WB, Karson CN, Bigelow LB. Increased urine volume in chronic schizophrenic patients. *Psychiat Res*, 14, 323-331 (1985)

2949 Lazzarino M, Orlandi E, Klersy C, et al. Serum CA 125 is of clinical value in the staging and follow-up of patients with non-Hodgkin's lymphoma: correlation with tumor parameters and disease activity. *Cancer*, 82, 576-582 (1998)

2950 Le Bouil A, Briand P, Allain P et al. Plasma selenium in congestive heart failure. *Clin Chem*, 38, 1192-1193 (1992)

2951 Leauti JB et al. Contribution to the early diagnosis of congenital toxoplasmosis. *Biomed Pharmacother*, 27, 283-284 (1977)

2952 Leavelle DE (ed). *Interpretive Handbook*. Rochester MN, Mayo Medical Laboratories (1994)

2953 Lebl J, Schober E, Frisch H et al. Urinary growth hormone secretion in diabetic children: relation to nocturnal course of blood glucose levels. *Horm Res*, 40, 204-208 (1993)

2954 Leblhuber F, Neubaeur C, Peichli M et al. Age and sex differences of dehydroepiandrosterone sulfate (DHEAS) and cortisol (CRT) plasma levels in normal controls and Alzheimer's disease (AD). *Psychopharmacology*, 111, 23-29 (1993)

2955 Lechin F, van der Dijs B, Lechin ME. Plasma neurotransmitters and functional illness. *Psychothher Psycosom*, 65, 293-318 (1996)

2956 Lechin F, van der Dijs B, Orozoco B, et al. Increased levels of free serotonin in plasma of symptomatic asthmatic patients. *Ann Allergy Asthma Immunol*, 77, 245-253 (1996)

2957 Lechleitner P, Genser N, Mair J et al. Plasma immunoreactive endothelin in the acute and subacute phases of myocardial infarction in patients undergoing fibrinolysis. *Clin Chem*, 39, 955-959 (1993)

2958 Leckman JF, Goodman WK, North WG et al. Elevated cerebrospinal fluid levels of oxytocin in obsessive-compulsive disorder: comparison with Tourette's syndrome and healthy controls. *Arch Gen Psychiat*, 51, 782-792 (1994)

2959 Lecomte E, Herbeth B, Clerc G et al. Cholesterol content of circulating immune complexes in patients with coronary stenosis and subjects without evidence of atherosclerosis. *Clin Chem*, 41, 1526-1531 (1995)

2960 Leda M et al. Ectopic production of a salivary type amylase by adenocarcinoma cells: demonstration by a culture technique. *Clin Chim Acta*, 80, 105-111 (1977)

2961 Ledue TB, Weiner DL, Sipe JD, et al. Analytical evaluation of particle-enhanced immunonephelometric assays for C-reactive protein, serum amyloid A and mannose-binding protein in human serum. *Ann Clin Biochem*, 35, 745-753 (1998)

2962 Ledwich JR. Chest pain in the early recognition of large infarcts. *Can Med Ass J*, 116, 38-43 (1977)

2963 Lee EJ, Kim KR, Lee HC, et al. Acipimox potentiates growth hormone response to growth-hormone-releasing hormone by decreasing serum free fatty acid levels in hyperthyroidism. *Metabolism*, 44, 1509-1512 (1995)

2964 Lee F-Y, Lin H-C, Tsai Y-T, et al. Plasma substance P levels in patients with liver cirrhosis: relationship to systemic and portal hemodynamics. *Am J Gastroenterol*, 92, 2080-2084 (1997)

2965 Lee HB, Yoo OJ, Ham JS et al. Serum α_1-antitrypsin in patients with hepatocellular carcinoma. *Clin Chim Acta*, 206, 225-230 (1992)

2966 Lee JB. Cardiovascular-renal effects of prostaglandins. *Arch Intern Med*, 133, 56 (1974)

2967 Lee JC et al. Calcitonin secretion in renal failure. *Calcif Tissue Int*, 22, Suppl, 154-157 (1977)

2968 Lee JG, Sahagun G, Oehlke MA, et al. Serious gastrointestinal pathology found in patients with serum ferritin < 50 ng/mL. *Am J Gastroenterol*, 93, 772-776 (1998)

2969 Lee MC et al. Cerebrospinal fluid in cerebral hemorrhage and infarction. *Stroke*, 6, 638-641 (1975)

2970 Lee MM, Donohoe PK, Silverman BL, et al. Measurements of serum Mullerian inhibiting substance in the evaluation of children with nonpalpable gonads. *N Engl J Med*, 336, 1480-1486 (1997)

2971 Lee PDK, Mistry J, Hintz RL. Active Insulin-like growth factor-I (IGF-I) assays. Diagnostic Systems Laboratories, Inc., Webster TX (1996)

2972 Lee SH, Nam SY, Chung BC. Altered profile of endogenous steroids in the urine of patients with prolactinoma. *Clin Biochem*, 31, 529-535 (1998)

2973 Lee SH, Suh JW, Chung BC, Kim SO. Polyamine profiles in the urine of patients with leukemia. *Cancer Lett*, 122, 1-8 (1998)

2974 Lee WC, Lin HC, Hou MC, et al. Serum uric acid levels in patients with cirrhosis: a re-evaluation. *J Clin Gastroenterol*, 29, 261-265 (1999)

2975 Lee W-L, Chen J-W, Ting C-T, et al. Changes of the insulin-like growth factor I system during acute myocardial infarction: implications on left ventricular remodeling. *J Clin Endocrinol Metab*, 84, 1575-1581 (1999)

2976 Lee Y-J, Shin S-J, Tsai J-H. Increased urinary endothelin-1-like immunoreactivity excretion in NIDDM patients with albuminuria. *Diabetes Care*, 17, 263-266 (1994)

2977 Lee YN et al. Peripheral B- and T- lymphocyte counts in patients with sarcoma and breast carcinoma. *Cancer*, 40, 667-672 (1977)

2978 Legakis I, Saramantis A, Voros D, et al. Dissociation of ACTH, β-endorphin and cortisol in graded sepsis. *Horm Metab Res*, 30, 570-574 (1998)

2979 Legido A, Lago P, Chung HJ et al. Serum prolactin in neonates with seizures. *Epilepsia*, 36, 682-686 (1995)

2980 Legovini P, De Menis E, Doroldi C et al. Parathormone levels during treatment of acromegaly with octreotide: one-year follow-up. *Clin Ther Res*, 53, 360-366 (1993)

2981 Legro RS, Gentzschein E, Carmina E et al. Alterations in androgen conjugate levels in women and men with alopecia. *Fertil Steril*, 62, 744-750 (1994)

2982 Lehmann M, Spori U, Keul J. The excretion of free catecholamines in relation to age, sex and blood pressure. *Z Kardiol*, 74, 294-297 (1985)

2983 Lehrner LM et al. An evaluation of the usefulness of amylase isoenzyme differentiation in patients with hyperamylasemia. *Am J Clin Pathol*, 66, 576-87 (1976)

2984 Lehtinen T, Lumio J, Dillner J et al. Increased risk of malignant lymphoma indicated by elevated Epstein-Barr virus antibodies, a prospective study. *Cancer Causes Control*, 4, 187-193 (1993)

2985 Lehto T, Honkanen E, Teppo A-M et al. Urinary excretion of protectin (CD59) complement SC_5b-9 and cytokines in membranous glomerulonephritis. *Kidney Int*, 47, 1403-1411 (1995)

2986 Leibovici L, Sharir T, Kalter-Leibovici O et al. An outbreak of measles amoung young adults. *J Adolesc Health*, 9, 203-207 (1988)

2987 Leighton B, Cooper GKS. The role of amylin in the insulin resistance of non-insulin dependent diabetes mellitus. *Trends Biochem Sci*, 15, 295-299 (1990)

2988 Lein M, Weiss S, Jung K, et al. Soluble CD44 variants in serum of patients with prostate cancer and other urological malignancies. *Prostate*, 29, 334-335 (1996)

2989 Lejeune P-J, Mallet B, Farnarier C et al. Changes in serum level and affinity for concanavalin A of human α_1-proteinase inhibitor in severe burn patients. Relationship to natural killer cell activity. *Biochim Biophys Acta*, 990, 122-127 (1989)

2990 Lejoyeux M, Dubois G, Turpin JC et al. Assays of arylsulfatase activity in psychotic patients: Review of the literature and results of a study of 22 patients. *Encephale*, 17, 87-92 (1991)

2991 Leme CE et al. Interaction of calcium ions with serum albumin in chronic renal failure. *Clin Chim Acta*, 77, 287-294 (1977)

2992 Lemke MR. Plasma magnesium decrease and altered calcium/magnesium ratio in severe dementia of the Alzheimer type. *Biol Psychiat*, 37, 341-343 (1995)

2993 Lemne C, Vesterqvist O, Egberg N et al. Platelet activation and prostacyclin release in essential hypertension. *Prostaglandins*, 44, 219-235 (1992)

2994 Lenders JWM, Keiser HR, Goldstein DS, et al. Plasma metanephrines in the diagnosis of pheochromocytoma. *Ann Intern Med*, 123, 101-109 (1995)

2995 Lenzo A, Wright R. Evaluation of a new amylase reagent for the Olympus DEMAND and REPLY. *Clin Chem*, 39, 1153 (1993)

2996 Lephart ED, Baxter CR, Parker CR Jr. Effect of burn trauma on adrenal and testicular steroid hormone production. *J Clin Endocrinol Metab*, 64, 842-848 (1987)

2997 Leppaluoto J, Vuolteenaho O, Arjamaa O. Plasma immunoreactive atrial natriuretic peptide and vasopressin after ethanol intake in man. *Acta Physiol Scand*, 144, 121-127 (1992)

2998 Lerner A, Gruener N, Iancu TC. Serum carnitine concentrations in coeliac disease. *Gut*, 34, 933-935 (1993)

2999 Lerner RG, Rapaport SI, Meltzer J. Thrombotic thrombocytopenic purpura: serial clotting studies. *Ann Intern Med*, 66, 1181 (1967)

3000 Lesem MD, Kaye WH, Bissette G et al. Cerebrospinal fluid TRH immunoreactivity in anorexia nervosa. *Biol Psychiat*, 35, 48-53 (1994)

3001 Leser HG, Gross V, Scheibenbogen C et al. Elevation of serum interleukin-6 concentration precedes acute-phase response and reflects severity in acute pancreatitis. *Gastroenterology*, 101, 782-785 (1991)

3002 Letizia C, Minisola S, Cerci S et al. Serum activity of angiotensin-converting enzyme and osteocalcin levels in hyperthyroidism. *Minerva Endocrinologia*, 17, 103-106 (1992)

3003 Letnansky K, Seelich F. Krebsartzt. *Klin Wschr*, 13, 80 (1958)

3004 Leto G, Tumminello FM, Pizzolanti G, et al. Cathepsin D serum mass concentrations in patients with hepatocellular carcinoma and/or liver cirrhosis. *Eur J Clin Chem Clin Biochem*, 34, 555-560 (1996)

3005 Leu SY, Wang SR. Clinical significance of arginase in colorectal cancer. *Cancer*, 70, 733-736 (1992)

3006 Leung HY, Lai LC, Day J, et al. Serum free prostate-specific antigen in the diagnosis of prostate cancer. *Br J Urol*, 80, 256-259 (1997)

3007 Leung T-N, Lam CWK, To K-F, Haines CJ. Changes in concentrations of lipoprotein (a) and other lipids and lipoproteins in pregnancies complicated by pregnancy-induced hypertension or intrauterine growth retardation. *Hypertens Preg*, 17, 157-168 (1998)

3008 Levin JH, Carmina E, Lobo RA. Is the inappropriate gonadotrophin secretion of patients with polycystic ovary syndrome similar to that of patients with adult-onset congenital adrenal hyperplasia? *Fertil Steril*, 56, 635-640 (1991)

3009 Levin PH et al. Health of the intensively treated hemophiliac, with special references to abnormal liver chemistries and splenomegaly. *Blood*, 50, 1-9 (1977)

3010 Levine B, Kalman J, Mayer L et al. Elevated circulating levels of tumor necrosis factor in severe chronic heart failure. *N Engl J Med*, 323, 236-241 (1990)

3011 Levine J, Ellis CJ, Furne JK, et al. Fecal hydrogen sulfide production in ulcerative colitis. *Am J Gastroenterol*, 93, 83-87 (1998)

3012 Levine J, Rapoport A, Mashiah M, Dolev E. Serum and cerebrospinal levels of calcium and magnesium in acute versus remitted schizophrenic patients. *Biol Psychiatr*, 33, 169-172 (1996)

3013 Levine PH, Ebbesen P, Ablashi DV et al. Antibodies to human herpes virus-6 and clinical course in patients with Hodgkin's disease. *Int J Cancer*, 51, 53-57 (1992)

3014 Levinson SS. Relationship between bilirubin, apolipoprotein B, and coronary artery disease. *Ann Clin Lab Sci*, 27, 185-192 (1997)

3015 Levital RD, Kaplan AS, Brown GM, et al. Low plasma cortisol in bulimia nervosa patients with reversed neurovegative symptoms of depression. *Biol Psychiat*, 41, 366-368 (1997)

3016 Levitan R et al. Serum enzyme activities in patients with polycythemia and myelofibrosis. *Cancer*, 13, 1218 (1960)

3017 Levy RI, Feinleib M. *Heart Disease*, Philadelphia PA, WB Saunders (1980)

3018 Lewczuk P, Reiber H, Ehrenreich H. Prothrombin in normal human cerebrospinal fluid originates from the blood. *Neurochem Res*, 23, 1027-1030 (1998)

3019 Lewczuk P, Reiber H, Tumani H. Intercellular adhesion molecule-1 in cerbrospinal fluid - the evaluation of blood-derived and brain-derived fractions in neurological diseases. *J Neuroimmunol*, 87, 156-161 (1998)

3020 Lewin KJ et al. Gastric morphology and serum gastrin levels in pernicious anemia. *Gut*, 17, 551-560 (1976)

3021 Lewis EJ et al. Serum complement levels in human glomerulonephritis. *Ann Intern Med*, 75, 555 (1971)

3022 Lewis SM. Red cell abnormalities in aplastic anemia. *Br J Haematol*, 8, 322 (1962)

3023 Lewis SM et al. Neutrophil (leukocyte) alkaline phosphatase in paroxysmal nocturnal hemoglobinuria. *Br J Haematol*, 11, 549 (1965)

3024 Lewison EF. The clinical value of the serum amylase test. *Surg Gynecol Obstet*, 72, 202-212 (1941)

3025 Leydon JJ. Low serum iron levels and moderate anemia in severe nodulocystic acne. *Arch Dermatol*, 121, 214 (1985)

3026 Lhotta K, Schlogl A, Kronenberg F, et al. Soluble intercellular adhesion molecule-1 (ICAM-1) in serum and urine: correlation with renal expression of ICAM-1 in patients with kidney disease. *Clin Nephrol*, 48, 85-91 (1997)

3027 Li CY et al. Acid phosphatase isoenzyme in human leukocytes in normal and pathologic conditions. *J Histochem Cytochem*, 18, 473 (1970)

3028 Li D, Keffer J, Corry K et al. Nonspecific elevation of troponin T levels in patients with chronic renal failure. *Clin Chem*, 41, S199 (1995)

3029 Li PKT, Leung JCK, Lai FM et al. Use of antineutrophil cytoplasmic autoantibodies in diagnosing vasculitis in a Chinese patient population. *Am J Nephrol*, 14, 99-105 (1994)

3030 Li Y-H, Teng J-K, Tsai W-C, et al. Elevation of soluble adhesion molecules is associated with the severity of myocardial damage in acute myocardial infarction. *Am J Cardiol*, 80, 1218-1221 (1997)

3031 Li Y-H, Teng J-K, Tsai W-C, et al. Prognostic significance of elevated hemostatic markers in patients with acute myocardial infarction. *J Am Coll Cardiol*, 33, 1543-1548 (1999)

3032 Lian EC, Deykin D. Diagnosis of von Willebrand's disease. *Am J Med*, 60, 344-356 (1976)

3033 Liang. Value of enzyme studies after prostatic surgery. *RI Med J*, 59, 457-458, 472 (1976)

3034 Liaw C-C, Wang C-H, Huang J-S, et al. Serum lactate dehydrogenase level in patients with nasopharyngeal carcinoma. *Acta Oncol*, 36, 159-164 (1997)

3035 Libertino JA, Zinman L. Renal cell carcinoma. *Med Clin North Am*, 59, 293-298 (1975)

3036 Licht A, Rachmilewitz EA. Myelofibrosis, osteolytic bone lesions and hypercalcemia in chronic myeloid leukemia. *Acta Haematol*, 49, 182 (1973)

3037 Lichtenfeld JL, Wiernik PH, Mardiney MR Jr et al. Abnormalities of complement and its components in patients with acute leukemia, Hodgkin's disease, and sarcoma. *Cancer Res*, 36, 3678-3680 (1976)

3038 Lieber CS. Interaction of alcohol with other drugs and nutrients: implications for the therapy of alcoholic liver disease. *Drugs*, 40, 23-44 (1990)

3039 Lieber CS (ed). *Metabolic Effects of Alcoholism*, Baltimore MD, University Park Press (1977)

3040 Lieberman J. Complement components in cystic fibrosis. *Lancet*, 1, 1230 (1974)

3041 Lieberman J. Elevation of serum angiotensin converting enzyme (ACE) level in sarcoidosis. *Am J Med*, 59, 365-372 (1975)

3042 Lieberman J, Bell DS. Serum angiotensin-converting enzyme as a marker for the chronic fatigue-immune dysfunction syndrome: a comparison to serum angiotensin-converting enzyme in sarcoidosis. *Am J Med*, 95, 407-412 (1993)

3043 Lieberman J, Sastre A. Serum angiotensin-converting enzyme: elevations in diabetes mellitus. *Ann Intern Med*, 93, 825-826 (1980)

3044 Lieberman J, Schleissner L, Tachik KH, Kling AS. Serum α1-antichymotrypsin level as a marker for Alzheimer-type dementia. *Neurobiol Aging*, 16, 747-753 (1995)

3045 Lieberman J, Schleissner LA, Nosal A et al. Clinical correlations of serum angiotensin-converting enzyme (ACE) in sarcoidosis. a longitudinal study of serum ACE, 67 gallium scans, chest roentgenograms, and pulmonary function. *Chest*, 84, 522-528 (1983)

3046 Lieberman JR, Hagay ZJ, Mazor M et al. Plasma and urine β-thromboglobulin in severe preeclampsia. *Arch Gynecol Obstet*, 243, 165-168 (1988)

3047 Liedtke RJ, Williams S, Kroon G. The performance of the vitamin B_{12} assay on the Access immunoassay system. *Clin Chem*, 41, S177 (1995)

3048 Lien E, Aukrust P, Sundan A, et al. Elevated levels of serum-soluble CD14 in human immunodeficiency virus type 1 (HIV-1) infection: correlation to disease progression and clinical events. *Blood*, 92, 2084-2092 (1998)

3049 Lieschke GJ, Burgess AW. Drug therapy: granulocyte colony-stimulating factor and granulocyte-macrophage colony-stimulating factor. *N Engl J Med*, 327, 28-35 (1992)

3050 Liewendahl K, Tikanoja S, Mahonen H et al. Concentrations of iodothyronines in serum of patients with chronic renal failure and other nonthyroidal illnesses: role of free fatty acids. *Clin Chem*, 33, 1382-1386 (1987)

3051 Lifton L et al. Ethanol-induced hypertriglyceridemia. prevalence and contributing factors. *Am J Clin Nutr*, 31, 614-618 (1978)

3052 Light RW. Pleural effusions. *Med Clin North Am*, 61, 1339-1352 (1977)

3053 Light RW. Pleural fluid analysis: how to interpret the tests. *Consultant*, 97 (1978)

3054 Light RW, Ball WC Jr. Glucose and amylase in pleural effusions. *J Am Med Ass*, 225, 257-259 (1973)

3055 Lightman A, Brandes JM, Binur N et al. Use of the serum copper/zinc ratio in the differential diagnosis of ovarian malignancy. *Clin Chem*, 32, 101-103 (1986)

3056 Lightsey AL et al. Platelet-associated immunoglobulin G in childhood idiopathic thrombocytopenic purpura. *J Pediatr*, 94, 201-204 (1979)

3057 Ligtenberg JJM, Van Tol A, Van Haeften TW, et al. Impaired suppression of plasma free fatty acids and triglycerides by acute hyperglycaemia-induced hyperinsulinaemia and alterations in high density lipoproteins in essential hypertension. *J Intern Med*, 240, 233-242 (1996)

3058 Liippo KK, Terho T. Concomitant monitoring of serum neuron-specific enolase and creatine kinase BB in small cell lung cancer. *Acta Oncol*, 30, 321-324 (1991)

3059 Lim K-H, Rice GE, de Groot CJM et al. Plasma type II phospholipase A_2 levels are elevated in severe preeclampsia. *Am J Obstet Gynecol*, 172, 998-1002 (1995)

3060 Lim P et al. Serum ionized calcium in nephrotic syndrome. *Q J Med*, 69, 421-426 (1976)

3061 Lin CC, Potter JJ, Mezey E. Erythrocyte aldehyde dehydrogenase activity in alcoholism. *Alcohol Clin Exp Res*, 8, 539-541 (1984)

3062 Lin C-L, Wu T-J, Machacek DA, Jiang N-S. Urinary free cortisol and cortisone determined by high performance liquid chromatography in the diagnosis of Cushing's syndrome. *J Clin Endocrinol Metab*, 82, 151-155 (1997)

3063 Lin X-Z, Chen T-W, Wang S-S et al. Pancreatic enzymes in uremic patients with or without dialysis. *Clin Biochem*, 21, 189-192 (1988)

3064 Lind T. Clinical Chemistry of Pregnancy. *Adv Clin Chem*, 21, 1-24 (1980)

3065 Linder R, Sziegoleit A, Brattstrom C et al. Pancreatic elastase 1 after pancreatic transplantation. *Pancreas*, 6, 31-36 (1990)

3066 Linderholm M, Ahim C, Settergren B, et al. Elevated plasma levels of tumor necrosis factor (TNF)-α, soluble TNF receptors, interleukin (IL)-6, and IL-10 in patients with hemorrhagic fever and renal syndrome. *J Infect Dis*, 173, 38-43 (1996)

3067 Lindgren A, Brattstrom L, Norrving B et al. Plasma homocysteine in the acute and convalescent phases after stroke. *Stroke*, 26, 795-800 (1995)

3068 Lindgren A, Swolin B, Nilsson O, et al. Serum methylmalonic acid and total homocysteine in patients with suspected cobalamin deficiency: a clinical study based on gastrointestinal histopathological findings. *Am J Hematol*, 56, 230-238 (1997)

3069 Lindholm J, Steiniche T, Rasmussen E et al. Bone disorder in men with chronic alcoholism: a reversible disease? *J Clin Endocrinol Metab*, 73, 118-124 (1991)

3070 Lindner MD, Gordon DD, Miller JM et al. Increased levels of truncated nerve growth factor receptor in urine of mildly demented patients with Alzheimer's disease. *Arch Neurol*, 50, 1054-1058 (1993)

3071 Lindqvist B et al. Differential count of urinary leucocytes and renal epithelial cells by phase contrast microscopy. *Acta Med Scand*, 198, 505-509 (1975)

3072 Lindqvist U. Is serum hyaluronan a helpful tool in the management of patients with liver disease? *J Intern Med*, 242, 67-71 (1997)

3073 Lindqvist U, Chichibu K, Delpech B et al. Seven different assays of hyaluronan compared to clinical utility. *Clin Chem*, 38, 127-132 (1992)

3074 Linker-Israeli M, Deans RJ, Wallace DJ, et al. Elevated levels of endogenous IL-6 in systemic lupus erythematosus: a putative role in pathogenesis. *J Immunol*, 147, 117-123 (1991)

3075 Linkola J et al. Renin-aldosterone axis in ethanol intoxication and hangover. *Eur J Clin Invest*, 6, 191-194 (1976)

3076 Linko-Lopponen S. Fluorometric measurement of urinary N-acetyl-β-N-glucosaminidase and its correlation to uremia. *Clin Chim Acta*, 160, 119-127 (1986)

3077 Linkowski P, Menlewicz J, Leclercq R et al. The 24-hour profile of adrenocorticotropin and cortisol in major depressive illness. *J Clin Endocrinol Metab*, 61, 429-438 (1985)

3078 Links TP, Monkelbaan JF, Dullaart RPF, van Haeften TW. Growth hormone-, α-subunit and thyrotropin -cosecreting pituitary adenoma in familial setting of pituitary tumour. *Acta Endocrinol*, 129, 516-518 (1993)

3079 Linnane SJ, Keatings VM, Costello CM, et al. Total sputum nitrate plus nitrite is raised during acute pulmonary infection in cystic fibrosis. *Am J Respir Crit Care Med*, 158, 207-212 (1998)

3080 Lio S, Albin M, Girelli G, et al. Abnormal thyroid function test results in patients with Fisher-Evans syndrome. *J Endocrinol Invest*, 16, 163-167 (1993)

3081 Liozon E, Volkov L, Comte L et al. AcSDKP serum concentrations vary during chemotherapy in patients with acute myeloid leukemia. *Br J Haematol*, 89, 917-920 (1995)

3082 Lipinski B et al. Abnormal fibrinogen heterogeneity and fibrinolytic activity in advanced liver disease. *J Lab Clin Med*, 90, 187-194 (1977)

3083 Lipman LM et al. Relationship of long-acting thyroid stimulator to the clinical features and course of Graves' disease. *Am J Med*, 43, 486 (1967)

3084 Lipsett MB et al. Hormonal syndromes associated with non-endocrine tumors. *Ann Intern Med*, 61, 733 (1964)

3085 Lipton A, Demers L, Daniloff Y et al. Increased urinary excretion of pyridinium cross-links in cancer patients. *Clin Chem*, 39, 614-618 (1993)

3086 Lipton A, Sheehan L, Mortel R et al. Urinary polyamine levels in patients with localized malignancy. *Cancer*, 38, 1344-1347 (1976)

3087 Lisowska-Myjak B, Pachecka J, Witak P, Radowicki S. Comparison of urinary excretion of albumin and α1-antitrypsin in patients with arterial hypertension. *Scand J Clin Lab Invest*, 59, 93-98 (1999)

3088 Lissoni P, Mengo S, Mandala M, et al. Physiopathology of IL-12 in human solid neoplasmss: blood levels of IL-12 in early or advanced cancer patients, and their variations with surgery and immunotherapy. *J Biol Reg Homeost Agents*, 12, 38-41 (1998)

3089 Lissoni P, Rovelli F, Pittalis S, et al. Interleukin-12 in early or advanced cancer patients. *Eur J Cancer*, 33, 1703-1705 (1997)

3090 Litten RZ, Allen JP, Fertig JB. γ-Glutamyltranspeptidase and carbohydrate deficient transferrin: alternative measures of excessive alcohol consumption. *Alcohol Clin Exp Res*, 19, 1541-1546 (1995)

3091 Liu C-S, Wu H-M, Kao S-H, Wei Y-H. Phenytoin-mediated oxidative stress in serum of female epileptics: a possible pathogenesis in the fetal hydantoin syndrome. *Hum Exp Toxicol*, 16, 177-181 (1997)

3092 Liu FJ, Buchsbaum RM II, Fritsche HA. Serum lactate dehydrogenase-3 (LD-3) isoenzyme in acute non-lymphocytic leukemia. *Clin Chem*, 39, 1186 (1993)

3093 Liuzzo G, Biasucci LM, Gallimore JR et al. The prognostic value of C-reactive protein and serum amyloid A protein in severe unstable angina. *N Engl J Med*, 331, 417-424 (1994)

3094 Liuzzo G, Biasucci LM, Rebuzzi AG, et al. Plasma protein acute-phase response in unstable angina is not induced by ischemic injury. *Circulation*, 94, 2373-2380 (1996)

3095 Ljungberg B, Grankvist K, Rasmuson T. Serum acute-phase reactants and prognosis in renal cell carcinoma. *Cancer*, 76, 1435-1439 (1995)

3096 Lloyd-Still JD, Bohan T, Hughes S, Wessel HU. Acylcarnitine is low in cord blood in cystic fibrosis. *Acta Paediat Scand*, 79, 427-430 (1990)

3097 Lluberas-Acosta G, Schumacher HR. Markedly elevated erythrocyte sedimentation rates: consideration of clinical implications in a hospital population. *Br J Clin Pract*, 50, 138-143 (1998)

3098 Lo Cigno M, Montanari F, Bercovich E et al. Prostate-specific antigen (PSA): diagnostic and prognostic implications in the evaluation of carcinomas of the prostate. *Arch Ital Urol Nefrol Androl*, 61, 29-36 (1989)

3099 Lobo A, Naso A, Arheart K, et al. Reduction of homocysteine levels in coronary artery disease by low-dose folic acid combined with vitamins B_6 and B_{12}. *Am J Cardiol*, 83, 821-825 (1999)

3100 Lock RJ, Unsworth DJ. Measurement of limmune complexes is not useful in routine clinical practice. *Ann Clin Biochem*, 37, 253-261 (2000)

3101 Lockwood DH et al. Insulin secretion in type I glycogen storage disease. *Diabetes*, 18, 755-758 (1969)

3102 Loewenstein MS et al. Carcinoembryonic antigen assay of ascites and detection of malignancy. *Ann Intern Med*, 88, 635-38 (1978)

3103 Lofberg M, Tahtela R, Harkonen M, somer H. Myosin heavy-chain fragments and cardiac troponins in the serum of rhabdomyolysis; diagnostic specificity of new biochemical markers. *Arch Neurol*, 52, 1210-1214 (1995)

3104 Loge JP et al. Characterization of anemia associated with chronic renal insufficiency. *Am J Med*, 24, 4 (1958)

3105 Logue FC, Perry B, Chapman RS, et al. A two-site immunoradiometric assay for PTH(1-84) using N and C terminal specific monoclonal antibodies. *Ann Clin Biochem*, 28, 160-166 (1991)

3106 Loguercio C, Taranto D, Vitale LM, et al. Effect of liver cirrhosis and age on the glutathione concentration in the plasma, erythrocytes, and gastric mucosa of man. *Free Rad Biol Med*, 29, 483-488 (1996)

3107 Lohr M, Spies B, Heptner G, Domschke S. Parameters of connective tissue metabolism as markers in acute and chronic pancreatitis. A retrospective study with a cohort of normal subjects. *Z Gastroenterol*, 29, 231-236 (1991)

3108 Loirat P et al. Increased glomerular filtration rate in patients with major burns. *N Engl J Med*, 299, 915-919 (1978)

3109 Loizate Toricaguena A, Lamiquiz Vallejo A, Dominguez Merru-Urrutia MJ et al. Tumor-associated trypsin inhibitor (TATI) in benign and malignant gastric disease. *Scand J Clin Lab Invest*, 51, 59-62 (1991)

3110 Lokech JJ. Leukocyte alkaline phosphatase activity in patients with malignant disease. *Cancer*, 40, 1202-1205 (1977)

3111 Loko F, Robic D, Bondiou M-T et al. Concentrations of N-acetyl-β-D-glucosaminidase and its intermediate isoenzymes in serum of patients with renal transplants. *Clin Chem*, 37, 583-584 (1991)

3112 Lombardi C, Tassi GF, Pizzocolo MD et al. Clinical significance of a multiple biomarker assay in patients with lung cancer. *Chest*, 97, 639-644 (1990)

3113 Lommi J, Kupari M, Koskinen P, et al. Blood ketone bodies in congestive heart failure. *J Am Coll Cardiol*, 28, 665-672 (1996)

3114 London et al. On low acid phosphatase values of patients with known metastatic cancer of the prostate. *Cancer Res*, 14, 718-724 (1954)

3115 Long PA et al. Importance of abnormal glucose tolerance (hypoglycemia and hyperglycemia) in the aetiology of pre-eclampsia. *Lancet*, 1, 923-925 (1977)

3116 Look MP, Rockstroh JK, Rao GS, et al. Serum selenium versus lymphocyte subsets and markers of disease progression and inflammatory response in human immunodeficiency vurus-1 infection. *Biol Trace Elem Res*, 56, 31-41 (1997)

3117 Lopes A, Daras V, Cross PA et al. Thrombocytosis in women with cancer of the cervix. *Cancer*, 74, 90-92 (1994)

3118 Lopes J et al. Heterogeneity of 5'-nucleotidase activity in lymphocytes in chronic leukemia. *J Clin Invest*, 52, 1297 (1973)

3119 Lopez EL, Contrini MM, Devoto S et al. Tumor necrosis factor concentrations in hemolytic uremic syndrome patients and children with bloody diarrhea. *Pediatr Infect Dis J*, 14, 594-598 (1995)

3120 Lopez JB, Thambyrajah V, Balasegaram M et al. Tumour markers in hepatocellular carcinoma and liver diseases. *Clin Biochem*, 14, 260 (1993)

3121 Lopez JB, Thambyrajah V, Balasegaram M, Satgunasingam N. Serum ferritin in hepatocellular carcinoma and benign liver diseases. *Diagn Oncol*, 4, 143-147 (1994-95)

3122 Lopez-Cortes LF, Cruz-Ruiz M, Gomez-Mateos J et al. Adenosine deaminase activity in the CSF of patients with aseptic meningitis: utility in the diagnosis of tuberculous meningitis or neurobrucellosis. *Clin Infect Dis*, 20, 525-530 (1995)

3123 Lopez-Cortes LF, Cruz-Ruiz M, Gomez-Mateos J, et al. Interleukin-6 in cerebrospinal fluid of meningitis is not a useful diagnostic marker in the differential diagnosis of meningitis. *Ann Clin Biochem*, 34, 165-169 (1997)

3124 Lopez-Llera M et al. Coagulation and fibrinolysis in molar pregnancy. *Am J Obstet Gynecol*, 127, 855-860 (1977)

3125 Lopponen T, Saukkonen A-L, Serlo W, et al. Reduced levels of growth hormone, insulin-like growth factor-1 and binding protein-3 in patients with shunted hydrocephalus. *Arch Dis Child*, 77, 32-37 (1997)

3126 Loraine JA. Bioassay of pituitary and placental gonadotropins in relation to clinical problems in man. *Vitamins Hormones*, 14, 305-357 (1956)

3127 Lorber A et al. Serum copper levels in rheumatoid arthritis. *Arth Rheum*, 11, 65-71 (1968)

3128 Lorber M. Adult-type Gaucher's disease: a secondary disorder of iron metabolism. *J Mt Sinai Hosp*, 37, 404

3129 Lorber M, Aviram M, Linn S et al. Hypocholesterolaemia and abnormal high-density lipoprotein in rheumatoid arthritis. *Br J Rheumatol*, 24, 250-255 (1985)

3130 Lorentzen B, Endresen MJ, Clausen T et al. Fasting serum free fatty acids and triglycerides are increased before 20 weeks of gestation in women who later develop preeclampsia. *Hypertens Pregnancy*, 13, 103-109 (1994)

3131 Loria A et al. Red cell life span in iron deficiency anaemia. *Br J Haematol*, 13, 294 (1967)

3132 Lorusso L Miniello VL, Francioso G, Aceto G et al. Antithrombin III in infantile nephrotic syndrome. *Boll Soc Ital Biol Sper*, 58, 1093 (1982)

3133 Loser C, Mollgaard A, Folsch UR. Fecal elastase 1: a novel, highly sensitive, and specific tubeless pancreatic function test. *Gut*, 39, 580-586 (1996)

3134 Losito R, Gattiker H, Bilodeau G et al. Levels of antithrombin III, α_2-macroglobulin, and α_1-antitrypsin in acute ischemic heart disease. *J Lab Clin Med*, 97, 241-50 (1981)

3135 Losowsky MS et al. Lipid metabolism in acute and chronic renal failure. *J Lab Clin Med*, 71, 736 (1968)

3136 Lotstra et al. Reduced CCK levels in CSF. *Ann NY Acad Sci*, 448, 507-517 (1985)

3137 Loun B, Astles R, Copeland KR et al. Leukocytes magnesium content in leukemia, infection, G-CSF treatment. *Clin Chem*, 41, S222 (1995)

3138 Loutit JF. Discussion on the life and death of the red corpuscle. *Proc Roy Soc Med*, 34, 755 (1946)

3139 Love PE, Santoro SA. Antiphospholipid antibodies: anticardiolipin and the lupus anticoagulant in systemic lupus erythematosus (SLE) and in non-SLE disorders. Prevalence and clinical significance. *Ann Intern Med*, 112, 682-698 (1990)

3140 Loviselli A, Calia MA, Murenu S et al. Circulating soluble IL-2 receptor levels are low in patients with hypothyroid autoimmune thyroiditis. *Horm Metab Res*, 26, 548-551 (1994)

3141 Lowe JR, Dixon JS, Guthrie JA, McWhinney P. Serum and synovial fluid levels of angiotensin converting enzyme in polyarthritis. *Ann Rheum Dis*, 45, 921-924 (1986)

3142 Lowell JR. Diagnosis: fluid and tissue examination. In:. *Pleural Effusions*, Baltimore MD, University Park Press, 45-73 (1977)

3143 Lowis EI, Oakey RE. Steroid sulphatase deficiency: identification of heterozygotes using hydrolysis of dehydroepiandrosterone sulphate by peripheral leukocytes. *Ann Clin Biochem*, 33, 219-226 (1996)

3144 Lowy C et al. Urinary excretion of insulin and growth hormone in subjects with renal failure. *Acta Endocrinol*, 67, 85 (1971)

3145 Lu L, Shen G. Detection of hyaluronic acid serum concentrations using microtiter EIA. *Clin Chem*, 39, 1261 (1993)

3146 Lubran M. The effects of drugs on laboratory values. *Med Clin North Am*, 53, 211 (1969)

3147 Lucas PA, Woodhead JS, Brown RC. Vitamin D_3 metabolites in chronic renal failure and after renal transplantation. *Nephrol Dial Transplant*, 3, 70-76 (1988)

3148 Lucca A, Lucini V, Piatti E et al. Plasma tryptophan levels and plasma tryptophan/neutral amino acid ratios in patients with mood disorder, patients with obsessive-compulsive disorder, and normal subjects. *Psychiat Res*, 44, 85-91 (1992)

3149 Lucky AW. Hormonal correlates of acne and hirsutism. *Am J Med*, 98, 89S-94S (1995)

3150 Ludwig M, Bauer O, Lopens A, et al. Serum concentration of vascular endothelial growth factor cannot predict the course of severe ovarian hyperstimulation syndrome. *Hum Reprod*, 13, 30-32 (1998)

3151 Luetscher JA et al. Aldosterone secretion and metabolism in hypertension and myxedema. *J Clin Endocrinol Metab*, 23, 873 (1963)

3152 Lugassy G, Plator I, Schlesinger M. Hypocomplementemia in multiple myeloma. *Leukemia Lymphoma*, 33, 365-370 (1999)

3153 Luhdorf K et al. Grand mal provoked hyperuricemia. *Acta Neurol Scand*, 58, 280-287 (1978)

3154 Luisetti M, Bulgheroni A, Bacchella L et al. Elevated serum procollagen III aminopeptide levels in sarcoidosis. *Chest*, 98, 1414-1420 (1990)

3155 Luisi M et al. Plasma steroid dynamics in Cushing's syndrome. *Ann Endocrinol*, 39, 107-115 (1978)

3156 Lukas R, Trif I, Cucuianu M. Plasma phospholipase A2 in children with malignant disorders. *Eur J Clin Chem Clin Biochem*, 30, 127-130 (1992)

3157 Lukert BP, Higgins JC, Stoskopf MM. Serum osteocalcin is increased in patients with hyperthyroidism and decreased in patients receiving glucocorticoids. *J Clin Endocrinol Metab*, 62, 1056-1058 (1986)

3158 Lukumsky P E, Oganov R G. Blood plasma catecholamines and their urinary excretion in patients with acute myocardial infarction. *Am Heart J*, 83, 182 (1972)

3159 Lum G. Hypomagnesemia in acute and chronic care patient populations. *Am J Clin Pathol*, 97, 827-830 (1992)

3160 Lum G. Significance of low serum alkaline phosphatase activity in a predominantly adult population. *Clin Chem*, 41, 515-518 (1995)

3161 Lum G et al. Serum γ-glutamyl transpeptidase activity as an indicator of disease of liver, pancreas, or bone. *Clin Chem*, 18, 358-362 (1972)

3162 Lund AM, Hansen M, Kollerup G, et al. Collagen-derived markers of bone metabolism in osteogenesis imperfecta. *Acta Paediatr*, 87, 1131-1137 (1998)

3163 Lundberg JM. Elevated plasma endothelin-1 concentrations are associated with the severity of illness in patients with sepsis. *Ann Surg*, 213, 261-264 (1991)

3164 Lundin A, Engstrom-Laurent A, Hallgren R et al. Circulating hyaluronate in psoriasis. *Br J Dermatol*, 112, 663-671 (1985)

3165 Lunel F, Musset L, Cacoub P, et al. Cryoglobulinemia in chronic liver disease: role of hepatitis C and liver damage. *Gastroenterology*, 106, 1291-1300 (1994)

3166 Luo J-C, Neugut AI, Garbowski G et al. Levels of p53 antigen in the plasma of patients with adenomas and carcinomas of the colon. *Cancer Lett*, 91, 235-240 (1995)

3167 Luo YP, Huang ZG, Qian HJ. Tumor necrosis factor and interleukin 6 in acute leukemia. *Chung Hua Nei Ko Tsa Chih*, 32, 85-87 (1993)

3168 Luoni R, Ucci G, Riccardi A et al. Serum thymidine kinase in monoclonal gammopathies: a prospective study. *Cancer*, 69, 1368-1372 (1992)

3169 Luparini RL, Ferri C, Santucci A et al. Atrial natriuretic peptide in non-modulating essential hypertension. *Hypertension*, 21, 803-809 (1993)

3170 Luppa P, Hauck S, Schwab I et al. 6α-Biotinylated estrone: novel tracer in competitive chemiluminescence immunoassay of estrone in serum. *Clin Chem*, 41, 564-570 (1995)

3171 Luppinger K et al. Klinefelter's syndrome, a clinical and cytogenetic study in twenty-two cases. *Acta Endocrinol*, 54, Suppl, 113 (1967)

3172 Lusher JM, Zuelzer WW. Idiopathic thrombocytopenic purpura in childhood. *J Pediatr*, 68, 971 (1966)

3173 Lutomski DM, Bower RH. The effect of thrombocytosis on serum potassium and phosphorus concentration. *Am J Med*, 307, 255-258 (1994)

3174 Lydiard RB, Ballenger JC, Laraia MT et al. CSF cholecystokinin concentrations in patients with panic disorder and in normal comparison subjects. *Am J Psychiat*, 149, 691-693 (1992)

3175 Lydiard RB, Brewerton TD, Fossey MD et al. CSF cholecystokinin octapeptide in patients with bulimia nervosa and in normal comparison subjects. *Am J Psychiat*, 151, 1098 (1994)

3176 Lynch A, Marlar R, Murphy J et al. Antiphospholipid antibodies in predicting adverse pregnancy outcome. A prospective study. *Ann Intern Med*, 120, 470-475 (1994)

3177 Lynch PJ, Miedler LJ. Erythropoietic porphyria: report of a family and clinical review. *Arch Dermatol*, 92, 351 (1965)

3178 Lynch PJ, Voorhees JJ, Harrell ER. Systemic sporotrichosis. *Ann Intern Med*, 73, 23-30 (1970)

3179 Macciardi F, Lucca A, Catalano M et al. Amino acid patterns in schizophrenia: some new findings. *Psychiat Res*, 32, 63-70 (1990)

3180 MacDonald TT et al. *Clin Exp Immunol*, 81, 301- (1990)

3181 MacGibbon BH, Mollin DL. Sideroblastic anaemia in man: observations on seventy cases. *Br J Haematol*, 11, 59 (1965)

3182 MacGowan GA, Mann DI, Kormos RL, et al. Circulating interleukin-6 in severe heart failure. *Am J Cardiol*, 79, 1128-1131 (1997)

3183 Machin ND, Chard MD, Paice EW. Serum angiotensin converting enzyme in Sjögren's syndrome--a case report and study of 21 further cases. *Postgrad Med J*, 60, 270-271 (1984)

3184 Mackay IR. Chronic hepatitis: effect of prolonged suppressive treatment and comparison of azathioprine with prednisolone. *Q J Med*, 37, 379 (1968)

3185 Mackay IR et al. Autoimmune hepatitis. *Ann NY Acad Sci*, 124, 767 (1965)

3186 Mackay IR, Larkin L. The significance of the presence in human serum of complement-fixing antibodies to human tissue antigens. *Aust Ann Med*, 7, 251 (1958)

3187 Mackenzie MR, Fudenberg HH. Macroglobulinemia: an analysis of forty patients. *Blood*, 39, 874 (1972)

3188 Mackinney AA Jr et al. Ascertaining genetic carriers of hereditary spherocytosis by statistical analysis of multiple laboratory tests. *J Clin Invest*, 41, 554 (1962)

3189 Mackintosh C, Dolan I, Li F et al. Biochemical bone markers in polymyalgia rheumatica and the effects of steroid treatment. *Proc ACB Natl Meet*, 72 (1994)

3190 Mackintosh C, Treasure J, Ward A et al. Biochemical bone markers in anorexia nervosa. *Proc ACB Natl Meet*, 68 (1995)

3191 Macrae FA. Faecal occult blood testing: sensitivity and specificity. *Br J Surg*, 72, S67-S74 (1985)

3192 Maddrey WC, Weber FL. Chronic hepatic encephalopathy. *Med Clin North Am*, 59, 937-944 (1975)

3193 Madeddu G, Casu AR, Costanza C et al. Serum thyroglobulin levels in the diagnosis and follow-up of subacute 'painful' thyroiditis. *Arch Intern Med*, 145, 243 (1985)

3194 Madersbacher S, Klieber R, Mann K et al. Free α-subunit, free β-subunit of human chorionic gonadotropin (hCG), and intact hCG in sera of healthy individuals and testicular cancer patients. *Clin Chem*, 38, 370-376 (1992)

3195 Madias JE, Sheth K, Choudry MA, et al. Admission serum magnesium level does not predict the hospital outcome of patients with acute myocardial infarction. *Arch Intern Med*, 156, 1701-1708 (1996)

3196 Madsen SN et al. Urinary cyclic AMP relation to albumin-corrected serum calcium in healthy persons and patients with primary hyperparathyroidism. *Acta Med Scand*, 200, 195-199 (1976)

3197 Madson KL, Moore TL, Lawrence JM III, et al. Cytokine levels in serum and synovial fluid of patients with juvenile rheumatoid arthritis. *J Rheumatol*, 21, 2359-2363 (1994)

3198 Mae M, Vandoolaeghe E, Ranjan R, et al. Increased serum interleukin-1-receptor-antagonist concentrations in major depression. *J Affect Disord*, 36, 29-36 (1995)

3199 Maeda K, Chung Y-S, Onoda N et al. Prognostic value of serum pepsinogen levels in patients with gastric carcinoma. *Int J Oncol*, 3, 437-440 (1993)

3200 Maeda K, Tsutamoto T, Wada A, et al. Plasma brain natriuretic peptide as a biochemical marker of high left ventricular end-diastolic pressure in patients with symptomatic left ventricular dysfunction. *Am Heart J*, 135, 825-832 (1998)

3201 Maeda K, Yasuda M, Kaneda H et al. Cerebrospinal fluid (CSF) neuropeptide Y- and somatostatin-like immunoreactivities in man. *Neuropeptides*, 27, 323-332 (1994)

3202 Maeda Y, Chihara J, Horiuchi F, et al. Elevated levels of soluble ICAM-1 in serum of patients with acute myeloid leukemia undergoing bone marrow transplantation. *Am J Hematol*, 52, 227-228 (1996)

3203 Maeno N, Takei S, Masuda K, et al. Increased serum levels of vascular endothelial growth factor in Kawasaki disease. *Pediatr Res*, 44, 596-599 (1998)

3204 Maes M, Bosmans E, Kenis G, De Jong R. In vivo immunomodulatory effects of clozapine in schizophrenia. *Schiz Res*, 26, 221-225 (1997)

3205 Maes M, Bosmans E, Ranjan R, et al. Lower plasma CC16, a natural anti-inflammatory protein, and increased plasma interleukin-1 receptor antagonist in schizophrenia: effects of antipsychotic drugs. *Schiz Res*, 21, 39-50 (1996)

3206 Maes M, Bosmans E, Scharpe S, et al. Plasma soluble interleukin-2-receptor in depression: relationships to plasma neopterin and serum IL-2 concentrations and HPA-axis activity. *Eur Psychiatr*, 10, 397-403 (1995)

3207 Maes M, De Meester I, Vanhoof G et al. Decreased serum dipeptidyl peptidase IV activity in major depression. *Biol Psychiat*, 30, 577-586 (1991)

3208 Maes M, Delange J, Ranjan R, et al. Acute phase proteins in schizophrenia, mania and major depression: modulation by psychotropic drugs. *Psychiat Res*, 66, 1-11 (1997)

3209 Maes M, D'Haese PC, Scharpe S et al. Hypozincemia in depression. *J Affect Disord*, 31, 135-140 (1994)

3210 Maes M, Lin A-H, Delmeire L, et al. Elevated serum interleukin-6 (IL-6) and IL-6 receptor concentrations in posttraumatic stress disorder following accidental man-made traumatic events. *Biol Psychiat*, 45, 833-839 (1999)

3211 Maes M, Meltzer HY, Bosmans E et al. Increased plasma concentrations of interleukin-6, soluble interleukin-6 and transferrin receptor in major depression. *J Affect Disord*, 34, 301-309 (1995)

3212 Maes M, Scharpe S, Meltzer HY, et al. Increased neopterin and interferon-γ secretion and lower availability of L-tryptophan in major depression: further evidence for an immune response. *Psychiatr Res*, 54, 143-160 (1994)

3213 Maes M, Scharpe S, Van Grootel L et al. Higher α_1-antitrypsin, haptoglobin, ceruloplamsin and lower retinol binding protein plasma levels during depression: further evidence for the existence of an inflammatory response during that illness. *J Affect Disord*, 24, 183-192 (1992)

3214 Maes M, Van der Planken M, Van Gastel A, Desnyder R. Blood coagulation and platelet aggregation in major depression. *J Affect Disord*, 40, 35-40 (1996)

3215 Maes M, Vandoolaeghe E, Neels H, et al. Lower serum zinc in major depression is a sensitive marker of treatment resistance and of the immune/inflammatory response in that illness. *Biol Psychiat*, 42, 349-358 (1997)

3216 Maes M, Wauters A, Neels H, et al. Total serum protein and serum protein fractions in depression: relationships to depressive symptoms and glucocorticoid activity. *J Affect Disord*, 34, 61-69 (1995)

3217 Maes M, Wauters A, Verkerk R, et al. Lower serum L-tryptophan availability in depression as a marker of a more generalized disorder in protein metabolism. *Neuropsychopharmacology*, 15, 243-251 (1996)

3218 Maestranzi S, Przeioslo R, Mitchell H, Sherwood RA. The effect of benign and malignant liver disease on the tumour markers CA 19-9 and CEA. *Ann Clin Biochem*, 35, 99-103 (1998)

3219 Magiakou MA, Mastorakos G, Gomez MT et al. Suppressed spontaneous and stimulated growth hormone secretion in patients with Cushing's disease before and after surgical cure. *J Clin Endocrinol Metab*, 78, 131-137 (1994)

3220 Magill GB et al. Serum lactic dehydrogenase and serum transaminase in human leukemia. *Blood*, 14, 870 (1959)

3221 Magnus IA. The cutaneous porphyrias. *Semin Hematol*, 5, 380 (1968)

3222 Magnus IA et al. Erythropoietic protoporphyria: a new porphyria syndrome with solar urticaria due to protoporphyrinaemia. *Lancet*, 2, 448 (1961)

3223 Magri G et al. Relationship between urine acidification and intracellular pH in respiratory acidosis. *Bronchopneμmologie*, 27, 293-300 (1977)

3224 Maguire TM, Gillian AM, O'Mahony D et al. A decrease in serum sialyltransferase levels in Alzheimer's disease. *Neurobiol Aging*, 15, 99-102 (1994)

3225 Maguire TM, O'Mahony D, Gillian AM et al. The serum expression of sialoglycoproteins and sialyltransferase in Alzheimer's disease: evidence for the altered expression of individual isoforms. *Neurodegeneration*, 3, 129-133 (1994)

3226 Maguire TM, Thakore J, Dinan TG , et al. Plasma sialyltransferase levels in psychiatric disorders as a possible indicator of HPA axis function. *Biol Psychiatr*, 41, 1131-1136 (1997)

3227 Mahajan RC et al. Significance of serum lactic dehydrogenase enzyme in hepatic amoebiasis. *Ind J Med Res*, 63, 1006-1009 (1975)

3228 Maharaj B, Pillay S, Padayschi T. Circulating CA-195 in hepatocellular carcinoma and metastatic hepatic carcinoma. *Trop Geog Med*, 43, 329-331 (1991)

3229 Maharajan G et al. Thyroxine, triiodothyronine and thyrotrophin levels in meningococcal meningitis, typhoid fever and other febrile conditions. *Clin Endocrinol*, 9, 401-406 (1979)

3230 Maheshwari HG, Butler J, Norman M. Growth hormone binding protein in patients with renal failure. *Acta Endocrinol*, 127, 485-488 (1992)

3231 Mahida YR, Kurlc L, Gallagher A et al. High circulating concentrations of interleukin-6 in active Crohn's disease but not ulcerative colitis. *Gut*, 32, 1531-1534 (1991)

3232 Mahmoud MY, Lugon M, Anderson CC. Unexplained macrocytosis in the elderly. *Age Ageing*, 25, 310-312 (1996)

3233 Main KM, Lindholm J, Vandeweghe M et al. Urinary growth hormone excretion in acromegaly: diagnostic value in mild disease activity. *Acta Endocrinol*, 129, 409-413 (1993)

3234 Mair DC, Whipkey R, Bruns DE et al. Potential use of the serum myoglobin in the emergency room. *Clin Chem*, 39, 1148 (1993)

3235 Mair J. Glycogen phosphorylase isoenzyme BB to diagnose ichaemic myocardial damage. *Clin Chim Acta*, 272, 79-86 (1998)

3236 Mair J, Wagner I, Leichieitner P et al. Release of cardiac troponin T in patients with acute myocardial infarction is related to scintigraphic estimates of myocardial scar. *Clin Chem*, 39, 1133 (1993)

3237 Maisel AS, Scott NA, Motulsky HJ et al. Elevation of plasma neuropeptide Y levels in congestive heart failure. *Am J Med*, 86, 43-48 (1989)

3238 Maisel JD et al. Fatal Mycoplasma pneumoniae infection with isolation of organisms from lung. *J Am Med Ass*, 202, 287 (1967)

3239 Major RH, Leger LH. Marked eosinophilia in Hodgkin's disease. *J Am Med Ass*, 112, 2601 (1939)

3240 Mak TWL, Ho SS, Ho CS, et al. Pleural fluid in malignant and benign pleural effusions. *Ann Clin Biochem*, 35, 94-98 (1998)

3241 Mako ME et al. Circulating proinsulin in patients with maturity onset diabetes. *Am J Med*, 63, 865-873 (1977)

3242 Malagelada JR, Iber FL, Linscheer WG. Origin of fat in chylous ascites of patients with liver cirrhosis. *Gastroenterology*, 67, 878-886 (1974)

3243 Malamitsi-Puchner A, Sarandakou A, Dafogianni C, et al. Serum angiogenin levels in children and adolescents with insulin-dependent diabetes mellitus. *Pediatr Res*, 43, 798-800 (1998)

3244 Malan C, Donald PR, Golden M et al. Adenosine deaminase levels in cerebrospinal fluid in the diagnosis of tuberculous meningitis. *J Trop Med Hyg*, 87, 33-40 (1984)

3245 Malaval L, Ffrench M, Delmas PD. Circulating levels of osteonectin in normal subjects and patients with thrombocytopenia. *Bone Miner*, 9, 129-135 (1990)

3246 Maldonado JE, Hanlon DG. Monocytosis: a current appraisal. *Mayo Clin Proc*, 40, 248 (1965)

3247 Malee MP, Malee KM, Azuma SD et al. Increases in atrial natriuretic peptide concentration antedate clinical evidence of preeclampsia. *J Clin Endocrinol Metab*, 74, 1095-1100 (1992)

3248 Malek-Ahmadi P. Cytokines in dementia of the Alzheimer's type (DAT): relevance to research and treatment. *Neurosci Behav Res*, 22, 389-394 (1998)

3249 Malesci A, Montorsi M, Mariani A et al. Clinical utility of the serum CA 19-9 test for diagnosing pancreatic carcinoma in symptomatic patients: a prospective study. *Pancreas*, 7, 497-502 (1992)

3250 Malette LE, Henkin RI. Altered copper and zinc metabolism in primary hyperparathyroidism. *Am J Med Sci*, 272, 167-174 (1976)

3251 Malinow MR, Levenson J, Giral P et al. Role of blood pressure, uric acid, and hemorheological parameters on plasma homocyst(e)ine concentration. *Atherosclerosis*, 114, 175-183 (1995)

3252 Malkasian GD, Knapp RC, Lavin PT et al. Preoperative evaluation of serum CA 125 levels in premenopausal and postmenopausal patients with pelvic masses: discrimination of benign from malignant disease. *Am J Obstet Gynecol*, 159, 341-346 (1988)

3253 Malkjaersig N et al. Reduction of coagulation factor XIII concentration in patients with myocardial infarction, cerebral infarction, and other thromboembolic disorders. *Thromb Haemostas*, 38, 863-873 (1977)

3254 Mallat Z, Philip I, Lebret M, et al. Elevated levels of 8-iso-prostaglandin F_{α} in pericardial fluid of patients with heart failure: a potential role for in vivo oxidant stress in ventricular dilatation and progression in heart failure. *Circulation*, 97, 1536-1539 (1998)

3255 Mallette LE et al. Primary hyperparathyroidism: clinical and biochemical features. *Medicine*, 53, 127-146 (1974)

3256 Mallmann P, Diedrich K, Mallmann R et al. Determination of TNFα, interferon-α, interleukin 2 and reactivity in the leukocyte migration inhibition test in breast cancer patients. *Anticancer Res*, 11, 1509-1515 (1991)

3257 Mallmann P, Mallmann R, Krebs D. Determination of tumor necrosis factorα (TNFα) and interleukin 2 (IL 2) in women with idiopathic recurrent miscarriage. *Arch Gynecol Obstet*, 249, 73-78 (1991)

3258 Malmatsi-Puchner A, Sarandakou A, Tziotis J, et al. Serum levels of basic fibroblast growth factor and vascular endothelial growth factor in children and adolescents with type 1 diabetes mellitus. *Pediatr Res*, 44, 873-875 (1998)

3259 Malmendier CL, Lontie J-F, Mathe D et al. Lipid and apolipoprotein changes after orthoptic liver transplantation for end-stage liver diseases. *Clin Chim Acta*, 209, 169-177 (1992)

3260 Malozowski S, Muzzo S, Burrows R et al. The hypothalamic-pituitary-adrenal axis in infantile malnutrition. *Clin Endocrinol*, 32, 461-465 (1990)

3261 Maly A. Oligoclonal immunoglobulins in cerebrospinal fluid. *Klin Biochem Metab*, 4, 191-194 (1996)

3262 Mamet R, Gafter U, Korzets A et al. Decreased uroporphyrinogen decarboxylase activity in patients with end-stage renal disease undergoing hemodialysis. *Nephron*, 70, 202-206 (1995)

3263 Man et al. The lipids of serum and liver in patients with hepatic diseases. *J Clin Invest*, 64, 623-643 (1945)

3264 Mandal S, Sarode R, Dash S et al. Hyperaggregation of platelets detected by whole blood platelet aggregometry in newly-diagnosed noninsulin-dependent diabetes mellitus. *Am J Clin Pathol*, 100, 103-107 (1993)

3265 Mandell JR et al. Amyotrophic lateral sclerosis: metabolism of central monoamines and treatment with L-dopa. *Trans Amer Neurol Ass*, 96, 284 (1972)

3266 Mandrup-Poulsen T, Pociot F, Molvig J et al. Monokine antagonism is reduced in patients with IDDM. *Diabetes*, 43, 1242-1247 (1994)

3267 Maneschi F, Geraci P, Barreca P et al. Estradiol, progesterone, 17-hydroxyprogesterone, androstenedione, and CA 125 in patients wtih ovarian carcinoma. *Gynecol Endocrinol*, 6, 25-30 (1992)

3268 Maneva A, Michailova D. Serum antioxidative enzyme activity and juvenile chronic arthritis. *Med Sci Res*, 22, 637-639 (1994)

3269 Manger WM, Steinsland OS, Nahas GG, Wakim KG. Comparison of improved fluorometric methods used to quantitate plasma catecholamines. *Clin Chem*, 15, 1101 (1969)

3270 Manglano CL, Diaz M, Seijas V et al. Biochemical analyses of proteins recovered by bronchoalveolar lavage (BAL) from normal subjects and patients with acquired immunodeficiency syndrome (AIDS). *Clin Biochem Rev*, 14, 203 (1993)

3271 Manicatide MA et al. Breathlessness and blood oxygen tension in patients with chronic bronchitis and emphysema. *Med Interne*, 14, 211-214 (1976)

3272 Manicatide MA et al. Hypoxemia in chronic bronchitis and pulmonary emphysema. *Med Interne*, 15, 41-48 (1977)

3273 Manicourt DH, Triki R, Fukuda K et al. Levels of circulating tumor necrosis factor alpha and interleukin-6 in patients with rheumatoid arthritis. Relationship to serum levels of hyaluronan and antigenic keratan sulfate. *Arth Rheum*, 36, 490-499 (1993)

3274 Manjula S, Aroor AR, Raja A et al. Serum immunoglobulins in brain tumours. *Acta Neurochir*, 115, 103-105 (1992)

3275 Manlet SE, Carter RD, Neil HAW et al. Abnormal triglyceride and HDL cholesterol levels at diagnosis of type II diabetes. *Proc ACB Natl Meet*, 60 (1995)

3276 Manley SE, Bassett P, Christopher P et al. Biochemical variables in type II diabetic patients at diagnosis compared with a normoglycaemic population. *Proc ACB Natl Meet*, 115 (1993)

3277 Manley SE, Burton ME, Fisher KE et al. Decreases in albumin/creatinine and N-acetyl-glucoaminidase/creatinine ratios in urine samples stored at -20 °C. *Clin Chem*, 38, 2294-2299 (1992)

3278 Mann NP, Johnston DI. Total glycosylated haemoglobin (HbA1) levels in diabetic children. *Arch Dis Child*, 57, 434-437 (1982)

3279 Mannello F, Sebastiani M, Amatl S, Gazzanelli G. Prostate-specific antigen expression in a case of intracystic carcinoma of the breast: characterization of immunoreactive protein and literature surveys. *Clin Chem*, 43, 1448-1454 (1997)

3280 Manning EMC, Fraser WD. A survey of diagnoses in patients with a low intact parathyroid hormone concentration. *Ann Clin Biochem*, 30, 252-255 (1993)

3281 Manroe BL et al. The differential leukocyte count in the assessment and outcome of early-onset neonatal group B streptococcal disease. *J Pediatr*, 91, 632-637 (1977)

3282 Mansfield CM, Kimler BF, Henderson SD et al. Angiotensin-I-converting enzyme in cancer patients. *J Clin Oncol*, 2, 452-6 (1984)

3283 Mansour M, Farouk N, Maragy A et al. Elevated plasma level of leukotrienes in bronchial asthma patients: a possible clinical relevance. *Dis Mark*, 12, 117-122 (1994)

3284 Mansour O, Motawi T, Khaled H et al. Clinical value of thymidine kinase and tissue polypeptide specific antigen in breast cancer. *Dis Mark*, 11, 171-177 (1993)

3285 Mantero-Atienza E, Sotoayor MG, Shor-Posner G et al. Selenium status and immune function in asymptomatic HIV-1 seropositive men. *Nutr Res*, 11, 1237-1250 (1991)

3286 Manyam BV, Giacobini E, Colliver JA. Cerebrospinal fluid choline levels are decreased in Parkinson's disease. *Ann Neurol*, 27, 683-685 (1990)

3287 Marchant A, Deviere J, Byl B et al. Interleukin-10 production during septicaemia. *Lancet*, 343, 707-708 (1994)

3288 Marchesi C, Terzi C, Delsignore R et al. Blunted GH response to nicotine from cigarette smoking in 4 week abstinent alcoholics. *Neuroendocrinol Lett*, 13, 349-354 (1991)

3289 Marcovina S, Kottke BA, Mao SJT. Monoclonal antibodies can precipitate low-density lipoprotein. III. radioimmunoassays with single and combined monoclonal antibodies for determining apolipoprotein B in serum of patients with coronary artery disease. *Clin Chem*, 31/10, 1659-1663 (1985)

3290 Marecek Z et al. The effect of long term treatment with penicillamine on the copper content in the liver in patients with Wilson's disease. *Acta Hepatogastroenterol*, 22, 292-296 (1975)

3291 Marel M, Stastny B, Melinova L et al. Diagnosis of pleural effusions: experience with clinical studies, 1986 to 1990. *Chest*, 107, 1598-1603 (1995)

3292 Marescau B, De Deyn PP, Holvoet J et al. Guanidino compounds in serum and urine of cirrhotic patients. *Metabolism*, 44, 584-588 (1995)

3293 Margolis ML, Hyzy JB, Schenken LL et al. Serum tumor markers in non-small cell lung cancer: a comparative analysis. *Cancer*, 73, 605-609 (1994)

3294 Margolis S, Homcy C. Systemic manifestations of hepatoma. *Medicine*, 51, 381 (1972)

3295 Marguerie C, Bunn CC, Black CM, et al. Anti-PL 4 in patients with systemic lupus erythematosus with severe renal and haematological disease. *Q J Med*, 90, 347-352 (1997)

3296 Marhoffer W, Schatz H, Stracke H et al. Serum osteocalcin levels in rheumatoid arthritis: a marker for accelerated bone turnover in late onset rheumatoid arthritis. *J Rheumatol*, 18, 1158-1162 (1991)

3297 Mariani G et al. Pathophysiology of hypoalbuminemia associated with carcinoid tumor. *Cancer*, 38, 854-860 (1976)

3298 Marie C, Losser M-R, Fitting C, et al. Cytokines and soluble cytokine receptors in pleural effusions from septic and nonseptic patients. *Am J Respir Crit Care Med*, 156, 1515-1522 (1997)

3299 Marino M, Chiovato L, Friedlander JA, et al. Serum antibodies against Megalin (GP330) in patients with autoimmune thyroiditis. *J Clin Endocrinol Metab*, 84, 2468-2474 (1999)

3300 Mariotti S, Caturegli P, Barbesino G et al. Glucose tolerance and insulin release in adolescent females. *J Endocrinol Invest*, 14, 751-756 (1991)

3301 Markianos M, Sfagos C, Bistolaki E. Platelet monoamine oxidase and plasma dopamine-β-hydroxylase activities in patients with multiple sclerosis. *Acta Neurol Scand*, 84, 511-533 (1991)

3302 Markus HS, Kapadia R, Sherwood RA. Relationship between lipoprotein (a) and both stroke and carotid atheroma. *Ann Clin Biochem*, 34, 360-365 (1997)

3303 Marner IL et al. Disease activity and serum proteins in ulcerative colitis. *Scand J Gastroenterol*, 10, 538 (1975)

3304 Marrelli D, Roviello F, De Stefano A, et al. Prognostic significance of CEA, CA 19-9 and CA 72-4 preoperative serum levels in gastric carcinoma. *Oncology*, 57, 55-62 (1999)

3305 Marsded S et al. Detection of occult metastatic melanoma by urine chromatography. *Cancer Res*, 36, 3317-3323 (1976)

3306 Marsh JC. Analysis of 106 patients with chronic myelocytic leukemia examined in the University of Utah Hematology Clinic, 1944-1963. *Unpublished*

3307 Marshall et al. Prostatic acid phosphatase levels. *Urology*, 4, 435-538 (1974)

3308 Martelletti P, Granata M, Giacovazzo M. Serum interleukin-1 beta is increased in cluster headache. *Cephalalgia*, 13, 343-345; discussion 307-308 (1993)

3309 Martens HF, Sheets PK, Tenover JS et al. Decreased testosterone levels in men with rheumatoid arthritis: effect of low dose prednisone therapy. *J Rheumatol*, 21, 1427-1431 (1994)

3310 Martin C, Boisson C, Haccoun M, et al. Patterns of cytokine evolution (tumor necrosis factor-α and interleukin-6) after septic shock, hemorrhagic shock, and severe trauma. *Crit Care Med*, 25, 1813-1819 (1997)

3311 Martin EW. *Hazards of Medication*. Philadelphia PA, JB Lippincott (1971)

3312 Martin HE et al. The fluid and electrolyte therapy of severe diabetic acidosis and ketosis. *Am J Med*, 20, 376-388 (1956)

3313 Martin JV et al. The association between serum triglycerides and γ-glutamyl transpeptidase activity in diabetes mellitus. *Clin Biochem*, 9, 208-211 (1976)

3314 Martin RJ et al. Pulmonary alveolar proteinosis. *Am Rev Resp Dis*, 117, 1059-1062 (1978)

3315 Martin TG III, Somberg KA, Meng YG, et al. Thrombopoietin levels in patients with cirrhosis before and after orthoptic liver transplantation. *Ann Intern Med*, 128, 285-288 (1997)

3316 Martin-Ancel A, Garcia-Alix A, Pascual-Salcedo D, et al. Interleukin-6 in the cerebrospinal fluid after perinatal asphyxia is related to early and late neurological manifestations. *Pediatrics*, 100, 789-794 (1997)

3317 Martinez L, Castilla JA, Gil T, et al. Thyroid hormones in fibrocystic breast disease. *Eur J Endocrinol*, 132, 673-676 (1995)

3318 Martinez M, Frank A, Hernanz A. Relationship of interleukin-1 beta and beta 2-microglobulin with neuropeptides in cerebrospinal fluid of patients with dementia of the Alzheimer type. *J Neuroimmunol*, 48, 235-240 (1993)

3319 Martinez ME, Gonzalez J, Sanchez-Cabezudo MJ et al. Evidence of absorptive hypercalciuria in tuberculosis patients. *Calcif Tissue Int*, 53, 384-387 (1993)

3320 Martinez-Brotons F, Oncins JR, Mestres J et al. Plasma kallikrein-kinin system in patients with uncomplicated sepsis and septic shock - comparison with cardiogenic shock. *Thromb Haemostas*, 58, 709-713 (1987)

3321 Martinez-Bru C, Ampudia X, Castrillo P et al. Urinary glycosaminoglycans in active Graves' ophthalmopathy. *Clin Chem*, 38, 2341 (1992)

3322 Martinez-Hernandez D, Barbero JA, Aroca JJ et al. Adenosine deaminase, acquired immunodeficiency syndrome (AIDS), and hepatitis B infection. *Clln Chem*, 38, 162-163 (1992)

3323 Martin-Mateo MC, Sanchez-Portugal M, Iglesias S, et al. Oxidative stress in chronic renal failure. *Renal Fail*, 21, 155-167 (1999)

3324 Martinoli L, Di Felice M, Seghieri G et al. Plasma retinol and α-tocopherol concentrations in insulin-dependent diabetes mellitus: their relationship to microvascular complications. *Int J Vitam Nutr Res*, 63, 87-92 (1993)

3325 Marumo F, Shichiri M, Emori T et al. Circulating and excreted forms of atrial natriuretic peptide in healthy subjects and patients with renal disease. *Clin Nephrol*, 38, 203-208 (1992)

3326 Marwaha G, Grace AA, Slade AKB et al. Plasma levels of brain natriuretic peptide are increased in hypertrophic cardiomyopathy. *Proc ACB Natl Meet*, 36-37 (1994)

3327 Marx JL. The HDL: the good cholesterol carriers? *Science*, 205, 677-679 (1979)

3328 Marz P, Heese K, Hock C, et al. Interleukin-6 (IL-6) and soluble forms of IL-† receptors are not altered in cerebrospinal fluid of Alzheimer's disease patients. *Neurosci Lett*, 239, 29-32 (1997)

3329 Masenko V, Lopatin Y, Mareyev V et al. Elevated plasma β-endorphin levels in congestive heart failure. *Clin Chem*, 39, 1136 (1993)

3330 Masoero G, Andriulli A, Recchia S et al. Trypsin-like immunoreactivity in the diagnosis of acute pancreatitis. *Scand J Gastroenterol*, 15, 21-25 (1980)

3331 Masoero G, Bruno M, Gallo L, et al. Increased serum pancreatic enzymes in uremia: relation with treatment modality and pancreatic involvement. *Pancreas*, 13, 350-355 (1996)

3332 Mason BH, Tatnell MA, Holdaway IM. Measurement of human IGF-II using Sephacryl extraction: a rapid and reliable assay method. *Ann Clin Biochem*, 33, 201-208 (1996)

3333 Mason J, Southwick S, Yehuda R et al. Elevation of serum free triiodothyronine, total triiodothyronne, thyroxine-binding globulin, and total thyroxine levels in combat-related posttraumatic stress disorder. *Arch Gen Psychiat*, 51, 629-641 (1994)

3334 Mason JE Jr et al. Thrombocytosis in chronic granulocytic leukemia: incidence and clinical significance. *Blood*, 44, 483 (1974)

3335 Masry BE et al. LDH isoenzymes in some haemopoietic diseases. *Haematologia*, 7, 405-411 (1973)

3336 Massaron S, Seregni E, Luksch R, et al. Neuron-specific enolase evaluation in patients with neuroblastoma. *Tumor Biol*, 19, 261-268 (1998)

3337 Massart C, Sonnet E, Gibassier J, et al. Clinical validity of intercellular adhesion molecule-1 (ICAM-1) and TSH receptor antibodies in sera from patients with Graves' disease. *Clin Chim Acta*, 265, 157-168 (1997)

3338 Massey SG et al. Calcium metabolism in patients with nephrotic syndrome. *Am J Clin Nutr*, 31, 1572-1580 (1978)

3339 Massey SG et al. Divalent ion metabolism in patients with acute renal failure. studies on the mechanism of acute renal failure. *Kidney Int*, 5, 437 (1974)

3340 Masson P, Palsson B, Andren-Sandberg A. Evaluation of CEA, CA 19-9, CA-50, CA-195, and TATI with special reference to pancreatic disorders. *J Pancreatol*, 8, 333-344 (1991)

3341 Mastroianni CM, Paoletti F, Lichtner M, et al. Cerebrospinal fluid cytokines in patients with tuberculous meningitis. *Clin Immunol Immunopathol*, 84, 171-176 (1997)

3342 Masuda E, Kawano S, Michida T, et al. Plasma and gastric mucosal endothelin-1 concentrations in patients with peptic ulcer. *Dig Dis Sci*, 42, 314-318 (1997)

3343 Masuda H, Kurita Y, Suzuki K, et al. Predictive value of serum immunosuppressive acidic protein for staging renal cel carcinoma: comparison with other tumor markers. *B J Urol*, 80, 25-29 (1997)

3344 Masuda I, Cardenal A, Ono W, et al. Nucleotide pyrophosphorylase in human synovial fluid. *J Rheumatol*, 24, 1588-1594

3345 Matas C, Cabre M, La Ville A et al. Limitations of the Friedewald formula for estimating low-density lipoprotein cholesterol in alcoholics with liver disease. *Clin Chem*, 40, 404-406 (1994)

3346 Mateo MCM, Martin B, Beneit MS, Rabadan J. Catalase activity in erythrocytes from colon and gastric cancer patients] Influence of nickel, lead, mercury and cadmium. *Biol Trace Elem Res*, 57, 79-90 (1997)

3347 Mathiak K, Gowin W, Hebebrand J, et al. Serum leptin levels, body fat deposition, and weight in females with anorexia or bulimia nervosa. *Horm Metab Res*, 31, 274-277 (1999)

3348 Mathiesen T, Andersson B, Loftenius A, von Holst H. Increased interleukin-6 levels in cerebrospinal fluid following subarachnoid hemorrhage. *J Neurosurg.*, 78, 562-567 (1993)

3349 Mathiot C, Galon J, Tartour E, et al. Soluble CD16 in plasma cell dyscrasias. *Leukemia Lymphoma*, 32, 467-474 (1999)

3350 Mathiot C, Mary JY, Tartour E, et al. Soluble CD16 (sCD16), a marker of malignancy in individuals with monoclonal gammopathy of undetermined significance (MGUS). *Br J Hamatol*, 95, 660-665 (1996)

3351 Mathis P, Schmitt L, Benatia M et al. Plasmatic amino acid levels and depression. *Encephale*, 14, 77-82 (1988)

3352 Mathison DA et al. Hypocomplementemia in chronic idiopathic urticaria. *Ann Intern Med*, 86, 534-538 (1977)

3353 Matinlauri I, Ekblad U, Maenpaa K et al. Total renin in pre-eclampsia. *Clin Chim Acta*, 234, 163-170 (1995)

3354 Matinlauri IH, Aalto MA, Ronnemaa T, et al. Elevated serum total renin is insensitive in detecting incipient diabetic nephropathy. *Diabetes Care*, 18, 1357-1361 (1995)

3355 Matsubara K, Yano J, Kitagawa H, et al. Serum platelet-activating factor acetylhydrolase activity in normal pregnancy and preeclampsia. *Hypertens Preg*, 15, 51-59 (1996)

3356 Matsubara N, Fuchimoto S, Iwagaki H et al. Plasma amino acid levels in patients with gastrointestinal cancer. *Cancer J*, 5, 35-37 (1992)

3357 Matsubara T. Interleukin 6 activities and tumor necrosis factor-α levels in serum. *Arerugi*, 40, 147-154 (1991)

3358 Matsubayashi S, Tamai H, Kobayashi N et al. Angiotensin-converting enzyme and anorexia nervosa. *Horm Metab Res*, 20, 761-764 (1988)

3359 Matsuda J, Gohchi K, Gotoh M et al. Plasma concentrations of total/free and functional protein S are not decreased in systemic lupus eryjthematosus patients with lupus anticoagulant and/or antiphospholipid antibodies. *Ann Hematol*, 69, 311-315 (1994)

3360 Matsuda J, Saitoh N, Gochi K et al. Detection of β-2-glycoprotein-I-dependent antiphospholipid antibodies and anti-β-2-glycoprotein-I antibody in patients with systemic lupus erythematosus and in patients with syphilis. *Int Arch Allergy Immunol*, 103, .239-244 (1994)

3361 Matsuda J, Tsukamoto M, Gohchi K et al. Effect of total-body cold exposure on plasma concentrations of von Willebrand factor, endothelin-1 and thrombomodulin in systemic lupus erythematosus patients with or without Raynaud's phenomenon. *Acta Haematol*, 88, 189-193 (1992)

3362 Matsuda M, Shikata K, Wada J, et al. Increased urinary excretion of macrophage-colony-stimulating factor (M-CSF) in patients with IgA nephropathy: tonsil stimulation enhances urinary M-CSF excretion. *Nephron*, 81, 264-270 (1999)

3363 Matsui H, Yudoh K, Tsuji H. Significance of serum levels of type I procollagen peptide and intact osteocalcin and bone marrow density in patients with ossification of posterior longitudinal ligaments. *Calcif Tissue Int*, 59, 397-400 (1996)

3364 Matsuishi T, Sakai T, Nagamitsu S et al. Decreased cerebrospinal fluid levels of β-endorphin in Japanese patients with Joseph disease. *Ann Neurol*, 36, 441-443 (1994)

3365 Matsumiya K, Shimizu T, Matsunaga T et al. Evaluation of a new assay kit of hyaluronic acid (hyaluronic acid "Chugai") and study of serum hyaluronic acid levels as a marker of hepatic fibrosis. *Clin Biochem Rev*, 14, 213 (1993)

3366 Matsumoto S, Hayashi Y, Kinoshita I, et al. immunoaffinity purification of prostaglandin E_2 and leukotriene C_4 prior to radioimmunoassay: application to human synovial fluid. *Ann Clin Biochem*, 30, 60-68 (1993)

3367 Matsumoto T, Iwasaki K. Clinical and laboratory parameters which affect soluble interleukin-2 receptor levels in the serum and synovial fluids of patients with rheumatoid arthritis. *Ann Rheum Dis*, 52, 876-880 (1993)

3368 Matsumoto T, Miike T, Nelson RP et al. Elevated serum levels of IL-8 in patients with HIV infection. *Clin Exp Immunol*, 93, 149-151 (1993)

3369 Matsumoto T, Miike T, Yamaguchi K et al. Serum levels of soluble IL-2 receptor, IL-4 and IgE-binding factors in childhood allergic diseases. *Clin Exp Immunol*, 85, 288-292 (1991)

3370 Matsushima H, Shimohama S, Tanaka S et al. Platelet protein kinase C levels in Alzheimer's disease. *Neurobiol Aging*, 15, 671-674 (1995)

3371 Matsuyoshi N, Tanaka T, Toda K, et al. Soluble E-cadherin: a novel cutaneous disease marker. *Br J Dermatol*, 132, 745-749 (1995)

3372 Matsuzono Y, Narita M, Akutsu Y et al. Interleukin-6 in cerebrospinal fluid of patients with central nervous system infections. *Acta Paediat*, 84, 879-883 (1995)

3373 Mattenheimer H. Enzymes in renal disease. *Ann Clin Lab Sci*, 7, 422 (1977)

3374 Mattsson L, Lindqvist U, Weiland O et al. Serum levels of the aminoterminal propeptide of type III procollagen and hyaluronan during resolving and nonresolving posttransfusion non-A, non-B hepatitis. *Scand J Infect Dis*, 22, 11-17 (1990)

3375 Mattyus I, Zimmerhackl LB, Schwarz A, et al. Elevated urinary excretion of endothelin in insulin-dependent diabetes mellitus: no influence of physical exrecise. *Acta Paediatr*, 85, 1058-1061 (1996)

3376 Maugeri D, Russo MS, Franze C, et al. Correlations between C-reactive protein, interleukin-6, tumor necrosis factor-α and body mass index during senile osteoporosis. *Arch Gerontol Geriat*, 27, 159-163 (1998)

3377 Mauri M, Pico AM, Alfayate R et al. Usefulness of urinary growth hormone (GH) measurement for evaluating endogenous GH secretion in acromegaly. *Horm Res*, 39, 13-18 (1993)

3378 Maury CP, Teppo AM, Froseth B, Wegelius O. α1-Antitrypsin and reactive systemic amyloidosis. *Clin Sci*, 64, 453-454 (1983)

3379 Maury CPJ, Teppo A-M. Comparative study of serum amyloid-related protein SAA, C-reactive protein, and β_2-microglobulin as markers of renal allograft rejection. *Clin Nephrol*, 22, 284-292 (1984)

3380 Maury CPJ, Teppo AM, Eklund B et al. Serum amyloid A levels in human renal allograft rejection. *Clin Sci*, 65, 547-550 (1983)

3381 Mauvais-Jarvis P et al. Benign breast disease: hormonal studies in 125 cases. *Nouv Presse Med*, 6, 4115-4118 (1977)

3382 Mauzerall D, Granick S. The occurrence and determination of δ-aminolevulinic acid and porphobilinogen in urine. *J Biol Chem*, 219, 435 (1956)

3383 Mavromatidis K, Fytil C, Kynigopoulou P, et al. Serum ferritin levels are increased in patients with acute renal failure. *Clin Nephrol*, 49, 296-298 (1998)

3384 Mayatepek E. 5-Oxoprolinuria in patients with and without defects in the γ-glutamyl cycle. *Eur J Pediatr*, 158, 221-225 (1999)

3385 Mayatepek E, Flock B. Increased urinary excretion of LTB_4, and w-carboxy-LTB_4 in patients with Zellweger syndrome. *Clin Chim Acta*, 282, 151-155 (1999)

3386 Mayatepek E, Pecher G. Increased excretion of endogenous urinary leukotriene E_4 in extrahepatic cholestasis. *Clin Chim Acta*, 218, 185-192 (1993)

3387 Mayoss-Hurd D, Izzard A. Retinol and total carotenoid levels in cystic fibrosis. *Proc ACB Natl Meet*, 59 (1993)

3388 Mazure R, Vazquez H, Gonzalez D et al. Bone mineral affection in asymptomatic adult patients with celiac disease. *Am J Gastroenterol*, 89, 2130-2134 (1994)

3389 Mazza DS, Grieco MH, Reddy MM, Meriney D. Serum IgE in patients with human immunodeficiency virus infection. *Ann Allergy Asthma Immunol*, 74, 411-414 (1995)

3390 McArdle B. Familial periodic paralysis. *Br Med Bull*, 12, 226 (1956)

3391 McBlack P. Diagnosis of pituitary tumor. *Hosp Med*, Oct, 43-69 (1985)

3392 McCance DR, Clarke KC, Kennedy L. Serum fructosamine in uraemia, myeloma and acute inflammatory disorders - relationship to serum glucose and albumin levels. *Ann Clin Biochem*, 26, 63-68 (1989)

3393 McCarthy K, Maguire T, McGreal G, et al. High levels of tissue inhibitor of metalloproteinase-1 predict poor outcome in patients with breast cancer. *Int J Cancer (Pred Oncol)*, 84, 44-48 (1999)

3394 McCarty KS, Dodson CE. Pituitary pathology associated with abnormalities of prolactin secretion. *Clin Obstet Gynecol*, 23, 367 (1980)

3395 McCarty MF. Hemostatic concomitants of syndrome X. *Med Hypotheses*, 44, 179-193 (1995)

3396 McClain C, Cohen D, Phillips R et al. Increased plasma and ventricular fluid interleukin-6 levels in patients with head injury. *J Lab Clin Med*, 118, 225-231 (1991)

3397 McClellan JE et al. Survival time of the erythrocyte in myxedema and hyperthyroidism. *J Lab Clin Med*, 51, 91 (1958)

3398 McClelland P, Yaqoob M, Bone JM, et al. Urinary dopamine excretion in chronic renal disease. *Ann Clin Biochem*, 29, 646-651 (1992)

3399 McClure PD. Idiopathic thrombocytopenic purpura in children: diagnosis and management. *Pediatrics*, 55, 68 (1975)

3400 McCormick JR, Thrall RS, Ward PA, Moore VL. Serum angiotensin-converting enzyme levels in patients with pigeon-breeder's disease. *Chest*, 80, 431-3 (1981)

3401 McCullough AJ, Bugianesi E, Marchesni G, Kalhan SC. Gender-dependent alterations in serum leptin in alcoholic cirrhosis. *Gastroenterology*, 115, 947-953 (1998)

3402 McCurdy PR, Sherman A S. Irreversibly sickled cells and red cell survival in sickle cell anemia. *Am J Med*, 64, 253-258 (1978)

3403 McDonnell MG, Archbold GPR. Plasma ubiquinol/cholesterol ratios in patients with hyperlipidaemia, those with diabetes mellitus and in patients requiring ialysis. *Clin Chim Acta*, 253, 117-126 (1996)

3404 McEwen J , Paterson C. Drugs and false-positive screening tests for porphyria. *Br Med J*, 1, 421 (1972)

3405 McFadyen IJ et al. Circulating hormone concentrations in women with breast cancer. *Lancet*, 1, 1100-1102 (1976)

3406 McFarlane I, Bomford A, Sherwood R, eds. *Liver Disease and Laboratory Medicine*. ACB Venture Publications, London (2000)

3407 McFarlane NP, Browning MCK, Quilty P et al. Interpretation of prostatic specific antigen results: some questions answered. *Proc ACB Natl Meet*, 90 (1991)

3408 McFarlin DE, Johnson JS. Studies of antimuscle factor in myasthenia gravis: III. reactions of fragments produced in enzymatic digestion. *J Immunol*, 106, 292 (1971)

3409 McGale EHF et al. Quantitative changes in plasma amino acids in patients with renal disease. *Clin Chim Acta*, 38, 395-403 (1972)

3410 McGowan GK et al. Diagnostic value of plasma amylase especially after gastrectomy. *Br Med J*, 1, 160 (1964)

3411 McGowan L, Bunnag B, Arias LF. Mesothelioma of the abdomen in women. monitoring of therapy by peritoneal fluid study. *Gynecol Oncol*, 3, 10-14 (1975)

3412 McGuckin MA, Layton GT, Bailey MJ et al. Evaluation of two new assays for tumor-associated antigens, CASA and OSA, found in the serum of patients with epithelial ovarian carcinoma - comparison with CA 125. *Gynecol Oncol*, 37, 165-171 (1990)

3413 McGuigan JE. Serum gastrin in health and disease. *Am J Dig Dis*, 22, 712-716 (1977)

3414 McGuinness BJ, Power MJ, Fottrell PF. Radioimmunoassay of 2-hydroxyestrone in urine. *Clin Chem*, 40, 80-85 (1994)

3415 McIlroy M et al. Glucose tolerance in viral hepatitis. *Ir J Med Sci*, 145, 3-9 (1976)

3416 McKay EJ. Measurement of complement as an aid in diagnosis: I. nephrites and collagen disease. *NZ Med J*, 87, 315-318 (1978)

3417 McKee PA et al. Incidence and significance of cryofibrinogenemia. *J Lab Clin Med*, 61, 203 (1963)

3418 McKenna R et al. Non-specific esterase positive acute leukemia. *Proc AAACR/ASCO*, 16, 61 (1974)

3419 McKenzie CG et al. Biochemical markers in bronchial carcinoma. *Br J Cancer*, 36, 700-707 (1977)

3420 McKenzie SW, Dallalio G, North M, et al. Serum chemokine levels in patients with non-progressing HIV infections. *AIDS*, 10, F29-F33 (1996)

3421 McLaren CF, et al. Distribution of transferrin saturation in an Australian population: relevance to the early diagnosis of hemochromatosis. *Gastroenterology*, 114, 543-549 (1998)

3422 McLaughlin P, Stanworth DR. A critical search for evidence of changes in levels in circulating IgE in patients with cancer. *Lancet*, 1, 64-65 (1975)

3423 McLaughlin R, O'Hanlon D, Kerin M, et al. Are elevated levels of the tumour marker CA 19-9 of any clinical significance? *Ir J Med Sci*, 168, 124-126 (1999)

3424 McLean AS. Early adverse effects of radiation. *Br Med Bull*, 29, 69 (1973)

3425 McLellan AC, Thornalley PJ, Benn J et al. Glyoxalase system in clinical diabetes mellitus and correlation with diabetic complications. *Clin Sci*, 87, 21-29 (1994)

3426 McMurray JJ, Ray SG, Abdullah I et al. Plasma endothelin in chronic heart failure. *Circulation*, 85, 1374-1379 (1992)

3427 McMurray W et al. Urinary copper excretion in rheumatoid arthritis. *Ann Rheum Dis*, 34, 340-5 (1975)

3428 McNeely MD, Sunderman FW, Nechay MW, Levine H. Abnormal concentrations of nickel in serum in cases of myocardial infarction, stroke, burns, hepatic cirrhosis, and uremia. *Clin Chem*, 17, 1123-1128 (1971)

3429 McNeely MJ, Chesler SD, Boyko EJ, et al. Association between baseline plasma leptin levels and subsequent development of diabetes in Japanese Americans. *Diabetes Care*, 22, 65-70 (1999)

3430 McNeil AB, Woollard CA. Uinary catecholamines and the diagnosis of pheochromocytoma in Auckland. *NZ Med J*, 110, 2175-2182 (1997)

3431 McNichol KN, Williams HE. Spectrum of asthma in children: i. clinical and physiological components. *Br Med J*, 4, 7 (1973)

3432 Meade TW, Dyer S, Howarth DJ, et al. Antithrombin III and procoagulant activity: sex differences and effects of the menopause. *Br J Haematol*, 74, 77-81 (1990)

3433 Meador CK et al. Cause of Cushing's syndrome in patients with tumors arising from nonendocrine tissue. *J Clin Endocrinol Metab*, 22, 693 (1962)

3434 Mecocci P, Cherubini A, Bregnocchi M, et al. Tau protein in cerebrospinal fluid: a new diagnostic and prognostic marker in Alzheimer's disease? *Alzheimer Dis Assoc Disord*, 12, 211-214 (1998)

3435 Mecz Y, Barak M, Stein A et al. Tumor necrosis factor and tissue polypeptide-specific antigen levels in monitoring bladder cancer. *Diag Oncol*, 4, 148-152 (1994-95)

3436 Mediene S, Hakem S, Bard JM et al. Serum lipoprotein profile in Algerian patients with celiac disease. *Clin Chim Acta*, 235, 189-196 (1995)

3437 Medrano NM, Luz MRMP, Cabello PH, et al. Acute Chagas' disease: plasma levels of α-2-macroglobulin and C-reactive protein in children under 13 years in a high endemic area of Bolivia. *J Trop Pediatr*, 42, 68-74 (1996)

3438 Medri G, Carella C, Padmanabhan V et al. Pituitary glycoprotein hormones in chronic renal failure: evidence for an uncontrolled α-subunit release. *J Endocrinol Invest*, 16, 169-174 (1993)

3439 Meggiato T, Plebiani M, Basso D, et al. Serum growth factors in patients with pancreatic cancer. *Tumor Biol*, 20, 65-71 (1999)

3440 Mehta et al. Leucocyte alkaline phosphatase activity--its utility in diagnosis. *Ind J Med Sci*, 28, 12-18 (1974)

3441 Mehta PD, Dalton AJ, Mehta SP, et al. Increased plasma amyloid β protein 1 - 42 levels in Down syndrome. *Neurosci Lett*, 241, 13-16 (1998)

3442 Meillet D, Labrousse F, Benoit M-O et al. Serum IgA subclasses and interleukin-6 in alcoholic liver disease. *Ann Clin Biol*, 50, 530 (1992)

3443 Meinhold H, Gramm H-J, Meissner W et al. Elevated serum diiodotyrosine (DIT) in severe infections and sepsis: DIT, a possible new marker of leukocyte activity. *J Clin Endocrinol Metab*, 72, 945-953 (1991)

3444 Melegos DM, Diamandis EP, Oda H, et al. Immunofluorometric assay of prostaglandin D synthase in human tissue extracts and fluids. *Clin Chem*, 42, 1984-1991 (1996)

3445 Melegos DN, Yu H, Ashok M, et al. Prostate-specific antigen in female serum, a potential new marker of androgen excess. *J Clin Endocrinol Metab*, 82, 777-780 (1997)

3446 Melichar B, Gregor J, Solichova D et al. Increased urinary neopterin in acute myocardial infarction. *Clin Chem*, 40, 338-339 (1994)

3447 Melichar B, Jandik P, Solichova D, et al. Urinary neopterin excretion in colorectal cancer. *Onkologie*, 17, 434-436 (1994)

3448 Melichar B, Jandik P, Tichy M, et al. Urinary zinc excretion and acute phase response in cancer patients. *Clin Investig*, 72, 1012-1014 (1994)

3449 Melissinos K et al. LDH activity of red cells in chronic renal failure. *Clin Chim Acta*, 40, 165 (1972)

3450 Melissinos K et al. Study of the activity of erythrocyte acid phosphatase in chronic renal failure. *Clin Chim Acta*, 43, 195-199 (1973)

3451 Meljic M, Gorisek B. C-reactive protein and the treatment of pelvic inflammatory disease. *Int J Gynecol Obstet*, 60, 143-150 (1998)

3452 Melmon KL. The endocrinologic manifestations of the carcinoid tumor. In:. *Textbook of Endocrinology*. RH Williams (ed), Philadelphia PA, WB Saunders, 161 (1968)

3453 Meltzer H et al. Serum-enzyme changes in newly admitted psychiatric patients. *Arch Gen Psychiat*, 21, 731-738 (1969)

3454 Menczer J, Schejter E, Geva D, et al. Ovarian carcinoma associated with thrombocytosis. Correlation with prognostic factors and with survival. *Eur J Gynecol Oncol*, 19, 82-84 (1998)

3455 Mendenhall CL, Chedid A, French SW et al. α-Fetoprotein alterations in alcoholics with liver disease. *Alcohol Alcoholism*, 26, 527-534 (1991)

3456 Menell S, Cesarman GD, Jacovina AT, et al. Annexin II and bleeding in acute promyelocytic leukemia. *N Engl J Med*, 340, 994-1004 (1999)

3457 Mennes P et al. Hypomagnesemia and impaired parathyroid hormone secretion in chronic renal disease. *Ann Intern Med*, 88, 206-209 (1978)

3458 Mercer et al. Acid phosphatase isoenzymes in Gaucher's disease. *Clin Chem*, 23, 631-635 (1977)

3459 Meria P, Toubert M-E, Cussenot O et al. Tumor-associated trypsin and renal cell carcinoma. *Eur Urol*, 27, 223-226 (1995)

3460 Merkel PA, Dooley MA, Dawson DV, et al. Interleukin-2 receptor levels in sera of patients with rheumatoid arthritis treated with sulfasalazine, parental gold, or placebo. *J Rheumatol*, 23, 1856-1861 (1996)

3461 Mertz LE et al. Ticks, spirochetes and new diagnostic tests for Lyme disease. *Mayo Clin Proc*, 60, 402-406 (1985)

3462 Messinezy M, Westwood NB, Woodcock SP, et al. Low serum erythropoietin - a strong diagnostic criterion of primary polycythemia even at normal hemoglobin levels. *Clin Lab Haematol*, 17, 217-220 (1995)

3463 Meter TE, Kassianides C, Bothwell TH et al. Effects of heavy alcohol consumption on serum ferritin concentrations. *S Afr Med J*, 66, 573-575 (1984)

3464 Meunier P, Filipe P, Emerit I et al. Adenosine deaminase in progressive systemic sclerosis. *Acta Derm Venereol*, 75, 297-299 (1995)

3465 Meyer D, Larrieu MJ. Factor VIII and IX variants. *Eur J Clin Invest*, 1, 425 (1971)

3466 Meyer LM et al. A study of cholinesterase activity of the blood of patients with pernicious anemia. *J Lab Clin Med*, 33, 1068 (1948)

3467 Meyer MS et al. Low levels of serum calcium, phosphorus and plasma 25-hydroxy vitamin D in cirrhosis of the liver. *Isr J Med Sci*, 14, 725-730 (1978)

3468 Meyer O. The ESR in viral hepatitis. *Pediatrics*, 61, 484-485 (1978)

3469 Meyer-Lehnert H, Bayer T, Predel H-G et al. Effects of atrial natriuretic peptide on systemic and renal hemodynamics and renal excretory function in patients with chronic renal failure. *Klin Wschr*, 69, 895-903 (1991)

3470 MGI Pharma, Inc. Manufacturer's literature on Didronel® . Minnetonka, MN 55343 (1994)

3471 Miale JB. *Laboratory Medicine: Hematology*, 2nd edition, St Louis MO, CV Mosby (1962)

3472 Miale JB. *Laboratory Medicine: Hematology,* 5th edition, St Louis MO, CV Mosby (1977)

3473 Michaels LA, Ohane-Frempong K, Zhao H, Douglas SD. Serum levels of substance P are elevated in patients with sickle cell disease and increase further during vaso-occlusive crisis. *Blood,* 92, 3148-3151 (1998)

3474 Michel U, Shintani Y, Nau R. Serum follistatin concentrations are increased in patients with septicaemia. *Clin Endocrinol,* 48, 413-417 (1998)

3475 Michelakis H, Spanou C, Kondyli A, et al. Plasma tumor necrosis factor-a (TNF-a) levels in Gaucher disease. *Biochim Biophys Acta,* 1317, 219-222 (1996)

3476 Michelis MF et al. Hypouricemia and hyperuricosuria in Laennec's cirrhosis. *Arch Intern Med,* 134, 681-683 (1974)

3477 Michelsen A, Laage M, Froscher W et al. Folic acid in epilepsy and depression. *Clin Biochem Rev,* 14, 350 (1993)

3478 Michener WM. Hyperuricemia and mental retardation with athetosis and self-mutilation. *Am J Dis Child,* 113, 195 (1967)

3479 Mier M et al. Acanthocytosis, pigmentary degeneration of the retina and atoxic neuropathy: a genetically determined syndrome with associated metabolic disorder. *Blood,* 5, 1586 (1960)

3480 Miesch F, Bieth J. The α-2 antitrypsin and α-2 macroglobulin content and the protease inhibiting capacity of normal and pathological sera. *Clin Chim Acta,* 31, 231-241 (1971)

3481 Migdalis MN, Iliopoulou V, Kalogeropoulou K et al. Elevated serum levels of angiotensin-converting enzyme in patients with diabetic retinopathy. *South Med J,* 83, 425-427 (1990)

3482 Migueres J et al. Value theorique et practique de certains dosages enzymatiques au cours des epanchements pleuraux. *J Fr Med Cher Thorac,* 23, 443-58 (1969)

3483 Miida T, Nakamura Y, Inano K, et al. Preβ_1-high-density lipoprotein increases in coronary artery disease. *Clin Chem,* 42, 1992-1995 (1996)

3484 Mikkelson WM. The possible association of hyperuricemia and/or gout with diabetes mellitus. *Arth Rheum,* 8, 853-859 (1965)

3485 Milhaud G et al. *Rencontre Biologique,* Paris, Expansion Scientific, 125 (1975)

3486 Milhaud G et al. Epithelioma de la thyroide secretant de la thryrocalcitonine. *Rend Acad Sci Ser D,* 266, 608 (1968)

3487 Milionis HJ, Elisaf MS, Tselepis A, et al. Apolipoprotein(a) phenotypes and lipoprotein(a) concentrations in patients with renal failure. *Am J Kid Dis,* 33, 1100-1106 (1999)

3488 Mill'AN N'Unez-Cortes J. Biological and clinical aspects of alpha 1-antitrypsin with special reference to malignant tumor processes. *Rev Esp Oncol,* 28, 591-641 (1981)

3489 Miller BF, Dubos RJ. Determination by a specific enzymatic method of the creatinine content of blood and urine. *J Biol Chem,* 121, 457 (1937)

3490 Miller EJ, Cohen AB, Matthay MA. Increased interleukin-8 concentrations in the pulmonary edema fluid of patients with acute respiratory distress syndrome from sepsis. *Crit Care Med,* 24, 1448-1454 (1996)

3491 Miller LC, Kaplan MM. Serum interleukin-2 and tumor necrosis factor-α in primary biliary cirrhosis: decrease by colchicine and relationship to HLA-DR4. *Am J Gastroenterol,* 87, 465-470 (1992)

3492 Miller LH et al. Hyponatremia in malaria. *Ann Trop Med Parasitol,* 61, 265 (1967)

3493 Miller PD et al. Dextrose phosphorus and iron metabolism in alcoholism. *Nutr Rev,* 36, 142-144 (1978)

3494 Miller TR, Anderson RJ, Linas SL et al. Urinary diagnostic indices in acute renal failure, a prospective study. *Ann Intern Med,* 89, 47-50 (1978)

3495 Miller WR, Dawes J. Platelet-associated proteins in human breast fluids. *Clin Chim Acta,* 152, 37-42 (1985)

3496 Miller WW et al. Oxygen releasing factor in hyperthyroidism. *J Am Med Ass,* 211, 1824 (1970)

3497 Milliner DS, Eickholt JT, Bergstralh EJ et al. Results of long-term treatment with orthophosphate and pyridoxine in patients with primary hyperoxaluria. *N Engl J Med,* 331, 1553-1558 (1994)

3498 Milman N, Senglov H, Dombernowsky P. Iron status in patients with small cell carcinoma of the lung. Relation to survival. *Br J Cancer,* 64, 895-898 (1991)

3499 Milne DB. Assessment of copper nutritional status. *Clin Chem,* 40, 1479-1484 (1994)

3500 Milosavljevic J et al. Diagnostic significance of α-fetoproteins in neonatal hyperbilirubinemias and primary cancer of the liver in adults. *Acta Hepatogastroenterol,* 24, 30-33 (1977)

3501 Miltenyi M, Korner A, Tulassay T, Szabo A. Tubular dysfunction in type I diabetes mellitus. *Arch Dis Child,* 60, 929-931 (1985)

3502 Mimic-Oka J, Simic T, Ekmescic V, Dragicevic P. Erythrocyte glutathione peroxidase and superoxide dismutase activities in different stages of chronic renal failure. *Clin Nephrol,* 44, 44-48 (1995)

3503 Mimori T, Ohosone Y, Hama N et al. Isolation and characterization of cDNA encoding the 80-kDa subunit protein of the human autoantigen Ku (p70/p80) recognized by autoantibodies from patients with scleroderma-polymyositis overlap syndrome. *Proc Natl Acad Sci USA,* 87, 1777-1781 (1990)

3504 Mimoz O, Edouard A, Beydon L, et al. Contribution of bronchoalveolar lavage to the diagnosis of posttraumatic pulmonary fat embolism. *Intensive Care Med,* 21, 973-980 (1995)

3505 Min W-K, Lee JO, Huh JW. Relation between lipoprotein(a) concentrations in patients with acute-phase response and risk analysis for coronary heart disease. *Clin Chem,* 43, 1891-1895 (1997)

3506 Minisola S, Romagnoli E, Scarnecchia L et al. Serum carboxy-terminal propeptide of human type I procollagen in patients with primary hyperparathyroidism: studies in basal conditions and after parathyroid surgery. *Eur J Endocrinol,* 130, 587-591 (1994)

3507 Minuz P, Barrow SE, Cockcroft JR et al. Prostacyclin and thromboxane biosynthesis in mild essential hypertension. *Hypertension,* 15, 469-474 (1990)

3508 Mir MA. Renal excretion of uric acid and its relation to relapse and remission in acute myeloid leukemia. *Nephron,* 19, 69-80 (1977)

3509 Mir MM et al. Hypokalaemia in acute myeloid leukaemia. *Ann Intern Med,* 82, 54-57 (1975)

3510 Miron MJ, Perrier A, Bounameaux H, et al. Contribution of noninvasive evaluation to the diagnosis of pulmonary embolism in hospitalized patients. *Eur Respir J,* 13, 1365-1370 (1999)

3511 Misaki F et al. Estimation of serum acid proteases at pH 1.8 and pH 3.5 in patients with duodenal ulcer, gastric ulcer and gastric carcinoma. *Gastroenterol Jpn,* 12, 202-208 (1977)

3512 Misaki M, Shima T, Yano Y et al. Serum transferrin as a marker of bone growth in boys: correlation with serum alkaline phosphatase activity, plasma insulin-like growth factor-I and rate of growth in height. *Horm Metab Res,* 23, 230-232 (1991)

3513 Missiroli A et al. Influence of autologous serum on in vitro reactivity of peripheral lymphocytes of patients with breast cancer. *Tumori,* 63, 129-135 (1977)

3514 Missov E, Mair J. A novel biochemical approach to congestive cardiac failure: cardiac troponin T. *Am Heart J,* 138, 5-9 (1999)

3515 Missow E, Calzolari C, Pau B. Circulating cardiac troponin I in severe congestive heart failure. *Circulation,* 96, 2953-2958 (1997)

3516 Mistilis SP et al. Plasma lipids in extra-hepatic biliary obstruction. *Aust NZ J Med,* 5, 540-543 (1975)

3517 Misumi K, Ogawa H, Yasue H, et al. Comparison of plasma tissue factor levels in unstable and stable angina pectoris. *Am J Cardiol,* 81, 22-24 (1998)

3518 Mitaka C, Hirata Y, Makita K et al. Endothelin-1 and atrial natriuretic peptide in septic shock. *Am Heart J,* 126, 466-468 (1993)

3519 Mitaka C, Hirata Y, Nagura T et al. Circulating endothelin-1 concentrations in acute respiratory failure. *Chest*, 104, 476-480 (1993)

3520 Mitaka C, Nagura T, Sakanishi N et al. Plasma α-atrial natriuretic peptide concentrations in acute respiratory failure associated with sepsis: Preliminary study. *Crit Care Med*, 18, 1201-1203 (1990)

3521 Mitch WE et al. Plasma renin and angiotensin II in acute renal failure. *Lancet*, 2, 328-330 (1977)

3522 Mitchell DN et al. Immunoglobulin levels in patients with sarcoidosis. *Z Erkrank Atm-Org*, 149, 247-252 (1977)

3523 Mitchell LE, Sprecher DL, Borecki IB et al. Evidence for an association between dehydroepiandrosterone sulfate and nonfatal, premature myocardial infarction in males. *Circulation*, 89, 89-93 (1994)

3524 Mitchell P, Smythe G. Hormonal responses to fenfluramine in depressed and control subjects. *J Affect Disord*, 19, 43-51 (1990)

3525 Mittman C et al. Smoking and chronic obstructive lung disease in α_1-antitrypsin deficiency. *Chest*, 60, 214-21 (1971)

3526 Mittman N, Avram MM. Dyslipidemia in renal disease. *Semin Nephrol*, 16, 202-213 (1996)

3527 Mitus WJ et al. Alkaline phosphatase of mature neutrophils in various polycythemias. *N Engl J Med*, 260, 1131 (1959)

3528 Miura H, Nakayama M, Sato T. Serum angiotensin converting enzyme (S-ACE) activity in patients with chronic renal failure on regular hemodialysis. *Jpn Heart J*, 25, 87-92 (1984)

3529 Miura N, Terai M, Meng WG, et al. Serum thrombopoietin levels in Kawasaki disease. *Br J Haematol*, 100, 387-388 (1998)

3530 Miwa A, Adachi J, Mizuno K, Tatsuno Y. Very long-chain fatty acid pattern in crush syndrome patients in the Kobe earthquake. *Clin Chim Acta*, 258, 125-135 (1997)

3531 Miwa K, Igawa A, Inoue H. Soluble E-selectin, ICAM-1 and VCAM-1 levels in systemic and coronary circulation in patients with variant angina. *Cardiovasc Res*, 36, 37-44 (1997)

3532 Miyagawa S et al. Characterization of cryoprecipitates in pemphigus: demonstration of pemphigus antibody activity in cryoprecipitates using the immuno fluorescent technique. *J Invest Dermatol*, 69, 373-375 (1977)

3533 Miyakawa I et al. Plasma levels of human chorionic somatomammotropin progesterone, unconjugated oestradiol and oestriol, and α-fetoprotein in patients with hydatidiform moles. *J Endocrinol*, 72, 371-378 (1977)

3534 Miyakita H, Puri P. Urinary levels of N-acetyl-β-D-glucosaminidase: a simple marker for predicting tubular damage in higher grades of vesicoureteric reflux. *Eur Urol*, 25, 135-137 (1994)

3535 Miyamori I, Takeda Y, Takasaki H et al. Determination of urinary 18-hydroxycortisol in the diagnosis of primary aldosteronism. *J Endocrinol Invest*, 15, 19-24 (1992)

3536 Miyao Y, Nishikimi T, Goto Y, et al. Increased plasma adrenomedullin levels in patients with acute myocardial infarction in proportion to the clinical severity. *Heart*, 79, 39-44 (1998)

3537 Mizutani S, Akiyama H, Kurauchi O et al. Plasma angiotensin I and serum placental leucine aminopeptidase (P-LAP) in pre-eclampsia. *Arch Gynecol*, 236, 165-172 (1984)

3538 Mizutani S, Tomoda Y. Plasma angiotensin I concentration and serum placental leucine aminopeptidase (P-LAP) activities in puerperal hypertension. *Res Comm Chem Pathol Pharmacol*, 81, 271-291 (1993)

3539 Mizutani S, Yamada R, Kurauchi O et al. Serum aminopeptidase A (AAP) in normal pregnancy and pregnancy complicated by pre-eclampsia. *Arch Gynecol Obstet*, 240, 27-31 (1987)

3540 Modahl C, Green L, Fein D, et al. Plasma oxytocin levels in autistic children. *Biol Psychiatr*, 43, 270-277 (1998)

3541 Modena MG, Molinari R, Rossi R, et al. Modification in serum concentrations of aminoterminal propeptide of type III procollagen in patients with previous transmural myocardial infarction. *Am Heart J*, 135, 287-292 (1998)

3542 Modigliani E, Krivitzky A, Guilevin L et al. Carcinoembryonic antigen: first sign of medullary thyroid cancer. *Rev Med Interne*, 12, S340 (1991)

3543 Moelby L, Rasmussen K, Hojgaard Rasmussen H. Serum methylmalonic acid in uraemia. *Scand J Clin Lab Invest*, 52, 351-354 (1992)

3544 Mofenson LM, Harris DR, Rich K, et al. Serum HIV-1 p24 antibody, HIV-1 RNA copy number and CD4 lymphocyte percentage are independently associated with risk of mortality in HIV-1 infected children. *AIDS*, 13, 31-39 (1999)

3545 Mogensen O, Mogensen B, Jakobsen A. Predictive value of CA 125 during early chemotherapy of advanced ovarian cancer. *Gynecol Oncol*, 37, 44-46 (1990)

3546 Moghetti P, Castello R, Magnani CM et al. Clinical and hormonal effects of the 5α-reductase inhibitor finasteride in idiopathic hirsutism. *J Clin Endocrinol Metab*, 79, 1115-1121 (1994)

3547 Mogi M, Harada M, Kojima K et al. Selective removal of β_2-microglobulin from plasma specimens of long-term hemodialysis patients by high-performance immunoaffinity chromatography. *Clin Chem*, 39, 277-280 (1993)

3548 Mogi M, Harada M, Riederer P et al. Tumor necrosis factor-α (TNF-α) increases both in the brain and in the cerebrospinal fluid from Parkinsonian patients. *Neurosci Lett*, 165, 208-210 (1994)

3549 Mohamed AO, Jansson A, Ronquist G. Increased activity of 5'-nucleotidase in serum of patients with sickle cell anaemia. *Scand J Clin Lab Invest*, 53, 701-704 (1993)

3550 Mohammed I et al. Multiple immune complexes and hypocomplementemia in dermatitis herpetiformis and celiac disease. *Lancet*, 2, 487 (1976)

3551 Mohammed S, Addae S, Suleiman S, et al. Serum calcium, parathyroid hormone, and vitamin D status in children and young adults. *Ann Clin Biochem*, 30, 45-51 (1993)

3552 Mohammed SM, Suleiman SA, Addae SK et al. Urinary hydroxyproline and serum alkaline phosphatase in sickle cell disease. *Clin Chim Acta*, 203, 285-294 (1991)

3553 Moirand R, Lescoat G, Delamaire D et al. Increase in glycosylated and nonglycosylated serum ferritin in chronic alcoholism and their evolution during alcohol withdrawal. *Alcohol Clin Exp Res*, 15, 963-969 (1991)

3554 Mokuno K, Riku S, Matsuoka Y et al. Serum carbonic anhydrase III in myotonic dystrophy. *Muscle Nerv*, 9, 257-260 (1986)

3555 Mokuno K, Riku S, Matsuoka Y et al. Serum carbonic anhydrase III in progressive muscular dystrophy. *J Neurol Sci*, 67, 223-228 (1985)

3556 Mol MJTM, de Rijke YB, Denmacker PNM, Stalenhoef AFH. Plasma levels of lipid and cholesterol oxidation products and cytokines in diabetes mellitus and cigarette smoking: effects of vitamin E treatment. *Atherosclerosis*, 129, 169-176 (1997)

3557 Moley KH, Massad LS, Mutch DG. Pelvic inflammatory disease: correlation of severity with CA 125 levels. *J Reprod Med*, 41, 341-346 (1996)

3558 Molina JA, Jimenez-Jimenez FJ, Fernandez-Calle P, et al. Serum lipid peroxides in patients with Parkinson's disease. *Neurosci Lett*, 136, 137-140 (1992)

3559 Molina R, Agusti C, Filella X, et al. Study of a new tumor marker, CYFRA 21-1, in malignant and nonmalignant disease. *Tumor Biol*, 15, 318-325 (1994)

3560 Molina R, Filella X, Bruix J, et al. Cancer antigen 125 in serum and ascites fluid of patients with liver disease. *Clin Chem*, 37, 1379-1383 (1991)

3561 Molina R, Filella X, Torres MD, et al. SCC antigen measured in malignant and nonmalignant diseases. *Clin Chem*, 36, 251-254 (1990)

3562 Molina R, Jo J, Filella X, et al. C-erbB-2 oncoprotein, CEA, and CA 15.3 in patients with breast cancer: prognostic value. *Breast Cancer Res Treat*, 51, 109-119 (1998)

3563 Molina R, Jo J, Filella X, et al. C-erbB-2 oncoprotein in the sera and tissue of patients with breast cancer. Utility in prognosis. *Anticancer Res*, 16, 2295-2300 (1996)

3564 Molina R, Jo J, Filella X, et al. Serum levels of c-erbB-2 (HER-2/neu) in patients with malignant and non-malignant diseases. *Tumor Biol*, 18, 188-196 (1997)

3565 Moliterno AR, Hankins WD, Spivak JL. Impaired expression of the thrombopoietin receptor by platelets from patients with polycythemia vera. *N Engl J Med*, 338, 572-580 (1998)

3566 Moller S, Emmeluth C, Henriksen JH. Elevated circulating plasma endothelin-1 concentrations in cirrhosis. *J Hepatol*, 19, 285-290 (1993)

3567 Moller S, Gulberg V, Henriksen JH, Gerbes AL. Endothelin-1 and endothelin-3 in cirrhosis: relations to systemic and splanchnic haemodynamics. *J Hepatol*, 23, 135-144 (1995)

3568 Moller S, Henriksen JH. Endothelins in chronic liver disease. *Scand J Clin Lab Invest*, 56, 481-490 (1996)

3569 Mollison PL. Measurement of survival and destruction of red cells in haemolytic syndromes. *Br Med Bull*, 15, 59 (1959)

3570 Molnar GB, Salgo L, Kovacs L. Fibronectin determination in pregnancy. *Clin Biochem*, 21, 123-125 (1988)

3571 Molo MW, Kelly M, Radwanska E et al. Preoperative serum CA-125 and CA-72 in predicting endometriosis in infertility patients. *J Reprod Med*, 39, 964-966 (1994)

3572 Molvalilar S, Kocak N. Excretion of vanillylmandelic acid in renal insufficiency. *Lancet*, 2, 1263 (1972)

3573 Moncayo R, Moncayo H. Serum levels of CA 125 are elevated in patients with active systemic lupus erythematosus. *Obstet Gynecol*, 77, 932-934 (1991)

3574 Mononen I, Mononen T, Ylikangas P et al. Enzymatic diagnosis of aspartylglycosaminuria by fluorometric assay of glycosylasparaginase in serum, plasma or lymphocytes. *Clin Chem*, 40, 385-388 (1994)

3575 Montagna MP, Laghi F, Cremona G et al. Influence of serum proteins on fructosamine concentration in multiple myeloma. *Clin Chim Acta*, 204, 123-130 (1991)

3576 Montalban C, Garcia-Unzueta G, de Francisco ALM, Amado JA. Serum interleukin-6 in renal osteodystrophy: relationship with serum PTH and bone remodeling markers. *Horm Metab Res*, 31, 14-17 (1999)

3577 Montalescot G, Ankri A, Chadefaux-Vekemans B, et al. Plasma homocysteine and the extent of atherosclerosis in patients with coronary artery disease. *Int J Cardiol*, 60, 295-300 (1997)

3578 Monteleone P, Maj M, Fusco M et al. Depressed nocturnal plasma melatonin levels in drug-free paranoid schizophrenics. *Schiz Res*, 7, 77-84 (1992)

3579 Montine TJ, Markesbery WR, Morrow JD, Roberts LJ II. Cerebrospinal fluid F_2-Isoprostane levels are increased in Alzheimer's disease. *Ann Neurol*, 44, 410-413 (1998)

3580 Montorsi P, Tonolo G, Polonia J et al. Correlates of plasma atrial natriuretic factor in health and hypertension. *Hypertension*, 10, 570-576 (1987)

3581 Moody BJ, Shakespeare PG, Batstone GF. The effects of septic complications upon the serum protein changes associated with thermal injury. *Ann Clin Biochem*, 22, 391-396 (1985)

3582 Mooradian AD, Morley JE. Endocrine dysfunction. *Arch Intern Med*, 144, 352 (1984)

3583 Mooradian AD, Morley JE, Levine AS et al. The effects of chronic renal failure and hemodialysis on human red and white cell calmodulin levels. *J Clin Endocrinol Metab*, 58, 1010-1013 (1984)

3584 Moore DF et al. Monoclonal γ-globulinemia in malignant lymphoma. *Ann Intern Med*, 72, 43 (1970)

3585 Moore JA, Noiva R, Wells IC. Selenium concentrations in plasma of patients with arteriographically defined coronary atherosclerosis. *Clin Chem*, 30/7, 1171-1173 (1984)

3586 Moore MR et al. Evaluation of human chorionic gonadotropin and α-fetoprotein in benign and malignant testicular disorders. *Surg Gynecol Obstet*, 147, 167-174 (1978)

3587 Moore T et al. Liver physiology and disease. *Gastroenterology*, 63, 88 (1972)

3588 Moore TL et al. Carcinoembryonic antigen assay in cancer of the colon and pancreas and other digestive tract disorders. *Am J Dig Dis*, 16, 1-7 (1971)

3589 Mora A, Perez-Mateo M, Viedma JA, Sanchez-Paya J. Serum β_2-microglobulin in acute pancreatitis. *Int J Pancreatol*, 21, 73-75 (1997)

3590 Mora F et al. An immunological study of nine proteins in CSF and serum of a group of epileptic patients. *Clin Chim Acta*, 80, 55-59 (1977)

3591 Moraglio D, Pagano M, Galeazi D et al. Tissue polypeptide specific antigen (TPS) in liver disease. *Clin Chim Acta*, 224, 209-214 (1994)

3592 Morales A, Bass NE, Verhulst SJ. Serum prolactin levels and neonatal seizures. *Epilepsia*, 36, 349-354 (1995)

3593 Moran A, Radley S, Neoptolemos J, et al. Detection of colorectal cancer by faecal α_1-antitrypsin. *Ann Clin Biochem*, 30, 28-33 (1993)

3594 Moran JP, Cohen L, Greene JM et al. Plasma ascorbic acid concentrations relate inversely to blood pressure in human subjects. *Am J Clin Nutr*, 57, 213-217 (1993)

3595 Moreau R, Hadengue A, Pussard E et al. Relationships between plasma atrial natriuretic peptide concentrations and hemodynamics and hematocrit in patients with cirrhosis. *Hepatology*, 14, 1035-1039 (1991)

3596 Morelli A et al. Dopamine uptake by platelets in hepatic encephalopathy; evidence for a possible depletion of brain dopamine. *Acta Hepatogastroenterol*, 24, 405-410 (1977)

3597 Morelli S, Ferri C, Polettini E, et al. Plasma endothelin-1 levels, pulmonary hypertension, and lung fibrosis in patients with systemic sclerosis. *Am J Med*, 99, 255-260 (1995)

3598 Morel-Maroger L et al. Pathology of the kidney in Waldenström's macroglobulinemia: study of 16 cases. *N Engl J Med*, 283, 123 (1970)

3599 Moreno-Reyes R, Suetens C, Mathieu F, et al. Kashin-Beck osteoarthropathy in rural Tibet in relation to selenium and iodine status. *N Engl J Med*, 339, 1112-1120 (1998)

3600 Morgan LR et al. Arylsulfatase and its relation to homovanillic acid in neuroblastomas. *Clin Chim Acta*, 37, 292-294 (1972)

3601 Morgan RE, Palinkas LA, Barrett-Connor E et al. Plasma cholesterol and depressive symptoms in older men. *Lancet*, 341, 75-79 (1993)

3602 Morganroth J et al. The biochemical, clinical and genetic features of type III hyperlipoproteinemia. *Ann Intern Med*, 82, 158-174 (1975)

3603 Mori M, Murai Y, Hirai M et al. Serum erythropoietin titers in the aged. *Mech Age Dev*, 46, 105-109 (1988)

3604 Mori T, Sasaki J, Kawaguchi H et al. Serum glycoproteins and severity of coronary atherosclerosis. *Am Heart J*, 129, 234-238 (1995)

3605 Morineau G, Boudi A, Barka A, et al. Radioimmunoassay of cortisone in serum, urine, and saliva to assess the status of the cortisol-cortisone shuttle. *Clin Chem*, 43, 1397-1407 (1997)

3606 Moris RS, Gentschein E, Wong IL, et al. Prorenin is elevated in polycystic ovary syndrome and may reflect hyperandrogenism. *Fertil Steril*, 64, 1099-1103 (1995)

3607 Morise T, Takeuchi Y, Takeda R et al. Increased plasma endothelin levels in Kawasaki disease: a possible marker for Kawasaki disease. *Angiology*, 44, 719-723 (1993)

3608 Morishima I, Kumada T, Nakano S et al. Serum levels of soluble interleukin-2 receptor in chronic hepatitis C treated with interferon-α. *Scand J Gastroenterol*, 30, 807-811 (1995)

3609 Morishita E, Saito M, Asakura H et al. Increased levels of plasma thrombomodulin in chronic myelogenous leukemia. *Am J Hematol*, 39, 183-187 (1992)

3610 Morley AA et al. Adrenal steroids and haemolysis in paroxysmal nocturnal haemoglobinuria. *Lancet*, 2, 448 (1967)

3611 Moro L, Gazzarrini C, Modricky C et al. High predictivity of galactosyl-hydroxylysine in urine as an indicator of bone metastases for breast cancer. *Clin Chem*, 36, 772-774 (1990)

3612 Moro L, Modricky C, Rovis L, de Bernard B. Determination of galactosyl hydroxylysine in urine as a means for the identification of osteoporotic women. *Bone Miner*, 3, 1271-1276 (1988)

3613 Moroz C, Bessler H, Katz M, et al. Elevated serum ferritin level in acute myocardial infarction. *Biomed Pharmacother*, 51, 126-130 (1997)

3614 Morrin PAF et al. Rapidly progressive glomerulonephritis. *Am J Med*, 65, 446-460 (1978)

3615 Morris MW et al. The zeta sedimentation ratio (ZSR) and activity of disease in rheumatoid arthritis. *Am J Clin Pathol*, 68, 760-762 (1977)

3616 Morris RS, Stanczyk FZ, Carmina E et al. Alterations in the sensitivity of serum insulin-like growth factor I and insulin-like growth factor binding protein-3 to octreotide in polycystic ovary syndrome. *Fertil Steril*, 63, 742-746 (1995)

3617 Morrison JC et al. Enzyme levels in the serum and cerebrospinal fluid in eclampsia. *Am J Obstet Gynecol*, 110, 619-624 (1971)

3618 Morse JO. α-1-Antitrypsin deficiency. *N Engl J Med*, 299, 1045-1105 (1978)

3619 Morsy MR, Adina H, Sharaf SA et al. Hyperammonemia in marasmic children. *J Trop Pediatr*, 40, 97-99 (1994)

3620 Mortimer G, Casey M. Serum acid phosphatase activities in patients with lung cancer: a biochemical and immunohistochemical analysis of 25 cases. *J Clin Pathol*, 34, 958-962 (1981)

3621 Mortola JF, Laughlin GA, Yen SSC. Melatonin rhythms in women with anorexia nervosa and bulimia nervosa. *J Clin Endocrinol Metab*, 77, 1540-1544 (1993)

3622 Morton JJ, Howe SF, Lowell JA et al. Influence of end-stage renal disease and renal transplantation on serum prostate-specific antigen. *Br J Urol*, 75, 498-501 (1995)

3623 Mosca A, Tagarelli A, Palcari R et al. Rapid determination of erythrocyte pyruvate kinase activity. *Clin Chem*, 39, 512-516 (1993)

3624 Mosekilde L et al. Decreased parathyroid function in hyperthyroidism. *Acta Endocrinol*, 84, 66-75 (1977)

3625 Moseley RH. Evaluation of abnormal liver function tests. *Med Clin N Am*, 80, 887-906 (1996)

3626 Moser PB, Borel J, Majerus T et al. Serum zinc and urinary zinc excretion of trauma patients. *Nutr Res*, 5, 253-261 (1985)

3627 Moses AM, Spencer H. Hypercalcemia in patients with malignant lymphoma. *Ann Intern Med*, 59, 531 (1963)

3628 Moses RG, Theile H, Colagiuri S. The clinical usefulness of 3α-androstanediol glucuronide in premenopausal women with hirsutism. *Aust NZ J Obstet Gynaecol*, 34, 208-210 (1994)

3629 Moshkin AV, Migalina LA. Neuron specific enolase and some other parameters in patients with severe brain injury. *Clin Biochem Rev*, 14, 245 (1993)

3630 Mosnaim MD, Wolf ME, Chevesich J et al. Plasma methionine enkephalin. A biological marker for migraine? *Headache*, 25, 259-261 (1985)

3631 Motojima S, Hirata A, Kushima A et al. Serum levels of soluble interleukin-2 receptor in asthma patients. *J Asthma*, 32, 151-158 (1995)

3632 Motyl T, Traczyk Z, Holska W et al. Comparison of urinary neopterin and pseudouridine in patients with malignant proliferative diseases. *Eur J Clin Chem Clin Biochem*, 31, 205-209 (1993)

3633 Mouly F, Janier M, Nordmann Y, Flageul B. Excretion des porphyrines urinaires au cours de l'infection par le virus de l'immunodeficience humaine. *Presse Med*, 25, 1541-1545 (1996)

3634 Mourdian MM, Heyes MP, Pan JB et al. No changes in central quinolinic acid levels in Alzheimer's disease. *Neurosci Lett*, 105, 233-238 (1989)

3635 Moustapha A, et al. Prospective study of hyperhomocysteinemia as an adverse cardiovascular risk factor in end-stage renal disease. *Circulation*, 97, 138-141 (1998)

3636 Mozas J, Castilla JA, Jimena P, et al. Serum CA-125 in the diagnosis of acute pelvic inflammatory disease. *Int J Gynecol Obstet*, 44, 53-57 (1994)

3637 Mraz W, Jacob K, Cremer P et al. Influence of the thyroid function on the serum concentration of lipoprotein(a). Comparison with low density and high density lipoproteins. *Clin Biochem*, 14, 255 (1993)

3638 Mrowka C, Sieberth HG. Determination of circulating adhesion molecules ICAM-1, VCAM-1 and E-selectin in Wegener's granulomatosis, systemic lupus erythematosus and chronic renal failure. *Clin Nephrol*, 43, 288-296 (1995)

3639 Mudge TJ, James MJ, Jones WR et al. Peritoneal fluid 6-keto prostaglandin F(1α) levels in women with endometriosis. *Am J Obstet Gynecol*, 152, 901-904 (1985)

3640 Mueller WK, Handschumacher R, Wade ME. Serum haptoglobin in patients with ovarian malignancies. *Obstet Gynecol*, 38, 427-435 (1971)

3641 Muggeo M, Zenti MG, Travia D et al. Serum retinol levels throughout 2 years of cholesterol-lowering therapy. *Metabolism*, 44, 398-403 (1995)

3642 Muggia FM et al. Lysozymuria and renal tubular dysfunction in monocytic and myelomonocytic leukemia. *Am J Med*, 47, 351 (1969)

3643 Mukasa H, Nakamura J, Yamada S et al. Platelet monoamine oxidase activity and personality traits in alcoholics and methamphetamine dependents. *Drug Alcohol Dep*, 26, 251-254 (1990)

3644 Mukoyama M, Nakao K, Obata K et al. Augmented secretion of brain natriuretic peptide in acute myocardial infarction. *Biochem Biophys Res Commun*, 180, 431-436 (1991)

3645 Mulder M, Ravid R, Swaab DF, et al. Reduced levels of cholesterol, phospholipids, and fatty acids in cere brospinal fluid of Alzheimer's disease patients are not related to apolipoprotein E4. *Alzheimer Dis Assoc Disord*, 12, 198-203 (1998)

3646 Mulder TPJ, Janssens AR, Verspaget HW et al. Plasma metallothionien concentration in patients with liver disorders: special emphasis on the relation with primary biliary cirrhosis. *Hepatology*, 14, 1008-1012 (1991)

3647 Muldoon MF, Marsland A, Flory JD, et al. Immune system differences in man with hypo- or hypercholesterolemia. *Clin Immunol Immunopathol*, 84, 145-149 (1997)

3648 Muldowney FP et al. The total red cell mass in thyrotoxcosis and myxoedema. *Clin Sci*, 16, 309 (1957)

3649 Muller F, Aukrust P, Nilssen DE et al. Reduced serum level of transforming growth factor-β in patients with IgA deficiency. *Clin Immunol Immunopathol*, 76, 203-208 (1995)

3650 Muller F, Savey L, Le Fiblec B, et al. Maternal serum human chorionic gonadotropin level at fifteen weeks is a predictor for preeclampsia. *Am J Obstet Gynecol*, 175, 37-40 (1996)

3651 Muller MM, Curtius H-C, Herold M et al. Neopterin in clinical practice. *Clin Chim Acta*, 201, 1-16 (1991)

3652 Muller T, Baum SS, Haussermann P, et al. Plasma levels of R- and S-salsolinol are not increased in "de novo" Parkinsonian patients. *J Neural Transm*, 105, 239-246 (1998)

3653 Muller TF, Vogl M, Neumann MC, et al. Noninvasive monitoring using serum amyloid A and serum neopterin in cardiac transplantation. *Clin Chim Acta*, 276, 63-74 (1998)

3654 Muller WA et al. Hyperglucagonemia in diabetic ketoacidosis: its prevalence and significance. *Am J Med*, 54, 52-57 (1973)

3655 Muller-Ladner U, Bosserhoff AK, Dreher K, et al. MIA (melanoma inhibitory activity): a potential serum marker for rheumatoid arthritis. *Rheumatology*, 38, 148-154 (1999)

3656 Mullner M, Sterz F, Binder M, et al. Creatine kinase and creatine kinase-MB after nontraumatic cardiac arrest. *Am J Cardiol*, 77, 581-585 (1996)

3657 Munck-Wikland E, Kuylenstierna R et al. Carcinoembryonic antigen, CA 19-9 and CA 50 in monitoring human squamous cell carcinoma of the esophagus. *Anticancer Res*, 10, 703-708 (1990)

3658 Mundal H-H, Hjemdahl P, Urdal P, et al. β-Thromboglobulin in urine and plasma: influence of coronary risk factors. *Thromb Res*, 90, 229-237 (1998)

3659 Mungan U, Kirkali G, Celebi I, Kirkali Z. Significance of serum laminin P_1 values in patients with transitional cell carcinoma of the bladder. *Urology*, 48, 496-500 (1996)

3660 Munoz MT, Barrios V, Pozo J, Argente J. Insulin-like growth factor I, its binding proteins 1 and 3, and growth hormone-binding protein in children and adolescents with insulin-dependent diabetes mellitus: clinical implications. *Pediatr Res*, 39, 992-998 (1996)

3661 Munroe WA, Southwick PC, Chang L et al. Tau protein in cerebrospinal fluid as an aid in the diagnosis of Alzhemer's disease. *Ann Clin Lab Sci*, 25, 207-217 (1995)

3662 Murakami S, Satomi A, Ishida K et al. Serum-soluble interleukin-2 receptor concentrations in patients with gastric cancer. *Cancer*, 74, 2745-2748 (1994)

3663 Murakami S, Satomi A, Ishida K et al. Serum soluble interleukin-2 receptor in colorectal cancer. *Acta Oncol*, 33, 19-21 (1994)

3664 Murakami S, Satomi A, Ishida K et al. Serum tumor necrosis factor-α and immunosuppressive acidic protein levels in patients with colorectal cancer. *J Jpn Cancer Ther*, 28, 1781-1788 (1993)

3665 Muraki M, Tohda Y, Iwanaga T, et al. Assessment of serum CYFRA 21-1 in lung cancer. *Cancer*, 77, 1274-1277 (1996)

3666 Murata M, Saito T, Takahashi S, et al. Plasma lipoprotein(a) levels are high in patients with central retinal artery occlusion. *Thromb Res*, 91, 169-175 (1998)

3667 Murawaki Y, Ikuta Y, Idobe Y, Kawasaki H. Characterization of tissue inhibitor of metalloproteinases-1 in plasma from patients with chronic liver disease. *Clin Chim Acta*, 254, 77-83 (1996)

3668 Murawaki Y, Ikuta Y, Kawasaki H. Clinical usefulness of serum tissue inhibitor of metalloproteinases (TIMP)-2 assay in patients with chronic liver disease in comparison with TIMP-1. *Clin Chim Acta*, 281, 109-120 (1999)

3669 Murawaki Y, Ikuta Y, Nishimura Y, et al. Serum markers for connective tissue turnover in patients with chronic hepatitis B and chronic hepatitis C: a comparative analysis. *J Hepatol*, 23, 145-152 (1995)

3670 Murawaki Y, Kusakabe Y, Hirayama C. Serum lysyl oxidase activity in chronic liver disease in comparison with serum levels of prolyl hydroxylase and laminin. *Hepatology*, 14, 1167-1173 (1991)

3671 Murdoch JM, Smith CC. Hematological aspects of systemic disease: infection. *Clin Lab Haematol*, 1, 619 (1972)

3672 Murialdo G, Filippi U, Costelli P et al. Urine melatonin in alcoholic patients: a marker of alcohol abuse? *J Endocrinol Invest*, 14, 503-507 (1991)

3673 Murman DL, Foster NL, Kilgore SP, et al. Apolipoprotein E and Alzheimer's disease: strength of association is related to age. *Dementia*, 7, 251-255 (1996)

3674 Murohisa T, Sugaya H, Tetsuka I et al. A case of common bile duct stone with cholangitis presenting an extraordinarily high serum CA 19-9 value. *Intern Med*, 31, 516-520 (1992)

3675 Murone M, Soldarinin A, Gaia P et al. Decrease of plasma concentrations of essential aminoacids and trace elements in HIV-1 infected individuals affected by wasting syndrome. *Clin Chem*, 41, S147 (1995)

3676 Murphy ED, Kallio P. Soluble CD antigen (cytokine) expression in various hyperthyroid states and use in the assessment of propylthiouracil treatment. *J Lab Clin Med*, 124, 255-262 (1994)

3677 Murphy GP et al. Comparison of total and prostatic fraction serum acid phosphatase levels in patients with differentiated and undifferentiated prostatic carcinoma. *Cancer*, 23, 1309-1314 (1969)

3678 Murphy JR. Hemoglobin CC erythrocytes: decreased intracellular pH and decreased affinity-anemia. *Semin Hematol*, 13, 177 (1976)

3679 Murray JF. Arterial studies in primary and secondary polycythemic disorders. *Am Rev Resp Dis*, 92, 435 (1965)

3680 Murray-Lyon IM et al. Prognostic value of serum α-fetoprotein in fulminant hepatic failure including patients treated by charcoal haemofusion. *Gut*, 17, 576-580 (1976)

3681 Murray-Lyon IM et al. Quantitative immunoelectrophoresis of serum proteins in cryptogenic cirrhosis, alcoholic cirrhosis, and active chronic hepatitis. *Clin Chim Acta*, 39, 215-220 (1972)

3682 Murthy VV. Alkaline phosphatase band-10 isoenzyme in serum, resolved by isoelectric focusing electrophoresis is a potential marker of HIV-1 infection in neonates. *Clin Chem*, 39, 1152 (1993)

3683 Murthy VV, Karmen A. Troponin-T as a serum marker for myocardial infarction. *J Clin Lab Anal*, 11, 125-128 (1997)

3684 Muscari A, Bozzoli C, Puddu GM et al. Increased serum IgA levels in subjects with previous myocardial infarction or other major ischemic events. *Cardiology*, 83, 383-389 (1993)

3685 Musoki S, Alitalo R, Stephens RW, Vaheri A. Blast cell-surface and plasma soluble urokinase receptor in acute leukemia patients: relationship to classification and response to therapy. *Thromb Haemost*, 81, 705-710 (1999)

3686 Musso P, Cox I, Vidano E, et al. Cardiac troponin elevations in chronic renal failure: prevalence and clinical significance. *Clin Biochem*, 32, 125-130 (1999)

3687 Mustafa MM, Ramilo O, Saez-Llorens X et al. Role of tumor necrosis factor - (cachectin) in experimental and clinical bacterial meningitis. *Pediatr Infect Dis J*, 8, 907-908 (1989)

3688 Musto P, Matera R, Minervini MM et al. Low serum levels of tumor necrosis factor and interleukin-1β in myelodysplastic syndromes responsive to recombinant erythropoietin. *Haematologica*, 79, 265-268 (1994)

3689 Mutti A, Alinovi R, Ghiggeri GM et al. Urinary excretion of brush-border antigen and plasma proteins in early stages of diabetic neuropathy. *Clin Chim Acta*, 188, 93-100 (1990)

3690 Muzzillo DA, Imoto M, Fukuda Y et al. Clinical evaluation of serum tissue inhibitor of metalloproteinases-1 levels in patients with liver diseases. *J Gastroenterol Hepatol*, 8, 437-441 (1993)

3691 Myerson RM, Frumin AM. Hyperkalemia associated with the myeloproliferative disorders. *Arch Intern Med*, 106, 479 (1960)

3692 Mygind N. Serial serum enzyme studies in infectious mononucleosis. *Scand J Infect Dis*, 8, 139-142 (1976)

3693 Myllyla VV et al. Cyclic AMP concentration and enzyme activities of cerebrospinal fluid in patients with epilepsy or central nervous system damage. *Eur Neurol*, 13, 123-130 (1975)

3694 Myrup B, Bregengard C, Faber J. Primary haemostasis in thyroid disease. *J Intern Med*, 238, 59-63 (1995)

3695 Myrup B, Rossing P, Jensen T et al. Procoagulant activity and intimal dysfunction in IDDM. *Diabetologia*, 38, 73-78 (1995)

3696 Naber THJ, Baadenhuysen H, Jansen JBMJ, et al. Serum alkaline phosphatase activity during zinc deficiency and long-term inflammatory stress. *Clin Chim Acta*, 249, 109-127 (1996)

3697 Naber THJ, van den Hamer CJA, Baadenhuysen H, Jansen JBMJ. The value of methods to determine zinc deficiency in patients with Crohn's disease. *Scand J Gasterol*, 33, 514-523 (1998)

3698 Nachold BS Jr, Kirschner N. The metabolism of adrenaline and noradrenaline in patients with basal ganglia disease. *Neurology*, 13, 753 (1963)

3699 Nachtigall LB, Boepple PA, Pralong FP, Crowley WF Jr. Adult onset idiopathic hypogonadotropic hypogonadism - a treatable form of male infertility. *N Engl J Med*, 336, 410-415 (1997)

3700 Nadal M, Wilkstrom I, Ruthstrom L. Secretory pattern of vasopressin in plasma and of patients with dementia and two control groups cerebrospinal fluid. *Eur J Endocrinol*, 130, 364-369 (1994)

3701 Naeije R et al. A low T3 syndrome in diabetic ketoacidosis. *Clin Endocrinol*, 8, 467-472 (1978)

3702 Naff GB, Byers PH. Possible implication of complement in acute gout. *J Clin Invest*, 46, 1099 (1967)

3703 Nagamine T, Saito S, Yamada S et al. Clinical evaluation of serum biotin levels and biotinidase activities in patients with various liver diseases. *Jpn J Gastroenterol*, 87, 1168-1174 (1990)

3704 Nagasawa T et al. Fibrinogen/fibrin degradation products in serum of patients with ITP. *Thromb Haemostas*, 35, 628 (1976)

3705 Nagataki S et al. Thyroid function in molar pregnancy. *J Clin Endocrinol Metab*, 44, 254-263 (1977)

3706 Nagaya N, Nishikimi T, Goto Y, et al. Plasma brain natriuretic peptide is a biochemical marker for the prediction of progressive ventricular remodeling after acute myocardial infarction. *Am Heart J*, 135, 21-28 (1998)

3707 Nagaya N, Uematsu M, Satoh T, et al. Serum uric acid levels correlate with the severity and the mortality of primary pulmonary hypertension. *Am J Respir Crit Care Med*, 160, 487-492 (1999)

3708 Nagele H, Bahlo M, Klapdor R, et al. CA 125 and its relation to cardiac function. *Am Hear J*, 137, 1044-1049 (1999)

3709 Nagy E, Chalmers IM, Baragar FD et al. Prolactin deficiency in rheumatoid arthritis. *J Rheumatol*, 18, 1662-1668 (1991)

3710 Najean Y et al. Blood volume in health and disease. *Clin Lab Haematol*, 6, 543-564 (1977)

3711 Najean Y, Legrand M, Poirier O et al. Clinical significance of serum pro-collagen III in chronic myeloproliferative disorders. *Eur J Haematol*, 45, 239-243 (1990)

3712 Nakamura RM. Clinical laboratory concepts and methods. In:. *Immunopathology* (1974)

3713 Nakamura RM, Dito WR, Tucker ES III. *Immunoassays in the Clinical Laboratory*, New York NY, Alan R Liss (1979)

3714 Nakamura S, Gohda E, Matsuo Y et al. Significant amount of hepatocyte growth factor detected in blood and bone marrow plasma of leukaemia patients. *Br J Haematol*, 87, 640-642 (1994)

3715 Nakamura T, Ebihara I, Shimada N, Koide H. Elevated levels of erythropoietin in cerebrospinal fluid of depressed patients. *Am J Med Sci*, 315, 199-201 (1998)

3716 Nakamura T, Shoji M, Harigaya Y, et al. Amyloid β protein levels in cerebrospinal fluid are elevated in early-onset Alzheimer's disease. *Ann Neurol*, 36, 903-911 (1994)

3717 Nakamura Y, Takeda T, Ishii M et al. Elevation of serum angiotensin-converting enzyme activity in patients with hyperthyroidism. *J Clin Endocrinol Metab*, 55, 931-934 (1982)

3718 Nakamuta M, Ohashi M, Tanabe Y et al. High plasma concentration of myeloperoxidase in cirrhosis: a possible marker of hypersplenism. *Hepatology*, 18, 1377-1383 (1993)

3719 Nakano I, Funakoshi A, Sumii T et al. Appearance mechanism and molecular heterogeneity of serum pancreatic secretory inhibitor (PSTI). *Gastroenterol Jpn*, 20, 354-360 (1985)

3720 Nakano K, Nakao T, Schram KH et al. Urinary excretion of modified nucleosides as biological marker of RNA turnover in patients with cancer and AIDS. *Clin Chim Acta*, 218, 169-183 (1993)

3721 Nakano T, Chahinian AP, Shinjo M, et al. Interleukin 6 and its relationship to clinical parameters in patients with malignant pleural mesothelioma. *Br J Cancer*, 77, 907-912 (1998)

3722 Nakashima I, Fujihara K, Endo M, et al. Clinical and laboratory features of myelitis patients with anti-neutrophil cytoplasmic antibodies. *J Neurol Sci*, 157, 60-66 (1998)

3723 Nakashima J, Sumitomo M, Miyajima A, et al. A transient increase in serum procollagen 1 carboxyterminal peptide following effective treatment in prostate cancer. *Urol Int*, 58, 236-238 (1997)

3724 Nakashima T, Tanaka M, Okamura S-I. Survey of immunosuppressive acidic protein and other immunological parameters in head and neck cancer patients. *J Laryngol Otol*, 105, 939-845 (1991)

3725 Nakata B, Chung KH-YS, Kato Y, et al. Serum CA 125 level as a predictor of peritoneal dissemination in patients with gastric carcinoma. *Cancer*, 83, 2488-2492 (1998)

3726 Nakata B, Chung KH-YS, Muguruma K, et al. Changes in tumor marker levels as a predictor of chemotherapeutiv effect in patients with gastric carcinoma. *Cancer*, 83, 19-24 (1998)

3727 Nakatsuka K. Serum anti-streptococcal IgA, IgG and IgM antibodies in IgA-associated. *Acta Paediat Jpn*, 35, 118-123 (1993)

3728 Nakayama T, Sonoda S, Urano T et al. Monitoring both serum amyloid protein A and C-reactive protein as inflammatory markers in infectious diseases. *Clin Chem*, 39, 293-297 (1993)

3729 Nakeeb A, Lipsett PA, Lillemore KD, et al. Biliary carcinoembryonic antigen levels are a marker for cholangiocarcinoma. *Am J Surg*, 171, 147-153 (1996)

3730 Nalpas B, Vassault A, Le Guillou A et al. Serum activity of mitochondrial aspartate aminotransferase: a sensitive marker of alcoholism with or without alcoholic hepatitis. *Hepatology*, 4, 893-896 (1984)

3731 Nankerves GA, Kumar M. Diseases produced by cytomegaloviruses. *Med Clin North Am*, 62, 1021-1035 (1978)

3732 Napal J, Amado JA, Riancho JA et al. Stress decreases the serum level of osteocalcin. *Bone Miner*, 21, 113-118 (1993)

3733 Narayanan I et al. Muscular dystrophy. part I: serum enzymes in the Duchenne muscular dystrophy and neuromuscular disorders. *Ind J Med Res*, 62, 598-604 (1974)

3734 Nardi GL et al. Serum trypsin. *N Engl J Med*, 265, 797-798 (1958)

3735 Nardone DA et al. Mechanisms in hypokalemia: clinical correlation. *Medicine*, 57, 435-446 (1978)

3736 Narin F, Narin N, Andac H, et al. Carnitine levels in patients with chronic rheumatic heart disease. *Clin Biochem*, 30, 643-645 (1997)

3737 Narin N, Kutukculer N, Ozyurek R, et al. Lymphocyte subsets and plasma IL-α, IL-2, and TNG-α concentrations in acute rheumatic fever and chronic rheumatic heart disease. *Clin Immunol Immunopathol*, 77, 172-176 (1995)

3738 Narita T, Funahashi H, Satoh Y et al. Procollagen type III N-peptide and type IV collagen 7S-domain in the sera of breast cancer patients. *Surg Today*, 23, 682-686 (1993)

3739 Naruse M, Kawana M, Hifumi S et al. Plasma immunoreactive endothelin-1, but not thrombomodulin, is increased in patients with essential hypertension and ischemic heart disease. *J Cardiovasc Pharmacol*, 17, S471-S474 (1991)

3740 Nasman B, Olsson T, Backstrom T et al. Serum dehydroepiandrosterone sulfate in Alzheimer's disease and in multi-infarct dementia. *Biol Psychiat*, 30, 684-690 (1991)

3741 Nastuk WL et al. Changes in serum complement activity in patients with myasthenia gravis. *Proc Soc Exp Biol Med*, 105, 177 (1960)

3742 Natowicz MR, Prence EM, Cajolet A. Marked variation in blood β-hexosaminidase in Gaucher disease. *Clin Chim Acta*, 203, 17-22 (1991)

3743 Natowicz MR, Wang Y. Plasmahyaluronidase activity in mucolipidoses II and III: marked differences from other lysosomal enzymes. *Am J Med Genet*, 65, 209-212 (1996)

3744 Naudin J, Mege JL, Azorin JM, Dassa D. Elevated circulating levels of IL-6 in schizophrenia. *Schiz Res*, 20, 269-273 (1996)

3745 Navarro JF, Macia ML, Gallego E, et al. Serum magnesium concentration and PTH levels. Is long-term chronic hypermagnesemia a risk factor for adynamic bone disease? *Scand J Urol Nephrol*, 31, 275-280 (1997)

3746 Navis G, Buter H, de Jong PE, et al. Effect of antiproteinuric treatment on the lipid profile in nondiabetic renal disease. *Contrib Nephrol*, 120, 88-96 (1997)

3747 Nawawi H, Samson D, Apperley J, Girgis S. Biochemical bone markers in patients with multiple myeloma. *Clin Chim Acta*, 253, 61-77 (1996)

3748 Neale et al. Effects of intrahepatic and extrahepatic infection on liver function. *Br Med J*, 1, 382-387 (1966)

3749 Necic D, Popovic O, Jolic N et al. Measurement of fecal α_1-antitrypsin excretion in patients with protein-losing enteropathies. *Clin Biochem Rev*, 14, 209 (1993)

3750 Needleman BW, Wigley FM, Stair RW. Interleukin-1, interleukin-2, interleukin-4, interleukin-6, tumor necrosis factor alpha, and interferon-γ levels in sera from patients with scleroderma. *Arth Rheum*, 35, 67-72 (1992)

3751 Neely CL et al. Lactic acid dehydrogenase activity and plasma hemoglobin elevations in sickle cell disease. *Am J Clin Pathol*, 52, 167-169 (1969)

3752 Neidel J, Zander D, Hackenbroch MH. No physiologic age-related increase of circulating somatomedin-C during early stage of Perthes' disease: a longitudinal study in 21 boys. *Arch Orthop Trauma Surg*, 111, 171-173 (1992)

3753 Neil GA, Summers RW, Cheyne BA et al. Analysis of T-lymphocyte subpopulations in inflammatory bowel diseases by three-color flow cytometry. *Dig Dis Sci*, 39, 1900-1908 (1994)

3754 Neilly IJ, Copland M, Haj M et al. Plasma nitrate concentrations in neutropenic and non-neutropenic patients with suspected septicaemia. *Br J Haematol*, 89, 199-202 (1995)

3755 Nelson CS. Review of fat embolism: special reference to cardiac and pulmonary fat embolectomy. In:. *Current Topics in Critical Care Medicine*. Shoemaker WC et al (eds), 153-160 (1976)

3756 Nelson KB, Dambrosia JM, Grether JK, Phillips TM. Neonatal cytokines and coagulation factors in children with cerebral palsy. *Ann Neurol*, 44, 665-675 (1998)

3757 Nelson PV et al. Diagnostic significance and source of lactate dehydrogenase and its isoenzymes in cerebrospinal fluid of children with a variety of neurologic disorders. *J Clin Pathol*, 28, 828-833 (1975)

3758 Nelson R, Jiang N-S, Shellum C. Simple and sensitive immunochemiluminescent assay for tumor necrosis factor-α. *Clin Chem*, 38, 1079-1080 (1992)

3759 Nemeroff CB, Simon JS, Haggerty JJ Jr et al. Antithyroid antibodies in depressed patients. *Am J Psychiat*, 142, 840-843 (1985)

3760 Nemeth A, Samuelson K, Strandvik B. Serum bile acids as markers of juvenile liver disease in α_1-antitrypsin deficiency. *J Pediatr Gastroenterol Nutr*, 1, 479-483 (1982)

3761 Neri B, Bartalucci S, Cataliotti L et al. Clinical utility of the combined use of plurime tumor markers in human breast cancer. *Cancer Detect Prevent*, 13, 115-121 (1988)

3762 Neri B, Bartalucci S, Gemelli MT et al. Creatine kinase isoenzyme BB: a lung cancer associated marker. *Int J Biol Mark*, 3, 19-22 (1988)

3763 Neugut AI, Johnsen CM, Fink DJ. Serum cholesterol levels in adenomatous polyps and cancer of the colon. *J Am Med Ass*, 255, 365 (1986)

3764 Neuhaus TJ, Shah V, Barratt TM. Salivary excretion of endogenous proteins in nephrotic syndrome in children. *Pediatr Nephrol*, 11, 411-414 (1997)

3765 Neumann et al. Distinct alkaline phosphatase in serum of patient with lymphatic leukemia and infectious mononucleosis. *Science*, 186, 151-153 (1974)

3766 Nevalainen TJ. Serum phospholipases A_2 in inflammatory diseases. *Clin Chem*, 39, 2453-2459 (1993)

3767 Nevalainen TJ, Gronroos JM. Serum phospholipase A_2 in inflammatory diseases. *Prog Surg*, 24, 104-109 (1997)

3768 Nevalainen TJ, Kortesuo PT, Rintala E et al. Immunochemical detection of group I and group II phospholipases A_2 in human serum. *Clin Chem*, 38, 1824-1829 (1992)

3769 Nevalainen TJ, Losacker W. Serum phospholipase A_2 in Dengue. *J Infect*, 35, 251-252 (1997)

3770 Newcombe DS, Cohen AS. Chylous synovial effusion in rheumatoid arthritis. *Am J Med*, 38, 156-164 (1965)

3771 Newell-Price J, Trainer P, Perry L, et al. A single sleeping midnight cortisol has 100% sensitivity for the diagnosis of Cushing's syndrome. *Clin Endocrinol*, 43, 545-550 (1995)

3772 Newland P, Yiannakou JY, Calder F et al. Tumour marker CAM 17.1 enzyme linked sandwich assay: value in the diagnosis and monitoring of pancreatic tumours. *Proc ACB Natl Meet*, 19 (1994)

3773 Neyses L, Nitsch J, Biegel T et al. Elevated levels of atrial natriuretic peptide and plasma catecholamines in arterial hypertension - a putative interaction. *Z Kardiol*, 77, 407-412 (1988)

3774 Neyses L, Nitsch J, Tuttenberg H-P et al. Elevated atrial natriuretic peptide (ANP) in essential hypertension - dependence on right atrial pressure. *Klin Wschr*, 67, 756-761 (1989)

3775 Ngan HYS, Chan SYW, Wong LC et al. Serum squamous cell carcinoma antigen in the monitoring of radiotherapy treatment response in carcinoma of the cervix. *Gynecol Oncol*, 37, 260-263 (1990)

3776 Niarchos AP, Resnick LM, Weinstein DL et al. Angiotensin I converting enzyme activity in hypertension. Relationship to blood pressure, renin-sodium profiles, and antihypertensive therapy. *Am J Med*, 79, 435-444 (1985)

3777 Nichols Institute. Professional Services Information. San Pedro, CA (1979)

3778 Nickel K. DHEA-S: new from Bio-Science. *Bio-Science Reports*, Van Nuys CA, Bio-Science Laboratories (1980)

3779 Niederau C, Niederau M, Strohmeyer G et al. Does acute consumption of large alcohol amounts lead to pancreatic injury? A prospective study of serum pancreatic enzymes in 300 drunken drivers. *Digestion*, 45, 115-120 (1990)

3780 Niejadlik DC. Hydroxyproline. *J Postgrad Med*, 51, 213-216 (1972)

3781 Nielsen HJ, Mynster T, Jensen S et al. Effect of ranitidine on soluble interleukin-2 receptors and CD8 molecules in surgical patients. *Br J Surg*, 81, 1747-1751 (1994)

3782 Nielsen HJ, Pappot H, Christensen IJ, et al. Association between plasma concentrations of plasminogen activator inhibitor-1 and survival in patients with colorectal cancer. *Br Med J*, 316, 829-830 (1998)

3783 Nielsen OH, Langholz E, Hendel J et al. Circulating soluble intercellular adhesion molecule-1 (sICAM-1) in active inflammatory bowel disease. *Dig Dis Sci*, 39, 1918-1923 (1994)

3784 Nielsen OJ, Andersen LS, Hansen NE et al. Serum transferrin receptor levels in anaemic patients with rheumatoid arthritis. *Scand J Clin Lab Invest*, 54, 75-82 (1994)

3785 Nielsen OJ, Thaysen JH. Erythropoietin deficiency in acute tubular necrosis. *J Intern Med*, 227, 373-380 (1990)

3786 Niemela O, Risteli L, Sotaniemi EA et al. Type IV collagen and laminin-related antigens in human serum in alcoholic liver disease. *Eur J Clin Invest*, 15, 132-137 (1985)

3787 Niemi M, Kervinen K, Rantala A, et al. The role of apolipoprotein E and glucose intolerance in gallstone disease in middle aged subjects. *Gut*, 44, 557-562 (1999)

3788 Niemi S, Maentausta O, Bolton NJ et al. Time-resolved immunofluorometric assay of sex-hormone binding globulin. *Clin Chem*, 34, 63-66 (1988)

3789 Nightingale S et al. The haematology of hyperthyroidism. *Q J Med*, 185, 35-47 (1978)

3790 Niihara Y, Zerez CR, Akiyama DS, Tanaka KB. Increased red cell glutamine availability in sickle cell anemia: demonstration of increased active transport, affinity, and increased glutamate level in intact red cells. *J Lab Clin Med*, 130, 83-90 (1997)

3791 Niimi A, Amitani R, Suzuki K, et al. Serum eosinophil cationic protein as a marker of eosinophilic inflammation in asthma. *Clin Exp Allergy*, 28, 233-240 (1998)

3792 Niitsu Y, Kohgo Y, Yokota M et al. Radioimmunoassay of serum ferritin in patients with malignancy. *Ann NY Acad Sci*, 450-452 (1990)

3793 Nikkila K, Hockerstedt K, Miettinen TA. Liver transplantation modifies serum cholestanol, cholesterol precursor and plant sterol levels. *Clin Chim Acta*, 208, 205-218 (1992)

3794 Nikkila K, Hockerstedt K, Miettinen TA. Serum and hepatic cholestanol, squalene and noncholesterol sterols in man: a study on liver transplantation. *Hepatology*, 15, 863-870 (1992)

3795 Nikkila M, Pitkajarvi T, Koivula T et al. Elevated high-density-lipoprotein cholesterol and normal triglycerides as markers of longevity. *Klin Wschr*, 69, 780-785 (1991)

3796 Niklinski J, Furman M, Burzykowski T, et al. Preoperative CYFRA 21-1 level as a prognostic indicator in resected primary squamous cell lung cancer. *Br J Cancer*, 74, 956-960 (1996)

3797 Niloff JM et al. CA 125 antigen levels in obstetric and gynecology patients. *Obstet Gynecol*, 64, 703-707 (1984)

3798 Nilsson C, Karlsson G, Blenow KAL, et al. Differences in the neuropeptide Y-like immunoreactivity of the plasma and platelets of human volunteers and depressed patients. *Peptides*, 17, 359-362 (1996)

3799 Nishida K, Kaneko T, Yoneda M, et al. Doubling time of serum CA 19-9 in the clinical course of patients with pancreatic cancer and its significant association with prognosis. *J Surg Oncol*, 71, 140-146 (1999)

3800 Nishida Y, et al. Hyperlipidemia in patients with Down's syndrome. *Arteriosclerosis*, 26, 369-372 (1977)

3801 Nishigaki K, Minatoguchi S, Seishima M, et al. Plasma Fas ligand, an inducer of apoptosis, and plasma soluble Fas, an inhibitor of apoptosis, in patients with chronic congestive heart failure. *J Am Coll Cardiol*, 29, 1214-1220 (1997)

3802 Nishikimi T, Morimoto A, Ishikawa K, et al. Different secretion patterns of adrenomedullin, brain natriuretic peptide, and atrial natriuretic peptide during exercise in hypertensive and normotensive subjects. *Clin Exp Hypertens*, 19, 503-518 (1997)

3803 Nishimura M, Ushiyama M, Ohtsuka K, et al. Serum hepatocyte growth factor as a possible indicator of vascular lesions. *J Clin Endocrinol Metab*, 84, 2475-2480 (1999)

3804 Nishioka K et al. The complement system in tumor immunity: significance of elevated levels of complement in tumor bearing hosts. *Ann NY Acad Sci*, 276, 303-315 (1976)

3805 Nishioka K, Romsdahl MM. Elevation of putrescine and spermidine in sera of patients with solid tumors. *Clin Chim Acta*, 57, 155-161 (1974)

3806 Nishiura T, Suzuki K, Kawaguchi T et al. Elevated serum manganese superoxide dismutase in acute leukemia. *Cancer Lett*, 62, 211-215 (1992)

3807 Nishiya K, Tanimoto N, Hashimoto K, et al. Serum and synovial fluid levels of interleukin-5 in a patient with eosinophilic fasciitis. *Ann Rheum Dis*, 55, 935-936 (1996)

3808 Nishiyama E, Iwamoto N, Kimura M, Arai H. Serum amyloid P component level in Alzheimer's disease. *Dementia*, 7, 256-259 (1996)

3809 Nisman B, Lafair J, Heching N, et al. Evaluation of tissue polypeptide specific antigen, CYFRA 21-1, an carcinoembryonic antigen in nonsmall cell lung cancer. *Cancer*, 82, 1850-1859 (1998)

3810 Nitsch RM, Rebeck GW, Deng M et al. Cerebrospinal fluid levels of amyloid β-protein in Alzheimer's disease: inverse correlation with severity of dementia and effect of apolipoprotein E genotype. *Ann Neurol*, 37, 512-518 (1995)

3811 Niwa T. Phenol and p-cresol accumulated in uremic serum measured by HPLC with fluorescence detection. *Clin Chem*, 39, 108-111 (1995)

3812 Niwa T, Dewald L, Sone J et al. Quantitation of serum 1,5-anhydroglucitol in uremic and diabetic patients by liquid chromatography/mass spectrometry. *Clin Chem*, 40, 260-264 (1994)

3813 Niwa T, Shiobara K, Hamada T et al. Serum pyridinolines as specific markers of bone resorption in hemodialyzed patients. *Clin Chim Acta*, 235, 33-40 (1995)

3814 Niwa T, Takeda N, Miyazaki T et al. Elevated serum levels of 3-deoxyglucosone, a potent protein-cross-linking intermediate of the Maillard reaction, in uremic patients. *Nephron*, 69, 438-443 (1995)

3815 Nixon LS, Yung B, Bell SC, et al. Circulating immunoreactive interleukin-6 in cystic fibrosis. *Am J Respir Crit Care Med*, 157, 1764-1769 (1998)

3816 Nockher WA, Bergmann L, Scherberich JE. Increased soluble CD14 serum levels and altered CD14 expression of peripheral blood monocytes in HIV-infected patients. *Clin Exp Immunol*, 98, 369-374 (1994)

3817 Noel LH et al. Long-term prognosis of idiopathic membranous glomerulonephritis. *Am J Med*, 66, 82-89 (1979)

3818 Noguchi S, Numano F, Gravanis MB, Wilcox JN. Increased levels of soluble forms of adhesion molecules in Takayasu arteritis. *Int J Cardiol*, 66 Suppl 1, S23-S33 (1998)

3819 Noh GW, Lee W, Lee W, Lee K. Effects of intravenous immunoglobulin on plasma interleukin-10 levels in Kawasaki disease. *Immunol Lett*, 63, 19-24 (1998)

3820 Nolph K et al. Antibodies to nuclear antigens in patients with renal failure. *J Lab Clin Med*, 91, 559-567 (1978)

3821 Nomura N, Zolla-Pazner S, Simberkoff M, et al. Abnormal serum porphyrin levels in patients with the acquired immunodeficiency syndrome with or without hepatitis C virus infection. *Arch Dermatol*, 132, 906-910 (1996)

3822 Nomura S et al. Reduced peripheral conversion of thyroxine to triiodothyronine in patients with hepatic cirrhosis. *J Clin Invest*, 56, 643-652 (1975)

3823 Nooijen PTGA, Schoonnderwaldt HC, Wevers RA, et al. Neuron-specific enolase, S-100 protein, myelin basic protein and lactate in CSF in dementia. *Dement Geriatr Cogn Disord*, 8, 169-173 (1997)

3824 Nordin BE, Morris HA, Need AG et al. Relationship between plasma calcium fractions, other bone-related variables, and serum follicle-stimulating hormone levels in premenopausal, perimenopausal and post menopausal women. *Am J Obstet Gynecol*, 163, 140-145 (1990)

3825 Nordman H, Koskinen H et al. Increased activity of serum angiotensin-converting enzyme in progressive silicosis. *Chest*, 86, 203-207 (1984)

3826 Nordoy I, Aukrust P, Muller F, Froland SS. Abnormal levels of circulating adhesion molecules in HIV-1 infection with characteristic alterations in opportunistic infections. *Clin Immunol Immunopathol*, 81, 16-21 (1996)

3827 Norfolk D, Child JA, Cooper EH, et al. Serum β_2-microglobulin in myelomatosis: potential value in stratification and monitoring. *Br J Cancer*, 42, 510-515 (1980)

3828 Norkin SA et al. Thrombotic thrombocytopenic purpura in siblings. *Am J Med*, 43, 294 (1967)

3829 Noronha IL, Daniel V, Schimpf K et al. Soluble IL-2 receptor and tumor necrosois factor-α in plasma of hemophilia patients infected with HIV. *Clin Exp Immunol*, 87, 287-292 (1992)

3830 North WG. Neuropeptide production by small cell carcinoma: vasopressin and oxytocin as plasma markers of disease. *J Clin Endocrinol Metab*, 73, 1316-1320 (1991)

3831 Northoff G, Demisch L, Wenke J, Pflug B. Plasma homovanillic acid concentrations in catatonia. *Biol Psychiatr*, 39, 436-443 (1996)

3832 Northoff H, Berg A. Immunologic mediators as parameters of the reaction to strenuous exercise. *Int J Sports Med*, 12, S9-S15 (1991)

3833 Norwood SH, Torma MJ, Fontenella L. Hyperamylasemia due to poorly differentiated adenosquamous carcinoma of the ovary. *Arch Surg*, 116, 225-226 (1981)

3834 Notman DD et al. Profiles of antinuclear antibodies in systemic rheumatic diseases. *Ann Intern Med*, 83, 464-469 (1975)

3835 Nowacznski W et al. A decreased metabolic benign essential hypertension. *J Clin Invest*, 50, 2184 (1971)

3836 Nowak G, Zieba A, Dudek D, et al. Serum trace elements in animal models and human depression. Part I. Zinc. *Hum Psychopharmacol*, 14, 83-86 (1999)

3837 Nowak J et al. B and T lymphocytes in viral hepatitis. *Pol Med Sci Hist Bull*, 15, 149-154 (1975)

3838 Numata Y, Morita A, Kosugi Y, et al. New sandwich ELISA for human urinary N-acetyl-β-D-glucosaminidase B as a useful clinical test. *Clin Chem*, 43, 569-574 (1997)

3839 NumataY, Dohi K, Furukawa A, et al. Immunoradiometric assay for the N-terminal fragment of proatrial natiuretic peptide in human plasma. *Clin Chem*, 44, 1008-1013 (1998)

3840 Nunez-Gornes JF, Tewksbury DA. Serum angiotensin-converting-enzyme in Crohn's disease. *Am J Gastroenterol*, 75, 384-385 (1981)

3841 Nurminen M, Dejmek A, Martensson G et al. Clinical utility of liquid-chromatographic analysis of effusions for hyaluronate content. *Clin Chem*, 40, 777-780 (1994)

3842 Nyberg A, Lindqvist U, Engstrom-Laurent A. Serum hyaluronan and aminoterminal propeptide of type III procollagen in primary biliary cirrhosis: relation to clinical symptoms, liver histopathology and outcome. *J Intern Med*, 231, 485-491 (1992)

3843 Nydegger UE et al. Circulating complement breakdown products in patients with rheumatoid arthritis. correlation between plasma C_3d, circulating immune complexes, and clinical activity. *J Clin Invest*, 59, 862-868 (1977)

3844 Nygard O, Nordrehaug JE, Refsum H, et al. Plasma homocysteine levels and mortality in patients with coronary artery disease. *N Engl J Med*, 337, 230-236 (1997)

3845 Nylander, Lunqvist E, Back O et al. Prevalence of anti-endothelial cell antibodies in patients with autoimmune diseases. *Clin Rheumatol*, 11, 248-253 (1992)

3846 Nyulassy S et al. Subacute (de Quervain's) thyroiditis: association with HLA-BW35 antigen and abnormalities of the complement system, immunoglobulins and other serum proteins. *J Clin Endocrinol Metab*, 45, 270-274 (1977)

3847 Oades RD, Daniels R, Rascher W. Plasma neuropeptide-Y levels, monoamine metabolism, electrolyte excretion and drinking behavior in children with attention deficit hyperactivity disorder. *Pyschiatr Res*, 80, 177-186 (1998)

3848 Oakley C. The diagnosis of acute pulmonary embolism. *Br J Hosp Med*, 18, 15-24 (1977)

3849 Obiekwe BC, Sturdee D, Cockrill BL et al. Human placental lactogen in pre-eclampsia. *Br J Obstet Gynaecol*, 91, 1077-1080 (1984)

3850 O'Brien JS et al. Tay-Sach's disease: detection of heterozygotes and homozygotes by hexosaminidase assay. *N Engl J Med*, 283, 15 (1970)

3851 O'Brien T, Dinneen SF, O'Brien PC et al. Hyperlipidemia in patients with primary and secondary hypothyroidism. *Mayo Clin Proc*, 68, 860-866 (1993)

3852 O'Brien T, Nguyen TT, Harrison JM et al. Lipids and Lp(a) lipoprotein levels and coronary artery disease in subjects with non-insulin-dependent diabetes mellitus. *Mayo Clin Proc*, 69, 430-435 (1994)

3853 O'Brien T, Nguyen TT, Zimmerman BR. Hyperlipidemia and diabetes mellitus. *Mayo Clin Proc*, 73, 969-976 (1998)

3854 Ockerman PA. Glucose glycerol and free fatty acids in glycogen storage disease type I: blood levels in the fasting and non-fasting state. *Clin Chim Acta*, 12, 370-382 (1965)

3855 O'Connor DT, Cervenka JH, Stone RA et al. Dopamine β-hydroxylase immunoreactivity in human cerebrospinal fluid: properties, relationship to central noradrenergic neuronal activity and variation in Parkinson's disease and congenital dopamine β-hydroxylase deficiency. *Clin Sci*, 86, 149-158 (1994)

3856 O'Connor TA, Ringer KM, Gaddis ML. Mean platelet volume during coagulase-negative staphylococcus sepsis in neonates. *Am J Clin Pathol*, 99, 69-71 (1993)

3857 O'Donnell MC, Catts SV, Ward PB, et al. Increased production of interleukin-2 (IL-2) but not soluble interleukin-2 receptors (sIL-2R) in unmedicated patients with schizophrenia and schizophreniform disorder. *Psychiat Res*, 65, 171-178 (1996)

3858 Oehler G, Budinger M, Heinrich D et al. Antithrombin III changes following myocardial infarct. *Klin Wschr*, 62, 832-836 (1984)

3859 Oen K, Danell G. Interleukin 6 and autoantibodies in juvenile rheumatoid arthritis. *J Rheumatol*, 20, 1949-1956 (1993)

3860 Ogawa H, Yasue H, Miyao Y, et al. Plasma soluble intercellular adhesion molecule-1 levels in coronary circulation in patients with unstable angina. *Am J Cardiol*, 83, 38-42 (1999)

3861 Ogawa K, Shiozu H, Mizuno K et al. Increased plasma cyclic nucleotide concentrations in congestive heart failure. *Br Heart J*, 52, 524-529 (1984)

3862 Ogbuawa O et al. Bacterial endocarditis in narcotic addicts: analysis of arterial blood gases. *South Med J*, 71, 813-814 (1978)

3863 Ogilvie D et al. Urinary outputs of oxalate, calcium, and magnesium in children with intestinal disorders: potential cause of renal calculi. *Arch Dis Child*, 51, 790-795 (1976)

3864 Ogiwara S, Kinchi K, Nagatsu T et al. Highly sensitive, specific enzyme-linked immunosorbent assay of neopterin and biopterin in biological samples. *Clin Chem*, 38, 1954-1958 (1992)

3865 Ogrodowski JL, Hebert LA, Sedmak D et al. Measurement of SCb5-9 in urine in patients with the nephrotic syndrome. *Kidney Int*, 40, 1141-1147 (1991)

3866 Ogunleye IO, Olusi SO. Properties of serum alcohol dehydrogenase in Nigerians with primary hepatoma. *Ann Clin Biochem*, 28, 606-612 (1992)

3867 O'Hanlon M, Salter S, Scull D, Labib M. Neopterin in alcohol-dependent patients. *Ann Clin Biochem*, 33, 536-59 (1996)

3868 Ohashi K, Yukioka H, Mayashi M, Asada A. Elevated methernoglobin in patients with sepsis. *Acta Anaesthesiol Scand*, 42, 713-716 (1998)

3869 Ohashi M, Fujio N, Nawata H et al. Human atrial natriuretic polypeptide in plasma of patients with anorexia nervosa. *Horm Metab Res*, 20, 705-708 (1988)

3870 Ohashi Y, Nakai H, Okamoto Y, et al. Serum level of interleukin-4 in patients with perennial allergic rhinitis during allergen speficic immunotherapy. *Scand J Immunol*, 43, 680-686 (1996)

3871 Ohashi Y, Tanaka A, Kakinoki Y, et al. Serum level of siloble interleukin-2 receptor in patients with seasonal allergic rhinitis. *Scand J Immunol*, 45, 315-321 (1997)

3872 Ohdama S, Matsubara O, Aoki N. Plasma thrombomodulin in Wegener's granulomatosis as an indicator of vascular injuries. *Chest*, 106, 666-671 (1994)

3873 Ohdama S, Takano S, Miyake S et al. Plasma thrombomodulin as a marker of vascular injuries in collagen vascular diseases. *Am J Clin Pathol*, 101, 109-113 (1994)

3874 Ohga E, Nagase T, Tomita T, et al. Increased levels of circulating ICAM-1. VCAM-1, and L-selectin in obstructive sleep apnea syndrome. *J Appl Physiol*, 87, 10-14 (1999)

3875 Ohishi K, Ueno R, Nishimo S et al. Increased level of salivary prostaglandins in patients with major depression. *Biol Psychiat*, 23, 326-334 (1988)

3876 Ohman KP, Karlberg BE. Circulating plasma prekallikrein and tissue kallikrein in normotensive and hypertensive humans: effects of angiotensin II infusion. *Clin Exp Hypertens*, 20, 313-318 (1998)

3877 Ohnishi A, Murakami S, Harada M et al. Renal and hormonal responses to repeated treatment with enalapril in non-azotemic cirrhosis with ascites. *J Hepatol*, 20, 223-230 (1994)

3878 Ohnishi K. Serum levels of thrombomodulin, intercellular adhesion molecule-1, vascular cell adhesion molecule-1, and E-selectin in the acute phase of Plasmodium vivax malaria. *Am J Trop Med Hyg*, 60, 248-250 (1999)

3879 Ohsaka A, Saionji K, Igari j. Granulocyte colony-stimulating factor administration increases serum concentrations of soluble selectins. *Br J Haematol*, 100, 66-69 (1998)

3880 Ohta M, Obayashi H, Takahashi K, et al. Radioimmunoprecipitation assay for glutamic acid decarboxylase antibodies evaluated clinically with sera from patients with insulin-dependent diabetes mellitus. *Clin Chem*, 42, 1975-1978 (1996)

3881 Oian P, Kjeldsen SE, Eide I et al. Adrenaline and preeclampsia. *Acta Med Scand*, 217, 29-32 (1985)

3882 Oian P, Kjeldsen SE, Eide I et al. Increased arterial catecholamines in pre-eclampsia. *Acta Obstet Gynecol Scand*, 65, 613-616 (1986)

3883 Oian P, Monrad-Hansen H-P, Maltau JM. Serum uric acid correlates with β_2-microglobulin in pre-eclampsia. *Acta Obstet Gynecol Scand*, 65, 103-106 (1986)

3884 Oida K, Takai H, Maeda H et al. Apolipoprotein(a) is present in urine and its excretion is decreased in patients with renal failure. *Clin Chem*, 38, 2244-2248 (1992)

3885 Oka N, Akiguchi I, Kawaaki T et al. Elevated serum levels of endothelial leukocyte adhesion molecules in Guillain-Barre syndrome and chronic inflammatory demyelinating polyneuropathy. *Ann Neurol*, 35, 621-624 (1994)

3886 Oka S, Ogino K, Matsuura S, Yoshimura S et al. Human serum immuno-reactive copper, zinc-superoxide dismutase assayed with an enzyme monoclonal immunosorbent in patients with digestive cancer. *Clin Chim Acta*, 182, 209-219 (1989)

3887 Okabe K, Kato I, Sato S et al. Clinical evaluation of tissue plasminogen activator (t-PA) levels in patients with liver diseases. *Gastroenterol Jpn*, 27, 61-68 (1992)

3888 Okada M, Miyazaki S, Hirasawa Y. Increase in plasma concentration of ubiquitin in dialysis patients: possible involvement in β_2-microglobulin amyloidosis. *Clin Chim Acta*, 230, 135-144 (1995)

3889 Okajima K, Fujise R, Motosato Y et al. Plasma levels of granulocyte elastase-α_1-proteinase inhibitor complex in patients with disseminated intravascular coagulation: pathophysiologic implications. *Am J Hematol*, 47, 82-88 (1994)

3890 Okajima K, Uchiba M, Murakami K, et al. Plasma levels of soluble E-selectin in patients with disseminated intravascular coagulation. *Am J Hematol*, 54, 219-224 (1997)

3891 O'Kane PD, McClune JA, Carter GD et al. Changes in serum testosterone and sex hormone binding globulin in male patients with myocardial infarction. *Proc ACB Natl Meet*, 69 (1992)

3892 Okano K, Yamamoto K, Ohba Y et al. Source of elevated serum mitochondrial creatine kinase activity in patients with malignancy. *Clin Chim Acta*, 169, 159-164 (1987)

3893 Okazaki I, Matsuyama S, Suzuki F et al. Endogenous urinary 3-hydroxyproline has 96% specificity and 44% sensitivity for cancer screening. *J Lab Clin Med*, 120, 908-920 (1992)

3894 Okazaki R, Matsuoka K, Atsumi Y et al. Serum concentrations of basement membrane proteins in NIDDM as a prognostic marker for nephropathy. *Diabetes Res Clin Pract*, 27, 39-49 (1995)

3895 Oksanen V, Fyhrquist F, Somer H et al. Angiotensin converting enzyme in cerebrospinal fluid: a new assay. *Neurology*, 35, 1220-1223 (1985)

3896 Okubo H, Yasue H, Ogawa H et al. Plasma lipoprotein(a) levels and fibrinolytic activity in patients with unstable angina. *Jpn Circ J*, 57, 947-954 (1993)

3897 Okuda H, Nakanishi T, Takatsu K, et al. Measurement of serum levels of des-γ-carboxy prothrombin in patients with hepatocellular carcinoma by a revised enzyme immunoassay kit with increased sensitivity. *Cancer*, 85, 812-818 (1999)

3898 Okuno T et al. Value of determination of serum fibrin-fibrinogen degradation products in acute myocardial infarction. *Am J Clin Pathol*, 61, 155-159 (1974)

3899 Olaison L, Hogevik H, Alestig K. Fever, C-reactive protein, and other acute-phase reactants during treatment of infective endocarditis. *Arch Intern Med*, 157, 885-892 (1997)

3900 Olatunbosun DA, Isaacs-Dodeye WA et al. Serum copper in sickle-cell anemia. *Lancet*, 1, 285-286 (1975)

3901 Olbrich HG, Evangeliou A, Tabatabaei SB et al. Correlation between long-chain acylcarnitine in serum and myocardium after heart transplantation in humans. *Am J Clin Nutr*, 60, 414-417 (1994)

3902 O'Leary JA, Feldman M. Serum copper alterations in genital cancer. *Surg Forum*, 21, 411-412 (1970)

3903 Oleesky DA, Rogers C. An investigation of complement activation in newly diagnosed insulin-dependent diabetes mellitus. *Proc ACB Natl Meet*, 119 (1993)

3904 Olivo D, D'Amore M, Mattace-Raso F, Mattace R. Clinical and laboratory features at onset of polymyalgia rheumatica (PMR) and elderly onset of rheumatoid arthritis in PMR-like presentation: a comparison of two groups of patients. *Arch Gerontol Geriatr*, Suppl 5, 527-533 (1996)

3905 Olivo J et al. Studies of protein-binding of testosterone in plasma in disorders of thyroid function. *J Clin Endocrinol Metab*, 31, 539 (1970)

3906 Olmedilla B, Granado F, Gil-Martinez E , et al. Reference values for retinol, tocopherol, and main carotenoids in serum of control and insulin-dependent diabetic Spanish subjects. *Clin Chem*, 43, 1066-1071 (1997)

3907 Olmos JM, Riancho JA, Amado JA et al. Vitamin D metabolism and serum binding proteins in anorexia nervosa. *Bone*, 12, 43-46 (1991)

3908 Olszewski AJ, Szostak WB, McCully KS. Plasma glucosamine and galactosamine in ischemic heart disease. *Atherosclerosis*, 82, 75-83 (1990)

3909 Olt G, Berchuck A, Bast Jr. RC. The role of tumor markers in gynecologic oncology. *Obstet Gynecol Surv*, 45, 570-577 (1990)

3910 Olusi SO et al. Complement components in children with protein-calorie malnutrition. *Trop Geog Med*, 28, 323-328 (1976)

3911 Omland T, Aarsland T, Aakvaag A et al. Prognostic value of plasma atrial natriuretic factor, norepinephrine and epinephrine in acute myocardial infarction. *Am J Cardiol*, 72, 255-259 (1993)

3912 Omland T, Opstad PK, Dickstein K. Plasma neuropeptide Y levels in the acute and early convalescent phase after myocardial infarction. *Am Heart J*, 127, 774-779 (1994)

3913 Ommen SR, Gibbons RJ, Hodge DO, et al. Usefulness of the lymphocyte concentrations as a prognostic marker in coronary artery disease. *Am J Cardiol*, 79, 812-614 (1997)

3914 Ommen SR, Hodge DO, Rodeheffer RJ, et al. Predictive value of the relative lymphocyte concentration in patients with advanced heart failure. *Circulation*, 97, 19-22 (1998)

3915 Onarheim H, Reed RK, Laurent TC. Elevated hyaluronan blood concentrations in severely burned patients. *Scand J Clin Lab Invest*, 51, 693-697 (1991)

3916 Onji M, Doi Y, Miyaoka H et al. Serum levels of soluble CD4 and CD8 in patients with chronic viral hepatitis. *Hepatogastroenterology*, 41, 377-379 (1994)

3917 Ono E, Siratori Y, Okudaira T, et al. Platelet count reflects stage of chronic hepatitis C. *Hepatol Res*, 15, 192-200 (1999)

3918 Ono J et al. Tryptophan and hepatic coma. *Gastroenterology*, 74, 196-200 (1978)

3919 Ono M, Sekiya C, Ohhira M et al. Elevated level of serum Mn-superoxide dismutase in patients with primary biliary cirrhosis: possible involvement of free radicals in the pathogenesis in primary biliary cirrhosis. *J Lab Clin Med*, 118, 476-483 (1991)

3920 Ono Y, Aoki S, Ohnishi K, et al. Increased serum levels of advanced glycation end-products and diabetic complications. *Diabetes Res Clin Pract*, 41, 131-137 (1998)

3921 Ooi BS et al. Serum transferrin levels in chronic renal failure. *Nephron*, 9, 200-207 (1972)

3922 Opatrny K Jr, Opatrny K, Vit L et al. What are the factors contributing to the changes in tissue-type plasminogen activator during hemodialysis? *Nephrol Dial Transplant*, 6, 26-30 (1991)

3923 Oppenheim DS, Kana AR, Sangha JS et al. Prevalence of α-subunit hypersecretion in patients with pituitary tumors: clinically nonfunctioning and somatotroph adenomas. *J Clin Endocrinol Metab*, 70, 859-864 (1990)

3924 Orazi G, Dufour PH, Puech F. Jaundice induced by hyperemesis gravidarum. *Int J Gynecol Obst*, 61, 181-183 (1998)

3925 Ordonez-Llanos J, Rodriguez-Espinosa J et al. Antibody binding serum T3 in a patient with hepatocarcinoma. *J Endocrinol Invest*, 7, 123-127 (1984)

3926 Orfanos AP, Naylor EW, Guthrie R. Micromethod for estimating adenosine deaminase activity in dried blood spots on filter paper. *Clin Chem*, 24, 591-594 (1978)

3927 Orgel HA. Genetic and developmental aspects of IgE. *Pediatr Clin North Am*, 22, 17 (1975)

3928 Orosz L, Udvardy M, Vincze P et al. Connection between plasma thromboxane and prostacyclin levels in the metabolic control of diabetic children. *Orvosi Hetilap*, 13, 125-128 (1989)

3929 Orrett FA. Comparison of CSF C-reactive protein with standard laboratory tests in the diagnosis of inadequately treated and untreated bacterial meningitis. *Med Sci Res*, 22, 843-845 (1994)

3930 Orriss DE. Serum C-reactive protein levels as an indicator of infection in cardiac transplant patients. *Med Lab Sci*, 45, 116-120 (1988)

3931 Orth SR, Ritz E. The nephrotic syndrome. *N Engl J Med*, 338, 1202-1211 (1998)

3932 Osada J, Dabrowska M, Piettruczuk M et al. Macrocytosis due to chronic alcohol consumption. *Diag Lab*, 27, 111 (1991)

3933 Osathanondh R et al. Total and free thyroxine and triiodothyronine in normal and complicated pregnancy. *J Clin Endocrinol Metab*, 42, 98-104 (1976)

3934 Oscarsson J, Wiklund O, Jakobsson K-E, et al. Serum lipoproteins in acromegaly before and 6-15 months after transsphenoidal adenectomy. *Clin Endocrinol*, 41, 603-608 (1994)

3935 O'Shea G. Plasma estriols. *Can J Med Technol*, 41, E132-E134 (1979)

3936 Oshima S, Uchida K, Yasu T et al. Transient increase of plasma lipoprotein(a) in patients with unstable angina pectoris: does lipoprotein(a) alter fibrinolysis? *Arterioslcer Thromb*, 11, 1772-1777 (1991)

3937 Oski FA et al. Use of the plasma acid phosphatase value in the differentiation of thrombocytopenic states. *N Engl J Med*, 268, 1423-1431 (1963)

3938 Osredkar J, Vrhovec I, Jesenovec N et al. Salivary free testosterone in hirsutism. *Ann Clin Biochem*, 522-526 (1989)

3939 Osselaer J-C, Jamart J, Scheif J-M. Platelet distribution width for differential diagnosis of thrombocytosis. *Clin Chem*, 43, 1072-1076 (1997)

3940 Osserman EF. Amyloidosis and plasma cell dyscrasia. *Fourth International Symposium*, 283 (1965)

3941 Osserman EF, Lawlor DP. Serum and urinary lysozyme (muramidase) in monocytic and monomyelocytic leukemia. *J Exp Med*, 124, 921 (1966)

3942 Oster O. Trace element concentrations (Cu, Zn, Fe) in sera from patients with dilated cardiomyopathy. *Clin Chim Acta*, 214, 209-218 (1993)

3943 Ostergaard PA. α-1-Antitrypsin levels and clinical symptoms in forty-eight children with selective IgA deficiency. *Eur J Pediatr*, 142, 276-278 (1984)

3944 Osundeko O, Tetlow L, Bundred N, Gowland E. Radioimmunoassay for serum apolipoprotein D, an atypical apolipoprotein: validation and clinical application. *Ann Clin Biochem*, 34, 537-542 (1997)

3945 Ota T, Katsuki I. Ferritin subunits in sera and synovial fluids from patients with rheumatoid arthritis. *J Rheumatol*, 25, 2315-2318 (1998)

3946 Otani S, Usuki S, Saitoh T et al. Comparison of endothelin-1 concentrations in normal and complicated pregnancies. *J Cardiovasc Pharmacol*, 17, S308-S312 (1991)

3947 O'Toole SM, Chiappelli F, Rubin RT. Plasma neopterin in major depression: relationship to basal and stimulated pituitary-adrenal cortical axis function. *Psychiat Res*, 79, 21-29 (1998)

3948 Otsuki M, Hashimoto K, Morimoto Y, et al. Circulating vascular cell adhesion molecule-1 (VCAM-1) in atherosclerotic NIDDM patients. *Diabetes*, 46, 2096-2101 (1997)

3949 Otsuki M, Oka T, Suehiro I et al. Serum pancreatic secretory trypsin inhibitor in pancreatic disease. *Clin Chim Acta*, 142, 231-240 (1984)

3950 Otto C, Pschierer V, Soennichsen AC, et al. Postprandial hemorrheology and apolipoprotein B metabolism in patients with familial hypertriglyceridemia. *Metabolism*, 46, 1299-1304 (1997)

3951 Oudart J L, Rey M. Proteinurie, protienemie et transaminasemies dans 23 cas de fievre jaune confirmie. *Bull WHO*, 42, 95-102 (1970)

3952 Ouellette DR, Kelly JW, Anders GT. Serum angiotensin-converting enzyme level is elevated in patients with human immunodeficiency virus infection. *Arch Intern Med*, 152, 321-324 (1992)

3953 Owen CA. *Mayo Medical Laboratories Handbook*. Mayo Medical Laboratories, Rochester MN (1977)

3954 Owen EE, Verner JV. Renal tubular diseases with muscle paralysis and hypokalemia. *Am J Med*, 28, 8 (1960)

3955 Ozan H, Wsmer A, Ko Nlsal, et al. Plasma ascorbic acid level and erythrocte fragility in preeclampsis and eclampsia. *Eur J Obstet Gynecol*, 71, 35-40 (1997)

3956 Ozata M, Bulur M, Bingol N, et al. Daytime plasma melatonin levels in male hypogonadism. *J Clin Endocrinol Metab*, 81, 1877-1881 (1996)

3957 Ozawa T, Ninomiya Y, Honma T et al. Increased serum angiotensin I-converting enzyme activity in patients with mixed connective tissue disease and pulmonary hypertension. *Scand J Rheumatol*, 24, 38-43 (1995)

3958 Ozben T. Elevated serum and urine sialic acid levels in renal diseases. *Ann Clin Biochem*, 28, 44-48 (1991)

3959 Ozben T, Nacitarhan S, Tuncer N. Plasma and urine sialic acid in non-insulin dependent diabetes mellitus. *Ann Clin Biochem*, 32, 303-306 (1995)

3960 Ozdemir A, Oygur N, Gultekin M et al. Neonatal tumor necrosis factor, interleukin-1α, interleukin-1β, and interleukin-6 response to infection. *Am J Perinatol*, 11, 282-285 (1994)

3961 Ozeki T, Imanishi K, Unoki H et al. Interleukin-1 and -2 in sera of patients with chronic hepatitis (type B). *Int J Exp Pathol*, 11, 815-821 (1990)

3962 Ozen S, Saatci U, Tinaztepe K et al. Urinary tumor necrosis factor levels in primary glomerulonephropathies. *Nephron*, 66, 291-294 (1994)

3963 Ozgunes H, Gurer H, Tuncer S. Correlation between plasma malondialdehyde and ceruloplasmin activity values in rheumatoid arthritis. *Clin Biochem*, 28, 193-194 (1995)

3964 Ozgunes H, Sinan Beksac M, Duru S et al. Instant effect of induced abortion on serum ceruloplasmin activity, copper and zinc levels. *Arch Gynecol Obstet*, 240, 21-25 (1987)

3965 Ozoran K, Aydintug O, Tokgoz G, et al. Serum levels of interleukin-8 in patients with Behcet's disease. *Br Med J*, 610

3966 Paarlberg KM, de Jong CLD, van Geijn HP, et al. Total plasma fibronectin as a marker of pregnancy-induced hypertensive disorders: a longitudinal study. *Obstet Gynecol*, 91, 383-388 (1998)

3967 Pacher R, Berger-Klein J, Globits S et al. Plasma big endothelin-1 concentrations in congestive heart failure patients with or without systemic hypertension. *Am J Cardiol.*, 71, 1293-1299 (1993)

3968 Paddock RK, Smith SE. The platelets in pernicious anemia. *Am J Med Sci*, 198, 372 (1939)

3969 Padova J et al. Hyperuricemia in diabetic ketoacidosis. *N Engl J Med*, 267, 530-534 (1962)

3970 Pagligra AS, Goodman AD. Elevation of plasma glutamate in gout, its possible role in the pathogenesis of hyperuricemia. *N Engl J Med*, 281, 767 (1969)

3971 Pahpiha et al. Serum alkaline phosphatase in patients with multiple sclerosis. *Clin Genet*, 7, 77-82 (1975)

3972 Pahwa et al. HTLV-III infection in children. *J Am Med Ass*, 255, 2301 (1986)

3973 Pai S, Pai L, Birkenfeldt R. Correlation of serum IgA rheumatoid factor levels with disease severity in rheumatoid arthritis. *Scand J Rheumatol*, 27, 252-256 (1998)

3974 Paiker JE, Raal FJ, von Arb M. Auto-antibodies against oxidized LDL as a marker of coronary artery disease in patients with familial hypercholesterolaemia. *Ann Clin Biochem*, 37, 174-178 (2000)

3975 Paimela L, Heiskanen A, Kurki P et al. Serum hyaluronate level as a predictor of radiologic progression in early rheumatoid arthritis. *Arth Rheum*, 34, 815-821 (1991)

3976 Palicka V, Vavrova J, Smahelova A et al. Carnitine concentration changes during hemodialysis. *Clin Biochem Rev*, 14, 260 (1993)

3977 Palicka V, Zivny P, Erben J et al. Concentration changes of some cytokines during hemodialysis. *Clin Biochem Rev*, 14, 217 (1993)

3978 Pall HS et al. Raised cerebrospinal-fluid copper concentrations in Parkinson's disease. *Lancet*, 2, 238 (1987)

3979 Pall RH, Kantor FS. Serum complement in eclamptogenic toxemia. *Am J Obstet Gynecol*, 95, 530 (1966)

3980 Pallas D, Koutras DA, Adamopoulos P et al. Increased mean serum thyrotropin in apparently euthyroid hypercholesterolemic patients: does it mean occult hypothyroidism? *J Endocrinol Invest*, 14, 743-746 (1991)

3981 Palmer AM, Sims NR, Bowen DM, Neary D. Monoamine metabolite concentrations in lumbar cerebrospinal fluid of patients with histologically verified Alzheimer's dementia. *J Neurol Neurosurg Psychiatry*, 47, 481-484 (1984)

3982 Palmer et al. The chloride-phosphate ratio in hypercalcemia. *Ann Intern Med*, 80, 200-204 (1974)

3983 Paloyan D et al. Carcinoembryonic antigen levels in pancreatic carcinoma. *Am Surg*, 43, 410 (1977)

3984 Palsson B, Andren-Sandberg A, Masson P. Plasma concentrations of CA-50 in relation to tumor burden in exocrine pancreatic cancer. *Eur J Cancer*, 27, 1279-1282 (1991)

3985 Paltiel O, Falutz J, Veilleux M, et al. Clinical correlates of subnormal vitamin B_{12} levels in patients infected with human immunodeficiency virus. *Am J Hematol*, 49, 318-322 (1995)

3986 Pandey GN, Fawcett J, Gibbons R et al. Platelet monoamine oxidase in alcholism. *Biol Psychiat*, 24, 15-24 (1988)

3987 Pandian MR, Morgan CH, Carlton E et al. Modified immunoradiometric assay of parathyroid hormone-related protein: clinical application in the differential diagnosis of hypercalcemia. *Clin Chem*, 38, 282-288 (1992)

3988 Pandolfino J, Hakimian D, Rademaker AW, Tallman MS. Hypocholesterolemia in hairy cell leukemia: a marker for proliferative activity. *Am J Hematol*, 55, 129-133 (1997)

3989 Pang S, Wang M, Jefferies S et al. Normal and elevated 3α-androstanediol glucuronide concentrations in women with various causes of hirsutism and its correlation with degree of hirsutism and androgen levels. *J Clin Endocrinol Metab*, 75, 243-248 (1992)

3990 Panidis D, Vavilis D, Rousso D et al. Danazol influences gonadotropin secretion at the hypothalamic level. *Int J Gynaecol Obstet*, 45, 241-246 (1994)

3991 Panidis D, Vavilis D, Rousso D et al. Provocative tests of prolactin before, during and after long-term danazol treatment in patients with endometriosis. *Gynecol Endocrinol*, 6, 19-24 (1992)

3992 Pansadero V, Emiliozzi P, Defido L, et al. Prostate-specific antigen and prostatitis in men under fifty. *Eur Urol*, 30, 24-27 (1996)

3993 Panteghini M. Electrophoretic fractionation of 5'-nucleotidase. *Clin Chem*, 40, 190-196 (1994)

3994 Panz VR, Wing JR, Raal FJ, et al. Improved glucose tolerance after effective lipid-lowering therapy with bezafibrate in a patient with lipoatrophic diabetes mellitus: a putative role for Randle's cycle in its pathogenesis. *Clin Endocrinol*, 46, 365-368 (1997)

3995 Panzer A, Viljoen M. Urinary 6-sulfatoxymelatonin levels in osteosarcoma: a case-control study. *Med Sci Res*, 26, 43-45 (1998)

3996 Panzer S, Kronik G, Lechner K, Bettelheim P. Glycosylated hemoglobins (GHB): an index of red cell survival. *Blood*, 59, 1348-1350 (1982)

3997 Paoli I, Dave M, Cohen BD. Pharmacodynamics of zidovudine in patients with end-stage renal disease. *N Engl J Med*, 326, 839 (1992)

3998 Papapoulos SE, Frolich M, Mudde AG et al. Serum osteocalcin in Paget's disease of bone: basal concentrations and response to bisphonate treatment. *J Clin Endocrinol Metab*, 65, 89-94 (1987)

3999 Papianicolaou DA, Wilder RL, Manolagos SC, Chrousos GP. The pathophysiologic roles of interleukin-6 in human disease. *Ann Intern Med*, 128, 127-137 (1998)

4000 Paradisi R, Capelli M, Mandini M, et al. Interleukin-2 in seminal plasma of fertile and infertile men. *Arch Androl*, 35, 35-41 (1995)

4001 Paradowski M, Lobos M, Kuydowicz J, et al. Acute phase proteins in serum and cerebrospinal fluid in the course of bacterial meningitis. *Clin Biochem*, 28, 459-466 (1995)

4002 Paragh G, Seres I, Balogh Z, et al. The serum paraoxonase activity in patients with chronic renal failure and hyperlipidemia. *Nephron*, 80, 166-170 (1998)

4003 Paramo JA, Panizo C, Montes , et al. Markers of fibrinolytic potency and clotting activation in stable angina pectoris: role of urokinase, assessment of artrioventricular differences and correlation with coronary patency. *Fibrinolysis Proteolysis*, 13, 133-138 (1999)

4004 Parida SK, Grau GE, Zaheer SA et al. Serum tumor necrosis factor and interleukin 1 in leprosy and during lepra reactions. *Clin Immunol Immunopathol*, 63, 23-27 (1992)

4005 Park CW, Song HC, Shin YS, et al. Urinary soluble HLA class I antigen in patients with minimal change disease: a predictor of steroid response. *Nephron*, 79, 44-49 (1998)

4006 Park Y-D, Yasui M, Yoshimoto T, et al. Changes in hemostatic parameters in hepatic veno-occlusive disease following bone marrow transplantation. *Bone Marrow Transplant*, 19, 915-920 (1997)

4007 Parke-Davis. Manufacturer's literature on Cerebyx® . Morris Plains, NJ 07950 (1996)

4008 Parke-Davis. Manufacturer's literature on Dilantin® . Morris Plains, NJ 07950 (1995)

4009 Parker CW, et al. Leukocyte and lymphocyte cyclic AMP responses in atopic eczema. *J Invest Dermatol*, 68, 302-306 (1977)

4010 Parker D, Bradley C, Bogle SM, et al. Serum albumin and CA 125 are powerful predictors of survival in epithelial ovarian cancer. *Br J Obstet Gynaecol*, 101, 888-893 (1994)

4011 Parker MD, et al. Comparison of the complement-fixing activity of antinuclear antibodies in lupus nephritis, mixed connective tissue disease, and scleroderma. *Arth Rheum*, 19, 857-861 (1976)

4012 Parkkila AK, Parkkila S, Reunanen M, et al. Carbonic anhydrase II in the cerebrospinal fluid: its value as a disease marker. *Eur J Clin Invest*, 27, 392-397 (1997)

4013 Parmar VP et al. A study of magnesium serum and urine in acute nephritis and nephrotic syndrome in childhood. *Ind J Pediatr*, 13, 701-706 (1976)

4014 Parrish RW, Williams JD, Davies BH. Serum β_2 microglobulin and angiotensin-converting enzyme activity in sarcoidosis. *Thorax*, 37, 936-940 (1982)

4015 Parson HA et al. Erythrokinetic studies in thalassemia trait. *J Lab Clin Med*, 56, 866 (1960)

4016 Parsons V et al. Use of dialysis in the treatment of renal failure in liver disease. *Postgrad Med J*, 51, 515-20 (1975)

4017 Partin AW, Criley SR, Steiner MS, et al. Serum ferritin as a clinical marker for renal cell carcinoma: influence of tumor volume. *Urology*, 45, 211-217 (1995)

4018 Partin AW, Simons JW, Criley SR et al. Serum ferritin as a clinical marker for renal carcinoma: influence of tumor volume. *Urology*, 45, 211-217 (1995)

4019 Parviainen MT, Jaaskelainen K, Kroger H, et al. Urinary bone resorption markers in monitoring treatment of symptomatic osteoporosis. *Clin Chim Acta*, 279, 145-154 (1999)

4020 Pasanen PA, Eskelinen M, Partanen K et al. Clinical evaluation of a new serum tumor marker CA 242 in pancreatic carcinoma. *Br J Cancer*, 65, 731-734 (1992)

4021 Pascual RS et al. Usefulness of serum lysozyme measurement in diagnosis and evaluation of sarcoidosis. *N Engl J Med*, 289, 1074-1075 (1973)

4022 Pasquall M, Dembure PP, Still MJ et al. Urinary pyridinium cross-links: a non-invasive diagnostic test for Ehlers-Danlos Syndrome Type VI. *N Engl J Med*, 331, 132-133 (1994)

4023 Passamonte. Hypouricemia. *Arch Intern Med*, 144, 1570 (1984)

4024 Pasternack A et al. Clearance ratios of amylase and isoamylase to creatinine in renal disease. *Clin Nephrol*, 9, 25-28 (1978)

4025 Pastor R, Gutierrez C, Vendrell J et al. Lipoprotein (a) levels in NIDDM population. *Clin Chem*, 39, 1128 (1993)

4026 Patel DD, Bhatavdekar JM, Ghosh N et al. Plasma prolactin in patients with colorectal cancer: value in follow-up and as a prognosticator. *Cancer*, 73, 570-574 (1994)

4027 Patel PS, Adhvaryu SG, Balar DB. Clinical significance of serum total and heat-stable alkaline phosphatase in leukemia patients. *Tumori*, 79, 352-356 (1993)

4028 Patel PS, Adhvaryu SG, Balar DB. Serum lactate dehydrogenase and its isoenzymes in leukemia patients: possible role in diagnosis and treatment monitoring. *Neoplasma*, 41, 55-59 (1994)

4029 Patel PS, Adhvaryu SG, Balar DB et al. Clinical application of serum levels of sialic acid, fucose and seromucoid fraction as tumour markers in human leukemias. *Anticancer Res*, 14, 747-752 (1994)

4030 Patel PS, Raval GN, Rawal RR et al. Assessing benefits of combining biochemical and immunological markers in patients with lung carcinoma. *Cancer Lett*, 82, 129-133 (1994)

4031 Patel PS, Rawal GS, Balar DB. Combined use of serum enzyme levels as tumor markers in cervical carcinoma patients. *Tumor Biol*, 15, 45-51 (1994)

4032 Patel S et al. Serum enzyme levels in alcoholism and drug dependency. *J Clin Pathol*, 28, 414-417 (1975)

4033 Paternoster DM, Stella A, Simioni P, et al. Fibronectin and antithrombin as markers of pre-eclampsia in pregnancy. *Eur J Obstet Gynecol*, 70, 33-39 (1996)

4034 Pateron D, Beyne P, Laperche T, et al. Elevated circulating cardiac troponin I in patients with cirrhosis. *Hepatology*, 29, 640-643 (1999)

4035 Paton A. Alcohol-induced Cushingoid syndrome. *Br Med J*, 2, 1504 (1976)

4036 Patrono C. Biosynthesis and pharmacological modulation of thromboxane in humans. *Circulation*, 81, 112-115 (1990)

4037 Patton RB, Horn RC. Primary liver carcinoma. *Cancer*, 17, 757-768 (1967)

4038 Pauksen K, Elfman L, Ulfgren A-K et al. Serum levels of granulocyte-colony stimulating factor (G-CSF) in bacterial and viral infections, and in atypical pneumonia. *Br J Haematol*, 88, 256-260 (1994)

4039 Paul MA, Visser JJ, van Kamp GJ. A simple extraction procedure for the determination of carcinoembryonic antigen in gallbladder bile. *Ann Clin Biochem*, 32, 332-333 (1995)

4040 Paul MA, Vissr JJ, Mulder C, et al. The use of biliary CEA measurements in the diagnosis of recurrent colorectal cancer. *Eur J Surg Oncol*, 23, 419-423 (1997)

4041 Paulson GW. Elevation of serum uric acid levels in patients with seizures. *Ohio State Med J*, 9, 245-252 (1978)

4042 Paunio M, Virtamo J, Giref C, et al. Serum high-density lipoprotein cholesterol, alcohol and coronary mortality in heavy smokers. *Br Med J*, 312, 1200-1203 (1996)

4043 Pavlidis N, Nicolaides C, Bairaktari E, et al. Soluble interleukin-2 receptors in patients with advanced colorectal carcinoma. *Int J Biol Mark*, 11, 6-11 (1996)

4044 Pavlidis NA, Bairaktrai E, Kalef-Ezra J et al. Serum soluble interleukin-2 receptors in epithelial ovarian cancer patients. *Int J Biol Mark*, 10, 75-80 (1995)

4045 Pavlovic-Kentera V et al. Erythropoietin levels in patients with acute leukemia. *Haematologia*, 10, 455-462 (1976)

4046 Pavri KM et al. Immunoglobulin E in sera of patients of dengue haemorrhagic fever. *Ind J Med Res*, 66, 537-543 (1977)

4047 Pawlotsky Y, Le Dantec P, Moirand R, et al. Elevated parathyroid hormone 44-68 and osteoarticular changes in patients with genetic hemochromatosis. *Arth Rheum*, 42, 799-806 (1999)

4048 Payne RB. Creatinine clearance: a redundant clinical investigation. *Ann Clin Biochem*, 23, 243-250 (1986)

4049 Pazos F, Alvarez JJ, Rubies-Prat J et al. Long term thyroid replacement therapy and levels of lipoprotein(a) and other lipoproteins. *J Clin Endocrinol Metab*, 80, 562-566 (1995)

4050 Pearce J et al. Uric acid and plasma lipids in cerebrovascular disease. part I. *Br Med J*, 4, 78-80 (1969)

4051 Pearson CM, Bohan A. The spectrum of polyarteritis and dermatomyositis. *Med Clin North Am*, 61, 439-457 (1977)

4052 Pearson HA. Erythrokinetic studies in thalassemia trait. *J Lab Clin Med*, 56, 866 (1960)

4053 Pearson HA et al. Screening for thalassemia trait by electronic measurement of mean corpuscular volume. *N Engl J Med*, 288, 351 (1973)

4054 Pedersen BJ, Ravn P, Bonde M. Type I collagen C-telopeptide degradation products as bone resorption markers. *J Clin Ligand Assay*, 21, 118-127 (1998)

4055 Pedersen EB, Danielsen H, Jensen T et al. Angiotensin II, aldosterone and arginine vasopressin in plasma in congestive heart failure. *Eur J Clin Invest*, 16, 56-60 (1986)

4056 Pedersen EB, Johannesen P, Kristensen S et al. Calcium, parathyroid hormone and calcitonin in normal pregnancy and preeclampsia. *Gynecol Obstet Invest*, 18, 156-164 (1984)

4057 Pedersen LM, Milman N. Prognostic significance of thrombocytosis in patients with primary lung cancer. *Eur J Respir Dis*, 9, 1826-1830 (1996)

4058 Pederson ED, Stanke SR, Whitener SJ, et al. Salivary levels of α_2-macroglobulin, α_1-antitrypsin, C-reactive protein, cathepsin G and elastase in humans with or without destructive periodontal disease. *Arch Oral Biol*, 40, 1151-1155 (1995)

4059 Pedro-Botet J, Senti M, Auguet T et al. Apolipoprotein(a) genetic polymorphism and serum lipoprotein(a) concentration in patients with peripheral vascular disease. *Atherosclerosis*, 104, 87-94 (1993)

4060 Peipert JF, Boardman L, Hogan JW, et al. Laboratory evaluation of acute upper genital tract infection. *Obstet Gynecol*, 87, 730-736 (1996)

4061 Pejme J. Infectious mononucleosis. *Acta Med Scand*, 413 (1964)

4062 Pekarek RS et al. Serum zinc, iron, and copper concentrations during typhoid fever in man: effect of chloramphenicol therapy. *Clin Chem*, 21, 528-32 (1975)

4063 Pekin TJ et al. Synovial fluid findings in systemic lupus erythematosus. *Arth Rheum*, 13, 777-785 (1970)

4064 Pekonen F, Rasi V, Ammala M et al. Platelet function and coagulation in normal and preeclamptic pregnancy. *Thromb Res*, 43, 553-560 (1986)

4065 Pelfrey CV, Seubert P, Barbour R et al. Elevation of microtubule-associated protein Tau in the cerebrospinal fluid of patients with Alzheimer's disease. *Neurology*, 45, 788-793 (1995)

4066 Pelkonen R et al. Hydroxyprolinemia. *N Engl J Med*, 283, 451 (1970)

4067 Pelletier LL et al. Infective endocarditis: a preview of 125 cases from the University of Washington hospitals, 1963-1972. *Medicine*, 56, 287-313 (1977)

4068 Peltier AP, Ester D. *Pathobiology Annual*. New York NY, Appleton-Century-Crofts (1972)

4069 Penarrubia MJ, Steegman JL, Lavilla E et al. Hypertriglyceridemia may be severe in CML patients treated with interferon-α. *Am J Hematol*, 49, 240-241 (1995)

4070 Pendleton N, Occleston NL, Walshaw MJ et al. Simple cytokeratins in the serum of patients with lung cancer: relationship to cell death. *Eur J Cancer*, 30A, 93-96 (1994)

4071 Penney MD, Oleesky DA. Renal tubular acidosis. *Ann Clin Biochem*, 36, 408-422 (1999)

4072 Pepersack T, Rossi C, Dupuis F. Hormonal status and clinical relevance of hirsutism in elderly women. *Acta Endocrinol*, 129, 307-310 (1993)

4073 Pepys J. Hypersensitivity diseases of the lungs due to fungi and organic dusts. *Monogr Allergy*, 4 (1969)

4074 Peralta V, Cuesta MJ, Mata I, et al. Serum iron in catatonic and noncatatonic psychotic patients. *Biol Psychiat*, 45, 788-790 (1999)

4075 Perasso A, Testino G. Advanced gastric cancer of the antrum: anatomic-functional correlation between chief cell mass and serum pepsinogen I. *Gastroenterol Jpn*, 26, 588-592 (1991)

4076 Percy ME, Dalton AJ, Markovic VD et al. Red cell superoxide dismutase, glutathione peroxidase and catalase in Down syndrome patients with and without manifestations of Alzheimer's disease. *Am J Med Genet*, 35, 459-467 (1990)

4077 Pereira BFG, Sundaram S, Snodgrass B, et al. Plasma lipopolysaccharide binding protein and bactericidal/permeability increasing factor in CRF and HD patients. *Am J Nephrol*, 7, 479-487 (1996)

4078 Perel JM, Stull S, Sloan S et al. Salivary cortisol in prepubertal major depression assessed by adaptation of plasma radioimmunoassay. *Clin Chem*, 39, 1183 (1993)

4079 Perillie PE et al. Significance of changes in serum muramidase activity in megaloblastic anemia. *N Engl J Med*, 277, 10-12 (1967)

4080 Perkash I, Martin DE, Warner H et al. Reproductive biology of paraplegics: results of semen collection, testicular biopsy and serum hormone evaluation. *J Urol*, 134, 284-288 (1985)

4081 Perkoff GT et al. Reversible acute muscular syndrome in chronic alcoholism. *N Engl J Med*, 274, 1277-1285 (1966)

4082 Perlmann P, Perlmann H, El Ghazali G, Blomberg NT. IgE and tumor necrosis factor in malaria infection. *Immunol Lett*, 65, 29-33 (1999)

4083 Perlmutter DH. α1-Antitrypsin deficiency: biochemistry and clinical manifestations. *Ann Med*, 28, 385-394 (1996)

4084 Perrella O, Carrieri PB, Guarnaccia D, Soscia M. Cerebrospinal fluid cytokines in AIDS dementia complex. *J Neurol*, 239, 387-388 (1992)

4085 Perrella O, Guerriero M, Izzo E et al. Interleukin-6 and granulocyte macrophage-CSF in the cerebrospinal fluid from HIV infected subjects with involvement of the central nervous system. *Arq Neuropsiquiatr*, 50, 180-182 (1992)

4086 Perrier A, Desmarais S, Goehring C, et al. D-dimer testing for suspected pulmonary embolism in outpatients. *Am J Respir Crit Care Med*, 156, 492-496 (1997)

4087 Perrin KJ et al. Quantitation of C_3 proactivator (properdin factor B) and other complement components in diseases associated with a low C_3 level. *Clin Immunol Immunopathol*, 2, 16 (1973)

4088 Perrin R, Brianicon S, Jeandel C et al. Blood activity of Cu/Zn superoxide dismutase, glutathione peroxidase and catalase in Alzheimer's disease: a case-control study. *Gerontology*, 36, 306-313 (1990)

4089 Persani L, Preziati D, Matthews CH, et al. Serum levels of carboxyterminal cross-linked telopeptide of type I collagen (ICTP) in the differential diagnosis of the syndromes of inappropriate secretion of TSH. *Clin Endocrinol*, 47, 207-214 (1997)

4090 Persky H et al. The effect of alcohol and smoking on testosterone function and aggression in chronic alcoholics. *Am J Psychiat*, 134, 621-625 (1977)

4091 Pertsemlidis D et al. Pheochromacytoma. *Ann Surg*, 169, 376 (1969)

4092 Peskind ER, Elrod R, Dobie DJ, et al. Cerebrospinal fluid epinephrine in Alzheimer's disease and normal aging. *Neuropsychopharmacology*, 19, 465-471 (1998)

4093 Peter JB. *Use and Interpretation of Tests in Clinical Immunology*. 8th edition, Specialty Laboratories, Santa Monica CA (1991)

4094 Peter JB. *Use and Interpretation of Tests in Neuroimmunology*. Specialty Laboratories, Santa Monica CA (1991)

4095 Peter JB, Reyes H. *Use and Interpretation of Tests in Allergy and Immunology*. Specialty Laboratories, Santa Monica CA (1992)

4096 Peters JE, Rehfeld N, Schneider I et al. Abgrenzung von nieren-und serumfraktion der alaninaminopeptidase. *Clin Chim Acta*, 24, 314-315 (1969)

4097 Peters SP et al. Gaucher's disease: a review. *Medicine*, 56, 425-442 (1977)

4098 Peterslund NA, Heinsvig EM, Dencker Christensen K. Creatine kinase in the serum of patients with acute infections of the central nervous system. *J Infect*, 10, 115-120 (1985)

4099 Peterson IF, Boegard T, Dahlstrom J, et al. Bone scan and serum markers of bone and cartilage in patients with knee pain and osteoarthritis. *Osteoarth Cartilage*, 6, 33-39 (1998)

4100 Peterson PK, Shepard J, Macres M et al. A controlled trial of intravenous immunoglobulin G in chronic fatigue syndrome. *Am J Med*, 89, 554-560 (1990)

4101 Petrovich G, Ursich-Jankovich J, Prijovich Z. Ratio of serum tartrate-inhibitable acid phosphatase to total serum protein in benign prostatic hypertrophy and prostatic carcinoma. *Clin Chem*, 38, 276-277 (1992)

4102 Pettersson A, Hedner J, Hedner T et al. Increased plasma levels of atrial natriuretic peptide in patients with congestive heart failure. *Eur Heart J*, 7, 693-696 (1986)

4103 Pettersson K, Eskelinen M, Pasanen P. Evaluation of serum tumour markers CA 242, CA 50 and CEA in gastrointestinal cancers. *Clin Biochem Rev*, 14, 262 (1993)

4104 Pettersson T et al. T and B lymphocytes in pleural effusions. *Chest*, 73, 49-51 (1978)

4105 Pettersson T, Weber TH, Ojala K. Creatine kinase isoenzyme BB as a tumor marker in pleural effusions. *Clin Chem*, 27, 1147-1148 (1981)

4106 Pettingale KW et al. Serum protein changes in breast cancer: a prospective study. *J Clin Pathol*, 30, 1048-1052 (1977)

4107 Petty F, Kramer GL, Fulton M et al. Stability of plasma GABA at four-year follow-up in patients with primary unipolar depression. *Biol Psychiat*, 37, 806-811 (1995)

4108 Peuravuori HJ, Funatomi H, Nevalainen TJ. Group I and group II phospholipases A2 in serum in uraemia. *Eur J Clin Chem Clin Biochem*, 31, 491-494 (1993)

4109 Peyron F, Burdin N, Ringwald P et al. High levels of circulating IL-10 in human malaria. *Clin Exp Immunol*, 95, 300-303 (1994)

4110 Pezzilli R, Andreone P, Morselli-Labate AM, et al. Serum pancreatic enzyme concentrations in chronic liver diseases. *Dig Dis Sci*, 44, 350-353 (1999)

4111 Pezzilli R, Billi P, Fiocchi M et al. Serum β-microglobulin in chronic diseases of the pancreas. *Int J Pancreatol*, 17, 161-166 (1995)

4112 Pezzilli R, Billi P, Gullo L et al. Behavior of serum soluble interleukin-2 receptor, soluble CD8 and soluble CD4 in the early phases of acute pancreatitis. *Digestion*, 55, 268-273 (1994)

4113 Pezzilli R, Billi P, Miniero R, Barakat B. Serum interleukin-10 in human acute pancreatitis. *Dig Dis Sci*, 42, 1469-1472 (1997)

4114 Pezzilli R, Billi P, Miniero R, et al. Serum interleukin-6, interleukin-8, and β_2-microglobulin in early assessment of severity of acute pancreatitis: comparison with serum C-reactive protein. *Dig Dis Sci*, 40, 2341-2348 (1995)

4115 Pezzilli R, et al. Simultaneous serum assays and lipase and interleukin-6 for early diagnosis and prognosis of acute pancreatitis. *Clin Chem*, 45, 1762-1767 (1999)

4116 Pfau A et al. The pH of the prostatic fluid in health and disease: implications of treatment in chronic bacterial prostatitis. *J Urol*, 119, 384 (1978)

4117 Pfeiffer A, Drewes C, Middelberg-Bisping K, Schatz H. Elevated plasma levels of transforming growth factor-β1 in NIDDM. *Diabetes Care*, 19, 1113-1117 (1996)

4118 Phelan JP, Ahn MO, Korst LM, et al. Nucleated red blood cells: a marker for fetal asphyxia. *Am J Obstet Gynecol*, 173, 1380-1384 (1995)

4119 Philip RN et al. A comparison for serologic methods for diagnosis of Rocky Mountain spotted fever. *Am J Epidemol*, 105, 56-67 (1977)

4120 Philipsen EK, Bondesen S, Andersen J et al. Serum immunoglobulin G subclasses in patients with ulcerative colitis and Crohn's disease of different disease activities. *Scand J Gastroenterol*, 30, 50-53 (1995)

4121 Phillip CS, Cisar LA, Kim H, et al. Association of hemostatic factors with peripheral vascular disease. *Am Heart J*, 134, 978-984 (1997)

4122 Phillipp E, Pirke KM, Kellner MB et al. Disturbed cholecystokinin secretion in patients with eating disorders. *Life Sci*, 48, 2443-2450 (1991)

4123 Phillips GB, Jing T-Y, Laragh JH et al. Serum sex hormone levels and renin-sodium profile in men with hypertension. *Am J Hypertens*, 8, 626-629 (1995)

4124 Phillips RW et al. Elevation of leucine aminopeptidase in disseminated malignant disease. *Cancer*, 26, 1006-1012 (1970)

4125 Phillipson OT et al. Plasma glucose, non-esterified fatty acids and amino acids in Huntington's chorea. *Clin Sci*, 52, 311-318 (1977)

4126 Phuarpradit W, Taeepankhskul S, Jetsawangsri T, et al. Serum ferritin levels in normal and HIV-1-infected pregnant women. *Aust NZ Obstet Gynecol*, 36, 24-26 (1996)

4127 Piantino P, Fusaro A, Randone A et al. Increased levels of CA 19-9, CA 50, and CA 195 in patients with benign diseases of the billiary tract and pancreas. *J Nucl Med Allied Sci*, 34, 97-102 (1990)

4128 Piccinini L, Zironi S, Cenci AM et al. Soluble interleukin-2 receptor and urinary neopterin concentrations in malignant lymphoma. *Eur J Clin Chem Clin Biochem*, 31, 567-574 (1993)

4129 Piccirillo G, Fimognari FL, Infantino V et al. High plasma concentrations of cortisol and thromboxane B_2 in patients with depression. *Am J Med Sci*, 307, 228-232 (1994)

4130 Pick AI. Diagnostic significance of CEA concentrations. *Am J Proctol*, 28, 37, 77 (1977)

4131 Pietila KO, Harmoinen AP, Jokiniitty J, et al. Serum C-reactive protein concentration in acute myocardial infarction and its relationship to mortality during 24 months following in patients under thrombolytic treatment. *Eur Heart J*, 17, 1345-1349 (1996)

4132 Pietschmann P, Pils P, Woloszczuk W et al. Increased serum osteocalcin levels in patients with paraplegia. *Paraplegia*, 30, 204-209 (1992)

4133 Pietschmann P, Resch H, Krexner E et al. Decreased serum osteocalcin levels in patients with postmenopausal osteoporosis. *Acta Med Austriaca*, 18, 114-116 (1991)

4134 Pietschmann P, Vychytil A, Wolosczcuk W et al. Bone metabolism in patients with functioning kidney grafts: increased serum levels of osteocalcin and parathyroid hormone despite normalisation kidney function. *Nephron*, 59, 533-536 (1991)

4135 Pietschumann P, Zielinski CH, Woloszczuk W. Serum osteocalcin levels in breast cancer patients. *J Cancer Res Clin Oncol*, 115, 456-458 (1989)

4136 Pilhen JA et al. Serum proteins in pulmonary tuberculosis. *Dis Chest*, 41, 174 (1962)

4137 Pin Lim et al. Elevated serum enzymes in patients with wasp/bee sting and their clinical significance. *Clin Chim Acta*, 66, 405-409 (1976)

4138 Pinna G, Hiedra L, Meinhold M, et al. 3,3'-Diidothyronine concentrations in the sera of patients with nonthyroidal illnesses and brain tumors and of healthy subjects during acute stress. *J Clin Endocrinol Metab*, 83, 3071-3077 (1998)

4139 Pinto MM, Kotta S. CA125 in fine-needle aspirates of solid tumors: comparison with cytologic diagnosis and carcinoembryonic antigen (CEA) assay. *Diagn Cytopathol*, 14, 121-125 (1996)

4140 Piovesan A, Berruti A, Torta M, et al. Comparison of assay of total and bone-specific alkaline phosphatase in the assessment of osteoblastic activity in patients with metastatic bone disease. *Calcif Tissue Int*, 61, 362-369 (1997)

4141 Piovesan A, Terzolo M, Reimondo G et al. Biochemical markers of bone and collagen turnover in acromegaly or Cushing's syndrome. *Horm Metab Res*, 26, 234-237 (1994)

4142 Piper D et al. Gastric juice lactic acidosis in the presence of gastric carcinoma. *Gastroenterology*, 58, 766 (1970)

4143 Pirisi M, Falleti E, Fabris C et al. Circulating intercellular adhesion molecule-1 (cICAM-1) concentration in liver disease: relationship with cholestasis and functioning hepatic mass. *Am J Clin Pathol*, 102, 600-604 (1994)

4144 Pirke KM, Friess E, Kellner MB et al. Somatostatin in eating disorders. *Int J Eat Disord*, 15, 99-102 (1994)

4145 Pirke KM, Pahl J, Cashweiger U et al. Metabolic and endocrine indices of starvation in bulimia: a comparison with anorexia nervosa. *Psychiat Res*, 15, 33-39 (1985)

4146 Pita M-L, Rubio J-M, Murillo M-L, et al. Chronic alcoholism decreases polyunsaturated fatty acid levels in human plasma, erythrocytes, and platelets - influence of chronic liver disease. *Thromb Haemost*, 78, 808-812 (1997)

4147 Pitney WR. The tropical splenomegaly syndrome. *Trans Roy Soc Trop Med Hyg*, 62, 717 (1968)

4148 Pitney WR et al. Observations on the bound form of vitamin B_{12} in human serum. *J Biol Chem*, 207, 143 (1954)

4149 Pittet J-F, Morel DR, Hemsen A et al. Elevated plasma endothelin-1 concentrations are associated with the severity of illness in patients with sepsis. *Ann Surg*, 213, 261-264 (1991)

4150 Pitts AF, Samuelson SD, Meller WH et al. Cerebrospinal fluid corticotropin-releasing hormone, vasopressin, and oxytocin concentrations in treated patients with major depression and controls. *Biol Psychiat*, 38, 330-335 (1995)

4151 Pizzolo G, Vinante F, Chilosi M et al. Serum levels of soluble CD30 molecule (K-1 antigen) in Hodgkin's disease: relationship with disease activity and clinical stage. *Br J Haematol*, 75, 282-284 (1990)

4152 Plassart F, Cynober L, Baudin B et al. Plasma fibronectin and angiotensin-converting enzyme: markers of primary pulmonary injury in burn patients. *Clin Chim Acta*, 227, 135-144 (1994)

4153 Plebani M, Basso D, Panozzo MP, et al. Tumor markers in the diagnosis, monitoring and therapy of pancreatic cancer: state of the art. *Int J Biol Mark*, 10, 189-199 (1995)

4154 Plebani M, Giacomini A, Floreani A et al. Biochemical markers of hepatic fibrosis in primary biliary cirrhosis. *Ric Clin Lab*, 20, 269-274 (1990)

4155 Plebani M, Mioni R, Melo M et al. Different steroidogenic pathways are involved in idiopathic and hyperandrogenic hirsute patients. *Clin Chem*, 39, 1168 (1993)

4156 Plevris JN, Dhariwal A, Elton RA et al. The platelet count as a predictor of variceal hemorrhage in primary biliary cirrhosis. *Am J Gastroenterol*, 90, 959-961 (1995)

4157 Pliopkys AV, Plioplys S. Serum levels of carnitine in chronic fatigue syndrome: clinical correlates. *Neuropsychobiology*, 32, 132-138 (1995)

4158 Plishker GA et al. Myotonic muscular dystrophy: altered calcium transport in erythrocytes. *Science*, 200, 323-325 (1978)

4159 Ploeckinger B, Dantendorfer K, Ulm M, et al. Rapid decrease of serum cholesterol concentration and postpartum depression. *Br Med J*, 313, 664 (1996)

4160 Plotz PH. Autoimmunity in hepatitis. *Med Clin North Am*, 59, 869-876 (1975)

4161 Plum CM, Hansen SE. Studies on variations in serum copper and serum copper oxidase activity together with studies on the copper content of the cerebrospinal fluid, with particular reference to the variations in multiple sclerosis. *Acta Psychiat Scand*, 35, 41-78 (1960)

4162 Pohl WR, Thompson AB, Kohn H et al. Serum procollagen III peptide levels in subjects with sarcoidosis: a 5-year follow-up study. *Am Rev Resp Dis*, 145, 412-417 (1992)

4163 Poirier J, Davignon J, Bouthillier D, et al. Apolipoprotein E polymorphism and Alzheimer's disease. *Lancet*, 342, 697-699 (1993)

4164 Pokora J, Berbec H, Zearo T. Blood serotonin level and 24 hour urinary excretion of 5-HIAA in patients with gastric and duodenal ulcer before and during treatment with Spasmophen. *Pol Tyg Lek*, 25, 1199-1201 (1970)

4165 Polak M, Toress DA, Costa AC. Diagnostic value of the estimation of glucose in ascitic fluid. *Digestion*, 8, 347-352 (1973)

4166 Poley S, Fateh-Moghadam A, Nussler V et al. Serum β_2-microglobulin for staging and monitoring of multiple myelomas and other non-Hodgkin lymphomas. *Onkologie*, 17, 428-432 (1994)

4167 Polisson RP, Dooley MA, Dawson DV et al. Interleukin-2 receptor levels in the sera of rheumatoid arthritis patients with methotrexate. *Arth Rheum*, 37, 50-56 (1994)

4168 Polley MJ, Bearn AG. Annotation: cystic fibrosis current concepts. *J Med Genet*, 11, 249 (1974)

4169 Pollycove M et al. Classification and evolution of patterns of erythropoiesis in polycythemia vera as studied by iron kinetics. *Blood*, 28, 807 (1966)

4170 Polmar SH et al. Immunoglobulin E in immunologic deficiency diseases. *J Clin Invest*, 51, 326 (1972)

4171 Polowe D. Blood amylase. *Am J Clin Pathol*, 13, 288 (1943)

4172 Pomeroy C, Eckert E, Hu S et al. Role of interleukin-6 and transforming growth factor-β in anorexia. *Biol Psychiat*, 36, 836-839 (1994)

4173 Ponting J, Howell A, Pye D, Kumar S. Prognostic relevance of serum hyaluronan levels in patients with breast cancer. *Int J Cancer*, 52, 873-876 (1992)

4174 Poole AR, Witter J, Roberts N et al. Inflammation and cartilage metabolism in rheumatoid arthritis. Studies of the blood markers hyaluronic acid, orosomucoid, and keratan sulfate. *Arth Rheum*, 33, 790-799 (1990)

4175 Popovic V, Spremovic S. The effect of sodium valproate on luteinizing hormone secretion in women with polycystic ovary disease. *J Endocrinol Invest*, 18, 104-108 (1995)

4176 Popper H, Schaffner F (eds). *Progress in Liver Disease*, New York NY, Grune and Stratton, 3 (1970)

4177 Porath A et al. Serum cholinesterase in tetanus. *Anesthesia*, 32, 1009-1011 (1977)

4178 Porcelli B, Frosi B, Rosi F, et al. Levels of folic acid in plasma and in red blood cells of colorectal cancer patients. *Biomed Pharmacother*, 50, 303-305 (1996)

4179 Portaluppi F, Bagni B, Cavallini AR et al. Plasma levels of atrial natriuretic peptide are increased in normotensive postmenopausal women as a function of age. *Cardiology*, 78, 317-322 (1991)

4180 Portaluppi F, Bagni B, degli Uberti E et al. Circadian rhythms of atrial natriuretic peptide, renin, aldosterone, cortisol, blood pressure and heart rate in normal and hypertensive subjects. *J Hypertens*, 8, 85-95 (1990)

4181 Porter JR, Brawer MK. Prostatic intraepithelial neoplasia and prostate-specific antigen. *World J Urol*, 11, 196-200 (1993)

4182 Porter WH, Jennnings CD Jr, Wilson HD. Measurement of α-glucosidase activity in serum from patients with cystic fibrosis or pancreatitis. *Clin Chem*, 32, 652-656 (1986)

4183 Portero-Otin M, Pamplona R, Bellmunt MJ, et al. Urinary pyrraline as a biochemical marker of non-oxidative Maillard reactions in vivo. *Life Sci*, 60, 279-287 (1997)

4184 Pos O, van der Stelt ME, Wolbink GJ et al. Changes in the serum concentration and the glycosylation of human alpha 1-acid glycoprotein and alpha 1-protease inhibitor in severely burned persons: relation to interleukin-6 levels. *Clin Exp Immunol*, 82, 579-582 (1990)

4185 Posey LE et al. Urine enzyme activities in patients with transitional cell carcinoma of the bladder. *Clin Chim Acta*, 74, 7-10 (1977)

4186 Post FA, Wood R, Maartens G. CD4 and total lymphocyte counts as predictors of HIV progression. *Quart J Med*, 89, 505-508 (1996)

4187 Pottathil R, Huang S-W, Chandrabose KA. Essential fatty acids in diabetes and systemic lupus erythematosus (SLE) patients. *Biochem Biophys Res Commun*, 128, 803-808 (1985)

4188 Potter BJ et al. Serum complement in chronic liver disease. *Gut*, 14, 451 (1973)

4189 Potter WZ, Manji HK. Catecholamines in depression: an update. *Clin Chem*, 40, 279-287 (1994)

4190 Potts DE et al. Pleural fluid pH in parapneumonic effusions. *Chest*, 70, 328-331 (1976)

4191 Poulakis N, Sarandakou A, Ritzos D et al. Soluble interleukin-2 receptors and other markers in primary lung cancer. *Cancer*, 68, 1045-1049 (1991)

4192 Poulos JE, Leggett-Frazier N, Khazanie P et al. Circulating insulin-like growth factor-I concentrations in clinically obese patients with and without NIDDM in response to weight loss. *Horm Metab Res*, 26, 478-480 (1994)

4193 Poupon RE, Gervaise G, Riant P et al. Blood thiamine and thiamine phosphate concentrations in excessive drinkers with or without peripheral neuropathy. *Alcohol Alcoholism*, 25, 605-611 (1990)

4194 Pouta AM, Vuolteenaho OJ, Laatikainen TJ. An increase of the plasma N-terminal peptide of proatrial natriuretic peptide in preeclampsia. *Obstet Gynecol*, 89, 747-753 (1997)

4195 Pouta AM, Vuolteenaho OJ, Laatikainen TJ. The association of plasma endothelin with clinical parameters in preeclampsia. *Hypertens Preg*, 17, 135-145 (1998)

4196 Pouw EM, Schols AMWJ, Deutz NEP, Wouters EFM. Plasma and muscle amino acid levels in relation to resting energy expenditures and inflammation in stable chronic obstructive pulmonary disease. *Am J Respir Crit Care Med*, 158, 797-801 (1998)

4197 Powell FC, Winkelmann RK et al. The anticentromere antibody: disease specificity and clinical significance. *Mayo Clin Proc*, 59, 700-706 (1984)

4198 Powell LW et al. Cirrhosis of the liver: a comparative study of the four major aetiological groups. *Med J Aust*, 1, 941-950 (1971)

4199 Powell LW et al. Haemolysis in liver disease: relationship to erythrocyte membrane function, serum bilirubin concentration and plasma electrolyte disturbances. *Aust NZ J Med*, 6, 3-6 (1976)

4200 Powell LW et al. Relationship between serum ferritin and total body iron stores in idiopathic haemochromatosis. *Gut*, 19, 538-42 (1978)

4201 Powell LW et al. The relationship of red cell membrane lipid content to red cell morphology and survival in patients with liver disease. *Aust NZ J Med*, 5, 101-107 (1975)

4202 Pozzilli C, Lenzi GL, Argentino C et al. Peripheral white blood cell count in cerebral ischemic infarction. *Acta Neurol Scand*, 71, 396-400 (1985)

4203 Pralong G, Calandra T, Glauser M-P et al. Plasminogen activator inhibitor 1: a new prognostic marker in septic shock. *Thromb Haemostas*, 61, 459-462 (1989)

4204 Pranzatelli MR, Huang Y, Tate E et al. Cerebrospinal fluid 5-hydroxyindoleacetic acid and homovanillic acid in the pediatric opsoclonus-myoclonus syndrome. *Ann Neurol*, 37, 189-197 (1995)

4205 Prasad C, Hilton CW, Lohr JB et al. Increased cerebrospinal fluid cyclo(His-Pro) content in schizophrenia. *Neuropeptides*, 20, 187-190 (1991)

4206 Preece MA, Green A. Abnormalities of plasma copper in tyrosinaemia type I. *Proc ACB Natl Meet*, 84 (1993)

4207 Pregant P, Schernthaner G, Legenstein E et al. Decreased plasma carnitine in Type I diabetes mellitus. *Klin Wschr*, 69, 511-516 (1991)

4208 Prell GD, Green JP, Elkashef AM, et al. The relationship between urine excretion and biogenic amines and their metabolites in cerebrospinal fluid of schizophrenic patients. *Schiz Res*, 19, 171-178 (1996)

4209 Prell GD, Green JP, Kaufman CA, et al. Histamine metabolites in cerebrospinal fluid of patients with chronic schizophrenia: their relationships to levels of other aminergic transmitters and ratings of symptoms. *Schiz Res*, 14, 93-104 (1995)

4210 Premert J, Larsson J, Westermark GT et al. Islet amyloid polypeptide in patients with pancreatic cancer and diabetes. *N Engl J Med*, 330, 313-318 (1994)

4211 Prestigiacomo AF, Stamey TA. Clinical usefulness of free and complexed PSA. *Scand J Clin Lab Invest*, 55, 32-34 (1995)

4212 Preti HA, Cabanillas F, Talpaz M, et al. Prognostic value of serum interleukin-6 in diffuse large cell lymphoma. *Ann Intern Med*, 127, 186-194 (1997)

4213 Preuss HG et al. Ammonia metabolism in renal failure. *Ann Intern Med*, 65, 54-61 (1966)

4214 Preuss HG et al. Electrolyte and acid-base disturbances in diabetes mellitus. *Compr Ther*, 4, 20-23 (1978)

4215 Prii D, Blanchet FB, Essig M, et al. Dipyridamole decreases renal phosphate leak and augments serum phosphorus in patients with low renal phosphate threshold. *J Am Soc Nephrol*, 9, 1264-1269 (1998)

4216 Price CP, Sammons. The nature of the serum alkaline phosphatases in liver diseases. *J Clin Pathol*, 27, 392-398 (1974)

4217 Price CP, Thompson PW. The role of biochemical tests in the screening and monitoring of osteoporosis. *Ann Clin Biochem*, 32, 244-260 (1995)

4218 Price FV, Chambers SK, Carcanglu ML, et al. CA 125 may not reflect disease status in patients with uterine serous carcinoma. *Cancer*, 82, 1720-1725 (1998)

4219 Price PA, Parthemore JG, Deftos LJ. New biochemical marker for bone metabolism. *J Clin Invest*, 66, 878-883 (1980)

4220 Priestley GC, Gawkrodger DJ, Seth J et al. Growth hormone levels in psoriasis. *Arch Dermatol Res*, 276, 147-150 (1984)

4221 Prinz RA, Sandberg L. Serum levels of α-1-antitrypsin in pancreatic islet cell tumors. *J Med*, 15, 177-83 (1984)

4222 Priosky B. *Infectious Disease and Autoimmune Hemolytic Anemia: Autoimmunization and the Autoimmune Hemolytic Anemias*, Baltimore MD, Waverly Press, 147 (1969)

4223 Pritchard JA, MacDonald PC. In: *Obstetrics*. 15th edition. Williams RJ (ed), New York NY, Appleton-Century-Crofts (1971)

4224 Prockop DJ, Davidson WD. A study of urinary and serum lysozyme in patients with renal disease. *N Engl J Med*, 240, 269 (1964)

4225 Prompt CA et al. High concentration of sweat calcium, magnesium and phosphate in chronic renal failure. *Nephron*, 20, 4-9 (1978)

4226 Proudler AJ, Crook D, Godsland IF et al. Serum angiotensin-I-converting enzyme activity in women with cardiological syndrome X: relation to blood pressure and lipid and carbohydrate metabolite risk markers for coronary heart disease. *J Clin Endocrinol Metab*, 80, 696-699 (1995)

4227 Prout GR et al. Alterations in serum lactic dehydrogenase and its fourth and fifth isozymes in patients with prostatic carcinoma. *J Urol*, 94, 451 (1965)

4228 Pruimboom WM, Bac DJ, van Dijk APM, et al. Levels of soluble intercellular adhesion molecule-1, eicosanoids and cytokines in ascites of patients with liver cirrhosis, peritoneal cancer and spontaneous bacterial peritonitis. *Int J Immunopharmacol*, 17, 375-384 (1995)

4229 Pruzansky W, Vadas P, Stefanski E et al. Phospholipase A2 activity in sera and synovial fluids in rheumatoid arthritis and osteoarthritis. *J Rheumatol*, 12, 211-216 (1985)

4230 Psathakis D, Wedemeyer N, Oevermann E, et al. Blood selenium and glutathione peroxidase status in patients with colorectal cancer. *Dis Colon Rectum*, 41, 328-335 (1998)

4231 Puchois P, Fontan M, Gentilini J-L et al. Serum apolipoprotein A-II, a biochemical indicator of alcohol abuse. *Clin Chim Acta*, 144, 185-189 (1984)

4232 Pudenz RH et al. The role of potassium in familial periodic paralysis. *J Am Med Ass*, 111, 2253 (1938)

4233 Pudil R, Pidrman V, Krejsek J, et al. Cytokines and adhesion molecules in the course of acute myocardial infarction. *Clin Chim Acta*, 280, 127-134 (1999)

4234 Pugeat M, Crave JC, Tourniaire J, Forest MG. Clinical utility of sex hormone-binding globulin measurement. *Horm Res*, 45, 148-155 (1996)

4235 Pui C-H, Hudson M, Luo X et al. Serum interleukin-2 receptor levels in Hodgkin's disease and other solid tumors of childhood. *Leukemia*, 7, 1242-1244 (1993)

4236 Puig JG, Ruilope LM. Uric acid as a cardiovascular risk factor in arterial hypertension. *J Hypertens*, 17, 869-872 (1999)

4237 Pujol M, Ribera A, Vilardell M et al. High prevalence of platelet autoantibodies in patients with systemic lupus erythematosus. *Br J Haematol*, 89, 137-141 (1995)

4238 Pulkki K, Tienhaara T, Mattila K et al. Comparison of serum immunoreactive interleukin-6 and C-reactive protein measurements as predictors of survival in patients with multiple myeloma. *Clin Biochem Rev*, 14, 261 (1993)

4239 Punnonen K, Irjala K, Rajamaki A. Iron-deficiency anemia is associated with high concentrations of transferrin receptor in serum. *Clin Chem*, 40, 774-776 (1994)

4240 Puskar D, Vuckovic I, Bedlov G et al. Urinalysis, ultrasound analysis, and renal dynamic scintiography in acute appendicitis. *Urology*, 45, 108-112 (1995)

4241 Putnam FW (ed). *The Plasma Proteins: Structure, Functions and Genetic Control*, New York NY, Academic Press, 1-3 (1977)

4242 Puzigaca Z, Prelevic GM, Stretenovic Z et al. Ovarian enlargement as a possible marker of androgen activity in polycystic ovary syndrome. *Gynecol Endocrinol*, 5, 167-174 (1991)

4243 Pyhala R et al. The value of complement fixation and haemagglutination inhibition tests in the diagnosis of influenza A. *Acta Virol*, 20, 66-69 (1976)

4244 Qasim W, Geritsen B, Veys P. Anticardiolipin antibodies and thromboembolism after BMT. *Bone Marrow Transplant*, 21, 845-847 (1998)

4245 Qi H, Koyama T, Nishida K, et al. Urinary procoagulant activity and tissue factor levels in patients with diabetes mellitus. *Haemostasis*, 27, 57-64 (1997)

4246 Qin Q-P, Christiansen M, Nguyen TH, et al. Schwangerschaftsprotein 1 (SP1) as a maternal serum marker for Down syndrome in the first and second trimester. *Prenatal Diagnosis*, 17, 101-108 (1997)

4247 Qiu S, Theroux P, Marcil M et al. Plasma endothelin-1 levels in stable and unstable angina. *Cardiology*, 82, 12-19 (1993)

4248 Quadros NP, Roberts-Thomson PJ et al. IgG and IgM anti-endothelial cell antibodies in patients with collagen-vascular disorders. *Rheumatol Int*, 10, 113-119 (1990)

4249 Quattrin T, Albini CH, Reiter EO et al. Urinary excretion of IGF-I and growth hormone in children with IDDM. *Diabetes Care*, 15, 490-494 (1992)

4250 Quattrin T, Albini CH, Sportsman C et al. Urinary insulin-like growth factor-II excretion in healthy infants and children with normal and abnormal growth. *Pediatr Res*, 34, 435-438 (1993)

4251 Qui S, Theroux P, Marcil M et al. Plasma endothelin-1 levels in stable and unstable angina. *Cardiology*, 82, 12-19 (1993)

4252 Quindos G. Diagnostic value of enzymatic detection of serum mannose in invasive cadidiasis. *Enfermedades Infecciosas y Microbiologia Clinica*, 10, 227-229 (1992)

4253 Quoix E, Charloux A, Popin E et al. Inability of serum neuron-specific enolase to predict disease extent in small cell lung cancer. *Eur J Cancer*, 29A, 2248-2250 (1993)

4254 Raab WP. The diagnostic value of urinary enzyme determinations. *Clin Chem*, 18, 5 (1972)

4255 Rabinwicz AL, Correale JD, Bracht KA et al. Neuron-specific enolase is increased after nonconvulsive status epilepticus. *Epilepsia*, 36, 475-479 (1995)

4256 Rabitzsch G, Mair J, Lechleitner P et al. Immunoenzymometric assay of human glycogen phosphorylase isoenzyme BB in diagnosis of ischemic myocardial injury. *Clin Chem*, 41, 966-978 (1995)

4257 Raccah D, Alessi MC, Scelles V et al. Plasminogen activator inhibitor activity in various types of endogenous hypertriglyceridemia. *Fibrinolysis*, 7, 171-176 (1993)

4258 Rachelefsky GS et al. Serum enzyme abnormalities in juvenile rheumatoid arthritis. *Pediatrics*, 58, 730-736 (1976)

4259 Radetti G, Mazzanti L, Paganini C et al. Frequency, clinical and laboratory features of thyroiditis in girls with Turner's syndrome. *Acta Paediat*, 84, 909-912 (1995)

4260 Radetti G, Paganani C, Antoniazzi F, et al. Growth hormone-binding proteins, IGF-1 and IGF-binding proteins in children and adolescents with type 1 diabetes mellitus mellitus. *Horm Res*, 47, 110-115 (1997)

4261 Raffensperger EC. Elevated serum pancreatic enzyme values without primary intrinsic disease. *Ann Intern Med*, 35, 342 (1951)

4262 Raffin-Sanson M-L, Massias J-F, Dumont C, et al. High plasma proopiomelanocortin in aggressive adrenocorticotropin-secreting tumors. *J Clin Endocrinol Metab*, 81, 4272-4277 (1996)

4263 Raftery AT. The value of the leucocyte count in the diagnosis of acute appendicitis. *Br J Surg*, 63, 143-144 (1976)

4264 Raganati M et al. Adenosine deaminase activity in serum of children with different diseases. *Pediatria (Napoli)*, 84, 247-52 (1976)

4265 Rainbow SJ, Tickner TR. Development and evaluation of an enhanced chemiluminescence assay for CA 19-9 using Enzymun-test reagents. *Clin Chem*, 39, 1191 (1993)

4266 Raine AEG, Anderson JV, Bloom Sr et al. Plasma atrial natriuretic factor and graft function in renal transplant patients. *Transplantation*, 48, 796-800 (1989)

4267 Rainwater LM, Morgan WR, Klee GG et al. Prostate-specific antigen testing in untreated and treated prostatic adenocarcinoma. *Mayo Clin Proc*, 65, 1118-1126 (1990)

4268 Raivio KO. Neonatal hyperuricemia. *J Pediatr*, 88, 625-630 (1976)

4269 Ramachandran S et al. pH of amoebic liver pus. *Trans Roy Soc Trop Med Hyg*, 70, 159-160 (1976)

4270 Ramadori G, Zohrens G, Manns M et al. Serum hyaluronate and type III NP procollagen aminoterminal propeptide concentration in chronic liver disease. Relationship to cirrhosis and disease activity. *Eur J Clin Invest*, 21, 323-330 (1991)

4271 Ramirez A et al. Daily urinary catecholamine profile in marasmus and kwashiorkor. *Am J Clin Nutr*, 31, 41-45 (1978)

4272 Ramirez G, Narvarte J, Bittle PA et al. Cyclosporine-induced alterations in the hypothalamic hypophyseal gonadal axis in transplant patients. *Nephron*, 58, 27-32 (1991)

4273 Ramos-Dias JC, Yateman M, Camacho-Huber C, et al. Low circulating IGF-I levels in hyperthyroidism are associated with decreased GH response to GH-releasing hormone. *Clin Endocrinol*, 43, 583-589 (1995)

4274 Ramu G et al. Plasma fibrinogen levels and fibrinolytic activity in lepromatous leprosy. *J Ass Physicians India*, 25, 133-138 (1977)

4275 Rannikko S, Adlercreutz H, Haapiainen R. Urinary oestrogen excretion in benign prostatic hyperplasia and prostatic cancer. *Br J Urol*, 64, 172-175 (1989)

4276 Rao JK, Weinberger M, Oddone EZ, et al. The role of antineutrophil cytoplasmic antibody (c-ANCA) testing in the diagnosis of Wegener's granulomatosis. *Ann Intern Med*, 123, 925-932 (1995)

4277 Rao ML, Gross G, Strebel B et al. Circadian rhythm of tryptophan, serotonin, melatonin, and pituitary hormones in schizophrenia. *Biol Psychiat*, 35, 151-163 (1994)

4278 Rapaport MH. Circulating lymphocyte surface markers in anxiety disorder patients and normal volunteers. *Biol Psychiat*, 43, 458-463 (1998)

4279 Rapaport MH, McAllister CG, Kim YS et al. Increased serum soluble interleukin-2 receptors in Caucasian and Korean schizophrenic patients. *Biol Psychiat*, 35, 767-771 (1994)

4280 Rar V et al. Blood histamine and histaminase in leprosy patients - a short communication. *Ind J Med Res*, 66, 978-982 (1977)

4281 Rascher W, Tulassay T, Lang RE. Atrial natriuretic peptide in plasma of volume-overloaded children with chronic renal failure. *Lancet*, 2, 303-305 (1985)

4282 Raskind MA, Peskind ER, Lampe TH et al. Cerebrospinal fluid vasopressin, oxytocin, somatostatin, and B-endorphin in Alzheimer's disease. *Arch Gen Psychiat*, 43, 382 (1986)

4283 Rasmussen K. Phosphoethanolamine and hypophosphatasia. *Dan Med Bull*, 15, 1 (1968)

4284 Rasmussen K, Moller J, Lyngbak M, et al. Age- and gender-specific reference intervals for total homocysteine and methylmalonic acid in plasma before and after vitamin supplementation. *Clin Chem*, 42, 630-636 (1996)

4285 Rasmusson T, Bjork GR, Damber L et al. Tumor markers in mammary carcinoma. An evaluation of carcinoembryonic antigen, placental alkaline phosphatase, pseudouridine and CA-50. *Acta Oncol*, 26, 261-267 (1987)

4286 Rassiga-Pidot AL et al. Paroxysmal nocturnal hemoglobinuria with elevated fetal hemoglobin. *Blood*, 43, 233 (1974)

4287 Ratnoff OD, Colopy JE. A familial hemorrhagic trait associated with a deficiency of a clot-promoting fraction of plasma. *J Clin Invest*, 34, 602 (1955)

4288 Rautonen J, Rautonen N, Martin NL et al. Serum interleukin-6 concentrations are elevated and associated with elevated tumor necrosis factor-α and immunoglobulin G and A concentrations in children with HIV infections. *AIDS*, 5, 1319-1325 (1991)

4289 Ravel R. *Clinical Laboratory Medicine,* 4th edition, Chicago IL, Year Book Medical Publishers (1984)

4290 Ravelli A, Caporali R, Di Fuccia G et al. Anticardiolipin antibodies in pediatric systemic lupus erythematosus. *Arch Pediat Adolesc Med*, 148, 398-402 (1994)

4291 Ravindran AV, Griffiths J, Kerall Z, Anisman H. Circulating lymphocyte subsets in major depression and dysthymia with typical or atypical features. *Psychosomat Med*, 60, 283-289 (1998)

4292 Rawat M, Vijayvargiya R. Serum copper estimation in lymphomas. *Ind J Med Res*, 66, 815-819 (1977)

4293 Rayfield EJ, Curnow RT, Beisel WR. Acute glucose intolerance during sandfly fever in man: metabolic interrelationships. *Am J Clin Nutr*, 26, 463 (1973)

4294 Rayfield EJ et al. Impaired carbohydrate metabolism during a mild viral illness. *N Engl J Med*, 289, 618 (1973)

4295 Raz R et al. Serum and urinary uric acid in infectious hepatitis. *Isr J Med Sci*, 13, 1219-1221 (1977)

4296 Recan L, Riggs P S. Thyroid function in nephrosis. *J Clin Invest*, 31, 789 (1952)

4297 Rector WG Jr, Lewis FW, Adair OV et al. Plasma renin activity in alcoholic liver disease. *Am J Med*, 92, 485-492 (1992)

4298 Reddi YR et al. Cerebrospinal fluid and blood sugar ratio in health and disease: diagnostic and prognostic significance in intracranial infections. *Ind J Pediatr*, 12, 401 (1975)

4299 Reddy BS et al. Fecal bile acids and cholesterol metabolites of patients with ulcerative colitis, a high-risk group for development of colon cancer. *Cancer Res*, 37, 1697-1701 (1977)

4300 Reddy BS et al. Fecal bile acids and neutral sterols in patients with familial polyposis. *Cancer*, 39, 1694-1698 (1976)

4301 Reddy BS et al. Metabolic epidemiology of colon cancer. fecal bile acids and neutral sterols in colon cancer patients with adenomatous polyps. *Cancer*, 39, 2533-2539 (1977)

4302 Reddy MM, Grieco MH. Changed circulating CD35 levels and unchanged CD71 levels in patients with human immunodeficiency virus infection. *Immunol Infect Dis*, 3, 249-252 (1993)

4303 Reddy MM, Grieco MH. Elevated levels of soluble CD54 (ICAM-1) in human immunodeficiency virus infection. *J Clin Lab Anal*, 7, 269-272 (1993)

4304 Reding MT, Hibbs JR, Morrison VA, et al. Diagnosis and outcome of 100 consecutive patients with extreme granulocyte leukocytosis. *Am J Med*, 104, 12-16 (1998)

4305 Redman CW et al. Plasma urate and serum deoxycytidylate deaminase measurements for the early diagnosis of pre-eclampsia. *Br J Obstet Gynaecol*, 84, 904-908 (1977)

4306 Redman CW et al. Plasma-urate measurements in predicting fetal death in hypertensive pregnancy. *Lancet*, 1, 1370-1373 (1976)

4307 Reed JS, Boyer JL. Viral hepatitis, epidemiologic, serologic and clinical manifestation. *DM*, 25, 1-61 (1979)

4308 Rees EG et al. Serum proteins in systemic lupus erythematosus. *Br Med J*, 5155, 795 (1959)

4309 Rees GW, Trull AK, Doyle S. Evaluation of an enzyme-immunometric assay for serum α-glutathione S-transferase. *Ann Clin Biochem*, 32, 575-583 (1995)

4310 Reeves B. Significance of joint fluid uric acid levels in gout. *Ann Rheum Dis*, 24, 569-571 (1965)

4311 Reeves et al. Differential diagnosis of hypercalcemia by the chloride: phosphate ratio. *Am J Surg*, 130, 166-171 (1975)

4312 Regland B, Gottfries CG, Oreland L. Vitamin B_{12}-induced reduction of platelet monoamine oxidase activity in patients with dementia and pernicious anaemia. *Eur Arch Psych Clin Neurosci*, 240, 288-291 (1991)

4313 Reibnegger G, Boonpucknavig V, Fuchs D et al. Urinary neopterin is elevated in patients with malaria. *Trans Roy Soc Trop Med Hyg*, 78, 545-546 (1984)

4314 Reichman RC, Dolin R. Viral pneumonias. *Med Clin North Am*, 64, 491-506 (1980)

4315 Reijonen TM, Korppi M, Kuikka L, et al. Serum eosinophil cationic protein as a predictor of wheezing bronchiolitis. *Pediatr Pulmonol*, 23, 397-403 (1997)

4316 Reincke M, Allolio B, Petzke F et al. Thyroid dysfunction in African trypanosomiasis: a possible role for inflammatory cytokines. *Clin Endocrinol*, 39, 455-461 (1993)

4317 Reinisch W, Heider K-H, Oberhuber G, et al. Poor diagnostic value of colonic CD44v6 expression and serum concentrations of its soluble form in the differentiation of ulcerative colitis from Crohn's disease. *Gut*, 43, 375-382 (1998)

4318 Reiss E, Canterbury J. Blood levels of parathyroid hormone in disorders of calcium metabolism. *Annu Rev Med*, 24, 217-232 (1973)

4319 Reljic M, Gorisek B. C-reactive protein and the treatment of pelvic inflammatory disease. *Int J Gynecol Obstet*, 60, 143-150 (1998)

4320 Remacha AF, Montserrat I, Santamaria A, et al. Serum erythropoietin in the diagnosis of polycythemia vera, a follow up study. *Haematologica*, 82, 406-410 (1997)

4321 Remes J. Neuroendocrine activation after myocardial infarction. *Br Heart J*, 72, 65-69 (1994)

4322 Remme WJ et al. Changes in purine nucleoside content in human myocardial efflux during pacing-induced ischemia. *Recent Adv Stud Cardiac Struct Metab*, 12, 409-413 (1976)

4323 Ren H, Zheng DF, Jia XP. Tumor necrosis factor and interleukin 6 in hepatitis C virus infection. *Chung Hua Nei Ko Tsa Chih*, 31, 344-346 (1992)

4324 Renkema TEJ, Kerstjens HAM, Schouten JP, et al. The importance of serum IgE for level and longitudinal change in airways hyperresponsiveness in COPD. *Clin Exp Allergy*, 28, 1210-1218 (1998)

4325 Rennie et al. The clinical significance of serum transaminase in infectious mononucleosis complicated by hepatitis. *N Engl J Med*, 257, 547-553 (1957)

4326 Repetto MG, Reides CG, Evelson P, et al. Peripheral markers of oxidative stress in probable Alzheimer patients. *Eur J Clin Invest*, 29, 643-649 (1999)

4327 Rerabek JE. Low density lipoproteins and immunoglobulins in human pleural effusions. *Clin Chim Acta*, 76, 363-369 (1977)

4328 Resnitzky P et al. Osmotic fragility of peripheral blood lymphocytes in chronic lymphatic leukemia and malignant lymphoma. *Blood*, 51, 645-651 (1978)

4329 Reverter JL, Pizarro E, Senti M et al. Relationship between lipoprotein profile and urinary excretion in type II diabetic patients with stable metabolic control. *Diabetes Care*, 17, 189-194 (1994)

4330 Revillion F, Hebbar M, Bonneterre J, Peyrat JP. Plasma c-erbB2 concentrations in relation to chemotherapy in breast cancer patients. *Eur J Cancer*, 32A, 231-234 (1996)

4331 Reynafarie C et al. The polycythemia of high altitude: iron metabolism and related studies. *Blood*, 14, 433 (1959)

4332 Reynafarje C, Ramos J. The hemolytic anemia of human bartonellosis. *Blood*, 17, 562 (1961)

4333 Reynolds C. Urine glucose measurement in the management of diabetes mellitus. *Compr Ther*, 4, 13-19 (1978)

4334 Reynolds EH. Multiple sclerosis and vitamin B_{12} metabolism. *J Neuroimmunol*, 40, 225-230 (1992)

4335 Reynolds MD et al. Copper-resistant serum acid phosphatase I. method and values in health and disease. *Cancer Res*, 16, 943-950 (1959)

4336 Reynolds RD, Natta CL. Depressed plasma pyridoxal phosphate concentrations in adult asthmatics. *Am J Clin Nutr*, 41, 684-688 (1985)

4337 Reynolds TB et al. Lupoid hepatitis. *Ann Intern Med*, 61, 650 (1964)

4338 Reynolds TM, Brain A, Marshall P. The vitamin B_6 status of patients with femoral fractures. *Proc ACB Natl Meet*, 48 (1992)

4339 Reza S, Shetty V, Dar S, et al. Tumor necrosis factor-α levels decrease with anticytokine therapy in patients with myelodysplastic syndromes. *J Interferon Cytokine Res*, 18, 871-877 (1998)

4340 Rhoads CP et al. Observations on etiology and treatment of anemia associated with hookworm infection. *Medicine*, 13, 317 (1934)

4341 Rhone et al. Isoenzymes of liver alkaline phosphatase in serum of patients with hepatobiliary disorders. *Clin Chem*, 19, 1142-1147 (1973)

4342 Ribalta J, LaVille AE, Girona J, et al. Low plasma vitamin A concentrations in familial combined hyperlipidemia. *Clin Chem*, 43, 2379-2383 (1997)

4343 Ricard-Blum S, Chevalier X, Grimaud JA et al. Detectable levels of pyridinoline are present in synovial fluid from various patients with knee effusion: preliminary results. *Eur J Clin Invest*, 25, 438-441 (1995)

4344 Ricci G, D'Ambrosi A, Resca D et al. Comparison of serum total sialic acid, C-reactive protein, α_1-acid glycoprotein and β_2-microglobulin in patients with non-malignant bowel diseases. *Biomed Pharmacother*, 5, 259-262 (1995)

4345 Richter et al. Acute myoglobinuria associated with heroin addiction. *J Am Med Ass*, 216, 1172-1176 (1971)

4346 Richterich R, Zuppinger K, Rossi E. Diagnostic significance of heterogeneous lactic dehydrogenases in malignant effusions. *Nature*, 191, 507-508 (1961)

4347 Rickies FF, O'Leary DS. The role of the coagulation system in the pathophysiology of sickle cell disease. *Arch Intern Med*, 133, 465 (1974)

4348 Rico H. Alcohol and bone disease. *Alcohol Alcoholism*, 25, 348-352 (1990)

4349 Riddoch D, Thompson R A. Immunoglobulin levels in the cerebrospinal fluid. *Br Med J*, 1, 396 (1970)

4350 Ridker PM, Cushman M, Stampfer MJ, et al. Plasma concentration of C-reactive protein and risk of developing peripheral vascular disease. *Circulation*, 97, 425-428 (1998)

4351 Rieckmann P, Martin S, Weichselbraun I et al. Serial analysis of circulating adhesion molecules and TNF receptor in serum from patients with multiple sclerosis: cICAM-1 is an indicator for relapse. *Neurology*, 44, 2367-2372 (1994)

4352 Riedler et al. Hypophosphataemia in septicaemia:higher incidence in gram-negative than in gram-positive infections. *Br Med J*, 1, 753-756 (1969)

4353 Riemens S, van Tol A, Sluiter W, Dullaart R. Elevated plasma cholesteryl ester transfer in NIDDM: relationships with apolipoprotein B-containing lipoproteins and phospholipid transfer protein. *Atherosclerosis*, 140, 71-79 (1998)

4354 Riemenschneider M, Buch K, Schmolke M, et al. Cerebrospinal protein tau is elevated in early Alzheimer's disease. *Neurosci Lett*, 212, 209-211 (1996)

4355 Riera A, Gimferrer E, Cadafalch J et al. Prevalence of high serum and red cell ferritin levels in HIV-infected patients. *Haematologica*, 79, 165-167 (1994)

4356 Riesen WF et al. *Arteriosclerosis*, 37, 197 (1980)

4357 Rieu M, Revue E, Bonete R, Nunez S. Relationships between plasma thyrotropin receptor antibodies and lipid or lipoprotein parameters in Graves' disease. *Eur J Endocrinol*, 135, 77-81 (1996)

4358 Rifkind BM, Levy RI. *Hyperlipidemia: Diagnosis and Therapy*, New York NY, Grune and Strattton (1977)

4359 Rigby AJ, Ray M, Basu TK. Biochemical status of vitamin A in patients with malignant and benign breast disease. *J Clin Biochem Nutr*, 13, 53-61 (1992)

4360 Riikonen RS, Soderstrom S, Vanhala R, et al. West syndrome: cerebrospinal fluid nerve growth factor and effect of ACTH. *Pediatr Neurol*, 17, 224-29 (1997)

4361 Riley V. Breast cancer patients: substance in blood causing acceleration of erythrocyte sedimentation rate. *Science*, 191, 86-88 (1976)

4362 Rimington C. The excretion of porphyrin-peptide conjugates in porphyria variegata. *Clin Sci*, 43, 299 (1972)

4363 Rinderknecht H et al. Serum creatine phosphokinase in acute pancreatitis. *Clin Biochem*, 3, 165-170 (1970)

4364 Ristamaki R, Joensuu H, Lappalainen K, et al. Elevated serum CD44 level is associated with unfavorable outcome in non-Hodgkin's lymphoma. *Blood*, 90, 4039-4045 (1997)

4365 Risteli L, Risteli J, Puistola U. Aminoterminal propeptide of type III procollagen in ovarian cancer. A review. *Acta Obstet Gynecol Scand Suppl.*, 155, 99-103 (1992)

4366 Ristell J, Elomaa I, Niemi S et al. Radioimmunoassay for the pyridinoline cross-linked carboxy-terminal telopeptide of type I collagen: a new serum marker of bone collagen degradation. *Clin Chem*, 39, 635-640 (1993)

4367 Ritland S et al. Hepatic copper content, urinary copper excretion, and serum ceruloplasmin in liver disease. *Scand J Gastroenterol*, 12, 81-88 (1977)

4368 Rittenhouse HG, Chan DW. Can complexed PSA be used as a single test for detecting prostate cancer? *Urology*, 54, 4-5 (1999)

4369 Rittgers RH et al. Carcinoembryonic antigen levels in benign and malignant effusions. *Ann Intern Med*, 88, 631-634 (1978)

4370 Rittmaster RS. Finasteride. *N Engl J Med*, 330, 120-125 (1994)

4371 Ritzmann SE, Daniels JC. *Serum Protein Abnormalities: Diagnostic and Clinical Aspects*, Boston MA, Little, Brown and Co (1975)

4372 Ritzmann SE, Tucker ES III. Electrophoresis assays. In:. *Clinical Medicine*. Spittell JA Jr. (ed), Hagerstown MD, Harper and Row (1980)

4373 Ritzmann SE, Tucker ES III. Protein analysis in disease-current concepts. *Workshop Manual*, Chicago IL, American Society of Clinical Pathologists (1979)

4374 Rivero SJ et al. Lymphopenia in systemic lupus erythematosus: clinical, diagnostic, and prognostic significance. *Arth Rheum*, 21, 295-305 (1978)

4375 Rizzoli R, Stoermann C, Ammann P et al. Hypercalcemia and hyperosteolysis in vitamin D intoxication: effects of clodronate therapy. *Bone*, 15, 193-198 (1994)

4376 Roa D, Turner E, Aguinaga MdP. Reference ranges for hemoglobin variants by HPLC in African Americans. *Ann Clin Lab Sci*, 25, 228-235 (1995)

4377 Rob PM, Erbsloh-Moller B, Steinhoff J, et al. Follow-up measurement of magnesium metabolism after renal transplantation and FK 506 treatment in man. *Trace Elem Elect*, 15, 5-7 (1998)

4378 Robak T, Gladalska A, Stepien H. The tumour necrosis factor family of receptor/Ligands in the serum of patients with rheumatoid arthritis. *Eur Cytokine Netw*, 9, 145-154 (1998)

4379 Robboy SJ et al. Mechanism of aspergillus-induced microangiopathic hemolytic anemia. *Arch Intern Med*, 128, 790 (1971)

4380 Roberti I, Dikman S, Spiera H, et al. Comparative value of urinalysis, urine cytology and urine sIL2R in the assessment of renal diseases in patients with systemic lupus erythematosus (SLE). *Clin Nephrol*, 46, 176-182 (1996)

4381 Roberts MM, Bathgate EM, Stevenson A. Serum immunoglobulin levels in patients with breast cancer. *Cancer*, 36, 221-224 (1975)

4382 Roberts NB, King D. Biochemical indices of nutrition in the elderly. *Proc ACB Natl Meet*, 49 (1993)

4383 Robins SP, Woitge H, Hesley R et al. Direct, enzyme-linked immunoassay for urinary deoxypyridinoline as a specific marker for measuring bone resorption. *J Bone Miner Res*, 9, 1643-1649 (1994)

4384 Robinson AD, Boyden KN, Hendrickson SM, Muirden KD. Antitrypsin activity and enzyme inhibitors in the rheumatoid joint. *J Rheumatol*, 8, 547-554 (1981)

4385 Robinson D, Whitehead TP. Effect of body mass and other factors on serum liver enzyme levels in men attending for well population screening. *Ann Clin Biochem*, 26, 393-400 (1989)

4386 Robinson et al. Clinical significance of increased serum 'acid' phosphatase in patients with bone metastases secondary to prostatic carcinoma. *J Urol*, 42, 602-618 (1939)

4387 Robinson H et al. A comparison of fasting plasma insulin and growth hormone concentrations in marasmic, kwashiorkor, and underweight children. *Pediatr Res*, 11, 637-640 (1977)

4388 Robinson J, Birkinshaw G, Dutton J et al. Urinary free PYR and DPYR excretion in the diagnosis and treatment of metabolic bone disease and hypercalcaemia of malignancy. *Proc ACB Natl Meet*, 67-68 (1995)

4389 Robinson N et al. Serum enzymes in Friedreich's ataxia. *Brain*, 88, 131 (1965)

4390 Roblot P, Morel F, Lelievre E, et al. Serum soluble CD23 levels in giant cell arteritis. *Immunol Lett*, 53, 41-44 (1996)

4391 Roccatello D, Mosso R, Ferro M et al. Urinary endothelin in glomerulonephritis patients with normal renal function. *Clin Nephrol*, 41, 323-330 (1994)

4392 Roche Pharmaceuticals, Inc. Manufacturer's literature on Roferon A® . Nutley, NJ 07110 (1996)

4393 Rocher HD et al. Diagnosis of primary and secondary hyperparathyroidism. *World J Surg*, 1, 709-720 (1977)

4394 Rochlitz C, Hasslacher C, Brocks DG et al. Serum concentration of laminin, and the course of the disease in patients with various malignancies. *J Clin Oncol*, 5, 1424-1429 (1987)

4395 Rock G, Kelton JG, Shumak KH, et al. Laboratory abnormalities in thrombotic thrombocytopenic purpura. *Br J Haematol*, 103, 1031-1036 (1998)

4396 Roda A et al. Serum primary bile acids in Gilbert's syndrome. *Gastroenterology*, 82, 77-83 (1982)

4397 Rodin A, Thakkar H, Taylor N et al. Hyperandrogenism in polycystic ovary syndrome - evidence of dysregulation of 11β-hydroxysteroid dehydrogenase. *N Engl J Med*, 330, 460-465 (1994)

4398 Rodnan GP. Primer on the rheumatic diseases. *J Am Med Ass*, 224, 661-812 (1973)

4399 Rodrguez-Garcia J, Requena JR, Rodrguez-Segade S. Increased concentrations of serum pentosidine in rheumatoid arthritis. *Clin Chem*, 44, 250-255 (1998)

4400 Rodriguez JF, Cordero J, Chantry C, et al. Plasma glutathione concentrations in children infected with human immunodeficiency virus. *Pediat Infect Dis J*, 17, 236-241 (1998)

4401 Rodriguez-Segade S, Alonso de la Pena C, Paz M et al. Carnitine concentrations in dialysed and undialysed patients with chronic renal insufficiency. *Ann Clin Biochem*, 23, 671-675 (1986)

4402 Rodwell RL, Taylor KM, Tudehope DI et al. Capillary plasma elastase α_1-proteinase inhibitor in infected and noninfected neonates. *Arch Dis Child*, 67, 436-439 (1992)

4403 Roe TF et al. The pathogenesis of hyperuricemia in glycogen storage disease, type I. *Pediatr Res*, 11, 664-669 (1977)

4404 Roelen CAM, Bolanowski M, Donker GH et al. Effect of treatment on plasma GHBP-II concentrations in patients with acromegaly. *Clin Biochem Rev*, 14, 248 (1993)

4405 Roguljic A, Safwan T, Separovic V. Creatine kinase-BB activity in malignant tumors and in sera from patients with malignant diseases. *Tumori*, 75, 537-541 (1989)

4406 Rohn RD, Pleban P, Jenkins LL. Magnesium, zinc and copper in plasma and blood cellular components in children with IDDM. *Clin Chim Acta*, 215, 21-28 (1993)

4407 Rohrbach MS, Deremee RA. Measurement of angiotensin converting enzyme activity in serum in the diagnosis and management of sarcoidosis. In:. *Clinical Laboratory Annual: 1982*, New York NY, Appleton-Century-Crofts, 1, 435-453 (1982)

4408 Rohrlich P, Sarfati J, Mariani P, et al. Prospective sandwich enzyme-linked immunosorbent assay for serum galactomannan: early predictive value and clinical use in invasive aspergillosis. *Pediatr Infect Dis*, 15, 232-237 (1996)

4409 Roijen SB, Worsaae U, Zlotnik G. Zinc in patients with anorexia nervosa. *Ugeskr Laeger*, 152, 721-723 (1991)

4410 Roine RP, Turpeinen U, Ylikahri R et al. Urinary dolichol - a new marker of alcoholism. *Alcohol Clin Exp Res*, 11, 525-527 (1987)

4411 Roizen NJ, Amarose AP. Hematologic abnormalities in children with Down syndrome. *Am J Med Genet*, 46, 510-512 (1993)

4412 Rolak LA, Beck RW, Paty DW, et al. Cerebrospinal fluid in acute optic neuritis : experience of the optic neuritis treatment trial. *Neurology*, 46, 368-372 (1996)

4413 Romas E, Paspaliaris B, d'Apice AJ et al. Autoantibodies to neutrophil cytoplasmic (ANCA) and endothelial cell surface antigens (AECA) in chronic inflammatory bowel disease. *Aust NZ J Med*, 22, 652-659 (1992)

4414 Romer FK. Angiotensin-converting enzyme and its association with outcome in lung cancer. *Br J Cancer*, 43, 135-42 (1981)

4415 Romer FK, Ahlbom G, Jensen JU. Relationship between angiotensin-converting enzyme and lysozyme in sarcoidosis. *Eur J Respir Dis*, 63, 330-336 (1982)

4416 Romer FK, Emmertsen K. Serum angiotensin-converting enzyme in malignant lymphomas, leukaemia and multiple myeloma. *Br J Cancer*, 42, 314-318 (1980)

4417 Romer FK, Schmitz O. Angiotensin-converting enzyme activity in renal disorders: influence of disease pattern, hemodialysis and transplantation. *Clin Nephrol*, 21, 178-183 (1984)

4418 Romero KM, Butcher BA, Boyle PJ et al. Decreased renal excretion of β-hexosaminidase in adults with insulin-dependent diabetes mellitus and normal renal function. *Clin Chim Acta*, 216, 125-133 (1993)

4419 Romics L, Nemesanscky E, Szalay F, et al. Lipoprotein(a) concentration and phenotypes in primary biliary cirrhosis. *Clin Chim Acta*, 255, 165-171 (1996)

4420 Romijn JA, Wiersinga WM. Decreased nocturnal surge of thyrotropin in nonthyroidal illness. *J Clin Endocrinol Metab*, 70, 35-42 (1990)

4421 Romppanen J, Mononen I. Age-related reference values for urinary excretion of sialic acid and deoxysialic acid: application to diagnosis of storage disorders of sialic acid. *Clin Chem*, 41, 544-547 (1995)

4422 Ronchi MC, Piragino C, Rosi E, et al. Role of sputum differential cell count in detecting airway inflammation in patients with chronic bronchial asthma or COPD. *Thorax*, 51, 1000-1004 (1996)

4423 Roncoroni AJ et al. Metabolic acidosis in status asthmaticus. *Respiration*, 33, 85-94 (1976)

4424 Ronquist G, Frithz G, Gunnarsson K, Arvidson G. Decreased erythrocyte cholesterol/phospholipid ratio in untreated patients with essential hypertension. *J Intern Med*, 232, 247-251 (1992)

4425 Rooney PJ et al. Serum immunoreactive gastrin in rheumatoid arthritis. *Ann Rheum Dis*, 35, 246 (1976)

4426 Rosahn P D, Pearce L. The blood cytology in untreated and treated syphilis. *Am J Med Sci*, 187, 88 (1934)

4427 Rosano TG, Peaston RT, Bone HG, Borg S. Urinary free deoxypyridinoline by chemiluminascence immunoassay: analytical and clinical evaluation. *Clin Chem*, 44, 2126-2132 (1998)

4428 Rose DP. Aspects of tryptophan metabolism in health and disease: a review. *J Clin Pathol*, 25, 17 (1972)

4429 Rose DP et al. Plasma thyroid-stimulating hormone and thyroxine concentrations in breast cancer. *Cancer*, 41, 666-669 (1978)

4430 Rose DP, Pruitt BT. Plasma prolactin levels in patients with breast cancer. *Cancer*, 48, 2687-2691 (1981)

4431 Rose NR, Friedman H. *Manual of Clinical Immunology*, 2nd edition, Washington DC, American Society for Microbiology (1980)

4432 Rose PG, Sommers RM, Reale FR et al. Serial serum CA 125 measurements for evaluation of recurrence in patients with endometrial carcinoma. *Obstet Gynecol*, 84, 12-16 (1994)

4433 Rose S, Hindmarsh JG, Steiger MJ et al. Plasma HVA levels following debrisoquine administration do not reflect cerebral dopamine loss in early Parkinson's disease. *Clin Neuropharmacol*, 17, 260-269 (1994)

4434 Rosen B. Multiple myeloma: a critical review. *Med Clin North Am*, 59, 375-386 (1975)

4435 Rosen C, Donahue LR, Hunter S et al. The 24/25-kDa serum insulin-like growth factor-binding protein is increased in elderly women with hip and spine fractures. *J Clin Endocrinol Metab*, 74, 24-27 (1992)

4436 Rosenbach LM, Xefteris ED. Erythrocytosis associated with carcinoma of the kidney. *J Am Med Ass*, 176, 136 (1961)

4437 Rosenberg M et al. Clinical and immunologic criteria for the diagnosis of allergic bronchopulmonary aspergillosis. *Ann Intern Med*, 86, 405-414 (1977)

4438 Rosenberg SA et al. Lymphosarcoma. *Ann Intern Med*, 53, 877 (1960)

4439 Rosenhein ML. Sodium. *Lancet*, 2, 505 (1951)

4440 Rosenkrantz JA et al. Paget's disease (osteitis deformans). *Arch Intern Med*, 90, 610-633 (1952)

4441 Rosenlund M et al. Dietary essential fatty acids in cystic fibrosis. *Pediatrics*, 59, 428-432 (1977)

4442 Rosenthal A et al. Hemoglobin-oxygen equilibrium in cystic fibrosis. *Pediatrics*, 59, 919-926 (1976)

4443 Rosenthal R. Blood coagulation in leukemia and polycythemia. *J Lab Clin Med*, 34, 1321 (1949)

4444 Rosing U, Carlstrom K. Serum levels of unconjugated and total oestrogens and dehydroepiandrosterone, progesterone and urinary oestriol excretion in preeclampsia. *Gynecol Obstet Invest*, 18, 190-205 (1984)

4445 Rosler A, Pohl M, Braune H-J, et al. Time course of chemokines in the cerebrospinal fluid and serum during herpes simplex type I encephalitis. *J Neur Sci*, 157, 82-89 (1998)

4446 Rosler A, Witztum E. Treatment of men with paraphilia with a long-acting analogue of gonadotropin-releasing hormone. *N Engl J Med*, 338, 416-422 (1998)

4447 Rosner F et al. Leukocyte alkaline phosphatase fluctuations with disease status in chronic granulocytic leukemia. *Arch Intern Med*, 130, 892-894 (1972)

4448 Rosner F, Schreiber Z. Serum vitamin B_{12} and vitamin B_{12} binding capacity in chronic myelogenous leukemia and other disorders. *Am J Med Sci*, 263, 473-480 (1972)

4449 Ross GA, Newbould EC, Thomas J, et al. Plasma and 24 h-urinary catecholamine concentrations in normal and patient populations. *Ann Clin Biochem*, 30, 38-44 (1993)

4450 Rosse F, Waldman TA. A comparison of some physical and chemical properties of erythropoiesis-stimulating factors from different sources. *Blood*, 24, 739 (1964)

4451 Rossen RD et al. Circulating immune complexes and antinuclear antibodies in juvenile rheumatoid arthritis. *Arth Rheum*, 20, 1485-1490 (1977)

4452 Rossi E, Casali B, Regolisti G, et al. Increased plasma levels of platelet-derived growth factor (PDGF-BB + PDGF-AB) in patients with never-treated mild essential hypertension. *Am J Hypertens*, 11, 1239-1243 (1998)

4453 Rostaing L, Oksman F, Izopet J, et al. Serological markers of autoimmunity in renal transplant patients before and after α-interferon therapy for chronic hepatitis C. *Am J Nephrol*, 16, 478-483 (1996)

4454 Rotenberg Z, Weinberger I, Fuchs Y et al. Elevation of serum lactate dehydrogenase levels as an early marker of occult malignant lymphoma. *Cancer*, 54, 1379-1381 (1984)

4455 Roth E, Zoch G, Schulz F et al. Amino acid concentrations in plasma and skeletal muscle of patients with acute hemorrhagic necrotizing pancreatitis. *Clin Chem*, 31/8, 1305-1309 (1985)

4456 Rothfield NF et al. Serum antinuclear antibodies in progressive systemic sclerosis (scleroderma). *Arth Rheum*, 11, 607-617 (1968)

4457 Rothschild AM, Reis ML, Melo VL, et al. Increased kininogen levels observed in plasma of diabetic patients are corrected by the administration of insulin. *Horm Metab Res*, 31, 326-328 (1999)

4458 Rotter JI et al. Duodenal-ulcer disease associated with elevated serum pepsinogen i. *N Engl J Med*, 300, 63-66 (1979)

4459 Rottino A et al. Behavior of total serum complement in Hodgkin's disease and other malignant lymphomas. *Blood*, 14, 246-253 (1959)

4460 Rovin BH, Doe N, Tan LC. Monocyte chemoattractant protein-1 levels in patients with glomerular disease. *Am J Kid Dis*, 27, 640-646 (1996)

4461 Roxborough HE, Mercer C, McMaster D, et al. Plasma glutathione peroxidase activity is reduced in hemodialysis patients. *Nephron*, 1999, 81 (278-283)

4462 Roy A, Agren H, Pickar D et al. Reduced CSF concentrations of homovanillic acid and homovanillic acid to 5-hydroxyindoleacetic acid ratios in depressed patients: relationship to suicidal behavior and dexamethasone nonsuppression. *Am J Psychiat*, 143, 1539-1545 (1986)

4463 Roy A, Pickar D, Paul S et al. CSF corticotropin-releasing hormone in depressed patients and normal control subjects. *Am J Psychiat*, 144, 641-645 (1987)

4464 Rozner F, Gorfien PC. Erythrocyte and plasma zinc and magnesium in health and disease. *J Lab Clin Med*, 72, 213-219 (1968)

4465 Rozniecki JJ, Hauser SL, Stein M et al. Elevated mast cell tryptase in cerebrospinal fluid of multiple sclerosis patients. *Ann Neurol*, 37, 63-66 (1995)

4466 Rubach M, Szymendera JJ, Kamiska J, Kowalska M. Serum CA 15.3, CEA and ESR patterns in breast cancer. *Int J Biol Markers*, 12, 168-173 (1997)

4467 Rubies-Prat J, Reverter JL, Senti M et al. Calculated low-density lipoprotein cholesterol should not be used for management of lipoprotein abnormalities in patients with diabetes mellitus. *Diabetes Care*, 16, 1081-1086 (1993)

4468 Rubin H, Solomon A. Cold agglutinins of anti-I specificity in alcoholic cirrhosis. *Vox Sang*, 12, 227 (1967)

4469 Rubin RT, Poland RE, Lesser IM et al. Neuroendocrine aspects of primary endogenous depression - IV. Pituitary-thyroid axis activity in patients and matched control subjects. *Psychoneuroendocrinology*, 12, 333-347 (1987)

4470 Rubins JB, Dunitz J, Rubins HB, et al. serum carcinoembryonic antigen as an adjunct to preoperative staging of lung cancer. *J Thorac Cardiovasc Surg*, 116, 412-416 (1998)

4471 Rudduck C, Franzen G, Hansson A et al. Properdin factor B (Bf) types in schizophrenia. *Hum Hered*, 34, 331-333 (1984)

4472 Rudge A, Niaz S, Palfrey S et al. Urinary neopterin as a marker of clinical activity in Crohn's disease. *Proc ACB Natl Meet*, 60 (1993)

4473 Rudolph G, Blum WF, Jenne EW et al. Growth hormone (GH), insulin-like growth factors (IGFs), and IGF-binding protein-3 (IGFBP-3) in a child with proteus syndrome. *Am J Med Genet*, 50, 204-210 (1994)

4474 Rudzite V, Skards JI, Fuchs D et al. Serum kynurenine and neopterin concentrations in patients with cardiomyopathy. *Immunol Lett*, 32, 125-130 (1992)

4475 Rudzki C et al. Chronic intrahepatic cholestasis of sarcoidosis. *Am J Med*, 59, 373-387 (1975)

4476 Ruiz C, Alegria A, Barbera R, et al. Lipid peroxidation and antioxidant enzyme activities in patients with type I diabetes. *Scand J Clin Lab Invest*, 59, 99-106 (1999)

4477 Rule AHE et al. Tumor-associated (CEA-reacting) antigen in patients with inflammatory bowel disease. *N Engl J Med*, 287, 24 (1972)

4478 Rumsby G, Weir T, Samuell CT. A semiautomated alanine:glyoxylate aminotransferase assay for the tissue diagnosis of primary hyperoxaluria type 1. *Ann Clin Biochem*, 34, 400-404 (1997)

4479 Rundles RA et al. Serum proteins in leukemia. *Am J Med*, 16, 842 (1954)

4480 Russell D et al. Biphasic response on oral glucose tolerance testing in myotonic dystrophy. *Acta Neurol Scand*, 53, 226-228 (1976)

4481 Russell IJ, Orr MD, Littman B et al. Elevated cerebrospinal fluid levels of substance P in patients with the fibromyalgia syndrome. *Arth Rheum*, 37, 1593-1601 (1994)

4482 Rust OA, Bofill JA, Zappe DH, et al. The origin of endothelin-1 in patients with severe preeclampsia. *Obstet Gynecol*, 89, 754-757 (1997)

4483 Rustin GSJ. The clinical value of tumour markers in the management of ovarian cancer. *Ann Clin Biochem*, 33, 284-289 (1996)

4484 Rutenburg AM et al. Serum γ-glutamyl transpeptidase activity in hepatobiliary pancreatic disease. *Gastroenterology*, 45, 43-48 (1963)

4485 Rutgeerts P. Clinical value of the detection of antibodies in the serum for diagnosis and treatment of inflammatory bowel disease. *Gastroenterology*, 115, 1006-1009 (1998)

4486 RY, Caveliere LF, Lorenzana FG et al. Pattern of C_3, iC_3b, and C_3d in patients hospitalized for acute asthma. *Ann Allergy*, 68, 324-330 (1992)

4487 Ryan WE, Ellefson RD, Ward LE. Clinical conference: lipid synovial effusion. unique occurrence in systemic lupus erythematosus. *Arth Rheum*, 16, 759-764 (1973)

4488 Ryder KW, Jay SJ, Jackson SA, Hoke SR. Characterization of a spectrophotometric assay for angiotensin converting enzyme. *Clin Chem*, 27, 530-534 (1981)

4489 Ryder KW, Jay SJ, Kiblawi SO, Hull MT. Serum angiotensin converting enzyme activity in patients with histoplasmosis. *J Am Med Ass*, 249, 1888-1889 (1983)

4490 Saad MJA, Morais SL, Saad STO. Reduced cortisol secretion in patients with iron deficiency. *Ann Nutr Metab*, 35, 111-115 (1991)

4491 Saatci U, Ozdemir S, Ozen et al. Serum concentration and urinary excretion of β_2-microglobulin and microalbuminuria in familial Mediterranean fever. *Arch Dis Child*, 70, 27-29 (1994)

4492 Saber MA, Mikkall N, Ibrahim MT et al. Serum procollagen type III peptide (PIIIP) in systemic and portal blood in chronic liver diseases. *Clin Biochem Rev*, 14, 215 (1993)

4493 Sabin SA. Pulmonary disease. In:. *Clinical Internal Medicine*. Keller LB et al (eds), Boston MA, Little Brown and Co, 100-107 (1979)

4494 Sachs C, Marsoner HJ, Ritter C, et al. Ionized magnesium measurement in serum. *Clin Biochem Rev*, 14, 196 (1993)

4495 Sacks DB. Amylin - a glucoregulatory hormone involved in the pathogenesis of diabetes mellitus. *Clin Chem*, 42, 494-495 (1996)

4496 Sacks DB, Berman MC. Hypophosphataemia in acute pancreatitis. *S Afr Med J*, 68, 87-90 (1985)

4497 Sadamori N. Clinical and biological significance of serum tumor markers in adult T-cell leukemia. *Leukemia Lymphoma*, 22, 415-419 (1996)

4498 Sadayasu T, Nakashima Y, Yashiro A et al. Heparin-releasable platelet factor 4 in patients with coronary artery disease. *Clin Cardiol*, 14, 725-729 (1991)

4499 Sadovsky Y, Pineda J, Collins JL. Serum CA-125 levels in women with ectopic and intrauterine pregnancies. *J Reprod Med Obstet Gynecol*, 36, 875-878 (1991)

4500 Saedi MS, Hill TM, Kuus-Reichel K, et al. The precursor form of the human kallikrein 2, a kallikrein homologous to prostate-specific antigen, is present in human sera and is increased in prostate cancer and benign prostatic hyperplasia. *Clin Chem*, 44, 2115-2119 (1998)

4501 Saeed AM, Khalil EAG, Elhassan AMA, et al. Serum erythropoietin concentration in anaemia of visceral leishmaniasis (kala-azar) before and during antimonial therapy. *Br J Haematol*, 100, 720-724 (1998)

4502 Saeed BO, Atabani GS, Bayoumi MA et al. Hypoglycaemia complicating cerebral malaria. *Proc ACB Natl Meet*, 123 (1993)

4503 Saeki T, Kuroda T, Morita T, et al. Significance of myeloperoxidase in rapidly progressive glomerulonephritis. *Am J Kid Dis*, 26, 13-21 (1995)

4504 Safa AM, Van Ordstrand HS. Pleural effusion due to multiple myeloma. *Chest*, 64, 246-248 (1973)

4505 Safi F, Kuhns V, Beger HG. Comparison of CA 72-4, CA 19-9 and CEA in the diagnosis and monitoring of gastric cancer. *Int J Biol Mark*, 10, 100-106 (1995)

4506 Safi F, Roscher R, Beger HG. The clinical relevance of the tumor marker CA 19-9 in the diagnosing and monitoring of pancreatic carcinoma. *Bull Cancer*, 77, 83-91 (1990)

4507 Safi F, Roscher R, Beger HG. Tumor markers in pancreatic cancer. Sensitivity and specificity of CA19-9. *Hepatogastroenterology*, 36, 419-423 (1989)

4508 Sager PM, Tayler OM, Cooper EH et al. The tumor marker CA 195 in colorectal and pancreatic cancer. *Int J Biol Mark*, 6, 241-246 (1991)

4509 Sagnella GA, Markandu ND, Buckley MG et al. Atrial natriuretic peptides in essential hypertension: basal plasma levels and relationship to sodium balance. *Can J Physiol Pharmacol*, 69, 1592-1600 (1991)

4510 Saha H, Harmoinen A, Nisula M, Pasternack A. Serum ionized versus total magnesium in patients with chronic renal disease. *Nephron*, 80, 149-152 (1998)

4511 Saha HHT, Salmela KT, Ahonen PJ et al. Sequential changes in vitamin D and calcium metabolism after successful renal transplantation. *Scand J Urol Nephrol*, 28, 21-27 (1994)

4512 Saha PK, Gupta I, Ganguly NK. Evaluation of serum creatine kinase as a diagnostic marker fo tubal pregnancy. *Aust NZ Obstet Gynecol*, 39, 366-367 (1999)

4513 Sahai J, Gallicano K, Swick L, et al. Reduced plasma concentrations of antituberculosis drugs in patients with HIV infection. *Ann Intern Med*, 128, 289-293 (1997)

4514 Sahi T et al. Serum lipids and proteins in lactose malabsorption. *Am J Clin Nutr*, 30, 476-481 (1977)

4515 Said ME, Campbell DM, Azzam ME et al. β-human chorionic gonadotrophin levels before and after the development of pre-eclampsia. *Br J Obstet Gynaecol*, 91, 772-775 (1984)

4516 Saito H, Tsujitani S, Ikeguchi M, et al. Serum level of a soluble receptor for interleukin-2 receptor as a prognostic factor in patients with gastric cancer. *Oncology*, 56, 253-258 (1999)

4517 Saito I, Itsuji S, Takeshita E, et al. Increased urinary dopamine excretion in young patients with essential hypertension. *Clin Exp Hypertens*, 16, 29-39 (1994)

4518 Saito K, Nagashima M, Iwata M, et al. The concentration of tissue plasminogen activator and urokinase in plasma and tissues of patients with ovarian and uterine tumors. *Thromb Res*, 58, 355-366 (1990)

4519 Saito Y, Kazuwa N, Shirakami G, et al. Endothelin in patients with chronic renal failure. *J Cardiovasc Pharmacol*, 17, S437-S439 (1991)

4520 Saito Y, Nakao K, Mukoyama M, et al. Application of monoclonal antibodies for endothelin to hypertensive research. *Hypertension*, 15, 734-738 (1990)

4521 Saitoh O, Sugi K, Matsuse R, et al. The forms and the levels of PMN-elastase in patients with colorectal diseases. *Am J Gastroenterol*, 90, 388-393 (1995)

4522 Sakaguchi S, Furuta Y, Kameda T. Haemopathological changes in recurrent deep venous thrombosis of the extremities. *J Cardiovasc Surg (Torino)*, 23, 117-122 (1982)

4523 Sakamoto Y, Shintani Y, Harada K, et al. Determination of free follistatin levels in sera of normal subjects and patients with various diseases. *Eur J Endocrinol*, 135, 345-351 (1996)

4524 Sakata M, Tasaka K, Kurachi H et al. Changes of bioactive luteinizing hormone after laparoscopic ovarian cautery in patients with polycystic ovarian syndrome. *Fertil Steril*, 53, 610-613 (1990)

4525 Saku K, Gartside PS, Hynd BA et al. Apolipoprotein AI and AII metabolism in patients with primary high-density lipoprotein deficiency associated with familial hypertriglyceridemia. *Metabolism*, 34, 754-764 (1985)

4526 Salah IA et al. Levels of some serum enzymes in patients with schistosomiasis. *J Trop Med Hyg*, 79, 270-4 (1976)

4527 Salaka LA. Serum electrolytes in hypertension in nigerians. *Clin Chim Acta*, 34, 105 (1971)

4528 Salaspuro M. Characteristics of laboratory markers in alcohol-related organ damage. *Scand J Gastroenterol*, 24, 769-780 (1989)

4529 Salat C, Holler E, Kolb H-J, et al. Plasminogen activator inhibitor-I confirms the diagnosis of hepatic veno-occlusive disease in patients with hyperbilirubinemia after bone marrow transplantation. *Blood*, 89, 2184-2189 (1997)

4530 Salih ST et al. Eosinophilia in Schistosoma mansoni infection. *East Afr Med J*, 54, 421-424 (1977)

4531 Salles GS, Bievenu J, Bastion Y, et al. Elevated circulating levels of TNFα and its p55 soluble receptor are associated with an adverse prognosis in lymphoma patients. *Br J Haematol*, 93, 352-359 (1996)

4532 Salman K, Spielvogel RL, Shulman LH et al. Serum androstanediol glucuronide in women with facial hirsutism. *J Am Acad Dermatol*, 26, 411-414 (1992)

4533 Salmayenli N, Genc S, Karan A, et al. Intterleukin-6 in chronic liver diseases. *Med Sci Res*, 26, 207-208 (1998)

4534 Salo E, Pesonen E, Viikari J. Serum cholesterol levels during and after Kawasaki disease. *J Pediatr*, 119, 557-561 (1991)

4535 Salojin KV, Le Tonqueze M, Saraux A, et al. Antiendothelial cell antibodies: useful markers of systemic sclerosis. *Am J Med*, 102, 178-185 (1997)

4536 Salt HB et al. On having no β-lipoprotein: a syndrome comprising a-β-lipoproteinemia, acanthocytosis and steatorrhea. *Lancet*, 2, 325 (1960)

4537 Salt WB II, Schenker S. Amylase - its clinical significance: a review of the literature. *Medicine*, 55, 269-290 (1976)

4538 Salvarani C, Boiardi L, Macchioni P et al. Serum soluble CD4 and CD8 levels in polymyalgia rheumatica. *J Rheumatol*, 21, 1865-1869 (1994)

4539 Salven P, Perhoniemi V, Tykka H, et al. Serum VEGF levels in women with a benign breast tumor or breast cancer. *Breast Cancer Res Treat*, 53, 161-166 (1999)

4540 Salven P, Ruotsalainen T, Mattson K, Joensuu H. High pre-treatment serum level of vascular endothelial growth factor (VEGF) is associated with poor outcome in small-cell lung cancer. *Int J Cancer (Pred Oncol)*, 79, 144-146 (1998)

4541 Salven P, Teerenhovi L, Joensuu H. A high pretreatment serum vascular endothelial growth factor concentration is associated with poor outcome in non-Hodgkin's lymphoma. *Blood*, 90, 3167-3172 (1997)

4542 Salvioni A, Marenzi G, Lauri G et al. β-Thromboglobulin plasma levels in the first week after myocardial infarction: influence of thrombolytic therapy. *Am Heart J*, 128, 472-476 (1994)

4543 Samama MM, Schlegel N, Cazenave B et al. Alpha 2 antiplasmin assay: amidolytic and immunological method. critical evaluation. *Synthetic Substrates in Clinical Blood Coagulation Assays*, 93-101 (1980)

4544 Sameshima Y, Chia D, Terasaki PJ et al. Appearance of the tumor marker CA 19-9 in liver transplant patients during rejection episodes. *Transplantation*, 53, 580-582 (1992)

4545 Samloff IM, Walsh JH. Unpublished observations

4546 Sammour MG et al. Serum and placental lactic dehydrogenase and alkaline phosphatase isoenzymes in normal pregnancy and in pre-eclampsia. *Acta Obstet Gynecol Scand*, 54, 393-400 (1975)

4547 Sampson B, Constantinescu MA, Chandarana I, Cussoms PD. Severe hypocupraemia in a patient with extensive burn injuries. *Ann Clin Biochem*, 33, 462-464 (1996)

4548 Sampson SE, Costello JF, Sampson AP. The effects of inhaled leukotriene B_4 in normal and asthmatic subjects. *Am J Resp Crit Care Med*, 155, 1789-1792 (1997)

4549 Samsonov M, Nassonov E, Dhzuzenova B et al. Serum neopterin in acute rheumatic fever. *Clin Chem*, 39, 693-695 (1993)

4550 Samsonov MY, Nassonov EL, Tilz GP, et al. Elevated serum levels of neopterin in adult patients with polymyositis/dematomyositis. *Br J Rheumatol*, 36, 656-660 (1997)

4551 Samter M (ed). *Immunological Diseases*, 3rd ed, Boston MA, Little Brown and Co (1978)

4552 Samuelson K, Aly A, Johansson C, Norman A. Serum and urinary bile acids in patients with primary biliary cirrhosis. *Scand J Gastroenterol*, 17, 121-128 (1982)

4553 Sanchez-Martin M et al. Dopamine beta hydroxylase in human synovial fluid. *Experientia*, 33, 650-651 (1977)

4554 Sanchez-Muniz FJ, Marcos A, Varela A. Serum lipids and apolipoprotein B values in, blood pressure and pulse rate in anorexia nervosa. *Eur J Clin Nutr*, 45, 33-36 (1991)

4555 Sanchez-Ubeda R et al. The significance of pancreatitis accompanying acute cholecystitis. *Ann Surg*, 144, 44 (1956)

4556 Sandberg AA et al. Studies on leukemia I. uric acid excretion. *Blood*, 11, 154 (1956)

4557 Sandberg T, Cooper EH, Lidin-Janson G et al. Fever and proximal tubular function in acute pyelonephritis. *Nephron*, 41, 39-41 (1985)

4558 Sandler M et al. Prostaglandins in amine-peptide secreting tumours. *Lancet*, 2, 1053 (1968)

4559 Sandock DS, Seftel AD, Resnick MI. The role of γ-glutamyl transpeptidase in the preoperative metastatic evaluation of renal cell carcinoma. *J Urol*, 137, 798-799 (1997)

4560 Sandoz Pharmaceuticals Corporation. Manufacturer's literature on Miacalcin® . East Hanover, NJ 07936 (1997)

4561 Sandron D, Lecossier D, Grodet A, Basset G. Diagnostic, prognostic and developmental value of serum angiotensin converting enzyme in sarcoidosis. *Ann Med Interne (Paris)*, 135, 46-50 (1984)

4562 Sandstead HH, Shukry AS, Prasad AS et al. Kwashiorkor in Egypt. I. clinical and biochemical studies with special reference to plasma zinc and serum lactic dehydrogenase. *Am J Clin Nutr*, 17, 15-26 (1965)

4563 Sandstrom H, Wahlin A, Eriksson M et al. Serum thymidine kinase in congenital dyserythropoietic anaemia type III. *Br J Haematol*, 87, 653-654 (1994)

4564 Sane AS, Chokshi SA, Mishra VV et al. Serum lipoperoxides in induced and spontaneous abortions. *Gynecol Obstet Invest*, 31, 172-175 (1991)

4565 Sanmarti R, Collado A, Gratacos J, et al. Reduced activity of serum creatine kinase in rheumatoid arthritis: a phenomenom linked to the inflammatory response. *Br J Rheumatol*, 33, 231-234 (1994)

4566 Sano H, Asano K, Minatoguchi S, et al. Plasma soluble Fas and soluble Fas ligand in chronic glomerulonephritis. *Nephron*, 80, 153-161 (1998)

4567 Sano M, Kushida K, Takahashi M et al. Urinary pyridinoline and deoxypyridinoline in prostate carcinoma patients with bone metastases. *Br J Cancer*, 70, 701-703 (1994)

4568 Santabarbara P, Molina R, Estape J, Ballesta AM. Phosphohexose isomerase and carcinoembryonic antigen in the sera of patients with primary lung cancer. *Int J Biol Mark*, 3, 113-122 (1988)

4569 Santiyanont R, Harnpanich S, Sitpreeja S. Comparative study of urinary N-acetyl-B-D-galactosidase and microalbuminuria in normals and diabetics. *Clin Biochem Rev*, 14, 249 (1993)

4570 Santos M, Kondo T, Wiezzorek A et al. Clinical utility of serum hyaluronic acid levels in liver disease. *Clin Chem*, 41, S71 (1995)

4571 Santos PG et al. Les lipides plasmatique dans l'insuffisance respiratoire: relation avec l'hypercapnie et l'hypoxemie. *Br J Cancer*, 12, 179-183 (1976)

4572 Saoji A et al. Electrophoresis and immunoelectrophoresis in leprosy. *Leprosy India*, 50, 161-165 (1978)

4573 Sapira JD, Domm BM. Cryofibrinogenemia and cirrhosis of the liver. *Tex Rep Biol Med*, 25, 156 (1967)

4574 Sappey C, Leclercq P, Coudray C, et al. Vitamin, trace element and peroxide status in HIV serpositive patients: asymptomatic patients present a severe β-carotene dficiency. *Clin Chim Acta*, 230, 35-42 (1994)

4575 Sarandakou A, Phocas I, Botsis D, et al. Vaginal fluid and serum CEA, CA125 and SCC in normal conditions and in benign and malignant diseases of the genital tract. *Acta Oncol*, 36, 755-759 (1997)

4576 Sarcione EJ et al. Ferritin synthesis by splenic tumor tissue of Hodgkin's disease. *Experientia*, 31, 1334-1335 (1975)

4577 Sarne AS et al. Renal clearances of amino acids in Indian childhood cirrhosis and portal cirrhosis. *Ind J Pediatr*, 13, 713-718 (1976)

4578 Sartorio A, Conti A, Ferrario S, et al. Serum bone Gla protein and carboxyterminal cross-linked telopeptide of type I collagen in patients with Cushing's syndrome. *Postgrad Med J*, 72, 419-422 (1996)

4579 Sartorio A, Conti A, Ferrero S, et al. Evaluation of markers of bone and collagen turnover in patients with active and preclinical Cushing's syndrome and in patients with adrenal incidentaloma. *Eur J Endocrinol*, 138, 146-152 (1998)

4580 Sartorio A, Conti A, Monzani M et al. Growth hormone treatment in adults with GH deficiency: effects of new biochemical markers of bone and collagen turnover. *J Endocrinol Invest*, 16, 893-898 (1993)

4581 Sartorius OW et al. The renal regulation of acid-base balance in man. *J Clin Invest*, 28, 423 (1949)

4582 Sasagawa T, Okita M, Murakami J, et al. Abnormal serum lysophospholipids in multiple myeloma patients. *Lipids*, 14, 17-21 (1999)

4583 Sasaki T, Hiwatashi N, Yamazaki I et al. The role of interferon-γ in the pathogenesis of Crohn's disease. *Gastroenterol Jpn*, 27, 29-36 (1992)

4584 Sasayuki T, Grmet FC, McDevitt HO. The association between genes in the major histocompatibility complex and disease susceptibility. *Annu Rev Med*, 28, 425-452 (1977)

4585 Sasco AJ, Rey F, Reynaud C, et al. Breast cancer prognostic significance of some modified urinary nucleosides. *Cancer Lett*, 108, 157-162 (1996)

4586 Sass-Kortsak A. Copper metabolism. *Adv Clin Chem*, 8, 1-67 (1965)

4587 Satake K, Chung Y-S, Umeyama K et al. The possibility of diagnosing small pancreatic cancer (less than 4.0 cm) by measuring various serum markers: a retrospective study. *Cancer*, 68, 149-152 (1991)

4588 Sategna-Guidetti C, Grosso S, Bruno M et al. Comparison of serum anti-gliadin, anti-endomyesium, and anti-jejuum antibodies in adult celiac sprue. *J Clin Gastroenterol*, 20, 17-21 (1995)

4589 Sato A, Shirota T, Shinoda T et al. Hyperuricemia in patients with hyperthyroidism due to Graves' disease. *Metabolism*, 44, 207-211 (1995)

4590 Sato S, Hasegawa M, Nagaoka T, et al. Autoantibodies against calpastatin in sera from patients with systemic sclerosis. *J Rheumatol*, 25, 2135-2139 (1998)

4591 Sato Y, Asoh T, Oizumi K. High prevalence of vitamin D deficiency and reduced bone mass in elderly women with Alzheimer's disease. *Bone*, 23, 555-557 (1998)

4592 Satoh K, Imaizumi T, Yoshida H et al. Increased levels of blood platelet-activating factor (PAF) and PAF-like lipids in patients with ischemic stroke. *Acta Neurol Scand*, 85, 122-127 (1992)

4593 Satomi A, Murakami S, Ishida K et al. Significance of increased neutrophils in patients with advanced colorectal cancer. *Acta Oncol*, 34, 69-73 (1995)

4594 Sattar N, Bendomir A, Berry C, et al. Lipoprotein subfraction concentrations in preeclampsia: pathogenic parallels to atherosclerosis. *Obstet Gynecol*, 89, 403-408 (1997)

4595 Sattar N, Blacklock C, O"Reilly D et al. Selenium containing proteins, acute phase reactants? *Proc ACB Natl Meet*, 87 (1995)

4596 Sauberlich HE, Dowdy RP, Skala JH. *Laboratory Tests for the Assessment of Nutritional Status*, Cleveland OH, CRC Press (1974)

4597 Saudek CD et al. Abnormal glucose tolerance in beta thalassemia major. *Metabolism*, 26, 43-52 (1977)

4598 Savage DG, Lindenbaum J, Stabler SP et al. Sensitivity of serum methylmalonic acid and total homocysteine determinations for diagnosing cobalamin and folate deficiencies. *Am J Med*, 96, 239-246 (1994)

4599 Savic J, Cernak I, Jevic M, et al. Glucose as an adjunct triage tool to the Red Cross wound classification. *J Trauma*, 40, S144-S147 (1996)

4600 Savige JA, Chang L, Smith CL et al. Myelodysplasia, vasculitis and anti-neutrophil cytoplasm antibodies. *Leukemia Lymphoma*, 9, 49-54 (1993)

4601 Savige JA, Davies DJ. Anti-neutrophil cytoplasm antibodies (ANCA). *Aust NZ J Med*, 20, 271-274 (1990)

4602 Savige JA, Smith CL, Chang L et al. Anti-neutrophil cytoplasmic antibodies (ANCA) in myelodysplasia and other haematological disorders. *Aust NZ J Med*, 24, 282-287 (1994)

4603 Sawczuk IS, Lee B. The mechanism and clinical applications of the NMP22 tumor marker immunoassay: a review. *Am Clin Lab*, April, 24-26 (1999)

4604 Saxena R, Sturfelt G, Nived O et al. Significance of anti-entactin antibodies in patients with systemic lupus erythematosus and related disorders. *Ann Rheum Dis*, 53, 659-665 (1994)

4605 Saxne T, Palladino MA, Heinegard D et al. Detection of tumor necrosis factor α but not tumor necrosis factor β in rheumatoid arthritis synovial fluid and serum. *Arth Rheum*, 31, 1041-1045 (1988)

4606 Saxon A, Shanahan F, Landers C et al. A distinct subset of anti-neutrophil cytoplasmic antibodies is associated with inflammatory bowel disease. *J Allerg Clin Immunol*, 718, 724-727 (1990)

4607 Sayinalp S, Gedik O, Koray Z. Increasing serum osteocalcin after glycemic control in diabetic men. *Calcif Tissue Int*, 57, 422-425 (1995)

4608 Scadding GK, Havard CW. Pathogenesis and treatment of myasthenia gravis. *Br Med J*, 283, 1008-1012 (1981)

4609 Scanlon MJ, Whorwood CB, Franks S et al. Serum androstanediol glucuronide concentrations in normal and hirsute women and in patients with thyroid dysfunction. *Clin Endocrinol*, 29, 529-538 (1988)

4610 Scanni A et al. Serum copper and ceruloplasmin levels in patients with neoplasias localized in the stomach, large intestine or lung. *Tumori*, 63, 175-180 (1977)

4611 Schaarschmidt H, Prange HW, Reiber H. Neuron-specific enolase concentrations in blood as a prognostic parameter in cerebrovascular diseases. *Stroke*, 25, 558-565 (1994)

4612 Schachter J et al. Lymphogranuloma venereum. I. comparison of the Frei test, complement-fixation test, and isolation of the agent. *J Infect Dis*, 120, 372 (1969)

4613 Schaffer AJ, Avery ME. *Diseases of the Newborn,* 4th edition, Philadelphia PA, WB Saunders (1977)

4614 Schaffer et al. Comparison of enzyme, clinical radiographic and radionuclide methods of detecting bone metastases from carcinoma of the prostate. *Radiology*, 121, 431-434 (1976)

4615 Schechter PJ et al. Distribution of serum zinc between albumin and α_2-macroglobulin in patients with decompensated hepatic cirrhosis. *Eur J Clin Invest*, 6, 147-150 (1976)

4616 Scheer WD, Boudreau DA, Cook CB. Lipoprotein(a) levels in African-Americans with NIDDM. *Diabetes Care*, 19, 1129-1133 (1996)

4617 Scheig R. Evaluation of tests used to screen patients with liver disorders. *Primary Care*, 23, 551-560 (1996)

4618 Scheja A, Akesson A, Horslev-Petersen K. Serum levels of aminoterminal type III procollagen peptide and hyaluronan predict mortality in systemic sclerosis. *Scand J Rheumatol*, 21, 5-9 (1992)

4619 Scheja A, Eskilsson J, Akesson A et al. Inverse relation between plasma concentration of von Willebrand factor and Cr-EDTA clearance in systemic sclerosis. *J Rheumatol*, 21, 639-642 (1994)

4620 Scheja A, Hellmer G, Wollheim FA et al. Carboxyterminal type I procollagen peptide concentrations in systemic sclerosis: higher levels in early diffuse disease. *Br J Rheumatol*, 32, 59-62 (1993)

4621 Schellenberg F, Martin M, Caces E, et al. Nephelometric determination of carbohydrate-deficient transferrin. *Clin Chem*, 42, 551-557 (1996)

4622 Schelp FP et al. Alterations of human serum proteins and other biochemical parameters after five to ten days of untreated acute falciparum malaria. *Tropenmed Parasitol*, 28, 319-322 (1977)

4623 Schelp FP et al. Serum proteinase inhibitors and other serum proteins in protein-energy malnutrition. *Br J Nutr*, 38, 31-38 (1977)

4624 Schelp FP, Thanangkul O, Supawan V et al. Serum proteinase inhibitors and acute-phase reactants from protein-energy malnutrition children during treatment. *Am J Clin Nutr*, 32, 1415-1422 (1979)

4625 Schena FP, Pertosa G, Germinario C. Plasma fibronectin levels in patients with chronic uremia. *Nephron*, 44, 320-323 (1986)

4626 Schenk S, Muser J, Vollmer G et al. Tenascin-C in serum: a questionable tumor marker. *Int J Cancer*, 61, 443-449 (1995)

4627 Scher H, Berman D, Weinberg EG, et al. Granulocyte proteins in serum in childhood asthma: relation to spirometry. *Clin Exp Allergy*, 26, 1131-1141 (1995)

4628 Schernthaner G, Schwarzer C, Kuzmits R et al. Increased angiotensin-converting enzyme activities in diabetes mellitus: analysis of diabetes type, state of metabolic control and occurrence of diabetic vascular complications. *J Clin Pathol*, 37, 307-312 (1984)

4629 Schiavi RC, Stimmel BB, Mandell J, White D. Chronic alcoholism and male sexual function. *Am J Psychiatr*, 152, 1045-1051 (1995)

4630 Schiff E, Ben-Baruch G, Peleg E et al. Immunoreactive circulating endothelin-1 in normal and hypertensive pregnancies. *Am J Obstet Gynecol*, 166, 624-628 (1992)

4631 Schiff E, Friedman SA, Sibai BM, et al. Plasma and placental calcitonin gene-related peptide in pregnancies complicated by severe preeclampsis. *Am J Obstet Gynecol*, 173, 1405-1409 (1995)

4632 Schiffer T, Zahavi I, Moroz C. Antimotochondrial antibodies after acute myocardial infarction. *Cardiology*, 87, 67-70 (1996)

4633 Schiffrin EL, Thibault G. Plasma endothelin in human essential hypertension. *Am J Hypertens*, 4, Pt 1, 303-308 (1991)

4634 Schild A, Pscheidl E, v Hintzenstern U. Phospholipase A - A parameter of sepsis? *Klin Wschr*, 67, 207-211 (1989)

4635 Schiller LR, Rivera LM, Santangelo WC et al. Diagnostic value of fasting plasma peptide concentrations in patients with chronic diarrhea. *Dig Dis Sci*, 39, 2216-2222 (1994)

4636 Schimizu T et al. Behcet's disease. *Semin Arth Rheum*, 8, 223 (1979)

4637 Schiodt FV, Ott P, Bondesen S, Tygstrup N. Reduced serum Gc-globulin concentrations in patients with fulminant hepatic failure : association with multiple organ failure. *Crit Care Med*, 25, 1366-1370 (1997)

4638 Schipper I, Rommerts FFG, Ten Hacken PM, et al. Low levels of follicle-stimulating hormone receptor-activation inhibitors in serum and follicular fluid from normal controls and anovulatory patients with or without polycystic ovary syndrome. *J Clin Endocrinol Metab*, 82, 1325-1331 (1997)

4639 Schlegel-Zawadzka M, Zieba A, Dudek D, et al. Serum trace elements in animal models and human depression. Part II. Copper. *Hum Psychopharmacol*, 14, 447-451 (1999)

4640 Schleiffer T, Hellstern P, Freitag M et al. Plasminogen activator inhibitor 1 activity and lipoprotein (a) in nephropathic patients with non-insulin-dependent diabetes mellitus versus patients with nondiabetic nephropathy. *Haemostasis*, 24, 49-54 (1994)

4641 Schliep G, Felgenhauer K. The α_2-macroglobulin level in cerebrospinal fluid; a parameter for the condition of the blood-CSF carrier. *J Neurol*, 207, 171-181 (1974)

4642 Schloesser LL et al. Thrombocytosis in iron deficiency anemia. *J Lab Clin Med*, 66, 107 (1965)

4643 Schlueter K, Lewis W, Schroeder T et al. Serum amyloid A (SAA) and soluble interleukin 2 receptor (sIL-2R) in heart transplant recipients: comparison to histopathologic changes. *Clin Chem*, 39, 1151 (1993)

4644 Schmid R et al. Erythropoietic (congenital) porphyria: a rare abnormality of the normoblasts. *Blood*, 10, 416 (1955)

4645 Schmid R et al. Porphyrin content of bone marrow and liver in the various forms of porphyria. *Arch Intern Med*, 93, 167 (1954)

4646 Schmid R, Hammaker L. Metabolism and disposition of C^{14} bilirubin in congenital nonhemolytic jaundice. *J Clin Invest*, 42, 1720 (1963)

4647 Schmidt JB, Lindmaier A, Spona J. Hyperprolactinemia and hypophyseal hypothyroidism as cofactors in hirsutism and androgen-induced alopecia in women. *Hautarzt*, 42, 168-172 (1991)

4648 Schmidt JB, Spona J. The levels of androgen in serum in female acne patients. *Endocrinol Exp*, 19, 17 (1985)

4649 Schmidt P, Zazgornik J, Kopsa H. Hypouricemia after renal transplantation. *N Engl J Med*, 289, 1373 (1973)

4650 Schmidt R et al. The course of multiple sclerosis with extremely high γ-globulin values in the CSF. *Eur Neurol*, 15, 241-248 (1977)

4651 Schmidt-Rhode P, Schulz K-D, Sturm G et al. C-reactive protein is a marker for the diagnosis of adnexitis. *Int J Gynaecol Obstet*, 32, 133-139 (1990)

4652 Schmitt WH, Heesen C, Csernok E et al. Elevated serum levels of soluble interleukin-2 receptor in patients with Wegener's granulomatosis. Association with disease activity. *Arth Rheum*, 35, 1088-1096 (1992)

4653 Schnabel A, Csernok E, Isenberg DA, et al. Antineutrophil cytoplasmic antibodies in systemic lupus erythematosus. *Arth Rheum*, 38, 633-637 (1995)

4654 Schneede J, Ueland PM. Automated assay of methylmalonic acid in serum and urine by derivatization with 1-pyrenyldiazomethane, liquid chromatography, and fluorescence detection. *Clin Chem*, 39, 392-399 (1993)

4655 Schneider J, Centeno M, Saez M, et al. Preoperative CA-125, CA 19-9 and nuclear magnetic resonance in endometrial carcinoma: correlation with surgical stage. *Tumor Biol*, 20, 25-29 (1999)

4656 Schoelmerich J, Becher MS, HoppeSeyler P et al. Zinc and vitamin A deficiency in patients with Crohn's disease is correlated with activity but not with localization or extent of the disease. *Hepatogastroenterology*, 32, 34-38 (1985)

4657 Schoen MS et al. Significance of serum level of 25-hydroxycholecalciferol in gastrointestinal disease. *Am J Dig Dis*, 23, 137-142 (1978)

4658 Schoen RE, Tangen CM, Kuller LH, et al. Increased blood glucose and insulin, body size, and incident colorectal cancer. *J Natl Cancer Inst*, 91, 1147-1154 (1999)

4659 Schoenfeld MR et al. Acid hyperphenylphosphatasia in thrombophlebitis and pulmonary embolism. *Ann Intern Med*, 57, 468-471 (1962)

4660 Schoenfeld MR et al. Acid phosphatase in serum: increase in acute myocardial infarction. *Science*, 139, 51-52 (1963)

4661 Schoenfeld MR et al. Increased serum phosphatase after arterial embolism. *Am Heart J*, 67, 92-94 (1964)

4662 Schoenfeld Y et al. Immunoglobulin changes in SLE. *Clin Immunol Immunopathol*, 39, 99-101 (1977)

4663 Schoffel U, Bonnaire F, van Specht BU et al. Monitoring the response to injury. *Injury*, 22, 377-382 (1991)

4664 Scholl GM, Wu CH, Leyden J. Androgen excess in women with acne. *Obstet Gynecol*, 64, 683 (1984)

4665 Scholl SM, Lidereau R, de la Rochefordiere A, et al. Circulating levels of the macrophage colony stimulating factor CSF-1 in primary and metastatic breast cancer patients. A pilot study. *Breast Cancer Res Treat*, 39, 275-283 (1996)

4666 Schoni MH, Turler K, Kaser H et al. Abnormal 3,4-dihydroxyphenylalanine (dopa) concentrations in plasma and urine of patients with cystic fibrosis. *Eur J Clin Invest*, 20, 272-278 (1990)

4667 Schoonbrood DFM, Out TA, Lutter R, et al. Plasma protein leakage and local secretion of proteins assessed in sputum in asthma and COPD: the effect of inhaled corticosteroids. *Clin Chim Acta*, 240, 163-178 (1995)

4668 Schrader J, Tebbe U, Borries M et al. Plasma endothelin in normal persons and in patients with various diseases. *Klin Wschr*, 68, 774-779 (1990)

4669 Schreiber S, Nikolaus S, Hampe J, et al. Tumour necrosis factor-α and interleukin-1β in relapse of Crohn's disease. *Lancet*, 353, 459-461 (1999)

4670 Schreiber W, Schweiger U, Werner D et al. Circadian pattern of large neutral amino acids, glucose, insulin, and food intake in anorexia nervosa and bulimia nervosa. *Metabolism*, 40, 503-507 (1991)

4671 Schreiner GE. The nephrotic syndrome. In:. *Diseases of the Kidney*. MB Strauss, LG Welt (eds). 2nd ed, Boston MA, Little Brown and Co, 1971, 503

4672 Schreiner GE, Maher JF. Toxic nephropathy: adverse renal effects caused by drugs and chemicals. *J Am Med Ass*, 191, 849 (1965)

4673 Schrezenmeier H, Noe G, Raghavachar A et al. Serum erythropoietin and serum transferrin receptor levels in aplastic anemia. *Br J Haematol*, 88, 286-294 (1994)

4674 Schrire V, Asherson RA. Arteritis of the aorta and its major branches. *Q J Med*, 33, 439 (1964)

4675 Schriver EE, Davidson JM, Sutcliffe MC et al. Comparison of elastin peptide concentrations in body fluids from healthy volunteer, smokers, and patients with chronic obstructive pulmonary disease. *Am Rev Resp Dis*, 145, 762-766 (1992)

4676 Schroder W, Ruppert C, Bender HG. Concomitant measurements of interleukin-6 (IL-6) in serum and peritoneal fluid of patients with benign and malignant ovarian tumors. *Eur J Obstet Gynecol*, 56, 43-46 (1994)

4677 Schror K. Thromboxane A2 and platelets as mediators of coronary arterial vasconstriction in myocardial ischaemia. *Eur Heart J*, 11, 27-34 (1990)

4678 Schulpis KH, Nounopoulos C, Scarpalezou A et al. Serum carnitine level in phenylketonuric children under dietary control in Greece. *Acta Paediat Scand*, 79, 930-934 (1990)

4679 Schultz JC, Shahidi NT. Detection of tumor necrosis factor-α in bone marrow plasma and peripheral blood plasma from patients with aplastic anemia. *Am J Hematol*, 45, 32-38 (1994)

4680 Schulze E, Hermann K, Haustein UF. N-procollagen(III) peptide and lysosomal β-galactosidase in progressive scleroderma and silicosis. *Dermatol Monatsschr*, 176, 687-693 (1990)

4681 Schumacher HR Jr. Laboratory diagnosis of degenerative joint disease. *Ann Clin Lab Sci*, 5, 242-247 (1975)

4682 Schur PH. Complement studies of sera and other biologic fluids. *Hum Pathol*, 14, 338-342 (1983)

4683 Schur PH et al. Complement in rheumatic diseases. *Bull Rheum Dis*, 26, 666-673 (1971)

4684 Schur PH et al. Immunologic factors and clinical activity in systemic lupus erythematosus. *N Engl J Med*, 278, 533 (1968)

4685 Schurmann G, Betzler M, Post S et al. Soluble interleukin-2 receptor, interleukin-6 and interleukin-1 beta in patients with Crohn's disease and ulcerative colitis: preoperative levels and postoperative changes of serum concentrations. *Digestion*, 51, 51-59 (1992)

4686 Schuster V, Herold M, Wachter H, Reibnegger G. Serum concentrations of interferon-γ, interleukin-6 and neopterin in patients with infectious mononucleosis and other Epstein-Barr virus-related lymphoproliferative diseases. *Infection*, 21, 210-213 (1993)

4687 Schwarcz R, Tamminga CA, Kurlan R, Shoulson I. Cerebrospinal fluid levels of quinolinic acid in Huntington's disease and schizophrenia. *Ann Neurol*, 24, 580-582 (1988)

4688 Schwartz JF et al. Bassen-Kornzweig syndrome: deficiency of serum β-lipoprotein. *Arch Neurol*, 8, 438 (1963)

4689 Schwartz MK. An evaluation of markers in the early detection of large bowel cancer. *Cancer*, 40, 2620-2624 (1977)

4690 Schwartz MK. Interferences in diagnostic biochemical procedures. *Adv Clin Chem*, 16, 1 (1973)

4691 Schwartz MK. Role of trace elements in cancer. *Cancer Res*, 35, 3481-3487 (1975)

4692 Schwartz MK et al. Laboratory aids to diagnosis: enzymes. *Cancer*, 37, Suppl, 542 (1976)

4693 Schwartz PE, Chambers SK, Chambers JT et al. Circulating tumor markers in the monitoring of gynecologic malignancies. *Cancer*, 60, 353-361 (1987)

4694 Schwarz-Eywill M, Heilig B, Bauer H et al. Evaluation of serum ferritin as a marker for adult Still's disease activity. *Ann Rheum Dis*, 51, 683-685 (1992)

4695 Schweiger U, Pirke K-M, Laessle RG et al. Gonadotropin secretion in bulimia nervosa. *J Clin Endocrinol Metab*, 74, 1122-1127 (1992)

4696 Schwick H-G, Haupt H. Chemistry and function of human plasma proteins. *Angew Chem*, 191, 87-99 (1980)

4697 Schwille PO et al. Urinary thyroxine in rats fed various diets and in renal calcium stone-forming patients. *Eur Urol*, 2, 196-199 (1976)

4698 Scioscia KA, Snyderman CH, Wagner R. Altered serum amino acid profiles in head and neck cancer. *Nutr Cancer Res*, 30, 144-147 (1998)

4699 Scott IV. The identification of high risk and practical strategies for a population based randomized trial of ovarian cancer screening. *Dis Mark*, 9, 133-152 (1991)

4700 Scott LV, Dinan TG. Urinary free cortisol excretion in chronic fatigue syndrome, major depression and in healthy volunteers. *J Afect Dis*, 47, 49-54 (1998)

4701 Scott P, Bruce C, Schofield D et al. Vitamin C status in patients with acute pancreatitis. *Br J Surg*, 80, 750-754 (1993)

4702 Scott R et al. Hypercalciuria related to cadmium exposure. *Urology*, 11, 462-465 (1978)

4703 Scudder PR et al. Serum copper and related variables in rheumatoid arthritis. *Ann Rheum Dis*, 37, 67-70 (1978)

4704 Scudder PR et al. Synovial fluid copper and related variables in rheumatoid and degenerative arthritis. *Ann Rheum Dis*, 37, 71-72 (1978)

4705 Seal US et al. Response of serum cholesterol and triglycerides to hormone treatment and the relation of pretreatment values to mortality in patients with prostatic cancer. *Cancer*, 38, 109-107 (1976)

4706 Seamonds B, Towfighi J, Arvan DA. Determination of ionized calcium in serum by use of an ion-selective electrode. *Clin Chem*, 18, 155 (1972)

4707 Searcy RL. *Diagnostic Biochemistry*. New York NY, McGraw-Hill (1969)

4708 Seed JR et al. The presence of agglutinating antibody in the IgM immunoglobulin fraction of rabbit antiserum during experimental African trypanosomiasis. *Parasitology*, 59, 283 (1969)

4709 Seedat YK, Bhoola KD, Muller R, et al. Urinary levels of tissue kallikrein in black and Indian hypertensives and their implications for therapy. *S Afr Med J*, 88 Cardiovasc Suppl 2, C73-C78 (1998)

4710 Seeldrayers P, Messina D, Desmedt D et al. CSF levels of neurotransmitters in Alzheimer-type dementia. Effects of ergoloid mesylate. *Acta Neurol Scand*, 71, 411-414 (1985)

4711 Seelig MS et al. Magnesium interrelationships in ischemic heart disease: a review. *Am J Clin Nutr*, 27, 59 (1974)

4712 Seely EW, Wood RJ, Brown EM, Graves SW. Lower serum ionized calcium and abnormal calciotropic hormone levels in preeclampsia. *J Clin Endocrinol Metab*, 74, 1436-1440 (1992)

4713 Seghieri G, Anichini R, Ciuti M, et al. Raised erythrocyte polyamine levels in non-insulin-dependent diabetes mellitus with great vessel disease and albuminuria. *Diabetes Res Clin Pract*, 37, 15-20 (1997)

4714 Segoloni G, Vercellone A, Manes M et al. Levels of tumor necrosis factor (TNF) in sera of renal allograft recipients. *Clin Transplant*, 5, 102-106 (1991)

4715 Seibel MJ, Cosman F, Shen V, et al. Urinary hydroxypyridinium crosslinks of collagen as markers of bone reabsorption and estrogen efficacy in postmenopausal osteoporosis. *J Bone Mineral Res*, 8, 881-889 (1993)

4716 Seibel MJ, Woitge HW, Pecherstorfer M, et al. Serum immunoreactive bone sialoprotein as a new marker of bone turnover in metabolic and malignant bone disease. *J Clin Endocrinol Metab*, 81, 3289-3294 (1996)

4717 Seidel A, Arolt V, Hunstiger M et al. Cytokine production and serum proteins in depression. *Scand J Immunol*, 41, 534-538 (1995)

4718 Seigneur M, Dufourcq P, Conri C et al. Levels of plasma thrombomodulin are increaed in atheromatous arterial disease. *Thromb Res*, 71, 423-431 (1993)

4719 Seigneur M, Freyburger G, Gin H, et al. Serum fatty acid profiles in type I and type II diabetes: metabolic alterations of fatty acids of the main serum lipids. *Diabet Res Clin Pract*, 23, 169-177 (1994)

4720 Seino Y et al. Hypergastrinemia in hyperthyroidism. *J Clin Endocrinol Metab*, 43, 852-855 (1976)

4721 Seip M et al. Serum cholesterol and triglycerides in children with anemia. *Scand J Haematol*, 19, 503-508 (1977)

4722 Seipelt G, Ganser A, Duranceyk H et al. Induction of soluble IL-2 receptor in patients with myelodysplastic syndromes undergoing high-dose interleukin-3 treatment. *Ann Hematol*, 68, 167-170 (1994)

4723 Seipelt G, Ganser A, Duranceyk H et al. Induction of TNF-α in patients with myelodysplastic syndromes undergoing treatment with interleukin-3. *Br J Haematol*, 84, 749-751 (1993)

4724 Seitanidis B et al. Serum immunoglobulin levels in white patients with sickle cell disease. *Clin Chim Acta*, 37, 531-532 (1972)

4725 Seitz R, Leugner F, Katschinski M et al. Ulcerative colitis and Crohn's disease: factor XIII, inflammation and haemostasis. *Digestion*, 55, 361-367 (1994)

4726 Seki T, Joh K, Oh-ishi T. Augmented production of interleukin-8 in cerebrospinal fluid in bacterial meningitis. *Immunology*, 80, 333-335 (1993)

4727 Sekiya S, Seki K, Nagai Y. Rise of serum CA 125 in patients with pure ovarian yolk sac tumors. *Int J Gynecol Obstet*, 58, 323-324 (1997)

4728 Sell S. Hepatocellular cancer markers. In:. *Cancer Markers*, Clifton NJ, Humana Press, II (1982)

4729 Selmaj K. Histamine release from leucocytes during migraine attack. *Cephalagia*, 4, 97-100 (1984)

4730 Selye H. *The Stress of Life,* 3rd Edition, New York NY, McGraw-Hill (1978)

4731 Senay LC Jr, Christensen ML. Changes in blood plasma during progressive dehydration. *J Appl Physiol*, 20, 1136 (1965)

4732 Seppa K, Silanaukee P, Koivula T. Abnormalities of hematologic parameters in heavy drinkers and alcoholics. *Alcohol Clin Exp Res*, 16, 117-121 (1992)

4733 Seppa K, Sillanaukee P. Women, alcohol, and red cells. *Alcohol Clin Exp Res*, 18, 1168-1171 (1994)

4734 Seppala M. Fetal pathophysiology of human AFP. *Gut*, 14, 939 (1977)

4735 Seppala M et al. Congenital nephrotic syndrome: prenatal diagnosis and genetic counselling by estimation of amniotic fluid and maternal serum α-fetoprotein. *Lancet*, 2, 123-125 (1976)

4736 Sepp'AL'AM, Ranta T, Rutanen EM et al. Improved diagnosis of pregnancy-related gynaecological emergencies by rapid human chorionic gonadotropin β-subunit assay. *Br J Obstet Gynaecol*, 88, 138-140 (1981)

4737 Sequeira W, Stinar D. Serum angiotensin-converting enzyme levels in sarcoid arthritis. *Arch Intern Med*, 146, 125 (1986)

4738 Sera RK, McBride JH, Higgins SA et al. Evaluation of reference ranges for fatty acids in serum. *J Clin Lab Anal*, 8, 81-85 (1994)

4739 Serby M, Richardson SB, Twente S et al. CSF somatostatin in Alzheimer's disease. *Neurobiol Aging*, 5, 187-189 (1984)

4740 Seregni E, Botti C, Bogni A et al. Tumour marker evaluation in patients with lung cancer. *Scand J Clin Lab Invest*, 53, 67-71 (1995)

4741 Seregni E, Luksch R, Crippa F et al. Evaluation of serum osteocalcin and myosin in pediatric patients affected by osteosarcoma and rhabdomyosarcoma. *Int J Biol Mark*, 9, 260-261 (1994)

4742 Serjeant GR, Galloway RE, Gueri MC. Serum-copper in sickle-cell anemia. *Lancet*, II, 891 (1970)

4743 Serno Y et al. Hypogastrinemia in hypothyroidism. *Am J Dig Dis*, 23, 189-191 (1978)

4744 Setsuta K, Seino Y, Takahasi N, et al. Clinical significance of elevated levels of cardiac troponin T in patients with chronic heart failure. *Am J Cardiol*, 84, 608-611 (1999)

4745 Seufert R, Casper F, Bauer H et al. Changes in the renin aldosterone system in preeclampsia. *Arch Gynecol Obstet*, 250, 546-548 (1991)

4746 Sfogliano L, Benigno R, Bonanno G et al. Effects of long-term administration of the calcium-antagonist nicardipine on kidney function parameters and renin-angiotensin/angiotensin-converting-enzyme/aldosterone system. *Curr Ther Res*, 44, 267-274 (1988)

4747 Shaarawy M, Darwish NA. Serum cytokines in gestational trophoblastic diseases. *Acta Oncol*, 34, 177-182 (1995)

4748 Shaarawy M, Youssef El Mallah S, Abd El-Monem El-Yamani A. Clinical significance of urinary human tissue non-specific alkaline phosphatase (hTNAP) in pre-eclampsia and eclampsia. *Ann Clin Biochem*, 34, 405-411 (1997)

4749 Shabana A, Onsrud M. Tissue polypeptide-specific antigen and CA 125 as serum tumor markers in ovarian carcinoma. *Tumor Biol*, 15, 361-367 (1994)

4750 Shahangian S, Ash KO, Wahlstrom NO Jr et al. Creatine kinase and lactate dehydrogenase isoenzymes in serum of patients suffering burns, blunt trauma, or myocardial infarction. *Clin Chem*, 30, 1332-1338 (1984)

4751 Shahangian S, Fritsche HA, Hughes JI. Carcinoembryonic antigen in serum of patients with colorectal polyps: correlation with histology and smoking status. *Clin Chem*, 37, 651-655 (1991)

4752 Shahid A, Siddiqui AA, Zuberi SJ et al. Serum α_1-antitrypsin and duodenal ulcer. *J Gastroenterol Hepatol*, 8, 505-507 (1993)

4753 Shahidi NT et al. Alkali-resistant hemoglobin in aplastic anemia of both acquired and congenital types. *N Engl J Med*, 266, 177 (1962)

4754 Shalel SM, Didi M, Ogilvy-Stuart AL, et al. Growth and endocrine function after bone marrow transplantation. *Clin Endocrinol*, 42, 333-339 (1995)

4755 Shambaugh GE et al. Insulin response during tularemia in man. *Diabetes*, 16, 369 (1967)

4756 Shannon IL et al. Human parotid saliva urea in renal failure and during dialysis. *Arch Oral Biol*, 22, 83-86 (1977)

4757 Sharief MK, Hentges R. Association between tumor necrosis factor-α and disease progression in patients with multiple sclerosis. *N Engl J Med*, 325, 467-472 (1991)

4758 Sharif M, George E, Dieppe PA. Correlation between synovial fluid markers of cartilage and bone turnover and scintigraphic scan abnormalities in osteoarthritis of the knee. *Arth Rheum*, 38, 78-81 (1995)

4759 Sharma A, Chandra M, Gujrati VR et al. Involvement of catecholamines and serotonin in human hypertension. *Pharmacol Res Commun*, 17, 565-574 (1985)

4760 Sharma GV et al. Pulmonary embolism: the great imitator. *DM*, 22, 16-21 (1976)

4761 Sharma RP, Faull K, Javaid JL, Davis JM. Cerebrospinal fluid levels of phenylacetic acid in mental illness: behavioral associations and response to neuroleptic treatment. *Acta Psychiatr Scand*, 91, 293-298 (1995)

4762 Sharma SC et al. Platelet adhesiveness, plasma fibrinogen, and fibrinolytic activity in young patients with ischaemic stroke. *J Neurol Neurosurg Psychiatry*, 41, 118-121 (1978)

4763 Sharp HL. α-1-Antitrypsin deficiency. *Hosp Pract*, 83-96 (1971)

4764 Shaw AB, Scholes MC. Reticulocytosis in renal failure. *Lancet*, 1, 799 (1967)

4765 Shaw PJ, Forrest V, Ince PG et al. CSF and plasma amino acid levels in motor neuron disease: elevation of CSF glutamate in a subset of patients. *Neurodegeneration*, 4, 209-216 (1995)

4766 Sheagren JN et al. Rheumatoid factor in bacterial endocarditis. *Arth Rheum*, 19, 887-890 (1976)

4767 Shearn MA. Sjögren's syndrome. *Med Clin North Am*, 61, 271-282 (1977)

4768 Shearn MA et al. Serum viscosity in the rheumatic diseases and macroglobulinemia. *Arch Intern Med*, 112, 684-687 (1963)

4769 Sheehy T W, Berman A. The anemia of cirrhosis. *J Lab Clin Med*, 56, 72 (1960)

4770 Sheffer Z, Peleg E, Landau-Salzberg M et al. Atrial natriuretic peptide in diabetic patients before and after control of blood sugar level. *J Cardiovasc Pharmacol*, 18, 878-881 (1991)

4771 Sheish S-C, Jap T-S, Chiang H. Serum neuron-specific enolase in patients with lung cancer. *Clin Biochem Rev*, 14, 263 (1993)

4772 Sheldon J, Riches PG, Soni N et al. Plasma neopterin as an adjunct to C-reactive protein in assessment of infection. *Clin Chem*, 37, 2038-2042 (1991)

4773 Sheldon J, Stearman M, James R et al. Measurement of connective tissue metabolism in saliva. *Proc ACB Natl Meet*, 127 (1995)

4774 Sheldon S et al. Plasma catecholamines in hypothyroidism and hyperthyroidism. *J Clin Endocrinol Metab*, 36, 587-589 (1973)

4775 Sheps SG, Kirkpatrick RA. Hypertension. *Mayo Clin Proc*, 50, 709-720 (1975)

4776 Sher G et al. Pregnancy, pre-eclampsia, and disseminated intravascular coagulation. *S Afr Med J*, 49, 1197 (1975)

4777 Shering SG, Sherry F, McDermott EW, et al. Preoperative CA 15-3 concentrations predict outcome of patients with breast carcinoma. *Cancer*, 83, 2521-2527 (1998)

4778 Sherlock S et al. Immunological disturbance in diseases of liver and thyroid. *Proc Roy Soc Med*, 70, 851-857 (1977)

4779 Sheron N, Bird G, Goka J et al. Elevated plasma interleukin-6 and increased severity and mortality in alcoholic hepatitis. *Clin Exp Immunol*, 84, 449-453 (1991)

4780 Sherwin AL, Norris JW, Bulcke JA. Spinal fluid creatine kinase in neurologic disease. *Neurology*, 19, 993-999 (1969)

4781 Sherwin R et al. Hyperglucagonemia in Laennec's cirrhosis: the role of portal systemic shunting. *N Engl J Med*, 290, 239-242 (1974)

4782 Sherwin RS et al. Hyperglucagonemia in cirrhosis: altered secretion and sensitivity to glucagon. *Gastroenterology*, 74, 1224-1228 (1978)

4783 Sherwin RW, Wentworth DN, Cutler JA et al. Serum cholesterol levels and cancer mortality in 361,662 men screened for the multiple risk factor intervention trial. *J Am Med Ass*, 257, 943 (1987)

4784 Sherwood RA, Pippard MJ, Peters TJ. Iron homeostasis and the assessment of iron status. *Ann Clin Biochem*, 35, 693-708 (1998)

4785 Sheth SG, Flamm SL, Gordon FD, et al. AST/ALT ratio predicts cirrhosis in patients with chronic hepatitis C virus infection. *Am J Gastroenterol*, 93, 44-48 (1998)

4786 Shetty KR, Sutton CH, Rudman IW et al. Lipid and lipoprotein abnormalities in young quadriplegic men. *Am J Med Sci*, 303, 213-216 (1992)

4787 Shi M, Taylor JMG, Fahey JL, et al. Early levels of CD4, neopterin, and β-microglobulin indicate future disease progression. *J Clin Immunol*, 17, 43-52 (1997)

4788 Shi YF, Liu ZM. The clinical manifestations and endocrine changes of anorexia nervosa. *Chung Kuo I Hsueh Ko Hsueh Yuan Hsueh Pao*, 11, 159-164 (1989)

4789 Shibata T, Magari Y, Kamberi P, et al. Significance of urinary fibrin/fibrinogen degradation products (FDP) D-dimer measured by a highly sensitive ELISA method with a new monoclonal antibody (D-D E72) in various renal diseases. *Clin Nephrol*, 44, 91-95 (1995)

4790 Shibata T, Magari Y, Mizunaga S, et al. Urinary fibrin/fibrinogen degradation product E (FDP-E) measured by a highly sensitive ELISA method in renal diseases. *Nephron*, 79, 494-495 (1998)

4791 Shibata T, Ogawa M, Takata N et al. Elevation of serum pancreatic secretory trypsin inhibitor following serious injury. *Resuscitation*, 16, 163-168 (1988)

4792 Shibata Y, Kotangi H, Andoh H, et al. Detection of circulating anti-p53 antibodies in patients with colorectal carcinoma and the antibody's relation to clinical factors. *Dis Colon Rectum*, 39, 1269-1274 (1996)

4793 Shield JPH, Carradus M, Stone JE et al. Urinary heparan sulphate proteoglycan excretion is abnormal in insulin dependent diabetes. *Ann Clin Biochem*, 32, 557-560 (1995)

4794 Shiesh S-C, Jap T-S, Chiang H. Serum neuron-specific enolase in patients with lung cancer. *Clin Biochem Rev*, 14, 236 (1993)

4795 Shifrine M, Fisher GL. Ceruloplasmin levels in sera from human patients with osteosarcoma. *Cancer*, 38, 244-248 (1976)

4796 Shigeta H, Fujii M, Yamaguchi M, et al. Serum autoantibodies against sulfatide and phospholipid in NIDDM patients with diabetic neuropathy. *Diabetes Care*, 20, 1896-1899 (1997)

4797 Shih J-Y, Yang S-C, Yu C-J, et al. Elevated serum levels of mucin-associated antigen in patients with acute respiratory distress syndrome. *Am J Respir Crit Care Med*, 156, 1453-1457 (1997)

4798 Shih V. *Laboratory Techniques for the Detection of Hereditary Metabolic Disorders*, Boca Raton FL, CRC Press (1973)

4799 Shilo R et al. Reevaluation of the polyvinylpyrrolidone sedimentation test in the diagnosis of ABO hemolytic disease of the newborn. *Vox Sang*, 31, 16-24 (1976)

4800 Shimada K, Koh CS, Yanagisawa N. Detection of interleukin-6 in serum and cerebrospinal fluid of patients with neuroimmunological diseases. *Arerugi*, 42, 934-940 (1993)

4801 Shimada M, Miyashimaki, Yavata. Increased calcium uptake in the red cells of unsplenectomized patients with hereditary spherocytosis. *Clin Chim Acta*, 142, 183-192 (1984)

4802 Shimamura J et al. Non-pancreatic hyperamylasemia in pancreatic cancer. *Gastroenterology*, 68, 985 (1975)

4803 Shimizu H, Kakizaki S, Tsuchiya T, et al. An increase of circulating leptin in patients with liver cirrhosis. *Int J Obesity*, 22, 1234-1238 (1998)

4804 Shimoda K, Okamura S, Omori F et al. Detection of granulocyte-macrophage colony-stimulating factor in cerebrospinal fluid of patients with aseptic meningitis. *Acta Haematol*, 86, 36-39 (1991)

4805 Shimomura H, Ogawa H, Arai H, et al. Serial changes in plasma levels of soluble P-selectin in patients with acute myocardial infarction. *Am J Cardiol*, 81, 397-400 (1998)

4806 Shimomura T, Araga S, Esumi E, Takahashi K. Decreased serum interleukin-2 level in patients with chronic headache. *Headache*, 31, 310-313 (1991)

4807 Shimura M, Wada H, Wakita Y, et al. Plasma tissue factor and tissue factor pathway inhibitor levels in patients with disseminated intravascular coagulation. *Am J Hematol*, 52, 165-170 (1996)

4808 Shinchi K, Kono S, Honjo S et al. Serum lipids and gallstone disease. A study of self-defense officials in Japan. *Ann Epidemiol*, 3, 614-618 (1993)

4809 Shine B, Gould J, Campbell C et al. Serum C-reactive protein in normal and infected neonates. *Clin Chim Acta*, 148, 97-103 (1985)

4810 Shirabe K, Takenaka K, Gion T, et al. Significance of α-fetoprotein levels for detection of early recurrence of hepatocellular carcinoma after hepatic resection. *J Surg Oncol*, 64, 143-146 (1997)

4811 Shirakami A, Hirai Y, Takeichi T et al. Changes in plasma fibronectin levels in thyroid diseases. *Horm Metab Res*, 18, 345-348 (1986)

4812 Shiroky JB, Cohen M, Ballachey M-L et al. Thyroid dysfunction in rheumatoid arthritis: a controlled prospective survey. *Ann Rheum Dis*, 52, 454-456 (1993)

4813 Shirota T, Shinoda T, Yamada T et al. Alteration of renal function in hyperthyroidism: increased tubular secretion of creatinine and decreased distal tubule delivery of chloride. *Metabolism*, 41, 402-405 (1992)

4814 Shirrock RD et al. Raised levels of complement inactivation products in ankylosing spondylitis. *J Rheumatol*, 1, 428 (1974)

4815 Shoenfeld Y, Grunebaum E, Laufer M, et al. Anti-topoisomerase-I and clinical findings in systemic sclerosis (scleroderma). *Isr J Med Sci*, 32, 537-542 (1996)

4816 Shoji S, Kanazawa H, Hirata K, et al. Clinical implication of protein levels of IL-5 in induced sputum of asthmatic patients. *J Asthma*, 35, 243-249 (1998)

4817 Short CL, Bauer W, Reynolds WE. *Rheumatoid Arthritis*, Cambridge MA, Harvard University Press (1957)

4818 Shotan A, Mehra A, Ostrzega E et al. Plasma cyclic guanosine monophosphate in chronic heart failure: hemodynamic and neurohumoral correlations and response to nitrate therapy. *Clin Pharmacol Ther*, 54, 638-644 (1993)

4819 Shou I, Tashiro K, Kurusu A, et al. Serum levels of soluble Fas and disease activity in patients with IgA nephropathy. *Nephron*, 81, 387-392 (1999)

4820 Shovlin CL, Hughes JMB, Simmonds HA et al. Adult presentation of adenosine deaminase deficiency. *Lancet*, 341, 1471 (1993)

4821 Shu K-H, Lu Y-S, Chen C-H et al. Serum immunoglobulin E in primary IgA nephropathy. *Clin Nephrol*, 44, 86-90 (1995)

4822 Shuster F et al. Dissociation of serum bilirubin and alkaline phosphatase in infectious mononucleosis. *J Am Med Ass*, 209, 267-268 (1969)

4823 Shuster J, Gold P. β-2 microglobulin levels in cancerous and other disease states. *Clin Chim Acta*, 67, 307-313 (1976)

4824 Shuster S et al. Small intestine in psoriasis. *Br Med J*, 3, 445-506 (1967)

4825 Sidenius JS, Pedersen SA, Jorgensen JOL et al. Effect of growth hormone (GH) on plasma Gla-protein in GH-deficient adults. *J Clin Endocrinol Metab*, 70, 916-919 (1990)

4826 Siebel MJ, Gartenberg F, Silverberg SJ et al. Urinary hydroxypyridinium cross-links of collagen in primary hyperparathyroidism. *J Clin Endocrinol Metab*, 74, 481-486 (1992)

4827 Siebers RWL, Carter JM, Maling TJB. Increase in haematocrit in borderline hypertensive men. *Clin Exp Pharmacol Physiol*, 21, 401-403 (1994)

4828 Sieg I, Doss MO, Kandels H et al. Effect of alcohol on δ-aminolevulinic acid dehydratase and porphyrin metabolism in man. *Clin Chim Acta*, 202, 211-218 (1991)

4829 Siegel JE, Swami VK, Glenn P, Peterson P. Effect (or lack of it) of severe anemia on PT and APTT results. *Am J Clin Pathol*, 110, 106-110 (1998)

4830 Siemes H et al. Oligoclonal γ-globulin banding of cerebrospinal fluid in patients with subacute sclerosing panencephalitis. Comparison of the electrophoretic pattern with that in multiple sclerosis and congenital. *J Neurol Sci*, 32, 395-409 (1977)

4831 Siemkowicz E et al. Changes in cisternal fluid potassium concentration following cardiac arrest. *Acta Neurol Scand*, 55, 137-44 (1977)

4832 Sierra C, Pastor MC, Bonal J et al. Hypervitaminosis A in uraemic patients. Effect of dialysis therapy. *Clin Biochem Rev*, 14, 222 (1993)

4833 Siever LJ, Tresiman RL, Coccaro EF et al. The growth hormone response to clonidine in acute and remitted depressed male patients. *Neuropsychopharmacology*, 6, 165-177 (1992)

4834 Sigurdsson et al. Calcium absorption and excretion in the gut in acromegaly. *Clin Endocrinol*, 2, 187-192 (1973)

4835 Sigurdsson G, Baldursdottir A, Sigvaldason et al. Predictive value of apolipoproteins in a prospective survey of coronary artery disease in men. *Am J Cardiol*, 69, 1251-1254 (1992)

4836 Silen A, Wiklund B, Norlen BJ et al. Evaluation of a new tumor marker for cytokeratin 8 and 18 fragments in healthy individuals and prostate cancer patients. *Prostate*, 24, 326-332 (1994)

4837 Sillanaukee P, Koivula T, Jokela H et al. Relationship of alcohol consumption to changes in HDL-subfractions. *Eur J Clin Invest*, 23, 486-491 (1993)

4838 Silverberg J, Volpe R. Rheumatoid factors in Graves' disease. *Ann Intern Med*, 88, 216-217 (1978)

4839 Silveri F, Brecciaroli D, Argentati F et al. Serum levels of insulin in overweight patients with osteoarthritis of the knee. *J Rheumatol*, 21, 1899-1902 (1994)

4840 Silverman BA, Rubinstein A. Serum lactate dehydrogenase levels in adults and children with acquired immune deficiency syndrome (AIDS) and AIDS-related complex: possible indicator of B cell lymphoproliferation and disease activity. Effect of intravenous γ-globulin on enzyme levels. *Am J Med*, 78, 728-736 (1985)

4841 Silverman LM, Chapman JF, Jones ME et al. Creatine kinase BB and other markers of prostatic carcinoma. *Prostate*, 2, 109-119 (1981)

4842 Silverman LM, Dermer GB, Zweig MH et al. Creatine kinase BB: a new tumor-associated marker. *Clin Chem*, 25, 1432-1435 (1979)

4843 Silverstein E, Brunswick J, Rao TK, Friedland J. Increased serum angiotensin-converting enzyme in chronic renal disease. *Nephron*, 37, 206-210 (1984)

4844 Silverstein E et al. Elevated serum and spleen angiotensin converting enzyme and serum lysozyme in Gaucher's disease. *Clin Chim Acta*, 74, 21-26 (1977)

4845 Silverstein E, Schussler GC, Friedland J. Elevated serum angiotensin-converting enzyme in hyperthyroidism. *Am J Med*, 75, 233-236 (1983)

4846 Silverstein MN et al. Leukocyte alkaline phosphatase in agnogenic myeloid metaplasia. *Am J Clin Pathol*, 61, 307 (1974)

4847 Silvis SE et al. Thrombocytosis in patients with lung cancer. *J Am Med Ass*, 211, 1852 (1970)

4848 Sim JM, Castellano I, Ferri N, et al. Evaluation of a homogeneous assay for high-density lipoprotein cholesterol: limitations in patients with cardiovascular, renal and hepatic disorders. *Clin Chem*, 44, 1233-1241 (1998)

4849 Sim SJ, Glassman AB, Ro JY, et al. Serum calcitonin in small cell carcinoma of the prostate. *Ann Clin Lab Sci*, 26, 487-494 (1996)

4850 Simionescu L, Dimitriu L, Dimitriu D et al. The serum osteocalcin levels in adult and aged hypothyroid patients. *Endocrinologie*, 26, 255-260 (1988)

4851 Simionescu L et al. The hormonal pattern in alcoholic disease. I. luteinizing hormone (LH), follicle-stimulating hormone (FSH) and testosterone. *Endocrinologie*, 15, 45-49 (1977)

4852 Simmen HP, Battaglia H, Giovanoli P, et al. Biochemical analysis of peritoneal fluid in patients with and without bacterial infection. *Eur J Surg*, 161, 23-27 (1996)

4853 Simmons P. Plasma Protein - Diagnostics. Somerville NJ, Behring Diagnostics (1974)

4854 Simon E, Paul J-L, Soni T, et al. Plasma and erythrocyte vitamin E content in asymptomatic hypercholesterolemic subjects. *Clin Chem*, 43, 285-289 (1997)

4855 Simon ER et al. Incubation hemolysis and red cell metabolism in acanthocytosis. *J Clin Invest*, 43, 1311 (1964)

4856 Simon RP. Neurosyphilis: an update. *West J Med*, 134, 87-91 (1981)

4857 Simone JV et al. Blood coagulation in thyroid dysfunction. *N Engl J Med*, 273, 1057 (1965)

4858 Simone JV et al. Initial features and prognosis in 363 children with acute lymphocytic leukemia. *Cancer*, 36, 2099-2108 (1975)

4859 Simons LA et al. Type V hyperlipoproteinaemia re-visited: findings in a Sydney population. *Aust NZ J Med*, 5, 210-219 (1975)

4860 Simpson H. CSF acid-base status and lactate and pyruvate concentrations after short (< 30 minutes) first febrile convulsions in children. *Arch Dis Child*, 52, 837-843 (1977)

4861 Singer FR et al. Hypercalcemia in reticulum cell sarcoma without hyperparathyroidism or skeletal metastases. *Ann Intern Med*, 78, 365 (1973)

4862 Singer K et al. The life span of the megalocyte and the hemolytic syndrome of pernicious anemia. *J Lab Clin Med*, 33, 1068 (1948)

4863 Singh J, Kulig K, Lucco L. Levels of serum β-2 microglobulin in human subjects by an automated method on Behring nephelometer (BN) using reagents from The Binding Site (TBS). *Clin Chem*, 39, 1137 (1993)

4864 Singh MM. Carbohydrate metabolism in pre-eclampsia. *Br J Obstet Gynaecol*, 83, 124-131 (1976)

4865 Singh SM, Dean HG, de Dombal FT et al. Concentrations of serotinin in plasma - a test for appendicitis? *Clin Chem*, 34, 2572-2574 (1988)

4866 Singh V et al. Prognostic value of serum uric acid in patients with acute myocardial infarction. *J Ind Med Ass*, 59, 97-99 (1977)

4867 Singh VS et al. Serum free fatty acids and arrhythmias after acute myocardial infarctions. *J Postgrad Med*, 23, 19-24 (1977)

4868 Singhal A, Cook JD, Skikne BS, et al. The clinical significance of serum transferrin receptor levels in sickle cell disease. *Br J Haematol*, 84, 301-304 (1993)

4869 Singsen BH et al. Systemic lupus erythematosus in childhood correlations between changes in disease activity and serum complement levels. *J Pediatr*, 89, 358-69 (1976)

4870 Sinha S et al. Serum calcium and magnesium in different types of leprosy. *Leprosy India*, 50, 54-56 (1978)

4871 Sinha SN, Gabrieli ER. Serum copper and zinc levels in various pathologic conditions. *Am J Clin Pathol*, 54, 570-577 (1970)

4872 Sinigaglia L, Varenna M, Binelli L et al. Urinary and synovial pyridinium crosslink concentrations in patients with rheumatoid arthritis and osteoarthritis. *Ann Rheum Dis*, 54, 144-147 (1995)

4873 Siriken F, Tokgozoglu SL, Renda N et al. Erythrocyte CuZn superoxide dismutase and the extent of coronary atherosclerosis. *Clin Chem*, 40, 1597 (1994)

4874 Sirinathsinghji DJS, Mills IH. Concentration patterns of plasma dehydroepiandrosterone, δ_5-androstenediol and their sulphates, testosterone and cortisol in normal healthy women and in women with anorexia nervosa. *Acta Endocrinol*, 108, 255-260 (1985)

4875 Sirinek KR, O'Dorisio TM, Gaskill HV et al. Chronic renal failure: effect of hemodialysis on gastrointestinal hormones. *Am J Surg*, 148, 732-735 (1984)

4876 Sise HS et al. Blood coagulation factors in total body irradiation. *Blood*, 18, 702 (1961)

4877 Sitas F, Carrara H, Beral V, et al. Antibodies against human herpes virus 8 in black South African patients with cancer. *N Engl J Med*, 340, 1863-1871 (1999)

4878 Sitprija V et al. Renal failure in malaria: a pathophysiologic study. *Nephron*, 18, 277-287 (1977)

4879 Sjejgaard A, Ryder LP. Association between HLA and disease. In:. *HLA and Disease*. Dausset J, Svejgaard A (eds), Baltimore MD, Williams and Wilkins, 46-71 (1977)

4880 Sjolund K, Nobin A. Increased levels of plasma serotonin in patients with coeliac disease. *Scand J Gastroenterol*, 20, 304-308 (1985)

4881 Skansberg P. Prognostic value of blood platelet counts, coagulation factors and serum fibrin/fibrinogen degradation products (FDP) in acute infections. *Scand J Infect Dis*, 10, 61-65 (1978)

4882 Skare S, Dahl-Jorgensen K, Hanssen K-F et al. Increased peripheral venous somatostatin concentration and decreased glucagon response to arginine to arginine in patients with insulin dependent diabetes mellitus without residual B-cell function. Increased plasma SRIF in IDDM. *Acta Endocrinol*, 109, 517-521 (1985)

4883 Skenderis BS II, Rodriguez-Bigas M, Weber TK, Petrelli NJ. Utility of routine postoperative laboratory studies in patients undergoing potentially curative resection for adenocarcinoma of the colon and rectum. *Cancer Invest*, 17, 102-109 (1999)

4884 Skiest DJ, Keiser P. Clinical significance of eosinophilia in HIV-infected individuals. *Am J Med*, 102, 449-453 (1997)

4885 Skjoldebrand L, Brundin J, Carlstrom A, et al. Thyroxine-binding globulin in spontaneous abortion. *Gynecol Obstet Invest*, 21, 187-192 (1986)

4886 Skogen W, Price G, Taylor C, et al. The clinical utility of C-reactive protein, WBC, and percent neutrophils as indicators for acute appendicitis. *Clin Chem*, 39, 1147 (1993)

4887 Skrha J, Hilgertova J. Relationship of serum N-acetyl-β-glucosaminidase activity to oxidative stress in diabetes mellitus. *Clin Chim Acta*, 282, 167-174 (1999)

4888 Skrha J, Hodinar A, Kvasnicka J et al. Early changes of serum N-acetyl-β-glucosaminidase, tissue plasminogen activator and erythrocyte superoxide dismutase in relation to retinopathy in type I diabetes mellitus. *Clin Chim Acta*, 229, 5-14 (1994)

4889 Skude G et al. Amylase, hepatic enzymes and bilirubin in serum of chronic alcoholics. *Acta Med Scand*, 201, 53-58 (1977)

4890 Slavinskie Z. Decreased synthesis of serum complement (C_3) in hypocomplementemic SLE. *Clin Exp Immunol*, 11, 21-29 (1972)

4891 Sleisenger MH, Fortran JS. *Gastrointestinal Disease*. Philadelphia PA, WB Saunders (1978)

4892 Slunga L, Asplund K, Johnson O et al. Lipoprotein (a) in a randomly selected 25-64 year old population: the northern Sweden Monica study. *J Clin Epidemiol*, 46, 612-624 (1993)

4893 Smalley MJ et al. Antinuclear factors and human leucocytes: reaction with granulocytes and lymphocytes. *Aust Ann Med*, 17, 28 (1968)

4894 Smallridge RC, Rodgers J, Verma PS. Serum angiotensin-converting enzyme. alterations in hyperthyroidism, hypothyroidism, and subacute thyroiditis. *J Am Med Ass*, 250, 2489-2493 (1983)

4895 Smals AG et al. The pituitary-thyroid axis in Klinefelter's syndrome. *Acta Endocrinol*, 84, 72-79 (1977)

4896 Smedsrod B, Einarsson M, Pertoft H. Tissue plasminogen activator is endocytosed by mannose and galactose receptors of rat liver cells. *Thromb Haemostas*, 59, 480-484 (1988)

4897 Smeenk R, Westgeest T, Swaak T. Antinuclear antibody determination: the present state of diagnostic and clinical relevance. *Scand J Rheumatol*, Suppl, 56, 78-92 (1985)

4898 Smirnov VV, Skorniakov VI, Popov AS et al. Creatine phosphokinase in the cerebrospinal fluid of patients with acute meningitis. *Vrachebnoe Delo*, 7, 112-113 (1989)

4899 Smith CE et al. Serological tests in the diagnosis and prognosis of coccidioidomycosis. *Am J Hyg*, 52, 1 (1950)

4900 Smith CH. Familial blood studies in cases of Mediterranean (Cooley's) anemia. *Am J Dis Child*, 65, 681 (1943)

4901 Smith DH, Goldwasser E, Vokes EE. Serum immunoerythropoietin levels in patients with cancer receiving cisplatin-based chemotherapy. *Cancer*, 68, 1101-1105 (1991)

4902 Smith EF. Thromboxane A2 in cardiovascular and renal disorders: is there a defined role for thromboxane receptor antagonists or thromboxane synthase inhibitors? *Eicosanoids*, 2, 199-212 (1989)

4903 Smith FB, Lee AJ, Rumley A et al. Tissue-plasminogen activator, plasminogen activator inhibitor and risk of peripheral arterial disease. *Atherosclerosis*, 115, 35-43 (1995)

4904 Smith GA, Mihalov L, Shields BJ. Diagnostic aids in the differentiation of pyloric stenosis from severe gastrointestinal reflux during early infancy. *Am J Emerg Med*, 17, 28-31 (1999)

4905 Smith GM, Ward RL, McGuigan L et al. Measurement of human phospholipase A2 in arthritis plasma using a newly developed sandwich ELISA. *Br J Rheumatol*, 31, 175-178 (1992)

4906 Smith GV. The anterior pituitary-like hormone in late pregnancy toxemia. *Am J Obstet Gynecol*, 38, 618 (1939)

4907 Smith GV et al. Estrogen and progestin metabolism in pregnant women, with especial reference to pre-eclamptic toxemia and the effect of hormone administration. *Am J Obstet Gynecol*, 39, 405 (1940)

4908 Smith J. The plasma phosphatase in rickets and scurvy. *Arch Dis Child*, 7, 149-158 (1932)

4909 Smith RG, Henry YK, Mattson MP, Appel SH. Presence of 4-hydoxynonenal in cerebrospinal fluid of patients with sporadic amyotrophic lateral sclerosis. *Ann Neurol*, 44, 696-699 (1998)

4910 Smith RM, Neuman TS. Elevation of serum creatine kinase in divers with arterial gas embolization. *N Engl J Med*, 330, 19-24 (1994)

4911 Smith RP, Lipworth BJ, Cree IA, et al. C-reactive protein: a clinical marker in community-acquired pneumonia. *Chest*, 108, 1288-1291 (1995)

4912 Smith SJ et al. Lowering of serum 4,4',5-triiodothyronine thyroxine ratio in patients with myocardial infarction: relationship with extent of tissue injury. *Eur J Clin Invest*, 8, 99-102 (1978)

4913 Smith SL, Novotny M. Elevation of certain polyols in the cerebrospinal fluid of patients with multiple sclerosis. *J Chromatog Biomed Appl*, 336, 351-355 (1984)

4914 Smith WGJ, Holden M, Benton M et al. Carbamylated haemoglobin in chronic renal failure. *Clin Chim Acta*, 178, 297-304 (1988)

4915 SmithKline Beecham Pharmaceuticals. Manufacturer's literature on Coreg® . Philadelphia, PA 19101 (1997)

4916 Smulders RA, Stehouwer CDA, Olthof CG et al. Plasma endothelin levels and vascular effects of intravenous L-arginine infusion in subjects with uncomplicated insulin-dependent diabetes mellitus. *Clin Sci*, 87, 37-43 (1994)

4917 Snaedal J, Kristinsson J, Gunnarsdottir S, et al. Copper, ceruloplasmin and superoxide dismutase in patients with Alzheimer's disease. *Dement Geriat Cogn Disord*, 9, 239-242 (1998)

4918 Snape WJ et al. Marked alkaline phosphatase elevation with partial common bile duct obstruction due to calcific pancreatitis. *Gastroenterology*, 70, 70-73 (1976)

4919 Snapper I et al. Determination of Bence-Jones protein in urine. *J Am Med Ass*, 173, 1137-1139 (1959)

4920 Snider GL. Pathogenesis of emphysema and chronic bronchitis. *Med Clin North Am*, 65, 647-651 (1981)

4921 Sniderman A, Shapiro S, Marpole D et al. Association of coronary atherosclerosis with hyperapolipoproteinemia I. increased protein but normal cholesterol levels in human plasma low density (β) lipoproteins. *Proc Natl Acad Sci USA*, 77, 604-608 (1980)

4922 Snodgrass PJ et al. Urea-cycle enzyme deficiencies and an increased nitrogen load producing hyperammonemia in Reye's syndrome. *N Engl J Med*, 294, 855-860 (1976)

4923 Snook JA, Chapman RW, Fleming K et al. Anti-neutrophil nuclear antibody in ulcerative colitis, Crohn's disease and primary sclerosing cholangitis. *Clin Exp Immunol*, 76, 30-33 (1989)

4924 Snower DP, Weil SC. Changing etiology of macrocytosis: zidovudine as a frequent causative factor. *Am J Clin Pathol*, 99, 57-60 (1993)

4925 Snyderman R, McCarty GA. Clinical usefulness of hemolytic complement determination. In:. *Clinical Aspects of the Complement System.* Opferkuch et al (ed) (1976)

4926 Solajic-Bozicevic N, Stavljenic-Rukavina A, Sesto M. Lecithin-cholesterol acyltransferase activity in patients with coronary artery disease examined by coronary angiography. *Clin Investig*, 72, 951-956 (1994)

4927 Solary E, Guiguet M, Zeller V et al. Radioimmunoassay for the measurement of serum IL-6 and its correlation with tumour cell mass parameters in multiple myeloma. *Am J Hematol*, 39, 163-171 (1992)

4928 Solinas A, Cossu P, Poddighe P et al. Changes of serum 2',5'-oligoadenylate synthetase activity during interferon treatment of chronic hepatitis C. *Liver*, 13, 253-258 (1993)

4929 Solomons NW et al. Zinc nutrition in celiac sprue. *Am J Clin Nutr*, 29, 371-375 (1976)

4930 Solovey A, Lin Y, Browne P, et al. Circulating activated endothelial cells in sickle cell anemia. *N Engl J Med*, 337, 1584-1590 (1997)

4931 Soma J, Saito T, Ootaka T, et al. Intercellular adhesion molecule-I, intercellular adhesion molecule-3, and leukocyte integrins in leukocyte accumulation in membranoproliferative glomerulonephritis type I. *Am J Kid Dis*, 28, 685-694 (1996)

4932 Somer T. Hyperviscosity syndrome in plasma cell dyscrasias. *Adv Microcirc*, 6, 1 (1975)

4933 Somers K, Fowler J N. Endomyocardial fibrosis: clinical diagnosis. *Cardiologia*, 52, 25 (1968)

4934 Song C, Vandewoude M, Stevens w, et al. Alterations in immune functions during normal aging and Alzheimer's disease. *Psychiat Res*, 85, 71-80 (1999)

4935 Song H et al. Usefulness of serum lipase, esterase, and amylase estimations in the diagnosis of pancreatitis. a comparison. *Clin Chem*, 16, 264 (1970)

4936 Song H, Seishima M, Saito K, et al. Apo A-I and apo E concentrations in cerebrospinal fluids of patients with acute meningitis. *Ann Clin Biochem*, 35, 408-414 (1998)

4937 Sonksen P, Salomon F, Cuneo R. Metabolic effects of hypopituitarism and acromegaly. *Horm Res*, 36, 27-31 (1991)

4938 Sorensen JV, Jensen HP, Rahr HB, et al. Hemostatic activation in patients with head injury with and without simultaneous multiple trauma. *Scand J Clin Lab Invest*, 53, 659-665 (1993)

4939 Sorensen JV, Rahr HB, Jensen HP et al. Markers of coagulation and fibrinolysis after fractures of the lower extremities. *Thromb Res*, 65, 479-486 (1992)

4940 Sorensen PJ, Knudsen F, Nielsen AH et al. Protein C activity in renal disease. *Thromb Res*, 38, 243-249 (1985)

4941 Sorenson B, Brunish R. Urinary excretion of acid mucopolysaccharides and hydroxyproline in psoriasis. *Dermatologica*, 130, 165 (1965)

4942 Soria C, Chadefaux B, Coude M et al. Concentrations of total homocysteine in plasma in chronic renal failure. *Clin Chem*, 36, 2137 (1990)

4943 Sorice M, Griggi T, Arcieri P et al. Protein S and HIV infection. The role of anticardiolipin and anti-protein S antibodies. *Thromb Res*, 73, 165-175 (1994)

4944 Sorva R, Thtel R, Turpeinen M, et al. Changes in bone markers in children with asthma during inhaled budesonide and nedocromil treatments. *Acta Paediat*, 85, 1176-1180 (1996)

4945 Souroujon M, Ashkenazi A, Lupo M. Serum ferritin levels in celiac disease. *Am J Clin Pathol*, 77, 82-86 (1982)

4946 Southern P M, Sanford J P. Relaping fever: a clinical and microbiological review. *Medicine*, 48, 129 (1967)

4947 Southgate HJ, Townsend J, Barron J. Cherubism: biochemistry and response to treatment with the diphosphonate etidronate. *Proc ACB Natl Meet*, 67 (1995)

4948 Souto JC, Martinez E, Roca M et al. Low levels of plasminogen activator inhibitor type 1 in patients with inflammatory bowel disease. *Fibrinolysis*, 8, 359-363 (1994)

4949 Sox HC, Liang Mit. The erythrocyte sedimentation rate. *Ann Intern Med*, 104, 515-523

4950 Soylemezoglu O, Sultan N, Gursel T, et al. Circulating adhesion molcules ICAM-1, E-selectin, and von Willebrand factor in Henoch-Schonlein purpura. *Arch Dis Child*, 75, 507-511 (1996)

4951 Spandrio S, Sleiman I, Scalvini T et al. Lipoprotein (a) in thyroid dysfunction before and after treatment. *Horm Metab Res*, 25, 586-589 (1993)

4952 Spati B, Child JA, Kerruish SM et al. Behavior of serum $\beta_{,2}$-microglobulin and acute phase reactant proteins in chronic lymphocytic leukaemia: a multicentre study. *Acta Haematol*, 64, 79-86 (1980)

4953 Specks U, Wheatley CL, McDonald TJ et al. Anticytoplasmic autoantibodies in the diagnosis and follow-up of Wegener's granulomatosis. *Mayo Clin Proc*, 64, 28-36 (1989)

4954 Spector DA et al. Thyroid function and metabolic state in chronic renal failure. *Ann Intern Med*, 85, 724-730 (1976)

4955 Spencer K, Carpenter P. Is prostate-specific antigen a marker for pregnancies affected by Down syndrome? *Clin Chem*, 44, 2362-2364 (1998)

4956 Spencer N, Hopkinson DA, Harris H. Adenosine deaminase polymorphism in man. *Ann Hum Genet*, 32, 9-14 (1968)

4957 Speranza V et al. Progress in the treatment of acute gastroduodenal mucosal lesions (AGML). *World J Surg*, 1, 35-44 (1977)

4958 Sperber SJ, Blevins DD, Francis JB. Hypercalcitoninemia, hypocalcemia, and toxic shock syndrome. *Rev Infect Dis*, 12, 736-739 (1990)

4959 Spies C, Haude V, Fitzner R, et al. Serum cardiac troponin T as a prognostic marker in early sepsis. *Chest*, 113, 1055-1063 (1998)

4960 Spiro HM. *Clinical Gastroenterology,* 1st edition, New York NY, MacMillan (1970)

4961 Spivak B, Vered Y, Graff E, et al. Low platelet-poor plasma concentrations of serotonin in patients with combat-related posttraumatic stress disorder. *Biol Psychiat*, 45, 840-845 (1999)

4962 Spivak JL. Felty's syndrome: an analytical review. *Johns Hopkins Med J*, 141, 156-162 (1977)

4963 Spranger M, Schwab S, Krempian S, et al. Excess glutamate levels in the cerebrospinal fluid predict clinical outcome of bacterial meningitis. *Arch Neurol*, 53, 992-996 (1996)

4964 Spronk PE, ter Borg EJ, Limburg PC, Kallenberg CG. Plasma concentration of IL-6 in systemic lupus erythematosus; an indicator of disease activity. *Clin Exp Immunol*, 90, 106-110 (1992)

4965 Srfontein WJ, Ubbink JB, De Villiers LS et al. Plasma pyridoxal-5-phosphate level as risk index for coronary artery disease. *Atherosclerosis*, 55, 357-361 (1985)

4966 Srichaikul T et al. Ferrokinetics in patients with malaria: haemoglobin synthesis and normoblasts in vitro. *Trans Roy Soc Trop Med Hyg*, 70, 244-246 (1976)

4967 Srinivasan SR, Freedman DS, Berenson GS. Are plasma apolipoproteins helpful as markers of coronary artery disease? *Intern Med Special*, 8, 195 (1987)

4968 Srivastava MD, Srivastava A, Srivastava BI. Soluble interleukin-2 receptor, soluble CD8 and soluble intercellular adhesion molecule-1 levels in hematologic malignancies. *Leuk Lymphoma*, 12, 241-251 (1994)

4969 St John A, Hoad K, Mallon D et al. Serum parathyroid hormone concentrations in patients with HIV infection. *Ann Clin Biochem*, 32, 94-95 (1995)

4970 Stabile BE, Braunstein GD, Passaro E Jr. Serum gastrin and human chorionic gonadotropin in the Zollinger-Ellison syndrome. *Arch Surg*, 115, 1090-1095 (1980)

4971 Stabile BE, Passaro E JR, Carlson HE. Elevated serum prolactin level in the Zollinger-Ellison syndrome. *Arch Surg*, 116, 449-453 (1981)

4972 Stachura Z, Kowalski J, Obuchowicz E, et al. Concentration of enkephalins in cerebrospinal fluid of patients after severe head injury. *Neuropeptides*, 31, 78-81 (1997)

4973 Stachura Z, Obuchowicz E, Herman ZS. Neuropeptide Y-like immunoreactivity in lumbar cerebrospinal fluid of patients after severe head trauma. *Neuropeptides*, 31, 12-14 (1997)

4974 Stahl WM. Acute phase protein response to tissue injury. *Crit Care Med*, 15, 545-550 (1987)

4975 Stahr K, Hubl W, Scheuch DW. Kinin excretion in urine in normal adults and patients with essential hypertension determined by an enzyme immunoassay. *Exp Clin Endocrinol*, 92, 106-110 (1988)

4976 Stalla GK, Doerr HG, Bidlingmaier F et al. Serum levels of eleven steroid hormones following motion sickness. *Aviat Space Environ Med*, 56, 995-999 (1985)

4977 Stampfer MJ, Malinow MR, Willett WC et al. A prospective study of plasma homocyst(e)ine and risk of myocardial infarction in US physicians. *J Am Med Ass*, 268, 877-881 (1992)

4978 Stampfer MJ, Sacks FM, Salvini S et al. A prospective study of cholesterol, apolipoproteins, and the risk of myocardial infraction. *N Engl J Med*, 325, 373-381 (1991)

4979 Stanbury JB et al. *The Metabolic Basis of Inherited Disease,* 3rd edition, New York NY, McGraw-Hill (1972)

4980 Standley CA, Whitty JE, Mason BA, Cotton DB. Serun ionized magnesium levels in normal and preeclamptic gestation. *Obstet Gynecol*, 89, 24-27 (1997)

4981 Stanwell-Smith R, Thompson SG, Haines AP et al. A comparative study of zinc, copper, cadmium, and lead levels in fertile and infertile men. *Fertil Steril*, 40, 670 (1983)

4982 Starcevic D, Jelic-Ivanovic Z, Kalimanosvka V. Plasma C! inhibitor in malignant diseases: functional activity versus concentration. *Ann Clin Biochem*, 28, 595-598 (1991)

4983 Starkweather WH et al. Alterations of erythrocyte lactate dehydrogenase in man. *Blood*, 26, 63-73 (1965)

4984 Stasi R, Stipa E, Masi M et al. Antiphospholipid antibodies: prevalence, clinical significance and correlation to cytokine levels in acute myeloid leukemia and non-Hodgkin's Lymphoma. *Thromb Haemostas*, 70, 568-572 (1993)

4985 Stasi R, Zinzani PL, Galieni P, et al. Clinical implications of cytokine and soluble receptor measurements in patients with newly-diagnosed aggressive non-Hodgkin's lymphoma. *Eur J Haematol*, 54, 9-17 (1995)

4986 Statland BE, Winkel P. Selected pre-analytical sources of variation. In:. *Reference values in Laboratory Medicine.* R Grasbeck, T Alstrom (eds), Chichester, Wiley, 127-137 (1981)

4987 Stearman M, Southgate HJ. The use of cytokine and C-reactive protein measurements in cerebrospinal fluid during acute infective meningitis. *Ann Clin Biochem*, 31, 255-261 (1994)

4988 Stearman M, Southgate HJ. The use of extended cytokine measurements in CSF during acute infective meningitis. *Proc ACB Natl Meet*, 83-84 (1993)

4989 Stefanini M. Enzymes, isozymes, and enzyme variants in the diagnosis of cancer: A short review. *Cancer*, 55, 1931-1936 (1985)

4990 Stefanis N, Mackintosh C, Abraha HD, et al. Dissociation of bone turnover in anorexia nervosa. *Ann Clin Biochem*, 35, 709-716 (1998)

4991 Steffanini M (ed). *Progress in Clinical Pathology*, New York NY, Grune and Stratton, 3 (1970)

4992 Stegeman CA, Tervaert JWC, Huitema MG et al. Serum levels of soluble adhesion molecules intercellular adhesion molecule 1, vascular cell adhesion molecule 1, and E-selectin in patients with Wegener's granulomatosis. *Arth Rheum*, 37, 1228-1235 (1994)

4993 Stehouwer CDA, Gall M-A, Hougaard P, et al. Plasma homocysteine concentration predicts mortality in non-insulin-dependent patients with and without albuminuria. *Kidney Int*, 55, 308-314 (1999)

4994 Steihoff J, Einecke G, Niederstadt C, et al. Renal graft rejection or urinary tract infection? *Transplantation*, 64, 443-447 (1997)

4995 Stein ID et al. Lactate dehydrogenase in megaloblastic anemia. *J Lab Clin Med*, 74, 331-339 (1969)

4996 Stein JA. Acute intermittent porphyria. *Medicine*, 49, 1 (1970)

4997 Stein MB, Uhde TW. Thyroid indices in panic disorder. *Am J Psychiat*, 145, 745-747 (1988)

4998 Steinberg WM, Gelfand R, Anderson KK et al. Comparison of the sensitivity and specificity of the CA19-9 and carcinoembryonic antigen assays in detecting cancer of the pancreas. *Gastroenterology*, 90, 343-349 (1986)

4999 Steiner S et al. Renal function and protein elimination of human subjects during carbon monoxide exposure. *Helv Med Acta*, 36, 39 (1972)

5000 Steinhoff J, Feddersen A, Wood WG et al. Glomerular proteinuria as an early sign of renal-transplant rejection. *Clin Nephrol*, 35, 255-262 (1991)

5001 Steinkamp RC et al. Long term experience with the use of P^{32} in the treatment of chronic lymphocytic leukemia. *J Nucl Med*, 4, 92 (1963)

5002 Stemmermann GN. An histologic and histochemical study of familial osteoectasia. *Am J Pathol*, 48, 641-648 (1966)

5003 Stenvinkel P, Berglund L, Ericsson S, et al. Low-density lipoprotein metabolism and its association to plasma lipoprotein(a) in the nephrotic syndrome. *Eur J Clin Invest*, 27, 169-177 (1997)

5004 Stenvinkel P, Berglund L, Heimburger O et al. Lipoprotein(a) in nephrotic syndrome. *Kidney Int*, 44, 1116-1123 (1993)

5005 Stenvinkel P, Heimburger O, Tuck CH, Berglund L. Apo(a)-isoform size, nutritional status and inflammatory markers in chronic renal failure. *Kid Int*, 53, 1336-1342 (1998)

5006 Stephens RW, Pedersen AN, Nielsen HJ, et al. ELISA determination of soluble urokinase receptor in blood from healthy donors and cancer patients. *Clin Chem*, 43, 1868-1876 (1997)

5007 Stephensen CB, Alvarez JO, Kohatsu J et al. Vitamin A is excreted in the urine during acute infection. *Am J Clin Nutr*, 60, 388-392 (1994)

5008 Sterkel RL et al. Serum isocitric dehydrogenase activity with particular reference to liver disease. *J Lab Clin Med*, 52, 176

5009 Stern JJ, Ng RH, Triplett DA et al. Incidence of antiphospholipid antibodies in patients with monoclonal gammopathy of undetermined significance. *Am J Clin Pathol*, 101, 471-474 (1994)

5010 Sterner G, Carlson J, Ekberg G. Raised platelet levels in diabetes mellitus complicated with nephropathy. *J Intern Med*, 244, 437-441 (1998)

5011 Stetter F, Gaertner HJ, Wiatr G et al. Urinary dolichol - a doubtful marker of alcoholism. *Alcohol Clin Exp Res*, 15, 938-941 (1991)

5012 Stevens TR, Harley SL, Groom JS et al. Anti-endothelial cell antibodies in inflammatory bowel disease. *Dig Dis Sci*, 38, 426-432 (1993)

5013 Stewart DJ, Kubac G, Costello KB et al. Increased plasma endothelin-1 in the early hours of acute myocardial infarction. *J Am Coll Cardiol*, 18, 38-43 (1991)

5014 Stewart JM, Kilpatrick ES, Cathcart S et al. Low-density lipoprotein particle size in type 2 diabetic patients and age matched controls. *Ann Clin Biochem*, 31, 153-159 (1994)

5015 Stewart S, Malto M, Sandberg L et al. Increased serum levels of anti-elastin antibodies in patients with Peyronie's disease. *J Urol*, 152, 105-106 (1994)

5016 Steyn ME, Viljoen M, Ubbink JB, et al. Whole blood serotonin levels in chronic renal failure. *Life Sci*, 51, 359-366 (1992)

5017 Stibler H, Borg S. Glycoprotein glycosyltransferase activities in serum in alcohol-abusing patients and healthy controls. *Scand J Clin Lab Invest*, 51, 43-51 (1991)

5018 Stibler H, von Dobelin U, Kristiansson B, Guthenberg C. Cabohydrate-deficient transferrin in galactosaemia. *Acta Paediatr*, 86, 1377-1378 (1997)

5019 Stichtenoth DO, Fauler J, Zeidler H et al. Urinary nitrate excretion in patients with rheumatoid arthritis and reduced by prednisolone. *Ann Rheum Dis*, 54, 820-824 (1995)

5020 Stiegler G, Stohlawetz P, Brugger S, et al. Elevated numbers of reticulated platelets in hyperthyroidism: direct evidence for an increase of thrombopoiesis. *Br J Haematol*, 101, 636-638 (1998)

5021 Stigbrand T, Holmgren PA, Jeppsson A, et al. On the value of placental alkaline phosphatase as a marker for gynecological malignancy. *Acta Obstet Gynecol Scand*, 64, 99-103 (1985)

5022 Stimac D, Lenac T, Marusic Z. A scoring system for early differentiation of the etiology of acute pancreatitis. *Scand J Gastroenterol*, 33, 209-211 (1998)

5023 Stinebaugh BT et al. Pathogenesis of distal renal tubular acidosis. *Kidney Int.*, 17, 1-7 (1981)

5024 Stockenhuber F, Gottsauner-Wolf M, Marosi L et al. Plasma endothelin in chronic renal failure and after renal transplantation: impact on hypertension and cyclosporin A-associated nephrotoxicity. *Clin Sci*, 82, 255-258 (1992)

5025 Stocks AE, Martin FIR. Pituitary function in haemochromatosis. *Am J Med*, 45, 839 (1968)

5026 Stocks AE, Powell L. Pituitary function in idiopathic hemochromatosis and cirrhosis of the liver. *Lancet*, 2, 298-300 (1972)

5027 Stokkel MPM, van Eck-Smith BL, Zwinderman AH, et al. Pretreatment serum LDH as additional staging parameter in small cell lung carcinoma. *Neth J Med*, 52, 65-70 (1998)

5028 Stolbach LL et al. Correlation of Regan isoenzyme and hCG in serum and malignant effusions of patients with ovarian cancer. *Proc Am Ass Cancer Res*, 78 (1974)

5029 Stolbach LL et al. Ectopic production of an alkaline phosphatase isoenzyme in patients with cancer. *N Engl J Med*, 281, 757-762 (1974)

5030 Stone JH. HELLP syndrome: hemolysis, elevated liver enzymes, and low platelets. *J Am Med Ass*, 280, 559-562 (1998)

5031 Stone NN, Clejan SJ. Response of prostate volume, prostate-specific antigen, and testosterone to flutamide in men with benign prostatic hyperplasia. *J Androl*, 12, 376-380 (1991)

5032 Stone PJ, Gottlieb DJ, O'Connor GT et al. Elastin and collagen degradation products in urine of smokers with and without chronic obstructive pulmonary disease. *Am J Resp Crit Care Med*, 151, 952-959 (1995)

5033 Stoving RK, Flyvbjerg A, Frystyk J, et al. Low serum levels of free and total insulin-like growth factor-I (IGF-I) in patients with anorexia nervosa are not associated with increased IGF-binding protein-3 proteolysis. *J Clin Endocrinol Metab*, 84, 1346-1350 (1999)

5034 Stowe CD, Phelps SJ. Altered clearance of theophylline in children with Down syndrome: a case series. *J Clin Pharmacol*, 39, 359-365 (1999)

5035 Straffen AM, Carmichael DJS, Fairney A et al. Calcium metabolism following renal transplantation. *Ann Clin Biochem*, 31, 125-128 (1994)

5036 Strand A. The function of the placenta and placental insufficiency with especial reference to the development of prolonged foetal distress. *Acta Obstet Gynecol Scand*, 45, 125-230 (1966)

5037 Strand LJ et al. Decreased red cell uroporphyrinogen I synthetase activity in intermittent acute porphyria. *J Clin Invest*, 51, 2530 (1972)

5038 Strand T, Marklund SL. Release of superoxide dismutase into cerebrospinal fluid as a marker of brain lesion in acute cerebral infarction. *Stroke*, 23, 515-518 (1992)

5039 Strandvik B, Samuelson K. Fasting serum bile acid levels in relation to liver histopathology in cystic fibrosis. *Scand J Gastroenterol*, 20, 381-384 (1985)

5040 Strasser-Vogel B, Blum WF, Past R et al. Insulin-like growth factor (IGF)-I and -II and IGF-binding proteins-1, -2, and -3 in children and adolescents with diabetes mellitus: correlation with metabolic control and height attainment. *J Clin Endocrinol Metab*, 80, 1207-1213 (1995)

5041 Straub FB, Stephaneck O, Aes G. *Biochimica*, 22, 118 (1957)

5042 Straub RH, Zeuner M, Antoniou E, et al. Dehydroepiandrosterone sulfate is positively correlated with soluble interleukin 2 receptor and soluble intercellular adhesion molecule in systemic lupus erythematosus. *J Rheumatol*, 23, 856-861 (1996)

5043 Strauss A et al. Exocrine disorder in asthmatics: demonstration of high sweat chloride levels in chronic patients and their relatives. *Allergol Immunopathol (Madr)*, 6, 19-24 (1978)

5044 Streffer JR, Schuster M, Zipp F, Weller M. Soluble CD95 (Fas/APO-1) in malignant glioma: (No) implications for CD95-based immunotherapy? *J Neuro-oncol*, 40, 233-235 (1998)

5045 Stremple, Watson. Serum calcium, serum gastrin, and gastric acid secretion before and after parathyroidectomy for hyperparathyroidism. *Surgery*, 75, 841-852 (1974)

5046 Strickland GT et al. Hypersplenism in Wilson's disease. *Gut*, 13, 220 (1972)

5047 Strickland GT, Leu M. Wilson's disease - clinical laboratory manifestations in 40 patients. *Medicine*, 54, 113-138 (1975)

5048 Strickland P, Morriss R, Wearden A, Deakin B. A comparison of salivary cortisol in chronic fatigue syndrome, community depression and healthy controls. *J Affect Disord*, 47, 191-194 (1998)

5049 Strickland RE et al. A reappraisal of the nature and significance of chronic atrophic gastritis. *Am J Dig Dis*, 18, 426-440 (1973)

5050 Strimlan CV et al. Lymphocytic interstitial pneumonitis. review of 13 cases. *Ann Intern Med*, 88, 616-621 (1978)

5051 Strojan P, Budihba M, Smid L, et al. Cathepsin D in tissue and serum of patients with squamous cell carcinoma of the head and neck. *Cancer Lett*, 130, 49-56 (1998)

5052 Stubbs P, Seed M, Moseley D, et al. A prospective study of the role of lipoprotein(a) in the pathogenesis of unstable angina. *Eur Heart J*, 18, 603-607 (1997)

5053 Stubbs TM, Lazarchick J, Horger EO III. Plasma fibronectin levels in preeclampsia: a possible biochemical marker for vascular endothelial damage. *Am J Obstet Gynecol*, 150, 885-887 (1984)

5054 Studd JWW. Immunoglobulins in normal pregnancy, pre-eclampsia and pregnancy complicated by the nephrotic syndrome. *Br J Obstet Gynaecol*, 78, 786-790 (1971)

5055 Studd JWW et al. A study of serum protein changes in late pregnancy and identification of the pregnancy zone protein using antigen antibody crossed immunoelectrophoresis. *Br J Obstet Gynaecol*, 77, 42-51 (1970)

5056 Studd JWW et al. Serum protein changes in the pre-eclampsia-eclampsia syndrome. *Br J Obstet Gynaecol*, 77, 796-801 (1970)

5057 Sturgeon P , Finch CA. Erythrokinetics in Cooley's anemia. *Blood*, 12, 64 (1959)

5058 Sturmer T, Sun Y, Sauerland S, et al. Serum cholesterol and osteoarthritis. The baseline examination of the ULM Osteoarthritis study. *J Rheumatol*, 25, 1827-1832 (1998)

5059 Sturniolo GC, Mestriner C, Lecis PE, et al. Altered plasma and mucosal concentrations of trace elements and antioxidants in active ulcerative colitis. *Scand J Gastroenterol*, 33, 644-649 (1998)

5060 Stutzman FL et al. Blood serum magnesium in portal cirrhosis and diabetes mellitus. *J Lab Clin Med*, 26, 215 (1953)

5061 Suberbielle-Boissel C, Legendre C, Kassentini M, et al. Anti-endothelial and epithelial antibodies in renal transplantation. *Transplant Proc*, 30, 2852 (1998)

5062 Subhash MN., Padmashree TS, Srinivas KL et al. Calcium and phosphorus levels in serum and CSF in dementia. *Neurobiol Aging*, 12, 267-269 (1991)

5063 Suchiro T, Yamamoto M, Yoshida K et al. Increase of plasma proapolipoprotein A-I in patients with liver cirrhosis and its relationship to circulating high-density lipoproteins 2 and 3. *Clin Chem*, 39, 60-65 (1995)

5064 Suda S, Weidmann P, Saxenhofer H et al. Atrial natriuretic factor in mild to moderate chronic renal failure. *Hypertension*, 11, 483-490 (1988)

5065 Sudo K. Exertional myoglobinuria. *Abstracts*, 5th APCCB, Kobe (1991)

5066 Sudo N, Kamoi K, Ishibashi M et al. Plasma endothelin-1 and big endothelin-1 levels in women with pre-eclampsia. *Acta Endocrinol*, 129, 114-120 (1993)

5067 Suer S, Ulutin T, Sonmez H, et al. Plasma Lp(a) and t-PA-PAI complex in coronary heart disease. *Thromb Res*, 83, 77-85 (1996)

5068 Sufrin G et al. Adenosine deaminase activity in patients with carcinoma of the bladder. *J Urol*, 119, 343 (1978)

5069 Sufrin G et al. Adenosine deaminase activity in patients with renal adenocarcinoma. *Cancer*, 40, 796-802 (1977)

5070 Sufrin G et al. Hormones in renal cancer. *J Urol*, 117, 433-438 (1977)

5071 Sugawara A, Nakao K, Kono T et al. Atrial natriuretic factor in essential hypertension and adrenal disorders. *Hypertension*, 11, I207-I211 (1988)

5072 Sugawara T, Honke K, Gasa S et al. Serum levels of steroid sulfatase protein in gynecologic carcinomas. *Clin Chim Acta*, 226, 13-20 (1994)

5073 Sugimoto K-I, Shionoiri H, Minamisawa K et al. Measurement of plasma total renin by the anti-human renin monoclonal antibodies. *Am J Med Sci*, 302, 342-346 (1991)

5074 Sugino H, Mitani I, Koike M et al. Detection of elevated levels of 2-5A synthetase in serum from children with various infectious diseases. *J Clin Microbiol*, 24, 478-481 (1986)

5075 Suh JW, Lee SH, Chung BC, Park J. Urinary polyamine evaluation for effective diagnosis of various cancers. *J Chromatog B*, 688, 179-196 (1997)

5076 Sullivan PS, Hanson DL, Chu SY, et al. Surveillance for thrombocytopenia in persons infected with HIV: results from the multistate adult and adolescent spectrum of disease project. *J Acquir Immune Defic Syn*, 14, 374-379 (1997)

5077 Sultan C, Oliel V, Audran F et al. Free and total plasma testosterone in men and women with acne. *Acta Derm Venereol (Stockh)*, 66, 301-304 (1986)

5078 Sumii K, Kimura M, Morikawa A et al. Recurrence of duodenal ulcer and elevated serum pepsinogen I levels in smokers and nonsmokers. *Am J Gastrointerol*, 85, 1493-1497 (1990)

5079 Sumimoto S, Kawai M, Kasajima Y et al. Increased plasma tumor necrosis factor-α concentration in atopic dermatitis. *Arch Dis Child*, 67, 277-279 (1992)

5080 Sun Y, Tokushige K, Isono E et al. Elevated serum interleukin-6 levels in patients with acute hepatitis. *J Clin Immunol*, 12, 197-200 (1992)

5081 Sundblad C, Bergman L, Eriksson E. High levels of free testosterone in women with bulimia nervosa. *Acta Psychiat Scand*, 90, 397-398 (1994)

5082 Sunderman FW et al. Clinical applications of the fractionation of serum proteins by paper electrophoresis. *Am J Clin Pathol*, 27, 125-128 (1957)

5083 Sunderman FW Jr. Current status of zinc deficiency in the pathogenesis of neurological, dermatological and musculoskeletal disorders. *Ann Clin Lab Sci*, 5, 132-145 (1975)

5084 Sunder-Plassmann G, Sedlacek PL, Sunder-Plassmann R et al. Anti-interleukin-1α autoantibodies in hemodialysis patients. *Kidney Int*, 40, 787-791 (1991)

5085 Suominen P, Punnonen K, Rajamki A, Irjala K. Evaluation of new immunoenzymometric assay for measuring soluble transferrin receptor to detect iron deficiency in anemic patients. *Clin Chem*, 43, 1641-1646 (1997)

5086 Surtees R, Clelland J, Heales S. Cerebrospinal fluid concentrations of nitrate plus nitrite during the treatment of acute lymphoblastic leukemia in childhood. *Leuk Res*, 22, 751-754 (1998)

5087 Suryaatmadia M, Hidayat EM. Prevalence of microalbuminuria in hypertensive patients. *Clin Biochem Rev*, 14, 356 (1993)

5088 Susheela AK, Jethanandani P. Serum haptoglobin and C-reactive protein in human skeletal fluorosis. *Clin Biochem*, 27, 463-468 (1994)

5089 Suskind R et al. Complement activity in children with protein-calorie malnutrition. *Am J Clin Nutr*, 29, 1089-1092 (1976)

5090 Sutherland WH, Walker RJ, Lewis-Barned NJ et al. Plasma cholesteryl ester transfer in patients with non-insulin dependent diabetes mellitus. *Clin Chim Acta*, 21, 29-38 (1994)

5091 Suzaki I, Hara T, Maegaki Y, et al. Nerve growth factor levels in cerebrospinal fluid from patients with neurologic disorders. *J Child Neurol*, 12, 205-207 (1997)

5092 Suzuki H, Sato S, Suzuki Y et al. Increased endothelin concentration in CSF from patients with subarachnoid hmorrhage. *Acta Neurol Scand*, 81, 553-554 (1990)

5093 Suzuki K, Kinoshita N, Matsuda Y et al. Elevation of immunoreactive serum Mn-superoxide dismutase in patients with acute myocardial infarction. *Free Rad Res Comm*, 15, 325-334 (1992)

5094 Suzuki M, Ohwada M, Sato I et al. Serum levels of macrophage colony-stimulating factor as a marker for gynecologic malignancies. *Oncology*, 52, 128-133 (1995)

5095 Suzuki S et al. Histamine contents of blood plasma and cells in patients with myelogenous leukemia. *Cancer*, 28, 384 (1971)

5096 Suzuki T, Koizumi J, Moroji T et al. Effects of long-term anticonvulsant therapy on copper, zinc, and magnesium in hair and serum of epileptics. *Biol Psychiat*, 31, 571-581 (1992)

5097 Svartman M et al. Immunoglobulins and complement components in the synovial fluid of patients with acute rheumatic fever. *J Clin Invest*, 56, 111 (1975)

5098 Swan SK. Role of lipids in chronic renal allograft rejection. *Contrib Nephrol*, 120, 62-67 (1997)

5099 Swano M, Dohi K, Hirata E et al. Urinary levels of IL-6 in patients with active lupus nephritis. *Clin Nephrol*, 40, 16-21 (1993)

5100 Swaroop AK et al. Uric acid levels in neurological and psychiatric disorders. *Neurol India*, 24, 100-103 (1976)

5101 Swartz CM. Albumin decrement in depression and cholesterol decrement in mania. *J Affect Disord*, 19, 173-176 (1990)

5102 Swartz CM, Breen KJ. Multiple muscle enzyme release with psychiatric illness. *J Nerv Ment Dis*, 178, 755-759 (1990)

5103 Swedlund HA, Hunder GG, Gleich GJ. α_1-Antitrypsin in serum and synovial fluid in rheumatoid arthritis. *Ann Rheum Dis*, 33, 162-164 (1974)

5104 Sweeney JD. Patterns of porphyrin excretion in South African porphyric patients. *S Afr J Lab Clin Med*, 9, 182 (1963)

5105 Sweeney KJ, Weiss AS. Hyaluronic acid in progeria and the aged phenotype. *Gerontology*, 38, 139-152 (1992)

5106 Sweeney VP et al. Acute intermittent porphyria: increased ALA-synthetase activity during an acute attack. *Brain*, 93, 369 (1970)

5107 Sweet RA, Pollock BG, Mulsant BH, et al. Asociation of plasma homovanillic acid with behavioral symptoms in patients diagnosed with dementia: a preliminary report. *Biol Psychiat*, 42, 1016-1023 (1997)

5108 Sybulski S et al. Relationship between cortisol levels in umbilical cord plasma and development of the respiratory distress syndrome in premature newborn infants. *Am J Obstet Gynecol*, 125, 239-243 (1976)

5109 Sybulski S et al. Umbilical cord plasma estradiol levels in relation to complication of pregnancy and newborn and to cortisol levels. *Biol Neonate*, 27, 302-307 (1974)

5110 Symonds EM et al. Changes in the renin-angiotensin system in primigravidae with hypertensive disease of pregnancy. *Br J Obstet Gynaecol*, 83, 643-650 (1975)

5111 Symons JA, Wood NC, DiGiovine FS et al. Soluble CD8 in patients with rheumatic diseases. *Clin Exp Immunol*, 80, 354-359 (1990)

5112 Syrjala H, Vuori J, Huttunen K et al. Carbonic anhydrase III as a serum marker for diagnosis of rhabdomyolysis. *Clin Chem*, 39, 696 (1993)

5113 Szegedi A, Czirjak L, Unkeless JC, Boros P. Serum cytokine and anti-FcgammaR autoantibody measurements in patients with systemic sclerosis. *Acta Derm Venereol*, 76, 21-23 (1996)

5114 Szekanecz Z, Strieter RM, Kunkel SL, Koch AE. Chemokines in rheumatoid arthritis. *Springer Semin Immupathol* (1998)

5115 Szinnyai M et al. Transaminase-utersuchungen bei fruher und spater schwangerschaftoxikose. *Zentralbl Gynakol*, 84, 1675-1678 (1962)

5116 Szurmowicz M, Tomkowski W, Fijalkowska A, et al. The role in pericardial fluid for the recognition of malignant pericarditis of carcinoembryonic antigen (CEA) and neuron-specific enolase (NSE) evaluation. *Int J Biol Markers*, 12, 96-101 (1997)

5117 Taberner DA. Acquired alpha 2-antiplasmin deficiency in patients with glomerular proteinuria. *Thromb Haemostas*, 46, 389 (1981)

5118 Tachiki et al. A rapid column chromatographic procedure for the routine measurement of taurine in plasma of normals and depressed patients. *Clin Chim Acta*, 75, 455-465 (1977)

5119 Tachimori Y, Watanabe H, Kato H et al. Hypercalcemia in patients with esophageal carcinoma: the physiologic role of parathyroid hormone-related protein. *Cancer*, 68, 2625-2629 (1993)

5120 Tadderni L, Watson C J. The clinical porphyrias. *Semin Hematol*, 5, 335 (1968)

5121 Tai D-I, Shen F-H, Liaw Y-F. Abnormal pre-drainage serum creatinine as a prognostic indicator for cholangitis. *Hepatogastroenterology*, 39, 47-50 (1992)

5122 Takabatake N, Nakamura H, Abe S, et al. Circulating leptin in patients with chronic obstructive pulmonary disease. *Am J Respir Crit Care Med*, 159, 1215-1219 (1999)

5123 Takacs O et al. Distribution of serum amylase isoenzymes in cystic fibrosis homozygotes and heterozygotes. *Acta Paediat Hung*, 18, 21-26 (1977)

5124 Takacse-Nagay L et al. Definition of clinical features and diagnosis of myelofibrosis. *Clin Lab Haematol*, 4, 291-308 (1977)

5125 Takada K, Nasu H, Hibi N, et al. Serum concentrations of free ubiquitin and multiubiquitin chains. *Clin Chem*, 43, 1188-1195 (1997)

5126 Takagi M, Yamamuchi M, Toda G, et al. Serum ubiquitin levels in patients with alcoholic liver disease. *Alcohol Clin Exp Res*, 23, 76S-80S (1999)

5127 Takahashi H, Hattori A, Shibata A. Profile of blood coagulation and fibrinolysis in chronic myeloproliferative disorders. *Tohoku J Exp Med*, 138, 71-80 (1982)

5128 Takahashi K et al. Pathological, histochemical and ultrastructural studies on sea-blue histiocytes and Gaucher-like cells in acquired lipidosis occurring in leukemia. *Acta Pathol Jpn*, 27, 775-779 (1977)

5129 Takahashi M, Kushida K, Hoshino H, et al. Comparson of bone and total alkaline phosphatase activity on bone turnover during menopause and in patients with established osteoporosis. *Clin Endocrinol*, 47, 177-183 (1997)

5130 Takahashi M, Kushida K, Kawana K et al. Quantification of the cross-link pentoside in serum from normal and uremic subjects. *Clin Chem*, 39, 2162-2165 (1993)

5131 Takahashi M, Suzuki M, Naitou K, et al. Comparison of free and peptide-bound pyridinoline cross-links excretion in rheumatoid arthritis and osteoarthritis. *Rheumatology*, 38, 133-138 (1999)

5132 Takahashi S, Yamamoto T, Moriwaki Y, et al. Decreased serum concentrations of 1,25-$(OH)_2$-vitamin D_3 in patients with gout. *Metabolism*, 47, 336-338 (1998)

5133 Takahashi S, Yamamoto T, Moriwaki Y et al. Increased concentrations of serum Lp(a) lipoprotein in patients with primary gout. *Ann Rheum Dis*, 54, 90-93 (1995)

5134 Takahashi T, Munakata M, Suzuki I, et al. Serum and bronchoalveolar fluid KL-6 levels in patients with pulmonary alveolar proteinosis. *Am J Respir Crit Care Med*, 158, 1294-1298 (1998)

5135 Takahashi Y, Suga T, Mai M. Clinical significance of serum CA 125 values in patients with gastric cancers -- especially correlation with peritonitis carcinomatosa. *Gan To Kagaku Ryoho*, 19, 975-979 (1992)

5136 Takala I et al. The activities of plasma membrane marker enzymes in rheumatoid synovial tissues and fluids. *Scand J Rheumatol*, 6, 33-36 (1977)

5137 Takami H. Measurement of serum PDN-21 (katacalcin) levels by radioimmunoassay in patients with various thyroid diseases. *Exp Clin Endocrinol*, 102, 370-373 (1994)

5138 Takase S, Yoshida M. Quantitative determination of immunoglobulins in cerebrospinal fluid. *Tohoku J Exp Med*, 98, 189 (1969)

5139 Takashi M, Zhu Y, Hasegawa S, Kato K. Serum creatine kinase B subunit in patients with renal cell carcinoma. *Urol Int*, 48, 144-148 (1992)

5140 Takayama N, Ogawa M, Nakano I et al. Changes of the urinary excretion of hydroxyproline and fibronectin fragment in acute pancreatitis. *Nippon Shokakibyo Gakkai Zasshi*, 88, 1579-1583 (1991)

5141 Takebayashi M, Kagaya A, Uchitomi Y, et al. Plasma dehydroepiandrosterone sulfate in unipolar major depression. *J Neural Transm*, 105, 537-542 (1998)

5142 Takeda M, Komeyama T, Tsutsu T et al. Changes in urinary excretion of endothelin-1-like immunoreactivity in patients with testicular cancer receiving high-dose cisplatin therapy. *Am J Kid Dis*, 24, 12-16 (1994)

5143 Takeda M, Komeyama T, Tsutsui T et al. Urinary endothelin-1-like immunoreactivity in young male patients with testicular cancer treated by cis-platinum: comparison with other urinary parameters. *Clin Sci*, 86, 703-707 (1994)

5144 Takeda Y, Chen AY. Fibrinogen metabolism and distribution in patients with the nephrotic syndrome. *J Lab Clin Med*, 70, 678 (1967)

5145 Takei Y, Kurobe M, Uchida A et al. Serum concentrations of basic fibroblast growth factor in breast cancer. *Clin Chem*, 40, 1980-1981 (1994)

5146 Takei Y, Minato K, Tsuchiya S, et al. CYFRA 21-1: an indicator of survival and therapeutic effect in lung cancer. *Oncology*, 54, 43-47 (1997)

5147 Takeuchi A, Haraoka H, Hashimoto T. Increased serum alkaline phosphatase activity in Behcet's disease. *Clin Exp Rheumatol*, 7, 619-621 (1989)

5148 Takikawa H, Beppu T, Seyama Y. Urinary concentrations of bile acid glucuronides and sulfates in hepatobiliary diseases. *Gastroenterol Jpn*, 19, 104-109 (1984)

5149 Takikawa H, Otsuka H, Beppu T, Seyama Y. Determination of 3 β-hydroxy-5-cholenoic acid in serum of hepatobiliary diseases--its glucuronidated and sulfated conjugates. *Biochem Med Metab Biol*, 33, 393-400 (1985)

5150 Talal N, Grey HM, Zvaifler N et al. Elevated salivary and synovial fluid β_2-microglobulin in Sjögren's syndrome and rheumatoid arthritis. *Science*, 187, 1196-1198 (1975)

5151 Talamini G, Uomo G, Pezzilli R, et al. Serum creatinine and chest radiographs in the early assessment of acute pancreatitis. *Am J Surg*, 177, 7-14 (1999)

5152 Talwar KK et al. Serum levels of thyrotropin, thyroid hormones and their response to thyrotropin releasing hormone in infective febrile illnesses. *J Clin Endocrinol Metab*, 44, 398-403 (1977)

5153 Taman M, Liu Y, Tolbert E, Dworkin LD. Increased urinary hepatocyte growth factor excretion in human acute renal failure. *Clin Nephrol*, 48, 241-245 (1997)

5154 Tamaoka A, Fukushima T, Sawamura N, et al. Amyloid β protein in plasma from patients with sporadic Alzheimer's disease. *J Neurol Sci*, 151, 65-68 (1996)

5155 Tamate K, Charleton M, Gosling JP, et al. Direct colorimetric monoclonal antibody enzyme immunoassay for estradiol-17β in saliva. *Clin Chem*, 43, 1159-1164 (1997)

5156 Tampellini M, Berruti A, Gerbino A, et al. Relationship between CA 15-3 serum levels and disease extent in predicting overall survival of breast cancer patients with newly diagnosed metastatic disease. *Br J Cancer*, 75, 698-702 (1997)

5157 Tanabe M, Ochi T, Tomita T et al. Remarkable elevation of interleukin-6 and interleukin-8 levels in bone marrow serum of patients with rheumatoid arthritis. *J Rheumatol*, 21, 830-835 (1994)

5158 Tanaka H, Abe S, Yamashita T, et al. Serum levels of cardiac troponin I and troponin T in estimating myocardial infarct size soon after reperfusion. *Coronary Artery Dis*, 8, 433-439 (1997)

5159 Tanaka K, Takeshita K, Suganuma I, Kasagi S. Low serum cholic acid concentration of Duchenne muscular dystrophy. *Brain Dev*, 5, 511-513 (1983)

5160 Taneda S, Monnier VM. ELISA of pentosidine, an advanced glycation end product, in biological specimens. *Clin Chem*, 40, 1766-1773 (1994)

5161 Tang MLK, Coleman J, Kemp AS. Interleukin-4 and interferon-γ production in atopic and non-atopic children with asthma. *Clin Exp Allergy*, 25, 515-521 (1995)

5162 Tani Y, Sato H, Tanaka N, et al. Serum IgA1 and IgA2 subclass antibodies against collagens in patients with ankylosing spondylitis. *Scand J Rheumatol*, 26, 380-382 (1997)

5163 Tarantino A et al. Serum complement pattern in essential mixed cryoglobulinemia. *Clin Exp Immunol*, 32, 77-85 (1978)

5164 Taraszkiewicz F. Badania nad aktywnoscia kreatynofosfokinazy i jej izoenzymow w surowicy krwi u drieci w ostrych choroback zakaznych ze szczegolnym uwzglednieniem odry. *Pol Tyg Lek*, 28, 1699-1701 (1973)

5165 Tarim O, et al. Effects of iron deficiency on hemoglobin A_{1c} in type 1 diabetes mellitus. *Pediat Int*, 41, 357-362 (1999)

5166 Tarng D-C, Lin H-Y, Shyong M-L et al. Renal function in gout patients. *Am J Nephrol*, 15, 31-37 (1995)

5167 Tassi G, Nava AM, Bettoncelli G, Dotti A. Determination of serum angiotensin-converting enzyme in sarcoidosis. *Ric Clin Lab*, 14, 621-627 (1984)

5168 Tateishi K, Shima K, Funakoshi A et al. Glucagon-like peptide-1 (GLP-1) molecular forms in human pancreatic endocrine tumors resemble those in intestine rather than pancreas. *Diabetes Res Clin Pract*, 25, 43-49 (1994)

5169 Tateossian S, Peynet JG, Legrand AG et al. Variations in HDL and VLDL levels in chronic alcoholics. Influence of the degree of liver damage and of withdrawal of alcohol. *Clin Chim Acta*, 148, 211-219 (1985)

5170 Tatsumura T et al. Clinical significance of fucose levels in glycoprotein fraction of serum in patients with malignant tumors. *Cancer Res*, 37, 4101-4103 (1977)

5171 Tauber C, Noff D, Noff M et al. Blood levels of active metabolites of vitamin D_3 in fracture repair in humans. A preliminary report. *Arch Orthop Trauma Surg*, 109, 265-267 (1990)

5172 Tauber MG, Moser B. Cytokines and chemokines in meningeal inflammation: biology and clinical implications. *Clin Infect Dis*, 28, 1-12 (1999)

5173 Taufield PA, Ales KL, Resnick LM et al. Hypocalciuria in preeclampsia. *N Engl J Med*, 316, 715-718 (1987)

5174 Taylor A. Detection and monitoring of disorders of essential trace elements. *Ann Clin Biochem*, 33, 486-510 (1996)

5175 Taylor HC Jr et al. Hormone factors in the toxemias of pregnancy, with special reference to quantitative abnormalities of prolan and estrogens in the blood and urine. *Am J Obstet Gynecol*, 37, 980 (1939)

5176 Taylor LM Jr, DeFrang RD, Harris EJ Jr et al. The association of elevated plasma homocyst(e)ine with progression of symptomatic peripheral arterial disease. *J Vasc Surg*, 13, 128-136 (1991)

5177 Taylor MA, Ragsdale MV, Ayers CA et al. Atrial natriuretic factor in essential hypertension. *Life Sci*, 44, 603-610 (1989)

5178 Taylor RN, Varma M, Teng NNH et al. Women with preeclampsia have higher plasma endothelin levels than women with normal pregnancies. *J Clin Endocrinol Metab*, 71, 1675-1677 (1990)

5179 Taylor SC, Shacks SJ, Mitchell RA, Banks A. Serum interleukin-6 levels in the steady state of sickle cell disease. *J Interferon Cytokine Res*, 15, 1061-1064 (1995)

5180 Taylor W. Urinary excretion of metabolites of steroid hormones by men with cancer of the stomach. *J Steroid Biochem*, 7, 929-934 (1976)

5181 Teal JF, Jeng JE, Chuang LY, et al. Elevated urinary transforming growth factor-β1 level as a tumour marker and predictor of poor survival in cirrhotic hepatocellular carcinoma. *Br J Cancer*, 76, 244-250 (1997)

5182 Teale JD, Marks V. The measurement of insulin-like growth factor -: clinical applications and significance. *Ann Clin Biochem*, 23, 413-424 (1986)

5183 Teare JP, Sherman D, Greenfield SM et al. Comparison of serum procollagen III peptide concentrations and PGA index for assessment of hepatic fibrosis. *Lancet*, 342, 895-898 (1993)

5184 Teculescu D et al. Ventilatory impairment and hypoxemia in chronic non-specific lung disease. *Bull Eur Physiopathol Respir*, 12, 735-745 (1976)

5185 Tedesco FJ et al. Serum amylase determinations and amylase to creatinine clearance ratios in patients with chronic renal insufficiency. *Gastroenterology*, 71, 594-8 (1976)

5186 Tefferi A, Ho TC, Ahmann GJ et al. Plasma interleukin-6 and C-reactive protein levels in reactive versus clonal thrombocytosis. *Am J Med*, 97, 374-378 (1994)

5187 Teger-Nilsson AC, Friberger P, Gyzander E. Determination of fast-acting plasmin inhibitor (alpha 2 - antiplasmin) in plasma from patients with tendency to thrombosis and increased fibrinolysis. *Haemostasis*, 7, 155-157 (1978)

5188 Telci A, Salmayenli N, Aydin AE et al. Serum lipids and apolipoprotein concentrations and plasma fibronectin concentrations in renal transplant patients. *Eur J Clin Chem Clin Biochem*, 30, 847-850 (1992)

5189 Teloh HA. Serum proteins in hepatic disease. *Ann Clin Lab Sci*, 8, 127-128 (1978)

5190 Tempfer C, Hefler L, Haeusler G, et al. Serum M3/M21 in ovarian cancer patients. *Br J Cancer*, 76, 1387-1389 (1997)

5191 Tempfer C, Hefler L, Heinzl H, et al. CYFRA 21-1 serum levels in women with adnexal masses and inflammatory diseases. *Br J Cancer*, 78, 1106-1112 (1998)

5192 Templeton AA et al. Arterial blood gases in pre-eclampsia. *Br J Obstet Gynaecol*, 84, 290-293 (1977)

5193 Tencer J, Thysell H, Westman K et al. Elevated plasma levels of acute phase proteins in mesangioproliferative glomerulonephritis, membranous nephropathy and IgA nephropathy. *Scand J Urol Nephrol*, 29, 5-9 (1995)

5194 Teni TR, Sheth AR, Kamath MR et al. Serum and urinary prostatic inhibin-like peptide in benign prostatic hyperplasia and carcinoma of prostate. *Cancer Lett*, 43, 9-14 (1988)

5195 Tepper R, Weizman A, Apter A et al. Elevated plasma immunoreactive β-endorphin in anorexia nervosa. *Clin Neuropharmacol*, 15, 387-391 (1992)

5196 Teree R M, Klein L. Hypophosphatasia: clinical and metabolic studies. *Pediatrics*, 72, 41 (1968)

5197 Territo, Tanaka. Hypophosphatemia in chronic alcoholism. *Arch Intern Med*, 134, 445-447 (1974)

5198 Terry PB et al. False-positive complement-fixation serology in histoplasmosis. a retrospective study. *J Am Med Ass*, 239, 2453-2456 (1978)

5199 Terzolo M., Piovesan A, Osella G et al. Serum levels of bone Gla protein (osteocalcin, BGP) and carboxyterminal propeptide of type I procollagen (PICP) in acromegaly: effects of long-term octreotide treatment. *Calcif Tissue Int.*, 52, 188-191 (1993)

5200 Testa M, Yeh M, Lee P, et al. Circulating levels of cytokines and their endogenous modulators in patients with mild to severe congestive heart failure due to coronary disease or hypertension. *J Am Coll Cardiol*, 28, 964-971 (1996)

5201 Testa R, Bonfigli AR, Piantanelli L, et al. Relationship between plasminogen activator inhibitor type-1 plasma levels and the lipoprotein(a) concentrations in non-insulin-dependent diabetes mellitus. *Diabetes Res Clin Pract*, 33, 111-118 (1996)

5202 Tetta C, Bussolino F, Modena V et al. Release of platelet-activating factor in systemic lupus erythematosus. *Int Arch Allergy Immunol*, 91, 244-250 (1990)

5203 Thaler MS, Klausner RD, Cohen HJ. *Medical Immunology*, Philadelphia PA, JB Lippincott (1977)

5204 Thatte L, Oster JR, Singer I, et al. Review of the literature: severe hyperphosphatemia. *Am J Med Sci*, 310, 167-174 (1995)

5205 Thayer WR et al. The subpopulations of circulating white blood cells in inflammatory bowel disease. *Gastroenterology*, 71, 379-384 (1976)

5206 Theodoraki TG, Tsoμkatos DC, Karabina S-A, et al. LDL subfractions in patients with myovardial infarction: effect of smoking and β-blocker treatment. *Ann Clin Biochem*, 37, 313-318 (2000)

5207 Thestrup-Pedersen K, Romer FK, Jensen JH et al. Serum angiotensin-converting enzyme in sarcoidosis and psoriasis. *Arch Dermatol Res*, 277, 16-18 (1985)

5208 Thiounn N Pages F, Flam T, et al. IL-6 is a survival prognostic factor in renal cell carcinoma. *Immunol Lett*, 58, 121-124 (1997)

5209 Thomas AG, Holly JMP, Taylor F et al. Insulin like growth factor-I, insulin like growth factor binding protein-1, and insulin in childhood Crohn's disease. *Gut*, 34, 944-947 (1993)

5210 Thomas ED et al. Homozygous hemoglobin C disease. *Am J Med*, 18, 832 (1955)

5211 Thomas MJ, Adebajo A, Chapel HM, et al. The use of rheumatoid factors in clinical practice. *Postgrad Med J*, 71, 674-677 (1995)

5212 Thomas MK, Lloyd-Jones DM, Thadhani RI, et al. Hypovitaminosis D in medical inpatients. *N Engl J Med*, 338, 777-783 (1998)

5213 Thomas PH, Karachalios T, Pearse M et al. Biochemical and endocrine parameters in males who have sustained a fracture of the hip. *Proc ACB Natl Meet*, 71-72 (1994)

5214 Thommesen P et al. Histiocytosis X. I. erythrocyte sedimentation rate correlated to prognosis and extent of disease. *Acta Radiol*, 16, 538-544 (1977)

5215 Thompson RHS, Johnson RE. Blood pyruvate in vitamin B_1 deficiency. *Biochem J*, 29, 694 (1935)

5216 Thompson SP, White DA, Hosking DJ et al. Changes in osteocalcin after femoral neck fracture. *Ann Clin Biochem*, 26, 487-491 (1989)

5217 Thomsen JK, Storm TL, Thamsborg G et al. Atrial natriuretic peptide concentrations in pre-eclampsia. *Br Med J*, 294, 1508-1510 (1987)

5218 Thomson ABR et al. Iron deficiency in inflammatory bowel disease. *Am J Dig Dis*, 23, 705-709 (1978)

5219 Thomson C et al. Changes in blood coagulation and fibrinolysis in the nephrotic syndrome. *Q J Med*, 43, 399 (1974)

5220 Thomson JM. *Blood Coagulation and Haemostasis,* 2nd edition, New York NY, Churchill-Livingstone (1980)

5221 Thomson RD, Clejan S. Digital rectal examination-associated alterations in serum prostate-specific antigen. *Am J Clin Pathol*, 97, 528-534 (1992)

5222 Thomson SP, Gibbons RJ, Smars PA et al. Incremental value of the leukocyte differential and the rapid creatine kinase-MB isoenzyme for the early diagnosis of myocardial infarction. *Ann Intern Med*, 122, 335-341 (1995)

5223 Thonar EJ, Manicourt DH, Triki R. Levels of circulating tumor necrosis factor alpha and interleukin-6 in patients with rheumatoid arthritis. Relationship to serum levels of hyaluronan and antigenic keratan sulfate. *Arth Rheum*, 36, 490-499 (1993)

5224 Thoren M, Hilding A, Baxter RC, et al. Serum insulin-like growth factor-I (IGF-I), IGF-binding protein-1 and -3, and the acid labile subunit as serum markers of body composition during growth hormone (GH) therapy in adults with GH deficiency. *J Clin Endocrinol Metab*, 82, 223-228 (1007)

5225 Thorling EB, Thorling K. The clinical usefulness of serum copper determinations in Hodgkin's disease. a retrospective study of 241 patients from 1963-1973. *Cancer*, 38, 225-231 (1976)

5226 Thornton CA et al. Factor VIII-related antigen and factor VIII coagulant activity in normal and pre-eclamptic pregnancy. *Br J Obstet Gynaecol*, 84, 919-923 (1977)

5227 Thougaard AV, Hogdall CK, Kjaer SK, et al. Determination of serum tetranectin: technical and clinical evaluation of three sandwich immunoassays. *Clin Chim Acta*, 276, 19-34 (1998)

5228 Tierney LM., McPhee SJ., Papadakis MA. *Current Medical Diagnosis and Treatment.* New York NY, Appleton and Lange (1994)

5229 Tietz NW. *Clinical Guide to Laboratory Tests*, Philadelphia PA, WB Saunders (1983)

5230 Tietz NW (ed). *Fundamentals of Clinical Chemistry,* 2nd edition, Philadelphia PA, WB Saunders (1976)

5231 Tietz NW, Shuey DF. Lipase in serum -- the elusive enzyme: an overview. *Clin Chem*, 39, 746-758 (1993)

5232 Tikkanen I, Fyhrquist F, Metsarinne K et al. Plasma atrial natriuretic peptide in cardiac disease and during infusion in healthy volunteers. *Lancet*, 2, 100-101 (1985)

5233 Tilg H, Ceska M, Vogel W et al. Interleukin-8 serum concentrations after liver transplantation. *Transplantation*, 53, 800-803 (1992)

5234 Tint GS, Irons M, Elias ER et al. Defective cholesterol biosynthesis associated with the Smith-Lemli-Opitz syndrome. *N Engl J Med*, 330, 107-113 (1994)

5235 Tischendorf FW, Brattig NW, Burchard GD, et al. Eosinophils, eosinophil cationic protein and eosinophil-derived neurotoxin in serum and urine of patients with onchocerciasis coinfected with intestinal nematodes and in urinary schistosomiasis. *Acta Tropica*, 72, 157-175 (1999)

5236 Tischendorf FW et al. Heavy lysozymuria after X-irradiation of the spleen in human chronic myelocytic leukemia. *Nature*, 235, 274 (1972)

5237 Tisdale WA et al. The significance of the direct-reacting fraction of serum bilirubin in hemolytic jaundice. *Am J Med*, 26, 214 (1959)

5238 Tishkov I et al. Diagnostic value of ceruloplasmin, haptoglobin and sialic acid in chronic pyelonephritis. *Int Urol Nephrol*, 8, 155-159 (1976)

5239 Tobiasson P, Boeryd B. Serum cholic and chenodeoxycholic acid conjugates and standard liver function tests in various morphological stages of alcoholic liver disease. *Scand J Gastroenterol*, 15, 657-63 (1980)

5240 Tobiume H, Kanzaki S, Hida S, et al. Serum bone alkaline phosphatase isoenzyme levels in normal children and children with growth hormone (GH) deficiency: a potential marker for bone formation and response to GH therapy. *J Clin Endocrinol Metab*, 82, 2056-2061 (1997)

5241 Todd D. Observations on the aminoaciduria in megaloblastic anemia. *J Clin Pathol*, 12, 238 (1959)

5242 Togashi K, Ando K, Hasegawa N et al. Concentrations of brain natriuretic peptide in treated congestive cardiac failure. *Clin Chem*, 37, 765 (1991)

5243 Tokoo M, Oguchi H, Kawa S et al. Eosinophilia associated with chronic pancreatitis: an analysis of 122 patients with definite chronic pancreatitis. *Am J Gastroenterol*, 87, 455-460 (1992)

5244 Tomas C, Penttinen J, Ristell J et al. Serum concentrations of CA 125 and aminoterminal propeptide of type III procollagen (PIIINP) in patients with endometrial carcinoma. *Cancer*, 66, 2399-2406 (1990)

5245 Tomino Y, Funabiki K, Ohmuro H et al. Urinary levels of interleukin-6 and disease activity in patients with IgA nephropathy. *Am J Nephrol*, 11, 459-464 (1991)

5246 Tomoda H. Plasma endothelin-1 in acute myocardial infarction with heart failure. *Am Heart J*, 125, 667-672 (1993)

5247 Tomokuni K et al. Erythrocyte protoporphyrin test for occupational lead exposure. *Arch Environ Health*, 30, 588-90 (1975)

5248 Tomsen TR. HELLP syndrome (hemolysis, elevated liver enzymes, and low platelets) presenting as generalized malaise. *Am J Obstet Gynecol*, 172, 1876-1880 (1995)

5249 Tomson T, Lindbom U, Nilsson BY et al. Serum prolactin during status epilepticus. *J Neurol Neurosurg Psychiatry*, 52, 1435-1437 (1989)

5250 Tonnesen H, Andersen JR, Pedersen AE et al. Lymphopenia in heavy drinkers - reversibility and relation to the duration of drinking episodes. *Ann Med*, 22, 229-231 (1990)

5251 Tonstad S, Aksnes L. Fat-soluble vitamin levels in familial hypercholesterolemia. *J Perdiatr*, 130, 274-280 (1997)

5252 Top FH, Wehrele PF (eds). *Communicable and Infectious Diseases.* 7th edition, St Louis MO, CV Mosby (1972)

5253 Topar G, Staudacher C, Geisen F, et al. Urticaria pigmentosa: a clinical, hematopathologic, and serological study of 30 adults. *Am J Clin Pathol*, 109, 279-285 (1998)

5254 Torlontano M, Chiodini I, Pileri M, et al. Altered bone mass and turnover in female patients with adrenal incidentaloma: the effect of subclinical hypercortisolism. *J Clin Endocrinol Metab*, 84, 2381-2385 (1999)

5255 Torr-Brown SR, Sobel BE. Plasminogen activator inhibitor is elevated in plasma and diminished in platelets with diabetes mellitus. *Thromb Res*, 75, 475-477 (1994)

5256 Torre D, Ferrario G, Matteelli A, et al. Levels of circulating nitrate/nitrite and γ-interferon not increased in uncomplicated maleria. *Infection*, 26, 301-303 (1998)

5257 Torre D, Ferrario G, Speranza F, et al. Increased levels of nitrite in the sera of children infected with human immunodeficiency virus type I. *Clin Infect Dis*, 22, 650-653 (1996)

5258 Torre D, Ferrario G, Speranza F, et al. Serum concentration of nitrite in patients with HIV-1 infection. *J Clin Pathol*, 49, 674-576 (1996)

5259 Torre D, Zeroli C, Giola M et al. Serum levels of interleukin-1α, interleukin-1β, interleukin-6, and tumor necrosis factor in patients with acute viral hepatitis. *Clin Infect Dis*, 18, 194-198 (1994)

5260 Torres M, Pacheco C, Valverde A et al. CA 549 and SP2 in postoperative breast cancer patients. Comparison with CA 15.3, CEA and TPA. *Int J Biol Mark*, 10, 94-99 (1995)

5261 Torres R, de la Piedra C, Rapado A. Osteocalcin and bone remodeling in Paget's disease of bone, primary hyperparathyroidism, hypercalcaemia of malignancy and involutional osteoporosis. *Scand J Clin Lab Invest*, 49, 279-285 (1989)

5262 Toschi V, Fiorini GF, Motta A et al. Clinical significance of endothelial damage markers in essential mixed cryoglobulinemia. *Acta Haematol*, 86, 90-94 (1991)

5263 Toss H, Lindahl B, Siegbahn A, et al. Prognostic influence of increased fibrinogen and C-reactive protein levels in unstable coronary disease. *Circulation*, 96, 4204-4210 (1997)

5264 Toth J et al. Eosinophil predominance in Hodgkin's disease. *Z Krebsforsch*, 89, 107-111 (1977)

5265 Totsune K, Takahashi K, Satoh F, et al. Urinary immunoreactive brain natriuretic peptide in patients with renal disease. *Reg Peptides*, 63, 141-147 (1996)

5266 Toulon P, Gris JC, Candia N et al. Increased plasmin generation and activity in HIV-infected patients: in vivo rather than in vitro activation of the fibrinolytic system. *Fibrinolysis*, 8, 128-131 (1994)

5267 Tountas Y, Sparos L, Theodropoulos C et al. α_1-Antitrypsin and cancer of the pancreas. *Digestion*, 31, 37-40 (1985)

5268 Tour Tellotte W E, Haerer A F. Lipids in cerebrospinal fluid. *Arch Neurol*, 20, 605 (1969)

5269 Toussirot E, Nguyen NU, Dumoulin G, et al. Insulin-like growth factor-I and insullin-like growth factor binding protein-3 serum levels in ankylosing spondylitis. *Br J Rheumatol*, 37, 1172-1178 (1998)

5270 Toussirot E, Ricard-Blum S, Dumoulin G, et al. Relationship between urinary pyridinium cross-links, disease activity and disease subsets of ankylosing spondylitis. *Rheumatology*, 38, 21-27 (1999)

5271 Tovey JA, Banning A, Buchalter M et al. Troponin T release following CABG surgery. *Proc ACB Natl Meet*, 114-115 (1995)

5272 Tovey JA, Oleesky DA. Troponin T levels in patients receiving haemodialysis and continuous ambulant peritoneal dialysis treatment. *Proc ACB Natl Meet*, 116 (1995)

5273 Townend J, Doran J, Jones S et al. Effect of angiotensin converting enzyme inhibition on plasma endothelin in congestive heart failure. *Int J Cardiol*, 43, 299-304 (1994)

5274 Townes AS. Complement levels in disease. *Johns Hcpkins Med J*, 120, 337 (1967)

5275 Toyozaki T, Saito T, Takano T, et al. Increased serum levels of circulating intercellular adhesion molecule-1 in patients with myocarditis. *Cardiology*, 87, 189-193 (1996)

5276 Tredger JM, Sherwood RA. The liver: new functional, prognostic and diagnostic tests. *Ann Clin Biochem*, 34, 121-141 (1997)

5277 Trenkwalder P, James GD, Laragh JH, Sealey JE. Plasma renin activity and plasma prorenin are not suppressed in hypertensives surviving to old age. *Am J Hypertens*, 9, 621-627 (1996)

5278 Triantafillidis JK, Kottaras G, Sgourous S, et al. A-β-lipoproteinemia: Clinical and laboratory features, theraputic manipulations, and follow-up studies of three members of a Greek family. *J Clin Gastroenterol*, 26, 207-211 (1998)

5279 Trichopoulos D, Tzonou A, Kalapothaki V et al. α_1-Antitrypsin and survival in pancreatic cancer. *Int J Cancer*, 45, 685-686 (1990)

5280 Trimarchi F, Benvenga S, Fenzi G et al. Immunoglobulin binding of thyroid hormones in a case of Waldenström's macroglobulinemia. *J Clin Endocrinol Metab*, 54, 1045-1050 (1982)

5281 Trimble EL, Saigo PE, Freeberg GW et al. Peritoneal sarcoidosis and elevated CA 125. *Obstet Gynecol*, 78, 976-977 (1991)

5282 Trimble M, Bell DA, Brien W et al. The antiphospholipid syndrome: prevalence among patients with stroke and transient ischemic attacks. *Am J Med*, 88, 593-597 (1990)

5283 Trivedi P, Cheeseman P, Mowat AP. Serum hyaluronic acid in healthy infants and children and its value as a marker of progressive hepatobiliary disease starting in infancy. *Clin Chim Acta*, 215, 29-39 (1993)

5284 Troffa C, Tonolo G, Manunta P et al. Prorenin is present in human red blood cells. *Can J Physiol Pharmacol*, 69, 1394-1397 (1991)

5285 Trojan J, Raedle J, Zeuzem S. Serum tests for diagnosis and follow-up of hepatocellular carcinoma after treatment. *Digestion*, 59 Suppl 2, 72-74 (1998)

5286 Trongone L et al. CEA assay in the follow-up of patients with extra- gastrointestinal malignancies. *Bull Cancer*, 63, 495-504 (1976)

5287 Trontzas P, Kamper EF, Potamianou A, et al. Comparaative study of serum and synovial fluid interleukin-11 levels in patients with various arthritides. *Clin Biochem*, 31, 673-679 (1998)

5288 Trotter JL, Collins KG, van der Veen RC. Serum cytokine levels in chronic progressive multiple sclerosis: interleukin-2 levels parallel tumor necrosis factor-α levels. *J Neuroimmunol*, 33, 29-36 (1991)

5289 Trotter JL, Van der Veen RC, Clifford DB. Serial studies of serum interleukin-2 in chronic progressive multiple sclerosis patients: occurrence of burst and effects of cyclosporine. *J Neuroimmunol*, 28, 9-14 (1990)

5290 Troughton PR, Platt R, Bird H, et al. Synovial fluid interleukin-9 and neutrophil function in rheumatoid arthritis and seronegative polyarthritis. *Br J Rheumatol*, 35, 1244-1251 (1996)

5291 Trouillas P et al. Multiple sclerosis with reduced and with normal levels of complement in the blood. clinical and genetic correlation. *Rev Neurol (Paris)*, 132, 684-704 (1976)

5292 Trull AK, Hughes V, Watanabe S. Serum hyaluronic acid as a marker of hepatic endothelial cell dysfunction associated with liver allograft rejection. *Proc ACB Natl Meet*, 151 (1995)

5293 Trulson A, Nilsson A, Venge P. The eosinophil granule proteins in serum, but not the oxidative metabolism of the blood eosinophils, are increased in cancer. *Br J Haematol*, 98, 312-314 (1997)

5294 Tryfiates GP. Adenosine-N6-diethylthioether-N1-pyridoxime 5'-phosphate. A novel marker for human cancer detection. *Anticancer Res*, 16, 2301-2304 (1996)

5295 Tsai C-Y, Wu T-H, Tsai S-T et al. Cerebrospinal fluid interleukin-6, prostaglandin E_2 and autoantibodies in patients with neuropsychiatric systemic lupus erythematosus and central nervous system infections. *Scand J Rheumatol*, 23, 57-63 (1994)

5296 Tsai LY, Lee KT, Tsai SM et al. Changes of lipid peroxide levels in blood and liver tissue of patients with obstructive jaundice. *Clin Chim Acta*, 215, 41-50 (1993)

5297 Tsai Y-T, Lin H-C, Yang MC-M, et al. Plasma endothelin levels in patients with cirrhosis and their relationships to the severity of cirrhosis and renal function. *J Hepatol*, 23, 681-688 (1995)

5298 Tsakiris DA, Kappos L, Reber G et al. Lack of association between antiphospholipid antibodies and migraine. *Thromb Haemostas*, 69, 415-417 (1993)

5299 Tsakiris DA, Marbet GA, Burkart F et al. Anticardiolipin antibodies and coronary heart disease. *Eur Heart J*, 13, 1645-1648 (1992)

5300 Tsau Y-K, Chen C-H. Urinary epidermal growth factor excretion in children with chronic renal failure. *Am J Nephrol*, 19, 400-404 (1999)

5301 Tsau Y-K, Sheu J-N, Chen C-H, et al. Decreased urinary epidermal growth factor in children with acute renal failure: epidermal growth factor/creatinine ratio not a reliable parameter for urinary epidermal growth factor excretion. *Pediatr Res*, 39, 20-24 (1996)

5302 Tsavaris N, Gogou L, Tzaninis D, et al. Comparison of tumor markers CEA, α-fetoprotein, CA 125, CA 19.9, CA 72.4 and CA 50 in patients with advanced gastric cancer. *Diagn Oncol*, 95, 165-169 (1994)

5303 Tsavaris N, Tsigalacis D, Kosmas C, et al. Preliminary evaluation of the potential prognostic value of serum levels of immunoglobulins (IgA, IgM, IgG, IgE) in patients with gastric cancer. *Int J Biol Mark*, 13, 87-91 (1998)

5304 Tso SC, Hua A. Erythrocytes in hepatocellular carcinoma: a compensatory phenomenon. *Br J Haematol*, 28, 497 (1974)

5305 Tstouras PD, Zhong Y-G, Spungen AM et al. Serum testosterone and growth hormone/insulin-like growth factor-I in adults with spinal cord injury. *Horm Metab Res*, 27, 287-292 (1995)

5306 Tsuchiya N, Shiota M, Yamaguchi A, Ito K. Elevated serum levels of soluble HLA class 1 antigens in patients with systemic lupus erythematosus. *Arth Rheum*, 39, 792-795 (1996)

5307 Tsuda K, Namba H, Nomura T et al. Automated measurement of urinary iodine with use of ultraviolet irradiation. *Clin Chem*, 41, 581-585 (1995)

5308 Tsuda Y, Satoh K, Kitadai M, Takahashi T. Effects of pravastatin sodium and simvastatin on plasma fibrinogen level and blood rheology in type II hyperlipproteinemia. *Atherosclerosis*, 122, 225-233 (1996)

5309 Tsukada N, Miyagi K, Matsuda M et al. Tumor necrosis factor and interleukin-1 in the CSF and sera of patients with multiple sclerosis. *J Neurol Sci*, 104, 230-234 (1991)

5310 Tsunoda K, Abe K, Yoshinaga K et al. Maternal and umbilical venous levels of endothelin in women with pre-eclampsia. *J Hum Hypertens*, 6, 61-64 (1992)

5311 Tsuruta T, Ogawa A, Ishii K, Ikado S. CA 19-9: a possible serum marker for embryonal carcinoma. *Urol Int*, 58, 20-24 (1997)

5312 Tsutamoto T, Hisanaga T, Fukai D, et al. Prognostic value of plasma soluble intercellular adhesion molecule-1 and endothelin-1 concentration in patients with chronic congestive heart failure. *Am J Cardiol*, 76, 803-808 (1995)

5313 Tsutsui K, Hasegawa M, Takata M, Takehara K. Increased plasma granulocyte elastase levels in Behcet's disease. *J Rheumatol*, 25, 326-328 (1998)

5314 Tsutsumi A, Matsuura E, Ichikawa K, et al. Antibodies to β_2-glycoprotein I and clinical manifestations in patients with systemic erythematosus. *Arth Rheum*, 39, 1466-1474 (1996)

5315 Tsutsumi M, Takase S, Urashima S, et al. Serum markers for hepatic fibrosis in alcoholic liver disease: which is the best marker, type III procollagen, type IV collagen, laminin, tissue inhibitor of metallopoteinase, or prolyl hydroxylase. *Alcohol Clin Exp Res*, 20, 1512-1517 (1996)

5316 Tu D-G, Wang S-T, Chang T-T, et al. The value of serum tissue polypeptide specific antigen in the diagnosis of hepatocellular carcinoma. *Cancer*, 85, 1039-1043 (1999)

5317 Tuchman et al. Studies of the nature of the increased serum acid phosphatase in Gaucher's disease. *Am J Med*, 27, 959-962 (1959)

5318 Tudhope GR, Wilson GM. Anemia in hypothyroidism incidence, pathogenesis and response to treatment. *Q J Med*, 29, 513 (1960)

5319 Tuinenberg AE, Van Veldhuisen DJ, Boomsma F, et al. Comparison of plasma neurohormones in congestive heart failure patients with atrial fibrillation versus patients with sinus rhythm. *Am J Cardiol*, 81, 1207-1210 (1998)

5320 Tulchinsky M, Zeller JA, Reba RC. Urinary fibrinopeptide A in evaluation of patients with suspected acute pulmonary embolism: a prospective pilot study. *Chest*, 100, 394-398 (1991)

5321 Tullgren O, Grimfors G, Holm G et al. Lymphocyte abnormalities predicting a poor prognosis in Hodgkin's disease: a long-term follow-up. *Cancer*, 68, 768-775 (1991)

5322 Tullus K, Escobar-Billing R, Fituri O, et al. Interleukin-1α and interleukin-1 receptor antagonist in the urine of children with acute pyelonephritis and relation to renal scarring. *Acta Paediatr*, 85, 158-162 (1996)

5323 Tumaru H, Reiber H, Nau R, et al. β-trace protein concentration in cerebrospinal fluid is decreased in patients with bacterial meningitis. *Neurosci Lett*, 242, 5-8 (1998)

5324 Tuncer AM, Hisönmez G, Gumruk F, et al. Serum TNF-α, γ-INF and GM-CSF levels in neutropenic children with acute leukemia treated with short-course, high dose methylprednisolone. *Leuk Res*, 20, 265-269 (1996)

5325 Tunny TJ, Gordon RD, Klemm SA et al. Inappropriately elevated levels of atrial natriuretic peptide may contribute to the pathophysiology of orthostatic hypotension. *Clin Exp Pharmacol Physiol*, 19, 283-286 (1992)

5326 Turanen EM et al. Carcinoembryonic antigen in gynecologic tumors. *Cancer*, 42, 581-590 (1978)

5327 Turk JL, Bryceson ADM. Immunological phenomena in leprosy and related diseases. *Adv Immunol*, 13, 209 (1971)

5328 Turkington RW et al. Insulin secretion in the diagnosis of adult-onset diabetes mellitus. *J Am Med Ass*, 240, 833-836 (1978)

5329 Turnbull A et al. Iron metabolism in porphyria cutanea tarda and in erythropoietic protoporphyria. *Q J Med*, 42, 341 (1973)

5330 Turner A et al. Hairy cell leukemia: a review. *Medicine*, 57, 477-500 (1978)

5331 Turner G, Coates P, Porter S et al. Urinary growth hormone measurements as a marker of renal tubular function in diabetes mellitus. *Clin Chim Acta*, 220, 19-30 (1993)

5332 Turner G, Skinner A, Woodhead JS. Urinary growth hormone measurements in children with renal insufficiency. *Ann Clin Biochem*, 30, 540-544 (1993)

5333 Turney JH, Cooper EH, Davison AM et al. Hyaluronic acid in end-stage renal failure treated by haemodialysis. *Clin Chem*, 37, 944 (1991)

5334 Tutor JC, Alvarez-Prechous A, Bernabeu F et al. Urinary D-glucaric acid and serum hepatic enzyme levels in chronic alcoholics. *Clin Biochem*, 21, 193-198 (1988)

5335 Tutuarima JA, Hische Eah, Van Trotsenburg L et al. Thromboplastic activity of cerebrospinal fluid in neurological disease. *Clin Chem*, 31/1, 99-100 (1985)

5336 Twomey JJ et al. Rheumatoid factor and tumor-host interaction. *Proc Natl Acad Sci USA*, 73, 2106-2108 (1976)

5337 Twomey JJ et al. Studies on the inheritance and nature of hemophilia B. *Am J Med*, 46, 372 (1969)

5338 Ucar G, Yildirim Z, Ataol E, et al. Serum angiotensin converting enzyme activity in pulmonary diseases: correlation with lung function parameters. *Life Sci*, 61, 1075-1082 (1997)

5339 Uchida Y, Watanabe M. Plasma endothelin-1 concentrations are elevated in acute hepatitis and liver cirrhosis but not in chronic hepatitis. *Gastroenterol Jpn*, 28, 666-672 (1993)

5340 Uchihara M, Izumi N, Sato C et al. Clinical significance of elevated plasma endothelin concentration in patients with cirrhosis. *Hepatology*, 16, 95-99 (1992)

5341 Uchihashi M, Hirata Y, Nakajima H et al. Urinary excretion of human epidermal growth factor (hEGF) in patients with malignant tumors. *Horm Metab Res*, 15, 261-262 (1983)

5342 Ueda S, Ikeda U, Iamamoto K, et al. C-reactive protein as a predictor of cardiac rupture after acute myocardial infarction. *Am Heart J*, 131, 857-860 (1996)

5343 Ueda S, Nishio K, Minamino N, et al. Increased plasma levels of adrenomedullin in patients with systemic inflammatory response syndrome. *Am J Respir Crit Care Med*, 160, 132-136 (1999)

5344 Ueda Y, Nagasawa K, Tsukamoto H, et al. Urinary C4 excretion in systemic lupus erythematosus. *Clin Chim Acta*, 243, 11-23 (1995)

5345 Uehara H. Reevaluation of the usefulness of serum free hydroxyproline as a parameter for assessing renal osteodystrophy. *Nippon Jinzo Gakkai Shi*, 35, 49-58 (1993)

5346 Ueland PM, Refsum H, Stabler SP et al. Total homocysteine in plasma or serum: methods and clinical applications. *Clin Chem*, 39, 1764-1779 (1983)

5347 Uemura M, Buchholz U, Kojima H et al. Cysteinyl leukotrienes in the urine of patients with liver disease. *Hepatology*, 20, 804-812 (1994)

5348 Uemura M, Masahiko Y, Yoshida S et al. An enzyme immunoassay for galactosyltransferase isoenzyme II, and its clinical application to cancer diagnosis. *Clin Chem*, 36, 598-601 (1990)

5349 Uemura M, Tsujii T, Kikuchi E, et al. Increased plasma levels of substance P and disturbed water excretion in patients with liver cirrhosis. *Scand J Gastroenterol*, 33, 860-866 (1998)

5350 Ueshiba H, Shimojo M, Miyachi Y. 18-hydroxycortisol and 18-oxocortisol in Cushing's syndrome. *Scand J Clin Lab Invest*, 57, 395-400 (1997)

5351 Ueyama M, Maruyama I, Osame M, Sawada Y. Marked increase in plasma interleukin-6 in burn patients. *J Lab Clin Med*, 120, 693-698 (1992)

5352 Uguccioni M, Meliconi R, Nesci S et al. Elevated interleukin-8 serum concentrations in β-thalassemia and graft-versus-host disease. *Blood*, 81, 2252-2256 (1993)

5353 Uguccioni M, Pulsatelli L, Grigolo B et al. Endothelin-1 in idiopathic pulmonary fibrosis. *J Clin Pathol*, 48, 330-334 (1995)

5354 Ukita C, Nishikawa M, Shouzu A et al. Urinary excretion of glycated protein determined with a specific radioimmunoassay. *Clin Chem*, 37, 504-507 (1993)

5355 Ultmann JE. Clinical features and diagnosis of Hodgkin's disease. *Cancer*, 9, 297 (1966)

5356 Ultmann JE et al. The clinical implications of hypogammaglobulinemia in patients with chronic lymphocytic leukemia and lymphocytic lymphosarcoma. *Ann Intern Med*, 51, 501 (1959)

5357 Undar L, Karadogan I, Ozturk F. Plasma protein Z levels inversely correlate with plasma interleukin-6 levels in patients with acute leukemia and non-Hodgkin's lymphoma. *Thromb Res*, 94, 131-134 (1999)

5358 Underman HE et al. Bacterial meningitis. *DM*, 24, 19-27 (1978)

5359 Underwood JC et al. Persistent diarrhea and hypoalbuminemia associated with cytomegalovirus enteritis. *Br Med J*, 1, 1029-1030 (1976)

5360 Ungerer JPJ, Oosthuizen HM, Bissbort SH et al. Serum adenosine deaminase: isoenzymes and diagnostic application. *Clin Chem*, 38, 1322-1326 (1992)

5361 Unkila-Kallio L, Kallio MJT, Eskola J et al. Serum C-reactive protein, erythrocyte sedimentation rate, and white blood cell count in acute hematogenous osteomyelitis of children. *Pediatrics*, 93, 59-62 (1994)

5362 Unkila-Kallio L, Kallio MJT, Peltola H et al. Acute haematogenous osteomyelitis in children in Finland. *Ann Med*, 25, 545-549 (1993)

5363 Unkila-Kallio L, Kallio MJT, Peltola H et al. The usefulness of C-reactive protein levels in the identification of concurrent septic arthritis in children who have acute hematogenous osteomyelitis. *J Bone Joint Surg*, 76A, 848-853 (1994)

5364 Unknown or lost reference

5365 Uno H, Shima T, Maeda K, et al. Hypercalcemia associated with parathyroid hormone-related protein produced by B-cell type primary malignant lymphoma of the kidney. *Ann Hematol*, 76, 221-224 (1998)

5366 Uohta K, Seno A, Shintani N et al. Increased levels of urinary interleukin-6 in Kawasaki disease. *Eur J Pediatr*, 152, 647-649 (1993)

5367 Uozumi K, Hanada S, Arima T. Elevated levels of soluble factors in the cerebrospinal fluid in patients with adult T-cell leukemia complicated with meningeal infiltration. *Br J Haematol*, 87, 641-64 (1994)

5368 Uozumi K, Hanada S, Ishitsuka K et al. Elevated soluble CD4 levels in the cerebrospinal fluid in patients with adult T-cell leukemia. *Am J Hematol*, 46, 95-100 (1994)

5369 Uozumi K, Uematsu T, Otsuka M, et al. Serum dehydroepiandrosterone and DHEA-sulfate in patients with adult T-cell leukemia and human T-lymphotropic virus type I carriers. *Am J Hematol*, 53, 165-168 (1996)

5370 Uppenkamp M, Makarova E, Petrasch S, Brittinger G. Thrombopoietin serum concentration in patients with reactive and myeloproliferative thrombocytosis. *Ann Hematol*, 77, 217-223 (1998)

5371 Ural AU, Valcin A, Beyan C et al. Plasma endothelin-1 concentrations in patients with Behcet's disease. *Scand J Rheumatol*, 23, 322-325 (1994)

5372 Urbaniak WJ et al. Circulating lymphocyte subpopulations in Hashimoto's thyroiditis. *Clin Exp Immunol*, 15, 345 (1973)

5373 Ureles AL. Diagnosis and treatment of malignant carcinoid syndrome. *J Am Med Ass*, 229, 10 (1974)

5374 Usher DJ et al. Serum lactate dehydrogenase isoenzyme activities in patients with asthma. *Thorax*, 29, 685-689 (1974)

5375 Usui A, Kato K, Sasa H et al. S-100ao protein in serum during acute myocardial infarction. *Clin Chem*, 36, 639-641 (1993)

5376 Uza G, Pavel O, Kovacs A et al. Serum concentration of Na, K, Ca, Mg, P, Zn and Cu in patients with essential arterial hypertension. *Clin Exp Hypertens Theory Pract*, 6, 1415-1429 (1984)

5377 Vaananen HK, Syrjaia H, Rahkila P et al. Serum carbonic anhydrase III and myoglobin concentrations in acute myocardial infarction. *Clin Chem*, 39, 635-638 (1993)

5378 Vacca JB et al. Pancreatic exocrine function in diabetes mellitus and cirrhosis of the liver. *J Lab Clin Med*, 52, 176 (1958)

5379 Vadasdi E, Jacobs E, Linekin P et al. The effect of hematocrit and uremia on whole blood glucose analysis. *Clin Chem*, 36, 1113 (1990)

5380 Vainionpaa L, Risteli L, Lanning M et al. Aminoterminal propeptide of type III procollagen in cerebrospinal fluid. Variation with age and in childhood leukemia. *Clin Chim Acta*, 203, 47-56 (1991)

5381 Vaisman N, Wolfhard D, Sklan D. Vitamin A metabolism in plasma of normal and anorectic women. *Eur J Clin Nutr*, 6, 873-878 (1992)

5382 Vakil BJ et al. Serum creatine phosphokinase in tetanus. *J Ass Physicians India*, 24, 417-421 (1976)

5383 Valcavi R, Diequez C, Zini M, et al. Influence of hyperthyroidism on growth hormone secretion. *Clin Endocrinol*, 38, 515-522 (1993)

5384 Valentine RJ, Grayburn PA, Vega GL et al. Lp(a) lipoprotein is an independent, discriminating risk factor for premature peripheral atherosclerosis among white men. *Arch Intern Med*, 154, 801-806 (1994)

5385 Valero M-A, Leon M, Ruiz Valdepenas MP et al. Bone density and turnover in Addison's disease: effect of glucocorticoid treatment. *Bone Miner*, 26, 9-17 (1994)

5386 Valsecchi R, Imberti G, Martino D et al. Alopecia areata and interleukin-2 receptor. *Dermatology*, 184, 126-128 (1992)

5387 van Beek EJR, Schenk BE, Michel BC, et al. The role of plasma D-dimer concentration in the exclusion of pulmonary embolism. *Br J Haematol*, 92, 725-732 (1996)

5388 Van Bodegraven AA, Tuynman HARE, Schoorl M et al. Fibrinolytic split products, fibrinolysis, and factor XIII activity in inflammatory bowel disease. *Scand J Gastroenterol*, 30, 580-585 (1995)

5389 van Dalen A. BR-MA, OM-MA, GI-MA and CEA: clinical evaluation using the IMMULITE analyzer. *Tumor Biol*, 20, 117-129 (1999)

5390 van Dalen A. TPS in breast cancer -- a comparative study with carcinoembryonic antigen and CA 15-3. *Tumor Biol*, 13, 10-17 (1992)

5391 van de Kar NCAJ, Sauerwein RW, Demacker PNM, et al. Plasma cytokine levels in hemolytic uremic syndrome. *Nephron*, 71, 309-313 (1995)

5392 Van Demmelen CKV, Klassen CHL. Cyanocobalamin-dependent depression on the serum alkaline phosphatase level in patients with pernicious anemia. *N Engl J Med*, 271, 541 (1964)

5393 Van den Berg MP, Crijns HJGM, Van Veldhuisen DJ, et al. Atrial natriuretic peptide in patients with heart failure and chronic atrial fibrillation: role of duration of atrial fibrillation. *Am Heart J*, 135, 242-244 (1998)

5394 Van Den Bergh M et al. Elevation in erythrocyte-1-glutamate in chronic hypoxia and hypercapnia. *Br J Cancer*, 12, 177-178 (1976)

5395 van der Dijs FPL, van der Klis FRM, Muskiet FD, Muskiet FAJ. Serum calcium and vitamin D status of patients with sickle cell disease in Curacao. *Ann Clin Biochem*, 34, 170-172 (1997)

5396 van der Gaast A, Kok TC, Kho BG, et al. Disease monitoring by the tumour markers CYFRA 21.1 and TPA in patients with non-small cell lung cancer. *Eur J Cancer*, 31A, 1790-1793 (1995)

5397 van der Gaast A, Schoenmakers CHH, Kok TC et al. Prognostic significance of tissue polypeptide-specific antigen (TPS) in patients with advanced non-small cell lung cancer. *Eur J Cancer*, 30A, 1783-1786 (1994)

5398 Van der Westhuyzen JM. Plasma-T3 assay in kwashiorkor. *Lancet*, 2, 965 (1973)

5399 van der Zee JM, Miltenburg AMM, Siegert CEH et al. Antiendothelial cell antibodies in systemic lupus erythematosus: enhanced antibody binding to interleukin-1-stimulated endothelium. *Int Arch Allergy Immunol*, 104, 131-136 (1994)

5400 van der Zee JM, Siegert CE, de Vreede C et al. Characterization of anti-endothelial cell antibodies in systemic lupus erythematosus (SLE). *Clin Exp Immunol*, 84, 238-244 (1991)

5401 Van Deuren M, van der Ven-Jongekrijg J, Vannier E, et al. The pattern of interleukin-1β (IL-1β) and its modulating agents IL-I receptor antagonist and soluble receptor type II in acute meningococcal infections. *Blood*, 90, 1101-1108 (1997)

5402 van Duijnhoven EM, Lustermans FAT, van Wersch JWJ. Evaluation of the coagulation/fibrinolysis balance in patients with colorectal cancer. *Haemostasis*, 23, 168-172 (1993)

5403 van Hilten JJ, Ferrari MD, Van der Meer JW et al. Plasma interleukin-1, tumour necrosis factor and ophthalmic-pituitary-adrenal axis responses during migraine attacks. *Cephalalgia*, 11, 65-67 (1991)

5404 van Hulst KL, Hackeng WHL, Hoppener JWM et al. An improved method for the determination of islet amyloid polypeptide levels in plasma. *Ann Clin Biochem*, 31, 165-170 (1994)

5405 Van Hunsel F, Wauters A, Vandoolaeghe E, et al. Lower total serum protein, albumin, and β- and γ-globulin in major and treatment resistant depression: effects of antidepressant treatments. *Psychiat Res*, 65, 159-169 (1996)

5406 van Kamp GJ, von Mensdorff-Pouilly S, Kenemans P et al. Evaluation of colorectal cancer-associated mucin CA M43 assay in serum. *Clin Chem*, 39, 1029-1032 (1993)

5407 Van Krugten M, Cobben NAM, Lamers RJS, et al. Serum LDH, a marker of disease activity and its response to therapy in idiopathic pulmonary fibrosis. *Neth J Med*, 48, 220-223 (1996)

5408 van Leeuwen MA, Westra J, Limburg PC et al. Clinical significance of interleukin-6 measurement in early rheumatoid arthritis: relation with laboratory clinical variables and radiological progression in a three year prospective study. *Ann Rheum Dis*, 54, 674-677 (1995)

5409 van Londen L, Goekoop JG, van Kempen GMJ, et al. Plasma levels of arginine vasopressin elevated in patients with major depression. *Neuropsychopharmacology*, 17, 284-292 (1997)

5410 Van Nagell JR et al. Carcinoembryonic antigen in carcinoma of the uterine cervix. *Cancer*, 42, 2428-2434 (1978)

5411 Van Norstrand WE, Wagner SL, Shankle WR et al. Decreased levels of soluble amyloid β-protein precursor in cerebrospinal fluid of live Alzheimer's disease patients. *Proc Natl Acad Sci USA*, 89, 2551-2555 (1992)

5412 van Papendorp DH, Theron JJ, Viljoen M et al. Plasma melatonin levels in patients with spinal cord lesions. *Med Sci Res*, 23, 189-190 (1995)

5413 van Pelt J, Azimi H. False-positive CDTect values in patients with low ferritin values. *Clin Chem*, 44, 2219-2220 (1998)

5414 Van Poppel H, Billen J, Goethuys H, et al. Serum tissue polypeptide antigen (TPA) as tumor marker for bladder cancer. *Anticancer Res*, 16, 2205-2208 (1996)

5415 van Rossum MAJ, Fiselier TJW, Franssen MJAM, et al. Sulfasalazine in the treatment of juvenile chronic arthritis: a randomized, double-blind, placebo-controlled multicenter study. *Arth Rheum*, 41, 808-816 (1998)

5416 van Stetten PA, van Hansbergh VWM, van den Heuvel LPW, et al. Monocyte chemotractant protein-1 and interleukin-8 levels in urine and serum of patients with hemolytic uremic syndrome. *Pediatr Res*, 43, 759-767 (1998)

5417 van Wersch JWJ. The behaviour of lipoprotein(a) in patients with various diseases. *Scand J Clin Lab Invest*, 54, 559-562 (1994)

5418 van Wersch JWJ, Peters C, Ubachs HMH. Haemostasis activation markers in plasma of patients with benign and malignant gynaecological tumours: a pilot study. *Eur J Clin Chem Clin Biochem*, 33, 225-229 (1995)

5419 Van Zandwijk N, Jassem E, Bonfrer JMG et al. Value of neuron specific enolase in early detection of relapse in small cell lung carcinoma. *Eur J Cancer*, 26, 373-376 (1990)

5420 van Zanten RAA, van Leeuwen RE, Wilson JHP. Serum procollagen III N-terminal peptide and laminin P1 fragment concentrations in alcoholic liver disease and primary biliary cirrhosis. *Clin Chim Acta*, 177, 141-146 (1988)

5421 Vancurova R, Kocinova F, Englis M. Cerebrospinal fluid (CSF) β-2-microglobulin (Sp-B_2M) levels: topographic and time dependency. *Clin Biochem Rev*, 14, 208 (1993)

5422 Vanderschueren-Lodeweyckx M et al. Decreased serum thyroid hormone levels and increased TSH response to TRH in infants with celiac disease. *Clin Endocrinol*, 6, 361-367 (1977)

5423 Vanderstraeten EF, De Vos MM, Versieck JM et al. Serum gastrin levels and colorectal neoplasia. *Dis Colon Rectum*, 38, 172-176 (1995)

5424 Vanek VW, Seballos RM, Chong D et al. Serum potassium concentrations in trauma patients. *South Med J*, 87, 41-46 (1994)

5425 Varagunam M, Nwosu AC, Adu D et al. Little evidence for anti-endothelial-cell antibodies in microscopic polyarteritis and Wegener's granulomatosis. *Adv Exp Med Biol*, 336, 419-422 (1993)

5426 Varalakshmi G et al. Blood lipids in renal stone disorder. *Ind J Med Res*, 66, 840-846 (1977)

5427 Vardi J, Kisch E, Bornstein N et al. CSF renin activity in hypertensive and normotensive patients. *Schweiz Arch Neurol Neurochir Psychiatr*, 129, 347-352 (1981)

5428 Various. Allergy and Immunology. *MKSAP VII*, Philadelphia PA, American College of Physicians (1986)

5429 Vassar MJ, Weber CJ, Holcroft JW. Measurement of 6-keto-PGF(1α) and thromboxane B_2 levels in critically ill surgical patients. *Prostaglandins Leukot Essent Fatty Acids*, 33, 129-135 (1988)

5430 Vassella F et al. The diagnostic value of serum creatine kinase in neuromuscular and muscular disease. *Pediatrics*, 35, 322-330 (1965)

5431 Vasson M-P, Paul J-L, Couderc R et al. Serum α-1 acid glycoprotein in chronic renal failure and hemodialysis. *Int J Artif Org*, 14, 92-96 (1991)

5432 Vasson MP, Roch-Arveiller M, Bargnoux PJ et al. Serum and urinary α-1 acid glycoprotein in the uremic patients. *Ann Clin Biol*, 50, 476 (1992)

5433 Vaubourdolle M, Chazouilleres O, Briaud I et al. Plasma α-glutathione S-transferase assessed as a marker of liver damage in patients with chronic hepatitis C. *Clin Chem*, 41, 1716-1719 (1995)

5434 Vawter MP, Dillon-Carter O, Issa F, et al. Transforming growth factors β1 and β2 in the cerebrospinal fluid of chronic schizophrenic patients. *Neuropsychopharmacology*, 16, 83-87 (1997)

5435 Vawter MP, Dillon-Carter O, Tourtellotte WW, et al. TGFβ1 and TGFβ2 concentrations are elevated in Parkinsn's disease in ventricular cerebrospinal fluid. *Exp Neurol*, 142, 313-332 (1996)

5436 Vaziri ND, Gonzales EC, Shayestehfar B et al. Plasma levels and urinary excretion of fibrinolytic and protease inhibitory proteins in nephrotic syndrome. *J Lab Clin Med*, 124, 118-124 (1994)

5437 Vaziri ND, Kaupke CJ, Barton CH et al. Plasma concentration and urinary excretion of erythropoietin in adult nephrotic syndrome. *Am J Med*, 92, 35-40 (1992)

5438 Vaziri ND, Paule P, Toohey J, Hung E. Acquired deficiency and urinary excretion of antithrombin III in nephrotic syndrome. *Arch Intern Med*, 144, 1802-1803 (1984)

5439 Veale DJ, Maple C, Kirk G, et al. Soluble cell adhesion molecules - P-selectin and ICAM-1, and disease activity in patients receiving sulphasalazine for active rheumatoid arthritis. *Scand J Rheumatol*, 27, 296-299 (1998)

5440 Vecino A, Navarro-Antolin J, Teruel J, et al. Lipid composition of platelets in patients with uremia. *Nephron*, 78, 271-273 (1998)

5441 Vedra B. Das renin-angiotensin-aldosteron-system in der pathogenese der gestoseodems. *Die Spatgestose Rippmann E T (Ed) Based Schwabe*, 1970, 152-156

5442 Veenstra J, te Wierik E, Kluft C. Alcohol and fibrinolysis. *Fibrinolysis*, 4, 64-68 (1990)

5443 Veglio F, Melchio R, Rabbia F et al. Plasma immunoreactive endothelin-1 in primary hyperaldosteronism. *Am J Hypertens*, 7, 559-561 (1994)

5444 Velardo A, Del Rio G, Zizzo G et al. Plasma catecholamines after thyrotropin-releasing hormone administration in hypothyroid patients before and during therapy. *Eur J Endocrinol*, 130, 220-223 (1994)

5445 Velayudhan A, Sunitha TA, Balachander S, et al. A study of platelet serotonin receptor in mania. *Biol Psychiatr*, 45, 1059-1062 (1999)

5446 Velazquez EM, Mendoza S, Hamer T et al. Metformin therapy in polycystic ovary syndrome reduces hyperinsulinemia, insulin resistance, hyperandrogenemia, and systolic blood pressure, while facilitating normal menses and pregnancy. *Metabolism*, 43, 647-654 (1994)

5447 Velazquez H, Perazella MA, Wright FS et al. Renal mechanism of trimethoprim-induced hyperkalemia. *Ann Intern Med*, 119, 296-301 (1993)

5448 Velde J et al. The eosinophilic fibrohistiocytic lesion of the bone marrow. a mastocellular lesion in bone disease. *Virchows Arch Pathol Anat*, 377, 277-85 (1978)

5449 Velentzas C et al. Abnormal vitamin D levels. *Ann Intern Med*, 86, 198 (1977)

5450 Velho G, Erlich D, Turpin E et al. Lipoprotein (a) in diabetic patients and normoglycemic relatives in familial NIDDM. *Diabetes Care*, 16, 742-747 (1993)

5451 Veltri RW, Miller MC, Zhao G, et al. Interleukin-8 serum levels in patients with benign prostatic hyperplasia and prostate cancer. *Urology*, 53, 139-147 (1999)

5452 Vendsalu A. Studies on adrenaline and noradrenaline in human plasma. *Acta Physiol Scand*, 49, Suppl 173, 1 (1966)

5453 Ventura S et al. La porfiria eritropoietica. nota. I. il comportamento del ricambio porfirinico. *Haematologica*, 44, 993 (1959)

5454 Verges BL, Lagrost L, Vaillant G et al. Apolipoprotein A-IV levels and phenotype distribution in NIDDM. *Diabetes Care*, 17, 810-817 (1994)

5455 Vergote IB, Abeler VM, Bormer OP et al. CA 125 and placental alkaline phosphatase as serum tumor markers in epithelial ovarian carcinoma. *Tumor Biol*, 13, 168-174 (1992)

5456 Verhagen H et al. Increase of serum complement levels in cancer patients with progressing tumors. *Cancer*, 38, 1608-1613 (1976)

5457 Verlooy H, Devos P, Janssens J et al. Clinical significance of squamous cell carcinoma antigen in cancer of the human uterine cervix: comparison with CEA and CA-125. *Gynecol Obstet Invest*, 32, 55-58 (1991)

5458 Vermes I, Beishuizen A, Hampsink RM et al. Dissociation of plasma adrenocorticotropin and cortisol levels in critically ill patients: possible role of endothelin and atrial natriuretic hormone. *J Clin Endocrinol Metab*, 80, 1238-1242 (1995)

5459 Vermes I, Hampsink RM, Haanen C. Dissociation of the pituitary and the adrenal functions in critical illness: possible role of endothelin and atriopeptin. *Clin Chem*, 41, S46 (1995)

5460 Versieck J, Barbier F, Speecke A, Hoste J. Manganese, copper, and zinc concentrations in serum and packed blood cells during acute hepatitis, chronic hepatitis, and posthepatic cirrhosis. *Clin Chem*, 20, 1141-1145 (1974)

5461 Versieck J, Cornelis R. Normal levels of trace elements in human blood, plasma or serum. *Anal Chim Acta*, 116, 217-254 (1980)

5462 Versieck J et al. Influence of myocardial infarction on serum manganese, copper, and zinc concentration. *Experientia*, 31, 280-281 (1975)

5463 Vgontzas AN, Papanicolaou DA, Bixler EO, et al. Elevation of plasma cytokines in disorders of excessive daytime sleepiness: role of sleep disturbance and obesity. *J Clin Endocrinol Metab*, 82, 1313-1318 (1997)

5464 Viani A, Rizzo G, Carrai M et al. Interindividual variability in the concentrations of albumin and α_1-acid glycoprotein in patients with renal or liver disease, newborns and healthy subjects: implications for binding of drugs. *Int J Clin Pharmacol Ther Toxicol*, 30, 128-133 (1992)

5465 Vicente V, Estelles A, Moraleda JM et al. Fibrinolytic changes during acute vascular damage induced by Mediterranean spotted fever. *Fibrinolysis*, 7, 324-329 (1993)

5466 Vicente-Gutierrez MM, Ruiz AD, Extremera BG et al. Low serum levels of α-interferon, γ-interferon, and interleukin-2 in alcoholic cirrhosis. *Dig Dis Sci*, 36, 1209-1212 (1991)

5467 Viedma JA, Perez-Mateo M, Dominguez JE, Carballo F. Role of interleukin-6 in acute pancreatitis. Comparison with C-reactive protein and phospholipase A. *Gut*, 33, 1264-1267 (1992)

5468 Vieira JG, Kasamatsu T, Nishida S. Monoclonal antibody-based immunofluorometric assay for free alpha subunit of glycoprotein. *Clin Chem*, 41, S36 (1995)

5469 Vieira JGH, Nishida SK, Lombardi MT, et al. Serum PSA levels in patients with different degrees of secondary hypogonadism. *Clin Chem*, 39, 1161 (1993)

5470 Vierhapper H, Raber W, Bieglmayer C, et al. Routine measurement of plasma calcitonin in nodular thyroid diseases. *J Clin Endocrinol Metab*, 82, 1589-1593 (1997)

5471 Vilaseca MA, Moyano D, Artuch R, et al. Selective screening for hyperhomocysteinemia in pediatric patients. *Clin Chem*, 44, 662-664 (1998)

5472 Vincent RG, Chu TM, Fergen TB et al. Carcinoembryonic antigen in 228 patients with carcinoma of the lung. *Cancer*, 36, 2069-2076 (1975)

5473 Vincent RG et al. Carcinoembryonic antigen in patients with carcinoma of the lung. *Int Thorac Card Surg*, 66, 320-327 (1973)

5474 Vindenes H, Ulvestad E, Bjerknes R. Increased levels of circulating interleukin-8 in patients with large burns: relation to burn size and sepsis. *J Trauma injury Infect Crit Care*, 39, 635-640 (1995)

5475 Vinke B, Donker AJM. The neutropenic (pancytopenic?) type of bacillary dysentery. *Acta Trop*, 23, 81 (1966)

5476 Vinuya RZ, Simon MR, Schwartz LB. Elevated serum tryptase levels in a patient with protracted anaphylaxis. *Ann Allergy*, 73, 232-234 (1994)

5477 Violi F, Leo R, Vezza E et al. Bleeding time in patients with cirrhosis: relation with degree of liver failure and clotting abnormalities. *J Hepatol*, 20, 531-540 (1994)

5478 Virdi NK, Huddart SN, Taylor GN et al. The value of biochemical tests in neuroblastoma. *Proc ACB Natl Meet*, 65-66 (1993)

5479 Virkkunen M, Rawlings R, Tokola R et al. CSF biochemistries, glucose metabolism, and diurnal activity rhythms in alcoholic, violent offenders, fire setters, and healthy volunteers. *Arch Gen Psychiat*, 51, 20-27 (1994)

5480 Vitale G, Mocciaro C, Malta R et al. Evaluation of serum levels of soluble CD4, CD8 and β_2-microglobulin in visceral Leishmaniasis. *Clin Exp Immunol*, 97, 280-283 (1994)

5481 Vitelli LL, et al. Glycosylated hemoglobin level and carotid intimal-medial thickening in nondiabetic individuals. *Diabetes Care*, 20, 1454-1458 (1997)

5482 Viti A, Maioli E, Billi M et al. Atrial natriuretic peptide and acute myocardial infarction: critical reappaisal. *Cardiology*, 83, 390-395 (1993)

5483 Vitoratos N, Gregoriou O, Papadias C, et al. Clinical value of creatine kinase in the diagnosis of ectopic pregnancy. *Gynecol Obstet Invest*, 46, 80-83 (1998)

5484 Vitto J et al. Further evaluation of the significance of urinary hydroxyproline determinations in the diagnosis of thyroid disorders. *Clin Chim Acta*, 22, 583 (1968)

5485 Vladutiu AO et al. Double spike in the electropherogram of a myeloma serum, from Bence Jones protein. *Clin Chem*, 23, 67-73 (1975)

5486 Vocanson C, Caudie C, Quincy C. Reference values for CSF albumin, IgG, IgA and IgM and their application in diagnosing inflammatory neurological disorders. *Clin Chem*, 39, 263 (1993)

5487 Vogel AV, Peake GT, Rada RT. Pituitary-testicular axis dysfunction in burned men. *J Clin Endocrinol Metab*, 60, 658-665 (1985)

5488 Vogelsang H, Hamwi A, Ferenci P. Elevated liver isoenzymes of alkaline phosphatase and disease activity in patients with Crohn's disease. *Digestion*, 57, 11-15 (1996)

5489 Vogl M, Andert SE, Muller MM. Tissue polypeptide specific antigen, neopterin, and CRP for monitoring heart transplant recipients. *Clin Biochem*, 28, 291-295 (1995)

5490 Voight D et al. Uber die blutkonzentrationen der leukozyten und thrombocyten ber eisenmangel. *Blut*, 14, 267 (1967)

5491 Voller A et al. Serological indices in Tanzania: II. antinuclear factor and malarial indices in populations living at different altitudes. *J Trop Med Hyg*, 75, 136 (1972)

5492 Volta U, De Franceschi L, Molinaro N, et al. Frequency and significance of anti-gliadin anti-endomysial antibodies in autoimmune hepatitis. *Dig Dis Sci*, 43, 2190-2195 (1998)

5493 von Herbay A, de Groot H, Hegi U et al. Low vitamin E content in plasma of patients with alcoholic liver disease, hemochromatosis and Wilson's disease. *J Hepatol*, 20, 41-46 (1994)

5494 von Knorring AL, Hallman J, von Knorring L, Oreland L. Platelet monoamine oxidase activity in type 1 and type 2 alcoholism. *Alcohol Alcoholism*, 26, 409-416 (1991)

5495 von Toorenenbergen AW, Balk AHMM, Vermeulen AM. Sustained decrease of serum total IgE in cardiac transplant recipients. *Int Arch Allergy Immunol*, 110, 163-165 (1996)

5496 Vonderheid EC, Zhang Q, Lessin SR, et al. Use of serum soluble interleukin-2 receptor levels to monitor the progression of cutaneous T-cell lymphoma. *J Am Acad Dermatol*, 38, 207-220 (1998)

5497 Voon BH, Romero R, Jun JK, et al. Amniotic fluid cytokines (interleukin-6, tumor necrosis factor-α, interleukin-1β, and interleukin-8) and the risk for the development of bronchopulmonary dysplasia. *Am J Obstet Gynecol*, 177, 825-830 (1997)

5498 Vorhaus et al. Serum cholinesterase in health and disease. *Am J Med*, 15, 707-711 (1953)

5499 Vucic M, Gavella M, Bozikov V, et al. Superoxide dismutase activity in lymphocytes and polymorphonuclear cells of diabetic patients. *Eur J Clin Chem Clin Biochem*, 35, 517-521 (1997)

5500 Vucic M, Rocic B, Bozikov V, Ashcroft SJH. Plasma uric acid and total antioxidant status in patients with diabetes mellitus. *Horm Metab Res*, 29, 355-357 (1997)

5501 Vuoristo M, Kesaaniemi VA, Gylling H et al. Metabolism of cholesterol and apolipoprotein B in celiac disease. *Metabolism*, 42, 1386-1391 (1993)

5502 Waage A, Brandtzweg P, Halstensen A. The complex pattern of cytokines in serum from patients with meningococcal septic shock. *J Exp Med*, 169, 333-338 (1989)

5503 Waage A, Halstensen A, Espevik T et al. Association between tumour necrosis factor in serum and fatal outcome in patients with meningococcal disease. *Lancet*, 1, 355-357 (1987)

5504 Waage A, Remick D, Steinshamn S et al. Interleukin 8 in serum in granulocytopenic patients with infections. *Br J Haematol*, 86, 36-40 (1994)

5505 Waalkes TP, Dinsmore SR, Mrochek JE. Urinary excretion by cancer patients of the nucleosides N^2,N^2-dimethylyguanosine, 1-methylinosine, and pseudouridine. *J Natl Cancer Inst*, 51, 271-274 (1972)

5506 Wacker et al. Metalloenzymes and myocardial infarction. *N Engl J Med*, 255, 449 (1956)

5507 Wacker WEC et al. Magnesium metabolism. *N Engl J Med*, 278, 712 (1968)

5508 Wada H, Kaneko T, Ohiwa M et al. Increased levels of vascular endothelial cell markers in thrombotic thrombocytopenic purpura. *Am J Hematol*, 44, 101-105 (1993)

5509 Wada H, Minamikawa K, Wakita Y et al. Increased vascular endothelial cell markers in patients with disseminated intravascular coagulation. *Am J Hematol*, 44, 85-88 (1993)

5510 Wada H, Mori Y, Kaneko T et al. Elevated plasma levels of vascular endothelial cell markers in patients with hypercholesterolemia. *Am J Hematol*, 44, 112-116 (1993)

5511 Wada H, Nakase T, Nakaya R et al. Elevated plasma tissue factor antigen level in patients with disseminated intravascular coagulation. *Am J Hematol*, 45, 232-236 (1994)

5512 Wada H, Sakuragawa N, Mori Y, et al. Hemostatic molecular markers before the onset of disseminated intravascular coagulation. *Am J Hematol*, 60, 273-278 (1999)

5513 Wada H, Tanigawa M, Wakita Y et al. Increased plasma level of interleukin-6 in disseminated intravascular coagulation. *Blood Coag Fibrinolysis*, 4, 583-590 (1993)

5514 Wada H, Wakita Y, Nakase T, et al. Increased plasma-soluble fibrin monomer levels in patients with disseminated intravascular coagulation. *Am J Hematol*, 51, 255-260 (1996)

5515 Wada M et al. Serum lipid and lipoprotein abnormalities in major clinical entities of renal disease. *Contrib Nephrol*, 9, 61-68 (1978)

5516 Wadman SK et al. Three new cases of histidinemia: clinical and biochemical data. *Acta Paediat Scand*, 56, 485 (1967)

5517 Wadstein J et al. Does hypokalaemia precede delirium tremens? *Lancet*, 2, 549-550 (1978)

5518 Wagener D et al. Total serum haemolytic complement activity, ESR and plasma fibrinogen as indicators of the stage in Hodgkin's disease. *Eur J Clin Invest*, 7, 289-294 (1977)

5519 Wagner OF, Jilma B. Putative role of adhesion molecules in metabolic disorders. *Horm Metab Res*, 29, 627-630 (1997)

5520 Wagner OF, Waldhausi W, Parzer S et al. Determination of endothelin-1 by RIA: disturbed pulmonary clearance in acute lung failure. *Clin Biochem Rev*, 14, 348 (1993)

5521 Wagner R, Hayatghebi S, Rosenkranz M et al. Increased serum neopterin levels in patients with Graves' disease. *Exp Clin Endocrinol*, 101, 249-254 (1994)

5522 Wahby V, Ibrahim G, Friedenthal S et al. Serum concentrations of circulating thyroid hormones in a group of depressed men. *Neuropsychobiology*, 22, 8-10 (1989)

5523 Waisman HA et al. Amino acid metabolism in patients with acute leukemia. *Pediatrics*, 10, 653 (1952)

5524 Wajima T et al. Low leukocyte alkaline phosphatase activity in sickle cell anemia. *J Lab Clin Med*, 72, 980 (1968)

5525 Wajsman WR et al. Evaluation of biological markers in bladder cancer. *J Urol*, 114, 879-893 (1975)

5526 Wakabayashi A et al. Serum amylase isozymes in patients with chronic pancreatitis with hyperamylasemia. *Gastroenterol Jpn*, 12, 269-274 (1977)

5527 Wald NJ, Watt HC, Wald J, et al. Homocysteine and ischemic heart disease: results of a prospective study with implications regarding prevention. *Arch Intern Med*, 158, 862-867 (1998)

5528 Waldenström J. Studien ueber porphyrie. *Acta Med Scand*, 82, Suppl (1937)

5529 Waldenström J G, Haeger-Aronsen B. The liver in porphyria and cutanea tarda. *Ann Intern Med*, 53, 286 (1960)

5530 Waldhauser F, Boepple PA, Schemper M et al. Serum melatonin in central precocious puberty is lower than in age-matched pubertal children. *J Clin Endocrinol Metab*, 73, 793-796 (1991)

5531 Waldman TA et al. The proteinuria of cystinosis: its pattern and pathogenesis. In:. *Cystinosis.* JD Schulman (ed), 72-249 (1973)

5532 Waldman TA, Mcintyre KR. Serum AFP levels in patients with ataxia-telangiectasia. *Lancet*, 2, 1112 (1972)

5533 Waldmann T et al. Albumin metabolism in patients with lymphoma. *J Clin Invest*, 42, 171 (1963)

5534 Waldmann TA, Bradley JE. Polycythemia secondary to a pheochromocytoma with production of an erythropoiesis stimulating factor tumor. *Proc Soc Exp Biol Med*, 108, 425 (1962)

5535 Waldvagel FA et al. Ostemyelitis: a review of clinical features, therapeutic considerations and unusual aspects. I. *N Engl J Med*, 282, 198 (1970)

5536 Walenga JM, Lietz H, Hoppensteadt D, et al. Positive anti-platelet factor 5-heparin antibody titers in non-heparin-induced thrombocytopenic patients not exposed to heparin. *Am J Clin Path*, 108, 347 (1997)

5537 Walenga JM, Pifarre R, Hoppensteadt D et al. Non-invasive diagnosis of heart transplant rejection as measured by plasma markers. *Clin Biochem Rev*, 14, 200 (1993)

5538 Walker R, Crebbin V, Stern J et al. Urinary gonadotropin peptide (UGP) as a marker of gynecologic malignancies. *Anticancer Res*, 14, 1703-1710 (1994)

5539 Walkoff A et al. Rotors syndrome: a distinct inheritable pathophysiologic entity. *Am J Med*, 60, 173 (1976)

5540 Wall AJ, Kirsner JB. Ulcerative colitis and Crohn's disease of the colon: symptoms, signs, and laboratory aspects. In:. *Inflammatory Bowel Disease*, Philadelphia PA, Lea and Febiger, 101 (1975)

5541 Wallace AM. Analytical support for the detection and treatment of congenital adrenal hyperplasia. *Ann Clin Biochem*, 32, 9-27 (1995)

5542 Wallace AM. Measurement of leptin and leptin binding in the human circulation. *Ann Clin Biochem*, 37, 244-252 (2000)

5543 Wallace JMW, Freeburn JC, Gilmore WS, et al. The assessment of platelet derived growth factor concentrations in post myocardial infarction and stable angina patients. *Ann Clin Biochem*, 35, 236-241 (1998)

5544 Wallach J. *Interpretation of Diagnostic Tests,* 2nd edition, Boston MA, Little Brown and Co (1974)

5545 Wallach J. *Interpretation of Diagnostic Tests,* 3rd edition, Boston MA, Little Brown and Co (1978)

5546 Wallach J. *Interpretation of Diagnostic Tests,* 5th edition, Boston MA, Little Brown Co

5547 Wallach S et al. Plasma and erythrocyte magnesium in health and disease. *J Lab Clin Med*, 59, 195-209 (1962)

5548 Wallberg-Jonsson S, Dahlen G, Johnson O, et al. Lipoprotein lipase in relation to inflammatory activity in rheumatoid arthritis. *J Intern Med*, 240, 373-380 (1996)

5549 Wallberg-Jonsson S, Uddhammar A, Dahlen G et al. Lipoprotein (a) in relation to acute phase reaction in patients with rheumatoid arthritis and polymyalgia rheumatica. *Scand J Clin Lab Invest*, 55, 309-315 (1995)

5550 Wallentin L et al. Studies on plasma lipid and phospholipid composition in pernicious anemia before and after specific treatment. *Acta Med Scand*, 201, 161-165 (1977)

5551 Wallerstedt S et al. Serum lipids and lipoproteins during abstinence after heavy alcohol consumption in chronic alcoholics. *Scand J Clin Lab Invest*, 37, 599-604 (1977)

5552 Walls J, Ratcliffe WA, Howell A et al. Parathyroid hormone and parathyroid hormone-related protein in the investigation of hypercalcaemia in two hospital populations. *Clin Endocrinol*, 41, 407-413 (1994)

5553 Walsh CH et al. A study of pituitary function in patients with idiopathic hemochromatosis. *J Clin Endocrinol Metab*, 43, 866-872 (1976)

5554 Walsh CH, Murphy AL, Cunningham S et al. Mineralocorticoid and glucocorticoid status in idiopathic haemochromatosis. *Clin Endocrinol*, 41, 439-443 (1994)

5555 Walter JE. The significance of antibodies in chronic histoplasmosis by immunoelectrophoretic and complement fixation test. *Am Rev Resp Dis*, 99, 50 (1969)

5556 Wan AT, Conyers RAJ, Coombs CJ et al. Determination of silver in blood, urine, and tissues of volunteers and burn patients. *Clin Chem*, 37, 1683-1687 (1991)

5557 Wands JR et al. Circulating immune complexes and complement activation in primary biliary cirrhosis. *N Engl J Med*, 298, 233-37 (1978)

5558 Wanebo HJ, Clarkson BD. Essential macroglobulinemia. *Acta Med Scand*, 170, Suppl, 367, 110 (1961)

5559 Wang CR, Chuang CY, Chen CY. Anticardiolipin antibodies and interleukin-6 in cerebrospinal fluid and blood of Chinese patients with neuro-Behcet's syndrome. *Clin Exp Rheumatol*, 10, 599-602 (1992)

5560 Wang DY, Stepniewska KA, Allen DS et al. Serum prolactin levels and their relationship to survival in women with operable breast cancer. *J Clin Epidemiol*, 48, 959-968 (1995)

5561 Wang G, Hansen H, Tatsis E, et al. High plasma levels of the soluble form of CD30 activation molecule reflect disease activity in patients with Wegener's granulomatosis. *Am J Med*, 102, 517-523 (1997)

5562 Wang H. An investigation on changes in blood Cu, Zn-superoxide dismutase contents in type I, II schizophrenics. *Chung Hua Shen Ching Ching Shen Ko Tsa Chih*, 25, 6-8 (1992)

5563 Wang MX, Walker RG, Kincaid-Smith P. Clinicopathologic associations of anti-endothelial cell antibodies in immunoglobulin A nephropathy and lupus nephritis. *Am J Kid Dis*, 22, 378-386 (1993)

5564 Wang S-R, Chen M-L, Huang M-H et al. Plasma arginase concentration measured by an enzyme-linked immunosorbent assay (ELISA) in normal adult population. *Clin Biochem*, 26, 455-460 (1993)

5565 Wang Y, Kay HH, Killam AP. Decreased levels of polyunsaturated fatty acids in preeclampsia. *Am J Obstet Gynecol*, 164, 812-818 (1991)

5566 Wangel AG, Kontiainen S, Melamies L et al. Hypothyroidism and anti-endothelial cell antibodies. *APMIS*, 101, 91-94 (1993)

5567 Wangel AG, Kontiainen S, Scheinin T, et al. Anti-endothelial cell antibodies in insulin-dependent diabetes mellitus. *Clin Exp Immunol*, 88, 410-413 (1992)

5568 Wannemacher RW et al. Effect of glucose infusion on the concentration of individual serum free amino acids during sandfly fever in man. *Am J Clin Nutr*, 30, 573-578 (1977)

5569 Wanner C, Bohler J, Eckardt HG et al. Effects of simvastin on lipoprotein (a) and lipoprotein composition in patients with nephrotic syndrome. *Clin Nephrol*, 41, 138-143 (1994)

5570 Wanner C, Rader D, Bartens W et al. Elevated plasma lipoprotein (a) in patients with the nephrotic syndrome. *Ann Intern Med*, 119, 263-269 (1993)

5571 Wanner C, Riegel W, Schaefer RM et al. Carnitine and carnitine esters in acute renal failure. *Nephrol Dial Transplant*, 4, 951-956 (1989)

5572 Ward AM et al. Acute-phase reactant protein profiles: an aid to monitoring large bowel cancer by CEA and serum enzymes. *Br J Cancer*, 35, 170 (1977)

5573 Ward JR, Atcheson S. Infectious arthritis. *Med Clin North Am*, 61, 313-329 (1977)

5574 Ward TT et al. Acidosis of synovial fluid correlates with synovial fluid leukocytosis. *Am J Med*, 64, 933-936 (1978)

5575 Wardener NE. Renal hemodynamics in primary polycythemia. *Lancet*, 2, 204 (1951)

5576 Warner A, Bencosme A, Healy D et al. Prognostic role of antioxidant enzymes in sepsis: preliminary assessment. *Clin Chem*, 41, 867-871 (1995)

5577 Warrell RP et al. Increased factor VIII/von Willebrand factor antigen and von Willebrand factor activity in renal failure. *Am J Med*, 66, 226-228 (1978)

5578 Warrens AN, Cassidy MJD, Takahishi K et al. Endothelin in renal failure. *Nephrol Dial Transplant*, 5, 418-422 (1990)

5579 Warshaw AL. On the cause of raised serum amylase in diabetic ketoacidosis. *Lancet*, 1, 929 (1977)

5580 Warshaw DL et al. Characteristic alterations of serum isoenzymes of amylase in diseases of liver, pancreas, salivary gland, lung, and genitalia. *J Surg Res*, 22, 362-369 (1977)

5581 Wartofsky L et al. Studies on the nature of thyroidal suppression during acute falciparum malaria: integrity of pituitary response to TRH and alterations in serum T3 and reverse T3. *J Clin Endocrinol Metab*, 44, 85-90 (1977)

5582 Wasada T, Inoue K, Fujimi S et al. Hypersomatostatinemia in chronic renal failure. *Endocrinol Jpn*, 34, 251-256 (1987)

5583 Washington JA. The role of the microbiology laboratory in the diagnosis and antimicrobial treatment of infective endocarditis. *Mayo Clin Proc*, 57, 22-32 (1982)

5584 Wasi P, Block M. The mechanism of the development of anemia in untreated chronic lymphatic leukemia. *Blood*, 17, 597 (1961)

5585 Wasowicz W, Neve J, Peretz A. Optimized steps in fluorometric determination of thiobarbituric acid-reactive substances in serum: importance of extraction pH and influence of sample preservation and storage. *Clin Chem*, 39, 2522-2526 (1993)

5586 Wasserheit C, Acaba L, Gulati S. Abnormal liver function in patients undergoing autologous bone marrow transplantation for hematological malignancies. *Czncer Invest*, 13, 347-354 (1995)

5587 Wasserman LR et al. Blood oxygen studies in patients with polycythemia and in normal subjects. *J Clin Invest*, 28, 60 (1940)

5588 Wasserman LR, Gilbert HS. Surgical bleeding in polycythemia vera. *Ann NY Acad Sci*, 115, 122 (1964)

5589 Wassif WS, Butterworth RJ, Gerges A et al. Serum carnosinase activity following cerebral infarction or haemorrhage. *Proc ACB Natl Meet*, 154 (1995)

5590 Wassif WS, Sherwood RA, Amir A et al. Serum carnosinase activities in central nervous system disorders. *Clin Chim Acta*, 225, 57-64 (1994)

5591 Wast DC, Yaqoob M. Serum hyaluronan levels follow disease activity in vasculitis. *Clin Nephrol*, 48, 9-15 (1997)

5592 Watanabe M et al. Aldosterone secretion rates in abnormal pregnancy. *J Clin Endocrinol Metab*, 25, 1665-1670 (1965)

5593 Watanabe N, Miyamoto M, Tokuda Y et al. Serum c-erbB-2 in breast cancer. *Acta Oncol*, 33, 901-904 (1994)

5594 Waters PJ, Lewry E, Pennock CA. Measurement of sialic acid in srum and urine: clinical applications and limitations. *Ann Clin Biochem*, 29, 625-637 (1992)

5595 Watschinger B, Hartter E, Traindl O et al. Increased levels of plasma amylin in advanced renal failure. *Clin Nephrol*, 37, 131-134 (1992)

5596 Watschinger B, Watzinger U, Templ H et al. Effect of recombinant human erythropoietin on anterior pituitary function in patients on chronic hemodialysis. *Horm Res*, 36, 22-26 (1991)

5597 Watson CJ. Porphyrin metabolism in the anemias. *Arch Intern Med*, 99, 323 (1957)

5598 Watson CJ. The problem of porphyria - some facts and questions. *N Engl J Med*, 263, 1205 (1960)

5599 Watson CJ et al. A simple test for urinary porphobilinogen. *Proc Soc Exp Biol Med*, 47, 393 (1941)

5600 Watson RR, Jackson JC, Sampliner R et al. Cellular immune functions, endorphins, and alcohol consumption in males. *Alcohol Clin Exp Res*, 9, 248-254 (1985)

5601 Watson RR, McMurray DN, Martin P et al. Effect of age, malnutrition and renutrition on free secretory component and IgA in secretions. *Am J Clin Nutr*, 42, 281-288 (1985)

5602 Wayman J, O'Hanlon D, Hayes N, et al. Fibrinogen levels correlate with stage of disease in patients with esophageal cancer. *Br J Surg*, 84, 185-188 (1997)

5603 Ways P et al. Red cell and plasma lipids in acanthocytosis. *J Clin Invest*, 42, 1248 (1963)

5604 Webb DJ, Cockcroft JR. Plasma immunoreactive endothelin in uraemia. *Lancet*, 1, 2211 (1989)

5605 Webb J et al. Analysis by pattern recognition techniques of changes in serum levels of 14 trace metals after acute myocardial infarction. *Exper Mol Pathol*, 25, 322-331 (1976)

5606 Wechsler M et al. The cancer associated antigen test as an index to failure of complete removal of urologic cancer. *J Urol*, 109, 699 (1973)

5607 Weeke B, Flenborg EW, Jacobsen L et al. Immunochemical quantitation of 18 serum proteins in sera from patients with cystic fibrosis: concentrations correlated to class of fibroblast metachromasia, clinical and radiological lung symptoms. *Dan Med Bull*, 23, 155-160 (1976)

5608 Weeke B, Jarnum S. Serum concentration of 19 serum proteins in Crohn's disease and ulcerative colitis. *Gut*, 12, 197-302 (1972)

5609 Wegner F, Dummler W, Kruger B et al. Soluble ICAM-1 in pancreas transplant recipients - preliminary results. *Clin Biochem Rev*, 14, 201 (1993)

5610 Wehr H, Czartoryska B, Gorska D et al. Serum β-hexosaminidase and α-mannosidase activities as markers of alcohol abuse. *Alcohol Clin Exp Res*, 15, 13-15 (1991)

5611 Wehr H, Rodo M, Szacka E et al. High density lipoprotein (HDL) composition in ethanol intoxication. *Diag Lab*, 27, 127 (1991)

5612 Wei J, Xu H, Ramchand CN et al. Low concentrations of serum tyrosine in neuroleptic-free schizophrenics with an early onset. *Schiz Res*, 14, 257-260 (1995)

5613 Wei LK. The clinical and laboratory studies of superoxide dismutase activity in the human whole blood with early gastric cancer. *Free Rad Res Comm*, 12-13, 759-760 (1991)

5614 Weight MJ, Coetzee HS, Smuts CM et al. Lecithin:cholesterol acyltransferase activity and high-density lipoprotein subfraction composition in type I diabetic patients with improving metabolic control. *Acta Diabetol*, 30, 159-165 (1993)

5615 Weinberger A et al. Increased uric acid clearance in patients with burns. *Biomed Pharmacother*, 27, 277-278 (1977)

5616 Weinberger MH et al. Sequential changes in the renin-antigotensin-aldosterone systems and plasma progesterone concentration in normal and abnormal human pregnancy. *Perspect Nephrol Hypertens*, 5, 263-269 (1976)

5617 Weiner CP, Kwaan H, Duboe F. Diagnosis of septic pelvic thrombophlebitis by measurement of fibrinopeptide A. *Am J Perinatol*, 2, 93-95 (1985)

5618 Weinstein A et al. Antibodies to native DNA and serum complement (C3) levels: applications to diagnosis and classification of systemic lupus erythematosus. *Am J Med*, 74 (1983)

5619 Weinstein AJ, Farkas S. Serologic tests in infectious diseases: clinical utility and interpretation. *Med Clin North Am*, 62, 1099-1118 (1978)

5620 Weir CJ, Murray GD, Dyker AG, et al. Is hyperglycaemia an independent predictor of poor outcome after acute stroke? *Br Med J*, 314, 1303-1306 (1997)

5621 Weir GC et al. The hypocalcemia of acute pancreatitis. *Ann Intern Med*, 83, 185-189 (1975)

5622 Weir RJ et al. Angiotensin, aldosterone, and DOC in hypertensive disease of pregnancy. *Scott Med J*, 18, 64 (1973)

5623 Weiss SH, Goedert JJ, Sarngadharan MG et al. Screening test for HTLV-III (AIDS agent) antibodies. *J Am Med Ass*, 253, 221 (1985)

5624 Weitzberg E, Lundberg JM, Rudehill A. Elevated plasma levels of endothelin in patients with sepsis syndrome. *Circ Shock*, 33, 222-227 (1991)

5625 Welch CE, Hedberg SE. *Polypoid Lesions of the Gastrointestinal Tract,* 2nd edition, Philadelphia PA, WB Saunders (1975)

5626 Welle S, Jozefowicz R, Forbes G et al. Effect of testosterone on metabolic rate and body composition in normal men and men with muscular dystrophy. *J Clin Endocrinol Metab*, 74, 332-335 (1992)

5627 Weller M, Stevens A, Sommer N et al. Cerebrospinal fluid interleukins, immunoglobulins, and fibronectin in neuroborreliosis. *Arch Neurol*, 48, 837-841 (1991)

5628 Welt LG et al. An ion transport defect in erythrocytes for uremic patients. *Arch Intern Med*, 126, 827 (1970)

5629 Weltzin TE, McConaha C, McKee M et al. Circadian patterns of cortisol, prolactin, and growth hormonal secretion during bingeing and vomiting in normal weight bulimic patients. *Biol Psychiat*, 30, 37-48 (1991)

5630 Wener MF, Vobach S, Svetlik D et al. Cortisol secretion and Alzheimer's disease progression: a preliminary report. *Biol Psychiat*, 34, 158-161 (1993)

5631 Weng X, Roederer GO, Beaulieu R, Cloutier G. Contribution of acute-phase proteins and cardiovascular risk factors to erythrocyte aggregation in normolipidemic and hyperlipidemic individuals. *Thromb Haemostas*, 80, 903-908 (1998)

5632 Wenham PR, Haddad L, Panarelli M, et al. Simplified detection of a mutation causing familial hypercholesterolaemia throughout Britain: evidence for an origin in a common distant ancestor. *Ann Clin Biochem*, 35, 226-235 (1998)

5633 Wenisch C, Bankl HC, Schonthal E et al. Serum levels of the carboxy-terminal cross-linked telopeptide of type I collagen and laminin are elevated in Graves' disease but not in toxic nodular goiter. *Clin Immunol Immunopathol*, 75, 225-230 (1995)

5634 Wenisch C, Myskiw D, Gessi A, Graninger W. Circulating selectins, intercellular adhesion molecule-1, and vascular cell adhesion molecule-1 in hyperthyroidism. *J Clin Endocrinol Metab*, 80, 2122-2126 (1995)

5635 Wenisch C, Myskiw D, Narzt E et al. Serum laminin in Graves' disease. *Eur J Clin Invest*, 25, 425-428 (1995)

5636 Wenisch C, Parschalk B, Burgmann H et al. Decreased serum levels of TGF-β in patients with acute Plasmodium falciparum malaria. *J Clin Immunol*, 15, 69-73 (1995)

5637 Wenisch C, Parschalk B, Narzt E, et al. Elevated serum levels of IL-10 and IFN-γ in patients with acute Plasmodium falciparum malaria. *Clin Immunol Immunopathol*, 74, 115-117 (1995)

5638 Wennberg A, Hyltander A, Sjoberg A et al. Prevalence of carnitine depletion in critically ill patients with undernutrition. *Metabolism*, 41, 165-171 (1992)

5639 Weredehoff SG, Moore RB, Hoff CJ, et al. Elevated plasma endothelin-1 levels in sickle cell anemia: relationships to oxygen saturation and left ventricular hypertrophy. *Am J Haematol*, 58, 195-199 (1998)

5640 Werener JA, Gottschlich S, Folz BJ, et al. p53 serum antibodies as prognostic indicator in head and neck cancer. *Cancer Immunol Immunother*, 44, 112-116 (1997)

5641 Werner M, Faser C, Silverberg M. Clinical utility and validation of emerging biochemical markers for mammary adenocarcinoma. *Clin Chem*, 39, 2386-2396 (1993)

5642 West CD, McAdams J. Serum and glomerular IgG in poststreptococcal glomerulonephritis are correlated. *Pediatr Nephrol*, 12, 392-396 (1998)

5643 Westcott JY, Thomas RB, Voelkel NF. Elevated urinary leukotriene E_4 excretion in patients with ARDS and severe burns. *Prostaglandins Leukot Essent Fatty Acids*, 43, 151-158 (1991)

5644 Westerhuis LWJJM, Venekamp WJRR. Serum lipoprotein-a levels and glyco-metabolic control in insulin and non-insulin dependent diabetes mellitus. *Clin Biochem*, 29, 255-259 (1996)

5645 Westerman MP et al. Hypocholesterolaemia and anaemia. *Br J Haematol*, 31, 87-94 (1975)

5646 Westhoff C, Gollub E, Patel J et al. CA 125 levels in menopausal women. *Obstet Gynecol*, 76, 428-431 (1990)

5647 Weston MW, Cintron GB, Giordano AT et al. Normalization of circulating atrial natriuretic peptides in cardiac transplant recipients. *Am Heart J*, 127, 129-142 (1994)

5648 Wettsberg L, Aberg H, Ross SB, Froden O. Plasma dopamine-β-hydroxylase activity in hypertension and various neuropsychiatric disorders. *Scand J Clin Lab Invest*, 30, 283 (1972)

5649 Whalley LJ, Christie JE, Bennie J et al. Selective increase in plasma luteinising hormone concentrations in drug free young men with mania. *Br Med J*, 290, 99-102 (1985)

5650 Wheelock EF et al. The participation of lymphocytes in viral infections. *Adv Immunol*, 16, 124 (1973)

5651 Whicher JT. The value of complement assays in clinical chemistry. *Clin Chem*, 24, 7-22 (1978)

5652 White et al. Histiocytic medullary reticulosis with parallel increases in serum acid phosphatase and disease activity. *Cancer*, 37, 1403-1411 (1976)

5653 Whitelaw A, Mowinckel M-C, Abildgaard U. Low plasminogen in cerebrospinal fluid after intraventricular haemorrhage: a limiting factor for clot lysis? *Acta Paediat*, 84, 933-936 (1995)

5654 Whitfield JB, Martin NG. Blood pressure and chemistry: some correlations and apparent correlations. *Ann Clin Biochem*, 21, 257-260 (1984)

5655 Whiting PH, Petersen J, Power DA, et al. Diagnostic value of urinary N-acetyl-β-D-glucosaminidase, its isoenzymes and the fractional excretion of sodium following renal transplantation. *Clin Chim Acta*, 130, 369-376 (1983)

5656 Whiting PH, Ross LS, Borthwick LJ. Serum and urine N-acetyl-β-D-glucosaminidase in diabetics on diagnosis and subsequent treatment, and stable insulin dependent diabetics. *Clin Chim Acta*, 97, 459-463 (1979)

5657 Whittaker JA, Cawood ML, Oakey RE. A method for the determination of sex hormone binding globulin using Concanavalin A-Sepharose. *Ann Clin Biochem*, 29, 168-171 (1992)

5658 Whittingham S et al. Smooth muscle autoantibody (SMA) in autoimmune hepatitis. *Gastroenterology*, 51, 499 (1966)

5659 Whyte MP, Chines A, Silva DP Jr, et al. Creatine kinase brain isoenzyme (BB-CK) presence in serum distinguishes ostepetroses among the sclerosing bone disorders. *J Bone Miner Res*, 11, 1438-1443 (1996)

5660 Wibe E, Paus E, Aamdal S. Neuron specific enolase (NSE) in serum of patients with malignant melanoma. *Cancer Lett*, 52, 29-31 (1990)

5661 Widecka K, Gozdzik J, Dutkiewic T et al. Atrial natriuretic factor in untreated hyperthyroidism. *Ann Clin Biochem*, 27, 313-317 (1990)

5662 Widomska-Czekajska T. Blood oxygenation and disturbances of the acid-base equilibrium in myocardial infarction. *Cor Vasa*, 18, 1-10 (1976)

5663 Wiener K. Plasma calcium in acute myocardial infarction. *Ann Clin Biochem*, 14, 553-54 (1977)

5664 Wiener K. Uraemia and hyperuricaemia in acute myocardial infarction. *Clin Chim Acta*, 73, 45-50 (1976)

5665 Wikkelso C, Ekman R, Wesergren I et al. Neuropeptides in cerebrospinal fluid in normal-pressure hydrocephalus and dementia. *Eur Neurol*, 31, 88-93 (1991)

5666 Wild RA, Alaupovic P, Parker IJ. Lipid and apolipoprotein abnormalities in hirsute women. I. The association with insulin resistance. *Am J Obstet Gynecol*, 167, 575 (1992)

5667 Wilden EG. Urinary and whole blood cadmium concentrations in renal disease. *Ann Clin Biochem*, 10, 107-110 (1973)

5668 Wilkins J, Gallimore JR, Tennent GA et al. Rapid automated enzyme immunoassay of serum amyloid A. *Clin Chem*, 40, 1284-1290 (1994)

5669 Wilkinson H, Horsley E. Changes in markers of bone collagen turnover in toxic and euthyroid states: a study of 22 patients. *Ann Clin Biochem*, 33, 454-455 (1996)

5670 Wilkinson H, Horsley E. PICP and ICTP as markers of bone collagen turnover: a study of 25 thyrotoxic patients. *Proc ACB Natl Meet*, 147 (1995)

5671 Wilkinson JH. *The Principles and Practice of Diagnostic Enzymology*, Chicago IL, Year Book Medical Publishers (1976)

5672 Wilkinson MR, Wagstaffe C, Delbridge L et al. Serum osteocalcin concentrations in Paget's disease of bone. *Arch Intern Med*, 146, 268 (1986)

5673 Wilkinson SP. Abnormalities of sodium excretion and other disorders of renal function in fulminant hepatic failure. *Gut*, 17, 501-505 (1976)

5674 Wilkinson SP et al. Renal retention of sodium in cirrhosis and fulminant hepatic failure. *Postgrad Med J*, 51, 527-531 (1975)

5675 Williams A, Sturman S, Steventon G, Waring R. Metabolic biomarkers of Parkinson's disease. *Acta Neurol Scand*, 136, Suppl, 19-23 (1991)

5676 Williams AT, Shearer MR, Oyeyi J et al. Serum osteocalcin in the management of myeloma. *Eur J Cancer*, 29A, 140-142 (1992)

5677 Williams JW et al. *Hematology,* 2nd edition, New York NY, McGraw-Hill (1977)

5678 Williams JW et al. *Hematology,* 3rd edition, New York NY, McGraw-Hill (1983)

5679 Williams RH. *Textbook of Endocrinology,* 5th edition, Philadelphia PA, WB Saunders (1974)

5680 Willis FR, Smith GC, Beattie TJ. Plasma E-selectin and ICAM-1 in acute Henoch-Schonlein purpura. *Arch Dis Child*, 76, 94 (1997)

5681 Wills MR, McGowan GK. Plasma chloride levels in hyperparathyroidism and other hypercalcemic states. *Br Med J*, 1, 1153 (1964)

5682 Wilmer A, Nolchen B, Tilg H et al. Serum neopterin concentrations in chronic liver disease. *Gut*, 37, 108-112 (1995)

5683 Wilmore DW et al. Impaired glucose flow in burned patients with gram-negative sepsis. *Surg Gynecol Obstet*, 143, 720-724 (1976)

5684 Wilschanski M, Chait P, Wade JA, et al. Primary sclerosing cholangitis in 32 children: clinical, laboratory, and radiographic features, with survival analysis. *Hepatology*, 22, 1415-1422 (1995)

5685 Wilson CB, Dixon FJ. Antiglomerular basement membrane antibody induced glomerulonephritis. *Kidney Int*, 3, 74 (1973)

5686 Wilson CB et al. Glomerulonephritis. *DM*, 22, 18-27 (1976)

5687 Wilson DM et al. Renal urate excretion in patients with Wilson's disease. *Kidney Int*, 4, 331-336 (1973)

5688 Wilson M et al. Comparison of the complement fixation, indirect immunofluorescence, and indirect hemagglutination tests for malaria. *Am J Trop Med Hyg*, 24, 755-759 (1975)

5689 Wilson MG, Melnyk J. Translocation: normal mosaicism in D trisomy. *Pediatrics*, 40, 842 (1967)

5690 Wilson RB, Lynch DR, Fischbeck KH. Normal serum iron and ferritin concentrations in patients with Friedreich's ataxia. *Ann Neurol*, 44, 132-134 (1998)

5691 Wilson RF, Farag A, Mammen EF et al. Sepsis and antithrombin III, prekallikrein, and fibronectin levels in surgical patients. *Am Surg*, 55, 450-456 (1989)

5692 Wilson T, Thong KJ, Howie PW. Decrease in human plasma gravidin levels after medical abortion. *Prostaglandins*, 48, 175-185 (1994)

5693 Wiman B. Plasminogen activator inhibitor 1 (PAI-1) in plasma: its role in thrombotic disease. *Thromb Haemostas*, 74, 71-76 (1995)

5694 Winawer SJ et al. Screening for colon cancer. *Gastroenterology*, 70, 783 (1976)

5695 Winkler G, Salamon F, Harmos G, et al. Elevated serum tumor necrosis factor-α concentrations and bioactivity in type 2 diabetics and patients with android type obesity. *Diabetes Res Clin Pract*, 42, 169-174 (1998)

5696 Winklhofer-Roob BM, Ellemunter H, Fruhwirth M, et al. Plasma vitamin C concentrations in patients with cystic fibrosis: evidence of associations with lung inflammation. *Am J Clin Nutr*, 65, 1858-1855 (1997)

5697 Winocour PH, Bhatnagar D, Ishola M et al. Lipoprotein (a) and microvascular disease in Type I (insulin-dependent) diabetes. *Diabetic Med*, 8, 922-927 (1991)

5698 Winston RM et al. Enzymatic diagnosis of megaloblastic anemia. *Br J Haematol*, 19, 587 (1970)

5699 Wintrobe MM et al. *Clinical Hematology,* 7th ed, Philadelphia PA, Lea and Febiger (1974)

5700 Wiseman C, McGregor RF, McCredie KB. Urinary amino acid excretion in acute leukemia. *Cancer*, 38, 219-224 (1976)

5701 Withers KL. Leukaemoid reactions in disseminated non-reactive tuberculosis: a review of the literature with report of a case. *Med J Aust*, 2, 142 (1964)

5702 Withold W, Degenhardt S, Grabensee B et al. Bone alkaline phosphatase (BAP) and the carboxy-terminal propeptide of type I procollagen (PICP) in patients following renal transplantation. *Clin Chem*, 41, S44 (1995)

5703 Withold W, Friedrich W, Reinaeur H. Comparison of biochemical markers of bone resorption in patients with metabolic and malignant bone diseases. *Ann Clin Biochem*, 33, 421-427 (1996)

5704 Witt BR, Miles R, Wolf GC et al. CA 125 levels in abruptio placentae. *Am J Obstet Gynecol*, 164, 1225-1228 (1991)

5705 Witteveen SA et al. The influence of plasma volume changes on enzymatic estimation of infarct size. *Recent Adv Stud Cardiac Struct Metab*, 12, 401-407 (1976)

5706 Witts LJ et al. Chronic granulocytic leukemia comparison of radiotherapy and busulphan therapy. report of the Medical Research Council's working party for therapeutic trials in leukaemia. *Br Med J*, 1, 201 (1968)

5707 Witztum J, Schonfeld G. High density lipoproteins. *Diabetes*, 28, 326-336 (1979)

5708 Wobbes T, Thomas CMG, Segers MFG et al. Evaluation of seven tumor markers (CA 50, CA 19-9, CA 19-9 TruQuant, CA 72-4, CA 195, carcinoembryonic antigen, and tissue polypeptide antigen) in the pretreatment sera of patients with gastric carcinoma. *Cancer*, 69, 2036-2041 (1992)

5709 Wochos DN et al. Serum lipids in chronic renal failure. *Mayo Clin Proc*, 51, 660-664 (1976)

5710 Wolff JM, Bares R, Jung PK, et al. Prostate-specific antigen as a marker of bone metastasis in patients with prostate cancer. *Urol Int*, 56, 169-173 (1996)

5711 Wolff JM, Fandel T, Borchers H, et al. Transforming growth factor-β1 serum concentration in patients with prostatic cancer and benign prostatic hyperplasia. *Br J Urol*, 81, 403-405 (1998)

5712 Wolff K, Nisell H, Carlstrom K, et al. Endothelin-1 and big endothelin-1 levels in normal pregnancy and in preeclampsia. *Regulat Peptide*, 67, 211-216 (1996)

5713 Wolintz AH et al. Serum and cerebrospinal fluid enzymes in cerebrovascular disease. *Arch Neurol*, 20, 54-61 (1969)

5714 Wolkoff AW et al. Inheritance of the Dubin-Johnson syndrome. *N Engl J Med*, 288, 113 (1973)

5715 Wong K, Beardshall K, Waters CM et al. Postprandial hypergastrinemia in patients with colorectal cancer. *Gut*, 32, 1352-1354 (1991)

5716 Wong KL, Wong RPO. Serum soluble interleukin 2 receptor in systemic lupus erythematosus: effects of disease activity and infection. *Ann Rheum Dis*, 50, 706-709 (1991)

5717 Wong RD, Goetz MB, Mathisen G et al. Clinical and laboratory features of measles in hospitalized adults. *Am J Med*, 95, 377-383 (1993)

5718 Wong TW, Jones TM. Hyperprolactinemia and male infertility. *Arch Pathol Lab Med*, 108, 35-39 (1984)

5719 Wong TYH, Szeto CC, Lai FFM, et al. Nephrotic syndrome in strongyloidosis: remission after eradication with anthelmintic agents. *Nephron*, 79, 333-336 (1998)

5720 Wonke B. Bone disease in β-thalassaemia major. *Br J Haematol*, 103, 897-901 (1998)

5721 Woo KT, Lee EJC, Lau YK et al. Antithrombin III in renal transplant recipients. *Thromb Res*, 38, 201-206 (1985)

5722 Wood PJ. The measurement of parathyroid hormone. *Ann Clin Biochem*, 29, 11-21 (1992)

5723 Wood PJ, Barth JH, Freedman DB, et al. Evidence for the low dose dexamethasone suppression test to screen for Cushing's syndrome - recommendations for a protocol for biochemistry laboratories. *Ann Clin Biochem*, 34, 222-229 (1997)

5724 Woodard HQ. Changes in blood chemistry associated with carcinoma metastatic to bone. *Cancer*, 6, 1219-1227 (1953)

5725 Woodbury J et al. Cerebrospinal fluid and serum levels of magnesium, zinc, and calcium in man. *Neurology*, 18, 700 (1968)

5726 Woodruff AW et al. Anemia in African trypanosomiasis and big spleen disease in Uganda. *Trans Roy Soc Trop Med Hyg*, 67, 329 (1973)

5727 Woodruff AW et al. The anaemia of kala azar. *Br J Haematol*, 22, 319 (1972)

5728 Woodward CG, Cox RA. Epstein-Barr virus serology in the chronic fatigue syndrome. *J infect*, 24, 133-139 (1992)

5729 Woody MC et al. Histidinemia. *Am J Dis Child*, 110, 606 (1965)

5730 Woolas RP, Xu F-J, Jacobs IJ et al. Elevation of multiple serum markers in patients with stage I ovarian cancer. *J Natl Cancer Inst*, 85, 1748-1751 (1993)

5731 Woolf PD, Hamill RW, Lee LA et al. Free and total catecholamines in critical illness. *Am J Physiol Endocrinol Metab*, 254, E287-E291 (1988)

5732 Worcester EM, Fellner SK, Nakagawa Y et al. Effect of renal transplantation on serum oxalate and urinary oxalate excretion. *Nephron*, 67, 414-418 (1994)

5733 Worgall S, Manz F, Kleschin K et al. Elevated urinary excretion of endothelin-like immunoreactivity in children with renal disease is related to urinary flow rate. *Clin Nephrol*, 41, 331-337 (1994)

5734 Wouters MG, Boers GH, Blom HJ , et al. Hyperhomocysteinemia: a risk factor in women with unexplained recurrent early pregnancy loss. *Fertil Steril*, 60, 820-825 (1993)

5735 Woyda J et al. Free adrenaline, noradrenaline and vanillylmandelic acid excretion with 24-hour urine in patients with chronic circulatory failure. *Pol Med Sci Hist Bull*, 15, 425-430 (1975)

5736 Wroblewski. The clinical significance of alterations in lactic dehydrogenase activity of body fluids. *Am J Med Sci*, 234, 301-312 (1957)

5737 Wroblewski. The clinical significance of alterations in transaminase activities of serum and other body fluids. *Adv Clin Chem*, 1, 313 (1958)

5738 Wroblewski. The significance of alterations in serum enzymes in the differential diagnosis of jaundice. *Arch Intern Med*, 100, 635-641 (1957)

5739 Wröbel K, Wröbel K, Garay-Sevilla M, et al. Novel analytical approach to monitoring advanced glycosylation end products in human serum with on-line spectrophotometric and spectrofluorometric detection in a flow system. *Clin Chem*, 43, 1563-1569 (1997)

5740 Wu AHB, Feng YJ, Contois JH, Pervaiz S. Comparison of myoglobin, creatine kinase-MB, and cardiac troponin-I for diagnosis of acute myocardial infarction. *Ann Clin Lab Sci*, 26, 291-300 (1996)

5741 Wu AHB, Gornet T, Apple F et al. Use of cardiac troponin-T in diagnosis of acute myocardial infarction: a multicenter clinical evaluation. *Clin Chem*, 39, 1159 (1993)

5742 Wu C-T, Lee J-N, Shen WW et al. Serum zinc, copper and ceruloplasmin levels in male alcoholics. *Biol Psychiat*, 19, 1333-1338 (1984)

5743 Wu JH, Kao J-T, Wen M-S et al. Coronary artery disease risk prediction by plasma concentrations of high-density lipoprotein cholesterol, apolipoprotein AI, apolipoprotein B, and lipoprotein(a) in a general Chinese population. *Clin Chem*, 39, 209-212 (1993)

5744 Wu JT, Carlisle P. Low frequency and low level of elevation of serum CA 72-4 in human carcinomas in comparison with established tumor markers. *J Clin Lab Anal*, 6, 59-64 (1992)

5745 Wu JT, Olson J, Walker K. Tumor markers CA 19-9 and CA 195 are also useful as markers for cystic fibrosis. *J Clin Lab Anal*, 6, 151-161 (1992)

5746 Wu LL, Wu J, Hunt SC et al. Plasma homocyst(e)ine as a risk factor for early familial coronary artery disease. *Clin Chem*, 40, 552-561 (1994)

5747 Wu T-H, Wu S-C, Huang T-P, et al. Increased excretion of tumor necrosis factor alpha and interleukin 1β in urine of patients with IgA nephropathy and Schonlein-Henoch purpura. *Nephron*, 74, 79-88 (1996)

5748 Wu TT, Lee YH, Tzeng WS et al. The role of C-reactive protein and erythrocyte sedimentation rate in the diagnosis of infected hydronephrosis and pyonephrosis. *J Urol*, 152, 26-28 (1994)

5749 Wuster C, Blum WF, Schlemilch S et al. Decreased serum levels of insulin-like growth factors and IGF binding protein 3 in osteoporosis. *J Intern Med*, 234, 249-255 (1993)

5750 Wu-Wang CY, Patel M, Feng J, et al. Decreased levels of salivary prostaglandin E_2 and epidermal growth factor in recurrent apthous stomatitis. *Arch Oral Biol*, 40, 1093-1098 (1995)

5751 Wyeth-Ayerst Laboratories. Manufacturer's literature on Inderal® LA. Philadelphia, PA 19101 (1990)

5752 Wyllie E, Luders H, MacMillan JP et al. Serum prolactin levels after epileptic seizures. *Neurology*, 34, 1601-1604 (1984)

5753 Wyngaarden JB. Uric acid. In:. *The Encyclopedia of Medicine Surgery Specialties*, 341 (1955)

5754 Xie B. A study on the serum biochemistry in carrier detection of Duchenne muscular dystrophy. *Chung Hua Shen Ching Ching Shen Ko Tsa Chih*, 24, 165-168 (1991)

5755 Xing RD, Wang ZS, Li CQ, et al. Total sialic acid as a tumor marker for oral cancer. *Int J Biol Mark*, 9, 239-242 (1994)

5756 Xu F-J, Ramakrishnan S, Daly L et al. Increased serum levels of macrophage colony-stimulating factor in ovarian cancer. *Am J Obstet Gynecol*, 165, 1356-1362 (1991)

5757 Xu SY, Pauksen K, Venge P. Serum measurements of human neutrophil lipocalcin (HNL) discriminate between acute bacterial and viral infections. *Scand J Clin Lab Invest*, 55, 125-131 (1995)

5758 Xu Y, Shen Z, Wiper DW, et al. Lysophosphatidic acid as a potential biomarker for ovarian and other gynecologic cancers. *J Am Med Ass*, 280, 719-723 (1998)

5759 Yachman et al. Clinical significance of the human α-feto protein. *Ann Clin Lab Sci*, 8, 84-90 (1978)

5760 Yagame M, Suzuki D, Jinde K, et al. Significance of urinary type IV collagen in patients with diabetic nephropathy using a highly sensitive one-step sandwich enzyme immunoassay. *J Clin Lab Anal*, 11, 110-116 (1997)

5761 Yahara O, Hashimoto K, Taniguchi N et al. Serum manganese-superoxide dismutase in patients with neuromuscular disorders as judged by an ELISA. *Res Comm Chem Path Pharmacol*, 72, 315-326 (1991)

5762 Yam LT et al. Impaired marrow granulocyte reserve and leukocyte mobilizations in leukemia reticuloendotheliosis. *Ann Intern Med*, 87, 444-446 (1977)

5763 Yamada K, Kono K, Umegaki H, et al. Decreased interleukin-6 level in the cerebrospinal fluid of patients with Alzheimer-type dementia. *Neurosci Lett*, 186, 219-221 (1995)

5764 Yamada S, Suou T, Kawasaki H. Plasma vitronectin concentrations in patients with chronic hepatitis C treated with interferon alpha. *Clin Chim Acta*, 261, 61-90 (1997)

5765 Yamada S, Suou T, Kawasaki H, et al. Clinical significance of serum 7S collagen in various liver diseases. *Clin Biochem*, 25, 467-470 (1992)

5766 Yamada T, et al. Activation of the kallikrein-kinin system in rocky mountain spotted fever. *Ann Intern Med*, 88, 764-766 (1978)

5767 Yamada T, Ozawa T, Geiyo F, et al. Decreased serum apolipoprotein AII/AI ratio in systemic amyloidosis. *Ann Rheum Dis*, 57, 249-251 (1998)

5768 Yamada Y, Ishizaki M, Kido T, et al. Elevations of serum angiotensin-converting enzyme and γ-glutamyltranspeptidase activities in hypertensive drinkers. *J Hum Hypertens*, 5, 183-188 (1991)

5769 Yamada Y, Ohmoto Y, Murata K, et al. Increased plasma M-CSF concentration in patients with adult T cell leukemia: clinical correlation. *Leukemia Lymphoma*, 14, 151-156 (1994)

5770 Yamagata S, et al. A case of congenital afibrinogenemia and review of reported cases in Japan. *Tohoku J Exp Med*, 96, 15 (1968)

5771 Yamaguchi A, Kurosaka Y, Ishida T, et al. Clinical significance of tumor marker NCC-ST 439 in large bowel cancers. *Dis Colon Rectum*, 34, 921-924 (1991)

5772 Yamaguchi M, Mori N. Urinary excretion of 6-keto prostaglandin $F_1\alpha$ in pre-eclampsia. *Arch Gynecol Obstet*, 244, 7-13 (1988)

5773 Yamaguchi T, Takahashi T, Yokota T, et al. Urinary pepsinogen I as a tumor marker of stomach cancer after total gastrectomy. *Cancer*, 68, 906-909 (1991)

5774 Yamaji T, Ishibashi M, Sekihara H, et al. Plasma levels of atrial natriuretic peptide in primary aldosteronism and essential hypertension. *J Clin Endocrinol Metab*, 63, 815-818 (1986)

5775 Yamakita N, Mune T, Morita H, et al. Plasma 18-oxocortisol levels in the patients with adrenocortical disorders. *Clin Endocrinol*, 40, 583-587 (1994)

5776 Yamamoto H, Ninomiya H, Yoshimatsu K, et al. Serum levels of major basic protein in patients with or without eosinophilia: measurement by enzyme linked immunosorbent assay. *Br J Haematol*, 86, 490-495 (1994)

5777 Yamamoto K, Ozaki I, Fukushima N, et al. Serum lipoprotein (a) levels before and after subtotal thyroidectomy in subjects with hypothyroidism. *Metabolism*, 44, 4-7 (1995)

5778 Yamamoto Y, Nakano S, Kawashima S, et al. Plasma and serum G4 isoenzyme of acetylcholinesterase in patients with Alzheimer-type dementia and vascular dementia. *Ann Clin Biochem*, 27, 321-326 (1990)

5779 Yamamura M, Yamada Y, Momita S, et al. Circulating interleukin-6 levels are elevated in adult T-cell leukemia/Lymphoma patients and correlate with adverse clinical features and survival. *Br J Haematol*, 100, 129-134 (1998)

5780 Yamane K, Kashiwagi H, Suzuki N, et al. Elevated plasma levels of endothelin-1 in systematic sclerosis (Letter). *Arth Rheum*, 34, 243-244 (1991)

5781 Yamanobe S, Nakagawa Y, Hishinuma T, et al. Analysis of urinary dehydrothromboxane B_2 in patients with occluded retinal vein using GC/SIM. *Prostaglandins, Leukotrienes Essent Fatty Acids*, 58, 65-68 (1998)

5782 Yamashiki M, Kosaka Y, Nishimura A, et al. Analysis of serum cytokine levels in primary biliary cirrhosis patients and healthy adults. *J Clin Lab Anal*, 12, 77-82 (1998)

5783 Yamashita J-I, Hideshima T, Shirakusa T, Ogawa M. Medroxyprogesterone acetate treatment reduces serum interleukin-6 levels in patients with metastatic breast carcinoma. *Cancer*, 78, 2346-2352 (1996)

5784 Yamauchi A, Fujii M, Shirai D, et al. Plasma concencentration and peritoneal clearance of oxalate in patients on continuous ambulatory peritoneal dialysis (CAPD). *Clin Nephrol*, 25, 181-185 (1986)

5785 Yamauchi M, Mizuhara Y, Takahashi A, et al. Increases in serum β_3 integrin in patients with chronic liver disease. *Clin Chim Acta*, 225, 71-76 (1994)

5786 Yamazaki M, Ito S, Usami A, et al. Urinary excretion rate of ceruloplasmin in non-insulin-dependent diabetic patients with different stages of nephropathy. *Eur J Endocrinol*, 132, 681-687 (1995)

5787 Yamazaki M, Uchiyama S, Maruyama S. Alterations of haemostatic markers in various subtypes and phases of stroke. *Blood Coag Fibrinolysis*, 4, 707-712 (1993)

5788 Yaneva M, Arnett FC.. Antibodies against Ku protein in sera from patients with autoimmune disease. *Clin Exp Immunol*, 76, 366-372 (1989)

5789 Yao Z. The production and significance of interleukin-4 in patients with idiopathic nephrotic syndrome. *So Chung Hua I Hsueh Tsa Chih*, 73, 317 (1993)

5790 Yasumura S, Aloia JF, Gundberg CM, et al. Serum osteocalcin and total body calcium in normal pre- and post-menopausal women and postmenopausal osteoporotic women. *J Clin Endocrinol Metab*, 64, 681-685 (1987)

5791 Yates CM, et al. Lysosomal enzymes, amino acid and acid metabolites of amines in Huntington's chorea. *Clin Chim Acta*, 44, 139 (1973)

5792 Yates CM, et al. Lysosomal enzymes in cerebral atrophy. *Clin Chim Acta*, 71, 215-219 (1976)

5793 Yazawa S, Tanaka S, Nishimura T, et al. Plasma α1,3-fucosyltransferase deficiency in schizophrenia. *Exp Clin Immunogenet*, 16, 125-130 (1999)

5794 Yazzie D, Adoga GI, Okolo A, et al. Decreased urinary excretion of β-glucuronidase in sickle cell anemia in Nigeria. *Renal Fail*, 17, 57-64 (1995)

5795 Yegin A, Ozben T. Serum glycated lipoproteins in type II diabetic patients with and without complications. *Ann Clin Biochem*, 32, 459-463 (1995)

5796 Yehuda R, Kahana B, Binder-Brynes K, et al. Low urinary cortisol excretion in Holocaust Survivors with posttraumatic stress disorder. *Am J Psychiat*, 152, 982-986 (1995)

5797 Yehuda R, Teicher MH, Trestman RL, et al. Cortisol regulation in posttraumatic stress disorder and major depression: a chronobiological study. *Biol Psychiatr* (1996)

5798 Yen TS, et al. Humoral components of immunological response in nephrotic syndrome. *Chin J Microbiol*, 10, 21-27 (1977)

5799 Yeo KHJ, Whitau WJ. ^{125}I radioimmunoassay for 17α-hydroxyprogesterone in plasma, for diagnosing and managing congenital adrenal hyperplasia. *Clin Chem*, 31/3, 454-456 (1985)

5800 Yetgin S, Hincal F, Basaran N, et al. Serum selenium status in children with iron deficiency anemia. *Acta Haematol*, 88, 185-188 (1992)

5801 Yeyati NL, Adrogue HJ. Inappropriately high plasma renin activity accompanies chronic loss of renal function. *Am J Nephrol*, 16, 471-477 (1996)

5802 Yocum MW, Butterfield JH, Gharib H. Increased plasma calcitonin levels in systemic mast cell disease. *Mayo Clin Proc*, 69, 987-990 (1994)

5803 Yokose N, Ogata K, Ito T, et al. Elevated plasma soluble interleukin 2 receptor level correlates with defective natural killer and CD8+ T-cells in myelodysplastic syndromes. *Leukemia Res*, 18, 777-782 (1994)

5804 Yokoyama A, Kohno N, Sakai K, et al. Circulating levels of soluble interleukin-6 receptor in patients with bronchial asthma. *Am J Resp Crit Care*, 156, 1688-1691 (1997)

5805 Yokoyama H, Jensen JS, Jensen T, et al. Serum sialic acid concentration is elevated in IDDM especially in early diabetic nephropathy. *J Intern Med*, 237, 519-523 (1995)

5806 Yokoyama M, et al. Amylase-producing lung cancer. *Cancer*, 40, 766-72 (1977)

5807 Yoneda K, Fujita S, Katayama Y, et al. A rapid assay of human plasma phosphoglyceric acid mutase activity and application for clinical evaluation of acute myocardial infarction. *Clin Biochem Rev*, 14, 351 (1993)

5808 Yoneda M, Takatsuki K, Yamauchi K, et al. Influence of thyroid function on serum bone Gla protein. *Endocrinol Jpn*, 35, 39-45 (1988)

5809 Yonemitsu H. Elevated serum lactate dehydrogenase and creatine kinase (CK) activities with high CK-BB percentage in a patient with acute myeloblastic leukemia. *Jpn J Clin Path*, 37, 431-435 (1989)

5810 Yoneyama T, Fowler HL, Pendleton JW, et al. Elevated levels of creatine. *N Engl J Med*, 320, 1284-1285 (1989)

5811 Yoon BH, Jun JK, Park KH, et al. Serum C-reactive protein, white blood cell count, and amniotic fluid white blood cell count in women with preterm rupture of membranes. *Obstet Gynecol*, 88, 1034-1040 (1996)

5812 Yoshibayashi M, Kamiya T, Saito Y, et al. Increased plasma levels of brain natriuretic peptide in hypertrophic cardiomyopathy. *N Engl J Med*, 329, 433-434 (1993)

5813 Yoshida K, Kiso Y, Kurihara H, et al. Erythrocyte carbonic anhydrase I concentration in patients receiving thyroxine. *Endocrinol Jpn*, 38, 363-367 (1991)

5814 Yoshimoto S, Kaku H, Shimogawa S, et al. Urinary trace amine excretion and platelet monoamine oxidase activity in schizophrenia. *Psychiat Res*, 21, 229-236 (1987)

5815 Yoshinari M, Yamamoto M, Wakisaka M, et al. Effect of bezafibrate on hypercoagulability assessed by fluorogenic prothrombin time in hyperlipidemic patients with non-insulin-dependent diabetes mellitus. *Thromb Res*, 86, 443-451 (1997)

5816 Yoshioka N, Takahashi K, Oshima T, Watanabe T. Serum haptoglobin deficiency in healthy adults. *ASEAN J Clin Sci*, 1, 232-234 (1980)

5817 Yoshitomi Y, Kojima S, Umemoto T, et al. Serum hepatocyte growth factor in patients with peripheral arterial occlusive disease. *J Clin Endocrinol Metab*, 84, 2425-2428 (1999)

5818 Yoshitomi Y, Nishikimi T, Kojima S, et al. Plasma levels of adrenomedullin in patients with acute myocardial infarction. *Clin Sci*, 94, 135-139 (1998)

5819 Yoshizawa M, Nagai Y, Ohsawa K, et al. Elevated serum levels of soluble vascular cell adhesion molecule-1 in NIDDM patients with proliferative retinopathy. *Diabet Res Clin Pract*, 42, 65-70 (1998)

5820 Yoshizawa T, Iwamoto H, Mizusawa H, et al. Cerebrospinal fluid endothelin-1 in Alzheimer's disease and senile dementia. *Neuropeptides*, 22, 85-88 (1992)

5821 Yosipovitch G, Shohat B, Bshara J, et al. Elevated serum interleukin 1 receptors and interleukin 1β in patients with Behcet's disease: correlations with disease activity and severity. *Isr J Med Sci*, 31, 345-348 (1995)

5822 Yotsumoto H, Imai Y, Kuzuya N, Uchimura H. Increased levels of serum angiotensin-converting enzyme activity in hyperthyroidism. *Ann Intern Med*, 96, 326-8 (1982)

5823 Younes A, Snell V, Consoli U, et al. Elevated levels of biologically active soluble CD40 ligand in the serum of patients with chronic lymphocytic leukemia. *Br J Haematol*, 100, 135-141 (1998)

5824 Young G, Driscoll MC. Coagulation abnormalities in the carbohydrate-deficient glycoprotein syndrome: case report and review of the literature. *Am J Haematol*, 60, 66-69 (1999)

5825 Young LE, Miller G. Differentiation between congenital and acquired forms of hemolytic anemia. *Am J Med Sci*, 226, 664 (1953)

5826 Yu TF. Secondary gout associated with myeloproliferative diseases. *Arth Rheum*, 8, 765 (1965)

5827 Yu TF, et al. Plasma and urinary amino acids in primary gout with special reference to glutamine. *J Clin Invest*, 48, 885 (1969)

5828 Yu W, Kuhara T, Inoue Y, et al. Increased urinary excretion of β-hydroxyisovaleric acid in ketotic and nonketotic type II diabetes mellitus. *Clin Chim Acta*, 188, 161-168 (1990)

5829 Yucel I, Arpaci F, Ozet A , et al. Serum copper and zinc levels and copper/zinc ratio in patients with breast cancer. *Biol Trace Elem Res*, 40, 31-38 (1994)

5830 Yuki H, Hashimoto K, Yoshida Y, et al. Determination of modified bases and nucleoside in urines of cancer patients and comparison of their molar ratio to creatinine with that of normal humans. *Clin Biochem Rev*, 14, 265 (1993)

5831 Zabay JM, Sempere JM, Benito JM, et al. Serum β_2-microglobulin and prediction of progression to AIDS in HIV-infected drug users. *J Acq Immun Defic Syndromes*, 8, 266-277 (1995)

5832 Zachariae H, Aslam HM, Bjerring P, et al. Serum aminoterminal propeptide of type III procollagen in psoriasis and psoriatic arthritis: relation to liver fibrosis and arthritis. *J Am Acad Dermatol*, 25, 50-53 (1991)

5833 Zachariae H, Heickendorff L, Bjerring P. Plasma endothelin in psoriasis: possible relations to therapy and toxicity. *Acta Derm Venereol*, 76, 442-443 (1996)

5834 Zagorski T, Dudek I, Berkan L, et al. Superoxide dismutase (SOD-1) activity in erythrocytes of patients with multiple sclerosis. *Neurol I Neurochir Polska*, 25, 725-730 (1991)

5835 Zaitsu M, Hamasaki Y, Ishii K, et al. Direct evidence that LTC_4 and LTB_4 but not TXA_2 are involved in asthma attacks in children. *J Asthma*, 35, 4445-448 (1998)

5836 Zaman A, et al. Factors predicting the presence of esophageal or gastric varices in patients with advanced liver disease. *Am J Gastroenterol*, 94, 3292-3296 (1999)

5837 Zaman AG, Edelsten C, Stanford MR, et al. Soluble intercellular adhesion molecule-1 (sICAM-!) as a marker of disease relapse in idiopathic uveoretinitis. *Clin Exp Immunol*, 95, 60-65 (1994)

5838 Zander M, Nagel F, Kerth P, et al. Diagnostic benefits of routine troponin T measurements in suspected myocardial infarction - results of the German troponin T multicenter study. *Clin Chem*, 39, 1150-1151 (1993)

5839 Zangerie R, Sarcletti M, Gallati H, et al. Decreased plasma concentrations of HDL cholesterol in HIV-infected individuals are associated with immune activation. *J Acq Immune Defic Syndromes*, 7, 1149-1156 (1994)

5840 Zangerle R, Steinhuber S, Sarcletti M, et al. Serum HIV-1 RNA levels compared to soluble markers of immune activation to predict disease progression in HIV-1-infected individuals. *Int Arch Allergy Immunol*, 116, 228-239 (1998)

5841 Zaniewski M, Jordan PH Jr, Yip B, et al. Serum gastrin level is increased by chronic hypercalcemia of parathyroid of parathyroid or nonparathyroid origin. *Arch Intern Med*, 146, 478 (1986)

5842 Zannos-Mariclea L, et al. Relationship between tocopherols and serum lipid levels in children with β-thalassemia major. *Am J Clin Nutr*, 31, 259-263 (1978)

5843 Zanussi S, Andrea MD, Simonelli C, et al. Serum levels of RANTES and MIP-1α in HIV-positive long-term survivors and progressor patients. *AIDS*, 10, 1431-1432 (1996)

5844 Zargar AH, Shah NA, Masoodi SR, et al. Copper, zinc, and magnesium levels in non-insulin dependent diabetes mellitus. *Postgrad Med J*, 74, 665-668 (1998)

5845 Zatloukal P, Glagolicova A, Linhart M, et al. Tissue polypeptide antigen in bronchogenic carcinoma. *Neoplasma*, 40, 301-303 (1993)

5846 Zavaroni I, Bonini L, Fantuzzi M, et al. Hyperinsulinemia, obesity and syndrome X. *J Intern Med*, 235, 31-36 (1994)

5847 Zazzo J-F, Troche G, Ruel P, et al. High incidence of hypophosphatemia in surgical intensive care patients: efficacy of phosphorus therapy on myocardial infarction. *Intensive Care Med*, 21, 826-831 (1995)

5848 Zeck R T, Cugell D. Diffuse infiltrative lung disease. *Med Clin North Am*, 61, 1251-1266 (1977)

5849 Zedan MM, el-Shennawy FA, Abou-Bakr HM, al-Basousy AM. Interleukin-2 in relation to T cell subpopulations in rheumatic heart disease. *Arch Dis Child*, 67, 1373-1375 (1992)

5850 Zeferos N, Digenis GE, Christophoaki M, et al. Tumor markers in patients undergoing hemodialysis or kidney transplantation. *Nephron*, 59, 618-620 (1991)

5851 Zeltzer PM. α-Fetoprotein in the differentiation of neonatal hepatitis and biliary atresia: current status and implications for the pathogenesis of these disorders. *J Pediatr Surg*, 13, 381-7 (1978)

5852 Zerez CR, Lachant NA, Tanaka KR. Decreased erythrocyte phosphoribosylpyrophosphate synthetase activity and impaired. *J Lab Clin Med*, 114, 43-50 (1989)

5853 Zerlotti H, Grotto W, Ferreira F, et al. Serum neopterin in patients with Chagas disease. *Trans Roy Soc Trop Med Hyg*, 88, 75 (1994)

5854 Zerr I, Bodemer M, Gefeller O, et al. Detection of 14-3-3 protein in the cerebrospinal fluid supports the diagnosis of Creutzfeldt-Jakob disease. *Ann Neurol*, 43, 32-40 (1998)

5855 Zhang X, Cornelis R, Mees L, et al. Chemical speciation of arsenic in serum of uraemic patients. *Analyst*, 123, 13-17 (1998)

5856 Zhong Y-G, Levy E, Bauman WA. The relationships among serum uric acid, plasma insulin, and serum lipoprotein levels in subjects with spinal cord injury. *Horm Metab Res*, 27, 283-286 (1995)

5857 Zhou D, Tian YP, He ZQ. Immunologic changes in serum Cu/Zn-containing superoxide dismutase in patients with lung cancer. *Chung Hua Nei Ko Tsa Chih*, 28, 421-422 (1989)

5858 Ziegenhagen MW, Benner UK, Zissel G, et al. Sarcoidosis: TNF-α release from alveolar macrophages and serum level of sIL-2R are prognostic markers. *Am J Respir Crit Care Med*, 156, 1586-1592 (1997)

5859 Ziegenhagen MW, Zabel P, Zissel G, et al. Serum level of interleukin 8 is elevated in idiopathic pulmonary fibrosis and indicates disease activity. *Am J Respir Crit Care Med*, 157, 762-768 (1998)

5860 Ziegler MG, Kennedy B, Morrissey E, et al. Norepinephrine clearance, chromogranin A and dopamine-β-hydroxylase in renal failure. *Kidney Int*, 37, 1357-1362 (1990)

5861 Zilberman-Kaufman M, Agam G, Moscowits L, et al. Raised monophosphatase in schizophrenic patients. *Clin Chim Acta*, 209, 89-93 (1992)

5862 Zilva JF, et al. Plasma phosphate and potassium levels in the hypercalcemia of malignant disease. *J Clin Endocrinol Metab*, 36, 1019 (1973)

5863 Zilva JF, Pannall P. *Clinical Chemistry in Diagnosis and Treatment, 2nd edition*, Chicago IL, Year Book Medical Publishers (1975)

5864 Zilversmit DB. In:. *Disturbances in Lipid and Lipoprotein Metabolism*. JA Dietschy, AM Gotto, JA Ontko (eds), Baltimore MD, Waverly Press, 69-81 (1978)

5865 Zimering MB, Eng J. Increased basic fibroblast growth factor-like substance in plasma from a subset of middle-aged or elderly male diabetic patients with microalbuminuria or proteinuria. *J Clin Endocrinol Metab*, 81, 4446-4452 (1996)

5866 Zimmer R, Teelken AW, Trieling WB, et al. γ-Aminobutyric acid and homovanillic acid concentration in the CSF of patients with senile dementia of Alzheimer's type. *Arch Neurol*, 41, 602-604 (1984)

5867 Zimmerman TS, et al. Immunologic differentiation of classic hemophilia (factor VIII deficiency) and von Willebrand's disease with observation on combined deficiencies of antihemophilic factor and proaccelerin (factor V). *J Clin Invest*, 50, 244 (1971)

5868 Zimmermann B, Baki S, Dengler TJ, et al. Troponin T release after heart transplantation. *Br Heart J*, 69, 395-398 (1993)

5869 Zini R, Riant P, Barre J, Tillement J-P. Disease-induced variations in plasma protein levels: Implications for drug dosage regimens (Part I). *Clin Pharmacokinet*, 19, 147-159 (1990)

5870 Zipp F, Weller M, Calabresi PA, et al. Increased serum levels of soluble CD95 (APO-1/Fas) in relapsing-remitting multiple sclerosis. *Ann Neurol*, 43, 116-120 (1998)

5871 Ziv I, Fleminger G, Djaldetti R, et al. Increased plasma endothelin-1 in acute ischemic stroke. *Stroke*, 23, 1014-1016 (1992)

5872 Zivny P, Palicka V, Pliskova L. Diagnostic value of cytokine estimation in the cerebrospinal fluid (CSF). *Clin Biochem Rev*, 14, 347 (1993)

5873 Zoccali C, Ciccarelli M, Mallamaci F, et al. Plasma met-enkephalin and leu-enkephalin in chronic renal failure. *Nephrol Dial Transplant*, 1, 219-222 (1987)

5874 Zonana-Nacach A, Salas M, Sanchez M, et al. Measurement of clinical activity of systemic lupus erythematosus and laboratory abnormalities: a 12-month prospective study. *J Rheumatol*, 22, 45-49 (1995)

5875 Zozaya JLC, Viloria MP, Castro A. Urinary excretion of zinc in patients with essential arterial hypertension. *Res Comm Chem Pathol Pharmacol*, 48, 445-453 (1985)

5876 Zubenko GS, Volicer L, Direnfeld LK, et al. Cerebrospinal fluid levels of angiotensin-converting enzyme in Alzheimer's disease, Parkinson's disease and progressive supranuclear palsy. *Brain Res*, 328, 215-221 (1985)

5877 Zucchelli GC, Clerico A, De Maria R, et al. Increased circulating concentrations of interleukin 2 receptor during rejection episodes in heart- or kidney-transplant recipients. *Clin Chem*, 36, 2106-2109 (1990)

5878 Zucker S, Lysik RM, Zarrabi MH, et al. Elevated plasma stromelysin levels in arthritis. *J Rheumatol*, 21, 2329-2333 (1994)

5879 Zuojun S, Zhiguo W, Yihua D, et al. Determination of γ-aminobutyric acid in serum by precolumn derivation with 9 fluorenylmethyl chlorformate and reverse-phase high performance liquid chromatography. *Clin Chem*, 41, S35 (1995)

5880 Zuppi C, Baroni S, Scribano D, et al. Choice of time for urine collection for detecting early kidney abnormalities in hypertensives. *Ann Clin Biochem*, 32, 373-378 (1995)

5881 Zusman J, et al. Hyperphosphatemia, hyperphosphaturia, and hypocalcemia in acute lymphoblastic leukemia. *N Engl J Med*, 289, 1335-40 (1973)

5882 Zuspan FP, et al. Urine amine excretion in pregnancy-induced hypertension. *Perspect Nephrol Hypertens*, 5, 339-447 (1976)

5883 Zuyderhoudt FM, et al. An enzyme linked immunoassay for ferritin in human serum and rat plasma and the influence of the iron in serum ferritin on serum iron measurement, during acute hepatitis. *Clin Chim Acta*, 88, 37-44 (1978)

5884 Zweig MH, van Sterteighem AC. Assessment by radioimmunoassay of serum creatine kinase BB (CK-BB) as a tumor marker: Studies in patients with various cancers and a comparison of CK-BB concentrations to prostate acid phosphatase concentrations. *J Natl Cancer Inst*, 66, 859-862 (1981)

5885 Zwicker H, Rittmaster RS. Androsterone sulfate: physiology and clinical significance in hirsute women. *J Clin Endocrinol Metab*, 76, 112-116 (1993)

NOTES

NOTES

NOTES

NOTES

NOTES

NOTES

NOTES

NOTES

NOTES

NOTES

NOTES

NOTES

NOTES

NOTES

NOTES

NOTES

NOTES

NOTES

NOTES

NOTES